FVC	forced vital capacity
FVS	full ventilatory support
f/V_T	rapid shallow breathing index (frequency divided by tidal volume)
G_{aw}	airway conductance
g/dl	grams per deciliter
$[H^+]$	hydrogen ion concentration
HAP	hospital-acquired pneumonia
Hb	hemoglobin
HCAP	health care–associated pneumonia
HCH	hygroscopic condenser humidifier
HCO_3^-	bicarbonate
H_2CO_3	carbonic acid
He	helium
He/O_2	helium/oxygen mixture; heliox
HFFI	high-frequency flow interrupter
HFJV	high-frequency jet ventilation
HFO	high-frequency oscillation
HFOV	high-frequency oscillatory ventilation
HFPV	high-frequency percussive ventilation
HFPPV	high-frequency positive pressure ventilation
HFV	high-frequency ventilation
HHb	reduced or deoxygenated hemoglobin
HMD	hyaline membrane disease
HME	heat and moisture exchanger
HMEF	heat and moisture exchange filter
H_2O	water
HR	heart rate
ht	height
Hz	hertz
IBW	ideal body weight
I	inspired
IC	inspiratory capacity
ICP	intracranial pressure
ICU	intensive care unit
ID	inner diameter
I : E	inspiratory-to-expiratory ratio
ILD	interstitial lung disease
IMPRV	intermittent mandat ventilation
IMV	intermittent mandat
INO	inhaled nitric oxide
IPAP	inspiratory positive a
IPPB	intermittent positive
IPPV	intermittent positive
IR	infrared
IRDS	infant respiratory dis
IRV	inverse ratio ventilati
IRV	inspiratory reserve vo
IV	intravenous
IVC	inspiratory vital capa
IVH	intraventricular hemo
IVOX	intravascular oxygena
kcal	kilocalorie
kg	kilogram
kg-m	kilogram-meters
kPa	kilopascal
L	liter
LAP	left atrial pressure
lb	pound
LBW	low birth weight
LED	light emitting diode
$LFPPV\text{-}ECCO_2R$	low-frequency positive with extracorporeal removal
LV	left ventricle
LVEDP	left ventricular end-di
LVEDV	left ventricular end-di
LVSW	left ventricular stroke
m^2	meters squared

MABP	mean ar
MAlvP	mean alv
MAP	mean arterial pressure
MAS	meconium aspiration syndrome
max	maximal
MDI	metered dose inhaler
MDR	multidrug resistant
mEq/L	milliequivalents per liter
MEP	maximum expiratory pressure
metHb	methemoglobin
mg	milligram
mg%	milligram percent
mg/dl	milligrams per deciliter
MICP	mobile intensive care paramedic
MI-E	mechanical insufflation-exsufflation
MIF	maximum inspiratory force
MIGET	multiple inert gas elimination technique
min	minute
MIP	maximum inspiratory pressure
ml	milliliter
MLT	minimal leak technique
mm	millimeter
MMAD	median mass aerodynamic diameter
mm Hg	millimeters of mercury
mmol	millimole
MMV	mandatory minute ventilation
mo	month
MOV	minimal occluding volume
$mP_{aw} - P_{\overline{aw}}$	mean airway pressure
MRI	magnetic resonance imaging
msec	millisecond
MV	mechanical ventilation
MVV	maximum voluntary ventilation
NaBr	sodium bromide
NaCl	sodium chloride
NAVA	neurally adjusted ventilatory assist
NBRC	National Board of Respiratory Care
NEEP	end expiratory pressure
	h-frequency oscillatory ventilation
	intensive care unit
	inspiratory force (also see MIP and
	Institutes of Health
	ive mechanical ventilation
	e
	er
	scular blocking agent
	e per liter
	de
	xide
	yngeal
	by mouth
	pressure ventilation
	ive positive pressure ventilation
	dal antiinflammatory drugs
	chronized intermittent mandatory tion
	itive airway pressure with periodic
	bilevel positive airway pressure
	or bilevel nasal continuous positive pressure
	d hemoglobin
	ions
	globin dissociation curve
	e sleep apnea
	pressure
	hich 50% saturation of hemoglobin

EGAN'S
Fundamentals of Respiratory Care

evolve
learning system

ELSEVIER

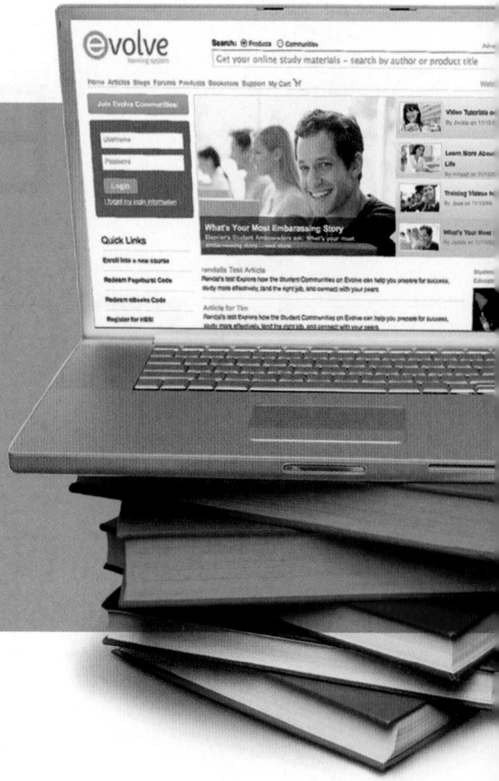

YOU'VE JUST PURCHASED MORE THAN A TEXTBOOK

ACTIVATE THE COMPLETE LEARNING EXPERIENCE THAT COMES WITH YOUR BOOK BY REGISTERING AT

http://evolve.elsevier.com/Egans/

Evolve Student Learning Resources for Egan's Fundamentals of Respiratory Care, 10th edition offers the following features

- Class, Exam Prep, etc.
- Image Collection
- Cross Reference for the NBRC Content Outlines
- Student Lecture Notes
- Body Spectrum Anatomy Coloring Book
- Common Respiratory Care Equations
- English/Spanish Glossary
- Acknowledgments

REGISTER TODAY!

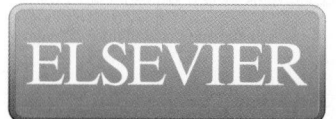

EGAN'S
Fundamentals of Respiratory Care

10TH EDITION

Robert M. Kacmarek, PhD, RRT
Professor of Anesthesiology
Harvard Medical School
Director, Respiratory Care
Massachusetts General Hospital
Boston, Massachusetts

James K. Stoller, MD, MS, FCCP, FACP, FAARC
Jean Wall Bennett Professor of Medicine
Cleveland Clinic Lerner College of Medicine of Case Western Reserve University
Chair, Education Institute
Head, Cleveland Clinic Respiratory Therapy
Cleveland Clinic
Cleveland, Ohio

Albert J. Heuer, PhD, MBA, RRT, RPFT
Associate Professor and Program Director
Respiratory Care Program
The University of Medicine and Dentistry of New Jersey
Newark, New Jersey

Consulting Editors

Robert L. Chatburn, MHHS, RRT-NPS, FAARC
Adjunct Associate Professor
Lerner College of Medicine of Case Western University
Clinical Research Manager
Respiratory Institute
Cleveland Clinic
Cleveland, Ohio

Richard H. Kallet, MS, RRT, FAARC, FCCM
Director of Quality Assurance
Respiratory Care Services
San Francisco General Hospital
University of California, San Francisco
San Francisco, California

Lucy Kester, MBA, RRT, FAARC
Education Coordinator
Section of Respiratory Therapy
Respiratory Institute
Cleveland Clinic
Cleveland, Ohio

With 826 illustrations

ELSEVIER

ELSEVIER
MOSBY

3251 Riverport Lane
St. Louis, Missouri 63043

EGAN'S FUNDAMENTALS OF RESPIRATORY CARE ISBN-13: 978-0-323-08203-7

Notices

Knowledge and best practice in this field are constantly changing. As new research and experience broaden our understanding, changes in research methods, professional practices, or medical treatment may become necessary.

Practitioners and researchers must always rely on their own experience and knowledge in evaluating and using any information, methods, compounds, or experiments described herein. In using such information or methods they should be mindful of their own safety and the safety of others, including parties for whom they have a professional responsibility.

With respect to any drug or pharmaceutical products identified, readers are advised to check the most current information provided (i) on procedures featured or (ii) by the manufacturer of each product to be administered, to verify the recommended dose or formula, the method and duration of administration, and contraindications. It is the responsibility of practitioners, relying on their own experience and knowledge of their patients, to make diagnoses, to determine dosages and the best treatment for each individual patient, and to take all appropriate safety precautions.

To the fullest extent of the law, neither the Publisher nor the authors, contributors, or editors assume any liability for any injury and/or damage to persons or property as a matter of products liability, negligence, or otherwise, or from any use or operation of any methods, products, instructions, or ideas contained in the material herein.

Library of Congress Cataloging-in-Publication Data

Egan's fundamentals of respiratory care.—10th ed. / [edited by] Robert M. Kacmarek, James K. Stoller, Albert J. Heuer ; consulting editors, Robert L. Chatburn, Richard H. Kallet, Lucy Kester.
p. ; cm.
Fundamentals of respiratory care
Includes bibliographical references and index.
ISBN 978-0-323-08203-7 (hardcover : alk. paper)
I. Kacmarek, Robert M. II. Stoller, James K. III. Heuer, Albert J. IV. Egan, Donald F., 1916- V. Title: Fundamentals of respiratory care.
[DNLM: 1. Respiratory Therapy–methods. 2. Respiratory Tract Diseases–therapy. WF 145]
615.8′36–dc23
2011048754

Content Manager: Billie Sharp
Senior Content Development Specialist: Kathleen Sartori
Content Coordinator: Andrea Hunolt
Publishing Services Manager: Catherine Jackson
Senior Project Manager: Rachel E. McMullen
Designer: Amy Buxton

Printed in China

Last digit is the print number: 9 8 7 6 5 4 3 2 1

For Robert, Julia, Katie, and Callie who all make it worthwhile.

RMK

I dedicate this work to the memory of my father, Alfred Stoller (1919-2011), who is my bastion of tenacity; to my wife, Terry Stoller, whose love and support is my bedrock; and to our son, Jake Fox Stoller, whose shining promise gives purpose and keeps us looking forward.

JKS

To Drs. Wilkins, Kacmarek, and Stoller for the privilege of working with them on this text; to my wife Laurel for her unwavering faith and support; and to my fellow respiratory therapists and faculty, as well as the students who provide inspiration in my pursuit of excellence.

AJH

Contributors

Loutfi S. Aboussouan, MD
Staff Physician
Respiratory Institute
Cleveland Clinic
Cleveland, Ohio

Alexander B. Adams, MPH, RRT
Research Associate
Pulmonary Research
Regions Hospital/Healthpartners
St. Paul, Minnesota

Neila Altobelli, BA, RRT
Clinical Scholar and Instructor
Respiratory Care Services
Massachusetts General Hospital
Boston, Massachusetts

Michael E. Anders, PhD, RRT
Associate Professor
Department of Respiratory and Surgical Technologies, College of Health Related Professions
University of Arkansas for Medical Sciences
Little Rock, Arkansas

Arzu Ari, PhD, RRT, PT, CPFT
Associate Professor
Division of Respiratory Therapy
Georgia State University
Atlanta, Georgia

Alejandro C. Arroliga, MD
Chairman and Professor
Dr. A. Ford Wolf and Brooksie Nell Boyd Wolf Centennial Chair of Medicine
Scott and White Hospital;
Texas A&M Health Science Center College of Medicine
Temple, Texas

Rendell W. Ashton, MD, FACP, FCCP
Program Director, Pulmonary and Critical Care Fellowship
Associate Director, Medical Intensive Care Unit
Cleveland Clinic
Cleveland, Ohio

Jami E. Baltz, RD, CNSD
Clinical Dietitian
San Francisco General Hospital and Trauma Center
San Francisco, California

Thomas A. Barnes, EdD, RRT, FAARC
Professor Emeritus of Cardiopulmonary Sciences
Department of Health Sciences
Bouve College of Health Sciences
Northeastern University
Boston, Massachusetts

Will Beachey, PhD, RRT, FAARC
Professor and Chair
Respiratory Therapy Department
University of Mary and St. Alexius Medical Center
Bismarck, North Dakota

Jeffrey T. Chapman, MD
Chairman, Department of Quality and Patient Safety
Cleveland Clinic Abu Dhabi
Abu Dhabi, United Arab Emirates

Robert L. Chatburn, MHHS, RRT-NPS, FAARC
Adjunct Associate Professor
Lerner College of Medicine of Case Western University
Clinical Research Manager
Respiratory Institute
Cleveland Clinic
Cleveland, Ohio

Daniel W. Chipman, BS, RRT
Assistant Director of Respiratory Care
Massachusetts General Hospital
Boston, Massachusetts

Elliott D. Crouser, MD
Associate Professor of Medicine
Division of Pulmonary, Allergy, Critical Care and Sleep Medicine
Department of Internal Medicine
Ohio State University Medical Center
Columbus, Ohio

Ehab G. Daoud, MD, FACP, FCCP
Program Director of Critical Care Medicine Fellowship
Respiratory Institute
Cleveland Clinic
Cleveland, Ohio

Douglas D. Deming, MD
Professor of Pediatrics
Chief, Division Neonatology
Medical Director, Neonatal Respiratory Care
Medical Director, Extracorporeal Membrane Oxygenation Program
Department of Pediatrics
Division of Neonatology
Loma Linda University Children's Hospital
Loma Linda, California

Anthony L. DeWitt, JD, RRT
Attorney at Law
Bartimus Frickleton, Robertson & Gorny, PC
Jefferson City, Missouri and Leawood, Kansas

Enrique Diaz-Guzman, MD
Assistant Professor of Medicine
University of Kentucky
Lexington, Kentucky

F. Herbert Douce, MS, RRT-NPS, RPFT, FAARC
Associate Professor Emeritus
Respiratory Therapy
The Ohio State University
Columbus, Ohio

Patrick J. Dunne, MEd, RRT, FAARC
President/CEO
HealthCare Productions, Inc.
Fullerton, California

Raed A. Dweik, MD
Professor of Medicine
Cleveland Clinic, Lerner College of Medicine
Director, Pulmonary Vascular Program
Department of Pulmonary, Allergy, & Critical Care Medicine
The Cleveland Clinic
Cleveland, Ohio

Patricia English, MS, RRT
Staff Therapist
Respiratory Care Department
Massachusetts General Hospital
Boston, Massachusetts

Matthew C. Exline, MD, FCCP
Assistant Professor
Division of Pulmonary, Allergy, Critical Care, and Sleep Medicine
Department of Internal Medicine
The Ohio State University
Columbus, Ohio

Ruairi J. Fahy, MD, FCCP, FRCPI
Consultant Pulmonary Physician
St. James Hospital;
Senior Lecturer, Trinity College Dublin
Dublin, Ireland

Jim Fink, PhD, RRT, FAARC, FCCP
Adjunct Professor
Georgia State University
Division of Respiratory Therapy
Atlanta, Georgia

Daniel F. Fisher, MS, RRT
Assistant Director
Respiratory Care Services
Massachusetts General Hospital
Boston, Massachusetts

Thomas G. Fraser, MD
Vice Chairman, Department of Infectious Disease
Medical Director for Infection Control, Quality and Patient Safety Institute
Cleveland Clinic
Cleveland, Ohio

Douglas S. Gardenhire, EdD, RRT-NPS
Director of Clinical Education
School of Health Professions
Division of Respiratory Therapy
Georgia State University
Atlanta, Georgia

Donna D. Gardner, MSHP, RRT-NPS, FAARC
Interim Chair
The University of Texas Health Science Center at San Antonio
School of Health Professions
Department of Respiratory Care
San Antonio, Texas

Albert J. Heuer, PhD, MBA, RRT, RPFT
Associate Professor and Program Director
Respiratory Care Program
The University of Medicine and Dentistry of New Jersey
Newark, New Jersey

George H. Hicks, MS, RRT
Instructor of Respiratory Care and Anatomy & Physiology
Allied Health and Science Divisions
Mt. Hood Community College
Gresham, Oregon

Christopher A. Hirsch, MPH, RRT
Pulmonary and Critical Care Services
Maine Medical Center
Portland, Maine

Robert M. Kacmarek, PhD, RRT
Professor of Anesthesiology
Harvard Medical School
Director, Respiratory Care
Massachusetts General Hospital
Boston, Massachusetts

Richard H. Kallet, MS, RRT, FAARC, FCCM
Director of Quality Assurance
Respiratory Care Services
San Francisco General Hospital
University of California, San Francisco
San Francisco, California

Lucy Kester, MBA, RRT, FAARC
Education Coordinator
Section of Respiratory Therapy
Respiratory Institute
Cleveland Clinic
Cleveland, Ohio

Euhan John
Assistant Professor of Medicine
Division of Pulmonary, Allergy, and Critical Care Medicine
University of Pittsburgh Medical Center
Pittsburgh, Pennsylvania

David L. Longworth, MD
Medical Director, Medical Institute
Cleveland Clinic
Cleveland, Ohio

Scott P. Marlow, BA, RRT
Pulmonary Rehabilitation Coordinator
Respiratory Institute
Cleveland Clinic
Cleveland, Ohio

Peter Mazzone, MD, MPH, FRCPC, FCCP
Staff
Director, Lung Cancer Program
Respiratory Institute
Cleveland Clinic
Cleveland, Ohio

Hilary Petersen, MPAS, PA-C
Physician Assistant
Cleveland Clinic
Cleveland, Ohio

Narciso Rodriguez, BS, RRT-NPS, RPFT, AE-C
Assistant Professor
Respiratory Care Program
University of Medicine and Dentistry of New Jersey
School of Health Related Professions
Newark, New Jersey

Steven K. Schmitt, MD
Staff Physician, Department of Infectious Disease
Vice Chair, Medicine Institute
Cleveland Clinic
Cleveland, Ohio

Mark S. Siobal, BS, RRT, FAARC
Clinical Specialist, Respiratory Care Services
San Francisco General Hospital;
Department of Anesthesia and Perioperative Care
University of California, San Francisco
San Francisco, California

N. Lennard Specht, MD
Assistant Professor of Medicine and Cardiopulmonary Sciences
Department of Medicine
Loma Linda University
Loma Linda, California

James K. Stoller, MD, MS, FCCP, FACP, FAARC
Jean Wall Bennett Professor of Medicine
Cleveland Clinic Lerner College of Medicine of Case Western Reserve University
Chair, Education Institute
Head, Cleveland Clinic Respiratory Therapy
Cleveland Clinic
Cleveland, Ohio

Charlie Strange, MD
Professor of Pulmonary and Critical Care Medicine
Department of Medicine
Medical University of South Carolina
Charleston, South Carolina

Patrick J. Strollo, Jr., MD
Professor of Medicine and Clinical and Translational Science
Medical Director, UPMC Sleep Medicine Center
Division of Pulmonary, Allergy, and Critical Care Medicine
University of Pittsburgh
Pittsburgh, Pennsylvania

Adriano R. Tonelli, MD
Associate Staff
Respiratory Institute
Cleveland Clinic
Cleveland, Ohio

David L. Vines, MHS, RRT, FAARC
Acting Chair and Program Director
Department of Respiratory Care
Rush University
Chicago, Illinois

Teresa A. Volsko, MHHS, RRT, FAARC
Director, Respiratory Care
Akron Children's Hospital
Akron, Ohio

Purris F. Williams, BS, RRT
Respiratory Care Services
Massachusetts General Hospital
Boston, Massachusetts

Kenneth A. Wyka, MS, RRT, AE-C, FAARC
Center Manager and Respiratory Care Patient Coordinator
Anthem Health Services
Queensbury, New York

Reviewers

Allen W. Barbaro, MS, RRT
Department Chairman, Respiratory Care Education
St. Lukes College
Sioux City, Iowa

Ellen Becker, PhD, RRT-NPS, RPFT, AE-C
Associate Professor
Respiratory Care Director
Brenda Pillors Asthma Education Program
Long Island University
Brooklyn, New York

Suellen Carmody-Menzer, BBA, RRT-NPS, AE-C
Clinical Coordinator and Instructor
Respiratory Care Program
Southeastern Community College
West Burlington, Iowa

William M. Cornelius, EdD, RRT-NPS
Chairman, Department of Respiratory Care
Temple College
Temple, Texas

Bradley H. Franklin, MEd, RRT, RCP
Department Chair, Allied Health
Crafton Hills College
Yucaipa, California

Valerie Greene, Ph
Director, Pharmacy Technician Program
St. Louis College of Health Careers
St. Louis, Missouri

Christine A. Hamilton, DHSc, RRT, AE-C
Program Director and Associate Professor
Nebraska Methodist College
Omaha, Nebraska

Robert L. Joyner, PhD, RRT, FAARC
Associate Dean, Henson School of Science and Technology
Director, Respiratory Therapy Program
Salisbury University
Salisbury, Maryland

Joel S. Livesay, MS, RRT, RVT
Department Chair, Respiratory Care
Spartanburg Community College
Spartanburg, South Carolina

Ronald P. Mlcak, PhD, RRT, FAARC
Director of Respiratory Care Services
Shriners Hospitals for Children
Galveston, Texas

James R. Sills, MEdRRT, CPFT
Professor Emeritus
Former Director, Respiratory Care Program
Rock Valley College
Rockford, Illinois

Stephen F. Wehrman, RRT, RPFT, AE-C
Professor
University of Hawaii
Program Director
Kapi'olani Community College
Honolulu, Hawaii

Richard Wettstein, MMEd, RRT
Director of Clinical Education
University of Texas Health Science Center at San Antonio
San Antonio, Texas

Preface

Donald F. Egan, MD, the original author of *Egan's Fundamentals of Respiratory Care,* sought to provide a foundation of knowledge for respiratory students learning the practice in 1969. However, the scope of the respiratory care profession is ever-expanding, and the skills and information needed to be an effective respiratory therapist have expanded with it. With improved technology and vast scientific and medical advances, the body of knowledge required for respiratory therapists has increased greatly since the first edition of the text was published.

Now in its tenth edition, *Egan's Fundamentals of Respiratory Care* encompasses the most relevant information to date and has provided a comprehensive knowledge base for students and professionals for more than 40 years. While these updated editions of *Egan's Fundamentals of Respiratory Care* still accomplish Dr. Egan's original goal—"to present what is felt to be the minimum knowledge for the safe and effective administration of inhalation therapy"—this text also goes far beyond the minimum, delving into important concepts and providing detailed information and resources to enhance student comprehension.

Every editor, guest editor, and contributor to the book is a leading figure in respiratory care, and the vast experience of these individuals ensures that critical content is covered accurately. Using the combined knowledge of these individuals, *Egan's Fundamentals of Respiratory Care* covers the role of respiratory therapists, the scientific bases for treatment, and clinical application skills. With 51 detailed chapters all focused on a unique aspect of respiratory care, *Egan's Fundamentals of Respiratory Care* is without equal in providing the prerequisite information required of a respiratory therapist today.

ORGANIZATION

This edition of the text is organized in a logical sequence of sections and chapters that build on each other to facilitate comprehension of the material. The earlier sections provide a basis for the profession and cover the physical, anatomic, and physiologic principles necessary to understand succeeding chapters. The later chapters address specific cardiopulmonary diseases and the diagnostic and therapeutic techniques that accompany them. Details on preventive and long-term care are also provided in the later chapters. In order of presentation, the seven sections are:

I. Foundations of Respiratory Care
II. Applied Anatomy and Physiology
III. Assessment of Respiratory Disorders
IV. Review of Cardiopulmonary Disease
V. Basic Therapeutics
VI. Acute and Critical Care
VII. Patient Education and Long-Term Care

FEATURES

There are many characteristic features throughout the book designed with the student in mind, making *Egan's Fundamentals of Respiratory Care* unique and engaging as a primary textbook. Each chapter begins in a similar manner, outlining the content and drawing attention to what should be mastered through the use of:

- Chapter Objectives
- Chapter Outlines
- Key Terms

The most important features within each chapter are accented by the ample use of figures and tables containing key information and by the use of:

- "Rules of Thumb"—"Pearls" of information highlighting rules, formulas, and key points necessary to the study of respiratory therapy and to future clinical practice
- "Mini-Clinis"—Critical thinking case studies illustrating potential problems that may be encountered during patient care
- Clinical Practice Guidelines—Statements of care extracted from the AARC list of guidelines defining evidence-based practice
- Therapist Driven Protocols—Examples of decision trees developed by hospitals and used by respiratory therapists to assess patients, initiate care, and evaluate outcomes.

Also, each chapter concludes with:

- A "Summary Checklist" of key points that the student should have mastered on completion of the chapter
- A complete list of references

NEW TO THIS EDITION

This edition has been updated to reflect the most current information in the National Board for Respiratory Care (NBRC) CRT Content Outline. Also featured is an expanded role for the NBRC Exam Matrix Correlation chart within all of the student and instructor offerings.

LEARNING AIDS

Workbook

The *Workbook for Egan's Fundamentals of Respiratory Care* is an exceptional resource for students. Offering a wide range of activities, it allows students to apply the knowledge they have gained using the core text. Presented in an engaging format, the workbook breaks down the more difficult concepts and guides students through the most important information. Beyond the many NBRC-style multiple-choice questions in the workbook, students are challenged with exercises such as fill-in-the-blanks, matching, crossword puzzles, case studies, short answers, and more.

Mosby's Respiratory Care Online

Designed to supplement the text, *Mosby's Respiratory Care Online,* now in its second edition, is a Web-based course designed to help reinforce text content, synthesize difficult concepts, and provide practice to students through a range of interactive audio and visual learning elements. Available as a separate purchase, *Mosby's Respiratory Care Online* offers unique learning opportunities beyond what is available in the text. Accommodating different learning styles and environments, the online course features:

- Videos, animations, and slideshows with audio narration
- Image enlarge function for heavily detailed illustrations
- Mini-Clini challenges with representative patient information and simulated electronic medical records
- Audio glossary with a comprehensive list of definitions and pronunciations
- Formulas organized by content area and printable
- Breath sounds
- Ventilator graphics
- Branching logic case studies
- Module examinations with correct and incorrect rationales
- Interactive learning exercises

This online course supplement is accessible only with purchase of an access code. For more information, visit http://evolve.elsevier.com/Egans/.

FOR THE INSTRUCTOR

Evolve Resources

Evolve is an interactive learning environment designed to work in coordination with this text. Instructors may use Evolve to provide an Internet-based course component that expands the concepts presented in class. Evolve can be used to publish the class syllabus, outlines, and lecture notes; set up "virtual office hours" and e-mail communication; and encourage student participation through chatrooms and discussion boards. Evolve also allows instructors to post exams and manage their grade books.

Created by the faculty and staff at The University of Medicine and Dentistry of New Jersey School of Health Related Professions, under the direction of Dr. Al Heuer, our Evolve Learning Resources provide instructors with valuable resources to use as they teach, including:

- More than 3000 test bank questions available in ExamView
- Comprehensive PowerPoint presentations for each chapter
- An image collection of the figures in the book

For more information, visit http://evolve.elsevier.com/Egans/ or contact an Elsevier sales representative.

Acknowledgments

We dedicate this book to the memory of Bob Wilkins, PhD, RRT. Bob was the consummate educator and a passionate editor of *Egan's Fundamentals of Respiratory Care* for the last several editions, to which he lent his extraordinary vision and leadership. He was a prolific and beloved educator of respiratory therapists worldwide, and the field both moved because of his presence and stalled in his passing.

Our hope is that this book, the continued legacy of his work, will continue to propel the world toward the excellence in respiratory therapy to which he dedicated his life. Bob is deeply missed, yet his presence lives in these pages.

Respectfully,
Bob Kacmarek, Jamie Stoller, and Al Heuer

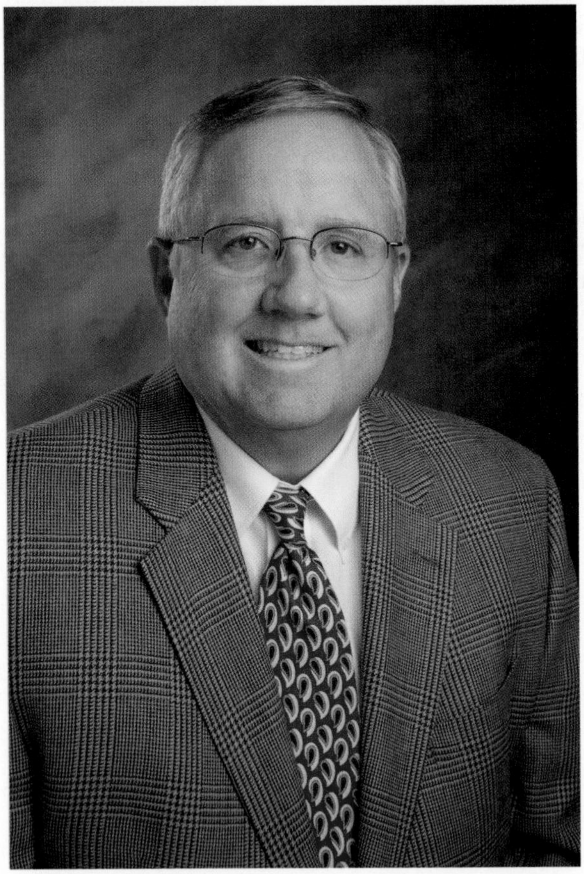

Contents

SECTION I

FOUNDATIONS OF RESPIRATORY CARE

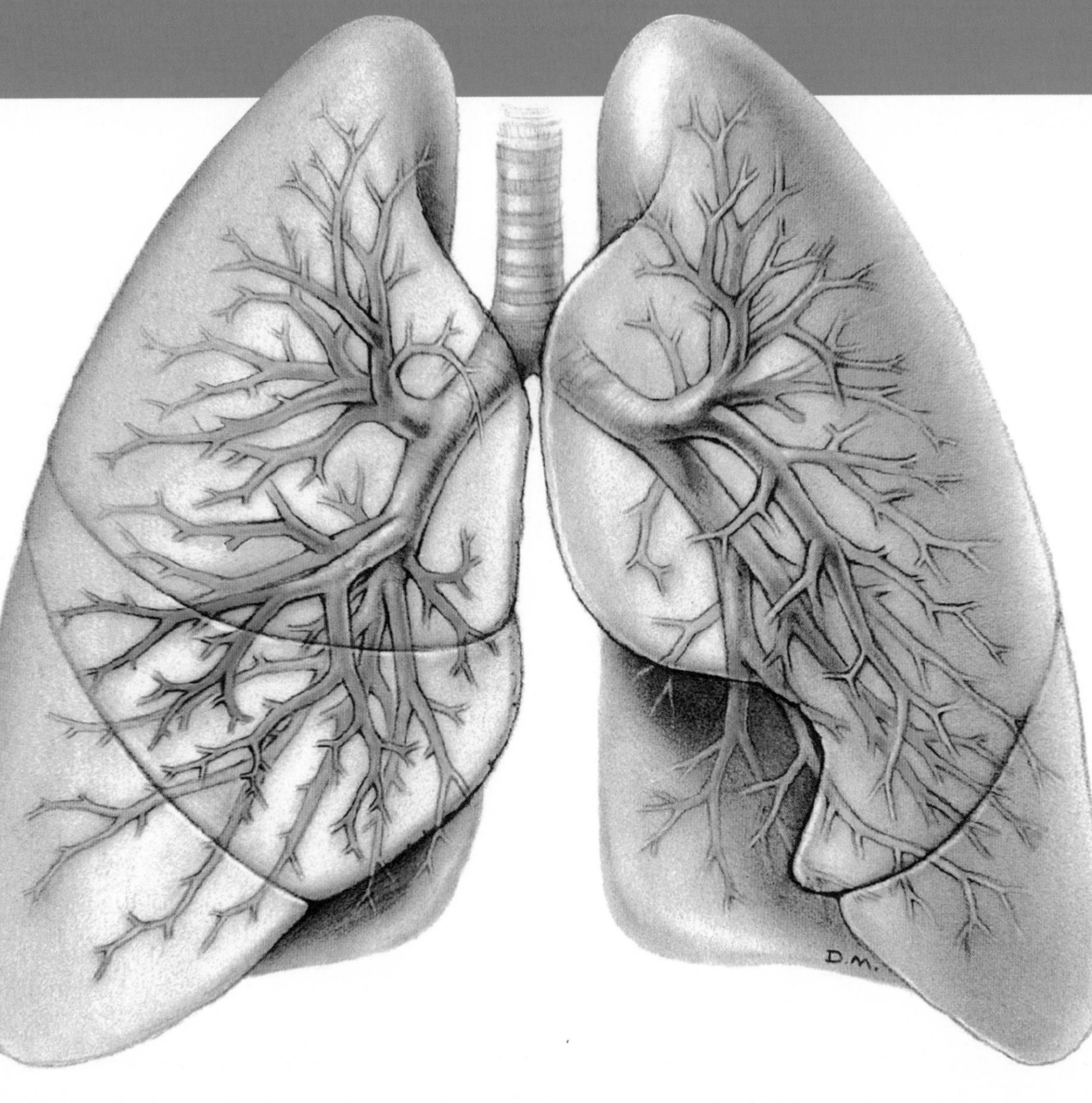

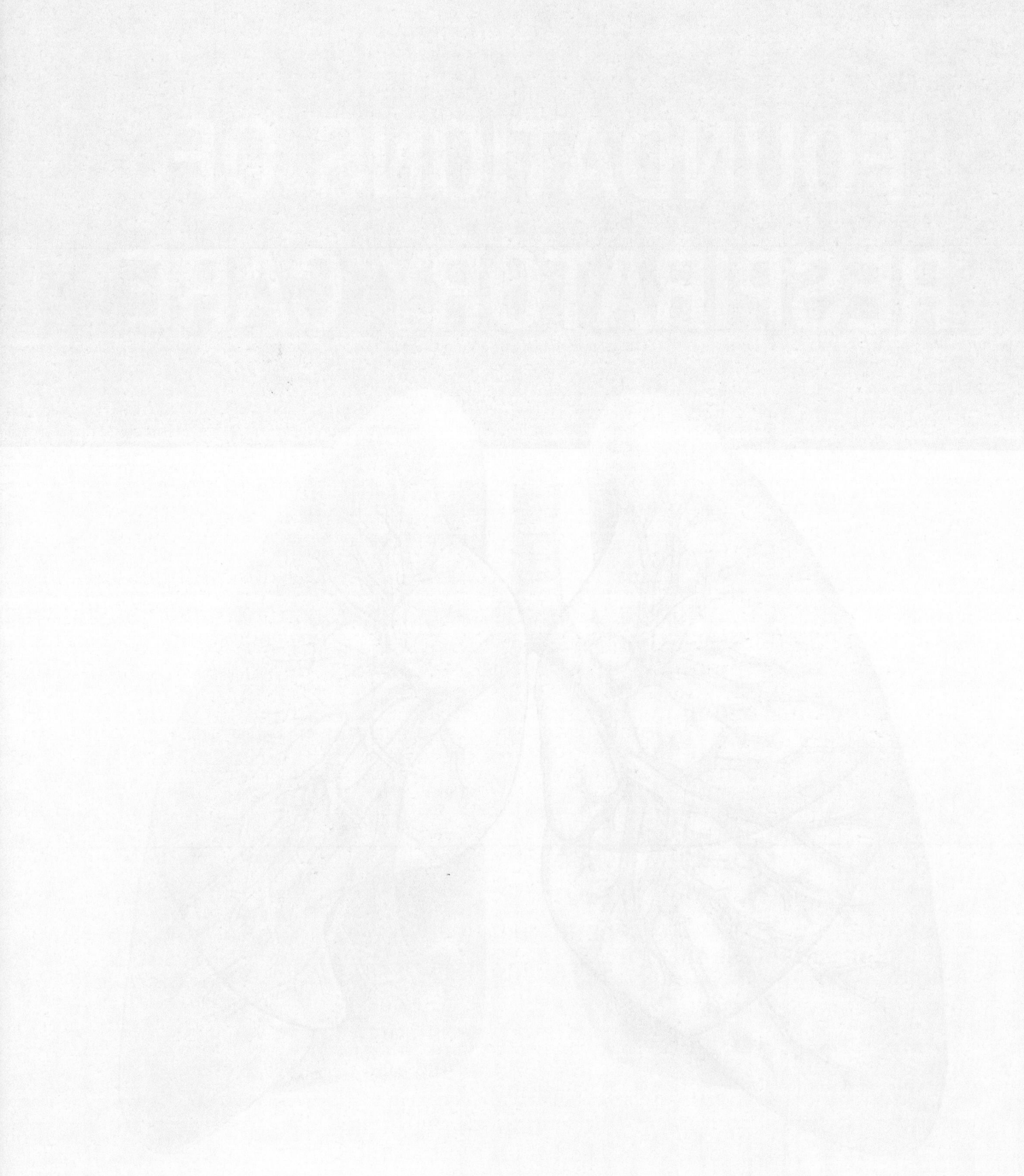

Chapter 1

History of Respiratory Care

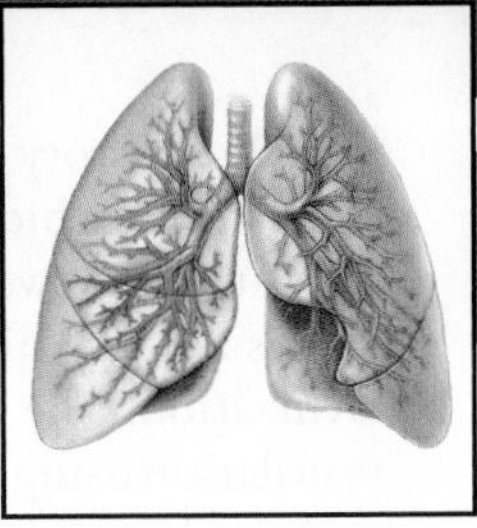

PATRICK J. DUNNE

CHAPTER OBJECTIVES

After reading this chapter you will be able to:

- Define respiratory care.
- Summarize some of the major events in the history of science and medicine.
- Explain how the respiratory care profession got started.
- Describe the historical development of the major clinical areas of respiratory care.
- Name some of the important historical figures in respiratory care.
- Describe the major respiratory care educational, credentialing, and professional associations.
- Explain how the important respiratory care organizations got started.
- Describe the development of respiratory care education.
- Predict future trends for the respiratory care profession.

CHAPTER OUTLINE

KEY TERMS

aerosol medications
airway management
American Association for Respiratory Care (AARC)
American Respiratory Care Foundation (ARCF)
Board of Medical Advisors (BOMA)
cardiopulmonary system
Committee on Accreditation for Respiratory Care (CoARC)
Fellow of the American Association for Respiratory Care (FAARC)
International Council for Respiratory Care (ICRC)
mechanical ventilation
National Board for Respiratory Care (NBRC)
oxygen therapy
physician assistant
pulmonary function testing
respiratory care
respiratory care practitioner(s)
respiratory therapist(s) (RTs)
respiratory therapy

The history of science and medicine is a fascinating topic, which begins in ancient times and progresses to the twenty-first century. Although respiratory care is a newer discipline, its roots go back to the dawn of civilization. The first written account of positive pressure ventilation using mouth-to-mouth resuscitation is thought to have been recorded more than 28 centuries ago.[1] Air was thought to be one of the four basic elements by the ancients, and the practice of medicine dates back to ancient Babylonia and Egypt. The progression of science and medicine continued through the centuries, and development of the modern disciplines of anesthesiology, pulmonary medicine, and respiratory care during the twentieth century was dependent on the work of many earlier scientists and physicians. This chapter describes the history and development of the field of respiratory care and possible future directions for the profession.

DEFINITIONS

Respiratory care, also known as **respiratory therapy,** has been defined as the health care discipline that specializes in the promotion of optimal cardiopulmonary function and health.[2] **Respiratory therapists (RTs)** apply scientific principles to prevent, identify, and treat acute or chronic dysfunction of the **cardiopulmonary system.**[2] Respiratory care includes the assessment, treatment, management, control, diagnostic evaluation, education, and care of patients with deficiencies and abnormalities of the cardiopulmonary system.[2] Respiratory care is increasingly involved in the prevention of respiratory disease, the management of patients with chronic respiratory disease, and the promotion of health and wellness.[2]

Respiratory therapists, also known as **respiratory care practitioners,** are health care professionals who are educated and trained to provide respiratory care to patients. About 75% of all respiratory therapists work in hospitals or other acute care settings.[3] However, many respiratory therapists are employed in clinics, physicians' offices, skilled nursing facilities, cardiopulmonary diagnostic laboratories, and public schools. Others work in research, disease management programs, home care, and industry. Some respiratory therapists work in colleges and universities, teaching students the skills they need to become respiratory therapists. Regardless of practice setting, all direct patient care services provided by respiratory therapists must be done under the direction of a qualified physician. Medical directors are usually physicians who are specialists in pulmonary or critical care medicine.

A human resources survey conducted in 2009 revealed that there were approximately 145,000 respiratory therapists practicing in the United States[3]; this represented a 9.3% increase over a similar study conducted 4 years earlier in 2005. As the incidence of chronic respiratory diseases continues to increase, the demand for respiratory therapists is expected to be even greater in the years ahead. Although the respiratory therapist as a distinct health care provider was originally a uniquely North American phenomenon, since the 1990s there has been a steady increase in interest of other countries in having specially trained professionals provide respiratory care. This trend is referred to as the "globalization of respiratory care."

HISTORY OF RESPIRATORY MEDICINE AND SCIENCE

Several excellent reviews of the history of respiratory care have been written, and the reader is encouraged to review these publications.[1,4-6] Summaries of notable historical events in science, medicine, and respiratory care are provided in Tables 1-1 and 1-2. A brief description of the history of science and medicine follows.

TABLE 1-1

Major Historical Events in Science, Medicine, and Respiratory Care from Ancient Times to the Nineteenth Century

Dates	Historical Event
Ancient Period	
1550 BC	What may be the world's oldest medical document, known as Ebers Papyrus, describes an ancient Egyptian inhalational treatment for asthma
800 BC	Biblical reference to what may be the first recorded episode of mouth-to-mouth resuscitation
500-300 BC	Hippocrates (460-370 BC; Greece) describes diseases as "humoral disorders" and speculates that an essential substance in air enters the heart and is distributed throughout the body
304 BC	Erasistratus of Alexandria describes the pneumatic theory of respiration, in which air travels through the lungs to the heart and then through the air-filled arteries to the tissues of the body
100-200 AD	Galen (130-199 AD) in Asia Minor identifies "pneuma" as the vital substance in inspired air that enters the heart and then the blood
Middle Ages (500-1500 AD) and Renaissance (1450-1600)	
500-1500 AD	The Middle Ages brings a period of little scientific progress in the West; however, this period coincides with the Golden Age of Arabian medicine (850-1050 AD)
1400s-1500s	da Vinci (1452-1519; Italy) performs human dissections and physiologic experiments on animals, learning that subatmospheric intrapleural pressures inflate the lungs and that there is a vital substance in air that supports combustion

TABLE 1-1

Major Historical Events in Science, Medicine, and Respiratory Care from Ancient Times to the Nineteenth Century—cont'd

Dates	Historical Event
1542	Vesalius (1514-1564; Belgium), one of the great early pioneers in human anatomy, performs a thoracotomy on a pig, placing a reed tracheotomy tube for ventilation of the animal, and resuscitates an apparently dead person
Seventeenth Century (1600s)	
1628	Harvey (1578-1657; England) describes the arterial and venous circulatory systems
1643	Torricelli (1608-1647; Italy) builds the world's first barometer for measurement of atmospheric pressure
1648	Pascal (1623-1662) describes the relationship between altitude and barometric pressure
1662; 1666	Boyle (1627-1691; England) explains the inverse relationship between gas pressure and volume (Boyle's law: pressure [P] $\times$ volume [V] = *k* or [P1V1] = [P2V2]). Boyle also describes a mysterious substance in air that supports combustion
1683	van Leewenhoek (1632-1723; Holland) improves the microscope and begins the science of microbiology
Eighteenth Century (1700s)	
1738	Bernoulli (1700-1782; Switzerland) determines that as the velocity of a liquid or gas increases, the pressure decreases (Bernoulli principle). Bernoulli also proposed that gases are composed of tiny particles in rapid, random motion. This idea became the basis of the modern kinetic theory of gases, which was developed further by Maxwell (1831-1879; Scotland) in 1860
1744	Fothergill (1712-1780; England) reports successful resuscitation methods
1754	Black (1728-1799; Scotland) rediscovers carbon dioxide, which he calls "fixed air" (prior work had been done by van Helmot in the 1600s)
1771	Scheele (1742-1786; Sweden) makes "fire air" (oxygen) by heating magnesium oxide; Scheele's findings are published in June 1774
1774	Priestley (1733-1804; England), usually credited with the discovery of oxygen, publishes his work on "dephlogisticated air" (oxygen) 3 months after Scheele's report
1775	Lavosier (1743-1794; France) renames "dephlogisticated air" "oxygen," or "acid maker" and shows that oxygen is absorbed by the lungs and consumed by the body, producing carbon dioxide and water vapor, which are exhaled
1776	Hunter (1728-1793; England) recommends use of a fireplace bellows for artificial ventilation
1787	Charles (1746-1823; France) describes the relationship between gas temperature and volume; Charles' law: volume (V)/temperature (T) = constant; or $(V_1/T_1) = (V_2/T_2)$
1794	Lavosier (1743-1794; France) describes oxygen absorption by the lungs and carbon dioxide production
1798	Beddoes (1760-1808; England) establishes the Pneumatic Institute in Bristol and uses oxygen to treat various disorders
Nineteenth Century (1800s)	
1800	Henry (1774-1836; England) determines that the amount of gas dissolved in a liquid is directly proportioned to its partial pressure (Henry's law)
1800s	Fick (1829-1911) describes a method to calculate cardiac output based on oxygen consumption and arterial and venous oxygen content: $Q_T = (\dot{V}O_2)/(CaO_2 - C\bar{v}O_2)$
1801-1808	Dalton (1766-1844; England) describes his atomic theory and the relationship between the partial pressures and total pressure of a gas mixture; Dalton's law: $P_1 + P_2 + P_3 \ldots P_N = P_{Total}$, where P = pressure
1806	de LaPlace (1749-1827; France) describes the relationship between pressure and surface tension in fluid droplets
1808	Gay-Lussac (1778-1850; France) describes the relationship between gas pressure and temperature; Gay-Lussac's law: pressure (P)/temperature (T) = constant; or $(P_1/T_1) = (P_2/T_2)$
1811	Avogadro (1776-1856; Italy) describes "Avogadro principle," where equal volumes of all gases (at the same temperature and pressure) contain the same number of molecules
1816	Laennec (1781-1826; France) invents the stethoscope for chest auscultation and lays the foundation for modern pulmonology with his book *Diseases of the Chest*
1831	Graham (1805-1869; Scotland) describes diffusion of gases (Graham's law)
1837	Magnus (1802-1870; Germany) measures arterial and venous blood oxygen and carbon dioxide content
1846	Hutchinson (1811-1861; England) develops the spirometer and measures the vital capacity of more than 2000 human subjects
1864	Jones (United States) patents a negative pressure device to support ventilation
1865	Pasteur (1822-1895; France) describes his "germ theory" of disease
1876	Woillez develops the spirophore negative pressure ventilator
1878	Bert (1833-1886; France) shows that low inspired oxygen levels cause hyperventilation
1880	MacEwen reports success with oral endotracheal intubation
1885	Miescher-Rusch demonstrates that carbon dioxide is the major stimulus for breathing
1886; 1904	Bohr (1855-1911; Danish) describes the oxyhemoglobin dissociation curve
1888	The Fell-O'Dwyer device combines a foot-operated bellows with a laryngeal tube for ventilatory support
1895	Roentgen (1845-1923; Germany) discovers the "x-ray." A direct vision laryngoscope is introduced by Jackson in the United States and Kirstein in Germany

Data from references 1, 3-13, and 16.

TABLE 1-2

Major Historical Events in Science, Medicine, and Respiratory Care in the Twentieth and Twenty-First Centuries

Twentieth Century	
Early 1900s	Bohr (1855-1911; Denmark), Hasselbach (1874-1962; Denmark), Krogh (1874-1940; Denmark), Haldane (1860-1936; Scotland), Barcroft (1872-1947; Ireland), Priestly (1880-1941; Britain), Y. Henderson (1873-1944; United States), L.J. Henderson (1878-1942; United States), Fenn (1893-1971; United States), Rahn (1912-1990; United States), and others make great strides in respiratory physiology and the understanding of oxygenation, ventilation, and acid-base balance
1904	Bohr, Hasselbach, and Krogh (1874-1940) describe the relationships between oxygen and carbon dioxide transport. Sauerbruch (1875-1951; Germany) uses a negative pressure operating chamber for surgery in Europe
1907	von Linde (1842-1934; Germany) begins large-scale commercial preparation of oxygen
1909	Melltzer (1851-1920; United States) introduces oral endotracheal intubation
1910	Oxygen tents are in use, and the clinical use of aerosolized epinephrine is introduced
1911	Drager (1847-1917; Germany) develops the Pulmotor ventilator for use in resuscitation
1913	Jackson develops a laryngoscope to insert endotracheal tubes
1918	Oxygen mask is used to treat combat-induced pulmonary edema
1919	Strohl (1887-1977; France) suggests the use of FVC as a measure of pulmonary function
1920	Hill develops an oxygen tent to treat leg ulcers
1926	Barach develops an oxygen tent with cooling and carbon dioxide removal
1928	Drinker develops his "iron lung" negative pressure ventilator
1938	Barach develops the meter mask for administering dilute oxygen. Boothby, Lovelace, and Bulbulian devise the BLB mask at the Mayo Clinic for delivering high concentrations of oxygen
1940	Isoproterenol, a potent beta-1 and beta-2 bronchodilator administered via aerosol, is introduced. Most common side effects are cardiac (beta-1)
1945	Motley, Cournand, and Werko use IPPB to treat various respiratory disorders
1947	The ITA is formed in Chicago, Illinois. The ITA later becomes the AARC
1948	Bennett introduces the TV-2P positive pressure ventilator
1948	FEV_1 is introduced as a pulmonary function measure of obstructive lung disease
1951	Isoetherine (Bronkosol), a preferential beta-2 aerosol bronchodilator with fewer cardiac side effects, is introduced
1952	Mørch introduces the piston ventilator
1954	The ITA becomes the AAIT
1958	Bird introduces the Bird Mark 7 positive pressure ventilator
1960	The Campbell Ventimask for delivering dilute concentrations of oxygen is introduced
1961	Jenn becomes the first registered respiratory therapist. Also, metaproterenol, a preferential beta-2 bronchodilator, is introduced
1963	Board of Schools is formed to accredit inhalation therapy educational programs
1964	The Emerson Postoperative Ventilator (3-PV) positive pressure volume ventilator is introduced
1967	The Bennett MA-1 volume ventilator is introduced, ushering in the modern age of mechanical ventilatory support for routine use in critical care units
1967	Combined pH-Clark-Severinghaus electrode is developed for rapid blood gas analysis
1968	Fiberoptic bronchoscope becomes available for clinical use. The Engström 300 and Ohio 560 positive pressure volume ventilators are introduced
1969	ARDS and PEEP are described by Petty, Ashblaugh, and Bigelow
1970	Swan-Ganz catheter developed for measurement of pulmonary artery pressures. The ARCF is incorporated. The JRCITE is incorporated to accredit respiratory therapy educational programs
1971	Continuous positive airway pressure is introduced by Gregory. *Respiratory Care* journal is named
1972	Siemens Servo 900 ventilator is introduced
1973	IMV is described by Kirby and Downs. The AAIT becomes the AART
1974	IMV Emerson ventilator is introduced
1974	NBRT is formed
1975	Bourns Bear I ventilator is introduced
1977	The JRCITE becomes the JRCRTE
1978	Puritan Bennett introduces the MA-2 volume ventilator. The *AAR Times* magazine is introduced
1979	AIDS is recognized by the Centers for Disease Control (CDC [later, Centers for Disease Control and Prevention])
1982	Siemens Servo 900C and Bourns Bear II ventilators are introduced
1983	The NBRT becomes the NBRC
1983	President Reagan signs proclamation declaring National Respiratory Care Week
1984	Bennett 7200 microprocessor controlled ventilator is introduced
1984	The AART is renamed the AARC
1991	Servo 300 ventilator is introduced
1992, 1993	The AARC holds national respiratory care education consensus conferences
1994	The CDC publishes the first guidelines for the prevention of VAP
1998	The CoARC is formed, replacing the JRCRTE

TABLE 1-2

Major Historical Events in Science, Medicine, and Respiratory Care in the Twentieth and Twenty-First Centuries—cont'd

Twenty-First Century	
2002	The NBRC adopts a continuing competency program for respiratory therapists to maintain their credentials
2002	The Tripartite Statements of Support are adopted by the AARC, NBRC, and CoARC to advance respiratory care education and credentialing
2003	The AARC publishes its white paper on the development of baccalaureate and graduate education in respiratory care. Asian bird flu appears in South Korea
2004	The Fiftieth AARC International Congress is held in New Orleans
2005	Number of working respiratory therapists in the United States reaches 132,651
2006	The National Heart, Lung and Blood Institute (NHLBI) of the U.S. Department of Health and Human Services begins national awareness and education campaign for COPD. The AARC works with government officials to recruit and train respiratory therapists for disaster response
2007	The first AARC president to serve a 2-year term begins term of office
2008	First of three conferences held for 2015 and Beyond strategic initiative of the AARC

Data from references 1, 3-13, and 16.

Ancient Times

Humans have been concerned about the common problems of sickness, disease, old age, and death since primitive times. Early cultures developed herbal treatments for many diseases, and surgery may have been performed in Neolithic times. Physicians practiced medicine in ancient Mesopotamia, Egypt, India, and China.[1,4,7] However, the foundation of modern Western medicine was laid in ancient Greece with the development of the Hippocratic Corpus.[1,4,7,8] This ancient collection of medical treatises is attributed to the "father of medicine," Hippocrates, a Greek physician who lived during the fifth and fourth centuries BC.[1,7,8] Hippocratic medicine was based on four essential fluids, or "humors"—phlegm, blood, yellow bile, and black bile—and the four elements—earth (cold, dry), fire (hot, dry), water (cold, moist), and air (hot, moist). Diseases were thought to be humoral disorders caused by imbalances in these essential substances. Hippocrates believed there was an essential substance in air that was distributed to the body by the heart.[1] The Hippocratic Oath, which admonishes physicians to follow certain ethical principles, is given in a modern form to many medical students at graduation.[1,8]

Aristotle (384-322 BC), a Greek philosopher and perhaps the first great biologist, believed that knowledge could be gained through careful observation.[1,8] Aristotle made many scientific observations, including observations obtained by performing experiments on animals. Erasistratus (about 330-240 BC), regarded by some as the founder of the science of physiology, developed a pneumatic theory of respiration in Alexandria, Egypt, in which air ("pneuma") entered the lungs and was transferred to the heart.[1,7] Galen (130-199 AD) was an anatomist in Asia Minor whose comprehensive work dominated medical thinking for centuries.[1,6,7] Galen also believed that inspired air contained a vital substance that somehow charged the blood through the heart.[1]

Middle Ages, the Renaissance, and the Enlightenment Period

The Romans carried on the Greek traditions in philosophy, science, and medicine. With the fall of the Western Roman Empire in 476 AD, many Greek and Roman texts were lost and Europe entered a period during which there were few advances in science or medicine. In the seventh century AD, the Arabians conquered Persia, where they found and preserved many of the works of the ancient Greeks, including the works of Hippocrates, Aristotle, and Galen.[1,7] A Golden Age of Arabian medicine (850-1050 AD) followed.

An intellectual rebirth in Europe began in the twelfth century.[1,7] Medieval universities were formed, and contact with the Arabs in Spain and Sicily reintroduced ancient Greek and Roman texts. Magnus (1192-1280) studied the works of Aristotle and made many observations related to astronomy, botany, chemistry, zoology, and physiology. The Renaissance (1450-1600) ushered in a period of scientific, artistic, and medical advances. da Vinci (1452-1519) studied human anatomy, determined that subatmospheric interpleural pressures inflated the lungs, and observed that fire consumed a vital substance in air without which animals could not live.[1,4] Vesalius (1514-1564), considered to be the founder of the modern field of human anatomy, performed human dissections and experimented with resuscitation.[1] In 1543, the date commonly given as the start of the modern Scientific Revolution, Copernicus observed that the Earth orbited the sun.[8] Before this time, it had been accepted that the Earth was the center of the universe.

The seventeenth century was a time of great advances in science. Accomplished scientists from this period include Kepler, Bacon, Galileo, Pascal, Hooke, and Newton. In 1628, Harvey fully described the circulatory system.[4,8] In 1662, the chemist Boyle published what is now known as Boyle's law, governing the relationship between gas volume and pressure.[8] Torricelli invented the barometer in 1650, and Pascal showed that atmospheric pressure decreases with altitude.[1,4] van Leeuwenhoek (1632-1723), known as the "father of microbiology," improved the microscope and was the first to observe and describe single-celled organisms, which he called "animalcules."[7]

The eighteenth-century Enlightenment Period brought further advances in the sciences. In 1754, Black described the properties of carbon dioxide, although the discovery of carbon dioxide should be credited to van Helmont, whose work occurred about 100 years earlier.[1] In 1774, Priestley described his discovery of oxygen, which he called "dephlogisticated air."[1,4] Before 1773, Scheele performed the laboratory synthesis of oxygen, which he called "fire air"; a general description of his discovery appeared in 1774, and a more thorough description appeared in 1777.[1,4] Shortly after the discovery of oxygen, Spallazani worked out the relationship between the consumption of oxygen and tissue respiration.[1] In 1787, Charles described the relationship between gas temperature and volume now known as Charles' law.[8] In experiments performed between 1775 and 1794, Lavoisier showed that oxygen was absorbed by the lungs and that carbon dioxide and water were exhaled.[1,4] In 1798, Beddoes began using oxygen to treat various conditions at his Pneumatic Institute in Bristol.[1,4]

Nineteenth and Early Twentieth Centuries

During the nineteenth century, important advances were made in physics and chemistry related to respiratory physiology. Dalton described his law of partial pressures for a gas mixture in 1801 and his atomic theory in 1808.[8] Young in 1805 and de LaPlace in 1806 described the relationship between pressure and surface tension in fluid droplets.[8] Gay-Lussac described the relationship between gas pressure and temperature in 1808, and in 1811, Avogadro stated that equal volumes of gases at the same temperature and pressure contain the same number of molecules.[1,8] In 1831, Graham described his law of diffusion for gases (Graham's law).[8]

In 1865, Pasteur advanced his "germ theory" of disease, which held that many diseases are caused by microorganisms.[8] Medical advances during this time included the invention of the spirometer and ether anesthesia in 1846, antiseptic techniques in 1865, and vaccines in the 1880s.[1,4,7] Koch, a pioneer in bacteriology, discovered the tubercle bacillus, which causes tuberculosis, in 1882 and the vibrio bacterium, which causes cholera, in 1883.[7] Respiratory physiology also progressed with the measurement in 1837 of blood oxygen and carbon dioxide content, the description around 1880 of the respiratory quotient, demonstration in 1885 that carbon dioxide is the major stimulant for breathing, and demonstration in 1878 that oxygen partial pressure and blood oxygen content were related.[1,4,9] In 1895, Roentgen discovered the x-ray, and the modern field of radiologic imaging sciences was born.[8] Pioneering respiratory physiologists of the early twentieth century described oxygen diffusion, oxygen and carbon dioxide transport, the oxyhemoglobin dissociation curve, acid-base balance, and the mechanics of breathing and made other important advances in respiratory physiology (see Table 1-2).

DEVELOPMENT OF THE RESPIRATORY CARE PROFESSION

Clinical Advances in Respiratory Care

The evolution of the respiratory care profession depended in many ways on developments in the various treatment techniques that matured in the twentieth century. As the scientific basis for oxygen therapy, mechanical ventilatory support, and administration of medical aerosols became well established, the need for a health care practitioner to provide these services became apparent. Concurrent with this need was the continuing development of specialized cardiopulmonary diagnostic tests and monitoring procedures, which also required health care specialists to perform.

The first health care specialists in the field were oxygen technicians in the 1940s.[1,4,5] The first inhalation therapists were oxygen technicians or oxygen orderlies who could haul cylinders of oxygen and related equipment around the hospital and set up oxygen tents, masks, and nasal catheters. The development of positive pressure breathing during World War II for breathing support of high-altitude pilots led to its use as a method to treat pulmonary patients and deliver aerosol medications during the 1950s, expanding the role of the inhalation therapist. Inhalation therapists began to be trained in the 1950s, and formal education programs began in the 1960s.[1,4,5] The development of sophisticated mechanical ventilators in the 1960s naturally led to a further expansion in the role of respiratory therapists, who soon also found themselves responsible for arterial blood gas and pulmonary function laboratories. In 1974, the designation "respiratory therapist" became standard, and the respiratory therapist became the allied health professional primarily concerned with the assessment, diagnostic testing, treatment, education, and care of patients with deficiencies and abnormalities of the cardiopulmonary system. The historical development of several clinical areas of respiratory care is described next, followed by an overview of the establishment of the major professional organizations in the field. The evolution of respiratory care education is also described.

RULE OF THUMB

When looking for information about the respiratory care profession, the best place to look is the AARC (see www.AARC.org).

Oxygen Therapy

Although the therapeutic administration of oxygen first occurred in 1798, and Bert showed that lack of oxygen caused hyperventilation in 1878, the physiologic basis and indications for **oxygen therapy** were not well understood until the twentieth century.[1,4] Large-scale production of oxygen was developed by von Linde in 1907. The use of a nasal catheter for oxygen administration was introduced by Lane in the same year.[1,4] Oxygen tents were in use in 1910, and an oxygen mask was used to treat combat gas-induced pulmonary edema in 1918.[1] In 1920, Hill developed an oxygen tent to treat leg ulcers, and in 1926, Barach introduced a sophisticated oxygen tent for clinical use. Oxygen chambers and whole oxygen rooms were designed.[1,4] In 1938, a meter mask was developed by Barach to administer dilute oxygen.[1,4] The BLB mask (named for Boothby, Lovelace, and Bulbulian) to administer 80% to 100% oxygen to pilots was introduced during World War II and later used on patients.[1,4] By the 1940s, oxygen was widely prescribed in hospitals, although there was still no good way to measure blood oxygen levels routinely until the mid-1960s, with the introduction of the Clark electrode, followed by the clinical use of the ear oximeter in 1974 and the pulse oximeter in the 1980s.[1,4,5] The Campbell Venti-mask, which allowed the administration of 24%, 28%, 35%, or 40% oxygen, was introduced in 1960, and modern versions of the nasal cannula, simple oxygen mask, partial rebreathing mask, and nonrebreathing mask were available by the late 1960s. Portable liquid oxygen systems for long-term oxygen therapy in the home were introduced in the 1970s, and the oxygen concentrator soon followed. Oxygen-conserving devices, including reservoir cannulas, demand pulse oxygen systems, and transtracheal oxygen catheters, were introduced in the 1980s.

The 2000s saw further advances in home oxygen therapy equipment with the introduction of oxygen concentrators used in conjunction with a pressure booster to allow for the transfilling of small, portable oxygen cylinders in the home. Smaller, lightweight portable oxygen concentrators were also introduced. Both of these advances have greatly enhanced the ability of patients receiving long-term oxygen therapy to ambulate beyond the confines of their home.

Aerosol Medications

Aerosol therapy is defined as the administration of liquid or powdered aerosol particles via inhalation to achieve a desired therapeutic effect. Bland aerosols (sterile water, saline solutions) or solutions containing pharmacologically active drugs may be administered. In 1802, the use of inhaled *Datura* leaf fumes, which contain atropine, to treat asthma was described.[10] Early use of **aerosol medications** dates to 1910, when the first use of aerosolized epinephrine was reported. Later, other short-acting bronchodilators such as isoproterenol (1940), isoetharine (1951), metaproterenol (1961), albuterol sulfate (1980), and levalbuterol (2000) were introduced, primarily for the emergency treatment of acute asthma attacks.[10] Oral and injectable steroids were first used in the treatment of asthma in the early 1950s, and the use of aerosolized steroids for the maintenance of patients with moderate to severe asthma began in the 1970s.[10] Since that time, numerous medications have been designed for aerosol administration, including long-acting bronchodilators, mucolytics, antibiotics, and antiinflammatory agents. Along with newer respiratory drugs, newer delivery devices such as dry powder inhalers and innovative designs for small volume nebulizers have been introduced.

Mechanical Ventilation

Mechanical ventilation refers to the use of a mechanical device to provide ventilatory support for patients. In 1744, Fothergill advocated mouth-to-mouth resuscitation for drowning victims.[1,6] During the mid to late 1700s, there was a great deal of interest in resuscitation, and additional procedures for cardiopulmonary resuscitation (CPR) were developed.[1,4,6] Positive pressure ventilation using a bag-mask system or bellows was suggested. However, the observation that a fatal pneumothorax may result caused this technique to be rejected around 1827.[1,4] Interest in negative pressure ventilation developed, and the first negative pressure tank ventilator was described in 1832.[6] Other negative pressure ventilators began to appear in the mid-1800s; in 1928, the iron lung was developed by Drinker, an industrial hygienist and faculty member at Harvard University.[1] Emerson developed a commercial version of the iron lung that was used extensively during the polio epidemics of the 1930s and 1950s (Figure 1-1).[1,11] The chest cuirass negative pressure ventilator was introduced in the early 1900s, and a negative pressure "wrap" ventilator was introduced in the 1950s.[12] Other early noninvasive techniques to augment ventilation included the rocking bed (1950) and the pneumobelt (1959).[12]

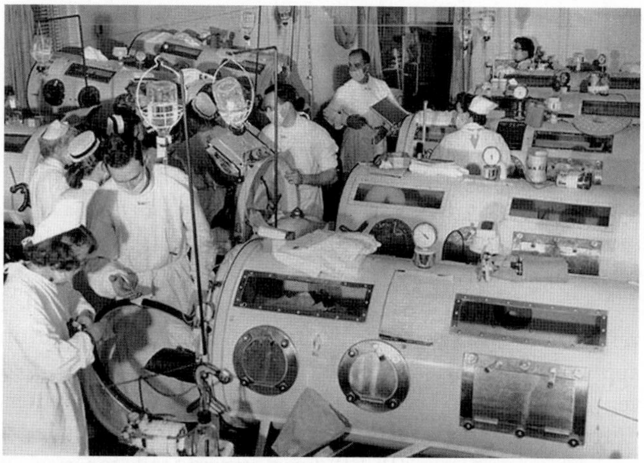

FIGURE 1-1 Iron lung patients in a 1950s polio ward. (From the Associated Press and Post-Gazette.com Health, Science and Environment. http://www.post-gazette.com/pg/05094/482468.stm.)

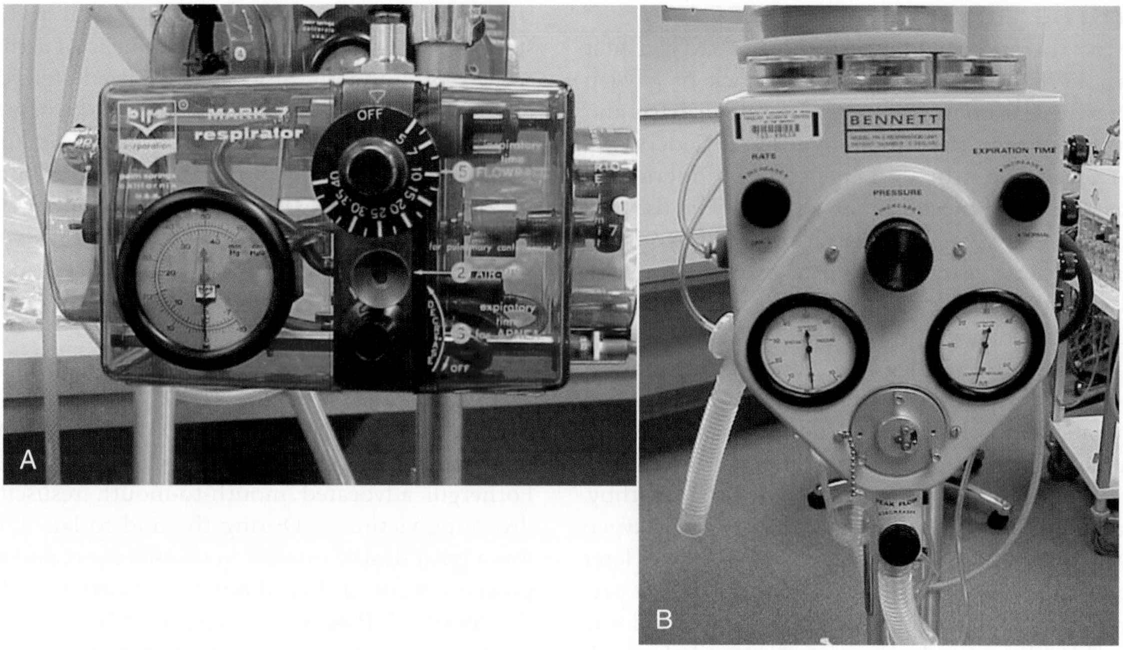

FIGURE 1-2 Bird Mark 7, introduced in 1958 by Bird **(A),** and Bennett PR-2, introduced in 1963 by Bennett **(B),** were pneumatically powered, pressure-limited positive pressure ventilators that could provide assist-control ventilation and were used to deliver IPPB treatments.

Originally, positive pressure ventilators were developed for use during anesthesia and later were altered for use on hospital wards.[13] Early positive pressure ventilators included the Drager Pulmotor (1911), the Spiropulsator (1934), the Bennett TV-2P (1948), the Morch Piston Ventilator (1952), and the Bird Mark 7 (1958) (Figure 1-2).[1,13] More sophisticated positive pressure volume ventilators were developed in the 1960s and included the Emerson Postoperative Ventilator, MA-1 (Figure 1-3), Engstrom 300, and Ohio 560.[1,13] A new generation of volume ventilators appeared in the 1970s that included the Servo 900, Bourns Bear I and II, and MA-II. By the 1980s, microprocessor-controlled ventilators began to appear, led by the Bennett 7200 in 1984, and in 1988, the Respironics BiPAP (bilevel positive airway pressure) device was introduced for providing noninvasive positive pressure ventilation in a wide variety of settings.[1] During the 1990s and early 2000s, new ventilators have continued to be developed, including the Hamilton Galileo, Servo-i, Bennett 840, and Drager Evita series (see Chapter 42). Since 1970, more than 50 new ventilators have been introduced with various characteristics for clinical use.[14,15]

Early mechanical ventilators provided only controlled ventilation. "Assist-control" as a mode of ventilation appeared with the early Bird and Bennett pressure-limited ventilators in the 1950s, which were often used for intermittent positive pressure breathing (IPPB). Positive end-expiratory pressure (PEEP) was introduced for use in patients with acute respiratory distress syndrome (ARDS) in 1967. The modern form of intermittent mandatory ventilation (IMV) was introduced in 1971, followed by synchronized intermittent mandatory ventilation in 1975 and mandatory minute volume ventilation in 1977.[1,4] Pressure support ventilation and pressure control ventilation were introduced in the 1980s, followed by airway pressure release ventilation and inverse ratio ventilation. In the

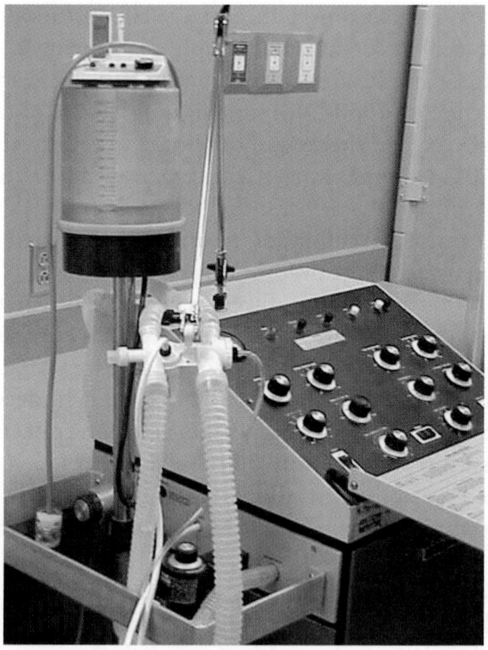

FIGURE 1-3 Bennett MA-1 ventilator, introduced in 1967, played a major role in making mechanical ventilatory support routinely available in intensive care units throughout the world.

1990s, volume support ventilation, pressure-regulated volume control, and adaptive support ventilation were introduced. The commercial implementation of proportional assist ventilation and other modes of ventilation occurred in the twenty-first century.

Because traditional short-term mechanical ventilation, regardless of mode, necessitates the use of an endotracheal tube, there is always the potential for a serious infection known as ventilator-associated pneumonia (VAP). VAP is a deadly and very costly consequence of invasive mechanical ventilation that develops when external microorganisms accidentally enter the airway. There has been a concerted effort to try to support inadequate ventilation noninvasively, by using a nasal or full-face mask, to avoid the need for endotracheal intubation. When noninvasive ventilation does not work and endotracheal intubation is necessary, respiratory therapists must be constantly vigilant in their efforts to prevent VAP.

Airway Management

Airway management refers to the use of various techniques and devices to establish or maintain a functional air passageway. Tracheotomies may have been performed to relieve airway obstruction in 1500 BC.[6] Galen, the Greek anatomist, described a tracheotomy and laryngeal intubation in 160 AD. Vesalius, the anatomist, described a tracheotomy in an animal in 1555.[1,6] In 1667, Hooke described a tracheotomy and use of a bellows for ventilation.[6] In 1776, tracheal intubation was suggested for resuscitation.[6] In 1880, MacEwen reported success with oral endotracheal intubation in patients.[6] O'Dwyer further described the technique for endotracheal tube placement. By 1887, Fell had developed a bellows-endotracheal tube system for mechanical ventilation, and this system was used in 1900 to deliver anesthesia.[6]

In 1913, the laryngoscope was introduced by Jackson. Additional early laryngoscopes were designed by Kirstein, Janeway, and others.[1,6] Endotracheal intubation for anesthesia administration was firmly established by World War I. After the war, Magill introduced the use of soft rubber endotracheal tubes, and this made blind nasal intubation possible, as described by Magill in 1930.[6] In 1938, Haight advocated nasotracheal suctioning for secretion removal, and in 1941, Murphy described the ideal suction catheter, which included side holes known as "Murphy eyes."[6] The double-lumen Carlen tube for independent lung ventilation was introduced in 1940, followed by a double-lumen tube developed by Robertshaw in 1962. Damage to the trachea by the tube cuff was reduced with the introduction of low-pressure cuffs in the 1970s.[6]

Cardiopulmonary Diagnostics and Pulmonary Function Testing

Pulmonary function testing refers to a wide range of diagnostic procedures to measure and evaluate lung function. The volume of air that can be inhaled in a single deep breath was first measured in 1679, and the measurement of the lung's residual volume was first performed in 1800.[9] In 1846, Hutchinson developed a water seal spirometer, with which he measured the vital capacity of more than 2000 subjects.[9,16] Hutchinson observed the relationship between height and lung volume and that vital capacity decreases with age, obesity, and lung disease. Hering and Breuer described the effects of lung inflation and deflation on breathing—the "Hering-Breuer reflex"—in 1868.[4] In 1919, Strohl suggested the use of forced vital capacity (FVC), and in 1948, forced expiratory volume in 1 second (FEV_1) was suggested as a measure of obstructive lung disease by Tiffeneau.[9]

Arterial and venous oxygen and carbon dioxide contents were measured in 1837, and methods to measure blood oxygen and carbon dioxide levels were available in the 1920s. These early methods for measuring blood oxygen, carbon dioxide, and pH were slow and cumbersome. In 1967, the combined pH, Clark, and Severinghaus electrodes produced a rapid and practical blood gas analyzer for routine clinical use.[1,4] The ear oximeter was introduced in 1974, and the pulse oximeter was introduced in the 1980s. Sleep medicine became well established in the 1980s, and polysomnography became a routine clinical test, often performed by respiratory therapists.

PROFESSIONAL ORGANIZATIONS AND EVENTS

American Association for Respiratory Care (AARC)

Founded in 1947 in Chicago, the Inhalational Therapy Association (ITA) was the first professional association for the field of respiratory care.[1,4,5] The purpose of the ITA was to provide for professional advancement, foster cooperation with physicians, and advance the knowledge of inhalation therapy through educational activities.[5] The ITA provided a forum to discuss the clinical application of oxygen therapy, improve patient care, and advance the art and science of the field.[1] There were 59 charter members of the ITA.[1] The ITA became the American Association for Inhalation Therapists (AAIT) in 1954, the American Association for Respiratory Therapy (ARRT) in 1973, and the **American Association for Respiratory Care (AARC)** in 1982.[4,5] By early 2011, membership in the AARC had reached 52,000 respiratory therapists, respiratory therapy students, physicians, nurses, and others interested in respiratory care. The AARC also has a formal affiliation with all 50 state respiratory societies (known as *Chartered Affiliates*) as well as with similar organizations in several foreign countries.[17]

During the 1980s, the AARC began a major push to introduce state licensure for respiratory therapists based

MINI CLINI

Preparing a Presentation for Respiratory Care Week

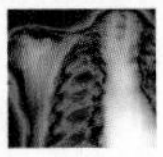

PROBLEM: You are a staff therapist in a 300-bed hospital. Your supervisor asks you to prepare a 20-minute presentation on the history and development of the respiratory care profession to be presented at the department's annual Respiratory Care Week luncheon. How would you gather the information needed and develop your presentation?

SOLUTIONS: First, review Chapter 1 in your textbook to get an overview of the history and development of the respiratory care profession. You may also want to read one or two of the supplemental references that are cited. Next, go to the AARC website (see www.AARC.org) and review the "Resources" and "Site Map" sections, which list many helpful resources. You should be able to find sections on "The History of the AARC," "Strategic Plan of the AARC," "Position Statements," and "White Papers." You should also find a section on Respiratory Care Week. Review the material that the AARC has provided and develop an outline for your presentation. Your outline may include a brief overview of the history of science and medicine, the development of the respiratory care profession, and the future of respiratory care in the twenty-first century. After you have your outline, decide on your delivery method. PowerPoint slides are easy to make and use. If you choose to do a PowerPoint presentation, a good rule of thumb is about one slide per minute, so you would need about 20 slides. Using your outline, begin to develop your presentation.

Box 1-1 AARC Specialty Sections

Adult Acute Care
Continuing Care/Rehabilitation
Diagnostics
Education
Home Care
Long-Term Care
Management
Neonatal/Pediatrics
Sleep
Surface and Air Transport

on the National Board for Respiratory Care (NBRC) credentials. As of 2011, 49 states, the District of Columbia, and Puerto Rico have state licensure or some other form of legal credentialing required for the practice of respiratory care. State licensing laws set the minimum educational requirements and the method of determining competence to practice. Competency is typically determined by obtaining a passing grade on a credentialing examination (administered by the NBRC) after graduation from an approved training program. State licensing boards also set the number of continuing education credits required to keep a license active.

The stated mission of the AARC is to "encourage and promote professional excellence, advance the science and practice of respiratory care, and serve as an advocate for patients, their families, the public, the profession and the respiratory therapist."[18] The AARC serves as an advocate for the profession to legislative and regulatory bodies, the insurance industry, and the general public. To fulfill its mission, the AARC sponsors many continuing educational activities, including international meetings, conferences and seminars, publications, and a sophisticated website (see www.AARC.org). In addition to the monthly science journal *Respiratory Care,* the AARC publishes the monthly news magazine *AARC Times* and numerous electronic newsletters. In the fall of each year, the AARC also sponsors the International Respiratory Congress, the largest respiratory care scientific meeting in the world. Finally, in an effort to ensure that the unique practice interests of AARC members are addressed (e.g., neonatal/pediatrics, adult acute care, management, home care, diagnostics), members are invited to join one or more of 10 Specialty Sections (Box 1-1) within the AARC, designed to facilitate networking and the free exchange of ideas.

The leadership and direction of the AARC is provided by a Board of Directors, which comprises members who volunteer their time and services. The executive officers of the Board of Directors include the president, immediate past-president, president-elect, vice-president for internal affairs, vice-president for external affairs, and secretary-treasurer. The remainder of the Board of Directors consists of a minimum of six members-at-large plus the chairpersons of the Specialty Sections having at least 1000 members. At the present time, 6 of the 10 Specialty Sections meet this requirement. All members of the Board of Directors, including Specialty Section chairpersons, are elected directly by the AARC membership. The AARC Board of Directors meets three times a year to conduct the official business of the association.

Each year, the incoming AARC president assigns interested members to chair or serve on more than 50 standing or temporary AARC committees. Many of the initiatives of the AARC are undertaken and eventually brought to completion through committee work. The AARC Board of Directors also receives input from each of the 50 Chartered Affiliates that constitute the House of Delegates. Each Chartered Affiliate elects two of their members to represent the interests of their state affiliate in the meetings of the House of Delegates. The 100 delegates elect their own leaders so that they can conduct the business of the House of Delegates. The House of Delegates meets twice a year. The efforts of the Board of Directors, the House of Delegates, and the numerous committees of the AARC are supported by a staff of more than 35 employees of the AARC who work fulltime in the association's executive offices located in Irving, Texas.

Many volunteers who have been elected to the AARC or House of Delegates leadership positions or have been asked to chair important committees started by volunteering at the affiliate level. Student members of the AARC are always welcomed as volunteers, especially at the affiliate level. Student members of the AARC have access to a wide array of resources that can greatly enhance the experience of becoming a professional respiratory therapist.

Respiratory Care Week

In November 1982, President Reagan signed a proclamation declaring the third week of each October as National Respiratory Care Week. Since then, Respiratory Care Week has become a yearly event to promote lung awareness and the work of respiratory therapists is all care settings. Respiratory therapists (and students) around the United States use Respiratory Care Week to celebrate their profession and dedication to quality patient care. Many respiratory care departments use the opportunity to conduct special events in their hospitals to help raise awareness of the vital role the respiratory therapist plays as a member of the health care team. Other departments plan community activities to help the public understand the importance of good lung health and the role respiratory therapists play in diagnosing and treating breathing disorders. Respiratory Care Week is also an excellent opportunity for respiratory therapy students to become ambassadors of the profession to the rest of the student body. Some respiratory therapy classes conduct free breathing tests on campus, in shopping malls, or in community centers.

Fellow of the American Association for Respiratory Care (FAARC)

In any given profession, there are always individuals who go above and beyond what is expected of the average practitioner. To recognize respiratory therapists and physician members who have done so in our profession, the AARC established the **Fellow of the American Association for Respiratory Care (FAARC)** award in 1998. To be considered for FAARC status, nominees must be either a registered respiratory therapist or a licensed physician and have a minimum of 10 consecutive years of membership in the AARC. Of greater importance, nominees for FAARC must show superior achievement in patient care and as a volunteer serving the profession. Individuals selected to receive this prestigious award are so noted by having "FAARC" appear after their name following educational degrees and credentials.

Board of Medical Advisors (BOMA)

Because respiratory therapists can practice only under medical direction, it is essential that the AARC leadership receive formal input from physicians on all matters and questions pertaining to patient care. The **Board of Medical Advisors (BOMA)** is the group of physicians who provide this valuable input. The BOMA comprises approximately 18 physicians who are appointed by their respective professional medical associations (e.g., American College of Chest Physicians, American Thoracic Society, Society for Critical Care Medicine) to serve this cause voluntarily. The BOMA meets annually, but the chairperson of the BOMA attends all meetings of the AARC Board of Directors. Individual members of the BOMA are assigned by the AARC president to serve as a medical liaison to each of the 10 Specialty Sections of the AARC. Effective medical direction at the hospital level is indispensable for the practice of safe, high-quality respiratory care.

American Respiratory Care Foundation (ARCF)

Established in 1970 by the AARC, the **American Respiratory Care Foundation (ARCF)** is a not-for-profit charitable foundation that helps promote and further the mission of the AARC. Commonly known as the Foundation, the ARCF collects and manages contributions from individuals, corporations, and other foundations to recognize individual achievements of excellence in clinical practice, chronic disease management, public respiratory health, scientific research, and literary excellence. The ARCF also provides research grants to establish the scientific basis of respiratory care further. Lastly, the ARCF oversees and distributes numerous scholarships for respiratory therapy students who are student members of the AARC. The ARCF awards and scholarships are presented at the awards ceremony held in conjunction with the annual International Respiratory Congress of the AARC. Respiratory therapy students who are interested in applying for an ARCF scholarship should visit the ARCF website (see www.arcfoundation.org) to learn more about this great opportunity.

International Council for Respiratory Care (ICRC)

The **International Council for Respiratory care (ICRC)** is an AARC-sponsored organization dedicated to the globalization of quality respiratory care. As mentioned previously, having formally trained professionals who were not physicians or nurses and who worked in a dedicated department assume full responsibility for providing respiratory care was a uniquely North American phenomenon, limited only to the United States and Canada. However, during the 1970s and 1980s, when many foreign physicians came to the United States to study, they became aware of what a respiratory therapist was and the important role the respiratory therapist played in hospitals nationwide. When these physicians returned to their native countries, they wished to have their own specialized team able to provide the same level of quality respiratory care.

However, because the health care delivery system is structured differently in each country, the specially trained teams were most often nurses, physicians, or physical therapists, not respiratory therapists.

Formed in 1991, the ICRC (in close collaboration with the International Committee of the AARC) began to offer fellowships to interested foreign clinicians that provide the opportunity to visit the United States for 2 weeks before the annual International Respiratory Congress to observe how practice respiratory care is practiced. The idea is to allow these international fellows to observe how the various components of respiratory care are practiced in several cities. The international fellows can take back to their home countries ideas and practices that can be integrated into their unique health care delivery systems. The program has been so successful that many countries (e.g., Mexico, Costa Rica, Taiwan) are starting to establish respiratory therapy training programs similar to the American model. As of 2010, 135 international fellows from 54 countries have participated in this program.

National Board for Respiratory Care (NBRC)

The credentialing body for registered respiratory therapists began in 1960 as the American Registry of Inhalation Therapists (to test and credential registered therapists), and a certification board was established in 1968 to certify technicians.[1,4] These two groups merged in 1974 as the National Board for Respiratory Therapy, which became the **National Board for Respiratory Care (NBRC)** in 1983.[1,4] Also in 1983, the National Board for Cardiopulmonary Technologists joined the NBRC, and the credentialing examinations for pulmonary function technology were brought in under the respiratory care umbrella.[1,4] Since 1968, there have been two levels of clinical practice credentialing examinations in the United States: the certified technician and the registered therapist (see www.NBRC.org).

> **RULE OF THUMB**
> For requirements for testing, examination schedules, study guides, and requirements for maintaining your CRT or RRT credential, check with the NBRC (see www.NBRC.org).

In 1998, the NBRC renamed the lower level certified respiratory therapist (CRT, or entry-level respiratory therapist); the advanced level remained registered respiratory therapist (RRT, or advanced-level respiratory therapist).[19] The NBRC began offering specialty examinations for pulmonary function technology in 1984 and neonatal/pediatrics in 1991. The NBRC is considering new specialty credentialing examinations in the areas of polysomnography and critical care.

Committee on Accreditation for Respiratory Care (CoARC)

In 1956, the first guidelines for respiratory care educational programs were published, followed by the formation of the Board of Schools to accredit programs in 1963.[1] The Board of Schools was replaced by the Joint Review Committee for Inhalation Therapy Education (JRCITE) in 1970, led by its first chairman, Helmholtz.[1,4] The JRCITE became the Joint Review Committee for Respiratory Therapy Education (JRCRTE) in 1977 and then the **Committee on Accreditation for Respiratory Care (CoARC)** in 1996 (see www.COARC.com).[4] Today, respiratory care educational programs in the United States are accredited by the CoARC in collaboration with the Association of Specialized and Professional Accreditors.[20-22]

RESPIRATORY CARE EDUCATION

The first formal educational course in inhalation therapy was offered in Chicago in 1950.[1] In the 1960s, numerous schools were developed to prepare students to become respiratory therapists. Early programs concentrated on teaching students the proper application of oxygen therapy, oxygen delivery systems, humidifiers, and nebulizers and the use of various IPPB devices. The advent of sophisticated critical care ventilators, blood gas analyzers, and monitoring devices in the 1960s and 1970s helped propel the respiratory therapist into the role of cardiopulmonary technology expert.

Respiratory care educational programs in the United States are offered at technical and community colleges, 4-year colleges, and universities. These programs are designed to prepare competent respiratory therapists to care for patients. The minimum degree required to become a respiratory therapist is an associate degree.[20] There are approximately 300 associate, 50 baccalaureate, and 3 graduate-level degree programs in the United States; 19 programs in Canada; and a handful of respiratory care educational programs in Mexico, South America, Japan, India, Taiwan, and other countries.[22-24]

> **RULE OF THUMB**
> Jobs in management, education, research, or advanced clinical practice may require bachelor or graduate level educational preparation.

The AARC completed a Delphi study and held two important Education Consensus Conferences in the early 1990s to assess the status of respiratory care education and recommend future direction for the field.[25-28] The first conference suggested that major trends affecting the field were advances in technology; demographic trends and the aging of the population; a need to provide better assessment, outcome evaluation, problem solving, and analytical skills; use of protocol-based care; and the need to increase the focus on patient education, prevention, and wellness, to include tobacco education and smoking cessation.[26] The conference concluded that the curriculum should encompass a broad scope of clinical practice, a significant arts and science component, emphasis on communication skills, and a minimum of an associate degree to enter practice. The second Educational Consensus Conference, held in the fall of 1993, focused on strategies to implement the recommendations made at the first conference.[28] Both conferences identified the need for more baccalaureate and graduate education in respiratory care. The view that programs should prepare students better in the areas of patient assessment, care plan development, protocols, disease management, pulmonary rehabilitation, research, and geriatrics/gerontology became well accepted.[29,30]

In 1997, Mishoe and MacIntyre[31] described a profession as "a calling or vocation requiring specialized knowledge, methods, and skills as well as preparation, in an institution of higher learning, in the scholarly, scientific, and historical principles underlying such methods and skills." These authors noted that professional roles are different and more complex than technical roles, which are oriented to performing specific tasks as ordered by the physician. Examples of professional roles in respiratory care include patient assessment and care plan development, ventilator management, disease management, pulmonary rehabilitation, and respiratory care consulting services. Technical roles may include basic task performance (e.g., oxygen, aerosol therapy, bronchial hygiene), routine diagnostic testing (e.g., electrocardiography, phlebotomy), and other routine tasks where little or no assessment is required and decisions are limited to device selection and fine-tuning therapy.[31] In professional practice, the therapist may function as a physician extender who applies protocols or guidelines.[31] Examples include making protocol-based ventilator adjustments, applying assessment-based care plans, and performance of advanced procedures such as arterial line insertion and management, intubation and extubation of patients, application of ventilator weaning protocols, and application of advanced cardiopulmonary technologies (e.g., extracorporeal membrane oxygenation, nitric oxide therapy, aortic balloon pumps).

According to Mishoe and MacIntyre, economic, educational, and institutional forces may limit respiratory care in certain settings to a task-oriented, technical role. There are many opportunities, however, for the respiratory therapist to function as a physician extender, in a role similar to the **physician assistant.** Working under the supervision of a physician, the physician assistant may perform many medical procedures that might otherwise be performed by a physician. In a similar way, the respiratory physician extender could improve the quality of care while controlling costs and minimizing unnecessary care. Many authorities believe that the critical thinking, assessment, problem-solving, and decision-making skills needed for advanced practice in the twenty-first century require advanced levels of education.[31]

In 1998, Hess[32] observed that a task orientation has coincided with a pattern of overordering and misallocation of respiratory care services. Therapist-driven protocols and the increasing use of the respiratory therapist as a consultant may allow physicians to order protocols as opposed to specific therapies. The therapist assesses the patient, develops a care plan, implements the plan, and evaluates and modifies care as appropriate.[32] Protocol-based care has been shown to be safe and effective, while reducing misallocation of care and helping to control costs.[32,33] Acceptance by physicians of respiratory therapists as consultants depends on the professionalism, education, and skill of the therapists at the bedside.[32]

In 2001, a report of the Conference Proceedings on Evidence-Based Medicine in Respiratory Care was published.[34] Evidence-based practice requires careful examination of the evidence for diagnosis, treatment, prognosis, and, in turn, practice using a formal set of rules.[35] The best evidence is used for clinical decision making, which should lead to optimal respiratory care.[35] Evidence-based practice has been advocated for all respiratory care delivered.

In 2002, the AARC, NBRC, and CoARC published their "Tripartite Statements of Support," which suggested that all respiratory therapists seek and obtain the RRT credential.[36] An AARC white paper followed in 2003, which encouraged the continuing development of baccalaureate and graduate education in respiratory care.[37]

FUTURE OF RESPIRATORY CARE

In 2001, Pierson, a prominent pulmonary physician and one of the many physician supporters of respiratory therapists, set out to describe the future of respiratory care.[38] Among other responsibilities, Pierson predicted a much greater use of patient assessment and protocols in chronic disease state management in all clinical settings. He also envisioned a more active role for respiratory therapists in palliative and end-of-life care, increasing emphasis on smoking cessation and prevention, early detection, and intervention in chronic obstructive pulmonary disease (COPD). Pierson also predicted an increase in the use of respiratory therapists acting as coordinators and caregivers in home care.

MINI CLINI

Educational Program Advisory Committee

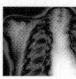

PROBLEM: You are asked to serve on your respiratory care educational program advisory committee. The committee wants to know how respiratory care education has developed and where it should be headed. You are appointed as a member of a subcommittee to research these issues. What should you do?

SOLUTIONS: You may want to read the sections in Chapter 1 that cover the history and development of respiratory care education to get an overview. You may wish to obtain copies of some of the reference materials that are cited. Items that may be helpful are the AARC Delphi Study,[26] reports of the AARC education consensus conferences,[27-29] and articles about the future of respiratory care.[30-33,37-41] You may wish to review the AARC strategic plan (see www.AARC.org) and AARC statements regarding respiratory care education and credentialing.[10,40,41] By reviewing these materials, you should be well prepared to discuss the future direction of your educational program.

2015 and Beyond

In 2005, recognizing that many national politicians were beginning to call for an overhaul of the U.S. health care delivery system, the AARC Board of Directors began to think strategically, which led to the formation in 2007 of a special task force called "2015 and Beyond." The task force was charged with the task of envisioning potential new roles and responsibilities of respiratory therapists by 2015 and beyond. The leadership of the task force decided to convene three strategic conferences to answer the following five key questions about the profession:

1. How will most patients receive health care services in the future?
2. How will respiratory care services be provided?
3. What new knowledge, skills, and attributes will respiratory therapists need to be able to provide care that is safe, efficacious, and cost-effective in 2015?
4. What education and credentialing systems will be needed to ensure respiratory therapists acquire the new knowledge, skills, and attributes?
5. How should the profession transition from traditional practice to the newer system without adversely impacting the existing workforce?[39]

The initial 2015 and Beyond conference was held in the spring of 2008, and a consensus was reached that there were likely to be:

- Eleven significant changes in how health care would be delivered (Box 1-2),
- Nine changes likely to occur in the U.S. health care workforce (Box 1-3), and

Box 1-2 2015 and Beyond: 11 Predicted Changes in Health Care

1. More patients will receive diagnoses of chronic and acute respiratory diseases
2. Cost increases will continue to grow creating challenges for all payers of health care services
3. Personal electronic health records will become more widely used in all health care settings
4. Health care consumers will pay a greater percentage of costs but will have new options for obtaining care
5. Retail storefront health care and the Internet will stimulate consumer-driven cost competition
6. Acute care hospitals will continue to provide episodic, cutting-edge respiratory life support technology; however, subacute and home care providers will continue to play important roles
7. Subacute and long-term care will increase in volume and complexity
8. The disconnect between prevention and acute care treatment will lessen but not disappear
9. All health care delivery will undergo increasing scrutiny for quality that will be linked to reimbursement under a new system called *Pay for Performance*
10. New models for the delivery of health care will emerge, such as *Accountable Care Organizations* and *Medical Home*
11. Reimbursement and costs will influence the development and success of these new models

From Bunch D: 2015 and Beyond. AARC Times 33:50, 2009.

Box 1-3 2015 and Beyond: Nine Likely Changes in the Health Care Workforce

1. There will be national and regional shortages of certain providers in all sectors of health care
2. There will be long-term competition for all health care professionals
3. The clinical demand will increase at a faster pace than the workforce will be able to expand
4. The imbalance in jobs and available workforce will be aggravated by the retirement of current providers
5. Brutal work hours requiring 24/7 staffing will dissuade many individuals from pursuing health care careers
6. Shortages of teaching faculty and a limited number of training programs will limit the number of entrants into allied health professional schools
7. Traditional clinical sites will be limited in number and variety and will need to be expanded to alternate sites, such as physicians' offices and patients' homes
8. Newer educational technologic resources will challenge traditional education
9. Health care delivery organizations will find reinvestment in education an attractive way to secure competent and loyal workers

From Bunch D: 2015 and Beyond. AARC Times 33:50, 2009.

- Five expected changes in how respiratory care services would be provided (Box 1-4).[40]

In the words of one conference organizer, "the take home message was that indeed the scope and depth of respiratory care practice will increase by 2015."[39] The second conference was held in the spring of 2009 and built on the findings of the 2008 conference by identifying the competencies needed by graduate respiratory therapists and the educational content and curriculum that would be needed to practice in 2015 and beyond. Conference participants agreed that there would be seven major competencies (Box 1-5) that future respiratory therapists would need to practice effectively by 2015.[40,41] The third conference was held in the summer of 2010 to determine how the educational programs for entry-level respiratory therapists would have to be structured to accomplish the seven major competencies identified during the 2009 conference. The recommendations of the third conference were published in 2011.[42]

Although the respiratory care profession is undergoing substantial change, there will be a continuing demand for respiratory care services well into the future because of advances in treatment and technology, increases in the general population, and increases in the elderly population (the baby boomers). A growing population will result in increases in asthma, COPD, and other chronic respiratory diseases. There will also be a continuing demand for controlling costs and ensuring that care provided is evidence-based, safe, and effective. Respiratory care will need to be provided using carefully designed protocols to ensure that patients get the appropriate care at the right time and that unnecessary care is reduced or eliminated. Aggressive steps to prevent disease and control the cost of chronic respiratory disease will be essential. Effective smoking cessation and tobacco education programs and aggressive disease management and pulmonary rehabilitation for patients with moderate to severe asthma, COPD, and other chronic respiratory disease will continue to be needed.

As exemplified by the 2015 and Beyond project, the knowledge, skills, and attributes needed by respiratory therapists will continue to expand, and it will become increasingly difficult to prepare respiratory therapists for expanded practice within the credit hour limitations of many existing programs. To alleviate this situation, associate degree programs may develop articulation agreements with 4-year colleges and universities to allow their graduates to complete the bachelor degree in respiratory care without leaving their home campus; distance education technology will play an important role and allow this to occur at minimal cost.

Bachelor degree programs often seek to provide students with a foundation for leadership in the profession in the areas of management, supervision, research, education, or clinical specialty areas. To meet the leadership needs of the profession, some baccalaureate programs have already implemented postbaccalaureate certificates or master degree programs. Clinical areas in which more graduate education programs could be beneficial include critical care, cardiopulmonary diagnostics, clinical research, sleep medicine, rehabilitation, and preparation as a pulmonary physician assistant. There will also be an increasing demand for respiratory therapists with master and doctoral degrees to serve as university faculty, educators, and researchers.

Box 1-4 2015 and Beyond: Five Changes Expected in Respiratory Care

1. The science of respiratory care will continue to evolve and increase in complexity, and clinical decisions will increasingly be data-driven
2. Patient care teams will become the standard throughout health care
3. New respiratory life-support technologies will be developed and deployed
4. Reimbursement changes will be the most important impetus for more recognition of the importance of health promotion and disease state management
5. Concerns over public health issues and military and disaster response will continue and require new skill sets for all respiratory care providers

From Bunch D: 2015 and Beyond. AARC Times 33:50, 2009.

Box 1-5 Seven Major Competencies Required by Respiratory Therapists by 2015

1. Diagnostics
2. Chronic disease state management
3. Evidence-based medicine and respiratory care protocols
4. Patient assessment
5. Leadership
6. Emergency and critical care
7. Therapeutics

From Barnes TA, Gale DD, Kacmarek RM, et al: Competencies needed by graduate respiratory therapists in 2015 and beyond. Respir Care 55:601, 2010.

SUMMARY CHECKLIST

- Respiratory therapists apply scientific principles to prevent, identify, and treat acute or chronic dysfunction of the cardiopulmonary system.
- Respiratory care includes the assessment, treatment, management, control, diagnostic evaluation, education, and care of patients with deficiencies and abnormalities of the cardiopulmonary system.
- The AARC is the professional association for the field.
- Respiratory therapists work under the direction of a physician who is specially trained in pulmonary medicine, anesthesiology, and critical care medicine.

Continued

- The NBRC, the credentialing board for respiratory therapists, was founded in 1974. The American Registry of Inhalation Therapists was founded in 1960.
- The CoARC accredits respiratory care educational programs. The first Board of Schools was established in 1963.
- As the physiologic basis for oxygen therapy became understood, use of oxygen to treat respiratory disease became established by the 1920s, and oxygen was used routinely in hospitals by the 1940s.
- Use of aerosolized medications for the treatment of asthma began in 1910, with numerous new drugs being developed in the twentieth century and continuing up to the present.
- Mechanical ventilation was explored in the 1800s. In 1928, Drinker developed his iron lung; this was followed by the Emerson iron lung in the 1930s, which was used extensively during the polio epidemics of the 1940s and 1950s, and the modern critical care ventilator, which became available in the 1960s.
- The ITA was founded in 1947, becoming the AAIT in 1954, the AART in 1973, and the AARC in 1982.
- The AARC now has 10 Specialty Sections to provide resources to members based on where they are employed and practice.
- The ARCF offers many scholarships and grants to respiratory therapy students.
- Although originally found only in the United States and Canada, the practice of respiratory therapy is quickly expanding around the world.
- Respiratory Care Week is a yearly event to promote the profession and raise awareness of the importance of good lung health.
- In the future, there will be an increase in demand for respiratory care because of advances in treatment and technology; increases in and aging of the population; and increases in the number of patients with asthma, COPD, and other cardiopulmonary diseases.
- The respiratory therapist of the future will be focused on patient assessment, care plan development, protocol administration, disease management and rehabilitation, and patient and family education, to include tobacco education and smoking cessation.

References

1. Ward JJ, Helmholtz HF: Roots of the respiratory care profession. In Burton GG, Hodgkin JE, Ward JJ, editors: Respiratory care: a guide to clinical practice, ed 4, Philadelphia, 1997, Lippincott.
2. American Association for Respiratory Care: Definition of respiratory care. December 2006. http://www.aarc.org/resources/position_statements/defin.html. Accessed April 4, 2007.
3. Dubbs WH: AARC's 2009 human resources survey. AARC Times 33, 2009.
4. Smith GA: Respiratory care: evolution of a profession, Lenexa, KS, 1989, AMP.
5. Weilacher RR: History of the respiratory care profession. In: Hess DR, MacIntyre NR, Mishoe SC, et al, editors: Respiratory care: principles and practice, Philadelphia, 2002, Saunders.
6. Stoller JK: The history of intubation, tracheotomy and airway appliances. Respir Care 44:595, 1999.
7. Medicine, history of. 2006. Encyclopaedia Britannica Premium Service. http://www.britannica.com/eb/article-9110313. Accessed April 4, 2007.
8. Verma S: The little book of scientific principles, theories and things, New York, 2005, Sterling Publishing.
9. Cotes JE: Lung function assessment and application in medicine, ed 4, Oxford, 1979, Blackwell Scientific Publications.
10. Rau JL: Respiratory care pharmacology, ed 5, St Louis, 1998, Mosby.
11. Branson RD: A tribute to John H Emerson. Respir Care 43:567, 1998.
12. Hill NS: Use of negative pressure ventilation, rocking beds and pneumobelts. Respir Care 39:532, 1994.
13. Mushin WW, Rendell-Baker L, Thompson PW, et al: Automatic ventilation of the lungs, ed 3, Oxford, 1980, Blackwell Scientific Publications, pp 184–249.
14. Chatburn RL: Mechanical ventilators. In Branson RD, Hess DR, Chatburn RL, editors: Respiratory therapy equipment, ed 2, Philadelphia, 1999, Lippincott Williams & Wilkins, pp 395–525.
15. Cairo JM, Pilbeam SP: Mosby's respiratory care equipment, ed 7, St. Louis, 2004, Elsevier.
16. Petty TL: John Hutchinson's mysterious machine revisited. Chest 121:219s, 2002.
17. American Association for Respiratory Care: Member services. www.aarc.org/member_services. Accessed February 23, 2011.
18. American Association for Care: Strategic plan. www.aarc.org/members_area/resources/strategic.asp. Accessed January 25, 2011.
19. Wilson BG: Delivering "the promise". NBRC Horizons 25:1, 3, 5, 1999.
20. Commission on Accreditation of Allied Health Education Programs: Standards and guidelines for the profession of respiratory care, Bedford, TX, 2003, Committee on Accreditation for Respiratory Care.
21. Committee on Accreditation for Respiratory Care: Respiratory care accreditation handbook, Bedford, TX, 2001, Committee on Accreditation for Respiratory Care.
22. Commission on Accreditation of Allied Health Education Programs: Respiratory therapy (advanced). http://www.caahep.org/Find_An_Accredited_Program.aspx. Accessed April 6, 2007.
23. American Association for Respiratory Care: Accredited programs. http://www.aarc.org/education/accredited_programs/. Accessed April 6, 2007.
24. Canadian Society for Respiratory Therapy: Education: respiratory therapy programs approved by a CSRC. http://csrt.com/accreditation.php?display&en&4. Accessed April 6, 2007.
25. O'Daniel C, Cullen DL, Douce FH, et al: The future educational needs of respiratory care practitioners: a Delphi study. Respir Care 37:65, 1992.
26. Douce HF: A critical analysis of respiratory care scope of practice and education: past, present, and future. In: American Association for Respiratory Care: Delineating the educational direction for the future respiratory care practitioner: proceedings of a National Consensus Conference on Respiratory Care Education, Dallas, 1992, AARC.
27. American Association for Respiratory Care: Delineating the educational direction for the future respiratory care

practitioner: proceedings of a National Consensus Conference on Respiratory Care Education, Dallas, 1992, AARC.
28. American Association for Respiratory Care: An action agenda: proceedings of the Second National Consensus Conference on Respiratory Care Education, Dallas, 1993, AARC.
29. Meredith RL, Pilbeam SP, Stoller JK: Is our educational system adequately preparing respiratory care practitioners for therapist-driven protocols? (editorial). Respir Care 39:709, 1994.
30. Kester L, Stoller JK: Respiratory care education: current issues and future challenges (editorial). Respir Care 41:98, 1996.
31. Mishoe SC, MacIntyre NR: Expanding professional roles for respiratory care practitioners. Respir Care 42:71, 1997.
32. Hess DR: Professionalism, respiratory care practice and physician acceptance of a respiratory care consult service (editorial). Respir Care 43:546, 1998.
33. Stoller JK, Mascha EJ, et al: Randomized controlled trial of physician-directed versus respiratory therapy consult service-directed respiratory care to adult non-ICU inpatients. Am J Respir Crit Care Med 158:1068, 1998.
34. Mishoe SC, Hess DR: Forward: evidence-based medicine in respiratory care. Respir Care 46:1200, 2001.
35. Montori VM, Guyatt GH: What is evidence-based medicine and why should it be practiced? Respir Care 46:1201, 2001.
36. American Association for Respiratory Care: Respiratory care: advancement of the profession tripartite statements of support. http://www.aarc.org/resources/cpgs_guidelines_statements/. Accessed April 4, 2007.
37. American Association for Respiratory Care, Barnes, TA, Black CP, Douce, FH, et al: A white paper from the AARC Steering Committee of the Coalition for Baccalaureate and Graduate Respiratory Therapy Education: development of baccalaureate and graduate degrees in respiratory care. Respir Care Educ Annu 12:29, 2003.
38. Pierson DJ: The future of respiratory care. Respir Care 46:705, 2001.
39. Bunch D. 2015 and Beyond, AARC Times 33:50, 2009.
40. Kacmarek RM, Durbin CG, Barnes TA, et al: Creating a vision for respiratory care in 2015 and beyond. Respir Care 54:375, 2009.
41. Barnes TA, Gale DD, Kacmarek RM, et al: Competencies needed by graduate respiratory therapists in 2015 and beyond. Respir Care 55:601, 2010.
42. Barnes TA, Kacmarek RM, Kageler WV, et al: Transitioning the respiratory therapy workforce for 2015 and beyond. Respir Care 56, 2011.

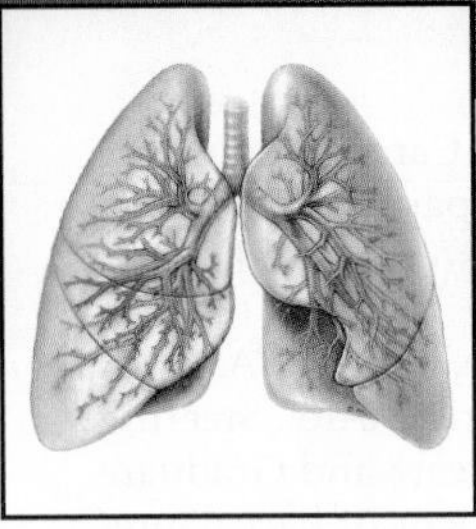

Chapter 2

Quality and Evidence-Based Respiratory Care

LUCY KESTER AND JAMES K. STOLLER

CHAPTER OBJECTIVES

After reading this chapter you will be able to:

- Describe the elements that constitute quality respiratory care.
- Explain methods used for monitoring the quality of respiratory care that is provided.
- Explain how respiratory care protocols enhance the quality of respiratory care services.
- Define disease management.
- Describe evidence-based medicine.

CHAPTER OUTLINE

KEY TERMS

algorithms
Committee on Accreditation for Respiratory Care (CoARC)
competencies
cross-training
disease management
evidence-based medicine
The Joint Commission (TJC)
misallocation
National Board for Respiratory Care (NBRC)
performance improvement
quality
quality assurance
respiratory care protocols
respiratory therapy consult service
therapist-driven protocols

Quality is defined as a characteristic reflecting a high degree of excellence, fineness, or grade. Ruskin, a nineteenth-century British author, stated, "Quality is never an accident. It is always the result of intelligent effort." Conclusions drawn from the assessment of quality are only temporary because the components of quality are constantly changing. Specifically, quality, as applied to the practice of respiratory care, is multidimensional. It encompasses the personnel who perform respiratory care, the equipment used, and the method or manner in which care is provided. Determining the quality of services provided by a respiratory care department requires intelligent efforts to establish guidelines for delivering quality care and a method for monitoring this care. The conclusions derived from monitoring the respiratory care provided change as clinical practice and expectations change. In the current cost-attentive era of health care, quality can be challenged by pressures to minimize cost, making the measurement and monitoring of quality even more important.

This chapter reviews issues related to the quality of respiratory care. First, we review the elements of a hospital-based respiratory care program, focusing on medical direction, practitioners, and technical direction. With the objective of quality being the competent delivery of indicated care, we discuss respiratory care protocols as one strategy to ensure quality. Methods for monitoring quality are discussed next, with attention to the role of **The Joint Commission (TJC)** and peer review organizations (PROs). We then discuss the effect of several health care delivery strategies on respiratory care quality. Finally, we review the concept of evidence-based medicine as it applies to the practice of respiratory care.

ELEMENTS OF A HOSPITAL-BASED RESPIRATORY CARE PROGRAM: ROLES SUPPORTING QUALITY CARE

Medical Direction

The medical director of respiratory care is professionally responsible for the clinical function of the department and provides oversight of the clinical care that is delivered (Box 2-1). Medical direction for respiratory care is usually provided by a pulmonary/critical care physician or an anesthesiologist. Whether the role of a respiratory care service medical director is designated as a full-time or part-time position, it is a full-time responsibility; the medical director must be available on a 24-hour basis for consultation with and to give advice to other physicians and the respiratory care staff. The current philosophy of cost containment and cost-effectiveness, dictated by medical care market forces, poses a challenge to the medical and technical leadership of respiratory care services to provide increasingly high-quality patient care at low cost. A medical director must possess administrative and medical skills.[1]

Box 2-1 Responsibilities of a Medical Director of Respiratory Care

- Medical supervision of RTs in the following areas
  - General medical, surgical, and respiratory nursing wards
  - ICUs
  - Ambulatory care (including rehabilitation)
  - Pulmonary function laboratory
- Development and approval of department clinical policies and procedures
- Supervision of ongoing quality assurance activities
- Medical direction for respiratory care in-service and training programs
- Education of medical and nursing staffs regarding respiratory therapy
- Participation in the selection and promotion of technical staff
- Participation in the preparation of the department budget

Perhaps the most essential aspect of providing quality respiratory care is to ensure that the care being provided is indicated and that it is delivered competently and appropriately. Traditionally, the physician has evaluated patients for respiratory care and has written the specific respiratory therapy orders for the respiratory therapist (RT) to follow. However, such traditional practices have often been shown to be associated with misallocation of respiratory care.[2-4] This **misallocation** may consist of ordering therapy that is not indicated, ordering therapy to be delivered by an inappropriate method, or failing to provide therapy that is indicated.[5] Table 2-1 reviews studies evaluating the allocation of respiratory care services and the frequency of misallocated care.[3,6-12] These studies provide ample evidence that misallocation of respiratory care occurs frequently. Such misallocation has led to the use of respiratory care protocols that are implemented by RTs (as described under Methods for Enhancing the Quality of Respiratory Care).

Respiratory Therapists

In addition to capable medical direction and the application of well-constructed respiratory care protocols (see p. 26), capable RTs are an indispensable element of a quality respiratory care program. The quality of RTs depends primarily on their training, education, experience, and professionalism. Training teaches students to perform tasks at a competent level, whereas clinical education provides students with a knowledge base they can use in evaluating a situation and making appropriate decisions.[13] Both adequate training and clinical education are required to produce qualified RTs for assessment of patients and implementation of respiratory care protocols.[14]

Designations and Credentials of Respiratory Therapists

There are two levels of general practice credentialing in respiratory care: (1) certified respiratory therapists (CRTs) and (2) registered respiratory therapists (RRTs). Students eligible to become CRTs and RRTs are trained and educated in colleges and universities. After completion of an approved respiratory care educational program, a graduate may become credentialed by taking the entry-level examination to become a CRT. A CRT may be eligible to sit for the registry examinations to become a credentialed RRT. Students who complete a 2-year program graduate with an associate degree, and students who complete a 4-year program receive a baccalaureate degree. Some RTs go on to complete a graduate degree (e.g., master or doctorate) with additional study in the areas of respiratory care, education, management, or health sciences. The further

TABLE 2-1

Frequency of Misallocation of Respiratory Care Services in Selected Series

Type of Service	Author	Date	Patient Type	No. Patients	Frequency of Overordering	Frequency of Underordering
Supplemental oxygen	Zibrak et al[6]	1986	Adults	NS	55% reduction in incentive spirometry after therapist supervision began	NA
	Brougher et al[7]	1986	Adult, non-ICU inpatients	77	38% ordered to receive oxygen despite adequate oxygenation	NA
	Small et al[8]	1992	Adult, non-ICU inpatients	47	72% of patients checked had $PaO_2 > 60$ mm Hg or $SaO_2 > 90\%$ but were prescribed oxygen	NA
	Kester and Stoller[3]	1992	Adult, non-ICU inpatients	230	28% for supplemental oxygen	8% for supplemental oxygen
	Albin et al[9]	1992	Adult, non-ICU inpatients	274	61% ordered to receive supplemental oxygen despite $SaO_2 \geq 92\%$	21% underordered, including 19% prescribed to receive inadequate O_2 flow rates
	Shelledy et al[12]	2004	Adults	75	0	5.3% indicated but not ordered
Bronchial hygiene techniques	Zibrak et al[6]	1986	Adults	NS	55% reduction in incentive spirometry after therapist supervision began	NA
	Shapiro et al[10]	1988	Adult, non-ICU inpatients	3400 evaluations	61% reduction of bronchial hygiene after system implemented	NA
	Kester and Stoller[3]	1992	Adult, non-ICU inpatients	230	32%	8%
	Shelledy et al[12]	2004	Adults	75	37.5%	8%
Bronchodilator therapy	Zibrak et al[6]	1986	Adults	NS	50% reduction in incentive aerosolized medication after therapist supervision began	NA
	Kester and Stoller[3]	1992	Adult, non-ICU inpatients	230	12%	12%
	Shelledy et al[12]	2004	Adults	75	34.4%	5.3%
	Kester and Stoller[3]	1992	Adult, non-ICU inpatient	230	40%	6.7%
ABGs	Browning et al[11]	1989	Surgical ICU inpatients	724 ABGs	42.7% inappropriately ordered before guidelines implemented	NA

Modified from Stoller JK: The rationale for therapist-driven protocols. Respir Care Clin N Am 2:1–14, 1996.
NS, Not stated; *NA,* not assessed.

development of graduate education in respiratory care has been encouraged by the American Association for Respiratory Care (AARC), and programs are both currently available and under development.[15]

Respiratory care education programs are reviewed by the **Committee on Accreditation for Respiratory Care (CoARC).** This committee is sponsored by four organizations: the AARC, the American College of Chest Physicians (ACCP), the American Society of Anesthesiologists (ASA), and the American Thoracic Society (ATS). The CoARC is responsible for ensuring that respiratory therapy educational programs follow accrediting standards or essentials as endorsed by the American Medical Association (AMA). Members of the CoARC visit respiratory therapy educational programs to judge applications for accreditation and make periodic reviews. The mission of the CoARC, in collaboration with the Association of Specialized and Professional Accreditors, is to promote quality respiratory therapy education through accreditation services. An annual listing of accredited respiratory therapy programs is published. As of November 2010, there were approximately 415 CoARC-approved respiratory care programs.

Credentialing is a general term that refers to the recognition of individuals in particular occupations or professions. Generally, the two major forms of credentialing in the health fields are state licensure and voluntary certification. Licensure is the process in which a government agency gives an individual permission to practice an occupation. Typically, a license is granted only after verifying that the applicant has demonstrated the minimum competency necessary to protect the public health, safety, or welfare. Licensure laws are normally made by state legislatures and enforced by specific state agencies, such as medical, nursing, and respiratory care boards. In states where licensure laws govern an occupation, practicing in the field without a license is considered a crime punishable by fines or imprisonment or both. Licensure regulations are based on a practice act that defines (and limits) what activities the professional can perform. Two other forms of state credentialing are less restrictive. States that use title protection simply safeguard the use of a particular occupational or professional title. Alternatively, states may request or require practitioners to register with a government agency (registration). Neither title protection nor state registration constitutes a true practice act, and because both title protection and registration are voluntary, neither provides strong protection against unqualified or incompetent practice.

Certification is a voluntary, nongovernment process whereby a private agency grants recognition to an individual who has met certain qualifications. Examples of qualifications are graduation from an approved educational program, completion of a specific amount of work experience, and acceptable performance on a qualifying examination. The term *registration* is often used interchangeably with the term *certification,* but it may also refer to a type of government credentialing. As a voluntary process, certification involves standards that are often higher than the minimum standards specified for entry-level competency. A major difference between certification and licensure is that certification generally does not prevent others from working in that occupation, as do most forms of licensure. Both types of credentialing apply in respiratory care.

The primary method of ensuring quality in respiratory care is voluntary certification or registration conducted by the **National Board for Respiratory Care (NBRC).** The NBRC is an independent national credentialing agency for individuals who work in respiratory care and related services. The NBRC is cooperatively sponsored by the AARC, the ACCP, the ASA, the ATS, and the National Society for Pulmonary Technology. Representatives of these organizations make up the governing board of the NBRC, which assumes the responsibility for all examination standards and policies through a standing committee. The NBRC provides the credentialing process for both the entry-level CRT and the advanced-practitioner RRT. As established in January 2006, to be eligible for either the CRT or the RRT examination, all candidates must have an associate degree or higher. An additional advanced-practitioner credential, the neonatal/pediatric specialist (NPS), has been established for the field of pediatrics. The NBRC also encourages professionals in the field to maintain and upgrade their skills through voluntary recredentialing. Both CRTs and RRTs may demonstrate ongoing professional competence by retaking examinations. Individuals who pass these examinations are issued a certificate recognizing them as "recredentialed" practitioners. In addition to the certification and registration of RTs, the NBRC provides credentialing in the area of pulmonary function testing for certified pulmonary function technologists (CPFTs) and registered pulmonary function technologists (RPFTs). Since its inception, the NBRC has issued more than 350,000 professional credentials to more than 209,000 individuals. As of 2010, there were approximately 206,150 active RTs, many of whom hold more than one credential. Table 2-2 shows the distribution of these credentialed individuals.

TABLE 2-2

Distribution of Credentialed Practitioners

Credential Type	No. Credentialed Practitioners
CRT	206,150
RRT	117,215
CPFT	12,393
RPFT	4192
NPS	10,060

As of October 14, 2010.
Note: Practitioners may hold more than one credential (i.e., RRTs are also CRTs and NPS are also CRTs and RRTs).

At the time of publication, 49 states, the District of Columbia, and Puerto Rico have some form of state licensure. Many states use the NBRC entry-level respiratory care examination for state licensing, whereas others simply verify NBRC credentials. Most licensure acts require the RT to attain a specified number of continuing education credits to maintain his or her license. Continuing education helps practitioners keep abreast of the changes and advances that occur in their health care field.

Licensure and certification help ensure that only qualified RTs participate in the practice of respiratory care. Many institutions conduct annual skills checks or competency evaluations in compliance with TJC requirements. Beyond TJC–required skills checks, experience with respiratory care protocols suggests the need to develop and monitor additional skills among RTs (Box 2-2). Assurance and maintenance of these skills require ongoing training and quality review programs, which are discussed in the section on Monitoring Quality Respiratory Care.

Box 2-2 Additional Respiratory Therapist Skills Required for Implementing Protocols

- Assess and evaluate patients regarding indications for therapy and for the most appropriate delivery method
- Be cognizant of age-related issues and how they affect the patient's ability to understand and use various treatment modalities
- Adapt hospital policies and procedures to alternative care sites
- Conduct and participate in research activities to ensure a scientific basis for advances in respiratory care technology
- Communicate effectively with all members of the health care team, and contribute to the body of literature concerning the field of respiratory care

Box 2-3 Professional Characteristics of a Respiratory Therapist

- Completes an accredited respiratory therapy program
- Obtains professional credentials
- Participates in continuing education activities
- Adheres to the code of ethics put forth by the institution or state licensing board or both
- Joins professional organizations

Professionalism

By definition, professionalism is a key attribute to which all RTs should aspire and that must guide respiratory care practice. *Webster's New Collegiate Dictionary* defines a *profession* as "a calling that requires specialized knowledge and often long and intensive academic preparation." A professional is characterized as an individual conforming to the technical and ethical standards of a profession. RTs demonstrate their professionalism by maintaining the highest practice standards, by engaging in ongoing learning, by conducting research to advance the quality of respiratory care, and by participating in organized activities through professional societies such as the AARC and associated state societies. Box 2-3 lists the professional attributes of the RT. We emphasize the importance of these attributes because the continued value and progress of the field depend critically on the professionalism of each practitioner.[16]

In the highly regulated careers of health care, professionalism also requires compliance with external standards, such as the standards set by TJC and by the government. One such standard is defined by the Health Insurance Portability and Accountability Act (HIPAA) of 1996. HIPAA sets standards regarding the way sensitive health care information is communicated and revealed in the transmission of medical records and in the written and verbal communication of information in the hospital. Some specific provisions of HIPAA are presented in Box 2-4. As with all hospital and health care personnel, standards of respiratory therapy professionalism require knowledge of HIPAA and compliance with its terms.

Box 2-4 Health Insurance Portability and Accountability Act of 1996 (HIPAA)

The use and disclosure of protected health information (PHI) by a covered entity are prohibited unless it is a permitted use or disclosure for purposes of treatment, payment, or health care operations or is authorized by the patient. When disclosure or use of PHI is permitted, ensure that only the minimum necessary information is disclosed.

DEFINITION OF TERMS

Use: Release of PHI within the institution
Disclosure: Release of PHI outside the institution
PHI: Individually identifiable health information
Covered entity: Health care provider, health plan, health care clearinghouse
Permitted: As long as there are reasonable safeguards in place regarding the Privacy Rule and the information given is the "minimum necessary"
Treatment: Necessary information can be disclosed to all involved in treatment (physicians, nurses, allied health personnel)
Payment: To allow for billing, for insurance purposes and third-party payers
Authorized: Patient's written agreement for permitted use
Minimum necessary: Reasonably necessary to accomplish intended purpose

Technical Direction

Another important element for delivering quality respiratory care is technical direction. Technical direction is often the responsibility of the manager of a respiratory care department, who must ensure the equipment and the associated protocols and procedures have sufficient quality to ensure the safety, health, and welfare of the patient using the equipment. Medical devices are regulated under the Medical Device Amendment Act of 1976, which comes under the authority of the U.S. Food and Drug Administration (FDA). The FDA also regulates the drugs delivered by RTs. The purpose of the FDA is to establish safety and effectiveness standards and to ensure that these standards are met by equipment and pharmaceutical manufacturers.

Procedures and protocols related to the use of equipment and medications must be written to provide a guide for the respiratory care staff. In addition, equipment must be safety checked, and specific maintenance procedures must be performed on a regular basis. Because of rapidly changing respiratory care technology, the job of the technical director poses significant challenges. Circuit boards and computers have replaced simpler mechanical devices. New medications and delivery devices for the treatment of asthma and new strategies for treating other respiratory diseases (e.g., low-stretch ventilatory approaches for acute respiratory distress syndrome [ARDS]) continue to evolve. Individuals responsible for technical direction must ensure that these new devices, methods, and strategies not only are effective but also deliver a benefit commensurate with the cost.

METHODS FOR ENHANCING QUALITY RESPIRATORY CARE

Respiratory Care Protocols

In an effort to improve the allocation of respiratory care services, **respiratory care protocols** (also known as **therapist-driven protocols**) have been developed and are in use in many hospitals in the United States, Canada, and other countries. Respiratory care protocols are guidelines for delivering appropriate respiratory care treatments and services (i.e., treatments and services that are indicated, delivered by the correct method, and discontinued when no longer needed). Protocols may be written in outline form or may use **algorithms** (an example of which is a branching logic flow diagram [Figures 2-1 and 2-2]).

Gaylin and colleagues[17] conducted a telephone survey in 1999 of 371 RT members of the AARC, of whom 51% were practitioners, 26% were clinical supervisors, and 23% were administrators. When asked if their organizations used guidelines or protocols, 98% of the respondents indicated that they did. Of the 2% who did not, 53% were planning their use.[17] A survey conducted by the AARC in 2005 indicated that of 681 responding hospitals, 73% were providing care by means of at least one protocol.[18] More recently, the 2009 AARC Human Resources Survey showed that of 2764 responders, about two-thirds (65.7%) indicated that they have delivered respiratory care by protocol.[19] The use of respiratory care protocols by qualified RTs is a logical practice based on the premise that well-trained RTs possess extensive knowledge of respiratory care modalities and have the assessment and communication skills required to execute the protocols effectively.[20]

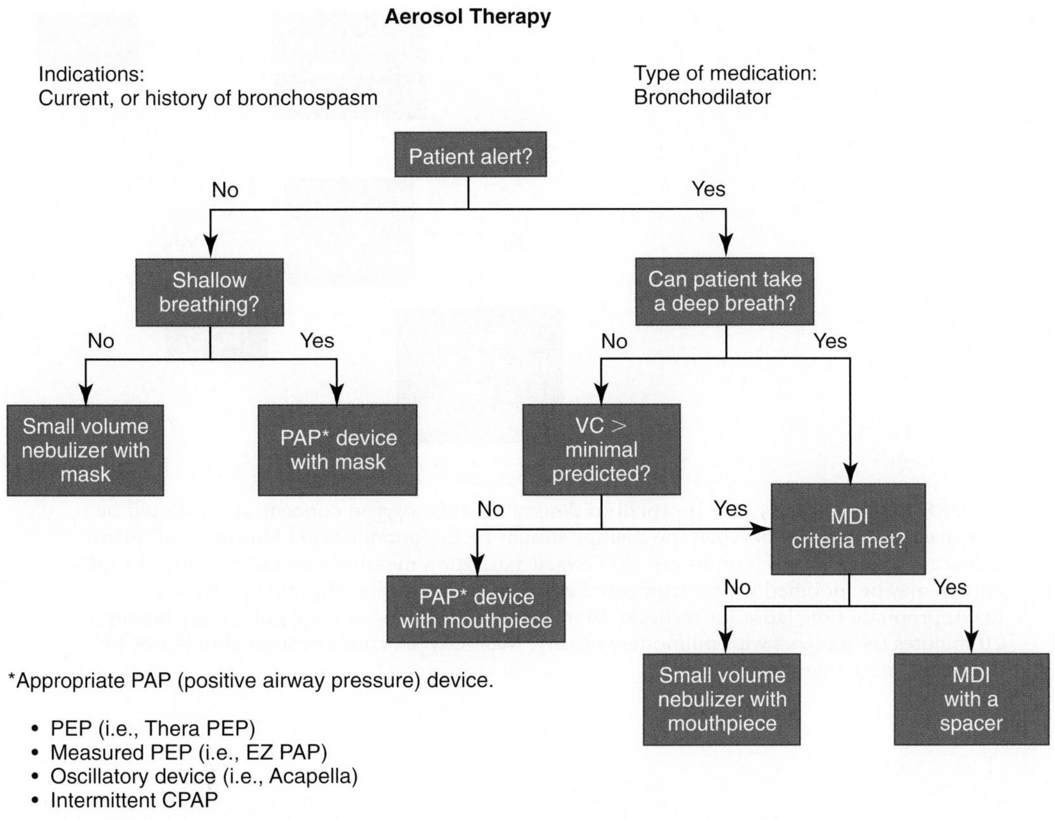

FIGURE 2-1 Respiratory care protocol. Aerosolized bronchodilator therapy algorithm for current or history of bronchospasm.

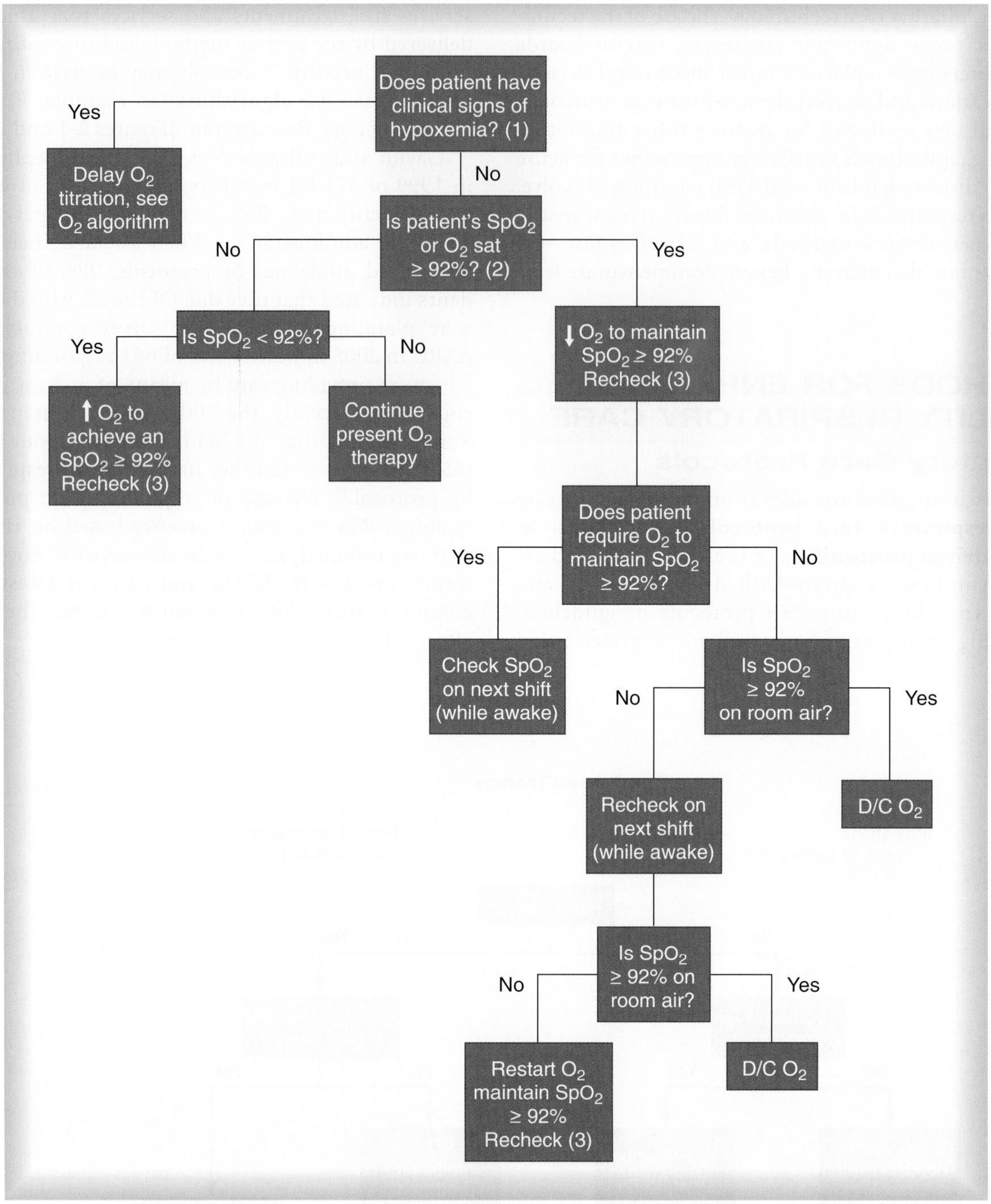

FIGURE 2-2 Respiratory care protocol to determine when oxygen concentration should be increased or decreased or when the therapy should be discontinued. *(1)* Shortness of breath, tachycardia, diaphoresis, confusion. *(2)* Oxygen saturation measured by pulse oximeter (SpO_2) criteria may be modified with documented evidence of preexisting chronic hypoxemia. *(3)* Appropriate time lapse for recheck: 10 minutes for patients without pulmonary history; 20 minutes for patients with pulmonary history. *Note:* Oxygen concentration should not be decreased more than once per shift.

MINI CLINI

A Specific Treatment Protocol: Aerosolized Bronchodilator Therapy

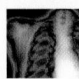

PROBLEM: A 54-year-old woman is admitted to the hospital with an exacerbation of COPD. She has a history of smoking one and one-half packs of cigarettes a day for 32 years. She is alert and oriented, and her respiratory rate is 32 breaths/min. On auscultation, she has bilateral wheezes on inspiration and exhalation. Her vital capacity (1.3 L) is greater than the predicted minimal volume for effective incentive spirometry, but she is unable to take in a slow, deep breath and hold it for longer than 5 seconds, which is the criterion sometimes used for appropriate MDI use. What should the RT do now?

SOLUTIONS: Following the aerosol therapy protocol algorithm, this patient would receive an aerosolized bronchodilator treatment from a small volume nebulizer with a mouthpiece. An algorithm for aerosolized bronchodilator therapy is shown in Figure 2-1.

MINI CLINI

A Specific Purpose Protocol: Oxygen Therapy Titration

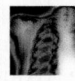

PROBLEM: A 42-year-old man has returned to a medical-surgical nursing unit from the recovery room after a cholecystectomy. He has no history of lung disease and is wearing a nasal cannula at 2 L/min. He is alert and oriented, and his respiratory rate is 18 breaths/min and heart rate is 82 beats/min. When the RT arrives to check his oxygen setup and pulse oximeter reading, his SpO_2 (pulse oximeter reading) is 97% on the 2 L/min nasal cannula. What should the RT do next?

SOLUTIONS: Following the oxygen therapy titration protocol algorithm, the RT removes the nasal cannula and returns in 15 minutes to recheck the patient's SpO_2 reading, which is now 93% on room air. The RT discontinues the oxygen therapy. An oxygen therapy titration algorithm is shown in Figure 2-2.

The success of a respiratory care protocol program requires several key elements, including active and committed medical direction, capable RTs, collaboration with physicians and nurses, careful monitoring, and a responsive hospital environment (Box 2-5). As further evidence of the widespread acceptance of protocols, the ACCP has identified the elements of an acceptable respiratory care protocol (Box 2-6). This document may serve as a guide for developing protocols. Protocols may be constructed for individual therapies, such as aerosol therapy, bronchopulmonary hygiene, oxygen therapy, hyperinflation techniques, suctioning, and pulse oximetry. Protocols also can be written for a specific purpose, such as arterial blood gas (ABG) sampling, weaning from mechanical ventilation, decannulating a tracheostomy, and titrating oxygen therapy.

Successful implementation of protocols requires acceptance by various stakeholder communities in the hospital, including the hospital administrators, physicians, nurses, and RTs themselves. Hospital administrators are likely to be accepting to the extent that they are convinced that protocols enhance patient care, improve allocation of respiratory care services, and reduce costs. Physicians are likely to accept RT protocols if they are convinced that protocols will enhance their patients' care, preserve the physician's ability to specify orders if desired, and maintain the physician's awareness of changes in a patient's condition and changes in the respiratory care plan. Physicians' acceptance also requires their having trust in the quality, professionalism, and competence of the respiratory therapy staff. Nurses are likely to accept protocols if they are persuaded that protocols will enhance the efficiency of care, help relieve sometimes excessive nursing workloads, and preserve communication with the bedside nurse regarding the patient's plan of treatment. Finally, successful implementation and acceptance of protocols by RTs requires a desire to be progressive, confidence in their

Box 2-5 Key Elements of a Respiratory Care Protocol Program

- Strong and committed medical direction
- Capable RTs
- Active quality monitoring
- Collaborative environment among RTs, physicians, and nurses
- Responsiveness of all participants to address and correct problems

Box 2-6 Elements of an Acceptable Respiratory Care Protocol as Described by the American College of Chest Physicians

- Clearly stated objectives
- Outline that includes an algorithm
- Description of alternative choices at decision and action points
- Description of potential complications and corrections
- Description of end points and decision points at which the physician must be contacted
- Protocol program

Box 2-7 "Highly Desired" Features of a Change-Avid Respiratory Therapy Department

1. Having a close and collegial working relationship between the medical director and the RTs
2. Having a strong and supportive champion for change in the hospital administrative structure (e.g., hospital leaders, medical director)
3. Using data and other evidence to define problems and to measure the effectiveness of proposed solutions
4. Using multiple and redundant types of communication to cascade information throughout the respiratory therapy department
5. Being attentive to the forces of resistance and obstacles to change and being able to navigate within institutional systems and people to achieve change
6. Being willing to confront, engage, and gain closure on tough issues
7. Having and maintaining a culture of internal, self-imposed, systematic, ongoing education and knowledge acquisition
8. Consistently rewarding and recognizing change-avid behavior among respiratory therapy department members
9. Fostering ownership for change rather than just complying with external policies and demands and, as part of this ownership, taking the time to identify and involve stakeholders in change (e.g., physicians, nurses, hospital thought leaders and decision makers)
10. Paying attention to leadership development and succession planning in the RTs
11. Having and communicating a vision in the department

From Stoller JK, Kester L, Roberts VT, et al: An analysis of features of respiratory therapy departments that are avid for change. Respir Care 53:871–884, 2008.

Box 2-8 Tactics for Implementing Respiratory Care Protocols

1. Select a planning team with diverse membership
2. Conduct an audit to assess the occurrence of misallocation of therapy to justify departure from usual care
3. Identify sources of resistance (e.g., physicians, nurses, administrators, RTs)
4. Design a protocol program that fits the individual hospital
5. Develop a training program for RTs
6. Develop an evaluation and quality monitoring system

own assessment and communication skills, "ownership" of the protocol process (e.g., by participating in drafting the protocol policies and strategies by which protocols are put in place), and willingness to change and to abandon antiquated task-driven practices in respiratory care.

Box 2-9 Sequence of Events for a Respiratory Care Consult

1. A physician writes an order for a respiratory care protocol or consult
2. A physician order entry system or the nursing unit secretary notifies an RT evaluator
3. The evaluator assesses the patient using specific guidelines
4. The evaluator writes a care plan using designated indications and algorithms and documents the care plan in the patient's chart for review by the physician
5. The RT covering the nursing unit delivers the care
6. The patient is assessed on a shift-by-shift basis for changes in status and indicated modifications for the care plan, which are also documented
7. The physician is notified of any deterioration in the patient's status
8. When indications for respiratory care no longer exist, respiratory care treatment is discontinued, and notification is placed in the patient's chart

Features of RT departments that are ready for and that embrace change have been studied[21] and are presented in Box 2-7. Steps and tactics to ensure successful implementation of respiratory care protocols are described in Box 2-8. Selecting a planning team with broad membership that includes physicians, nurses, and administrators is a key element in developing a protocol implementation process that avoids potential barriers and satisfies the institution's specific and unique requirements. Once protocols have been designed, it is often advisable to pilot them either individually or on a single hospital floor or unit. This staged rollout with an initial pilot trial allows an opportunity to work out unanticipated problems and obtain helpful feedback from the individuals involved before using the protocols on a hospital-wide basis.

A comprehensive approach for using protocols is to combine specific protocols to form a **respiratory therapy consult service** or an evaluate-and-treat program, which is used in institutions such as the University of California at San Diego and the Cleveland Clinic. With the use of a respiratory therapy consult service, the sequence of events for a respiratory therapy consult may occur as shown in Box 2-9.

A carefully structured assessment tool and care plan form (Figures 2-3 and 2-4) are essential elements for a comprehensive protocol program. These tools help ensure consistency among therapist evaluators. The following Mini Clini on Writing a Respiratory Care Plan shows how an assessment tool and care plan document, used in conjunction with corresponding algorithms, can guide therapists in formulating an appropriate respiratory care plan.

The Cleveland Clinic Foundation
Department of Pulmonary Disease
Respiratory Therapy Evaluation

Date: ___/___/___ Age: 40
Time: ____________ Ht: 5' 7"
Diagnosis: ____________
____
Respiratory therapist ____________

Inpatient ID label

Chart Assessment

Clinical findings	0	X	1	X	2	X	3	X	4	X	Points
Pulmonary status	(−) History (−)Smoking		Smoking history <1 pk a day		Smoking history ≥1 pk a day		Pulmonary impairment (acute or chronic)	X	Severe or chronic with exacerbation		3
Surgical status	No surgery	X	General surgery		Lower abdominal		Thoracic or upper abdominal		Thoracic with pulmonary disease		0
Chest x-ray	Clear or not indicated		Chronic changes or x-ray pending		Infiltrates, atelectasis or pleural effusions	X	Infiltrations in more than one lobe		Infiltrate + atelectasis ±pleural effusion		2

Lab test: Date: ___/___/___ WBC 10.2 Hb 11.6 Plts 260k	Date: ___/___/___	pH	$PaCO_2$	PaO_2	HCO_3	Sat/FIO_2

Pulmonary function test: Minimal pred. VC 0.927L VC 1.35L Peak flow ______	SpO_2/FIO_2 96% RA	Vital signs: HR 84 BP 110/70 RR 20 Temperature (24 hr max)

Patient Assessment

Clinical findings											
Respiratory pattern	Regular pattern RR 12-20	X	Increased RR 21-25		Dyspnea on exertion, irregular pattern RR 26-30		Decreased vital capacity* RR 31-35		Severe SOB, use of accessory muscles RR > 35		0
Mental status	Alert, oriented, cooperative	X	Lethargic, follows commands		Confused, does not follow commands		Obtunded		Comatose		0
Breath sounds	Clear to auscultation		Decreased unilaterally		Decreased bilaterally	X	Crackles in the bases		Wheezing and/or rhonchi	X	4
Cough effectiveness	Strong, spontaneous, non-productive		Strong, productive		Weak, non-productive	X	Weak, productive or weak with rhonchi		No spontaneous cough or may require suctioning		2
Level of activity	Ambulatory	X	Ambulatory with assistance		Temporarily non-ambulatory		Bed rest, able to position self		Bed rest, unable to position self		0
Oxygen required for $SpO_2 < 92\%$	No oxygen	X	1-3 liters		4-6 liters		>50% <100%		100%		0

Total points 11

*VC × 10 minimal predicted:

Predicted ideal body weight
(males: 50 + 2.54 x inches >60)
(females 45 + 2.54 × inches >60)
Multiply above ideal body wt. × 15 cc for min. pred. VC

Triage 1 >20	Triage 2 (16-20)	Triage 3 (11-15)	Triage 4 (6-10)	Triage 5 (0-5)

Triage # 3

FIGURE 2-3 Evaluation form for guiding a standardized patient assessment and assigning a severity of respiratory illness score. The score for the greatest degree of dysfunction for each assessment category is written in the right-hand column and tallied to determine the severity of respiratory illness (triage) score. (Courtesy Cleveland Clinic Respiratory Institute, Cleveland, Ohio.)

Respiratory Therapy Consult/Evaluation

Your patient has been evaluated by the Respiratory Therapy Consult Service. Based on the patient's clinical indicators, the Care Plan designated below will be implemented.

IMPRINT/LABEL

Date of Evaluation ____________

Time of Evaluation ____________

Diagnosis(es) GI dysmotility
Hx asthma

Post Thoracic Surgery Protocol ☐

Clinical Indications

Aerosol Therapy	Broncho/Pulm Hygiene	Hyperinflation	Oxygen Therapy	Respiratory Monitoring	Suctioning
☒ Bronchospasm	☐ Productive cough	☒ Atelectasis	☐ $SpO_2 < 92\%$ on room air	☐ O_2 titration (pulse ox.)	☐ Presence of secretions
☒ History of bronchospasm	☐ Rhonchi on auscultation	☐ Upper abdominal or thoracic surgery, or COPD & surgery	☐ $PaO_2 <$ 55 mm Hg on room air	☐ Unstable resp. status	☐ Unable to cough effectively
☐ Inflammation/ mucosal edema	☐ History of mucous prod. disease	☐ Restrictive disease associated with quadriplegia and/ or dysfunctional diaphragm	☐ Clinical signs of hypoxemia	☐ $SpO_2 < 92\%$ on room air or 4 Lpm O_2 (ABGs)	☐ Altered consciousness
☐ Proteinaceous secretions	☐ Patient unable to deep breathe and cough spontaneously				
☐ Home regimen					
☐ Physician order					

Oximetry sat/FIO_2	Vital capacity
96%/RA	1.35 l

Care Plan

Aerosol Therapy

	DPI	Neb.	MDI	Frequency
Albuterol			X	QID and prn
				at night

				Frequency
bph	☐ Pos. drainage	☐ Percussion/vibration	☐ Coughing techniques	
Hyperinflation	☒ Incen. spiro.	☐ CPAP/PEP	☐ IPPB	To be used q1hr
Oxygen Therapy	☐ FIO_2 % _____	☐ Liters/minute_______		
Monitoring	☐ Pulse oximetry	☐ ABGs	☐ Resp. mechanics	
Suctioning	☐ Nasal-tracheal	☐ Tracheal		

Comments Patient needs encouragement to cough effectively.

Triage Number 3

Signature: Respiratory Therapy Evaluator

Print Name: ____________ /Beeper: ____________

Care plan modifications, made in response to changes in the patient's condition, are available for your review through the Phamis Last Word computer system.

FIGURE 2-4 Care plan form for recording a patient's indications for therapy and the therapeutic modalities for treating the indications. (Courtesy Cleveland Clinic Respiratory Institute, Cleveland, Ohio.)

MINI CLINI

Writing a Respiratory Care Plan

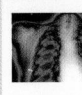

PROBLEM: A 40-year-old woman with a history of asthma was admitted to the hospital for gastrointestinal dysmotility with abdominal distention. Her chest radiograph showed an elevated diaphragm with accompanying atelectasis in the bases of the lung fields. Her laboratory test results were as follows: white blood cell count 10,200 cells/mcl, hemoglobin 11.6 g/dl, and platelet count 260,000/mm^3. Her pulse oximetry reading was 96% on room air; no ABGs were drawn. Her heart rate was 84 beats/min, blood pressure was 110/78 mm Hg, respiratory rate was 20 breaths/min, and temperature was 36.8° C. She was alert and oriented, and her vital capacity was 1.35 L. She is 5 feet 7 inches tall and has a predicted minimal vital capacity of 0.927 L (15 ml/kg of ideal body weight). On auscultation, her breath sounds were decreased bilaterally, and she had slight inspiratory wheezes in the apices of her lung fields. She had a weak, nonproductive cough and was able to ambulate on her own. Perform a respiratory care evaluation for this patient.

SOLUTIONS: The patient's assessment score sheet and her respiratory therapy care plan, using the respiratory therapy consult protocol and treatment algorithms currently in use at the Cleveland Clinic, are shown (see Figures 2-3 and 2-4).

Demonstrated advantages of respiratory care protocols include better allocation of respiratory care services without an increased frequency of respiratory care treatments and cost savings. Other advantages include more dynamic respiratory care with more adjustment of respiratory care services to keep pace with patients' changing clinical status and more versatile use of respiratory care services.[12,22-25]

Monitoring Quality Respiratory Care

Beyond ensuring that all elements of a high-quality respiratory care program are in place, quality must be monitored to ensure that it is being maintained. Strategies to monitor quality include intrainstitutional monitoring practices, centralized government monitoring bodies, such as the Centers for Medicare and Medicaid Services (CMS), and voluntary agencies such as TJC.

Intrainstitutional quality assurance often uses skills checks or **competencies.** Competence, or the quality of being competent, can be defined as having suitable or sufficient skill, knowledge, and experience for the purposes of a specific task.[26] Competence for a specific skill is frequently determined by observation of the practitioner's performance of the skill according to a prescribed checklist. Annual competency checks are documented for skills and procedures that carry some degree of patient risk (e.g., arterial puncture, aerosol therapy, bilevel positive airway pressure setup). An example of a skills checklist is shown in Figure 2-5.

Box 2-10 Nine Steps for a Quality Assurance Plan

1. Identify problem
2. Determine cause of problem
3. Rank problem
4. Develop strategy for resolving problem
5. Develop appropriate measurement techniques
6. Implement problem-resolution strategy
7. Analyze and compile results of intervention
8. Report results to appropriate personnel
9. Evaluate intervention outcome

Although skills checks have traditionally been done in person or with direct supervision of patient care activities, a new dimension of skills training and certification that is being widely implemented is the use of clinical simulation, using either low-fidelity or high-fidelity simulation trainers. Such simulation training (see Chapter 7), in which RTs use technology that attempts to reproduce reliably a true patient or true patient scenario, is similar to the flight simulator training that commercial airline pilots undergo to achieve certification to fly various airplanes. Uses of simulation training in respiratory therapy involve intubation, ventilator management, arterial line placement, and optimizing teamwork in acute resuscitation scenarios.[27]

Many health care organizations, including hospitals, subacute facilities, and outpatient clinics, seek voluntary accreditation as a way to improve their service and assure the public that they maintain high standards. In health care, TJC is a very important organization. TJC was formed in 1951 by the American College of Surgeons, the American Hospital Association, and the AMA. Accreditation by TJC is based on satisfying specific standards established by professional and technical advisory committees.

TJC requires a hospital service to have a **quality assurance** plan to provide a system for controlling quality. Nine generally recognized steps for a quality assurance plan are used as the basis for quality assurance programs (Box 2-10).

Current standards of TJC for accreditation emphasize organization-wide efforts for **performance improvement.** Despite increased emphasis on cost containment, quality care remains the first goal of hospitals and respiratory care services. Performance improvement, also commonly called continuous quality improvement, is an ongoing process designed to detect and correct factors hindering the provision of quality and cost-effective health care. This process crosses department boundaries and follows the continuum of the patient's care. In 2009, TJC

Skills Checklist

Suctioning

Date ____________ First name ____________ Last name ____________ Employee number ____________
mm/dd/yyyy
Use your employee number only, Do NOT use any letters.

Supervisor ____________ Observed by ____________
(Last name, first name)

Patient or simulation? ☐ Patient ☐ Simulation
Last 4 digits of patient MRN ____________ (If applicable)
Unit ____________ (Enter as unit-bed number ex. H81-15 or G111-09)

Age (If applicable) ☐ Neonate/infant (0-18 mos.) ☐ Child (19 mos.-8 yrs.) ☐ Adolescent (9-18 yrs.) ☐ Adult (19-69 yrs.) ☐ Geriatric (70+yrs.)

Did the RT interact appropriately with the patient with regard to the specific age category listed above? (If applicable) ☐ Yes ☐ No

According to section standards

Prepare equipment and assess patient ☐ Yes ☐ No

1. Verify order, verifies patient using at least 2 patient identifiers (Name, MRN, DOB)
2. Introduce self and explains procedure (If applicable)
3. Correctly assemble the equipment per procedure manual, suction kit, manual resuscitator, oxygen, saline for lavage, suction source (wall outlet: 80-120 mm Hg portable: 3-5 inches Hg), lubricating jelly for nasotracheal route

Observe OSHA standards for universal precautions ☐ Yes ☐ No

Pre-assesses patient ☐ Yes ☐ No

1. Heart rate
2. Respiratory rate
3. Breath sounds
4. Pulse oximetry

Perform suctioning procedure ☐ Yes ☐ No

1. Maintain sterile technique
2. Pre-oxygenate
3. Hyper-inflate at least 5-6 times with artificial airways
4. Suction
5. Lubricate catheter for nasotracheal route
6. Insert catheter smoothly as far as possible, careful to stop on encountering resistance
7. Apply suction intermittently as catheter is withdrawn
8. Suction period should not exceed 15 seconds
9. Oxygenate and hyper-inflate after each pass with the catheter
10. Lavage as needed
11. Repeat until airways are clear or as the patient tolerates
12. Note amount, color, and consistency of any secretions

Post treatment assessment ☐ Yes ☐ No

1. Heart rate
2. Respiratory rate
3. Breath sounds
4. Cough
5. Sputum
6. Mental status
7. Activity

Assures patient safety and clean environment ☐ Yes ☐ No

1. Removes all other trash from bed and area
2. Verifies medical support systems are intact (ex. oxygen)
3. Ensures patient safety (ex. bedrails are up)

Charts appropriately ☐ Yes ☐ No

1. Charts correctly in Mediserve in a timely manner
2. Includes any complications and/or adverse events and informs physician

Comments

FIGURE 2-5 Example of a skills checklist for suctioning.

Box 2-11 TJC Standards for Performance Improvement

- The hospital collects data to monitor its performance
- The hospital compiles and analyzes data
- The hospital improves performance on an ongoing basis

Compiled from The Joint Commission, Oakbrook Terrace, IL.

Box 2-12 Quality Monitoring Benchmarks

- Monitoring the correctness of respiratory care plans
- Monitoring the consistency of formulating respiratory care plans among therapist evaluators
- Evaluating the efficacy of algorithms or protocols
- Evaluating the overall effectiveness of the protocol program

set forth three standards for monitoring performance improvement along with associated elements of performance detailing how the monitoring is to be conducted. These standards are listed in Box 2-11. Meeting quality goals is increasingly being tied to reimbursement rates by the CMS and insurers to hospitals; this phenomenon has been called "pay for performance."[28] Beyond general monitoring goals for respiratory care, use of respiratory care protocols creates the need for additional quality monitoring benchmarks regarding correctness, consistency, efficacy, and effectiveness (Box 2-12).

At the present time, specific methods to monitor the quality of respiratory care protocol programs include conducting care plan audits in real time and ensuring practitioner training by using case study exercises. Evolving innovations include using simulation exercises to enhance and to measure the performance of RTs.

Monitoring correctness of respiratory care plans can be accomplished by using a care plan audit system. Care plan auditors must be therapists who are experienced in providing respiratory care and patient assessment. The auditors must also be practiced in using the institution's protocol system and in writing care plans. With an auditing system, the auditor writes a care plan for a patient and compares it with the care plan written by the therapist evaluator to determine correctness. A specified number of audits should be performed monthly, with results tabulated and reported monthly or quarterly, depending on the size of the hospital. Feedback must be provided to the evaluators whose care plans are being audited to show their proficiency or to indicate areas that require improvement. Figure 2-6 shows a form used at the Cleveland Clinic to provide feedback to evaluators.

Another monitoring method found useful for respiratory therapy consult services is the case study exercise (or simulated patient scenario exercise). Simulated patient exercises can help determine the consistency of respiratory care plans among therapist evaluators. The scores of individual therapists may be tracked over time to identify problems and to assess improvement.

Simulated patient exercises may consist of a set of three or four patient scenarios. All RTs working under the protocol system, whether or not they are evaluators, complete an assessment sheet and, following the associated algorithms, write a care plan for each scenario. The assessment sheets and the care plans are compared with the "gold standard," or correct assessments and care plans as determined by the consensus of the education coordinator and the supervisors. Scores are tabulated for the individual therapists, and the number of errors for each therapy is examined. If a particular therapy consistently has a large number of associated errors, the algorithm is reviewed for errors or vagueness. To facilitate administering and grading patient simulation exercise results, a computer-based system that scores the assessments and care plans and provides feedback to the RT has been used. Performance data of individual RTs are maintained in a database to calculate and track aggregate performance statistics.

Peer Review Organizations

In addition to the voluntary accreditation process that health care organizations use to help ensure that patients are receiving quality care, the federal government has established an elaborate system of PROs to evaluate the quality and appropriateness of care given to Medicare beneficiaries. PROs evaluate care provided to individual patients in real time to assess and ensure compliance with federal guidelines.

In recent years, health care organizations have attempted to improve the quality of patient care while reducing costs by implementing several innovative health care models. Historically, models that were commonly implemented were hospital restructuring and redesign and patient-focused care. Protocols and disease management represent continuing solutions. Accountable care organizations (ACOs)[29] have also been proposed as a solution to enhance quality and lessen cost. An ACO can be broadly thought of as an emerging model in which a group of health care providers aligns and agrees together to try to meet quality and care targets and to receive payments as a collective entity, from which individual payments can then be disbursed. The ACO can benefit as a group from its success and can absorb losses as a group related to its failure to meet the targets.

Restructuring and redesign involved changing the basic organization of health care services in an attempt to do more with less while increasing value. Approaches for restructuring commonly included cross-training employees, using unlicensed assistive staff, and decentralizing services.[30] When respiratory care departments are decentralized and respiratory care management is eliminated, RTs are deployed to individual nursing units and report

Stamp Here

Care Plan Audit

Date: ______________________

Auditor: ______________________

Therapist: ______________________

Diagnosis: ______________________

A = Auditor
T = Therapist

Triage Score

	0	1	2	3	4
Pulmonary Status					
Surgical Status					
Chest X-Ray					
Respiratory Pattern					
Mental Status					
Breath Sounds					
Cough					
Level of Activity					
Oxygen Requirement					

The triage score was __________% correct.* Total A____ T____

*"% Correct" defined as the percent of auditor's scores (for each of the eight axes) with which the therapist's score agrees.

Care Plan

	Aerosol	bph	Hyperinflation	Oxygen	Pulse Ox	Suctioning
A = Auditor						
T = Therapist						

The care plan was ______% correct.*

*"% Correct" defined as (number of agreements)/six (total items for therapy).

Care plan complete? Yes No

Evaluation on time? Yes No

Frequencies correct? Yes No

Comments: ______________________

FIGURE 2-6 Form for providing feedback to therapist evaluators on their patient assessment and care plan writing performance. Agreement is indicated by an *A* (auditor) and a *T* (therapist) in the same triage scoring box or therapeutic category. (Courtesy Cleveland Clinic Respiratory Institute, Cleveland, Ohio.)

to nursing supervisors. When complete decentralization occurs, the responsibilities of equipment purchase and maintenance, continuing education, and quality improvement may be assigned to nursing personnel, who often are uncomfortable with these additional burdens.[30]

Although less commonly practiced, another aspect of restructuring and redesign is **cross-training** personnel and using assistive staff. Cross-training among professional health care workers can be attempted by teaching activities normally performed by a specific discipline but not restricted by licensing to personnel of another discipline. Nurses might cross-train RTs to perform phlebotomy, whereas RTs might cross-train nurses to perform meter dose inhaler (MDI) therapy. Although theoretically appealing, this strategy has fallen into disfavor because of the substantial associated challenges in implementation.

Cross-training assistive personnel involves on-the-job training of unlicensed personnel, who may not have an educational background in health care, to perform basic technical functions. These assistive personnel may learn to perform some nursing functions, such as taking vital signs, measuring intake and output, and inserting urinary catheters; laboratory technician activities, such as phlebotomy and simple urinalysis; and respiratory therapy activities, such as incentive spirometry follow-up and oxygen checks. The intent of using cross-trained assistive personnel, whose compensation is lower than licensed health care workers, is to enable an institution to reduce the number of nurses, laboratory technicians, and RTs that they employ, reducing costs. Although some aspects of hospital restructuring and redesign have been implemented and persist, others (e.g., cross-training and decentralization) have been abandoned.

Protocols

As described previously, protocols are guided pathways to help direct specific aspects of a patient's treatment regimen. The primary purpose of respiratory care protocols is to provide therapy to patients needing and likely to benefit from therapy but to avoid delivering services to patients not likely to benefit. A comprehensive protocol program using clinical practice guidelines can provide a dynamic system for modifying the respiratory care regimen in response to a patient's changing clinical status.

The widespread use and acceptance of respiratory care protocols have been encouraged by studies reporting reduced misallocation of respiratory care and the cost savings associated with protocols. In addition to observational studies,[22] the benefits of RT protocols have been shown in randomized, controlled trials for weaning patients from mechanical ventilation[31-34] and for allocating respiratory therapy to adult inpatients not in intensive care units (ICUs).[24,25] Table 2-3 presents selected studies showing the effect of respiratory care protocols on the misallocation of respiratory therapy. Most studies show a significant decrease in overordering respiratory care services, whereas only a few address underordering services, which is a phenomenon more difficult to assess. Table 2-4 reviews studies addressing the cost savings associated with using protocols, which suggest that respiratory care protocols can effect savings by enhancing appropriate allocation of respiratory care services.[12,24,25,35-41] Table 2-5 summarizes the results of five randomized, controlled trials on the effectiveness of respiratory care protocols. These studies establish the efficacy of respiratory care protocols in weaning patients from mechanical ventilation[30-32] and in enhancing the allocation of services to adult patients not in ICUs.[23,24]

TABLE 2-3

Changes in Modalities After Protocol Implementation

Author and Year Published	Observed Reductions in Misallocated Therapy After Implementation of Protocols	Change from Preprotocol to Current Status
Hart et al,[35] 1989	37% (aerosol, hyperinflation)	48%-11%
Walton et al,[36] 1990	49.1% (aerosol, chest physiotherapy)	
Beasley et al,[37] 1992	11.9% (blood gas use)	42.7%-30.8%
Ford,[38] 1994	57% (aerosol, chest physiotherapy)	7000-4000 treatments
Orens,[39] 1993	35% (aerosol, bronchopulmonary, hygiene, hyperinflation oxygen, oximetry)	

From Haney DJ: Therapist-driven protocols for adult non-intensive care unit patients: availability and efficacy. Respir Care Clin N Am 2:93–104, 1996.

TABLE 2-4

Cost Savings Associated With Respiratory Care Protocols

Author	Date	Duration of Study	Cost Savings
Hart et al[35]	1989	3 mo	$4316 (decrease in actual costs)
Walton et al[36]	1990	6 yr	9.7% (decrease in charges)
Orens[39]	1993	1 yr	$81,826 (decrease in costs for one nursing unit)
Ford[38]	1994	1 yr	$150,000 (decrease in costs)
Komara and Stoller[41]	1995	40 patients	53.3% (decrease in costs)
Shrake et al[40]	1996	2 yr, 4420 patients; cost comparisons: 3 mo postprotocol	$15,337 for 3 study mo, annualized to $61,348/yr
Stoller et al[24]	1998	1 yr, 145 patients	$20 (decrease in true costs/patient)
Kollef et al[25]	2000	9 mo, 694 patients	$186 (decrease in charges/patient)
Shelledy et al[12]	2004	3 mo, 75 patients	$75,395 (estimated annual decrease)

Modified from Haney DJ: Therapist-driven protocols for adult non-intensive care unit patients: availability and efficacy. Respir Care Clin N Am 2:93–104, 1996.

TABLE 2-5

Summary of Available Randomized Trials on the Effectiveness of Respiratory Care Protocols

Clinical Activity	Author	Date	No. Patients	Findings
Weaning from mechanical ventilation	Kollef et al[31]	1997	357	Use of protocols was associated with shorter duration of mechanical ventilation
	Ely et al[32]	1996	300	Routine daily trials of spontaneous breathing trials were associated with shorter duration of mechanical ventilation
	Marelich et al[33]	2000	253	Use of protocols shortened duration of mechanical ventilation
Respiratory care protocol service	Stoller et al[24]	1998	145	Use of respiratory therapy consult service was associated with improved allocation of respiratory care service with lower costs and no adverse events
	Kollef et al[25]	2000	694	Use of respiratory protocol service was associated with fewer orders discordant with guidelines and lower charges

From Stoller JK: Are respiratory therapists effective? Assessing the evidence. Respir Care 46:56, 2001.

Disease Management

Disease management refers to an organized strategy of delivering care to a large group of individuals with chronic disease to improve outcomes and reduce cost. Disease management has been defined as a systematic population-based approach to identify persons at risk, intervene with specific programs of care, and measure clinical and other outcomes.[42,43] Disease management programs comprise four essential components: (1) an integrated health care system that can provide coordinated care across the full range of patients' needs; (2) a comprehensive knowledge base regarding the prevention, diagnosis, and treatment of disease that guides the plan of care; (3) sophisticated clinical and administrative information systems that can help assess patterns of clinical practice; and (4) a commitment to continuous quality improvement. Disease management programs may be developed for chronic conditions such as asthma, diabetes, chronic obstructive pulmonary disease (COPD), and congestive heart failure.

A disease management program for COPD might be adopted by a health care provider, insurance company, or health maintenance organization in defining its practice approach to individuals with COPD. The disease management program might contain algorithms addressing when to suspect COPD, tests to perform (e.g., spirometry, $alpha_1$-antitrypsin level, diffusing capacity), medications to prescribe based on disease severity, management of exacerbations, and indications for rehabilitation. Disease management programs are often outlined in documents containing branched logic algorithms that specify care, similar to respiratory care protocols; however, disease management protocols often address large groups and are based on an underlying diagnosis rather than on individual signs and symptoms. Other dimensions of the COPD disease management program include a data collection activity regarding the number of patients served, the outcomes of care, and, perhaps, the associated costs. In addition, ongoing review and periodic updating and revision of the care algorithms are important dimensions of the program.

EVIDENCE-BASED MEDICINE

Another important concept regarding quality care is evidence-based medicine. **Evidence-based medicine** refers to an approach to determining optimal clinical management based on several practices, as follows:[43-47] (1) a rigorous and systematic review of available evidence, (2) a critical analysis of available evidence to determine what management conclusions are most sound and applicable, and (3) a disciplined approach to incorporating the literature with personal practice and experience. In a broader context, evidence-based medicine can be thought of as understanding and using the best quality evidence available (i.e., the best-designed, most rigorous clinical trials) to support the most appropriate and correct possible clinical decisions.

In rating the quality of scientific evidence, it is important to recognize the various designs and types of study designs from which scientific evidence comes.[48] The simplest and least rigorous design is a single case report, in which a new clinical issue or problem is described in a single patient. A description of the favorable outcome of using a new mode of mechanical ventilation in one patient with refractory hypoxemia would be a single case report. Although single case reports have value in pointing out new insights and new possibilities for treatment, disease associations, or disease causation, they cannot prove the effectiveness of a treatment or the causality of a risk factor because they, by nature, lack a control or comparison group (i.e., a group that is similar to the patient or patients described, differing only in whether the risk factor of interest was present or the treatment of interest was applied). Collecting a group of patients with similar clinical features is called a case series and may have greater impact in that it suggests that the issue is more general than in a single patient alone. However, similar to a single case report, a case series cannot prove the efficacy of a treatment or the causality of a risk factor because no comparison or control group is included.

Cohort studies, which compare the clinical outcomes in two compared groups (or cohorts), generally have greater scientific rigor than case studies or case series and consist of two broad types of study designs: observational cohort studies and randomized controlled trials. In trying to establish whether a treatment works (i.e., has efficacy), an observational cohort study would compare the outcomes between two groups of patients when the treatment was allocated to one group but not the other by either physician or patient choice. More specifically, an observational cohort study of a new mode of mechanical ventilation would compare the outcomes between two groups of similar patients (i.e., especially similar with regard to their risk of developing the outcome measure that is being studied) when the mode of mechanical ventilation was determined either by physician choice (i.e., the physician decided to use this treatment in this patient) or by patient choice. In contrast, a randomized controlled trial, sometimes regarded as the most methodologically rigorous study design (when well conducted), would compare the outcomes of two similar groups of patients when the use of the new mode of mechanical ventilation was determined by chance alone (randomization) rather than by patient or physician choice. In the ideal situation, a randomized controlled treatment trial eliminates all sources of bias that would prevent attributing differences in outcomes between the compared groups to anything other than the treatment itself, "isolating" the effect of the treatment. Said differently, at its best, a randomized controlled treatment trial provides rigorous evidence regarding the efficacy of the treatment when all other potentially confounding variables (e.g., features of the compared patient groups, other medications or treatments used) are eliminated from consideration, allowing the investigators and the readers of the clinical trial results to ascribe confidently outcome differences between the compared groups to the treatment itself.

Variants of the randomized controlled trial include the parallel-control study and the crossover study (Figure 2-7). Parallel-control treatment studies compare two groups: one receives the treatment being studied, and the other receives the control treatment. Sometime after the end of the treatment, outcomes of the two groups are assessed and compared regarding the main outcomes of interest in the study. A parallel-control randomized trial of low-stretch ventilation for ARDS would compare one group of patients receiving low-stretch ventilation with another (otherwise similar) group receiving conventional, higher stretch ventilator settings, and the two groups would be compared after a prespecified time period with regard to key outcomes, such as survival, discharge from the ICU, and organ system failures. This design was used in the ARDS Net clinical trial showing the superiority of using a tidal volume of 6 ml/kg (ideal body weight) in managing patients with acute lung injury or ARDS.[49]

In the other type of randomized controlled trial—the crossover trial—the study treatment is first administered to one group of study subjects while the other group receives the control or comparison treatment, and then, after measuring outcomes and a subsequent "washout period" (in which the effects of the initial treatment decay and wear off fully), the group initially given the study

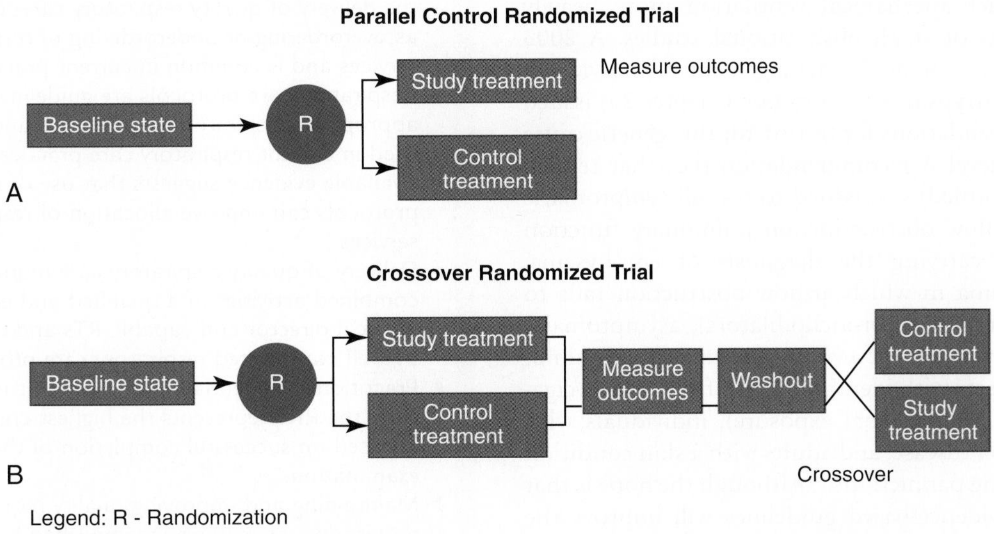

FIGURE 2-7 Study design of the two types of randomized controlled trial: parallel-control and crossover. In a parallel-control trial, after randomization (R), one group receives the study treatment, while the control group receives the comparison treatment (possibly a placebo). At the end of the subsequent observation period, study outcomes are measured, and the trial is over. In a crossover trial, one group initially receives the study treatment, and the other group receives the comparison treatment; outcomes are measured; and after a washout period (see text), each group receives the alternative treatment for another interval of time, after which outcomes are measured again.

treatment receives the control treatment and vice versa. The crossover study design offers a statistical advantage of greater power to detect a difference between the compared groups if a difference exists, but crossover studies can be performed only when the effects of the initial treatment administered to the first study group can be assured to wear off completely, allowing the study group to return to its baseline state before the alternative treatment is administered.

Evidence-based medicine requires knowledge of how to analyze carefully the results of clinical trials (e.g., randomized controlled trials and observational cohort studies) and how to incorporate the results of such research into high-quality clinical practice. Other tools of evidence-based medicine include systematically reviewing the available literature, or what is called meta-analysis of the literature.[28] A meta-analysis of a clinical issue (e.g., does a low-stretch mechanical ventilation strategy improve survival in ARDS?[49]) identifies, analyzes, and summarizes the body of literature about this topic by assessing the quality of the available evidence and giving greater weight to better designed, more rigorous studies. Sometimes, meta-analyses pool the actual data from different trials together when pooling is scientifically and statistically permissible. In other instances (called narrative analyses), the meta-analysis simply evaluates the quality of the data from each available trial (based on explicit methodologic criteria) to offer a conclusion about the clinical issue.

A meta-analysis performed as part of an evidence-based approach to determining the optimal ventilatory approach for ARDS might weigh the results of large randomized clinical trials of low-stretch versus conventional tidal volume approach mechanical ventilation more heavily than the results of small observational studies. A 2003 evidence-based review of the management of individuals with alpha$_1$-antitrypsin deficiency (see Chapter 23) issued graded recommendations for testing for this genetic cause of COPD.[50] A level A recommendation (i.e., that testing should be performed) was issued to test all symptomatic adults with airflow obstruction on pulmonary function tests (whether carrying the diagnosis of emphysema, COPD, or asthma in which airflow obstruction fails to reverse completely with bronchodilators), asymptomatic individuals with persistent airflow obstruction on pulmonary function tests with identifiable risk factors (e.g., cigarette smoking, occupational exposure), individuals with unexplained liver disease, and adults with a skin condition called necrotizing panniculitis.[50] Although the hope is that issuing such evidence-based guidelines will improve the care that such individuals receive by allowing clinicians to access efficiently the best available information, experience suggests that clinicians may be slow to adopt the best available evidence in caring for their patients.[51]

Although some authors point out that evidence-based medicine does not differ from prior practice in which clinicians were always called on to analyze carefully available data and make clinical judgments based on the best-quality information available, evidence-based medicine does specify precise methods for analyzing available information and allowing the clinician to judge best the available evidence. As a measure of the importance of evidence-based medicine in respiratory care, several articles in *Respiratory Care* considered the effectiveness of RTs and of various respiratory care treatment modalities using an evidence-based approach.[45-47] The Clinical Practice Guidelines of the American Association for Respiratory Care are being systematically reviewed to reflect the rigorous techniques of evidence-based medicine and to ensure that guidelines for respiratory care management reflect the best available evidence.[47] The proof that low-stretch ventilation is associated with improved survival in patients with ARDS and the methods used to enhance awareness of this best practice are further examples of evidence-based medical practice.

SUMMARY CHECKLIST

- Quality respiratory care can be defined as the competent delivery of indicated respiratory care services.
- Crucial elements for quality respiratory care include:
  - Energetic and competent medical direction
  - Methods for providing indicated and appropriate respiratory care
  - Educated, competent respiratory care personnel
  - Adequate, well-maintained equipment
  - Intelligent system for monitoring performance improvement
- Misallocation of respiratory care services, which hinders the delivery of quality respiratory care, can be defined as overordering or underordering of respiratory care services and is common in current practice.
- Respiratory care protocols are guidelines for delivering appropriate respiratory care services and are widely used in current respiratory care practice.
- Available evidence suggests that use of respiratory care protocols can improve allocation of respiratory care services.
- Delivery of quality respiratory care requires the combined activities of a qualified and committed medical director and capable RTs and can be enhanced by well-constructed respiratory care protocols.
- Practitioner credentialing is important in respiratory care; the RRT represents the highest credential and is based on successful completion of the NBRC examination.
- Maintaining and improving quality requires ongoing monitoring, as may be accomplished by quality audits and repeated competence testing of RTs.
- Evidence-based medicine is an approach to determining optimal patient management based on critically assessing the available evidence. It is recommended that RTs use this approach as they assess the support for respiratory care management strategies.

References

1. Stoller JK: Medical direction of respiratory care: past and present. Respir Care 43:217–223, 1998.
2. Stoller JK: Misallocation of respiratory care services: time for a change (editorial). Respir Care 38:263, 1993.
3. Kester L, Stoller JK: Ordering respiratory care services for hospitalized patients: practices of overuse and underuse. Cleve Clin J Med 59:581, 1992.
4. Malloy R, Pierce M, Friel D, et al: Reduction of unnecessary care through utilization of a respiratory care plan (abstract). Respir Care 37:1277, 1992.
5. Stoller JK: Why therapist-driven protocols? A balanced view (editorial). Respir Care 39:706, 1994.
6. Zibrak JD, Rossetti P, Wood E: Effect of reductions in respiratory therapy on patient outcomes. N Engl J Med 315:292, 1986.
7. Brougher LI, Blackwelder AK, Grossman GD, et al: Effectiveness of medical necessity guidelines in reducing cost of oxygen therapy. Chest 39:646, 1986.
8. Small D, Duha A, Weiskopf B, et al: Uses and misuses of oxygen in hospitalized patients. Am J Med 92:591, 1992.
9. Albin RJ, Criner GJ, Thomas S, et al: Pattern of non-ICU inpatient supplemental oxygen utilization in a university hospital. Chest 102:1672, 1992.
10. Shapiro BA, Cane RD, Peterson J, et al: Authoritative medical direction can assure cost-beneficial bronchial hygiene therapy. Chest 93:1038, 1988.
11. Browning JA, Kaiser DL, Durbin CG: The effect of guidelines on the appropriate use of arterial blood gas analysis in the intensive care unit. Respir Care 34:269, 1989.
12. Shelledy DC, LeGrand TS, Peters JI: An assessment of the appropriateness of respiratory care delivered at a 450 bed acute care Veterans Affairs hospital. Respir Care 49:907–916, 2004.
13. Kester L, Stoller JK: Respiratory care education: current issues and future challenges (editorial). Respir Care 41:98, 1996.
14. Stoller JK: Are respiratory therapists effective? Assessing the evidence. Respir Care 46:56, 2001.
15. Stoller JK. The future of respiratory therapy (RT) research and scholarship: when you're finished changing, you're finished. Can J Respir Therapy 2010; 46:8–9.
16. Beachey WD. A comparison of problem-based learning and traditional curricula in baccalaureate respiratory therapy education. Respir Care 52:1497–1506, 2007.
17. Gaylin DS, Shapiro JR, Mendelson DN, et al: The role of respiratory care practitioners in a managed healthcare system: emerging areas of clinical practice. Am J Manag Care 5:749, 1999.
18. Dubbs W: By the numbers: results from the AARC's 2005 Human Resources Study. AARC Times 30:37–43, 2005.
19. American Association for Respiratory Care: 2009 human resources survey of respiratory therapists. American Association for Respiratory Care, 2009, www.aarc.org.
20. Stoller JK: The rationale for therapist-driven protocols. Respir Care Clin N Am 2:1–14, 1996.
21. Stoller JK, Kester L, Roberts VT, et al. An analysis of features of respiratory therapy departments that are avid for change. Respir Care 2008;53:871–884.
22. Stoller JK, Haney D, Burkhart J, et al: Physician-ordered respiratory care vs. physician-ordered use of a respiratory therapy consult service: early experience at the Cleveland Clinic Foundation. Respir Care 38:1143, 1993.
23. Stoller JK, Skibinski C, Giles D, et al: Physician-ordered respiratory care vs. physician-ordered use of a respiratory therapy consult service: results of a prospective observational study. Chest 110:422, 1996.
24. Stoller JK, Mascha EJ, Kester L, et al: Randomized controlled trial of physician-directed versus respiratory therapy consult service-directed respiratory care to adult non-ICU inpatients. Am J Respir Crit Care Med 158:1068, 1998.
25. Kollef MH, Shapiro SD, Clinkscale D, et al: The effect of respiratory therapist-initiated treatment protocols on patient outcomes and resource utilization. Chest 117:467, 2000.
26. Mish FC, Gilman WW, editors: Webster's ninth new collegiate dictionary. Springfield, Mass, 1985, Merriam-Webster Inc.
27. Harder BN. Use of simulation in teaching and learning in health sciences: a systematic review. J Nurs Educ 49:23–28, 2010.
28. Van Herck P, De Smedt D, Annemans L, et al. Systematic review: effects, design choices, and context of pay-for-performance in health care. BMC Health Services Research 10:247, 2010.
29. Lowell KH, Bertko J. The accountable care organization (ACO) model: building blocks for success. J Ambul Care Manage 33:81, 2010.
30. Kester L, Stoller JK: Respiratory care in the adult non-ICU setting. Respir Care 42:101, 1997.
31. Kollef MH, Shapiro SD, Silver P, et al: A randomized, controlled trial of protocol-directed versus physician-directed weaning from mechanical ventilation. Crit Care Med 25:567, 1997.
32. Ely EW, Baker AM, Dunagan DP, et al: Effect on the duration of mechanical ventilation of identifying patients capable of breathing spontaneously. N Engl J Med 335:1864, 1996.
33. Marelich GP, Murin S, Battistella F, et al: Protocol weaning of mechanical ventilation in medical and surgical patients by respiratory care practitioners and nurses. Chest 118:459, 2000.
34. Haney DJ: Therapist-driven protocols for adult non-intensive care unit patients: availability and efficacy. Respir Care Clin N Am 2:93–104, 1996.
35. Hart SK, Dubbs W, Gil A, et al: The effects of therapist-evaluation of orders and interaction with physicians on the appropriateness of respiratory care. Respir Care 34:185, 1989.
36. Walton JR, Shapiro BA, Harrison EH: Review of a bronchial hygiene evaluation program. Respir Care 35:1214, 1990.
37. Beasley K, Darin J, Durbin C: The effect of respiratory care department management of a blood gas analyzer on the appropriateness of arterial blood gas utilization. Respir Care 37:343, 1992.
38. Ford R: The University of California San Diego experience with patient-driven protocols. Presented at AARC State-of-the-Art Conference: therapist-driven protocols, Dallas, May 1994.
39. Orens DK: A manager's perspective on a respiratory therapy consult service (editorial). Respir Care 38:884, 1993.
40. Shrake KL, Scaggs JE, England KR, et al: A respiratory care assessment-treatment program: results of a retrospective study. Respir Care 41:703, 1996.
41. Komara JJ, Stoller JK: The impact of a postoperative oxygen therapy protocol on use of pulse oximetry and oxygen therapy. Respir Care 40:1125, 1995.
42. Epstein RS, Sharwood LM: From outcomes research to disease management: a guide for the perplexed. Ann Intern Med 124:832, 1996.
43. Elrodt G, Cook DJ, Lee J, et al: Evidence-based disease management. JAMA 278:1687, 1997.
44. Stoller JK: 2000 Donald F. Egan Scientific Lecture: are respiratory therapists effective? Assessing the evidence. Respir Care 46:56, 2001.

45. Respiratory Care Special Issue: Evidence-based medicine in respiratory care, Part I. Respir Care 46(11), 2001.
46. Respiratory Care Special Issue: Evidence-based medicine in respiratory care, Part II. Respir Care 46(12), 2001.
47. Hess DR: Evidence-based clinical practice guidelines: where's the evidence and what do I do with it? Respir Care 48:838–839, 2003.
48. Feinstein AR. Randomized clinical trials. In: Feinstein AR, editor: Clinical epidemiology: the architecture of clinical research. Philadelphia, 1985, Saunders, pp 683–718.
49. The ARDS Network. Ventilation with lower tidal volumes as compared with traditional tidal volumes for acute lung injury and the ARDS. N Engl J Med 342:1301–1308, 2000.
50. American Thoracic Society/European Respiratory Society: Standards for the diagnosis and management of individuals with alpha-1 antitrypsin deficiency. Am J Respir Crit Care Med 168:816–900, 2003.
51. Carlbom DJ, Rubenfeld GD. Barriers to implementing protocol-based sepsis resuscitation in the emergency department—results of a national survey. Crit Care Med 35:2525–2532, 2007.

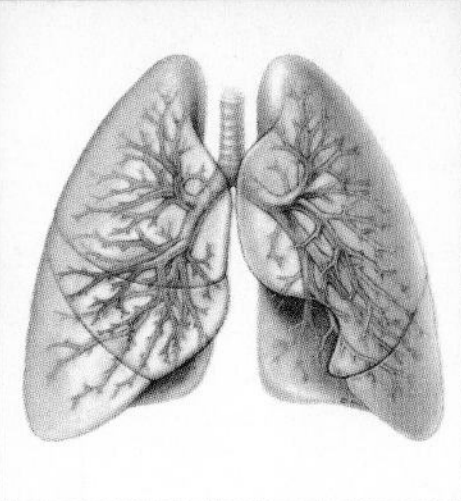

Chapter 3

Patient Safety, Communication, and Recordkeeping

SCOTT P. MARLOW

CHAPTER OBJECTIVES

After reading this chapter you will be able to:
- Describe how to apply good body mechanics and posture to moving patients.
- Describe how to ambulate a patient and the potential benefits of ambulation.
- Write definitions of key terms associated with electricity, including voltage, current, and resistance.
- Identify the potential physiologic effects that electrical current can have on the body.
- State how to reduce the risk of electrical shock to patients and yourself.
- Identify key statistics related to the incidence and origin of hospital fires.
- List the conditions needed for fire and how to minimize fire hazards.
- Identify impediments to care and risk in the direct patient environment.
- State how communication can affect patient care.
- Describe the two patient identifier system.
- List the factors associated with the communication process.
- Describe how to improve your communication effectiveness.
- Describe how to recognize and help resolve interpersonal or organizational sources of conflict.
- List the common components of a medical record.
- State the legal and practical obligations involved in recordkeeping.
- Describe how to maintain a problem-oriented medical record.

CHAPTER OUTLINE

KEY TERMS

ambulation
ampere
attending
auditory
channel
current
feedback
ground
macroshock
microshock
ohm
problem-oriented medical record (POMR)
resistance
SOAP
voltage

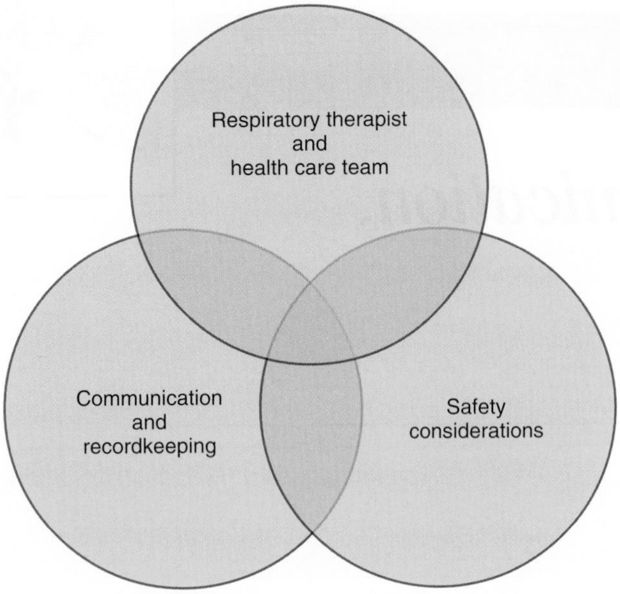

FIGURE 3-1 Patient safety continuum.

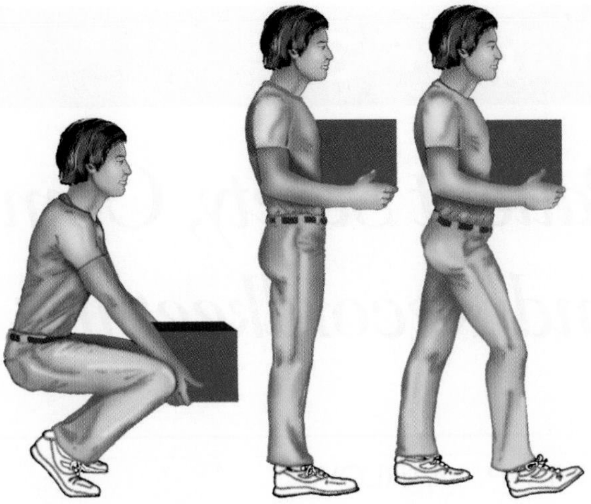

FIGURE 3-2 Body mechanics for lifting and carrying objects.

Respiratory therapists (RTs) share the general responsibilities for providing a safe and effective health care environment with nurses and other members of the health care team. The continuum of patient safety requires that the RT have specific technical knowledge of the environment of direct patient care. In addition to technical skills, all health care professionals must be able to communicate effectively with each other and with patients and patients' families and to document pertinent information. Figure 3-1 shows this relationship for patient safety. This chapter provides the foundation knowledge needed to assume these general aspects of patient care effectively.

SAFETY CONSIDERATIONS

Patient safety is always the first consideration in respiratory care. Although the RT usually does not have full control over the patient's environment, efforts must be made to minimize potential hazards associated with respiratory care. The key areas of potential risk are patient movement and ambulation, electrical hazards, fire hazards, and general safety concerns.

Patient Movement and Ambulation

Basic Body Mechanics

Posture involves the relationship of the body parts to each other. A person needs good posture to reduce the risk of injury when lifting patients or heavy equipment. Poor posture may place inappropriate stress on joints and related muscles and tendons. Figure 3-2 illustrates the correct body mechanics for lifting a heavy object. The correct technique calls for a straight spine and use of the leg muscles to lift the object.

Moving the Patient in Bed

Conscious people assume positions that are the most comfortable. Bedridden patients with acute or chronic respiratory dysfunction often assume an upright position, with their arms flexed and their thorax leaning forward. This position helps decrease their work of breathing. In other cases, patients may have to assume certain positions for therapeutic reasons such as when postural drainage is applied.

Figure 3-3 shows the correct technique for lateral movement of a bed-bound patient. Figure 3-4 illustrates the ideal method for moving a conscious patient toward the head of a bed. Figure 3-5 shows the proper technique for assisting a patient to the bedside position for dangling his or her legs or transfer to a chair.

Ambulation

Ambulation (walking) helps maintain normal body function. Extended bed rest can cause numerous problems, including bed sores and atelectasis (low lung volumes). Ambulation should begin as soon as the patient is physiologically stable and free of severe pain. Ambulation has been shown to reduce the length of hospital stay after surgery and in patients recovering from community-acquired pneumonia.[1,2] Safe patient movement includes the following steps:

1. Place the bed in a low position and lock its wheels.
2. Place all equipment (e.g., intravenous [IV] equipment, nasogastric tube, surgical drainage tubes) close to the patient to prevent dislodgment during ambulation.
3. Move the patient toward the nearest side of bed.
4. Assist the patient to sit up in bed (i.e., arm under nearest shoulder and one under farthest armpit).
5. Place one hand under the patient's farthest knee, and gradually rotate the patient so that his or her legs are dangling off the bed.

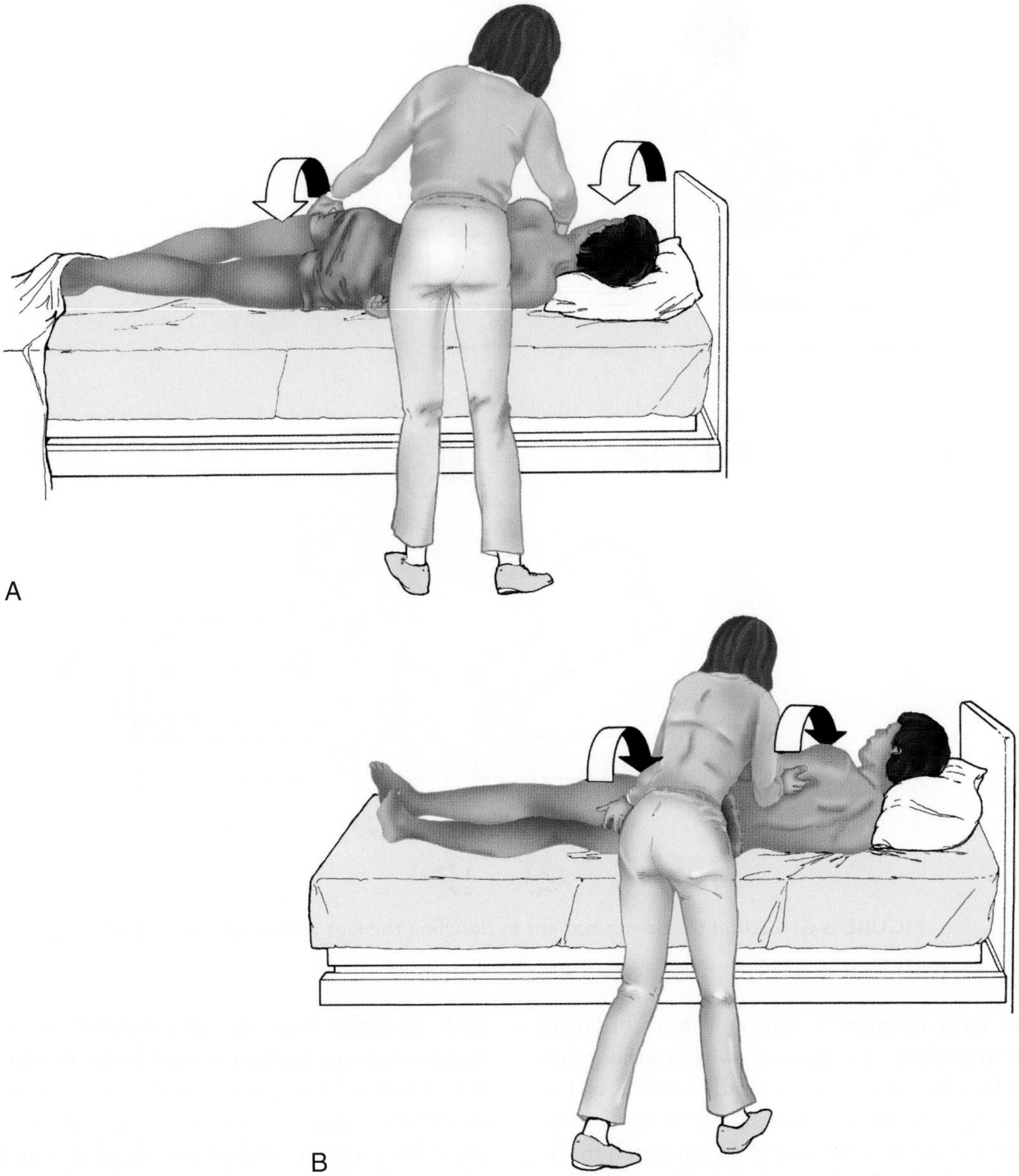

FIGURE 3-3 **A,** Method to pull a bed-bound patient. **B,** Method to push a bed-bound patient.

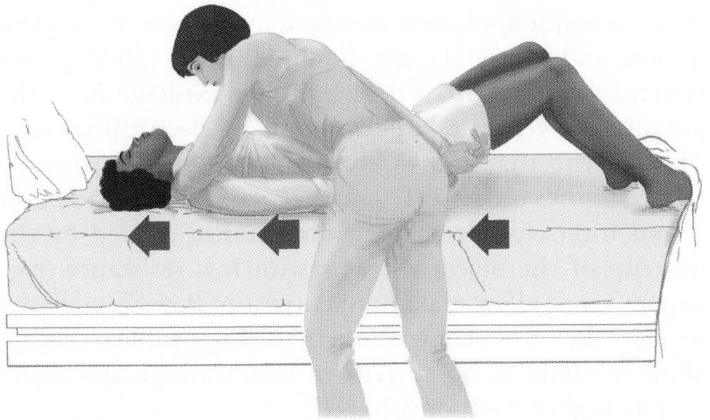

FIGURE 3-4 Method to move a patient up in bed with the patient's assistance.

6. Let the patient remain in this position until dizziness or lightheadedness lessens (encouraging the patient to look forward rather than at the floor may help).
7. Assist the patient to a standing position.
8. Encourage the patient to breathe easily and unhurriedly during this initial change to a standing posture.
9. Walk with the patient using no, minimal, or moderate support (moderate support requires the assistance of two practitioners, one on each side of the patient).
10. Limit walking to 5 to 10 minutes for the first exercise.

Monitor the patient during ambulation. Note the patient's level of consciousness, color, breathing, strength or weakness, and complaints such as pain or shortness of breath throughout the activity. Ask the patient about his

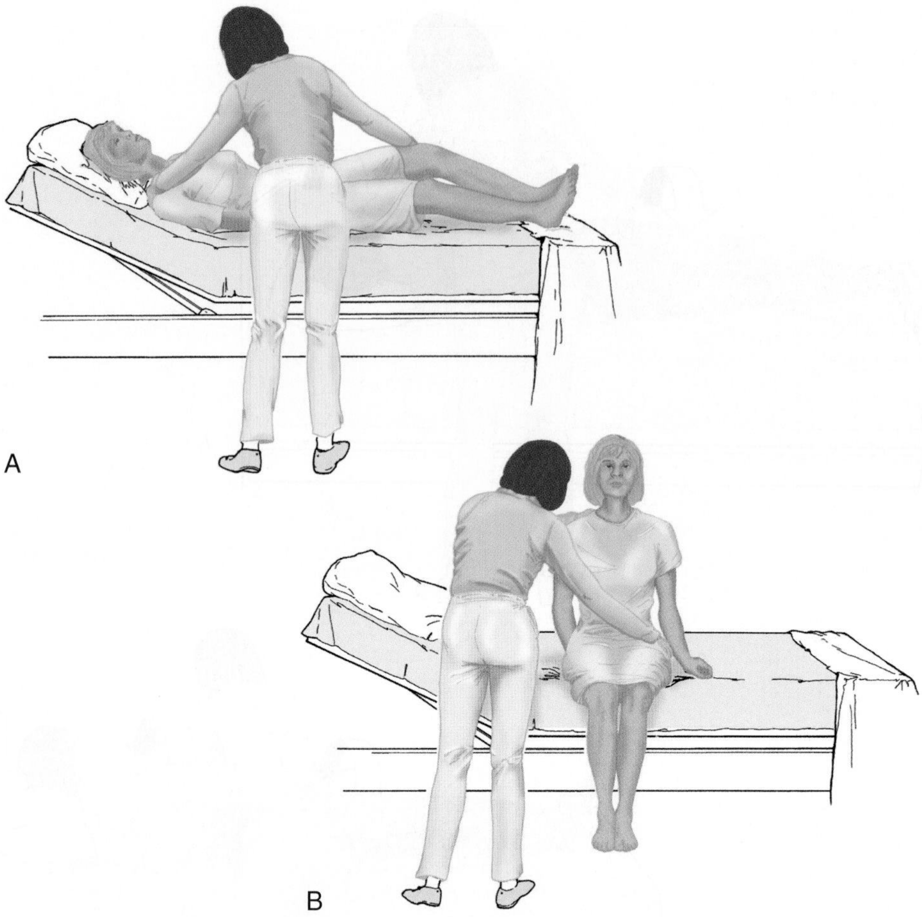

FIGURE 3-5 Method to assist a patient in dangling the legs at the side of the bed.

or her comfort level frequently during the ambulation period. Ensure that chairs are present so that emergency seats are available if the patient becomes distressed. Ambulation is increased gradually until the patient is ready to be discharged. Each ambulation session is documented in the patient chart and includes the date and time of ambulation, length of ambulation, and degree of patient tolerance.

Electrical Safety

The potential for accidental shocks of patients or personnel in the hospital exists because of the frequent use of electrical equipment. The presence of invasive devices, such as internal catheters and pacemakers, may add to the risk of serious harm from electrical shock. Although this risk is present, it has been significantly reduced in recent years through a combination of education and more rigid standards for wiring, especially in patient care areas. RTs must understand the fundamentals of electrical safety because respiratory care often involves the use of electrical devices.

Fundamentals of Electricity

The ability of humans to create and harness electricity is one of the most important developments in modern times. Because controlled electricity is available on a 24-hour-a-day basis, we can depend on it to power the equipment and appliances that make modern life comfortable and productive. Despite the fact that electricity is one of the most popular sources of power, most people who use it have a poor understanding of it. This lack of knowledge is often a major factor in cases of electrocution.

Electricity moves from point *A* to point *B* owing to differences in voltage. **Voltage** is the power potential behind the electrical energy. Low-voltage batteries (e.g., 9 V) are sufficient to power a small flashlight but inadequate to power a major appliance such as a microwave oven. Most homes and hospitals are powered with 120-V power sources. Power sources that have high voltage have the potential to generate large amounts of electrical current. The current that moves through an object is directly related to the voltage difference between point *A* and point *B* and inversely related to the resistance offered by the makeup of the object. Objects with low resistance (e.g., copper wires) allow maximum current to flow through the object. Objects with high resistance (e.g., rubber tubing) allow minimal or no current to flow through the object despite higher levels of voltage.

The simple analogy of water flowing through a piping system is useful to understand electricity. The water

MINI CLINI

"Tingling" Equipment

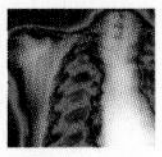

PROBLEM: An RT is caring for a patient on a mechanical ventilator that requires both electrical and pneumatic power for operation. When the RT touches the metal housing of the ventilator, a shock is felt. How should the RT handle the situation based on this observation?

DISCUSSION: All therapeutic instruments used in patient care, including mechanical ventilators, should be connected to grounded outlets (three-wire). Because the ground wire is a protection device only and not part of the main circuit, equipment may continue to operate without the clinician being aware that a problem exists. Because the RT felt a tingling sensation when touching the ventilator, this could represent an improper ground and possible serious current leakage. In this situation, the RT should immediately take the equipment out of service and get it replaced (while providing backup ventilation). All electrical equipment used in patient care should be routinely checked for appropriate grounding.

pressure level at the source is equivalent to the voltage. Higher water pressure provides the potential for greater water flow or current. The friction **(resistance)** offered by the pipe across the length of the pipe influences the flow exiting the other end. Pipes with lots of friction reduce the water flow (current) greatly. If the friction (resistance) is minimal, the water flow (current) is maximal. Similarly, when voltage is high and resistance is low, electrical current flows easily through the object.

The difference in resistance between two people or two objects explains why the same voltage applied to both can seriously damage one and cause no effect to the other. Two people accidentally touching a "hot" wire with 120 V can experience two completely different sensations. A person with wet skin offers little resistance, and the 120 V passes through the person with high current and can cause serious injury or death. A person with dry skin, which offers high resistance, may not even feel a shock and experiences no injury. The degree of resistance offered by the skin varies from person to person based on the chemistry of the person's skin, the cleanliness of the skin, and the amount of moisture on the surface. For this reason, it is never wise to touch a potentially hot wire even though your skin is dry.

As stated before, voltage is the energy potential from an electrical source, and it is measured with a voltmeter. **Current** is the flow of electricity from a point of higher voltage to one of lower voltage and is reported in **amperes** (amps). Current is measured with an ampmeter. The resistance to electrical current is reported in **ohms.** We can determine the resistance to current for any object by the following equation:

$$\text{Resistance (ohms } [\Omega]) = \text{Voltage (V)/Current (amps [A])}$$

Current represents the greatest danger to you or your patients when electrical shorts occur. Voltage and resistance are important only because they determine how much current potentially can pass through the body. High voltage provides greater potential for high currents, but if resistance is also very high, current would be minimal or nonexistent. Current represents the potential danger to the patient. The harmful effects of current depend on (1) the amount of current flowing through the body, (2) the path it takes, and (3) the duration the current is applied. Higher currents (>100 milliamps [mA]) that pass through the chest can cause ventricular fibrillation, diaphragm dysfunction (owing to severe, persistent contraction), and death.

Because current is most important, you should be familiar with the equation used to calculate it:

$$\text{Current (A)} = \text{Voltage (V)/Resistance } (\Omega)$$

For example, as long as a person is insulated by normal clothing and shoes and is in a dry environment, a 120-V shock may hardly be felt because the resistance is high in this situation (10,000 Ω). Current can be calculated as:

$$\text{Current (A)} = 120\ \text{V}/10{,}000\ \Omega = 0.012\ \text{A or } 12\ \text{mA}$$

Currents of 12 mA would cause a tingling sensation but no physical damage.

However, if the same person is standing without shoes on a wet floor, a much higher current occurs because the resistance is much lower (1000 Ω). The current is now calculated as:

$$\text{Current (A)} = 120\ \text{V}/1000\ \Omega = 0.12\ \text{A or } 120\ \text{mA}$$

Because the heart is susceptible to any current level greater than 100 mA, 120 mA represents a potentially fatal shock; this is in sharp contrast to the first example, where the same voltage caused only a tingling sensation.

A shock hazard exists only if the electrical "circuit" through the body is complete, meaning that two electrical connections to the body are required for a shock to occur. In the previous example, the person standing in water with no shoes has "grounded" himself. The finger touching the hot wire provides the input source while the feet standing in water provide the exit to ground. If the same person is wearing rubber boots, the connection to ground does not exist, and the current cannot flow through the individual.

In electrical devices, these two connections typically consist of a "hot" wire and a "neutral" wire. The neutral

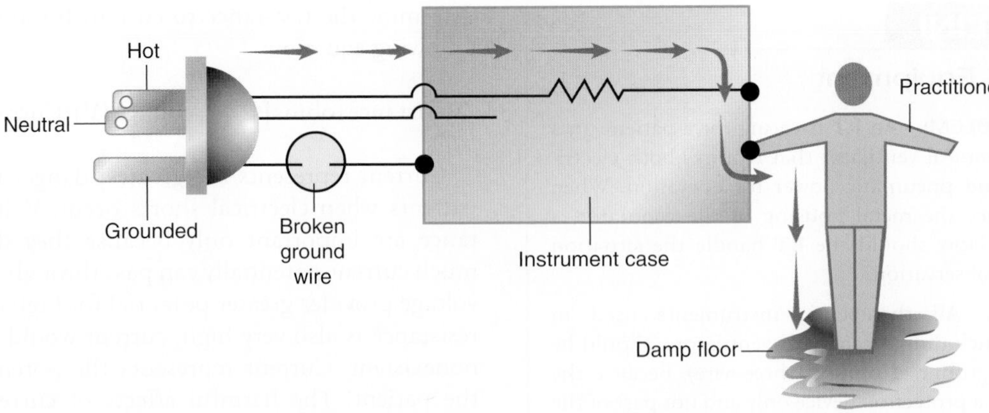

FIGURE 3-6 Hazard created by broken ground wire.

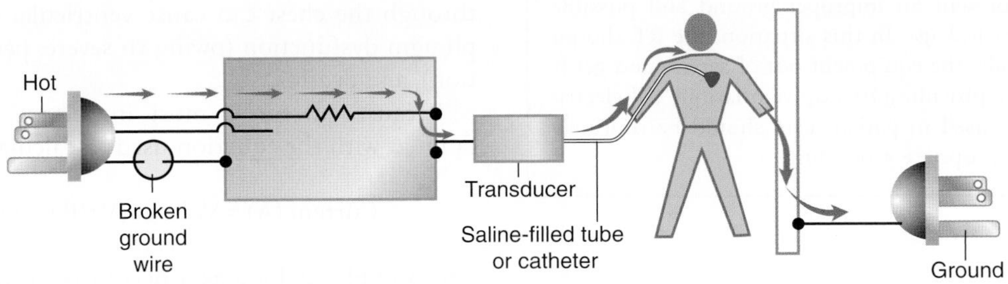

FIGURE 3-7 Possible microshock hazard caused by patient grounding.

wire completes the circuit by taking the electrical current to a ground. A **ground** is simply a low-resistance pathway to a point of zero voltage, such as the earth (hence the term "ground").

Figure 3-6 shows how current can flow through the body. In this case, a piece of electrical equipment is connected to AC line power via a standard three-prong plug. However, unknown to the practitioner, the cord has a broken ground wire. Normally, current leakage from the equipment would flow back to the ground through the ground wire. However, this pathway is unavailable. Instead, the leakage current finds a path of low resistance through the practitioner to the damp floor (an ideal ground).

Current can readily flow into the body, causing damage to vital organs when the skin is bypassed via conductors such as pacemaker wires or saline-filled intravascular catheters (Figures 3-7 and 3-8). Even urinary catheters can provide a path for current flow. The heart is particularly sensitive to electrical shock. Ventricular fibrillation can occur when currents of 20 μA (20 microamperes, or 20 millionths of 1 ampere) are applied directly to the heart.

Electrical shocks are classified into two types: macroshock and microshock. A **macroshock** exists when a high current (usually >1 mA) is applied externally to the skin. A **microshock** exists when a small, usually imperceptible current (<1 mA) bypasses the skin and follows a direct, low-resistance path into the body. Patients susceptible to microshock hazards are termed *electrically sensitive* or *electrically susceptible*. Table 3-1 summarizes the different effects of these two types of electrical shock.

Preventing Shock Hazards

Most shock hazards are caused by inappropriate or inadequate grounding. Shock hazards can be eliminated or minimized if wiring in patient care areas is appropriate and if all equipment brought into the patient care area has been UL approved and checked on a regular basis by a qualified person.

Ground Electrical Equipment Near the Patient. All electrical equipment (e.g., lights, electrical beds, ventilators, monitoring or therapeutic equipment) should be connected to grounded outlets with three-wire cords. In these cases, the third (ground) wire prevents the dangerous buildup of voltage that can occur on the metal frames of some electrical equipment.

Modern electrical devices used in hospitals are designed so that their frames are grounded, but their connections to the patient are not. In this manner, all electrical devices in reach of the patient are grounded, but the patient remains isolated from ground. Because the ground wire is simply a protection device and not part of the main circuit, equipment continues to operate normally even if the ground wire is broken. All electrical equipment, particularly devices used with electrically susceptible patients, must be checked for appropriate grounding on a regular basis by a qualified electrical expert.

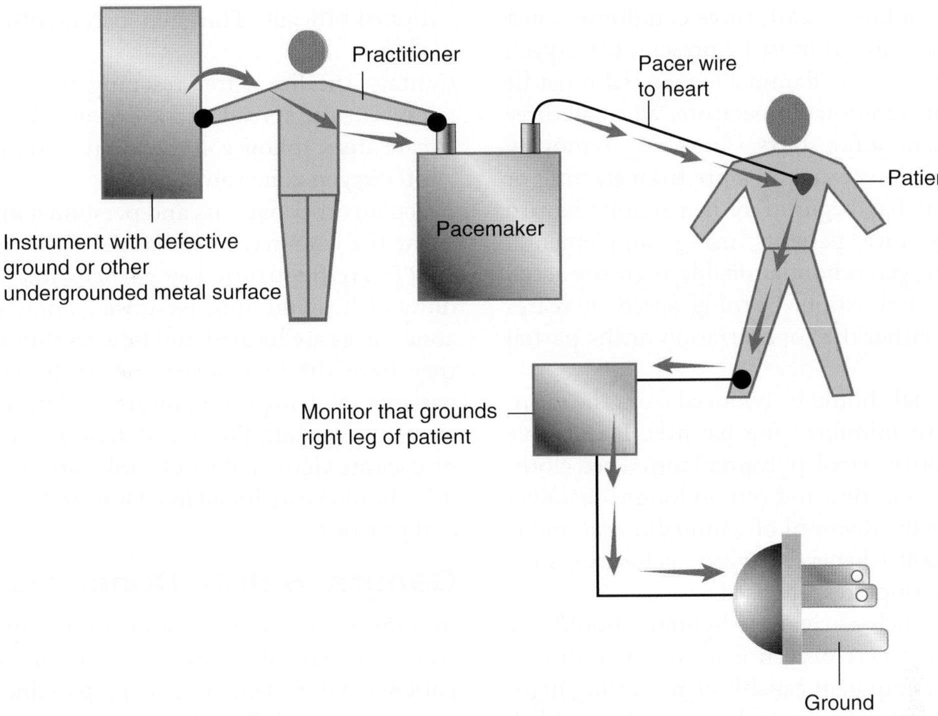

FIGURE 3-8 Possible hazard through use of certain cardiac monitors and a pacemaker.

TABLE 3-1
Effects of Electrical Shock*

Amperes (A)	Milliamperes (mA)	Microamperes (μA)	Effects
Applied to Skin (Macroshock)			
≥6	>6000	>6,000,000	Sustained myocardial contraction followed by normal rhythm; temporary respiratory paralysis; burns, if small area of contact
0.1-3	100-3000	100,000	Ventricular fibrillation; respiratory center intact
0.050	50	50,000	Pain; fainting; exhaustion; mechanical injury; heart and respiratory function intact
0.016	16	16,000	"Let go" current; muscle contraction
0.001	1	1000	Threshold of perception; tingling
Applied to Myocardium (Microshock)			
0.001	0.1	100	Ventricular fibrillation

Duration of exposure and current pathway are major determinants of human response to electrical shock.
*Physiologic effects of AC shocks applied for 1 second to the trunk or directly to the myocardium.

Fire Hazards

In 1980, approximately 13,000 health care facility fires were officially reported in the United States.[3] During the period 2004-2006, the average annual number of fires in health care facilities was 6400.[4] This significant reduction in health care facility fires is primarily due to education and enforcement of strict fire codes.

About 23% of fires in health care facilities occur in hospitals, and 44% occur in nursing homes; the most common site of origin of the fire is the kitchen.[3] About 15% of hospital fires start in patient care rooms and are usually due to patients or visitors smoking or using open flames to light tobacco products. Medical facility fires cause an annual average of five civilian deaths and approximately $34 million in damage.[4]

Hospital fires can be very serious, especially when they occur in patient care areas and when supplemental oxygen is in use. Fires in oxygen-enriched atmospheres (OEAs) are larger, more intense, faster burning, and more difficult to extinguish. In addition, some material that would not burn in room air would burn in OEAs. Hospital fires are also more serious because evacuation of critically ill patients is difficult and slow. For these reasons, hospital fires often cause more injuries and deaths per fire than do residential fires. For a fire to start, three conditions must exist: (1) flammable material must be present, (2) oxygen must be present, and (3) the flammable material must be heated to or above its ignition temperature. When all three conditions are present, a fire starts. Conversely, removing any one of the conditions can stop a fire from starting or extinguish it after it has begun. Fire is a serious hazard around respiratory care patients using supplemental oxygen. Although oxygen is nonflammable, it greatly accelerates the rate of combustion. Burning speed increases with an increase in either the concentration or the partial pressure of oxygen.

Flammable material should be removed from the vicinity of oxygen use to minimize fire hazards. Flammable materials include cotton, wool, polyester fabrics, bed clothing, paper materials, plastics, and certain lotions or salves such as petroleum jelly. Removal of flammable material is particularly important whenever oxygen enclosures, such as oxygen tents or croupettes, are used.

Ignition sources, such as cigarette lighters, should not be allowed in rooms where oxygen is in use. In addition, the use of electrical equipment capable of generating high-energy sparks, such as exposed switches, must be avoided. All appliances that transmit house current should be kept out of oxygen enclosures. Children should not play with toys that may create a spark when oxygen is in use. RTs must be diligent in educating patients and visitors about the dangers associated with spark-producing items, open flames, and burning cigarettes in the hospital environment, especially in OEAs.

A frequent source of concern is the presence of static electrical sparks generated by friction. Even in the presence of high oxygen concentrations, the overall hazard from static sparks with the materials in common use is very low. Solitary static sparks generally do not have sufficient heat energy to raise common materials to their flash points. The minimal risk that may be present can be reduced further by maintaining high relative humidity (>60%).

If you identify a fire in a patient care area, you must know what to do. Each hospital must have a core fire plan that identifies the responsibilities of hospital personnel. The plan should be taught to all hospital personnel and practiced with fire drills to reinforce the education. Requirements may include routinely walking the fire exits and reviewing proper fire extinguisher training. Fire extinguisher training includes following the acronym ***PASS***:

*P*ull the pin—there may be an inspection tag attached

*A*im the nozzle—aim low at the bottom of the fire

*S*queeze the handle—the extinguisher has less than 30 seconds of spray time

*S*weep the nozzle across the base of the fire.

The core fire plan follows the acronym ***RACE:***

*R*escue patients in the immediate area of the fire. The person discovering the fire should perform the rescue.

*A*lert other personnel about the fire so that they can assist in the rescue and can relay the location of the fire to officials. This step also involves pulling the fire alarm.

*C*ontain the fire. After rescuing patients, shut doors to prevent the spread of the fire and the smoke. In patient care areas, follow your hospital policy regarding turning off oxygen zone valves.

*E*vacuate other patients and personnel in the areas around the fire who may be in danger if the fire spreads.

RTs are frequently key participants in successful handling of hospital fires. First, they know where the oxygen zone valves are located and how to shut them off. Second, they have the knowledge and skills needed to evacuate patients receiving mechanical ventilation or supplemental oxygen to sustain life. Third, they know how to treat and resuscitate victims of smoke inhalation. For these reasons, RTs should be included in all hospital evacuation planning and practices.

General Safety Concerns

In addition to electrical and fire safety, RTs need to be aware of general safety concerns, including the direct patient environment, disaster preparedness, magnetic resonance imaging (MRI) safety, and medical gas safety. Medical gas safety is discussed in more detail in Chapter 37.

Direct Patient Environment

The immediate environment around the patient can create risk for patient safety. Because RTs use medical equipment and participate in direct patient care, it is necessary for RTs to be cognizant of the patient's immediate environment.

To reduce the risk of patient falls and allow easy access to care, the patient care environment should be as free of impediments to care as possible. Use of respiratory supplies and medical equipment by the RT creates an environment that could impede access to care and create a fall risk. It is the responsibility of the RT to position equipment, tubing, and treatments in a way that does not impede access to care and that reduces risk of falls. In addition, when care is completed, the RT should ensure that the patient has easy access to the patient call system.

Disaster Preparedness

A key component of disaster preparedness involves learning to transport and transfer critically ill patients. Another component includes preparing for a loss of electricity, whether it is due to an internal or external disaster. In these emergencies, hospitals have backup generators to power essential equipment. All electrical outlets may not function on the backup generator. Some hospitals designate emergency outlets with a red outlet or red dot on an outlet, whereas others may power an entire wing, such as a medical intensive care unit, with the backup generator power. It is incumbent on the RT to know the specific hospital policy for power failures and other potential disasters.

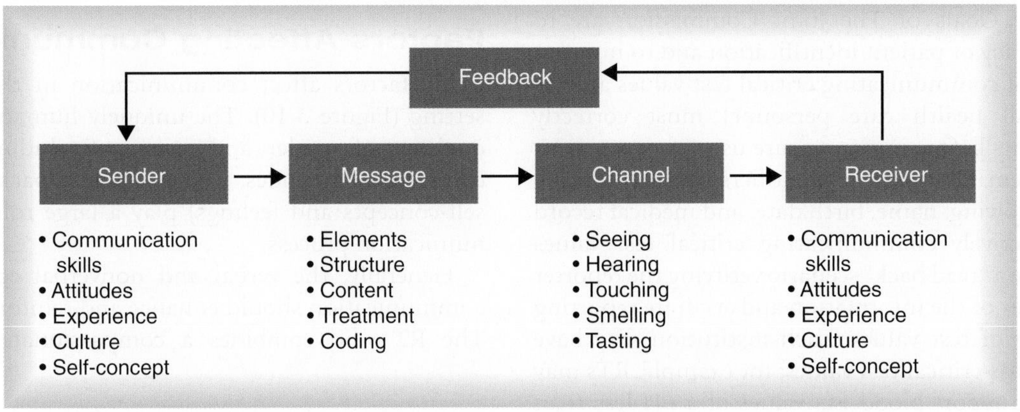

FIGURE 3-9 Elements of human communication. See text on pp. 49-51.

Magnetic Resonance Imaging Safety

MRI exposes the body to powerful magnetic fields and a small amount of radiofrequency. This powerful magnetic field can create a risk to patients, health care workers, and equipment if metal objects are brought within specified proximity to the field. There are safe proximity areas referred to as *safety zones* or *Gauss lines*. Metal objects can be so forcefully attracted to the magnetic field that they can mimic a missile, causing physical harm. Reports of accidents associated with MRI include oxygen cylinders, stethoscopes, scissors, and IV poles. RTs need to become familiar with MRI-compatible ventilators, oxygen supplies, and ancillary equipment. Each radiology department has specific rules and safety precautions that need to be communicated to all patients, caregivers, and health care personnel.

Medical Gas Cylinders

Use of compressed gas cylinders by RTs requires special handling. The physical hazards resulting from improper storage or handling of cylinders include increased risk of fire, explosive release of high-pressure cylinders, and the toxic effect of some gases. It is important to store and transport cylinders in appropriate racks or chained containers. Compressed gas cylinders should never be stored without support.

Storage of medical grade gases is regulated by National Fire Protection Association Standards 99 Health Care Facilities (2005 edition) and monitored by the Joint Commission on Accreditation of Healthcare Organizations. Quantities of oxygen or nitrous oxide of 300 cubic feet or less (about 12 E-cylinders) in a patient care area not to exceed 2100 m^2 are required to be secured properly but do not have special storage room requirements.[5] Storing 300 to 3000 cubic feet of oxygen or nitrous oxide requires noncombustible or limited combustible storage rooms with self-closing doors and at least a ½ hour fire rating.[5] Cylinders must be stored 20 feet from any combustibles (5 feet if room is equipped with a sprinkler system).[5] Follow your hospital policies and procedures when handling, transporting, or storing medical gas cylinders.

COMMUNICATION

Communication is a dynamic human process involving sharing of information, meanings, and rules. Communication has five basic components: sender, message, channel, receiver, and feedback (Figure 3-9).

The sender is the individual or group transmitting the message. The message is the information or attitude communicated by the sender. Messages may be verbal or nonverbal. Verbal messages are voiced or written. Examples of different kinds of messages are lectures, letters, and e-mail memos. Nonverbal communication is any communication that is not voiced or written. Nonverbal communication includes gestures, facial expressions, eye movements and contact, voice tone, space, and touch.

The **channel** of communication is the method used to transmit messages. The most common channels involve sight and hearing, such as written and oral messages. However, other sensory input, such as touch, may be used with visual or **auditory** communication. In addition, communication channels may be formal (memos or letters) or informal (conversation).

The receiver is the target of the communication and can be an individual or a group. One-on-one communication is often more effective because both parties can respond to each other. Communication with a group can be more challenging but is a more efficient way to get information to numerous individuals.

The last essential part of communication is **feedback.** Human communication is a two-way process in which the receiver serves an active role. Feedback from the receiver allows the sender to measure communication success and provide additional information when needed.

Communication in Health Care

Effective communication is the most important aspect of providing safe patient care. The first two 2010 National

Patient Safety Goals of The Joint Commission are to improve accuracy of patient identification and to improve effectiveness of communicating critical test values among caregivers.[6] All health care personnel must correctly identify patients before initiating care using a two patient identifier system. The patient identifiers can include any two of the following: name, birth date, and medical record number. Effectively communicating critical test values should include a "read back" scenario verifying the reporter and the receiver of the information and accurate reporting and recording of test values. Each institution may have specific values as critical test values; for example, RTs may be expected to report blood gas values of a pH less than 7.2 or a PO_2 less than 50 mm Hg. The process of the "read back" scenario is described in Box 3-1.

As an RT, you will have many opportunities to communicate with patients, other RTs, nurses, physicians, and other members of the health care team. Success as an RT depends on your ability to communicate with these key people. Poor communication skills can limit your ability to treat patients, work well with others, and find satisfaction in your employment.

RTs can communicate empathy to their patients through the use of key words and eye contact and the proper use of touch. Communicating empathy to patients is an effective way of letting them know you care for their well-being and are willing to provide respiratory care to help their breathing. Techniques involve asking the patient about his or her breathing on a regular basis, making good eye contact when the patient is speaking, and using gentle touch on the arm or hand when comforting the patient.

Factors Affecting Communication

Many factors affect communication in the health care setting (Figure 3-10). The uniquely human or "internal" qualities of sender and receiver (including their prior experiences, attitudes, values, cultural backgrounds, and self-concepts and feelings) play a large role in the communication process.

Generally, the verbal and nonverbal components of communication should enhance and reinforce each other. The RT who combines a compassionate-toned verbal

Box 3-1 "Read Back" Process to Ensure Accurate Communication of Information

PRESCRIBER/REPORTER

- Orders or critical test results are read and clearly enunciated, using two patient identifiers
- Avoid abbreviations
- Ask receiver to "read back" the information if this is not done voluntarily
- Verify with the receiver that the information is correct

RECEIVER

- Record the order or value
- Ask "prescriber/reporter" to repeat if information is not understood
- "Read back" the information, including two patient identifiers
- Receive confirmation from the "prescriber/reporter" that the information is correct; if incorrect, repeat the process

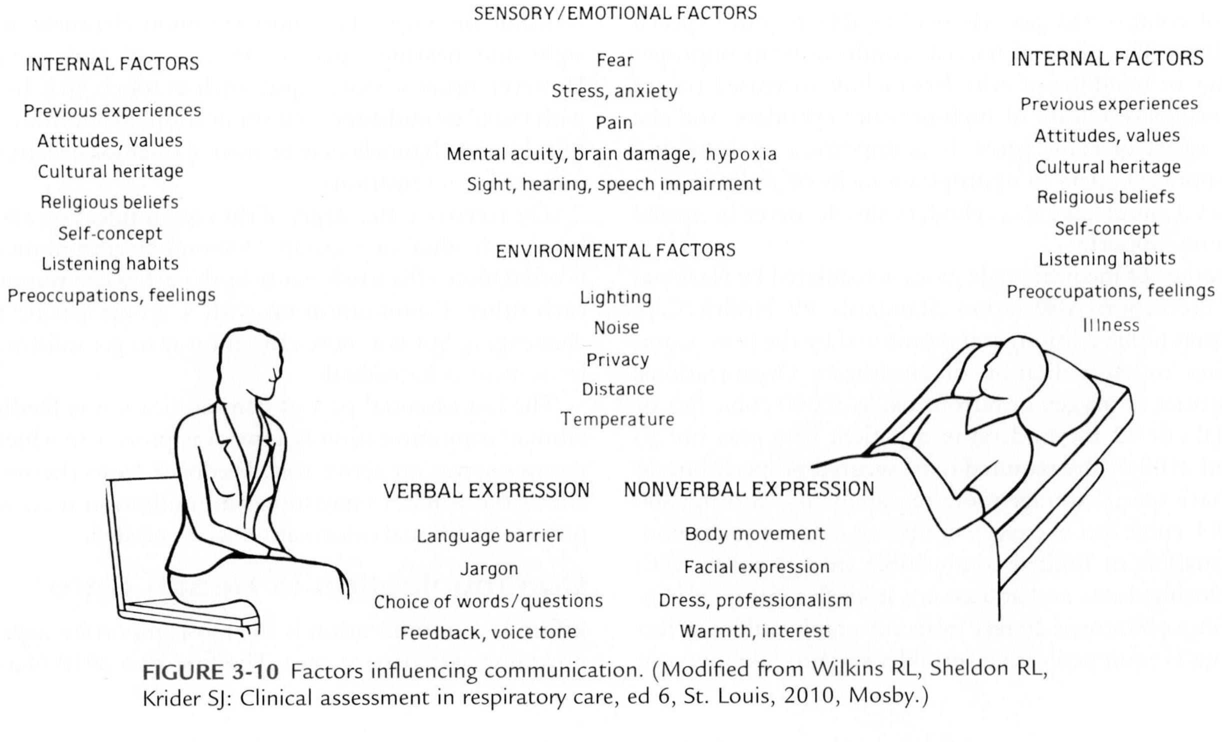

FIGURE 3-10 Factors influencing communication. (Modified from Wilkins RL, Sheldon RL, Krider SJ: Clinical assessment in respiratory care, ed 6, St. Louis, 2010, Mosby.)

message such as, "You're going to be all right now," with a confirming touch of the hand is sending a much stronger message to an anxious patient than the message provided by either component alone.

MINI CLINI

Patient Communication

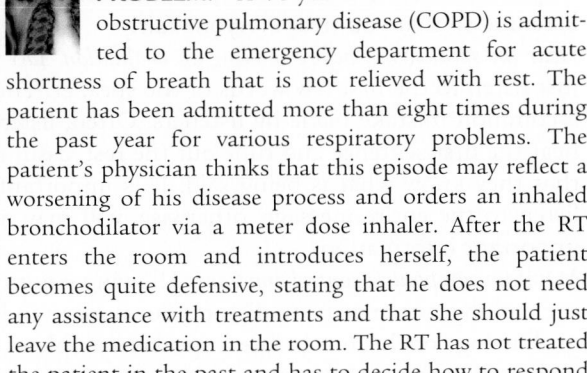

PROBLEM: A 73-year-old man with chronic obstructive pulmonary disease (COPD) is admitted to the emergency department for acute shortness of breath that is not relieved with rest. The patient has been admitted more than eight times during the past year for various respiratory problems. The patient's physician thinks that this episode may reflect a worsening of his disease process and orders an inhaled bronchodilator via a meter dose inhaler. After the RT enters the room and introduces herself, the patient becomes quite defensive, stating that he does not need any assistance with treatments and that she should just leave the medication in the room. The RT has not treated the patient in the past and has to decide how to respond to the patient's request.

DISCUSSION: Although this patient exhibited reluctance in allowing the RT to administer the therapy, enough verbal and perhaps nonverbal communication (message) was expressed by the patient (sender) for the RT (receiver) to determine a plan of action. Because human communication is a two-way process, the RT serves an active role for further messages and interaction. This is a key concept for RTs to master because it helps in identifying a patient's problems, evaluating progress, and recommending further respiratory care. The RT must recognize that when an individual verbalizes disagreement with a treatment order and exhibits defensive behavior, the RT must attempt to understand what the patient is saying and not overreact. The RT could try to put the patient at ease by making eye contact, gesturing effectively, and maintaining a safe distance from the patient when talking. The RT should seek feedback from the patient to ensure that the message was understood as it was intended. In this situation, it may be appropriate for the RT to review and demonstrate meter dose inhaler use and ask the patient to "teach back" proper inhaler use and observe the patient self-administer the medication. This process (message) can be repeated until the patient can demonstrate proper technique. Allowing the patient to participate actively in medical care when feasible may serve to help him maintain a sense of control over his disease process.

Effective Communication in Health Care

RTs must be effective communicators. Effective communication occurs when the intent or purpose of the interaction is achieved. Several key purposes of communication are summarized in Box 3-2. The RT must consider the roles involved, the message, the channel, and the appropriate feedback to help achieve these purposes when communicating.

Box 3-2 Purposes of Communication in the Health Care Setting

- To establish rapport with another individual, such as a colleague, a patient, or a member of the patient's family
- To comfort an anxious patient by explaining the unknown
- To obtain information, such as during a patient interview
- To relay pertinent information, as when charting the results of a patient's treatment
- To give instructions, as when teaching a patient how to perform a lung function test
- To persuade others to take action, as when attempting to convince a patient to quit smoking
- To educate and confirm understanding as in a "teach back" scenario

Roles

The RT may be primarily the sender or the receiver. When the RT is teaching a patient how to perform a lung function test, the RT's role of sender is paramount. When the RT is interviewing a patient to obtain information, the RT's role as receiver is most important. When an RT is instructing a patient on a particular piece of equipment, such as a home continuous positive airway pressure or a meter dose inhaler with a spacer, the RT serves as both a sender and a receiver. In this case, a "teach back" scenario would be helpful in which the RT sends information to the patient and receives confirmation of understanding by having the patient "teach back" his or her understanding. This process can be repeated until the RT is satisfied with the patient's understanding.

Message and Channel

Charting the results of a patient's treatment (to inform other health care professionals) requires formality, objectivity, brevity, accuracy, and consistency in the use of medical jargon. This type of message or channel would not be used to establish rapport with a patient. Instead, a less formal channel would be used; jargon would be avoided; and feelings and feedback, both verbal and nonverbal, would be emphasized.

Feedback

The central role played by feedback is evident in all of the listed purposes of communication. When instructing a patient to perform a lung function test, it is only by judging the patient's understanding and actual performance that the RT can assess the effectiveness of the teaching effort. Likewise, the feedback received by an RT while trying to establish rapport with a patient's family indicates the success of that effort and can provide clues as to how to improve the relationship.

Improving Communication Skills

To enhance your ability to communicate effectively, focus on improving sending, receiving, and feedback skills. In addition, identify and overcome common barriers to effective communication.

Practitioner as Sender

Your effectiveness as a sender of messages can be improved in several ways. These suggestions may be applied to the clinical setting as follows:

- *Share information rather than telling.* Health professionals often provide information in an authoritative manner by telling colleagues or patients what to do or say. This approach can cause defensiveness and lead to uncooperative behavior. Conversely, sharing information creates an atmosphere of cooperation and trust.
- *Seek to relate to people rather than control them.* This is of particular significance during communication with patients. Health care professionals often attempt to control patients. Few people like to be controlled. Patients feel much more important if they are treated as an equal partner in the relationship. Explaining procedures to patients and asking their permission to proceed is a way to make them feel a part of the decision making regarding their care.
- *Value disagreement as much as agreement.* When individuals express disagreement, make an attempt to understand what they are saying and do not become defensive. Be prepared for disagreement and be open to the input of others.
- *Use effective nonverbal communication techniques.* The nonverbal communication that you use is just as important as what you say. Nonverbal techniques include good eye contact, effective gesturing, facial expressions, and voice tone. It is important that your nonverbal communication matches what you are saying. If you are trying to establish rapport with a patient but do not look him or her in the eye, your communication will not be as effective. Your eye contact and facial expressions help convey what you are trying to say and cause your words to have more impact. Appropriate eye contact also conveys to the patient that you are a professional who is self-confident.

Practitioner as Receiver and Listener

Receiver skills are just as important as sender skills. Messages sent are of no value unless they are received as intended. Active listening on the part of the receiver is required. Learning to listen requires a strong commitment and great effort. A few simple principles can help improve your listening skills, as follows:

- *Work at listening.* Listening is often a difficult process. It takes effort to hear what others are saying. Focus your attention on the speaker and on the message.
- *Stop talking.* Practice silent listening and avoid interrupting the speaker during an interaction. Interrupting the patient is a sure way to diminish effective communication.
- *Resist distractions.* It is easy to be distracted by surrounding noises and conversations. This is particularly true in a busy environment such as a hospital. When you are listening, try to tune out other distractions and give your full attention to the person who is speaking.
- *Keep your mind open; be objective.* Being open-minded is often difficult. All people have their own opinions that may influence what they hear. Try to be objective in your listening so that you treat everyone fairly.
- *Hear the speaker out before making an evaluation.* Do not just listen to the first few words of the speaker. This is a common mistake made by listeners. Often, listeners hear the first sentence and tune out the rest, assuming that they know what is being said. It is important to listen to the entire message; otherwise, you may miss important information.
- *Maintain composure; control emotions.* Allowing emotions, such as anger or anxiety, to distort your understanding or drawing conclusions before a speaker completes his or her thoughts or arguments is a common error in listening.

Active listening is a key component in health care communication. Many of the messages being sent are vital to patient care. If you do not listen effectively, important information may be lost, and the care of your patients may be jeopardized.

Providing Feedback

To enhance communication with others, effective feedback needs to be provided. Examples of effective feedback mechanisms in oral communication with patients include attending, paraphrasing, requesting clarification, perception checking, and reflecting feelings:

- *Attending.* **Attending** involves the use of gestures and posture that communicates one's attentiveness. Attending also involves confirming remarks, such as, "I see what you mean."
- *Paraphrasing.* Paraphrasing, or repeating the other's response in one's own words, is a technique useful in confirming that understanding is occurring between the parties involved in the interaction. However, overuse of paraphrasing can be irritating.
- *Requesting clarification.* Requesting clarification begins with an admission of misunderstanding on the part of the listener, with the intent being to understand the message better through restating or using alternative examples or illustrations. Overuse of this technique, as with paraphrasing, can hamper effective communication, especially if it is used in a condescending or patronizing manner. Requests for clarification should be used only when truly necessary and should always be nonjudgmental in nature.
- *Perception checking.* Perception checking involves confirming or disproving the more subtle components of a

communication interaction, such as messages that are implied but not stated. For example, the RT might sense that a patient is unsure of the need for a treatment. In this case, the RT might check this perception by saying, "You don't seem to be sure that you need this treatment. Is that correct?" By verifying or disproving this perception, both the health care professional and the patient understand each other better.

- *Reflecting feelings.* Reflecting feelings involves the use of statements to determine better the emotions of the other party. Nonjudgmental statements, such as, "You seem to be anxious about (this situation)," provide the opportunity for patients to express and reflect on their emotions and can help them confirm or deny their true feelings.

Minimizing Barriers to Communication

There are many potential barriers to effective communication. A skillful communicator tries to identify and eliminate or minimize the influence of these barriers in all interactions. By minimizing the influence of these barriers, the sender can help ensure that the message will be received as intended. Key barriers to effective communication are the following:

- *Use of symbols or words that have different meanings.* Words and symbols (including nonverbal communication) can mean different things to different people. These differences in meaning derive from differences in the background or culture between the sender and receiver and the context of the communication. For example, RTs often use the letters "COPD" to refer to patients with chronic obstructive pulmonary disease caused by long-term smoking. Patients may hear "COPD" used in reference to them and be confused about the meaning and interpret COPD to mean a fatal lung disease. Never assume that the patient has the same understanding as you in the interpretation of commonly used symbols or phrases.
- *Different value systems.* Everyone has his or her own value system, and many people do not recognize the values held by others. A large difference between the values held by individuals can interfere with communication. A clinical supervisor may inform students of the penalties for being late with clinical assignments. If a student does not value timeliness, he or she may not take seriously what is being said.
- *Emphasis on status.* A hierarchy of positions and power exists in most health care organizations. If superiority is emphasized by individuals of higher status, communication can be stifled. Everyone has experienced interactions with professionals who make it clear who is in charge. Emphasis on status can be a barrier to communication not only among health care professionals but also between health care professionals and patients.
- *Conflict of interest.* Many people are affected by decisions made in health care organizations. If people are afraid that a decision will take away their advantage or invade their territory, they may try to block communication. An example might be a staff member who is unwilling to share expertise with students. This person may feel that a student is invading his or her territory.
- *Lack of acceptance of differences in points of view, feelings, values, or purposes.* Most of us are aware that people have different opinions, feelings, and values. These differences can thwart effective communication. To overcome this barrier, an effective communicator allows others to express their differences. Encouraging individuals to communicate their feelings and points of view benefits everyone. Most of us think we are always correct. Accepting input from others promotes growth and cooperation.
- *Feelings of personal insecurity.* It is difficult for people to admit feelings of inadequacy. Individuals who are insecure do not offer information for fear that they appear ignorant, or they may be defensive when criticized, blocking clear communication. Many of us have worked with individuals who are insecure, realizing the difficulty in communicating with them.

To become an effective communicator, identify the purpose of each communication interaction and your role in it. Use specific sending, receiving, and feedback skills in each interaction. Finally, minimize any identified barriers to communication with patients or peers, to ensure that messages are received as intended.

CONFLICT AND CONFLICT RESOLUTION

Conflict is sharp disagreement or opposition among people over interests, ideas, or values. Because no two people are exactly alike in their backgrounds or attitudes, conflict can be found in every organization. Health care professionals experience a great deal of conflict in their jobs. Rapid changes occurring in health care have made everyone's jobs more complex and often more stressful. Because conflict is inevitable, all health care professionals must be able to recognize its sources and help resolve or manage its effect on people and on the organization.

Sources of Conflict

The first step in conflict management is to identify its potential sources. The four primary sources of conflict in organizations are (1) poor communication, (2) structural problems, (3) personal behavior, and (4) role conflict.

Poor Communication

Poor communication is the primary source of conflict in organizations. The previously discussed barriers to communication all are potential sources of conflict. If a supervisor is unwilling to accept different points of view for dealing with a difficult patient, an argument may occur. The importance of good communication cannot be overemphasized.

Structural Problems

The structure of the organization itself can increase the likelihood of conflict. Conflict tends to grow as the size of an organization increases. Conflict is also greater in organizations whose employees are given less control over their work and in organizations where certain individuals or groups have excessive power. Structural sources of conflict are the most rigid and are often difficult to control.

Personal Behavior

Personal behavior factors are a major source of conflict in organizations. Different personalities, attitudes, and behavioral traits create the possibility of great disagreement among health care professionals and between health care professionals and patients.

Role Conflict

Role conflict is the experience of being pulled in several directions by individuals who have different expectations of a person's job functions. A clinical supervisor is often expected to function both as a staff member and as a student supervisor. Trying to fill both roles simultaneously can cause stress and create interpersonal conflict.

Conflict Resolution

Conflict resolution or management is the process by which people control and channel disagreements within an organization. There are five basic strategies for handling conflict:

1. Competing
2. Accommodating
3. Avoiding
4. Collaborating
5. Compromising

Competing

Competing is an assertive and uncooperative conflict resolution strategy. Competing is a power-oriented method of resolving conflict. A supervisor who uses rank or other forces to attempt to win is using the competing strategy. This strategy may be useful when an unpopular decision must be made or when one must stand up for his or her rights. However, because it often causes others to clam up and feel inferior, competing should be used cautiously.

Accommodating

Accommodating is the opposite of competing. Accommodating is unassertive and cooperative. When people accommodate others involved in conflict, they neglect their own needs to meet the needs of the other party. Accommodation is a useful strategy when it is essential to maintain harmony in the environment. Accommodation is also appropriate when an issue is much more important to one party or the other in a dispute.

Avoiding

Avoiding is both an unassertive and an uncooperative conflict resolution strategy. In avoiding conflict, one or both parties decide not to pursue their concerns. Avoidance may be appropriate if there is no possibility of meeting one's goals. In addition, if one or both of the parties are hostile, avoidance may be a good strategy, at least initially. However, too much avoidance can leave important issues unattended or unresolved.

Collaborating

As a conflict resolution strategy, collaborating is the opposite of avoiding. Collaborating is assertive and cooperative. In collaboration, the involved parties try to find mutually satisfying solutions to their conflict. Collaboration usually takes more time than other methods and cannot be applied when the involved parties harbor strong negative feelings about each other.

Compromising

Compromising is a middle-ground strategy that combines assertiveness and cooperation. People who compromise give up more than individuals who compete but give up less than individuals who accommodate. Compromise is best used when a quick resolution is needed that both parties can accept. However, because both parties often feel they are losing, compromise should not be used exclusively.

Deciding which type of conflict resolution strategy to use requires knowledge of the context, the specific underlying problem, and the desires of the involved parties.

RECORDKEEPING

By 2014, the U.S. government would like all medical recordkeeping to be done electronically. The electronic medical record (EMR) is changing the way health care practitioners document care, but the overall content and concept of what we record remains the same. A medical record or chart presents a written picture of occurrences and situations pertaining to a patient throughout his or her stay in a health care institution. Medical records are the property of the institution and are strictly confidential. This information is protected under the Health Insurance Portability and Accountability Act (HIPAA) of 1996. The content of a patient's medical records, health insurance, or billing are not to be read or discussed by anyone except the individuals directly caring for the patient in a hospital or medical care facility. In addition, the medical record is a legal document.

MINI CLINI

Legal Aspects of Recordkeeping

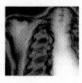

PROBLEM: A patient was given a respiratory treatment by a respiratory care student, who forgot to chart that the therapy was given. The student reasoned that because he did not observe any adverse effects during or immediately after the treatment and he knew that the treatment was given, not documenting the treatment in the medical record this one time would be acceptable. What are the problems associated with this student's judgment and subsequent actions?

DISCUSSION: The medical record is a legal document intended to identify types of care given to a patient and to serve as a source of information to the physician, RT (including the student), and other health care providers in developing an individualized plan of care. It further serves as a tool for evaluating the effectiveness in reaching the goals of therapy. Hospitals and other health care agencies critically evaluate the medical records of patients to maintain high-quality patient care. Failure to document care rendered, such as a respiratory treatment, hinders the process of providing high-quality care in several ways.

First, information that is important to the physician and other caregivers interested in the patient's respiratory status is missing from the medical record. In this situation, although the student observed a lack of response by the patient during and immediately after the treatment, a delayed effect could still have occurred. Consequently, the physician or RT would have difficulty in establishing the cause of a condition change in the patient related to the respiratory treatment. From a legal perspective, patient care not documented may be viewed as care not rendered, making the hospital or institution vulnerable to charges of patient neglect, which would be difficult to defend in a court of law.

Because the law requires that a record be kept of the patient's care, a patient's chart is also a legal document. For this reason, charting or recordkeeping must be done so that it is meaningful for days, months, or years, in case it must be used in court.

Components of a Traditional Medical Record

Each health care facility has its own specification for the medical records it keeps. Although the forms themselves vary among institutions, most acute care medical records share common sections (Box 3-3).

Figure 3-11 provides an example of a desaturation study for home oxygen therapy qualification. Documentation sheets are designed to report data briefly and to decrease time spent in documentation. Entries can include many

Box 3-3 General Sections Found in a Patient Medical Record

ADMISSION SHEET
Records pertinent patient information (e.g., name, address, religion, nearest of kin), admitting physician, and admission diagnosis

HISTORY AND PHYSICAL EXAMINATION
Records the patient's admitting history and physical examination, as performed by the attending physician or resident

HEALTH MAINTENANCE AND IMMUNIZATIONS
Records the dates of administration

PHYSICIAN'S ORDERS
Records the physician's orders and prescriptions

PROGRESS SHEET
Keeps a continuing account of the patient's progress for the physician

NURSES' NOTES
Describes the nursing care given to the patient, including the patient's complaints (subjective symptoms), the nurses' observations (objective signs), and the patient's response to therapy

MEDICATION RECORD
Notes drugs and IV fluids that are given to the patient

ALLERGIES
Notes reaction, severity, type, and date noted

VITAL SIGNS GRAPHIC SHEET
Records the patient's temperature, pulse, respirations, and blood pressure over time

I/O SHEET
Records patient's fluid intake (I) and output (O) over time

LABORATORY SHEET
Summarizes the results of laboratory tests

CONSULTATION SHEET
Records notes by physicians who are called in to examine a patient to make a diagnosis

SURGICAL OR TREATMENT CONSENT
Records the patient's authorization for surgery or treatment

ANESTHESIA AND SURGICAL RECORD
Notes key events before, during, and immediately after surgery

SPECIALIZED THERAPY RECORDS AND PROGRESS NOTES
Records specialized treatments or treatment plans and patient progress for various specialized therapeutic services (e.g., respiratory care, physical therapy)

SPECIALIZED FLOW SHEETS
Records measurement made over time during specialized procedures (e.g., mechanical ventilation, kidney dialysis)

ADVANCED DIRECTIVES
Records wishes and documents regarding living wills, power of attorney, and do not resuscitate orders

Date: ______________ Weaning Day #______ Patient Name: ________________________

Current Ventilator Settings		Spont. Resp. Mechanics		Pre-wean ABG	Post-wean ABG
Mode		Min. Volume (V_E)	L	pH	pH
Resp. Rate		Rest. Rate		$PaCO_2$	$PaCO_2$
Tidal Volume	mL	Tidal Volume	mL	PaO_2	PaO_2
Peak Pressure	cm H_2O	Max. Insp. Pressure	cm H_2O	HCO_3	HCO_3
FiO_2		Vital Capacity	mL	BE	BE
PEEP	cm H_2O	f/V_t ratio		SaO_2	SaO_2
PSV	cm H_2O	Static Comp.	mL/cm H_2O	PaO_2/FiO_2	PaO_2/FiO_2
AutoPEEP	cm H_2O	Plateau Pressure	cm H_2O	FiO_2	FiO_2

No Spontaneous Mechanics due to: ☐ Hemodynamic instability ☐ ICP ☐ Paralytics ☐ Sedation Other ________________
No Weaning due to: ☐ Hemodynamic instability ☐ ICP ☐ Paralytics ☐ Sedation ☐ Poor Spont Mechs ☐ Other ________________

Weaning Mode Guidelines			Weaning Guideline	Extubation Guidelines
	Criteria	Objectives	Reduce PSV to 75%, 50%, 25% of initial setting	Pressure Support
Rapid	Vent <5 days	Vent adjustment Q 30 mins		Rapid PSV <5 cm $H_2O \times 2$ hrs ⇨ extubate
Slow	Vent >5 days	Vent adjustment Q 1 hour		Slow PSV <5 cm $H_2O \times 4$ hrs ⇨ extubate

Time	Duration	PSV Level	PSV/Spont V_t	V_E	RR	HR	SpO_2/ SaO_2	BP	MAP (mm Hg)	PEEP	FiO_2	RCP initials

Total Weaning Time: ________________ Last successfully weaned PSV level: ____________ cmH_2O

Weaning Failure Guidelines

1. MAP change ≥ 20 mm Hg? Yes No
2. HR change ≥ 20 bpm? Yes No
3. $PaCO_2$ ⇧ by 10 – 20 mm Hg and is 10 over pt. projected baseline? Yes No
4. PaO_2 ⇩ by 10 – 20 mm Hg despite ⇧ FiO_2 to .45? Yes No
5. pH < 7.30? Yes No
6. RR > 30 – 35 bpm? Yes No
7. SpO_2 < 90% on FiO_2 ≥ .50? Yes No
8. f/V_t > 105? Yes No

Actions

- Successful wean? Yes No (if No, comment) ________________________
- Extubated? Yes No (if No, comment) ________________________

Practitioner #1: ________________________

Practitioner #2: ________________________

Loma Linda University Medical Center
Loma Linda University Community Medical Center
Department of Respiratory Care

FIGURE 3-11 Documentation form for fast or slow weaning tolerance. (Courtesy Loma Linda University Medical Center, Loma Linda, California.)

TABLE 3-2

The Joint Commission "Do Not Use" List*

Do Not Use	Potential Problem	Use Instead
U (unit)	Mistaken for 0 (zero), the number 4 (four) or cc	Write "unit"
IU (international unit)	Mistaken for IV (intravenous) or the number 10 (ten)	Write "international unit"
Q.E., QD, q.d., qd (daily); Q.O.D., POD, q.o.d, qod (every other day)	Mistaken for each other; period after the Q mistaken for I and the O mistaken for I	Write "daily" or "every other day"
Trailing zero (X.0 mg)†; lack of leading zero (.X mg)	Decimal point is missed	Write "X mg" or "0.X mg"
MS	Can mean morphine sulfate or magnesium sulfate	Write "morphine sulfate"
MSO_4, $MgSO_4$	Confused for one another	Write "magnesium sulfate"
Additional Abbreviations, Acronyms, and Symbols for *Possible* Future Inclusion in the Official "Do Not Use" List		
> (greater than); < (less than)	Misinterpreted as the number 7 (seven) or the letter L; confused for one another	Write "greater than" or "less than"
Abbreviations for drug names	Misinterpreted owing to similar abbreviations for multiple drugs	Write drug names in full
Apothecary units	Unfamiliar to many practitioners; confused with metric units	Use metric units
@	Mistaken for the number "2" (two)	Write "at"
cc	Mistaken for U (units) when poorly written	Write "mL" or "ml" or "milliliters" ("mL" is preferred)
μg	Mistaken for mg (milligrams) resulting in 1000-fold overdose	Write "mcg" or "micrograms"

From The Joint Commission: 2010 TJC "Do Not Use" list. http://www.jointcommission.org/ accessed December 17, 2010.

*Applies to all orders and all medication-related documentation that is handwritten (including free-text computer entry) or on preprinted forms.

†*Exception:* A "trailing zero" may be used only where required to show the level of precision of the value being reported, such as for laboratory results, imaging studies that report size of lesions, or catheter/tube sizes. It may not be used in medication orders or other medication-related documentation.

measurements, and review of a sequence of entries can reveal trends in patient status.

Legal Aspects of Recordkeeping

Legally, documentation of the care given to a patient means that care was given; no documentation means that care was not given. Hospital accreditation agencies critically evaluate the medical records of patients. If the RT does not document care given (i.e., patient assessment data, interventions, and evaluation of care rendered), the practitioner and the hospital may be accused of patient neglect.

Adequate documentation of care is valuable only in reference to standards and criteria of care. Similar to all departments in health care facilities, respiratory care departments must generate their own standards of patient care. For each standard, criteria must be outlined so that the adequacy of patient care can be measured. Documentation must reflect these standards.

Practical Aspects of Recordkeeping

Recordkeeping is one of the most significant duties that a health care professional performs. Documentation is required for each medication, treatment, or procedure. Accounts of the patient's condition and activities must be charted accurately and in clear terms. Brevity is essential, although a complete account of each patient encounter is needed. The use of standardized terms and abbreviations is acceptable; however, The Joint Commission has published a "Do Not Use" abbreviation list developed to reduce potential errors (Table 3-2).[7] Documentation of consultations with the attending physician that include the date and time of the conversation is recommended.

Accounts of care and the patient's condition are generally printed by hand or handwritten. In some institutions, computerized patient information systems facilitate data entry by selection from menus of choices or direct typing. In either case, you must document only what is—not an interpretation or a judgment. Assessments of data must be clearly within one's professional domain. When a practitioner cannot interpret the data obtained, he or she should state so in the record and contact another health care professional for advice or referral and document the referral in the patient's medical record. Other general rules for medical recordkeeping are listed in Box 3-4. In addition to these general rules, each institution has its own policies governing medical recordkeeping.

Problem-Oriented Medical Record

The **problem-oriented medical record (POMR)** is an alternative documentation format used by some health care institutions. The POMR contains four parts: (1) the

Box 3-4 General Rules for Medical Recordkeeping

Entries on the patient's chart should be printed or handwritten. After completing the account, sign the chart with one initial and your last name and your title (CRT, RRT, Resp Care Student; e.g., S. Smith, CRT). Institutional policy may require that supervisory personnel countersign student entries.

Do not use ditto marks.

Do not erase. Erasures provide reason for question if the chart is used later in a court of law. If a mistake is made, a single line should be drawn through the mistake and the word "error" printed above it. Then continue your charting in a normal manner.

Record after completing each task for the patient, and sign your name correctly after each entry.

Be exact in noting the time, effect, and results of all treatments and procedures.

Chart patient complaints and general behavior. Describe the type, location, onset, and duration of pain. Describe clearly and concisely the character and amount of secretions.

Leave no blank lines in the charting. Draw a line through the center of an empty line or part of a line. This prevents charting by someone else in an area signed by you.

Use standard abbreviations.

Use the present tense. Never use the future tense, as in "Patient to receive treatment after lunch."

Spell correctly. If you are unsure about the spelling of a word, look it up in a dictionary.

Document conversations with the patient or other health care providers that you think are important (e.g., you informed the patient's physician or nurse that the patient seems confused or more short of breath).

Box 3-5 Example of SOAP Entry

6/29/07

PROBLEM 1

Difficult breathing

SUBJECTIVE

"I can't catch my breath."

OBJECTIVE

Awake; alert; oriented to time, place, and person; sitting upright in bed with arms leaning over the bedside stand; pale, dry skin; respirations 26 breaths/min and shallow; pulse 98 beats/min, regular and faint to palpation; blood pressure 112/68 mm Hg, left arm, sitting position; body temperature 101° F; bronchial breath sounds in lower posterior lung fields; occasionally expectorating small volumes of mucopurulent sputum. Chest x-ray shows left lower lung infiltrate.

ASSESSMENT

Retained mucus and possible infection

PLAN

Therapeutic: Assist with coughing and deep breathing at least every 2 hours; postural drainage and percussion every 4 hours; assist with ambulation as per physician orders and patient tolerance.

Diagnostic: Continue to monitor lung sounds before and after each treatment.

Education: Teach patient to cough and deep breathe and evaluate return demonstration.

database, (2) the problem list, (3) the plan, and (4) the progress notes. The precise forms these records take vary among institutions.

The database contains routine information about the patient. A general health history, physical examination results, and results of diagnostic tests are included.

In the POMR, a problem is something that interferes with a patient's physical or psychologic health or ability to function. The patient's problems are identified and listed on the basis of the information provided by the database. The list of problems is dynamic; new problems are added as they develop, and problems are removed as they are resolved.

The POMR progress notes contain the findings (subjective and objective data), assessment, plans, and orders of the physicians, nurses, and other practitioners involved in the care of the patient. The format used is often referred to as *SOAP* (*S* = subjective information, *O* = objective information, *A* = assessment, *P* = plan of care). Figure 3-12 shows a representative SOAP form for respiratory care progress notes. Box 3-5 provides an example of a SOAP entry. Table 3-3 lists common objective data gathered by RTs and examples of applicable assessments and plans. In many institutions, all caregivers chart on the same form, using the SOAP format.

RULE OF THUMB

Charting Progress Notes Using the SOAP Format

SOAP stands for *S*ubjective, *O*bjective, *A*ssessment, *P*lan.

- Subjective information obtained from the patient, his or her family members, or a similar source
- Objective information based on caregivers' observations of the patient, the physical examination, or diagnostic or laboratory tests such as arterial blood gases or pulmonary function tests
- Assessment, which refers to the analysis of the patient's problem
- Plan of action to be taken to resolve the problem

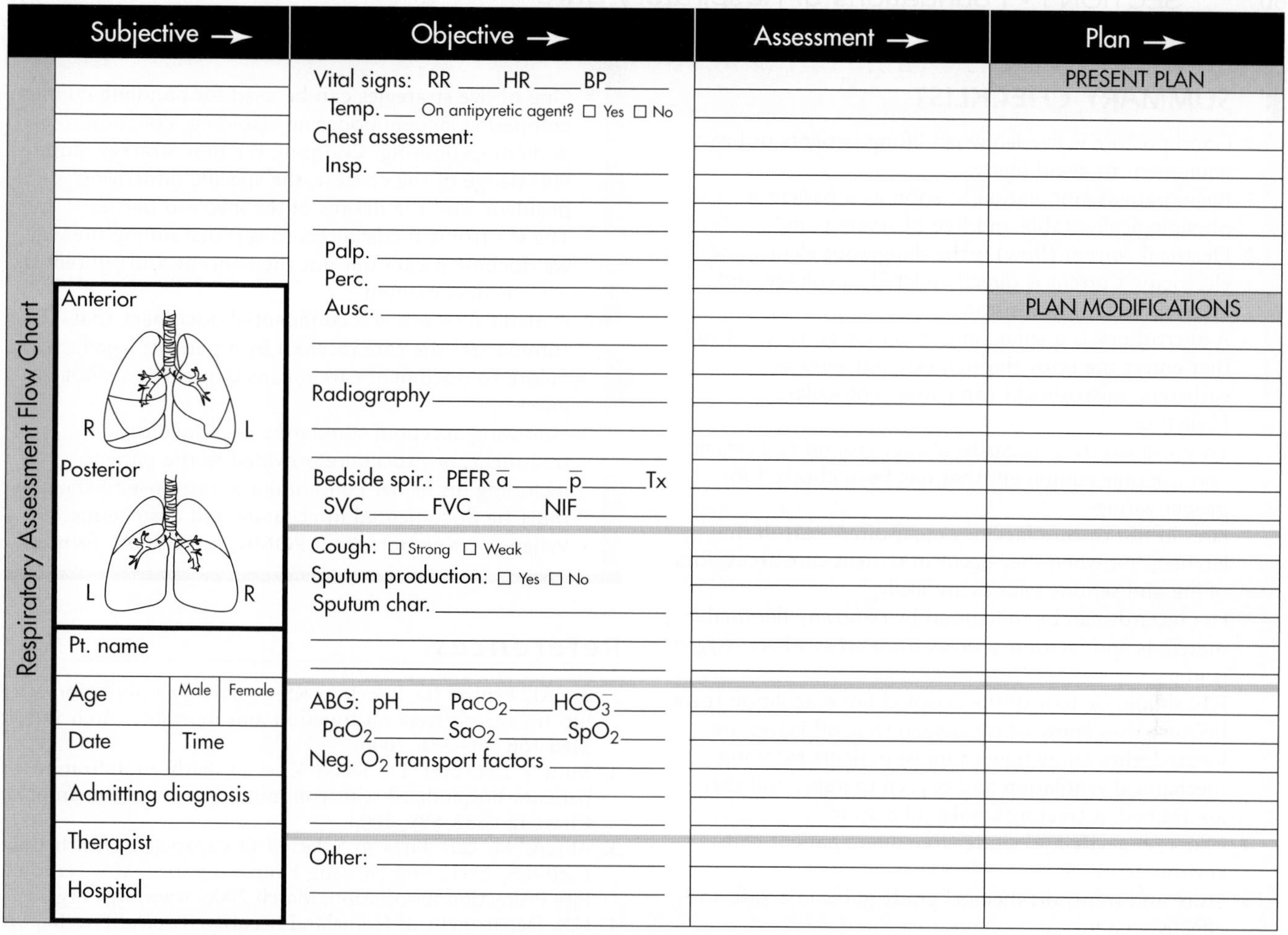

Subjective →	Objective →	Assessment →	Plan →

Respiratory Assessment Flow Chart

Vital signs: RR ___ HR ___ BP ___
Temp. ___ On antipyretic agent? ☐ Yes ☐ No
Chest assessment:
Insp. ___
Palp. ___
Perc. ___
Ausc. ___
Radiography ___
Bedside spir.: PEFR $\bar{a}$ ___ $\bar{p}$ ___ Tx
SVC ___ FVC ___ NIF ___
Cough: ☐ Strong ☐ Weak
Sputum production: ☐ Yes ☐ No
Sputum char. ___
ABG: pH ___ $PaCO_2$ ___ HCO_3^- ___
PaO_2 ___ SaO_2 ___ SpO_2 ___
Neg. O_2 transport factors ___
Other: ___

Pt. name
Age | Male | Female
Date | Time
Admitting diagnosis
Therapist
Hospital

PRESENT PLAN

PLAN MODIFICATIONS

FIGURE 3-12 Example of a SOAP form for respiratory care progress notes. (From Des Jardins T, Burton GG: Clinical manifestations and assessment of respiratory disease, ed 6, St. Louis, 2011, Mosby.)

TABLE 3-3

Examples of Objective Data, Assessments, and Plans Typical for Documentation Using SOAP Notes

Objective Data	Assessment	Plan
Sputum Production		
Thick, purulent	Respiratory infection	Humidity therapy, antibiotics
Auscultation		
Expiratory wheezing	Bronchospasm	Bronchodilator
Stridor	Upper airway obstruction	Racemic epinephrine, possible intubation
Late-inspiratory crackles	Atelectasis	Lung expansion therapy
Breathing Pattern		
Prolonged expiratory time	Bronchospasm	Bronchodilators
Prolonged inspiratory time	Upper airway obstruction	Racemic epinephrine; consider need for intubation
Rapid and shallow	Restrictive lung disease	Notify physician, perform additional assessment, consider lung expansion therapy
Vital Signs		
Acute tachycardia/tachypnea	Acute respiratory failure	Get ABGs, chest radiograph; call physician
Abnormal sensorium	Acute hypoxia	Assess patient further; oxygen therapy
ABGs		
PaO_2 40-60 mm Hg	Moderate hypoxemia	Give oxygen via cannula or mask
PaO_2 < 40 mm Hg	Severe hypoxemia	Give high concentration oxygen as needed and consider positive pressure ventilation with PEEP or CPAP
Chest Radiograph		
Low lung volumes or infiltrates	Atelectasis	Lung expansion therapy
Air in pleural space	Pneumothorax	Insert chest tube

ABGs, Arterial blood gas analysis; *CPAP,* continuous positive airway pressure; *PEEP,* positive end-expiratory pressure.

SUMMARY CHECKLIST

- Good posture is needed when lifting patients or heavy equipment to avoid injury.
- Begin patient ambulation as soon as a patient is physiologically stable and free of severe pain.
- Electrical current (flow) is the dangerous element of electricity. Current is directly related to voltage and inversely related to resistance.
- A microshock is a small, imperceptible current (<1 mA) that enters the body through external wires or catheters; microshocks can cause ventricular fibrillation.
- To avoid electrical hazards, always ground equipment and use only equipment that has been checked for proper wiring.
- Fires in health care facilities most often start in the kitchen, but when they occur in patient care areas, loss of life and serious injuries are likely.
- Fire hazards can be minimized by removing flammable materials and ignition sources from areas where oxygen is in use.
- RTs should be part of the hospital fire evacuation team because they know where oxygen shut-off valves are located, they know how to move patients receiving mechanical ventilation and oxygen therapy, and they are trained at treating smoke inhalation.
- Maintain a safe and clutter-free direct patient care environment.
- Store and transport medical grade gases in a safe and effective manner.
- Communication skills play a key role in the ability to identify a patient's problems, to evaluate the patient's progress, to make recommendations for respiratory care, and to achieve desired patient outcomes.
- Individuals' prior experiences, attitudes, values, cultural backgrounds, self-concepts, and feelings play a large role in the communication process.
- To enhance communication ability, focus on improving sending, receiving, and feedback skills; in addition, be able to identify and overcome common barriers to effective communication.
- One of five strategies can be used for handling conflict: competing, accommodating, avoiding, collaborating, and compromising. Choosing the best strategy requires knowledge of the context, the specific underlying problem, and the desires of the involved parties.
- The electronic medical record is transforming the way we document care but not the concept and content of what is documented.
- A medical record is a confidential document that summarizes the care received by a patient; legally, a failure to document care means that care was not given.
- Following accepted standards, each medication, treatment, or procedure provided to the patient, including his or her condition and response to therapy, must be documented in accurate and clear terms.
- When entering notes in a POMR, use a SOAP format.

References

1. Siu AL, Penrod JD, Boockvar KS, et al: Early ambulation after hip fracture: effects on function and mortality. Arch Intern Med 166:766–771, 2006.
2. Mundy LM, Leet TL, Darst K, et al: Early mobilization of patients hospitalized with community-acquired pneumonia. Chest 124:883–889, 2003.
3. Ahrens M: U.S. Fires in Selected Occupancies. Health Care Facilities, Excluding Nursing Homes. Quincy, MA, National Fire Protection Association, March 2006. www.nfpa.org.
4. U.S. Department of Homeland Security. Topical Fire Report Series (TFRS) Volume 9, Issue 4, May 2009. Emmitsburg, MD, U.S. Fire Administration National Fire Data Center, 2009.
5. National Fire Protection Association: Health Care Facilities 99; Standard for Health Care Facilities, 2005 Edition. Quincy, MA, National Fire Protection Association, 2005.
6. Joint Commission on Accreditation of Health Care Organizations National Patient Safety Goals 2010. http://www.jointcommission.org/hospitals_2010npsgs/. Accessed December 17, 2010.
7. Joint Commission on Accreditation of Health Care Organizations: 2010 JCAHO "Do Not Use" list. http://www.jointcommission.org/hospitals. Accessed December 17, 2010.

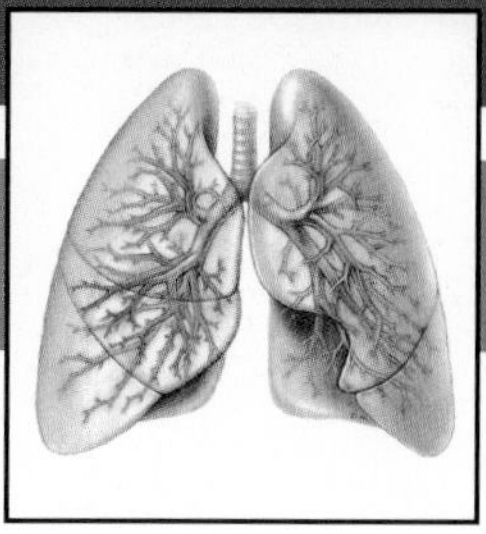

Chapter 4

Principles of Infection Prevention and Control

THOMAS G. FRASER

CHAPTER OBJECTIVES

After reading this chapter you will be able to:

- Define health care–associated infections and state how often they occur.
- Describe why infection prevention is important in respiratory care.
- Identify and describe the three elements that must be present for transmission of infection within a health care setting.
- List the factors associated with an increased risk of a patient acquiring a nosocomial infection.
- State the three major routes for transmission of human sources of pathogens in the health care environment.
- Describe strategies to control the spread of infection in the hospital.
- Describe how to select and apply chemical disinfectants for processing respiratory care equipment.
- Describe equipment-handling procedures that help prevent the spread of pathogens.
- State when to use general barrier measures during patient care.
- Describe surveillance with regard to infection control.

CHAPTER OUTLINE

Spread of Infection
- Sources of Infectious Agents
- Susceptible Hosts
- Modes of Transmission

Infection Prevention Strategies
- Creating a Safe Culture
- Decreasing Host Susceptibility
- Eliminating the Source of Pathogens
- Interrupting Transmission
- Standard Precautions
- Hand Hygiene
- Gloves
- Mouth, Nose, Eye, and Face Protection
- Respiratory Protection
- Gowns, Aprons, and Protective Apparel
- Transmission-Based Precautions
- Airborne Infection Isolation
- Protective Environment
- Patient Placement
- Transport of Infected Patients

Disinfection and Sterilization
- Spaulding Approach to Disinfection and Sterilization of Patient Care Equipment
- Cleaning
- Disinfection
- Sterilization

Equipment Handling Procedures
- Maintenance of In-Use Equipment
- Processing Reusable Equipment
- Disposable Equipment
- Fluids and Medications Precautions
- Handling Contaminated Articles and Equipment
- Using Needles and Syringes
- Handling Laboratory Specimens

Surveillance for Hospital-Acquired Infections

KEY TERMS

antiseptics
bactericidal
bacteriostatic
cohorting
contact precautions
disinfection
droplet nuclei
droplet precautions
fomites

health care–associated infections (HAIs)
Health Care Infection Control Practices Advisory Committee (HICPAC)
high-efficiency particulate air/aerosol (HEPA) filters
hospital-acquired or nosocomial infections
immunocompromised hosts
Occupational Safety and Health Administration (OSHA)
respiratory hygiene/cough etiquette
sporicidal
standard precautions
sterilization
surveillance
virucidal

Health care–associated infections (HAIs) are infections that patients acquire during the course of medical treatment. In 2002, there were an estimated 1.7 million HAIs in U.S. hospitals accounting for 99,000 excess deaths.[1] Approximately 5% of all patients admitted to a hospital develop an HAI, and 15% of HAIs are pneumonias.[2,3] Approximately 25% of patients undergoing mechanical ventilation develop pneumonia as a complication, and approximately 30% of these patients die as a result of lung infection.[4]

The seminal Institute of Medicine report identified that medical errors may be the fifth leading cause of death in the United States, with up to 100,000 deaths annually.[3] At the present time, there is increasing legislative and regulatory interest in patient safety, including a focus on HAIs. Health care professionals are giving increased attention to handwashing and protecting patients against infection. The emergence of *severe acute respiratory syndrome (SARS)* in China in 2002 and global spread with outbreaks in health care settings and transmission to large numbers of health care personnel and patients underscore the importance of consistent adherence to infection control precautions. Similarly, infection control practices were tested in 2009 by pandemic H1N1 influenza A, reinforcing the reality that new challenges continually arise.

Protecting patients and health care professionals against infections requires strict adherence to infection control procedures. Infection control procedures aim to eliminate the sources of infectious agents, create barriers to their transmission, and monitor and evaluate the effectiveness of control. Infection prevention is a major and ongoing responsibility of all health care workers, including respiratory therapists (RTs). To fulfill this responsibility, RTs must be able to select and apply various infection control procedures. This chapter provides the foundation needed to assume this important responsibility.

SPREAD OF INFECTION

Three elements must be present for transmission of infection within a health care setting: (1) a *source* (or reservoir) of pathogens, (2) a *susceptible host,* and (3) a *route* of transmission for the pathogen (Figure 4-1).[2]

Sources of Infectious Agents

Humans (patients, personnel, or visitors) are the primary source for infectious agents in the health care setting, but inanimate objects (e.g., contaminated medical equipment, linen, medications) have also been implicated in transmission. A person may have an acute infection with symptoms, may be in the asymptomatic or incubation period of the disease, or may be colonized by pathogens without symptoms. People may also serve as their own source of infection, via endogenous flora. This latter process is called *autogenous infection.*

Susceptible Hosts

Susceptibility and resistance to infection vary greatly. Some individuals may be immune to infection or able to resist colonization. Others exposed to the same organism may carry it but show no symptoms. Other individuals may develop clinical disease. Host factors, such as poorly controlled diabetes mellitus, extremes of age, and underlying acquired (HIV infection) or iatrogenic (through chemotherapy or anti–tumor necrosis factor inhibitors) immunodeficiency, can enhance susceptibility to infection. Surgical incisions and radiation therapy impair defenses of the skin and organ space. Medical devices, such as urinary tract catheters, central venous catheters, and endotracheal tubes, allow pathogens to increase the risk of infection by impeding local host defenses and providing biofilms that may facilitate adherence of pathogens.

Hospital-acquired or nosocomial infections are infections that are acquired in the hospital. The high incidence of nosocomial gram-negative bacterial pneumonia is associated with factors that promote colonization of the pharynx with these organisms. Gram-negative colonization dramatically increases in critically ill patients, which increases the likelihood of the development of these pneumonias.[4] Most nosocomial pneumonias occur in surgical patients, especially patients who have had chest or abdominal procedures. In these patients, normal swallowing and clearance mechanisms are impaired, allowing bacteria to enter and remain in the lower respiratory tract. Intubations, anesthesia, surgical pain, and use of narcotics and sedatives impair host defenses further. The risk of pneumonia is not the same for all surgical patients. Patients at

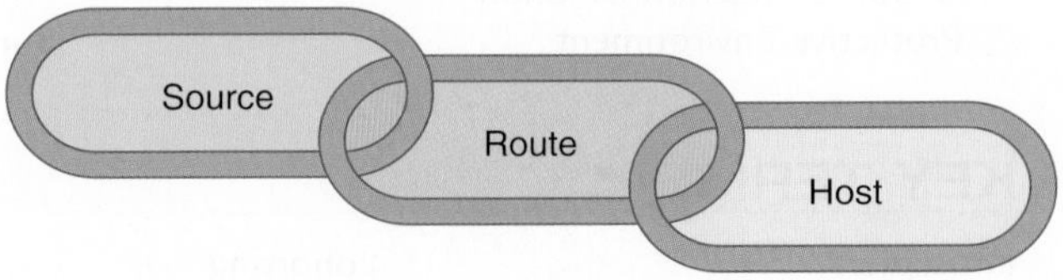

FIGURE 4-1 Elements that must be present for infection to spread.

the highest risk include elderly patients, severely obese patients, patients with chronic obstructive pulmonary disease (COPD) or a history of smoking, and patients with an artificial airway in place for long periods.[5]

Patients with an artificial tracheal airway are at high risk for nosocomial pneumonia for several reasons. Typically, patients requiring prolonged intubation already have one or more factors predisposing to infection, such as severe COPD. Another risk factor may be increased upper airway colonization with gram-negative bacteria. Because the tube bypasses the normal protective mechanisms of the upper airway, bacteria have easy access to the lower respiratory tract. Finally, handling of these tubes increases the likelihood of cross contamination, particularly during suctioning.

Some pneumonias occur primarily in immunocompromised hosts. Physicians may purposefully suppress a patient's immune response with drugs, as in organ transplant cases. Alternatively, immunosuppression may be a result of underlying disease, as with AIDS. **Immunocompromised hosts,** regardless of cause, are highly susceptible to infections, especially infections caused by opportunistic bacteria, fungi, or viruses.

Modes of Transmission

The three major routes for transmission of human sources of pathogens in the health care environment are *contact* (direct and indirect), *respiratory droplets,* and *airborne droplet nuclei* (respirable particles <5 μm). Table 4-1 provides examples of the common transmission routes for selected microorganisms.[6]

TABLE 4-1

Routes of Infectious Disease Transmission

Mode	Type	Examples
Contact	Direct	Hepatitis A HIV *Staphylococcus* Enteric bacteria
	Indirect	*Pseudomonas aeruginosa* Enteric bacteria Hepatitis B and C HIV
Droplet	Rhinovirus SARS-associated coronavirus	*Haemophilus influenzae* (type B) pneumonia and epiglottitis *Neisseria meningitidis* pneumonia
	Monkeypox	Diphtheria Pertussis Streptococcal pneumonia Influenza Mumps Rubella Adenovirus
Vehicle	Water-borne	Shigellosis Cholera
	Foodborne	Salmonellosis Hepatitis A
Airborne	Aerosols Droplet nuclei	Legionellosis Tuberculosis Varicella Measles Smallpox
Vector-borne	Ticks and mites	Rickettsia Lyme disease
	Mosquitoes	Malaria
	Fleas	Bubonic plague

Contact Transmission

Contact transmission is the most common route of transmission and is divided into two subgroups: direct and indirect. *Direct contact transmission* occurs when a pathogen is transferred directly from one person to another. Direct contact transmission occurs less frequently than indirect contact in the health care environment but is more efficient. An example of direct contact transmission would be development of respiratory syncytial virus bronchiolitis in a bone marrow transplant recipient owing to transmission of the virus from an ill health care worker who did not perform appropriate handwashing before providing care.

Indirect contact transmission is the most frequent mode of transmission in the health care environment and involves the transfer of a pathogen through a contaminated intermediate object or person. The most common indirect contact transmission in health care involves unwashed hands of health care personnel that touch an infected or a colonized body site on one patient or a contaminated inanimate object and subsequently touch another patient. Inanimate objects that may serve to transfer pathogens from one person to another are called **fomites.** Indirect contact transmission involving fomites can occur when instruments have been inadequately cleaned between patients before disinfection or sterilization.

Droplet Transmission

Droplet transmission is a form of contact transmission, but the mechanism of transfer of the pathogen is distinct, and additional prevention measures are required. Organisms that are transmitted by respiratory droplets include influenza and *Neisseria meningitidis*. Respiratory droplets are generated when an infected individual discharges large contaminated liquid droplets into the air by coughing, sneezing, or talking. Respiratory droplets are also generated during procedures such as suctioning, bronchoscopy, and cough induction. Transmission occurs when infectious droplets are propelled (usually ≤3 feet through the air) and are deposited on another person's mouth or nose. Using the distance of 3 feet or less as a threshold for donning a mask has been effective in preventing transmission of infectious agents. However, experimental studies with smallpox and investigations of outbreaks of SARS suggest that droplets from infected patients rarely are able to reach a person 6 feet away.[7] A distance of 3 feet or less around the patient is considered a short distance and is not used as a criterion for deciding when a mask should be donned to protect from exposure. Current **Health Care Infection Control Practices Advisory Committee (HICPAC)** guidelines state it may be prudent to don a mask when within 6 feet of a patient or on entry into the room of a patient who is on droplet isolation.[6]

Airborne Transmission

Airborne transmission occurs via the spread of airborne **droplet nuclei.** These are small particles (≤5 μm) of evaporated droplets containing infectious microorganisms that can remain suspended in air for long periods. Microorganisms carried in this manner may be dispersed widely by air currents because of their small size and inhaled by susceptible hosts over a longer distance from the source patient compared with droplet transmission. Examples of pathogens transmitted via the airborne route include *Mycobacterium tuberculosis,* varicella-zoster virus (chickenpox), and rubeola virus (measles). Airborne transmission of variola (smallpox) has been documented, and airborne transmission of SARS, monkeypox, and viral hemorrhagic fever virus has been reported, although it has not been proved conclusively.[6]

Special air handling and ventilation and respiratory protection are required to prevent airborne transmission because microorganisms may remain suspended in air and be widely dispersed by air currents before contacting a susceptible host. In addition to airborne infection isolation rooms, personal respiratory protection with National Institute for Occupational Safety and Health (NIOSH)–approved N-95 or higher respirators is required to prevent airborne transmission.[6] A surgical mask, used for droplet precautions, is insufficient.

Miscellaneous Types of Aerosol Transmission. Three novel categories of aerosol transmission have been proposed following investigations of SARS transmission, as follows[6]:

Obligate transmission: Under natural conditions, disease occurs after transmission of the microorganism through small-particle aerosols.

Preferential transmission: Natural infection results from transmission through multiple routes, but small-particle aerosols predominate.

Opportunistic transmission: Microorganisms that cause disease through other routes but under certain environmental conditions may be transmitted via fine-particle aerosol (e.g., SARS transmission via an aerosol plume that originated from sewage in the Amoy Gardens housing complex).[7]

Other Sources of Infection Not Involving Person-to-Person Transmission

Common vehicle transmission occurs via exposure to pathogens in contaminated food, water, or medications (e.g., heparin solution). Vector-borne transmission of infectious diseases from insects and rats and other vermin occurs but is of less significance in U.S. health care facilities.

INFECTION PREVENTION STRATEGIES

Creating a Safe Culture

Infection prevention programs are charged with identifying and categorizing HAIs and providing guidance to their organizations so that they can break the chain of events leading to these HAIs. Guidance and prevention efforts are directed at overall organizational structure and systems ("this is what we do as an institution to prevent infection") and at the individual caregiver level ("this is what I do to prevent infection"). Infection prevention efforts can be divided into efforts that decrease host susceptibility, efforts that eliminate the source of pathogens, and efforts that interrupt the transmission routes. From an organizational perspective, a crucial step is the creation by leadership of a culture of safety wherein there is a shared commitment to patient and health care worker safety.

Organizations also endorse best practices for infection prevention by ensuring that the bedside caregiver has the appropriate time, equipment, and training to provide the best possible care. Effective health care workers execute appropriate practice on a daily basis, such as attention to hand hygiene and adherence to infection prevention bundles of care. The presence of appropriate systems to deliver care and a committed workforce consistently executing best practice are necessary for an organization to prevent infections reliably.

Decreasing Host Susceptibility

Decreasing inherent host susceptibility to infection is the most difficult and least feasible approach to infection control. Hospital efforts at this level focus mainly on employee immunization and chemoprophylaxis. Certain immunizations are recommended for susceptible health care personnel to decrease the risk of infection and the potential for transmission to patients and coworkers within the health care facility. The **Occupational Safety and Health Administration (OSHA)** mandates that employers offer hepatitis B vaccination. Vaccinations of health care workers in the absence of evidence of immunity against varicella, rubella, and measles should be encouraged.[8] In addition, health care personnel in facilities that care for young infants and children should receive the adult acellular pertussis vaccine. Health care personnel without medical contraindications should also receive an annual influenza vaccination.[9]

Antimicrobial agents and topical **antiseptics** may be used to prevent outbreaks of selected pathogens. Postexposure chemoprophylaxis is recommended under defined circumstances for *Bordetella pertussis* (whooping cough), *N. meningitidis* (meningococcal meningitis), *Bacillus*

Box 4-1 Central Line Bundle

- Hand hygiene before line insertion
- Use of maximal sterile barrier precautions during line placement
- Chlorhexidine-based skin antisepsis at insertion site
- Daily review of line necessity

Box 4-2 Ventilator-Associated Pneumonia Bundle

- Elevate the head of the bed
- Daily sedation vacation
- Peptic ulcer disease prophylaxis
- Deep venous thrombosis prophylaxis
- Daily oral care with chlorhexidine

anthracis (anthrax), influenza virus, HIV, and group A streptococci.[6]

A large percentage of HAIs are due to device-related infections, including ventilator-associated pneumonia (VAP), catheter-related bloodstream infection, and catheter-associated urinary tract infection. The best way to decrease host susceptibility to a device-related infection is first to limit device use and second to ensure that devices are placed and maintained appropriately. Prevention bundles—defined as the use of multiple different evidence-based best practices to prevent device-related infection—have been shown to decrease the incidence of HAIs significantly.[10,11] Boxes 4-1 and 4-2 list the components of the central line bundle for vascular catheter placement and the VAP bundle. Institutions should be committed to these processes of care, and individual health care workers should be familiar with these practices and execute them on a routine basis.[12,13]

RULE OF THUMB

All health care workers with patient contact should undergo immunization for hepatitis B and varicella (if not immune), pertussis booster, and annual influenza vaccination.

Eliminating the Source of Pathogens

It is impossible to eliminate all pathogens from any working environment. Nonetheless, standard infection control procedures always include efforts to eliminate pathogens, and recommended practices for cleaning and disinfecting noncritical surfaces in patient care areas should be followed. Infection control procedures designed to remove environmental pathogens fall into two major categories: *general sanitation measures* and *specialized equipment processing*.

If the environment is dirty, all other infection control efforts are futile. General sanitation measures help to keep the overall environment clean. General sanitation aims to reduce the number of pathogens to a safe level. This reduction is achieved through sanitary laundry management, food preparation, and housekeeping. Environmental control of the air (using specialized ventilation systems) and water complements these efforts.

The goal of specialized equipment processing is to decontaminate equipment capable of spreading infection. Equipment processing involves cleaning, disinfection, and sterilization (when necessary). Methods that kill bacteria are **bactericidal,** whereas methods and techniques that inhibit the growth of bacteria are **bacteriostatic.** Methods that destroy spores are **sporicidal,** and methods that destroy viruses are **virucidal.**

Interrupting Transmission

General sanitation measures and equipment processing have limits. To prevent the spread of infections between patients and to keep themselves healthy, health care personnel also must take measures to stop infection. There are two tiers of HICPAC and Centers for Disease Control and Prevention (CDC) transmission precautions: standard precautions and transmission-based precautions.[6]

Standard Precautions

Standard precautions are intended to be applied to the care of all patients in all health care settings all the time. This is the primary strategy for the prevention of health care–associated transmission of infections among patients and health care personnel. From a health care worker protection perspective, application of standard precautions on a routine basis is recognition that all blood, body fluids, secretions, and excretions with the exception of sweat and urine may contain transmissible infectious agents. To mitigate against this risk, a health care worker should employ personal protective equipment (PPE). PPE refers to various barriers and respirators used alone or in combination to protect mucous membranes, skin, and clothing from contact with infectious agents. Gloves, gowns, masks, eye protection, and face shields should be employed depending on the anticipated exposure.

The application of standard precautions by health care personnel during patient care depends on the nature of the interaction and the extent of anticipated blood, body fluid, or pathogen contact. For some patient care situations, only gloves are required. In other cases, gloves, gowns, and face shield may be required. Box 4-3 describes standard precautions, including hand hygiene; use of gloves, masks, and eye protection; equipment handling; and patient placement.

Hand Hygiene

The importance of hand hygiene to reduce the transmission of infectious agents cannot be overemphasized and is an essential element of standard precautions.[14] Hand hygiene includes handwashing with either plain or antiseptic-containing soap and water for at least 15 seconds and the use of alcohol-based products (gels, rinses,

Box 4-3 Standard Precautions

HAND HYGIENE

Perform hand hygiene before and after patient contacts, immediately after removing gloves, and when otherwise indicated to avoid cross contamination.

Perform hand hygiene after touching blood, body fluids, secretions, excretions, and contaminated items, even if wearing gloves.

Perform hand hygiene between tasks and procedures on the same patient if cross contamination of different body sites is possible (e.g., tracheostomy care following assistance with a bedpan).

Use an approved alcohol-based product for routine hand hygiene. If hands are visibly soiled, use soap and water.

GLOVES

Perform hand hygiene before and after removing gloves.

Wear clean gloves when touching blood, body fluids, secretions, excretions, and contaminated items.

Don clean gloves just before touching mucous membranes and nonintact skin.

Change gloves between tasks and procedures on the same patient after contact with infectious material.

Remove gloves promptly after use, before touching noncontaminated items and environmental surfaces, and before going to another patient.

MASKS, EYE PROTECTION, FACE SHIELDS

Wear a mask and eye protection or a face shield to protect mucous membranes of the eyes, nose, and mouth during procedures and patient care activities that are likely to generate splashes or sprays of blood, body fluids, secretions, and excretions.

GOWNS

Wear a clean gown to protect skin and to prevent soiling of clothing during procedures and patient care activities that are likely to generate splashes or sprays of blood, body fluids, secretions, or excretions.

Remove a soiled gown as promptly as possible and perform hand hygiene to avoid transfer of microorganisms to other patients or environments.

PATIENT CARE EQUIPMENT

Handle used patient care equipment soiled with blood, body fluids, secretions, and excretions in a manner that prevents skin and mucous membrane exposures, contamination of clothing, and transfer of microorganisms to other patients and environments.

Do not use reusable equipment to care for another patient unless it has been cleaned and reprocessed appropriately.

Discard single-use items properly.

OCCUPATIONAL HEALTH AND BLOOD-BORNE PATHOGENS

Exercise extreme caution when handling needles, scalpels, and other sharp instruments or devices; when cleaning used instruments; and when disposing of used needles.

Never recap used needles, handle them using both hands, or point toward any part of the body.

Do not remove used needles from disposable syringes by hand, and do not bend, break, or otherwise manipulate used needles by hand.

Place used disposable syringes and needles, scalpel blades, and other sharp items in appropriate puncture-resistant containers; place reusable syringes and needles in a puncture-resistant container for transport to the reprocessing area.

Use mouthpieces, resuscitation bags, or other ventilation devices as an alternative to mouth-to-mouth resuscitation methods in areas where the need for resuscitation is predictable.

PATIENT PLACEMENT

Place patients who contaminate the environment or who do not (or cannot be expected to) assist in maintaining appropriate hygiene or environmental control in a private room.

If a private room is unavailable, consult with infection control specialists regarding patient placement.

and foams) containing an emollient that does not require the use of water. In the absence of visible soiling of hands, approved alcohol-based products are preferred over antimicrobial or plain soap and water because of their superior microbicidal activity, reduced drying of skin, and convenience. The quality of performing hand hygiene can be affected by the type and length of fingernails and by wearing jewelry. Artificial fingernails and extenders are discouraged because of their association with infections.[14] Figure 4-2 illustrates the proper technique for handwashing.

Gloves

Gloves protect both patients and health care workers from exposure to pathogens that may be carried on the hands of health care workers. Gloves protect caregivers from contamination when contacting blood, body fluids, secretions, excretions, mucous membranes, and nonintact skin of patients and when handling or touching visibly or potentially contaminated patient care equipment and environmental surfaces.[14]

Caregivers should wear sterile gloves whenever performing invasive procedures. A single pair of nonsterile disposable gloves (e.g., latex, vinyl, nitrile) may be used for routine patient care. Gloves should be changed, regardless of use, between each patient contact and after any direct contact with infectious material, even if in the middle of a procedure. After removing the gloves, caregivers must always wash their hands. Gloves may have small, invisible defects or may be torn during use. The hands can be contaminated during removal of the gloves. For these reasons, the wearing of gloves should never be used as a substitute for handwashing.

Mouth, Nose, Eye, and Face Protection

Face protection is an important component of standard precautions because the mucous membranes of the eyes, nose, and mouth are particularly vulnerable to some types of pathogens. Masks protect mucosal surfaces against splashes or sprays but should not be confused with particulate respirators that are recommended for protection from small particles (as described subsequently for airborne isolation [AI]). The wearing of masks, eye protection, and face shields in specified circumstances when exposures are likely to occur (e.g., bronchoscopy suite) is mandated by the OSHA Blood-borne Pathogen Standard.

Respiratory Protection

Respiratory protection (use of NIOSH-approved N-95 or higher level respirator) is intended for diseases (e.g., *M. tuberculosis,* SARS, smallpox) that could be transmitted through the airborne route.[6] The term *respiratory protection*

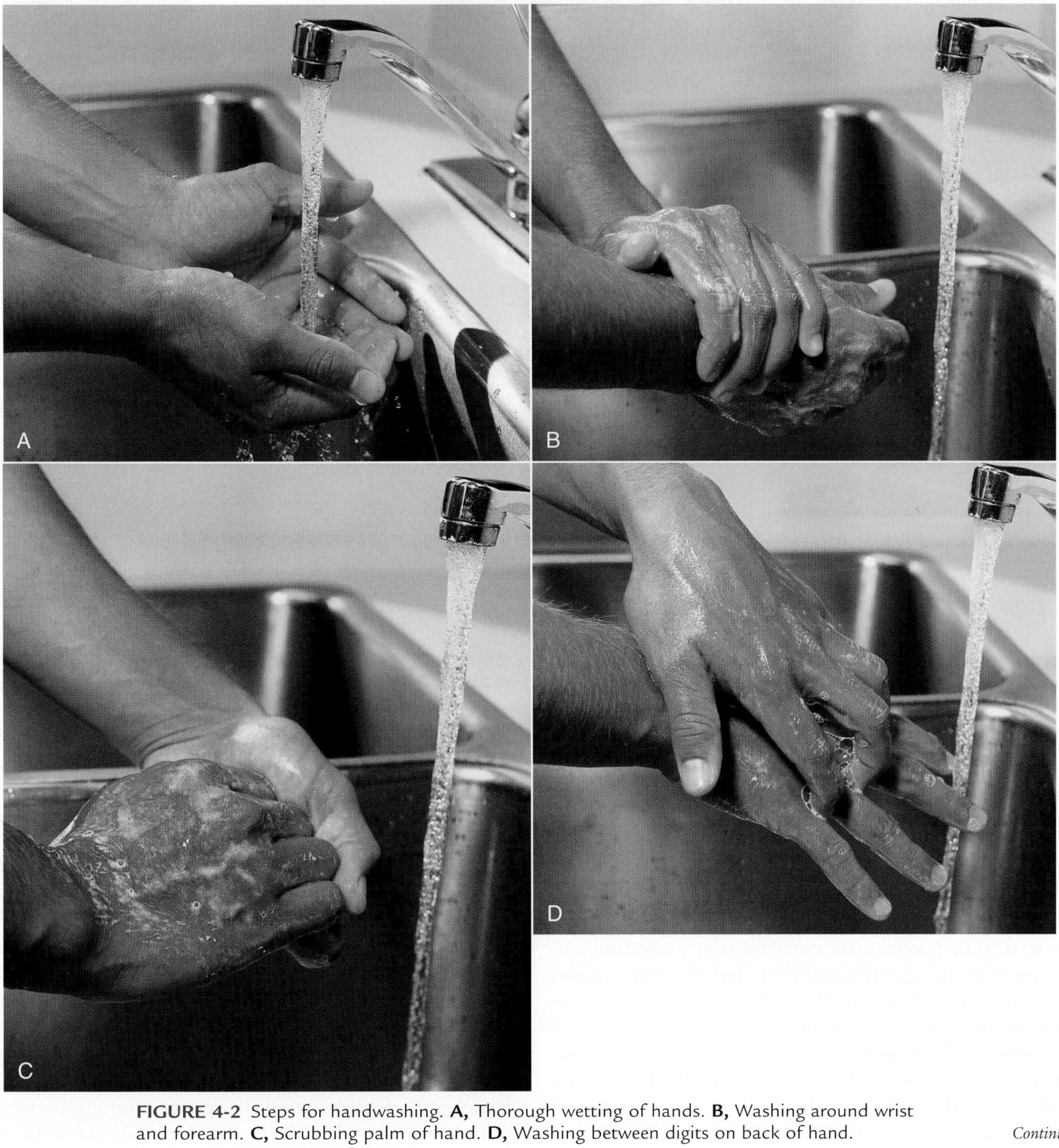

FIGURE 4-2 Steps for handwashing. **A,** Thorough wetting of hands. **B,** Washing around wrist and forearm. **C,** Scrubbing palm of hand. **D,** Washing between digits on back of hand.

Continued

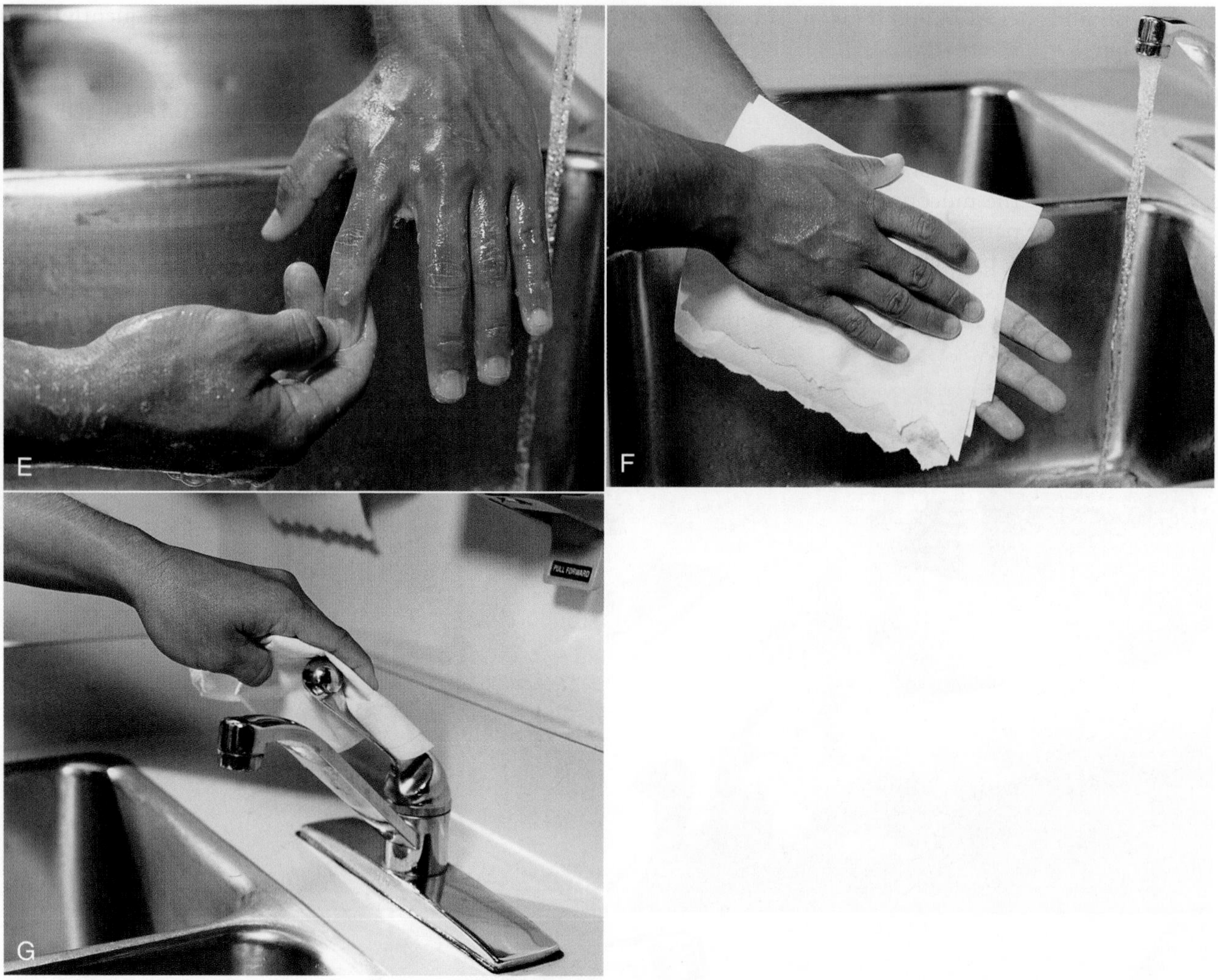

FIGURE 4-2, cont'd **E,** Washing around the cuticle. **F,** Drying hands with clean towel. **G,** Using towel to turn off faucet.

has a regulatory context that includes components of a program required by OSHA to protect workers: (1) medical clearance to wear a respirator, (2) provision and use of appropriate NIOSH-approved fit-tested respirators, and (3) education in respirator use. Information on types of respirators can be found at www.cdc.gov/niosh/npptl/respirators/respsars.html.

Gowns, Aprons, and Protective Apparel

Isolation gowns and other apparel (aprons, leg coverings, boots, or shoe covers) also provide barrier protection and can prevent the contamination of clothing and exposed body areas from blood and body fluid contact and transmissible pathogens (e.g., respiratory syncytial virus and *Clostridium difficile*). Selection of protective apparel is dictated by the nature of the interaction of the health care worker with the patient, including anticipated degree of body contact with infectious material.[6] In most instances, gowns are worn only if contact with blood and body fluid is likely. Clinical coats and jackets worn over clothing are not considered protective apparel. Isolation gowns should always be donned with gloves and other protective equipment as indicated. As with gloves and masks, a gown should be worn only once and then discarded. In most situations, aseptically clean, freshly laundered, or disposable gowns are satisfactory.

The emergence of SARS and the ongoing concerns for pandemic infection have led to a strategy of preventing transmission of respiratory infections at the first point of contact within a health care setting (e.g., physician's office) termed **respiratory hygiene/cough etiquette** that is intended to be incorporated into infection control practices as one component of standard precautions.[6] The elements of respiratory hygiene/cough etiquette include (1) education of health care personnel, patients, and visitors; (2) posted signs in language appropriate to the population served with instructions for patients and accompanying family members or friends; (3) source control measures (covering the mouth and nose with a tissue when coughing or placing a surgical mask on a coughing person when possible); (4) hand hygiene after contact with respiratory secretions; and (5) spatial separation (≥3 feet from persons with respiratory infections in common waiting areas).

Transmission-Based Precautions

Transmission-based precautions are for patients who are known or suspected to be infected with pathogens that require additional control measures to prevent transmission. There are three categories of transmission-based precautions: contact precautions, droplet precautions, and airborne infection isolation. Whether used singularly or in combination, these precautions are always used in addition to standard precautions.[6]

Contact precautions are intended to reduce the risk of transmission by direct or indirect contact with the patient or the patient's environment. Contact precautions intend for spatial separation of infected or colonized patients (≥3 feet between beds), and health care personnel and visitors wear gowns and gloves for all interactions that may involve contact with the patient or the patient's environment. Contact precautions are most commonly employed to decrease the spread of multidrug-resistant organisms such as *C. difficile*. Contact precautions are described in Box 4-4.

MINI CLINI

Isolation Methods

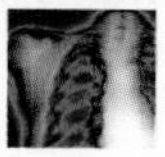

PROBLEM: A serious influenza outbreak occurs in a local long-term care facility. You are called to the emergency department because four of the sickest patients are being admitted together to your hospital for treatment. Currently, no private rooms are available for these patients. Outline the key isolation methods you would apply to help prevent the spread of influenza in your institution.

DISCUSSION: Influenza spreads via the droplet route. Both standard and droplet precautions must be applied for these patients. When transporting these patients out of the emergency department, you must be sure that they wear surgical masks. Because private rooms are unavailable, these patients need to be cohorted. If this is not feasible, the patients must be separated from other patients by at least 3 feet. Special air handling and ventilation are unnecessary, and the door may remain open. In addition to following standard precautions, all caregivers and visitors should wear surgical masks when within 3 feet of these patients (or entering the room). All remaining patients at the long-term care facility should be immunized with the flu vaccine (if not already) and be given antiviral prophylaxis.

Droplet precautions are used to prevent a form of contact transmission that occurs when droplets are propelled short distances (≤3 feet through the air). Droplets are often generated with coughing, sneezing, suctioning, bronchoscopy, and cough induction. Health care personnel and visitors should don a mask during all interactions that may involve contact with such patients. Droplet precautions are employed for patients with presumed or confirmed infection with organisms known to be transmitted by respiratory droplets such as influenza. Droplet precautions are described in Box 4-5. Precautions for use when performing cough-inducing and aerosol-producing procedures are described in Box 4-6.

Airborne Infection Isolation

AI refers to isolation techniques intended to reduce the risk of selected infectious agents transmitted by "small droplets" of aerosol particles (e.g., *M. tuberculosis*).[6] Persons

Box 4-4 Contact Precautions (Used *in Addition to* Standard Precautions)

- Place the patient in a private room; if a private room is unavailable, cohorting is acceptable
- Perform hand hygiene and don gown and gloves to enter room whether or not direct patient contact is anticipated. Wear clean gloves when entering the room
- Remove gown and gloves before leaving the patient's environment and perform hand hygiene
- After glove removal and handwashing, ensure that hands do not touch potentially contaminated environmental surfaces or items in the patient's room
- Limit transport of the patient from the room to essential purposes only
- When possible, dedicate the use of noncritical patient care equipment to a single patient or patient cohort
- If use of common equipment or items cannot be avoided, ensure that it is adequately cleaned and disinfected before use on another patient

Box 4-5 Droplet Precautions (Used *in Addition to* Standard Precautions)

- Place the patient in a private room; if a private room is unavailable, cohorting is acceptable
- Special air handling and ventilation are unnecessary, and the door may remain open

MASK

- Perform hand hygiene and put on a surgical mask before entering the room
- Remove mask before exiting the room, and perform hand hygiene
- Limit movement and transport of the patient from the room to essential purposes only
- If transport or movement is necessary, minimize droplet transmission by having the patient wear a surgical mask

Box 4-6 Guidelines for Cough-Inducing and Aerosol-Generating Procedures

Cough-inducing procedures include endotracheal intubation and suctioning, diagnostic sputum induction, aerosol treatments (e.g., pentamidine therapy), and bronchoscopy.

Cough-inducing procedures should not be performed on patients who may have infectious tuberculosis, unless the procedures are essential and can be performed with appropriate precautions.

All cough-inducing procedures performed on patients who may have infectious tuberculosis should be performed using booths or special enclosures; if this is not feasible, a room that meets the ventilation requirements for AI can be used.

After completion of cough-inducing procedures, patients who may have infectious tuberculosis should remain in their isolation rooms or enclosures until coughing subsides. They should be required to cover their mouths and noses with tissues when coughing.

Before the enclosure or room is used for another patient, enough time should be allowed to pass for at least 99% of airborne contaminants to be removed (this time varies according to the efficiency of the ventilation or filtration system).

Box 4-7 Airborne Precautions (Used *in Addition to* Standard Precautions)

- Place the patient in a private negative pressure room that has 6 to 12 air changes per hour and either safe external air discharge or HEPA filtration of recirculated air
- Keep the room door closed and the patient in the room
- If a private room is unavailable, cohorting is acceptable
- Perform hand hygiene and don respiratory protection when entering the room of a patient with known or suspected infectious pulmonary tuberculosis
- Remove respiratory protection and perform hand hygiene after leaving the room
- Susceptible persons should not enter the room of patients known or suspected to have measles (rubeola) or varicella (chickenpox) if other immune caregivers are available; individuals who are immune to measles or varicella need not wear respiratory protection
- Limit transport of the patient from the room to essential purposes only
- If transport or movement is necessary, minimize patient dispersal of droplet nuclei by having the patient wear a surgical mask

who enter an AI room must wear respiratory protection (an NIOSH-approved N-95 or higher respirator). Patients should be placed in a single-patient AI room that is equipped with special air handling and ventilation capacity that meets the American Institute of Architects/Facility Guidelines Institute standards (monitored negative pressure relative to surrounding area, two air exchanges per hour, and air exhausted directly to the outside or recirculated through high-efficiency particulate air/aerosol [HEPA] filtration). In settings where AI cannot be implemented because of limited resources, one should implement physical separation, mask patients, and provide respiratory protection for health care personnel to reduce the likelihood of airborne transmission. Box 4-7 describes airborne precautions that should be used in addition to standard precautions.

Protective Environment

A specialized engineering approach to protect highly immunocompromised patients is a protective environment. A protective environment is used for patients with allogeneic hematologic stem cell transplants to minimize fungal spore counts in the air.[15] The rationale for such controls has been studies showing outbreaks of aspergillosis associated with construction. Air quality for patients with hematologic stem cell transplants is improved through a combination of environmental controls that include (1) HEPA filtration of incoming air, (2) directed room airflow, (3) positive room air pressure relative to the corridor, (4) well-sealed rooms to prevent infiltration of outside air, (5) ventilation to provide 12 or more air changes per hour, (6) strategies to reduce dust, and (7) prohibition of dried and fresh flowers and potted plants in rooms.

Patient Placement

It is increasingly thought that single-occupancy rooms increase patient safety; reduce infection, injuries, falls, and medical errors; and reduce sources of environmental stress (e.g., noise). However, most facilities are not single occupancy only, and patient placement in private rooms is prioritized for patients who have conditions that may result in the transmission of infections to other patients or who are at increased risk for acquisition of HAIs.

Single-patient rooms are always indicated for patients on AI and in a protective environment. Single-patient rooms are preferred for patients who require contact precautions (e.g., *C. difficile*) or droplet precautions (e.g., influenza).

Cohorting is a practice of grouping patients with the same infection (or colonized with the same organism) together to confine care geographically and prevent transmission to other patients. Cohorting based on the presenting clinical syndrome is commonly used in pediatric hospitals during respiratory syncytial virus/influenza season. Cohorting health care workers to care only for patients infected or colonized with a particular transmissible pathogen may also limit transmission to uninfected patients.

Transport of Infected Patients

By limiting the transport of patients with contagious disease, the risk of cross infection can be reduced. However, infected patients sometimes do need to be transported, and when that occurs, the patient needs to wear appropriate barrier protection (mask, gown, impervious dressings) consistent with the route and risk for transmission.[6] Health care personnel receiving the patient need to be notified of the patient's impending arrival and what infection control measures are required.

RULE OF THUMB

Apply standard precautions when caring for all patients.

1. Wash your hands after touching blood, body fluids, or contaminated items (even if wearing gloves).
2. Wear fresh, clean gloves for all tasks and procedures involving potential contact with blood, body fluids, or contaminated items.
3. Exercise extreme caution when handling "sharps."
4. Handle soiled equipment in a manner that prevents skin and mucous membrane exposures, contamination of clothing, and transfer of microorganisms to other patients and environments.[6]

MINI CLINI

Spread of Infection

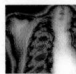

PROBLEM: You work in the neonatal intensive care unit (NICU) of a large urban hospital. Over the last 2 days, many infants in the unit have developed serious *Staphylococcus aureus* infections. Identify the most likely source and route of transmission and suggest ways to prevent spread of this serious infection.

DISCUSSION: In hospitals, *S. aureus* commonly colonizes the skin of both health care professionals and visitors. Neonates are also very susceptible hosts because of their poor immunity. *Staphylococcus* infections spread mainly via direct contact transmission (see Table 4-1). To help prevent the spread of this infection to the newborn infants, you should try to disrupt the transmission route. Meticulous attention to hand hygiene and use of gloves would help. In addition, you could isolate the infected neonates from uninfected infants (cohorting) and begin swabbing the umbilicus and nares of all infants in the NICU and all new admissions to identify who may be colonized with *S. aureus*.

DISINFECTION AND STERILIZATION

Medical instruments are used in tens of millions of procedures in the United States every year. When properly performed, cleaning, disinfection, and sterilization procedures can reduce the risk of infection associated with the use of invasive and noninvasive medical instruments. Although a detailed review of disinfection and sterilization is beyond the scope of this chapter, overall principles are discussed, particularly as they pertain to the use of bronchoscopes. The interested reader is referred to detailed guidance available from the CDC.[16] Table 4-2 lists definitions of the steps involved in equipment reprocessing.

TABLE 4-2

Equipment Processing Definitions

Term	Definition
Cleaning	Removal of all foreign material (e.g., soil, organic material) from objects
Disinfection (general term)	Inactivation of most pathogenic organisms, excluding spores
Disinfection, low-level	Inactivation of most bacteria, some viruses, and fungi, without destruction of resistant microorganisms such as *Mycobacterium tuberculosis* or bacterial spores
Disinfection, intermediate-level	Inactivation of all vegetative bacteria, most viruses, most fungi, and *M. tuberculosis,* without destruction of bacterial spores
Disinfection, high-level	Inactivation of all microorganisms *except* bacterial spores (with sufficient exposure times, spores may also be destroyed)
Sterilization	Complete destruction of all forms of microbial life

Bronchoscopes routinely become contaminated with high levels of organisms during a procedure because of the body cavities in which they are used. The benefits of these medical devices are numerous; however, proper reprocessing is crucial because numerous outbreaks and pseudooutbreaks owing to improper procedures have been described. Individuals responsible for bronchoscope reprocessing should receive initial and annual training, and their competency should be ensured. The five key components to bronchoscope reprocessing are cleaning, disinfecting, rinsing, drying, and storage (Box 4-8).[16] Automated bronchoscope reprocessors (ABRs) offer many advantages over manual disinfection because they automate several steps. Regardless of whether disinfection is done manually or with an ABR, personnel responsible for this task need to ensure reprocessing is done per device manufacturer and reprocessor guidelines with products approved by the U.S. Food and Drug Administration (FDA).

Spaulding Approach to Disinfection and Sterilization of Patient Care Equipment

In 1968, Spaulding published his approach to disinfection and sterilization, which was based on the degree of risk of infection involved in the use of the item in patient care.[17] The three categories he described were critical, semicritical, and noncritical (Table 4-3). *Critical* items are categorized based on the high risk of infection if such an item is contaminated with pathogens, including bacterial spores (e.g., items that enter sterile tissue or the vascular system). Critical devices enter normally sterile tissues. Most of these items should be purchased sterile or be sterilized, by steam sterilization if possible. *Semicritical* items come into contact with mucous membranes or nonintact skin; this includes most respiratory equipment. These items should be free of all microorganisms before use (bacterial spores may be present). Semicritical items require at least high-level disinfection using chemical disinfectants. *Noncritical* items come into contact with intact skin (an effective barrier to most microbes) but not mucous membranes. Most noncritical reusable devices may be decontaminated where they are used (e.g., bedpans, patient bed rails).

Box 4-8 Key Components of Bronchoscope Sterilization or Disinfection

Clean: Mechanically clean external surfaces, including brushing internal channels and flushing each internal channel with water and a detergent or enzymatic cleaner

1. *Disinfect:* Immerse bronchoscope in high-level disinfectant and perfuse disinfectant into the suction/biopsy channel and air/water channel and expose for at least 20 minutes (or FDA-cleared exposure time)
2. *Rinse:* The bronchoscope and all channels should be rinsed with sterile water, filtered water, or tap water
3. *Dry:* Rinse insertion tube and inner channels with alcohol, and dry with forced air after disinfection and before storage
4. *Store:* The bronchoscope should be stored in a way that prevents recontamination (e.g., hung vertically in an enclosed cabinet, the bronchoscope should not touch any surface of the cabinet)

Data from Rutala WA, Weber DJ and the Healthcare Infection Control Practices Advisory Committee (HICPAC), Centers for Disease Control and Prevention: Guidelines for sterilization and disinfection in healthcare facilities, Atlanta, GA, 2008, www.edu.gov./hicpac/.pdf/guidelines.

Cleaning

Medical equipment must be cleaned and maintained according to the manufacturer's instructions. Noncritical items, such as commodes, intravenous pumps, and ventilator surfaces, must be thoroughly cleaned and disinfected before use with another patient. Cleaning is the first step in all equipment processing. Cleaning involves removing dirt and organic material from equipment, usually by washing (see Table 4-3).[16] Failure to clean equipment properly can render all subsequent processing efforts ineffective. Cleaning should occur in a designated facility with separate dirty and clean areas. Before being cleaned, the equipment should be disassembled and examined for worn parts. Complete disassembly helps ensure good exposure to the cleaning agent. After disassembly, the parts should be placed in a clean basin filled with hot water and soap, detergent, or enzymatic cleaners.

Because water alone cannot dissolve organic matter, soaps or detergents should be used to clean equipment. Soaps act by reducing surface tension and forming an emulsion with organic matter. Soaps have little bactericidal activity and work poorly in hard water. A *detergent* refers to a substance (usually a chemical agent but

TABLE 4-3

Processing of Medical Equipment According to Infection Risk Categories

Category	Description	Examples	Processing
Critical	Devices introduced into the bloodstream or other parts of the body	Surgical devices Intravascular catheters Implants Heart-lung bypass components Dialysis components Bronchoscope forceps/brushes	Sterilization
Semicritical	Devices that directly or indirectly contact mucous membranes	Bronchoscopes Oral, nasal, and tracheal airways Ventilator circuits/humidifiers PFT mouthpieces and tubing Nebulizers and their reservoirs Resuscitation bags Laryngoscope blades/stylets Pressure, gas, or temperature probes	High-level disinfection
Noncritical	Devices that touch only intact skin or do not contact patient	Face masks Blood pressure cuffs Ventilators	Detergent washing Low- to intermediate-level disinfection

Modified from Chatburn RL, Kallstrom TJ, Bajasouzian S: A comparison of acetic acid with a quartinary ammonium compound for disinfection of hand-held nebulizers. Resp Care 34:98-109, 1989.
PFT, Pulmonary function testing.

sometimes a physical one) applied to inanimate objects that destroys disease-causing pathogens but not spores. Detergents work in hard water but can be inactivated by proteins. Most detergents are weakly bactericidal but against gram-positive bacteria only. Some commercial products combine a germicide with a detergent, providing the dual action of cleaning and disinfection. Although careful cleaning removes most pathogens from the equipment, it cannot eliminate the risk of infection. For this reason, most equipment must undergo either disinfection or sterilization.

Disinfection

Disinfection describes a process that destroys the vegetative form of all pathogenic organisms on an inanimate object except bacterial spores. By definition, *disinfection* differs from *sterilization* by its lack of sporicidal activity.[16] However, a few disinfectants kill spores with prolonged exposure times (hours) and are called *chemical sterilants*. Disinfection can involve either physical or chemical methods. The most common physical method of disinfection is *pasteurization*. Many chemical methods are used to disinfect respiratory care equipment.

Chemical Disinfection

Chemical disinfection involves the application of chemical solutions to contaminated surfaces or equipment. For disinfection, the equipment is immersed in the solution. After a set "contact" time, the equipment is removed, rinsed in sterile water (to remove toxic residues), and dried. Equipment must be handled aseptically, with sterile gloves and towels, to prevent recontamination during subsequent reassembly and packaging. The FDA provides a list of cleared chemical disinfectants that can be used for high-level disinfection of medical devices. Cleared agents include agents that are 2.4% or greater glutaraldehyde, 0.55% ortho-phthaladehyde (OPA), 0.95% glutaraldehyde with 1.64% phenolphenate, 7.35% hydrogen peroxide with 0.23% peracetic acid, 1.0% hydrogen peroxide with 0.08% peracetic acid, and 7.5% hydrogen peroxide.[16] The choice of agent is dictated by device and in many cases recommendations of the ABR manufacturer.

The U.S. Environmental Protection Agency groups disinfectants based on whether the product label claims "limited," "general," or "hospital" disinfection.[16] Numerous disinfectants are used alone or in combination in the health care setting, including alcohol, chlorine and chlorine products, glutaraldehyde, iodophors, phenolics, quaternary ammonium compounds, peracetic acid, and hydrogen peroxide. In most cases, a given product is designed for a specific purpose and should be used in a certain manner; the label should be read carefully. Table 4-4, excerpted from the CDC guideline for sterilization and disinfection, summarizes common chemical disinfectants and their activity against various pathogens.[16] Health care facilities should select disinfectant agents that best meet their overall needs. Recommendations for the amount, dilution, and contact time of disinfectants should be followed. A comprehensive overview of disinfectants in the hospital can be found in the updated CDC guidelines for disinfection and sterilization in health care facilities.[16]

MINI CLINI

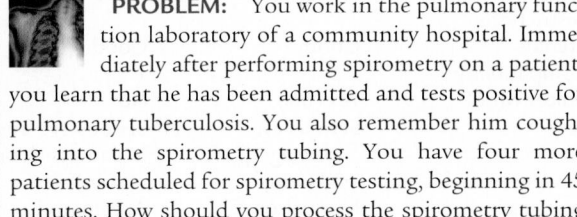

Selection of a Disinfectant

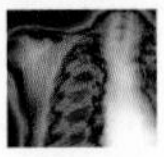

PROBLEM: You work in the pulmonary function laboratory of a community hospital. Immediately after performing spirometry on a patient, you learn that he has been admitted and tests positive for pulmonary tuberculosis. You also remember him coughing into the spirometry tubing. You have four more patients scheduled for spirometry testing, beginning in 45 minutes. How should you process the spirometry tubing to prevent transmission of the tuberculosis?

DISCUSSION: Ideally, you would have a backup set of tubing to deal with this type of problem. If not, you need to disinfect or sterilize the tubing quickly. Because permanent spirometry tubing is made from heat-labile plastics, you cannot use steam (damage). EtO gas is an option, but aeration would take too long. Instead, you should select a broad-spectrum, quick-acting disinfectant solution that works well in the presence of organic matter and does not damage rubber or plastic. Glutaraldehyde is a good choice, with a minimum exposure time of 20 minutes. A stabilized hydrogen peroxide–based compound or a 1:50 sodium hypochlorite solution might also be considered.

Sterilization

Sterilization destroys all microorganisms on the surface of an article or in a fluid, which prevents transmission of pathogens associated with the use of that item. Both physical and chemical means can achieve sterilization. Physical methods include various forms of heat (steam) and ionizing radiation. Chemical methods of sterilization include low-temperature sterilization technologies such as ethylene oxide (EtO) gas. Table 4-5, excerpted from the CDC guideline for sterilization and disinfection, compares and contrasts the major methods of sterilization.[16]

Medical devices that have contact with sterile body tissues or fluids are crucial items and should be sterile before use. If the object is heat resistant, steam sterilization is usually recommended. However, increases in the use of medical devices that are heat and moisture sensitive have necessitated the development of low-temperature sterilization technology. These include, but are not limited to, EtO, hydrogen peroxide gas plasma, and peracetic acid. A review of the commonly used sterilization technologies with a summary of advantages and disadvantages can be found

TABLE 4-4

Comparison of the Characteristics of Selected Chemicals Used as High-Level Disinfectants or Chemical Sterilants

	HP (7.5%)	PA (0.2%)	Glut (≥2.0%)	OPA (0.55%)	HP/PA (7.35%/0.23%)
HLD claim	30 min at 20° C	NA	20-90 min at 20°-25° C	12 min at 20° C, 5 min at 25° C in AER	15 min at 20° C
Sterilization claim	6 hr at 20° C	12 min at 50°-56° C	10 hr at 20°-25° C	None	3 hr at 20° C
Activation	No	No	Yes (alkaline glut)	No	No
Reuse life[a]	21 days	Single use	14-30 days	14 days	14 days
Shelf life stability[b]	2 yr	6 mo	2 yr	2 yr	2 yr
Disposable restrictions	None	None	Local[c]	Local[c]	None
Materials compatibility	Good	Good	Excellent	Excellent	No data
Monitor MEC[d]	Yes (6%)	No	Yes (≥1.5%)	Yes (0.3% OPA)	No
Safety	Serious eye damage (safety glasses)	Serious eye and skin damage (conc soln)[e]	Respiratory	Eye irritant, stains skin	Eye damage
Processing	Manual or automated	Automated	Manual or automated	Manual or automated	Manual
Organic material resistance	Yes	Yes	Yes	Yes	Yes
OSHA exposure limit	1 ppm TWA	None	None[f]	None	HP-1 ppm TWA
Cost profile (per cycle)[g]	+ (manual), ++ (automated)	++++ (automated)	+ (manual), ++ (automated)	++ (manual)	++ (manual)

Data from Rutala WA, Weber DJ and the Healthcare Infection Control Practices Advisory Committee (HICPAC), Centers for Disease Control and Prevention: Guidelines for sterilization and disinfection in healthcare facilities, Atlanta, GA, 2008, www.edu.gov./hicpac/.pdf/guidelines.

HLD, High level-disinfectant; *HP,* hydrogen peroxide; *NA,* not applicable; *OPA,* ortho-phthalaldehyde (FDA cleared as a high-level disinfectant, included for comparison with other chemical agents used for high-level disinfection); *PA,* peracetic acid; glut, glutaraldehyde; *PA/HP,* peracetic acid and hydrogen peroxide; *TWA,* time-weighted average for a conventional 8-hour workday.

[a]Number of days a product can be reused as determined by reuse protocol.

[b]Time a product can remain in storage (unused).

[c]No U.S. Environmental Protection Agency regulations, but some states and local authorities have additional restrictions.

[d]Minimum effective concentration (MEC) is the lowest concentration of active ingredients at which the product is still effective.

[e]Conc soln, concentrated solution.

[f]The ceiling limit recommended by the American Conference of Governmental Industrial Hygienists is 0.05 ppm.

[g]Per cycle cost profile considers cost of the processing solution (suggested list price to health care facilities in August 2001) and assumes maximum use life (e.g., 21 days for hydrogen peroxide, 14 days for glutaraldehyde), five reprocessing cycles per day, 1-gallon basin for manual processing, and 4-gallon tank for automated processing. + = least expensive; ++++ = most expensive.

in the updated CDC guidelines for disinfection and sterilization in health care facilities.[16] Following is an overview of a few of these technologies.

Steam Sterilization

Moist heat in the form of steam under pressure is the most common, most efficient, and easiest sterilization method. Generally, the higher the temperature, the shorter is the time needed for sterilization. Autoclaving (steam sterilization) is the application of steam under pressure. Autoclaving is efficient, quick, cheap, clean, and reliable. The higher the temperature and pressure, the shorter is the time needed for sterilization. The combination most commonly used for autoclaving is 15 psi at 121° C. Equipment must be cleaned before autoclaving. Clean equipment is wrapped in muslin, linen, or paper, all of which is easily penetrated by steam. Items must be properly packed in the autoclave to ensure exposure. In addition, chamber air must be evacuated before steam is introduced. After sterilization, the packaging prevents recontamination during handling and storage.

Flash Sterilization

Flash "steam sterilization" is a modification of conventional steam sterilization in which the item is placed in an open tray or a specially designed container to allow for rapid penetration of steam.[16] It is considered an acceptable practice for processing cleaned patient care items that cannot be packaged, sterilized, and stored before use. Its use only for reasons of convenience (e.g., to save time) should be discouraged.

Low-Temperature Sterilization Technologies

Low-temperature (<60° C) sterilants are needed for sterilizing temperature-sensitive and moisture-sensitive medical devices and equipment. Low-temperature sterilant technology includes EtO, hydrochlorofluorocarbon, hydrogen peroxide gas plasma, and peracetic acid.[16] We review the most commonly used process—EtO.

EtO is a colorless, toxic gas and potent sterilizing agent. Because it is active at ambient temperatures and is harmless to rubber and plastics, EtO is a good sterilant for

TABLE 4-5

Advantages and Disadvantages of Accepted Methods for Equipment Sterilization

Sterilization Method	Advantages	Disadvantages
Steam	Nontoxic to patient, staff, environment Cycle easy to control and monitor Rapidly microbial Least affected by organic/inorganic soils among sterilization processes listed Rapid cycle time Penetrates medical packing, device lumens	Deleterious for heat-sensitive instruments Microsurgical instruments damaged by repeated exposure May leave instruments wet, causing them to rust Potential for burns
Hydrogen peroxide gas plasma	Safe for the environment Leaves no toxic residuals Cycle time is 28-75 min (varies with model type) and no aeration necessary Used for heat- and moisture-sensitive items because process temperature <50° C Simple to operate, install (208 V outlet), and monitor Compatible with most medical devices Requires electrical outlet only	Cellulose (paper), linens, and liquids cannot be processed Sterilization chamber size from 1.8-9.4 ft^3 total volume (varies with model type) Some endoscopes or medical devices with long or narrow lumens cannot be processed at this time in the United States (see manufacturer's recommendations for internal diameter and length restrictions) Requires synthetic packaging (polypropylene wraps, polyolefin pouches) and special container tray Hydrogen peroxide may be toxic at levels >1 ppm TWA
100% EtO	Penetrates packaging materials, device lumens Single-dose cartridge and negative pressure chamber minimizes potential for gas leak and EtO exposure Simple to operate and monitor Compatible with most medical materials	Requires aeration time to remove EtO residue Sterilization chamber size 4.0-7.9 ft^3 total volume (varies with model type) EtO is toxic, a carcinogen, and flammable EtO emission regulation by states but catalytic cell removes 99.9% of EtO and converts it to CO_2 and H_2O EtO cartridges should be stored in flammable liquid storage cabinet Lengthy cycle/aeration time
EtO mixtures: 8.6% EtO/91.4% HCFC; 10% EtO/90% HCFC; 8.5% EtO/91.5% CO_2	Penetrates medical packaging and many plastics Compatible with most medical materials Cycle easy to control and monitor	Some states (e.g., California, New York, Michigan) require EtO emission reduction of 90%-99.9% CFC (inert gas that eliminates explosive hazard) banned in 1995 Potential hazards to staff and patients Lengthy cycle/alteration time EtO is toxic, a carcinogen, and flammable
Peracetic acid	Rapid cycle time (30-45 min) Low temperature (50°-55° C) liquid immersion sterilization Environmentally friendly by-products Sterilant flows through endoscope, which facilitates salt, protein, and microbe removal	Point-of-use system, no sterile storage Biologic indicator may be unsuitable for routine monitoring Used for immersible instruments only Some material incompatibility (e.g., aluminum anodized coating becomes dull) One scope or a small number of instruments processed in a cycle Potential for serious eye and skin damage (concentrated solution) with contact

Data from Rutala WA, Weber DJ and the Healthcare Infection Control Practices Advisory Committee (HICPAC), Centers for Disease Control and Prevention: Guidelines for sterilization and disinfection in healthcare facilities, Atlanta, GA, 2008, www.edu.gov./hicpac/.pdf/guidelines.
CFC, Chlorofluorocarbon; *HCFC,* hydrochlorofluorocarbon.

items that cannot be autoclaved. Similar to steam, EtO penetrates most packaging materials, permitting prewrapping. Were it not for its many hazards, EtO would be the ideal sterilant.[18] Acute exposure to EtO gas can cause airway inflammation, nausea, diarrhea, headache, dizziness, and convulsions. Chronic exposure to the gas is associated with respiratory infections, anemia, and altered behavior. Residual EtO left on processed equipment can cause tissue inflammation and hemolysis. When combined with water, EtO forms ethylene glycol, which also can irritate tissues. Other potential problems include carcinogenic, mutagenic, and teratogenic effects. EtO concentrations greater than 3% are explosive.

EtO requires special attention to general safety precautions, equipment preparation, and sterilization cycle parameters. In addition, because of its toxicity, residual

EtO must be removed from equipment after sterilization via a process called *aeration*. EtO is used to sterilize critical (and sometimes semicritical) items that cannot be steam sterilized.

EQUIPMENT HANDLING PROCEDURES

Equipment handling procedures that help prevent the spread of pathogens include maintenance of in-use equipment, processing of reusable equipment, application of one-patient-use disposables, and fluid and medication precautions.

Maintenance of In-Use Equipment

In-use respiratory care equipment that can spread pathogens includes nebulizers, ventilator circuits, bag-valve-mask devices (manual resuscitators), and suction equipment. Oxygen therapy and pulmonary function equipment are also implicated as potential sources of nosocomial infections.

Nebulizers

Small volume medication nebulizers (SVNs) can also produce bacterial aerosols. SVNs have been associated with nosocomial pneumonia, including Legionnaires' disease, resulting from either contaminated medications or contaminated tap water used to rinse the reservoir. Procedures designed to prevent nebulizers from spreading pathogens are presented in Box 4-9.

Box 4-9 Procedures to Minimize Infection Risk With Nebulizers

LARGE VOLUME NEBULIZERS AND MIST TENTS

- Always fill nebulizers with sterile distilled water
- Fill fluid reservoirs immediately before use; do not add fluid to replenish partially filled reservoirs. If fluid is to be added, discard the remaining old fluid first
- Drain tubing condensate away from the patient, and discard as contaminated waste; do not allow condensate to drain back into reservoir
- Sterilize or high-level disinfect large volume nebulizers between patients and after every 24 hours of use on the same patient
- Use mist tent nebulizer and reservoirs that have undergone sterilization or high-level disinfection, and replace them between patients
- Do not use large volume room air humidifiers that create aerosols unless they can be sterilized or subjected to high-level disinfection at least daily and filled only with sterile water

SMALL VOLUME NEBULIZERS

- Between treatments on the same patient, disinfect, rinse with sterile water, and air dry SVNs
- Between patients, replace SVNs with sterile or high-level disinfected units
- Use only sterile fluids for nebulization, and dispense these fluids aseptically
- When possible, use single-use medication vials; if using multidose vials, handle, dispense, and store them according to manufacturer's instructions and checking expiration dates

Ventilators and Ventilator Circuits

The internal workings of ventilators are uncommon sources for infection; this is partly a result of the widespread use of **high-efficiency particulate air/aerosol (HEPA) filters,** which have an efficiency rate of 99.97%, and the use of ensheathed suction catheters, which help reduce endotracheal tube contamination. An inspiratory HEPA filter (placed between the machinery and the external circuit, proximal to any humidifier) can eliminate bacteria from the driving gas and prevent retrograde contamination back into the machine. An expiratory filter using a heated thermistor to prevent condensation performs the same function and still protects the internal ventilator components. Expiratory filters also prevent pathogens from being expelled into the surroundings from the patient's expired air.

The external ventilator circuitry poses the most significant contamination risk, particularly in systems using heated humidifiers. The humidifiers themselves are rarely the problem. Bubble or wick designs produce little or no aerosol and pose minimal infection risk. In addition, heating the humidifier reduces or eliminates growth of most bacterial pathogens. However, because tap water or distilled water may harbor heat-resistant pathogens, sterile water should still be used to fill bubble-type humidifiers.

The primary problem stems from contaminated condensate in the inspiratory limb of the ventilator circuit. Most often, the source of this contamination is the patient. Spillage of contaminated condensate into the patient circuit and the patient occurs when moving the tubing or the patient, increasing the risk of autogenous infection. In addition, microorganisms in this condensate can be transmitted to other patients via the hands of the health care worker handling the fluid, if he or she is negligent. This is another reason why it is crucial for RTs to practice hand hygiene before and after contact with every ventilated patient. Contact with the patient's ventilator is considered contact with the patient's body.

One way to address this problem is by reducing or eliminating circuit condensation. This reduction or elimination is easily achieved using heated wire circuits or a *heat-and-moisture exchanger (HME)*. Evidence suggests that to prevent bacterial colonization, even if the HME remains free of secretions, the maximal duration that it may be used is 96 hours (4 days).[19]

Based on current knowledge, both the CDC and the American Association for Respiratory Care (AARC) developed guidelines addressing ventilator-associated infection control. Box 4-10 provides general procedures for minimizing nosocomial infection associated with ventilator use. Mechanical ventilation exposes the patient to the risk of VAP, and the frequency of circuit changes and the relationship to VAP have been investigated.[20,21] Current guidelines suggest that ventilator circuits should not be changed routinely for infection control purposes; however, they should be changed when visibly soiled or malfunctioning.

Bag-Mask Devices

Bag-mask devices are a source for colonizing both the airways of intubated patients and the hands of medical personnel.[22] Nondisposable bag-mask devices should be sterilized or high-level disinfected between patients. In addition, the exterior surface of any bag-mask device should be cleaned of visible debris and disinfected at least once a day.

Suction Systems

Tracheal suctioning increases the risk of infection. Proper handwashing and gloving help minimize this risk. Although much has been made of the infection control advantages of ensheathed suction systems over open

Box 4-10 Procedures to Minimize Infection Risk With Mechanical Ventilators

- Do not routinely sterilize or disinfect the internal workings of ventilators
- Do not routinely change ventilator circuit more often than every 48 to 72 hours with HMEs
- Sterilize or high-level disinfect reusable breathing circuits and humidifiers
- Periodically drain tubing condensate away from patient and discard
- Wash hands after draining tubing condensate or handling the fluid
- Do not place bacterial filters distal to humidifier reservoirs
- Use sterile water to fill bubble humidifiers
- Use sterile, distilled water to fill wick humidifiers
- Change HMEs according to manufacturer's recommendation and when you observe evidence of gross contamination or mechanical dysfunction
- Do not routinely change HME breathing circuits while in use

4-1 Care of the Ventilator Circuit and Its Relationship to Ventilator-Associated Pneumonia

AARC Clinical Practice Guideline (Excerpts)*

INTRODUCTION

A concern related to the care of a mechanically ventilated patient is the development of VAP. For many years, this concern focused on the ventilator circuit and humidifier. The circuit and humidifier have been changed on a regular basis in an attempt to decrease the VAP rate. However, as the evidence evolved, it became apparent that the origin of VAP is more likely from sites other than the ventilator circuit, and the prevailing practice has become one of changing circuits less frequently. If this practice is safe, it would offer substantial cost savings. Other issues related to the components of the circuit and VAP have also become more important recently. Humidification systems can be either active or passive. Increasingly, in-line suction is used, and this becomes part of the ventilator circuit.

QUESTIONS

A systematic review of the literature was conducted with the intention of making recommendations for change frequency of the ventilator circuit and additional components of the circuit. Specifically, the Writing Committee wrote these evidence-based clinical practice guidelines to address the following questions:

1. Do ventilator circuits need to be changed at regular intervals?
2. What is the economic impact of decreasing the frequency of ventilator circuit changes?
3. What are the issues related to circuit type?
4. Does the choice of active versus passive humidification affect ventilator circuit change frequency?
5. Do passive humidifiers need to be changed at regular intervals?
6. Do in-line suction catheters need to be changed at regular intervals?
7. Are there specific populations for which the recommendations should be altered?

RECOMMENDATIONS

Recommendation #1

Ventilator circuits should not be changed routinely for infection control purposes. The available evidence suggests no patient harm and considerable cost savings associated with extended ventilator circuit change intervals. The maximum duration of time that circuits can be used safely is unknown. (Evidence Grade A)

Continued

4-1 Care of the Ventilator Circuit and Its Relationship to Ventilator-Associated Pneumonia—cont'd

AARC Clinical Practice Guideline (Excerpts)*

Recommendation #2

Evidence is lacking related to VAP and issues of heated versus unheated circuits, type of heated humidifier, method for filling the humidifier, and technique for clearing condensate from the ventilator circuit. It is prudent to avoid excessive accumulation of condensate in the circuit. Care should be taken to avoid accidental drainage of condensate into the patient's airway and to avoid contamination of caregivers during ventilator disconnection or during disposal of condensate. Care should be taken to avoid breaking the ventilator circuit, which could contaminate the interior of the circuit. (Evidence Grade D)

Recommendation #3

Although the available evidence suggests a lower VAP rate with passive humidification than with active humidification, other issues related to the use of passive humidifiers (e.g., resistance, dead space volume, airway occlusion risk) preclude a recommendation for the general use of these devices. The decision to use a passive humidifier should not be based solely on infection control considerations. (Evidence Grade A)

Recommendation #4

Passive humidifiers do not need to be changed daily for reasons of infection control or technical performance. They can be safely used for at least 48 hours, and with some patient populations, some devices may be able to be used for up to 1 week. (Evidence Grade A)

Recommendation #5

The use of closed suction catheters should be considered part of a VAP prevention strategy. When closed suction catheters are used, they do not need to be changed daily for infection control purposes. The maximum time that closed suction catheters can be used safely is unknown. (Evidence Grade A)

Recommendation #6

Clinicians (e.g., respiratory therapists, nurses, and physicians) caring for mechanically ventilated patients should be aware of risk factors for VAP (e.g., nebulizer therapy, manual ventilation, and patient transport). (Evidence Grade B)

EVIDENCE GRADES

Grade A: Scientific evidence provided by randomized, well-designed, well-conducted, controlled trials with statistically significant results that consistently support the guideline recommendation; supported by Level 1 or 2 evidence

Grade B: Scientific evidence provided by well-designed, well-conducted observational studies with statistically significant results that consistently support the guideline recommendation; supported by Level 3 or 4 evidence

Grade C: Scientific evidence from bench studies, animal studies, and case studies; supported by Level 5 evidence

Grade D: Expert opinion provides the basis for the guideline recommendation, but scientific evidence either provided inconsistent results or was lacking

For the complete guidelines, see AARC Clinical Practice Guidelines, Care of the ventilator circuit and its relation to ventilator-associated pneumonia. Respir Care 48:569–879, 2003.

tracheal suction systems, evidence shows neither system to be clearly superior.[4] To minimize the risk of cross contamination during suctioning with an open system, a fresh, sterile single-use catheter should be used on each patient. In addition, only sterile fluid should be used to remove secretions from the catheter. Last, both the suction collection tubing and collection canister should be changed between patients except in short-term care units, where only the collection tubing needs to be changed.

Oxygen Therapy Apparatus

Oxygen therapy devices pose much less risk than other in-use equipment but are still a potential infection hazard. In-use nondisposable oxygen humidifiers have a contamination rate of 33%. Conversely, prefilled, sterile disposable humidifiers present a negligible infection risk.[23] On the basis of this knowledge, procedures that can help prevent oxygen therapy apparatus from spreading pathogens are outlined in Box 4-11.

Pulmonary Function Equipment

The inner parts of pulmonary function testing equipment are not a major source for spread of infection. However, contamination of external tubing, connectors, rebreathing valves, and mouthpieces can occur during testing. These components should be cleaned and subjected to high-level

Box 4-11 Procedures to Minimize Infection Risk With Oxygen Therapy Apparatus

- Humidifiers are not needed with flows less than 4 L/min
- When needed and whenever possible, prefilled, sterile disposable humidifiers should be used
- With reusable humidifiers, fluid reservoirs should be filled immediately before use with sterile distilled water
- Fluid must not be added to replenish partially filled reservoirs. If fluid is to be added, discard the remaining old fluid first, then clean and dry reservoir before refilling
- The tubing and oxygen delivery device should be changed between patients; prefilled, sterile, disposable humidifiers do not need to be changed between patients in high-use areas such as the recovery room
- Prefilled, disposable humidifiers can be used safely for 30 days

Box 4-12 Factors to Consider in Processing Reusable Equipment

- Infection risk (critical, semicritical, noncritical)
- Material and equipment configuration
- Available hospital disinfection resources
- Relative cost (labor and materials)

disinfection or sterilization between patients.[4] The common practice of using HEPA filters to isolate the spirometer from the patient makes sense logically but has yet to be proven either effective or necessary in preventing nosocomial infection.

Other Respiratory Care Devices

Use of other respiratory care equipment, including oxygen analyzers, the hand-held bedside respirometer, and circuit probes, has been linked with hospital outbreaks of gram-negative bacterial infections.[4] The most likely transmission route is direct patient-to-patient contact via either the device itself or the contaminated hands of caregivers. The best way to control this problem is with proper handwashing and sterilization or high-level disinfection of the devices between patients.

Processing Reusable Equipment

Improperly processed reusable equipment is another potential source for pathogens. General principles for cleaning, disinfection, and sterilization were provided previously. This section presents specific guidelines for processing reusable respiratory care equipment and a special section on bronchoscope disinfection.

Respiratory Care Equipment

Several factors must be considered in selecting a processing method for reusable respiratory care equipment (Box 4-12). When a device's risk category is known, its composition must be matched to the resources available for hospital disinfection and sterilization. In this manner, each reusable device undergoes the most effective and least costly processing approach available.

MINI CLINI

Selection of Equipment Processing Methods

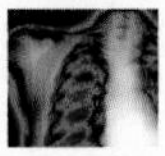

PROBLEM: A patient is discharged from the intensive care unit after extubation from mechanical ventilatory support. The following contaminated nondisposable items are returned to the respiratory care department for processing: the ventilator, the ventilator circuit and humidifier, a resuscitation bag, a mechanical (vane-type) respirometer, and a laryngoscope with blades. Outline what processing you would select for each item and why.

DISCUSSION: First, the circuit, humidifier, and resuscitation bag should be disassembled and cleaned, using a soap or detergent combined with a low-level or intermediate-level disinfectant. Because the ventilator, respirometer, and laryngoscope and blades cannot be immersed in water, they should immediately undergo surface disinfection, using 70% ethyl alcohol or the equivalent.

After cleaning and initial disinfection, you should sort the items according to risk category and heat sensitivity. No items from this patient are a critical infection risk. The ventilator circuit, humidifier, resuscitation bag, respirometer, and laryngoscope are semicritical items, whereas the ventilator itself is a noncritical item. The ventilator circuit, humidifier, and resuscitation bag are also plastic and probably heat labile. The respirometer and laryngoscope are heat stable.

When possible, semicritical items should be sterilized between patients; the heat-stable items should be autoclaved, and heat-labile items should undergo EtO sterilization. The ventilator (a noncritical item) need undergo only low-level to intermediate-level surface disinfection. The inner parts of the ventilator need not be sterilized or disinfected between patients.

HAIs associated with bronchoscopes have been most commonly reported with *M. tuberculosis,* nontuberculosis mycobacteria, and *Pseudomonas aeruginosa.*[22] The most common reasons for transmission include failure to adhere to recommended cleaning and disinfection procedures, failure of automated endoscope reprocessors, and flaws in design. Flexible endoscopes are particularly difficult to disinfect, and meticulous cleaning must precede any sterilization or high-level disinfection process.

Disposable Equipment

An important alternative to reprocessing equipment continually is the use of single-patient-use disposable devices. In the past, only oxygen therapy devices (i.e., masks, cannulas), suction apparatus (i.e., catheters, tubing), and some supplies were disposable. Today, manufacturers provide a whole range of disposable devices, including humidifiers, nebulizers, incentive spirometers, ventilator circuits, bag-valve-masks, and monitoring transducers.

Three major issues are involved in using disposable devices: *cost, quality,* and *reuse.* Cost issues boil down to straightforward dollar comparisons between purchasing and processing reusable devices versus stocking and distributing disposable devices. Good comparisons take into account direct and indirect costs (e.g., personnel, inventory, maintenance) and risk factors. Most recent findings support the cost-effectiveness of disposable devices over reusable devices in respiratory care.

Cost savings notwithstanding, many quality issues persist. Although disposable devices generally perform well, poor quality control remains a problem.[23] Respiratory care managers need to evaluate carefully disposable devices being considered for bulk purchase before actual clinical use.[24] To ensure reliability, this evaluation should include physical testing of multiple units of each model being assessed. Finally, bedside clinicians need to inspect carefully and confirm the operation of any disposable device before use.

Reusing high-cost, high-volume disposable equipment saves hospitals money. The practice of reusing devices labeled by the manufacturer for "single-use only" raises significant safety concerns and issues of negligence.[25] The CDC recommends that single-use devices be considered for reuse only if there is good evidence that reprocessing poses no threat to the patient and does not alter the function of the device.[4] Individuals responsible for reusing disposable equipment bear a significant burden of proof. Without such proof, users of reprocessed single-use devices may be transferring legal liability for the safe performance of the product from the manufacturer to themselves or their employer.[26]

Fluids and Medications Precautions

Unit dosing has decreased but has not eliminated the infection hazard associated with medications. Box 4-13 outlines several simple procedures designed to help prevent cross contamination while using fluids and medications.

Handling Contaminated Articles and Equipment

Contaminated items, whether reusable or disposable, should be enclosed in an impervious bag before removal from a patient's room. Bagging helps prevent accidental exposure of both personnel and the environment to contaminated articles. A single bag is satisfactory if (1) the bag is strong and impervious, and (2) the contaminated items can be bagged without contaminating the outer surface of the bag. Otherwise, the contaminated items should be double-bagged. Bags used for contaminated articles or waste materials should be clearly labeled or color-coded for this purpose.

After bagging, reusable patient care equipment must be returned to the applicable processing area. Contaminated reusable equipment should remain bagged until ready for decontamination or sterilization. When contaminated waste is being discarded, both OSHA procedures and any applicable local, state, or federal regulations must be followed.

Box 4-13 Fluids and Medications Precautions

Sterile fluids should always be used for tracheal suctioning and to fill nebulizers and bubble humidifiers. These fluids should be dispensed aseptically.

Sterile water should be used when rinsing equipment. If tap water must be used, either an alcohol rinse must follow or the equipment must thoroughly air dry before use.

If a large stock bottle of sterile fluid must be reused, the container must be resealed and dated after opening. Remaining fluid should be discarded within 24 hours.

When multidose medication vials are being used, they must be handled, dispensed, and stored according to manufacturer's instructions (on the label or package insert). Medication must not be used after its expiration date.

Using Needles and Syringes

Needlestick injuries are a growing area of concern among health care personnel because accidental skin puncture with a contaminated sharp can transmit blood-borne pathogens such as hepatitis C and HIV to the health care worker.[2] All health care workers should exercise extreme caution when handling any sharp instruments, including needles and syringes.

Handling Laboratory Specimens

When gathering laboratory specimens (e.g., sputum), extreme care needs to be taken to prevent contamination of the external surface of the container. If the outside of the container is contaminated, the caregiver must either disinfect it or place it in an impervious bag. To minimize the likelihood of laboratory specimens leaking during transport, they should always be placed in a sturdy container with a secure lid. When gathering a specimen from a patient on isolation precautions, the container must be placed in an appropriately labeled, impervious bag before it is removed from the room.

SURVEILLANCE FOR HOSPITAL-ACQUIRED INFECTIONS

Surveillance is an ongoing process of monitoring patients and health care personnel for acquisition of infection or colonization of pathogens, or both. It is one of the five key recommended components of an infection prevention program; the others are *investigation, prevention, control,* and *reporting.*[2] Surveillance is a tool to provide HAI data on patients to provide outcome measurements either to ensure that there is no ongoing problem or to detect problems and intervene to prevent transmission of pathogens in the health care environment.

Generally, an infection prevention committee establishes surveillance policies, and an infection control nurse or epidemiologist administers them. The surveillance program may be centralized or decentralized (to the various service departments). The following principles should be a part of any infection prevention surveillance program[2]: (1) use of standard definitions for HAIs, (2) use of microbiology-based data (when available) including resistance patterns for pathogens of significance (e.g., *Staphylococcus aureus*), (3) establishment of risk stratification for infection risk when available (e.g., ventilator days, device days), (4) monitoring of results prospectively and identifying trends that indicate unusual rates of infection or transmission within the facility, and (5) provision of feedback to stakeholders within the institution (e.g., surgical site infection rates reported back to individual surgeons). It is also common for infection prevention programs to oversee hand hygiene and standard precautions adherence observations. Increasingly, data on adherence to infection prevention processes such as the VAP bundle and patient and health care influenza vaccination rates are available.

The hospital microbiology laboratory fulfills a central role in surveillance for HAIs and community-acquired pathogens (e.g., influenza) that is important for the infection control practitioner. In addition, the increased incidence of multidrug-resistant organisms makes it essential that clinicians have up-to-date information on the resistance patterns of pathogens they are treating in the hospital.

Microbiology personnel work closely with infection control professionals in support of the surveillance program; regular diagnostic activities often reveal patterns of infection with certain microorganisms that can precede widespread outbreaks. The combination of diagnostic activities with ongoing surveillance can help prevent or minimize large-scale in-hospital epidemics.

The surveillance activities of an infection control program are most effective when they generate actionable data that are communicated to the bedside caregiver in a timely fashion. These data can become the springboard for continuous improvement in the delivery of care. Infection control practitioners communicate the results of surveillance activities to bedside caregivers in a meaningful way so that continuous improvements in care occur based on local data. All health care workers should be aware of the rates of adherence in their area to bundles, hand hygiene, and HAI and should seek out their infection control practitioner with any questions, observations, and suggestions on how care could be improved.

SUMMARY CHECKLIST

- The five major routes for transmission of pathogens are contact, droplet, airborne, common vehicle, and vector-borne.
- Infection control procedures involve (1) eliminating the sources of infectious agents, (2) creating barriers to their transmission, and (3) monitoring and evaluating the effectiveness of control.
- Failure to clean equipment properly can render all subsequent processing efforts ineffective.
- Physical or chemical disinfection destroys the vegetative form of pathogenic organisms but cannot kill bacterial spores.
- Glutaraldehyde (20 minutes) is the most common option for high-level disinfection of semicritical respiratory care equipment.
- EtO is best suited for sterilization of critical moisture-sensitive or heat-sensitive items; heat-stable critical items should be autoclaved (steam-sterilized).
- Among respiratory care equipment, large volume nebulizers have the greatest potential to spread infection.
- Ventilator circuits should be changed when visibly soiled or malfunctioning.
- HMEs may be used up to 96 hours before they need to be changed.
- Single-use items should be reused only if there is hard documented evidence that reprocessing poses no threat to the patient and does not alter the function of the device.
- Sterile fluids must always be used for tracheal suctioning and for filling nebulizers and humidifiers.
- Hands need to be thoroughly washed after any patient contact, even when gloves are used.
- Standard precautions must be used in caring for all patients, regardless of their diagnosis or infection status.
- The use of gloves is part of routine basic care when there is skin contact with a patient.
- Masks, goggles, or a face shield must be worn during any procedure that can generate splashes or sprays of blood, body fluids, secretions, or excretions.
- RTs must be familiar with the overall infection control program of OSHA, including surveillance policies and procedures.

References

1. Klevens RM, Edwards JR, Richards CL, et al: Estimating healthcare associated infections and deaths in U.S. hospitals, 2002. Public Health Rep 122:160–165, 2007.
2. Centers for Disease Control and Prevention (CDC), Health Care Infection Control Practices Advisory Committee (HICPAC): Guidelines for environmental infection control in health-care facilities, Atlanta, 2003, CDC.
3. Institute of Medicine: To err is human: building a safer health care system, Washington D.C., 2000, Institute of Medicine.

4. Centers for Disease Control: Guideline for prevention of health care associated pneumonia, 2003: recommendations of CDC and the HICPAC. MMWR Morb Mortal Wkly Rep 53(RR-3):1–40, 2004.
5. Stephen F: Pulmonary complications following lung resection. Chest 118:1263, 2000.
6. Siegel JD, Rhinehart E, Jackson M, et al; Healthcare Infection Control Practices Advisory Committee: 2007 guideline for isolation precautions: preventing transmission of infectious agents in healthcare settings, 2007, www.cdc.gov/ncidod/dhqp/pdf/isolation2007.pdf.
7. Yi IT, Li Y, Wong TW, et al: Evidence of airborne transmission of the severe acute respiratory syndrome virus. N Engl J Med 350:1731–1739, 2004.
8. Centers for Disease Control and Prevention: Guidelines for infection control in healthcare personnel. 1998 HICPAC. Infect Control Hosp Epidemiol 19:407–463, 1998.
9. Centers for Disease Control and Prevention: Prevention and control of influenza with vaccines. MMWR Morb Mortal Wkly Rep 59(RR-8):1–62, 2010.
10. Pronovost P, Needham D, Berenholtz S, et al. An intervention to decrease catheter related bloodstream infections in the ICU. N Engl J Med 355:2725–2732, 2006.
11. Bonten MJ, Kollef MH, Hall JB: Risk factors for ventilator-associated pneumonia: from epidemiology to patient management. Clin Infect Dis 38:1141–1149, 2004.
12. Marschall J, Mermel LA, Classen D, et al: Strategies to prevent central line-associated bloodstream infections in acute care hospitals. Infect Control Hosp Epidemiol 29:S22-S30, 2008.
13. Coffin SB, Klompas M, Classen D, et al: Strategies to prevent ventilator associated pneumonia in acute care hospitals. Infect Control Hosp Epidemiol 29:S31-S40, 2008.
14. Centers for Disease Control and Prevention: Guideline for hand hygiene in healthcare settings: recommendations of the Healthcare Infection Control Practices Advisory Committee and the HICPAC/SHEA/IDSA/APIC Hand Hygiene Task Force. MMWR Morb Mortal Wkly Rep 51(RR-16):1–47, 2002.
15. Centers for Disease Control: Guidelines for preventing opportunistic infections among hematopoietic stem cell transplant recipients. Recommendations of CDC, the Infectious Disease Society of America and the American Society of Blood and Marrow Transplantation. MMWR Morb Mortal Wkly Rep 49(RR-10):1–125, 2000.
16. Rutala WA, Weber DJ and the Healthcare Infection Control Practices Advisory Committee (HICPAC), Centers for Disease Control and Prevention: Guidelines for sterilization and disinfection in healthcare facilities, Atlanta, GA, 2008, www.edu.gov./hicpac/.pdf/guidelines.
17. Spaulding EH: Chemical disinfection of medical and surgical materials. In Lawrance C, Block SS, editors, Disinfection, sterilization, and preservation, Philadelphia, 1968, Lea & Febiger, pp 517–531.
18. Haney PE, Raymond BA, Lewis LC: Ethylene oxide: an occupational health hazard for hospital workers. AORN J 51:480, 1990.
19. Thomachot L, Boisson C, Arnaud S, et al: Changing heat and moisture exchangers after 96 hours rather than after 24 hours: a clinical and microbiological evaluation. Crit Care Med 28:714, 2000.
20. Kollef MH: The prevention of ventilator-associated pneumonia. N Engl J Med 340:627, 1999.
21. Han JN, Liu YP, Ma S, et al: Effects of decreasing the frequency of ventilator circuit changes to every 7 days on the rate of ventilator-associated pneumonia in a Beijing hospital. Respir Care 46:891, 2001.
22. Weber DJ, Wilson MB, Rutala WA, et al: Manual ventilation bags as a source for bacterial colonization of intubated patients. Am Rev Respir Dis 142:892, 1990.
23. AARC Guideline: Oxygen therapy for adults in acute care facilities. Respir Care 47:717–720, 2002.
24. Alvine GF, Rodgers P, Fitzsimmons KM, et al: Disposable jet nebulizers: how reliable are they? Chest 101:316, 1992
25. Kissoon N, Nykanen D, Tiffin N, et al: Evaluation of performance characteristics of disposable bag-valve resuscitators. Crit Care Med 19:102, 1991.
26. Ball CK, Schafer EM, Thorne D: Reusing disposables: same old story—more characters added, Insight.

Chapter 5

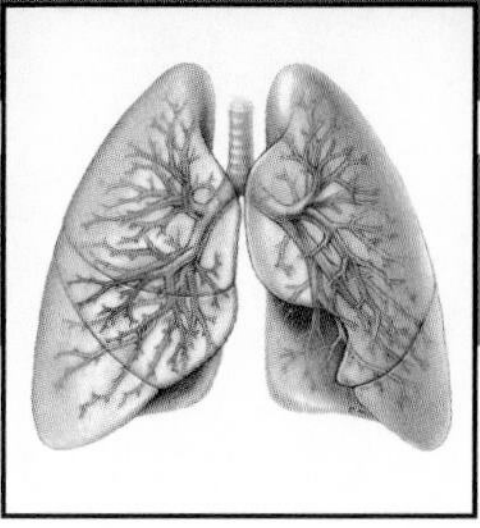

Ethical and Legal Implications of Practice

ANTHONY L. DEWITT

CHAPTER OBJECTIVES

After reading this chapter you will be able to:

- Summarize the philosophical foundations of ethics.
- Explain what constitutes an ethical dilemma and how such dilemmas arise in health care.
- Describe how professional codes of ethics apply to ethical decision making.
- Explain how traditional ethical principles are useful in resolving ethical dilemmas.
- Describe the information that should be gathered before making an ethical decision.
- Explain how the systems of civil and criminal law differ.
- Describe what constitutes professional malpractice and negligence.
- Explain how a respiratory therapist can become liable for wrongful acts.
- List the elements that constitute a practice act.
- Explain how licensing affects legal responsibility and liability.
- Describe how changes in health care delivery have shaped the ethical and legal aspects of practice.
- Summarize the basic elements of the Health Insurance Portability and Accountability Act of 1996 (HIPAA)
- Describe the role of advance directives and living wills in health care.

CHAPTER OUTLINE

Philosophical Foundations of Ethics
Ethical Dilemmas of Practice
Codes of Ethics
Ethical Theories and Principles
- Autonomy
- Veracity
- Nonmaleficence
- Beneficence
- Confidentiality
- Justice
- Role Duty

Ethical Viewpoints and Decision Making
- Formalism
- Consequentialism
- Mixed Approaches
- Virtue Ethics
- Intuitionism
- Comprehensive Decision-Making Models

Legal Issues Affecting Respiratory Care
- Systems of Law
- Health Insurance Portability and Accountability Act of 1996
- Medical Supervision

Interaction of Ethics and the Law
Professional Licensure Issues
- Licensure Statute
- Understanding the Causes of Discipline
- Engaging Counsel

Respiratory Therapists Who Speak Out About Wrongdoing
- Patient Protection and Affordable Care Act
- National Labor Relations Act
- False Claims Act

Health Care and Change
- Health Care Advance Directives

KEY TERMS

advance directives
assault
autonomy
axiology
battery
beneficence
benevolent deception
breach of contract
compensatory justice
confidentiality
consequentialism
defendant
distributive justice
double effect
formalism
informed consent
intuitionism
justice
libel
living will
malpractice
negligence
nonmaleficence
plaintiff
res ipsa loquitur
respondeat superior
rule utilitarianism
slander
strict liability
tort
veracity
virtue ethics

An effective respiratory therapist (RT) must possess excellent clinical skills and an understanding of the business of health care. The health care industry, similar to all industries, must deliver services in an atmosphere in which ethical and legal considerations are an integral part of the organizational culture. RTs regularly encounter circumstances that require them to make choices or take actions that have ethical and legal implications. In society, ethics and law help maintain order and stability. In professional practices, ethics guide RTs in carrying out their duties in a morally defensible way. Law establishes the minimum legal standards to which practitioners must adhere. Although not always the case, ethical practice may require a standard above that of legal practice.

The force behind law is twofold: (1) statutory punishment, ranging from reparations and fines to licensure suspension and incarceration; and (2) civil judgments for violations of duties that cause harm to others. Sanctions for ethical misconduct involve censorship or expulsion from the profession. In some cases, ethical misconduct and legal misbehavior may result from the same incident. The distinction between illegal acts and unethical behavior is not always straightforward. A given act may fit any one of the following categories, depending on the circumstances and the ethical orientation of the person involved: ethical and legal, unethical but legal, ethical but illegal, or unethical and illegal. This chapter provides a foundation of principles related to the ethical and legal practice of respiratory care.

PHILOSOPHICAL FOUNDATIONS OF ETHICS

Although an in-depth discussion of philosophy is beyond the scope of this chapter, it is important to note that ethics has its origins in philosophy. *Philosophy* may be defined as the love of wisdom and the pursuit of knowledge concerning humankind, nature, and reality.[1] *Ethics* is one of the disciplines of philosophy, which include ontology (the nature of reality), metaphysics (the nature of the universe), epistemology (the nature of knowledge), **axiology** (the nature, types, and criteria of values), logic, and aesthetics. Ethics is primarily concerned with the question of how we should act. Although ethics may share common origins with the disciplines of law, theology, and economics, as an applied practice, ethics is clearly different from these disciplines.[1] Ethics can be described philosophically as a moral principle that supplements the golden rule and can be summed up by a commitment to "respect the humanity in persons."[2]

ETHICAL DILEMMAS OF PRACTICE

The growth of respiratory care has paralleled the development of advanced medical technology and treatment protocols. At the same time, during the 1970s through the 1990s, an ever-growing and sophisticated patient population, fueled by medical benefit packages from the government and employers, developed rising expectations about acceptable standards of care. In the latter part of the 1990s, managed care strategies and other cost-containment methods adopted by most third-party payers slowed the growth of the health care industry. The ethical and legal issues faced by practitioners, although changed in many cases, continued to grow. In the earlier period, RTs faced ethical dilemmas and legal issues associated with patient expectations, staffing, and quality of care, among others. RTs continue to face ethical dilemmas and legal issues at the present time; however, such dilemmas may now include the rationing of care, dealing with conflicts associated with third-party standards of care, and delivery of the appropriate standard of care in the face of cost constraints. Staffing issues continue to be a problem and are at the root of many of the ethical and legal concerns faced by RTs. As respiratory care continues to mature as a profession, these challenges are likely to increase. The twenty-first century has brought one particular challenge, although not new to health care or to RTs: a heightened awareness of the patient's right to privacy. The Health Insurance Portability and Accountability Act of 1996 (HIPAA), discussed later in this chapter, is now a major consideration for RTs as they perform their jobs.

RTs work in complex health care settings, making it difficult to predict definitively the range of ethical dilemmas likely to be experienced on a regular basis. The clinical aspects and the management aspects of health care are rife with possibilities for ethical dilemmas. In addition, the ethical orientation of the RT plays a role in recognition and identification of ethical dilemmas. The health care industry continues to be in a period of dynamic change bringing many new challenges. New technologic and management methodologies are continuously being introduced to accomplish the missions and goals of health care organizations. Over the past decade, there has been an almost complete change from a relatively open fee-for-service system to one in which care is managed in some fashion, and the fees are in some form of capitated payment. These changes often pose serious ethical dilemmas.

For example, managed care uses a concept known as "restrictive gatekeeping." Restrictive gatekeeping requires patients to obtain prior approval from their third-party payer, usually an insurance company, before hospitalization and before certain procedures. When the hospital admission or procedure is approved, specific requirements or limitations are usually associated with the patient's care. As a result, health care workers, including RTs, may find themselves engaged in clinical processes that are dictated more by the third-party payers than by patient needs. Under these circumstances, health care workers may feel frustrated and helpless if they believe that a patient needs care beyond that approved by the third-party payer.

The rationing of care continues to be a side effect of staffing patterns created by managed care. Although all businesses must carefully balance staffing patterns against productivity, managed care has brought this concept home in a major way to health care facilities. An RT working in an understaffed department may decide that Patient A can really forego therapy because the department is short staffed and Patient A is really not going to get better anyway. Although this may sound at first like a case of simple neglect of duty, it is also an ethical dilemma.

The approaches used to address ethical issues in health care range from the specific to the general. Specific guidance in resolving ethical dilemmas is usually provided by a professional code of ethics. General approaches involve the use of ethical theories and principles to reach a decision.[3]

CODES OF ETHICS

A *code of ethics* is an essential part of any profession that claims to be self-regulating. The adoption of a code of ethics is one way in which an occupational group establishes itself as a profession. A code may try to limit competition, restrict advertisement, or promote a particular image in addition to setting forth rules for conduct.[4]

The first American medical code of ethics (established in 1847) was as much concerned with separating orthodox practitioners from nontraditional ones as it was with regulating behavior. Even modern codes tend to be vague regarding what is prescribed and what is to be avoided.

The American Association for Respiratory Care (AARC) has also adopted a Statement of Ethics and Professional Conduct. The current code appears in Box 5-1. This code represents a set of general principles and rules that have been developed to help ensure that the health needs of the public are provided in a safe, effective, and caring manner. Codes for different professions might differ from the code governing respiratory care because they may seek different goals. However, all codes of ethics seek to establish parameters of behavior for members of the chosen profession. Professional codes of ethics often represent overly simplistic or prohibitive notions of how to deal with open misbehavior or flagrant abuses of authority.

Box 5-1 AARC Statement of Ethics and Professional Conduct (Revised 7/04)

In the conduct of professional activities, the respiratory therapist shall be bound by the following ethical and professional principles. Respiratory therapists shall:

- Demonstrate behavior that reflects integrity, supports objectivity, and fosters trust in the profession and its professionals. Actively maintain and continually improve their professional competence and represent it accurately
- Perform only those procedures or functions in which they are individually competent and which are within the scope of accepted and responsible practice
- Respect and protect the legal and personal rights of patients they treat, including the right to informed consent and refusal of treatment
- Divulge no confidential information regarding any patient or family unless disclosure is required for responsible performance of duty, or required by law
- Provide care without discrimination on any basis, with respect for the rights and dignity of all individuals
- Promote disease prevention and wellness
- Refuse to participate in illegal or unethical acts, and shall refuse to conceal illegal, unethical, or incompetent acts of others
- Follow sound scientific procedures and ethical principles in research
- Comply with state or federal laws that govern and relate to their practice
- Avoid any form of conduct that creates a conflict of interest and shall follow the principles of ethical business behavior
- Promote health care delivery through improvement of the access, efficacy, and cost of patient care
- Encourage and promote appropriate stewardship of resources

The most difficult ethical decisions arise from situations in which two or more right choices are incompatible, in which the choices represent different priorities, or in which limited resources exist to achieve a desired end. Ethicists readily admit that reducing these issues to simple formulations is not an easy task. The number and complexity of ethical dilemmas continue to grow as the complexity of life and health care increases. For health care, difficult ethical dilemmas continue to involve concerns about the practical limits on financial resources, the growing emphasis on individual autonomy, and more research advances such as cloning and stem cell research. Resolution of these more complex problems requires a more general approach than that provided by a code of ethics. This more general perspective is provided by ethical theories and principles.

In addition to the moral obligations that ethical duties impose on RTs, ethical obligations are often cited in legal proceedings as a tool of cross-examination. If an RT expresses opinions or is accused of actions that would violate the ethical duties of the profession, the RT's ignorance of ethical standards during cross-examination can have a powerful effect on a jury.

MINI CLINI

Conflicting Obligations

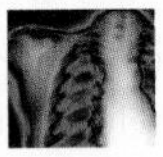

PROBLEM: Therapist H, a registered RT with 18 years' experience, has worked for a large regional medical center for the past 10 years. She is generally happy with her work but is concerned about the financial stability of the hospital. As a result, she has signed on with a temporary agency to ensure that she will have work if the hospital decides to initiate a reduction in force. On one of her scheduled days off, Therapist H agrees to work a shift for the temporary agency at another hospital. Two hours before her shift is scheduled to begin, she receives a telephone message from the medical center where she is employed. Her supervisor asks Therapist H to report to work at the medical center because the only experienced therapist on the shift has been in an automobile accident. Therapist H is torn between her obligation to the medical center where she has worked for 10 years and the agency.

DISCUSSION: Professionalism and ethics generally require a commitment to one's duties. In this situation, Therapist H must consider not only her duty but also the consequences of each decision that she might make. In either case, there is the possibility that her decision will leave a staffing shortage at one of the hospitals.

DISCUSSION QUESTIONS: Should Therapist H cancel her shift with the agency, although she has agreed to give the agency a 4-hour notice except in an emergency? Should she work the shift at the agency as scheduled, using the rationale that she did not create the staffing problem at the medical center? Should she call her supervisor and explain the situation and ask for help in making the right decision, realizing that the final decision would still be hers? Should she call her supervisor and tell the supervisor that she is ill and cannot come in and report to the agency job?

ETHICAL THEORIES AND PRINCIPLES

Ethical theories and principles provide the foundation for all ethical behavior. Contemporary ethical principles have evolved from many sources, including Aristotle's and Aquinas' natural law, Judeo-Christian morality, Kant's universal duties, and the values characterizing modern democracy.[5,6] Although controversy exists, most ethicists agree that autonomy, veracity, nonmaleficence, beneficence, confidentiality, justice, and role fidelity are the primary guiding principles in contemporary ethical decision making.[1,5]

Each of these ethical principles, as applied to professional practice, consists of two components: a *professional duty* and a *patient right* (Figure 5-1). The principle of autonomy obliges health care professionals to uphold the freedom of will and freedom of action of others. The principle of beneficence obliges health care professionals to further the interests of others either by promoting their good or by actively preventing their harm. The principle of justice obliges health care professionals to ensure that others receive what they rightfully deserve or legitimately claim.

Expressed in each duty is a reciprocal patient right. Reciprocal patient rights include the right to autonomous choice, the right not to be harmed, and the right to fair and equitable treatment. More specific rules can be generated from these general principles of rights and obligations, such as those included in a code of ethics.

Autonomy

The principle of **autonomy** acknowledges the personal liberty of patients and their right to decide their own course of treatment and follow through a plan on which they freely agree. It is from this principle that rules about

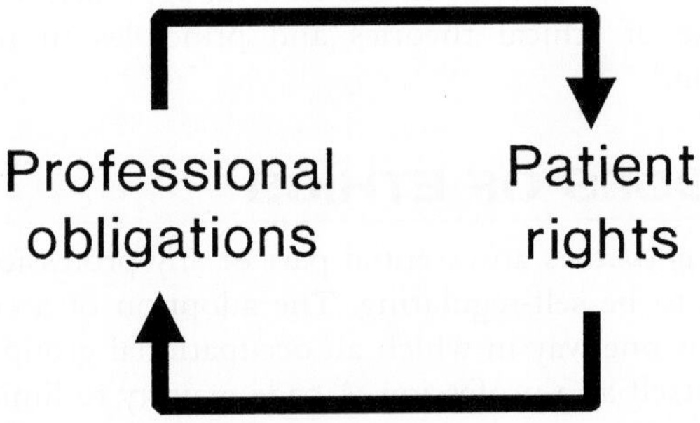

FIGURE 5-1 Reciprocal relationship between professional obligations and patient rights.

informed consent are derived. Under the principle of autonomy, the use by an RT of deceit or coercion to get a patient to reverse the decision to refuse a treatment is considered unethical. Likewise, it is unethical and illegal to threaten a patient who is unwilling to sign a consent form.

Veracity

The principle of **veracity** is often linked to autonomy, especially in the area of informed consent. Generally, veracity binds the health care provider and the patient to tell the truth. The nature of the health care delivery process is such that both parties involved are best served in an environment of trust and mutual sharing of all information. Problems with the veracity principle revolve around such issues as benevolent deception. In actions of **benevolent deception,** the truth is withheld from the patient for his or her own good.

When the physician decides to withhold the truth from a conscious, well-oriented adult, the decision affects the interactions between health care providers and the patient and has a chilling effect on the rapport that is so necessary for good care. In a poll conducted by the Louis Harris group, 94% of Americans surveyed indicated that they wanted to know everything about their cases, even the dismal facts. Other than with pediatrics and rare cases in which there is evidence that the truth would lead to a harm (e.g., suicide), the truth, provided in as pleasant a manner as possible, is probably the best policy.[7]

Truth telling can also involve documentation and medical recordkeeping. This type of dilemma is occurring more frequently under strict managed care reimbursement protocols. The accompanying Mini Clini provides a good example of this type of dilemma.

Nonmaleficence

The principle of **nonmaleficence** obligates health care providers to avoid harming patients and to prevent harm actively where possible. It is sometimes difficult to uphold this principle in modern medicine because in many cases drugs and procedures have secondary effects that may be harmful in varying degrees. For example, an RT might ask whether it is ethical to give a high dose of steroids to an asthmatic patient, knowing the many harmful consequences of these drugs. One solution to these dilemmas is based on the understanding that many helping actions inevitably have both a good and a bad effect, or *double effect.* The key is the first intent. If the first intent is good, the harmful effect is viewed as an unintended result. The **double effect** brings us to the essence of the definition of the word *dilemma.* The word comes from the Greek terms *di,* meaning "two," and *lemma,* meaning "assumption" or "proposition."[8]

Beneficence

The principle of **beneficence** raises the "do no harm" requirement to an even higher level. Beneficence requires that health care providers go beyond doing no harm and contribute actively to the health and well-being of their patients. Many quality-of-life issues are included within this dictum. Practitioners of medicine today possess the technology to keep some individuals alive well beyond any likelihood of meaningful recovery. This technology presents dilemmas for practitioners who have the ability to prolong life but not the ability to restore any uniquely human qualities.

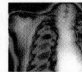

MINI CLINI

Patient Rights

PROBLEM: An RT working at a hospital receives a physician order to administer an aerosolized bronchodilator treatment to a 26-year-old female asthmatic patient admitted for suspected pneumonia. The patient refuses the treatment on entering the room, stating that she is having a "bad day" today and does not want to be bothered by anyone. The patient is regarded as being competent and fully capable of making health care decisions for herself. How could the RT handle this situation?

DISCUSSION: The RT must acknowledge and respect the patient's right to decide freely whether or not to allow the respiratory care treatment. According to the principles of ethical theory and conduct, health care professionals have an obligation to promote patient autonomy by permitting freedom of will and freedom of action. An additional requirement on the part of the practitioner is that coercion or deceit not be used to get a patient to reverse his or her decision to refuse a treatment. According to the American Hospital Association statement entitled "The Patient Care Partnership," the patient has the right to refuse treatment and to be informed of the medical consequences of her action.

The RT could talk to the patient and explore what the term "bad day" meant to her. It might be that she is not feeling well because of breathing problems from her asthma condition and worsening symptoms of possible pneumonia. The RT has an important role in ensuring that the patient understands the benefits of the respiratory treatment and the health consequences of refusal so that the patient can make a well-informed decision. If the RT approaches the patient in a professional, nonthreatening manner, she may feel more at ease and be willing to discuss in greater depth why she does not want to take the treatment. It is common for a patient to refuse therapy initially only to change his or her mind after communication with the RT. Should the patient still refuse the treatment after discussion with the RT, the RT should remain nonjudgmental, even if he or she disagrees with the patient's decision. Appropriate documentation in the medical record and physician notification should then occur.

MINI CLINI

Veracity

PROBLEM: Jon performs pulmonary function testing, including blood gases, for his hospital. Many of the patients he sees are attempting to qualify or requalify for continuous reimbursement for home oxygen use. To qualify, the patient's PaO_2 must be less than 60 mm Hg. Patient A, who has home oxygen therapy, is attempting to requalify, although her condition has improved from what it was 1 year earlier. Her blood gas results show a PaO_2 of 63 mm Hg. The patient's husband asks Jon if there is anything he can do, while relating how greatly his wife benefits from the oxygen. Jon tells the husband that there is nothing that he can do and assists the husband in taking the patient out to her car. At the car, the husband pulls out his wallet, shows it to Jon, and repeats the question.

DISCUSSION POINTS: RTs have an obligation to carry out their duties in the most competent and professional manner possible. Failure to do so may constitute both an ethical dilemma and a legal issue.

DISCUSSION QUESTIONS: What is the potential ethical dilemma in this situation? What other ways could Jon have chosen to handle this situation?

In these cases, some individuals interpret the principle of beneficence to mean that they must do everything to promote a patient's life, regardless of how useful the life might be to that individual. Other professionals in the same situation might believe they are allowing the principle to be better served by doing nothing and allowing death to occur without taking heroic measures to prevent it. In an attempt to allow patients to participate in resolving this dilemma, legal avenues, called **advance directives,** have been developed.[9] Advance directives allow a patient to give direction to health care providers about treatment choices in circumstances in which the patient may no longer be able to provide that direction. The two types of advance directives available at the present time and widely used are the *living will* and the *durable power of attorney for health care.* A durable power of attorney for health care allows the patient to identify another person to carry out his or her wishes with respect to health care, whereas a **living will** states a patient's health care preferences in writing. As a result of the Patient Self-Determination Act of 1990, most states require that all health care agencies receiving federal reimbursement under Medicare/Medicaid legislation provide adult clients with information on advance directives.[9,10]

Confidentiality

The principle of **confidentiality** is founded in the Hippocratic Oath; it was later reiterated by the World Medical Association in 1949. It obliges health care providers to "respect the secrets which are confided even after the patient has died."[11] Confidentiality, as with the other axioms of ethics, must often be balanced against other principles, such as beneficence.

The main ethical issue surrounding confidentiality is whether more harm is done by occasionally violating its mandate or by always upholding it, regardless of the consequences. This limitation to confidentiality is known as the *harm principle*. This principle requires that practitioners refrain from acts or omissions in which foreseeable harm to others could result, especially when the others are vulnerable to risk. This principle would require that confidentiality be maintained for a patient with AIDS in matters involving his or her landlord. In this case, confidentiality is justified because the landlord is not particularly vulnerable. However, if the patient was planning to marry, the harm principle would require that confidentiality be broken because of the special vulnerability of the spouse.

Confidentiality is usually considered a qualified, rather than an absolute, ethical principle in most health care provider–patient relationships. These qualifications are often written into codes of ethics. The American Medical Association Code of Ethics, Section 9, provides the following guidelines: "A physician may not reveal the confidences entrusted to him in the course of medical attendance or the deficiencies he may observe in the character of patients, unless he is required to do so by law or unless it becomes necessary in order to protect the welfare of the community or a vulnerable individual." Under the requirements of public health and community welfare, there is often a legal requirement to report such things as child abuse, poisonings, industrial accidents, communicable diseases, blood transfusion reactions, narcotic use, and injuries caused with knives or guns.[12] In many states, child abuse statutes protect the health care practitioner from liability in reporting even if the report should prove false as long as the report was made in good faith. Failure to report a case of child abuse can leave the practitioner legally liable for additional injuries that the child may sustain after being returned to the hostile environment.

Breaches of confidentiality more often result from careless slips of the tongue than from rational decision making. Such social trading in gossip about patients is unprofessional, unethical, and, in certain cases, illegal. Risks of inadvertent disclosure increase exponentially with membership on social networking sites such as Facebook where RTs may exchange information that sometimes violates the rights of individual patients.

RULE OF THUMB

Patient information should be discussed only in private and with persons who have a legitimate reason and need to know.

Because of the widespread use of computerized databases, confidential information, previously highly protected, is now relatively easy to obtain. Clinical data are available for close scrutiny by the clerical staff, laboratory personnel, and other health care providers. The widespread use of these data systems is a threat to patient confidentiality. In an attempt to reduce this threat, most clinical databases are restricted to use by only the health care workers who have a need to know. In addition to being unethical, an RT who reads the file of a patient whom he or she is not treating would likely be in violation of institutional policy. The accompanying Mini Clini below provides an example.

MINI CLINI

Confidentiality

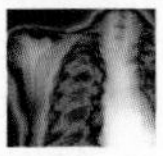

PROBLEM: Mary, an RT, is working the evening shift at a large urban medical center when she receives a telephone call from a friend telling her that her next door neighbor has been admitted to the medical center. Mary's first thought is to check the neighbor's file on the computer system to see why her neighbor has been hospitalized.

DISCUSSION POINT: Mary knows that the medical center has a policy that employees are to access only the charts for which they have a reason to do so.

DISCUSSION QUESTIONS: Should Mary access this chart via the computer system? If she does, what kind of violation will she be committing–ethical, legal, or both? What ethical principles, if any, would apply here? What is the harm in simply checking the computer on this patient? Is anyone likely to know if Mary accesses this patient's information?

Despite medical and sociologic advances, potential violations of the individual's right to privacy in certain populations, such as patients with AIDS, pose a special risk because disclosure may result in economic, psychologic, or physical harm to the patient. RTs would do well to adhere to the dictum found in the Hippocratic Oath: "What I may see or hear in the course of the treatment or even outside of treatment of the patient in regard to the life of men, which on no account one must spread abroad, I will keep to myself, holding such things to be shameful to be spoken about."[13]

Justice

The principle of **justice** involves the fair distribution of care. Rising health care expectations, coupled with the decreased availability of care because of cost, is making this principle an important one for health care workers. Population trends and the financial shortfalls in programs such as Medicaid and Medicare will contribute to the continuing importance of this principle.

The United States is rapidly approaching the point at which a balance must be found between health care expenses and the revenue available to pay for them. Efforts to achieve this balance will inevitably lead to some form of rationing of the delivery of health care services. This type of justice is properly referred to as **distributive justice.**

A second form of justice seen in health care is **compensatory justice.** This form of justice calls for the recovery for damages that were incurred as a result of the action of others. Damage awards in civil cases of medical malpractice or negligence are examples of compensatory justice. Compensatory justice has often been cited as playing a major role in increasing the cost of health care. However, the Congressional Budget Office estimates that less than 2% of the cost of health care is related to medical malpractice. Studies by Zurich Insurance Company,[14] Harvard University, and Dartmouth University showed little to no impact on the cost of health care and generally debunk the myth that physicians always practice defensive medicine. The Harvard study showed that patients were uncompensated in the presence of actual malpractice more frequently than physicians were held accountable in the absence of actual malpractice. Other studies generally confirm that the civil justice system does a good job of protecting the rights of health care workers and patients in negligence litigation.

Role Duty

Because no single individual can be solely responsible for providing all of a patient's health care needs, modern health care is a team effort by necessity. There are more than 100 allied health professions, and allied health workers (excluding nursing and physicians) provide about 60% of all patient care. Each of the allied health professions has its own practice niche, defined by tradition or by licensure law. Practitioners have a duty to understand the limits of their role and to practice with fidelity. For example, because of differences in *role duty,* an RT might be ethically obliged not to tell a patient's family how critical the situation is, instead having the attending physician do so.[3] The previous Mini Clinis addressed role duty, and the accompanying Mini Clini presents another example of the ethics of role duty.

ETHICAL VIEWPOINTS AND DECISION MAKING

In deciding ethical issues, some practitioners try to adhere to a strict interpretation of one or more ethical principles, such as those just described. Other practitioners seek to decide the issue solely on a case-by-case basis, considering only the potential good (or bad) consequences. Still other

MINI CLINI

Role Duty

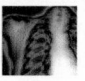

PROBLEM: Sue, an RT, receives a request to perform a blood gas analysis for a patient on a ventilator because, as reported by the nurse, the patient's oxygen saturation is only 61%. The patient has an order for blood gases as needed. As the nurse and RT look at the blood gas results, they both are surprised because the saturation is now 93%. The nurse suggests repeating the blood gases. The RT is about to comply until she notes the oximeter display on which the nurse is relying shows the patient with an oxygen saturation of 93% and a pulse rate of 61 beats/min.

DISCUSSION POINT: Teamwork and role delineation are both essential components of good patient care. Each practitioner also has an obligation to perform his or her duties in the most competent and professional manner possible.

DISCUSSION QUESTIONS: What kind of issue or dilemma exists here—legal, ethical, or both? What should the RT do at this point? Should an incident report be written and, if so, by whom?

MINI CLINI

Role Duty

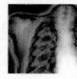

PROBLEM: Courtney is the lone RT on duty on the midnight shift in a small, 65-bed rural hospital. She likes working at the small hospital and knows most of the patients and their conditions from memory. The night is quiet and uneventful until 2:00 AM, when a code is called for a patient in the intensive care unit (ICU). Courtney immediately heads for the ICU while mentally noting the patient's condition on which the code has been called. She remembers that the patient is 78 years old and has chronic obstructive pulmonary disease. Just as she nears the ICU, a second code is called for a patient in a room just outside of the ICU. Courtney quickly jogs her memory and remembers that this patient is a 25-year-old diabetic who has just given birth to a baby girl.

DISCUSSION POINT: The lone RT can attend to only one code, although she has an obligation to provide the best care possible to all patients. There is no protocol of which the RT is aware that would provide guidance as to which patient she should seek to assist with first. At the time the second code is called, she is at an equal distance from both patients.

DISCUSSION QUESTIONS: Is this RT facing an ethical dilemma? If so, what guiding principle or principles should be relied on to determine the best course of action? Which patient should the RT assist with first?

practitioners would appeal to the image of a "good practitioner," asking themselves what a virtuous person would do in a similar circumstance. Finally, many practitioners acknowledge that they largely follow their intuition for making ethical decisions. These different viewpoints represent the four dominant theories underlying modern ethics.[5,15] The viewpoint that relies on rules and principles is called **formalism,** or duty-oriented reasoning. The viewpoint in which decisions are based on the assessment of consequences is called **consequentialism.** The viewpoint that asks what a virtuous person would do in a similar circumstance is called **virtue ethics.** When intuition is involved in the decision-making process, the approach is called *intuitionism*.

Formalism

Formalist thought asserts that certain features of an act itself determine its moral rightness. In this framework, ethical standards of right and wrong are described in terms of rules or principles. These rules function apart from the consequences of a particular act. An act is considered morally justifiable only if it upholds the rules or principles that apply.

The major objection to this duty-oriented approach lies in its potential for inconsistency. Critics of formalist reasoning insist that no principle or rule can be framed that does not have exceptions. These critics claim that no principle or rule can be framed that does not conflict with other rules.

Consequentialism

For the consequentialist, an act is judged to be right or wrong based on its consequences. Each possible act is assessed in terms of the relative amount of good (over evil) that it would bring into being. The most common application of consequentialism judges acts according to the *principle of utility*. The principle of utility, in its simplest form, aims to promote the greatest general good for most people.

Critics of this approach claim that it has two fundamental flaws. First, the "calculus" involved in projecting and weighing the amount of good over evil that might occur is not always possible. Second, reliance on the principle of utility to the exclusion of all else can result in actions that are incompatible with ordinary judgments about right and wrong. A classic example of this problem can be seen in the true World War II case of the battle for North Africa. In this scenario, there were two groups of soldiers but only enough antibiotics for one group. One group required the medication for syphilis contracted in the local brothels; the other group needed antibiotics for wounds sustained in battle. The dilemma arose as to who should receive the antibiotics. Formalist or duty-oriented reasoning would base the decision about who should receive the antibiotics on some concept of justice, such as giving priority to the sickest or to the individuals most in need. However, the actual decision in this case was a consequentialist one, based not on the desire to distribute the drug justly but rather on the need to obtain a quick victory with as few casualties as possible. The scarce medication was given to the soldiers who were "wounded" in the brothels rather than in battle because these soldiers could be restored quickly and returned to the frontlines to aid the war effort.

Mixed Approaches

Mixed approaches to moral reasoning try to capitalize on the strengths inherent in these two major lines of ethical thought. One approach, called **rule utilitarianism,** is a variation of consequentialism. Under this framework, the question is not which act has the greatest utility but which rule would promote the greatest good if it were generally followed.

The rule utilitarian would agree with the formalist that truth telling is a necessary ethical principle but for a different reason. To the rule utilitarian, truth telling is a needed principle not because it has any underlying moral rightness but because it promotes the greatest good in professional-patient relationships. Specifically, if truth telling were not followed consistently, trusting relationships between patients and health care professionals would be impossible.

The rule utilitarian approach is probably the most appealing and useful to health care professionals. This approach is appealing because it addresses both human rights and obligations and the consequences of actions. Rule utilitarianism seems best able to account for the modern realities of human experience that so often affect the day-to-day practice of health care. However, although it has some value as an ethical framework, it has the disadvantage of being quite variable among caregivers. Where caregivers have different values and different educational levels, ethical decision making using this tool frequently is inconsistent.

Virtue Ethics

A theory of *virtue ethics* has evolved based in part on the limits of both formalism and consequentialism. Virtue ethics is founded not in rules or consequences but in personal attributes of character or virtue. Under this formulation, the first question is not, "How do I act in this situation?" but rather, "How should I carry out my life if I am to live well?" or "How would the good RT act?"

Virtue-oriented theory holds that professions have historical traditions. Individuals entering a profession enter into a relationship not only with current practitioners but also with the practitioners who have come before them. With these traditions comes a history of character standards set by the individuals who have previously distinguished themselves in that profession.

According to this perspective, the established practices of a profession can give guidance, without an appeal to either the specific moral principles or the consequences of an act.[3] When the professional is faced with an ethical dilemma, he or she need only envision what the "good practitioner" would do in a similar circumstance. It is hard to imagine the good RT stealing from the patient, charging for services not provided, or smothering a patient with a pillow.

Rapidly changing fields such as respiratory care pose some problems for virtue ethics. What might be considered good ethical conduct at one time might be deemed wrong the next time. An example of this change over time is an RT who is asked not only to disconnect a brain-dead patient from a ventilator but also to remove the feeding tubes and intravenous lines.

In addition to the difficulty with changing values in virtue ethics, it provides no specific directions to aid decision making. The heavy reliance of virtue ethics on experience rather than on reason makes creative solutions less likely. Finally, practitioners often find themselves in conflicting role situations for which virtue ethics has no answers. A good example is an RT who practices the virtue of being a good team player but is confronted with the need to "blow the whistle" on a negligent or incompetent team member.[3] Despite these limitations, virtue ethics is probably the way most practitioners make their ethical decisions.

Intuitionism

Intuitionism is an ethical viewpoint that holds that there are certain self-evident truths, usually based on moral maxims such as "treat others fairly." The easiest way to understand intuitionism is to think of as many timeless maxims as you can, which form the basis for intuitionism. These maxims may range from "do not kill" to "look before you cross the street."[6] As a decision-making tool, intuitionism is unhelpful in large measure because it depends on the intuitional abilities of the specific caregiver.

Comprehensive Decision-Making Models

To aid in the process of decision making in bioethics, several comprehensive models have been developed. Figure 5-2 depicts one example of a comprehensive decision-making model that combines the best elements of formalism, consequentialism, and virtue ethics. As is evident in this approach, the ethical problem is framed in terms of the conditions and who is affected. Initially, an action is chosen based on its predicted consequences. The potential consequences of this decision are compared with the human values underlying the problem. The short test of this comparison is a simple restatement of the golden rule that is, "Would I be satisfied to have this action performed on me?" The initial decision is considered ethical if, and only if, it passes this test of human values. A simpler but

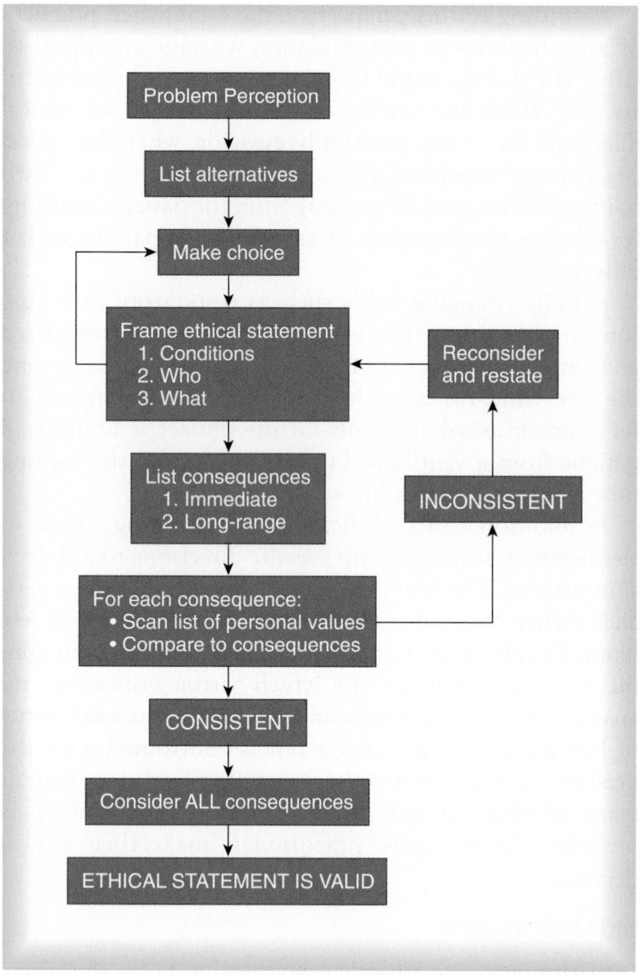

FIGURE 5-2 Comprehensive ethical decision-making model. (Redrawn from Brody H: Ethical decisions in medicine, ed 2, Boston, 1981, Little, Brown.)

Box 5-2 Ethical Decision-Making Model

1. Identify the problem or issue
2. Identify the individuals involved
3. Identify the ethical principle or principles that apply
4. Identify who should make the decision
5. Identify the role of the practitioner
6. Consider the alternatives (long-term and short-term consequences)
7. Make the decision (including the decision not to act)
8. Follow the decision to observe its consequences

nonetheless comprehensive model is used by many ethicists. The model uses eight key steps (Box 5-2).

With or without these models, RTs are often at a double disadvantage in ethical decision making because RTs not only must live with their own decisions but also must support (and act on) the decisions of their physician colleagues. Unless excellent communication exists, misunderstandings can occur. Such misunderstandings may be an essential factor in the high job stress, burnout, and attrition in respiratory care.

Classes in ethics, decision making, and communication skills are crucial components of the preparation of RTs for the often confusing and frustrating practice in today's medical settings. The specialty requires practitioners who can go beyond simple assertions of right or wrong and provide justifications that are both right and reasoned. Many hospitals have ethics boards or committees to review and set policy and to assist in making informed ethical decisions. In addition to administrators and medical staff members, these committees may include a member of the lay public, a chaplain, and one or more experts in bioethics.

A major factor in the disciplinary decisions of professional boards is frequently whether the acts of the RT conformed to the ethical standards of the profession. Nearly every Respiratory Care Practice Act has ethical principles embedded in the statute and codified in state regulations. Every RT should be aware of what his particular state dictates in terms of ethical practice.

RULE OF THUMB

Never attempt to make ethical decisions for others. You can only make them for yourself.

LEGAL ISSUES AFFECTING RESPIRATORY CARE

Sometimes decisions cannot be made in the confines of the medical community and with the help of the patients it serves. These problems often go to the courts. The problem of professional liability in the delivery of health care is immense and plays a key role in skyrocketing health care costs. Limits on medical liability have been key factors in recent legislation.

Practitioners are caught in the middle. On one hand, they are required to keep costs down by avoiding overuse of technology and therapeutics. On the other hand, they are faced with a level of consumerism that holds them accountable as never before. The costs, losses, frustration, and distraction brought about by the current level of legal intervention in health care practice are a national crisis.

Systems of Law

Under our legal system, the law is divided into two broad classes: *public law* and *civil law.* Public law deals with the relationships of private parties and the government. Civil law is concerned with the recognition and enforcement of the rights and duties of private individuals and organizations.

Public (Criminal and Administrative) Law

The two major divisions of public law are *criminal law* and *administrative law*. Criminal law deals with acts or offenses against the welfare or safety of the public. Offenses against criminal law are punishable by fines, imprisonment, or both. In these cases, the accuser is the state, and the person prosecuted is the **defendant.**

Administrative law is the second major branch of public law. Administrative law consists of the countless regulations set by government agencies. Health care facilities are inundated by a host of administrative and agency rules that affect almost every aspect of operation. RTs are obligated to abide by these rules and regulations.

Civil Law

Private or civil law protects private citizens and organizations from others who might seek to take unfair and unlawful advantage of them. If an individual believes that his or her rights have been compromised, the individual can seek redress in the civil courts. In these cases, the individual bringing the complaint is known as the **plaintiff,** and the individual accused of wrong is the defendant. Civil courts decide between the two parties with regard to the degree of wrong and the level of reparation required. The category of civil law best related to respiratory care is tort law.

Tort Law. A **tort** is a civil wrong, other than a breach of contract, committed against an individual or property, for which a court provides a remedy in the form of an action for damages. Causes for the complaints may range from assault and battery to invasion of privacy. The basic functions of torts are to keep the peace between individuals and to substitute a remedy for personal injury instead of vengeance.

There are three basic forms of torts: *negligent torts, intentional torts,* and torts in which liability is assessed regardless of fault (as in the case of manufacturers of defective products). The basic difference between negligent and intentional torts is the element of intent. An intentional tort always involves a willful act that violates another's interest. A negligent tort does not have to involve any action at all. Instead, a negligent tort can consist of an omission of an action.

Professional Negligence. **Negligence,** in its simplest terms, is the failure to perform one's duties competently. Negligence may involve acts of commission or omission. The tort of negligence is concerned with the compensation of an individual for loss or damages arising from the unreasonable behavior of another. The normal standard for the claim is the duty imposed on individuals not to cause risk or harm to others, the standard being what a reasonable and prudent person should have foreseen and avoided.

In negligence cases, the breach of duty often involves the matter of foreseeability. Cases in which the patient falls, is burned, is given the wrong medication, or is harmed by defects in an apparatus often revolve around the duty of the health care provider to anticipate the harm. Duty can be defined as an obligation to do a thing, a human action exactly conformable to the law that requires us to obey. For the tort of negligence to be a valid claim, the four conditions listed in Box 5-3 must be met.

Box 5-3 Elements of Negligence

- The practitioner owes a duty to the patient
- The practitioner breaches that duty
- The breach of duty was the cause of damages
- Damage or harm came to the patient

The assessment of what is reasonable and prudent for an RT can be determined by guidelines established by a professional group (e.g., the AARC), by direct expert testimony, or by circumstantial evidence. In the last case, the legal principle ***res ipsa loquitur*** (the thing speaks for itself) may apply. *Res ipsa loquitur* is sometimes invoked to show that the harm would not ordinarily have happened if the individuals in control had used appropriate care. In these cases, negligence is established by inference.

For a claim of *res ipsa loquitur* to be supported, three basic conditions must be met: (1) The harm was such that it would not normally occur without someone's negligence. (2) The action responsible for the injury was under the control of the defendant. (3) The injury did not result from any contributing negligence or voluntarily assumed risk on the part of the injured party. An example of *res ipsa loquitur* might be the failure to recognize that a patient's right main stem bronchus had been intubated with a resultant pneumothorax. For negligence to occur, the breach in duty must also cause damage or injury to the individual. The injured party must file the lawsuit within the time frame set by the statute of limitations. The term *injury,* in this sense, may include not only physical harm but also mental anguish and other invasions of the patient's rights and privileges. The claim must be supported by a preponderance of evidence to prevail.

For the tort of negligence to be sustained, the breach of duty must be shown to be the cause of the injury. *Causation* revolves around whether the acts of negligence were the cause in fact and the legal cause of the damages. *Causation in fact* means simply that the negligent act of the caregiver caused the damages. *Proximate causation* or *legal causation* usually turns on foreseeability and whether it is fair to impose damages on a defendant.

Factual causation usually is a question for the jury. It is best illustrated in the context of a motor vehicle accident. If a car runs a stop sign but does not hit anyone, the driver may well be negligent, but no one could sue because the driver did not cause any harm. If there is a collision, there is harm flowing directly from the failure to stop. For that reason, the mere failure to provide the appropriate standard of care is insufficient to necessitate payment of damages unless injury occurs as a result of the action or omission. In most states, the act of negligence does not have to be the only cause; it only has to be one cause. Sometimes this is referred to in jury instructions as a requirement that the defendant's actions "caused or contributed to cause" the injury. Ordering oxygen turned off on a severely hypoxemic patient might be the direct cause of the patient's injury, but the therapist's acting on that order instead of questioning it could be thought of as a contributing cause.

Proximate causation turns on foreseeability. It tends to be a retrospective analysis. If an RT fails to check a ventilator as required, it is foreseeable that the patient could develop a compromised airway and sustain brain damage or die. The RT's failure would be both the factual and the legal cause of the injury. Proximate causation also comes into play, however, when there are multiple wrongdoers. For example, a nurse requests a therapist's help to place a patient on the bedside commode. The therapist is unaware that the patient's blood pressure is 60 mm Hg by Doppler. The patient bears down, experiences a cardiac arrest, and dies. Although the actions of the therapist in helping to move the patient to the commode are the cause in fact, the therapist might escape liability because it was not foreseeable that helping the nurse move the patient would result in the patient's death.

Damages are another factor in negligence lawsuits. There are three kinds of damages: economic, noneconomic, and punitive. Economic damages are awarded for economic loss. For example, a working wife and mother killed in a vehicular accident leaves a family without a caregiver for the children and without the $45,000 a year salary she earned. Her economic damages include both the salary figure (adjusted for inflation and wage increases over her work life) and the cost of replacing the home care she rendered to her family.

Noneconomic damages include pain, suffering, disability, disfigurement, and loss of the enjoyment of life. Although economic damages can be guided by hard numbers, juries are often left to decide what the value of a person's pain or suffering is. Many states have limited the amounts that can be awarded for these elements of damage.

Punitive damages are damages that are awarded to punish wrongful conduct and deter future unlawful conduct. These damages are quite rare in medical negligence cases except for rare cases that involve alcohol or drug use by caregivers or systemic negligence that is equivalent to intentional conduct. Some states also limit these damages.

Malpractice. Malpractice, as a form of negligence, can involve professional misconduct, unreasonable lack of skill or fidelity in professional duties, evil practice, or unethical conduct. There are three classifications of malpractice: (1) *Criminal* malpractice includes crimes such as assault and battery or euthanasia (handled in criminal court). (2) *Civil* malpractice includes negligence or practice below a reasonable standard (handled in civil court). (3) *Ethical* malpractice includes violations of professional ethics and may result in censure or disciplinary actions by licensure boards.

Intentional Torts. An intentional tort is a wrong perpetrated by someone who intends to break the law. In contrast, in negligence, the professional fails to exercise adequate care in doing what is otherwise permissible. The acts must be intentionally performed to produce the harm or must be performed with the belief that the result was likely to follow. These torts are more serious than the tort of negligence, in that the defendant intended to commit the wrong. Consequently, punitive and actual damages may be awarded. Examples of intentional torts are acts that involve defamation of character, invasion of privacy, deceit, infliction of mental distress, and assault and battery.

In the hospital, the unwarranted discussion of the patient's condition, diagnosis, or treatment for purposes other than the exchange of information is always deemed suspect in regard to defamation of character. Under the general title of defamation of character are the torts of libel and slander. **Slander** is the verbal defamation of an individual by false words by which his or her reputation is damaged. **Libel** is printed defamation by written words, cartoons, and such representations to cause the individual to be avoided or held in contempt. Libel and slander do not exist unless they are seen or heard by a third person. If the practitioner directed such remarks only to the individual involved, it would not be slanderous; if the remark was made in the presence of a third party, it might constitute slander.

Caution in regard to unauthorized disclosure of patient information is especially critical in cases involving diseases such as AIDS, which often carries a high degree of medical and social stigma. Patients have the legal right to expect that all information about their illness would be held in strict confidence. Several states now have civil liability and criminal penalties for the release of confidential HIV test results in which the breach of confidence results in economic, psychologic, or bodily harm to the patient.

An **assault** is an intentional act that places another person in fear of immediate bodily harm. Threatening to injure someone is considered an act of assault. **Battery** represents unprivileged, nonconsensual physical contact with another person. In the classic act of assault and battery, one individual threatens and injures another.

Although battery is an unusual charge against a clinician (because of the nature of the work), it is one that creates special problems. The major element of battery is physical contact without consent. When a practitioner performs a procedure without the patient's consent, this contact may be considered battery. In most instances, there is an implied consent, created when the patient solicits care from the physician. This implied consent allows the performance of ordinary procedures without written consent. In all cases of unusual, difficult, or dangerous procedures, such as surgery, the courts require written consent. For this reason, to avoid being accused of battery, RTs should always explain all procedures involving physical contact to their patients before they proceed.

There are two general defenses against intentional torts. The first defense is that there was a lack of intent to harm and that only clinicians who engage in intentional conduct are liable. For example, if a practitioner fainted during a procedure and caused the patient injury, he or she would not be liable because the action was involuntary. The second defense is that the patient gave consent to the procedure. If the patient consented to the action, knowing the risks involved, the practitioner would not be liable. Consent by the patient for both nonroutine and routine procedures should be obtained before care is rendered.

Strict Liability. **Strict liability** is a theory in tort law that can be used to impose liability without fault, even in situations where injury occurs under conditions of reasonable care. The most common cases of strict liability are cases involving the use of dangerous products or techniques. Courts have imposed this principle on medical equipment manufacturers and on hospitals. However, strict liability generally has not been extended to professional services.

Breach of Contract. **Breach of contract** is a much rarer malpractice claim than negligence. This claim is based on the theory that when a health care professional renders care, an implicit or explicit professional-patient "contract" is established. Essentially, the contract binds the health care professional to place the patient's welfare as the foremost concern, to act only in the patient's behalf, to protect the patient's life, to preserve the patient's health, to relieve suffering, and to protect privacy. When the patient is injured as a result of the services rendered under this contract, the patient may claim that the failure of the health care professional to perform the service competently is a breach of the contract.

RTs are responsible for their actions, as are members of all other professions. When these actions result in the injury of another, the injured party may turn to the courts for redress. If the RT, while acting for the physician, injures the patient through some negligent act, the patient may sue both the RT and the physician.

Civil Suits. Civil action can be brought for many reasons, such as to challenge a law or to enjoin an activity. However, as in the case of malpractice suits, most civil suits seek monetary damages. The following scenario is an example of a situation that might involve the RT: The physician intends to order 0.5 ml of a bronchodilator for a 3-year-old asthmatic patient but inadvertently prescribes 5.0 ml of the drug. Because of the overdose given by the RT, the child dies.

A clearly articulated legal principle in negligence is that the duty owed to the patient is commensurate with the patient's needs. In short, the more vulnerable the patient, the greater is the caregiver's duty to protect. When the order is unclear or seems inappropriate under this principle, clinicians have an obligation to clarify rather than risk harm.

The suit could be brought against the physician for negligence for ordering the overdose, against the nurses and RT for failing to recognize that the dose was incorrect for the child, and, possibly, against the pharmacist for failing to gain adequate information as to the nature of the patient so that an appropriate dosage could be calculated. The plaintiff would base the secondary charges against the nurses and allied health practitioners on the theory that liability would be incurred by the individuals who missed an opportunity to correct the first wrongdoer's mistake. The hospital's risk management department and legal counsel can sometimes provide direction and counsel to the RT in the case of a civil suit. However, every respiratory care professional should have his or her own policy of malpractice insurance. Such insurance is available through the AARC, and it provides RTs with an attorney not only to represent them in the case of a malpractice lawsuit, but also in those rare instances where a professional board questions the conduct of the RT. Should a judgment result, it protects the RT not only from the plaintiff, but also from any settling defendant who attempts to point the finger at the RT. It is crucial that the RT adhere to professional legal advice and not try to "go it alone" in a malpractice case.

Avoiding Lawsuits

There is no foolproof formula for avoiding lawsuits because the right to bring suit cannot be denied under the U.S. legal system. From a legal perspective, a practitioner should always adhere to the goal of delivering and documenting care in such a manner that (1) a legal cause of action would be difficult to develop, and (2) if a lawsuit were filed, the success of the lawsuit would be highly unlikely. Key components of this goal include being aware of and conforming to all legal requirements of licensure, institutional practice policies and procedures, and acceptable standards of care. In addition, institutional risk management processes should be an ongoing component of departmental operation and professional development. If the possibility of a lawsuit becomes a certainty, an alternative such as mediation might be an option. However, when any potential legal action surfaces, decisions should be made with full input of institutional risk management and legal counsel.

In recent years, the experience of several large hospital systems has suggested that active risk management practices and appropriate guest relations policies are two of the most effective tools in preventing malpractice litigation. Unhappy patients are identified quickly, and corrective action is implemented immediately. Good guest relations programs encourage listening that often results in better clinical decision making, preventing the malpractice that is at the heart of every medical malpractice lawsuit. The best malpractice policy money cannot buy is a good sound relationship with the patient that communicates to the patient that he or she is important and valued.

Health Insurance Portability and Accountability Act of 1996

In August 1996, the U.S. Congress enacted HIPAA, which required, among other things, the establishment of Standards for Privacy of Individually Identifiable Health Information. These standards, which have become known as simply the Privacy Rule, added a major dimension to the need to treat medical records and information as confidential. The Privacy Rule was developed, with public comment and input, in the years following the enactment of HIPAA. The final rule was issued in March 2002. Updates to the Privacy Rule are likely to continue, making it imperative that the practitioner remain up-to-date with the latest requirements of the rule. The primary goal of the rule was to strike a balance between protecting individuals' health information and not impeding the exchange of information needed to provide quality health care and protect the public's health and well-being.[16]

The Privacy Rule applies to all health care providers, health plan providers (with some exceptions, such as small employer plans with <50 participants administered solely by the employer), and health care clearinghouses. An example of a health care clearinghouse is an entity that processes insurance claims for payment. Some of the exceptions are complex and are beyond the scope of this chapter. The practitioner in clinical practice need not be concerned with particular exceptions because, in most cases, basic patient confidentially requires a standard at least equal to the strictest interpretation of the Privacy Rule.[16]

The basic goal of the Privacy Rule is to protect all "individually identifiable health information," commonly referred to as *protected health information (PHI)*. Protected information includes any record or information that would or could identify or reveal (1) an individual's past, present, or future physical or mental health or condition; (2) the provision of health care to the individual; or (3) the past, present, or future payment for the provision of health care to the individual. PHI includes information in any format, which may include patient charts (electronic or paper), faxes, e-mails, or other records. The Privacy Rule provides avenues for the normal and appropriate conduct of health care treatment and business for all "covered entities" and individuals and organizations that have a legitimate need to access and use the information. Consent of the individual is not required for these covered entities.[16]

Medical Supervision

RTs are required by their scope of practice to work under competent medical supervision. This requirement creates not only a professional relationship but also a legal one. If the RT is employed by the physician, the physician is liable for the RT's actions. If the RT is employed by the hospital, the hospital is liable for the RT's actions. Under the laws of some states, the supervising physician may still be liable even if the RT is employed by the hospital where the legal theory involves a failure to supervise. The legal framework for this liability is rooted in centuries-old common law. When tradesmen had apprentices and masters had servants, the negligence of the apprentice or servant was imputed to the master who controlled the action of the servants. Under modern law, an employer is deemed a master, and an employee is deemed a servant. This principle, sometimes called vicarious liability, is premised on this centuries-old concept expressed in Latin as ***respondeat superior*** ("let the master answer").

MINI CLINI

HIPAA

PROBLEM: You, the RT, are in Ms. Smith's room tending to her respiratory equipment when the telephone rings. Ms. Smith as well as some of her family members are well known to you because of her many previous hospitalizations. During this hospitalization, Ms. Smith's condition has progressively worsened and today has been a particularly bad day for her. At this point, she is having serious difficulty moving and even talking. As the telephone rings, she looks at you and in a barely audible voice asks you to please answer the telephone. You do so, and the person on the other end identifies herself as Ms. Smith's granddaughter. You tell Ms. Smith that her granddaughter is on the telephone, but Ms. Smith simply looks away. You tell the granddaughter that Ms. Smith cannot talk right now and to call back later. The granddaughter asks you why Ms. Smith cannot talk, along with a series of specific questions about her condition.

DISCUSSION: As the RT, how should you handle this situation?

1. What HIPAA guidelines, if any, are applicable in this case?
2. Because you know Ms. Smith and her family, is it permissible to answer the granddaughter's questions?
3. To avoid alarming the granddaughter, should you say Ms. Smith is asleep or in the bathroom?

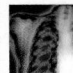

Under this doctrine, the physician assumes responsibility for the wrongful actions of the RT as long as such negligence occurred in the course of the employer-employee relationship. For this liability to be incurred, two conditions must be met: (1) The act must be within the scope of employment, and (2) the injury caused must be the result of an act of negligence. If the RT acted outside of his or her scope of practice, as outlined by licensure laws or by institutional regulations, the court would have to decide whether the physician would still be liable. If the

RT, while in the patient's room to deliver an aerosol treatment, went beyond the normal scope of practice and adjusted cervical traction, causing injury, it is doubtful that the physician could be held fully responsible. However, under the principle of *respondeat superior,* the hospital, as a corporate entity, could be held responsible for the actions of its employees.

Historically, RTs have not been named individually as defendants in malpractice cases because the law generally has not focused on their role as specialized health care providers separate from the health care facility. Either the hospital or the physician is usually named as the defendant for the acts of the practitioner. RTs in these cases have been viewed simply as employees, merely carrying out the orders of a superior. However, with the increased application of state licensure regulations governing respiratory care, and especially with the development of respiratory care protocols giving RTs more autonomy, this relative protection from liability is changing rapidly. As RTs are given more discretion and are permitted to exercise independent judgment, their decision making is likely to be more frequently called into question in court.

Scope of Practice

One measure of professionalism is the extent to which the group is willing to direct its own development and regulate its own activities. This self-direction is carried out mainly through professional associations and state licensure boards, which attempt to ensure that professionals exhibit minimum levels of competence.

Basic Elements of a Practice Act. Some practice acts emphasize one area over another, but most acts address the following elements:

- Scope of professional practice
- Requirements and qualifications for licensure
- Exemptions
- Grounds for administrative action
- Creation of examination board and processes
- Penalties and sanctions for unauthorized practice

Licensure Laws and Regulations. In licensure legislation, there is always a clause specifying a scope of practice. The scope-of-practice statutes give general guidelines and parameters for the clinician's practice. Deviation from these statutes could be a source of legal problems as the specialty seeks to add new duties. Practitioners must know the limits of their scope of care and seek amendments to the licensure regulations as they expand their practice. Ideally, the original language of a licensure law should be broad enough to account for changes in practice without requiring continual amendment. Continuing education and regular review of the practice act are essential to ensure compliance with both the statute and evolving rules of the practice act.

Providing Emergency Care Without Physician Direction. One unique area that allows practice without the direction of a competent physician is that of rendering emergency medical care to injured persons. Good Samaritan laws protect citizens from civil or criminal liability for any errors they make while attempting to give emergency aid. Most states have legislated Good Samaritan statutes to encourage individuals to give needed emergency medical assistance. It is necessary for this aid to be given in good faith and free of gross negligence or willful misconduct. However, it is unlikely that the RT would be protected for giving aid that went beyond the expected skills of the individual or aid that went beyond that which could be defined as first aid, such as performing a tracheostomy. Good Samaritan rules generally apply only to roadside accidents and emergency situations outside the hospital, although this is not always the case. The doctrine has sometimes been used by physicians inside a health care organization who respond to an emergency on a patient who is not their own. However, in California, the statute for respiratory care practitioners specifically extends protection only where the acts of the RT are "outside both the place and the course of employment..." (Cal. Bus. & Prof. Code § 3706).

INTERACTION OF ETHICS AND THE LAW

A good example of the interaction of ethics and the law in respiratory care is the diversification of the field into home care and durable medical equipment supply. This diversification has led to new relationships between these elements of the health care system and has created the potential for unethical and unlawful activity. If a practitioner accepts some remuneration, such as a finder's fee or percentage of the total lease costs for referring patients to a particular home care company or equipment service, he or she should be prepared to face charges of unethical and perhaps illegal practice.

Several federal statutes address the legality of these types of transactions. Many states also have statutes. Generally, these statutes state that anyone who knowingly or willfully solicits, receives, offers, or pays directly or indirectly any remuneration in return for Medicare business is guilty of a criminal offense. Violation of these statutes carries the potential for prison or a substantial fine, or both. In addition, violation of the statutes by an organization can result in exclusion from Medicare and other federal health care programs.

In recent years, hospitals have been encouraged to appoint a corporate compliance officer (CCO) to oversee the hospital's business practices and ensure that they conform to the law. In most hospitals with a working compliance plan, the CCO is freely available to discuss legal or ethical issues arising in the course of care. Appointed by the board of directors and reporting both to the hospital administration and to the board, the CCO can often address legal issues quickly and competently. Most hospitals use a toll-free anonymous number to allow employees who wish to remain anonymous to report wrongful activity. Most employees feel a loyalty to their organization and frequently use this method to address serious wrongdoing inside a facility. If the practitioner is aware of others who are engaged in these practices, he or she should report these activities to the appropriate state or federal health care agency. To aid the clinician in maintaining an ethical stance on these new issues, the AARC has established a position statement about ethical performance of respiratory home care.

PROFESSIONAL LICENSURE ISSUES

Because nearly every state has now passed some form of licensure for respiratory care practitioners, more RTs are being disciplined for various offenses related to the practice of respiratory care. Most RTs serve their entire professional careers and never have a problem with their professional boards. There are four significant things that RTs can be aware of now that would help prevent problems with their professional boards later.

Licensure Statute

All RTs should know in detail the requirements of their Respiratory Care Practice Act. They should know what is expected of them in terms of obtaining licensure and in the requirements to remain licensed. After receiving licenses, many professionals never look at their statute and never evaluate what actions are mandated by the rules and regulations enacted by their board. Some states by statute require that RTs report certain behavior.

§ 3758.5. Reporting Violations

If a licensee has knowledge that another person may be in violation of, or has violated, any of the statutes or regulations administered by the board, the licensee shall report this information to the board in writing and shall cooperate with the board in furnishing information or assistance as may be required.

California Respiratory Care Practice Act

Some states also require that employers make reports not only on individuals terminated for cause but also on the supervisors of the RTs.

§ 3758.6. Report on Supervisor

1. (a) In addition to the reporting required under Section 3758, an employer shall also report to the board the name, professional licensure type and number, and title of the person supervising the licensee who has been suspended or terminated for cause, as defined in subdivision (b) of Section 3758. If the supervisor is a licensee under this chapter, the board shall investigate whether due care was exercised by that supervisor in accordance with this chapter. If the supervisor is a health professional, licensed by another licensing board under this division, the employer shall report the name of that supervisor and any and all information pertaining to the suspension or termination for cause of the person licensed under this chapter to the appropriate licensing board.
2. (b) The failure of an employer to make a report required by this section is punishable by an administrative fine not to exceed $10,000 per violation.

The second thing all RTs should do to protect themselves against licensure issues is to purchase an insurance policy that covers professional discipline. Most policies available for purchase by RTs provide for coverage of both malpractice liability and professional discipline.

Understanding the Causes of Discipline

A review of professional discipline cases available from publicly available sources, including the California Board for Respiratory Care, reveals that the most frequent causes of professional discipline are as follows:

- Substance abuse
- Domestic violence
- Sexual abuse
- Gross incompetence

Even in cases where the cause of discipline is rooted in domestic violence or sexual abuse of another person, some form of substance abuse is a contributing factor. Alcohol violations (DWI [driving while impaired]) are often the most frequent violation that brings an RT face-to-face with his or her professional board. RTs with alcoholism or a significant drug habit are almost certain to come before their professional board. Sometimes employers and supervisors take the position that as long as such a problem does not affect a person's work at the facility, they should not address it. However, even in cases where an RT does not use drugs or alcohol at work, the disease process is affecting their judgment and decision making and should be addressed. A supervisor who fails to report a substance abuser of any kind is asking for legal trouble, in the form of either a damages lawsuit or a visit from the professional board. Academic respiratory care practitioners should be especially vigilant with students and should insist on substance abuse counseling for any student who appears to have such a problem.

Sometimes human resources personnel and administrators do not see the value in addressing these kinds of problems and may counsel against discipline for impaired workers. Sometimes supervisors, needing a warm body to fill positions, ignore the behaviors that should be red flags. Sometimes the human resources department may have made exceptions for other workers and fears that these exceptions may permit an inference of discrimination. None of these excuses would sound good to a jury.

Any good attorney would tell you that it is far better to defend a wrongful termination lawsuit than a wrongful death lawsuit. If you are wrong about the termination, the employee can be rehired. There is no remedy for the patient when an employee's substance abuse leads to that patient's death.

Engaging Counsel

If approached by the professional board, an RT should never talk to investigators without an attorney present. Every investigation is by its nature oppressive and burdensome, and an attorney ensures that the RT's rights are respected and protected. Often in cases in which an RT has violated the professional code or engaged in conduct that merits discipline, an attorney can help negotiate a better resolution than the RT could without the help of a professional.

RESPIRATORY THERAPISTS WHO SPEAK OUT ABOUT WRONGDOING

RTs are in a unique position to help protect patients from multiple harms. Sometimes they have a duty to speak out about problems or issues in the department. Usually a CCO is the most effective way to effect change inside an organization. However, sometimes the person who speaks out and identifies a problem still faces retaliation. Several federal laws protect RTs who, because of their respect for ethical issues, speak out about wrongdoing.

Patient Protection and Affordable Care Act

In 2010, Congress passed the Patient Protection and Affordable Care Act (PPACA) in an attempt to reform health care. Challenges to the PPACA are still finding their way through the state and federal courts, and results to date have been mixed. One thing that the statute did was improve whistleblower protections for hospital workers. Section 1558 of the PPACA amends the Fair Labor Standards Act of 1938 (FLSA) by adding Section 18C, which provides that an employer cannot discriminate "against any employee with respect to his or her compensation, terms, conditions, or other privileges of employment" because the employee, among other things:

1. Provided, caused to be provided, or is about to provide or cause to be provided to the employer, the Federal Government, or the attorney general of a State information relating to the violation of, or any act or omission the employee reasonably believes to be a violation of, any provision of this title;
2. Actually did or is about to assist, participate, or testify in a proceeding about such violation; or
3. Objected to or refused to participate in any activity or task that the employee "reasonably believed" to be in violation of the statute or any rule or regulation promulgated under the statute.

Any employee who believes that he or she has been discharged or discriminated against in violation of Section 18C of the FLSA is entitled to seek relief using the same procedures provided in 15 U.S.C. §2087(b), which contains the extensive whistleblower protections contained in the Consumer Product Safety Improvement Act of 2008. These procedures include filing a complaint concerning discrimination or retaliation with the Department of Labor, going through an administrative process to determine whether the employee's conduct protected by Section 18C was "a contributing factor in the unfavorable personnel action" alleged by the employee, and providing for the filing of a civil action in federal court after exhaustion of the administrative remedies provided by the statute.

Section 1558 explicitly limits application of Section 18C only to violations of the statute's central provisions related to medical care in hospital and clinic settings. Employees who report fraud, waste, or violations in traditional health care settings fall under the protections afforded by Section 1558. In most cases, an employee needs legal advice to pursue remedies under this section of the FLSA.

National Labor Relations Act

Although the National Labor Relations Act (NLRA) is usually thought of as a "union" statute, the NLRA provides protections to hospital workers whether they are organized into a union or not. Specifically, the NLRA provides for protection where a worker engages in actions for the benefit of all employees. For example, when an RT approaches the supervisor on behalf of all the workers on the second shift to request that shift differentials be increased, that RT—who is engaged in what is called "protected concerted activity"—cannot be discharged for acting on behalf of the other RTs in the department. When an RT is discharged for such an offense, the RT has 180 days in which to make a complaint to the local office of the National Labor Relations Board. No attorney is necessary to make such a complaint.

False Claims Act

Buried in the banking section of the United States Code is a little-known statute called the False Claims Act (FCA) (31 USC § 3729). The statute forbids making false claims against the government and provides for severe sanctions for people who do. Someone making a false claim against a government health care program can be made to repay three times the amount of the false claim plus a civil penalty of $5500 to $11,000 per false claim. Similar to the whistleblower protections built into the PPACA, the FCA contains language that prevents retaliation against an employee who gathers information or supports a government case against his or her employer. Remedies may include reinstatement and back pay.

Perhaps the most powerful part of the statute is the part that permits an employee with knowledge of fraud or false billing to file a lawsuit against the company or organization engaging in fraud. For example, when an emergency medical technician (EMT) knows that his employer is giving away free ambulance services to nursing homes in exchange for the Medicare business of the nursing homes, the EMT could file an FCA case against the employer.

The government investigates such lawsuits and frequently intervenes in them. Where the government intervenes, the employee who blows the whistle stands to receive an award of up to 25% of the amount the government recovers. In recent years, the United States has recovered greater than $3 billion in fraudulently paid claims, most of which came from employees who blew the whistle on the fraud of their employers or competitors.

HEALTH CARE AND CHANGE

The health care industry is experiencing rapid change relating to how services are funded and how patients and health care workers interact. These changes are occurring at the same time that ethical considerations are reemerging as significant components of how health care should be structured and delivered. Managed care affects the ethical decision-making process. Although the effect is not negative, it forces health care workers to take a new look at ethical dilemmas to arrive at both the best ethical outcome and the best managed care outcome. Patients no longer freely choose who will deliver health care services to them. Health care practitioners must consider not only the best services to deliver to patients but also the best managed care outcome.

If ethical reasoning is to be of any value, it must account for the reality of human experience and take into account changes in the health care system. Specific considerations include (1) factual premises and beliefs, such as the definition of death; (2) legal concepts, such as tort laws; (3) externally imposed mandates or expectations, such as hospital accreditation standards; and (4) the best managed care outcome. In many instances, such considerations uphold our moral convictions and provide support for a given action. The real challenge to RTs arises when moral principles dictate one course of action and factual knowledge, legal concepts, or external expectations dictate another.

Socrates demanded that professionals acknowledge the social context of their activities and that they recognize their obligations toward the segment of society that they profess to serve. As our analysis of ethical reasoning and the law has made clear, only by identifying, justifying, and prioritizing basic principles of human values can the RT resolve the difficult questions of professional behavior consistently. To the extent that clearly articulated principles guide our choices and actions, all involved will be well served.

RULE OF THUMB

The letters *RCP* are used to indicate respiratory care practitioner. They also suggest three important characteristics of the RT when confronted with ethical dilemmas:

*R*espect
*C*ompassion
*P*rofessionalism

Health Care Advance Directives

In recognition of the right of competent adults to exercise choices concerning their health care, all 50 states and the District of Columbia have adopted some form of health care advance directives. Although the federal government acknowledged the need for advance directives with the 1991 Patient Self-Determination Act by requiring that all hospitals receiving Medicaid or Medicare funds ascertain whether patients have or wish to have advance directives, the advance directive instruments are state regulated.

SUMMARY CHECKLIST

- Ethical dilemmas occur when there are two equally desirable or equally undesirable choices. Ethical dilemmas may involve situations that are either legal or illegal.
- Ethical dilemmas in respiratory care involve scope of practice, confidentiality, working within levels of professional responsibility, professional development issues, staffing patterns, or recordkeeping.
- Professional codes of ethics are general guidelines established to identify ideal behavioral parameters by members of a professional group. These codes are often simplistic and tend to deal with behavior over which there is little disagreement.
- Traditional ethical principles are rooted in philosophical thought and include autonomy, beneficence, confidentiality, role fidelity, justice, nonmaleficence, and veracity. These principles are used in the ethical decision-making process.
- There are two basic ethical theories: formalism and consequentialism. The most commonly used ethical decision-making model is the mixed approach. The mixed approach combines components of formalism, consequentialism, and modern decision-making theory.
- The basic information that must be identified before a reasoned ethical decision is made includes the problem or issue, the individuals involved, and the ethical principle or principles that apply; a determination of who should make the decision; and the role of the practitioner.
- Public law deals with the relationships of private parties and the government. Civil law is concerned with the recognition and enforcement of the rights and duties of private individuals and organizations.
- Professional malpractice is negligence in which a professional has failed to provide the care expected,

resulting in harm to someone. Examples of situations that RTs might encounter include attempting procedures beyond the practitioner's skill level, failure to perform a duty as assigned, or failure to perform the duty correctly.

- RTs, similar to members of other professions, are responsible for their actions. If their actions result in injury to others, the injured party or parties are entitled to seek redress in the courts.
- A professional license provides a framework under which a licensee carries out his or her duties. Because licensure acts define who can perform specified duties, it is expected that the duties will be performed in a responsible manner, and the professional will be responsible for his or her actions. The purpose of licensure is to provide for the public's safety. Practitioners must carry out their duties with an eye toward defending themselves in the case of legal action.
- Patients today are better educated and hold higher expectations from health care practitioners. Many patients are assuming responsibility for their own health care, placing the health care practitioner into the role of consultant.

References

1. Brincat CA, Wike VS: Morality and the professional life: values at work, Upper Saddle River, NJ, 2000, Prentice Hall.
2. Bowie, NE: Respecting the humanity in a person. In Ciulla JB, et al, editors: Honest work: a business ethics reader, New York, 2007, Oxford University Press.
3. Carroll C: Legal issues and ethical dilemmas in respiratory care, Philadelphia, 1996, FA Davis.
4. Edge R, Groves R: The ethics of health care: a guide for practice, Albany, NY, 1994, Delmar.
5. Beauchamp TL, Childress JF: Principles of biomedical ethics, ed 4, New York, 1994, Oxford University Press.
6. Boylan M: Business ethics: basic ethics in action, Upper Saddle River, NJ, 2001, Prentice Hall.
7. Husted GL, Husted JH: Ethical decision making in nursing, St Louis, 1991, Mosby.
8. Pickett JP, et al: The American Heritage Dictionary of the English Language, ed 4, Boston, 2000, Houghton Mifflin.
9. Logue B: Rights: death control and the elderly in America, New York, 1993, Macmillan.
10. Hill TP, Shirley D: A good death: taking more control at the end of your life, Reading, MA, 1992, Addison-Wesley.
11. World Medical Association Code of Medical Ethics, www.wma.net/en/30publications/10policies/c8/index.html.
12. Pozgar G: Legal aspects of health care administration, Gaithersburg, MD, 1990, Aspen Publishers.
13. Hippocrates: The oath. In Jones WHS, translator: The Loeb classical library: Hippocrates, no. 147–150, Cambridge, MA, 1948, Harvard University Press.
14. Sernick-Weinstein TH: Risk manager's practical guide to bringing a forward looking approach to a hospital risk management program, http://www.zurichna.com/internet/zna/SiteCollectionDocuments/en/Products/healthcare/PerspectivesHCnwsltrFall.pdf/ accessed August 14, 2011.
15. Ross WD: The right and the good, Oxford, 1930, Clarendon Press.
16. U.S. Department of Health and Human Services: Summary of the HIPAA Privacy Rule. Revised 2003. http://www.hhs.gov/ocr/privacysummary.pdf.

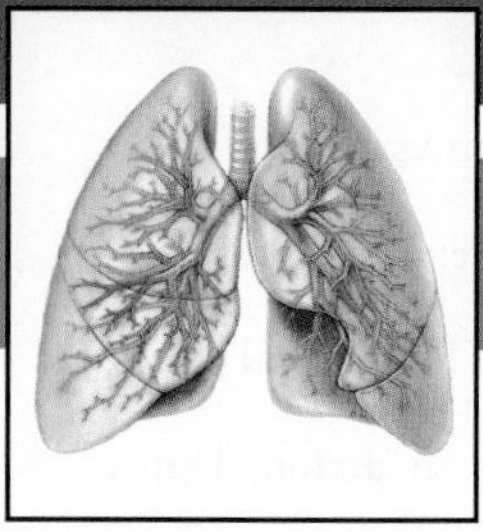

Chapter 6

Physical Principles of Respiratory Care

DANIEL F. FISHER

CHAPTER OBJECTIVES

After reading this chapter you will be able to:

- Describe the properties that characterize the three states of matter.
- Describe how heat transfer occurs among substances.
- Identify the three common temperature scales and explain how to use them.
- Describe how substances undergo change of state.
- Identify the factors that influence the vaporization of water.
- Describe how water vapor capacity, absolute humidity, and relative humidity are related.
- Describe how to predict gas behavior under changing conditions, including at extremes of temperature and pressure.
- Describe the principles that govern the flow of fluids.

CHAPTER OUTLINE

States of Matter
- Internal Energy of Matter
- Heat and the First Law of Thermodynamics
- Heat Transfer
- Laws of Thermodynamics

Change of State
- Liquid-Solid Phase Changes (Melting and Freezing)
- Properties of Liquids
- Liquid-Vapor Phase Changes
- Properties of Gases

Gas Behavior Under Changing Conditions
- Gas Laws
- Effect of Water Vapor
- Properties of Gases at Extremes of Temperature and Pressure
- Critical Temperature and Pressure

Fluid Dynamics
- Pressures in Flowing Fluids
- Patterns of Flow
- Flow, Velocity, and Cross-Sectional Area
- Bernoulli Effect
- Fluid Entrainment
- Venturi and Pitot Tubes
- Fluidics and Coanda Effect

KEY TERMS

absolute humidity
adhesion
ATPS
Avogadro's law
BTPS
Coanda effect
cohesion
condensation
conduction
convection
critical temperature
Dalton's law
dew point
evaporation
flow resistance
fluid entrainment
Graham's law
Henry's law
kinetic energy
laminar flow
Laplace's law
latent heat of fusion
latent heat of vaporization
law of continuity
laws of thermodynamics
melting point
Pascal's principle
Poiseuille's law
potential energy
radiation

relative humidity (RH)
Reynold's number (NR)
solubility coefficient
specific gravity
STPD
strain-gauge pressure transducers
surface tension
thermal conductivity
thermodynamics
turbulent flow
vaporization
viscosity
water vapor pressure

STATES OF MATTER

There are three primary states of matter: solid, liquid, and gas. Figure 6-1, *A-C* depicts simplified models of these states of matter.

Solids have a fixed volume and shape. The molecules that make up the solid have the shortest distance to travel until they collide with one another. This motion has been referred to as a "jiggle." Solids have a high degree of internal order; their atoms or molecules are limited to back-and-forth motion about a central position, as if held together by springs (see Figure 6-1, *A*). Solids maintain their shape because their atoms are kept in place by strong mutual attractive forces, called *van der Waals forces.*[1]

Liquids have a fixed volume, but adapt to the shape of their container. If a liquid is not held within a container, the shape is determined by numerous internal and external forces. Liquid molecules exhibit mutual attraction. However, because these forces are much weaker in liquids than in solids, liquid molecules can move about freely (see Figure 6-1, *B*). This freedom of motion explains why liquids take the shape of their containers and are capable of flow. However, similar to solids, liquids are dense and cannot be compressed easily.

In a *gas,* molecular attractive forces are very weak. Gas molecules, which lack restriction to their movement, exhibit rapid, random motion with frequent collisions (see Figure 6-1, *C*). Gases have no inherent boundaries and are easily compressed and expanded. Similar to liquids, gases can flow. For this reason, both liquids and gases are considered fluids. Gases have no fixed volume or shape. Both of these qualities depend on local conditions for the gas.

Plasma has been referred to as a fourth state of matter. Plasma is a combination of neutral atoms, free electrons, and atomic nuclei. Plasmas can react to electromagnetic forces and flow freely similar to a liquid or a gas (see Figure 6-1, *D*). Although mentioned here for the sake of completeness, plasmas are not discussed further because at this time they are not known to be relevant to the practice of respiratory care.

Internal Energy of Matter

All matter possesses energy. The energy matter possesses is called *internal energy*. There are two major types of internal energy: (1) the energy of position, or **potential energy,** and (2) the energy of motion, or **kinetic energy.**

The atoms of all matter, at ordinary temperatures, are in constant motion.[2] All matter has some kinetic energy. However, most internal energy in solids and liquids is potential energy. This potential energy is a result of the strong attractive forces between molecules. These intermolecular forces cause rigidity in solids and cohesiveness and

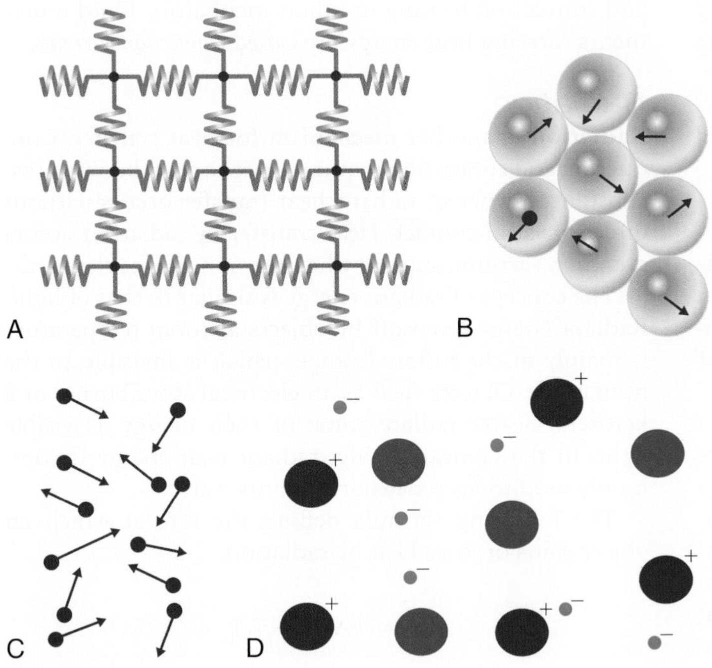

FIGURE 6-1 Simplified models of the four states of matter. **A,** Solid. **B,** Liquid. **C,** Gas. **D,** Plasma.

viscosity in liquids. In contrast, because these attractive forces are so weak in gases, most internal energy in gases is kinetic energy.

Heat and the First Law of Thermodynamics

The term **thermodynamics** can refer to either the science studying the properties of matter at various temperatures or the kinetics (speed) of reactions of matter at various temperatures. From the science of thermodynamics, various principles have been described **(laws of thermodynamics).** Knowing the basics of these principles is helpful in understanding other aspects of respiratory care.

According to the *first law of thermodynamics,* energy can be neither created nor destroyed, only transformed in nature. Any energy a substance gains must exactly equal the energy lost by its surroundings. Conversely, if a substance loses energy, this loss must be offset by an equal gain in the energy of its surroundings. This is stated as a simple formula:

$$U = E + W$$

where U is the internal energy of an object, E is the energy transferred to or from the object, and W is the external work performed on the object. In this sense, the quantity E is equivalent to heat. Heating is the transfer of internal energy from a high-temperature object to a low-temperature object. Based on this formula, you can increase the internal energy of an object by heating it or by performing work on it.

Heat Transfer

When two objects exist at different temperatures, the first law of thermodynamics tells us that heat will move from the hotter object to the cooler object until the objects' temperatures are equal. This is an example of transitioning from a higher state of order to a lower state. Two objects with the same temperature exist in thermal equilibrium. This heat transfer can be affected in four ways: (1) *conduction,* (2) *convection,* (3) *radiation,* and (4) *evaporation and condensation.*

Conduction

Heat transfer in solids occurs mainly via conduction. **Conduction** is the transfer of heat by direct contact between hot and cold molecules. How well heat transfers by conduction depends on both the number and the force of molecular collisions between adjoining objects.

Heat transfer between objects is quantified by using a measure called **thermal conductivity.** Table 6-1 lists the thermal conductivities of selected substances in cgs (centimeter-gram-second) system units. As is evident, solids, in particular, metals, tend to have high thermal conductivity. This is why metals feel cold to the touch even when at room temperature. In this case, the high thermal conductivity of metal quickly draws heat away from the skin, creating a feeling of "cold." In contrast, with fewer molecular collisions than in solids and liquids, gases exhibit low thermal conductivity.

TABLE 6-1

Thermal Conductivities in (cal/sec)/(cm² °C/cm)

Material	Thermal Conductivity (k)
Silver	1.01
Copper	0.99
Aluminum	0.50
Iron	0.163
Lead	0.083
Ice	0.005
Glass	0.0025
Concrete	0.002
Water at 20° C	0.0014
Asbestos	0.0004
Hydrogen at 0° C	0.0004
Helium at 0° C	0.0003
Snow (dry)	0.00026
Fiberglass	0.00015
Cork board	0.00011
Wool felt	0.0001
Air at 0° C	0.000057

From Nave CR, Nave BC: Physics for the health sciences, ed 3, Philadelphia, 1985, WB Saunders.

Convection

Heat transfer in both liquids and gases occurs mainly by convection. **Convection** involves the mixing of fluid molecules at different temperatures. Although air is a poor heat conductor (see Table 6-1), it can efficiently transfer heat by convection. To do so, the air is first warmed in one location and then circulated to carry the heat elsewhere; this is the principle behind forced-air heating in houses and convection heating in infant incubators. Fluid movements carrying heat energy are called *convection currents.*

Radiation

Radiation is another mechanism for heat transfer. Conduction and convection require direct contact between two substances, whereas radiant heat transfer occurs without direct physical contact. Heat transfer by radiation occurs even in a vacuum, such as when the sun warms the earth.

The concept of radiant energy is similar to that of light. Radiant energy given off by objects at room temperature is mainly in the infrared range, which is invisible to the human eye. Objects such as an electrical stove burner or a kerosene heater radiate some of their energy as visible light. In the clinical setting, radiant heat energy is commonly used to keep newborn infants warm.

The following formula defines the rate at which an object gains or loses heat by radiation:

$$\frac{E}{t} = ekA\,(T_2 - T_1)$$

In this formula, E/t is the heat loss or gain per unit time. The symbol *e* is the emissivity of the object, or its relative effectiveness in radiating heat. The constant *k* is the Stefan-Boltzmann constant (based on mass and surface area). A is the area of the radiating object, and T_1 and T_2 are the temperatures of the environment and the object. In simple terms, for an object with a given emissivity, the larger the surface area (relative to mass) and the lower the surrounding temperature, the greater is the radiant heat loss per unit time.

Evaporation and Condensation

Vaporization is the change of state from liquid to gas. Vaporization requires heat energy. According to the first law of thermodynamics, this heat energy must come from the surroundings. In one form of vaporization, called **evaporation,** heat is taken from the air surrounding the liquid, cooling the air. In warm weather or during strenuous exercise, the body takes advantage of this principle of *evaporation cooling* by producing sweat. The liquid sweat evaporates and cools the skin.

Condensation is the opposite of evaporation. During condensation, a gas turns back into a liquid. Because vaporization takes heat from the air around a liquid (cooling), condensation must give heat back to the surroundings (warming). A refrigerator works on the principle of repeated vaporization cycles. As the food in the cooler passes its warmth to the cooler condensed refrigerant, it provides enough heat to cause it to vaporize. Sufficient energy is provided for the material to vaporize and expand, which cools the system, and the cycle repeats. The next section expands on the concept of change of state and provides more detail on the processes of vaporization and condensation.

Laws of Thermodynamics

Three physical principles describe how energy is handled and transferred. These principles are known as the laws of thermodynamics.[3,4]

1. The law of *conservation of energy* states that energy cannot be created or destroyed. This law is usually stated as follows: The total amount of energy in a system is equal to the amount of heat put into the system minus the work.
2. The principle of *thermodynamic equilibrium* is that given time all systems achieve the lowest possible energy state (entropy).
3. The third law is a statistical law describing the *impossibility of achieving absolute zero*. As stated in the third law, at absolute zero all processes cease, and entropy is at a minimum value.

Internal Energy and Temperature

Two interrelated terms are significant when discussing thermodynamics: entropy and enthalpy. *Entropy* is the amount of energy in a system that is unavailable for work. Entropy is the lowest amount of organization that a system can achieve (chaos). *Enthalpy* is the total measure of energy in the system. Enthalpy can be considered to be the order of a system. Temperature and kinetic energy are closely related.[2] Temperature is a measurement of heat. Heat is the result of molecules colliding with one another. The temperature of a gas, with most of its internal energy spent keeping molecules in motion, is directly proportional to its kinetic energy. In contrast, the temperatures of solids and liquids represent only part of their total internal energy.

Absolute Zero

In concept, absolute zero is the lowest possible temperature that can be achieved. That is the temperature at which there is no kinetic energy. Because there is no energy, the molecules cease to vibrate, and the object has no heat that can be measured. This temperature is defined to be absolute zero. Although researchers have come close to attaining absolute zero, no one has actually achieved it; this is due to the third law of thermodynamics, which states absolute zero is impossible to achieve.

Temperature Scales

Multiple scales can be used to measure temperature. The Fahrenheit and Celsius scales are based on a property of water. A third scale, the Kelvin scale, is based on molecular motion. Absolute zero provides a logical zero point on which to build a temperature scale. The SI (International System of Units) units for temperature are measured in kelvin (K) with a lower case "k," with a zero point equal to absolute zero (0° K).[5-7] Because the Kelvin scale has 100 degrees between the freezing and boiling points of water, it is a centigrade, or 100-step, temperature scale. The Kelvin scale has the unique quality of being based on the triple point definition for water (the temperature where all three phases of water exist). This temperature happens to be approximately 273° K (0.0° C).[5-7]

The cgs temperature system is based on Celsius (C) units. Similar to the Kelvin scale, the Celsius scale is a centigrade scale (100 degrees between the freezing and boiling points of water). However, 0° C is not absolute zero but instead is the freezing point of water.

In Celsius units, kinetic molecular activity stops at approximately −273° C. Therefore 0° K equals −273° C, and 0° C equals 273° K. To convert degrees Celsius to degrees Kelvin, simply add 273:

$$^\circ K = ^\circ C + 273$$

For example:

$$25^\circ C = 25 + 273 = 298^\circ K$$

Conversely, to convert degrees Kelvin to Celsius, you simply subtract 273. For example:

$$310^\circ K = 310 - 273 = 37^\circ C$$

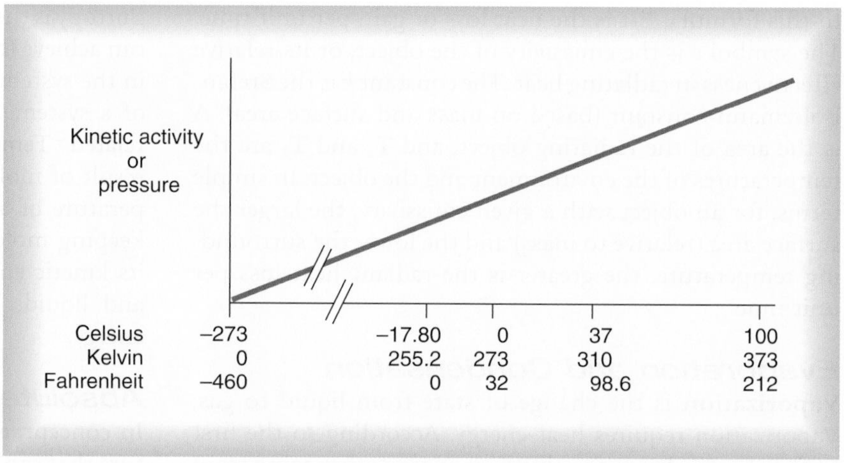

FIGURE 6-2 Linear relationship between gas molecular activity, or pressure, and temperature. The graph shows comparable readings on three scales for five temperature points.

The Fahrenheit scale is the primary temperature scale in the fps (foot, pound, and second) or British system of measurement. Absolute zero on the Fahrenheit scale equals –460° F.

To convert degrees Fahrenheit to degrees Celsius, use the following formula:

$$^\circ C = \frac{5}{9}(^\circ F - 32)$$

For example:

$$^\circ F = 98.6$$
$$^\circ C = \frac{5}{9} \times (98.6 - 32)$$
$$^\circ C = 37$$

To convert degrees Celsius to degrees Fahrenheit, simply reverse this formula:

$$^\circ F = \left(\frac{9}{5} \times {^\circ C}\right) + 32$$

For example:

$$^\circ C = 100$$
$$^\circ F = \left(\frac{9}{5} \times 100\right) + 32$$
$$^\circ F = 212$$

Figure 6-2 shows the relationship between the kinetic activity of matter and temperature on all three common temperature scales. For ease of reference, five key points are defined: the zero point of each scale, the freezing point of water (0° C), body temperature (37° C), and the boiling point of water (100° C).

CHANGE OF STATE

All matter can change state. Because respiratory therapists (RTs) work extensively with both liquids and gases, they must have a good understanding of the key characteristics of these states and the basic processes underlying their phase changes.

Liquid-Solid Phase Changes (Melting and Freezing)

When a solid is heated, its molecular kinetic energy increases. This added internal energy increases molecular vibrations. If enough heat is applied, these vibrations eventually weaken the intermolecular attractive forces. At some point, molecules break free of their rigid structure, and the solid changes into a liquid.

Melting

The changeover from the solid to liquid state is called *melting*. The temperature at which this changeover occurs is the **melting point.**[2] The range of melting points is considerable. For example, water (ice) has a melting point of 0° C, carbon has a melting point of greater than 3500° C, and helium has a melting point of less than –272° C.

Figure 6-3 depicts the phase change caused by heating water. At the left origin of –50° C, water is solid ice. As the ice is heated, its temperature increases. At its melting point of 0° C, ice begins to change into liquid water. However, the full change to liquid water requires additional heat. This additional heat energy changes the state of water but does not immediately change its temperature.

The extra heat needed to change a solid to a liquid is the **latent heat of fusion.** In cgs units, the latent heat of fusion is defined as the number of calories required to change 1 g of a solid into a liquid without changing its temperature. The latent heat of fusion of ice is 80 cal/g, whereas the latent heat of fusion of oxygen is 3.3 cal/g. This change of state, compared with simply heating a solid, requires enormous energy.

Freezing

Freezing is the opposite of melting. Because melting requires large amounts of externally applied energy, you would expect freezing to return this energy to the surroundings, and this is exactly what occurs. During

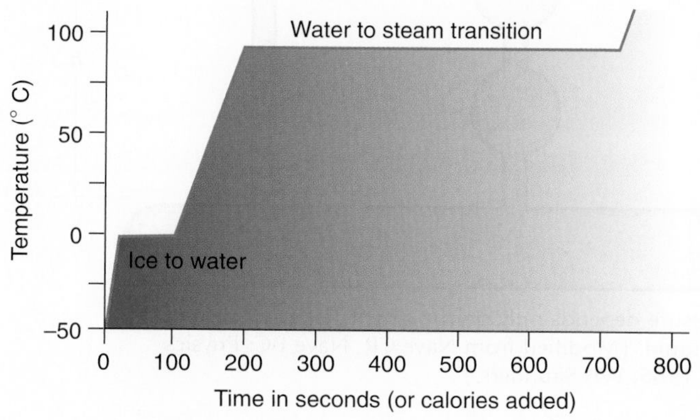

FIGURE 6-3 Temperature as a function of time for 1 g of water heated at the rate of 1 cal/sec. (Modified from Nave CR, Nave BC: Physics for the health sciences, ed 3, Philadelphia, 1985, WB Saunders.)

freezing, heat energy is transferred from a liquid back to the environment, usually by exposure to cold.

As the kinetic energy of a substance decreases, its molecules begin to regain the stable structure of a solid. According to the first law of thermodynamics, the energy required to freeze a substance must equal that needed to melt it. The freezing and melting points of a substance are the same.

Sublimation is the term used for the phase transition from a solid to a vapor without becoming a liquid as an intermediary form. An example of sublimation is dry ice (frozen carbon dioxide [CO_2]). Dry ice sublimates from its solid form into gaseous CO_2 without first melting and becoming liquid CO_2. This sublimation occurs because the vapor pressure is low enough for the intermediate liquid not to appear.

Properties of Liquids

Liquids exhibit flow and assume the shape of their container. Liquids also exert pressure, which varies with depth and density. Variations in liquid pressure within a container produce an upward supporting force, called *buoyancy.*

Although melting weakens intermolecular bonding forces, liquid molecules still attract one another. The persistence of these cohesive forces among liquid molecules helps explain the physical properties of viscosity, capillary action, and surface tension.

Pressure in Liquids

Liquids exert pressure. The *pressure* exerted by a liquid depends on both its *height* (depth) and *weight density* (weight per unit volume), which is shown in equation form:

$$P_L = h \times d_w$$

P_L is the static pressure exerted by the liquid, h is the height of the liquid column, and d_w is the liquid's weight density.

For example, to compute the pressure at the bottom of a 33.9-ft (1034-cm)-high column of water (density = 1 g/cm^3), you would use this equation:

$$\begin{aligned} P_L &= h \times d_w \\ &= 1034\ \text{cm} \times (1\ \text{g/cm}^3) \\ &= 1034\ \text{g/cm}^2 \end{aligned}$$

The answer (1034 g/cm^2) also equals 1 atmosphere of pressure (atm), or approximately 14.7 lb/in^2. This figure does not account for the additional atmospheric pressure (P_B) acting on the top of the liquid. The total pressure at the bottom of the column equals the sum of the atmospheric and liquid pressures. In this case, the total pressure is 2068 g/cm^2, equal to 29.4 lb/in^2, or 2 atm.

As shown in Figure 6-4, the pressure of a given liquid is the same at any specific depth (h), regardless of the container's shape. This is because the pressure of a liquid acts equally in all directions. This concept is called **Pascal's principle.**

Buoyancy (Archimedes' Principle)

Thousands of years ago, Archimedes showed that an object submersed in water appeared to weigh less than in air. This effect, called *buoyancy,* explains why certain objects float in water. Liquids exert buoyant force because the pressure below a submerged object always exceeds the pressure above it. This difference in liquid pressure creates an upward or supporting force. According to Archimedes' principle, this buoyant force must equal the weight of the fluid displaced by the object. Because the weight of fluid displaced by an object equals its weight density times its volume (d_w = V), the buoyant force (B) may be calculated as follows:

$$B = d_w \times V$$

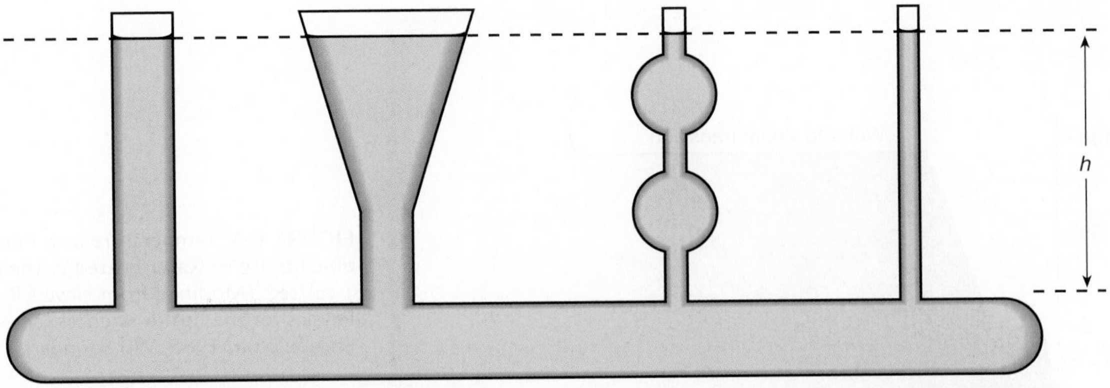

FIGURE 6-4 Pascal's principle. Liquid pressure depends only on the height (h) and not on the shape of the vessel or the total volume of liquid. (Modified from Nave CR, Nave BC: Physics for the health sciences, ed 3, Philadelphia, 1985, WB Saunders.)

If the weight density of an object is less than that of water (1 g/cm^3), it will displace a weight of water greater than its own weight. In this case, the upward buoyant force will overcome gravity, and the object will float. Conversely, if an object's weight density exceeds the weight of water, the object will sink.

Clinically, Archimedes' principle is used to measure the specific gravity of certain liquids. The term **specific gravity** refers to the ratio of the density of one fluid compared with the density of another reference substance, which is typically water. Figure 6-5 shows the use of a hydrometer to measure the specific gravity of urine. The specific gravity of gases also can be measured. In this case, oxygen or hydrogen is used as the standard instead of water.

Gases also exert buoyant force, although much less than that provided by liquids. Buoyancy helps keep solid particles suspended in gases. These suspensions, called *aerosols,* play an important role in respiratory care. More detail on the characteristics and use of aerosols is provided in Chapter 35.

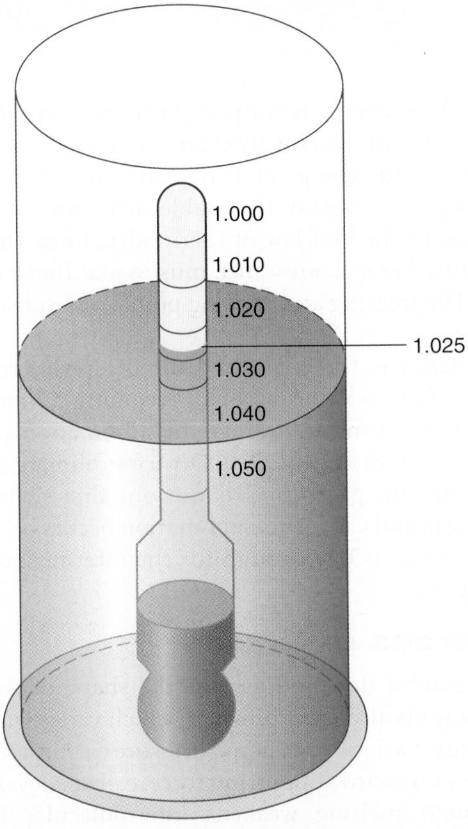

FIGURE 6-5 Using a hydrometer to measure the specific gravity of a urine specimen. The scale value of 1.025 indicates that this urine sample has a weight density 1.025 times greater than that of water.

Viscosity

Viscosity is the force opposing a fluid's flow. Viscosity in fluids is similar to friction in solids. The viscosity of a fluid is directly proportional to the cohesive forces between its molecules. The stronger these cohesive forces are, the greater the fluid's viscosity. The greater a fluid's viscosity, the greater its resistance to deformation, and the greater its opposition to flow.

Viscosity is most important when fluids move in discrete cylindrical layers, called *streamlines.* This pattern of motion is called **laminar flow.** As shown in Figure 6-6, frictional forces between the streamlines and the tube wall impede movement of the outer layers of a fluid. Each layer, moving toward the center of the tube, hinders the motion of the next inner layer less and less. Laminar flow consists of concentric layers of fluid flowing parallel to the tube wall at velocities that increase toward the center.

The difference in the velocity among these concentric layers is called the *shear rate.* The shear rate is simply a measure of how easily the layers separate. How easily the layers separate depends on two factors: (1) the pressure pushing or driving the fluid, called the *shear stress;* and (2) the viscosity of the fluid. Shear rate is directly proportional to shear stress and inversely proportional to viscosity.

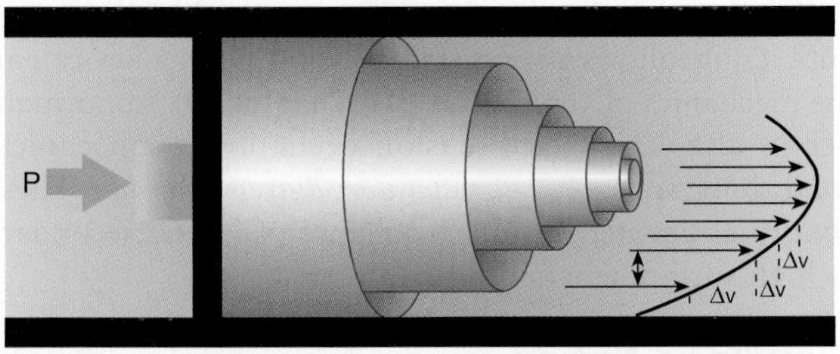

FIGURE 6-6 Effects of shear stress or pressure (P) on shear rate (velocity gradient [v]) in a Newtonian fluid. (Modified from Winters WL, Brest AN, editors: The microcirculation, Springfield, IL, 1969, Charles C Thomas.)

In uniform fluids such as water or oil, viscosity varies with temperature. Because higher temperatures weaken the cohesive forces between molecules, heating a uniform fluid reduces its viscosity. Conversely, cooling a fluid increases its viscosity. This is why a car's engine is so hard to start on a cold winter morning. The oil becomes so viscous that it impedes movement of the engine's parts.

Blood, in contrast to water or oil, is a complex fluid that contains not only liquid (plasma, which is 90% water) but also cells in suspension. For this reason, blood has a viscosity approximately five times greater than the viscosity of water. The greater the viscosity of a fluid, the more energy is needed to make it flow. The heart works harder to pump blood than it would if it were pumping water. The heart must perform even more work when blood viscosity increases, as occurs in *polycythemia* (an increase in red blood cell concentration in the blood).

Cohesion and Adhesion

The attractive force between like molecules is called **cohesion.** The attractive force between unlike molecules is called **adhesion.** These forces can be observed at work by placing a liquid in a small-diameter tube. As shown in Figure 6-7, the top of the liquid forms a curved surface, or *meniscus*. When the liquid is water, the meniscus is concave because the water molecules at the surface adhere to the glass more strongly than they cohere to each other (see Figure 6-7A). In contrast, a mercury meniscus is convex (see Figure 6-7B). In this case, the cohesive forces pulling the mercury atoms together exceed the adhesive forces trying to attract the mercury to the glass.

Surface Tension

Surface tension is a force exerted by like molecules at the surface of a liquid. A small drop of fluid provides a good illustration of this force. As shown in Figure 6-8, cohesive forces affect molecules inside the drop equally from all directions. However, only inward forces affect molecules on the surface. This imbalance in forces causes the surface film to contract into the smallest possible surface area, usually a sphere or curve (meniscus). This phenomenon explains why liquid droplets and bubbles retain a spherical shape.

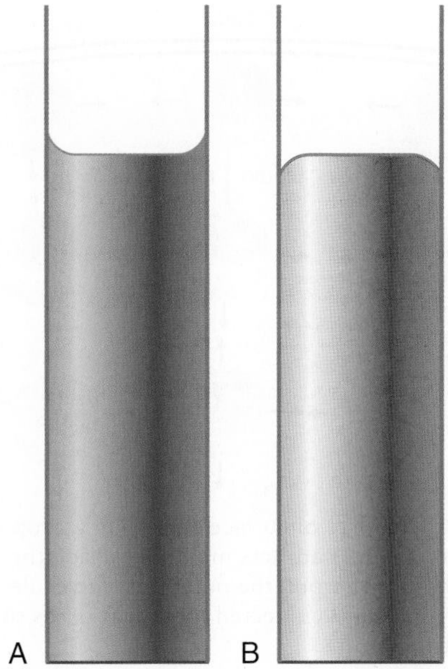

FIGURE 6-7 The shape of the meniscus depends on the relative strengths of adhesion and cohesion. **A,** Water: Adhesion stronger than cohesion. **B,** Mercury: Cohesion stronger than adhesion.

TABLE 6-2

Examples of Surface Tension

Substance	Temperature (° C)	Surface Tension (dynes/cm)
Water	20° C	73
Water	37° C	70
Whole blood	37° C	58
Plasma	37° C	73
Ethyl alcohol	20° C	22
Mercury	17° C	547

Surface tension is quantified by measurement of the force needed to produce a "tear" in a fluid surface layer. Table 6-2 lists the surface tensions of selected liquids in dynes/cm (cgs). For a given liquid, surface tension varies inversely with temperature: The higher the temperature, the lower is the surface tension.

Surface tension, similar to a fist compressing a ball, increases the pressure inside a liquid drop or bubble. According to **Laplace's law,** this pressure varies directly with the surface tension of the liquid and inversely with its radius. The equation for a liquid bubble follows:

$$P = \frac{2ST}{r}$$

P is the pressure in the bubble, ST is the surface tension, and r is the bubble radius. Figure 6-9 shows this relationship for two bubbles of different sizes, each with the same surface tension.

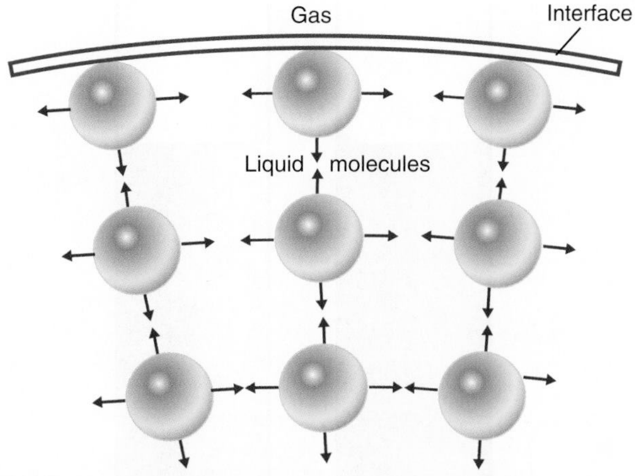

FIGURE 6-8 The force of surface tension in a drop of liquid. Cohesive force *(arrows)* attracts molecules inside the drop to one another. Cohesion can pull the outermost molecules inward only, creating a centrally directed force that tends to contract the liquid into a sphere.

Because the alveoli of the lungs resemble clumps of bubbles, it follows that surface tension plays a key role in the mechanics of ventilation (see Chapter 10). Abnormalities in alveolar surface tension occur in certain clinical conditions, such as *acute respiratory distress syndrome.* These abnormalities may result in collapse of alveoli secondary to high surface tension.

Capillary Action

Capillary action is a phenomenon in which a liquid in a small tube moves upward, against gravity. Capillary action involves both adhesive and surface tension forces. As shown in Figure 6-10, *A*, the adhesion of water molecules to the walls of a thin tube causes an upward force on the edges of the liquid and produces a concave meniscus.

Because surface tension acts to maintain the smallest possible liquid-gas interface, instead of just the edges of the liquid moving up, the whole surface is pulled upward.

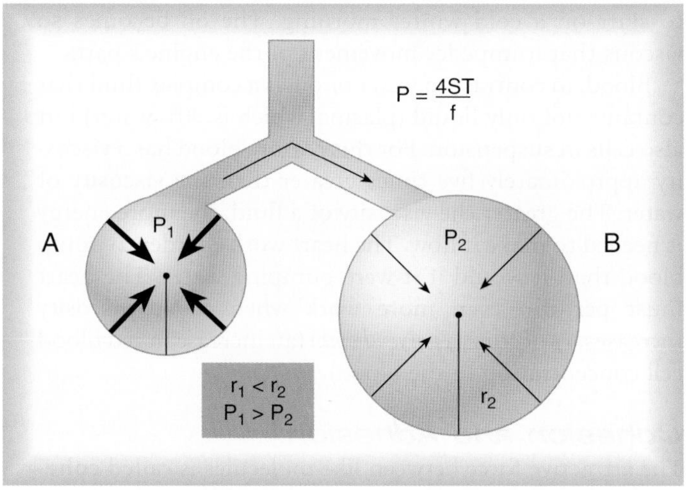

FIGURE 6-9 Laplace's relationship. Two bubbles of different sizes with the same surface tension. Bubble *A*, with the smaller radius, has the greater inward or deflating pressure and is more prone to collapse than the larger bubble *B*. Because the two bubbles are connected, bubble *A* would tend to deflate and empty into bubble *B*. Conversely, because of the greater surface tension of bubble *A*, it would be harder to inflate than bubble *B*.

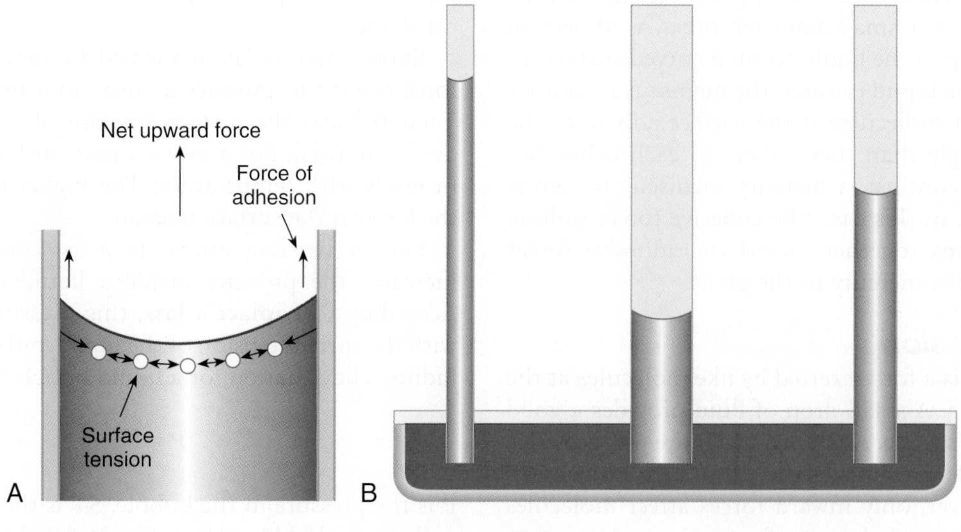

FIGURE 6-10 Capillary action. **A,** Adhesion and surface tension contribute to capillary action (capillarity). **B,** The liquid rises highest in the smallest tube. (Modified from Nave CR, Nave BC: Physics for the health sciences, ed 3, Philadelphia, 1985, WB Saunders.)

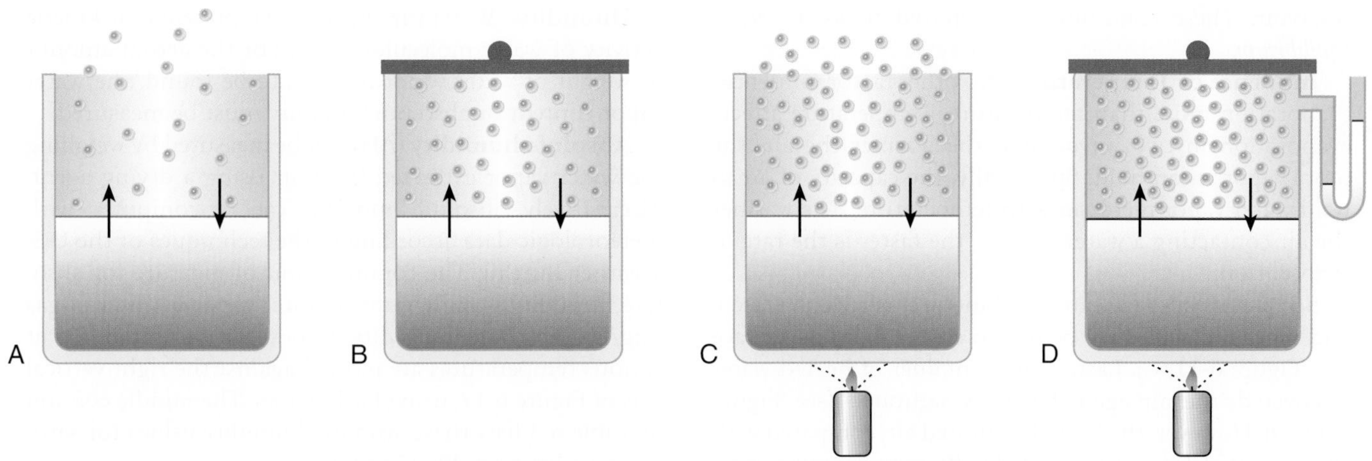

FIGURE 6-11 Factors influencing vaporization of water. See text for details.

How strong this force is depends on the amount of liquid that contacts the tube's surface. Because a small capillary tube creates a more concave meniscus and a greater area of contact, liquid rises higher in tubes with smaller cross-sectional areas (see Figure 6-10, *B*).

Capillary action is the basis for blood samples obtained by use of a capillary tube. The absorbent wicks used in some gas humidifiers are also an application of this principle, as are certain types of surgical dressings.

Liquid-Vapor Phase Changes

Only after ice completely melts does additional heat increase the temperature of the newly formed liquid (see Figure 6-3). As the water temperature reaches 100° C, a new change of state begins—from liquid to vapor. This change of state is called *vaporization.* There are two different forms of vaporization: *boiling* and *evaporation.*

Boiling

Boiling occurs at the boiling point. The *boiling point* of a liquid is the temperature at which its vapor pressure exceeds atmospheric pressure. When a liquid boils, its molecules must have enough kinetic energy to force themselves into the atmosphere against the opposing pressure. Because the weight of the atmosphere retards the escape of vapor molecules, the greater the ambient pressure, the greater is the boiling point. Conversely, when atmospheric pressure is low, liquid molecules escape more easily, and boiling occurs at lower temperatures. This is why cooking times must be increased at higher altitudes.

Although boiling is associated with high temperatures, the boiling points of most liquefied gases are very low. At 1 atm, oxygen boils at −183° C.

Energy is also needed to vaporize liquids, as with other phase changes. The energy required to vaporize a liquid is the **latent heat of vaporization.** In cgs units, the latent heat of vaporization is the number of calories required to vaporize 1 g of a liquid at its normal boiling point.

Melting weakens attractive forces between molecules, whereas vaporization eliminates them. Elimination of these forces converts essentially all of the internal energy of a substance into kinetic energy. For this reason, vaporization requires substantially more energy than melting. As shown in Figure 6-3, almost seven times more energy is needed to convert water to steam (540 cal/g) than is needed to melt ice.

Evaporation, Vapor Pressure, and Humidity

Boiling is only one type of vaporization. A liquid also can change into a gas at temperatures lower than its boiling point through a process called *evaporation.* Water is a good example (Figure 6-11). When at a temperature lower than its boiling point, water enters the atmosphere via evaporation. The liquid molecules are in constant motion, as in the gas phase. Although this kinetic energy is less intense than in the gaseous state, it allows some molecules near the surface to escape into the surrounding air as water vapor (see Figure 6-11, *A*).

After water is converted to a vapor, it acts like any gas. To be distinguished from visible particulate water, such as mist or fog, this invisible gaseous form of water is called *molecular water.* Molecular water obeys the same physical principles as other gases and exerts a pressure called **water vapor pressure.**

Evaporation requires heat. The heat energy required for evaporation comes from the air next to the water surface. As the surrounding air loses heat energy, it cools. This is the *principle of evaporative cooling,* which was previously described.

If the container is covered, water vapor molecules continue to enter the air until it can hold no more water (see Figure 6-11, *B*). At this point, the air over the water is saturated with water vapor. However, vaporization does not stop when saturation occurs. Instead, for every molecule escaping into the air, another returns to the water reservoir. These conditions are referred to as a *state of equilibrium*.

Influence of Temperature. No other factor influences evaporation more than temperature. Temperature affects evaporation in two ways. First, the warmer the air, the more vapor it can hold. Specifically, the capacity of air to hold water vapor increases with temperature. The warmer the air contacting a water surface, the faster is the rate of evaporation.

Second, if water is heated, its kinetic energy is increased, and more molecules are helped to escape from its surface (see Figure 6-11, *C*). Last, if the container of heated water is covered, the air again becomes saturated (see Figure 6-11, *D*). However, the heated saturated air, compared with the unheated air (see Figure 6-11, *B*), now contains more vapor molecules and exerts a higher vapor pressure (as shown by the manometer in Figure 6-11, *D*). The temperature of a gas affects both its capacity to hold molecular water and the water vapor pressure.

The relationship between water vapor pressure and temperature is shown graphically in Figure 6-12. The left vertical axis plots water vapor pressure in both mm Hg and kPa (kilopascal). The horizontal axis plots temperatures between 0° C and 70° C. This graph shows that the greater the temperature, the greater the saturated water vapor pressure (bold red dots). Table 6-3 lists actual water vapor pressures in saturated air in the clinical range of temperatures (20° C to 37° C).

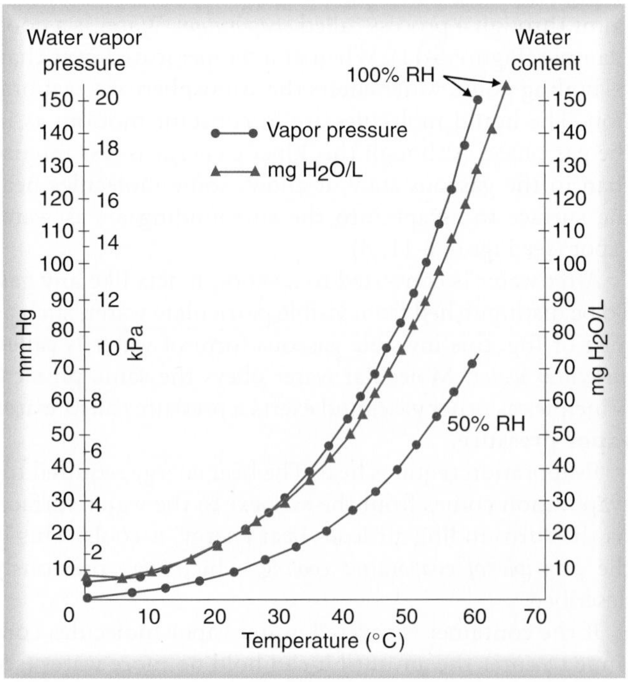

FIGURE 6-12 Water vapor pressure (P_{H_2O}) and absolute humidity (mg H_2O/L) curves for gas that is fully saturated (relative humidity [RH] = 100%) and gas that is half saturated (RH = 50%).

Humidity. Water vapor pressure represents the kinetic activity of water molecules in air. For the actual amount or weight of water vapor in a gas to be found, the water vapor content or absolute humidity must be measured.

Absolute humidity (AH) can be measured by weighing the water vapor extracted from air using a drying agent. Alternatively, absolute humidity can be computed with meteorologic data according to the techniques of the U.S. Weather Bureau. The common unit of measure for absolute humidity is milligrams of water vapor per liter of gas (mg/L). Absolute humidity values for saturated air at various temperatures are plotted against the right vertical axis of Figure 6-12, using hash marks. The middle column of Table 6-3 lists these absolute humidity values for saturated air between 20° C and 37° C.

A gas does not need to be fully saturated with water vapor. If a gas is only half saturated with water vapor, its water vapor pressure and absolute humidity are only half that in the fully saturated state. Air that is fully saturated with water vapor at 37° C and 760 mm Hg has a water vapor pressure of 47 mm Hg and an absolute humidity of 43.8 mg/L (see Table 6-3). However, if the same volume of air were only 50% saturated with water vapor, its water vapor pressure would be 0.50 × 47 mm Hg, or 23.5 mm Hg, and its absolute humidity would be 0.50 × 43.8 mg/L, or 21.9 mg/L.

When a gas is not fully saturated, its water vapor content can be expressed in relative terms using a measure called **relative humidity (RH).** The RH of a gas is the ratio of its actual water vapor content to its saturated capacity at a

TABLE 6-3

Water Vapor Pressures and Contents at Selected Temperatures

Temperature (° C)	Vapor Pressure (mm Hg)	Water Vapor Content (mg/L)	ATPS to BTPS Correction Factor*
20	17.50	17.30	1.102
21	18.62	18.35	1.096
22	19.80	19.42	1.091
23	21.10	20.58	1.085
24	22.40	21.78	1.080
25	23.80	23.04	1.075
26	25.20	24.36	1.068
27	26.70	25.75	1.063
28	28.30	27.22	1.057
29	30.00	28.75	1.051
30	31.80	30.35	1.045
31	33.70	32.01	1.039
32	35.70	33.76	1.032
33	37.70	35.61	1.026
34	39.90	37.57	1.020
35	42.20	39.60	1.014
36	44.60	41.70	1.007
37	47.00	43.80	1.000

*Correction factors are based on 760 mm Hg pressure.

given temperature. RH is expressed as a percentage and is derived with the following simple formula:

$$\%RH = \frac{\text{Content (absolute humidity)}}{\text{Saturated capacity}} \times 100$$

For example, saturated air at a room temperature of 20° C has the capacity to hold 17.3 mg/L of water vapor (see Table 6-3). If the absolute humidity is 12 mg/L, the RH is calculated as follows:

$$\%\ RH = \frac{12\ mg/L}{17.3\ mg/L} \times 100$$
$$\%RH = 0.69 \times 100$$
$$\%RH = 69\%$$

Actual water vapor content does not have to be measured for RH to be computed. Simple instruments called *hygrometers* allow direct measurement of RH without extracting and weighing the water in air.

When the water vapor content of a volume of gas equals its capacity, the RH is 100%. When the RH is 100%, a gas is fully saturated with water vapor. Under these conditions, even slight cooling of the gas causes its water vapor to turn back into the liquid state, a process called *condensation.*

Condensed moisture deposits on any available surface, such as on the walls of a container or delivery tubing or on particles suspended in the gas. Condensation returns heat to and warms the surrounding environment, whereas vaporization of water cools the adjacent air.

If air that is at an RH of 90% is cooled, its capacity to hold water vapor decreases. Although the water vapor capacity of the air decreases, its content remains constant. With a lower capacity but the same content, the RH of the air must increase. Continued cooling decreases the air's water vapor capacity until it eventually equals the water vapor content (RH = 100%). When content equals capacity, the air is fully saturated and can hold no more water vapor.

Because RH never exceeds 100%, any further decrease in temperature causes condensation. The temperature at which condensation begins is called the **dew point.** Cooling a saturated gas below its dew point causes increasingly more water vapor to condense into liquid water droplets.

Figure 6-13 provides a useful analogy of the relationship between water vapor content, capacity, and RH. The various-sized glasses represent the capacity of a gas to hold water vapor. The larger the glass, the greater is its capacity. The water in the glasses represents the actual water vapor content. A glass that is half full is at 50% capacity, or 50% RH. A full glass represents the saturated state, which is equivalent to 100% RH.

Figure 6-13, *A* shows what happens when a saturated gas is heated. Warming a gas increases its capacity to hold water vapor but does not change its content. This is equivalent to pouring the contents of the full glass on the left in Figure 6-13, *A* into progressively larger glasses. The amount of water does not change, but as the glasses get larger, they become less full. We started with a full glass (100% RH) but end up with one that is only one-third full (33% RH).

A decrease in capacity would have the opposite effect. In Figure 6-13, *B*, we start with a large glass, which is half full (50% RH). The capacity of the glass is decreased by pouring the water into progressively smaller glasses (equivalent to decreasing the gas temperature). Eventually, the water volume is enough to fill a smaller glass (100% RH). What happens if we try to empty this full glass into an even

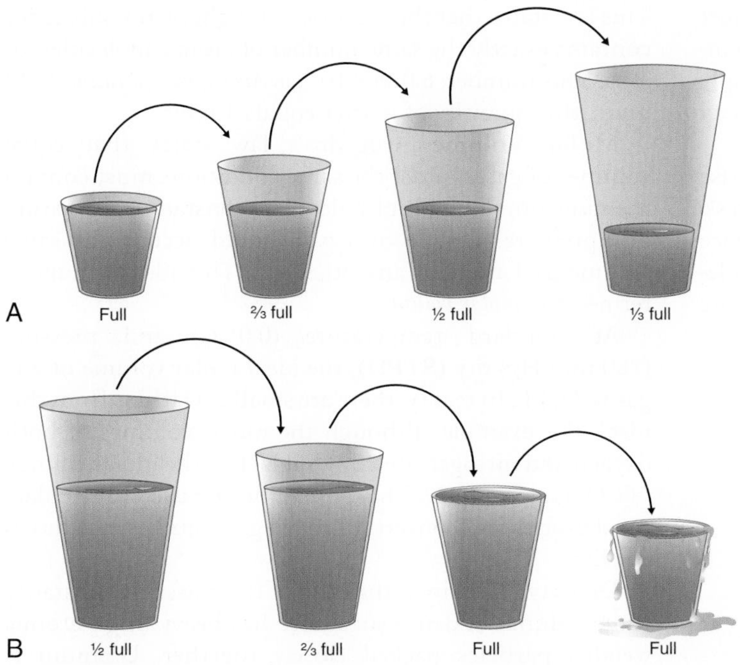

FIGURE 6-13 Relative humidity analogy. **A,** The effect of increasing capacity without changing content, as when heating a saturated gas. **B,** The effect of decreasing capacity, as when cooling a gas. See text for details.

smaller one? Because the smaller glass has less capacity, the excess content must spill over. This spillover is analogous to the condensation occurring when a saturated gas cools below its dew point. However, although condensation has removed the excess moisture from the air, the smaller glass is still full (100% RH).

MINI CLINI

Condensation and Evaporation

A good clinical example of condensation and evaporation is the hygroscopic condenser humidifier, a form of artificial nose (Figure 6-14). These devices consist of layers of water-absorbent material encased in plastic. When a patient exhales into an artificial nose, the warm, saturated expired gas cools, causing condensation on the absorbent surfaces. As condensation occurs, heat is generated in the device. When the patient inhales through the device, the inspired gases are warmed, and the previously condensed water now evaporates, aiding in airway humidification. Chapter 35 provides more detail on humidification devices, including the artificial nose.

In clinical practice, two additional measures of humidity are used: *percent body humidity* (%BH) and *humidity deficit.* The %BH of a gas is the ratio of its actual water vapor content to the water vapor capacity in saturated gas at body temperature (37° C). The %BH is the same as RH except that the capacity (or denominator) is fixed at 43.8 mg/L:

$$\%BH = \frac{AH}{43.8} \times 100$$

The humidity deficit associated with a %BH less than 100% represents the amount of water vapor the body must add to the inspired gas to achieve saturation at body temperature (37° C). To compute the humidity deficit, simply subtract the actual water vapor content from its capacity at 37° C (43.8 mg/L).

Influence of Pressure. High temperatures increase vaporization, whereas high pressures impede this process. Water molecules trying to escape from a liquid surface must push their way out against the opposing air molecules. If the surrounding air pressure is high, there are more opposing air molecules, and vaporization decreases. Conversely, low atmospheric pressures increase vaporization.

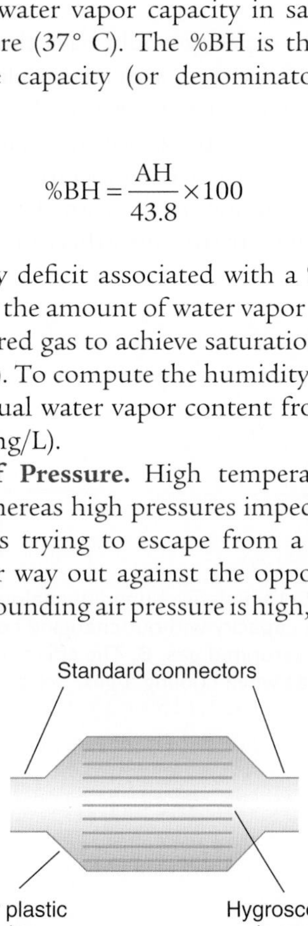

FIGURE 6-14 Hygroscopic condenser humidifier.

Influence of Surface Area. The greater the available surface area of the gas in contact with air, the greater is the rate of liquid evaporation. This statement can be easily proved by comparing how quickly equal volumes of water evaporate under dry conditions from a flat plate versus from a tall, narrow glass. The water spread over a flat plate evaporates more quickly compared with the same amount of liquid in a tall, narrow glass. This principle is applied to the design of certain humidifiers to increase their ability to put water vapor in the passing gas.

Properties of Gases

Gases share many properties with liquids. Specifically, gases exert pressure, are capable of flow, and exhibit the property of viscosity. However, in contrast to liquids, gases are readily compressed and expanded and fill the spaces available to them through diffusion.

Kinetic Activity of Gases

Because the intermolecular forces of attraction of a gas are so weak, most of the internal energy of a gas is kinetic energy. *Kinetic theory* says that gas molecules travel about randomly at very high speeds and with frequent collisions.

The velocity of gas molecules is directly proportional to temperature. As a gas is warmed, its kinetic activity increases, its molecular collisions increase, and its pressure increases. Conversely, when a gas is cooled, molecular activity decreases, particle velocity and collision frequency decrease, and the pressure decreases.

Molar Volume and Gas Density

A major principle governing chemistry is **Avogadro's law.** This law states that the 1-g atomic weight of any substance contains exactly the same number of atoms, molecules, or ions. This number, 6.023×10^{23}, is *Avogadro's constant.* In SI units, this quantity of matter equals 1 mole.

Molar Volume. Avogadro's law states that equal volumes of gases under the same conditions must contain the same number of molecules. At a constant temperature and pressure, 1 mole of a gas should occupy the same volume as 1 mole of any other gas. This ideal volume is termed the *molar volume.*

At standard temperature (0.0° C) and pressure (760 mm Hg) dry **(STPD),** the ideal molar volume of any gas is 22.4 L. In reality, there are small deviations from this ideal. For example, although the molar volumes of both oxygen and nitrogen are 22.4 L at STPD, the molar volume of CO_2 is closer to 22.3 L. These values are used to calculate gas densities and convert dissolved gas volumes into moles per liter.

Density. Density is the ratio of the mass of a substance to its volume. A dense substance has heavy (high atomic weight) particles packed closely together. Uranium is

Box 6-1 Examples of Gas Densities d_w at STPD

$$d_wO_2 = \frac{gmw}{22.4} = \frac{32}{22.4} = 1.43\ g/L$$
$$d_wN_2 = \frac{gmw}{22.4} = \frac{28}{22.4} = 1.25\ g/L$$
$$d_wHe = \frac{gmw}{22.4} = \frac{4}{22.4} = 0.179\ g/L$$
$$d_wCO_2 = \frac{gmw}{22.4} = \frac{44}{22.4} = 1.97\ g/L$$

a good example of a dense substance. Conversely, a low-density substance has a low concentration of light atomic particles per unit volume. Hydrogen gas is a good example of a low-density substance.

In clinical practice, weight is often substituted for mass, and weight density (weight per unit volume, or d_w) is actually measured. Solid or liquid weight density is commonly measured in grams per cubic centimeter (cgs). For gases, the most common unit is grams per liter. Because weight density equals weight divided by volume, the density of any gas at STPD can be computed easily by dividing its molecular weight (gmw) by the universal molar volume of 22.4 L (22.3 for CO_2). Box 6-1 provides examples of gas density calculations.

For the density of a gas mixture to be calculated, the percentage or fraction of each gas in the mixture must be known. To calculate the density of air at STPD, the following equation is used:

$$d_w air = \frac{(FN_2 \times gmw\ N_2) + (FO_2 \times gmw\ O_2)}{22.4\ L}$$
$$d_w air = \frac{(0.79 \times 28) + (0.21 \times 32)}{22.4}$$
$$d_w air = 1.29\ g/L$$

FN_2 and FO_2 equal the fractional concentrations of nitrogen and oxygen in air.

Gaseous Diffusion

Diffusion is the process whereby molecules move from areas of high concentration to areas of lower concentration. *Kinetic energy* is the driving force behind diffusion. Because gases have high kinetic energy, they diffuse most rapidly. However, diffusion also occurs in liquids and can occur in solids. Gas diffusion rates are quantified using **Graham's law.** Mathematically, the rate of diffusion of a gas (D) is inversely proportional to the square root of its gram molecular weight:

$$D_{gas} \propto \frac{1}{\sqrt{gmw}}$$

According to this principle, light gases diffuse rapidly, whereas heavy gases diffuse more slowly. Because diffusion is based on kinetic activity, anything that increases molecular activity quickens diffusion. Heating and mechanical agitation speed diffusion.

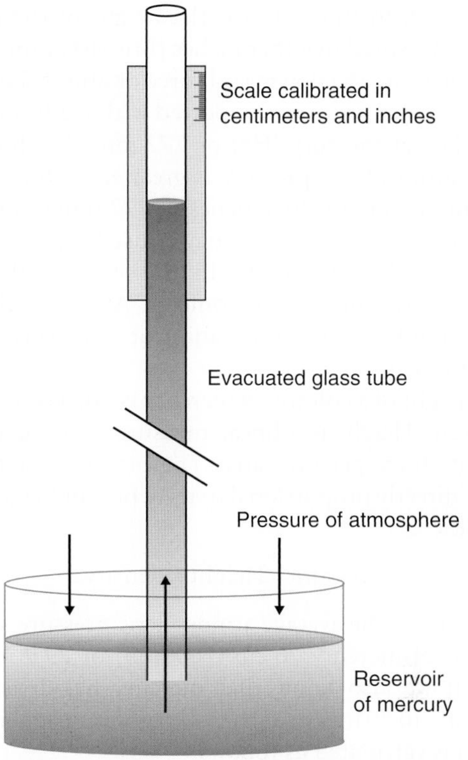

FIGURE 6-15 Major components of a mercury barometer.

Gas Pressure

Whether free in the atmosphere, enclosed in a container, or dissolved in a liquid such as blood, all gases exert pressure. In physiology, the term *tension* is often used to refer to the pressure exerted by gases when dissolved in liquids. The pressure or tension of a gas depends mainly on its kinetic activity. In addition, gravity affects gas pressure. Gravity increases gas density, increasing the rate of molecular collisions and gas tension; this explains why atmospheric pressure decreases with altitude.

Pressure is a measure of force per unit area. The SI unit of pressure is the N/m^2, or pascal (Pa). Pressure in the cgs system is measured in $dynes/cm^2$, whereas pounds per square inch (lb/in^2 or psi) is the British fps pressure unit. Pressure can also be measured indirectly as the height of a column of liquid, as is commonly done to determine atmospheric pressure.

Measuring Atmospheric Pressure. Atmospheric pressure is measured with a barometer. A barometer consists of an evacuated glass tube approximately 1 m long. This tube is closed at the top end, with its lower, open end immersed in a mercury reservoir (Figure 6-15). The pressure of the atmosphere on the mercury reservoir forces the mercury up the vacuum tube a distance equivalent to the force exerted. In this manner, the height of the mercury column (measured in either inches [British] or millimeters [cgs]) represents the downward force of atmospheric pressure. Barometer pressure is reported with readings such as 30.4 inches of mercury (Hg) or 772 mm Hg; this means that the atmospheric pressure is great enough to support a column of mercury 30.4 inches or 772 mm in height.

Alternatively, the term *torr* may be used in pressure readings. Torr is short for Torricelli, the seventeenth-century inventor of the mercury barometer. At sea level, 1 torr equals 1 mm Hg. A pressure reading of 772 torr is the same as 772 mm Hg.

The height of a column of mercury is not a true measure of pressure. Height is a linear measure, whereas pressure represents force per unit area. The pressure exerted by a liquid is directly proportional to its depth (or height) times its density:

$$\text{Pressure} = \text{Height} \times \text{density}$$

At sea level, the average atmospheric pressure supports a column of mercury 76 cm (760 mm) or 29.9 inches in height. If we also know that mercury has a density of 13.6 g/cm^3 (0.491 lb/in^3), the average atmospheric pressure (P_B) is calculated as follows:

$$\text{cgs units: } P_B = 76 \text{ cm} \times 13.6 \text{ g/cm}^3 = 1034 \text{ g/cm}^2$$
$$\text{fps units: } P_B = 29.9 \text{ in} \times 0.491 \text{ lb/in}^3 = 14.7 \text{ lb/in}^2$$

These two measures, 1034 g/cm^2 and 14.7 lb/in^2, are considered standards in the cgs and British fps systems, each being equivalent to 1 atm.

Similar to any solid material, a barometer's housing reacts to temperature changes by expanding and contracting. In addition, the mercury column acts like a large thermometer. Both pressure and temperature affect the mercury level of a barometer. For accuracy, the reading must be corrected for temperature changes. The U.S. Weather Bureau provides temperature correction factors for barometric readings. To correct the reading, subtract the applicable table value from the observed reading. For pressures between those listed in the table, use simple linear interpolation.

Clinical Pressure Measurements. Mercury is the most common fluid used in pressure measurements both in barometers and at the bedside. Because of the high density (13.6 g/cm^3) of mercury, it assumes a height that is easy to read for most pressures in the clinical range. Water columns can also be used to measure pressure (in cm H_2O) but only low pressures. Because water is 13.6 times less dense than mercury, 1 atm would support a water column 33.9 feet high, or about as tall as a two-story building.

Both mercury and water columns are still used in clinical practice, especially when vascular pressures are being measured. However, these traditional tools are rapidly being replaced by mechanical or electronic pressure-measuring devices. Even so, these new instruments must be calibrated against a mercury or water column before making measurements.

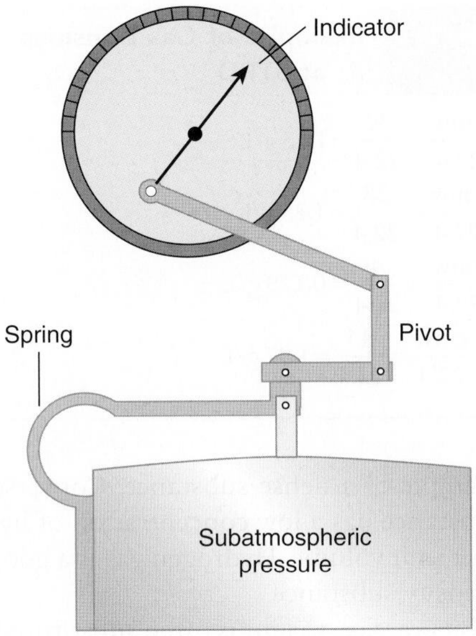

FIGURE 6-16 Aneroid barometer.

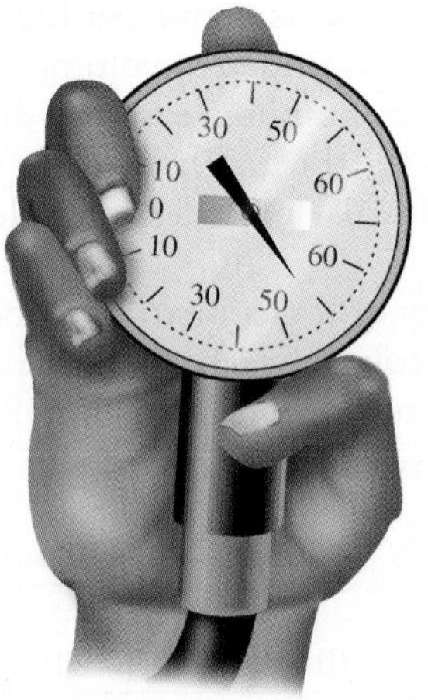
FIGURE 6-17 Mechanical manometer used to measure a patient's airway pressure.

The simplest mechanical pressure gauge is the *aneroid barometer,* which is common in homes. An aneroid barometer consists of a sealed evacuated metal box with a flexible, spring-supported top that responds to external pressure changes (Figure 6-16). This motion activates a geared pointer, which provides a scale reading analogous to pressure.

This same concept underlies the simple mechanical manometers used to measure blood or airway pressure at the bedside (Figure 6-17). However, rather than the pressure acting externally on the sealed chamber, the inside is connected to the pressure source. In this manner, the flexible chamber wall expands and contracts as pressure increases or decreases.

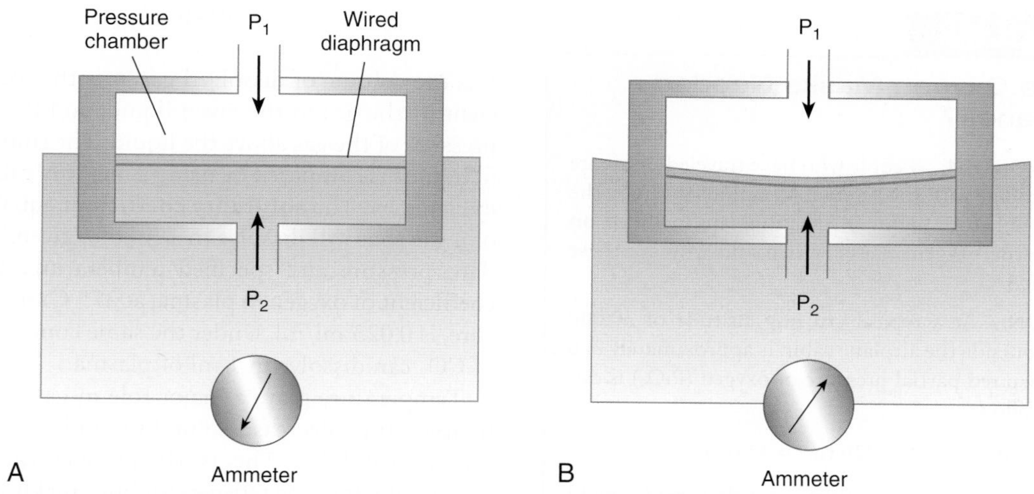

FIGURE 6-18 Strain-gauge pressure transducer. **A,** No pressure is applied. **B,** Pressure is applied to the transducer. An ammeter shows a change in electrical current proportional to the magnitude of pressure applied.

A flexible chamber can also be used to measure pressure electronically. These devices are called **strain-gauge pressure transducers.** In these devices, pressure changes expand and contract a flexible metal diaphragm connected to electrical wires (Figure 6-18). The physical strain on the diaphragm changes the amount of electricity flowing through the wires. By measuring this change in electrical flow, we are indirectly measuring changes in pressure.

Although mm Hg and cm H_2O are still the most common pressure units used at the bedside, they do not represent the SI standard. The SI unit of pressure is the kPa; 1 kPa equals approximately 10.2 cm H_2O or 7.5 torr. To convert between these pressure units accurately, use the factors provided in the rear inside cover of this book.

RULE OF THUMB

One kilopascal equals approximately 10.2 cm H_2O. A pressure of 10 kPa equals approximately 100 cm H_2O. Conversely, a pressure of 60 cm H_2O equals approximately 6 kPa.

Partial Pressures (Dalton's Law)

Many gases exist together as mixtures. Air is a good example of a gas mixture, consisting mainly of oxygen and nitrogen. A gas mixture, similar to a solitary gas, exerts pressure. The pressure exerted by a gas mixture must equal the sum of the kinetic activity of all its component gases. The pressure exerted by a single gas in a mixture is called its *partial pressure.*

Dalton's law describes the relationship between the partial pressure and the total pressure in a gas mixture. According to this law, the total pressure of a mixture of gases must equal the sum of the partial pressures of all component gases. The principle states that the partial pressure of a component gas must be proportional to its percentage in the mixture.[8]

A gas making up 25% of a mixture would exert 25% of the total pressure. For consistency, the percentage of a gas in a mixture is usually expressed in decimal form, using the term *fractional concentration*. A gas that is 25% of a mixture has a fractional concentration of 0.25. For example, air consists of approximately 21% O_2 and 79% N_2. To compute the partial pressure of each component, simply multiply the fractional concentration of each component by the total pressure. Assuming a normal atmospheric pressure of 760 torr, the individual partial pressure is computed as follows:

$$\text{Partial pressure} = \text{Fractional concentration} \times \text{total pressure}$$
$$PO_2 = 0.21 \times 760 \text{ torr} = 160 \text{ torr}$$
$$PN_2 = 0.79 \times 760 \text{ torr} = 600 \text{ torr}$$

As predicted by Dalton's law, the sum of these partial pressures equals the total pressure of the gas mixture.

What if the total pressure changed? Barometric pressure changes, in addition to minor fluctuations caused by weather, are mainly a function of altitude. Considering only oxygen, we know that its fractional concentration, or fractional inspired oxygen (FiO_2), remains constant at approximately 0.21. At a P_B of 760 torr, the PO_2 is equal to 0.21 × 760, or 160 torr. At 25,000 feet, the FiO_2 of air is still 0.21. However, the P_B is only 282 torr, and the resulting PO_2 is 0.21 × 282, or 59 torr, just more than one-third of that available at sea level. Because the PO_2 (not its percentage) determines physiologic activity, high altitudes can impair oxygen uptake by the lungs. Mountain climbers must sometimes use supplemental oxygen at high altitudes for this reason. By increasing the amount of O_2 more than 0.21, we can raise its partial pressure and increase uptake by the lungs. For a practical application of this principle, see the accompanying Mini Clini.

MINI CLINI

Why Are Oxygen Masks Needed on Airplanes?

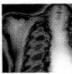

PROBLEM: People who have traveled by air are familiar with the safety instructions given by the crew before flight. Instructions are included on how to use the oxygen masks. When and why are these masks needed?

DISCUSSION: At a typical cruising altitude of 30,000 feet, the P_B outside the airplane cabin is approximately 226 torr. The inspired partial pressure of oxygen (PiO_2) is calculated as follows:

$$PiO_2 = 0.21 \times 226 \text{ torr} = 47 \text{ torr}$$

If the cabin were to depressurize, travelers inside would be exposed to this low PiO_2. At this PiO_2, most people become unconscious within seconds and eventually die of lack of oxygen (anoxia).

To overcome this problem, emergency oxygen masks are available when the cabin depressurizes. These masks, assuming a tight fit, probably provide approximately 70% oxygen, or an FiO_2 of 0.70. The PiO_2 of a person wearing a mask under these conditions is calculated as follows:

$$PiO_2 = 0.70 \times 226 \text{ torr} = 158 \text{ torr}$$

This PiO_2 (about the same as at sea level) is sufficient to keep the passengers alive until the crew can bring the plane down to a safe altitude.

In contrast, high atmospheric pressures increase the partial pressure of inspired oxygen (PiO_2) in an air mixture. Pressures above atmospheric are called *hyperbaric pressures*.[9] Hyperbaric pressures commonly occur only in underwater diving and in special hyperbaric chambers.[9] For example, at a depth of 66 feet under the sea, water exerts a pressure of 3 atm, or 2280 mm Hg (3 × 760). At this depth, the oxygen in an air mixture breathed by a diver exerts a PO_2 of 0.21 × 2280, or approximately 479 mm Hg. This is nearly three times the PO_2 at sea level.

The same conditions can be created on dry land in a *hyperbaric chamber*. The U.S. Navy uses hyperbaric chambers for controlled depressurization of deep-sea divers and to treat certain types of diving accidents. Clinically, hyperbaric chambers and oxygen are used together to treat various conditions, including carbon monoxide poisoning and gangrene. Chapter 38 provides more details on this use of high-pressure oxygen.

Solubility of Gases in Liquids (Henry's Law)

Gases can dissolve in liquids. Carbonated water and soda are good examples of a gas (CO_2) dissolved in a liquid (water). **Henry's law** predicts how much of a given gas will dissolve in a liquid. According to this principle, at a given temperature, the volume of a gas that dissolves in a liquid is equal to its solubility coefficient times its partial pressure:

$$V = \alpha \times P_{gas}$$

V is the volume of dissolved gas, α is the solubility coefficient of the gas in the given liquid, and P_{gas} is the partial pressure of the gas above the liquid. The solubility of gases in liquids is compared by using a measure called the *solubility coefficient*. The **solubility coefficient** equals the volume of a gas that will dissolve in 1 ml of a given liquid at standard pressure and specified temperature. The solubility coefficient of oxygen in plasma, at 37° C and 760 torr pressure, is 0.023 ml/ml. Under the same conditions, 0.510 ml of CO_2 can dissolve in 1 ml of plasma.

Temperature plays a major role in gas solubility. High temperatures decrease solubility, and low temperatures increase solubility. This is why an open can of soda may still fizz if left in the refrigerator but quickly goes flat when left out at room temperature.

The effect of temperature on solubility is a result of changes in kinetic activity. As a liquid is warmed, the kinetic activity of any dissolved gas molecules is increased. This increase in kinetic activity increases the escaping tendency of the molecules and partial pressure. As an

MINI CLINI

Blood Gases versus Patient Temperature

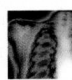

PROBLEM: RTs frequently need to sample and measure the partial pressures of oxygen and carbon dioxide in patients' arterial blood. These samples are called arterial blood gases (ABGs). Typically, ABG samples are measured in analyzers kept at a normal body temperature of 37° C. However, not all patients have normal body temperatures. Many are feverish (hyperpyrexia), and some have low body temperatures (hypothermia). What effect does this have on the measurements?

DISCUSSION: The direct relationship between temperature and partial pressure causes higher arterial PO_2 and PCO_2 readings at higher temperatures. At 37° C, the arterial PO_2 in a normal adult is approximately 100 torr. However, at 47° C, the PO_2 would be nearly twice as high. A smaller increase from 37° C to 39° C increases the arterial PO_2 less markedly from 100 torr to approximately 110 torr. Likewise, an increase in temperature increases the arterial PCO_2. Arterial PCO_2 values increase approximately 5% per degree Celsius. An increase in temperature from 37° C to 39° C increases the PCO_2 by approximately 10%, from 40 torr to 44 torr.

The reverse is also true. Decreased temperatures decrease the arterial partial pressures of oxygen and carbon dioxide. Nomograms are available to help compute these corrections; however, they correct only for the relationship between temperature and pressure. Nomograms do not take into account metabolic and cardiovascular changes that accompany a change in a patient's temperature. For this reason, the use of corrected PO_2 and PCO_2 readings remains controversial.

increasing number of gas molecules escape, the amount left in a solution decreases rapidly. For a practical application of this principle, see the accompanying Mini Clini, which discusses blood gases and patient temperature.

GAS BEHAVIOR UNDER CHANGING CONDITIONS

Gases, with large distances between their molecules, are easily compressed and expanded. When a gas is pressurized, the molecules are squeezed closer together. If a gas-filled container could be enlarged, the gas would expand to occupy the new volume. Figure 6-19 illustrates the concepts of gas compression and expansion.

Gas Laws

Several laws help define the relationship among gas pressure, temperature, mass, and volume (Table 6-4). Using these laws, the behavior of gases under changing conditions can be predicted. Underlying all these laws are three basic assumptions: (1) No energy is lost during molecular collisions, (2) the volume of the molecules themselves is negligible, and (3) no forces of mutual attraction exist between these molecules. These three assumptions describe the behavior of an "ideal gas." Under normal conditions, most gases exhibit ideal behavior.

Effect of Water Vapor

In clinical practice, most gas law calculations must take into account the presence of water vapor. Water vapor, similar to any gas, occupies space. The dry volume of a gas at a constant pressure and temperature is always smaller than its saturated volume. The opposite is also true. Correcting from the dry state to the saturated state always yields a larger gas volume.

The pressure exerted by water vapor is independent of the other gases with which it mixes, depending only on the temperature and RH. The addition of water vapor to a gas mixture always lowers the partial pressures of the other gases present. This fact becomes relevant when discussing the partial pressure of gases in the lung where the gases are saturated with water vapor at body temperature.

Corrected Pressure Computations

To compute the new or corrected partial pressure of a gas after saturation with water vapor, the following formula is applied:

$$P_C = F_{gas} \times (P_T - P_{H_2O})$$

P_C is the corrected gas pressure, F_{gas} is the fractional concentration of the gas in the gas mixture, P_T is the total gas pressure of the mixture, and P_{H_2O} is the water vapor

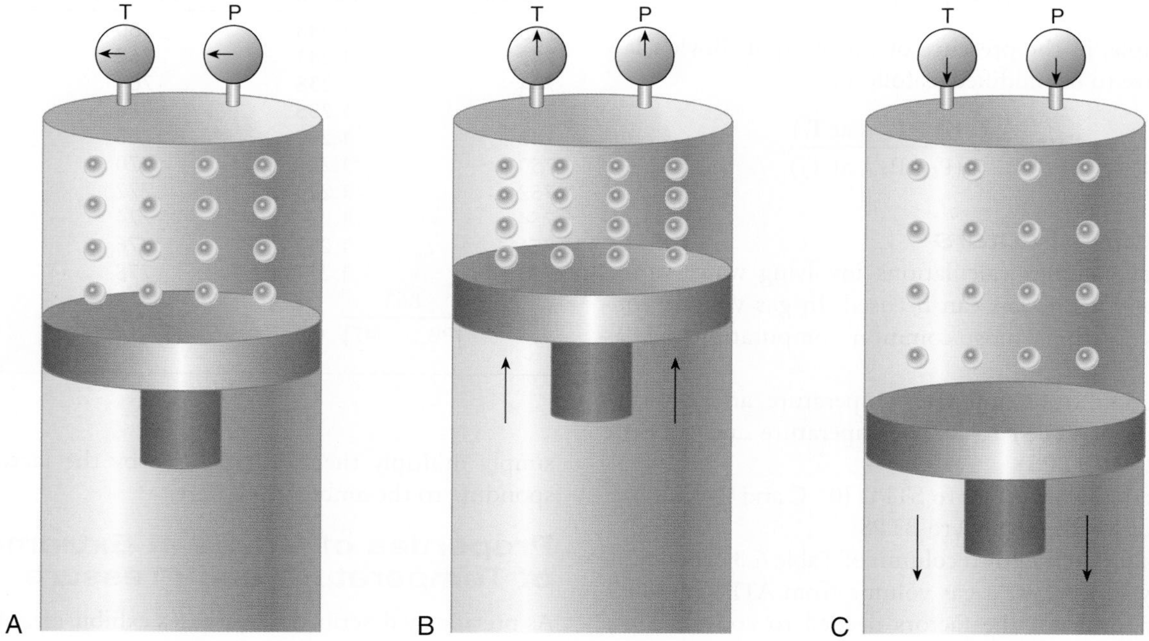

FIGURE 6-19 A mass of gas in the resting state exerts a given pressure *(P)* at a given temperature *(T)* in cylinder **A.** In cylinder **B,** as the piston compresses the gas, the molecules are crowded closer together, and the increased energy of molecular collisions increases both the temperature and the pressure. Conversely, as the gas expands in cylinder **C,** molecular interaction decreases, and the temperature and pressure decrease.

TABLE 6-4

Laws Describing Gas Behavior Under Changing Conditions

Gas Law	Basic Relationship	Constants	Description	Working Formula*	Clinical Applications
Boyle's law	$P \times V = k$	Temperature, mass	Volume of a gas varies inversely with its pressure	$P_1V_1 = P_2V_2$	Ventilation (see Chapter 10) Body plethysmography (see Chapter 19) Compressed volume (see Chapter 38)
Charles' law	$\frac{V}{T} = k$	Pressure, mass	Volume of gas varies directly with changes in its temperature (° K)	$\frac{V_1}{T_1} = \frac{V_2}{T_2}$	ATPS to BTPS corrections (see this chapter)
Gay-Lussac's law	$\frac{P}{T} = k$	Volume, mass	Pressure exerted by a gas varies directly with its absolute temperature	$\frac{P_1}{T_1} = \frac{P_2}{T_2}$	Cylinder pressures (see Chapter 37)
Combined gas law	$PV = nRT$	—	Interaction of above (none held constant)	$\frac{P_1V_1}{nT_1} = \frac{P_2V_2}{nT_2}$	Complex interactions of variables

*Use the working formulas to calculate the new value of a parameter when a gas undergoes a change in P, V, n, or T. For example, to solve for a new volume (V_2) using Boyle's law, you would simply rearrange its working equation as follows:

$$V_2 = V_1 \times \frac{P_1}{P_2}$$

n, Mass; *P*, pressure; *R*, the gas constant (a combined constant of proportionality); *T*, temperature (° K); *V*, volume.

pressure at the given temperature (see Table 6-3). If only a single gas is present, F_{gas} equals 1, and the formula can be simplified:

$$P_C = (P_T - P_{H_2O})$$

For example, in the presence of water vapor, Boyle's law would have to be modified as follows:

$$V_2 = V_1 \times \frac{(P_1 - P_{H_2O} \text{ at } T_1)}{(P_2 - P_{H_2O} \text{ at } T_2)}$$

Correction Factors

Instead of complex calculations involving water vapor, simple *correction factors* can be used. In gas volume conversions, the three most common computations are as follows:

1. Correction from ambient temperature and pressure saturated **(ATPS)** to body temperature and pressure saturated **(BTPS)**
2. Correction from ATPS to STPD (0° C and 760 torr)
3. Correction from STPD to BTPS

The values in the third column of Table 6-3, when multiplied by V_1, convert a gas volume from ATPS to BTPS. Table 6-5 provides the factors needed to convert a gas volume from ATPS to STPD. To use Table 6-5, simply multiply the ATPS volume by the factor corresponding to the specified temperature and uncorrected barometric pressure. Finally, Table 6-6 provides the factors needed to correct volumes from STPD to BTPS. To use Table 6-6, simply multiply the STPD volume by the factor corresponding to the ambient pressure.

TABLE 6-5

Factors to Convert Gas Volumes from STPD to BTPS at Given Barometric Pressures

Pressure	Factor	Pressure	Factor
740	1.245	760	1.211
742	1.241	762	1.208
744	1.238	764	1.203
746	1.235	766	1.200
748	1.232	768	1.196
750	1.227	770	1.193
752	1.224	772	1.190
754	1.221	774	1.188
756	1.217	776	1.183
758	1.214	778	1.181

$$\text{Factor} = \frac{863}{[PB_{amb} - 47]}$$

Properties of Gases at Extremes of Temperature and Pressure

As previously described, most gases exhibit ideal behavior under normal conditions. However, gases can deviate from these expectations, especially at the extremes of pressure and temperature. The accompanying Mini Clini provides two good clinical examples of how gas behavior can deviate from the ideal.

TABLE 6-6

Factors to Convert Gas Volumes from ATPS to STPD

Observed Pa	15°	16°	17°	18°	19°	20°	21°	22°	23°	24°	25°	26°	27°	28°	29°	30°	31°	32°
700	0.855	851	847	842	838	834	829	825	821	816	812	807	802	797	793	788	783	778
702	857	853	849	845	840	836	832	827	823	818	814	809	805	800	795	790	785	780
704	860	856	852	847	843	839	834	830	825	821	816	812	807	802	797	792	787	783
706	862	858	854	850	845	841	837	832	828	823	819	814	810	804	800	795	790	785
708	865	861	856	852	848	843	839	834	830	825	821	816	812	807	802	797	792	787
710	867	863	859	855	850	846	842	837	833	828	824	819	814	809	804	799	795	790
712	870	866	861	857	853	848	844	839	836	830	826	821	817	812	807	802	797	792
714	872	868	864	859	855	851	846	842	837	833	828	824	819	814	809	804	799	794
716	875	871	866	862	858	853	849	844	840	835	831	826	822	816	812	807	802	797
718	877	873	869	864	860	856	851	847	842	838	833	828	824	819	814	809	804	799
720	880	876	871	867	863	858	854	849	845	840	836	831	826	821	816	812	807	802
722	882	878	874	869	865	861	856	852	847	843	838	833	829	824	819	814	809	804
724	885	880	876	872	867	863	858	854	849	845	840	835	831	826	821	816	811	806
726	887	883	879	874	870	866	861	856	852	847	843	838	833	829	825	818	813	808
728	890	886	881	877	872	868	863	859	854	850	845	840	836	831	826	821	816	811
730	892	888	884	879	875	870	866	861	857	852	847	843	838	833	828	823	818	813
732	895	891	886	882	877	873	868	864	859	854	850	845	840	836	831	825	820	815
734	897	893	889	884	880	875	871	866	862	857	852	847	843	838	833	828	823	818
736	900	895	891	887	882	878	873	869	864	859	855	850	845	840	835	830	825	820
738	902	898	894	889	885	880	876	871	866	862	857	852	848	843	838	833	828	822
740	905	900	896	892	887	883	878	874	869	864	860	855	850	845	840	835	830	825
742	907	903	898	894	890	885	881	876	871	867	862	857	852	847	842	837	832	827
744	910	906	901	897	892	888	883	878	874	869	864	859	855	850	845	840	834	829
746	912	908	903	899	895	890	886	881	876	872	867	862	857	852	847	842	837	832
748	915	910	906	901	897	892	888	883	879	874	869	864	860	854	850	845	839	834
750	917	913	908	904	900	895	890	886	881	876	872	867	862	857	852	847	842	837
752	920	915	911	906	902	897	893	888	883	879	874	869	864	859	854	849	844	839
754	922	918	913	909	904	900	895	891	886	881	876	872	867	862	857	852	846	841
756	925	920	916	911	907	902	898	893	888	883	879	874	869	864	859	854	849	844
758	927	923	918	914	909	905	900	896	891	886	881	876	872	866	861	856	851	846
760	930	925	921	916	912	907	902	898	893	888	883	879	874	869	864	859	854	848
762	932	928	923	919	914	910	905	900	896	891	886	881	876	871	866	861	856	851
764	934	930	926	921	916	912	907	903	898	893	888	884	879	874	869	864	858	853
766	937	933	928	925	919	915	910	905	900	896	891	886	881	876	871	866	861	855
768	940	935	931	926	922	917	912	908	903	898	893	888	883	878	873	868	863	858
770	942	938	933	928	924	919	915	910	905	901	896	891	886	881	876	871	865	860
772	945	940	936	931	926	922	917	912	908	903	898	893	888	883	878	873	868	862
774	947	943	938	933	929	924	920	915	910	905	901	896	891	886	880	875	870	865
776	950	945	941	936	931	927	922	917	912	908	903	898	893	888	883	878	872	867
778	952	948	943	938	934	929	924	920	915	910	905	900	895	890	885	880	875	869
780	955	950	945	941	936	932	927	922	917	912	908	903	898	892	887	882	877	872

$$\text{Factor} = \frac{[PB_{abs} \text{ corrected for } t_{amb} - PH_2O \text{ at } t_{amb}] \times 0.359}{[t_{amb} + 273]}$$

As previously discussed, weak attractive forces (van der Waals forces) between gas molecules oppose their kinetic activity. Both temperature and pressure affect these forces. At high temperatures, the increased kinetic activity of gas molecules far overshadows these forces. However, at very low temperatures, kinetic activity lessens, and these forces become more important. Likewise, very low pressures permit gas molecules to move freely about with little mutual attraction. In contrast, high pressures crowd molecules together, increasing the influence of these forces.

The actual space occupied by gas molecules also can influence their behavior. At low pressure, the total mass of matter in a gas is a negligible fraction of the total volume. However, at very high pressures, molecular density becomes important, altering the expected relationship between pressure and volume.

Critical Temperature and Pressure

For every liquid, there is a temperature above which the kinetic activity of its molecules is so great that the attractive forces cannot keep them in a liquid state. This temperature is called the **critical temperature.** The critical temperature is the highest temperature at which a substance can exist as a liquid. The pressure needed to maintain equilibrium between the liquid and gas phases of a substance at this critical temperature is the *critical pressure*.

MINI CLINI

Variations from Ideal Gas Behavior: Expansion Cooling and Adiabatic Compression

Boyle's law describes gas behavior under constant temperature, or isothermal conditions.[10] During isothermal conditions, the temperature of an ideal gas should not change with either expansion or contraction. For example, if an ideal gas were to escape rapidly from a high-pressure cylinder into the atmosphere, its temperature should not change. The rapid expansion of real gases causes substantial cooling. This phenomenon of expansion cooling is called the *Joule-Thompson effect.*

A rapidly expanding gas cools because the attractive force between its molecules is broken. Because the energy needed to break these forces must come from the gas itself, the temperature of the gas must decrease. This decrease in temperature, depending on the pressure drop that occurs, can be large enough to liquefy the gas. This is the primary method used to liquefy air for the production of oxygen.

Isothermal processes keep gas temperature constant, whereas adiabatic compression and expansion have no such restrictions. During an adiabatic process, heat energy of a gas is allowed to increase or decrease as it undergoes changes in pressure or volume. Adiabatic compression of a gas can cause rapid increases in temperature. A diesel engine uses this principle to ignite fuel without a spark. Adiabatic compression can also occur in gas delivery systems where rapid compression occurs within a fixed container. The increase in temperature caused by this rapid compression can ignite any combustible material in the system. For this reason, RTs must clear any combustible matter from high-pressure gas delivery systems before pressurization.

Together, the critical temperature and pressure represent the critical point of a substance.

The critical temperature of water is 374° C. At this temperature, a pressure of 218 atm is needed to maintain equilibrium between the liquid and gaseous forms of water. No pressure can return water vapor to its liquid form at a temperature greater than 374° C.

Compared with liquids, gases have much lower critical points. Table 6-7 lists the critical points of four gases used in clinical practice: oxygen, helium, CO_2, and nitrous oxide (N_2O). The critical temperatures of oxygen and helium are well below the normal room temperature of 20° C (68° F), whereas the critical temperatures of CO_2 and N_2O are above room temperature.

The concept of critical temperature can be applied to distinguish between a true gas and a vapor. A true gas, such as oxygen, has a critical temperature so low that at room temperature and pressure it cannot exist as a liquid. In contrast, a vapor is the gaseous state of a substance coexisting with its liquid or solid state at room temperature and pressure. This is why molecular water is referred to as *water vapor.*

TABLE 6-7

Critical Points of Three Gases

Gas	° C	° F	Atmosphere
Helium (He)	−267.9	−450.2	2.3
Oxygen (O_2)	−118.8	−181.1	49.7
Carbon dioxide (CO_2)	31.1	87.9	73.0
Nitrous oxide (N_2O)	36.5	97.7	71.8

The concept of critical temperature and pressure also helps explain how gases are liquefied. A gas can be liquefied by being cooled to below its boiling point. Alternatively, a gas can be liquefied by being cooled to less than its critical temperature and then being compressed. The more a gas is cooled below its critical temperature, the less pressure will be needed to liquefy it. However, under no circumstances can pressure alone liquefy a gas existing above its critical temperature.

According to these principles, any gas with a critical temperature above ambient should be able to be liquefied simply by having pressure applied. Both CO_2 and N_2O have critical temperatures above normal room temperature (see Table 6-7). Both gases can be liquefied by simple compression and stored as liquids at room temperature without cooling. However, both liquefied gases still need to be stored under pressure, usually in strong metal cylinders.

Liquid oxygen is produced by separating it from a liquefied air mixture at a temperature below its boiling point (−183° C or −297° F). After it is separated from air, the oxygen must be maintained as a liquid by being stored in insulated containers below its boiling point. As long as the temperature does not exceed −183° C, the oxygen remains liquid at atmospheric pressure. If higher temperatures are needed, higher pressures must be used. If at any time the liquid oxygen exceeds its critical temperature of −118.8° C, it converts immediately to a gas.

FLUID DYNAMICS

So far, liquids and gases have been presented under static, or nonmoving, conditions. However, both liquids and gases can flow. *Flow* is the bulk movement of a substance through space. The study of fluids in motion is called *hydrodynamics.* Because many respiratory care devices use hydrodynamic principles, the RT must have a good understanding of the basic concepts governing fluids in motion.

Pressures in Flowing Fluids

As we have seen, the pressure of a static liquid depends solely on the depth and density of the fluid. In contrast, the pressure exerted by a liquid in motion depends on the nature of the flow itself. As shown in Figure 6-20, *A,* the pressure exerted by a static fluid is the same at all points

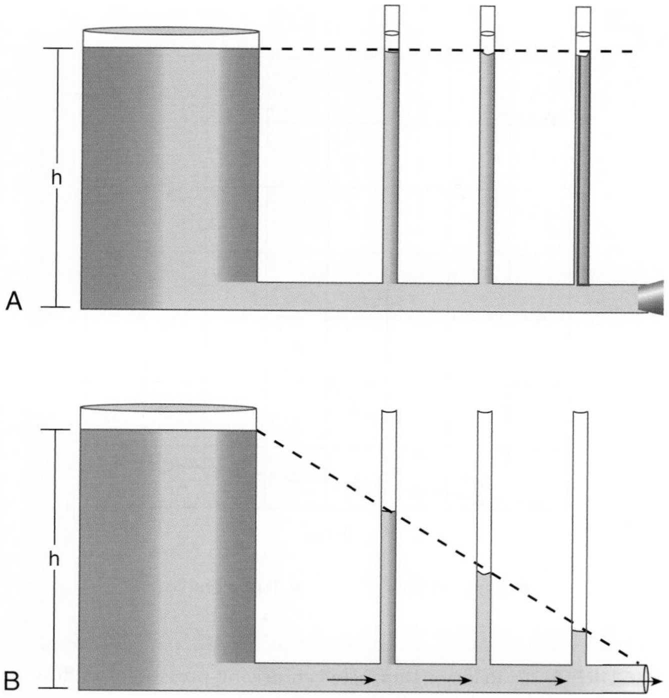

FIGURE 6-20 **A,** The pressure is the same at all points along the horizontal tube when there is no flow. **B,** A progressive decrease in pressure occurs as the fluid flows. (Modified from Nave CR, Nave BC: Physics for the health sciences, ed 3, Philadelphia, 1985, WB Saunders.)

along a horizontal tube, depending only on the height (h) of the liquid column. However, when the fluid flows out through the bottom tube, the pressure progressively decreases all along the tube length (see Figure 6-20, *B*). In addition, the decrease in pressure between each of the equally spaced vertical tubes is the same.

The decrease in fluid pressure along the tube reflects a cumulative energy loss, as predicted by the second law of thermodynamics. In simple terms, this law states that in any mechanical process, there will always be a decrease in the total energy available to do work. Available energy decreases because frictional forces oppose fluid flow. Frictional resistance to flow exists both within the fluid itself (viscosity) and between the fluid and the tube wall. Generally, the greater the viscosity of the fluid and the smaller the cross-sectional area of the tube, the greater is the decrease in pressure along the tube.

For any given tube length, **flow resistance** equals the difference in pressure between the two points along the tube divided by the actual flow. This is expressed as a formula:

$$R = \frac{(P_1 - P_2)}{\dot{V}}$$

where R is the total flow resistance, P_1 is the pressure at the upstream point (point 1), P_2 is the pressure at the downstream point (point 2), and $\dot{V}$ is the flow (volume per unit time). This formula has wide application in pulmonary physiology and respiratory care. The accompanying Mini Clini provides a good example of such application.

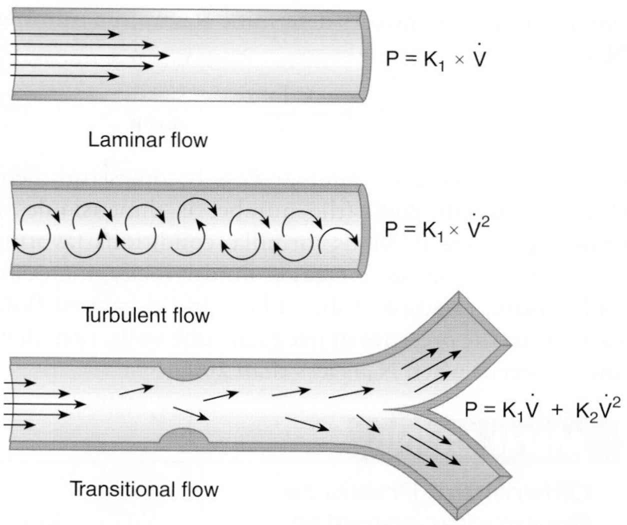

FIGURE 6-21 Three patterns of flow—laminar, turbulent, and transitional. (Modified from Moser KM, Spragg RG: Respiratory emergencies, ed 2, St Louis, 1982, Mosby.)

Patterns of Flow

The pressure difference that results from flow also varies with the pattern of flow. There are three primary patterns of flow through tubes: *laminar, turbulent,* and *transitional* (Figure 6-21).

Laminar Flow

As discussed earlier, during laminar flow, a fluid moves in discrete cylindrical layers or streamlines. The difference in pressure required to produce a given flow, under conditions of laminar flow through a smooth tube of fixed size, is defined by **Poiseuille's law:**

$$\Delta P = \frac{8nl\dot{V}}{\pi r^4}$$

where ΔP is the driving pressure gradient, n is the viscosity of the fluid, l is the tube length, $\dot{V}$ is the fluid flow, r is the tube radius, and π and 8 are constants.

According to this formula, for fluids flowing in a laminar pattern, the driving pressure increases whenever the fluid viscosity, tube length, or flow increases. In addition, greater pressure is required to maintain a given flow if the tube radius decreases.

Turbulent Flow

Under certain conditions, the pattern of flow through a tube changes significantly, with a loss of regular streamlines. Instead, fluid molecules form irregular eddy currents in a chaotic pattern called **turbulent flow** (see Figure 6-21). This changeover from laminar to turbulent flow depends on several factors, including fluid density (d), viscosity (h), linear velocity (v), and tube radius (r). In combination, these factors determine **Reynold's number (N_R).**

$$N_R = \frac{v \times d \times 2r}{h}$$

In a smooth-bore tube, laminar flow becomes turbulent when N_R exceeds 2000 (the number is dimensionless). According to the previous formula, conditions favoring turbulent flow include increased fluid velocity, increased fluid density, increased tube radius, and decreased fluid viscosity. In the presence of irregular tube walls, turbulent flow can occur when N_R is less than 2000.

MINI CLINI

Differential Pressure Pneumotachometer

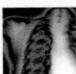

PROBLEM: It is often necessary to measure and record changes in airflow as a patient breathes. How can we apply the formula for resistance to measure and record airflow?

DISCUSSION: Airflow can be measured by using a device called a *pneumotachometer*. One of the simplest designs is the differential pressure pneumotachometer. A differential pressure pneumotachometer incorporates a flow tube with a known and constant resistance (R). If the formula for resistance is rearranged to solve for flow, it appears as follows:

$$\dot{V} = \frac{(P_1 - P_2)}{R}$$

Flow through a tube with constant resistance is directly proportional to the pressure difference across the tube. By measuring this pressure difference (using a strain-gauge transducer, such as described in Figure 6-18), we can measure flow. To ensure linearity between pressure and flow, the flow pattern through the tube must remain laminar.

When flow becomes turbulent, Poiseuille's law no longer applies. Instead, the pressure difference across a tube is defined as follows:

$$\Delta P = \frac{fl\dot{V}^2}{4\pi^2 r^5}$$

where ΔP is the driving pressure, f is a friction factor based on the density and viscosity of the fluid and the tube wall roughness, l is the tube length, and $\dot{V}$ is the fluid flow.

Figure 6-22 compares the relationship between pressure and flow under laminar and turbulent conditions. As can be seen, when flow is laminar (Poiseuille's law), the relationship between driving pressure and flow is linear. However, when flow becomes turbulent, driving pressure varies with the square of the flow ($\dot{V}^2$). To double flow under laminar conditions, we need only double the driving pressure. To double flow under turbulent conditions, we would have to increase the driving pressure fourfold.

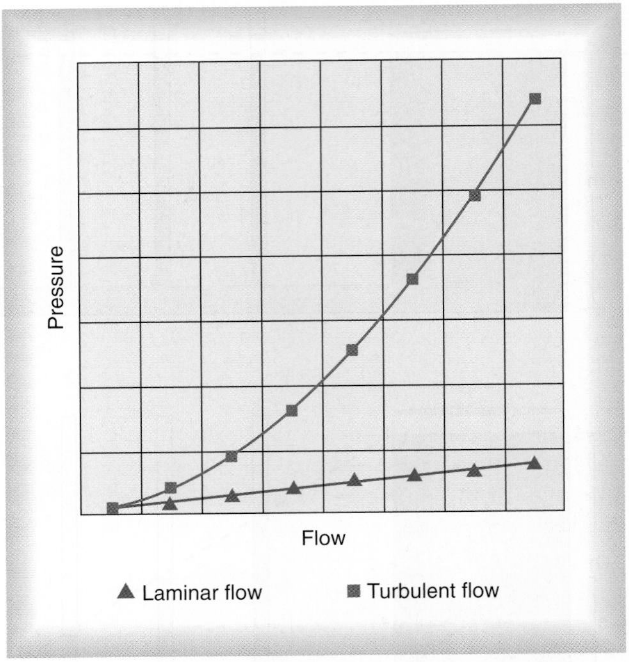

FIGURE 6-22 Relationship between driving pressure and flow under laminar and turbulent conditions.

Transitional Flow

Transitional flow is a mixture of laminar and turbulent flow. Flow in the respiratory tract is mainly transitional in nature. When flow is transitional, the total driving pressure equals the sum of the pressures resulting from laminar and turbulent flow:

$$\Delta P = (k_1 \times \dot{V}) + (k_2 \times \dot{V}^2)$$

k_1 and k_2 are factors indicating the respective contribution of laminar and turbulent flow to overall driving pressure. When flow is mainly laminar, the pressure varies linearly with the flow. When flow is mainly turbulent, driving pressure varies exponentially with the flow. With all else equal, pressures generated during laminar flow are most affected by fluid viscosity, whereas fluid density is the key factor when flow is turbulent.

Flow, Velocity, and Cross-Sectional Area

Flow is the bulk movement of a volume of fluid per unit of time. Clinically, the most common units of flow are liters per minute (L/min) or liters per second (L/sec). In contrast, velocity is a measure of linear distance traveled by the fluid per unit of time. Centimeters per second (cm/sec) is a common velocity unit used in pulmonary physiology.

Although fluid flow and velocity are different measures, the two concepts are closely related. The key factor relating velocity to flow is the cross-sectional area of the conducting system. Figure 6-23 shows this relationship.

Throughout the tube, the fluid flows at a constant rate of 5 L/min. At *point A,* with a cross-sectional area of 5.08 cm^2, the velocity of the fluid is 16.4 cm/sec. At *point B,* the cross-sectional area of the tube decreases to 2.54 cm^2, half its prior value. At this point, the velocity of the fluid doubles to 32.8 cm/sec. At *point C,* the passage divides into eight smaller tubes. Although each tube is smaller than its "parent," together they provide a 10-fold increase in the cross-sectional area available for flow compared with *point B.* The velocity of the fluid decreases proportionately, from 32.8 cm/sec to 3.28 cm/sec.

These observations show that the velocity of a fluid moving through a tube at a constant flow varies inversely with the available cross-sectional area. This relationship is called the **law of continuity.** Mathematically, the equation is as follows:

$$(A_1 \times v_1) + (A_2 \times v_2) + (A_n \times v_n) = k$$

where A is the cross-sectional area of the tube; v is the velocity of the fluid; 1, 2, and n are different points in the tube; and *k* is a constant value.

Although the principle holds true only for incompressible liquids, the qualitative features are similar for gas flow.

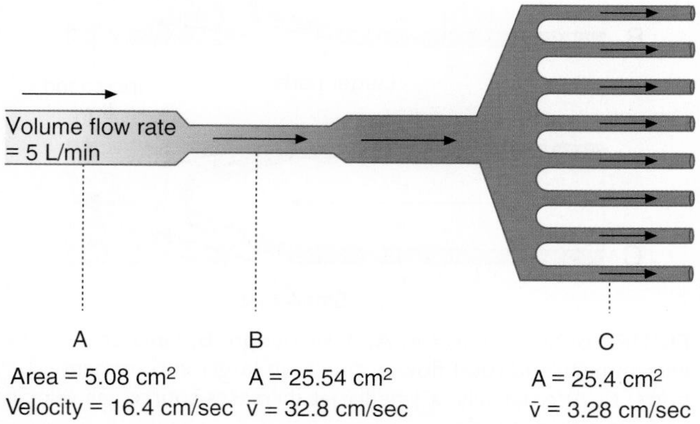

FIGURE 6-23 Fluid velocity, at a constant flow, varies inversely with the cross-sectional area of the tube. (Modified from Nave CR, Nave BC: Physics for the health sciences, ed 3, Philadelphia, 1985, WB Saunders.)

This principle also underlies the application of nozzles or jets in fluid streams. Nozzles and jets are simply narrow passages in a tube designed to increase fluid velocity. A garden-hose nozzle is a good example of this principle in action. Clinically, jets are used in many types of respiratory care equipment, including pneumatic nebulizers (see Chapter 36) and gas entrainment or mixing devices (see Chapter 38).

Bernoulli Effect

When a fluid flows through a tube of uniform diameter, pressure decreases progressively over the tube length.[11] The first three water columns in Figure 6-24 show this continuous pressure decrease. However, when the fluid passes through a constriction, the decrease in pressure is much greater. This large pressure decrease can be observed in the fourth water column in Figure 6-24. The eighteenth-century scientist Bernoulli was the first to study this effect carefully, which now bears his name. Bernoulli explained the pressure decrease depicted in Figure 6-24 by showing how the potential, kinetic, and pressure energies of a fluid interact.

A fluid's position determines its potential energy. The common adage that "water always seeks its lowest level" is actually an expression of potential energy. At the top of a tilted tube, gravity gives any fluid the potential energy to flow "downhill." In this case, the fluid's potential energy is proportional to the difference between the height of the tube's inlet and outlet. If a tube is level, the fluid's potential energy remains constant and can be disregarded.

Kinetic energy is the amount of work performed by matter in motion. The kinetic energy of a moving fluid is directly proportional to both its velocity and its mass. The greater the velocity and mass (density) of a fluid, the greater its kinetic energy. If mass is constant, kinetic energy varies directly with velocity only.

Although potential and kinetic energy are common physical concepts, the principle of pressure energy is unique to fluid flow. The pressure energy of a fluid is the *radial* or *outward force* exerted by the moving fluid. This radial force is measured as the fluid's lateral pressure.

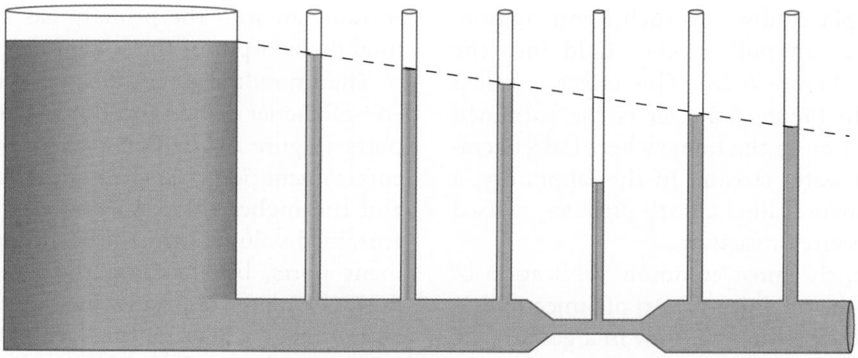

FIGURE 6-24 The Bernoulli effect. (Modified from Nave CR, Nave BC: Physics for the health sciences, ed 3, Philadelphia, 1985, WB Saunders.)

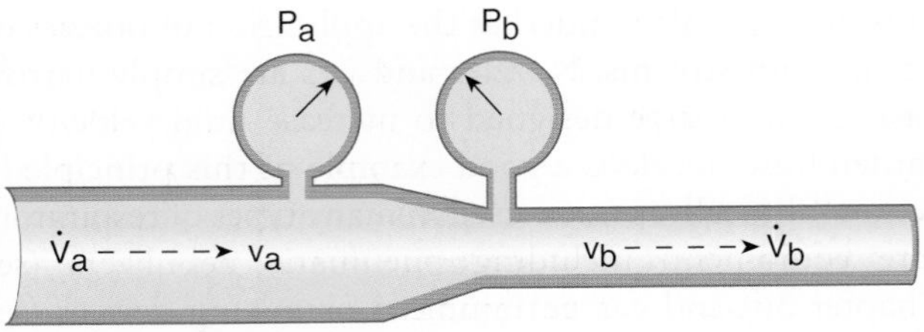

FIGURE 6-25 According to the Bernoulli theorem, lateral pressure of a flowing fluid must vary inversely with its velocity. $\dot{V}_a$, flow in tube "a"; v_a, velocity in tube "a"; v_b, velocity in tube "b"; $\dot{V}_b$, flow in tube "b"; P_a, lateral wall pressure in tube "a"; P_b, lateral wall pressure after restriction (see text).

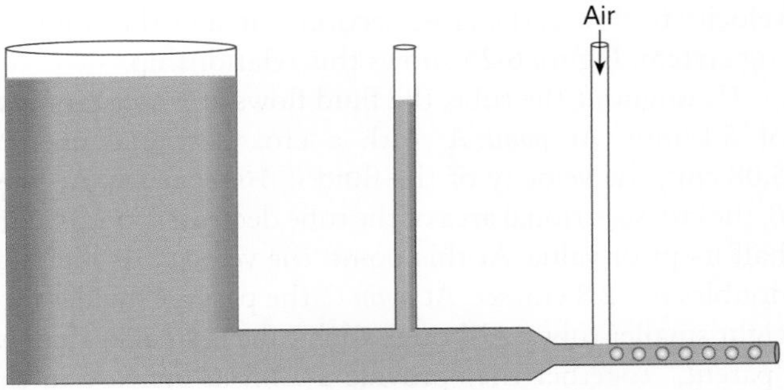

FIGURE 6-26 Fluid entrainment based on the Bernoulli effect. (Modified from Nave CR, Nave BC: Physics for the health sciences, ed 3, Philadelphia, 1985, WB Saunders.)

According to the first law of thermodynamics, the total energy at any given point in a fluid stream must be the same throughout the tube. If potential energy is held constant (a level tube), the sum of the kinetic and pressure energies at any given point in a fluid stream must equal their sum at any other point.

Velocity is equivalent to the kinetic energy of a fluid, whereas lateral force equates to pressure energy. Because a moving fluid's velocity and lateral pressure sum must always be equal, they must vary inversely with each other. In other words, if additional energy is applied to increase velocity, the energy available to exert pressure must decrease. As velocity increases, lateral pressure decreases. Conversely, as velocity decreases, lateral pressure increases.

Figure 6-25 shows this relationship. Fluid is flowing through a tube at a point with a certain velocity (v_a) and a lateral pressure (P_a). According to the law of continuity, as the fluid moves into the narrow or constricted portion of the tube, its velocity must increase ($v_b > v_a$). According to the Bernoulli theorem, the higher velocity at point b should result in a lower lateral pressure at that point ($P_b < P_a$). As a fluid flows through the constriction, its velocity increases, and its lateral pressure decreases.

Fluid Entrainment

When a flowing fluid encounters a very narrow passage, its velocity can increase greatly. In some cases, the increase in velocity can be so great as to cause the fluid's lateral pressure to fall below that exerted by the atmosphere (i.e., to become negative).

If an open tube is placed distal to such a constriction, this negative pressure can pull another fluid into the primary flow stream (Figure 6-26). This effect is called **fluid entrainment.** In Figure 6-26, air is the entrained fluid. This use is common in the home where faucet aerators mix air into the water stream. In the laboratory, a similar faucet attachment, called a *water aspirator,* is used to create negative pressure or vacuum.

In respiratory care, the most common application of fluid entrainment is the air injector. An air injector is a device designed to increase the total flow in a gas stream. In this case, a pressurized gas, usually oxygen, serves as the primary flow source. This pressurized gas passes through a nozzle or jet, beyond which is an air entrainment port. The negative lateral pressure created at the jet orifice entrains air into the primary gas stream, increasing the total flow output of the system.

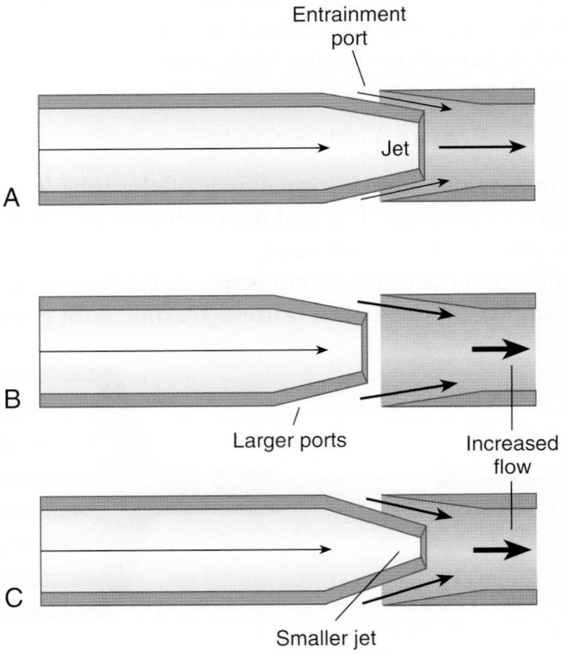

FIGURE 6-27 Air injector. **A,** Basic design. **B,** Greater entrainment and total flow occurs with larger entrainment ports. **C,** Alternatively, a smaller jet increases source gas velocity and entrains more air.

The amount of air entrained depends on both the diameter of the jet orifice and the size of the air entrainment ports (Figure 6-27). For a fixed jet size, the larger the entrainment ports, the greater the volume of air entrained and the higher the total flow (see Figure 6-27, *B*). The entrained volume can still be altered, with fixed entrainment ports, by changing the jet diameter (see Figure 6-27, *C*). A large jet results in a lower gas velocity and less entrainment, whereas a small jet boosts velocity, entrained volume, and total flow.

Venturi and Pitot Tubes

A *Venturi tube* is a modified entrainment device, developed approximately 200 years ago by Venturi.[12] A Venturi tube widens just after its jet or nozzle (Figure 6-28). As long as the angle of dilation is less than 15 degrees, this widening helps restore fluid pressure back toward prejet levels.

Compared with a simple air injector, the Venturi tube provides greater entrainment. This design helps keep the percentage of entrained fluid constant, even when the total flow varies. However, the Venturi tube has one major drawback: Any buildup of pressure downstream from the entrainment port decreases fluid entrainment. An alternative design, called a *Pitot tube,* partly overcomes this problem. Rather than restoring fluid pressure, a Pitot tube restores fluid velocity. This lessens the effect of downstream pressure on fluid entrainment.

Fluidics and Coanda Effect

Fluidics is a branch of engineering that applies hydrodynamic principles in flow circuits for purposes such as switching, pressure and flow sensing, and amplification. Because fluidic devices have no moving parts, they are very dependable and require little maintenance.

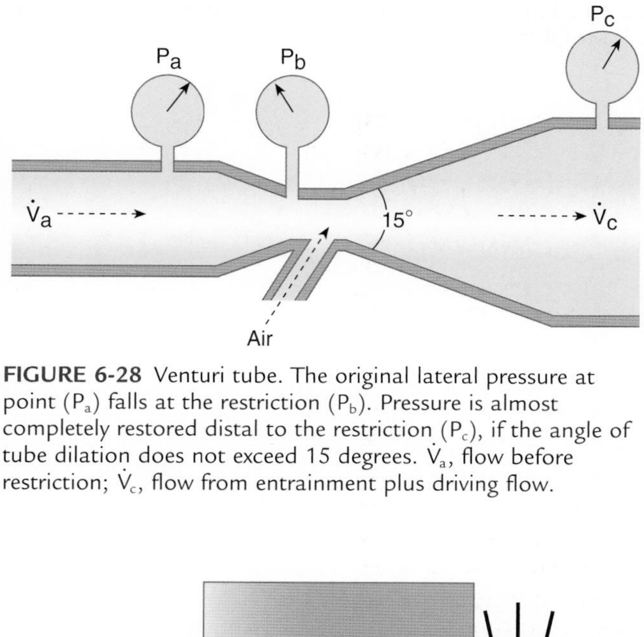

FIGURE 6-28 Venturi tube. The original lateral pressure at point (P_a) falls at the restriction (P_b). Pressure is almost completely restored distal to the restriction (P_c), if the angle of tube dilation does not exceed 15 degrees. $\dot{V}_a$, flow before restriction; $\dot{V}_c$, flow from entrainment plus driving flow.

The primary principle underlying most fluidic circuitry is a phenomenon called *wall attachment,* or the **Coanda effect.** This effect is observed mainly when a fluid flows through a small orifice with properly contoured downstream surfaces.[13]

Based on the Bernoulli effect, we know that the negative pressure created at a jet or nozzle entrains any surrounding fluid, such as air, into the primary flow stream (Figure 6-29, *A*). If a carefully contoured curved wall is added to one side of the jet (see Figure 6-29, *B*), the pressure near the wall becomes negative relative to atmospheric. The atmospheric pressure on the other side of the gas stream pushes it against the wall, where it remains "locked" until interrupted by some counterforce. By carefully extending the wall contour, we can deflect the fluid stream through a full 180-degree turn.

Various fluidic devices can be designed using this principle, including on/off switches, pressure and flow sensors, and flow amplifiers. These individual components can be combined into *integrated fluidic logic circuits,* which function much like electronic circuit boards but without the need for electrical power.

SUMMARY CHECKLIST

- Gases have no inherent boundary, are readily compressed and expanded, and can flow.
- Three temperature scales are in common use: Kelvin (SI), Celsius (cgs), and Fahrenheit (fps); conversion among these scale units can be done by using simple formulas.
- Transfer of heat energy can occur by conduction, convection, radiation, and evaporation.
- Liquids exert pressure and exhibit the properties of flow, buoyant force, viscosity, capillary action, and surface tension.
- The pressure exerted by a liquid depends on both its height (depth) and weight density.
- Surface tension forces increase the pressure inside a liquid drop or bubble; this pressure varies directly with the surface tension of the liquid and varies inversely with the radius.

Continued

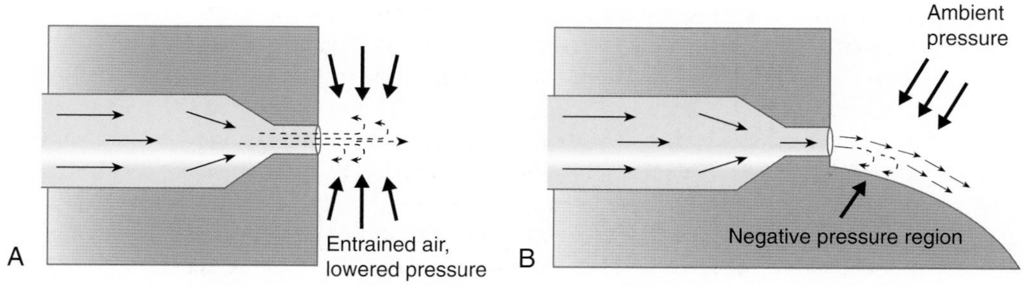

FIGURE 6-29 Coanda wall effect. **A,** Entrainment into the fluid stream. **B,** Wall attachment initiated by negative pressure near wall.

- A liquid can vaporize by either boiling or evaporation; in evaporation, the required heat energy is taken from the air surrounding the liquid, cooling the air.
- Vaporization causing cooling and condensation causes warming of the surroundings.
- The capacity of air to hold water vapor increases with temperature.
- Relative humidity (RH) is the ratio of water vapor content (absolute humidity) to saturated water vapor capacity; for a constant content, cooling increases RH and warming decreases RH.
- The rate of diffusion of a gas is inversely proportional to its molecular weight.
- The total pressure of a mixture of gases must equal the sum of the partial pressures of all component gases.
- The volume of a gas that dissolves in a liquid equals its solubility coefficient times its partial pressure; high temperatures decrease gas solubility, and low temperatures increase gas solubility.
- Volume and pressure of a gas vary directly with temperature; however, with constant temperature, gas volume and pressure vary inversely.
- The critical temperature of a substance is the highest temperature at which it can exist as a liquid; gases with critical temperatures higher than room temperature can be stored under pressure as liquids without cooling.
- Under conditions of laminar flow, the difference in pressure required to produce a given flow is defined by Poiseuille's law.
- The velocity of a fluid flowing through a tube at a constant rate of flow varies inversely with the available cross-sectional area; this allows entrainment of other fluids at jets or nozzles.

References

1. McNaught AD, Wilkinson A: Compendium of chemical terminology, IUPAC Gold Book, 2010.
2. Debenedetti PG, Stillinger FH: Supercooled liquids and the glass transition. Nature 410(8 March):259–267, 2001.
3. Ojovan MI: Configurons: thermodynamic parameters and symmetry changes at glass transition. Entropy 10(3):334–364, 2008.
4. TW Leland Jr: Basic principles of classical and statistical thermodynamics www.uic.edu/lobs/trl/1.onlinematerials/basicprinciplosbytwleland.pdf.
5. International System of Units (SI), Bureau International des Poids et Mesures (BIPM); 2006.
6. Mills I, Cvitas T, Homann K, Kallay N, Kuchitsu K. Quanities, units, and symbols in physical chemistry www.inpac.org/publications/books/gbook/green_book_2ed.pdf.
7. Fundamental Physical Constants: National Institute for Standards and Technology (NIST) http://physics.nist.gov/cuu/Units/kelvin.html |Accessed February 6, 2011|.
8. National Aeronautics and Space Administration (NASA) Animated Gas Lab: http://www.grc.nasa.gov/WWW/K-12/airplane/Animation/frglab.html Accessed February 2011.
9. Thom SR: Hyperbaric oxygen: its mechanisms and efficacy. Plastic and reconstructive surgery 127:131S–141S, 2011.
10. West JB: Robert Boyle's landmark book of 1660 with the first experiments on rarified air. Journal of Applied Physiology 98(1):31–39, 2004.
11. Eastlake CN: An aerodynamicist's view of lift, Bernoulli, and Newton. The Physics Teacher 40(March):166–176, 2002.
12. Bossart P: Venturi atomizers as potential sources of patient cross-infection. American Journal of Infection Control 31(7):441–444, 2003.
13. Ginghină C: The Coanda effect in cardiology. J Cardiovasc Med 8:411–413, 2007.

Chapter 7

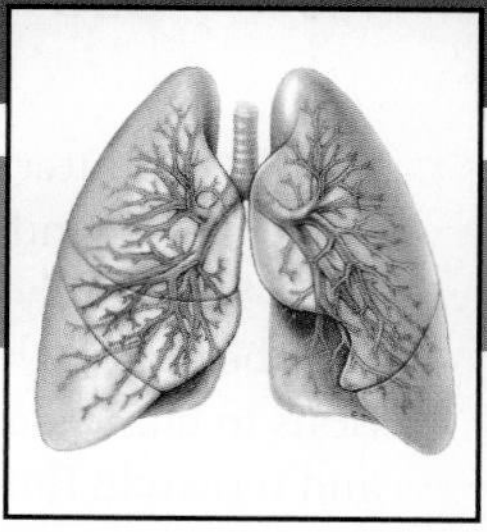

Computer Applications in Respiratory Care

MICHAEL E. ANDERS

CHAPTER OBJECTIVES

After reading this chapter you will be able to:

- Describe computer applications in clinical care, management, education, and research
- Retrieve evidence-based information
- Outline steps to maintain security and confidentiality

CHAPTER OUTLINE

Applications in Clinical Care
- Mechanical Ventilators
- Patient-Driven Protocols
- Clinical Decision Support
- Telemedicine
- Treatment of Tobacco Use and Dependence
- Management of Chronic Respiratory Diseases

Applications in Diagnostics
- Hemodynamic Monitoring
- Blood Gas Laboratories
- Pulmonary Function Laboratories

Information Retrieval
- World Wide Web
- Google Scholar
- PubMed and MEDLINE
- Ovid
- Information Retrieval by Patients

Applications in Management and Administration
- Respiratory Care Management Information Systems
- Benchmarking
- Hospital Information System
- Electronic Health Records

Applications in Education
- Clinical Simulation
- DataARC
- National Board for Respiratory Care Credentialing
- Distance Education
- Continuing Education
- Pulmonary Artery Catheter Education Project

Applications in Research
- Data Sources
- Data Collection
- Statistical Software
- Citations and Bibliographies
- Protection of Human Research Subjects

Security and Confidentiality
- Security
- Confidentiality

KEY TERMS

benchmarking
clinical decision support
Clinical Queries search filter in PubMed
clinical simulation
DataArc
eHealth
electronic health records
information retrieval
respiratory care management information systems
telemedicine

Computer applications are universal in respiratory care, and their impact continues to advance exponentially. Respiratory therapists (RTs) and other members of the health care team rely on computer applications in clinical care, diagnostics, management, education, and research. Emerging computer technology, or **eHealth,** applications aim to improve the processes of care and the performance of health care providers, engage patients, facilitate care from a distance, and manage information, improving health outcomes. Abundant, accessible, and up-to-date information from the government, universities, publishers, professional organizations, and industry is available to health care providers and patients on the World Wide Web. As established by a task force of the American Association for Respiratory Care (AARC) to chart a vision for the future, RTs will benefit from knowing how to retrieve information efficiently from the best available evidence-based resources.[1] RTs have compelling reasons to learn about computer applications.

APPLICATIONS IN CLINICAL CARE

Mechanical Ventilators

Conventional mechanical ventilators use microprocessors to control flow and pressure for triggering, limiting, and cycling breaths. Some modes of ventilation are closed-loop or adaptive, with predetermined algorithms that take actions automatically within preset limits. Breath-by-breath, microprocessors equilibrate measured values with target values. Based on the lung compliance measured during the previous breath, some modes adjust inspiratory pressure to attain a target tidal volume set by the clinician. New advanced adaptive systems, such as proportional assist ventilation and neurally adjusted ventilatory assist, aim to enhance the patient-ventilator synchrony via automation that is highly responsive to the patient.[2]

Microprocessors perform additional functions. They control ventilator alarms and archive the history of set and measured values, which can be uploaded to a computer. Current conventional ventilators allow for updating and adding new modes of ventilation via uploading new software, rather than purchasing new ventilators.

Protocols for ventilator weaning and management of acute respiratory distress syndrome can improve patients' outcomes; complete, accurate, and consistent documentation of ventilator settings is key. However, manual ventilator charting is frequently incomplete, inaccurate, and inconsistent.[3] Computerized ventilator charting applications have the potential to improve the quality and consistency of ventilator charting. Automated ventilator charting, verified by RTs, takes ventilator charting a step further, with the potential to improve completeness, accuracy, consistency, and efficiency.[4] Figure 7-1 is an example of a computer screen for automated charting.

Patient-Driven Protocols

Evidence-based, patient-driven protocols can improve health outcomes.[5,6] Under medical direction and based on patient assessment, RTs use protocols to allocate and titrate respiratory care. Consistency and timeliness of implementation are keys to the effectiveness of protocols. Automation of protocols at the point of care can help RTs address these concerns. An automated protocol for

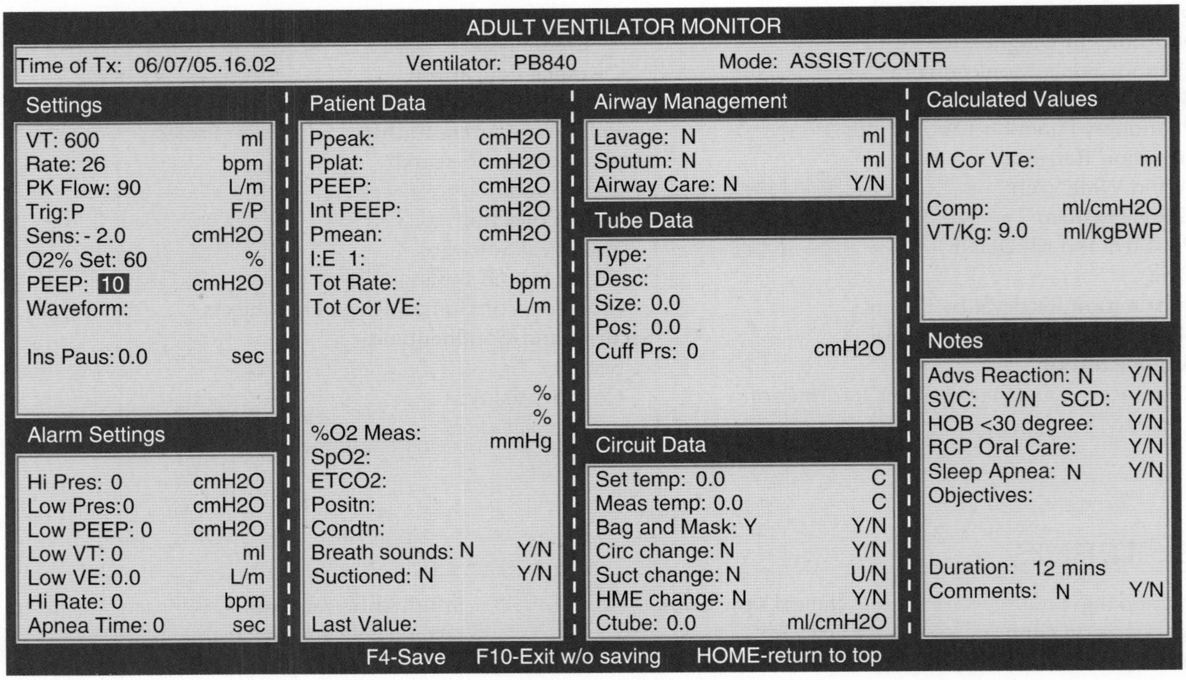

FIGURE 7-1 Automated ventilator charting.

discontinuation of the mechanical ventilation program on hand-held computers can decrease the time to the first spontaneous breathing trial and the length of stay in the intensive care unit (ICU) compared with a protocol without automation.[7] At least once a shift, RTs enter information about each mechanically ventilated patient via a hand-held computer. When patients meet preset criteria, the computer program prompts the RTs to conduct a spontaneous breathing trial to help determine the patients' readiness for ventilator discontinuation.

Clinical Decision Support

Information technology has the potential to assist clinicians actively with preventive measures, diagnosis, drug dosing, response to critical laboratory values, evidence-based care clinical practice guidelines, and chronic disease management. **Clinical decision support** systems match the characteristics of individual patients and their clinical interventions, drugs, and diagnostic tests to databases of scientific evidence and drug calculations and generate tailored recommendations, reminders, or even standing orders. These systems can optimally communicate these recommendations to clinicians via hospital information systems (HIS), e-mails, pagers, mobile phones, or printouts without the clinicians having to activate the system.

Clinical decision support systems are associated with improved clinician performance, decreased unnecessary care, and adherence to evidence-based clinical practice guidelines.[8,9] These systems are particularly useful in preventive care. Computerized reminders increased the proportion of indicated influenza vaccinations, rates of screening, counseling, and adherence to medications. They have also resulted in decreased unnecessary hospital admissions for inappropriately diagnosed cardiac ischemia, appropriately decreased tidal volume and more consistent monitoring of plateau pressure in patients with acute respiratory distress syndrome, and decreased exacerbations in asthma patients.[8] Clinical decision support is instrumental in improving clinical outcomes of patients by determining optimal drug dosages. Beneficial outcomes include the following:

- Faster time to achieve therapeutic drug levels
- Reduced toxic drug levels
- Decreased adverse drug reactions
- Decreased hospital length of stay[10]

Telemedicine

Telemedicine is the use of telecommunication and computer technology to promote access to diagnosis, monitoring, clinical decision support, and treatment for patients at medically underserved sites that are distant from health care providers. Telemedicine has been effectively implemented in various clinical settings, including home care, emergency departments, and ICUs, and is well accepted by patients.[11] Clinical outcomes have generally been similar to traditional health care delivery models; however, in the ICU setting, supplemental telemedicine has been associated with improved clinical outcomes, particularly among the most critically ill patients.[12,13] From a distance, on computers either within the hospital or at home, intensive care physicians can see the vital signs, ventilator data, medical record, and diagnostic images of the remote patients. Supplemental telemedicine helps to provide additional support that can potentially result in more rapid recognition of problems and timely, appropriate interventions.[14]

Treatment of Tobacco Use and Dependence

In the United States, tobacco use and dependence is the leading preventable cause of death and chronic diseases.[15] Health care costs attributable to tobacco use are unsustainable. Effective evidence-based treatments are available, but their implementation by health care providers is lagging.[16] RTs can play a vital role in the treatment of tobacco-related diseases and should aid in the pursuit of cost-effective ways to help tobacco users.

Emerging applications of computer technology, or eHealth applications, are exciting new components of treatment for tobacco use and dependence. With the extensive reach of the Internet and the demonstrated efficacy of some applications, the potential impact on health outcomes is immense. More than 10 million Internet users have searched for online information about how to quit smoking.[17]

Internet-based treatment programs can recruit tobacco users via search engines, or they can be an adjunct to telephone quitline counseling. Figure 7-2 is a screen

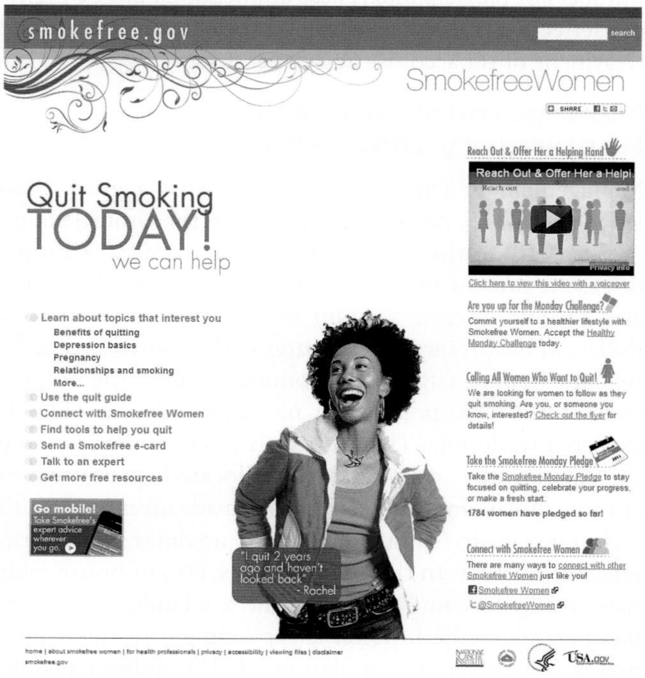
smokefree.gov
SmokefreeWomen
Quit Smoking TODAY!
we can help
Learn about topics that interest you
Benefits of quitting
Depression basics
Pregnancy
Relationships and smoking
More...
Use the quit guide
Connect with Smokefree Women
Find tools to help you quit
Send a Smokefree e-card
Talk to an expert
Get more free resources
Go mobile!
"I quit 2 years ago and haven't looked back" - Rachel
Reach Out & Offer Her a Helping Hand
Are you up for the Monday Challenge?
Calling All Women Who Want to Quit!
Take the Smokefree Monday Pledge
1784 women have pledged so far!
Connect with Smokefree Women

FIGURE 7-2 Example of an internet-based program: (http://women.smokefree.gov).

TABLE 7-1

Websites Related to the Treatment of Tobacco Use and Dependence

Website	Organization
SmokeFree.gov	U.S. Department of Health and Human Services
QuitNet.com	QuitNet
WHO.int/tobacco	World Health Organization, Tobacco Free Initiative
ITCProject.org	International Tobacco Control Policy Evaluation Project
ATTUD.org	Association for the Treatment of Tobacco Use and Dependence
TreaTobacco.net	Society for Research on Nicotine and Tobacco
TobaccoFreeKids.org	Tobacco Free Kids

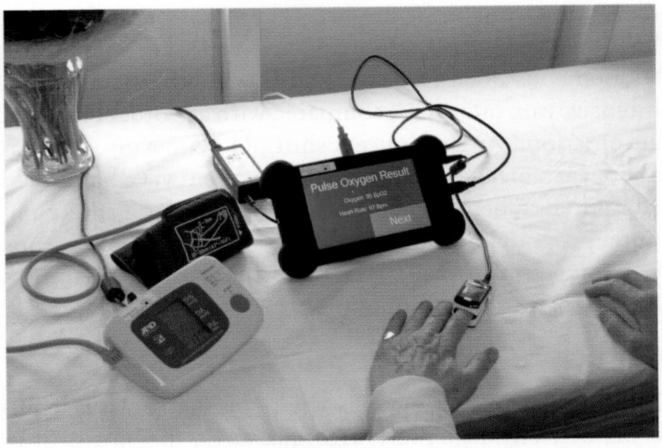

FIGURE 7-3 Telehealth Homepod. (Courtesy Tele Health Ltd. Dublin, Ireland.)

shot from the smokefree.gov tobacco treatment website. When eHealth applications are tailored to individual tobacco users, with frequent automated contacts via e-mail or text messages, rates of long-term abstinence from tobacco use are similar to other evidenced-based interventions.[18-22]

Consistent with the U.S. Public Health Service clinical practice guideline recommendation for a high-intensity, multicomponent approach, an Internet-based application has the capacity to provide both counseling that promotes tailored quit strategies and tobacco cessation medications that have been approved by the U.S. Food and Drug Administration (FDA).[16] Internet-based applications can provide unlimited, sustained access to virtually limitless numbers of participants. These applications can be highly cost-effective. Table 7-1 lists some websites related to the treatment of tobacco use and dependence.

Management of Chronic Respiratory Diseases

Management of chronic diseases presents a grave challenge to the U.S. health care system. In the United States, 7 out of 10 deaths are due to chronic disease.[23] Chronic disease is present in 8 out of 10 Americans on Medicare, and chronic diseases account for three out of every four dollars of health care expenditures in the United States.[24,25] As baby boomers age in the coming decades, the proportion of the U.S. population 65 years old and older is expected to double. There is much interest in addressing the historically disjointed, misallocated processes of chronic disease management through advances in eHealth technologies, to improve health outcomes in a cost-effective manner. In the United States, 60% of households have access to computers, and the availability of broadband access to the Internet is expanding.[17] In the United States, which has a population of 311 million people, there are more than 307 million wireless mobile phone connections.[26,27]

Asthma

eHealth applications for asthma include interactive Internet applications, such as games for children, Internet applications linked to cell phones for personalized or automated voice or text messaging, and other telemonitoring devices. Many of these applications use monitored patient data to tailor the adjustment of the plan of care. Some provide for personalized goals, calendars, and reminders. Educational tools include audiovisuals and quizzes. In patients with persistent asthma, evidence from research studies shows that these eHealth applications can result in an improvement in asthma knowledge, self-management skills, peak flow rates, and adherence to inhaled corticosteroid controller medications and fewer symptoms, missed school days, nighttime awakenings, activity limitations, emergency department visits, and hospitalizations.[28-33] These applications are well received by patients.[30]

A cornerstone of asthma disease management is assessing patients' level of control of the disease over time. One validated measure of impairment, recommended by the National Asthma Education and Prevention Program, is the Asthma Control Test.[34] This free questionnaire is available in an online format (see www.asthmacontrol.com), which patients can complete and take to a health care provider.

Chronic Obstructive Pulmonary Disease

Increasingly, chronic obstructive pulmonary disease (COPD) is being managed in the home. Internet-based telemonitoring systems, smartphones, and mobile phones with computer applications extend the reach of health care providers into the home. eHealth applications for patients with COPD facilitates education, self-management, and timely feedback from health care providers (Figure 7-3). Patients generally have a positive attitude about the role of this technology, and the quality of the transmitted data is good.[35] Improved outcomes include earlier identification of deteriorating symptoms, better response to exacerbations, increased rate of sustained exercise after pulmonary rehabilitation, and decreased emergency department visits and hospitalizations.[35-37] Additionally, eHealth applications can help detect comorbidities, such as sleep apnea.[35]

APPLICATIONS IN DIAGNOSTICS

Hemodynamic Monitoring

In hemodynamic monitoring via pulmonary artery catheters, computers calculate cardiac output, using the thermodilution technique. The thermistor port of the pulmonary artery catheter is linked to a computer. After the health care provider injects room air or iced solution into the catheter, the computer reads the subsequent change in the temperature of the solution and deduces the amount of blood flow or cardiac output.

Blood Gas Laboratories

The accuracy and precision of blood gas data influence clinical decisions and patient safety. Computerized blood gas analyzers and computer-assisted quality assurance measures in a blood gas laboratory are crucial functions in a respiratory care department. Quality assurance data are necessary for accreditation of blood gas laboratories by the College of American Pathologists, the Clinical Laboratory Improvement Amendments, or The Joint Commission. Manual backup procedures must be in place in the event of computer system failure or downtime because of the critical nature of timely reporting of blood gas results and the need to be able to assess archived data at all times. Blood gas laboratories interface analyzers with HIS to make blood gas results immediately available at the point of care; additionally, this enables storage, retrieval, billing, and quality assurance.

Pulmonary Function Laboratories

Some hospitals interface their pulmonary function testing system with the HIS. Alternatively, other hospitals connect their desktop or notebook computer–based pulmonary function testing system to a local area network, which allows clinicians to access reports and graphics from multiple workstations. Most cardiopulmonary exercise and metabolic measurement systems use desktop or notebook computers.

Interpretation of Pulmonary Function Tests

Computer algorithms use standard reference predicted values to aid in the interpretation of pulmonary function tests (PFTs), including spirometry, lung volume, diffusing capacity, and bronchodilator response. The algorithms compare the patterns of the patient's measured values with reference values based on age, height, gender, and race. The computer classifies the patterns of the patient's measured values as either normal or abnormal with degrees of severity. However, qualified interpreters must consider the effect of patient effort on the computer-assisted interpretation of PFTs.

The American Thoracic Society recommended pulmonary function reference standards based on the National Health and Nutrition Examination Survey (NHANES). These standards for prediction of normal PFT values may differ from other reference values. This difference can confound the interpretation of successive PFTs in an individual patient when clinicians focus on the computer-assisted interpretation of percent-of-predicted values, rather than the actual observed values.[38] Clinicians should have a clear understanding of which reference values were used for each test and interpret PFT results accordingly.

MINI CLINI

Computer-Assisted Interpretations of Pulmonary Function Tests in an Individual Patient

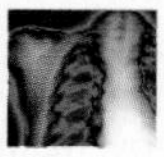

PROBLEM: A patient with alpha$_1$-antitrypsin deficiency has repeat PFTs, including a diffusing capacity of the lung for carbon monoxide (DLCO). Based on a computer-assisted interpretation, there appears to be a remarkable decrease in the percent-of-predicted value for DLCO. It was previously normal; now it is 68% of predicted, indicative of emphysema. An effective therapy, pooled human plasma alpha$_1$-antitrypsin, is available but expensive. What additional information should the clinicians evaluate?

DISCUSSION: The clinicians should determine (a) the actual observed DLCO values of the previous and repeat tests and (b) whether the computer-assisted interpretations are based on unannounced different reference values. If the computer-assisted percent of predicted values for each test were based on different sets of reference values, it could account for the change in DLCO.

INFORMATION RETRIEVAL

Effective **information retrieval** is essential to evidence-based respiratory care. It enhances clinical expertise by providing information for the development of evidence-based, patient-driven protocols, and it aids in clinical decisions for individual patients.

Although assessment skills of RTs generally sharpen with experience, their knowledge of the most up-to-date therapies may diminish over time.[39] However, the best available medical evidence is dynamic rather than static, and the amount of available information is staggering. A search with the Google search engine using the search word "smoking" yielded more than 169 million results in

TABLE 7-2
Helpful Websites for Respiratory Therapists

Organization	Website
American Academy of Allergy, Asthma, and Immunology	www.aaaai.org
American Academy of Pediatrics	www.aap.org
American Academy for Sleep Medicine	www.aasmnet.org
American College of Allergy, Asthma, and Immunology	www.acaai.org
American Association for Respiratory Care	www.aarc.org
American Cancer Society	www.cancer.org
American College of Chest Physicians	www.chestnet.org
American Heart Association	www.heart.org/heartorg
American Lung Association	www.lungusa.org
American Thoracic Society	www.thoracic.org
ARDS Network	www.ardsnet.org
Centers for Disease Control and Prevention	www.cdc.gov
Cochrane Collaboration	www.cochrane.org
Committee on Accreditation for Respiratory Care	www.coarc.com
Cystic Fibrosis Foundation	www.cff.org
Global Initiative for COPD	www.goldcopd.com
National Board for Respiratory Care	www.nbrc.org
National Heart, Lung and Blood Institute	www.nhlbi.nih.gov/health/indexpro.htm
Society for Critical Care Medicine	www.sccm.org
U.S. Surgeon General	www.surgeongeneral.gov

a fraction of a second. RTs need to be knowledgeable about efficient ways to access, filter, and retrieve information effectively. They must also be prepared to guide increasingly sophisticated patients, many of whom actively seek medical information on the Internet, in retrieving reliable information.

World Wide Web

The World Wide Web is a far-reaching, rich source of information. RTs can "bookmark" helpful websites for clinical practice guidelines, evidence-based systematic reviews of clinical questions, accrediting agencies, or other relevant sites for rapid retrieval of important information (Table 7-2). For example, the Cochrane Collaboration (see www.cochrane.org), well respected for rigorously conducted systematic evidence-based reviews, provides free access to abstracts and summaries pertaining to relevant clinical questions, including questions related to "airways."

Google Scholar

Google Scholar (see scholar.google.com) is a search engine for scholarly publications in a wide range of fields. It includes peer-reviewed manuscripts, abstracts, theses, and books from academic publishers, professional societies, and university libraries. Google Scholar uses a special algorithm to rank and determine the order of the search results. Variables in the algorithm include analyses of citations, authors, publications, and full texts.

Google Scholar is fast, yields wide-ranging search results, and provides citation data. Additionally, by virtue of agreements with certain publishers, search results sometimes include articles that are otherwise unavailable. The optimal application of Google Scholar may be for initial searches to find a relevant article quickly or when users know either an author or the title of a specific article that they are seeking.

Box 7-1 Examples of Using Boolean Connector Terms for Search Phrases

SENSITIVE SEARCHES

The search phrase "surfactant OR bronchopulmonary dysplasia" yields citations that pertain to *either* search term.

SPECIFIC SEARCHES

The search phrase "surfactant AND bronchopulmonary dysplasia" yields only citations that pertain to *both* of these terms.

PubMed and MEDLINE

PubMed (see www.pubmed.com) is the free search engine of the National Library of Medicine for health information. It searches several databases, including MEDLINE, the database of the National Library of Medicine of millions of references from thousands of journals related to medicine, nursing, the health care system, and science. The National Library of Science updates MEDLINE references in PubMed almost daily. Each MEDLINE citation in PubMed generally has the following information: title, authors, an abstract, journal, language, type of publication, and Medical Subject Headings (MeSH).

A unique feature of PubMed is that it maps users' search terms to MeSH. PubMed uses Boolean logic, in which users can combine search words or phrases with connectors such as AND or OR to narrow or broaden searches. Box 7-1 provides examples to illustrate the use of Boolean connector terms.

PubMed Clinical Queries Filter

The **Clinical Queries search filter in PubMed** is easy to use and very effective in retrieving valid research studies. To access it, on the PubMed home page, in the center column, under "PubMed Tools," click "Clinical Queries" (Figure 7-4). On the Clinical Queries page, select one of the "Clinical Studies Categories," such as "Therapy" or "Diagnosis." Then select the scope of the search, as either "Broad" or "Narrow." A "Broad" search is more sensitive, providing

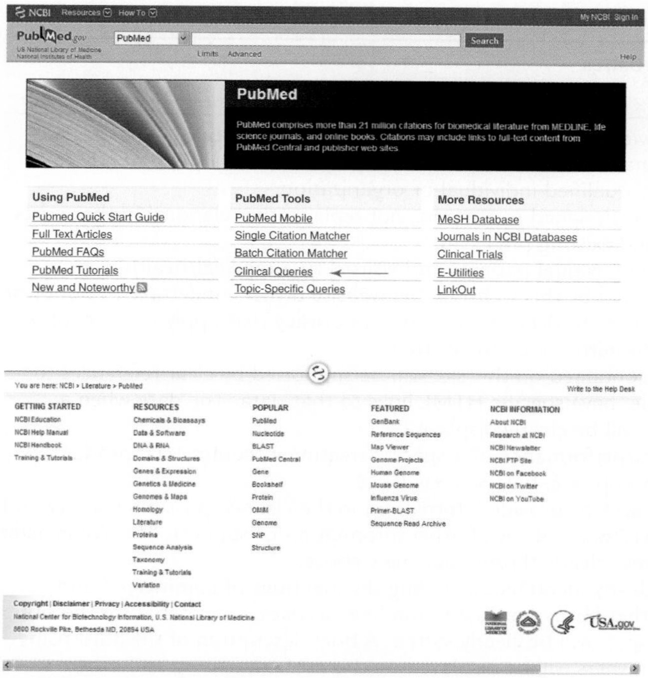

FIGURE 7-4 PubMed home page. Clinical queries is under PubMed Tools. (From US National Library of Medicine; National Institutes of Health, Bethesda, Maryland.)

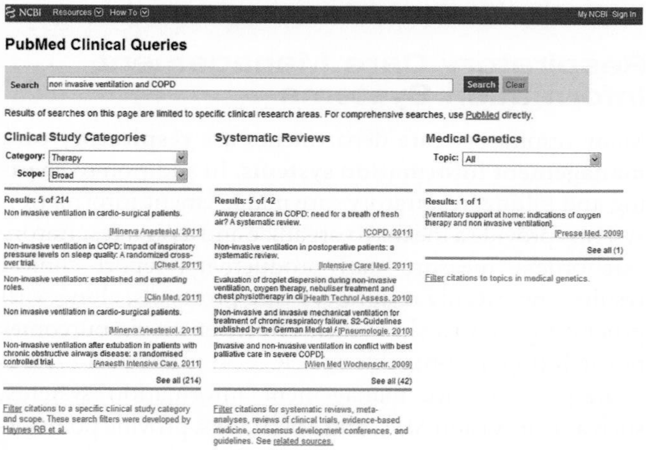

FIGURE 7-5 PubMed Clinical Queries page, with search results. (US National Library of Medicine; National Institute of Health, Bethesda, Md.)

more search results; a "Narrow" search is more specific, providing fewer search results. Selection of "Broad" versus "Narrow" depends on the reason for the search. Search results include clinical research studies in the left column and systematic reviews in the center column, or the user can elect to include only systematic reviews in the search results (Figure 7-5). When the user selects "Therapy" from the "Clinical Study Categories" with a "Narrow" scope, the Clinical Queries filter automatically searches for randomized controlled trials and systematic reviews.

RULE OF THUMB

When developing evidence-based patient-driven protocols, the user might elect to start with a "Broad," sensitive search that is more comprehensive.

When time efficiency is a high priority, such as when retrieving information to assist in the care of an individual patient, the user might select a "Narrow," specific search strategy.

The Clinical Queries search filter is very sensitive (true positives/true positives + false negatives) and specific (true positives/true positives + false positives) in the retrieval of the best available scientific evidence. A validation study of this search filter yielded 93% sensitivity and 97% specificity.[40] The Clinical Queries search filter effectively retrieves valid research studies, while eliminating nonrelevant information and poorly designed studies. Compared with Google Scholar, which lacks any way to filter a large volume of information, PubMed Clinical Queries filter is equally sensitive but considerably more specific, reducing the time it takes to find the best available evidence.[41]

Additional Features of PubMed

PubMed has additional convenient features. By completing a free registration, users may save search results and receive automatic e-mail updates. The "Send to" feature allows users to print or e-mail search results or send multiple search results to a clipboard. Several modular and interactive tutorials are available.

Ovid

Ovid is an extensive collection of Web-based information resources, including databases, journals, books, and searching software. Many medical libraries and large hospitals in the United States purchase and use Ovid in some form. An institution can customize Ovid content and resources to meet its particular needs. Among hundreds of available databases in Ovid, medical databases include Medline, Evidence-Based Medicine Reviews, and CINAHL. The Evidence-Based Reviews databases include the Cochrane Database of Systematic Reviews and the ACP Journal Club by the American College of Physicians. The ACP Journal Club features reviews of clinically relevant research studies that were conducted in a rigorous manner. The CINHAL (Cumulative Index to Nursing and Allied Health Literature) database features literature from nursing and 17 allied health professions, including respiratory care.

Information Retrieval by Patients

With the advent of extensive available information on the Web, patients increasingly seek knowledge about diseases and treatments on their own. Eight in 10 Internet users have searched the Web for health information.[17] However,

TABLE 7-3

Health on the Net Code of Conduct for Medical and Health Websites

Principle	Code
Authority	Any medical or health advice provided and hosted on this site will be given only by medically trained and qualified professionals unless a clear statement is made that a piece of advice offered is from a non-medically qualified individual or organization.
Complementarity	Information provided on this site is designed to support, not replace, the relationship that exists between a patient/site visitor and existing physician.
Confidentiality	Confidentiality of data relating to individual patients and visitors to a medical/health website, including their identity, is respected by this website. The website owners undertake to honor or exceed the legal requirements of medical/health information privacy that apply in the country and state where the website and mirror sites are located.
Attribution	Where appropriate, information contained on this site will be supported by clear references to source data and, where possible, have specific HTML links to that data. The date when a clinical page was last modified will be clearly displayed.
Justifiability	Any claims relating to the benefits/performance of a specific treatment, commercial product, or service will be supported by appropriate, balanced evidence.
Transparency of authorship	The designers of this website will seek to provide information in the clearest possible manner and provide contact addresses for visitors that seek further information or support. The Webmaster will display his/her e-mail address clearly throughout the website.
Transparency of sponsorship	Support for this website will be clearly identified, including the identities of commercial and noncommercial organizations that have contributed funding, services, or material for the site.
Honesty in advertising and editorial policy	If advertising is a source of funding, it will be clearly stated. A brief description of the advertising policy adopted by the website owners will be displayed on the site. Advertising and other promotional material will be presented to viewers in a manner and context that facilitates differentiation between it and the original material created by the institution operating the site.

From www.hon.ch/HONcode/Conduct.html.

many Web users neglect to scrutinize the quality or source of the information, which is largely unregulated.[42] RTs should be able to offer guidance to patients about appropriate information sources. Table 7-3 presents the Health on the Net criteria for evaluating the quality of medical and health websites. Selected resources for patients include the AARC site for patients (see www.yourlunghealth.org), the website of the National Lung Health Program (see www.nlhep.org) dedicated to COPD patients, and MedlinePlus.gov of the National Library of Medicine. MedlinePlus features online interactive tutorials, practical instructional handouts for patients, a medical encyclopedia, and videos of surgical procedures.

APPLICATIONS IN MANAGEMENT AND ADMINISTRATION

Computer applications are important to respiratory care managers and administrators. Respiratory care managers use computer applications to plan, organize, direct, and evaluate. Health care administrators rely on information systems for communication and processing information. There is widespread enthusiasm and support for further development and implementation of **electronic health records** to make patients' medical records available across the continuum of care of geographic locations.

Respiratory Care Management Information Systems

Many respiratory care departments use **respiratory care management information systems.** In addition to charting and billing, respiratory care management information systems provide a means to organize and assign respiratory care orders, measure staff productivity, report clinical results, and execute respiratory care protocols, along with generating data to show their effectiveness via outcomes research (Figure 7-6).

Respiratory care management information systems, such as CliniVision MPC and MediLinks, provide point-of-care, mobile, charting capabilities via hand-held computers, with wireless transmission of data to HIS. These hand-held computers integrate the AARC Uniform Reporting Manual, which includes time standards for respiratory care procedures, billing codes, and clinical practice guidelines. Additionally, they function as pagers and telephones, provide access to the Internet, and interface with mechanical ventilators and blood gas analyzers.

Hand-held computers offer several advantages compared with paper charts. Hand-held computers facilitate the organization and assignment of workload, facilitate the fulfillment of physicians' orders, and improve documentation.[43,44] Documentation of patient assessment becomes immediately available to other members of the health care team in the HIS. Incomplete or lack of patient information, which is more likely to occur with paper

Bennett Memorial Hospital

Workload Estimate for 3 Shifts by Zone

Procedure Name	Time Standard	Number of Orders	------Shift One------ # of Txs	------Shift One------ Work Units	------Shift Two------ # of Txs	------Shift Two------ Work Units	------Shift Three------ # of Txs	------Shift Three------ Work Units
CCU								
ABG	20	3	3	60	3	60	3	0
AIRWAY CARE	25	1	1	0	1	0	1	0
ASSESSMENT	30	1	1	30	1	0	1	0
CPAP	5	1	1	5	1	5	1	5
EKG	22	1	1	22	1	22	1	0
EQUIPMENT CHANGE	10	1	1	10	1	0	1	0
MED NEB	13	2	2	26	2	26	2	26
METER DOSE INHALER	7	3	3	42	3	35	3	35
O2/LPM	5	1	1	15	1	10	1	10
O2/VENTI MASK	5	1	1	5	1	5	1	5
SPONTANEOUS MECHS	25	1	1	25	1	25	1	0
VENT CARE/ADULT	12	2	2	0	2	0	2	0
Total by Zone		18	18	240	18	188	18	81
# of Therapists Required for Zone				0.53		0.42		0.18
PEDS								
MED NEB	13	1	1	26	1	26	1	26
Total by Zone		1	1	26	1	26	1	26
# of Therapists Required for Zone				0.06		0.06		0.06
RICU								
AIRWAY CARE	25	1	1	0	1	0	1	0
CPT	20	1	1	40	1	40	1	0
EKG	22	1	1	22	1	22	1	0
MED NEB	13	1	1	26	1	26	1	26
METER DOSE INHALER	7	1	1	0	1	0	1	0
O2/AEROSOL	5	1	1	5	1	5	1	5
O2/LPM	5	1	1	5	1	5	1	5
Total by Zone		7	7	98	7	98	7	36
# of Therapists Required for Zone				0.22		0.22		0.08
SICU								
ABG	20	2	2	40	2	40	2	0
AIRWAY CARE	25	2	2	0	2	0	2	0
CPR	30	1	1	30	1	30	1	0
CPT	20	1	1	40	1	40	1	40
INCENT SPIROMETER	10	1	1	20	1	20	1	0
METER DOSE INHALER	7	3	3	49	3	42	3	14
O2/AEROSOL	5	1	1	5	1	5	1	5
O2/LPM	5	1	1	5	1	5	1	5
VENT CARE/ADULT	12	2	2	0	2	0	2	0
Total by Zone		14	14	189	14	182	14	64
# of Therapists Required for Zone				0.42		0.40		0.14

FIGURE 7-6 Clinivision Mobile Patient Charting (MPC): Workload Estimate for 3 Shifts by Zone. This report is grouped by Zone and then Procedure to show the estimate for the number of procedures, work units, and therapists required. (Image used by permission from Nellcor Puritan Bennett LLC, Boulder, Colorado, doing business as Covidien.)

charts, is associated with numerous medical errors that cause adverse events, including prolonged hospitalization and death.[45]

Benchmarking

Benchmarking is valuable for each of the primary functions of respiratory care managers, including planning, organizing, directing, and evaluating. The AARC provides an online benchmarking system (Figure 7-7) in which managers can compare the performance of their department with other similar departments. Managers can compare the ratio of ventilator days with the number of patients or the number of missed treatments in a given time frame. Benchmarking helps to show the productivity of the department and establish best practices.

Additionally, many respiratory care managers benchmark the incidence of ventilator-associated pneumonia in their hospital to that reported to the National Nosocomial Infections Surveillance system. This type of benchmarking can lead to increased efforts to implement evidence-based interventions to reduce the rate of ventilator-associated pneumonia, improving patients' outcomes.

Hospital Information System

An HIS is a comprehensive system for communication and information processing. It encompasses networks, computer hardware and software, and computerized patient records. The HIS supports both the administrative and the clinical missions of hospitals. For administrative purposes, it facilitates patient billing, reimbursement, and communication. For clinical purposes, key functions of an HIS are to serve as a data repository and a means to report results.

The HIS can permit chart review of clinical data at both central and remote locations. Ideally, patient data are accessible across the continuum of care, from outpatient clinics, emergency departments, and hospitals to rehabilitation centers. Patient data may include chest x-rays, bronchoscopy videos or images, sputum culture results, blood gases, and PFT results. Because hospitals consist of many different clinical units and allied health departments, being able to share data between different devices and computer systems is an important characteristic of an HIS.

Electronic Health Records

Electronic health records can improve access to patients' updated health information for both clinicians and patients and assist clinicians with clinical decision support. Many investigators have begun to focus attention on the development of a seamless network of transferable, widely accessible, longitudinal electronic health records. A comprehensive national health information infrastructure would result in interconnectivity among health information systems in the United States.[46] Core functions are shown in Box 7-2.

The electronic health record would become the central component of health care information systems, satisfying the information needs of health care providers, public health officials, and individuals, and potentially reduce medical errors and elimination of redundant diagnostic tests (Figure 7-8). It would support health systems planning and development of policies. Major barriers and

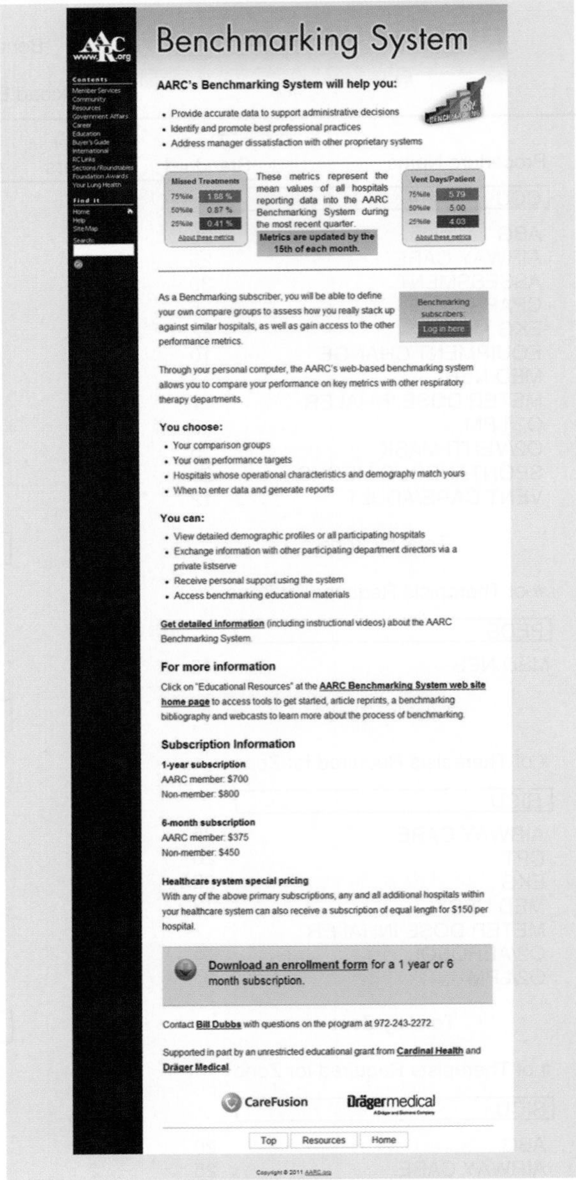

FIGURE 7-7 American Association for Respiratory Care, online Benchmarking System. (Courtesy AARC, Irving Texas.)

Box 7-2	Core Functions of Electronic Health Records

- Medical records
- Results reporting
- Computerized physician order entry
- Clinical decision support
- Electronic communication
- Channels between health care providers and patients
- Patient-entered data

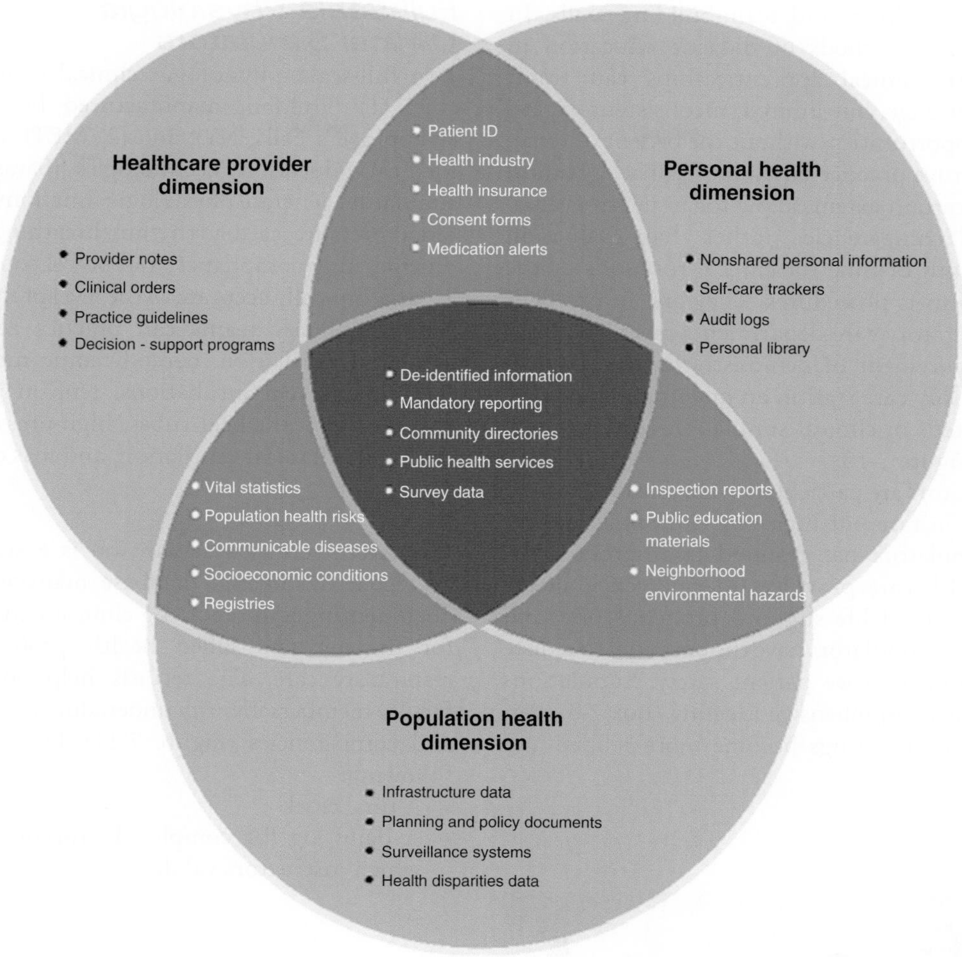

FIGURE 7-8 Electronic health records: dimensions of the national health information structure. (From United States Department of Health and Human Services. Information for health: a strategy for building the national health information infrastructure. Available at: http://aspe.hhs.gov/sp/NHII/Documents/NHIIReport 2001/default. htm. Accessed Sept. 25, 2006.)

challenges for the development and implementation of electronic health records are costs, the lack of uniformity of data, the inability to establish an interface among different health information systems, and accounting for the needs of various health professional disciplines.

APPLICATIONS IN EDUCATION

Computing plays a central role in the education of respiratory care students, credentialing of graduates of educational programs, and continuing education for practitioners.

Clinical Simulation

Computerized **clinical simulation** is a powerful learning aid. Computer-based simulation is a long-standing principal educational method for hazardous occupations that have shown remarkably low rates of failure (e.g., airline pilots, members of the military, astronauts, and nuclear power plant operators). Health care education has progressed to include the use of computer-based, full-body manikins and high-fidelity clinical simulators. These devices feature software to program clinical scenarios and simulated vital signs and physical examination findings that either improve or deteriorate in response to the actions of the learners. The simulators can reproduce situations requiring complex airway management or advanced life support. In virtual surgical simulators, haptic devices allow learners to exert force against simulated tissue that offers realistic resistance, and in virtual bronchoscopy simulators, vocal cord movements are exhibited that are synchronous with the phases of breathing and cough.

Learners are able to suspend disbelief, immersing themselves in carefully planned case scenarios and performing in a manner similar to that of real clinical situations (Figure 7-9). They develop psychomotor, critical thinking, decision-making, and team-building skills. In contrast, traditional methods of didactic education in combination with clinical apprenticeships can result in increased knowledge, but limited, inconsistent experiential learning opportunities, without the benefit of remediation and extensive practice based on feedback. Clinical simulators, to a certain extent, allow for in-depth evaluation of learners' competencies, rather than evaluation based on the length of time for clinical rotations or the number of performed procedures. They are an excellent tool to help respiratory care departments meet The Joint Commission requirement of demonstrating the competencies of respiratory care staff in an ongoing manner.[47,48] Recommended steps in clinical simulation education are diagrammed in Figure 7-10.

Clinical simulators are particularly valuable for learning how to function in rare but high-risk clinical situations. Training via simulators has resulted in improved performance of health care providers in emergency airway management, advanced life support, bronchoscopy, and surgery.[49-53] Clinical simulators have the potential to reduce medical errors and improve patient safety. Simulations promote relatively comprehensive learning (Box 7-3). Performances in clinical settings become more refined and automatic.

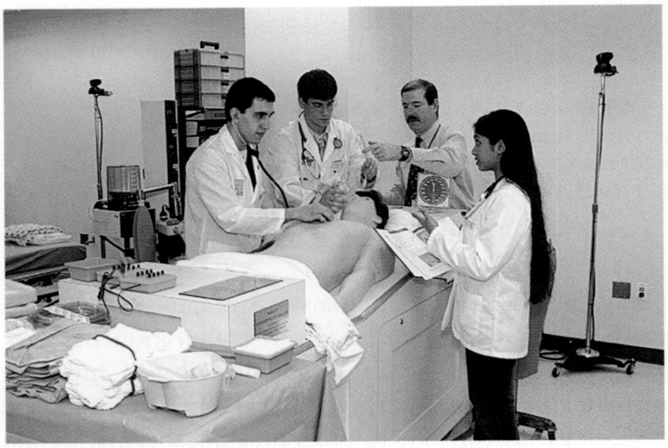

FIGURE 7-9 Clinical simulation benefits students. (From Cummings CW, et al: Cummings otolaryngeal: head and neck surgery, ed 2, St Louis, 2005, Mosby.)

Full-Scale Physiologic Clinical Simulators

Two full-scale, physiologic, clinical simulators are available: (1) SimMan, manufactured by Laerdal Medical (Wappingers Falls, NY); and (2) METI, manufactured by Medical Education Technologies (Sarasota, FL). These simulators generate physiologic functions including pulse, blood pressure, cardiac rhythm, breathing, exhaled carbon dioxide, lung compliance, and bowel sounds. The airways are anatomically accurate to the level of the lung segments. Interdisciplinary teams can practice scenarios such as cardiac defibrillation, hemodynamic monitoring, apnea, right main stem intubations, tension pneumothoraces, occluded endotracheal tubes, high-pressure alarm limits during mechanical ventilation, and loss of medical gas.

DataARC

DataARC (see www.dataarc.ws) is a secured, password-protected, Web-based database management system for documenting and reporting clinical educational activities for nursing and allied health professions, including respiratory care. The records help both students and faculty members identify underaddressed clinical activities and competencies (Figure 7-11). Functions include the following:

- A time clock
- A daily log for completed procedures and activities, which instructors validate

Box 7-3 Learner Objectives in Clinical Simulation

- Interpret data
- Recognize and prioritize problems
- Make decisions
- Observe consequences of decisions
- Develop leadership skills
- Develop interpersonal communication skills
- Develop team-building skills
- Use available resources
- Manage stress and crisis

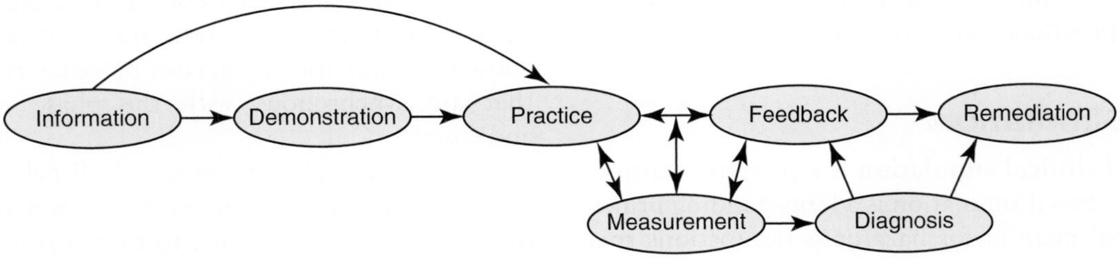

FIGURE 7-10 Steps in clinical simulation education.

Student name and initiator name	Date and IP address View record	Submission date Delete record	Patient and competency and summary	Clinical instructor	Clinical site and location	Area device
Kumar Patel Tonya Cook	Wednesday, December 16, 2009 144.30.0.221	Wednesday, January 6, 2010 at 1:42 PM 144.30.0.221	Adult vital signs Satisfactory	Tonya Cook	Baptist Health Clinic	Adult floor web
Kumar Patel Heather Neal-Rice	Saturday, April 3, 2010 144.30.0.221	Saturday, April 3, 2010 at 4:37 PM 144.30.0.221	Adult x-ray interpretation Satisfactory	Michael Anders	St. Vincent Infirmary Medical Center Clinic	Medical ICU web
Kumar Patel Tonya Cook	Tuesday, October 20, 2009 144.30.0.221	Tuesday, January 5, 2010 at 3:57 PM 144.30.0.221	Adult nasal cannula Satisfactory	Tonya Cook	Baptist Health Clinic	Adult floor web

FIGURE 7-11 DataArc documentation of clinical competencies. (Courtesy DataArc LLC. League City, Tex.)

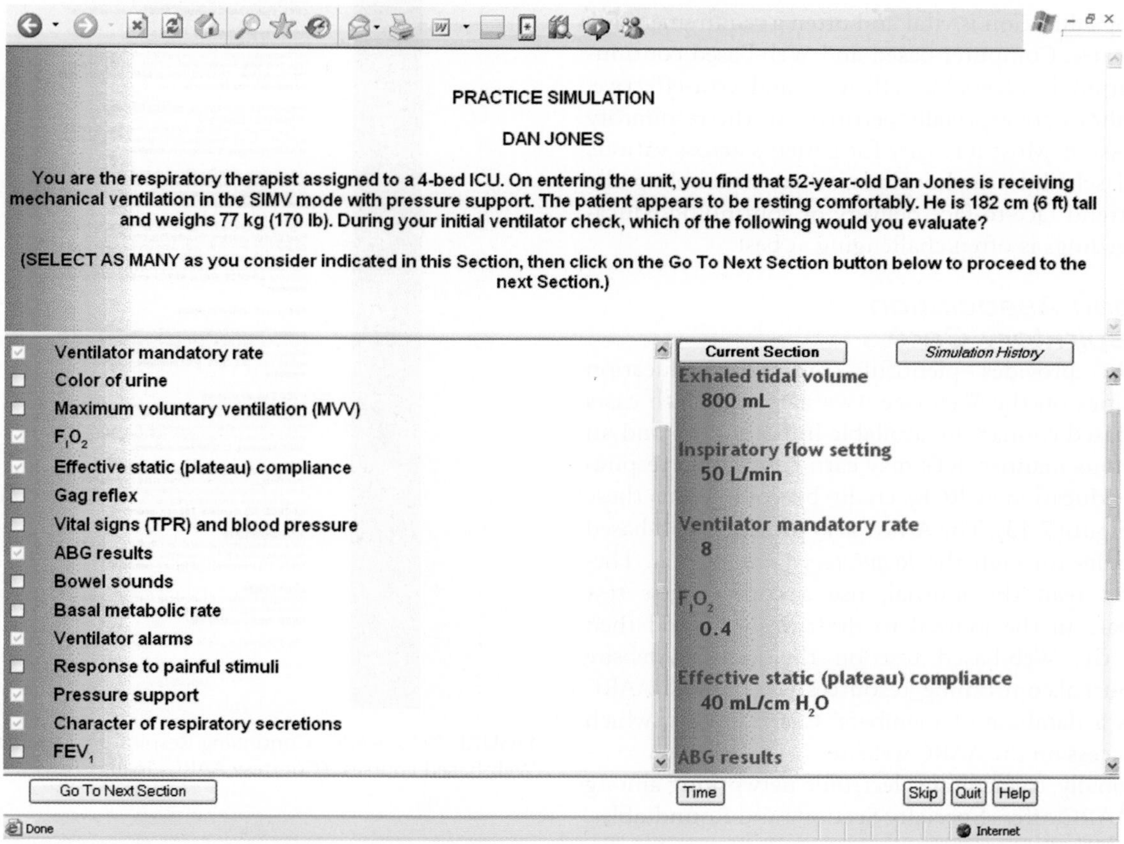

FIGURE 7-12 National Board for Respiratory Care, Practice Simulation Problem. (Courtesy NBRC, Olathe, Kan.)

- Competency evaluations
- Automated surveys to accommodate questionnaires for students, graduates, and clinical affiliates

Students and faculty can use hand-held computers or personal digital assistants to access it. DataARC archives data daily.

National Board for Respiratory Care Credentialing

The National Board for Respiratory Care (NBRC) uses computerized credentialing examinations. NBRC credentialing for the registry for advanced RTs consists of two distinct examinations—the written examination and the clinical simulation (Figure 7-12).

Distance Education

Respiratory care educators use interactive video networks and the Internet to deliver distance education courses. This technology improves access to a respiratory care education for students in rural areas. Asynchronous Web courses enable practicing RTs to advance their education to the baccalaureate or master level, by allowing for flexibility in coordinating completion of coursework with their work schedule. Wimba Classroom is an adjunct to the Blackboard learning system, in which Web-based classes are live and interactive. Students can talk to their instructor and classmates via live audio or chat or asynchronously access archived classes via streamed video or mp3 or mp4 files downloaded to their computers or smartphones.

Continuing Education

Continuing education is vital and often a requirement for state licensure. Computer-based and Web-based continuing education is accessible, efficient, and cost-effective. These qualities are especially pertinent to the respiratory care profession. Most RTs care for patients across various shifts and schedules in hospitals, where assembling the staff to attend face-to-face delivery of continuing education proceedings is often challenging at best.

American Association for Respiratory Care

The AARC provides plentiful continuing education opportunities on the Web (see www.aarc.org). Web casts and text-based courses are available in both a live and an asynchronous manner. RTs may earn continuing respiratory care education (CRCE) credit by completing these courses (Figure 7-13). The AARC also provides Web-based CRCE credits through the *Respiratory Care* journal. Therapists can read the journal, use a copy of the test that appears in the journal to draft answers, and then complete the Web-based test on the journal website (www.rcjournal.com/online_resources/crce). The AARC maintains a database of members' CRCE credits, which RTs can access on the AARC website.

Additionally, to facilitate electronic networking among RTs, the AARC offers Specialty Sections and Roundtables. Each Specialty Section features an e-mail listserv for discussions, e-newsletters, e-bulletins, and a website. Roundtables feature e-mail listserv for discussion.

Pulmonary Artery Catheter Education Project

The Pulmonary Artery Catheter Education Project (see www.pacep.org) provides excellent online training in hemodynamic monitoring. It includes Web casts with audio and slides and pretesting and posttesting for each module and case studies for many of the modules.

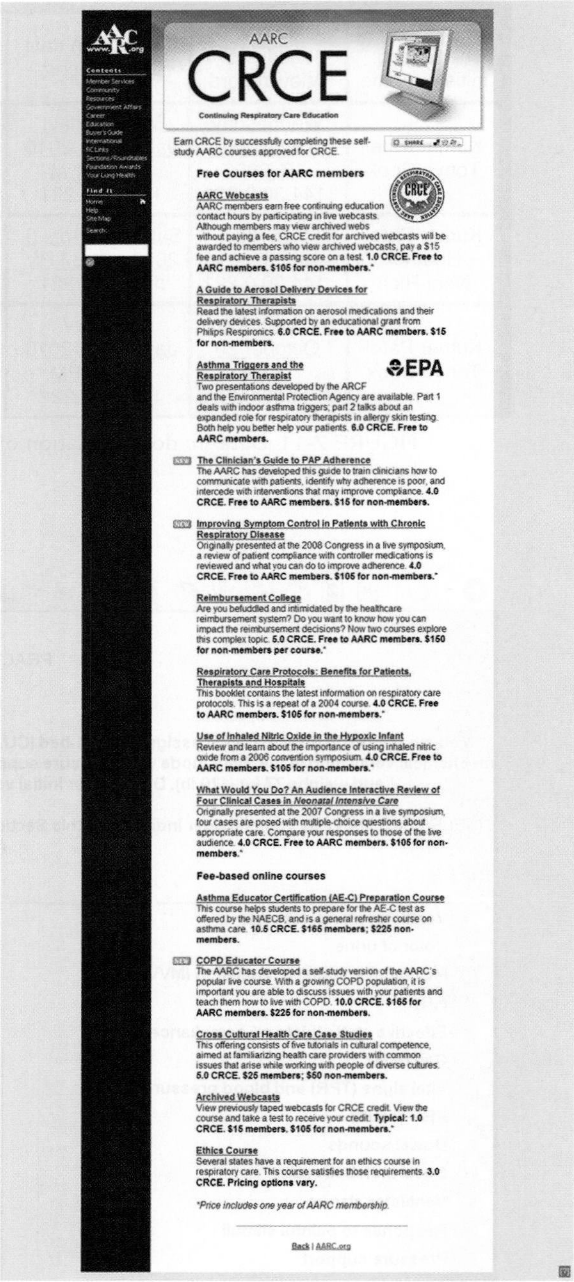

FIGURE 7-13 AARC, Continuing Respiratory Care Education, Web-based courses. (Courtesy AARC, Irving, Tex.)

APPLICATIONS IN RESEARCH

Computers are indispensable in research. Some of the more common functions are presented in Box 7-4.

Data Sources

Clinical databases are rich data sources for outcomes research. In a tobacco cessation program, clinicians can compare rates of tobacco consumption and abstinence from intake and follow-up patient interviews.

Additionally, public data sources are available on the Web to support descriptive and analytic research. The

Box 7-4 Common Functions of Computer Applications in Research

- Data sources
- Data collection
- Statistical testing
- Displaying study results
- Managing citations and references
- Managing ethical considerations

National Center for Health Statistics (see www.cdc.gov/nchs), the principal health statistics agency in the United States, oversees birth and mortality data, the National Maternal and Infant Health Survey, the Longitudinal Studies on Aging, the National Asthma Survey, and the NHANES. The NHANES is a comprehensive survey and examination of a nationally representative sample and includes data concerning demographics, tobacco use and other behaviors, pulmonary diseases, laboratory data, physical examination, and spirometry. State public health agencies are sources of public data available to researchers from instruments such as the Youth Behavioral Risk Survey.

Data Collection

Computers facilitate data collection via either hand-held computers or Web-based survey software. Compared with traditional paper methods of data collection, hand-held computers improve adherence to instructions, are faster, are preferred by research subjects, and may improve data accuracy.[54]

Web-based survey software, such as Survey Monkey (see www.surveymonkey.com) and Questionmark Perception (see www.questionmark.com/us/perception/index.htm), is a cost-effective approach for data collection. These tools enable researchers to create secured, Web-based, questionnaires with the capacity for adaptive branching of questions, tracking respondents, and downloading data into spreadsheets or statistical software.

Statistical Software

Statistical software programs, such as SPSS, SAS, and Statistica, are instrumental in research. In the hands of RTs with knowledge of statistics, these powerful programs can perform laborious and complex statistical tests for descriptive, analytic, and inferential analyses and reporting.

Citations and Bibliographies

Web-based software (see www.EndNote.com; www.RefWorks.com) automates the otherwise unwieldy and sometimes exhausting task of generating and formatting citations and bibliographies in research manuscripts. With relative ease, researchers can search for, import, organize, manage, and share databases of references.

Protection of Human Research Subjects

Research that features human subjects must have the ongoing approval of an institutional review board, which is responsible for protection of human subjects in research. Institutional review boards use information technology systems to help regulate the researchers' compliance with regulatory requirements for submission and monitoring of human and animal research.

SECURITY AND CONFIDENTIALITY

Security

RTs must be good stewards of computers by protecting against risks to security and confidentiality. Malicious software, such as viruses, can infiltrate a computer without the user's consent and harm or ravage a computer, server, or an entire network. Individuals in health care organizations must exercise caution to help prevent infiltration by malicious software.

To safeguard against infiltration by malicious software, hospitals and health care organizations use firewalls that filter the exchange of data between the Internet and local networks by verifying users' identification, passwords, and registered Internet addresses and restricting certain types of communication. Still, individual users must help prevent the infiltration of malicious software. Common sense is the best preventive measure.

RULE OF THUMB

Users can take steps to help prevent computer infiltration by malicious software.

1. *Users should regularly update their computers with security patches from authorized sources. For example, patches for Windows operating systems are available on the Microsoft website (see www.microsoft.com/microsoftupdate)*
2. *Users should install a virus scanning program and regularly update it*
3. *Most importantly, users should be discriminate when opening e-mail file attachments and refrain from downloading applications from unknown sources*

Confidentiality

Health Insurance Portability and Accountability Act of 1996 (HIPAA) regulations concerning confidentiality are pertinent to electronic medical records and research data that contain personal health information (see Chapter 5). To emphasize two important points concerning electronic personal health information, users of hospital and respiratory care information management systems and researchers must (1) refrain from sharing passwords and (2) access personal health information only on a need-to-know basis. Some respiratory care information management systems now feature thumbprint protected security.

SUMMARY CHECKLIST

- The role of computer applications in clinical care, diagnostics, management, education, and research is essential and continues to expand.
- The World Wide Web is a rich source of information for RTs and patients when the quality and source of information are appropriate.
- The PubMed search engine Clinical Queries filter is easy to use and yields valid, evidence-based results.
- Common sense is the best prevention against infiltration by malicious software.
- Emerging computer applications are expected to support management of chronic disease and potentially reduce medical errors.

References

1. Kacmarek RM, Durbin CG, Barnes TA, et al: Creating a vision for respiratory care in 2015 and beyond. Respir Care 54:375-389, 2009.
2. Kacmarek RM: Proportional assist ventilation and neurally adjusted ventilatory assist. Respir Care 56:140-148, 2011.
3. Akhtar SR, Weaver J, Pierson DJ, et al: Practice variation in respiratory therapy documentation during mechanical ventilation. Chest 124:2275-2282, 2003.
4. Vawdrey DK, Gardner RM, Evans RS, et al: Assessing data quality in manual entry of ventilator settings. J Am Med Inform Assoc 14:295-303, 2007.
5. Blackwood B, Alderdice F, Burns KE, et al: Protocolized versus non-protocolized weaning for reducing the duration of mechanical ventilation in critically ill adult patients. Cochrane Database Syst Rev (5):CD006904, 2010.
6. Kollef MH, Shapiro SD, Clinkscale D, et al: The effect of respiratory therapist-initiated treatment protocols on patient outcomes and resource utilization. Chest 117:467-475, 2000.
7. Iregui M, Ward S, Clinikscale D, et al: Use of a handheld computer by respiratory care practitioners to improve the efficiency of weaning patients from mechanical ventilation. Crit Care Med 30:2038-2043, 2002.
8. Garg AX, Adhikari NK, McDonald H, et al: Effects of computerized clinical decision support systems on practitioner performance and patient outcomes: a systematic review. JAMA 293:1223-1238, 2005.
9. Black AD, Car J, Pagliari C, et al: The impact of eHealth on the quality and safety of health care: a systematic overview. PLoS Med 8:e1000387, 2011.
10. Walton RT, Harvey E, Dovey S, et al: Computerised advice on drug dosage to improve prescribing practice. Cochrane Database Syst Rev (2), 2006.
11. Currell R, Urquhart C, Wainwright P, et al: Telemedicine versus face to face patient care: effects on professional practice and health care outcomes. Cochrane Database Syst Rev (2), 2006.
12. Breslow MJ, Rosenfeld BA, Doerfler M, et al: Effect of a multiple-site intensive care unit telemedicine program on clinical and economic outcomes: an alternative paradigm for intensivist staffing. Crit Care Med 32:31-38, 2004.
13. Thomas EJ, Lucke JF, Wueste L, et al: Association of telemedicine for remote monitoring of intensive care patients with mortality, complications, and length of stay. JAMA 302:2671-2678, 2009.
14. Rosenfeld BA, Dorman T, Breslow MJ, et al: Intensive care unit telemedicine: alternate paradigm for providing continuous intensivist care. Crit Care Med 28:3925-3931, 2000.
15. Centers for Disease Control and Prevention: Smoking-attributable mortality, years of potential life lost, and productivity losses—United States, 2000-2004. MMWR Morb Mortal Wkly Rep 57:1226-1228, 2008.
16. Fiore MC, Jaén CR, Baker TB, et al: Treating tobacco use and dependence: 2008 update. Clinical Practice Guideline. U.S. Department of Health and Human Services, Rockville, MD, 2008, Public Health Service.
17. Pew Internet and American Life Project: Health Information Online. http://www.pewinternet.org. Accessed March 18, 2011.
18. Civljak M, Sheikh A, Stead LF, et al: Internet-based interventions for smoking cessation. Cochrane Database Syst Rev (9):CD007078, 2010.
19. Whittaker R, Borland R, Bullen C, et al: Mobile phone-based interventions for smoking cessation. Cochrane Database Syst Rev (4):CD006611, 2009.
20. Myung SK, McDonnell DD, Kazinets G, et al: Effects of Web- and computer-based smoking cessation programs: meta-analysis of randomized controlled trials. Arch Intern Med 169:929-937, 2009.
21. Shahab L, McEwen A: Online support for smoking cessation: a systematic review of the literature. Addiction 104:1792-1804, 2009.
22. Graham AL, Cobb NK, Papandonatos GD, et al: A randomized trial of Internet and telephone treatment for smoking cessation. Arch Intern Med 171:46-53, 2011.
23. Centers for Disease Control and Prevention: Chronic disease prevention and health promotion. http://www.cdc.gov/chronicdisease. Accessed March 18, 2011.
24. Centers for Disease Control and Prevention: Chronic disease overview: costs of chronic disease, Atlanta: CDC, 2005. http://www.cdc.gov/nccdphp/overview.htm. Accessed March 18, 2011.
25. Anderson GF: Medicare and chronic conditions. N Engl J Med 353:305-309, 2005.
26. U.S. Census Bureau: http://www.census.gov/main/www/popclock.html10323. Accessed March 26, 2011.
27. CTIA Cellular Telecommunications and Internet Association: http://www.ctia.org/advocacy/research/index.cfm/AID/10323. Accessed March 26, 2011.
28. Bartholomew LK, Gold RS, Parcel GS, et al: Watch, Discover, Think, and Act: evaluation of computer-assisted instruction to improve asthma self-management in inner-city children. Patient Educ Couns 39:269-280, 2000.
29. Guendelman S, Meade K, Benson M, et al: Improving asthma outcomes and self-management behaviors of inner-city children: a randomized trial of the Health Buddy interactive device and an asthma diary. Arch Pediatr Adolesc Med 156:114-120, 2002.
30. Jan RL, Wang JY, Huang MC, et al: An internet-based interactive telemonitoring system for improving childhood asthma outcomes in Taiwan. Telemed J E Health 13:257-268, 2007.
31. Krishna S, Boren SA, Balas EA: Healthcare via cell phones: a systematic review. Telemed J E Health 15:231-240, 2009.
32. Krishna S, Francisco BD, Balas EA, et al: Internet-enabled interactive multimedia asthma education program: a randomized trial. Pediatrics 111:503-510, 2003.

33. McLean S, Chandler D, Nurmatov U, et al: Telehealthcare for asthma. Cochrane Database Syst Rev (10):CD007717, 2010.
34. U.S. Department of Health and Human Services, National Institutes of Health, National Heart, Lung and Blood Institute: Expert Panel Report 3: Guidelines for the diagnosis and management of asthma (EPR-3 2007). NIH Item No. 08-4051. http://www.nhlbi.nih.gov/guidelines/asthma/asthgdln.htm. Accessed March 24, 2011.
35. Jaana M, Paré G, Sicotte C: Home telemonitoring for respiratory conditions: a systematic review. Am J Manag Care 15:313-320, 2009.
36. Nguyen HQ, Donesky-Cuenco D, Wolpin S, et al: Randomized controlled trial of an internet-based versus face-to-face dyspnea self-management program for patients with chronic obstructive pulmonary disease: pilot study. J Med Internet Res 10:e9, 2008.
37. Polisena J, Tran K, Cimon K, et al: Home telehealth for chronic obstructive pulmonary disease: a systematic review and meta-analysis. J Telemed Telecare 16:120-127, 2010.
38. Stoller JK, McCarthy K: On the power and risks of the percent of predicted. Respir Care 51:722-725, 2006.
39. Hess DR: What is evidence-based medicine and why should I care? Respir Care 49:730-741, 2004.
40. Haynes RB, McKibbon KA, Wilczynski NL, et al: Hedges Team: Optimal search strategies for retrieving scientifically strong studies of treatment from Medline: analytical survey. BMJ 330:1179, 2005.
41. Anders ME, Evans PE: Comparison of PubMed and Google Scholar Literature Searches. Respir Care 55:578-583, 2010.
42. Eysenbach G, Powell J, Kuss O, et al: Empirical studies assessing the quality of health information for consumers on the world wide web: a systematic review. JAMA 287:2691-2700, 2002.
43. Wu RC, Straus SE: Evidence for handheld electronic medical records in improving care: a systematic review. BMC Med Inform Decis Mak 6:26, 2006.
44. Stoller JK, Kester L, Orens DK, et al: Impact of a radio frequency management information system on the process and timing of providing respiratory care services. Respir Care 47:893-897, 2002.
45. Koln LT, Corrigan JM, Donaldson M, editors: To err is human: building a safer health system. Institute of Medicine, Washington DC: National Academy Press; 2000.
46. United States Department of Health and Human Services: Information for health: a strategy for building the national health information infrastructure. http://aspe.hhs.gov/sp/NHII/Documents/NHIIReport2001/default.htm. Accessed March 24, 2011.
47. Tuttle RP, Cohen MH, Augustine AJ, et al: Utilizing simulation technology for competency skills assessment and a comparison of traditional methods of training to simulation-based training. Respir Care 52:263-270, 2007.
48. Salas E, Rosen MA, Burke CS, et al: Markers for enhancing team cognition in complex environments: the power of team performance diagnosis. Aviat Space Environ Med 78(5 Suppl):B77-B85, 2007.
49. Kory PD, Eisen LA, Adachi M, et al: Initial airway management skills of senior residents: simulation training compared with traditional training. Chest 132:1927-1931, 2007.
50. Wayne DB, Butter J, Siddall VJ, et al: Simulation-based training of internal medicine residents in advanced cardiac life support protocols: a randomized trial. Teach Learn Med 17:202-208, 2005.
51. Wayne DB, Didwania A, Feinglass J, et al: Simulation-based education improves quality of care during cardiac arrest team responses at an academic teaching hospital: a case-control study. Chest 133:56-61, 2008.
52. Ost D, DeRosiers A, Britt EJ, et al: Assessment of a bronchoscopy simulator. Am J Respir Crit Care Med 164:2248-2255, 2001.
53. Gallagher AG, Ritter EM, Champion H, et al: Virtual reality simulation for the operating room: proficiency-based training as a paradigm shift in surgical skills training. Ann Surg 241:364-372, 2005.
54. Lane SJ, Heddle NM, Arnold E, et al: A review of randomized controlled trials comparing the effectiveness of hand held computers with paper methods for data collection. BMC Med Inform Decis Mak 6:23, 2006.

SECTION II

APPLIED ANATOMY AND PHYSIOLOGY

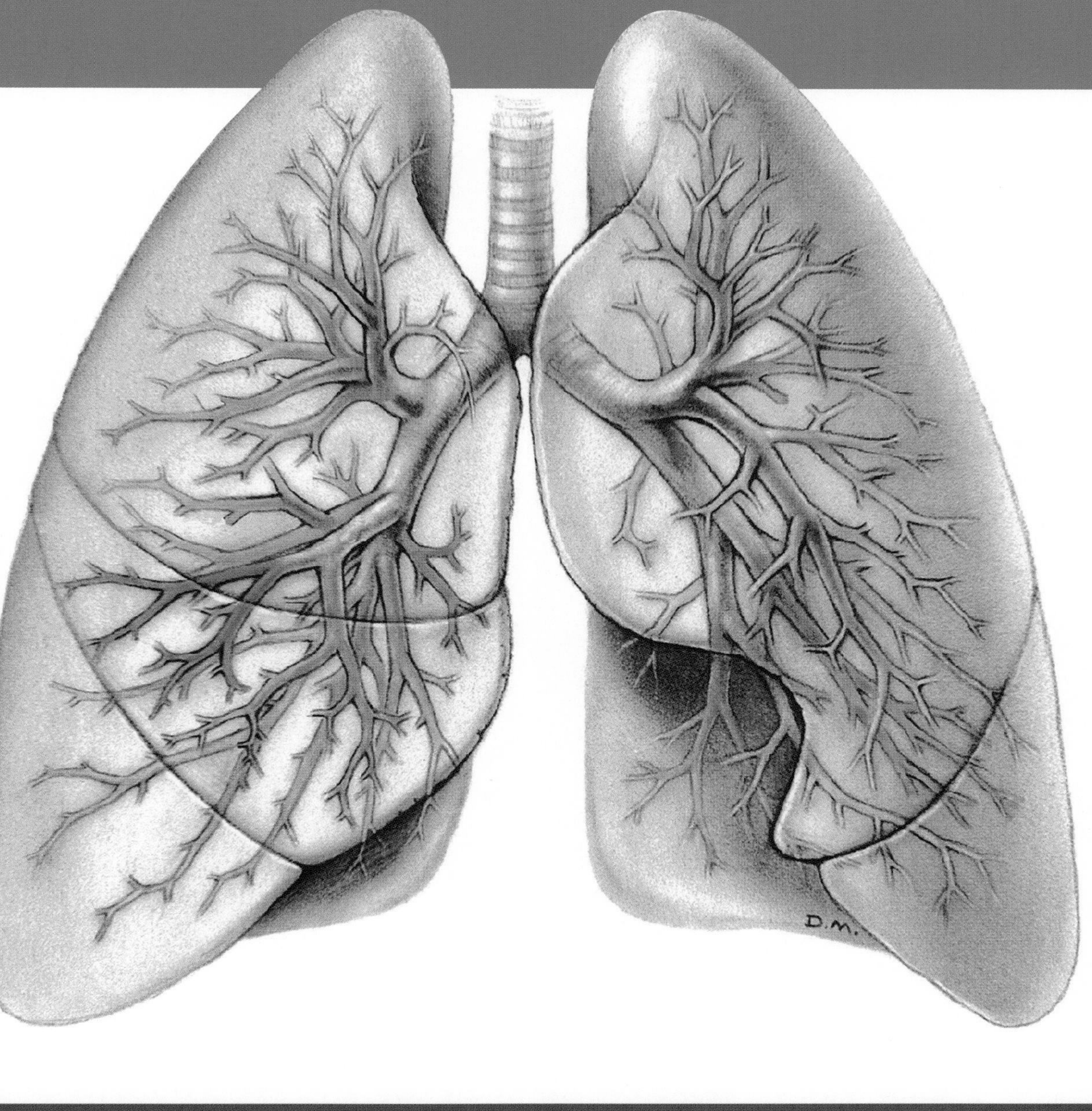

Chapter 8

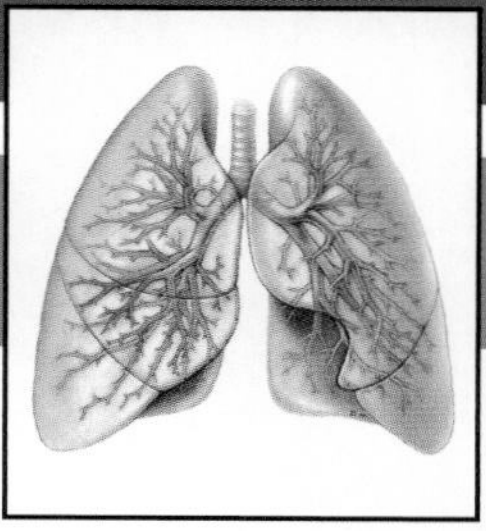

The Respiratory System

GEORGE H. HICKS

CHAPTER OBJECTIVES

After reading this chapter you will be able to:

- State the major developmental events of the respiratory system.
- Describe how genes control lung development.
- Describe the key elements of normal fetal circulation.
- State what happens to the respiratory system at birth.
- Describe the developmental events in the respiratory system that continue after birth.
- Identify the main structures in the thorax and describe their functions.
- Identify and describe the primary and accessory muscles of breathing.
- Describe how the pulmonary and bronchial circulations are organized and their functions.
- Describe how somatic and autonomic nervous systems connect to and control the lungs and respiratory muscles.
- Identify the major structures of the upper respiratory tract and how they function.
- Describe how the lungs are organized into lobes and segments and the airways that supply them with ventilation.
- Describe how and why airways produce and move mucus.
- Describe how the structures in the respiratory bronchioles and alveoli are organized.
- Describe the blood-gas barrier.

CHAPTER OUTLINE

KEY TERMS

accessory muscles of breathing
acinus
alae
alveolar-capillary membrane
alveoli
angle of Louis
anterior nares
apices
carina
cilia
costal cartilage
costophrenic angle
cricoid cartilage
diaphragm
ductus arteriosus
ductus venosus
epiglottis
eustachian tubes

external nares
external oblique
external respiration
false ribs
fissures
floating ribs
foramen ovale
gladiolus
glottis
hilum
hypopharynx
intercostal muscles
intercostal nerves
internal oblique
internal respiration
laryngopharynx
larynx
lobes
manubrium
mediastinum
mucociliary escalator
nasopharynx
oropharynx
palate
parietal pleura
pharynx
phrenic nerves
pores of Kohn
primary lobule
pseudostratified epithelia
pulmonary surfactant
rectus abdominis muscles
scalene muscles
segments
soft palate
sternal angle
sternocleidomastoid muscles
sternum
suprasternal notch
trachea
true ribs
turbinates
type I pneumocyte
type II pneumocyte
uvula
vallecula
visceral pleura
xiphoid process

The primary function of the respiratory system is the continuous absorption of oxygen (O_2) and the excretion of carbon dioxide (CO_2). This exchange between the gas of the atmosphere and blood is termed **external respiration.** This process supports **internal respiration,** which is the exchange of gases between blood and tissues. To carry out external respiration, the respiratory system brings gas into close proximity with flowing blood in the pulmonary circulatory system. This close "match" of gas and blood across a large but extremely thin blood-gas barrier membrane enables efficient gas exchange to occur via simple diffusion.

The various organs that support gas exchange and make up the respiratory system include the upper airways, chest wall, respiratory muscles, lower airways, pulmonary blood vessels, and support nerves and lymphatics. These organs begin to form early in the developing human and undergo dramatic functional changes at the time of birth, when the system begins its primary role of breathing and external respiration.

From the moment of conception, the human body, including the respiratory system, undergoes tremendous growth and development—from embryo to fetus to infant and child, through puberty, and into young adulthood. The mature lung continues its primary function with relatively little change through midlife and then begins a gradual loss of lung tissue and functional changes that continue through the elderly years until the time of death. During the typical life span of a human, the respiratory system maintains external respiration by matching phenomenal amounts of air with a similar amount of blood flow: Approximately 250 million L of each are moved and matched during a 75-year life span. The respiratory system normally moves this staggering amount of air and blood flow with a minimal amount of work and is equipped to filter out inhaled contaminants while warming and humidifying inspired gas and simultaneously to filter out various chemicals and small blood clots that are deposited or formed in the blood. The respiratory system is regulated by the nervous system and is capable of increasing function in response to elevated demands brought on by stressful conditions such as exercise and disease.

A functional understanding of the "normal" anatomy and physiology of the respiratory system is crucial to proper understanding of pulmonary disease and its treatment. The role of the respiratory care practitioner in assessment and treatment of various cardiopulmonary disorders requires a well-developed understanding of the structural and functional nature of the respiratory system.

DEVELOPMENT OF THE RESPIRATORY SYSTEM

After the fertilization of an oocyte by a spermatocyte, the developing human, similar to all other animals, undergoes a remarkable transformation from a single cell to an individual with a nearly complete set of organ systems. The developmental phases between fertilization and birth are generally divided into the *embryonic* and *fetal periods.* The embryonic period of human development occurs during the first 8 weeks and is traditionally organized into 23 stages, known as the Carnegie stages. During the embryonic period, all major organs begin their development. The fetal period occurs during the remaining 32 weeks of gestation. During this period, the organs continue to develop and refine their structure and function.

The respiratory system develops during these periods as a fluid-filled structure that plays no role in gas exchange yet must be developed sufficiently to assume this crucial activity at the time of birth. Its development is a continuous process that begins in the early stages of the embryonic period and extends for years after birth. A mass of cells forms between the yolk sac and amniotic cavity 17 days after fertilization (Carnegie stage 6). This mass is composed of three embryologically distinct germinal tissue layers that ultimately form all tissues and organs: *endoderm, mesoderm,* and *ectoderm.* The epithelium lining layer, which forms the mucous and gas exchange membranes, of the entire

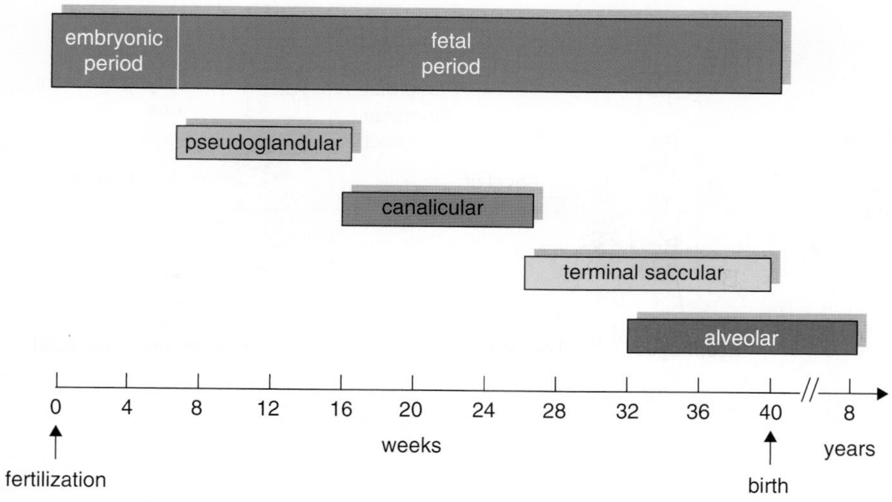

FIGURE 8-1 Major phases of respiratory development.

TABLE 8-1

Developmental Events of the Cardiopulmonary System

Gestational Age	Developmental Event
Embryonic Period	
20-22 days	Primordial pharyngeal arches form
21-23 days	Primordial respiratory cells form on fourth pharyngeal pouch, primordial heart starts forming
26th day	Laryngotracheal bud forms
4th wk	Primitive trachea develops
5th wk	Primary bronchial buds form, laryngeal structures develop
Fetal Period	
Pseudoglandular Stage	
6th wk	Segmental and subsegmental bronchioles form
7th wk	Diaphragm complete
8th wk	Heart complete, fetal circulatory pattern begins to develop
10th wk	Pulmonary lymphatic structures develop
12th wk	Major arteries formed
13th wk	Major airway epithelia and mucus-producing cells formed, smooth muscle cells developing
14th wk	Principal arteries formed
16th wk	Terminal bronchioles and associated pulmonary vessels form
Canalicular Stage	
16th-17th wk	Respiratory bronchioles and immature acini begin to form
20th-24th wk	Type I and II pneumocytes begin to appear and replicate
24th-26th wk	Pulmonary capillaries develop at surface of acinus, immature surfactant begins to appear in lung fluid
Terminal Saccular Stage	
26th wk-birth	Terminal saccules increase in number, pulmonary capillary density and proximity increase, type I and II pneumocytes continue to multiply, surfactant production increases, extrauterine life possible with support
Alveolar Stage	
32th-40th wk	Immature alveoli begin to form and increase in number; surfactant production matures
40th week	50 million immature alveoli formed
Period After Birth	
Birth	First breath and lung fluid cleared, adult circulatory pattern established
8-10 yr	470 million mature alveoli formed

respiratory system arises from the endoderm, whereas the supporting structures of the tracheobronchial tree, including muscle and connective tissues, develop from the mesoderm that surrounds the developing lung bud. The nervous system of the respiratory tract forms from the cells of the ectoderm that grow within the mesoderm layer.

Based on cellular differentiation and tissue architecture, development of the respiratory system has been categorized into various stages.[1] Figure 8-1 shows the various stages of lung development, and Table 8-1 summarizes the major developmental events in each phase. Respiratory development begins in the embryonic period on or about

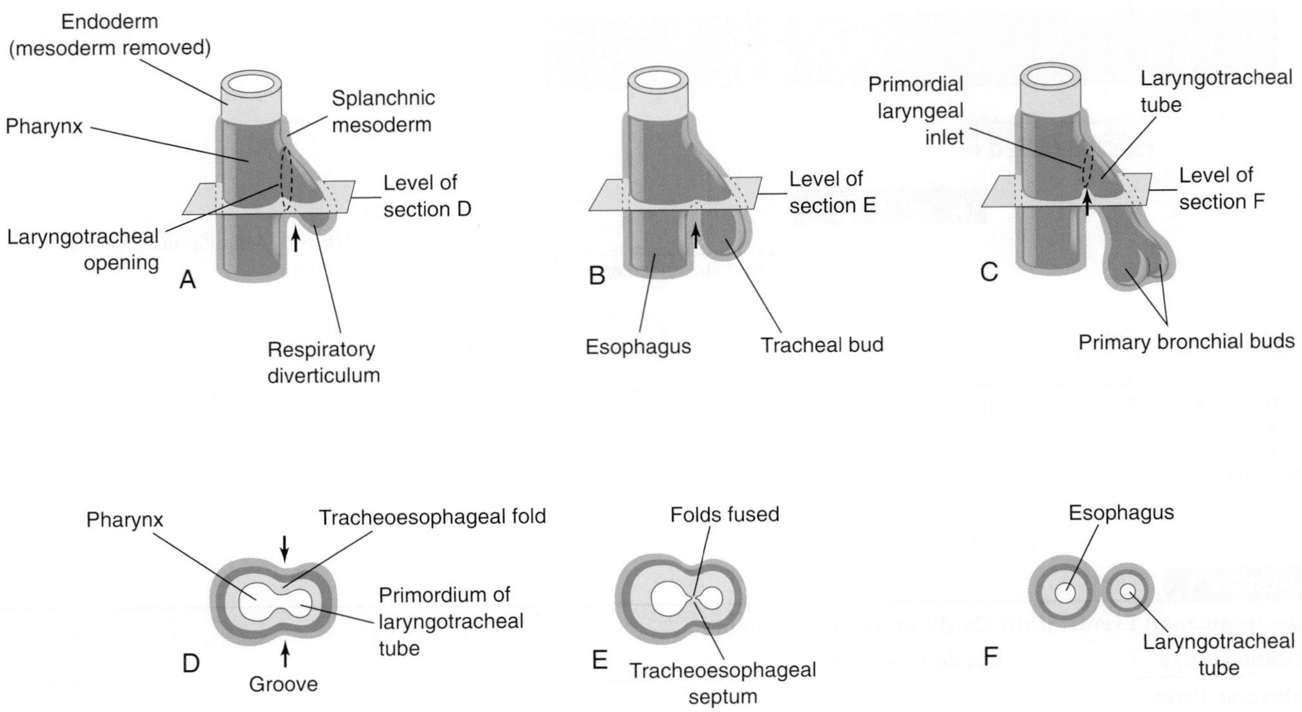

FIGURE 8-2 Successive stages in the development of the respiratory system from the primitive foregut. **A-C,** Lateral views of the caudal part of the primordial pharynx showing the respiratory diverticulum and partitioning of the foregut into the esophagus and laryngotracheal bud. **D-F,** Transverse sections illustrating the formation of the tracheoesophageal septum and showing how it separates the foregut into the laryngotracheal bud and esophagus. (From Moore KL, Persaud TVN: The respiratory system. In Moore KL, Persaud TVN, editors: The developing human—clinically oriented embryology, ed 8, Philadelphia, 2008, WB Saunders.)

day 22 after fertilization, when a small mass of cells, the respiratory primordium, begins to develop near the ventral region of the fourth pharyngeal arch of the primitive pharynx. This mass of cells forms a pouchlike bud, the respiratory diverticulum, on about day 26 (Carnegie stage 9) that continues to grow to form a laryngotracheal tube (Figure 8-2). The laryngotracheal tube forms from a groove in the fourth pharyngeal pouch. From the laryngotracheal tube, a tracheal bud forms by the end of the fourth week of life. The dorsal portion of the primitive foregut develops into the primordial esophagus and is separated from the tracheal bud by the formation of a tracheoesophageal septum. During week 5 of development, the tracheal bud continues to develop and bifurcates into left and right primary bronchial buds. The laryngeal structures develop at the superior end of the laryngotracheal bud.

The tracheal bud soon bifurcates into two main stem bronchial buds. The bronchial buds continue to grow and branch into secondary bronchi that form lobar, segmental, and subsegmental bronchi. As the bronchi form, plates of cartilage develop from the surrounding mesoderm to support these airways. During this same period, the vascular components of the respiratory system begin their development from the mesoderm. The pulmonary circulation and nervous system develop in parallel as the airways form. The pulmonary arteries form as buds off of the sixth pair of aortic arches, and primitive pulmonary veins emerge from the developing heart. Injury to the embryo or genetic dysregulation during this crucial phase of development can lead to many congenital anomalies, including tracheoesophageal fistulas, esophageal atresia, choanal atresia, pulmonary hypoplasia, and complex heart and vascular anomalies.

The developmental branching process of the airways and blood vessels of the lung is highly regulated by the timely activation of various genes in different locations. Of the approximate 22,000 genes in the human genome, about 40 are required for normal respiratory development.[2-4] Table 8-2 lists many of these genes and the process in which they play an important role. The initial step in the development of the respiratory system is the localized expression of the *NKX2-1* gene (also known as *thyroid-specific transcription factor, TTF-1*) in the anterior wall of the foregut, which stimulates the primary lung bud formation. Failure or mutation of the *NKX2-1* gene can lead to failure of lung bud formation and various tracheoesophageal malformations.[5] Lung bud elongation and the repetitive airway branching process is stimulated and directed by the highly choreographed expression of other key genes, including *FGF10, FGFR2IIB, GATA-6, HNF-3, SPROUTY2,*

TABLE 8-2

Genes Implicated in Pulmonary Development

Event	Factors and Genes
Early lung bud development and airway branching	Thyroid transcription factor 1 *(NKX2-1)* *FGF10* and *FGF9* *FGFR2IIIB* and *FGFR2IIIC* *GATA-6* *HNF-3* alpha and beta Vitamin A (retinoic acid) and receptor *LEFTY 1* and *2* Sprouty *(SPROUTY2)* Sonic hedgehog *(SHH)* Bone morphogenetic protein 4 (BMP-4) *NOGGIN* *N*-Acetylglucosaminyltransferase 1
Secondary dichotomous branching	Transforming growth factor alpha and beta (TGF-α and TGF-β) *WNT 5* and *7* Platelet-derived growth factor (PDGF)
Alveolar development	PDGF Tropoelastin 1 Fibrillin 1 Cyclin-dependent kinase inhibitors *(p57* and *p21)* Type 1 cell alpha transmembrane protein Ephrin B2
Surfactant formation	Surfactant protein A, B, and C *(SFTPA, SFTPB,* and *SFTPC)* ATP-binding cassette subfamily *(ABCA3)* *NKX2-1* *HNF-3*
Pulmonary vascular development	Activin receptor–like kinases TGF Vascular endothelial growth factors (VEGF) Forkhead box transcription factors *(Fox)* Integrin alpha forms Caveolin 1 and 2

SHH, BMP-4, and *NOGGIN* as well as numerous other genes (see Table 8-2). Mutations of the *FGF10* gene can result in tracheal development but fatal failure of further lung formation.[6]

At approximately 6 weeks of development, lung and airway growth has the appearance of a glandular structure—hence the name of the second phase of development, the *pseudoglandular stage* (Figure 8-3). For the next 10 weeks, the growth and branching of the tracheobronchial tree and pulmonary vasculature continue, under the direction of the various genes described earlier, and culminate with formation of the terminal and respiratory bronchioles. The distinction between these two types of bronchioles is important. Terminal bronchioles, similar to bronchi and the trachea, are conducting airways only and do not participate in gas exchange with blood. Respiratory bronchioles have much more superficial capillaries and are capable of gas exchange with blood and become more elaborate as development continues.

Branching and dividing of the tracheobronchial tree occur in several ways as the result of differential gene expression. A single bud that develops off of an existing structure is termed a *monopodial bud.* Airways that divide into two or more airways do so through *dichotomous branching.* Most of the divisions of airways occur in a nonsymmetric fashion termed *irregular dichotomous branching.*[7,8] The epithelial lining of the airways begins to differentiate into columnar epithelia in the proximal airways and differentiates into cuboidal epithelium in the more distal bronchioles (Figure 8-4, *A*). Development of *cilia, mucous glands,* and *goblet cells* occurs at this time, and these are found lining most of the conducting airways.

Below the basement membrane of the epithelia, growth of smooth muscle cells, connective tissue, and blood vessels continues as the airways continue to branch. Mesoderm-derived cartilage provides rigidity, especially for the trachea and main stem bronchi. Beginning with the trachea and moving distally, the amount of cartilage supporting the airway decreases as smooth muscle cells, in the middle layer of the airway, increase in number. Altered development of smooth muscle, cartilage, and vascular structures can lead to other congenital pulmonary disorders, such as tracheomalacia, anomalous pulmonary arteries, and vascular rings that can grow around and pinch the airway.

The third phase of development is termed the *canalicular stage* (see Figure 8-4, *B*). It begins at week 16 and continues until week 26. The canalicular stage overlaps with the pseudoglandular stage because the superior regions of the lung are developing slightly faster than the inferior regions. During this phase, primary changes include the development of two to four more generations of respiratory bronchioles from each terminal bronchiole, the formation of blind tubular alveolar ducts from each respiratory bronchiole, and greater blood vessel development. In the last several weeks of this stage, the region beyond each terminal bronchiole forms the functional structure called the **acinus,** the basic gas-exchanging unit of the lung. At this time, the two principal epithelial cell types that cover the gas exchange surface begin to appear, type I and type II pneumocytes. At the end of the canalicular period (24 to 26 weeks of gestation), the fetus, if born, is capable of sufficient gas exchange and is viable if supported with supplemental O_2, ventilatory support, and surfactant administration.

During the fourth phase, the *terminal saccular stage* (see Figure 8-4, *C*), more terminal bronchioles and their associated acini form, and their structure continues to develop from 26 weeks to birth. The formation of the total number of terminal bronchioles is complete at the end of this phase.[8] The cuboidal epithelia that line the blind tubules of the acinus continue to differentiate into rounded secretory cells **(type II pneumocytes)** and flatter squamous epithelial cells **(type I pneumocytes).** Mounting evidence shows that an important source of type I pneumocytes during both development and after lung injury are type II

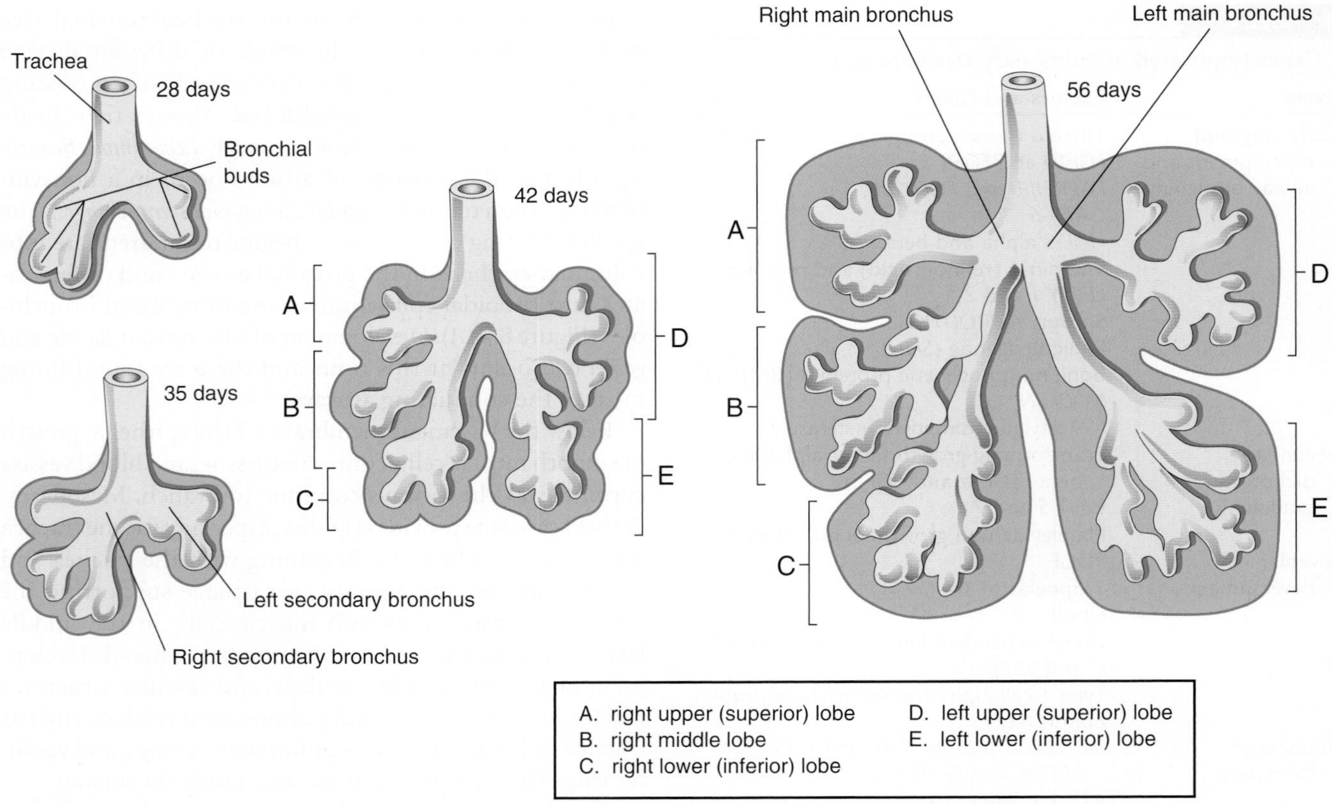

FIGURE 8-3 A-E, Various stages in the growth of the bronchi as the lungs enter the pseudoglandular period of development. (From Moore KL, Persaud TVN: The respiratory system. In Moore KL, Persaud TVN, editors: The developing human—clinically oriented embryology, ed 8, Philadelphia, 2008, WB Saunders.)

cells that can proliferate and differentiate.[9,10] Capillaries continue to form near and bulge from the surface of the acinus. Although some type II pneumocytes form by 20 weeks' gestation, they are in such small numbers and of such primitive function that their impact on lung function is marginal. From this point until birth, there is rapid proliferation of alveolar ducts and sacs, formed from the respiratory bronchioles. The type I pneumocytes of the saccule walls thin and elongate to cover the walls of this region. Type I cells become the primary gas-exchange cells in the lung with close approximation to developing pulmonary capillaries. Type II pneumocytes form and secrete the vital pulmonary surfactants that are necessary to alter surface tension and help keep the lungs inflated.

The development of mature alveoli, accompanied by capillary proliferation within the walls, marks the final phase of lung development and is known as the *alveolar period* (see Figure 8-4, *D*). This phase begins at about week 32 of gestation and continues for years after birth. During this phase, the terminal saccules develop pouchlike regions called *alveoli* in their walls that are hexagonal in shape. The process of alveolarization occurs through the formation of crests along the immature airway wall, which develop further into septa that lengthen into the terminal saccule lumen; this effectively divides up the terminal airspace and results in greater numbers of alveoli that enlarge to a mature state with time.

RULE OF THUMB

The development of mature alveoli marks the final stage of lung development and is known as the alveolar period. This period begins at about 32 weeks of gestation and continues for years after birth. Premature infants with gestational ages of less than 32 weeks are at greater risk for developing respiratory distress.

A full-term newborn infant has about 50 million alveoli, and the number continues to increase for about 2 to 3 years after birth.[11,12] The alveoli are lined with type I and II pneumocytes covering the pulmonary capillaries that have formed just below the basement membrane.

Human **pulmonary surfactant,** which promotes lung inflation and protects the alveolar surface, begins to be produced around 24 to 25 weeks of development by type II pneumocytes. It is composed primarily of phospholipids, a small amount of protein (types SP-A, SP-B, and SP-C), and a trace of carbohydrates.[13] Early research in

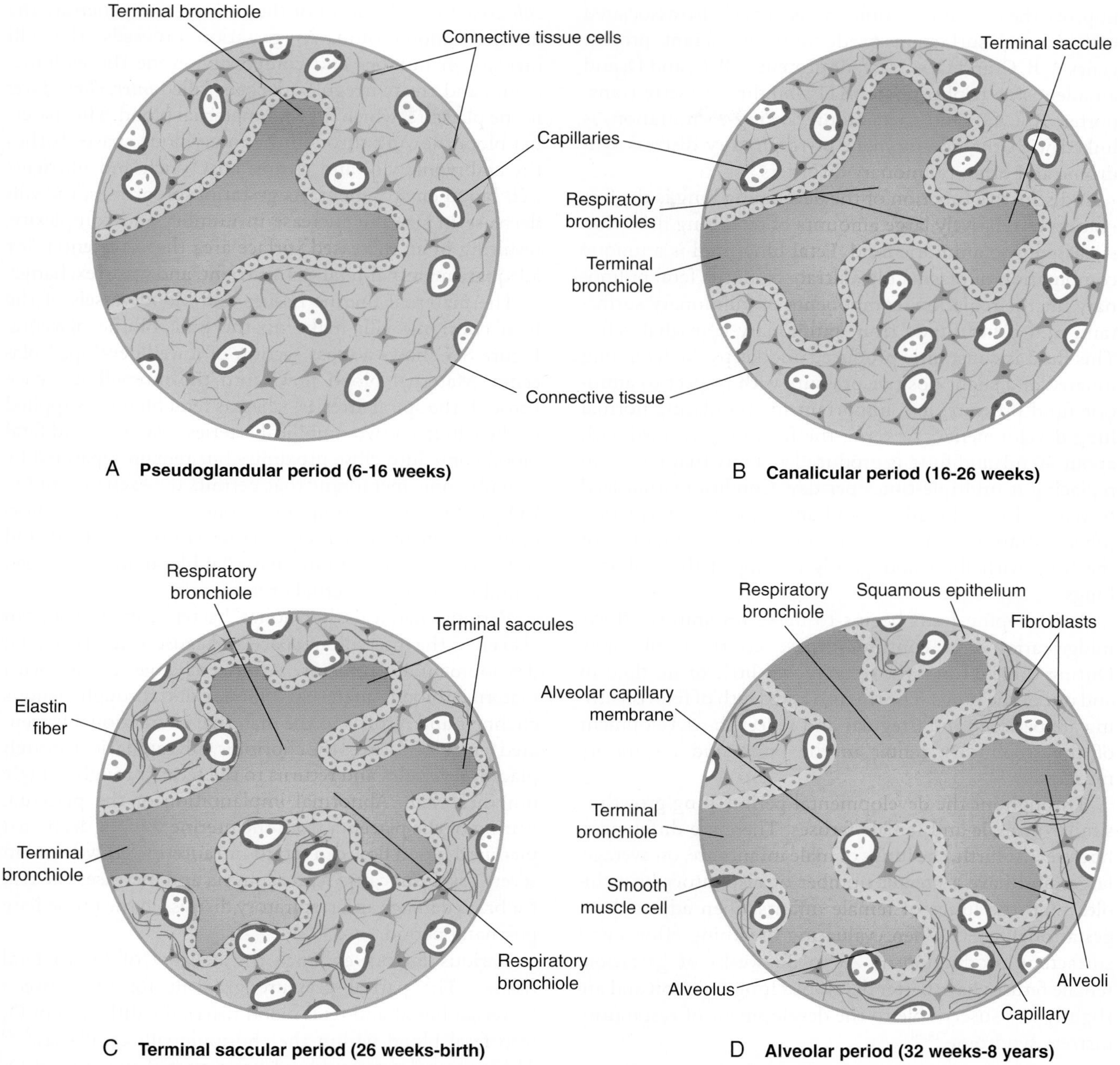

FIGURE 8-4 Histologic changes that illustrate various periods of airway development. **A** and **B,** There is considerable distance between the air within the airways and blood within the capillaries. **C** and **D,** The air-blood distance is considerably thinner and more supportive of effective air breathing. (From Moore KL, Persaud TVN: The respiratory system. In Moore KL, Persaud TVN, editors: The developing human—clinically oriented embryology, ed 8, Philadelphia, 2008, WB Saunders.)

pulmonary surfactants centered on the phospholipid components, mainly phosphatidylcholine (lecithin [L] and sphingomyelin [S]) and phosphatidylglycerol (PG). Quantification of these phospholipids (the *L/S ratio* and *PG concentration*) provides a predictive index of the lung maturity in a fetus before birth and the risks of the development of respiratory distress.[14] An L/S ratio of 2 or more indicates a relatively low risk for the development of respiratory distress syndrome, whereas an L/S ratio of less than 1.5 is associated with a high risk.

Surfactant synthesis is regulated by numerous hormones and factors, including glucocorticoids, prolactin, insulin, estrogens, androgens, thyroid hormones, and catecholamines.[15] Glucorticosteroid production increases at the end of gestation and stimulates receptors in type II pneumocytes to increase surfactant production and improve the L/S ratio. Various key genes are also associated with normal surfactant production (surfactant protein genes A, B, C, and D; surfactant protein A, B, C, and D; and an adenosine triphosphate (ATP)–binding cassette transporter, *ABCA3*), and their failure, owing to mutation, is linked with the development of respiratory distress syndrome and other pulmonary disorders.[16]

A distinctive function of the developing lung is the formation of relatively large amounts of fetal lung fluid that is passed into amniotic fluid. Fetal lung fluid is a unique combination of plasma ultrafiltrate from the fetal pulmonary microcirculation, components of pulmonary surfactant, and other fluids from pulmonary epithelial cells.[7] This fluid is constantly produced and keeps the fetal lung inflated at a slight positive pressure with respect to amniotic fluid pressure; it is important in stimulating normal lung development.[17] At term, the fetal lung is filled with about 40 ml, and fluid is produced at a rate that results in replacing it multiple times per day. Conditions that lead to reduced fetal breathing and amniotic fluid formation (oligohydramnios) are linked to incomplete inflation of the lung with fluid and poorly developed (hypoplastic) lungs.

A developing fetus begins to make respiratory efforts midgestation and continues these efforts until birth. During these efforts, the fetus moves little or no fluid in and out of the lungs. The rhythm and depth of fetal breathing are periodic and irregular and reflect the development of the respiratory center in the brain and respiratory muscles.

Throughout the developmental period, lung growth is similar in male and female fetuses. There are differences, however. At birth, the lungs of male infants are, on average, larger and have a greater number of respiratory bronchioles than the lungs of female infants when adjusted for gestational age.[18] When evaluating breathing efforts and surfactant production at 26 to 36 weeks of gestation, female fetuses have better developed lung function and are slightly less susceptible to the development of respiratory distress syndrome.[19,20]

TRANSITION FROM UTERINE TO EXTRAUTERINE LIFE

At birth, the lungs undergo a rapid and remarkable transition from being a liquid-filled organ that possesses very little circulation and is incapable of sufficient gas exchange to an air-filled organ that receives the entire cardiac output from the right heart and carries out all of the necessary gas exchange to sustain life.

Placental Structure and Function

Survival of the embryo and then fetus requires an effective circulatory interface with the circulation of the mother, which is provided by the placenta.[21] Within 1 week of uterine implantation, vascular projections called *chorionic villi* arise from the aorta of the embryo and penetrate the uterine endometrium. As gestation proceeds, the villi increase in number and complexity; erode the endometrium; and create irregular pockets called *intervillous spaces* in the placenta, which fill with maternal blood. The maternal blood flowing through the intervillous spaces bathes the embryonic villi and creates an O_2-rich and nutrient-rich blood environment. As gestation progresses, the villi decrease in size but increase in number and complexity, resulting in an increased surface area that is essential for adequate maternal-fetal gas, nutrient, and waste exchange.

The maternal uterine tissues and blood vessels of the fetal chorionic villi make up the bulk of the placenta. Figure 8-5 shows a cross section of a well-developed placenta. Maternal blood flows into the intervillous space through the spiral arteries, whereas fetal blood is supplied to the villi from two umbilical arteries. Maternal and fetal blood come into close proximity but remain separated by an embryonic membrane that permits the exchange of O_2, CO_2, water, ions, various metabolic molecules, and hormones. Some maternal cells do move into fetal blood, and some fetal cells move into maternal blood and have been found in various maternal organs.

Various chemicals, hormones, bacteria, and viruses can also cross the intervillous space and cause a variety of fetal developmental problems. After exchange occurs with maternal blood, maternal blood exits through venous channels and returns to the maternal circulation. Oxygenated fetal blood leaves the chorionic villi capillaries through placental venules and returns to the fetus through a single umbilical vein. Abnormal implantation of the placenta, tearing of the placenta from the uterine wall, or decreased placental blood flow can retard intrauterine growth and in severe cases can cause fetal asphyxia and increases the risk for brain damage and respiratory distress in the immediate postnatal period.

Various factors enhance the delivery of O_2 to fetal tissues. The partial pressure gradient for O_2 between maternal blood and fetal blood drives the diffusion of O_2 into fetal blood within the chorionic villi capillaries.[22,23] The maternal arterial blood has a partial pressure of O_2 (PaO_2) of approximately 100 mm Hg, which mixes with the blood in the intervillous space to produce a mean PO_2 of approximately 50 mm Hg. Fetal blood that enters the villi has a PO_2 of approximately 19 mm Hg, and the pressure gradient between maternal and fetal blood PO_2 ($50 - 19 = 31$ mm Hg) causes O_2 to diffuse into fetal blood. Blood leaving the villi and entering the umbilical vein has a PO_2 of approximately 30 mm Hg. Table 8-3 summarizes the normal gas and acid-base values in normal fetal umbilical arteries and veins and maternal intervillous blood. Assessment of umbilical vein blood gas data shortly after birth is a method of determining the degree of fetal asphyxiation during the birth process.

The O_2 content and delivery by fetal blood are almost the same as adult blood despite the much lower PO_2; this

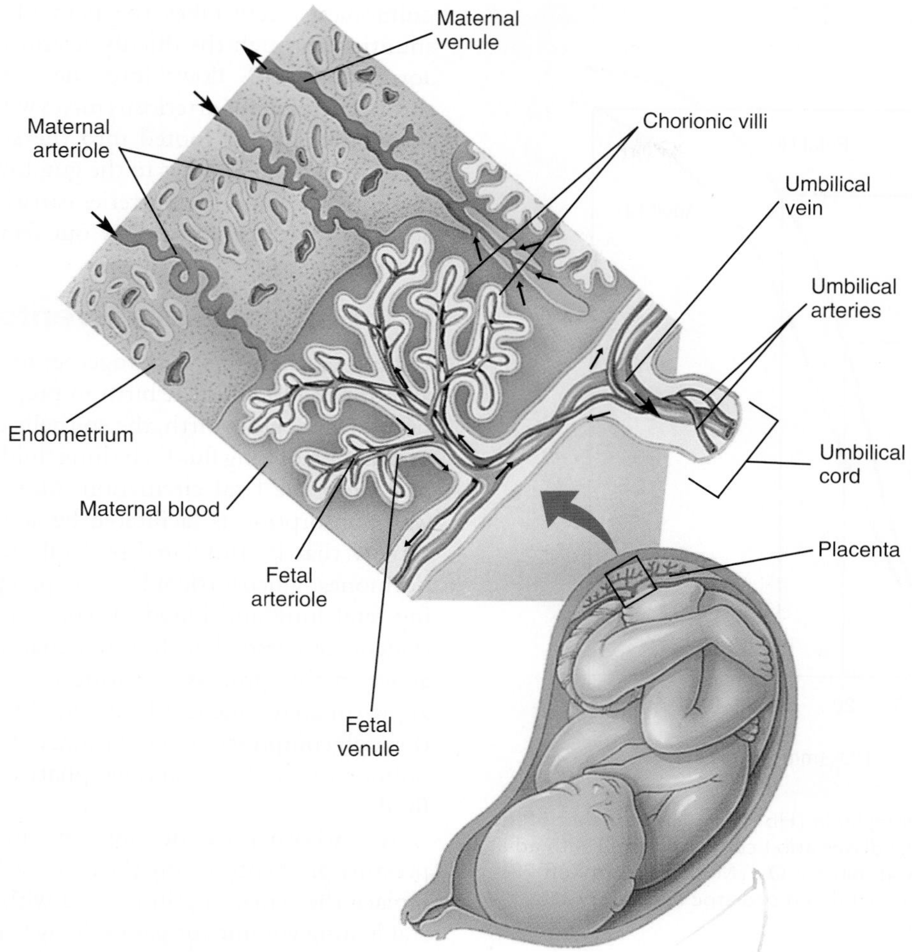

FIGURE 8-5 Cross-sectional view through the placenta showing the spiral arteries that supply maternal blood to the intervillous spaces. The fetal villi, immersed in maternal blood, are supplied with blood from the umbilical arteries and drain their blood back through the umbilical vein. (From Thibodeau GA, Patton KT: Anatomy and physiology, ed 7, St Louis, 2010, Mosby.)

TABLE 8-3

Approximate Normal Values of Blood Gases and Acid-Base in Fetal and Maternal Blood

Value	Maternal Intervillous Blood	Fetal Umbilical Artery Blood	Fetal Umbilical Venous Blood
pH	7.38	7.36	7.39
PCO_2 (mm Hg)	42	47	43
PO_2 (mm Hg)	50	19	30

is due to several factors, including relatively higher content of hemoglobin (18 g/dl) and hematocrit (54%) in fetal blood and the presence of fetal hemoglobin (HbF), which has an increased affinity for O_2 and a more pronounced Bohr effect (reduced oxyhemoglobin affinity with acidosis) to enhance O_2 release.[23] Figure 8-6 illustrates how the increased O_2 affinity is manifested by a leftward shift of the fetal oxyhemoglobin dissociation curve. The P_{50} (PO_2 that saturates 50% of the hemoglobin) is 6 to 8 mm Hg less than the P_{50} for adult hemoglobin (HbA), which indicates the degree of the shift toward higher affinity. At birth, approximately 70% of circulating hemoglobin is HbF. HbA gradually replaces HbF during the first 6 months of extrauterine life as HbA genes in bone marrow switch on and HbF genes in the liver (major site of fetal erythrocyte development) are switched off.

Fetal Circulation

Fetal circulation is different than the circulation of the neonate after birth.[24] Three important bypass pathways function in the developing fetus to enhance the flow of blood to the developing organs: **ductus venosus, ductus arteriosus,** and **foramen ovale.** Oxygenated blood from

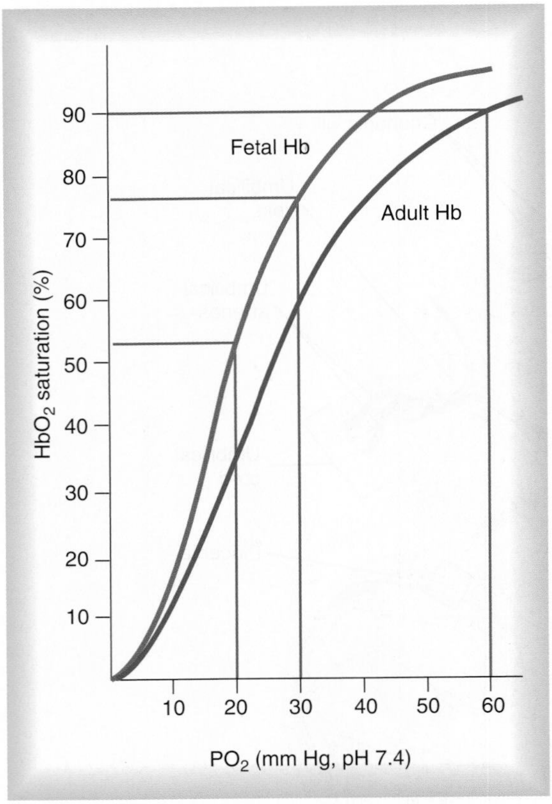

FIGURE 8-6 Fetal hemoglobin (Hb) has a leftward shift of the oxyhemoglobin (HbO_2) dissociation curve compared with adult Hb, indicating greater affinity for O_2. (Modified from Koff PB, Eitzman DV, Neu J: Neonatal and pediatric respiratory care, St Louis, 1988, Mosby.)

the placenta is carried in the umbilical vein back to the fetal circulation via the hepatic circulatory system (Figure 8-7). Approximately one-third of this blood flows to the lower trunk and extremities. The other two-thirds flows through the *ductus venosus,* which bypasses the liver's circulation and flows to the inferior vena cava. This better oxygenated blood in the inferior vena cava mixes with the venous blood returning from the lower trunk and extremities and enters the right atrium. Approximately 50% of this blood is shunted from the right atrium into the left atrium through an opening in the interatrial septum called the *foramen ovale.* Left atrial blood flows to the left ventricle and then to the ascending aorta, where it continues on to the brain, brachiocephalic trunk, and descending aorta. Venous blood from the superior vena cava is directed downward through the right atrium into the right ventricle and then into the main pulmonary artery.

The relatively low PO_2 and various prostaglandins in fetal blood cause the *ductus arteriosus,* a muscular vessel attached to the trunk of the pulmonary artery and the aorta, to dilate and the pulmonary arteries to constrict; this leads to increased pulmonary vascular resistance and higher pulmonary artery pressure than aortic blood pressure. As a result, 90% of the blood flow entering the pulmonary artery takes the path of least resistance by shunting through the ductus arteriosus and flows to the aorta. Only 10% flows into the lungs. Blood flowing through the ductus arteriosus mixes with the blood flowing through the aorta routed into the systemic circulation. Some of this blood flows to the gut, lower extremities, and placenta. Two umbilical arteries carry blood from the fetal aorta to the placenta to carry out fetal-maternal gas and nutrient exchange.

Cardiopulmonary Events at Birth

Various mechanisms work together to reduce and clear the amount of lung fluid at birth in preparation for air inflation.[25] Days before birth, the epithelia of the lung stop the production of lung fluid. The lung fluid is actively absorbed back into the fetal circulation. Most of the active lung water absorption is facilitated by active sodium channel activity that is stimulated by fetal and maternal thyroid hormones, glucocorticoids, and epinephrine and increasing fetal lung and blood O_2 content. In addition, some evidence suggests that the water channel aquaporin is also active in this process.[26] During normal vaginal delivery, approximately one-third of the lung fluid is cleared through compression of the thorax in the birth canal. The pulmonary capillaries and lymphatics clear the remaining fluid.

A newborn must develop very high transpulmonary pressure gradients during the first few breaths to open and replace the remaining lung fluid with air and establish a stable lung volume for gas exchange. These large pressure gradients overcome the opposing forces of fluid viscosity in the airways and surface tension in the alveoli. The stimulus for these initial respiratory efforts is apparently sent via peripheral and central chemoreceptors and augmented further by skin thermoreceptors.

The newborn infant is stimulated by new tactile and thermal stimuli, all of which stimulate breathing. In addition, as placental gas transfer is suddenly interrupted, the newborn quickly becomes hypoxemic, hypercapnic, and acidotic. This situation triggers strong inspiratory efforts (Figure 8-8). At first, no air enters the newborn lung until the transpulmonary pressure gradient exceeds 40 cm H_2O. As lung volume increases in a stepwise fashion with each breath, increasingly less pressure is needed to overcome the opposing forces. The volume trapped in the lung stabilizes quickly and is crucial to adequate gas exchange.

Figure 8-9 summarizes the major cardiopulmonary changes that occur during the transition from a fluid-filled lung to an air-filled lung. As the lung expands with air, and gas exchange starts within the lung, pulmonary blood PO_2 increases, PCO_2 decreases, and pH increases; this results in pulmonary vasodilation, lower pulmonary vascular resistance, and constriction of the ductus arteriosus, which facilitates greater blood flow through the pulmonary circulation. Ductus arteriosus closure is stimulated further by the loss of maternal prostaglandins. The combination

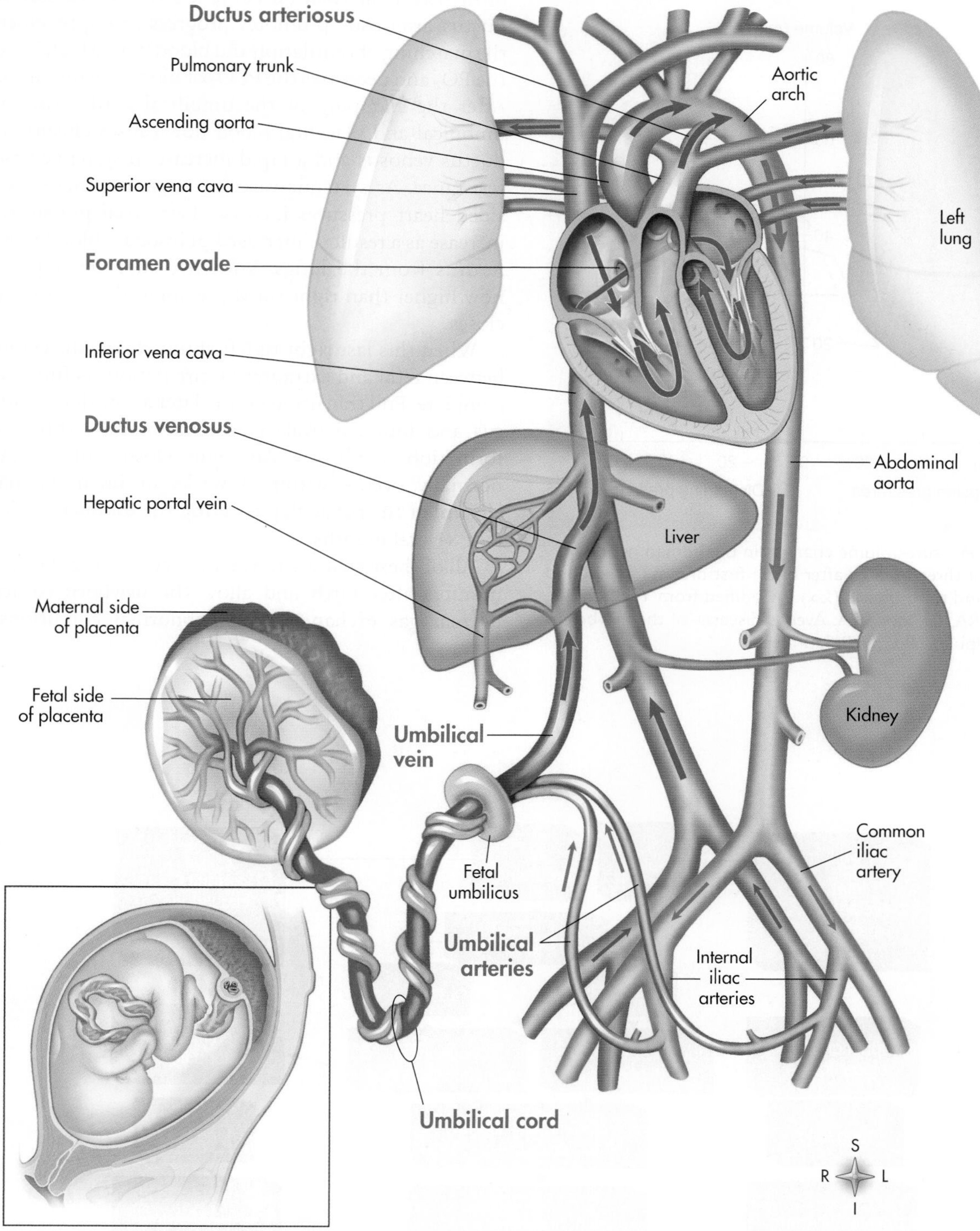

FIGURE 8-7 Fetal circulation before birth. Special features (shown in red) include the umbilical cord, two umbilical arteries, one umbilical vein, ductus venosus, foramen ovale, and ductus arteriosus. (From Thibodeau GA, Patton KT: Anatomy and physiology, ed 7, St Louis, 2010, Mosby.)

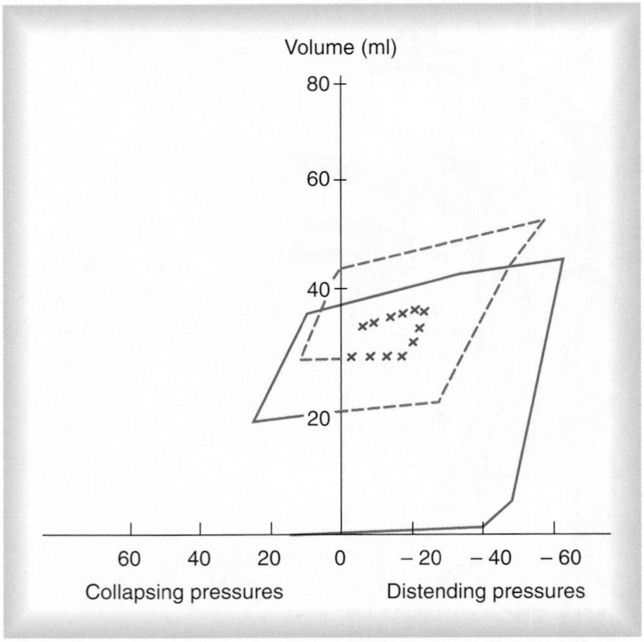

FIGURE 8-8 Pressure-volume changes in the human neonate during the first three breaths after birth: first breath (—), second breath (---), and third breath (xxx). (Modified from Taeusch WH, Ballard RA, Gleason, CA: Avery's diseases of the newborn, ed 8, Philadelphia, 2005, WB Saunders.)

of increasing alveolar air content and constriction of the ductus arteriosus promotes progressive improvement in the matching of ventilation and blood flow, which increases the PO_2 and decreases the PCO_2 of blood leaving the lungs. After the clamping of the umbilical cord, cessation of umbilical and placental blood flow causes closure of the ductus venosus and a rapid increase in systemic vascular resistance. As systemic vascular resistance increases, left-sided heart pressures increase. Left atrial pressures also increase as a result of increased pulmonary blood flow that returns from the lungs. With left-sided heart pressures now higher than right-sided pressures, the foramen ovale closes.

When this last right-to-left shunt closes, the transition between fetal and extrauterine circulations is functionally complete. Full transition occurs later as the ductus arteriosus and foramen ovale close anatomically through the formation of fibrosis. Anatomic closure of the ductus normally occurs within 3 weeks of birth. Permanent closure of the tissue flap covering the foramen ovale may take several months.

All of these changes normally occur during the first few minutes after birth and allow the newborn to achieve normal gas exchange. Many abnormal conditions can

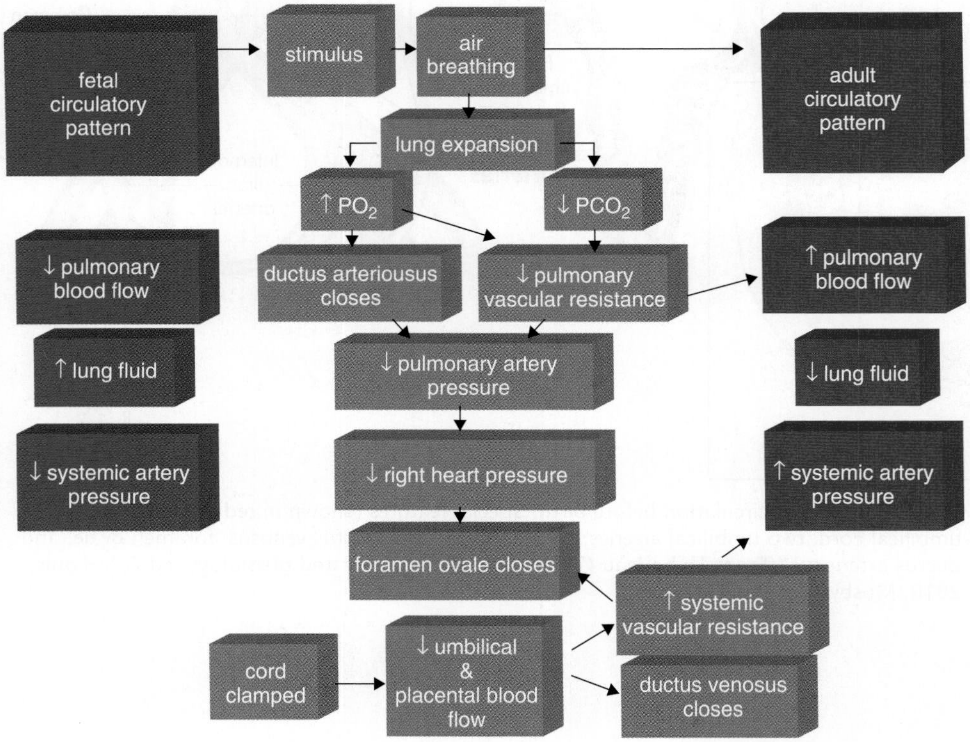

FIGURE 8-9 Major cardiopulmonary changes during the transition from the fetal to the adult circulatory pattern.

interfere with these transition events and can lead to persistence of the fetal circulation and cardiorespiratory failure.

POSTNATAL LUNG DEVELOPMENT

Upper Airway

The infant lung is a unique structure and not a mere miniaturization of the adult lung. The airways, distal lung tissue, and pulmonary capillary bed all continue to grow and develop after birth. Although the general pattern is well developed at birth, both the upper and the lower airways continue to change and are relatively unique in each person.

Figure 8-10 shows the relative differences of the upper airway in relation to body size in an infant and an adult. The greater relative weight of the head can cause acute flexion of the cervical spine in infants with poor muscle tone. Infant neck flexion causes acute airway obstruction. Although the head is larger, an infant's nasal passages are proportionately smaller than those of an adult. In addition, the infant's jaw is much rounder, and the tongue is much larger relative to the size of the oral cavity.[27] These anatomic differences increase the likelihood of airway obstruction when an infant becomes unconscious and loses muscle tone.

Most infants breathe through the nose. However, most term newborn infants shift to oral breathing in response to nasal occlusion and hypoxia.[28] As normal infants mature, they begin to use the oral breathing route more and are more capable of shifting to oral breathing when nasal obstruction is present.[29] At approximately 4 to 5 months of age, most infants are capable of full oral ventilation.

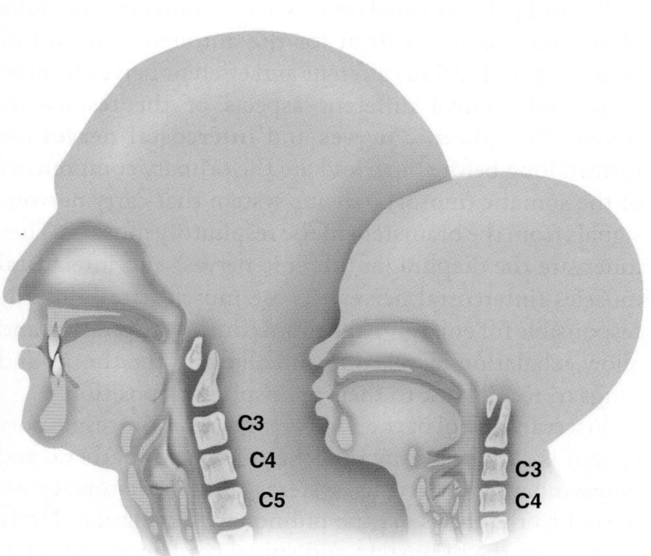

FIGURE 8-10 Adult and pediatric upper airways.

A newborn's larynx lies higher in the neck compared with the larynx of an adult, with the glottis located between C3 and C4, and is more funnel-shaped than that of an adult. In a child, the narrowest region of the upper airway is through the **cricoid cartilage,** rather than the **glottis,** as it is in adults. The **epiglottis** of an infant is longer and less flexible than the epiglottis of an adult and lies higher and in a more horizontal position. During swallowing, the infant's larynx provides a direct connection to the nasopharynx. This connection creates two nearly separate pathways, one for breathing and one for swallowing, allowing infants to breathe and suckle at the same time. Anatomic descent of the epiglottis begins at 2½ to 3 months of age. Mechanical and chemical irritant laryngeal reflexes develop at birth and can initiate protective laryngeal closure; these reflexes can trigger prolonged apnea in some and may be a cause of sudden infant death syndrome.[30] In addition, infections in this area or repeated attempts at intubation or suctioning can easily cause swelling and obstruction of this area.

The large conducting airways of infants are shorter and narrower than the airways of adults. The normal newborn trachea is approximately 5 to 6 cm long and 4 mm in diameter, whereas in small preterm infants, it may be only 2 cm long and 2 to 3 mm wide. Because of the smaller airways, a newborn's anatomic dead space is proportionately smaller than the anatomic dead space of an adult, being approximately 1.5 ml/kg of body weight. Figure 8-11 compares the tracheal anatomy in an adult and a newborn. The main stem bronchi branch off from the trachea in the infant at less acute angles than in the adult. However, similar to adults, the right main stem bronchus of the

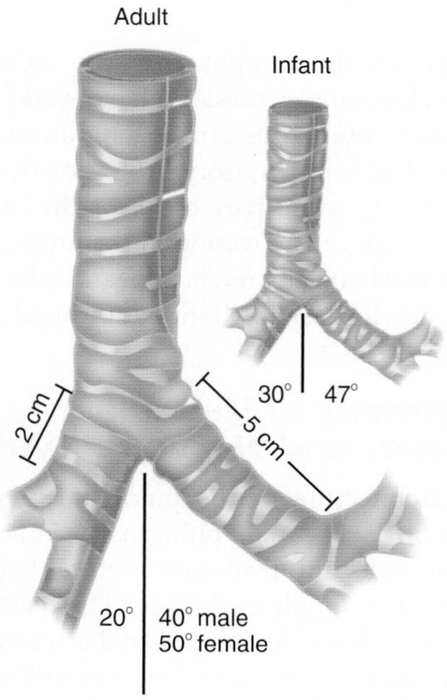

FIGURE 8-11 Adult and infant tracheas showing the different angles of main stem bifurcation.

infant is still more in line with the trachea, which promotes right main stem intubation when airways or suction catheters are inserted to deeply. Mean airway diameter, from main bronchi to respiratory bronchioles, increases about two to three times from birth to adulthood.[31]

Smooth muscle is present in the airways of a neonate down to the level of the respiratory bronchioles and continues to increase until the infant is approximately 8 months old. After this age, smooth muscle proliferation occurs primarily in the proximal airways, whereas chondrocytes producing cartilage predominate in the proximal airways. Distinct C-shaped rings of cartilage are found in the trachea and main stem bronchi of the neonate. The amount of cartilage progressively decreases in the more distal bronchi and eventually disappears in airways smaller than 2 mm in diameter.

Despite the presence of cartilage in the central airways of an infant, the trachea and larger bronchi of a neonate lack the rigidity of adult central airways. The compliant nature of these airways makes them prone to compression and collapse.

Lower Airway and Alveoli

The human lung continues to develop alveoli for years until it reaches a stable stage, at which the total number has increased to approximately 480 million alveoli.[32] All development is generally complete by 10 years of age with most occurring in the first 1½ postnatal years.[33] This development largely occurs by the formation of increasing numbers of septa in the terminal airspaces that continue to subdivide the airspace into shallow immature alveoli. These immature alveoli enlarge in size and undergo further refinement of pulmonary capillaries over the ensuing months and years.[34] By adulthood, the alveolar-capillary membrane has a gas exchange surface area of approximately 140 m^2.[35]

It was previously thought that the above-described alveolar development process ended several years after birth. However, numerous studies in various mammals have shown that compensatory lung growth can rapidly occur in the lung when part or all of the other lung is removed.[36-38] Stem cell activation in the lungs, in response to gene and mechanical stretch, appears to be responsible for alveolar development well into adulthood after loss of lung tissue.[39]

Development of Vascular, Lymphatic, and Nervous Systems

The basic architecture of the pulmonary circulation is complete at birth. The main pulmonary trunk arises from the right ventricle and divides into left and right pulmonary arteries that supply each lung. These arteries divide further to form direct or conventional arteries and supernumerary arteries. Conventional arteries follow the airway branching, whereas supernumerary arteries follow an irregular pattern that allows substantial collateralization of flow between different regions of lung. Both types of pulmonary arteries come together to supply blood to large clusters of alveoli that are supplied by a single bronchiole. Most of the growth in the vascular system that occurs after birth includes further smooth muscle growth within the walls of arteries and arterioles and greater density and refinement of the arterioles and capillaries in the distal airway region.[33,34]

The respiratory system is a unique organ in that it receives a double blood supply: one from the left ventricle and one from the right ventricle. The right heart supplies the bulk of the flow to the pulmonary circulation. The left heart supplies a smaller amount of flow (approximately 1% to 2% of cardiac output) to the bronchial arteries, which arise from the aorta and supply oxygenated blood to the tracheobronchial tree. The bronchial arteries supply O_2 to the airway tissue, blood vessels, nerves, lymphatics, and visceral pleura. In addition, O_2 is directly absorbed across the airway lumen. Although the pulmonary and bronchial circulations have entirely different origins and purposes, they mix and supply blood flow to the microcirculation of the alveoli; this provides some collateral circulation and allows the shunting of blood. The lung's double circulation benefits the entire lung in health and helps compensate for deficiencies or disease processes that can affect either circulation.

Paralleling the development of the pulmonary vascular circulation is a network of lymphatic vessels and blind lymphatic capillaries. The lymphatic vessels are located in the connective tissue tracts of the lung that surround the bronchi, bronchioles, blood vessels, nerves, and pleural membrane. They play a central role in the control of fluid and protein balance within the lung and house various defensive cells. Fluid collected from the pleural space and interstitium is carried by the pleural capillaries and vessels through the lymphatic system back to the root of the lung **(hilum)** where numerous lymph nodes are located.

Before birth, neuronal centers in the brainstem (medulla oblongata and pons) form for the automatic control of breathing, and various afferent and efferent nerves form to sense and control different aspects of the respiratory system. The **phrenic nerves** and **intercostal nerves** are formed long before birth and are the primary components of the somatic (motor) nervous system that carry nervous signals from the brainstem to the respiratory muscles. They innervate the diaphragm (phrenic nerves) and intercostal muscles (intercostal nerves). These muscles are primarily responsible for enlarging the thorax during inspiration and allow exhalation by relaxing and allowing the thorax and lungs to recoil back to their preinspiratory position.

Visceral control of the smooth muscle of the respiratory system is carried out by branches of the sympathetic and parasympathetic nervous systems and mediators transported to the lungs via the pulmonary circulation. Nerve fibers from the brainstem and spinal cord enter the lungs and grow in the same connective tissue tracts that surround the airways and house the blood and lymphatic vessels long before birth. Their development parallels airway and vessel development. These nervous fibers innervate the smooth muscles of the bronchioles to cause bronchodilation (sympathetic fibers), the mucous glands to produce mucus (parasympathetic), and the blood vessels to cause vasoconstriction (sympathetic). Cranial nerve X (*vagus* nerve) carries motor and sensory signals of the parasympathetic system. Branches from each thoracic spinal nerve carry sympathetic motor and sensory signals to and from the lungs.

Chest Wall Development, Diaphragm, and Lung Volume

The thoracic wall in infants is more compliant, and their muscles are less developed than the muscles of adults and provide little structural support. The infant thoracic cage is also more boxlike, with the ribs being horizontally oriented or elevated (Figure 8-12). In addition, the diaphragm inserts into the thoracic cage in a horizontal plane, which decreases the effective ability to enlarge the thorax.

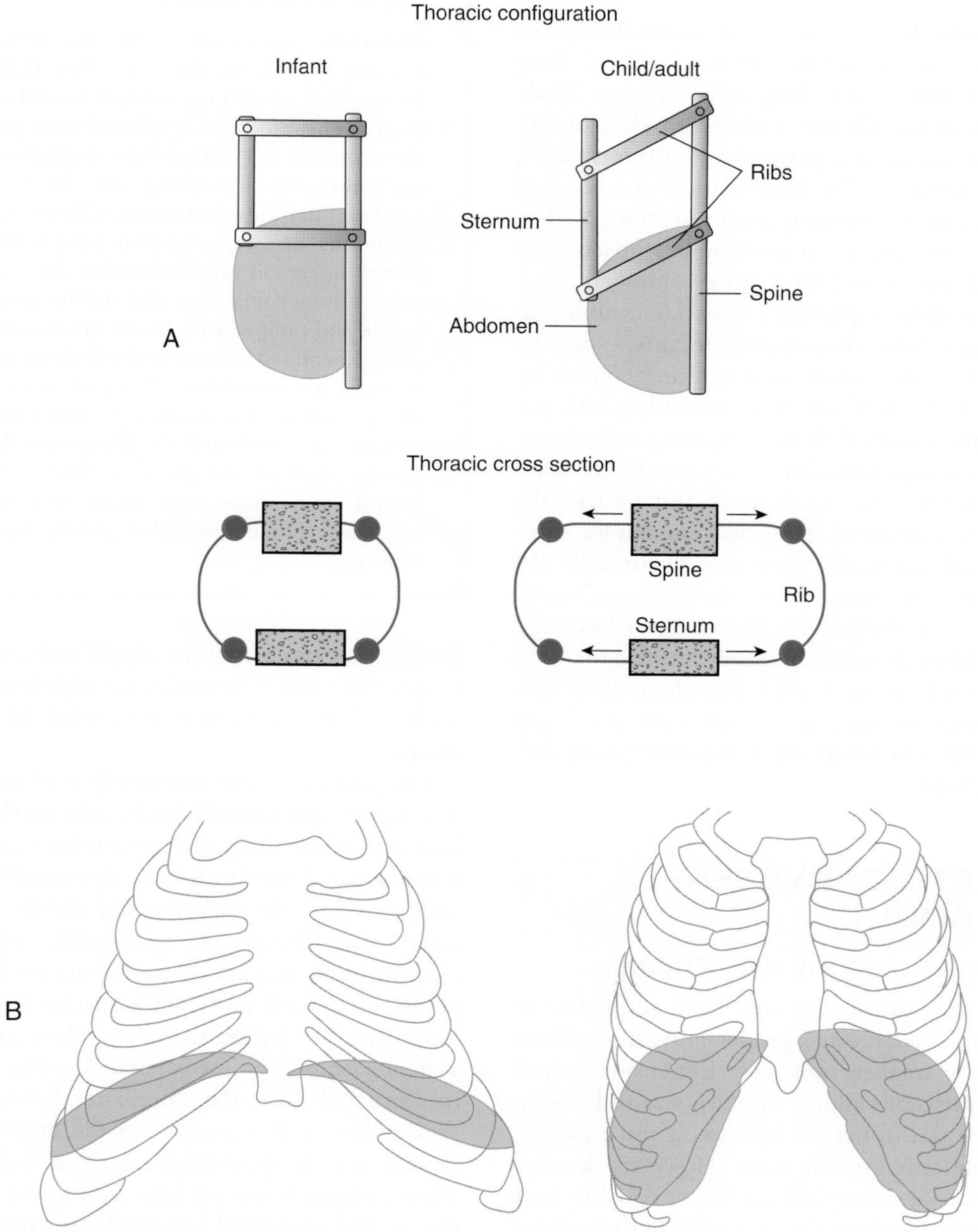

FIGURE 8-12 A, Changes in angularity of ribs and spine and cross-sectional shape of the thorax from an infant to an older child and adult. **B,** Anterior views of a newborn *(left)* and adult *(right)* rib cage and the relative position of the diaphragm *(shaded portions)*. (Modified from Taussig LM, Landau LI, editors: Pediatric and respiratory medicine, ed 2, St Louis, 2008, Mosby.)

As an infant inhales, the diaphragm moves down, but the flexible chest wall moves very little in the anteroposterior dimension as the chest wall muscles attempt to pull it upward and outward. Compounding this situation is a proportionately larger abdominal visceral content that restricts the vertical motion of the diaphragm. The ribs take on a progressively downward slope as a child grows, and by 10 years of age, the rib cage has the configuration seen in adults. Ossification of the ribs and sternum is normally complete by 25 years of age, and this, combined with muscular development, results in a stiffer chest wall that moves more in the anteroposterior dimension with inspiratory effort.

With a more compliant thorax, the resultant balance of these static forces in an infant favors a reduced lung volume. Proportionately lower lung volumes in an infant can lead to early airway closure, widespread alveolar collapse (atelectasis), ventilation/perfusion ($\dot{V}/\dot{Q}$) mismatch, and resultant hypoxemia. The combination of a reduced lung volume and high O_2 consumption in an infant renders the infant more susceptible to profound hypoxemia in situations that disturb ventilation, lung volume, or $\dot{V}/\dot{Q}$ matching further. Infants possess a remarkable ability to elevate their lung volume dynamically. Infants, especially infants in distress, can actively increase lung volume by trapping gas, which improves $\dot{V}/\dot{Q}$ matching and gas exchange. Infants accomplish gas trapping actively by using the diaphragm during exhalation to slow expiration and to adduct (close) the vocal cords and narrow the glottis. The combination of these two maneuvers effectively regulates volume in the lung and dynamically elevates lung volume. The narrowing of the glottis or larynx during exhalation is referred to as "laryngeal braking." Infants in respiratory distress commonly grunt, a manifestation of laryngeal braking. A more compliant chest wall contributes to suprasternal, substernal, intercostal, and subcostal retractions in distressed infants and young children (see Mini Clini).

MINI CLINI

Significance of Thoracic Soft Tissue Retractions

Supraclavicular and intercostal retractions are inward movements of the soft tissues above the clavicle and between the ribs of the chest wall during inspiration. This inward movement causes the clavicle and ribs to stand out prominently during inspiratory efforts.

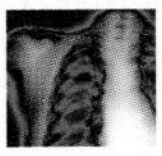

PROBLEM: Why do infants and adults in respiratory distress with severe airway obstruction or reduced compliant ("stiff") lungs exhibit thoracic soft tissue retractions?

ANSWER: The pressure within the intrapleural space is normally slightly negative (e.g., −5 cm H_2O) as a result of the tendency of the lung to recoil inward and the rib cage to recoil outward. The intrapleural space pressure becomes more negative (e.g., −8 cm H_2O) during inspiration as the respiratory muscles enlarge the chest, the diaphragm descends, and the intrathoracic volume increases. During conditions that cause severely obstructed airways (e.g., partial upper airway obstruction from epiglottitis) or reduced lung compliance and stiff lungs (e.g., viral pneumonia and pulmonary edema), much greater inspiratory effort is required because of the high resistance to airflow or stiffer lung condition. This increased effort translates into a much greater decrease in intrathoracic and pleural pressures (e.g., −40 cm H_2O). This greater decrease in intrathoracic and pleural pressure "sucks" the soft tissues inward and causes soft tissue retractions. Thoracic soft tissue retractions signal greatly increased work of breathing.

RESPIRATORY SYSTEM IN THE ADULT

Surface Features of the Thorax

Thoracic shape and dimension vary from individual to individual and are linked to age, gender, and race. At birth, the thorax has a smaller transverse dimension, which widens with the onset of walking. Thoracic size and volume continue to increase throughout childhood and especially during the adolescent growth spurt. However, development of the thorax and lung volume is not equal in both sexes. When evaluating lung size and volume throughout puberty and into adulthood, boys and men are consistently found to have larger lungs than age-matched and height-matched girls and women.[40] Some races have a proportionately larger thorax-to-height ratio than others. In females, the location of the nipple varies with the size and shape of the breast. In males, the nipple is usually located in the midclavicular line at the level of the fourth intercostal space.

Imaginary lines are commonly used to establish reference points and identify landmarks on the thorax. These lines and points help identify the location of underlying structures and the location of abnormal findings. On the anterior chest, the *midsternal line* divides the thorax into equal halves. The left and right *midclavicular lines* are parallel to the *midsternal line*. These are drawn through the midpoints of the left and right clavicles (Figure 8-13). The *midaxillary line* divides the lateral chest into equal halves. The *anterior axillary* line is parallel to the midaxillary line. It is situated along the anterolateral chest. The posterior axillary line is also parallel to the midaxillary line. It is located on the posterolateral chest wall (Figure 8-14). Three imaginary vertical lines are located on the posterior thorax. The midspinal line divides the posterior chest into two equal halves. The left and right midscapular lines are parallel to the midspinal line. They pass through the inferior angles of the scapulae in a relaxed upright subject (Figure 8-15).

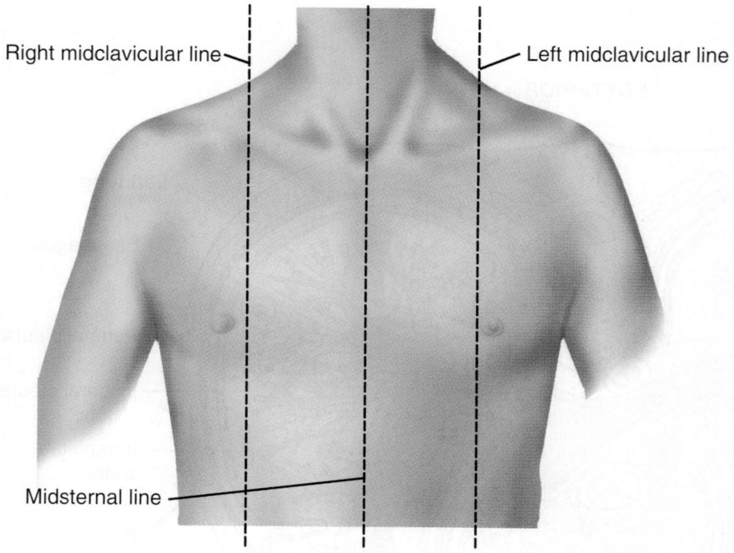

FIGURE 8-13 Anatomic reference lines on the anterior chest wall.

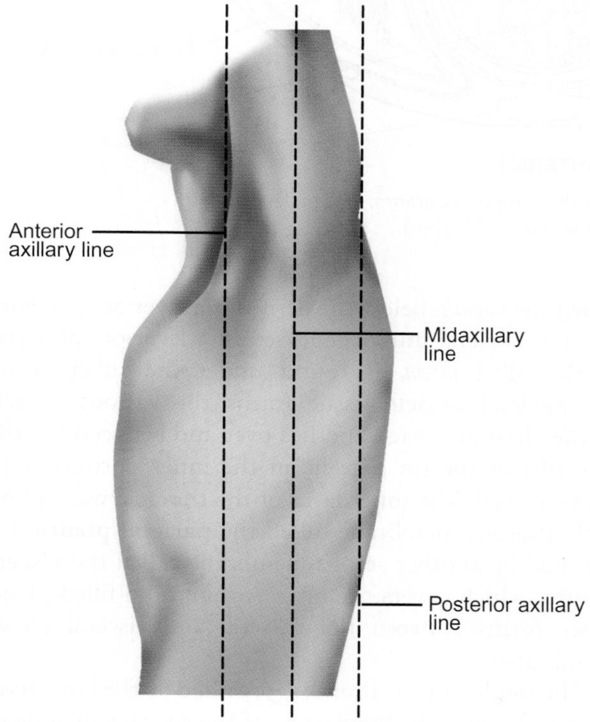

FIGURE 8-14 Anatomic reference lines on the lateral chest wall.

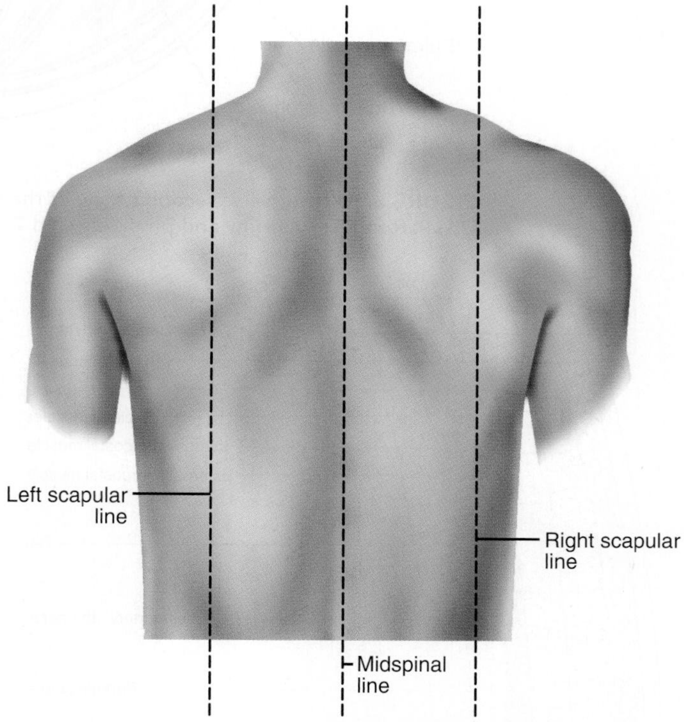

FIGURE 8-15 Anatomic reference lines on the posterior chest.

RULE OF THUMB

Anatomical Directions

Descriptions of various anatomical structures often use the following terms:

Anterior, anteriorly	Front of the body, toward the front
Posterior, posteriorly	Back of the body, toward the back
Anteroposterior	In a direction from the front to the back
Lateral, laterally	Side of the body, toward the side
Medial, medially	Midline of the body, toward the midline

Components of the Thoracic Wall

The thoracic cavity is formed by the tissues of the chest, upper back, and diaphragm.[41] It is a cone-shaped cavity that houses the lungs and the contents of the mediastinum (Figure 8-16). It functions to protect the vital organs within and is capable of changing shape to enable air to be moved into and out of the lungs. The thoracic cavity is formed from epithelial, connective, and muscle tissues.

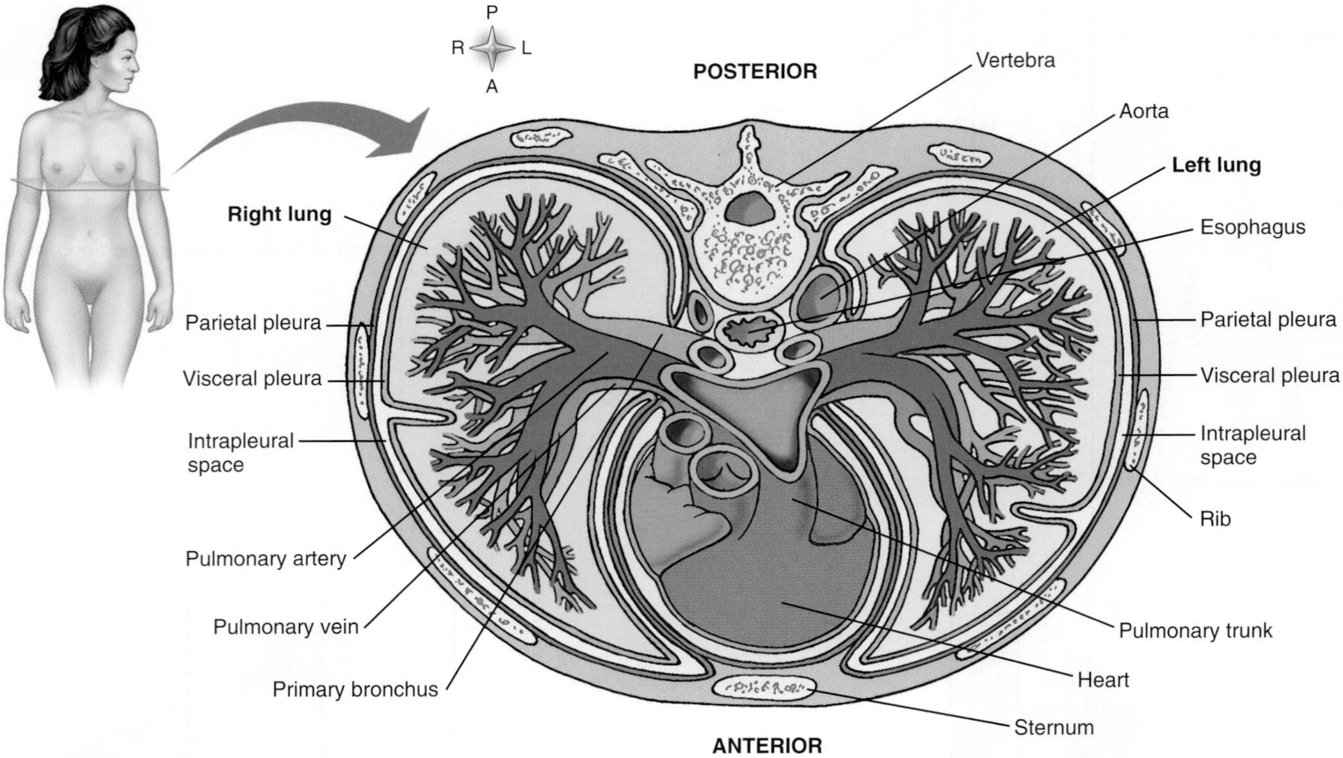

FIGURE 8-16 Transverse sectional view of the thorax showing its contents. (From Thibodeau GA, Patton KT: Anatomy and physiology, ed 7, St Louis, 2011, Mosby.)

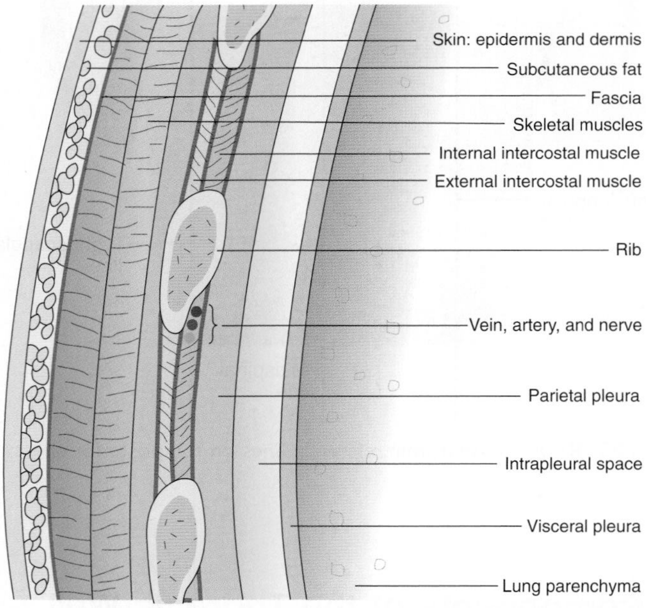

FIGURE 8-17 Sectional view of the thoracic wall. (From Hicks GH: Cardiopulmonary anatomy and physiology, Philadelphia, 2000, WB Saunders.)

The various parts of the thoracic wall are shown in Figure 8-17. The outer covering of the thorax is formed by the integumentary system, which includes skin, hair, subcutaneous fat, and breast tissues. Skin is a composite of an outer epidermis and an inner connective tissue layer called the *dermis.* Below the dermis is a layer of subcutaneous fat. Skeletal muscle, encased in a layer of connective tissue called *fascia,* is found under the subcutaneous fat. Skeletal muscle tissue forms the various muscles of the chest and back and lies over and between the ribs. The ribs of the rib cage lie in the inner portion of the thoracic wall. The inner layer of the thoracic wall is lined with a serous membrane called the **parietal pleura.** It is apposed by another serous membrane called the **visceral pleura,** which covers the lung. A thin, fluid-filled pleural space forms between the parietal and visceral pleural membranes.

The rigidity of the thorax is provided by the bone tissue of the rib cage. The bony parts of the rib cage include the sternum, ribs, thoracic vertebral bones, scapula, and clavicle (Figure 8-18). The **sternum** is a long, vertical flat bone found on the anterior side that is composed of three bones: the **manubrium,** the body (or **gladiolus**), and the **xiphoid process.** The superior edge of the manubrium forms a shallow depression that is known as the **suprasternal** (or jugular) **notch.** The fused connection between the manubrium and the body is known as the **sternal angle;** it is also known as the **angle of Louis.** The sternal angle is an external marker of the point where the trachea divides into the left and right main stem bronchi. A cartilaginous joint called the **costal cartilage** is on the lateral edges of the manubrium and sternal body and forms the attachment between the ribs and sternum. This joint allows the rib

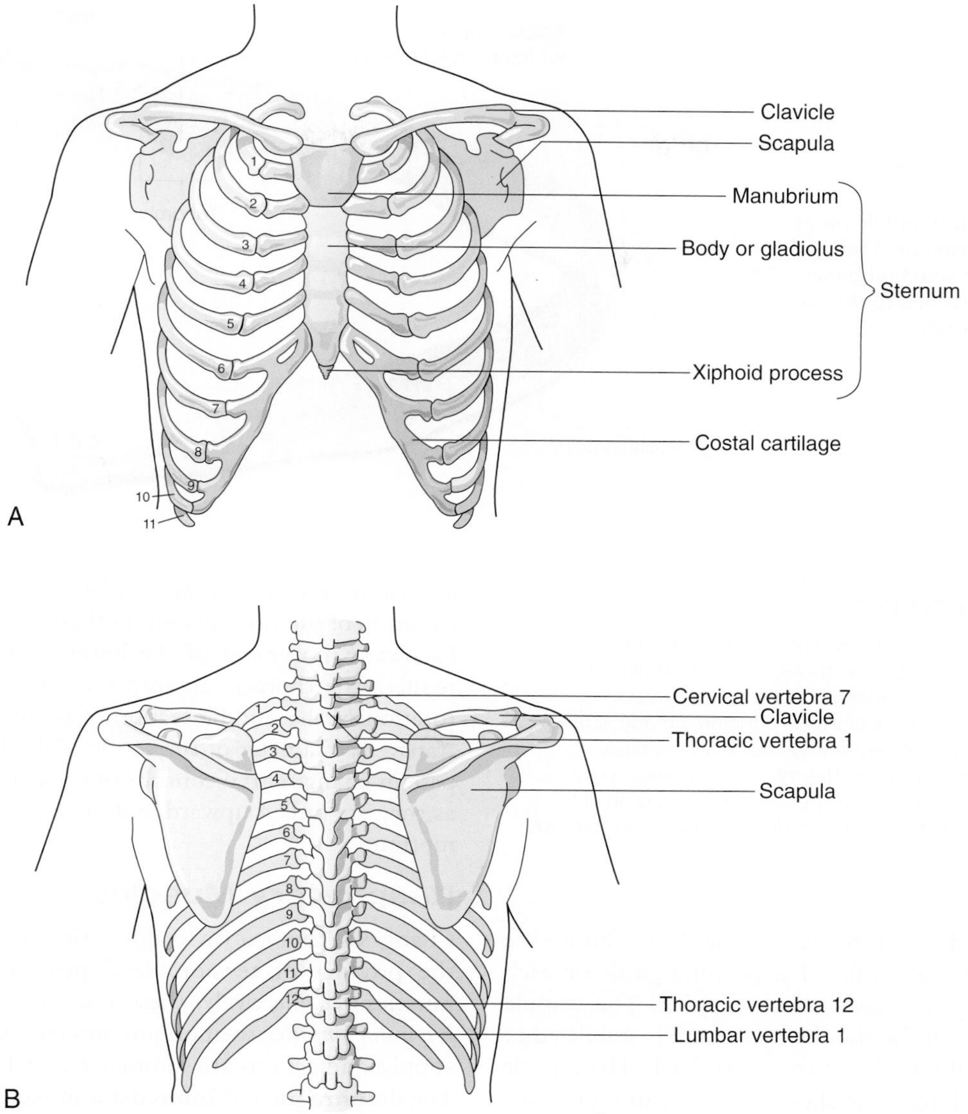

FIGURE 8-18 Anterior **(A)** and posterior **(B)** views of the bones of the thorax. (From Hicks GH: Cardiopulmonary anatomy and physiology, Philadelphia, 2000, WB Saunders.)

cage to bend and permits the thorax to increase and decrease in size.

RULE OF THUMB

Where the manubrium and body of the sternum meet, the anterior chest wall shows a slight depression that forms an oblique angle (when viewed from the side). This depression is referred to as the angle of Louis. *Beneath this important landmark, the trachea divides into the right and left main stem bronchi.*

The rib cage is formed by 12 pairs of ribs.[41] Rib pairs 1 through 7 are known as the **true ribs** because they are attached directly to the sternum. The first ribs and the upper sternum form the opening into the thorax that is called the *thoracic inlet,* or *operculum.* Ribs 8 through 12 are called **false ribs** because they are either indirectly attached to the sternum or not attached at all. The vertebrochondral ribs include rib pairs 8, 9, and 10, which are indirectly attached to the sternum through a common cartilaginous strap. Rib pairs 11 and 12 are called **floating ribs** because they are not attached to the sternum. Each rib has a sternal end; a long, curved, and relatively flat body; and a head that articulates with the thoracic vertebrae (Figure 8-19). Intercostal muscles lie between the ribs and hold them together. Just below each rib is a thoracic artery, vein, and nerve that supply blood flow and nerve communications to that region of the chest wall (see Figure 8-17).

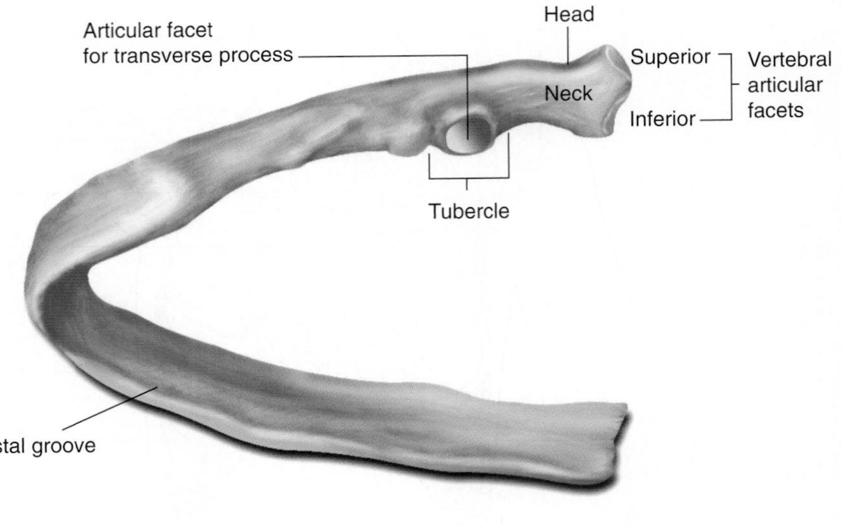

FIGURE 8-19 Typical middle rib as viewed from the posterior. The head end articulates with the vertebral bones, and the distal end is attached to the costal cartilage of the sternum.

RULE OF THUMB

Numerous procedures require entry into the pleural cavity, such as thoracentesis to drain fluid or pus and placement of chest tubes to treat pneumothorax. Incisions or punctures made during such procedures are always done immediately above a selected rib. The intercostal nerves, veins, and arteries all lie in a groove below each rib. To avoid these structures, needles and tubes are placed above a rib.

The upper and lateral regions of the thorax house the bones of the pectoral girdles. The pectoral girdle on each side is formed by the clavicle and scapula.[41] The scapula forms the socket for the shoulder joint and is stabilized or moved by skeletal muscles of the upper back. The clavicle supports and stabilizes the shoulder joint through a flexible attachment to the manubrium of the sternum.

Rib Movement

The various ribs move in different ways, and some may move more than others at different times. The first rib moves slightly, raising and lowering the sternum. Its slight motion increases the anteroposterior diameter of the chest. This action is not used during quiet breathing and becomes active only under conditions that require increased ventilation or deep breathing. Ribs 2 through 7 move simultaneously about two axes (Figure 8-20). As each rib rotates about the axis of its neck, its sternal end rises and falls. This movement increases the anteroposterior thoracic diameter in what is commonly referred to as a "pump handle"-like motion. At the same time, the rib moves about its long axis from its angle at the sternum. This motion causes the middle part of the rib to move up and down in what is commonly described as a "bucket handle." The compound action of ribs 2 through 7 changes both the anteroposterior and the transverse dimensions in an upward and outward motion. Ribs 8 through 10 rotate in a pattern similar to that of ribs 2 through 7. However, elevation of the anterior ends of these ribs produces a small backward movement of the lower sternum that slightly reduces the thoracic anteroposterior diameter. Outward rotation of the middle section of these ribs increases the transverse diameter of the thorax. Ribs 11 and 12 participate in changing the contour of the chest in a minor way as they are pulled upward and outward in a "caliper"-like motion.

Respiratory Muscles

Changes in thoracic cavity dimension during breathing are the product of tension developed by various skeletal muscles.[42] Collectively, these muscles are known as the *respiratory muscles;* their origins, insertions, somatic nervous supply, and actions are summarized in Tables 8-4 and 8-5. The **diaphragm** and **intercostal muscles** are the primary muscles of ventilation. They are active both while at rest and when the individual exhibits stress-induced increases in breathing. The accessory muscles of ventilation assist the diaphragm and intercostal muscles when ventilatory demand increases. The scalene, sternocleidomastoid, pectoral, and abdominal wall muscles are the predominant accessory muscles. Other abdominal and chest wall muscles may also function as accessory muscles.

The diaphragm is a thin, musculotendinous, dome-shaped structure that separates the thoracic and abdominal cavities (Figure 8-21).[43] It originates from the chest and abdominal wall and converges in a central tendon at the top of its dome. The posterior portion arises from the first three lumbar vertebrae. The lateral costal portions arise from the inner surface of ribs 7 through 12 and transverse abdominal muscles on each side. The anterior portion arises from the inner surface of the xiphoid process of the sternum. The best estimates of muscle fiber composition in the adult human diaphragm indicate that there are about 55% slow oxidative-type, 21% fast oxidative-type, and 24% fast glycolytic-type muscle fibers.[44] These findings

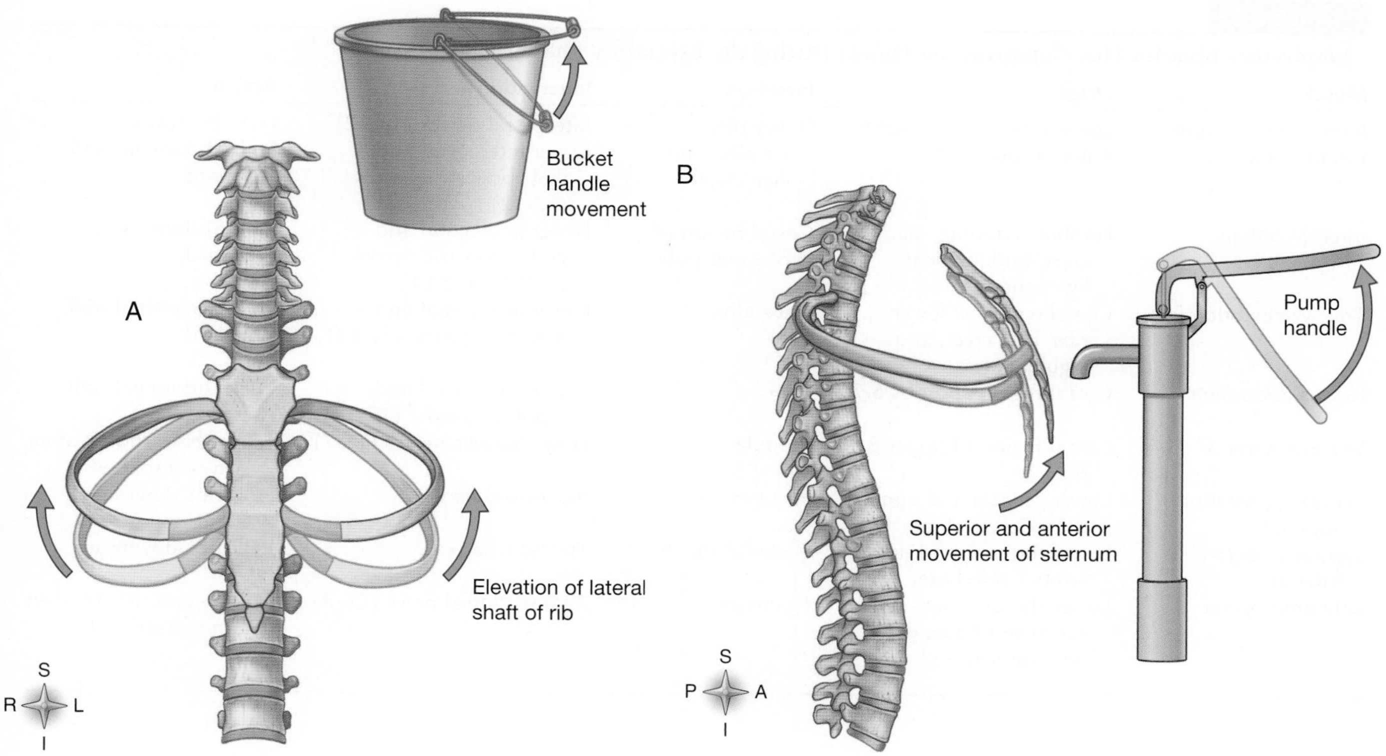

FIGURE 8-20 "Bucket handle"-type and "pump handle"-type rib motions. (From Thibodeau GA, Patton KT: Anatomy and physiology, ed 7, St Louis, 2011, Mosby.)

TABLE 8-4

Respiratory Muscles That Expand the Thorax During the Inspiratory Phase

Muscle	Origin	Insertion	Innervation	Action
Diaphragm	Xiphoid process, lower lateral ribs, lumbar vertebra	Central tendon of dome	Phrenic nerves (C3-5)	Diaphragm moves downward, abdominal wall forced outward
External intercostals	Upper ribs	Lower ribs	Intercostal nerves (T1-12)	Lift ribs upward
Scalene	Lower 5 cervical vertebrae	Ribs 1 and 2	Cervical nerves (C5-8)	Lifts ribs 1 and 2
Sternocleidomastoids	Manubrium and clavicle	Mastoid process of occipital bone	Accessory nerves (cranial nerve XI)	Lift sternum
Trapezius	Occipital bone, C7-T12 vertebrae	Scapula and clavicle	Accessory nerves (cranial nerve XI)	Stabilizes head
Pectoralis minor	Anterior region of ribs 3-5	Scapula	Pectoral nerves (C6-8)	Lifts upper ribs
Pectoralis	Clavicle and sternum	Humerus	Pectoral nerves (C5-C8)	Lifts sternum

coupled with an abundant blood supply throughout the breathing cycle help to explain in part why the diaphragm is so highly aerobic and fatigue-resistant compared with other skeletal muscles and more capable of long-term rhythmic contraction.

In an upright position and with the diaphragm relaxed, the liver forces the dome of the right hemidiaphragm upward approximately 1 cm higher than the left hemidiaphragm at the end of a quiet exhalation. The highest portion of the right dome sits at the eighth or ninth thoracic vertebra posteriorly and at the fifth rib anteriorly. The left diaphragmatic dome sits at the ninth or tenth thoracic vertebra posteriorly and the sixth rib anteriorly. Movements of the hemidiaphragms are synchronous in healthy subjects. When lying down in a supine position, the weight of the abdominal contents forces the diaphragm farther up into the thoracic cavity. During quiet breathing, the diaphragm is responsible for approximately 75% of the change in thoracic volume.[45] When the muscle fibers of the diaphragm are tensed during inspiration, the dome of the diaphragm is pulled down 1 to 2 cm; this results in enlargement of the thoracic cavity and compression of the

TABLE 8-5

Respiratory Muscles That Compress the Thorax During the Expiratory Phase

Muscle	Origin	Insertion	Innervation	Action
Internal intercostals	Lower ribs	Upper ribs	Intercostal nerves (T1-12)	Pull ribs down
External oblique	Anterior lower 8 ribs	Linea alba and iliac crest	Lower intercostal and iliohypogastric nerves (T7-12)	Pulls abdominal wall inward
Internal oblique	Lumbar vertebrae, iliac crest, and inguinal ligaments	Costal region of ribs and pubis	Lower intercostal and iliohypogastric nerves (T10-12 and L1)	Pulls abdominal wall inward
Transverse abdominis	Costal region of lower ribs, iliac crest, and inguinal crest	Linea alba	Lower intercostal and iliophypogastric (T7-L1)	Pulls abdominal wall inward
Rectus abdominis	Costal region and ribs 5-7	Pubis	Lower intercostal and iliophypogastric (T7-12)	Pulls abdominal wall inward
Serratus anterior	Costal region of upper 8 ribs	Scapula	Long thoracic nerves (T5-7)	Compresses thorax when arm is stabilized
Serratus, posterior superior	Lower cervical and upper thoracic vertebrae	Posterior ribs 2-5	Intercostal nerves	Pulls ribs downward
Serratus, posterior inferior	Lower thoracic and upper lumbar vertebrae	Posterior ribs 9-12	Thoracic nerves	Pulls ribs downward
Latissimus dorsi	Lower thoracic, lumbar, sacral vertebrae, ilium, and lower ribs	Humerus	Thoracodorsal nerve (C6-8)	Compresses thorax when arm is stabilized

abdominal contents. During maximal inspiration, the diaphragm can be pulled down approximately 10 cm. Exhalation results when diaphragmatic tension decreases, and the diaphragm returns to its relaxed position.

Increased lung volume causes the diaphragm to flatten out. Contraction of a flattened diaphragm can result in tension on the lower ribs that causes them to be pulled inward, resulting in compression of the thoracic cavity. This condition can occur in individuals with severe gas trapping as a result of emphysema or asthma. To compensate, these individuals must recruit other muscles to enlarge the thorax. Less efficient breathing and excessive muscle work result. Nonpulmonary diseases can also affect diaphragm function. Abdominal wall muscle tensioning *(splinting)* owing to pain, abdominal distention with fluid *(ascites)*, or other causes of rigidity of the abdominal wall can interfere with diaphragmatic descent during inspiration.

MINI CLINI

Lung Hyperinflation in Emphysema

Emphysema is a disease characterized by the destruction of the alveolar region of the lungs. This destruction causes the emphysematous lung to have less elastic recoil than a normal lung.

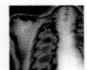

PROBLEM: Why do patients with severe emphysema have enlarged or overinflated lungs? How does hyperinflation interfere with breathing? What can be done to alleviate the problem?

ANSWER: Cigarette smoking promotes the development of emphysema. The pathologic findings of emphysema include the destruction of elastic fibers in the alveolar region, reduced lung recoil, and expansion of the remaining lung tissue. As the disease progresses, the collapsing forces of the lung become less than the normal outward expanding forces of the rib cage. The stronger outward expanding force of the rib cage expands the lungs, increases their volume, and results in overinflated lungs at the end of a normal, resting exhalation. Hyperinflation "flattens" the diaphragm for similar reasons, making it less effective during inspiration. Loss of elastic tissue allows small airways to collapse, resulting in air trapping, exaggerating hyperinflation further. Therapy for emphysema is directed at reducing the effects of air trapping. Administration of bronchodilators and corticosteroids may improve airway opening, reducing trapped gas and the work of breathing. Maneuvers such as pursed-lip exhaled breathing may also assist in reducing gas trapping by splinting open the airways and facilitating exhalation. Surgical removal of overdistended lung tissue (bullae) is known as *lung volume reduction surgery*. Surgical removal of nonfunctional hyperexpanded tissue may allow the remaining lung tissue to be better ventilated and improve gas exchange at the alveolar level.

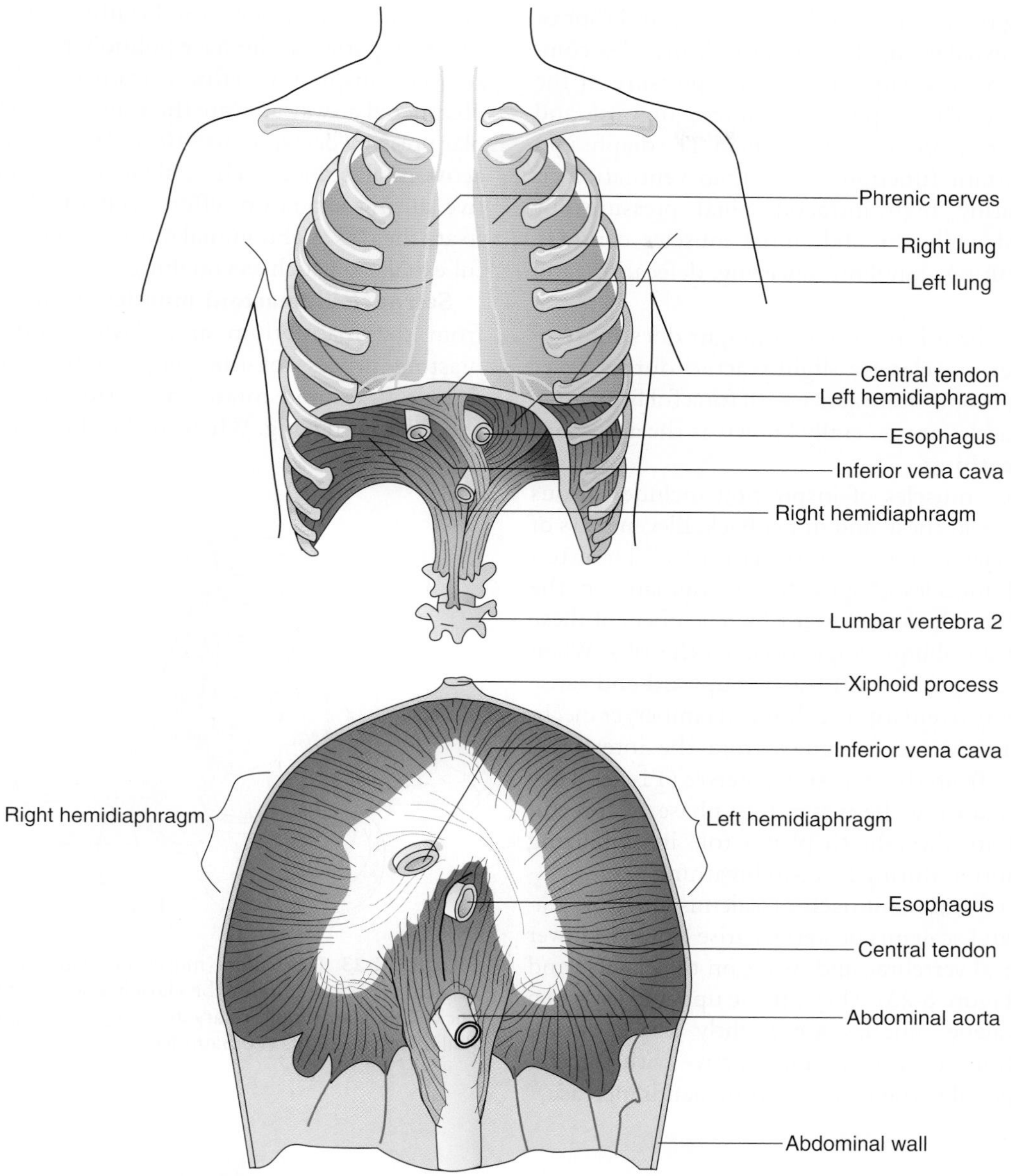

FIGURE 8-21 The diaphragm originates from the lumbar vertebrae, lower ribs, xiphoid process, and abdominal wall and converges in a central tendon. Note the locations of the phrenic nerves and openings for the inferior vena cava, esophagus, and abdominal aorta. (From Hicks GH: Cardiopulmonary anatomy and physiology, Philadelphia, 2000, WB Saunders.)

Functionally, the diaphragm is divided into a right and a left hemidiaphragm. Each hemidiaphragm is innervated by a phrenic nerve that arises from branches of spinal nerves C3, C4, and C5.[43] Spinal cord injuries at or above the level of the third cervical vertebrae result in diaphragmatic paralysis. In this situation, the individual has lost *all* nervous control of the respiratory muscles and is unable to breathe. Unilateral phrenic nerve injury or disease to one side can spare the other nerve and permit unilateral ventilation.

Although the diaphragm is the primary ventilatory muscle, it is not essential for survival. Limited, short-term ventilation is possible using accessory muscles, even if the diaphragm is paralyzed. If either or both of the hemidiaphragms are paralyzed, the affected component or components remain in a resting position. During deep inspiration, the paralyzed diaphragm rises as other ventilatory muscles reduce the intrathoracic pressure. During quiet breathing, the paralyzed diaphragm may remain immobile or may move in either direction. The pressures above and below a paralyzed diaphragm tend to make it rise during inspiration.

The diaphragm normally does not actively participate in exhalation. During exhalation, it returns to its resting position during the passive recoil of the lungs and thorax. During forced exhalation, abdominal wall muscles compress the abdominal cavity and increase pressure in the abdominal cavity. The diaphragm is forced upward, and the lungs compress, forcing gas from them. The diaphragm performs important functions other than ventilation; it aids in generating high intraabdominal pressures by remaining fixed while the abdominal muscles contract, facilitating vomiting, coughing, sneezing, defecation, and parturition.

During quiet breathing, the diaphragm does most of the work. Other muscles are slightly active during quiet breathing and become more active with forceful breathing. These other muscles are generally known as the **accessory muscles of breathing.**

The accessory muscles of inspiration include various muscles in the neck, chest, and upper back. Eleven pairs of intercostal muscles are found between the ribs.[46] The external intercostal muscles (Figure 8-22) originate on the upper ribs and attach to the lower ribs. The fibers of these muscles run at an oblique angle between the ribs. When they generate tension, they lift the ribs upward and cause the thoracic cavity to enlarge the thorax (Hamberger mechanism). They receive nerve signals from the intercostal nerves that arise from thoracic spinal nerves (T1-12). They are more active during the inspiratory phase of forceful breathing and are thought to play a role in stabilizing excessive rib motion during forceful breathing.[47]

Three pairs of **scalene muscles** (scalenus anterior, scalenus medius, and scalenus posterior) arise from the lower five or six cervical vertebrae and insert on the clavicle and first two ribs (Figure 8-23). They lift the upper chest when active. The scalene muscles are slightly active during resting inhalation and become more active with forceful inspiration, especially when ventilatory demands increase.[48] Such instances may occur in healthy subjects during exercise or in patients who have pulmonary disease. In healthy subjects, inspiratory efforts against a closed glottis or obstructed airway activate the scalene muscles. When alveolar pressure decreases to −10 cm H_2O, scalene muscles are active in all subjects. The scalene muscles are largely inactive during expiratory efforts but can become active to fixate the ribs as abdominal muscles contract during forceful exhalation such as coughing.

Sternocleidomastoid muscles (Figure 8-24) originate from the manubrium and clavicle and insert on the mastoid process of the temporal bone. Normally, this muscle flexes and rotates the head and is active during shoulder shrugging. When the head is held in an upright

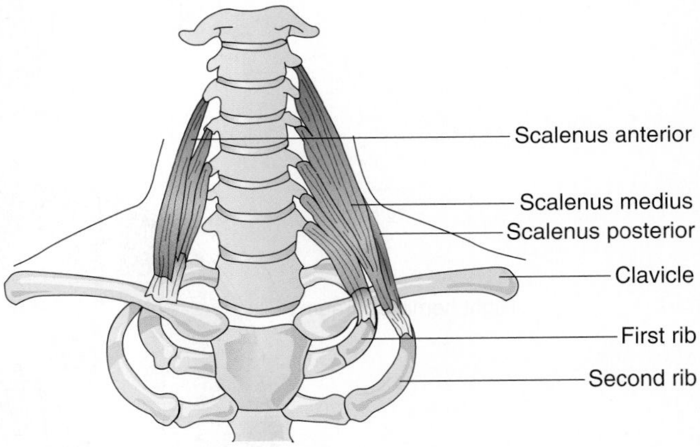

FIGURE 8-23 The scalene muscles originate from the lower cervical vertebrae and lift the clavicle and first two ribs. (From Hicks GH: Cardiopulmonary anatomy and physiology, Philadelphia, 2000, WB Saunders.)

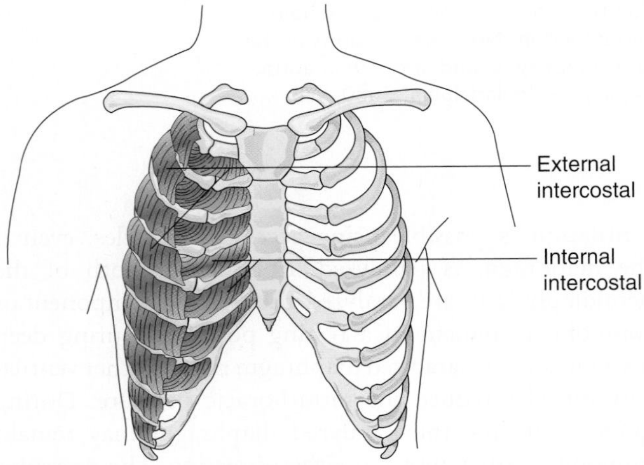

FIGURE 8-22 The external intercostal muscles lift the inferior ribs and enlarge the thoracic cavity. The internal intercostal muscles compress the thoracic cavity by pulling together the ribs. (From Hicks GH: Cardiopulmonary anatomy and physiology, Philadelphia, 2000, WB Saunders.)

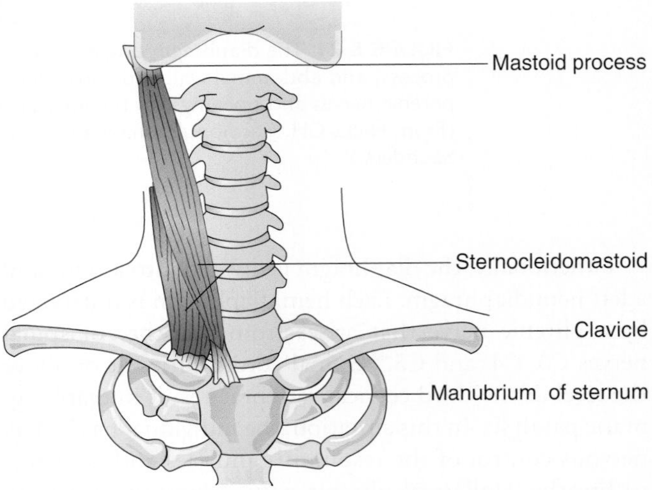

FIGURE 8-24 The sternocleidomastoid muscles originate from the manubrium and clavicle and insert on the mastoid process of the temporal bone. They lift the upper thorax when the trapezius stabilizes the head. (From Hicks GH: Cardiopulmonary anatomy and physiology, Philadelphia, 2000, WB Saunders.)

position by tensing the trapezius muscle of the upper back and neck, the sternocleidomastoid muscles can function to lift the upper chest. They receive nerve impulses from branches of the accessory nerves (cranial nerve XI) and cervical nerves C1 and C2. These muscles are active during forceful inspiration and become visible as thick bands on either side of the neck during the inspiratory phase in an individual who is in respiratory distress. This motion increases the anteroposterior diameter of the chest.[49]

RULE OF THUMB

Patients with advanced chronic obstructive pulmonary disease (COPD) often use accessory muscles to assist the flattened diaphragm and to help relieve their work of breathing. The muscle groups used include shoulder and neck muscles normally used to move the arms and head. To use these muscles, the shoulder girdle must be stabilized. Patients with COPD often do this by supporting their arms on a stationary object in front of them to form the "tripod" position to immobilize the shoulders so that the accessory muscles can raise the anterior chest wall.

The major and minor pectoralis muscles are broad fan-shaped muscles of the upper anterior chest (Figure 8-25). The pectoralis major originates on the humerus and inserts onto the clavicle and sternum. The pectoralis minor originates from the anterior region of the ribs 3 through 5 and inserts onto the scapula. When these muscles receive impulses from the pectoral nerves, they normally function to adduct the arms in a hugging motion. They are also capable of generating some anterior thoracic lift when the arms are braced on a surface in front of a subject. Individuals who have chronic shortness of breath often use these muscles by sitting in a "tripod" position. This position is generated by sitting upright and leaning forward with both arms braced on a table or other stationary object.

The trapezius muscles are flat triangular muscles that are located on the upper back and neck (Figure 8-26). They arise from the occipital bone, seventh cervical vertebra, and all of the thoracic vertebrae. They insert onto the scapulae and lateral third of the clavicles. Their action is to rotate the scapulae, lift the shoulders, and flex the head up and back. They become active during forceful inspiration by helping to brace the head and allowing the sternocleidomastoid muscles to lift the thorax.

The accessory muscles of exhalation become active during forceful breathing (see Table 8-5). Generally, these muscles act to compress the thoracic cavity and facilitate exhalation. The internal intercostal muscles (see Figure 8-22) lie between the ribs and just behind the external intercostal muscles. They originate along the inferior border of the upper ribs and insert into the superior border of the lower ribs. The muscle fibers of the internal intercostal muscles run downward and less obliquely than the external intercostal muscle fibers. This orientation causes these muscles to pull the ribs together, which results in compression of the thoracic cavity. They are stimulated by branches of the intercostal nerves and are most active during forceful exhalation. They also become active toward the end of deep inhalation and act to antagonize the lifting effect of the external intercostal muscles, which effectively stabilizes rib motion during forceful exhalation.[49]

When the abdominal wall muscles contract, they compress the abdominal cavity. This compression forces the diaphragm upward, compressing the thoracic cavity. The abdominal muscles include pairs of **external oblique, internal oblique,** transverse abdominis, and **rectus abdominis muscles** (Figure 8-27).[50] The external oblique

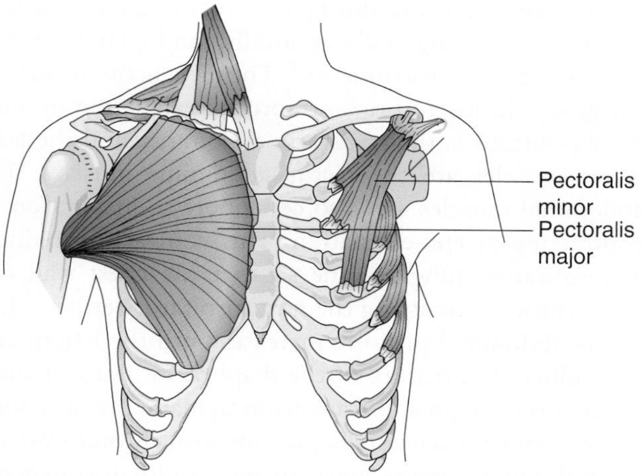

FIGURE 8-25 The pectoralis major and minor can lift and enlarge the thorax when the arms are braced by leaning forward on the elbows (tripod position). (From Hicks GH: Cardiopulmonary anatomy and physiology, Philadelphia, 2000, WB Saunders.)

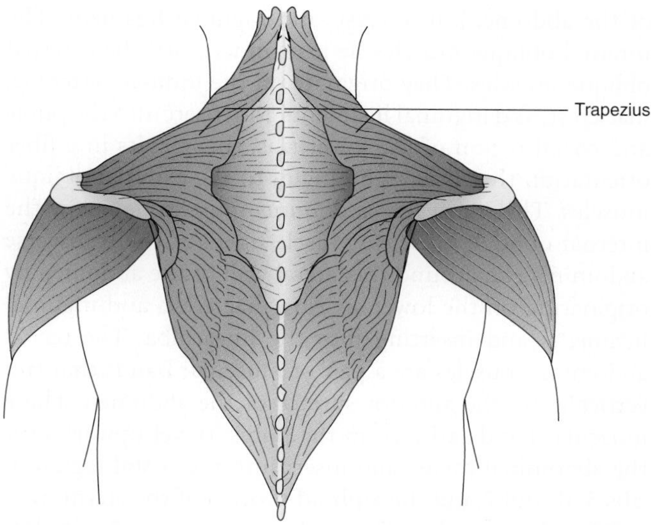

FIGURE 8-26 The trapezius assists forceful inspiration primarily by stabilizing the head, which allows the sternocleidomastoid to lift the anterior thorax. (From Hicks GH: Cardiopulmonary anatomy and physiology, Philadelphia, 2000, WB Saunders.)

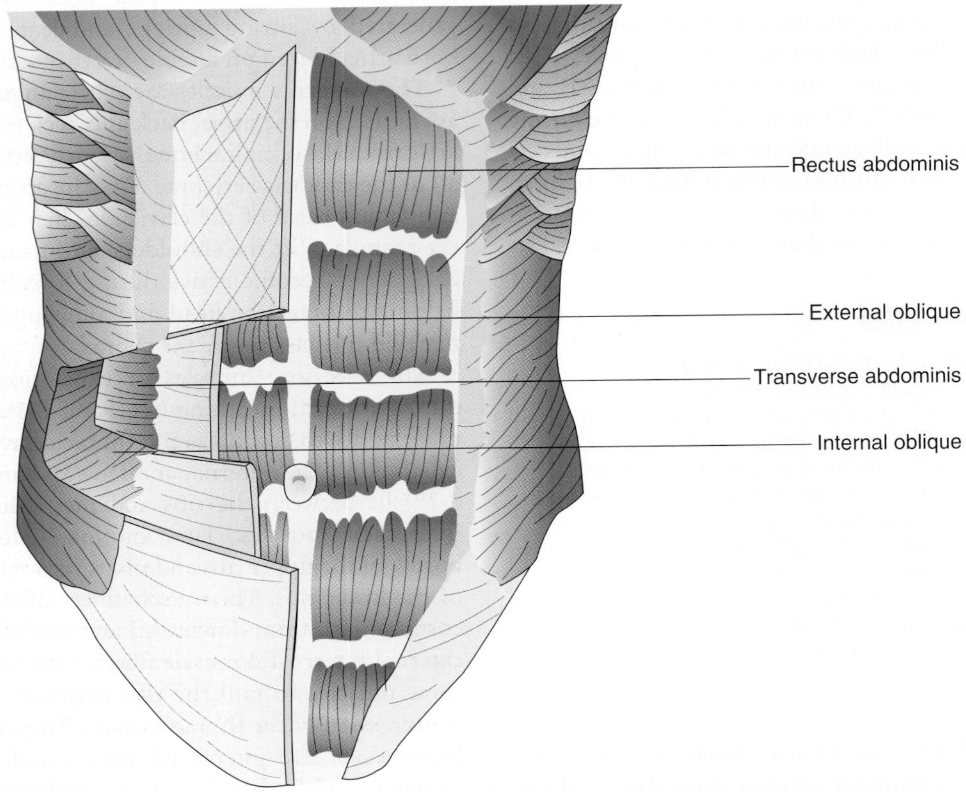

FIGURE 8-27 The abdominal wall muscles compress the thoracic cavity by compressing the abdominal wall and forcing the diaphragm upward. (From Hicks GH: Cardiopulmonary anatomy and physiology, Philadelphia, 2000, WB Saunders.)

muscles are the outermost layer of abdominal wall muscle and lie over the lateral aspects of the abdominal cavity. They originate on the anterior surface of the lower eight ribs and abdominal aponeurosis and insert into the linea alba (a connective tissue band on the midanterior surface of the abdomen), iliac crest, and inguinal ligament. The internal oblique muscles lie just underneath the external oblique muscles. They originate on the lumbar vertebrae, iliac crest, and inguinal ligaments and insert into the pubis and costal region of the lower ribs; this results in a fiber orientation that is at right angles to the external oblique muscles. The transverse abdominis muscles lie below the internal oblique muscles. Muscle fibers of the transverse abdominis run around the lateral wall of the abdomen by originating on the lower six ribs, iliac crest, and inguinal ligaments and inserting into the linea alba. The rectus abdominis muscles are a pair of muscular bands that run vertically on the anterior surface of the abdomen. These muscular bands arise from the pubis, travel upward over the abdominal cavity, and insert into the costal region of ribs 5, 6, and 7 and the xiphoid process of the sternum.

The abdominal wall muscles receive nerve impulses from branches of the lower intercostal and iliohypogastric nerves. When forceful contraction of the abdominal wall muscle group occurs, it results in increasing intraabdominal pressure, which forces the diaphragm upward and compresses the thorax.

Myographic analysis of each of the different abdominal wall muscles reveals that they are active during resting and forceful exhalation.[51] They become more active when the elastic recoil of the lung and thorax cannot provide the needed expiratory flow during forceful exhalation, such as coughing, sneezing, talking loudly, and playing wind-powered musical instruments.[52] The most active muscle of the group during resting and forceful exhalation in most body positions is the transverse abdominis, and the least active muscles are the rectus abdominis muscles. The abdominal muscles can also contribute to inspiration by contracting at end-exhalation. This contraction reduces end-expiratory lung volume so that the chest wall can recoil outward, assisting the next inspiratory effort.[53] Elevating abdominal pressure increases both the length and the radius of curvature of the diaphragm. Both of these effects result in greater transdiaphragmatic pressure for a given contractile tension. In patients with chronic obstructive pulmonary disease, any increase in ventilatory demand significantly increases the use of the abdominal muscles. Loss of effective use of the abdominal wall muscles results in a marked inability to exhale forcefully and to cough effectively.

Pleural Membranes, Space, and Fluid

The thoracic cavity is subdivided into the mediastinum and the left and right pleural cavities. The centrally located mediastinum contains the trachea, esophagus, heart, great vessels, and other organs.[54] The left and right pleural cavities contain the lungs. The surfaces of the inner thoracic wall, mediastinum, and lungs are covered with serous membranes called the *pleural membranes* (see Figure 8-17). The parietal pleural membrane lines the chest wall and mediastinum, whereas the lungs are covered by the visceral pleura. Both membranes are constructed from a thin surface layer of mesothelial cells, and below the layer of mesothelial cells is a layer of connective tissue that houses blood vessels, lymphatic vessels, and nerve fibers.[55] Numerous microscopic openings, called *stomata,* are found in the surface of the pleura and are surrounded by mesothelial cells. The stomata open into the lymphatic drainage system of the pleural membrane. The parietal pleura contains sensory fibers that are responsible for the painful sensation that is associated with inflammation of the pleura—a condition called *pleurisy*.

The space between the membranes is called the *pleural space* and is filled with approximately 0.26 ml/kg, or about 18 ml in a 70-kg adult, of pleural fluid.[56] Pleural fluid is a clear fluid with a pH of 7.60 to 7.65 that has few cells, a small amount of protein (about 1 g/dl), and glucose and electrolytes in concentrations that approximate those of plasma. The small volume of pleural fluid is spread out over the entire surface of both lungs and functions as a lubricant to reduce friction as the lungs move within the thorax and as an airtight seal that adheres together the two pleural membranes. Pleural fluid is secreted and reabsorbed by the two pleural membranes. A little more than half of the pleural fluid is thought to be produced by the parietal pleura according to Starling forces of filtration. Pleural fluid is formed from the systemic blood flow to each pleura. Blood pressure–driven filtration is supplied to the parietal pleura by blood flow from the intercostal arteries, and the bronchial circulation of the lung supplies most of the blood flow to the visceral pleura.

It is estimated that the pleurae produce 150 to 250 ml of pleural fluid per day.[57] Most of the fluid is thought to be absorbed by the visceral pleura capillaries (according to Starling forces), and the rest is cleared by drainage through the lymphatic stomata of parietal pleura, by solute-coupled liquid absorption, and through some transcytosis. Fluid and solutes or cells cleared by lymphatic drainage are carried by the pulmonary lymphatics to the hilar region, where they enter the major lymphatic vessels that drain back to the subclavian veins and right heart.

The angle where the costal parietal pleura joins the diaphragmatic parietal pleura is known as the **costophrenic angle.** It is located in the right and left lateral and inferior regions of the thoracic cavities. This angle is clearly visible and is an important landmark in the normal chest radiograph. Normally, it is a sharp angle of about 30 to 45 degrees. Excess fluids between the visceral and parietal pleura tend to pool here in an upright individual. This pooling of fluid causes the angle to appear blunted or flattened to 90 degrees when viewed in the chest radiograph.

Mediastinum

The **mediastinum** lies between the left and right pleural cavities that contain the lungs (see Figure 8-16). The mediastinum is bounded on either side by the pleural cavities, anteriorly by the sternum, posteriorly by the thoracic vertebrae, inferiorly by the diaphragm, and superiorly by the thoracic inlet. The mediastinum can be subdivided into three subcompartments.[54] Between the sternum and pericardium is an anterior compartment, which contains the thymus gland and lymph nodes. The middle compartment contains the pericardium, heart, great vessels, phrenic and upper portions of the vagus nerves, trachea, portions of the right and left main stem bronchi, and lymph nodes. The posterior compartment contains the thoracic aorta, esophagus, and thoracic duct. Also found in the posterior mediastinum are the sympathetic nervous system ganglionic chains and lower portions of the vagus nerve and lymph nodes.

MINI CLINI

Penetrating Chest Injury

Normally, the parietal and visceral pleurae are in physical contact with one another and are separated only by a thin, liquid film or fluid. This liquid film allows these two pleural membranes to slide over one another with little friction. This film also provides a cohesive force that resists separation of the membranes. When the respiratory muscles move the rib cage outward in an inspiratory effort, the lung is literally pulled by the cohesive forces between the parietal and visceral pleurae. The elastic recoil forces of the lung resist this outward movement.

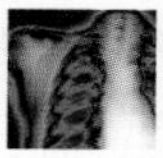

PROBLEM: A person sustains blunt force traumatic injury to the left chest. The fractured ribs are forced through the chest wall and parietal pleura, puncture the visceral pleura, and lacerate the lung. What happens to the lungs?

ANSWER: The lung on the affected side collapses as air and blood leak from the lacerated lung. As air and blood enter the pleural space (hemopneumothorax), the parietal and visceral pleurae separate. The chest wall expands outward, and the elastic recoil of the lung causes it to collapse. Both structures recoil in opposite directions as the pleural space between them separates. Treatment of a hemopneumothorax involves inserting a tube into the chest cavity (a chest tube) and applying vacuum to remove the air and blood to reexpand the lung.

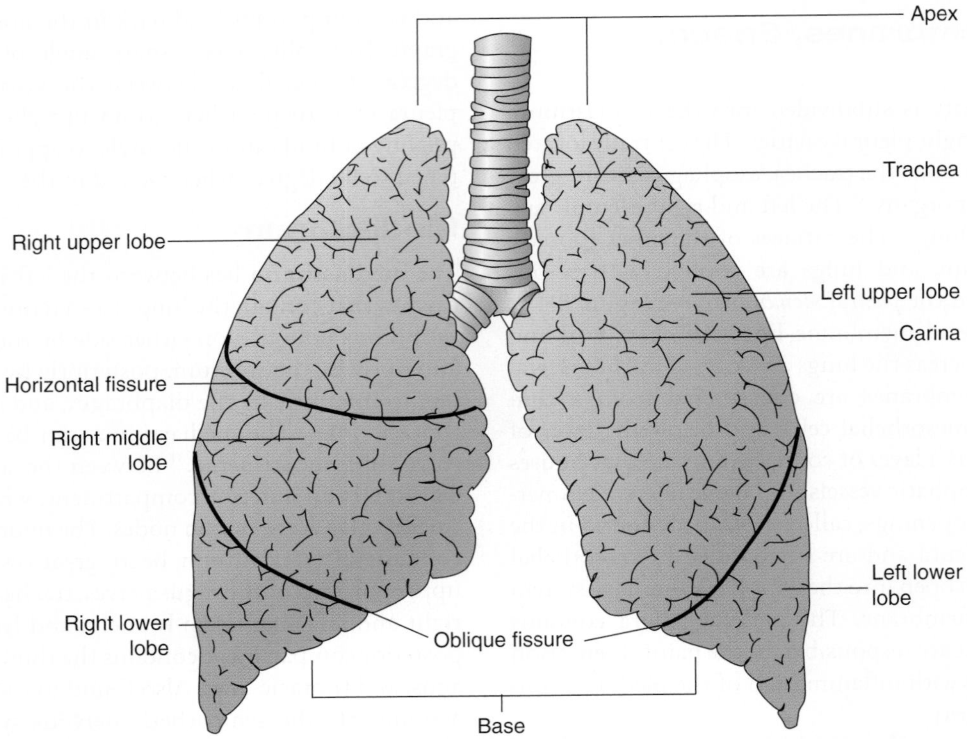

FIGURE 8-28 Anterior view of the lungs showing the lobes and fissures. (From Hicks GH: Cardiopulmonary anatomy and physiology, Philadelphia, 2000, WB Saunders.)

Lungs

The lungs are multilobed, cone-shaped, spongelike organs that lie within the pleural cavities (Figure 8-28). They are pink at birth and develop a gray coloration with age. Average adult lungs are hollow low-density organs that occupy a volume of approximately 3.5 L and weigh approximately 900 g.[55] The organs within the mediastinum bulge into the left hemithorax, resulting in a narrower and slightly smaller left lung. The liver below the right lung elevates the right diaphragm and results in a slightly shorter right lung.

The lungs extend from the diaphragm to a point 1 to 2 cm above the medial third of the clavicles. The uppermost regions are called the **apices.** At end-expiration, the anterior lower lung borders extend to approximately the sixth rib at the midclavicular line. Laterally, the lower lung border is at the eighth rib at the midaxillary line. The top of the lungs, viewed posteriorly, extends upward from the eighth or ninth thoracic vertebra to the first thoracic vertebra. The diaphragm rises and falls with resting breathing between the ninth and twelfth thoracic vertebrae.

The anterior, lateral, and posterior lung surfaces lie and move against the thoracic inner wall. The medial surfaces of the lungs lie in close contact to the mediastinal surfaces. Figure 8-29 shows the medial surfaces of the lungs and the opening in this region, which is called the *hilum*. The main stem bronchi, blood vessels, lymphatics, and nerves that enter or exit the lung all pass through the hilum.

Each lung is divided into two or three **lobes** (see Figure 8-28), which are separated by one or more **fissures.** The right lung has upper, middle, and lower lobes. The left lung has only an upper and a lower lobe. Both lungs have an oblique fissure that begins on the anterior chest at approximately the sixth rib at the midclavicular line. These fissures extend laterally and upward until they cross the fifth rib on the lateral chest in the midaxillary line. The fissures continue to the posterior chest to approximately the third thoracic vertebra. The right lung also has a horizontal or "minor" fissure that separates the upper and middle lobes. This horizontal fissure extends from the fourth rib at the sternal border to the fifth rib at the midaxillary line.

The lungs are elastic organs that can expand when inflated with air and recoil back to their resting volume when exhalation occurs. Lung elasticity stems from surface tension forces in the alveoli and from the elastic properties of the tissues and various connective tissue fibers. Three different fiber systems form a scaffold that supports the structure of the lungs as tension develops in them with inflation.[58] The axial system, primarily composed of collagen and reticulin fibers, originates in the hilum and extends outward in all of the airway walls almost all the way to the alveolar region. The septal fiber system, composed of collagen, reticulin, and elastin, supports the alveolar walls and capillaries. The peripheral fiber system, primarily composed of collagen, originates in the outer

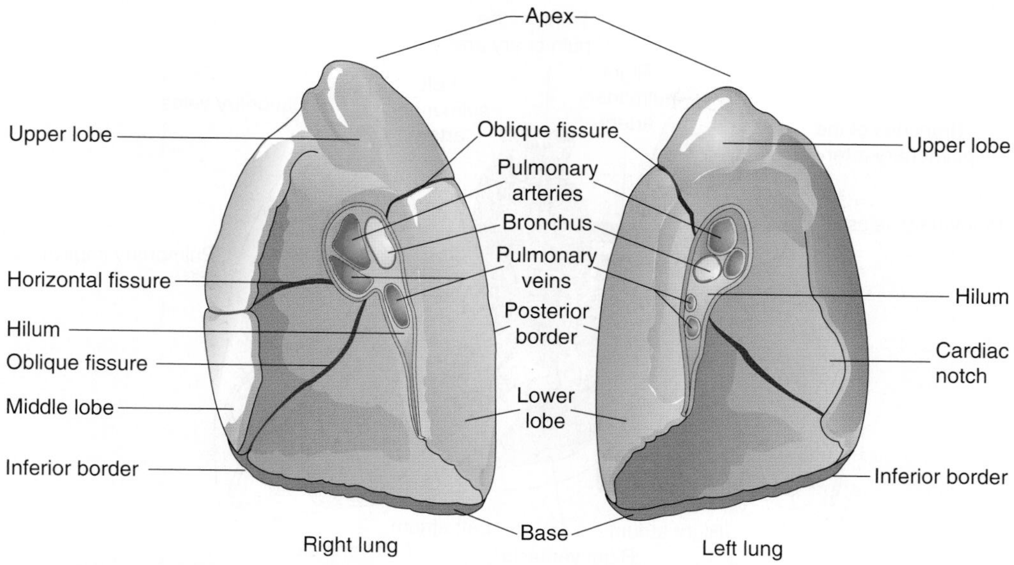

FIGURE 8-29 The medial surfaces of the lungs. (From Hicks GH: Cardiopulmonary anatomy and physiology, Philadelphia, 2000, WB Saunders.)

viscera and extends into the lung tissue to divide up the lung tissue effectively into interlobular regions.

Collectively, these connective tissue fibers function to provide support to the airway walls, lungs, and effective gas exchange membrane as it is stretched during inflation. When a lung is removed from the chest cavity, it quickly collapses to a smaller size. The same occurs if air or fluid enters into the pleural space; it is possible that individual lobes can collapse as the result of airway obstruction and gradual diffusion of air from the lobe. This tendency of the lung to collapse is counteracted by the tendency of the thoracic wall to spring outward and to hold the lung inflated. The "tension" developed by these two opposing tendencies results in the development of subatmospheric intrapleural pressure.

PULMONARY VASCULAR, LYMPHATIC, AND NERVOUS SYSTEMS

The vascular supply of the lungs is composed of the pulmonary and bronchial circulations. The pulmonary circulation carries mixed venous blood from the systemic circuit to the lungs to increase O_2 and reduce CO_2 content of blood. The bronchial circulation provides systemic arterial blood to the airways and pleura to support their metabolic needs. A network of lymphatics is also involved in fluid transport from the lungs. The lymphatic system removes fluid from the lung tissue and pleural space and returns it to the systemic circulation. The nervous system of the lungs acts to sense and modify lung function to help defend and improve its function.

Pulmonary Circulation

The pulmonary circulation is supplied with blood from the right heart (Figure 8-30) at a flow rate that is equal to the entire blood volume each minute at rest.[59] O_2-reduced systemic venous blood flows to the right heart via the inferior and superior venae cavae. This blood is pumped to the lungs by the right ventricle through the pulmonic semilunar valve and on to the trunk of the pulmonary artery. The trunk of the pulmonary artery passes upward and divides into right and left pulmonary arteries just below the point of tracheal bifurcation into left and right main stem bronchi (the **carina**). The pulmonary arteries accompany the right and left main stem bronchi through the hilar opening into the lungs and continue to divide along with the airways. The pulmonary arteries divide to form two types of arteries: conventional arteries, which continue to follow the airway branching, and supernumerary arteries, which branch at 90-degree angles from the conventional arteries and travel outside the common path. Supernumerary arteries account for about 25% of the cross-sectional area of the pulmonary arterial system. As the arteries continue to divide and become more numerous, they become smaller in diameter and possess greater smooth muscle in their medial walls. Both sets of arteries form arterioles that connect to and supply blood to the microcirculation of the respiratory zone of the lung.

The pulmonary arterial system continues to divide into increasing numbers all the way to the distal airspaces, where they subdivide and form dense "sheetlike" beds of alveolar capillaries that are located within the walls of the alveoli and just below approximately 90% of the alveolar surface (Figure 8-31). The wall of the pulmonary capillary is formed by endothelial cells. At rest, the pulmonary

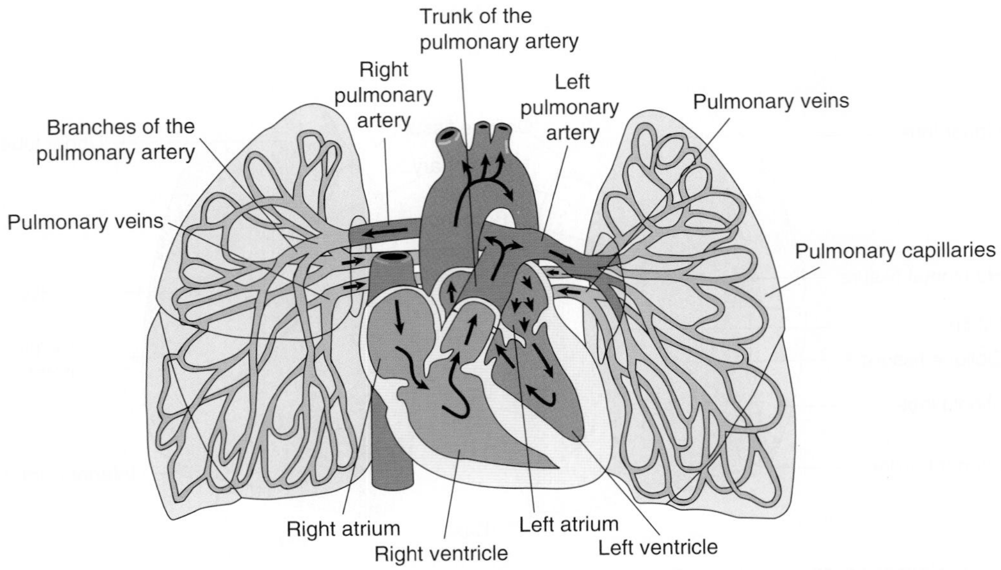

FIGURE 8-30 The pulmonary circulation. (From Hicks GH: Cardiopulmonary anatomy and physiology, Philadelphia, 2000, WB Saunders.)

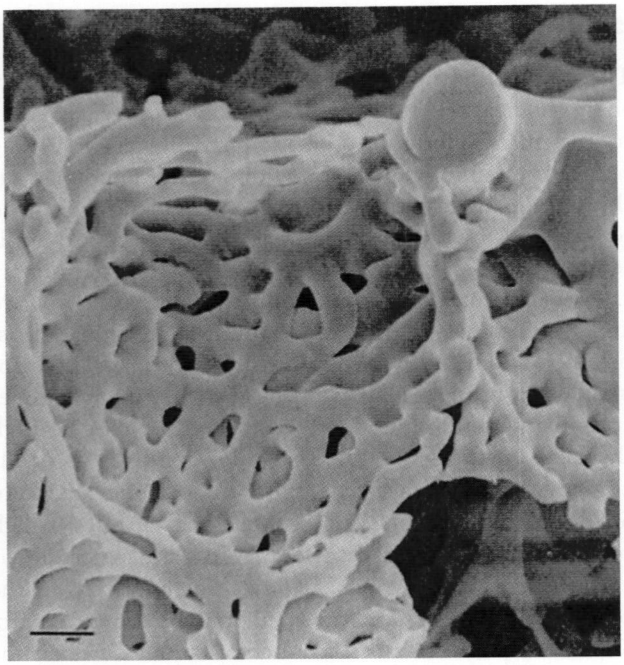

FIGURE 8-31 Scanning electron photomicrograph at high magnification of plastic cast of alveolar capillaries of the pulmonary circulation (black bar, 10 μm). (From Thibodeau GA, Patton KT: Anatomy and physiology, ed 7, St Louis, 2010, Mosby.)

capillary bed contains 60 to 80 ml of blood and can expand to 200 ml through dilation and recruitment of collapsed capillaries during conditions of higher cardiac output (e.g., exercise).[60] Pulmonary blood is collected from the capillaries by the pulmonary venules, which combine into larger veins. Similar to their arterial counterparts, the veins also form conventional and supernumerary types of veins that drain blood from the pulmonary capillary beds. The pulmonary veins possess less smooth muscle in their medial walls and have thinner walls than similar-sized pulmonary arteries. The veins follow the same connective tissue path that houses the bronchi and arteries and coalesce into larger and fewer vessels. Four major pulmonary veins—superior and inferior veins from each lung—exit through the hila and return arterialized blood to the left atrium of the heart for delivery to the systemic circulation (see Figure 8-30).

RULE OF THUMB

The pulmonary artery and its branches are the only arteries in the body to carry deoxygenated blood. Similarly, the pulmonary veins are the only veins that carry oxygenated blood back to the left side of the heart.

Respiratory Function of Pulmonary Circulation

The pulmonary circulation has several different functions.[59] The primary function of the pulmonary circulation is to deliver blood to the alveolar-capillary bed for the exchange of O_2 and CO_2 with alveolar gas and then to deliver it to the left heart. The second function is to serve as a barrier between the interstitial spaces and airspaces of the lung on one side and the blood within the capillaries on the other. Although less than 0.3 μm thick, the endothelial capillary membrane is an active barrier that controls the exchange of fluid and solutes that cross it. In doing so, it plays a crucial role in the regulation of the fluid balance

TABLE 8-6

Resting Hemodynamic Values in Adult Systemic and Pulmonary Vascular Systems

	Systemic Circuit	Pulmonary Circuit
Blood flow (cardiac output, L/min)	5	5
Arterial blood pressure (mm Hg)	120/80	25/10
Vascular resistance (dynes/sec/cm^{-5})	1200	120

within the lungs. Injury to the pulmonary capillary often disrupts the fluid balance and can result in excessive fluid leaks and the formation of pulmonary edema. The third function is nonrespiratory and involves the production, processing, and clearance of a large variety of chemicals and blood clots.

Table 8-6 compares the hemodynamics of the systemic and pulmonary circulatory systems.[61] Although the entire cardiac output passes through both pulmonary and systemic circuits, the pulmonary circulation offers much lower resistance and consequently has a much lower blood pressure. The low vascular pressures within the pulmonary circuit are essential in maintenance of fluid balance at the alveolar-capillary interface. The pulmonary capillaries are exposed to vascular pressures of about 7 to 10 mm Hg. Increased pressure in the pulmonary circulation, which can occur with mitral valve disease or congestive heart failure, can disrupt fluid balance and lead to excessive fluid leakage, fluid accumulation, and alveolar congestion, which can impair gas exchange and lead to hypoxia.

The low vascular pressures of the pulmonary circulation result in regional blood flow within the lungs that is highly influenced by gravity, airway pressure, and gas exchange.[59] In the upright lung, blood pressure in the pulmonary arteries increases approximately 1 cm H_2O for each 1 cm traversed downward from the apex to the base. As a consequence of having a low blood pressure and being susceptible to gravity, blood flow is much higher in the lung bases in resting upright subjects. Gravity-related effects also occur in recumbent positions but are less pronounced. The distribution of pulmonary blood flow is also closely related to local airway gas pressure and pulmonary gas exchange. Areas that experience higher airway pressure (e.g., during positive pressure ventilation) that equals or exceeds local arteriole and capillary pressure have reduced blood flow as a result of the opposing airway pressure (zone 1 airways). Regions where blood pressure is greater than the surrounding air pressure, such as in the bases of the upright lung during spontaneous breathing, have greater blood flow (zone 3 airways). Areas of regional lung hypoxia, because of reduced ventilation, congestion, or airway obstruction, can result in local pulmonary arterial vasoconstriction and cause blood flow to be shifted from these areas toward areas of higher O_2 content and pulmonary vasodilation.[60]

Nonrespiratory Function of the Pulmonary Circulation

The pulmonary circulation also serves as a blood reservoir for the left ventricle.[59,60] This reservoir maintains stable left ventricular volumes despite small changes in cardiac output. The pulmonary blood volume (approximately 600 ml) is sufficient to maintain normal left ventricle filling for several cardiac cycles. This reservoir is important if filling of the right heart is temporarily decreased or interrupted.

The pulmonary circulation also acts as a filter for the systemic circulation. The capillaries have an inner diameter of about 7 to 10 μm and theoretically trap particles (e.g., blood clots) down to this size before they enter the systemic circulation, where blockages could be life-threatening. Studies in animals have shown, however, that glass beads that are 500 μm in diameter can pass through the pulmonary circulation and probably do so through pulmonary arteriovenous shunts.[62]

The lungs also play an active role in the clearance and activation and release of various biochemical factors.[59,60] They are responsible for synthesis, activation, inactivation, and detoxification of many bioactive substances. Adenosine, norepinephrine, bradykinin, endothelins, atrial natriuretic peptide, and various leukotrienes and certain prostaglandins are removed by the pulmonary circulation. Angiotensin I is converted to its active form (angiotensin II) as it circulates through the lung. Various proinflammatory cytokines are released from the lung when it is injured or repetitively overinflated during mechanical ventilation.[63]

Bronchial Circulation

A separate arterial supply called the *bronchial circulation* supplies blood to the airways from the trachea to the bronchioles and to most of the visceral pleurae.[64] The metabolic needs of the lung are comparatively low, and much of the lung parenchyma is oxygenated by direct contact with inspired gas. The bronchial circulation is a branch of the systemic circuit and is supplied with blood from the aorta via minor thoracic branches. Blood flow through the bronchial circulation constitutes about 1% to 2% of the total cardiac output.

A single right bronchial artery, which supplies the right lung, arises from the upper intercostal artery, the right subclavian artery, or an internal mammary artery. Two bronchial arteries supply the left lung, and they branch directly from the upper thoracic aorta. Bronchial arteries follow their respective bronchi. Two or three branches accompany each subdivision of the conducting airway. The bronchial arterial circulation terminates in a plexus of capillaries that anastomose with the alveolar-capillary bed. Bronchial venous blood drains through the *azygos, hemiazygos,* and *intercostal* veins to the right atrium, and some drains through the pulmonary capillaries to the pulmonary veins and to the right left atrium. Figure 8-32 shows

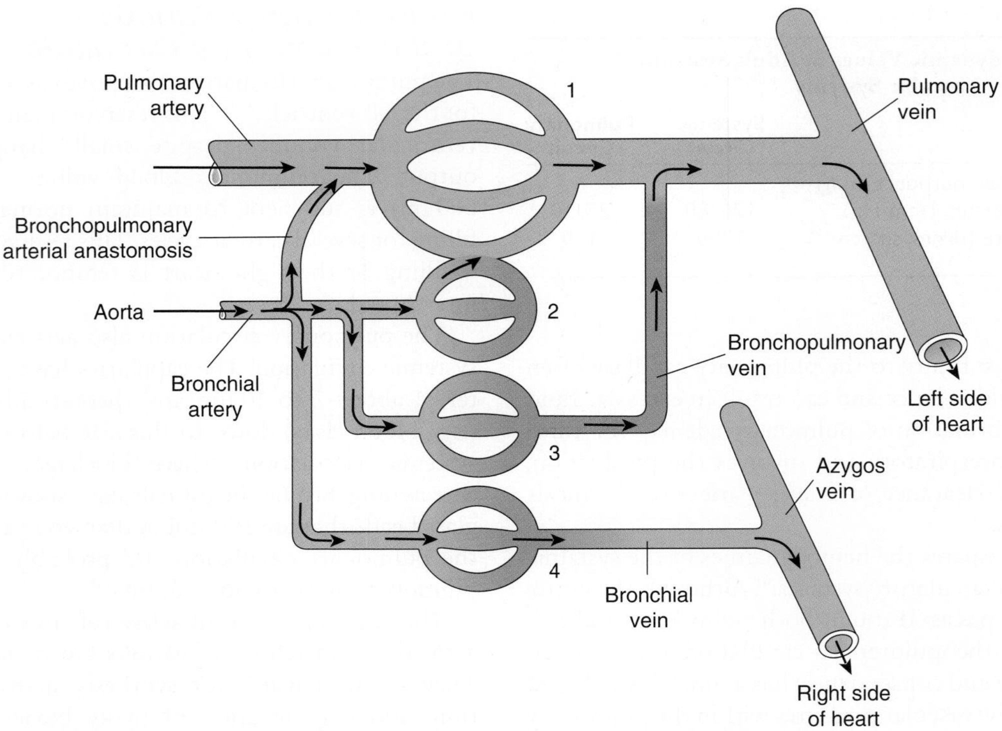

FIGURE 8-32 Schematic depiction of the interconnection of pulmonary and bronchial circulations. Bronchial blood flows to the pulmonary artery *(1),* through the capillary bed of the large airways and pleura and into pulmonary capillaries *(2),* through the bronchopulmonary veins and into the pulmonary veins *(3),* and through the bronchial vein and on to the azygos vein *(4)*. The route through the bronchopulmonary vein allows less oxygenated blood to mix with the better oxygenated blood, which returns to the left side of the heart. (From Hicks GH: Cardiopulmonary anatomy and physiology, Philadelphia, 2000, WB Saunders.)

the interrelationship and comingling of the pulmonary and bronchial circulatory systems.

The bronchial and pulmonary circulations share an important compensatory relationship.[65] Decreased pulmonary arterial blood pressure tends to cause an increase in bronchial artery blood flow to the affected area. This compensation minimizes the danger of pulmonary infarction, as sometimes occurs when a blood clot (pulmonary embolus) enters the lung. Similarly, loss of bronchial circulation can be partially offset by increases in pulmonary arterial perfusion. The adult lung does not require the bronchial circulation to remain viable, as evidenced by the success of lung transplantation, which does not preserve the bronchial circulation. However, this circulation apparently plays a more important role in lung development, helps to preserve gas exchange during various congenital cardiac conditions, and appears to compensate in certain pulmonary diseases (e.g., pulmonary fibrosis) for the gradual obstruction of the pulmonary circulation.

Lymphatics

The lymphatic system of the lungs is an extensive system of lymphatic vessels, lymph nodes, the tonsils, and the thymus gland.[66] The primary function of the lymphatic system is to clear fluid from the interstitial and pleural spaces to help maintain the fluid balance in the lungs. The lymphatic system also plays an important role in the specific defenses of the immune system. It removes bacteria, foreign material, and cell debris via the lymph fluid and through the action of various phagocytic cells (e.g., macrophages) that provide defense against foreign material and cells that are able to penetrate deep into the lung. It also produces various lymphocytes and plasma cells to aid in defense. Both roles are essential for maintaining normal function of the respiratory system.

Most of the pulmonary lymphatic system consists of superficial and deep vessels.[67] The superficial (pleural) vessels that drain the lung surface and pleural space are more numerous over the lower half of the upright lung. Many of these vessels are broad ribbon-like, reservoir-type vessels that are closely associated with the blind lymphatic capillaries. The deep (peribronchovascular) conduit-like vessels contain bicuspid valves to direct flow and travel through the connective tissue tracts that house the larger pulmonary vessels in the deeper lung tissue. Both drain the blind lymphatic capillaries in the respective regions. The deeper lymph vessels are closely associated with the small airways but do not extend into the walls of the alveolar-capillary membranes. The lymphatic vessels are thin-walled vessels that contain little connective and muscle tissue in their walls.

Lymph fluid is collected by the loosely formed lymphatic capillaries and drains through the lymph vessels toward the hilum. The fluid is propelled through the lymphatic system by the collective actions of the valves that direct flow toward the hilum and by the combined milking actions of smooth muscle contractions in the deeper conduit-like vessels and ventilation, which squeezes the lymphatic vessels.[68] Lymph fluid flow from the lungs can be increased after an injury to the pulmonary capillaries that results in increased leakage (e.g., acute respiratory distress syndrome) or from pulmonary capillary hypertension secondary to heart disease (e.g., left-sided heart failure).

The lymph vessels emerge from the hilum of each lung and drain lymph fluid through a series of lymph nodes that are clustered about each hilum and the mediastinum. From there, lymph travels through various inferior, superior tracheobronchial and paratracheal lymph nodes within the mediastinum (Figure 8-33). The lymph fluid rejoins the general circulation after passing through the right lymphatic or thoracic duct, which drains into the jugular, subclavian, or innominate veins. The lymph fluid mixes with blood and returns to the heart.

Lymphatic channels are not usually visible on chest radiographs. They may be detected if they are distended or thickened by disease. The "butterfly" pattern that radiates from the hilar region of both lungs during acute development of pulmonary edema is thought to be largely the result of interstitial and lymph vessel distention with fluid. In this situation, the lymphatic drainage system has been overwhelmed by a sudden and excessive surge of fluid from the circulation. The development of a pleural effusion is also evidence that the lymphatic system is unable to remove excess fluid in the lung.

Nervous Control of the Lungs

All of the major structures of the respiratory system are innervated by branches of the peripheral nervous system: the autonomic and somatic branches (Figure 8-34).[69] The somatic system provides voluntary and automatic motor

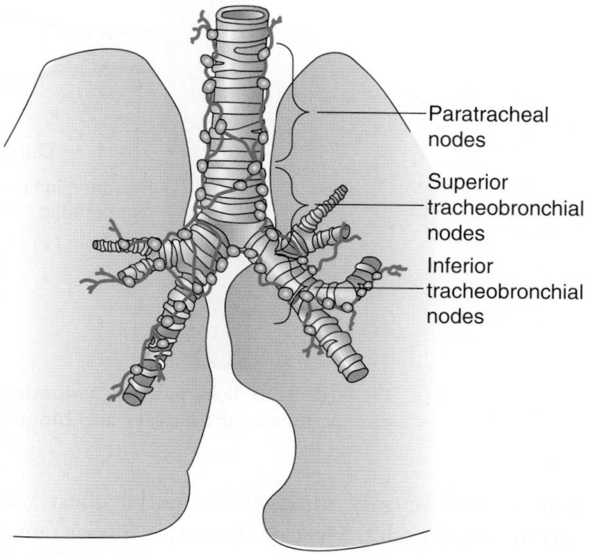

FIGURE 8-33 Mediastinal and paratracheal pulmonary lymph nodes. (From Hicks GH: Cardiopulmonary anatomy and physiology, Philadelphia, 2000, WB Saunders.)

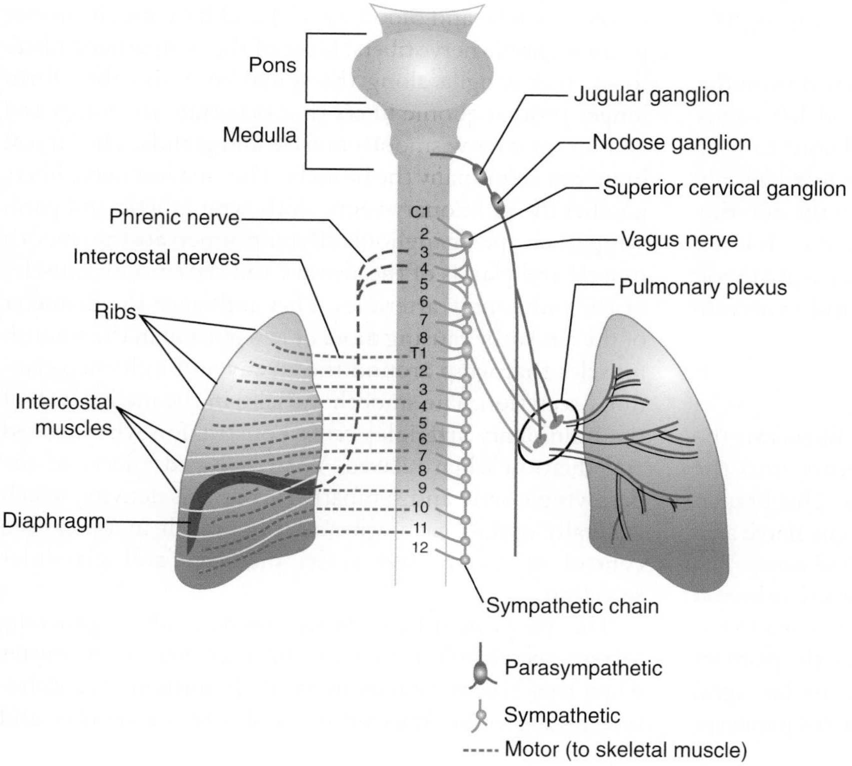

FIGURE 8-34 Schematic of the autonomic innervation (motor and sensory) of the lung and the somatic (motor) nerve supply to the intercostal muscles and diaphragm. (Modified from Murray JF: The normal lung, ed 2, Philadelphia, 1986, WB Saunders.)

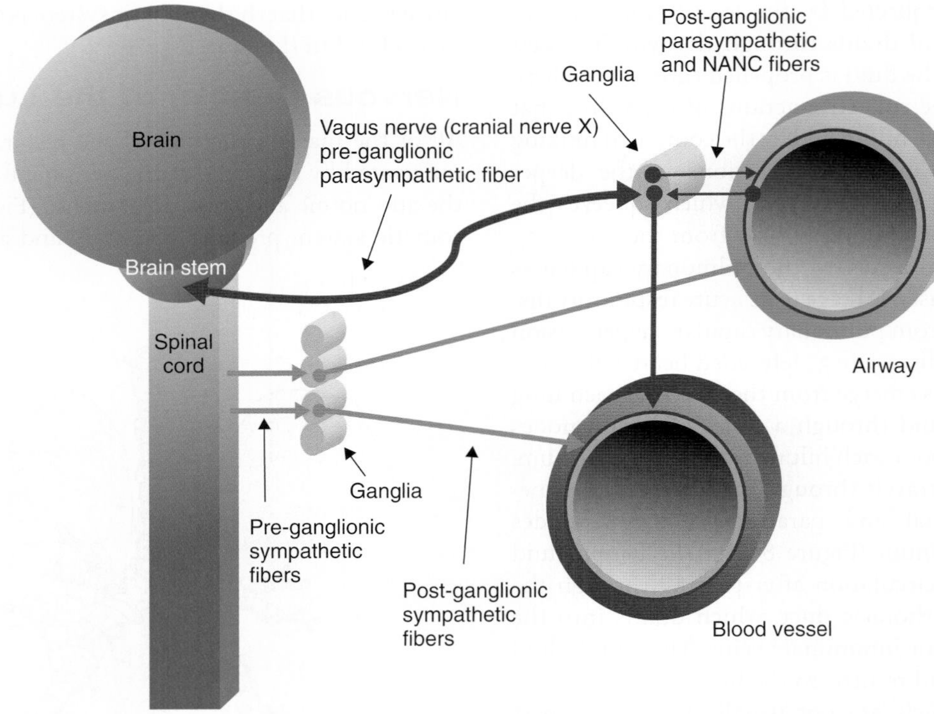

FIGURE 8-35 Schematic of sympathetic, parasympathetic, and NANC neural fiber connections to the airways and blood vessels of the lungs.

control and sensory innervation to the chest wall and respiratory muscles. Most of the major motor nerves that carry nervous signaling to the respiratory muscles are summarized in Tables 8-4 and 8-5. The autonomic nervous system signaling to and from the lungs is carried through efferent and afferent pathways. These pathways carry unconscious autonomic nervous system motor signals to smooth muscles and glands and various sensory signals back to the brain.

Autonomic innervation of the lungs is carried from the brainstem through branches of the right and left vagus nerves (cranial nerve X) and from the spinal cord to four or five thoracic sympathetic ganglia that lie just laterally to the spinal cord.[70] Both contribute fibers to the anterior and posterior pulmonary plexus at the root of each lung. From these plexus, sympathetic and parasympathetic fibers enter the lung through the hilum and innervate various structures.

Efferent Pathways

The parasympathetic nervous preganglionic fibers exit the brainstem via the two vagus nerves. On entry into the chest, the vagus nerve branches to the larynx. This branch is called the *recurrent laryngeal nerve.* Each vagus nerve also develops a branch called the *superior laryngeal nerve.* The external branch of this nerve supplies the cricothyroid muscle. The internal branch provides sensory fibers to the larynx. The recurrent laryngeal nerves provide the primary motor innervation to the larynx. Damage to laryngeal nerves can cause unilateral or bilateral vocal cord paralysis, depending on which branches are involved. Hoarseness, loss of voice, and an ineffective cough may result.

After forming ganglia and postganglionic nerve fibers, parasympathetic and sympathetic nerve fibers enter the lung through the hilum and run parallel to the airways as they branch (Figure 8-35). Parasympathetic fibers form their ganglia much closer to the target tissues (e.g., bronchioles, glands, and blood vessels) and have much shorter postganglionic nerve fibers. Most of the sympathetic fibers form their ganglia along the spinal cord and then form longer postganglionic fibers that penetrate the lungs and end on the airway smooth muscle and glands. The largest branches accompany the bronchi. The smallest nerve fibers parallel the pulmonary veins. Both sympathetic and parasympathetic postganglionic efferents innervate the smooth muscle and glands of the airways and the smooth muscles of the pulmonary arterioles. They influence the diameter of the airway by causing more or less tension in the smooth muscles that wrap around the airway and influence glandular secretion. The smooth muscles in the medial wall of the pulmonary arterioles cause constriction when tensed and dilation when relaxed. The combined effects of the parasympathetic and sympathetic nervous activity, which generally oppose each other's action, result in a balanced control of airway and vessel diameter and glandular secretion.

The parasympathetic postganglionic fibers generally secrete acetylcholine as their primary neurotransmitter when they receive signals from the brainstem. Acetylcholine binds to M_3 muscarinic cholinergic receptors and causes airway smooth muscle constriction, blood vessel dilation, and glandular secretion. The sympathetic postganglionic fibers are much less developed in comparison. The sympathetic postganglionic fibers in the lung primarily secrete norepinephrine, and the adrenal glands release epinephrine into the circulation when they receive sympathetic signals from the spinal cord. Epinephrine and norepinephrine bind to alpha-adrenergic receptors of blood vessels to cause constriction and to beta-adrenergic receptors of the bronchial airway and vessel smooth muscles to cause relaxation and dilation of the airways and blood vessels.

The airways are provided with a third autonomic pathway that is neither parasympathetic nor sympathetic in action.[58] The nonadrenergic, noncholinergic (NANC) system nerve fibers travel within the vagus nerve to each lung. When active, the NANC nerve endings release a neurotransmitter that promotes the production of nitric oxide, which causes the relaxation of airway smooth muscle and dilation. The NANC system is also thought to be capable of causing bronchoconstriction through the local reflex release of substance P and neurokinin A.

Afferent Pathways

Most afferent fibers follow pathways from the lungs to the central nervous system in the vagus nerve. The vagus afferent pathways are activated by a variety of different receptors within the lung that are sensitive to inflation, deflation, and chemical stimulation.[71] Slow adapting stretch receptors (SARs) are concentrated in the small and medium-sized airways and are closely associated with the airway smooth muscle. Lung inflation and airway stretch stimulate the SARs, and they continue to signal and do not adapt and drop their signaling rate—hence their name. In the mucosal layer of the airway, rapid adapting receptors (RARs) sense changes in tidal volume, respiratory rate, and changes in lung compliance and respond to a wide variety of mechanical and chemical irritants. In addition, a variety of other chemical and congestion sensors, when active, seem to modify the sensation of breathing and modify the breathing pattern (e.g., cough reflex and response to alveolar congestion). Additional receptors are located outside the lungs; they include respiratory muscle proprioceptors that sense the stretch state of the muscles and peripheral chemoreceptors that sense the chemical condition of blood (e.g., O_2, CO_2, and H^+ concentration) that are involved in the control of ventilation.

Pulmonary stretch SARs and RARs progressively discharge during lung inflation and are linked to inhibition of further inflation. This is a type of negative feedback known as the *inflation reflex*. It was originally described by Hering and Breuer and continues to bear their names. The inflation reflex is thought to be actively involved with controlling the depth of breathing. Studies in animals indicate that these receptors influence the duration of the expiratory pause between breaths. The inflation reflex is probably very weak or absent during quiet breathing in healthy adults, but there appears to be evidence of its activity in newborns.[72]

Another reflex that is associated with SAR and RAR activity is the Head paradoxical reflex.[73] This reflex stimulates a deeper breath rather than inhibiting further inspiration. It may be the basis for occasional deep breaths or gasps. Deep breaths or sighs occur with normal breathing, presumably preventing alveolar collapse. Head reflex may also be responsible for gasping in newborn infants as they progressively inflate their lungs.

Irritant or mechanical RARs are found mainly in the posterior wall of the trachea and at bifurcations of the larger bronchi. These receptors respond to various mechanical, chemical, and physiologic stimuli and behave as irritant receptors. The stimuli include physical manipulation or irritation, inhalation of noxious gases, histamine-induced bronchoconstriction, asphyxia, and microembolization of the pulmonary arteries. Stimulation of the irritant RARs can result in bronchoconstriction, hyperpnea, glottic closure, cough, and sneeze.[74] Stimulation of these receptors can also cause a reflex slowing of the heart rate (bradycardia). This response is referred to as the vagovagal reflex. It may occur during tracheobronchial suctioning, intubation of the airway, or bronchoscopy. These procedures can cause significant mechanical irritation of the airway.

Unmyelinated slow-conducting *C-fiber endings* (also known as *juxtacapillary* or *J receptors*), which are present in the walls of the bronchial and terminal airway region, have been linked to a breathing reflex pattern associated with mechanical stretch, pulmonary congestion, and exposure to various chemicals (e.g., capsaicin, phenylbiguanide, CO_2, and autacoids).[75,76] When C-fibers become activated, signals are sent back to the brainstem via the vagus nerve. Rapid, shallow breathing results. C-fiber activation has also been shown to cause bradycardia, hypotension, bronchoconstriction, mucus production, and apnea in experimental animals.[77] Stimulation of these receptors may contribute to the sensation of dyspnea and, in severe cases, the vagovagal reflex, which can complicate pulmonary edema, pulmonary embolism, and pneumonia.

ANATOMY OF THE RESPIRATORY TRACT

Upper Respiratory Tract

The *upper respiratory tract* is defined as the airways that start at the nose and mouth and extend down to the trachea (Figure 8-36).[78,79] The upper airway is open to the outside environment through the external nares or nostrils of the nose and the mouth of the oral cavity. Most of the air moved through the respiratory tract during resting breathing enters through the nares and nasal cavity. Mouth breathing is used during exercise to reduce the resistance

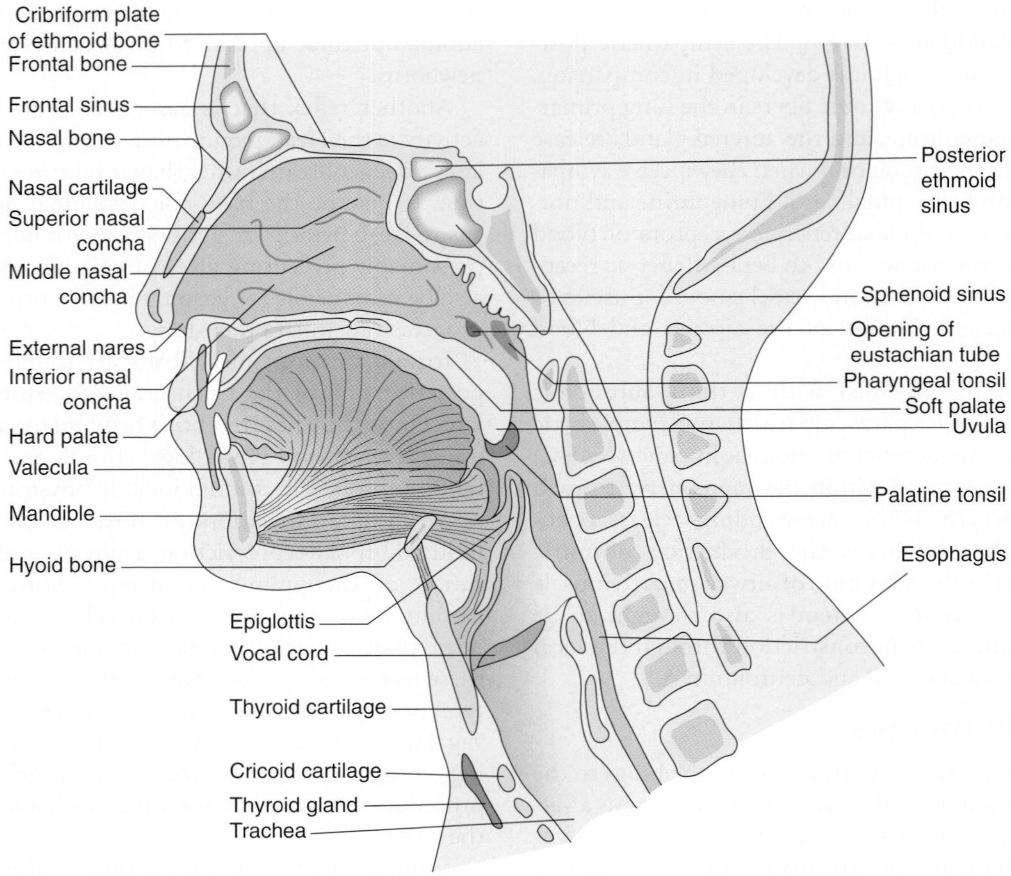

FIGURE 8-36 Midsagittal section through the upper airway. (From Hicks GH: Cardiopulmonary anatomy and physiology, Philadelphia, 2000, WB Saunders.)

Box 8-1 Functions of the Upper Airway

- Passageway for gas flow
- Filter
- Heater
- Humidification
- Sense of smell and taste
- Phonation
- Protection of the lower airways

to gas flow at higher ventilation rates. The functions of the upper airway are summarized in Box 8-1.

Nasal Cavity and Sinuses

There are two flared openings called **alae** that form the **external nares.** The alae enclose a space on each side called the *vestibule.* The vestibules have hairs that act as a gross filter. Located posterior to the vestibules are the openings to the internal nose, or the **anterior nares.** The left and right nasal cavities are formed by cartilage and numerous skull bones. The roof is formed by the nasal, frontal, sphenoid, and ethmoid bones. The septum separating the two cavities is formed by cartilage and the ethmoid and vomer bones. The lateral walls are created by the maxilla, lacrimal, and palatine bones. The floor of the cavity, or **palate,** is primarily formed by the maxilla. Three shelflike bones protrude into the cavity from the lateral walls. These bony shelves are called the superior, middle, and inferior *conchae,* or **turbinates.**

The conchae function to increase the surface area and complexity of the nasal cavity, enabling the nasal cavity to work as a passageway, filter, humidifier, and heater of inhaled airway. The posterior openings of the nasal cavity are called the *internal nares* and are formed in part by the flexible soft palate.

The surface of the nasal cavity is covered with epithelia. The anterior portion is covered with stratified squamous cells and possesses hair follicles and hair. This is the same type of tissue that forms the epidermis of skin. The middle portion of the cavity is covered with a mucous membrane that is composed of ciliated **pseudostratified epithelia** and goblet cells. The mucous membrane functions to secrete mucus, to humidify inhaled air, and to trap inhaled particles. Just below the mucous membrane is an extensive network of veins that form a venous plexus. These vessels supply water and heat to the gas within the nasal cavity. Inflammation of this mucous membrane is brought on by irritation or infection. This is produced by vasodilation and increased vessel leakage. The consequence of nasal cavity inflammation is partial or complete blockage of the air passage. The vessels of the venous plexus can rupture as a result of breathing dry air or the passage of foreign bodies through the nose. Rupture of these vessels can cause considerable nasal bleeding. The posterior portion of the nasal cavity is covered with stratified squamous epithelium similar to the tissue covering of the nearby oral cavity.

Within the skull bones and around the nasal cavity are the *sinuses* (Figure 8-37). These hollow spaces are named for the bones in which they are found.[80] The sinuses are lined with a mucous membrane and drain into the nasal cavity through numerous ducts. They function to reduce the weight of the skull, to strengthen the skull, and to modify the voice during phonation.

The nasal cavity functions to conduct air to and from the respiratory tract, to condition inhaled gas, to act as a region to which sinus and eye fluid drain, and to contain olfactory sensors for the sensation of smell. Conditioning inhaled gas helps to defend the respiratory tract and involves filtering, heating, and humidifying air. Filtration of inhaled air is carried out by the hair in the anterior portion of the cavity and the sticky mucous membrane that covers the complex surface of the cavity. Filtration is enhanced by the flow pattern through the nasal cavity. Inspired gas is accelerated to a high velocity through the anterior nares. It changes direction sharply as it enters the internal nasal cavity. This pattern causes particles larger than 10 μm in diameter to have an impact on the nasal mucosa. Ciliary action or nose blowing clears these particles. Past the external nares, the cross-sectional area increases; this results in a decrease in gas velocity. Turbulence increases because of the narrow convolutions of the passages. Low velocity and turbulence combine to remove any remaining particles. Filtration is based on impaction, sedimentation, and diffusion of various sized particles.

Surface fluids originate from the goblet cells and submucosal glands. This fluid lining has mild antibacterial properties. Mucosal fluids also remove water-soluble irritant gases such as sulfur dioxide. Ciliary activity in the nasal mucous membranes helps to transport the mucus produced so that it can be cleared. Foreign matter is typically cleared from the nasal cavity by sniffing and swallowing. During exhalation, the heated and moist expired air passes over the concha and is cooled, and the excess moisture deposits on the concha as condensation to help retain and recycle water. These defense and conditioning mechanisms help to ensure that inspired air is free from particulate and bacterial contamination and that it is heated and humidified to 37° C and 100% relative humidity by the time it reaches the trachea. In addition, the mucous membrane contains chemoreceptors that send signals to the olfactory nerve for the sensation of smell in the superior portion of the cavity just above each of the superior conchae.

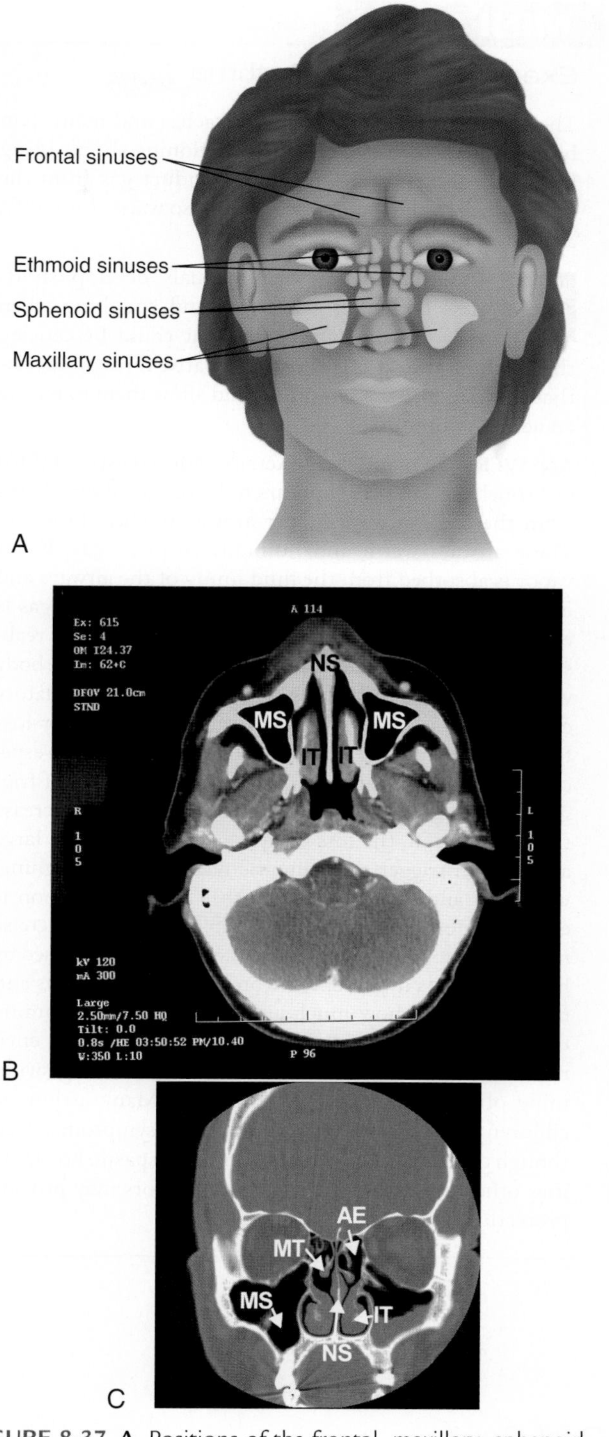

FIGURE 8-37 **A,** Positions of the frontal, maxillary, sphenoid, and ethmoid sinuses; the nasal sinuses are named for the bones in which they occur. **B,** Axial computed tomography (CT) scan at the approximate level of the inferior turbinates (IT) and maxillary sinuses (MS). The nasal septum (NS) is also well defined. **C,** Coronal CT scan showing the anterior ethmoid sinuses (AE) and the middle turbinates (MT) in addition to the structures seen in **B.**

MINI CLINI

Exercise-Induced Asthma

The upper airway, along with the trachea and main stem bronchi, plays a crucial role in conditioning the air being breathed. These airways not only conduct gas from the atmosphere to the lower airways but also warm, humidify, and filter it.

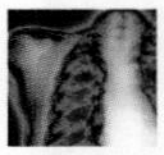

PROBLEM: Some individuals develop shortness of breath, wheezing, and coughing when they exercise outdoors. What could be causing their asthma attack? Is there an alternative form of exercise that could reduce the symptoms and allow them to receive an aerobic workout?

ANSWER: In many cases, exercise-induced asthma (EIA) or bronchospasm (EIB) appears to be triggered by reflexes from the large airways (upper airway, trachea, bronchi). These airways warm and humidify inspired gas. Water vapor is absorbed from the fluid lining of the airways and is replenished from the cells lining the airways. As gas is expired, it cools, and some of the water vapor is reabsorbed. Only a small amount of water is lost from the body via this mechanism. Exercise (with its increased ventilatory demands) causes an increase in the heat and water loss from the airways. The airways in some individuals are especially sensitive (hyperresponsive) to a wide variety of triggering agents. When these individuals exercise and increase their ventilation, the loss of heat or water from the large airways can trigger an asthmatic reaction (i.e., coughing, wheezing, and shortness of breath). The phenomenon is especially noticeable when susceptible individuals exercise in cold, dry conditions. Asthma is sometimes diagnosed by having patients hyperventilate breathing cold, dry gas and then measuring how much airflow decreases. Swimming usually involves exercise in a warm, high-humidity environment. The preconditioned air breathed during swimming often reduces or eliminates EIB. Many asthmatic children can swim vigorously with few symptoms, even though other sports trigger their bronchospasm. For activities other than swimming, bronchodilators may provide protection from EIB.

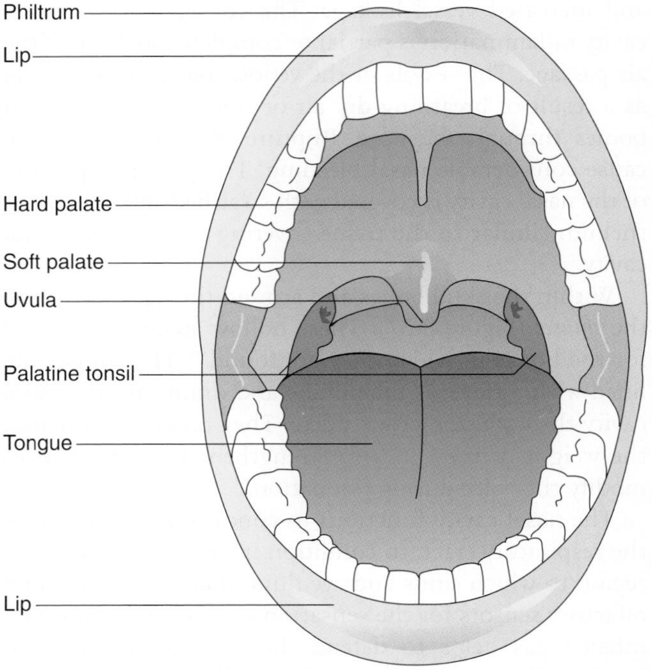

FIGURE 8-38 Frontal view into the open mouth showing the major structures within. (From Hicks GH: Cardiopulmonary anatomy and physiology, Philadelphia, 2000, WB Saunders.)

Oral Cavity

Air can also enter and exit from the respiratory tract through the oral cavity (Figure 8-38). The anterior roof of the oral cavity is called the *hard palate* and is formed by the maxillary bone. The posterior portion is known as the **soft palate** because of its soft tissue composition and ability to move upward to seal off the nasal cavity. The end of the soft palate hangs down into the posterior portion of the oral cavity. This part of the soft palate is called the **uvula.** The walls of the oral cavity are formed by the cheeks, and the floor is dominated by the tongue.

The uvula and the surrounding walls control the flow of air and fluid and food during eating, drinking, sneezing, coughing, and vomiting. The tongue is involved in mechanical digestion, taste, and phonation. The posterior surface of the tongue is supplied with many sensory nerve endings. These nerves produce a vagal gag reflex when stimulated, which protects the lungs from aspiration. This reflex must be considered when passing tubes or instruments through the mouth in conscious or semiconscious patients. The lingual tonsils are located at the base of the tongue.

The mucosal surfaces of the oral cavity also provide humidification and warming of inspired air. These surfaces are much less efficient than the nose. Saliva is produced by major and minor salivary glands. Saliva functions primarily as a wetting and digestive agent for food but provides some humidification of inspired gas. The oral cavity ends at a double web on each side, called the *palatine folds.* The palatine tonsils sit between these folds on each side (see Figure 8-38). The palatine tonsils are vascularized lymphoidal tissues that play an immunologic role, especially in childhood.

Reflexes of the mouth, pharynx, and larynx help to protect the lower respiratory tract during swallowing.[81] These protective functions can be severely compromised during anesthesia or unconsciousness. Loss or compromise of these important reflexes can result in aspiration of bacteria-colonized saliva or food and can cause pulmonary infection and asphyxiation in severe cases.

Pharynx

The posterior portion of the nasal and oral cavities opens into a region called the **pharynx.** The entire pharynx is lined with stratified squamous epithelium. The pharynx is subdivided into the **nasopharynx, oropharynx,** and **hypopharynx,** or **laryngopharynx.** The nasopharynx lies at the posterior end of the nasal cavity and extends to the tip of the uvula. Numerous foreign particles impact the surface of the nasopharynx. Located in this region are the two pharyngeal tonsils (also called the *adenoids*) that are on either side of the lateral and posterior walls of the pharynx. They function to monitor and interact with the particles inhaled through the actions of the lymphoid cells located here. In the same region, there are two openings into the left and right **eustachian tubes** that link the upper airway with the middle ear (see Figure 8-36). The eustachian tubes drain fluid out of the middle ear and allow gas to move in or out of the middle to equalize pressure on either side of the tympanic membrane.

The oropharynx is located in the posterior region of the oral cavity that spans the space between the uvula and the upper rim of the epiglottis. This region is also equipped with a pair of palatine tonsils that are located on the lateral walls of the oropharynx. These tonsils can become chronically swollen and cause partial airway obstruction. If the swelling is excessive and the individual has numerous repeat throat and ear infections, these tonsils can be removed by the surgical procedure known as a *tonsillectomy.*

The region below the oropharynx is known as the *hypopharynx.* It extends from the upper rim of the epiglottis to the opening between the vocal cords. The tissues of the nasopharynx and hypopharynx can move and undergo large changes of shape during speech and swallowing. Immediately below the hypopharynx, the digestive and respiratory tracts separate.

During unconsciousness, the muscles of the tongue and hypopharynx can relax and allow the tongue and other soft tissues to collapse and occlude the opening of the hypopharynx. This condition can result in partial to complete blockage of the upper airway and limit air movement to and from the respiratory tract. This condition is a primary cause of obstructive sleep apnea.

Larynx

The **larynx** lies below the hypopharynx and is formed by a complex arrangement of nine cartilages and numerous muscles (Figure 8-39).[82] Generally, it functions to protect the respiratory tract during eating and drinking and in phonation. The *thyroid cartilage* forms most of the upper portion of the larynx and is generally referred to as the *Adam's apple.* This cartilage is named for the thyroid gland that lies over its outer surface. Just below the thyroid cartilage is the *cricoid cartilage,* which is the only laryngeal structure that forms a complete ring of cartilage around the airway and is the most narrow region of the upper airway in infants. A membrane of connective tissue called the *cricothyroid ligament* spans the space between the thyroid and cricoid cartilage. This membrane is occasionally used as the location for placement of an emergency prosthetic airway in patients who have a life-threatening blockage of the upper airway.

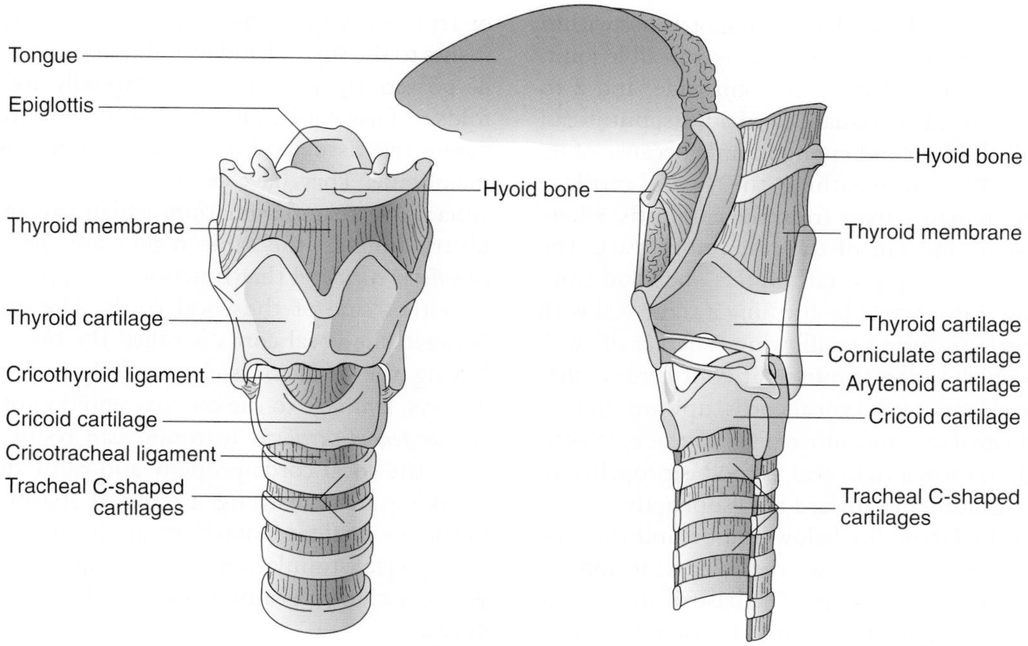

FIGURE 8-39 Anterior and lateral views of the larynx. (From Hicks GH: Cardiopulmonary anatomy and physiology, Philadelphia, 2000, WB Saunders.)

MINI CLINI

Snoring and Sleep Apnea

The upper airway in adults and children primarily functions as an open pathway to convey gas to and from the respiratory zone for gas exchange. The position, size, and shape of the upper airway also contribute to "protect" the lower airways.

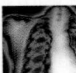

PROBLEM: Can abnormalities of upper airway anatomy lead to obstructive sleep apnea (OSA) and to sleep disturbances, chronic fatigue, and hypertension?

ANSWER: Snoring and breath holding during sleep are often associated with OSA. Snorers usually exhibit narrowing of the oropharyngeal, retropalatal, or hypopharyngeal airways. This narrowing is often observed in obese people; people with short, thick necks; people with large tongues and soft palates; and people with small, receding jaws (micrognathia). During sleep, the upper airway muscles relax, and the tissues of the upper airway can partially or completely obstruct the airway. Airway obstruction can lead to apnea, the development of hypoxia, gasping, and arousal after 10 to 20 seconds, and this cycle can be repeated multiple times to the point of disturbing the quality and quantity of sleep and inducing stress-related hypertension. Sleep studies can document partial and complete airflow obstruction. Management of OSA includes weight loss (to reduce anatomic narrowing of the airway), nasal continuous positive airway pressure to hold open the airway, surgical correction (uvulopalatopharyngoplasty) to remove obstructing tissue, and oral appliances that modify the shape of the oropharynx.

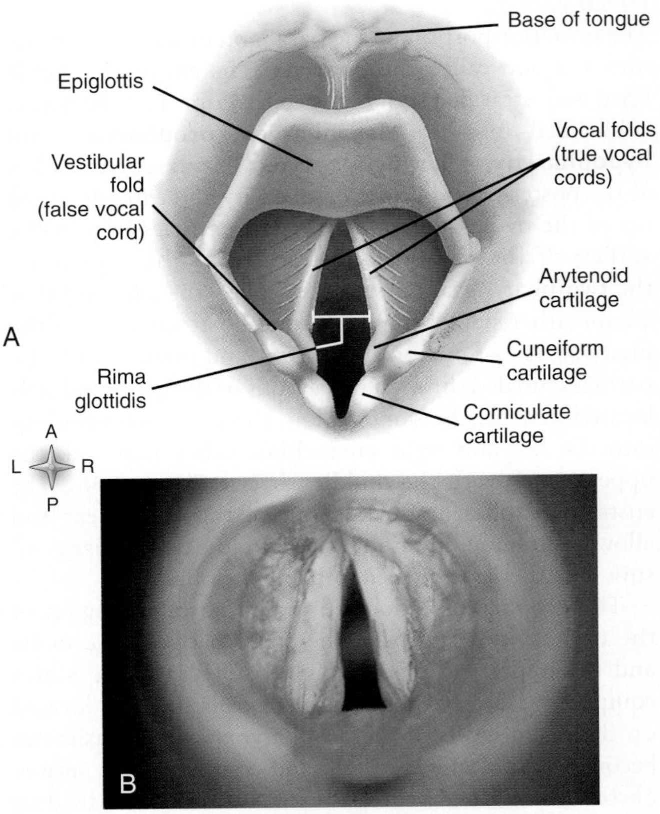

FIGURE 8-40 **A,** Superior view of true vocal cords, glottis (rima glottidis), epiglottis, and other structures within the larynx. **B,** Endoscopic photograph showing vocal cords in the open position. (From Thibodeau GA, Patton KT: Anatomy and physiology, ed 7, St Louis, 2011, Mosby.)

The cartilaginous and leaf-shaped epiglottis lies within and is attached to the thyroid cartilage by a flexible joint. In adults, it is 2 to 4 cm long, 2 to 3 cm wide, and 2 to 5 mm deep. It is not easily visualized in adults, but it can be seen in small children and crying infants because of its higher position. While air breathing, the thyroid cartilage slides down and remains apart from the epiglottis, allowing air to move in and out of the respiratory tract. The *epiglottis* functions to help prevent liquids and food from entering the respiratory tract by forming a tight seal with the thyroid cartilage during swallowing. The act of swallowing is a complex series of muscular contractions that results in early closure of the vocal cords, upward motion of the thyroid cartilage, and movement of the epiglottis down and back to form a tight seal as food is propelled to the back of the mouth and toward the esophagus.[82,83]

The inlet to the larynx lies below and behind the base of the tongue. Figure 8-40 shows the inlet as it appears when viewed with a laryngoscope. The base of the tongue is attached to the epiglottis by three folds. These folds form a space between the tongue and the epiglottis called the **vallecula,** which is a key landmark in oral intubation (see Figure 8-36).

Within the thyroid cartilage and just above the cricoid cartilage are the arytenoid cartilages. The vocal ligaments or true cords span the opening in the larynx by attachments to the thyroid and movable arytenoid cartilages that lie posteriorly. Just above and laterally are the vestibular folds or false cords. The true vocal cords are composed of connective tissue and muscle and covered with a mucous membrane. They have poor lymphatic drainage and are susceptible to inflammation, which can result in airway obstruction. In the same region are the *corniculate* and *cuneiform cartilages* that function to support the soft tissue on either side of the vocal cords. The opening formed between the vocal cords is called the *glottis.* During swallowing, the vocal cords close to help to protect the lower airways. Damage to the cricoarytenoid joint, which allows the *arytenoid cartilages* to rotate, can result in inability to open the vocal cords properly and cause difficulties with speaking and breathing. Laryngeal spasm and resultant partial or total temporary airway closure is brought about by laryngeal stimulation and reflex spasm of various laryngeal muscles that cause closure of the false and true vocal cords.

The muscles of the larynx are innervated by the *inferior laryngeal nerve,* which is also called the *recurrent laryngeal nerve.* It is a motor nerve that branches from the vagus nerve. Impulses carried by this nerve are important in phonation and swallowing. Injuries to this nerve can cause partial or complete paralysis of the vocal cords and inability to swallow correctly. This nerve injury results in difficulty with speech and in severe cases can cause airway obstruction as a result of vocal cord closure.

Speech. The laryngeal component of speech is called *phonation*. It requires the adjustment of vocal cord tension and position relative to one another.[84] The action of the posterior cricoarytenoid muscles causes the arytenoid cartilages to rotate and opens the vocal cords. Closure of the vocal cords is accomplished by rotating the arytenoids in the opposite direction through the action of the lateral cricoarytenoid and oblique arytenoid muscles. On closure of the vocal cords, the expiratory muscles of breathing (e.g., abdominal wall muscle group) compress the thoracic cavity and can increase intrapulmonary pressures to 35 cm H_2O during forceful speech. To form sound, the cricothyroid muscles tilt the cricoid and arytenoid cartilages posteriorly with respect to the thyroid cartilage, and this elongates and tenses the vocal cords. Simultaneously, this action is opposed by the thyroarytenoid muscles, which act to pull the arytenoid cartilages anteriorly and relax vocal cord tension. Release of pressurized airflow through the tensed vocal cords causes vocal cord vibration and the production of audible sound waves, which resonate in the upper airway and sinuses. By careful adjustment of thyroarytenoid muscle tension and mandible and tongue position, fine control over sound production is achieved. Swelling of the vocal cords or the adjacent tissues increases their mass and disturbs their ability to vibrate; this can result in hoarseness and the inability to phonate.

Breath Hold, Effort Closure, and Cough. Tight closure of the larynx and the buildup of intrapulmonary pressure through muscular effort are called *effort closure*. Effort closure of the larynx is necessary to generate loud sounds and for effective coughing and sneezing. It is generated by closure of the false and true vocal cords of the larynx. The vocal cords are closed by the action of the cricothyroid, aryepiglottic, and arytenoid muscles. This action effectively "clamps" the airway closed and enables the intraairway pressures to climb to greater than 100 cm H_2O when the various expiratory muscles compress the thorax. Sudden opening of the larynx results in the immediate release of high-flow gas that is necessary for coughing and sneezing. Patients who have artificial airways have difficulty producing an effective cough because the artificial airway prevents closure of the larynx.

Patent Upper Airway

The relative positions of the oral cavity, pharynx, and larynx are crucial to the patency of the upper airway in unconscious patients. In upright subjects, the head and neck form a 90-degree angle with the axis of the pharynx and larynx (Figure 8-41, *B*). With loss of consciousness, the head flexes forward and decreases this angle (see Figure 8-41, *A*). This positional change can partially or completely obstruct the upper airway. Extension of the head and lower jaw into the "sniff" position alleviates this obstruction (see Figure 8-41, *C*). Extension of the head moves the tongue away from the rear of the pharynx. This technique is used to maintain the airway in unconscious patients and facilitates placement of artificial airways.

Lower Respiratory Tract

The airways of the tracheobronchial tree extend from the larynx down to the airways that participate in gas exchange. Types of airways and their dimensions are summarized in Table 8-7. Each branching of an airway produces subsequent generations of smaller airways. The first 15 generations are known as *conducting airways* because they function to convey gas from the upper airway to the structures that participate in gas exchange with blood. The microscopic airways beyond the conducting airways that carry out gas exchange with blood are classified as the *respiratory airways*.

Trachea and Bronchi

The **trachea** extends from its connection to the cricoid cartilage down through the neck and into the thorax to the articulation point between the manubrium and body of the sternum (angle of Louis). At this point, it divides into two main stem bronchi (Figure 8-42). The adult trachea is approximately 12 cm long and has an inner diameter of about 2 cm. Figure 8-43 shows the different layers of tissue that form the trachea. The outermost layer is a thin connective tissue sheath. Below the sheath are numerous C-shaped cartilaginous rings that provide support and maintain the trachea as an open tube. The typical adult trachea has 16 to 20 of these rings. The inner surface of the trachea is covered with a mucous membrane. In the posterior wall of the trachea is a thin band of tissue, called the *trachealis muscle,* that supports the open ends of the tracheal rings. The esophagus lies just behind the trachea.

The trachea moves normally. The cartilaginous rings armor the trachea so that it does not collapse during exhalation. Some compression occurs when the pressure around the trachea becomes positive. During a strong cough, the trachea is capable of some compression and even collapse. The negative pressure generated around the trachea during inhalation causes it to expand and lengthen slightly.

The trachea lies midline in the upper mediastinum and branches into right and left main stem bronchi (see Figure 8-42). At the base of the trachea, the last cartilaginous ring that forms the bifurcation for the two bronchi is called the *carina*. The carina is an important landmark that is used to identify the level where the two main stem bronchi branch off from the trachea; this is normally at the base of the aortic arch. The right bronchus branches off from the trachea at an angle of about 20 to 30 degrees, and the left bronchus branches with an angle of about 45 to 55 degrees (Figure 8-44). The lower angle of branching of the right bronchus results in a greater frequency of foreign body passage into the right lung because of the more direct pathway.

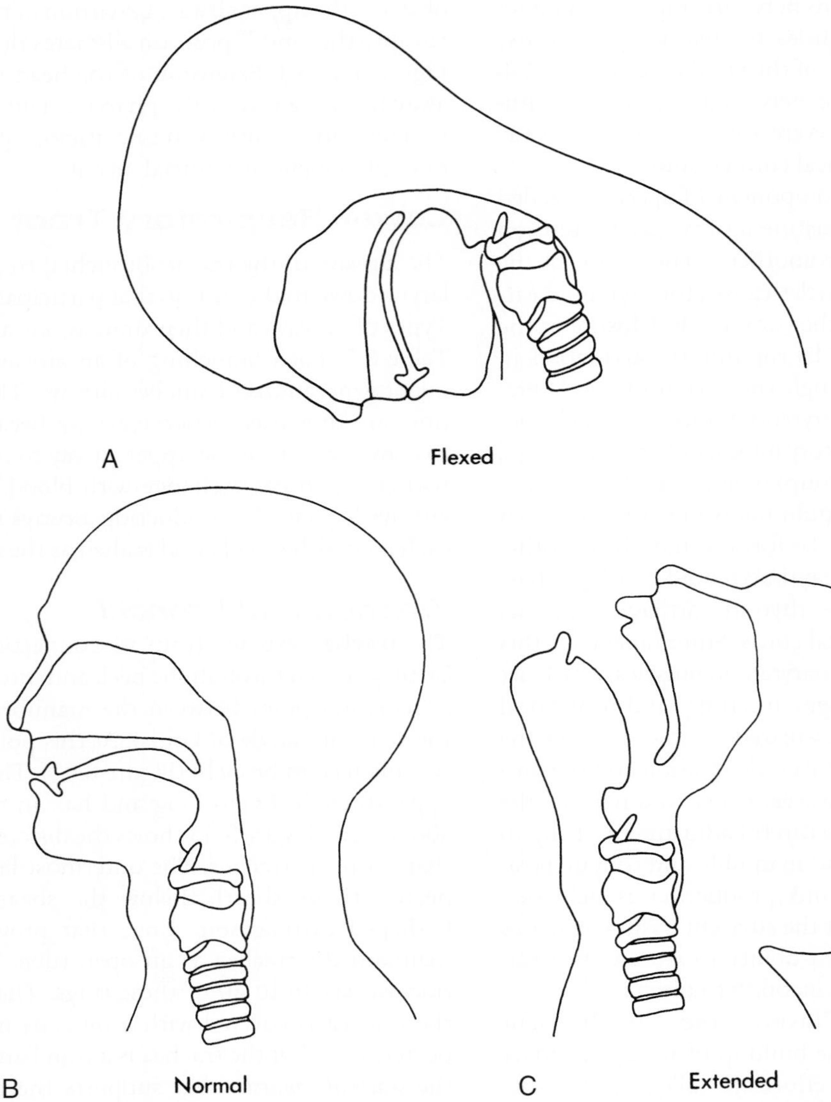

FIGURE 8-41 The position of the head affects patency of airway. **A,** With the head flexed, the airway may be kinked, making breathing or intubation difficult. **B,** Normal upright relationship of the head and neck to the chest. **C,** Extension of the head straightens the airway, making breathing, clearance of material, or intubation easier.

MINI CLINI

Only Ventilating the Right Lung

The placement of an endotracheal tube through the upper airway and into the trachea is a common airway management technique to facilitate mechanical ventilation.

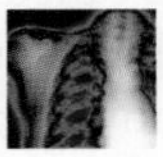

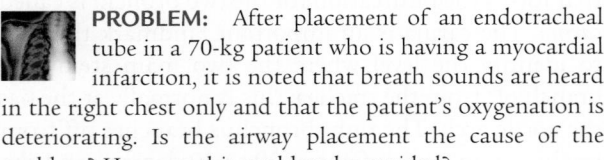

PROBLEM: After placement of an endotracheal tube in a 70-kg patient who is having a myocardial infarction, it is noted that breath sounds are heard in the right chest only and that the patient's oxygenation is deteriorating. Is the airway placement the cause of the problem? How can this problem be avoided?

ANSWER: Ideally, an endotracheal tube of proper diameter should be placed in the trachea so that the distal end of the airway is 3 to 5 cm above the carina. If the endotracheal tube is advanced too far, as in this case, it more often enters the right main stem bronchus because of the straighter path that this bronchus offers. The left main stem bronchus branches from the trachea at a greater angle and is less likely to be intubated. A right main stem intubation results in right lung ventilation only, and the left lung continues to receive pulmonary blood flow but does not oxygenate it adequately. To avoid the problem in this patient, the airway should not be advanced more than 24 cm past the lips. This is the typical depth that the endotracheal tube is advanced in a 70-kg patient. At this point, the patient is auscultated with a stethoscope to confirm breath sounds in both lungs, and then a chest radiograph can be taken to confirm the airway position.

TABLE 8-7

Bronchial and Bronchiolar Divisions

Structure	Trachea	Segmental Bronchus	Terminal Bronchiole	Number	Diameter of Individual Structures	Total Cross-Sectional Area
Cartilaginous Conducting Structures						
Trachea	0			1	2.5 cm	5.0 cm^2
Main bronchi	1			2	11-19 mm	3.2 cm^2
Lobar	2-3			5	4.5-13.5 mm	2.7 cm^2
Segmental	3-6	0		19	4.5-6.5 mm	3.2 cm^2
Subsegmental	4-7	1		38	3-6 mm	6.6 cm^2
Bronchi		2-6		Varies	Varies	Varies
Terminal bronchi		3-7		1000	1.0 mm	7.9 cm^2
No Cartilage in Walls						
Bronchioles		5-14		Varies	Varies	Varies
Terminal bronchioles		6-15	0	35,000	0.65 mm	116 cm^2
Respiratory bronchioles			1-8	Varies	0.5-0.3 mm	Varies
Terminal respiratory bronchioles			2-9	630,000	0.45 mm	1000 cm^2
Alveolar ducts/sacs			4-12	4×10^6	0.40 mm	1.71 m^2
Alveoli				300×10^6	0.25-0.30 mm	140 m^2

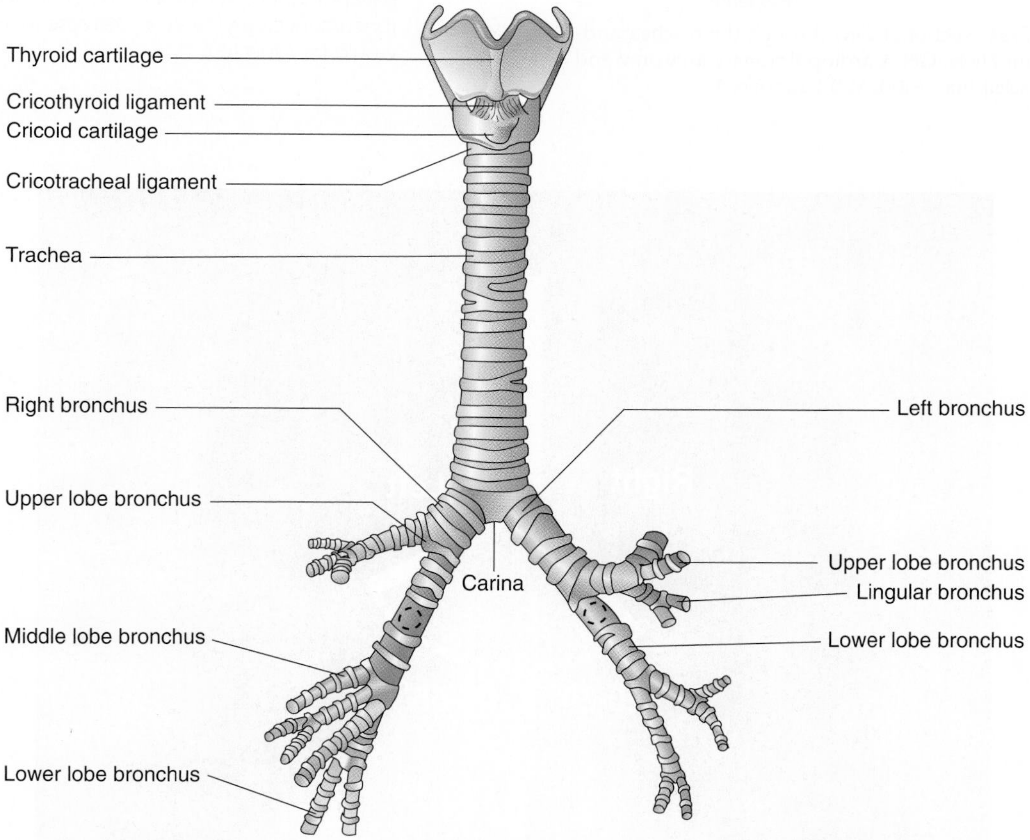

FIGURE 8-42 Major airways of the tracheobronchial tree. (From Hicks GH: Cardiopulmonary anatomy and physiology, Philadelphia, 2000, WB Saunders.)

Each bronchus carries gas to and from one lung. It enters the lung with the pulmonary vessels, lymph vessels, and nerves through the hilum. The bronchus branches repeatedly within each lung to supply gas to separate regions of each lung.

Lobar and Segmental Pulmonary Anatomy

The lungs have an apex and a base and are subdivided by fissures into lobes.[55] The lobes are subdivided further into bronchopulmonary **segments** (Table 8-8 and Figure 8-45).

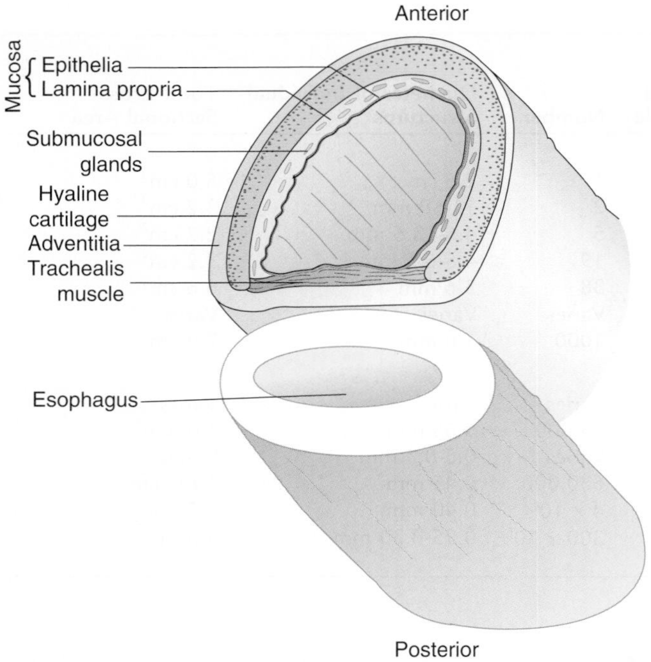

FIGURE 8-43 Cross-sectional view through the trachea and esophagus. (From Hicks GH: Cardiopulmonary anatomy and physiology, Philadelphia, 2000, WB Saunders.)

Each segment is supplied with gas from a single segmental bronchus. Controversy exists over the exact number of segments; some anatomists accept that each lung has 10 segments, whereas others maintain that the right has 10 and the left has 8. Knowledge of segmental anatomy is important in the physical examination of a patient to identify the location of a defect such as an infection site or a tumor mass in the lungs.

RULE OF THUMB

The 60-to-40 Rule

The right lung is slightly larger than the left lung because of the location of the heart. The right lung has a sizable middle lobe, and the left lung has a smaller lingular segment in the left upper lobe. For purposes of estimating the contribution of the right and left lungs to ventilation and to gas exchange, the 60-to-40 rule is sometimes used. The right lung is assumed to provide 60% of the ventilation/gas-exchange capacity, and the left lung is assumed to provide the remaining 40%. For example, if a patient required removal of the entire left lung (pneumonectomy), a 40% decrease in lung volume would be expected.

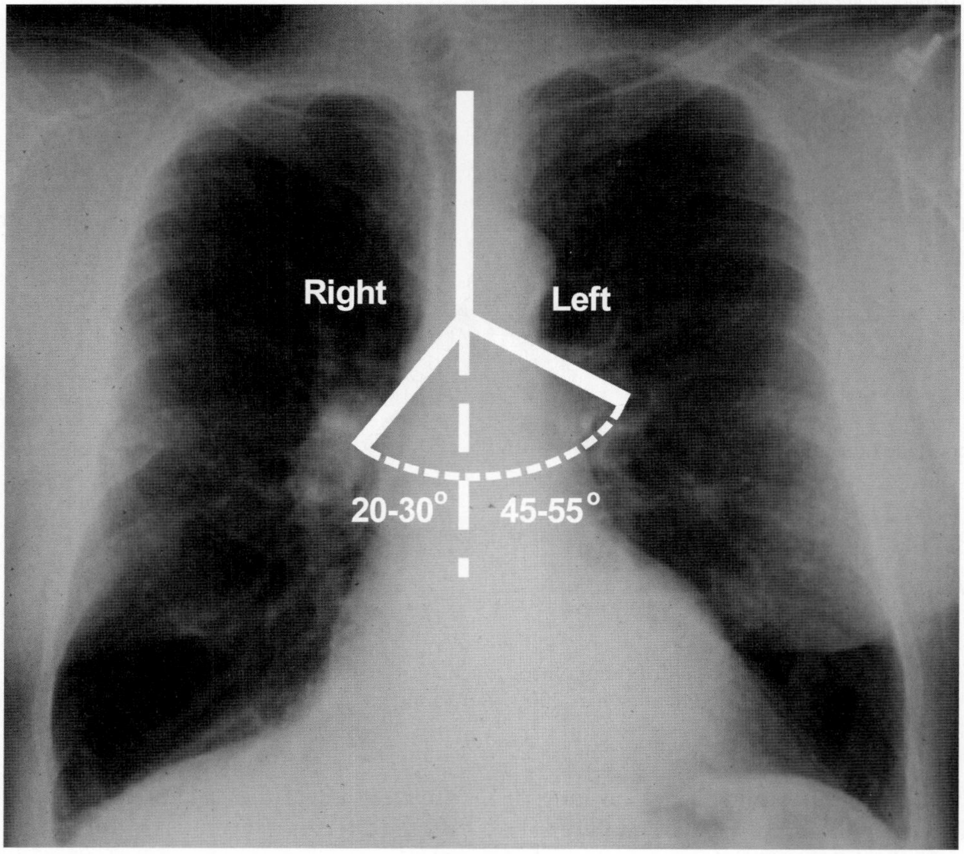

FIGURE 8-44 Course of trachea and right and left main stem bronchi, superimposed on a standard chest radiograph. The right main stem bronchus continues on a straighter course from midline than the left main stem bronchus.

TABLE 8-8

Bronchopulmonary Segments*

Segment	Number	Segment	Number
Right Upper Lobe		**Left Upper Lobe**	
Apical	1	Upper division	
Posterior	2	Apical-posterior	1 and 2†
Anterior	3	Anterior	3
Right Middle Lobe		Lower division (lingula)	
Lateral	4	Superior lingula	4
Medial	5	Inferior lingula	5
Right Lower Lobe		**Left Lower Lobe**	
Superior	6	Superior	6
Medial basal	7	Anterior basal	7 and 8
Anterior basal	8	Lateral basal	9
Lateral basal	9	Posterior basal	10
Posterior basal	10		

*The subdivisions of the lung and bronchial tree are fairly constant. Slight variations between right and left sides are noted by combined names and numbers.

†Some authors believe that the left lung should be numbered so that there are eight segments, where the apical-posterior is numbered 1 and the anteromedial is numbered 6.

The airways continue to divide as they penetrate deeper into the lungs. The segmental bronchi bifurcate into about 40 subsegmental bronchi, and these divide into hundreds of smaller bronchi. Thousands of bronchioles branch from the smaller bronchi. Bronchioles do not possess cartilage in their walls. Tens of thousands of terminal bronchioles arise from the bronchioles. *Terminal bronchioles* are the smallest conducting airways and function to supply gas to the respiratory zone of the lung.

With further divisions, the number of airways increases tremendously. The cross-sectional area of the conducting system increases exponentially. At the level of the terminal bronchioles, the cross-sectional area is approximately 20 times greater than that at the trachea. Gas flow in these airways conforms to the laws of fluid physics. Increased cross-sectional area reduces the velocity of gas flow during inspiration. When inspired gas reaches the level of the terminal bronchiole, its average velocity has fallen to about the same rate as the speed of diffusing gas molecules.[85] Low-velocity gas movement at the level of the terminal bronchiole and beyond is physiologically important for two reasons. First, laminar flow develops, which minimizes resistance in the small airways and decreases the work associated with inspiration. Second, low gas velocity facilitates rapid mixing of alveolar gases. This mixing provides a stable partial pressure of O_2 and CO_2 in the alveolar environment that supports stable diffusion and gas exchange.[86]

Histology of the Airway Wall

All of the conducting airways from the trachea to the bronchioles have walls that are constructed of three layers (Figures 8-46 and 8-47): an inner layer that forms a mucous membrane called the *mucosa,* which is primarily composed of epithelia; a submucosa composed of connective tissue, bronchial glands, and smooth fibers that wrap around the airway; and an outer covering of connective tissue called the *adventitia.*[87] The cartilaginous rings and plates found in larger airways are located in the adventitia.

The mucosa is composed of many different types of specialized epithelial cells that sit on top of a basement membrane. The most common type of epithelia are the numerous pseudostratified, ciliated, columnar epithelia.[88] The pseudostratified epithelial cells are held together toward their surface or apical end through three types of junctions—apical tight junctions, zonal adherens junctions, and desmosome-type junctions—and they anchored in place to the basement membrane.[89] The junctions, especially the tight junctions, play an important role in the maintenance of fluid and electrolyte (e.g., Cl^-) transport across the mucous membrane. These junctions prevent the movement of fluids and electrolytes between the apical surface and basal surfaces of the airway. Disturbances in this transport (e.g., Cl^- transport malfunction in cystic fibrosis transport receptor membrane channels) can lead to mucus and mucus transport abnormalities.

Near the base of the pseudostratified cells are large numbers of basal cells. The basal cells contribute to the appearance of a "pseudostratified" cellular layer. Basal cells mature into pseudostratified cells and are thought to play an important role in repair of the mucous membrane after diseases and injury. Dispersed between the pseudostratified epithelia are mucus-producing goblet cells and serous cells (in newborns) and the openings of submucosal bronchial glands. The bronchial glands are exocrine glands formed by secretory epithelial cells that sit on the basement membrane, which extends down into the lamina propria and into the submucosa. The bronchial glands are wrapped with myoepithelial cells. Myoepithelial cells contract and squeeze the bronchial gland when they receive signals from parasympathetic nerve fibers. In this region are neuroendocrine cells (also known as *Kulchitsky cells*) that are often organized into small clusters called neuroepithelial bodies.[90] Neuroendocrine cells are connected to the vagus nerve and are thought to function during lung development, are hypoxia and stress-strain sensors, and secrete various bioactive chemicals (e.g., serotonin, calcitonin, and gastrin-releasing peptide). Lymphocytes are also found intermixed with these cells, and it is thought that they may be migratory in nature.

Below the epithelial and basement membrane of the mucosa is the *lamina propria.*[89] The lamina propria is composed of loose fibroelastic connective tissue, lymphoid tissue, and a dense layer of elastic fibers. Below the lamina propria lies the submucosa. The submucosa of large airways contains bronchial glands, a capillary network, smooth muscle, some elastic tissue, and cartilage in larger airways. Bronchial glands vary in size up to 1 mm in length and connect to the bronchial surface via long, narrow ducts. The number of these glands increases significantly

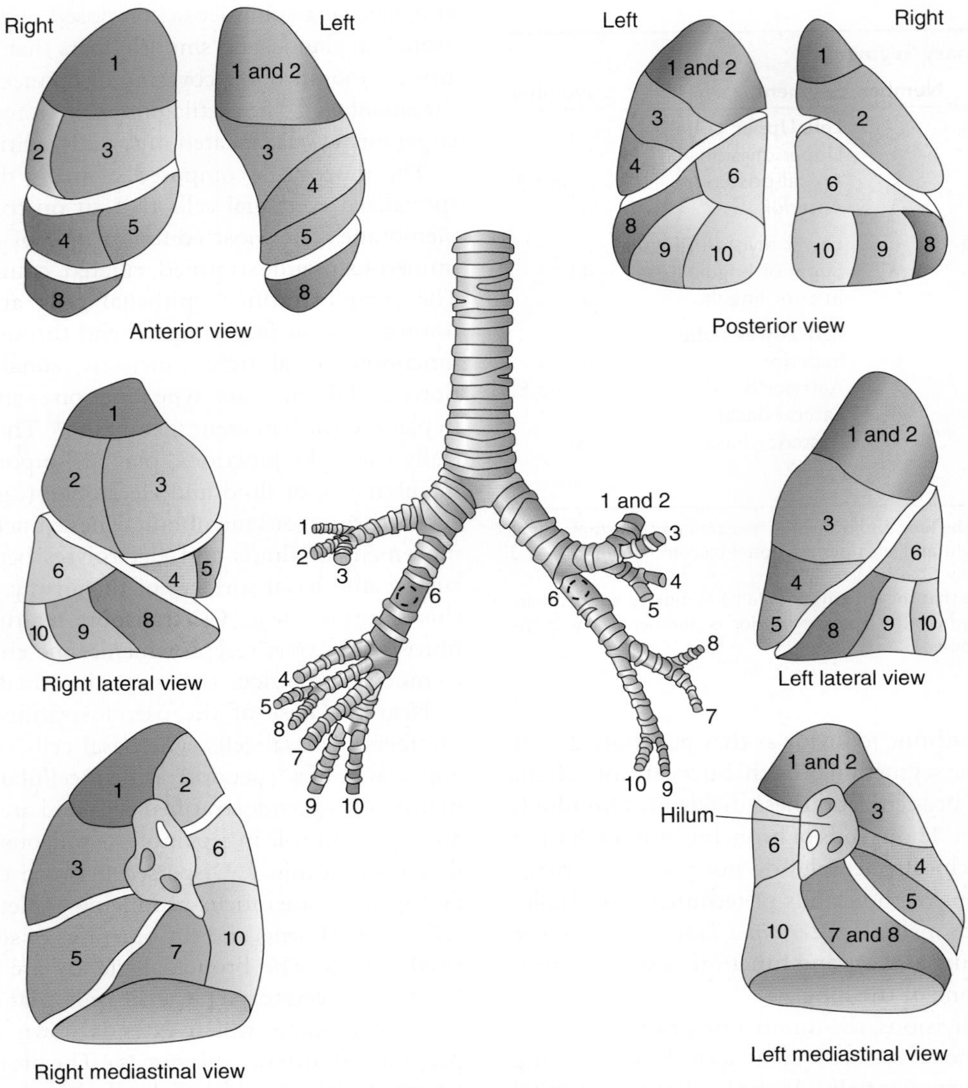

FIGURE 8-45 Bronchopulmonary segmental divisions of the lungs (see Table 8-8). (From Hicks GH: Cardiopulmonary anatomy and physiology, Philadelphia, 2000, WB Saunders.)

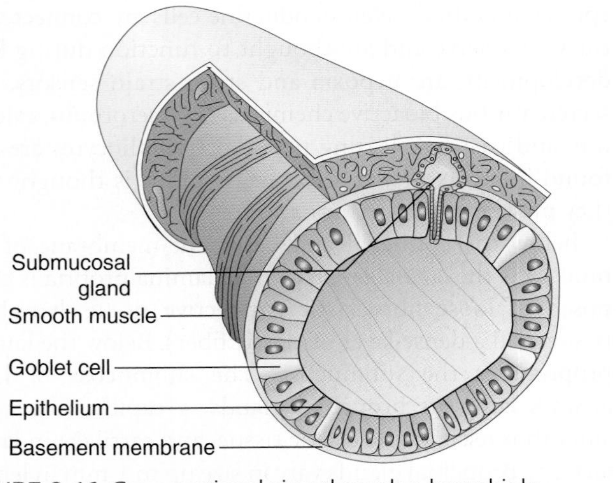

FIGURE 8-46 Cross-sectional view through a bronchiole. (From Hicks GH: Cardiopulmonary anatomy and physiology, Philadelphia, 2000, WB Saunders.)

in diseases such as chronic bronchitis. Mast cells are also found in the submucosa and release numerous and potent vasoactive and bronchoactive substances such as histamine.[91] Histamine causes vasodilation and bronchoconstriction, acting directly on smooth muscle. The triggering of mast cell release of its various substances and the resultant inflammation and bronchospasm of the airway are characteristic of the pathologic changes of asthma.

The various secretory cells (primarily goblet cells) of the mucosa and bronchial glands of the submucosa contribute to the production of mucus.[92] Normally, the respiratory tract produces about 100 ml of mucus per day. Most of the mucus formed in the larger airways is produced by the bronchial glands. Goblet cells contribute more in the smaller airways. The amount and composition of mucus produced can increase and change with airway irritation and diseases such as chronic bronchitis and asthma.[93]

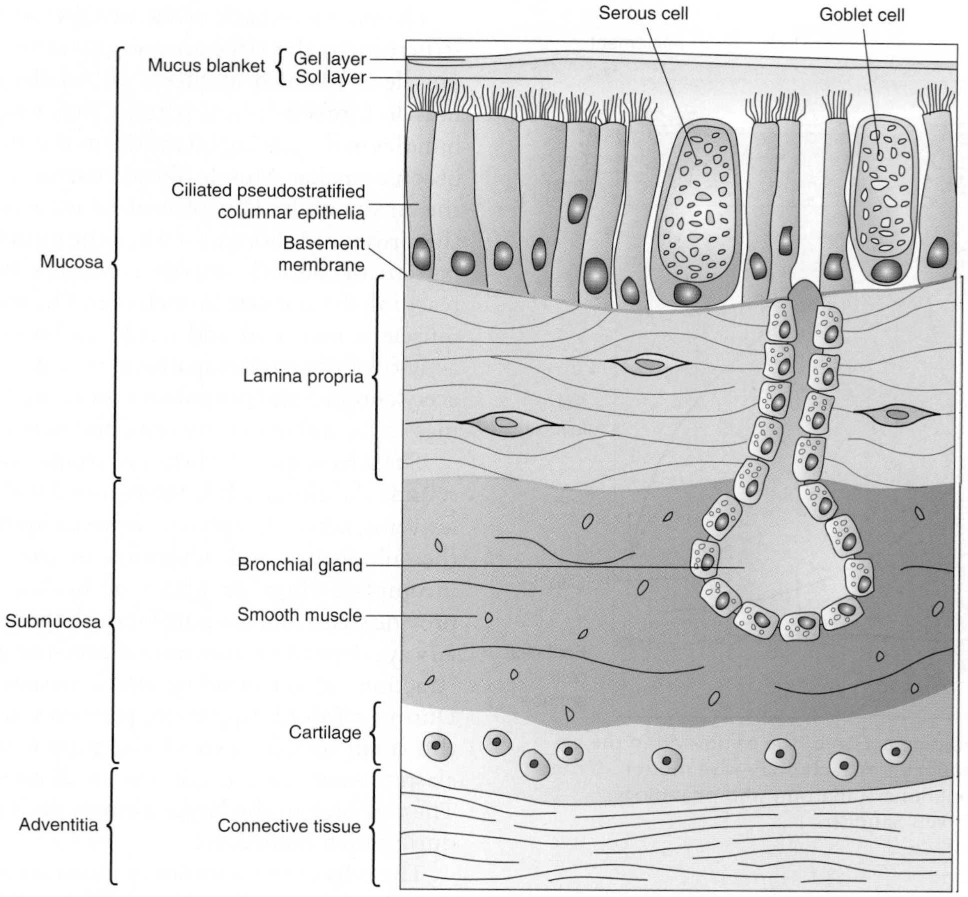

FIGURE 8-47 Microscopic view of mucous membrane. (From Hicks GH: Cardiopulmonary anatomy and physiology, Philadelphia, 2000, WB Saunders.)

Mucus is spread over the surface of the mucus membrane to a depth of about 7 μm and is propelled by the ciliated epithelia toward the pharynx. The outer layer of mucus is more gelatinous and is called the *gel layer*. The inner layer is much more fluid-like and is referred to as the *sol layer*. The mucus normally produced is a nearly clear fluid with greater viscosity than water. It is a mixture of 97% water and 3% solute.[92] The solute portion is produced primarily by goblet cells and bronchial glands; it is called *mucin* and is composed of protein (predominantly glycoproteins, proteoglycans, and IgA and IgG), lipids (primarily neutral lipids), and minerals (mainly inorganic electrolytes). The glycoprotein, lipid, and water content of mucus provides its viscoelastic gel nature. *Viscoelastic* refers to the ability of mucus to deform and spread when force is applied to it.

Mucus functions to protect the underlying tissue. It helps to prevent excessive amounts of water from moving into and out of the epithelia.[92] It shields the epithelia from direct contact with potentially toxic materials and microorganisms. It acts like sticky flypaper to trap particles that make contact with it. This makes mucus an important part of the pulmonary defenses. The production of mucus is stimulated by local mechanical and chemical irritation, release of proinflammatory mediators (e.g., cytokines), and parasympathetic (vagal) stimulation.

The ciliated pseudostratified epithelia play a crucial role in the defense of the respiratory tract by propelling mucus toward the pharynx. Ciliated cells are found in the nasal cavity and all the airways from the larynx to the terminal bronchioles. Each of the pseudostratified cells possesses about 200 **cilia** on its luminal surface.[89] Under the electron microscope, the surface of the mucus membrane looks like a "shag carpet" of cilia with about 1 to 2 billion cilia per square centimeter. Each cilium is an extension of the cell with an average length of about 6 μm and diameter of about 0.2 μm. A cross-sectional view through the cilium reveals it to be constructed of one inner and nine outer pairs of microtubules that are encased in the cell membrane. The outer pairs of microtubules are interlinked by a filamentous protein called *nexin*. From each of the outer pairs of microtubules, protein filaments called *dynein* extend toward the adjacent pair of microtubules. Each of the outer pairs also extends a protein spoke toward the central pair of microtubules. The presence of Mg^{2+} and ATP within the cilium causes the dynein arms and spokes to attach and slide along the outer and inner microtubules,

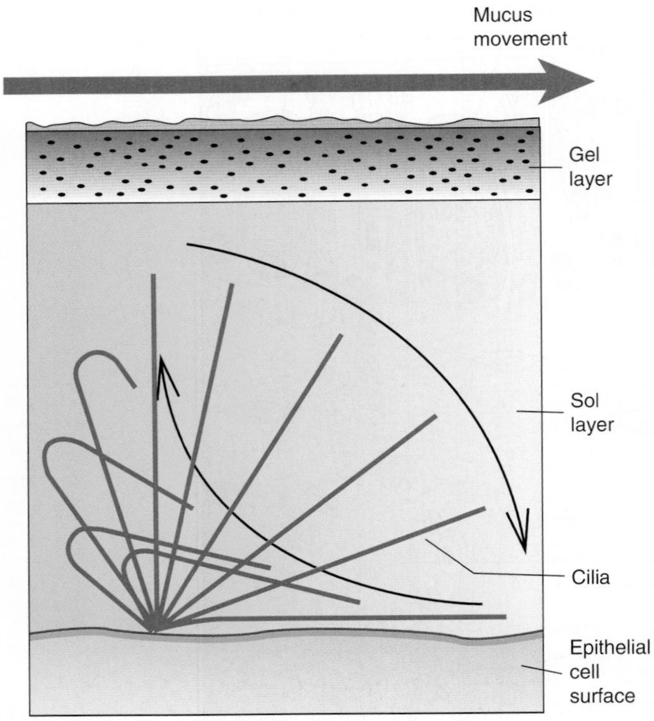

FIGURE 8-48 Whipping action of the cilium within the sol layer of mucus produces a metachronal wave motion. (From Hicks GH: Cardiopulmonary anatomy and physiology, Philadelphia, 2000, WB Saunders.)

similar to the action of actin and myosin. This action results in rapid bending of the cilium that resembles a whipping motion (Figure 8-48).

The cilia "stroke" at a rate of about 15 times per second, which produces a sequential motion of the cilia called a *metachronal wave.*[94] The metachronal "wavelength" is approximately 20 μm and propels surface material in a specific direction. In the nose, this motion propels material back to the pharynx. From the bronchioles up to the larynx, it moves material toward the pharynx. The stroking action of millions of cilia propels the surrounding mucus at a speed of about 2 cm/min. This action is commonly referred to as the **mucociliary escalator.** In healthy lungs, this mechanism allows inhaled particles to be removed within 24 hours. The control and coordination of ciliary motion are not totally understood and represent some of the many fascinating properties of pulmonary tissues.

The production of mucus and the rate of ciliary beating are sensitive to various conditions and chemicals. Mucus production increases when the respiratory tract is irritated by particles and by various chemicals and during increased parasympathetic nervous stimulation.[93] Ciliary beating can be effectively slowed or stopped if the viscosity of the sol layer is increased by exposure to dry gas. Ciliary motion is also slowed or stopped after exposure to smoke, high concentrations of inhaled O_2, and drugs such as atropine.

The smooth muscle of the airways varies in location and structure. In the large airways (e.g., the trachea), smooth muscle is bundled in sheets. In smaller airways, smooth muscle forms a helical pattern that wraps the airway in bundles in decreasing quantities as the airways branch and become smaller. Muscle fibers crisscross and spiral around the airway walls. This placement reduces the diameter of the airway and shortens it when the muscle contracts. This pattern of smooth muscle continues but thins out on reaching the smallest bronchioles. The tone of the smooth muscle is increased and results in bronchospasm by the activity of the parasympathetic nervous system (release of acetylcholine) and proinflammatory mediator release from mast cells, inflammatory cells, and neuroendocrine cells.

The adventitia is a sheath of connective tissue that surrounds the airways. It is interspersed with bronchial arteries, veins, nerves, lymph vessels, and adipose tissue. Between the submucosa and adventitia of the large airways are incomplete rings or plates of hyaline cartilage, which provide structural support for the larger airways. The small airways depend on transmural pressure gradients and the "traction" of surrounding elastic tissues to remain open. During a forced expiration, pressures across the walls of the small airways exceed the supporting forces of the elastic tissues. As a result, the small airways can collapse. The cartilage in the larger airways prevents their collapse during such maneuvers.

The cells of the respiratory mucosa change as they progress into the smaller airways (Figure 8-49). As the thickness of the airway walls decreases, bronchial glands become fewer in number. At the bronchiolar level, the number of ciliated cells decreases. Simple columnar and cuboidal epithelial cells begin to predominate and are interspersed with goblet cells. In this region, large numbers of *Clara cells,* nonciliated cuboidal cells with apical granules, are found. It is thought that these cells play a role in degrading various xenobiotic oxidants via cytochrome P-450, contribute proteins for surfactant production, synthesize various lipids, and play a role in lung repair by being able to differentiate into other important epithelial cells in the mucosa after injury.[95]

Respiratory Zone Airways

The terminal bronchioles begin about 12 to 15 generations beyond the trachea (Figure 8-50).[96] There are about 16,000 terminal bronchioles with airway opening diameters of about 700 μm. This yields a combined cross-sectional area opening that is almost 100 times that of the main stem bronchi. All of the airways down to and including the terminal bronchioles carry or conduct gas flow to and from the airways that participate in gas exchange with blood. The airways from the nares to and including the terminal bronchioles constitute the *conducting zone airways,* which do not participate in gas exchange. These airways constitute the anatomic dead space of the respiratory system, which is rebreathed with each breath. In an adult human,

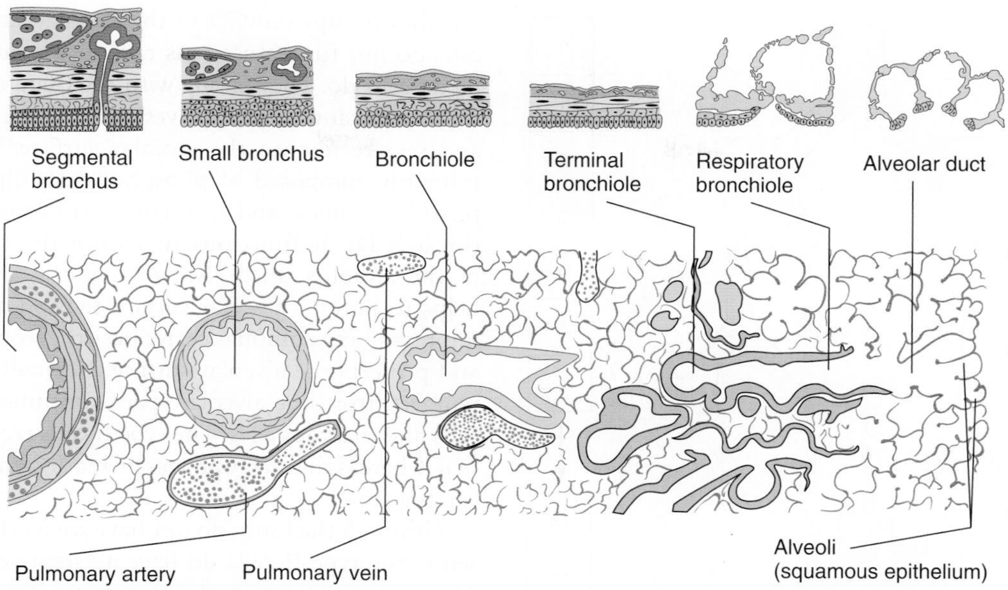

FIGURE 8-49 Histologic diagram of airways from the segmental bronchus to the alveolus. (Modified from Freeman WH, Bracegridle B: An atlas of histology, London, 1966, Heinemann Educational.)

the volume filling the airways of the anatomic dead space is approximately 2 ml/kg of lean body weight, or about 150 ml in a typical adult.

Branching of the terminal bronchioles gives rise to unique airways called *respiratory bronchioles.* Respiratory bronchioles are approximately 0.4 mm in diameter and have walls that are formed largely from flattened squamous epithelia and a thin outer layer of connective tissue. They have some ciliated cells at the connection with the terminal bronchiole, generally lack mucus-producing cells, and have rings of smooth muscles where they branch to form alveolar ducts. Respiratory bronchioles have a dual function. Similar to conducting airways, they not only conduct gas flow but also have small outpouchings known as *alveoli* in their walls. The alveoli and their pulmonary capillary bed enable the respiratory bronchioles to carry out gas exchange. The respiratory bronchioles constitute a transitional zone type of airway.

A single terminal bronchiole supplies a cluster of respiratory bronchioles. Collectively, this unit is referred to as the acinus, or **primary lobule.** Each acinus comprises numerous respiratory bronchioles, alveolar ducts, and approximately 10,000 alveoli (Figure 8-51). The adult lung is thought to contain more than 30,000 acini. Each acinus is supplied with pulmonary blood flow from a pulmonary arteriole, and blood is drained away from several acini through a pulmonary venule. In addition, each acinus is equipped with a lymphatic drainage vessel and nervous fibers. These features make the primary lobule the functional unit of the lungs. Gas molecule movement in this region is largely via diffusion rather than convective flow, which occurs in larger airways.

Millions of alveolar ducts branch from the respiratory bronchioles (Figure 8-52). Alveolar ducts are tiny airways only 0.3 mm in diameter, and their walls are composed entirely of alveoli. Each alveolar duct ends in a cluster of alveoli, which is frequently referred to as an *alveolar sac.* Each alveolar sac opens into about 16 or 17 **alveoli,** and about one-half of the total number of alveoli are found in this region.

Alveoli

More recent estimates suggest that the number of alveoli in adult lungs range from 270 to 790 million, with an average of about 480 million.[32] The number of alveoli increases with the height of the subject. Alveolar size varies with lung volume and averages about 0.2 mm in diameter when the lung is inflated to its functional residual volume. Figure 8-53 shows alveoli in a normal rat lung at different states of inflation and how their shapes change. When inflated at and beyond the functional residual volume (see Figure 8-53A-C), alveoli have a polyhedral shape that results from numerous flat walls rather than a curved spherical structure. Alveoli found in the apical regions of the vertical lung have greater diameters than alveoli in the basal regions as a result of the gravitational effects. Alveoli in the basal regions are partially collapsed as a result of the weight of the organ.

The alveolar walls or septa are formed by various cell types that are arranged to provide a thin surface for gas exchange and strength.[97] The alveolar septa are covered with extremely flat squamous epithelia called *type I pneumocytes* (Figure 8-54). Although they represent only about 8% of all the cells found in the alveolar region, type I cells

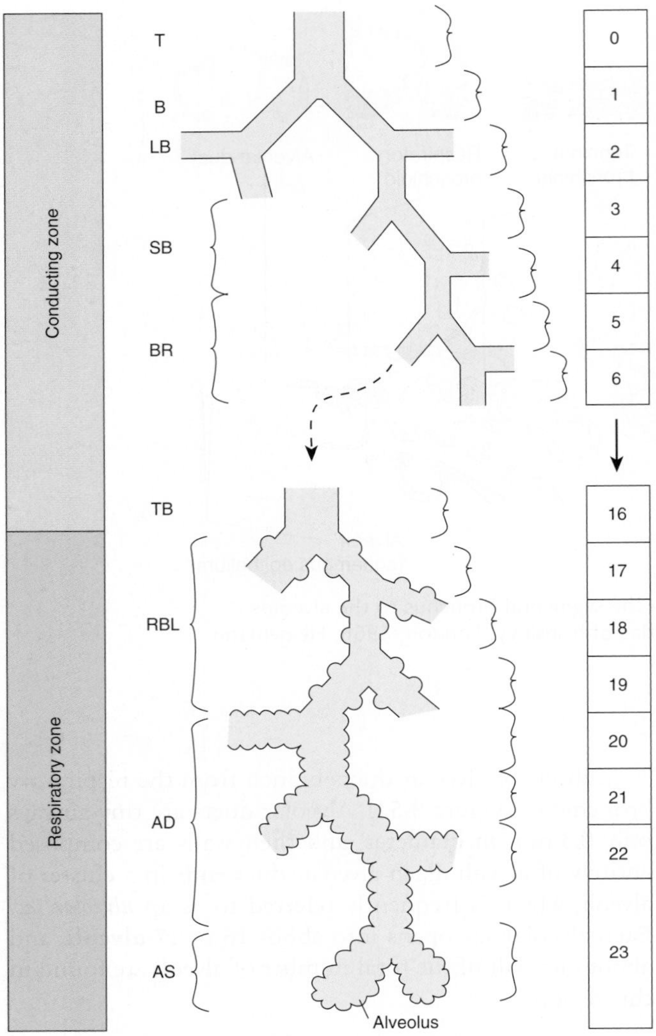

FIGURE 8-50 Airways of the conducting (generation *0* through *16*) and respiratory (generation *17* through *23*) zones: *T,* trachea; *B,* right and left bronchi; *LB,* lobar bronchi; *SB,* segmental and subsegmental bronchi; *BR,* bronchioles; *TB,* terminal bronchioles; *RBL,* respiratory bronchioles; *AD,* alveolar ducts; and *AS,* alveolar sacs. (From Hicks GH: Cardiopulmonary anatomy and physiology, Philadelphia, 2000, WB Saunders.)

cover about 93% of the alveolar surface.[98] These cells form a "patchwork"-like surface that covers the alveolar capillaries and forms the gas exchange surface of the alveolus. At their edges where they meet one another, they form tight junctions that help to limit the movement of material into the alveolar airspace from the interstitial space just below. They are held in place and supported from below by a network of collagen and elastin fibers. They are susceptible to injury and apoptosis (programmed cell death) from inhaled particles (e.g., cigarette smoke), bacterial infection, and excessive concentrations of inhaled O_2.

Interspersed on the alveolar surface and concentrated in the corners of the alveolar septa are type II pneumocytes, which are cuboidal epithelia with apical microvilli (Figure 8-55). These cells are twice as numerous as the type I cells, but they occupy only 7% of the alveolar surface.[98] Type II cells do not function as gas exchange membranes as the type I cells do. They (along with the Clara cells) manufacture surfactant, store it in vesicles called *lamellated bodies,* and secrete it onto the alveolar surface.[99] Surfactant is primarily composed of phospholipids (dipalmitoylphosphatidylcholine) and proteins (surfactant proteins A through D). It functions to reduce the surface tension of the alveolus, sheds water from the alveolar surface, helps to prevent alveolar surface tension-driven collapse, improves lung compliance, reduces the work of breathing, and protects the alveolar surface. Normally, surfactant is removed from the alveolar space continuously by type II cells and macrophages. The type II cells recycle about 50% of it, whereas the macrophages primarily remove it through catabolism.[100]

Although the lungs do not have stem cells in the classic sense, the type II cells do have a "stem cell"–like action. They can proliferate and differentiate into type I cells to repopulate and repair the alveolar surface after injury.[101] They are also involved in alveolar defense through surfactant production and the release of some cytokines that trigger inflammation.

Macrophages are another common cell found in the alveolar region.[98] They can move from the pulmonary capillary circulation by squeezing through openings in the alveolar septa and then move out onto the alveolar surface. They are defensive cells that patrol the alveolar region and phagocytize foreign particles and cells (e.g., bacteria). They can present portions of the foreign particles and bacteria to lymphocytes as part of the immune response and contain various digestive enzymes (e.g., trypsin) that break down the material they engulf.

Within the interalveolar septum is an interstitial space that contains matrix material and the pulmonary capillaries. Also found in the interstitial space are bands of elastin fibers and a collagen fiber matrix.[58] These fibers support the alveolar cells and the shape of the alveolus. Small openings are located in the alveolar septa. Some of the openings allow gas to move from one alveolus to another. These are called the **pores of Kohn.** Other openings connect alveoli with secondary respiratory bronchioles. These passageways are called the *canals of Lambert.* All of these alveolar openings and passageways facilitate the collateral movement of gas and help maintain alveolar volume.[102]

Blood-Gas Barrier

Gas exchange between alveolar gas and pulmonary capillary blood occurs across the **alveolar-capillary membrane.** In a typical adult, this blood-gas barrier stretches over a surface area of approximately 140 m^2 and is less than 1 μm thick over most of that area.[103] This makes the membrane more than 50 times larger than the area covered by skin and more than 2000 times thinner.

The blood-gas barrier is composed of many different layers through which O_2 and CO_2 diffuse (Figure 8-56).

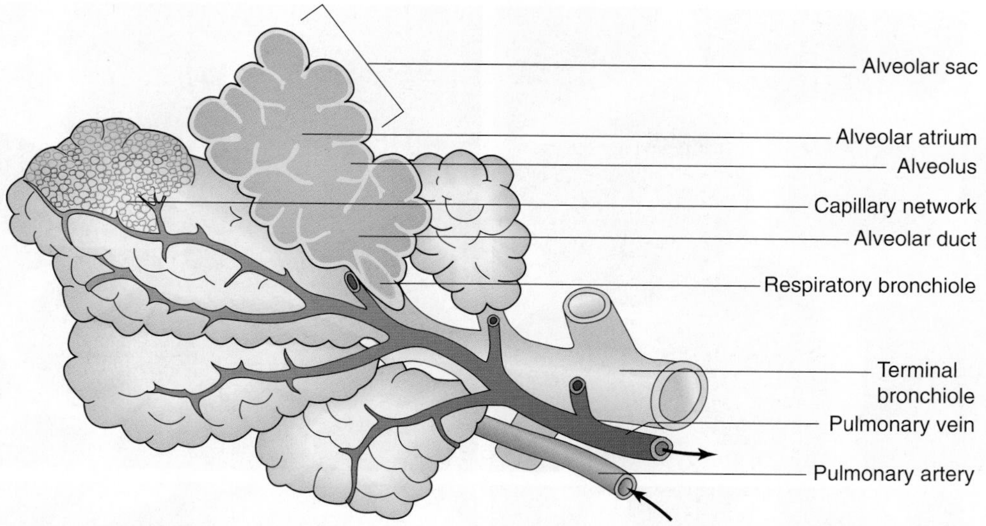

FIGURE 8-51 The acinus (primary lobule) of the lung is composed of a single terminal bronchiole, numerous respiratory bronchioles, alveolar ducts, sacs of alveoli, and about 10,000 alveoli. Pulmonary blood flow is delivered to the acinus by a pulmonary arteriole and drained from it by a pulmonary venule. (From Hicks GH: Cardiopulmonary anatomy and physiology, Philadelphia, 2000, WB Saunders.)

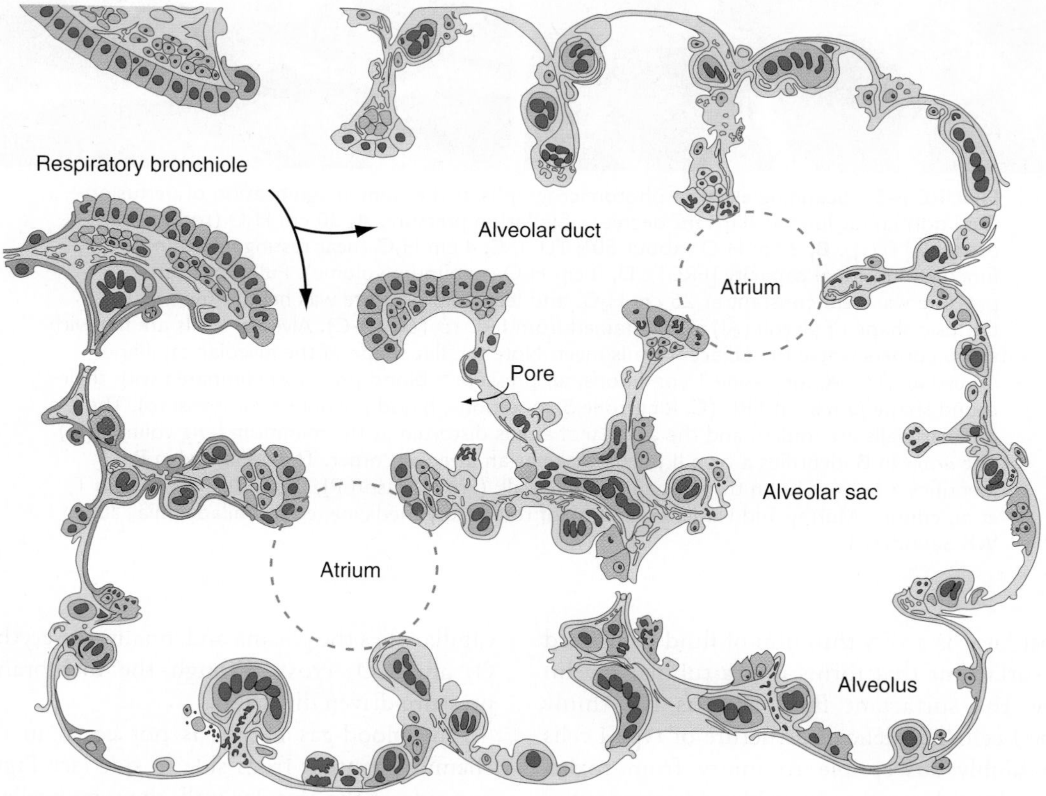

FIGURE 8-52 Microscopic view of respiratory zone airways. (Modified from Sorokin SP: The respiratory system. In Greep RO, Weiss L, editors: Histology, New York, 1973, McGraw-Hill.)

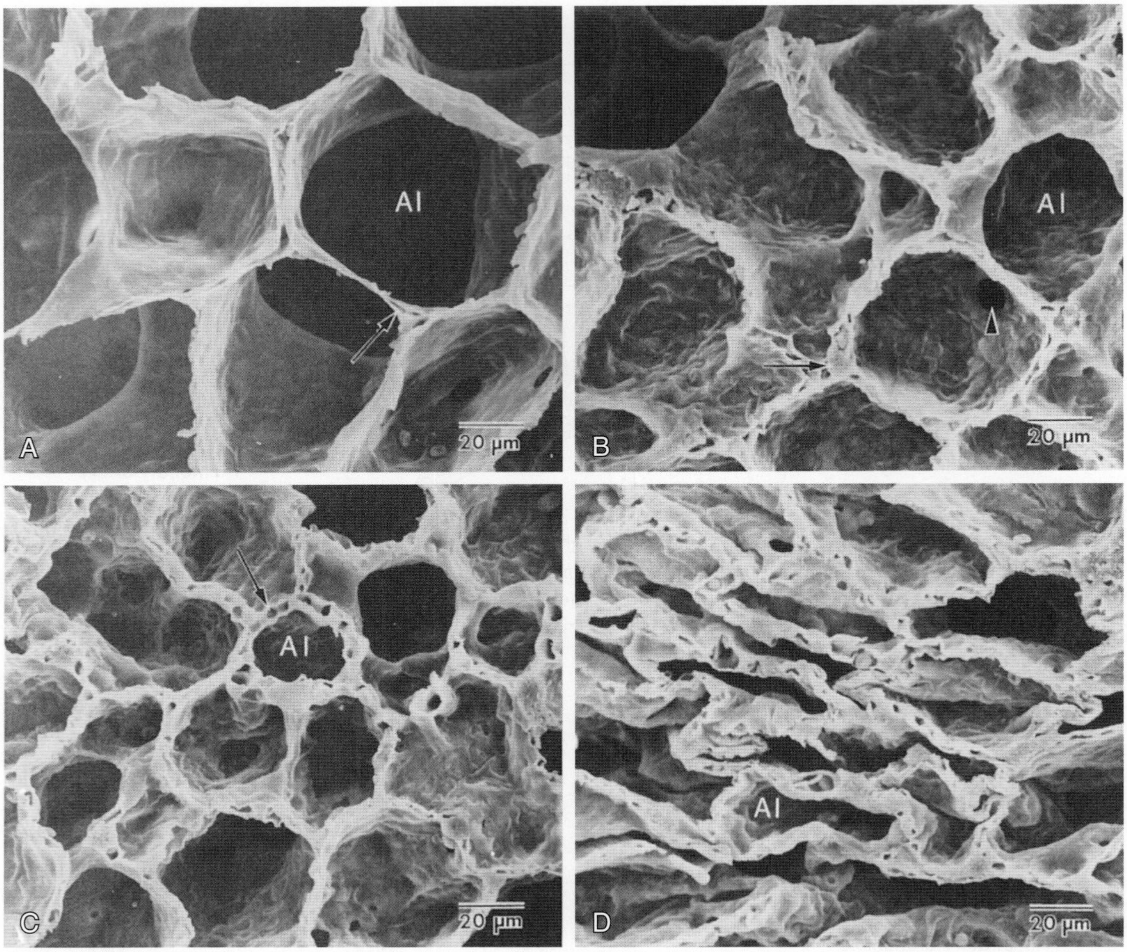

FIGURE 8-53 Scanning electron photomicrographs at the same magnification of perfusion-fixed normal rat lung at different degrees of inflation pressure. **A,** 30 cm H_2O (total lung capacity [TLC]). **B,** 8 cm H_2O (about 50% TLC). **C,** 4 cm H_2O (near resting inflation or functional residual capacity [FRC]). **D,** 0 cm H_2O (minimum volume). Pulmonary artery pressure was held constant at 25 cm H_2O, and left atrial pressure was held at 6 cm H_2O. Intrinsic shape of alveoli (Al) is maintained from FRC to TLC **(A-C).** Alveolar walls are flat with sharp corners where the adjacent walls meet. Note the flat shape of the alveolar capillaries *(arrow)* at TLC (**A,** lung zone 1 conditions, air pressure > blood pressure) compared with their round shape *(arrow)* at FRC (**C,** lung zone 3 conditions, blood pressure > air pressure). The alveolar walls are folded, and the alveolar shape is distorted at the minimum lung volume **(D).** The *arrow* in **B** identifies a type II pneumocyte at an alveolar corner. The *arrowhead* in **B** identifies a pore of Kohn through an alveolar wall. (From Mason RJ, Broaddus VC, Martin T, et al, editors: Murray and Nadel's textbook of respiratory medicine, ed 4, Philadelphia, 2011, WB Saunders.)

The outermost layer is a very thin film of fluid composed primarily of surfactant that forms into a tubular myelin matrix. Below the surfactant fluid layer is the thinly stretched type I cell. The delicate structure of type I cells makes them highly susceptible to injury from toxins carried to them by either airborne or blood-borne routes. The interstitial space and its contents lie below. Within this space are basement membranes, matrix material connective tissue fibers, and the alveolar capillary.[58] The capillary wall is formed from thin, flat squamous epithelia called *endothelial cells* that form a thin tube by connecting together at their edges with tight junctions. Within the capillary lies the plasma and, finally, the erythrocytes. Both O_2 and CO_2 cross through the membrane via partial pressure-driven diffusion.

The blood-gas barrier is not equal in thickness and chemical content from side to side (see Figure 8-56). On one side of the alveolar wall, the type I cells and capillary endothelial cells lie close together with a thin interstitial space. This part of the blood-gas barrier is, on average, 0.2 to 0.3 µm thick, and it is where the alveolar capillary bulges into the alveolar space.[103] On the other side, where there is a thicker interstitial space with greater fiber, matrix, and nuclear material content, the barrier can be more

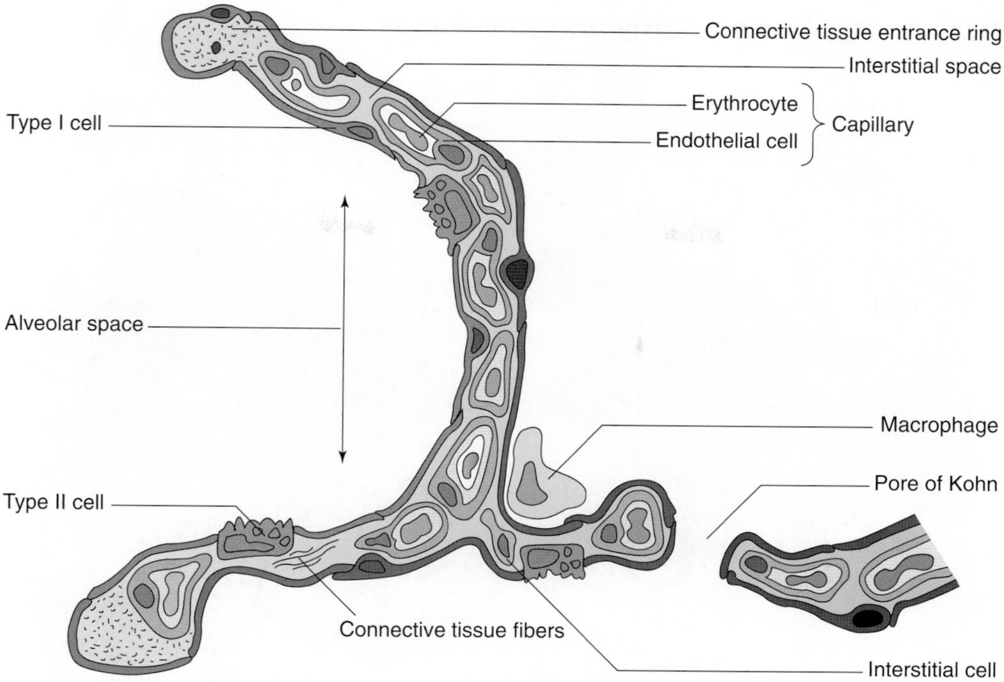

FIGURE 8-54 Highly magnified cross-sectional sketch of the cells and organization of the alveolar septa. (From Hicks GH: Cardiopulmonary anatomy and physiology, Philadelphia, 2000, WB Saunders.)

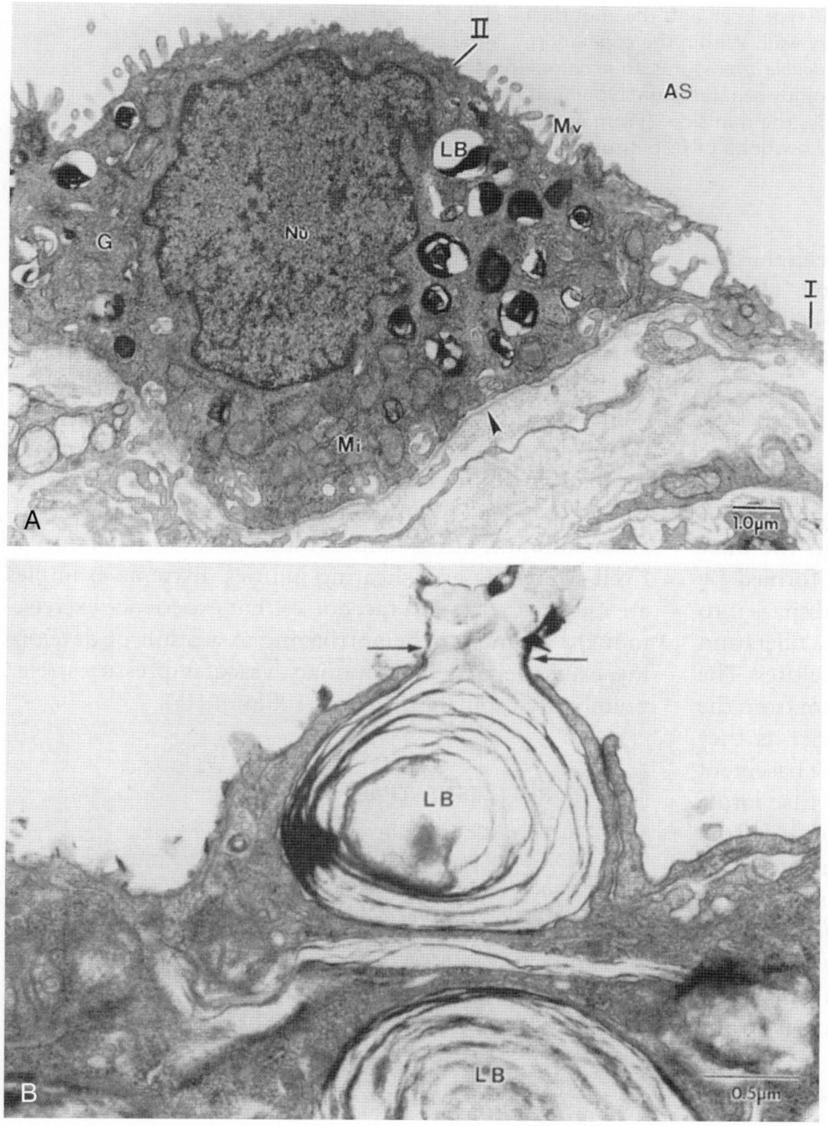

FIGURE 8-55 Transmission electron photomicrograph of human lungs at high magnification. **A,** Type II pneumocytes are cuboidal epithelial cells that contain characteristic lamellar bodies *(LB)* in their cytoplasm and have stubby microvilli *(Mv)* that extend from their apical surface into the alveolar airspace *(AS)*. Other prominent organelles within the type II cells are mitochondria *(Mi)*, a single nucleus *(Nu)*, and a Golgi apparatus *(G)*, which forms the lamellar bodies. Adjacent to the type II cell is a portion of a type I pneumocyte (I). The abluminal side of the epithelial cells of the alveolus rests on a continuous basal lamina *(arrowhead)*. **B,** Apical region of a type II cell contains two lamellar bodies *(LB)*, one of which has been fixed in the process of secreting its contents *(arrows)*. The lamellar bodies are believed to be the source of surfactant. Type II cells are more often found in the corners of the alveolar walls. (From Mason RJ, Broaddus VC, Martin, T, et al, editors: Murray and Nadel's textbook of respiratory medicine, ed 4, Philadelphia, 2011, WB Saunders.)

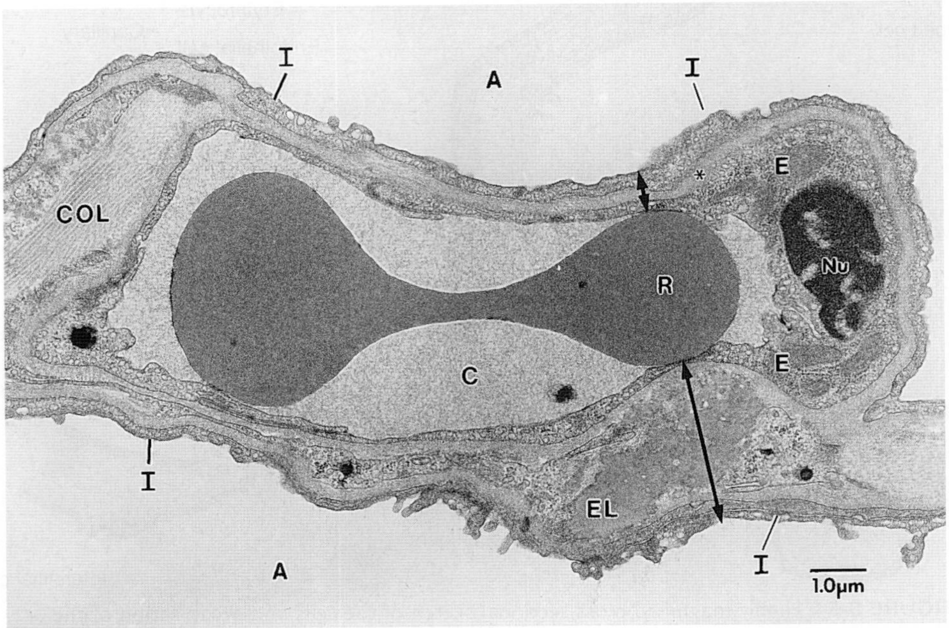

FIGURE 8-56 High-magnification transmission electron photomicrograph of a human lung showing a cross section of an alveolar wall through which O_2 and CO_2 diffuse. Air *(A)* in the alveolar space is seen on either side of the wall. The thin side of the alveolar-capillary membrane *(short double arrow)* consists of type I pneumocytes *(I)*, interstitium *(*)* formed by the fused basement membranes of the type I cell and the endothelial cells *(E)*, and its nucleus *(Nu)* that forms the pulmonary capillary wall. Within the capillary *(C)* is the erythrocyte *(R)*. The thick side of the membrane *(long double arrows)* has an accumulation of elastin *(EL)*, collagen *(COL)*, and matrix material that jointly separates the type I cell from the capillary endothelial cell. Greater diffusion occurs across the thin side. (From Mason RJ, Broaddus VC, Martin T, et al, editors: Murray and Nadel's textbook of respiratory medicine, ed 4, Philadelphia, 2011, WB Saunders.)

than 3 to 10 times thicker. This difference between the two sides functionally results in "faster-weaker" and "slower-stronger" diffusion sides of the blood-gas barrier.

The interstitial space within the alveolar septum contains a network of fibers that form a kind of connective tissue skeleton that holds the alveolar structures in place and together.[104] The fibers within the alveolar septum are part of the continuum of connective tissue fibers that are found in the pleural surface and in the airway walls that extends all the way to the root of the lung in the hilar region. Elastin and collagen fiber bands are formed by fibroblasts into a network within the interstitial space into which the capillaries are woven. Also around the fibers and capillaries is a nonliving matrix of fluid and solutes. The weaving path taken by the capillaries passes them from the thick to the thin sides of the blood-gas barrier as they extend through the septum. In the thin side, the basement membranes of the endothelial and type I cells fuse into a structure called the *lamina densa,* which is formed from type IV collagen.[105] In the thick side, thick bands of type I collagen and elastin are found. The type I cells and endothelial cells are attached to either side of the *lamina densa* by a series of protein fibers collectively known as *laminins.* Laminins effectively bind together the blood-gas barrier into a three-part laminate that results in a relatively strong and thin structure that can normally, with the additional support offered by the capillary network, withstand the everyday stress of alveolar and capillary stretch.[106]

However, conditions of pulmonary hypertension (e.g., capillary pressure >30 mm Hg during congestive heart failure and high-altitude pulmonary edema) and excessive tidal volume and airway pressure during positive pressure ventilation (e.g., tidal volume >6 ml/kg and airway pressures >30 cm H_2O) can result in stress failure of the blood-gas membrane. Stress failure results in endothelial or type I cell stretching and shearing injuries. Extreme examples are known to occur in racehorses that experience exercise-induced pulmonary hemorrhaging as a result of developing excessively high pulmonary vascular pressures (e.g., pulmonary capillary pressures 100 mm Hg).

RULE OF THUMB

The 30:30 Rule

Pulmonary hypertension (e.g., capillary pressure >30 mm Hg) and excessive tidal volume and airway pressure during positive pressure ventilation (e.g., tidal volume >6 ml/kg and airway pressures >30 cm H_2O) can result in stress failure of the blood-gas membrane.

SUMMARY CHECKLIST

- Many different genes regulate the development of the respiratory system from conception through adult life. Many pulmonary diseases are caused by genetic abnormalities.
- The development of the respiratory system follows a well-defined schedule; interruptions or insults in the course of development can result in respiratory disease at birth and in adulthood.
- Fetal circulation and respiration differ markedly from circulation and respiration in the postnatal period.
- The transition from intrauterine to extrauterine life involves a nonaerated, fluid-filled lung converting to an efficient air-filled organ of gas exchange.
- Closure of the foramen ovale and ductus arteriosus are important events in the transition to extrauterine life.
- The thorax houses and protects the lungs; it is also a movable shell that makes ventilation possible.
- The diaphragm is the primary muscle of ventilation; together with the accessory muscles and thoracic structures, it provides the ability to move large volumes of gas into and out of the lungs.
- The lungs receive blood flow from the pulmonary circulation for gas exchange and the bronchial circulation to support airway and pleural tissue metabolism.
- The pulmonary circulation is capable of acting as a reservoir, removing blood clots and numerous mediators and activating important vasoactive agents.
- Motor and sensory neurons innervate the muscles of ventilation and various lung tissues. Autonomic neurons conduct motor and sensory signaling to control various tissues and sense various activities.
- The upper respiratory tract heats and humidifies inspired air. Its various structures also protect the lungs against foreign substances.
- The lower respiratory tract conducts respired gases from the upper airway to the respiratory zones of the lung. It contains many structures that help clear and defend the lung.
- The airways branch into lobes in both the right and the left lungs; these lobes consist of various segments.
- The respiratory bronchioles, alveolar ducts, and alveoli provide a large, yet extremely thin membrane for the exchange of O_2 and CO_2 between air and blood. Disruption of the blood-gas barrier can occur from excessive capillary pressures and lung inflation and from exposure to various toxins (e.g., 100% O_2).

References

1. Moore KL, Persaud TVN: The respiratory system. In Moore KL, Persaud TVN, editors: The developing human—clinically oriented embryology, ed 7, Philadelphia, 2003, WB Saunders.
2. Maeda Y, Dave V, Whitsett JA: Transcriptional control of lung morphogenesis. Physiol Rev 87:219-244. 2007.
3. De Langhe S, Del Moral P, Tefft D, et al: The genetic, molecular, and cellular basis of lung development. In Fishman A, Elias J, Fishman J, et al, editors: Fishman's pulmonary diseases and disorders, ed 4, New York, 2008, McGraw-Hill.
4. Morrisey EE, Hogan BLM: Preparing for the first breath: genetic and cellular mechanisms in lung development. Dev Cell 18:8-23, 2010.
5. Minoo P, Su G, Drum H, et al: Defects in tracheoesophageal and lung morphogenesis in Nkx2.1(−/−) mouse embryos. Dev Biol 209:60-71, 1999.
6. Min H, Danilenko DM, Scully SA, et al: Fgf-10 is required for both limb and lung development and exhibits striking functional similarity to Drosophila branchless. Genes Dev 12:3156-3161, 1998.
7. Murray JF: Postnatal growth and development of the lung. In Murray JF, editor: The normal lung, ed 2, Philadelphia, 1986, WB Saunders.
8. Beech DJ, Sibbons PD, Howard CV, et al: Terminal bronchiolar duct ending number does not increase post-natally in normal infants. Early Hum Dev 59:193-200, 2000.
9. Adamson I, Bowden C: The type 2 cell as progenitor of alveolar epithelial regeneration: a cytodynamic study in mice after exposure to oxygen. Lab Invest 30:35-42, 1974.
10. Stanley MW, Henry-Stanley MJ, Gajl-Peczalska K, et al: Hyperplasia of type II pneumocytes in acute lung injury: cytologic findings of sequential bronchoalveolar lavage, Am J Clin Pathol 97:669-677, 1992.
11. Langston C, Kida K, Reed M, et al: Human lung growth in late gestation and in the neonate, Am Rev Respir Dis 129:607-613, 1984.
12. Merkus PJ, ten Have-Opbroek AA, Quanjer PH. Human lung growth: a review. Pediatr Pulmonol 21:383-397, 1996.
13. Frerking I, Gunther A, Seeger W, et al: Pulmonary surfactant: functions, abnormalities and therapeutic options, Intensive Care Med 27:1699-1717, 2001.
14. Gluck L, Kulovich MV, Borer RC, et al: Diagnosis of the respiratory distress syndrome by amniocentesis, Am J Obstet Gynecol 109:440-445, 1971.
15. Mendelson CR, Boggaram V: Hormone control of the surfactant system in fetal lung, Annu Rev Physiol 53: 415-440, 1991.
16. Whitsett JA: Genetic disorders of surfactant homeostasis. Paediatr Respir Rev 7:S240-S242, 2006.
17. Harding R, Hooper SB: Regulation of lung expansion and lung growth before birth, J Appl Physiol 8:209-224, 1996.
18. Thurlbeck WM: Postnatal growth and development of the lung, Am Rev Respir Dis 111:803-844, 1975.
19. Hepper PG, Shannon EA, Dornan JC: Sex differences in fetal mouth movements. Lancet 350:1820, 1997.
20. Torday JS, Nielsen HC: The sex difference in fetal lung surfactant production, Exp Lung Res 12:1-19, 1987.
21. Taeusch WH, Ballard RA, Gleason CA, editors: Avery's diseases of the newborn, ed 8, Philadelphia, 2004, WB Saunders.
22. Blackburn S: Fetal assessment. In Maternal, fetal, and neonatal physiology: a clinical perspective, ed 3, Philadelphia, 2007, WB Saunders.
23. Longo L: Fetal gas exchange. In Crystal R, West J, editors: The lung: scientific foundations, New York, 1991, Raven Press.
24. Czervinske MP: Fetal gas exchange and circulation. In Walsh B, Czervinske MP, DiBlasi R, editors: Perinatal and pediatric respiratory care, ed 3, Philadelphia, 2009, WB Saunders.
25. Barker PM, Oliver RE: Clearance of lung fluid during the perinatal period. J Appl Physiol 93:I542-I548, 2002.

26. Helve O, Pitkänen O, Janér C, et al: Pulmonary fluid balance in the human newborn infant. Neonatology. 95:347–352, 2009.
27. Hazinski, M, van Stralen D: Physiological and anatomical differences between children and adults. In Levin D, Morriss F, Fletcher J, editors: Essentials of pediatric intensive care, ed 2, St Louis, 1997, Churchill Livingstone.
28. Cozzi F, Morini F, Tozzi C, et al: Effect of pacifier use on oral breathing in healthy newborn infants. Pediatr Pulmonol 33:368–373, 2002.
29. Miller MJ, Carlo WA, Strohl KP, et al: Effect of maturation on oral breathing in sleeping premature infants. J Pediatr 109:515–519, 1986.
30. Praud JP, Reix P: Upper airways and neonatal respiration, Respir Physiol Neurobiol 149:131–141, 2005.
31. Gaultier C, Denjean A: Developmental anatomy and physiology of the respiratory system. In Taussig LM, Landau LI, editors: Pediatric respiratory medicine, ed 2, St Louis, 2008, Mosby.
32. Ochs M, Nyengaard JR, Jung L, et al: The number of alveoli in the human lung, Am J Respir Crit Care Med 169:120–124, 2004.
33. Zeltner TB, Burri PH: The postnatal development and growth of the human lung. II. Morphology, Respir Physiol 67:269–282, 1987.
34. Burri PH: Structural aspects of postnatal lung development—alveolar formation and growth. Biol Neonate 89:313–322, 2006.
35. Gehr P, Bachofen M, Weibel ER: The normal human lung ultrastructure and morphometric estimation of diffusion capacity. Respir Physiol 32:121–140, 1978.
36. Brown LM, Rannels SR, Rannels DE: Implications of post-pneumonectomy compensatory lung growth in pulmonary physiology and disease, Respir Res 2:340–347, 2001.
37. Hsia CC: Signals and mechanisms of compensatory lung growth. J Appl Physiol 97:1992–1998, 2004.
38. Hsia CC, Johnson RL: Further examination of alveolar septal adaptation to left pneumonectomy in the adult lung, Respir Physiol Neurobiol 151:167–177, 2006.
39. Warburton D, Perin L, Defilippo R, et al: Stem/progenitor cells in lung development, injury repair, and regeneration. Proc Am Thorac Soc 5:703–706, 2008.
40. Hibbert M, Lannigan A, Raven J, et al: Gender differences in lung growth. Pediatr Pulmonol 19:129–134, 1995.
41. Gatzoulis M, Tsiridis E: Chest wall and breast. In Standring S, editor: Gray's anatomy: the anatomic basis of clinical practice, ed 40, St Louis, 2009, Elsevier.
42. De Troyer A: Respiratory muscle function. In Brewis RAL, Corrin B, Gedded DM, et al, editors: Respiratory medicine, London, 1995, WB Saunders.
43. Gatzoulis M, Pepper J: Diaphragm and phrenic nerve. In Standring S, editor: Gray's anatomy: the anatomic basis of clinical practice, ed 40, St Louis, 2009, Elsevier.
44. Polla B, D'Antona G, Bottinelli R, et al: Respiratory muscle fibres: specialisation and plasticity. Thorax 59:808–817, 2004.
45. Celli B: The diaphragm and respiratory muscles. Chest Surg Clin North Am 8:207–224, 1998.
46. Wilson TA, De Troyer A: The two mechanisms of intercostal muscle action on the lung. J Appl Physiol 96:483–488, 2004.
47. DeTroyer A: Mechanics of intercostal space and actions of external and internal intercostal muscles. J Clin Invest 75:850–857, 1985.
48. DeTroyer A, Estenne M: Coordination between ribcage muscles and diaphragm during quiet breathing in humans. J Appl Physiol 57:899–906, 1984.
49. Celli BR: Clinical and physiologic evaluation of respiratory muscle function. Clin Chest Med 10:199–214, 1989.
50. Borley NR: Anterior abdominal wall. In Standring S, editor: Gray's anatomy: the anatomic basis of clinical practice, ed 40, St Louis, 2009, Elsevier.
51. Abe T, Kusuhara N, Yoshimura N, et al: Differential respiratory activity of four abdominal muscles in humans. J Appl Physiol 80:1379–1389, 1996.
52. Iscoe S: Control of abdominal muscles. Prog Neurobiol 56:433–506, 1998.
53. Mier A, Brophy C, Estenne M, et al: Action of the abdominal muscles on the ribcage in humans. J Appl Physiol 58:1438–1443, 1985.
54. Gatzoulis M, Padley S, Shah P, et al: Mediastinum. In Standring S, editor: Gray's anatomy: the anatomic basis of clinical practice, ed 40, St Louis, 2009, Elsevier.
55. Gatzoulis M, Padley S, Shah P, et al: Pleura, lungs and bronchi. In Standring S, editor: Gray's anatomy: the anatomic basis of clinical practice, ed 40, St Louis, 2009, Elsevier.
56. Noppen M. Normal volume and cellular contents of pleural fluid. Curr Opin Pulm Med 7:180–182, 2001.
57. Agostoni E, Zocchi L: Pleural liquid and its exchanges. Respir Physiol Neurobiol 159:311–323, 2007.
58. Weibel ER: What makes a good lung? Swiss Med Wkly 139:375–386, 2009.
59. Lumb AB: The pulmonary circulation. In Lumb AB, editor: Nunn's applied respiratory physiology, Philadelphia, 2010, Elsevier.
60. Murray JF: Pulmonary circulation. In Murray JF, editor: The normal lung: the basis for diagnosis and treatment of pulmonary disease, ed 2, Philadelphia, 1986, WB Saunders.
61. Smith JJ, Kampine JP: Cardiovascular physiology, ed 3, Philadelphia, 1990, Williams & Wilkins.
62. Niden AH, Aviado DM: Effects of pulmonary embolism on the pulmonary circulation with special reference to arteriovenous shunts in the lung. Circ Res 4:67–73, 1956.
63. Halbertsma FJ, Vaneker M, Scheffer GJ, et al: Cytokines and biotrauma in ventilator-induced lung injury: a critical review of the literature. Neth J Med 63:382–392, 2005.
64. McCullagh A, Rosenthal M, Wanner A, et al: The bronchial circulation—worth a closer look: a review of the relationship between the bronchial vasculature and airway inflammation. Pediatr Pulmonol 45:1–13, 2010.
65. Deffebach ME, Charan NB, Lakshminarayan S, et al: The bronchial circulation: small, but a vital attribute of the lung. Am Rev Respir Dis 135:463–481, 1987.
66. Murray JF: Lymphatics and nervous systems. In Murray JF, editor: The normal lung: the basis for diagnosis and treatment of pulmonary disease, ed 2, Philadelphia, 1986, WB Saunders.
67. Fraser RS, Müller NL, Colman N, et al: Fraser and Pare's diagnosis of diseases of the chest, vol 1, ed 4, Philadelphia, 1999, WB Saunders.
68. Drake RE, Dhother S, Oppenlander VM, et al: Lymphatic pump function curves in awake sheep. Am J Physiol 270:R486–R488, 1996.
69. Jordan D: Central nervous pathways and control of the airways. Respir Physiol 125:67–81, 2001.
70. Canning BJ, Fischer A: Neural regulation of airway smooth muscle tone. Respir Physiol 125:113–127, 2001.
71. Widdicombe J: Airway receptors. Respir Physiol 125:3–15, 2001.
72. Rabbette PS, Fletcher ME, Dezateux CA, et al: Hering-Breuer reflex and respiratory system compliance in the first year of life: a longitudinal study. J Appl Physiol 76:650–656, 1994.

73. Coleridge HM, Coleridge JC: Pulmonary reflexes: neural mechanisms of pulmonary defense. Annu Rev Physiol 56:69–91, 1994.
74. Karlsson JA, Sant'Ambrogio G, Widdicombe JG: Afferent neural pathways in cough and reflex bronchoconstriction. J Appl Physiol 65:1007–1023, 1988.
75. Coleridge JCG, Coleridge HM: Afferent vagal C fiber innervation of the lungs and airways and its functional significance. Rev Physiol Biochem Pharmacol 99:1–110, 1984.
76. Kubin L, Alheid GF, Zuperku EJ, et al: Central pathways of pulmonary and lower airway vagal afferents. J Appl Physiol 101:618–627, 2006.
77. Carr MJ, Undem BJ: Bronchopulmonary afferent nerves. Respirology 8:291–301, 2003.
78. Proctor DF: The upper airways: I. nasal physiology and defense of the lung. Am Rev Respir Dis 115:97–129, 1977.
79. Proctor DF: The upper airways: II. the larynx and trachea. Am Rev Respir Dis 115:315–342, 1977.
80. Jafeck B, Jones N: Nose, nasal cavity, and paranasal sinuses. In Standring S, editor: Gray's anatomy: the anatomic basis of clinical practice, ed 40, St Louis, 2009, Elsevier.
81. Wheatey JR, Amis TC: Mechanical properties of the upper airway, Curr Opin Pulm Med 4:363–369, 1998.
82. Standring S: Larynx. In Standring S, editor: Gray's anatomy: the anatomic basis of clinical practice, ed 40, St Louis, 2009, Elsevier.
83. Shaker R, Dodds WJ, Dantas RO, et al: Coordination of deglutitive glottic closure with oropharyngeal swallowing. Gastroenterology 98:1478–1484, 1990.
84. Bannister LH: Anatomy of speech. In Williams PL, editor: Gray's anatomy, London, 1995, Churchill Livingstone.
85. Fisher S, Dubois AE: The lung: physiologic basis of pulmonary function tests, ed 3, St Louis, 1986, Mosby.
86. Engle LA: Gas mixing within the acinus of the lung, J Appl Physiol 54:609–618, 1983.
87. Rhodin JA: Ultrastructure and function of the human tracheal mucosa. Am Rev Respir Dis 93(Suppl):1–15, 1966.
88. Breeze RG, Wheeldon EB: The cells of the pulmonary airways, Am Rev Respir Dis 116:705–777, 1977.
89. Albertine KH, Williams MC, Hyde DM: Anatomy of the lungs. In Mason RJ, Broaddus VC, Murray JF, et al, editors: Murray and Nadel's textbook of respiratory medicine, ed 4, Philadelphia, 2005, WB Saunders.
90. Cutz E, Yeger H, Pan J, et al: Pulmonary neuroendocrine cell system in health and disease. Curr Respir Med Rev 4:174–186, 2008.
91. Schulman ES: The role of mast cells in inflammatory responses in the lung. Crit Rev Immunol 13:35–70, 1993.
92. Fahy JV, Dickey BF: Airway mucus function and dysfunction. N Engl J Med 363:2233–2247, 2010.
93. Rogers DF: Physiology of airway mucus secretion and pathophysiology of hypersecretion. Respir Care 52:1134–1146, 2007.
94. Salathe M: Regulation of mammalian ciliary beating. Annu Rev Physiol 69:401–422, 2007.
95. Reynolds SD, Malkinson AM: Clara cell: progenitor for the bronchiolar epithelium. Int J Biochem Cell Biol 42:1–4, 2010.
96. Haefeli-Bleurer B, Weibel ER: Morphometry of the human pulmonary acinus. Anat Rec 220:401–414, 1988.
97. Johnson D, section editor: Microstructure of trachea, bronchi and lungs. In Standring S, editor: Gray's anatomy: the anatomic basis of clinical practice, ed 39, St Louis, 2005, Elsevier.
98. Crapo JD, Barry BE, Gehr P, et al: Cell number and cell characteristics of the normal human lung. Am Rev Respir Dis 125:740–745, 1982.
99. Tzortzaki EG, Vlachaki E, Siafakas NM: Pulmonary surfactant. Pneumon 4:364–371, 2007.
100. Ikegami M: Surfactant catabolism. Respirology 11:S24–S27, 2006.
101. Fels AO, Cohn ZA: The alveolar macrophage. J Appl Physiol 60:353–369, 1986.
102. Topol M: Collateral respiratory pathways of pulmonary acini in man. Folia Morphol 54:61–66, 1995.
103. Weibel ER: The pathway for oxygen, Cambridge, 1984, Harvard University Press.
104. Dudek SM, Garcia JGN: Cytoskeletal regulation of pulmonary vascular permeability. J Appl Physiol 91:1487–1500, 2001.
105. West JB: Thoughts on the pulmonary blood-gas barrier. Am J Physiol Lung Cell Mol Physiol 285:L501–L513, 2003.
106. Maina JN, West JB: Thin and strong! The bioengineering dilemma in the structural and functional design of the blood-gas barrier. Physiol Rev 85:811–844, 2005.

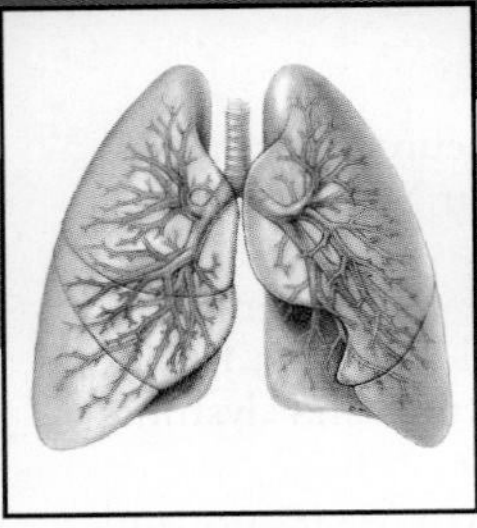

Chapter 9

The Cardiovascular System

NARCISO RODRIGUEZ

CHAPTER OBJECTIVES

After reading this chapter you will be able to:

- Describe the anatomy of the heart and vascular systems.
- State the key characteristics of cardiac tissue.
- Calculate systemic vascular resistance given mean arterial pressure, central venous pressure, and cardiac output.
- Describe how local and central control mechanisms regulate the heart and vascular systems.
- Describe how the cardiovascular system coordinates its functions under normal and abnormal conditions.
- Calculate cardiac output given stroke volume and heart rate.
- Calculate ejection fraction given stroke volume and end-diastolic volume.
- Identify how the electrical and mechanical events of the heart relate to a normal cardiac cycle.

CHAPTER OUTLINE

KEY TERMS

afterload
arteriovenous anastomosis
automaticity
baroreceptors
cardiac output
cardiac tamponade
chemoreceptors
congestive heart failure
contractility
end-diastolic volume (EDV)
end-systolic volume (ESV)
Frank-Starling law
heart rate (HR)
negative feedback loop
negative inotropism
pericardium
positive inotropism
preload
regurgitation
stenosis
stroke volume (SV)
vasoconstriction
vasodilation

FUNCTIONAL ANATOMY

Heart

Anatomy of the Heart

The heart is a hollow, four-chambered muscular organ approximately the size of a fist. It is positioned obliquely in the middle compartment of the mediastinum of the chest, just behind the sternum (Figure 9-1). Approximately two-thirds of the heart lies to the left of the midline of the sternum between the points of attachment of the second through the sixth ribs. The apex of the heart is formed by the tip of the left ventricle and lies just above the diaphragm at the level of the fifth intercostal space to the left. The base of the heart is formed by the atria and projects to the patient's right lying just below the second rib. It is level with the second rib below the sternum. Posteriorly, the heart rests on the bodies of the fifth to the eighth thoracic vertebrae. Because of its position between the sternum and the spine, rhythmic compression of the heart can maintain blood flow during cardiopulmonary resuscitation.

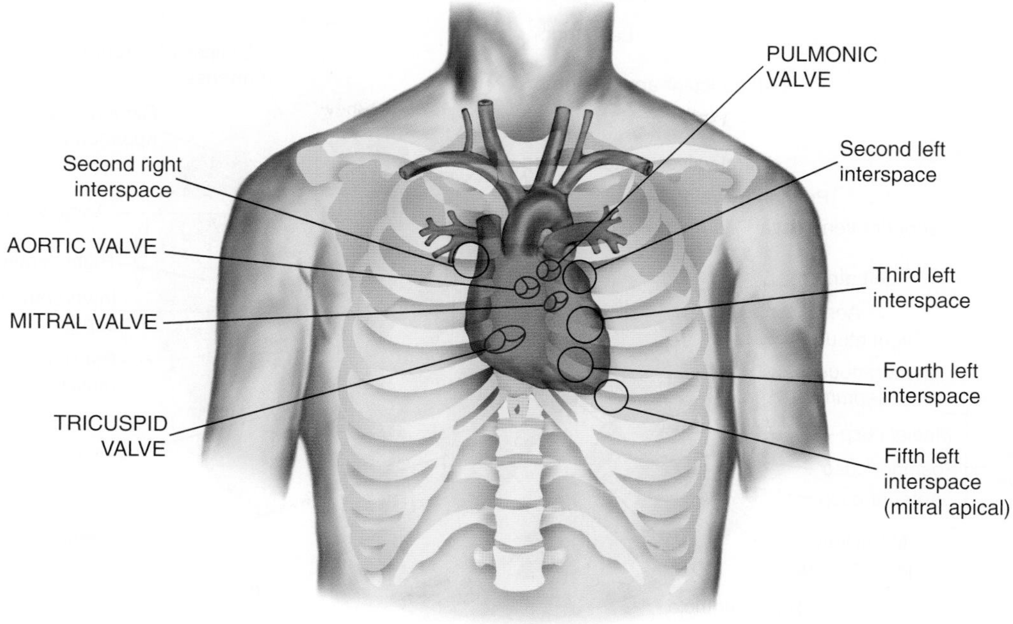

FIGURE 9-1 Anterior view of the thorax showing the position of the heart in relationship to the ribs, sternum, diaphragm, and position of the heart valves. (From Seidel HM, et al: Mosby's guide to physical examination, ed 2, St Louis, 1991, Mosby.)

Externally, surface grooves called *sulci* mark the boundaries of the heart chambers. Compared with the ventricles, the atria are small, thin-walled chambers that contribute little to the total pumping activity of the heart.

The heart is enclosed in a double-walled sac called the **pericardium.** The outer fibrous layer consists of tough connective tissue. The inner serous layer is thinner and more delicate. The structure of the pericardium can be summarized as follows:

1. *Fibrous pericardium:* Tough, loose-fitting, and inelastic sac surrounding the heart
2. *Serous pericardium:* Consisting of two layers:
   a. *Parietal layer:* Inner lining of the fibrous pericardium
   b. *Visceral layer or epicardium:* Covering the outer surface of the heart and great vessels

A thin layer of fluid called the *pericardial fluid* separates the two layers of the serous pericardium. This layer of fluid helps minimize friction as the heart contracts and expands within the pericardium. Inflammation of the pericardium results in a clinical condition called *pericarditis*. An abnormal amount of fluid can accumulate between the layers resulting in a *pericardial effusion*. A large pericardial effusion may affect the pumping function of the heart resulting in a **cardiac tamponade.** A cardiac tamponade compresses the heart muscle leading to a serious decrease in blood flow to the body, which ultimately may lead to shock and death.

The heart wall consists of three layers: (1) outer epicardium, (2) middle myocardium, and (3) inner endocardium. The myocardium composes the bulk of the heart muscle and consists of bands of involuntary striated muscle fibers. The contraction of these muscle fibers creates the pumplike action needed to move blood throughout the body.

Support for the four interior chambers and valves of the heart is provided by four atrioventricular rings, which form a fibrous "skeleton." Each ring is composed of dense connective tissue termed *anulus fibrosus cordis.* This connective tissue, besides providing an anchoring structure for the heart valves, electrically isolates the atria from the ventricle. No impulses can be transmitted through the heart tissue from the atria to the ventricles.

The two atrial chambers are thin-walled "cups" of myocardial tissue, separated by an interatrial septum. On the right side of the interatrial septum is an oval depression called the *fossa ovalis cordis,* which is the remnant of the fetal foramen ovale, the shunt that allowed blood to enter the left atrium from the right atrium before birth. In addition, each atrium has an appendage, or auricle, the function of which is unknown. In the presence of cardiac dysrhythmias, blood flow can become stagnant on these appendages leading to the formation of thrombi.

The two lower heart chambers, or ventricles, make up the bulk of the heart's muscle mass and do most of the pumping that circulates the blood (Figure 9-2). The mass of the left ventricle is normally about two-thirds larger than the mass of the right ventricle and has a spherical appearance when viewed in anteroposterior cross section. The right ventricle is thin-walled and oblong, forming a pocket-like attachment to the left ventricle. Because of this relationship, contraction of the left ventricle pulls in the

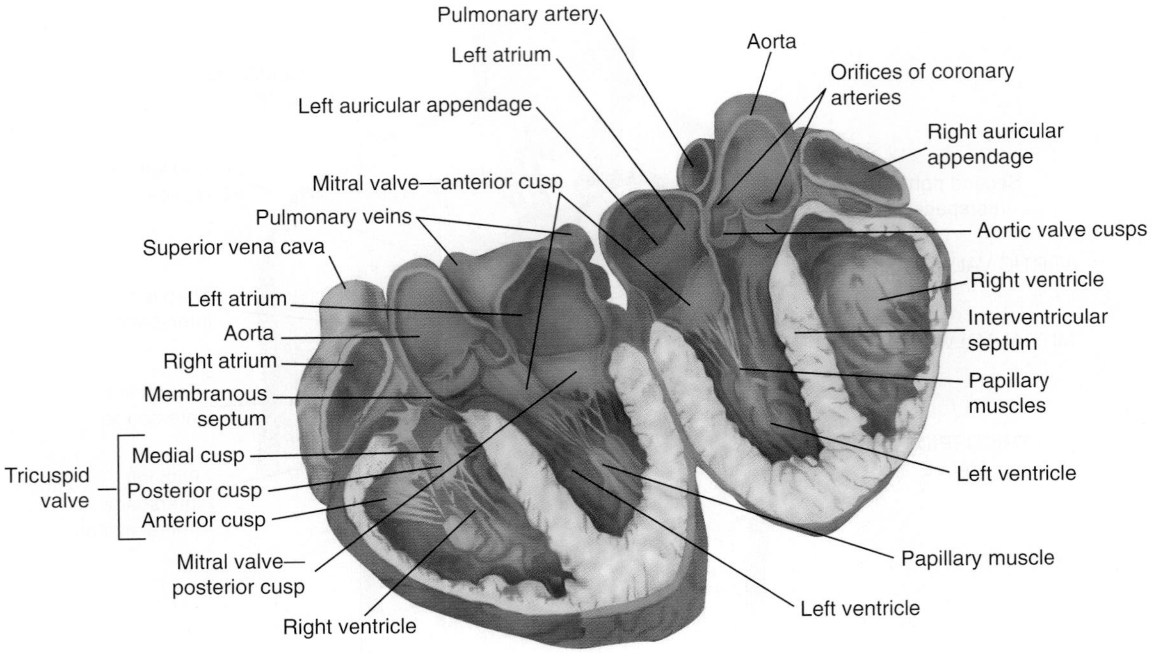

FIGURE 9-2 Drawing of the heart split perpendicular to the interventricular septum to illustrate anatomic relationships of the heart. (From Berne RM, Levy MN, editors: Physiology, ed 5, St Louis, 2004, Mosby.)

right ventricular wall, aiding its contraction. The effect, termed *left ventricular aid,* explains why some forms of right ventricular failure are less harmful than might be expected. The right and left ventricles are separated by a muscle wall termed the *interventricular septum* (see Figure 9-2).

RULE OF THUMB

Left ventricular contraction aids right ventricular contraction.

The valves of the heart are flaps of fibrous tissue firmly anchored to the *anulus fibrosus cordis* (Figure 9-3). Because they are located between the atria and ventricles, they are called atrioventricular valves. The valve between the right atrium and ventricle is called the *tricuspid valve.* The valve between the left atrium and ventricle is the *bicuspid,* or *mitral, valve.* The atrioventricular valves close during systole (contraction of the ventricles), preventing backflow of blood into the atria. Closure of these valves provides a critical period of isovolemic contraction, during which chamber pressures quickly increase just before ejection of the blood.

The free ends of the atrioventricular valves are anchored to papillary muscles of the endocardium by the *chordae tendineae cordis* (see Figure 9-2). During systole, papillary muscle contraction prevents the atrioventricular valves from swinging upward into the atria. Damage to either the chordae tendineae cordis or the papillary muscles can impair function of the atrioventricular valves and cause leakage upward into the atria.

Common valve problems include regurgitation and stenosis. **Regurgitation** is the backflow of blood through an incompetent or a damaged valve. **Stenosis** is a pathologic narrowing or constriction of a valve outlet, which causes increased pressure in the proximal chamber and vessels. Both conditions affect cardiac performance. In mitral stenosis, high pressures in the left atrium back up into the pulmonary circulation. This can cause pulmonary edema and a diastolic murmur (see Chapter 15).

A set of semilunar valves separates the ventricles from their arterial outflow tracts, the pulmonary artery and the aorta (see Figure 9-3). Consisting of three half-moon–shaped cusps attached to the arterial wall, these valves prevent backflow of blood into the ventricles during diastole (or when the chambers of the heart fill with blood). The pulmonary valve is at the outflow tract of the right ventricle. During the cardiac contraction (systole), blood is ejected out of the heart and to the lungs through the right valves and to the body through the left valves. Similar to the atrioventricular valves, the semilunar valves can leak (regurgitation) or become obstructed (stenosis).

Similar to the lungs, the heart has its own circulatory system, which is called the *coronary circulation.* However, in contrast to the lungs, the heart has a high metabolic rate, which requires more blood flow per gram of tissue weight than any other organ except the kidney. To meet these needs, the coronary circulation provides an extensive network of branches to all myocardial tissue (Figure 9-4).

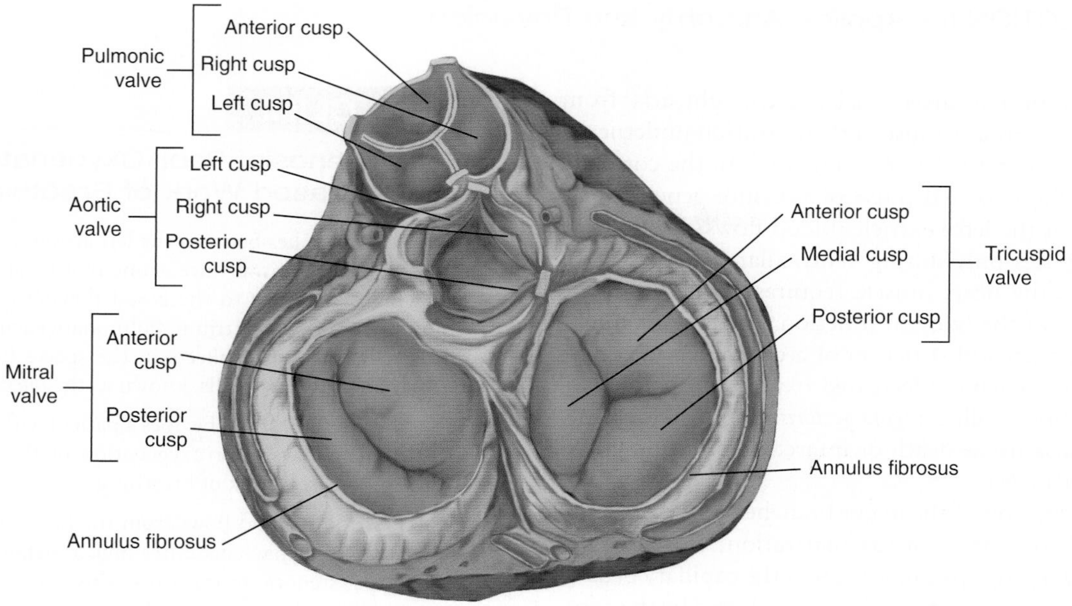

FIGURE 9-3 Four cardiac valves as viewed from the base of the heart. Note how the leaflets overlap in the closed valves.

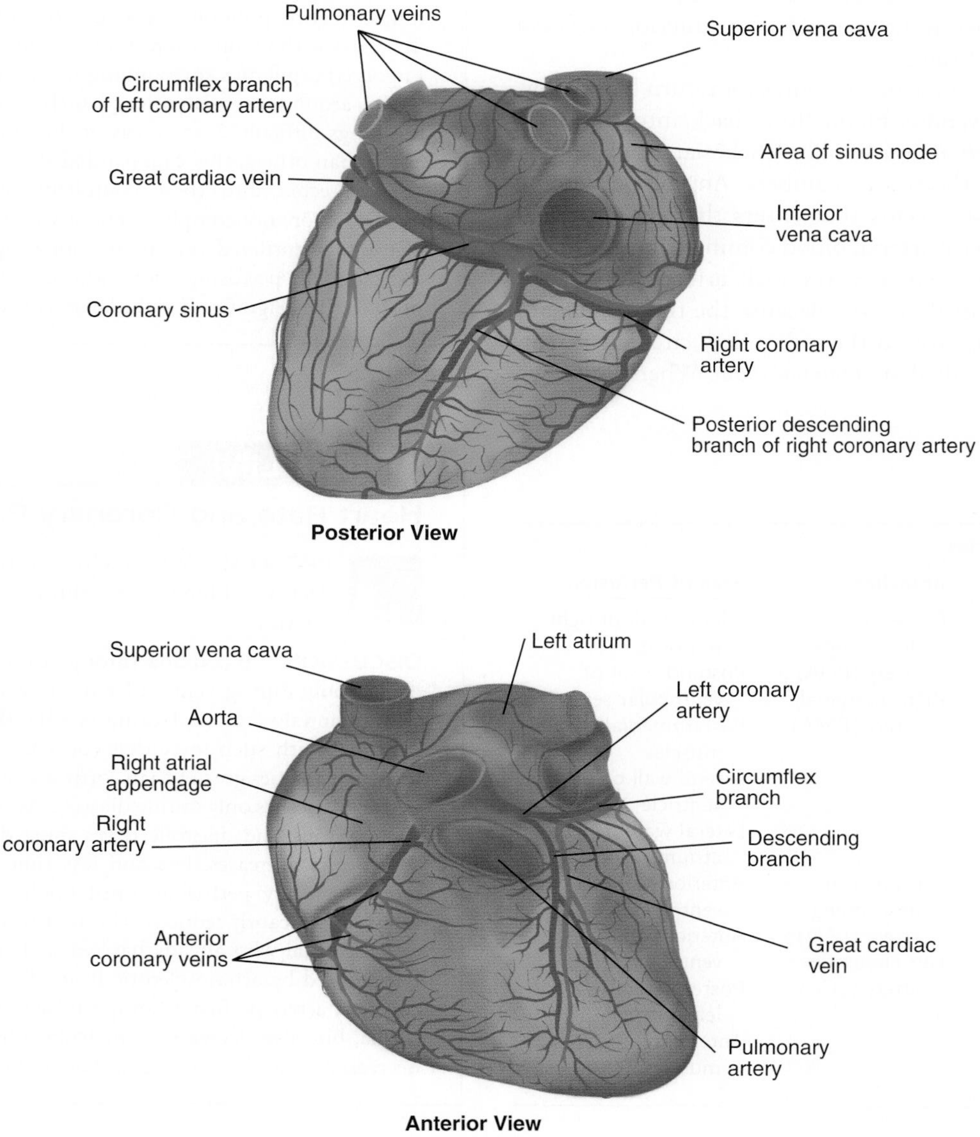

FIGURE 9-4 Coronary circulation as seen on anterior and posterior surfaces of the heart, illustrating the location and distribution of the principal coronary vessels.

Two main coronary arteries, a left and a right, arise from the root of the aorta. Because of their position underneath the aortic semilunar valves (see Figure 9-4), the coronary arteries get the maximal pulse of pressure generated by contraction of the left ventricle. Blood flows through the coronary arteries only during ventricular diastole (relaxation). A healthy heart muscle requires about $\frac{1}{20}$ of the blood supply of the body to function properly. As might be expected, partial obstruction of a coronary artery may lead to tissue ischemia (decreased oxygen [O_2] supply), a clinical condition called *angina pectoris*. Complete obstruction may cause tissue death or infarct, a condition called *myocardial infarction*.

For a description of the major branches of the coronary arteries and their areas of vascularization, see Table 9-1 and Figure 9-4. After passing through the capillary beds of the myocardium, the venous blood is collected by the coronary veins that closely parallel the arteries (see Figure 9-4). These veins gather together into a large vessel called the *coronary sinus,* which passes left to right across the posterior surface of the heart. The coronary sinus empties into the right atrium between the opening of the inferior vena cava and the tricuspid valve.

In addition to these major routes for return blood flow, some coronary venous blood flows back into the heart through the *thebesian veins.* The thebesian veins empty directly into all the heart chambers. Any blood coming from the thebesian veins that enters the left atrium or ventricle mixes with arterial blood coming from the lungs. Whenever venous blood mixes with arterial blood, the overall O_2 content decreases. Because the thebesian veins bypass, or shunt, around the pulmonary circulation, this phenomenon is called an *anatomic shunt.* When combined

TABLE 9-1

Coronary Arteries

Coronary Artery	Branches	Area of Perfusion
Right coronary artery	Posterior descending artery (PDA) Right marginal artery (RMA)	Inferior wall of right ventricle Posterior wall of ventricular septum Posteromedial papillary muscles Lateral wall of right ventricle Lateral wall of right atrium
Left coronary artery	Left anterior descending artery (LAD) Left circumflex artery (LCA)	Anterior wall of both ventricles Anterior wall of ventricular septum Posterolateral wall of left ventricle Anterolateral papillary muscles

MINI CLINI

Mitral Stenosis, Poor Oxygenation, and Increased Work of Breathing

The mitral valve lies between the left atrium and left ventricle. A stenotic mitral valve is one that is narrowed and offers high resistance to the blood flowing into the left ventricle from the left atrium. Pulmonary edema is a condition in which fluid collects in the spaces between the alveolar and capillary walls, known as the *interstitial spaces.*

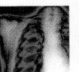

PROBLEM: Why does a patient with mitral stenosis have poor oxygenation of the blood and increased work of breathing?

DISCUSSION: Blood flows from the lungs into the left atrium, where it may encounter high resistance through a narrowed, stenotic mitral valve; this causes high pressure to build in the left atrium. Pressure in the pulmonary veins and eventually in the pulmonary capillaries also increases. This high pressure within the capillaries engorges them and forces fluid components of the blood plasma out of the vessels into the interstitial spaces of the lungs, creating pulmonary edema. This collection of fluid interferes with O_2 diffusion from the lung into the blood. Engorged capillaries surrounding the alveoli create a stiff "web" around each alveolus, which makes expanding the lungs difficult. Some areas of the lung expand more easily than others; this causes inhaled air to be preferentially directed into these compliant regions, whereas "stiffer," more noncompliant regions are underventilated. The underventilated regions do not properly oxygenate the blood as perfusing them. Mitral stenosis, a cardiac problem, has significant pulmonary consequences.

MINI CLINI

Heart Rate and Coronary Perfusion

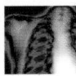

PROBLEM: Why might an extremely high HR decrease blood flow through the coronary arteries?

DISCUSSION: Blood flow through the coronary arteries occurs only during ventricular diastole when the aortic semilunar valves close. During systole, the myocardium contracts with such force that coronary artery pressures increase to values greater than aortic pressures. Myocardial perfusion occurs only during diastole. As the HR increases, both systolic and diastolic times must decrease. As diastolic time decreases, less and less time is available for coronary artery perfusion, until finally coronary blood flow is significantly reduced. This is critically important in an individual who already has reduced coronary circulation caused by arteriosclerotic heart disease. Not only is coronary artery perfusion compromised with severe tachycardia, but also decreased ventricular filling time causes decreased SV and decreased cardiac output.

with a similar bypass in the bronchial circulation (see Chapter 8), these normal anatomic shunts account for approximately 2% to 3% of the total cardiac output.

Properties of the Heart Muscle

The performance of the heart as a pump depends on its ability to (1) initiate and conduct electrical impulses and to (2) contract synchronously the heart's muscle fibers quickly and efficiently. These actions are possible only because myocardial tissue possesses four key properties:

- Excitability
- Inherent rhythmicity
- Conductivity
- Contractility

Excitability is the ability of cells to respond to electrical, chemical, or mechanical stimulation. The myocardial property of *excitability* is the same as that exhibited by other muscles and tissues. Electrolyte imbalances and certain drugs can increase myocardial excitability and produce abnormalities in electrical conduction that may lead to cardiac arrhythmias.

Inherent rhythmicity, or **automaticity,** is the unique ability of the cardiac muscle to initiate a spontaneous electrical impulse. Although such impulses can arise from anywhere in the cardiac tissue, this ability is highly developed in specialized areas called *heart pacemaker,* or *nodal tissues.* The sinoatrial node and the atrioventricular node are good examples of specialized heart tissues that are designed to initiate electrical impulses (see Chapter 17). An electrical impulse from any source other than a normal heart pacemaker is considered abnormal and represents one of the many causes of *cardiac arrhythmias.*

Conductivity is the ability of myocardial tissue to spread, or radiate, electrical impulses. This property is similar to that of smooth muscle in that it allows the myocardium to contract without direct neural innervation (as required by skeletal muscle). The rate at which electrical impulses spread throughout the myocardium is extremely variable. These differences in conduction velocity are needed to ensure synchronous contraction of the cardiac chambers. Abnormal conductivity can affect the timing of chamber contractions and decrease cardiac efficiency.

Contractility, in response to an electrical impulse, is the primary function of the myocardium. In contrast to the contractions of other muscle tissues, however, cardiac contractions cannot be sustained or tetanized because myocardial tissue exhibits a prolonged period of inexcitability after contraction. The period during which the myocardium cannot be stimulated is called the *refractory period,* and it lasts approximately 250 msec, nearly as long as the heart contraction or systole.

Microanatomy of the Heart Muscle

Understanding how cardiac muscle contracts requires knowledge of the microanatomy of the heart. In contrast to the long, cylindrical, multinucleated skeletal muscle fibers, cardiac cells are short, fat, branched, and interconnected. As seen under the microscope, myocardial muscle fibers are approximately 15 μm wide × 100 μm long. Individual fibers are enclosed in a membrane called the *sarcolemma,* which is surrounded by a rich capillary network (Figure 9-5).

Cardiac fibers are separated by irregular transverse thickenings of the sarcolemma called *intercalated discs.* These discs provide structural support and aid in electrical conduction between fibers. Each muscle fiber consists of many smaller units called *myofibrils,* which contain repeated structures approximately 2 μm in size termed *sarcomeres.* Within the sarcomeres are contractile protein filaments responsible for shortening the myocardium during systole. These proteins are of two types: thick filaments composed mainly of myosin and thin filaments composed mostly of actin.

According to the sliding filament theory, myocardial cells contract when actin and myosin combine to form reversible bridges between these thick and thin filaments. These bridges cause filaments to slide over one another, shortening the sarcomere and muscle fibers as a whole.

In principle, the tension developed during myocardial contraction is directly proportional to the number of cross-bridges between the actin and myosin filaments. The number of cross-bridges is directly proportional to the length of the sarcomere. This principle underlies Starling's law of the heart, also known as the **Frank-Starling law.** According to this law, the more a cardiac fiber is stretched, the greater the tension it generates when contracted.

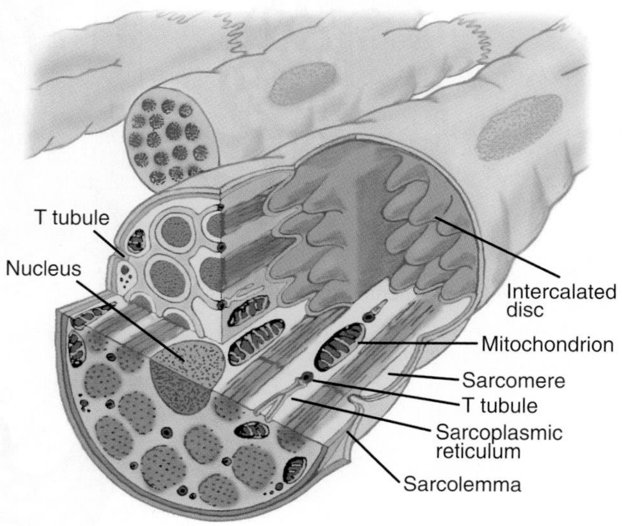

FIGURE 9-5 Major structural features of cardiac muscle fibers. Note the presence of intercalated discs connecting successive sarcomeres. (Modified from Moffett DF, Moffett SB, Schauf CL: Human physiology: foundations and frontiers, ed 2, St Louis, 1993, Mosby.)

The Frank-Starling law holds true up to a sarcomere length of 2.2 μm. Beyond this length, the actin and myosin filaments become partially disengaged, and fewer cross-bridges can be formed. With fewer cross-bridges, the overall tension developed during contraction is less. This relationship is extremely important and is explored later in the discussion of the heart as a pump.

Vascular System

The vascular system has two major subdivisions: the *systemic vasculature* and the *pulmonary vasculature*. The systemic vasculature begins with the aorta on the left ventricle and ends in the right atrium. The pulmonary vasculature begins with the pulmonary trunk out of the right ventricle and ends in the left atrium. The blood flow to and from the heart is depicted in Figure 9-6.

Venous, or deoxygenated, blood from the head and upper extremities enters the right atrium from the superior vena cava, and blood from the lower body enters from the inferior vena cava. From the right atrium, blood flows through the tricuspid valve into the right ventricle. The right ventricle pumps the blood through the pulmonary valve, into the pulmonary arteries, and on to the lungs.

Arterial, or oxygenated, blood returns to the left atrium through the pulmonary veins. The left atrium pumps blood through the mitral valve into the left ventricle. The blood is pumped through the aortic valve and into the aorta. From the aorta, the blood flows out to the tissues of the upper and lower body. From the capillary network of the various body tissues, the deoxygenated venous blood returns to the right ventricle through the superior and inferior venae cavae.

Systemic Vasculature

The systemic vasculature has three major components: (1) arterial system, (2) capillary system, and (3) venous system. These vessels regulate not only the amount of

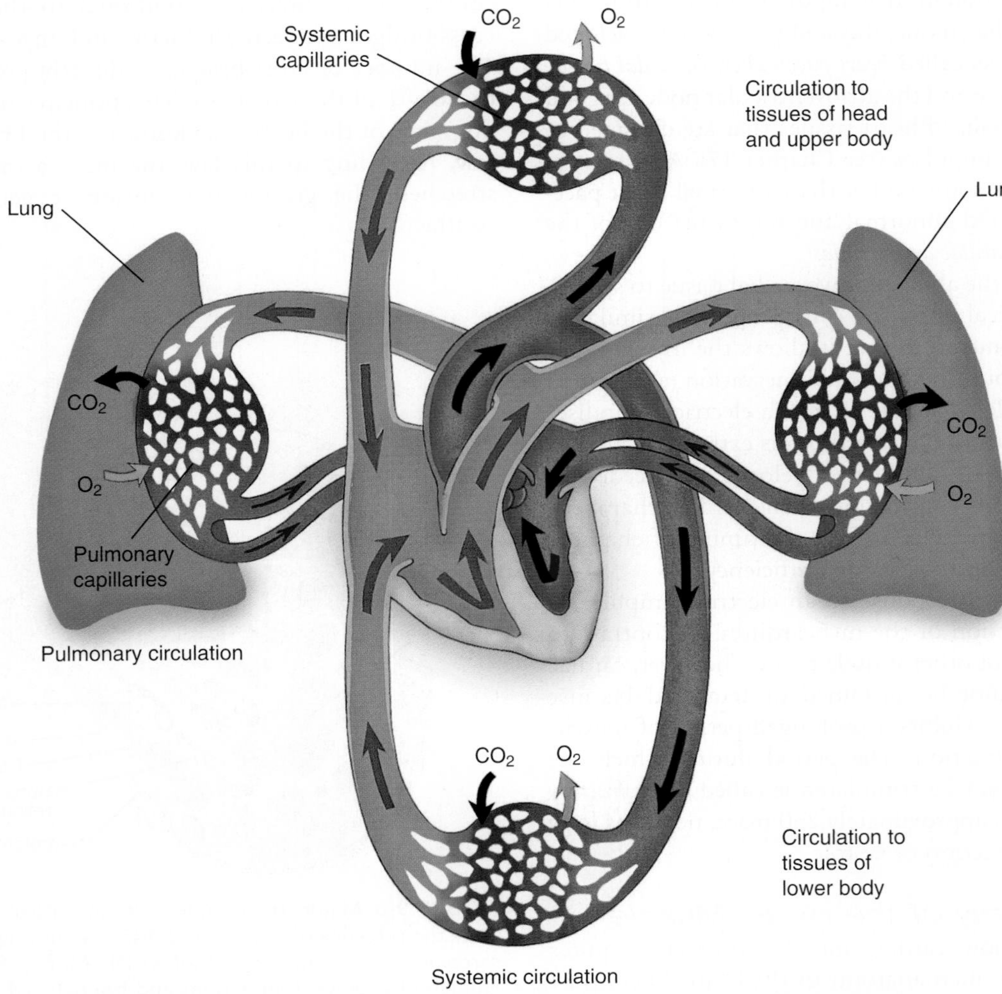

FIGURE 9-6 Generalized circulatory pathways between the heart, lung, and extremities.

blood flow per minute (cardiac output) but also the distribution of blood to organs and tissues. To achieve this function, each component has a unique structure and plays a different role in the circulatory system as a whole.

The *arterial system* consists of large, highly elastic, low-resistance arteries and small, muscular arterioles of varying resistance. With their high elasticity, the large arteries help transmit and maintain the head of pressure generated by the heart. Together, the large arteries are called *conductance vessels*. Just as faucets control the flow of water into a sink, the smaller arterioles control blood flow into the capillaries. Arterioles provide this control by varying their flow resistance. Arterioles play a major role in the distribution and regulation of blood pressure and are referred to as *resistance vessels*.

The vast *capillary system*, or microcirculation, maintains a constant exchange of nutrients and waste products for the cells and tissues of the body. For this reason, the capillaries are commonly referred to as *exchange vessels*. Figure 9-7 shows the structure of a typical capillary network. Blood flows into the network by an arteriole and out through a venule. A direct communication between these vessels is called an **arteriovenous anastomosis.** When open, an arteriovenous anastomosis allows arterial blood to shunt around the capillary bed and flow directly into the venules. Downstream from the arteriovenous anastomosis, the arteriole divides into terminal arterioles, which branch further into thoroughfare channels and true capillaries.

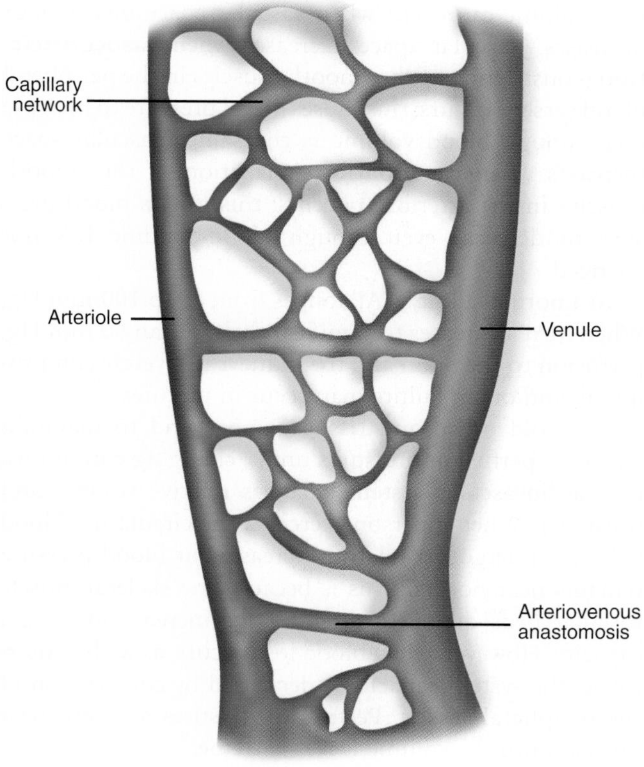

FIGURE 9-7 Components of a microcirculatory network. Blood flows from arteriolar to venular vessels through a network of capillaries. Opening of the arteriovenous anastomosis directs blood flow out of the capillary network. (Modified from Stevens A, Lowe J: Human histology, ed 2, St Louis, 1997, Mosby.)

Capillaries have smooth muscle rings at their proximal ends, called *precapillary sphincters*. Contraction of these sphincters decreases blood flow in that area, whereas relaxation increases perfusion. In combination, these various channels, sphincters, and bypasses allow precise control over the direction and amount of blood flow to a given area of tissue.

The *venous system* consists of small, expandable venules and veins and larger, more elastic veins. Besides conducting blood back to the heart, these vessels act as a reservoir for the circulatory system. At any given time, the veins and venules hold approximately three-fourths of the body's total blood volume. The volume of blood held in this reservoir can be rapidly changed as needed simply by altering the tone of these vessels. By quickly changing its holding capacity, the venous system can match the volume of circulating blood to that needed to maintain adequate tissue perfusion. The components of the venous system, especially the small, expandable venules and veins, are termed *capacitance vessels*.

The venous system must overcome gravity to return blood to the heart. The following four mechanisms combine to aid venous return to the heart: (1) sympathetic venous tone; (2) skeletal muscle pumping, or "milking" (combined with venous one-way valves); (3) cardiac suction; and (4) thoracic pressure differences caused by respiratory efforts.

The last mechanism is often called the *thoracic pump*. As an aid to venous return, the thoracic pump is particularly important to respiratory therapists (RTs) because artificial ventilation with positive pressure reverses normal thoracic pressure gradients. Positive pressure ventilation impedes, rather than assists, venous return. As long as blood volume, cardiac function, and vasomotor tone are adequate, positive pressure ventilation has a minimal effect on venous return. Patients who are hypovolemic or in cardiac failure are vulnerable to a reduction in cardiac output when positive pressure ventilation is applied to the lungs.

Although the heart is a single organ, it functions as two separate pumps. The right side of the heart generates a pressure of approximately 25 mm Hg to drive blood through the low-resistance, low-pressure pulmonary circulation. The left side of the heart normally generates pressures of about 120 mm Hg to propel blood through the higher pressure, high-resistance systemic circulation.

Vascular Resistance

Similar to the movement of any fluid through tubes, blood flow through the vascular system is opposed by frictional forces (based on Poiseuille's law). The sum of all frictional forces opposing blood flow through the systemic circulation is called *systemic vascular resistance (SVR)*. SVR must equal the difference in pressure between the beginning and the end of the circuit, divided by the flow. The beginning pressure for the systemic circulation is the mean aortic pressure; ending pressure equals right atrial pressure or *central venous pressure (CVP)*. Flow for the system as a whole equals the cardiac output. SVR can be calculated by the following formula:

$$\text{SVR} = \frac{\text{Mean aortic pressure} - \text{Right atrial pressure}}{\text{Cardiac output}}$$

Given a normal mean aortic pressure of 90 mm Hg, a mean right atrial pressure of approximately 4 mm Hg, and a normal cardiac output of 5 L/min, normal SVR is computed as follows:

$$\text{SVR} = \frac{90\text{ mm Hg} - 4\text{ mm Hg}}{5\text{ L/min}}$$
$$= 17.2\text{ mm Hg/L/min*}$$

The same concepts can be used to compute flow resistance in the pulmonary circulation. Beginning pressure for the pulmonary circulation is the mean pulmonary artery pressure; ending pressure equals left atrial pressure. Flow for the pulmonary circulation is the same as it is for the systemic system, which equals the cardiac output. *Pulmonary vascular resistance (PVR)* can be calculated by using the following formula:

$$\text{PVR} = \frac{\text{Mean pulmonary artery pressure} - \text{Left atrial pressure}}{\text{Cardiac output}}$$

Given a normal mean pulmonary artery pressure of approximately 16 mm Hg and a normal mean left atrial pressure of 8 mm Hg, normal PVR is computed as follows:

$$\text{PVR} = \frac{16\text{ mm Hg} - 8\text{ mm Hg}}{5\text{ L/min}}$$
$$= 1.6\text{ mm Hg/L/min*}$$

Resistance to blood flow in the pulmonary circulation is normally much less than it is in the systemic circulation. The pulmonary vasculature is characterized as a low-pressure, low-resistance circulation.

Determinants of Blood Pressure

A healthy cardiovascular system maintains sufficient pressure to propel blood throughout the body. The first priority of the cardiovascular system is to keep perfusion pressures to tissues and organs normal, even under changing conditions. If the equation for computing SVR is rearranged by deleting the normally low atrial pressure, the average blood pressure in the circulation is directly related to both cardiac output and flow resistance:

$$\text{Mean arterial pressure (MAP)}$$
$$= \text{Cardiac output} \times \text{Vascular resistance}$$

With a constant rate and force of cardiac contractions, cardiac output (blood flow per minute) is approximately equal to the circulating blood volume. Under similar conditions, vascular resistance varies inversely with the size of the blood vessels (i.e., the capacity of the vascular system). All else being constant, MAP is directly related to the volume of blood in the vascular system and inversely related to its capacity:

$$\text{MAP} = \frac{\text{Volume}}{\text{Capacity}}$$

Based on this relationship, MAP is regulated by the following: changing the volume of circulating blood, changing the capacity of the vascular system, or changing both. Volume changes can reflect absolute changes in total blood volume, such as changes resulting from hemorrhagic shock or blood transfusion. Alternatively, changes in "relative" volume can occur when vascular space increases or decreases. Vascular space decreases when **vasoconstriction** (constriction of the smooth muscles in the peripheral blood vessels) occurs; this causes blood pressure to increase even though blood volume is the same. Vascular space increases when **vasodilation** (relaxation of the smooth muscles in the arterioles) occurs; this causes blood pressure to decrease even though blood volume has not changed.

In a normal adult, MAP ranges from 80 to 100 mm Hg. When MAP decreases to significantly less than 60 mm Hg, perfusion to the brain and the kidneys is severely compromised, and organ failure may occur in minutes.

To avoid organ and tissue damage and to maintain adequate perfusion pressures under changing conditions, the cardiovascular system balances relative volume and resistance. When a person exercises, the circulating blood volume undergoes a relative increase, but blood pressure remains near normal; this is because the skeletal muscle vascular beds dilate, causing a large increase in system capacity. However, when blood loss occurs, as with hemorrhage, the system capacity is decreased by constriction of the peripheral vessels. Perfusion pressures are kept near normal until the volume loss is extreme.

Regulation of blood flow and pressure is much more complex than is suggested by these simplified equations. Cardiovascular control is achieved by a complex array of integrated functions. Some of these functions are explained subsequently.

*Multiply by 80 to convert to dynes-sec/cm^5.

CONTROL OF THE CARDIOVASCULAR SYSTEM

The cardiovascular system is responsible for transporting metabolites to and from the tissues under various conditions and demands. It must act in a highly coordinated fashion. Coordination is achieved by integrating the functions of the heart and vascular system. The goal is to maintain adequate perfusion to all tissues according to their needs.

The cardiovascular system regulates blood flow mainly by altering the capacity of the vasculature and the volume of blood it holds. The heart plays only a secondary role in regulating blood flow. In essence, the vascular system tells the heart how much blood it needs, rather than the heart dictating what volume of blood the vascular system will receive.

These integrated functions involve local and central neural control mechanisms. Local, or *intrinsic,* controls operate independently, without *central nervous system* control. Intrinsic control alters perfusion under normal conditions to meet metabolic needs. Central, or *extrinsic,* control involves both the central nervous system and circulating *humoral agents.* Extrinsic control mechanisms maintain a basal level of vascular tone. However, central control mechanisms take over when the competing needs of local vascular beds must be coordinated. Knowledge of vascular regulatory mechanisms and factors controlling cardiac output is essential to understanding how the cardiovascular system responds under both normal and abnormal conditions.

Regulation of Peripheral Vasculature

A basal level of vascular muscle tone is normally maintained throughout the vascular system at all times. Basal muscle tone must be present to allow for effective regulation. If blood vessels remained in a completely relaxed state, further dilation would be impossible, and local increases in perfusion could not occur.

Local vascular tone is maintained by the smooth muscle of the precapillary sphincters of the microcirculation and can function independently of neural control at the local tissue level according to metabolic needs. Central control of vasomotor tone involves either direct central nervous system innervation or circulation hormones. Central control mainly affects the high-resistance arterioles and capacitance veins.

Local Control

Local regulation of tissue blood flow includes both myogenic and metabolic control mechanisms. *Myogenic control* involves the relationship between vascular smooth muscle tone and perfusion pressure. Myogenic control ensures relatively constant flows to the capillary beds despite changes in perfusion pressures.

Metabolic control involves the relationship between vascular smooth muscle tone and the level of local cellular metabolites. High amounts of carbon dioxide (CO_2) or lactic acid, low pH levels, low partial pressures of O_2, histamines (released during inflammatory response), endothelium-derived relaxing factor, and some prostaglandins all cause relaxation of the smooth muscle and vasodilation, increasing flow to the affected area.

The influence of myogenic and metabolic control mechanisms varies in different organ systems. The brain is the most sensitive to changes in the local metabolite levels, particularly CO_2 and pH. In contrast, the heart shows a strong response to both myogenic and metabolic factors.

Central Control

Central control of blood flow is achieved primarily by the sympathetic division of the autonomic nervous system. The level of central control varies among organs and tissues. Although skeletal muscle and skin are mainly regulated by central control, the brain also is minimally regulated by this mechanism.

Smooth muscle contraction and increased flow resistance are mostly caused by adrenergic stimulation and the release of norepinephrine. Smooth muscle relaxation and vessel dilation occur as a result of stimulation of either *cholinergic* or specialized *beta-adrenergic* receptors. Although the contractile response is distributed throughout the entire vascular system, dilation response appears to be limited to the precapillary vessels. In addition to the sympathetic control, blood flow through the large veins can also be affected by abdominal and intrathoracic pressure changes.

Regulation of Cardiac Output

The heart, similar to the vascular system, is regulated by both intrinsic and extrinsic factors. These mechanisms act together, along with vascular control, to ensure that the output of the heart matches the different needs of the tissues.

The total amount of blood pumped by the heart per minute is called the **cardiac output.** Cardiac output is simply the product of the *heart rate (HR)* and the volume ejected by the left ventricle on each contraction, or **stroke volume (SV):**

$$\text{Cardiac output} = \text{HR} \times \text{SV}$$

A normal resting cardiac output of approximately 5 L/min can be calculated by substituting a normal HR (70 contractions/min) and SV (75 mL, or 0.075 L, per contraction):

$$\text{Cardiac output} = 70\ \text{beats/min} \times 0.075\ \text{L/beat} = 5.25\ \text{L/min}$$

This is a hypothetical average because actual cardiac output varies considerably in health and disease states and according to a subject's sex, height, and weight.

Regardless of an individual's state of health or disease, a change in cardiac output must involve a change in SV, a

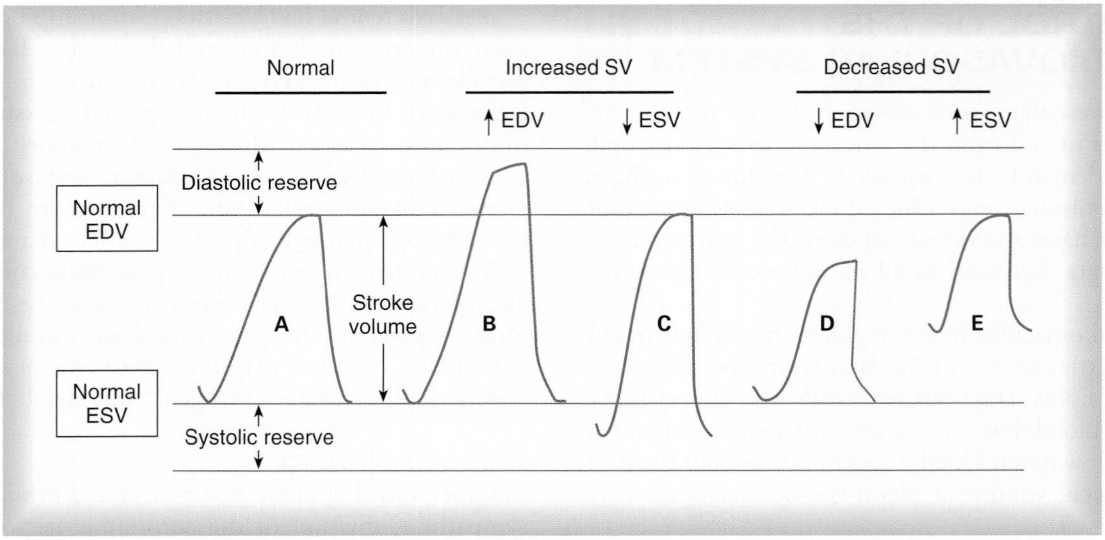

FIGURE 9-8 Relationship between SV, EDV, and ESV. Normal relationship between EDV, ESV, and SV *(A)*; increased SV resulting from increased EDV *(B)*; increased SV resulting from decreased ESV *(C)*; decreased SV resulting from decreased EDV (hypovolemia) *(D)*; and decreased SV resulting from increased ESV (poor contractility) *(E)*.

change in HR, or both. SV is affected primarily by intrinsic control of three factors: (1) preload, (2) afterload, and (3) contractility (all three factors are discussed subsequently). HR is affected primarily by extrinsic or central control mechanisms.

Changes in Stroke Volume

SV is the volume of blood ejected by the left ventricle during each contraction, or systole. The heart does not eject all of the blood it contains during systole. Instead, a small volume, called the **end-systolic volume (ESV),** remains behind in the ventricles. During the resting phase, or diastole, the ventricles fill to a volume called the **end-diastolic volume (EDV).**

SV equals the difference between the EDV and the ESV:

$$SV = EDV - ESV$$

In a healthy man at rest, the EDV ranges from 110 to 120 mL. Given a normal SV of approximately 70 mL, a normal ejection fraction (EF), or proportion of the EDV ejected on each stroke, can be calculated as follows:

$$\begin{aligned} EF &= \frac{SV}{EDV} \\ &= \frac{70\ \text{ml}}{110\ \text{ml}} \\ &= 0.64 \text{ or } 64\% \end{aligned}$$

On each contraction, a healthy heart ejects approximately two-thirds of its stored volume. Decreases in EF are normally associated with a weakened myocardium (heart failure) or decreased contractility or both. When the EF decreases to 30% or less, a person's exercise tolerance becomes severely limited.

As shown in Figure 9-8, an increase in SV occurs when either the EDV increases or the ESV decreases. Conversely, a decrease in SV occurs when either the EDV decreases or the ESV increases. This relationship is key to understanding regulation of cardiac output.

The heart's ability to change SV solely according to the EDV is an intrinsic regulatory mechanism based on the Frank-Starling law. Because the EDV corresponds to the initial stretch, or tension, placed on the ventricle, the greater the EDV (up to a point), the greater the tension developed on contraction, and vice versa. This concept is similar to stretching a rubber band—the greater the stretch (up to a point), the greater the contractile force.

In clinical practice, this initial ventricular stretch is called **preload,** whereas the tension of contraction is equivalent to SV. Figure 9-9 applies the Frank-Starling law to ventricular function by plotting ventricular stretch against SV. Ventricular stretch is directly proportional to EDV, and EDV is directly related to the pressure difference across the ventricle wall. Preload can be measured indirectly as the ventricular end-diastolic pressure.

RULE OF THUMB

Increases in preload result in increased SV in the healthy heart.

Another major factor affecting SV is the force against which the heart must pump, which is called **afterload.** Afterload represents the sum of all external factors that oppose ventricular ejection. The factors can be summarized as (1) the tension in the ventricular wall and (2) peripheral resistance or impedance. In clinical practice,

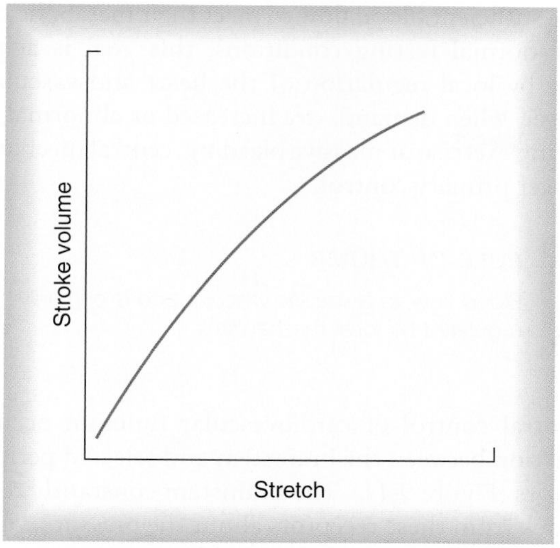

FIGURE 9-9 The Frank-Starling law—SV as a function of ventricular end-diastolic stretch. An increase in the stretch of the ventricles immediately before contraction (end-diastole) results in an increase in SV. Ventricular end-diastolic stretch is synonymous with the concept of preload.

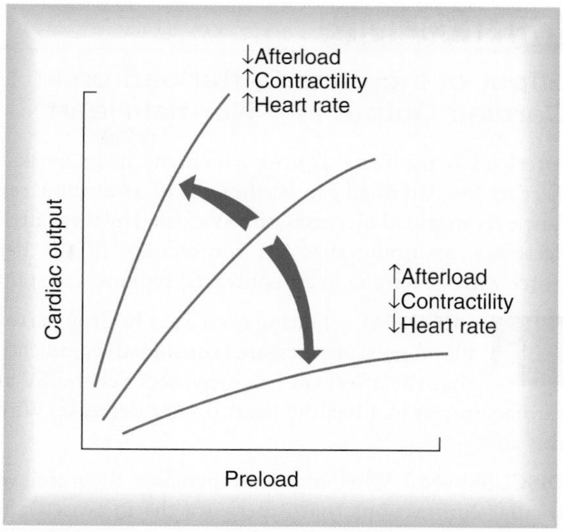

FIGURE 9-10 Effects of preload, afterload, contractility, and HR on cardiac output function curve. (Modified from Green JF: Fundamental cardiovascular and pulmonary physiology, ed 2, Philadelphia, 1987, Lea & Febiger.)

PVR on the right and SVR on the left are indirect indicators of ventricular afterload. In other words, the greater the resistance to blood flow out of the ventricles, the greater is the afterload.

All else being constant, the greater the afterload on the ventricles, the harder it is for the ventricles to eject their volume. For a given EDV, an increase in afterload causes the volume remaining in the ventricle after systole (ESV) to increase. If the EDV remains constant while the ESV increases, the SV (EDV − ESV) decreases (see Figure 9-8). Normally, however, the healthy heart muscle responds to increased afterload by altering its contractility.

> **RULE OF THUMB**
>
> Increases in afterload can decrease SV, especially in the failing heart.

Contractility represents the amount of systolic force exerted by the heart muscle at any given preload. At a given preload (EDV), an increase in contractility results in an increased EF, a decreased ESV, and an increased SV. Conversely, a decrease in contractility results in a decreased EF, an increased ESV, and a decreased SV.

Changes in contractility affect the slope of the ventricular function curve (Figure 9-10; see Figure 9-9). A higher SV for a given preload (increased slope) indicates a state of increased contractility, often referred to as **positive inotropism.** The opposite is also true. A lower SV for a given preload indicates decreased contractility, referred to as **negative inotropism.** Drugs that increase contractility of the heart muscle are called *positive inotropes;* drugs that decrease contractility are negative inotropes.

In addition to local mechanisms, cardiac contractility is influenced by neural control, circulating hormonal factors, and certain medications. Whether local or central in origin, these factors all influence the reactivity of contractile proteins, mainly by affecting calcium metabolism in the sarcomere. Typically, neural or drug-mediated *sympathetic* stimulation has a positive inotropic effect. Conversely, *parasympathetic* stimulation exerts a negative inotropic effect. *Profound hypoxia* and *acidosis* impair myocardial metabolism and decrease cardiac contractility.

> **RULE OF THUMB**
>
> Hypoxia and acidosis decrease cardiac contractility and output.

Changes in Heart Rate

The last factor influencing cardiac output is **heart rate (HR).** In contrast to the factors controlling SV, the factors affecting HR are mainly of central origin (i.e., neural or hormonal). Factors that increase HR are called *positive chronotropic* factors. Likewise, factors that decrease HR are called *negative chronotropic* factors.

As expected, cardiac output increases and decreases with similar changes in HR. However, this relationship is maintained only up to approximately 160 to 180 beats/min in a healthy heart. At higher HRs, there is not enough time for the ventricles to fill completely between each heart beat. An excessive HR causes a decrease in EDV, a decrease in SV, and a decrease in cardiac output. The decrease in EDV associated with an elevated HR usually occurs at significantly less than 160 beats/min in the failing heart.

MINI CLINI

Effect of Increased Afterload on Cardiac Output in a Normal Heart

Afterload is the force against which the heart works to eject its SV. Afterload can be thought of as outflow resistance. As afterload increases, the SV ejected by the ventricle decreases, assuming that the contractility of the heart (force with which the heart contracts) remains constant.

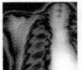

PROBLEM: During exercise, a healthy person's blood pressure increases considerably, indicating that the afterload has increased. Yet the SV and cardiac output in a healthy heart do not decrease. Why is this so?

DISCUSSION: When afterload increases, the initial ventricular contractions that experience the increased afterload produce smaller SVs; this causes more blood to remain in the ventricle at the end of systole (i.e., ESV is increased). During the subsequent diastole, blood rushes in from the atria to fill the ventricles, and because of the higher than normal ESV, the ventricle becomes more distended and stretched than before. Healthy heart muscle responds to increased stretch in a way described by the Frank-Starling law; that is, the heart now contracts with greater force than before, ejecting a greater SV. By increasing contractility in this fashion, SV and cardiac output are not compromised by increased afterload in a healthy heart.

RULE OF THUMB

Increase in HR increases cardiac output in a healthy heart up to a rate of 160 to 180 beats/min.

The combined effects of preload, afterload, contractility, and HR on cardiac performance are graphically portrayed in Figure 9-10. The middle ventricular function curve represents the normal state. The upper, steeper curve represents a hyperdynamic heart. In the hyperdynamic heart, a given preload results in a greater than normal cardiac output. Factors contributing to this state include decreased afterload, increased contractility (decreased ESV), and increased HR. The bottom curve has less slope than normal, indicating a hypodynamic heart. Factors contributing to this state include increased afterload, decreased contractility (increased ESV), and decreased rate. When the pumping efficiency of the heart is so low that cardiac output is inadequate to meet tissues needs, the heart is said to be in **congestive heart failure.**

Cardiovascular Control Mechanisms

Cardiovascular control is achieved by integrating local and central regulatory mechanisms that affect both the heart and the vasculature. The goal is to ensure that all tissues receive sufficient blood flow to meet their metabolic needs. Under normal resting conditions, this goal is achieved mostly by local regulation of the heart and vasculature. However, when demands are increased or abnormal, such as during exercise or massive bleeding, central mechanisms take over primary control.

RULE OF THUMB

Blood flow to a specific vascular bed is primarily regulated by local mechanisms.

Central control of cardiovascular function occurs by interaction between the brainstem and selected peripheral receptors (Figure 9-11). The brainstem constantly receives feedback from these receptors about the pressure, volume, and chemical status of the blood. The brainstem also receives input from higher brain centers, such as the hypothalamus and cerebral cortex. All these inputs are integrated with the inputs coming from the heart and blood vessels to maintain adequate blood flow and pressure under all but the most abnormal conditions.

MINI CLINI

Heart Rate and the Administration of Bronchodilator Drugs

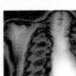

PROBLEM: You are giving a bronchodilator aerosolized drug to a patient, and you notice a significant increase in the patient's HR. Would you expect increased HR to be a common side effect of drugs that cause bronchodilation?

DISCUSSION: The discharge rate of the sinus node and the HR are increased by sympathetic nervous stimulation and decreased by parasympathetic nervous stimulation. The airways of the lung are dilated by sympathetic nervous stimulation and constricted by parasympathetic stimulation. Drugs that cause bronchodilation either mimic sympathetic stimulation (sympathomimetic) or block parasympathetic stimulation (parasympatholytic). Both of these drug actions also cause the HR to increase. Parasympatholytic drugs bring about effects similar to sympathetic stimulation because by inhibiting parasympathetic activity, they allow sympathetic impulses to predominate, ultimately causing a sympathetic-like response.

Cardiovascular Control Centers

Figure 9-11 is a simplified diagram of the cardiovascular regulatory centers. Areas in the medulla receive input from higher brain centers, peripheral pressure, and chemical receptors. Stimulation of the vasoconstrictor area within the medulla causes vasoconstriction and increased vascular resistance. A vasodepressor area works mainly by inhibiting the vasoconstrictor center.

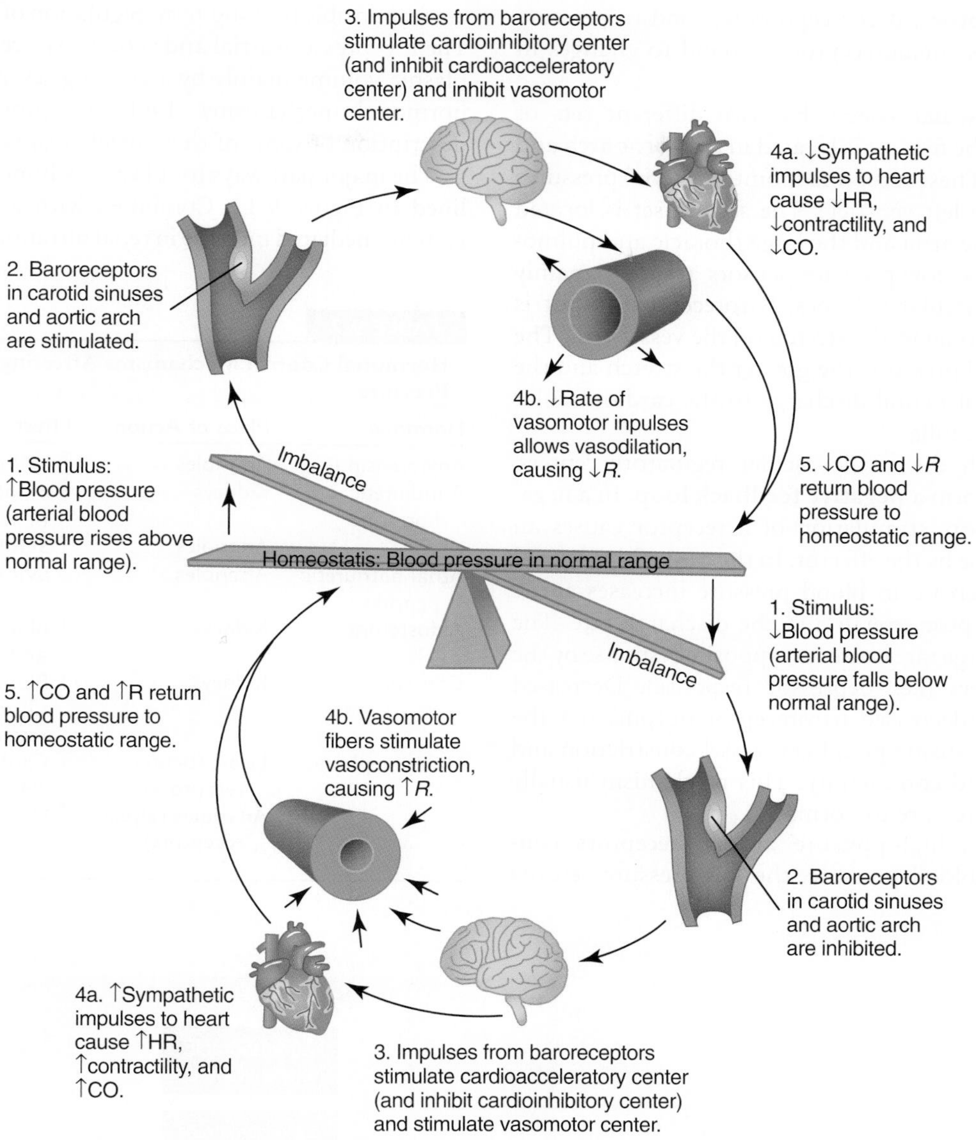

FIGURE 9-11 Simplified diagram of cardiovascular regulatory centers. (Modified from Marieb EN, Hoehn KN: Anatomy and physiology, ed 4, San Francisco, 2011, Pearson Benjamin Cummings.)

Closely associated with the vasoconstrictor center is a cardioaccelerator area. Stimulation of this center increases HR by increasing sympathetic discharge to the sinoatrial and atrioventricular nodes of the heart. A cardioinhibitory area plays the opposite role. Stimulation of this center decreases HR by increasing vagal (parasympathetic) stimulation to the heart.

Higher brain centers also influence the cardiovascular system, both directly and through the medulla. Signals coming from the cerebral cortex in response to exercise, pain, or anxiety pass directly through the cholinergic fibers to the vascular smooth muscle, causing vasodilation. Signals from the hypothalamus, in particular, its heat-regulating areas, indirectly affect HR and vasomotor tone through the cardiovascular centers.

The cardiovascular centers also are affected by local chemical changes in the surrounding blood and cerebrospinal fluid. Decreased levels of CO_2 tend to inhibit the medullary centers. General inhibition of these centers causes a decrease in vascular tone and a decrease in blood pressure. A local decrease in O_2 tension has the opposite effect. Mild hypoxia in this area increases sympathetic discharge rates; this tends to elevate both HR and blood pressure. Severe hypoxia has a depressant effect.

Peripheral Receptors

In addition to high-level and local input, the cardiovascular centers receive signals from peripheral receptors (see Figure 9-11). There are two types of peripheral cardiovascular receptors: **baroreceptors,** or stretch receptors, and **chemoreceptors.** Baroreceptors respond to pressure changes, whereas chemoreceptors respond to changes in blood chemistry.

The cardiovascular system has two different sets of baroreceptors. The first set is located in the aortic arch and carotid sinuses. These receptors monitor arterial pressures generated by the left ventricle. The second set is located in the walls of the atria and the large thoracic and pulmonary veins. These low-pressure sensors respond mainly to changes in vascular volumes. Baroreceptor output is directly proportional to the stretch on the vessel wall. The greater the blood pressure, the greater the stretch and the higher the rate of neural discharge to the cardiovascular centers in the medulla.

Together with the cardiovascular regulatory centers, these receptors form a **negative feedback loop.** In a negative feedback loop, stimulation of a receptor causes an opposite response by the effector. In the case of the arterial receptors, an increase in blood pressure increases aortic and carotid receptor stretch and the discharge rate. The increased discharge rate causes an opposite response by the medullary centers (i.e., depressor response). Decreased blood pressure (decreased baroreceptor output) has the opposite effect, causing peripheral vessel constriction and increased HR and contractility. This mechanism usually restores blood pressure to normal.

Although the high-pressure arterial receptors constantly control blood pressure, the low-pressure sensors are responsible for long-term regulation of plasma volume. The low-pressure atrial and venous baroreceptors regulate plasma volume mainly by activating several chemical and hormonal mechanisms. Table 9-2 provides a detailed description of some of these mechanisms.

The major pathways for plasma volume control are outlined in Figure 9-12. Combined with a central nervous system–mediated increase in renal filtration, these humoral

TABLE 9-2

Hormonal Control Mechanisms Affecting Blood Pressure

Hormone	Place of Action	Effect
Angiotensin II	Arterioles	↑ SVR (vasoconstriction)
Antidiuretic hormone	Kidneys	↑ Blood volume (↑ water retention)
	Arterioles	↑ SVR (vasoconstriction)
Atrial natriuretic peptide	Arterioles	↓ SVR (vasodilation)
Aldosterone	Kidneys	↑ Blood volume (↑ water and salt retention)
Cortisol	Kidneys	↑ Blood volume (↑ water and salt retention)
Norepinephrine	Heart (beta-1 receptors)	↑ Cardiac output (HR and contractility)
	Arterioles (alpha receptors)	↑ SVR (vasoconstriction)

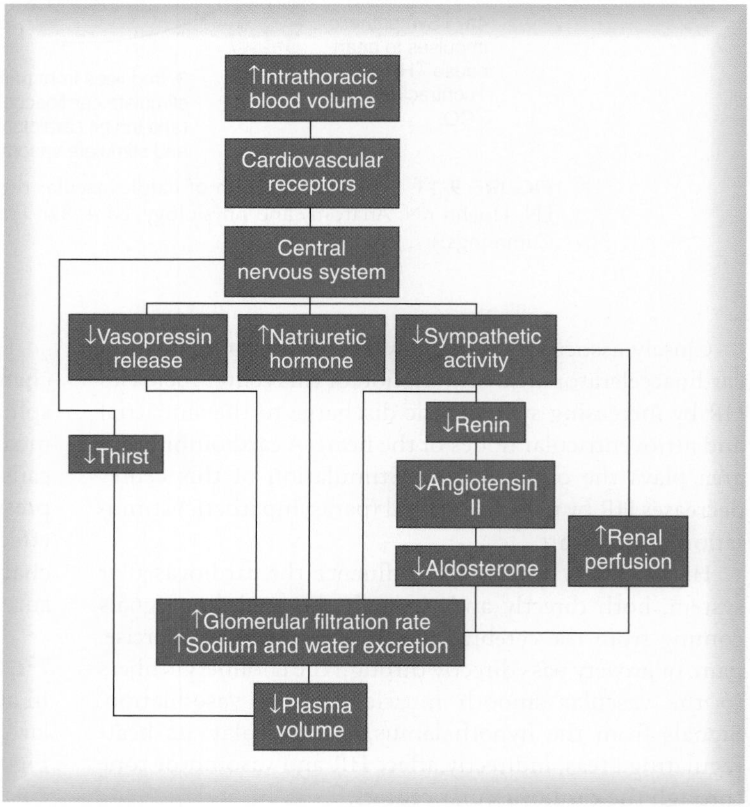

FIGURE 9-12 Major pathways for plasma volume control. See text for details. (Modified from Smith JJ, Kampine JP: Circulatory physiology: the essentials, ed 3, Baltimore, 1990, Williams & Wilkins.)

mechanisms decrease the overall plasma volume. A decrease in blood volume has the opposite effect (i.e., sodium and water retention and an increase in plasma volume).

Chemoreceptors are small, highly vascularized tissues located near the high-pressure sensors in the aortic arch and carotid sinus. Baroreceptors respond to pressure changes, whereas chemoreceptors are sensitive to changes in blood chemistry. They are strongly stimulated by decreased O_2 tensions, although low pH or high levels of CO_2 also can increase their discharge rate. It is important for the RT to know that the major cardiovascular effects of chemoreceptor stimulation are vasoconstriction and increased HR.

Because these changes occur only when the cardiopulmonary system is overtaxed, the chemoreceptors probably have little influence under normal conditions. However, their influence on respiration is clinically important. For this reason, the peripheral chemoreceptors are discussed in greater detail in Chapter 8.

Response to Changes in Overall Volume

The coordinated response of the cardiovascular system is best shown under abnormal conditions. Among the most common clinical conditions in which all essential regulatory mechanisms come into play is the large blood loss that occurs with hemorrhage. Figure 9-13 illustrates changes in these key factors during progressive blood loss in an animal model.

With 10% blood loss, the immediate decline in the CVP causes a 50% decrease in the discharge rate of the low-pressure (atrial) baroreceptors. There is little change in the activity of the high-pressure (arterial) receptors. The initial response, mediated through the medullary centers, is an increase in sympathetic discharge to the sinus node; this causes a progressive increase in HR. At the same time, plasma levels of antidiuretic hormone (vasopressin) begin to increase. These two initial changes are sufficient to maintain normal arterial blood pressure.

As the blood loss becomes more severe (20%), atrial receptor activity decreases further; this increases the intensity of sympathetic discharge from the cardiovascular centers. Plasma antidiuretic hormone and HR continue to increase, as does peripheral vasculature tone. An increase in vascular tone occurs through constriction of the capacitance vessels in the venous system, slowing the decrease in CVP.

The arterial pressure does not start to decrease until blood loss approaches 30%. At this point, arterial receptor activity begins to decrease, resulting in a marked increase in systemic vascular tone. Despite the magnitude of blood loss, CVP levels off. As long as no further hemorrhage occurs, blood pressure and tissue perfusion can be maintained at adequate levels.

If blood loss continues, central control mechanisms begin to take over. Massive vasoconstriction occurs in the resistance vessels, shunting blood away from skeletal muscle to maintain blood flow to the brain and heart. Increasing levels of local metabolites in these areas, especially CO_2 and other acids, override central control and cause further vessel dilation and increased blood flow. As these metabolites build up and as the tissues become hypoxic, cardiac function becomes impaired, and vasodilation occurs throughout the body. This vasodilation signals the onset of a state of irreversible shock, after which death ensues.

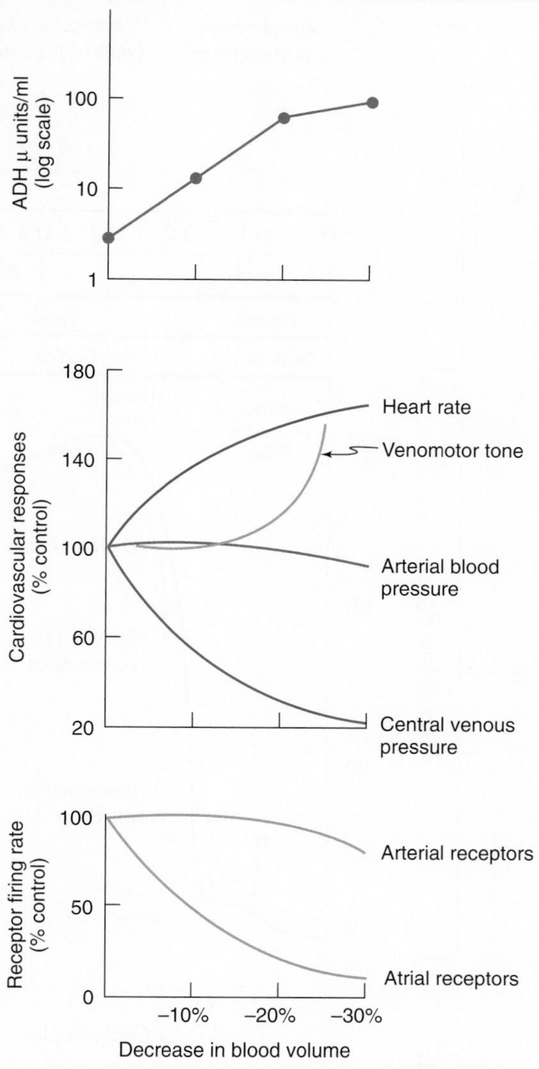

FIGURE 9-13 Plasma levels of antidiuretic hormone (ADH), cardiovascular responses, and receptor firing rates in response to graded hemorrhage in the dog. See text for details. (Sources: Richardson DR: Basic circulatory physiology, Boston, 1976, Little, Brown & Co. Venomotor tone data are those of W. J. Sears as cited in Gauer OH, Henry JP, Behn C: The regulation of extracellular fluid volume. Annu Rev Physiol 32:547, 1970. All other data are from Henry JP, et al: Can J Physiol Pharmacol 46:287, 1968.)

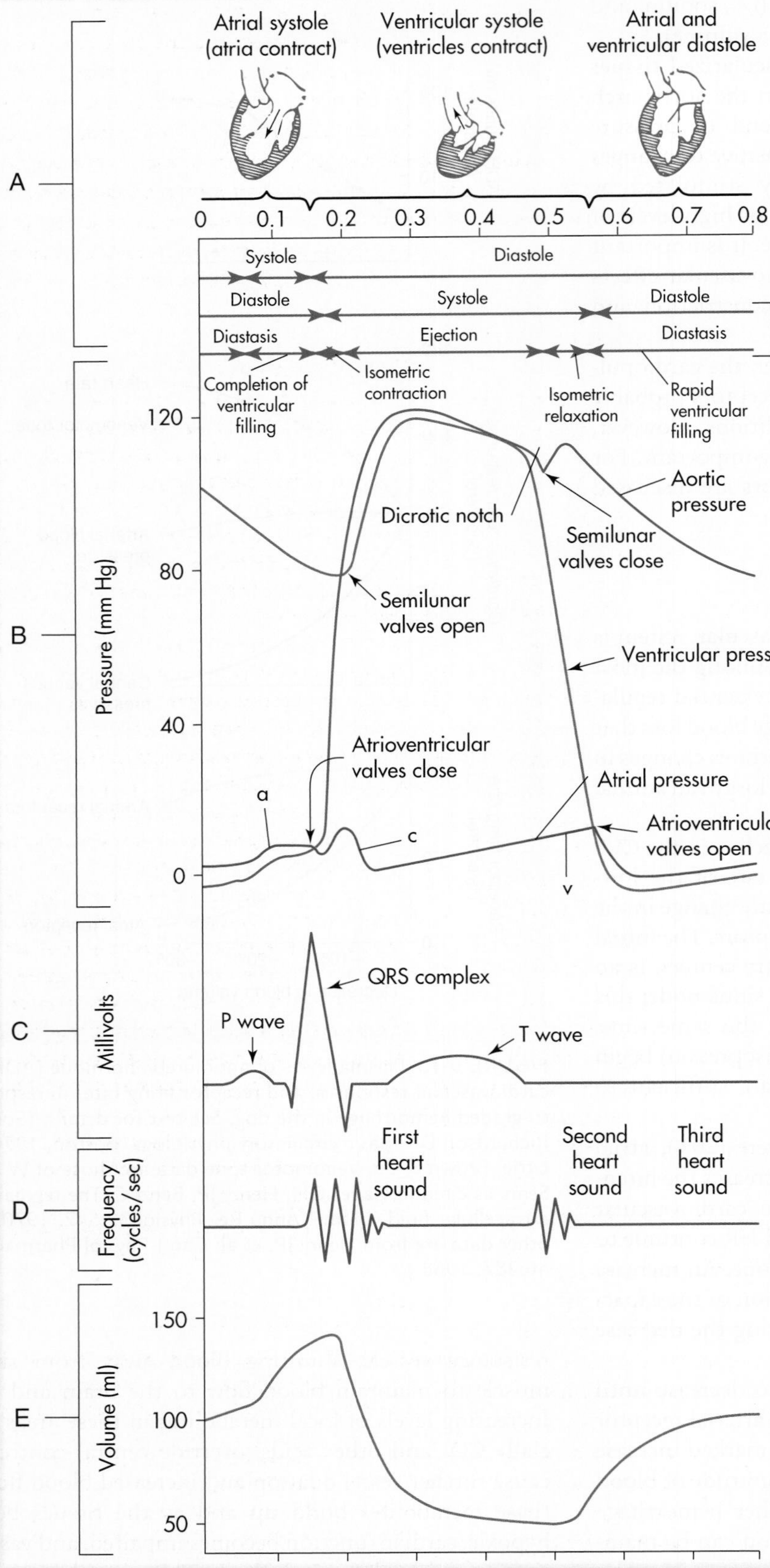

FIGURE 9-14 Cardiac cycle. **A,** Timing of cardiac events. **B,** Simultaneous pressures created in the aorta, left ventricle, and right atrium during the cardiac cycle. **C,** Electrical activity during the cardiac cycle. **D,** Heart sounds corresponding to the cardiac cycle. **E,** Ventricular blood volume during the cardiac cycle. (Modified from Moffett DF, Moffett SB, Schauf CL: Human physiology: foundations and frontiers, ed 2, St Louis, 1993, Mosby.)

EVENTS OF THE CARDIAC CYCLE

This chapter has focused on the mechanical properties of the heart, and the electrical activities of the heart are discussed in Chapter 17. Although they are discussed separately, the mechanical and electrical events are interdependent. Given the crucial role of RTs in dealing with cardiovascular problems, an in-depth knowledge of how these events relate is essential.

The events of the cardiac cycle are depicted in Figure 9-14. The top of the figure shows a time axis scaled in tenths of a second. Next are the timing bars for ventricular systole and diastole and pressure events in the atria, ventricles, and aorta. These are followed by an electrocardiogram (ECG), heart sounds, and ventricular flow (see Chapter 17 for an explanation of the ECG waves).

Going from left to right, the P wave (atrial depolarization) begins the ECG. Earlier, the ventricles have been passively filling with blood through the open atrioventricular valves. Within 0.1 second, the atria contract, causing a slight increase in both atrial and ventricular pressures (the *a waves*). This atrial contraction helps preload the ventricles, increasing their volume by 25%. This help from the atria to ventricular filling is called the *atrial kick*. Toward the end of diastole, the electrical impulses from the atria reach the atrioventricular node and bundle branches, and ventricular depolarization (the QRS complex) is initiated. Within a few hundredths of a second after depolarization, the ventricles begin to contract. As soon as ventricular pressures exceed pressures in the atria, the atrioventricular valves close. Closure of the mitral valve occurs first, followed immediately by closure of the tricuspid valve. This closure marks the end of ventricular diastole, producing the first heart sound on the phonocardiogram.

Immediately after atrioventricular valve closure, the ventricles become closed chambers. During this short isovolemic phase of contraction, ventricular pressures increase rapidly. Upward bulging of the atrioventricular valves during this phase causes a slight upswing in atrial pressure graphs, called the *c wave*. Within 0.05 second, ventricular pressures increase to exceed the pressures in the aorta and pulmonary artery opening the semilunar valves.

Toward the end of systole, as repolarization starts (indicated by the T wave), the ventricles begin to relax. Consequently, ventricular pressures decrease rapidly. When arterial pressures exceed pressures in the relaxing ventricles, the semilunar valves shut. Closure of the semilunar valves generates the second heart sound.

Rather than immediately dropping off, aortic and pulmonary pressures increase again after the semilunar valves close. The *dicrotic notch* is caused by the elastic recoil of the arteries. This recoil provides the extra "push" that helps maintain the head of pressure created by the ventricles.

As the ventricles continue to relax, their pressures decrease to less than the pressures in the atria. This decline in pressure reopens the atrioventricular valves. As soon as the atrioventricular valves open, the blood collected in the atria rushes to fill the ventricles, causing a rapid decrease in atrial pressures (the *v wave*). Thereafter, ventricular filling slows as the heart prepares for a new cycle.

Knowledge of these normal events helps one understand many of the diagnostic and monitoring procedures used for patients with cardiopulmonary disorders. Among the most common are the measurement of CVP, balloon-directed pulmonary artery catheterization, and direct arterial pressure monitoring.

SUMMARY CHECKLIST

- The cardiovascular system consists of the heart and a complex vascular network that work together to maintain homeostasis by continually distributing and regulating blood flow throughout the body.
- Specialized mechanical and electrical properties of cardiac tissue, combined with internal and external control mechanisms, provide the basis for coordinated cardiac function.
- The vascular system is regulated by local and central control mechanisms.
- Cardiac output is primarily determined by four factors: preload, afterload, contractility, and HR.
- Increased HR decreases cardiac output by decreasing filling times (decreasing EDV) and decreasing contraction times—hence increasing ESV.
- The vascular network assumes an active role in the control and distribution of blood flow.
- The heart and the vascular systems work together in a coordinated fashion to ensure that all body tissues receive sufficient blood to meet their metabolic needs.
- In a healthy subject, blood pressure is regulated by changing the volume of circulating blood, changing the capacity of the vascular system, or changing both.
- Under conditions of increased demand, special compensatory mechanisms are called on to maintain stable blood flow.
- Failure of cardiovascular control mechanisms often requires the intervention of RTs to help restore and maintain normal function.

References

1. Andreoli CC, et al: Cecil essentials of medicine, ed 8, Philadelphia, 2010, WB Saunders.
2. Berne RM, Levy MN, editors: Physiology, ed 6, St Louis, 2010, Mosby.
3. Barret KE, et al: Ganong's review of medical physiology, ed 23, New York, 2009, McGraw-Hill.
4. Des Jardins T: Cardiopulmonary anatomy and physiology, ed 5, New York, 2008, Delmar Cengage Learning.
5. Guyton AC, Hall JE: Textbook of medical physiology, ed 11, Philadelphia, 2006, WB Saunders.
6. Hess DR, et al: Respiratory care principles and practice, ed 2, Boston, 2011, Jones & Bartlett Learning.

7. Marieb EN, Hoehn KN: Anatomy and physiology, ed 4, San Francisco, 2011, Pearson Benjamin Cummings.
8. Moses KP, et al: Atlas of clinical gross anatomy, St Louis, 2005, Mosby.
9. Stevens A, Lowe J: Human histology, ed 3, St Louis, 2005, Mosby.
10. Thibodeau GA, Patton KT: Anatomy and physiology, ed 7, St Louis, 2011, Mosby.
11. Wilkins RL, Sheldon RL, Krider SJ: Clinical assessment in respiratory care, ed 6, St Louis, 2010, Elsevier.

Chapter 10

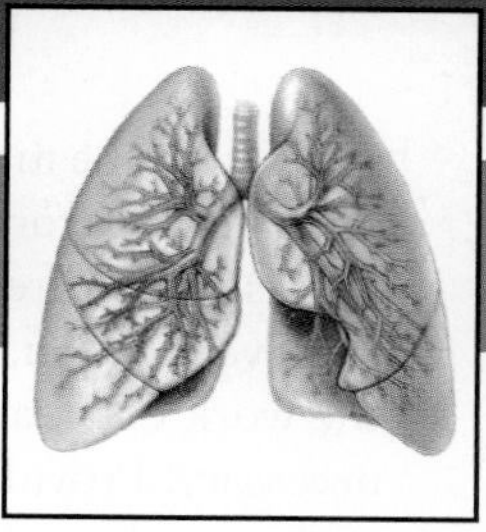

Ventilation

ROBERT L. CHATBURN AND EHAB G. DAOUD

CHAPTER OBJECTIVES

After reading this chapter you will be able to:

- Describe the physiologic functions provided by ventilation.
- Describe the pressure gradients responsible for gas flow, diffusion, and lung inflation.
- Identify the forces that oppose gas movement into and out of the lungs.
- Describe how surface tension contributes to lung recoil.
- Describe how lung, chest wall, and total compliance are related.
- State the factors that affect resistance to breathing.
- Describe how various lung diseases affect the work of breathing.
- State why ventilation is not evenly distributed throughout the lung.
- Describe how the time constants affect alveolar filling and emptying.
- Identify the factors that affect alveolar ventilation.
- State how to calculate alveolar ventilation, dead space, and the V_D/V_T ratio.

CHAPTER OUTLINE

KEY TERMS

airway resistance
alveolar dead space
compliance
dynamic compression
dynamic hyperinflation (air trapping)
elastance
elasticity
equal pressure point (EPP)
hyperventilation
hypoventilation
hysteresis
physiologic dead space
plethysmograph
pneumotachometer
pressure gradient
subatmospheric
surface tension
tidal volume (V_T)
time constant
transairway pressure (P_{TAW})
transalveolar pressure (P_{TA})
trans-chest wall pressure (P_{TCW})
transpulmonary
transpulmonary pressure difference (P_{TP})
transrespiratory
transrespiratory pressure (P_{TR})
transthoracic
transthoracic pressure difference (P_{TT})
ventilation

The primary functions of the lungs are to supply the body with oxygen (O_2) and to remove carbon dioxide (CO_2). To perform these functions, the lungs must be adequately ventilated. **Ventilation** is the process of moving gas (usually air) in and out of the lungs. Ventilation is to be distinguished from respiration, which involves complex physiologic processes at the blood and cellular levels.

In health, ventilation is regulated to meet the body's needs under a wide range of conditions. In disease, this process can be markedly disrupted. Inadequate ventilation or increased work of breathing often results. Respiratory care is often directed toward restoring adequate and efficient ventilation. Respiratory care modalities try to reduce the work of breathing and provide artificial ventilation if necessary. Providing effective respiratory care requires an understanding of normal ventilatory processes and of how various diseases may affect ventilation.

MECHANICS OF VENTILATION

Normal ventilation is a cyclic activity that has two phases: inspiration and expiration. During each cycle, a volume of gas moves in and out of the respiratory tract. This volume, measured during either inspiration or expiration, is called the **tidal volume (V_T).** The normal V_T refreshes the gas present in the lung removing CO_2 and supplying O_2 to meet metabolic needs. The V_T must be able to meet changing metabolic demands, such as during exercise or sleep. The *vital capacity* and its subdivisions provide the necessary reserves for increasing ventilation (see Chapter 19).

Ventilation can be related to a simplified version of the equation of motion for the respiratory system:

$$\text{Pressure} = \frac{\text{Volume}}{\text{Compliance}} + (\text{Resistance} \times \text{Flow})$$

where:

Pressure = Force generated by the respiratory muscles or a mechanical ventilator, or both, during inspiration
Volume = Volume change (e.g., V_T)
Elastance = Distensibility of the lungs and thorax (Δpressure/Δvolume); elastance is the reciprocal of compliance (Δvolume/Δpressure)
Resistance = Airflow and tissue resistance (Δpressure/Δflow)
Flow = Volume change per unit of time

In this equation, the terms *(elastance × volume)* and *(resistance × flow)* have units of pressure and represent the elastic and resistive loads against which the respiratory muscles or ventilator must work to ventilate the lungs. In healthy lungs, this work is minimal and performed during the inspiratory phase. Expiration is normally passive (i.e., no muscle force involved).

Pressure Differences During Breathing

The equation of motion is a mathematical model describing the behavior of a graphic model of the lungs. The graphic model is shown in Figure 10-1.[1] The model lumps all the resistive properties of the many airways into a single flow-conducting tube and lumps all the elastic properties of the alveoli and airways into a single elastic compartment. Surrounding the "lungs" is another elastic compartment representing the chest wall. This graphic representation of the respiratory system allows us to define points in space where pressures may be measured (or inferred) as defined in Table 10-1. Mathematical models relating pressure, volume, and flow corresponding to this graphic model are constructed using pressure differences between the points. The various components of the graphic model are

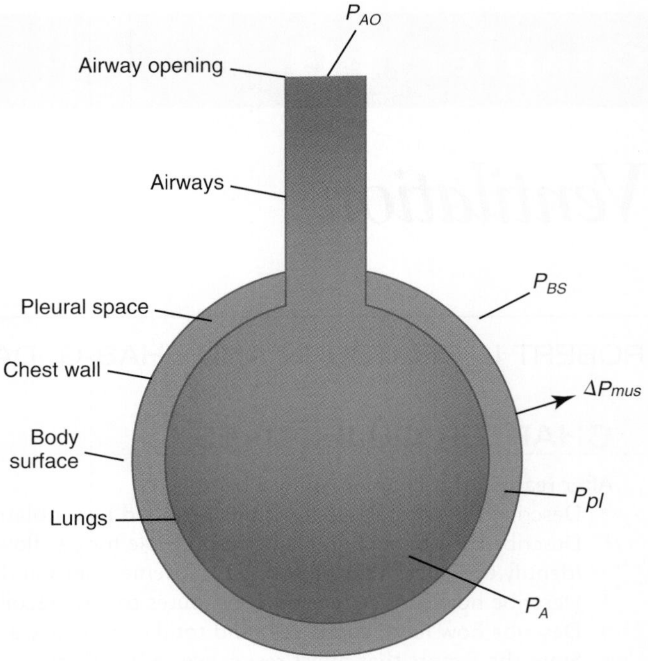

FIGURE 10-1 Schematic representation of the respiratory system consisting of a flow-conducting tube (representing the airways) connected to a single elastic compartment (representing the lungs) surrounded by another elastic compartment (representing the chest wall). ΔP_{mus}, Muscle pressure difference; P_A, alveolar pressure; P_{AO}, pressure at the airway opening; P_{BS}, pressure on the body surface; P_{pl}, pressure in the intrapleural space. (From Primiano FP Jr, Chatburn RL: Zen and the art of nomenclature maintenance: a revised approach to respiratory symbols and terminology. Respir Care 51:1458–1470, 2006.)

TABLE 10-1
Measurable Pressures Used in Describing Respiratory System Mechanics

Name	Symbol	Definition
Pressure at the airway opening	P_{AO}	Pressure measured at the opening of the respiratory system airway (e.g., mouth and nose, tracheostomy opening, and distal end of endotracheal tube)
Pleural pressure	P_{pl}	Pressure measured in the pleural space, changes in which are often estimated by measuring pressure changes in the esophagus
Alveolar pressure	P_A	Pressure in the alveolar (gas space) region of the lungs
Body surface pressure	P_{BS}	Pressure measured at the body surface

defined as everything that exists between these points in space. The *respiratory system* is everything that exists between the pressure measured at the airway opening (P_{AO}) and the pressure measured at the body surface (P_{BS}). The associated pressure difference is **transrespiratory pressure (P_{TR}):**

$$P_{TR} = P_{AO} - P_{BS}$$

The term P_{AO} comes before the term P_{BS} in the equation. This order is dictated by the direction of flow. For inspiration, P_{AO} is higher than P_{BS}, and P_{TR} is calculated by subtracting P_{BS} from P_{AO}. The same general principle applies to all the other pressure differences described subsequently.

The components of transrespiratory pressure correspond to the components of the graphic model (i.e., airways, lungs, and chest wall). The airways are whatever exists between pressure measured at the airway opening and pressure measured in the alveoli of the lungs (P_A). The graphic model makes the lungs look like one giant alveolus, which means that alveolar pressure represents an average pressure over all alveoli in real lungs. The associated pressure difference is **transairway pressure (P_{TAW}):**

$$P_{TAW} = P_{AO} - P_A$$

The alveolar region is whatever exists between pressure measured in the model alveolus and pressure measured in the pleural space (P_{pl}). The associated pressure difference is **transalveolar pressure (P_{TA}):**

$$P_{TA} = P_A - P_{pl}$$

The chest wall exists between pressure measured in the pleural space and the pressure on the body surface. The associated pressure difference is **trans–chest wall pressure (P_{TCW}):**

$$P_{TCW} = P_{pl} - P_{BS}$$

Some of these components can be combined to get respiratory subsystems. Most commonly, the pulmonary system (airways and alveolar region) is defined in terms of the **transpulmonary pressure difference (P_{TP}):**

$$P_{TP} = P_{AO} - P_{pl}$$

The literature is very confused regarding the definition of transpulmonary pressure. Authors often define P_{TP} as $P_A - P_{pl}$. The confusion arises from the fact that $P_{TA} = P_A - P_{pl}$ *but only under static conditions.* Static conditions can be imposed during mechanical ventilation by using an inspiratory hold maneuver. This situation should be considered a special case of P_{TP}, however; the general case is $P_{TP} = P_{AO} - P_{pl}$, which shows what pressures must be measured to derive the mechanical properties of the pulmonary system under either static or dynamic (breathing) conditions. If we want to evaluate the elastance and resistance of the pulmonary system, we substitute P_{TP} for P in the equation of motion. Alternatively, if we want to evaluate total respiratory system elastance and resistance, we substitute P_{TR} for P.

Sometimes it is useful to define **transthoracic pressure difference (P_{TT})** as:

$$P_{TT} = P_A - P_{BS}$$

Table 10-2 summarizes these equations.

The transrespiratory **pressure gradient** causes gas to flow into and out of the alveoli during breathing. For a spontaneously breathing subject, P_A is **subatmospheric** in the beginning of inspiration compared with P_{AO} causing air to flow into the alveoli. The opposite happens in the beginning of exhalation; P_A is higher than P_{AO} causing air to flow out of the airway opening.

During a normal breathing cycle, the glottis remains open. P_{BS} and P_{AO} remain at zero (i.e., atmospheric) throughout the cycle; only changes in P_A and P_{pl} are of interest. Before inspiration, pleural pressure is approximately −5 cm H_2O (i.e., 5 cm H_2O below atmospheric pressure), and alveolar pressure is 0 cm H_2O. The transpulmonary pressure gradient is also approximately 5 cm H_2O in the resting state, that is, $P_{TP} = P_{AO} - P_{pl} = 0 - (-5) = 5$. This positive end expiratory P_{TP} maintains the lung at its resting volume (i.e., functional residual capacity [FRC]). Airway opening and alveolar pressures are both zero, so the transairway pressure gradient also is zero. No gas moves into or out of the respiratory tract.

Inspiration begins when muscular effort expands the thorax. Thoracic expansion causes a *decrease* in pleural pressure. This decrease in pleural pressure causes a positive change on expiratory P_{TP} and P_{TA}, which induces flow into the lungs. The inspiratory flow is proportional to the positive change in transairway pressure difference; the higher the change in P_{TA}, the higher the flow.

Pleural pressure continues to decrease until the end of inspiration. Alveolar filling slows when alveolar pressure approaches equilibrium with the atmosphere, and inspiratory flow decreases to zero (Figure 10-2). At this point,

TABLE 10-2

Pressure Differences Used in Describing Respiratory System Mechanics

Definition	Name	Symbol
$P_{AO} - P_{BS}$	Transrespiratory pressure difference	ΔP_{TR}
$P_{AO} - P_A$	Transairway pressure difference	ΔP_{TAW}
$P_{AO} - P_{pl}$	Transpulmonary pressure difference	ΔP_{TP}
$P_A - P_{pl}$	Transalveolar pressure difference	ΔP_{TA}
$P_A - P_{BS}$	Transthoracic pressure difference	ΔP_{TT}
$P_{pl} - P_{BS}$	Trans–chest wall pressure difference	ΔP_{TCW}
	Global muscle pressure difference	ΔP_{mus}

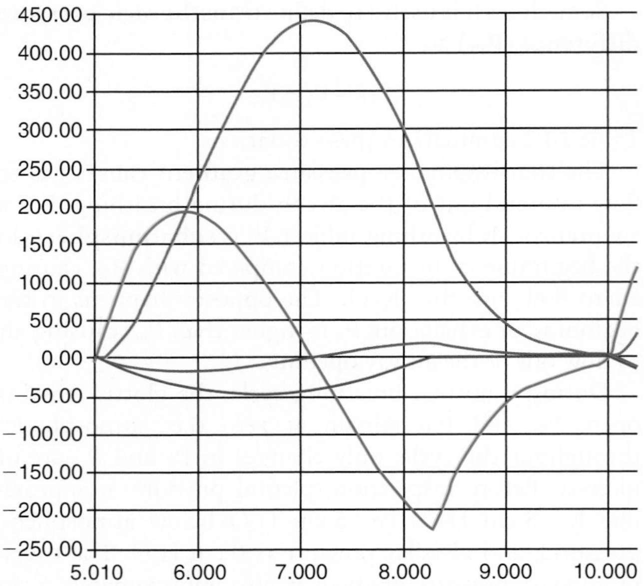

FIGURE 10-2 Waveforms for normal breathing. *Red,* change in pleural pressure relative to end expiratory value (cm H_2O, scaled times ten); *blue,* alveolar pressure (cm H_2O, scaled times ten); *green,* flow (L/min, scaled times ten); *purple,* volume (ml).

called *end-inspiration,* alveolar pressure has returned to zero, and the intrapleural pressure–and hence transpulmonary pressure gradient–reaches the maximal value (for a normal breath) of approximately 10 cm H_2O.

As expiration begins, the thorax recoils, and P_{pl} starts to increase, and the transpulmonary pressure difference starts to decrease. Because transpulmonary pressure difference is decreasing (e.g., from 10 cm H_2O to 5 cm H_2O), the opposite of inspiration, flow is in the opposite (negative) direction. The equation of motion shows this, setting the driving pressure, P_{mus}, to zero:

$$P_{mus} = 0 = (\text{Elastance} \times \text{Volume}) + (\text{Resistance} \times \text{Flow})$$

Rearranging, we get:

$$\begin{aligned}(\text{Elastance} \times \text{Volume}) &= -(\text{Resistance} \times \text{Flow}) \\ &= \text{Resistance} \times (-\text{Flow})\end{aligned}$$

This equation says two important things: (1) Flow is negative, indicating expiration, and (2) the driving force (transthoracic pressure, equal to elastance × volume) for expiratory flow is the energy stored in the combined elastances of lungs and chest wall (the total elastance is the sum of the chest wall and lung elastances).

These events occur during normal V_T excursions. Similar pressure changes accompany deeper inspiration and expiration. The magnitude of the pressure changes is greater with deeper breathing. Pleural pressures are always negative (subatmospheric) during normal inspiration and exhalation. During forced inspiration with a big down movement of the diaphragm, the pleural pressure can decrease to −50 cm H_2O, whereas during a forced expiration, pleural pressure may increase above atmospheric pressure to 50 to 100 cm H_2O.

Forces Opposing Inflation of the Lung

The lungs have a tendency to recoil inward, whereas the chest wall tends to move outward; these opposing forces keep the lung at its resting volumes (FRC). To generate the above-described pressure gradients, the lungs must be distended. This distention requires several opposing forces to be overcome for inspiration to occur. Normal expiration is passive, using the energy stored during inspiration. As indicated in the equation of motion, the forces opposing lung inflation may be grouped into two categories: *elastic forces* and *frictional forces.* Elastic forces involve the tissues of the lungs, thorax, and abdomen, along with surface tension in the alveoli. Frictional forces include resistance caused by gas flow through the airways (natural and artificial) and tissue movement during breathing.

Elastic Opposition to Ventilation

Elastin and *collagen* fibers are found in the lung parenchyma. These tissues give the lung the property of elasticity. **Elasticity** is the physical tendency of an object to return to an initial state after deformation. When stretched, an elastic body tends to return to its original shape. The tension developed when an elastic structure is stretched is proportional to the degree of deformation produced (Hooke's law). An example is a simple spring (Figure 10-3). When tension on a spring is increased, the spring lengthens. However, the ability of the spring to stretch is limited. When the point of maximal stretch is reached, further tension produces little or no increase in length. Additional tension may break the spring.

In the respiratory system, inflation stretches tissue. The elastic properties of the lungs and chest wall oppose inflation. To increase lung volume, pressure must be applied. This property may be shown by subjecting an excised lung to changes in transpulmonary pressure and measuring the associated changes in volume (Figure 10-4). To simulate the pressures during breathing, the lung is placed in an airtight jar. The force to inflate the lung is provided by a pump that varies the pressure around the lung inside the jar, simulating P_{pl}. This action mimics the pleural pressure changes associated with thoracic expansion and contraction. The changes in transpulmonary pressure are made in discrete steps, allowing the lungs to come to rest in between so that all of the applied pressure opposes elastic forces and none of it opposes resistive forces (i.e., flow is zero when the measurements are made). The amount of stretch (inflation) is measured as volume by a spirometer. Changes in volume resulting from changes in transpulmonary pressure are plotted on a graph.

During inspiration in this model, increasingly greater negative pleural pressures are required to stretch the lung to a larger volume. As the lung is stretched to its maximum

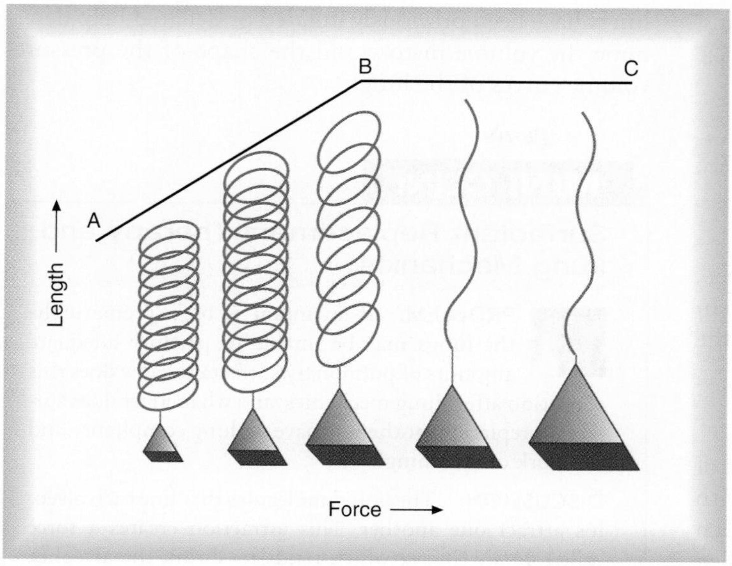

FIGURE 10-3 Graphic representation of the force-length relationship applied to a simple spring (increase in length with increase in force). With increasing force, or weight in this example, the spring lengthens from *A* to *B,* but at the point of maximal stretch, further force produces no additional increase in length (*B* to *C*).

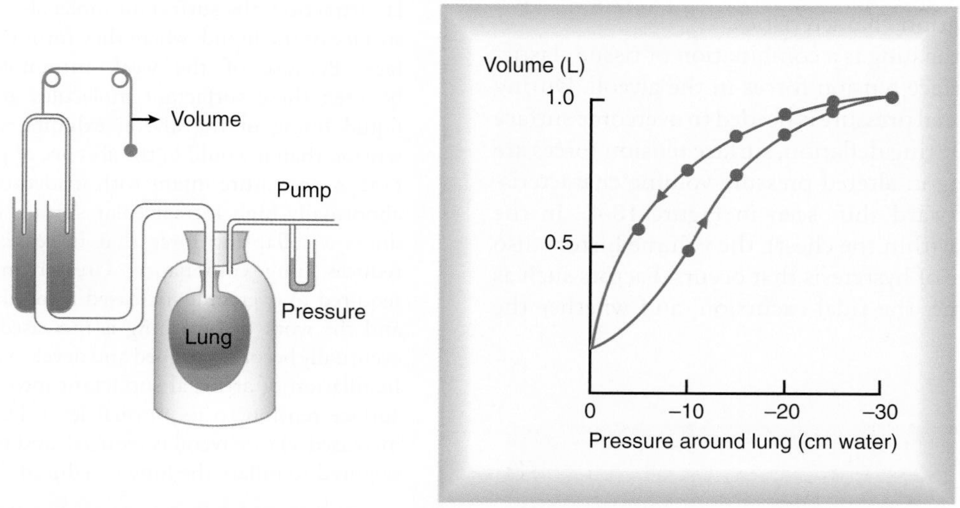

FIGURE 10-4 Measurement of the pressure-volume curve of an excised lung. The lung is placed in a sealed jar and connected to a spirometer (to measure volume). A pump generates subatmospheric pressure around the lung while its volume is measured. The curve plotting the relationship between pressure and volume is nonlinear and flattens at high expanding pressures (subatmospheric). The inflation and deflation curves are not the same. This difference is called *hysteresis.* (Modified from West JB: Respiratory physiology: the essentials, ed 7, Baltimore, 2005, Williams & Wilkins.)

(total lung capacity [TLC]), the inflation "curve" becomes flat. This flattening indicates *increasing* opposition to expansion (i.e., for the same change in transpulmonary pressure, there is less change in volume).[2]

As with a spring when tension is removed, deflation occurs passively as pressure in the jar is allowed to return toward atmospheric. Deflation of the lung does not follow the inflation curve exactly. During deflation, lung volume at any given pressure is slightly greater than it is during inflation. This difference between the inflation and deflation curves is called **hysteresis.**[2] Hysteresis indicates that factors other than simple elastic tissue forces are present. The major factor, particularly in sick lungs, is the opening of collapsed alveoli during inspiration that tend to stay open during expiration until very low lung volumes are reached.

Chest wall and lung elastances are connected in series, meaning that they both experience the same flow and change in volume, but they do not have the same pressure differences. Series elastances are simply additive.

The elastance of the respiratory system is the sum of lung (pulmonary) elastance (E_L) and chest wall elastance (E_{CW}):

$$E_{RS} = E_L + E_{CW}$$

Expressed in terms of **compliance:**

$$C_{RS} = \frac{C_L \times C_{CW}}{C_L + C_{CW}}$$

The resistance of the natural and artificial airways (e.g., endotracheal tube) is also in series so that the total system resistance is simply the sum of resistance of the components.

Surface Tension Forces

Part of the hysteresis exhibited by the lung is a result of **surface tension** forces in the alveoli. If a lung is filled with fluid such as saline, the pressure-volume curves look much different than the pressure-volume curves of an air-filled lung (Figure 10-5). Less pressure is needed to inflate a fluid-filled lung to a given volume. This phenomenon indicates that a gas-fluid *interface* in the air-filled lung changes its inflation-deflation characteristics.

The recoil of the lung is a combination of tissue elasticity and these surface tension forces in the alveoli. During inflation, additional pressure is needed to overcome surface tension forces. During deflation, surface tension forces are reduced, resulting in altered pressure-volume characteristics (i.e., the leftward shift seen in Figure 10-4). In the intact lung (i.e., within the chest), the volume history also affects the degree of hysteresis that occurs. Factors such as the initial volume, the tidal excursion, and whether the lungs have been previously inflated or deflated help determine the volume history and the shape of the pressure-volume curves of the lung.

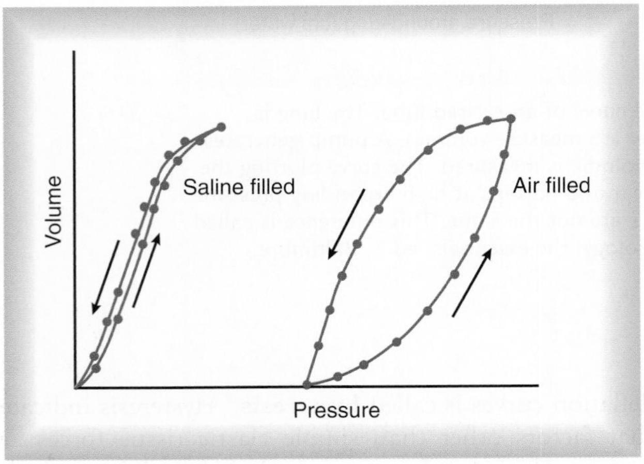

FIGURE 10-5 Static pressure-volume curves of saline-filled and air-filled excised lungs. In the saline-filled lung, the distending pressure is the same during inflation and deflation. The air-filled lung shows hysteresis (i.e., higher pressure for a given volume on inflation compared with deflation). The hysteresis results in part from the effects of surface tension forces caused by the air-liquid interface in the alveoli. (Modified from Slonim NB, Hamilton LH: Respiratory physiology, ed 5, St Louis, 1987, Mosby.)

MINI CLINI

Surfactant Replacement Therapy and Lung Mechanics

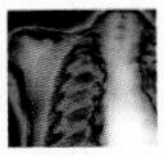

PROBLEM: If an infant is born prematurely, the lungs may be unable to produce adequate amounts of pulmonary surfactant. How does this condition affect lung mechanics, and what effect does surfactant replacement therapy have on lung compliance and the work of breathing?

DISCUSSION: The liquid molecules that line each alveolus attract one another. This attraction creates a force called *surface tension,* which tends to shrink the alveolus. Pulmonary surfactant molecules have weak intramolecular attractive forces. When surfactant molecules are mixed with other liquid molecules that have higher intramolecular attraction, the surfactant molecules are pushed to the surface of the liquid, where they form the air-liquid interface. Because of the weak intramolecular attraction between these surfactant molecules at the surface, the liquid lining of the alveoli exhibits much less surface tension than it would in the absence of pulmonary surfactant. A premature infant with inadequate surfactant has abnormally high intraalveolar surface tension; this produces a collapsing force that increases lung recoil and reduces lung compliance. Greater muscular effort is required to overcome increased recoil during inspiration, and the work of breathing is increased. The infant may eventually become fatigued and develop ventilatory failure. Instillation of artificial surfactant into the lungs reduces surface tension to its normal level. Lung compliance is increased, elastic recoil is reduced, and the muscular work required to inflate the lung is reduced.

A phospholipid called *pulmonary surfactant* reduces surface tension in the lung. Alveolar type II cells probably produce pulmonary surfactant (see Chapter 8). In contrast to typical surface-active agents, pulmonary surfactant changes surface tension according to its area.[3] The ability of pulmonary surfactant to reduce surface tension decreases as surface area (i.e., lung volume) increases. Conversely, when surface area decreases, the ability of pulmonary surfactant to reduce surface tension increases. This property of changing surface tension to match lung volume helps stabilize the alveoli. Any disorder that alters or destroys pulmonary surfactant can cause significant changes in the work of distending the lung.

Lung Compliance

Tissue elastic forces and surface tension oppose lung inflation. Compliance is the reciprocal of elastance:

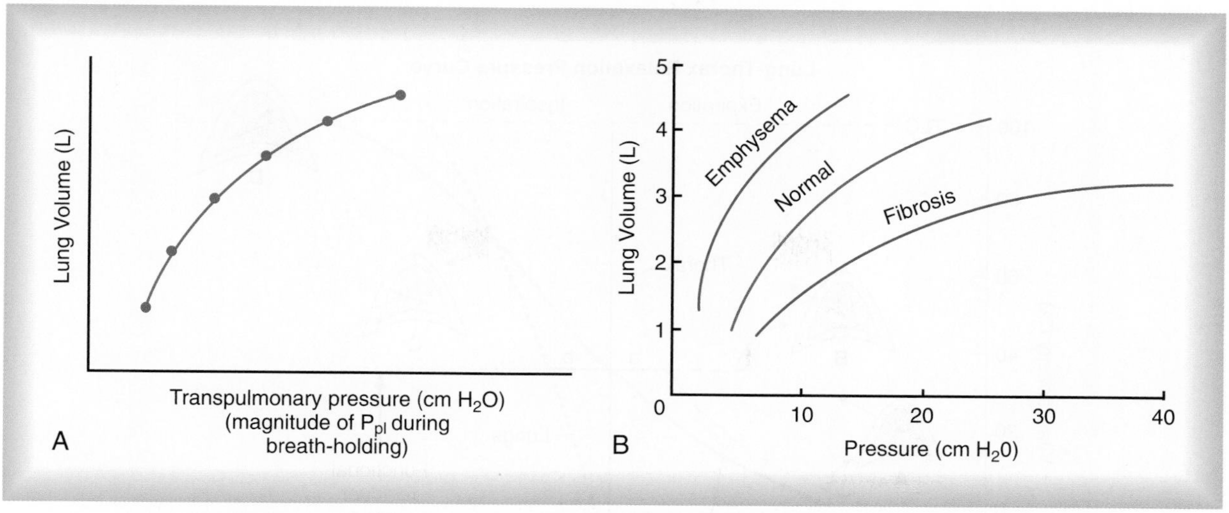

FIGURE 10-6 **A,** Compliance measurement (deflation curve). After swallowing an esophageal balloon, the subject inhales a full breath and then exhales slowly. At specific lung volumes, he holds his breath with the glottis open, ensuring an alveolar pressure of zero. Lung volume is plotted against esophageal pressure (which essentially equals P_{pl}), generating a compliance curve. **B,** Compliance curves. Normal lung compliance is approximately 0.2 L/cm H_2O (measured from the lower portion of the curve, near resting lung volume). Compliance is increased in emphysema because of the destruction of elastic tissue; conversely, it is decreased in pulmonary fibrosis because of increased elastic recoil. (Modified from Martin L: Pulmonary physiology in clinical practice: the essentials for patient care and evaluation, St Louis, 1987, Mosby.)

$$\text{Compliance} = \frac{1}{\text{Elastance}} = \frac{\Delta V}{\Delta P}$$

Compliance is defined as volume change per unit of change in the pressure difference across the structure. It is usually measured in milliliters per centimeter of water.

A graph of change in lung volume versus change in transpulmonary pressure (Figure 10-6, *A*) is the compliance curve of the lungs. Figure 10-6, *B* compares a normal lung compliance curve with curves that might be observed in patients who have emphysema (obstructive lung disease) or pulmonary fibrosis (restrictive lung disease). The curve from a patient with emphysema is steeper and displaced to the left. The shape and position of this curve represent large changes in volume for small pressure changes (increased compliance). Increased compliance results primarily from loss of elastic fibers, which occurs in emphysema. The lungs become more distensible so that the normal transpulmonary pressure results in a larger lung volume. The term *hyperinflation* is used to describe an abnormally increased lung volume. A distinctly opposite pattern is seen in pulmonary fibrosis. Interstitial fibrosis is characterized by an increase in connective tissue. The compliance curve of a patient with pulmonary fibrosis is flatter than the normal curve, shifted down and to the right. As a result, there is a smaller volume change for any given pressure change (decreased compliance). Consequently, the lungs become stiffer, usually with a reduced volume.

Chest Wall Compliance

Inflation and deflation of the lung occur with changes in the dimensions of the chest wall (see Chapter 8). The relationship between the lungs and the chest wall can be illustrated by plotting their relaxation pressure curves separately and combined (Figure 10-7). In the intact thorax, the lungs and chest wall recoil against each other. The point at which these opposing forces balance determines the resting volume of the lungs, or *functional residual capacity*. This is also the point at which alveolar pressure equals atmospheric pressure. The normal FRC is approximately 40% of the TLC. If the normal lung–chest wall relationship is disrupted, the lung tends to collapse to a volume less than the FRC, and the thorax expands to a volume larger than the FRC.

RULE OF THUMB

The lungs and chest wall each have their own compliance, or distensibility. In healthy adults, the compliance of the lungs and chest wall are approximately equal at 0.2 L/cm H_2O. However, because the lungs are contained within the thorax, the two systems act as springs pulling against each other. This action reduces the compliance of the system to approximately half that of the individual components, or 0.1 L/cm H_2O. This rule has many practical implications, particularly for mechanical ventilation of the lungs. Any disease process that alters the compliance of the lungs or chest wall can seriously disrupt the normal mechanics of ventilation.

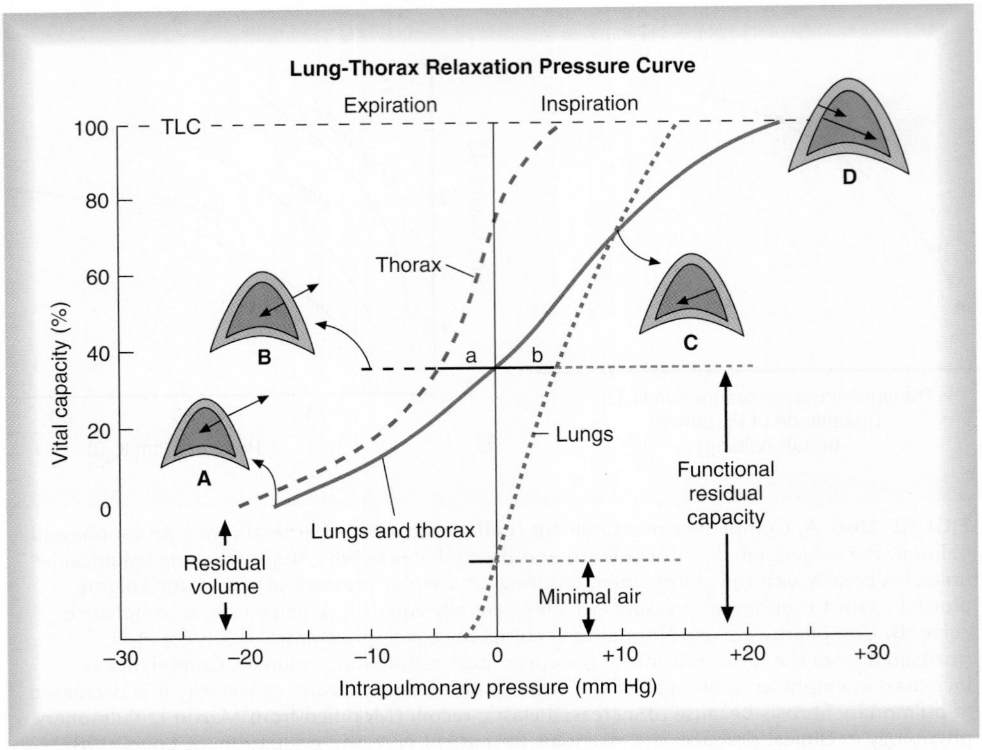

FIGURE 10-7 Relationship between the lungs and chest wall. Volumes of the lungs, thorax, and lungs and thorax combined are plotted as a percentage of vital capacity against intrapulmonary pressure (recoil pressure). The combined lung-thorax relaxation curve *(solid line)* is the sum of the individual lung and thorax curves. Equilibrium (zero pressure) occurs where the lung and thoracic recoil forces balance (a + b = 0). This point determines the FRC (lung *B*). Lung *A* represents low lung volume with greater recoil pressure exerted by the chest wall. Lung *C* shows a chest wall recoil of zero at approximately 70% of TLC. When lung volume is greater than 70% of TLC, greater pressures are required to distend both the lungs and the thorax (lung *D*). (Modified from Beachey W: Respiratory care anatomy and physiology, ed 2, St Louis, 2007, Mosby.)

The lung–chest wall system may be compared with two springs that are pulling against each other. The chest wall spring tends to expand, whereas the lung spring tends to contract. At the resting level, the forces of the chest wall and lungs balance. The tendency of the chest wall to expand is offset by the contractile force of the lungs. This balance of forces determines the resting lung volume, or FRC. The opposing forces between the chest wall and lungs are partially responsible for the subatmospheric pressure in the intrapleural space. Diseases that alter the compliance of either the chest wall or the lung often disrupt the balance point, usually with a change in lung volume.

Inhalation occurs when the balance between the lungs and chest wall shifts. Energy from the respiratory muscles (primarily the diaphragm) overcomes the contractile force of the lungs. At the beginning of the breath, the tendency of the chest wall to expand facilitates lung expansion. When lung volume nears 70% of the vital capacity, the chest wall reaches its natural resting level. To inspire to a lung volume greater than about 70% of TLC, the inspiratory muscles must overcome the recoil of both the lungs and the chest wall (see Figure 10-7).

For exhalation, potential energy "stored" in the stretched lung (and chest wall at high volumes) during the preceding inspiration causes passive deflation. To exhale below the resting level (FRC), muscular effort is required to overcome the tendency of the chest wall to expand. The expiratory muscles (see Chapter 8) provide this energy.

Compliance of the chest wall, similar to lung compliance, is a measure of distensibility. The compliance of the normal chest wall is similar to that of the lungs (0.2 L/cm H_2O). Obesity, kyphoscoliosis, ankylosing spondylitis, and many other abnormalities can reduce chest wall compliance and lung volumes.

Frictional (Nonelastic) Opposition to Ventilation

Frictional forces also oppose ventilation. Frictional opposition forces differ from the elastic properties of the lungs and thorax. Frictional opposition occurs only when the system is in motion. Frictional opposition to ventilation has the following two components: tissue viscous resistance and airway resistance.

Tissue Viscous Resistance

Tissue viscous resistance is the impedance of motion caused by displacement of tissues during ventilation. Displaced tissues include the lungs, rib cage, diaphragm, and abdominal organs. The energy to displace these structures is comparable to the impedance caused by friction in any dynamic system. Tissue resistance accounts for only approximately 20% of the total resistance to lung inflation. Obesity, fibrosis, and ascites can alter tissue viscous resistance, increasing the total impedance to ventilation.

Airway Resistance

Gas flow through the airways also causes frictional resistance. Impedance to ventilation by the movement of gas through the airways is called **airway resistance.** Airway resistance accounts for approximately 80% of the frictional resistance to ventilation.

Airway resistance is the ratio of driving pressure responsible for gas movement to the flow of the gas, calculated as follows:

$$R_{aw} = \frac{\Delta P_{TA}}{\Delta \dot{V}} = P_{AO} - \frac{P_A}{\Delta \dot{V}}$$

where R_{aw} is resistance, P_{TA} is transairway pressure difference, $\dot{V}$ is flow, P_{AO} is pressure at the airway opening, and P_A is alveolar pressure.

Driving pressure is measured in centimeters of water (cm H_2O), and flow is measured in liters per second (L/sec). Airway resistance (R_{aw}) is recorded in cm H_2O/L/sec or, more accurately, cm $H_2O \cdot sec \cdot L^{-1}$. Airway resistance in healthy adults ranges from approximately 0.5 to 2.5 cm H_2O/L/sec. To cause gas to flow into or out of the lungs at 1 L/sec, a healthy subject needs to lower his or her alveolar pressure only 0.5 to 2.5 cm H_2O below atmospheric pressure.

R_{aw} in nonventilated patients is usually measured in a pulmonary function laboratory (see Chapter 19). Flow ($\dot{V}$) is measured with a **pneumotachometer.** Alveolar pressures are determined in a body **plethysmograph,** an airtight box in which the patient sits. By momentarily occluding the patient's airway and measuring the pressure at the mouth, alveolar pressure can be estimated (i.e., mouth pressure equals alveolar pressure under conditions of no flow). By relating flow and alveolar pressure to changes in plethysmograph pressure, airway resistance can be calculated.

Factors Affecting Airway Resistance. Two patterns characterize the flow of gas through the respiratory tract: *laminar flow* and *turbulent flow.* A third pattern, *tracheobronchial flow,* is a combination of laminar and turbulent flow. When flow is laminar, gas moves in discrete layers, or streamlines. Layers near the center of an airway move faster than layers close to the wall of the airway; this results from friction between gas molecules and the wall.

MINI CLINI

HeO_2 Therapy for Large Airway Obstruction

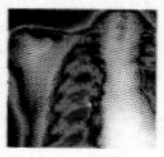

PROBLEM: Patients with significant obstruction in the upper airway, trachea, or main stem bronchi expend a large amount of energy overcoming the resistance to breathing. What type of gas therapy would be most advantageous in this situation?

DISCUSSION: Because most (approximately 80%) of the resistance to breathing occurs in the upper and large airways, disease processes that increase resistance in these airways cause tremendous increases in the work of breathing. Traumatic injuries to the vocal cords or trachea, along with tumors or foreign bodies in the trachea or main stem bronchi, are examples of the types of clinical conditions that can markedly increase the work of breathing. Patients who must breathe against high levels of resistance are prone to respiratory muscle fatigue and failure. Gas flow in the upper and large airways is predominantly turbulent. Turbulent flow is highly influenced by gas density. Patients with large airway obstruction can often be treated with a mixture of helium and oxygen (heliox or HeO_2). HeO_2, usually an 80/20 or 70/30 mixture, can be administered to reduce the work of breathing until the obstructive process can be treated. HeO_2 mixture does little for patients with small airway obstruction, as occurs in emphysema or asthma. Flow in the small airways is mainly laminar and largely independent of the density of the gas breathed. However, heliox therapy can be used for patients with small airway obstruction to allow them to exercise longer and more strenuously with less dyspnea and dynamic hyperinflation.

Poiseuille's law (see Chapter 6) defines laminar flow through a smooth, unbranched tube of fixed dimensions (i.e., length and radius). The pressure required to cause a specific flow of gas through a tube is calculated as follows:

$$\Delta P = \frac{\eta 8 l \dot{V}}{\pi r^4}$$

where:

ΔP = Driving pressure (dynes/cm^2)
η = Coefficient of viscosity of the gas
l = Tube length (cm)
$\dot{V}$ = Gas flow (ml/sec)
r = Tube radius (cm)
(π and 8 are constants.)

By eliminating factors that remain constant, such as viscosity, length, and known constants, this equation can be rearranged as follows to solve for ΔP:

$$\Delta P = \frac{\dot{V}}{r^4}$$

This equation says that for gas flow to remain constant, delivery pressure must vary *inversely* with the fourth power of the airway's radius. Reducing the radius of a tube by half requires a 16-fold pressure increase to maintain a constant flow. To maintain ventilation in the presence of narrowing airways, large increases in driving pressure may be needed. The energy necessary to generate these pressures can markedly increase the work of breathing.

RULE OF THUMB

A change in the caliber of an airway by a factor of 2 causes a 16-fold change in resistance. This rule applies to human airways and artificial airways (i.e., endotracheal and tracheostomy tubes). If the size of a patient's airway is reduced from 2 mm to 1 mm, airway resistance increases by a factor of 16. Similarly, if a 4.5-mm endotracheal tube is replaced with a 9-mm tube, the pressure required to cause a flow of 1 L/sec through the tube decreases 16-fold. This rule has many practical consequences. It is the basis for bronchodilator therapy and for using the largest practical size of artificial airway.

Another way to express the relationship between pressure and flow is as follows:

$$\dot{V} = \Delta P r^4$$

This equation shows that if the gas delivery pressure ventilating the lung remains constant, gas flow varies directly with the fourth power of the airway's radius. Reducing the airway radius by half decreases the flow 16-fold at a constant pressure. Small changes in bronchial caliber can markedly change gas flow through an airway.

Under certain conditions, gas flow through a tube changes significantly. The orderly pattern of concentric layers is no longer maintained. Gas molecules form irregular currents. This pattern is called *turbulent flow*. Transition from laminar to turbulent flow depends on the following factors: gas density (d), viscosity (h), linear velocity (v), and tube radius (I). Table 10-3 compares changes in flow and pressure resulting from laminar and turbulent flow.

TABLE 10-3

Comparison of Driving Pressures, Laminar versus Turbulent Flow

Flow	Laminar	Turbulent
1	1	1
2	2	4
4	4	16
8	8	64
16	16	256

Values are nondimensional units showing proportional effect.

RULE OF THUMB

Patients who have emphysema can directly influence the EPP in their airways to reduce airway collapse and closure. Airway collapse may occur in patients who have emphysema because the normal support structure for small airways has been destroyed. By exhaling through "pursed lips," a patient with emphysema changes the pressure at the airway opening. The gentle back pressure created counters the tendency for small airways to collapse by moving the EPP toward larger airways.

Distribution of Airway Resistance. Approximately 80% of the resistance to gas flow occurs in the nose, mouth, and large airways, where flow is mainly turbulent. Only about 20% of the total resistance to flow is attributable to airways smaller than 2 mm in diameter, where flow is mainly laminar. This fact seems to contradict the fact that resistance is inversely related to the radius of the conducting tube.

Branching of the tracheobronchial tree increases the cross-sectional area with each airway generation (Figure 10-8). As gas moves from the mouth to the alveoli, the

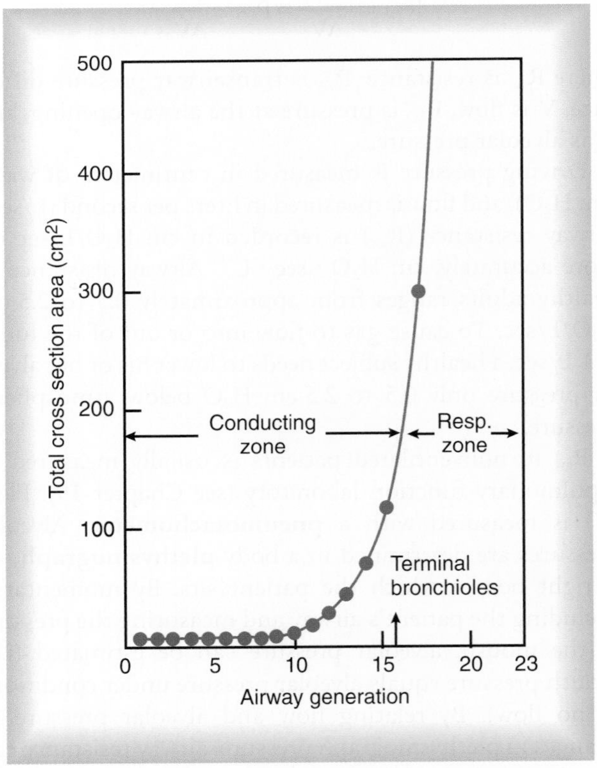

FIGURE 10-8 Cross-sectional area of the airways plotted against airway generation. The first 15 or 16 airway generations represent a conducting zone in which gas moves primarily by bulk flow, and no gas exchange takes place. These airways make up the anatomic dead space (see Chapter 8). The gas exchange surface increases markedly at the level of the terminal bronchiole. (Modified from West J: Respiratory physiology: the essentials, ed 7, Baltimore, 2005, Williams & Wilkins.)

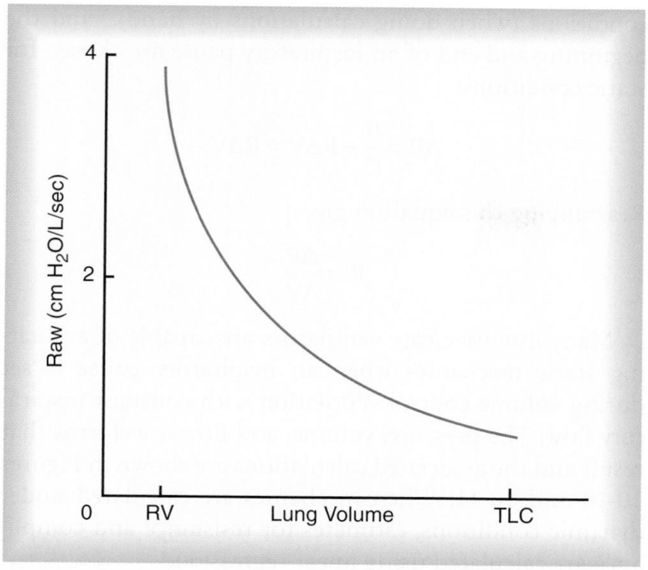

FIGURE 10-9 Change in airway resistance (R_{aw}) related to lung volume. Resistance to airflow is highly dependent on lung volume. At low lung volumes, near residual volume *(RV)*, the airways are compressed, and resistance increases markedly. At high lung volumes, near total lung capacity *(TLC)*, the airways are distended, and resistance decreases. See text for discussion.

TABLE 10-4

Distribution of Airway Resistance

Location	Total Resistance (%)
Nose, mouth, upper airway	50
Trachea and bronchi	30
Small airways (<2 mm)	20

combined cross-sectional area of the airways increases exponentially (see Chapter 8). According to the laws of fluid dynamics, this increase in cross-sectional area causes a decrease in gas velocity. The decrease in gas velocity promotes a laminar flow pattern, particularly in smaller (i.e., <2 mm) airways.

Turbulent flow predominates in the mouth, trachea, and primary bronchi (Table 10-4). Gas velocity is high in the bigger airways, favoring turbulent flow patterns. At the level of the terminal bronchioles, the cross-sectional area increases more than 30-fold. Gas velocity is very low here. In normal small airways, flow is laminar. The driving pressure across these airways is less than 1% of the total driving pressure for the system.

The diameter of the airways is not constant. During inspiration, the stretch of surrounding lung tissue and widening transpulmonary pressure gradient increase the diameter of the airways. The higher the lung volume, the more that these factors influence airway caliber (Figure 10-9). The increase in airway diameter with increasing lung volume decreases airway resistance. As lung volume decreases toward residual volume, airway diameters also decrease; this explains why wheezing (see Chapter 15) is most often heard during exhalation. Airway resistance increases dramatically at low lung volumes.

STATIC VERSUS DYNAMIC MECHANICS

Resistance and compliance can be evaluated under static or dynamic conditions.[4] The term *static* implies that flow throughout the respiratory system has ceased and all ventilatory muscle activity is absent (P_{mus} = 0). Static conditions can be imposed with an inspiratory pause when a patient is sedated and being mechanically ventilated. In contrast, the term *dynamic* means that flow at the airway opening is zero. Mechanics are evaluated under dynamic conditions, for example, when a nonintubated patient breathes spontaneously. In this case, the pressure difference used to calculate lung resistance and elastance is P_{TP}, and the driving pressure is P_{mus} instead of the ventilator.

In a single-compartment model (see Figure 10-1), estimation of resistance and compliance under static and dynamic conditions yields the same values. However, in a real respiratory system, composed of multiple compartments with different time constants (each compartment being a resistance in series with a compliance), mechanics estimated during static conditions yield different values than when evaluated during dynamic conditions. For a multiple-compartment system, when flow is zero at the airway opening, there may still be flow between compartments (pendelluft). As a result, dynamic mechanics become dependent on the respiratory frequency.[5,6] Typically, both compliance and resistance decrease as frequency increases.

For either the static or the dynamic method, the basic model is still the equation of motion described earlier. Written with symbols using compliance instead of elastance:

$$P(t) = \frac{V(t)}{C} + R\dot{V}(t)$$

where P(t) is the pressure difference across the system of interest as a function of time, t; C is compliance (a constant); V(t) is volume as a function of time; R is resistance (a constant); and $\dot{V}(t)$ is flow as a function of time. Usually P is either transrespiratory pressure difference or transpulmonary pressure difference. Because only one pressure difference can be measured, the effect of compliance has to be separated out from the effect of resistance.

To calculate compliance, the definition of compliance is $C = \Delta V/\Delta P$. The Δ sign indicates that we need to calculate a difference in volume and pressure between two points in time. The two points in time are when flow is zero, such as the beginning and end of inspiration. The volume change, ΔV, between the beginning and end of inspiration is the

V_T. If $\dot{V}(1) = 0$ and $\dot{V}(2) = 0$, $\Delta\dot{V} = 0 - 0 = 0$, and the equation of motion simplifies to:

$$\Delta P = \frac{\Delta V}{C} + R(0) = \frac{V_T}{C} + 0$$

Rearranging this equation gives the equation for compliance:

$$C = \frac{V_T}{\Delta P}$$

If P is transrespiratory system pressure, C is respiratory system compliance. Similarly, if P is transpulmonary pressure, C is pulmonary (lung) compliance.

To calculate resistance, we use a similar logic and eliminate the term $\Delta V/C$ by selecting two points in time when volumes are equal (i.e., V at time 1 equals V at time 2) so that $\Delta V = V(2) - V(1) = 0$. In this case, we cannot select the two times as the beginning and end of inspiration because the flow term would be zero. Typically, times corresponding to midinspiration are chosen for dynamic conditions (when doing calculations by hand),[7] and the beginning and end of an inspiratory pause are chosen for static conditions:

$$\Delta P = \frac{0}{C} + R\Delta\dot{V} = R\Delta\dot{V}$$

Rearranging this equation gives:

$$R = \frac{\Delta P}{\Delta\dot{V}}$$

Many intensive care ventilators are capable of evaluating static mechanics when an inspiratory pause is set during volume control ventilation with constant inspiratory flow. The pressure, volume, and flow waveforms that result and the associated calculations are shown in Figures 10-10 and 10-11. When mechanics are calculated under dynamic conditions, estimates for resistance and compliance are calculated using linear regression.[8]

A simplified conceptual explanation of how linear regression could be used to calculate resistance under

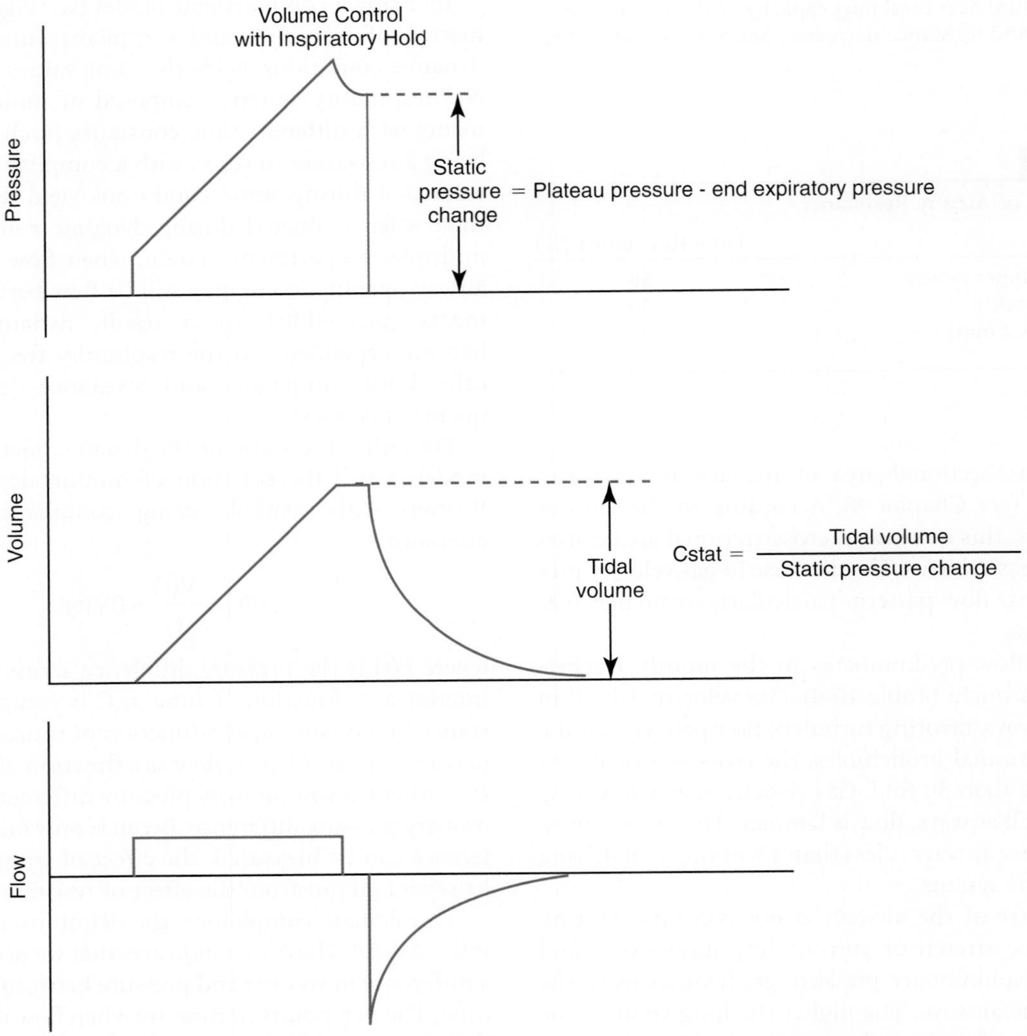

FIGURE 10-10 Calculation of respiratory system compliance under static conditions using an inspiratory pause during volume control mechanical ventilation with constant inspiratory flow.

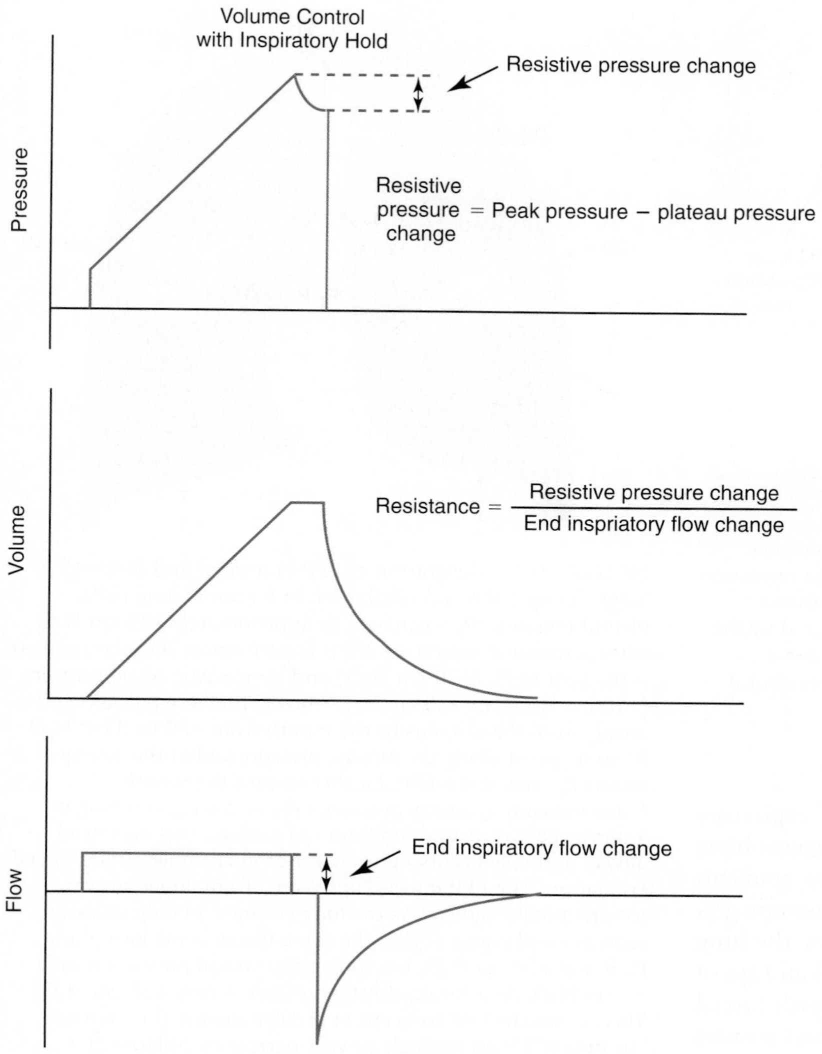

FIGURE 10-11 Calculation of respiratory system resistance under static conditions using an inspiratory pause during volume control mechanical ventilation with constant inspiratory flow.

dynamic conditions is shown in Figure 10-12. Measurements of pressure and flow are made every few milliseconds and plotted as shown. Using linear regression, a straight line is fit to the data that minimizes the squared distances from the line to individual data points (shown by the arrows). The slope of the line, $\Delta P/\Delta \dot{V}$, is the resistance. A similar procedure can be performed to calculate elastance if the horizontal axis is volume (or compliance if the vertical axis is volume and the horizontal axis is pressure). In practice, data for pressure, volume, and flow are fit to the equation of motion all at once. Conceptually, the equation represents a plane in three dimensions (i.e., pressure, volume, and flow). The projection of the plane on the pressure-volume axis is a straight line whose slope is elastance, whereas the projection on the pressure-flow axis is also a straight line whose slope is resistance. Dynamic respiratory mechanics evaluation may be more appropriate than static mechanics for guiding lung protective ventilation strategies in patients with acute lung injury and acute respiratory distress syndrome (ARDS).[9]

MECHANICS OF EXHALATION

Airway caliber is determined by several factors, including anatomic (i.e., physical) support provided to the airways and pressure differences across their walls. Anatomic support comes from cartilage in the wall of the airway and from "traction" provided by surrounding tissues. The larger airways depend mainly on cartilaginous support. Because smaller airways lack cartilage, they depend on support provided by surrounding lung parenchyma.[10]

The airways are also supported by the pressure difference across their walls. This transpulmonary pressure gradient helps stabilize the airways, particularly the small ones. During quiet breathing, pleural pressure is normally subatmospheric. Airway pressure varies minimally and is usually close to zero. The transmural pressure gradient during normal quiet breathing is negative, even during exhalation. It ranges from −5 to −10 cm H_2O. This negative transmural pressure gradient helps maintain the caliber of the small airways.

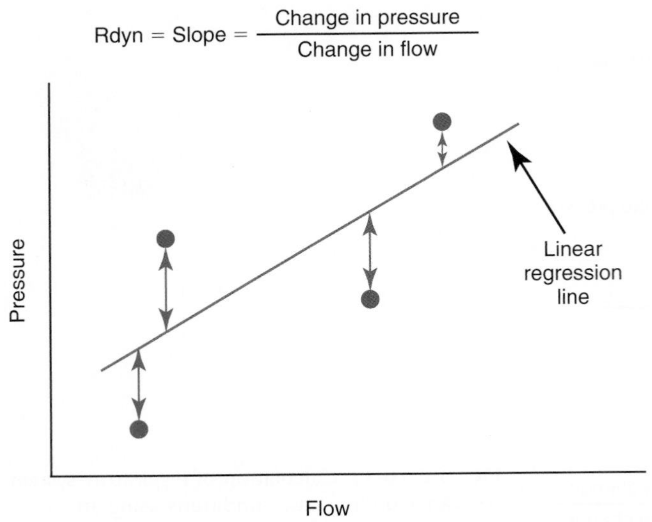

FIGURE 10-12 Calculation of respiratory system resistance under dynamic conditions using linear regression. The regression line is fitted to the data by minimizing the vertical distance between individual data points and the line as indicated by the *double arrows*. The slope of the line is resistance. The same technique can be used to calculate elastance if the horizontal axis is volume.

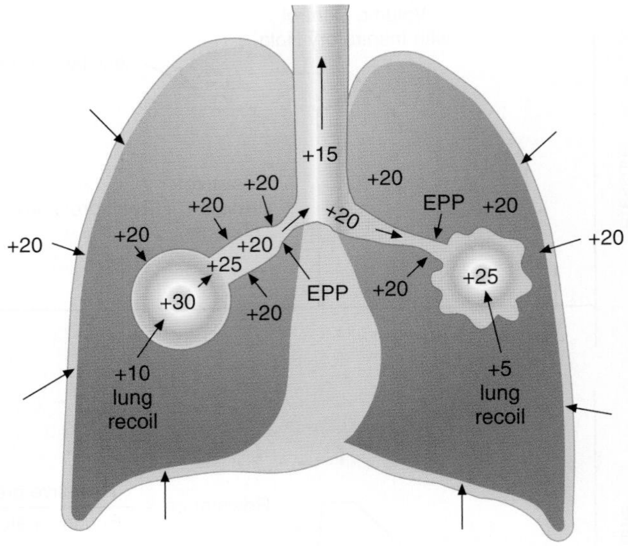

FIGURE 10-13 Generation of EPP in normal and diseased lungs during a forceful exhalation. In a normal lung *(left)*, pleural pressure (P_{pl}) increases to approximately +20 cm H_2O when a maximal expiratory effort is performed. Alveolar pressure is the sum of P_{pl} (+20 cm H_2O) and lung elastic recoil pressure (+10 cm H_2O), or +30 cm H_2O. Airway pressure falls along the airway from the alveolus to the mouth from +30 to 0 cm H_2O. At some point along the airway, pressure within the airway equals P_{pl}; this is the EPP. Further toward the mouth ("downstream"), airway pressure falls below P_{pl}, resulting in a narrowed airway and limitation of airflow. This narrowed airway normally occurs in healthy individuals only during forced exhalation. The EPP moves "upstream" from larger airways toward smaller airways as the lung empties. In lung diseases such as emphysema *(right)*, the same forces come into play. P_{pl} is still +20 cm H_2O, but lung elastic recoil pressure is only +5 cm H_2O. As a result, driving pressure is only +25 cm H_2O. This causes the EPP to occur in smaller airways (i.e., farther "upstream") than normal; airways narrow or collapse at a higher lung volume than in healthy lungs. In patients with emphysema, airway collapse is complicated further by loss of support for the small airways. (Modified from Martin L: Pulmonary physiology in clinical practice: the essentials for patient care and evaluation, St Louis, 1987, Mosby.)

During a forced exhalation, contraction of expiratory muscles can increase pleural pressure above atmospheric pressure; this reverses the transmural pressure gradient, making it positive. If the positive transmural pressure gradient exceeds the supporting force provided by the lung parenchyma, the small airways may collapse. In airways of healthy subjects, airway collapse occurs only with forced exhalation and at low lung volumes. In diseased airways (e.g., emphysema), it may occur with normal breathing and at much higher lung volumes.

Forceful contraction of the expiratory muscles causes pleural pressure to increase from its normal negative value to above atmospheric (Figure 10-13). Alveolar pressure during forced exhalation equals the sum of pleural pressure and the elastic recoil pressure of the lung itself.[11]

The pressure along the airway decreases as gas flows from the alveoli toward the mouth. Moving "downstream" (toward the mouth), transmural pressure (the pressure difference between inside and outside the airway wall) decreases continually. At some point along the airway, the pressure inside equals the pressure outside in the pleural space (transmural pressure equals zero). This point is referred to as the **equal pressure point (EPP).** Downstream from this point, pleural pressure exceeds the airway pressure. The resulting negative transmural pressure gradient causes airway compression and can lead to collapse. Airway compression increases expiratory airway resistance and limits flow. At the EPP, greater expiratory effort increases pleural pressure, restricting flow further.[12] Once the transmural pressure has increased sufficiently to cause this flow limitation (at the EPP), airflow becomes effort independent with airway caliber and elastic recoil pressure determining flow. **Dynamic compression** of the airways (narrowing of the airways owing to an increase in surrounding pressures) is responsible for the characteristic flow patterns observed in forced expiratory tests of pulmonary function (see discussion of flow-volume curves in Chapter 19).

In healthy individuals, dynamic airway compression occurs only at lung volumes well below the resting expiratory level. Additional anatomic support is provided by the surrounding lung parenchyma. This tissue support opposes the collapsing force created by negative transmural pressure gradients. In pulmonary emphysema, the elastic tissue responsible for supporting the small airways is damaged. Destruction of elastic tissue has multiple outcomes. It increases the compliance of the lung (i.e., elastic recoil decreases; see Figure 10-13). Emphysema also obliterates the anatomic structures responsible for small airway support.[12] This combination of decreased elastic recoil and loss of support for the small airways allows the airways to collapse during exhalation. Airway collapse causes air trapping and increase in the resting volume of the lung. Expiratory flow is limited by airway collapse during exhalation and can occur during tidal breathing when emphysematous changes in the lung are severe.[13]

WORK OF BREATHING

The respiratory muscles do the work for normal breathing. This work requires energy to overcome the elastic and frictional forces opposing inflation. Assessment of mechanical work involves measurement of the physical parameters of force and distance as they relate to moving air into and out of the lung. Assessment of metabolic work involves measurement of the O_2 cost of breathing.

During normal quiet breathing, inhalation is active, and exhalation is passive. The work of exhaling is recovered from potential energy "stored" in the expanded lung and thorax during inhalation. However, forced exhalation requires additional work by the expiratory muscles. The actual work of forced expiration depends on the mechanical properties of the lungs and thorax.

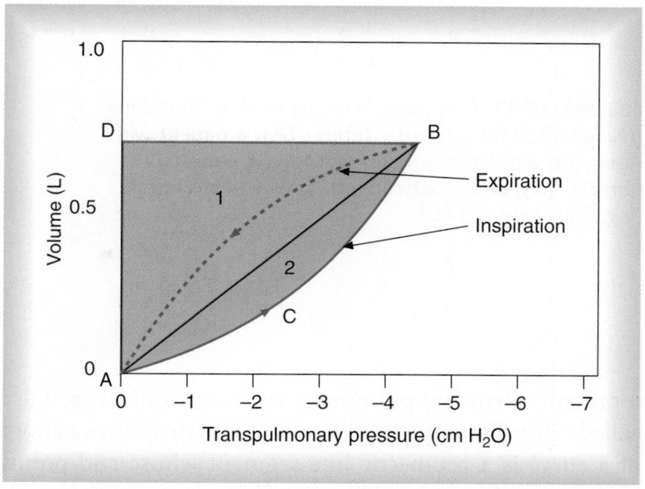

FIGURE 10-14 Factors involved in the work of breathing. Point *A* is the resting lung volume (FRC), and *B* is end-inspiration. The *straight solid line A-B* represents the pressure required to overcome simple elastic forces, and the *curved line A-C-B* represents the additional pressure required to overcome frictional resistance (airway and tissue). At *B,* where airflow momentarily ceases, frictional resistance is inactive. Area *1* represents the work (P × V) required to overcome elastic forces; area *2* represents the work required to overcome frictional forces. The work of breathing (inspiration) is the sum of these two areas. The *curved dashed line* within area *1* represents the pressure-volume curve of passive exhalation using energy stored during inspiration.

Mechanical

Work done on an object is the result of the force (F) exerted on the object and the distance (x) it is moved. The general equation for work is:

$$W = \int F dx$$

Work may be expressed in units of either dyne-centimeters (dyne-cm) or joules (J). For a constant applied force, this equation simplifies to:

$$\text{W} = \text{Force} \times \text{Distance}$$

In physiology, work is expressed in terms of pressure difference across a structure (P) and the volume change of the structure (V). Because pressure is equal to force/area and volume is equal to area × distance, work can have the dimensions of P × V:

$$\begin{aligned}\text{Pressure} \times \text{Volume} &= \frac{\text{Force}}{\text{Area}} \times (\text{Area} \times \text{Distance}) \\ &= \text{Force} \times \text{Distance} \\ &= \text{Work}\end{aligned}$$

In general:

$$W = \int P dV$$

Graphically, the integral of pressure difference with respect to volume is the area between the pressure-volume curve and the volume axis (Figure 10-14). P represents a pressure difference across a structure (i.e., inside pressure minus outside pressure), and the pressure difference *defines the structure* for which work is evaluated. The work the muscles do to inflate the pulmonary system is defined by the transpulmonary pressure, P_{TP}:

$$W_{TP} = \int P_{TP} dV$$

Similarly, the work done by a ventilator to inflate the respiratory system is defined in terms of the transrespiratory system pressure, P_{TR}:

$$W_{TR} = \int P_{TR} dV$$

For constant applied pressure difference across a structure (i.e., an instantaneous change from baseline, ΔP), work can be calculated as:

$$\text{W} = \text{P} \times \text{V}$$

Also, because of the equivalence of work and energy, the energy stored in a rigid wall container holding compressed gas is simply the product of the volume of the container and the pressure inside the container (relative to the outside). The higher the pressure, the more energy stored in the container. When the pressure is released, useful work can be recovered. This is the principle used in air rifles.

Figure 10-14 shows a graph of transpulmonary pressure versus lung volume derived from measurements taken during dynamic conditions (e.g., during a normal inspiration). The line *AB* connects two points in time when flow is zero. As discussed earlier, the slope of this line ($\Delta V/\Delta P_{TP}$)

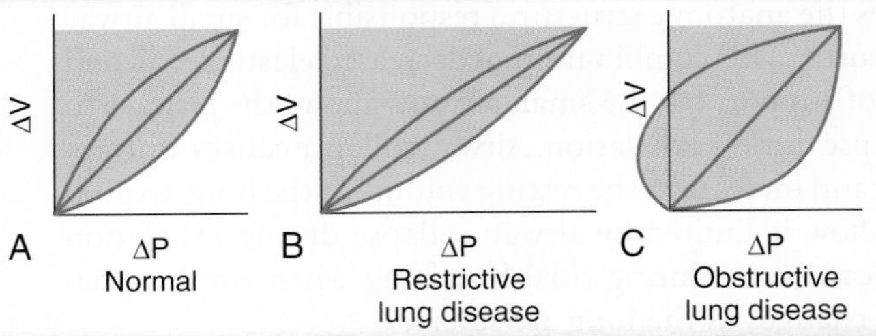

FIGURE 10-15 Comparison of the work of breathing *(shaded areas)* for a healthy subject **(A),** a patient with restrictive ventilatory impairment (e.g., pulmonary fibrosis) **(B),** and a patient with airway obstruction (e.g., emphysema) **(C).**

represents dynamic pulmonary or lung compliance (also called "chord" compliance because in mathematics a chord of a curve is a geometric line segment whose end points both lie on the curve). The work done overcoming purely elastic forces opposing inflation is represented by the triangular area 1 in Figure 10-14. The work required to overcome flow resistive forces is represented by area 2. The total mechanical work for one breath is the sum of the work overcoming both the elastic and the resistive forces opposing inflation; this is represented as the sum of areas 1 and 2. In healthy adults, approximately two-thirds of the work of breathing can be attributed to elastic forces opposing ventilation. The remaining one-third is a result of frictional resistance to gas and tissue movement.

Traditionally, static pressure-volume curves have been created by injecting the lungs with discreet volume steps using a large calibrated syringe ("super syringe").[14] Alternatively, the line *AB* can be approximated under clinical conditions using a very slow inspiratory flow (with the patient heavily sedated) producing what is called a *quasistatic* pressure-volume curve.[15] Evaluation of this type of pressure-volume curve can be useful for setting optimal positive end expiratory pressure (PEEP).[16] Ventilators made by Hamilton Medical, Inc., (Reno, NV) offer what they call the "PV Tool," which generates a quasistatic pressure-volume curve using a slow pressure ramp rather than a slow inspiratory flow. This method allows evaluation of both compliance and lung recruitability.[17]

In the presence of pulmonary disease, work of breathing can increase dramatically (Figure 10-15). The areas of the volume-pressure curves for patients with obstruction or restriction are greater than in healthy subjects.[18] The reasons for these increases in the mechanical work are quite different. In restrictive lung disease, the area of the volume-pressure curve is greater because the slope of the static component (compliance) is less than normal. The area of the volume-pressure curve in obstructive lung disease is increased because the portion associated with frictional resistance is markedly widened. The leftward "bulge" of the loop indicates positive pleural pressure that can occur during expiration, notably when lung compliance is increased (see Figure 10-15, *C*).

In healthy individuals, the mechanical work of breathing depends on the pattern of ventilation. Large V_T increases the elastic component of work. High breathing rates (and high flows) increase frictional work. When changing from quiet breathing to exercise ventilation, a healthy subject adjusts V_T and breathing frequency to minimize the work of breathing.

Similar adjustments occur in individuals who have lung disease (Figure 10-16). Patients with "stiff lungs" (i.e., increased elastic work of breathing), such as in pulmonary fibrosis, often assume a rapid, shallow breathing pattern. This pattern minimizes the mechanical work of distending the lungs but at the expense of more energy to increase breathing rate. Patients who have airway obstruction may assume a ventilatory pattern that reduces the frictional work of breathing. Breathing slowly and using pursed lip breathing during exhalation minimize airway resistance.

Increased work of breathing is often complicated by *respiratory muscle weakness,* which may result from electrolyte imbalance, *acidemia,* shock, *sepsis,* or diseases affecting the muscles themselves.[18] When increased work of breathing occurs with respiratory muscle weakness, inspiratory muscles can fatigue. V_T decreases and respiratory rate increases as the muscles fatigue and fail. Gas exchange may be compromised by ventilation/perfusion imbalances and increased dead space resulting from the low V_T (see the section on Efficiency and Effectiveness of Ventilation later).

Metabolic

To perform work, the respiratory muscles consume O_2. The rate of O_2 consumption ($\dot{V}O_2$) by the respiratory muscles reflects their energy requirements. It also provides an indirect measure of the work of breathing.

The O_2 cost of breathing is assessed by measuring $\dot{V}O_2$ at rest and at increased levels of ventilation. If no other factors increase O_2 consumption, the additional O_2 uptake is a result of respiratory muscle metabolism. The O_2 cost of breathing in healthy individuals averages 0.5 to 1.0 ml of O_2 per liter of increased ventilation. This range represents less than 5% of the O_2 consumption of the body. At high levels of ventilation (i.e., >120 L/min), the O_2 cost of breathing increases tremendously and may exceed 30% of the O_2 consumption of the body.

The $\dot{V}O_2$ of the respiratory muscles is closely related to the inspiratory pressures generated by the diaphragm. This

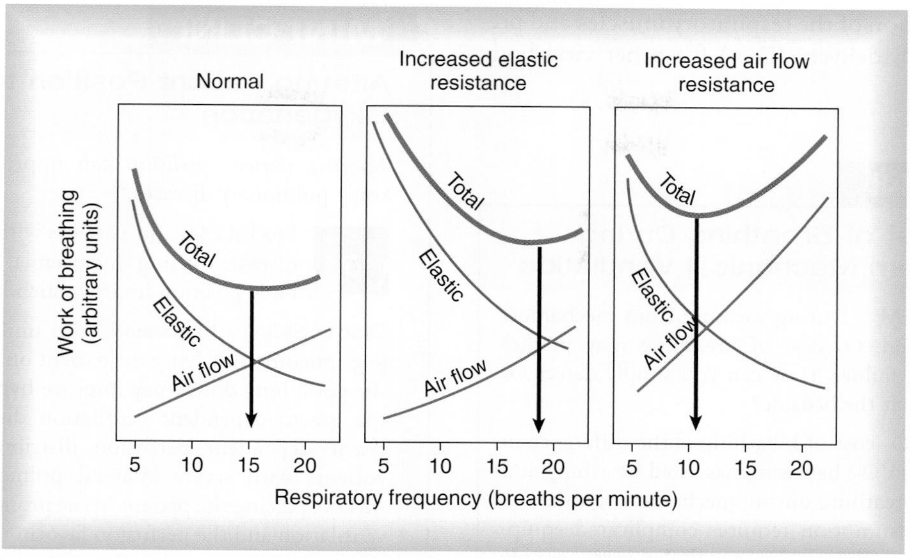

FIGURE 10-16 Work required to overcome airflow plus elastic resistance equals total work. In normal lungs, total work of breathing is minimal at approximately 15 breaths/min *(left)*. To achieve the same minute volume with stiff lungs (increased elastic resistance), minimum work is performed at higher frequencies *(middle)*. However, with increased airflow resistance (obstructive lung disease), minimum work requires lower rates of breathing *(right)*. (Modified from Nunn JF: Applied respiratory physiology, ed 2, London, 1977, Butterworth.)

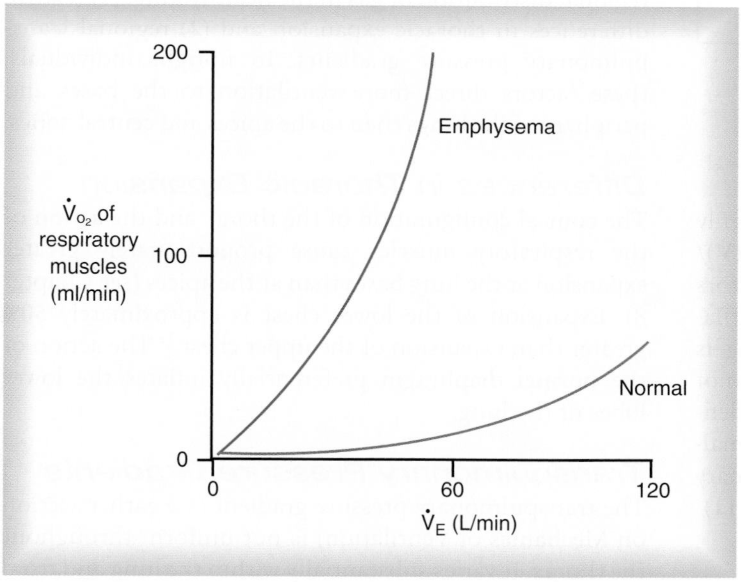

FIGURE 10-17 Relationship of oxygen cost of breathing to minute ventilation during maximum exercise for a healthy subject and for a patient with emphysema. Oxygen consumption ($\dot{V}O_2$) of the respiratory muscles is minimal at levels of ventilation up to about 100 L/min in normal subjects. The metabolic demand is significantly higher in obstructive lung disease (e.g., emphysema) even at low and moderate levels of ventilation.

transdiaphragmatic pressure (P_{di}) can be measured by a technique similar to the technique used for measuring intrapleural pressure (see earlier section on Lung Compliance). A thin catheter with two small balloons is advanced into the esophagus. One balloon remains in the esophagus (above the diaphragm), and the balloon at the tip is placed in the stomach. The pressure difference between the balloons measures the pressure across the diaphragm. The greater the pressure required to overcome inspiratory resistance, the higher the O_2 consumption of the respiratory muscles.

In the presence of pulmonary disease (either obstructive or restrictive), the O_2 cost of breathing may increase dramatically with increasing ventilation (Figure 10-17). In an obstructive disease such as emphysema, increased ventilation causes the O_2 consumption of the respiratory muscles to increase rapidly. This abnormally high O_2 cost of breathing is one factor that limits exercise in such patients. Increased O_2 consumption by the respiratory muscles may also contribute to the failure to wean patients from mechanical ventilation.[19] Intubation and mechanical ventilation in cases of shock may be indicated to decrease the excess O_2 consumption of the respiratory muscles and preserve the limited O_2 delivery (DO_2) for other vital body organs.

MINI CLINI

Oxygen Cost of Breathing During Weaning from Mechanical Ventilation

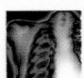

PROBLEM: During weaning from mechanical ventilation, O_2 cost of breathing may predict weaning failure. How can you simply detect O_2 cost of breathing at the bedside?

DISCUSSION: O_2 cost of breathing is the difference in O_2 consumption ($\dot{V}O_2$) between unassisted breathing and passive assisted breathing during mechanical ventilation. Although O_2 consumption requires complicated equipment (indirect calorimetry or metabolic cart), simply looking at the mixed venous O_2 saturation ($S\bar{v}O_2$) before and after initiation of weaning may be a good surrogate for O_2 cost of breathing. If the $S\bar{v}O_2$ was 75% (normal) before initiation of weaning, and after 30 minutes of spontaneous breathing trial the value is 60% without other reason for increased O_2 consumption, it is fair to assume that the O_2 cost of breathing has increased significantly, and failure of weaning or extubation is possible.

DISTRIBUTION OF VENTILATION

Neither ventilation nor perfusion is distributed evenly in healthy lungs, resulting in uneven ventilation ($\dot{V}$)/perfusion ($\dot{Q}$) ratio ($\dot{V}/\dot{Q} = 0.8$). Regional and local factors account for this unevenness in the distribution of ventilation. Uneven ventilation helps explain why the lung is imperfect for gas exchange. In disease, the distribution of ventilation can worsen dramatically. The resulting deficiencies in gas exchange can be life-threatening. The maldistribution of ventilation in disease represents a primary cause of impaired O_2 and CO_2 exchange (see Chapter 11).

RULE OF THUMB

Gravity, to a large extent, determines where ventilation goes in the lungs. In an upright lung, the weight of the lung tissues causes alveoli at the bases to be smaller but more easily distended. Alveoli at the top of the lung are larger but distend less easily. Gravity also causes most blood flow through pulmonary capillaries to go to the bases. The pressure-volume characteristics of the upright lung direct most ventilation to these dependent portions, matching ventilation and blood flow to promote gas exchange. This phenomenon can be useful clinically when localized lesions (e.g., lobar pneumonia) cause ventilation/perfusion abnormalities.

MINI CLINI

Altering Patient Position to Improve Oxygenation

Altering patient position can improve oxygenation in some pulmonary diseases.[20]

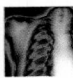

PROBLEM: In patients with severe pulmonary disease causing hypoxemia, how can altering body position improve such hypoxemia?

DISCUSSION: In patients with unilateral lung disease (e.g., pneumonia), lying the patient on his or her side with the good lung down may improve hypoxemia by altering the gravity-dependent ventilation distribution and the gravity-dependent perfusion distribution. Similarly in patients with severe bilateral pulmonary disease (e.g., ARDS), placing the patient in the prone position alters the ventilation and the perfusion favoring the ventral areas of the lungs and improving the hypoxemia.

Regional Factors

Two factors interact with the effects of gravity to affect regional distribution of gas in the healthy lung: (1) relative differences in thoracic expansion and (2) regional transpulmonary pressure gradients. In upright individuals, these factors direct more ventilation to the bases and periphery of the lungs than to the apices and central zones.

Differences in Thoracic Expansion

The conical configuration of the thorax and the action of the respiratory muscles cause proportionately greater expansion at the lung bases than at the apices (see Chapter 8). Expansion of the lower chest is approximately 50% greater than expansion of the upper chest.[21] The action of the normal diaphragm preferentially inflates the lower lobes of the lung.

Transpulmonary Pressure Gradients

The transpulmonary pressure gradient (see earlier section on Mechanics of Ventilation) is not uniform throughout the thorax. It varies substantially within the lung and from the top to the bottom of the lung. At a given level of alveolar inflation, the transpulmonary pressure gradient is directly related to the pleural pressure. Pleural pressure represents the pressure on the outer surface of the lung. Its effect lessens toward more centrally located alveoli. Changes in the transpulmonary pressure gradient are greatest in peripheral alveoli (i.e., near the surface of the lung). The changes are least in the alveoli of the central zones. Peripheral alveoli expand proportionately more than their more central counterparts.

Top-to-bottom differences in pleural pressure have an even greater effect on the distribution of ventilation, especially in the upright lung.[3] Pleural pressure increases by approximately 0.25 cm H_2O for each 1 cm, from the lung apex to its base for the average-sized adult lung. This increase in pressure results from the weight of the lung itself and the effect of gravity. In an adult-sized lung (approximately 30 cm from apex to base), pleural pressure at the apex is approximately −10 cm H_2O. At the base, pleural pressure is only about −2.5 cm H_2O. Because of these differences, the transpulmonary pressure gradient at the top of the upright lung is greater than it is at the bottom. As a result, alveoli at the apices have a larger resting volume than do alveoli at the bases.

Because of their larger volume, alveoli at the apices expand less during inspiration than alveoli at the bases. Apical alveoli rest on the upper portion of the lung's pressure-volume curve (Figure 10-18). This part of the curve is relatively flat. Each unit of pressure change causes only a small change in volume. Alveoli at the lung bases are positioned on the steeper middle portion of the pressure-volume curve. For each unit of pressure change, there is a larger change in volume (greater compliance). For a given transpulmonary pressure gradient, alveoli at the bases expand more than alveoli at the apices. The bases of the upright lung receive approximately four times as much ventilation as the apices.

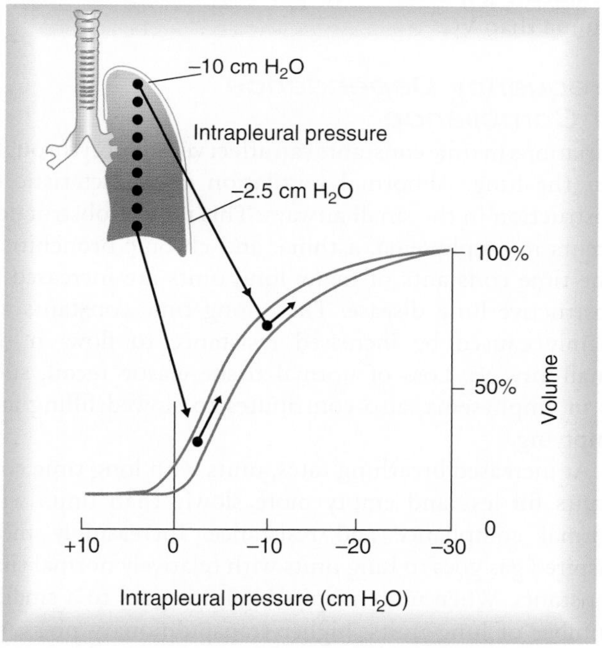

FIGURE 10-18 Causes of regional differences in ventilation from the apex to the base of an upright lung. Because of the weight of the lung and the influence of gravity, intrapleural pressure at the apex is more negative (subatmospheric) than at the base. Alveoli at the apex are maintained at a higher resting inflation volume than are further at the base. However, alveoli at the apex reside on the flatter upper portion of the pressure-volume curve. Alveoli at the base are positioned on the lower, steeper portion. For an equal change in intrapleural pressure, alveoli at the base expand more during inspiration than alveoli at the apex. This causes more ventilation to go to the bases in the upright lung. (Modified from West JB: Respiratory physiology: the essentials, ed 7, Baltimore, 2005, Williams & Wilkins.)

These gravity-dependent differences also are observed in recumbent individuals. The magnitude of the differences is less than in the upright lung because the top-to-bottom distance is less. Ventilation is still greatest in the dependent zones of the lung. In recumbent subjects, the posterior regions are dependent. Lying on the side causes more ventilation to go to whichever lung is lower. This gravity dependence can be exploited to direct ventilation toward healthy lung segments or away from diseased segments by appropriate positioning of the patient.

Local Factors

Alveolar filling and emptying are affected by local factors. Individual respiratory units and their associated airways may differ from each other. These local factors contribute to uneven ventilation in healthy lungs. Their influence on gas distribution becomes particularly important in disease.

Each respiratory unit has an elastic element, the alveolus, and a resistive element, the airway. Change in alveolar volume and the time required for the change to occur depend on the compliance and resistance of each respiratory unit.[3] In terms of compliance, the more distensible the lung unit, the greater the volume change at a given transpulmonary pressure. Lung units with high compliance have less elastic recoil than normal. These units fill and empty more slowly than normal units. Lung units with low compliance (high elastic recoil) increase their volume less. They fill and empty faster than normal. Alveolar surfactant helps to stabilize alveoli of different sizes and even out the filling and emptying times.

Airway resistance also affects emptying and filling. The size of the airway influences how much driving pressure reaches distal lung units. In healthy airways, the pressure decrease between the airway opening (i.e., the mouth) and the alveolus is minimal. Most of the driving pressure is available for alveolar inflation. If the airway is obstructed, high resistance to gas flow can occur in a local area. The pressure decrease across the obstruction may be substantial. Less driving pressure is available for alveolar inflation; there is less alveolar volume change.

Time Constants

Compliance and resistance determine local rates of alveolar filling and emptying. This relationship can be shown using the equation of motion where P(t) is set to a constant value, representing a step change (i.e., a sudden change from one level to another, as in from PEEP to inspiratory pressure during pressure control ventilation). For example:

$$\Delta P = PIP - PEEP = \frac{V(t)}{C} + R\dot{V}(t)$$

When this equation is solved for volume as a function of time (using calculus techniques), the result for passive inspiration is:

$$V(t) = C\Delta P(1 - e^{-t/RC})$$

For passive expiration (with any mode of ventilation), it is:

$$V(t) = C\Delta P(e^{-t/RC})$$

where e is the base of the natural logarithms (approximately 2.72). The product of resistance and compliance (RC in the equation) has units of time (usually seconds) and is called the *time constant.* It is referred to as a "constant" because for any value of resistance and compliance, the time constant always equals the time necessary for the lungs to fill or empty by 63%. For unit of inspiratory or expiratory time equal to the time constant, lung volume changes by 63%. After two time constants, lung volume has changed 86%; after three time constants, it has changed 95%. This relationship relates to ventilator settings in that for pressure control modes, inspiratory time must be at least three time constants long to deliver 95% of the volume that is possible with the given pressure settings and lung mechanics. For any mode, expiratory time must be set to at least three time constants for the lungs to empty passively to 95% (i.e., 5% of inspired volume still remains) (Figure 10-19).

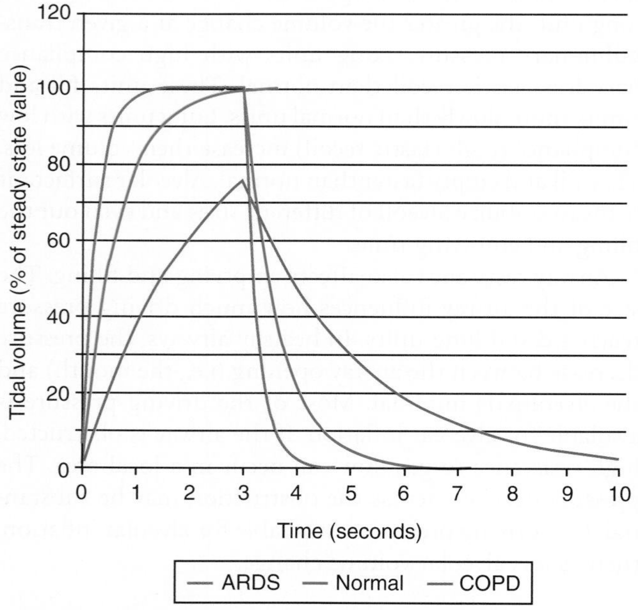

FIGURE 10-19 Graph illustrates the effect of the time constant on the time to exhale a V_T. The time constant for a ventilated patient with ARDS is short (in this example, 0.26 second) owing to normal resistance but low compliance. A person with normal lungs has a longer time constant (e.g., 0.65 second) owing to normal resistance and normal compliance. A patient with chronic obstructive pulmonary disease (COPD) has the longest time constant (e.g., 2.13 seconds) owing to high resistance and high compliance. The horizontal axis shows the expiratory time, and the vertical axis shows the percent of the V_T that remains at each moment. The curve representing the COPD time constant indicates significant gas trapping even after an expiratory time of 5 seconds.

A lung unit has a long time constant if resistance or compliance is high. Units with long time constants take longer to fill and to empty than units with normal compliance and resistance (see Figure 10-19). Lung units have a short time constant when resistance or compliance is low. Lung units with short time constants fill and empty more rapidly than lung units with normal compliance and resistance.

Time constants affect local distribution of ventilation in the lung. The effects of unequal time constants within the lung are different for volume control (VC) ventilation (with constant inspiratory flow) compared with pressure control (PC) ventilation (with constant inspiratory pressure). For lung units with equal resistance and compliance, both VC and PC result in equal distribution of volume. For lung units with different resistance and compliance but with equal time constants, the distribution of volume depends only on the ratio of resistance or compliance for both modes of ventilation. For lung units with different time constants but equal resistances, VC gives more uniform volumetric expansion and perhaps lower risk of volutrauma than PC. For lung units with different time constants but equal compliances, PC gives more uniform volumetric expansion and possibly lower risk of volutrauma than VC.[22]

Frequency Dependence of Compliance

Variations in time constants can affect ventilation throughout the lung. Abnormal ventilation is characteristic of obstruction in the small airways. This type of obstruction occurs in emphysema, asthma, and chronic bronchitis.[23] The time constants of many lung units are increased in obstructive lung disease. These long time constants are mainly caused by increased resistance to flow in the small airways. Loss of normal tissue elastic recoil, such as in emphysema, also contributes to slowed filling and emptying.

At increased breathing rates, units with long time constants fill less and empty more slowly than units with normal compliance and resistance. Increasingly more inspired gas goes to lung units with relatively normal time constants. When more inspired volume goes to a smaller number of lung units, higher transpulmonary pressures must be generated to maintain alveolar ventilation. Compliance of the lung seems to decrease as breathing frequency increases. This phenomenon is called *frequency dependence of compliance.*[5] If dynamic compliance decreases as the respiratory rate increases, some lung units must have abnormal time constants. Any stimulus to increase ventilation, such as exercise, may redistribute inspired gas. Mismatching of ventilation and perfusion can result in hypoxemia, severely limiting an individual's ability to perform daily activities.

Abnormal time constants in lung units and frequency dependence of compliance can have significant effects on patients requiring mechanical ventilation. When ventilation is controlled in terms of volume or flow along with inspiratory-expiratory times, **dynamic hyperinflation (air trapping)** can result. Lung volume can increase with mechanical ventilation in a manner similar to that occurring during exercise. Increased ventilation (i.e., breathing rates or flows or both) exaggerates the differences between lung units with long or short time constants.

EFFICIENCY AND EFFECTIVENESS OF VENTILATION

To be effective, ventilation must meet the body's needs for O_2 uptake and CO_2 removal. To be efficient, ventilation should consume little O_2 and should produce the minimum amount of CO_2.

MINI CLINI

Breathlessness and Dynamic Hyperinflation in Obstructive Airway Disease

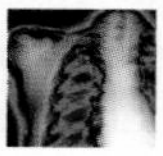

PROBLEM: Patients who have obstructive airway disease often complain of breathlessness (dyspnea). This breathlessness cannot be easily predicted from simple tests of lung function. Some patients with mild obstruction have debilitating dyspnea, whereas other patients with severe obstruction often have little sensation of breathlessness. Why does expiratory flow limitation cause dyspnea of varying degrees in patients who have obstructive lung disease?

DISCUSSION: Dynamic hyperinflation is an acute increase in the end expiratory lung volume (EELV) as a result of insufficient expiratory time. This increase in EELV occurs because the rate of lung emptying, which is determined by the time constant, is prolonged while the expiratory time is shortened by the increase in ventilatory frequency. As a result, the inspiratory capacity decreases. Breathing at higher EELV increases the loading on the respiratory muscles and restricts the normal V_T expansion during exercise. There is a strong correlation between the sensation of dyspnea and the EELV. Patients with obstructive lung disease describe the sensation of dyspnea differently than normal exercising subjects. Terms such as "difficulty inspiring" and "can't get the air in" are commonly used to identify the breathlessness associated with airflow limitation. These specific sensations suggest that patients with airway obstruction receive discordant sensory information from the receptors in the lungs and chest wall. The intensity of these sensations depends on the degree of dynamic hyperinflation that occurs. The use of bronchodilators and lung volume reduction surgery both relieve dyspnea by "deflating" the lungs and reducing hyperinflation. Both therapies improve dynamic airway function by improving lung emptying (more normal time constants). Patients are able to achieve the required ventilation at a lower operating lung volume with a lower O_2 cost of breathing.

Efficiency

Even in healthy lungs, ventilation is not entirely efficient. A substantial volume of inspired gas is wasted with each breath; this wasted ventilation is referred to as *dead space.* Gases must move in and out through the same airways leading to the gas exchange units (alveoli). For each inspiration, the gas left in the conducting airways *(anatomic dead space)* does not participate in gas exchange and is, in effect, wasted. Alveoli that are ventilated but have no perfusion contribute what is called *alveolar dead space.* The sum of anatomic and alveolar dead space is called *physiologic dead space.* The relationship between V_T, dead space volume (V_D), and alveolar volume (V_A) is expressed as:

$$V_T = V_A + V_D$$

Because only alveolar volume participates in gas exchange, this equation shows that the larger the dead space, the less efficient the V_T would be in eliminating CO_2. That is, if efficiency is defined as output/input, CO_2 output would be less for a given input V_T as dead space increases.

Minute Ventilation

Ventilation is usually expressed in liters per minute of fresh gas entering the lungs. The total volume moving in or out of the lungs per minute is called *minute ventilation.* Minute ventilation (exhaled) is denoted by $\dot{V}_E$, which is calculated as the product of frequency of breathing (f_B) times the expired tidal volume:

$$\dot{V}_E = f_B \times V_T$$

For a healthy adult breathing 12 breaths/min and having a VT of 500 ml:

$$\dot{V}_E = 12 \times 500\text{ ml} = 6000\text{ ml/min, or } 6\text{ L/min}$$

Minute ventilation is normally driven by the production of CO_2 and depends on the size of the subject and his or her metabolic rate. $\dot{V}_E$ values range from 5 to 10 L/min in healthy adult subjects at rest.

Alveolar Ventilation

The efficiency of ventilation depends on the volume of fresh gas reaching the alveoli (V_A). Rearranging the previously presented equation for calculating V_T yields the following:

$$V_A = V_T - V_D$$

Alveolar ventilation, $\dot{V}_A$, is the product of breathing frequency (f_B) and alveolar volume per breath (V_A):

$$\dot{V}_A = f_B \times V_A$$

In a healthy adult with a respiratory rate of 12, V_T of 500 ml, and dead space (V_D) of 150 ml, alveolar ventilation is calculated as follows:

$$\dot{V}_A = 12 \times (500\text{ ml} - 150\text{ ml})$$
$$= 12 \times 350\text{ ml}$$
$$= 4200\text{ ml/min}$$

Compare this volume with that described for minute ventilation. $\dot{V}_A$ is always less than $\dot{V}_E$ because of the effect of dead space.

Dead Space Ventilation

Estimation of wasted ventilation is essential to assess the efficiency of ventilation. Dead space can be subdivided into the following two components: anatomic dead space and alveolar dead space. When these are considered together, they often are referred to as *physiologic dead space.*

Anatomic Dead Space

The volume of the conducting airways (including the nasopharynx and oropharynx) is called the *anatomic dead space,* or V_{Danat}. V_{Danat} averages approximately 1 ml per pound of ideal body weight (2.2 ml/kg). For a subject who weighs 150 lb (68 kg), V_{Danat} is approximately 150 ml. V_{Danat} does not participate in gas exchange because it is rebreathed. During exhalation of a 500-ml tidal breath, the first 150 ml of gas exhaled comes from the V_{Danat}. The remaining 350 ml is alveolar gas. At the end of exhalation, the airways contain 150 ml of alveolar gas. During the next inhalation, this 150-ml volume is rebreathed. Only approximately 350 ml of fresh gas reaches the alveoli per breath.

The common estimation of V_D based on body weight goes back to a study published in 1955.[24] More recent research has shown poor agreement between an individual patient's measured dead space and dead space estimated by this and other "rule of thumb" equations.[25] Dead space to tidal volume ratio (V_D/V_T) can be more accurately estimated for mechanically ventilated adult patients using more data available at the bedside[26]:

$$\frac{V_D}{V_T} = 0.32 + 0.0106(PaCO_2 - P_{ET}CO_2) + 0.003(RR) + 0.0015(age)$$

where $PaCO_2$ is arterial O_2 tension (mm Hg), $P_{ET}CO_2$ is end-tidal CO_2 tension (mm Hg), RR is respiratory rate (breaths/min), and age is in years.

Alveolar Dead Space

In addition to the ventilation wasted on the conducting airways, some alveoli may not participate in gas exchange. These alveoli are ventilated but not perfused with mixed venous blood. Without perfusion, gas exchange cannot occur. Any gas that ventilates unperfused alveoli is also wasted *(dead space effect)*. Some alveoli have ventilation out of proportion to their perfusion (high $\dot{V}/\dot{Q}$ ratios; see Chapter 11). These alveoli also contribute to the inefficiency of ventilation because ventilation in excess of what is needed to arterialize the blood in an alveolus is wasted.

The volume of gas ventilating unperfused alveoli is called **alveolar dead space,** or V_{Dalv}. Significant amounts of V_{Dalv} are pathologic. V_{Dalv} is usually related to defects in the pulmonary circulation. A common clinical example of such a defect is a pulmonary embolism. A pulmonary embolus blocks a portion of the pulmonary circulation; this obstructs perfusion to ventilated alveoli, creating alveolar dead space. Alveolar dead space occurs in addition to the anatomic dead space. In a normal upright subject at rest, alveoli at the apices of the lungs have minimal or no perfusion and contribute to the total volume of dead space ventilation.

Physiologic Dead Space

The sum of anatomic and alveolar dead space is called **physiologic dead space** (V_{Dphy}):

$$V_{Dphy} = V_{Danat} + V_{Dalv}$$

The total volume of wasted ventilation, or physiologic dead space, equals the sum of the conducting airways and the alveoli that are ventilated but not perfused (Figure 10-20).

Physiologic dead space includes both the normal and the abnormal components of wasted ventilation. V_{Dphy} is the preferred clinical measure of ventilation efficiency. Measuring V_{Dphy} more accurately assesses alveolar ventilation:

$$\dot{V}_A = f_B \times (V_T - V_{Dphy})$$

Or:

$$\dot{V}_A = \dot{V}_E - \dot{V}_{Dphy}$$

Physiologic dead space is measured clinically by using a modified form of the Bohr equation.

Dead Space/Tidal Volume Ratio

In clinical practice, V_{Dphy} is often expressed as a ratio to V_T. This ratio (V_D/V_T) provides an index of the wasted ventilation (anatomic plus alveolar dead space) per breath. Measurement of the V_D/V_T ratio requires measurement (or estimation) of the arterial CO_2 ($PaCO_2$) and the mixed expired CO_2 ($P_{\bar{E}}CO_2$). $PaCO_2$ is usually measured by obtaining an arterial blood gas specimen but can be estimated from an end-tidal gas sample ($P_{ET}CO_2$). $P_{\bar{E}}CO_2$ may be collected in a sampling bag or balloon or estimated by means of capnography (see Chapter 18). The ratio is calculated using a modified form of the Bohr equation, which assumes that there is no CO_2 in inspired gas:

$$\frac{V_D}{V_T} = \frac{(PaCO_2 - P_{\bar{E}}CO_2)}{PaCO}$$

where $PaCO_2$ is arterial CO_2 tension and is the average CO_2 tension in exhaled gas.

In a normal adult subject who has a $PaCO_2$ of 40 mm Hg and an average expired (mixed expired) CO_2 of 28 mm Hg,

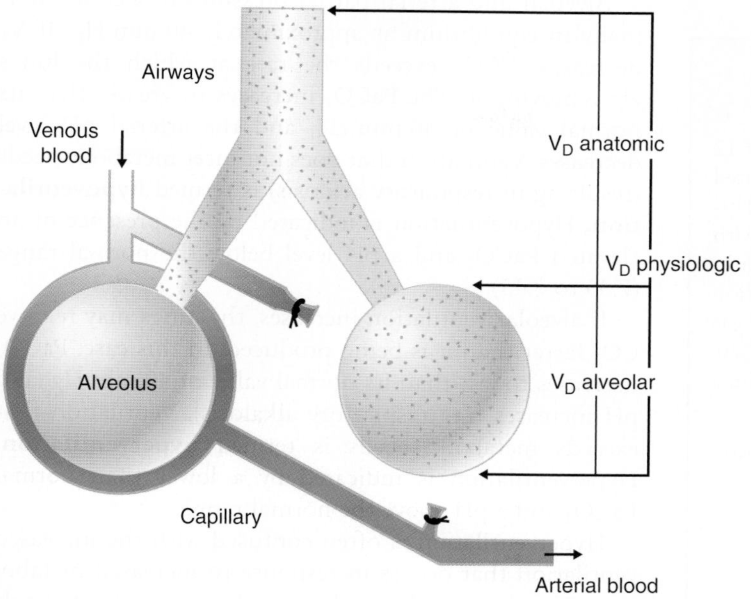

FIGURE 10-20 Three types of dead space. Anatomic dead space is composed of the conducting tubes leading to both alveoli. *Left,* Alveolus is normally perfused and ventilated. *Right,* Alveolus is ventilated but not perfused. The volume represents alveolar dead space. Physiologic dead space is the sum of the two components.

TABLE 10-5

Changes in Alveolar Ventilation (ml) Associated With Changes in Rate, Volume, and Physiologic Dead Space

Ventilatory Pattern	Rate of Breathing (breaths/min)	Tidal Volume (ml)	Minute Ventilation (ml)	Physiologic Dead Space (ml)	Alveolar Ventilation (ml)
Normal	12	500	6000	150	4200
High rate, low volume	24	250	6000	150	2400
Low rate, high volume	6	1000	6000	150	5100
Increased dead space	12	500	6000	300	2400
Compensation for increased dead space	12	650	7800	300	4200

$$\frac{V_D}{V_T} = \frac{(40-28)}{40} = 0.30$$

This equation indicates that the normal dead space ratio is about 30%. This equation assumes that all of the CO_2 in expired gas comes from ventilated alveoli. If all lung units contributed CO_2 equally to the expired gas and there was no anatomic dead space, $P_{\bar{E}}CO_2$ would equal $PaCO_2$, and the V_D/V_T ratio would be zero. Because of anatomic and alveolar dead space, the $P_{\bar{E}}CO_2$ is always less than $PaCO_2$. In a healthy adult, physiologic dead space is approximately one-third of the V_T, with a normal range of 0.2 to 0.4. The V_D/V_T ratio normally decreases with exercise. Both V_T and V_D increase with increased ventilation during exertion, but the V_T normally increases to a greater degree; the ratio decreases (in healthy subjects). V_D/V_T increases with diseases that cause significant dead space, such as pulmonary embolism.

Clinical Significance

Table 10-5 lists the effects of changes in the parameters that determine alveolar ventilation ($\dot{V}_A$). In healthy individuals, $\dot{V}_A$ changes with breathing rate and V_T because dead space is relatively fixed. High respiratory rate and low V_T result in a high proportion of wasted ventilation per minute (low $\dot{V}_A$). Generally, the most efficient breathing pattern is slow, deep breathing.

In pulmonary disease, increased V_{Dphy} causes a decrease in $\dot{V}_A$, unless compensation occurs. An increased breathing rate by itself worsens the problem. Effective compensation for increased V_{Dphy} requires an increased V_T. Elevating V_T increases the elastic work of breathing, however; this increases O_2 consumption by the respiratory muscles. In some patients, these increased demands cannot be met. In such cases, $\dot{V}_A$ may be inadequate to meet body needs, and CO_2 is not removed as rapidly as it is produced. CO_2 retention causes respiratory acidosis, often requiring mechanical support of ventilation.

Effectiveness

Ventilation is effective when it removes CO_2 at a rate that maintains a normal pH. Under resting metabolic conditions, a healthy adult produces approximately 200 ml of CO_2 per minute. Alveolar ventilation must match CO_2 production per minute to ensure acid-base balance.

MINI CLINI

Minute Ventilation, Dead Space, and $PaCO_2$

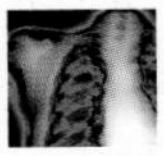

PROBLEM: A patient breathing at a rate of 12 breaths/min has a V_T of 600 ml and a measured physiologic dead space (V_{Dphy}) of 200 ml. This ventilatory pattern produces a $PaCO_2$ of 40 mm Hg with a pH of 7.39. Several hours later, the patient has a breathing rate of 24 breaths/min, but the minute ventilation ($\dot{V}_E$) has remained the same as before. Arterial blood gas analysis reveals a $PaCO_2$ of 72 mm Hg with a pH of 7.20. Why has the $PaCO_2$ increased even though the $\dot{V}_E$ remained constant?

DISCUSSION: The initial $\dot{V}_E$ and alveolar ventilation ($\dot{V}_A$) were as follows:

$$\begin{aligned}\dot{V}_E &= 600 \times 12\\ &= 7200 \text{ ml/min}\\ \dot{V}_A &= (600 - 200) \times 12\\ &= 4800 \text{ ml/min}\end{aligned}$$

The $\dot{V}_A$ of 4800 ml/min was responsible for maintaining a $PaCO_2$ of 40 mm Hg. When respiratory rate increased to 24 breaths/min and $\dot{V}_E$ remained at 7200 ml/min, V_T must have decreased:

$$\begin{aligned}V_T &= 7200 \div 24\\ &= 300 \text{ ml}\end{aligned}$$

However, if dead space remained at 200 ml, $\dot{V}_A$ subsequently decreased:

$$\begin{aligned}\dot{V}_A &= (300 - 200) \times 24\\ &= 2400 \text{ ml/min}\end{aligned}$$

The reduction in $\dot{V}_A$ (from 4800 ml/min to 2400 ml/min) explains the increase in $PaCO_2$ from 40 mm Hg to 72 mm Hg. $PaCO_2$ is inversely proportional to $\dot{V}_A$. Because $\dot{V}_A$ was reduced by half, $PaCO_2$ should have doubled. This approximates the data actually observed. Normally, increased CO_2 tension in the blood resulting in acidemia causes an increase in $\dot{V}_A$. This patient, although tachypneic, is hypoventilating.

The equilibrium between CO_2 production ($\dot{V}CO_2$) and $\dot{V}_A$ determines the PCO_2 in the lungs and arterial blood. This balance also plays a key role in determining the pH of arterial blood. The partial pressure of CO_2 in the alveoli and blood is directly proportional to its production ($\dot{V}CO_2$) and inversely proportional to its rate of removal by alveolar ventilation ($\dot{V}_A$):

$$P_ACO_2 = \frac{\dot{V}CO_2(P_B - P_{H_2O})}{\dot{V}_A} \approx PaCO_2$$

where P_ACO_2 is alveolar CO_2 tension, $\dot{V}CO_2$ is CO_2 production (ml/min), $\dot{V}_A$ is alveolar ventilation (ml/min), P_B is barometric pressure, P_{H2O} is the water vapor tension in the alveoli, and $PaCO_2$ is arterial CO_2 tension.

Alveolar and arterial partial pressures of CO_2 are normally in equilibrium at approximately 40 mm Hg. If $\dot{V}_A$ decreases, $\dot{V}CO_2$ exceeds the rate at which the lungs are removing it. The $PaCO_2$ increases to greater than its normal value of 40 mm Hg, and the arterial pH level decreases. Ventilation that does not meet metabolic needs (resulting in respiratory acidosis) is termed **hypoventilation.** Hypoventilation is indicated by the presence of an elevated $PaCO_2$ and a pH level below the normal range (7.35 to 7.45).

If alveolar ventilation increases, the lungs may remove CO_2 faster than it is being produced. In this case, $PaCO_2$ decreases to less than its normal value of 40 mm Hg, and pH increases (i.e., respiratory alkalosis). Ventilation that exceeds metabolic needs is termed **hyperventilation.** Hyperventilation is indicated by a lower than normal $PaCO_2$ and a pH above the normal range.

Hyperventilation is often confused with the increased ventilation that occurs in response to increased metabolism. The changes observed during low or moderate levels of exercise are an example. Ventilation increases in proportion to the increased $\dot{V}CO_2$ from exercise. The $PaCO_2$ remains in the normal range of 35 to 45 mm Hg, and the pH level remains near 7.4. The increase in ventilation that occurs with increased metabolic rates is termed *hyperpnea.*

Effectiveness of ventilation is determined by the partial pressure of CO_2 and the resulting pH, specifically in arterial blood. Ventilation is effective when the $PaCO_2$ is maintained at a level that keeps the pH within normal limits.

SUMMARY CHECKLIST

- Ventilation occurs because of pressure differences across the lung during breathing. Gas flows into the lung when the diaphragm creates a subatmospheric pressure in the lung; gas flows out of the lung when the recoil properties of the lung create a slight positive pressure.
- The forces that oppose lung inflation may be grouped into two categories: elastic forces and frictional forces.
- Resting lung volume is determined by the opposing elastic forces of the lungs and chest wall.
- Frictional forces opposing ventilation include airway and tissue resistance.
- Airway resistance accounts for 80% of the frictional resistance to ventilation in a healthy adult lung.
- Exhalation is normally passive but may become active when airway resistance is abnormally high.
- The work of breathing is performed by the muscles of breathing.
- Obstructive lung disease increases the frictional work of breathing, whereas restrictive lung disease increases the elastic work of breathing.
- Respiratory muscle fatigue causes a decrease in the tidal volume and an increase in the respiratory rate.

- Even a healthy lung does not distribute ventilation evenly throughout the lungs; greater ventilation normally occurs in the bases.
- The total volume of gas moving in and out of the lungs each minute is called the minute volume. It is determined by multiplying the V_T times the breathing frequency.
- Homeostasis is present when the alveolar ventilation matches CO_2 production.
- The portion of the V_T that does not come into contact with pulmonary blood flow is called dead space ventilation.
- Normally about 30% of the V_T is dead space. Most of this is called anatomic dead space because it is made up of the larger airways that serve to conduct gas to the alveolar sacs.
- Alveoli that are ventilated but have no blood perfusion are called alveolar dead space. Normally, alveolar dead space is minimal.
- The combination of anatomic and alveolar dead space is called physiologic dead space.

References

1. Primiano FP, Jr, Chatburn RL: Zen and the art of nomenclature maintenance: a revised approach to respiratory symbols and terminology. Respir Care 51:1458–1470, 2006.
2. Harris RS: Pressure-volume curves of the respiratory system. Respir Care 50:78–98, 2005.
3. West JB: Respiratory physiology: the essentials, ed 7, Baltimore, 2007, Lippincott Williams & Wilkins.
4. Lucangelo U, Bernabé F, Blanch L: Respiratory mechanics derived from signals in the ventilator circuit. Respir Care 50:55–65, 2005.
5. Otis AB, McKerrow CB, Bartlett RA, et al: Mechanical factors in distribution of pulmonary ventilation. J Appl Physiol 8:427–443, 1956.
6. Chatburn RL: Dynamic respiratory mechanics. Respir Care 31:703–711, 1986.
7. Davis GM, Lands LC: Measurement of infant pulmonary mechanics: comparative analysis of techniques. Pediatr Pulmonol 23:105–113, 1997.
8. Guttmann J, Eberhard L, Wolff G, et al: Maneuver-free determination of compliance and resistance in ventilated ARDS patients. Chest 102:1235–1242, 1992.
9. Stahl CA, Möller K, Schumann S, et al: Dynamic versus static respiratory mechanics in acute lung injury and acute respiratory distress syndrome. Crit Care Med 34:2090–2098, 2006.
10. Lumb AB: Nunn's applied respiratory physiology, ed 6, London, 2005, Butterworth-Heinemann Medical.
11. Zach MS: The physiology of forced expiration. Paediatr Respir Rev 1:36–39, 2000.
12. Thurlbeck WM: Pathophysiology of chronic obstructive pulmonary disease. Clin Chest Med 11:389, 1990.
13. O'Donnell DE: Hyperinflation, dyspnea, and exercise intolerance in chronic obstructive pulmonary disease. Proc Am Thorac Soc 3:180–184, 2006.
14. Venegas JG, Harris RS, Simon BA: A comprehensive equation for the pulmonary pressure-volume curve. J Appl Physiol 84:389–395, 1998.
15. Hata JS, Simmons JS, Kumar AB, et al: The acute effectiveness and safety of the constant-flow, pressure-volume curve to improve hypoxemia in acute lung injury. J Intensive Care Med 2011, in press.
16. Caramez MP, Kacmarek RM, Helmy M, et al: A comparison of methods to identify open-lung PEEP. Intensive Care Med 35:740–747, 2009.
17. Grooms DA, Sibole SH, Tomlinson JR, et al: Customization of an open lung ventilation strategy to treat a case of life threatening acute respiratory distress syndrome. Respir Care 2011, in press.
18. Rochester DF: Respiratory muscles and ventilatory failure: 1993 perspective, Am J Med Sci 305:394, 1993.
19. Mitsuoka M, Kinninger KH, Jacobson KL, et al: Utility of measurements of oxygen cost of breathing in predicting success or failure in trials of reduced mechanical ventilatory support. Respir Care 6:902–910, 2001.
20. Charron C, Bouferrache K, Caille V, et al: Routine prone positioning in patients with severe ARDS: feasibility and impact on prognosis. Intensive Care Med 2011, in press.
21. Martin L: Pulmonary physiology in clinical practice: the essentials for patient care and evaluation, St Louis, 1987, Mosby.
22. Chatburn RL, El Khatib M, Smith P: Respiratory system behavior with constant inspiratory pressure or flow. Respir Care 39:979–988, 1994.
23. Hogg JC: Pathophysiology of airflow limitation in chronic obstructive pulmonary disease. Lancet 364:709–721, 2004.
24. Radford EP, Jr: Ventilation standards for use in artificial respiration. J Appl Physiol 7:451–460, 1955.
25. Brewer LM, Orr JA, Pace NL: Anatomic dead space cannot be predicted by body weight. Respir Care 53:885–891, 2008.
26. Frankenfield DC, Alam S, Bekteshi E, et al: Predicting dead space ventilation in critically ill patients using clinically available data. Crit Care Med 38:288–291, 2010.

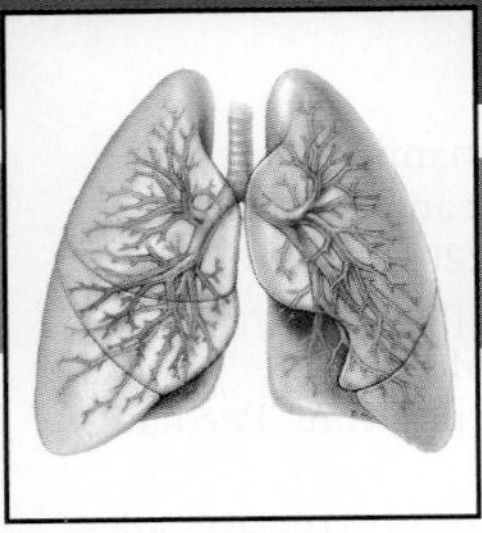

Chapter 11

Gas Exchange and Transport

CHRISTOPHER A. HIRSCH

CHAPTER OBJECTIVES

After reading this chapter you will be able to:

- Describe how oxygen and carbon dioxide move between the atmosphere and tissues.
- Identify what determines alveolar oxygen and carbon dioxide pressures.
- Calculate the alveolar partial pressure of oxygen at any given barometric pressure and fraction of inspired oxygen.
- State the effects that normal regional variations in ventilation and perfusion have on gas exchange.
- Describe how to compute total oxygen content for arterial blood.
- State the factors that cause the arteriovenous oxygen content difference to change.
- Identify the factors that affect oxygen loading and unloading from hemoglobin.
- Describe how carbon dioxide is carried in the blood.
- Describe how oxygen and carbon dioxide transport are interrelated.
- Describe the factors that impair oxygen delivery to the tissues and how to distinguish among them.
- State the factors that impair carbon dioxide removal.

CHAPTER OUTLINE

KEY TERMS

acute chest syndrome
alveolar shunts
Bohr effect
carboxyhemoglobin (HbCO)
dead space
dysoxia
fetal hemoglobin (HbF)
Fick equation
Fick's first law of diffusion
Haldane effect
Hamburger phenomenon
hypoxemia
hypoxia
methemoglobin
methemoglobinemia
oxyhemoglobin
P_{50}
right-to-left anatomic shunts
sickle cell hemoglobin
venous admixture
ventilation/perfusion ratio ($\dot{V}/\dot{Q}$)

Respiration is the process of getting oxygen (O_2) into the body for tissue use and removing carbon dioxide (CO_2) into the atmosphere. This complex process involves both gas exchange (at the lungs and at the cellular level) and transport of the gases. O_2 must be moved into the lungs, where it diffuses into the pulmonary circulation and is transported in the blood to the tissues. CO_2 builds up in the tissues because of metabolism and diffuses into the capillary blood before being carried to the lung for exchange with alveolar gases. Normally, these processes are well integrated. However, in disease states, impaired gas exchange or transport can cause physiologic imbalances, which can alter function or threaten survival. At such times, respiratory care intervention may be the only way to maintain or restore a level of function consistent with life. This chapter provides the background knowledge that respiratory therapists (RTs) need to understand and treat patients with diseases that affect gas exchange.

DIFFUSION

Whole-Body Diffusion Gradients

Gas movement between the lungs and tissues occurs via simple diffusion (see Chapters 6 and 8). Figure 11-1 shows the normal diffusion gradients for O_2 and CO_2. For O_2, there is a stepwise downward "cascade" of partial pressures from the normal atmospheric inspired partial pressure of O_2 (PiO_2) of 159 mm Hg to a low point of 40 mm Hg or less in the capillaries. The intracellular PO_2 (approximately 5 mm Hg) provides the final gradient for O_2 diffusion into the cell.

The diffusion gradient for CO_2 is the opposite of the diffusion gradient for O_2. The partial pressure of CO_2 (PCO_2) is highest in the cells (approximately 60 mm Hg) and lowest in room air (1 mm Hg). This reverse cascade causes CO_2 movement from the tissues into the venous blood, which is transported to the lungs and—with the aid of ventilation—out to the atmosphere.

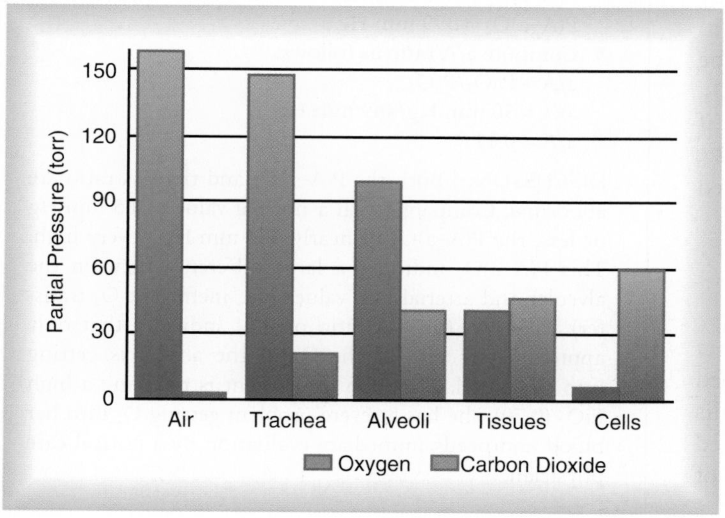

FIGURE 11-1 Normal diffusion gradients for O_2 and CO_2. There is a downward cascade for O_2 from air to cells, with a reverse gradient for CO_2.

Determinants of Alveolar Gas Tensions

Alveolar Carbon Dioxide

The alveolar partial pressure of CO_2 (P_ACO_2) varies directly with the body's production of CO_2 ($\dot{V}CO_2$) and inversely with alveolar ventilation ($\dot{V}_A$). The relationship is expressed by the following formula:

$$P_ACO_2 = \frac{\dot{V}CO_2 \times 0.863}{\dot{V}_A}$$

Where:

P_ACO_2 = Alveolar CO_2 tension (mm Hg)

$\dot{V}CO_2$ = Rate of CO_2 produced (in ml/min standard temperature and pressure, dry [STPD])

$\dot{V}_A$ = Alveolar ventilation (ml/min body temperature and pressure, saturated [BTPS])

Because $\dot{V}CO_2$ is expressed as a flow of dry gas at 0° C and 760 mm Hg, and $\dot{V}_A$ is reported as saturated gas at body temperature and ambient pressure, the factor 863 is employed to correct the measurement for comparison under the same conditions. It confers the units of pressure to the resulting dimensionless ratio of flow rates.

As an example, given $\dot{V}CO_2$ of 200 ml/min and alveolar ventilation of 4315 ml/min, application of this formula yields a P_ACO_2 of approximately 40 mm Hg:

$$P_ACO_2 = (863 \text{ mm Hg} \times 200 \text{ ml/min}) \div 4315 \text{ ml/min} = 40 \text{ mm Hg}$$

P_ACO_2 increases above this level if CO_2 production increases while alveolar ventilation remains constant or if alveolar ventilation decreases while $\dot{V}CO_2$ remains constant. An increase in **dead space,** the portion of inspired air that is exhaled without being exposed to perfused alveoli, can also lead to an increased P_ACO_2:

$$\dot{V} = (V_T - V_D) \times f$$

Where:
$\dot{V}_A$ = Alveolar ventilation
V_T = Tidal volume
V_D = Dead space volume
f = Ventilatory frequency

Likewise, P_ACO_2 decreases if CO_2 production decreases or alveolar ventilation increases. Normally, complex respiratory control mechanisms maintain P_ACO_2 within a range of 35 to 45 mm Hg under various conditions (see Chapter 14). If CO_2 production increases, as with exercise or fever, ventilation automatically increases to maintain P_ACO_2 within normal range.

Alveolar Oxygen Tensions

Many factors determine the alveolar partial pressure of O_2 (P_AO_2). Most important is PiO_2. In addition, when O_2 is in the lungs, it is diluted by both water vapor and CO_2. To account for all these factors, the following alveolar air equation is applied:

$$P_AO_2 = FiO_2 \times (P_B - 47) - (P_ACO_2 \div 0.8)$$

Where:
FiO_2 = Fraction of inspired O_2 (decimal)
P_B = Barometric pressure (mm Hg)
47 = Water vapor tension (in mm Hg) at 37° C
P_ACO_2 = Alveolar PCO_2
0.8 = Normal respiratory exchange ratio (R)

The equation component $FiO_2 \times (P_B - 47)$ is a simple application of Dalton's law:

Partial pressure = Fractional concentration × Total pressure

However, under BTPS conditions in the lungs, the total pressure available for O_2 is reduced by an amount equal to the saturated water vapor pressure at 37° C, or 47 mm Hg.

The equation component ($PaCO_2 \div 0.8$) accounts for the alveolar CO_2. However, $PaCO_2$ cannot simply be subtracted, as was done for water vapor. Instead, the equation must be corrected for the difference between O_2 and CO_2 movement into and out of the alveoli, which is done by dividing the P_ACO_2 by R. R is the ratio of CO_2 excretion to O_2 uptake, which normally averages 0.8 throughout the lung. In addition, because $PaCO_2$ nearly equals P_ACO_2, $PaCO_2$ can be substituted for P_ACO_2. For example, if FiO_2 is 0.21, P_B is 760 mm Hg, and $PaCO_2$ is 40 mm Hg, the normal alveolar partial pressure of O_2 can be estimated as follows:

$$P_AO_2 = 0.21 \times (760\text{ mm Hg} - 47) - (40\text{ mm Hg} \div 0.8) = 99.73\text{ mm Hg}$$

In clinical practice, if a patient is breathing 60% or more O_2 ($FiO_2 \geq 0.60$), the correction for R can be dropped because the magnitude of the correction to $PaCO_2$ falls below significance relative to the much larger calculated FiO_2 ($P_B - 47$). This yields the following simplified form of the alveolar air equation:

$$P_AO_2 = FiO_2\,(P_B - 47) - PaCO_2$$

The accompanying Mini Clini provides an example of how to use the alveolar air equation.

MINI CLINI

Alveolar-Arterial PO_2 Difference and a/A Ratio

Not all of the O_2 from the alveoli gets into the blood. Why this occurs is discussed later in this chapter. This Mini Clini considers how the efficiency of O_2 transfer from the alveoli to the blood can be computed.

Several bedside computations can be used to estimate the efficiency of pulmonary O_2 transfer. The most common computation is the difference between the alveolar and arterial PO_2, called the A-a gradient ($P[A–a]O_2$). Normally, this difference is small—only 5 to 10 mm Hg when air is breathed and no more than 65 mm Hg when 100% O_2 is breathed.

Another common bedside computation is the ratio of arterial to alveolar PO_2, called the a/A ratio. The a/A ratio should be thought of as the proportion of O_2 getting from the alveoli to the blood. Normally, this proportion is at least 90% (a ratio of 0.9).

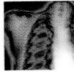

PROBLEM: Compute and interpret the $P(A–a)O_2$ and a/A ratio for a 45-year-old woman breathing 70% O_2 at sea level, with the following blood gas values: PaO_2, 50 mm Hg; $PaCO_2$, 50 mm Hg.

DISCUSSION:

1. Compute P_AO_2 using one form of the alveolar O_2 equation as follows: $P_AO_2 = FiO_2 \times (P_B - 47) - P_ACO_2$ (patient breathing >60% O_2)
   P_AO_2 = Alveolar O_2 tension (mm Hg)
   FiO_2 = Inspired O_2 fraction (decimal)
   P_ACO_2 = Alveolar CO_2 tension (mm Hg, often estimated by arterial CO_2 tension)
   $P_AO_2 = 0.7 \times (760\text{ mm Hg} - 47\text{ mm Hg}) - 50\text{ mm Hg}$
   $P_AO_2 = 449\text{ mm Hg}$
2. Compute $P(A–a)O_2$ as follows:
   $P(A–a)O_2 = P_AO_2 - PaO_2$
   PaO_2 = Arterial O_2 tension (mm Hg)
   $P(A–a)O_2 = 449\text{ mm Hg} - 50\text{ mm Hg}$
   $P(A–a)O_2 = 399\text{ mm Hg}$
3. Compute a/A ratio as follows:
   $a/A = PaO_2/P_AO_2$
   $a/A = 50\text{ mm Hg}/449\text{ mm Hg}$
   $a/A = 0.11$

DISCUSSON: Both the $P(A–a)O_2$ and the a/A ratio are abnormal. Compared with a normal value of 65 mm Hg or less, the $P(A–a)O_2$ of nearly 400 mm Hg is very high. This $P(A–a)O_2$ indicates a large difference between the alveolar and arterial PO_2 values (i.e., inefficient O_2 transfer). Likewise, the a/A ratio of 0.11 indicates that only approximately 11% of the O_2 in the alveoli is getting into the blood. Although the patient is receiving a high FiO_2 (0.70), she has a severe problem getting O_2 into her blood and needs immediate evaluation by a critical care physician.

Changes in Alveolar Gas Partial Tensions

In addition to CO_2, O_2, and water vapor, alveoli normally contain nitrogen. Nitrogen is inert and plays no role in gas exchange; however, it occupies space and exerts pressure. According to Dalton's law, the partial pressure of alveolar nitrogen (P_AN_2) must equal the pressure it would exert if it alone were present. To compute P_AN_2, subtract the pressures exerted by all the other alveolar gases, as follows:

$$P_AN_2 = P_B - (P_AO_2 + P_ACO_2 + P_{H2O})$$
$$P_AN_2 = 760\text{ mm Hg} - (100\text{ mm Hg} + 40\text{ mm Hg} + 47\text{ mm Hg})$$
$$P_AN_2 = 760\text{ mm Hg} - 187\text{ mm Hg}$$
$$P_AN_2 = 573\text{ mm Hg}$$

Because both water vapor tension and P_AN_2 remain constant, the only partial pressures that change in the alveolus are O_2 and CO_2. Based on the alveolar air equation, if FiO_2 remains constant, P_AO_2 must vary inversely with P_ACO_2.[2-4]

RULE OF THUMB

When the patient is breathing room air, the sum of P_AO_2 and P_ACO_2 equals about 140 mm Hg (100 mm Hg and 40 mm Hg). Changes in ventilation that cause P_ACO_2 to vary also vary the resulting P_AO_2 to keep the total at 140 mm Hg. If P_ACO_2 of a patient breathing room air increases from 40 mm Hg to 60 mm Hg (an increase of 20 mm Hg), P_AO_2 should decrease by approximately 20 mm Hg. This equation assumes a constant value for R.

P_ACO_2 itself varies inversely with the level of alveolar ventilation. For a constant CO_2 production, a decrease in $\dot{V}_A$ simultaneously increases P_ACO_2 and decreases P_AO_2, whereas an increase in $\dot{V}_A$ has the opposite effect (Figure 11-2). However, ventilation can be increased only so much. Neural control mechanisms and the increased work of breathing prevent decreases in P_ACO_2 much below 15 to 20 mm Hg. Whenever a patient is breathing room air at sea level, the RT should not expect to see a PaO_2 greater than 120 mm Hg during hyperventilation. PaO_2 values greater than 120 mm Hg indicate that the patient is breathing supplemental O_2. The accompanying Mini Clini presents a clinical application of these principles.

Mechanism of Diffusion

As described in Chapter 6, *diffusion* is the process whereby gas molecules move from an area of high partial pressure to an area of low partial pressure. To diffuse into and out of the lung and tissues, O_2 and CO_2 must move through significant barriers.

MINI CLINI

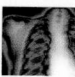

Assessing Arterial Gas Partial Pressures

PROBLEM: The RT is given the following arterial blood gas report for a patient who was just admitted to the emergency department: PaO_2 = 170 mm Hg; $PaCO_2$ = 23 mm Hg. Without additional data, what conclusions can the RT draw about the FiO_2 in this case?

DISCUSSION: In room air, the total pressure exerted by O_2 and CO_2 in the alveoli (and blood) should be approximately 140 mm Hg. In this case, the total is 170 mm Hg (PaO_2) + 23 mm Hg ($PaCO_2$), or 193 mm Hg. Whenever total pressure significantly exceeds 140 mm Hg and PaO_2 is greater than 120 mm Hg, the RT can be assured that the patient is breathing supplemental O_2.

Barriers to Diffusion

The barrier to gaseous diffusion in the lung is the alveolar-capillary membrane. For CO_2 or O_2 to move between the alveoli and the pulmonary capillary blood, the following three barriers must be penetrated: (1) alveolar epithelium, (2) interstitial space, and (3) capillary endothelium. In addition, to pass into and out of the red blood cells (RBCs), these gases also must traverse the erythrocyte membrane.[5,6]

Fick's First Law of Diffusion

The bulk movement of a gas through a biologic membrane ($\dot{V}_{gas}$) is described by **Fick's first law of diffusion:**

$$\dot{V}_{gas} = [(A \times D) \div T](P_1 - P_2)$$

In this formula, A is the cross-sectional area available for diffusion, D is the diffusion coefficient of the gas, T is the thickness of the membrane, and ($P_1 - P_2$) is the partial pressure gradient across the membrane.

According to Fick's law, the greater the surface area, diffusion constant, and pressure gradient, the more diffusion occurs. Conversely, with greater the distance across the membrane (thickness), less diffusion occurs. Given that the area of and distance across the alveolar-capillary membrane are constant in healthy people, diffusion in the normal lung mainly depends on gas pressure gradients.

Pulmonary Diffusion Gradients

For gas exchange to occur between the alveoli and pulmonary capillaries, a difference in partial pressures ($P_1 - P_2$) must exist. Figure 11-3 shows the size and direction of these gradients for O_2 and CO_2. In the normal lung, the alveolar PO_2 averages approximately 100 mm Hg, whereas the mean PCO_2 is approximately 40 mm Hg. Venous blood returning to the lungs has a lower PO_2 (40 mm Hg) than alveolar gas. The pressure gradient for O_2 diffusion into

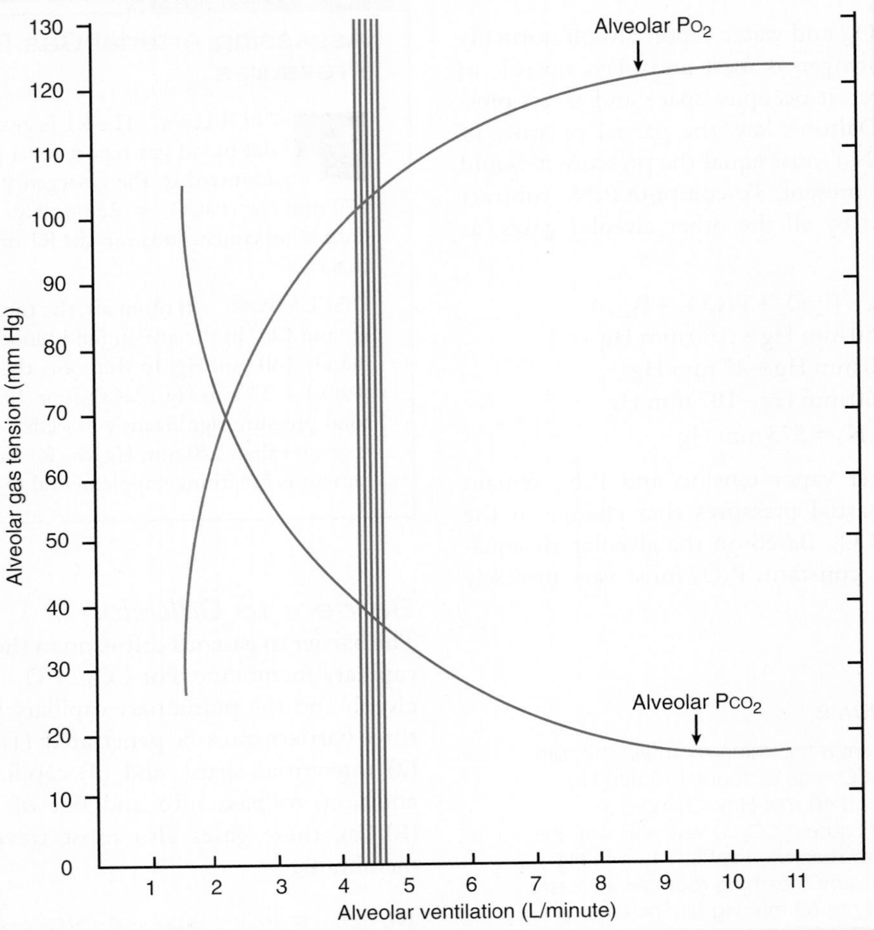

FIGURE 11-2 Effect of alveolar ventilation on alveolar gases. (Modified from Pilbeam SP: Mechanical ventilation, ed 4, St Louis, 2006, Mosby.)

the blood is approximately 60 mm Hg (100 mm Hg − 40 mm Hg). As blood flows past the alveolus, it takes up O_2 and moves to the left atrium with a PO_2 close to 100 mm Hg in healthy people.

Because venous blood has higher PCO_2 than alveolar gas (46 mm Hg vs. 40 mm Hg), the pressure gradient for CO_2 causes it to diffuse in the opposite direction, from the blood into the alveolus. This diffusion continues until capillary PCO_2 equilibrates with the alveolar level, at approximately 40 mm Hg.

Although the pressure gradient for CO_2 is approximately one-tenth of the pressure gradient for O_2, CO_2 has little difficulty diffusing across the alveolar-capillary membrane. CO_2 diffuses approximately 20 times faster across the alveolar-capillary membrane than O_2 because of its much higher solubility in plasma. Disorders that impair the diffusion capacity of the lung (D_L) can affect O_2 movement into the blood, especially when blood flow through the lung is rapid because the time the RBCs are in contact with the alveoli is reduced.

Time Limits to Diffusion

For blood leaving the pulmonary capillary to be adequately oxygenated, it must spend sufficient time in contact with the alveolus to allow equilibration.[5,8] If the time available for diffusion is inadequate, blood leaving the lungs may not be fully oxygenated. The diffusion time in the lung depends on the rate of pulmonary blood flow. As depicted in Figure 11-4, blood normally takes approximately 0.75 second to pass through the pulmonary capillary. This time is more than enough to ensure complete diffusion of O_2 across the alveolar-capillary membrane normally.

If blood flow increases, such as during heavy exercise, capillary transit time can decrease to 0.25 second. This short time frame is adequate to ensure that equilibration occurs as long as no other factors impair diffusion.

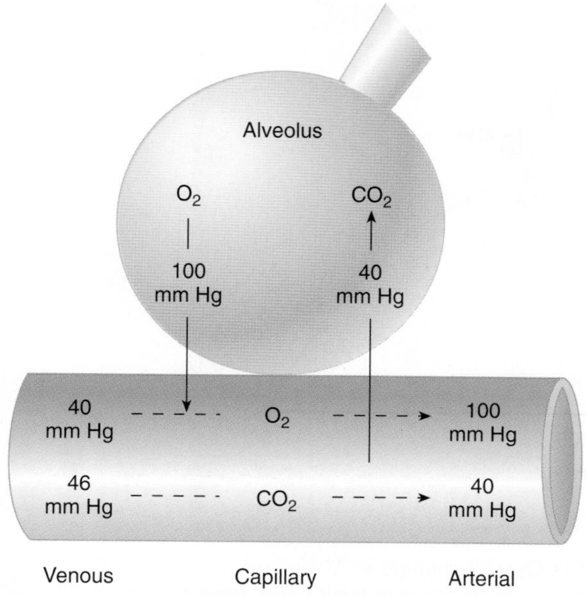

FIGURE 11-3 Ventilation maintains mean alveolar gas pressures for O_2 and CO_2 at approximately 100 mm Hg and 40 mm Hg. As blood enters the venous end of the capillary, it gives up CO_2 and loads O_2 until these two gases are in equilibrium with alveolar pressures. At this point, the blood is "arterialized."

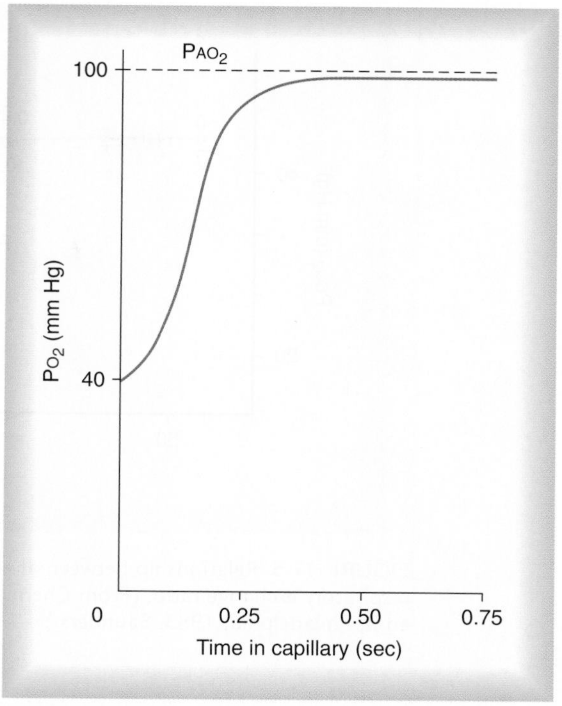

FIGURE 11-4 Alveolar-capillary PO_2 gradient. Normal transit time for RBC in the pulmonary capillary is approximately 0.75 second. Normally, blood PO_2 equilibrates with the alveolar PO_2 well before it reaches the end of the capillary.

However, in the presence of a diffusion limitation, rapid blood flow through the pulmonary circulation can result in inadequate oxygenation. High fever and septic shock, which often cause increased cardiac output, are good examples of conditions that limit diffusion time because of increased blood flow.

In clinical practice, knowledge of D_L can be helpful in evaluating certain diseases. D_L is the bulk flow of gas (ml/min) that diffuses into the blood for each 1-mm Hg difference in the pressure gradient. Although O_2 can be used to measure D_L, low concentrations (0.1% to 0.3%) of carbon monoxide are used more commonly. Chapter 19 provides details on the technique for measuring D_L and its diagnostic use.

Systemic Diffusion Gradients

Partial pressure gradients in the tissues are the opposite of the partial pressure gradients in the lung. As cellular metabolism depletes its O_2, intracellular PO_2 decreases to less than PO_2 of the blood entering the tissue capillary. O_2 diffuses from the tissue capillary blood ($PO_2 = 100$ mm Hg) to the cells ($PO_2 < 40$ mm Hg). Simultaneously, CO_2 diffuses from the cells ($PCO_2 > 46$ mm Hg) into the capillary blood ($PCO_2 = 40$ mm Hg). After equilibration, blood leaves the tissue capillaries with PO_2 of approximately 40 mm Hg and PCO_2 of approximately 46 mm Hg.

Just as arterial blood reflects pulmonary gas exchange, venous blood reflects events occurring in the tissues. The use of venous blood to assess tissue oxygenation is discussed in Chapter 46.

NORMAL VARIATIONS FROM IDEAL GAS EXCHANGE

This chapter has focused so far almost entirely on gas pressures in a perfect alveolus (i.e., one with ideal ventilation and blood flow). In reality, the normal lung is an imperfect organ of gas exchange. Clinically, this imperfection becomes clear, PaO_2 is measured in the average individual. Rather than equaling P_AO_2 of 100 mm Hg, PaO_2 of healthy individuals breathing air at sea level is approximately 5 to 10 mm Hg less than the calculated PaO_2. Two factors account for this difference: (1) right-to-left shunts in the pulmonary and cardiac circulation and (2) regional differences in pulmonary ventilation and blood flow.

Anatomic Shunts

A shunt is the portion of the cardiac output that returns to the left heart without being oxygenated by exposure to ventilated alveoli. Two **right-to-left anatomic shunts** exist in normal humans: (1) bronchial venous drainage and (2) thebesian venous drainage (see Chapters 8 and 9). A right-to-left shunt causes poorly oxygenated venous blood to move directly into the arterial circulation **(venous admixture),** reducing the O_2 content of arterial blood. Together, these normal shunts account for approximately three-fourths of the normal difference between

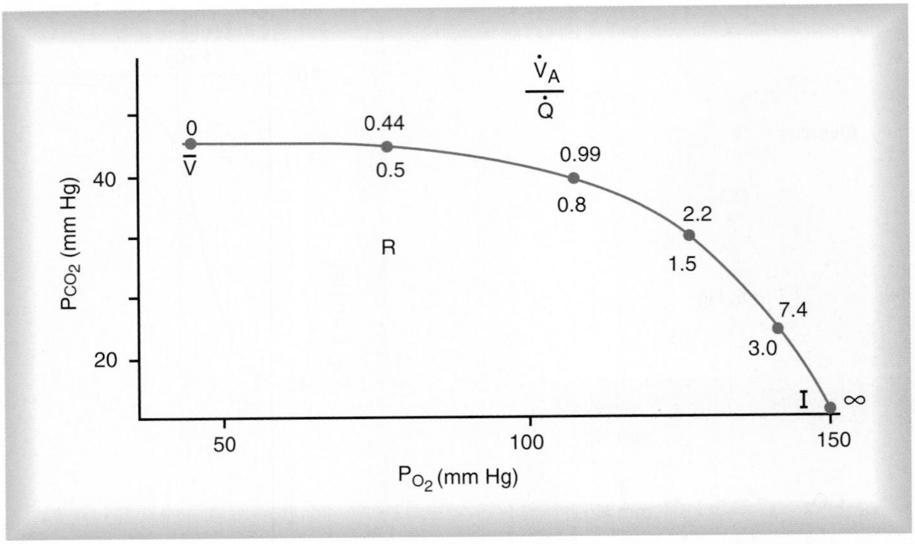

FIGURE 11-5 Relationship between alveolar PO_2 and PCO_2 with changes in $\dot{V}/\dot{Q}$ and respiratory exchange ratio. (From Cherniak RM, Cherniak L: Respiration in health and disease, ed 3, Philadelphia, 1983, Saunders.)

P_AO_2 and PaO_2. The remaining difference is a result of normal inequalities in pulmonary ventilation and perfusion.[5]

Regional Inequalities in Ventilation and Perfusion

The normal respiratory exchange ratio of 0.8 assumes that ventilation and perfusion in the lung are in balance, with every liter of alveolar ventilation ($\dot{V}_A$) matched by approximately 1 L of pulmonary capillary blood flow ($\dot{Q}_C$). Any variation from this perfect balance alters gas tensions in the affected alveoli. As previously discussed, changes in $\dot{V}_A$ affect P_ACO_2, which alters P_AO_2. Changes in blood flow also alter alveolar gas pressures. If blood flow to an area of the lung increases, CO_2 coming from the tissues is delivered faster, causing an increase in P_ACO_2 if minute ventilation remains the same. At the same time, O_2 is taken up by the capillaries faster than restored by ventilation, causing a decrease in alveolar P_AO_2. Decrease in pulmonary capillary blood flow has the opposite effect (i.e., decrease in P_ACO_2 and increase in P_AO_2) assuming minute ventilation remains the same.[5,7,8]

Ventilation/Perfusion Ratio

Changes in $\dot{V}_A$ and $\dot{Q}_C$ are expressed as a ratio called the **ventilation/perfusion ratio ($\dot{V}/\dot{Q}$).** An ideal ratio of 1.0 indicates that ventilation and perfusion are in perfect balance. A high $\dot{V}/\dot{Q}$ indicates that ventilation is greater than normal, perfusion is less than normal, or both. In the presence of a high $\dot{V}/\dot{Q}$, PO_2 is greater and PCO_2 is less than normal. Conversely, a low $\dot{V}/\dot{Q}$ indicates that ventilation is less than normal, perfusion is greater than normal, or both. In areas with a low $\dot{V}/\dot{Q}$, P_AO_2 is less than normal and P_ACO_2 is greater than normal.

Effect of Alterations in Ventilation/Perfusion Ratio

Figure 11-5 shows graphs of the effect of $\dot{V}/\dot{Q}$ changes on the respiratory exchange ratio (R), plotting all possible values of P_AO_2 and P_ACO_2. When ventilation and perfusion are in perfect balance ($\dot{V}/\dot{Q} = 0.99$), R equals 0.8. At this point, P_AO_2 and P_ACO_2 values equal the ideal values of 100 mm Hg and 40 mm Hg.

As the $\dot{V}/\dot{Q}$ increases above 1.0 (following the curve to the right), R increases. The result is a higher P_AO_2 and lower P_ACO_2. At the extreme right of the graph, perfusion is zero ($\dot{V}/\dot{Q} = \infty$). Areas with ventilation but no blood flow represent alveolar dead space (see Chapter 10). The makeup of gases in these areas is similar to that of inspired air (PO_2 = 150 mm Hg; PCO_2 = 0 mm Hg).

As the $\dot{V}/\dot{Q}$ decreases below 1.0 (following the curve to the left), R decreases. The result is a lower P_AO_2 and higher P_ACO_2. At the extreme left of the graph, there is perfusion but no ventilation ($\dot{V}/\dot{Q} = 0$). With no ventilation to remove CO_2 and restore fresh O_2, the makeup of gases in these areas is similar to mixed venous blood ($P\bar{v}O_2$ = 40 mm Hg; $P\bar{v}CO_2$ = 46 mm Hg).

Venous blood entering areas with $\dot{V}/\dot{Q}$ values of zero cannot pick up O_2 or unload CO_2 and leave the lungs unchanged. As this venous blood returns to the left side of the heart, it mixes with well-oxygenated arterial blood, diluting its O_2 contents in a manner similar to that described for a right-to-left anatomic shunt. To distinguish such areas from true anatomic shunts, exchange

TABLE 11-1

Summary of Variations in Gas Exchange in the Upright Lung, by Region

Lung Region	$\dot{V}/\dot{Q}$ Ratio	Mean P_AO_2 (mm Hg)	Mean P_ACO_2 (mm Hg)	Blood Flow
Apexes	3.3	132	32	Low
Middle	1.0	100	40	Moderate
Bases	0.66	89	42	High

units with $\dot{V}/\dot{Q}$ values of zero are called **alveolar shunts.** Although small anatomic shunts are normal, alveolar shunts are not.

Causes of Regional Differences in Ventilation/Perfusion Ratio

Regional variations in $\dot{V}/\dot{Q}$ in a normal lung are mainly caused by gravity and are most evident in the upright posture. Because the pulmonary circulation is a low-pressure system, blood flow in the upright lung varies considerably from top to bottom (see Chapter 8). Farther down the lung, perfusion increases linearly in proportion to the hydrostatic pressure so that the lung bases receive nearly 20 times as much blood flow as the apexes.

Regional differences in ventilation throughout the lung also occur, but they are less drastic than the differences in perfusion. Similar to perfusion, ventilation also is increased in the lung bases, with approximately four times as much ventilation going to the bases than to the apexes of the upright lung. These regional differences in ventilation are caused by the effect of gravity on pleural pressures (see Chapter 10).

Table 11-1 summarizes the relationships between ventilation and perfusion by lung region.[8] At the lung apexes, ventilation exceeds blood flow, resulting in a high $\dot{V}/\dot{Q}$ (approximately 3.3), high PO_2 (132 mm Hg), and low PCO_2 (32 mm Hg). Farther down the lung, blood flow increases more than ventilation owing to gravity. Toward the middle, the two are approximately equal ($\dot{V}/\dot{Q} = 1.0$). At the bottom of the lung, blood flow is greater than ventilation, resulting in a low $\dot{V}/\dot{Q}$ (approximately 0.66), low PO_2 (89 mm Hg), and slightly higher PCO_2 (42 mm Hg).

As shown in Table 11-1, because of gravity, most blood flows to the lung bases, where PO_2 is less than normal and PCO_2 is greater than normal. After leaving the lung, this large volume of blood combines with the smaller volume coming from the middle and apical regions. The result is a mixture of blood with less O_2 and more CO_2 than would come from an ideal gas exchange unit.

OXYGEN TRANSPORT

Blood carries O_2 in two forms. A small amount of O_2 exists in a simple physical solution, dissolved in the plasma and erythrocyte intracellular fluid. However, most O_2 is carried in a reversible chemical combination with hemoglobin (Hb) inside the RBC.

Physically Dissolved Oxygen

As gaseous O_2 diffuses into the blood, it immediately dissolves in the plasma and erythrocyte fluid. By applying Henry's law (see Chapter 6), the amount of dissolved O_2 in the blood (at 37° C) can be computed with the following simple formula:

$$\text{Dissolved } O_2 \text{ (ml/dl)} = PO_2 \times 0.003$$

This equation is plotted in Figure 11-6, which shows that the relationship between partial pressure and dissolved O_2 is direct and linear. In normal arterial blood with PaO_2 of approximately 100 mm Hg, there is approximately 0.3 ml/dl of dissolved O_2. However, if an individual with normal arterial blood breathes pure O_2, PaO_2 increases to approximately 670 mm Hg. In this case, the dissolved O_2 would increase to approximately 2.0 ml/dl. The blood of someone breathing pure O_2 in a hyperbaric chamber at 3 atm (2280 mm Hg) would carry nearly 6.5 ml/dl dissolved O_2 in the plasma. This amount is enough to supply most tissue needs at rest by itself.

Chemically Combined Oxygen (Oxyhemoglobin)

Hemoglobin and Oxygen Transport

Most blood O_2 is transported in chemical combination with Hb in the erythrocytes. Hb is a conjugated protein, consisting of four linked polypeptide chains (the *globin* portion), each of which is combined with a porphyrin complex called *heme*. The four polypeptide chains of Hb are coiled together into a ball-like structure, the shape of which determines its affinity for O_2.[5,8]

As shown in Figure 11-7, each heme complex contains a centrally located ferrous iron ion (Fe^{++}). When Hb is not carrying O_2, this ion has four unpaired electrons. In this deoxygenated state, the molecule exhibits the characteristics of a weak acid. Deoxygenated Hb serves as an important blood buffer for hydrogen ions, a crucial factor in CO_2 transport.

O_2 molecules bind to Hb by way of the ferrous iron ion, one for each protein chain. With complete O_2 binding, all electrons become paired, and Hb is converted to its oxygenated state (**oxyhemoglobin** [HbO_2]).

In whole blood, 1 g of normal Hb can carry approximately 1.34 ml of O_2. Given an average blood Hb content of 15 g/dl, the O_2-carrying capacity of the blood can be calculated as follows:

$$1.34 \text{ ml/g} \times 15 \text{ g/dl} = 20.1 \text{ ml/dl}$$

The addition of Hb increases the O_2-carrying capacity of the blood nearly 70-fold compared with plasma alone. The amount of O_2 bound to Hb depends on its level of saturation with O_2 (see later).

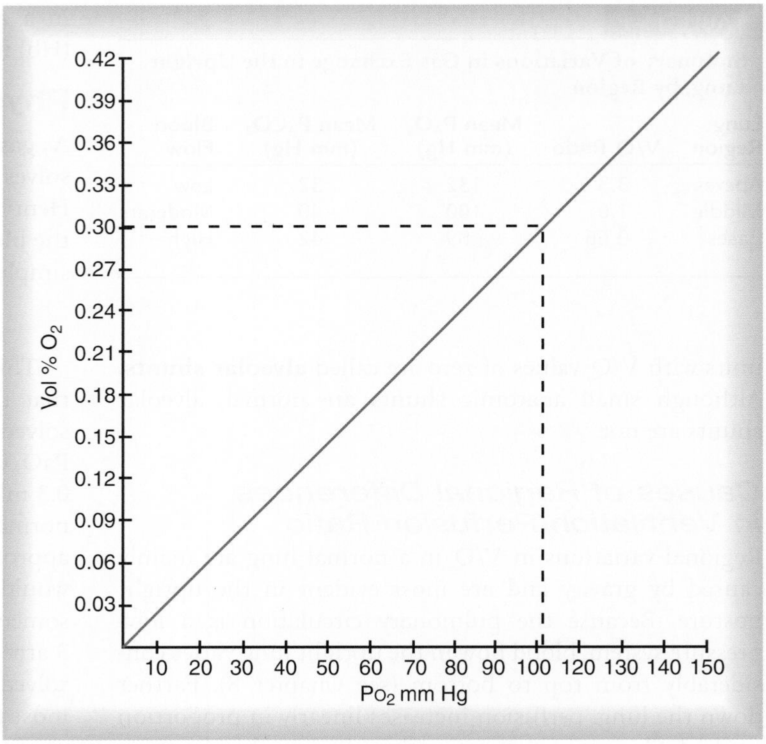

FIGURE 11-6 Relationship between PO_2 and dissolved O_2 contents of plasma at 37° C. The *dashed line* emphasizes the fact that arterial blood, with average PO_2 of 100 mm Hg, has 0.3 ml of O_2 dissolved in each deciliter (100 ml).

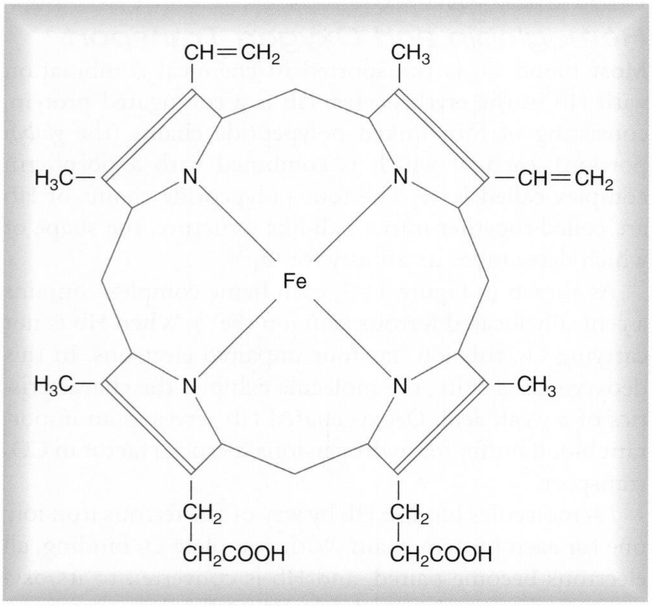

FIGURE 11-7 Structure of heme.

Hemoglobin Saturation

Saturation is a measure of the proportion of available Hb that is carrying O_2. Saturation is computed as the ratio of HbO_2 (content) to total Hb (capacity). Hb arterial oxygen saturation (SaO_2) is always expressed as a percentage of this ratio and calculated according to the following formula:

$$SaO_2 = [HbO_2 \div \text{Total Hb}] \times 100$$

Where $[HbO_2]$ equals the oxyhemoglobin content. If there were a total of 15 g/dl Hb in the blood, of which 7.5 g was HbO_2, the SaO_2 would be calculated as follows:

$$SaO_2\ (\%) = [7.5 \div 15] \times 100 = 50\%$$

In this example, Hb is said to be 50% saturated: Only half of the available Hb is carrying O_2, and the remainder is unoxygenated. In clinical practice, both SaO_2 and total Hb content are measured directly to derive the HbO_2. Normal SaO_2 is 95% to 100% depending on the age of the patient.

Oxyhemoglobin Dissociation Curve

Hb saturation with O_2 varies with changes in PO_2. Plotting the saturation (*y*-axis) against PO_2 (*x*-axis) yields the HbO_2 dissociation curve (Figure 11-8). In contrast to dissolved O_2, Hb saturation is not linearly related to PO_2.[4] Instead, the relationship forms an S-shaped curve. The flat upper part of this curve represents the normal operating range for arterial blood. Because the slope is minimal in this area, minor changes in PaO_2 have little effect on SaO_2, indicating a strong affinity of Hb for O_2. With a normal PaO_2 of 100 mm Hg, SaO_2 is approximately 97%. If some abnormality (e.g., lung disease) reduced PaO_2 to 65 mm Hg, SaO_2 would still be approximately 90%.

However, with PO_2 less than 60 mm Hg, the curve steepens dramatically, which is why it is beneficial to keep

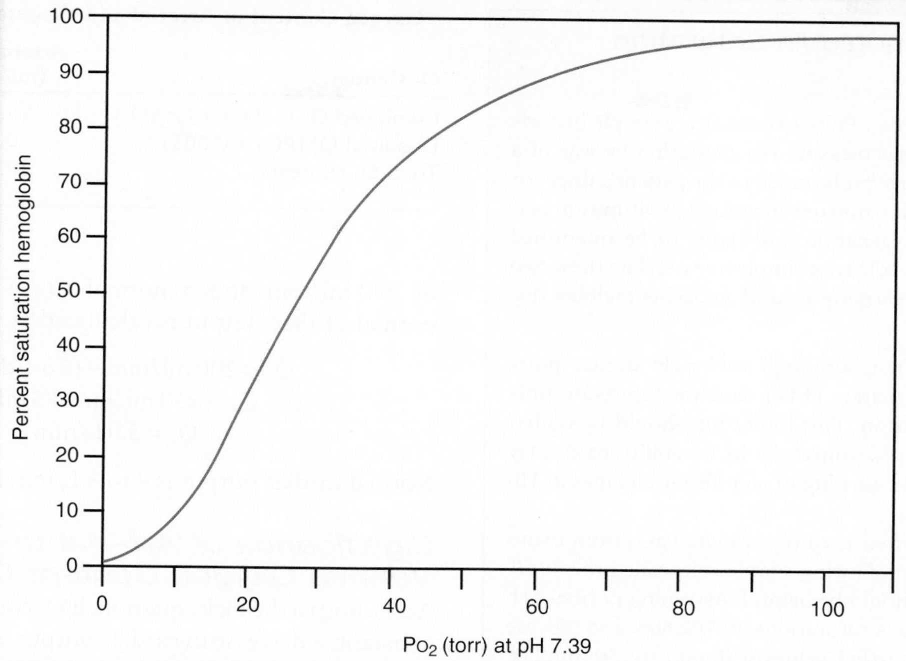

FIGURE 11-8 O_2 dissociation curve plots the relationship between plasma PO_2 (*x*-axis) and Hb saturation (*y*-axis).

PaO_2 greater than 60 mm Hg in clinical practice. With PO_2 less than 60 mm Hg, a small decrease in PO_2 causes a large increase in SaO_2, indicating a lessening affinity for O_2. This normal decrease in the affinity of Hb for O_2 helps release large amounts of O_2 to the tissues, where PO_2 is low.

Total Oxygen Content of the Blood

Total O_2 content of the blood equals the sum of O_2 dissolved and chemically combined with Hb.[2,7] For total O_2 content to be calculated, the following three values must be known: (1) PO_2, (2) total Hb content (g/dl), and (3) Hb saturation. Given these values, the following equation can be applied:

$$CaO_2 = (0.003 \times PO_2) + (Hb_{tot} \times 1.34 \times SO_2)$$

Where:
CaO_2 = Total O_2 content
PO_2 = Partial pressure of O_2 in the blood
Hb_{tot} = Total Hb content (in g/dl)
SO_2 = Hb saturation with O_2 (as a decimal)

Typically, clinicians want to know the O_2 content of arterial blood (CaO_2). The ($0.003 \times PO_2$) component of the equation represents dissolved O_2, whereas the ($Hb_{tot} \times 1.34 \times SO_2$) component represents the chemically combined oxyhemoglobin. For example, the RT obtains a sample of normal arterial blood with PO_2 of 100 mm Hg containing 15 g/dl of Hb that is 97% saturated with O_2. To compute the total O_2 content, the RT can apply the aforementioned equation as follows:

$$CaO_2 = (0.003 \times PaO_2) + (Hb_{tot} \times 1.34 \times SaO_2)$$
$$CaO_2 = (0.003\ \text{ml} \times 100\ \text{mm Hg}) + (15\ \text{g/dl} \times 1.34 \times 0.97)$$
$$CaO_2 = (0.3\ \text{ml}) + (19.5\ \text{g/dl})$$
$$CaO_2 = 19.8\ \text{ml/dl}$$

The normal CaO_2 concentration is 16 to 20 ml/dl.

Normal Loading and Unloading of Oxygen (Arteriovenous Differences)

Figure 11-9 uses the oxyhemoglobin dissociation curve to show the effects of O_2 loading and unloading in the lungs and tissues. *Point A* represents freshly arterialized blood leaving the pulmonary capillaries, with PO_2 of approximately 100 mm Hg and Hb saturation of approximately 97%. As blood perfuses body tissues, O_2 uptake causes a decrease in both PO_2 and saturation, such that venous blood leaving the tissues *(point V)* has PO_2 of approximately 40 mm Hg, with Hb saturation of approximately 73%.

Using a normal Hb content of 15 g/dl and knowing the saturation at each possible PO_2, the total O_2 content can be calculated at any PO_2 in the manner previously described. The *y*-axis of Figure 11-9 provides this information in SaO_2 increments of 10%. Table 11-2 summarizes the difference between the O_2 content of these normal arterial and venous points.

MINI CLINI

Relating Hemoglobin Saturation and PaO_2

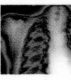

PROBLEM: Pulse oximeters are simple bedside devices that measure Hb saturation by way of a noninvasive probe taped to the patient's finger or forehead. Although oximeters measure Hb saturation percentage, blood oxygenation still tends to be quantified according to PaO_2. Is there a simple way to relate these two measures without carrying around an oxyhemoglobin dissociation curve?

DISCUSSION: First, although extremely useful, pulse oximeters are inaccurate (±4%), and they measure only normal Hb saturation. This limitation should be understood. The value of oximetry is in its ability to display trends and provide warning of significant changes in Hb saturation with O_2.

Even so, RTs often need to estimate PaO_2 from oximeter readings. The following simple rule, called the *40-50-60/70-80-90 rule,* should be helpful. Assuming normal pH, PCO_2, and Hb values, saturations of 70%, 80%, and 90% are roughly equivalent to PO_2 values of 40 mm Hg, 50 mm Hg, and 60 mm Hg:

Hb Saturation (%)	Approximate PaO_2 (mm Hg)
70	40
80	50
90	60

A patient with a pulse oximeter reading of 90% has a PaO_2 of approximately 60 mm Hg. If the saturation decreased to 80%, the PaO_2 would decrease to approximately 50 mm Hg. This rule works only in the middle range of PO_2 values, where the curve is most linear; it should not be applied with saturations greater than 90%. A saturation of 100% may represent a PaO_2 of 200 mm Hg.

As indicated in Table 11-2, the difference between the arterial and venous O_2 contents is normally approximately 5 ml/dl. This is the arterial-to-mixed venous O_2 content difference ($C(a-\bar{v})O_2$). $C(a-\bar{v})O_2$ is the amount of O_2 given up by every 100 ml of blood on each pass through the tissues.

Fick Equation

$C(a-\bar{v})O_2$ indicates O_2 extraction in proportion to blood flow. If this measure is combined with total-body O_2 consumption, cardiac output can be calculated. The basis for this calculation is the classic **Fick equation:**

$$\dot{Q}_t = \dot{V}O_2 \div [C(a-\bar{v})O_2 \times 10]$$

In this equation, $\dot{Q}_t$ is cardiac output (L/min), $\dot{V}O_2$ is the whole-body O_2 consumption (ml/min), and $C(a-\bar{v})O_2$ is the arteriovenous O_2 content difference (ml/dl). The factor of 10 converts ml/dl to ml/L. Given a normal $\dot{V}O_2$ of 250 ml/min and a normal $C(a-\bar{v})O_2$ of 5 ml/dl, a normal cardiac output is calculated as follows:

$$\dot{Q}_t = 200\text{ ml/min} \div (5\text{ ml/dl} \times 10)$$
$$\dot{Q}_t = 250\text{ ml/min} \div 5\text{ ml/L}$$
$$\dot{Q}_t = 5.0\text{ L/min}$$

Normal cardiac output is 4 to 8 L/min in an adult patient.

TABLE 11-2

Oxygen Content of Arterial and Venous Blood

O_2 Content	Arterial O_2 (ml/dl)	Venous O_2 (ml/dl)
Combined O_2 ($1.34 \times 15 \times SO_2$)	19.5	14.7
Dissolved O_2 ($PO_2 \times 0.003$)	0.3	0.1
Total O_2 content	19.8	14.8

Significance of Arterial-to-Mixed Venous Oxygen Content Difference

According to the Fick equation, if O_2 consumption remains constant, a decrease in cardiac output increases $C(a-\bar{v})O_2$. Conversely, if the cardiac output increases and O_2 consumption remains constant, $C(a-\bar{v})O_2$ decreases proportionately. Although the Fick equation for calculating cardiac output has been replaced by other techniques, the principle relating $C(a-\bar{v})O_2$ to perfusion is used to monitor tissue oxygenation at the bedside. More details on these methods are provided in Chapter 46.

Factors Affecting Oxygen Loading and Unloading

In addition to the shape of the HbO_2 curve, many other factors affect O_2 loading and unloading. Among the most important factors in clinical practice are blood pH, body temperature, and erythrocyte concentration of certain organic phosphates.[5] Variations in the structure of Hb also affect O_2 loading and unloading, as can chemical combinations of Hb with substances other than O_2, such as carbon monoxide.

pH (Bohr Effect)

The impact of changes in blood pH on Hb affinity for O_2 is called the **Bohr effect.** As shown in Figure 11-10, the Bohr effect alters the position of the HbO_2 dissociation curve. A low pH (acidity) shifts the curve to the right, whereas a high pH (alkalinity) shifts it to the left. These changes are a result of variations in the shape of the Hb molecule caused by fluctuations in pH.

As blood pH decreases and the curve shifts to the right, the Hb saturation for a given PO_2 decreases (decreased Hb affinity for O_2). Conversely, as blood pH increases and the curve shifts to the left, the Hb saturation for a given PO_2 increases (increased affinity of Hb for O_2).[4,5,8]

These changes enhance O_2 loading in the lungs and O_2 unloading in the tissues. As blood in the tissue picks up

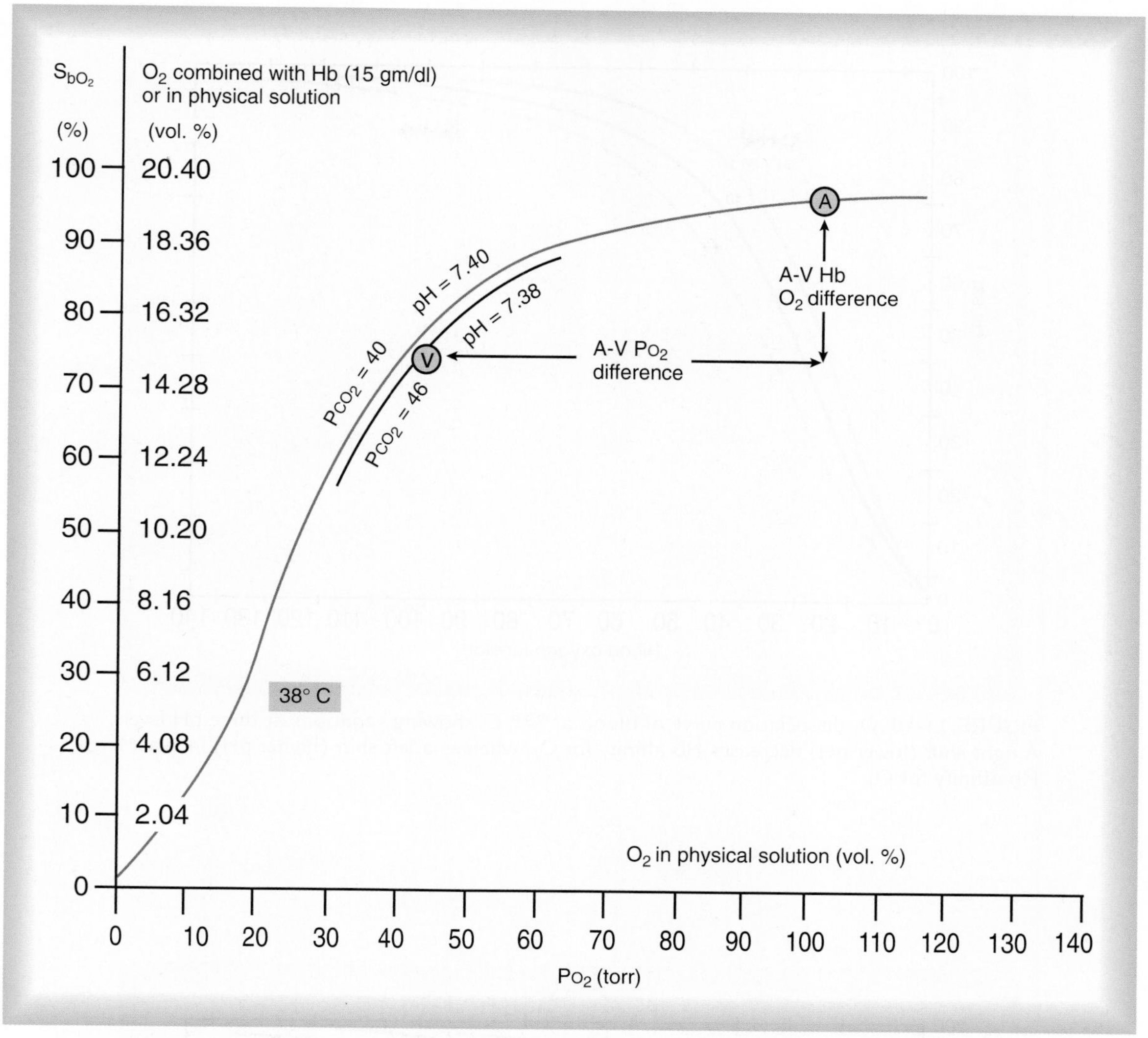

FIGURE 11-9 Normal oxyhemoglobin dissociation curve, showing the basic relationship of blood O_2 transport. Point "sA" represents normal values for arterial blood leaving the lungs (loading point). Point "sV" represents normal values for venous blood leaving the tissues (unloading point). The slight difference in curve position resulting from pH and CO_2 changes helps O_2 unloading at the tissues. Differences between O_2 content at these two points represent the amount of O_2 taken up by the tissues on one pass through the systemic circulation. (Modified from Slonim NB, Hamilton LH: Respiratory physiology, ed 5, St Louis, 1987, Mosby.)

CO_2, pH decreases from 7.40 to approximately 7.37. The HbO_2 curve shifts to the right, lowering the affinity of Hb for O_2. With lower affinity for O_2, Hb more readily gives up O_2 to the tissues. Conversely, when venous blood returns to the lungs, the pH increases again to 7.40. This change in pH shifts the HbO_2 curve back to the left, increasing the affinity of Hb for O_2 and enhancing its uptake from the alveoli.

Body Temperature

Variations in body temperature also affect the HbO_2 dissociation curve. As shown in Figure 11-11, a decrease in body temperature shifts the curve to the left, increasing Hb affinity for O_2. Conversely, as body temperature increases, the curve shifts to the right, and the affinity of Hb for O_2 decreases. As with the Bohr effect, these changes enhance normal O_2 uptake and delivery. At the tissues, temperature changes are directly related to metabolic rate, such that areas of high metabolic activity have higher temperatures. In exercising muscle, higher temperatures decrease Hb affinity for O_2, enhancing its release to the tissues. Conversely, in hypothermia, the O_2 demands of the tissues are greatly reduced, and Hb need not give up as much of its O_2.[2]

Organic Phosphates (2,3-Diphosphoglycerate)

The organic phosphate 2,3-diphosphoglycerate (2,3-DPG) is found in abundance in the RBCs, where it forms a loose chemical bond with the globin chains of deoxygenated

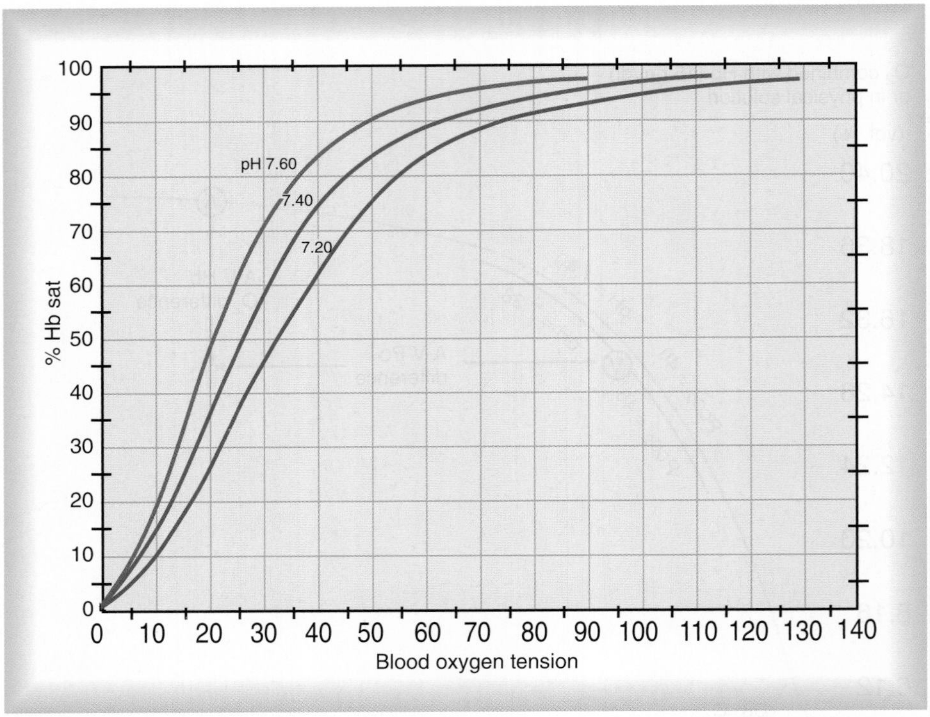

FIGURE 11-10 O_2 dissociation curve of blood at 37° C, showing variations at three pH levels. A right shift (lower pH) decreases Hb affinity for O_2, whereas a left shift (higher pH) increases Hb affinity for O_2.

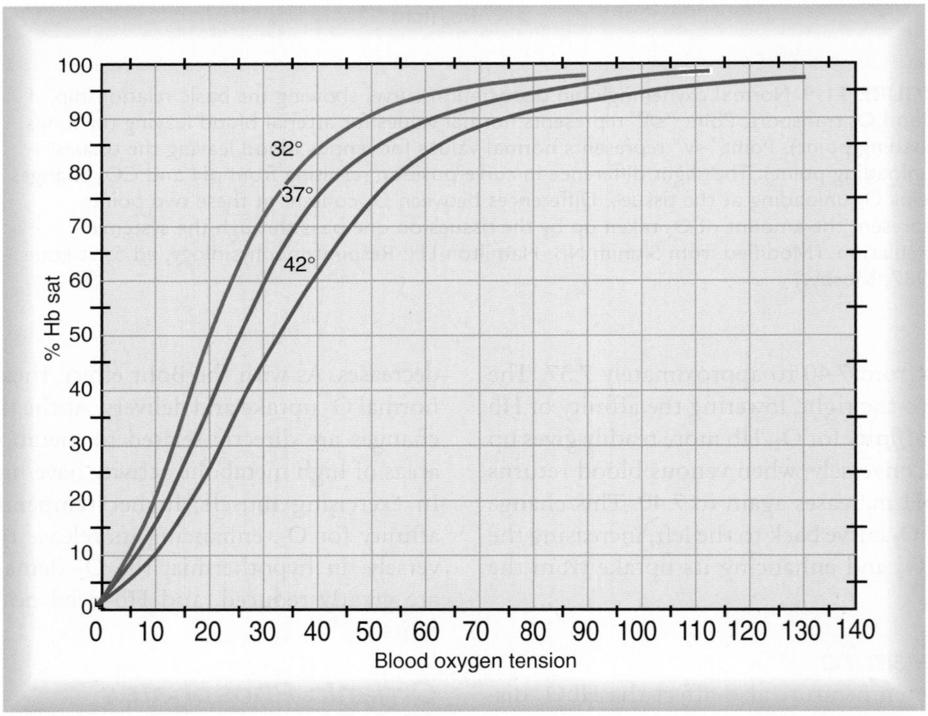

FIGURE 11-11 O_2 dissociation curve of blood at pH of 7.40, showing variations at three temperatures. For a given O_2 tension, the lower the temperature, the more the Hb holds onto O_2, maintaining a higher saturation.

Hb. In this configuration, 2,3-DPG stabilizes the molecule in its deoxygenated state, reducing its affinity for O_2.[5-7] Without 2,3-DPG, Hb affinity for O_2 would be so great that normal O_2 unloading would be impossible. Increased 2,3-DPG concentrations shift the HbO_2 curve to the right, promoting O_2 unloading. Conversely, low 2,3-DPG concentrations shift the curve to the left, increasing Hb affinity for O_2.

Alkalosis, chronic hypoxemia, and anemia all tend to increase 2,3-DPG concentrations and promote O_2 unloading. Conversely, acidosis results in a lower intracellular level of 2,3-DPG and a greater affinity of Hb for O_2.

Erythrocyte concentrations of 2,3-DPG in banked blood decrease over time. After 1 week of storage, the 2,3-DPG level may be less than one-third of the normal value. This change shifts the HbO_2 curve to the left, decreasing the availability of O_2 to the tissues. Large transfusions of banked blood that is more than a few days old can severely impair O_2 delivery, even in the presence of normal PO_2. Improved maintenance levels of 2,3-DPG can be achieved with newer blood storage techniques.

Abnormal Hemoglobin

Abnormalities in the Hb molecule also can affect O_2 loading and unloading. Structural abnormalities occur when the amino acid sequence in the polypeptide chains of the molecule varies from normal.[5] Changes in amino acid sequences alter the shape of the molecule, increasing or decreasing its O_2 affinity. More than 120 abnormal hemoglobins have been identified. In healthy individuals, 15% to 40% of the circulating Hb may be abnormal.

HbS **(sickle cell hemoglobin)** is less soluble than normal Hb, which causes it to become susceptible to polymerization and precipitation when deoxygenated. Certain events such as dehydration, hypoxia, and acidosis cause HbS to crystallize and the RBC to become hardened and curved like a sickle. Erythrocyte fragility is increased (leading to hemolysis), and the risk of thrombus formation is increased. Patients with sickle cell disease are prone to vasoocclusive disease and anemia. Some patients with sickle cell anemia develop **acute chest syndrome.** Acute chest syndrome is the most common cause of death in patients with sickle cell anemia. Patients usually complain of acute chest pain, cough, and shortness of breath. A new infiltrate is usually seen on the chest radiograph, and the patient often develops progressive anemia and hypoxemia. The causes of acute chest syndrome are multiple; the term *acute chest syndrome* does not indicate a definite diagnosis but rather indicates the clinical difficulty of defining a specific cause in most of such episodes.

Methemoglobin (metHb) is an abnormal form of the molecule, in which the heme-complex normal ferrous iron ion (Fe^{++}) loses an electron and is oxidized to its ferric state (Fe^{++}). In the ferric state, the iron ion cannot combine with O_2. The result is a special form of anemia called **methemoglobinemia.** As with HbCO, clinical abnormalities come from the associated increased affinity for O_2 and loss of O_2-binding capacity. The most common cause of methemoglobinemia is the therapeutic use of oxidant medications such as nitric oxide, nitroglycerin, and lidocaine. When using these therapeutic agents, frequent monitoring for metHb is important to weigh the risk against the benefit. The presence of metHb turns the blood brown, which can produce a slate-gray skin coloration that is often confused with cyanosis. The presence of metHb is confirmed by spectrophotometry (see Chapter 18). Methemoglobinemia is treated with reducing agents such as methylene blue or ascorbic acid when the blood level exceeds approximately 30%.

Carboxyhemoglobin (HbCO) is the chemical combination of Hb with carbon monoxide. The affinity of Hb for carbon monoxide is more than 200 times greater than it is for O_2. Extremely low concentrations of carbon monoxide can quickly displace O_2 from Hb, forming HbCO. Carbon monoxide partial pressure of 0.12 mm Hg can displace half the O_2 from Hb. Because HbCO cannot carry O_2, each 1 g of Hb saturated with carbon monoxide represents a loss in carrying capacity. The combination of carbon monoxide with Hb shifts the HbO_2 curve to the left, impeding O_2 delivery to the tissues further. Treatment for carbon monoxide poisoning involves giving the patient as much O_2 as possible because O_2 reduces the half-life of HbCO (Table 11-3). Sometimes a hyperbaric chamber is required to reverse rapidly the binding of CO with Hb.

During fetal life and for up to 1 year after birth, the blood has a high proportion of an Hb variant called **fetal hemoglobin (HbF).** HbF has a greater affinity for O_2 than normal adult Hb, as manifested by a leftward shift of the HbO_2 curve. Given the low PO_2 values available to the fetus in utero, this leftward shift aids O_2 loading at the placenta. Because of the relatively low pH of the fetal environment, O_2 unloading at the cellular level is not greatly affected. However, after birth, this enhanced O_2 affinity is less advantageous. Over the first year of life, HbF is gradually replaced with normal Hb.

Measurement of Hemoglobin Affinity for Oxygen

Variations in the affinity of Hb for O_2 are quantified by a measure called the $\mathbf{P_{50}}$.[2,8] The P_{50} is the partial pressure of O_2 at which the Hb is 50% saturated, standardized to a pH level of 7.40. A normal P_{50} is approximately 26.6 mm Hg.

TABLE 11-3

Half-Life of Carboxyhemoglobin (HbCO) at Different Oxygen Exposures

HbCO Half-life (min)	Inhaled FiO_2	PaO_2 (mm Hg)
280-320	0.21 at 1 atm	100
80-90	1.0 at 1 atm	673
20-30	1.0 at 3 atm	2193

Conditions that cause a decrease in Hb affinity for O_2 (a shift of the HbO_2 curve to the right) increase the P_{50} to a value higher than normal. Conditions associated with an increase in affinity (a shift of the HbO_2 curve to the left) decrease the P_{50} to lower than normal. With 15 g/dl Hb, a 4-mm Hg increase in P_{50} results in approximately 1 to 2 ml/dl more O_2 being unloaded in the tissues than when the P_{50} is normal. Figure 11-12 shows the effect of changes in P_{50} and summarizes how the major factors previously discussed affect Hb affinity for O_2.

CARBON DIOXIDE TRANSPORT

Figure 11-13 shows the physical and chemical events of gas exchange at the systemic capillaries. In the pulmonary capillaries, all events occur in the opposite direction. Although the primary focus is on CO_2 transport, Figure 11-13 also includes the basic elements of O_2 exchange. O_2 exchange is included here for completeness and to show that the exchange and transport of these two gases are closely related.

Transport Mechanisms

Approximately 45 to 55 ml/dl of CO_2 is normally carried in the blood in the following three forms: (1) dissolved in physical solution, (2) chemically combined with protein, and (3) ionized as bicarbonate.[5,7]

Dissolved in Physical Solution

As with O_2, CO_2 produced by the tissues dissolves in the plasma and erythrocyte intracellular fluid. However, in contrast to O_2, dissolved CO_2 plays an important role in transport, accounting for approximately 8% of the total released at the lungs; this is because of the high solubility of CO_2 in plasma.

Chemically Combined With Protein

Molecular CO_2 has the capacity to combine chemically with free amino groups (NH_2) of protein molecules (Prot), forming a carbamino compound:

$$\text{Prot-NH}_2 + CO_2 \Leftrightarrow \text{Prot-NHCOO}^- + H^+$$

A small amount of the CO_2 leaving the tissues combines with plasma proteins to form these carbamino compounds.

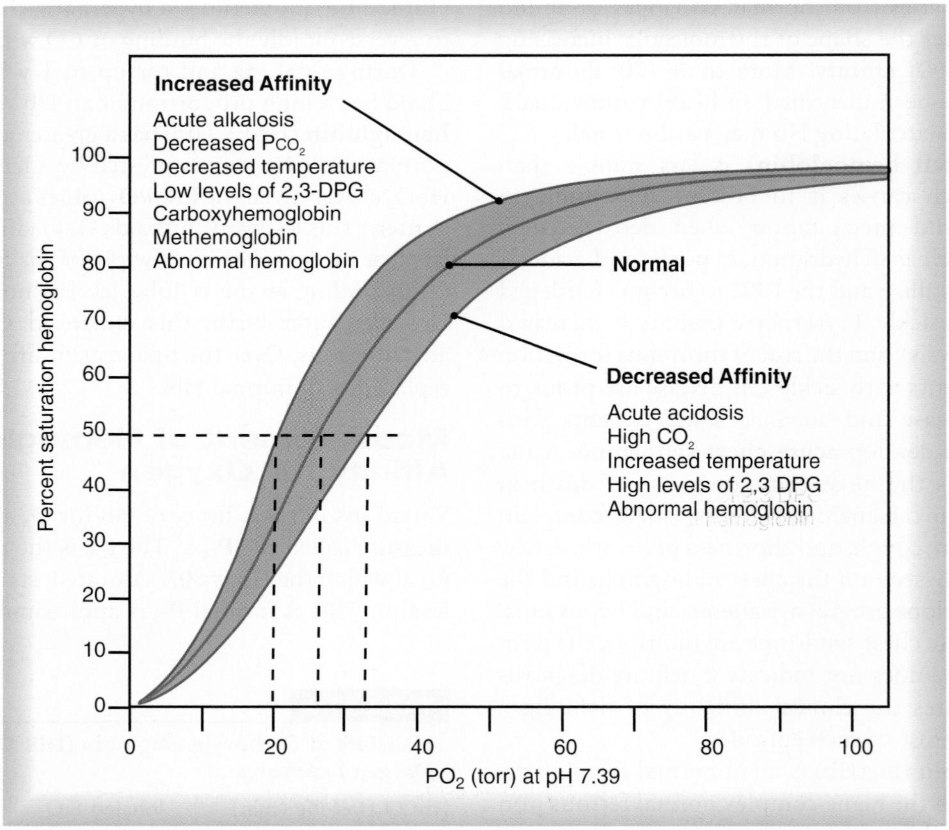

FIGURE 11-12 Conditions associated with altered affinity of Hb for O_2. P_{50} is PaO_2 at which Hb is 50% saturated (normally 26.6 mm Hg). A lower than normal P_{50} represents increased affinity of Hb for O_2. A high P_{50} is seen with decreased affinity. (Modified from Lane EE, Walker JF: Clinical arterial blood gas analysis, St Louis, 1987, Mosby.)

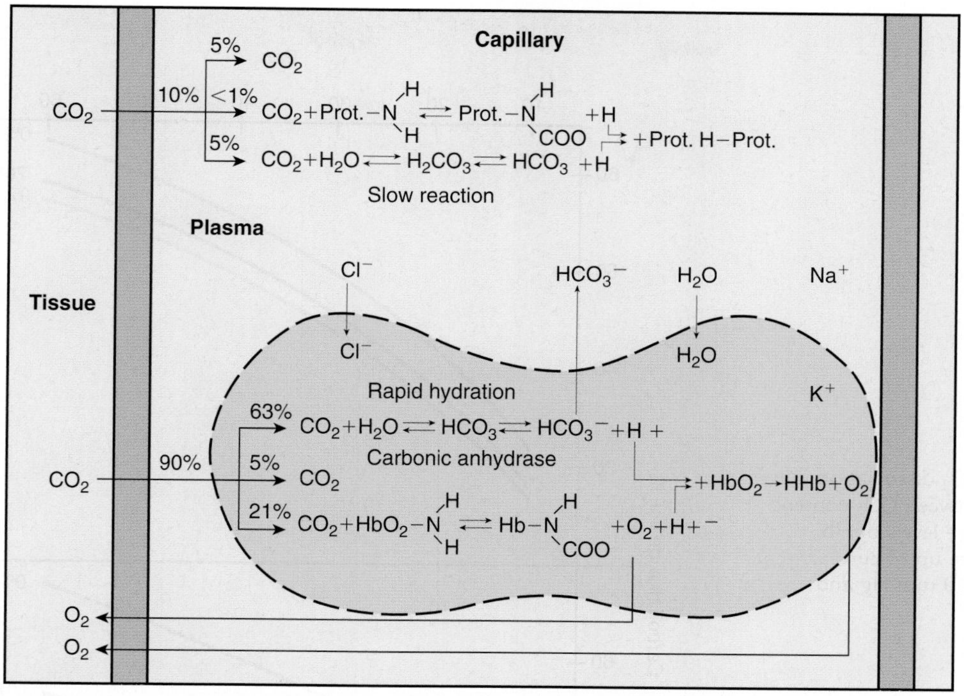

FIGURE 11-13 Summary diagram of various fates of CO_2 as it diffuses from the cells and interstitial spaces into the peripheral capillaries before its transport toward the venous circulation. (Modified from Martin DE, Youtsey JW: Respiratory anatomy and physiology, St Louis, 1988, Mosby.)

A larger fraction of CO_2 combines with erythrocyte Hb to form a carbamino compound called *carbaminohemoglobin*. As indicated in the previous equation, this reaction produces H^+ ions. These H^+ ions are buffered by the reduced Hb, which is made available by the concurrent release of O_2.

The availability of additional sites for H^+ buffering increases the affinity of Hb for CO_2. Because reduced Hb is a weaker acid than HbO_2, pH changes associated with the release of the H^+ ions in the formation of carbaminohemoglobin are minimized. Carbaminohemoglobin constitutes approximately 12% of the total CO_2 transported.

Ionized as Bicarbonate

Approximately 80% of CO_2 in the blood is transported as bicarbonate. Of the CO_2 that dissolves in plasma, a small portion combines chemically with water in a process called *hydrolysis*. Hydrolysis of CO_2 initially forms carbonic acid, which quickly ionizes into hydrogen and bicarbonate ions:

$$CO_2 + H_2O \Leftrightarrow H_2CO_3 \Leftrightarrow HCO_3^- + H^+$$

The H^+ ions produced in this reaction are buffered by the plasma proteins in much the same way as Hb buffers H^+ in the RBC. However, the rate of this plasma hydrolysis reaction is extremely slow, producing minimal amounts of H^+ and HCO_3^-.

Most CO_2 undergoes hydrolysis inside the erythrocyte. This reaction is greatly enhanced by an enzyme catalyst called *carbonic anhydrase*. The resulting H^+ ions are buffered by the imidazole group (R-NHCOO$^-$) of the reduced Hb molecule. The concurrent conversion of HbO_2 to its deoxygenated form helps buffer H^+ ions, enhancing the loading of CO_2 as carbaminohemoglobin.

As the hydrolysis of CO_2 continues, HCO_3^- ions begin to accumulate in the erythrocyte. To maintain a concentration equilibrium across the cell membrane, some of these anions diffuse outward into the plasma. Because the erythrocyte is not freely permeable by cations, electrolytic equilibrium must be maintained by way of an inward migration of anions. This migration is achieved by the shifting of chloride ions (Cl^-) from the plasma into the erythrocyte—a process called the *chloride shift,* or the **Hamburger phenomenon.**

Carbon Dioxide Dissociation Curve

As with O_2, CO_2 has a dissociation curve. The relationship between blood PCO_2 and CO_2 content is depicted in Figure 11-14. The first point to note is the effect of Hb saturation with O_2 on this curve. As previously discussed, CO_2 levels, through their influence on pH, modify the O_2 dissociation curve (Bohr effect). Figure 11-14 shows that oxyhemoglobin saturation also affects the position of the CO_2 dissociation curve. The influence of oxyhemoglobin saturation on CO_2 dissociation is called the **Haldane effect.** As previously explained, this phenomenon is a result of changes in the affinity of Hb for CO_2, which occur as a result of its buffering of H^+ ions.[4-7]

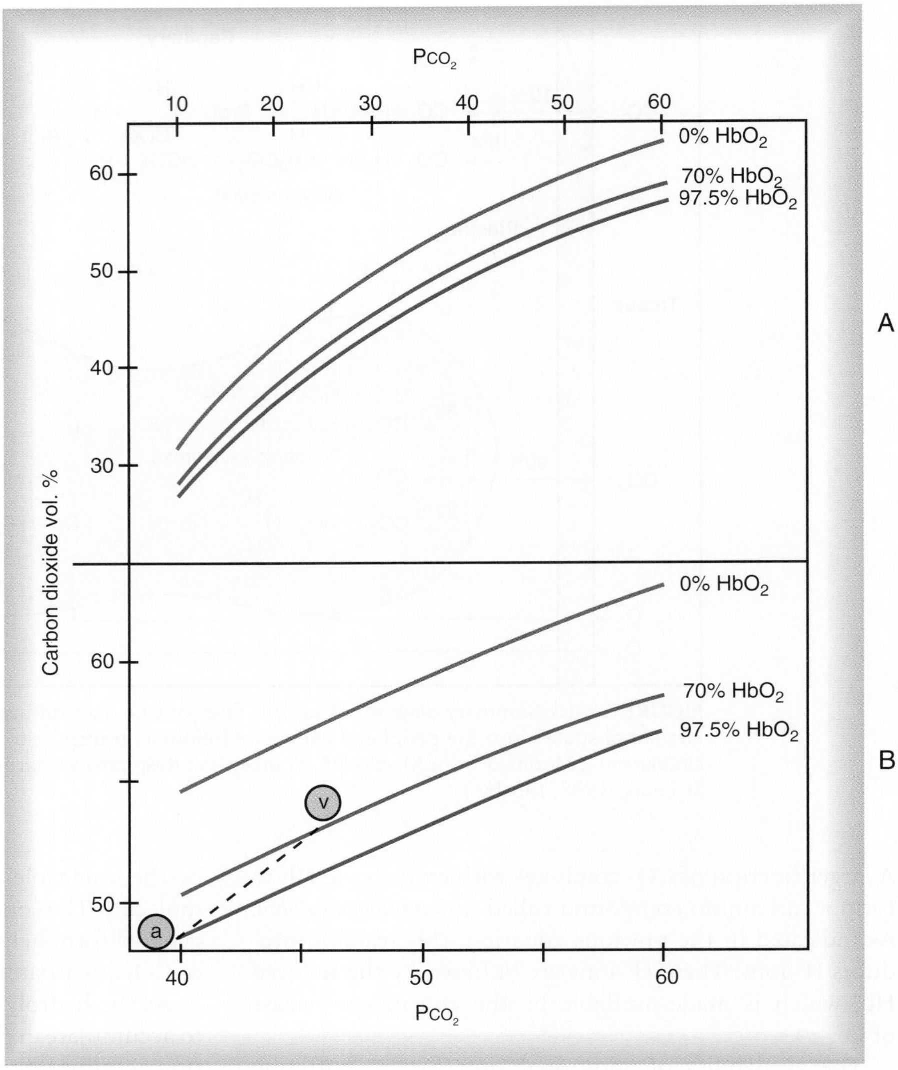

FIGURE 11-14 CO_2 dissociation curves. **A,** Relationship between CO_2 content and tension at three levels of Hb saturation. **B,** Close-up of curves between PCO_2 of 40 mm Hg and 60 mm Hg.

Figure 11-14, *A* shows CO_2 dissociation curves for three levels of blood O_2 saturation. The first two are physiologic values, and the third extreme value is provided for contrast. Figure 11-14, *B* amplifies selected segments of these curves in the physiologic range of PCO_2. Note first the arterial point "a" lying on the curve representing SaO_2 of 97.5%. At this point, PCO_2 is 40 mm Hg, and CO_2 content is approximately 48 ml/dl. The venous point "v" falls on the curve, representing SaO_2 of approximately 70%. At this point, PCO_2 is 46 mm Hg, and CO_2 content is approximately 52 ml/dl. Because O_2 saturation changes from arterial to venous blood, the true physiologic CO_2 dissociation curve must lie somewhere between these two points. This physiologic curve is represented as the dashed line in Figure 11-14, *B*.

At point "a," the high SaO_2 decreases the capacity of the blood to hold CO_2, helping unload this gas at the lungs. At point "v," the lower mixed venous O_2 saturation ($S\bar{v}O_2$) increases the capacity of the blood for CO_2, aiding uptake at the tissues.

TABLE 11-4

Carbon Dioxide Content of Arterial and Venous Blood

Unit of Measure	Arterial	Venous
mmol/L	21.53	23.21
ml/dl	48.01	51.76

The total CO_2 content of arterial and venous blood is compared in Table 11-4. The amounts of CO_2 are expressed in gaseous volume equivalents (ml/dl) and as millimoles per liter (mmol/L). This latter measure of the chemical combining power of CO_2 in solutions is critical in understanding the role of this gas in acid-base balance.

ABNORMALITIES OF GAS EXCHANGE AND TRANSPORT

Gas exchange is abnormal when either tissue O_2 delivery or CO_2 removal is impaired.

Impaired Oxygen Delivery

O_2 delivery ($\dot{D}O_2$) to the tissues is a function of arterial O_2 content (CaO_2) times cardiac output ($\dot{Q}t$):

$$\dot{D}O_2 = CaO_2 \times \dot{Q}t$$

When O_2 delivery is inadequate for cellular needs, **hypoxia** occurs. According to the preceding equation, hypoxia occurs if (1) the arterial blood O_2 content is decreased, (2) cardiac output or perfusion is decreased (*shock* or *ischemia*), or (3) abnormal cellular function prevents proper uptake of O_2. Table 11-5 summarizes causes, common clinical indicators, mechanisms, and examples of hypoxia.

Hypoxemia

Hypoxemia occurs when the partial pressure of O_2 in the arterial blood (PaO_2) is decreased to less than the predicted normal value based on the age of the patient. Impaired O_2 delivery also occurs in the presence of abnormalities that prevent saturation of Hb with O_2 (see subsequent discussion).

Decreased Partial Pressure of Oxygen in Arterial Blood. Decreased PaO_2 may be caused by a low ambient PO_2, hypoventilation, impaired diffusion, $\dot{V}/\dot{Q}$ imbalances, and right-to-left anatomic or physiologic shunting. PO_2 also decreases normally with aging. The normal predicted PaO_2 decreases steadily with age, and the average is approximately 85 mm Hg at age 60 years (see later discussion).

Breathing gases with a low O_2 concentration at sea level or breathing air at pressures less than atmospheric lowers the alveolar O_2 tension, decreasing PaO_2. A common example of this problem occurs during travel to high altitudes, where the visitor often experiences the ill effects of hypoxia for several days. This condition is called *mountain sickness*. In such cases, although PaO_2 is reduced, the pressure gradient between the alveoli and the arterial blood for O_2 ($P[A-a]O_2$) remains normal.

Assuming a constant FiO_2, alveolar PO_2 varies inversely with alveolar PCO_2. An increase in the alveolar PCO_2 (hypoventilation) is always accompanied by a proportionate decrease in alveolar PO_2. $P(A-a)O_2$ is normal in such cases. Conversely, hyperventilation decreases P_ACO_2 and helps compensate for hypoxemia.

Even when alveolar PO_2 is normal, disorders of the alveolar-capillary membrane may limit diffusion of O_2 into the pulmonary capillary blood, decreasing PaO_2. Examples are pulmonary fibrosis and interstitial edema. However, as previously noted, a pure diffusion limitation is an uncommon cause of hypoxemia at rest.

$\dot{V}/\dot{Q}$ imbalances are the most common cause of hypoxemia in patients with lung disease. A $\dot{V}/\dot{Q}$ imbalance is an abnormal deviation in the distribution of ventilation to perfusion in the lung. The normal lung has some $\dot{V}/\dot{Q}$ mismatch; however, in disease states, the degree of $\dot{V}/\dot{Q}$ imbalances becomes much greater.

A physiologic shunt is the portion of venous blood that travels from the right heart to the left heart without being involved in adequate gas exchange with ventilated portions of the lung. This includes capillary or absolute anatomic shunts and relative shunts where perfusion exceeds ventilation as seen in disease states that diminish pulmonary ventilation. Relative shunts can be caused by chronic

TABLE 11-5

Causes of Hypoxia

Cause	Primary Indicator	Mechanism	Example
Hypoxemia			
Low PiO_2	Low P_AO_2 Low PaO_2	Reduced P_B	Altitude
Hypoventilation	High $PaCO_2$	Decreased $\dot{V}_A$	Drug overdose
$\dot{V}/\dot{Q}$ imbalance	Low PaO_2 High $P(A-a)O_2$ on air; resolves with O_2	Decreased $\dot{V}_A$ relative to perfusion	COPD, aging
Anatomic shunt	Low PaO_2 High $P(A-a)O_2$ on air; does not resolve with O_2	Blood flow from right to left side of heart	Congenital heart disease
Physiologic shunt	Low PaO_2 High $P(A-a)O_2$ on air; does not resolve with O_2	Perfusion without ventilation	Atelectasis
Diffusion defect	Low PaO_2 High $P(A-a)O_2$ on air; resolves with O_2	Damage to alveolar-capillary membrane	ARDS
Hb deficiency			
Absolute	Low Hb content Reduced CaO_2	Loss of Hb	Hemorrhage
Relative	Abnormal SaO_2 Reduced CaO_2	Abnormal Hb	Carboxyhemoglobin
Low blood flow	Increased $C(a-\bar{v})O_2$	Decreased perfusion	Shock, ischemia
Dysoxia	Normal CaO_2 Decreased $C(a-\bar{v})O_2$	Disruption of cellular enzymes	Cyanide poisoning

ARDS, Acute respiratory distress syndrome; *COPD,* chronic obstructive pulmonary disease.

obstructive pulmonary disease (COPD), restrictive disorders, or any condition resulting in hypoventilation.

The shunt equation quantifies the portion of blood included in the $\dot{V}/\dot{Q}$ mismatch. It is usually expressed as a percentage of the total cardiac output:

$$\frac{\dot{Q}s}{\dot{Q}t} = \frac{Cc'O_2 - CaO_2}{Cc'O_2 - C\bar{v}O_2}$$

Where:

$\dot{Q}s$ = Blood entering systemic blood without being oxygenated in the lungs

$\dot{Q}t$ = Total cardiac output

$Cc'O_2$ = O_2 content at the end of the ventilated and perfused pulmonary capillaries

CaO_2 = Arterial O_2 content

$C\bar{v}O_2$ = Mixed venous O_2 content

Although arterial O_2 content can be directly measured from a systemic artery and mixed venous O_2 content can be directly measured from the pulmonary artery, the end capillary content must be derived from an additional calculation requiring use of the alveolar air equation and the Hb concentration.

Conversely, *dead space ventilation* refers to ventilation that does not participate in gas exchange. This can be considered wasted ventilation because it consumes energy to move gases into and out of the lung but without any resulting gas exchange. Dead space ventilation can be separated into two categories: alveolar and anatomic.

Alveolar dead space is ventilation that enters into alveoli that are without any perfusion or without adequate perfusion. Conditions that can lead to alveolar dead space include pulmonary emboli, partial obstruction of the pulmonary vasculature, destroyed pulmonary vasculature (as can occur in COPD), and reduced cardiac output.

Anatomic dead space is the portion of inspired ventilation that never reaches the alveoli for gas exchange. Normal individuals have a portion of inspired gases that never reach the alveoli before exhalation. This is usually a fixed volume. It becomes problematic in conditions where tidal volumes decrease to the point where a significant percentage of the inspired gas remains in the anatomic dead space.

Dead space is generally expressed as a ratio to total tidal volume:

$$\frac{V_D}{V_T} = \frac{PaCO_2 - P_{\bar{E}}CO_2}{PaCO_2}$$

Where:

V_D = Physiologic dead space (anatomic + alveolar)

V_T = Tidal volume

$PaCO_2$ = Partial pressure of arterial CO_2

$P_{\bar{E}}CO_2$ = Mean partial pressure of exhaled CO_2

The clinical significance of increased physiologic dead space is that it is wasted ventilation in that, by definition, it does not contribute to gas exchange. In the face of increased dead space, normal ventilation must increase to achieve homeostasis. This additional ventilation comes at a cost with an increase in the work of breathing, which consumes additional O_2 further adding to the burden of external ventilation.

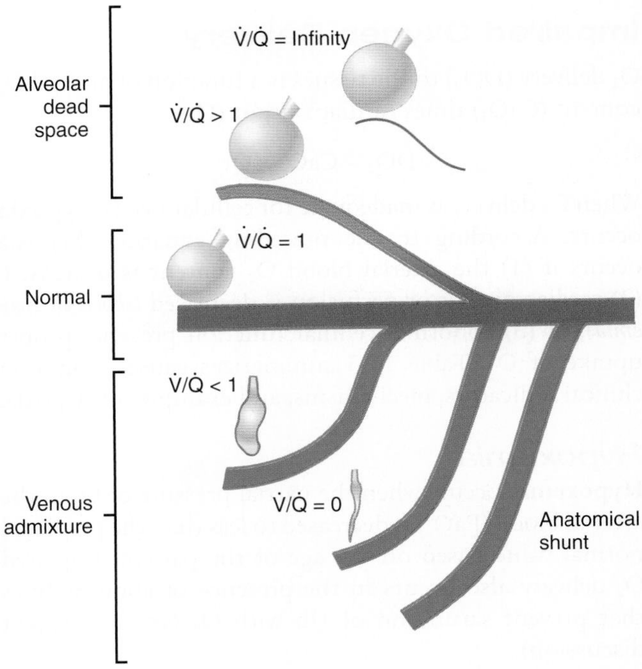

FIGURE 11-15 Range of $\dot{V}/\dot{Q}$ ratios. (Modified from Martin L: Pulmonary physiology in clinical practice: the essentials for patient care and evaluation, St Louis, 1987, Mosby.)

Figure 11-15 shows the possible range of $\dot{V}/\dot{Q}$. As shown in the top two units, when ventilation is greater than perfusion (high $\dot{V}/\dot{Q}$), there is wasted ventilation, or alveolar dead space. Conversely, when ventilation is less than perfusion, $\dot{V}/\dot{Q}$ is low (bottom two lung units). In this case, blood leaves the lungs with an abnormally low O_2 content. In lung disease, $\dot{V}/\dot{Q}$ imbalances usually cause both excess wasted ventilation and poor oxygenation. Because $\dot{V}/\dot{Q}$ imbalance impairs O_2 exchange, PaO_2 is reduced.

To understand how $\dot{V}/\dot{Q}$ imbalance causes hypoxemia, reinspect the normal oxyhemoglobin dissociation curve, with PO_2 plotted against O_2 content (Figure 11-16). The curve is nearly flat in the physiologic range of PaO_2 (>70 mm Hg) but falls steeply when PaO_2 is less than 60 mm Hg. Points representing O_2 content of three separate lung units also are shown. These units have $\dot{V}/\dot{Q}$ of 0.1, 1.0, and 10.0.

Blood leaving the normal unit ($\dot{V}/\dot{Q} = 1$) has a normal O_2 content (19.5 ml/dl). Blood leaving the unit with poor ventilation ($\dot{V}/\dot{Q} = 0.1$) has a low O_2 content (16.0 ml/dl). Because Hb is almost fully saturated at a normal PO_2 of 100 mm Hg, blood leaving the over ventilated unit ($\dot{V}/\dot{Q} = 10$) has an O_2 content that is just slightly greater than normal (20.0 ml/dl). When the blood from all three units mixes together, the result is O_2 content that is reduced (18.5 ml/dl). The decrease in oxygenation caused by the

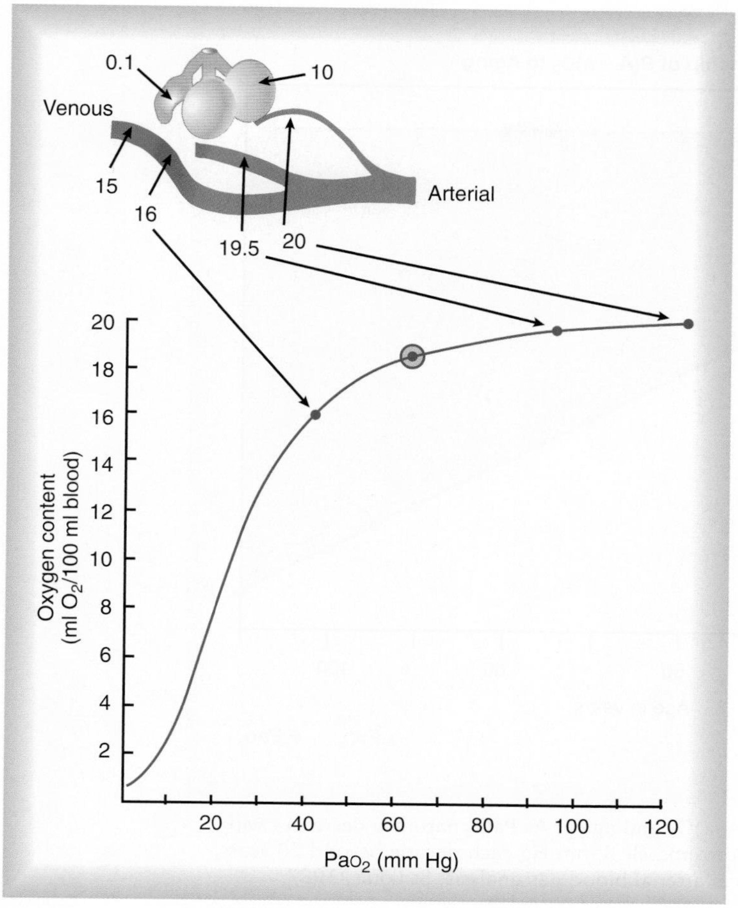

FIGURE 11-16 O_2 dissociation curve: PaO_2 versus O_2 content. O_2 content from alveolar-capillary units with $\dot{V}/\dot{Q}$ of 0.1, 1, and 10 is 16 ml/dl, 19.5 ml/dl, and 20.0 ml/dl. Lines are drawn for each O_2 content to its point on the dissociation curve. The average O_2 content, 18.5 ml/dl, is represented by a *circle* on the dissociation curve. (Modified from Martin L: Pulmonary physiology in clinical practice: the essentials for patient care and evaluation, St Louis, 1987, Mosby.)

poorly ventilated unit is not fully compensated for by the high $\dot{V}/\dot{Q}$ unit.

$\dot{V}/\dot{Q}$ of zero represents a special type of imbalance. When $\dot{V}/\dot{Q}$ is zero, there is blood flow but no ventilation. The result is equivalent to a right-to-left anatomic shunt, shown at the bottom of Figure 11-15. Venous blood bypasses ventilated alveoli and mixes with freshly oxygenated arterial blood, resulting in what is called a *venous admixture*. Right-to-left physiologic shunting results in a more severe form of hypoxemia than a simple $\dot{V}/\dot{Q}$ imbalance, as seen in conditions such as pulmonary edema, pneumonia, and atelectasis.

RULE OF THUMB

Although $\dot{V}/\dot{Q}$ imbalances are the most common cause of hypoxemia in patients with respiratory diseases, physiologic shunting also can occur commonly, especially in patients who are critically ill. To differentiate between hypoxemia caused by a $\dot{V}/\dot{Q}$ imbalance and hypoxemia caused by shunting, apply the following 50/50 rule: If O_2 concentration is greater than 50 (%) and PaO_2 is less than 50 (mm Hg), significant shunting is present; otherwise, the hypoxemia is mainly caused by a simple $\dot{V}/\dot{Q}$ imbalance.

When a low PaO_2 is observed, the RT must take into account the normal decrease in arterial O_2 tension that occurs with aging. As shown in Figure 11-17, for an individual breathing air at sea level, the "normal" $P(A\text{–}a)O_2$ increases in a near-linear fashion with increasing age (shaded area). This increase in $P(A\text{–}a)O_2$ results in a gradual decline in PaO_2 over time and is probably caused by reduced surface area in the lung for gas exchange and increases in $\dot{V}/\dot{Q}$ mismatching. PaO_2 of 85 mm Hg in a 60-year-old adult would be interpreted as normal, but the same PaO_2 in a 20-year-old adult would indicate hypoxemia. The expected PaO_2 in older adults may be estimated by using the following formula:

$$\text{Expected } PaO_2 = 100.1 - (0.323 \times \text{Age in years})$$

Hemoglobin Deficiencies. Normal PaO_2 does not guarantee adequate arterial O_2 content or delivery. For arterial O_2 content to be adequate, there also must be enough normal Hb in the blood. If the blood Hb is low—even when PaO_2 is normal—hypoxia can occur because of low O_2 content in the arterial blood.

Hb deficiencies, or anemias, can be either absolute or relative. Absolute Hb deficiency occurs when the Hb concentration is lower than normal. Relative Hb deficiencies are caused by either the displacement of O_2 from normal Hb or the presence of abnormal Hb variants. A low blood

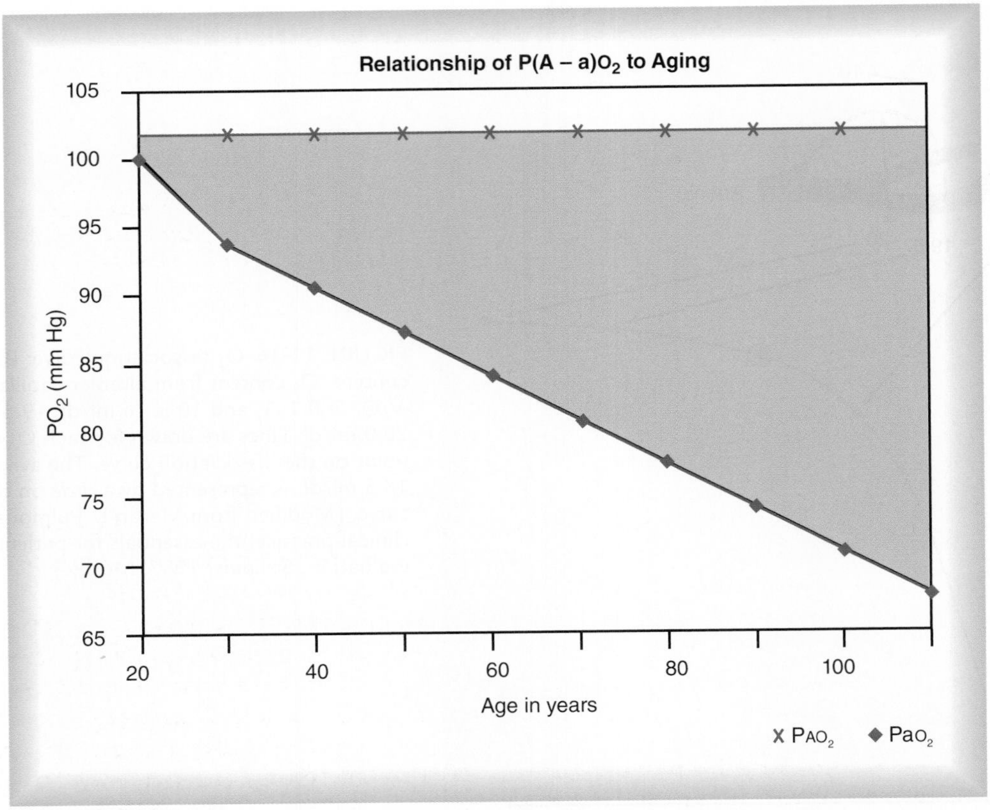

FIGURE 11-17 Relationship between $P(A–a)O_2$ and aging. As PaO_2 naturally decreases with age, $P(A–a)O_2$ increases at the rate of approximately 3 mm Hg each decade beyond 20 years. (Modified from Lane EE, Walker JF: Clinical arterial blood gas analysis, St Louis, 1987, Mosby.)

Hb concentration may be caused either by a loss of RBCs, as with hemorrhage, or by inadequate erythropoiesis (formation of RBCs in the bone marrow). Regardless of the cause, a low Hb content can seriously impair the O_2-carrying capacity of the blood, even in the presence of a normal supply (PaO_2) and adequate diffusion.[5]

Figure 11-18 plots the relationship between arterial O_2 content and PaO_2 as a function of Hb concentration. As can be seen, progressive decreases in blood Hb content cause large decreases in arterial O_2 content (CaO_2). A 33% decrease in Hb content (from 15 g/dl to 10 g/dl) reduces CaO_2 as much as would a decrease in PaO_2 from 100 mm Hg to 40 mm Hg.

Relative Hb deficiencies are caused by abnormal forms of Hb. As previously discussed, both carboxyhemoglobinemia and methemoglobinemia can cause abnormal O_2 transport, as can abnormal Hb variants. In carboxyhemoglobinemia and methemoglobinemia, each 1 g of affected Hb is comparable to the loss of 1 g of normal Hb. Abnormal hemoglobins have variable effects on O_2 transport. Hemoglobins causing left shifts in the dissociation curve impede O_2 unloading and are most likely to cause hypoxia.

Reduction in Blood Flow (Shock or Ischemia)

Because O_2 delivery depends on both arterial O_2 content and cardiac output, hypoxia can still occur when the CaO_2 is normal if blood flow is reduced. There are two types of reduced blood flow: (1) circulatory failure *(shock)* and (2) local reductions in perfusion *(ischemia)*.

Circulatory Failure (Shock). In circulatory failure, tissue O_2 deprivation is widespread. Although the body tries to compensate for the lack of O_2 by directing blood flow to vital organs, this response is limited. Prolonged shock ultimately causes irreversible damage to the central nervous system and eventual cardiovascular collapse.

Local Reductions in Perfusion (Ischemia). Even when whole-body perfusion is adequate, local reductions in blood flow can cause localized hypoxia. Ischemia can result in anaerobic metabolism, metabolic acidosis, and eventual death of the affected tissue. Myocardial infarction and stroke (cerebrovascular accident) are examples of ischemic conditions that can cause hypoxia and tissue death.

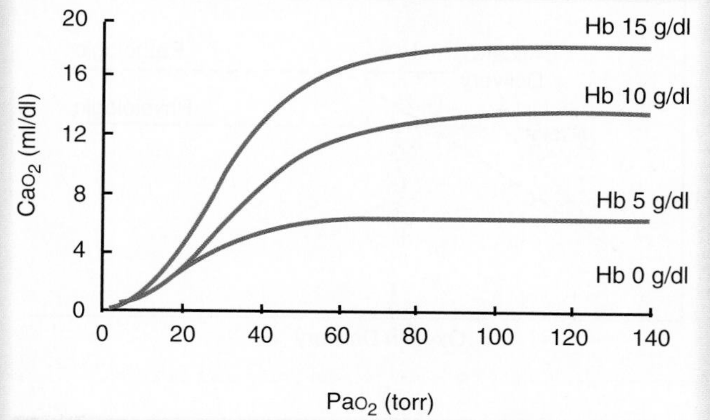

FIGURE 11-18 Relationship between CaO_2 and PaO_2 as a function of blood Hb concentration. Progressive decreases in Hb cause large decreases in CaO_2.

MINI CLINI

Effect of Anemia on Oxygen Content

In its most common form, anemia is a clinical disorder in which the number of RBCs is decreased. Because RBCs carry Hb, anemia decreases the amount of this O_2-carrying protein.

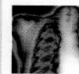

PROBLEM: What effect would anemia that causes a progressive decrease in Hb from (1) 15 g/dl to (2) 12 g/dl to (3) 8 g/dl to (4) 4 g/dl have on the amount of O_2 carried in a patient's blood? Assume that PO_2 and saturation stay normal at 100 mm Hg and 97%.

DISCUSSION:

1. Calculate dissolved O_2 the same way for all four examples as follows:
   $$\text{Dissolved } O_2 = 100 \times 0.003 = 0.30 \text{ ml/dl}$$
2. Compute chemically combined O_2 as follows: Chemically combined O_2 = Hb (g/dl) × 1.34 ml/g × SaO_2
   a. 15 g/dl × 1.34 ml/g × 97% = 19.50 ml/dl
   b. 12 g/dl × 1.34 ml/g × 97% = 15.60 ml/dl
   c. 8 g/dl × 1.34 ml/g × 97% = 10.40 ml/dl
   d. 4 g/dl × 1.34 ml/g × 97% = 5.20 ml/dl
3. Compute total O_2 content as follows:
   $$CaO_2 = \text{Dissolved } O_2 + \text{Chemically combined } O_2$$
   a. 0.30 + 19.50 = 19.80 ml/dl
   b. 0.30 + 15.60 = 15.90 ml/dl
   c. 0.30 + 10.40 = 10.70 ml/dl
   d. 0.30 + 5.20 = 5.50 ml/dl

Loss of Hb decreases the amount of O_2 carried in a patient's blood, even though PO_2 and saturation remain normal. With Hb concentration of 4 g/dl, the amount of O_2 carried in a patient's blood is only approximately one-fourth the normal concentration (5.50 vs. 19.80 ml/dl).

Dysoxia

Dysoxia is a form of hypoxia in which the cellular uptake of O_2 is abnormally decreased. The best example of dysoxia is cyanide poisoning. Cyanide disrupts the intracellular cytochrome oxidase system, preventing cellular use of O_2. Dysoxia also may occur when tissue O_2 consumption becomes dependent on O_2 delivery.

Figure 11-19 plots tissue O_2 consumption ($\dot{V}O_2$) against O_2 delivery ($\dot{D}O_2$) in both normal and pathologic states. Normally, the tissues extract as much O_2 as they need from what is delivered, and O_2 consumption equals O_2 demand (flat portion of solid line). However, if delivery decreases, conditions begin to change (solid line). At a level called the *point of critical delivery,* tissue extraction reaches a maximum. Further decreases in delivery result in an O_2 "debt," which occurs when O_2 demand exceeds O_2 delivery. Under conditions of O_2 debt, O_2 consumption becomes dependent on O_2 delivery (sloped line). This dependence leads to lactic acid accumulation and metabolic acidosis.

In pathologic conditions such as septic shock and acute respiratory distress syndrome (dotted line), this critical point may occur at levels of O_2 delivery considered normal. In addition, the slope of the curve below the point of critical delivery may be less than normal, indicating a decreased extraction ratio ($\dot{V}O_2/\dot{D}O_2$).[6] In combination, these findings indicate that O_2 demands are not being met and that a defect exists in the cellular mechanisms regulating O_2 uptake.

Impaired Carbon Dioxide Removal

Any disorder that decreases alveolar ventilation ($\dot{V}_A$) relative to metabolic need impairs CO_2 removal. Impaired CO_2 removal by the lung causes hypercapnia and respiratory acidosis (see Chapter 13). A decrease in alveolar ventilation occurs when (1) the minute ventilation is inadequate, (2) the dead space ventilation per minute is increased, or (3) a $\dot{V}/\dot{Q}$ imbalance exists.[4-8]

Inadequate Minute Ventilation

Clinically, inadequate minute ventilation usually is caused by decreased tidal volumes. Inadequate minute ventilation occurs in restrictive conditions, such as atelectasis, neuromuscular disorders, or impeded thoracic expansion (e.g.,

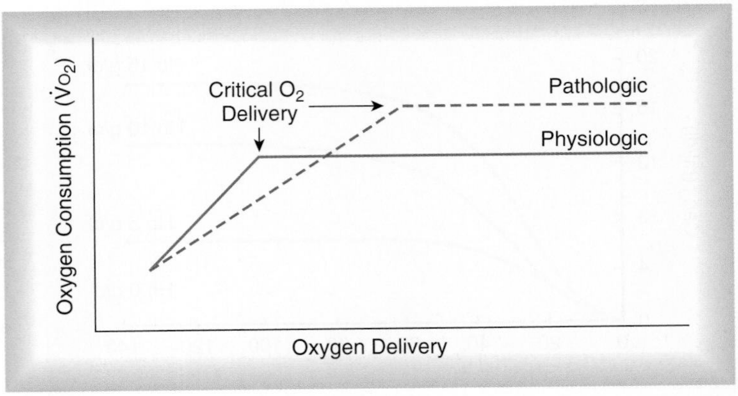

FIGURE 11-19 Physiologic versus pathologic O_2 consumption–delivery relationship. Critical O_2 delivery occurs at higher O_2 delivery in a pathologic state. The slope of the pathologic consumption curve below the critical delivery point reflects the decrease in O_2 extraction ratio that exists in these situations. (Modified from Pasquale MD, Cipolle MD, Cerra FB: Oxygen transport: does increasing supply improve outcome? Respir Care 38:800, 1993.)

kyphoscoliosis). A decrease in respiratory rate is less common but may be present with respiratory center depression, as in drug overdose.

Increased Dead Space Ventilation

An increase in dead space ventilation, or V_D/V_T, is caused by either (1) decreased tidal volume (as with rapid, shallow breathing) or (2) increased physiologic dead space as in pulmonary embolus. In either case, wasted ventilation increases. Without compensation, alveolar ventilation per minute is decreased, and CO_2 removal is impaired.

Ventilation/Perfusion Imbalances

Theoretically, any $\dot{V}/\dot{Q}$ imbalance should cause an increase in $PaCO_2$. However, $PaCO_2$ does not always increase in these cases. Many patients who are hypoxemic because of a $\dot{V}/\dot{Q}$ imbalance have a low or normal $PaCO_2$. This common clinical finding suggests that $\dot{V}/\dot{Q}$ imbalances have a greater effect on oxygenation than on CO_2 removal.

Careful inspection of the O_2 and CO_2 dissociation curves supports this finding. The O_2 and CO_2 dissociation curves are plotted on the same scale in Figure 11-20. The upper CO_2 curve is nearly linear in the physiologic range. The lower O_2 curve is almost flat in the physiologic range. Point "a" on each curve is the normal arterial point for both content and partial pressure. To the right of the graph are two lung units, one with a low $\dot{V}/\dot{Q}$ and the other with a high $\dot{V}/\dot{Q}$. The blood O_2 and CO_2 contents from each unit are plotted on the curves.

The final CO_2 content, arrived at by averaging the high and low $\dot{V}/\dot{Q}$ points, is shown as point "a" on the CO_2 curve. This point is the same as the normal arterial point for CO_2.

The final O_2 content, also arrived at by averaging the high and low $\dot{V}/\dot{Q}$ points, is shown as point "X" on the O_2 curve. Although the averaged value for CO_2 was normal, the PaO_2 resulting from averaging the O_2 content of the high and low $\dot{V}/\dot{Q}$ units is well below normal (point "a" on the O_2 curve).

The effect of low $\dot{V}/\dot{Q}$ units is decreased PaO_2 and increased $PaCO_2$. The effect of high $\dot{V}/\dot{Q}$ units is the

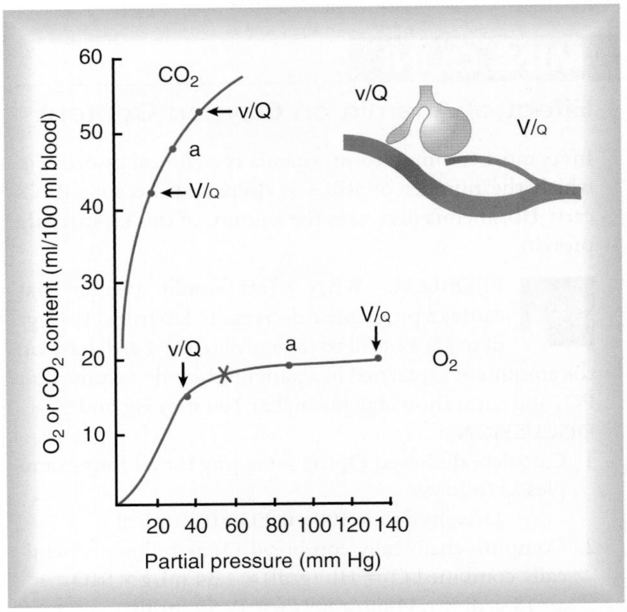

FIGURE 11-20 $\dot{V}/\dot{Q}$ imbalance and dissociation curves for CO_2 and O_2. $\dot{V}/\dot{Q}$ represents low $\dot{V}/\dot{Q}$ units, and V/q represents high $\dot{V}/\dot{Q}$ units. See text for discussion.

opposite (i.e., increased PO_2 and decreased PCO_2). However, the shape of the dissociation curves dictates that a high $\dot{V}/\dot{Q}$ unit can reverse the high PCO_2 but not the low PO_2. Any increase in PCO_2 from low $\dot{V}/\dot{Q}$ units can be corrected by a reduction in PCO_2 from high $\dot{V}/\dot{Q}$ units. However, these same high $\dot{V}/\dot{Q}$ units cannot compensate for the reduced O_2 content because the O_2 curve is nearly flat when PO_2 is higher than normal.

Patients with $\dot{V}/\dot{Q}$ imbalances still must compensate for high PCO_2 coming from underventilated units. To compensate for these high PCO_2 values, the patient's minute ventilation must increase (Figure 11-21). Patients who can increase their minute ventilation tend to have either normal or low $PaCO_2$, combined with hypoxemia.

Conversely, patients with a $\dot{V}/\dot{Q}$ imbalance who cannot increase their minute ventilation are hypercapnic.

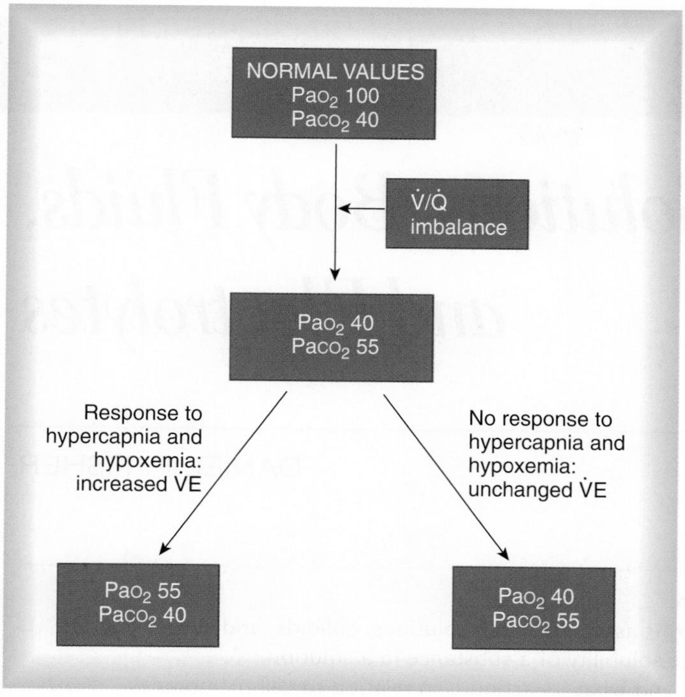

FIGURE 11-21 Changes in PaO_2 and $PaCO_2$ caused by $\dot{V}/\dot{Q}$ imbalance. All values are given in millimeters of mercury (mm Hg).

Hypercapnia generally occurs only when the $\dot{V}/\dot{Q}$ imbalance is severe and chronic, as in COPD. Such a patient must sustain a higher than normal minute ventilation just to maintain normal $PaCO_2$. If the energy costs required to sustain a high minute ventilation are prohibitive, the patient opts for less work—and hence elevated $PaCO_2$.

SUMMARY CHECKLIST

- Movement of gases between the lungs and the tissues depends mainly on diffusion.
- P_ACO_2 varies directly with CO_2 production and inversely with alveolar ventilation.
- P_AO_2 is computed using the alveolar air equation.
- With a constant FiO_2, P_AO_2 varies inversely with P_ACO_2.
- Normal P_AO_2 averages 100 mm Hg, with mean P_ACO_2 of approximately 40 mm Hg.
- Normal mixed venous blood has PO_2 of approximately 40 mm Hg and PCO_2 of approximately 46 mm Hg
- Ventilation and perfusion must be in balance for pulmonary gas exchange to be effective. Because of normal anatomic shunts and $\dot{V}/\dot{Q}$ imbalances, pulmonary gas exchange is imperfect.
- In disease, $\dot{V}/\dot{Q}$ can range from zero (perfusion without ventilation or physiologic shunting) to infinity (pure alveolar dead space).
- Blood carries a small amount of O_2 in physical solution, and larger amounts are carried in chemical combination with erythrocyte Hb.
- Hb saturation is the ratio of oxyhemoglobin to total Hb, expressed as a percentage.
- To compute total O_2 contents of the blood, add the dissolved O_2 content ($0.003 \times PO_2$) to the product of Hb content × Hb saturation × 1.34.
- $C(a-\bar{v})O_2$ is the amount of O_2 given up by every 100 ml of blood on each pass through the tissues. All else being equal, $C(a-\bar{v})O_2$ varies inversely with cardiac output.
- Hb affinity for O_2 increases with high PO_2, high pH, low temperature, and low levels of 2,3-DPG.
- Hb abnormalities can affect O_2 loading and unloading and can cause hypoxia.
- Most CO_2 (about 80%) is transported in the blood as ionized bicarbonate; other forms include carbamino compounds in physical solution.
- Changes in CO_2 levels modify the O_2 dissociation curve (Bohr effect). Changes in Hb saturation affect the CO_2 dissociation curve (Haldane effect). These changes are mutually beneficial, assisting in gas exchange at the lung and the cellular level.
- Hypoxia occurs if (1) the arterial blood O_2 content is decreased, (2) blood flow is decreased, or (3) abnormal cellular function prevents proper uptake of O_2.
- Decreased PaO_2 level may be a result of a low ambient PO_2, hypoventilation, impaired diffusion, $\dot{V}/\dot{Q}$ imbalances, and right-to-left anatomic or physiologic shunting.
- A decrease in alveolar ventilation occurs when (1) the minute ventilation is inadequate, (2) dead space ventilation is increased, or (3) a $\dot{V}/\dot{Q}$ imbalance exists.

References

1. Forster RE, Dubois AB, Brisoe WA, et al: The lung-physiologic basis of pulmonary function tests, ed 3, St Louis, 1986, Year Book Medical Publishers, Inc.
2. Shapiro BA, Peruzzi WT, Templin R: Clinical application of blood gases, ed 5, St Louis, 1994, Mosby.
3. Rose BD, Post TW: Clinical physiology of acid-base and electrolyte disorders, ed 5, New York, 2001, McGraw-Hill.
4. Malley WJ: Clinical blood gases—assessment and intervention, ed 2, St Louis, 2005, Elsevier Saunders.
5. Lump A, Pearl RG: Nunn's applied respiratory physiology, ed 7, St Louis, 2010, Elsevier.
6. West JB: Pulmonary physiology and pathophysiology—an integrated, case-based approach, ed 2, Philadelphia, 2007, Lippincott Williams and Williams.
7. Des Jardins T: Cardiopulmonary anatomy and physiology, essentials for respiratory care, ed 5, Clifton Park, NY, 2008, Delmar Publications.
8. West JB: Respiratory physiology—the essentials, ed 8, Philadelphia, 2008, Lippincott Williams and Williams.

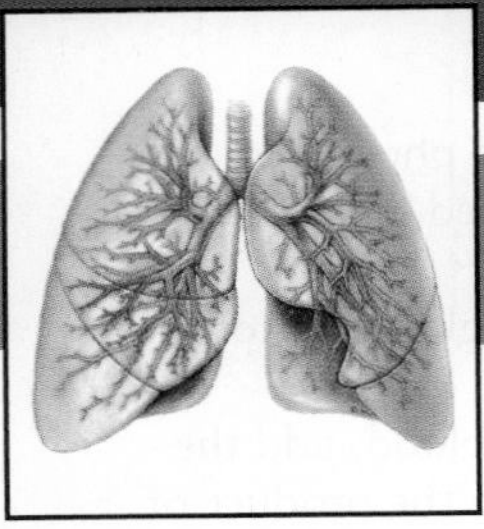

Chapter 12

Solutions, Body Fluids, and Electrolytes

DANIEL F. FISHER

CHAPTER OBJECTIVES

After reading this chapter you will be able to:

- Describe the characteristics of and key terms associated with solutions, colloids, and suspensions.
- Describe the five factors that influence the solubility of a substance in a solution.
- Describe how osmotic pressure functions and what its action is in relation to cell membranes.
- Describe how to calculate the solute content of a solution using ratio, weight/volume, and percent methods.
- State the ionic characteristics of acids, bases, and salts.
- Describe how proteins can function as bases.
- Describe how to calculate the pH of a solution when given the $[H^+]$ in nanomoles per liter.
- Identify where fluid compartments are located in the body and what their volumes are.
- Describe how water loss and replacement occur.
- Define the roles played by osmotic and hydrostatic pressure in edema.
- Identify clinical findings associated with excess or deficiency of the seven basic electrolytes.

CHAPTER OUTLINE

KEY TERMS

acid
active transport
anions
base
buffering
cations
colloids
diluent
dilute solution
dilution equation
equivalent weight
hydrostatic pressure
hyperkalemia
hypertonic
hypotonic
ionic
interstitial fluid
isotonic
law of mass action
nanomole
normal solution
osmolality
osmotic pressure (oncotic pressure)
plasma colloid osmotic pressure (oncotic pressure)
saturated solution
solute
solution
solvent
Starling equilibrium
suspensions

In healthy individuals, body water and various chemicals are regulated to maintain an environment in which biochemical processes can continue. Imbalances in the amount or concentration of chemicals in the body occur in many diseases. The nature and importance of body fluids and electrolytes require an understanding of physiologic chemistry. This chapter provides the reader with the background knowledge needed to understand body chemistry.

SOLUTIONS, COLLOIDS, AND SUSPENSIONS

Definition of a Solution

The body is based on liquid water chemistry and the interaction of various substances either dissolved or suspended within the fluid. Water itself is a polar covalent molecule and is referred to in chemistry as a *universal solvent.* Water is the primary component of any liquid within the body and has a great influence on the behavior of other materials as they are introduced. These substances and particles combine with water in the following three ways: as (1) colloids, (2) suspensions, or (3) solutions.

A **solution** is a stable mixture of two or more substances in a single phase that cannot be separated using a centrifuge. One substance is evenly distributed between the molecules of the other. The substance that dissolves is called the **solute.** The medium in which it dissolves is called the **solvent.** Gases, liquids, and solids all can dissolve to become solutes. The process of dissolving involves breaking the (relatively weak) bonds between the solute-solute molecules and the solvent-solvent molecules. These intermolecular forces must be broken before a new solute-solvent bond can be formed. A solute dissolves in a solvent if the solute-solvent forces of attraction are great enough to overcome the solute-solute and solvent-solvent forces of attraction. If the solute-solvent force is less than the solute-solute or solvent-solvent force, the solute does not dissolve. When all three sets of forces are approximately equal, the two substances typically are soluble in each other. The electrical properties of the solvent molecules determine how soluble a substance is for a particular solvent. Polar solvents, such as water, dissolve other polar covalent bonds; nonpolar solvents dissolve nonpolar solutes: "Like dissolves like."

Colloids (sometimes called *dispersions* or *gels*) consist of large molecules that attract and hold water (*hydrophilic:* "water loving"). These molecules are uniformly distributed throughout the dispersion, and they tend not to settle. The protoplasm inside cells is a common example of a colloid. Physiologically, colloids provide very little free water to the patient's system, and care should be taken not to create a hypotonic environment.[1]

Suspensions are composed of large particles that float in a liquid. Suspensions can be physically separated by centrifugation and do not possess the same interactions between solvent and solute that are found in a true solution. Red blood cells in plasma are an example of a suspension. Dispersion of suspended particles depends on physical agitation. Particles settle because of gravity when the suspension is motionless.

The ease with which a solute dissolves in a solvent is its *solubility,* which is influenced by the following five factors:

1. *Nature of the solute.* The ease with which substances go into a solution (dissociation) in a given solvent depends on the forces of the solute-solute molecules and varies widely.
2. *Nature of the solvent.* The ability of a solvent to dissolve a solute depends on the bonds of the solvent-solvent molecules and varies widely.
3. *Temperature.* Solubility of most solids increases with increased temperature. However, the solubility of gases varies inversely with temperature.
4. *Pressure.* The solubility of solids and liquids is not greatly affected by pressure. However, the solubility of gases in liquids varies directly with pressure.
5. *Concentration.* The concentration of a solute or available solvent affects how much of the substance goes into solution.

The effects of temperature and pressure on the solubility of gases are important. More gas dissolves in a liquid at lower temperatures. As the temperature of a liquid increases, gas dissolved in that liquid comes out of solution. Henry's law describes the effect of pressure on solubility of a gas in a liquid. At a given temperature, the volume of a gas that dissolves in a liquid is proportional to the solubility coefficient of the gas and the partial pressure of gas to which the liquid is exposed. Oxygen (O_2) and carbon dioxide (CO_2) transport can change significantly with changes in body temperature or atmospheric pressure (see Chapter 6).

Concentration of Solutions

The term *concentration* refers to the amount of solute dissolved into the solvent. Concentration can be described either qualitatively or quantitatively. Calling something a **dilute solution** is an example of a qualitative description. Stating that a specific container holds 50 ml of 0.4 molar solution of sodium hydroxide (NaOH) is a quantitative description (Figure 12-1, *A*). **Saturated solutions** occur when the solvent has dissociated the maximal amount of solute into itself. Additional solute added to a saturated solution does not dissociate into solution but remains at the bottom of the container (see Figure 12-1, *B*). Solute particles precipitate into the solid state at the same rate at which other particles go into solution. This equilibrium characterizes a saturated solution.

A solution is characterized as being *supersaturated* when the solvent contains more solute than a saturated solution at the same temperature and pressure. If a saturated solution is heated, the solute equilibrium is upset, and more solute goes into solution. If undissolved solute is removed

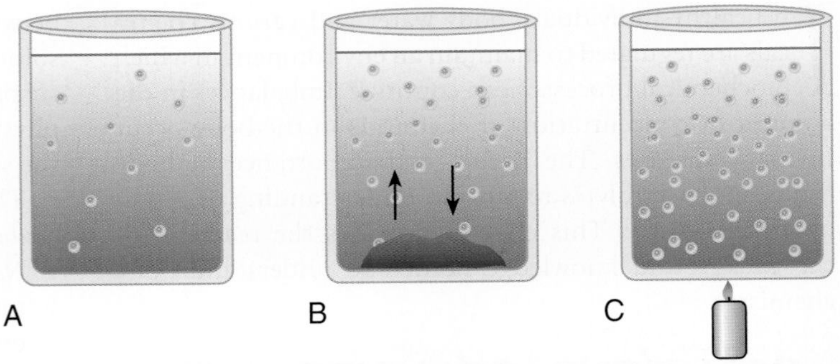

FIGURE 12-1 **A,** In the dilute solution, there are relatively few solute particles. **B,** In the saturated solution, the solvent contains all the solute it can hold in the presence of excess solute. **C,** Heating the solution dissolves more solute particles, which may remain in the solution if cooled gently, creating a state of supersaturation.

and the solution is cooled gently, there is an excess of dissolved solute (see Figure 12-1, *C*). The excess solute of supersaturated solutions may be precipitated out if the solution is disturbed or if a "seed crystal" is introduced.

Starling Forces

Starling was a nineteenth-century British physiologist who studied fluid transport across membranes. His hypothesis states that the fluid movement secondary to filtration across the wall of a capillary depends on both the hydrostatic and the oncotic pressure gradients across the capillary.[2] The driving force for fluid filtration across the wall of the capillary is determined by four separate pressures: hydraulic (hydrostatic) and colloid osmotic pressure both within the vessel and in the tissue space.[3] This process can be described mathematically using the following equation:

$$Jv = Lp\,[Pc - Pi - s\,(pc - pi)]$$

Where:

J_v = Fluid filtration flux across the capillary wall per unit area
L_p = Permeability of the capillary wall
s = Oncotic reflection coefficient
P_c, P_i, p_c, p_i = Global values for the hydrostatic and colloid osmotic pressures in the capillary and interstitial compartments.

Osmotic Pressure of Solutions

Most of the solutions of physiologic importance in the body are dilute. Solutes in dilute solution show many of the properties of gases. This behavior results from the relatively large distances between the molecules in dilute solutions. The most important physiologic characteristic of solutions is their ability to exert pressure.

Osmotic pressure (oncotic pressure)[4] is the force produced by solvent particles under certain conditions. A membrane that permits passage of solvent molecules but not solute is called a *semipermeable membrane.* If such a membrane divides a solution into two compartments, molecules of solvent can pass through it from one side to the other (Figure 12-2, *A*). The number of solvent molecules passing (or diffusing) in one direction must equal the number of solute molecules passing in the opposite direction. An equal ratio of solute to solvent particles (i.e., the concentration of the solution) is maintained on both sides of the membrane. A capillary wall is an example of a semipermeable membrane.[5,6]

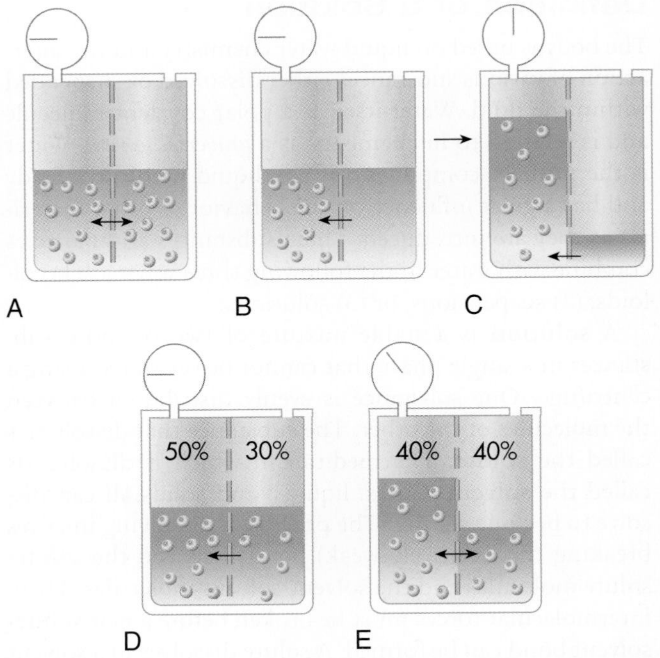

FIGURE 12-2 **A-E,** Osmotic pressure is illustrated by the solutions in the five containers. Each container is divided into two compartments by a semipermeable membrane, which permits passage of solvent molecules but not solute *(circles).* The number of solute particles represents relative concentrations of the solutions. Solute particles are fixed in number and are confined by the membranes. Volume changes are a function of the diffusible solvent. Solvent movement is indicated by *arrows* through the membranes. Container **A** shows a state of equilibrium, in which solute and solvent are equally distributed on either side of the membrane. Containers **B** and **C** show diffusion of solvent through the membrane as a result of solvent on only one side of the membrane and the resulting pressure change (osmotic pressure indicated by the gauge). Containers **D** and **E** show what happens when different concentrations exist on either side of a semipermeable membrane. Solvent moves from the lower concentration toward the higher concentration to establish an equilibrium secondary to osmotic pressure.

If a solution is placed on one side of a semipermeable membrane and pure solvent is placed on the other, solvent molecules move through the membrane into the solution. The force driving solvent molecules through the membrane is called *osmotic pressure*. Osmotic pressure tries to redistribute solvent molecules so that the same concentration exists on both sides of the membrane. Osmotic pressure may be measured by connecting a manometer to the expanding column of the solution (see Figure 12-2, *B* and *C*).

Osmotic pressure can also be visualized as an attractive force of solute particles in a concentrated solution. If 100 ml of a 50% solution is placed on one side of a membrane and 100 ml of a 30% solution is placed on the other side, solvent molecules move from the dilute to the concentrated side (see Figure 12-2, *D* and *E*). The particles in the concentrated solution attract solvent molecules from the dilute solution until equilibrium occurs. Equilibrium exists when the concentrations (i.e., ratio of solute to solvent) in the two compartments are equal (40% in Figure 12-2).

Osmolality is defined as the ratio of solute to solvent. In physiology, the solvent is water.[1,5,7] Osmotic pressure depends on the number of particles in solution but not on their charge or identity. A 2% solution has twice the osmotic pressure of a 1% solution under similar pressures. For a given amount of solute, osmotic pressure is inversely proportional to the volume of solvent. Most cell walls are semipermeable membranes. Through osmotic pressure, water is distributed throughout the body within certain physiologic ranges. Tonicity describes how much osmotic pressure is exerted by a solution. Average body cellular fluid has a tonicity equal to a 0.9% solution of sodium chloride (NaCl; sometimes referred to as *physiologic saline*). Solutions with similar tonicity are called **isotonic.** Solutions with more tonicity are **hypertonic,** and solutions with less tonicity are **hypotonic.** Most cells reside in a hypotonic environment in which the concentration of water (solute) is lower inside the cell than in the surroundings. Water flows into the cell causing it to expand until the cell membrane restricts further expansion. Pressure increases inside the cell to counteract osmotic pressure. This pressure is called *turgor,* and it is what prevents more water from entering the cell. The equilibrium that develops allows the cell to maintain a gradient across the cell membrane. Some cells have selective permeability, allowing passage not only of water but also of specific solutes. Through these mechanisms, nutrients and physiologic solutions are distributed throughout the body.

RULE OF THUMB

Solutions that have osmotic pressures equal to the average intracellular pressure in the body are called *isotonic.* This is roughly equivalent to a saline solution (NaCl) of 0.9%. Solutions with higher osmotic pressure are called *hypertonic,* whereas solutions with lower osmotic pressure are called *hypotonic.* Administration of isotonic solutions usually causes no net change in cellular water content. Hypertonic solutions draw water out of cells. Hypotonic solutions usually cause water to be absorbed from the solution into cells.

In electrochemical terms, there are three basic types of physiologic solutions. Depending on the solute, solutions are **ionic** (electrovalent), *polar covalent,* or *nonpolar covalent* (Table 12-1). In ionic and polar covalent solutions, some of the solute ionizes into separate particles known as *ions.* A solution in which this dissociation occurs is called an *electrolyte solution* (Figure 12-3). If an electrode is placed in such a solution, positive ions migrate to the negative pole of the electrode. These ions are called **cations.** Negative ions migrate to the positive pole of the electrode; they are called **anions.** In nonpolar covalent solutions, molecules of solute remain intact and do not carry electrical charges; these solutions are referred to as *nonelectrolytes.* These nonelectrolytes are not attracted to either the positive or the negative pole of an electrode (hence the designation *nonpolar*). All three types of solutions coexist in the body. These solutions also serve as the media in which colloids and simple suspensions are dispersed. Gases such as O_2 and CO_2 are nonpolar molecules (along with N_2) and do not dissolve very well in water, which is a polar solvent.

TABLE 12-1

Types of Physiologic Solutions

Type	Characteristics	Physiologic Example
Ionic (electrovalent)	Ionic compounds dissolved from crystalline form, usually in water (hydration); form strong electrolytes with conductivity dependent on concentration of ions	Saline solution (0.9% NaCl)
Polar covalent	Molecular compounds dissolved in water or other solvents to produce ions (ionization); electrolytes may be weak or strong, depending on degree of ionization; solutions polarize and are good conductors	Hydrochloric acid (HCl) (strong electrolyte); acetic acid (CH_3COOH) (weak electrolyte)
Nonpolar covalent	Molecular compounds dissolved into electrically neutral solutions (do not polarize); solutions are not good conductors; nonelectrolytes	Glucose ($C_6H_{12}O_6$)

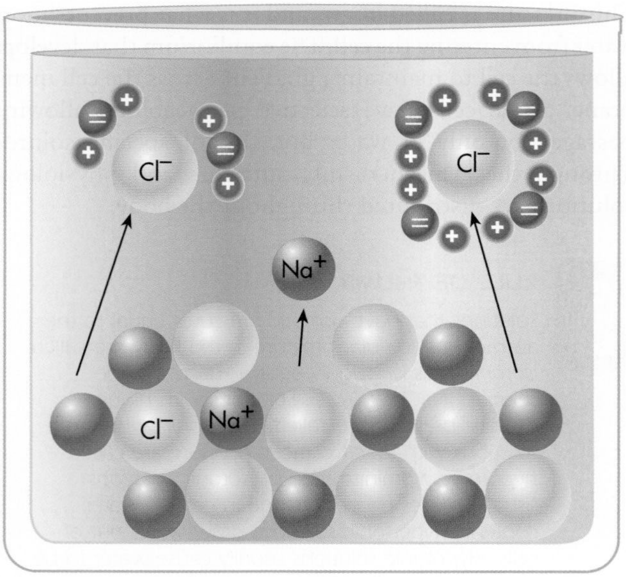

FIGURE 12-3 Sodium chloride (NaCl) is shown as a crystalline mass of ions being dissociated by the attraction of water dipoles.

MINI CLINI

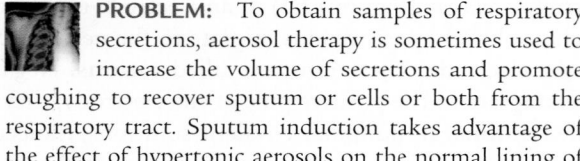

Sputum Induction and Hypertonic Saline

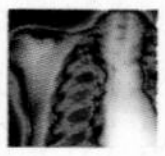

PROBLEM: To obtain samples of respiratory secretions, aerosol therapy is sometimes used to increase the volume of secretions and promote coughing to recover sputum or cells or both from the respiratory tract. Sputum induction takes advantage of the effect of hypertonic aerosols on the normal lining of the respiratory tract and the normal cough reflex.

SOLUTION: Sputum induction is usually performed by having the patient inhale a sterile hypertonic saline solution. Isotonic saline is approximately 0.9% (i.e., normal saline); concentrations greater than 0.9% are considered hypertonic. In clinical practice, concentrations of 3% to 10% have been used. The exact mechanism by which hypertonic saline increases the sputum volume has not been completely elucidated. However, when the particles of hypertonic saline are deposited in the airway, osmotic pressure is assumed to play a key role. When hypertonic saline comes into contact with the respiratory mucosa, water moves from the cells lining the airway into the sol-gel matrix that lines the airways, increasing its volume. The combination of increased volume of respiratory secretions with irritation of the epithelial cells themselves promotes reflex coughing. The volume of sputum and the rate of clearance from the lungs seem to depend on the osmolarity of the inhaled aerosol. Exposure of mast cells normally present in the airways to hypertonic aerosols results in the release of mediators (e.g., histamine) and bronchospasm. These effects may be related to the stimulation of the cough reflex. For the same reason, hypertonic saline is also sometimes used for bronchial challenge testing.

Quantifying Solute Content and Activity

The amount of solute in a solution can be quantified in two ways: (1) by actual weight (grams or milligrams) and (2) by chemical combining power. The weight of a solute is easy to measure and specify. However, it does not indicate chemical combining power. The sodium ion (Na^+) has a gram ionic weight of 23. The bicarbonate ion (HCO_3^-) has a gram ionic weight of 61. Because the gram atomic weight of every substance has 6.023×10^{23} particles, these ions have the same chemical combining power in solution. The number of chemically reactive units is usually more meaningful than their weight.

Equivalent Weights

In medicine, it is customary to refer to physiologic substances in terms of chemical combining power. The measure commonly used is **equivalent weight.** Equivalent weights are amounts of substances that have equal chemical combining power. For example, if chemical *A* reacts with chemical *B,* by definition, 1 equivalent weight of *A* reacts with exactly 1 equivalent weight of *B.* No excess reactants of *A* or *B* remain.

Two magnitudes of equivalent weights are used to calculate chemical combining power: gram equivalent weight (gEq) and milligram equivalent weight, or milliequivalent (mEq). One milliequivalent (1 mEq) is $\frac{1}{1000}$ of 1 gEq.

Gram Equivalent Weight Values. A gEq of a substance is calculated as its gram molecular (formula) weight divided by its valence. *Valence* refers to the number of electrons that need to be added or removed to make the substance electrically neutral. The valence signs (+ or −) are disregarded.

$$gEq = \frac{\text{Gram molecular weight}}{\text{Valence}}$$

The gEq of sodium (Na^+), with a valence of 1, equals its gram atomic weight of 23 g. The gEq of calcium (Ca^{++}) is its atomic weight (i.e., 40) divided by 2, or 20 g. The gEq of ferric iron (Fe^{+++}) is its atomic weight (i.e., 55.8) divided by 3, or approximately 18.6 g.

For radicals such as sulfate (SO_4^{2-}), the formula for sulfuric acid (H_2SO_4) shows that one sulfate group combines with two atoms of hydrogen. Half (0.5) of a mole of sulfate is equivalent to 1 mole of hydrogen atoms. The gEq of SO_4^{2-} is half its gram formula weight, or 48 g. If an element has more than one valence, the valence must be specified or must be apparent from the observed chemical combining properties.

Gram Equivalent Weight of an Acid. The gEq of an acid is the weight of the acid (in grams) that contains 1 mole of replaceable hydrogen. The gEq of an acid may be calculated by dividing its gram formula weight by the number of hydrogen atoms in its formula, as shown in the following reaction:

$$HCl + Na^+ \rightarrow NaCl + H^+$$

The single H^+ of hydrochloric acid (HCl) is replaced by Na^+. In 1 mole of HCl, there is 1 mole of replaceable hydrogen. By definition, the gEq of HCl must be the same as its gram formula weight, or 36.5 g. The two hydrogen atoms of sulfuric acid (H_2SO_4) are both considered to be replaceable. In 1 mole of sulfuric acid, there are 2 moles of replaceable hydrogen, and the gEq of H_2SO_4 is half its gram formula weight, or 48 g.

Acids in which hydrogen atoms are not completely replaceable are exceptions to the rule. In some acids, H^+ replacement varies according to specific reactions. Carbonic acid (H_2CO_3) and phosphoric acid (H_3PO_4) are examples of such exceptions. Their equivalent weights are determined by the conditions of their chemical reactions.

For example, H_2CO_3 has two hydrogen atoms. In physiologic reactions, only one is considered replaceable:

$$H_2CO_3 + Na^+ \rightarrow NaHCO_3 + H^+$$

Only one hydrogen atom is released; the other remains bound. In 1 mole of carbonic acid, there is only 1 mole of replaceable hydrogen. The gEq of carbonic acid is the same as its gram formula weight, or 61 g.

Gram Equivalent Weight of a Base. The equivalent weight of a base is its weight (grams) containing 1 mole of replaceable hydroxyl (OH^-) ions. Similar to acids, the gEq of bases is calculated by dividing gram formula weight by the number of OH^- groups in its formula.

Conversion of Gram Weight to Equivalent Weight. To determine the number of gEqs in a substance, the gram weight is divided by its calculated equivalent weight, as shown in the following example:

$$\frac{58.5\text{ g NaCl}}{\text{gEq } 58.5\text{ g}} = 1\text{ gEq}$$
$$\frac{29.25\text{ g NaCl}}{\text{gEq } 58.5} = 0.5\text{ gEq}$$

Milligram Equivalent Weights. The concentrations of most chemicals in the body are quite small. The term *milligram equivalent weight (milliequivalent)* is preferred for expressing these minute values; 1 mEq is simply 0.001 gEq:

$$\text{mEq} = \frac{\text{gEq}}{1000}$$

The normal concentration of potassium (K^+) in plasma ranges from 0.0035 to 0.005 gEq/L. These values may be converted to milliequivalents by multiplying by a factor of 1000. The normal concentration of K^+ in the plasma would be expressed as ranging from 3.5 to 5.0 mEq/L.

Solute Content by Weight

The measurement of many electrolytes is based on actual weight rather than on milliequivalents. This weight is often expressed as milligrams per 100 ml of blood or body fluid. The units for this measurement are abbreviated as mg% (mg percent) or mg/dl (milligrams per deciliter). This text uses the modern designation *mg/dl*. Some substances present in blood or body fluid are present in extremely small amounts and are expressed in *micrograms* ($\frac{1}{1000}$ of a milligram) per deciliter (μg/dl or mcg/dl).

Values stated in mg/dl may be converted into their corresponding equivalent weights and reported as mEq/L. Conversion between mEq/L and mg/dl may be calculated as follows:

(1) $$\text{mEq/L} = \frac{\text{mg/dl} \times 10}{\text{Equivalent weight}}$$

(2) $$\text{mEq/L} = \frac{\text{mEq/L} \times \text{Equivalent weight}}{10}$$

To convert a serum Na^+ value of 322 mg/dl to mEq/L, the equation is used as follows:

$$\text{mEq/L} = \frac{\text{mg/dl} \times 10}{\text{Equivalent weight}} = \frac{322 \times 10}{23} = 140\text{ mEq/L}$$

In clinical practice, electrolyte replacement is common when a laboratory test identifies a significant deficiency. The electrolyte content of intravenous solutions is usually stated in milligrams per deciliter or in mEq per liter. Lactated Ringer's solution is one such infusion used for electrolyte replacement (Table 12-2).

Calculating Solute Content

In addition to gEq, mEq, mg/dl, and μg/dl (mcg/dl), several other methods of calculating solute content exist. These common chemical standards are used to compute solute content and dilution of solutions.

Quantitative Classification of Solutions

The amount of solute in a solution may be quantified by the following six methods:

1. *Ratio solution.* The amount of solute to solvent is expressed as a proportion (e.g., 1:100). Ratio solutions are sometimes used in describing concentrations of drugs.

TABLE 12-2

Concentration of Ingredients in Lactated Ringer's Solution

Substance	mg/dl	Approximate mEq/L
NaCl (sodium chloride)	600 Na	130
	310 Cl	109
$NaC_3H_5O_3$ (sodium lactate)	30 $C_3H_5O_3$	28
KCl (potassium chloride)	30 K	4
$CaCl_2$ (calcium chloride)	20 Ca	27

2. *Weight-per-volume solution (W/V).* The W/V solution is commonly used for solids dissolved in liquids. It is defined as weight of solute per volume of solution. This method is sometimes erroneously described as a percent solution. W/V solutions are commonly expressed in grams of solute per 100 ml of solution. For example, 5 g of glucose dissolved in 100 ml of solution is properly called a 5% solution, according to the W/V scheme. A liquid dissolved in a liquid is measured as volumes of solute to volumes of solution.
3. *Percent solution.* A percent solution is weight of solute per weight of solution. For example, 5 g of glucose dissolved in 95 g of water is a true percent solution. The glucose is 5% of the total solution weight of 100 g.
4. *Molal solution.* A molal solution contains 1 mole of solute per kilogram of solvent, or 1 mmol/g solvent. The concentration of a molal solution is independent of temperature.
5. *Molar solution.* A molar solution has 1 mole of solute per liter of solution, or 1 mmol/ml of solution. Solute is measured into a container, and solvent is added to produce the solution volume desired.
6. *Normal solution.* A **normal solution** has 1 gEq of solute per liter of solution, or 1 mEq/ml of solution. For all monovalent solutes, normal and molar solutions are the same. The equivalent weights of their solutes equal their gram formula weights. Equal volumes of solutions of the same normality contain chemically equivalent amounts of their solutes. If the solutes react chemically with one another, equal volumes of the solutions react completely. Neither substance remains in excess. In the analytic process of titration, normal solutions are often used as standards to determine the concentrations of other solutions.

Dilution Calculations

Dilute solutions are made from a stock preparation. Preparation of medications often involves dilution. Dilution calculations are based on the weight-per-unit volume principle (the aforementioned W/V solution method).

Diluting a solution increases its volume without changing the amount of solute it contains, and this reduces the concentration of the solution. The amount of solute in a solution can be expressed as volume times concentration. For example, 50 ml of a 10% solution (10 g/dl) contains 50 × 0.1, or 5 g. In the dilution of a solution, initial volume (V_1) multiplied by initial concentration (C_1) equals final volume multiplied by final concentration. This can be expressed as follows:

$$V_1C_1 = V_2C_2$$

This equation is sometimes referred to as the **dilution equation.** Whenever three of the variables are known, the fourth can be calculated as in the following examples:

1. Diluting 10 ml of a 2% (0.02) solution to a concentration of 0.5% (0.005) requires finding the new volume (V_2) by rearranging the dilution equation as follows:

$$V_2 = \frac{V_1C_1}{C_2}$$

$$V_2 = \frac{10\ \text{ml} \times 0.02}{0.005}$$

$$V_2 = 40\ \text{ml}$$

2. If 50 ml of water is added to 150 ml of a 3% (0.03) solution, the new concentration is calculated by rearranging the dilution equation to find C_2 as follows:

$$C_2 = \frac{V_1C_1}{V_2}$$

$$C_2 = \frac{150\ \text{ml} \times 0.02}{(50\ \text{ml} + 150\ \text{ml})}$$

$$C_2 = 0.0225\ (2.25\%)$$

3. To dilute 50 ml of a 0.33 normal (N) solution to a 0.1N concentration, concentration is given as normality, but it can be used similar to a percentage. The new volume (V_2) can be calculated by rearranging the dilution equation as follows:

$$V_2 = \frac{V_1C_1}{C_2}$$

$$V_2 = \frac{50\ \text{ml} \times 0.33}{0.1}$$

$$V_2 = 165\ \text{ml}$$

In the last example, the volume needed to produce a 0.1N solution would be 165 ml − 50 ml (the original volume), or 115 ml. In other words, 115 ml of solvent would have to be added to the original 50 ml of 0.33N solution to produce the desired concentration. The added solvent is called the **diluent** because it dilutes the original concentration to a lower concentration.

ELECTROLYTIC ACTIVITY AND ACID-BASE BALANCE

Acid-base balance depends on the concentration and activity of electrolytic solutes in the body. Clinical application of acid-base homeostasis is discussed in detail in Chapter 13.

Characteristics of Acids, Bases, and Salts

Acids

The term **acid** refers to either compounds that can donate [H^+] (Brönsted-Lowry acid) or any compound that accepts an electron pair (Lewis acid). Although these two theories of acids differ in which is being transferred, both theories

MINI CLINI

Methacholine Dilution

The dilution equation ($V_1C_1 = V_2C_2$) is commonly used to calculate volumes or concentrations of medications when a specific dosage needs to be administered to a patient. If three of the variables are known, the fourth can be determined.

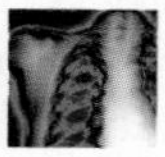

PROBLEM: Methacholine is a drug used to challenge the airways of patients suspected to have asthma. In healthy subjects, only higher doses of methacholine cause bronchospasm. In asthmatics, very low doses can precipitate a 20% decrease in the forced expiratory volume in 1 second (FEV_1). The methacholine challenge test begins with a low dose and increases the concentration (either doubling or quadrupling) until the patient has a significant change in FEV_1 or the highest dose has been given. Methacholine is supplied in vials that contain 100 mg of the active substance to which 6.25 ml of diluent (saline) can be added to produce a concentration of 16 mg/ml.* This is the highest dosage that is administered to the patient. How can you make serial dilutions of the drug so that five different dosages are available and each one is four times more concentrated than the previous dose?

SOLUTION: Starting with a 16 mg/ml stock solution of methacholine, how much diluent needs to be added to 3 ml of the stock to make a 4 mg/ml dose (one-fourth of the original concentration)?

Using the dilution equation:

$$C_1V_1 = C_2V_2$$
$$(16)(3.0) = (4)V_2$$
$$\frac{48}{4} = V_2$$
$$12 = V_1$$

Because there was 3 ml of the stock solution to begin with, the amount of diluent to add is the difference between 12 (V_2) and 3, or 9 ml. Adding 9 ml of diluent to the original 3 ml of stock (16 mg/ml) provides 12 ml of methacholine with a concentration of 4 mg/ml, exactly one-fourth of the highest dose. Additional dilutions can be prepared using 3 ml of solution according to the following table:

Start With	Add Diluent	To Make
3 ml of 4 mg/ml	9 ml	1 mg/ml
3 ml of 1 mg/ml	9 ml	0.25 mg/ml
3 ml of 0.25 mg/ml	9 ml	0.0625 mg/ml

Each of these dilutions uses the same proportions used in the first dilution as determined by the dilution equation. Methacholine is administered by nebulizer to the patient starting with the lowest concentration (0.0625 mg/ml) and increasing until a change in FEV_1 is observed. (See Chapter 19 for additional information on pulmonary function testing.)

*Only trained individuals should prepare and label solutions of methacholine.

attempt to describe how reactive groups perform within an aqueous solution[8,9]:

$$NH_4Cl + NaOH \rightarrow NH_3 + NaCl + HOH$$

In this reaction, sodium and chloride ions are not involved in the proton transfer. The equation can be rewritten ionically as follows to show the acidity of the ammonium ion:

$$NH_4^+ + OH^- \rightarrow NH_3 + HOH$$

The ammonium ion donates a hydrogen ion (proton) to the reaction. The H^+ combines with the hydroxide ion (OH^-), and this converts the former into ammonia gas and the latter into water.

Acids With Single Ionizable Hydrogen. Simple compounds such as HCl ionize into one cation and one anion:

$$HCl \rightarrow H^+ + Cl^-$$

Acids With Multiple Ionizable Hydrogens. The H^+ ions in an acid may become available in stages. The degree of ionization increases as an electrolyte solution becomes more dilute. Concentrated sulfuric acid ionizes only one of its two hydrogen atoms per molecule, as follows:

$$H_2SO_4 \rightarrow H^+ + HSO_4^-$$

With further dilution, second-stage ionization occurs:

$$H_2SO_4 \rightarrow H^+ + H^+ + SO_4^-$$

Bases

A **base** is a compound that yields hydroxyl ions (OH^-) when placed into aqueous solution. A substance capable of inactivating acids is also considered a base. These compounds, called *hydroxides,* consist of a metal that is ionically bound to a hydroxide ion or ions. The hydroxide may also be bound to an ammonium cation (NH_4^+). An example of this type of base is sodium hydroxide (NaOH). The Brönsted-Lowry definition of a base is any compound that accepts a proton; bases are paired with acids that donate the proton, and these are called *conjugate pairs.* This definition includes substances other than hydroxides, such as ammonia, carbonates, and certain proteins.

Hydroxide Bases. In aqueous solution, the following are typical dissociations of hydroxide bases:

$$Na^+OH \rightarrow Na^+ + OH^-$$
$$K^+OH \rightarrow K^+ + OH^-$$
$$Ca^{++}(OH^-)_2 \rightarrow Ca^{++} + 2(OH^-)$$

Inactivation of an acid is part of the definition of a base. This inactivation is accomplished by OH^- reacting with H^+ to form water:

$$NaOH + HCl \rightarrow NaCl + HOH$$

Nonhydroxide Bases. Ammonia and carbonates are examples of nonhydroxide bases. Proteins, with their amino groups, also can serve as nonhydroxide bases.

Ammonia. Ammonia qualifies as a base because it reacts with water to yield OH^-:

$$NH_3 + HOH \rightarrow NH_4^+ + OH^-$$

and neutralizes H^+ directly:

$$NH_3 + H^+ \rightarrow NH_4^+$$

In both instances, NH_3 accepts a proton to become NH_4^+. Ammonia plays an important role in renal excretion of acid (see Chapter 13).

Carbonates. The carbonate ion, CO_3^{2-}, can react with water in the following way to produce OH^-:

$$(1) \quad Na_2CO_3 \Leftrightarrow 2Na^+ + CO_3^{2-}$$

$$(2) \quad CO_3^{2-} + HOH \Leftrightarrow HCO_3^- + OH^-$$

In this reaction, the carbonate ion accepts a proton from water, becoming the bicarbonate ion. It simultaneously produces a hydroxide ion. The carbonate ion also can react directly with H^+ to inactivate it:

$$CO_3^{2-} + H^+ \Leftrightarrow HCO_3^-$$

Protein Bases. Proteins are composed of amino acids bound together by peptide links. Physiologic reactions in the body occur in a mildly alkaline environment. This environment allows proteins to act as H^+ receptors, or bases. Cellular and blood proteins acting as bases are transcribed as $prot^-$.

The imidazole group of the amino acid histidine is an example of an H^+ acceptor on a protein molecule (Figure 12-4). The ability of proteins to accept hydrogen ions limits H^+ activity in solution, which is called **buffering.** The buffering effect of hemoglobin is produced by imidazole groups in the protein. Each hemoglobin molecule contains 38 histidine residues. Each oxygen-carrying component (heme group) of hemoglobin is attached to a histidine residue. The ability of hemoglobin to accept (i.e., buffer) H^+ ions depends on its oxygenation state. Deoxygenated (reduced) hemoglobin is a stronger base (i.e., a better H^+ acceptor) than oxygenated hemoglobin. This difference partially accounts for the ability of reduced hemoglobin to buffer more acid than oxygenated hemoglobin can (see Chapter 13). Plasma proteins also act as buffers, although with less buffering power than hemoglobin, which contains more histidine.

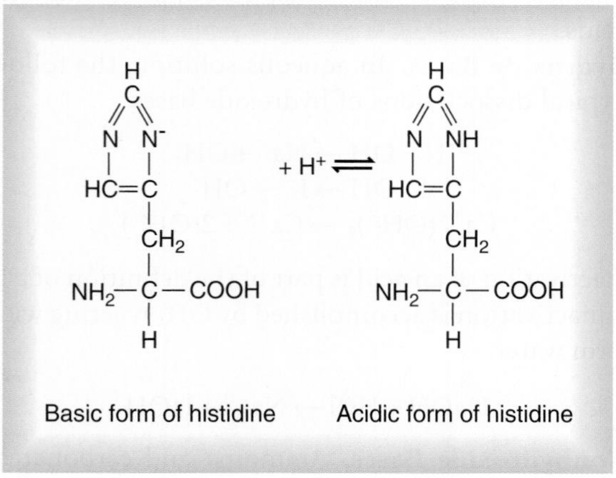

FIGURE 12-4 Histidine portion of a protein molecule (at *top*) serving as a proton acceptor (base).

Designation of Acidity and Alkalinity

Pure water can be used as a reference point for determining acidity or alkalinity. The concentration of both H^+ and OH^- in pure water is 10^{-7} mol/L. A solution that has a greater H^+ concentration or lower OH^- concentration than water acts as an acid. A solution that has a lower H^+ concentration or a greater OH^- concentration than water is alkaline, or basic.

The H^+ concentration $[H^+]$ of pure water has been adopted as the standard for comparing reactions of other solutions. Electrochemical techniques are used to measure the $[H^+]$ of unknown solutions. Acidity or alkalinity is determined by variation of the $[H^+]$ greater than or less than 1×10^{-7}. For example, a solution with a $[H^+]$ of 89.2×10^{-4} has a higher $[H^+]$ than water and is acidic. A solution with a $[H^+]$ of 3.6×10^{-8} has fewer hydrogen ions than water and is by definition alkaline. Two related techniques are used for expressing the acidity or alkalinity of solutions using the $[H^+]$ of water (i.e., 10^{-7}) as a neutral factor: (1) the $[H^+]$ in nanomoles per liter and (2) the logarithmic pH scale.

Nanomolar Concentrations

The acidity or alkalinity of solutions may be reported using the molar concentration of H^+ compared with that of water. The $[H^+]$ of water is 1×10^{-7} mol/L, or 0.0000001 (one ten-millionth of a mole). The unit for one-billionth of a mole is a **nanomole** (nmol). The $[H^+]$ of water can be expressed as 100 nmol/L. A solution that has a $[H^+]$ of 100 nmol/L is neutral. A solution with an $[H^+]$ greater than 100 nmol/L is acidic; one with an $[H^+]$ less than 100 nmol/L is alkaline. This system is limited because of the wide range of possible $[H^+]$ but is applicable in clinical medicine because the physiologic range of $[H^+]$ is narrow. $[H^+]$ in healthy individuals is usually 30 to 50 nmol/L.

pH Scale

The pH scale is used to describe the concentration of H^+, ($[H^+]$), (i.e., Brönsted-Lowry acid) in a solution. Rather than expressing the $[H^+]$ as a very small number or in nanomoles, it is more convenient to describe it in terms of the inverse logarithm of the nanomolar $[H^+]$. pH is defined as:

$$pH = -\log[H^+]$$

pH is always represented as a positive number and is derived by converting the value for $[H^+]$ to a negative exponent of 10 and calculating its logarithm. The $[H^+]$ of water is 1×10^{-7} mol/L. Because the negative logarithm of 1×10^{-7} is 7, the pH of water is 7.

Using this scheme, in a solution with a pH of 7.00, the $[H^+]$ is the same as would be seen in pure water, so by definition this is called "neutral." As the pH decreases to less than 7.00, the solution is termed more acidic, and when the pH increases to greater than 7.00, the solution is considered to be basic. With a whole number change in pH (i.e., pH decreasing from 7.00 to 6.00), the $[H^+]$ is a factor of 10 less. With a pH increase from 7.00 to 8.00, the $[H^+]$ is 10 times greater (Figure 12-5).

All fluids in the body are aqueous in origin. pK is the inverse logarithm of the dissociation constant for each solute. A pH of 7.00 is equivalent to a $[H^+]$ of 100 nmol. A pH of 8.00 is equivalent to a $[H^+]$ concentration of 10 nmol. Similarly, a change in pH of 0.3 unit equals a twofold change in $[H^+]$.

The **law of mass action** states that acids and bases freely dissociate and r-associate in a solution at a constant rate relative to the structure of the acid and the temperature of the system.[10] Using the Henderson-Hasselbalch equation, which describes the ratio of $[H^+]$ to base, we can calculate expected pH (see Chapter 13).

$$pH = pK + \log[H^+]$$

Where:

pH = Inverse log value $[H^+]$

pK = Inverse log of dissociation constant of solution

log $[H^+]$ = Logarithm of $[H^+]$, which can be expressed as the ratio between conjugate acid and total acid concentration

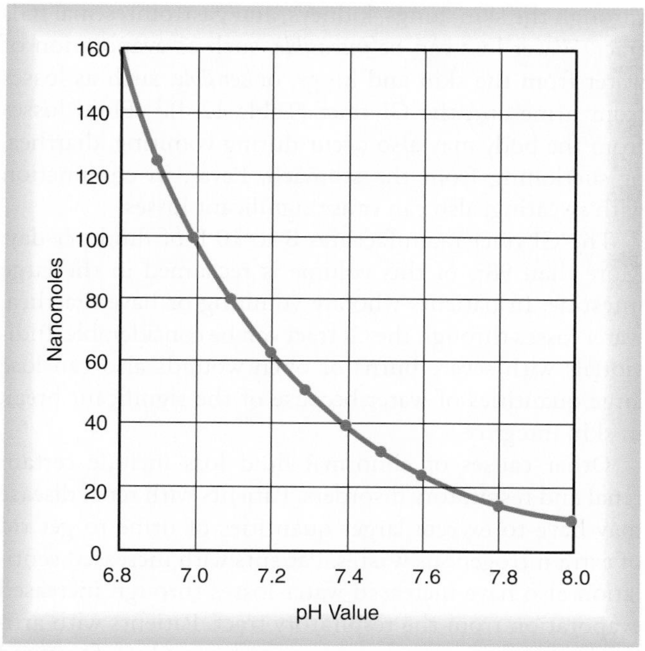

FIGURE 12-5 Relationship between pH scale and $[H^+]$ concentrations in nanomoles per liter (nmol/L). pH of 7.00 equals 100 nmol/L H^+, whereas the normal human pH (arterial blood) of 7.40 is equal to about 40 nmol/L.

Applying these concepts in an example pertinent to clinical medicine yields the following:

$$\begin{aligned}[H^+] &= 4.0\times10^{-8}\ \text{mol/L}\\ pH &= -\log(4.0\times10^{-8})\\ &= -\log 4.0 + -\log 10^{-8}\\ &= -\log 4.0 + \log 10^{8}\\ &= -0.602 + 8\\ &= 7.40\end{aligned}$$

In this example, the $[H^+]$ in arterial blood of a healthy adult is approximately 4.0×10^{-8} mol/L, or 40 nmol/L.

RULE OF THUMB

The pH scale is logarithmic. pH is a positive number representing the negative log of the hydrogen ion concentration $[H^+]$ of a solution. To visualize changes in acidity or alkalinity, the following two rules are helpful:

1. *A pH change of 0.3 unit equals a 2-fold change in $[H^+]$.*
2. *A pH change of 1 unit equals a 10-fold change in $[H^+]$.*

For example, if a patient's blood pH decreased from 7.40 (normal) to 7.10, the $[H^+]$ concentration would be twice as high. If a patient's urine pH decreased from 7.00 to 6.00, the $[H^+]$ would have increased by 10 times.

BODY FLUIDS AND ELECTROLYTES

Body Water

Water is a major component of the body. It constitutes 45% to 80% of an individual's body mass, depending on the mass, gender, and age of the individual. Leanness is associated with higher body water content. Obese individuals have a lower percentage of body water (≤30% less) than normal-weight individuals. Men have a slightly higher percentage of total body water than women. Total percentage of body water in infants and children is substantially greater than in adults. In a newborn, water accounts for 80% of the total body weight (Table 12-3).

TABLE 12-3

Distribution of Body Fluids

Body Water	Man (% body weight)	Woman (% body weight)	Infant (% body weight)
Total body Water	60 ± 15	50 ± 15	80
Intracellular	45	40	50
Extracellular	15-20	15-20	30
Interstitial	11-15	11-15	24
Intravascular	4.5	4.5	5.0
Transcellular	<1	<1	<1

Distribution

Total body water is divided into the following two major compartments: (1) *intracellular* ("within the cells") and (2) *extracellular* ("outside the cells"). Intracellular water accounts for approximately two-thirds of the total body water, and extracellular water accounts for the remaining one-third. Extracellular water is found in three subcompartments: (1) intravascular water (plasma), (2) interstitial water, and (3) transcellular fluid. Intravascular water constitutes approximately 5% of the body weight. Interstitial water is water in the tissues between the cells. It constitutes approximately 15% of the body weight. The proportion of *transcellular fluid* is quite small in proportion to plasma and **interstitial fluid.** Interstitial fluid is a matrix—a collagen/gel substance that allows the interstitium to provide structural support during times of extracellular volume depletion.[11] Examples of transcellular fluid include cerebrospinal fluid, digestive juices, and mucus. Transcellular fluid can become an important third space in some pathologic conditions, such as *ascites* (excess fluid in the peritoneal cavity) or *pleural effusion* (fluid collection in the pleural space).

Composition

The concentration of ionic solutes in intracellular and extracellular fluids differs significantly. Sodium (Na^+), chloride (Cl^-), and bicarbonate (HCO_3^-) are predominantly extracellular electrolytes. Potassium (K^+), magnesium (Mg^{++}), phosphate (PO_4^{3-}), sulfate (SO_4^{2-}), and protein constitute the main intracellular electrolytes. Although protein does not dissociate ionically, it can create hydrogen and other weak bonds and distribute net extra charge within its molecule. Intravascular and interstitial fluids have similar electrolyte compositions. However, plasma contains substantially more protein than interstitial fluid. Proteins, chiefly albumin, account for the high osmotic pressure of plasma. Osmotic pressure is an important determinant of fluid distribution between vascular and interstitial compartments.

Regulation

Movement of certain ions and proteins between body compartments is restricted. However, water diffuses freely. Control of total body water occurs through regulation of water intake (thirst) and water excretion (urine production, insensible loss, and stool water). The kidneys are mainly responsible for water excretion. If water intake is low, the kidneys reduce urine volume. Solutes in the urine can be concentrated up to four times the concentration of solutes in the plasma. If water intake is high, the kidneys can excrete large volumes of dilute urine.

The kidneys maintain the volume and composition of body fluids via two related mechanisms. First, filtration and reabsorption of sodium adjust urinary sodium excretion to match changes in dietary intake. Second, water excretion is regulated by osmoreceptors which are located in the hypothalamus and modulate secretion of antidiuretic hormone (ADH, also known as vasopressin).[7,12,13] These receptors are exceptionally sensitive; in vivo studies have shown that a single neuron can respond to either an osmotic or a nonosmotic baroreceptor simulus.[13] These mechanisms allow the kidneys to maintain the volume and concentration of body fluid despite variations in salt and water intake. Analysis of the urine (urinalysis) often provides diagnostic clues in disorders of body fluid volume.

TABLE 12-4

Daily Water Exchange

Regulation	Average Daily Volume (ml)	Maximum Daily Volume
Water Losses		
Insensible		
Skin	700	1500 ml
Lung	200	
Sensible		
Urine	1000-1200	>2000 ml/hr
Intestinal	200	8000 ml
Sweat	0	>2000 ml/hr
Water Gain		
Ingestion		
Fluids	1500-2000	1500 ml/hr
Solids	500-600	1500 ml/hr
Body metabolism	250	1000 ml

Water Losses. Water may be lost from the body through the skin, lungs, kidneys, and gastrointestinal (GI) tract. Water loss can be *insensible,* such as evaporation of water from the skin and lungs, or *sensible,* such as losses from urine and the GI tract (Table 12-4).[14] Fluid losses from the body may also occur during vomiting, diarrhea, or suctioning from the stomach. Fever, in conjunction with sweating, also can cause significant losses.

The GI tract manufactures 8 to 10 L of fluid per day. More than 98% of this volume is reclaimed in the large intestine. In patients who are vomiting or have diarrhea, water losses through the GI tract can be considerable. Individuals with severe burns or open wounds also can lose large quantities of water because of the significant break in skin integrity.

Other causes of abnormal fluid loss include certain renal and respiratory disorders. Patients with renal disease may have to excrete larger quantities of urine to get rid of extra nitrogenous wastes. Patients with increased ventilation also have increased water losses through increased evaporation from the respiratory tract. Patients with artificial airways are prone to evaporative water loss if inspired air is not adequately humidified. Infants have a greater proportion of body water than adults, particularly in the extracellular compartments (see Table 12-3). Water loss in infants may be twice of the water loss in adults. Infants also have a greater body surface area (in proportion to body volume) than adults, making their basal heat production twice as high. Higher metabolic rates in infants necessitate greater urinary excretion. Infants turn over approximately one-half of their extracellular fluid volume daily; adults turn over approximately one-seventh. Fluid loss or lack of intake can rapidly deplete an infant of water.

Water Replacement. Water is replenished in two major ways: ingestion and metabolism (see Table 12-4).

Ingestion. Water is replaced mainly by ingestion, through the consumption of liquids. An average adult drinks 1500 to 2000 ml of water per day. An additional 500 to 600 ml of water is ingested from solid food.

Metabolism. Water also is gained from the oxidation of fats, carbohydrates, and proteins in the body; the destruction of cells also releases some water. During total starvation, 2000 ml of water can be produced daily by the metabolism of 1 kg of fat. Recovery after surgery or trauma may be similar to starvation; under such conditions, approximately 500 mg of protein and a similar amount of fat are metabolized. This metabolism yields approximately 1 L of water per day.

Transport Between Compartments

Homeostasis depends largely on the total volume of body fluids and on fluid transport between body compartments. The first stage of homeostasis is fluid exchange between systemic capillaries and interstitial fluid via passive diffusion. Capillary walls are permeable to crystalline electrolytes. This allows equilibrium between the two extracellular compartments to occur quickly. Except for the large protein molecules, plasma can also move through capillary walls into the tissue spaces. Because water and small molecules can cross the capillary membranes, they produce little or no osmotic effect.

Movement of fluid and solutes from capillary blood to interstitial spaces is enhanced by the difference in **hydrostatic pressure** between compartments. Hydrostatic pressure difference depends on blood pressure, blood volume, and the vertical distance of the capillary from the heart (i.e., the effects of gravity). Hydrostatic pressure tends to cause fluid to leak out of capillaries into the interstitial spaces.

Osmotic pressure differences between interstitial and intravascular compartments oppose hydrostatic pressure; that is, osmotic pressure tends to keep fluid in the capillaries. Proteins with molecular weights greater than about 70,000 in colloidal suspension in the plasma cause this difference in osmotic pressure. Proteins such as albumin are too large to pass through the pores of the capillary. Instead, these proteins remain in the intravascular compartment and exert osmotic pressure, which draws water and small solute molecules back into the capillaries; this is called **plasma colloid osmotic pressure (oncotic pressure).** Because these large proteins are negatively charged, they attract (but do not bind) an equivalent amount of cations to the intravascular compartment. These cations have the effect of increasing osmotic pressure within the capillary *(Donnan effect)*.

In a typical capillary, blood pressure is approximately 30 mm Hg at the arterial end and approximately 20 mm Hg at the venous end (Figure 12-6). Colloid osmotic pressure of the intravascular fluid remains constant at approximately 25 mm Hg. Hydrostatic pressure along the capillary continually decreases. At the arterial end, hydrostatic pressure normally exceeds osmotic pressure, and water flows out of the vascular space into the interstitial space. At the venous end, colloidal osmotic pressure exceeds hydrostatic forces. Water is pulled back into the vascular compartment.

The outflow of water and electrolytes from the capillary at the arterial end is not completely balanced by the return on the venous end. Slightly more water diffuses out than is reabsorbed. This slight outward excess is balanced by fluid return through the lymphatic circulation (see Chapter 8). Fluid return via lymphatic channels also depends on pressure differences. The pressure in the interstitial space is determined by the volume of interstitial fluid and its electrolyte content. Interstitial fluid moves from a region of higher pressure (interstitial space) to a region of lower pressure (lymphatic channels). This lymph fluid moves into larger lymphatic spaces, where the pressure is continuously decreasing.

These relationships may be expressed by the Starling equilibrium equation:

$$Q_f = K_1(P_{ch} - P_{ih}) - K_2(P_{co} - P_{io})$$

Where:

Q_f = Bulk flow of fluid between intravascular and interstitial compartments

P_{ch} = Capillary hydrostatic pressure

P_{ih} = Interstitial fluid hydrostatic pressure

P_{co} = Capillary osmotic pressure

P_{io} = Interstitial osmotic pressure

K_1 = Capillary permeability coefficient for fluids and electrolytes

K_2 = Capillary permeability coefficient for proteins

Three examples of the forces in this equation are fluid return from gravity-dependent areas of the body, fluid exchange in the lung, and tissue edema.

Because of hydrostatic effects, capillary pressure in the feet can reach 100 mm Hg when an individual is standing. Reabsorption of tissue fluid can be accomplished, although hydrostatic pressure greatly exceeds colloidal osmotic pressure. Three factors favor reabsorption under these circumstances:

1. High intravascular hydrostatic pressure is balanced by a proportionally greater interstitial pressure.
2. The "pumping" action of the skeletal muscles surrounding leg veins reduces venous pressures.

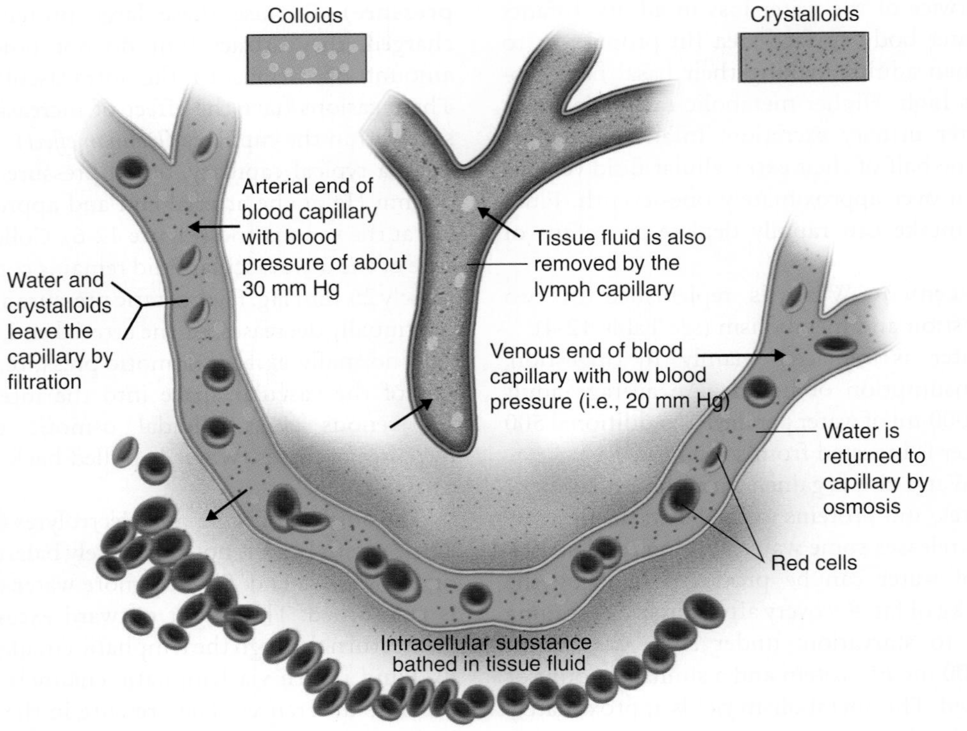

FIGURE 12-6 Tissue fluid is formed by a process of filtration at the arterial end of a systemic capillary *(left)*, where blood pressure exceeds colloid osmotic pressure. The fluid is absorbed by the blood capillaries and lymphatic vessels. It returns to the venous end of the capillary *(right)* when colloid osmotic pressure exceeds blood pressure. Fluid is absorbed into the lymphatic capillary system when interstitial fluid pressure is greater than the pressure within the lymphatic capillary. Normally, little colloid escapes from the capillary. Colloid that does escape is returned to the blood circulation by the lymphatic vessels. (Modified from Burke SR: The composition and function of body fluids, ed 3, St Louis, 1980, Mosby.)

3. Lymph flow back to the thorax is enhanced via a similar mechanism; this facilitates clearance of excess interstitial fluid.

However, when an imbalance results from changes in the basic pressures (e.g., arterial hypertension), edema tends to occur in the dependent limbs.

The lungs present a different situation. In systemic tissues, a constant exchange of interstitial fluid is essential. In the lungs, the alveoli must be kept relatively dry. Otherwise, interstitial fluid in the alveolar-capillary spaces would impede the diffusion of gas. Colloid osmotic pressure in pulmonary blood vessels is the same as it is in the systemic circulation. To minimize interstitial fluid in the alveolar-capillary region, the hydrostatic pressure difference must be kept low. The pulmonary circulation is a low-pressure system. The mean pulmonary vascular pressures are approximately one-sixth of those in the systemic circulation. Colloid osmotic pressure exceeds hydrostatic forces across the entire length of the pulmonary capillaries in healthy individuals. The alveoli are relatively free of excess interstitial water.

If hydrostatic pressure increases in the pulmonary circulation, this balance can be upset. This causes fluid movement into the alveolar-capillary spaces. Excess fluid in the interstitial space is called *edema*. In the lungs, edema caused by increased hydrostatic pressure often is a result of backpressure from a failing left ventricle (e.g., in congestive heart failure).

Edema can be caused by other factors. The **Starling equilibrium** equation given earlier shows that edema can be caused by a decrease in colloid osmotic pressure or an increase in capillary permeability. If albumin is depleted in the blood, the balance of forces is upset, favoring increased movement of fluid into the interstitium. Likewise, an increase in capillary permeability results in more fluid leaving the capillaries. Increased capillary permeability is a major factor in certain types of acute lung injuries (see Chapter 27).[15]

Electrolytes

Electrolytes in the various body fluids are not passive solutes. Electrolytes maintain the internal environment while making possible essential chemical and physiologic events. There are seven major electrolytes: sodium, chloride, bicarbonate, potassium, calcium, magnesium, and phosphorus (phosphate).

Sodium (Na^+)

Sodium is the major circulating cation within the body.[16] Regulation of sodium concentration in plasma and urine is related to regulation of total body water. Of the total body stores of sodium, 50% are extracellular. The remaining sodium is found in bone (40%) and in cells (10%). The normal serum concentration of sodium is 136 to 145 mEq/L. In cells, the sodium concentration is much lower, averaging only 4.5 mEq/L.

The average adult ingests and excretes approximately 100 mEq of sodium every 24 hours. Children require approximately half this amount, and infants typically exchange 20 mEq of sodium per day. Most sodium is reabsorbed through the kidney. Approximately 80% of the sodium in the body is reclaimed passively in the proximal tubules. The remainder is actively reabsorbed in the distal tubules. Sodium reabsorption in the kidneys is governed mainly by the level of aldosterone, which is secreted by the adrenal cortex. Na^+ reabsorption in the distal tubules of the kidney occurs in exchange for other cations. Sodium balance is involved in acid-base homeostasis (i.e., H^+ exchange) and the regulation of potassium (K^+). Abnormal losses of sodium can lead to *hyponatremia* (low sodium concentration in the plasma) and may occur for numerous reasons, as shown in Table 12-5.

Hyponatremia, which is the most common electrolyte imbalance found in hospitalized patients, is defined as having serum sodium levels less than 135 mEq/L.[7] Previously considered to be benign, mild hyponatremia has been shown in more recent studies to have a significant impact on a patient's cognitive function and gait stability, and it is thought to be a contributing factor in falls.[17] Hyponatremia can lead to cerebral edema owing to a change in osmotic pressure; the two most common causes for acute hyponatremia are postoperative iatrogenic and self-induced secondary to water intoxication.[17] One type of normal-volume (euvolemic) hyponatremia is known as

TABLE 12-5

Electrolyte Disorders and Clinical Findings

Electrolyte	Imbalance	Causes	Symptoms
Sodium (Na^+)	**Hyponatremia**	GI loss, sweating, fever, diuretics, ascites, congestive heart failure, kidney failure	Weakness, lassitude, apathy, headache, orthostatic hypotension, tachycardia
	Hypernatremia	Net sodium gain, net water loss, increased aldosterone, steroid therapy	Tremulousness, irritability, ataxia, confusion, seizures, coma
Chloride (Cl^-)	**Hypochloremia**	GI loss, diuretics	Metabolic alkalosis, muscle spasm, coma (severe cases)
	Hyperchloremia	Dehydration, metabolic acidosis, respiratory alkalosis	(Minimal)
Potassium (K^+)	**Hypokalemia**	Diuretics, steroid therapy, renal tubular disease, vomiting, diarrhea, malnutrition, trauma	Muscle weakness, paralysis, ECG abnormalities, supraventricular arrhythmias, circulatory failure, cardiac arrest
	Hyperkalemia	Chronic renal disease, hemorrhage, tissue necrosis, nonsteroidal antiinflammatory drugs, ACE inhibitors, cyclosporine, K^+-sparing diuretics	ECG changes, ventricular arrhythmias, cardiac arrest
Calcium (Ca^{++})	**Hypocalcemia**	Hyperparathyroidism, pancreatitis, renal failure, trauma	Hyperactive tendon reflexes, muscle twitching, spasm, abdominal cramps, ECG changes, convulsions (rarely)
	Hypercalcemia	Hyperthyroidism, hyperparathyroidism, metastatic bone cancer, sarcoidosis	Fatigue, depression, muscle weakness, anorexia, nausea, vomiting, constipation
Magnesium (Mg^{++})	**Hypomagnesemia**	Inadequate intake/impaired absorption of Mg^{++}, pancreatitis, alcoholism	Muscle weakness, irritability, tetany, ECG changes, arrhythmias, delirium, convulsions
	Hypermagnesemia	Dehydration, renal insufficiency, tissue trauma, lupus erythematosus	ECG changes (along with hyperkalemia, cardiac arrest, respiratory muscle paralysis)
Phosphate (HPO_4^{2-})	**Hypophosphatemia**	Starvation, malabsorption, hyperparathyroidism, hyperthyroidism, uncontrolled diabetes mellitus	Diaphragmatic weakness
	Hyperphosphatemia	Endocrine disorders, acromegaly, chronic renal insufficiency, acute renal failure, tissue trauma	(Minimal)

ACE, Angiotensin-converting enzyme; *ECG,* electrocardiogram.

syndrome of inappropriate antidiuretic hormone secretion (SIADH).[5,7,13,16-18]

Treatment of hypovolemic hyponatremia can have dire consequences as well. If fluid is administered too quickly, damage to the central nervous system occurs. With significant fluid shifts in Na^+ concentrations, rapid changes in cellular volume can lead to cell damage and cell death (apoptosis).[7] Osmotic demyelination syndrome occurs when serum sodium concentration changes more than 10 mEq/L in chronic hyponatremia or 18 mEq/L over 48 hours.[17]

Chloride (Cl^-)

Chloride is the most prominent anion in the body. Two-thirds of the body's store of chloride is extracellular; the remainder is intracellular. Intracellular chloride is present in significant amounts in red and white blood cells. It also is present in cells that have excretory functions, such as the GI mucosa.

Normal serum levels of chloride (Cl^-) are 98 to 106 mEq/L. The concentration of extracellular chloride is inversely proportional to the concentration of the other major anion, bicarbonate (HCO_3^-). Cl^- is regulated by the kidney in much the same manner as Na^+ (80% reabsorbed in the proximal tubules and 20% reabsorbed in the distal tubules). Cl^- is usually excreted with potassium in the form of KCl. An imbalance in one of these electrolytes usually affects both. Replacement therapy usually includes both K^+ and Cl^-. The stomach and the small bowel also affect the balance of Cl^-, and sweat contains hypotonic quantities of Cl^-. Abnormal Cl^- levels may occur for various reasons (see Table 12-5).

Bicarbonate (HCO_3^-)

After chloride, bicarbonate (HCO_3^-) is the most important body fluid anion. It plays an important role in acid-base homeostasis and is the strong base in the bicarbonate–carbonic acid buffer pair (see Chapter 13). HCO_3^- is the primary means for transporting CO_2 from the tissues to the lungs. The ratio of HCO_3^- to carbonic acid in healthy individuals is maintained near 20 : 1; this results in a pH of close to 7.40. HCO_3^- stores are evenly divided between intracellular and extracellular compartments. Normal serum HCO_3^- levels in arterial blood range from 22 to 26 mEq/L. HCO_3^- levels are slightly higher in venous blood as CO_2 is being transported to the lungs.

In acid-base disorders, the kidneys regulate HCO_3^- levels to maintain a near-normal pH. In healthy individuals, more than 80% of blood HCO_3^- is reabsorbed in the proximal tubules of the kidney. The remainder is reclaimed in the distal tubules. In respiratory acidosis, the kidneys retain or produce HCO_3^- to buffer the additional acid caused by CO_2 retention. In respiratory alkalosis, the opposite occurs. A reciprocal relationship exists between Cl^- and HCO_3^- concentrations. HCO_3^- retention is associated with chloride excretion, and vice versa (see Chapter 13).

MINI CLINI

Water, Salt, and Congestive Heart Failure

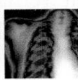

PROBLEM: Why do patients who have congestive heart failure (CHF) need to adhere to a low-salt diet?

SOLUTION: CHF occurs when the left ventricle cannot pump all of the blood presented to it. This situation leads to pooling of blood in the lungs and venous circulation and an increase in peripheral venous pressure. Normally, the ventricle pumps most of the blood entering it. This volume is the "preload" of the heart. The volume of extracellular water partially determines the preload of the ventricle.

The ventricle can fail as a pump either because of intrinsic heart disease, such as infarction or ischemia, or because of elevated distal pressures against which it must pump (hypertension). In addition to pooling of blood in the systemic venous circulation, blood can back up in the lungs, resulting in congestion and edema.

The most important determinant of the extracellular water volume is its sodium (Na^+) content. Changes in extracellular water are dictated by the net gain or loss of sodium, with an accompanying gain or loss of water. To reduce the work of the heart, fluid volume must be carefully regulated. By restricting salt intake, extracellular fluid volume can be reduced, allowing the heart to function more effectively as a pump. Treatment of CHF must address not only excess fluid volume but also the underlying cause.

Diuretics are often used to help reduce fluid volume. Many diuretics cause the kidney to excrete sodium, causing water to follow and reducing the extracellular fluid load. Because some diuretics also cause potassium (K^+) to be excreted, care must be taken in the management of CHF not to cause electrolyte imbalances. Potassium supplements may be used so that diuresis does not result in hypokalemia. Because of the central role of extracellular water in CHF, weighing the patient is a simple yet sensitive means of detecting excess fluid volume.

Potassium (K^+)

Potassium (K^+) is the main cation of the intracellular compartment. Most of the K^+ (98%) in the body is found in cells. **Active transport** of K^+ into the cells occurs through an ionic pump mechanism. An electrical differential across the cell membrane also facilitates K^+ movement into the cell. For every three K^+ ions that enter a cell, two Na^+ ions and one H^+ ion must leave. This transfer maintains electrical neutrality in the cell.

The difference in K^+ distribution is evident when comparing concentrations between fluid compartments. Intracellular K^+ concentration is approximately 150 mEq/L, whereas serum K^+ concentration normally ranges from 3.5 to 5.0 mEq/L. Serum K^+ is an indirect indicator only of the total body potassium. Serum potassium is usually analyzed by assessing both intake and excretion.

The average adult excretes 40 to 75 mEq of potassium in the urine every 24 hours. An additional 10 mEq is excreted in the stool. The average dietary intake of potassium ranges from 50 to 85 mEq/day. Patients who have undergone surgery, have sustained trauma, or have renal disease often have greater K^+ losses. Consequently, such patients may need K^+ replacement averaging 100 to 120 mEq/day.

Serum K^+ concentration is determined primarily by the pH of extracellular fluid and the size of the intracellular K^+ pool. In extracellular acidosis, excess H^+ ions are exchanged for intracellular K^+. Movement of K^+ from intracellular to extracellular spaces may produce dangerous levels of *hyperkalemia* (elevated potassium). Alkalosis has the opposite effect. When pH increases, K^+ moves into cells. In the absence of acid-base disturbances, serum K^+ reflects total body potassium. With excessive loss of K^+ from the GI tract, serum K^+ decreases. A 10% loss of total body K^+ causes the serum K^+ level to decrease approximately 1 mEq/L.

Renal excretion of K^+ is controlled by aldosterone levels.[19] Aldosterone inhibits the enzyme responsible for K^+ transport in the distal renal tubular cells of the kidney. Metabolic acidosis also inhibits the transport system. Na^+ and H^+ ions enter cells at the expense of increased K^+ excretion. Alkalosis has the reverse effect. It stimulates cellular retention of K^+. Kidney failure results in potassium retention and hyperkalemia.

Hypokalemia (reduced serum potassium) disturbs cellular function in numerous organ systems, including the GI, neuromuscular, renal, and cardiovascular systems (see Table 12-5), and is one of the most common electrolyte abnormalities within the hospital environment.[19] Management of hypokalemia involves replacement of K^+ losses and treatment of the underlying disorder. To manage the associated Cl^- deficit, K^+ is given with Cl^-. Caution is required in the administration of intravenous K^+ because cardiac muscle is very sensitive to extracellular concentrations of this electrolyte.

Hyperkalemia (elevated serum potassium) is most common in patients with renal insufficiency (see Table 12-5). The primary treatment of hyperkalemia is restriction of K^+ intake. The processes that precipitated the hyperkalemia also must be controlled. Temporary measures for reducing serum K^+ levels include administration of insulin, calcium gluconate, sodium salts, or large volumes of hypertonic glucose. Cation exchange resins may be given orally or rectally. If these measures fail, peritoneal or renal dialysis can aid in K^+ removal.

Calcium (Ca^{++})

Calcium is an important mediator of neuromuscular function and cell enzyme processes. Most of the calcium in the body is contained in the bones. The normal serum calcium is 8.7 to 10.4 mg/dl, or about 4.5 to 5.25 mEq/L. This concentration is maintained by the interaction of parathyroid hormone, vitamin D (calcitriol), and calcitonin.

Calcium is present in the blood in the following three forms: ionized, protein bound, and complex. The proportion of calcium in each form is affected by blood pH, concentration of plasma proteins, and presence of calcium-combining anions (e.g., HCO_3^- and HPO_4^{2-}). Approximately 50% of serum calcium is ionized (Ca^{++}) and is physiologically active. An additional 10% forms calcium-anion complexes. The remaining 40% is bound to plasma proteins, primarily albumen. Ionized calcium is physiologically active in processes such as enzyme activity, blood clotting, neuromuscular irritability, and bone calcification. Acidemia increases the concentration of Ca^{++} in the serum, and alkalemia decreases the concentration.

Abnormal levels of calcium can cause various serious symptoms (see Table 12-5). Treatment of *hypocalcemia* (low serum levels of calcium) consists of correcting the underlying cause and replacing Ca^{++} either orally or intravenously. *Hypercalcemia* (increased levels of calcium) can result from numerous disorders. The most common causes are hyperparathyroidism and malignancies (e.g., multiple myeloma, lung cancer). Acute hypercalcemia requires emergency treatment because death may occur quickly if serum Ca^{++} increases to more than 17 mg/L (8.5 mEq/L). In such cases, there is usually an associated deficit of extracellular fluid. Volume replacement reduces serum Ca^{++} by dilution. Steroids and loop diuretics are sometimes helpful in reducing serum calcium.

Magnesium (Mg^{++})

Magnesium (Mg^{++}) is the second most abundant intracellular cation after potassium. Magnesium plays an important role in cellular functions, including energy transfer; metabolism of protein, carbohydrate, and fat; and maintenance of normal cell membrane function (see Table 12-5). Systemically, magnesium decreases blood pressure and alters peripheral vascular resistance. Abnormalities of magnesium levels can result in disturbances in nearly every organ system and can cause potentially fatal complications (e.g., ventricular arrhythmia, coronary artery vasospasm, sudden death). Hypomagnesemia is also associated with multiple neuromuscular symptoms, such as muscular weakness, tetany, coma, and seizures. There is some evidence that intercellular magnesium levels may be related to bronchial hyperresponsiveness.

Normal values for serum Mg^{++} range from 1.7 to 2.1 mg/dl (1.7 to 1.4 mEq/L) in healthy adults. Most (99%) of the magnesium in the body is intracellular. Of the small portion in extracellular spaces, 80% is ionized or bound to other ions (e.g., phosphate) with the remaining 20% bound to proteins. Extracellular magnesium is in equilibrium with magnesium in the bone, kidneys, intestine, and other soft tissues. In contrast to most electrolytes, magnesium excretion in urine is not regulated hormonally, and circulating magnesium in the extracellular fluid does not exchange readily with its main repository—the bones. Serum levels of magnesium may remain normal even if total body stores are depleted by 20%. Conversely, when there is a negative magnesium balance, most of the losses come from the extracellular spaces. Equilibration with bone stores may take several weeks.

Phosphorus (P)

An average adult has approximately 1 kg (1000 g) of phosphorus, of which 80% to 90% is in bone and teeth in the form of apatite. The remaining phosphate is mostly present in the viscera and skeletal muscle, with a very small amount (<0.1%) in the extracellular fluids.[20] Of this total, 10% to 17% is combined with proteins, carbohydrates, and lipids in muscle tissue and blood, and the remainder is incorporated into complex organic compounds. Only about 1% of the total body phosphorus is available as free serum compounds, so the serum level (1.2 to 2.3 mEq/L) does not reflect total body content. Serum phosphate levels are influenced by several factors (see Table 12-5), including the serum calcium concentration and the pH of blood.

Organic phosphate (HPO_4^{2-}) is the main anion within cells with 20% present in the mitochondria. Approximately 30% of cellular phosphate is stored in the endoplasmic reticulum and is used in the phosphorylation of various proteins.[20] Inorganic phosphate plays a primary role in the metabolism of cellular energy, being the source from which adenosine triphosphate is synthesized. In acid-base homeostasis, phosphate is the main urinary buffer for titratable acid excretion (see Chapter 13).

Phosphorus homeostasis depends on balance between GI absorption and urinary excretion. The parathyroid hormone provides hormonal regulation. *Hyperphosphatemia* (elevated serum levels of phosphorus) can occur when the load (e.g., GI absorption, cellular release) exceeds renal excretion and tissue uptake. Hyperphosphatemia precipitates calcium, causing hypocalcemia, which can be life-threatening if severe. Central nervous system symptoms such as altered mental status, paresthesias, and seizures can result from hyperphosphatemia. Prolonged hyperphosphatemia can result in abnormal deposition of calcium phosphate in previously healthy connective tissues, such as cardiac valves, and in solid organs, such as muscles.

SUMMARY CHECKLIST

- The body is a water-based organism in which chemical substances and particles exist in solution or suspension.
- The concentration of solutes in a solution may be quantified (1) by actual weight (grams, milligrams, or micrograms) or (2) by chemical combining power (equivalents or milliequivalents). The weight of a solute does not give an indication of its chemical combining power, but gram equivalent weights do.
- Solutions commonly involve the action of osmotic pressure. Body cell membranes are semipermeable, and osmotic pressure maintains the distribution of water and solutes in physiologic ranges.
- Concentrations of solutions may be calculated using ratio, weight/volume, or percent methods. These techniques are useful in the preparation of medications and therapeutic fluids.
- Physiologically active compounds in the body are mostly weak electrolytic covalent substances. In aqueous solutions, some molecules ionize, leaving the remainder intact. Equilibrium is maintained between the ions and un-ionized molecules.
- Proteins made up of amino acids can function as bases in the mildly alkaline environment of the body; this allows hemoglobin and plasma proteins to function as buffers.
- Acidity or alkalinity is determined by variation of $[H^+]$ greater than or less than $1 \times 10^{-}7$ mol/L. Two methods for recording acidity or alkalinity use H^+ concentration of water as the neutral standard: (1) the actual measured molar concentration of H^+ in nanomoles per liter and (2) the logarithmic pH scale.
- Water makes up 45% to 80% of an individual's body weight. Percentage of total body water depends on weight, gender, age, and adipose tissue. Total body water is divided into intracellular and extracellular water. Extracellular water is divided further into intravascular and interstitial water, with a small component of transcellular fluids.
- Control of total body water is regulated by water intake and excretion. The kidneys maintain the volume and composition of body fluids by two related mechanisms: (1) filtration and reabsorption of sodium and (2) regulation of water excretion in response to changes in secretion of antidiuretic hormone.
- A balance between hydrostatic and osmotic pressure keeps water in the appropriate body compartments. Plasma proteins account for the high colloid osmotic pressure of plasma. Colloid osmotic pressure determines distribution of fluid between vascular and interstitial compartments. Imbalances in osmotic and hydrostatic pressures can result in edema.
- Electrolytes help maintain the internal environment and make important chemical and physiologic events possible. The concentrations of electrolytes in the intracellular and extracellular fluid compartments differ markedly. Sodium, chloride, bicarbonate, potassium, calcium, magnesium, and phosphorus are essential to homeostasis. Increased or decreased concentrations of any of these electrolytes can result in disease and sometimes death.

References

1. Kaplan LJ, Kellum JA: Fluids, pH, ions and electrolytes. Curr Opin Crit Care 16:323–331, 2010.
2. Brandis K: Fluid physiology. http://wwwanaesthesiamcqcom/FluidBook/fl4_2php. Accessed April 30, 2011.
3. Hu X, Adamson RH, Liu B, et al: Starling forces that oppose filtration after tissue oncotic pressure is increased. Am J Physiol Heart Circ Physiol 279:H1724–H1736, 2000.

4. Kramer GC: Hypertonic resuscitation: physiologic mechanisms and recommendations for trauma care. J Trauma 54:S89–S99, 2003.
5. Lewis CA, Martin GS: Understanding and managing fluid balance in patients with acute lung injury. Curr Opin Crit Care 10:13–17, 2004.
6. Levick JR, Michel CC: Microvascular fluid exchange and the revised Starling principle. Cardiovasc Res 87:198–210, 2010.
7. Lin M, Liu S, Lim I: Disorders of water imbalance. Emerg Med Clin North Am 23:749–770, 2005.
8. McNaught AD, Wilkinson A: Compendium of chemical terminology, Oxford, 2010, IUPAC.
9. Muller P: Glossary of terms used in physical organic chemistry. Pure Appl Chem 66:1077–1184, 1994.
10. Kudryavtsev AB, Jameson RF, Linert W: The law of mass action, New York, 2001, Springer.
11. Friedman A: Fluid and electrolyte therapy: a primer. Pediatr Nephrol 25:843–846, 2009.
12. Schrier RW, Bansal S: Diagnosis and management of hyponatremia in acute illness. Curr Opin Crit Care 14:627–634, 2008.
13. Bekheirnia M, Schrier R: Pathophysiology of water and sodium retention: edematous states with normal kidney function. Curr Opin Pharmacol 6:202–207, 2006.
14. Dries DJ: Hypotensive resuscitation. Shock 6:311–316, 1996.
15. Morissette MP: Colloid osmotic pressure: its measurement and clinical value. Can Med Assoc J 116:897–900, 1977.
16. Ball SG: Hyponatraemia. J R Coll Physicians Edinb 40:240–245, 2010.
17. Sterns RH, Hix JK, Silver S: Treatment of hyponatremia. Curr Opin Nephrol Hypertens 19:493–498, 2010.
18. Adrogue HJ, Madias NE: Hyponatremia. N Engl J Med 342:1581–1589, 2000.
19. Buckley MS, LeBlanc JM, Cawley MJ: Electrolyte disturbances associated with commonly prescribed medications in the intensive care unit. Crit Care Med 38:S253-S264, 2010.
20. Razzaque MS: Phosphate toxicity: new insights into an old problem. Clin Sci 120:91–97, 2011.

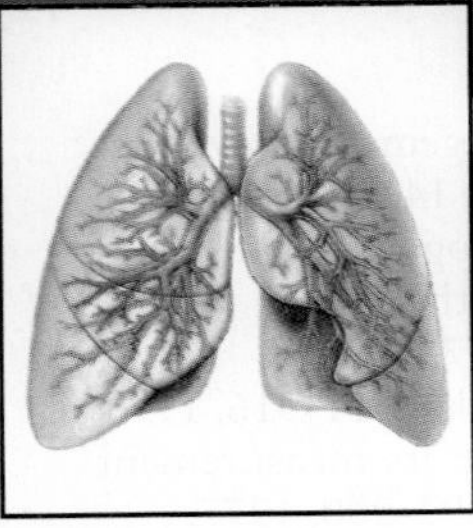

Chapter 13

Acid-Base Balance

WILL BEACHEY

CHAPTER OBJECTIVES

After reading this chapter you will be able to:

- Describe how the lungs and kidneys regulate volatile and fixed acids.
- Describe how the equilibrium constant of an acid is related to its ionization and strength.
- State what constitutes open and closed buffer systems.
- Explain why open and closed buffer systems differ in their ability to buffer fixed and volatile acids.
- Explain how to use the Henderson-Hasselbalch equation in hypothetical clinical situations.
- Describe how the kidneys and lungs compensate for each other when the function of one is abnormal.
- Explain how renal absorption and excretion of electrolytes affect acid-base balance.
- Classify and interpret arterial blood acid-base results.
- Explain how to use arterial acid-base information to decide on a clinical course of action.
- Explain why acute changes in the carbon dioxide level of the blood affect the blood's bicarbonate ion concentration.
- Calculate the anion gap and use it to determine the cause of metabolic acidosis.
- Describe how standard bicarbonate and base excess measurements are used to identify the nonrespiratory component of acid-base imbalances.
- State how Stewart's strong ion difference approach to acid-base regulation differs from the Henderson-Hasselbalch approach.

CHAPTER OUTLINE

KEY TERMS

acidemia
alkalemia
base excess (BE)
buffer base
closed buffer system
conjugate base
equilibrium constant
fixed (nonvolatile) acids
Henderson-Hasselbalch (H-H) equation
hypercapnia
hypocapnia

isohydric buffering
metabolic acidosis
metabolic alkalosis
open buffer system
paresthesia
respiratory acidosis
respiratory alkalosis
standard bicarbonate
volatile acid

Even small changes in hydrogen ion concentration [H^+] can cause vital metabolic processes in the body to fail. Normal metabolism continually generates H^+, and H^+ regulation is of utmost biologic importance. Various physiologic mechanisms work together to keep [H^+] of body fluids in a range compatible with life. This chapter helps the clinician understand how these mechanisms work and how to detect abnormalities in their function. With this knowledge, the clinician can make informed decisions about treating the underlying causes of acid-base disturbances.

HYDROGEN ION REGULATION IN BODY FLUIDS

Acid-base balance refers to physiologic mechanisms that keep [H^+] of body fluids in a range compatible with life. Hydrogen ions react readily with the protein molecules of vital cellular catalytic enzymes. Such reactions change the physical contour of the protein molecule and may render the enzyme inactive. To sustain life, the body must maintain the pH of fluids within a narrow range, from 7.35 to 7.45 (corresponding to a [H^+] of 45 to 35 nmol/L).

Hydrogen ions formed in the body come from either *volatile* or *fixed* (nonvolatile) acids. A **volatile acid** is one that is in equilibrium with a dissolved gas. The only volatile acid of physiologic significance in the body is carbonic acid (H_2CO_3), which is in equilibrium with dissolved carbon dioxide (CO_2). Normal aerobic metabolism generates approximately 13,000 mmol/L of CO_2 each day, producing an equal amount of H^+:

$$\underset{\substack{\uparrow \\ \text{Aerobic metabolism}}}{CO_2} + H_2O \rightarrow H_2CO_3 \rightarrow HCO_3^- + H^+$$

As CO_2 diffuses into the blood at the tissue level, this reaction occurs primarily in the erythrocyte where it is catalyzed by carbonic anhydrase, an intracellular enzyme. In a process called **isohydric buffering,**[1] most H^+ produced in this fashion causes no change in pH because hemoglobin (Hb) in the erythrocyte immediately buffers the H^+. When blood reaches the lungs, Hb releases H^+ to form CO_2 as shown:

$$\overset{\substack{\text{Ventilation} \\ \uparrow}}{CO_2} + H_2O \leftarrow H_2CO_3 \leftarrow HCO_3^- + \underset{\substack{\uparrow \\ HHb \rightarrow H^+ + Hb^-}}{H^+}$$

In this way, ventilation eliminates carbonic acid, keeping pace with its production. Isohydric buffering and ventilation are the two major mechanisms responsible for maintaining a stable pH in the face of massive CO_2 production.

Catabolism of proteins continually produces **fixed (nonvolatile) acids** such as sulfuric and phosphoric acids. In addition, anaerobic metabolism produces lactic acid. In contrast to carbonic acid, these nonvolatile acids are not in equilibrium with a gaseous component. However, H^+ of fixed acids can be buffered by bicarbonate ions (HCO_3^-) and converted to CO_2 and water (H_2O) (see the previous reaction); the CO_2 formed is eliminated in exhaled gas. Compared with daily CO_2 production, fixed acid production is small, averaging only about 50 to 70 mEq/day.[2] Certain diseases, such as untreated diabetes, increase fixed acid production. Hydrogen ions produced in this way stimulate respiratory centers in the brain. The resulting increase in ventilation eliminates more CO_2, pulling the hydration reaction to the left:

$$\overset{\substack{\text{Increased } \dot{V}_A \\ \uparrow}}{CO_2} + H_2O \leftarrow H_2CO_3 \leftarrow HCO_3^- + \underset{\substack{\uparrow \\ \text{Fixed acid } H^+}}{H^+}$$

In this way, the respiratory system compensates for fixed acid production, preventing a significant increase in [H^+].

Strong and Weak Acids and Bases: Equilibrium Constants

Strong acids and bases ionize almost completely in an aqueous solution. Weak acids and bases ionize only to a small extent. An example of a strong acid is hydrochloric acid (HCl). Nearly 100% of the HCl molecules dissociate to form H^+ and Cl^-:

$$HCl \longrightarrow H^+ + Cl^- \quad (1)$$

At *equilibrium,* the concentration of HCl is extremely small compared with either [H^+] or [Cl^-]. There is no arrow pointing to the left in Reaction 1, emphasizing that HCl ionizes almost completely in solution. In contrast, carbonic acid is an example of a relatively weak acid:

$$H_2CO_3 \rightleftarrows HCO_3^- + H^+ \quad (2)$$

The long arrow pointing to the left indicates that at *equilibrium,* the concentration of undissociated H_2CO_3 molecules is far greater than the concentration of HCO_3^- or H^+.

The **equilibrium constant** of an acid is a measure of the extent to which the acid molecules dissociate (ionize). At equilibrium, the number of dissociating H_2CO_3 molecules in Reaction 2 is equal to the number of associating HCO_3^- and H^+, even though the concentrations of reactants and products are unequal. In this state, no further change occurs in $[H_2CO_3]$, $[HCO_3^-]$, or $[H^+]$. At equilibrium, the following is true:

$$\frac{[H^+]\times[HCO_3^-]}{[H_2CO_3]} = K_A\ (Small) \quad (3)$$

Where K_A is the equilibrium constant for H_2CO_3. (K_A is also known as the acid's *ionization* or *dissociation* constant.)

K_A is small because the H_2CO_3 concentration is quite large with respect to the numerator of Reaction 3. The value of K_A is always the same for H_2CO_3 at equilibrium, regardless of the initial concentration of H_2CO_3.

A strong acid, such as HCl, has a *large* K_A because the denominator [HCl] is extremely small compared with the numerator ($[H^+] \times [Cl^-]$):

$$\frac{[H^+]\times[Cl^-]}{[HCl]} = K_A\ (Large) \quad (4)$$

As shown by Equations 3 and 4, K_A indicates the strength of an acid.

Buffer Solution Characteristics

A buffer solution resists changes in pH when an acid or a base is added to it. Buffer solutions are mixtures of acids and bases. The acid component is the H^+ cation, formed when a weak acid dissociates in solution. The base component is the remaining anion portion of the acid molecule, known as the **conjugate base.** An important blood buffer system is a solution of carbonic acid and its conjugate base, HCO_3^-:

$$H_2CO_3\,(Acid) \rightleftharpoons HCO_3^-\ (Conjugate\ base) + H^+$$

In the blood, HCO_3^- combines with sodium ions (Na^+) to form sodium bicarbonate ($NaHCO_3$). If hydrogen chloride, a strong acid, is added to the $H_2CO_3/NaHCO_3$ buffer solution, HCO_3^- reacts with the added H^+ to form weaker carbonic acid molecules and a neutral salt:

$$HCl + H_2CO_3/Na^+HCO_3^- \rightarrow 2H_2CO_3 + NaCl$$

The strong acidity of HCl is converted to the relatively weak acidity of H_2CO_3, preventing a large decrease in pH.

Similarly, if sodium hydroxide, a strong base, is added to this buffer solution, it reacts with the carbonic acid molecule to form the weak base, $NaHCO_3$, and H_2O:

$$NaOH + H_2CO_3/NaHCO_3 \rightarrow 2NaHCO_3 + H_2O$$

The strong alkalinity of NaOH is changed to the relatively weak alkalinity of $NaHCO_3$. pH change is minimized.

Bicarbonate and Nonbicarbonate Buffer Systems

Blood buffers are classified as bicarbonate or nonbicarbonate buffer systems. The bicarbonate buffer system consists of H_2CO_3 and its conjugate base, HCO_3^-. The nonbicarbonate buffer system consists mainly of phosphates and proteins, including Hb. The blood buffer base is the sum of bicarbonate and nonbicarbonate bases measured in millimoles per liter of blood.

The bicarbonate system is called an **open buffer system** because H_2CO_3 is in equilibrium with dissolved CO_2, which is readily removed by ventilation. That is, when H^+ is buffered by HCO_3^-, the product, H_2CO_3, is broken down into H_2O and CO_2 as long as ventilation removes CO_2. The removal of CO_2 from the reaction prevents it from reaching equilibrium with the reactants. For this reason, buffering activity can continue without being slowed or stopped:

$$HCO_3^- + H^+ \rightarrow H_2CO_3 \rightarrow H_2O + CO_2\ (Exhaled\ gas)$$

A nonbicarbonate buffer system is called a **closed buffer system** because all the components of acid-base reactions remain in the system. (In the following discussions, nonbicarbonate buffer systems are collectively represented as *Hbuf/Buf⁻*, where Hbuf is the weak acid, and Buf^- is the conjugate base.) When H^+ is buffered by Buf^-, the product, HBuf, accumulates and eventually reaches equilibrium with the reactants, preventing further buffering activity:

$$Buf^- + H^+ \leftrightarrow Hbuf$$

Box 13-1 summarizes the characteristics and components of bicarbonate and nonbicarbonate buffer systems.

Open and closed buffer systems play different roles in buffering fixed and volatile acids, and they differ in their ability to function in wide-ranging pH environments. Volatile acid (H_2CO_3) accumulates only if ventilation cannot eliminate CO_2 fast enough to keep up with the body's CO_2 production. In such a case, the reaction between CO_2 and H_2O moves continually to the right, creating more H_2CO_3 and, ultimately, more H^+ and HCO_3^-. The HCO_3^- produced in this way is incapable of buffering the H^+ with which it was coproduced. The only buffer system that can buffer the H^+ of volatile acid is the nonbicarbonate buffer system. Both nonbicarbonate and bicarbonate buffer systems can

Box 13-1 Classification of Whole Blood Buffers

OPEN SYSTEM

BICARBONATE

Plasma

Erythrocyte

CLOSED SYSTEM

NONBICARBONATE

Hemoglobin

Organic phosphates

Inorganic phosphates

Plasma proteins

From Beachey W: Respiratory care anatomy and physiology: foundations for clinical practice, ed 2, St Louis, 2007, Mosby.

buffer the H^+ produced by fixed acids; this is true of the bicarbonate buffer system only if ventilation is not impaired and CO_2 can be adequately eliminated. Both systems are physiologically important, each playing a unique and essential role in maintaining pH homeostasis. Table 13-1 summarizes the approximate contributions of various blood buffers to the total buffer base. Bicarbonate buffers have the greatest buffering capacity because they function in an open system.

Bicarbonate and nonbicarbonate buffer systems do not function in isolation from one another but are intermingled in the same solution (whole blood), in equilibrium with the same $[H^+]$ (Figure 13-1). Increased ventilation increases the CO_2 removal rate, causing nonbicarbonate buffers (Hbuf) to release H^+. Decreased ventilation ultimately causes Hbuf to accept more H^+.

TABLE 13-1

Individual Buffer Contributions to Whole Blood Buffering

Buffer Type	Total Buffering (%)
Bicarbonate	
Plasma bicarbonate	35
Erythrocyte bicarbonate	18
Total bicarbonate buffering	*53*
Nonbicarbonate	
Hemoglobin	35
Organic phosphates	3
Inorganic phosphates	2
Plasma proteins	7
Total nonbicarbonate buffering	*47*
Total	*100*

From Beachey W: Respiratory care anatomy and physiology: foundations for clinical practice, ed 2, St Louis, 2007, Mosby.

pH of a Buffer System: Henderson-Hasselbalch Equation

Buffer solutions in body fluids consist of mostly undissociated acid molecules and only a small amount of H^+ and conjugate base anions. The $[H^+]$ of a buffer solution can be calculated if the concentrations of the buffer's components and the acid's equilibrium constant are known. Consider the bicarbonate buffer system. As described earlier, the equilibrium constant (K_A) for H_2CO_3 is as follows:

$$K_A = \frac{[H^+]\times[HCO_3^-]}{[H_2CO_3]}$$

$[H^+]$ can be calculated by algebraic rearrangement of this equation, as follows:

$$[H^+] = K_A \times \frac{[H_2CO_3]}{[HCO_3]}$$

$[H^+]$ is determined by the ratio between undissociated acid molecules $[H_2CO_3]$ and base anions $[HCO_3^-]$. This equation is the basis for deriving the **Henderson-Hasselbalch (H-H) equation:**

$$pH = 6.1 + \log\frac{[HCO_3^-]}{Pa_{CO_2} \times 0.03}$$

pH is a logarithmic expression of $[H^+]$, and the term *6.1* is the logarithmic expression of the H_2CO_3 equilibrium constant. Because dissolved carbon dioxide ($P_{CO_2} \times 0.03$) is in equilibrium with and directly proportional to blood $[H_2CO_3]$, and because blood P_{CO_2} is more easily measured than $[H_2CO_3]$, dissolved CO_2 is used in the denominator of the H-H equation. The H-H equation is specific for calculating the pH of the bicarbonate buffer system of the blood. The calculation of this pH is important because it equals the pH of blood plasma; because all buffer systems in the blood are in equilibrium with the same pH, the pH

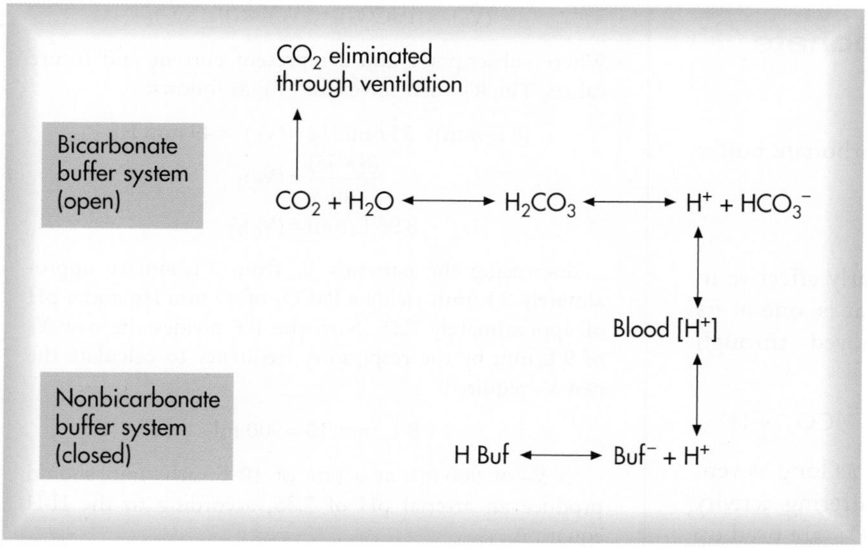

FIGURE 13-1 The bicarbonate and nonbicarbonate buffer systems exist in equilibrium in the plasma. (Modified from Beachey W: Respiratory care anatomy and physiology: foundations for clinical practice, ed 2, St Louis, 2007, Mosby.)

of one buffer system is the same as the pH of the entire plasma solution (the isohydric principle).[1]

Clinical Use of Henderson-Hasselbalch Equation

The H-H equation allows the pH, $[HCO_3^-]$, or PCO_2 to be computed if two of these three variables are known (shown as follows for PCO_2 and HCO_3^-):

$$[HCO_3^-] = \text{antilog}\,(pH - 6.1) \times (PCO_2 \times 0.03)$$

$$PCO_2 = \frac{[HCO_3^-]}{(\text{antilog}\,[pH - 6.1] \times 0.03)}$$

Blood gas analyzers *measure* pH and PCO_2 but *compute* $[HCO_3^-]$. Assuming a normal arterial pH of 7.40 and a $PaCO_2$ of 40 mm Hg, arterial $[HCO_3^-]$ can be calculated as follows:

$$pH = 6.1 + \log\left(\frac{[HCO_3^-]}{PCO_2 \times 0.03}\right)$$

$$7.40 = 6.1 + \log\left(\frac{[HCO_3^-]}{[40 \times 0.03]}\right)$$

$$7.40 = 6.1 + \log\left(\frac{[HCO_3^-]}{1.2}\right)$$

Solving for $[HCO_3^-]$:

$$\begin{aligned}[HCO_3^-] &= \text{antilog}\,(7.40 - 6.1) \times 1.2\\ &= \text{antilog}\,(1.3) \times 1.2\\ &= 20 \times 1.2\\ &= 24\ \text{mEq/L}\end{aligned}$$

The H-H equation is useful for checking a clinical blood gas report to see if the pH, PCO_2, and $[HCO_3^-]$ values are compatible with one another. In this way, transcription errors and analyzer inaccuracies can be detected. It is also clinically useful to predict what effect changing one H-H equation component will have on the other components. For example, a clinician may want to know how low the arterial blood pH will fall for a given increase in $PaCO_2$.

Physiologic Roles of Bicarbonate and Nonbicarbonate Buffer Systems

The functions of bicarbonate and nonbicarbonate buffer systems are summarized in Table 13-2.

Bicarbonate Buffer System

The bicarbonate buffer system is particularly effective in the body because it is an open system—that is, one of its components (CO_2) is continually removed through ventilation:

$$(\text{Exhaled gas}) \leftarrow CO_2 + H_2O \leftarrow H_2CO_3 \leftarrow HCO_3^- + H^+$$

In this way, HCO_3^- continues to buffer H^+ as long as ventilation continues. Hypothetically, this buffering activity can continue until all body sources of HCO_3^- are used up in binding H^+.

TABLE 13-2

Buffering Functions

Buffer	Type of System	Acids Buffered
Bicarbonate	Open	Fixed (nonvolatile)
Nonbicarbonate	Closed	Volatile (carbonic) Fixed

From Beachey W: Respiratory care anatomy and physiology: foundations for clinical practice, ed 2, St Louis, 2007, Mosby.

MINI CLINI

Applying the Henderson-Hasselbalch Equation in a Clinical Setting

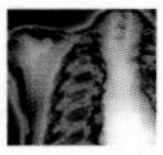

PROBLEM: The respiratory therapist (RT) is caring for a mechanically ventilated patient. The patient has a tidal volume (V_T) of 800 ml and a breathing frequency of 10/min, yielding a minute ventilation ($\dot{V}_E$) of 8 L/min. The patient's $PaCO_2$ is 55 mm Hg, pH is 7.30, and bicarbonate is 26 mEq/L, and the therapist wishes to maintain a pH of 7.35. How much does the RT need to change the $PaCO_2$ to achieve this desired pH, and what change in the patient's V_T does this require?

SOLUTION: First, the therapist needs to calculate the $PaCO_2$ required to achieve a pH of 7.35 using the known values:

$$PaCO_2 = \frac{26\ \text{mEq/L}}{0.03 \times \text{antilog}\,(7.35 - 6.1)}$$

$$PaCO_2 = \frac{26}{0.53}$$

$$PaCO_2 = 49\ \text{mm Hg}$$

Next, the RT must calculate the $\dot{V}_E$ required to produce a $PaCO_2$ of 49 mm Hg. Because $\dot{V}_E$ is inversely proportional to $PaCO_2$, the following can be stated:

$$(\dot{V}_E)_1 \times (PaCO_2)_1 = (\dot{V}_E)_2 \times (PaCO_2)_2$$

Where subscripts 1 and 2 represent current and future values. The RT then solves for $(\dot{V})_2$ as follows:

$$(8\ \text{L/min}) \times 55\ \text{mm Hg} = (\dot{V}_E)^2 \times 49\ \text{mm Hg}$$

$$\frac{(8 \times 55)}{49} = (\dot{V}_E)_2$$

$$8.98\ \text{L/min} = (\dot{V}_E)_2$$

Increasing the patient's $\dot{V}_E$ from 8 L/min to approximately 9 L/min yields a $PaCO_2$ of 49 mm Hg and a pH of approximately 7.35. Now the RT divides the new $\dot{V}_E$ of 9 L/min by the respiratory frequency to calculate the new V_T required:

$$9\ \text{L/min}/10 = 900\ \text{ml}$$

A V_T of 900 mL at a rate of 10 breaths/min should produce an arterial pH of 7.35, according to the H-H equation.

The bicarbonate buffer system can buffer only fixed acid. An increased fixed acid load in the body (e.g., lactic acid) reacts with HCO_3^- of the bicarbonate buffer system:

$$\underset{\substack{\uparrow \\ \text{Fixed acid}}}{H^+} + HCO_3^- \rightarrow H_2CO_3 \rightarrow H_2O + \overset{\substack{\text{Ventilation} \\ \uparrow}}{CO_2}$$

As shown, the process of buffering fixed acid produces CO_2, which is eliminated in exhaled gas. Large amounts of acid are buffered in this fashion. If the ability to ventilate is impaired, this type of buffering cannot occur.

The bicarbonate buffer system cannot buffer carbonic (volatile) acid, which accumulates in the blood whenever ventilation fails to eliminate CO_2 as fast as it is produced (hypoventilation). The resulting accumulation of CO_2 drives the hydration reaction in the direction that produces more carbonic acid, H^+, and HCO_3^-, as shown:

$$\overset{\substack{\text{Hypoventilation} \\ \downarrow}}{CO_2} + H_2O \rightarrow H_2CO_3 \rightarrow HCO_3^- + H^+$$

H^+ produced by dissociating H_2CO_3 molecules cannot be buffered by the simultaneously produced HCO_3^- because hypoventilation prevents the reaction from reversing its direction. The closed nonbicarbonate buffer systems are the only buffers that can buffer carbonic acid.

Nonbicarbonate Buffer System

Table 13-1 lists the nonbicarbonate buffers in the blood. Of these, *Hb* is the most important because it is the most abundant. As mentioned, these buffers are the only ones available to buffer carbonic acid. However, they can buffer H^+ produced by any acid, fixed or volatile. Because nonbicarbonate buffers (Buf^-/HBuf) function in closed systems, the products of their buffering activity eventually accumulate, slowing or stopping further buffering activity:

$$H^+ + Buf^- \leftrightarrow HBuf$$

This slowing or stopping of buffering activity means that not all of the Buf^- is available for buffering activity. At equilibrium (denoted by the *double arrow*), Buf^- still exists in solution but cannot combine further with H^+. In contrast, most of the HCO_3^- in the bicarbonate buffer system is available for buffering activity because it functions in an open system where equilibrium between reactants and products does not occur. Both open and closed systems function in a common fluid compartment (blood plasma) as illustrated in the following equation:

$$\begin{array}{l}
\quad(CO_2 \text{ removed by ventilation}) \quad (\text{from body's } HCO_3^- \text{ stores}) \\
\qquad\qquad \uparrow \qquad\qquad\qquad\qquad\qquad \downarrow \\
\text{Open system: } CO_2 + H_2O \leftarrow H^+ + HCO_3^- \\
\qquad\qquad\qquad\qquad\qquad\quad \uparrow \\
\qquad\qquad\qquad\qquad \text{Added fixed acid} \\
\qquad\qquad\qquad\qquad\qquad\quad \downarrow \\
\text{Closed system: } HBuf \leftrightarrow H^+ + Buf^- \\
\qquad\qquad\qquad\qquad\qquad\qquad\quad \uparrow \\
\qquad\qquad\qquad (\text{from body's } Buf^- \text{ stores})
\end{array}$$

Most of the added fixed acid is buffered by HCO_3^- because ventilation continually pulls the reaction to the left. Smaller amounts of H^+ react with Buf^- because equilibrium is approached, slowing the reaction.

ACID EXCRETION

Bicarbonate and nonbicarbonate buffer systems are the immediate defense against the accumulation of H^+. However, if the body fails to eliminate the remaining acids, these buffers are soon exhausted, and the pH of body fluids quickly decreases to life-threatening levels.

The lungs and kidneys are the primary acid-excreting organs. The lungs can excrete only volatile acid (i.e., the CO_2 from dissociating H_2CO_3). However, as discussed previously, bicarbonate buffers effectively buffer the H^+ originating from fixed acid, converting it to H_2CO_3 and to CO_2 and H_2O. By eliminating the CO_2, the lungs can rapidly remove large quantities of fixed acid from the blood. The kidneys also remove fixed acids but at a slow pace. In healthy individuals, the acid excretion mechanisms of lungs and kidneys are delicately balanced. In individuals affected by disease, failure of one system can be partially offset by a compensatory response of the other.

Lungs

Because the volatile acid H_2CO_3 is in equilibrium with dissolved CO_2, the lungs can decrease blood H_2CO_3 concentration through ventilation. The elimination of CO_2 is crucial because normal aerobic metabolism produces large quantities of CO_2, which reacts with H_2O to form large quantities of H_2CO_3. The reaction between fixed acids and bicarbonate buffers also produces H_2CO_3. H_2CO_3 generated by both pathways is eliminated as CO_2 through the lungs. Approximately 24,000 mmol/L of CO_2 is removed from the body daily through normal ventilation. CO_2 excretion of the lungs does not remove H^+ from the body. Instead, the chemical reaction that breaks down H_2CO_3 to form CO_2 binds H^+ in the harmless H_2O molecule:

$$H^+ + HCO_3^- \rightarrow H_2CO_3 \rightarrow H_2O + CO_2$$

Kidneys

The kidneys physically remove H^+ from the body. The following terms refer to certain kidney functions:

- *Excretion* is the elimination of substances from the body in the urine.
- *Secretion* is the process by which renal tubule cells actively transport substances into the fluid of the tubule lumen, or filtrate.
- *Reabsorption* is the active or passive transport of filtrate substances back into the tubule cell and into the blood of nearby capillaries.

The amount of H^+ the kidney tubules secrete into the filtrate depends on the blood's pH. Secreted H^+ may originate from H_2CO_3 (when the blood PCO_2 is increased) or from fixed acids. The kidneys excrete less than 100 mEq of fixed acid per day, which is a small amount compared with volatile H_2CO_3 elimination by the lungs.[3] In addition to excreting H^+, the kidneys influence blood pH by retaining or excreting HCO_3^-. If the blood PCO_2 is high, creating high levels of H_2CO_3, the kidneys excrete greater amounts of H^+ and reabsorb all of the tubule filtrate's HCO_3^- back into the blood. The opposite happens when the blood PCO_2 is low. The kidneys excrete less H^+ and more HCO_3^-. Compared with the ability of the lungs to change blood PCO_2 in seconds, the renal process is slow, requiring hours to days.

Basic Kidney Function

To understand how the kidneys determine whether to excrete acidic or basic urine, some fundamental facts about renal function must be understood. The *glomerulus* is the component of the renal nephron responsible for filtering the blood. Hydrostatic blood pressure forces water, electrolytes, and other nonprotein substances through semipermeable glomerular capillary endothelium. The resulting filtrate is greatly modified in volume and composition as it flows through the nephron tubules. Excreted filtrate is called *urine.*

HCO_3^- is one of the electrolytes filtered from the blood at the glomerulus to become part of the tubular filtrate. In this way, base (HCO_3^-) is removed from the blood. This loss of base is offset by the simultaneous secretion of the nephron tubular epithelium of H^+ into the tubular lumen and into the filtrate. Under normal conditions, the rate of H^+ secretion is almost the same as the rate of HCO_3^- filtration.[4] In this way, the kidneys titrate H^+ and HCO_3^- against each other to form CO_2 and H_2O.

H^+ secretion begins with the diffusion of blood CO_2 into the tubule cell (Figure 13-2). Aided by the enzyme carbonic anhydrase, CO_2 reacts with H_2O to form carbonic acid, which forms HCO_3^- and H^+. The tubule cell actively secretes H^+ into the filtrate by means of *countertransport,* in which Na^+ and H^+ are simultaneously transported in opposite directions. That is, Na^+ and H^+ combine with opposite ends of a carrier protein in the luminal border of the tubule cell membrane. Sodium ions move into the cell down its high concentration gradient, providing the energy to secrete H^+ into the tubular filtrate (see Figure 13-2).[4]

The rate of tubular H^+ secretion increases if the concentration of H^+ in the blood plasma increases. Conversely, the rate of H^+ secretion decreases if blood plasma $[H^+]$ decreases (Figure 13-3). Any factor that increases $PaCO_2$, such as hypoventilation, increases H^+ secretion, and any factor that decreases $PaCO_2$, such as hyperventilation, decreases H^+ secretion.

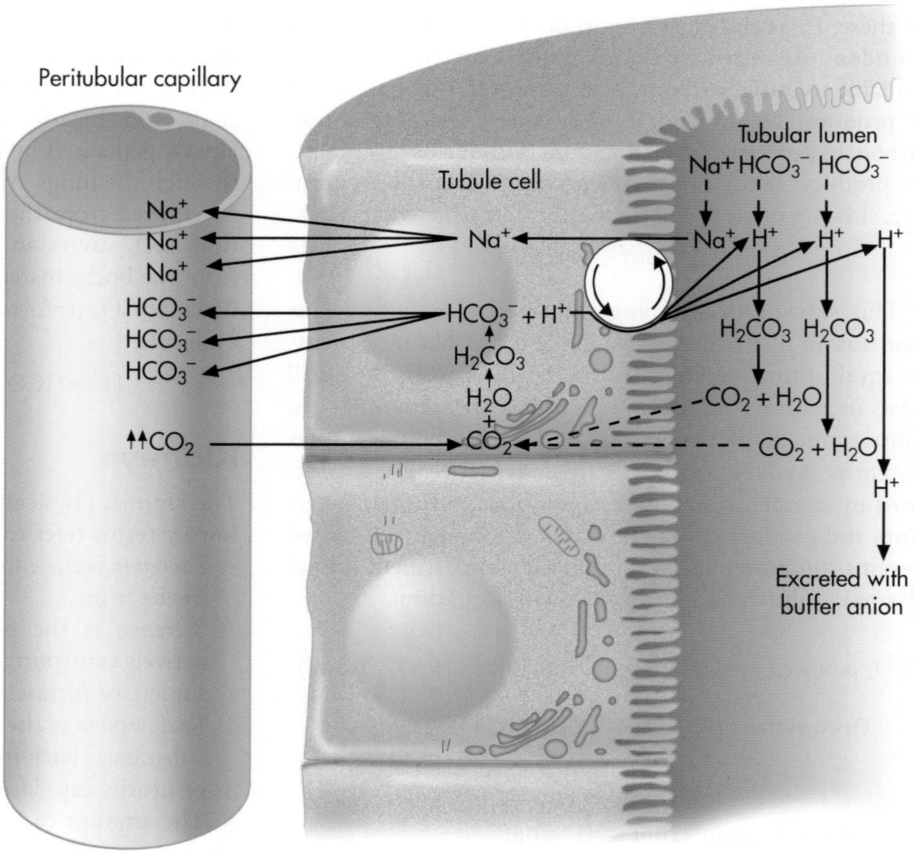

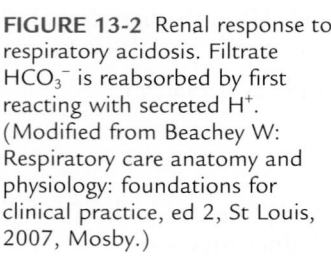

FIGURE 13-2 Renal response to respiratory acidosis. Filtrate HCO_3^- is reabsorbed by first reacting with secreted H^+. (Modified from Beachey W: Respiratory care anatomy and physiology: foundations for clinical practice, ed 2, St Louis, 2007, Mosby.)

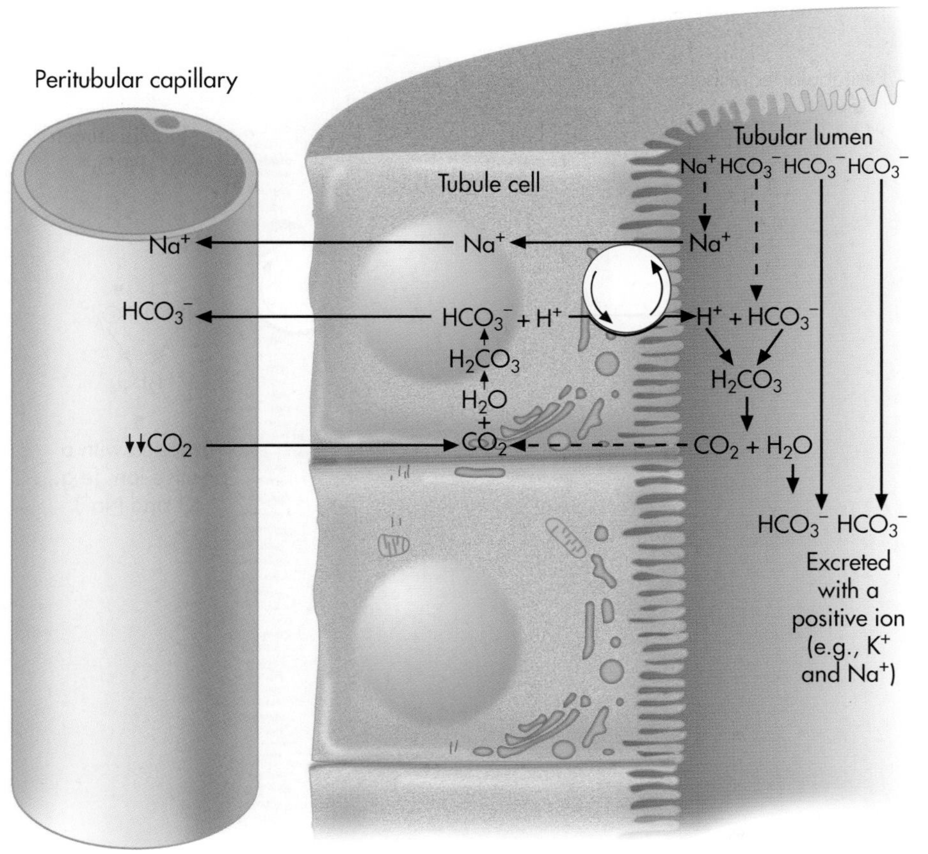

FIGURE 13-3 Renal response to respiratory alkalosis. Excess HCO_3^- is excreted in the urine with a positive ion. (Modified from Beachey W: Respiratory care anatomy and physiology: foundations for clinical practice, ed 2, St Louis, 2007, Mosby.)

HCO_3^- formed in the tubule cell from the reaction between CO_2 and H_2O (see Figure 13-2) diffuses back into the blood plasma because the luminal side of the tubule cell is relatively impermeable to HCO_3^-. HCO_3^- and Na^+ are reabsorbed whenever H^+ is secreted into the tubular filtrate.

Reabsorption of Bicarbonate Ion

Because the luminal side of the renal tubule cell is relatively impermeable to HCO_3^-, these ions are reabsorbed indirectly, as shown in Figure 13-2. The HCO_3^- in the filtrate reacts with the H^+ secreted by the tubular cells. The resulting carbonic acid breaks down into CO_2 and H_2O. Because CO_2 is extremely diffusible through biologic membranes, it diffuses instantly into the tubule cell. There, CO_2 reacts rapidly with H_2O in the presence of carbonic anhydrase, rapidly forming HCO_3^- and H^+. The HCO_3^- diffuses back through the nonluminal side of the tubule cell into the blood. The reabsorbed HCO_3^- ion is not the same HCO_3^- ion that existed in the tubular fluid. If the tubule cells secrete sufficient H^+, all HCO_3^- in the tubular fluid is reabsorbed in this manner.

The net effect of secreting H^+ (caused by high blood CO_2 or *hypoventilation,* as shown in Figure 13-2) is to reabsorb all filtrate HCO_3^-, increasing the quantity of HCO_3^- in the blood. According to the H-H equation, this brings blood pH up toward the normal range.

If blood CO_2 is low, as is the case in a state of *hyperventilation* (see Figure 13-3), the ratio of HCO_3^- to dissolved CO_2 molecules increases, and the renal filtrate has more HCO_3^- than H^+. Because HCO_3^- cannot be reabsorbed without first reacting with H^+, the excess HCO_3^- is excreted in the urine, carrying positive ions such as Na^+ or K^+ in the filtrate. The net effect of secreting less H^+ is to increase the quantity of HCO_3^- (base) lost in the urine. According to the H-H equation, this brings blood pH down toward the normal range. These renal responses to high and low blood PCO_2 are the mechanisms by which the kidneys compensate for respiratory acid-base disturbances.

Excess Hydrogen Ion Excretion and Role of Urinary Buffers

If no buffers existed in the filtrate to react with H^+, the H^+-secreting mechanism would soon cease to function because when the filtrate pH decreases to 4.5, H^+ secretion stops.[4] Buffers in the tubular fluid are essential for the secretion and elimination of excess H^+ in acidotic states.

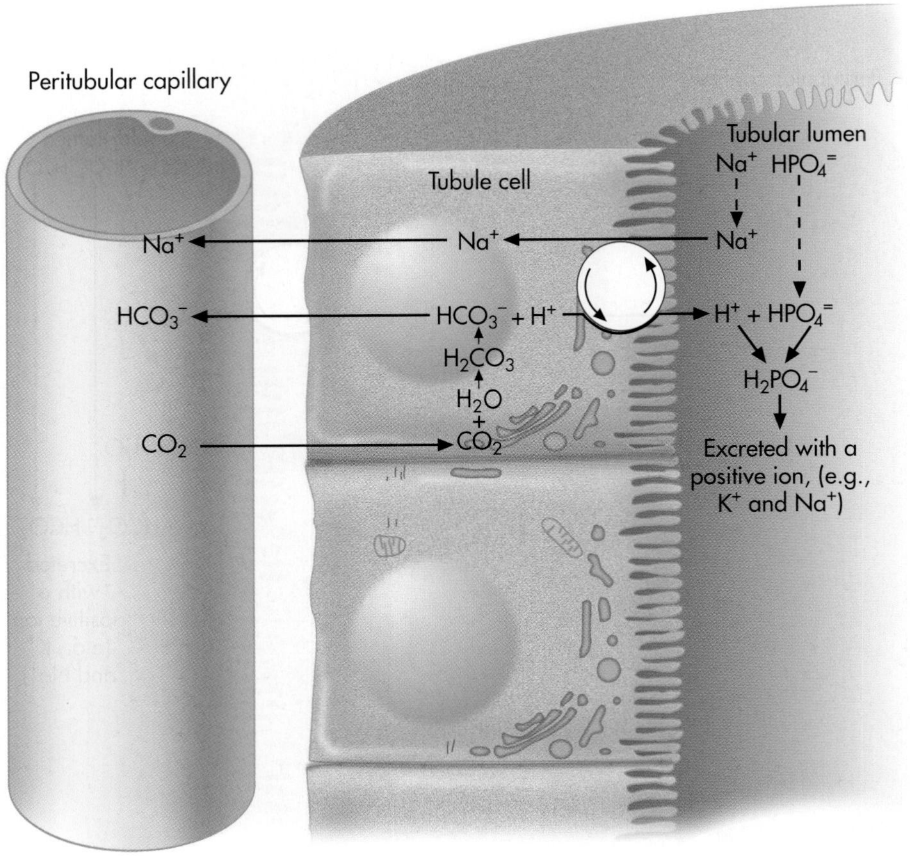

FIGURE 13-4 Phosphate buffer system. After bicarbonate buffers are exhausted, the remaining H^+ reacts with urinary phosphate buffers. (Modified from Beachey W: Respiratory care anatomy and physiology: foundations for clinical practice, ed 2, St Louis, 2007, Mosby.)

In Figure 13-2, more H^+ than HCO_3^- is present in the filtrate. After all available HCO_3^- reacts with H^+, the remaining H^+ reacts with two other filtrate buffers, phosphate and ammonia, as illustrated in Figures 13-4 and 13-5. In Figure 13-4, phosphate and H^+ react to form $H_2PO_4^-$, which must be excreted with a positive ion to maintain tubular electroneutrality. Figure 13-5 shows that when urinary buffers are depleted, the resulting fall in filtrate pH stimulates the tubules to secrete ammonia. The NH_3 molecule buffers H^+ by reacting with it to form the ammonium ion (NH_4^+). To maintain electroneutrality, the kidney excretes a negatively charged ion to accompany NH_4^+. This negative ion is chloride (Cl^-), the most abundant filtrate anion.

When NH_4^+ reacts with H^+, HCO_3^- diffuses from the tubule cell into the blood (see Figure 13-5). The net effect of ammonia buffer activity is to cause more bicarbonate to be reabsorbed into the blood, counteracting the acidic state of the blood. Figure 13-5 shows that when Cl^- is excreted in combination with NH_4^-, the blood gains HCO_3^-. Blood [Cl^-] and [HCO_3^-] are reciprocally related (i.e., when one is high, the other is low). This relationship explains why people with chronically high blood PCO_2 tend to have low blood [Cl^-] or *hypochloremia*. Activation of the ammonia buffer system enhances Cl^- loss and HCO_3^- gain.

ACID-BASE DISTURBANCES

In healthy individuals, the body buffer systems, the lungs, and the kidneys work together to maintain acid-base homeostasis under various conditions.

Normal Acid-Base Balance

Normally, the kidneys maintain an arterial bicarbonate concentration of approximately 22 to 26 mEq/L, whereas lung ventilation maintains an arterial PCO_2 of approximately 35 to 45 mm Hg. These normal values produce an arterial pH of 7.35 to 7.45, as shown by the H-H equation as follows:

$$pH = 6.1 + \log\frac{[HCO_3^-]}{PCO_2 \times 0.03}$$

$$pH = 6.1 + \log\frac{24}{1.2}$$

$$pH = 6.1 + \log[20]$$

$$pH = 7.40$$

The pH is determined by the ratio of [HCO_3^-] to dissolved CO_2, rather than by the absolute values of these components. As long as the ratio of HCO_3^- buffer to dissolved CO_2 is 20 : 1, the pH is normal, or 7.40. Because the kidneys control blood [HCO_3^-] and the lungs control

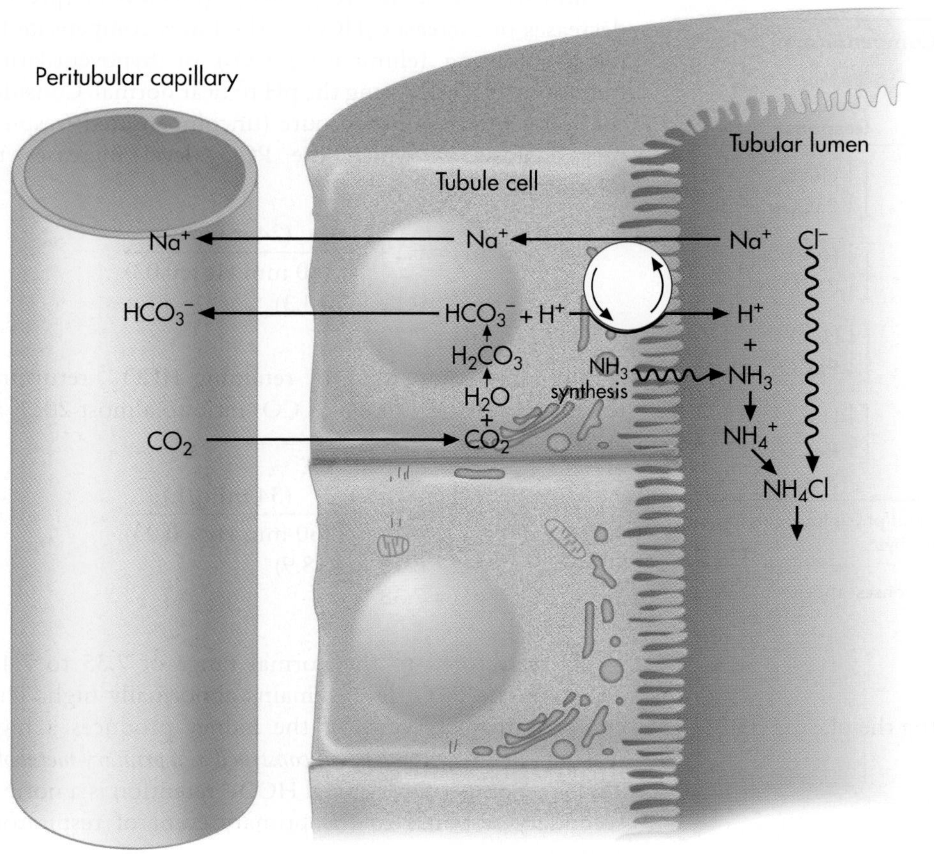

FIGURE 13-5 Tubule cells secrete ammonia in response to low-filtrate pH. NH_3 molecules buffer H^+, forming NH_4^+, which is excreted with Cl^-. (Modified from Beachey W: Respiratory care anatomy and physiology: foundations for clinical practice, ed 2, St Louis, 2007, Mosby.)

blood CO_2 levels, the H-H equation can be conceptually rewritten as follows:

$$pH \propto \frac{\text{Kidney control of } [HCO_3^-]}{\text{Lung control of } PCO_2}$$

An increase in $[HCO_3^-]$ or a decrease in PCO_2 increases the pH, leading to **alkalemia.** This condition produces an $[HCO_3^-]/(PCO_2 \times 0.03)$ ratio greater than 20:1 (e.g., 25:1). A decreased $[HCO_3^-]$ or an increased PCO_2 decreases the pH, leading to **acidemia.** This condition produces an $[HCO_3^-]/(PCO_2 \times 0.03)$ ratio less than 20:1 (e.g., 15:1). The normal ranges for arterial pH, PCO_2, and $[HCO_3^-]$ are as follows:

$$pH = 7.35 \text{ to } 7.45$$
$$PaCO_2 = 35 \text{ to } 45 \text{ mm Hg}$$
$$[HCO_3^-] = 22 \text{ to } 26 \text{ mEq/L}$$

Alkalemia is defined as a blood pH greater than 7.45. *Acidemia* is defined as a blood pH less than 7.35. *Hyperventilation* is defined as $PaCO_2$ less than 35 mm Hg. *Hypoventilation* is defined as $PaCO_2$ greater than 45 mm Hg.

Primary Respiratory Disturbances

Abnormal arterial pH levels caused by changes in $PaCO_2$ are *primary respiratory disturbances* because the lungs control $PaCO_2$. Respiratory disturbances affect the denominator of the H-H equation. A high $PaCO_2$ increases dissolved CO_2, decreasing the pH:

$$\downarrow pH \propto \frac{\rightarrow HCO_3^-}{\uparrow PaCO_2}$$

Where ↓ means *decreased,* → means *no change,* and ↑ means *increased.* Respiratory disturbance causing acidemia is called **respiratory acidosis.** A low $PaCO_2$ decreases dissolved CO_2, raising the pH; this is called **respiratory alkalosis:**

$$\uparrow pH \propto \frac{\rightarrow HCO_3^-}{\downarrow PaCO_2}$$

*Hypo*ventilation causes respiratory acidosis, whereas *hyper*ventilation causes respiratory alkalosis.

Primary Metabolic (Nonrespiratory) Disturbances

Nonrespiratory processes change arterial pH by changing $[HCO_3^-]$. These are called *primary metabolic disturbances.* In this context, the term *metabolic* is arbitrary, but by convention, it refers to all nonrespiratory acid-base disturbances. These kinds of disturbances involve a gain or loss of fixed acids or HCO_3^-. Such processes affect the numerator of the H-H equation. An accumulation of fixed acid in the body

TABLE 13-3

Primary Acid-Base Disorders and Compensatory Responses

Acid-Base Disorder	Primary Defect	Compensatory Response
Respiratory acidosis	$\left[\begin{matrix}\rightarrow HCO_3^- \\ \uparrow \mathbf{PaCO_2}\end{matrix}\right] = \downarrow pH$	$\left[\begin{matrix}\uparrow \mathbf{HCO_3^-} \\ \uparrow PaCO_2\end{matrix}\right] = \rightarrow pH$
Respiratory alkalosis	$\left[\begin{matrix}\rightarrow HCO_3^- \\ \downarrow \mathbf{PaCO_2}\end{matrix}\right] = \uparrow pH$	$\left[\begin{matrix}\downarrow \mathbf{HCO_3^-} \\ \downarrow PaCO_2\end{matrix}\right] = \rightarrow pH$
Metabolic acidosis	$\left[\begin{matrix}\downarrow \mathbf{HCO_3^-} \\ \rightarrow PaCO_2\end{matrix}\right] = \downarrow pH$	$\left[\begin{matrix}\downarrow HCO_3^- \\ \downarrow \mathbf{PaCO_2}\end{matrix}\right] = \rightarrow pH$
Metabolic alkalosis	$\left[\begin{matrix}\uparrow \mathbf{HCO_3^-} \\ \rightarrow PaCO_2\end{matrix}\right] = \uparrow pH$	$\left[\begin{matrix}\uparrow HCO_3^- \\ \uparrow \mathbf{PaCO_2}\end{matrix}\right] = \rightarrow pH$

From Beachey W: Respiratory care anatomy and physiology: foundations for clinical practice, ed 2, St Louis, 2007, Mosby.
→, No change; ↓, decrease; ↑, increase.
Note: Primary defects and compensatory responses appear in boldface type.

is buffered by bicarbonate, decreasing the plasma $[HCO_3^-]$ and the pH:

$$\downarrow pH \propto \frac{\downarrow HCO_3^-}{\rightarrow PaCO_2}$$

The same effect is created by a loss of HCO_3^-. Nonrespiratory processes causing acidemia are traditionally called **metabolic acidosis.**

In contrast, ingesting too much alkali (e.g., $NaHCO_3$ or other antacids) increases $[HCO_3^-]$ and pH:

$$\uparrow pH \propto \frac{\uparrow HCO_3^-}{\rightarrow PaCO_2}$$

Plasma $[HCO_3^-]$ can be increased by its *addition,* as in the previous example, or by its *generation,* as occurs when fixed acid is lost from the body.[5] An individual may lose HCl from the body by vomiting large amounts of gastric juice. This loss generates HCO_3^-, as discussed later (see Figure 13-8 further on).

Processes that increase arterial pH by losing fixed acid or gaining HCO_3^- produce a condition called **metabolic alkalosis.** Table 13-3 shows the four primary acid-base disturbances causing alkalemia and acidemia.

Compensation: Restoring pH to Normal

When any primary acid-base defect occurs, the body immediately initiates a compensatory response. In hypoventilation (respiratory acidosis), the kidneys restore the pH toward normal by reabsorbing HCO_3^- into the blood. In contrast, the compensatory renal response to hyperventilation (respiratory alkalosis) is urinary elimination of HCO_3^- (bicarbonate diuresis).

Similarly, if a nonrespiratory (metabolic) process decreases or increases $[HCO_3^-]$, the lungs compensate by hyperventilating (eliminating CO_2) or hypoventilating (retaining CO_2), restoring the pH to near normal. Consider the following example of pure (uncompensated) respiratory acidosis in which the PCO_2 level increases to 60 mm Hg:

$$\begin{aligned} pH &= 6.1 + \log\frac{(24\ mEq/L)}{(60\ mm\ Hg \times 0.03)} \\ pH &= 6.1 + \log(13.3) \\ pH &= 7.22 \end{aligned}$$

The kidneys compensate by retaining HCO_3^-, returning the plasma HCO_3^-/dissolved CO_2 ratio to almost 20:1, as shown:

$$\begin{aligned} pH &= 6.1 + \log\frac{(34\ mEq/L)}{(60\ mm\ Hg \times 0.03)} \\ pH &= 6.1 + \log(18.9) \\ pH &= 7.38 \end{aligned}$$

pH is restored to the normal range of 7.35 to 7.45, although the PCO_2 level remains abnormally high. This compensatory response of the kidney produces a high plasma $[HCO_3^-]$, *not to be misconstrued as a primary metabolic alkalosis.* Compensatory renal HCO_3^- retention is a normal secondary response to the primary event of respiratory acidosis.

The lungs normally compensate quickly for metabolic acid-base defects because ventilation can change the $PaCO_2$ within seconds. The kidneys require more time to retain or excrete significant amounts of HCO_3^- and compensate for respiratory defects at a much slower pace. Table 13-3 summarizes the four primary acid-base disturbances and the body's compensatory responses.

Effect of Carbon Dioxide Hydration Reaction on $[HCO_3^-]$

In the previous examples of pure (uncompensated) respiratory acidosis and alkalosis, it was assumed that $[HCO_3^-]$ did not change as the $PaCO_2$ level increased or decreased. Arterial $[HCO_3^-]$ does increase slightly as the $PaCO_2$ increases because the CO_2 hydration reaction generates HCO_3^-. This reaction occurs primarily in the red blood cell because the catalytic enzyme, carbonic anhydrase, is present:

$$\begin{aligned} &CO_2 + H_2O - (\text{carbonic anhydrase}) \rightarrow H_2CO_3 \\ &\quad \rightarrow H^+ + HCO_3^- \end{aligned}$$

As H^+ and HCO_3^- are rapidly produced, Hb immediately buffers H^+, generating HCO_3^- in the process:

$$CO_2 + H_2O \rightarrow H_2CO_3 \rightarrow H^+ + HCO_3^-\ \textit{(HCO}_3^-\textit{ generation)}$$
$$\downarrow$$
$$Hb^- + H^+ \rightarrow HHb\ \textit{(Hb buffering of H}^+\textit{)}$$

The amount of HCO_3^- increase depends on the amount of nonbicarbonate buffer that is available to accept the H^+

produced by the hydration reaction. Generally, when the nonbicarbonate buffer concentration is normal, and the PCO_2 increase is acute, the hydration reaction increases the plasma [HCO_3^-] approximately 1 mEq/L for every 10-mm Hg increase in PCO_2 higher than 40 mm Hg. Figure 13-6 illustrates this hydration reaction effect. Normal status is represented by point *A:* $PaCO_2$ of 40 mm Hg, pH of 7.40, and plasma HCO_3^- of 24 mEq/L. An acute increase in $PaCO_2$ from 40 mm Hg to 80 mm Hg proceeds from point *A,* moving to the left, up the normal blood buffer line (line *BAC*) to point *D,* where the buffer line intersects the $PaCO_2$ = 80 mm Hg isopleth. Point *D* indicates an HCO_3^- of approximately 28.5 mEq/L and a pH of approximately 7.18. This small change in [HCO_3^-] should not be erroneously interpreted as early renal compensation.

RULE OF THUMB

For an acute increase in PCO_2, the plasma [HCO_3^-] increases by about 1 mEq/L for every 10 mm Hg PCO_2 increment greater than 40 mm Hg.

CLINICAL ACID-BASE STATES

Systematic Acid-Base Classification

In analyzing an acid-base problem, it is helpful to use a series of systematic steps. Consistently applying them to all acid-base disturbances helps avoid the tendency to jump to conclusions. Four steps in acid-base classification are outlined in Box 13-2. The order of the steps is not as

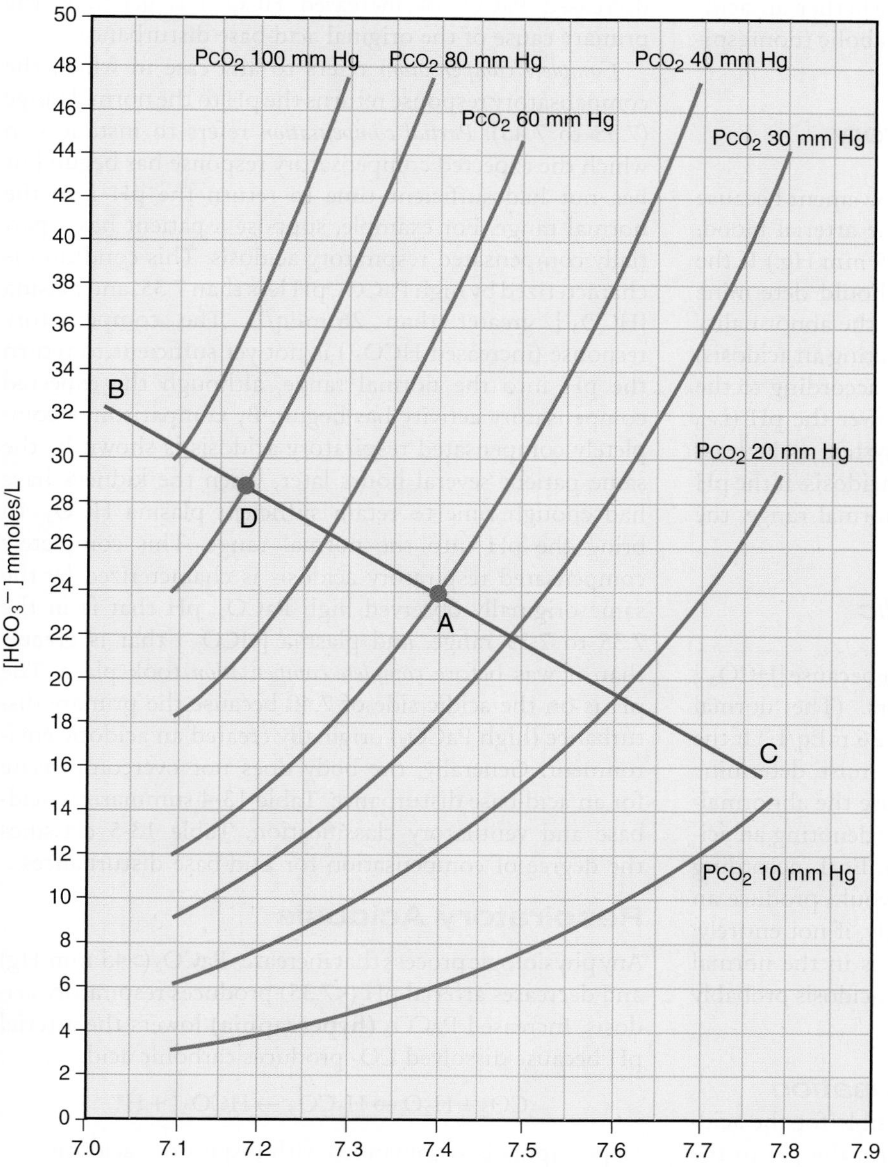

FIGURE 13-6 pH-PCO_2 diagram. Because of the hydration reaction between CO_2 and H_2O, acute increases in PCO_2 increase the plasma HCO_3^- concentration along line *CADB*. An acute increase in PCO_2 from 40 mm Hg to 80 mm Hg (point *A* to point *D*) increases [HCO_3^-] from 24 mEq/L to approximately 29 mEq/L. (Modified from Masoro EJ, Siegel PD: Acid-base regulation: its physiology and pathophysiology, Philadelphia, 1971, Saunders.)

Box 13-2 Systematic Acid-Base Classification

- Inspect the pH (acidemia, alkalemia, or normal).
- Inspect $PaCO_2$ (respiratory component). Can it explain the pH?
- Inspect HCO_3^- (metabolic component). Can it explain the pH?
- Check for compensation. Did the noncausative component respond appropriately?

From Beachey W: Respiratory care anatomy and physiology: foundations for clinical practice, ed 2, St Louis, 2007, Mosby.

important as following the same procedure for each situation.

Step 1: Categorize pH

If the pH is greater than 7.45, a state of alkalosis exists. If the pH is less than 7.35, a state of acidosis exists. Steps 2 through 4 help the clinician determine whether an acid-base abnormality is of respiratory or metabolic (nonrespiratory) origin.

Step 2: Determine Respiratory Involvement

$PaCO_2$ is the indicator of respiratory involvement because the lungs control the level of CO_2 in the arterial blood. (The normal range for $PaCO_2$ is 35 to 45 mm Hg.) If the arterial pH is abnormal, the clinician should determine whether the observed $PaCO_2$ could cause the abnormality by itself. If the pH was less than 7.35 (denoting an acidosis) and $PaCO_2$ was greater than 45 mm Hg, according to the H-H equation, the high $PaCO_2$ would lower the pH (i.e., produce an acidosis). The respiratory system is at least partly, if not entirely, responsible for the acidosis. If the pH is less than 7.35 and $PaCO_2$ is in the normal range, the acidosis probably is of metabolic origin.

Step 3: Determine Metabolic Involvement

Plasma $[HCO_3^-]$ is the metabolic indicator because $[HCO_3^-]$ is controlled by nonrespiratory factors. (The normal plasma $[HCO_3^-]$ of arterial blood is 22 to 26 mEq/L.) If the arterial pH is abnormal, the clinician must determine whether the observed $[HCO_3^-]$ could cause the abnormality by itself. If the pH was less than 7.35 (denoting an acidosis) and the $[HCO_3^-]$ was less than 22 mEq/L, according to the H-H equation, the low $[HCO_3^-]$ would produce an acidosis. Nonrespiratory factors are partly, if not entirely, responsible for the acidosis. If $[HCO_3^-]$ is in the normal range in the presence of this acidosis, the acidosis probably is of respiratory origin.

Step 4: Assess for Compensation

The system that is not primarily responsible for the acid-base imbalance usually attempts to return the pH to the normal range. Compensation may be complete (pH is brought into the normal range) or partial (pH is still out of the normal range but is in the process of moving toward the normal range). In a pure respiratory acidosis, the kidneys compensate by increasing the plasma $[HCO_3^-]$, restoring the pH to normal. Similarly, respiratory alkalosis elicits a compensatory decrease in plasma $[HCO_3^-]$. A pure metabolic acidosis normally stimulates a compensatory increase in ventilation, decreasing $PaCO_2$. A pure metabolic alkalosis causes a compensatory decrease in ventilation, increasing the $PaCO_2$. All compensatory responses work to restore the pH to the normal range.

In cases in which compensation has occurred, if the pH is on the acidic side of 7.40 (7.35 to 7.39), the component that would cause an acidosis (either increased $PaCO_2$ or decreased plasma HCO_3^-) is generally the primary cause of the original acid-base imbalance. If compensation is present but pH is on the alkalotic side of 7.40 (7.41 to 7.45), the component that would cause an alkalosis (either decreased $PaCO_2$ or increased HCO_3^-) is generally the primary cause of the original acid-base disturbance.

Complete compensation refers to any case in which the compensatory response returns the pH to the normal range (7.35 to 7.45). *Partial compensation* refers to instances in which the expected compensatory response has begun but has not had sufficient time to return the pH into the normal range. For example, suppose a patient has a partially compensated respiratory acidosis. This condition is characterized by high $PaCO_2$, pH less than 7.35, and plasma $[HCO_3^-]$ greater than 26 mEq/L. The compensatory response (increased HCO_3^-) is not yet sufficient to return the pH into the normal range, although the expected compensatory activity has begun. By comparison, a completely compensated respiratory acidosis is shown by the same patient several hours later, when the kidneys have had enough time to retain sufficient plasma HCO_3^- to bring the pH into the normal range. This completely compensated respiratory acidosis is characterized by the same originally observed high $PaCO_2$, pH that is in the 7.35 to 7.39 range, and plasma $[HCO_3^-]$ that is greater than it was before *complete compensation* took place. The pH is on the acidic side of 7.40 because the primary disturbance (high $PaCO_2$) originally created an acidotic environment. Generally, the body does not overcompensate for an acid-base disturbance. Table 13-4 summarizes acid-base and ventilatory classification. Table 13-5 classifies the degree of compensation for acid-base disturbances.

Respiratory Acidosis

Any physiologic process that increases $PaCO_2$ (>45 mm Hg) and decreases arterial pH (<7.35) produces respiratory acidosis. Increased $PaCO_2$ **(hypercapnia)** lowers the arterial pH because dissolved CO_2 produces carbonic acid:

$$CO_2 + H_2O \rightarrow H_2CO_3 \rightarrow HCO_3^- + H^+$$

Hypercapnia is synonymous with respiratory acidosis.

TABLE 13-4

Acid-Base and Ventilatory Classification

Component	Classification	Range
pH (arterial)	Normal status	7.35-7.45
	Acidemia	<7.35
	Alkalemia	>7.45
$PaCO_2$ (mm Hg)	Normal ventilatory status	35-45
	Respiratory acidosis (hypoventilation)	>45
	Respiratory alkalosis (hyperventilation)	<35
HCO_3^- (mEq/L)	Normal metabolic status	22-26
	Metabolic acidosis	<22
	Metabolic alkalosis	>26

From Beachey W: Respiratory care anatomy and physiology: foundations for clinical practice, ed 2, St Louis, 2007, Mosby.

TABLE 13-5

Degrees of Acid-Base Compensation

Compensating (Noncausative Component)	pH	Classification
Within normal range	Abnormal	Noncompensated (acute)
Out of normal range in the expected direction	Abnormal	Partially compensated
Out of normal range in the expected direction	Normal	Compensated (chronic)

From Beachey W: Respiratory care anatomy and physiology: foundations for clinical practice, ed 2, St Louis, 2007, Mosby.

MINI CLINI

Acute (Uncompensated) Respiratory Acidosis

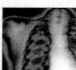

PROBLEM: A 35-year-old woman was admitted to the emergency department with a diagnosis of heroin overdose. Her breathing was shallow and slow. Arterial blood gas analysis showed a pH of 7.30, PCO_2 of 55 mm Hg, and HCO_3^- of 27 mEq/L. How would the RT assess this patient's respiratory condition?

SOLUTION: The RT should follow these steps:

1. Categorize the pH. The pH is below normal, indicating the presence of acidemia.
2. Determine respiratory involvement. $PaCO_2$ is elevated above normal, consistent with a low pH, indicating hypoventilation as a contributing factor to acidemia (respiratory acidosis).
3. Determine metabolic involvement. HCO_3^- is elevated slightly above normal. However, this is in the expected range for acute respiratory acidosis (1 mEq for each 10-mm Hg increase in PCO_2).
4. Assess for compensation. As explained in step 3, HCO_3^- is within the expected range for acute respiratory acidosis. There is no evidence of metabolic compensation.

Box 13-3 Common Causes of Respiratory Acidosis

NORMAL LUNGS

Central Nervous System Depression

Anesthesia
Sedative drugs
Narcotic analgesics

Neuromuscular Disease

Poliomyelitis
Myasthenia gravis
Guillain-Barré syndrome

Trauma

Spinal cord
Brain
Chest wall
Severe restrictive disorders
Obesity (pickwickian syndrome)
Kyphoscoliosis

ABNORMAL LUNGS

Chronic obstructive pulmonary disease
Acute airway obstruction (late phase)

Causes

Any process in which alveolar ventilation fails to eliminate CO_2 as rapidly as the body produces it causes respiratory acidosis. This acidosis could occur in different ways. A person's ventilation may be decreased from a drug-induced central nervous system depression, or a person with limited ventilatory reserve may have a normal $PaCO_2$ at rest but cannot accommodate the increased CO_2 production associated with increased physical activity. Box 13-3 summarizes causes of respiratory acidosis.

If hypercapnia is uncompensated, respiratory acidosis occurs with decreased pH, increased $PaCO_2$, and normal or slightly increased $[HCO_3^-]$. In this instance, the *slightly* increased $[HCO_3^-]$ is not a sign that the kidneys have started compensatory activity; it merely reflects the effect of CO_2 hydration reaction on $[HCO_3^-]$.

Compensation

Renal compensation for respiratory acidosis begins as soon as $PaCO_2$ increases. The kidney reabsorbs HCO_3^- from the renal tubular filtrate, bringing the arterial pH into the normal range (see Figure 13-2). However, this process cannot keep pace with an acutely increasing $PaCO_2$. Full compensation may take several days.

Partly compensated respiratory acidosis is characterized by increased $PaCO_2$, increased $[HCO_3^-]$, and an acid pH—still not quite up in the normal range. *Fully compensated* respiratory acidosis is characterized by a pH on the acidic side of the normal range (<7.40 but >7.35), increased $PaCO_2$, and increased $[HCO_3^-]$. Increased $[HCO_3^-]$ in the presence of increased $PaCO_2$ is a sign that the $PaCO_2$ has been elevated for a considerable time (i.e., the kidneys have had sufficient time to compensate). The underlying pathologic process producing hypercapnia is still present; the kidneys simply mask the problem by maintaining a normal-range pH. Because of hypercapnia, the term *acidosis* is retained in classifying this condition (compensated respiratory acidosis). This term emphasizes that lung function is still abnormal, and, if unopposed by the renal compensatory mechanism, it would produce an acidosis.

Correction

The main goal in correcting respiratory acidosis is to improve alveolar ventilation. Various respiratory care modalities may be employed ranging from bronchial hygiene and lung expansion techniques to noninvasive positive pressure ventilation to endotracheal intubation and mechanical ventilation. If hypoventilation is chronic and compensation has restored pH within the normal range, corrective action aimed at decreasing $PaCO_2$ is inappropriate and possibly harmful. In this instance, rapidly decreasing $PaCO_2$ to normal would induce an alkalosis because of the compensatory $[HCO_3^-]$ retention by the kidneys (Table 13-6).

TABLE 13-6

Expected Effect of Acute Changes in PaCO2 on Arterial pH

$PaCO_2$ Change	pH Change
Decrease	*Increase*
1 mm Hg	0.01
10 mm Hg	0.10
Increase	*Decrease*
1 mm Hg	0.006
10 mm Hg	0.06
Expected pH when measured $PaCO_2$ < 40 mm Hg	
Expected pH = 7.40 + (40 mm Hg − Measured $PaCO_2$)0.01	
Expected pH when measured $PaCO_2$ > 40 mm Hg	
Expected pH = 7.40 − (Measured $PaCO_2$ − 40 mm Hg)0.006	

MINI CLINI

Chronic (Compensated) Respiratory Acidosis

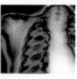

PROBLEM: A 73-year-old man is being treated on an outpatient basis for pulmonary emphysema, which was diagnosed 7 years earlier. His breathing is labored at rest, with marked use of accessory muscles. Arterial blood gas analysis showed a pH of 7.36, PCO_2 of 64 mm Hg, and HCO_3^- of 35 mEq/L. How would the RT assess this patient's respiratory condition?

SOLUTION: The RT should follow these steps:

1. Categorize the pH. The pH is on the acidic side of the normal range, but it is still normal.
2. Determine respiratory involvement. $PaCO_2$ is higher than normal, indicating hypoventilation as a contributing factor to the low-normal pH (respiratory acidosis).
3. Determine metabolic involvement. HCO_3^- is substantially elevated. By itself, this would cause alkalemia, but because pH is on the acidic side of normal, primary metabolic alkalosis is ruled out. Compensation for the respiratory acidosis has occurred.
4. Assess for compensation. HCO_3^- is approximately 8 to 10 mEq higher than normal. This is consistent with a compensatory response by the kidneys. In addition, the expected pH for a $PaCO_2$ of 64 mm Hg is [7.40 − (64 mm Hg − 40 mm Hg) 0.006], or 7.26 (see Table 13-6). Because the actual pH is 7.36, metabolic compensation (retention of HCO_3^-) must have occurred.

Respiratory Alkalosis

Any physiologic process that decreases $PaCO_2$ (<35 mm Hg) and increases arterial pH (>7.45) produces respiratory alkalosis. A low $PaCO_2$ **(hypocapnia)** forces the hydration reaction to the left, decreasing carbonic acid concentration and increasing the pH:

$$CO_2 + H_2O \leftarrow H_2CO_3 \leftarrow HCO_3^- + H^+$$

Hypocapnia is synonymous with respiratory alkalosis.

MINI CLINI

Acute (Uncompensated) Respiratory Alkalosis

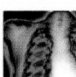

PROBLEM: A distraught 77-year-old man experiencing anxiety of apparent psychosomatic origin was brought to the hospital by his wife. The patient exhibited rapid and deep breathing, had slurred speech, and complained about tingling in his extremities. Arterial blood gas analysis showed a pH of 7.57, PCO_2 of 23 mm Hg, and HCO_3^- of 21 mEq/L. How would the RT assess this patient's acid-base condition?

SOLUTION: The RT should follow these steps:

1. Categorize the pH. The pH is substantially higher than normal, indicating the presence of an alkalemia.
2. Determine respiratory involvement. $PaCO_2$ is well below normal, which is consistent with the high pH, indicating hyperventilation as a contributing factor in alkalemia (respiratory alkalosis).
3. Determine metabolic involvement. HCO_3^- is slightly lower than normal. However, this is within the expected range for acute respiratory alkalosis (hydrolysis effect).
4. Assess for compensation. The decrease in HCO_3^- is within the expected range for acute respiratory alkalosis (1 mEq for each 5-mm Hg decline in PCO_2).

Causes

Any process in which ventilatory elimination of CO_2 exceeds production of CO_2 causes respiratory alkalosis. The most common cause of hyperventilation in patients

Box 13-4 Common Causes of Respiratory Alkalosis

NORMAL LUNGS
Anxiety
Fever
Stimulant drugs
Central nervous system lesion
Pain
Sepsis

ABNORMAL LUNGS
Hypoxemia-causing conditions
Acute asthma
Pneumonia
Stimulation of vagal lung receptors
Pulmonary edema
Pulmonary vascular disease

EITHER NORMAL OR ABNORMAL LUNGS
Iatrogenic hyperventilation

with pulmonary disease is decreased PaO_2 (hypoxemia). Hypoxemia causes specialized neural structures to signal the brain, increasing ventilation (see Chapter 14). Anxiety, fever, stimulatory drugs, pain, and central nervous system injuries are possible causes of hyperventilation. Other possible causes include stimulation of irritant receptors in the lung parenchyma, which may occur in pneumonia or pulmonary edema.

Hyperventilation and respiratory alkalosis also may be *iatrogenically* induced (induced by medical treatment). Iatrogenic hyperventilation is most commonly associated with overly aggressive mechanical ventilation. It may also be associated with aggressive deep breathing and lung expansion respiratory care procedures. Decreased $PaCO_2$, increased pH, and normal-range $[HCO_3^-]$ characterize acute respiratory alkalosis. A slight decrease in $[HCO_3^-]$ is expected from the effect of the hydration reaction. Box 13-4 summarizes causes of respiratory alkalosis.

Clinical Signs

An early sign of respiratory alkalosis is **paresthesia** (numbness or a tingling sensation in the extremities). Severe hyperventilation is associated with hyperactive reflexes and possibly tetanic convulsions. The low $PaCO_2$ may constrict cerebral vessels sufficiently to impair cerebral circulation, causing light-headedness and dizziness.

Compensation

The kidneys compensate for respiratory alkalosis by excreting HCO_3^- in the urine (bicarbonate diuresis; see Figure 13-3). This activity brings arterial pH down into the normal range. As with respiratory acidosis, renal compensation is a slow process. Complete compensation may take days.

Partly compensated respiratory alkalosis is characterized by decreased $PaCO_2$, decreased $[HCO_3^-]$, and alkaline pH—still not quite down in the normal range. Fully compensated respiratory alkalosis is characterized by decreased $PaCO_2$, decreased $[HCO_3^-]$, and pH on the alkaline side of normal (pH > 7.40 but ≤ 7.45). Compensated respiratory alkalosis is sometimes called *chronic respiratory alkalosis*. The underlying hyperventilation and hypocapnia are still present. The term *alkalosis* is used in classifying this condition, although the pH is within the normal range.

Correction

Correcting respiratory alkalosis involves removing the stimulus causing the hyperventilation. If hypoxemia is the stimulus, oxygen (O_2) therapy is needed.

MINI CLINI

Compensated (Chronic) Respiratory Alkalosis

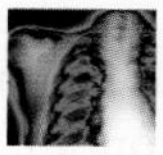

PROBLEM: A 27-year-old man was admitted to the hospital with a persistent case of bacterial pneumonia, which had not responded to 6 days of ambulatory care with antimicrobial drugs. He exhibited mild cyanosis and labored breathing. Arterial blood gas analysis (with the patient breathing room air) showed a pH of 7.44, $PaCO_2$ of 26 mm Hg, HCO_3^- of 17 mEq/L, and PaO_2 of 53 mm Hg. How would the RT assess this patient's acid-base condition?

SOLUTION: The RT should follow these steps:

1. Categorize the pH. The pH is on the alkalotic side of the normal range, but it is still normal.
2. Determine respiratory involvement. PCO_2 is well below normal, indicating hyperventilation as a contributing factor to the high-normal pH (respiratory alkalosis).
3. Determine metabolic involvement. HCO_3^- is substantially lower than normal, but because the pH is on the alkalotic side of normal, primary metabolic acidosis is ruled out. Compensation for the respiratory alkalosis has occurred.
4. Assess for compensation. HCO_3^- is approximately 7 mEq below normal. This is consistent with a compensatory response by the kidneys. In addition, the expected pH for $PaCO_2$ of 26 mm Hg is [7.40 + (40 mm Hg − 26 mm Hg) 0.01], or 7.54 (see Table 13-6). Because the actual pH is 7.44, metabolic compensation (excretion of HCO_3^-) must have occurred.

Alveolar Hyperventilation Superimposed on Compensated Respiratory Acidosis

Consider a patient with a compensated respiratory acidosis who has an arterial pH of 7.38, $PaCO_2$ of 58 mm Hg, and HCO_3^- of 33 mEq/L. If this patient becomes severely hypoxic, the hypoxia may stimulate increased alveolar ventilation if lung mechanics are not too severely deranged. This increased alveolar ventilation would acutely lower $PaCO_2$, possibly increasing the pH to the alkalotic side of normal. For example, the patient's blood gas values might now be as follows: pH of 7.44, $PaCO_2$ of 50 mm Hg, and HCO_3^- of 33 mEq/L.

The novice might erroneously interpret these values as compensated metabolic alkalosis. This example shows that blood gas data alone are insufficient for rational acid-base assessment. Knowledge of the patient's medical history and the nature of the current problem is essential to evaluate this problem accurately. The blood gas values in this example are described as acute hyperventilation (although $PaCO_2$ is >45 mm Hg) superimposed on compensated respiratory acidosis.

Metabolic (Nonrespiratory) Acidosis

Any nonrespiratory process that decreases plasma $[HCO_3^-]$ causes metabolic acidosis. Reducing the $[HCO_3^-]$ decreases blood pH because it decreases the amount of base relative to the amount of acid in the blood.

Causes

Metabolic acidosis can occur in one of the following two ways: (1) fixed (nonvolatile) acid accumulation in the blood or (2) an excessive loss of HCO_3^- from the body. An example of fixed acid accumulation is a state of low blood flow in which tissue hypoxia and anaerobic metabolism produce lactic acid. The resulting H^+ accumulates and reacts with HCO_3^-, reducing blood $[HCO_3]$. An example of bicarbonate loss is severe diarrhea, in which large stores of HCO_3^- are eliminated from the body, also producing a nonrespiratory acidosis.

Because these two kinds of metabolic acidosis are treated differently, it is important to identify the underlying cause. Analysis of the plasma electrolytes is helpful in distinguishing between these two types of metabolic acidosis. Specifically, measuring the anion gap is helpful in making this distinction.

Anion Gap

The *law of electroneutrality* states that the total number of positive charges must equal the total number of negative charges in the body fluids. *Cations* (positively charged ions) in the plasma produce a charge exactly balanced by plasma *anions* (negatively charged ions). Plasma electrolytes (cations and anions) *routinely* measured in clinical medicine are Na^+, K^+, Cl^-, and HCO_3^-. Normal plasma concentrations of these electrolytes are such that the cations (Na^+ and K^+) outnumber the anions (Cl^- and HCO_3^-), leading to the so-called *anion gap.* Generally, K^+ is ignored in calculating the anion gap:

$$\text{Anion gap} = [Na^+] - ([Cl^-] + [HCO_3^-])$$

Figure 13-7, *A* shows that normal concentrations of these ions in the plasma are as follows: 140 mEq/L for Na^+, 105 mEq/L for Cl^-, and 24 mEq/L for HCO_3^-, yielding an anion gap of 11 mEq/L (140 mEq/L − [105 mEq/L + 24 mEq/L] = 11 mEq/L). The normal anion gap range is 9 to 14 mEq/L.[6]

An increased anion gap (>14 mEq/L) is caused by metabolic acidosis in which fixed acids accumulate in the body.

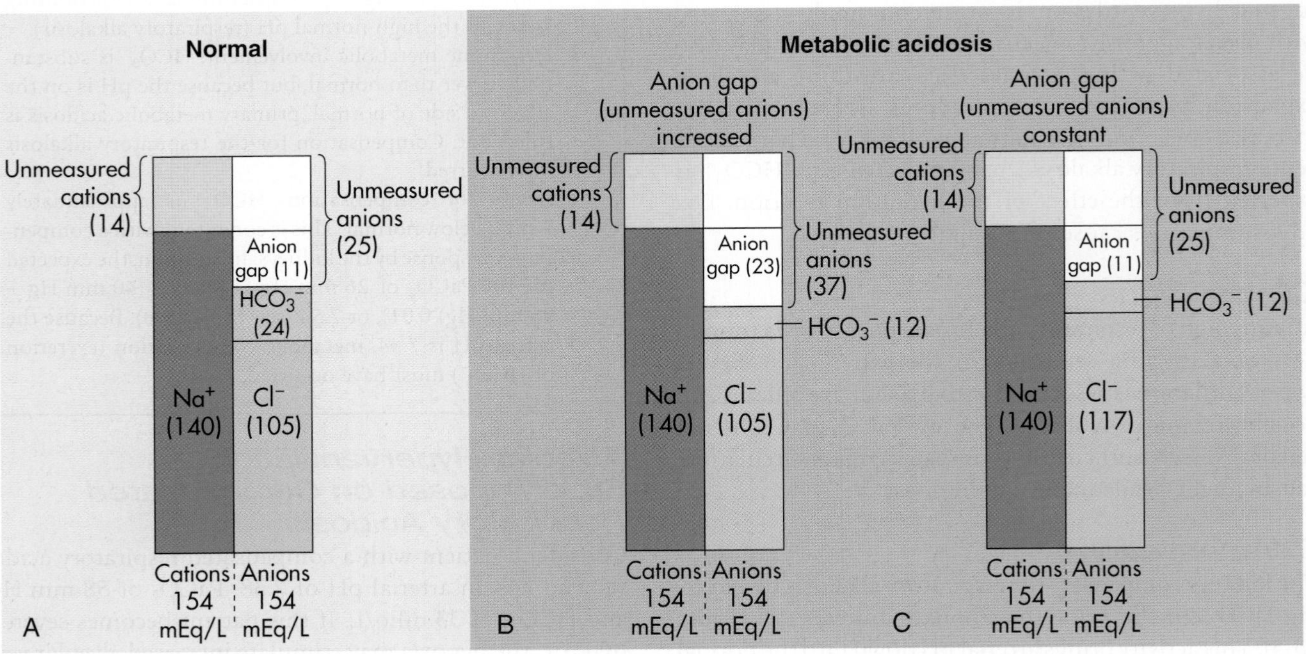

FIGURE 13-7 The anion gap in normal **(A)** and metabolic acidosis (**B** and **C**). Fixed acid accumulation increases the anion gap **(B),** whereas HCO_3^- loss is accompanied by an equal Cl^- gain, keeping the anion gap within the normal range. (Modified from Beachey W: Respiratory care anatomy and physiology: foundations for clinical practice, ed 2, St Louis, 2007, Mosby.)

Box 13-5 Causes of Anion Gap and Non–Anion Gap Metabolic Acidosis

HIGH ANION GAP

Metabolically Produced Acid Gain
Lactic acidosis
Ketoacidosis
Renal failure (e.g., retained sulfuric acid)

Ingestion of Acids
Salicylate (aspirin) intoxication
Methanol (formic acid)
Ethylene glycol (oxalic acid)

NORMAL ANION GAP (HYPERCHLOREMIC ACIDOSIS)

Gastrointestinal Loss of HCO_3^-
Diarrhea
Pancreatic fistula

Renal Tubular Loss: Failure to Reabsorb HCO_3^-
Renal tubular acidosis

Ingestion
Ammonium chloride
Hyperalimentation intravenous nutrition

From Beachey W: Respiratory care anatomy and physiology: foundations for clinical practice, ed 2, St Louis, 2007, Mosby.)

The H^+ of these acids reacts with plasma HCO_3^-, lowering its concentration; this leads to an increased anion gap (i.e., an increase in *unmeasured anions*) (see Figure 13-7, *B*). (When the H^+ of fixed acids is buffered by HCO_3^-, the anion portion of the fixed acid remains in the plasma, increasing unmeasured anion concentration.) A high anion gap indicates that fixed acid concentration in the body has increased.

Metabolic acidosis caused by HCO_3^- loss from the body does not cause an increased anion gap. Bicarbonate loss is accompanied by Cl^- gain, which keeps the anion gap within normal limits (see Figure 13-7, *C*). The law of electroneutrality helps explain the reciprocal nature of $[HCO_3^-]$ and $[Cl^-]$ in this instance. With a constant cation concentration, losing HCO_3^- means that another anion must be gained to maintain electroneutrality. In this case, the kidney increases its reabsorption of the most abundant anion in the tubular filtrate, the Cl^-. The kind of metabolic acidosis in which HCO_3^- is lost from the body is sometimes called *hyperchloremic acidosis* because of the characteristic increase in plasma $[Cl^-]$. Box 13-5 summarizes causes of anion gap and non–anion gap metabolic acidosis.

RULE OF THUMB

Metabolic acidosis accompanied by a high anion gap means that the body has accumulated an unusual fixed acid. A metabolic acidosis accompanied by a normal anion gap means that the body has lost a greater than normal number of bicarbonate ions.

Compensation

Hyperventilation is the main compensatory mechanism for metabolic acidosis. The increased plasma $[H^+]$ of metabolic acidosis is buffered by plasma HCO_3^-, reducing the plasma $[HCO_3^-]$ and the pH. A low pH activates sensitive receptors in the brain, signaling the respiratory muscles to increase ventilation. This increased ventilation lowers the blood's volatile acid (H_2CO_3) and dissolved CO_2 levels, returning pH toward the normal range. Uncompensated metabolic acidosis suggests that a ventilatory defect is present. Metabolic acidosis accompanied by $PaCO_2$ of 40 mm Hg means that something prevents the lungs from responding appropriately to the brain's stimulation. The defect may lie in nerve impulse transmission, the respiratory muscles, or the lungs themselves.

MINI CLINI

Partially Compensated Metabolic Acidosis

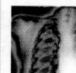

PROBLEM: A 42-year-old woman in a diabetic coma was taken to the emergency department. She exhibited gasping and deep respirations. Arterial blood gas analysis showed a pH of 7.22, PCO_2 of 20 mm Hg, HCO_3^- of 8 mEq/L, and BE of −16 mEq/L. How would the RT assess this patient's acid-base condition?

SOLUTION: The RT should follow these steps:

1. Categorize the pH. The pH is below the normal range, indicating the presence of acidemia.
2. Determine respiratory involvement. $PaCO_2$ is well below normal, indicating severe hyperventilation. By itself, this would cause alkalosis, but the presence of acidemia rules out primary respiratory alkalosis. The low $PaCO_2$ is probably a compensatory response to primary metabolic acidosis, although this response is insufficient to restore pH to the normal range.
3. Determine metabolic involvement. HCO_3^- is severely reduced, consistent with the low pH. In the presence of low pH and low $PaCO_2$, a low HCO_3^- signals primary metabolic acidosis. This is confirmed by the large BE.
4. Assess for compensation. The severe hyperventilation represents a compensatory response to primary metabolic acidosis, although compensation is far from complete. Nevertheless, the pH level would be even lower if $PaCO_2$ were normal.

Symptoms

Respiratory compensation in metabolic acidosis may result in a great increase in minute ventilation, causing patients to complain of dyspnea. Hyperpnea (increased tidal volume depth) is a common finding during physical examination of patients with metabolic acidosis. In patients with severe diabetic ketoacidosis, a very deep, gasping type of breathing develops, called *Kussmaul respiration.* Neurologic symptoms of severe metabolic acidosis range from lethargy to coma.

MINI CLINI

Compensated Metabolic Acidosis

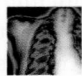

PROBLEM: A 38-year-old man had severe diarrhea for weeks without receiving medical attention. Arterial blood gas analysis showed a pH of 7.36, PCO_2 of 24 mm Hg, HCO_3^- of 13 mEq/L, and a BE of −11 mEq/L. How would the RT assess this patient's acid-base condition?

SOLUTION: The RT should follow these steps:

1. Categorize the pH. The pH is on the acidic side of the normal range, but it is still normal.
2. Determine respiratory involvement. $PaCO_2$ is below normal, indicating hyperventilation. By itself, this would cause alkalosis; however, because the pH is on the acidic side of normal, the presence of primary respiratory alkalosis is ruled out. The low $PaCO_2$ is likely a compensatory response to a primary metabolic problem (possible metabolic acidosis).
3. Determine metabolic involvement. HCO_3^- level is substantially lower than normal, consistent with a low pH. Given that the pH level is on the acidic side of normal, the low HCO_3^- level signals a possible metabolic acidosis. This is confirmed by the large BE.
4. Assess for compensation. The hyperventilation previously described must represent a compensatory response to primary metabolic acidosis. The pH is in the normal range.

Correction

The initial goal in severe acidemia is to increase the arterial pH greater than 7.20, a level below which serious cardiac arrhythmias are likely.[7] If respiratory compensation maintains the pH at or above this level, immediate corrective action is usually not indicated. Treatment of the underlying cause of acid gain or base loss is the rational approach.

In cases of severe metabolic acidosis, intravenous infusion of $NaHCO_3$ may be indicated. If respiratory compensation is under way, only small amounts of $NaHCO_3$ are required to attain an arterial pH of 7.20. In any case, rapid correction of arterial pH greater than 7.20 by $NaHCO_3$ infusion is undesirable.

Metabolic Alkalosis

Metabolic alkalosis is characterized by increased plasma $[HCO_3^-]$ or a loss of H^+ and a high pH. Increased $[HCO_3^-]$ is not always diagnostic of a primary metabolic alkalosis because it may be caused by renal compensation for respiratory acidosis.

Causes

Metabolic alkalosis can occur in one of the following two ways: (1) loss of fixed acids or (2) gain of blood buffer base. Both processes increase plasma $[HCO_3^-]$. To explain why losing fixed acid increases the plasma $[HCO_3^-]$, consider a situation in which vomiting removes gastric HCl from the body (Figure 13-8). In response to HCl loss, H^+ diffuses out of the gastric cell into the gastric fluid, where Cl^- accompanies it; this forces the CO_2 hydration reaction

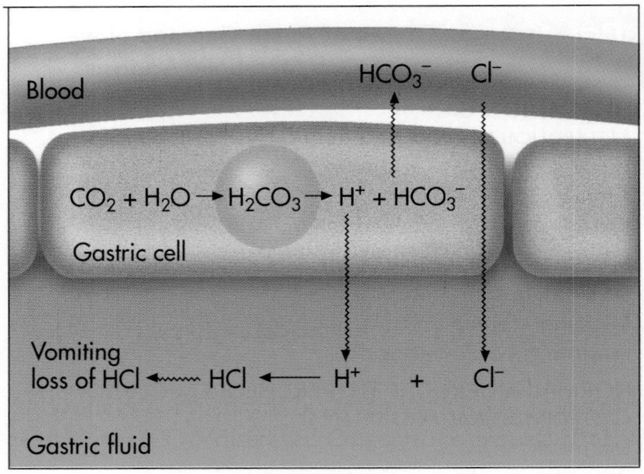

FIGURE 13-8 Gastric H^+ loss generates HCO_3^-, creating metabolic alkalosis. (Modified from Beachey W: Respiratory care anatomy and physiology: foundations for clinical practice, ed 2, St Louis, 2007, Mosby.)

MINI CLINI

Metabolic Alkalosis

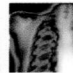

PROBLEM: An 83-year-old woman with heart disease had been taking a powerful diuretic to remove excess edematous fluid from her legs and to help keep her free of pulmonary edema. Blood gas and serum electrolyte analyses showed a pH of 7.58, $PaCO_2$ of 48 mm Hg, HCO_3^- of 44 mEq/L, BE of +19 mEq/L, serum K^+ of 2.5 mEq/L, and serum Cl^- of 95 mEq/L. How would the RT assess this patient's acid-base condition?

SOLUTION: The RT should follow these steps:

1. Categorize the pH. The pH level is substantially above normal, indicating the presence of alkalemia.
2. Determine respiratory involvement. $PaCO_2$ is slightly higher than normal, indicating mild hypoventilation. However, because alkalemia is present, the existence of primary respiratory acidosis is ruled out. The elevated $PaCO_2$ may be a compensatory response to a primary metabolic problem (possible metabolic alkalosis).
3. Determine metabolic involvement. HCO_3^- is substantially higher than normal. Given the high pH, the elevated HCO_3^- signals a metabolic alkalosis. This is confirmed by the large BE. In addition, the low serum K^+ and Cl^- values indicate hypokalemic/hypochloremic metabolic alkalosis.
4. Assess for compensation. Although $PaCO_2$ is slightly elevated, compensation for metabolic alkalosis is minimal. This lack of compensation is consistent with the presence of hypokalemic metabolic alkalosis.

in the gastric cell to the right, which generates HCO_3^-. The HCO_3^- enters the blood in exchange for the Cl^-. The plasma gains an HCO_3^- for each Cl^- (or H^+) that is lost (see Figure 13-8).[7]

The causes of metabolic alkalosis are summarized in Box 13-6. Metabolic alkalosis is common in acutely ill patients and is probably the most complicated acid-base imbalance to treat because it involves fluid and electrolyte imbalances. Metabolic alkalosis is often iatrogenic, resulting from the use of diuretics, low-salt diets, and gastric drainage.

Box 13-6 Causes of Metabolic Alkalosis (Increased Plasma HCO_3^-)

LOSS OF HYDROGEN IONS

Gastrointestinal

Vomiting
Nasogastric drainage

Renal

Diuretics (loss of Cl^-, K^+ fluid volume)
Hypochloremia (increased H^+ secretion and HCO_3^- reabsorption)
Hypokalemia (increased H^+ secretion and HCO_3^- reabsorption)
Hypovolemia (increased H^+)

RETENTION OF BICARBONATE ION

$NaHCO_3$ infusion or ingestion

From Beachey W: Respiratory care anatomy and physiology: foundations for clinical practice, ed 2, St Louis, 2007, Mosby.

To understand how the loss of Cl^-, K^+, and fluid volume may cause alkalosis, one needs to understand how the kidney regulates Na^+. Approximately 26,000 mEq of Na^+ passes through the glomerular membrane daily, but the body's daily Na^+ intake averages only approximately 150 mEq.[4] The kidney's main job is to reabsorb Na^+, not to excrete it. For this reason, and because Na^+ has a major role in maintaining fluid balance, the kidney places a greater priority on reabsorbing Na^+ than on maintaining Cl^-, K^+, or acid-base balance.

Normally, Na^+ is reabsorbed through *primary active transport* (Figure 13-9), in which the sodium-potassium-adenosine triphosphatase (Na^+,K^+-ATPase) pump actively transports Na^+ out of the renal tubule cell into the blood. This process causes Na^+ to diffuse continually from the filtrate into the tubule cell. Cl^- must accompany Na^+ to maintain electroneutrality in the filtrate. If blood Cl^- concentration is low (hypochloremia), less Cl^- is present in the filtrate, which means that the kidney relies more on other mechanisms to reabsorb Na^+. These mechanisms, called *secondary active secretion,* require the kidney to secrete H^+ or

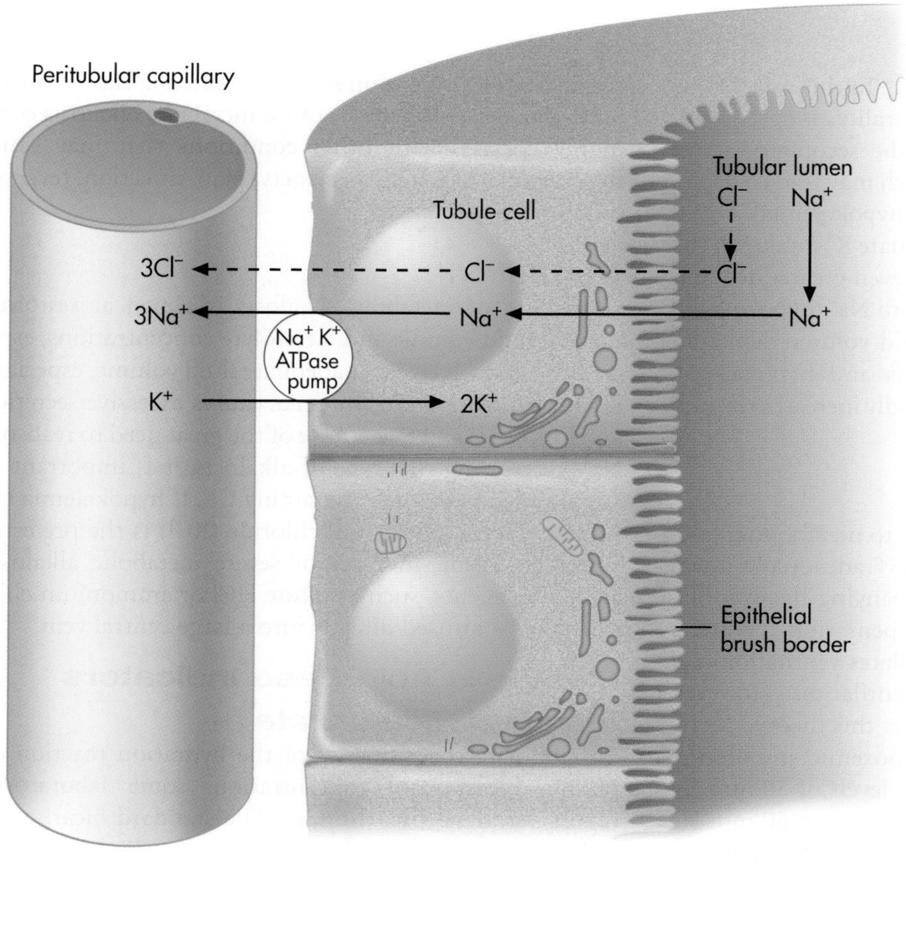

FIGURE 13-9 Sodium reabsorption through primary active transport. The sodium-potassium-adenosine triphosphatase (Na^+,K^+-ATPase) pump generates tubular cell electronegativity by pumping out more Na^+ than it pumps in K^+. This creates both electrostatic and concentration gradients favoring Na^+ diffusion from the filtrate into the tubular cell. Normally, negatively charged Cl^- passively follows Na^+ (cotransport). (Modified from Beachey W: Respiratory care anatomy and physiology: foundations for clinical practice, ed 2, St Louis, 2007, Mosby.)

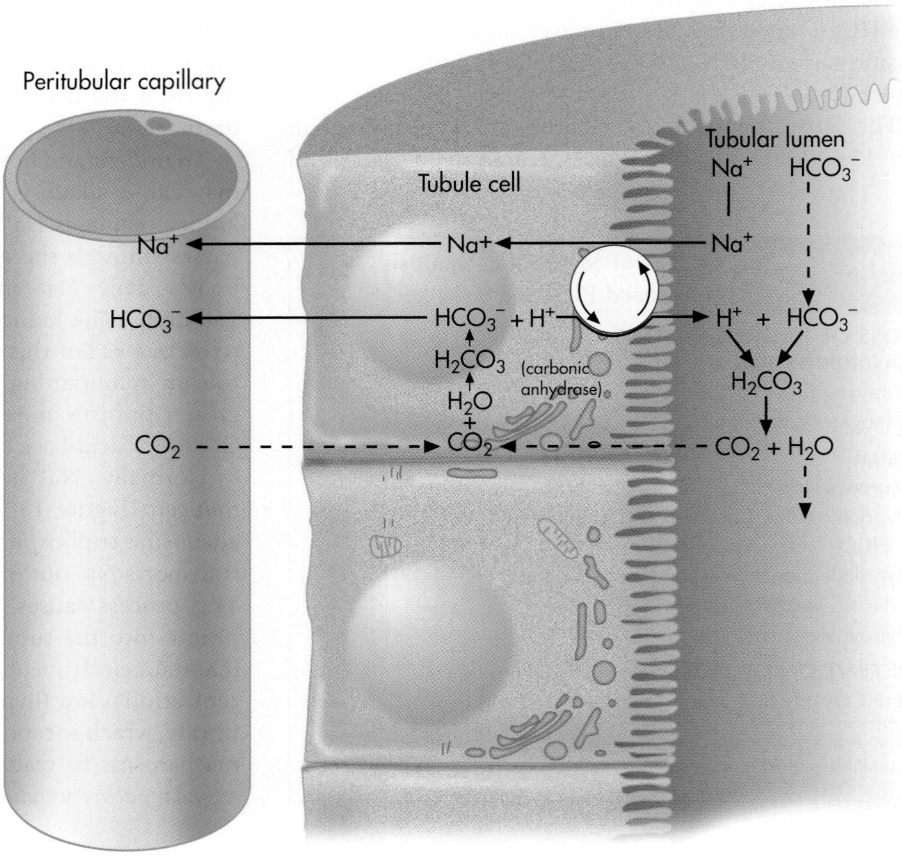

FIGURE 13-10 Sodium reabsorption through secondary active H^+ secretion. Through the countertransport process, Na^+ is reabsorbed as H^+ is secreted into the filtrate. HCO_3^- ion is reabsorbed with Na^+ instead of Cl^-. This process becomes more predominant when Cl^- is scarce, and it leads to alkalosis. (Modified from Beachey W: Respiratory care anatomy and physiology: foundations for clinical practice, ed 2, St Louis, 2007, Mosby.)

K^+ into the filtrate in exchange for Na^+. In this way, Na^+ is reabsorbed, and filtrate electroneutrality is preserved. Figures 13-10 and 13-11 illustrate the secondary active secretion process for H^+ and Na^+, which may lead to depletion of blood H^+ (alkalemia) and K^+ (hypokalemia). Preexisting hypokalemia (e.g., from inadequate K^+ intake) in the presence of hypochloremia places an even greater demand on the kidney to secrete H^+ to reabsorb Na^+; hypokalemia produces alkalosis. Dehydration (fluid volume depletion or hypovolemia) aggravates alkalosis and hypokalemia further because hypovolemia profoundly increases the kidney's stimulus to reabsorb Na^+.

Compensation

The expected compensatory response to metabolic alkalosis is hypoventilation (CO_2 retention). Traditionally, it was thought that the hypoxemia accompanying hypoventilation greatly limited respiratory compensation for metabolic alkalosis (i.e., hypoxemia stimulates ventilation and should prevent compensatory hypoventilation). However, more recent evidence does not support this theory.[6] Metabolic alkalosis apparently blunts hypoxemic stimulation to ventilation. Individuals with PaO_2 levels of 50 mm Hg may still hypoventilate to $PaCO_2$ levels of 60 mm Hg to compensate for metabolic alkalosis. Nevertheless, significant CO_2 retention is not seen often in cases of metabolic alkalosis, probably because metabolic alkalosis commonly coexists with other conditions that may cause hyperventilation, such as anxiety, pain, infection, fever, or pulmonary edema.

Correction

Correction of metabolic alkalosis is aimed at restoring normal fluid volume and electrolyte concentrations, especially K^+ and Cl^- levels. Inadequate fluid volume, especially if coupled with hypochloremia, causes excessive secretion and loss of H^+ and K^+ because of the great need to reabsorb Na^+. In treating this type of alkalosis, it is important to supply adequate fluids containing Cl^-. If hypokalemia is a primary factor, potassium chloride (KCl) is the preferred corrective agent. In cases of severe metabolic alkalosis, acidifying agents, such as dilute HCl or ammonium chloride may be infused directly into a large central vein.[8]

Metabolic Acid-Base Indicators

Standard Bicarbonate

To eliminate the influence of the hydration reaction on plasma bicarbonate concentration, some laboratories report **standard bicarbonate.** The standard bicarbonate is the plasma concentration of HCO_3^- (in mEq/L) obtained

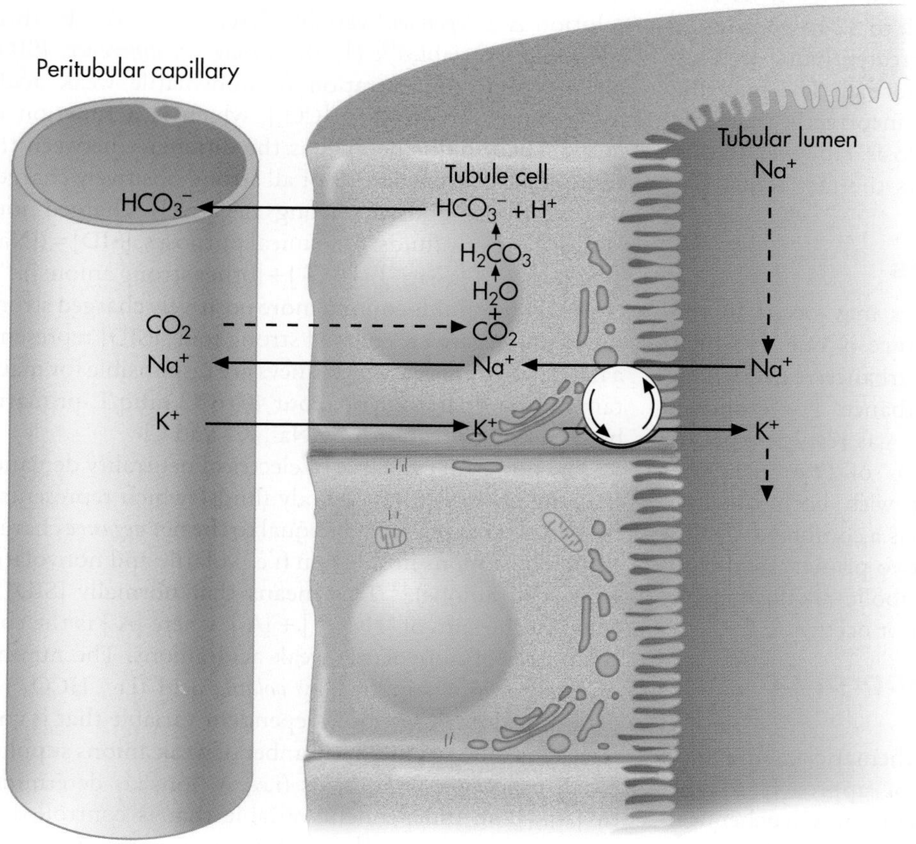

FIGURE 13-11 Sodium reabsorption through secondary active K^+ secretion. This mechanism is more likely to occur when Cl^- is scarce and an alkalemia (low H^+) exists. In such instances, hypokalemia develops. (Modified from Beachey W: Respiratory care anatomy and physiology: foundations for clinical practice, ed 2, St Louis, 2007, Mosby.)

from a blood sample that has been equilibrated (at body temperature) with a PCO_2 of 40 mm Hg. This HCO_3^- measurement presumably reflects only the metabolic component of acid-base balance, unhampered by the influence that CO_2 changes have on HCO_3^-. However, the process of standardizing the bicarbonate under in vitro laboratory conditions creates an artificial situation not present in the patient's body. The blood in the patient's vascular system is separated from the extravascular fluid (fluid outside of the vessels) by a thin capillary endothelial membrane, readily permeable to HCO_3^-. When a patient hypoventilates and the blood $PaCO_2$ increases, the plasma HCO_3^- also increases because of the hydration reaction. Consequently, plasma HCO_3^- diffuses out of the capillary into the extravascular fluid until HCO_3^- equilibrium is established between the blood and extravascular fluid. If the patient were now to hyperventilate so that the $PaCO_2$ again was 40 mm Hg, blood HCO_3^- would decrease, and extravascular HCO_3^- would diffuse down its concentration gradient back into the blood until an HCO_3^- equilibrium was established again. This diffusion of HCO_3^- between vascular and extravascular spaces cannot occur in a laboratory blood sample when the blood PCO_2 of a hypercapnic patient is artificially lowered to 40 mm Hg. Even the standard bicarbonate is not a perfect measure of purely nonrespiratory factors that influence blood pH.

Base Excess

Base excess (BE) is determined by equilibrating a blood sample in the laboratory to a PCO_2 of 40 mm Hg (at 37° C) and recording the amount of acid or base needed to titrate 1 L of blood to a pH of 7.40. A normal BE is ±2 mEq/L. A "positive BE" (>+2 mEq/L) indicates a gain of base or loss of acid from nonrespiratory causes. A "negative BE" (<−2 mEq/L) indicates a loss of base or a gain of acid from nonrespiratory causes. The BE has the same limitation as the standard bicarbonate in that it is an in vitro, rather than in vivo, measurement. That is, in hypercapnia, the **buffer base** that diffused into the extravascular fluid in vivo cannot be recovered during laboratory in vitro titrations.

The reliance on BE to quantify metabolic acid-base abnormalities can be misleading. In cases of acute (uncompensated) respiratory acidosis, the BE commonly would be within the normal range, indicating correctly that the disturbance is purely respiratory in origin. However, when renal compensation has occurred to offset chronic hypercapnia, the BE measurement is elevated above the normal range because of the compensatory increase in plasma HCO_3^-.

To illustrate, consider the Mini Clini in the left-hand column on p. 304 in which the patient has respiratory acidosis for which the body has compensated by renal retention of HCO_3^-. If this patient's blood were equilibrated in vitro to a $PaCO_2$ of 40 mm Hg, the HCO_3^- would decrease by only 2 to 3 mEq/L to 32 to 33 mEq/L, and the pH would increase to much greater than 7.45. This patient's BE would be well above normal. The high BE may lead the clinician to conclude incorrectly that this patient has a primary metabolic alkalosis. However, in this instance, the high BE merely reflects the fact that renal compensation has occurred.

Mixed Acid-Base States

Combinations of acid-base disorders may occur in the same patient. A combined disturbance is one in which both respiratory and metabolic disturbances exist, which promote the same acid-base disturbance. For example, consider the following arterial blood gas results: a pH of 7.62, $PaCO_2$ of 32 mm Hg, and HCO_3^- of 29 mEq/L. The pH indicates alkalemia, consistent with both the low $PaCO_2$ and the elevated HCO_3^-. This is a combined alkalosis, indicating that the patient has two primary acid-base problems (i.e., respiratory and metabolic alkalosis combined) for which compensation cannot occur.

Stewart's Strong Ion Approach to Acid-Base Balance

In the early 1980s, Stewart, a mathematician and biophysicist, introduced the *strong ion* approach to the study of acid-base physiology. This physicochemical perspective is controversial because it refutes the venerable Henderson-Hasselbalch approach. Although the Henderson-Hasselbalch approach to acid-base analysis is appropriate from a practical clinical standpoint, a basic overview of the strong ion approach is presented here to acquaint the reader with the concepts involved.

In the strong ion approach, substances that affect acid-base balance in body fluids are classified into three groups, based on their degree of dissociation in an aqueous solution: (1) strong ions, (2) weak ions, (3) and nonelectrolytes. Strong ions such as Na^+ and Cl^- are always fully dissociated, existing only in their charged forms in aqueous solutions. This means the number of strong ions in body fluids can never be converted back to the parent compound (e.g., NaCl or KCl), as occurs with weak ions. Weak ions are produced from compounds that only partially dissociate in solution, such as volatile carbonic acid ions (HCO_3^- and H^+) and nonvolatile acid ions such as phosphates and proteins.[9] As explained earlier in this chapter, weak acid molecules dissociate until they reach equilibrium with the concentrations of their component ions, each acid in accordance with its unique equilibrium constant. Nonvolatile weak acids include protein and inorganic phosphate molecules. Nonelectrolytes are substances that never dissociate in solution but contribute to the solution's osmotic pressure and affect the movement of ions and water across biologic membranes that separate body fluids.

Stewart distinguished between independent and dependent variables involved in acid-base regulation. Through a series of complex equations, he showed that the $[H^+]$ of a solution is a *dependent* variable determined *solely* by three *independent* variables[10]: (1) the *strong ion difference,* [SID]; (2) the total concentration of nonvolatile weak acids, $[A_{TOT}]$; and (3) dissolved $[CO_2]$, which is a function of PCO_2. The [SID] is defined as the difference between the summative concentrations of all strong positively charged ions (cations) and all strong negatively charged ions (anions) in body fluids; for clinical purposes, $[SID] = ([Na^+] + [K^+] + [Ca^{++}] + [Mg^{++}]) - ([Cl^-] + [\text{other strong anions}])$.[10,11] Normal body fluids contain more positively charged strong ions than negatively charged strong ions; [SID] represents a net positive charge. The kidneys are responsible for maintaining a normal [SID] of about 40 to 42 mEq/L, primarily by excreting or reabsorbing Na^+, K^+, and Cl^-.

The powerful principle of electrical neutrality demands that the normal [SID] of body fluids—which represents a net *positive* charge—must be equal to the net *negative* charges of all weak anions in solution (i.e., volatile and nonvolatile weak acid anions).[10] This means that normally [SID] is equal to the sum of $[HCO_3^-] + [A^-]$, where $[A^-]$ is the concentration of nonvolatile weak acid anions. The number of weak anions supplied by *volatile* acid (i.e., HCO_3^-) is determined by PCO_2, an independent variable that is controlled by ventilation. The number of weak anions supplied by all *nonvolatile* weak acids (i.e., A^- ions) is determined by $[A_{TOT}]$, an independent variable that is controlled by its temperature-dependent dissociation constant. At any given point in time, ventilation and body temperature are relatively constant, and PCO_2 and the dissociation of $[A_{TOT}]$ are relatively constant. With these two independent variables predetermined, a change in [SID] generates powerful electrochemical forces that affect the H_2O molecule's dissociation such that electrical neutrality is maintained. In this way, changes in [SID] affect the solution's $[H^+]$; a fall in [SID] (a decrease in net positive charges) increases H_2O dissociation, liberating more H^+ to maintain electrical neutrality, whereas an increase in [SID] (an increase in net positive charges) has the opposite effect.[10]

In Stewart's scheme, *metabolic* (nonrespiratory) acid-base disturbances can be caused only by changes in [SID] and the nonvolatile weak acid concentration $[A_{TOT}]$, *not* by changes in $[HCO_3^-]$. In Stewart's model, $[HCO_3^-]$ and $[H^+]$ are *dependent* variables (i.e., dependent on [SID], $[A_{TOT}]$, and PCO_2). In this scheme, the kidneys manipulate [SID] to change the plasma $[H^+]$ through the excretion or reabsorption of Na^+, K^+, and Cl^-.

Stewart's perspective is a departure from the Henderson-Hasselbalch concept of acid-base balance in which $[HCO_3^-]$ is treated as though it varies *independently* of dissolved $[CO_2]$, *independently* influencing pH or $[H^+]$. On closer inspection, however, $[HCO_3^-]$ and $[CO_2]$ *cannot* vary independently of each other as the CO_2 hydrolysis reaction clearly shows; instead, both $[HCO_3^-]$ and $[H^+]$ *depend* on $[CO_2]$[10]:

$$CO_2 + H_2O \leftrightarrow H_2CO_3 \leftrightarrow HCO_3^- + H^+$$

Changes in [HCO_3^-] cannot *cause* changes in [H^+]; changes in [HCO_3^-] and [H^+] are merely *correlated* with each other. It would seem that [HCO_3^-] cannot be a valid indicator of metabolic acid-base disturbances.

Nevertheless, clinicians generally agree that the complex nature of the equations involved in Stewart's strong ion approach make this method unwieldy. $PaCO_2$ and arterial pH are easy, direct measurements in the clinical setting, and [HCO_3^-] can be calculated with sufficient precision from these values; there is no need to calculate [HCO_3^-] and pH from the concentrations of electrolytes and weak acids, which are often unknown.[12] Although the strong ion approach is conceptually more correct, it is not sufficiently superior to the Henderson-Hasselbalch approach to merit its universal adoption. It is reasonable and clinically appropriate to explain metabolic acid-base physiology in terms of [H^+] and [HCO_3^-] from the Henderson-Hasselbalch perspective,[9,11,12] and so the Henderson-Hasselbalch approach is retained in this chapter.

SUMMARY CHECKLIST

- The lungs regulate the volatile acid content (CO_2) of the blood, and the kidneys control the fixed acid concentration of the blood.
- The larger the equilibrium constant of an acid, the more the acid molecule dissociates and yields H^+.
- In the *open* bicarbonate buffer system, H^+ is buffered to form the volatile acid, H_2CO_3, which is exhaled into the atmosphere as CO_2. In the *closed* nonbicarbonate buffer system, H^+ is buffered to form fixed acids, which accumulate in the body.
- Bicarbonate buffers can buffer only fixed acids, but nonbicarbonate buffers can buffer both fixed and volatile acids.
- The ratio between the plasma [HCO_3^-] and dissolved CO_2 determines the blood pH, according to the H-H equation; a 20 : 1 [HCO_3^-]/dissolved CO_2 ratio always yields a normal arterial pH of 7.40.
- The kidneys respond to hypoventilation by reabsorbing bicarbonate, and they respond to hyperventilation by excreting bicarbonate.
- The lungs respond to metabolic acidosis by hyperventilating, and they respond to metabolic alkalosis by hypoventilating.
- $PaCO_2$ abnormalities characterize respiratory acid-base disturbances, and [HCO_3^-] abnormalities characterize metabolic acid-base disturbances.
- Hypochloremia forces the kidneys to excrete increased amounts of H^+ and K^+ to reabsorb Na^+, causing alkalosis and hypokalemia.
- Hypokalemia forces the kidneys to excrete increased amounts of H^+ to reabsorb Na^+, causing alkalosis.
- Standard bicarbonate and BE measurements are made under conditions of a normal $PaCO_2$ (40 mm Hg), which means that any abnormality in these measurements reflects only nonrespiratory influences.
- Although Stewart's strong ion difference may be the most conceptually accurate approach to acid-base physiology, the Henderson-Hasselbalch approach is nevertheless clinically appropriate and more practical in the context of patient care.

References

1. Masoro EJ, Siegel PD: Acid-base regulation: its physiology and pathophysiology, Philadelphia, 1971, Saunders.
2. Comroe JH: Physiology of respiration, ed 2, Chicago, 1974, Year Book.
3. West JB: Respiratory physiology: the essentials, ed 8, Baltimore, 2008, Lippincott Williams & Wilkins.
4. Hall JE: Guyton and Hall: Textbook of medical physiology, ed 12, Philadelphia, 2010, Saunders.
5. Filley GF: Acid-base and blood gas regulation, Philadelphia, 1971, Lea & Febiger.
6. Rose BD: Clinical physiology of acid-base and electrolyte disorders, ed 3, New York, 1989, McGraw-Hill.
7. Javaheri S, Kazemi H: Metabolic alkalosis and hypoventilation in humans. Am Rev Respir Dis 136:1011, 1987.
8. Malley WJ: Clinical blood gases: assessment and intervention, ed 2, St Louis, 2005, Saunders.
9. Kellum JA: Determinants of blood pH in health and disease. Crit Care 4:6, 2000.
10. Morfei J: Stewart's strong ion difference approach to acid-base analysis. Respir Care 44:45, 1999.
11. Swenson ER: The strong ion difference approach: can a strong case be made for its use in acid-base analysis? Respir Care 44:26, 1999.
12. Effros RM, Swenson ER: Acid-base balance. In Mason RJ, Broaddus VC, Martin TR, et al, editors: Murray and Nadel's textbook of respiratory medicine, ed 5, Philadelphia, 2010, Saunders.

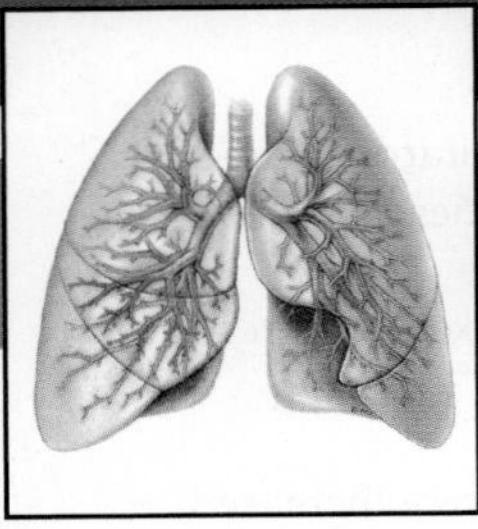

Chapter 14

Regulation of Breathing

WILL BEACHEY

CHAPTER OBJECTIVES

After reading this chapter you will be able to:

- Identify where the structures that regulate breathing are located.
- Describe how the inspiratory and expiratory neurons in the medulla establish the basic pattern of breathing.
- Describe the effect that impulses from the pneumotaxic and apneustic centers in the pons have on the medullary centers of breathing.
- Identify the effect of various reflexes on breathing.
- Describe how the central and peripheral chemoreceptors differ in the way they regulate breathing.
- State how the central chemoreceptors respond differently to respiratory and nonrespiratory acid-base disorders.
- Describe how the regulation of breathing in individuals with chronic hypercapnia differs from the regulation of breathing in healthy individuals.
- Describe why administering oxygen to patients with chronic hypercapnia poses a special risk that is not present in healthy individuals.
- Describe why ascending to a high altitude has different immediate and long-term effects on ventilation.
- State why mechanically ventilated patients with head injuries may benefit from deliberate hyperventilation.
- Describe the characteristics of abnormal breathing patterns.

CHAPTER OUTLINE

Medullary Respiratory Center
- Dorsal Respiratory Groups
- Ventral Respiratory Groups
- Inspiratory Ramp Signal

Pontine Respiratory Centers
- Apneustic Center
- Pneumotaxic Center

Reflex Control of Breathing
- Hering-Breuer Inflation Reflex
- Deflation Reflex
- Head Paradoxical Reflex
- Irritant Receptors
- J-Receptors
- Peripheral Proprioceptors
- Muscle Spindles

Chemical Control of Breathing
- Central Chemoreceptors
- Peripheral Chemoreceptors
- Control of Breathing in Chronic Hypercapnia
- Oxygen-Associated Hypercapnia

Ventilatory Response to Exercise

Abnormal Breathing Patterns

Carbon Dioxide and Cerebral Blood Flow

KEY TERMS

apnea
apneustic breathing
apneustic center
Biot respiration
blood-brain barrier
chemoreceptors
Cheyne-Stokes respiration
dorsal respiratory groups (DRGs)
Hering-Breuer inflation reflex
J-receptors
pneumotaxic center
vagovagal reflexes
ventral respiratory groups (VRGs)

Breathing, similar to the heartbeat, is an automatic activity requiring no conscious awareness. In contrast to the heartbeat, breathing patterns can be consciously changed, although powerful neural control mechanisms overwhelm conscious control soon after one willfully stops breathing. The normal unconscious cycle of breathing is regulated by complex mechanisms that continue to elude complete understanding. The rhythmic cycle of breathing originates in the brainstem, mainly from neurons located in the medulla. Higher brain centers and many systemic receptors and reflexes modify the output of the medulla. These different structures function in an integrated manner, precisely controlling ventilatory rate and depth to accommodate the gas exchange needs of the body. This chapter helps the clinician understand basic physiologic mechanisms that regulate breathing; with this knowledge, the clinician can anticipate the effects that various therapeutic interventions and disease processes have on ventilation.

MEDULLARY RESPIRATORY CENTER

Animal experiments show that transecting the brainstem just below the medulla (Figure 14-1, level IV) stops all ventilatory activity. However, breathing continues rhythmically after the brainstem is transected just above the pons (see Figure 14-1, level I). Until more recently, physiologists thought that separate inspiratory and expiratory neuron "centers" in the medulla were responsible for the cyclic pattern of breathing. Researchers believed that inspiratory and expiratory neurons fired by self-excitation and that they mutually inhibited one another. More recent evidence shows that inspiratory and expiratory neurons are anatomically intermingled and do not inhibit one another.[1] No clearly separate inspiratory and expiratory centers exist. Instead, the medulla contains several widely dispersed respiratory-related neurons, as shown in Figure 14-1. The **dorsal respiratory groups (DRGs)** contain mainly inspiratory neurons, whereas the **ventral respiratory groups (VRGs)** contain both inspiratory and expiratory neurons.

Dorsal Respiratory Groups

As shown in Figure 14-1, DRG neurons are mainly inspiratory neurons located bilaterally in the medulla. These neurons send impulses to the motor nerves of the diaphragm and external intercostal muscles, providing the main inspiratory stimulus.[1] Many DRG nerves extend into the VRGs, but few VRG fibers extend into the DRGs. Reciprocal inhibition is an unlikely explanation for rhythmic, spontaneous breathing.[1]

The vagus and glossopharyngeal nerves transmit many sensory impulses to the DRGs from the lungs, airways, peripheral chemoreceptors, and joint proprioceptors. These impulses modify the basic breathing pattern generated in the medulla.

Ventral Respiratory Groups

VRG neurons are located bilaterally in the medulla in two different nuclei and contain inspiratory and expiratory neurons (see Figure 14-1). Some inspiratory VRG neurons send motor impulses through the vagus nerve to the laryngeal and pharyngeal muscles, abducting the vocal cords and increasing the diameter of the glottis. Other VRG inspiratory neurons transmit impulses to the diaphragm and external intercostal muscles. Still other VRG neurons have mostly expiratory discharge patterns and send impulses to the internal intercostal and abdominal expiratory muscles.

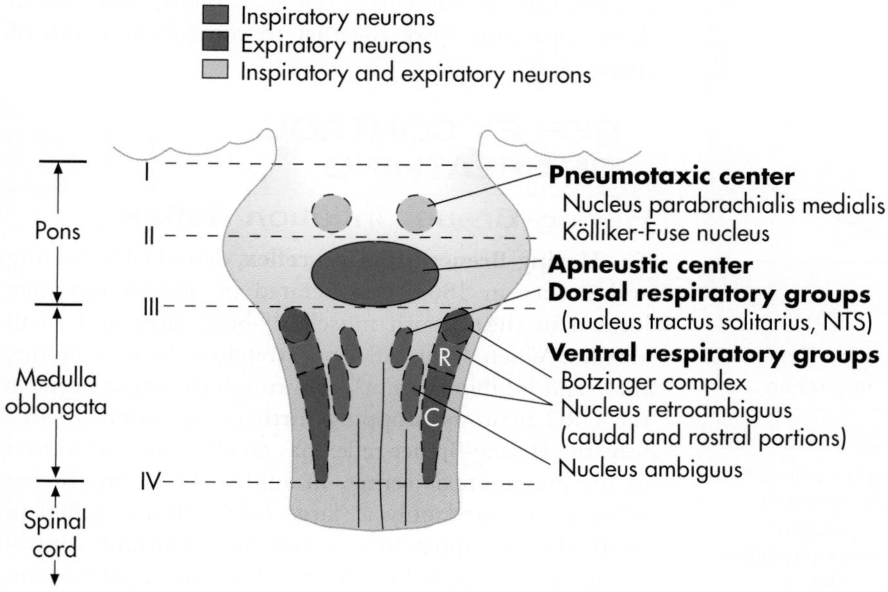

FIGURE 14-1 Dorsal view of the brainstem. Dashed lines *I* to *IV* refer to transections at different levels. (Modified from Beachey W: Respiratory care anatomy and physiology: foundations for clinical practice, ed 2, St Louis, 2007, Mosby.)

The exact origin of the basic rhythmic pattern of ventilation is unknown. No single group of pacemaker cells has been identified. Two predominant theories of rhythm generation are the *pacemaker hypothesis* and the *network hypothesis*.[2] The pacemaker hypothesis holds that certain medullary cells have intrinsic pacemaker properties (i.e., rhythmic self-exciting characteristics) and that these cells drive other medullary neurons. The network hypothesis suggests that rhythmic breathing is the result of a particular pattern of interconnections between neurons dispersed throughout the rostral VRG, the pre-Bötzinger complex, and the Bötzinger complex. This hypothesis assumes that certain populations of inspiratory and expiratory neurons inhibit one another and that one of the neuron types fires in a self-limiting way, such that it becomes less responsive the longer it fires. There is no definitive proof of either hypothesis; the precise origin of respiratory rhythm generation remains elusive.[2]

Inspiratory Ramp Signal

The inspiratory muscles do not receive an instantaneous burst of signals from the dorsal and ventral inspiratory neurons. Rather, the firing rate of DRG and VRG inspiratory neurons increases gradually at the end of the expiratory phase, creating a ramp signal (Figure 14-2). The inspiratory muscles contract steadily and smoothly, gradually expanding the lungs rather than filling them in an abrupt inspiratory gasp. During exercise, various reflexes and receptors influence the medullary neurons, steepening the ramp signal and filling the lungs more rapidly.

During quiet breathing, inspiratory neurons fire with increasing frequency for approximately 2 seconds and then abruptly switch off, allowing expiration to proceed for approximately 3 seconds.[3] At the start of expiration, inspiratory neurons again fire briefly, retarding the early phase of expiration (see Figure 14-2). The inhibitory neurons that switch off the inspiratory ramp signal are controlled by the pneumotaxic center and pulmonary stretch receptors, which are discussed later in this chapter.

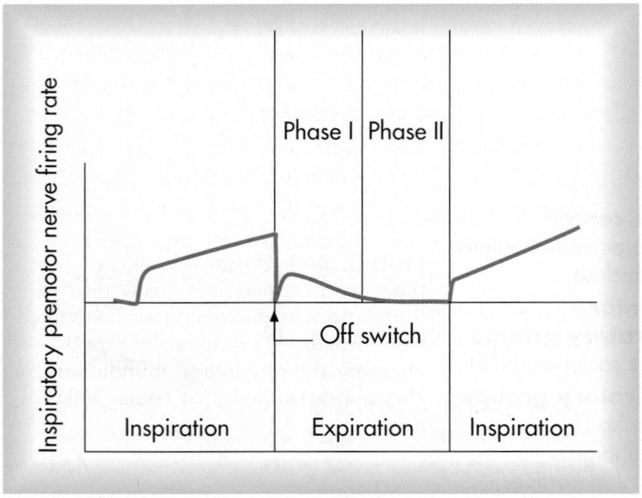

FIGURE 14-2 Inspiratory neural activity during breathing. Note the inspiratory ramp signal *(left)* and the braking action of inspiratory signals in the early part *(phase I)* of expiration. (Redrawn from Leff AR, Shumacher PT: Respiratory physiology: basics and applications, Philadelphia, 1993, Saunders.)

PONTINE RESPIRATORY CENTERS

If the brainstem is transected above the medulla (see Figure 14-1, level III), spontaneous respiration continues, although in a more irregular pattern. The pons does not promote rhythmic breathing; rather, it modifies the output of the medullary centers. Figure 14-1 shows two groups of neurons in the pons: (1) the apneustic center and (2) the pneumotaxic center.

Apneustic Center

The **apneustic center** is anatomically ill defined; its existence and function can be shown only if its connections to the higher pneumotaxic center and vagus nerves are severed. Under such circumstances, the DRG inspiratory neurons fail to switch off, causing prolonged inspiratory gasps interrupted by occasional expirations **(apneustic breathing).** Vagal and pneumotaxic center impulses hold the apneustic center's stimulatory effect on DRG neurons in check.

Pneumotaxic Center

The **pneumotaxic center** is a bilateral group of neurons located in the upper pons (see Figure 14-1). The pneumotaxic center controls the "switch-off" point of the inspiratory ramp, controlling inspiratory time. Strong pneumotaxic signals increase the respiratory rate, and weak signals prolong inspiration and increase tidal volumes. The exact nature of the interaction between the pneumotaxic and apneustic centers is poorly understood. They apparently work together to control the depth of inspiration.[3]

REFLEX CONTROL OF BREATHING

Hering-Breuer Inflation Reflex

The **Hering-Breuer inflation reflex,** described by Hering and Breuer in 1868, is generated by stretch receptors located in the smooth muscle of both large and small airways. When lung inflation stretches these receptors, they send inhibitory impulses through the vagus nerve to the DRG neurons, stopping further inspiration. In this way, the Hering-Breuer reflex has an effect similar to that of the pneumotaxic center. In adults, the Hering-Breuer reflex is activated only at large tidal volumes (≥800 to 1000 ml) and apparently is not an important control mechanism in quiet breathing.[2] This reflex is important, however, in regulating respiratory rate and depth during moderate to strenuous exercise.

Deflation Reflex

Sudden collapse of the lung stimulates strong inspiratory effort. This inspiratory effort may be the result of decreased stretch receptor activity, or it may be caused by the stimulation of other receptors, such as the irritant receptors and J-receptors (discussed later). Although it is unclear which receptors are involved, it is clear that the vagus nerve is the pathway (as it is for the Hering-Breuer reflex) and that the effect is hyperpnea.[1] The deflation reflex is probably responsible for the hyperpnea observed with pneumothorax (air in the pleural space).

Head Paradoxical Reflex

In 1889, Head observed that if the Hering-Breuer reflex is blocked by cooling the vagus nerve, lung hyperinflation causes a further increase in inspiratory effort—the opposite of the Hering-Breuer reflex. The receptors for this reflex are called *rapidly adapting receptors* because they stop firing promptly after a volume change occurs. The Head reflex may help maintain large tidal volumes during exercise and may be involved in periodic deep sighs during quiet breathing. Periodic sighs help prevent alveolar collapse, or atelectasis. The Head reflex also may be responsible for the first breaths of a newborn.[1]

Irritant Receptors

Rapidly adapting irritant receptors in the epithelium of the larger conducting airways have vagal sensory nerve fibers. Their stimulation, whether by inhaled irritants or by mechanical factors, causes reflex bronchoconstriction, coughing, sneezing, tachypnea, and narrowing of the glottis. Some of these reflexes, called **vagovagal reflexes,** have both sensory and motor vagal components; they are responsible for laryngospasm, coughing, and slowing of the heartbeat. Endotracheal intubation, airway suctioning, and bronchoscopy readily elicit vagovagal reflexes. Physical stimulation of the conducting airways, as with suctioning or bronchoscopy, may cause a severe case of bronchospasm, coughing, and laryngospasm.

J-Receptors

C fibers in the lung parenchyma near the pulmonary capillaries are called *juxtacapillary receptors,* or **J-receptors.** Alveolar inflammatory processes (pneumonia), pulmonary vascular congestion (congestive heart failure), and pulmonary edema stimulate these receptors. This stimulation causes rapid, shallow breathing; a sensation of dyspnea; and expiratory narrowing of the glottis.

Peripheral Proprioceptors

Proprioceptors in muscles, tendons, and joints and pain receptors in muscles and skin send stimulatory signals to the medullary respiratory center. Such stimuli increase medullary inspiratory activity and cause hyperpnea.[4] For this reason, moving the limbs, slapping or splashing cold water on the skin, and other painful stimuli stimulate ventilation in patients with respiratory depression.

Proprioceptors in joints and tendons may be important in initiating and maintaining increased ventilation at the beginning of exercise. Passive limb movement around a joint increases breathing rate in both anesthetized animals and unanesthetized humans.[4]

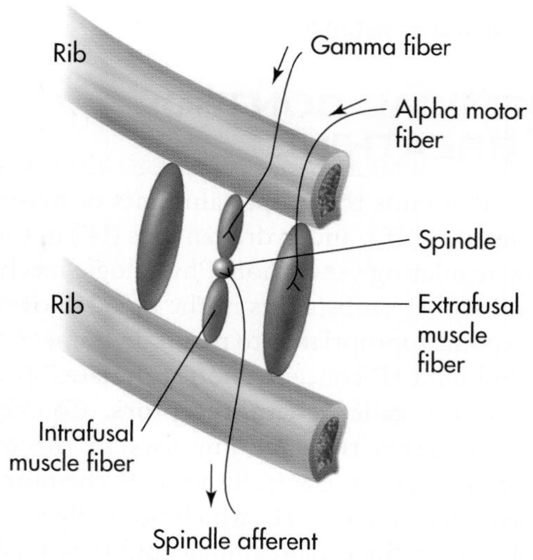

FIGURE 14-3 Stretch-sensitive muscle spindle located on the intrafusal fibers of intercostal muscles. Motor innervation for intrafusal fibers (gamma nerve fibers) is different than for extrafusal fibers (alpha nerve fibers). Spindle afferent nerve fibers synapse with alpha motor neurons in the spinal cord, creating a single synapse reflex arc.

Muscle Spindles

Muscle spindles in the diaphragm and intercostal muscles are part of a reflex arc that helps the muscles adjust to an increased load. Muscle spindles are sensing elements located on intrafusal muscle fibers, arranged parallel to the main extrafusal muscle fibers (Figure 14-3). The extrafusal fibers that elevate the ribs are innervated by different motor fibers (alpha fibers) than the fibers that innervate the intrafusal spindle fibers (gamma fibers). When the main extrafusal muscle fiber and the intrafusal fibers contract simultaneously, the sensing element *(spindle)* of the intrafusal muscle fiber stretches and sends impulses over spindle afferent nerves directly to the spinal cord (see Figure 14-3). The spindle's afferent (sensory) nerve synapses directly with the alpha motor neuron in the spinal cord, sending impulses back to the main extrafusal muscle. A single synapse reflex arc is created. Alpha motor neuron impulses cause the main extrafusal muscle fibers to contract with greater force, shortening the nearby intrafusal fibers. The stretch-sensitive spindle is unloaded, and its impulses cease. In this way, inspiratory muscle force adjusts to the load imposed by decreased lung compliance or increased airway resistance.

CHEMICAL CONTROL OF BREATHING

The body maintains the proper amounts of oxygen (O_2), carbon dioxide (CO_2), and hydrogen ions (H^+) in the blood mainly by regulating ventilation. Physiologic mechanisms that monitor these substances in the blood allow ventilation to respond appropriately to maintain homeostasis. An increase in blood H^+ concentration stimulates specialized nerve structures called **chemoreceptors.** Consequently, the chemoreceptors transmit impulses to the medulla, increasing ventilation. Centrally located chemoreceptors in the medulla respond to H^+, which normally arises from dissolved CO_2 in the cerebrospinal fluid (CSF). Peripherally located chemoreceptors in the fork of the common carotid arteries and the aortic arch are also sensitive to H^+ and indirectly to CO_2. These receptors are also indirectly sensitive to hypoxemia because hypoxemia increases the sensitivity of the peripheral chemoreceptors to H^+.[2]

Central Chemoreceptors

Hydrogen ions, not CO_2 molecules, stimulate highly responsive chemosensitive nerve cells, located bilaterally in the medulla. Nevertheless, these central chemoreceptors are extremely sensitive to CO_2 in an indirect fashion. The chemoreceptors are not in direct contact with arterial blood (Figure 14-4). Instead, they are bathed in the CSF, separated from the blood by a semipermeable membrane called the **blood-brain barrier.** This membrane is almost impermeable to H^+ and HCO_3^-, but it is freely permeable to CO_2. When $PaCO_2$ increases, CO_2 diffuses rapidly through the blood-brain barrier into the CSF. In the CSF, CO_2 reacts with water (H_2O) to form H^+ and HCO_3^- (see Figure 14-4). The H^+ generated in this fashion stimulates the central chemoreceptors, which stimulate the medullary inspiratory neurons. $PaCO_2$ is indirectly the primary minute-to-minute controller of ventilation. CO_2 diffusing from the blood into the CSF increases [H^+] almost instantly, exciting the chemoreceptors within seconds. Alveolar ventilation increases by approximately 2 to 3 L/min for each 1-mm Hg increase in $PaCO_2$.[5]

The stimulatory effect of chronically high CO_2 on the central chemoreceptors gradually declines over 1 or 2 days because the kidneys retain bicarbonate ions in response to respiratory acidosis, bringing the blood pH level back toward normal. The increased number of bicarbonate ions in the blood eventually diffuses across the blood-brain barrier into the CSF, where they buffer H^+ and bring the CSF pH level back to normal. This activity removes the stimulus to the chemoreceptors, and ventilation decreases. An acute increase in $PaCO_2$ has a powerful effect on ventilation, which is greatly weakened after 1 or 2 days of adaptation.

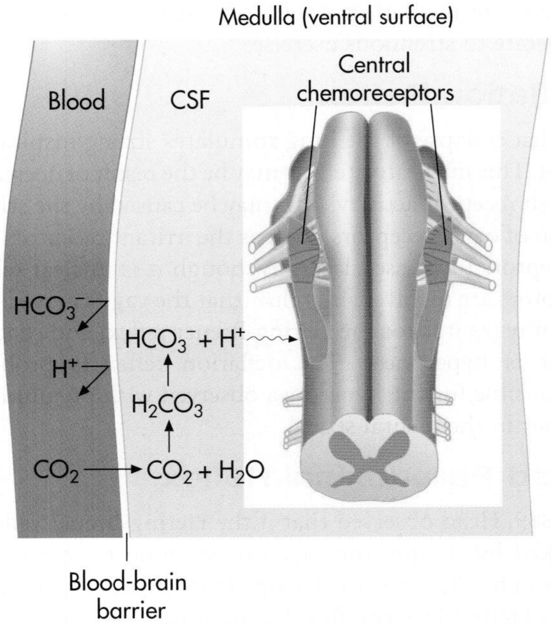

FIGURE 14-4 CO_2 stimulates the medullary chemoreceptors by forming H^+ in the CSF. The blood-brain barrier is almost impermeable to H^+ and HCO_3^- but is freely permeable to CO_2. (Modified from Beachey W: Respiratory care anatomy and physiology: foundations for clinical practice, ed 2, St Louis, 2007, Mosby.)

Peripheral Chemoreceptors

The peripheral chemoreceptors are small, highly vascular structures known as the *carotid* and *aortic bodies*. The carotid bodies are located bilaterally in the bifurcations of the common carotid arteries. The aortic bodies are found in the arch of the aorta. These neural structures increase their firing rates in response to increased arterial [H^+] regardless of its origin (i.e., whether from fixed acid accumulation or increased CO_2). The carotid bodies send their impulses to the respiratory centers in the medulla via the glossopharyngeal nerve, whereas the aortic bodies send their impulses over the vagus nerve. The carotid bodies exert much more influence over the respiratory centers than the aortic bodies do, especially with respect to arterial hypoxemia and acidemia.[1]

Because the carotid bodies receive an extremely high rate of blood flow, they have little time to remove O_2 from the blood. Consequently, venous blood leaving the carotid bodies has almost the same O_2 content as the arterial blood entering them. The carotid bodies are exposed at all times to arterial blood, not venous blood, and they sense arterial (not venous) [H^+].

Response to Decreased Arterial Oxygen

Traditionally, it was believed that the carotid bodies directly sense low PaO_2, implying that arterial hypoxemia represents an independent drive to breathe—the "hypoxic drive." Although the peripheral chemoreceptors fire more frequently in the presence of arterial hypoxemia, they do so only because hypoxemia makes them more sensitive to H^+.[2] That is, when PaO_2 is low, carotid body sensitivity to a given $[H^+]$ increases; in this way, hypoxia increases ventilation for any given pH. Conversely, elevated PaO_2 (hyperoxia) decreases carotid body sensitivity to $[H^+]$. The carotid bodies respond to arterial hypoxemia only because hypoxia makes them more sensitive to $[H^+]$. This means that if the arterial $[H^+]$ is extremely low (high pH), as in severe alkalemia, hypoxemia has little effect on the carotid bodies.[2] Simply stated, the ultimate effect of hypoxemia is to increase the sensitivity of the peripheral chemoreceptors to the given blood $[H^+]$, which increases their firing rate and brings about increased ventilation.

Because of their extremely high blood flow rates, the carotid bodies respond to decreased arterial *partial pressure* of O_2 (in the indirect way just described) rather than to an actual decrease in arterial O_2 *content*. That is, the extraction of O_2 by the carotid bodies from each unit of rapidly flowing blood is so small that their O_2 needs are met entirely by dissolved O_2 in the plasma. This is why conditions associated with low arterial O_2 content but normal PaO_2 (e.g., anemia and carbon monoxide poisoning) do not stimulate ventilation.[5]

When pH and $PaCO_2$ are normal (pH = 7.40 and $PaCO_2$ = 40 mm Hg), the nerve-impulse transmission rate of the carotid bodies does not increase significantly until the PaO_2 decreases to about 60 mm Hg.[5] If PaO_2 decreases further from 60 mm Hg to 30 mm Hg, the rate of impulse transmission increases sharply and linearly because hypoxemia makes the carotid bodies much more sensitive to a pH of 7.40. A decrease in PaO_2 from 60 mm Hg to 30 mm Hg corresponds to the sharpest decrease in O_2 content on the O_2-hemoglobin equilibrium curve (i.e., the steepest part of the curve). Arterial hypoxemia does not stimulate ventilation greatly until the PaO_2 decreases to less than 60 mm Hg. O_2 plays no role in the drive to breathe in healthy individuals at sea level. High altitude causes a healthy person's ventilation to increase because low barometric pressure decreases the inspired PO_2 and the arterial PO_2, which increases the sensitivity of peripheral chemoreceptors to their H^+ environment. The resulting increase in ventilation is less than expected, however, because hyperventilation decreases $PaCO_2$ and increases arterial pH. The increased pH depresses the medullary respiratory center, counteracting the excitatory effect of a low PaO_2 on peripheral chemoreceptors. Hypoxemia-mediated hyperventilation may be impossible in certain conditions, such as severe chronic obstructive pulmonary disease (COPD), in which lung mechanics are so deranged that the stimulatory effect of hypoxemia on ventilation fails to decrease $PaCO_2$ regardless of the patient's effort. In such instances, there is no alkalosis to counteract the stimulatory effects of hypoxemia on ventilation.

RULE OF THUMB

Hypoxemia is not associated with an increased drive to breathe until PaO_2 is less than 60 mm Hg, after which the drive to breathe increases proportionally with the decrease in PaO_2.

Response to Increased $PaCO_2$ and Hydrogen Ions

For a given increase in $PaCO_2$ or $[H^+]$, the carotid bodies are less responsive than the central chemoreceptors. The peripheral chemoreceptors account for only 20% to 30% of the ventilatory response to hypercapnia.[5] However, they respond to increased arterial $[H^+]$ more rapidly than do the central chemoreceptors. The explanation is that, in contrast to the central chemoreceptors, the carotid bodies are exposed directly to arterial blood. The body's initial ventilatory response to metabolic acidosis is fairly quick, even though H^+ crosses the blood-brain barrier with difficulty.

As stated earlier, hypoxemia increases the sensitivity of the peripheral chemoreceptors to H^+ and to $PaCO_2$. Conversely, high PaO_2 (hyperoxia) *decreases* the peripheral chemoreceptors' PCO_2 sensitivity to almost zero.[2] This means that when the PaO_2 is high, the ventilatory response to $PaCO_2$ is mainly due to the central chemoreceptors, which are unaffected by hypoxemia.

Because the only effect of hypoxia on the peripheral chemoreceptors is to increase their sensitivity to arterial $[H^{++}]$—and indirectly to $PaCO_2$—the following statements are true: (1) High PO_2 renders the peripheral chemoreceptors almost unresponsive to PCO_2, and (2) low $PaCO_2$ renders the peripheral chemoreceptors almost unresponsive to hypoxemia.[2] Coexisting arterial hypoxemia, acidemia, and high $PaCO_2$ (i.e., asphyxia) maximally stimulate the peripheral chemoreceptors.

Individuals with chronic hypercapnia secondary to advanced COPD have depressed ventilatory responses to acute increases in arterial CO_2, partly because of their altered acid-base status and partly because their deranged lung mechanics prevents them from increasing their ventilation adequately.[1] The altered acid-base status arises from the preexisting high levels of blood buffer base, a compensatory response to chronic respiratory acidosis (see Chapter 13).

Control of Breathing in Chronic Hypercapnia

A sudden increase in arterial PCO_2 causes an immediate increase in ventilation because CO_2 rapidly diffuses from the blood into the CSF, increasing the $[H^+]$ surrounding central chemoreceptors. If $PaCO_2$ increases gradually over many years, as might occur in the development of severe COPD and worsening lung mechanics, the kidneys compensate by increasing the plasma bicarbonate concentration, keeping the arterial pH within normal limits. As plasma bicarbonate levels increase, these ions slowly diffuse

MINI CLINI

Delayed Hyperventilation at High Altitude

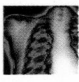

PROBLEM: If a person ascends to an elevation of 10,000 feet above sea level, his or her inspired PO_2 decreases because of low barometric pressure. Consequently, the peripheral chemoreceptors become excited and stimulate an increase in ventilation. Why must a day or so pass at this altitude before ventilation increases to its maximal level?

SOLUTION: Hypoxia-induced hyperventilation reduces $PaCO_2$ and creates alkalemia. This condition produces an alkalotic CSF because the blood-brain barrier is nearly impermeable to bicarbonate ions (HCO_3^-); that is, as CO_2 diffuses out of the CSF in response to the low arterial blood PCO_2, HCO_3^- remains behind in the CSF. The central chemoreceptors are exposed to an alkalotic environment, diminishing the effect of the hypoxic ventilatory stimulus on peripheral chemoreceptors. In other words, the development of respiratory alkalosis limits the magnitude of hypoxia-induced hyperventilation. Over the first 24 hours or so of hyperventilation, HCO_3^- gradually diffuses out of the CSF across the blood-brain barrier, restoring the CSF pH level to normal. In addition, the kidneys excrete HCO_3^- to compensate for the respiratory alkalemia. Consequently, the blood pH level decreases toward normal, and the hypoxic ventilatory stimulus keeps the $PaCO_2$ low. As the CSF pH level returns to normal, the progressively unrestrained hypoxic stimulus increases ventilation further. It takes approximately 24 hours of high-altitude exposure before ventilation increases to its maximal level.

RULE OF THUMB

The ventilatory response to hypoxemia is greatly enhanced by hypercapnia and acidemia.

across the blood-brain barrier, keeping CSF pH within its normal range. The central chemoreceptors respond to $[H^+]$, not the CO_2 molecule; they sense a normal pH environment, even though the $PaCO_2$ is abnormally high.

This adaptation explains why the chronically high $PaCO_2$ of people with severe COPD does not overly stimulate their ventilation. Instead, the hypoxemia that accompanies chronic hypercapnia becomes the minute-to-minute breathing stimulus in the roundabout way discussed previously: Hypoxemia increases the sensitivity of the peripheral chemoreceptors to $[H^+]$, increasing the nerve impulses they transmit to the medulla and stimulating ventilation. Patients with severe COPD are invariably hypoxemic when breathing room air because their lungs have mismatches in ventilation and blood flow. It stands to reason that breathing supplemental O_2 would increase the PaO_2 and make the carotid bodies less sensitive to $[H^+]$, which would decrease ventilation further and increase the $PaCO_2$.

Oxygen-Associated Hypercapnia

$PaCO_2$ of chronically hypercapnic patients with COPD often increases acutely after these patients are given O_2. The reason for this phenomenon continues to be a subject of much debate and misunderstanding. The traditional explanation for this phenomenon is that O_2 breathing removes the hypoxic ventilatory stimulus and induces hypoventilation, but this explanation is probably overly simplified. (This explanation has been challenged only in the context of *chronically* hypercapnic and hypoxemic patients with COPD; no investigator has suggested a different kind of explanation for why severely hypoxemic, hyperventilating patients with no history of chronic hypercapnia decrease their ventilation and increase their $PaCO_2$ values after breathing supplemental O_2. That is, if one accepts that hypoxemia stimulates ventilation as earlier described, it logically follows that the removal of that stimulus via O_2 administration would cause ventilation to decrease and $PaCO_2$ to increase; however, when a chronically hypercapnic patient is involved, many investigators completely discount this mechanism as playing a causative role.) Nevertheless, the reduction in minute ventilation after O_2 breathing in patients with advanced COPD is not always severe enough to account for the increased $PaCO_2$.[6,7] Some investigators suggest that O_2 breathing worsens the ventilation/perfusion ratio ($\dot{V}/\dot{Q}$) relationships in the lungs and is responsible for the increase in $PaCO_2$.[6,7] Other investigators have suggested that O_2-induced hypercapnia is caused by the combined effects of hypoxic stimulus removal and redistribution of $\dot{V}/\dot{Q}$ relationships in the lungs.[8,9]

Breathing O_2 worsens the already poor $\dot{V}/\dot{Q}$ relationships in patients with COPD because it abolishes hypoxic pulmonary vasoconstriction in poorly ventilated lung regions. As a result, vascular resistance of underventilated regions decreases, and they receive more blood flow, drawing blood away from well-ventilated regions (Figure 14-5). At the same time that poorly ventilated regions receive more blood flow, they become even less ventilated as O_2-rich inspired gas washes out resident nitrogen gas, making these alveoli more subject to absorption atelectasis (i.e., O_2 may be absorbed by the pulmonary circulation more rapidly than the slowed ventilation can replenish it—notice the further decreased $\dot{V}$ in Figure 14-5, *B*). As a result, inspired gas tends to flow preferentially to the already well-ventilated alveoli (see Figure 14-5, *B*), increasing their $\dot{V}/\dot{Q}$. The increased $\dot{V}/\dot{Q}$ in these alveoli is exaggerated further as a greater proportion of the cardiac output than before is redirected to poorly ventilated alveoli, whose vascular resistance is reduced by O_2 breathing.

O_2 breathing causes more blood flow to be directed to poorly ventilated alveoli, which takes blood flow away from well-ventilated alveoli. The key point is that already underventilated alveoli receive additional blood flow, which causes blood PCO_2 to increase further. These events can occur without a decrease in overall minute ventilation.

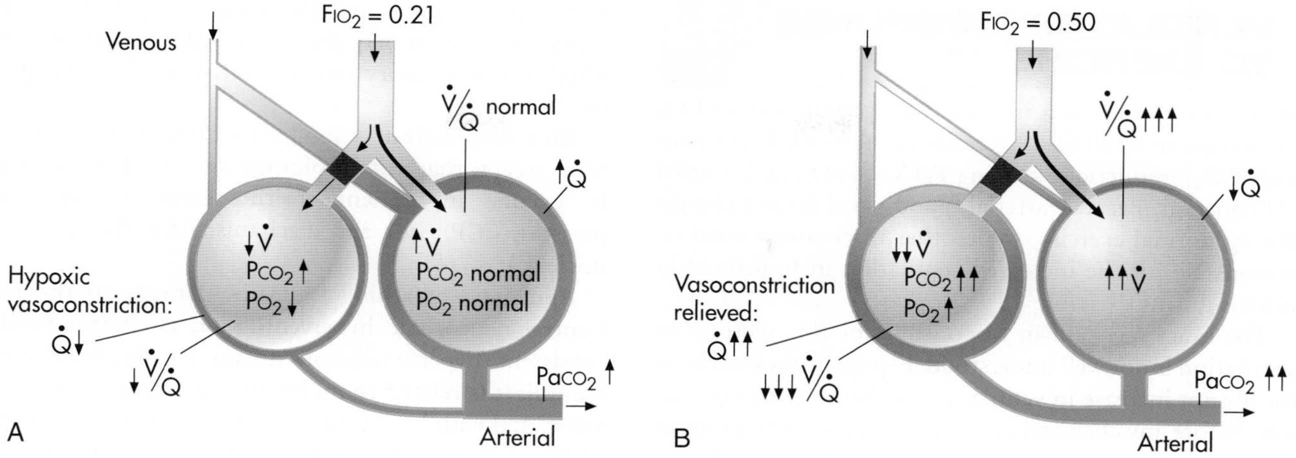

FIGURE 14-5 Proposed mechanism whereby O_2 administration in chronically hypercapnic individuals induces further hypercapnia by creating $\dot{V}/\dot{Q}$ mismatches. **A,** Low $\dot{V}/\dot{Q}$ unit *(left)* is hypoxic and hypercapnic while breathing ambient air; this induces pulmonary vasoconstriction. **B,** Breathing 50% O_2 predisposes the poorly ventilated unit to absorption atelectasis, further decreasing its ventilation, and simultaneously relieves hypoxic vasoconstriction, increasing its blood flow. These events (1) lower the poorly ventilated unit's $\dot{V}/\dot{Q}$ ratio further and (2) divert blood flow away from and ventilation toward already well-ventilated units. The latter increases alveolar dead space (high $\dot{V}/\dot{Q}$). (Modified from Beachey W: Respiratory care anatomy and physiology: foundations for clinical practice, ed 2, St Louis, 2007, Mosby.)

Although some investigators believe the mechanisms just described explain why O_2 administration is associated with hypercapnia in COPD, other studies support an equally important role for O_2 suppression of the hypoxic ventilatory stimulus.[8,9] These studies show that O_2 administration in acutely ill, chronically hypercapnic patients with COPD significantly reduces ventilation and increases the $PaCO_2$ level needed to stimulate ventilation.

The diagnosis of COPD on a patient's medical record does not automatically mean the patient has a chronically high $PaCO_2$ or that O_2 administration may be associated with hypercapnia. These characteristics are present only in severe end-stage disease, which includes only a small percentage of patients with COPD. Concern about O_2-associated hypercapnia and acidemia is not warranted in most patients with a diagnosis of COPD. O_2 should never be withheld from acutely hypoxemic patients with COPD for fear of inducing hypoventilation and hypercapnia. Tissue oxygenation is an overriding priority; O_2 must never be withheld from exacerbated, hypoxemic patients with COPD for any reason. The clinician must be prepared to support ventilation mechanically if O_2 administration is accompanied by severe hypoventilation.

Central Chemoreceptor Response to Acute Carbon Dioxide Increase in Chronic Hypercapnia

As discussed earlier, the kidneys compensate for the acidic effects of chronic hypercapnia by increasing the plasma bicarbonate level, keeping the medullary chemoreceptor pH environment in the normal range. This does not mean that the medullary chemoreceptors cannot respond to further *acute* increases in $PaCO_2$. A sudden elevation in $PaCO_2$ immediately crosses the blood-brain barrier into the CSF, generating H^+ that subsequently stimulates the medullary chemoreceptors. The resulting ventilatory response is depressed, however, for chemical and mechanical reasons: (1) The blood's increased buffering capacity (high HCO_3^- level) in chronic hypercapnia prevents arterial pH from decreasing as sharply as it would in normal conditions, and (2) abnormal breathing mechanics impair the lung's ability to increase ventilation appropriately. To illustrate the blood's changed buffering capacity, compare a healthy person (pH = 7.40, $PaCO_2$ = 40 mm Hg, HCO_3^- = 24 mEq/L) with a chronically hypercapnic person (pH = 7.38, $PaCO_2$ = 60 mm Hg, HCO_3^- = 34 mEq/L). A sudden 30-mm Hg increase in $PaCO_2$ of both individuals causes the healthy person's arterial pH to decrease to 7.21 and the hypercapnic person's pH to decrease to only 7.24. (These values are calculated using the Henderson-Hasselbalch equation, assuming a 1-mEq/L increase in plasma HCO_3^- concentration for each acute 10-mm Hg increase in $PaCO_2$.) The central chemoreceptors of a chronically hypercapnic patient experience less stimulation than the central chemoreceptors of normal individuals for the same increase in $PaCO_2$. Several investigators have confirmed the reduced ventilatory response to CO_2 in chronic hypercapnia.[10,11]

RULE OF THUMB

Tissue oxygenation is of overriding importance and must not be sacrificed because of undue concern about hypercapnia and acidemia in a patient with exacerbated COPD.

VENTILATORY RESPONSE TO EXERCISE

Strenuous exercise can increase CO_2 production and O_2 consumption by 20-fold.[3] Ventilation normally keeps pace with CO_2 production, keeping $PaCO_2$, PaO_2, and arterial pH constant. Because arterial blood gases do not change during normal exercise, some other mechanism must be responsible for the increased ventilation in healthy individuals during exertion.

The exact mechanism responsible for this increase in ventilation is not well understood. Especially mysterious is the abrupt increase in ventilation at the onset of exercise, long before any chemical or humoral changes can occur in the body. Two predominating theories for this phenomenon are the following: (1) When the cerebral motor cortex sends impulses to exercising muscles, it apparently sends collateral excitatory impulses to the medullary respiratory centers; (2) exercising limbs moving around their joints stimulate proprioceptors, which transmit excitatory impulses to the medullary centers.[1,3] Evidence also suggests that the sudden increase in ventilation at the onset of exercise is a learned response.[1,3] With repeated experience, the brain may learn to anticipate the proper amount of ventilation required to maintain normal blood gases during exercise.

ABNORMAL BREATHING PATTERNS

Commonly described abnormal breathing patterns include Cheyne-Stokes respiration, Biot respiration, apneustic breathing, and central neurogenic hypoventilation and hyperventilation. In **Cheyne-Stokes respiration,** respiratory rate and tidal volume gradually increase and then gradually decrease to complete **apnea** (absence of ventilation), which may last several seconds. Tidal volume and breathing frequency gradually increase again, repeating the cycle. This pattern occurs when cardiac output is low, as in congestive heart failure, delaying the blood transit time between the lungs and the brain.[4] In this instance, changes in respiratory center PCO_2 lag behind changes in $PaCO_2$.

For example, when an increased $PaCO_2$ from the lungs reaches the respiratory neurons, ventilation is stimulated; this lowers the $PaCO_2$ level. By the time the reduced $PaCO_2$ reaches the medulla to inhibit ventilation, hyperventilation has been in progress for an inappropriately long time. When blood from the lung finally does reach the medullary centers, the low $PaCO_2$ greatly depresses ventilation to the point of apnea. $PaCO_2$ increases, but an increase in respiratory center PCO_2 is delayed because of low blood flow rate. The brain eventually does receive the high $PaCO_2$ signal, and the cycle is repeated. Cheyne-Stokes respiration may also be caused by brain injuries in which the respiratory centers overrespond to changes in the PCO_2 level.

Biot respiration is similar to Cheyne-Stokes respiration except that tidal volumes are of identical depth. It occurs in patients with increased intracranial pressure (ICP), but the mechanism for this pattern is unclear.[4]

Apneustic breathing indicates damage to the pons. Central neurogenic hyperventilation is characterized by persistent hyperventilation driven by abnormal neural stimuli. It is related to midbrain and upper pons damage associated with head trauma, severe brain hypoxia, or lack of blood flow to the brain.[12] Conversely, central neurogenic hypoventilation means the respiratory centers do not respond appropriately to ventilatory stimuli, such as CO_2. It also is associated with head trauma and brain hypoxia as well as narcotic suppression of the respiratory center.[12]

CARBON DIOXIDE AND CEREBRAL BLOOD FLOW

CO_2 plays an important role in regulating cerebral blood flow. Its effect is mediated through the formation of H^+ by CO_2.[13] Increased PCO_2 dilates cerebral vessels, increasing cerebral blood flow, whereas decreased PCO_2 constricts cerebral vessels and reduces cerebral blood flow. In patients with traumatic brain injury (TBI), the brain swells acutely; this increases the ICP in the rigid skull to such high levels that blood supply to the brain might be cut off, causing cerebral hypoxia *(ischemia)*. That is, high ICP may exceed cerebral arterial pressure and stop blood flow to the brain.

Mechanical hyperventilation has been used for many years in patients with TBI to decrease $PaCO_2$ and reduce the cerebral blood flow and ICP. In patients with TBI, a cerebral blood volume reduction of only 0.5 to 0.7 ml reduces the ICP by 1 mm Hg; for every 1-mm Hg acute reduction in $PaCO_2$ (between 20 mm Hg and 60 mm Hg), there is a 3% reduction in cerebral blood flow. Although an acute reduction in $PaCO_2$ reduces ICP, it also reduces cerebral blood flow and potentially causes cerebral ischemia. For this reason, the practice of inducing mechanical hyperventilation in patients with TBI is controversial; it seems counterintuitive to reduce blood flow and O_2 to an injured organ intentionally. In any event, *hypoventilation* in a head trauma patient with a preexisting high ICP is especially dangerous because the resulting hypercapnia dilates cerebral vessels and elevates the ICP even more.

MINI CLINI

Mechanical Hyperventilation of a Patient With Traumatic Brain Injury

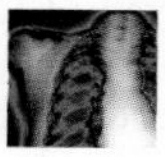

PROBLEM: An automobile accident victim, previously healthy, sustained a closed head injury with accompanying high ICP. Mechanical ventilation in the intensive care unit is required. In ventilating this patient's lungs, you can control the $PaCO_2$. What is your goal in establishing an appropriate $PaCO_2$?

DISCUSSION: More than 40 years ago, clinical investigators showed that the volume of the swollen brain could be reduced by decreasing the $PaCO_2$. Since then, mechanical hyperventilation has been a cornerstone in managing increased ICP associated with TBI.[13] Hyperventilation decreases ICP by causing cerebral vasoconstriction, ultimately reducing cerebral blood volume. This subject is not without controversy; hyperventilation-induced cerebral vasoconstriction has the potential to reduce cerebral blood flow to levels that cause cerebral hypoxia *(ischemia)*. Over the last decade, this concern has dampened enthusiasm for hyperventilation in TBI. Both the proponents and the opponents of hyperventilation recognize that TBI poses an ischemic threat to the brain; proponents believe that the reduction of cerebral blood flow ultimately improves cerebral oxygenation by reducing the ICP, which helps sustain the cerebral perfusion pressure. Opponents point out that no other hypoxic organ in the body is treated by reducing its blood flow and O_2 supply. (Hyperventilation in this context is generally defined as $PaCO_2 < 35$ mm Hg.[13])

The debate centers around the question of whether a hyperventilation-induced decrease in cerebral blood flow creates an additional hypoxic insult to the already ischemic brain and whether patients managed in this way have better clinical outcomes than patients in whom hyperventilation is not instituted. A comprehensive review of the subject published in 2005 concluded that hyperventilation produced no advantage in long-term clinical outcome of TBI compared with ventilation that maintained $PaCO_2$ in the normal range.[13] The authors concluded that in TBI, hyperventilation therapy should be considered only for patients with high ICPs; no benefit can be expected if ICP is normal. They further concluded that hyperventilation is most appropriate in the second or third day after injury because cerebral blood flow is lowest in the first 24 hours after injury, and the risk of inducing ischemia through hyperventilation is greatest during this time. The authors advise against the hyperventilation of TBI patients to $PaCO_2$ less than 30 mm Hg because of the increased danger of cerebral ischemia. Finally, hyperventilation is effective for only about 24 to 48 hours because compensatory renal elimination of bicarbonate in the face of alkalemia restores the acid-base balance, negating the vasoconstrictive effect of hypocapnia. In any case, *hypoventilation* in patients with head trauma and increased ICPs is especially dangerous because hypercapnia dilates cerebral vessels and increases ICP further. Even opponents of hyperventilation generally maintain $PaCO_2$ of TBI patients in the low-normal range around 35 mm Hg.

SUMMARY CHECKLIST

- The DRGs and VRGs of neurons in the medulla generate the basic cyclic breathing pattern.
- Apneustic center impulses prevent medullary inspiratory neurons from switching off, creating a prolonged, gasping inspiration.
- Impulses from the pneumotaxic center inhibit the apneustic center, shortening inspiratory time and increasing respiratory rate.
- Various reflexes from peripheral sources affect the breathing pattern by altering the output of the medullary center.
- Central chemoreceptors in the medulla are bathed in the CSF, separated from arterial blood by a semipermeable membrane called the blood-brain barrier.
- The blood-brain barrier is almost impermeable to arterial H^+ and bicarbonate ions, but it is freely permeable to arterial CO_2.
- Central chemoreceptors stimulate increased ventilation in response to the H^+ formed in the CSF by the reaction between arterial CO_2 and H_2O.
- Peripheral chemoreceptors, located mainly in the carotid bodies, respond to arterial $[H^+]$; hypoxemia increases the sensitivity of chemoreceptors to a given arterial pH.
- The peripheral chemoreceptors are indirectly stimulated by arterial CO_2 to the extent that CO_2 reacts with H_2O to form H^+.
- The primary stimulus for breathing in healthy individuals is arterial CO_2, mediated through the central chemoreceptors via H^+ formed by the reaction between H_2O and CO_2 molecules.
- The secondary stimulus for breathing in healthy individuals is arterial hypoxemia, which is not clinically significant until PaO_2 is less than 60 mm Hg.
- Breathing of patients with chronic, compensated hypercapnia is driven more by the hypoxic stimulus than when acid-base status is normal.
- O_2 therapy is associated with acute arterial CO_2 retention and acidosis in patients with chronic hypercapnia.
- O_2 should never be withheld for any reason from patients with severe hypoxemia.
- CO_2 dilates cerebral blood vessels and increases ICP; reducing arterial CO_2 constricts cerebral vessels and decreases ICP.

References

1. Levitzky MG: Pulmonary physiology, ed 7, New York, 2007, McGraw-Hill Medical.
2. Philipson EA, Duffin J: Hypoventilation and hyperventilation syndromes. In Mason RJ, Broaddus VC, Martin TR, et al, editors: Murray and Nadel's textbook of respiratory medicine, ed 5, Philadelphia, 2010, Saunders.
3. Hall JE: Guyton and Hall: textbook of medical physiology, ed 12, Philadelphia, 2010, Saunders.

4. Comroe JH: Physiology of respiration, ed 2, Chicago, 1974, Year Book.
5. West JB: Respiratory physiology: the essentials, ed 8, Philadelphia, 2008, Lippincott Williams & Wilkins.
6. Crossley DJ, McGuire GP, Barrow PM, et al: Influence of inspired oxygen concentration on deadspace, respiratory drive, and $PaCO_2$ in intubated patients with chronic obstructive pulmonary disease. Crit Care Med 25:1522, 1997.
7. Gomersall CD, Joynt GM, Freebairn RC, et al: Oxygen therapy for hypercapnic patients with chronic obstructive pulmonary disease and acute respiratory failure: a randomized, controlled pilot study. Crit Care Med 30:113, 2002.
8. Robinson TD, Freiberg DB, Regnis JA, et al: The role of hypoventilation and ventilation-perfusion redistribution in oxygen-induced hypercapnia during acute exacerbations of chronic obstructive pulmonary disease. Am J Respir Crit Care Med 161:1524, 2000.
9. Calverley PM: Oxygen-induced hypercapnia revisited (editorial). Lancet 356:1538, 2000.
10. Heyer L, Lorino H, Delclaux C, et al: Carbon dioxide respiratory response during positive inspiratory pressure in COPD patients. Respir Physiol 109:29, 1997.
11. Scano G, Spinelli A, Duranti R, et al: Carbon dioxide responsiveness in COPD patients with and without chronic hypercapnia. Eur Respir J 8:78, 1995.
12. Bleck TP: Levels of consciousness and attention. In Goetz CG, editor: Textbook of clinical neurology, ed 2, Philadelphia, 2003, Saunders.
13. Stocchetti N, Maas AI, Chieregato A, et al: Hyperventilation in head injury: a review. Chest 127:1812, 2005.

SECTION III

ASSESSMENT OF RESPIRATORY DISORDERS

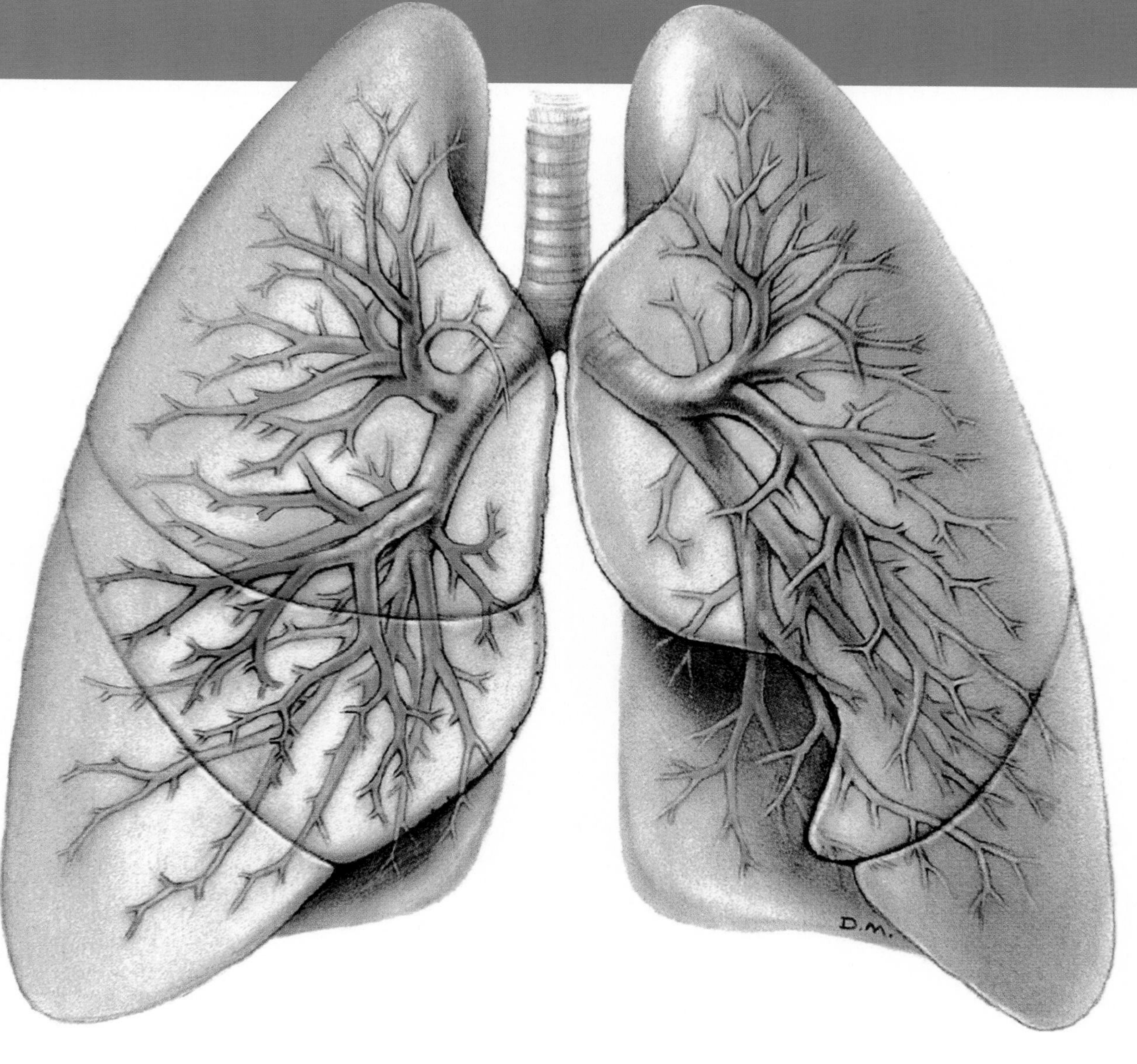

Chapter 15

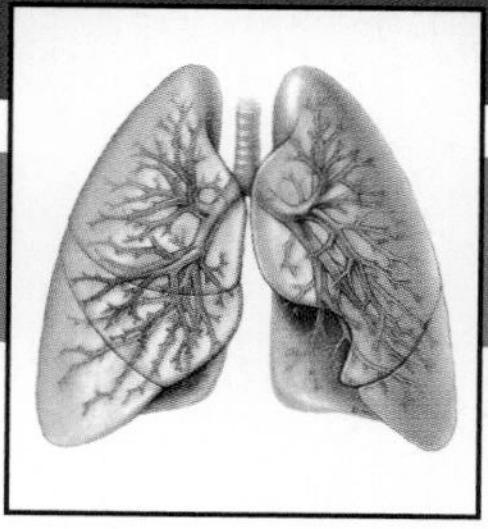

Bedside Assessment of the Patient

RICHARD H. KALLET

CHAPTER OBJECTIVES

After reading this chapter you will be able to:

- Describe why patient interviews are necessary and the appropriate techniques for conducting an interview.
- Identify abnormalities in lung function associated with common pulmonary symptoms.
- Identify breathing patterns associated with underlying pulmonary disease.
- Differentiate between dyspnea and breathlessness.
- Identify terms used to describe normal and abnormal lung sounds.
- Describe the mechanisms responsible for normal and abnormal lung sounds.
- Explain why it is necessary to examine the precordium, abdomen, and extremities in patients with cardiopulmonary disease.
- Describe some common abnormalities found during the examination of the precordium, abdomen, and extremities in patients with cardiopulmonary disease.

CHAPTER OUTLINE

KEY TERMS

abdominal compartment syndrome
abdominal paradox
advance directive
adventitious lung sounds
angina
barrel chest
bradycardia
bradypnea
breathlessness
bronchophony
cachexia
clubbing
cough
crackles
cyanosis
diaphoresis
diastolic pressure
dyspnea
febrile
fetid
fever
gallop rhythm
heave
hematemesis
hemoptysis
hepatomegaly
Hoover sign
hypertension
hypotension
hypothermia
hypovolemia
jugular venous distention
Kussmaul breathing
Kussmaul sign
loud P_2
lymphadenopathy
mucoid
murmurs
orthodeoxia
orthopnea
pack-years
pedal edema
phlegm
platypnea
pneumothorax
postural hypotension
pulse deficit
pulse pressure
pulsus alternans
pulsus paradoxus
purulent
respiratory alternans
retractions

sensorium
shock
sputum
stridor
subcutaneous emphysema
syncope
systolic pressure
tachycardia
tachypnea
thrills
tracheal tugging
tripodding
wheezes

Progress in the field of respiratory care has placed increasing demands on respiratory therapists (RTs) to develop competent bedside assessment skills. Decisions regarding when to initiate, change, or discontinue therapy depend on accurate clinical assessment. Although the physician has the ultimate responsibility for these decisions, RTs often participate in the clinical decision-making process. To fulfill this role effectively, the RT must assume responsibility for gathering and interpreting relevant bedside patient data.

Bedside assessment is the process of interviewing and examining a patient for signs and symptoms of disease and the effects of treatment. It is a cost-effective way of obtaining pertinent information about the patient's health status. In many cases, bedside assessment provides the initial evidence that something is wrong and often helps establish the severity of the problem. In contrast to some diagnostic tests, bedside assessment techniques are of little risk to the patient.

Two key sources of patient data are the medical history and the physical examination. Data gathered initially by interview and physical examination help identify the need for subsequent diagnostic tests. After a tentative diagnosis is made, these assessment procedures also help the clinician to select the best approach to therapy. After a treatment regimen begins, these assessment procedures are repeated to monitor patient progress toward predefined goals.

The patient initially is assessed to identify the correct diagnosis. This initial assessment is most often performed by a physician. Exceptions may occur in emergency situations in which a physician is unavailable. In such cases, other health care personnel, such as nurses and RTs, may need to evaluate the patient rapidly to implement appropriate lifesaving treatment (e.g., cardiopulmonary resuscitation). After a tentative diagnosis is reached and the physician orders specific treatment, subsequent evaluations are made by health care personnel to monitor the patient during the hospital stay and to evaluate treatment results.

The skills of bedside assessment described here are not difficult to learn; however, mastery requires practice. Initially, students should practice the skills on healthy individuals. This practice helps improve technique and provides an understanding of normal variations. The ability to discriminate abnormal from the range of possible normal findings is an important skill that requires experience to master.

INTERVIEWING THE PATIENT AND TAKING A MEDICAL HISTORY

Interviewing furnishes unique information because it provides the patient's perspective. It serves the following three related purposes:

1. To establish a rapport between the clinician and patient
2. To obtain essential diagnostic information
3. To help monitor changes in the patient's symptoms and response to therapy

MINI CLINI

Bedside Assessment of the Postoperative Patient

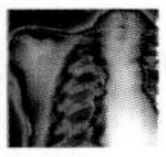

PROBLEM: The RT is called to the surgical ward to see a 54-year-old woman who underwent abdominal surgery 2 days earlier. She is currently afebrile, alert, and oriented but is complaining of dyspnea. Her resting respiratory rate is 34 breaths/min, and the breaths are shallow. Her heart rate is 110 beats/min. She is 5 feet tall and weighs approximately 185 lb. During the brief interview, the RT identifies that the dyspnea has gradually increased over the past 12 hours and increases with exertion. During auscultation, the RT identifies diminished breath sounds in the bases, with some fine, late inspiratory crackles. The remainder of the physical examination is normal. What is the most likely cause of this patient's dyspnea, and what should be done?

SOLUTION: The findings indicate a loss of lung volume as the cause of the sudden dyspnea. The rapid, shallow breathing; fine, late inspiratory crackles; and history of recent abdominal surgery suggest atelectasis. Patients who undergo abdominal surgery are prone to developing atelectasis in the postoperative period. Other concerns include CHF and pulmonary thromboembolism. The RT should ask the attending physician to order a chest radiograph and begin lung expansion therapy if the chest film confirms the presence of atelectasis.

For these reasons, interviewing is a crucial aspect of general patient assessment.

Principles of Interviewing

Interviewing is a way of "connecting" with the patient. This connection is especially important for the patient who is under the stress of an illness because meaningful human contact lessens the patient's sense of isolation. The factors that affect communication between the RT and the patient include the following:

- Sensory and emotional factors
- Environmental factors
- Verbal and nonverbal components of the communication process
- Cultural and other internal values, beliefs, feelings, habits, and preoccupations of both the health care professional and the patient

Because of the above-listed factors, no two interviews are the same.

Although developing interviewing skills takes time and experience, beginners can get a head start by following a few basic guidelines and by becoming knowledgeable about the causes and characteristics of common cardiopulmonary symptoms. The following discussion provides some of the guidelines for interviewing and discusses common symptoms associated with diseases of the chest.

Structure and Technique for Interviewing

The ideal interview is one in which the patient feels secure and free to talk about important personal matters. Each interview should begin with the RT introducing himself or herself to the patient and stating the purpose of the visit. The introduction is done in the *social space,* approximately 4 to 12 feet from the patient. It begins the process of establishing a rapport with the patient and helps the patient feel more comfortable about answering personal questions. Pulling the curtain between the beds of a semiprivate room also may be helpful in making the patient feel more at ease with the interview (Box 15-1).

Next, the RT moves into the *personal space* (2 to 4 feet from the patient) to begin the interview. In this space, the patient does not have to speak loudly in response to questions. The RT should assume a physical position at the same level with the patient (e.g., by sitting in a chair) before beginning the formal interview. Standing over the patient

Box 15-1 Guidelines for Effective Patient Interviewing

PROJECT A SENSE OF UNDIVIDED INTEREST IN THE PATIENT

- Provide for privacy and do not permit interruptions.
- Review records and prepare materials before entering the room.
- Listen and observe carefully.
- Use appropriate eye contact.
- Be attentive and respond to the patient's priorities, concerns, feelings, and comfort.

ESTABLISH YOUR PROFESSIONAL ROLE DURING THE INTRODUCTION

- Dress and groom professionally.
- Enter the room with a smile and unhurried manner.
- Make immediate eye contact.
- If the patient is well enough, introduce yourself with a firm handshake.
- State your role and the purpose of your visit, and define the patient's involvement in the interaction.
- Address adult patients by title (e.g., Mr., Mrs., Ms.) and their last name. Using these formal terms of address alerts the patient to the importance of the interaction.

SHOW YOUR RESPECT FOR THE PATIENT'S BELIEFS, ATTITUDES, AND RIGHTS

- Ensure the patient is appropriately covered.
- Position yourself so that eye contact is comfortable for the patient. (Ideally, patients should be sitting up, with their eye level at or slightly above yours.)
- Avoid standing at the foot of the bed or with your hand on the door because this may send the nonverbal message that you do not have time for the patient.
- Ask the patient's permission before moving any personal items or making adjustments in the room.
- Remember that the patient's dialog with you and his or her medical record are confidential. Share this information only with other health care providers who need to know about it, and do not share the information in a place where others can overhear the conversation.
- Be honest; never guess at an answer or information that you do not know; do not provide information beyond your scope of practice; providing new information to the patient is the privilege and responsibility of the attending physician.
- Make no moral judgments about the patient; set your values for patient care according to the patient's values, beliefs, and priorities.
- Expect the patient to have an emotional response to illness and the health care environment.
- Listen, and then clarify and teach, but never argue.
- Adjust the time, length, and content of the interview to the patient's needs.

USE A RELAXED, CONVERSATIONAL STYLE

- Ask questions and make statements that communicate empathy.
- Encourage the patient to express his or her concerns.
- Expect and accept some periods of silence.
- Close even the briefest interview by asking whether there is anything the patient needs or wants to discuss.
- Tell the patient when you will return.

should be avoided because this position makes the patient feel inferior. Appropriate eye contact with the patient is essential for a quality interview. Eye contact gives the patient more confidence in the interviewer. Eye contact also allows the interviewer to see confusion, anger, frustration, and other emotions that may be expressed by the patient in response to questions.

Using neutral questions and avoiding leading questions during the interview is important. Asking the patient, "Is your breathing better now?" leads the patient toward a desired response and may elicit false information. Asking the patient, "How is your breathing now?" is a better way to get accurate information about the patient's breathing (Box 15-2).

Common characteristics of symptoms can be identified by asking questions such as the following during the interview:

Box 15-2 Types of Questions Used in Patient Interviews

- *Open-ended questions* encourage patients to describe events and priorities as they see them, helping to bring out concerns and attitudes and to promote understanding. Questions such as "What brought you to the hospital?" or "What happened next?" encourage conversational flow and rapport, while giving patients enough direction to know where to start.
- *Closed questions,* such as "When did your cough start?" or "How long did the pain last?" focus on specific information and provide clarification.
- *Direct questions* can be open-ended or closed and always end in a question mark. Although they are used to obtain specific information, a series of direct questions or frequent use of the question "Why?" can be intimidating and cause the patient to minimize his or her responses to questions.
- *Indirect questions* are less threatening than direct questions because they sound like statements (e.g., "I gather your doctor told you to take the treatments every 4 hours"). Inquiries of this type also work well to confront discrepancies in the patient's statements (e.g., "If I understood you correctly, it is harder for you to breathe now than it was before your treatment").
- *Neutral questions* and statements are preferred for all interactions with the patient. "What happened next?" and "Can you tell me more about ...?" are neutral, open-ended questions. A neutral, closed question may give the patient a choice of responses, while focusing on the type of information desired (e.g., "Would you say there was a teaspoon, a tablespoon, or a half cup?"). Leading questions, such as "You didn't cough up blood, did you?" should be avoided because they imply an answer.

- When did it start?
- How severe is it? (This can be rated on a scale of 1 to 10.)
- Where on the body is it? (This is especially important for chest pain.)
- What seems to make it better or worse?
- Has it occurred before? (If so, how long did it last?)

Identifying these characteristics of any new symptom can be helpful in recognizing the cause and potential therapy; this is primarily the role of the attending physician but sometimes falls to other clinicians in certain settings. Once the symptom or symptoms are established and therapy is started, other questions are used to evaluate the changes in the symptoms over the course of the hospital stay. For example, the clinician may ask, "Has the symptom changed in any way since admission?" or, "Does the therapy seem to make a difference?"

The best interview techniques are of no value if the interviewer is not knowledgeable about the pathophysiology and characteristics of common cardiopulmonary symptoms. The interview is a series of focused questions that pursue specific information related to a tentative diagnosis. The ability to ask the key questions at the right time comes from experience and familiarity with the signs and symptoms of lung disease.

Common Cardiopulmonary Symptoms

Dyspnea

Dyspnea is a *general term* describing the sensation of breathing discomfort. It is the most important symptom that the RT is called on to assess and treat. Dyspnea is a *subjective experience* and should not be inferred from observing the patient's breathing pattern. Analogies often have been made between dyspnea and pain. Both sensations possess qualitatively distinct features and varying intensity. Similar to pain, dyspnea causes suffering. *As breathing is the primordial sensation of life,* dyspnea often is perceived as life-threatening and may provoke a profound sense of dread.

The term *dyspnea* also is used *specifically* to describe *difficulty in the mechanical act of breathing.* The simplest explanation is that the effort to breathe is proportionally greater than the tidal volume achieved. A person's perception of breathing is a complex balance between the following three factors:

1. The neural drive to breathe
2. The tension developed in the respiratory muscles
3. The corresponding displacement of the lungs and chest wall

When the neuronal signals governing these sensations become unbalanced, breathing is perceived to be abnormal and unpleasant. The technical name for this imbalance is *neuromechanical dissociation.* Individuals normally experience this form of dyspnea only in unusual circumstances, such as when trying to breathe through a straw or when wearing a restrictive garment.

Breathlessness. Breathlessness is the specific sensation of an *unpleasant urge to breathe*. It is believed to be the conscious perception of intense neural discharge to the respiratory muscles. Breathlessness can be triggered by acute hypercapnia and acidosis and by hypoxemia. A normal experience of breathlessness is the unpleasant throbbing sensation that accompanies prolonged breath holding or feeling "winded" during strenuous physical exercise. However, it is not known how closely normal encounters with breathlessness resemble the sensation that arises during disease because dyspnea in patients with cardiopulmonary disease also is affected by other stimuli that contribute to both the quality and the intensity of the sensation. These include stimuli arising from hypoxemia, irritant receptors in the lungs and airways, and receptors in the blood vessels and heart.

Ultimately, dyspnea and breathlessness are magnified by the emotional distress that accompanies them. This distress is influenced by situation, knowledge, and control. In other words, a healthy person can quickly identify the source of breathlessness and arrest the symptom simply by stopping exercise or the breath hold. In contrast, a patient with cardiopulmonary disease may be unable to control the symptom, let alone be able to identify the source. These factors have a profound emotional impact that must be appreciated by the RT.

Positional Dyspnea. Dyspnea may be present only when the patient assumes the reclining position, in which case it is referred to as **orthopnea.** Orthopnea is common in patients with congestive heart failure (CHF); it apparently is caused by the sudden increase in venous return that occurs with reclining. The failing left ventricle is unable to accommodate the increased venous return, resulting in pulmonary vascular congestion and dyspnea. Orthopnea is also a symptom of bilateral diaphragmatic paralysis.

Dyspnea in the upright position is known as **platypnea.** This unusual symptom may accompany arteriovenous malformations in the lung, such as occur in chronic liver disease (hepatopulmonary syndrome), and some hereditary conditions. Platypnea may be accompanied by **orthodeoxia,** which is oxygen desaturation on assuming an upright position.

Language of Dyspnea. Dyspnea is a subjective experience, and patients possess a nuanced language to describe their sensations. RTs should ask specific questions about the quality and characteristics of the patient's dyspnea. In this way, the RT might gain insight into the mechanism provoking dyspnea. As the patient describes the sensations, the RT should try to categorize each according to a particular aspect of breathing such as inspiration, expiration, respiratory drive, or lung volume. A remark such as, "I feel that my breath stops," reflects a problem with inspiration, whereas the remark, "my breath does not go all the way out," suggests a problem with expiration. Statements such as, "I can't catch my breath," suggest that respiratory drive is elevated (i.e., breathlessness).

Different types of lung diseases often evoke unique sensations that may provide clues about the underlying pathophysiology. Patients with asthma frequently complain of chest tightness. In contrast, patients with interstitial lung disease tend to focus on the sensations of increased work of breathing, shallow breathing, and gasping. Patients with CHF are seemingly unique in frequently feeling suffocated. Although the language used to describe dyspnea provides helpful clues, the RT should keep in mind that many lung diseases evoke common sensations.

Patients with cardiopulmonary disease frequently experience several unpleasant breathing sensations simultaneously. A particular sensation may be more prominent than others and may change over time. As mentioned previously, patients with asthma typically complain first about the sensation of chest tightness. However, as bronchoconstriction worsens and the lungs become more hyperinflated, patients often begin to focus more on the sensation of excessive work of breathing, air hunger, and the inability to take a deep breath.

Assessing Dyspnea in the Interview. The assessment of dyspnea is largely determined by the situation. When conducting an interview, the RT should pay particular attention to whether the patient can speak in full sentences. It may be very difficult for patients with severe dyspnea from any cause to speak more than a few words at a time. In this situation, the initial interview should be curtailed, and treatment should be initiated as soon as possible. Questions should be brief and limited to the quality and intensity of dyspnea and the circumstances of symptom onset. Also, the assessment of dyspnea should occur simultaneously with a gross examination of the patient's breathing pattern (see later section of this chapter). Assessment of dyspnea that arises acutely in patients without a prior history of cardiopulmonary disease typically does not require the same detail as assessment in patients with long-standing cardiopulmonary or neurologic disease.

In patients with chronic cardiopulmonary disease, a detailed and systematic history should cover four major areas, as follows:

1. The RT should ask what activities of daily living tend to trigger episodes of dyspnea. For example, is dyspnea triggered by walking on flat surfaces, by climbing stairs, by bathing, by dressing?
2. The RT should ask how much exertion is required for the patient to stop to catch his or her breath with different activities. Does the patient need to stop after walking up one flight of stairs or one step? Dyspnea provoked by less strenuous activities indicates more advanced disease.
3. The RT should ask whether the quality or the sensation of breathing discomfort varies with different activities.
4. To gain a better understanding of the patient's history, the RT should ask the patient to recall when dyspnea first began and how it has evolved over time. Has

Modified Borg Scale

Number	Verbal Description
10	Severe
9	
8	Moderately severe
7	
6	
5	Moderate
4	
3	
2	Slight
1	
0	None

A

Visual Scale

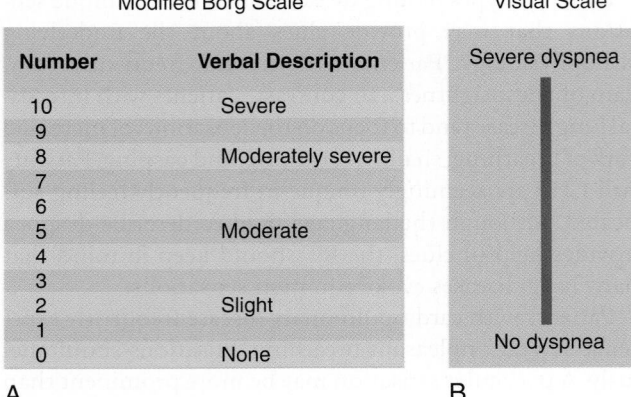

B

FIGURE 15-1 A, Modified Borg scale. **B,** Visual analog scale for measuring the degree of dyspnea.

dyspnea progressed slowly or rapidly? How long has this progression taken place: over a period of months or years? Has there been a dramatic change in the intensity of dyspnea over recent months, weeks, days, or even within the past few hours?

Beyond the information gleaned, a detailed conversation about a patient's struggle with dyspnea allows the patient to share his or her experience and decreases the patient's sense of isolation.

The intensity of dyspnea can be documented using a numeric intensity or visual analog scale (Figure 15-1). Such scales provide a way to evaluate the patient's response to treatment over time. These scales are important because objective lung function measurements (e.g., pulmonary function tests, PaO_2) seldom correlate with the degree of dyspnea in many patients.

Psychogenic Dyspnea: Panic Disorders and Hyperventilation. There are perplexing situations in which patients with normal cardiopulmonary function complain of intense dyspnea or suffocation. This condition is known as *psychogenic hyperventilation syndrome* and is associated with panic disorders. Hyperventilation may coincide with other symptoms such as chest pain, anxiety, palpitations and *paresthesia* (the sensation of tingling and numbness in the extremities that often accompanies respiratory alkalosis). This syndrome may be either sporadic or chronic and often is self-perpetuating.

Anxiety often is accompanied by breathlessness and hyperventilation. The resulting respiratory alkalosis amplifies the sensation of breathlessness and provokes more anxiety, increasing the intensity of hyperventilation. The classic homespun remedy of having the patient slowly rebreathe into a paper bag holds merit because this can arrest the respiratory alkalosis and help break the cycle. However, rebreathing techniques may require formal behavioral therapy and may not be appropriate in the hospital setting. This condition usually is treated clinically by administering judicious amounts of anxiolytic agents.

The RT *always* must approach any situation involving hyperventilation or dyspnea as if it had a pathophysiologic basis. The first priority is to measure the vital signs, including arterial oxygen saturation, and perhaps a 12-lead electrocardiogram and arterial blood gases. A psychogenic source should be considered only after a pathogenic source for hyperventilation or dyspnea has been ruled out. Intense pain or fear may provoke anxiety and hyperventilation. The RT must work in concert with nursing and physician colleagues to determine the root cause of any hyperventilation syndrome.

Cough

A **cough** is the most common, yet nonspecific symptom seen in patients with pulmonary disease. Coughing is a forceful expiratory maneuver that expels mucus and foreign material from the airways. It usually occurs when the cough receptors are stimulated by inflammation, mucus, foreign materials, or noxious gases. The cough receptors are located primarily in the larynx, trachea, and larger bronchi.

The effectiveness of a cough depends on the ability of the individual to take a deep breath, lung elastic recoil, expiratory muscle strength, and level of airway resistance. The ability to take a deep breath or exhale forcefully is often impaired in patients with neuromuscular disease. An effective cough also is impaired secondary to pain; this is typically seen in the early postoperative period in patients following upper abdominal surgery or thoracic surgery or after trauma. Often expiratory flow is limited by factors such as bronchospasm (e.g., asthma) and reduced lung elastic recoil (as in emphysema). Patients with an inadequate ability to cough because of impairment of these factors often have problems with retained secretions and are more prone to the development of pneumonia.

Important characteristics of the patient's cough to identify include whether it is dry or loose, productive or nonproductive, and acute or chronic and whether it occurs more frequently at particular times (i.e., day or night). Knowledge of such details may help in determining the cause of the cough. A dry, nonproductive cough is typical for restrictive lung diseases such as CHF or pulmonary fibrosis. A loose, productive cough is more often associated with inflammatory obstructive diseases such as bronchitis and asthma. The most common cause of an acute, self-limited cough is a viral infection of the upper airway. Common causes of chronic coughing include asthma, postnasal drip, chronic bronchitis, and gastroesophageal reflux,[1] although combinations of these often exist.[2] Cough is also associated with the use of certain medications for hypertension (e.g., angiotensin-converting enzyme inhibitors).[3]

Sputum Production

Healthy airways produce mucus daily. Normally, the quantity of this mucus is minimal, and it is not enough to stimulate the cough receptors. Mucus is gradually moved to the hypopharynx by the mucociliary escalator, where it is either swallowed or expectorated. Disease of the airways may cause the mucous glands, which line the airways, to produce an abnormally increased amount of mucus, which usually stimulates the cough receptors and causes the patient to generate a loose, productive cough. This cough is seen in acute bronchitis or asthma attacks brought on by airway infection.

RTs need to be aware of the terminology associated with sputum. Technically, mucus from the tracheobronchial tree that has not been contaminated by oral secretions is called **phlegm.** Mucus that comes from the lung but passes through the mouth as it is expectorated is **sputum.** Because this is how most mucus samples from the lung are obtained, the term *sputum* is used in this chapter. Sputum that contains pus cells is said to be **purulent,** suggesting a bacterial infection. Purulent sputum appears thick, colored, and sticky. Sputum that is foul-smelling is said to be **fetid.** Sputum that is clear and thick is **mucoid** and is commonly seen in patients with airways disease (i.e., asthma). Changes in the color, viscosity, or quantity of sputum produced are often signs of infection and must be documented and reported to the physician.

Hemoptysis

Coughing up blood or blood-streaked sputum from the lungs is referred to as **hemoptysis.** Blood-streaked sputum is common in patients with pulmonary disease. *Frank hemoptysis* is the presence primarily of blood in the expectorant. Hemoptysis is characterized as massive when more than 300 ml of blood is expectorated over 24 hours, and this represents a medical emergency. Hemoptysis must be distinguished from **hematemesis,** which is vomiting blood from the gastrointestinal tract. Blood from the lung is often seen in patients with a history of pulmonary disease and may be mixed with sputum. Blood from the stomach may be mixed with food particles and occurs most often in patients with a history of gastrointestinal disease.

Nonmassive hemoptysis is caused most often by infection of the airways but also is seen in lung cancer, tuberculosis, blunt or penetrating chest trauma, and pulmonary embolism. Hemoptysis associated with infection usually is seen as blood-streaked, purulent sputum. Hemoptysis commonly is found in patients with bacterial pneumonia. Hemoptysis from bronchogenic carcinoma often is chronic and may be associated with a monophonic wheeze and cough. Common causes of massive hemoptysis include bronchiectasis, lung abscess, and acute or old tuberculosis.

Chest Pain

Most chest pain can be categorized as either *pleuritic* or *nonpleuritic. Pleuritic chest pain* usually is located laterally or posteriorly. It worsens when the patient takes a deep breath, and it is described as a *sharp, stabbing* type of pain. It is associated with diseases of the chest that cause the pleural lining of the lung to become inflamed, such as pneumonia or pulmonary embolism.

Nonpleuritic chest pain is located typically in the center of the anterior chest and may radiate to the shoulder or back. It is not affected by breathing, and it is described as a *dull ache* or *pressure* type of pain. A common cause of nonpleuritic chest pain is **angina,** which classically is a pressure sensation with exertion or stress and results from coronary artery occlusion. Other common causes of nonpleuritic chest pain include gastroesophageal reflux, esophageal spasm, chest wall pain (e.g., costochondritis), and gallbladder disease.

MINI CLINI

Sudden Onset of Chest Pain

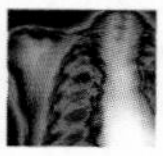

PROBLEM: The RT is called to the emergency department to see a 47-year-old man who came to the hospital with anxiety and chest pain. He is certain he is having a heart attack and demands immediate treatment. The attending physician is on the way to the hospital but has asked the nurse to call the RT in the interim. The RT places the patient on oxygen per protocol and asks him for details about the chest pain. The patient states that the pain is located laterally on the left side and increases with each inspiratory effort. The pain is sharp in nature. The patient's vital signs are normal (including respiratory rate) except for a slight increase in heart rate. What is the most likely cause of this patient's chest pain, given its characteristics? What should be done until the physician arrives?

SOLUTION: Chest pain is a worrisome symptom because it can indicate a life-threatening problem or a less serious problem. Among the most serious problems are acute heart attack, pulmonary embolism, aortic dissection, and pneumothorax. In this case, the pain seems to be pleuritic. Angina, acute myocardial infarction, and aortic dissection are not likely causes. The pleuritic character of the pain is consistent with pulmonary embolism and pneumothorax, but the normal respiratory rate suggests that pulmonary embolism is not the likely cause of the chest pain. If pneumothorax is present, it must be small. The RT should continue oxygen therapy and monitor the patient until the attending physician arrives. The RT should ask the nurse to attach chest leads to monitor the patient's heart rate and rhythm just in case the chest pain is related to heart disease. In addition, the RT should try to comfort the patient as much as possible.

Fever

Fever (an elevated body temperature secondary to disease) is a common complaint of patients with an infection of the airways or lungs. Fever may occur with a viral infection of the upper airway or bacterial pneumonia or tuberculosis. All patients with a fever need further assessment to determine the cause. When infection causes fever, the magnitude of temperature elevation may indicate the type and virulence of the infection. Low-grade fever typically accompanies common upper respiratory tract infections, whereas a high fever occurs with viral influenza infection.

Fever that occurs with a cough suggests a respiratory infection. An infection is even more likely to be the cause of the fever if the patient is producing purulent sputum. In this situation, a persistent fever of at least 38.9° C (102° F) for 2 days accompanied by chills is suggestive of pneumonia. However, the absence of coughing or sputum production does not rule out lung infection. Noninfectious causes of fever include head trauma (secondary to damage of the hypothalamus), cancer, immunologic disorders (e.g., sarcoidosis), an adverse reaction to certain medications (e.g., sulfa drugs), and thromboembolic disorders such as pulmonary embolism.

It was believed for many years that there was a link between fever and atelectasis in postoperative surgical patients. However, more recent evidence has shown no link between the formation of atelectasis and the development of fever (>101.3° F [>38.5° C]) during the first 72 hours after surgery.[4]

Patients with a significant fever have an increased metabolic rate and an increased oxygen (O_2) consumption and carbon dioxide (CO_2) production. The increased need for O_2 intake and CO_2 removal may cause tachypnea. The increased ventilatory demand caused by fever is particularly dangerous for patients with severe chronic cardiopulmonary disease because it may cause acute respiratory failure.

Pedal Edema

Swelling of the lower extremities is known as **pedal edema.** It most often occurs with heart failure, which causes an increase in the hydrostatic pressure of the blood vessels in the lower extremities. This increase in hydrostatic pressure causes fluid to leak into the interstitial spaces and leads to pedal edema, the degree of which depends on the level of heart failure. There are two subtypes of pedal edema. When pressure is applied with a finger on a swollen extremity, an indentation mark left on the skin is called *pitting edema*. *Weeping edema* is when a small fluid leak occurs at the point where pressure is applied.

Patients with chronic hypoxemic lung disease are especially prone to right-sided heart failure (cor pulmonale) because of the heavy demands placed on the right ventricle when hypoxemia causes severe pulmonary vasoconstriction. Eventually, the right side of the heart begins to fail and results in a backup of pressure into the venous blood vessels, especially in the dependent regions such as the lower extremities. This situation promotes high intravascular venous hydrostatic pressures and pedal edema. The patient often complains of "swollen ankles" in such cases.

Format for the Medical History

All health care practitioners must be familiar with the medical history of the patients they are treating, even if their reason for contact is simply to provide intermittent therapy. The medical history familiarizes clinicians with the signs and symptoms the patient exhibited on admission and the reason the therapy is being administered.

The RT should begin reviewing the patient's chart by reading about the patient's current medical problems. This information is found under the headings of *chief complaint* and *history of present illness*. This section of the medical history represents a detailed account of each of the patient's major complaints. It is written by the physician after his or her interview with the patient at admission to the hospital.

The next step is to review the patient's *past medical history*, which describes all past major illnesses, injuries, surgeries, hospitalizations, allergies, and health-related habits. This information provides a basic understanding of the patient's previous experiences with illness and health care and may have an impact on decisions made during the current hospitalization. This section of the health history may be the place the interviewer records the patient's history of cigarette and alcohol consumption.

An accurate determination of a patient's smoking history is an extremely important aspect of assessing pulmonary health. The smoking history is often recorded in **pack-years,** which is determined by *multiplying the number of packs smoked per day by the number of years smoked*. Typically, a patient is asked how many cigarettes (on average) he or she smokes per day. Some patients express this in terms of packs of cigarettes, whereas others state the number of cigarettes. If a patient states that he or she has smoked a pack of cigarettes a day for 20 years, the patient has a 20 pack-year smoking history.

If patients describe their smoking in terms of the number of cigarettes, or fractions of a pack, the calculation is slightly more difficult. Two examples may help illustrate how to calculate pack-years of smoking. There are 20 cigarettes per pack. If a patient states he or she has smoked a pack and a half of cigarettes per day for 20 years, the smoking history is calculated as follows:

$$30 \text{ cigarettes}/20 \text{ cigarettes per pack} = 1.5 \text{ packs} \times 20 \text{ years} = 30 \text{ pack-years smoking history}$$

If the patient states that he or she has smoked 15 cigarettes per day for 20 years:

$$15 \text{ cigarettes}/20 \text{ cigarettes per pack} = 0.75 \text{ packs} \times 20 \text{ years} = 15 \text{ pack-years smoking history}$$

Next, the *family* and *social/environmental history* should be reviewed. This part of the medical history focuses on potential genetic or occupational links to disease and the patient's current life situation. Pulmonary disorders such as asthma, lung cancer, cystic fibrosis, and chronic obstructive pulmonary disease (COPD) are believed to have a genetic link in many cases. A detailed occupational history is important in assessing pulmonary disorders that may result from inhaling dusts in the workplace, either organic (i.e., containing protein) or nonorganic (e.g., asbestos, silica). There is a strong link between asthma and poverty.

The *review of systems* is designed to uncover problem areas the patient forgot to mention or omitted. This information is usually obtained in a head-to-toe review of all body systems. For each body system, the interviewer obtains information about current, pertinent symptoms. During a review of the respiratory system, questioning would determine the presence or history of cough, hemoptysis, sputum production, chest pain, shortness of breath, and fever (Box 15-3).

Finally, the medical record should be examined for information indicating any limits on the extent of care to be provided in the event of cardiac or respiratory arrest. This information is known as an **advance directive,** whereby the patient (or a legally authorized representative) has formalized his or her wishes for resuscitative efforts; this is typically referred to as the *DNR status* ("do not resuscitate") or may be expressed as DNI ("do not intubate"). This information may be found either in the admission note or within the body of the physician progress notes. In addition to this descriptive note, there must be an order written by the physician clearly specifying how care should be limited in the event of a medical emergency.

The first priority of the RT reviewing the medical record is to ensure that all respiratory care procedures are supported by a physician order that is current, clearly written, and complete.

Box 15-3 Outline of a Complete Health History

Demographic data (obtained from admission interview): Name, address, age, birth date, place of birth, race, nationality, marital status, religion, occupation, and source of referral

Date and source of history and estimate of the reliability of the historian

Brief description of the patient's condition at the time the history or patient profile was taken

Chief complaint and reason for seeking treatment

History of present illness: Chronologic description of each symptom
- Onset: Time, type, source, setting
- Frequency and duration of symptoms
- Location and radiation of pain
- Severity (quantity)
- Quality (character)
- Aggravating and alleviating factors
- Associated manifestations

Past medical history
- Childhood diseases and development
- Hospitalizations, surgeries, injuries, accidents, and major illnesses
- Allergies
- Medications

Family history
- Familial disease history
- Marital history
- Family relationships

Social and environmental history
- Education
- Military experience
- Occupational history
- Religious and social activities
- Alcohol and cigarette consumption
- Living arrangements
- Hobbies and recreation
- Satisfaction with and stresses of life situation, finances, and relationships
- Recent travel or other event that might affect health

Review of systems: Respiratory system
- Cough
- Hemoptysis
- Sputum (amount and consistency)
- Chest pain
- Shortness of breath
- Hoarseness or changes in voice
- Dizziness or fainting
- Fever or chills
- Peripheral edema

Patient's printed name and signature

PHYSICAL EXAMINATION

A careful physical examination of the patient is essential for evaluating the patient's problem and determining the effects of therapy. The physical examination consists of the following four general steps: (1) inspection (visually examining), (2) palpation (touching), (3) percussion (tapping), and (4) auscultation (listening with a stethoscope).

General Appearance

The first few seconds of an encounter with the patient usually helps reveal the severity of the current problem. For an experienced clinician, these initial impressions determine the course of subsequent assessment. If the patient's general appearance indicates an acute problem, the rest of the examination may be abbreviated and focused until the patient's condition is stabilized. If the initial impressions indicate that the patient is stable and not in immediate danger, a more complete assessment can be conducted (Box 15-4). Several indicators are important in assessing the patient's overall appearance, including the patient's level of consciousness (see later), facial expression, level of anxiety or distress, positioning, and personal hygiene.

The RT should look for specific characteristics when observing the body as a whole. Does the patient appear well nourished or emaciated? Weakness and emaciation **(cachexia)** are signs of general ill health and malnutrition. Is the patient sweating? **Diaphoresis** (sweating) can indicate fever, pain, severe stress, increased metabolism, or acute anxiety.

The general facial expression may help reveal pain or anxiety. Facial expression also can help in evaluating

Box 15-4 Typical Format for Recording the Physical Examination

INITIAL IMPRESSION
- Age, height, weight, sensorium, and general appearance

VITAL SIGNS
- Pulse rate, respiratory rate, temperature, and blood pressure

HEAD, EARS, EYES, NOSE, AND THROAT
- Inspection findings

NECK
- Inspection and palpation findings

THORAX
- Lungs: Inspection, palpation, percussion, and auscultation findings
- Heart: Inspection, palpation, and auscultation findings

ABDOMEN
- Inspection, palpation, percussion, and auscultation findings

EXTREMITIES
- Inspection and palpation findings

Box 15-5 Levels of Consciousness

CONFUSED
The patient
- Exhibits slight decrease of consciousness
- Has slow mental responses
- Has decreased or dulled perception
- Has incoherent thoughts

DELIRIOUS
The patient
- Is easily agitated
- Is irritable
- Exhibits hallucinations

LETHARGIC
The patient
- Is sleepy
- Arouses easily
- Responds appropriately when aroused

OBTUNDED
The patient
- Awakens only with difficulty
- Responds appropriately when aroused

STUPOROUS
The patient
- Does not awaken completely
- Has decreased mental and physical activity
- Responds to pain and exhibits deep tendon reflexes
- Responds slowly to verbal stimuli

COMATOSE
The patient
- Is unconscious
- Does not respond to stimuli
- Does not move voluntarily
- Exhibits possible signs of upper motor neuron dysfunction, such as Babinski reflex or hyperreflexia
- Loses reflexes with deep or prolonged coma

alertness, mood, general character, and mental capacity. More specific facial signs also can indicate respiratory distress. Simple observation of the patient's anxiety level can indicate the severity of the current problem and whether cooperation can be expected. The patient's position also may be useful in assessing the severity of the problem and the patient's response to it. For example, a patient with severe pulmonary hyperinflation tends to sit upright while bracing his or her elbows on a table. This position helps the accessory muscles gain a mechanical advantage for breathing and is called **tripodding.** Finally, personal hygiene indicators can help determine both the duration and the impact of the illness on the patient's daily activities.

Level of Consciousness

While observing the patient's overall appearance, the RT should assess the patient's level of consciousness (alertness). Evaluating the patient's alertness is a simple but important task. If the patient appears conscious, the RT should assess the patient's orientation to time, place, person, and situation. This assessment often is called evaluating the **sensorium.** An alert patient who can correctly tell the interviewer the current date, location, his or her name, and his or her situation (e.g., "I'm in the hospital because I fell and broke my hip") is said to be "oriented × 4," and the patient's sensorium is considered normal. If the patient is not alert, the level of consciousness is assessed. The simple rating scale shown in Box 15-5 allows clinicians to describe the patient's level of consciousness objectively, using common clinical terms.

Depressed consciousness may occur with poor cerebral blood flow (e.g., hypotension) or when poorly oxygenated blood perfuses the brain. As cerebral oxygenation acutely decreases, the patient initially becomes restless, confused, or disoriented. If hypoxia worsens, the patient may become comatose. However, patients with chronic hypoxia may adapt well and may have normal mental status despite significant hypoxemia. Abnormal consciousness also may occur in chronic degenerative brain disorders, as a side effect of certain medications, and in cases of drug overdose. Additional information on the evaluation of neurologic function is presented in Chapter 46 (see Glasgow Coma Scale score).

Vital Signs

Vital signs—the body temperature, pulse rate, respiratory rate, and blood pressure—are the most frequently used clinical measurements because they are easy to obtain and provide useful information about the patient's clinical condition. Abnormal vital signs may reveal the first clue of adverse reactions to treatment. In addition, improvement in a patient's vital signs is strong evidence that a treatment is having a positive effect. For example, a decrease in the patient's breathing and heart rate toward normal after the application of O_2 therapy suggests a beneficial effect.

Body Temperature

The average body temperature for adults is approximately 37° C (98.6° F), with daily variations of approximately 0.5° C (1° F). Body temperature normally varies over a 24-hour day and usually is lowest in the early morning and highest in the late afternoon. Metabolic functions occur optimally when the body temperature is normal.

Body temperature is kept normal by balancing heat production with heat loss. If the body were unable to discharge the heat generated by metabolism, the temperature would increase approximately 2° F (−16.7° C) per hour. The hypothalamus plays an important role in regulating heat loss and can initiate peripheral vasodilation and sweating *(diaphoresis)* to dissipate body heat. The respiratory system also helps remove excess heat through ventilation by warming the inspired air, which is subsequently exhaled.

An elevated body temperature (*hyperthermia* or *hyperpyrexia*) can result from disease or from normal activities such as exercise. Temperature elevation caused by disease is called fever, and the patient is said to be **febrile.** Fever increases the body's metabolic rate, increasing both O_2 consumption and CO_2 production. This increase in metabolism must be matched by an increase in both circulation and ventilation to maintain homeostasis; this is why febrile patients often have increased heart and breathing rates. However, not all patients can easily accommodate the need for increased circulation and ventilation, and respiratory failure can result.

A body temperature below normal is called **hypothermia.** The most common cause of hypothermia is prolonged exposure to cold, to which the hypothalamus responds by initiating shivering (to generate heat) and vasoconstriction (to conserve heat). Other, less common causes of hypothermia include head injury or stroke, causing dysfunction of the hypothalamus; decreased thyroid activity; and overwhelming infection, such as sepsis.

Because hypothermia reduces O_2 consumption and CO_2 production, patients with hypothermia may exhibit slow, shallow breathing and reduced pulse rate. Mechanical ventilators in the control mode may need appropriate adjustments in the depth and rate of delivered tidal volumes as the body temperature of the patient varies above and below normal.

Body temperature is measured most often at one of the following four sites: mouth, axilla, ear (tympanic membrane), or rectum. The oral site is the most acceptable for an alert, adult patient, but it cannot be used with infants, comatose patients, or orally intubated patients. If a patient ingests hot or cold liquid or has been smoking, oral temperature measurement should be delayed for 10 to 15 minutes for accuracy. The axillary site is acceptable for infants or small children who do not tolerate rectal thermometers, but this site may underestimate core temperature by 33.8° F to 35.6° F (1° C to 2° C). The body temperature can also be assessed accurately with the use of a hand-held device to measure the temperature of the eardrum (tympanic membrane). Rectal temperatures are closest to actual core body temperature.

Box 15-6 Key Characteristics of the Pulse

- Is the pulse rate normal, high, or low?
- Is the rhythm regular, consistently irregular, or irregularly irregular?
- Are there any changes in the amplitude (strength) of the pulse in relation to respiration? Are there changes in amplitude from one beat to another?
- Are there any other abnormalities, such as palpable vibrations (thrills or bruits)?

Pulse Rate

The peripheral pulse is evaluated for rate, rhythm, and strength (Box 15-6). The normal adult pulse rate is 60 to 100 beats/min, with a regular rhythm. A condition in which the pulse rate exceeds 100 beats/min is called **tachycardia.** Common causes of tachycardia are exercise, fear, anxiety, low blood pressure, anemia, fever, reduced arterial blood O_2 levels, and certain medications. A condition in which the pulse rate is less than 60 beats/min is called **bradycardia.** Bradycardia is less common than tachycardia but can occur with hypothermia, as a side effect of medications, with certain cardiac arrhythmias, and with traumatic brain injury.

The amount of O_2 delivered to the tissues depends on the ability of the heart to pump oxygenated blood. The amount of blood circulated per minute (cardiac output) is a function of heart rate and stroke volume. Pulmonary disease almost always causes a decrease in arterial O_2 content and an increase in O_2 consumption. In this situation, the heart tries to maintain adequate O_2 delivery to the tissues by increasing cardiac output. Cardiac output is increased primarily by increasing the heart rate.

The radial artery is the most common site used to palpate the pulse. The second and third fingertip pads (but not the thumb) are used to palpate the radial pulse. Ideally, the pulse rate is counted for 1 minute, especially if the pulse is irregular. Essential pulse characteristics that should be noted and documented are described in Box 15-6.

Spontaneous ventilation can influence pulse strength, or amplitude. Normally, a slight decrease in pulse pressure is present with each inspiratory effort. This decrease is caused by negative intrathoracic pressure from respiratory muscle contraction during inspiration. The decrease in blood pressure is the result of decreased left ventricular filling from two mechanisms. First, negative intrathoracic pressure pools blood in the pulmonary circulation, which impedes left heart filling. Second, it simultaneously increases venous return (which increases right ventricular volume and pressure) and limits expansion of the left heart during diastole. This mechanism briefly reduces left ventricular stroke volume and decreases systolic blood pressure during inspiration. The slight decrease in pulse pressure (normally <10 mm Hg) with inspiration may not be noticeable with palpation. A *significant* decrease in pulse strength (>10 mm Hg) during spontaneous inhalation is called **pulsus paradoxus,** or *paradoxical pulse*. Pulsus paradoxus can be quantified with a blood pressure cuff (see later section) and is common in patients with acute obstructive pulmonary disease, especially patients experiencing an asthma attack. During respiratory distress, vigorous inspiratory efforts decrease stroke volume by impeding the strength of left ventricular contraction.[5] Pulsus paradoxus also may signal a mechanical restriction of the pumping action of the heart, as can occur with constrictive pericarditis or cardiac tamponade.

Pulsus alternans is an alternating succession of strong and weak pulses. Pulsus alternans suggests left-sided heart failure and usually is not related to respiratory disease. The pulse also may be assessed by palpating the carotid, brachial, femoral, temporal, popliteal, posterior tibial, and dorsalis pedis pulses. The more centrally located pulses (e.g., the carotid and femoral) should be used when the blood pressure is abnormally low. If the carotid site is used, great care must be taken to avoid the carotid sinus area. Pressure on the carotid sinus area may cause strong parasympathetic stimulation resulting in bradycardia.

Respiratory Rate

The normal resting adult rate of breathing is 12 to 18 breaths/min. **Tachypnea** is defined as a respiratory rate greater than 20 breaths/min. Rapid respiratory rates are associated with exertion, fever, arterial hypoxemia, metabolic acidosis, anxiety, pulmonary edema, lung fibrosis, and pain. A respiratory rate less than 10 breaths/min is called **bradypnea.** Although uncommon, bradypnea may occur with traumatic brain injury or hypothermia, as a side effect of certain medications such as narcotics, with severe myocardial infarction, and in cases of drug overdose. In addition to respiratory rate, the pattern of breathing (see later section) is assessed.

The respiratory rate is counted by watching the abdomen or chest wall move in and out. With practice, even subtle breathing movements of a healthy individual at rest can be identified easily. In some cases, the RT may need to place a hand on the patient's abdomen to confirm the breathing rate. Ideally, the patient should be unaware that the respiratory rate is being counted. One successful method for accomplishing this is for the RT to count the respiratory rate immediately after evaluating the patient's pulse, while keeping the fingers on the patient's wrist, giving the impression that the pulse rate is being counted.

Blood Pressure

The arterial blood pressure is the force exerted against the wall of the arteries as the blood moves through them. Arterial **systolic pressure** is the peak force exerted in the major arteries during contraction of the left ventricle. Arterial blood pressure typically increases with age. Generally, the normal range for systolic blood pressure in an adult is 90 to 140 mm Hg. **Diastolic pressure** is the force in the major arteries remaining after relaxation of the ventricles; it is normally 60 to 90 mm Hg. **Pulse pressure** is the difference between the systolic and diastolic pressures. A normal pulse pressure is 30 to 40 mm Hg. When the pulse pressure is less than 30 mm Hg, the peripheral pulse is difficult to detect.

Blood pressure is determined by the interaction of the force of left ventricular contraction, the systemic vascular resistance, and the blood volume (see Chapter 9). The blood pressure is recorded by listing systolic pressure over diastolic pressure (e.g., 120/80 mm Hg).

Hypertension is defined as arterial blood pressure persistently greater than 140/90 mm Hg. Hypertension is a common medical problem in adults, and in approximately 90% of cases the cause is unknown (primary hypertension). There are two subcategories of hypertension.[6] *Stage I* hypertension occurs when the systolic blood pressure is 140 to 159 mm Hg or the diastolic blood pressure is 90 to 99 mm Hg. *Stage II* hypertension occurs when the systolic blood pressure is 160 mm Hg or greater or the diastolic blood pressure is 100 mm Hg or greater. In addition, there is a third category known as *prehypertension,* which is a systolic blood pressure between 120 mm Hg and 139 mm Hg or a diastolic blood pressure between 80 mm Hg and 89 mm Hg. This last category is not a disease state and does not require treatment but rather is used to assess the risk of eventually developing hypertension.

Mechanically, hypertension results from increased systemic vascular resistance or an increased force of ventricular contraction. Sustained hypertension can cause central nervous system abnormalities, such as headaches, blurred vision, and confusion. Other potential consequences of hypertension include uremia (renal insufficiency), CHF, and cerebral hemorrhage, leading to stroke. Acute, severe elevation of blood pressure can cause acute neurologic, cardiac, and renal failure and is called *acute hypertensive crisis*.

Hypotension is defined as a systolic arterial blood pressure less than 90 mm Hg or a mean arterial pressure less than 65 mm Hg.[7] Hypotension also can be defined as a decrease of more than 40 mm Hg from baseline. This expanded definition acknowledges that patients with baseline hypertension may have inadequate tissue perfusion at a blood pressure that may be considered normal for most patients.

Shock is defined precisely as the inadequate delivery of O_2 and nutrients to the vital organs relative to their metabolic demand.[7] Hypotension is not synonymous with shock. In shock, vital body organs are in imminent danger of receiving inadequate blood flow (underperfusion) and impaired O_2 delivery to the tissues (i.e., tissue hypoxia). For this reason, shock is usually treated aggressively with fluids, blood products, or vasoactive drugs, or a combination of these, depending on the cause and severity of shock.

There are two broad categories of hypotension and shock based on whether they are caused by a *hypodynamic* or *hyperdynamic* cardiovascular state.[8] Hypodynamic states includes left ventricular failure *(cardiogenic)* and reduced blood volume (**hypovolemia** or *hypovolemic*) caused by either hemorrhage or severe fluid loss. Hyperdynamic states occur with profound systemic vasodilation *(peripheral vascular failure)* associated with overwhelming infection *(septic shock)*, systemic allergic reaction *(anaphylaxis)*, or severe liver failure.

When healthy individuals sit or stand up, there is little change in blood pressure. However, similar postural changes may produce an abrupt decrease in the blood pressure in hypovolemic patients. This condition is called **postural hypotension** and can be confirmed by measuring the blood pressure in both the supine and the sitting positions or on standing up. Postural hypotension is commonly caused by hypovolemia. A rapid decrease in arterial blood pressure caused by postural hypotension can reduce cerebral blood flow and lead to **syncope** (fainting). Postural hypotension generally is treated by administration of fluid.

A common technique for measuring arterial blood pressure requires a blood pressure cuff (sphygmomanometer) and a stethoscope (Figure 15-2). When the cuff is applied to the upper arm and pressurized to exceed systolic blood pressure, the brachial artery blood flow stops. As the cuff pressure is slowly released to a point just below the systolic pressure, blood flows intermittently past the obstruction. Partial obstruction of the blood flow creates turbulence and vibrations called *Korotkoff sounds.* Korotkoff sounds are heard with a stethoscope over the brachial artery distal to the cuff.

To measure the blood pressure, a deflated cuff is wrapped snugly around the patient's upper arm, with the lower edge of the cuff 1 inch above the antecubital fossa. While palpating the brachial pulse, the clinician inflates the cuff to approximately 30 mm Hg above the point at which the pulse can no longer be felt. The clinician places the diaphragm of the stethoscope over the artery and deflates the cuff at a rate of 2 to 3 mm Hg/sec while observing the manometer.

The systolic pressure is recorded at the point at which the first Korotkoff sounds are heard. The point at which the sounds become muffled is the diastolic pressure. This muffling is the final change in the Korotkoff sounds just before they disappear. At this point, cuff pressure equals

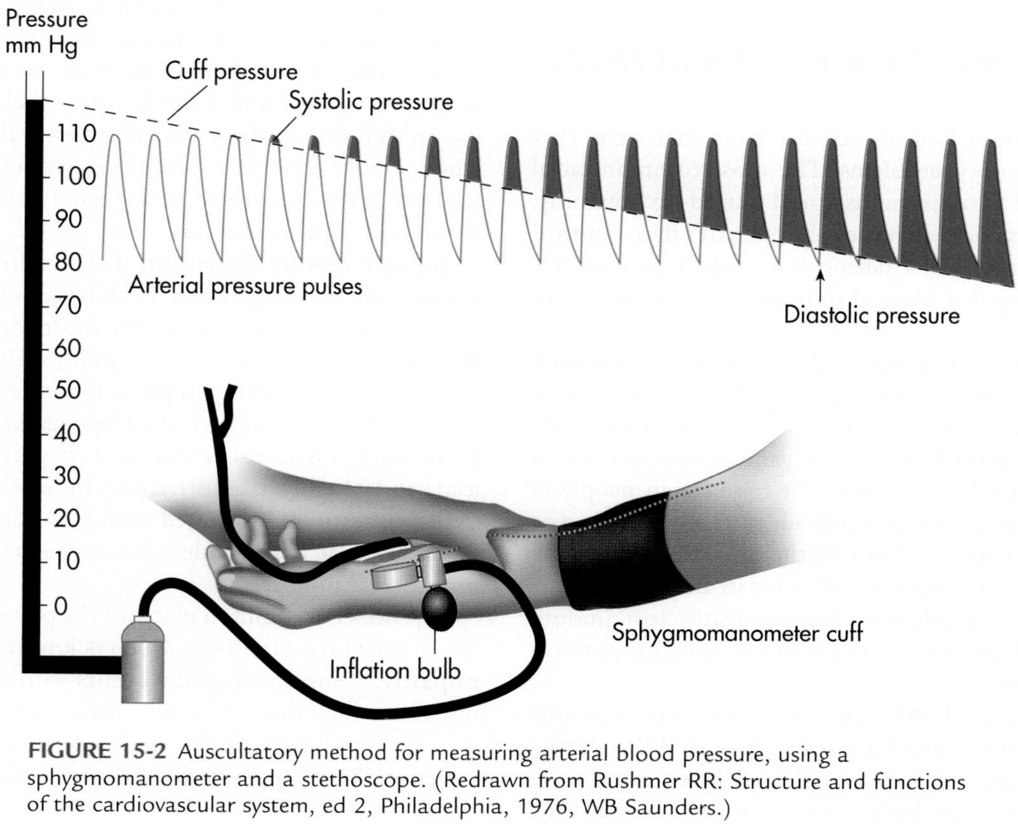

FIGURE 15-2 Auscultatory method for measuring arterial blood pressure, using a sphygmomanometer and a stethoscope. (Redrawn from Rushmer RR: Structure and functions of the cardiovascular system, ed 2, Philadelphia, 1976, WB Saunders.)

diastolic pressure, and turbulence ceases. When muffling begins and the sounds disappear at a wide interval, all three pressures are recorded (e.g., 120/80/60 mm Hg). The clinician must perform the procedure rapidly because the pressurized cuff impairs circulation to the forearm and hand.

The systolic blood pressure usually decreases slightly with normal inhalation. However, a decrease in systolic pressure of more than 6 to 8 mm Hg during a resting inhalation is abnormal and is called *paradoxical pulse,* or *pulsus paradoxus* (see Chapter 9). Although simple palpation may be adequate to signal the presence of paradoxical pulse, it can be quantified only by auscultatory measurement. To obtain this measurement, the clinician inflates the cuff until the radial or brachial pulse can no longer be palpated. The clinician slowly deflates the cuff until sounds are heard on exhalation only (point 1). Next, the clinician reduces the cuff pressure until sounds are heard throughout respiration (point 2). The difference between points 1 and 2 indicates the degree of paradoxical pulse.

Most hospitals and clinics have adopted use of the digital blood pressure measuring devices. These devices do not require the health care provider to listen for the Korotkoff sounds and eliminate variances in recorded blood pressures based on human perception. They are considered to be very accurate and simply require the clinician to apply the blood pressure cuff correctly and press the start button. Subsequently, the device takes over and inflates and deflates the cuff automatically. The blood pressure and pulse rate are displayed on a digital screen.

Examination of the Head and Neck

Head

The patient's face is inspected for abnormal signs that indicate respiratory problems. The most common facial signs are nasal flaring, cyanosis, and pursed-lip breathing. Nasal flaring occurs when the external nares flare outward during inhalation. This flaring is prevalent in neonates with respiratory distress and indicates an increased work of breathing.

When respiratory disease reduces arterial O_2 content, **cyanosis** (a bluish discoloration of the tissues) may be detected, especially around the lips and in the oral mucosa of the mouth (central cyanosis). Cyanosis may be difficult to detect, especially in a poorly lit room or in people of color. Although central cyanosis suggests inadequate oxygenation (respiratory failure), further investigation is indicated. However, the absence of cyanosis does not ensure that oxygenation is adequate because a sufficient amount of desaturated hemoglobin (5 g) must exist before cyanosis can be identified.

Patients with COPD may use pursed-lip breathing during exhalation. Breathing through pursed lips during exhalation creates resistance to flow. The increased resistance creates a slight back pressure in the small airways during exhalation, which prevents their premature collapse and allows more complete emptying of the lung.

Neck

Inspection and palpation of the neck help determine the position of the trachea and the jugular venous pressure (JVP). Normally, when the patient faces forward, the trachea is located in the middle of the neck. The midline of the neck can be identified by palpating the suprasternal notch. The midline of the trachea should be directly below the center of the suprasternal notch.

The trachea can shift away from the midline in certain thoracic disorders. Generally, the trachea shifts *toward* an area of collapsed lung. Conversely, the trachea shifts *away* from areas with increased air or fluid (e.g., tension pneumothorax or large pleural effusion). Abnormalities in the lung bases generally do not shift the trachea.

JVP is estimated by determining how high the jugular vein extends above the level of the sternal angle. JVP reflects the volume and pressure of venous blood in the right side of the heart. Typically, the internal vein is assessed because it is more reliable. Individuals with obese necks may not have visible neck veins, even when the veins are distended.

When lying in a supine position, a healthy individual has neck veins that are full. When the head of the bed is elevated gradually to a 45-degree angle, the level of the blood column descends to a point no more than a few centimeters above the clavicle. With elevated venous pressure, the neck veins may be distended as high as the angle of the jaw, even when the patient is sitting upright.

JVP may vary with breathing. Under normal circumstances, the blood column descends toward the thorax during inhalation and ascends with exhalation. For this reason, JVP should always be estimated at the end of exhalation. Under abnormal conditions (e.g., cardiac tamponade), the JVP may increase during inhalation. This is called **Kussmaul sign** and is rare.

Jugular venous distention (JVD) is present when the jugular vein is enlarged and it can be seen more than 3 to 4 cm above the sternal angle. The most common cause of JVD is right heart failure (cor pulmonale). Right heart failure frequently occurs in patients with advanced COPD because of chronic hypoxemia. Hypoxemia causes chronic pulmonary vasoconstriction and hypertension, which leads to right heart failure from the excessive workload. Other conditions associated with JVD include left heart failure, cardiac tamponade, tension pneumothoraces, and mediastinal tumors.

The neck is a common place for the physician to palpate for enlarged lymph nodes, which is known as **lymphadenopathy.** Lymphadenopathy occurs with various medical disorders, including infection, malignancy, and sarcoidosis. Tender lymph nodes in the neck suggest a nearby infection. The lymph nodes are not tender when malignancy is the cause.

Examination of the Thorax and Lungs

Inspection

The chest should be inspected visually to assess the thoracic configuration and the pattern and effort of breathing. For adequate inspection, the room must be well lit, and the patient should be sitting upright. When the patient is too ill to sit up, the clinician should carefully roll the patient to one side to examine the posterior chest. Inspection, palpation, percussion, and auscultation of the patient's chest require that the patient be disrobed. Consequently, the clinician should make every effort to respect the patient's modesty (especially for female patients) and drape the chest when possible.

Thoracic Configuration. The anteroposterior (AP) diameter of the average adult thorax is less than the transverse diameter. Normally, the AP diameter increases gradually with age but may prematurely increase in patients with COPD. This abnormal increase in AP diameter is called **barrel chest** and is associated with emphysema. When the AP diameter increases, the normal 45-degree angle of articulation between the ribs and spine is increased, becoming more horizontal (Figure 15-3). Other abnormalities of the thoracic configuration are listed in Table 15-1.

Breathing Pattern and Effort. At rest, a healthy adult has a consistent rate and rhythm of breathing. Breathing effort is minimal on inhalation and passive on exhalation. Abnormal breathing patterns can be broken down into two broad categories. First are breathing patterns directly associated with thoracic or pulmonary diseases that increase work of breathing. Second are patterns primarily associated with neurologic disease (see Chapter 14). Table 15-2 describes common abnormal patterns of breathing.

Cardiopulmonary or thoracic diseases that increase work of breathing typically cause recruitment of the accessory muscles of ventilation. Common causes of an increase in the work of breathing include narrowed airways (e.g.,

TABLE 15-1

Abnormalities of Thoracic Configuration

Name	Condition
Pectus carinatum	Abnormal protrusion of sternum
Pectus excavatum	Depression of part or entire sternum, which can produce a restrictive lung defect
Kyphosis	Spinal deformity in which the spine has an abnormal AP curvature
Scoliosis	Spinal deformity in which the spine has a lateral curvature
Kyphoscoliosis	Combination of kyphosis and scoliosis, which may produce a severe restrictive lung defect as a result of poor lung expansion

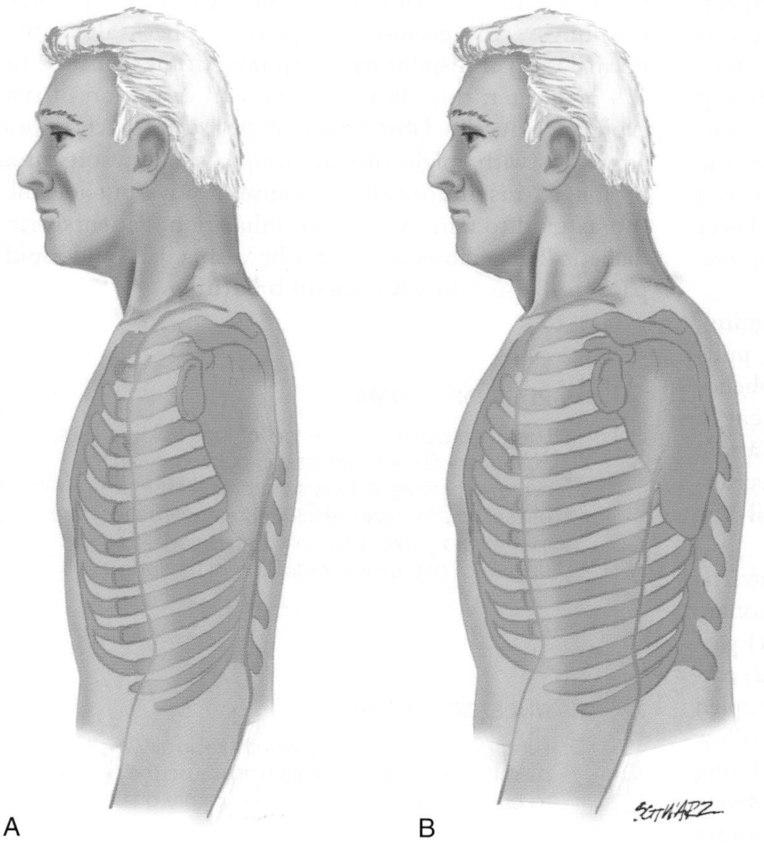

FIGURE 15-3 **A,** Patient with normal thoracic configuration. **B,** Patient with increased AP diameter. Note contrasts in the angle of slope of the ribs and development of accessory muscles.

TABLE 15-2
Abnormal Breathing Patterns

Breathing Pattern	Characteristics	Causes
Apnea	No breathing	Cardiac arrest, narcotic overdose, severe brain trauma
Apneustic breathing	Deep, gasping inspiration with brief, partial expiration	Damage to upper medulla or pons caused by stroke or trauma; sometimes observed with hypoglycemic coma or profound hypoxemia
Ataxic breathing	Completely irregular breathing pattern with variable periods of apnea	Damage to medulla
Asthmatic breathing	Prolonged exhalation with recruitment of abdominal muscles	Obstruction to airflow out of the lungs
Biot's respiration	Clustering of rapid, shallow breaths coupled with regular or irregular periods of apnea	Damage to medulla or pons caused by stroke or trauma; severe intracranial hypertension
Cheyne-Stokes respiration	Irregular type of breathing; breaths increase and decrease in depth and rate with periods of apnea; variant of "periodic breathing"	Most often caused by severe damage to bilateral cerebral hemispheres and basal ganglia (usually infarction); also seen in patients with CHF owing to increased circulation time and in various forms of encephalopathy
Kussmaul breathing	Deep and fast respirations	Metabolic acidosis
Paradoxical breathing	*Abdominal paradox:* Abdominal wall moves inward on inspiration and outward on expiration	*Abdominal paradox:* Diaphragmatic fatigue or paralysis
	Chest paradox: Part or all of the chest wall moves in with inhalation and out with exhalation	*Chest paradox:* Typically observed in chest trauma with multiple rib or sternal fractures Also found in patients with high spinal cord injury with paralysis of intercostal muscles
Periodic breathing	Breathing oscillates between periods of rapid, deep breathing and slow, shallow breathing *without* periods of apnea	Same causes as Cheyne-Stokes respiration

COPD, asthma), "stiff lungs" (e.g., severe pneumonia, pulmonary edema), or a stiff chest wall (e.g., ascites, anasarca, pleural effusions). Increased work of breathing also can result in retractions. **Retractions** are an intermittent sinking inward of the skin overlying the chest wall during inspiration. They occur when the ventilatory muscles contract forcefully enough to cause a large decrease in the intrathoracic pressure. Retractions may be seen between the ribs, above the clavicles, or below the rib cage. These are called *intercostal, supraclavicular,* or *subcostal retractions.* Retractions are difficult to see in obese patients.

Another form of retraction is **tracheal tugging,** which is caused by extreme negative pressure that pulls the trachea downward during inspiration. This phenomenon is noted by observing the downward movement of the thyroid cartilage toward the chest during inspiration. Typically, this movement occurs in concert with recruitment of the accessory muscles of inspiration, primarily the sternocleidomastoid muscles of the neck.

Generally, two archetypal abnormal breathing patterns exist that provide clues about the underlying pulmonary problem. These patterns fall into two categories: (1) patterns characterized by rapid, shallow breathing and (2) patterns marked by a relatively brief inspiratory phase coupled with an abnormally prolonged exhalation. Rapid, shallow breathing typically occurs in patients with increased lung stiffness, such as patients with pulmonary edema or severe pneumonia. Obstruction of the intrathoracic airways slows lung emptying and results in a prolonged expiratory phase as patients attempt to minimize gas trapping inside the lungs. This prolonged expiratory phase alters the normal ratio of inspiratory to expiratory time from 1:2 to 1:4 or greater; this always occurs with activation of the expiratory muscles. Obstruction of the extrathoracic upper airway (as with epiglottitis or croup) usually results in a prolonged inspiratory time because airways outside the thorax tend to narrow more on inhalation. Patients with diabetic ketoacidosis often breathe with a deep and rapid pattern that is called **Kussmaul breathing.**

RULE OF THUMB

Lung diseases that cause loss of lung volume (e.g., pulmonary fibrosis, atelectasis, pulmonary edema, acute respiratory distress syndrome) cause the patient to take rapid, shallow breaths. The increase in respiratory rate is typically proportional to the degree of gas volume reduction in the lung.

RULE OF THUMB

Lung diseases that cause intrathoracic airways to narrow (e.g., asthma, bronchitis) cause the patient to breathe with a prolonged expiratory phase.

> **RULE OF THUMB**
>
> *Lung diseases that cause the upper airway to narrow (e.g., croup, epiglottitis) cause the patient to breathe with a prolonged inspiratory phase.*

The diaphragm may be nonfunctional in patients with spinal injuries or neuromuscular disease and may be severely limited in patients with COPD. When the diaphragm is nonfunctional or limited, the accessory muscles of ventilation become active to maintain adequate gas exchange. Heavy use of accessory muscles is reliable evidence of significant cardiopulmonary disease.

In patients with emphysema, the lungs lose their elastic recoil and become hyperinflated. Over time, the hyperinflation forces the diaphragm into a low, flat position. Contraction of a flat diaphragm tends to draw in the lateral costal margins instead of expanding them **(Hoover sign)** and does little to help move air into the thorax. Ventilation eventually must be achieved by other means and involves heavy use of the accessory muscles. The accessory muscles must assist ventilation by raising the anterior chest in an effort to increase thoracic volume. The severity of lung disease in this situation is often reflected by the magnitude of accessory muscle activity.

Diaphragmatic fatigue is found in many types of chronic and acute pulmonary diseases. When it occurs acutely, diaphragmatic fatigue often manifests with distinctive breathing patterns.[9] The first sign of acute diaphragmatic fatigue is tachypnea. Sometimes tachypnea is followed by a breathing pattern in which the diaphragm and rib cage muscles alternately power breathing in an attempt to give each muscle group some rest **(respiratory alternans).** This pattern is noted by the upward motion of the diaphragm during inspiration on a *series of breaths,* followed by diaphragmatic contractions and inward movement of the abdominal wall on the following series of breaths. When the diaphragm is relaxed, contraction of the rib cage muscles sucks the diaphragm upward and the abdomen inward during inspiration. The opposite phenomenon occurs on breaths when the diaphragm is active. When the rib cage muscles are relaxed, the chest wall may appear to sink in as the abdomen protrudes during diaphragmatic contraction; this often gives the impression that the chest has a rocking motion. Finally, **abdominal paradox** occurs with complete diaphragmatic fatigue, as the diaphragm is drawn upward into the thoracic cavity with *each* inspiratory effort of the rib cage muscles. An abdominal paradox also occurs when the diaphragm is paralyzed.

These patterns are not always associated with impending muscle fatigue. Rather, they may be adaptations to high workloads when the respiratory muscle strength is normal.[10] Also, patients with respiratory distress often have tachypnea, along with recruitment of the expiratory muscles. This situation can make it difficult to discern accurately the presence and type of abnormal breathing pattern. The RT must be careful about offering definitive therapeutic suggestions (e.g., absolute need for mechanical ventilation) when he or she perceives the presence of these abnormal breathing patterns.

Palpation

Palpation is the art of touching the chest wall to evaluate underlying structure and function. It is used in selected patients to confirm or rule out suspected problems suggested by the history and initial examination findings. Palpation is performed to evaluate vocal fremitus, estimate thoracic expansion, and assess the skin and subcutaneous tissues of the chest.

Vocal and Tactile Fremitus. The term *vocal fremitus* refers to the vibrations created by the vocal cords during speech. These vibrations are transmitted down the tracheobronchial tree and through the lung to the chest wall. When these vibrations are felt on the chest wall, it is called *tactile fremitus.* Assessing vocal fremitus requires a conscious, cooperative patient. Both vocal and tactile fremitus increase in intensity when the lung becomes consolidated (e.g., filled with inflammatory exudate) as in pneumonia. However, if the consolidated area is not in communication with an open airway, speech cannot be transmitted, and fremitus is absent or decreased. In addition, fremitus is reduced in patients who are obese or overly muscular.

Vocal and tactile fremitus decrease in intensity when either fluid or air collects in the pleural space (e.g., pleural effusion or pneumothoraces). Similarly, in patients with emphysema, the lungs become hyperinflated, which reduces the density of lung tissue. Because the density is low, speech vibrations transmit poorly through the lung, resulting in a bilateral reduction in fremitus.

To assess for tactile fremitus, the RT asks the patient to repeat the word "ninety-nine" while the RT systematically palpates the thorax. The palmar aspect of the fingers or the ulnar aspect of the hand can be used for palpation. If one hand is used, it should be moved from one side of the chest to the corresponding area on the other side. The anterior, lateral, and posterior portions of the chest wall are evaluated.

Thoracic Expansion. The normal chest wall expands symmetrically during deep inhalation. This expansion can be evaluated on the anterior and posterior chest. To evaluate expansion anteriorly, the RT places his or her hands over the anterolateral chest, with the thumbs extended along the costal margin toward the xiphoid process. To evaluate posteriorly, the RT positions the hands over the posterolateral chest with the thumbs meeting at the T8 vertebra (Figure 15-4). The patient is instructed to exhale slowly and completely. When the patient has exhaled maximally, the RT gently secures his or her fingertips against the sides of the patient's chest and extends the thumbs toward the midline until the tip of each thumb meets at

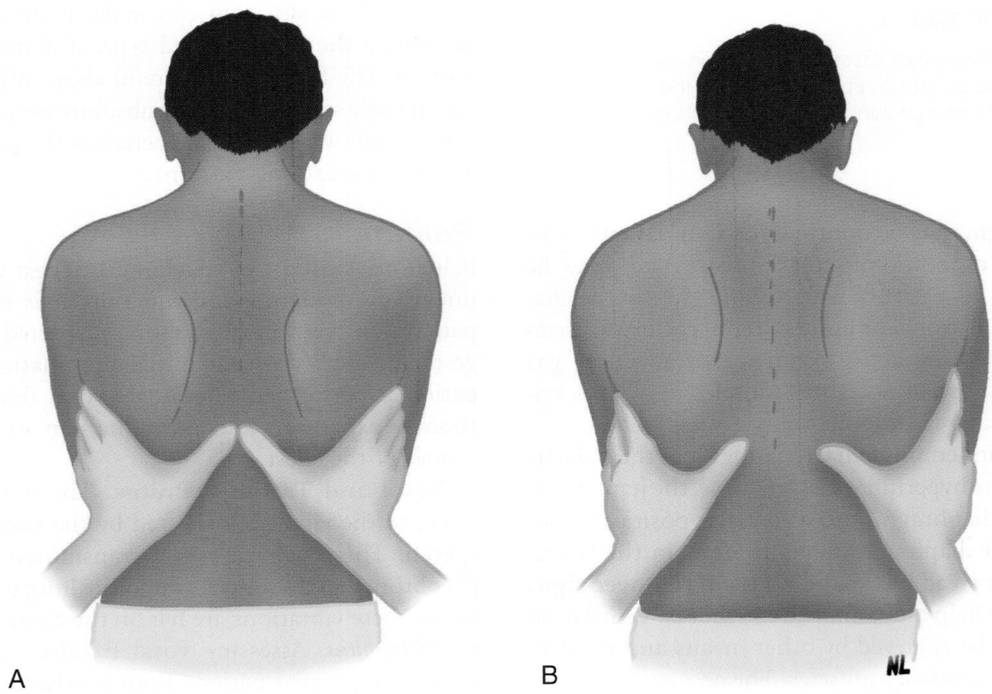

FIGURE 15-4 Estimation of thoracic expansion. **A,** Exhalation. **B,** Maximal inhalation.

the midline. The RT next instructs the patient to take a full, deep breath and notes the distance the tip of each of the thumbs moves from midline. Normally, each thumb moves an equal distance of approximately 3 to 5 cm.

Diseases that affect the expansion of both lungs cause a bilateral reduction in chest expansion. Reduced expansion commonly is seen in neuromuscular disorders and COPD. Unilateral reduction in chest expansion occurs with respiratory diseases that reduce the expansion of one lung or a major part of one lung. This condition can occur with lobar consolidation, atelectasis, pleural effusion, or pneumothorax.

Skin and Subcutaneous Tissues. The chest wall can be palpated to determine the general temperature and condition of the skin. When air leaks from the lung into the subcutaneous tissues, fine air bubbles produce a crackling sound and sensation when palpated. This condition is referred to as **subcutaneous emphysema.** The sensation produced on palpation is called *crepitus.* Crepitus is a classic sign of barotrauma and can be felt over the chest of a patient who develops this condition as a result of receiving mechanical ventilation with high airway pressures and end inspiratory volumes.

Percussion of the Chest

Percussion is the art of tapping on a surface to evaluate the underlying structure. Percussion of the chest wall produces a sound and a palpable vibration useful in evaluating underlying lung tissue. The vibration created by percussion penetrates the lung to a depth of 5 to 7 cm below the chest wall. This assessment technique is not performed routinely on all patients but is reserved for patients with suspected conditions for which percussion could be helpful (e.g., pneumothorax).

The technique most often used in percussing the chest wall is called *mediate,* or *indirect,* percussion. A right-handed RT places the middle finger of the left hand firmly against the patient's chest wall, parallel to the ribs, with the palm and other fingers held off the chest. The RT uses the tip of the middle finger of the right hand or the lateral aspect of the right thumb to strike the finger against the chest near the base of the terminal phalanx with a quick, sharp blow. Movement of the hand striking the chest is generated at the wrist, not at the elbow or shoulder.

The percussion note is clearest if the RT remembers to keep the finger on the patient's chest firmly against the chest wall and to strike this finger and then immediately withdraw. The two fingers should be in contact for only an instant. As one gains experience in percussion, the feel of the vibration becomes as important as the sound in evaluating lung structures.

Percussion Over Lung Fields. Percussion of the lung fields is performed systematically, consecutively testing comparable areas on both sides of the chest. Percussion over the bony structures and over the breasts of female patients has no diagnostic value and should not be performed. Asking patients to raise their arms above their shoulders helps move the scapulae laterally and minimize their interference with percussion on the posterior chest wall.

The sounds generated during percussion of the chest are evaluated for intensity (loudness). Percussion over normal lung fields produces a moderately low-pitched sound that can be heard easily. This sound is described as normal resonance or *tympanic.* When the percussion note is louder and lower than normal, the sound is said to be increased resonance or *hypertympanic.* Percussion may produce a sound with characteristics just the opposite of resonance, referred to as decreased resonance, *dampened,* or *dull.*

Clinical Implications. By itself, percussion of the chest is of little value in making a diagnosis. However, when considered along with other findings, percussion can provide essential information. In modern practice, chest percussion enables rapid bedside assessment of abnormalities inside the chest and may aid in the decision to obtain chest radiographic studies.

Any abnormality that increases lung tissue density, such as pneumonia, tumor, or atelectasis, results in a loss of resonance and decreased resonance to percussion over the affected area. Pleural spaces filled with fluid, such as blood or water, also produce decreased resonance to percussion. Increased resonance can be detected either when the lungs are hyperinflated (e.g., asthma or emphysema) or when the pleural space contains large amounts of air **(pneumothorax).**

Unilateral problems are easier to detect than bilateral problems because the normal side provides a normal standard for immediate comparison. The unilateral decrease in resonance heard when percussing an area of consolidation is easier to detect than the subtle bilateral increase in resonance heard with bilateral hyperinflation.

Percussion of the chest has clinically important limitations. Abnormalities that are small or deep below the surface are not likely to be detected during percussion of the chest. Many clinicians do not routinely use chest percussion to evaluate lung resonance.

Auscultation of the Lungs

Auscultation is the process of listening for bodily sounds. Auscultation over the thorax is performed to identify normal and abnormal lung sounds and to evaluate the effects of therapy. Because auscultation can be performed quickly and is noninvasive, it is a particularly useful tool in many clinical situations. Auscultation is performed with a stethoscope to enhance sound transmission from the patient's lungs to the examiner's ears. The clinician always must ensure that the room is as quiet as possible whenever performing auscultation.

Stethoscope. A stethoscope has the following four basic parts: (1) a bell, (2) a diaphragm, (3) tubing, and (4) earpieces (Figure 15-5). The bell detects a broad spectrum of sounds and is very useful for listening to low-pitched sounds (e.g., heart sounds). Proper technique for listening to heart sounds is to place the bell lightly against the chest; this avoids stretching the skin, which makes auscultating heart sounds more difficult by inadvertently filtering out low-frequency sounds. Using the bell to auscultate the lungs is also helpful when emaciation causes rib protrusion that restricts placement of the diaphragm flat against the chest.

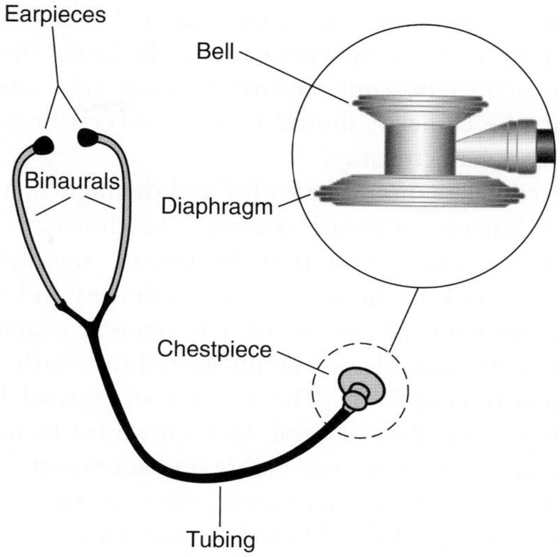

FIGURE 15-5 Acoustic stethoscope.

The diaphragm is preferred for auscultation of the lungs because most lung sounds are high frequency. The ideal tubing should be thick enough to exclude external noises and approximately 25 to 35 cm (11 to 16 inches) in length. Longer tubing may impair sound transmission.

The clinician should examine his or her stethoscope regularly for cracks in the diaphragm, wax or dirt in the earpieces, and other defects that may interfere with the transmission of sound. The stethoscope should always be cleaned with hospital-approved disinfectant after every patient contact to minimize contamination with microorganisms.[11,12] Patients who are placed in contact isolation and patients who are in protective isolation because of immunosuppression should have a dedicated stethoscope in the room to prevent cross infection.

Technique. When possible, the patient should be sitting upright in a relaxed position. The patient should be instructed to breathe a little more deeply than normal through an open mouth. Exhalation should be passive. The bell or diaphragm is placed directly against the chest wall when possible because clothing may produce distortion. The tubing must not be allowed to rub against any objects because this may produce extraneous sounds, which could be mistaken for adventitious lung sounds (discussed later).

Auscultation of the lungs should be systematic and include all lobes on the anterior, lateral, and posterior chest. Auscultation should begin at the lung bases with comparison of breath sounds side to side, working upward toward the lung apexes (Figure 15-6). It is important to begin at the bases because certain abnormal sounds that occur only in the lower lobes may be altered by several deep breaths. At least one full ventilatory cycle should be evaluated at each stethoscope position. If abnormal sounds are present, the clinician should listen to several breaths to clarify the characteristics.

The clinician should listen for and distinguish among the key features of breath sounds. The clinician should identify the pitch (vibration frequency), the intensity (loudness), and the duration of the inspiratory and expiration components of the sound. The acoustic characteristics of breath sounds can be illustrated in breath sound diagrams (Figure 15-7). The features of normal breath sounds are described in Table 15-3. One must be familiar with normal breath sounds before one can expect to identify the subtle changes that may signify respiratory disease.

Terminology. In healthy individuals, the sounds heard over the trachea have a loud, tubular quality. These are referred to as *tracheal breath sounds.* Tracheal breath sounds are loud sounds with an expiratory component equal to or slightly longer than the inspiratory component.

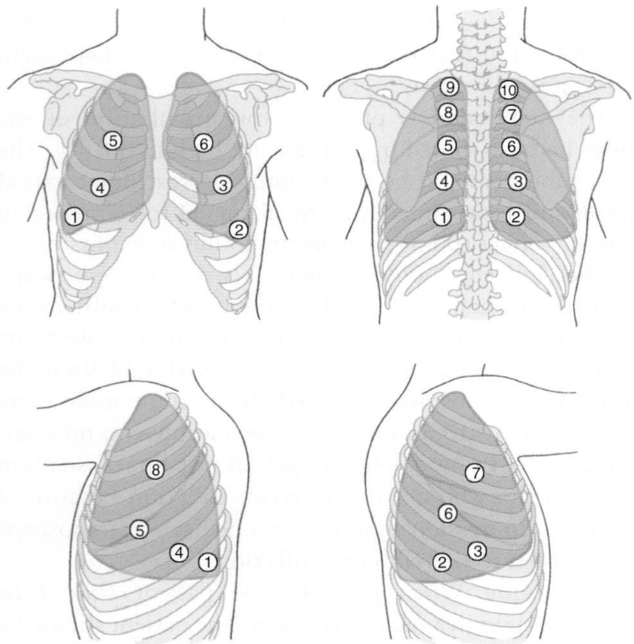

FIGURE 15-6 Sequencing for auscultation technique. (Modified from Wilkins RL, Dexter JR, editors: Respiratory diseases: a case study approach to patient care, ed 3, Philadelphia, 2007, FA Davis.)

A variation of the tracheal breath sounds can be heard around the upper half of the sternum on the anterior chest and between the scapulae on the posterior chest. These sounds are not as loud as tracheal breath sounds, are slightly lower in pitch, and have equal inspiratory and expiratory components. They are referred to as *bronchovesicular breath sounds.*

MINI CLINI

Terminology for Adventitious Lung Sounds

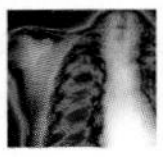

PROBLEM: The RT is auscultating a patient in the intensive care unit who has severe pneumonia. He hears low-pitched, discontinuous sounds with inspiration and exhalation. He documents this as "coarse crackles," but his supervisor instructs him to describe them as "rales and rhonchi." Who is right, and what pathologic condition is indicated by these sounds?

SOLUTION: The American Thoracic Society and American College of Chest Physicians Joint Committee on Pulmonary Nomenclature has endorsed the term *crackles* for discontinuous abnormal lung sounds. The same committee also has suggested that the term *rhonchi* be used to describe low-pitched, continuous sounds. The term *rhonchi* is not to be used to describe discontinuous sounds. Many clinicians have been trained to describe all secretion sounds as "rales and rhonchi," but this terminology is outdated and inaccurate. The RT's supervisor is mistaken, but diplomacy probably is needed in this case. Coarse inspiratory and expiratory crackles indicate that excessive airway secretions are present.

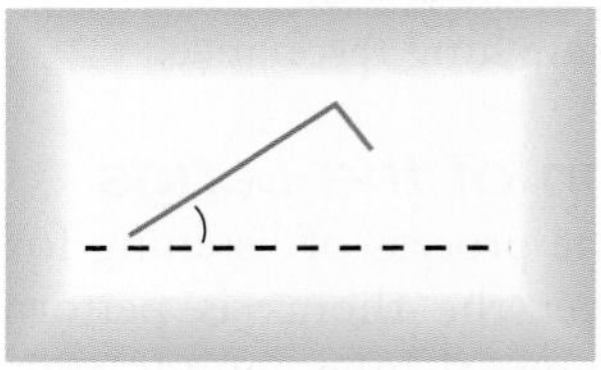

FIGURE 15-7 Diagram of normal breath sound. Upstroke represents inhalation, and downstroke represents exhalation; length of upstroke represents duration; thickness of stroke represents intensity; angle between upstroke and horizontal line represents pitch.

TABLE 15-3

Characteristics of Normal Breath Sounds

Breath Sound	Pitch	Intensity	Location	Diagram
Vesicular	Low	Soft	Peripheral lung areas	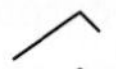
Bronchovesicular	Moderate	Moderate	Around upper part of sternum, between the scapulae	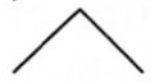
Tracheal	High	Loud	Over the trachea	

When auscultating over the lung parenchyma of a healthy individual, soft, muffled sounds are heard. These normal breath sounds, referred to as *vesicular breath sounds,* are lower in pitch and intensity than bronchovesicular breath sounds. Vesicular sounds are heard primarily during inhalation, with an exhalation component approximately one-third the duration of inhalation (see Table 15-3).

Respiratory disease may alter the intensity of normal breath sounds heard over the lung fields. Breath sounds are described as *diminished* when the intensity decreases and as *absent* in extreme cases. They are described as *harsh* when the intensity increases. When the expiratory component of harsh breath sounds equals the inspiratory component, they are described as *bronchial breath sounds.*

Adventitious lung sounds are added sounds or vibrations produced by the movement of air through abnormal airways. Adventitious lung sounds are classified as either discontinuous or continuous. Discontinuous adventitious lung sounds are intermittent, crackling, or bubbling sounds of short duration. Discontinuous adventitious lung sounds are referred to as **crackles,** whereas continuous adventitious lung sounds are described with the term **wheezes;** a wheeze is a quasimusical sound. The term *rhonchi* is encountered frequently. *Rhonchi* is derived from the Latin word meaning "wheezing." This term has had a confusing history in clinical practice, and its use is not recommended.

Another continuous type of adventitious lung sound, heard primarily over the larynx and trachea during inhalation, is **stridor.** Stridor is a loud, high-pitched sound and sometimes can be heard without a stethoscope. Most common in infants and small children, stridor is a sign of obstruction in the trachea or larynx. Stridor is most often heard during inspiration.

When abnormal lung sounds are heard, their location and specific features should be documented. Abnormal lung sounds may be high-pitched or low-pitched, loud or faint, scant or profuse, and inspiratory or expiratory (or both). Faint or low-intensity crackles are often referred to as *fine crackles;* more pronounced or more intense crackles are referred to as *coarse crackles.*

Mechanisms and Significance of Lung Sounds. The exact mechanisms that produce normal and abnormal lung sounds are not fully known. However, there is sufficient agreement among investigators to allow a general description.

Normal Breath Sounds. Lung sounds heard over the chest of a healthy individual are generated primarily by turbulent airflow in the larger airways. Turbulent airflow creates audible vibrations in the airways, producing sounds that are transmitted through the lungs and chest wall. As this sound travels to the lung periphery and the chest wall, it is altered by the filtering properties of normal lung tissue. Normal lung tissue acts as a low-pass filter, which means it preferentially passes low-frequency sounds. If you place the diaphragm portion of your stethoscope over the chest wall of a friend and listen while he or she speaks, this filtering (attenuation) effect will be evident. The voice sounds are muffled and difficult to understand because of attenuation. This filtering effect explains the characteristic differences between tracheal breath sounds, heard directly over the trachea, and vesicular sounds, heard over the lung periphery. Normal vesicular lung sounds essentially are attenuated tracheal breath sounds.

Bronchial Breath Sounds. Bronchial breath sounds are considered abnormal when they are heard over peripheral lung regions. Normal vesicular sounds are replaced with bronchial sounds when lung tissue density increases, and the attenuation is reduced. When normal air-filled lung tissue becomes atelectatic or consolidated (e.g., pneumonia), the resulting breath sounds are similar to the sounds normally heard over large upper airways.

Diminished Breath Sounds. Diminished breath sounds occur when the sound intensity at the site of generation (larger airways) is reduced, or when the sound transmission through the lung or chest wall is decreased. Sound intensity is reduced with shallow or slow breathing patterns that cause less turbulence in the larger airways, resulting in diminished breath sounds over the entire chest. Sound transmission through the chest wall also is diminished by airways plugged with mucus, hyperinflated lung tissue (e.g., COPD, asthma), air or fluid in the pleural space (e.g., pneumothorax, hemothorax, pleural effusion), and obesity.

Wheezes and Stridor. Wheezes and stridor represent vibrations of airway wall that are caused when air flows at high velocity through a narrowed airway. Airway diameter can be reduced by bronchospasm, mucosal edema, inflammation, tumors, foreign bodies, and pulmonary edema. This narrowing initially causes an increase in the velocity of airflow, which causes the lateral wall pressure to decrease. This decrease in pressure causes the lateral walls of the narrowed airway to pull closer together, and airflow stops. When airflow stops, the lateral wall pressure increases, and the airway opens back to the previous position. This cycle repeats many times per second and causes the airway walls to vibrate and make a musical type of adventitious lung sound similar to a reed instrument.

RULE OF THUMB

Generally, expiratory wheezes indicate obstruction of intrathoracic airways such as occurs with lung diseases (e.g., bronchitis, asthma). Wheezes in such cases are polyphonic. A monophonic wheeze suggests one airway is narrowed and the cause is not likely to be asthma.

It is useful to monitor the pitch and duration of wheezing. Improved expiratory flow is associated with a decrease in the pitch and length of the wheezing. If high-pitched wheezing is present during the entire expiratory time before treatment but becomes lower pitched and occurs only late in exhalation after therapy, the pitch and duration of the wheeze have diminished. This change suggests that the degree of airway obstruction has decreased.

Wheezing may be monophonic (single note) or polyphonic (multiple notes). A monophonic wheeze indicates that a single airway is partially obstructed. Monophonic wheezing may be heard during inhalation and exhalation or during exhalation only. Polyphonic wheezing suggests that many airways are obstructed, such as with asthma, and is heard only during exhalation. Bronchitis and CHF with pulmonary edema can also cause polyphonic wheezing.

Stridor is a serious adventitious lung sound that indicates that the upper airway is compromised. It may occur in patients of any age but most often is heard from the neck of children. In children, laryngomalacia is the most common cause of chronic stridor, whereas croup is the most common cause of acute stridor. Generally, inspiratory stridor is consistent with narrowing above the glottis, whereas expiratory stridor indicates narrowing of the lower trachea.

Crackles. Crackles occur when airflow moves secretions or fluid in the airways. In this situation, coarse crackles are usually heard during inspiration and expiration. These crackles often clear when the patient coughs or when the upper airway is suctioned. Crackles also may be heard in patients without excess secretions. These crackles occur when collapsed airways pop open during inspiration. Airway collapse or closure can occur in peripheral bronchioles or in larger, more proximal bronchi.

Larger, more proximal bronchi may close during expiration when there is an abnormal increase in bronchial compliance or when the retractile pressures around the bronchi are low. In this situation, crackles usually occur early in the inspiratory phase and are referred to as *early inspiratory crackles* (Figure 15-8). Early inspiratory crackles are usually scant but may be loud or faint. They often are transmitted to the mouth and are not silenced by a cough or a change in position. They frequently occur in patients with COPD (chronic bronchitis, emphysema, or asthma) and usually indicate severe airway obstruction.

Peripheral airways may close during exhalation when the surrounding intrathoracic pressure increases and when surfactant levels are diminished. *Fine, late inspiratory crackles* are produced by the sudden opening of peripheral airways, usually late in the inspiratory phase. They are more common in the dependent lung regions, where the peripheral airways are most prone to collapse during exhalation. They may clear with changes in posture or if the patient performs several deep inspirations. Late inspiratory crackles are most common in patients with respiratory disorders that reduce gas volume of the lung, such as atelectasis, pneumonia, pulmonary edema, and pulmonary fibrosis (Table 15-4).

RULE OF THUMB

Fine, late inspiratory crackles suggest restrictive lung diseases such as pulmonary fibrosis.

Pleural Friction Rub. A pleural friction rub is a creaking or grating sound that occurs when the pleural surfaces become inflamed, and the roughened edges rub together during breathing, as in pleurisy. It may be heard only

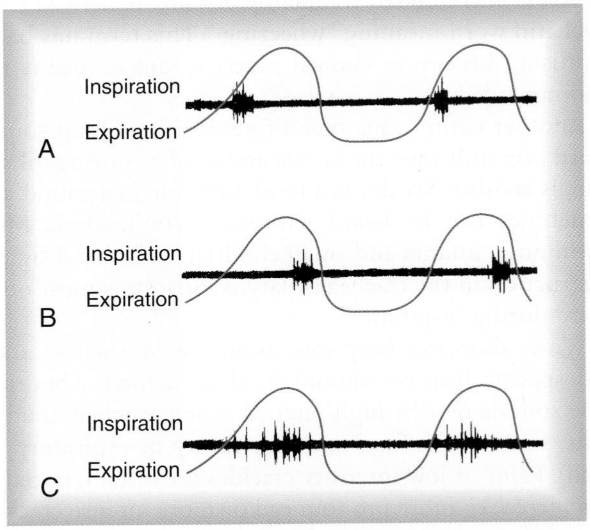

FIGURE 15-8 Timing of inspiratory crackles. **A,** Early inspiratory crackles. **B,** Late inspiratory crackles. **C,** Pan-inspiratory crackles.

TABLE 15-4

Application of Adventitious Lung Sounds

Lung Sound	Possible Mechanism	Characteristics	Causes
Wheezes	Rapid airflow through obstructed airways	High-pitched, usually expiratory	Asthma, CHF
Stridor	Rapid airflow through obstructed upper airway	High-pitched, monophonic	Croup, epiglottitis, postextubation laryngeal edema
Coarse crackles	Excess airway secretions moving through airways	Coarse, inspiratory and expiratory	Severe pneumonia, bronchitis
Fine crackles	Sudden opening of peripheral airways	Fine, late inspiratory	Atelectasis, fibrosis, pulmonary edema

during inhalation but often is identified during both phases of breathing. The rub usually is localized to a certain site on the chest wall. It sounds similar to coarse crackles but is not affected by coughing. The intensity of pleural rubs may increase with deep breathing.

Voice Sounds. If chest inspection, palpation, percussion, or auscultation suggests a lung abnormality, evaluation of vocal resonance may be useful in further assessment. Vocal resonance is produced by the same mechanism as vocal fremitus. Vibrations created by the vocal cords during speech travel down the airways and through the peripheral lung units to the chest wall. The patient is instructed to repeat the words "one," "two," "three," or "ninety-nine" while the clinician listens over the chest wall with a stethoscope, comparing one side with the other side. Normal, air-filled lung tissue filters the voice sounds, producing a significant reduction in intensity and clarity. Pathologic abnormalities in lung tissue alter the transmission of voice sounds, causing either increased or decreased vocal resonance. Increased vocal resonance occurs with lung consolidation, whereas decreased vocal resonance occurs with hyperinflated lung or with pneumothorax.

Bronchophony. An increase in the intensity and clarity of vocal resonance produced by enhanced transmission of vocal vibrations is called **bronchophony.** Bronchophony indicates increased lung tissue density, such as occurs in the consolidation phase of pneumonia. Bronchophony is easier to detect when it is unilateral. It often accompanies bronchial breath sounds, a dull percussion note, and increased vocal fremitus.

Vocal resonance is reduced when the transmission of voice sounds through the lung or chest wall is impeded. Hyperinflation, pneumothorax, bronchial obstruction, and pleural effusion all impede transmission of voice sounds and decrease vocal resonance. Decreased vocal resonance usually occurs together with reduced breath sounds and decreased tactile fremitus.

Cardiac Examination

Because of the close relationship between the heart and lungs, chronic lung diseases often cause cardiac problems. The techniques for physical examination of the chest wall overlying the heart (precordium) include inspection, palpation, and auscultation. Most clinicians examine the precordium at the same time they assess the lungs.

Inspection and Palpation

Inspection and palpation of the precordium help identify normal or abnormal pulsations. Pulsations on the precordium are created by ventricular contraction. Detection of pulsations depends on the force of ventricular contraction, the thickness of the chest wall, and the quality of the tissue through which the vibrations travel.

Normally, left ventricular contraction is the most forceful and generates a visible, palpable pulsation during systole. This pulsation is called the *point of maximal impulse* (PMI). In healthy individuals who are not obese (or overly muscular), the PMI can be felt and visualized near the left midclavicular line in the fifth intercostal space. The PMI shifts laterally with left ventricular hypertrophy.

Right ventricular hypertrophy (a common finding in COPD) often produces a systolic thrust called a **heave** that is felt (and possibly visualized) near the lower left sternal border. To identify the PMI, the clinician places the palmar aspect of the right hand over the lower left sternal border. Right ventricular hypertrophy may be the result of chronic hypoxemia, pulmonary valve disease, or primary pulmonary hypertension.

In patients with chronic pulmonary hyperinflation (emphysema), the PMI may be difficult to locate. Because of the increase in AP diameter and the changes in lung tissue, systolic vibrations are not well transmitted to the chest wall.

The PMI may shift either left or right, following deviations in the position of the lower mediastinum, which may be caused by pneumothorax or lobar collapse. Typically, the PMI shifts toward lobar collapse but away from a tension pneumothorax. The PMI in patients with emphysema and low flat diaphragms may be shifted centrally to the epigastric area.

The second left intercostal space near the sternal border is referred to as the *pulmonic area* and is palpated to identify accentuated pulmonary valve closure. Strong vibrations may be felt in this area with the presence of pulmonary hypertension or valvular abnormalities (Figure 15-9). Rapid blood flow through a narrowed valve or backflow through an incompetent valve may produce palpable vibrations known as **thrills.** Thrills are usually accompanied by a murmur (see discussion later).

Auscultation of Heart Sounds

Normal heart sounds are created by closure of the heart valves (see Chapter 9). The first heart sound (S_1) is produced by closure of the mitral and tricuspid (atrioventricular [AV]) valves during contraction of the ventricles. When systole ends, the ventricles relax, and the pulmonic and aortic (semilunar) valves close, creating the second heart sound (S_2). Because pressures in the left side of the heart are higher, mitral valve closure is louder and contributes more to S_1. For the same reason, closure of the aortic valve usually is more significant in producing S_2. If either the AV valves or the semilunar valves do not close together, a split heart sound is heard. A slight splitting of S_2 is normal; it occurs because of increased venous return during spontaneous breathing.

A third heart sound (S_3) can be heard during diastole and is produced by rapid ventricular filling immediately after systole. S_3 is a low-intensity, low-pitched sound best heard over the apex of the heart. In young, healthy children, S_3 is considered normal and is called *physiologic* S_3. Otherwise, S_3 is abnormal. In older patients with heart disease, S_3 may signify CHF.

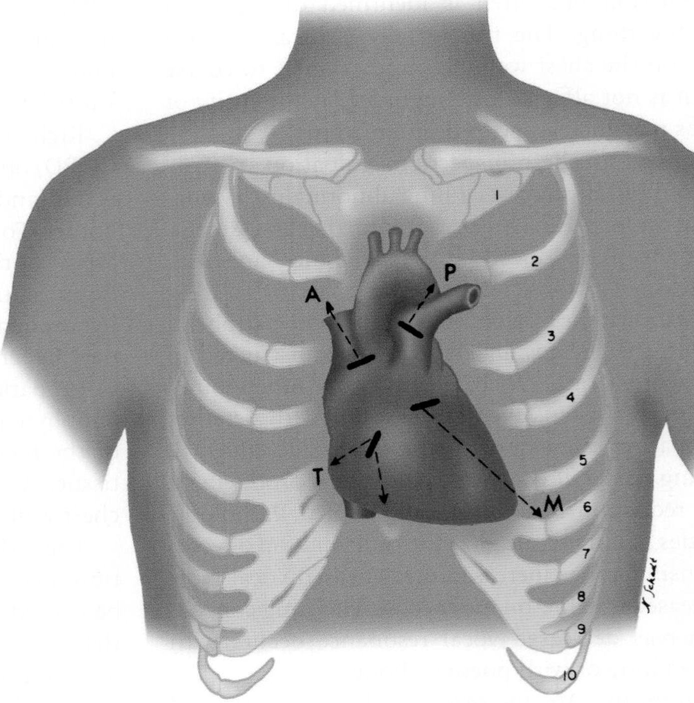

FIGURE 15-9 Anatomic and auscultatory valve area. Location of anatomic valve sites is represented by *solid bars*. *Arrows* designate transmission of valve sounds to their respective auscultatory valve areas. *A,* Aortic valve; *M,* mitral valve; *P,* pulmonic valve; *T,* tricuspid valve.

A fourth heart sound (S_4) is produced by mechanisms similar to the mechanisms that produce S_3. S_4 may occur in healthy individuals or may be considered a sign of heart disease. S_4 differs from S_3 only in its timing during the cardiac cycle. S_4 occurs later, just before S_1, whereas S_3 occurs just after S_2. A patient with heart disease who has S_3 and S_4 is said to have a **gallop rhythm.**

RULE OF THUMB

The presence of a gallop heart rhythm in an adult patient is consistent with CHF.

Abnormal Heart Sounds

Reduced intensity of heart sounds may result from cardiac or extracardiac abnormalities. Extracardiac factors include alteration in the tissue between the heart and the surface of the chest. Pulmonary hyperinflation, pleural effusion, pneumothorax, and obesity make identification of both S_1 and S_2 difficult. The intensity of S_1 and S_2 also decreases when the force of ventricular contraction is poor, as in heart failure, or when valvular abnormalities exist.

Pulmonary hypertension may cause two abnormalities in heart sounds. First, it increases the intensity of S_2 from a more forceful closure of the pulmonic valve (this is also referred to as a **loud P_2**). Second, S_2 splitting may be absent. An increased P_2 is identified best over the pulmonic area of the chest (see Figure 15-9).

Cardiac **murmurs** occur whenever the heart valves are incompetent or stenotic. Murmurs are classified as either systolic or diastolic. *Systolic murmurs* are produced by an incompetent AV valve or a stenotic semilunar valve. An incompetent AV valve typically produces a high-pitched "whooshing" noise simultaneously with S_1. This noise is caused by a backflow of blood through the AV valve into the atrium. In contrast, a stenotic semilunar valve produces a crescendo-decrescendo sound created by an obstruction of blood flow out of the ventricle during systole.

Diastolic murmurs are created by either an incompetent semilunar valve or a stenotic AV valve. An incompetent semilunar valve allows a backflow of blood into the ventricle simultaneously with, or immediately after, S_2. A stenotic AV valve obstructs blood flow from the atrium into the ventricles during diastole and creates a turbulent murmur.

A murmur also may be created by rapid blood flow across normal valves, such as occurs with heavy exertion. Murmurs are created by the following: (1) a backflow of blood through an incompetent valve, (2) a forward flow of blood through a stenotic valve, and (3) a rapid flow of blood through a normal valve.

Heart sounds can be auscultated by using the bell or diaphragm pieces of the stethoscope. The heart sounds may be easier to identify when the patient leans forward or lies on the left side. This positioning moves the heart closer to the chest wall. When peripheral pulses are difficult to identify, auscultation over the precordium may provide important additional information. Normally, the rate heard over the precordium (the apical rate) should be the same as the palpated peripheral pulse. In patients with atrial fibrillation, the apical rate often is higher than the peripheral pulse **(pulse deficit).** During atrial fibrillation, the irregular rhythm causes frequent weak ventricular contractions that cannot be detected at peripheral locations.

Abdominal Examination

The abdomen should be inspected and palpated for evidence of distention and tenderness. Abdominal distention and pain impair diaphragmatic movement and may contribute to or cause respiratory insufficiency. Abdominal dysfunction may inhibit deep breathing and coughing and promote atelectasis. Of particular concern is the presence of intraabdominal hypertension, which is defined as intraabdominal pressure greater than 12 mm Hg and is found in 18% of critically ill patients.[13] **Abdominal compartment syndrome** occurs when intraabdominal pressures are greater than 20 mm Hg and often requires emergency decompressive surgery. This syndrome causes profound atelectasis and hypoxemia, hypotension, and renal failure.

Intraabdominal hypertension is a common finding in patients with blunt or penetrating abdominal trauma, ruptured aortic aneurysm, bowel infarction, and end-stage liver failure. It is suspected when gross examination of the abdomen reveals very pronounced abdominal distention. Intraabdominal pressure is measured by connecting an intraarterial pressure catheter to the culture port of a Foley urine catheter.

The presence of an enlarged liver **(hepatomegaly)** is a frequent cause of right lower lobe atelectasis and pleural effusion. Hepatomegaly is a common finding in patients with liver disease and patients with cor pulmonale.

Examination of the Extremities

Respiratory disease may cause several abnormalities of the extremities, including digital clubbing, cyanosis, and pedal edema.

Clubbing

Clubbing of the digits is a significant manifestation of cardiopulmonary disease. **Clubbing** is a painless enlargement of the terminal phalanges of the fingers and toes that develops over time. As the process advances, the angle of the fingernail to the nail base increases, and the base of the nail feels "spongy." The profile view of the digits allows easier recognition of clubbing (Figure 15-10), but sponginess of the nail bed is the most important sign. Causes of clubbing include infiltrative or interstitial lung disease, bronchiectasis, various cancers (particularly lung cancer),[14] congenital heart problems that cause cyanosis, chronic liver disease, and inflammatory bowel disease. COPD alone, even when hypoxemia is present, does not lead to clubbing. Clubbing of the digits in a patient with COPD indicates that something other than obstructive lung disease is occurring.

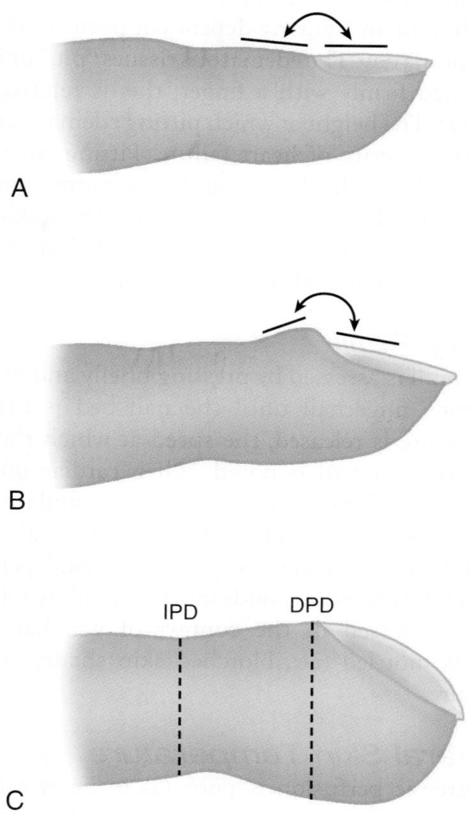

FIGURE 15-10 A, Normal digit configuration. **B,** Mild digital clubbing with increased hyponychial angle. **C,** Severe digital clubbing; the depth of the finger at the base of the nail *(DPD)* is greater than the depth of the interphalangeal joint *(IPD)* with clubbing.

Cyanosis

Examination of the digits for cyanosis is part of the initial assessment and is done whenever hypoxemia is suspected. Cyanosis can be detected easily because of the transparency of the fingernails and skin.

Cyanosis becomes visible when the amount of unsaturated hemoglobin in the capillary blood exceeds 5 to 6 g/dl; this may be caused by a reduction in arterial or venous O_2 content, or both. Cyanosis of the digits is referred to as *peripheral cyanosis* or *acrocyanosis* and may involve extensive portions of limbs. This condition is mainly the result of poor perfusion, especially in the extremities. When capillary blood flow is poor, the tissues extract more O_2, reducing the venous O_2 content and increasing the amount of reduced hemoglobin. The extremities are usually cool to the touch when peripheral cyanosis is a sign of poor perfusion.

Pedal Edema

Pedal edema most often results from heart failure, which causes an increase in the hydrostatic pressure of the venous system and leaking of fluid from the vessels into the surrounding tissues. The ankles are affected most often because they are in a gravity-dependent position throughout most of the day. The edematous tissues "pit," or indent, when pressed firmly with a finger; this is referred to as *pitting edema*. The height at which pitting edema occurs can indicate the severity of heart failure. Pitting edema that extends to above the knee signifies a more significant problem than edema limited to around the ankles. Any patient who is suspected to have right-sided or left-sided heart failure is examined for pedal edema.

Capillary Refill

Capillary refill is assessed by pressing briefly and firmly on the patient's fingernail until the nail bed is blanched. When pressure is released, the speed at which the blood flow and color return is noted. When cardiac output is reduced and the digital perfusion is poor, capillary refill is slow, taking several seconds to complete. In healthy individuals with good cardiac output and digital perfusion, capillary refill time is 2 seconds or less. Capillary refill time should be assessed in the context of whether or not the skin is mottled (i.e., blotched skin shade) and skin temperature.

Peripheral Skin Temperature

When systemic perfusion is poor (as in heart failure or shock), compensatory vasoconstriction in the extremities helps shunt blood to the vital organs. This reduction in peripheral perfusion causes the extremities to become cool to the touch. The extent to which the coolness to touch extends back toward the torso is an indication of the degree of circulatory failure. In contrast, patients with high cardiac output and peripheral vascular failure (as occurs in septic shock) may have warm, dry skin.

SUMMARY CHECKLIST

- The interview is used to obtain important diagnostic information and to build a rapport between the health care provider and the patient.
- Dyspnea is the sensation that occurs when breathing effort is excessive relative to the tidal volume achieved. The work of breathing increases with reduced lung compliance and narrowed airways. Breathlessness is the unpleasant urge to breathe and is the sensation associated with a heightened drive to breathe.
- Cough is one of the most common symptoms of lung disease and occurs when the cough receptors that line the larger airways are stimulated by foreign material, mucus, noxious gases, or inflammation.
- The most common cause of hemoptysis (spitting up blood from the lung) is infection.
- Vital signs provide reliable assessment information about the general condition of the patient and the patient's response to therapy.
- Rapid, shallow breathing indicates pathologic changes in the lung consistent with a reduction in the gas volume of the lungs.
- A prolonged expiratory phase suggests that the intrathoracic airways are narrowed.
- Normal breath sounds are generated by turbulent airflow in the larger airways.
- Crackles are generated by the sudden opening of closed airways or by the movement of excessive airway secretions with breathing.
- Wheezes are produced by the rapid vibration of narrow airways as gas passes through at high velocity.
- Cor pulmonale causes jugular venous distention, hepatomegaly, a loud P_2, and pedal edema.
- Central cyanosis is a sign of hypoxemia caused by respiratory failure, whereas peripheral cyanosis indicates circulatory failure.

References

1. Irwin RS: Chronic cough due to gastroesophageal reflux. Chest 129:80S–94S, 2006.
2. Palombini BC, Villanova CA, Araújo E, et al: A pathogenic triad in chronic cough: asthma, postnasal drip syndrome, and gastroesophageal reflux disease. Chest 116:279, 1999.
3. Sica DA, Brath L: Angiotensin-converting enzyme inhibition—emerging pulmonary issues relating to cough. Congest Heart Fail 12:223–226, 2006.
4. Engoren M: Lack of association between atelectasis and fever. Chest 107:81–84, 1995.
5. Buda AJ, Pinsky MR, Ingels NB, Jr, et al: Effect of intrathoracic pressure on left ventricular performance. N Engl J Med 301:453–459, 1979.
6. National High Blood Pressure Education Program: The 7th report of the Joint National Committee on Prevention, Detection, Evaluation and Treatment of High Blood Pressure, Besthesda, MD, 2004, National Institutes of Health National Heart, Lung and Blood Institute.
7. Antonelli M, Levy M, Andrews PJD, et al: Hemodynamic monitoring and shock and implications for management. International consensus conference, Paris, France. 27th-28th April 2006. Intensive Care Med 33:575–590, 2007.
8. Astiz ME: Pathophysiology and classification of shock states. In Fink MP, Abraham E, Vincent J-L, Kochanek PM, editors: Textbook of critical care, ed 5, Philadelphia, 2005, Saunders, pp 897–904.
9. Cohen CA, Zagelbaum G, Gross D, et al: Clinical manifestations of inspiratory muscle fatigue. Am J Med 73:316, 1982.
10. Tobin MJ, Perez W, Guenther SM, et al: Does rib cage-abdominal paradox signify respiratory muscle fatigue. J Appl Physiol 63:851–860, 1987.
11. Zachary KC, Bayne PS, Morrison VJ, et al: Contamination of gowns, gloves, and stethoscopes with vancomycin-resistant enterococci. Infect Control Hosp Epidemiol 22:560–564, 2001.
12. Cohen HA, Amir J, Matalon A, et al: Stethoscopes and otoscopes: a potential vector of infection. Fam Pract 14:446–449, 1997.
13. Malbrain M: Abdominal pressure in the critically ill. Curr Opin Crit Care 6:17–29, 2000.
14. Sridhar KS, Lobo CF, Altman RD: Digital clubbing and lung cancer. Chest 114:1535–1537, 1998.

Bibliography

Bickley LS: Bate's guide to physical examination and history taking, ed 10, Philadelphia, 2008, Lippincott.

Booth S, Dudgeon D: Dyspnoea in advanced disease: a guide to clinical management, Oxford, 2006, Oxford University Press.

Bowers AC, Thompson JM: Clinical manual of health assessment, ed 4, St Louis, 1992, Mosby.

Gardner WN: The pathophysiology of hyperventilation syndrome. Chest 109:516–534, 1996.

Mahler DA, O'Donnell DE: Dyspnea: mechanisms, measurement and management, ed 2, Boca Raton, FL, 2005, Taylor & Francis.

Ropper AH, Brown RH: Adams and Victor's principles of neurology, ed 8, New York, 2005 McGraw-Hill.

Seidel HM, Ball JW, Dains JE, et al: Mosby's guide to physical examination, ed 7, St Louis, 2011, Mosby.

Wilkins RL, Dexter JM, Heuer AJ: Clinical assessment in respiratory care, ed 6, St Louis, 2010, Mosby.

Wilkins RL, Hodgkin JE, Lopez B: Lung sounds: a practical guide, ed 3, St Louis, 2004, Mosby.

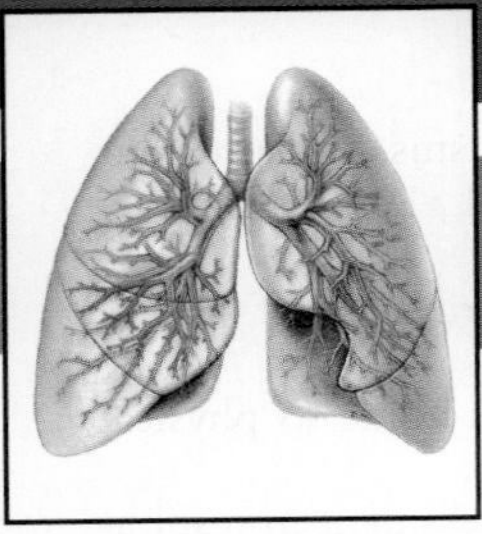

Chapter 16

Interpreting Clinical and Laboratory Data

RICHARD H. KALLET

CHAPTER OBJECTIVES

After reading this chapter you will be able to:

- Describe what a critical value is, and state its importance in clinical practice.
- Define the following terms related to clinical laboratory tests: leukocytosis, leukopenia, anemia, polycythemia, and thrombocytopenia.
- Identify which electrolyte disturbances interfere with normal respiratory function.
- Describe clinical tests used to identify cardiac stress and myocardial infarction.
- Identify the three main tests used to diagnose coagulation disorders.
- Describe how the sputum Gram stain and culture are used to diagnose pulmonary infections.

CHAPTER OUTLINE

KEY TERMS

acid-fast bacterium
anemia
bands
basic chemistry panel
complete blood count
critical test value
erythrocytes
hematology
homeostasis
hyperglycemia
hyperkalemia
hypernatremia
hypoglycemia
hypokalemia
lactate
leukocytes
leukocytosis
leukopenia
neutropenia
polycythemia
reference range
segs
thrombocytes
thrombocytopenia
troponin
troponin I

INTERPRETING CLINICAL LABORATORY TESTS

This chapter primarily discusses common blood tests performed on patients admitted to the hospital. These tests are done to evaluate the general health status of the patient, identify organ system dysfunction, detect the presence of infection, and determine the effects of therapy. The respiratory therapist (RT) must be familiar with these tests to understand the overall clinical status of patients under their care. The RT must be able to recognize how some abnormalities influence pulmonary function specifically. Sometimes the RT must alter his or her approach to practice based on abnormal laboratory test results.

This chapter also presents a brief review of fundamental physiologic concepts related to these tests. Comprehensive tables provide detailed information that can be used as a quick reference for each test. The chapter text provides a more general explanation on the significance of these tests and how they fit into an overall assessment of a patient's status.

Introduction to Laboratory Medicine

Laboratory medicine involves the study of patient tissue and fluid specimens. It is divided into five major disciplines. *Clinical biochemistry* involves the analysis of blood, urine, and other bodily fluids primarily for electrolytes and proteins; **hematology** analyzes the cellular components of blood. The analysis of blood and other bodily fluids for the presence of infectious agents is the purview of *clinical microbiology;* this includes the subspecialties of identifying bacteria *(bacteriology),* viruses *(virology),* fungi *(mycology),* and parasites *(parasitology).* A closely related discipline involves the analysis of the immune system *(immunology)* focusing on autoimmune and immunodeficiency diseases. Finally, the analysis of tissue for diagnosing diseases is the purview of the *anatomic pathology* service.

Reference Range

Laboratory tests are employed to determine a patient's health status and aid medical decisions. It is important to determine whether a specific test result falls within an expected range of values considered to be "normal." The notion of normal is problematic, however. Early on in the history of laboratory medicine, tests to determine the normal range for blood chemistry and hematology were done primarily on small convenience samples of subjects who were not representative of the larger population in terms of age, gender, race, and ethnicity. An additional problem is that the term *normal* is not the same as *healthy.* The best example is cholesterol. A normal range of cholesterol found in most Americans puts them at risk of cardiovascular disease and cannot be considered healthy.

Beginning in the 1970s,[1] the term *normal ranges* was slowly replaced with more appropriate terms such as *reference ranges, biologic reference intervals,* and *expected value.*[2] This change in terminology acknowledged that what we consider normal must take into account variations related to age, gender, race, and ethnicity, which change over time as the demographic composition of society changes. A **reference range** sets the boundaries for any analyte (e.g., electrolyte, blood cell, protein, enzyme) that would likely be encountered in healthy subjects. This range would encompass the variability reflected in the larger, presumably healthy population.

Reference ranges vary from laboratory to laboratory for various reasons, including differences in measurement techniques, the populations of healthy individuals used to establish the reference intervals, or analytic imprecision when the intervals were constructed. Most differences in reference ranges are relatively small, with reasonably close agreement between most laboratories.[2] The reference ranges and critical values given in this chapter are from a single institution, and they serve as representative examples. RTs must become familiar with the reference ranges used at their institutions.

Critical Test Value

A **critical test value** is a result *significantly* outside the reference range and represents a pathophysiologic condition. A critical value may be *potentially* life-threatening unless corrective action is taken promptly. Critical values are reported in the hospital to alert caregivers as well to decrease medical errors and protect patients.

Typically, critical values are communicated by telephone from the clinical laboratory to the general ward or intensive care unit where the patient is situated. The nurse or RT who receives these results is required to read-back the critical value to the clinical laboratory. This requirement is to ensure that the correct information has been communicated. It is the responsibility of the nurse or RT to communicate the critical value in a timely fashion to the physician caring for the patient. The same read-back procedure is used. All communication of critical test values is documented in the medical record.

In this chapter, critical values are listed along with common pathophysiologic states with which they commonly occur. Not all clinical analytes have an associated critical value. For some tests, there is no general agreement on what a critical value would be. Others have only a one-sided value that exists below or above a critical threshold; this is true particularly for substances that do not normally appear in the blood. For example, certain enzymes and proteins are released only after extensive cellular damage following injury (see later section on enzyme tests). Under normal circumstances, these proteins or enzymes may be virtually undetectable in the serum or plasma.

When interpreting derangements for *any* test result, the clinician must consider the *context* of the change. In a patient with chronic renal disease, a serum creatinine of 3.0 mg/dl (approximately twice the upper limit of normal) would not be considered urgent. However, in a patient who presents with a bloodstream infection (i.e., sepsis) and hypotension, a sudden increase in serum creatinine to 3.0 mg/dl would be considered critical because it indicates acute kidney injury in the context of rapidly developing clinical instability.

Complete Blood Count

The **complete blood count** (CBC) provides a detailed description of the number of circulating white blood cells (WBCs), called **leukocytes;** red blood cells (RBCs), called **erythrocytes;** and platelets, called **thrombocytes.** The WBC count is made up of five different types of cells and is reported under the differential. RBCs are evaluated for size and hemoglobin content. The platelets are evaluated for number present. Table 16-1 lists the normal CBC results for adults.

Elevation of the WBC count is termed **leukocytosis.** It results from numerous problems, including stress, infection, and trauma. The degree of leukocytosis reflects the severity of infection. A significantly elevated WBC count ($>20 \times 10^3$/mcl) suggests the presence of a serious infection and that the patient's immune system is generating a significant response. In contrast, **leukopenia** (or leukocytopenia) is a WBC count below normal that often occurs when the patient's immune system is overwhelmed by infection. Other important causes of leukopenia include bone marrow diseases (e.g., leukemia, lymphoma), influenza, systemic lupus erythematosus, tuberculosis, and acquired immunodeficiency syndrome (AIDS). Also, chemotherapy and radiation therapy given to cancer patients frequently causes leukopenia.

TABLE 16-1

Reference Range Values for Complete Blood Count in an Adult

Test	Reference Range
Red blood cell count	
Men	$4.4\text{-}5.9 \times 10^6$/mcl
Women	$3.8\text{-}5.2 \times 10^6$/mcl
Hemoglobin	
Men	13.3-17.7 g/dl
Women	11.7-15.7 g/dl
Hematocrit	
Men	40%-52%
Women	35%-47%
White blood cell count	$3.9\text{-}11.7 \times 10^3$/mcL
White blood cell differential	
Segmented neutrophils	40%-75%
Bands	0%-6%
Eosinophils	0%-6%
Basophils	0%-1%
Lymphocytes	20%-45%
Monocytes	2%-10%
Platelet count	$150\text{-}400 \times 10^3$/mcL

Values for reference ranges and critical test results are from the University of California San Francisco Moffit-Long Hospital and San Francisco General Hospital. http://pathology.ucsf.edu/labmanual/mftlng-mtzn/test/test-index.html and http://pathology.ucsf.edu/sfghlab/test/ReferenceRanges.html. Accessed January 1, 2011.

White Blood Cell Count

White Blood Cell Count Differential. The differential of the WBC count determines the exact number of each type of WBC present in the circulating blood (Table 16-2). Most circulating WBCs are either neutrophils or lymphocytes. Because leukocytosis usually results from only one of the five cell types responding to a problem, significant elevation of the WBC count ($>15 \times 10^3$/mcl) occurs only when either neutrophils or lymphocytes are responding to an abnormality. Because basophils, eosinophils, and monocytes make up such a small proportion of the circulating WBCs, they are not likely to cause a major increase in the WBC count when responding to disease.

The WBC count differential is best interpreted by determining the absolute count of each WBC; this is calculated by multiplying the percentage of the WBCs under study by the total WBC count. This calculation prevents misinterpretation of the WBC count differential when any one cell type changes in absolute numbers and causes a relative change in the percentage of the other four cell types. For example, if the WBC count doubles because of an increase in neutrophils, the relative value of the other four cells would decrease by half, although their absolute value would not change. Many laboratories report the absolute value for each of the five WBCs to avoid this confusion.

The subanalysis of lymphocytes is important for identifying infection with HIV, the causative agent of AIDS. HIV targets and destroys CD4 T lymphocytes. Opportunistic infections, in particular, *Pneumocystis jiroveci* pneumonia, generally occur when these lymphocytes decrease to less than 200×10^6/L, and this information is used in making the diagnosis of AIDS.

Elevation of the absolute value of neutrophils is termed *neutrophilia.* Immature neutrophils are known as **bands** because of the banded shape of the nucleus. Most bands are located in the bone marrow where they continue to mature. Mature neutrophils are known as **segs** because of the segmented shape of their nucleus. Severe infection causes the bone marrow to release stores of any available neutrophils, and both bands and segs enter the circulating blood volume. When bands and segs are elevated in the CBC, the patient is likely experiencing a more severe bacterial infection.

A reduced number of circulating neutrophils is termed **neutropenia.** Although uncommon, neutropenia is characteristic of patients with bone marrow disease (e.g., lymphoma, leukemia), patients undergoing treatment for cancer with chemotherapy or radiation or both, patients with some autoimmune disorders, and HIV-infected

TABLE 16-2

Reference Range Values for White Blood Cell Count Differential and Common Causes for Abnormalities

Cell Type	Relative Value	Absolute Value	Causes for Abnormalities
Neutrophils	40%-75%	$1.8\text{-}6.8 \times 10^9/L$	Increased with bacterial infection and trauma; reduced with bone marrow diseases (critical value <1.0)
Lymphocytes	20%-45%	$1.0\text{-}3.4 \times 10^9/L$	Increased with viral and other infections; reduced with immunodeficiency problems
CD4 T lymphocytes	31%-60%*	$410\text{-}1590 \times 10^6/L$	HIV disease; diagnostic threshold <200
Eosinophils	0%-6%	$0\text{-}0.4 \times 10^6/L$	Increased with allergic reactions and parasitic infections
Basophils	0%-1%	$0\text{-}0.1 \times 10^6/L$	Increased with allergic reactions
Monocytes	2%-10%	$0.2\text{-}0.8 \times 10^6/L$	Increased with invasion of foreign material

Values for reference ranges and critical test results are from the University of California San Francisco Moffit-Long Hospital and San Francisco General Hospital. http://pathology.ucsf.edu/labmanual/mftlng-mtzn/test/test-index.html and http://pathology.ucsf.edu/sfghlab/test/ReferenceRanges.html. Accessed January 1, 2011.
*Percentage of lymphocyte.

patients. Neutropenia puts the patient at risk for the development of infection.

RULE OF THUMB

Elevation of the WBC count is usually caused by an increase in either neutrophils or lymphocytes in response to infection.

RULE OF THUMB

When bacterial pneumonia is present, the severity of the infection can be assessed by evaluation of the degree of increase in neutrophils.

Red Blood Cell Count

The primary function of RBCs or erythrocytes is to supply oxygen to the tissues. The RBC count helps determine the ability of the blood to carry oxygen. An abnormally low RBC count is referred to as **anemia** and suggests that either RBC production by the bone marrow is inadequate or excessive blood loss has occurred. In either case, the oxygen-carrying capacity of the blood is reduced, and the patient is more likely to experience tissue hypoxia. There are several types of anemia with different causes. Some are related to dietary deficiencies in iron or vitamins (e.g., vitamin B_{12} and folate). Other causes are related to chronic inflammatory diseases, such as Crohn disease, HIV/AIDS, lymphoma, and autoimmune diseases that result in the destruction of erythrocytes (hemolytic and aplastic anemia). A hereditary cause is sickle cell anemia, which is common in African-Americans. For most forms of anemia, a blood transfusion may be needed if the RBC count is too low. The trigger point for transfusion is based on the hemoglobin or hematocrit measurement rather than the RBC count.

MINI CLINI

White Blood Cell Count Differential

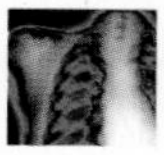

PROBLEM: A patient has been admitted to the hospital for acute shortness of breath. A chest x-ray reveals pneumonia, and the patient's temperature is elevated. The CBC shows an increased WBC count of 15×10^3/mcl with 75% neutrophils but only 10% lymphocytes. Given that the normal lymphocyte differential is 20% to 45%, does the value of 10% suggest a problem with lymphocyte production by the immune system? What type of pneumonia is probably present in this case?

SOLUTION: The 10% differential for the lymphocytes represents a relative value. Because the total WBC count is markedly elevated, the 10% in relative terms represents 1500 lymphocytes in absolute value, which is well within normal range. If the total WBC count was reduced to less than normal and the differential showed a lymphocyte count of 10%, an abnormal absolute value would be present and would suggest an immunologic problem. This patient probably has bacterial pneumonia, given the elevated number of neutrophils.

An abnormally elevated RBC count is known as **polycythemia.** It occurs most often when the bone marrow is stimulated to produce extra RBCs in response to chronically low blood oxygen levels (secondary polycythemia). Polycythemia counteracts the negative side effects of reduced PO_2 in the blood by increasing the oxygen-carrying capacity of the blood. Patients who live at a high altitude and patients with chronic lung disease are most likely to experience chronic hypoxia and to develop secondary polycythemia.

In addition to the RBC count, the clinical laboratory reports hemoglobin and hematocrit levels. Hemoglobin is a protein substance with the unique ability to bind with oxygen. Each healthy RBC contains 200 million to 300 million molecules of hemoglobin, for a hemoglobin level of 12 to 17 g/dl in a healthy adult. Patients with an inadequate hemoglobin concentration have reduced oxygen-carrying capacity. In this condition, the RBCs are smaller than normal (microcytic anemia) and lack normal color (hypochromic anemia). The necessity for RBC transfusion depends on the cause of anemia and the patient's overall condition. Usually a transfusion is triggered by a hemoglobin concentration of approximately 7.0 g/dl or a hematocrit of approximately 21%.

The hematocrit level is the ratio of RBC volume to whole blood. It is determined by spinning a blood sample in a centrifuge to separate the blood cells from the plasma. The proportion of the sample represented by the packed cells is the hematocrit. A low hematocrit reading occurs with anemia, and a high hematocrit reading is common with polycythemia. The hematocrit level is also a reflection of the hydration status of the patient. Dehydration causes the hematocrit to increase, whereas overhydration causes it to decrease.

RULE OF THUMB

The threshold for blood transfusion typically is a hematocrit of 21% or a hemoglobin of 7.0 g/dl.

Electrolyte Tests

Basic Concepts for Understanding Electrolyte Balance

Normal cellular function depends on homeostasis of fluids, electrolytes, and acid-base balance. **Homeostasis** is the ability of complex organisms to maintain a *dynamic balance* or *equilibrium* in their internal environments by making constant adjustments. The guiding principle is that the total amount of water, electrolytes, acid, and base gained each day must be balanced by the total amount lost.

Electrolytes are positively or negatively charged ions that influence the functioning of enzymes. The concentration of any electrolyte is determined by the amount of water in which it is suspended. Electrolytes always must be interpreted within the context of fluid balance. Enzymes are proteins that regulate all chemical reactions occurring within cells, such as metabolism and protein synthesis. All cellular functions operate within very narrow parameters of electrolyte concentrations. Disturbances in electrolyte balance may disrupt normal cellular functioning.

Two important points must be kept in mind when interpreting these blood tests. First, blood samples provide a one-time "snapshot" of processes that are constantly in flux. These "snapshots" provide the clinician with valuable but time-limited insight into cellular processes. Often, the most important information comes from serial measurements, whereby both the degree of abnormalities and the directional changes can be assessed. Changes over time provide vital information about the severity and progression of disease as well as judging the effectiveness of therapy.

Second, the intravascular blood compartment is remote from the intracellular environment. Analyzing serum electrolyte levels gives the clinician only an indirect view of what might be occurring inside the cells of the body. The intracellular fluid compartment represents approximately two-thirds of total body fluid compared with approximately one-third that exists outside in the extracellular fluid compartment. Blood plasma is just a small component of the extracellular environment. Monitoring abnormalities in the extracellular fluid compartment via blood samples provides important but indirect information in assessing intracellular functioning.

Basic Chemistry Panel

The **basic chemistry panel** (BCP) or *basic metabolic panel* includes the predominant electrolytes sodium (Na^+), potassium (K^+), chloride (Cl^-), and total carbon dioxide/bicarbonate (CO_2) and glucose. Because the body's electrolyte balance is controlled by the kidneys, excretion of renal-mediated waste products is included in the panel: creatinine and blood urea nitrogen. A more comprehensive metabolic panel would include other important electrolytes, such as magnesium (Mg^{++}), phosphorus (PO_4^-), and calcium (Ca^{++}). Each electrolyte plays a crucial role in maintaining normal cellular function. Specific information on the reference range and physiologic significance of each electrolyte and waste product can be found in Table 16-3. Information regarding the terminology used to describe abnormal test values for electrolytes, diseases associated with these disturbances, and sample critical test results are provided in Table 16-4.

The respiratory therapist needs to be aware of subtle differences in how electrolytes are reported as this may cause confusion. The concentration of electrolytes in solution is reported either by the number of molecules (millimoles: mmol) or their associated valence or electrical charge (milliequivalents: mEq). Although customary practice has been to report electrolytes as mEq/L, many laboratories report electrolytes as mmol/L. In an electrolyte solution milliequivalents is simply millimoles per liter multiplied by the valence. For example, sodium possesses a valence of 1, so that the expression as either mmol/L or mEq/L is the same. For calcium and magnesium, which both possess a valence of 2, then the mEq value is twice the mmol value.

Glucose

The breakdown of carbohydrates results in the production of serum glucose, which is metabolized by the cells for energy. Insulin, which comes from the pancreas, is necessary for cells to use the glucose circulating in the blood. Abnormal elevation of blood glucose level is termed **hyperglycemia** and is most often the result of diabetes. An abnormally reduced serum glucose level is termed

TABLE 16-3

Components of Basic Metabolic Panel and Common Electrolyte Tests With Sample Reference Ranges and Physiologic Significance

Test	Reference Range*	Physiologic Importance
Sodium (Na^+)	136-145 meq/L	Primary extracellular cation; crucial for maintaining fluid balance and nerve impulse conduction
Potassium (K^+)	3.5-5.0 meq/L	Primary intracellular cation; crucial for maintaining normal heart and kidney function and acid-base balance
Chloride (Cl^-)	98-106 meq/L	Primary extracellular anion; crucial for maintaining serum osmolarity and acid-base balance
Total carbon dioxide (CO_2)	22-29 meq/L	Primary metabolic end product of aerobic metabolism; crucial for maintaining acid-base balance
Calcium (Ca)	4.5-5.25 meq/L	Most abundant mineral in the body; essential for bone strength, muscular contraction, nerve impulse conduction, and coagulation
Ionized calcium (Ca^{++})	2.2-2.7 meq/L	The approximately 50% of calcium not bound to circulating proteins; represents the biologically active portion
Glucose (Glu)	70-139 mg/dl	Primary cellular energy source
Creatinine (Cr)	0.7-1.3 mg/dl	Waste product from muscle catabolism excreted by the kidneys; one of the key markers of kidney function because it provides a gross estimation of glomerular filtration rate
Blood urea nitrogen (BUN)	8-23 mg/dl	Waste product from metabolism of amino acids; a key marker of kidney function
Magnesium (Mg^{++})	1.7-2.1 meq/L	Essential for regulation of most biochemical processes; important for: normal muscle and neuronal functioning, regulating heart rate and blood pressure, glucose levels, bone strength, and immune function
Phosphorus (PO_4^-)	1.2-2.3 meq/L	Main intracellular anion (phosphate), exists as phosphorus in serum; combined with calcium in teeth and bones; serum levels inversely related to serum calcium
Lactate	0.7-2.1 meq/L	End product of glucose metabolism under anaerobic conditions; clinically significant levels coincide with regional or systemic tissue hypoxia
Osmolarity	275-295 mOsm/kg	Tonicity or ability to attract water molecules; indicates overall ionic concentration in the serum

*Reference ranges vary among clinical laboratories. See text for explanation.
Values for reference ranges and critical test results are from the University of California San Francisco Moffit-Long Hospital and San Francisco General Hospital. http://pathology.ucsf.edu/labmanual/mftlng-mtzn/test/test-index.html and http://pathology.ucsf.edu/sfghlab/test/ReferenceRanges.html. Accessed January 1, 2011.

TABLE 16-4

Sample Critical Test Results Reflecting Abnormalities in Electrolyte and Other Common Laboratory Tests

Test	Sample Critical Test Result*	Common Pathologic Conditions Associated With *Abnormally High Levels*	Common Pathologic Conditions Associated With *Abnormally Low Levels*
Sodium (Na^+)	>155 meq/L; <125 meq/L	*Hypernatremia:* Dehydration from excessive water loss or fluid restriction; excessive administration of saline fluids or diuretics (usually ≥180 mmol)	*Hyponatremia:* Overhydration or abnormal secretion of antidiuretic hormone; severe vomiting or diarrhea; congestive heart failure, renal or hepatic failure, Addison disease
Potassium (K^+)	>6.0 meq/L; <3.0 meq/L	*Hyperkalemia:* Acute or chronic kidney disease, Addison disease, severe alcoholism, rhabdomyolysis; values ≥6 mmol are life-threatening	*Hypokalemia:* Severe vomiting or diarrhea; chronic renal disease; high-dose beta-agonist therapy
Chloride (Cl^-)	>120 meq/L; <70 meq/L	*Hyperchloremia:* Excessive chloride administration (usually saline resuscitation during shock); metabolic acidosis, diabetes insipidus	*Hypochloremia:* Severe vomiting or diarrhea; metabolic alkalosis, adrenal insufficiency, severe burns, excessive intravenous dextrose administration
Total carbon dioxide (CO_2)	>40 meq/L; <15 meq/L	Ventilatory failure	Metabolic acidosis; hyperventilation syndrome; severe diarrhea

Continued

TABLE 16-4

Sample Critical Test Results Reflecting Abnormalities in Electrolyte and Other Common Laboratory Tests—cont'd

Test	Sample Critical Test Result*	Common Pathologic Conditions Associated With *Abnormally High Levels*	Common Pathologic Conditions Associated With *Abnormally Low Levels*
Calcium (Ca)	>13.5 meq/L; <6.5 meq/L	*Hypercalcemia:* Hyperparathyroidism, lithium or thiazide diuretic therapy, metastatic cancer, multiple myeloma	*Hypocalcemia:* Hypoparathyroidism, blood transfusions, acute pancreatitis, vitamin D deficiency
Ionized calcium (Ca^{++})	>1.5 meq/L; <0.8 meq/L		
Glucose (Glu)	>500 mg/dl; <50 mg/dl	*Hyperglycemia:* Diabetes mellitus, severe sepsis	*Hypoglycemia:* Excessive insulin administration, inadequate dietary intake of carbohydrates
Creatinine (Cr)	>10 mg/dl	Acute kidney injury, chronic renal failure	Protein starvation, liver disease
Blood urea nitrogen (BUN)	>100 mg/dl	Acute kidney injury, chronic renal failure, dehydration	Liver disease, malnutrition
Magnesium (Mg^{++})	>3.7 meq/L; <0.8 meq/L	*Hypermagnesemia:* Chronic renal failure, Addison disease, diabetic ketoacidosis, dehydration	*Hypomagnesemia:* Cirrhosis, pancreatitis, severe alcoholism, hemodialysis, toxemia of pregnancy, ulcerative colitis
Phosphorus (PO_4^-)	<1.0 meq/L; >2.5 meq/L	*Hyperphosphatemia:* Commonly found in patients with renal failure, hepatic failure, bone metastasis, hypocalcemia, hypoparathyroidism	*Hypophosphatemia:* Most often seen in chronic hyperventilation syndrome; also caused by hypercalcemia, hyperparathyroidism, and malnutrition
Lactate	>4 meq/L		Primarily causes anaerobic metabolism; frequently found in patients with hemorrhagic or septic shock; may also be due to reduced hepatic clearance, dehydration, or trauma
Osmolarity	>320 mOsm/kg; <240 mOsm/kg		

Values for reference ranges and critical test results are from the University of California San Francisco Moffit-Long Hospital and San Francisco General Hospital. http://pathology.ucsf.edu/labmanual/mftlng-mtzn/test/test-index.html and http://pathology.ucsf.edu/sfghlab/test/ReferenceRanges.html. Accessed January 1, 2011.

*Reference ranges and critical test results vary among clinical laboratories. See text for explanation.

hypoglycemia and may be drug-induced or associated with digestive problems, inadequate dietary intake of carbohydrates, or overtreatment of diabetes with insulin.

Diabetes is diagnosed by measuring fasting blood glucose levels (i.e., a glucose measurement taken after 12 hours without food). A blood glucose level greater than 140 mg/dl on two occasions usually indicates diabetes. Severe hyperglycemia occurring with metabolic acidosis is consistent with diabetic ketoacidosis and represents a potentially life-threatening condition if not treated immediately.

In critically ill patients, insulin resistance and hyperglycemia are common. This condition is associated with a higher incidence of multiorgan failure and increased mortality. The condition can be ameliorated with a regimen of intensive insulin therapy to keep blood glucose levels at approximately 110 mg/dl.[3] For intensive insulin therapy to be effective, blood glucose levels must be monitored frequently with a bedside (point-of-care) measuring device to facilitate rapid titration of insulin.

Anion Gap

As discussed in Chapter 13, metabolic acidosis is caused by either the addition of nonvolatile acids or a primary loss of HCO_3^-. The anion gap provides a quick method for determining whether a decrease in HCO_3^- is caused by a disruption of normal anion balance or the presence of an abnormal acid anion. A balance normally exists between cations and anions in the serum. The normal anion gap occurs because sulfate, phosphate, and organic anions such as lactate are not routinely measured, whereas most cations are measured. The anion gap is calculated by adding the CO_2 and Cl^- values and then subtracting this total from the serum Na^+. The normal anion gap is approximately 8 to 14 meq/L, and *gap acidosis* usually coincides with an anion gap of 16 mmol/L or greater. However, serum proteins are an important determinant of the anion gap. *Hypoalbuminemia* (decreased serum albumin) is a common finding in critically ill patients and significantly reduces the anion gap. As a rule, for every 1-g reduction in serum albumin below 4 g/dl, the anion gap is corrected upward by 3 meq/L.

RULE OF THUMB

An anion gap greater than 16 is consistent with the presence of metabolic acidosis.

Lactate

Lactate is the end product of anaerobic glucose metabolism. Blood lactate concentration is dependent on the production of lactate in muscle cells and erythrocytes and the rate of metabolism by the liver. Lactic acidosis results from either overproduction of or insufficient metabolism of lactate. Abnormal levels of lactate can be found in diverse conditions such as diabetes mellitus; malignancies; and toxic ingestion of ethanol, methanol, or salicylates. However, the most common cause of lactic acidosis is anaerobic metabolism from tissue hypoxia associated with shock. Initial values of serum lactate greater than 4 meq/L are associated with higher mortality in patients with septic shock. Also, the inability to clear high lactate levels rapidly is associated with poorer outcomes in critically ill patients.

RULE OF THUMB

In patients with septic shock, a serum lactate level greater than 4 meq/L is associated with higher mortality.

Enzyme Tests

Liver Function Tests

The liver is primarily responsible for converting food into substrates essential for cellular metabolism, protein synthesis, and detoxifying substances in the body. Liver damage is assessed by abnormal increases in the hepatic enzymes *alanine aminotransferase, aspartate aminotransferase, alkaline phosphatase*. *Total bilirubin* is produced by the liver from the breakdown of destroyed RBCs. It is a crucial component of the liver panel test because it assesses one of the primary functions of the liver. Protein synthesis is another vital aspect of liver function and is assessed by measuring concentrations of total protein and albumin. Liver disease is characterized by the inability to remove toxins from the bloodstream. One of the primary toxins associated with altered mental function in patients with liver disease is the accumulation of *ammonia,* which forms in the body from the breakdown of proteins.

MINI CLINI

Anion Gap

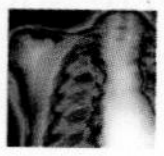

PROBLEM 1: A patient in the intensive care unit is being treated for shock and acute renal failure. No ABGs have been drawn yet, but the RT suspects the respiratory system is involved because the patient has been breathing more rapidly over the past 12 hours. The electrolyte panel reveals a serum Na^+ of 146 meq/L, a total CO_2 of 20 meq/L, and a serum Cl^- of 100 meq/L. Does the electrolyte panel suggest any problems, and what should be done if there are any?

SOLUTION: The electrolytes are normal except for a decrease in the serum CO_2. The anion gap is calculated by subtracting the sum of CO_2 and Cl^- from the Na^+ (146 – [100 + 20]). In this case, the anion gap is elevated (26 meq/L) and is consistent with a metabolic acidosis. An ABG analysis is needed to evaluate the acid-base status of the patient further. The patient's rapid breathing probably is related to the metabolic acidosis because hyperventilation decreases CO_2 levels and promotes acid-base compensation.

PROBLEM 2: A patient in the trauma intensive care unit is undergoing large fluid resuscitation with normal saline solution. The patient is in hemorrhagic and hypovolemic shock following a motor vehicle accident. An initial ABG reveals a pH of 7.25, PCO_2 of 25 mm Hg, and HCO_3^- of 10.6 with a base deficit of −14.9 meq/L. The trauma surgeons are debating increasing the amount of normal saline solution infused. They suspect their resuscitation efforts are inadequate, and metabolic acidosis is worsening from continued lactate accumulation. What additional information can be provided by obtaining a BCP to help guide therapy?

SOLUTION: If the BCP reveals a Na^+ of 140 meq/L, Cl^- of 95 meq/L, and CO_2 of 20 meq/L (anion gap of 25 meq/L), the surgeons would be correct in assuming that their resuscitation efforts were inadequate. The anion gap of 25 likely represents a worsening lactic acidosis. However, if the BCP reveals a Na^+ of 150 meq/L, CO_2 of 20 meq/L, and Cl^- of 122 meq/L, the anion gap would be normal (8 meq/L). The metabolic acidosis would be caused by an abnormally high serum chloride concentration from excessive normal saline administration. This example represents a common problem in emergency and critical care practice: the overresuscitation of trauma patients from severe shock.

Pancreatic and Muscle Enzyme Tests

Other diseases also produce abnormal amounts of enzymes in the serum. Patients with pancreatitis have abnormal levels of the pancreatic enzymes *lipase* and *amylase*. *Creatine phosphokinase* (CPK) or *creatinine kinase* is an enzyme found mainly in heart, brain, and skeletal muscle tissue. Patients who have sustained ischemic damage to these tissues have elevated CPK levels. Three types of CPK are associated with each tissue. CPK-1 (CPK-BB) is released primarily from the lungs or brain after injury. Patients who have sustained extensive crush injuries involving the skeletal muscles or with myositis have elevated levels of CPK-3 (CPK-MM). The third type of CPK is associated with cardiac injury and is discussed subsequently.

Lactate dehydrogenase is the enzyme that catalyzes the conversion of pyruvate into lactate. Elevated serum levels of lactate dehydrogenase are associated with tissue breakdown. This breakdown often occurs with numerous diverse conditions, such as rhabdomyolysis, cancer, meningitis, hemolytic anemia, acute pancreatitis, acute myocardial infarction, and HIV disease. Moderate increases in lactate dehydrogenase are associated with myocardial infarction or hemolytic anemia (880 U/L), whereas large increases are seen in extensive cancers, rhabdomyolysis, severe shock, and anoxia (8800 U/L).

Cardiac Enzyme and Protein Tests

The most common CPK enzyme test is CPK-2 (CPK-MB), which is released from the heart after myocardial infarction. Peak levels occur 12 to 24 hours after injury. Serial CPK-2 measurements are monitored in patients with suspected myocardial infarction and patients with cardiac contusion from chest trauma, open heart surgery, or myocarditis. **Troponin** is a complex protein that plays an important role in the regulation of skeletal and cardiac muscle contractility. The protein fragment **troponin I** is associated with cardiac muscle damage. Similar to CPK-2, troponin I levels peak 12 to 16 hours after myocardial infarction. Reference values for these enzyme tests are presented in Table 16-5.

B-type natriuretic peptide (BNP) is a substance secreted by the heart in response to increased stretch in the cardiac muscle. The BNP test primarily is used to evaluate patients for heart failure, in particular, patients who present to the emergency department with dyspnea and pulmonary edema.[4] Generally, values greater than 300 pg/ml indicate mild heart failure, whereas values greater than 600 pg/ml are found in patients with moderate heart failure, and values greater than 900 pg/ml are found in patients with severe heart failure.[4] Other conditions such as acute respiratory distress syndrome and severe sepsis also cause increased stretch of the cardiac muscle. In these cases, the BNP levels typically are lower (300 to 500 pg/ml) than what is found commonly in critically ill patients with primary heart failure (700 to –1200 pg/ml).[5]

TABLE 16-5

Liver Function and Other Enzymatic Tests

Test	Reference Range	Sample Critical Test Result*
Total bilirubin (T Bil)	0.1-1.1 mg/dl	≥15 mg/dl
Alanine aminotransferase (ALT)	7-56 U/L	†
Aspartate aminotransferase (AST)	10-50 U/L	†
Alkaline phosphatase (ALK)	40-125 U/L	†
Total protein (TP)	15-45 mg/dl	†
Albumin (ALB)	3.3-5.2 g/dl	†
Ammonia	18-54 μmol/L	≥500 mcg/dl
Amylase (serum)	20-110 U/L	>330 U/L
Lipase	10-140 U/L	>420 U/L
Creatinine phosphokinase (CPK)	20-220 U/L	>10,000 U/L
Troponin I	0 ng/ml	>0.05 ng/ml
B-type natriuretic peptide	<100 pg/ml	†
Lactate dehydrogenase (LDH)	110-220 U/L	>880 (moderate); >8800 (severe)

Values for reference ranges and critical test results are from the University of California San Francisco Moffit-Long Hospital and San Francisco General Hospital. http://pathology.ucsf.edu/labmanual/mftlng-mtzn/test/test-index.html and http://pathology.ucsf.edu/sfghlab/test/ReferenceRanges.html. Accessed January 1, 2011.

*Critical test results vary among clinical laboratories based on instrumentation and calibration procedures. Not all tests have an associated critical result that can be reported.

†No critical value established.

Sweat Chloride

Patients with cystic fibrosis have increased levels of Cl^- in their sweat because of an inability to reabsorb it. These patients have abnormally elevated sweat Cl^- levels of greater than 60 mmol/L. Values between 40 mmol/L and 60 mmol/L are considered borderline for cystic fibrosis, whereas values less than 40 mmol/L are considered unlikely to confirm the diagnosis. Although the sweat electrolyte test is an important tool for diagnosing cystic fibrosis, it must be combined with other tests.

Coagulation Studies

Coagulation is the process by which the blood and vascular tree form clots to stop bleeding and repair damage to the injured blood vessels. In brief, damage to the internal vascular wall (endothelium) exposes the blood to tissue factors that attract and activate platelets, which begin the clotting process. **Thrombocytopenia** (low platelets) and *thrombasthenia* (abnormal platelet functioning) lead to excessive bleeding, whereas *thrombocytosis* (excessive platelets) causes excessive clotting. In addition to direct measurement of platelets, the functionality of the entire process of coagulation is measured by the *prothrombin time* (PT) and *partial thromboplastin time* (PTT). These tests assess the two different pathways by which fibrin clots are formed.

PT is defined as the time in seconds required by plasma to form a fibrin clot after exposure to tissue factors. It assesses the extrinsic coagulation pathway and reflects the function of clotting factors I, II, V, VII, and X. In contrast, PTT primarily assesses the intrinsic coagulation pathway. It is used to evaluate abnormalities in blood clotting and to monitor the effects of anticoagulation therapy. Abnormalities in PTT are associated with clotting factors I through VI and factors VIII through XII. Clinically, abnormal increases in PT and PTT are found in patients with vitamin K deficiencies and patients receiving anticoagulation therapy such as warfarin or heparin. Increases in PT and PTT are also seen frequently in patients with *disseminated intravascular coagulation* (DIC) and patients with end-stage liver disease.

Because PT test results (Table 16-6) depend on manufactured animal tissue factors, which have unavoidable variability, PT is accompanied by an additional measurement known as the *international normalized ratio* (INR). The INR expresses PT relative to an established sample value. The reference range for INR is 0.9 to 1.3. INR values of approximately 5.0 indicate a high likelihood for

TABLE 16-6

Coagulation Studies

Test	Reference Range	Critical Test Result
Prothrombin time (PT)	12-15 sec	>30 sec
Partial thromboplastin time (PTT)	25-39 sec	>50 sec
International normalized ratio (INR)	0.8-1.2	>5 sec
Fibrin D-dimer	<200 ng/ml	*
Platelet count	150,000-400,000/mm^3	<25,000/mm^3

Values for reference ranges and critical test results are from the University of California San Francisco Moffit-Long Hospital and San Francisco General Hospital. http://pathology.ucsf.edu/labmanual/mftlng-mtzn/test/test-index.html and http://pathology.ucsf.edu/sfghlab/test/ReferenceRanges.html. Accessed January 1, 2011.
*No critical value established.

bleeding. Values of 0.5 are associated with a tendency toward increased clotting.

D-dimer is a small protein fragment found in the blood when fibrin clots are dissolving. It belongs to a larger group of substances generally referred to as *fibrin degradation products*. Clinically, D-dimer levels are measured to help diagnose the presence of deep vein thrombosis, pulmonary embolism, or disseminated intravascular coagulation. Unless significant clotting has occurred in the body, the D-dimer test is normal.

Protein C has an integral role in the regulation of coagulation. In its activated state (activated protein C), it inhibits coagulation and promotes the degradation of clots. Protein C levels are greatly reduced in patients with severe sepsis and acute respiratory distress syndrome. Low protein C promotes abnormal clot formation and damages blood vessels in the microcirculation throughout the body (disseminated intravascular coagulation). Significant deficiencies in protein C levels (<40% of normal) are associated with increased risk of death in patients with severe sepsis.[6] Protein C levels are measured in patients with severe sepsis to assess the appropriateness of therapy with pharmacologic preparations of activated protein C.

Infection Monitoring

Procalcitonin (PCT) is an inactive protein of the hormone calcitonin that is released in response to bacterial infections. PCT levels are directly related with the severity of infection. Because PCT does not increase appreciably in response to viral infections, it is a unique marker for bacterial infections. PCT levels typically increase within 12 hours of infection and promptly decrease once the infection is controlled with appropriate antibiotic therapy. PCT inceasingly is being used to titrate antibiotic therapy. In general, a cutoff value between 0.25-0.50 mcg/L is used to initiate antibiotic therapy. Measurements of PCT are repeated every 1-2 days to evaluate antibiotic therapy. When PCT decreases by approximately 90% from peak values antibiotic therapy is usually terminated.[6]

Sweat Chloride

Patients with cystic fibrosis have increased levels of Cl^- in sweat because of an inability to reabsorb it. These patients will have abnormally elevated sweat Cl^- levels of greater than 60 Eq/L. Values between 40-60 mEq/L are considered borderline for systic fibrosis, whereas values less than 40 mEq/L are considered unlikely to confirm the diagnosis. Although the sweat electrolyte test is an important tool for diagnosing systic fibrosis, it must be combined with other tests.

Microbiology Tests

Sputum Gram Stain

A patient who is suspected to have an infection in the lungs or airways may benefit from analysis of a sputum sample. The purpose of such an analysis is to determine the specific microorganism causing the infection, which indicates the most appropriate antibiotic to be given. The first step in evaluating the sputum sample is the Gram stain, which is performed in the clinical laboratory by a technician who smears the sputum sample on a glass slide, applies a staining solution, and examines it through a microscope.

Initially, the technician uses the Gram stain to determine the quality of the sputum sample. Some patients have difficulty producing an adequate sputum sample from the lung and may expectorate only saliva into the sputum cup. In such cases, the Gram stain shows few (<25 per low-power field) or no pus cells and numerous epithelial cells. This result indicates that the sample is merely saliva and should be discarded. A sample with numerous pus cells and few or no epithelial cells is most likely a true sample from the lung and is reflective of the infection source.

RULE OF THUMB

A legitimate sputum sample has few epithelial cells and many pus cells (leukocytes).

After the sample has been verified, the laboratory technician identifies the Gram stain reaction (either positive or negative) and the shape of any bacteria present (rods vs. cocci). Such results are presumptive, and a definitive diagnosis is made only by isolation and culture of the specific organism present. *Streptococcus pneumoniae,* a common bacterium associated with pneumonia, stains as encapsulated, lancet-shaped, gram-positive diplococci. These results are consistent with the diagnosis of streptococcal pneumonia and allow the physician to begin an appropriate course of antibiotic therapy before the results of the sputum culture are available, perhaps days later.

Sputum Culture

If the Gram stain reveals an adequate sample, the technician prepares a portion of the sputum for culture. The sputum sample is placed in a medium consistent with growth of the organism. When the organism has matured, it is examined microscopically to determine its exact type and sensitivity to antibiotic therapy. This information allows the physician to prescribe the most effective antibiotic. These same procedures for Gram staining and culturing can be applied to samples of blood, pleural fluid, or any other body fluid involved in an infection.

Acid-Fast Testing

Pulmonary tuberculosis is caused by a mycobacterium *(Mycobacterium tuberculosis)* and is a highly communicable disease. The rapid identification and isolation of patients with suspected tuberculosis infection is an extremely important infection control measure to protect other patients and health care providers. A rapid and effective method for detecting tuberculosis infection is to perform a Gram stain of a slide containing a sample of sputum followed by an acid wash. A characteristic of all mycobacteria is that after staining, the subsequent acid wash does not weaken the cell wall sufficiently to remove the color dye. This resistance to decolorization classifies the organism as an **acid-fast bacterium.**

CLINICAL APPLICATION OF LABORATORY DATA

The RT has a unique position in the health care team. Respiratory therapy is a highly specialized profession focused primarily on the pulmonary system. One disadvantage is that the day-to-day practice does not entail dealing directly with other organ systems, as nurses and physicians do. RTs normally do not have the integrated global perspective that these caregivers must have. However, it behooves the RT to have a general understanding of a patient's overall condition and illness trajectory. This understanding can be gained by becoming familiar with laboratory tests and their implications. Disruption in other organ systems has a direct impact on the practice of respiratory care. The primary focus of the RT is on the oxygen-carrying capacity of the blood. Anemia and insufficient hemoglobin levels result in overall weakness that often stymies the ability of patients to participate effectively in respiratory care.

Coagulation Disorders

In patients requiring arterial blood gas (ABG) testing or nasotracheal suctioning, the RT must evaluate the clotting characteristics of the blood. For ABG testing, patients with an abnormally low platelet count or an elevated PT and INR need to have the puncture site compressed for a longer time after the arterial sample is obtained to prevent bleeding and hematoma development. Patients with an extremely low platelet count should have an arterial puncture performed (or undergo nasotracheal suctioning) *only* when it is essential because of the extremely high risk of bleeding.

In addition, RTs are intimately involved in assessing patients with suspected pulmonary embolism. Patients with pulmonary embolism present with some of the same symptoms as patients with myocardial infarction (e.g., dyspnea and chest pain), and it is important for the RT to be familiar with tests such as D-dimers, troponin I, CPK-1, and CPK-2, which help make the differential diagnosis.

Electrolyte Disorders

Severe electrolyte disorders have a profound impact on pulmonary function. The primary concern of the RT is the effect of electrolyte disorders on respiratory muscle function. Many electrolyte disorders cause generalized skeletal muscle weakness. This weakness may limit ambulation and increases the risk for patients developing pneumonia and venous thromboembolism that can lead to pulmonary embolism. In a patient with pulmonary disease, respiratory muscle weakness impairs the ability to sustain spontaneous ventilation and the ability to maintain pulmonary hygiene through deep breathing and adequate cough.

Primary electrolyte disorders causing respiratory muscle weakness include low serum levels of calcium, magnesium, and phosphate.[7,8] A patient with hypoglycemia often complains of weakness, so that weaning from a ventilator is unlikely to be successful in the patient with hypoglycemia. In addition, abnormally high serum potassium levels, or **hyperkalemia** (>8.0 mmol/L), and abnormally low serum potassium, or **hypokalemia** (<2.0 mmol/L), or phosphorus, or hypophosphatemia (<1.0 mg /dl), can lead to respiratory muscle paralysis. In addition, severe hyperkalemia (>6.0 mmol/L) increases the likelihood of cardiac arrhythmias. Severe hypocalcemia (<6.5 mmol/L)sometimes leads to laryngeal stridor and dyspnea.

Electrolyte disorders and other toxins in the bloodstream can depress neurologic function. Pulmonary function is profoundly affected because decreased mental functioning may depress respiratory drive, prevent patients from cooperating with therapy, and suppress the ability of patients to protect their airway and clear secretions by depressing the cough mechanism. In severe cases, **hypernatremia** is a major cause of central nervous system depression, which can lead to lethargy, coma, and respiratory arrest.[9] In patients with severe liver disease, elevated ammonia levels also depress neurologic function.

Lastly, laboratory tests are used by physicians to assess the overall likelihood of survival of a critically ill patient. RTs care for patients with primary pulmonary failure. Survival is intimately related to the prevention or amelioration of secondary organ failures. Following trends in creatinine, total bilirubin, and platelets is crucial in monitoring the development or progression of renal, hepatic, and hematologic failure. Patients with primary respiratory failure have less chance of survival with each additional organ system dysfunction that develops.

SUMMARY CHECKLIST

- The three formed elements of the blood are the WBCs (leukocytes), RBCs (erythrocytes), and platelets (thrombocytes).
- Elevation of the WBC count is known as leukocytosis. It often occurs with infection, stress, or trauma.
- A reduced WBC count is known as leukopenia. It puts the patient at risk for serious infection.
- Abnormal elevation of the RBC count is known as polycythemia, and an abnormal reduction in the RBC count is known as anemia.
- Anemia reduces the oxygen-carrying capacity of the blood and increases the risk of tissue hypoxia. It also contributes to weakness that prevents patients from participating effectively in respiratory therapy.
- Severe electrolyte abnormalities, including low calcium, magnesium, and phosphorus, cause respiratory muscle weakness. This weakness may limit the ability of the patient to breathe spontaneously or maintain adequate pulmonary hygiene.
- Severe hyperkalemia (>6 mmol/L) greatly increases the risk of cardiac arrhythmias.
- Troponin I and CPK-MM tests are used to help diagnose myocardial infarction.
- To minimize the risk of bleeding, respiratory care procedures such as arterial punctures and nasotracheal suctioning should be done with extreme caution in patients with thrombocytopenia, elevated PT, and increased INR.
- A sputum Gram stain is useful for determining the quality of the sample and the type of organism present. Samples with many epithelial cells and few pus cells are of no value and probably are saliva from the mouth.

References

1. Grasbeck R: The evolution of the reference value concept. Clin Chem Lab Med 42:692-697, 2004.
2. Friedberg RC, Soures R, Wagar EA, et al: The origin of reference intervals. Arch Pathol Lab Med 131:348-357, 2007.
3. van den Berghe G, Wouters P, Weekers F, et al: Intensive insulin therapy in critically ill patients. N Engl J Med 345:1359-1367, 2001.
4. Karmpaliotis D, Kirtane AJ, Ruisi CP, et al: Diagnostic and prognostic utility of brain natriuretic peptide in subjects admitted to the ICU with hypoxic respiratory failure due to non-cardiogenic and cardiogenic pulmonary edema. Chest 131:964-971, 2007.
5. Levitt JE, Binayak AG, Gehlbach BK, et al: Diagnostic utility of B-type natriuretic peptide in critically ill patients with pulmonary edema: a prospective cohort study. Crit Care 12: 1-9, 2008.
6. Shorr AF, Bernard GR, Dhainaut J-F: Protein C concentrations in severe sepsis: an early directional change in plasma levels predicts outcome. Crit Care 10:1-8, 2006.
7. Gravelyn TR, Brophy N, Siegert C, et al: Hypophosphatemia-associated respiratory muscle weakness and a general inpatient population. Am J Med 84:870-876, 1988.
8. Fiaccadori E, Del Canale S, Coffrini E, et al. Muscle and serum magnesium in pulmonary intensive care unit patients. Crit Care Med 16:751-760, 1988.
9. Riggs JE: Neurologic manifestations of electrolyte disturbances. Neurol Clin 20:227-239, 2002.

Bibliography

Clinical Laboratory reference ranges and critical values: http://pathology.ucsf.edu/labmanual/mftlng-mtzn/test/test-index.html and http://pathology.ucsf.edu/sfghlab/test/Referemce Ranges.html

Conversion factors for clinical laboratory tests between conventional and standardized international units: University of North Carolina at Chapel Hill http://www.unc.edu/~rowlett/units/sclaes/clinical_data.html

Hoffman R, Benz PJ, Shattil SJ, et al: Hematology basic principles and practice, ed 4, Philadelphia, 2005, Saunders.

McPherson RA, Pincus MR: Henry's clinical diagnosis and management by laboratory methods, ed 21, Philadelphia, 2007, Saunders.

Moffit-Long Hospital and San Francisco General Hospital: Clinical laboratory reference ranges and critical values. http://pathology.ucsf.edu/sfghlab/test/ReferenceRanges.html.

University of California San Francisco: Clinical laboratory reference ranges and critical values. http://pathology.ucsf.edu/labmanual/mftlng-mtzn/test/test-index.html.

Wu AHB. Tietz's Clinical guide to laboratory tests, ed 4, St Louis, 2006, Saunders.

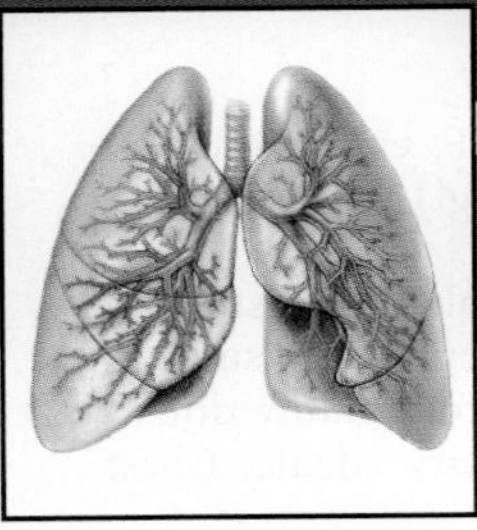

Chapter 17

Interpreting the Electrocardiogram

ALBERT J. HEUER

CHAPTER OBJECTIVES

After reading this chapter you will be able to:
- Describe the value and limitations of the electrocardiogram.
- Describe the electrophysiology of cardiac cells.
- Describe how the cardiac impulse is conducted through the different structures of the heart.
- Recognize various abnormal electrocardiographic recordings.

CHAPTER OUTLINE

KEY TERMS

automaticity
depolarization
ectopic beat
ectopic foci
impulse-conducting system
repolarization

Electrocardiography is an important tool used by health care practitioners. In some settings, the electrocardiogram (ECG) is obtained by the respiratory therapist (RT), which places the RT at the bedside in a prime position to recognize and respond to life-threatening arrhythmias. For this reason, RTs must be familiar with the electrocardiographic results and must be able to interpret them accurately. This chapter emphasizes the basics of cardiac physiology, lead placement, ECG interpretation, and the identification and key points in the treatment of dysrhythmias. More details of the cardiopulmonary anatomy and emergency cardiovascular life support are presented in Chapters 9 and 34.

The most diagnostic value can be garnered from a standard 12-lead ECG, although some settings may dictate otherwise, such as the use of a 3-lead ECG for telemetry. A 12-lead ECG provides a more complete assessment of the electrical activity of the heart by viewing it from 12 different angles. The focus of this chapter is the 12-lead ECG.

The ECG is a popular evaluation tool because it is inexpensive, noninvasive, and easy to obtain. It is used primarily to evaluate a patient with an acute clinical condition suggestive of myocardial disease. A physician would order an ECG for most adult patients complaining of certain types of chest pain, shortness of breath, dyspnea with palpitations, weakness, lethargy, or syncope. These are classic clinical symptoms associated with heart disease for which the ECG is used. In addition, the ECG is routinely used by physicians for evaluating the general health status of middle-aged or older patients before major surgery or for periodic health screening. A resting ECG has little or no value as a predictor of future heart problems, however. It is useful only for detecting abnormalities that are occurring or have already occurred, such as a myocardial infarction (MI). In addition, certain abnormalities, such as valvular defects, cannot be identified directly by an ECG.[1]

BASIC PRINCIPLES OF ELECTROPHYSIOLOGY

Understanding the ECG requires a basic knowledge of physiology related to the contraction and relaxation of the heart muscle. The muscle cells of the heart normally are stimulated and paced by the electrical activity of the cardiac

impulse-conducting system. The impulse-conducting system cells have the ability to stimulate the heart without the influence of the nervous system. However, the autonomic nervous system normally plays a major role in controlling heart function (see subsequent discussion).[1]

Cardiac muscle cells normally generate an electrical imbalance across the cell membrane with a positive charge on the outside and a negative charge on the inside. This is the resting or polarized state in which there is no electrical activity. Stimulation of the "polarized" cells causes an influx of sodium into the interior portion of the cell; this is called **depolarization** (Figure 17-1). Depolarization causes the cardiac muscle cells to contract momentarily, which is seen as a shortening of the muscle. Depolarization is immediately followed by **repolarization,** which is a rapid return of the cell to the "polarized" position in which the electrical imbalance across the membrane is reestablished.

The impulse-conducting system has three types of cardiac cells capable of electrical excitation: pacemaker cells (e.g., sinoatrial [SA] node, atrioventricular [AV] node), specialized rapidly conducting tissue (e.g., Purkinje fibers), and atrial and ventricular muscle cells. The ability of these cells to depolarize without stimulations is known as **automaticity.** Each of these cardiac cell groups varies in their degree of automaticity.[1-3]

Impulse-Conducting System

The impulse-conducting system is responsible for initiating the heartbeat and controlling the heart rate. It also coordinates the contraction of the heart chambers, which is essential to move blood effectively. A defect in the impulse-conducting system may lead to inadequate cardiac output and decreased tissue perfusion. Normally, the SA node, which is located in the upper portion of the right atrium, has the greatest degree of automaticity and paces the heart (Figure 17-2). Any heartbeat originating outside the SA node is considered an **ectopic beat.**[2] The SA node is innervated by the autonomic nervous system, which allows the sympathetic and parasympathetic nervous systems to influence heart rate. Stimulation of the sympathetic nervous system increases the heart rate, whereas activation of the parasympathetic nervous system slows the heart rate by influencing the degree of automaticity within the SA node.

The electrical impulse generated by the SA node travels rapidly across the right atrium, through intraatrial pathways, to the left atrium by way of Bachmann bundle; this causes a wave of depolarization to occur over the atria, producing atrial contraction. Next, the impulse moves to the AV node, located in the intraventricular septum in the inferior aspect of the right atrium (see Figure 17-2). The AV node is the "backup" pacemaker because it has the second greatest degree of automaticity in the healthy heart. In most cases, if the SA node fails to function properly, the AV node paces ventricular activity at a lower heart rate of 40 to 60 beats/min, which is generally sufficient to maintain adequate cardiac output.[2]

The electrical impulse is temporarily delayed at the AV node to allow the ventricles time to fill with blood. That brief delay also limits the rate of the ventricular stimulation during excessively fast atrial rhythms that, if passed to the ventricles, would lead to inadequate cardiac output.[3,4]

The impulse exits the AV node, enters the bundle of His, and rapidly moves to the bundle branches. The bundle branches carry the impulse rapidly into the right and left ventricles. The bundle branches terminate in the Purkinje fibers, which are small, finger-like projections that penetrate the myocardium (see Figure 17-2). These fibers stimulate contraction of the myocardium from the apex of the heart upward toward the base of the heart, causing a coordinated contraction of the ventricles, which normally is effective in moving blood. The impulse travels the most rapidly in the Purkinje fibers, which is essential if contraction of the ventricles is to occur in a coordinated fashion. Immediately after depolarization of the ventricles, repolarization occurs in preparation for the next impulse.[3,4]

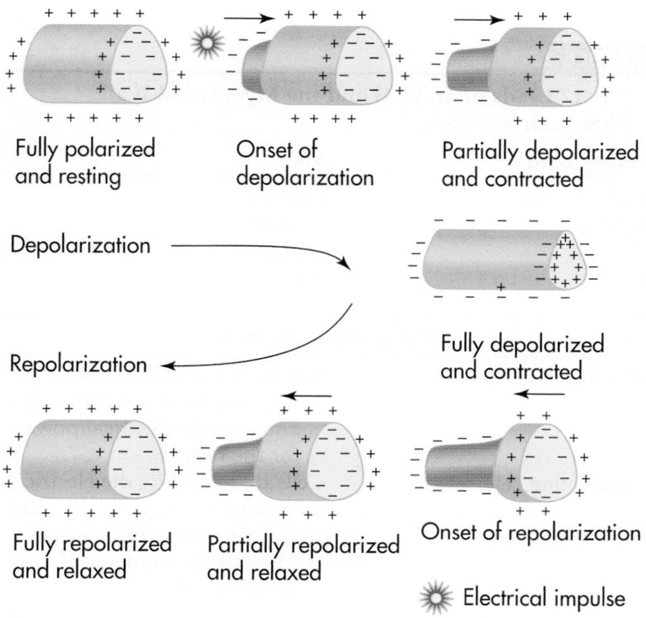

FIGURE 17-1 Depolarization and repolarization of a cardiac cell. (Modified from Huszar RH: Basic dysrhythmias and acute coronary syndromes: interpretation and management, ed 4, St Louis, 2012, Mosby.)

ELECTROCARDIOGRAM PROCEDURAL SUMMARY

The ECG procedure is noninvasive and can generally be done in less than about 5 minutes by the RT or other qualified health professional. Once the physician orders a 12-lead ECG, the RT gathers the equipment, which includes the portable ECG unit, lead wires, and electrodes. This procedure is only as useful as the equipment and technique, so fully functional equipment operated by a

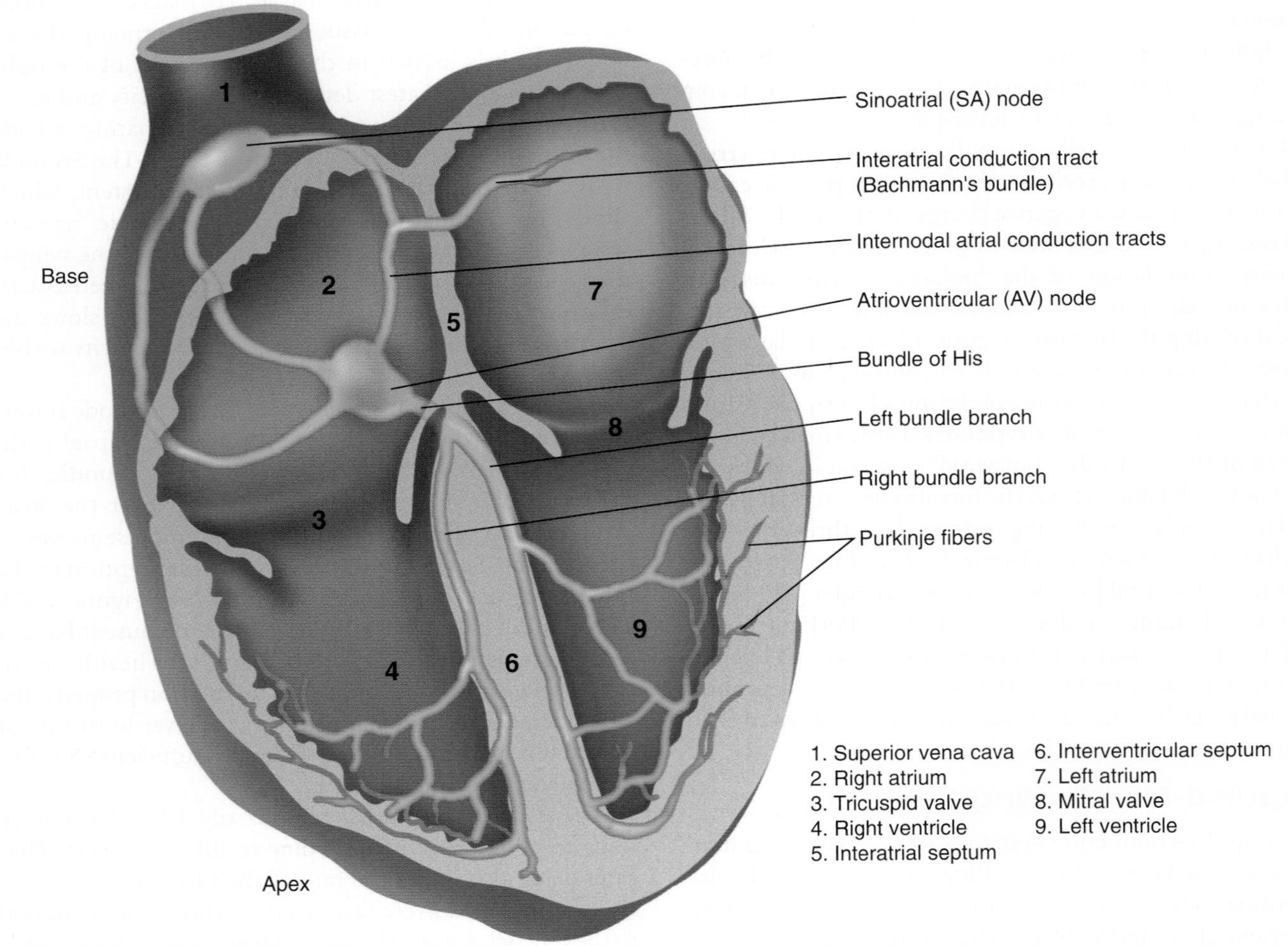

FIGURE 17-2 Anatomy of the impulse-conducting system of the human heart.

competent clinician and proper lead placement are essential.

The lead wires permit the connection between the ECG unit and the electrodes, which have adhesive permitting temporary attachment to the skin. Generally, the lead wires should be attached to the electrodes before being placed on the skin to avoid unnecessary pressure while being attached to the skin's surface. The lead wires are often marked to help ensure proper placement on the patient's body.

The 12 leads can be subdivided into two groups: 6 extremity (limb) leads and 6 chest (precordial) leads. To obtain the six limb leads, four electrodes are placed on the extremities, one on each wrist and one on each ankle. These leads are bipolar, which permits the measurement of electrical activity in two different directions. Additionally, the ECG unit can vary the orientation of these four electrodes to create six different views. Any electrical activity of the heart that is directed up, down, left, or right is recorded by the limb leads. The limb leads are called leads *I, II, III, aV_R, aV_L,* and *aV_F* (Table 17-1).

TABLE 17-1

The 12 Leads of an ECG and the Myocardial Wall That Each Set Views

Facing Lead*	View
I, aV_L, V_5, V_6	Lateral
II, III, aV_F	Inferior
V_1, V_2	Septal
V_3, V_4	Anterior

CELLS AND FUNCTION

Pacemaker cells	Specialized cells that have a high degree of automaticity and provide electrical power for the heart
Conducting cells	Cells that conduct the electrical impulse throughout the heart
Myocardial cells	Cells that contract in response to electrical stimuli and pump blood

From Wilkins RL, Dexter JR, Heuer AJ: Clinical assessment in respiratory care, ed 6, St Louis, 2010, Mosby.

*Excludes aV_R, which faces the interior, endocardial surface of the ventricles.

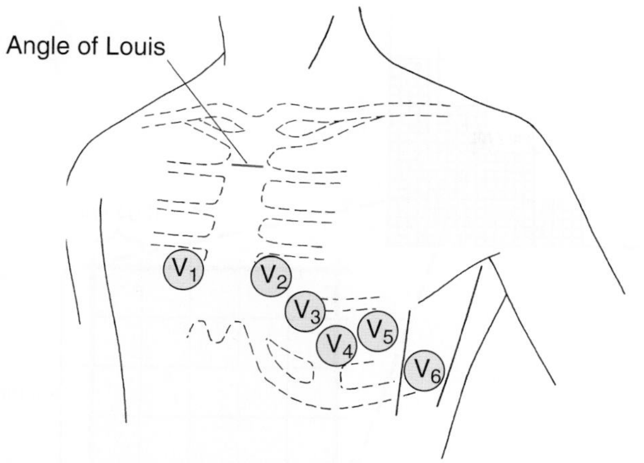

FIGURE 17-3 Proper precordial lead placement. (From Wilkins RL, Dexter JR, Heuer AJ: Clinical assessment in respiratory care, ed 6, St Louis, 2010, Mosby.)

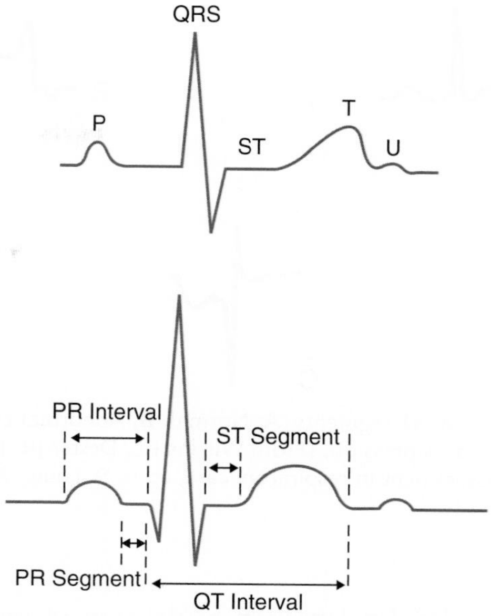

FIGURE 17-4 Normal configuration of electrocardiographic waves, segments, and intervals. (From Wilkins RL, Dexter JR, Heuer AJ: Clinical assessment in respiratory care, ed 6, St Louis, 2010, Mosby.)

The six chest or precordial leads are called leads V_1, V_2, V_3, V_4, V_5, and V_6. These leads are unipolar, which means that they measure electrical activity in only one direction. These leads are placed in a horizontal plane across the chest, starting with V_1 in the fourth intercostal space to the right of the sternum. The rest of the chest leads are on the left side, starting with V_2, which is placed in the fourth intercostal space just to the left of the sternum, and ending with V_6, which is placed at the fifth intercostal space at the left midaxillary line (V_6). Figure 17-3 illustrates proper placement of ECG leads. The view from each chest lead provides its own angle of orientation to measure cardiac electrical activity moving anteriorly or posteriorly.[2,4]

After all leads are properly placed and the ECG unit is activated, the six limb and six chest leads together provide a comprehensive view of the electrical activity of the heart. Given that an array of conditions, including cardiac ischemia and acute MI, can alter electrical conduction through the heart, the ECG has considerable diagnostic value in ruling in or out such conditions. The balance of this chapter focuses mainly on how electrocardiographic waves are generated, interpreting ECGs, identifying abnormal rhythms, and some treatment considerations.

Basic Electrocardiographic Waves

The wave of depolarization occurring in the atria is seen as the P wave on the ECG (Figure 17-4). The normal P wave is no more than 2.5 mm high or 3 mm long. Atrial hypertrophy may cause the P wave to enlarge to a height and length beyond the normal parameters. Atrial repolarization is not seen on the electrocardiographic tracing because it is obscured by the electrical activity occurring in the ventricles at the same time.

The wave of depolarization occurring over the ventricles is seen as the QRS complex on the electrocardiographic tracing. The QRS complex is normally larger than the P wave because the muscle mass of the ventricles is much greater than that of the atria. The normal QRS complex is not wider than 3 mm (0.12 second) because of the rapid movement of the impulse through the ventricles by the bundle branches and Purkinje fibers. Abnormalities in the ventricular conduction system may lead to irregular QRS complexes that are wider than normal.

The QRS complex usually consists of several distinct waves, each of which has a letter assigned to it as a label. If the first wave of the complex is negative (downward), it is labeled the *Q wave*. The initial positive (upward) deflection is electrocardiographically referred to as the *R wave*, and the next negative deflection after the R wave is labeled the *S wave*. Not all QRS complexes have all three components present, but the waves making up ventricular depolarization are electrocardiographically referred to as the *QRS complex*, regardless of its exact makeup. The wave of repolarization occurring in the ventricles immediately after depolarization is the *T wave* (see Figure 17-4).

Two important segments of the electrocardiographic pattern must be observed and measured. The first is the *PR interval*, which refers to the distance (time) between the start of atrial depolarization and the start of ventricular depolarization. The PR interval represents the time in which the impulse begins in the SA node and travels across the atria to the AV node, where it is held briefly before passing on to the ventricles. Normally, the PR interval represents a period no longer than 0.20 second. PR intervals longer than 0.20 second suggest that the impulse is abnormally delayed at the AV node and a "block" is present; this may mean that there is a serious defect in the impulse-conducting system that needs immediate attention.

The next important part of the ECG to evaluate is the *ST segment*, which represents the time from the end

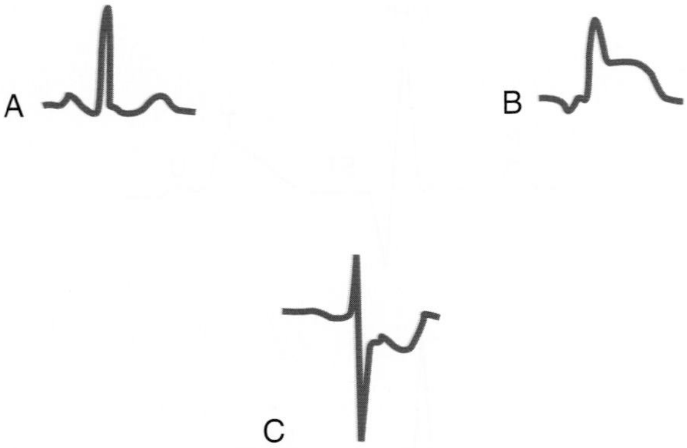

FIGURE 17-5 ST segments. **A,** Normal. **B,** Abnormal elevation. **C,** Abnormal depression. (From Wilkins RL, Dexter JR, Heuer AJ: Clinical assessment in respiratory care, ed 6, St Louis, 2010, Mosby.)

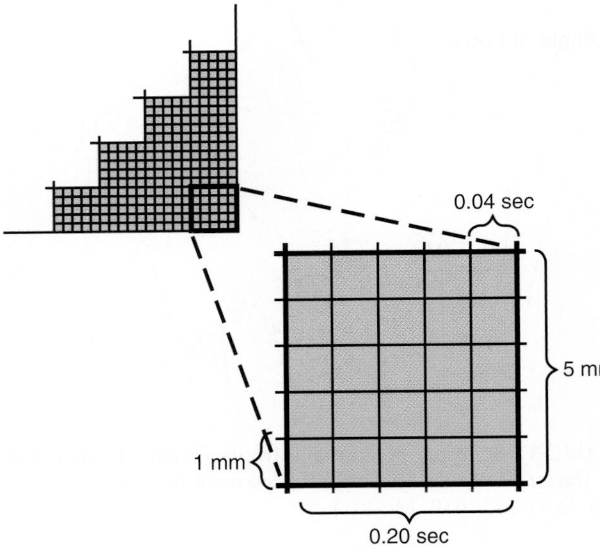

FIGURE 17-6 Gridlike boxes of electrocardiographic paper illustrating the 1 × 1 mm and 5 × 5 mm boxes. (From Wilkins RL, Dexter JR, Heuer AJ: Clinical assessment in respiratory care, ed 6, St Louis, 2010, Mosby.)

of ventricular depolarization to the start of ventricular repolarization. The normal ST segment is isoelectric, which is seen as a flat line that is not above or below the neutral baseline. Certain pathologic abnormalities in the myocardium cause the ST segment configuration to become abnormal; this is seen as an elevated or depressed ST segment and is common in cardiac ischemia and MI (Figure 17-5). Because this configuration represents a potentially life-threatening arrhythmia, abnormal ST segments must be identified as soon as possible.[3-5]

RULE OF THUMB

A negative QRS complex in lead I is consistent with right-axis deviation, which is often caused by cor pulmonale.

Electrocardiographic Paper and Measurements

Electrocardiographic paper is made up of gridlike boxes that define time on the horizontal axis and voltage on the vertical axis. Dark lines circumscribe larger boxes that are 5 mm × 5 mm, and lighter lines define smaller boxes that are 1 mm × 1 mm (Figure 17-6). Because the paper passes through the electrocardiograph at a set speed of 25 mm/sec, each large box represents 0.20 second, and each small box represents 0.04 second on the horizontal axis. The standard ECG is calibrated so that 1 mV causes an upward deflection of 10 small boxes or 2 large boxes on the vertical axis; this allows measurement of the exact voltage occurring during depolarization of the cardiac muscle fibers.[1,4,6]

Interpreting the Electrocardiogram

Official interpretation of the ECG is generally performed by a cardiologist or by the patient's attending physician. The official interpretation is not always rendered in a timely fashion, however. In some circumstances, RTs need to recognize serious arrhythmias and respond appropriately. For example, the RT performing a routine ECG on a patient scheduled for surgery the next day is in a good position to recognize an arrhythmia that may need immediate attention before the surgery can be conducted safely. The RT who simply obtains the ECG and does not recognize the arrhythmia may cause a delay in appropriate therapy and indirectly contribute to an adverse clinical outcome or even the death of the patient. The following steps for interpreting the ECG ensure that all abnormalities are detected.

MINI CLINI

Weaning Complications

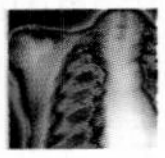

PROBLEM: The clinician is in the intensive care unit attending to a 65-year-old woman who is being weaned from the ventilator after 2 weeks of mechanical ventilation. After 15 minutes of T-piece weaning, the patient complains of mild shortness of breath, and the bedside ECG shows an increase in heart rate, inverted T waves, and acute elevation of the ST segment. What do the inverted T waves and ST segment elevation indicate? What should be done?

SOLUTION: The inverted T waves and elevated ST segment suggest that the heart is experiencing acute hypoxia, probably caused by the stress of weaning. Changes in $\dot{V}/\dot{Q}$ matching in the lung are probably causing acute hypoxemia and inadequate tissue oxygenation. T wave inversion and ST segment elevation are serious signs indicating that the patient is not tolerating the weaning. She should be put back on the ventilator at an elevated FiO_2 and monitored closely. Weaning should not be attempted again until the patient's clinical condition improves significantly. The attending physician should be notified.

Steps to Follow

Step 1. *Identify the atrial and ventricular rates.* Normally, the rate of the atria and ventricles is the same, but they may differ when a defect in the conduction system is present. The clinician can identify the heart rate by counting the number of QRS complexes (for the ventricular rate) or the number of P waves (for the atrial rate) in 6 seconds (30 large boxes) and multiplying this number by 10. The clinician also can count the number of large boxes between two successive complexes and divide this number into 300 to obtain the heart rate. This is a reasonable technique when the heart rate is regular.

Step 2. *Measure the PR interval.* This is done by determining the number of small boxes between the start of the P wave and the start of the QRS complex. Normally, this interval is less than 0.20 second (five small boxes) and is consistently the same for each complex. PR intervals that are longer than 0.20 second or that vary from one complex to the next indicate an abnormality in the impulse-conducting system.

Step 3. *Evaluate the QRS complex.* Normally, the QRS complex is shorter than 0.12 second. If it is longer, there is an abnormality in the impulse-conducting system within the ventricles, which often leads to a decrease in cardiac output and blood pressure and may cause the patient to experience symptoms such as fainting spells.

Step 4. *Evaluate the T wave.* Normally, the T wave is upright and rounded. Inverted T waves suggest ischemia of the heart muscle, and abnormal configuration of the T wave occurs with electrolyte abnormalities such as hyperkalemia.

Step 5. *Evaluate the ST segment.* The ST segment should be flat or at least no more than 1 mm above or below baseline. As stated earlier, significant elevation or depression of the ST segment indicates serious problems with oxygenation of the myocardium and must be recognized as soon as possible.

Step 6. *Identify the R-R interval.* The R-R interval is identified to assess regularity of the rhythm. The distance, in millimeters or time, is measured between the R waves of several successive QRS complexes. Normally, there is little variance in the R-R interval between QRS complexes, but if the variance between the different R-R intervals exceeds 0.12 second, an abnormal rhythm exists.

Step 7. *Identify the mean QRS axis.* The limb lead exhibiting the largest amount of voltage is identified. If the lead shows a positive QRS complex, the axis is very close to the position on the hexaxial reference circle where that limb lead is labeled. If the QRS complex with the most voltage is negative, the mean axis is moving in the opposite direction from where that lead is labeled on the hexaxial reference circle.[1-3]

Axis Evaluation

A less understood area of ECG interpretation for RTs is the axis evaluation and the identification of related deviations from normal. Axis evaluation is used to determine the general direction of current flow during ventricular depolarization; this is helpful to know when hypertrophy of one of the ventricles is suspected, which would cause the direction of current flow to deviate from normal. Normally, the mean QRS axis (vector) points leftward (patient's left) and downward, between 0 and +90 degrees in the frontal plane (Figure 17-7). The normal position of the QRS axis results from the slight tilt of the heart to the left and from the large muscle mass of the left ventricle compared with the right ventricle.

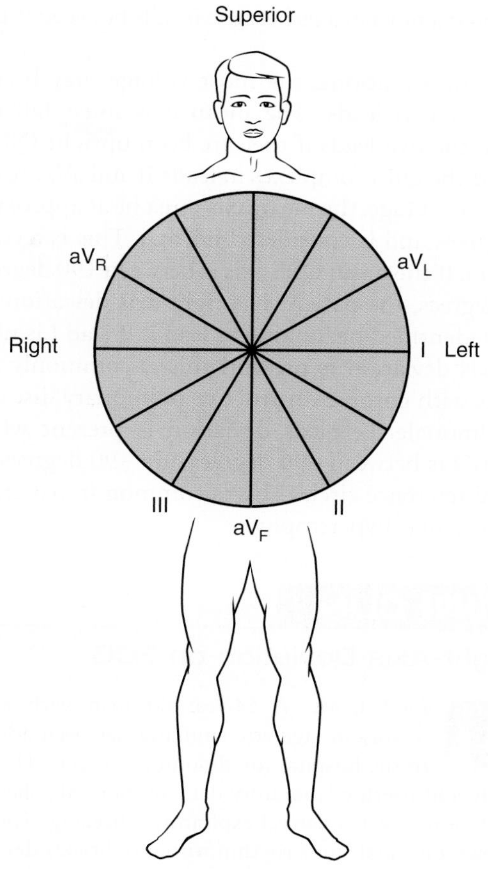

FIGURE 17-7 Hexaxial reference circle used for axis evaluation. (From Wilkins RL, Dexter JR, Heuer AJ: Clinical assessment in respiratory care, ed 6, St Louis, 2010, Mosby.)

The clinician identifies the mean QRS axis by using the hexaxial reference circle (see Figure 17-7) with the position of each limb lead labeled on the circle. Next, the clinician identifies the limb lead with the most voltage (either positive or negative) from the ECG being evaluated. If the lead with the most voltage is positive (upright), the clinician locates the position of that lead on the hexaxial reference circle. The mean axis must be very close to that position on the circle. If the lead with the most voltage is negative (downward), the mean axis points in the opposite direction from that lead. If the lead with the most voltage is lead II and it is positive, the mean QRS axis must be approximately +60 degrees because this is where lead II is located on the hexaxial reference circle (see Figure 17-7). This is considered a normal axis because it falls between 0 and +90 degrees.[5,6]

In some situations, the most voltage may be equally present in two leads. The mean axis must fall equally between the two leads if they are both upright QRS complexes. If the QRS complexes in leads II and aV_F are equally positive in voltage, the mean axis must be at approximately +75 degrees and is considered normal. This is a common situation. If the mean QRS axis is between +90 degrees and +180 degrees, the patient has right-axis deviation; this is quickly identified by looking at lead I. If lead I is negative, right-axis deviation is present; this is commonly seen in patients with chronic obstructive pulmonary disease with cor pulmonale. Left-axis deviation is present when the mean axis is between +90 degrees and −90 degrees on the hexaxial reference circle. This is common in patients with left ventricular hypertrophy.

MINI CLINI

Right-Axis Deviation on ECG

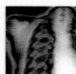

PROBLEM: A 54-year-old man with a long history of cigarette smoking has been admitted to the hospital for abdominal surgery. His chest x-ray and routine laboratory data are normal. Chest auscultation reveals bilateral expiratory wheezing. The ECG shows a normal sinus rhythm with a right-axis deviation. What does the right-axis deviation suggest, and is there any connection between it and the long smoking history? How is the right-axis deviation detected on the ECG?

SOLUTION: Normally, the mean axis (summary of electrical activity) of the heart travels from top to bottom and from right to left. This results in the mean axis of 0 to +90 degrees in the healthy heart. The slight leftward shift of the normal axis results from the angle at which the heart is situated in the chest and the fact that the left ventricle is normally larger than the right one. Right-axis deviation indicates that the electrical activity of the heart has been abnormally shifted to the patient's right side, between +90 degrees and +180 degrees. This is most commonly the result of right ventricle enlargement, such as occurs with cor pulmonale (right heart failure caused by chronic hypoxic lung disease).

In this patient, the long history of cigarette smoking provides more evidence that he may have cor pulmonale. Further investigation of the patient's respiratory system with pulmonary function testing is needed before surgery is performed. Right-axis deviation is detected by noting a negative deflection of the QRS in lead I.

Recognizing Arrhythmias

Normal Sinus Rhythm. Recognizing abnormal rhythms from an electrocardiographic strip is easier if you have an appreciation for the normal tracing. The normal sinus rhythm begins with an upright P wave that is identical from one complex to the next. The PR interval is consistent throughout the rhythm strip and is 0.12 to 0.20 second. The QRS complexes are identical and no longer than 0.12 second. The ST segment is flat. The R-R interval is regular and does not vary more than 0.12 second between QRS complexes. The heart rate is between 60 beats/min and 100 beats/min (Figure 17-8).[2,3]

Sinus Tachycardia. Heart rates exceeding 100 beats/min are abnormal in resting adult patients and are electrocardiographically referred to as *sinus tachycardia* when a P wave is appropriately present before each QRS complex (Figure 17-9). Other than the rate exceeding 100 beats/min, sinus tachycardia does not differ from a normal sinus rhythm. This abnormality is common and can be caused by numerous problems. Most often, sinus tachycardia is caused by anxiety, pain, fever, hypovolemia, or hypoxemia. It may also be a side effect of certain medications, such as bronchodilators. Treatment typically involves eliminating the underlying cause.[5,6]

Sinus Bradycardia. A heart rate of less than 60 beats/min that is otherwise normal is electrocardiographically referred to as *sinus bradycardia*. Other than the rate being too slow, sinus bradycardia does not differ from a normal sinus rhythm (Figure 17-10). This abnormal rhythm is not as common as sinus tachycardia, but it represents a significant clinical problem if it causes the patient's blood pressure to decrease significantly or impairs tissue perfusion causing symptoms such as fatigue, lightheadedness, or syncope. It is most often caused by hypothermia or abnormalities in the SA node and in some cases may simply be the result of intense athletic conditioning. Numerous medications, such as atropine, are available to stimulate the heart rate when clinical bradycardiac symptoms occur.[5,6]

Sinus Arrhythmia. Sinus arrhythmia is a common arrhythmia and is recognized by the irregular spacing between QRS complexes. The spacing is measured by identifying the intervals between the R waves of successive QRS complexes, which are normally consistent. When the R-R interval varies more than 0.12 second throughout the rhythm strip, sinus arrhythmia is present (Figure 17-11). This arrhythmia may occur with the effects of breathing on the heart or as a side effect of medications such as digoxin. Most cases of sinus arrhythmia are benign and do not need treatment. If the arrhythmia is severe, the underlying cause must be identified and eliminated.[5,6]

First-Degree Heart Block. In first-degree heart block, the PR interval is longer than 0.20 second. In addition, there is one P wave before each QRS complex (Figure 17-12). This tracing indicates that the impulse from the SA node is getting through to the ventricles but is abnormally delayed in passing through the AV node or bundle of His. Typically, the QRS complex has a normal configuration, and the R-R intervals are regular. First-degree heart block is common after an MI that damages the AV node, or it may be a complication of certain medications, such as digoxin or beta blockers. Treatment usually is not needed for first-degree heart block if the patient is able to maintain an adequate blood pressure.[6,7]

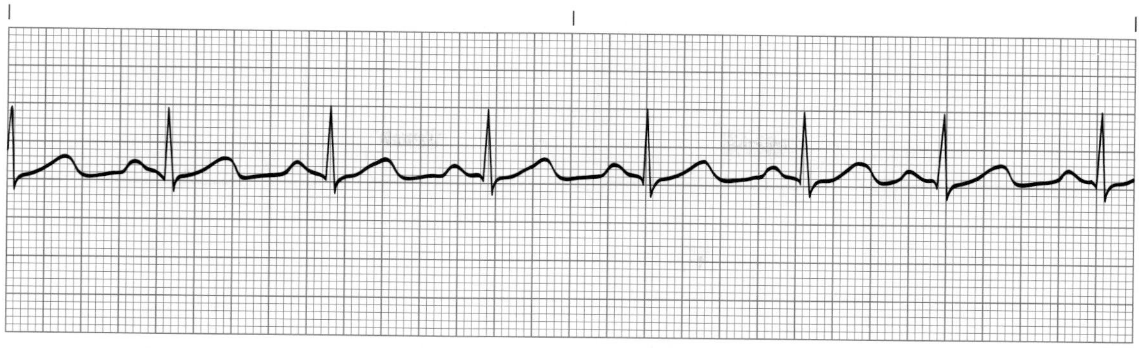

FIGURE 17-8 Electrocardiographic tracing showing a normal sinus rhythm. (Modified from Atwood S, Stanton C, and Storey Davenport J: Introduction to basic cardiac dysrhythmias, ed 4, St. Louis, 2009, Mosby/JEMS.)

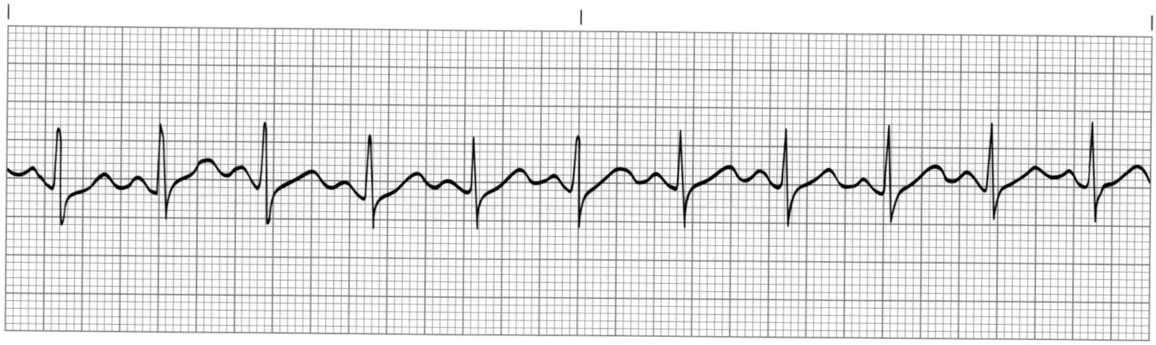

FIGURE 17-9 Electrocardiographic tracing showing sinus tachycardia. (Modified from Atwood S, Stanton C, and Storey Davenport J: Introduction to basic cardiac dysrhythmias, ed 4, St. Louis, 2009, Mosby/JEMS.)

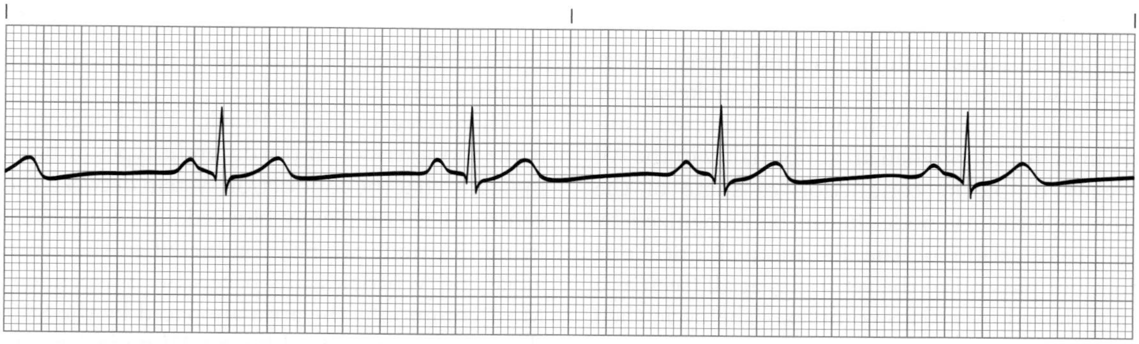

FIGURE 17-10 Electrocardiographic tracing showing sinus bradycardia with first-degree heart block. (Modified from Atwood S, Stanton C, and Storey Davenport J: Introduction to basic cardiac dysrhythmias, ed 4, St. Louis, 2009, Mosby/JEMS.)

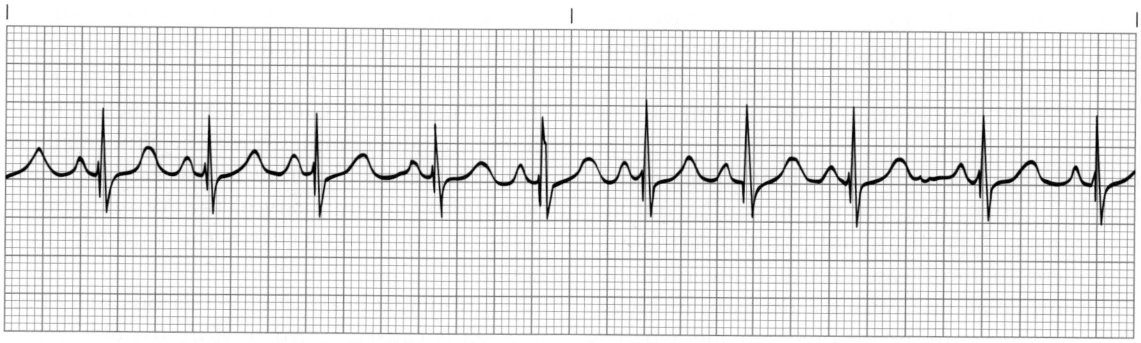

FIGURE 17-11 Electrocardiographic tracing showing sinus arrhythmia. (Modified from Atwood S, Stanton C, and Storey Davenport J: Introduction to basic cardiac dysrhythmias, ed 4, St. Louis, 2009, Mosby/JEMS.)

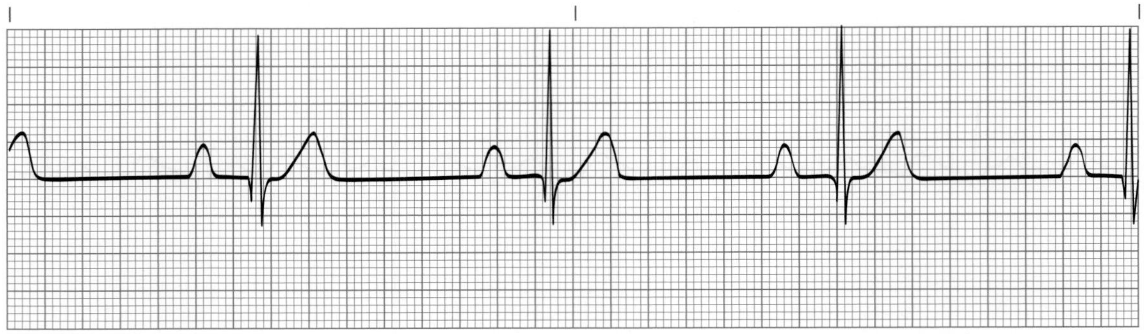

FIGURE 17-12 Electrocardiographic tracing showing first-degree heart block. (Modified from Atwood S, Stanton C, and Storey Davenport J: Introduction to basic cardiac dysrhythmias, ed 4, St. Louis, 2009, Mosby/JEMS.)

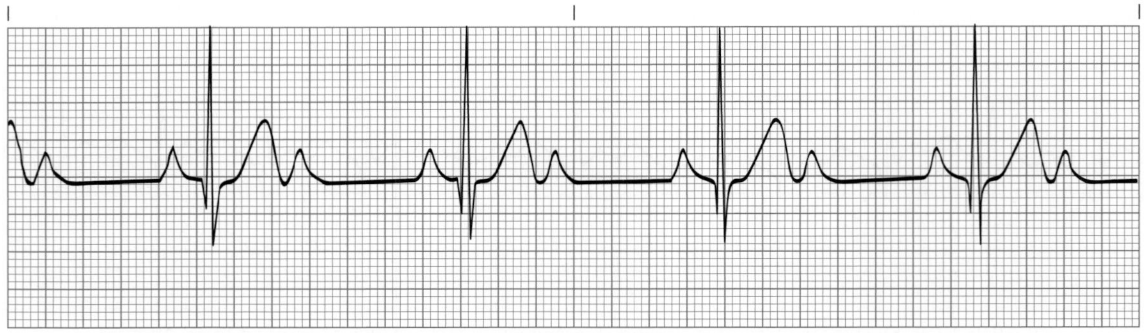

FIGURE 17-13 Electrocardiographic tracing showing second-degree heart block type II. (Modified from Atwood S, Stanton C, and Storey Davenport J: Introduction to basic cardiac dysrhythmias, ed 4, St. Louis, 2009, Mosby/JEMS.)

Second-Degree Heart Block. Second-degree heart block comes in two different types. Type I (Wenckebach or Mobitz type I) block is a relatively benign and often transient arrhythmia. It occurs when an abnormality in the AV junction delays or blocks conduction of some of the impulses through the AV node. It can be recognized by progressive prolongation of the PR interval until one impulse does not pass on to the ventricles at all (seen as a P wave not followed by a QRS complex). The cycle then repeats itself.

Second-degree heart block type II (Mobitz type II) is less common and is more often the result of serious problems such as MI or ischemia. Type II heart block is seen as a series of nonconducted P waves followed by a P wave that is conducted to the ventricles (Figure 17-13). Sometimes the ratio of nonconducted to conducted P waves is fixed at 3:1 or 4:1. The PR interval for the conducted impulses is consistent.[6,7]

Treatment for type I second-degree heart block is not needed because it usually does not impair cardiac output or cause symptoms. Type II second-degree heart block requires treatment in most cases because the resulting reduction in ventricular rate causes a decrease in blood pressure. Medications such as atropine provide a better cardiac output until a pacemaker can be inserted. Because type II block may progress to third-degree heart block without warning, a pacemaker is indicated even if the patient is asymptomatic.[8,9]

Third-Degree Heart Block. Third-degree heart block is the most serious of the different types of heart block. It indicates that the conduction system between the atria and ventricles is completely blocked, and impulses generated in the SA node are not conducted to the ventricles. The atria and ventricles are paced by independent sources. Most commonly, the atria are paced by the SA node, and the ventricles are paced by the AV node. This arrhythmia can be recognized when it is established that there is no relationship between the P waves and the QRS complexes. The P-P intervals are regular, and the R-R intervals are regular, but they have no correlation with one another. In addition, the QRS complexes are normal in configuration if the ventricles are paced by the AV node (Figure 17-14). If the ventricles are paced by an ectopic site in the myocardium, the QRS complexes may be abnormally wide. Typically, the ventricular rate is slower than the atrial rate because the automaticity of the AV node or other latent points is much slower than the automaticity of the SA node.[6,7]

Third-degree heart block is a serious arrhythmia because it often is caused by MI or drug toxicity (especially digitalis), and it may render the heart unable to meet the normal metabolic demands of the body. In almost all cases,

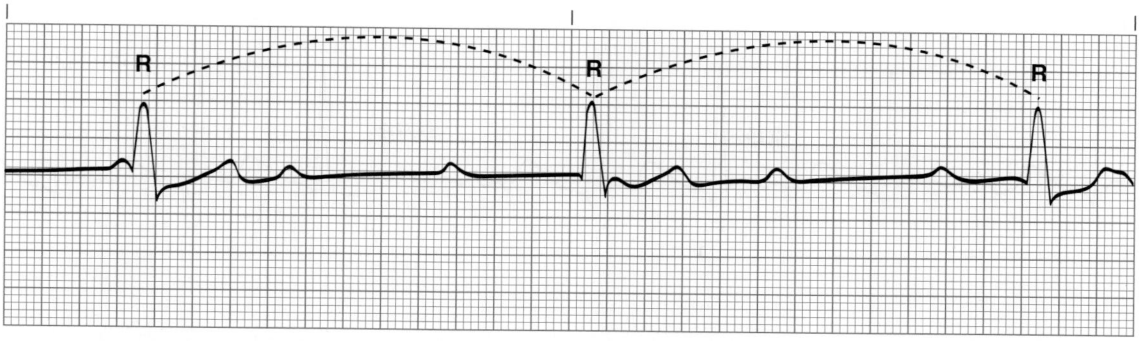

FIGURE 17-14 Electrocardiographic tracing showing third-degree heart block. (Modified from Atwood S, Stanton C, and Storey Davenport J: Introduction to basic cardiac dysrhythmias, ed 4, St. Louis, 2009, Mosby/JEMS.)

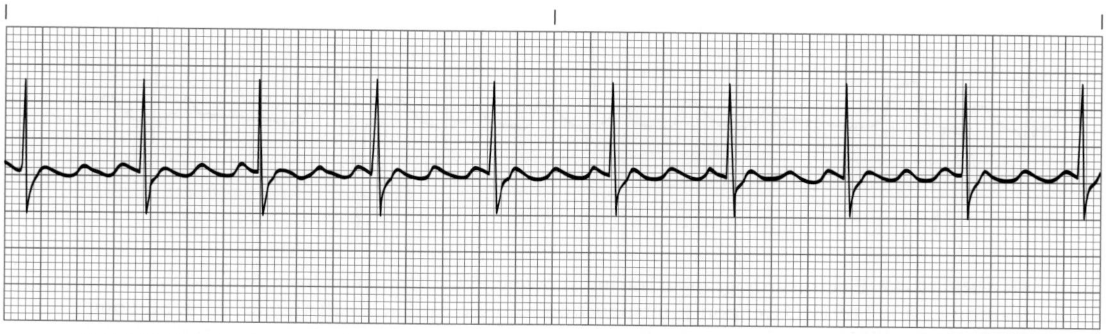

FIGURE 17-15 Electrocardiographic tracing showing atrial flutter. (Modified from Atwood S, Stanton C, and Storey Davenport J: Introduction to basic cardiac dysrhythmias, ed 4, St. Louis, 2009, Mosby/JEMS.)

treatment usually includes medication to speed up the ventricles and a temporary external pacemaker until a permanent pacemaker can be surgically placed.[8,9]

Atrial Flutter. Atrial flutter is the rapid depolarization of the atria resulting from an ectopic focus that depolarizes at a rate of 250 to 350 times per minute. Typically, only one ectopic focus is causing the arrhythmia, which results in each P wave appearing similar. The result is a characteristic saw-toothed baseline pattern (Figure 17-15). Numerous P waves are present for every QRS complex, and the QRS complexes are normal in configuration. The R-R interval may be regular or it may vary, depending on the ability of the atrial impulse to pass through the AV node.[1,3,4]

Various conditions can produce atrial flutter, including rheumatic heart disease, coronary heart disease, stress, renal failure, and hypoxemia. This arrhythmia is not considered life-threatening, but it may lead to atrial fibrillation if untreated. Treatment usually includes medications such as digoxin, beta blockers, or calcium channel blockers. Once the rate is significantly slowed, cardioversion is attempted to return the heart rhythm back to a normal sinus rhythm.[8,9]

Atrial Fibrillation. Atrial fibrillation is present when the atrial muscle quivers in an irregular pattern that does not result in a coordinated contraction. The baseline electrical activity appears erratic, and no true P waves are seen in atrial fibrillation (Figure 17-16). The AV node determines the ventricular response to the atrial activity by controlling which impulses pass through and which do not. The ventricular rate is often very irregular and results in an abnormal R-R interval.[1,3,4]

The causes of atrial fibrillation are similar to the causes of atrial flutter. However, atrial fibrillation is a more serious arrhythmia because it can lead to a significant reduction in cardiac output resulting from the loss of the atrial kick that helps fill the ventricles before systole. It also can lead to formation of thrombi in the atria caused by the stagnation of blood. Emboli may occur if the thrombi break free and enter the pulmonary artery or aorta. Treatment for atrial fibrillation is similar to the treatment for atrial flutter. However, if the length of time the patient has been in atrial fibrillation cannot be determined, the patient may be put on anticoagulants or antithrombolytic medications for a period concurrently with medications to slow the heart rate before cardioversion is attempted. This treatment decreases the chance of accidentally releasing a thrombus that may have formed in the atria, which could potentially cause a life-threatening embolic event.[8,9]

Premature Ventricular Contractions. Premature beats can occur when a portion of the impulse-conducting

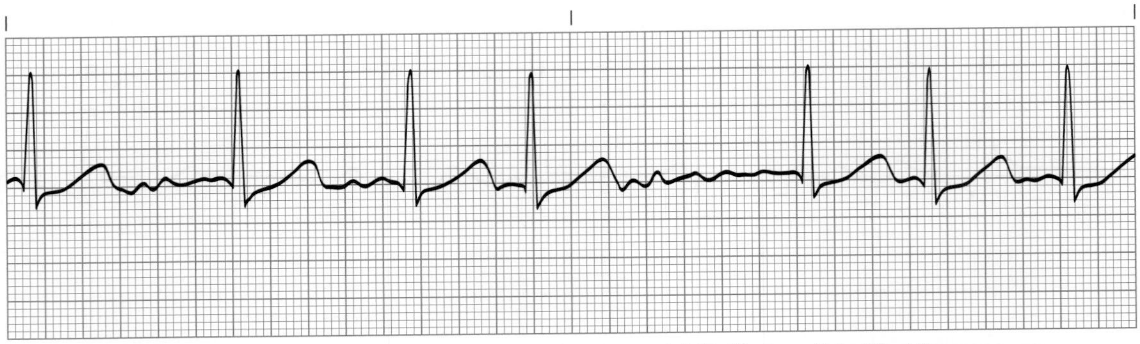

FIGURE 17-16 Electrocardiographic tracing showing atrial fibrillation. (Modified from Atwood S, Stanton C, and Storey Davenport J: Introduction to basic cardiac dysrhythmias, ed 4, St. Louis, 2009, Mosby/JEMS.)

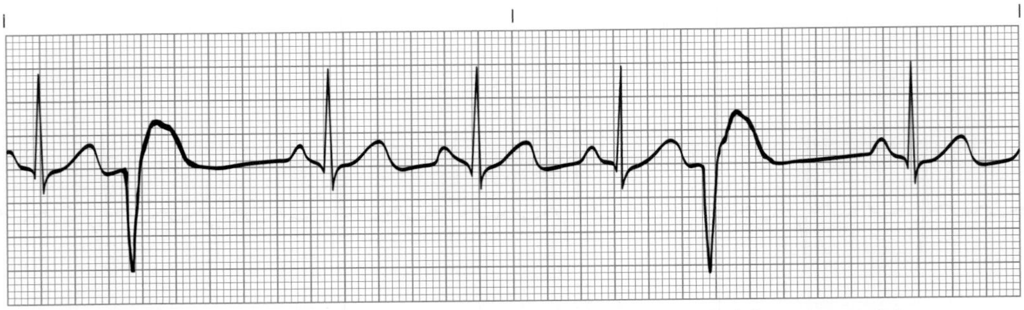

FIGURE 17-17 Electrocardiographic tracing showing PVCs. (Modified from Atwood S, Stanton C, and Storey Davenport J: Introduction to basic cardiac dysrhythmias, ed 4, St. Louis, 2009, Mosby/JEMS.)

system or myocardium other than the SA node becomes diseased and triggers depolarization of the surrounding cardiac cells. Sources for the impulse outside the SA node are called **ectopic foci.** Ectopic foci occur when hypoxia, acid-base imbalances, or electrolyte abnormalities are present and cause the cardiac cells to become abnormally excited. Premature ventricular contractions (PVCs) are an example of ectopic foci that originate in the ventricles. PVCs are easy to recognize because they cause a unique and bizarre QRS complex that is much wider than normal (Figure 17-17). The QRS complex of a PVC is wider than normal because the ectopic focus is using channels outside the normal conduction system to move the impulse throughout the myocardium. PVCs have no P wave preceding them and may occur as a singular event or, more commonly, as a temporary run of PVCs. They also may occur at every other beat (bigeminy) or every third beat (trigeminy).[1,3,4]

An occasional PVC is not of major concern and may occur as a result of stress, caffeine intake, nicotine use, or electrolyte imbalance. However, frequent PVCs are more serious and most often occur in response to ischemia of the myocardium. They also are commonly seen as a side effect of some medications. Treatment is based on the frequency and cause of the PVCs and is needed when the PVCs are frequent (more than six per minute), paired together, or multifocal (appear differently because they come from more than one ectopic focus) or when they land directly on the T wave *(R on T phenomenon)*. In such cases, treatment must be prompt because the problem may progress rapidly to ventricular tachycardia (VT) and ventricular fibrillation (VF) (see subsequent discussion). A complete cardiac evaluation is usually needed to identify the appropriate plan of action. Antiarrhythmic medications (e.g., lidocaine) may offer a temporary solution until the underlying cause can be identified and treated.[8,9]

Ventricular Tachycardia. VT is a run of three or more PVCs. It usually is easy to recognize as a series of wide, bizarre QRS complexes that have no preceding P wave. The ventricular rate is usually 100 to 250 beats/min (Figure 17-18). It is considered sustained VT if it lasts longer than 30 seconds.

Sustained or symptomatic VT is a serious arrhythmia because it indicates that an ectopic focus is rapidly firing from the ventricles, which results from increased automaticity. It suggests a significant pathologic defect in the myocardium and often leads to VF if untreated. MI, coronary artery disease, and hypertensive heart disease are the most common causes.[1,3,4]

Treatment must be prompt and specific and usually consists of cardioversion followed by long-term antiarrhythmic drugs for long-term suppression. Patients at high risk for recurrent VT may have an internal cardioverter-defibrillator (ICD) placed so that if VT occurs it can be

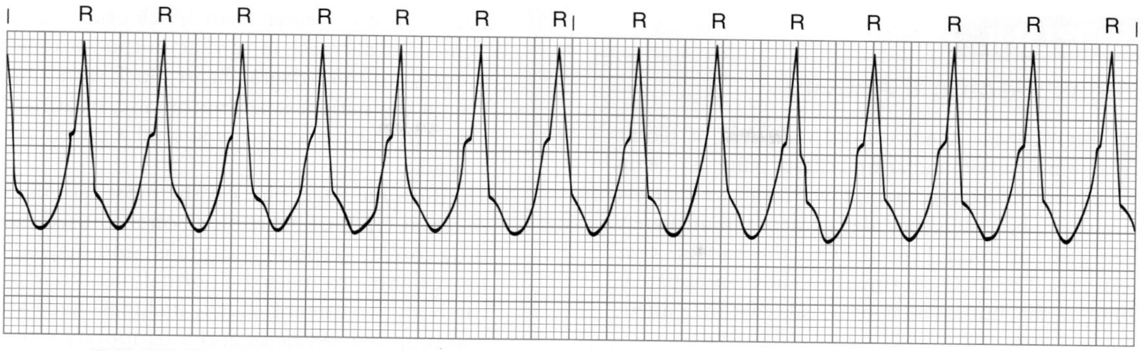

FIGURE 17-18 Electrocardiographic tracing showing VT. (Modified from Atwood S, Stanton C, and Storey Davenport J: Introduction to basic cardiac dysrhythmias, ed 4, St. Louis, 2009, Mosby/JEMS.)

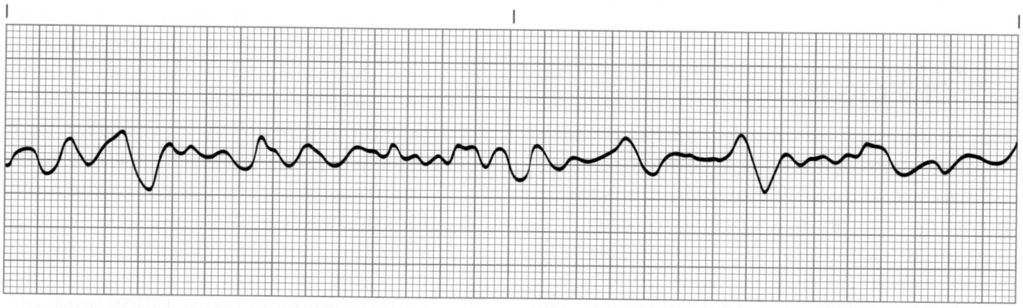

FIGURE 17-19 Electrocardiographic tracing showing VF. (Modified from Atwood S, Stanton C, and Storey Davenport J: Introduction to basic cardiac dysrhythmias, ed 4, St. Louis, 2009, Mosby/JEMS.)

treated automatically and promptly. Asymptomatic patients with recurrent nonsustained VT and ventricular ectopic beats may be treated with beta blockers to reduce symptoms of non–life-threatening ventricular arrhythmias. Symptomatic or sustained VT is considered a medical emergency, and the patient must be treated and monitored continuously in the intensive care unit until his or her condition is stabilized.[8-12]

RULE OF THUMB

Ventricular tachycardia causes the cardiac output to decrease significantly because the ventricles do not have time to fill between contractions. This places the patient in danger of cardiac arrest and death.

Ventricular Fibrillation. VF is the most life-threatening arrhythmia and is defined as erratic quivering of the ventricular muscle mass. It causes the cardiac output to drop to zero; the patient becomes unconscious and represents a true medical emergency. The electrocardiographic tracing of VF shows grossly irregular fluctuations with a zigzag pattern (Figure 17-19). This pattern is caused by the same problems associated with VT.

Treatment calls for rapid defibrillation, cardiopulmonary resuscitation, and administration of oxygen and antiarrhythmic medications; treatment of the underlying cause of the ischemia is also warranted. Survivors of VF usually receive an internal cardioverter-defibrillator.[8-12]

Pulseless Electrical Activity

In addition to the arrhythmias noted throughout this chapter, pulseless electrical activity (PEA) is a serious condition characterized by a disassociation between the electrical and mechanical activity of the heart. In essence, the ECG pattern on the monitor does not generate a pulse. PEA is relatively rare and generally does not occur without a precipitating event, such as a tension pneumothorax, MI, drug overdose, or severe electrolyte or acid-base disturbances.

Treatment involves emergency life support and the immediate reversal of the cause. PEA also illustrates why RTs and other clinicians should never "treat the monitor" and underscores the importance of using ECGs as just one of several clinical indicators in assessing patients.[10-12] The prompt recognition and response to VT, VF, and PEA are discussed in detail in Chapter 34, which covers the broader topic of emergency cardiovascular life support.

MINI CLINI

Pulseless Electrical Activity

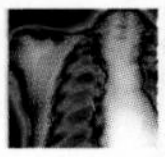

PROBLEM: A 68-year-old man with a recent complaint of radiating chest pain is being placed on oxygen therapy with a nasal cannula at 2 L/min in the emergency department. Immediately after being set up on a 12-lead ECG, the patient loses consciousness. The ECG continues to show an apparent sinus bradycardia, but assessment reveals that the patient is pulseless.

SOLUTION: This is an apparent case of PEA, which should be treated as a potentially life-threatening emergency. Cardiopulmonary resuscitation should be started immediately, and potential causes, including in this instance MI, should be considered and treated.

SUMMARY CHECKLIST

- The ECG is an inexpensive, noninvasive, and easy way to evaluate patients with acute clinical conditions suggestive of myocardial disease. However, it has no value as a predictor of future heart problems or in identifying certain abnormalities (i.e., valvular defects).
- Official interpretation of the ECG is always done by a cardiologist or by the patient's attending physician. The official interpretation is not always rendered in a timely fashion, however, and RTs need to be able to recognize serious arrhythmias and respond quickly and appropriately.
- The impulse-conducting system has three types of cardiac muscle cells capable of electrical excitation: pacemaker cells (e.g., SA node, AV node), specialized rapidly conducting tissue (e.g., Purkinje fibers), and atrial and ventricular muscle cells. Each of these cardiac muscle cell groups varies in their degree of automaticity.
- A defect in the impulse-conducting system leads to inadequate cardiac output.
- An elevated or depressed ST segment is common in MI and is a potentially life-threatening arrhythmia. Abnormal ST segments must be identified and reported as soon as possible.
- Axis evaluation is used to determine the general direction of current flow during ventricular depolarization and is helpful in identifying hypertrophy of one of the ventricles.
- Sinus bradycardia is a significant clinical problem only if it causes the patient's blood pressure to decrease significantly or the patient becomes symptomatic.
- Frequent, paired together, multifocal PVCs or the R on T phenomenon with PVCs is serious because it most often occurs in response to ischemia of the myocardium. The rhythm may progress rapidly to ventricular tachycardia and fibrillation; antiarrhythmic medications (e.g., lidocaine) may offer a temporary solution until an urgent complete cardiac evaluation is performed to identify and treat the underlying cause.
- Type II second-degree heart block usually causes a significant decrease in cardiac output. It may also progress to third-degree heart block without warning. Even if the patient is asymptomatic, treatment calls for medication such as atropine until a pacemaker can be placed.
- Third-degree heart block is the most serious of the different types of heart block often caused by MI or drug toxicity (especially digitalis) and may render the heart unable to meet the normal metabolic demands of the body. Treatment usually includes medication to speed up the ventricles and a temporary external pacemaker until a permanent pacemaker can be surgically placed.
- Atrial fibrillation is a serious arrhythmia that can lead to a significant reduction in cardiac output. In addition, if untreated, over time it can potentially cause an embolic event. Treatment entails medications to control the rate, antithrombolytics or anticoagulants, and potential cardioversion depending on the length of time the patient has been in atrial fibrillation.
- Sustained or symptomatic VT is a serious arrhythmia that often leads to VF if untreated. Prompt treatment usually consists of cardioversion, antiarrhythmic drugs, and transferring the patient to the intensive care unit for continuous monitoring until he or she is stabilized.
- VF is the most life-threatening arrhythmia, requiring emergent treatment with rapid defibrillation, cardiopulmonary resuscitation, and administration of oxygen and antiarrhythmic medications.
- The clinician must always treat the patient, not the rhythm on the ECG monitor. Patients with PEA often have a seemingly productive rhythm on the ECG but are pulseless and require immediate emergency life support.

References

1. Goldberger AL: Clinical electrocardiography: a simplified approach, ed 7, St Louis, 2006, Mosby.
2. Conover M: Understanding electrocardiography, ed 8, St Louis, 2002, Mosby.
3. Thaler MS: The only EKG book you'll ever need, ed 5, Philadelphia, 2006, Lippincott-Raven.
4. Aehlert B: ECGs made easy, ed 3, St Louis, 2005, Mosby.
5. Huszar R: Basic dysrhythmias and acute coronary syndromes: interpretation and management, ed 4, St Louis, 2012, Mosby.
6. Walraven G: Basic arrhythmias, ed 6, Upper Saddle River, NJ, 2005, Prentice Hall.
7. Phalen T, Aehlert B: The 12-lead ECG in acute coronary syndromes, ed 2, St. Louis, 2006, Mosby.
8. Barrett D, Gretton M, Quinn T: Cardiac care: an introduction for healthcare professionals, Indianapolis, 2006, Wiley.
9. Hazinski MF, Field JM, editors: 2010 guidelines for cardiopulmonary resuscitation and emergency cardiovascular care, Dallas, 2010, American Heart Association.
10. Darovic GO: Hemodynamic monitoring: invasive and noninvasive clinical application, ed 3, Philadelphia, 2002, Saunders.
11. Huff J: ECG workout exercises in arrhythmia interpretation, ed 5, Philadelphia, 2005, Lippincott Williams & Wilkins.
12. Wilkins RL, Dexter JR, Heuer AJ: Clinical assessment in respiratory care, ed 6, St Louis, 2010, Mosby.

Chapter 18

Analysis and Monitoring of Gas Exchange

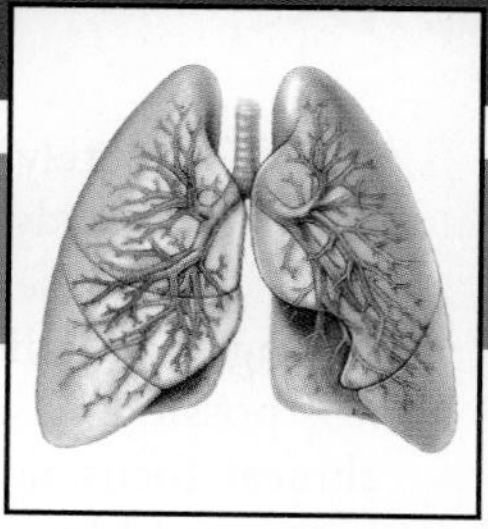

MARK S. SIOBAL

CHAPTER OBJECTIVES

After reading this chapter you will be able to:

- Describe the difference between monitoring and analysis.
- Describe the two types of electrochemical oxygen analyzers.
- Describe calibration and problem-solving techniques for oxygen analyzers.
- State how to obtain, process, and analyze arterial and capillary blood gas samples.
- List the quality control procedures applied to blood gas analysis.
- List the potential advantages of point-of-care testing.
- Describe how to obtain and interpret transcutaneous oxygen and carbon dioxide monitoring.
- Describe the basic principles used by an oximeter to monitor oxygen saturation.
- State when and how to perform pulse oximetry.
- Identify true statements related to interpretation of pulse oximetry results.
- Describe how to perform capnometry and interpret capnograms.

CHAPTER OUTLINE

KEY TERMS

analyte
analyzer
arterialized blood
bias
calibration media
capnography
capnometry
collateral circulation
cuvette
electrochemical
ex vivo
imprecision
invasive
in vivo
modified Allen test
monitor
needle capping device
noninvasive
optical fluorescence
optode
oximetry
photoplethysmography
point-of-care testing
preanalytic error
precision
proficiency testing
pulse cooximetry
quality control
random error
spectrophotometry
systematic error

Ultimately, gas exchange takes place inside each of the body's cells, where complex metabolic pathways use oxygen (O_2) to create energy, while producing carbon dioxide (CO_2) as a waste product. Although it is possible to analyze gas exchange at the cellular level, clinical focus normally is on gas exchange between the lungs and blood or between the blood and tissues. Gas exchange between the lungs and blood is usually analyzed by measuring O_2 and CO_2 levels in the arterial blood. Clinicians also can measure CO_2 levels in the expired air to monitor ventilation. The most common approach to analyzing gas exchange between the blood and tissues is to measure O_2 levels in the mixed venous (pulmonary artery [PA]) blood. This chapter focuses on these important concepts and the parameters that reflect gas exchange.

ANALYSIS VERSUS MONITORING

Although the term *analysis* is defined broadly as *study* or *interpretation,* analysis conducted in a clinical laboratory has a special meaning, as does the term *monitoring.* In clinical practice, *laboratory analysis* refers to discrete measurements of fluids or tissue that must be removed from the body. Such measurements are made by a laboratory **analyzer.** Conversely, monitoring is an ongoing process by which clinicians obtain and evaluate dynamic physiologic processes in a timely manner, usually at the bedside. A **monitor** is a device that provides the important data to the clinician in real time, usually without removal of samples from the body.

INVASIVE VERSUS NONINVASIVE PROCEDURES

Invasive procedures require insertion of a sensor or collection device into the body, whereas **noninvasive** monitoring is a means of gathering data externally.[1] Because laboratory analysis of gas exchange requires blood samples, it is usually considered invasive. Monitoring can be either invasive or noninvasive. Generally, invasive procedures tend to provide more accurate data than noninvasive methods, but they carry greater risk.

When both approaches are available, the need for measurement accuracy should dictate which is chosen. However, clinicians can sometimes combine the two approaches—using the invasive approach to establish accurate baseline information, while applying the noninvasive method for ongoing monitoring of a stable patient. After the gradient between the invasive and noninvasive method is established, trends in the change of the noninvasive method can be useful in making clinical decisions.

MEASURING FRACTIONAL INSPIRED OXYGEN

Analysis of gas exchange begins with knowledge of the system inputs—the inspired O_2 and CO_2 concentrations. Healthy individuals breathe air that contains a fixed O_2 concentration (21%) and negligible amounts of CO_2. Patients who are ill often have hypoxemia and are given supplemental O_2. O_2 analyzers are used to measure the fractional inspired O_2 concentration (FiO_2).

Instrumentation

Although many methods exist for measuring O_2 concentrations, most bedside systems apply electrochemical principles. There are two common types of **electrochemical** O_2 analyzers: (1) the polarographic (Clark) electrode and (2) the galvanic fuel cell. Under ideal conditions of temperature, pressure, and relative humidity, both types are accurate to within ± 2% of the actual concentration.[1]

The Clark electrode is similar to electrodes used in blood gas analyzers and transcutaneous monitors (see later section on Transcutaneous Blood Gas Monitoring). This system typically consists of a platinum cathode and a silver–silver chloride anode (Figure 18-1). O_2 molecules diffuse through the sensor membrane into the electrolyte,

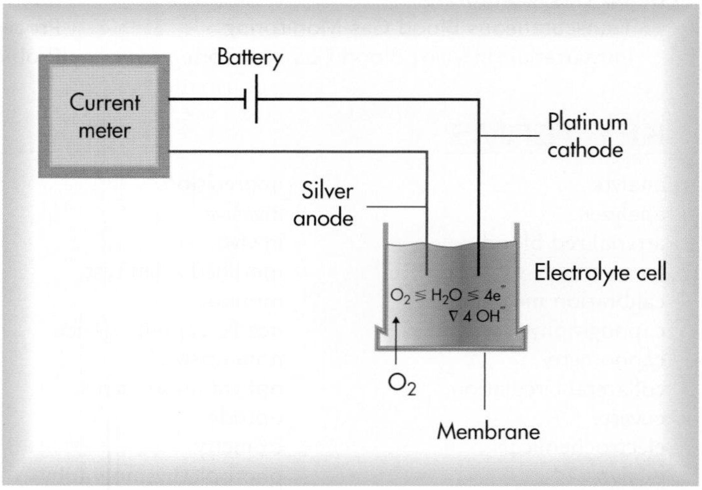

FIGURE 18-1 The basic principle underlying a Clark polarographic analyzer. (Modified from Kacmarek RM, Hess D, Stoller JK, editors: Monitoring in respiratory care, St Louis, 1993, Mosby.)

where a polarizing voltage causes electron flow between the anode and cathode. While silver is oxidized at the anode, the flow of electrons reduces O_2 (and water) to hydroxyl ions (OH^-) at the cathode. The more O_2 molecules that are reduced, the greater is the electron flow across the poles (current). The resulting change in current is proportional to the PO_2, with its value displayed on a galvanometer, calibrated in percent O_2. Response times for Clark electrode O_2 analyzers range from 10 to 30 seconds.

Most galvanic fuel cells use a gold anode and a lead cathode. In contrast to the Clark electrode, current flow across these poles is generated by the chemical reaction itself. Unless accessories such as alarms are included, a galvanic cell needs no external power; this means that galvanic cells respond more slowly than Clark electrodes, sometimes taking 60 seconds.

The Clark electrode and galvanic cell are suitable for basic FiO_2 monitoring. When greater accuracy or faster response times are needed (e.g., when performing indirect calorimetry), a paramagnetic, zirconium cell, Raman scattering, or mass spectroscopy analyzer should be selected.

Procedure

To obtain accurate results with an O_2 analyzer, the clinician first must calibrate it. Although procedures differ according to the manufacturer, the basic steps are similar, requiring exposure of the sensor to two gases with different O_2 concentrations, usually 100% O_2 and room air (21% O_2). In one common procedure, the sensor is first exposed to 100% O_2. If the analyzer fails to read 100%, the device's *calibration,* or balance control, must be adjusted until it reads 100%. Then the clinician exposes the sensor to room air and confirms a second reading of 21% (± 2%). The clinician should use the analyzer to measure a patient's FiO_2 only after confirming both readings.

Problem Solving and Troubleshooting

Because O_2 analyzers include replaceable components that deteriorate over time (batteries, electrodes, membranes, electrolytes), the best way to avoid problems is through preventive maintenance, which should include both scheduled parts replacement and routine operational testing by biomedical engineering personnel. As with any preventive maintenance program, it is essential that detailed records be kept on each piece of equipment.

Even with the best preventive maintenance, O_2 analyzers sometimes malfunction. The clinician would know that an analyzer is not working if it fails to calibrate or gives an inconsistent reading during use. The most common causes of analyzer malfunction are low batteries (Clark electrode systems), sensor depletion, and electronic failure. Because a low battery condition is so common with Clark electrode systems, the first step in troubleshooting is to replace the batteries. If the analyzer still does not calibrate on fresh batteries, the problem is probably a depleted sensor. With most analyzers, a depleted sensor must be replaced (some Clark electrodes can be recharged). If an analyzer still fails to calibrate after battery and sensor replacement, the most likely problem is an internal failure of its electrical system. In this case, the device should be taken out of service and repaired.

Inaccurate readings also can occur with electrochemical analyzers, resulting from either condensed water vapor or pressure fluctuations. Galvanic cells are particularly sensitive to condensation. To avoid this problem during continuous use in humidified circuits, the clinician should place the analyzer sensor proximal to any humidification device.

Fuel cell and Clark electrode readings also are affected by ambient pressure changes. Under conditions of low pressure (high altitude), these devices read lower than the actual O_2 concentration. Conversely, higher pressures, such as pressures that occur during positive pressure ventilation, cause these devices to read higher than the actual FiO_2. These observations are consistent with the fact that both devices measure the PO_2 but report a percent concentration scale.

SAMPLING AND ANALYZING BLOOD GASES

In the clinical setting, it is common for the collection of blood specimens (sampling) to be performed separately from their analysis. Each procedure involves different knowledge and skill. For these reasons, these topics are covered separately.

Sampling

Clinicians have been using blood samples to assess gas exchange parameters for more than 50 years.[2] The definition of *respiratory failure* still is based largely on blood gas measurements. Depending on the need, blood gas samples can be obtained by percutaneous puncture of a peripheral artery, from an indwelling catheter (arterial, central venous, or PA), or by capillary sampling.

Arterial Puncture and Interpretation

Results obtained from sampling arterial blood gas (ABG) are the cornerstone in the diagnosis and management of oxygenation and acid-base disturbances. ABGs are considered the "gold standard" of gas exchange analysis, against which all other methods are compared.

Arterial puncture involves drawing blood from a peripheral artery (radial, brachial, femoral, or dorsalis pedis) through a single percutaneous needle puncture (Figure 18-2). The radial artery is the preferred site for arterial blood sampling for the following reasons:

- It is near the surface and relatively easy to palpate and stabilize.
- Effective **collateral circulation** normally exists in the ulnar artery.

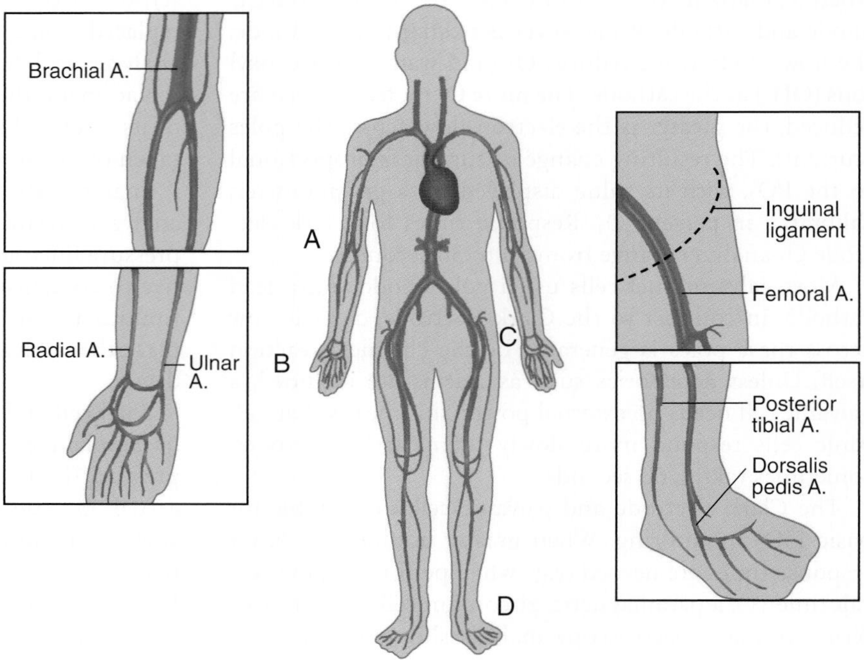

FIGURE 18-2 Arteries used for arterial puncture. **A,** Brachial artery. **B,** Radial artery (with collateral flow through the ulnar arteries). **C,** Femoral artery. **D,** Dorsalis pedis (with collateral flow through the posterior tibial artery). The radial artery is the preferred site.

- The artery is not near any large veins.
- The procedure is relatively pain-free.

Other sites (brachial, femoral, and dorsalis pedis) are riskier and should be used only by clinicians specifically trained in their use. Likewise, arterial puncture in infants (through either the radial or the temporal artery) requires advanced training. Arterial cannulation sites with indwelling catheters include radial, brachial, femoral, dorsalis pedis, umbilical (in neonates), and axillary arteries. The focus here is on radial artery puncture.

To guide practitioners in providing quality care, the American Association for Respiratory Care (AARC) has published Clinical Practice Guideline: Sampling for Arterial Blood Gas Analysis.[3] Complementary recommendations have been published by the National Committee for Clinical Laboratory Standards.[4] Modified excerpts from the AARC guideline appear in Clinical Practice Guideline 18-1.

Equipment. Box 18-1 lists the equipment needed to perform an arterial puncture. Commercial vendors provide kits containing most of the equipment listed. If provided, the **needle capping device** serves two purposes. First, it isolates the sample from air exposure (to ensure accurate results). Second, it helps prevent inadvertent needlestick injuries. There are many different capping device designs; devices that allow single-handed recapping are preferred. If a capping safety device is not provided, the clinician should use the single-handed "scoop" method to cap the needle before removing it and plugging the syringe.

Procedure. Box 18-2 outlines the basic procedure for radial artery puncture of adults. Before radial artery puncture is performed, a **modified Allen test** (Figure 18-3) is recommended. The test is normal (indicating adequate collateral circulation) if the palm, fingers, and thumb flush pink within 5 to 10 seconds after pressure on the ulnar artery is released. A normal test result indicates the presence of collateral circulation but may not predict the development of complications after radial artery puncture or cannulation.

The modified Allen test has been a widely used clinical method to assess adequacy of ulnar artery collateral blood

Box 18-1 Recommended Equipment for Percutaneous Arterial Blood Sampling

- Standard precautions barrier protection (gloves, safety goggles)
- Preheparinized blood gas kit syringe (1-3 ml)
- Short-bevel 20-gauge to 22-gauge needle with a clear hub (23-gauge to 25-gauge for children and infants)
- Patient/sample label
- Isopropyl alcohol (70%), povidone-iodine (Betadine) (check patient for iodine sensitivity), or chlorhexidine swabs
- Sterile gauze squares, tape, bandages
- Puncture-resistant container
- Ice slush (if specimen is not analyzed within 10-30 minutes)
- Towels
- Sharps container
- Local anesthetic (0.5% lidocaine)*
- Hypodermic needle (25-gauge or 26-gauge)*
- Needle capping device

*Optional.

18-1 Sampling for Arterial Blood Gas Analysis

AARC Clinical Practice Guidelines (Excerpts)*

INDICATIONS

- The need to evaluate ventilation ($PaCO_2$), acid-base balance (pH and $PaCO_2$), oxygenation status (PaO_2 and SaO_2), and oxygen-carrying capacity of blood (PaO_2, HbO_2, total Hb, and dyshemoglobins)
- The need to assess the patient's response to therapy or diagnostic tests (e.g., O_2 or exercise testing)
- The need to monitor the severity and progression of a documented disease process

CONTRAINDICATIONS

- Abnormal results of a modified Allen test (lack of collateral circulation) may be indicative of inadequate blood supply to the hand and suggest the need to select another puncture site.
- Arterial puncture should not be performed through a lesion or distal to a surgical shunt. For example, arterial puncture should not be performed on a patient undergoing dialysis. If there is evidence of infection or peripheral vascular disease involving the selected limb, an alternative site should be selected.
- Because of the need for monitoring the femoral puncture site for an extended period, femoral punctures should not be performed outside the hospital.
- Coagulopathy or medium-dose to high-dose anticoagulation therapy, such as heparin or warfarin (Coumadin), streptokinase, and tissue plasminogen activator (but not aspirin), may be a relative contraindication.

PRECAUTIONS AND POSSIBLE COMPLICATIONS

- Arteriospasm
- Hemorrhage
- Air or clotted blood emboli
- Trauma to the vessel
- Anaphylaxis from local anesthetic
- Arterial occlusion
- Patient or sampler contamination
- Vasovagal response
- Hematoma
- Pain

ASSESSMENT OF NEED

The following may make it easier to decide whether arterial blood sampling is needed:

- History and physical indicators, such as positive smoking history, recent onset of difficulty breathing independent of activity level, or trauma
- Presence of other abnormal diagnostic tests or indices, such as abnormal pulse oximetry reading or chest x-ray examination
- Initiation, change, or discontinuation of therapy (e.g., oxygen therapy or mechanical ventilation)
- Projected enrollment in a pulmonary rehabilitation program

FREQUENCY

The frequency with which sampling is repeated should depend on the clinical status of the patient and the indication for performing the procedure. Because repeated punctures at a single site can cause injury, clinicians should consider either finding alternative sites or using an indwelling catheter.

MONITORING

The following should be monitored as part of arterial blood sampling:

- FiO_2 (analyzed) or prescribed flow
- Patient's respiratory rate
- Proper application of oxygen device
- Patient's temperature
- Mode of ventilatory support and settings
- Patient's position and level of activity
- Pulsatile blood return
- Patient's clinical appearance
- Presence of air bubbles or clots in the syringe or sample
- Ease or difficulty in obtaining a blood sample
- Appearance of the puncture site (for hematoma) after application of pressure and before dressing

*For the complete guideline, see American Association for Respiratory Care: Clinical practice guideline: sampling for arterial blood gas analysis. Respir Care 37:891, 1992.

Box 18-2 Procedure for Radial Artery Puncture

- Check the medical record to (1) confirm the order and indications and (2) determine the patient's primary diagnosis, history (especially bleeding disorders or blood-borne infections), current status, respiratory care orders (especially oxygen therapy or mechanical ventilation), and anticoagulant or thrombolytic therapy.
- Confirm steady-state conditions (20-30 minutes after changes).
- Obtain and assemble necessary equipment and supplies.
- Wash hands and don barrier protection (e.g., gloves, eyewear).
- Identify the patient using current patient safety standards.
- Explain the procedure to the patient.
- Position the patient, extending the patient's wrist to approximately 30 degrees.
- Perform a modified Allen test, and confirm collateral circulation.
- Clean site thoroughly with 70% isopropyl alcohol or an equivalent antiseptic.
- Inject a local anesthetic subcutaneously and periarterially (wait 2 minutes for effect).*
- Use a preheparinized blood gas kit syringe, or heparinize a syringe and expel the excess (fill dead space only).
- Palpate and secure the artery with one hand.
- Insert the needle, bevel up, through the skin at a 45-degree angle until blood pulsates into the syringe.
- Allow 1 ml of blood to fill syringe (the need to aspirate indicates a venous puncture).
- Apply firm pressure to puncture site with sterile gauze until the bleeding stops.
- Expel any air bubbles from the sample, and cap or plug the syringe.
- Mix the sample by rolling and inverting the syringe.
- Place the sample in a transport container (ice slush) if specimen is not to be analyzed within 10-30 minutes.
- Dispose of waste materials and sharps properly.
- Document the procedure and patient status in the chart and on the specimen label.
- Check the site after 20 minutes for hematoma and adequacy of distal circulation.

From Malley WJ: Clinical blood gases: application and noninvasive alternatives, Philadelphia, 1990, Saunders; Shapiro BA, Peruzzi WT, Kozelowski-Templin R: Clinical application of blood gases, ed 5, St Louis, 2005, Mosby.

*Optional.

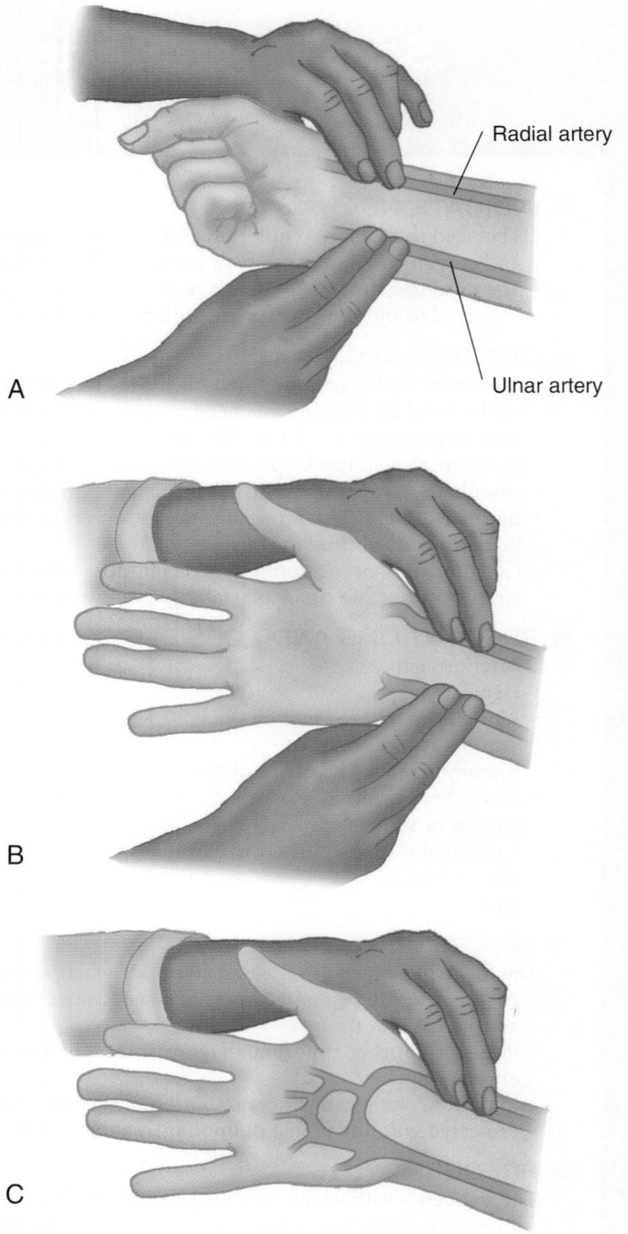

FIGURE 18-3 Modified Allen test. **A,** The hand is clenched into a tight fist, and pressure is applied to the radial and ulnar arteries. **B,** The hand is opened (but not fully extended); the palm and fingers are blanched. **C,** Removal of pressure on the ulnar artery should result in flushing of the entire hand (within 5 to 10 seconds) indicative of adequate collateral circulation or a normal modified Allen test.

flow despite the lack of evidence that it can predict ischemic complications in the setting of complete radial artery occlusion.[5] The criteria for an abnormal test result are not agreed on, which renders the significance of an abnormal test unclear. The test result may be inaccurate in predicting postcannulation hand ischemia, has poor interrater reliability, and is known to yield a high incidence of false normal and abnormal results. The modified Allen test cannot be performed on most critically ill patients who are either uncooperative or unconscious. In addition, prior radial artery cannulation, severe circulatory insufficiency, wrist or hand burns, or jaundice makes interpreting the results difficult. Performance of a modified Allen test before radial artery puncture or cannulation should not be considered a "standard of care," but the need for its use and appropriate application should be well recognized.[6]

In patients who have undergone previous radial artery cannulation, the modified Allen test can provide documentation of possible arterial thrombosis and should be used to direct catheter placement. In that circumstance, it is imprudent to ignore totally the utility of the modified Allen test, especially if another arterial site is available for cannulation.[7]

In most cases, a sample volume of 0.5 to 1 ml of blood is adequate. The actual sample volume needed depends on the following: (1) the anticoagulant used, (2) the requirements of the specific analyzer used, and (3) whether other tests are to be performed on the sample.

The following rules for careful handling of the needle help avoid transmission of blood-borne diseases:

- Never recap a used needle without a safety device; never handle a used needle using both hands; never point a used needle toward any part of the body.
- Never bend, break, or remove used needles from syringes by hand.
- Always dispose of used syringes, needles, and other sharp items in appropriate puncture-resistant sharps containers.

Indications for Blood Gas Sampling. Knowing when to obtain a blood gas sample is just as important as knowing how to perform the procedure. See Clinical Practice Guideline 18-1 for the general indications for ABG sampling. Box 18-3 lists common clinical situations associated with the need for ABG analysis.

Problem Solving and Troubleshooting. There are two major problem areas associated with arterial puncture. The first problem area involves difficulties in getting a good sample. The second problem area involves preanalytic error.

Getting a Good Sample. Problems with getting a good sample include an inaccessible artery, absent pulse, deficient sample return, and alteration of test results caused by the patient's response. If the selected artery cannot be located, another site should be considered. Likewise, if an adequate pulse cannot be palpated at the chosen site, another site should be selected, or an acceptable noninvasive approach should be considered as an alternative (e.g., pulse oximetry).

If the clinician gets only a small spurt of blood, the needle has probably passed through the artery. In this situation, the needle is slowly withdrawn until a pulsatile flow fills the syringe. The tip of the needle is never redirected without it first being withdrawn to the subcutaneous tissue. If the needle must be withdrawn completely and the clinician does not have an adequate sample, the procedure is repeated with a fresh blood gas kit.

Small sample volumes or the need to apply syringe suction also may indicate that venous blood has been obtained. However, when drawing arterial blood from hypotensive patients or when using small needles (<23-gauge), the clinician may need to pull gently on the syringe barrel. Excessive suction can alter the blood gas results. If the clinician suspects that pain or anxiety during the procedure may have altered the results (most typically causing hyperventilation), he or she should consider using a local anesthetic for subsequent sampling attempts.

Preanalytic Error. **Preanalytic errors** are problems occurring before sample analysis that can alter the accuracy of the blood gas results. Table 18-1 summarizes the most common errors associated with arterial blood sampling, including recommendations on how to recognize and avoid these problems.[8,9] Clinicians can avoid most preanalytic errors by ensuring that the sample is obtained anaerobically, is properly anticoagulated (with immediate expulsion of air bubbles), and is analyzed within 10 to 30 minutes.

The traditional method used to avoid preanalytic errors caused by blood cell metabolism is to chill the sample quickly by placing it in an ice slush. Chilling is needed if the sample is not to be analyzed within 10 to 30 minutes.[3] Chilled samples should be discarded if they are not analyzed within 60 minutes. PaO_2 of samples drawn from subjects with elevated white blood cell counts may decrease rapidly, and immediate chilling is recommended. Chilled samples can result in potassium transport between blood cells and plasma and can result in erroneous elevation in potassium measured from a blood gas sample. Use of a glass syringe or a plastic syringe with low diffusibility minimizes the risk of room air gases contaminating the sample. Pneumatic tube transport of samples containing small air bubbles can have a noticeable effect on increasing PaO_2.[9]

Interpretation of Arterial Blood Gases. Given that gas exchange is a dynamic process, looking at results from a single blood sample is akin to looking at a single frame in a feature-length movie. If the scene is changing rapidly, the single frame can be misleading. Conversely, if the scene is relatively stable, a single frame can provide useful information. Blood gas results must be interpreted in light of the patient status at the time the sample was obtained.

Box 18-3 Clinical Indications for Arterial Blood Gas Analysis

- Sudden, unexplained dyspnea
- Cyanosis
- Abnormal breath sounds
- Severe, unexplained tachypnea
- Heavy use of accessory muscles
- Changes in ventilator settings
- Cardiopulmonary resuscitation
- New appearance of diffuse infiltrates in chest radiograph
- Sudden appearance or progression of cardiac arrhythmias
- Acute hypotension
- Acute deterioration in neurologic function

TABLE 18-1

Preanalytic Errors Associated With Arterial Blood

Error	Effect on Parameters	How to Recognize	How to Avoid
Air in sample	↓ PCO_2 ↑ pH ↑ low PO_2 ↓ high PO_2	Visible bubbles or froth Low PCO_2 inconsistent with patient status	Discard frothy samples Fully expel bubbles Mix only after air is expelled Cap syringe quickly
Venous admixture	↑ PCO_2 ↓ pH Can greatly lower PO_2	Failure of syringe to fill by pulsations Patient has no symptoms of hypoxemia	Avoid brachial and femoral sites Do not aspirate sample Use short-bevel needles Avoid artery "overshoot" Cross-check with SpO_2
Excess anticoagulant (dilution)	↓ PCO_2 ↑ pH ↑ low PO_2 ↓ high PO_2	Visible heparin remains in syringe before sampling	Use premade lyophilized (dry) heparin blood gas kits Fill dead space only Collect >2 ml (adults) and >0.6 ml (infants)
Metabolic effects	↑ PCO_2 ↓ pH ↓ PO_2	Excessive time lag since sample collection Values inconsistent with patient status	Analyze within 15 min Place sample in ice slush

Any major change in either patient condition or therapy disrupts the patient's steady state. However, over time, a steady state normally returns. The time needed to restore a steady state varies with the patient's pulmonary status. Patients with healthy lungs achieve a steady state in only 5 minutes after changes, whereas patients with chronic obstructive pulmonary disease (COPD) may require 20 to 30 minutes. If a patient's FiO_2 is changed, the measured PaO_2 would accurately reflect the patient's gas exchange status within 5 minutes in healthy individuals but may require 20 to 30 minutes in patients with COPD.

To document the patient's status, the following need to be recorded: (1) date, time, and site of sampling; (2) results of the modified Allen test, when performed; (3) patient's body temperature, position, activity level, and respiratory rate; and (4) FiO_2 concentration or flow and all applicable ventilatory support settings. Noting such information may prove useful in interpretation of the results.

RULE OF THUMB

To ensure a steady state, wait 20 to 30 minutes after any major change in ventilatory support before sampling and analyzing the blood gases of a critically ill patient.

In the first step of interpretation of the results, the clinician must ensure he or she is looking at the results of the correct patient. The name and patient identification number from the blood gas report must match the patient. Interpretation of the results can be divided into two basic steps: (1) interpretation of the oxygenation status and (2) interpretation of the acid-base status.

The oxygenation status is determined by examination of the PaO_2, arterial O_2 saturation (SaO_2), and arterial O_2 content (CaO_2) The PaO_2 represents the partial pressure of O_2 in the plasma of the arterial blood and is the result of gas exchange between the lung and blood. The PaO_2 is reduced in various settings but most often when lung disease is present. PaO_2 of less than 40 mm Hg is called *severe* hypoxemia, PaO_2 of 40 to 59 mm Hg is called *moderate* hypoxemia, and PaO_2 of 60 mm Hg to the predicted normal is called *mild* hypoxemia.

SaO_2 represents the degree to which the hemoglobin (Hb) is saturated with O_2 (see Chapter 11). Normally, the Hb saturation with O_2 is 95% to 100% with healthy lungs. When the lungs cannot transfer O_2 into the blood at normal levels, the SaO_2 decreases in most cases in proportion to the degree of lung disease present. Blood gas analyzers report a calculated SaO_2. Measurement of SaO_2 by hemoximetry and Hb content is required for accurate determination of CaO_2.

CaO_2 represents the content of O_2 in 100 ml of arterial blood and is a function of the amount of Hb present and the degree to which it is saturated. A normal CaO_2 is 18 to 20 ml of O_2 per 100 ml of arterial blood. A reduced CaO_2 is often the result of low PaO_2 and SaO_2, reduced Hb level, or both.

The acid-base status of the patient is determined by evaluating the pH, $PaCO_2$, and plasma HCO_3^-. The steps for interpreting the acid-base status of the ABG results are described in Chapter 13.

Indwelling Catheters (Arterial and Central Venous Pressure and Pulmonary Artery Lines)

Indwelling catheters provide ready access for blood sampling and allow continuous monitoring of vascular pressures, without the traumatic risks associated with repetitive percutaneous punctures. However, infection and thrombosis are more likely with indwelling catheters than they are with intermittent punctures.

The most common routes for indwelling vascular lines are a peripheral artery (usually radial, brachial, or less commonly dorsalis pedis and axillary) or femoral artery, a central vein (usually the vena cava), and the PA. In neonates, the umbilical artery is cannulated for arterial blood sampling. Table 18-2 summarizes the usefulness of these various sites in providing relevant clinical information. Chapter 46 provides details on the use of these systems for hemodynamic pressure and flow monitoring.

Equipment. Figure 18-4 shows the basic setup used for an indwelling vascular line, in this case, a brachial artery catheter. The catheter connects to a disposable continuous-flush device (Delta-flow; Utah Medical Products, Midvale, UT). This device keeps the line open by providing a continuous low rate of flow (2 to 4 ml/hr) of intravenous saline solution through the system.

Heparinized saline flush solution has been commonly used with indwelling vascular catheters. However, it has been shown that heparin does not significantly improve arterial catheter function, extend the duration of use, or decrease the number of manipulations required. Additionally, results of coagulation studies can be affected by heparinized flush solution, and unnecessary exposure to heparin may increase the risk of heparin-induced thrombocytopenia.[10] Because arterial pressures are much higher than venous pressures, the intravenous bag supplying these systems must be pressurized, usually by using a hand bulb pump. A strain-gauge pressure transducer connected to the flush device provides an electrical signal to an amplifier or monitor, which displays the corresponding pressure waveform.

Procedure. Access for sampling blood from most intravascular lines is provided by a three-way stopcock (Figure 18-5). Equipment and supplies are the same as specified for arterial puncture, with the addition of a second "waste" syringe. Box 18-4 outlines the proper

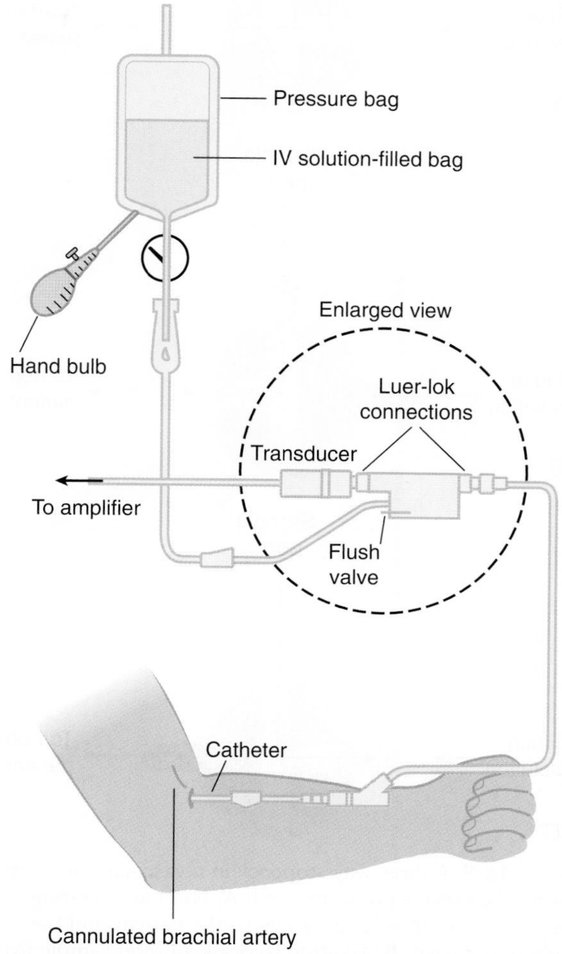

FIGURE 18-4 An indwelling vascular line (brachial artery catheter) used to monitor blood pressure and obtain a blood sample.

TABLE 18-2

Common Sites for Indwelling Vascular Catheters and the Information They Provide

	Blood Collection		Pressure Monitoring	
Location	**Sample**	**Reflects**	**Pressure**	**Reflects**
Peripheral, umbilical artery	Arterial blood	Pulmonary gas exchange (O_2 uptake/CO_2 removal)	Systemic arterial pressure	LV afterload; vascular tone; blood volume
Central vein	Venous blood (unmixed)	Not useful for assessing gas exchange; can be used for some other laboratory tests	CVP	Fluid volume; vascular tone; RV preload
Pulmonary artery	Mixed venous blood (balloon deflated)	Gas exchange at tissues (O_2 consumption/CO_2 production)	PAP; PCWP	RV afterload; vascular tone; blood volume; LV preload

CVP, Central venous pressure; *LV,* left ventricular; *PAP,* pulmonary artery pressure; *PCWP,* pulmonary capillary wedge pressure; *RV,* right ventricular.

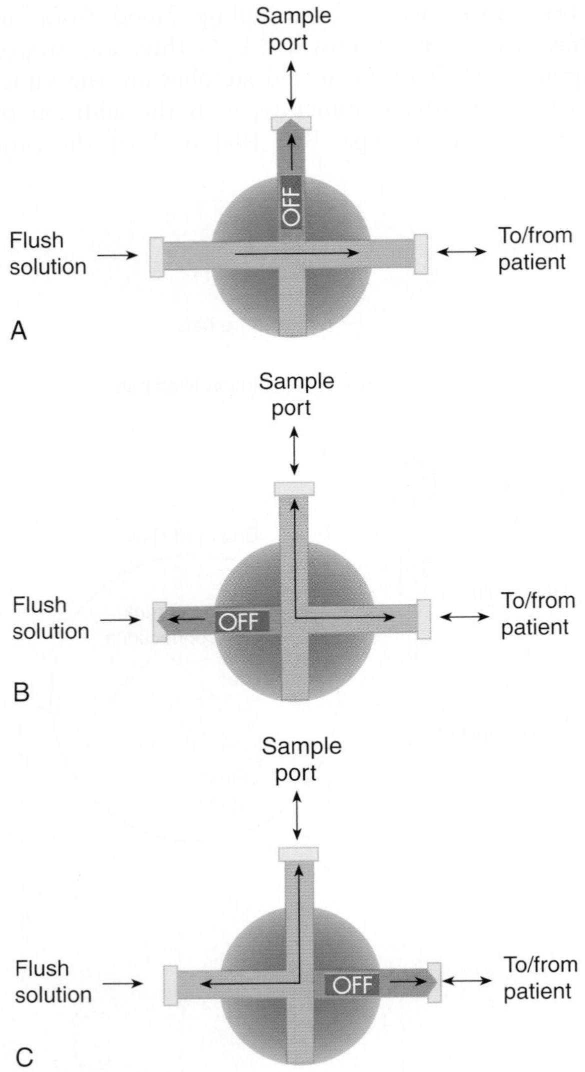

FIGURE 18-5 A three-way stopcock in a vascular line system showing the various positions used. **A,** Normal operating position, with flush solution going to the patient and the sample port closed. **B,** Position to draw a blood sample from the vascular line (closed to flush solution). **C,** Position to flush sample port (closed to patient). In any intermediary position, all ports are closed.

procedure for taking an arterial blood sample from a three-way stopcock system.

The procedure is slightly different when obtaining mixed venous blood samples from PA catheters because PA catheters have separate sampling and intravenous infusion ports and a balloon at the tip is used to measure pulmonary capillary wedge pressure. The clinician must ensure that the balloon is deflated and withdraw the sample slowly (e.g., approximately 3 ml/min or 1 ml in 20 seconds). If the clinician fails to deflate the balloon or withdraws the sample too quickly, the venous blood may be "contaminated" with blood from the pulmonary capillaries. The result is always a falsely high O_2 level. In addition, close attention must be paid to the infusion rate through the catheter. Rapid flow of IV fluid can dilute the blood sample and affect O_2 content measurements.

Problem Solving and Troubleshooting. With the exception of venous admixture, the preanalytic errors that occur when sampling blood from a vascular line are the same as the errors that occur with intermittent puncture, as are the ways to avoid them. For clinicians, the challenge with vascular lines is to maintain their function properly and troubleshoot the many potential problems that can occur. Because these are key components of bedside monitoring skills, they are discussed in the section on hemodynamics in Chapter 46.

Box 18-4 Procedure for Sampling Arterial Blood from an Indwelling Catheter

- Check the medical record to affirm order (as per arterial puncture).
- Confirm steady-state conditions (20-30 minutes after changes).
- Obtain and assemble needed equipment and supplies.
- Wash hands and don barrier protection (e.g., gloves, eyewear).
- Identify the patient using current patient safety standards.
- Explain the procedure to the patient.
- Attach the waste syringe to the stopcock port.
- Position the stopcock so that blood flows into the syringe and the IV bag port is closed.
- Aspirate at least 1-2 ml, or five to six times the tubing volume, of fluid or blood.
- Reposition the stopcock handle to close off all ports.
- Disconnect and properly discard waste syringe.
- Attach new heparinized syringe to the sampling port.
- Position the stopcock so that blood flows into the sample syringe and the IV bag port is closed.
- Fill syringe with 1 ml of blood.
- Reposition the stopcock handle to close off the sampling port and open the IV bag port.
- Disconnect the syringe, expel air bubbles from sample, and cap or plug the syringe.
- Flush the line and stopcock with the IV solution.
- Mix the sample by rolling and inverting the syringe.
- Confirm that the stopcock port is open to the IV bag solution and catheter.
- Confirm undampened pulse pressure waveform on the monitor graphic display.
- Place the sample in a transport container (ice slush) if specimen is not to be analyzed within 10-30 minutes.
- Dispose of waste materials properly.
- Document the procedure and patient status in the chart and on the specimen label.

IV, Intravenous.

Capillary Blood Gases

Capillary blood gas sampling is used as an alternative to direct arterial access in infants and small children. Properly obtained capillary blood from a well-perfused patient can accurately reflect and provide clinically useful estimates of arterial pH and PCO_2 levels.[6] However, capillary PO_2 is of no value in estimating arterial oxygenation, and O_2 saturation by pulse oximetry must also be evaluated when a capillary blood gas sample is obtained. Respiratory therapists (RTs) must exercise extreme caution when using capillary blood gases to guide clinical decisions. Direct arterial access is still the preferred approach for assessing gas exchange in infants and small children with severe acute respiratory failure.

Capillary blood values are meaningful only if the sample site is properly warmed. Warming the skin (to approximately 42° C) causes dilation of the underlying blood vessels, which increases capillary flow well above tissue needs. Blood gas values resemble the values in the arterial circulation; this is why a sample obtained from a warmed capillary site is often referred to as **arterialized blood.** It has been shown that capillary blood samples from the earlobe reflect arterial PCO_2 and PO_2 better than samples drawn from a finger stick.[11] The posterior medial or lateral curvature of the heel is the recommended site for capillary puncture specimens in infants less than 1 month old to avoid nerve and bone damage.

To guide practitioners in providing quality care, the AARC has published Clinical Practice Guideline: Capillary Blood Gas Sampling for Neonatal and Pediatric Patients.[12] Modified excerpts from the AARC guideline appear in Clinical Practice Guideline 18-2.

Equipment. Equipment needed for capillary blood sampling includes a lancet, preheparinized glass or plastic capillary tubes, small metal stirrer bar (metal flea), a magnet, clay or wax sealant or caps, gauze or cotton balls, bandages, ice, gloves, skin antiseptic, warming pads (42° C), sharps container, and labeling materials.

Procedure. Box 18-5 outlines the basic procedure for capillary blood sampling. The most common site for sampling is the heel, specifically the lateral aspect of the plantar surface.

Problem Solving and Troubleshooting. Sampling of capillary blood is useful for patient management only if the procedure is performed according to an established quality assurance program. The most common technical errors in capillary sampling are inadequate warming of the capillary bed and squeezing of the puncture site. Squeezing the puncture site may result in venous and lymphatic contamination of the sample.[13]

Both errors invalidate the test results. Other preanalytic errors are essentially the same as the errors described for arterial puncture. Because of the small sample volume (75 to 100 mcl or 0.075 to 0.1 ml) and collection tube size, the clinician must ensure an adequate sample collection while avoiding air contamination and clotting.

Analyzing

The primary **analytes** or parameters of pH, PCO_2, and PO_2 in a blood sample are measured with a blood gas analyzer. Typically, analyzers use these measures to compute several secondary values, such as plasma bicarbonate, base excess or deficit, and Hb saturation. If actual measurement of total Hb saturation (oxyhemoglobin [HbO_2], methemoglobin [metHb], and carboxyhemoglobin [HbCO]) is required, the sample usually must be analyzed separately using hemoximetry (see p. 401). Some analyzers combine the blood gas and hemoximetry measurements, which may require a larger sample size (usually 100 mcl).

Blood gas analysis and hemoximetry are moderately complex laboratory procedures. Clinicians performing these tests must have documented training and must demonstrate proficiency in performing the procedures, preventive maintenance, troubleshooting, and instrument calibration. In addition, clinicians must be skilled in validating test results using rigorous **quality control** methods.[14]

To guide practitioners in providing quality care, the AARC has published Clinical Practice Guideline: Blood Gas Analysis and Hemoximetry.[15] Related recommendations have been published by the National Committee for Clinical Laboratory Standards.[9] Modified excerpts from the AARC guideline appear in Clinical Practice Guideline 18-3.

Box 18-5 Procedure for Capillary Blood Sampling

- Check the chart (as per arterial puncture).
- Confirm steady-state conditions (20-30 minutes after changes).
- Obtain and assemble necessary equipment and supplies.
- Wash hands and don barrier protection (e.g., gloves, eyewear).
- Select site (e.g., heel, earlobe, great toe, finger).
- Warm site to 42° C for 10 minutes using a compress, heat lamp, or commercial hot pack.
- Clean skin with an antiseptic solution.
- Puncture the skin (<2.5 mm) with the lancet.
- Wipe away the first drop of blood and observe free flow (do not squeeze).
- Fill the sample tube from the middle of the blood drop until it is completely full (75-100 mcl).
- Place the metal flea in the capillary tube, and then seal the tube ends.
- Tape sterile cotton or a bandage over the puncture wound.
- Mix the sample by moving the magnet back and forth along the capillary tube.
- Sample should be immediately chilled or analyzed within 10-15 minutes if left at room temperature.
- Dispose of waste materials properly.
- Document the procedure and patient status in the chart and on the specimen label.

18-2

Capillary Blood Gas Sampling for Neonatal and Pediatric Patients

AARC Clinical Practice Guideline (Excerpts)*

■ INDICATIONS

Capillary blood gas sampling is indicated when:

- ABG analysis is indicated, but arterial access is unavailable
- Noninvasive monitor readings (e.g., $PtcCO_2$: $P_{ET}CO_2$, SpO_2) are abnormal
- Assessment of initiation, administration, or change in therapy (e.g., mechanical ventilation) is indicated
- A change in patient status is detected by history or physical assessment
- Monitoring the severity and progression of a documented disease process is desirable

■ CONTRAINDICATIONS

Capillary punctures should not be performed at or through the following:

- The posterior curvature of the heel (because it can puncture the bone)
- The heel of a patient who has begun walking and has callus development
- The fingers of neonates (because it can cause nerve damage)
- Previous puncture sites
- Inflamed, swollen, or edematous tissues
- Cyanotic or poorly perfused tissues
- Localized areas of infection
- Peripheral arteries

Capillary punctures should not be performed:

- On patients less than 24 hours old (because of poor peripheral perfusion)
- When there is a need for direct analysis of oxygenation
- When there is a need for direct analysis of arterial blood

Relative contraindications include:

- Peripheral vasoconstriction
- Polycythemia (caused by shorter clotting times)
- Hypotension

■ PRECAUTIONS AND POSSIBLE COMPLICATIONS

- Contamination and infection of the patient, including calcaneus osteomyelitis and cellulitis
- Inappropriate patient management may result from reliance on capillary PO_2 value
- Inadvertent puncture or incision and consequent infection
- Tibial artery laceration (puncture of posterior sample of medial aspect of heel)
- Burns
- Hematoma
- Bone calcification
- Nerve damage
- Bruising
- Scarring
- Pain
- Bleeding

■ ASSESSMENT OF NEED

Capillary blood gas sampling is an intermittent procedure and should be performed only when a documented need exists and arterial access is unavailable or contraindicated. Documented need exists in response to initiation, administration, or change in therapy and is determined by history and physical assessment or results of noninvasive respiratory monitoring.

■ MONITORING

The following should be monitored and documented in the medical record as part of the capillary sampling procedure:

- FiO_2 or prescribed oxygen flow
- Appearance of puncture site
- Oxygen modality or ventilator settings
- Complications or adverse reactions to the procedure
- Ease or difficulty of obtaining the sample
- Results of blood gas analysis
- Free flow of blood, without the necessity for "milking"
- Patient's temperature, respiratory rate, position or level of the foot or finger to obtain a sample of activity, and clinical appearance
- Presence or absence of air or clot in the sample
- Date, time, and sampling site
- Noninvasive monitoring values (e.g., SpO_2)

For the complete guideline, see American Association for Respiratory Care: Clinical practice guideline: capillary blood gas sampling for neonatal and pediatric patients. Respir Care 46:506, 2001.

18-3 Blood Gas Analysis and Hemoximetry

AARC Clinical Practice Guideline (Excerpts)*

■ INDICATIONS

- The need to evaluate the adequacy of a patient's ventilation ($PaCO_2$), oxygenation (PaO_2 and HbO_2), or acid-base balance (pH, $PaCO_2$, HCO_3^-)
- The need to quantify the response to therapeutic intervention (e.g., oxygen therapy, mechanical ventilation) or diagnostic evaluation (e.g., exercise desaturation)
- The need to monitor the severity and progression of documented disease processes

■ CONTRAINDICATIONS

Contraindications to pH and blood gas analysis and hemoximetry include the following:

- An improperly functioning analyzer
- An analyzer for which the performance has not been validated by quality control or proficiency testing procedures
- Any specimen gathered with *known* or suspected preanalytic errors (e.g., air contamination, improper anticoagulation, improper storage or handling)
- An incomplete requisition that precludes adequate interpretation and documentation of results
- An inadequately labeled specimen lacking the patient's full name or other unique identifier, such as the medical record number, date, and time of sampling

■ PRECAUTIONS AND POSSIBLE COMPLICATIONS

- Infection of specimen handler from blood (HIV, hepatitis B, other blood-borne pathogens)
- Inappropriate patient medical treatment based on an improperly analyzed blood specimen, on analysis of an unacceptable specimen, or on incorrect reporting of results

■ ASSESSMENT OF NEED

Presence of the above-listed indications in a patient to be tested supports the need for sampling and analysis.

■ FREQUENCY

The frequency with which pH–blood gas analysis is repeated (on different samples from the same patient) should depend on the clinical status of the patient and not on an arbitrarily designated time or frequency. The frequency of reanalysis of single specimens depends on laboratory protocol and technologist suspicion that preliminary results may not reflect the clinical status of the patient (e.g., because of preanalytic or instrument error).

■ MONITORING

The following aspects of analysis should be monitored, and corrective action should be taken as indicated:

- Presence of air bubbles or clots in the specimen, with evacuation before mixing and sealing the syringe
- Assurance that a continuous sample is aspirated (or injected) into the analyzer and that all the electrodes are covered by the sample (confirmed by direct visualization if possible)
- Assurance that 8-hour quality control and calibration procedures have been completed and that instrumentation is functioning properly before patient sample analysis
- Assurance that the specimen was properly labeled, stored, and analyzed within an acceptable period
- Participation in an accredited (recognized) proficiency testing program
- As part of any quality assurance program, indicators must be developed to monitor potential sources of error:
  - There must be evidence of active review of quality control; proficiency testing; and physician alert, or "panic values" on a level commensurate with the number of tests performed
  - Personnel who do not meet acceptable performance thresholds should not be allowed to participate independently further, until they have received remedial instruction and have been reevaluated

**For the complete guideline, see American Association for Respiratory Care: Clinical practice guideline: in vitro pH and blood gas analysis and hemoximetry. Respir Care 46:498, 2001.*

Instrumentation

Many instrumentation companies manufacture laboratory blood gas analyzers. Although available in a range of designs, these devices typically share the following key components:

- Operator interface (e.g., operating controls, light-emitting diode [LED] or cathode ray tube [CRT] displays, touch screen keypads, software)
- Measuring chamber incorporating the typical three-electrode system
- Calibrating gas tanks
- Reagent containers (buffers used for calibration, rinse solutions)
- Waste container
- Results display, storage, and transmittal system (e.g., screen, printer, disk storage device, network interface)

Measurement of the three primary parameters—pH, PCO_2, and PO_2—is accomplished using three separate electrodes. To measure PO_2, blood gas analyzers use the Clark polarographic electrode (see Figure 18-1).

The pH electrode consists of two electrodes or half-cells (Figure 18-6). The measuring half-cell contains a silver-silver chloride rod surrounded by a solution of constant pH and enclosed by a pH-sensitive glass membrane. As the sample passes this membrane, the difference in H^+ concentration on either side of the glass changes the potential of the measuring electrode. The reference half-cell (here mercury-mercurous chloride) produces a constant potential, regardless of sample pH. The difference in potential between the two electrodes is proportional to the H^+ concentration of the sample, which is displayed on a voltmeter calibrated in pH units.

To measure PCO_2, blood gas analyzers use the Severinghaus electrode, which is essentially a pH electrode exposed to an electrolyte solution that is in equilibrium with the sample through a CO_2-permeable membrane. As CO_2 diffuses through this membrane into the electrolyte solution, it undergoes the following hydration reaction:

$$CO_2 + H_2O \leftrightarrow H_2CO_3 \leftrightarrow H^+ + HCO_3^-$$

The greater the partial pressure of CO_2, the more H^+ produced by this reaction, and the more pH of the electrolyte solution changes. The measuring electrode detects the pH change as a change in electrical potential, which is proportional to the PCO_2 of the sample.

In addition to electrochemical electrodes, a sensor technology based on optical fluorescence and the process of photoluminescence is available to measure pH, PCO_2, and PO_2. **Optical fluorescence** sensors use fluorescent dyes that are illuminated with light of a specific wavelength. The illuminating light is transmitted, reflected, absorbed, and reemitted to varying degrees depending on the concentration of O_2, CO_2, and hydrogen ions. These photochemical alterations in light illumination are used to calculate pH, PCO_2, and PO_2 values. Compared with electrochemical sensors, optical sensors do not require electrical connections, making them less affected by electrical interference and drift. The sensor reactions are reversible so that the analyte is not consumed. These features make them easier to miniaturize for intravascular measurement of blood gases.[16,17]

Procedure

To provide accurate and clinically useful data, blood gas analysis must be performed as follows:

- On a sample free of preanalytic errors
- With a properly functioning analyzer (validated by quality control procedures)
- Using a procedure that follows the manufacturer's recommendations

Prior discussion addressed how to avoid preanalytic errors. Subsequent discussion focuses on blood gas quality control and key elements involved in the analysis procedure.

Box 18-6 outlines the steps commonly used in most established procedures for laboratory blood gas analysis. One should always refer to the manufacturer's literature for the particular steps to use with a specific analyzer.

Rigorous application of U.S. Centers for Disease Control and Prevention (CDC) standard precautions is essential. In addition, the Occupational Safety and Health Administration (OSHA) requires personnel to wear gloves when handling all laboratory specimens. Although splashes are rare during analysis, some manufacturers provide extra protection by mounting splash shields on their instruments. If splashes are anticipated, the operator can wear a face shield.

Waste fluids are potentially infectious and should be handled as if they were blood samples. In addition, the National Committee for Clinical Laboratory Standards recommends adding a strong disinfectant, such as 2% glutaraldehyde or a 1:4 solution of sodium hypochlorite, to

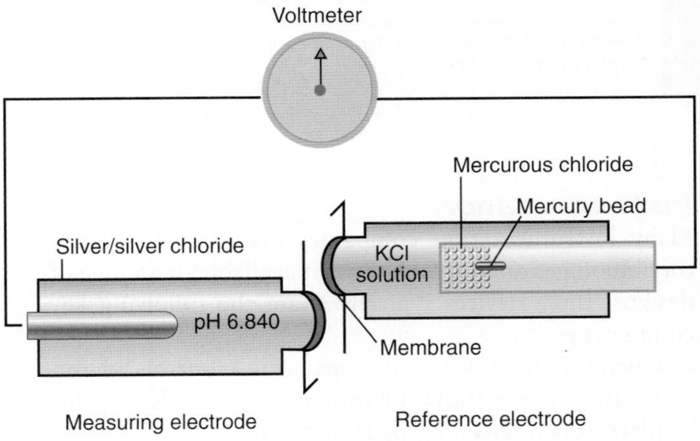

FIGURE 18-6 Blood gas analyzer pH electrode system, consisting of both a measurement and a reference electrode. (Modified from Shapiro BA, Peruzzi WT, Kozelowski-Templin R: Clinical application of blood gases, ed 5, St Louis, 1994, Mosby.)

Box 18-6 Basic Procedure for Analyzing a Blood Gas Sample

- Apply standard precautions.
- Confirm that the instrument and its electrodes are operating properly.
- Identify the specimen, and confirm all relevant information provided on the request slip.
- Note the time at which the sample was obtained (discard sample if >60 minutes has passed).
- Inspect the sample for obvious signs of preanalytic error (e.g., air bubbles, gross dilution, clotting, air exposure).
- Mix the sample (critical for Hb and hematocrit measurements).
- Uncap the syringe, and expel and discard a drop or two of blood from the syringe tip.
- Introduce the sample (manually or by automatic aspiration).
- Confirm the readings.
- Remove the syringe and clear the system.
- Dispose of waste materials properly.
- Transmit the results.
- Contact the responsible clinician if the results warrant.

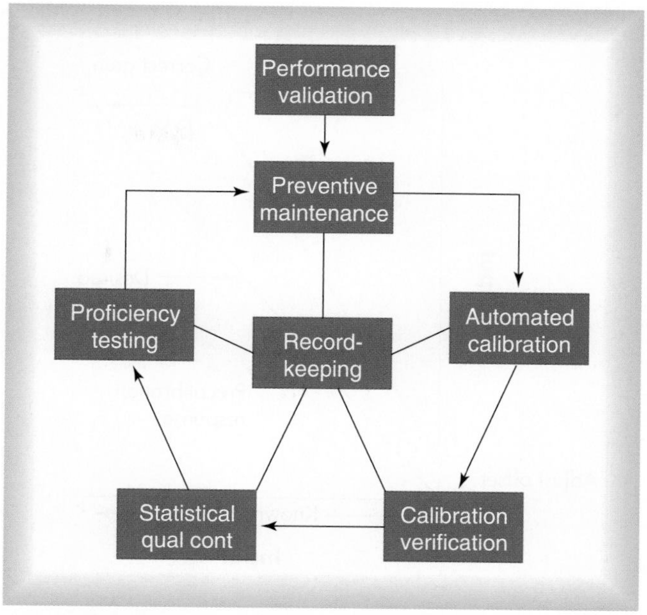

FIGURE 18-7 Blood gas analysis quality control program. (Data from Kozelowski-Templin R: Blood gas analyzers. Respir Care Clin North Am 1:35–46, 1995.)

the waste container of the instrument either during use or before disposal.

Quality Assurance

Quality patient care depends on consistently accurate blood gas results. Modern laboratory analyzers are often automated, computer-controlled, self-calibrating systems. This sophistication has led to the false assumption that accurate results are "automatic," with clinicians needing only to input the sample properly and record the results. Nothing could be further from the truth. As with all diagnostic laboratory procedures, the accuracy of blood gas testing depends on rigorous quality control.

The Clinical Laboratory Standards Institute (CLSI), formerly the National Committee for Clinical Laboratory Standards (NCCLS), establishes guidelines and standards for blood gas analysis and quality assurance. Government regulatory agencies collaborate to update the Clinical Laboratory Improvement Amendments (CLIA) that establish proficiency testing requirements.[18] Although an in-depth review of laboratory quality control is beyond the scope of this text, all RTs must understand the key elements.[19]

Figure 18-7 depicts the key components of laboratory quality control. A brief description of each element follows.

Recordkeeping. Meticulous recordkeeping and clearly written and comprehensive policies and procedures are the hallmark of a comprehensive quality control program. Both statutory law and professional accreditation requirements emphasize this component as the basis for demonstrating and ensuring quality.

Performance Validation. Performance validation is the process of testing a new instrument to confirm a manufacturer's claims. Typically, this process involves using samples with known values to assess both the accuracy (comparing the value from the tested instrument with a known value) and the **precision** (examining the repeatability of results) of the instrument.

Preventive Maintenance and Function Checks. Many components used in blood gas analyzers, such as filters, membranes, electrolyte solution, and single-test and multitest cartridges, have a limited life and can deteriorate, be consumed, or fail over time, resulting in faulty analysis. The best way to avoid these problems is to schedule regular preventive maintenance. Preventive maintenance should include scheduled parts replacement and routine function tests, as recommended by the manufacturer.

Automated Calibration. Calibration is the only fully automated element of blood gas quality control. Blood gas analyzers regularly calibrate themselves by adjusting the output signal of each electrode when exposed to media having known values. In most units, the media used to calibrate the gas electrodes are precision mixtures of O_2 and CO_2. For the pH electrode, standard pH buffer solutions are used. **Calibration media** must meet the requirements set by nationally recognized standards organizations. Users are responsible for ensuring that calibration media are properly stored and that in-use life and expiration dates are strictly enforced.

Calibration is performed to ensure that the output of the analyzer is both accurate and linear across the range of

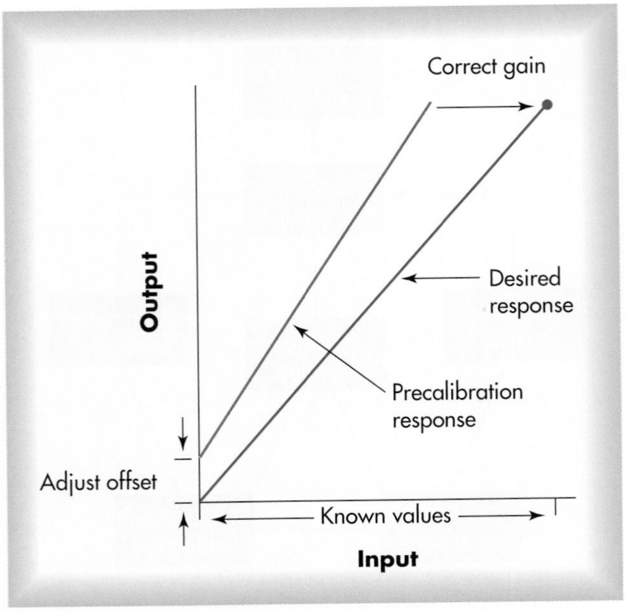

FIGURE 18-8 Two-point calibration procedure. (Modified from Chatburn RL: Fundamentals of metrology: evaluation of instrument error and method agreement. In Kacmarek RM, Hess D, Stoller JK, editors: Monitoring in respiratory care, St Louis, 1993, Mosby.)

measured values. Parameters must be measured with known input values representing at least two points, usually a low and a high value. Figure 18-8 shows a typical two-point calibration procedure. In this example, the instrument's initial precalibration response indicates that the output readings are consistently higher than the actual input, with this positive **bias** worsening at higher levels. Calibration is performed first by adjusting the offset (or balance) of the instrument so that the low output equals the low input (in this case zero). Next, the gain (or slope) of the device is adjusted to ensure that the high output equals the high input. When both offset and gain are adjusted against known inputs, the instrument is properly calibrated and can undergo calibration verification with control samples.

Calibration Verification by Control Media. Calibration verification establishes and periodically confirms the validity of blood gas analyzer results. Calibration verification requires analysis of at least three materials with known values spanning the entire range of values expected for clinical samples. Ideally, these materials, called *controls,* should mimic real blood samples chemically and physically. Because requirements for use of control media currently vary among regulatory agencies, users should consult the applicable regulations directly. As a general recommendation, at least two levels of control media should be analyzed during every 8-hour shift. Rotation among the three levels should ensure that all three levels are analyzed at least once every 24 hours.

MINI CLINI

Blood Gas Quality Control

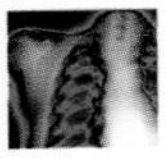

PROBLEM: The RT is responsible for the quality control of a blood gas analyzer in the intensive care unit. Using control media for calibration verification, he notes that the readings on the "high PCO_2" control have increased progressively over the last four quality control analyses from 60 ± 1 SD mm Hg to 66 ± 1 SD mm Hg. What is the likely problem, and what actions should the RT take?

SOLUTION: The observed problem indicates a trending, or systematic, error (bias). If the analyzer solutions and calibrating gases have not been changed during the error period, the likely problem is component failure—probably the PCO_2 electrode. The electrode should be checked, and any faulty components should be replaced.

Internal Statistical Quality Control. Internal quality control takes calibration verification a step further by applying statistical and rule-based procedures (Westgard rules)[20,21] to help detect, respond to, and correct instrument error. In one common approach, the results of control media analyses are plotted on a graph and compared with statistically derived limits, usually ±2 standard deviation (SD) ranges (Figure 18-9). Control results that fall outside these limits indicate analytic error.

There are two categories of analytic error: (1) **random error** and (2) **systematic error.** Random error is observed when sporadic, out-of-range data points occur (see Figure 18-9, point *A*). Random errors are errors of precision or, more precisely, **imprecision.** Conversely, either a trending or an abrupt shift in data points outside the statistical limits (see Figure 18-9, point *B*) is sometimes observed. This phenomenon is called *systematic error* or sometimes *bias.* Bias plus imprecision equals total instrument error, or *inaccuracy.* Table 18-3 outlines the major factors causing these two types of error and suggests some common corrective actions.

External Quality Control (Proficiency Testing). The federal government mandated a rigorous program of external quality control for analytic laboratories. CLIA were established in 1988. To meet these standards, analytic laboratories must undergo regular proficiency testing designed to evaluate their operating procedures and the competence of their personnel.[22] **Proficiency testing** requires analysis and reporting on externally provided control media with unknown values, usually three times per year, with five samples per test. There are many CLIA-approved proficiency testing providers.[23] A commonly used provider is the College of American Pathologists (CAP) proficiency testing survey. Proficiency testing survey analyses must be performed along with the regular workload by the personnel

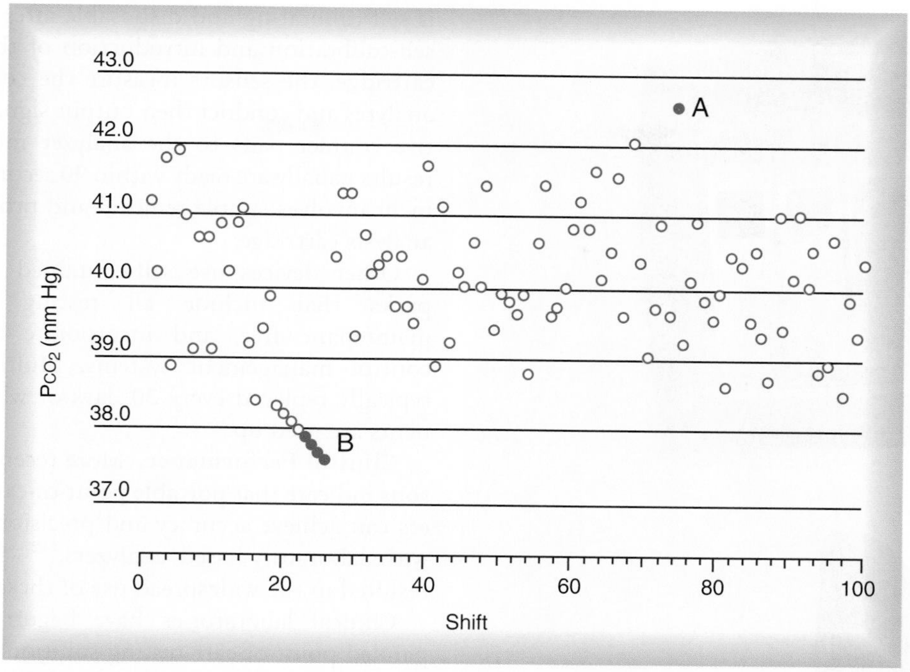

FIGURE 18-9 Schematic representation of a quality control plot for PCO_2. The horizontal axis depicts time. *White circles* represent values within 2 standard deviations of the mean; *blue circles* represent values outside 2 standard deviations of the mean. Point *A* represents a random error; point *B* represents systematic errors. (Modified from Shapiro BA, Peruzzi WT, Kozelowski-Templin R: Clinical application of blood gases, ed 5, St Louis, 1994, Mosby.)

TABLE 18-3

Correction of Analytic Errors

Error Type	Common Contributing Factors	Common Corrective Actions
Imprecision (random) errors	Statistical probability Sample contamination Sample mishandling	Rerun control Repeat analysis on different instrument
Bias (systematic) errors	Contaminated buffers Incorrect gas concentrations Incorrect procedures Component failure	Perform function check of suspected problem area Repair or replace failed components

routinely responsible for testing, following the laboratory's standard testing practices.

Criteria for acceptable performance specify a range around a target value, such as ±0.04 for pH. A single incidence of unsatisfactory performance requires documentation of remedial action. Multiple or recurring incidences of poor performance can result in severe sanctions, including suspension of Medicare and Medicaid reimbursement or the loss of the laboratory's operating license and accreditation.

Remedial Action. Remedial action is the ongoing process of applying appropriate measures to correct errors identified through the quality assurance cycle. Analytic errors include calibration and internal quality control failures, actual sample errors, and unsatisfactory proficiency test results. A comprehensive quality assurance program also tries to identify and correct both preanalytic and postanalytic errors, such as clerical misreporting.

Examples of remedial action include procedural changes, staff training and retraining, closer supervision, and more frequent preventive maintenance checks. The remedial action chosen should be appropriate for the identified problem. As with all other components of the process, meticulous documentation is necessary.

Point-of-Care Testing

Point-of-care testing takes blood gas analysis from the specialized laboratory to the patient's bedside.[24] Point-of-care testing reduces turnaround time, which should improve care and reduce costs. Theoretically, cost savings can be accrued by eliminating delays in therapy, decreasing patient length of stay in the hospital and emergency

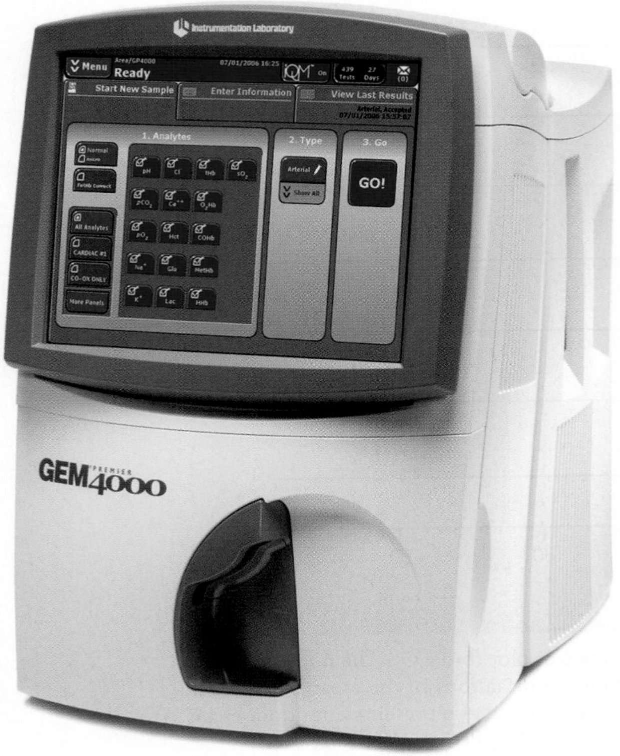

FIGURE 18-10 GEM Premier 4000 critical care analyzer for blood gas, electrolyte, metabolite, and integrated cooximetry testing; the device also performs continuous automated quality assurance. (Courtesy Instrumentation Laboratory, Bedford, MA.)

department.[25] Additional cost savings may occur if point-of-care testing decreases the need for specialized laboratory personnel. Point-of-care testing is used increasingly in the hospital and physician office settings.[26]

Instrumentation. Figure 18-10 shows a typical point-of-care blood gas analyzer (GEM 4000; Instrumentation Laboratory, Bedford, MA). In addition to blood gas analysis, such devices can be used to measure several chemistry and hematology parameters, including serum electrolytes, blood glucose levels, blood urea nitrogen, hematocrit, hemoximetry, lactate, bilirubin, and prothrombin and partial thromboplastin times.

These devices are portable, and some can perform 900 tests on a single set of batteries. They typically include a display screen for accessing menu functions and viewing results. Most devices include a simple keypad or touch screen for data and command entry. Analysis occurs using disposable cartridges or inside a chamber in the body of the unit.

Some devices employ single-use sample cartridges that differ according to the array of tests being performed. Each cartridge contains the necessary calibration solution, a sample handling system, a waste chamber, and miniaturized electrochemical or photochemical sensors. The cartridge system requires no operator oversight because it is self-calibrating and disposable after a single use. After self-calibration and introduction of the sample into the cartridge, the sensors measure the concentration of the analytes and conduct their output signal through conductive contact pads to the analyzer microprocessor. Test results usually are ready within 90 seconds. Waste management involves simple removal and proper disposal of the analysis cartridge.

Other devices use self-contained multiuse cartridge packs that include all testing components, are maintenance-free, and incorporate automated quality control management systems. Multiuse cartridges are typically replaced every 30 days or when testing components are used up.

Clinical Performance. More recent method comparisons indicate that portable point-of-care blood gas analyzers can achieve accuracy and precision levels comparable with laboratory-based analyzers.[14,27] Such findings have resulted in the widespread use of these systems.

Clinical laboratories have begun implementing expanded point-of-care testing solutions to improve operational costs, streamline workflow in the clinical laboratory and critical care setting, and provide blood analysis results more quickly.[28,29] Guidelines for providers who are considering adoption of this new technology have been published in the clinical laboratory literature.[30]

BLOOD GAS MONITORING

A blood gas monitor is a bedside tool (usually dedicated to a single patient) that can provide measurements either continuously or at appropriate intervals without permanently removing blood from the patient. Four systems are in current clinical use: (1) transcutaneous blood gas monitor, (2) intraarterial **(in vivo)** blood gas monitor, (3) extraarterial **(ex vivo)** blood gas monitor, and (4) tissue O_2 monitor.

Transcutaneous Blood Gas Monitoring

Transcutaneous blood gas monitoring provides continuous, noninvasive estimates of arterial PO_2 and PCO_2 through a surface skin sensor. As with capillary sampling, the device arterializes the underlying blood by heating the skin. Warming also increases the permeability of the skin to O_2 and CO_2, which allows them to diffuse more readily from the capillaries to the sensor, where they are measured as transcutaneous partial pressures ($PtcO_2$ and $PtcCO_2$).

Numerous factors influence the agreement between arterial blood and transcutaneous gas measurements, with O_2 levels being affected most. The two most important factors are age and perfusion status. Table 18-4 summarizes these relationships using the ratio of $PtcO_2$ to PaO_2. A ratio of 1 : 1 indicates "perfect" agreement between $PtcO_2$ and PaO_2. As can be seen, this level of agreement occurs only in neonates.

TABLE 18-4

Ratios Correlating $PtcO_2$ With PaO_2

Age Group	$PtcO_2/PaO_2$ Ratio	Perfusion Status	$PtcO_2/PaO_2$
Premature infants	1.14:1	Stable	0.79:1
Neonates	1.00:1	Moderate shock	0.48:1
Children	0.84:1	Severe shock	0.12:1
Adults	0.79:1		
Older adults	0.68:1		

From Tobin MJ: Respiratory monitoring. JAMA 264:244–251, 1990.

In terms of age, the younger the patient, the better is the agreement between PaO_2 and $PtcO_2$; this is mainly because of age-related differences in skin composition. With regard to perfusion status, PaO_2 and $PtcO_2$ are similar only in patients with normal cardiac output and fluid balance because accurate transcutaneous measures require adequate skin perfusion. Low cardiac output, shock, and dehydration all cause peripheral vasoconstriction and impair capillary flow, which decreases the $PtcO_2$ level. Some clinicians use $PtcO_2$ not to monitor oxygenation as a surrogate for PaO_2 but to assess blood flow changes during procedures such as vascular surgery and resuscitation.

Agreement between $PaCO_2$ and $PtcCO_2$ is better because CO_2 is more diffusible. $PaCO_2$ changes of 5 mm Hg can be monitored or "trended" by transcutaneous blood gas analysis.

Based on these factors, $PtcCO_2$ monitoring is a reasonable choice when there is a need for continuous, noninvasive analysis of trends in ventilation and $PaCO_2$. In hemodynamically stable infants and children, PaO_2 can be "correlated" against $PtcO_2$, decreasing the need for repeated arterial samples. Because pulse oximetry cannot provide accurate estimates of excessive blood O_2, the transcutaneous monitor may be useful for monitoring hyperoxia in neonates. However, prevention of hyperoxia in premature neonates is more often achieved by maintaining pulse oximetry saturation between 85% and 93%.[31]

Transcutaneous blood gas monitoring of $PtcCO_2$ can also be useful in adult patients during deep sedation and mechanical ventilation in the emergency department and intensive care unit and during surgery.[32-37] $PtcCO_2$ is a more accurate reflection $PaCO_2$ than both $P_{ET}CO_2$ and nasal ETCO2 in intubated and spontaneously breathing adult patients. The use of $PtcCO_2$ in conjunction with pulse oximetry reduces the need for repeated arterial blood gas sampling.[38]

To guide practitioners in providing quality care, the AARC has published Clinical Practice Guideline: Transcutaneous Blood Gas Monitoring for Neonatal and Pediatric Patients.[39] Modified excerpts from the AARC guideline appear in Clinical Practice Guidelines 18-4.

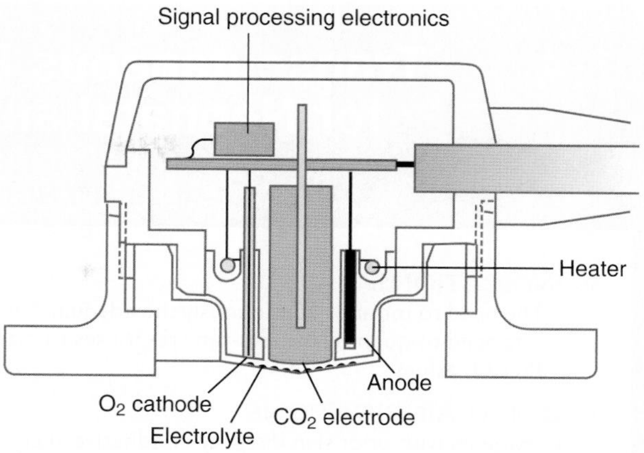

FIGURE 18-11 Schematic diagram of transcutaneous O_2-CO_2 sensor. (Modified from Mahutte CK, Michiels TM, Hassell KT, et al: Evaluation of a single transcutaneous PO_2-PCO_2 sensor in adult patients. Crit Care Med 12:1063–1066, 1984.)

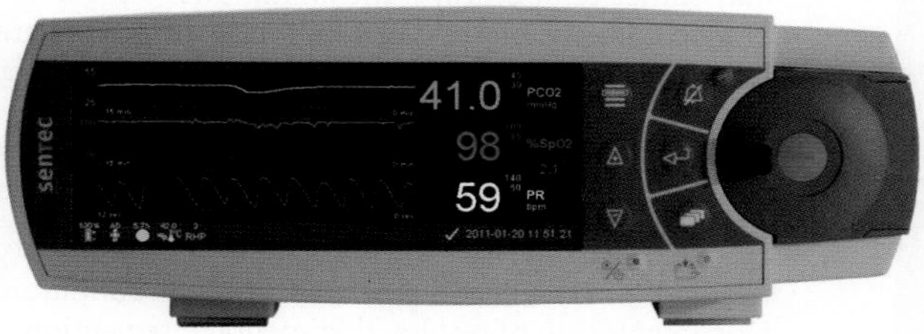

FIGURE 18-12 SenTec Digital Monitoring System, combined $PtcCO_2$ and SpO_2 sensor suitable for neonatal, pediatric, and adult patients. (Courtesy SenTec AG, Therwil, Switzerland.)

Instrumentation

Figure 18-11 shows a simplified diagram of a transcutaneous blood gas monitor sensor. Included are a heating element and two electrodes, one for O_2 and one for CO_2. These electrodes are similar in design to the electrodes found in bench-top analyzers. However, instead of measuring gas tensions in a blood sample, transcutaneous electrodes measure PO_2 and PCO_2 in an electrolyte gel between the sensor and the skin. When properly set up, the response time for these electrodes is 20 to 30 seconds, a bit slower than the response time for pulse oximetry.

Figure 18-12 shows a transcutaneous monitor with digital signal processing. A Severinghaus-type $PtcCO_2$ electrode and two-wavelength reflectance SpO_2 are combined into a single sensor. The sensor can be applied to the skin surface in neonates and infants or to the earlobe of pediatric and adult patients for combined noninvasive monitoring of ventilation and oxygenation.

Procedure

Box 18-7 outlines the basic procedure for setting up a transcutaneous blood gas monitor. The most common sites for electrode placement in infants and children are the abdomen, chest, and lower back. Once the electrodes are properly set up, the clinician should compare the

18-4 Transcutaneous Blood Gas Monitoring for Neonatal and Pediatric Patients

AARC Clinical Practice Guideline (Excerpts)*

INDICATIONS

- The need to monitor continuously the adequacy of arterial oxygenation or ventilation
- The need to quantify the real-time responses to diagnostic and therapeutic interventions, as evidenced by $PtcO_2$ or $PtcCO_2$ values

CONTRAINDICATIONS

In patients with poor skin integrity or adhesive allergy, transcutaneous monitoring may be relatively contraindicated.

PRECAUTIONS AND POSSIBLE COMPLICATIONS

- False-negative or false-positive results may lead to inappropriate treatment.
- Tissue injury (e.g., erythema, blisters, burns, skin tears) may occur at the measuring site.

ASSESSMENT OF NEED

- When direct measurement of arterial blood is unavailable or not readily accessible, $PtcO_2$ or $PtcCO_2$ measurements may suffice temporarily if the limitations of the data are appreciated.
- Transcutaneous blood gas monitoring is appropriate for continuous and prolonged monitoring (e.g., during mechanical ventilation, continuous positive airway pressure [CPAP], and supplemental oxygen administration) of infants and children.
- $PtcO_2$ values can be used for diagnostic purposes, such as in the assessment of functional shunts or in determining the response to oxygen challenge in the assessment of congenital heart disease.

ASSESSMENT OF OUTCOME

- Results should reflect the patient's clinical condition (i.e., they should validate the basis for ordering the monitoring).
- Documentation of results, therapeutic intervention (or lack thereof), and clinical decisions based on the transcutaneous measurements should be noted in the medical record.

MONITORING

The schedule of patient and equipment during transcutaneous monitoring should be integrated into assessment of the patient and determination of vital signs. Results should be documented in the patient's medical record and should detail the following conditions:

- Date and time of measurement, transcutaneous reading, patient's position, respiratory rate, and activity level
- Inspired oxygen concentration or supplemental oxygen flow, specifying the type of oxygen delivery device
- Mode of ventilatory support, ventilator, or CPAP settings
- Electrode placement site, electrode temperature, and time of placement
- Results of simultaneously obtained PaO_2, $PaCO_2$, and pH, when available
- Clinical appearance of the patient and subjective assessment of perfusion, pallor, and skin temperature

**For the complete guideline, see American Association for Respiratory Care: Clinical practice guideline: transcutaneous blood gas monitoring for neonatal and pediatric patients. Respir Care 49:1070, 2004.*

monitor readings with the readings obtained with a concurrent ABG. Consistency between values validates monitor performance under the existing conditions. This validation should be repeated anytime the patient's status undergoes a major change. During validation studies of patients with anatomic shunts, the electrode site and arterial sampling site should be on the same "side" of the shunt.

Problem Solving and Troubleshooting

Transcutaneous blood gas monitoring is a complex and labor-intensive activity that requires ongoing training and careful quality control. Table 18-5 lists the major factors that can affect the accuracy or limit the performance of a transcutaneous monitor. In terms of technical limitations, the lengthy stabilization time needed by transcutaneous monitors precludes their use during short procedures or in emergencies. In such cases, the pulse oximeter is a better choice.

Sensors must be calibrated and maintained using methods similar to the methods described for bench-top analyzers. Improper calibration yields erroneous patient information. Improper calibration can be difficult to detect on some systems. Meticulous care of the sensor membranes is also essential for proper maintenance.

Because the sensor is heated, clinicians must take care to avoid thermal injury to the patient's skin. Thermal

Box 18-7 Procedure for Using a Transcutaneous Monitor

- Place the unit at bedside, and provide manufacturer-specified warm-up time.
- Check the membrane to ensure that it is free of bubbles or scratches, and change it if necessary.
- Select the monitoring site by evaluating perfusion, skin thickness, and absence of bones.
- Prepare the sensor with an adhesive ring and electrolyte gel.
- Set the appropriate probe temperature (per the manufacturer's recommendations).
- Prepare the site by removing excess hair and cleaning the skin.
- Securely attach probe to the patient.
- Allow for stabilization time (10-20 minutes).
- Schedule site change time (2-6 hours, depending on patient).
- Set the high and low alarms.
- Monitor and document the results per institutional protocol.
- Change the site at appropriate intervals.
- Validate the reading against ABG values.

From Koff PB, Hess D: Transcutaneous oxygen and carbon dioxide measurements. In Kacmarek RM, Hess D, Stoller JK, editors: Monitoring in respiratory care, St Louis, 1993, Mosby.

MINI CLINI

Selecting a Monitoring System

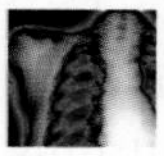

PROBLEM: A neonatologist, concerned about retinopathy of prematurity, asks the RT to set up a noninvasive system to monitor a preterm infant for hyperoxia. What type of system should the RT choose and why?

SOLUTION: Because the neonatologist wants the infant to be monitored for hyperoxia, a system that provides continuous data would be the best choice. Because hyperoxia is best assessed using PO_2 (as opposed to hemoglobin saturation), the RT needs to use a PO_2 electrode system. A transcutaneous PO_2 electrode system would provide the needed measurement noninvasively.

injury can be avoided by (1) careful monitoring of sensor temperature (the safe upper limit is approximately 42° C) and (2) regularly rotating the sensor site.

Proper sensor-electrolyte contact is essential, as is proper application to the skin surface. A loosely applied sensor may have air leaks or may become dislodged. In either case, the resulting measurements would approach those in room air:

$$PO_2 = 159 \text{ mm Hg}$$
$$PCO_2 = 0 \text{ mm Hg}$$

TABLE 18-5
Factors Affecting Transcutaneous Blood Gas Monitors

Technical Factors	Clinical Factors
Labor-intensive, high-skill procedure	Poor perfusion
Lengthy stabilization time	Hyperoxemia
Improper calibration can be difficult to detect	Improper sensor application or placement
Heating required to obtain valid PO_2 results	Use of vasoactive drugs
Proper sensor-electrolyte contact is essential	Variation in skin characteristics

Conversely, excessive pressure on the sensor compresses the underlying capillaries and produces a falsely low $PtcO_2$. Even with proper application and placement, $PtcO_2$ measures can vary by 10% at different sites, with values from the extremities generally being lower than values obtained from the chest or abdomen.[39]

When arterial and transcutaneous blood gas values are inconsistent with each other or with the clinical status of the patient, the clinician should explore possible causes before reporting any results. Often, discrepancies can be reduced by switching the monitoring site or recalibrating the instrument. If these steps fail to resolve the inconsistencies, the clinician should recommend an alternative method for assessing gas exchange, such as pulse oximetry or more frequent ABG analysis.

Intraarterial (In Vivo) Blood Gas Monitoring

Over the past 20 years, the desire for continuous in vivo blood gas analysis has led to remarkable strides in technology. However, the clinical requirements for such systems (Box 18-8) are extremely demanding and have yet to be fully met. Potential benefits of continuous blood gas analysis include real-time monitoring and a reduction in therapeutic decision-making time, less blood loss and the need for transfusion (especially in pediatric patients), lower infection risk to the patient and blood exposure to the health care provider, improved accuracy by reducing preanalytic errors, and elimination of specimen transport.

Early research focused on miniaturized versions of standard blood gas analyzer electrodes. However, problems with instrument drift, fouling of electrode surfaces, wire breakage, current leakage, and corrosion have limited clinical application of these systems. Better success has been achieved using indwelling fiberoptic photochemical sensors, or *optodes.*

Instrumentation

Rather than using electrochemical electrodes, miniaturized optical fluorescence sensors, called **optodes,** measure blood gas parameters by photochemical reactions and changes in the intensity of light transmission through

Box 18-8 Requirements for an Intraarterial Blood Gas Monitor

- Should accurately measure pH, PCO_2, PO_2, and temperature with a rapid response time
- Must operate within a 20-gauge catheter without affecting (1) continuous pressure measurement, (2) blood sampling procedures, (3) routine function of the arterial catheter system
- Must be biocompatible and nonthrombogenic
- Must be simple to operate and maintain
- Should withstand abuse and rigors of clinical conditions common in the intensive care unit and operating room
- Should remain stable and operate consistently for at least 72 hours
- Should not be adversely affected by a reduction in local blood flow or temperature
- Should not be adversely affected by hemodynamic changes
- Should be cost-effective

From Peruzzi WT, Shapiro BA: Blood gas monitors. Respir Care Clin North Am 1:143–156, 1995.

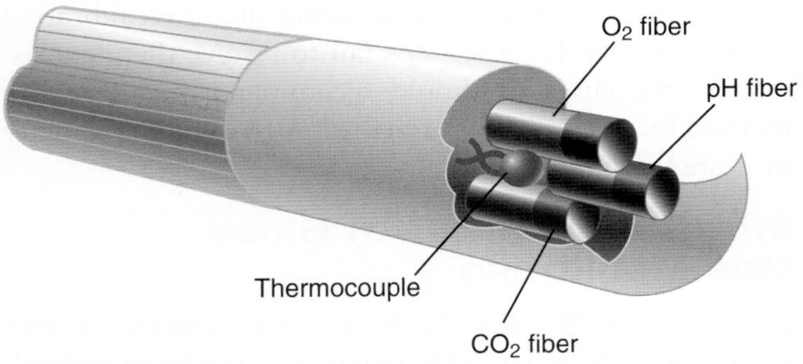

FIGURE 18-13 Simplified diagram of an indwelling optode-based arterial blood gas catheter showing O_2, CO_2, pH, and thermocouple fibers.

optical fibers. Figure 18-13 shows how optodes are combined (with a thermocouple) at the tip of a flexible fiber-optic catheter that is inserted into a peripheral artery. Several optode-based systems have been developed and validated for commercial use for continuous intraarterial blood gas assessment and monitoring of PaO_2 during cardiopulmonary bypass.[40,41]

Clinical Performance and Usefulness

Despite technical improvements, the actual performance of in vivo blood gas monitors falls short of the clinical requirements previously specified. Compared with standard blood gas analysis, accuracy is improved.[42,43] However, concerns about bias in PO_2 measurement,[44] sensor accuracy over extended periods in divergent patient groups,[45] the need for femoral artery insertion because of blood pressure waveform dampening in the radial artery,[46] high acquisition cost of the monitor and sensor catheters, dedication of a monitor to a single patient,[47] and lack of evidence showing an impact on patient care have prevented widespread adoption and use of this technology.

Extraarterial (Ex Vivo) Blood Gas Monitoring

Extraarterial (ex vivo) on-demand blood gas monitoring systems are a logical compromise between bench-top and in vivo blood gas analysis. Ex vivo systems eliminate all the problems associated with indwelling sensors, while still providing quick results. In concept, the only major shortcoming of ex vivo systems is their inability to provide real-time continuous data.

Instrumentation and Procedure

Both optode-based and electrochemical-based systems have been developed. Figure 18-14 depicts an optode-based, ex vivo blood gas monitoring system. The optodes are located in a sensor cassette inserted in-line with the arterial catheter near the patient's wrist. To measure pH, PCO_2, and PO_2, the system is closed to the intravenous fluid source at the stopcock (Figure 18-14, *A*). Subatmospheric pressure is created in the syringe attached to the stopcock (see Figure 18-14, *A*), which functions as an aspirating reservoir (Figure 18-14, *B*); this causes arterial blood to flow into the sensor cassette for analysis. During analysis, the stopcock (see Figure 18-14, *A*) is returned to its original position (off to the aspirating syringe). The connection through the line to the pressure transducer is restored, and blood pressure monitoring is able to continue. Blood gas parameter results are displayed in approximately 1 to 2 minutes. When analysis is complete, the blood sample is returned to the patient by emptying the aspirating reservoir (see Figure 18-14, *B*) and flushing the system through the flow valve (Figure 18-14, *D*).

Clinical Performance and Usefulness

In clinical trials, ex vivo on-demand systems performed as well as laboratory blood gas analyzers in adults, neonates, and infants.[48-50] Measurements could be obtained every 3 to 5 minutes from a peripheral or umbilical artery, and the intermittent errors commonly associated with in vivo systems were not observed. A commercially available system for blood gas monitoring in neonates and infants also incorporates electrolyte, hematocrit, and Hb measurements.[50]

Ex vivo blood gas monitoring systems share many of the requirements, advantages, and disadvantages related to in vivo systems stated in the previous section. Further justification of the costs associated with monitoring weighed against potential patient benefit are needed before widespread use of this technology occurs.

Tissue Oxygen

Tissue O_2 (PtO_2) can be measured by probes inserted directly into organs, tissue, and body fluids. Ease of probe placement and the sensitivity of PtO_2 as an indicator of

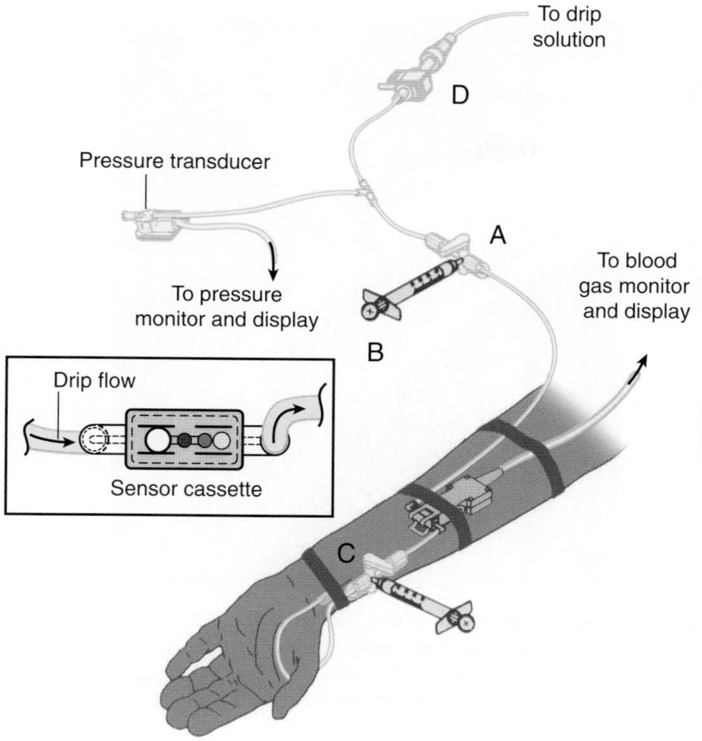

FIGURE 18-14 Schematic representation of an ex vivo blood gas monitoring system in place on a patient. The *inset* depicts a longitudinal section through the sensor cassette showing the three optodes (pH, PCO_2, PO_2) and the thermistor. *A,* "Upstream" stopcock, which permits function of the aspirating reservoir. *B,* Syringe used as an aspirating reservoir. *C,* Stopcock to permit blood sampling. *D,* Tubing flush valve connected to a pressure transducer. (Modified from Shapiro BA, Mahutte CK, Cane RD, et al: Clinical performance of a blood gas monitor: a prospective, multicenter trial. Crit Care Med 21:487–494, 1993.)

tissue perfusion make tissue O_2 monitoring attractive for clinical research applications. Clinical indications for measuring PtO_2 include monitoring brain tissue O_2 as an early sign of ischemia, assessing brain blood flow autoregulation, and monitoring the adequacy of brain perfusion in patients with traumatic brain injury.[51] In patients with traumatic brain injury, brain PtO_2 values when intracranial pressure and cerebral perfusion are normal are between 25 mm Hg and 30 mm Hg. The critical threshold for ischemic brain damage and poor outcome is suspected to be around a brain PtO_2 of 10 to 15 mm Hg.[51]

Instrumentation

Both electrochemical and optical fluorescence tissue O_2 probes have been developed for clinical use and research applications. Figure 18-15 shows a Clarke-type polarographic sensor and its insertion into brain tissue through an intracranial bolt. Optode probes capable of monitoring tissue pH, CO_2, and O_2 have also been developed.[52]

OXIMETRY

Oximetry is the measurement of blood Hb saturations using **spectrophotometry.** According to the principles of spectrophotometry, every substance has a unique pattern of light absorption, similar to a fingerprint. The pattern of light absorption of a substance varies predictably with the amount present; this is known as the *Lambert-Beer law*. By measuring the light absorbed and transmitted by a substance, scientists can identify its presence and determine its concentration.

The particular pattern of light absorption exhibited by a substance at different wavelengths is called its *absorption spectrum*. As shown in Figure 18-16, each form of Hb (e.g., Hb, HbO_2, HbCO, metHb) has its own unique pattern. By comparison of the amount of light transmitted through (or reflected from) a blood sample at two or more specific wavelengths, the relative concentrations of two or more forms of Hb can be measured. For example, oxygenated Hb absorbs less red light (600 to 750 nm) and more infrared light (850 to 1000 nm) than deoxygenated or reduced Hb does. Comparing a blood sample's light absorption with red and infrared light yields the $\%HbO_2$ and %Hb. For measurement of the concentration of additional forms of Hb, additional (more than two) wavelengths of light need to be used.

Several types of oximetry are used in clinical practice, including hemoximetry (also called cooximetry), pulse oximetry, venous oximetry, and tissue oximetry. Hemoximetry is a laboratory analytic procedure requiring invasive sampling of arterial blood. Pulse oximetry is a noninvasive monitoring technique performed at the bedside. Venous oximetry requires invasive monitoring through a fiberoptic catheter placed in the vena cava or pulmonary artery. Tissue oximetry is a noninvasive method of measuring the saturation of Hb at the tissue level.

Hemoximetry

Hemoximetry is an analytic method of oximetry and is covered in the AARC Clinical Practice Guideline: Blood Gas Analysis and Hemoximetry[15] (see Clinical Practice

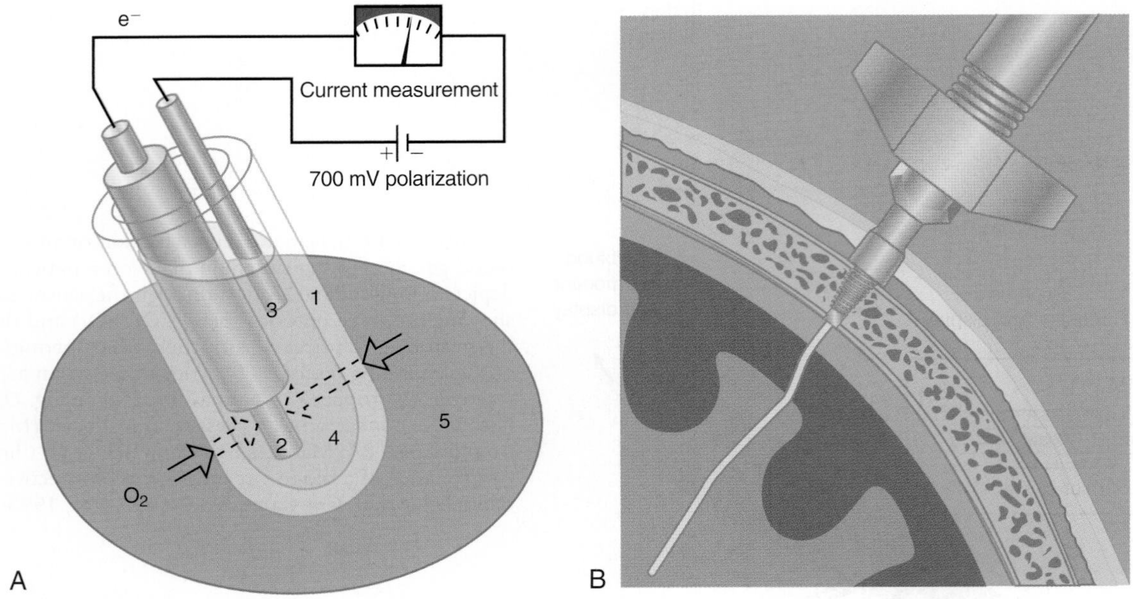

FIGURE 18-15 A, Schematic of Clark-type polarographic tissue oxygen probe. Polyethylene membrane *(1)*, gold cathode *(2)*, silver anode *(3)*, electrolyte solution *(4)*, cerebral tissue *(5)*. **B,** Insertion into cerebral tissue. (From Mulvey JM, Dorsch NW, Mudaliar Y, et al: Multimodality monitoring in severe traumatic brain injury: the role of brain tissue oxygenation monitoring. Neurocrit Care 1:391–402, 2004.)

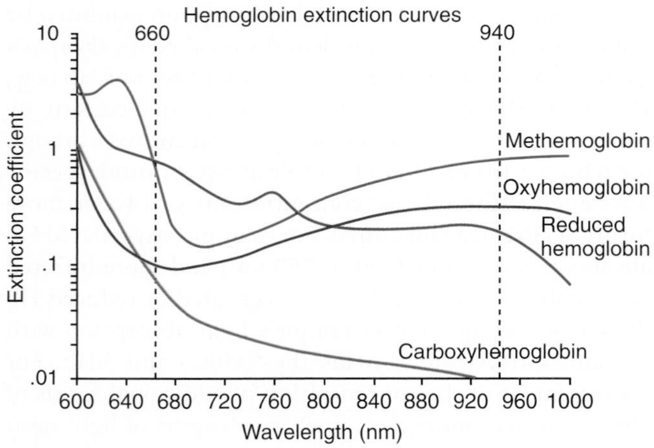

FIGURE 18-16 Principle of spectrophotometric oximetry. Different forms of hemoglobin (e.g., Hb, HbO_2, HbCO, metHb) absorb light differently at different wavelengths. By comparing points of equal absorbance (isobestic points) between pairs of Hb forms (e.g., Hb vs. HbO_2, Hb vs. HbCO), the relative proportion of each can be measured.

Guideline 18-3). Related recommendations have been published by CLSI).[9]

Instrumentation

Figure 18-17 is a simplified diagram showing the key components of a laboratory hemoximeter. Light generated by a thallium cathode lamp passes through a series of lenses and filters, yielding the specific wavelengths needed for analysis. A beam splitter divides the light into two portions, directing one through a reference solution and the other through a sample chamber, or **cuvette.** Photodetection sensors measure the amount of light transmitted through these two sources. By comparing the difference in light transmission through the reference and sample solutions, a microprocessor computes the relative amount of Hb present, with its output sent to the calibrated device meter or display. Because a laboratory hemoximeter uses four or more different wavelengths of light, it can simultaneously compute the relative concentrations of multiple forms of Hb, such as Hb, HbO_2, HbCO, and metHb.

Procedure and Quality Assurance

Similar to modern blood gas analyzers, laboratory hemoximeters are highly automated and simple to use. Some devices now combine both technologies into a single instrument. However, the caveats remain the same. Accurate and clinically useful hemoximetry results can be expected only if an error-free sample is assessed on a calibrated analyzer, using the manufacturer's protocol.

Although variations exist among devices, the basic procedure is similar. First, the blood is introduced into the sampling port of the analyzer, usually either by aspiration or injection. Required sample sizes vary from approximately 200 μL to 40 μL (microanalysis). Once introduced, erythrocyte Hb is released into the solution by hemolysis (incomplete hemolysis can cause erroneous results). After hemolysis, the sample is transported to the cuvette for analysis. On completion of the analysis, the sampling system (cuvette and tubing) is flushed and cleaned. As with blood gas analysis, operators must follow CDC Standard

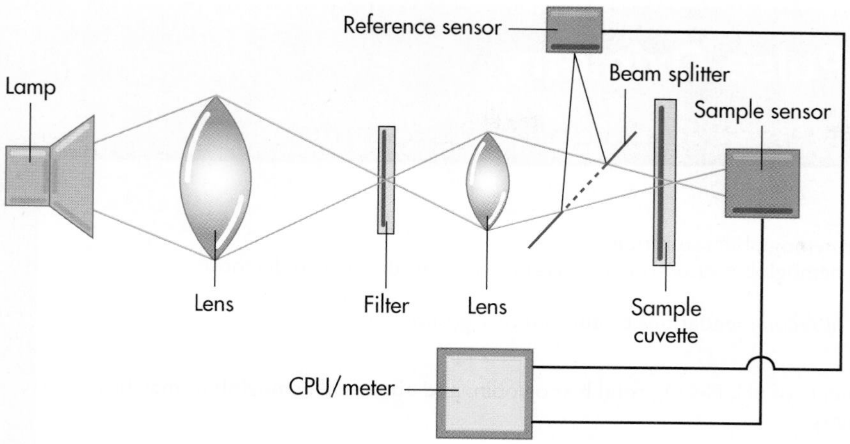

FIGURE 18-17 Simplified diagram showing key components of a laboratory hemoximeter. (Modified from Lane EE: Clinical arterial blood gas analysis, St Louis, 1987, Mosby.)

Precautions and ensure proper disposal of syringes and waste materials.

Quality assurance procedures for hemoximetry are essentially the same as the procedures used for blood gas analysis, differing only with regard to the control materials used. In addition, careful cleaning and maintenance of the cuvette chamber is essential because clouding of its walls decreases absorbance and can cause falsely elevated values.[53]

Problem Solving and Troubleshooting

A major assumption underlying hemoximetry is that the measured changes in light absorbance result only from variations in the relative concentrations of various hemoglobins. In practice, this assumption does not always hold true. Table 18-6 outlines some of the potential problems and resulting errors that can occur with hemoximetry.

TABLE 18-6

Problems Causing Measurement Errors With Hemoximeters

Problem	Potential Error
Incomplete hemolysis	Falsely low total Hb, HbO_2
Sickle cell anemia (caused by incomplete hemolysis)	Falsely low HbO_2
Presence of vascular dyes (e.g., methylene blue)	Falsely low total Hb, HbO_2
High lipid levels (e.g., from parenteral nutrition)	Falsely low total Hb, HbO_2
Presence of high levels of fetal hemoglobin	Falsely high HbCO
Elevated bilirubin levels (>20 mg/dl)	Falsely high total Hb, HbO_2, metHb
Dirty cuvette chamber	Falsely high total Hb, HbO_2

Pulse Oximetry

A pulse oximeter is a portable noninvasive monitoring device that provides estimates of arterial blood oxyhemoglobin saturation levels. So as not to confuse these estimates with actual SaO_2 measures obtained by hemoximetry, the abbreviation SpO_2 is used to refer to pulse oximetry readings.

No other device in recent medical history has been so widely and quickly adopted into clinical practice. With this widespread use have come equally widespread misconceptions regarding the appropriate applications and limitations of this technology.[54] In addition, the true benefit of pulse oximetry related to patient outcomes is unknown.[55]

To guide practitioners in providing quality care, the AARC has published Clinical Practice Guideline: Pulse Oximetry.[56] Modified excerpts from the AARC guideline appear in Clinical Practice Guideline 18-5.

Instrumentation

The pulse oximeter combines the principle of spectrophotometry, as used by hemoximeters, with **photoplethysmography.** Photoplethysmography uses light to detect the tiny volume changes that occur in living tissue during pulsatile blood flow. However, compared with a hemoximeter, the pulse oximeter usually uses only two wavelengths of light, one red (approximately 660 nm) and one infrared (approximately 940 nm) (see Figure 18-16). In addition, rather than measuring light transmission through a blood sample in a glass cuvette, the pulse oximeter measures transmission through living tissue, such as a finger or earlobe, or reflectance through the skin surface.

Figure 18-18, *A* provides a schematic block diagram of a pulse oximeter, consisting of a transmission sensor, processor, and display unit. The sensor has two sides. From one side, separate red and infrared LEDs alternately transmit light through the tissue. The transmitted light intensity is measured by a photodetector on the other side. The resulting output signal is filtered and amplified by instrument electronics, with processing and display functions controlled by a microprocessor.

Figure 18-18, *B* shows a schematic of a reflectance pulse oximeter sensor. This type of sensor has only one side, which contains both the LED light sources and the photodetector. The principle of operation is identical to a

18-5 Pulse Oximetry

AARC Clinical Practice Guideline (Excerpts)*

INDICATIONS
- To monitor the adequacy of arterial oxyhemoglobin saturation
- To quantify the response of arterial oxyhemoglobin saturation to therapeutic intervention or to diagnostic procedures, such as bronchoscopy
- To comply with mandated regulations or recommendations by authoritative groups

CONTRAINDICATIONS
- The ongoing need for actual measurements of pH, $PaCO_2$, total hemoglobin, and abnormal hemoglobins may be a relative contraindication to pulse oximetry.

PRECAUTIONS
- Device limitations causing false-negative results for hypoxemia or false-positive results for normoxemia or hyperoxemia may lead to inappropriate treatment of the patient.
- Factors that may affect the accuracy of the SpO_2 reading include motion artifact, abnormal hemoglobins, intravascular dyes, low perfusion states, skin pigmentation, and nail polish.

ASSESSMENT OF NEED
- When direct measurement of SaO_2 is unavailable or not accessible in a timely fashion, a pulse oximetry measurement may temporarily suffice if the limitations of the data are appreciated.
- SpO_2 is appropriate for continuous and prolonged monitoring (e.g., during sleep, exercise, or bronchoscopy).
- SpO_2 may be adequate when assessment of acid-base status or PaO_2 is not required.

ASSESSMENT OF OUTCOME

The following should be used to evaluate the benefits of pulse oximetry:
- SpO_2 results should reflect the patient's clinical condition (i.e., validate the basis for ordering the test).
- Documentation of results, therapeutic intervention (or lack thereof), and clinical decisions based on the SpO_2 measurements should be noted in the medical record.

FREQUENCY

After agreement has been established initially between SaO_2 and SpO_2, the frequency of SpO_2 monitoring (i.e., continuous vs. spot check) depends on the clinical status of the patient, the indications for performing the procedure, and recommended guidelines. For example, continuous SpO_2 monitoring may be indicated throughout a bronchoscopy to detect desaturation, whereas a spot check may suffice for evaluating the efficacy of oxygen therapy in a stable postoperative patient. Direct measurement of SaO_2 is needed whenever SpO_2 does not confirm or verify suspicions about the patient's clinical state.

MONITORING

During continuous pulse oximetry, the monitoring schedule for both the patient and the equipment should be correlated with the bedside assessment and determination of vital signs.

For the complete guideline, see American Association for Respiratory Care: Clinical practice guideline: sampling for arterial blood gas analysis. Respir Care 37:891, 1992.

transmission sensor except that the sensor is placed on the skin surface, usually the forehead, and reflected light from the tissue back to the sensor is used to calculate SpO_2.

Figure 18-19 shows a typical output signal generated by the photodetector (the pulsatile component can be observed on instruments that have a plethysmographic display). A baseline component represents the stable absorbance of the tissue bed, which mainly is the result of venous and capillary blood. At the top is the pulsatile component, caused by intermittent arterial flow through the tissues. By comparing light absorbance during the pulsatile phase with the baseline value at each wavelength, a pulse-added measure is obtained that is independent of incident light. Arterial oxyhemoglobin saturation is computed as the ratio of the pulse-added absorbances at the two different wavelengths.

In terms of accuracy, the pulse oximetry readings of sick patients usually fall within ±3% to 5% of the readings obtained with invasive hemoximetry.[56,57] Generally, the lower the actual SaO_2, the less accurate and reliable is the SpO_2 measurement. Most clinicians consider pulse oximeter readings unreliable at saturations less than 80%. Instrument response times vary by manufacturer, sensor location, and the patient's hemodynamic status from 10 seconds to 1 minute or longer.

Procedure

The actual procedure used to measure SpO_2 varies according to the device used, sensor site selected, and whether a spot check or continuous monitoring is required. Box 18-9 lists key points to be considered when performing pulse oximetry.

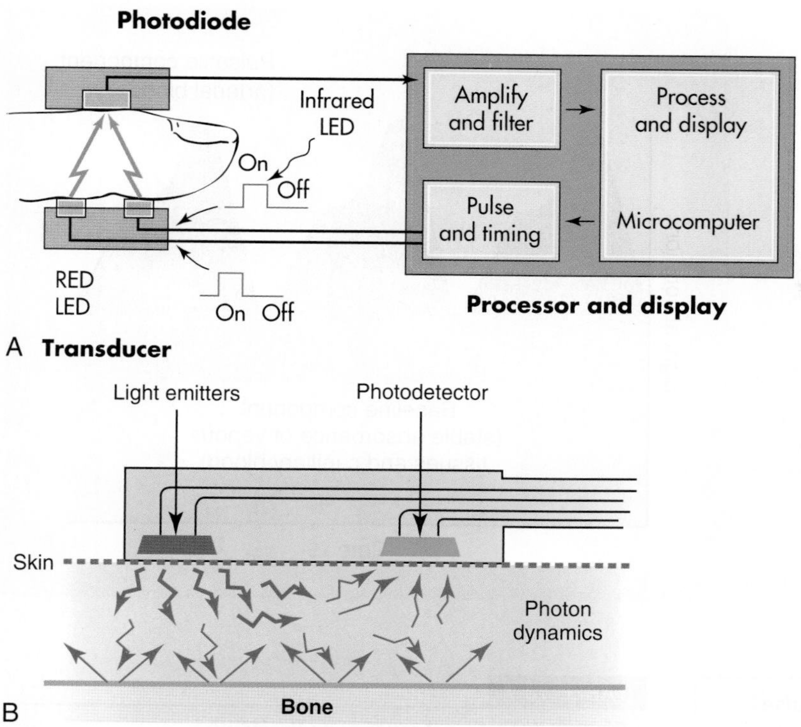

FIGURE 18-18 A, Schematic block diagram of a transmission pulse oximeter sensor and monitor. **B,** Schematic of a reflectance pulse oximeter sensor. (**A,** Modified from Gardner R: Pulse oximetry: is it monitoring's "silver bullet"? J Cardiovasc Nurs 1:79-83, 1987; **B,** from Keogh BF, Kopotic RJ: Recent findings in the use of reflectance oximetry: a critical review. Curr Opin Anaesthesiol 18:649-654, 2005.)

Given the limits of this technology, meticulous documentation is a must. Specifically, all SpO_2 results should be recorded in the patient's medical record. The following details should be documented:

- Date, time of measurement, and reading
- Patient's position, activity level, and location during monitoring
- FiO_2 or O_2 flow and O_2 delivery device
- Probe type and placement site
- Model of device (if more than one device is available for use)
- Results of simultaneously obtained ABGs and hemoximetry (if available)
- Stability of readings (length of observation time and range of fluctuation)
- Patient's clinical appearance, including assessment of perfusion at the measuring site (e.g., cyanosis, skin temperature)
- Agreement between oximeter and actual patient heart rate, as determined by palpation or electrocardiogram

RULE OF THUMB

When using a pulse oximeter to warn of hypoxemia in otherwise healthy adults, never set the low alarm below 92%. Generally, this level ensures that the alarm is activated before true arterial saturation drops below the critical value of 90%.

MINI CLINI

Troubleshooting Pulse Oximetry

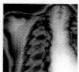

PROBLEM: The RT draws an ABG sample from a conscious and alert patient in a postsurgical unit who also is being monitored with a pulse oximeter, which reads 80% saturation. The patient is breathing 35% oxygen through an air-entrainment mask. The patient's extremities are pink and warm. After running the blood sample through a calibrated ABG analyzer with a hemoximeter, the RT obtains the following values:

PO_2 = 90 mm Hg
Hb = 12 g/dl
SaO_2 = 98%
metHb = 0.5%
HbCO = 1%

Explain the difference between the pulse oximeter and hemoximeter readings of this patient's blood oxygen levels and what action the RT should take.

SOLUTION: Given that a calibrated hemoximeter provides more accurate results than a pulse oximeter and that the patient exhibits no signs of hypoxemia, it is likely that the pulse oximeter reading is falsely low. Because the Hb and metHb levels are not grossly abnormal, potential problems include motion artifact, poor sensor placement, or device malfunction. The oximeter and sensor should be rechecked, and if found to be malfunctioning, they should be replaced.

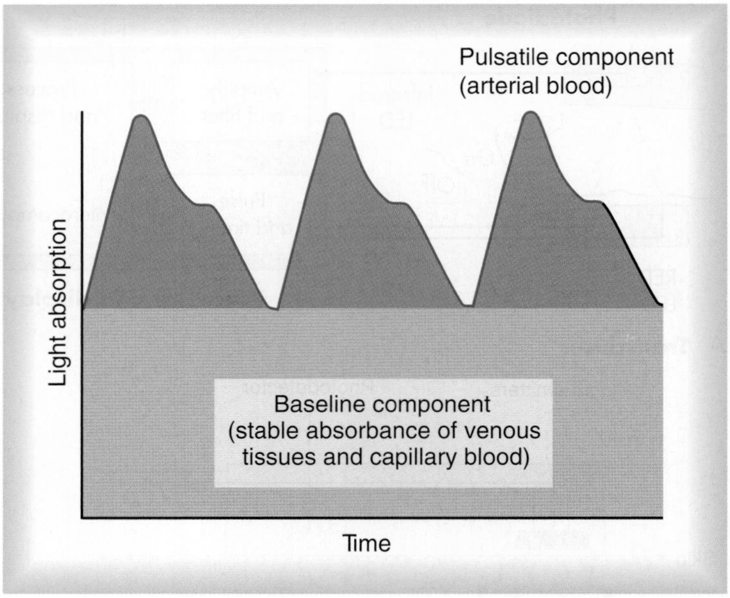

FIGURE 18-19 Output signal generated by pulse oximeter. Saturation is based on the ratio of light absorption between two or more wavelengths during pulsatile and baseline phases.

Box 18-9 Key Points for Performing Pulse Oximetry

- Always follow manufacturer's recommended protocol.
- Never mix sensors among different devices.
- Ensure the sensor is the correct size for the site chosen.
- Ensure the sensor is properly applied (not too tight or loose).
- Before taking or recording a reading, confirm the adequacy and accuracy of the pulse signal.
- When doing spot checks, allow sufficient response time before taking a reading because response times vary greatly.
- For continuous monitoring of adults and children, set the low alarm at 88% to 92%.
- Whenever possible, validate the initial SpO_2 reading against the actual SaO_2.
- Clean multiuse sensors and disinfect the instrument housing between patients.
- Inspect the sensor site frequently throughout the duration of continuous monitoring, and change it as needed.
- Never act on SpO_2 readings alone.
- Avoid using pulse oximetry to monitor hyperoxia in neonates.

TABLE 18-7
Factors Affecting Accuracy or Precision of Pulse Oximeters

Factor	Potential Error
Presence of HbCO	Falsely high $\%HbO_2$
Presence of high levels of metHb	Falsely low $\%HbO_2$ if SaO_2 >85% Falsely high $\%HbO_2$ if SaO_2 <85%
Presence of fetal hemoglobin	No effect
Anemia (very low hematocrit, <10%)	Falsely low CaO_2 and high $\%HbO_2$
Vascular dyes (e.g., methylene blue)	Falsely low $\%HbO_2$
Elevated bilirubin levels	No effect
Dark skin pigmentation	Falsely high $\%HbO_2$ (3%-5%)
Nail polish (especially black)	Falsely high $\%HbO_2$
Ambient light	Varies (e.g., falsely high $\%HbO_2$ in sunlight); also may cause falsely high pulse reading
Poor perfusion (vasoconstriction)	Inadequate signal; unpredictable results
Motion artifact	Unpredictable, spurious readings
Electrocautery	Falsely low HbO_2
Magnetic resonance imaging	Falsely low HbO_2

Problem Solving and Troubleshooting

Problems with pulse oximetry fall into the following two categories: (1) problems inherent in the technology itself and (2) problems associated with clinical interpretation and use of data. Dozens of technical factors may affect the readings, limit the precision, or alter the performance of pulse oximeters. Table 18-7 summarizes the most important of these factors and the types of errors they cause.

Motion artifact probably is the most common source of error and false alarms. Although new technologies promise to reduce motion artifact, relocation of the sensor to the earlobe, toe, or forehead can minimize the problem. Falsely elevated readings can occur with dark skin pigmentation at low saturation levels; this can be compensated for by setting oximeter low alarms 3% to 5% higher in applicable cases.

Early studies of the effect of nail polish found significant differences in lowering SpO_2 readings. More recent studies have found no effect or small differences that are not considered to be clinically relevant; this may be due to improvements in LED light sources.[58] It has been suggested that the effect of nail polish could be minimized either by using a different site or by rotating the sensor so that the light path does not cross the fingernails.

If ambient light interference is creating problems, the sensor can be loosely covered with an opaque towel or cloth. Problems that occur during procedures producing electromagnetic interference (e.g., electrocautery, magnetic resonance imaging) need only be recognized. Careful monitoring of the patient during episodes of false low alarms is essential.

Regarding problems with the use and interpretation of pulse oximetry data, rule number one is to treat the patient, not the monitor. The clinician should never interpret or act on monitoring data without first assessing the patient and verifying proper sensor placement and signal quality. A related problem is simple confusion over the relationship between oxyhemoglobin saturation and PO_2. Many clinicians rely solely on PaO_2 readings to assess oxygenation and do not understand oxyhemoglobin saturation. To these clinicians, an SpO_2 reading of 80% might be confused easily with PaO_2 of 80 mm Hg. The latter measure of partial pressure is normal, whereas a saturation of 80% indicates moderate to severe hypoxemia, equivalent to PaO_2 of approximately 50 mm Hg.

A similar interpretation error (PaO_2 vs. SpO_2) occurs because of the limited accuracy of most pulse oximeters. It is common practice to set the low alarm of a monitoring oximeter to 90%. In theory, this practice makes sense because an SaO_2 reading of 90% normally corresponds to a PO_2 reading of approximately 60 mm Hg, which is the lower limit of clinically acceptable oxygenation. However, with the accuracy of some oximeters being only ±4%, an SpO_2 reading of 90% could mean an actual SaO_2 reading of 86%, corresponding to a PO_2 level of 55 mm Hg or less.

At the high end, oximetry data can be even less meaningful. Because of the characteristics of the oxyhemoglobin dissociation curve (see Chapter 11), a patient with an SpO_2 reading of 100% could represent a PaO_2 level anywhere between 100 mm Hg and 600 mm Hg. The lesson here is not to use the pulse oximeter for monitoring hyperoxia (as may be important for neonates).

The pulse oximeter does not measure PCO_2. A patient breathing an elevated FiO_2 can have normal SpO_2 readings despite severe hypercarbia. ABG analysis is needed when acute ventilatory failure may be present.

SpO_2 can read falsely high when carbon monoxide poisoning or methemoglobinemia is present. This false reading is due to the fact that the two-wavelength pulse oximeter measures only saturation of the Hb and not specifically saturation with O_2. HbCO and metHb cannot be distinguished from HbO_2 with a pulse oximeter. A falsely high SpO_2 reading occurs when significant HbCO is present. When metHb is elevated, the SpO_2 reading is higher than the actual measured SaO_2. As metHb level increases, SpO_2 decreases and plateaus at approximately 85% when the metHb level reaches 30%.[59]

To address these limitations, pulse oximeters using seven or more wavelengths of light have been developed. Use of multiwavelength pulse oximeters capable of measuring Hb, HbO_2, HbCO, and metHb has been referred to as **pulse cooximetry.** The accuracy of measurements does not equal the accuracy of conventional hemoximetry, but pulse cooximetry may be useful for trend monitoring in some clinical situations.[60]

As with transcutaneous monitoring, if pulse oximetry and blood gas values are inconsistent with each other or the clinical status of the patient, the RT should explore possible causes before reporting, interpreting, or acting on results. Often, discrepancies can be reduced by switching sites or replacing the sensor probe. If these steps fail to resolve the inconsistencies, the RT should document the problem and recommend obtaining an ABG with hemoximetry if indicated.

Venous Oximetry

Continuous central venous (vena cava) and mixed venous (pulmonary artery) O_2 saturation monitoring ($S\bar{v}O_2$) is performed to assess the balance between O_2 delivery and use as an indirect index of global tissue oxygenation and perfusion. Decreased $S\bar{v}O_2$ has been found to be indicative of cardiac failure in patients with myocardial infarction and to predict poor prognosis in patients after cardiovascular surgery, in patients with severe cardiopulmonary disease, and in patients with septic or cardiogenic shock.[61] Regional and organ-specific $S\bar{v}O_2$ monitoring has been performed via catheters placed in the coronary sinus, hepatic vein, and cranial jugular venous bulb for cerebral perfusion monitoring. Normal values for $S\bar{v}O_2$ range from 60% to 80%.

Instrumentation

Figure 18-20 shows a diagram of an $S\bar{v}O_2$ monitoring system. Venous oximetry is measured through a fiberoptic catheter by reflectance spectrophotometry. Two or three wavelengths of light are emitted from LEDs through fiberoptic filaments into the venous blood. Some of this light is reflected back and received through another fiberoptic channel, which is read by a photodetector. The amount of light that is absorbed by the venous blood and reflected back is determined by the amount of O_2 that is saturated or bound to Hb. This information is processed by the monitor, updated, and displayed as $S\bar{v}O_2$.

Clinical Usefulness

Continuous $S\bar{v}O_2$ can be monitored through an $S\bar{v}O_2$-equipped pulmonary artery catheter or venous catheter. Mixed venous oximetry from the pulmonary artery is an indication of global O_2 delivery and use. Central venous

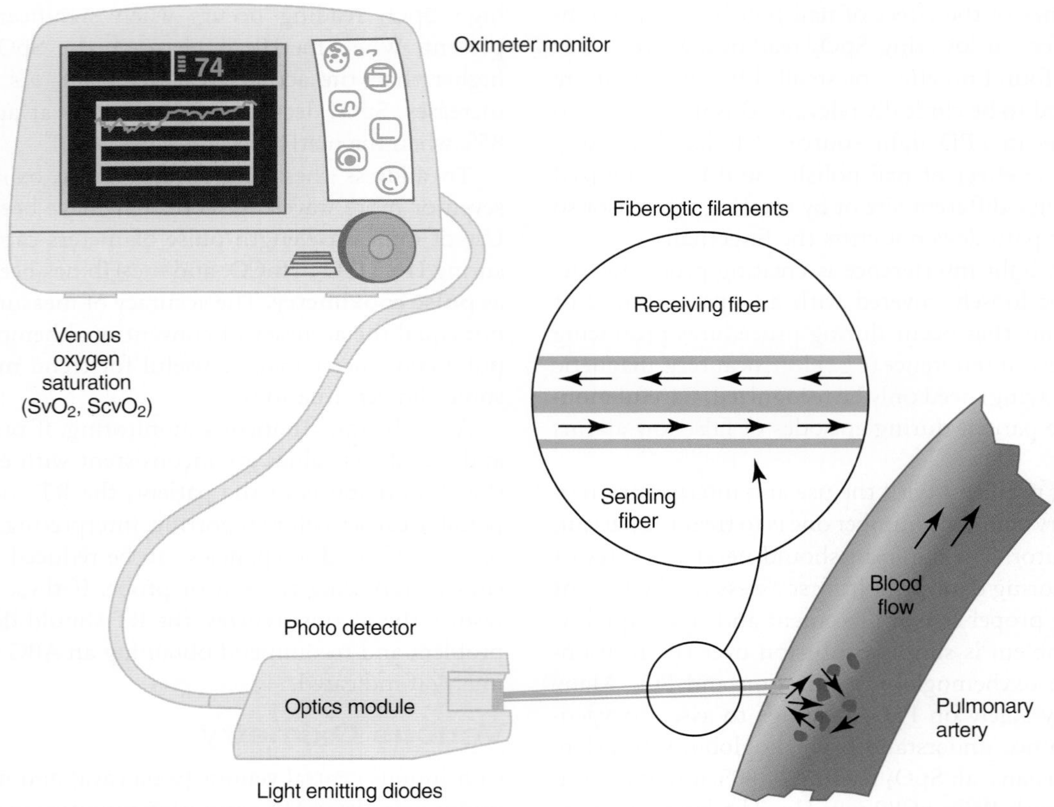

FIGURE 18-20 Diagram of a venous oximetry monitoring system using reflectance oximetry. (Courtesy Edwards Life Science, Irvine, CA.)

oximetry is nearly interchangeable with mixed venous oximetry. Both correlate with mixed venous saturation measured by hemoximetry with an accuracy within ±3% to 5%. Accuracy of venous oximetry monitoring depends on the frequency of calibration with measured $S\bar{v}O_2$ and Hb, the position of the catheter free floating in the vein, the absence of wall artifact, damage to the fiberoptic filaments, and clot formation at the catheter tip.[62,63]

Tissue Oximetry

O_2 saturation at the tissue level (StO_2) assesses the adequacy of circulation and O_2 delivery. Early detection of low StO_2 can be used as method of early detection of tissue hypoperfusion in patients with traumatic injuries.[64,65] Cerebral StO_2 monitoring can also be used to monitor brain oxygenation and detect cerebral ischemia during neurosurgical or cardiovascular procedures.[66-68]

Instrumentation

Tissue oximetry is essentially a reflectance oximeter that uses near-infrared spectroscopy to measure StO_2. Multiwavelengths of light in the near-infrared spectrum transilluminate muscle tissue in the hand or brain through the forehead. Because biologic tissue, including the skull, is relatively transparent in the near-infrared range, the absorbance and reflectance characteristics of HbO_2 and Hb concentrations in the tissue being monitored is used to calculate StO_2. To date, a clear role for monitoring StO_2 has not been found in routine clinical practice.

CAPNOMETRY AND CAPNOGRAPHY

Capnometry is the measurement of CO_2 in respiratory gases. A capnometer is the device that measures CO_2. **Capnography** is the graphic display of CO_2 levels as they change during breathing.

Although capnography can be applied to any patient, its primary clinical use is for monitoring during either general anesthesia (where it is a standard of care) or mechanical ventilation. The remainder of this section assumes application during mechanical ventilation. To guide practitioners in providing quality care, the AARC has published Clinical Practice Guideline: Capnography/Capnometry During Mechanical Ventilation.[69] Modified excerpts from the AARC guideline appear in Clinical Practice Guidelines 18-6.

Instrumentation

The key component in a capnograph is a rapidly responding CO_2 analyzer. Rapid CO_2 analysis can be achieved using infrared absorption, Raman scattering, mass spectroscopy,

18-6 Capnography and Capnometry During Mechanical Ventilation

AARC Clinical Practice Guideline (Excerpts)*

INDICATIONS

Based on available evidence, capnography may be indicated for the following:

- Evaluation of exhaled CO_2, especially end-tidal CO_2 levels (P_{ETCO_2})
- Monitoring severity of pulmonary disease and evaluating the patient's response to therapy, especially that intended to do the following:
  Improve the V_D/V_T ratio
  Improve the matching of $\dot{V}/\dot{Q}$
  Increase coronary blood flow
- Determining that tracheal, rather than esophageal, intubation has taken place
- Continued monitoring of the integrity of the ventilatory circuit, including the artificial airway
- Evaluation of the efficiency of mechanical ventilatory support (by [$PaCO_2 - P_{ETCO_2}$])
- Monitoring adequacy of pulmonary, systemic, and coronary blood flow
- Monitoring inspired CO_2 when CO_2 gas is being therapeutically administered
- Graphic evaluation of ventilator-patient interface
- Measurement of the volume of CO_2 elimination to assess metabolic rate or alveolar ventilation

CONTRAINDICATIONS

There are no absolute contraindications to capnography in mechanically ventilated adults, provided that the data obtained are evaluated with consideration given to the patient's clinical condition.

PRECAUTIONS AND POSSIBLE COMPLICATIONS

- Misunderstanding of the data provided may lead to inappropriate treatment of the patient.
- With mainstream analyzers, too large a sampling window can excessively increase the mechanical dead space circuit.
- The sampling window or the sampling lines can place additional weight on the circuit and increase traction on the patient's artificial airway.

ASSESSMENT OF NEED

Capnography is a standard of care during anesthesia. The Society of Critical Care Medicine has suggested that capnography be available for patients with acute ventilatory failure on mechanical ventilatory support. The American College of Emergency Physicians recommends capnography as an adjunctive method to ensure proper endotracheal tube position.

Assessment of the need to use capnography with a specific patient should be guided by the clinical situation. The patient's primary cause of respiratory failure and the acuteness of his or her condition should be considered.

ASSESSMENT OF OUTCOME

Results should reflect the patient's condition and should validate the basis for ordering the monitoring. Documentation of results (along with all ventilatory and hemodynamic variables available), therapeutic interventions, and clinical decisions made based on the capnogram should be included in the patient's chart.

MONITORING

During capnography, the following should be considered and monitored:

- *Ventilatory variables:* Tidal volume, respiratory rate, positive end expiratory pressure, inspiratory/expiratory time ratio, peak airway pressure, and concentrations of respiratory gas mixture
- *Hemodynamic variables:* Systemic and pulmonary blood pressures, cardiac output, shunt, and ventilation/perfusion imbalances

**For the complete guideline, see American Association for Respiratory Care: Clinical practice guideline: capnography/capnometry during mechanical ventilation. Respir Care 48:534, 2003.*

or photoacoustic technology, with the infrared capnometer being the most common.

Figure 18-21 provides a simple schematic of a double-beam infrared capnometer. A filtered infrared light source passes through a sample chamber. (Because glass absorbs infrared radiation, the chamber "windows" usually are constructed of sodium chloride or sodium bromide.) After the infrared light passes through the sample chamber, a lens focuses the remaining, unabsorbed radiation onto an electrical photodetector. Because CO_2 absorbs infrared radiation, the greater the concentration of CO_2 in the sample, the less infrared light arrives at the detector.

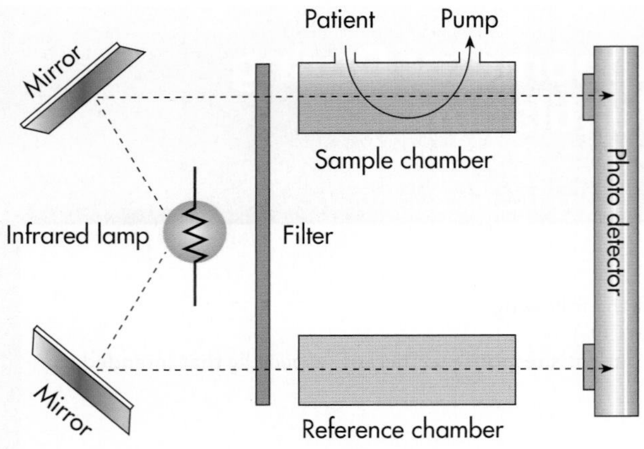

FIGURE 18-21 Schematic representation of infrared capnometer.

Variations in the concentration of CO_2 alter the electrical output signal of the detector. This signal is used either to display the CO_2 concentration with LEDs (capnometer) or to generate a real-time graphic display (capnogram).[70]

Capnometers use two different methods to sample the respiratory gases: mainstream sampling and sidestream sampling (Figure 18-22). The mainstream analyzer places an in-line analysis chamber between the patient's airway and the ventilator circuit. The sidestream analyzer uses a sampling tube to pump a small volume of gas continually from the ventilator circuit into the analysis chamber within the device. Table 18-8 lists the advantages and disadvantages of these two approaches. Differences notwithstanding, clinicians should use the method best suited to the patient's needs and the device with which they are most experienced and familiar.

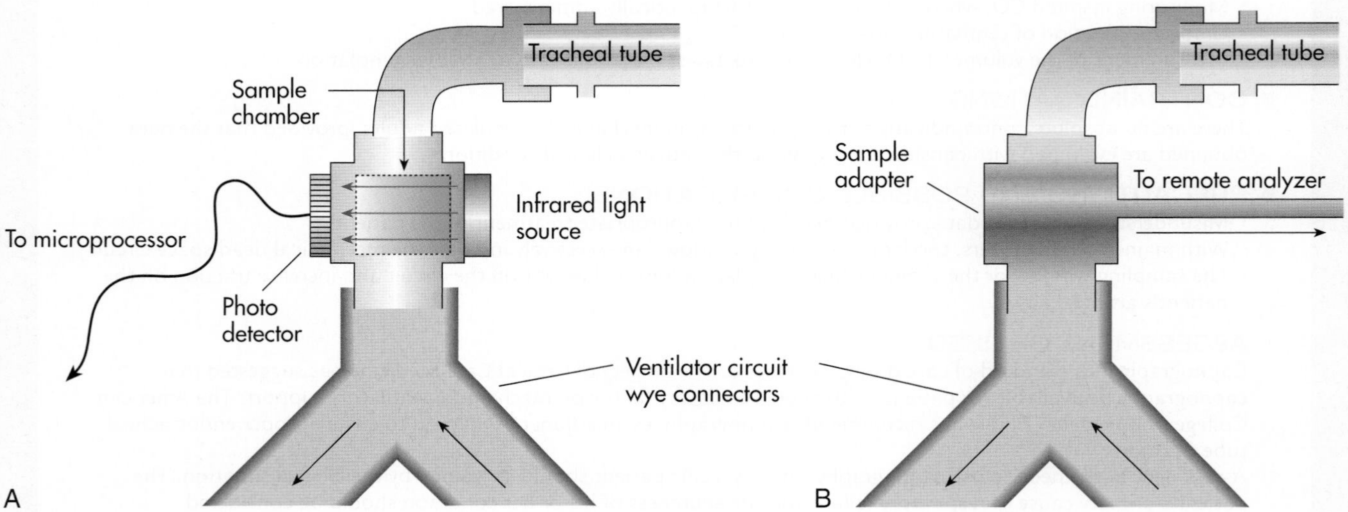

FIGURE 18-22 A, Mainstream CO_2 sampling. The sample chamber, light source, and photodetector are attached to the breathing circuit, with the output signal sent to a microprocessor for analysis and display. **B,** Sidestream CO_2 sampling through an in-line sampling adapter with a small-bore connector. A small sample of expired gas is drawn continuously through the tubing and analyzed inside a remote capnometer.

TABLE 18-8

Advantages and Disadvantages of Mainstream and Sidestream Capnometers

	Mainstream	Sidestream
Advantages	Sensor at patient airway	No bulky sensors or heaters at airway
	Fast response (crisp waveform)	Ability to measure N_2O
	Short lag time (real-time readings)	Disposable sample line
	No sample flow to reduce tidal volume	Ability to use with nonintubated patients
Disadvantages	Secretions and humidity can block sensor window	Secretions block sample tubing
	Sensor requires heating to prevent condensation	Trap required to remove water from sample
	Requires frequent calibration	Frequent calibration required
	Bulky sensor at patient airway	Slow response to CO_2 changes
	Does not measure N_2O	Lag time between CO_2 change and measurement
	Difficult to use with nonintubated patients	Sample flow may decrease tidal volume
	Reusable adapters require cleaning and sterilization	

From Kacmarek RM, Hess D, Stoller J, editors: Monitoring in respiratory care, St Louis, 1993, Mosby.

Interpretation

Interpretation of the capnogram can be useful in assessing trends in alveolar ventilation and detecting ventilation/perfusion ratio ($\dot{V}/\dot{Q}$) imbalance caused by either pulmonary disease or cardiovascular disorders. Capnometry also has been used to estimate physiologic dead space, to detect esophageal intubation, to assess blood flow during cardiac arrest, and to determine positive end expiratory pressure levels. To interpret abnormal events, clinicians first must understand the normal capnogram.

Normal Capnogram

Figure 18-23 shows a typical normal single-breath capnogram. Initially, the expired PCO_2 is 0 mm Hg, indicating exhalation of pure dead space gas (*A*, phase I). Soon after, alveolar gas begins mixing with dead space gas, causing a rapid increase in expired PCO_2 (*A* to *B*, phase II). Later in expiration, the CO_2 concentration begins leveling off. This plateau indicates exhalation of gas coming mainly from ventilated alveoli (*B* to *C*, phase III). Gas sampled at the end of exhalation is called *end-tidal gas,* with its partial pressure of CO_2 abbreviated as $P_{ET}CO_2$. In healthy individuals, $P_{ET}CO_2$ averages 3 to 5 mm Hg less than $PaCO_2$, or 35 to 43 mm Hg (approximately 5% to 6% CO_2). The sharp downstroke and return to baseline that normally occurs after the end-tidal point indicates inhalation of fresh gas with zero CO_2.

MINI CLINI

Interpreting Capnometry Data

PROBLEM: The RT is monitoring an intubated, mechanically ventilated patient in the intensive care unit with a capnograph. She notices the expired CO_2 level suddenly drop to near zero. On auscultation, the patient exhibits good bilateral breath sounds, and all connections between the airway and capnograph are tight. What is the likely problem?

SOLUTION: The most common causes of a zero $P_{ET}CO_2$ are extubation and ventilator or monitoring system disconnection. However, a $P_{ET}CO_2$ of zero can also occur with shock or cardiac arrest (no CO_2 returns to the lungs for exhalation). The RT should check this patient's cardiovascular status immediately. If the patient's cardiovascular system is functioning within normal limits, the RT should check the position of the endotracheal tube.

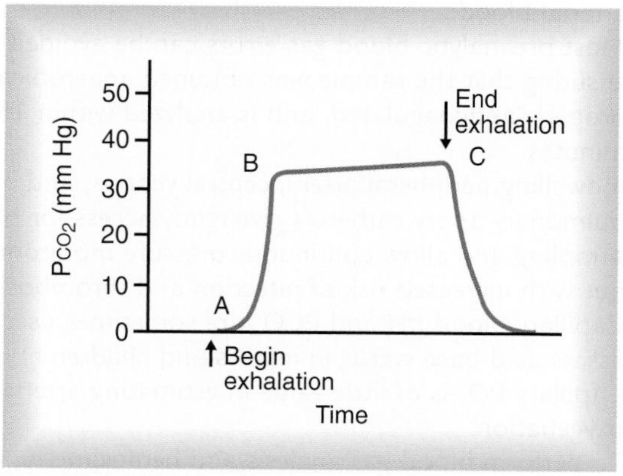

FIGURE 18-23 Normal single-breath capnograph tracing.

Abnormal Capnogram

The first step in assessing the capnogram is to determine the actual $P_{ET}CO_2$ and whether it has changed over time. Table 18-9 differentiates between the causes of high and low $P_{ET}CO_2$ readings by the suddenness of the change. A $P_{ET}CO_2$ of zero usually indicates a system leak, esophageal intubation, or cardiac arrest.

After the capnogram has been assessed for changes in $P_{ET}CO_2$, the waveform and its pattern should be analyzed. A normal capnogram starts with a sharp upstroke, followed by a plateau and then a rapid downstroke. As indicated in Figure 18-24, changes in this normal contour may indicate a ventilation/perfusion abnormality. Such patterns, although not diagnostic, can indicate the severity of the $\dot{V}/\dot{Q}$ disturbance and can warn of developing problems, such as acute pulmonary emboli.

Waveform changes also may occur with equipment malfunction. Because the normal inspired CO_2 level is zero, the capnogram baseline also should be at zero. An elevated baseline (>0 mm Hg) indicates rebreathing. However, an expired CO_2 level of zero might indicate patient disconnect. (For more information on the use of capnography during mechanical ventilation, see Chapter 46.)

Procedure

Bedside capnography procedures vary according to the type of equipment used and the manufacturer's recommended protocol. Generally, a capnograph should be

TABLE 18-9

Conditions Associated With Changes in $P_{ET}CO_2$

Change	High $P_{ET}CO_2$	Low $P_{ET}CO_2$
Sudden	Sudden increase in cardiac output Sudden release of a tourniquet Injection of sodium bicarbonate	Sudden hyperventilation Sudden decrease in cardiac output Massive pulmonary embolism Air embolism Disconnection of ventilator Obstruction of endotracheal tube Leakage in the circuit
Gradual	Hypoventilation Increase in CO_2 production	Hyperventilation Decrease in oxygen consumption Decreased pulmonary perfusion

Note: An absent $P_{ET}CO_2$ means that a system leak, esophageal intubation, or cardiac arrest has occurred.

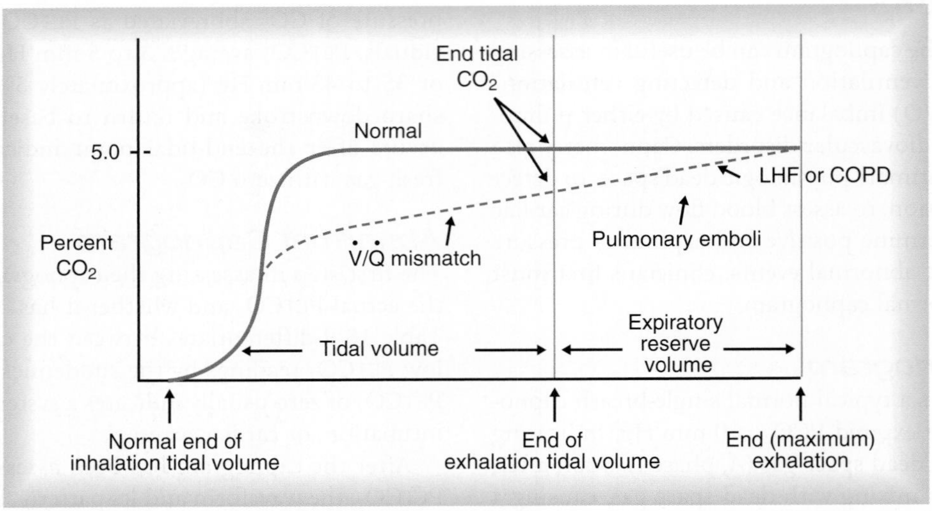

FIGURE 18-24 Normal and abnormal capnogram waveforms. For a healthy individual *(solid line)*, the end-tidal CO_2 at the completion of normal tidal exhalation is equal to end-tidal CO_2 at maximum exhalation. With shock caused by left ventricular heart failure *(LHF)* or chronic obstructive pulmonary disease *(COPD)*, the CO_2 level increases more slowly and does not reach a true end-tidal plateau. The end-tidal CO_2 is less than normal at the completion of a normal exhalation (but may increase slightly with a maximum exhalation). Similar findings can be noted with a pulmonary embolus except that the low end-tidal CO_2 does not increase with a maximum exhalation. (Modified from Darin J: Curr Rev Resp Ther 3:146, 1981; Erickson L, Wollmer P, Olsson CG, et al: Chest 96:357, 1989; Hatte CJ, Rokseth R: Chest 66:352, 1974. In Pilbeam SP, Cairo JM: Mechanical ventilation, ed 4, St Louis, 2006, Mosby.)

calibrated as recommended by its manufacturer, using precision CO_2 mixtures in the clinical range of measurement.

In terms of infection control, nondisposable components that contact the patient's airway or ventilator circuit should undergo high-level disinfection between patients. The monitor should be cleaned as needed, according to the manufacturer's recommendations.

Problem Solving and Troubleshooting

Monitoring a patient with a capnograph that is properly calibrated and operating according to the manufacturer's specifications presents few major problems. The most significant error is assuming that the end-expired CO_2 levels can substitute for actual $PaCO_2$ measurements. The most common problem is contamination or obstruction of the sampling system or monitor by secretions or condensate.[27] Proper use of water traps and regular changing of sample tubing or chambers can help prevent this problem. Other potential problems include the following:

- False reading caused by the presence of gases with infrared absorption spectra similar to CO_2 (e.g., nitrous oxide)
- Inaccurate readings with high frequencies of breathing (this is more of a problem with sidestream systems)
- Misinterpreting low or absent cardiac output as a disconnect or possible esophageal intubation (all three can result in a $P_{ET}CO_2$ of zero)

SUMMARY CHECKLIST

- To measure the inspired O_2 concentration, a properly calibrated electrochemical O_2 analyzer should be used.
- The most common causes of O_2 analyzer malfunction are low batteries, sensor depletion, and electronic failure.
- As the "gold standard" of gas exchange analysis, ABG results help the clinician assess ventilation, acid-base balance, oxygenation, and the O_2-carrying capacity of blood.
- The radial artery is the preferred site for adult arterial blood sampling. Before radial puncture, a modified Allen test to confirm collateral circulation is performed.
- For critically ill patients, the clinician waits 20 to 30 minutes after a change in treatment before sampling arterial blood.
- Most preanalytic blood gas errors can be avoided by ensuring that the sample was obtained anaerobically, is properly anticoagulated, and is analyzed within 15 minutes.
- Indwelling peripheral artery, central venous, and pulmonary artery catheters give ready access for blood sampling and allow continuous pressure monitoring but with increased risk of infection and thrombosis.
- Capillary blood pH and PCO_2 are sometimes used to assess acid-base status in infants and children. Capillary PO_2 is of little value in estimating arterial oxygenation.
- To perform blood gas analysis and hemoximetry, the clinician must be proficient in performing procedures,

preventive maintenance, troubleshooting, instrument calibration, and quality control.

- A blood gas analyzer measures pH, PCO_2, and PO_2 using three separate electrodes.
- To obtain accurate blood gas results, the clinician ensures that the sample is free of preanalytic error and follows the manufacturer's recommended analysis protocol.
- Blood gas analysis quality control involves a cycle of performance validation for new instruments, preventive maintenance and function checks, automated calibration, calibration verification with control media, internal statistical quality control, external proficiency testing, and thorough recordkeeping of all processes.
- Portable point-of-care blood gas analyzers can achieve accuracy and precision levels comparable with laboratory-based analyzers.
- A blood gas monitor provides bedside measurements either continuously or at appropriate intervals, without permanently removing blood from the patient; this may be accomplished transcutaneously or with either in vivo or ex vivo blood analysis.
- Transcutaneous blood gas monitoring provides continuous noninvasive analysis of gas exchange, but it is useful only for hemodynamically stable infants or children.
- Current in vivo blood gas monitors are not yet reliable enough to replace traditional blood gas analysis, but they may provide information at a level of accuracy and reliability sufficient for trend analysis.
- Oximetry is the measurement of blood Hb saturations using spectrophotometry. Hemoximetry is a laboratory procedure that requires an arterial blood sample. Pulse oximetry combines spectrophotometry with photoplethysmography to obtain a noninvasive measure of blood Hb saturations.
- At best, pulse oximetry readings fall within ±3% to 5% of readings obtained by hemoximetry.
- Dozens of technical factors affect the readings, limit the precision, or alter the performance of pulse oximeters. To interpret test results properly, clinicians must have in-depth knowledge of these factors.
- Capnometry is the measurement of CO_2 in respiratory gases. A capnometer is the device that measures the CO_2. Capnography is the graphic display of CO_2 levels as they change during breathing.
- A capnogram may be used to assess trends in alveolar ventilation, to identify $\dot{V}/\dot{Q}$ imbalance caused by cardiopulmonary disorders, to estimate physiologic dead space, to detect esophageal intubation, and to determine the amount of blood flow during cardiac arrest.

References

1. Wahr JA, Tremper KK: Noninvasive oxygen monitoring techniques. Crit Care Clin 11:199, 1995.
2. Severinghaus JW: The invention and development of blood gas analysis apparatus. Anesthesiology 97:253–256, 2002.
3. American Association for Respiratory Care: Clinical practice guideline: sampling for arterial blood gas analysis. Respir Care 37:891, 1992.
4. Blonshine S: Procedures for the collection of arterial blood specimens: approved standard, H11-A4, ed 2, Wayne, PA, 2004, National Committee for Clinical Laboratory Standards.
5. Brzezinski M, Luisetti T, London MJ: Radial artery cannulation: a comprehensive review of recent anatomic and physiologic investigations. Anesth Analg 109:1763–1781, 2009.
6. Barone JE, Madlinger RV: Should an Allen test be performed before radial artery cannulation? J Trauma 61:468–470, 2006.
7. Durbin CG, Jr: Radial arterial lines and sticks: what are the risks? Respir Care 46:229–231, 2001.
8. Szaflarski NL: Preanalytic error associated with blood gas/pH measurement. Crit Care Nurse 16:89, 1996.
9. D'Orazio P: Blood gas and pH analysis and related measurements: approved guideline, C46-A2, ed 2, Wayne, PA, 2009, Clinical Laboratory Standards Institute.
10. Del Cotillo M, Grané N, Llavoré M, et al: Heparinized solution vs. saline solution in the maintenance of arterial catheters: a double blind randomized clinical trial. Intensive Care Med 34:339–343, 2008.
11. Zavorsky GS, Cao J, Mayo NE, et al: Arterial versus capillary blood gases: a meta analysis. Respir Physiol Neurobiol 155:268–279, 2007.
12. American Association for Respiratory Care: Clinical practice guideline: capillary blood gas sampling for neonatal and pediatric patients. Respir Care 46:506, 2001.
13. Meites S: Skin puncture and blood collecting techniques for infants: update and problems. In: Meites S, ed. Pediatric clinical chemistry, 3rd ed, Washington, DC, 1989, American Association for Clinical Chemistry, pp 5–15.
14. MacIntyre NR, Lawlor B, Castere D, et al: Accuracy and precision of a point-of-care blood gas analyzer incorporating optodes. Respir Care 41:800, 1996.
15. American Association for Respiratory Care: Clinical practice guideline: in vitro pH and blood gas analysis and hemoximetry. Respir Care 46:498, 2001.
16. Mahutte CK: On-line arterial blood gas analysis with optodes: current status. Clin Biochem 31:119–130, 1998.
17. Ganter M, Zollinger A: Continuous intravascular blood gas monitoring: development, current techniques, and clinical use of a commercial device. Br J Anaesth 91:397–407, 2003.
18. Centers for Disease Control and Prevention: http://wwwn.cdc.gov/clia/default.aspx, accessed Oct 26, 2011.
19. Berte L: Application of a quality management system model for laboratory services: approved guideline, GP26-A3, ed 3, Wayne, PA, 2004, National Committee for Clinical Laboratory Standards.
20. Westgard JO, Barry PL, Hunt MR, et al: A multi-rule Shewhart chart for quality control in clinical chemistry. Clin Chem 27:493–501, 1981.
21. Westguard SC: http://www.westgard.com/westgard-rules, accessed Oct 26, 2011.
22. Centers for Disease Control and Prevention: http://wwwn.cdc.gov/clia/default.aspx, accessed Oct 26, 2011.
23. Center for Medicare and Medicine Services: https://www.cms.gov/CLIA/14_Proficiency_Testing_Providers.asp, accessed Oct 26, 2011.
24. Smith BL, Vender JS: Point-of-care testing. Respir Care Clin North Am 1:133, 1995.
25. Singer AJ, Ardise J, Gulla J, et al: Point-of-care testing reduces length of stay in emergency department chest pain patients. Ann Emerg Med 45:587–591, 2005.
26. Scalise D: Poised for growth: point-of-care testing. Hosp Health Netw 80:77–83, 2006.
27. Wahr JA: Accuracy and precision of a new, portable, handheld blood gas analyzer: the IRMA. J Clin Monit 12:317, 1996.

28. Schimke I: Quality and timeliness in medical laboratory testing. Anal Bioanal Chem 393:1499–1504, 2009.
29. Giuliano KK, Grant ME: Blood analysis at the point of care: issues in application for use in critically ill patients. AACN Clin Issues 13:204–220, 2002.
30. Jacobs E: Point-of-care in vitro diagnostic (IVD) testing: approved guideline, POCT4-A2, Wayne, PA, 2006, Clinical Laboratory Standards Institute.
31. Finer N, Leone T: Oxygen saturation monitoring for the preterm infant: the evidence basis for current practice. Pediatr Res 65:375–380, 2009.
32. De Oliveira GS, Jr, Ahmad S, Fitzgerald PC, et al: Detection of hypoventilation during deep sedation in patients undergoing ambulatory gynaecological hysteroscopy: a comparison between transcutaneous and nasal end-tidal carbon dioxide measurements. Br J Anaesth 104:774–778, 2010.
33. McVicar J, Eager R: Validation study of a transcutaneous carbon dioxide monitor in patients in the emergency department. Emerg Med J 26:344–346, 2009.
34. Rodriguez P, Lellouche F, Aboab J, et al: Transcutaneous arterial carbon dioxide pressure monitoring in critically ill adult patients. Intensive Care Med 32:309–312, 2006.
35. Roediger R, Beck-Schimmer B, Theusinger OM, et al: The revised digital transcutaneous PCO2/SpO2 ear sensor is a reliable noninvasive monitoring tool in patients after cardiac surgery. J Cardiothorac Vasc Anesth 25:243–249, 2011.
36. Chakravarthy M, Narayan S, Govindarajan R, et al: Weaning mechanical ventilation after off-pump coronary artery bypass graft procedures directed by noninvasive gas measurements. J Cardiothorac Vasc Anesth 24:451–455, 2010.
37. Xue Q, Wu X, Jin J, et al: Transcutaneous carbon dioxide monitoring accurately predicts arterial carbon dioxide partial pressure in patients undergoing prolonged laparoscopic surgery. Anesth Analg 111:417–420, 2010.
38. Hirabayashi M, Fujiwara C, Ohtani N, et al: Transcutaneous PCO2 monitors are more accurate than end-tidal PCO2 monitors. J Anesth 23:198–202, 2009.
39. American Association for Respiratory Care: Clinical practice guideline: transcutaneous blood gas monitoring for neonatal and pediatric patients. Respir Care 49:1070, 2004.
40. Ganter M, Zollinger A: Continuous intravascular blood gas monitoring: development, current techniques, and clinical use of a commercial device. Br J Anaesth 91:397–407, 2003.
41. Schaarschmidt J, Seeburger J, Borger MA, et al: Clinical evaluation of the new BMU 40 in-line blood analysis monitor. Perfusion 24:277–286, 2009.
42. Ganter M, Zollinger A: Continuous intravascular blood gas monitoring: development, current techniques, and clinical use of a commercial device. Br J Anaesth 91:397–407, 2003.
43. Coule LW, Truemper EJ, Steinhart CM, et al: Accuracy and utility of a continuous intra-arterial blood gas monitoring system in pediatric patients. Crit Care Med 29:420–426, 2001.
44. Ganter MT, Hofer CK, Zollinger A, et al: Accuracy and performance of a modified continuous intravascular blood gas monitoring device during thoracoscopic surgery. J Cardiothorac Vasc Anesth 18:587–591, 2004.
45. Mahutte CK: On-line arterial blood gas analysis with optodes: current status. Clin Biochem 31:119–130, 1998.
46. Coule LW, Truemper EJ, Steinhart CM, et al: Accuracy and utility of a continuous intra-arterial blood gas monitoring system in pediatric patients. Crit Care Med 29:420–426, 2001.
47. Hess D: Detection and monitoring of hypoxemia and oxygen therapy. Respir Care 45:65–83, 2000.
48. Shapiro BA, Mahutte CK, Cane RD, et al: Clinical performance of a blood gas monitor: a prospective, multicenter trial. Crit Care Med 21:487–494, 1993.
49. Mahutte CK, Sasse SA, Chen PA, et al: Performance of a patient-dedicated, on-demand blood gas monitor in medical ICU patients. Am J Respir Crit Care Med 150:865–869, 1994.
50. Billman GF, Hughes AB, Dudell GG, et al: Clinical performance of an in-line, ex vivo point-of-care monitor: a multicenter study. Clin Chem 48:2030–2043, 2002.
51. Mulvey JM, Dorsch NW, Mudaliar Y, et al: Multimodality monitoring in severe traumatic brain injury: the role of brain tissue oxygenation monitoring. Neurocrit Care 1:391–402, 2004.
52. Mellstrom A, Mansson P, Jonsson K, et al: Measurements of subcutaneous tissue PO2 reflect oxygen metabolism of the small intestinal mucosa during hemorrhage and resuscitation: an experimental study in pigs. Eur Surg Res 42:122–129, 2009.
53. Mathews PJ: Co-oximetry. Respir Care Clin North Am 1:47, 1995.
54. Moyle JT: Uses and abuses of pulse oximetry. Arch Dis Child 74:77, 1996.
55. Ochroch EA, Russel MW, Hanson WC, 3rd: The impact of continuous pulse oximetry monitoring on intensive care unit admissions from a postsurgical care floor. Anesth Analg 102:868–875, 2006.
56. American Association for Respiratory Care: Clinical practice guideline: pulse oximetry. Respir Care 37:891, 1992.
57. Wahr JA, Tremper KK, Diab M: Pulse oximetry. Respir Care Clin North Am 1:77, 1995.
58. Yamamoto LG, Yamamoto JA, Yamamoto JB, et al: Nail polish does not significantly affect pulse oximetry measurements in mildly hypoxic subjects. Respir Care 53:1470–1474, 2008.
59. Barker SJ, Tremper KK, Hyatt J: Effects of methemoglobinemia on pulse oximetry and mixed venous oximetry. Anesthesiology 70:112–117, 1989.
60. Feiner JR, Bickler PE: Improved accuracy of methemoglobin detection by pulse CO-oximetry during hypoxia. Anesth Analg 111:1160–1167, 2010.
61. Reinhart K, Kuhn HJ, Hartog C, et al: Continuous central venous and pulmonary artery oxygen saturation monitoring in the critically ill. Intensive Care Med 30:1572–1578, 2004.
62. Cariou A, Monchi M, Dhainaut JF: Continuous cardiac output and mixed venous oxygen saturation monitoring. J Crit Care 13:198–213, 1998.
63. Molnar Z, Umgelter A, Toth I, et al: Continuous monitoring of ScvO2 by a new fibre-optic technology compared with blood gas oximetry in critically ill patients: a multicentre study. Intensive Care Med 33:1767–1770, 2007.
64. Cohn SM, Nathens AB, Moore FA, et al: Tissue oxygen saturation predicts the development of organ dysfunction during traumatic shock resuscitation. J Trauma 62:44–55, 2007.
65. Santora RJ, Moore FA: Monitoring trauma and intensive care unit resuscitation with tissue hemoglobin oxygen saturation. Crit Care 13(Suppl 5):S10, 2009.
66. Murkin JM, Arango M: Near-infrared spectroscopy as an index of brain and tissue oxygenation. Br J Anaesth 103 (Suppl 1):i3–i13, 2009.
67. Bhatia R, Hampton T, Malde S, et al: The application of near-infrared oximetry to cerebral monitoring during aneurysm embolization: a comparison with intraprocedural angiography. J Neurosurg Anesthesiol 19:97–104, 2007.
68. Nortje J, Gupta AK: The role of tissue oxygen monitoring in patients with acute brain injury. Br J Anaesth 97:95–106, 2006.
69. American Association for Respiratory Care: Clinical practice guideline: capnography/capnometry during mechanical ventilation. Respir Care 48:534, 2003.
70. Stock MC: Capnography for adults. Crit Care Clin 11:219, 1995.

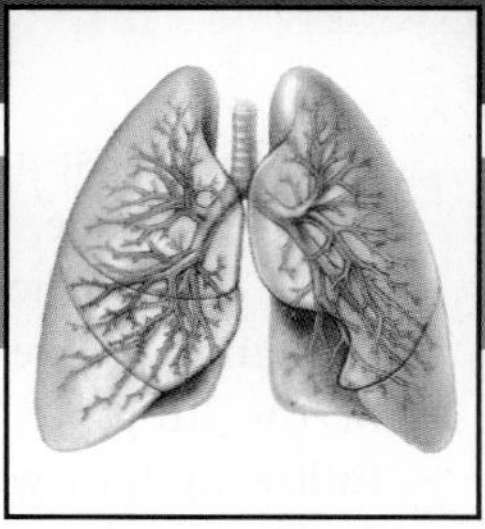

Chapter 19

Pulmonary Function Testing

F. HERBERT DOUCE

CHAPTER OBJECTIVES

After reading this chapter you will be able to:

- List the three categories of pulmonary function tests.
- State the primary purposes of pulmonary function testing.
- Describe the pathophysiologic patterns associated with obstructive and restrictive lung disease.
- State what is meant by the term *spirometer,* and list the parameters that can be measured by it.
- List and describe the four general principles that should be considered for pulmonary function tests.
- List and describe the measurements that indicate pulmonary mechanics.
- Describe the purpose and technique for the bronchial challenge test.
- List and describe the four volumes and four capacities that can be measured with pulmonary function testing.
- Describe the purpose and techniques used to measure diffusion capacity.
- Interpret pulmonary function reports.

CHAPTER OUTLINE

Pulmonary Function Testing
- Purposes
- Pathophysiologic Patterns
- Infection Control
- Equipment

Principles of Measurement and Significance
- Spirometry
- Lung Volumes and Capacities
- Diffusing Capacity

Interpretation of the Pulmonary Function Report

KEY TERMS

compliance
diffusing capacity of the lung (DL)
diffusing capacity of the lung for carbon monoxide (DLCO)
diffusing capacity of the lung-to-effective total lung capacity ratio ($DLCO/V_A$)
effective total lung capacity (V_A)
expiratory reserve volume (ERV)
forced expiratory flow between 25% and 75% of FVC ($FEF_{25\%-75\%}$)
forced expiratory flow between 75% and 85% of FVC ($FEF_{75\%-85\%}$)
forced expiratory flow between 200 ml and 1200 ml of FVC ($FEF_{200-1200}$)
forced expiratory volume in 1 second (FEV_1)
forced expiratory volume in 1 second-to-vital capacity ratio (FEV_1/FVC)
forced expiratory volume in half of a second ($FEV_{0.5}$)
forced vital capacity (FVC)
functional residual capacity (FRC)
inspiratory capacity (IC)
inspiratory reserve volume (IRV)
maximal voluntary ventilation (MVV)
minute ventilation ($\dot{V}_E$)
obstructive pulmonary disease
peak expiratory flow (PEF) rate
residual volume (RV)
restrictive pulmonary disease
thoracic gas volume (TGV)
tidal volume (V_T)
total lung capacity (TLC)
vital capacity (VC)

The most important function of the lungs is gas exchange. As mixed venous blood passes through the pulmonary circulation, the lungs add oxygen (O_2) and remove excess carbon dioxide (CO_2). The ability of the lungs to perform gas exchange depends on the following four general physiologic functions:

1. The diaphragm and thoracic muscles must be capable of expanding the thorax and lungs to produce a subatmospheric pressure.
2. The airways must be unobstructed to allow gas to flow into the lungs and reach the alveoli.
3. The cardiovascular system must circulate blood through the lungs and ventilated alveoli.
4. O_2 and CO_2 must be able to diffuse through the alveolar-capillary membrane.

Pulmonary function tests can provide valuable information about these important individual processes that support gas exchange. Various measurements are available to aid in the diagnosis and assessment of pulmonary diseases, to determine the need for therapy, and to evaluate the effectiveness of respiratory care. For respiratory therapists (RTs), knowledge of these tests and the ability to interpret the measurements are essential for assessing patients objectively and for planning and implementing effective patient care. The key terms used in this chapter are terms adopted and defined by the pulmonary medical community and should become the standard vocabulary of all RTs.[1]

PULMONARY FUNCTION TESTING

A complete evaluation of the respiratory system includes a patient history, physical examination, chest x-ray examination, arterial blood gas analysis, and tests of pulmonary function. Test results become most meaningful when considered in the context of a complete evaluation. Although diagnostic pulmonary function testing is performed in a laboratory setting and usually only on patients in a stable condition, RTs also perform many of these tests at the bedside on patients who are acutely ill. There are three categories of pulmonary function tests, measuring (1) dynamic flow rates of gases through the airways, (2) lung volumes and capacities, and (3) the ability of the lungs to diffuse gases. A combination of these measurements provides a quantitative picture of lung function. Although pulmonary function tests do not diagnose specific pulmonary diseases, these tests identify the presence and type of pulmonary impairments and the degree of pulmonary disease present. Some basic tests of pulmonary function are often performed at the bedside to provide immediate information about the need for respiratory therapy and its effectiveness.

Purposes

Generally, the primary purposes of pulmonary function testing are to identify pulmonary impairment and to quantify the severity of pulmonary impairment if present.[2] Pulmonary function testing has diagnostic and therapeutic roles and helps clinicians answer some general questions about patients with lung disease (Box 19-1).

Box 19-1 Basic Diagnostic and Therapeutic Questions for Clinical Pulmonary Function Testing

DIAGNOSTIC
- Is lung disease present?
- What type of lung impairment is present?
- What is the degree of lung impairment?
- Is more than one type of lung impairment present?
- Can multiple lung diseases be separated?

THERAPEUTIC
- Is therapy indicated?
- What treatments are most effective?
- To what degree is the disease reversible?
- Can treatments be evaluated?
- Is rehabilitation feasible?

The indications for pulmonary function testing are as follows:

- *To identify and quantify changes in pulmonary function.* The most common purposes of pulmonary function testing are to detect the presence or absence of pulmonary disease, to classify the type of disease as either obstructive or restrictive, and to quantify the severity of pulmonary impairment as mild, moderate, severe, or very severe. Over time, pulmonary function tests help quantify the progression or the reversibility of the disease.[3]
- *To evaluate need and quantify therapeutic effectiveness.*[4] Pulmonary function tests may aid clinicians in selecting or modifying a specific therapeutic regimen or technique (e.g., bronchodilator medication, airway clearance therapy, rehabilitation exercise protocol). Clinicians and researchers use pulmonary function tests to measure changes in lung function objectively before and after treatment.
- *To perform epidemiologic surveillance for pulmonary disease.* Screening programs may detect pulmonary abnormalities caused by disease or environmental factors in general populations, in people in occupational settings, in smokers, or in other high-risk groups. In addition, researchers have determined what normal pulmonary function is by measuring the pulmonary function of healthy people.[5]
- *To assess patients for risk of postoperative pulmonary complications.* Preoperative testing can identify patients who may have an increased risk of pulmonary complications after surgery.[6] Sometimes the risk of complications can be reduced by preoperative respiratory care, and sometimes the risk may be significant enough to rule out surgery.

- *To determine pulmonary disability.*[7] Pulmonary function tests can also determine the degree of disability caused by lung diseases, including occupational diseases such as pneumoconiosis of coal workers. Some federal entitlement programs and insurance policies rely on pulmonary function tests to confirm claims for financial compensation.

There are also contraindications to pulmonary function testing.[4] Patients with acute, unstable cardiopulmonary problems, such as hemoptysis, pneumothorax, myocardial infarction, and pulmonary embolism, and patients with acute chest or abdominal pain should not be tested. Testing could be harmful if needed treatment would be delayed. Patients who have nausea and who are vomiting should not be tested because there is a risk of aspiration. Testing for patients who have had recent cataract removal surgery should be delayed because changes in ocular pressure may be harmful to the eye. Pulmonary function testing requires patient effort and cooperation. Patients with dementia or confusion may not achieve optimal or repeatable results. Pulmonary function testing should not be performed if valid and reliable results cannot be predicted. In patients who are acutely ill or who have recently smoked a cigarette, the test validity of measuring the **forced vital capacity (FVC)** may be hindered.

Pathophysiologic Patterns

Pulmonary function testing provides the basis for classifying pulmonary diseases into two major categories, **obstructive pulmonary disease** and **restrictive pulmonary disease.** These two types of lung diseases sometimes occur together as a mixed impairment. Obstructive and restrictive types of lung diseases differ in several important ways. Figure 19-1 shows normal lungs with the pathophysiologic aspects of obstructive lung diseases and restrictive lung diseases, and the differences are summarized in Table 19-1. The primary problem in obstructive pulmonary disease is an increased airway resistance (R_{aw}). R_{aw} is the difference in pressure between the ends of the airways divided by the flow rate of gas moving through the airway, according to the following formula: $R_{aw} = \Delta P/\dot{V}$.

There is an inverse relationship between R_{aw} and flow rates ($\dot{V}$). If the pressure difference is constant, a reduced flow rate indicates an increase in R_{aw}. Because the radius of the airways normally lessens slightly during expiration, flow rates are usually measured during expiration. By rearranging the symbols in Poiseuille's law (see Chapter 6), R_{aw} is inversely related to the radius of the airways according to the following formula: $R_{aw} = \Delta P/\dot{V} = \eta 8l/r^4$.

When airway radius (r) decreases, R_{aw} increases, while the flow rate of gas through the airways ($\dot{V}$) decreases. Airway radius can be reduced by excessive contraction of the bronchial and bronchiolar muscles (bronchospasm), excessive secretions in the airways, swelling of the airway mucosa, airway tumors, collapse of the bronchioles, and other causes. By measuring flow rates, pulmonary function tests measure indirectly the size of the airways, R_{aw}, and the presence of obstructive disease.

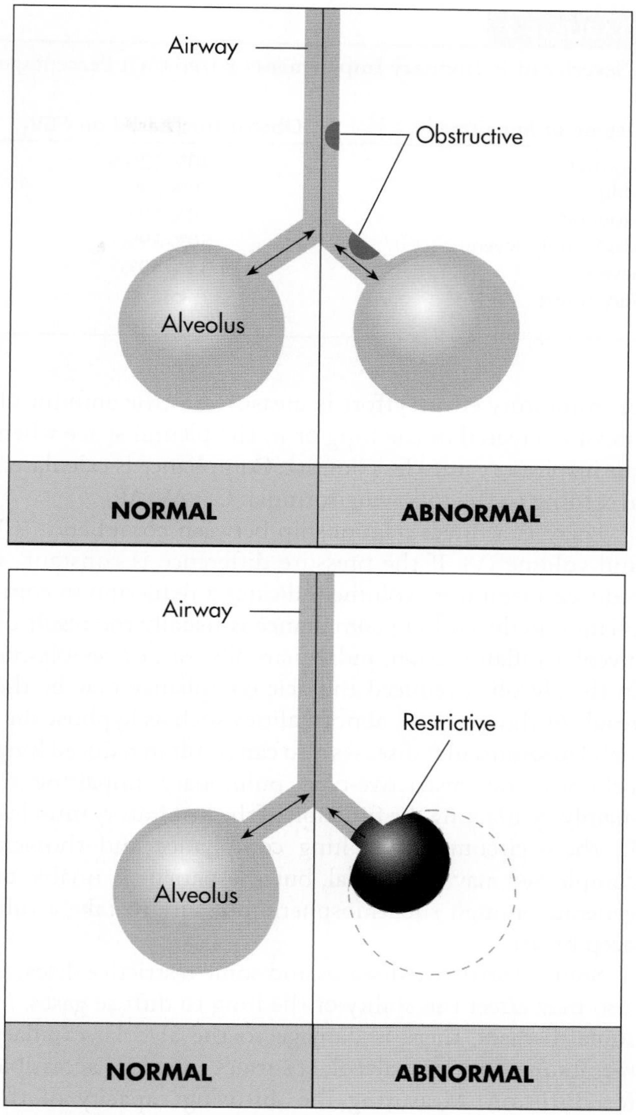

FIGURE 19-1 Pathophysiologic aspects of lung disease.

TABLE 19-1

Comparison of Obstructive and Restrictive Types of Pulmonary Diseases

Characteristic	Obstructive Disease	Restrictive Disease
Anatomy affected	Airways	Lung parenchyma, thoracic pump
Breathing phase difficulty	Expiration	Inspiration
Pathophysiology	Increased airway resistance	Decreased lung or thoracic compliance
Useful measurements	Flow rates	Volumes or capacities

The primary problem in restrictive lung disease is reduced lung compliance, thoracic compliance, or both. **Compliance** is the volume of gas inspired per the amount

TABLE 19-2

Severity of Pulmonary Impairments Based on a Percentage of Predicted Normal Values

Degree of Impairment	Obstruction based on FEV_1	Restriction or Obstruction Based on TLC, FRC, RV	Gas Exchange Based on DLCO
Normal	80%-120%	80%-120%	80%-120%
Mild	70%-79%	70%-79% or 121%-130%	61%-79%
Moderate	60%-69%	60%-69% or 131%-140%	40%-60%
Moderately severe	50%-59%	50%-59% or 141%-150%	
Severe	35%-49%	35%-49% or 151%-165%	<40%
Very severe	<35%	<35% or >165%	

of inspiratory effort; effort is measured as the amount of pressure created in the lung or in the pleural space when the inspiratory muscles contract. Compliance is calculated according to the following formula: $C = \Delta V/\Delta P$.

There is a direct relationship between compliance (C) and volume (V). If the pressure difference is constant, a reduced inspiratory volume indicates a reduction in compliance. Reduced lung compliance is usually the result of alveolar inflammation, pulmonary fibrosis, or neoplasms in the alveoli; a reduced thoracic compliance may be the result of thoracic wall abnormalities such as kyphoscoliosis. Neuromuscular diseases also can result in reduced lung volumes and restrictive-type pulmonary impairments, mainly by affecting the function of the inspiratory muscles. In these circumstances, lung compliance and thoracic compliance may be normal, but the patient is unable to generate enough subatmospheric pressure to take a full, deep breath.

Some obstructive diseases and some restrictive diseases also may affect the ability of the lung to diffuse gases. In some diseases, there is damage to the alveolar-capillary membrane, or less alveolar surface area is accessible for diffusion. Measuring the diffusing capacity of the lung for carbon monoxide (DLCO) can identify the destruction of alveolar tissue or the loss of functioning alveolar surface area.

For each measurement of pulmonary function, there is a normal value and a lower limit of normal (LLN). Measurements less than the LLN indicate the presence of an abnormality. The severity of pulmonary impairment is based on a comparison of each patient's measurement with the predicted normal value for the patient. Several methods are used for comparison with the normal value. A common method of comparison is to compute a percentage of the predicted normal value according to the following equation:

$$\%\ \text{Predicted} = \frac{\text{Measured value}}{\text{Predicted normal value}} \times 100$$

Determining if the patient's value is within 1 or 2 standard deviations of the predicted normal value is an alternative method used in some laboratories. The predicted percentage or the number of standard deviations from the predicted normal value can be used to quantify severity of impairment. Typical degrees of severity are listed in Table 19-2.

Infection Control

Pulmonary function testing is considered safe, but there is potential to transmit infective microorganisms to patients and technologists.[8] Transmission can occur by direct or indirect contact. Standard precautions should be applied because of the potential exposure to saliva or mucus, which could possibly contain blood or other potentially hazardous microorganisms. Patients with oral lesions pose the greatest potential hazard, and patients with compromised immune systems are at the greatest risk. Practitioners should wear gloves when handling potentially contaminated mouthpieces, valves, tubing, and equipment surfaces. When performing procedures on patients with potentially infectious airborne diseases, practitioners should wear a personal respirator or a close-fitting surgical mask, especially if the testing induces coughing. Practitioners should always wash their hands between testing patients and after contact with testing equipment. Although it is unnecessary to clean the interior surfaces of the testing instruments routinely between patients,[9] the mouthpiece, nose clips, tubing, and any parts of the instrument that come into direct contact with a patient should be disposed, sterilized, or disinfected between patients. Any equipment surface showing visible condensation from exhaled air should be discarded, disinfected, or sterilized before reuse. When testing instruments are disassembled for cleaning and disinfecting, manufacturer recommendations should be considered, and recalibration may be necessary before testing resumes. The routine use of low-resistance, in-line barrier filters is controversial.[10-12] Filters may be appropriate when internal surfaces of manifolds and valves proximal to mouthpieces are inaccessible or difficult to disassemble for cleaning and disinfecting. Filters provide visible evidence to reassure patients that their protection has been considered.

Equipment

Pulmonary function testing requires measurement of gas volume or flow, and various instruments and measurement principles are used to make these measurements. There are two general types of measuring instruments: instruments that measure gas volume and instruments that measure gas flow. Both types of instruments simultaneously measure time, and both compute various volumes and flow rates used in pulmonary function testing. The term *spirometer* is sometimes used as a generic term for all volume-measuring and flow-measuring devices.

Volume-measuring devices are specifically called *spirometers* and include water-sealed, bellows, and dry rolling seal types. These devices expand as they collect gas volumes. The magnitude of the expansion is the *volume* measured, and the speed of expansion represents the *flow rate*. In the absence of leaks and with low momentum forces, volume-measuring devices can be extremely accurate for measuring volumes, and with low inertia and friction forces, volume-measuring devices can be extremely accurate when computing flow rates.

Flow-measuring devices are commonly called *pneumotachometers,* although some practitioners reserve this term for only the device originally designed by Fleisch. These devices measure flow using a variety of unique principles. The Fleisch-type pneumotachometer measures the change in pressure as gas flows through a minimal, constant resistance according to the formula: $\dot{V} = \Delta P \div R$. Different manufacturers have used several materials to provide the resistance, including screens, capillary tubes, and fiber sheets made of silk, nylon, or filter paper. With multiple uses, condensation from exhaled air can collect in these devices and alter the resistance and accuracy of the device; some devices are heated to body temperature to prevent condensation. Known as *thermistors* or *mass flowmeters,* another type of flow-measuring device measures the temperature change created by gas flowing through it. There are also *tubinometers,* which use rotation of a fan or blades similar to a windmill. The number of rotations indicates volume, and the speed of the rotations indicates flow. How gas flow affects the transmission of sound waves and the force of flow stretching a spring have also been used to measure flow. Detailed descriptions and examples of each type of device are beyond the scope of this chapter and are available elsewhere.[13]

Regardless of the type of device or the principle of measurement used, several important characteristics are common to all volume-measuring and flow-measuring devices. Having an understanding of these common characteristics provides RTs the ability to select and use these devices properly. Every measuring instrument has capacity, accuracy, error, resolution, precision, linearity, and output.[14,15] The ideal instrument would have unlimited capacity to measure every pulmonary parameter, and it would have perfect accuracy and precision over its entire measurement range; there are no ideal instruments.

The *capacity* of an instrument refers to the range or limits of how much it can measure. Most instruments are designed with capacities to measure volumes and flow rates of all adults. The *accuracy* of a measuring instrument is how well it measures a known reference value. For volume measurements, standard reference values are provided by a graduated 3.0-L calibration syringe.[16] No measuring instrument is perfect, and there usually is an arithmetic difference between reference values and measured values. This difference is called the *error. Accuracy* and *error* are opposing terms; the greater the accuracy, the smaller is the error. Accuracy and error are commonly expressed as percentages, with their sum always equaling 100%. To determine percent accuracy and percent error, several reference values are measured, and the mean of the measured values is computed and compared with the reference values according to the following equations:

$$\% \text{ Accuracy} = \frac{\text{Mean measured value}}{\text{Reference value}} \times 100$$

or

$$\% \text{ Error} = \frac{\text{Mean measured value} - \text{Reference value}}{\text{Reference value}} \times 100$$

Resolution is the smallest detectable measurement; instruments with high resolution can measure the smallest volumes, flows, and times. *Precision* is synonymous with reliability of measurements and the opposite of variability. When multiple known reference values are measured, the standard deviation of the mean measured reference value is the statistic that indicates the precision of an instrument. A small standard deviation indicates low variability and high precision. *Linearity* refers to the accuracy of the instrument over its entire range of measurement, or its *capacity*. Some devices may accurately measure large volumes or high flow rates but may be less accurate when measuring small volumes or low flow rates. To determine linearity, accuracy and precision are calculated at different points over the range (capacity) of the device.

Output includes the specific measurements made or computed by the instrument. Most volume-measuring and flow-measuring devices measure the FVC and **forced expiratory volume in 1 second (FEV_1).** Others calculate various forced expiratory flow (FEF) rates, and some measure tidal volume (V_T) and **minute ventilation ($\dot{V}_E$).** Diagnostic spirometers usually measure and calculate **vital capacity (VC),** FVC, FEV_1, **peak expiratory flow (PEF) rate,** and FEF rates. Some measure and calculate **maximal voluntary ventilation (MVV).** Some of these instruments may be a component of a laboratory system providing the volume-measuring or flow-measuring capability for other diagnostic tests of pulmonary function. For example, they may be used with gas analyzers to measure **functional residual capacity (FRC)** and **total lung capacity (TLC)** or the inspiratory VC during *single-breath diffusing capacity (DLCOSB)*. Whether a spirometer or pneumotachometer is used in a diagnostic laboratory, a physician's office, or at the bedside in an intensive care unit, it should meet or exceed the national performance standards for volume-measuring and flow-measuring devices.

In 1978, the American Thoracic Society (ATS) adopted the initial standards for diagnostic spirometers. These standards have been adopted by other medical organizations and government agencies. Updated most recently in 2005 in collaboration with the European Respiratory Society (ERS), the standards are now recognized internationally as the standards for the industry.[17] Some instruments have been independently evaluated against the standards or compared with instruments that meet those standards. Regardless of the measuring principle used by the instrument or the purpose of the patient testing, RTs should use only devices that meet or exceed current ATS/ERS performance standards. According to the ATS/ERS standards, when measuring a slow VC, the spirometer should be able to measure for up to 30 seconds, and for the FVC, the time capacity should be at least 15 seconds. When measuring the VC, FVC, and forced expiratory volumes, a volume-measuring spirometer should have a capacity of at least 8 L and should measure volumes with less than a 3% error or within 50 ml of a reference value, whichever is greater. These standards, including the 8-L standard for capacity, also apply to children. A diagnostic spirometer that measures flow should be at least 95% accurate (or within 0.2 L/sec, whichever is greater) over the entire 0 to 14 L/sec range of gas flow. The standards are summarized in Table 19-3.

The spirometer standards also require spirometers to have a thermometer or to produce values corrected for body temperature, ambient pressure, and fully saturated with water vapor (BTPS). Standards also require that graphic outputs be of sufficient size and scale of display and recording to allow for visual inspection during testing, validation, and hand measurements. For visual display on a computer monitor, the resolution required is 0.050 L, and the scale of the volume axis must be 5 mm/L; the scale for the time axis must be at least 10 mm/sec. For validation and hand measurement functions from graph paper, the resolution must be 0.025 L, and the scale of the volume axis must be 10 mm/L; the scale for the time axis must be at least 20 mm/sec. Most manufacturers have designed their spirometers to meet or exceed the validation and hand measurement standards.

For quality control, the standards include verifying volume accuracy with a 3.0-L calibration syringe at least daily, although best practice in many laboratories is to verify accuracy before each test subject. The 2005 standards recognize that 3.0-L calibration syringes may have up to 0.5% error, and error may be acceptable if in the ±3.5% range. Volume linearity should be verified quarterly using 1.0-L increments over the entire volume range; flow linearity should be checked weekly using at least three different flow ranges. Recorder speed should be checked with a stopwatch quarterly. When new versions of software are installed, testing known subjects and comparing results is recommended. For comprehensive quality assurance of pulmonary function testing, there are three equally important aspects to consider: verifying the accuracy and precision of the measuring instruments, the performance of the technologist, and the test results when measuring a standard.

Most modern pulmonary function laboratories use computers for data acquisition and reduction. Computer-assisted testing decreases the time necessary to complete the tests and enhances the effectiveness of pulmonary function testing by increasing accuracy, increasing patient acceptance, and monitoring patient performance. Although computer-assisted testing and interpretations of test results are often applied by a computer, pulmonary function testing always requires a trained and competent RT to administer the tests, and computer analysis should not replace human analysis.

PRINCIPLES OF MEASUREMENT AND SIGNIFICANCE

For tests of pulmonary function, four important general principles should be considered: test specificity, sensitivity, validity, and reliability. Most tests of pulmonary function are not *specific* because several different diseases may cause the test result to be abnormal. This limitation of many pulmonary function tests explains why these tests identify a pattern of impairment rather than diagnose specific diseases. Some tests are extremely *sensitive,* and apparently healthy individuals may have an abnormal test result. However, some tests are not sensitive; individuals must be extremely sick to have an abnormal test result. To be

TABLE 19-3

2005 Spirometer Performance Standards of the American Thoracic Society/European Respiratory Society (ATS/ERS) Task Force

Test	Volume (L)	Flow (L/sec)	Accuracy	Time (sec)	Back Pressure (cm H_2O/L/sec)
VC	0.5-8 L	0-14	≤3% or 0.05 L*	30	
FVC	0.5-8 L	0-14	≤3% or 0.05 L*	15	<1.5%scm H_2O/L/sec at 14 L/sec
FEV_1	0.5-8 L	0-14	≤3% or 0.05 L*	1	<1.5%scm H_2O/L/sec at 14 L/sec
PEF		0-14	≤10% or 0.3 L/sec*		<1.5%scm H_2O/L/sec at 14 L/sec
FEF		±14	≤5% or 0.2 L/sec*		<1.5%scm H_2O/L/sec at 14 L/sec
MVV	250 L/min at 2 L/breath		±10% or 15 L/min*	12-15	<1.5%scm H_2O/L/sec at 14 L/sec

From Miller MR, Hankinson J, Brusasco V, et al: Standardisation of spirometry. Eur Respir J 26:319-338, 2005.
*Whichever is greater.

meaningful, each test must be *valid,* or the test is not measuring what it is intended to measure. When performing pulmonary function testing, strictly following testing procedures, ensuring patient effort and performance, and ensuring equipment accuracy and calibration establish test validity. Test *reliability* is the consistency of the test results. A reliable test produces consistent test results with minimal variability. To be reliable, each test must be performed more than once. Ensuring test validity and reliability is the most important role of the RT. Test results that are invalid or unreliable can lead to misdiagnosis, mistreatment, and poor outcomes.

RULE OF THUMB

Never report test results that are invalid or unreliable.

In most pulmonary function laboratories, there are three components to pulmonary function testing: (1) performing spirometry for measuring airway mechanics, (2) measuring lung volumes and capacities, and (3) measuring the **diffusing capacity of the lung (DL).** For each component, there are various techniques and different types of equipment that make the measurements. When the purpose of the testing is to identify the presence and the degree of pulmonary impairment and the type of pulmonary disease, all three testing components are required. When the purpose of the testing is more limited, such as to assess postoperative pulmonary risk or to evaluate and quantify therapeutic effectiveness, the scope of measurement also is limited. Many pulmonary function laboratories also perform arterial blood gas analysis (see Chapter 18), and some laboratories provide more specialized and advanced tests, such as bronchial challenge tests and exercise stress tests.

Spirometry

Spirometry includes the tests of pulmonary mechanics—the measurements of FVC, FEV_1, several FEF values, forced inspiratory flow rates, and MVV. Measuring pulmonary mechanics is assessing the ability of the lungs to move large volumes of air quickly through the airways to identify airway obstruction. Some measurements are aimed at large intrathoracic airways, some are aimed at small airways, and some assess obstruction throughout the lungs. Measuring flow rates is a surrogate for measuring airways resistance according to the formula: $Raw = \Delta P \div \dot{V}$. A decrease in flow rate signifies an increase in airways resistance and the presence of airway obstruction when patient effort creating the difference between mouth pressure and lung pressure is constant (see Clinical Practice Guideline 19-1).[17]

Although performing tests of pulmonary mechanics is considered safe, some adverse reactions have occurred, including pneumothorax,[18] syncope, chest pain, paroxysmal coughing, and bronchospasm associated with exercise-induced asthma.[19] The contraindications for pulmonary function testing are primarily for testing mechanics. The

19-1 Spirometry

AARC Clinical Practice Guideline (Excerpts)*

INDICATIONS

The indications for spirometry include the need to do the following:

- Detect the presence or absence of lung dysfunction suggested by history or physical signs and symptoms or the presence of other abnormal diagnostic tests (e.g., chest radiograph, ABGs)
- Quantify the severity of known lung disease
- Assess the change in lung function over time or after administration of or change in therapy
- Assess the potential effects or response to environmental or occupational exposure
- Assess the risk for surgical procedures known to affect lung function
- Assess impairment or disability (e.g., for rehabilitation, legal reasons, military)

CONTRAINDICATIONS

Circumstances listed here could affect the reliability of spirometry measurements. In addition, forced expiratory maneuvers may aggravate these conditions, which may make test postponement necessary until the medical condition resolves. The following are some relative contraindications to performing spirometry:

- Hemoptysis of unknown origin (forced expiratory maneuver may aggravate the underlying condition)
- Pneumothorax
- Unstable cardiovascular status (forced expiratory maneuver may worsen angina or cause changes in blood pressure) or recent myocardial infarction or pulmonary embolus
- Thoracic, abdominal, or cerebral aneurysms (danger of rupture resulting from increased thoracic pressure)
- Recent eye surgery (e.g., cataract)
- Presence of an acute disease process that might interfere with test performance (e.g., nausea, vomiting)
- Recent surgery of thorax or abdomen

Continued

19-1 Spirometry—cont'd

AARC Clinical Practice Guideline (Excerpts)*

■ HAZARDS AND COMPLICATIONS

Although spirometry is a safe procedure, untoward reactions may occur, and the value of the test data should be weighed against potential hazards. The following have been reported anecdotally:

- Pneumothorax
- Paroxysmal coughing
- Increased intracranial pressure
- Contraction of nosocomial infections
- Syncope, dizziness, lightheadedness
- O_2 desaturation resulting from interruption of O_2 therapy
- Chest pain
- Bronchospasm

■ ASSESSMENT OF NEED

Need is assessed by determining that valid indications are present.

■ ASSESSMENT OF TEST QUALITY

Spirometry performed for the listed indications is valid only if the spirometer functions acceptably and the subject is able to perform the maneuvers in an acceptable and reproducible fashion. All reports should contain a statement about the technician's assessment of test quality and specify which acceptability criteria were not met.

■ QUALITY CONTROL

- *Volume verification (i.e., calibration):* At least daily before testing, use a calibrated known-volume syringe with a volume of at least 3 L to ascertain that the spirometer reads a known volume accurately. The known volume should be injected or withdrawn at least three times, at flows that vary between 2 L/sec and 12 L/sec (3-L injection times of approximately 1 second, 6 seconds, and between 1 seconds and 6 seconds). The tolerance limits for an acceptable calibration are ±3% of the known volume. For a 3-L calibration syringe, the acceptable recovered range is 2.91 to 3.09 L. The practitioner is encouraged to exceed this guideline whenever possible (i.e., reduce the tolerance limits to less than ±3%).
- *Leak test:* Volume-displacement spirometers must be evaluated for leaks daily. One recommendation is that any volume change of more than 10 ml/min while the spirometer is under at least 3 cm H_2O pressure be considered excessive.
- A spirometry procedure manual should be maintained.
- A log that documents daily instrument calibration, problems encountered, corrective action required, and system hardware or software changes should be maintained.
- Computer software for measurement and computer calculations should be checked against manual calculations if possible. In addition, biologic laboratory standards (i.e., healthy, nonsmoking individuals) can be tested periodically to ensure historic reproducibility, to verify software upgrades, and to evaluate new or replacement spirometers.
- The known-volume syringe should be checked for accuracy at least quarterly using a second known-volume syringe, with the spirometer in the patient-test mode; this validates the calibration and ensures that the patient-test mode operates properly.
- For water-seal spirometers, water level and paper tracing speed should be checked daily. The entire range of volume displacement should be checked quarterly.

■ QUALITY ASSURANCE

- Each laboratory or testing site should develop, establish, and implement quality assurance indicators for equipment calibration and maintenance and patient preparation.
- Methods should be devised and implemented to monitor technician performance (with appropriate feedback) while obtaining, recognizing, and documenting acceptability criteria.

■ MONITORING

- The following should be evaluated during the performance of spirometric measurements to ascertain the validity of the results:
  Acceptability of maneuver and reproducibility of FVC and FEV_1
  Level of effort and cooperation by the subject
  Equipment function or malfunction (e.g., calibration)
- The final report should contain a statement about test quality.
- Spirometry results should be subject to ongoing review by a supervisor, with feedback to the technologist.
- Quality assurance or quality improvement programs should be designed to monitor technician competency initially and in an ongoing fashion.

**For the complete guideline, see American Association for Respiratory Care: Clinical practice guideline: spirometry. 1996 update, Respir Care 41:629, 1996.*

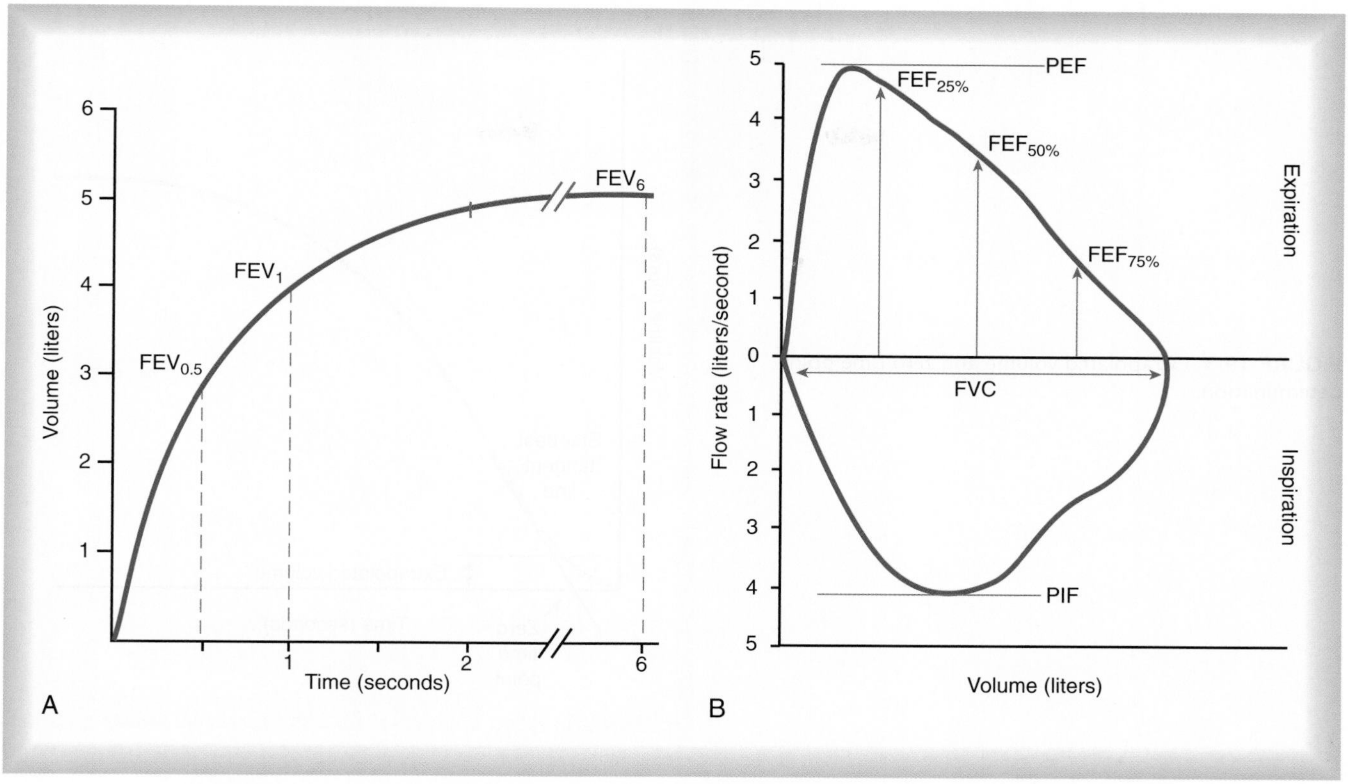

FIGURE 19-2 Forced vital capacity, forced expiratory volumes, and flow rates. **A,** Forced vital capacity on a volume-time graph. **B,** Forced vital capacity on a flow-volume graph.

ATS/ERS 2005 standards for spirometry[17] specify the validity and reliability criteria of the measurements and accuracy and precision limits of the measuring equipment. These standards have been incorporated into the clinical practice guidelines of the AARC, medical societies, and government agencies.[4,20-22]

Forced Vital Capacity

FVC is the most commonly performed test of pulmonary mechanics, and many measurements are made while the patient is performing the FVC maneuver (Figure 19-2). Measuring FVC often occurs under baseline or untreated conditions. For baseline testing, patients should temporarily abstain from bronchodilator medications. Short-acting bronchodilators (e.g., β-agonist albuterol, anticholinergic agent ipratropium bromide) should not be used for 4 hours before baseline spirometry, whereas long-acting β-agonist bronchodilators and oral therapy with aminophylline should be stopped for 12 hours. When a patient's baseline results show airway obstruction, performing FVC after treatment (e.g., albuterol bronchodilator aerosol or metered dose inhaler) can help determine if the treatment is effective. The FVC maneuver is also performed repeatedly during bronchial provocation testing.

FVC may be measured on a spirometer that measures volumes or flows, that presents a graph of volume and time or flow and volume, that is mechanical or electronic, and that has a calculator or computer. The forced expiratory VC sometimes is followed by a forced inspiratory VC to produce a complete image of forced breathing called a *flow-volume loop*.[23]

FVC is an effort-dependent maneuver that requires careful patient instruction, understanding, coordination, and cooperation. Spirometry standards for FVC specify that patients must be instructed in the FVC maneuver, that the appropriate technique be demonstrated, and that enthusiastic coaching occur. When measuring FVC, the RT needs to coach the preceding inspiratory capacity (IC) as enthusiastically as the FVC. According to the standards, nose clips are encouraged, but not required, and patients may be tested in the sitting or standing position. Although standing usually produces a larger FVC compared with sitting, sitting is considered safer in case of lightheadedness. It is recommended that the position be consistent for repeat testing of the same patient. FVC should be converted to body temperature conditions and reported as liters under BTPS conditions.

RULE OF THUMB

If you don't inhale it, you can't exhale it. So, coach the preceding IC as enthusiastically as the FVC.

To ensure validity, each patient must perform a minimum of three acceptable FVC maneuvers. To ensure reliability, the largest FVC and second largest FVC from the acceptable trials should not vary by more than 0.150 L. To

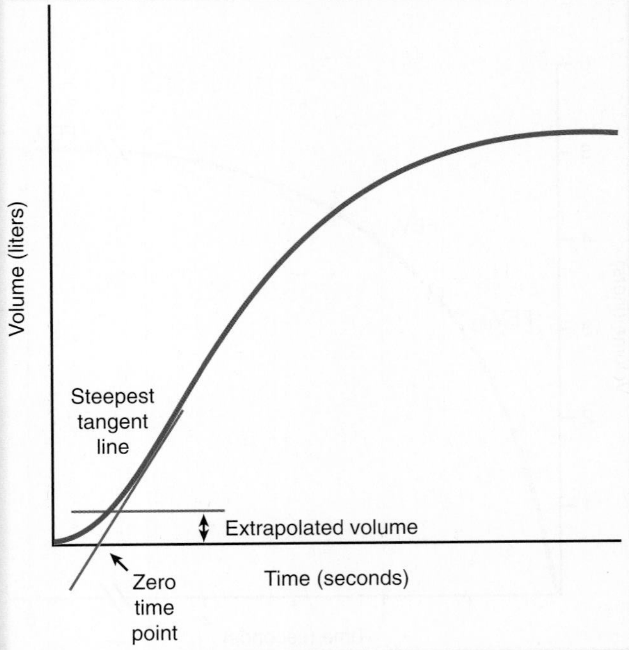

FIGURE 19-3 Extrapolated volume and zero time point determination.

perform an FVC trial, the patient should inhale rapidly and completely to TLC from the resting FRC level. The forced exhalation of an acceptable FVC trial should begin abruptly and without hesitation. A satisfactory start of expiration is defined as an extrapolated volume at the zero time point less than 5% of FVC or 0.150 L, whichever is greater (Figure 19-3). The volume exhaled before the zero time point is called the *extrapolated volume.* To be valid, no more than 5% of the VC or 0.150 L is allowed to be exhaled before the zero time point. An acceptable FVC trial also is smooth, continuous, and complete. A cough, an inspiration, a Valsalva maneuver, a leak, or an obstructed mouthpiece while an FVC maneuver is being performed disqualifies the trial. FVC must be completely exhaled or an exhalation time of at least 6 seconds must occur for adults and children older than 10 years (longer times are commonly needed for patients with airway obstruction). A 3-second exhalation is acceptable for children younger than 10 years old. An end expiratory plateau must be obvious in the volume-time curve; the objective standard is less than 0.025 L exhaled during the final second of exhalation. Consistent with its definition, the largest acceptable FVC (BTPS) measured from the set of three acceptable trials is the patient's FVC.

Forced Expiratory Volume in 1 Second

During FVC testing, several other measurements are also made. FEV_1 is a measurement of the volume exhaled in the first second of FVC (see Figure 19-2, *A*). To ensure validity of FEV_1, the measurement must originate from a set of three acceptable FVC trials. The first second of forced exhalation begins at the zero time point (see Figure 19-3). To ensure reliability of FEV_1, the largest FEV_1 and second largest FEV_1 from the acceptable trials should not vary by more than 0.150 L. Consistent with its definition, the largest FEV_1 (BTPS) measured is the patient's FEV_1. The largest FEV_1 sometimes comes from a different trial than the largest FVC.

The %FEV_1/FVC, also called the **forced expiratory volume in 1 second-to-vital capacity ratio (FEV_1/FVC),** is calculated by dividing the patient's largest FEV_1 by the patient's largest VC and converting it to a percentage (by multiplying by 100). The two values do not have to come from the same trial; the VC should be the largest VC measured, even if measured as a slow VC or during inspiration.

Except for PEF rate, all other measurements that originate from FVC come from the "best curve"—these include **forced expiratory flow between 200 ml and 1200 ml of FVC ($FEF_{200\text{-}1200}$); forced expiratory flow between 25% and 75% of FVC ($FEF_{25\%\text{-}75\%}$); forced expiratory flow between 75% and 85% of FVC ($FEF_{75\%\text{-}85\%}$);** and instantaneous $FEF_{25\%}$, $FEF_{50\%}$, and $FEF_{75\%}$. The *best test curve* is defined as the trial that meets the acceptability criteria and gives the largest sum of FVC plus FEV_1. The validity and reliability of these other measurements of pulmonary mechanics are based on their origin from a valid and reliable FVC.

Forced Expiratory Flow Between 200 ml and 1200 ml of Forced Vital Capacity and Forced Expiratory Flow Between 25% and 75% of Forced Vital Capacity

$FEF_{200\text{-}1200}$ and $FEF_{25\%\text{-}75\%}$ represent average flow rates that occur during specific intervals of FVC. Both measurements can be made on a volume-time spirogram as the slope of a

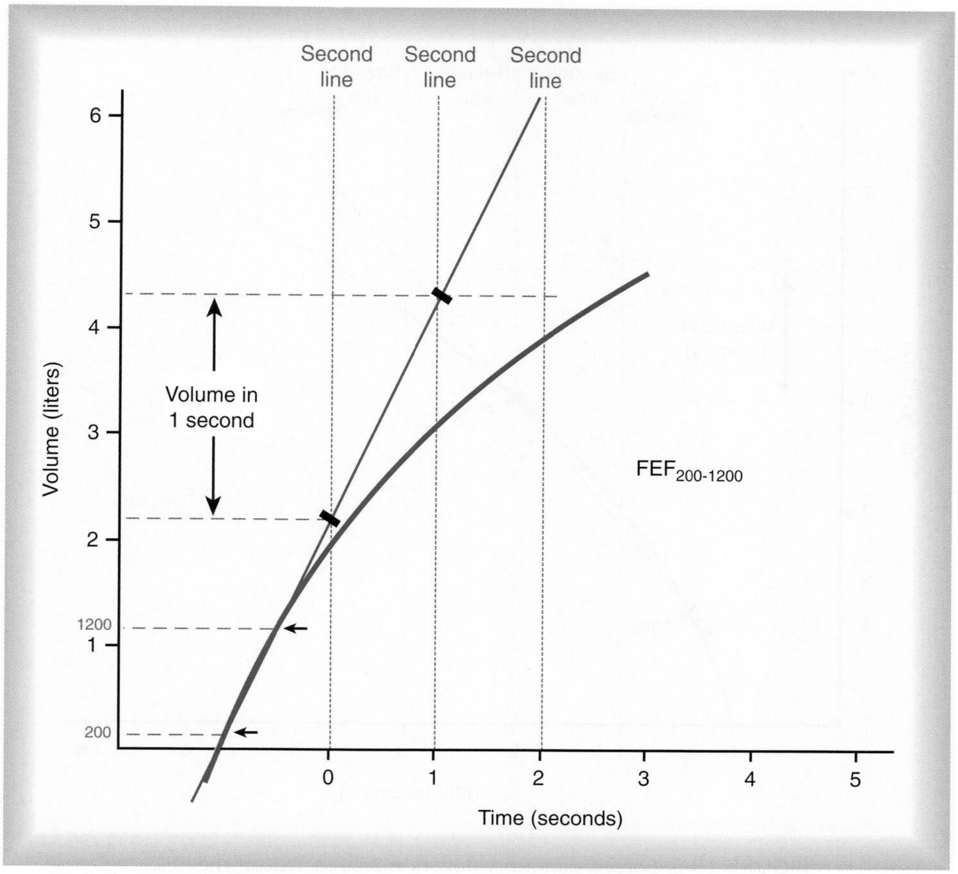

FIGURE 19-4 Forced expiratory flow rate 200 to 1200 ml.

line connecting the two points in their subscripts. For $FEF_{200\text{-}1200}$, the 200-ml point and the 1200-ml point are identified. A straight line is drawn connecting these points, and the line is extended to intersect two vertical time lines 1 second apart on the graph (Figure 19-4). The volume of air measured between the two time lines is $FEF_{200\text{-}1200}$ in liters per second. The volume measured must be corrected to BTPS.

$FEF_{25\%\text{-}75\%}$ is a measure of the flow during the middle portion of FVC, or the time necessary to exhale the middle 50%. For $FEF_{25\%\text{-}75\%}$, the VC of the best curve is multiplied by 25% and 75%, and the points are identified on the tracing. A straight line is drawn connecting these points, and the line is extended to intersect two vertical time lines 1 second apart on the graph. The volume of air measured between the two time lines is $FEF_{25\%\text{-}75\%}$ in liters per second. The volume measured must be corrected to BTPS (Figure 19-5).

Peak Expiratory Flow

PEF is difficult to identify on a volume-time graph of FVC. The peak flow is the slope of the tangent to the steepest portion of the FVC curve. PEF is easy to identify on a flow-volume graph as the highest point on the graph (see Figure 19-2, *B*).[23] PEF is sometimes measured independently of FVC with a peak flowmeter. These devices are designed to indicate only the greatest expiratory flow rate. The validity of PEF rate is based on a preceding inspiration to TLC and a maximal effort. The FVC principles of ensuring reliability should apply to measurements of PEF rate. The two largest repeated measurements should agree within 5%.

In addition to PEF rate, the other instantaneous flow rates, such as forced expiratory flow at 25% ($FEF_{25\%}$) of FVC, forced expiratory flow at 50% ($FEF_{50\%}$) of FVC, and forced expiratory flow at 75% ($FEF_{75\%}$) of FVC, during FVC are graphed on a flow-volume curve. When FVC is followed by a forced inspiratory VC, a flow-volume loop is produced (see Figure 19-2, *B*). On the flow-volume loop, the maximal forced inspiratory flow rate at 50% ($FIF_{50\%}$) of VC can be measured and compared with $FEF_{50\%}$.

Maximal Voluntary Ventilation

Another measurement of pulmonary mechanics is MVV. MVV is another effort-dependent test for which the patient is asked to breathe as deeply and as rapidly as possible for at least 12 seconds. MVV is a test that reflects patient cooperation and effort, the ability of the diaphragm and thoracic muscles to expand the thorax and lungs, and airway patency. Because of the potential for acute hyperventilation and fainting or coughing, the patient

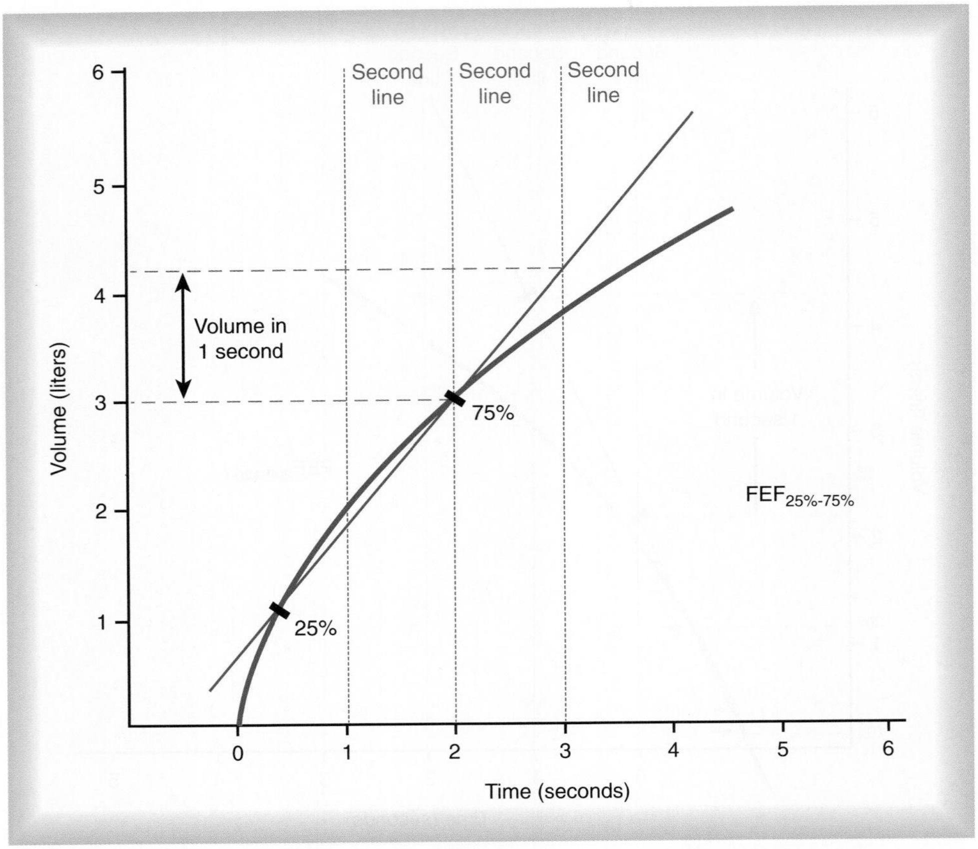

FIGURE 19-5 Forced expiratory flow rate 25% to 75% of the FVC.

should be seated. Measuring systems that incorporate rebreathing may minimize hyperventilation. After a demonstration of the expected breathing pattern is performed, the patient should be instructed to breathe as rapidly and as deeply as possible for at least 12 seconds. The patient's breathing is measured on a spirogram (Figure 19-6) or electronically for the specific number of seconds (t) and the volume (V) breathed when the MVV is converted to liters per minute. As with all volumes measured on a spirometer, the recorded values should be in BTPS conditions. The validity of MVV depends on the duration of the maneuver, which should be at least 12 seconds; the breathing frequency, which should be at least 90/min; and the average volume, which should be at least 50% of FVC. Patients should perform at least two MVV trials when the first trial does not exceed 80% of the subject's $FEV_1 \times 40$, which may indicate less than maximal effort, or 80% of the predicted normal value, which may indicate disease. Reliability is shown when there is less than 20% variability between the two largest trials. The largest MVV (BTPS) should be reported.

Quality Assurance

For comprehensive quality assurance of spirometry, the accuracy and precision of the volume or flow measuring device must be verified with a 3.0-L syringe using multiple full strokes at various injection speeds to mimic fast and slow flow rates. The average volume should meet the ±3% standard; the standard deviation should be small, and the 95% confidence interval or expected performance range should be determined. Subsequent individual checks of accuracy with the 3.0-L syringe should be compared with the ±3% standard and the expected performance range to ensure that the device is measuring consistently. The performance of the technologist to coach subjects during spirometric testing should be observed and reviewed periodically. Technologists successfully achieving testing acceptability and repeatability criteria should be monitored and feedback to the technologist should be provided periodically.

Significance

The normal values for the spirometric measurements of pulmonary mechanics are based on height, age, gender, and ethnicity. Table 19-4 provides common regression equations to predict normal values for the measurements of pulmonary mechanics for individuals of specific height (in centimeters), age (in years), and gender.[24-26] A positive correlation exists between measurements of pulmonary mechanics and height, and a negative correlation exists

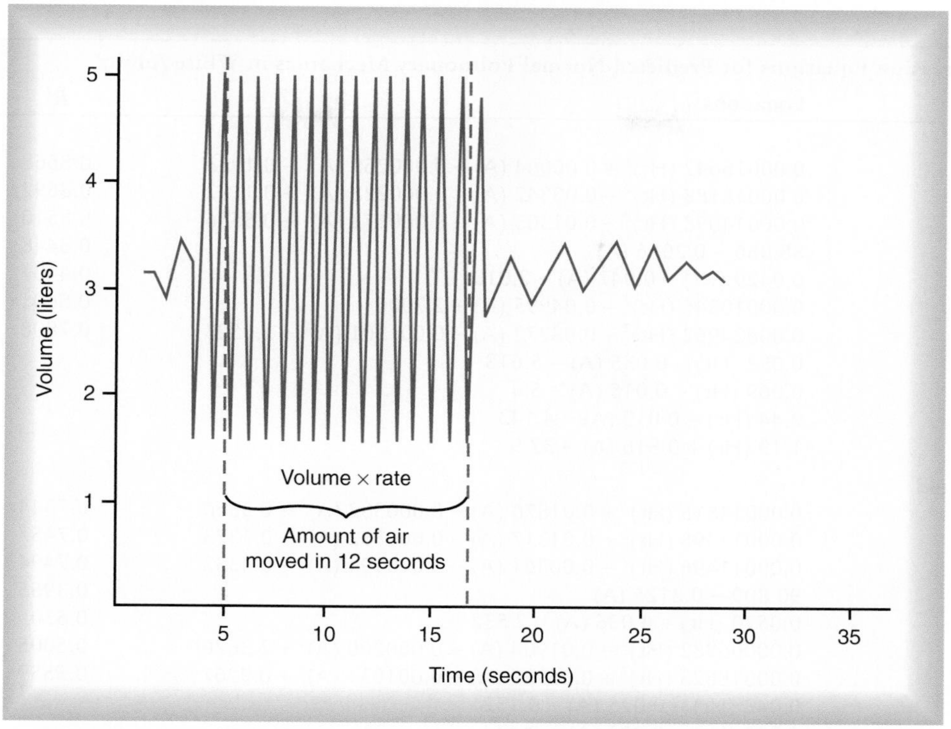

FIGURE 19-6 Maximal voluntary ventilation tracing. Actual ventilations recorded during a 12-second period.

MINI CLINI

Decreased Forced Vital Capacity and Forced Expiratory Volume in 1 Second: Is It Obstruction or Restriction?

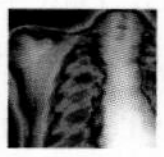

PROBLEM: Both obstructive and restrictive diseases may exhibit decreased FVC and FEV_1. How can the two kinds of patterns be differentiated?

SOLUTION: FVC and FEV_1 are reduced in both obstructive and restrictive diseases for different reasons. With restrictive disease, lung expansion is reduced. If a person can inhale only a small volume, he or she can exhale only a small volume. All lung volumes are smaller than normal, including TLC, FVC, and FEV_1.

With obstructive disease, there is airway obstruction, which slows expiratory flow. FEV_1 is reduced because of the increased airway resistance, which decreases expiratory flow rates. FVC is reduced because airway obstruction in the bronchioles causes air trapping in the lung. If a person cannot exhale all of his or her air because some is trapped in the lungs, the volume the person does exhale is reduced.

To differentiate between obstructive and restrictive patterns of impairment, compare FEV_1 with FVC using the FEV_1/FVC ratio. Only individuals with airway obstruction exhale less than 70% of FVC in the first second. Individuals with restrictive disease or healthy lungs are able to exhale more than 70% of FVC during the first second.

between measurements of pulmonary mechanics and age for patients older than 20 years. Male values are larger than female values when height and age are equal. The populations that were studied to determine the normal values of pulmonary mechanics were predominantly white. To account for ethnic differences of nonwhites, the predicted normal values for whites commonly are reduced by 12% to 15% when applied to nonwhites. Ethnic-specific equations for special populations, such as African-Americans and Mexican-Americans, have also been developed.[24]

Although traditional textbooks suggest the typical normal VC is 4.80 L, the predicted normal FVC for a 20-year-old, 180-cm man approaches 5.60 L. A reduced FVC may occur with obstructive or restrictive impairments. Figure 19-7 shows FVC from volume-time spirometer tracings for normal, obstructive, and restrictive conditions. The FVC values in both the obstructed and the restricted curves are shown as reduced volumes compared with the normal curve. The primary difference between the curve in the restricted patient compared with the curve in the obstructed patient is the slope of the tracing; obstructive diseases produce flattened slopes and smaller FEV_1.

Figure 19-8 displays the FVC from flow-volume tracings for obstructive and restrictive conditions. The shapes of these tracings are different; obstructive diseases produce lower peaks and lower flow rates at all lung volumes. Forced inspiratory flow rates sometimes are useful for identifying extrathoracic airway obstructions. In moderate and severe obstructive lung diseases, the FVC is reduced if

TABLE 19-4

Examples of Regression Equations for Predicted Normal Pulmonary Mechanics in White Adults

Parameters	Equations	R^2	Reference
Men ≥20 years old			
FVC (L)	$0.00018642\ (Ht)^2 + 0.00064\ (A) - 0.000269\ (A)^2 - 0.1933$	0.8668	24
FEV_6 (L)	$0.00018188\ (Ht)^2 - 0.00842\ (A) - 0.000223\ (A)^2 + 0.1102$	0.8692	24
FEV_1 (L)	$0.00014098\ (Ht)^2 - 0.01303\ (A) - 0.000172\ (A)^2 + 0.5536$	0.8510	24
% FEV_1/FVC	$88.066 - 0.2066\ (A)$	0.3448	24
$FEF_{200\text{-}1200}$ (L/sec)	$0.0429\ (Ht) - 0.047\ (A) + 2.010$	0.440	25
$FEF_{25\%\text{-}75\%}$ (L/sec)	$0.00010345\ (Ht)^2 - 0.04995\ (A) + 2.7006$	0.5601	24
PEF (L/sec)	$0.00024962\ (Ht)^2 + 0.08272\ (A) - 0.001301\ (A)^2 + 1.0523$	0.7808	24
$FEF_{25\%}$ (L/sec)	$0.088\ (Ht) - 0.035\ (A) - 5.618$		23
$FEF_{50\%}$ (L/sec)	$0.069\ (Ht) - 0.015\ (A) - 5.4$		23
$FEF_{75\%}$ (L/sec)	$0.44\ (Ht) - 0.012\ (A) - 4.143$		23
MVV (L/min)	$1.19\ (Ht) - 0.816\ (A) - 37.9$		26
Women ≥18 years old			
FVC (L)	$0.00014815\ (Ht)^2 + 0.01870\ (A) - 0.000382\ (A)^2 - 0.3560$	0.7344	24
FEV_6 (L)	$0.00014395\ (Ht)^2 + 0.01317\ (A) - 0.000352\ (A)^2 - 0.1373$	0.7457	24
FEV_1 (L)	$0.00011496\ (Ht)^2 - 0.00361\ (A) - 0.000194\ (A)^2 + 0.4333$	0.7494	24
% FEV_1/FVC	$90.809 - 0.2125\ (A)$	0.3955	24
$FEF_{200\text{-}1200}$ (L/sec)	$0.0570\ (Ht) - 0.036\ (A) - 2.532$	0.530	25
$FEV_{25\%\text{-}75\%}$ (L/sec)	$0.00006982\ (Ht)^2 - 0.01904\ (A) - 0.000200\ (A)^2 + 2.3670$	0.5005	24
PEF (L/sec)	$0.00018623\ (Ht)^2 + 0.06929\ (A) - 0.001031\ (A)^2 + 0.9267$	0.5559	24
$FEF_{25\%}$ (L/sec)	$0.043\ (Ht) - 0.025\ (A) - 0.132$		23
$FEF_{50\%}$ (L/sec)	$0.035\ (Ht) - 0.013\ (A) - 0.444$		23
$FEF_{75\%}$ (L/sec)	$3.042 - 0.014\ (A)$		23
MVV (L/min)	$0.84\ (Ht) - 0.685\ (A) - 4.87$		26

A, Years; *Ht,* cm; *L,* liters at BTPS.

weakened bronchioles collapse and trap air in the lungs, creating an increase in RV. Some laboratories compare the volumes of slow vital capacity (SVC) and FVC to identify air trapping. VC is reduced in restrictive lung diseases because the patient's inhaled volume is reduced.

Forced expiratory volume in half of a second ($FEV_{0.5}$) is an indicator of patient effort during the initial phase of the FVC maneuver. With good effort, a patient should exhale at least 50% of his or her VC in the initial half of a second.

Although FEV_1 is measured as a volume, FEV_1 is considered a flow rate. The predicted normal FEV_1 for a 20-year-old, 180-cm man approaches 4.70 L. FEV_1 may be reduced with obstructive or restrictive impairments. For patients with airway obstruction, FEV_1 measures the general severity of airway obstruction. For patients with restrictive impairment, FEV_1 may be reduced when the patient's VC is smaller than the predicted FEV_1.

The *FEV_1/FVC* ratio separates patients with airway obstruction from individuals with normal pulmonary function and from patients with restrictive impairment. The LLN can be determined or the predicted normal %FEV_1/FVC can be calculated by dividing the predicted normal FEV_1 by the predicted normal VC. Generally, individuals without airway obstruction are able to exhale at least 70% of their VC in the first second, and individuals with airway obstruction exhale less than 70% of their VC in the first second.

To interpret other flow rates, a generalization may be helpful. Gas exhaled during the early portion of the FVC reflects the resistance in the larger airways, and gas exhaled during the later portion of the FVC reflects the resistance in the smaller airways. As exhalation of FVC proceeds, flow decreases, and the airways reflected in the measurements get smaller. Any flow measured in the first half of the FVC reflects on the bronchi; any flow measured beyond 50% of the VC reflects on the bronchioles.

PEF, $FEF_{200\text{-}1200}$, and $FEF_{25\%}$ occur near the onset of FVC. Typical normal values are similar; PEF is 9.5 L/sec, $FEF_{200\text{-}1200}$ is 8.5 L/sec, and $FEF_{25\%}$ is 9.0 L/sec. A reduced PEF rate, $FEF_{200\text{-}1200}$, or $FEF_{25\%}$ may occur as a result of a large airway obstruction and from lack of sufficient effort to inhale maximally and exhale forcibly. $FEF_{25\%\text{-}75\%}$ and $FEF_{50\%}$ occur in the middle of FVC. Because $FEF_{25\%\text{-}75\%}$ is an average of half the VC and $FEF_{50\%}$ is an instantaneous flow, the typical normal values are less similar; $FEF_{25\%\text{-}75\%}$ is 4.5 L/sec, and $FEF_{50\%}$ is 6.5 L/sec. Reduced $FEF_{25\%\text{-}75\%}$ or $FEF_{50\%}$ may occur because of small airway obstruction and from lack of effort to sustain a maximal exhalation. $FEF_{75\%}$ and $FEF_{75\%\text{-}85\%}$ occur late in FVC and reflect on the smallest airways. Typical values are 3.5 L/sec for $FEF_{75\%}$ and 1.5 L/sec for $FEF_{75\%\text{-}85\%}$. Sometimes patients who are

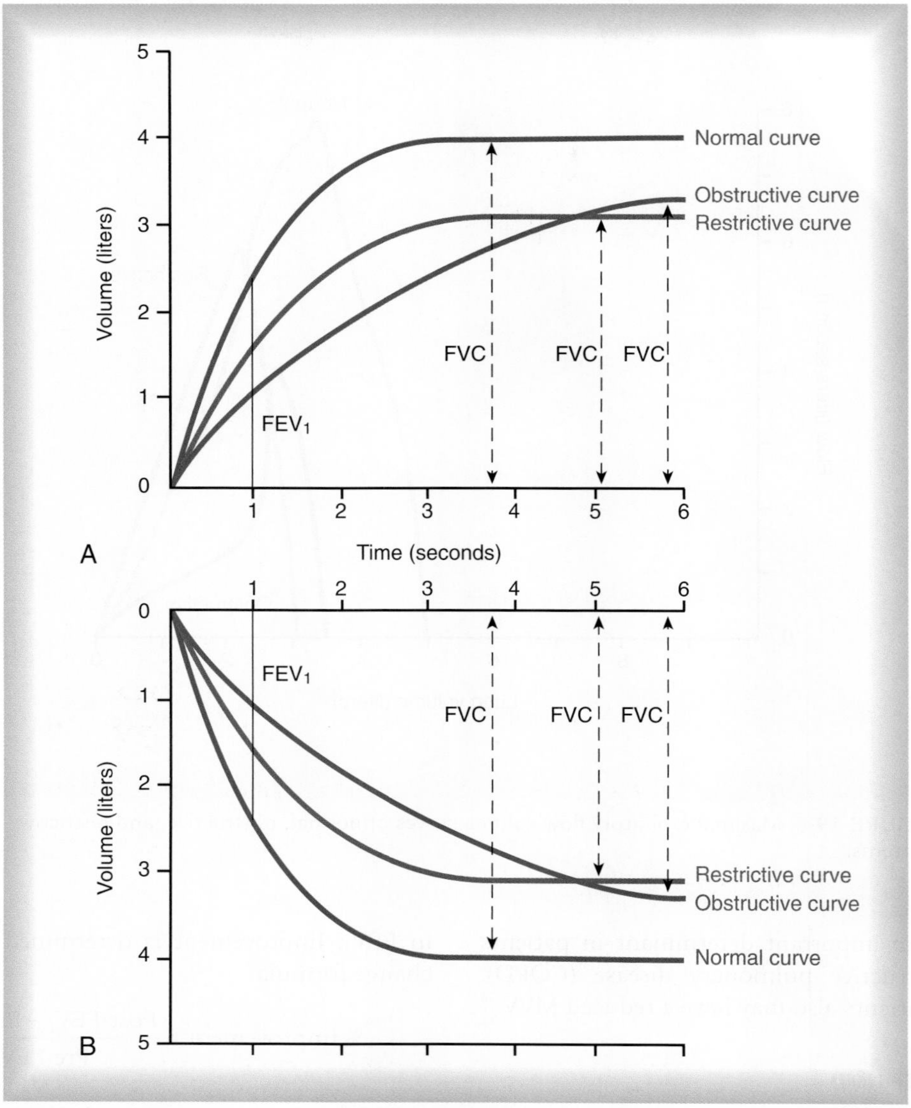

FIGURE 19-7 Forced vital capacity curves comparing normal, obstructive, and restrictive disorders. **A,** Curves as they appear on commonly available spirometers with tracings beginning at the bottom left corner. **B,** The same curves as they appear on some spirometers with tracings beginning at upper left corner.

asymptomatic for cough, sputum production, or dyspnea may have reduced flow in the small airways. A singular reduction in small airway flow may indicate nothing at all or may be an early indicator of obstruction.

The shape of the flow-volume loop and the $FEF_{50\%}/FIF_{50\%}$ ratio provide additional information about upper airway obstruction. Compared with the normal flow-volume loop, a fixed upper airway obstruction produces a curve that appears box-shaped. In Figure 19-9, both expiratory and inspiratory flows are decreased and limited by the solid obstruction; the $FEF_{50\%}/FIF_{50\%}$ ratio remains normal. Variable upper airway obstructions produce two different shapes depending on the site of the obstruction. Because the intraairway pressure during a forced inspiration is less than atmospheric outside the thorax, a variable extrathoracic upper airway obstruction limits inspiratory flow, and the $FEF_{50\%}/FIF_{50\%}$ ratio is greater than 1.0. Because the intraairway pressure during a forced inspiration is greater than atmospheric pressure inside the thorax, a variable intrathoracic upper airway obstruction limits expiratory flow, and the $FEF_{50\%}/FIF_{50\%}$ ratio is less than 1.0.

Similar to other spirometric measurements of pulmonary mechanics, normal values of MVV are based on gender, age, and height. MVV is reduced in patients with moderate and severe airway obstruction. A measured value less than 75% of predicted is significant. The normal for men is approximately 160 to 180 L/min; it is slightly lower in women. In restrictive lung disease, MVV may be normal or only slightly reduced. Respiratory muscle strength is a primary determinant of MVV in patients with interstitial

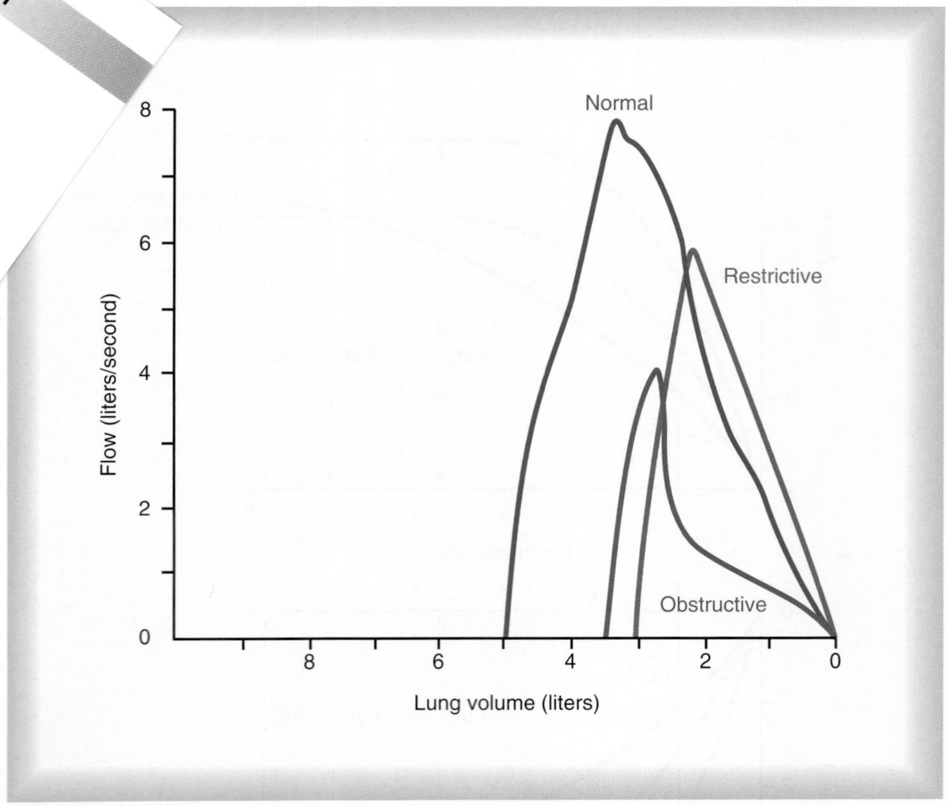

FIGURE 19-8 Maximal expiratory flow volume curves of normal, obstructive, and restrictive patterns.

lung disease and an important determinant in patients with chronic obstructive pulmonary disease (COPD). Undernourished patients also may have a reduced MVV.[26]

> **RULE OF THUMB**
>
> If a person cannot exhale at least 70% of his or her VC in 1 second, there must be obstruction. An FEV_1/FVC of less than 70% indicates an obstructive impairment.

Reversibility

Based on the initial results of baseline spirometry, additional testing of pulmonary mechanics is often desirable. If the baseline test indicates airway obstruction, determining the reversibility of the obstruction is indicated. RTs also use the concept of reversibility when evaluating routine therapy by performing spirometry before and after therapy. In the laboratory, the FVC maneuver is often repeated after the patient has received a bronchodilator administered by small volume nebulizer or metered dose inhaler. This laboratory protocol is commonly known as *spirometry before and after bronchodilator*. Reversibility of the airway obstruction indicates effective therapy. Although improvement in other measurements of pulmonary function is sometimes used, reversibility is defined as a 15% or greater improvement in FEV_1 and at least a 200-ml increase in FEV_1. Improvement is determined using the percent change formula:

$$\%\ \text{Improvement} = \frac{\text{Post-FEV}_1 - \text{Pre-FEV}_1}{\text{Pre-FEV}_1} \times 100$$

> **RULE OF THUMB**
>
> A "change in percent" (A% – B%) is not the same as a "percent change" (B% – A%)/A%.

Bronchial Challenge

When the patient's history suggests episodic symptoms of hyperreactive airways and airway obstruction, such as seasonal or exercise-induced wheezing, and the results of baseline spirometry are normal, performing a bronchial provocation may be indicated.[27] Bronchial provocation testing uses an agent to stimulate a hyperreactive airway response and to create airway obstruction. Although several types of provocations are possible, such as inhaling histamine or cold air or exercising, provoking a hyperreactive airway response by inhaling methacholine is the most popular technique with the most predictable results. The procedure usually begins with the patient inhaling a normal saline aerosol and then repeating the FVC maneuver. Some very sensitive patients exhibit hyperreactive airways with saline alone; a positive response to saline is defined as a

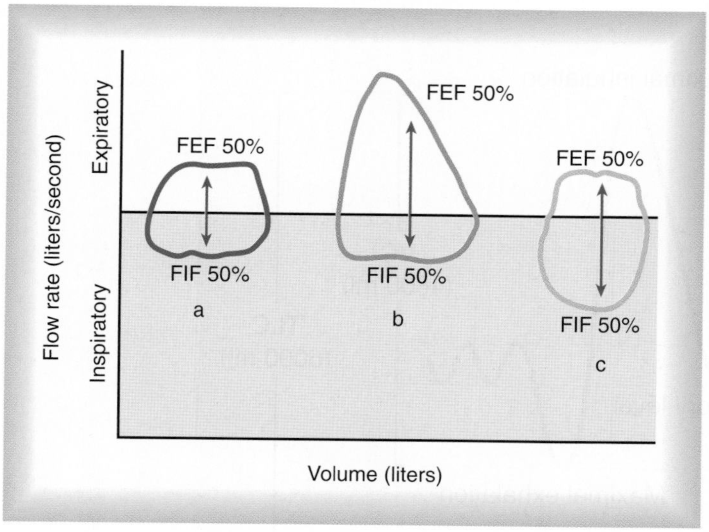

FIGURE 19-9 Flow-volume loops of fixed upper airway obstruction *(a)*, variable extrathoracic upper airway obstruction *(b)*, and variable intrathoracic upper airway obstruction *(c)*.

decrease in FEV_1 of 10% or greater. The methacholine provocation protocol systematically exposes the patient to increasing dosages of methacholine. Usually starting with a low dose of 0.03 mg/ml, patients inhale methacholine aerosol and then repeat the FVC maneuver. A *positive response* to methacholine is defined as a decrease in FEV_1 of 20% or greater (another example of percent change). If a positive response does not occur, the methacholine dose is doubled to 0.06 mg/ml, and the FVC maneuver is repeated. The process of "double-dosing" and performing FVC maneuvers continues until there is a positive response or until the full dose, 16 mg/ml, is given. If a positive response occurs, treatment with a fast-acting bronchodilator is indicated, and sometimes administering O_2 is helpful. The final test report should include the concentration of methacholine that caused the 20% decrease in FEV_1 in the form of PD%FEV_1. For example, $PD_{22}FEV_1$ = 4 mg/ml indicates that the provocation dose of 4 mg/ml resulted in a 22% decrease in FEV_1.

RULE OF THUMB

Normal pulmonary function values are predictably based on the subject's age, height, gender, ethnicity, and sometimes weight. Normal pulmonary function predictably declines with age older than 20 years.

Lung Volumes and Capacities

There are four lung volumes and four lung capacities. A lung capacity consists of two or more lung volumes. The lung volumes are **tidal volume (V_T), inspiratory reserve volume (IRV), expiratory reserve volume (ERV),** and **residual volume (RV).** The four lung capacities are TLC, IC, FRC, and VC. These volumes and capacities are shown in Figure 19-10. The lung volumes that can be measured directly with a spirometer or pneumotachometer include V_T, IC, IRV, ERV, and VC. Because the RV cannot be exhaled, the RV, FRC, and TLC must be measured using indirect methods.

Knowing TLC is necessary to identify patients with a restrictive pattern of pulmonary impairment. Measuring FRC is necessary to quantify hyperinflation, which may be associated with obstructive impairment. Calculating RV is necessary to gauge any air trapping present. Measurements of V_T, IC, ERV, IRV, and VC may be used in calculations of TLC or be useful to clinicians considering weaning parameters such as the rapid-shallow-breathing index (f/V_T) or inspiration goals of hyperinflation therapy. Standards for measuring lung volumes and capacities were initially published in 2005; these standards focus primarily on the techniques to measure FRC.[28] Following the measurement of FRC, measurements of ERV and VC enable calculation of TLC according to the formulas: TLC = (FRC − ERV) + VC and TLC = FRC + IC.

The V_T is measured directly from a spirogram (see Figure 19-10). For the purposes of ensuring test validity and standardization, the patient should be in a sitting or reclining position and wearing a nose clip. It sometimes takes the patient 1 to 2 minutes to be at rest and become accustomed to the nose clip and mouthpiece. The patient breathes through a tight-fitting mouthpiece until a normal, rhythmic breathing pattern is established. Because V_T varies normally from breath to breath, an average V_T is a more reliable measurement. In the laboratory, an average V_T sometimes is measured during 3 minutes of quiet breathing while the spirometer records volumes and graphs volume and time. At the bedside, an average V_T usually is measured over 1 minute; the patient breathes normally into a spirometer that stores in memory each volume exhaled for 1 minute and computes an average. An alternative approach is to measure the total volume of air exhaled for 1 minute ($\dot{V}_E$) and divide by the breathing

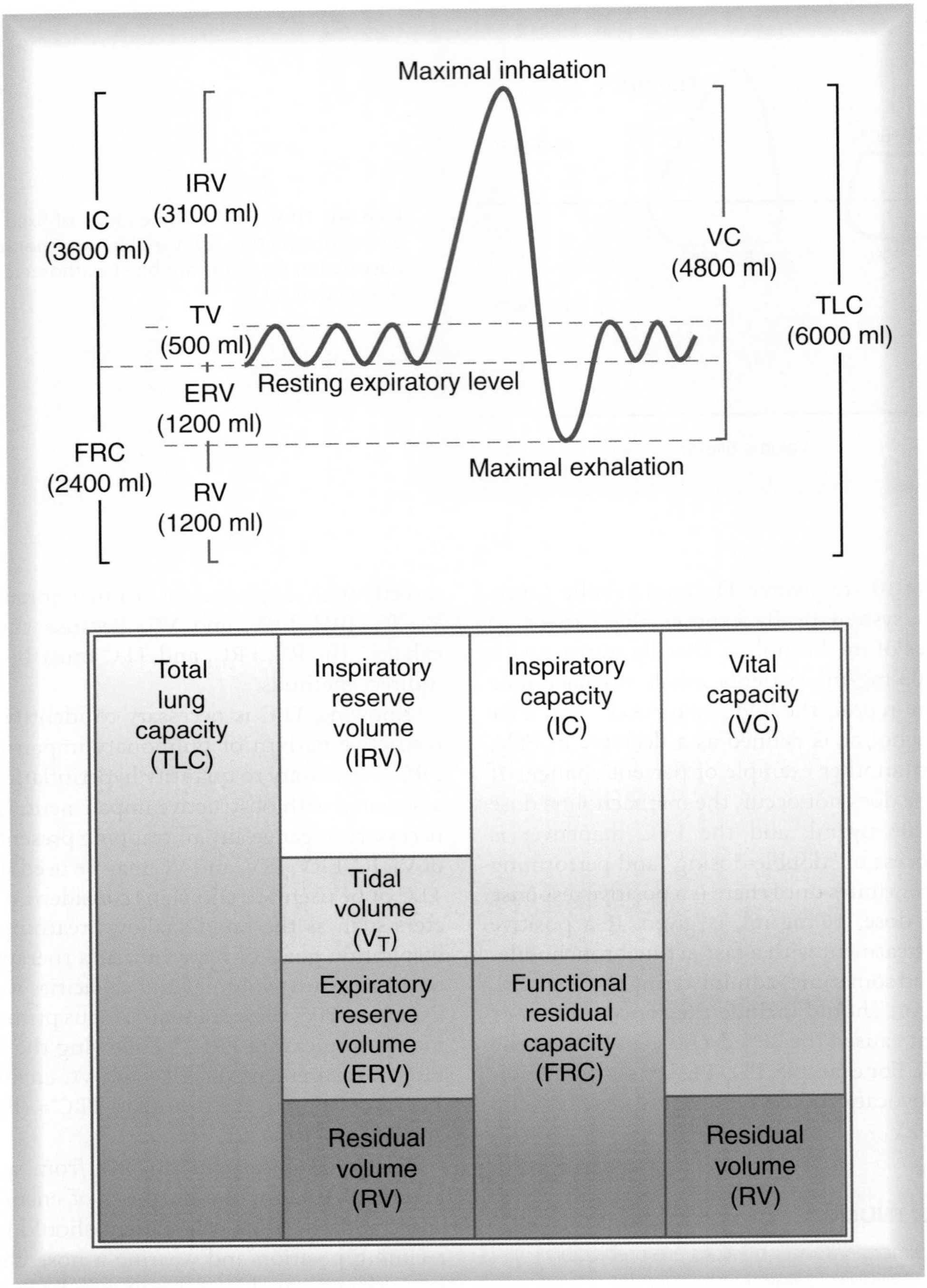

FIGURE 19-10 Lung volumes and capacities. Volumes listed are average normal values for a young, healthy adult man.

frequency (f) counted during the same period. The following formula can be used to calculate the V_T: $V_T = \dot{V}_E \div f$.

The **inspiratory capacity (IC)** is also measured directly from a spirogram. The patient is asked to inhale maximally from the resting FRC at the end of a normal effortless exhalation. To ensure validity, a consistent resting expiratory level should be obvious on the spirogram before inhaling. To ensure reliability, the IC should be measured at least twice, and the two largest measurements should agree within 5%. Because the definition of IC is the maximal volume inhaled, the largest measurement is the patient's IC. (See Clinical Practice Guidelines 19-2 and 19-3.)

The expiratory reserve volume (ERV) is measured directly from the spirogram (see Figure 19-10). The patient is asked to breathe normally for a few breaths and then exhale maximally. The ERV is the volume of air exhaled between the resting expiratory level and the maximal exhalation level on the spirogram. To ensure validity, a

MINI CLINI

Why Are Functional Residual Capacity and Residual Volume Increased in Emphysema?

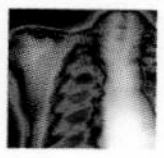

PROBLEM: In the advanced stages of pulmonary emphysema, FRC and RV are increased; in addition, VC is often decreased. Why do these changes occur?

SOLUTION: When the ventilatory muscles relax, the opposing forces of lung recoil and chest wall expansion determine the size of FRC. Emphysema is characterized by a destruction of elastic tissue in the lung, which causes a lower lung recoil force. When lung recoil forces decrease, as in emphysema, chest wall expansion forces predominate, and the chest wall expands outward, pulling the lung with it. As the lung stretches to a larger volume, its recoil force increases, and eventually equilibrium is reestablished between the lung and chest wall. This new equilibrium occurs at an increased lung volume, so FRC is increased. RV is increased in emphysema because VC is decreased owing to small airway obstruction. When a person with emphysema tries to exhale completely, the bronchioles collapse, trapping air in the lungs and increasing RV. Increased FRC is called *hyperinflation,* and increased RV is called *air trapping.*

consistent resting expiratory level should be obvious on the spirogram before exhaling maximally. To ensure reliability, the ERV should be measured at least twice and the two largest measurements should agree within 5%. Because the definition of ERV is the maximal volume exhaled, the largest measurement is the patient's ERV.

The VC is the most commonly measured lung volume. There are several methods of measuring the VC. The VC can be measured during inspiration or during a slow prolonged expiration when air trapping is of concern. To measure the VC during inspiration, the patient exhales maximally and then inhales as deeply as possible. The volume of the maximal inspiration is the inspiratory VC. To measure the VC during expiration, the patient inhales maximally and then exhales maximally, taking all the time necessary to exhale completely. The exhaled volume is the slow VC. An alternative method is to measure the IC and the ERV and add these volumes together for a "combined" VC, but this method should be reserved only for patients who cannot otherwise execute the VC. The VC also is measured when it is exhaled forcefully and as rapidly as possible. This technique is called the FVC, and it is used to assess pulmonary mechanics under the section spirometry.

Because the RV cannot be exhaled, RV, FRC, and TLC cannot be measured directly with a spirometer or pneumotachometer. There are three indirect techniques to measure these lung volumes: helium dilution, nitrogen washout, and body plethysmography. The helium dilution and nitrogen washout techniques measure whatever gas is in the lungs at the beginning of the test, if the gas is in contact with unobstructed airways. The body plethysmographic technique measures all the gas in the thorax at the resting expiratory volume. Because the plethysmographic technique measures all gas in the thorax, including gas that is trapped distal to obstructed airways or gas in the pleural space, the lung volume measured by this technique is called the **thoracic gas volume (TGV)** (V_{TG}, or FRC_{Pleth}). In patients with obstructive lung disease with gas trapping, TGV is often larger than FRC measured by helium dilution or nitrogen washout. In healthy individuals, TGV is identical to FRC measured by both the gas dilution and the washout techniques. When FRC is known, RV can be calculated as the difference between FRC and ERV. TLC also can be calculated by adding RV to VC.

Helium Dilution

The helium dilution technique for measuring lung volumes uses a closed, rebreathing circuit (Figure 19-11).[29] This technique is based on the assumptions that a known volume and concentration of helium in air begin in the closed spirometer, that the patient has no helium in his or her lungs, and that an equilibration of helium can occur between the spirometer and the lungs. For the helium dilution procedure to be performed, a measurable volume of helium is added into the spirometer circuit, and the initial concentration of helium (F_iHe) is measured. Next, the valve is turned to connect the patient to the breathing circuit usually at the resting expiratory level of the FRC. Starting the test at RV requires maximal expiratory effort by the patient and is not considered a reliable starting point. Although starting the test at the TLC level requires a maximal inspiration, TLC may be a reliable alternative beginning point.

The patient is connected to the helium-air mixture, and the concentration of helium is diluted slowly by the patient's lung volume. Wearing nose clips, the patient breathes normally in the closed circuit. Exhaled CO_2 is absorbed with soda lime, and O_2 is added at a rate equal to the patient's O_2 consumption. A constant volume is maintained to ensure accurate helium concentration measurements. The patient rebreathes the gas in the system until equilibrium of helium concentration is established. In healthy patients and patients with a small FRC, equilibration occurs in 2 to 5 minutes. Patients with obstructive lung disease may require 20 minutes to equilibrate because of slow gas mixing in the lungs. The helium dilution time or the duration of the test is a gross index of the distribution of ventilation.

For FRC to be calculated using the helium dilution technique, several observations must be made: the volume of helium added (vol He) to the closed spirometer, the initial helium concentration (F_iHe) before the patient is connected to the breathing circuit, the final helium

19-2 Methacholine Challenge Testing

AARC Clinical Practice Guideline (Excerpts)*

INDICATIONS

Indications for testing include the need to do the following:

- Exclude the diagnosis of airway hyperreactivity
- Evaluate occupational asthma
- Assess the severity of hyperresponsiveness
- Determine the relative risk of developing asthma
- Assess the response to therapeutic interventions

CONTRAINDICATIONS

The following are absolute contraindications to methacholine challenge testing:

- Presence of severe ventilatory impairment, defined as $FEV_1 < 50\%$ predicted normal or <1.0 L
- Heart attack or stroke within last 3 months
- Known aortic or cerebral aneurysm
- Uncontrolled hypertension, defined as systolic pressure >200 mm Hg or diastolic pressure >110 mm Hg

Relative contraindications include the following:

- Presence of moderate ventilatory impairment, defined as $FEV_1 > 50\%$ predicted normal or >1.5 L, but <60% predicted
- Inability to perform spirometry
- Significant response to inhaling the diluent
- Recent respiratory tract infection (defined as within 2 to 6 weeks)
- Current use of cholinesterase-inhibitor medication
- Pregnancy and lactation
- Recent ingestion of foods or medications that contain caffeine or other factors that may confound the test results

HAZARDS AND COMPLICATIONS

Possible hazards or untoward reactions include the following:

- Bronchoconstriction
- Chest pain
- Hyperinflation
- Nosocomial infection contracted from improperly cleaned tubing, mouthpieces, and pneumotachographs
- Severe coughing
- Dizziness, lightheadedness

ASSESSMENT OF NEED

Need is assessed by determining that valid indications are present.

ASSESSMENT OF OUTCOME AND TEST QUALITY

- Outcome and test quality are determined by ascertaining that the desired information has been generated for the specific indication and that validity and reproducibility have been ensured.
- Results are valid if the equipment functions acceptably and the subject is able to perform the maneuvers in an acceptable and reproducible fashion.
- Report of test results should contain a statement by the technician performing the test about test quality (including patient understanding of directions and effort expended) and, if appropriate, which recommendations were not met.
- Equipment calibration and quality control measures specific to methacholine challenge should be applied and documented.

MONITORING

- FEV_1 is the primary variable to be monitored. Breath sounds, pulse rate, pulse oximetry, or blood pressure should be monitored. Patients should not be left unattended.
- Test data of repeated efforts (i.e., reproducibility of results) to ascertain the validity of results.
- Monitor the patient for a positive response to provocation, defined as a decrease in $FEV_1 > 20\%$ from baseline.

**For the complete guideline, see American Association for Respiratory Care: Clinical practice guideline: methacholine challenge testing: 2001 revisions and updates, Respir Care 46:523–530, 2001.*

19-3 Static Lung Volumes

AARC Clinical Practice Guideline (Excerpts)*

INDICATIONS

Indications include the need to do the following:

- Diagnose restrictive disease patterns
- Differentiate between obstructive and restrictive disease patterns
- Assess response to therapeutic interventions (e.g., transplantation, radiation, chemotherapy, lobectomy)
- Aid in the interpretation of other lung function tests
- Make preoperative assessments in patients with impaired lung function that would be affected by surgery
- Evaluate pulmonary disability
- Quantify the amount of gas trapping by comparing results of different techniques

CONTRAINDICATIONS

- No apparent absolute contraindications exist; relative contraindications for spirometry include hemoptysis of unknown origin, untreated pneumothorax, unstable cardiovascular status, and thoracic and abdominal or cerebral aneurysms.
- With respect to whole-body plethysmography, factors such as claustrophobia, upper body paralysis, obtrusive body casts, or other conditions that immobilize or prevent the patient from fitting into or gaining access to the "body box" are a concern. In addition, the procedure may necessitate stopping intravenous therapy or supplemental O_2.

HAZARDS AND COMPLICATIONS

- Nosocomial infection contracted from improperly cleaned tubing, mouthpieces, and pneumotachographs
- Hypoxemia from interruption of O_2 therapy with the body box
- Depressed ventilatory drive in susceptible subjects (i.e., CO_2 retainers) as a consequence of breathing 100% O_2 during the nitrogen washout; such patients should be carefully observed
- Hypercapnia and hypoxemia during helium-dilution FRC determinations as a consequence of failure to remove CO_2 or add O_2 adequately

ASSESSMENT OF NEED

Determine that valid indications are present.

ASSESSMENT OF OUTCOME AND TEST QUALITY

- Outcome and test quality are determined by ascertaining that the desired information has been generated for the specific indication and that validity and reproducibility have been ensured.
- Results are valid if the equipment functions acceptably and the subject is able to perform the maneuvers in an acceptable and reproducible fashion.
- Report of test results should contain a statement by the technician performing the test about test quality (including patient understanding of directions and effort expended) and, if appropriate, which recommendations were not met.
- Equipment calibration and quality control measures specific to measuring lung volumes should be applied and documented.

MONITORING

The following should be monitored during lung-volume determinations:

- Test data of repeated efforts (i.e., reproducibility of results) to ascertain the validity of results
- The patient for any adverse effects of testing (patients on supplemental O_2 may require periods of time to rest on O_2 between trials)

**For the complete guideline, see American Association for Respiratory Care: Clinical practice guideline: static lung volumes: 2001 revisions and updates, Respir Care 46:531–539, 2001.*

concentration (F_fHe) after helium equilibrium between the spirometer and patient is established, the spirometer temperature, and the time necessary for helium equilibration to occur. If the patient is connected to the circuit at the resting level, the FRC can be calculated with the following equation:

$$FRC = (vol\ He \div F_iHe) \times [(F_iHe - F_fHe) \times F_fHe]$$

Corrections for temperature and helium absorption are normally applied. All lung volumes and capacities must be reported under BTPS conditions. Volumes measured by spirometers are at ambient temperature, pressure, and saturated (ATPS) conditions and must be adjusted for the temperature difference between the spirometer and the patient's body temperature. This ATPS to BTPS adjustment can increase volumes 5% to 10%, and the difference

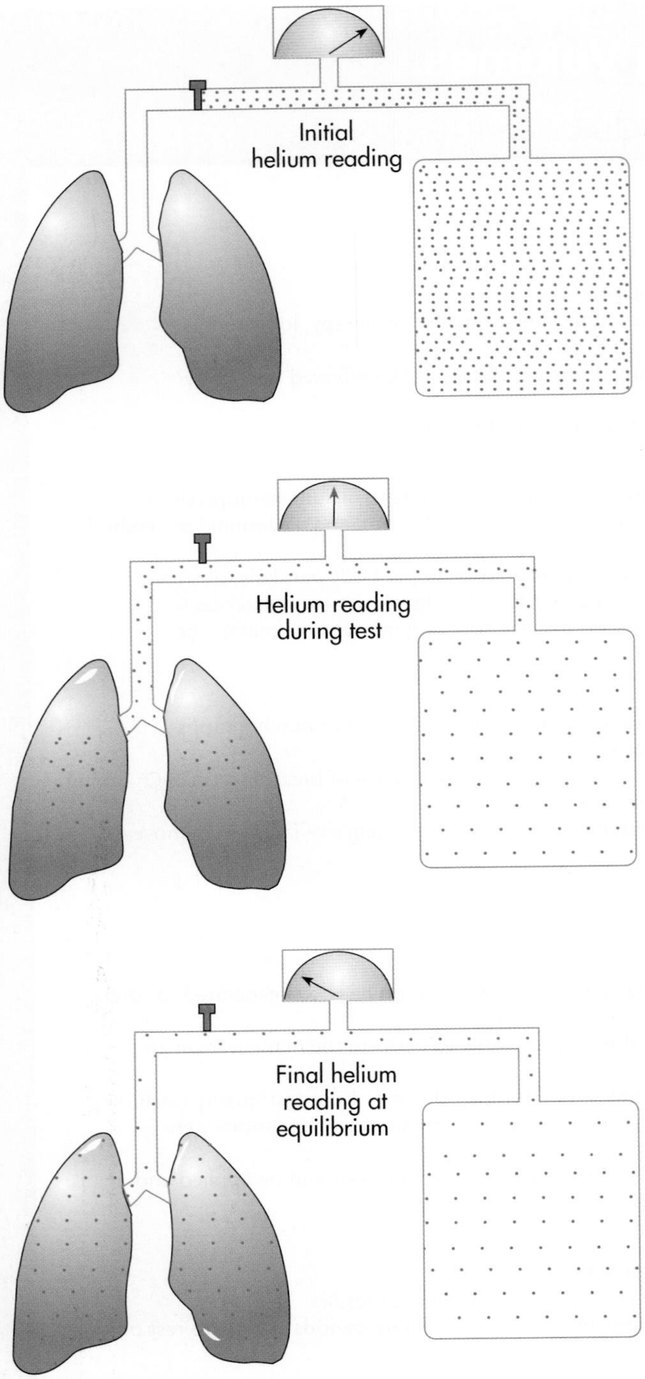

FIGURE 19-11 Helium dilution method for measuring functional residual capacity, residual volume, and total lung capacity.

is large enough to invalidate the test results, unless the correction is made.

Although helium is an inert gas with a negligible solubility in plasma, another correction is sometimes applied. A small amount of helium is thought to diffuse across the alveolar-capillary membrane and is lost in the measurement of final helium concentration. To account for the loss, 30 ml of BTPS-corrected volume is subtracted for each minute of helium breathing, up to 200 ml for a 7-minute test.[30] Once these corrections are made, RV can be calculated by subtracting ERV from FRC according to the equation: RV = FRC − ERV.

Nitrogen Washout

The nitrogen washout technique uses a nonrebreathing or open circuit (Figure 19-12).[31] The technique is based on the assumptions that the nitrogen concentration in the lungs is 78% and in equilibrium with the atmosphere, that the patient inhales 100% O_2, and that the O_2 replaces all of the nitrogen in the lungs. Similar to the helium dilution technique, the patient is connected to the system at either the resting expiratory level or the TLC. The patient's exhaled gas is monitored, and its volume and nitrogen percentage are measured.

Generally, two types of circuits are used to measure lung volumes with this technique. In one type of circuit, all of the exhaled gases are collected in a large container, where the volume and concentration of nitrogen are measured. In the second type of circuit, the volume and concentration of each exhaled breath are measured separately and stored in a memory; the sum of the volumes and the weighted average of the nitrogen concentration are calculated by a computer.

Wearing nose clips, the patient breathes 100% O_2 until nearly all of the nitrogen has been washed out of the lungs, leaving less than 1.5% nitrogen in the lungs. When the peak exhaled concentration of nitrogen is less than 1.5%, the patient exhales completely, and the fractional concentration of alveolar nitrogen (F_AN_2) is noted. Similar to the helium technique, the time it takes to wash out the nitrogen is approximately 2 to 5 minutes in healthy individuals and longer in patients with obstructive lung disease. The test must occur in a leakproof circuit because the presence of any air increases the measured nitrogen percentages and results in grossly elevated measurements of lung volume.

For FRC or TLC to be calculated by the nitrogen washout technique, several measurements must be made: the total volume of gas exhaled during the test (V_E), the fractional concentration of exhaled nitrogen in the total gas volume (F_EN_2), the fractional concentration of nitrogen in the alveoli at the end of the test (F_AN_2), and the spirometer temperature. FRC (or TLC, if the test began at TLC) can be calculated with the following equation:

$$FRC = (V_E \times FEN_2) \div (0.78 - FAN_2)$$

The calculated FRC (or TLC, if connection to the breathing circuit occurred after inspiring maximally) must be adjusted for the temperature difference between the spirometer and the patient's body temperature using the BTPS correction factor. During the test, some nitrogen from the plasma and body tissues is usually excreted and exhaled with lung nitrogen. For this reason, another correction is needed. The volume of tissue nitrogen excreted (V_{tis} in milliliters) is directly related to the duration (t in

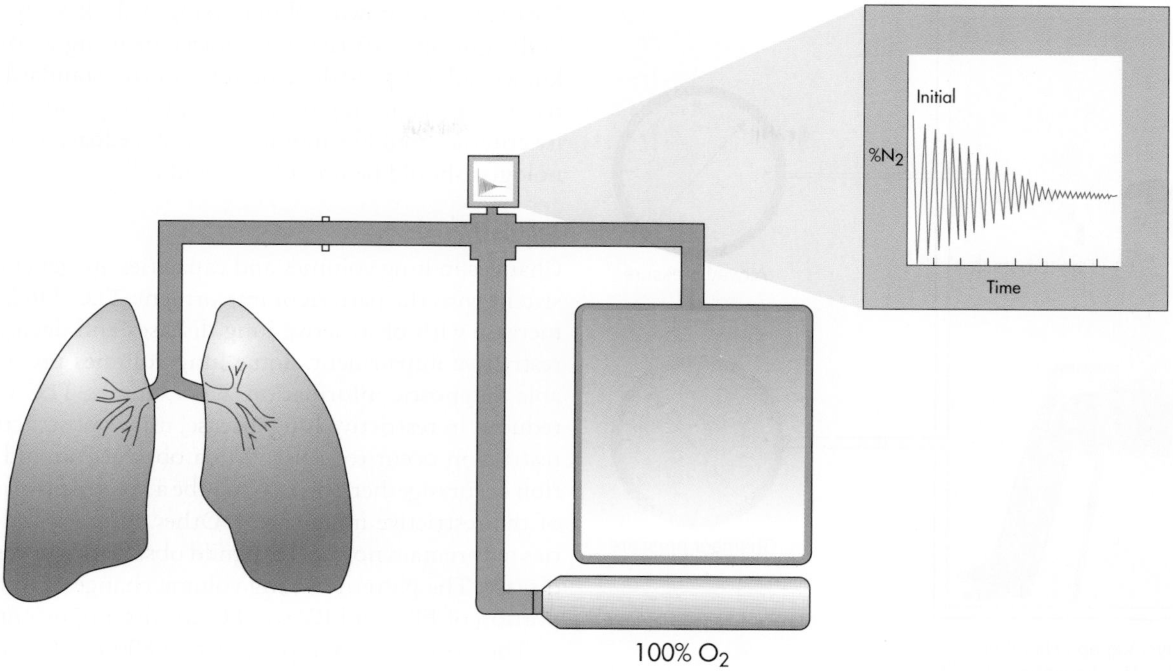

FIGURE 19-12 Nitrogen washout method for measuring functional residual capacity, residual volume, and total lung capacity.

minutes) of the test and weight (W in kilograms) of the patient. A correction for this extra nitrogen should be made according to the following formula: V_{tis} (ml) = $(0.1209\ t^{-1/2} - 0.0665) \times (W \div 70)$. V_{tis} (ml) is subtracted from the BTPS-corrected lung volume. RV is the difference between ERV and FRC.

The validity of the helium dilution and nitrogen washout techniques can be ensured by measuring known volumes accurately, such as a 3.0-L syringe, while recognizing that this method would not include O_2 consumption and O_2 titration for the helium method or tissue nitrogen excretion for the nitrogen method. The reliability of these techniques can be established by repeated measurements of known volumes or healthy patients that agree within 5%. Establishing reliability of these measurements on patients requires repeating tests after reestablishing baseline lung gases. For patients with severe obstructive lung disease, waiting up to 1 hour may be necessary. When the FRC is measured by either He dilution or N_2 washout, any leak anywhere in the patient, tubing, or gas analyzers would increase the measured FRC and may be falsely interpreted as hyperinflation.

Plethysmography

The plethysmography technique applies Boyle's law and uses measurements of volume and pressure changes to determine lung volume, assuming temperature is constant.[32] The plethysmography technique measures the volume of all compressible gas in the thorax, including gas trapped behind airway obstructions or in the pleural space. Gas in the abdomen may also be included in the measurement. The whole-body plethysmograph consists of a sealed chamber in which the patient sits (Figure 19-13). Pressure transducers (electronic manometers) measure pressure at the mouth and in the chamber. An electronically controlled shutter near the mouthpiece allows the airway to be occluded periodically, measuring airway pressure changes under conditions of no airflow. Without air flow, pressure changes measured at the mouth are pressure changes in the alveoli. According to Boyle's law ($V \times P = k$), when temperature is constant, volume changes in the thorax create volume changes in the chamber, which are reflected by pressure changes in the chamber. The pressure and volume changes are included in the equation:

$$V_{TG1} \times P_{alv1} = V_{TG2} \times P_{alv2}$$

When measurement of TGV is being done, the patient sits in the chamber and initially breathes normal tidal volumes through the mouthpiece. When the patient is near FRC, the shutter is closed at end expiration for 2 to 3 seconds. The patient holds his or her cheeks and performs gentle panting at 1 Hz or one pant per second.[33] During panting, changes in airway pressure (ΔP) and changes in chamber volume (ΔV) are measured. Because the panting maneuver occurs with small pressure changes around barometric pressure, the simplified equation used to calculate TGV is $V_{TG} = P_B \times (\Delta V \div \Delta P)$, where P_B is the barometric pressure in cm H_2O. A series of three to five panting maneuvers should be performed. After panting, the patient should exhale completely to record ERV and then inhale maximally to record the inspiratory vital capacity.

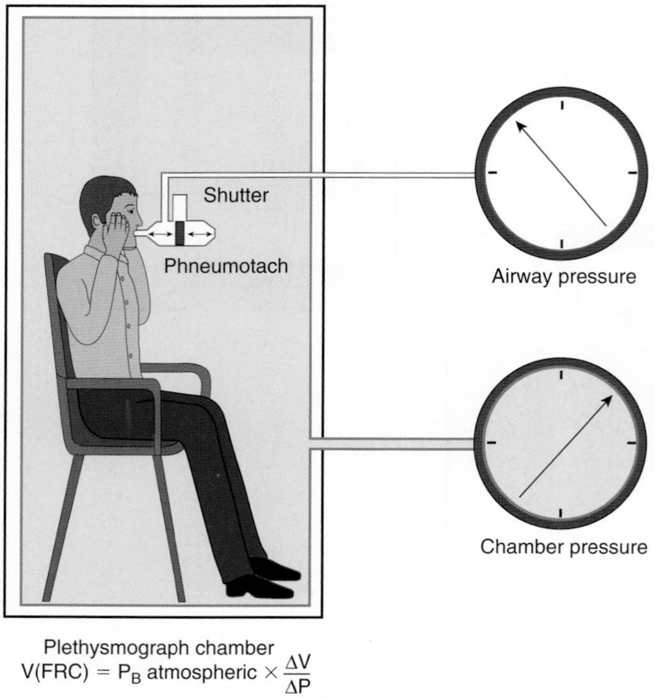

FIGURE 19-13 Body plethysmography method for measuring lung volumes. *V* is the change in gas volume in the lungs, as sensed by the chamber pressure manometer. *P* is the change in pressure produced by the respiratory efforts of breathing against the shutter, as sensed by the airway pressure manometer.

Because the body plethysmographic method of measuring FRC actually measures TGV, the value obtained for some patients may be larger than values resulting from either the helium dilution or nitrogen washout techniques. Such a difference occurs whenever there is gas in the thorax that is not in communication with patent airways, as might be the case in patients with pneumothorax, pneumomediastinum, or emphysema. The RV is the difference between TGV and ERV, and the TLC is the sum of RV and VC, or the sum of TGV and IC.

Quality Assurance

Comprehensive quality assurance for measuring lung volumes depends on the measuring technique. For helium dilution and nitrogen washout techniques, the accuracy and precision of the volume or flow measuring device must be ensured as in spirometry; the accuracy and linearity of the gas analyzer must be verified, and the leak test must be acceptable while monitoring change in volume and gas concentrations over at least 1 minute. Technologists successfully identifying the subject's breath-to-breath resting level and complying with retest waiting periods should be monitored. Correctly measuring the volume of the 3.0-L syringe provides a quality control standard. For the plethysmographic technique, the box and mouth pressure transducers must be calibrated and accurate. The technologist's choice of the best-fit line of the relationship between box and mouth pressures should be monitored. Measuring a known volume using a flask with squeeze bulb connected to the mouthpiece or using a consistent known subject provides a quality control standard. For all techniques, achieving testing acceptability and repeatability criteria should be monitored, and feedback to the technologist should be provided periodically.

Significance

Changes in lung volumes and capacities are generally consistent with the pattern of impairment. TLC, FRC, and RV increase with obstructive lung diseases and decrease with restrictive impairment. Some lung volumes provide valuable diagnostic information. For example, TLC is always reduced in restrictive lung disease, unless obstruction and restriction occur together. When obstruction and restriction occur together, the TLC may be a less sensitive measure of the restrictive impairment. Other volumes and capacities may remain normal with mild obstructive or restrictive disease. The pattern of lung volume changes and the proportion of FRC and RV to TLC are also important.

The normal V_T is approximately 500 to 700 ml for an average healthy adult. In the normal population, great variation of tidal volumes and measurements beyond the normal range are not indicative of a disease process. Normal V_T is often observed in both restrictive and obstructive lung diseases. V_T alone is not a valid indicator of the type of lung disease.

The normal IC is approximately 3600 ml, with a significant variation in the normal population. IC may be normal or reduced in restrictive and obstructive lung diseases. A reduction of IC occurs in restrictive lung diseases because the patient's inhaled volume is reduced, and there is a reduction in TLC. In mild obstructive lung diseases, IC is usually normal. In moderate and severe obstructive diseases, IC can be reduced because the resting expiratory level of FRC has increased owing to hyperinflation of the lungs. An increase in IC may occur when the patient inhales from below the resting expiratory level when the measurement is performed; athletes and musicians who play wind instruments may also have increased inspiratory capacities. RTs use the measurement of IC in clinical protocols to decide between methods of lung expansion therapy (see Chapter 39).

IRV is not commonly measured. Similar to V_T and IC, IRV can be normal in both restrictive and obstructive diseases and is not a useful diagnostic measurement. The normal value for IRV is 3.10 L.

The normal ERV is approximately 1.20 L and represents approximately 20% to 25% of the VC. It can be either normal or reduced in obstructive and restrictive lung diseases. ERV is subtracted from FRC to calculate RV.

The normal value of the VC is 4.80 L and represents approximately 80% of TLC. Normal values for VC can vary significantly depending on age, gender, height, and ethnicity. A reduction of VC occurs in restrictive lung diseases because the patient's inhaled volume is reduced and there is a reduction in TLC. In mild obstructive lung diseases, the slow VC is usually normal if the patient exhales leisurely and has had enough time to exhale completely or if the VC is measured during inspiration. Measurements made from FVC provide valuable data for pulmonary mechanics.

RV, FRC, and TLC are the most important measurements of lung volumes. Age, height, gender, ethnicity, and sometimes weight or body surface area correlate with normal values for these lung volumes.[34] Table 19-5 provides common regression equations to predict the lung volumes for individuals of specific height (in centimeters), age (in years), and gender. A positive correlation exists between lung volumes and height, and a negative correlation exists between lung volumes and age for patients older than 20 years. Male values are larger than female values when height and age are equal.

The typical normal TLC is 6.00 L. The normal RV is approximately 1.20 L and represents approximately 20% of TLC. FRC is approximately 2.40 L, which represents approximately 40% of the TLC. RV and FRC are usually enlarged in acute and chronic obstructive lung diseases because of hyperinflation and air trapping (Figure 19-14).

TLC may also be enlarged in COPD. TLC is always reduced in restrictive lung diseases because of a loss of lung volume; RV and FRC are often reduced proportionately. Certain acute disorders, such as pulmonary edema, atelectasis, and consolidation, also cause a reduction of TLC and FRC.

Diffusing Capacity

The third major category of pulmonary function testing is measuring the ability of the lungs to transfer gases across the alveolar-capillary membrane. The diffusing capacity of the lung (DL) is sometimes called the *transfer factor*. Carbon monoxide (CO) is the gas normally used to measure the DL. The **diffusing capacity of the lung for carbon**

TABLE 19-5

Examples of Regression Equations for Predicting Normal Lung Volumes and Capacities in Adults

Lung Volumes	Equations
Men	
FRC (L)	0.0234 (Ht) + 0.01 (A) − 1.09
RV (L)	0.0131 (Ht) + 0.022 (A) − 1.23
TLC (L)	0.0799 (Ht) − 7.08
FRC/TLC%	43.8 + 0.21 (A)
RV/TLC%	14.0 + 0.39 (A)
Women	
FRC (L)	0.0224 (Ht) + 0.001 (A) − 1.00
RV (L)	0.0181 (Ht) + 0.016 (A) − 2.00
TLC (L)	0.0660 (Ht) − 5.79
FRC/TLC%	45.1 + 0.16 (A)
RV/TLC%	19.0 + 0.34 (A)

A, Years; *Ht*, cm; *L*, liters at BTPS.
Stocks J, Quanjer PH: Reference values for residual volume, functional residual capacity and total lung capacity. Eur Respir J 8:492–497, 1995.

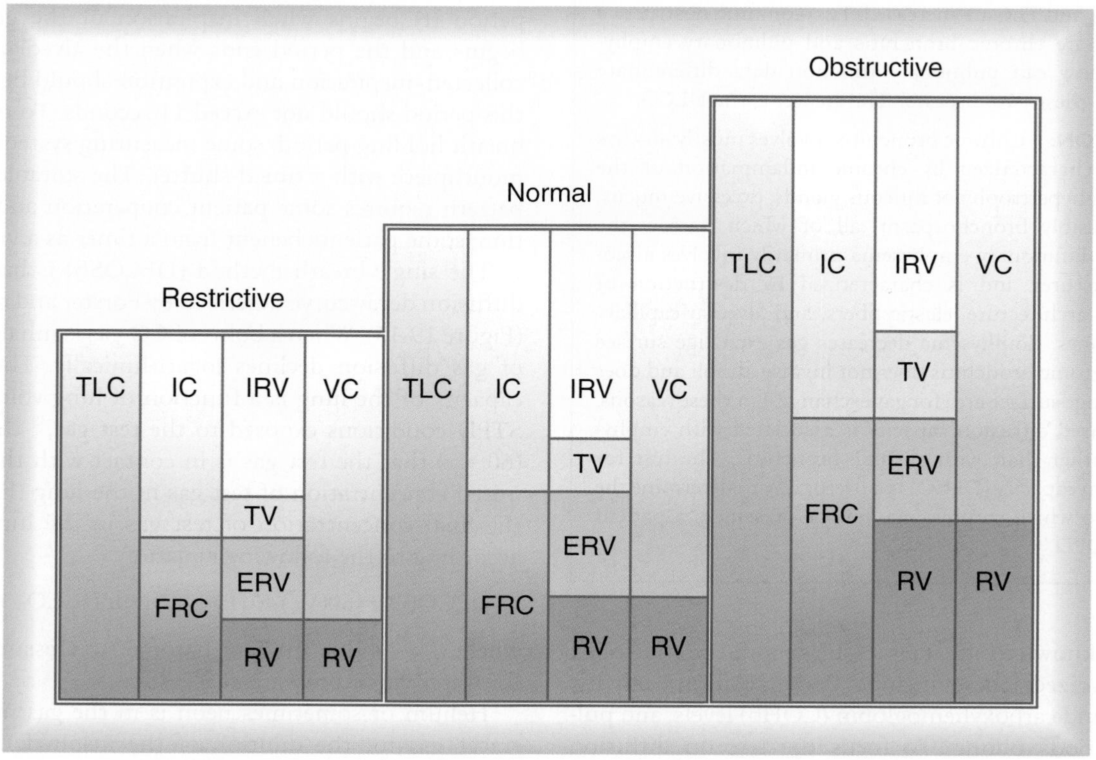

FIGURE 19-14 Changes in lung volumes and capacities with pulmonary disease.

monoxide (DLCO) is expressed in ml/min/mm Hg under standard temperature and pressure and dry conditions (STPD). Generally, DLCO is the difference between the volume of CO inhaled and the volume of CO exhaled, considering the partial pressure of CO in the lung at the time of measurement. The general equation used to explain the diffusing capacity is DLCO = V_E (F_iCO − F_eCO) ÷ (P_ACO). The difference between CO inhaled and exhaled is attributed to CO diffusing into the pulmonary capillary blood.

CO is used as the transfer gas because CO is similar to O_2 in important ways. CO and O_2 have similar molecular weights and solubility coefficients. Similar to O_2, CO also chemically combines with hemoglobin (Hb). CO has a very high affinity for Hb and diffuses rapidly into the pulmonary blood. CO has an affinity for Hb nearly 210 times greater than O_2, and the high affinity keeps the *pulmonary capillary partial pressure of CO (PcCO)* near zero. Consequently, the diffusion of CO across the alveolar-capillary membrane is membrane limited and not limited as much by the partial pressure gradient.

MINI CLINI

Diffusing Capacity of the Lung for Carbon Monoxide in Chronic Obstructive Pulmonary Disease

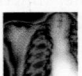

PROBLEM: A patient has spirometry and lung volumes typical of the obstructive pattern. FEV_1, FEV_1/FVC, and FEFs are significantly reduced, and FRC and TLC are increased. Two common obstructive diseases are chronic bronchitis and pulmonary emphysema. How can pulmonary function data differentiate between these two diseases? The answer is the DLCO.

SOLUTION: Chronic bronchitis involves mostly airways and is characterized by chronic inflammation of the mucosa, hypertrophy of mucous glands, excessive mucus, and possibly bronchospasm, all of which narrow the airways. Pulmonary emphysema primarily involves alveolar structures and is characterized by destruction of alveolar architecture, elastic fibers, and alveolar-capillary membranes. Emphysema decreases gas exchange surface area. Chronic bronchitis does not involve alveoli and does not change surface area for gas exchange. For these reasons, a decreased diffusion capacity is associated with emphysema rather than with chronic bronchitis. The test for diffusion capacity (DLCO) is a useful way to determine the extent to which emphysema may be present in a patient with COPD.

Factors known to affect test results should be controlled or standardized; these include body position, activity, P_AO_2, Hb and carboxyhemoglobin (COHb) levels, and pulmonary blood volume. To focus the test on diffusion through the alveolar-capillary membrane, the patient should be tested at rest in a seated position, should not breathe supplemental O_2 for 10 minutes before testing, and should not have an abnormal level of COHb before the test. Mathematical corrections can be applied for patients who cannot abstain from O_2. Performing the diffusing capacity on patients who have recently smoked a cigarette or who have been exposed to environmental CO may hinder test validity.[35] Patients should refrain from smoking on the day of the test. Hb of all patients undergoing diffusing capacity should be measured, and a mathematical correction should be applied if Hb level is abnormal.

Single-Breath Technique

There are several techniques to measure the diffusing capacity of the lung for CO, including steady-state, intrabreath, and rebreathing techniques, but the single-breath method (DLCOSB) is the most common measurement technique because it is quick and reproducible. Standards for measuring diffusing capacity of the lung were initially published in 1995 and updated in 2005; these standards focus primarily on the DLCOSB.[36,37] The entire test can be performed in just slightly longer than 10 seconds. The patient exhales completely to RV, rapidly inspires a VC of a gas mixture containing 0.3% CO and an inert tracer gas such as He in air, maintains breath holding for 10 seconds, and then exhales rapidly at least 1.0 L. Inspiring at least 85% of VC measured during spirometry is expected. After a predesignated volume of 0.75 to 1.0 L is exhaled, a sample of alveolar gas is collected and analyzed for expired CO (F_eCO_t) and helium (F_eHe). Because the breath holding period (t) begins when inspiration of the gas mixture begins and the period ends when the alveolar sample is collected, inspiration and expiration should be rapid, and this period should not exceed 11 seconds. To regulate the breath holding period, some measuring systems close the mouthpiece with a timed shutter. The suitable breathing pattern requires some patient cooperation and coordination; some patients benefit from a timer as a visual aid.

The single-breath method (DLCOSB) is based on the diffusion decay curve described by Forster and colleagues[38] (Figure 19-15). When a bolus of CO gas is inhaled, the rate of gas diffusion declines logarithmically. The diffusing capacity of the lung is a function of lung volume (V_A) in STPD conditions exposed to the test gas,[39] the duration (60 ÷ t) that the test gas is in contact with the lung, the initial concentration of test gas in the lung (F_ACO_0), and the final concentration of test gas in the lung (F_ACO_t), according to the following equation:

$$\text{DLCOSB} = [60(V_A) \div t(P_B - 47)] \times \ln(F_ACO_0 \div F_ACO_t)$$

where (P_B − 47) is ambient barometric pressure corrected for water vapor pressure at 37° C.

Helium or sometimes neon is in the gas mixture as a tracer gas for the dilution of the inspired CO concentration by RV and to measure the effective TLC by a

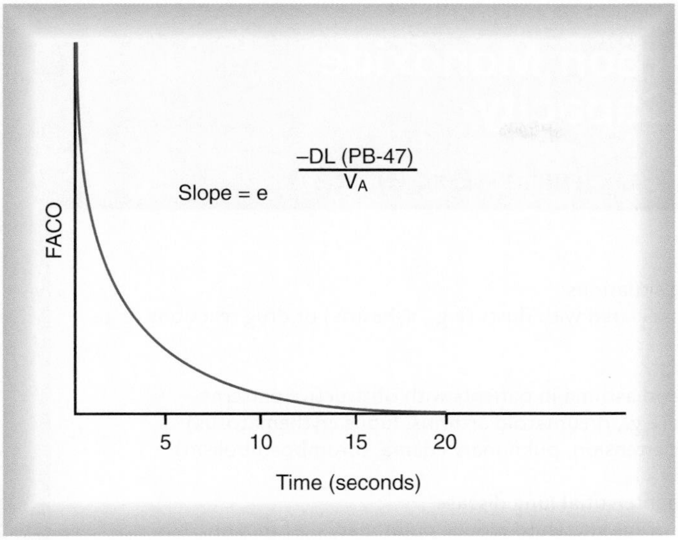

FIGURE 19-15 Concentration of alveolar carbon monoxide following a single breath to total lung capacity.

single-breath helium dilution. The inspired CO concentration of 0.3% is not the concentration of CO received by the lungs because the inspired volume is diluted by RV of the patient. The dilution of CO is reflected by the dilution of helium, and the F_ACO_0 can be calculated according to the following equation:

$$F_ACO_0 = F_iCO \times (F_eHe \div F_iHe)$$

The F_ACO_0 is the concentration of CO in the lung at "zero time" before any diffusion occurs. The single-breath technique distributes the gas mixture through unobstructed airways to an alveolar volume that is also called the effective total lung capacity. The **effective total lung capacity (V_A)** can be calculated according to the following equation:

$$V_A = VC \times (F_iHe \div F_eHe)$$

The V_A is necessary to calculate the DLCO, and it is used in the determination of the diffusing capacity of the lung-to-alveolar volume ratio ($DLCO/V_A$).

The reliability of the DLCO is based on repeatability of the test. At least 4 minutes should be allowed between tests to allow an adequate elimination of CO from the lungs. In patients with obstructive airway disease, a longer period (e.g., 10 minutes) may be necessary. The actual DLCO reported should be the mean of 2 acceptable tests. An acceptable test is defined as one that is reproducible to within 10% or 3 ml of the CO/min/mm Hg value, whichever is greater. (See Clinical Practice Guideline 19-4.)

Quality Assurance

For comprehensive quality assurance for measuring diffusing capacity, the accuracy and precision of the volume or flow measuring device must be ensured as in spirometry; the accuracy and linearity of the gas analyzer must

TABLE 19-6

Examples of Regression Equations for Predicting Normal Diffusing Capacity in Adults

Parameter	Regression Equations
Men	
DLCOSB (ml/min/mm Hg)	0.0416 (Ht) − 0.219 (A) − 26.34
DLCOSB/V_A (ml/min/mm Hg/L)	6.61 − 0.034 (A)
Women	
DLCOSB (ml/min/mm Hg)	0.0256 (Ht) − 0.144 (A) − 8.36
DLCOSB/V_A (ml/min/mm Hg/L)	7.34 − 0.032 (A)

A, Years; *Ht*, cm; *L*, Liters at BTPS; *ml*, milliliters at STPD.
Crapo RO, Morris AM: Standardized single breath normal values for carbon monoxide diffusing capacity. Am Rev Respir Dis 123:185, 1981.

be verified as in measuring lung volumes. Technologists successfully achieving testing acceptability and repeatability criteria should be monitored, and feedback should be provided to the technologist periodically. Measuring the diffusing capacity of the 3.0-L syringe or using a consistent known subject provides a quality control standard.

Significance

Normal values for the DLCO using the single-breath technique are based primarily on a patient's age, height, and gender (Table 19-6). A typical normal value for a 20-year-old healthy man is 40 ml/min/mm Hg.[40] Before interpretation of the test result, corrections for abnormal Hb level, breathing supplemental O_2 or testing at altitude, and elevated COHb levels may be necessary, if these conditions apply. Initially, all Hb levels were corrected to 15 g/dl.[41] More recent and more specific corrections have been advocated. For men and adolescents, if the Hb level varies from 14.6 g/dl, the predicted normal value should be adjusted using the following equation:[42]

$$\text{Predicted DLCO for Hb} = \text{Predicted DLCO} \times (1.7\ \text{Hb}/10.22 + \text{Hb})$$

For women and children, the normal Hb level is 13.4 g/dl, and the equation is[42]:

$$\text{Predicted DLCO for Hb} = \text{Predicted DLCO} \times (1.7\ \text{Hb}/9.38 + \text{Hb})$$

If the patient's P_AO_2 differs from 100 mm Hg because of breathing supplemental O_2 or performing the test at altitude, the DLCO would be affected by approximately 0.31% to 35% per mm Hg difference from 100 mm Hg.[43,44] The predicted normal value should be adjusted using the following equations:

$$\text{Predicted DLCO for elevated } P_AO_2 = \text{Predicted DLCO}/[1.0 + 0.0035\,(P_AO_2 - 100)]$$

$$\text{Predicted DLCO for altitude} = \text{Predicted DLCO}/[1.0 + 0.0031\,(P_iO_2 - 150)]$$

19-4 Single-Breath Carbon Monoxide Diffusing Capacity

AARC Clinical Practice Guideline (Excerpts)*

■ INDICATIONS

Tests of diffusing capacity may be indicated in the following situations:

- Evaluation and follow-up of parenchymal lung diseases associated with dusts (e.g., asbestos) or drug reactions (e.g., amiodarone) or related to sarcoidosis
- Evaluation and follow-up of emphysema and cystic fibrosis
- Differentiation between chronic bronchitis, emphysema, and asthma in patients with obstructive patterns
- Evaluation of pulmonary involvement in systemic diseases (e.g., rheumatoid arthritis, lupus erythematosus)
- Evaluation of cardiovascular diseases (e.g., pulmonary hypertension, pulmonary edema, thromboembolism)
- Prediction of arterial desaturation during exercise in COPD
- Evaluation and quantification of disability associated with interstitial lung disease
- Evaluation of the effects of chemotherapy agents or other drugs known to induce pulmonary dysfunction
- Evaluation of hemorrhagic disorders

■ CONTRAINDICATIONS

The following are relative contraindications to performing a diffusing capacity test:

- Mental confusion or incoordination preventing the subject from adequately performing the maneuver
- A large meal or vigorous exercise immediately before the test
- Smoking within 24 hours of test administration (may have effect on DLCO independent of COHb)

■ HAZARDS AND COMPLICATIONS

- DLCOSB requires breath holding at TLC; some patients may perform either a Valsalva (high intrathoracic pressure) or Müller (low intrathoracic pressure) maneuver. Either of these maneuvers can result in alteration of venous return to the heart.
- Transmission of infection is possible via improperly cleaned mouthpieces or from the inadvertent spread of droplet nuclei or body fluids (patient to patient or patient to technologist).

■ ASSESSMENT OF NEED

The need for DLCO testing exists when any of the aforementioned indications are present.

■ ASSESSMENT OF TEST QUALITY

Individual test maneuvers and results should be evaluated according to the American Thoracic Society recommendations. In particular, the following recommendations are pertinent:

- The inspiratory volume should exceed 90% of the largest previously measured vital capacity (FVC or VC).
- Breath hold time should be between 9 seconds and 11 seconds, with a rapid inspiration.
- The washout volume (dead space) should be 0.75 to 1 L, or 0.50 L if the subject's VC is <2 L. If a washout volume other than 0.75 to 1 L is used, it should be noted.
- Two or more acceptable tests should be averaged. The maneuvers should be reproducible to within 10% or 3 ml of CO/min/mm Hg, whichever is greater.
- The subject should have refrained from smoking for 24 hours before the test.
- Corrections for Hb and COHb should be included; correction for tests performed at high altitude is recommended.
- If Hb correction is made, both the corrected and the uncorrected DLCO values should be reported.
- Equipment calibration and quality control measures specific to measuring diffusing capacity should be applied and documented.

■ MONITORING

- The final report should contain a statement about test quality.
- The final report should contain the DLCO, the corrected DLCO (Hb, COHb, altitude), and the Hb value used for correction. The alveolar volume (V_A) and DL/V_A (i.e., the ratio of diffusing capacity to the lung volume at which the measurement was made) may be included in the report. These values are helpful for purposes of interpretation.

For complete guideline, see American Association for Respiratory Care: Clinical practice guideline: single-breath carbon monoxide diffusing capacity, 1999 update, Respir Care 44:539–546, 1999.

Box 19-2 Effect of Various Factors on Diffusing Capacity of the Lung for Carbon Monoxide (DLCO)

FACTORS THAT DECREASE DLCO

- Anemia
- Carboxyhemoglobin
- Pulmonary embolism
- Diffuse pulmonary fibrosis
- Pulmonary emphysema

FACTORS THAT INCREASE DLCO

- Polycythemia
- Exercise
- Congestive heart failure

The DLCO may be reduced from the predicted normal in patients with obstructive or restrictive lung diseases. With destruction of alveoli in pulmonary emphysema, with small lung volumes, and with fibrosis of alveoli in asbestosis, the DLCO may be less than normal. Pulmonary embolism also may decrease the DLCO. The DLCO may be useful in identifying which patients with obstructive impairment are likely to desaturate during exercise and which may benefit from O_2 therapy. The DLCO may be increased in patients with polycythemia, congestive heart failure (resulting from an increase in pulmonary vascular blood volume), and elevated cardiac output. Factors that can alter the DLCO above or below the normal value are summarized in Box 19-2.

The **diffusing capacity of the lung-to-effective total lung capacity ratio ($DLCO/V_A$)** differentiates between diffusion abnormalities caused by having a small lung volume compared with diffusion abnormalities caused by alveolar-capillary membrane pathologies. Patients whose only problem is small lungs would have a decreased DLCO, but their $DLCO/V_A$ ratio would be normal. Patients with pulmonary emphysema or fibrosis would have a decreased DLCO and a decreased $DLCO/V_A$ ratio.

INTERPRETATION OF THE PULMONARY FUNCTION REPORT

Interpretive strategies for pulmonary function testing abound. Most computer-based pulmonary function testing systems have algorithms in their software programs for computer-assisted interpretations of the pulmonary function report.[45] A consensus for interpreting test results is growing.[46,47] Table 19-7 summarizes pulmonary function changes that may occur in advanced obstructive and restrictive patterns of lung diseases, and Figure 19-16 presents a simple algorithm to assess pulmonary function test results in clinical practice.[47]

TABLE 19-7 Pulmonary Function Changes in Advanced Lung Diseases

Measurement	Normal*	Obstructive	Restrictive
V_T	500%smL	N or ↑	N or ↓
IRV	3.10 L	N or ↓	↓
ERV	1.20 L	N or ↓	↓
RV	1.20 L	↑	↓
IC	3.60 L	N or ↓	↓
FRC	2.40 L	↑	↓
TLC	6.00 L	N or ↑	↓
FVC	4.80 L	↓	↓
FEV_1	4.20 L	↓	N or ↓
FEV_1/FVC	>70%	↓	N or ↑
$FEF_{200-1200}$	8.5 L/sec	↓	N
$FEF_{25\%-75\%}$	4.5 L/sec	↓	N
PEF	9.5 L/sec	↓	N
$FEF_{25\%}$	9.0 L/sec	↓	N
$FEF_{50\%}$	6.5 L/sec	↓	N
$FEF_{75\%}$	3.5 L/sec	↓	N
MVV	160 L/min	↓	N or ↓
DLCO	40%smL/min/mm Hg	N or ↓	N or ↓
$DLCO/V_A$	6.6%smL/min/mm Hg/L	N or ↓	N or ↓

N, No change.
*Values for 20-year-old, 70-kg man.

When considering a pulmonary function report, the $\%FEV_1/VC$ ratio is a good place to start because it provides an initial focus as normal, restrictive, or obstructive impairment. When the $\%FEV_1/FVC$ is less than the LLN, there is airway obstruction. When the $\%FEV_1/FVC$ is greater than the LLN, there is no airway obstruction. The LLN $\%FEV_1/FVC$ can be determined directly for various populations using regression equations in Table 19-8 or simply estimated at 70%. If the $\%FEV_1/FVC$ ratio is greater than the LLN or 70% and if the TLC is less than the LLN, often defined as less than 80% predicted normal, the patient has a restrictive impairment according to this algorithm. The severity of the restriction is based on the percent predicted or on the number of standard deviations below the LLN TLC according to Table 19-2. If the $\%FEV_1/FVC$ ratio is less than 70%, the patient likely has an obstructive impairment; the severity of the obstruction is based on the percent predicted normal FEV_1 according to Table 19-2. If the percent predicted normal DLCO is less than 80%, the patient has a diffusion impairment. Some laboratories also report the $DLCO/V_A$ ratio, which indexes the DLCO for lung volume measured during the single-breath test. If the $DLCO/V_A$ ratio is also less than 80% of the indexed value, the cause of the diffusion impairment is considered to be within the lung, and if the $DLCO/V_A$ ratio is greater than 80% of the indexed value, the cause of the diffusion impairment is considered to be due to small lung volume.

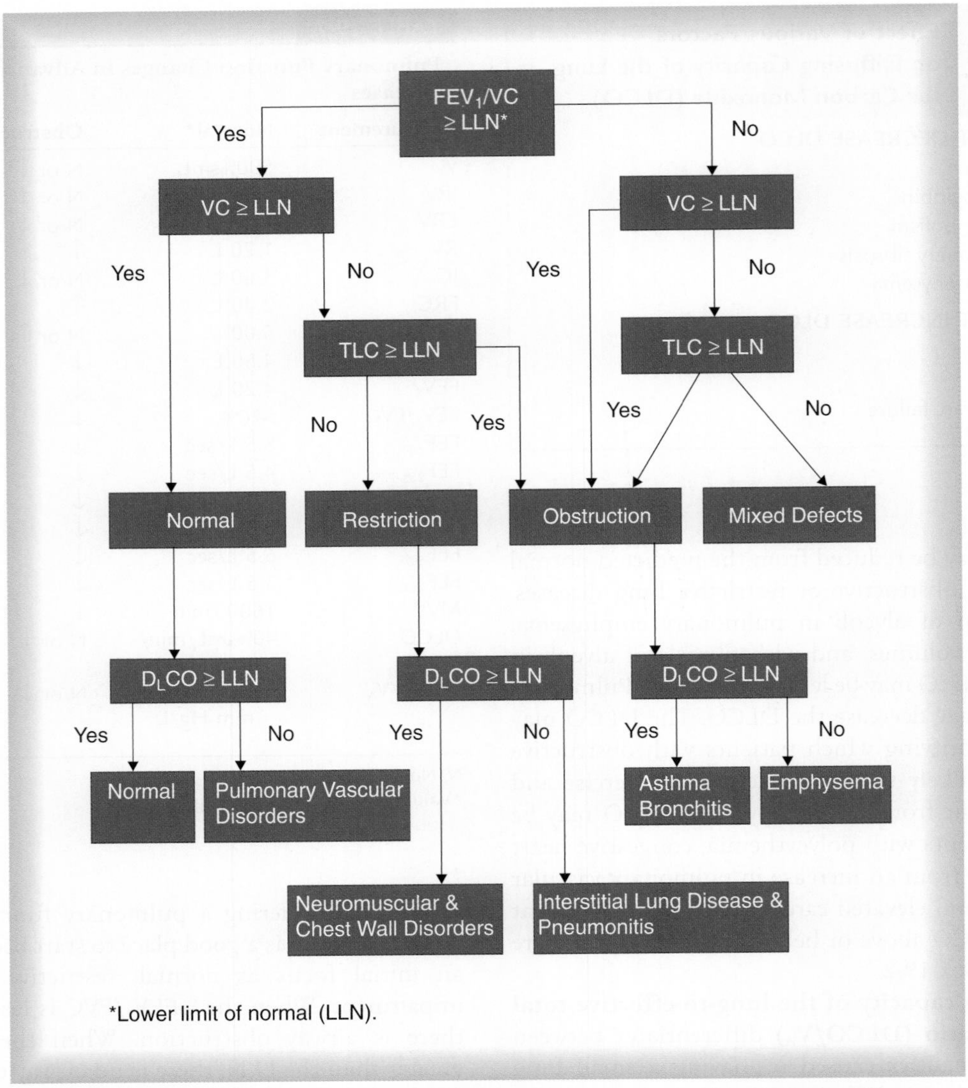

FIGURE 19-16 A simple algorithm to assess pulmonary function test results in clinical practice. (From Gardner RM, Crapo RO, Morris AH, et al: Computer guidelines for pulmonary laboratories. Am Rev Respir Dis 134:628, 1986.)

TABLE 19-8

Examples of Regression Equations for Determining Lower Limit of Normal of Forced Expiratory Volume in 1 Second-to-Vital Capacity Ratio (%FEV1/FVC) in Adults

Population	Equations	R^2
Men		
White	78.388 – 0.2066 (A)	0.3448
African-American	78.822 – 0.1828 (A)	0.1538
Mexican-American	80.925 – 0.2186 (A)	0.2713
Women		
White	81.015 – 0.2125 (A)	0.3955
African-American	80.978 – 0.2039 (A)	0.2284
Mexican-American	83.044 – 0.2248 (A)	0.3352

A, Years.

Hankinson JL, Odencratz JR, Fedan KB: Spirometric reference values from a sample of the general U.S. population. Am J Respir Crit Care Med 159:179, 1999.

MINI CLINI

Identifying Patterns of Pulmonary Impairment

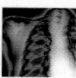

PROBLEM: Following are three pulmonary function reports that show three distinct examples of pulmonary impairment. Using the algorithm in Figure 19-16, identify the patterns typical of asthma, pulmonary fibrosis, and COPD.

PULMONARY FUNCTION REPORT 1

Pulmonary Measurements	Predicted Normal Value	Measured Baseline Conditions	Percent Predicted Baseline	Measured After Bronchodilator Treatment	Percent Predicted After Treatment
SVC (L)	5.00	3.00	60%		
FVC (L)	5.00	3.00	60%		
FEV_1 (L)	4.00	2.80	70%		
$\%FEV_1/FVC$	80%	94%	—		
$FEF_{25\%-75\%}$ (L/sec)	4.00	3.75	94%		
PEF (L/sec)	8.00	8.25	103%		
TLC (L)	7.20	3.96	55%		
FRC (L)	4.10	2.00	49%		
RV (L)	2.20	1.40	60%		
DLCO (ml/min/mm Hg)	34.0	15.9	47%		
$DLCO/V_A$ (ml/min/mm Hg/L)	7.20	3.50	49%		

SOLUTION REPORT 1: Although FEV_1 is less than 80% of predicted, because the FEV_1/FVC is greater than 70%, there is no apparent airway obstruction. FEV_1 is reduced because FVC is reduced. The patient's measured FVC is less than the predicted FEV_1. Because TLC is less than 80% predicted, the data suggest a restrictive impairment, and because DLCO is less than 80% predicted, there is also a diffusion impairment. The low $DLCO/V_A$ suggests that the diffusion impairment is out of proportion to the lung volume. This finding implies that the impairment to normal diffusion is the lung tissue. Overall, this report shows a moderate restrictive pattern consistent with pulmonary fibrosis.

PULMONARY FUNCTION REPORT 2

Pulmonary Measurements	Predicted Normal Value	Measured Baseline Conditions	Percent Predicted Baseline	Measured After Bronchodilator Treatment	Percent Predicted After Treatment
SVC (L)	5.00	3.50	70%	4.25	85%
FVC (L)	5.00	3.30	66%	4.00	80%
FEV_1 (L)	4.00	2.00	50%	2.50	62%
$\%FEV_1/FVC$	80%	57%	—	62%	—
$FEF_{25\%-75\%}$ (L/sec)	4.00	1.00	25%	2.00	50%
PEF (L/sec)	8.00	6.00	75%	6.50	81%
TLC (L)	5.27	5.51	105%	5.36	102%
FRC (L)	3.11	4.55	146%	3.60	116%
RV (L)	1.67	2.60	156%	2.00	120%
DLCO (ml/min/mm Hg)	28.7	25.25	88%	—	—
$DLCO/V_A$ (ml/min/mm Hg/L)	5.45	5.17	96%	—	—

SOLUTION REPORT 2: The FEV_1/FVC is less than 70%; there is airway obstruction. FEV_1 is 50% of predicted; the obstruction is moderate. Because the $FEF_{25\%-75\%}$ is 25% of predicted, the major site of obstruction is in the bronchioles. After bronchodilator inhalation, FEV_1 improved by 24% (remember to compute percent change), showing effective treatment and partial reversibility of the obstruction. The large FRC and RV show hyperinflation and air trapping, which also improved after bronchodilator therapy. Diffusing capacity is in the normal range, indicating no diffusion impairment and no alveolar problems. Overall, this report shows a moderate obstructive pattern with hyperinflation and air trapping responsive to bronchodilators and consistent with acute hyperreactive airways disease, such as asthma.

Continued

MINI CLINI

Identifying Patterns of Pulmonary Impairment—cont'd

PULMONARY FUNCTION REPORT 3

Pulmonary Measurements	Predicted Normal Value	Measured Baseline Conditions	Percent Predicted Baseline	Measured After Bronchodilator Treatment	Percent Predicted After Treatment
SVC (L)	5.00	4.00	80%	4.25	85%
FVC (L)	5.00	3.50	70%	4.00	80%
FEV_1 (L)	4.00	2.00	50%	2.20	55%
$\%FEV_1/FVC$	80%	57%	—	55%	—
$FEF_{25\%-75\%}$ (L/sec)	4.00	1.75	50%	2.00	50%
PEF (L/sec)	8.00	6.00	75%	6.50	80%
TLC (L)	5.27	5.51	105%	5.36	102%
FRC (L)	3.11	4.55	146%	3.79	122%
RV (L)	1.67	2.60	156%	2.24	134%
DLCO (ml/min/mm Hg)	28.7	14.25	56%	—	—
$DLCO/V_A$ (ml/min/mm Hg/L)	5.45	3.17	58%	—	—

SOLUTION REPORT 3: This case is similar to case 2, but there are some important differences. The FEV_1/FVC is less than 70%; there is airway obstruction. FEV_1 is 50% of predicted; the obstruction is moderate. After a single bronchodilator treatment, FEV_1 improved by 10% (remember to compute percent change)—not enough to show that bronchodilator therapy was immediately effective. The large FRC and RV show hyperinflation and air trapping, which did improve after bronchodilator therapy. DLCO and $DLCO/V_A$ are reduced, suggesting alveolar involvement. This report shows a moderate obstructive pattern with hyperinflation and air trapping not responsive to bronchodilators. There is diffusion impairment and alveolar disease. Overall, this report is consistent with COPD, the combination of chronic bronchitis and pulmonary emphysema.

PULMONARY FUNCTION REPORT 4

Pulmonary Measurements	Predicted Normal Value	Measured Baseline Conditions	Percent Predicted Baseline	Measured After Bronchodilator Treatment	Percent Predicted After Treatment
SVC (L)	5.38	4.84	90%		
FVC (L)	5.38	4.92	92%	5.16	109%
FEV_1 (L)	4.33	2.95	68%	3.24	75%
$\%FEV_1/FVC$	80%	54%	—	63%	
$FEF_{25\%-75\%}$ (L/sec)	5.23	1.20	23%	1.08	21%
PEF (L/sec)	9.96	6.32	63%	7.53	76%
TLC (L)	7.51	6.38	85%		
FRC (L)	4.10	3.51	86%		
RV (L)	2.10	1.58	75%		
DLCO (ml/min/mm Hg)	37.22	29.60	89%		
$DLCO/V_A$ (ml/min/mm Hg/L)	4.96	4.06	82%		

SOLUTION REPORT 4: This case is similar to case 3, but there are some important differences. The FEV_1/FVC is less than 70%; there is airway obstruction. FEV_1 is 68% of predicted; the obstruction is mild. After a single bronchodilator treatment, FEV_1 improved by only 9.8% (remember to compute percent change)—not enough to show that the bronchodilator therapy was immediately effective. Lung volumes and diffusing capacity are within the normal range, so there is no hyperinflation, air trapping, or diffusion impairment. This report shows a mild obstructive pattern not responsive to bronchodilators. Overall, this report is consistent with chronic bronchitis.

MINI CLINI

Identifying Patterns of Pulmonary Impairment—cont'd

PULMONARY FUNCTION REPORT 5

Pulmonary Measurements	Predicted Normal Value	Measured Baseline Conditions	Percent Predicted Baseline	Measured After Bronchodilator Treatment	Percent Predicted After Treatment
SVC (L)	3.85	1.93	50%		
FVC (L)	3.85	2.01	52%		
FEV_1 (L)	3.01	1.66	55%		
$\%FEV_1/FVC$	78%	86%	—		
$FEF_{25\%-75\%}$ (L/sec)	3.40	1.85	55%		
PEF (L/sec)	6.50	4.55	70%		
TLC (L)	5.65	3.39	60%		
FRC (L)	3.01	2.11	70%		
RV (L)	1.80	1.35	75%		
DLCO (ml/min/mm Hg)	22.13	13.28	60%		
$DLCO/V_A$ (ml/min/mm Hg/L)	3.91	3.60	92%		

SOLUTION REPORT 5: The FEV_1/FVC is greater than 70%, so there is no apparent airway obstruction even though the FEV_1 is less than 80% of predicted. The patient's measured FVC is less than the predicted FEV_1, and FEV_1 is reduced because FVC is reduced. Because TLC is less than 80% predicted, the data suggest a moderate restrictive impairment. Although DLCO is less than 80% predicted, there is no apparent diffusion impairment involving lung tissue because the $DLCO/V_A$ suggests that the diffusion impairment is proportional to the low lung volume. This finding implies that the diffusion impairment is due to the subject having small lungs. Overall, this report shows a moderate restrictive pattern consistent with neuromuscular weakness or other extrapulmonary restriction.

SUMMARY CHECKLIST

- Pulmonary function testing includes measurements of airway mechanics, lung volumes and capacities, and the diffusing capacity of the lung.
- The results of pulmonary function testing can aid in the diagnosis of disease and include patterns of obstructive and restrictive impairments.
- Pulmonary function testing provides objective data on which decisions may be made regarding the status of the patient, the selection of appropriate therapy, and the evaluation of therapeutic outcomes.
- Patients with obstructive lung disease exhibit reduced expiratory flows and possibly lung hyperinflation, whereas patients with restrictive lung disease exhibit reduced lung volumes and capacities.

References

1. Pulmonary terms and symbols: a report of the ACCP-ATS Joint Committee on Pulmonary Nomenclature. Chest 67:583, 1975.
2. Zibrak JD, O'Donnell CR, Marton K: Indications for pulmonary function testing. Ann Intern Med 112:793, 1990.
3. American Thoracic Society: Evaluation of impairment/disability secondary to respiratory disorders. Am Rev Respir Dis 133:1205, 1986.
4. American Association for Respiratory Care: Clinical practice guideline: spirometry, 1996 update. Respir Care 41:629, 1996.
5. Ferris BG: Epidemiology standardization project: recommended standardized procedures for pulmonary function testing. Am Rev Respir Dis 118:1, 1978.
6. Hodgkin JE: Preoperative assessment of respiratory function. Respir Care 29:496, 1984.
7. Evaluation of impairment/disability secondary to respiratory disorders. American Thoracic Society. Am Rev Respir Dis 133:1205, 1986.
8. Tabalan OC, Williams WW, Martone WJ: Infection control in pulmonary function laboratories. Infect Control 6:442, 1985.
9. Tokars JI, McKinley GF, Otten J: Use and efficacy of tuberculosis infection control practices at hospitals with previous outbreaks of multidrug-resistant tuberculosis. Infect Control Hosp Epidemiol 22:449-455, 2001.
10. Johns DP, Imgram C, Booth H, et al: The effect of a microaerosol barrier filter on the measurement of lung function. Chest 107:1045, 1995.
11. Side EA, Harrington G, Thien F, et al: A cost-analysis of two approaches to infection control in a lung function laboratory. Aust N Z J Med 29:9, 1999.
12. Leeming JP, Pryce-Roberts DM, Kendrick AH, et al: The efficacy of filters used in respiratory function apparatus. J Hosp Infect 31:205, 1995.
13. Douce FH: Flow and volume measuring devices. In Branson R, Hess D, Chatburn R, editors: Respiratory care equipment, Philadelphia, 1995, Lippincott.
14. Shigeoka JW: Calibration and quality control of spirometer systems. Respir Care 28:747, 1983.
15. Norton A: Accuracy in pulmonary measurements. Respir Care 24:131, 1979.
16. American Thoracic Society: Quality assurance in pulmonary function laboratories. Am Rev Respir Dis 134:6257, 1986.

17. Miller MR, Hankinson J, Brusasco V, et al: Standardisation of spirometry. Eur Respir J 26:319, 2005.
18. Varkey B, Kory RC: Mediastinal and subcutaneous emphysema following pulmonary function tests. Am Rev Respir Dis 108:1393, 1973.
19. Stanescu DC, Teculescu DB: Exercise and cough induced asthma. Respiration 27:273, 1970.
20. Taussig LM, Chernick V, Wood R, et al: Standardization of lung function testing in children. Proceedings and Recommendations of the GAP Conference Committee, Cystic Fibrosis Foundation. J Pediatr 97:668, 1980.
21. Zamel N, Altose MD, Speir WA Jr: ACCP Scientific Section Recommendations: statement of spirometry: a report of the section on respiratory pathophysiology. Chest 83:547, 1983.
22. U.S. Department of Labor: Pulmonary function standards for cotton dust standard: 29 Code of Federal Regulations: 1910.1043 Appendix D. Occupational Safety and Health Administration 808832, 1980.
23. Knudson RJ, Slatin RC, Lebowitz MD, et al: The maximal expiratory flow volume curve: normal standards, variability, and effects of age. Am Rev Respir Dis 113:587, 1976.
24. Hankinson JL, Odencratz JR, Fedan KB: Spirometric reference values from a sample of the general U.S. population. Am J Respir Crit Care Med 159:179, 1999.
25. Crapo RO, Morris AH, Gardner RM: Reference spirometric values using techniques and equipment that meet ATS recommendations. Am Rev Respir Dis 123:659, 1981.
26. Aldrich TK, Arora NS, Rochester DF: The influence of airway obstruction and respiratory muscle strength on maximal voluntary ventilation in lung disease. Am Rev Respir Dis 126: 1959, 1982.
27. American Thoracic Society: Guidelines for methacholine and exercise challenge testing—1999. Am J Respir Crit Care Med 161:309-329, 2000.
28. Wanger J, Clausen JL, Coates A, et al. Standardisation of the measurement of lung volumes. Eur Respir J 26:511-522, 2005.
29. Hathirat S, Renzetti AD, Mitchell M: Measurement of the total lung capacity by helium dilution in a constant volume system. Am Rev Respir Dis 102:760, 1970.
30. Birath G, Swenson EW: A correction factor for helium absorption in lung volume determination. Scand J Clin Lab Invest 8:155, 1956.
31. Boren HG, Kory RC, Snyder JC: The Veterans Administration-Army cooperative study of pulmonary function, II: the lung volume and its subdivisions in normal men. Am J Med 41:96, 1966.
32. Dubois AB, Botelho SY, Bedell GN, et al: A rapid plethysmographic method for measuring thoracic gas volume: a comparison with a nitrogen washout method for measuring FRC in normal patients. J Clin Invest 35:322, 1956.
33. Habib MP, Engel LA: Influence of the panting technique on the plethysmographic measurement of thoracic gas volume. Am Rev Respir Dis 117:265, 1978.
34. Stocks J, Quanjer PH: Reference values for residual volume, functional residual capacity and total lung capacity. Eur Respir J 8:492, 1995.
35. Knudson RJ, Kaltenborn WT, Burrows B: The effects of cigarette smoking and smoking cessation on the carbon monoxide diffusing capacity of the lung in asymptomatic patients. Am Rev Respir Dis 140:645, 1989.
36. American Thoracic Society: Single breath carbon monoxide diffusing capacity (transfer factor): recommendations for a standard technique. Am J Respir Crit Care Med 152:2185, 1995.
37. MacIntyre N, Crapo R, Viegi G, et al: Standardization of the single breath determination of carbon monoxide uptake in the lung. Eur Respir J 26:720, 2005.
38. Forster RE, Fowler WS, Bates DV, et al: The absorption of carbon monoxide by the lungs during breathholding. J Clin Invest 33:1135, 1954.
39. Ogilvie CM, Forster RE, Blakemore WS, et al: A standardized breath holding technique for the clinical measurement of the diffusing capacity of the lung for carbon monoxide. J Clin Invest 36:117, 1957.
40. Crapo RO, Morris AM: Standardized single breath normal values for carbon monoxide diffusing capacity. Am Rev Respir Dis 123:185, 1981.
41. Dinakara P, Blumenthal WS, Johnston RF, et al: The effect of anemia on pulmonary diffusing capacity with derivation of a correction equation. Am Rev Respir Dis 102:965, 1970.
42. Marrades RM, Diaz O, Roca J, et al: Adjustment of DLCO for hemoglobin concentration. Am J Respir Crit Care Med 155:236, 1997.
43. Kanner RE, Crapo RO: The relationship between alveolar oxygen tension and the single-breath carbon monoxide diffusing capacity. Am Rev Respir Dis 133:676-678, 1986.
44. Gray C, Zammel N, Crapo RO: The effect of a simulated 3048 meter altitude on single breath transfer factor. Bull Eur Physiopathol Respir 22:429, 1986.
45. Gardner RM, Clousen JL, Crapo RO, et al: Computer guidelines for pulmonary laboratories. Am Rev Respir Dis 134:628, 1986.
46. American Thoracic Society: Lung function testing: selection of reference values and interpretative strategies. Am Rev Respir Dis 144:1202, 1991.
47. Pelligrino R, Viegi G, Brusasco V, et al: Interpretive strategies for lung function testing. Eur Respir J 26:948, 2005.

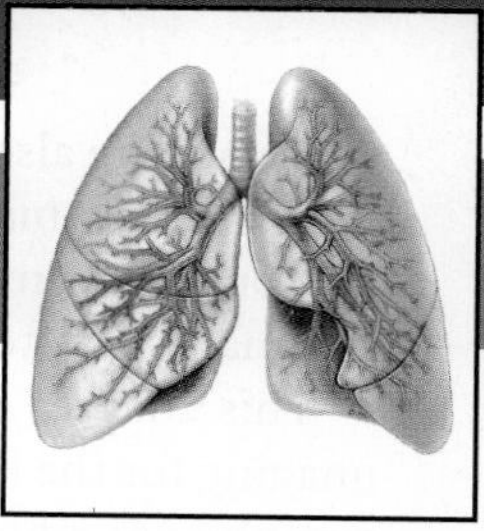

Chapter 20

Review of Thoracic Imaging

N. LENNARD SPECHT AND JAMES K. STOLLER

CHAPTER OBJECTIVES

After reading this chapter you will be able to:

- List the four tissue densities seen on a chest radiograph.
- Define the terms *radiolucent* and *radiopaque.*
- Describe how to evaluate the technical quality of a chest radiograph.
- State the differences between a posteroanterior chest film and an anteroposterior chest film.
- List the anatomic structures seen on a chest radiograph.
- List the steps used to interpret thoracic imaging studies.
- Identify the value of a computed tomography (CT) scan, high-resolution CT scan, and CT angiogram.
- Describe the common radiographic abnormalities seen in the pleura, lung parenchyma, and mediastinum.

CHAPTER OUTLINE

KEY TERMS

air bronchograms
cephalization
chest radiograph
computed tomography (CT)
empyema
gantry
hydropneumothorax
hydrothorax
infiltrates
interstitial lung disease
Kerley B lines
plate (or platelike) atelectasis
pneumomediastinum
pneumothorax
radiograph
radiolucent
radiopaque
roentgenogram
solitary pulmonary nodule

Chest imaging is crucial in the practice of pulmonary and critical care medicine. It is essential that the respiratory therapist (RT) have a solid understanding of chest imaging to facilitate patient assessment. Various chest imaging modes exist, including conventional chest film (more accurately called a **radiograph** or **roentgenogram** after Roentgen, who first discovered the x-ray beam), computed tomography (CT) scanning, ultrasound, and magnetic resonance imaging (MRI).

Scanning radioactive material within a patient after inhalation or injection of a radioisotope is a separate radiographic technique. Radioisotopes are used for ventilation/perfusion ($\dot{V}/\dot{Q}$) scans, which have been historically used in the diagnosis of pulmonary embolism. Radioisotope injections are also used for positron emission tomography (PET), which may help localize tumors and metastases. The branch of medicine that uses radioisotopes to generate images is often called *nuclear medicine*.

This chapter summarizes important concepts in chest imaging for the RT. The basic elements of plain chest radiography are addressed first, and then the role of various imaging techniques used to evaluate the different components of the chest (e.g., pleura, mediastinum, lung tissue [*parenchyma*]) is described. Examples of abnormal findings are shown, including some images obtained with the more sophisticated techniques such as ultrasound, CT, and MRI.

OVERVIEW OF PLAIN CHEST RADIOGRAPH

Passing an x-ray beam through part of a person's body to a photographic film creates an x-ray film. The resulting image is formed as x-rays strike the film and darken it. A radiograph is similar to a negative from an old-fashioned black and white film camera. X-rays that pass directly through low-density tissue (e.g., lung) strike the film more directly and cause the resulting shadow to turn darker. X-rays that strike denser tissue (e.g., bone) are more absorbed and leave the exposed film lighter. The shadows on the radiograph vary in shades of gray based on the density of the tissue through which the x-ray beam has passed.

Four different tissue densities are visible on a normal **chest radiograph.** The tissue types that generate these densities are *air, fat, soft tissue* (*water density* because soft tissues, similar to muscle, are mainly composed of water), and *bone.* Each tissue absorbs different amounts of the x-ray beam, which varies the shade of the shadow on the final film. Air in the lung, stomach, or intestines absorbs the least energy and appears virtually black on a film **(radiolucent).** Soft tissue absorbs a small amount of the x-ray beam and is usually seen as a medium gray shadow. Bone absorbs a large amount of the x-ray beam and is seen as a nearly white **(radiopaque)** shadow. Fat absorbs a slightly smaller amount of x-ray energy than soft tissue and appears just slightly darker than soft tissue.

X-ray images have traditionally been recorded on film. Once developed, x-ray films can be displayed by placing the film over a viewbox that illuminates the film for the observer. At the present time, most x-ray films are recorded and displayed in a digital format. To record a digital image, an x-ray detector (digital film) replaces the photographic film. A computer takes the data from the x-ray detector and creates the image. The resulting image is projected on a computer monitor.

Compared with images recorded on traditional film, digital images have advantages regarding the interpretation of the image and its retrieval. The display of digital images can be manipulated by adjusting contrast, brightness, and magnification. These adjustments allow findings that would be subtle and hard to see on traditional film to be seen more easily. Digital images also allow multiple people to see the image at the same time on large plasma screen viewing stations or multiple people in different locations to see the image. For example, an RT in a critical care unit, a radiologist in the imaging department, and a critical care physician in another hospital may collaborate by all viewing at the same time an x-ray image on a rapidly deteriorating patient. Digital images can also be easily copied and recorded on compact discs so that patients can get digital copies of films to take to their physicians. One can easily imagine a time when such images will be kept by individuals on their own digital files of medical information or transmitted from one facility to another as patients move or travel.

The structures visible on a chest radiograph are seen only when tissue of one density is next to tissue of another density. The heart is visible as a soft tissue density in the middle of the chest because the lungs, which are primarily air density, normally surround it. If the chest on either side of the heart were filled with water (pulmonary consolidation or pleural effusion), the normal heart shadow would be invisible on the radiograph. This obscuring of the margin of adjacent structures of the same density is called the *silhouette sign* and can be useful to localize abnormalities within the lung anatomically.

When to obtain a chest radiograph is ultimately the decision of the attending physician. However, the RT may be able to suggest that a chest x-ray should be obtained in certain circumstances, such as when a patient in the intensive care unit suddenly deteriorates for no apparent reason. The RT needs to be familiar with the common clinical indications for obtaining a chest radiograph (Box 20-1).

A chest radiograph is extremely valuable in many patients with lung disease, but it does have limitations. A

Box 20-1 Clinical Indications for Obtaining a Chest Radiograph

OUTPATIENT
- Unexplained dyspnea
- Severe persistent cough
- Hemoptysis
- Fever and sputum production
- Acute severe chest pain
- Positive tuberculosis skin test

INPATIENT
- Placement of endotracheal tube
- Placement of pulmonary artery catheter
- Placement of central venous pressure catheter
- Sudden onset of dyspnea or chest pain
- Elevated or changing plateau pressure during mechanical ventilation
- Sudden decline in oxygenation

chest radiograph may appear normal even though the patient is in respiratory failure; this is common in patients with acute (e.g., pulmonary embolism) or chronic obstructive lung disease (e.g., emphysema that is not apparent on a plain chest x-ray). In addition, the chest radiograph may lag behind the clinical condition of the patient. This situation is common in pneumonia, where the patient may present with high fever and cough typical for pneumonia, but an infiltrate may not appear on a chest film until 12 to 24 hours later. Similarly, the infiltrate on the chest film may persist for days to weeks after symptoms of pneumonia have resolved.

Approach to Reading a Plain Chest Radiograph

A disciplined approach is required to obtain the maximal value out of any diagnostic imaging study. A plain chest radiograph may best exemplify this statement. An obvious abnormality such as a 6-cm mass is easily spotted, even by the untrained eye. Such an abnormality tends to monopolize the observer's attention immediately, which causes more subtle abnormalities, often with equal or even greater diagnostic importance, to go unnoticed. To avoid this pitfall, the observer must develop a step-by-step approach that is applied to reading a plain chest x-ray in a disciplined fashion until it becomes second nature. The following suggestions are broad guidelines, and each observer must formulate an approach that he or she finds comfortable.

In broad terms, the steps in reviewing a chest film are as follows:

- Identify the name on the radiograph.
- Review the technique and quality of the film: Is the film well centered (i.e., the spinous processes are right in the middle of the trachea on a posteroanterior [PA] film), and is the amount of penetration of the beam adequate, too high (i.e., the lung parenchyma is too dark to see subtle changes), or too low (i.e., the lung parenchyma is too white, causing normal lung markings to appear abnormal)?
- Systematically review the anatomic structures on the chest film to assess their normality or abnormality.

In subsequent sections, to discuss common abnormalities that the RT should recognize, the following areas are reviewed: (1) evaluation of the technical quality and adequacy of the film, (2) normal anatomic structures on a chest radiograph, (3) more sophisticated imaging techniques, and (4) major anatomic components seen on the radiograph.

Chest Radiograph Technique and Quality

Several technical factors should be routinely assessed when reading a chest film:

1. Is the film appropriately labeled?
2. Is the film PA with a lateral view, or is it an anteroposterior (AP) portable film?
3. Is the entire chest imaged on the film (i.e., are any structures cut off from the film)?
4. Was the patient properly positioned for the film?
5. Were the optimal settings for the x-ray beam selected when the film was taken (the term used is *penetration,* which is similar to *exposure* on camera film)?

As the first step, the RT should check the patient's identity on the film or image file and all labels visible on the film. This check helps avoid the mistake of interpreting a chest radiograph for a patient different than the patient being considered and establishes which side is which because labels are often placed to indicate the patient's left or right side; such labeling of the side is important in cases where the patient's chest or abdominal contents are reversed—known as *situs inversus* or *dextrocardia.*

MINI CLINI

Evaluating the Heart Size on a Portable Chest Radiograph

A standard chest film is obtained with the patient standing and facing the film cassette. The x-ray beam penetrates the patient's back first and then passes through the anterior chest and finally to the film. This standard technique is called the *posteroanterior (PA) chest film.* The heart is located very close to the film with the standard PA view, and magnification of the heart shadow is minimal.

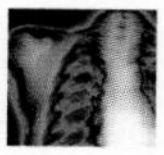

PROBLEM: In the intensive care unit, patients are generally too ill for a PA chest film to be obtained. The chest film is obtained with the patient lying in bed and the film cassette placed behind the patient. The x-ray beam passes from anterior to posterior, producing an anteroposterior (AP) portable chest film. In examining an AP portable chest film, how is the appearance of the heart size affected?

ANSWER: An AP portable radiograph is obtained with the patient's heart farther from the film, producing a heart shadow that is artificially magnified compared with the shadow produced with a PA chest film; this may give the appearance of an enlarged heart in some cases. The clinician interpreting an AP portable radiograph must keep this in mind to avoid misinterpreting the film as erroneously showing an enlarged heart (cardiomegaly). To illustrate this point, hold a flashlight 3 feet from a wall and turn it on. While holding the flashlight steady, place one hand in line with the beam. The shadow created by the hand becomes smaller as the hand is moved closer to the wall and farther from the light source.

A plain chest radiograph is taken using one of two techniques: the PA view or the AP view. The views are named for the path of the x-ray beam. In the PA view, the patient puts his or her back to the x-ray source and the chest against the film. The x-ray beam leaves the source, passes through the posterior (P) side of the patient, through the patient and then through the patient's anterior (A) surface,

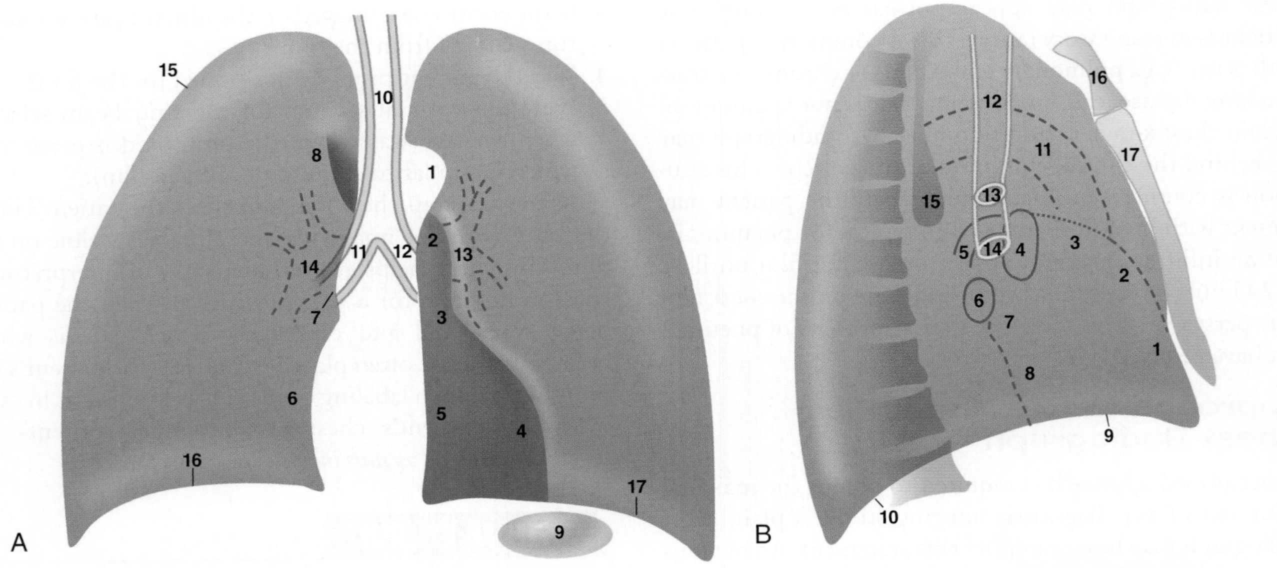

1. Aortic arch
2. Main pulmonary artery
3. Left atrium
4. Left ventricle
5. Descending aorta
6. Right atrium
7. Ascending aorta
8. Superior vena cava
9. Gastric bubble
10. Trachea
11. Right main bronchus
12. Left main bronchus
13. Left pulmonary artery
14. Right pulmonary artery
15. Pleural line
16. Right hemidiaphragm
17. Left hemidiaphragm

1. Right ventricle
2. Pulmonary outflow tract
3. Main pulmonary artery
4. Right pulmonary artery
5. Left pulmonary artery
6. Pulmonary veins
7. Left atrium
8. Left ventricle
9. Right hemidiaphragm
10. Left hemidiaphragm
11. Aortic arch
12. Trachea
13. Right upper lobe bronchus
14. Left upper lobe bronchus
15. Scapulae
16. Manubrium
17. Sternum

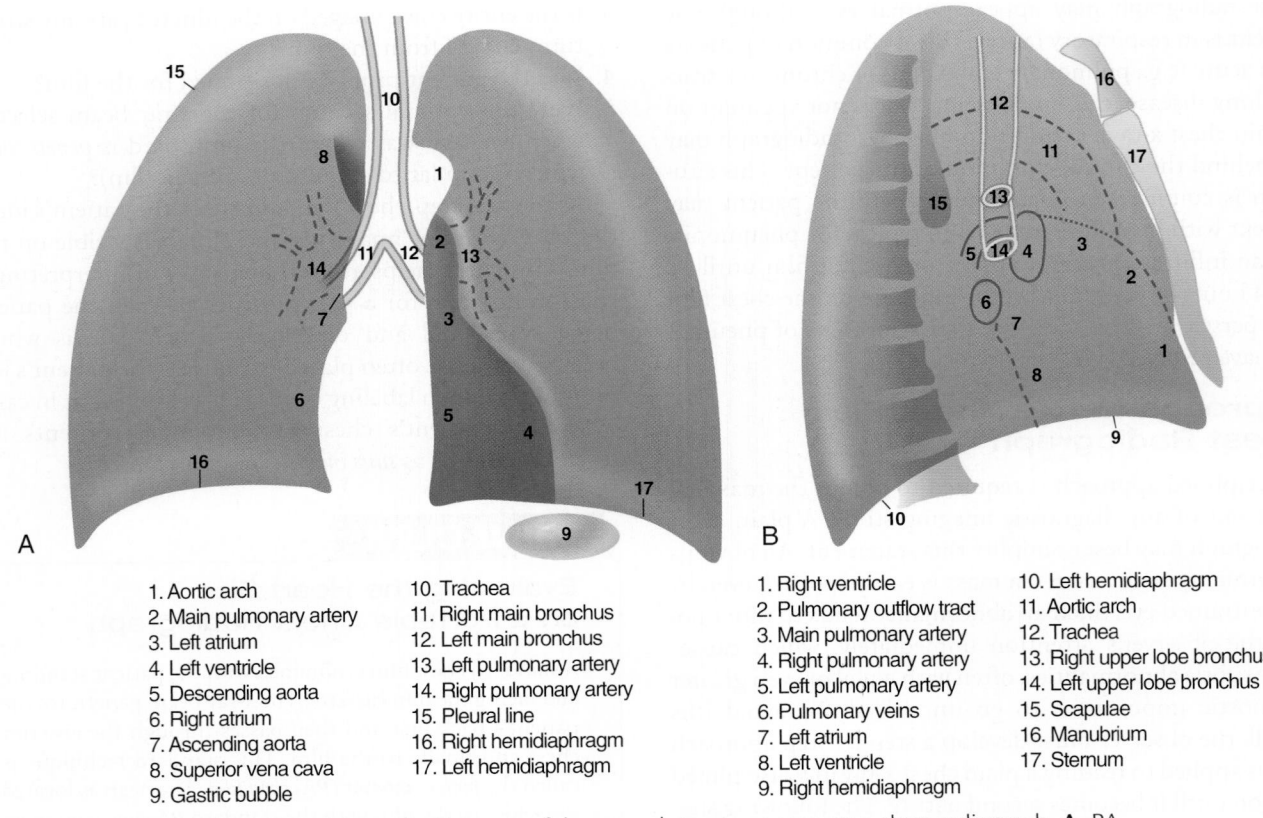

FIGURE 20-1 Schematic diagrams of the normal structures seen on a chest radiograph. **A,** PA view. **B,** Lateral view.

and finally to the film. The PA view is usually performed in the radiology department with equipment that standardizes the distance from the x-ray source to the film and where the x-ray technician can maximize the quality of each film. In addition, as noted, taking the film with the anterior chest closest to the film minimizes magnification of the heart.

The AP film is usually taken with a portable x-ray machine. The AP technique puts the x-ray source in front of the patient with the film behind the patient's back. The source of the x-ray beam is usually much closer to the patient than with a PA film, although the distance varies from patient to patient. The closer x-ray source and the position of the patient both lead to a slight magnification of the heart shadow. The AP film is usually taken in the intensive care unit because these patients are too ill to go out of the intensive care unit to the radiology department. Overall, AP portable films are usually of lesser quality compared with PA films. During the reading of the chest radiograph, the RT needs to take into account the view (AP or PA) as he or she interprets the heart size and subtle findings that may be influenced by film quality and technique.

When a chest film is taken using the portable AP technique, it is sometimes difficult to align the patient properly, and a portion of the chest may be missed. Although these problems are seen far more often with portable films, they may occur with PA and lateral films as well. The RT should ask the following questions: (1) Is the whole chest visible on the film? (2) Is the patient well positioned?

Patient rotation can make interpretation more difficult by projecting *midline* structures (e.g., the trachea) to the right or left. The observer can assess for rotation by comparing anterior structures such as the *medial* (toward the middle) ends of the clavicles with a posterior structure such as the spinous process (midline structure of the spine). In a perfectly positioned or aligned chest film, the spinous process should be seen midway between the medial ends of the clavicles and in the middle of the tracheal air column (Figure 20-1). Patient rotation makes the mediastinum appear unusually wide and obscures or distorts the appearance of the pulmonary arteries as they emerge from the mediastinum into the lung parenchyma.

The RT also must ensure that the film is adequately penetrated. An improperly penetrated film may conceal important details. A chest radiograph with proper exposure should show the intervertebral disc spaces through the shadow of the heart and should allow the blood vessels in the peripheral regions of the lungs to be visualized. A chest radiograph that is underexposed or underpenetrated (i.e., owing to too-low kilovoltage of the x-ray beam) does not allow visualization of the intervertebral discs through the heart shadow and may make identification of pathology in soft tissue areas such as the mediastinum more

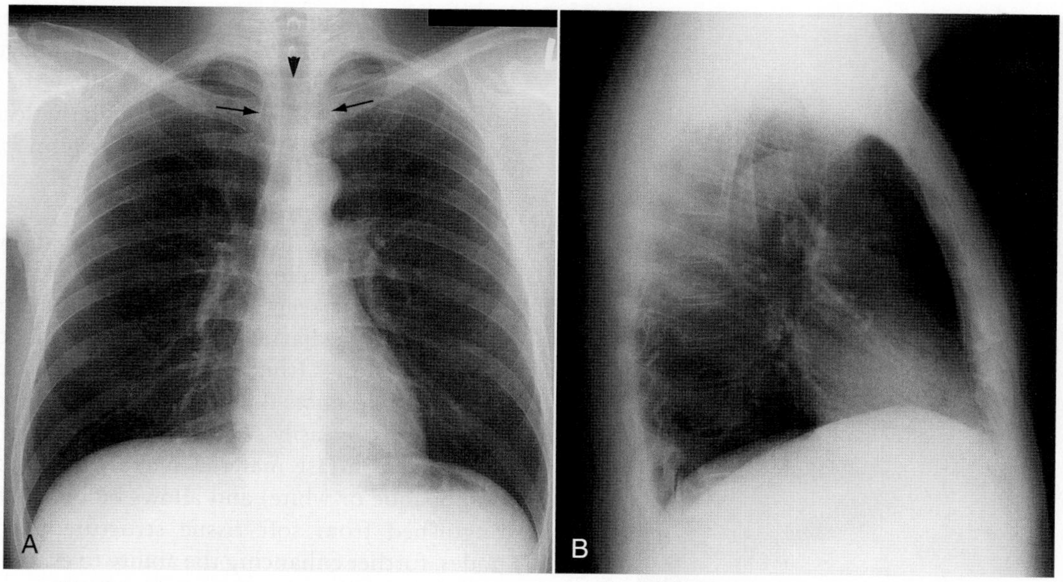

FIGURE 20-2 Normal frontal **(A)** and normal lateral **(B)** chest films. Note the medial ends of the clavicles *(arrows)* with the spinous process *(arrowhead)* framed between them **(A).**

difficult. Specifically, an underpenetrated film may cause the normal branching of the pulmonary arteries in the lung to appear abnormal and be misinterpreted as evidence of interstitial infiltrates. Similarly, an overpenetrated radiograph overexposes the film, leaving the lung parenchyma black and no ability to visualize the peripheral blood vessels or abnormalities that may be present (e.g., infiltrates secondary to pneumonia, pulmonary nodules). This overpenetration makes evaluation of the lung parenchyma far more difficult. Adjustment of the contrast and brightness of the chest film on the computer display improves the ability to see certain aspects of a chest x-ray with improper penetration. However, adjusting the display cannot completely overcome the loss of important details caused by an improperly penetrated film.

Anatomic Structures Seen on a Chest Radiograph

After the RT has reviewed the technical aspects of the chest radiograph, it is time to review the anatomic findings in the film. The main structures imaged on a routine chest radiograph are listed next and illustrated in Figure 20-2:

1. Bones (e.g., ribs, clavicles, scapulae, vertebrae)
2. Soft tissues (e.g., tissues of the chest wall, upper abdomen, lymph nodes)
3. Lungs (including the trachea, bronchi, and lung tissue or parenchyma)
4. Pleura (membranous coverings of the lung, including the *visceral pleura* [the part attached to the lungs] and the *parietal pleura* [the part lining the inside of the chest wall]; although normally occupied by only a small amount of fluid, the space between the parietal and visceral pleura is called the *pleural space*)
5. Heart, great vessels, and mediastinum (i.e., the tissues between the two lungs in the center of the chest, bordered by the sternum and the vertebral column in the AP dimension and by the thoracic inlet [where the trachea enters the thorax] and the diaphragm in the cephalocaudal direction)
6. Upper abdomen
7. Lower neck

The anatomy seen on the film should be reviewed in a thorough, systematic manner. All of the above-listed anatomic structures must be individually assessed. When first beginning to read films, it is helpful for the RT to create a list of the anatomic structures that must be assessed and to check off the structures as they are reviewed. As the reader gains experience, the checklist becomes second nature and automatic.

Assessment of the chest wall should include looking for symmetry, rib fractures, or other bone changes. Lung evaluation begins by assessing the size and density. Any obvious differences in symmetry must be explained. Of the lung parenchyma, 80% to 90% is overlaid with bone in the form of ribs, clavicles, and spine. The overlying bone may conceal some lung abnormalities. A lateral film is helpful in clarifying the presence or absence of suspicious lung abnormalities on frontal projections. The RT must pay specific attention to areas where subtle abnormalities may be hiding; these include the lung tissue behind the clavicles (especially medially), the area of lung that projects behind the heart, and part of the lung that lies deep in the posterior sulcus (the extreme bottom of the lung projecting behind the dome of the diaphragm on the frontal view).

Review of the lung edge on both frontal and lateral films discloses any pleural abnormalities, such as fluid in the

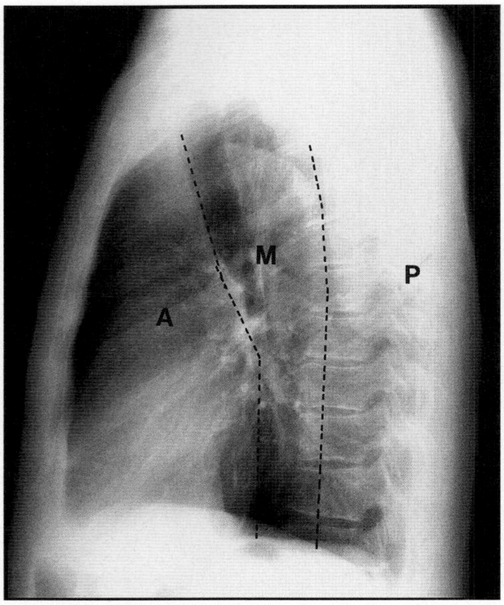

FIGURE 20-3 Lateral view of the chest, indicating the divisions of the mediastinum: anterior *(A)*; middle *(M)*; posterior *(P)*.

pleural space (e.g., hydrothorax, hemothorax [blood in the pleural space]) and air in the pleural space (pneumothorax). Evaluation of the mediastinum should include assessment of heart size. In the PA projection, the diameter of the heart shadow should not exceed one-half the diameter of the chest. An enlarged heart may occur with congestive heart failure or with a large pericardial effusion (accumulation of fluid within the space that surrounds the heart encased within the pericardium). The lateral contours of the mediastinum should correspond to normal anatomic structures as outlined in Figure 20-3.

Advanced Chest Imaging Techniques

Computed Tomography of the Chest

Computed tomography (CT) scanning is a very helpful chest imaging technique because it can visualize structures in cross section and can visualize great detail and miniscule structures (e.g., approximately 2 mm) within the lungs. To perform a CT scan, a patient lies on an examination table called a **gantry.** The gantry is passed into a circular opening in the CT scanner. X-ray sources and detectors surround the opening in the scanner. When the scanning begins, the x-ray source and detectors pass quickly around the patient in a circular motion with the x-ray beam passing through the patient to the detector on the opposite side. The information from the detector is sent to a computer, which calculates the two-dimensional image from the data sent to it. The image created by the scan looks like a slice of the patient. Originally after each CT image was made, the gantry and patient were advanced 1 cm for the next image. The scanning and stepwise advancement of the patient were repeated until the entire chest was imaged.

Newer CT scanners use many x-ray sources and detectors, all connected to a highly capable image processing computer. These new CT scanners allow the patient and the examination table to pass through the scanner rapidly without stopping for each image. The term *spiral* or *helical* is often applied to these high-powered CT scanners, which can gather complete images in seconds.

Conventional CT scanning provides an excellent view of the chest and allows imaging of portions of the chest that are poorly seen on plain chest radiographs. Areas such as the mediastinum, the apices and costophrenic sulci of the lungs (the normally sharp shadows where the diaphragm contacts the rib cage laterally), and the pleural surfaces all are easily seen with CT scanning. Injection of iodinated contrast material makes blood appear denser (radiopaque or white) and allows blood vessels to be distinguished from soft tissue structures such as lymph nodes, further enhancing the ability to evaluate areas such as the mediastinum. Conventional CT scanning of the chest is commonly performed to evaluate the following: lung nodules and masses, great vessels of the chest, mediastinum, and pleural disease.

Conventional CT scans display images as slices every 3 to 7 mm. Each slice displays everything within the 3- to 7-mm slice of tissue. CT scans can also evaluate the delicate structures of lung parenchyma. To see lung parenchyma optimally, images need to be displayed with extremely thin slices, often 1 mm thick or less. To limit the number of images to be reviewed, thin-slice CT scans often provide images at intervals of 5 mm or 10 mm. When displayed this way, thin-cut CT scan images provide great detail of lung parenchyma but just a sampling of lung tissue rather than displaying the entire chest. The term *high-resolution CT scanning* (HRCT) is associated with CT scans designed to evaluate the lung parenchyma using thin-slice images. High-quality CT scanners often acquire much more image data than are displayed. Image data can be easily formatted into either conventional or thin-slice (HRCT) format. If the original image data are saved, a radiologist can easily go back and generate thin-slice images even if the CT scan was first displayed as a "conventional" CT scan. Thin-slice displays are especially helpful in imaging small nodules or the details of parenchymal infiltrates (e.g., interstitial lung disease) because such thin slices allow maximal spatial resolution (i.e., the ability to separate objects that are close together).

Computed Tomography Angiography

The rapid scanning that can be performed on helical CT scanners has made CT angiography possible. To perform CT angiography, a large amount of contrast dye is injected into the patient's vein. The CT technician monitors the movement of contrast material so the scan can be started when the contrast material has entered the area to be studied. CT angiography of the chest has been used for years to identify pulmonary thromboemboli

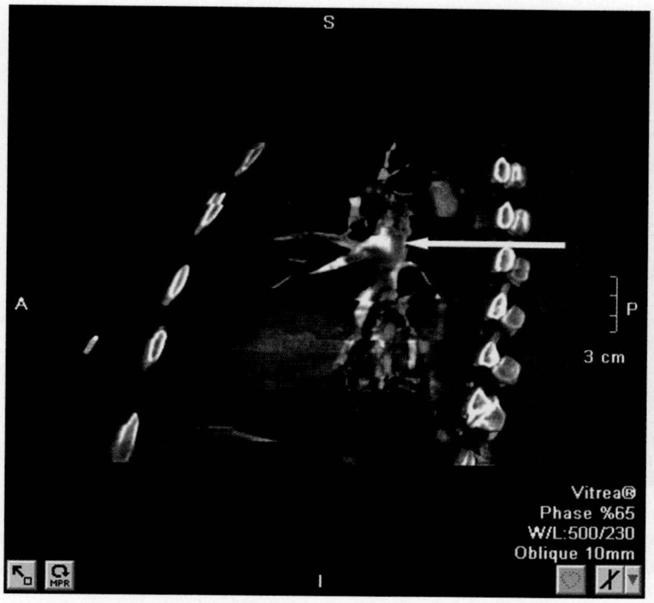

FIGURE 20-4 CT angiogram of a patient with acute pulmonary thromboembolism. The embolism is seen as the dark area within the white contrast-enhanced blood vessels *(arrow)*. (Courtesy G. Foster.)

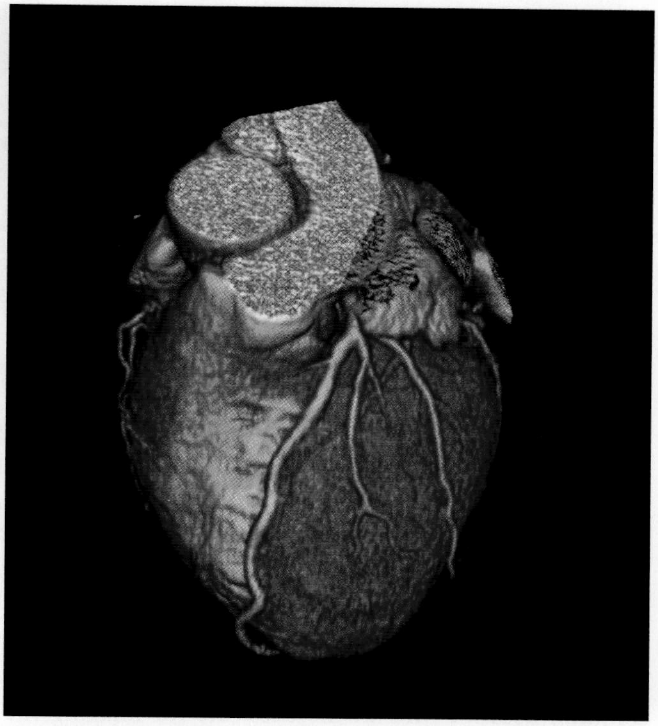

FIGURE 20-5 Three-dimensional reconstruction of the heart from a CT angiogram. (Courtesy G. Foster.)

(Figure 20-4).[1] More recently, CT angiography of the coronary artery has been evaluated; this seems to provide an alternative to routine coronary angiography in many patients.

Three-Dimensional Reconstruction

The imaging processing capabilities of modern CT scanners allow reconstruction of the chest in any direction and production of three-dimensional representations of some areas of the body (Figure 20-5). The term *virtual bronchoscopy* is used when these reconstructions simulate the view of the airways that a physician would have during bronchoscopy.

Magnetic Resonance Imaging of the Chest

MRI is occasionally useful in evaluating chest pathology. When a patient is placed into a strong magnetic field, a portion of the nuclei of their atoms with nonzero spin numbers (nuclei that have an odd number of protons and neutrons), such as the hydrogen atom, align themselves with the magnetic field. Because hydrogen atoms are present in so many molecules in the body, they provide an excellent target for MRI evaluation. Hydrogen is in water, sugars, fats, and amino acids. A brief pulse of a radio wave causes the alignment of hydrogen nuclei to flip 180 degrees. After the radio signal is stopped, the nuclei flip back to their original alignment and release their own radio wave. MRI uses the radio waves from the realigning nuclei to generate an image. The strength of the released radio waves is typically measured at less than 100 msec (T2) and 1 second (T1) after the radio signal is stopped.

MRI has advantages over other imaging techniques, especially for imaging vascular structures. MRI does not use x-rays; bone has very little hydrogen in it so it appears dark on MRI and does not obscure soft tissue detail. Blood vessels often appear black on T1-weighted images because the blood that was treated with radio waves has been moved out of the image when it was created 1 second later. This phenomenon helps differentiate between large blood vessels and nearby soft tissue.

MRI also has significant limitations when applied to imaging the chest. The large magnet required for the study makes it impossible for patients with pacemakers or other significant metal objects in their bodies to undergo MRI. A patient with a small metal object, such as a surgical clip, in the brain or eye cannot undergo MRI. The powerful magnet also prevents RTs from taking metal-containing respiratory care equipment such as ventilators or gas cylinders near the MRI machine. It is crucial to avoid taking conventional metal objects near the MRI machine because the powerful magnet would pull the metallic object into the magnet with great force, exposing patients and health care providers in its path to life-threatening risk. Deaths have been reported when oversight has allowed metal objects (e.g., oxygen cylinders) to come within the magnetic field of the MRI, and RTs must be especially vigilant about this issue. Another limitation is the slow nature of the MRI process means that respiratory and cardiac motion limits its value in chest imaging. The most

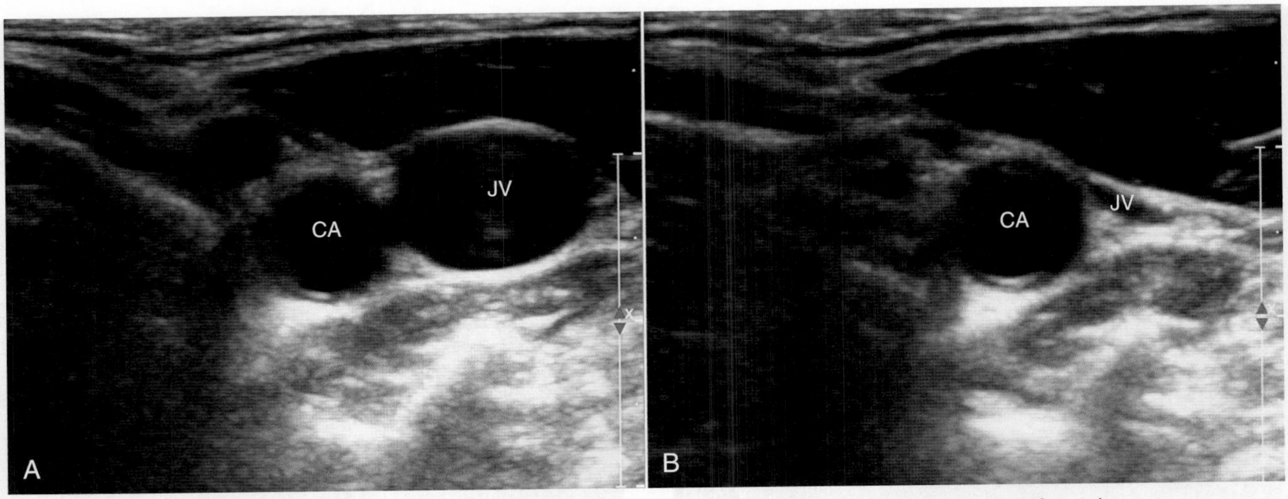

FIGURE 20-6 Two ultrasound images of the carotid artery *(CA)* and jugular vein *(JV)* from the same subject. In the first image, the jugular vein is distended; in the second image, the jugular vein is collapsed as would be seen by pressing gently with the ultrasound transducer. The carotid artery did not compress. (Courtesy G. Foster.)

common uses for MRI in the chest are for imaging the mediastinum, large vessels in the lung,[2] and hilar regions of the lungs.

Ultrasound

Ultrasound imaging is created by passing high-frequency sound waves into the body and detecting the sound waves that bounce back (echo) from the tissues of the body. The pattern of the returning sound waves is used to generate an image of the tissue studied. Ultrasound of the chest is excellent for evaluating the heart or pleural fluid.[3] Ultrasound evaluation of the lung itself is rarely useful because of the poor ability of ultrasound to transmit through the air-filled lungs.

Ultrasound imaging using small portable machines has become common in critical care units. Portable ultrasound units allow rapid assessment of heart function and volume status and are used to assist in many critical care procedures.[4] Ultrasound is also commonly used to guide the placement of central and arterial catheters. Blood vessels can be easily identified using ultrasound. The compressibility of veins is used to differentiate veins from arteries (Figure 20-6). Because the path the needle is taking is clearly seen on the ultrasound screen, using ultrasound guidance for venous and arterial puncture allows the procedure to be more easily accomplished with less time, risk, and patient discomfort.

The remainder of the chapter outlines commonly encountered abnormalities involving the pleura, lung parenchyma, and mediastinum. The reader is encouraged to fine-tune his or her observational powers for assessment of imaging studies because, as noted by Pasteur, "In the field of observation, chance favors the prepared mind."

RULE OF THUMB

Three general steps to assessing a chest film are as follows:

1. Content assurance: Is the entire chest visible on the film?
2. Quality assurance: Is the chest radiograph properly exposed and centered?
3. Disciplined application of personalized search pattern

PLEURA

The lungs are surrounded by two thin pleural membranes. The outer membrane, known as the *parietal pleura,* adheres to the inside of the chest wall, the upper surface of the diaphragm, and the lateral aspect of the mediastinum. The inner pleural membrane, or *visceral pleura,* closely adheres to the surface of each lung. The visceral pleura extends along the fissures that separate the lobes. The pleural membranes around the lung cannot be seen on a plain (or conventional) chest radiograph because they blend into the water density of the chest wall, diaphragm, and mediastinum. However, the visceral pleura separating the lobes can be seen if the pleural surface is parallel to the x-ray beam (as with the "minor" or "horizontal" fissure separating the right upper lobe from the right middle lobe on a PA chest x-ray). Although very thin, the visceral pleura separating the lobes is visible because it is contrasted with aerated lung on either side.

Hydrothorax

In healthy individuals, it is estimated that 1 to 8 ml of pleural fluid is normally present.[5] **Hydrothorax** (also

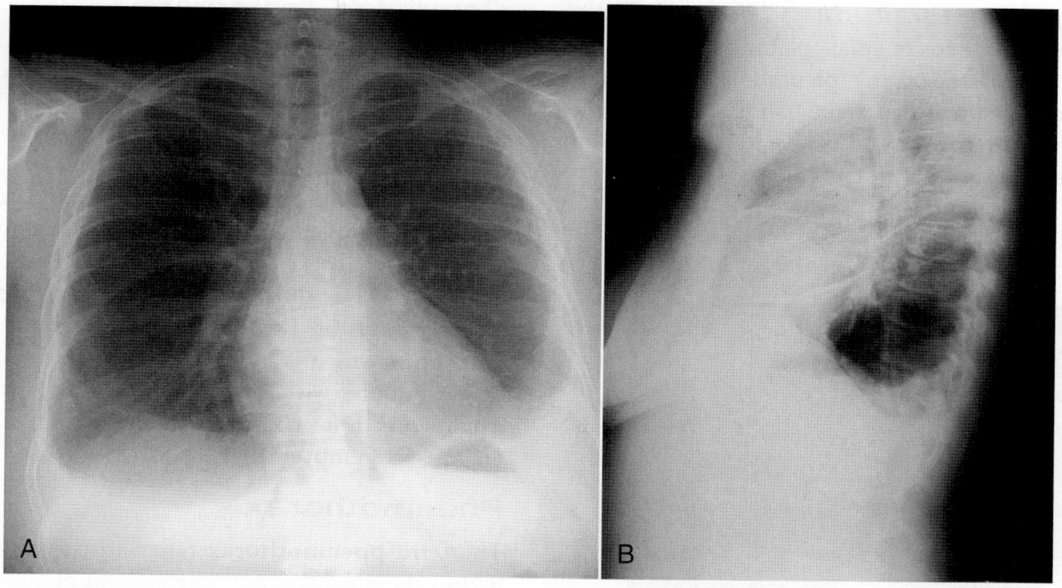

FIGURE 20-7 Pleural effusion. PA **(A)** and lateral **(B)** chest films in a 43-year-old patient with long-standing bilateral pleural effusions resulting from rheumatoid arthritis. Note the bilateral meniscus sign is also visualized posteriorly on the lateral view.

called *pleural effusion*) refers to the accumulation of excessive fluid within the pleural space. Normally, the diaphragm forms a dome that curves down to attach to the chest wall on the lower ribs and thoracic vertebra. On a chest radiograph, the arch of the diaphragm and the chest wall meet to form a point called the *costophrenic angle.* The costophrenic angle is seen on both PA and lateral views (see Figure 20-2). If the point of the costophrenic angle is rounded rather than sharp, it usually indicates a pleural effusion is present (Figure 20-7).[6] For a pleural effusion to cause blunting of the costophrenic angle on the frontal view, at least 175 to 200 ml of pleural fluid must have accumulated. The lateral film detects smaller pleural effusions than are detected with the frontal view. The posterior costophrenic angle becomes blunted with 75 to 100 ml of fluid. The best film for detecting small amounts of pleural fluid is the lateral decubitus view, which is a frontal view taken as the patient is lying on the side of the suspected effusion; 5 ml of pleural fluid can be detected on a decubitus radiograph.[7]

Sometimes, fluid can accumulate between the lung and the diaphragm and maintain a sharp costophrenic angle, hiding 500 ml of fluid.[8] Fluid that accumulates between the lung and the diaphragm is said to be in a *subpulmonic* location. The subpulmonic location is the first place pleural effusions accumulate in an upright patient.[9] The earliest sign of a left-sided pleural effusion on an upright chest radiograph is an increased distance between the inferior margin of the left lung and the stomach gas bubble. With a subpulmonic effusion, there may be an associated slight lateral shift of the point at which the diaphragm dips downward on the frontal chest radiograph (i.e., similar to a hockey stick with the blade toward the lateral chest wall).

If both air and fluid are contained within the same space, the interface between the air and the fluid forms a soft tissue density with a straight, level border that has air density above it. The interface may have a small meniscus on both sides. These straight, level interfaces between air and fluid are called *air-fluid levels.* An air-fluid level in the pleural space indicates a **hydropneumothorax** (Figure 20-8).

Occasionally, fluid occupies an unusual position, such as within an interlobar fissure (which separates lobes of the lung). Fluid is most commonly seen in the minor fissure, which is between the right middle lobe and the right upper lobe. Fluid within a fissure can be diagnosed on a chest radiograph by a characteristic lenslike, elliptic shape on either the PA or the lateral projection (Figure 20-9).

An increased volume of fluid generally is categorized as either a *transudate* or an *exudate* (see Chapter 25), but an exudate cannot be distinguished from a transudate on a chest radiograph. This distinction requires analyzing a sample of the pleural fluid. *Loculation* of pleural fluid (or trapping so that the fluid does not move freely with changing positions) is more commonly seen in exudative effusions, hemothorax (blood in the pleural space), and empyema (infection of the pleural fluid).

Clues as to whether a pleural exudate results from inflammation or from cancer may be present on the chest radiograph. Clues that favor a malignant cause for a pleural effusion include surgical absence of a breast shadow (breast cancer), evidence of prior axillary (armpit) node dissection (breast cancer), a pulmonary parenchymal mass (lung cancer), or multiple lung masses (metastatic disease).

Ultrasound for Evaluating Pleural Fluid

Ultrasound reliably detects small pleural effusions. It is also very useful in separating pleural fluid from solid tissue[10] and readily identifies tissue bands associated with loculated effusions. Ultrasound is also helpful in guiding thoracentesis, in particular, for small or loculated pleural effusions.

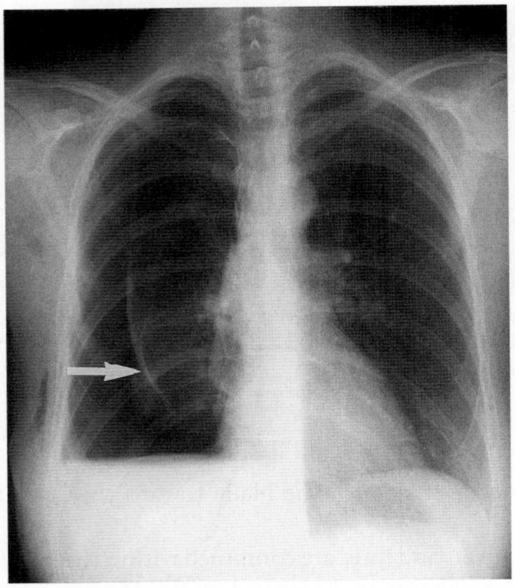

FIGURE 20-8 Hydropneumothorax. Single PA view of the chest in a patient with a hydropneumothorax. Note the air-fluid level in the pleural space. The visceral pleura is slightly thickened *(arrow)* from prior surgery on the right.

Computed Tomography

Pleural fluid can be identified easily on CT scans of the chest. In a supine patient, free fluid accumulates in the most dependent area of the pleura, which is posterior. Pleural fluid that does not flow to the posterior thorax is loculated.

The pleural lining is enhanced by contrast media with some forms of pleural disease. Pleural thickening and nodularity are well seen with contrast-enhanced CT scan. An elliptic pleural fluid collection with thickening and enhancement of the surrounding pleura suggests an **empyema,** which is infected pleural fluid.[11] The presence of gas bubbles within the fluid without prior surgery or needle insertion (which can introduce air) establishes the diagnosis of empyema (Figure 20-10).

Pneumothorax

The term **pneumothorax** refers to the collection of air within the pleural space. The visceral pleura surrounding the lung becomes visible when air accumulates in the pleural space. Pneumothorax may occur spontaneously because of rupture of a *bleb* (a gas-containing space within the visceral pleura of the lung—a form of pulmonary air cyst) or may result from trauma or an invasive procedure that punctures the pleura, such as a transbronchial biopsy or percutaneous aspiration lung biopsy. Pneumothorax may also occur as a complication of positive pressure ventilation (which is called *barotrauma*). When the patient is upright, the intrapleural air accumulates over the top of the lung (apex) and pushes the lung away from the chest wall. The clinician can easily detect a pneumothorax by

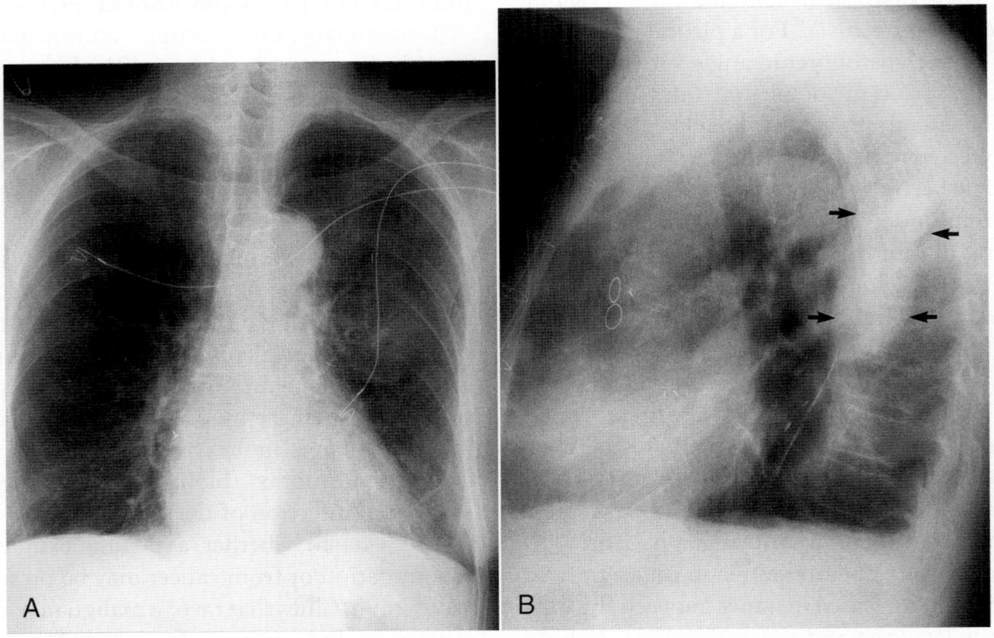

FIGURE 20-9 Intrafissural fluid. Two views of the chest showing fluid accumulating within the superior portion of the major fissure. In the PA view, the fluid is seen as vague increased density in the left upper lobe. Note the typical elliptic shape of the fluid on the lateral projection *(arrows)*.

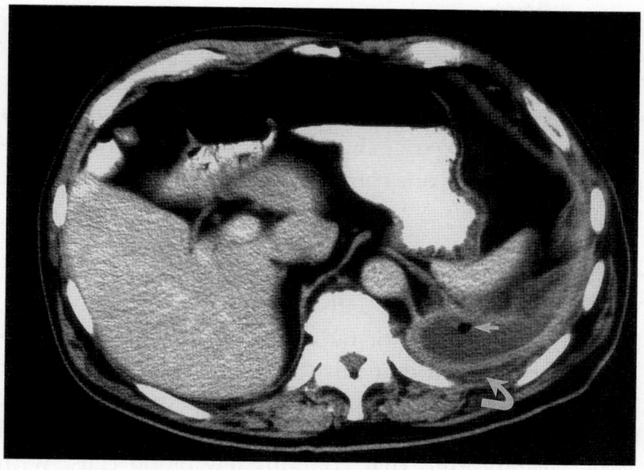

FIGURE 20-10 Empyema. Cross-sectional CT image shows an elliptic pleural fluid collection surrounded by thickened enhancing pleura (split pleural sign). The presence of the gas bubble *(short arrow)* within the fluid and the thickened extrapleural subcostal tissues *(curved arrow)* is strongly suggestive of empyema.

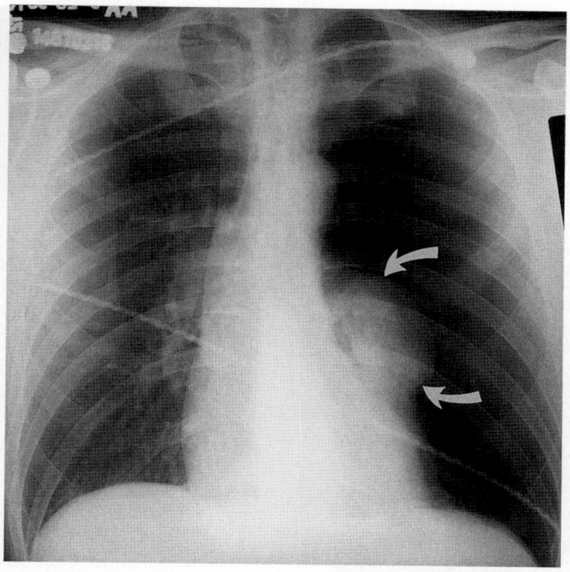

FIGURE 20-11 Pneumothorax. Complete atelectasis of the left lung *(curved arrows)* resulting from a large left pneumothorax.

seeing the thin pleural line at the lung margin and noting the absence of bronchovascular markings between the lung margin and the inner aspect of the chest wall (Figure 20-11). If a diagnosis of pneumothorax is suspected, an upright chest radiograph should be obtained. Visualizing a small pneumothorax may be assisted by taking the chest radiograph when the patient exhales.

When the patient is supine, the free air in the pleural space moves to the highest point in the chest, which is the anterior cardiophrenic sulcus (see Figure 20-1).[12] Because air in this region does not create a visible edge between the pleura and the x-ray beam, radiographic clues to the presence of pneumothorax are more subtle in a supine patient.[12] A supine patient with a pneumothorax may have a *deep sulcus sign* (Figure 20-12),[13] which refers to air accumulating anteriorly and outlining the heart border below the dome of the diaphragm. In addition, the upper abdomen on the same side often shows increased lucency. If the diagnosis remains in doubt, a decubitus radiograph or a cross-table lateral radiograph (in which the patient lies face up while the x-ray is directed across the body) can help make the diagnosis of pneumothorax.

A pneumothorax may be difficult to diagnose if a patient has bullous emphysema. If after carefully examining the chest film, there is uncertainty about the presence of a pneumothorax, a CT scan of the chest can resolve the question. Skin folds can mimic a pneumothorax. To avoid mistaking a skin fold for a pneumothorax, the clinician needs to look carefully at what appears to be the lung margin. The absence of the pleural line at the lung margin and the presence of bronchovascular markings between the lung margin and the chest wall suggest a skin fold rather than a pneumothorax.

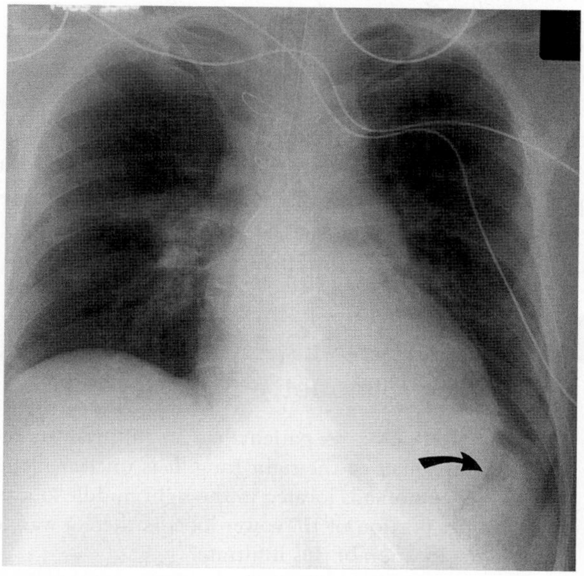

FIGURE 20-12 Deep sulcus sign. Portable supine radiograph in a patient status-post median sternotomy. Note the increased lucency in the left upper quadrant. The highest portion of the thorax in a supine patient is the anterior cardiophrenic sulcus; this accounts for the well-defined low cardiac border *(arrow)* and the adjacent fat pad.

Occasionally, air within the pleural space may be under pressure or tension (Figure 20-13); this is called a *tension pneumothorax*. Tension pneumothorax is an emergency that occurs when the tear in the pleura (which allows air to leave the lung and enter the pleural space) opens on inspiration but closes on expiration. Air continues to accumulate in the pleural space and can compress the heart and adjacent lung. A tension pneumothorax is suggested on

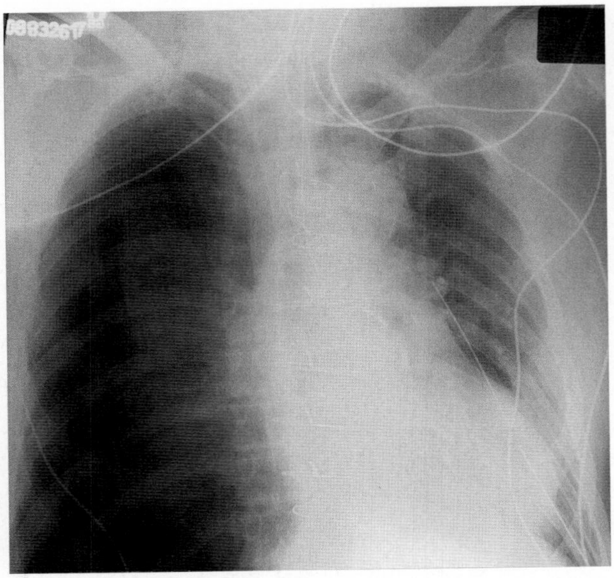

FIGURE 20-13 Tension pneumothorax. Portable chest radiograph in a patient status-post median sternotomy and coronary artery bypass graft surgery. Note the large right pneumothorax displacing the mediastinum to the left and the right hemidiaphragm inferiorly. These findings indicate the presence of a tension pneumothorax on the right requiring immediate chest tube placement.

chest films when the hemidiaphragm is pushed down inferiorly or when the mediastinum is shifted toward the opposite lung. A tension pneumothorax requires immediate decompression with a chest tube, Heimlich valve, or needle aspiration of the trapped air.

MINI CLINI

Use of the Silhouette Sign

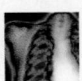

PROBLEM: A patient has an infiltrate in the lower half of the right lung. It is unclear if this pneumonia is located in the right middle lobe or in the upper portion of the lower lobe. Is there a way to identify the location of this infiltrate?

ANSWER: If the right heart border is visible next to the infiltrate, the pneumonia is located in the lower lobe behind the heart. If the right heart border is invisible, the infiltrate must be located in the right middle lobe next to the right side of the heart. The disappearance of the right heart border in this circumstance is due to the silhouette sign. In this instance, pneumonia is considered a water density, and when two structures of similar density are touching each other in the same plane, the border between the two structures (or the silhouette of the heart border) is not seen. Pneumonia in the upper segments of the lower lobe appears to be next to the heart on the PA chest film but does not obliterate the heart border in such cases because the water density of the pneumonia in the lower lobe is not adjacent to the water density of the heart. In this instance, the heart border or silhouette is seen because the silhouette sign is not present.

LUNG PARENCHYMA

The lung parenchyma is made up of two components: air sacs (alveoli) and interstitium (the supporting structures of the lung). Lung parenchymal disease involves both components, although one component is usually affected more than the other.

Alveolar Disease

When alveoli are filled with something denser than air, they have a characteristic radiographic appearance regardless of the material that fills them. The type of fluid that fills the alveoli varies depending on the disease process. In the case of pulmonary edema, the alveoli are flooded with a watery fluid that contains few blood cells. With bacterial pneumonia, the alveoli are filled with an exudative fluid containing numerous white blood cells (pus). In the case of pulmonary hemorrhage, the alveoli fill with blood. In the condition known as *pulmonary alveolar proteinosis,* the alveoli fill with a fat-rich material derived from pulmonary surfactant. Both pneumonia and a bleeding lung can cause identical-appearing patchy, increased density shadows that tend to coalesce over time on the chest radiograph. These shadows are often referred to as **infiltrates.**

These *shadows,* or *opacities,* often have lucent tubular visible structures running through them that represent **air bronchograms** (Figure 20-14). Normally, patent airways are invisible in the outer two-thirds of the lung on a chest radiograph. There is no contrast between air in the airway and air in the lung. However, the increased contrast produced by filling of the surrounding alveoli with fluid makes the airways more visible and causes the air bronchogram sign. Air bronchograms are the hallmark of infiltrates that fill alveoli (so-called *airspace disease*) (Figure 20-15 and Box 20-2).

RULE OF THUMB

Air bronchograms indicate that the opacification is located in the lung parenchyma and not in the pleural space. They suggest pulmonary infiltrates such as pneumonia.

Pulmonary Edema

Pulmonary edema is one of the most common chest film findings in critically ill patients. Pulmonary edema can be caused by vascular congestion, loss of integrity of the pulmonary capillaries, or some combination of both factors. Edema from vascular congestion can be caused by failure of the left heart (cardiogenic pulmonary edema), renal failure, or fluid overload. Breakdown in the integrity of the lung capillaries can also cause pulmonary edema as in acute respiratory distress syndrome (ARDS; see Chapter 27).

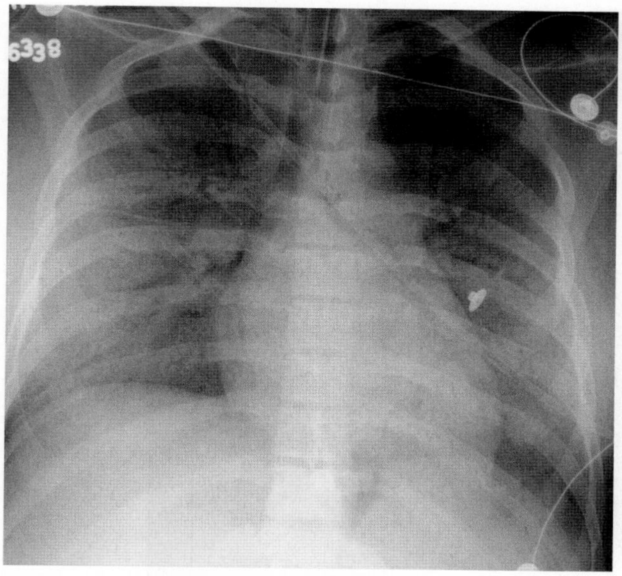

FIGURE 20-14 Air bronchograms. This portable radiograph shows diffuse increased density throughout both lungs highlighted by tubular lucencies. These are air bronchograms. They are visualized because of the alveolar filling that surrounds them. This typical alveolar filling pattern (airspace disease) suggests acute pneumonia, pulmonary hemorrhage, or pulmonary edema.

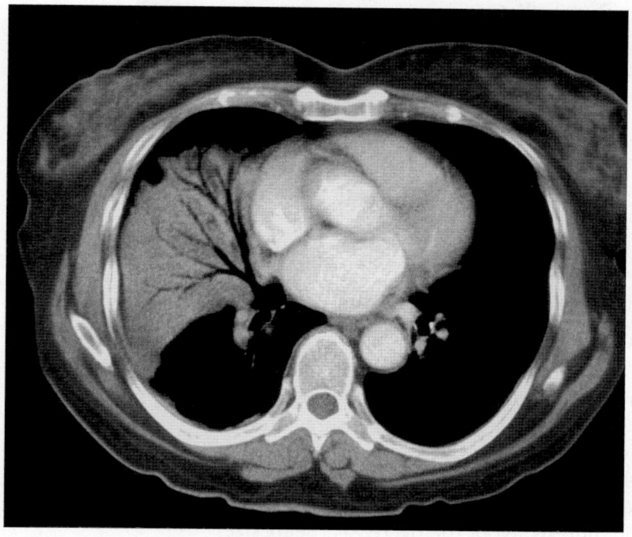

FIGURE 20-15 Right middle lobe pneumonia. CT slice shows an alveolar filling process in the right middle lobe with tubular air bronchograms running through it. The patient is a 73-year-old woman with right middle lobe pneumonia.

The development of cardiogenic pulmonary edema can be described through a series of changes on the chest film. Before pulmonary edema develops, the pressure in the pulmonary veins increases. The increasing pressure in the pulmonary veins can be seen on the chest film as enlarging blood vessels to the apices of the lungs. If the blood vessels to the apices of the lungs are the same size or larger than the blood vessels to the base, the vessels are said to be "cephalized" (Figure 20-16). **Cephalization** of the pulmonary blood flow is often caused by left-sided heart failure.

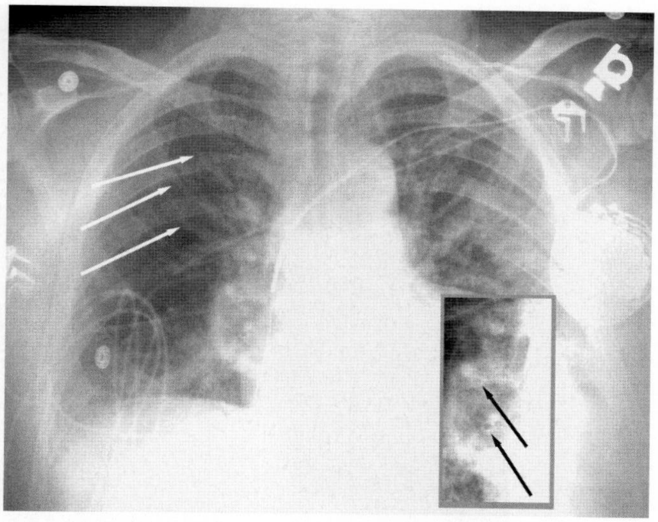

FIGURE 20-16 Moderate pulmonary edema. Cephalization of blood flow is visible *(white arrows)*. The blood vessels to the apex of the lung are enlarged and similar in size to the blood vessels to the base of the lungs. The *inset* displays peribronchial cuffing *(black arrows);* the *inset* is from the right hilum of the same film but is enhanced to make the peribronchial cuffing easier to see.

Box 20-2 Radiographic Features of Alveolar versus Interstitial Processes

Alveolar (Airspace) Disease	Interstitial Disease
Air bronchograms	Nodules
Fluffy opacities	Linear/reticular opacities
Rapid coalescence	Septal lines
Acinar nodules	Cysts
Segmental/lobar distribution	Honeycombing

As fluid builds up from the high venous pressures, thickening of bronchial walls *(peribronchial cuffing)* (see Figure 20-16) and edema in the septa that separate the lung lobules become evident. The thickened septa are most clearly seen as thin lines against the pleural edge that run perpendicularly away from the pleural edge. These lines are called **Kerley B lines** (Figure 20-17).

RULE OF THUMB

Radiographic signs of cardiac decompensation include the following:

- *Cardiac enlargement*
- *Pleural effusion*
- *Redistribution of blood flow to the upper lobes*
- *Poor definition to central vessels (perihilar haze)*
- *Kerley B lines*
- *Alveolar filling*

Note: These findings are seen in Figure 20-17.

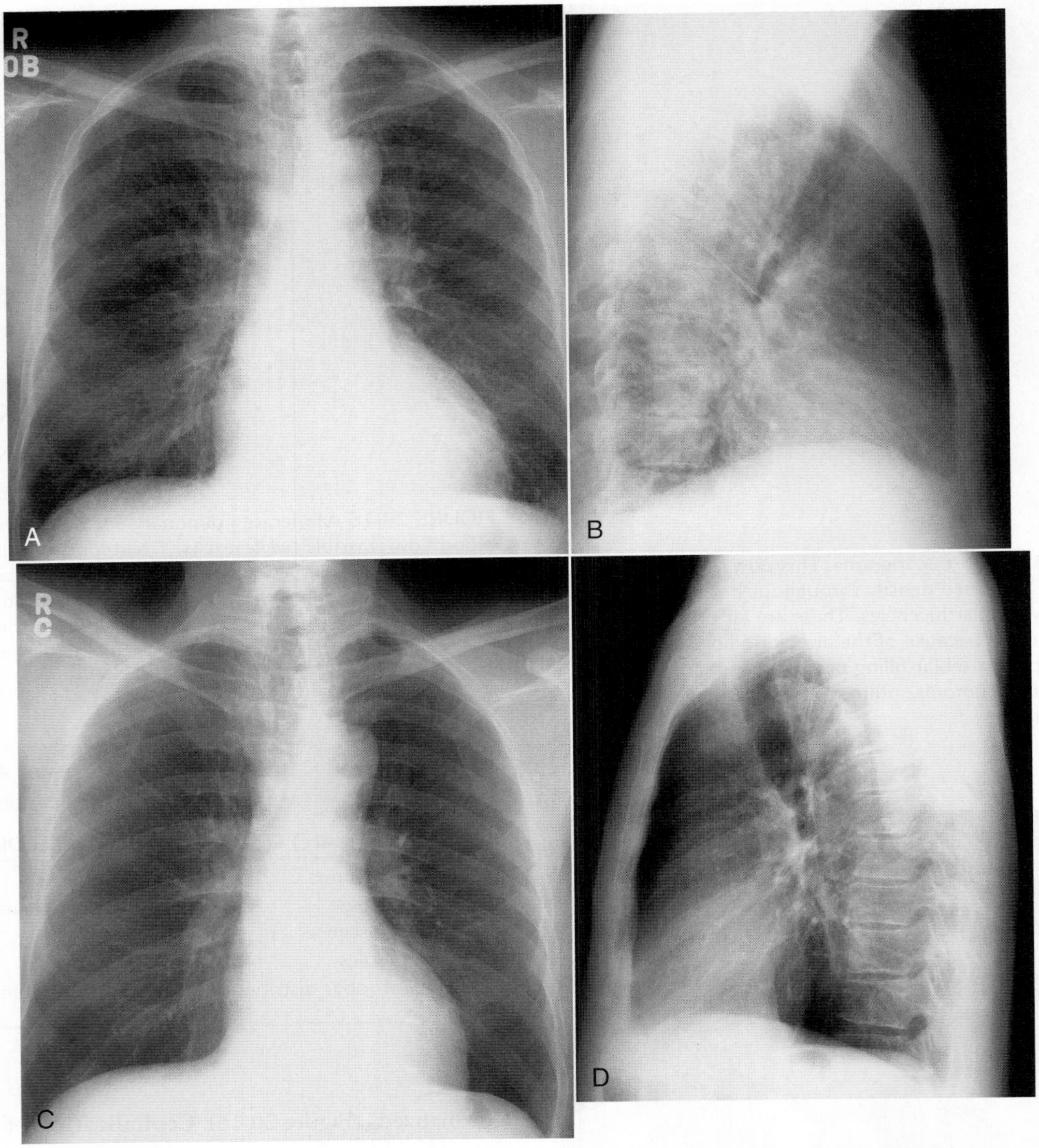

FIGURE 20-17 PA **(A)** and lateral **(B)** chest films show an enlarged cardiac silhouette. The lateral lung margins are slightly displaced away from the inner chest wall in both costophrenic angles, which is consistent with bilateral effusions. There is thickening of the fissures on the lateral projection, indicating that the pleural fluid is extending into the interlobar fissures. Numerous Kerley B lines are seen as linear densities extending to the pleural surface in the right lower chest. The definition of the central vessels is suboptimal, indicating interstitial edema. **C** and **D,** The same patient after therapeutic diuresis. Note the decreased heart size, disappearance of Kerley B lines, and improved definition of the central pulmonary vasculature.

The development of edema in the lung itself is seen first in the hila of the lungs by blurring the normally distinct walls of the hilar blood vessels; this is followed by blurring and increased haziness caused by the edema progressing outward toward the pleura. The term *bat's wing appearance* is applied to the predominance of edema in the hilar regions of both lungs with progressively less edema in the more peripheral areas of the lungs (Figure 20-18).

In addition to the above-mentioned classic signs of pulmonary edema, many patients with long-standing heart failure have enlargement of the heart or a pleural effusion. Pleural effusions from heart failure are usually bilateral. If the effusion is visible only on one side, it is more commonly on the right side than the left.

The appearance of ARDS is sometimes similar to the appearance of other forms of pulmonary edema. However similar they may appear at first, there are some key differences to help distinguish ARDS from pulmonary edema caused by high vascular pressures. The edema of ARDS is patchy and bilateral and does not predominate in the

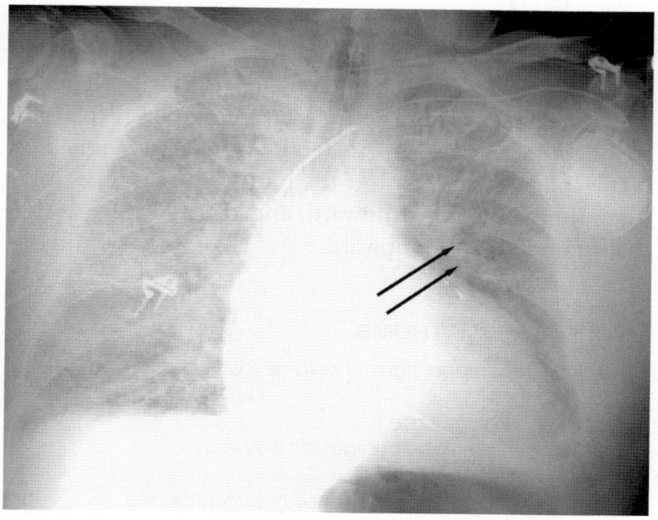

FIGURE 20-18 Severe pulmonary edema. Both lungs are opacified in a bat's wing distribution. The hilar vessels are invisible because of the edema in the lung tissue surrounding these vessels. Peribronchial cuffing is indicated by the *black arrows*.

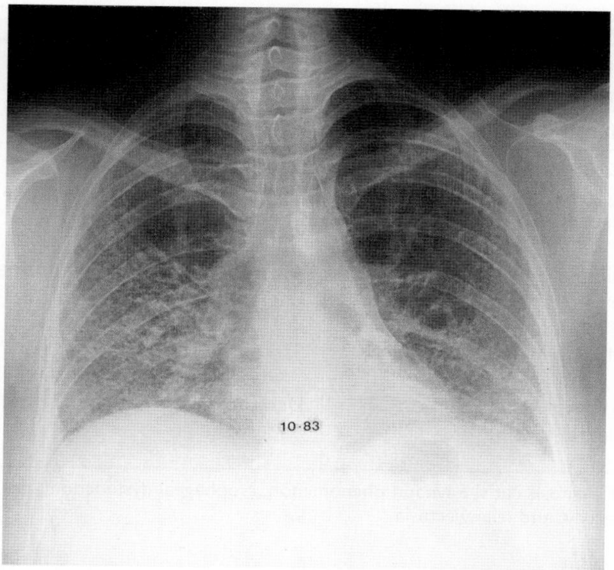

FIGURE 20-19 PA view of the chest in a patient complaining of shortness of breath. The radiograph shows interstitial lung disease. The lung volumes are diminished. Several small cystic lucencies are visualized between the increased basilar interstitial markings representing honeycombing. The diagnosis is scleroderma lung. No esophageal abnormalities are evident on this film.

central hilar regions. A chest film of a patient with ARDS also lacks cardiomegaly, cephalization, and Kerley B lines, which are often seen in cardiogenic pulmonary edema.

Interstitial Disease

Diseases that mainly involve the interstitium of the lung have a different radiographic appearance than alveolar diseases (see Box 20-2). The interstitium of the lung represents the part of the lung that frames the airspaces and supports the vessels and bronchi as they travel through the lung. A pulmonary lobule is the smallest functional unit of the lung.[14] A *pulmonary lobule* contains alveoli and alveolar ducts built around a central pulmonary arteriole and bronchiole, all surrounded by a thin sheet of fibrous connective tissue called the *intralobular septa.* Intralobular septa are invisible on a normal chest radiograph. Pulmonary edema secondary to poor left-sided heart function causes edema of the intralobular septa. As noted, short thin lines from the edematous intralobluar septa can be seen perpendicular to the pleura (see Figure 20-16); these are Kerley B lines.

Interstitial lung disease (see Chapter 24) refers to a group of diseases that involve the lower respiratory tract. Chest radiographs of patients with interstitial lung disease may have several different appearances, depending on the stage and type of interstitial lung disease (see Box 20-2). A chest radiograph of a patient with interstitial lung disease usually has diffuse, bilateral infiltrates. The infiltrates may resemble scattered, ill-defined nodules (nodular); a collection of scattered lines (reticular); a combination of both nodules and lines (reticular-nodular); or *honeycombing,* which is the development of cystic spaces with well-defined walls seen in the periphery of the lung and resembling a bee's honeycomb. Honeycombing is thought to represent irreversible scarring and indicates end-stage lung disease (Figure 20-19).

There are many types of interstitial lung disease. Causes include *infectious* (e.g., viral pneumonia) or *occupational* exposures (e.g., to asbestos [asbestosis] or to silica [silicosis]). The two most common interstitial lung diseases, *sarcoidosis* and *idiopathic pulmonary fibrosis,* have no known cause.[15] Because many different types of interstitial lung diseases have the same appearance on a chest radiograph, the chest film rarely helps establish the specific cause of interstitial disease. Clues to specific causes of interstitial lung disease on a plain chest film are reviewed in Table 20-1. HRCT has become an important tool in establishing the specific form of interstitial lung disease that a patient may have. HRCT is particularly helpful in diagnosing idiopathic pulmonary fibrosis.[16]

Assessing Lung Volume

Volume loss, or *atelectasis,* is a common abnormality on chest radiographs, and the location and extent of volume loss produce characteristic chest radiograph patterns. Atelectasis may be localized to a subsegmental portion of the lung, where it has a classic radiographic appearance called **plate (or platelike) atelectasis** (Figure 20-20).[17] Plate atelectasis is seen occasionally on chest films of normal individuals but is often associated with ventilatory disturbance, including restricted diaphragmatic motion, sometimes with resultant alveolar hypoventilation; retained secretions, producing small airway obstruction; and diminished

TABLE 20-1

Clues on Plain Chest Radiograph That Indicate the Specific Cause of Interstitial Lung Disease

Clues on Radiograph	Cause of Disease
Pneumothorax	Lymphangioleiomyomatosis, Langerhans cell histiocytosis
Pleural effusion	Rheumatoid arthritis, systemic lupus erythematosus
Dilated esophagus	Scleroderma, CREST syndrome*
Erosive arthropathy (shoulder joints, clavicles)	Rheumatoid arthritis
Mediastinal adenopathy	Sarcoidosis, scleroderma, metastatic cancer
Soft tissue calcification	Dermatomyositis, scleroderma
Pleural plaque	Asbestosis

*Calcinosis cutis, *R*aynaud phenomenon, *e*sophageal dysfunction, *s*clerodactyly, and *t*elangiectasia.

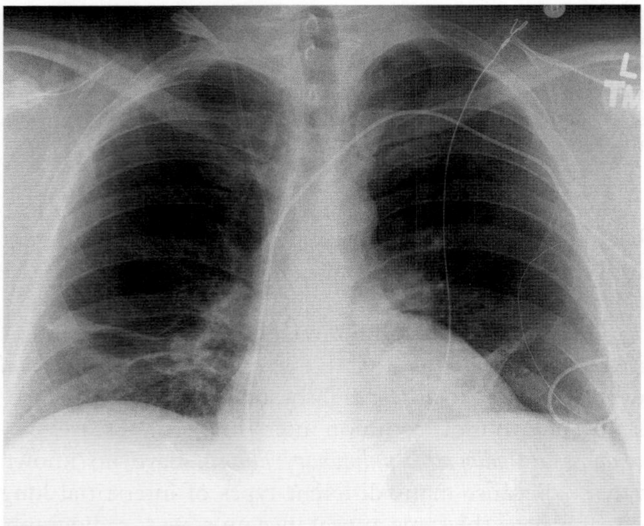

FIGURE 20-20 Plate atelectasis. PA chest radiograph shows linear areas of plate atelectasis in both lower lobes.

surfactant production.[18] Atelectasis commonly occurs after abdominal or thoracic surgery, with pleurisy, or after pleural irritation from rib fracture or pulmonary infarction.

Volume loss involving a whole lobe is usually caused by central airway obstruction.[19] The collapsed lobe assumes the shape of a wedge with the apex of the wedge at the hilum and the base of the wedge on the pleural surface. This wedge is visible on a PA or lateral x-ray film, depending on which lobe is collapsed (Figure 20-21). The central bronchial obstruction may be caused by cancer, a foreign body, or a mucous plug (Figure 20-22). As shown in Figure 20-23, a bulging convexity to the apex of the wedge indicates a central tumor.

Atelectasis of a segment or lobe of the lung causes changes to surrounding structures. As lung volumes decrease, surrounding tissues collapse in to fill the space the collapsed segment or lobe usually fills. The diaphragm becomes elevated on the side of the atelectasis, the mediastinum shifts toward the atelectasis, and poor expansion of the chest causes narrowing of the space between the ribs. If the collapsed segment of the lung is in the upper lobe, the hilum is displaced upward, and the minor fissure on the right is displaced upward.

RULE OF THUMB

Radiographic signs of volume loss include the following:
- Lobar collapse
- Unilateral diaphragmatic elevation
- Mediastinal shift
- Narrowing of the space between the ribs
- Hilar displacement

See Figures 20-19, 20-20, and 20-21.

Assessment of lung volumes on a chest radiograph requires several observations. Rib counting is a popular method to assess lung volume. With a good inspiration, the sixth and sometimes the seventh anterior rib should project above the diaphragm. If more than seven anterior ribs are visible above the diaphragm, *hyperinflation* is present. Obstructive pulmonary disease is classically associated with increased lung volumes (hyperinflation). In patients with chronic obstructive pulmonary disease, there may also be an increase in the AP diameter of the chest, with associated enlargement of the retrosternal and retrocardiac airspaces and flattening of the hemidiaphragms. These all are secondary signs of *pulmonary emphysema*. The only primary signs of emphysema are loss or shifting of pulmonary vessel markings and the appearance of the walls of bullous airspaces (Figure 20-24).

RULE OF THUMB

A good inspiratory effort by the patient is needed to obtain a good-quality chest film. Visualization of 6 anterior or 10 posterior ribs above the level of the diaphragm indicates a good inspiratory effort by the patient.

Because radiographic signs of emphysema are apparent only with more advanced disease, the chest radiograph is generally considered insensitive for detecting obstructive lung disease. However, HRCT is far more sensitive and may show evidence of emphysema even when pulmonary function test results are normal.[20] Figure 20-25 shows a case of upper lobe paraseptal emphysema, characterized by cysts on the pleural surface. A chest CT scan may prove useful to help define which patients may benefit from treatments such as lung volume reduction surgery.

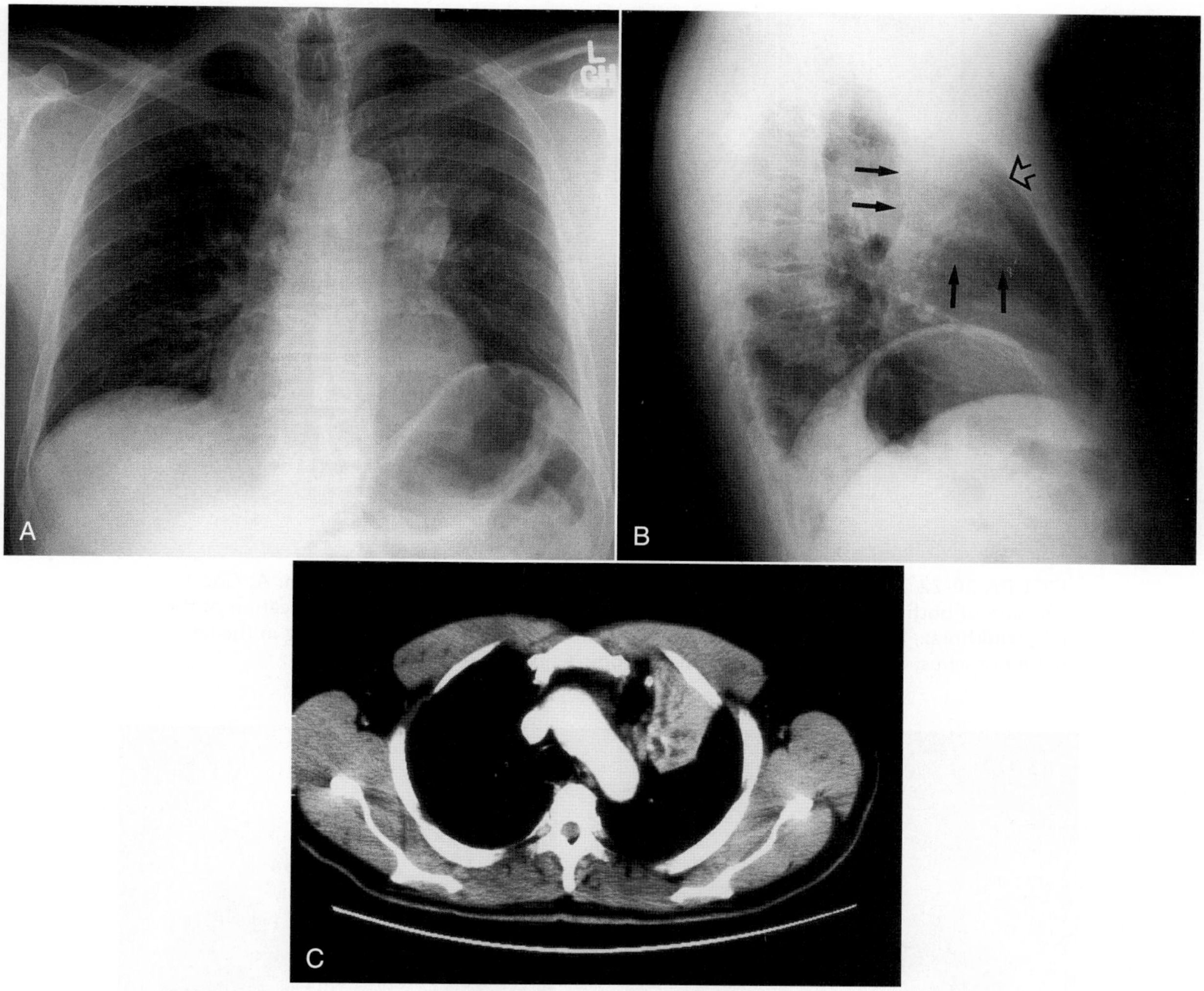

FIGURE 20-21 **A,** PA view of the chest shows an elevated left hemidiaphragm, a left hilar mass, and increased density in the left upper chest. **B,** Lateral projection shows elevation of the left hemidiaphragm and a wedge of increased density *(black arrows)*, with its apex at the hilum and its base on the pleural surface. The lucency *(open arrow)* between the sternum and the wedge is herniated right upper lobe. **C,** CT slice shows the wedge of atelectatic left upper lobe. The tubular lucencies within it are mucus-filled bronchi.

Solitary Pulmonary Nodule

A **solitary pulmonary nodule** (SPN) is a parenchymal opacity smaller than 3 cm in diameter that is totally surrounded by aerated lung. One or two SPNs are encountered in every 1000 chest radiographs. SPNs are important to identify because they may be caused by lung cancer. The reported prevalence of malignancy in SPN ranges from 3% to 6% in large surveys of the general population. In patients with SPN who have surgical resection, 30% to 60% of the nodules are malignant.[21]

When first encountered, SPN should be assessed for features listed in Table 20-2 that may help establish a nonmalignant cause. The goal of imaging SPNs is to avoid resecting benign nodules, while encouraging surgical removal of all potentially curable cancers. The axial anatomic display of CT coupled with better density-discriminating powers make CT a favored tool for evaluating SPN. CT provides a detailed evaluation of the shape and edges of pulmonary nodules, in addition to helping to identify whether calcification is present and, if so, the pattern of its calcification (Figure 20-26).

Central, or lamellar (swirls of concentric rings), calcification strongly suggests a benign cause of SPN or a granuloma. Eccentric (off-center), speckled, or amorphous calcification may be seen in cancers. A smooth-edged, round nodule more often is benign, whereas a lobulated or spiculated (having a spikelike appearance) edge is more likely to be a malignant nodule (see Figure 20-26). PET is often very helpful in evaluating SPNs. Nodules with greater than 1 cm diameter that are avid for the isotope used in PET (fluorodeoxyglucose) and "light up" on the scan generally are more likely to be malignant than nodules without uptake.

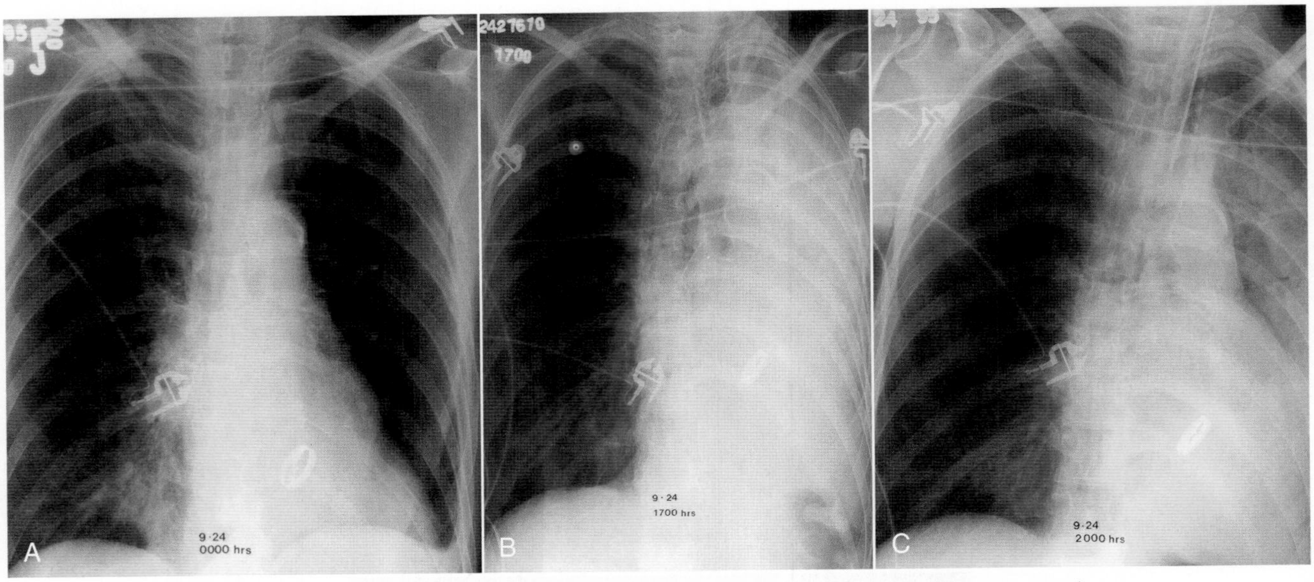

FIGURE 20-22 Three portable chest films obtained within a 20-hour time span. **A,** Good aeration of both lungs. **B,** Film obtained 17 hours later shows complete opacification of the left hemithorax. Bronchoscopy performed after this film revealed a mucous plug in the left main bronchus. It was removed at bronchoscopy. **C,** Partial reexpansion.

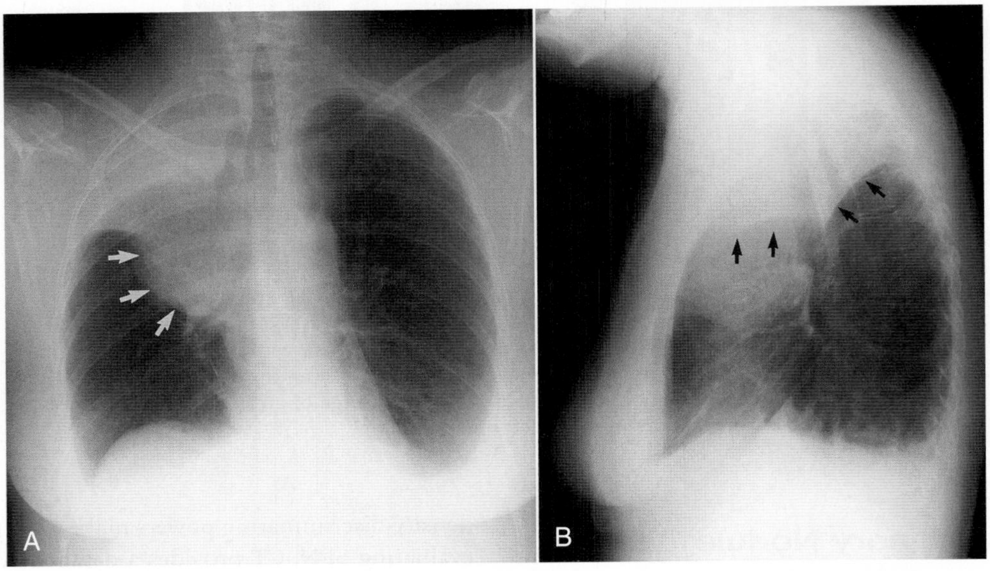

FIGURE 20-23 PA **(A)** and lateral **(B)** views of the chest in a patient with right upper lobe collapse. **A,** Note the wedge opacity of the right upper lobe. Note the inferior bulge *(arrows)* of the minor fissure on the PA film. This bulge indicates the presence of a central mass. **B,** The wedge shape of right upper lobe atelectasis *(arrows)* is well seen on the lateral film.

MEDIASTINUM

The mediastinum consists of the heart, great vessels, trachea, and other soft tissue structures that lie between the lungs. The mediastinum is divided into three compartments: anterior, middle, and posterior. When a mediastinal abnormality has been found, determining the precise portion of the mediastinum that is affected helps determine possible causes. The mediastinal compartments are best defined on a lateral chest film (see Figure 20-3). A line extending from the diaphragm along the posterior margin of the heart and the anterior margin of the trachea to the neck divides the anterior mediastinum from the middle compartment. A second line traversing the vertebral bodies 1 cm behind their anterior margins and extending from the neck to the diaphragm divides the middle from the posterior compartment. Most mediastinal masses are visible on both front and lateral projections, and the specific location within the mediastinum offers the first clue to diagnosis.

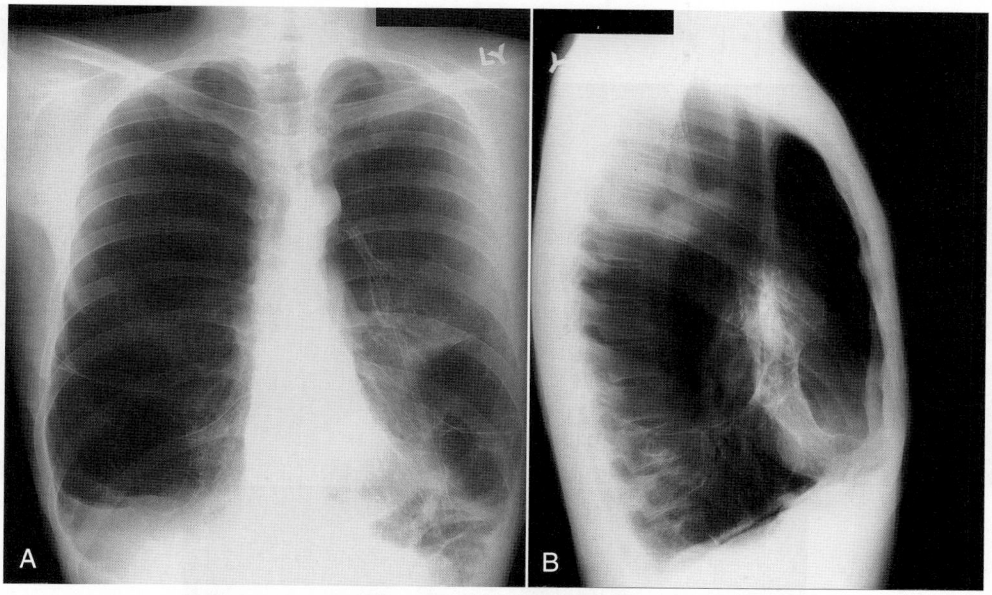

FIGURE 20-24 PA **(A)** and lateral **(B)** views of the chest of a patient with bullous emphysema. Marked pulmonary hyperinflation is worse on the right. The asymmetric hyperinflation is producing mediastinal shift to the left. There is flattening of the diaphragm, prominence of the clear spaces, and large areas in the upper lung zones that are devoid of any vascular markings. The walls of these bullous airspaces are well visualized.

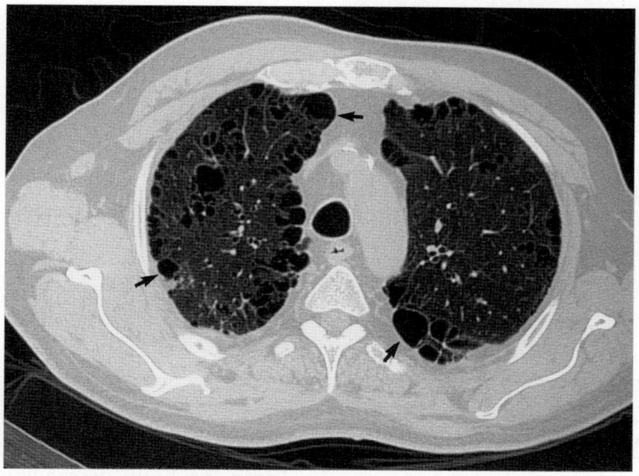

FIGURE 20-25 CT slice through the upper lungs in a patient with pulmonary emphysema. Numerous cystic lucencies are present in both lungs. Note the absence of bronchovascular markings within the lucencies. Most of the emphysematous areas are located in a peripheral distribution *(arrows)* along the pleural surface (paraseptal).

Table 20-3 lists the common causes of masses in the three mediastinal compartments. CT is the best type of imaging for assessing most mediastinal masses. Figure 20-27 shows the normal axial anatomic display on contrast-enhanced CT scan at the levels of the great vessels, aortic arch, carina, and cardiac chambers. The CT appearance of an anterior mediastinal mass (thymoma) is shown in Figure 20-28. Figure 20-29 shows a middle mediastinal mass (bronchogenic cyst) on both axial CT and MRI scans.

TABLE 20-2

Features Useful in Distinguishing Benign from Malignant Solitary Pulmonary Nodules

Feature	Favoring Malignant Nodule	Favoring Benign Nodule
Patient age	>40 years old	<40 years old
Smoking status	Current or former smoker	Lifetime nonsmoker
Size of nodule	>3 cm	<3 cm
Shape of nodule	Lobulated	Spherical
Margins of nodule	Spiculated	Well defined
If cavity	Thick-walled	Thin-walled
Doubling time*	7-465 days	<7 or >465 days
Calcification	Rare, usually eccentric	Central, lamellar, popcorn

*Time necessary for the nodule to double in volume.

A large hiatal hernia in the posterior mediastinum can easily be confused with a mass on the frontal chest film but is easily seen on CT in Figure 20-30.

Pneumomediastinum

Pneumomediastinum, a form of barotrauma, may result from movement of air into the mediastinum, as may also be seen in cases of esophageal rupture (Figure 20-31). This condition usually occurs in the distal portion of the esophagus in patients who undergo procedures to stretch or dilate the esophagus. Chest trauma may cause rupture of a main bronchus, also allowing movement of air into the mediastinum. Rarely, air dissects down from the soft

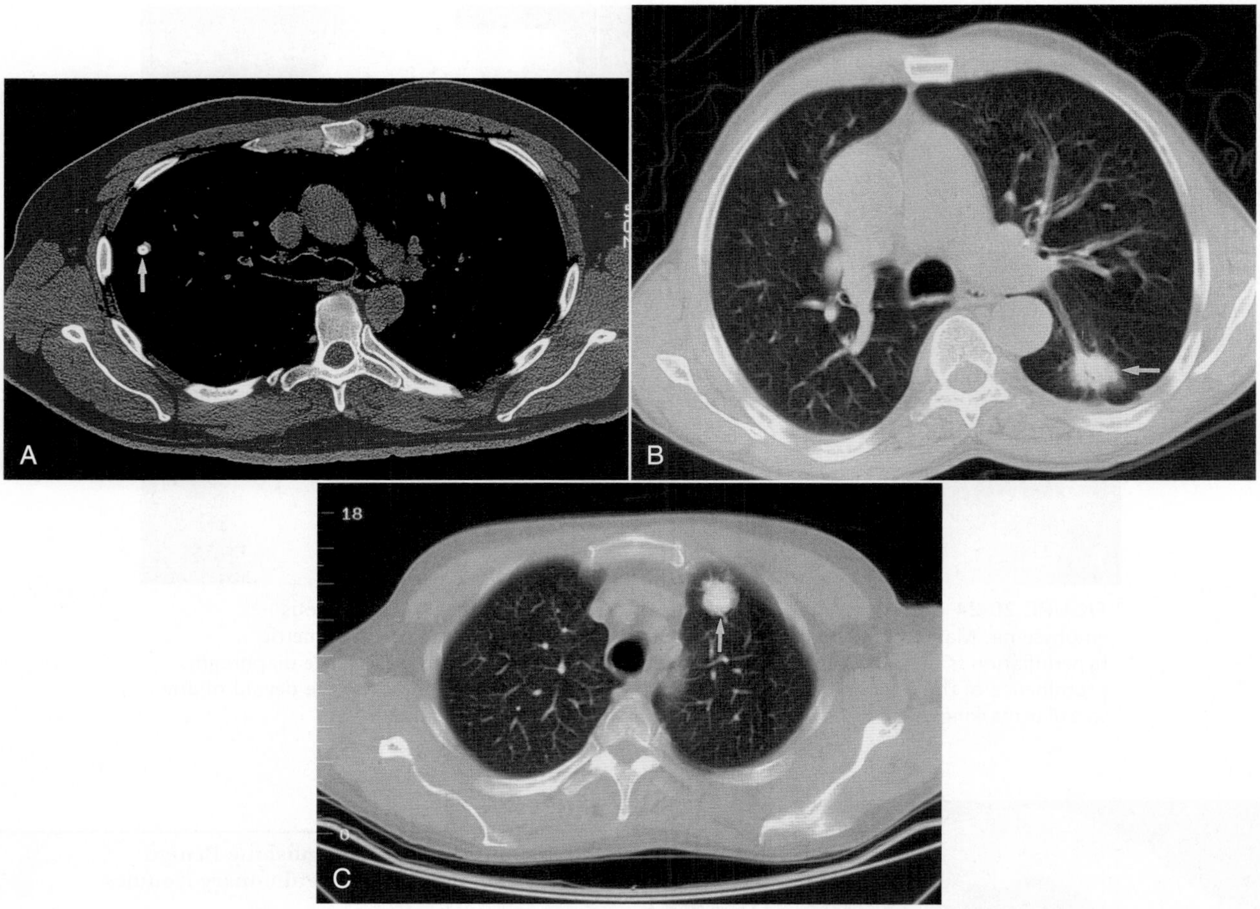

FIGURE 20-26 CT examples of SPNs. **A,** Ringlike calcification in a right upper lobe SPN. This lamellar calcification indicates a granuloma (a benign nodule usually caused by an inhaled infectious agent, such as fungus) *(arrow)*. **B,** Note the spiculated edge of this left lower lobe pulmonary nodule *(arrow)*; this is a lung cancer. **C,** The lobulated edge of this nodule *(arrow)* indicates different growth rates within different areas of this bronchogenic carcinoma.

TABLE 20-3

Mediastinal Abnormalities by Compartment

Anterior Mediastinum	Middle Mediastinum	Posterior Mediastinum
Thyroid or parathyroid mass	Aortic aneurysm (ascending/arch)	Aortic aneurysm (descending)
Thymic lesions	Lymphadenopathy	Neurogenic tumors
Lymphoma	Bronchogenic cyst	Lymphoma
Pericardial cyst/fat pad	Tracheoesophageal masses	Neurenteric cyst
Teratoma	Hiatal hernia	Bochdalek hernia*
Morgagni hernia*		
Ventricular aneurysm		

*Hernia in which the abdominal contents press through a gap in the diaphragm.

tissues of the neck after thyroid, parathyroid, or tonsillar surgery. Gas associated with a retrotonsillar abscess may also move down to the mediastinum through the fascial planes of the neck. Air that accumulates in the retroperitoneum may enter the mediastinum via openings in the diaphragm for the aorta or esophagus.

Catheters, Lines, and Tubes

A common use of a chest radiograph is to check on the position of catheters, lines, and tubes after they have been inserted. RTs must be skilled at examining the chest radiograph to determine the position of the endotracheal tube, chest tubes, and hemodynamic monitoring lines.

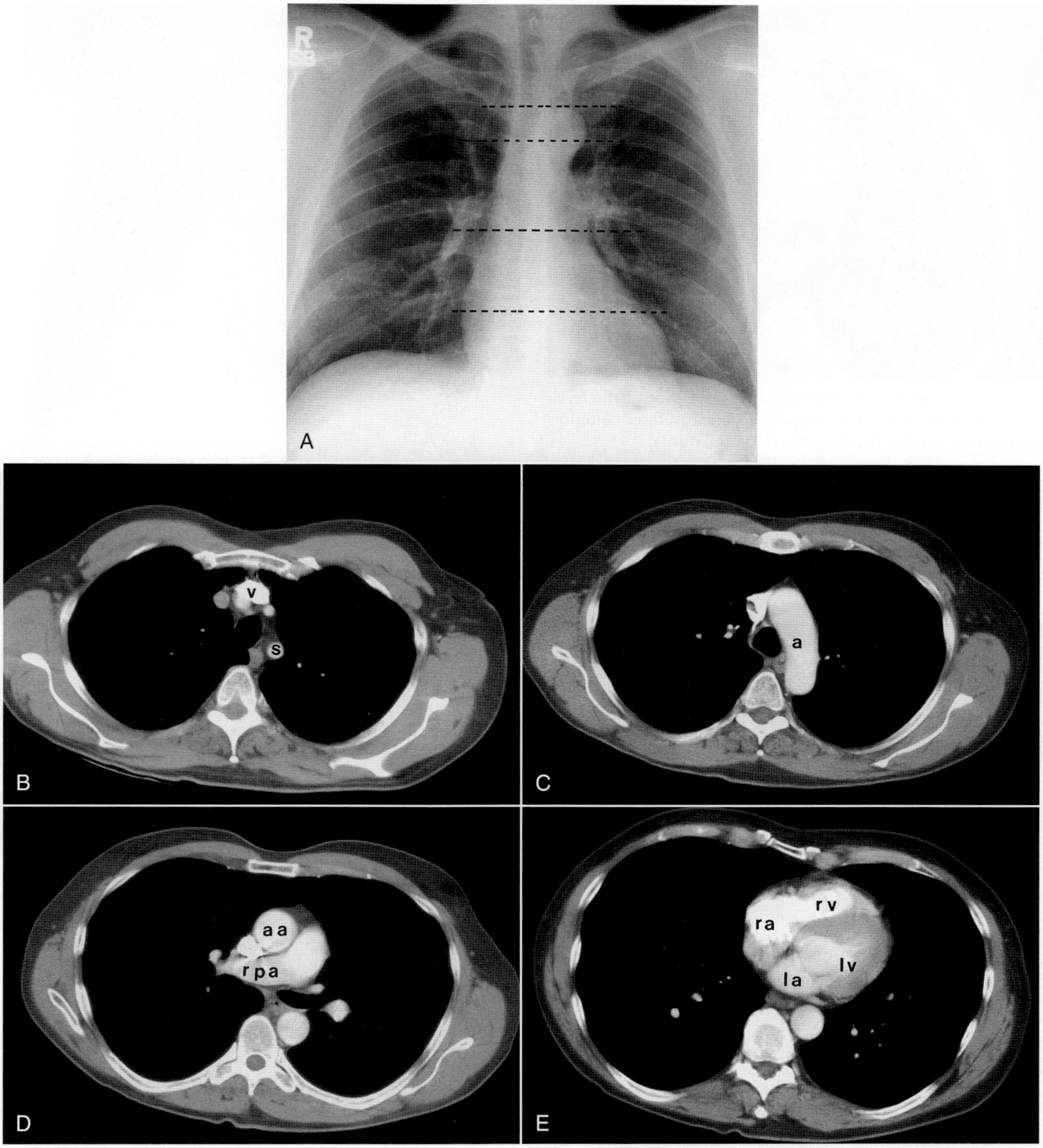

FIGURE 20-27 **A,** PA chest film indicating the four levels at which CT scan slices **B-E** were obtained. **B,** The most superior image is at the level of the great vessels. Contrast material fills the left brachiocephalic vein *(v)* as it courses across the anterior mediastinum to meet the right brachiocephalic vein and form the superior vena cava. The innominate artery and left common carotid are in front of the trachea behind the veins. The left subclavian artery *(s)* sits on the left of the airway next to the esophagus. **C,** At this level, the arch of the aorta *(a)* lies on the left side of the airway. The esophagus is seen in front of the vertebral body behind the airway. The opacified superior vena cava lies to the right of the arch anteriorly. **D,** At the carina, the airway bifurcates, and the right pulmonary artery *(rpa)* crosses the mediastinum anterior to the right main bronchus. The vena cava lies to the right of the ascending aorta *(aa)*. The lower lobe branch of the left pulmonary artery sits behind the left main bronchus. The descending aorta is seen next to the vertebral body. **E,** At the level of the heart, contrast material is seen filling the right atrium *(ra)* and crossing the atrioventricular valve into the right ventricle *(rv)*. The thick, muscular left ventricular *(lv)* wall is visualized as it contracts. The left atrium *(la)* is seen anterior to the esophagus.

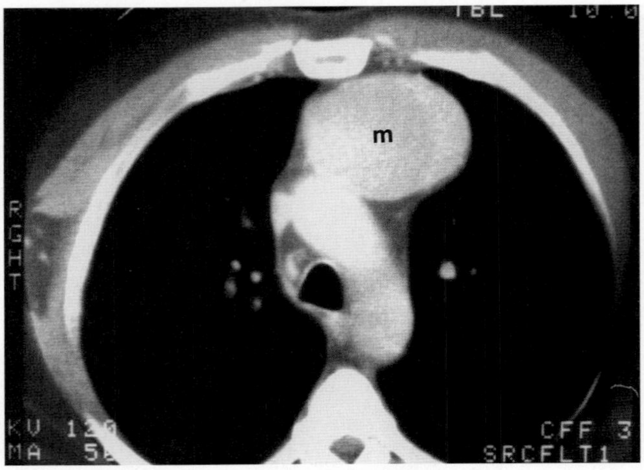

FIGURE 20-28 Anterior mediastinal mass. CT slice at the level of the aortic arch shows a homogeneous encapsulated anterior mediastinal mass *(m)*. The diagnosis was thymoma.

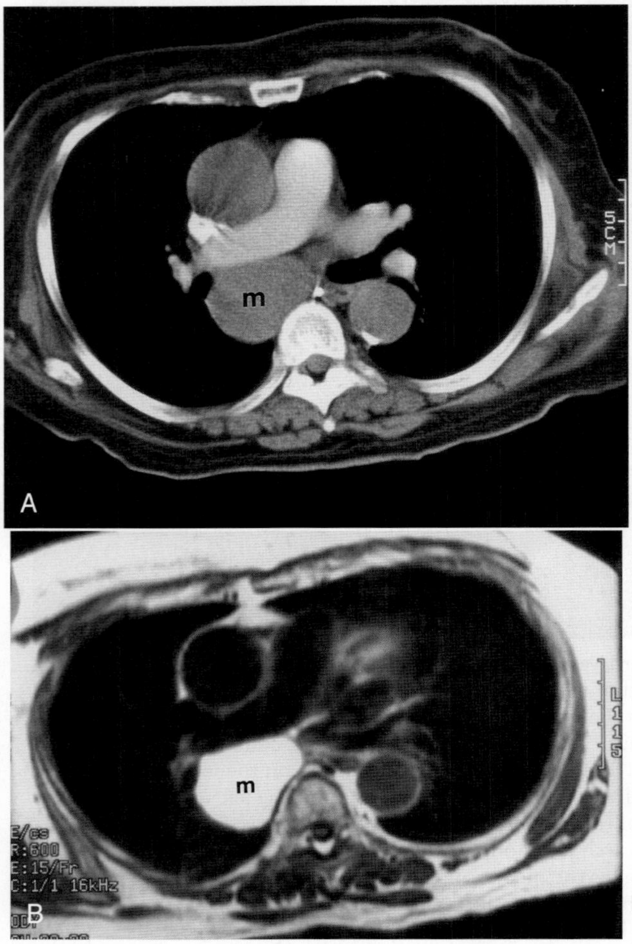

FIGURE 20-29 Middle mediastinal mass. CT **(A)** and MRI **(B)** scans at the subcarinal level show a large cystic mass *(m)* in the middle mediastinum. The diagnosis was bronchogenic cyst.

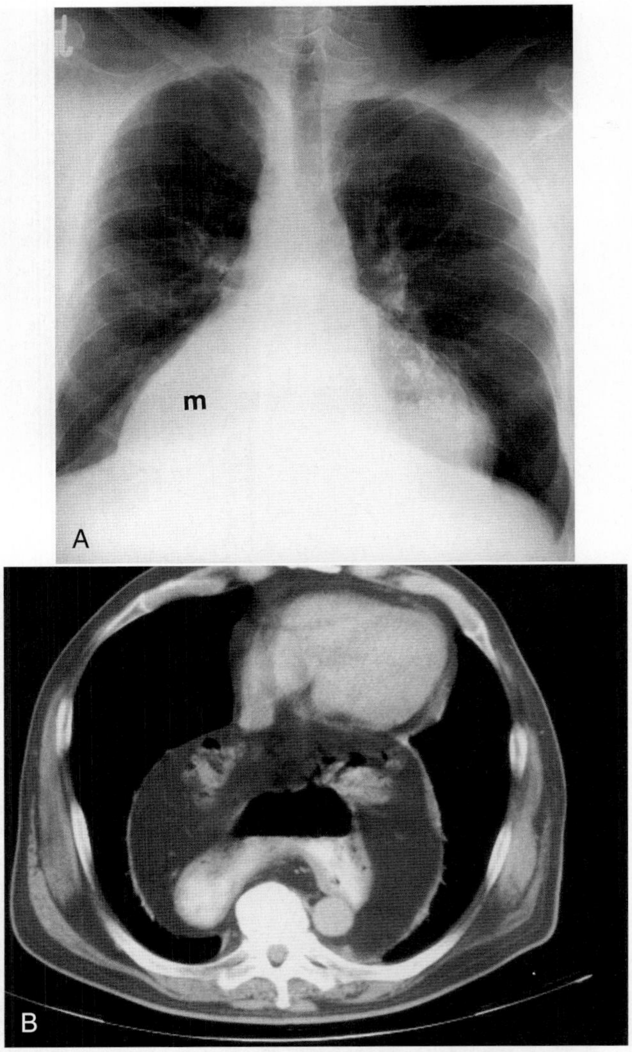

FIGURE 20-30 Posterior mediastinal mass. **A,** PA chest film shows a large soft tissue density *(m)* obscuring the right heart border and the right hemidiaphragm. **B,** CT image at this level shows a large retrocardiac diaphragmatic hernia containing omentum and stomach.

Endotracheal Tube

Endotracheal tubes are radiopaque or have an opaque marker indicating the end of the tube. Radiographs are routinely obtained at the bedside after intubation to assess correct tube position. The radiograph shows the distal tip of the endotracheal tube and the carina.[22] The position of the patient's neck is important. The neck position usually is neutral, but the position of the tip of the endotracheal tube can vary with neck position. Specifically, the endotracheal tube position can move 4 cm toward the main carina as the neck moves from full extension (high position) to full neck flexion (low position), which is one-third the length of the average adult trachea. Goodman and Putman[23] suggested that when the head and neck are in the neutral position, the endotracheal tube should be

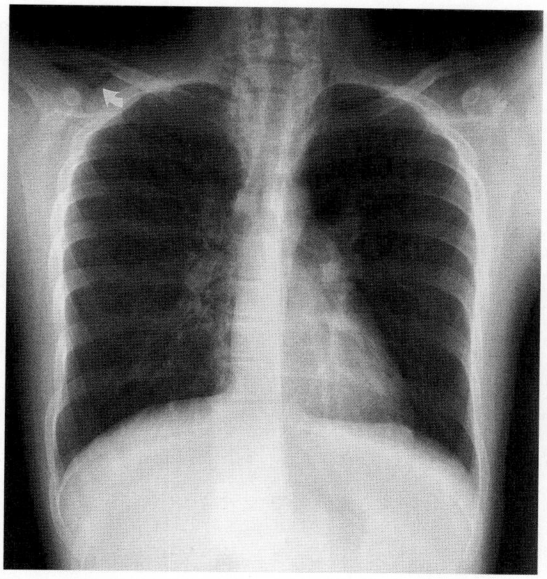

FIGURE 20-31 Pneumomediastinum. PA view of the chest of an 11-year-old child with asthma shows linear lucencies (free air) in the mediastinum and extending into the soft tissues of the neck bilaterally. Note the free air around the lateral aspect of the right clavicle *(arrow)*.

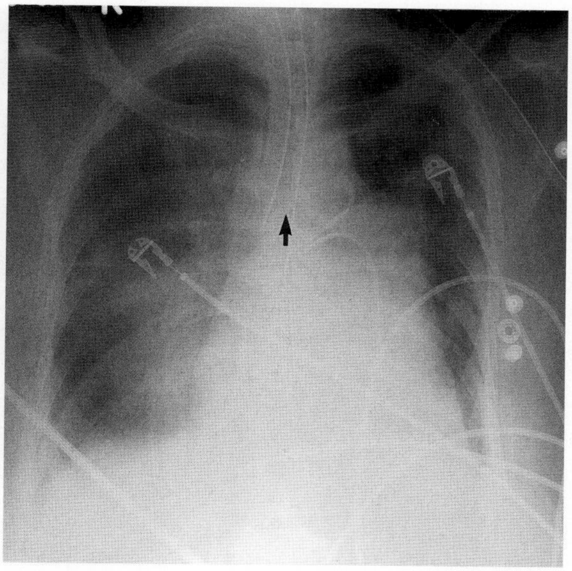

FIGURE 20-32 Portable supine chest film shows malposition of an endotracheal tube in the right main stem bronchus *(arrow)*.

positioned in the midtrachea (5 to 7 cm from the carina). Placement below the thoracic inlet ensures that the tube is beyond the vocal cords (usually at C5-6). Figure 20-32 shows a malpositioned endotracheal tube in the right main stem bronchus.

RULE OF THUMB

The distal tip of the endotracheal tube should be positioned approximately 5 to 7 cm above the level of the carina in an adult patient.

Tracheostomy Tube

Tracheostomy tubes should be two-thirds the diameter of the trachea and should project within the borders of the trachea on the radiograph. The tip should extend beyond half the distance from the stoma to the carina.

Central Line

A central venous pressure catheter is often placed via the internal jugular veins or subclavian veins. A chest radiograph should be obtained after placement to assess the position and to exclude procedural complications (e.g., pneumothorax, hemothorax). Ideally, the tip of the central venous pressure catheter should be in the superior vena cava. This vessel usually forms at the level of the first anterior intercostal space where the brachiocephalic veins come together. The brachiocephalic veins contain valves, and these catheters ideally should be placed central to any valves.

Pulmonary Artery (Swan-Ganz) Catheter

A Swan-Ganz catheter is used to measure hemodynamic and central pressure variables such as pulmonary artery occlusion pressure. Pulmonary artery catheters are placed at the bedside and ideally should reside in the proximal right or left main pulmonary arteries. They are floated into position using an inflatable balloon on the catheter tip. Because of this floating, they are placed in the right pulmonary artery more than 90% of the time. When measuring the so-called wedge or pulmonary artery occlusion pressure, the balloon is inflated, and the catheter moves out into a more peripheral vessel. As soon as the reading is accomplished, the balloon should be deflated, and the catheter should be pulled back to a central location. Persistent peripheral placement (i.e., when the catheter tip is far out in the lung parenchyma) can cause infarction of lung distal to the wedged catheter (Figure 20-33).

Chest Tube

Chest tubes are small-bore to large-bore tubes placed into the pleural space from outside the chest wall. The most common indications for a chest tube are pneumothorax (air in the pleural space) and empyema (pus in the pleural space), although chest tubes may also be used to drain blood *(hemothorax)* or fluid *(hydrothorax)* or to install a sealant (e.g., the antibiotic doxycycline) to achieve closure of the pleural space, preventing recurrent pneumothorax or hydrothorax. Radiographically, most chest tubes have radiopaque stripes along their axis so that they can be seen on the plain chest radiograph. The chest tube should be within the pleural space; it usually follows the contour of the chest wall or diaphragm on one chest radiograph view.

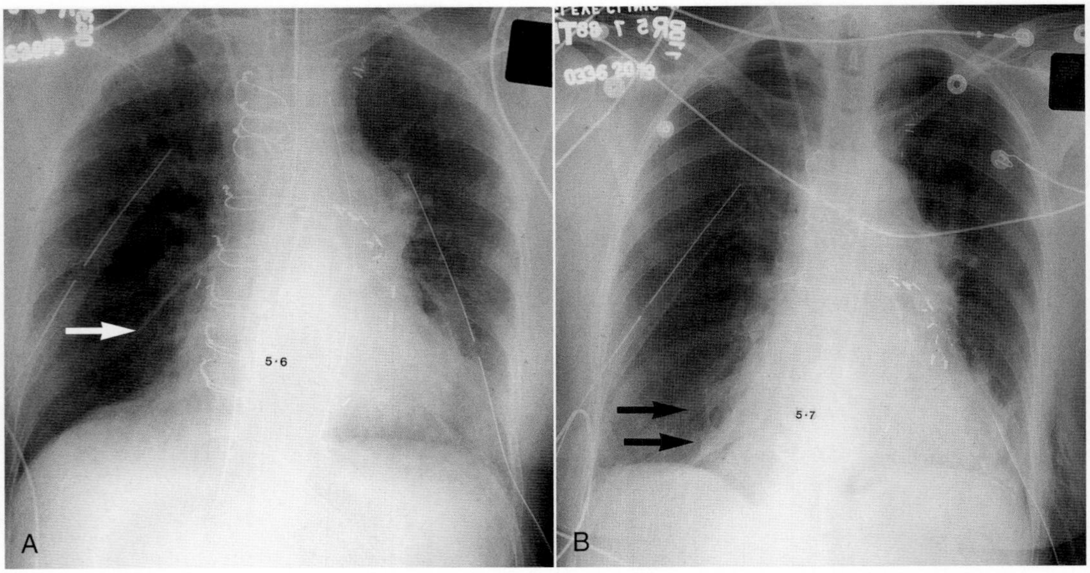

FIGURE 20-33 Two portable supine chest films obtained 30 hours apart. **A,** Wedged Swan-Ganz (pulmonary artery) catheter in the right lower lobe *(arrow)*. **B,** Film obtained after retraction of the catheter shows increased density at the site, reflecting an area of infarction caused by prolonged inadvertent wedging of the catheter *(arrows)*.

Intraaortic Balloon Pump

The intraaortic balloon pump is a counterpulsation device that is used to improve cardiac output and blood pressure in patients with cardiogenic shock. It is inserted through the femoral artery and advanced into the thoracic aorta. The device is approximately 26 cm long, and a radiopaque tip on the top allows radiographic verification of position. The pump inflates the balloon during diastole, and it deflates during systole to enhance perfusion of the coronary arteries and cardiac output. The radiopaque tip should reside just beyond the origin of the left subclavian artery.

SUMMARY CHECKLIST

- Thoracic imaging is an important tool for evaluating the cause and degree of various pulmonary diseases. Various thoracic imaging techniques are available to assist assessment of patients with lung disease.
- The steps to interpretation of the chest film include (1) reviewing the technique and quality of the chest film and (2) taking a disciplined approach to review of all anatomy seen on the chest film.
- The lungs are considered radiolucent, and the bones are radiopaque.
- The chest film is useful for detecting pleural diseases such as pleural effusion or pneumothorax.
- Infiltrates in the lung represent alveolar filling secondary to edema fluid, blood, or pus. Lung infiltrates appear as white segments in the involved lung tissue and may represent pus, blood, fat, or water in the lung.
- Air bronchograms are seen when air-filled airways are surrounded by consolidated (infiltrated) lung.
- Radiographic signs of pulmonary edema secondary to heart failure include (1) redistribution of blood flow to the upper lobes, (2) Kerley B lines, and (3) alveolar filling.
- Signs of long-standing heart failure include cardiac enlargement and pleural effusion.
- Signs of volume loss in the lungs include (1) lobar collapse, (2) unilateral diaphragmatic elevation, (3) mediastinal shift lobar collapse, (4) narrowing of the space between the ribs, (5) hilar displacement, and (6) fissure displacement.
- The chest film is useful in identifying the position of catheters and tubes. The tip of the endotracheal tube should be 5 to 7 cm above the carina when the neck is in a neutral position.

References

1. Perrier A, Bounameaux H: Accuracy of outcome in suspected pulmonary embolism. N Engl J Med 354:2383, 2006.
2. Gefter WB, Hatabu H: Evaluation of pulmonary vascular anatomy and blood flow by magnetic resonance. J Thorac Imaging 8:122, 1993.
3. McLoud TC, Flower CD: Imaging the pleura: sonography, CT and MR imaging. AJR Am J Roentgenol 156:1145, 1991.
4. Nicolaou S, Talsky A, Khashoggi K, et al: Ultrasound-guided interventional radiology in critical care. Crit Care Med 35:s186, 2007.
5. Black LF: The pleural space and pleural fluid. Mayo Clin Proc 47:493, 1972.
6. Raasch BN, Carsky EW, Lane EJ, et al: Pleural effusion: explanation of some typical appearances. AJR Am J Roentgenol 139:899, 1982.
7. Moskowitz H, Platt RT, Schachar R, et al: Roentgen visualization of minute pleural effusions: an experimental study to

determine the minimum amount of pleural fluid visible on a radiograph. Radiology 109:33, 1973.
8. Collins JD, Burwell D, Furmanski S, et al: Minimum detectable pleural effusions: a roentgen pathology model. Radiology 105:51, 1972.
9. Hessen I: Roentgen examination of pleural fluid: a study of the localization of free effusions, the potentialities of diagnosing minimal quantities of fluid and its existence under physiological conditions. Acta Radiol 86:1, 1951.
10. Lipscomb DJ, Flower CDR, Hadfield JW: Ultrasound of the pleura: an assessment of its clinical value. Clin Radiol 32:289, 1981.
11. Tocino IM: Pneumothorax in the supine patient: radiographic anatomy. Radiographics 5:557, 1985.
12. Chiles C, Ravin C: Radiographic recognition of pneumothorax in the intensive care unit. Crit Care Med 14:677, 1986.
13. Gordon R: The deep sulcus sign. Radiology 136:25, 1980.
14. Bergin C, Roggli V, Coblentz C, et al: The secondary pulmonary lobule: normal and abnormal CT appearances. AJR Am J Roentgenol 151:21, 1988.
15. Lynch DA: Radiology of interstitial lung disease. In Newell JD Jr, Tarver RD, editors: Thoracic Radiology, New York, 1993, Raven Press.
16. American Thoracic Society: Idiopathic pulmonary fibrosis: diagnosis and treatment. International consensus statement. American Thoracic Society (ATS), and the European Respiratory Society (ERS). Am J Respir Crit Care Med 161:646, 2000.
17. Wescott JL, Cole S: Plate atelectasis. Radiology 155:1, 1985.
18. Fraser RG, Pare JA: Diagnosis of diseases of the chest, Philadelphia, 1977, WB Saunders.
19. Woodring JH, Reed JC: Types and mechanisms of pulmonary atelectasis. J Thorac Imaging 11:92, 1996.
20. Gurney JW, Jones KK, Robbins RA, et al: Regional distribution of emphysema: correlation of high-resolution CT with pulmonary function tests in unselected smokers. Radiology 183:457, 1992.
21. Steele JD: The solitary pulmonary nodule. J Thorac Cardiovasc Surg 46:21, 1963.
22. Studer SM, Meade A, Combs AH: Management of airway difficulties in the intensive care unit. Hosp Physician 31:15, 1995.
23. Goodman LR, Putman CE: Radiological evaluation of patients receiving assisted ventilation. JAMA 245:858, 1981.

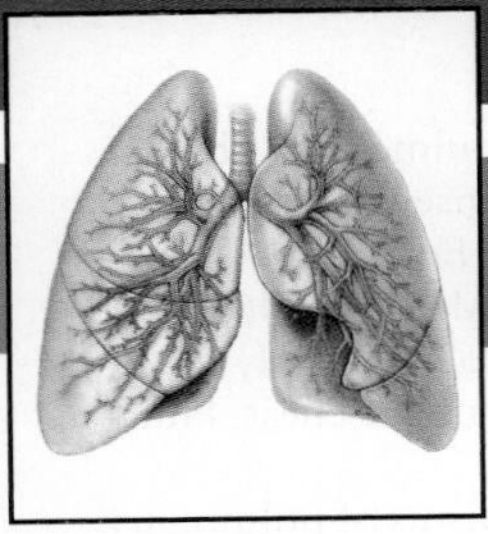

Chapter 21

Nutrition Assessment

JAMI E. BALTZ

CHAPTER OBJECTIVES

After reading this chapter you will be able to:

- Describe how a comprehensive nutrition assessment is conducted.
- Describe how to calculate and interpret body mass index.
- Describe how to distinguish two forms of protein-energy malnutrition from each other.
- List the biochemical indicators of nutrition status.
- State what to observe clinically in a malnourished patient.
- Describe how to obtain and evaluate a nutrition history.
- Describe how to estimate daily resting energy expenditure.
- List the indications, contraindications, hazards, and limitations of indirect calorimetry.
- Describe how to prepare a patient properly for indirect calorimetry.
- Describe how to interpret the results of indirect calorimetry.
- Describe how resting energy expenditure values are adjusted to reflect the actual energy needs of a patient.
- State the effects of malnutrition on the respiratory system.
- Describe how to identify patients at high risk for malnutrition.
- Identify the effect of too much protein, carbohydrate, or fat on a patient.
- State when enteral nutrition and parenteral nutrition are needed.
- Describe how to identify and minimize the common respiratory complications of enteral feedings.
- State specific nutrition guidelines that apply to patients with specific pulmonary diseases.
- Explain how common pulmonary medications affect nutrition.

CHAPTER OUTLINE

Nutrition Assessment
- Anthropometrics
- Biochemical Indicators
- Pulmonary Function
- Clinical Indicators
- Dietary Measures
- Subjective Global Assessment
- Considerations Throughout the Life Span

Outcomes of Nutrition Assessment
- Base Recommendations on Major Guidelines

Macronutrients and Energy Requirements
- Estimating Energy Requirements
- Indirect Calorimetry
- Alternative Resting Energy Expenditure Measures

General Aspects of Nutrition Support
- Meeting Overall Energy Needs
- Respiratory Consequences of Malnutrition
- Providing the Appropriate Combination of Substrates
- Routes of Administration

Nutrition Support in Specific Circumstances
- General Guidelines for Critically Ill Patients
- Systemic Inflammatory Response Syndrome
- Mechanical Ventilation
- Chronic Obstructive Pulmonary Disease
- Asthma
- Cystic Fibrosis

KEY TERMS

anergy
anthropometrics
azotemia
basal metabolic rate (BMR)
body mass index (BMI)
cachexic
indirect calorimetry
kwashiorkor
marasmus
normometabolic
protein-energy malnutrition (PEM)
resting energy expenditure (REE)

Nutrition is vital to life, health, and a sense of well-being. Second to the provision of oxygen (O_2) to a living organism is the necessity for the provision of nutrients to sustain the function, growth, maintenance, and repair of the human body. A human deprived of air for minutes can no longer function. Similarly, a human deprived of food for days to weeks can no longer function.

Adequate nutrition is essential for health. The relationship between nutrition and respiratory status is reciprocal. A balanced supply of nutrients is needed for proper respiratory function; O_2 is required for adenosine triphosphate synthesis and muscle function, including the respiratory muscles. Poor or inadequate nutrient intake disrupts energy use and impairs normal organ function. Conversely, disease can impair nutrient intake or alter metabolism, causing malnutrition.

To heal, traumatized tissue requires the provision of the substrates for healing—that is, nutrients. To achieve a sense of vibrant living for a long life requires daily, consistent attention to providing essential nutrients. A patient with a respiratory condition is particularly challenged to ensure adequate nutrition because it is difficult to breathe and swallow at the same time. This chapter focuses on nutrition assessment—determining the nutrient needs of individuals.

NUTRITION ASSESSMENT

The process of collecting and evaluating data to determine the nutrition status of an individual is termed *nutrition assessment*. A registered dietitian or physician trained in clinical nutrition gathers data to compare various social, pharmaceutical, environmental, physical, and medical factors to evaluate the nutrient needs of an individual. The purpose of nutrition assessment is to gather data to develop a *nutrition care plan* that ensures adequate nutrition for health and well-being when implemented.

Registered dietitians or physicians obtain data from numerous sources for nutrition assessment. Interviewing the individual or the caregiver to determine past and current eating practices is most helpful. Medical charts reveal additional information regarding social, pharmaceutical, environmental, and medical issues. In particular, the *ABCDs* of nutrition assessment—anthropometrics, biochemical tests, clinical observations, and dietary analyses (described subsequently)—lead to nutrition care plans.[1]

The social history of an individual includes marital status, employment, education, and economic status. Drug-nutrient interactions may be identified from prescribed medications that lead to potential nutrient deficiencies. Environmental issues could point out the difficulties the individual has in procuring, storing, or preparing food. The education attained by the individual could determine the potential for understanding and applying nutrition counseling. The economic status of the individual may drive certain food choices.[2] Box 21-1 presents an overview of the information to incorporate into a nutrition assessment.

Box 21-1 Components of a Comprehensive Nutrition Assessment

MEDICAL CHART
- History and physical examination
- Present diseases
- Current medications
- Activity level
- Physical assessment
- Social history

ANTHROPOMETRICS
- Usual weight and height
- History of weight loss
- Actual vs. ideal body weight
- BMI
- Body composition (triceps skinfold, arm muscle area)

CLINICAL LABORATORY TESTS
- Visceral proteins
- Creatinine-height index
- Immune-related tests
- Nitrogen balance

DIETARY HISTORY
- Usual food intake
- Food likes and dislikes
- Appetite

TOTAL CALORIC REQUIREMENTS
- REE predictive equations (Harris-Benedict equation)
- Indirect calorimetry

ACCESS TO FOOD
- Income
- Education
- Mobility
- Mechanical impediments

Anthropometrics

Anthropometrics refers to measurements of the body. The most frequently used measurements are height and weight. Skinfold thicknesses, arm muscle measurements, waist and hip measurements, head circumference, and wrist diameter are body composition measurements that may be useful when assessing nutrition status.

Height and Weight

A measured height and weight is preferred, but the clinician may ask the patient or caregiver for the height and weight. When the data are recorded, a notation should be made of the date and whether the height and weight were stated or measured. The height and weight can be evaluated to determine weight status by comparing actual body weight with ideal body weight. Table 21-1 shows healthy weights for adults. Ideal body weight may also be determined using the Hamwi formulas. To estimate ideal body weight in pounds, the following simple formulas (Hamwi method) can be used:

Men: 106 lb for the first 5 ft + 6 lb for each 1 in >5 ft
Women: 100 lb for the first 5 ft + 5 lb for each 1 in >5 ft

TABLE 21-1

Healthy Adult Weights

	Weight (lb)*	
Height*	**Midpoint**	**Range**
4′10″	105	91-119
4′11″	109	94-124
5′0″	112	97-128
5′1″	116	101-132
5′2″	120	104-137
5′3″	124	107-141
5′4″	128	111-146
5′5″	132	114-150
5′6″	136	118-155
5′7″	140	121-160
5′8″	144	125-164
5′9″	149	129-169
5′10″	153	132-174
5′11″	157	136-179
6′0″	162	140-184
6′1″	166	144-189
6′2″	171	148-195
6′3″	176	152-200
6′4″	180	156-205
6′5″	185	160-201
6′6″	190	164-216

From Report of the Dietary Guidelines Advisory Committee on the Dietary Guidelines for Americans, Washington, DC, 1995, Government Printing Office.

Note: The higher weights in the ranges generally apply to men, who tend to have more muscle and bone; the lower weights more often apply to women, who have less muscle and bone.

*Without shoes or clothes.

A more useful number, the **body mass index (BMI),** may also be calculated. This number is a handy tool for determining the category of body weight: underweight, healthy weight, overweight, obese, or morbidly obese (Figures 21-1 and 21-2). BMI numerically states the relationship of weight to height. The formula used to calculate BMI is as follows for measurements in kilograms and meters:

$$\text{BMI} = \frac{\text{Actual body weight (kg)}}{\text{height}^2\ (\text{m}^2)}$$

The following formula is used when the weight and height measurements are in pounds and inches:

$$\text{BMI} = \frac{\text{Actual body weight (lb)} \times 703}{\text{height}^2\ (\text{in}^2)}$$

An Internet calculator for BMI is available at: http://www.nhlbisupport.com/bmi/.

Body Mass Index Categories. A *healthy weight* is defined as a BMI between 18.5 and 24.9 for adults or a BMI-for-age between the 10th and 85th percentiles for children.[2] A BMI of 25.0 to 29.9 indicates *excessive weight* in adults and a BMI-for-age between the 85th and 95th percentiles indicates excessive weight in children. *Obesity* is defined as a BMI greater than 30 in adults and greater than the 95th percentile in boys and girls 2 to 20 years old. Adults who are categorized as *underweight* have a BMI less than 18.5, and underweight children have a BMI-for-age in the 10th percentile (see Figures 21-1 and 21-2).[3,4]

Overweight and Obesity. Simply defined, overweight and obesity occur over time with the consumption of too many calories or too little expenditure of calories through activity or exercise or both overconsumption and underexpenditure. Other factors may contribute to the accumulation of stored calories, including rare diseases, genes yet to be clearly identified, and loss of mobility through trauma or disease. In any case, too many calories have been ingested for the amount of energy (calories) expended.

Kwashiorkor and Marasmus. Undernutrition classifications include kwashiorkor and marasmus. Typically seen in children 6 to 18 months old in deprived areas of the world, **marasmus** results from an extreme lack of calories and protein over a long time. "Matchstick" arms and obvious lack of muscle and fat characterize a child or adult with marasmus. **Kwashiorkor** results from a more sudden lack of protein and calories, as in a first-born infant weaned suddenly on the arrival of a new sibling, when a diet of nutrient-rich breast milk is traded for a nutrient-poor, cereal-based diet.[2] The protruding belly and edematous face and limbs that are characteristics of kwashiorkor result from a lack of circulating proteins needed to maintain fluid balance and to transport fat out of the liver. Numerous sequelae accompany changes in the liver. Infections and parasites may also cause the enlarged belly seen in kwashiorkor.[2] Some patients exhibit combined

Are you at a healthy weight?

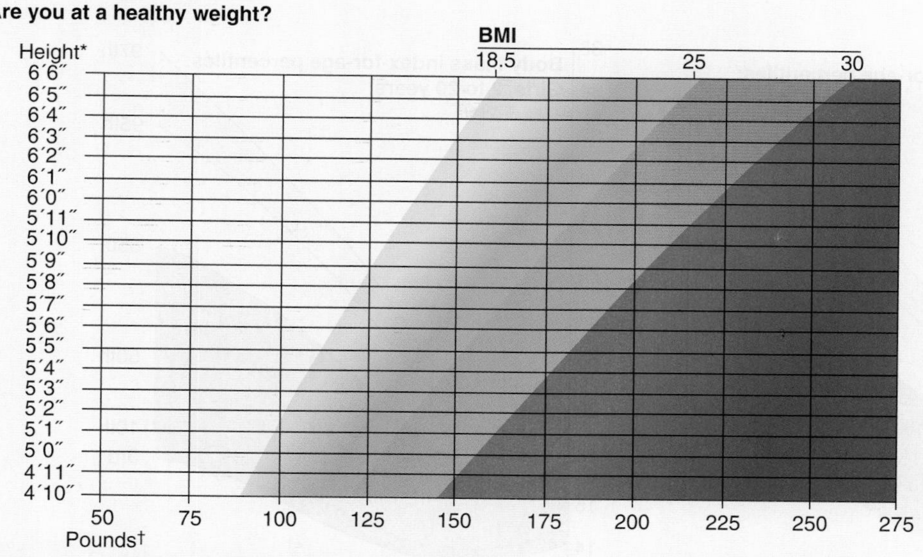

Healthy Weight **Overweight** **Obesity** * Without shoes. † Without clothes

The BMI (weight-for-height) ranges shown above for adults. They are not exact ranges of healthy and unhealthy weights. However, they show that health risk increases at higher levels of overweight and obesity. Even within the healthy BMI range, weight gains can carry health risks for adults.

Directions: Find your weight on the bottom of the graph. Go straight up from that point until you come to the line that matches your height. Then look to find your weight group.

- BMI of 25 defines the upper boundary of healthy weight
- BMI of higher than 25 to 30 defines overweight
- BMI of higher than 30 defines obesity

FIGURE 21-1 BMI categories for adults. (Modified from U.S. Department of Agriculture and U.S. Department of Health and Human Services: Report of the Dietary Guidelines Advisory Committee for Americans, Washington, DC, 2005, U.S. Government Printing Office.)

kwashiorkor and marasmus from protein and calorie deprivation over an extended period. A mixture of loss of muscle and fat and circulating albumin is evident in the extreme wasting and edema that are present.

Body Composition

Other anthropometric measurements useful in nutrition assessment are *arm muscle area* (index for muscle) and *skinfolds* (measures of fat), bioelectric impedance analysis devices, and more sophisticated imaging technologies. These methods are generally expensive and time-consuming and are not relevant in the clinical setting but may be more useful in research settings.[5]

Triceps Skinfold. Measurement of the triceps skinfold is done on the right arm at the midpoint between the acromion process of the scapula and the inferior margin of the olecranon process of the ulna. The arm should be bent at a 90-degree angle at the elbow to mark the midpoint. The arm hangs by the side with the palm facing anteriorly as a caliper is used to measure a pinch of skinfold. The thumb and index finger of the left hand of the measurer grasp the skinfold while the caliper is placed approximately ½ inch from the fingers. When the caliper is perpendicular to the skinfold, the dial can be easily read.[5]

Arm Muscle Area. The triceps skinfold (TSF) measurement is used to calculate the arm muscle area (AMA). The result indicates muscle stores available for protein synthesis or energy needs. Changes over time in AMA show whether the patient has been deprived of protein or calories; AMA is one of the markers of nutrition status and can be a predictor of mortality.[6] The formula to calculate AMA is as follows:

$$\text{AMA} = [\text{MAC (cm)} - (\pi \times \text{TSF cm})]^2 - 10\ \text{cm}^2\ \text{(males) or } 6.5\ \text{cm}^2\ \text{(females)}/4\pi$$

where MAC equals midarm circumference. A factor for sex is included for a corrected AMA formula because this accounts for bone area and provides a more accurate assessment of bone-free muscle area.[7] Standards have been established for age groups throughout the life span.[5]

Biochemical Indicators

Laboratory values of particular significance used in assessing nutrition status include serum proteins. PEM may be reflected in low values for albumin, transferrin, transthyretin, and retinol-binding protein. Blood levels of these markers indicate the level of protein synthesis and yield information on overall nutrition status. However, inadequate intake may not be the cause of low values; certain disease states, level of hydration, liver function, pregnancy, infection, and medical therapies may alter laboratory values for each of the circulating proteins.[8] Other visceral

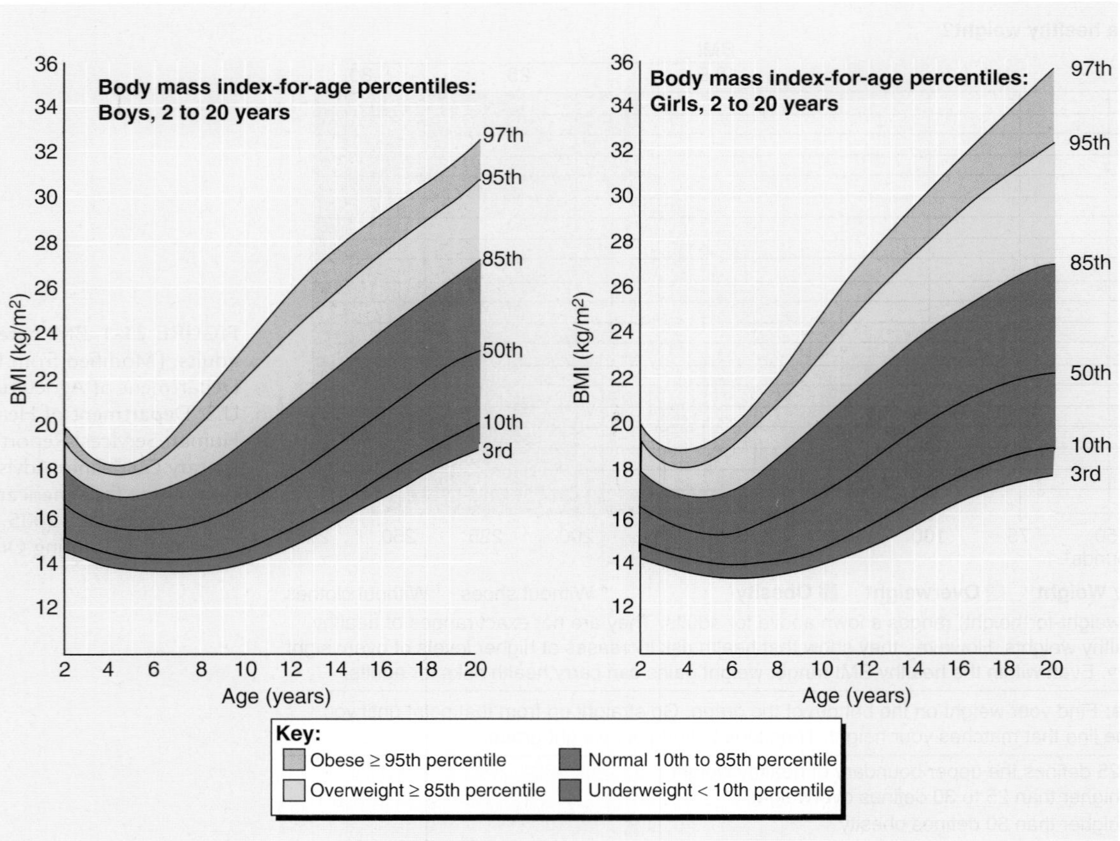

FIGURE 21-2 BMI categories for children. (Modified from Whitney EN, Cataldo CB, Rolfes SR: Understanding normal and clinical nutrition (with Info Trac), ed 6, Monteray, CA, 2002, Brooks Cole. Reprinted with permission of Brooks/Cole, a division of Thomson Learning; www.thomsonrights.com.)

proteins that may help evaluate nutrition risk are positive acute phase reactants and include fibronectin, insulinlike growth hormone, and C-reactive protein.

Albumin

Albumin constitutes most protein in plasma and is commonly measured at minimal cost. The half-life of albumin is 14 to 21 days, which reduces its usefulness for monitoring the effectiveness of nutrition in the critical care setting.[8] The general availability and stability of albumin levels from day to day make it one of the most useful tests for assessing *long-term* trends (Table 21-2). It is important to determine an albumin value before the onset of disease or insult of injury. In combination with other findings, such as hair pluckability, edema, and poor wound healing, a serum albumin level less than 2.8 g/dl helps differentiate kwashiorkor from marasmus.[9] Table 21-3 compares the two forms of PEM.[10,11]

Transferrin

Transferrin is the transport protein for iron. It has a half-life of 8 to 10 days and is a better indicator of improved nutrition status than albumin. However, lack of iron influences transferrin values along with numerous other factors, including hepatic and renal disease, inflammation, and congestive heart failure.[8,12]

TABLE 21-2

Assessment of Serum Albumin

Level (g/dl)	Interpretation
3.5-5.0	Normal
2.8-3.5	Mild depletion
2.1-2.7	Moderate depletion
<2.1	Severe depletion

Transthyretin and Retinol-Binding Protein

Transthyretin, also called prealbumin, has a half-life of 2 to 3 days, and retinol-binding protein has a half-life of 12 hours. Each of these proteins responds to nutrition changes more quickly than either albumin or transferrin. However, numerous metabolic states, diseases, therapies, and infections influence the laboratory values.[13]

These two tests are more costly than testing for albumin. Levels of each protein are influenced by many factors other than nutrition status. Because these conditions are so

TABLE 21-3

Comparison of Two Primary Forms of Protein-Energy Malnutrition

Parameter	Starvation (Marasmus)	Hypercatabolism (Kwashiorkor)
Etiology	Inadequate energy intake	Response to injury or infection
Examples	Cancer, pulmonary emphysema	Sepsis, burns
Body habitus	Thin, wasted, cachexic	May be normal, edematous
Rate of malnutrition	Slow	Rapid
Metabolic rate	Decreased	Increased
Fuel	Glucose/fat	Mixed
Catabolism	Decreased	Increased
Gluconeogenesis	Increased	Markedly increased
Glucagon	Increased	Markedly increased
Insulin	Decreased	Increased
Ketogenesis	Increased	Slightly increased
Catecholamines	Unchanged	Increased
Cortisol	Unchanged	Increased
Growth hormone	Increased	Increased
Visceral proteins	Normal	Decreased
Cytokines	Variable	Increased
Immune function	Normal	Impaired
Clinical course	Adequate responsiveness to short-term stress	Infections, poor wound healing, decubitus ulcers, skin breakdown
Mortality	Low unless related to underlying disease	High

common among critically ill patients, visceral protein markers are of limited usefulness for assessing nutrition deficiency and of greater usefulness in assessing the severity of illness and the risk for future malnutrition.[14] Inflammatory metabolism causes a 25% decrease in the synthesis of these visceral proteins and causes lean body mass depletion and anorexia. It is important to evaluate their values with positive acute phase reactants (fibronectin, insulin-like growth hormone, C-reactive protein) where there is a reverse relationship.

Fibronectin, Insulinlike Growth Hormone, and C-Reactive Protein

Fibronectin, a glycoprotein with a half-life of 15 hours, plays an important role in wound healing. Because it is less affected by acute stress than other visceral proteins, it may become an important marker of nutrition status and an indicator of the efficacy of nutrition support.

Insulinlike growth hormone type 1, also called somatomedin C, is not routinely used in the clinical setting at this time in nutrition assessment. However, insulinlike growth hormone type 1 is used to measure protein status routinely in research settings. It may be more effective than other means in measuring nutrition status in the acute phase of stress, and its usefulness may increase.

C-reactive protein is an acute phase protein released with infection and inflammation. As transport proteins (albumin and prealbumin) decrease, levels of the acute phase proteins increase. Increased levels of C-reactive protein during stress, illness, and trauma have been linked to increased nutrition risk.[12]

Creatinine-Height Index

Because the rate of creatinine formation in skeletal muscle is constant, the amount of creatinine excreted in the urine every 24 hours reflects skeletal muscle mass. Predicted values are based on gender and height, with reference values of approximately 18 mg/kg body weight/day for women and approximately 23 mg/kg body weight/day for men. Values of 60% to 80% of predicted indicate a mild deficit of muscle mass, values of 40% to 60% of predicted indicate a moderate deficit, and values less than 40% of predicted indicate a severe depletion of muscle mass.[5] Factors that influence creatinine excretion and complicate interpretation of this index include age, diet, exercise, stress, trauma, fever, and sepsis.[12]

Nitrogen Balance (Protein Catabolism)

Approximately 16% of protein is nitrogen, a useful factor in determining nitrogen balance. Because nitrogen is a major by-product of protein catabolism, its rate of urinary excretion can be used to assess protein adequacy. Nitrogen balance is calculated as follows:

$$\text{Nitrogen balance} = \text{Nitrogen intake} - \text{Nitrogen losses}$$

$$\text{Nitrogen intake} = \frac{\text{Protein intake}}{6.25}$$

$$\text{Nitrogen losses} = \text{UUN excretion in grams} + \text{3-5 g (for insensible losses)}$$

The conversion factor for dietary protein is 6.25 g of nitrogen per 1 g of protein. The amount of nitrogen excretion in the urine is typically measured as the 24-hour urinary urea nitrogen (UUN). Between 3 g/day and 5 g/day is added to the 24-hour urinary urea nitrogen for an estimate of the average daily unmeasured nitrogen lost through other sources (skin and gastrointestinal [GI] sloughing, hair loss, sweat, feces). Theoretically, by increasing exogenous protein, loss of endogenous protein is reduced. However, because of invalid 24-hour urine collections, alterations in renal or liver function, large immeasurable insensible losses (burns, high-output fistulas, wounds, or ostomies), and inflammatory conditions (generally occurring in critically ill patients), nitrogen balance calculations are inaccurate.

Immune Status

Impaired immunity **(anergy)** is a common finding in malnutrition, especially the kwashiorkor type. Two laboratory values, white blood cells and percentage of lymphocytes, have been used as measures of a compromised immune system. The result is often a reduction in lymphocytes, as measured by the total lymphocyte count (TLC): TLC = white blood cells × % lymphocytes. Many nonnutrition variables influence these laboratory values, and their usefulness in assessing nutrition status is questioned.[15]

Malnourished patients also may exhibit signs of depressed immunity when challenged by certain hypersensitivity skin tests. Because many disease states and drugs are associated with anergy, the value of this test also is limited.[16]

Pulmonary Function

Pulmonary function test results may change with malnutrition. Weakness of the diaphragm and other muscles of inspiration can lead to reduced vital capacity and peak inspiratory pressures. The strength and endurance of respiratory muscles are affected, in particular, the diaphragm. Healthy lung function has been correlated with dietary antioxidant intake, such as vitamins C and E, beta-carotene, and selenium.[17]

Clinical Indicators

The physical signs of malnutrition often appear first in selected tissues, such as the hair, eyes, lips, mouth and gums, skin, and nails. Hair that is shiny and firmly in the scalp; bright clear eyes that adjust to light easily; an appropriately red tongue without swelling; gums without bleeding or swelling; skin of good color that is smooth and firm; and nails that are pink, smooth, and firm all are signs of acceptable nutrition status. In addition to malnutrition, other causes of these abnormalities might be medical therapies, anemia, allergies, sunburn, medications, poor hygiene practices, aging, or various pathologies.[8] Patients with persistent malnutrition often appear very thin to the point that their ribs and bony structures of the chest are very visible. A patient is said to be **cachexic** in such cases.

Dietary Measures

Past dietary practices need to be identified in the nutrition assessment process. Numerous means are available to determine food consumed by an individual. A registered dietitian may use a 24-hour recall or a usual daily intake recall, a food diary or food record, or a food frequency questionnaire. Each method has advantages and disadvantages.

Twenty-four-Hour Recall

The 24-hour recall may be used in an interview in which the patient states the foods and the amount of each food consumed in the previous 24 hours. It is a straightforward commonly used technique that may easily be incorporated into a patient interview. Accuracy of the recall depends on the patient's memory, the perception of serving size, and the skill of the interviewer to elicit complete information. Spreads, gravies, dressings, beverages, or snacks may be forgotten rendering a nutrient analysis inaccurate (i.e., especially total calories). Patients often report that the previous 24 hours were an aberration in their food intake.

Usual Intake Recall

To improve accuracy, patients may be asked to recall their usual daily food intake. However, neither the 24-hour recall nor usual intake recall method makes allowances for weekends, holidays, celebrations, or other major changes in food intake.

Food Diary or Food Record

The food diary or food record may be used to discover what a patient has been eating. In this case, the patient is asked to write down daily everything he or she has eaten. The patient may record food intake over an extended time, most frequently, a 3-day or 7-day period. Patients arrive with the dietary history in place rather than the interview time being used to reveal dietary practices. However, the act of recording everything eaten influences food choices, reducing the accuracy of a diet history.

Food Frequency Questionnaire

Patients may complete a multiple-item questionnaire choosing foods, serving size, and frequency in which the food was typically eaten to identify their food intake history. Such forms may cover a wide spectrum of foods or foods specifically of interest to current issues. Food frequency questionnaires list commonly used foods in typical serving sizes and often are linked to computer software for ease of analysis of the nutrient content of a patient's diet. Accuracy of the nutrient analysis depends on the patient's memory of foods eaten over an extended time and the patient's perception of the serving size listed versus the serving size consumed.

Evaluation of Nutrition History

A 24-hour recall or usual recall, food diary or record, or a food frequency questionnaire may be evaluated for nutrient intake using the food guide pyramid My Pyramid, a nutrient analysis handbook, or a nutrient analysis software package.

Food Guide Pyramid. The U.S. Department of Agriculture and the U.S. Department of Health and Human Services have cooperated through the years to recommend balanced nutrition for U.S. citizens. The current graphic showing recommendations, *My Pyramid,*[18] divides foods into groups based on the nutrient contribution of the grouping. For example, the grains group consists of breads, pasta, and rice, which all contribute B vitamins, folate, iron, and protein to the diet. The measure (ounces or cups) of servings is recommended for multiple calorie levels of each of the food groups: grains, protein, dairy, fruits, and vegetables. Consuming the recommended amounts of each should provide balanced, adequate nutrition for a healthy person (Table 21-4). The calorie level is based on

TABLE 21-4

Dietary Guidelines for Americans—2005

Guideline	Application
Adequate nutrients with calorie needs	Consume a variety of nutrient-dense foods and beverages within and among the basic food groups while choosing foods that limit the intake of saturated and *trans* fats, cholesterol, added sugars, salt, and alcohol
	Meet recommended intakes within energy needs by adopting a balanced eating pattern, such as the USDA Food Guide or the DASH Eating Plan
Weight management	Maintain body weight in a healthy range, balance calories from food and beverage calories, and increase physical activity
	To prevent gradual weight gain, make small reductions in calorie intake and increase physical activity
Physical activity	Engage in regular physical activity
	Achieve physical fitness through cardiovascular conditioning, stretching, and resistance exercises
Food groups to encourage	Consume sufficient amounts of fruits and vegetables
	Choose a variety of fruits and vegetables every day
	Consume ≥3 oz equivalents of whole-grain products per day; half of the grains should be whole
	Consume 3 cups per day of fat-free or low-fat milk or equivalent milk products
Fats	Consume 10% of calories from saturated fats and <300 mg/day of cholesterol, and keep *trans* fats as low as possible
	Keep total fat intake between 20% and 35% of calories
	Choose lean, low-fat, or fat-free meat, poultry, dry beans, milk, and milk products
	Limit intake of fats and oils high in saturated and *trans* fats, and choose products low in such fats and oils
Carbohydrates	Choose fiber-rich fruits, vegetables, and whole grains often
	Choose and prepare foods and beverages with little added sugars
	Reduce incidence of dental caries by practicing good oral hygiene and consuming sugars and starches less often
Sodium and potassium	Consume <2300 mg of sodium per day (approximately 1 tsp of salt)
	Choose and prepare foods with little salt
	Consume potassium-rich foods (i.e., fruits and vegetables)
Alcoholic beverages	Alcohol should be consumed in moderation
	Pregnant and lactating women, individuals who cannot restrict their intake of alcohol, patients taking medications that interact with alcohol, and patients with specific medical conditions should not consume alcohol
Food safety	Clean your hands, food contact surfaces, and fruits and vegetables; meats and poultry should *not* be rinsed
	Separate raw, cooked, and ready-to-eat foods while shopping, preparing, or storing foods
	Cook foods to a safe temperature to kill microorganisms
	Refrigerate perishable food promptly, and defrost foods properly
	Avoid raw (unpasteurized) milk or any products made from unpasteurized milk, raw or partially cooked eggs or foods containing raw eggs, raw or undercooked meat and poultry, unpasteurized juices, and raw sprouts[4]

Compiled from U.S. Department of Agriculture and U.S. Department of Health and Human Services: Nutrition and your health: dietary guidelines for Americans, Washington, DC, 2005, U.S. Government Printing Office.

age, gender, and activity level. The clinician or patient can go to http://mypyramid.gov to enter an individual's data and be given the recommended calorie level. A comparison of a 24-hour recall with My Pyramid (Figure 21-3) gives an estimation of the adequacy of the patient's diet.[18] Individuals choosing meatless meals may select foods and number of servings from *My Vegetarian Food Pyramid* (Figure 21-4).[19]

Nutrient Analysis Handbook. A handbook listing the nutrient content of specific foods may be used to calculate manually the adequacy of a 24-hour recall. This is a tedious and time-consuming task.

Nutrient Analysis Software. Computer programs are used to determine total calories, percent of calories of the macronutrients (protein, carbohydrate, and fat), and units of micronutrients and fiber. The patient's individual foods and serving size may be entered into a computer file to determine quickly the nutrient content of a diet history. Total number of foods listed in the software packages differ, as do the usefulness of their printed reports and user-friendly characteristics of the software.

Subjective Global Assessment

Nutrition assessment may be accomplished through a process referred to as *subjective global assessment*. This process uses patient information regarding weight changes, food intake, various symptoms, functional capacity in numerous areas, the disease and its nutrient requirements, and numerous physical traits. Scores are given in each category to determine the subjective global assessment rating of

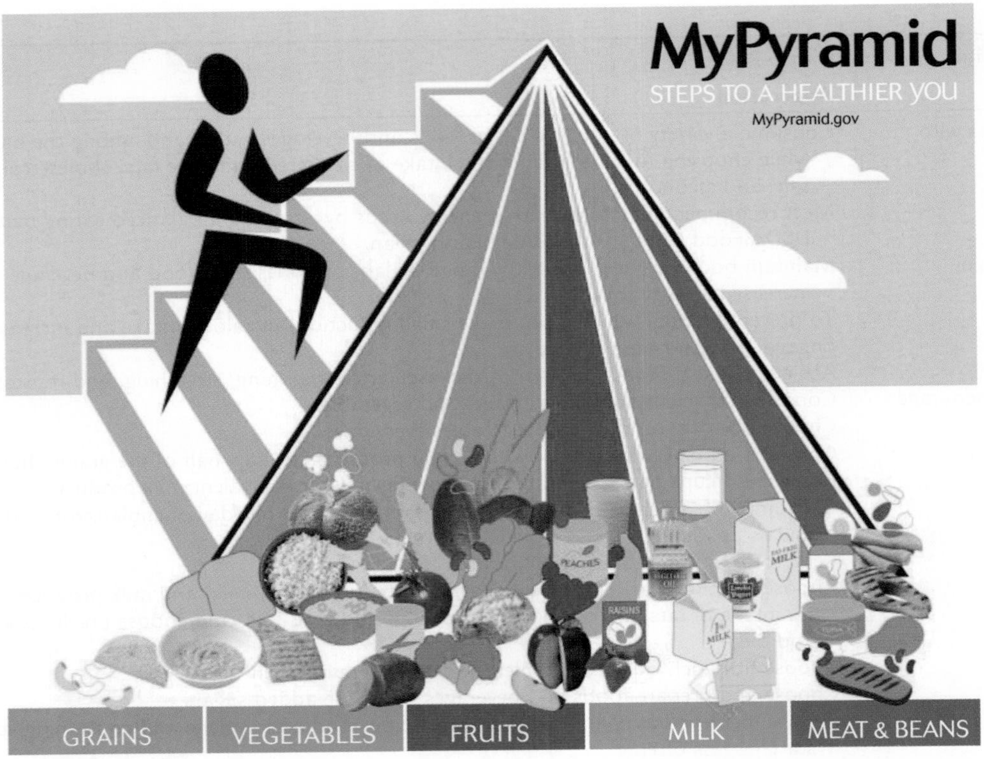

FIGURE 21-3 My Pyramid food guide pyramid. (From U.S. Department of Agriculture, Center for Nutrition Policy and Promotion, April 2005.)

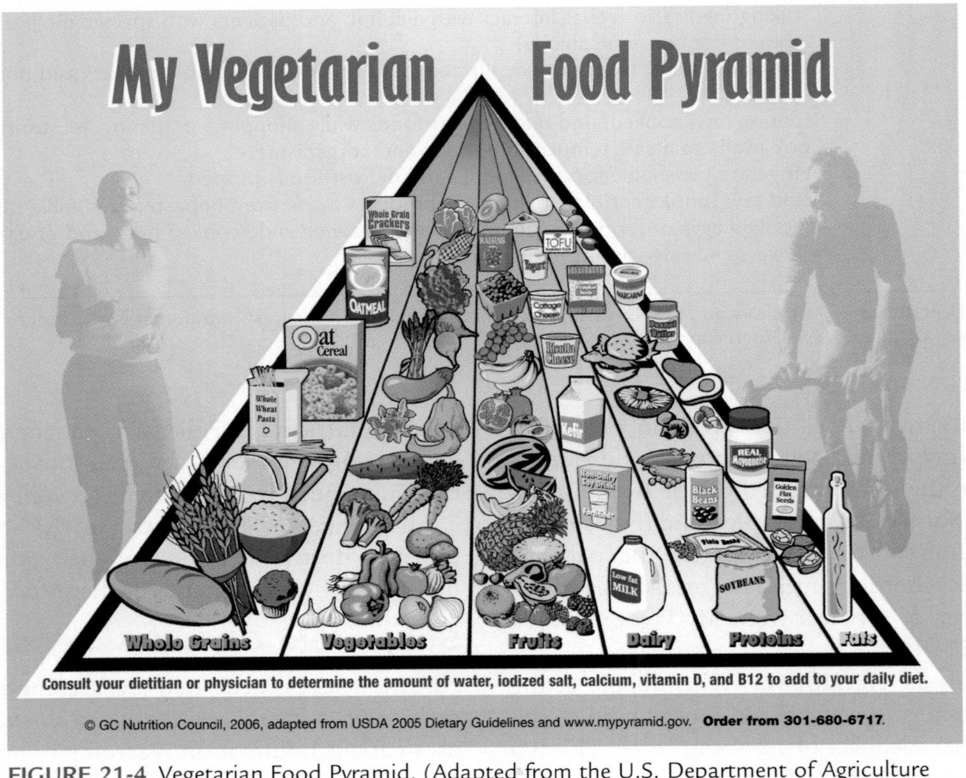

FIGURE 21-4 Vegetarian Food Pyramid. (Adapted from the U.S. Department of Agriculture and U.S. Department of Health and Human Services: Nutrition and your health: dietary guidelines for Americans, Washington, DC, 2005, U.S. Government Printing Office; http://mypyramid.gov; and General Conference [of Seventh-day Adventists] Nutrition Council: My vegetarian food pyramid, Silver Spring, MD, 2006, GC Department of Health.)

well-nourished, moderately malnourished, or severely malnourished clients.[20,21]

Considerations Throughout the Life Span

Pregnancy and Lactation

A healthful diet with added nutrients is essential to a successful pregnancy and to lactation. The demands of the growing fetus and of the nursing infant add to the calorie and protein needs of the mother.[22] Ensuring adequate vitamin and mineral intake to support pregnancy and lactation requires a modest increase in all vitamins and minerals compared with the requirements for 19- to 30-year-old women with the exceptions of magnesium; phosphorus; vitamins D, E, and K; and biotin for certain age groups.[23-26]

Children

The rapid growth seen in infancy slows during the toddler and school-age years. Nutrition must provide the nutrients for the steady growth of childhood. During these years, eating habits for a lifetime form, influenced by peers, parents, other relatives, television, and advertising. Children, especially an ill child, use food to manipulate parents and caregivers.[27]

Adolescents

Adolescents continue to grow in spurts. Nutrient needs reflect growth and activity levels at this stage, which may be met by varying the number of servings of the same foods fed to the rest of the family. Food choices need to be based on the *U.S. Dietary Guidelines* and the *Food Guide Pyramid,* rather than on advertising or peer pressure. Food is an area where teens may express their growing independence by choosing new food patterns. Some patterns are based on needs or perceived needs, whereas others are based on image (e.g., pregnancy, muscle-building, calorie restricted or calorie excessive, fast foods, multiple snacks with skipped meals). Other adolescents choose vegetarian meal patterns.[27,28]

Adults

Previous adult nutrition recommendations aimed to decrease nutrient deficiencies. Beriberi, pellagra, and scurvy are no longer the primary health concerns of Americans. Heart disease, strokes, cancer, diabetes, and diseases that result from obesity drive the current recommendations. The *U.S. Dietary Guidelines,* the *Food Guide Pyramid,* and the *food label* together recommend meal patterns low in total fat, saturated fat, cholesterol, sodium, and sugar, while including abundant fruits, vegetables, and whole grains in food choices.[4,18,19,29]

Elderly Adults

The percentage of the U.S. population older than 65 years has increased from 4% in 1900 to 12.8% in 2000. This group of citizens is a very heterogeneous group ranging from very active individuals to institutionalized individuals. As the years pass, weight loss becomes a prime concern. Loss of total lean body mass (muscle) and an increase in total body fat secondary to a decrease in activity result in a decrease in the total calories needed. With the exception of increases from adult years in vitamins D and B_6 and minerals calcium and chromium,[23-26] nutrient needs for elderly adults remain the same even though total calories have decreased. Often, elderly adults choose to consume fewer calories than previously consumed because of changes in the ability to taste, to smell, and to discern brightly colored foods; because of taste alterations from medications; and because of lack of interest in food procurement or food preparation. Socioeconomic issues may limit the ability to purchase food. In addition, the enjoyment of food decreases when eating alone.[30]

OUTCOMES OF NUTRITION ASSESSMENT

Registered dietitians focus much of their professional effort toward nutrition assessment with the goal to develop a nutrition care plan. Implementation of the care plan requires the cooperation of the patient, family or caregivers, and health care professionals including the respiratory therapist (RT). All members of the health care team benefit patients through their intentional support of recommended dietary changes. Reinforcement of the food choices patients are to make has multiple positive outcomes.

With nutrition intervention, patients improve their nutrient intake and reduce mortality and morbidity. Improved nutrition status increases the patient's tolerance of therapeutic regimens in the treatment of disease and decreases recovery time. The resulting economic benefits are multifactorial and include reduced hospital stays, reduced need for medication or medical care or extended care, and increased years of productivity.[31]

Base Recommendations on Major Guidelines

Past dietary practices may be evaluated using recommendations from many sources. U.S. government agencies, nongovernment groups, and professional organizations have developed recommendations for the public to improve the nutrition status of Americans. Basic to a national nutrition policy are the Dietary Guidelines for Americans,[4] MyPyramid,[18,19] and the food label.[29] Recommendations have come from other sources as well.

MACRONUTRIENTS AND ENERGY REQUIREMENTS

The purpose of nutrition assessment is to determine a nutrition care plan for the patient or client. Calorie or energy needs are fundamental to the recommendations of

Box 21-2 Factors Influencing Energy and Macronutrient Needs

ENERGY NEEDS
- Height, weight
- Activity level
- Growth state: Infants through teens, pregnancy, lactation
- Presence of infection or fever
- Surgery
- Trauma, fractures
- Presence of infection or inflammation

PROTEIN NEEDS
- State of growth
- Surgery, trauma, fractures, infection
- Renal (kidney) function
- Liver function
- Corticosteroid administration

FAT NEEDS
- Total energy needs
- Hyperlipidemia, diabetes mellitus
- Liver, gallbladder, and pancreatic disorders
- Cardiovascular disease

the nutrition care plan. Several means are available to determine calorie needs. These means include calculating total calories using the Harris-Benedict formula and applying a stress factor to it.

Macronutrients supply the energy requirements of the body. The three macronutrients are *protein, carbohydrate,* and *fat.* Each contributes to calorie intake with 4, 4, and 9 calories (kcal) per gram. Alcohol is the only other calorie source with approximately 7 kcal/g. Box 21-2 outlines the factors influencing energy and macronutrient needs.

Estimating Energy Requirements

An individual's energy requirement represents the ratio of energy intake to energy expenditure relative to body weight, activity level, and stressors (Table 21-5). The classic measure of energy expenditure is the **basal metabolic rate (BMR).** Obtained after 10 hours of fasting, the BMR measures the number of calories (kcal) expended at rest per square meter of body surface per hour (kcal/m^2/hr). BMR varies by body size, age, and sex. Calorie needs for energy expenditure increase beyond the BMR based on activity level, stage of growth (pregnancy, lactation), and extent of injury.

In clinical practice, clinicians are more interested in a patient's *daily* energy requirements (kcal/day). Multiple methods are available for estimating daily energy needs. The "quick method" estimates daily energy needs based on a simple body weight factor of 20 to 35 kcal/kg.[31] Alternatively, predictive equations such as the *Harris-Benedict equation* can be used to estimate daily **resting energy expenditure (REE):**

TABLE 21-5
Adjustments of Harris-Benedict Predicted Resting Energy Expenditure (REE) for Stress and Activity Levels

Instructions: Multiply REE times (1) the most relevant stress factor, then (2) the appropriate activity factor

Condition	Factor
Stress Factors	
Malnutrition	0.7
Chronic renal failure, nondialyzed	1.00
Maintenance hemodialysis	1.00-1.05
Elective surgery, uncomplicated	1.0
Peritonitis	1.15
Soft tissue trauma	1.15
Fracture	1.20
Infection, mild	1.00
Infection, moderate	1.20-1.30
Infection, severe	1.40-1.50
Burns, 0%-20% BSA	1.00-1.50
Burns, 20%-40% BSA	1.50-1.80
Burns, 40%-100% BSA	1.80-2.00
Activity Factors	
Confined to bed	1.2
Out of bed	1.3

Example: A bedridden patient with a moderately severe infection has a Harris-Benedict predicted REE of 1100 kcal/day; estimate this patient's actual energy needs

Actual energy needs = predicted REE × stress factor × activity factor

Actual energy needs = 1100 kcal × 1.25 × 1.2

Actual energy needs = 1650 kcal

BSA, Body surface area.

$$\text{REE kcal/day (male)} = 66.5 + [13.8 \times \text{weight (kg)}] + [5 \times \text{height (cm)}] - 6.8 \times \text{Age (in years)}$$

$$\text{REE kcal/day (female)} = 655.1 + [9.6 \times \text{weight (kg)}] + [1.9 \times \text{height (cm)}] - 4.7 \text{ Age (in years)}$$

An Internet calculator for REE is located at http://www.brianmac.demon.co.uk/predictrdee.htm; height in inches is converted to centimeters by multiplying by 2.54, and weight in pounds is converted to kilograms by dividing by 2.2. REE is multiplied by an activity factor to determine daily calorie needs. Although the predicted REE averages approximately 10% higher than the BMR, it still tends to underestimate actual energy needs.

To overcome the limitations of estimating formulas, energy needs can be measured at the bedside. To do so, a procedure called **indirect calorimetry** is used. Indirect calorimetry involves measurement of a patient's O_2 consumption and carbon dioxide (CO_2) production. From these data, an actual REE can be quickly computed. Indirect calorimetry is described in more detail later.

Energy needs vary according to activity level and state of health. Energy needs of sick patients can be significantly greater than predicted normal values. Energy needs for obese individuals are less because adipose tissue uses less energy than muscle. Energy needs should be reevaluated and adjusted whenever weight changes more than 5 to 10 lb.

RULE OF THUMB

To estimate the energy needs of an average adult in kcal/day, identify the goal and multiply the individual's actual body weight in kilograms times the factor listed as follows:

Goal	Energy Needs (kcal/kg)
Weight maintenance	25-30
Weight gain	30-35
Weight loss	20-25

Indirect Calorimetry

Indirect calorimetry is the estimation of energy expenditure by measurement of O_2 consumption and CO_2 production. Data obtained can be used to assess a patient's metabolic state, to determine nutrition needs, or to assess response to nutrition therapy.[32] To guide practitioners in using indirect calorimetry, the American Association for Respiratory Care (AARC) has published Clinical Practice Guideline: Metabolic Measurement Using Indirect Calorimetry During Mechanical Ventilation. Excerpts appear in Clinical Practice Guideline 21-1.[33]

In regard to the indications for indirect calorimetry, the determination of energy and protein needs by an empiric formula is sufficient for most patients. Given the cost and

21-1 Metabolic Measurement Using Indirect Calorimetry During Mechanical Ventilation

AARC Clinical Practice Guideline (Excerpts)*

INDICATIONS

Metabolic measurements may be indicated:
- In patients with known nutrition deficits or derangements
- When patients fail attempts at weaning from mechanical ventilation to measure the O_2 cost of breathing in mechanically ventilated patients
- When the need exists to assess the $\dot{V}O_2$ to evaluate the hemodynamic support of mechanically ventilated patients

CONTRAINDICATIONS

When a specific indication is present, there are no contraindications to performing a metabolic measurement using indirect calorimetry, unless short-term disconnection of ventilatory support for connection of measurement lines results in hypoxemia, bradycardia, or other adverse effects.

HAZARDS AND COMPLICATIONS

Performing metabolic measurements using an indirect calorimeter is a safe, noninvasive procedure with few hazards or complications. Under certain circumstances and with particular equipment, the following hazards or complications may be seen:
- Closed circuit calorimeters may cause a reduction in alveolar ventilation secondary to increased compressible volume of the breathing circuit
- Closed circuit calorimeters may decrease the trigger sensitivity of the ventilator and result in increased patient work of breathing
- Short-term disconnection of the patient from the ventilator for connection of the indirect calorimetry apparatus may result in hypoxemia, bradycardia, and patient discomfort
- Inappropriate calibration or system setup may result in erroneous results causing incorrect patient management

ASSESSMENT OF NEED

Metabolic measurements should be performed only on the order of a physician after review of indications (see above) and objectives.

ASSESSMENT OF TEST QUALITY

Test quality can be evaluated by determining whether:
- RQ is consistent with the patient's nutrition intake
- RQ is in the normal physiologic range (0.67-1.3)
- Variability of the measurements of $\dot{V}O_2$ and $\dot{V}CO_2$ should be ≤5% for a 5-minute data collection
- The measurement is of sufficient length to account for variability in $\dot{V}O_2$ and $\dot{V}CO_2$ if the conditions above are not met

Outcome may be assessed by comparing the measurement results with the patient's condition and nutrition intake.
Outcome may be assessed by observation of the patient before and during the measurement to determine if the patient is at steady state.

Continued

21-1 Metabolic Measurement Using Indirect Calorimetry During Mechanical Ventilation—cont'd

AARC Clinical Practice Guideline (Excerpts)*

MONITORING

The following should be evaluated during the performance of a metabolic measurement to ascertain the validity of the results:

- Clinical observation of the resting state
- Patient comfort and movement during testing
- Values in concert with the clinical situation
- Equipment function
- Results within the specifications of test quality (see above)
- FiO_2 stability

Measurement data should include a statement of test quality and list the current nutrition support, ventilator settings, FiO_2 stability, and vital signs.

**For the complete guidelines, see American Association of Respiratory Care: Clinical practice guideline. Respir Care 49:1073, 2004. Accessed at www.rcjournal.com/contents/09.04/09.04.1073.pdf on June 1, 2007.*

complexity of this procedure, its routine use cannot be justified.[34] Specific clinical conditions supporting the need for indirect calorimetry as a tool in nutrition assessment are listed in Box 21-3.[10,11,34,35]

Box 21-3 Clinical Situations in Which Indirect Calorimetry May Be Indicated

- Patients with morbid obesity
- Patients who are difficult to wean from ventilatory support
- Patients for whom weight estimates are uncertain
- Patients with severe malnutrition
- Patients with high level of stress
- Patients at the extremes of weight or age
- Patients failing to respond to nutrition support

Equipment and Technique

Good calorimetry results require extensive preparation. Box 21-4 outlines the key preparatory steps to be taken before testing.[10] Indirect calorimetry can be performed with a Douglas bag, a Tissot spirometer, and CO_2 and O_2 gas analyzers. The patient's expired gas is collected in the Douglas bag where it is sampled for O_2 and CO_2 concentrations; the Tissot spirometer measures expired volume. Commercially available metabolic carts are much easier to use. These automated systems either use a mixing chamber or perform breath-by-breath analysis. The breath-by-breath method provides real-time data, which may aid in ensuring optimal measurement conditions, particularly in mechanically ventilated patients.[36]

Figure 21-5 shows the basic configuration for open-circuit indirect calorimetry during mechanical ventilation using a metabolic cart with mixing chamber. Gas sampled from the inspiratory limb of the ventilator circuit is assessed for fractional inspired oxygen (FiO_2) using a paramagnetic or zirconium oxide O_2 analyzer. Volume exhaled by the patient is measured using a flow transducer. The patient's exhaled gas enters a mixing chamber, from which a sample is drawn to measure $FeCO_2$ (usually by infrared analysis) and FeO_2. Exhaled gas is returned to the ventilator after volume and gas concentration measurements. After all measurements are obtained, O_2 consumption, CO_2 production, and *respiratory quotient (RQ)* are computed using the equations shown in Box 21-5. *All measurements must be corrected to standard temperature and pressure and dry conditions (STPD) before computation.*[38] The values are used in the abbreviated Weir equation to determine REE:

$$REE = [(O_2 \times 3.9) + (CO_2 \times 1.1)] \times 1.44$$

Indirect calorimetry is more difficult to perform on spontaneously breathing patients, especially patients breathing supplemental O_2. Although a mouthpiece with nose clips or a mask can be used to collect expired gas, these items tend to alter the patient's steady state and invalidate results.[36] Instead, most clinicians recommend using a plastic canopy that covers the patient's head. Expired gases are cleared from the canopy by a preset flow of air; expired gas concentrations are sampled and corrected for the air dilution.

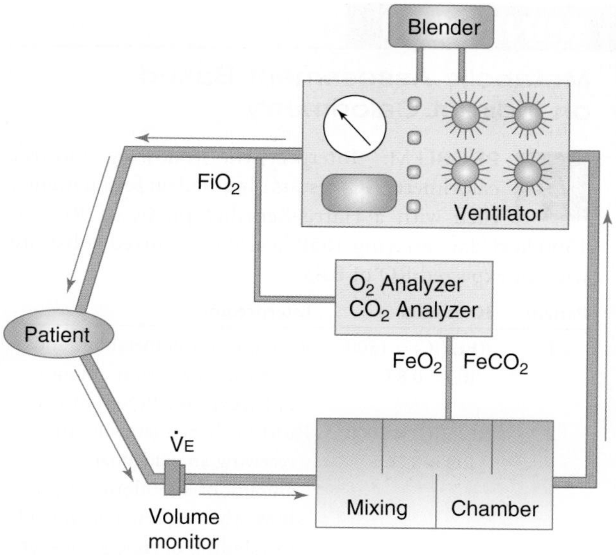

FIGURE 21-5 Open-circuit indirect calorimetry in a mechanically ventilated patient. Inspiratory gas is sampled for determination of FiO_2, volume is measured in the expiratory limb of the ventilator circuit, and mixed exhaled gas is drawn from the mixing chamber for analysis of FeO_2 and $FeCO_2$. *Arrows* indicate direction of gas flow. (Modified from Witte MK: Metabolic measurements during mechanical ventilation in the pediatric intensive care unit. Respir Care Clin N Am 2:573, 1996.)

Box 21-4 Preparation for Indirect Calorimetry

30 HOURS BEFORE TEST
- 24-hour urine urea nitrogen collection (with sufficient time to receive result) if determination of carbohydrate, fat, and protein use desired

10 HOURS BEFORE TEST
- Patient fasting if measuring energy requirements; if feeding is continued, results will reflect the patient's energy expenditure in response to feeding (may be spuriously high if patient is being overfed)

4 HOURS BEFORE TEST
- Patient resting and avoiding physical activity, physical therapy, dressing changes

2 HOURS BEFORE TEST
- Endotracheal tube suctioned for the last time before test; further ventilator changes or suctioning avoided

1 HOUR BEFORE TEST
- Supine position, complete rest; analgesic or sedative administered if needed

Box 21-5 Equations Used to Calculate $\dot{V}O_2$ and $\dot{V}CO_2$ Using the Gas Exchange Method

$\dot{V}O_2 = \dot{V}E \times [3\ FiO_2 4] - (\dot{V}E \times FeO_2)$
$\dot{V}CO_2 = \dot{V}E \times FeCO_2$
$RQ = \dot{V}CO_2/\dot{V}O_2$

Because standard modes of O_2 therapy do not deliver a consistent FiO_2 to spontaneously breathing patients, special delivery systems must be used. To overcome this problem, the clinician can substitute a precise O_2 mixture for the air used to clear the canopy. Alternatively, one can place a large gas reservoir (e.g., a Douglas bag) between an O_2 flow source and the subject[36]; this ensures that the FiO_2 remains stable throughout the test procedure.

Problems and Limitations

Indirect calorimetry is a technically complex procedure that requires rigorous attention to both instrument and procedure quality control. Regarding instrumentation, small errors in measurements can result in large errors in calculated O_2, CO_2, and energy expenditure. For this reason, the calorimeter's gas analyzers and volume measurement device must be properly calibrated before each patient use. Gas analyzers should be accurate to the hundredth percent and linear over the clinical range of O_2 concentrations.[38,39]

Regarding procedure quality control, it is essential that measurements be made during steady-state conditions. Although proper patient preparation (see Box 21-4) is helpful in this regard, steady-state conditions can be confirmed only during the test procedure itself. A common standard for ensuring steady-state conditions is five consecutive 1-minute averages with a variability of 5% or less.[36]

Perhaps the most significant problem in performing indirect calorimetry on mechanically ventilated patients is the presence of leaks (circuit, tracheal tube cuff, chest tubes).[33] Because any leak would invalidate test results, no procedure should begin until a leak-free patient-ventilator-calorimeter system is confirmed. Other sources of error during open-circuit indirect calorimetry of mechanically ventilated patients are listed in Box 21-6.[33]

Interpretation and Use of Results

Results obtained from indirect calorimetry are used to assess metabolic status and to plan nutrition support. In regard to assessing metabolic status, the first step is to compare the REE obtained by calorimetry with the REE predicted by the Harris-Benedict equations. If the calorimetry REE is within 10% of the predicted value, the patient is considered **normometabolic.** Measured REEs greater than 10% above predicted values indicate a hypermetabolic state, whereas values less than 90% of predicted indicate hypometabolism.

The second step in metabolic assessment is to interpret the RQ. The RQ is the ratio of moles of CO_2 expired to

Box 21-6 Sources of Error During Open-Circuit Indirect Calorimetry of Mechanically Ventilated Patients

- Instability of FiO_2 because of changes in source gas pressure or ventilator/blender variability
- Delivery of high FiO_2 levels (>0.60)
- Inability to separate inspired and expired gases because of bias flow from flow-triggering systems, intermittent mandatory ventilation systems, or specific ventilator characteristics
- Presence of anesthetic gases or gases other than O_2, CO_2, and nitrogen in the ventilation system
- Presence of water vapor resulting in sensor malfunction
- Inappropriate calibration
- Adverse effect on functions of some ventilators (triggering, expiratory resistance, pressure measurement)
- Total circuit flow exceeding internal calorimeter flow (if using dilutional principle)
- Concurrent peritoneal dialysis or hemodialysis

TABLE 21-6

Interpretation and Use of the Respiratory Quotient (RQ)

Value	Interpretation	General Nutrition Strategy
>1.00	Overfeeding	Decrease total kcal
0.9-1.00	Carbohydrate oxidation	Decrease carbohydrates or increase lipids
0.8-0.9	Fat, protein, and carbohydrate oxidation	Target range for mixed substrate
0.7-0.8	Fat and protein oxidation Starvation	Increase total kcal

Note: Acute hyperventilation or acute metabolic acidosis increases RQ and can lead to misinterpretation. Metabolism of ketones or ethyl alcohol decreases RQ to <0.7.

moles of O_2 consumed. The RQ correlates to the ratio of percent calories provided to the percent calories required. Traditionally, the RQ has been used to determine substrate use, where carbohydrates have an RQ of 1.0, protein has an RQ of 0.82, and fat has an RQ of 0.7. Table 21-6 outlines the basic significance of the RQ relative to substrate use and traditional nutrition strategies.[36] The RQ has been shown more recently to have low sensitivity and reduced specificity in critically ill patients.[37] This finding limits the RQ as an indicator for substrate use. The RQ may be low in an overfed patient because of a shift in substrates secondary to inflammatory mediators. If the RQ is outside its physiologic range of 0.67 to 1.3, this should alert the clinician to assess the validity of the study.

MINI CLINI

Metabolic Assessment Based on Indirect Calorimetry

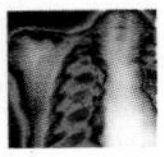

PROBLEM: Interpret the following indirect calorimetry (IC) results obtained on four patients, each with a Harris-Benedict predicted REE of 1500 kcal/day receiving 1850 kcal/day of mixed substrate with an expected RQ of 0.85.

Patient	IC Results	Interpretation
1	REE (IC) = 1500; RQ = 0.85	Patient is normometabolic and receiving the correct amount of kilocalories. RQ is normal.
2	REE (IC) = 2000; RQ = 0.76	Patient is hypermetabolic and receiving an inadequate amount of kilocalories. RQ is lower than expected because of metabolism of endogenous fat and protein sources.
3	REE (IC) = 1200; RQ = 0.95	Patient is hypometabolic and receiving too many kilocalories. RQ is high, reflecting lipogenesis caused by overfeeding.
4	REE (IC) = 1500; RQ = 0.94	Patient is normometabolic and receiving the correct amount of kilocalories, but RQ is higher than expected. Possible causes include the patient is receiving more kilocalories from carbohydrates than expected, acute hyperventilation, acute metabolic acidosis, or inaccurate measurement.

From McArthur C: Indirect calorimetry. Respir Care Clin N Am 3:291, 1997.

Alternative Resting Energy Expenditure Measures

In patients with pulmonary artery catheters, REE can be measured using a modification of the Fick equation:

$$REE\ (kcal/day) = \text{Cardiac output} \times \text{Hemoglobin} \times (SaO_2 - S\bar{v}O_2) \times 95.18$$

In a patient with cardiac output of 4.2 L, hemoglobin of 11 g/dl, SaO_2 of 89%, and $S\bar{v}O_2$ of 69%, the REE would be computed as follows:

$$REE = 4.2 \times 11 \times (0.89 - 0.69) \times 95.18$$
$$REE = 4.2 \times 11 \times (0.20) \times 95.18$$
$$REE = 879\ kcal/day$$

GENERAL ASPECTS OF NUTRITION SUPPORT

The primary goal of nutrition support is the maintenance or restoration of lean body (skeletal muscle) mass. This goal is accomplished by (1) meeting the patient's overall energy needs and (2) providing the appropriate combination of substrates to do so. The route of administration used to provide the support is also important.

Meeting Overall Energy Needs

When the patient's REE is derived, it needs to be adjusted to account for variations in activity and stress levels. If using the Harris-Benedict equations, it is recommended that the predicted REE be corrected for both stress and activity levels (see Table 21-5).[11] When the REE is derived from indirect calorimetry, a stress or activity factor should not be used.

Insufficient Energy Consumed

Malnutrition results from insufficient energy (calorie) intake over time. This insufficient intake leads to a state of impaired metabolism in which the intake of essential nutrients falls short of the body's needs. Certain factors may place a patient at risk for malnutrition (Box 21-7).

Protein-Energy Malnutrition

Protein-energy malnutrition (PEM) has adverse effects on respiratory musculature and the immune response.[15] PEM may be either primary or secondary. Primary PEM results from inadequate intake of calories or protein or both and is typically seen only in developing countries.[10]

Secondary PEM is due to underlying illness. Illness may cause (1) decreased caloric or protein intake (e.g., anorexia, dysphagia); (2) increased nutrient losses (e.g., malabsorption or diarrhea); and (3) increased nutrient demands (e.g., injury or infection).[32] Secondary PEM may be present in 50% of hospital patients.

When PEM is due to inadequate nutrient intake or excessive loss, the body responds by decreasing its metabolic rate, ventilatory drive, thyroid function, and adrenergic activity.[34] As calorie intake decreases, energy for metabolic processes is initially supplied by converting liver glycogen stores into glucose *(gluconeogenesis)*. However, liver reserves of glycogen are adequate for less than 1 day at rest and only a few hours during exercise.[8] Thereafter, endogenous fat stores are mobilized in the form of free fatty acids *(ketogenesis)*. When fat stores are depleted, nutrient needs must be met by catabolizing skeletal muscle protein. This type of PEM usually manifests as a gradual wasting process, as seen in patients with chronic diseases such as cancer and emphysema. The primary clinical sign is progressive weight loss.

When PEM is due to increased demand for nutrients, metabolism, thyroid function, and adrenergic activity all increase. Visceral protein levels tend to decrease early in the course of illness and are associated with impaired immunity.[34] This type of PEM typically occurs with acute catabolic disease, such as in sepsis, burns, or trauma. Weight loss and depletion of muscle and fat stores generally do not occur because of the rapidity of onset of the underlying disease.[11] The two types of PEM are often referred to as *marasmus* and *kwashiorkor*,[2,10,11] as previously described (see Table 21-3).

Box 21-7 Patients at High Risk for Malnutrition

- Underweight (% ideal body weight <90%) or recent loss of ≥10% of usual body weight
- Poor intake: Anorexia, food avoidance (e.g., psychiatric condition), "nothing allowed by mouth" (NPO) status for >5-7 days
- Protracted nutrient losses: Malabsorption, enteric fistulas, draining abscesses or wounds, renal dialysis
- Hypermetabolic states: Sepsis, protracted fever, extensive trauma, or burns
- Chronic use of alcohol or drugs with antinutrient or catabolic properties: Steroids, antimetabolites (e.g., methotrexate), immunosuppressants, antitumor agents
- Impoverishment, isolation, advanced age, limited mobility

Micronutrient Malnutrition

The same problems that lead to PEM can produce deficiencies in micronutrients. Deficiencies of nutrients that are stored only in small amounts (e.g., water-soluble vitamins) or are lost through external secretions (e.g., zinc in diarrhea fluid or burn exudate) are quite common.[10] Although the causes and results of micronutrient deficiencies are beyond the scope of this chapter, a few of the most common problems are described.

Signs of scurvy (vitamin C deficiency) may be observed in chronically ill patients and patients with alcoholism hospitalized for acute illnesses. Low folic acid blood levels are common wherever illness, alcoholism, or poverty is present. Alcoholism is also associated with thiamin deficiency. Zinc deficiencies can impair clotting, slow wound healing, and impair immunity. Magnesium deficiencies can result in cardiac, vascular, neurologic, and electrolyte abnormalities (hypocalcemia, hypokalemia) and in decreases in respiratory muscle strength. Hypophosphatemia is seen frequently with cachexia or alcoholism, especially in patients receiving intravenous glucose or taking antacids. Severe hypophosphatemia can result in decreased muscle strength and contractility and acute cardiopulmonary failure.

Box 21-8 Respiratory Consequences of Malnutrition

RESPIRATORY MUSCLE DYSFUNCTION
- Loss of diaphragmatic mass and contractility
- Loss of accessory muscle mass and contractility

EFFECT ON CONTROL OF VENTILATION
- Decreased hypoxic and hypercapnic response

INCREASED INCIDENCE OF RESPIRATORY INFECTIONS
- Decreased lung clearance mechanisms
- Decreased secretory IgA
- Increased bacterial colonization

CHANGES IN LUNG PARENCHYMAL STRUCTURE
- Unopposed enzymatic digestion
- Reduced production of surfactant

Respiratory Consequences of Malnutrition

Malnutrition affects all organ systems. In addition, malnutrition seems to interact with disease processes to increase the morbidity and mortality of respiratory, cardiac, and renal failure.[34] Specific effects of malnutrition on the respiratory system are listed in Box 21-8.[11,13]

Approximately one-third of all patients with acute respiratory failure have malnutrition. In these patients, the underlying diseases (e.g., sepsis, burns, trauma) increase energy expenditure and promote skeletal muscle catabolism. These patients are prone to hypercapnia and can be difficult to wean from ventilatory support. Malnourished patients who require mechanical ventilatory support also have higher mortality rates than patients with normal nutrition status.[11]

Malnutrition also plays a role in chronic obstructive pulmonary disease (COPD). The combined effect of increased energy expenditure (because of high work of breathing) and inadequate caloric intake contributes to a marasmus-type malnutrition. The resulting progressive muscle weakness and dyspnea can limit caloric intake further, as can several profound psychosocial factors. Box 21-9 summarizes the factors contributing to malnutrition in patients with COPD.[15,17] The RT may notice signs that could lead to malnutrition in patients for whom they provide care (Box 21-10).

Providing the Appropriate Combination of Substrates

After energy requirements are estimated, the patient's physician or registered dietitian determines the appropriate combination of macronutrients (protein, carbohydrate, fat) needed.

Box 21-9 Underlying Causes of Malnutrition in Patients With Chronic Obstructive Pulmonary Disease

INCREASED ENERGY EXPENDITURE
- Increased caloric cost of breathing
- Increased systemic inflammation
- Thermogenic effect of medications (e.g., bronchodilators)

INADEQUATE CALORIC INTAKE
- Dyspnea while eating
- Chewing and swallowing difficulties
- Early satiety
- Taste alterations from medications, nasal cannulas, or a tracheostomy
- Suppressed appetite from medications (e.g., theophylline)

PSYCHOSOCIAL FACTORS
- Depression
- Poverty
- Difficulty shopping
- Tire easily when preparing food

Box 21-10 Nutrition Status Changes Observable by Respiratory Therapists

- Mechanics of breathing impacted by cachexia, obesity, pregnancy
- Increased coughing effort may indicate poor nutrition
- Viscosity of sputum, jugular venous pressure, ascites, edema suggest fluid imbalance
- Lung crackles relate to fluid overload or oncotic pressure changes (loss of blood protein)
- Wheezing may be associated with food intolerances, alcohol, aspirated food particles
- Late inspiratory crackles of atelectasis may result from decreased surfactant production from malnutrition
- S_3 heart sounds of congestive heart failure may indicate fluid imbalance
- S_4 heart sounds may be associated with severe anemia
- Pulmonary function measures may be related to:

FVC or FEV_1 decrease—severe malnutrition
FVC—excess fat weight
PEP and PIP decrease—poor nutrition
Lung compliance—fluid and serum albumin changes acutely or chronic malnutrition

- Arterial blood gas values may be related to:

$PaCO_2$ increases—excess glucose, inadequate ventilation from lack of muscle energy
O_2 saturation, O_2 content, hemoglobin—nutrition status

- Meal acceptance may be related to visible equipment—suction bottles, sputum specimens
- Lack of O_2 may increase difficulty of eating—ensure availability of O_2 via cannula if needed

FEV_1, Forced expiratory volume in 1 second; *FVC,* forced vital capacity; *PEP,* positive expiratory pressure; *PIP,* peak inspiratory pressure.

Protein

Amino acids or proteins are essential to maintaining or restoring lean body mass. Because illness usually increases protein catabolism and protein requirements, the Recommended Dietary Allowance (RDA) of 0.8 g/kg/day is generally insufficient for sick patients. Based on the assessment of the protein catabolism rate (see previous equations for nitrogen balance), protein intake may need to be doubled or tripled above the RDA (1.5 to 2.5 g/kg/day).[15,40] Ideally, approximately 20% of a patient's estimated calorie needs should be provided by protein. Higher percentages of protein may be needed in cachexic patients, critically ill patients, and patients with severe infections. However, whenever high protein intakes are given, the patient should be monitored for progressive **azotemia** (blood urea nitrogen >100 mg/dl).

Too much protein is harmful, especially for patients with limited pulmonary reserves. Excess protein can increase O_2 consumption, REE, minute ventilation, and central ventilatory drive.[41] In addition, overzealous protein feeding may lead to symptoms such as dyspnea in patients with chronic pulmonary disease.

Carbohydrate

Adequate amounts of carbohydrates and fat help prevent protein catabolism. Glucose (dextrose) is the most commonly administered intravenous carbohydrate. For critically ill patients, 50% to 60% of the total daily calories can be in the form of simple carbohydrate.[16,40,42] In an average-sized patient, daily glucose provision should be 300 to 400 g/day or less. Glucose blood levels should be monitored and maintained at less than 200 mg/dl.[16]

For patients with pulmonary disease or patients requiring mechanical ventilation, high carbohydrate loads can cause problems. High carbohydrate loads increase CO_2 production and the RQ, resulting in increased ventilatory demand, O_2 consumption, and work of breathing.[40] Although the observed effects are usually modest, some patients with limited functional reserves cannot tolerate these changes, resulting in development or worsening of ventilatory failure. More recent evidence indicates that this problem is probably more closely related to total calorie load (overfeeding) than to the proportion of carbohydrate in the diet.[10] Based on this knowledge, overfeeding should be carefully avoided in patients with pulmonary disease and patients requiring mechanical ventilation.

Fat

The remaining calories (20% to 30%) should be provided from fat.[39,40] In critically ill patients, current guidelines support increased levels of omega-3 fatty acid intake to modulate inflammation, to enhance immune response, and ultimately to support recovery.[41,42] Fat intakes greater than 50% of energy needs have been associated with fever, impaired immune function, liver dysfunction, and hypotension.

The initiation of nutrition support is determined by the patient's nutrition status and the estimated length of time the patient will be unable to consume a diet by mouth to meet his or her nutrition needs. To ensure a satisfactory nutrition and metabolic response, early enteral nutrition begun within 24 to 48 hours provides significant benefits to critically ill patients, including reduced infectious complications and lengths of stay.[42]

Routes of Administration

There are two primary routes for supplying nutrients to patients: *enteral* (oral and tube feeding) and *parenteral* (peripheral or central venous alimentation). Box 21-11 provides guidelines for initiating nutrition support as recommended by the American Society for Parenteral and Enteral Nutrition.[46-48]

Enteral Feeding

Enteral feedings are the route of choice: "If the gut works, use it." The enteral route is safer and cheaper to use than the parenteral route. Enteral feeding stimulates gut hormones, subjects nutrients to the absorptive and metabolic controls of the intestinal tract and liver, and produces less

Box 21-11 Guidelines for Initiation of Nutrition Support

CLINICAL SETTINGS WHERE ENTERAL NUTRITION SHOULD BE PART OF ROUTINE CARE

- Protein-calorie malnutrition (>10% loss of usual weight or serum albumin <3.5 g/dl) with inadequate oral intake of nutrients for previous 5-7 days
- Normal nutritional status with <50% of required nutrient intake orally for previous 7-10 days
- Severe dysphagia
- Burns of >15% total BSA in infants and children and >25% total BSA in older children and adults
- Massive small bowel resection in combination with administration of total parenteral nutrition
- Low output (<500 ml/day) enterocutaneous fistulas

CLINICAL SETTINGS WHERE PARENTERAL NUTRITION SHOULD BE PART OF ROUTINE CARE

- Patients with inability to absorb nutrients by the GI tract
- Patients undergoing high-dose chemotherapy, radiation, and bone marrow transplantation
- Moderate to severe pancreatitis (bowel rest anticipated beyond 5-7 days)
- Severe malnutrition in the face of a nonfunctional GI tract (within 1-3 days)
- Severely catabolic patients with or without malnutrition when the GI tract is not usable within 7-10 days

From Merritt RJ, editor: The A.S.P.E.N. nutrition support practice manual, Silver Spring, MD, 2005, ASPEN.
BSA, Body surface area.

hyperglycemia (providing for better immune function) than the parenteral route. In addition, the buffering capacity of enteral feeding can improve resistance against stress ulcers. Finally, enteral feeding maintains a more normal intestinal mucosa than the parenteral route (the intestinal mucosa may undergo atrophy during parenteral nutrition).[10]

Enteral Tube Routes. There are six primary sites for enteral tube feeding: nasogastric, nasoduodenal, nasojejunal, gastrostomy, jejunostomy, and esophagotomy. Site selection depends on GI function, respiratory status, surgical state, and anticipated length of time the patient will be receiving tube feeding.

Gastric feedings are indicated if there are no physiologic factors affecting GI function, such as gastroparesis, delayed gastric emptying, or obstruction or surgery in the upper GI tract. Small bowel (duodenum and jejunal) feedings are indicated if the upper GI tract cannot be used. Intestinal feeding tube placement is often recommended to minimize the risk of aspiration because it is believed to decrease the risk of gastric distention and gastroesophageal reflux; however, this has not yet been convincingly shown.[49]

Nasogastric and *nasoenteric* tubes are indicated if the duration of enteral therapy is anticipated to be short (<30 days). The tubes can be placed at the bedside and generally have a large internal diameter, which helps deliver viscous feedings and medications. *Nasoduodenal* and *nasojejunal* tubes are placed through the nose past the pylorus.

Long-term feeding tubes can be placed endoscopically and surgically. Percutaneous endoscopic placement of a feeding tube can be done to establish gastric (percutaneous endoscopic gastrostomy) or intestinal (percutaneous endoscopic jejunostomy) access. This method is generally preferred to surgical placement because it is associated with reduced costs, lack of need for operating room time, and lack of need for anesthesia.[50] Surgical laparotomy is indicated if endoscopy is contraindicated.

Tube Feeding Administration. There are three basic methods of tube feeding administration: bolus, intermittent, and continuous drip. *Bolus* feedings involve the rapid infusion of 250 to 500 ml of feeding several times daily. Feedings are provided by a syringe into the feeding tube port. There is an increased risk of aspiration associated with bolus feedings because of the rapid infusion of formula into the stomach. Nausea, vomiting, abdominal pain, and distention can develop in conjunction with this feeding route. This feeding method can be used only with gastric tubes and is primarily applied to patients who are stable and patients receiving enteral nutrition support at home.

Intermittent feedings are also administered several times per day, but they are infused over at least a 30-minute period. Feedings can be given only into the gastric cavity. Intermittent feedings are associated with the same problems as bolus feedings.

Continuous drip infusion provides a constant, steady flow of formula at a predetermined rate for a set period, generally 12 to 24 hours per day. Drip regulators, roll clamps, or pumps are used to control rates. Because the small bowel lacks storage capacity, feedings delivered beyond the pylorus must be provided by the continuous drip method. This method is generally preferred for critically ill patients because it is usually associated with less gastric residual volume, less abdominal distention, less gastroesophageal reflux, and a decreased incidence of aspiration.[49]

Enteral Formula Selection. Selection of an enteral formula depends on the patient's medical and surgical state, GI function, energy and nutrient needs, and route of administration. There are eight broad categories of enteral formulas: oral supplements, blenderized, whole protein lactose-free, fiber containing, nutrient dense, elemental, disease specific, and modular. Table 21-7 describes the indications for the various formulas and lists examples of commercial preparations.

Complications of Enteral Therapy. Complications occurring in patients receiving enteral nutrition are categorized as GI, mechanical, or metabolic. Complications may be avoided by careful selection of formulas, proper administration, and consistent monitoring of the patient.

Pulmonary aspiration is of particular concern in a critically ill patient with respiratory disease. Aspiration can occur if the patient is lying flat, has a depressed gag reflux, has delayed gastric emptying, or has improper tube placement. The incidence of pulmonary aspiration varies depending on the patient population and technique used to identify aspiration in the tube-fed patient. The two most important ways to minimize the likelihood of aspiration are (1) to raise the head of the bed at least 45 degrees and (2) to deliver the feeding beyond the pylorus using the continuous drip method in patients at risk for gastric atony or with gastroesophageal reflux. Tube placement always should be verified by x-ray examination before feeding.

Aggressive suctioning of oropharyngeal secretions can help prevent aspiration. The greatest risk is in patients with endotracheal tubes. Endotracheal tubes increase aspiration risk because they alter sensation, impair glottic closure, increase secretion volume, and act as "wicks" to allow secretions to enter the airway.[49] The use of special endotracheal tubes that provide continuous aspiration of subglottic secretions may help overcome the leakage-type aspiration that is so common in tube-fed patients.[51] The use of blue dye to detect aspiration is no longer a standard practice because of numerous problems surrounding the practice including a U.S. Food and Drug Administration Public Health Advisory issued in 2003. Blue discoloration of body parts and fluids followed by refractory hypotension, metabolic acidosis, and death were reported in some patients receiving blue food dye.

TABLE 21-7

Enteral Product Reference Guide

Category	Indications	Examples
Oral supplements	Given with an oral diet to increase calorie and protein intake	Boost*†, Carnation Instant Breakfast*
Blenderized	Made from natural foods and usually lower in sucrose and corn syrup than other formulas; beneficial if intolerance to synthetic formulas exists	Compleat*, Compleat Modified*†
Fiber containing	Dietary fiber can increase stool bulk and transit time, decrease intraluminal pressure, and improve bowel motility	Jevity*†, FiberSource*†, Nutren 1.0 with Fiber*†
Nutrient dense	Increased calories in a limited volume; useful in hypermetabolic states (burns, trauma, sepsis, major surgery) and congestive heart failure	Two Cal HN*†, Ensure Plus*†, Deliver*†, Nutren 2.0*†
Elemental	Impaired GI function with impaired ability to digest or absorb intact nutrients	Peptamen†, Vital HN†, Criticare†, Vivonex TEN†, Subdue Plus†, Alitraq†
Disease specific	Liver disease; renal disease; pulmonary disease; glucose intolerance; fat modified, trauma; immune-enhancing	Nutrihep*†, Deliver 2.0*†; Nepro*†, Magnacal Renal*†, NovaSource Renal*†; Pulmocare*†, NutriVent*†, Respalor*†; Diabetisource*†, Glucerna*†, Choice DMTF*†, Glytrol*†; Travasorb MCT, Portagen, Advera*†, Lipisorb*†; TraumaCal*†; Impact*†, Advera*†, Lipisorb*†
Modular	Need to modify a single nutrient (carbohydrate, protein, fat)	Polycose, Promod, Microlipid, MCT oil

*Intact nutrients.
†Lactose-free.

Parenteral Nutrition Support

When it is impossible to provide nutrition support through the GI tract, intravenous or parenteral nutrition support may be needed. Parenteral nutrition support can be administered through a peripheral or central vein. Ideally, the vascular access line should be isolated and maintained as a sterile route and not used for any other purpose. Because the volume and concentration of nutrients given through a small vein are limited, peripheral parenteral nutrition is generally considered only for short-term support. Mechanical, infectious, and metabolic complications have been reported in patients fed parenterally.[52]

NUTRITION SUPPORT IN SPECIFIC CIRCUMSTANCES

Details on the appropriate nutrition support provided to all the various types of patients seen by RTs are beyond the scope of this chapter. This section emphasizes key points related to nutrition support and management of the most common conditions encountered by practitioners.

General Guidelines for Critically Ill Patients

The general goals of nutrition support in critically ill patients are to (1) provide for energy needs; (2) maintain nitrogen balance; (3) provide adequate (not excessive) calories to preserve lean body mass (muscle); (4) provide a positive nitrogen balance; (5) provide adequate vitamins, minerals, and fat; and (6) provide appropriate fluid.[53] Table 21-8 outlines the general guidelines recommended to achieve these goals.[53]

Systemic Inflammatory Response Syndrome

The *systemic inflammatory response syndrome* underlies many critical illnesses, including *sepsis* and *acute respiratory distress syndrome (ARDS)*. Metabolism in systemic inflammatory response syndrome is characterized by increased total caloric requirements, hyperglycemia, triglyceride intolerance, increased net protein catabolism, and increased macronutrient and micronutrient requirements.[16] Caloric requirements may need to be increased by 10% to 20%. If blood glucose level exceeds 225 mg/dl, glucose intake must be reduced, insulin must be given, or both. Because of the hypercatabolic state, protein administration may need to be increased to 1.7 to 2.0 g/kg/day. If serum triglycerides exceed 500 mg/dl, total calories or the dose of polyunsaturated fatty acids, or both, should be reduced.[15] Enteral supplementation with omega-3 fatty acid may have a beneficial effect in treatment for ARDS. Omega-3 fatty acids have been observed to reduce inflammation, improve oxygenation, and improve outcomes in these patients.[44,45]

Requirements for micronutrients are also increased in systemic inflammatory response syndrome. Because of the potential high losses of potassium, zinc, magnesium, calcium, and phosphorus, serum levels of these minerals need to be closely monitored and maintained within the normal range.[16]

TABLE 21-8

General Nutrition Guidelines for Chronically Critically Ill Patients

Category	Guideline
Energy need	Provide 25-30 kcal/kg/day for men and 20-25 kcal/kg/day for women in volume consistent with total fluid needs of the patient (approximately 1 ml H_2O/kcal) or use Harris-Benedict equations times a stress factor of 1.2-1.4
Protein	20% of total calories/day; 1-2 g/kg/day and adjust by periodic monitoring of nitrogen balance
Carbohydrate	60%-70% total calories/day. Fat 20%-30% total calories/day; provide essential fatty acids
Micronutrients	Adequate vitamins and minerals such as vitamins A, B_6, C, E; potassium; magnesium; zinc; iron; selenium; phosphate
Fluid	Approximately 1 ml/kcal
Specialized nutrients	Glutamine (may improve nitrogen stores), arginine (may improve immune system), and omega-3 fatty acids (may reduce inflammatory processes)
Route of delivery	Use enteral nutrition unless the gut is not functioning, then choose total parenteral nutrition

Compiled from Pingleton SK: Nutrition in chronic critical illness. Clin Chest Med 22:149, 2001.

Mechanical Ventilation

Adequate nutrition support is crucial for ventilator-dependent patients. During acute illness, proper nutrition helps prevent the loss of lean body mass. After the resolution of the acute phase of illness, good nutrition helps the muscles regain strength and improves the likelihood of successful ventilator weaning.[43]

For most patients requiring ventilatory support, following the general guidelines provided in Table 21-8 suffices. As always, care must be taken to avoid overfeeding and the increased ventilatory demands that follow. Patients with COPD present a special situation, in terms of both nutrition needs and ventilatory support. More details regarding these patients are provided in the next section.

Nutrition support alone is insufficient to ensure weaning of ventilator-dependent patients. For these patients, appropriate nutrition may need to be combined with a tailored exercise program designed to strengthen and retrain muscles. Methods used to wean ventilator-dependent patients are discussed in detail in Chapter 47.

Chronic Obstructive Pulmonary Disease

Malnutrition occurs in 70% of patients with COPD,[54] and it is most evident in patients with pulmonary emphysema. Progressive weight loss is common. Malnutrition seems to have two causes: an insufficient intake for a prolonged period and increased nutrient needs because of chronic increases in metabolism. Malnutrition and low body weight seem to be independent factors associated with a poor prognosis.[55]

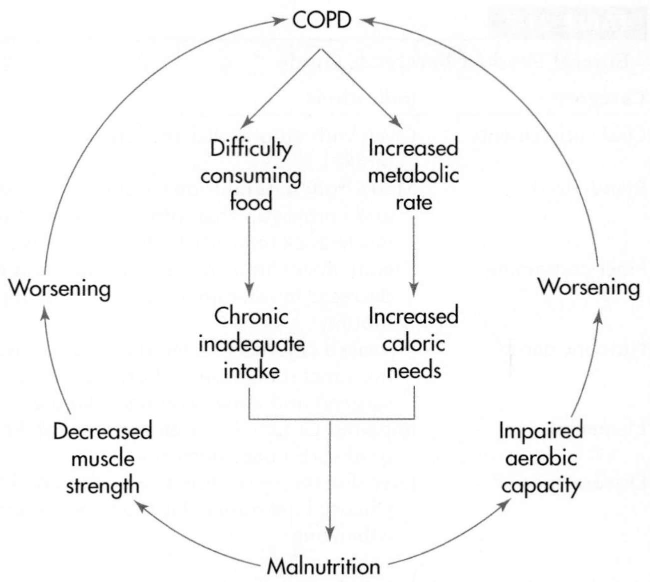

FIGURE 21-6 The vicious cycle of respiratory impairment and malnutrition in COPD.

The degree of weight loss generally correlates with deterioration of pulmonary function values. COPD can create a cycle in which respiratory dysfunction promotes weight loss, and weight loss further hinders respiratory function.[10] Figure 21-6 illustrates the cycle.

Factors contributing to poor intake include fatigue, shortness of breath, frequent coughing, early fullness because of pressure on the abdominal cavity, increased dyspnea during eating, side effects from medications (nausea, vomiting, diarrhea, dry mouth, taste changes), and depression. The increased metabolic rate is due to the added effort to breathe and frequent respiratory infections, both of which increase calorie and fluid needs.

The goal for the health care team is to increase nutrient intake carefully without overfeeding the patient. For most COPD patients, 1.2 to 1.5 times the REE for energy and 1.2 to 1.7 g/kg body weight for protein are sufficient. If the patient is malnourished, additional calories and protein are needed to replenish body stores. Cachexic patients with COPD should be refed cautiously.[56] Functional capacity and the patient's overall health status may improve with an anabolic stimulus, such as exercise, along with nutrition supplementation.[57]

In patients with COPD without hypercapnia, conventional macronutrient allocations are satisfactory (15% to 20% as protein, 50% to 60% as carbohydrates, and 20% to 30% as fat). For patients with hypercapnia, the diet should be individually tailored to provide the lowest percentage of fat that maintains an acceptable $PaCO_2$.[10] However, as

Box 21-12 Sample Foods and Methods to Increase Nutrient Intake

- Dried fruits, nuts, popsicles, milkshakes
- Whole milk or skim milk powder added to milk, soup, gravies
- Nutrition supplements
- Rich desserts—cheesecake, pie, cake, pastries
- Puddings, custards, yogurt, ice cream
- Cream soups
- Added butter or margarine or cheese to vegetables
- Casseroles and egg dishes with sauces and gravies
- Fried foods
- Peanut butter or other nut butters, spread on bananas, celery, crackers, apple slices, breads

FOOD PREPARATION SUGGESTIONS

- Pan fry in oil rather than broil
- Use prepared meals for the microwave
- Add skim milk powder, sour cream, cream, cheese to mashed potatoes

Box 21-13 Nutrition Support for Patients With Pulmonary Disease

- Perform a complete nutrition assessment
- Evaluate energy needs and provide an appropriate amount (do not overfeed or underfeed)
- Ensure protein balance
- Monitor fluids and electrolytes, especially phosphorus
- Evaluate vitamin and mineral status as indicated
- Consider high-fat, low-carbohydrate feedings in patients with hypercapnia

previously stated, setting an appropriate total calorie load is more important than fine-tuning the ratio of carbohydrates to fat.

Given the positive link between dietary intake and knowledge of diet and health, good patient education is crucial.[58] Patients should be taught to select easy-to-consume, calorically dense foods (Box 21-12). Emphasis should be placed on small, frequent feedings, and use of high-calorie, high-protein nutrition supplements should be encouraged. Because many of the listed foods are not consistent with publicly disseminated guidelines, health care team members need to explain and justify the differences. Other considerations in providing nutrition support to patients with COPD are listed in Box 21-13.[10] Medications prescribed for patients with respiratory disease may influence food intake or interact with foods. Common medications with their effects on nutrition are listed in Table 21-9.[59,60]

TABLE 21-9 Common Respiratory Medication Interactions With Food

Medication*	Interactions With Food
Beta-2 Agonists	
Albuterol	Peculiar taste, sore/dry throat, nausea/vomiting, dyspepsia, diarrhea, increased appetite or anorexia, limit caffeine
Proventil	
Ventolin	
Salmeterol xinafoate	Dental pain, decreased salivation, candidiasis, pharyngitis, throat irritation, nausea/vomiting, stomachache, diarrhea
Advair Diskus	
Serevent Diskus	
Metaproterenol sulfate	
Alupent	Dry mouth/throat, nausea/vomiting, dyspepsia, diarrhea, limit caffeine
Terbutaline	
Brethaire	Dry mouth/throat and unusual taste (inhalant), nausea/vomiting, dyspepsia, limit caffeine
Anticholinergics	
Ipratropium bromide	
Atrovent	Dry mouth/throat, metallic/bitter taste, nausea, dyspepsia. Do not use inhaler with soy or peanut allergy. Caution with lactation
Inhaler	
Nasal spray	
Tiotropium bromide	
Spiriva HandiHaler	Dry mouth, dyspepsia, abdominal pain, constipation, nausea/vomiting. Caution with lactation
Mucolytic Agents	
Dornase alfa	
Pulmozyme	Sore throat, laryngitis
Corticosteroids	
Beclomethasone	Dry mouth, decreased sense of taste, oral candidiasis, sore throat, nausea/vomiting
Beconase nasal inhaler	Rinse mouth after use and do not swallow rinse water. Nasal: Caution with lactation
Beconase AQ nasal spray	Oral: Do not use with lactation
Vancenase Pockethaler nasal inhaler	
Vancenase AQ nasal spray	
Qvar oral inhalant CFC-free (chlorofluorocarbons free)	
Triamcinolone acetonide	

Continued

TABLE 21-9

Common Respiratory Medication Interactions With Food—cont'd

Medication*	Interactions With Food
Azmacort	Oral candidiasis, dry mouth, toothache, sore throat, pharyngitis with aerosol, nausea, abdominal pain, diarrhea. Rinse mouth after use and do not swallow rinse water
Flunisolide	Nausea/vomiting, sore throat, unpleasant taste, loss of smell, abdominal pain, heartburn, constipation, gas
AeroBid	
Fluticasone propionate	Nausea/vomiting, diarrhea, dyspepsia, stomach disorder
Advair Diskus	
Flovent	
Budesonide	
Pulmicort	Oral candidiasis, dyspepsia, gastroenteritis, nausea/vomiting, diarrhea
Mediator Antagonists	
Cromolyn sodium	
Intal	Take 30 min before meals and snacks. Open capsule and dissolve powder in 4 oz hot water; add 4 oz cold water (not juice, milk, or food). Unpleasant aftertaste, nausea. With aerosol/nebulizer: Dry mouth/throat, sore throat. With oral capsule: Abdominal pain, diarrhea
Zafirlukast	
Accolate	Take 1 hr before or 2 hr after food. Nausea/vomiting, dyspepsia, diarrhea, abdominal pain. Food decreased bioavailability of drug 40%
Zileuton	
Zyflo	Dyspepsia, nausea/vomiting, abdominal pain, constipation, flatulence; limit alcohol
Montelukast	
Singulair	Chew tablet well; caution with grapefruit juice—may increase side effects; dyspepsia
Aerosolized Antiinfective Agents	
Ribavirin	
Rebetol	Taste changes, nausea/vomiting, dyspepsia, dry mouth, abdominal pain
Copegus	Do not use with lactation
Tobramycin sulfate	Ensure adequate fluid intake/hydration. Anorexia, weight loss
TOBI (inhalation solution)	Stomatitis, increased salivation, nausea/vomiting

Compiled from the Physicians' desk reference, ed 60, Montvale, NJ, 2006, Medical Economics (www.pdr.net, Accessed August 24, 2006); and Pronsky Z: Food medication interactions, ed 14, Birchrunville, PA, 2006, Food-Medication Interactions.
*The generic name is followed by brand names of the drug.

When patients with COPD are hospitalized for ventilatory failure, the clinical outcome is affected by nutrition support. Patients who receive adequate nutrition support are more readily weaned from mechanical ventilators than patients whose diets are deficient in protein and energy. In patients who are not catabolic, reducing energy intake to a level equal to or just below the REE may also aid weaning.[10] Nutrition support may be ineffective in some patients.[61] Factors associated with such outcomes include aging, anorexia, and elevated inflammatory response.[62]

Asthma

Bronchial asthma is subdivided into allergic asthma and nonallergic asthma. Nutrient-dense small meals are recommended that are high in quality protein, calories, vitamins, and minerals during prolonged asthma attacks. The patient should avoid foods identified as allergens; most often, these foods are milk, eggs, seafood, and fish. Fluid intake should be generous, unless contraindicated. Saturated fats may aggravate the airway, and monounsaturated fats may be inversely related.[63] Omega-3 fatty acids may be beneficial; these are available in walnuts and flaxseed if the patient is allergic to fish.[21]

Cystic Fibrosis

The exocrine gland dysfunction seen in cystic fibrosis (CF) may cause chronic lung disease with recurrent infections. The same disturbance may cause pancreatic insufficiency. Metabolic problems in patients with CF are similar to metabolic problems in patients with COPD, with reduced intake and increased metabolic needs. However, pancreatic insufficiency causes malabsorption of all nutrients, especially fat. The administration of pancreatic enzyme supplements with meals enhances absorption but requires trial and error and intense education on how to balance the amount of food and the intake of enzymes. In addition, the time spent in various treatment programs reduces the ability to consume small frequent feedings.

The goals of nutrition management in CF are to (1) maximize a nutrition intake through calorically dense foods (see Box 21-12), (2) balance intake with pancreatic enzymes to maximize absorption, and (3) provide a nutrition plan that meets the changing clinical and psychosocial needs of the patient.[64] Use of calorically dense nutrition supplements (see Table 21-7) consumed throughout the day has proved helpful in achieving weight gain.[65,66] Because of the malabsorption of micronutrients, vitamin and mineral supplementation is encouraged, especially of fat-soluble vitamins.[15] Evidence suggests that the progressive pulmonary dysfunction seen in CF is partly attributable to nutrition deficiencies that can be readily corrected.[67] Helping CF patients achieve optimal nutritional health may minimize the decline in pulmonary function and improve their quality of life.[68]

SUMMARY CHECKLIST

- Nutrition assessment is the basis for developing a nutrition care plan.
- The ABCDs of nutrition assessment include anthropometry, biochemical indicators, clinical indicators, and dietary history of the patient.
- Body mass index is a comparison of weight to height used to determine underweight, healthy weight, overweight, obesity, or morbid obesity.
- Classifications of undernutrition, called protein-energy malnutrition, include kwashiorkor, marasmus, and a combination of the two (lack of circulating protein, starvation, and a mixture of the two).
- Laboratory values of albumin, transferrin, transthyretin, and retinal-binding protein may indicate malnutrition.
- The creatinine-height index reflects skeletal muscle mass.
- Nitrogen balance compares protein intake to nitrogen excretion in the urine.
- Observable signs in hair, eyes, lips, mouth and gums, skin, and nails may indicate malnutrition.
- Resting energy expenditure (REE) may be determined by the Harris-Benedict equations or indirect calorimetry.
- Estimation of total caloric need involves multiplying the REE by a factor that accounts for activity and stressors.
- Indirect calorimetry involves measurement of whole-body $\dot{V}O_2$, $\dot{V}CO_2$, and respiratory quotient (RQ); results are used to assess a patient's metabolic state, determine nutrition needs, or assess response to nutrition therapy.
- RQ greater than 1.00 indicates overfeeding and the need to decrease total calories; values between 0.7 and 0.8 indicate fat and protein oxidation secondary to starvation and the need to increase total calories.
- Malnutrition is a state of impaired metabolism in which the intake of essential nutrients is less than the body's needs; marasmus is malnutrition associated with inadequate nutrient intake (starvation), and kwashiorkor is the hypercatabolic form.
- Malnutrition can affect the respiratory system by causing loss of respiratory muscle mass and contractility, decreased ventilatory drive, impaired immune response, and alterations in lung parenchymal structure.
- About one-third of all patients with acute respiratory failure have malnutrition, mainly the hypercatabolic form; these patients are prone to hypercapnia, can be difficult to wean from ventilatory support, and have higher mortality rates than patients with a normal nutrition status.
- In chronic lung disease, the combined effect of increased energy expenditure (secondary to increased work of breathing) and inadequate caloric intake contributes to a marasmus-type malnutrition.
- The primary goal of nutrition support is to maintain or restore lean body (skeletal muscle) mass by (1) meeting the overall energy needs of the patient and (2) providing the appropriate combination of macronutrients (protein, carbohydrate, and fat) and micronutrients (vitamins and minerals).
- Predicted REEs should be corrected for both stress and activity levels; typical factors range from 0.7 (for starvation) to 2.0 (for severe burns) of REE calories.
- For most patients, a balance of 20% of daily calorie needs from protein, 50% to 60% from simple carbohydrate, and 20% to 30% from fat is adequate.
- For a patient with pulmonary disease, high carbohydrate loads can increase CO_2 production and the RQ, resulting in increased ventilatory demand, O_2 consumption, and work of breathing.
- Nutrients can be supplied enterally (oral and tube feeding) or parenterally (peripheral or central venous alimentation); the enteral route should be used whenever possible.
- The likelihood of aspiration during tube feedings can be minimized by delivering the feeding beyond the pylorus using the continuous drip method and raising the head of the bed at least 45 degrees.
- Nutrition support should be individualized according to patient needs and condition or disease process; accepted guidelines for systemic inflammatory response syndrome, COPD, mechanical ventilation, asthma, and cystic fibrosis should be followed.

References

1. Insel P, Turner RE, Ross D: Discovering nutrition, Sudbury, MA, 2003, Jones & Bartlett.
2. Whitney EN, Cataldo CB, Rolfes SR: Understanding normal and clinical nutrition, ed 6, Belmont, CA, 2002, Wadsworth.
3. U.S. Department of Agriculture and U.S. Department of Health and Human Services: Report of the Dietary Guidelines Advisory Committee on the dietary guidelines for Americans, Washington, DC, 1995, U.S. Government Printing Office.
4. U.S. Department of Agriculture and U.S. Department of Health and Human Services: Nutrition and your health: dietary guidelines for Americans, Washington, DC, 2005, U.S. Government Printing Office.
5. Lee RD, Neiman DC: Nutritional assessment, ed 4, Boston, 2007, McGraw-Hill.
6. Soler-Cataluna JJ, Sanchez-Sanchez L, Martinez-Garcia MA, et al: Mid-arm muscle area is a better predictor of mortality than body mass index in COPD. Chest 128:2108–2115, 2005.
7. Heymsfield SB, McManus C, Smith J, et al: Anthropometric measurement of muscle mass: revised equations for calculating bone-free arm muscle area. Am J Clin Nutr 1982;66: 289–295.
8. Rolfes SR, Pinna K, Whitney E: Understanding normal and clinical nutrition, ed 7, Belmont, CA, 2006, Thomson & Wadsworth.
9. Heimburger DC: Adulthood. In Shils ME, Shike M, Ross AC, et al, editors: Modern nutrition in health and disease, ed 10, Philadelphia, 2006, Lippincott Williams & Wilkins.
10. Heimburger DC, Weinsier RI: Handbook of clinical nutrition, ed 3, St Louis, 1997, Mosby.

11. Mizock BA, Troglia S: Nutritional support of the hospitalized patient. Dis Mon 43:349–426, 1997.
12. Nelms M: Assessment of nutrition status and risk. In Nelms M, Sucher K, Long S, editors: Nutrition therapy and pathophysiology, Belmont, CA, 2007, Thomson.
13. Carlson TH: Laboratory data in nutrition assessment. In Mahan LK, Escott-Stump S, editors: Krauses's food, nutrition, and diet therapy, ed 11, Philadelphia, 2004, Saunders.
14. Bloch AS, Maillet J, Howell WH, et al, editors: Issues and choices in clinical nutrition practice, Philadelphia, 2007, Lippincott Williams & Wilkins.
15. Hodgkin GE, Maloney S, editors: Loma Linda University diet manual, a handbook supporting vegetarian nutrition, Loma Linda, CA, 2003, Loma Linda University Press.
16. American College of Chest Physicians: Applied nutrition in ICU patients (consensus statement). Chest 111:769, 1997.
17. Bergman EA, Buergel NS: Diseases of the respiratory system. In Nelms M, Sucher K, Long S, editors: Nutrition therapy and pathophysiology, Belmont, CA, 2007, Thomson.
18. U.S. Department of Agriculture: My Pyramid. http://mypyramid.gov. Accessed June 3, 2007.
19. General Conference (of Seventh-day Adventists) Nutrition Council: My vegetarian food pyramid, Silver Spring, MD, 2006, GC Department of Health.
20. Detsky A, McLaughlin JR, Baker JP, et al: Subjective global nutritional assessment. JPEN J Parenter Enteral Nutr 11:8–13, 1987.
21. Escott-Stump S: Nutrition and diagnosis-related care, ed 5, Philadelphia, 2002, Lippincott Williams & Wilkins.
22. Institute of Medicine of the National Academies: Dietary reference intakes for energy, carbohydrate, fiber, fat, fatty acids, cholesterol, protein, and amino acids, Washington, DC, 2002, National Academy Press.
23. Institute of Medicine of the National Academies: Dietary reference intakes for calcium, phosphorous, magnesium, vitamin D, and fluoride, Washington, DC, 1997, National Academy Press.
24. Institute of Medicine of the National Academies: Dietary reference intakes for thiamine, riboflavin, niacin, vitamin B_6, folate, vitamin B_{12}, pantothenic acid, biotin, and choline, Washington, DC, 1998, National Academy Press.
25. Institute of Medicine of the National Academies: Dietary reference intakes for vitamin C, vitamin E, selenium, and carotenoids, Washington, DC, 2000, National Academy Press.
26. Institute of Medicine of the National Academies: Dietary reference intakes for vitamin A, vitamin K, arsenic, boron, chromium, copper, iodine, iron, manganese, molybdenum, nickel, silicon, vanadium, and zinc, Washington, DC, 2001, National Academy Press.
27. Kleinman RE, editor: Pediatric nutrition handbook, ed 5, Elk Grove Village, IL, 2004, American Academy of Pediatrics.
28. Treuth MS, Griffin IJ: Adolescence. In Shils ME, Shike M, Ross AC, et al, editors: Modern nutrition in health and disease, ed 10, Philadelphia, 2006, Lippincott Williams & Wilkins.
29. U.S. Food and Drug Administration: Food label. www.cfsan.fda.gov/label.html. Accessed March, 2007.
30. Morley JE: Nutrition in the older person. In Shils ME, Shike M, Ross AC, et al, editors: Modern nutrition in health and disease, ed 10, Philadelphia, 2006, Lippincott Williams & Wilkins.
31. Grant A, DeHoog S: Nutrition assessment support and management, ed 5, Seattle, WA, 1999, Grant & DeHoog.
32. Kudsk KA, Sacks GA: Nutrition in the care of the patient with surgery, trauma, and sepsis. In Shils ME, Shike M, Ross AC, et al, editors: Modern nutrition in health and disease, ed 10, Philadelphia, 2006, Lippincott Williams & Wilkins.
33. American Association of Respiratory Care: Clinical practice guideline. Respir Care 49:1073, 2004.
34. Grossman GD: Nutritional assessment of critically ill patients. Respir Care 30:463, 1985.
35. McClave SA, McClain CJ, Snider HL: Should indirect calorimetry be used as part of nutritional assessment? J Clin Gastroenterol 33:14, 2001.
36. McArthur C: Indirect calorimetry. Respir Care Clin North Am 3:291, 1997.
37. McClave SA, Lowen CC, Kleber MJ, et al: Clinical use of the respiratory quotient obtained from indirect calorimetry. J Parenter Enteral Nutr 2003;27:21–26.
38. Witte MK: Metabolic measurements during mechanical ventilation in the pediatric intensive care unit. Respir Care Clin N Am 2:573, 1996.
39. Ritz R, Cunningham J: Indirect calorimetry. In Kacmarek RM, Hess DAY, Stoller JK, editors: Monitoring in respiratory care, St Louis, 1993, Mosby.
40. Grant JP: Nutrition care of patients with acute and chronic respiratory failure. Nutr Clin Pract 9:11, 1994.
41. Shikora SA, Benotti PN: Nutritional support of the mechanically ventilated patient. Respir Care Clin North Am 3:69, 1997.
42. Askanazi J: Nutrition for the patient with respiratory failure: glucose versus fat. Anesthesiology 54:373, 1981.
43. Mizock BA: Nutritional support in acute lung injury and acute respiratory distress syndrome. Nutr Clin Pract 2001; 16:319–328.
44. McClave SA, Martindale RG, Vanek VW, et al: Guidelines for the Provision and Assessment of Nutrition Support Therapy in the Adult Critically Ill Patient: Society of Critical Care Medicine (SCCM) and American Society for Parenteral and Enteral Nutrition (A.S.P.E.N.). JPEN J Parenter Enteral Nutr 2009;33:277.
45. Singer P, Theilla M, Fisher H, et al: Benefit of an enteral diet enriched in eicosapentaenoic acid and gamma-linolenic acid in ventilated patients with acute lung injury. Crit Care Med. 2006;34:1033–1038.
46. ASPEN: Standards of practice for nutrition support dietitians. Nutr Clin Pract 22:558, 2007.
47. Gottschlich MM, Mayer T, Khoury J, et al, editors: The science and practice of nutritional support, a case-based core curriculum, Silver Spring, MD, 2007, ASPEN.
48. Merritt RJ, editor: The A.S.P.E.N. nutrition support practice manual, Silver Spring, MD, 2005, ASPEN.
49. Elpern EH: Pulmonary aspiration in hospitalized adults. Nutr Clin Pract 12:5, 1997.
50. Lipman TO, Cass OW, Ho CS, et al: Group I: choosing the appropriate method of placement of an enteral feeding tube in the high-risk population. Nutr Clin Pract 12(1 Suppl):S54, 1997.
51. Valles J, Artigas A, Rello J, et al: Continuous aspiration of subglottic secretions in preventing ventilator-associated pneumonia. Ann Intern Med 122:179, 1995.
52. von Allmen DAY, Fischer JE: Metabolic complications in total parenteral nutrition, ed 2, New York, 1991, Little, Brown.
53. Pingleton SK: Nutrition in chronic critical illness. Clin Chest Med 22:149, 2001.
54. Gray-Donald K, Gibbons L, Shapiro SH, et al: Nutritional status and mortality in chronic obstructive pulmonary disease. Am J Respir Crit Care Med 153:961, 1996.

55. Lando C, Prescott E, Lange P, et al: Prognostic value of nutritional status in chronic obstructive pulmonary disease. Am J Respir Crit Care Med 160:1856, 1999.
56. Thorsditter I, Gunnarsditter I: Energy intake must be increased among recently hospitalized patients with chronic obstructive pulmonary disease to improve nutritional status. J Am Diet Assoc 102:247, 2002.
57. Schols AM: Nutritional abnormalities and supplementation in chronic obstructive pulmonary disease. Clin Chest Med 21:753, 2000.
58. Mackay L: Health education and COPD rehabilitation: a study. Nurs Stand 10:34, 1996.
59. Pronsky ZM: Food medication interactions, ed 14, Birchrunville, PA, 2006, Food-Medication Interactions.
60. Murray L, editor: Physicians' desk reference, Montvale, NJ, 2006, Thomson.
61. Ferreira IM, Brooks D, Lacasse Y, et al: Nutritional support for individuals with COPD: a meta-analysis. Chest 117:672, 2000.
62. Creutzberg EC, Schols AM, Weling-Scheepers CA, et al: Characterization of nonresponse to high caloric oral nutritional therapy in depleted patients with chronic obstructive pulmonary disease. Am J Respir Crit Care Med 161(3 Pt 1): 745, 2000.
63. Huang S, Pan W: Dietary fats and asthma in teenagers: analyses of the first Nutrition and Health Survey in Taiwan (NAHSIT). Clin Exp Allergy 31:1875, 2001.
64. MacDonald A: Nutritional management of cystic fibrosis. Arch Dis Child 74:81, 1996.
65. Rettammel AL, Marcus MS, Farrell PM, et al: Oral supplementation with a high-fat, high-energy product improves nutritional status and alters serum lipids in patients with cystic fibrosis. J Am Diet Assoc 95:454, 1995.
66. Mora Gandarillas I, Orejas Rodríguez-Arango G, et al: Nutritional status assessment in a group of cystic fibrosis patients. An Esp Pediatr 44:40, 1996.
67. Thomson MA, Quirk P, Swanson CE, et al: Nutritional growth retardation is associated with defective lung growth in cystic fibrosis: a preventable determinant of progressive pulmonary dysfunction. Nutrition 11:350, 1995.
68. Zemel BS, Jawad AF, FitzSimmons S, et al: Longitudinal relationship among growth, nutritional status, and pulmonary function in children with cystic fibrosis: analysis of the Cystic Fibrosis Foundation National CF Patient Registry. J Pediatr 137:374, 2000.

SECTION IV

REVIEW OF CARDIOPULMONARY DISEASE

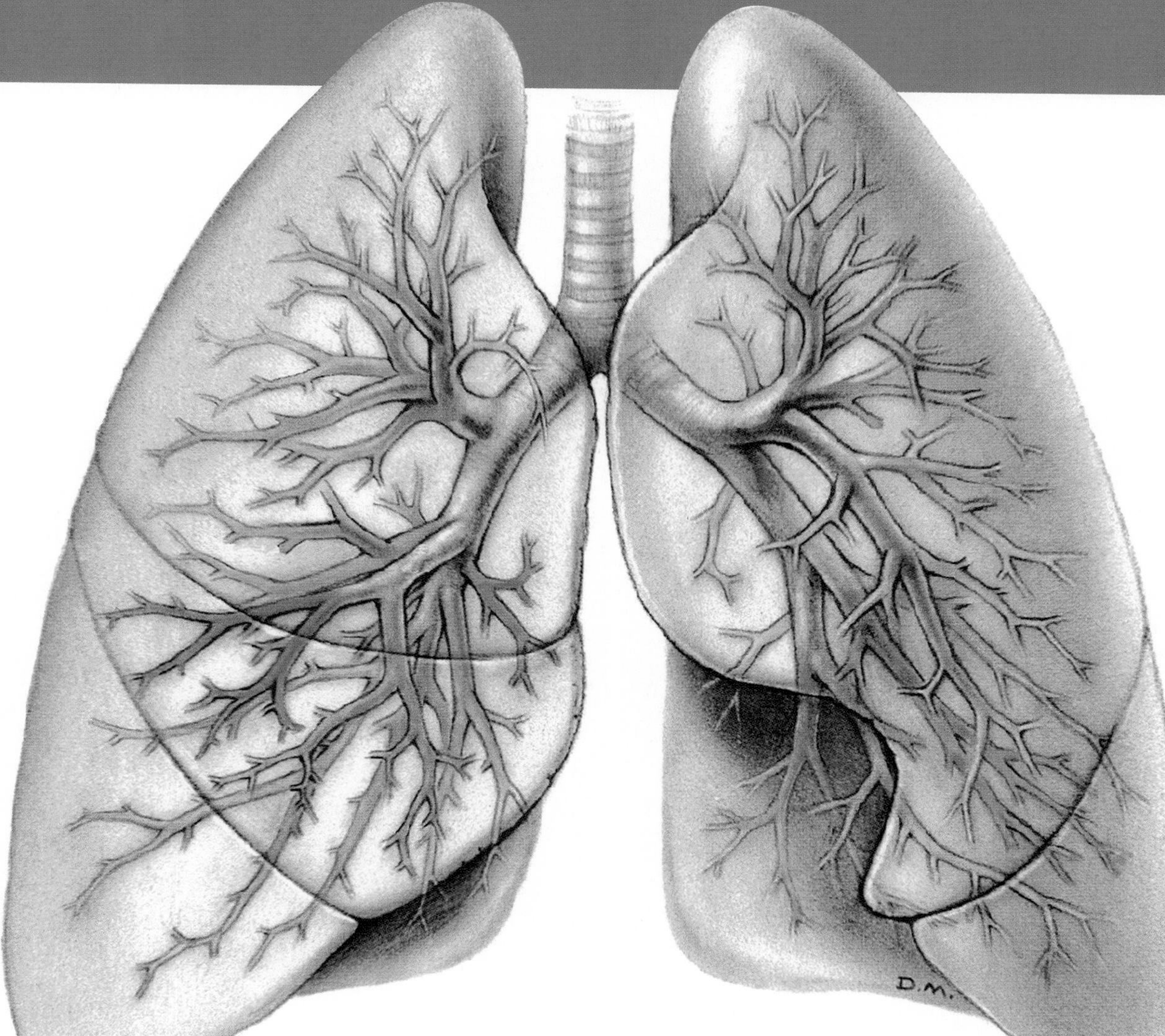

Chapter 22

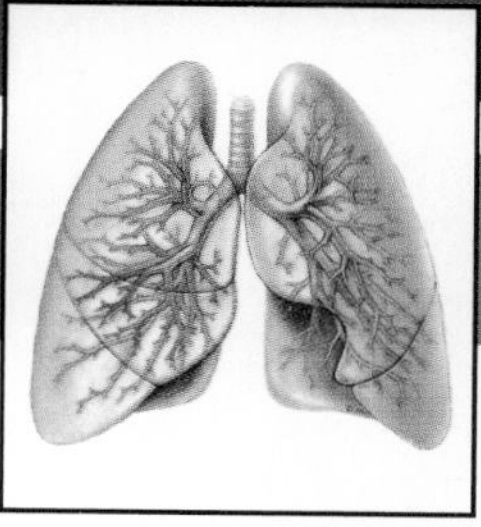

Pulmonary Infections

STEVEN K. SCHMITT AND DAVID L. LONGWORTH

CHAPTER OBJECTIVES

After reading this chapter you will be able to:

- State the incidence of pneumonia in the United States and its economic impact.
- Discuss the current classification scheme for pneumonia and be able to define hospital-acquired pneumonia, health care–associated pneumonia, and ventilator-associated pneumonia.
- Recognize the pathophysiology and common causes of lower respiratory tract infections in specific clinical settings.
- List the common microbiologic organisms responsible for community-acquired and nosocomial pneumonias.
- Describe the clinical findings seen in patients with pneumonia.
- State the radiographic findings seen in patients with pneumonia; state why some patients with pneumonia may have a normal chest radiograph.
- Describe the risk factors associated with increased morbidity and mortality in patients with pneumonia.
- State the criteria used to identify an adequate sputum sample for Gram stain and culture.
- Describe the techniques used to identify the organism responsible for nosocomial pneumonia.
- List the latest recommendations regarding empiric and pathogen-specific antibiotic regimens used to treat various types of pneumonia.
- Discuss strategies that can be used to prevent pneumonia.
- Describe how the respiratory therapist aids in diagnosis and management of patients with suspected pneumonia.

CHAPTER OUTLINE

KEY TERMS

antibiotic therapy
atypical pathogens
community-acquired pneumonia
fomites
health care–associated pneumonia (HCAP)
hospital-acquired pneumonia (HAP)
lower respiratory tract infection
nosocomial pneumonia
pneumonia
tuberculosis
ventilator-associated pneumonia (VAP)

Infection involving the lungs is termed **pneumonia** or **lower respiratory tract infection** and is a common clinical problem in the practice of respiratory care. In the late 1800s, Osler remarked that pneumonia is "captain of the men of death" because of its poor prognosis in the preantibiotic era. More than a century later, pneumonia remains a major cause of morbidity and mortality in the United States and around the world. Each year, 5 million people die from pneumonia worldwide. In the United States, it is estimated that 5 million cases of pneumonia occur annually, of which approximately 1 million require hospitalization, at a projected yearly cost of more than $20 billion.[1] Pneumonia is the seventh leading cause of death in the United States and the most common cause of infection-related mortality.[2]

CLASSIFICATION

Pneumonia can be classified based on the clinical setting in which it occurs (Table 22-1). This classification is useful because it predicts the likely microbial causes and determines empiric antimicrobial chemotherapy while a definitive microbiologic diagnosis is awaited. (The term *empiric therapy* refers to treatment that is initiated based on the most likely cause of infection when the specific causative organism is still unknown.)

Community-acquired pneumonia can be divided into two types—acute and chronic—based on its clinical presentation. *Acute* pneumonia generally appears as an illness of relatively sudden onset over a few hours to several days. The clinical presentation may be typical or atypical, depending on the pathogen. The onset of *chronic* pneumonia is more insidious than acute pneumonia, often with gradually escalating symptoms over days, weeks, or months.

Pneumonia acquired in health care settings is often caused by different microorganisms than community-acquired pneumonia. Previously termed **nosocomial pneumonia,** this clinical entity has been further classified as **health care–associated pneumonia (HCAP), hospital-acquired pneumonia (HAP),** and **ventilator-associated pneumonia (VAP).**[3] HCAP is defined as pneumonia occurring in any patient hospitalized for 2 or more days in the past 90 days in an acute care setting or who in the past 30 days has resided in a long-term care or nursing facility; attended a hospital or hemodialysis clinic; or received intravenous antibiotics, chemotherapy, or wound care. HAP is defined as lower respiratory tract infection that develops in hospitalized patients more than 48 hours after admission and excludes community-acquired infections that are incubating at the time of admission. VAP is defined as lower respiratory tract infection that develops more than 48 to 72 hours after endotracheal intubation.

HAP is a common clinical problem and represents the second most common nosocomial infection in the United

TABLE 22-1

Classifications and Possible Causes of Pneumonia

Classification	Likely Organisms
Community-acquired: acute	
Typical	*S. pneumoniae* *H. influenzae* *Moraxella catarrhalis* *S. aureus*
Atypical	*L. pneumophila* *C. pneumoniae* *M. pneumoniae* Viruses *Coxiella burnetii*
Community-acquired: chronic	*M. tuberculosis* *H. capsulatum* *B. dermatitidis* *C. immitis*
Health care–associated	Mixed aerobic and anaerobic mouth flora *S. aureus* Enteric gram-negative bacilli Influenza *M. tuberculosis*
Immunocompromised host	*P. jiroveci* Cytomegalovirus *Aspergillus* species *Cryptococcus neoformans* Reactivation tuberculosis or histoplasmosis
Nosocomial	
Aspiration	Mixed aerobes and anaerobes Gram-negative bacilli
Health care–associated	*S. aureus*
Ventilator-associated	*P. aeruginosa* *Acinetobacter* species *Enterobacter* species *Klebsiella* species *S. maltophilia* *S. aureus*

States, accounting for 15% to 18% of all such infections.[4,5] Current estimates suggest that more than 250,000 individuals develop this complication each year. HAP increases hospital length of stay 7 to 9 days at an average incremental per-patient cost of $40,000. In selected patient populations, such as patients in the intensive care unit (ICU) and bone marrow transplant recipients, the crude mortality rate from HAP may approach 30% to 70%, with attributable mortality of 33% to 50%. Certain microorganisms, such as *Pseudomonas aeruginosa* and *Acinetobacter* species, are associated with higher rates of mortality.[6]

PATHOGENESIS

Six pathogenetic mechanisms may contribute to the development of pneumonia (Table 22-2). To minimize nosocomial spread, knowledge of these mechanisms is important to the understanding of the various disease processes and to the formulation of effective infection control strategies within the hospital. The fact that tuberculosis is acquired by inhalation of infectious particles is the basis for a policy whereby patients with suspected or proven tuberculosis who are coughing are placed in respiratory isolation, minimizing the risk of disease transmission within the hospital setting.

TABLE 22-2

Pathogenetic Mechanisms Responsible for the Development of Pneumonia

Mechanism of Disease	Examples of Specific Infections
Inhalation of aerosolized infectious particles	Tuberculosis Histoplasmosis Cryptococcosis Blastomycosis Coccidioidomycosis Q fever Legionellosis
Aspiration of organisms colonizing the oropharynx	Community-acquired bacterial pneumonia Aspiration pneumonia Hospital-acquired pneumonia Ventilator-associated pneumonia
Direct inoculation of organisms into the lower airway	Hospital-acquired pneumonia Ventilator-associated pneumonia
Spread of infection to the lungs from adjacent structures	Mixed anaerobic and aerobic pneumonia from subdiaphragmatic abscess Amebic pneumonia from rupture of amebic liver abscess into the lung
Spread of infection to the lung through the blood	*S. aureus* pneumonia arising from right-sided bacterial endocarditis Parasitic pneumonia: strongyloidiasis, ascariasis, hookworm
Reactivation of latent infection, usually resulting from immunosuppression	*P. jiroveci* pneumonia Reactivation tuberculosis Cytomegalovirus

Aspiration of oropharyngeal secretions is the second mechanism that may contribute to the development of lower respiratory tract infection. Healthy individuals may aspirate periodically, especially at night during sleep, and a small volume of oropharyngeal secretions, which are colonized with potential pathogens such as *Streptococcus pneumoniae* and *Haemophilus influenzae,* may contribute to the development of community-acquired pneumonia. Certain patient populations are at risk of large volume aspiration, such as patients with impaired gag reflexes from narcotic use, alcohol intoxication, or prior stroke. Aspiration also may occur as a result of seizure disorder, cardiac arrest, or syncope.

Aspiration seems to be the major mechanism responsible for the development of some types of mixed aerobic and anaerobic, gram-negative, and staphylococcal HAP. In intubated patients, chronic aspiration of colonized secretions through a tracheal cuff has been linked to the subsequent occurrence of pneumonia,[4] which has led to the development of novel strategies to prevent HAP, such as continuous suctioning of subglottic secretions in mechanically ventilated patients and elevation of the head of the bed.[7,8]

Direct inoculation of microorganisms into the lower airway is a less common cause of lower respiratory tract infection that may contribute to the development of nosocomial pneumonia in mechanically ventilated patients who undergo frequent suctioning of lower airway secretions. In this instance, passage of a suction catheter through the oropharynx may result in inoculation of colonizing organisms into the trachea.

Contiguous spread of microorganisms to the lungs or pleural space from adjacent areas of infection, such as subdiaphragmatic or liver abscesses, is an infrequent cause of pneumonia. This pathogenetic mechanism may occur in patients with pyogenic or amebic liver abscesses involving the dome of the liver in whom rupture of the abscess through the diaphragm leads to the development of pulmonary infection or empyema.

The spread of infection through the bloodstream from a remote site is called *hematogenous dissemination*. Hematogenous dissemination is an uncommon cause of pneumonia, which may occur in patients with right-sided bacterial endocarditis in whom fragments of an infected heart valve break off and produce either pneumonia or septic pulmonary infarcts after embolization through the pulmonary arteries to the lungs. Certain parasitic pneumonias, including strongyloidiasis, ascariasis, and hookworm, arise through hematogenous dissemination. In such cases, migrating parasite larvae travel to the lungs through the bloodstream from remote sites of infection, such as the skin or the gastrointestinal tract.

Pneumonia also may develop when a latent infection, acquired earlier in life, is reactivated. This reactivation may occur for no apparent reason, as in the case of reactivation pulmonary tuberculosis, but most often it is attributable to the development of cellular immunodeficiency. *Pneumocystis jiroveci* (previously called *Pneumocystis carinii*) pneumonia is a prime example of lower respiratory tract infection arising as a result of this mechanism. In developed countries, most healthy individuals have acquired *P. jiroveci* by age 3 years and show serologic evidence of prior infection. The organism remains dormant in the lung but may reactivate later in life and produce pneumonia in individuals with compromised cell-mediated immunity, such as patients with human immunodeficiency virus (HIV) infection or recipients of long-term immunosuppressive therapy. Cytomegalovirus pneumonia is another example of a latent infection that can reactivate during chronic immunosuppression, especially in solid organ and bone marrow transplant recipients. Immunosuppressive drugs used to modify inflammatory diseases, such as tumor necrosis factor inhibitors, have been associated with pulmonary and extrapulmonary tuberculosis.[9]

MICROBIOLOGY

The microbiology of community-acquired and nosocomial pneumonia has been studied extensively. Knowledge of which organisms are most commonly associated with pneumonia in different settings is essential because the microbial differential diagnosis guides the diagnostic evaluation and the selection of empiric antimicrobial therapy.

In most studies, *S. pneumoniae,* also called pneumococcus, has been the most commonly identified cause of community-acquired pneumonia, accounting for 20% to 75% of cases (Table 22-3). Various other organisms have been implicated with varying frequencies. *H. influenzae, Staphylococcus aureus,* and gram-negative bacilli each account for 3% to 10% of isolates in many reports.[10] *Legionella* species, *Chlamydophila pneumoniae,* and *Mycoplasma pneumoniae* together account for 10% to 20% of cases. These latter organisms, called **atypical pathogens,** vary in frequency in more recent reports, depending on the age of the patient population, the season of the year, and geographic locale. Legionellosis and *C. pneumoniae,* in particular, seem to exhibit significant geographic variation in incidence.

TABLE 22-3

Frequency of Pathogens in Community-Acquired Pneumonia

Cause	Cases (%)
S. pneumoniae	20-75
Aspiration	6-10
C. pneumoniae	4-11
H. influenzae	3-10
Gram-negative bacilli	3-10
S. aureus	3-5
Legionella species	2-8
Viruses	2-16
Moraxella catarrhalis	1-3
M. pneumoniae	1-24
P. jiroveci	0-13
M. tuberculosis	0-5
No diagnosis	25-50

Many studies examining the epidemiology and microbiology of community-acquired pneumonia are potentially biased because they focus on patients requiring hospitalization. In patients with less severe illnesses not requiring hospitalization, more recent studies suggest that organisms such as *M. pneumoniae* and *C. pneumoniae* account for 38% of cases and may be more common than typical bacterial pathogens such as pneumococcus and *H. influenzae.*[11] In patients who are ill enough to require admission to the ICU, *Legionella* species, gram-negative bacilli, and pneumococcus are disproportionately more common.[1] A virulent strain of methicillin-resistant *S. aureus* (MRSA) has emerged as a cause of severe necrotizing community-acquired pneumonia.[12]

In urban settings that have a high incidence of endemic HIV infection, *P. jiroveci* may be a more common cause of community-acquired pneumonia and, according to one report, may account for 13% of cases.[13] Viruses such as influenza, respiratory syncytial virus, and adenovirus are occasional causes of community-acquired pneumonia, especially in patients with milder illnesses not requiring hospitalization and encountered in the late fall and winter months. A worldwide pandemic of H1N1 influenza during 2009-2010[14] and ongoing sporadic cases of transmission of H5N1 influenza from birds to humans have led to heightened international awareness of influenza epidemiology, pathogenesis, and prevention.

Mixed aerobic and anaerobic aspiration pneumonia may account for 10% of cases. This pneumonia is an important consideration for nursing home residents and for individuals with impaired gag reflexes or recent loss of consciousness.

The outbreak in 2000-2001 of inhalation anthrax in the United States adds another microbial differential diagnostic consideration in patients with fulminant community-acquired lower respiratory tract infection.[15] To date, inhalation anthrax remains a rare disease. However, it must be considered in selected clinical and epidemiologic settings (see later). A new human pathogen, *severe acute respiratory syndrome*–associated coronavirus, emerged and spread worldwide in 2002-2003. No cases have been identified since 2004, but this virus should also be considered in the appropriate clinical and epidemiologic setting.[16]

In most published series, no microbiologic diagnosis is established in 50% of patients. This situation is attributable to many factors, including the following:

- Inability of many patients to produce sputum
- Failure to perform numerous serologic studies routinely in all patients
- The fact that many organisms (e.g., viruses and anaerobic bacteria) were not routinely sought
- Failure, until more recently, to recognize "new" pneumonia pathogens, such as *C. pneumoniae*

The common microbial agents producing HCAP, HAP, and VAP are summarized in Table 22-1 and include gram-negative bacilli, *S. aureus, Legionella* species, and, rarely, viruses such as influenza or respiratory syncytial virus. The last-mentioned viruses are considerations only during the winter months, when they are endemic in the community and may be brought into the hospital by health care workers, visitors, or patients with incubating or active infections.

The relative frequencies and antimicrobial susceptibilities of these respective bacteria may vary considerably from one institution to another. Knowledge of which nosocomial isolates are most common within one's own institution and community, along with their drug-sensitivity profiles, has important implications with regard to selection of **antibiotic therapy,** formulation of infection control policies, investigation of potential outbreaks, and selection of antimicrobial agents for the hospital formulary. For example, patients developing severe VAP in ICUs with a high prevalence of carbapenem resistance among gram-negative organisms such as *Klebsiella pneumoniae* and *Acinetobacter baumannii* may warrant empiric antimicrobial therapy for these organisms pending culture information. Similarly, nosocomial legionellosis is so uncommon in some institutions that empiric therapy in critically ill patients with nosocomial lower respiratory tract infection does not require coverage of this pathogen. However, in other institutions, nosocomial legionellosis occurs more frequently, and patients with HAP may require empiric treatment for this organism.

Nosocomial pathogens capable of producing HAP can be transmitted directly from one patient to another, as in the case of tuberculosis. However, transmission from health care workers (including respiratory therapists [RTs]), contaminated equipment, or **fomites** (objects capable of transmitting infection through physical contact with them) is more common, especially for gram-negative bacilli, *S. aureus,* and viruses. The RT has an important role to play in preventing the transmission and development of nosocomial pneumonia (see further discussion later).

CLINICAL MANIFESTATIONS

Patients with community-acquired pneumonia typically have fever and respiratory symptoms, such as cough, sputum production, pleuritic chest pain, and dyspnea. Not all of these symptoms are present all the time, especially in elderly patients in whom the presentation may be subtle. Other problems, such as hoarseness, sore throat, headache, and diarrhea, may accompany certain pathogens. Fever, cough, and sputum production may occur in other illnesses such as acute bronchitis or flare-ups of chronic bronchitis.

In the past, clinicians often distinguished between typical and atypical clinical syndromes as a means of predicting the most likely microbial causes. A typical presentation consisted of the sudden onset of high fever, shaking, chills, and cough with purulent sputum. Such a presentation was considered more common with bacterial pathogens such as pneumococcus and *H. influenzae.* An atypical presentation was an illness characterized by the gradual onset of fever, headache, constitutional symptoms, diarrhea, and cough, often with minimal sputum production. Coughing was often a relatively minor symptom at the outset, and the illness was initially dominated by nonrespiratory symptoms. Such a presentation was thought to be more common with pathogens such as *M. pneumoniae, C. pneumoniae, Legionella* species, and viruses. More recent studies have shown that these distinctions are not ironclad and that considerable overlap exists in the clinical presentations of pneumonia with typical and atypical pathogens.[17] The occurrence of concomitant diarrhea, previously considered indicative of legionellosis, is now known to be common in pneumococcal and mycoplasmal pneumonia.

Despite the limitations in predicting with certainty the microbial diagnosis based on the clinical presentation, clinicians use certain historical clues and physical findings at the bedside to determine the likely cause of pneumonia in patients presenting from the community. In patients presenting with high fever, teeth-chattering chills, pleuritic pain, and a cough producing rust-colored sputum, pneumococcal pneumonia is the most likely diagnosis. Patients with pneumonia accompanied by foul-smelling breath, an absent gag reflex, or recent loss of consciousness are most likely to have a mixed aerobic and anaerobic infection as a consequence of aspiration. Community-acquired pneumonia accompanied by hoarseness suggests that the culprit is *C. pneumoniae.* Pneumonia in a patient with a history of splenectomy suggests infection with an encapsulated pathogen such as pneumococcus or *H. influenzae.* Epidemics of pneumonia occurring within households or closed communities, such as dormitories or military barracks, suggest pathogens such as *M. pneumoniae* or *C. pneumoniae.* Pneumonia accompanied by splenomegaly prompts consideration of psittacosis or Q fever. Bullous myringitis and erythema multiforme are associated with *Mycoplasma* infection. Relative bradycardia (defined as a heart rate <100 beats/min) in the presence of fever and the absence of preexisting cardiac conduction system disease or beta-blocker therapy, may suggest infection with an atypical pathogen. Pneumonia accompanied by conjunctivitis suggests adenovirus infection.

The clinical presentation of community-acquired pneumonia in elderly patients warrants special mention because it may be subtle. Older individuals with pneumonia may not have a fever or cough and may simply present with shortness of breath, confusion, worsening congestive heart failure (CHF), or failure to thrive.

As noted previously, inhalation anthrax is a rare disease, but it warrants mention because of the small epidemic believed to have been an act of bioterrorism.[15] This outbreak affected mainly postal workers who were exposed to mail containing anthrax spores. Most patients presented with a febrile flulike illness of several days' duration accompanied by dry cough and shortness of breath. Some patients in whom the diagnosis was not quickly considered went on to develop septic shock, meningitis, and disseminated intravascular coagulation over several days, culminating in death.

Because of a lack of prior host immunity or unique viral virulence factors, patients infected with pandemic influenza strains may have unusually severe presentations. During the 2009-2010 pandemic of H1N1 influenza, clinical presentations varied from mild upper respiratory syndromes to fulminant pneumonias with acute respiratory distress syndrome (ARDS) and shock.[14] Severe acute respiratory syndrome manifests with high fever and myalgia for 3 to 7 days followed by nonproductive cough and progressive hypoxemia with progression to mechanical ventilation in 20%.[16]

HCAP, HAP, and VAP usually manifest with new onset of fever in hospitalized or institutionalized patients. Nonintubated patients may have a recent history of vomiting, seizure, or syncope, during which aspiration of oropharyngeal or gastric secretions may have occurred. In intubated patients, VAP traditionally manifests with new onset of fever, purulent endotracheal secretions, and a new pulmonary infiltrate. The diagnosis of HCAP, HAP, or VAP can be extremely difficult to make in patients with preexisting abnormalities on the chest radiograph, such as CHF or ARDS. In mechanically ventilated patients, purulent tracheobronchitis may be accompanied by fever, and in patients with preexisting abnormalities on chest x-ray, the distinction between bronchitis and pneumonia can be especially difficult.

CHEST RADIOGRAPH

In patients with a compatible clinical syndrome, the diagnosis of community-acquired pneumonia is established by the presence of a new pulmonary infiltrate on the chest radiograph. Not all healthy outpatients with suspected pneumonia require a chest radiograph, and physicians may elect to forego radiography and treat empirically for community-acquired pneumonia in individuals with mild illnesses who are at low risk for morbidity or mortality.

A normal chest radiograph does not exclude the diagnosis of pneumonia. The chest radiograph may be normal in patients with early infection, dehydration, or *P. jiroveci* infection. The pattern of radiographic abnormality is not diagnostic of the causative agent, although specific radiographic findings should suggest specific microbial differential diagnoses (Table 22-4).

TABLE 22-4

Radiographic Patterns Produced by Pathogens in Community-Acquired Pneumonia

Pattern	Pathogens
Lobar consolidation	Bacterial
Bronchopneumonia	Bacterial
Pleural effusion	Bacterial Inhalation anthrax
Interstitial infiltrates	Viruses *P. jiroveci*
Cavities	Mycobacteria Fungi *Nocardia* species *S. aureus* Gram-negative bacilli Polymicrobial aerobic and anaerobic lung abscess *P. jiroveci* (rare)
Mediastinal widening without infiltrates	Inhalation anthrax
Rapidly progressive multilobar	*Legionella* species *S. pneumoniae* Endobronchial tuberculosis

Consolidation involving an entire lobe is called *lobar consolidation,* whereas *bronchopneumonia* refers to the presence of a patchy infiltrate surrounding one or more bronchi, without opacification of an entire lobe. Both radiographic patterns suggest the presence of a bacterial pathogen. Pleural effusions are common in patients with bacterial pneumonia and uncommon in patients with viral, *P. jiroveci, C. pneumoniae,* or fungal pneumonia. Pleural effusions are seen in approximately 10% of patients with *M. pneumoniae* and *Legionella pneumophila* pneumonia, and they occur occasionally in patients with reactivation pulmonary tuberculosis. Interstitial infiltrates, especially if diffuse, suggest viral disease, *P. jiroveci,* or miliary tuberculosis in patients with community-acquired pneumonia. Cavitary infiltrates are seen in reactivation pulmonary tuberculosis; fungal pneumonias, such as histoplasmosis and blastomycosis; nocardiosis; pyogenic lung abscess; and, rarely, *P. jiroveci* pneumonia. Patients with severe staphylococcal or gram-negative pneumonias may develop small cavities called *pneumatoceles.* Legionellosis should be seriously considered in sicker patients with pneumonia of a single lobe, which quickly spreads to involve multiple lobes over 24 to 48 hours. Inhalation anthrax manifests with widening of the mediastinal silhouette resulting from mediastinal lymphadenopathy. Parenchymal pulmonary infiltrates are typically absent, and pleural effusions are common.

The chest radiograph may be helpful in diagnosing HCAP or HAP in nonintubated patients with a suspected aspiration event and a previously normal chest film. In such cases, development of a new infiltrate may confirm the clinical suspicion of aspiration pneumonia. The chest radiograph is often less helpful in the diagnosis of VAP because mechanically ventilated patients often have other reasons for radiographic abnormalities, such as ARDS, CHF, pulmonary thromboembolism, alveolar hemorrhage, or atelectasis. In these patients, the accurate diagnosis of a new nosocomial lower respiratory tract infection can be difficult. *Clinical diagnosis,* defined as the presence of fever, purulent respiratory secretions, new leukocytosis, and a new pulmonary infiltrate, is sensitive but not specific for the diagnosis of VAP. Other strategies to diagnose VAP more accurately have been investigated.

RISK FACTORS FOR MORTALITY AND ASSESSING THE NEED FOR HOSPITALIZATION

Many cases of community-acquired pneumonia can be managed successfully on an outpatient basis. The challenge for the clinician is to identify individuals at higher risk of morbidity and mortality for whom hospitalization is indicated. Over the past 20 years, numerous studies have analyzed risk factors for mortality in patients with community-acquired pneumonia.[17-19] Risk factors predictive of a high risk of death are summarized in Box 22-1.

Fine and associates[19] performed a meta-analysis of 127 cohorts of patients with community-acquired pneumonia. The study examined risk factors for fatal outcome. The overall mortality for the 33,148 patients in these cohorts was 13.7%. Eleven prognostic variables were significantly associated with mortality, including male sex, absence of pleuritic chest pain, hypothermia, systolic hypotension, tachypnea, diabetes mellitus, cancer, neurologic disease, bacteremia, leukopenia, and multilobar infiltrates on chest radiograph. Mortality varied according to the infecting agent and was highest for *P. aeruginosa* (61.1%), *Klebsiella* species (35.7%), *Escherichia coli* (35.3%), and *S. aureus* (31.8%). Mortality rates for more common pathogens were lower but still substantial and included *Legionella* species (14.7%), *S. pneumoniae* (12.3%), *C. pneumoniae* (9.8%), and *M. pneumoniae* (1.4%).

Because some variables are unknown at the time a patient seeks treatment for pneumonia, such as the causative agent and whether bacteremia is present, more recent studies have sought to assess the risk of fatal outcome by using clinical and laboratory data that are readily available at the time of the initial evaluation. Based on an analysis of more than 40,000 patients regarding 30-day mortality, Fine and associates[20] proposed a prediction rule to identify low-risk and high-risk patients with community-acquired pneumonia. Their algorithm uses the demographic, clinical, and laboratory data available at presentation to stratify the risk of fatal outcome and the criteria for hospitalization in outpatient groups. Points are assigned for the presence of numerous variables, and cumulative point scores are used to stratify patients into one of five different risk groups with predictable mortality rates (Tables 22-5 and 22-6). In this model, which has been validated in large prospective cohorts of patients, the patients at the lowest risk of death fall into groups I and II. In most instances, these patients may be treated successfully as outpatients, unless they are hypoxic, vomiting and unable to take oral antibiotics, noncompliant, or

Box 22-1 Risk Factors for Mortality in Community-Acquired Pneumonia from Multiple Studies

I. Patient variables
   A. Age >50 years
   B. Male sex
   C. Comorbid illnesses
      1. Cerebrovascular disease
      2. Cancer
      3. CHF
      4. Renal disease
      5. Liver disease
      6. Immunosuppression
      7. Alcoholism
      8. Diabetes mellitus
      9. Chronic lung disease
II. Clinical parameters at presentation
   A. Altered mentation
   B. Systolic hypotension <90 mm Hg
   C. Tachypnea >30 breaths/min
   D. Hypothermia (temperature <35° C)
   E. Fever (temperature >40° C)
   F. Pulse rate >125 beats/min
   G. Extrapulmonary site of infection
III. Laboratory and radiographic findings at presentation
   A. Arterial pH <7.35
   B. Blood urea nitrogen >30 mg/dl
   C. Serum sodium <130 mmol/L
   D. Glucose >250 mg/dl
   E. Hematocrit <30%
   F. Hypoxia (PaO_2 < 60 mm Hg) or hypercarbia (PCO_2 > 50 mm Hg) on room air
   G. White blood cell count $<4 \times 10^9$/L or $>30 \times 10^9$/L or an absolute neutrophil count $<1 \times 10^9$
   H. Multilobar infiltrate
   I. Bacteremia
   J. Pleural effusion
   K. High-risk cause
      1. Gram-negative bacilli
      2. *Staphylococcus aureus*
      3. Postobstructive pneumonia
      4. Aspiration

From Fine MJ, Smith MA, Carson CA, et al: Prognosis and outcomes of patients with community-acquired pneumonia: a meta-analysis. JAMA 275:134–141, 1996.

TABLE 22-5

Scoring System for Stratifying Risk of 30-Day Mortality in Adults With Community-Acquired Pneumonia

Variable	Points Assigned
Age	
Men	Age (yr)
Women	Age (yr) − 10
Nursing home resident	+10
Comorbid illnesses	
Cancer	+30
Liver disease	+20
Kidney disease	+10
Cerebrovascular disease	+10
CHF	+10
Physical findings	
Altered mentation	+20
Tachypnea >30 breaths/min	+20
Systolic hypotension <90 mm Hg	+20
Temperature <35° C or >40° C	+15
Heart rate >125 beats/min	+10
Laboratory and radiographic findings	
Acidemia (arterial pH <7.35)	+30
Azotemia (BUN >30 mg/dl)	+20
Hyponatremia (sodium <130 mmol/L)	+20
Hypoxia (PaO_2 < 60 mm Hg)	+10
Hyperglycemia (glucose >250 mg/dl)	+10
Anemia (hematocrit <30%)	+10
Pleural effusion	+10

Modified from Fine MJ, Auble TE, Yealy DM, et al: A prediction rule to identify low-risk patients with community-acquired pneumonia. N Engl J Med 336:243–250, 1997.
BUN, Blood urea nitrogen.
Note: Plus sign (+) denotes adding points; minus sign (−) denotes subtracting points (e.g., for women, points assigned equal age in years − 10).

TABLE 22-6

Risk Class Mortality Rates Using Prediction Model Cumulative Point Scores in Patients With Community-Acquired Pneumonia

Risk Class (Cumulative Point Score)	Mortality Rate (%)
I	0.1
II (≤70)	0.6
III (71-90)	2.8
IV (91-130)	8.2
V (>130)	29.2

Modified from Fine MJ, Auble TE, Yealy DM, et al: A prediction rule to identify low-risk patients with community-acquired pneumonia. N Engl J Med 336:243–250, 1997.
Note: Patients in risk class I are <50 years old and lack existing illness or physical findings listed in Table 19-5. Points are assigned to patients in risk classes II and higher.

immunocompromised. Patients in group I are patients younger than 50 years without comorbid illnesses and abnormal physical findings at presentation (see Box 22-1 and Table 22-5). This group of patients has a risk of fatal outcome of 0.1%.

Because of the complexity of the pneumonia severity index (PSI), many practitioners prefer a simpler stratification system, the Confusion, Urea, Respiratory rate, Blood pressure, age >65 (CURB-65). Risk criteria in this system include confusion, blood urea nitrogen greater than 20 mg/dl, respiratory rate greater than 30 breaths/min, systolic blood pressure less than 90 mm Hg or diastolic blood pressure less than 60 mm Hg, and age older than 65 years. Based on mortality in the derivation and validation cohorts, the authors recommend that patients with one or two risk criteria be treated outside the acute care setting, patients with two criteria be treated on general hospital wards, and patients with three or more criteria be admitted to the ICU.[21]

Patients with HAP are, by definition, already hospitalized at the time pneumonia develops, and a decision regarding the need for hospitalization is unnecessary. Many studies have examined risk factors for the development of HAP and VAP, which in broad terms can be divided into (1) factors that interfere with host defense and (2) factors that facilitate exposure to large numbers of bacteria.[6] Examples of the factors that interfere with host defense include the following:

- Underlying illnesses such as diabetes mellitus, malignancy, chronic heart and lung disease, and renal failure
- Critical illnesses such as sepsis syndrome and ARDS
- Therapeutic interventions such as endotracheal intubation, tracheostomy, and administration of medications such as sedatives and corticosteroids

Factors that promote exposure of the lung to large numbers of microorganisms or smaller numbers of virulent pathogens include the following:

- Use of endotracheal or nasogastric tubes
- Contaminated ventilator equipment or water supplies
- Prior antibiotic therapy
- Neutralization of gastric pH

Although numerous studies have highlighted the substantial mortality rate (20% to 50%) for patients who develop HAP or VAP, few studies have examined the specific risk factors associated with mortality in hospital-acquired lower respiratory tract infection. For nonventilated patients, risk factors for mortality include bilateral infiltrates, respiratory failure, and infection with high-risk organisms.[22,23] In mechanically ventilated patients, factors associated with fatal outcome include the following:[23,24]

- Infection with high-risk organisms such as *P. aeruginosa*, *Acinetobacter* species, and *Stenotrophomonas maltophilia*
- Multisystem organ failure
- Nonsurgical diagnosis
- Therapy with antacids or H_2-receptor antagonists
- Transfer from another hospital or ward
- Renal failure
- Prolonged mechanical ventilation
- Coma or shock
- Inappropriate antibiotic therapy
- Hospitalization in a noncardiac ICU

MINI CLINI

Estimating Risk from Pneumonia

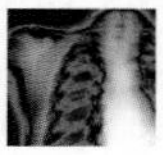

PROBLEM: The RT is called to the emergency department to perform an arterial blood gas analysis on a 70-year-old woman who has been sent from a nursing home with confusion and shortness of breath. Her history is notable for end-stage renal disease caused by hypertension and a recent stroke, which has resulted in left-sided hemiplegia. The emergency physician ordered a chest x-ray, which revealed a right lower lobe infiltrate and a right pleural effusion.

On physical examination, the patient is somnolent. Her vital signs are temperature 35° C, blood pressure 85/50 mm Hg, and heart rate 130 beats/min. Additional findings are as follows:

- Absent gag reflex
- Right basilar rales and left hemiplegia
- Peripheral white blood cell count 3000 cells/mm^3
- Blood urea nitrogen 100 mg/dl
- Hematocrit 31%
- Blood glucose 110 mg/dl
- Serum sodium 144 mmol/L

The RT collects the arterial blood gas on room air, which discloses a pH of 7.30, PaO_2 of 58 mm Hg, and PCO_2 of 25 mm Hg. Should the patient be admitted to the hospital, or should she be sent back to the nursing home? What is her risk of 30-day mortality?

DISCUSSION: This patient is at substantial risk of dying of pneumonia and should be admitted to the hospital. The Fine prediction rule[15] may be used as follows to estimate the risk of 30-day mortality (see Tables 22-5 and 22-6):

Variable	Points
Age 70 years	+70
Sex female	−10
Nursing home resident	+10
Cerebrovascular disease	+10
Renal disease	+10
Altered mentation	+20
Systolic hypotension	+20
Hypothermia	+15
Tachycardia	+10
Acidemia	+30
Renal failure	+20
Hypoxemia, with PaO_2 < 60 mm Hg	+10
Pleural effusion	+10
Total	*225*

Her cumulative point score is 225, she belongs in risk class V, and her estimated risk of mortality is 29.2% (see Table 22-6). She should be admitted to the hospital for treatment.

DIAGNOSTIC STUDIES

Community-Acquired Pneumonia

Many patients with community-acquired pneumonia who are treated as outpatients never have an established microbiologic diagnosis. Many are treated based on the history and on compatible findings on physical examination, with or without a chest radiograph to confirm the presence of an infiltrate. Patients who are sick enough to warrant hospitalization or consideration of hospitalization should undergo numerous studies to stratify risk of mortality and to establish a microbiologic diagnosis (Box 22-2). Complete blood count, blood glucose, serum sodium, and blood urea nitrogen all are necessary to derive a point score for estimating the risk of mortality. An arterial blood gas analysis is used to detect the presence of hypoxemia and acidemia, which indicate a more serious illness.

The value of Gram stain and culture of expectorated sputum has been debated for years.[25] Many patients lack a productive cough, making collection of an adequate specimen difficult. Prior antibiotic therapy reduces the yield

Box 22-2 Recommended Tests for Adults With Community-Acquired Pneumonia Warranting Consideration of Hospitalization

- Chest radiograph
- Complete blood count
- Blood chemistries
  - Glucose
  - Serum sodium
  - Blood urea nitrogen
- Arterial blood gas
- Sputum Gram stain and culture
- Additional sputum studies as clinically indicated
  - Acid-fast stains and culture for mycobacteria
  - Potassium hydroxide examination and fungal culture
  - Stain for *Pneumocystis jiroveci*
  - Direct fluorescent antibody stain for *Legionella* species
- Blood cultures
- Pleural fluid analysis if sizable effusion is present
  - Cell count with differential
  - Glucose, protein, and lactate dehydrogenase
  - pH
  - Gram stain and routine aerobic and anaerobic culture
  - Acid-fast stain and culture for mycobacteria
- Additional other studies as clinically indicated
  - *Legionella* urinary antigen
  - Pneumococcal urinary antigen
  - Acute and convalescent sera for *M. pneumoniae, Legionella* species, and *C. pneumoniae*
  - Fungal serologies
  - HIV test for individuals 13-64 years old or for individuals engaging in high-risk behavior

from both of these tests. Only approximately 50% of patients with bacteremic pneumococcal pneumonia have a positive sputum culture.[26] Nevertheless, the finding of a predominant organism on Gram stain in an appropriately collected specimen has a high predictive value for the selection of appropriate antibiotic therapy.[27] In addition, isolation of penicillin-resistant pneumococci from sputum has important implications for therapy. A routine sputum culture can be interpreted only within the context of the sputum Gram stain. Specimens contaminated with oropharyngeal epithelial cells are unsatisfactory for analysis.

RULE OF THUMB

A routine sputum culture can be interpreted only within the context of the sputum Gram stain.

The RT has an important role in the collection of an appropriate specimen of expectorated sputum. Patients should be advised to rid the mouth of contaminating saliva, either by rinsing with water or by spitting, and then to expectorate a specimen from deep within the tracheobronchial tree into a collection container. Prompt transportation to the laboratory is essential and improves the diagnostic yield from culture.[11] Most microbiology laboratories screen the adequacy of the specimen by cytologic examination. A satisfactory specimen contains more than 25 leukocytes and less than 10 squamous epithelial cells per high-power field.[28] In routine sputum culture, the isolation of bacteria, such as *S. pneumoniae* and *H. influenzae,* must be interpreted within the context of the Gram stain because these organisms can colonize the oropharynx, and their presence in culture may not signify true lower respiratory tract infection. The culture isolation of other organisms, such as *Mycobacterium tuberculosis, Histoplasma capsulatum, Blastomyces dermatitidis, Coccidioides immitis,* and *Legionella* species is diagnostic of disease because these organisms almost never colonize the respiratory tract.

RULE OF THUMB

The presence of *Candida* species on sputum smear or culture is almost never clinically significant.

Other stains and cultures of expectorated sputum should be obtained as dictated by the clinical circumstance, when management would be changed, or for purposes of tracking unusual or resistant organisms in an institution or population. In patients with suspected tuberculosis, the finding of acid-fact bacilli in stained specimens of sputum often prompts initiation of antituberculous therapy because culture isolation of *M. tuberculosis* may take 6 weeks. A direct fluorescent antibody stain of sputum for *Legionella* species may reveal the organism in 25% to 80% of individuals with Legionnaire's disease, and cultures are positive in 50% to 70% of these individuals.[29] Toluidine blue O stains of sputum may disclose the organism in 80% of patients with *P. jiroveci* pneumonia. Potassium hydroxide preparations of sputum disclose fungi in a few patients with histoplasmosis, blastomycosis, or coccidioidomycosis but are very helpful if positive. In inhalation anthrax, patients typically do not produce sputum, and the organism is usually absent if they do.

Blood cultures should be obtained in hospitalized patients with community-acquired pneumonia and may be helpful in establishing the diagnosis in patients with typical bacterial pathogens. Blood cultures are positive in approximately 30% of patients with pneumococcal pneumonia and 70% of patients with *H. influenzae* pneumonia.[30] Blood cultures are often positive in patients with inhalation anthrax and should be collected if the diagnosis is suspected. They are not helpful in patients with legionellosis or *M. pneumoniae, C. pneumoniae, P. jiroveci,* or most viral infections. Collection of blood cultures within 24 hours of hospitalization in elderly patients with pneumonia has been associated with improved survival.[31]

Parapneumonic pleural effusions are common; they occur in 30% to 50% of cases of community-acquired pneumonia.[8] Hemorrhagic pleural effusions are typically present in patients with inhalation anthrax. Thoracentesis is indicated for patients with large pleural effusions and for patients with smaller effusions who fail to respond to therapy or for whom the microbiologic diagnosis is not established. Pleural fluid should also be sampled in patients with suspected inhalation anthrax. Pleural fluid should be tested for cell count, glucose, protein, pH, lactate dehydrogenase, Gram and acid-fast bacilli stains, and routine (aerobic and anaerobic) and mycobacterial cultures. Patients with effusions with a pH less than 7.30 or an elevated white blood cell count require tube thoracostomy for drainage.[32]

Other studies may be helpful in establishing a microbiologic diagnosis in the appropriate clinical setting. *L. pneumophila* serogroup 1 accounts for 80% of cases of legionnaires disease.[33] The urinary antigen test for *L. pneumophila* serogroup 1 is a sensitive and rapid test and usually becomes positive within 3 days of onset of illness. The test has limitations. First is its inability to detect the non-serogroup 1 *L. pneumophila* and non–*L. pneumophila* species that account for 20% of cases of Legionnaire's disease. Second, the test may remain positive for 1 year, obviating the ability to distinguish new from remote infection in patients with a recent history of pneumonia.

Serologic tests for IgM and IgG antibodies to *M. pneumoniae, Legionella* species, or *C. pneumoniae* are rarely helpful during the initial stages of pneumonia, but convalescent titers 3 to 4 weeks later may permit a retrospective microbiologic diagnosis by showing a fourfold increase in IgG titer or the development of IgM antibody against a specific pathogen. Acute sera should be analyzed in patients who are critically ill with pneumonia and for whom microbiologic diagnosis is unavailable. Fungal serologies are occasionally helpful in supporting the diagnosis of blastomycosis, histoplasmosis, or coccidioidomycosis, pending culture isolation of the organism.

Because pneumococcal and *H. influenzae* pneumonia occur with higher frequency in patients with HIV infection than in the average population, an HIV test is recommended for patients with community-acquired pneumonia who are 13 to 64 years old. HIV testing also is recommended for other individuals who engage in behaviors that put them at risk for HIV infection.

Molecular techniques, such as DNA probes and polymerase chain reaction, used for detecting specific organisms such as *M. pneumoniae* or *M. tuberculosis* or for confirming identity in culture isolates, are being developed and are coming into use in some larger centers.

MINI CLINI

Importance of Clinical Setting for Determining the Cause of Pneumonia

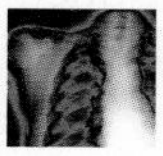

PROBLEM: The RT is caring for a 32-year-old man admitted to the hospital 24 hours earlier with fever, shaking chills, and a new left lower lobe infiltrate. His white blood cell count on admission was 3500 cells/mm^3, with 96% neutrophils and 4% lymphocytes. A sputum Gram stain disclosed many polymorphonuclear leukocytes and lancet-shaped, gram-positive diplococci. Blood cultures have grown *S. pneumoniae* at 24 hours. He remains febrile 24 hours into therapy with penicillin G. While checking pulse oximetry, the RT notes that the patient is emaciated and that multiple needle tracks are present in each antecubital fossa. He tells the RT that he uses intravenous heroin. What other tests are indicated?

DISCUSSION: This patient, who is an intravenous drug user, has bacteremic pneumococcal pneumonia. These findings, along with the presence of cachexia and leukopenia with lymphopenia, should suggest the possibility of underlying HIV infection. An HIV test is indicated and should be performed after the patient's consent is obtained.

Both pneumococcal and *H. influenzae* pneumonia occur with higher frequency in HIV-infected individuals than in the general population. Occasionally, an HIV-infected patient has his or her first contact with the health care system as a result of one of these infections. Individuals 13 to 64 years old with these infections should be offered HIV testing.

The RT would also want to know the antibiotic susceptibility profile of this patient's pneumococcus. Although fever at 24 hours into therapy for pneumococcal pneumonia is not unusual, penicillin resistance to *S. pneumoniae* is becoming increasingly common. If this patient's isolate were penicillin resistant, he would likely require therapy with vancomycin or a respiratory fluoroquinolone.

Flexible bronchoscopy is usually reserved for severe cases of community-acquired pneumonia, for immunocompromised individuals in whom opportunistic pathogens must be excluded, or for cases in which HIV or *P. jiroveci* infection is suspected. The yield from flexible bronchoscopy is higher if performed before the initiation of antibiotic therapy in patients with bacterial pneumonia. Open lung biopsy is rarely indicated for patients with community-acquired pneumonia.

Health Care–Associated Pneumonia, Hospital-Acquired Pneumonia, and Ventilator-Associated Pneumonia

The accurate diagnosis of nosocomial pneumonia is fraught with difficulty and has been the subject of intense investigation over the past 2 decades. Numerous techniques have been extensively reviewed (Box 22-3)[34,35]; none is absolutely sensitive and specific. *Clinical diagnosis* has been defined as the development of a new infiltrate on chest radiograph in the setting of fever, purulent tracheal secretions, and leukocytosis in a hospitalized patient. Clinical diagnosis lacks specificity because many other causes of pulmonary infiltrates exist in hospitalized patients, especially patients on mechanical ventilation.[36] In addition, the upper airway commonly is colonized with nosocomial gram-negative bacilli and staphylococci, even in the absence of pneumonia. The qualitative culture isolation of these organisms from tracheal secretions correlates poorly with the presence or absence of pneumonia.

Direct visualization by bronchoscopy of the lower airway in ventilated patients is sometimes helpful in supporting the diagnosis of VAP. In one study, the presence of distal, purulent secretions; persistence of secretions surging from distal bronchi during exhalation; and a decrease in the PaO_2/FiO_2 ratio of less than 50 were independently associated with the presence of pneumonia. The presence

Box 22-3 Techniques for Diagnosing Nosocomial Pneumonia

- Clinical diagnosis
- Direct visualization of the airway by bronchoscopy
- Quantitative cultures of endotracheal aspirates
- Quantitative cultures of protected brush-bronchoscopy specimens
- Quantitative cultures of nonbronchoscopic distally protected specimens
- Quantitative cultures of conventional or protected BAL specimens, plus microscopic examination of recovered cells
- Quantitative cultures of PSB and BAL specimens, plus microscopic examination of BAL fluid cells
- RT-directed mini-BAL
- Transthoracic fine-needle aspiration

of two of three of these factors had a sensitivity of 78% in the diagnosis of nosocomial pneumonia, and these factors were absent 89% of the time when there was no pneumonia (89% specific).[37]

Because the specificity of qualitative sputum cultures has been unreliable, several studies have examined the role of quantitative cultures of endotracheal aspirates using various breakpoints ranging from 10^3 to 10^7 *colony-forming units (CFU)* per milliliter of respiratory secretions. Results with this technique have been best using a breakpoint of 10^6 CFU/ml, but sensitivities have been only 68% to 82% with specificities of 84% to 96% with this modality.[38,39]

Protected specimen brush (PSB) was developed in the 1970s and uses a special double-catheter brush system to minimize contamination by upper airway flora. Specimens obtained with this technique are cultured quantitatively. Numerous studies have validated the sensitivity of PSB in the diagnosis of nosocomial pneumonia.[40,41] However, the usefulness of PSB may be suboptimal for cases in which antibiotic therapy has already been initiated, in cases of early infection, and in cases in which the wrong lobe is sampled.[34]

Nonbronchoscopic techniques using telescoping protected catheters have been developed to obtain specimens for quantitative culture from the lower airway. In most studies, sensitivity has been comparable with bronchoscopic techniques, but discordant results, compared with bronchoscopy, have been noted in 20% of cases.[34]

Bronchoalveolar lavage (BAL), in which a lung segment is lavaged with sterile saline through the bronchoscope and recovered fluid is quantitatively cultured, has been studied extensively as a tool for diagnosing nosocomial pneumonia. Some studies have supported the usefulness of this technique, whereas others have questioned its specificity because of upper airway contamination.[40,41] BAL has proved useful for obtaining alveolar cells for microscopic analysis, and several studies have suggested that the presence of intracellular bacteria in 3% to 5% of BAL cells distinguishes patients with nosocomial pneumonia from patients without pneumonia.[40,41] In one study, the combination of PSB cultures and microscopic examination of BAL cells for intracellular bacteria was 100% sensitive and 96% specific in identifying patients with nosocomial pneumonia.[40]

Mini-BAL performed by RTs has been advocated for diagnosing VAP. In one study, results obtained using this technique were comparable with results obtained by bronchoscopy using PSB.[42] Some centers use this technique as the primary method of sampling respiratory secretions in suspected nosocomial pneumonia. Transthoracic ultrathin needle aspiration of the lung in nonventilated patients with nosocomial pneumonia also has been studied and in one report was found to have a sensitivity of 60%, a specificity of 100%, and a positive predictive value of 100%.[43]

The accurate diagnosis of HAP, HCAP, and VAP remains a challenge for the physician and the RT. None of the available diagnostic techniques is 100% sensitive or specific, and all of them are limited in the populations at the greatest risk for contracting nosocomial pneumonia—mechanically ventilated patients and patients receiving prior antibiotic therapy.

ANTIBIOTIC THERAPY

Community-Acquired Pneumonia

The selection of antibiotic therapy for patients with community-acquired pneumonia should be guided by several considerations, including the age of the patient, severity of the illness, presence of risk factors for specific organisms, and results of initial diagnostic studies. Pathogen-specific therapy should be used when clinical circumstances and initial evaluation strongly suggest the microbiologic diagnosis or when cultures or other studies confirm the cause. In many instances, initial studies fail to establish a diagnosis, and empiric therapy must be initiated. Major classes of antibiotics used to treat pneumonia are listed in Table 22-7. Consensus guidelines for therapy have been published by the American Thoracic Society (ATS) and the Infectious Disease Society of America (IDSA) (Table 22-8).[44-46] Therapy initiated within 4 hours of hospital admission has been associated with improved survival.[31]

TABLE 22-7

Major Classes of Antibiotics Used in the Treatment of Pneumonia

Antibiotic Class	Representative Drugs
Penicillins	Penicillin G, ampicillin
Ureidopenicillins	Ticarcillin, piperacillin, mezlocillin
Semisynthetic penicillins	Oxacillin, nafcillin
First-generation cephalosporins	Cefazolin
Second-generation cephalosporins	Cefuroxime
Third-generation cephalosporins	Cefotaxime, ceftriaxone, ceftizoxime
Antipseudomonal cephalosporins	Ceftazidime, cefepime
Carbapenems	Imipenem, meropenem, ertapenem
Monobactams	Aztreonam
Beta-lactam/beta-lactamase inhibitor combinations	Ticarcillin/clavulanate, piperacillin/tazobactam, ampicillin/sulbactam
Quinolones	Ciprofloxacin, levofloxacin, moxifloxacin, gemifloxacin
Macrolides	Erythromycin, clarithromycin, azithromycin
Tetracyclines	Doxycycline
Glycopeptides	Vancomycin
Oxazolidinones	Linezolid

TABLE 22-8

Empiric Regimens for Treatment of Hospitalized Adults With Community-Acquired Pneumonia

Patient Group	Likely Pathogens	Empiric Regimens
Hospitalized on ward	*S. pneumoniae, H. influenzae, C. pneumoniae, S. aureus, M. pneumoniae,* anaerobes, viruses	Respiratory fluoroquinolone (levofloxacin, moxifloxacin, gemifloxacin) alone or beta-lactam (cefotaxime, ceftriaxone, ampicillin, ertapenem) and macrolide
Critically ill, ICU	*S. pneumoniae, Legionella* species, *S. aureus,* gram-negative bacilli, *M. pneumoniae, C. pneumoniae*	If *P. aeruginosa* unlikely: beta-lactam (cefotaxime, ceftriaxone, ampicillin-sulbactam) plus either azithromycin or a respiratory fluoroquinolone If *P. aeruginosa* possible: IV antipseudomonal beta-lactam (piperacillin-tazobactam, cefepime, imipenem, meropenem) plus fluoroquinolone (ciprofloxacin or levofloxacin) or IV antipseudomonal beta-lactam plus aminoglycoside plus either IV macrolide or fluoroquinolone

Adapted from Mandell MA, Wunderink RG, Anzueto A, et al: Infectious Disease Society of America/American Thoracic Society consensus guidelines on the management of community-acquired pneumonia in adults. Clin Infect Dis 44:S27–S72, 2007.
IV, Intravenous; *PO,* by mouth.

For hospitalized patients who are not critically ill and who are admitted to the ward, an empiric regimen of a respiratory fluoroquinolone alone or an advanced macrolide plus a beta-lactam (cefotaxime, ceftriaxone, or ampicillin) is recommended (see Table 22-8). For critically ill patients requiring admission to the ICU, the IDSA and ATS recommend as empiric therapy a beta-lactam (cefotaxime, ceftriaxone, or ampicillin-sulbactam) plus either an advanced macrolide or a respiratory fluoroquinolone. Certain pathogens require specific consideration in the ICU setting. If *Pseudomonas* is a concern, recommended regimens include an antipseudomonal beta-lactam (piperacillin-tazobactam, cefepime, imipenem, or meropenem) and ciprofloxacin or levofloxacin; an antipseudomonal beta-lactam, an aminoglycoside, and azithromycin; or an antipseudomonal beta-lactam, an aminoglycoside, and a respiratory fluoroquinolone (see Table 22-8). When MRSA is a concern, addition of vancomycin or linezolid is recommended.

The duration of therapy of community-acquired pneumonia is guided by the specific pathogen and the patient's clinical course. Recommendations have evolved from the traditional 14 days to a minimum of 5 days of therapy with clinical stability except in cases of legionnaires disease or staphylococcal pneumonia.

When a microbiologic diagnosis is established, the antimicrobial regimen should be tailored to the isolated pathogen. Pathogen-specific treatment recommendations from the IDSA and ATS are summarized in Table 22-9. For isolates of *S. pneumoniae* susceptible to penicillin, penicillin remains the preferred agent. Many strains of *H. influenzae* produce beta-lactamase, rendering them resistant to penicillin. Second-generation or third-generation cephalosporins and amoxicillin/clavulanate are the agents of choice. Legionellosis should be treated with a macrolide or with a fluoroquinolone alone. Pneumonia caused by

TABLE 22-9

Pathogen-Specific Treatment Recommendations for Adults With Community-Acquired Pneumonia: Infectious Disease Society of America Guidelines

Pathogen	Recommended Regimen
S. pneumoniae	
Penicillin susceptible	Penicillin G or amoxicillin
Penicillin resistant	Ceftriaxone, cefotaxime, fluoroquinolone, or vancomycin
H. influenzae	Second- or third-generation cephalosporin, azithromycin, or TMP-SMX
Legionella species	Macrolide ± rifampin or fluoroquinolone alone
M. pneumoniae	Macrolide or doxycycline
C. pneumoniae	Macrolide or doxycycline
S. aureus	
Methicillin susceptible	Semisynthetic penicillin ± rifampin or gentamicin
Methicillin resistant	Vancomycin or linezolid
Enterobacteriaceae	Third-generation cephalosporin ± aminoglycoside or carbapenem
P. aeruginosa	Aminoglycoside + antipseudomonal beta-lactam or carbapenem
Influenza with suspected secondary pneumococcal or staphylococcal infection	Neuraminidase inhibitor (oseltamivir or zanamivir) and vancomycin or linezolid

From Mandell MA, Wunderink RG, Anzueto A, et al: Infectious Disease Society of America/American Thoracic Society consensus guidelines on the management of community-acquired pneumonia in adults. Clin Infect Dis 44:S27–S72, 2007.
TMP-SMX, Trimethoprim-sulfamethoxazole.

M. pneumoniae and *C. pneumoniae* should be treated with a macrolide or doxycycline. Trimethoprim-sulfamethoxazole is the drug of choice for *P. jiroveci* pneumonia. However, 50% of HIV-infected patients may develop fever or a rash while taking this medication. Pentamidine is an acceptable alternative. Treatment for staphylococcal or gram-negative pneumonias is dictated by the antibiotic susceptibility profiles of the offending organism. For patients with staphylococcal pneumonia, vancomycin is preferred, pending antibiotic susceptibility results. If the isolate is methicillin susceptible, a semisynthetic penicillin, such as oxacillin or nafcillin, should be used; in seriously ill patients, rifampin or an aminoglycoside may be added. In patients with suspected or proven inhalation anthrax, doxycycline, ciprofloxacin, or levofloxacin should be administered along with one or two of the following antibiotics: penicillin, ampicillin, vancomycin, rifampin, chloramphenicol, imipenem, clindamycin, or clarithromycin.

A detailed discussion of antibiotic therapy for the treatment of pulmonary tuberculosis is beyond the scope of this chapter. In general, three drugs are initiated in patients with suspected or confirmed tuberculosis, unless a multidrug-resistant strain is suspected. In this case, four or five drugs usually are administered.

The duration of therapy of community-acquired pneumonia is guided by the specific pathogen and the patient's clinical course. Recommendations have evolved from the traditional 14 days to a minimum of 5 days of therapy with clinical stability. Exceptions include Legionnaire's disease or staphylococcal pneumonia, for which a minimum of 2 weeks of therapy is recommended. Older individuals and patients with comorbidities may also require longer courses of treatment. When fever has resolved and patients begin to improve clinically, oral therapy may be used to complete the treatment program. Failure of the patient's temperature to normalize within 4 or 5 days suggests the following possibilities: a missed pathogen, a metastatic or closed-space infection (e.g., empyema), drug fever, or the presence of an obstructing endobronchial lesion. Empyema should be treated with tube thoracostomy. Abnormal findings on physical examination may persist beyond 1 week in 20% to 40% of patients, despite clinical improvement. By 1 month, radiographic resolution occurs in 90% of individuals younger than 50 years.[47] After 1 month, radiographic abnormalities may persist in 70% of cases involving older individuals or in patients with significant underlying illnesses.[47]

RULE OF THUMB

Empyema should be ruled out in patients with community-acquired pneumonia and a large pleural effusion who fail to respond to therapy. In cases of community-acquired pneumonia, patients often get better before the chest radiograph shows any improvement.

MINI CLINI

Evaluating Persisting Fever in Pneumonia

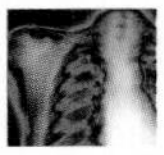

PROBLEM: The RT is caring for a 68-year-old man admitted 1 week ago with bacteremic *H. influenzae* pneumonia. His admitting chest radiograph disclosed right lower lobe consolidation and a large right pleural effusion. He has a history of chronic obstructive pulmonary disease (COPD) and reports a 100 pack-year smoking history. He was treated initially with erythromycin and ceftizoxime until his blood cultures became positive. The organism was susceptible to ceftizoxime, which was continued as monotherapy. Despite treatment, the patient has remained persistently febrile (39° C), and his chest radiograph has not improved. Why is he not responding to therapy?

DISCUSSION: Patients with community-acquired pneumonia who have comorbid illnesses such as alcoholism or COPD may recover more slowly than healthy individuals despite appropriate therapy. Nevertheless, persistent fever 7 days into optimal treatment should prompt several considerations.

The two most likely concerns for this patient are (1) an undrained empyema and (2) an obstructing endobronchial malignancy, given his substantial smoking history. Other, less likely considerations are drug fever; a new nosocomial infection; a missed pathogen, which is not responsive to ceftizoxime, contributing to his pneumonia; or a deep venous thrombosis resulting from bed rest.

The next step should be to repeat the history and physical examination. If these do not reveal a cause of the persistent fever, a thoracentesis should be performed to exclude empyema. If thoracentesis is negative, further investigation in search of an occult endobronchial-obstructing lesion should be considered.

Health Care–Associated Pneumonia, Hospital-Acquired Pneumonia, and Ventilator-Associated Pneumonia

Empiric and definitive therapy of nosocomial pneumonia is dictated by institution-specific data regarding the most common organisms and their antibiotic-susceptibility profiles and by patient-specific risk factors. Although general guidelines have been published,[3] the importance of local data cannot be overemphasized because considerable geographic and institutional variability exists regarding the prevalence and susceptibility profiles of specific pathogens.

Generally, in-hospital aspiration should be treated with a regimen that provides coverage against anaerobes and gram-negative bacilli, such as a beta-lactam/beta-lactamase inhibitor combination or clindamycin with a third-generation cephalosporin. Although vancomycin has been the traditional treatment agent of choice for MRSA pneumonia, evolving data suggest that linezolid may be superior to vancomycin in this role.[48] For VAP, empiric coverage may be targeted at organisms known to colonize the patient's oropharynx or pathogens endemic to the ICU. Patients with *P. aeruginosa* pneumonia usually are treated with two agents, such as ureidopenicillin or antipseudomonal cephalosporin together with an aminoglycoside or fluoroquinolone. Other gram-negative pneumonias generally are treated with a single agent except in cases involving critically ill patients, for whom a second drug is sometimes added. If legionellosis is endemic as a nosocomial infection within an institution, a macrolide may be added to the empiric regimen.

Similar to community-acquired pneumonia, the duration of therapy for cases of nosocomial pneumonia is dictated by the clinical course. A study comparing 8 days versus 15 days of therapy in patients with VAP found that short-course therapy was associated with comparable outcomes to long-course therapy, although the rate of relapse was slightly higher in patients with *Pseudomonas* or *Acinetobacter* infections.[48] More prolonged courses of therapy may be required in patients slow to respond but are associated with a greater risk of new colonization with other organisms. Failure of the patient to improve should prompt the following considerations: the presence of an occult empyema; an unrecognized pathogen; a new, unrelated nosocomial infection; or other noninfectious causes of fever common in the ICU, such as deep venous thrombosis, drug fever, occult pancreatitis, or acalculous cholecystitis (gallbladder inflammation without gallstones).

Some organisms, such as *P. aeruginosa* and *Acinetobacter* species, are associated with a poor prognosis in VAP despite optimal therapy.[49] The mortality rate for these organisms may approach 90% despite appropriate treatment.

The RT has an important role in the diagnosis and management of patients with community-acquired and nosocomial pneumonia. Ensuring mobilization of infected secretions facilitates clinical improvement, and maintenance of adequate oxygenation is essential. The usefulness of chest physiotherapy in the treatment of pneumonia is still unproved, but some patients seem to benefit from it.

PREVENTION

Community-Acquired Pneumonia

Preventive strategies for community-acquired pneumonia have focused on immunization of high-risk individuals against influenza and *S. pneumoniae*. Influenza is a risk factor for subsequent development of community-acquired pneumonia during the fall and winter months. Immunization is indicated for individuals older than 60 years because it reduces the incidence of illness for this age group by half.[50] Immunization also is indicated for individuals with chronic lung or heart disease or for whom the morbidity of influenza may be substantial. More recent studies have suggested that widespread immunization of healthy working adults may be cost-effective because the number of sick days taken and the number of visits to a physician are reduced.[51] Health care workers, including RTs, should be immunized annually to prevent transmission of influenza to patients.

Currently available pneumococcal vaccines provide protection against the 23 serotypes of *S. pneumoniae*, which cause 85% to 90% of invasive pneumococcal infections in the United States. Vaccination is indicated for all individuals older than 65 years and for individuals older than 2 years who have functional or anatomic asplenia. Vaccination is also indicated in patients with chronic illnesses such as CHF, chronic lung disease, or chronic liver disease; alcoholism; cerebrospinal fluid leaks; or conditions characterized by impaired immunity.[52] Routine pneumococcal vaccination of all health care workers is not currently recommended; pneumococcal vaccination is recommended to health care workers who possess one of the specific indications for vaccination outlined previously.

Immunity against *Bordetella pertussis* wanes over time, leading to transmission from older adults to other adults and infants. Because secondary bacterial pneumonia occurs in a significant number of cases of pertussis, the Advisory Committee on Immunization Practices has recommended that the tetanus-diphtheria-acellular pertussis (Tdap) vaccine replace the tetanus-diphtheria (Td) vaccine in the adult immunization schedule.[53]

Health Care–Associated Pneumonia, Hospital-Acquired Pneumonia, and Ventilator-Associated Pneumonia

The prevention of nosocomial pneumonia has been an area of intense investigation over the past 20 years. Table 22-10 summarizes currently available strategies and their relative efficacy. No preventive strategy is uniformly effective. Many institutions now employ a "ventilator bundle" including several of these measures.

TABLE 22-10

Strategies for Prevention of Nosocomial Pneumonia

Strategy	Efficacy
Handwashing	Probably effective
Isolation of patients with resistant organisms	Probably effective
Infection control and surveillance	Probably effective
Enteral feeding, rather than TPN	Possibly effective
Semierect position	Possibly effective
Sucralfate for bleeding prophylaxis	Possibly effective
Careful handling of respiratory therapy equipment	Possibly effective
Subglottic secretion aspiration	Possibly effective
Selective digestive decontamination	Unproved efficacy
Topical tracheobronchial antibiotics	Unproved efficacy

TPN, Total parenteral nutrition.

Handwashing is an important but frequently neglected measure that can reduce transmission of nosocomial bacteria from one patient to another. Handwashing is especially important for RTs who may be caring for several ventilated patients in the ICU. Failure to wash the hands between patient contacts may result in transmission of respiratory pathogens from one patient to another. Handwashing is important even if gloves are worn. Gloves should be changed between patient contacts because they also can become contaminated with and transmit bacteria.

Infection control surveillance to detect outbreaks of nosocomial pneumonia with specific pathogens and to monitor antibiotic resistance patterns is an important strategy. Isolation and cohorting of infected patients can limit the scope and duration of outbreaks, especially in ICUs.

In patients requiring nutrition support, the use of enteral feeding via jejunostomy has been associated with a lower risk of nosocomial pneumonia than the use of total parenteral nutrition.[54] In addition, patients who are fed enterally have a lower incidence of pneumonia if kept semierect rather than recumbent.[7]

Two studies have suggested that gastrointestinal bleeding prophylaxis with sucralfate is associated with a lower risk of pneumonia compared with antacid or H_2-blockers.[55,56] Careful handling of respiratory therapy equipment may reduce the risk of lower respiratory tract infection in ventilated patients. Condensate within the tubing may be colonized with bacteria and should be drained away from the patient because passage of this material into the airway may facilitate colonization with nosocomial pathogens. One study found that continuous subglottic aspiration of secretions was effective in reducing the incidence of nosocomial pneumonia in intubated patients.[57] Many studies have failed to show the efficacy of selective digestive decontamination in the prevention of nosocomial pneumonia, a strategy that uses topical antibiotics in the oropharynx and gastrointestinal tract along with a brief course of systemic therapy. A meta-analysis suggested that topical oral decontamination may reduce the incidence of VAP but not mortality, duration of mechanical ventilation, or length of ICU stay.[58]

Prevention of nosocomial pneumonia remains a challenge to the RT. Careful attention to basic infection control practices, such as frequent handwashing, using new gloves with each patient contact, and careful handling of respiratory care equipment, is important in the prevention of nosocomial pneumonia.

TUBERCULOSIS

Tuberculosis, which is caused by *M. tuberculosis,* can sometimes mimic community-acquired pneumonia and poses special management challenges for the RT. Knowledge of the epidemiology, clinical manifestations, diagnosis, infection control management, and treatment of patients with suspected or proven tuberculosis is essential.

Epidemiology

The epidemiology of tuberculosis in the United States has changed over the past 25 years. After the introduction of effective drugs to treat tuberculosis in the 1950s, the incidence of tuberculosis steadily declined. Tuberculosis increasingly became a disease affecting elderly patients, and most cases represented reactivation of old latent disease. With the emergence of the acquired immunodeficiency syndrome (AIDS) epidemic in the early 1980s, however, there was a resurgence of tuberculosis in the United States and worldwide. This resurgence began in 1985 and peaked in 1992. Since 1992, the incidence of tuberculosis has again declined. This resurgence of tuberculosis was accompanied by dramatic shifts in the patients at risk and the clinical manifestations of the disease. Drug-resistant tuberculosis, defined as resistance of *M. tuberculosis* to both isoniazid and rifampin, emerged as a major public health problem in some populations and areas. Compared with the era before AIDS, tuberculosis now more often manifests in younger individuals with HIV infection, especially inner-city minority populations with a history of injection drug use. Foreign-born nationals residing in the United States have also contributed to the resurgence of disease and have accounted for half of cases reported annually in recent years.

Tuberculosis has increasingly become a disease affecting individuals of lower socioeconomic status in whom homelessness or crowded living conditions, poor access to health care, and unemployment have contributed to the resurgence of the disease.[59] Other risk factors for tuberculosis include the presence of hematologic malignancies, head and neck cancer, or celiac disease (a bowel disease characterized by poor absorption) and the receipt of certain medications such as corticosteroids and tumor necrosis factor-alpha antagonists.[59-62]

Pathophysiology

Tuberculosis is acquired by inhalation of airborne droplets containing the responsible microorganism, *M. tuberculosis,* and the lungs are the major site of infection. Microorganism-laden droplets are deposited in the terminal airways and incite a host immune response. Most exposed individuals successfully contain the infection and remain asymptomatic, although they remain at risk for reactivation of infection later in life, especially in the setting of immunosuppression. The 5 tuberculin unit purified protein derivative (5 TU PPD) skin test becomes positive 3 to 8 weeks after acquisition of infection.

Patients with tuberculosis can present with pulmonary or extrapulmonary manifestations. The major syndromes of pulmonary tuberculosis include primary, reactivation, and endobronchial tuberculosis and tuberculoma.

Primary Tuberculosis

Symptomatic primary tuberculosis occurs in a few individuals shortly after exposure. Primary tuberculous pneumonia is a more common clinical presentation in children and in HIV-infected individuals compared with non–HIV-infected adults. Fever is the most common symptom and occurs in 70% of patients; it persists for 14 to 21 days on average.[63] Chest pain occurs in about 25%; cough is even less common. The chest radiograph shows hilar lymphadenopathy (enlargement of the lymph nodes in the area where the pulmonary arteries emerge from the mediastinum) in 65%, pleural effusion in one-third, and an infiltrate in about 25%. The disease may be difficult to diagnose given the infrequency of cough and a pulmonary infiltrate.

Reactivation and Endobronchial Tuberculosis

Reactivation tuberculosis develops months to years after acquisition of infection and may occur spontaneously or in the setting of immunosuppression. In individuals without HIV infection, reactivation disease accounts for 90% of cases of tuberculosis. The most common symptoms include fever, cough, night sweats, and weight loss. Sputum production increases as the infection progresses and is occasionally accompanied by hemoptysis, which is seldom massive. Older patients may present with a more indolent illness in which fever and night sweats are absent. Physical examination is often unrevealing in patients with reactivation tuberculosis. Chest radiograph shows apicoposterior upper lobe disease in 80% to 90% of patients, and cavities are present in 20% to 40%.

Endobronchial tuberculosis involves the airways and may be seen in both primary and reactivation tuberculosis. In primary tuberculosis, hilar nodal enlargement may impinge on the bronchi, resulting in compression and ultimately ulceration. In patients with reactivation disease, endobronchial involvement may occur as a result of direct extension from the parenchyma or pooling of secretions from upper lobe cavities in the dependent distal airways. Symptoms of endobronchial tuberculosis include a barking cough in two-thirds of patients, sputum production, wheezing, and hemoptysis. On physical examination, wheezing is common. Chest radiograph most often shows an upper lobe cavitary infiltrate with an ipsilateral (same side) lower lobe infiltrate. Extensive endobronchial disease may produce bronchiectasis.

Tuberculomas

Tuberculomas are rounded solitary mass lesions and may occur in primary or reactivation tuberculosis. They are often asymptomatic and may mimic malignancy. Tuberculoma is in the differential diagnosis of solitary pulmonary nodule and may be difficult to diagnose without biopsy or excision because expectorated sputum in patients with tuberculoma rarely shows *M. tuberculosis* on smear or culture. Complications of pulmonary tuberculosis include tuberculous empyema, bronchiectasis, extensive pulmonary parenchymal destruction, spontaneous pneumothorax, and massive hemoptysis from rupture of a Rasmussen aneurysm in the wall of a cavity.

Extrapulmonary tuberculosis is defined as spread of *M. tuberculosis* infection beyond the lung and may involve virtually any organ. The central nervous system, musculoskeletal system, genitourinary tract, and lymph nodes (scrofula) are the most common sites of extrapulmonary tuberculosis. Patients coinfected with HIV who acquire tuberculosis present with unique clinical manifestations compared with non–HIV-infected patients. Patients with HIV infection may develop rapidly progressive primary infection and may present with both pulmonary and extrapulmonary disease. In patients with advanced AIDS, tuberculosis may manifest as disseminated disease with involvement of multiple organs, including lymph nodes, bone marrow, liver, and spleen. Symptoms in this setting may include high fevers, sweats, progressive weight loss, and inanition (wasting). Findings on physical examination may include hectic fever, wasting, and hepatosplenomegaly (enlargement of the liver and spleen). Laboratory testing may show pancytopenia (decreased cell counts in white blood cells, red blood cells, and platelets) and advanced immunodeficiency. Imaging studies often show mediastinal and abdominal lymphadenopathy and hepatosplenomegaly.

Assessment

The history is vital in the diagnosis and management of patients with suspected tuberculosis. In addition to eliciting the patient's symptoms, the clinician should inquire about any prior history of tuberculosis, about the presence of risk factors for acquiring infection as discussed earlier, about the presence of risk factors for HIV infection, about any history of travel, and about potential contacts with individuals with known or suspected tuberculosis. In patients with a prior history of tuberculosis, outside medical records, including drug susceptibility results of prior isolates, should be obtained. If previously treated, the drugs chosen, duration of treatment, and adherence to therapy should be evaluated. Risk factors for drug-resistant tuberculosis should be sought, which include prior treatment for tuberculosis, exposure to individuals with known drug-resistant disease, exposure to individuals with active tuberculosis who have been previously treated, and travel to parts of the world with a high prevalence of drug resistance or exposure to individuals with active tuberculosis from those areas.

Precautions

Patients hospitalized with suspected or proven active pulmonary tuberculosis should be placed in respiratory isolation in private negative pressure airflow rooms because they pose a risk of transmitting infection to others by coughing up aerosolized droplets containing *M. tuberculosis*. Individuals entering the patient's room should wear fit-tested National Institute for Occupational Safety and Health–approved N-95 or higher masks or respirators. A surgical mask should be placed on a patient with suspected or proven active pulmonary tuberculosis during transport outside the negative pressure room.

The "gold standard" for the diagnosis of tuberculosis from pulmonary and extrapulmonary sites is culture isolation of the organism on solid or liquid media. The major disadvantage of culture is that *M. tuberculosis* may take 4 to 6 weeks to grow, delaying diagnosis. Acid-fast staining of expectorated sputum, bronchoscopic specimens, and other body fluids or tissues may be used in patients with suspected pulmonary or extrapulmonary disease. In patients with pulmonary tuberculosis, it is estimated that 10^4 organisms/ml is required for smear positivity. The sensitivity of sputum smear and of acid-fast smears from other body sites is less than culture methods. The presence of acid-fast bacilli on smear is not synonymous with a diagnosis of *M. tuberculosis* because nontuberculous mycobacteria can produce pulmonary and extrapulmonary disease in selected populations. More rapid diagnostic techniques for identification of *M. tuberculosis* in clinical specimens and for confirmation of the identity of the organism in culture are being developed and are available in some centers. These techniques include nucleic acid amplification, nucleic acid probes, polymerase chain reaction genomic analysis, and molecular tests for chromosomal mutations associated with drug resistance.

A 5 TU PPD may be performed in individuals with suspected tuberculosis. A positive skin test supports the diagnosis in the appropriate clinical setting, but a negative skin test does not exclude the diagnosis. Patients with HIV infection, other causes of immunodeficiency, advanced age, or other comorbidities may be anergic (i.e., have decreased immune responsiveness to skin tests) and unable to mount a positive skin test. Interferon gamma release assays may be used to support diagnosis of tuberculosis when clinical suspicion is high, but decreased sensitivity in immunocompromised persons limits their usefulness in diagnosis of active tuberculosis.[64]

Treatment

Treatment recommendations for tuberculosis have been published by the ATS, U.S. Centers for Disease Control (CDC), and IDSA.[65] The goals of therapy are to cure the patient and to prevent transmission of *M. tuberculosis* to others. Treatment must address clinical and social issues and should be customized to the patient's circumstance. At the outset, daily observed therapy should be part of the treatment program; this consists of observing the patient taking his or her antituberculous medications. Treatment programs that use comprehensive case management and daily observed therapy have a higher rate of successful completion of therapy than other treatment strategies. Social service support, housing assistance, and treatment for substance abuse may be required for selected individuals with tuberculosis and should be part of the treatment plan. Patients with tuberculosis must be promptly reported to the local department of public health so that contact tracing can be performed. Contact tracing includes identification, if possible, of the index case from whom the patient has contracted the infection and identification of close personal contacts to whom the patient may have transmitted *M. tuberculosis*. Identification of key contacts should also occur at the time of the patient's hospitalization, and appropriate counseling and referral for medical evaluation should be provided to potential at-risk individuals.

Isoniazid, rifampin, pyrazinamide, and ethambutol are first-line antituberculous medications. Pending antimicrobial susceptibility results, treatment with four drugs at the outset is recommended. In patients with drug-susceptible pulmonary tuberculosis, many 6- to 9-month treatment regimens have been shown to be effective as outlined in guidelines by the ATS, CDC, and IDSA.[65] Patients with multidrug-resistant tuberculosis may require more prolonged courses of therapy with multidrug regimens.

ROLE OF THE RESPIRATORY THERAPIST IN PULMONARY INFECTIONS

The RT plays a key role in managing patients with pulmonary infections, including helping to diagnose and treat the illnesses. Diagnostically, RTs may participate in the collection of sputum, either by expectoration or perhaps by assisting physicians during bronchoscopy. In some settings, RTs may perform mini-BAL.

RTs often administer chest physiotherapy when indicated, as in patients with bronchiectasis and cystic fibrosis. They may also be involved in counseling patients in other clearance techniques, such as autogenic drainage and positive expiratory pressure (PEP) therapy. RTs also play key roles in modeling optimal infection control and prevention practices (e.g., handwashing, implementing and complying with respiratory precautions, vaccination) and in advising patients about preventive interventions, such as influenza, pneumococcal, and Tdap vaccines.

SUMMARY CHECKLIST

- Community-acquired pneumonia and nosocomial pneumonia are common and important clinical problems with significant morbidity and mortality.
- In most studies, *S. pneumoniae* remains the most common cause of community-acquired pneumonia.
- Gram-negative bacilli and *S. aureus* are the most common pathogens that produce nosocomial pneumonia, but their relative incidence and antimicrobial susceptibility profiles may vary from one institution to another.
- The mortality risk can be quantified at presentation for most patients with community-acquired pneumonia, which may help in determining the need for hospitalization.
- Routine sputum cultures for patients with community-acquired pneumonia must be interpreted within the context of the sputum Gram stain, which provides valuable information regarding the adequacy of the specimen and the predominance of potential pathogens.
- The accurate diagnosis of nosocomial pneumonia remains a challenge, and none of the diagnostic methods currently available is completely reliable.
- Guidelines exist for the treatment of community-acquired pneumonia and nosocomial pneumonia. To whatever extent possible, pathogen-specific antibiotic therapy should be used.
- Immunization of high-risk individuals against influenza and *S. pneumoniae,* although imperfect, is the major strategy in the prevention of community-acquired pneumonia.
- Strategies for preventing nosocomial pneumonia are not uniformly effective. Pulmonary tuberculosis may mimic community-acquired pneumonia, and the recognition and appropriate isolation, diagnostic evaluation, and management of individuals with possible pulmonary tuberculosis are essential.
- The RT can help prevent nosocomial pneumonia by careful attention to basic infection control procedures such as handwashing.

References

1. Schmitt S: Community-acquired pneumonia, www.clevelandclinicmeded.com/medicalprbs/diseasemanagement/infections-disease/community-acquiredpneumonia, accessed October 2011.
2. Xu J, Kochanek, KD, Murphy SL, et al: Deaths: final data for 2007. Natl Vital Stat Rep 58:1–135, 2010.
3. American Thoracic Society: Guidelines for the management of adults with hospital-acquired, ventilator-associated, and healthcare-associated pneumonia. Am J Respir Crit Care Med 171:388–416, 2005.
4. Craven DE, Steger KA, Barber TW: Preventing nosocomial pneumonia: state of the art and perspectives for the 1990s. Am J Med 91:44S–53S, 1991.
5. Wiblin RT, Wenzel RP: Hospital-acquired pneumonia. Curr Clin Top Infect Dis 16:194–214, 1996.
6. Bassin A, Niederman MS: New approaches to prevention and treatment of nosocomial pneumonia. Semin Thorac Cardiovasc Surg 7:70–77, 1995.
7. Torres A, Serra-Batlles J, Ros E, et al: Pulmonary aspiration of gastric contents in patients receiving mechanical ventilation: the effect of body position. Ann Intern Med 116:540–543, 1992.
8. Valles J, Artigas A, Rello J, et al: Continuous aspiration of subglottic secretions in preventing ventilator-associated pneumonia. Ann Intern Med 122:179–186, 1995.
9. Wallis RS, Broder MS, Wong JY, et al: Granulomatous infectious diseases associated with tumor necrosis factor antagonists. Clin Infect Dis 38:1261–1265, 2004.
10. Bartlett JG, Mundy LM: Community-acquired pneumonia. N Engl J Med 333:1618–1624, 1995.
11. Marrie TJ, Peeling RW, Fine MJ, et al: Ambulatory patients with community-acquired pneumonia: the frequency of atypical agents and clinical course. Am J Med 101:508–515, 1996.
12. Kollef MH, Micek ST: Methicillin-resistant *Staphylococcus aureus*—a new community-acquired pathogen? Curr Opin Infect Dis 19:161–168, 2006.
13. Mundy LM, Auwaerter PG, Oldach D, et al: Community-acquired pneumonia: impact of immune status. Am J Respir Crit Care Med 152:1309–1315, 1995.
14. World Health Organization: Clinical management of human infection with avian influenza A (H5N1) virus. August 2007. http://www.who.int/csr/disease/avian_influenza/guidelines/Clinical Management07.pdf. Accessed January 2011.
15. Bush LM, Abrams BH, Beall A, et al: Index case of fatal inhalational anthrax due to bioterrorism in the United States. N Engl J Med 345:1607–1610, 2001.
16. Christian MD, Poutanen SM, Loutfy MR, et al: Severe acute respiratory syndrome. Clin Infect Dis 38:1420–1427, 2004.
17. Fang GD, Fine M, Orloff J, et al: New and emerging etiologies for community-acquired pneumonia with implications for therapy: a prospective multicenter study of 359 cases. Medicine 69:307–316, 1990.
18. Fine MJ, Smith DN, Singer DE: Hospitalization decision in patients with community-acquired pneumonia: a prospective cohort study. Am J Med 89:713–721, 1990.
19. Fine MJ, Smith MA, Carson CA, et al: Prognosis and outcomes of patients with community-acquired pneumonia: a meta-analysis. JAMA 275:134–141, 1996.
20. Fine MJ, Auble TE, Yealy DM, et al: A prediction rule to identify low-risk patients with community-acquired pneumonia. N Engl J Med 336:243–250, 1997.
21. Lim WS, van der Erden MM, Laing R, et al. Defining community acquired pneumonia severity on presentation to hospital: an international derivation and validation study. Thorax 58:377–382, 2003.
22. Torres A, Aznar R, Gatell JM, et al: Incidence, risk, and prognosis factors of nosocomial pneumonia in mechanically ventilated patients. Am Rev Respir Dis 142:523–528, 1990.
23. Craven DE, Steger KA: Epidemiology of nosocomial pneumonia: new perspectives on an old disease. Chest 108:1S–16S, 1995.
24. Kollef MH, Silver P, Murphy DM, et al: The effect of late-onset ventilator-associated pneumonia in determining patient mortality. Chest 108:1655–1662, 1995.
25. Rein MF, Gwaltney JM, Jr, O'Brien WM, et al: Accuracy of Gram's stain in identifying pneumococci in sputum. JAMA 239:2671–2673, 1978.

26. Barrett-Connor E: The nonvalue of sputum culture in the diagnosis of pneumococcal pneumonia. Am Rev Respir Dis 103:845–848, 1971.
27. Gleckman R, DeVita J, Hibert D, et al: Sputum Gram's stain assessment in community-acquired bacteremic pneumonia. J Clin Microbiol 26:846–849, 1988.
28. Murray PR, Washington JA: Microscopic and bacteriologic analysis of expectorated sputum. Mayo Clin Proc 50:339–344, 1975.
29. Nguyen ML, Yu VL: *Legionella* infection. Clin Chest Med 12:257–268, 1991.
30. Farley MM, Stephens DS, Harvey RC, et al: Invasive *Haemophilus influenzae* disease in adults. Ann Intern Med 116:806–812, 1992.
31. Houck PM, Bratzler DW, Nsa W, et al: Timing of antibiotic administration and outcomes for Medicare patients hospitalized with pneumonia. Arch Intern Med 164:637–644, 2004.
32. Heffner JE, Brown LK, Barbieri C, et al: Pleural fluid chemical analysis in parapneumonic effusions: a meta-analysis. Am J Respir Crit Care Med 151:1700–1708, 1995.
33. Kohler RB: Antigen detection for the rapid diagnosis of mycoplasma and *Legionella* pneumonia. Diagn Microbiol Infect Dis 4:47S–59S, 1986.
34. Chastre J, Fagon JY, Trouillet JL: Diagnosis and treatment of nosocomial pneumonia in patients in intensive care units. Clin Infect Dis 21(Suppl 3):S226–S237, 1995.
35. Garrard CS, A'Court CD: The diagnosis of pneumonia in the critically ill. Chest 108(Suppl 2):17S–25S, 1995.
36. Fagon JY, Chastre J, Hance AJ, et al: Evaluation of clinical judgment in the identification and treatment of nosocomial pneumonia in ventilated patients. Chest 103:547–553, 1993.
37. Timsit JF, Misset B, Azoulay E, et al: Usefulness of airway visualization in the diagnosis of nosocomial pneumonia in ventilated patients. Chest 110:172–179, 1996.
38. Marquette CH, Georges H, Wallet F, et al: Diagnostic efficacy of endotracheal aspirates with quantitative bacterial cultures in intubated patients with suspected pneumonia. Am Rev Respir Dis 148:138–144, 1993.
39. Jourdain B, Novara A, Joly-Guillou ML, et al: Role of quantitative cultures of endotracheal aspirates in the diagnosis of nosocomial pneumonia. Am J Respir Crit Care Med 152:241–246, 1995.
40. Chastre J, Fagon JY, Soler P, et al: Quantification of BAL cells containing intracellular bacteria rapidly identifies ventilated patients with nosocomial pneumonia. Chest 95:S190–S192, 1989.
41. Chastre J, Fagon JY, Soler P, et al: Diagnosis of nosocomial bacterial pneumonia in intubated patients undergoing ventilation: comparison of the usefulness of bronchoalveolar lavage and the protected specimen brush. Am J Med 85:499–506, 1988.
42. Kollef MH, Bock KR, Richards RD, et al: The safety and diagnostic accuracy of minibronchoalveolar lavage in patients with suspected ventilator-associated pneumonia. Ann Intern Med 122:743–748, 1995.
43. Dorca J, Manresa F, Esteban L, et al: Efficacy, safety, and therapeutic relevance of transthoracic aspiration with ultrathin needle in nonventilated nosocomial pneumonia. Am J Respir Crit Care Med 151:1491–1496, 1995.
44. Mandell MA, Wunderink RG, Anzueto A, et al. Infectious Disease Society of America/American Thoracic Society consensus guidelines on the management of community-acquired pneumonia in adults. Clin Infect Dis 44:S27–S72, 2007.
45. Bartlett JG, Dowell SF, Mandell LA, et al: Practice guidelines for the management of community-acquired pneumonia in adults. Clin Infect Dis 31:347–382, 2000.
46. Mandell LA, Bartlett JG, Dowell SF, et al: Update of practice guidelines for the management of community-acquired pneumonia in immunocompetent adults. Clin Infect Dis 37:1405–1433, 2003.
47. Mittl RL, Jr, Schwab RJ, Duchin JS, et al: Radiographic resolution of community-acquired pneumonia. Am J Respir Crit Care Med 149:630–635, 1994.
48. Kunkel M, Chastre JE, Kollef M, et al: Linezolid vs vancomycin in the treatment of nosocomial pneumonia proven due to methicillin-resistant *Staphylococcus aureus* (abstract LB-49). Presented at 48th Annual Meeting of the Infectious Diseases Society of America, Vancouver, 2010.
49. Fagon JY, Chastre J, Domart Y, et al: Nosocomial pneumonia in patients receiving continuous mechanical ventilation. Am Rev Respir Dis 139:877–884, 1989.
50. Govaert TM, Thijs CT, Masurel N, et al: The efficacy of influenza vaccination in elderly individuals: a randomized double-blind placebo-controlled trial. JAMA 272:1661–1665, 1994.
51. Nichol KL, Lind A, Margolis KL, et al: The effectiveness of vaccination against influenza in healthy, working adults. N Engl J Med 333:889–893, 1995.
52. Centers for Disease Control and Prevention: Prevention of pneumococcal disease: recommendations of the Advisory Committee on Immunization Practices (ACIP). MMWR CDC Surveill Summ 46(RR-8):1–24, 1997.
53. Centers for Disease Control and Prevention: ACIP votes to recommend use of combined tetanus, diphtheria and pertussis (Tdap) vaccine for adults. http://www.cdc.gov/nip/vaccine/tdap/tdap_adult_recs.pdf. Accessed January 22, 2010.
54. Moore FA, Moore EE, Jones TN, et al: TEN versus TPN following major abdominal trauma: reduced septic mortality. J Trauma 29:916–922, 1989.
55. Tryba M: Sucralfate versus antacids or H_2-antagonists for stress ulcer prophylaxis: a meta-analysis on efficacy and pneumonia rate. Crit Care Med 19:942–949, 1991.
56. Cook DJ, Laine LA, Guyatt GH, et al: Nosocomial pneumonia and the role of gastric pH: a meta-analysis. Chest 100:7–13, 1991.
57. Valles J, Artigas A, Rello J, et al: Continuous aspiration of subglottic secretions in preventing ventilator-associated pneumonia. Ann Intern Med 122:179–186, 1995.
58. Chan EY, Ruest A, O'Meade M, et al. Oral decontamination for prevention of pneumonia in mechanically ventilated adults: systematic review and meta-analysis. BMJ 334:889, 2007.
59. Centers for Disease Control and Prevention: Trends in tuberculosis—United States, 2005. MMWR Morb Mortal Wkly Rep 55:305, 2006.
60. Kamboj M, Sepkowitz KA: The risk of tuberculosis in patients with cancer. Clin Infect Dis 42:1592–1595, 2006.
61. Jick SS, Lieberman ES, Rahman MU, et al. Glucocorticoid use, other associated factors, and the risk of tuberculosis. Arthritis Rheum 55:19–26, 2006.
62. Ludvigsson JF, Wahlstrom J, Grunewald J, et al: Coeliac disease and risk of tuberculosis: a population based cohort study. Thorax 62:23–28, 2007.
63. Poulson A: Some clinical features of tuberculosis. 2. Initial fever. 3. Erythema nodosum. 4. Tuberculosis of lungs and pleura in primary infection. Acta Tuberc Scand 33:37, 1951.
64. Mazurek GH, Jereb J, Vernon A, et al. Updated guidelines for using interferon gamma release assays to detect *Mycobacterium tuberculosis* infection—United States, 2010. MMWR Recomm Rep 59(RR-5):1–25, 2010.
65. Blumberg HM, Burman WJ, Chaisson RE, et al: ATS/CDC/IDSA: treatment of tuberculosis. Am J Respir Crit Care Med 167:603–662, 2003.

Chapter 23

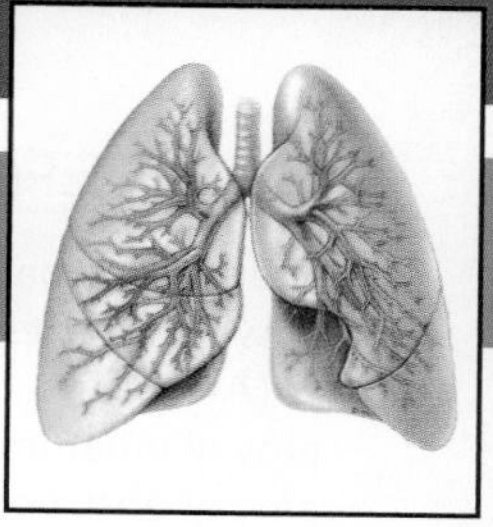

Obstructive Lung Disease: Chronic Obstructive Pulmonary Disease (COPD), Asthma, and Related Diseases

ENRIQUE DIAZ-GUZMAN, RAED A. DWEIK, AND JAMES K. STOLLER

CHAPTER OBJECTIVES

After reading this chapter you will be able to:

- State definitions of chronic obstructive pulmonary disease (COPD), asthma, and bronchiectasis.
- Identify how many Americans are diagnosed with COPD and how many deaths from COPD occur each year.
- Understand the major risk factors associated with the onset of COPD.
- Identify the common signs and symptoms associated with COPD.
- Describe a treatment plan for a patient with stable COPD and for a patient with an acute exacerbation.
- State the factors associated with the onset of asthma.
- Describe the typical clinical presentation of a patient with asthma.
- Identify the treatment currently available for a patient with acute asthma.
- Describe the treatment currently available for patients with bronchiectasis.

CHAPTER OUTLINE

KEY TERMS

acute exacerbation of COPD
airway hyperresponsiveness (AHR)
airway inflammation
airway obstruction
asthma
bronchiectasis
bronchodilator
bronchospasm
chronic bronchitis
cystic fibrosis
emphysema
noninvasive ventilation
supplemental oxygen

The spectrum of obstructive lung diseases is broad and includes chronic obstructive pulmonary disease (COPD) and **asthma** as the most common components and less common entities such as **bronchiectasis** and **cystic fibrosis.** This chapter reviews the major obstructive lung diseases, emphasizing their defining features, epidemiology, pathophysiology, clinical signs and symptoms, prognosis, and management.

CHRONIC OBSTRUCTIVE PULMONARY DISEASE

Overview and Definitions

The term *chronic obstructive pulmonary disease (COPD)*, or sometimes *chronic obstructive lung disease (COLD)*, refers to a disease state characterized by the presence of incompletely reversible airflow obstruction. New guidelines by the American Thoracic Society (ATS) and the Global Initiative for Chronic Obstructive Lung Disease (GOLD) guidelines recommend the use of the term COPD to encompass both chronic bronchitis and emphysema. The ATS guidelines statement regarding COPD define this entity as follows[1]:

> Chronic obstructive pulmonary disease (COPD) is a preventable and treatable disease state characterized by airflow limitation that is not fully reversible. The airflow limitation is usually progressive and is associated with an abnormal inflammatory response of the lungs to noxious particles or gases, primarily caused by cigarette smoking. Although COPD affects the lungs, it also produces significant systemic consequences.

Similarly, the GOLD guidelines define COPD as "a disease state characterized by airflow limitation that is not fully reversible, is usually progressive, and is associated with an abnormal inflammatory response of the lungs to noxious particles or gases."[2]

The spectrum of COPD is shown in Figure 23-1, which presents a nonproportional Venn diagram representing the major components of COPD—chronic bronchitis and emphysema. Although asthma is no longer conventionally considered to be part of the spectrum of COPD, the diagram shows that considerable overlap between asthma and COPD exists. In actual practice, individuals with a history of asthma but with incompletely reversible airflow obstruction may be indistinguishable from patients with COPD.

The two major entities constituting COPD—emphysema and chronic bronchitis—are defined in different ways. **Emphysema** is defined in anatomic terms as a condition characterized by abnormal, permanent enlargement of the airspaces beyond the terminal bronchiole, accompanied by destruction of the walls of the airspaces without fibrosis. **Chronic bronchitis** is defined in clinical terms as a condition in which chronic productive cough is present for at

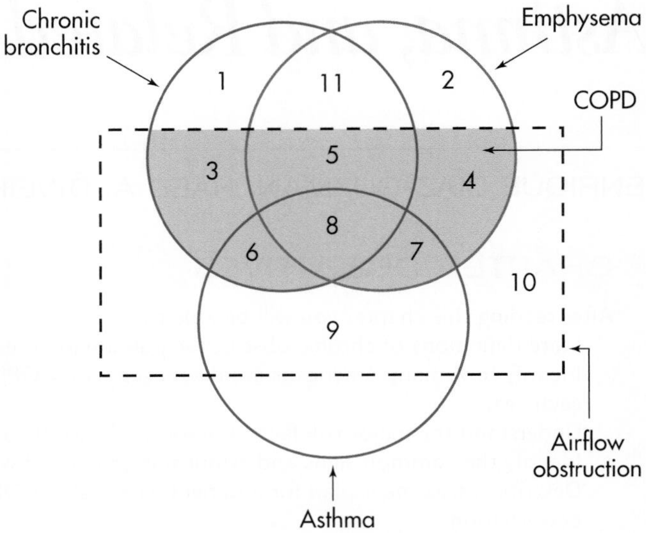

FIGURE 23-1 Schema of COPD. This nonproportional Venn diagram shows subsets of patients with chronic bronchitis, emphysema, and asthma. The subsets constituting COPD are shaded. Subset areas are not proportional to actual relative subset sizes. Asthma is by definition associated with reversible airflow obstruction, although in variant asthma special maneuvers may be necessary to make the obstruction evident. Patients with asthma whose airflow obstruction is completely reversible *(subset 9)* are not considered to have COPD. Because in many cases it is virtually impossible to differentiate patients with asthma whose airflow obstruction does not remit completely from patients with chronic bronchitis and emphysema who have partially reversible airflow obstruction with airway hyperreactivity, patients with unremitting asthma are classified as having COPD (*subsets 6, 7,* and *8*). Chronic bronchitis and emphysema with airflow obstruction usually occur together *(subset 5),* and some patients may have asthma associated with these two disorders *(subset 8).* Individuals with asthma who are exposed to chronic irritation, as from cigarette smoke, may develop a chronic, productive cough, a feature of chronic bronchitis *(subset 6).* Such patients are often referred to as having *asthmatic bronchitis* or the *asthmatic form of COPD.* Individuals with chronic bronchitis or emphysema without airflow obstruction (*subsets 1, 2,* and *11*) are not classified as having COPD. Patients with airway obstruction caused by diseases with a known etiology or specific pathology, such as cystic fibrosis or obliterative bronchiolitis *(subset 10)*, are not included in this definition.

least 3 months per year for at least 2 consecutive years. The definition specifies further that other causes of chronic cough (e.g., gastroesophageal reflux, asthma, and postnasal drip) have been excluded. Figure 23-1 shows considerable overlap between chronic bronchitis and emphysema and some overlap with asthma—that is, when airflow obstruction is incompletely reversible. Figure 23-1 also shows that chronic bronchitis and emphysema can occur without airflow obstruction, although the clinical significance of these diseases usually stems from obstruction to airflow.

Epidemiology

COPD is one of the most frequent causes of morbidity and mortality worldwide.[3] The World Health Organization predicts that COPD will become the fifth most prevalent disease in the world and the fourth leading cause of worldwide mortality by 2020. In the United States, COPD is currently the third leading cause of death; it was responsible for 145,075 deaths in 2008.[4] Estimates suggest that 24 million Americans are affected.[4-6] Data from the National Health and Nutrition Examination Survey (NHANES) suggest that among adults 25 to 75 years old in the United States, mild COPD (defined as forced expiratory volume in 1 second [FEV_1]/forced vital capacity [FVC] <70%, and FEV_1 >80% predicted) occurs in 6.9% and moderate COPD (defined as FEV_1/FVC <79% and FEV_1 ≤80% predicted) occurs in 6.6%.[3] COPD prevalence increases with aging, with a fivefold increased risk for adults older than 65 years compared with adults younger than 40 years, and some studies estimate a prevalence of 20% to 30% in adults older than 70 years.[7]

The growing health burden from COPD is caused in part by the aging of the population but mainly by the continued use of tobacco. The socioeconomic burden of COPD is also substantial. In 2000, COPD caused 726,000 hospitalizations (which accounted for 1.9% of all hospitalizations in the United States), 7,997,000 office visits to physicians, and 1,549,000 emergency department visits, and, in 2002, COPD resulted in a total health expenditure of $32.1 billion.[3] In this regard, COPD is a problem that is a frequent challenge for the respiratory clinician.

Risk Factors and Pathophysiology

Although many risk factors exist for COPD (Box 23-1), the two most common are *cigarette smoking* (which has been estimated to account for 80% to 90% of all COPD-related deaths) and *alpha$_1$-antitrypsin (AAT) deficiency*.[8] Evidence linking cigarette smoking to the development of COPD is strong and includes the following:

- Symptoms of COPD (e.g., chronic cough and phlegm production) are more common in smokers than in nonsmokers.
- Impaired lung function with evidence of an obstructive pattern of lung dysfunction is more common in smokers than in nonsmokers.

Box 23-1 Causes of Chronic Obstructive Pulmonary Disease*

COMMON CAUSES
- Cigarette smoking
- AAT deficiency
- Outdoor air pollution
- Long-standing asthma
- Biomass and occupational exposure

LESS COMMON CAUSES
- Hypocomplementemic urticarial vasculitis
- Intravenous Ritalin abuse
- Ehlers-Danlos syndrome, Marfan syndrome
- Salla disease†
- Alpha$_1$-antichymotrypsin deficiency†
- HIV (emphysemalike illness)

*Multiple causes (e.g., cigarette smoking and alpha$_1$-antitrypsin deficiency) may coexist in a single patient.
†Putative cause; firm evidence is unavailable.

- Pathologic changes of airflow obstruction and chronic bronchitis are evident in the lungs of smokers.
- So-called susceptible smokers, who represent approximately 15% of all cigarette smokers, experience more rapid rates of decline of lung function than nonsmokers.

Information from the Lung Health Study (Figure 23-2) highlighted the accelerated rate of decrease of FEV_1 in smokers compared with former smokers who have achieved sustained quitting.[9,10] Overall, the strength of evidence implicating cigarette smoking as a cause of COPD has allowed the U.S. Surgeon General to conclude, "Cigarette smoking is the major cause of chronic obstructive lung disease in the United States for both men and women. The contribution of cigarette smoking to chronic obstructive lung disease morbidity and mortality far outweighs all other factors."[11]

As the second well-recognized cause of emphysema, AAT deficiency, sometimes called *genetic emphysema,* is a condition characterized by a deficient amount of the protein AAT, which may result in the early onset of emphysema and which is inherited as a so-called autosomal codominant condition. Accounting for 2% to 3% of all cases of COPD, AAT deficiency is severely underrecognized by health care providers but affects an estimated 100,000 Americans. In one 1995 survey, the mean interval between the first onset of pulmonary symptoms and initial diagnosis of AAT deficiency was 7.2 years, and 43% of individuals with severe deficiency of AAT reported seeing at least three physicians before the diagnosis of AAT deficiency was first made.[12] More recent studies suggested that underrecognition of AAT deficiency persisted as of 2003 and that the diagnostic delay interval had not decreased significantly.[12-14]

The importance of early identification is emphasized by the need to test (by simply sending a serum level for AAT)

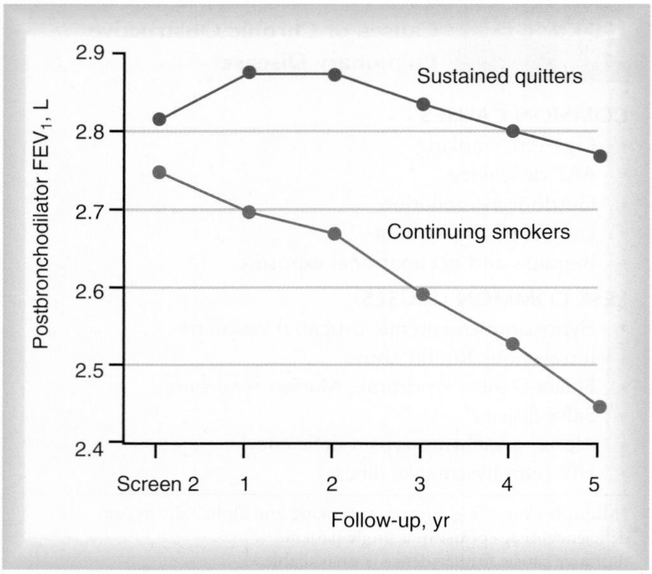

FIGURE 23-2 Mean postbronchodilator FEV_1 for participants in the smoking intervention and placebo groups who were sustained quitters *(red circles)* and continuing smokers *(purple circles)*. The two curves diverge sharply after baseline. (From Anthonisen SR, Connett JE, Kiley JP, et al: Effects of smoking intervention and the use of an anticholinergic bronchodilator on the rate of decline of FEV_1: the Lung Health Study. JAMA 272:1497–1504, 1994.)

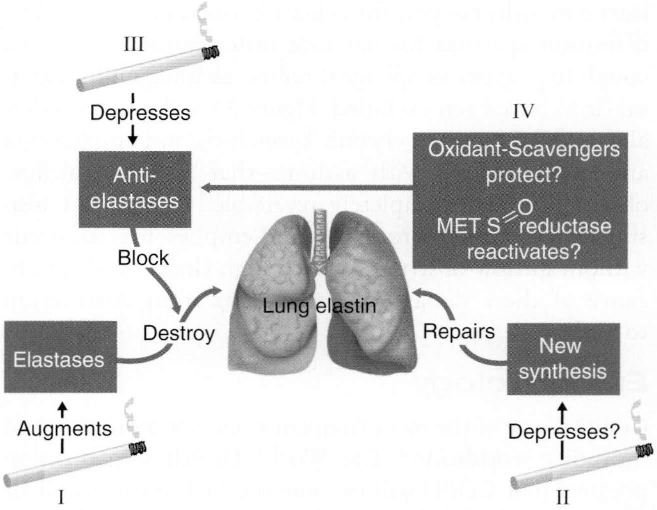

FIGURE 23-3 Proposed biochemical links between cigarette smoking and the pathogenesis of emphysema. *(I)* Smoking recruits monocytes, macrophages, and (through macrophage chemotactic factors) polymorphonuclear neutrophils to the lung, elevating the connective tissue "burden" of elastolytic serine and metalloproteases. *(III)* At the same time, oxidants in smoke plus oxidants produced by smoke-stimulated lung phagocytes (and oxidizing products of chemical interactions between these two) inactivate bronchial mucus proteinase inhibitor and AAT, the latter representing the major antielastase "shield" of the respiratory units. *(II)* Other, unidentified water-soluble, gas-phase components of cigarette smoke (cyanide, copper chelators) inhibit lysyl oxidase–catalyzed oxidative deamination of epsilon-amino groups in tropoelastin and block formation of desmosine and presumably other cross-links during elastin synthesis, decreasing connective tissue repair. *(IV)* Antioxidants (ceruloplasmin, methionine-sulfoxide-reductase) may protect or reactivate elastase inhibitors, and other unidentified factors may modulate the chemical lesions induced in the lung by smoking to influence the risk of developing COPD. (Modified from Janoff A, Carp H, Laurent P, et al: The role of oxidative processes in emphysema. Am Rev Respir Dis 127[Suppl]:S31, 1983.)

first-degree relatives (e.g., siblings, parents, and children), by the favorable effect of primary prevention of smoking among individuals identified early, and by the availability of a specific therapy called *intravenous augmentation therapy*. The risk of developing emphysema for individuals with AAT deficiency increases as the serum AAT level decreases to less than 11 μmol/L, or less than approximately 57 mg/dl using nephelometry, and is enhanced by cigarette smoking.[14]

Study of AAT deficiency has helped formulate the protease-antiprotease hypothesis of emphysema.[14,15] In this explanatory model (Figure 23-3), lung elastin, a major structural protein that supports the alveolar walls of the lung, is normally protected by AAT, a protein that opposes the degradative threat of neutrophil elastase. Neutrophil elastase is a protein contained within neutrophils that is released when neutrophils are attracted to the lung during inflammation or infection. Under normal circumstances of an adequate amount of AAT, neutrophil elastase is counteracted so as not to digest lung elastin. However, in the face of a severe deficiency of AAT (i.e., when serum levels decrease below a "protective threshold" value of 11 μmol/L, or 57 mg/dl), neutrophil elastase may go unchecked, causing breakdown of elastin and resulting in dissolution of alveolar walls. This protease-antiprotease model explains the pathogenesis of emphysema in AAT deficiency, but evidence suggesting its role in COPD in individuals with normal amounts of AAT is conflicting. Also, other proteases (e.g., matrix metalloproteinases and inflammation) are thought to contribute to the proteolysis that produces emphysema.[16]

COPD may occur in the absence of active cigarette smoking or AAT deficiency (see Box 23-1).[17,18] Factors such as passive smoking, air pollution, occupational exposure, and airway hyperresponsiveness may contribute to fixed airflow obstruction.

The mechanisms of airflow obstruction in COPD include inflammation and obstruction of small airways (<2 mm in diameter); loss of elasticity, which keeps small airways open when elastin is destroyed in emphysema; and active **bronchospasm.** Although traditionally considered to be characteristic of asthma, some reversibility of airflow obstruction has been observed in up to two-thirds of COPD patients when tested serially with inhaled bronchodilators.[19]

TABLE 23-1

Clinical Features of COPD: Distinctions Between Chronic Bronchitis and Emphysema, With Emphasis on Distinguishing Features of Alpha$_1$-Antitrypsin Deficiency

Features	Chronic Bronchitis	Emphysema	Severe Alpha$_1$-Antitrypsin Deficiency
Symptoms and Signs			
Chronic cough, phlegm	Common	Less common	Less common, but may be present
Dyspnea on exertion	Less common	Common	Common
Cor pulmonale	Present (often with multiple exacerbations)	Present (but often in end-stage emphysema)	Present (but often in end-stage emphysema)
Age of patient at symptom onset	6th-7th decade	6th-7th decade	4th-5th decade (although late onset is possible)
Family history of COPD	Possible but not characteristic	Possible but not characteristic	Common in parents, children, and siblings
History of cigarette smoking	Present, often heavy	Present, often heavy	May be present, but COPD can occur in the absence of smoking
Physiologic Function			
Airflow (FEV_1, FEV_1/FVC)	Decreased	Decreased	Decreased
Lung volumes, residual volume	Normal	Increased, suggesting air trapping	Increased
Gas exchange, diffusion PaO_2	Often decreased	Often preserved until advanced stage	Often preserved until advanced stage
$PaCO_2$	May be increased	Often preserved until advanced disease, then elevated	Often preserved until advanced disease, then elevated
Diffusion capacity	Often normal	Decreased	Decreased
Static lung compliance	Normal	Increased	Increased
Chest radiograph	"Dirty lungs" with peribronchial cuffing, suggesting thickened bronchial walls	Hyperinflation, with evidence of emphysema; greater at lung apex than at lung base	Hyperinflation, with evidence of emphysema; frequently greater at lung base than at lung apex (basilar hyperlucency)

Clinical Signs and Symptoms

Common symptoms of COPD include cough, phlegm production, wheezing, and shortness of breath, typically on exertion. Dyspnea is often slow but progressive in onset and occurs later in the course of the disease, characteristically in the late sixth or seventh decade of life. One notable exception is AAT deficiency, in which dyspnea characteristically begins sooner (mean age approximately 45 years).[8]

Table 23-1 reviews the characteristic features of emphysema and chronic bronchitis and emphasizes traits that should suggest the possibility of AAT deficiency, including early onset of emphysema, emphysema in a nonsmoker, or a family history of emphysema. Suspicion of AAT deficiency should lead to a simple blood test by which the serum level can be established.[8,14]

Physical examination of the chest early on in a patient with COPD may show wheezing or diminished breath sounds. Later, signs of hyperinflation may be evident—that is, increased anteroposterior diameter (sometimes called a *barrel chest*), diaphragm flattening, and dimpling inward of the chest wall at the level of the diaphragm on inspiration (called *Hoover sign*). Other late signs of COPD include use of accessory muscles of respiration (e.g., sternocleidomastoid), edema from cor pulmonale, mental status changes caused by hypoxemia or hypercapnia (especially in acute exacerbations of chronic, severe disease), or asterixis (i.e., involuntary flapping of the hands when held in an extended position, as in "stopping traffic").

RULE OF THUMB

In patients with COPD, $PaCO_2$ is usually preserved until airflow obstruction is severe (i.e., $FEV_1 < 1$ L), when $PaCO_2$ may increase.

RULE OF THUMB

Digital clubbing is not caused by COPD alone, even if hypoxemia is present. Clubbing in a patient with COPD warrants consideration of another cause (e.g., bronchogenic cancer, bronchiectasis).

Management

In managing patients with chronic, stable COPD, the following goals must guide the clinician[1,2]:

- Establish the diagnosis of COPD.
- Optimize lung function.
- Maximize the patient's functional status.
- Simplify the medical regimen as much as possible.
- Prolong survival whenever possible.

In managing an **acute exacerbation of COPD,** additional considerations are to reestablish the patient to baseline status as quickly and with as little incidence of morbidity and mortality as possible.[20,21] Each of the treatments discussed in this section is considered in the context of these goals, recognizing differences in management between patients with chronic, stable COPD versus an acute exacerbation of COPD. In patients with COPD, $PaCO_2$ usually is generally preserved until airflow obstruction is severe (FEV_1 < 1 L), when the $PaCO_2$ level may increase.

Establishing the Diagnosis

Although a spectrum of diseases can give rise to obstructive lung disease, including some unusual entities such as chronic eosinophilic pneumonia, bronchiectasis, and allergic bronchopulmonary aspergillosis, the major challenge facing the clinician who encounters a patient with airflow obstruction is to distinguish COPD (i.e., emphysema or chronic bronchitis or both) from asthma. Distinguishing asthma from COPD may be very difficult in practice; features that tend to favor COPD include chronic daily phlegm production, which establishes the diagnosis of chronic bronchitis; diminished vascularity on chest radiograph; and a decreased diffusing capacity. The diagnosis of asthma is favored if the diminished FEV_1 obtained on spirometry can be normalized after use of an inhaled **bronchodilator.**

After the diagnosis of COPD is established, a secondary issue is for the clinician to consider whether the patient has an underlying predisposition to COPD, such as AAT deficiency or other cause listed in Box 23-1.[17,18] Underlying causes are present in fewer than 5% of patients with COPD, with AAT deficiency being the most common (2% to 3% of all patients with COPD).

MINI CLINI

Determining the Severity of Chronic Obstructive Pulmonary Disease

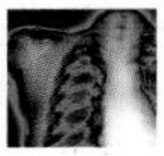

PROBLEM: You are called to see a patient with COPD (FEV_1 40% predicted) and are asked to describe the severity of the patient's illness to a colleague. How do you characterize the severity of COPD?

DISCUSSION: The severity of COPD is described by the degree of airflow obstruction. Traditional descriptors such as hypoxemia and hypercapnia are useful for characterizing COPD. The Global Initiative for Chronic Obstructive Lung Disease (GOLD) has proposed a staging system for COPD.[2] According to this staging system, patients are categorized into one of the following four stages:

Stage	Description
I	Patients with FEV_1/FVC < 70% and FEV_1 > 80% predicted
II	Patients with FEV_1/FVC < 70% and FEV_1 50%-79% predicted
III	Patients with FEV_1/FVC < 70% and FEV_1 30%-49% predicted
IV	Patients with FEV_1/FVC < 70% and FEV_1 < 30% or FEV_1 < 50% predicted plus chronic respiratory failure

This patient would be described as having stage III COPD. The stages generally correspond to other physiologic features of COPD. Patients with stage I COPD do not usually have severe hypoxemia. Also, hypercapnia from airflow obstruction would not be expected in patients with stage I COPD, and an arterial blood gas analysis usually is not recommended. Patients with stage III or IV COPD may require supplemental O_2. A blood gas analysis may be helpful in assessment of these patients.

Optimizing Lung Function

Stable Chronic Obstructive Pulmonary Disease

Although airflow obstruction from emphysema itself is irreversible, most (up to two-thirds) patients with stable COPD exhibit a reversible component of airflow obstruction, defined as a 12% and 200-ml increase in postbronchodilator FEV_1 or FVC or both. For this reason, as indicated in an algorithm developed by GOLD (Figure 23-4),[2,22-24] bronchodilator therapy is recommended for patients with COPD.

Bronchodilators produce smooth muscle relaxation resulting in improved airflow obstruction, improved symptoms and exercise tolerance, and decrease in the frequency and severity of exacerbations, but they do not enhance survival. The results of the Lung Health Study,[9] which compared the effects of inhaled ipratropium bromide (two puffs four times daily) with placebo in patients with mild, stable COPD, showed that regular, long-term use of ipratropium did not change the rate of decline of lung function but offered a one-time, small increase in FEV_1.

Both anticholinergic and adrenergic (beta agonist) bronchodilators can improve airflow in patients with COPD, although some clinicians favor an inhaled anticholinergic medication (e.g., ipratropium bromide or tiotropium[22-24]) as first-line therapy (Figure 23-5). More recent concerns about the possible adverse cardiovascular effects of anticholinergic therapy in patients with COPD[25] have been dismissed by the results of a multicenter trial (UPLIFT [Understanding Potential Long-Term Impacts on Function with Tiotropium]), which found a significantly lower rate of cardiac adverse events and cardiovascular death in patients who received tiotropium.[26]

The GOLD guidelines[2] recommend the use of short-acting beta-adrenergic agents (≤6 hours) for symptomatic management of all patients with COPD. Also, the use of a long-acting beta agonist (e.g., salmeterol) or a long-acting

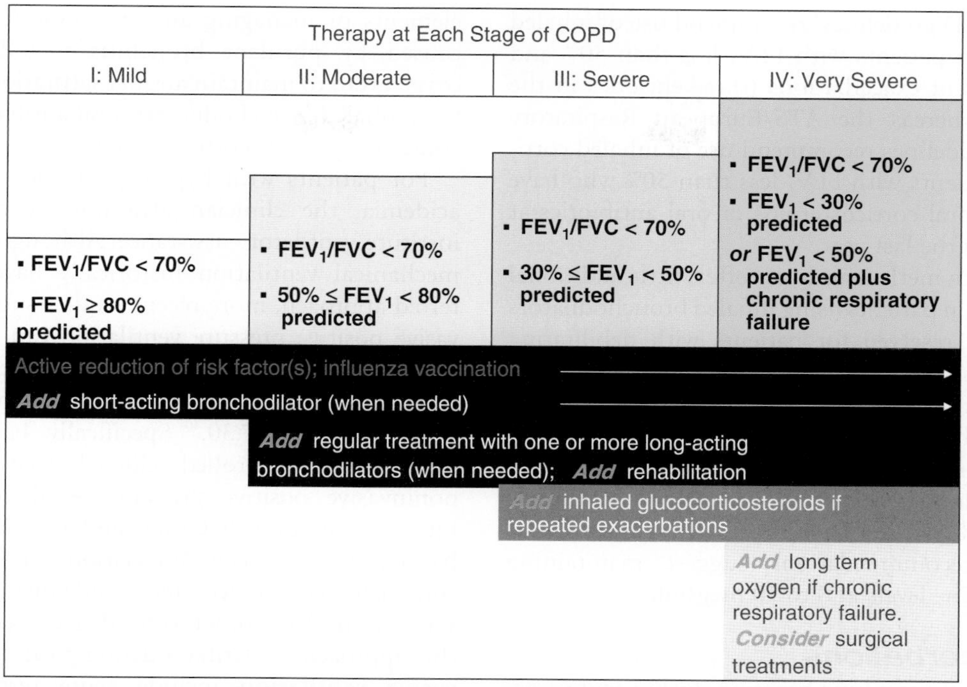

FIGURE 23-4 COPD management algorithm. (From The Global Strategy for the Diagnosis, Management and Prevention of COPD. Global Initiative for Chronic Obstructive Lung Disease [GOLD], 2006. http://www.goldcopd.com.)

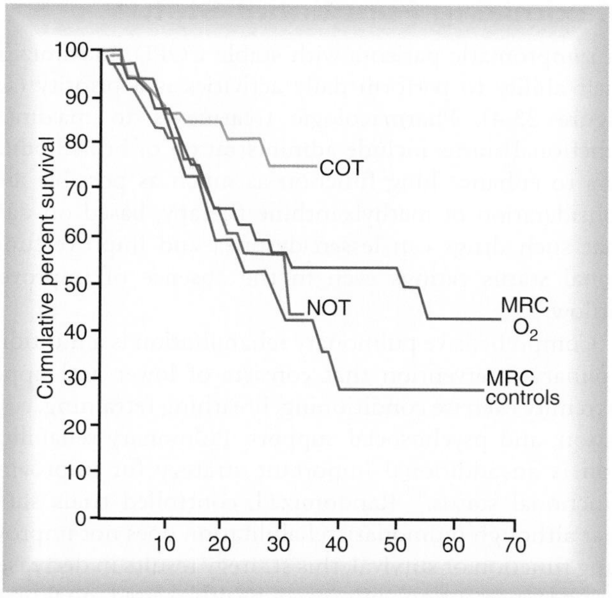

FIGURE 23-5 Cumulative percent survival of patients in the Nocturnal Oxygen Therapy Trial (NOTT) and Medical Research Council (MRC) controlled trials of long-term domiciliary O_2 therapy for men older than 70 years. MRC control subjects *(red line)* received no O_2. NOTT subjects *(purple line)* received O_2 for 12 hours in the 24-hour day, including the sleeping hours. MRC O_2 subjects *(blue line)* received O_2 for 15 hours in the 24-hour day, including the sleeping hours, and continuous O_2 therapy (COT) subjects *(green line)* received O_2 for 24 hours in the 24-hour day (on average, 19 hours). (Modified from Flenley DC: Long-term oxygen therapy. Chest 87:99–193, 1985.)

anticholinergic drug (e.g., tiotropium) can lessen the frequency of acute exacerbations of COPD.[25]

Other treatment options to optimize lung function include administering corticosteroids and methylxanthines. Systemic corticosteroids can produce significant improvements in airflow in a few (6% to 29%) patients with stable COPD.[27] To assess whether airflow obstruction is completely reversible (i.e., the patient has asthma) and whether a patient with COPD is responsive to steroids, a brief course of corticosteroids (20 to 40 mg/day of prednisone or equivalent for 10 to 14 days) is often recommended. Patients with a significant clinical response often are treated with long-term inhaled corticosteroids or rarely with the smallest necessary dose of systemic corticosteroids, recognizing that long-term systemic steroid therapy has risks.[28] Also, results of several major clinical trials (e.g., Lung Health Study II, Euroscop, ISOLDE, and Copenhagen City Study but not TORCH) agree that inhaled corticosteroids do not change the rate of decline of FEV_1 in patients with COPD, although their use is associated with a decreased frequency of acute exacerbations.[29,30]

Studies of combined salmeterol and fluticasone versus placebo in patients with COPD suggest that adding an inhaled corticosteroid (fluticasone) to the long-acting beta agonist (salmeterol) can improve FEV_1 and can reduce the frequency of acute exacerbations of COPD but does not improve survival.[29,30] The finding of a higher rate of pneumonia in inhaled corticosteroid users is concerning.

Overall, the GOLD guidelines[2] recommend use of inhaled corticosteroids in patients with FEV_1 less than 50% and history of recurrent exacerbations (three episodes in the last 3 years), whereas the ATS/European Respiratory Society (ERS) guidelines recommend use of inhaled corticosteroids in patients with FEV_1 less than 50% who have required use of oral corticosteroids or oral antibiotics at least once within the last year.[31]

Treatment with methylxanthines offers little additional bronchodilation in patients using inhaled bronchodilators and generally is reserved for patients with debilitating symptoms from stable COPD despite optimal inhaled bronchodilator therapy. Controlled trials show lessened dyspnea in methylxanthine recipients despite a lack of measurable increases in airflow.[32] Side effects of methylxanthines include anxiety, tremulousness, nausea, cardiac arrhythmias, and seizures. To minimize the chance of toxicity, current recommendations suggest maintaining serum theophylline levels at 8 to 10 mcg/ml.

Acute Exacerbations

Strategies for improving lung function during acute exacerbations of COPD generally include inhaled bronchodilators (especially beta-2 agonists), antibiotics, and systemic corticosteroids. Because of their rapid onset of action and efficacy, short-acting beta-2 agonists are first-line therapy for patients with COPD exacerbation. Inhaled beta-2 agonists are frequently administered through a nebulizer, although metered dose inhaler devices may have equal efficacy if administered appropriately.[2] A common practice is to administer 2.5 mg of albuterol by nebulizer every 1 to 4 hours as needed. Higher doses of albuterol (i.e., 5 mg) do not produce further improvement in pulmonary function and may cause cardiac side effects.[33] Similarly, continuous nebulization of short-acting beta-2 agonists in patients with COPD exacerbation is not recommended.

In addition to inhaled bronchodilator therapy, short-term systemic corticosteroids are recommended to reduce inflammation and improve lung function. An early randomized, controlled trial of intravenous methylprednisolone for patients with acute exacerbations showed accelerated improvement in FEV_1 within 72 hours.[34] Larger, more recent trials have confirmed the benefits of systemic corticosteroids in acute exacerbations and have shown that short-term oral courses (i.e., approximately 2 weeks) are as effective as longer courses (i.e., 8 weeks) with fewer adverse steroid effects.[35] For patients with acute exacerbations characterized by purulent phlegm, oral antibiotics (e.g., trimethoprim-sulfamethoxazole, amoxicillin, or doxycycline) administered for 7 to 10 days have produced accelerated improvement of peak flow rates compared with placebo recipients.[20,36,37]

Finally, intravenous methylxanthines offer little benefit in the setting of acute exacerbations of COPD and have fallen into disfavor.[38,39] Taken together, important elements of managing an acute exacerbation of COPD caused by purulent bronchitis include supplemental oxygen (O_2) to maintain arterial saturation at greater than 90%, inhaled bronchodilators, oral antibiotics, and a brief course of systemic corticosteroids.[20]

For patients with hypercapnia and acute respiratory acidemia, the clinician also must decide whether to institute ventilatory assistance. Although intubation and mechanical ventilation historically have been the preferred approach, more recent studies suggest that noninvasive positive pressure ventilation can be an appealing alternative for patients with acute exacerbations of COPD, especially with severe exacerbations characterized by pH less than 7.30.[40] Specifically, based on available randomized, controlled clinical trials showing that noninvasive positive pressure ventilation can shorten intensive care unit (ICU) stay and avert the need for intubation, the American Association for Respiratory Care consensus conference and guidelines on noninvasive ventilation from other official societies have endorsed this approach.[41,42] Criteria defining candidacy for **noninvasive ventilation** include acute respiratory acidosis (without frank respiratory arrest); hemodynamic stability; ability to tolerate the interface needed for noninvasive ventilation; ability to protect the airway; and lack of craniofacial trauma or burns, copious secretions, or massive obesity.[41]

Maximizing Functional Status

In symptomatic patients with stable COPD, maximizing their ability to perform daily activities is a priority (see Figure 23-4). Pharmacologic treatments to maximize functional status include administration of bronchodilators to enhance lung function as much as possible and consideration of methylxanthine therapy, based on data that such drugs can lessen dyspnea and improve functional status ratings even in the absence of improved airflow.[32]

Comprehensive pulmonary rehabilitation is a multidisciplinary intervention that consists of lower and upper extremity exercise conditioning, breathing retraining, education, and psychosocial support. Pulmonary rehabilitation is an additional important strategy for improving functional status.[43] Randomized, controlled trials show that although pulmonary rehabilitation does not improve lung function or survival, this strategy results in decreased dyspnea perception, improved health-related quality of life, fewer days of hospitalization, and decreased health care usage.[44,45]

Finally, transcutaneous neuromuscular electrical stimulation is a new experimental therapy that has been successfully used to stimulate peripheral muscles in patients with COPD. Studies have shown significant improvements in quadriceps muscle function, exercise tolerance (including walk distance), and health status in patients with severe COPD.[46]

MINI CLINI

Recognizing and Managing an Acute Exacerbation of Chronic Obstructive Pulmonary Disease

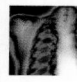

PROBLEM: A 70-year-old man with long-standing COPD is admitted to the hospital with an acute exacerbation. On physical examination, he is not dehydrated, and examination shows diminished breath sounds bilaterally without wheezing. Pertinent laboratory values show a hematocrit of 54% (normal is 40%-47%). An arterial blood gas analysis taken on room air revealed the following:

PaO_2 = 47 mm Hg
PCO_2 = 67 mm Hg
pH = 7.30
HCO_3^- = 34 mEq/L

How do you describe his current status, what do his current laboratory values suggest about his long-term gas exchange status, and what treatment should be considered?

SOLUTION: The patient has an acute exacerbation of COPD. The acidemia (pH 7.30) on his arterial blood gas analysis suggests an acute increase in PCO_2 superimposed on chronic hypercapnia, which is suggested by the elevated serum bicarbonate (HCO_3^-), indicating renal compensation for chronic respiratory acidosis. Although his current hypoxemia may be due to worsened gas exchange accompanying the current flare-up of COPD, his elevated hematocrit, in the absence of dehydration, suggests chronic hypoxemia and secondary erythrocytosis. The goal of therapy is to restore his gas exchange to baseline and to avoid invasive or high-risk interventions, while optimizing survival.

To achieve these goals, treatment would consist of aggressive use of bronchodilators, intravenous corticosteroids, supplemental O_2, and antibiotics (if there is evidence of acute lung infection, either bronchitis or pneumonia). In view of the patient's acute chronic respiratory acidemia, ventilatory support should be implemented. As indicated by several randomized, controlled trials, noninvasive positive pressure ventilation is an effective alternative to intubation.

Preventing Progression of Chronic Obstructive Pulmonary Disease and Enhancing Survival

Cigarette smoking is widely recognized as the major risk factor for accelerating airflow obstruction in smokers who are "susceptible." For these individuals, smoking cessation can slow the rate of decline of FEV_1 and restore the rate of lung decline to that seen in healthy, age-matched nonsmokers.

Follow-up data from the Lung Health Study[9] confirm that a comprehensive smoking cessation program (including instruction, group counseling, and nicotine replacement therapy) can achieve sustained smoking cessation in 22% of participants and that the rate of annual FEV_1 decline in these sustained nonsmokers was significantly less than it was for continuing smokers, even over 11 years of follow-up.[10] Participation in aggressive smoking cessation can enhance survival rates in patients with COPD.[10]

Critical elements in achieving successful abstinence from smoking include identifying "teachable moments" (i.e., during episodes of illness where smoking can be identified as a contributing factor[47]), identifying the role of smoking in adverse health outcomes, negotiating a "quit date," and providing frequent follow-up reminders from health care providers.[48] A helpful strategy during counseling is to use the five *A*'s of smoking cessation[2]:

*A*sk if they are smoking
*A*dvise to quit
*A*ssess willingness to quit
*A*ssist by providing a plan
*A*rrange a follow up

In this regard, the respiratory therapist (RT), who sees the patient frequently, has a special responsibility to provide frequent, constructive reminders about the advisability of smoking cessation.[49]

Among available treatments for COPD, **supplemental oxygen** is important because, similar to smoking cessation and lung volume reduction surgery in selected individuals (see later), it can prolong survival.[50-53] Box 23-2 reviews the indications for supplemental O_2, and Figure 23-5 shows the results of the American Nocturnal Oxygen Therapy Trial[50] and the British Medical Research Council trial of domiciliary O_2 (1980-1981).[51,52] Survival was improved when eligible patients used supplemental O_2 for as close to 24 hours as possible; survival improved less for patients using O_2 only 15 hours per day. No survival advantage was observed when O_2 use was confined to the sleeping hours. Patients should be assessed for supplemental O_2 use only after receiving optimal bronchodilator therapy because one-third of potential O_2 candidates can experience sufficient improvement with aggressive bronchodilation to avoid the need for long-term supplemental O_2. Also, patients prescribed to receive supplemental O_2 during acute exacerbations should be reassessed several months later to determine whether their candidacy and need for supplemental O_2 continue.[54] RTs can play a key role in ensuring compliance with this recommendation and optimizing O_2 therapy.[54,55]

Finally, preventive strategies such as annual influenza and pneumococcal vaccinations are recommended for all patients with chronic debilitating conditions such as COPD.[56] Specific indications for pneumococcal vaccination are presented in Box 23-3.

Additional Therapies

Additional therapies for individuals with end-stage COPD include lung transplantation[57] and lung volume reduction surgery (LVRS),[58-60] in which small portions of emphysematous lung are removed to reduce hyperinflation and

Box 23-2 Indications for Long-Term Oxygen Therapy

I. Continuous O_2
  A. Resting $PaO_2 \leq 55$ mm Hg
  B. Resting PaO_2 56-59 mm Hg or SaO_2 89% in the presence of any of the following:
    1. Dependent edema, suggesting congestive heart failure
    2. *P. pulmonale* on the electrocardiogram (P wave >3 mm in standard lead II, III, or aV_F)
    3. Erythrocytosis (hematocrit >56%)
      (a) Reimbursable only with additional documentation justifying O_2 prescription and a summary of more conservative therapy that has failed

II. Noncontinuous O_2
  A. O_2 flow rate and number of hours per day must be specified
    1. During exercise: $PaO_2 \leq 55$ mm Hg or $SaO_2 \leq 88\%$ with a low level of exertion
    2. During sleep: $PaO_2 \leq 55$ mm Hg or $SaO_2 \leq 88\%$ with associated complications, such as pulmonary hypertension, daytime somnolence, or cardiac arrhythmias

From Tarpy SP, Celli BR: Long-term oxygen therapy. N Engl J Med 333:710-714, 1995.

Box 23-3 Indications for Pneumococcal Vaccine Administration

Vaccination is recommended for the following adults:
- Adults age 65 years and older and adults of all ages with long-term illnesses that are associated with a high risk of contracting pneumococcal disease, including heart or lung diseases, diabetes, alcoholism, cirrhosis, or cerebrospinal fluid leaks
- Adults with diseases or conditions that lower the body's resistance to infections, including abnormal function of the spleen or removed spleen, Hodgkin disease, lymphoma, multiple myeloma, kidney failure, nephrotic syndrome, or organ transplantation, and adults who are taking drugs that lower the body's resistance to infections
- Adults with HIV/AIDS infection, with or without symptoms

Revaccination should be considered for the following groups:
- Individuals at the highest risk of fatal pneumococcal infection, such as individuals with abnormal function or removal of the spleen, who received the original pneumococcal vaccination (from 1979-1983) or who received the current vaccine (1983 to present) ≥6 years ago
- Individuals shown to lose protection rapidly (e.g., individuals with nephrotic syndrome, kidney failure, or transplants), who received the current vaccine ≥6 years ago
- Children ≤10 years old with nephrotic syndrome, abnormal function or removal of the spleen, or sickle cell anemia, who received the vaccine 3-5 years ago

improve lung mechanics of the remaining tissue. COPD is the most common current indication for lung transplantation. Lung transplantation is a consideration for patients with severe airflow obstruction (i.e., $FEV_1 < 20\%$ predicted) who are younger than 65 years old, who lack major dysfunction of other organs, and who are psychologically and motivationally suitable. Given the scarcity of available lungs to transplant, single-lung transplantation usually is performed for individuals with COPD. Although lung transplantation may be associated with significantly improved quality of life and functional status, major risks include rejection (manifested as bronchiolitis obliterans and progressive, debilitating airflow obstruction), infection with unusual opportunistic organisms, and death from these and other complications. The 5-year actuarial survival rate after single-lung transplantation is approximately 54% (Figure 23-6).

LVRS has regained popularity after initial experiences were reported in 1957.[58] Results of randomized controlled trials of LVRS, including the large National Emphysema Treatment Trial, indicate that in selected subsets of patients with COPD (i.e., patients with heterogeneous emphysema that is upper lobe predominant and who have low exercise capacity after pulmonary rehabilitation), LVRS can prolong survival, improve quality of life, and increase exercise capacity.[59,60] LVRS should not be considered in individuals with very severe COPD (i.e., characterized by $FEV_1 < 20\%$ predicted with either a homogeneous pattern of emphysema or a diffusing capacity <20% predicted) because the mortality rate of LVRS is higher in such individuals than in medically treated patients.[61]

Given the positive results associated with LVRS in selected patients with COPD, nonsurgical bronchoscopic techniques have been developed in an attempt to reduce costs and expand treatment options for patients with high operative risk.[62] With the use of the bronchoscope, deployment of unidirectional endobronchial valves into the airways results in collapse of the targeted lung parenchyma. Other techniques include application of biodegradable gel to induce lung collapse or application of bronchial stents to create fenestrations and allow gas escape from hyperinflated areas of the lung. None of the aforementioned devices is currently approved by the U.S. Food and Drug Administration (FDA) for treatment of emphysema in the United States.[63]

Finally, for patients with AAT deficiency and established COPD, so-called intravenous augmentation with a purified preparation of AAT from human blood donors is recommended.[14] Although no definitive randomized, controlled trials are available,[64,65] observational studies suggest that for individuals with severe AAT deficiency and moderate degrees of airflow obstruction (i.e., FEV_1 35% to 60%

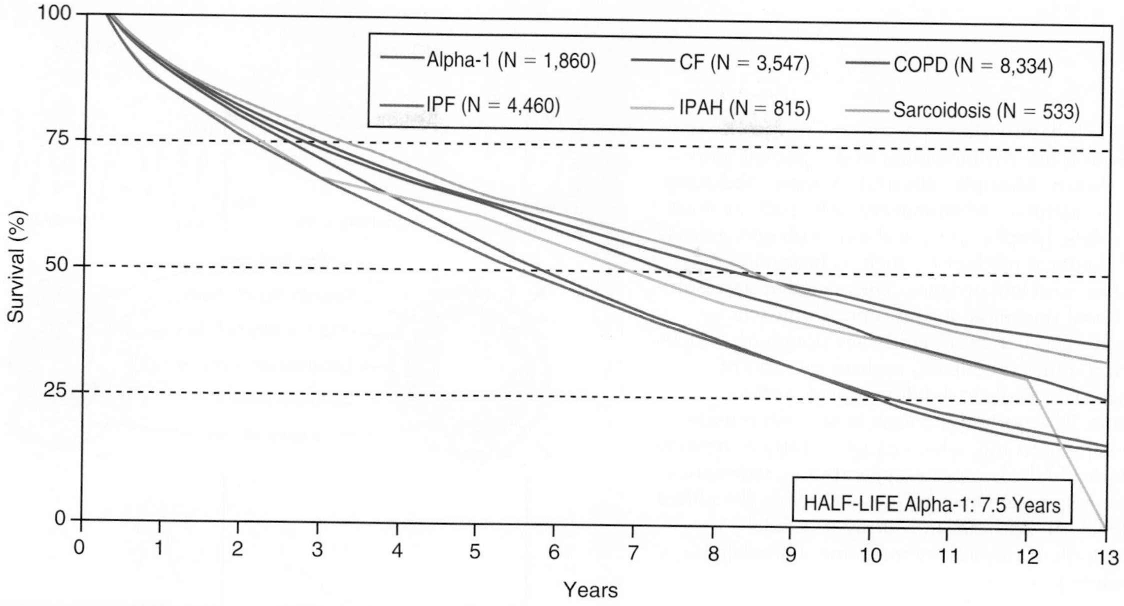

Survival comparisons
All comparisons with Alpha-1, CF and IPAH are statistically significant at 0.01 except Alpha-1 vs. Sarcoidosis p = 0.1099 and CF vs. IPAH p = 0.8588

COPD vs. IPF: p = 0.0087
IPF vs. Sarcoidosis: p = 0.0162

FIGURE 23-6 Actuarial survival curves according to pretransplant diagnosis. The overall survival rate of patients with emphysema (including AAT deficiency) is significantly higher than the survival rate of patients with idiopathic pulmonary fibrosis. (From Christie JD, Edwards LB, Kucheryavaya AY, et al: 27th offical adult lung and heart-lung transplant report, 2010 in the Registry of the International Society for Heart and Lung Transplantation. www.ishlt.org. Accessed January 6, 2010.)

predicted), weekly augmentation therapy may be associated with a slower rate of decline of lung function and improved survival. Difficulties with intravenous augmentation therapy include the substantial expense (approximately $100,000 per year); the inconvenience of frequent intravenous infusions for life; and the infusion itself, which confers a theoretical risk of transmitting a blood-borne infection. Despite these drawbacks, the facts that augmentation therapy can slow the rate of FEV_1 decline, can possibly slow the rate of computed tomography (CT) density loss, and is currently the only specific therapy for AAT deficiency have led to its endorsement in official guidelines from the ATS, the ERS, and the Canadian Thoracic Society.[14,48,66]

ASTHMA

Definition

Asthma is a clinical syndrome characterized by **airway obstruction,** which is partially or completely reversible either spontaneously or with treatment; **airway inflammation;** and **airway hyperresponsiveness (AHR)** to various stimuli.[67-69] Past definitions of asthma emphasized AHR and reversible obstruction; however, newer and more accurate definitions of asthma focus on asthma as a primary inflammatory disease of the airways, with clinical manifestations of increased airway hyperreactivity and airflow obstruction caused by the inflammation.

Incidence

Asthma is a chronic illness that has been increasing in prevalence in the United States since 1980. In 2007, asthma accounted for 3447 deaths, approximately 456,000 hospitalizations, and approximately 13.3 million emergency department or physician office visits among persons of all ages. Approximately 7.7% of U.S. adults, or 17.5 million Americans, have asthma currently.[67-70]

Etiology and Pathogenesis

In the genetically susceptible host, allergens, respiratory infections, certain occupational and environmental exposures, and many unknown hosts or environmental stimuli can produce the full spectrum of asthma, with persistent airway inflammation, bronchial hyperreactivity, and subsequent airflow obstruction. When inflammation and bronchial hyperreactivity are present, asthma can be triggered by additional factors, including exercise; inhalation of cold, dry air; hyperventilation; cigarette smoke; physical

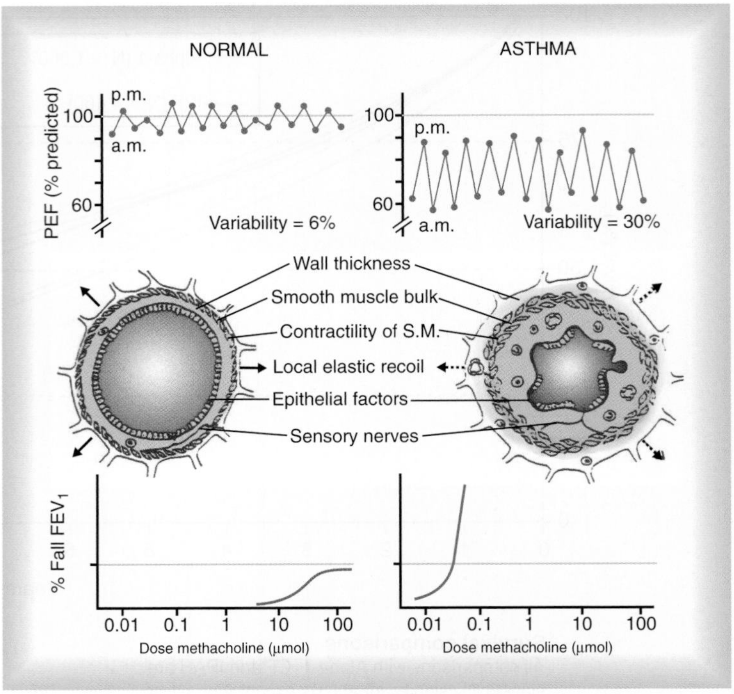

FIGURE 23-7 Inflammation in asthma. Cross sections of an airway from a healthy individual and a patient with asthma are shown. Multiple cells and multiple mediators are involved in asthma. Inflammatory cells, such as mast cells, eosinophils, lymphocytes, and macrophages, release a variety of chemical mediators, such as histamine, prostaglandins, and leukotrienes. These mediators result in increased wall thickness, airway smooth muscle hypertrophy and constriction, epithelial sloughing, mucus hypersecretion, mucosal edema, and stimulation of nerve endings. *Top,* Daily variability in peak airflow measurements. The normal increase in smooth muscle tone in the early morning, which causes airway narrowing in healthy individuals, is more exaggerated in asthmatics. *Bottom,* Dose-response curves to methacholine. (Modified from Woolcock AJ: Asthma. In Murray JF, Nadel JA, editors: Textbook of respiratory medicine, Philadelphia, 1994, Saunders.)

or emotional stress; inhalation of irritants; and pharmacologic agents, such as methacholine and histamine.[71-73]

When a patient with asthma inhales an allergen to which he or she is sensitized, the antigen cross-links to specific IgE molecules attached to the surface of mast cells in the bronchial mucosa and submucosa. The mast cells degranulate rapidly (within 30 minutes), releasing multiple mediators including leukotrienes (previously known as slow-reacting substance of anaphylaxis [SRS-A]), histamine, prostaglandins, platelet-activating factor, and other mediators. These mediators lead to smooth muscle contraction, vascular congestion, and leakage resulting in airflow obstruction, which can be assessed clinically as a decline in FEV_1 or *peak expiratory flow rate* (PEFR) (Figure 23-7). This is the *early (acute) asthmatic response,* which is an immediate hypersensitivity reaction that usually subsides in about 30 to 60 minutes. In approximately 50% of asthmatic patients, however, airflow obstruction recurs in 3 to 8 hours.[73] This *late asthmatic response* is usually more severe and lasts longer than the early asthmatic response (Figure 23-8).[74] The late asthmatic response is characterized by increasing influx and activation of inflammatory cells such as mast cells, eosinophils, and lymphocytes.[74,75]

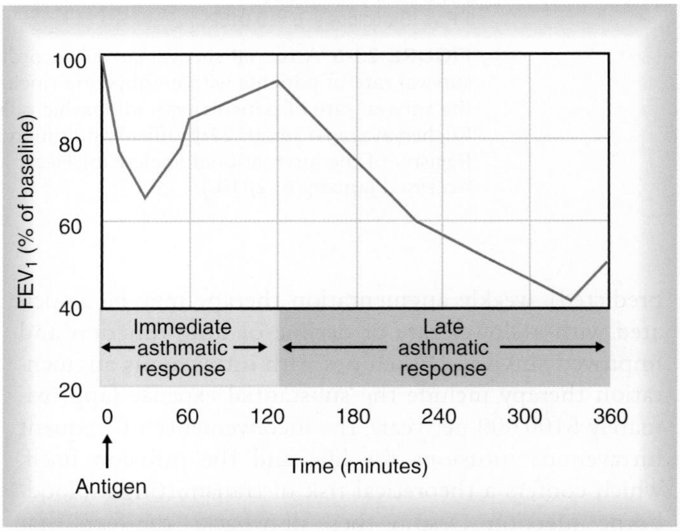

FIGURE 23-8 Early and late asthmatic responses. When a person with asthma is exposed to an allergen to which he or she is sensitized, the challenge results in a biphasic decline in respiratory function. An early asthmatic response occurs within minutes and usually subsides within 2 hours. In about half of asthmatic patients, a late asthmatic response occurs within 3 to 8 hours and may last for 24 hours or longer. (Modified from Wiedemann HP, Kavuru MS: Diagnosis and management of asthma, Caddo, OK, 1994, Professional Communications.)

Clinical Presentation and Diagnosis

The diagnosis of asthma requires clinical assessment supported by laboratory evaluation. Because no single measurement can establish the diagnosis with certainty and physical examination can be entirely normal between episodes, the history plays a key role in suggesting, and later establishing, the diagnosis of asthma. The classic symptoms of asthma are episodic wheezing, shortness of breath, chest tightness, and cough. The absence of wheezing does not exclude asthma, and sometimes a cough can be the only manifestation (cough-variant asthma). Not all wheezing is due to asthma, however. Obstruction of the upper airway by tumors, laryngospasm, aspirated foreign objects, tracheal stenosis, or functional laryngospasm (vocal cord dysfunction) can mimic the wheezing of asthma.

Confirmation of the diagnosis of asthma requires demonstration of reversible airflow obstruction. Pulmonary function tests may be normal in asymptomatic patients with asthma, but more commonly they reveal some degree of airway obstruction manifested by decreased FEV_1 and FEV_1/FVC ratio. By convention, improvement in the FEV_1 by at least 12% and 200 ml after administration of a bronchodilator is considered evidence of reversibility. Spontaneous variation in self-recorded PEFR by 15% or more also can provide evidence of reversibility of airway obstruction (see Figure 23-7).

Asthmatics evaluated in a symptom-free period may have a normal chest x-ray examination and normal pulmonary function tests. Under these circumstances, provocative testing can be used to induce airway obstruction. Bronchoprovocation is a well-established method to detect and quantify AHR. Pharmacologic agents, including acetylcholine, methacholine, histamine, cysteinyl leukotrienes, and prostaglandins, and physical stimuli such as exercise and isocapnic hyperventilation with cold, dry air have been used to detect, quantify, and characterize nonspecific AHR in asthma.

The most commonly used stimulus for bronchoprovocation is methacholine. The generally accepted criterion for hyperresponsiveness is a decrease in FEV_1 by 20% or more below the baseline value after inhalation of methacholine (see Figure 23-7).

The methacholine provocation test has few false-negative results (<5%), but a false-positive result may be found in 7% to 8% of the average population and patients with other obstructive lung diseases. Elevated IgE levels and eosinophilia may be present in patients with asthma, but their presence is not specific, and their absence does not exclude asthma, rendering them not useful for the diagnosis.[67-69] Although arterial blood gas analysis is not helpful or necessary in diagnosing asthma, it can be helpful in assessing the severity of an acute asthma attack.

A patient experiencing an acute asthma attack usually has a low $PaCO_2$ as a result of hyperventilation. A normal $PaCO_2$ in such a situation indicates a severe attack and impending respiratory failure.

Management

The goal of asthma management is to maintain a high quality of life for the patient, uninterrupted by asthma symptoms, side effects from medications, or limitations on the job or during exercise. This goal can be accomplished by preventing acute exacerbations, with their potential mortality and morbidity, or by returning the patient to a stable baseline when exacerbations occur. Asthma management relies on the following four integral components recommended by the National Asthma Education Program (NAEP) expert panel[67]:

1. Objective measurements and monitoring of lung function
2. Pharmacologic therapy
3. Environmental control
4. Patient education

Table 23-2 outlines the stepwise approach currently recommended for long-term management of asthma. This approach provides a framework for an individually tailored dose of medication based on the severity of asthma in any patient at a particular time. This approach acknowledges that asthma is a chronic and dynamic disease, which needs optimum control. Control of asthma is defined as minimal to no chronic diurnal or nocturnal symptoms, infrequent exacerbations, minimal to no need for beta-2 agonists, no limitation to exercise activity, PEFR or FEV_1 greater than 80% predicted with less than 20% diurnal variation, and minimal to no adverse effects of medication.[67-69]

MINI CLINI

Diagnosis of Wheezing

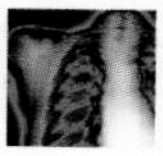

PROBLEM: You are asked to see a patient with a history of wheezing. The patient notes that the wheezing has been continuous, has been present for several months, and has been unresponsive to bronchodilator medications, including systemic corticosteroids and various inhaled bronchodilators.

SOLUTION: The patient has either refractory asthma or a condition mimicking asthma. The aphorism "all that wheezes is not asthma" applies here, and the clinician should suspect alternative diagnoses. Features that are atypical for asthma in this patient are the continuous nature of the wheezing and its complete refractoriness to medication. With this in mind, consideration of other "wheezy" disorders should include abnormalities of the upper airway. Specifically, tracheal stenosis or fixed upper airway obstruction (e.g., caused by tracheal tumors) could account for the patient's symptoms. Another condition that mimics asthma is vocal cord dysfunction. Characteristically, vocal cord dysfunction causes stridor with convergence of the vocal cords on inspiration (a paradoxical response). However, vocal cord dysfunction also can cause expiratory wheezing, with closure of the vocal cords on expiration. Further assessment of this patient might include a flow-volume loop or a fiberoptic examination of the upper airway, observing both the vocal cords and the trachea to the level of the main stem bronchi.

Objective Measurement and Monitoring

Objective measurement of lung function is particularly important in asthma because subjective measures, such as patient reports of the degree of dyspnea and physical examination findings, often do not correlate with the variability and severity of airflow obstruction. It is

TABLE 23-2

Stepwise Approach to Long-Term Management of Asthma Based on Severity

Severity*	Clinical Features Before Treatment†	PEFR or FEV_1	Long-Term Preventive Medications	Quick-Relief Medications
Step 4				
Severe persistent	Continuous symptoms	≤60% predicted	Inhaled corticosteroids ≥800-2000 mcg/day	Inhaled beta-2 agonist as needed for symptoms
Red zone	Frequent exacerbations Nocturnal symptoms Symptoms limit activity	>30% variability	Long-acting bronchodilator‡ Oral corticosteroids	
Step 3				
Moderate persistent	Daily symptoms	>60%-<80% predicted	Inhaled corticosteroids ≥800-2000 mcg/day	Inhaled beta-2 agonist as needed for symptoms, not to exceed 3-4 times per day
Yellow zone	Exacerbations affect activity and sleep Nocturnal symptoms more than once per week Daily use of short-acting beta-2 agonist	>30% variability	Long-acting bronchodilator,‡ especially for nocturnal symptoms	
Step 2				
Mild persistent	Symptoms at least once per week but <1 time per day	≥80% predicted	Inhaled corticosteroid, 200-500 mg/day, cromolyn, or nedocromil	Inhaled beta-2 agonist as needed for symptoms, not to exceed 3-4 times per day
Yellow zone	Exacerbations may affect activity or sleep Nocturnal symptoms more than twice per month	20%-30% variability	Long-acting bronchodilator‡ for nocturnal symptoms	
Step 1				
Intermittent	Intermittent symptoms less than once per week	≥80% predicted	None needed	Inhaled beta-2 agonist needed for symptoms but less than once per week
Green zone	Nocturnal symptoms not more than twice per month Asymptomatic with normal lung function between exacerbations	<20% variability		Inhaled beta-2 agonist or cromolyn before exercise or exposure to allergen

Modified from Global Initiative for Asthma: Asthma management and prevention: a practical guide for public health officials and health care professionals, NIH publication no. 96-3659A, Bethesda, MD, 1995, National Institutes of Health, National Heart, Lung, and Blood Institute, and World Health Organization.

**Step-down:* Review treatment every 3-6 months. If control is sustained for at least 3 months, consider a gradual stepwise reduction in treatment. *Step-up:* If control is not achieved, consider step-up, but first review patient medication technique, compliance, and environmental control.

†The presence of one of the features of severity is sufficient to place a patient in that category.

‡Long-acting beta-2 agonist or sustained-release theophylline.

recommended that spirometry be performed as part of the initial assessment of all patients being evaluated for asthma and periodically thereafter as needed.

Either spirometry or PEFR measurement can be used to assess response to therapy in the outpatient setting, emergency department, or hospital. NAEP guidelines also recommend that home PEFR measurement be used for patients with moderate to severe asthma.

When patients learn how to take PEFR measurements at home, the clinician is better able to recommend effective treatment. Daily monitoring of PEFR helps detect early stages of airway obstruction. All PEFR measurements are compared with the patient's personal best value, which can be established during a 2- to 3-week asymptomatic period when the patient is being treated optimally.[67-69]

To help patients understand home PEFR monitoring, a zonal system corresponding to the traffic light system may be helpful (see Table 23-2). A PEFR measurement of 80% to 100% of the personal best is considered to be in the *green zone*. No asthma symptoms are present, and maintenance medications can be continued or tapered. A PEFR in the 60% to 80% range of the personal best is in the *yellow zone* and may indicate an acute exacerbation and requires a temporary step-up in treatment. A PEFR less than 60% of the personal best is in the *red zone* and signals a medical alert, requiring immediate medical attention if the patient does not return to the yellow zone or green zone with bronchodilator use.[69]

Pharmacotherapy

Pharmacotherapy for asthma reflects the basic understanding that asthma is a chronic inflammatory airway disease that requires long-term antiinflammatory therapy for adequate control.[67-76] Antiinflammatory agents, such as corticosteroids and cromolyn, suppress the primary disease process and its resultant airway hyperreactivity. Bronchodilators, such as beta-2-adrenergic agonists, anticholinergics, and theophylline, relieve asthma symptoms. Because asthma is a disease of the airways, inhalation therapy is preferred to oral or other systemic therapy. Inhaled therapy using metered dose inhalers or powders allows high concentration of the medication to be delivered directly to the airways, resulting in fewer systemic side effects. Spacer devices can be used to improve delivery of inhaled medication, but training and coordination are still required for patients using metered dose inhalers. Table 23-3 lists commonly used medications in the treatment of asthma.

Corticosteroids

Corticosteroids are the most effective medication currently available for the treatment of asthma. Although their mode of action is still uncertain, corticosteroids probably act on various components of the inflammatory response in asthma.[76] Inhaled corticosteroids are effective locally, and regular use suppresses inflammation in the airways, decreases bronchial hyperreactivity and airflow obstruction, and reduces the symptoms of and mortality from asthma. Long-term, high-dose inhaled corticosteroids have far fewer side effects than oral corticosteroids. Side effects such as oropharyngeal candidiasis and dysphonia are controllable with spacer use and by rinsing the mouth after each treatment.

Oral corticosteroids are effective for treating asthma, but the potential for devastating side effects during long-term use restricts their use to patients not responding to other forms of asthma therapy. Short-term, high-dose (0.5 to 1.0 mg/kg/day) oral corticosteroid therapy during exacerbation reduces the severity and duration, decreases the need for emergency department visits and hospitalization, and reduces mortality.[76]

Cromolyn

Cromolyn sodium is a noncorticosteroid antiinflammatory medication. Its mechanism of action is not completely understood, but it has a protective effect against provocative stimuli such as allergens, cold air, and exercise. The drug is most effective when administered prophylactically. Cromolyn does not dilate smooth muscle and is not useful for treating the symptoms of an acute asthma attack. Cromolyn is useful in cough-variant and exercise-induced asthma but otherwise has only limited usefulness in the treatment of adult asthmatics. However, many experts believe that cromolyn is the drug of choice for atopic children with asthma.[72]

Nedocromil

In 1993, nedocromil was approved in the United States for use in metered dose inhalers. It is structurally different from cromolyn but has similar pharmacologic activity and is 4 to 10 times more potent in preventing acute allergic bronchospasm. Nedocromil can be used as an alternative to cromolyn, but neither nedocromil nor cromolyn has a clear advantage over inhaled corticosteroids.[72]

Leukotriene Inhibitors

Leukotrienes are mediators of inflammation and bronchoconstriction and are thought to play a role in the pathogenesis of asthma. Three leukotriene antagonists are currently available for the treatment of asthma. Montelukast (Singulair; Merck, Whitehouse Station, NJ) and zafirlukast (Accolate; Astra Zeneca, London, United Kingdom) are leukotriene receptor antagonists, and zileuton (Zyflo; Abbott Laboratories, Chicago, IL) is a leukotriene synthesis inhibitor. These agents all are modestly effective for maintenance of mild to moderate asthma, but their exact role in asthma therapy remains to be determined. Inhaled steroids remain the antiinflammatory drugs of choice for the treatment of asthma.[77]

Beta-2-Adrenergic Agonists

Inhaled beta-2-adrenergic agents are the most rapid and effective bronchodilators for the treatment of asthma. They are the drugs of choice for all types of acute bronchospasm, and they provide protection from all bronchoconstrictor challenges when given prophylactically. However, they do not prevent the late asthmatic response. Beta-2 agonists are the drugs of choice for exercise-induced asthma. They exert their action by attaching to beta receptors on the cell to produce smooth muscle relaxation and by blocking mediator release from mast cells.

The effectiveness of beta-2 agonists as bronchodilators is not disputed, and they are the drug of choice for acute emergency management of asthma. However, there is concern that they may worsen asthma control if used regularly and that excessive use may increase the risk of death from asthma, which makes the role of beta-2 agonists in long-term maintenance therapy questionable.

Although there is sufficient concern regarding fenoterol to justify avoiding its use, it remains unclear whether the association between excessive beta-2 agonist use and death from asthma is a genuine or spurious association.[77] It is clear, however, that excessive beta-2 agonist use by asthmatics indicates an increased risk of death from asthma and indicates the need for more effective antiinflammatory therapy. There is currently little definitive evidence to establish that treatment with conventional doses of the short-acting beta-2 agonists available in the United States is harmful to asthmatic patients.[75,76,78] The NAEP

TABLE 23-3

Medications Commonly Used in the Treatment of Asthma and COPD

Medication	Trade Names	Available Preparations	Usual Dosage
Inhaled Corticosteroids			
Beclomethasone	Beclovent, Vanceril	MDI 42 mcg/puff, 200 puffs/canister	2 puffs tid-qid, maximum 20 puffs/day
Triamcinolone	Azmacort	MDI 100 mcg/puff, 240 puffs/canister	2-4 puffs qid, maximum 16 puffs/day
Flunisolide	AeroBid	MDI 250 mg/puff, 100 puffs/canister	2 puffs bid, maximum 8 puffs/day
Fluticasone	Flovent	MDI 44, 110, 220 mcg/puff	88-880 mcg/day
Mometasone	Asmanex	DPI 220 mcg/spray	1-2 sprays qd-bid, maximum 4 puffs/ day
Budesonide	Pulmicort	DPI 90, 180 mcg/puff	360-720 mcg/day
Systemic Corticosteroids			
Prednisone	Many	Tablets 1, 5, 20, 50 mg	5-50 mg/day
Methylprednisolone	Medrol	Tablets 2, 4, 8, 16, 24, 32 mg	4-48 mg/day
	Solu-Medrol	IV 40, 125, 500, 1000 mg	1-2 mg/kg q4-6h
Hydrocortisone	Solu-Cortef	IV 100, 250, 500, 1000 mg	4 mg/kg q4-6h
Beta-2 Agonists			
Albuterol	Proventil	MDI 90 mcg/puff, 200 puffs/canister	2-4 puffs q4-6h, maximum 20 puffs/day
	Ventolin	Solution for nebulizer 0.083% and 0.5%	2.5-10 mg q6-8h
		Tablets 2, 4 mg	2-4 mg q6-8h
	Volmax	Sustained-release tablets 4, 8 mg	4-8 mg q12h
Metaproterenol	Alupent	MDI 650 mcg/puff, 200 puffs/canister	2-3 puffs q3-4h, maximum 12 puffs/day
	Metaprel	Solution 0.5%	2.5-10 mg q4-6h
		Tablets 10, 20 mg	10 mg q6-8h
Pirbuterol	Maxair	MDI 200 mcg/puff, 300 puffs/canister	1-2 puffs q4-6h, maximum 12 puffs/day
Terbutaline	Breathaire	MDI 200 mcg/puff, 300 puffs/canister 1-2 puffs q4-6h	
	Bricanyl	Tablets 2.5, 5 mg	2.5-5 mg tid, maximum 15 mg/day
		Solution 1 mg/ml	0.25 mg SC q15-30min
Salmeterol	Serevent	MDI 50 mcg/puff	2 puffs q12h
Formoterol	Foradil	DPI 12 mcg/capsule	1 capsule inhaled q12h
Arformoterol	Brovana	Solution 15 mcg/ml	15 mcg inhaled bid
Anticholinergics			
Ipratropium bromide	Atrovent	MDI 18 mcg/puff, 200 puffs/canister	2-4 puffs q6h
		Solution for nebulizer 0.02%	
		0.5 mg/2.5 ml vial, 0.5 mg qid	
Tiotropium	Spiriva	DPI 18 mcg/capsule	1 capsule inhaled/day
Methylxanthines			
Aminophylline		IV	Load 5-6 mg/kg, maintenance
		Tablets or capsules	0.5-0.9 mg/kg/hr
Theophylline	Theo-Dur		300-1200 mg/day divided q6-8h for immediate and q12-24h for sustained
	Slo-bid		
	Theovent		
	Uniphyl (immediate or sustained release)		
Leukotriene Inhibitors			
Zafirlukast	Accolate	Tablets 20 mg	20 mg bid
Zileuton	Zyflo	Tablets 600 mg	600 mg qid
Montelukast	Singulair	Tablets 10 mg	10 mg qd
Other			
Cromolyn	Intal	MDI 800 mcg/puff, 112 puffs/canister	2 puffs qid
		Spinhaler 20 mg/capsule	20 mg qid
Nedocromil	Tilade	MDI 1.75 mg/puff, 112 puffs/canister	2 puffs bid-qid

DPI, Dry powder inhaler; *IV,* intravenous; *MDI,* metered dose inhaler; *SC,* subcutaneous.

guidelines recommend that inhaled beta-2 agonists be used as needed. If a patient needs more than 3 or 4 puffs a day of a beta-2 agonist, additional antiinflammatory therapy should be considered.[77]

Newer, longer acting (12 to 24 hours) beta-2 agonists, such as salmeterol and formoterol, are available in the United States. Their mechanism of action is different from the shorter acting beta-2 agonists discussed earlier. Long-acting beta-2 agonists have use in treating nocturnal asthma.[67-69,78]

Monotherapy with beta agonists has been shown to be inferior to use of inhaled corticosteroids, which are recommended as first-line treatment for asthma. When added to inhaled corticosteroids, long-acting beta agonists have been found to improve asthma control, symptoms, and exacerbations. However, a meta-analysis of randomized controlled clinical trials examining outcomes for asthma control found that long-acting beta agonists increase the risk for hospitalization from asthma, life-threatening asthma attacks, and asthma-related deaths compared with placebo.[79] Several mechanisms need to be considered to explain such reactions, including paradoxical bronchospasm, increased bronchial responsiveness, and tolerance. Racial and genetic factors may also influence these outcomes.

The FDA requested manufacturers of Serevent Diskus (salmeterol xinafoate inhalation powder), Advair Diskus (fluticasone propionate and salmeterol inhalation powder), and Foradil Aerolizer (formoterol fumarate inhalation powder) to update their existing product labels with new warnings and a medication guide for patients to alert health care professionals and patients that these medicines may increase the chance of severe asthma episodes and death when such episodes occur.[80] Inhaled corticosteroids remain the first choice of therapy in asthma, and careful monitoring is required when long-acting beta agonists are used for asthma control.

Methylxanthines

The role of theophylline and similar drugs in the treatment of acute asthma is controversial. The NAEP expert panel did not recommend using theophylline routinely in the emergency treatment of asthma but did recommend its use orally or intravenously for patients admitted to the hospital for an acute asthma attack. Sustained-release theophyllines added to long-term asthma management therapy may be helpful in controlling nocturnal asthma symptoms because they maintain therapeutic plasma concentrations overnight. They also are helpful in soothing the symptoms of labile asthmatics. However, the efficacy of theophylline is limited by its side effects of nausea, vomiting, headache, insomnia, seizures, and cardiac arrhythmias. Toxicity increases with blood levels greater than 15 mcg/ml, but levels of 8 to 10 mcg/ml are adequate for long-term therapy and are associated with fewer side effects.

Several factors affect the plasma levels of theophylline by increasing or decreasing hepatic metabolism of the drug. Conditions that tend to increase plasma concentrations include acute viral infections, cardiac failure, hepatic disease, and concomitant use of certain medications such as erythromycin or cimetidine. In these cases, the maintenance dose should be halved, and the theophylline blood levels should be monitored. Conditions that tend to decrease plasma levels of theophylline include cigarette smoking and use of medications that increase hepatic clearance, such as phenobarbital.[67-69,72]

Anticholinergics

Inhaled anticholinergic agents, such as ipratropium bromide, are effective dilators of airway smooth muscles. Although the regular use of these agents seems to be effective in patients with COPD, their benefit in the day-to-day management of asthma has not been established. Ipratropium produces bronchodilation by reduction of intrinsic vagal tone and by blocking vagal reflex bronchospasm. However, ipratropium does not stabilize mast cells or prevent mediator release and is a less potent bronchodilator than beta-2 agonists. Ipratropium has few side effects, is safe because it is poorly absorbed, adds a bronchodilator effect to beta-2 agonists, and is useful for treating cough-variant asthma. Ipratropium also can be used in treating acute asthma when first-line bronchodilators are ineffective. The long-acting anticholinergic agent, tiotropium, has been shown to enhance asthma control (e.g., improved peak expiratory flow, increased FEV_1, and improved symptoms) when added to an inhaled corticosteroid compared with doubling the inhaled steroid dose.[81]

Anti-IgE Therapy

IgE plays a key role in the pathogenesis of asthma, and many asthmatic patients have elevated levels of IgE.[82] Corticosteroids do not inhibit synthesis of IgE by activated lymphocytes. Omalizumab, an antibody that binds IgE and blocks its biologic effects, has been approved by the FDA for patients with a history of allergy and with moderate to severe asthma that is poorly controlled with inhaled corticosteroids.[83] Studies have shown that treatment with omalizumab results in a reduction in the dose of inhaled glucocorticoids required to control symptoms and a reduction in the number of asthma exacerbation episodes.[84] For this reason, the NAEP asthma guidelines recommended that omalizumab should be considered as adjunctive therapy for patients with severe persistent asthma.[67]

Emergency Department and Hospital Management

Emergency management of acute asthma should include early and frequent administration of aerosolized beta-2 agonists and therapy with systemic corticosteroids. Frequent assessment for response with PEFR should be performed. The NAEP guidelines recommend that only selective beta-2 agonists (i.e., albuterol, levalbuterol, pirbuterol) should be used in high doses to avoid cardiotoxicity.[67] It is unclear which subset of patients may benefit from continuous aerosolized beta-2 agonists.

Hospital and ICU care for patients with asthma should be aggressive. The goal is to decrease mortality and morbidity and to return the patient to preadmission stability and function as quickly as possible. Management includes O_2 supplementation, frequent administration of high doses of aerosolized beta-2 agonists (limited only by tachycardia or tremor), high-dose parenteral corticosteroids (>0.5 to 1.0 mg/kg/day), and antibiotics if there is evidence of infection. Sedatives and hypnotics should be avoided. Symptoms, PEFR, and arterial blood gases should be monitored.

Patients with severe asthma and respiratory failure (hypoxemia, hypercapnia, increased work of breathing) need ventilatory support and present special challenges. Mortality rates for these patients can reach 22%, and complications are common, especially barotrauma. These complications can be minimized by limiting peak inspiratory pressure to less than 50 cm H_2O and by the use of small tidal volumes, allowing "permissive hypercapnia" if necessary. When asthma control is achieved, hospital discharge criteria include being off O_2, with PaO_2 greater than 60 mm Hg; stable PEFR or FEV_1, with values close to the patient's best or greater than 70% of predicted; asthma symptoms returning to preadmission levels; no nocturnal symptoms; and 12- to 24-hour stability on discharge medications.[67-69]

RULE OF THUMB

In a patient presenting with an acute asthma attack, $PaCO_2$ is usually low because of hyperventilation. A normal $PaCO_2$ in this situation indicates a severe attack and impending respiratory failure.

Bronchial Thermoplasty

Bronchial thermoplasty is a recently approved addition to treatment options for adults whose asthma remains uncontrolled despite use of inhaled steroids and long-acting beta agonists.[85] Bronchial thermoplasty is a procedure in which a probe is introduced into the central airways through a bronchoscope and heat is applied (through radiofrequency waves) to airways of 3 to 10 mm diameter with the goal to reduce the airway smooth muscle mass, reducing the ability of the airways to constrict. Studies have shown that bronchial thermoplasty improves asthma-specific quality of life and reduces the number of severe asthma exacerbation episodes and emergency department visits.[86,87] Although bronchial thermoplasty is a promising new treatment for patients with difficult to control asthma, the long-term side effects of this procedure have not been well studied, and more studies are needed before it can be recommended to all patients with poorly controlled asthma.

MINI CLINI

Assessing the Severity of an Acute Asthma Attack

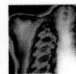

PROBLEM: You have just obtained an arterial blood gas (ABG) analysis on a patient who sought treatment at the emergency department for an acute attack of asthma. How would the ABG analysis help you assess the severity of the attack?

SOLUTION: In the early stages of an asthma attack, the ABG analysis shows a low $PaCO_2$ caused by hyperventilation. As the asthma attack progresses, and the FEV_1 decreases to less than 25% of predicted, the $PaCO_2$ returns to normal. When the FEV_1 decreases to less than 15% of predicted, carbon dioxide retention begins to occur. Changes in the pH reflect changes in the $PaCO_2$ level. The following table summarizes the ABG abnormalities based on the severity of an asthma attack:

Asthma Severity	Stage	PaO_2	$PaCO_2$	pH
Mild	I	Normal	Decreased	Increased
Moderate	II	Decreased	Decreased	Increased
Severe	III	Decreased	Normal	Normal
Very severe (respiratory failure)	IV	Decreased	Increased	Decreased

Immunotherapy

Immunotherapy is based on the theoretical rationale that part of the immunologic response to an administered allergen is the production of IgG-specific antibody to the allergen injected. This newly generated IgG does not affix to most cells but can react with the allergen diffusing into the tissues and "neutralize" it. Although immunotherapy is acceptable in the treatment of allergic rhinitis, its use in the treatment of asthma is not standardized and remains controversial. However, a meta-analysis of 88 randomized controlled trials of injection allergen immunotherapy for asthma reported that immunotherapy is effective, with evidence of significant reductions in asthma medications and symptoms and a reduction in the degree of bronchial hyperreactivity.[88]

Environmental Control

The association between asthma and allergy has long been recognized. Of patients with asthma, 75% to 85% are reported to have positive immediate skin test reaction to common inhalant allergens. A thorough history is essential to diagnosing whether a patient's asthma has an allergic component and to determining the relationship between exposure to an allergen and the occurrence of symptoms. Skin tests are more helpful for excluding an allergen as a cause of asthma symptoms because clinical sensitivity to an aeroallergen is rare in the absence of a positive skin test, whereas many positive skin tests do not have clinical relevance.

To prevent allergic reactions in asthma patients, environmental control measures to reduce exposure to indoor and outdoor allergens and irritants are essential. Patients should be advised to avoid outdoor antigens, primarily ragweed, grass, pollens, and molds. Exposure to outdoor allergens is best reduced by staying indoors, with the windows closed, in an air-conditioned environment, particularly during the midday and afternoon, when pollen and some mold counts are highest. Patients who are allergic to indoor allergens, primarily house-dust components and indoor molds, should implement strategies for eliminating these allergens from the home environment (e.g., single room air purifier). All warm-blooded pets, including small rodents and birds, should be removed from the house because they produce dander, urine, and saliva that can cause allergic reactions. House-dust mites depend on atmospheric moisture and human dander for survival. Essential house-dust mite control measures include encasing mattresses and pillows in airtight covers, washing the bedding in water of 130° F weekly, avoiding sleeping on upholstered furniture, and removing carpets that are laid on concrete.

Additional helpful control measures include reducing the indoor humidity to less than 50%, removing carpets from the bedroom, and using chemical agents to kill mites. Indoor air-cleaning devices, especially high-efficiency particulate air/aerosol filters, may be useful, but they cannot substitute for controlling the allergen source. Humidifiers are potentially harmful because they can harbor and aerosolize mold spores, and the increased humidity they generate may encourage production of both mold and house-dust mites.[67-69]

Patient Education

Much of the day-to-day responsibility for managing asthma falls on the patient and the patient's family. Patient education is a powerful motivational tool, helping patients attain the skills and gain the confidence to control their asthma. Patient education involves helping patients understand asthma and learning and practicing the skills necessary to manage it. Patient education includes providing information; developing a partnership with the patient; involving the patient in decision making; and demonstrating and observing asthma management practices such as the proper use of inhalers, nebulizers, and peak flowmeters.[78]

Special Considerations in Asthma Management

Exercise-Induced Asthma

Exercise-induced asthma is common in asthmatics, especially after participation in outdoor activities in cold weather. The causes are not fully understood, but heat loss from the airways seems to be one of the causes.[74] Treatment consists of prophylactic inhalation of a beta-2 agonist or cromolyn before exercise. Leukotriene inhibitors also may have a role in treatment of exercise-induced asthma.[67,68]

Occupational Asthma

An estimated 2% to 5% of all asthma episodes may be caused by exposure to a specific sensitizing agent in the workplace. Occupational asthma is the most common form of occupational lung disease in many industrialized countries. In an attempt to distinguish occupational from preexisting asthma, occupational asthma is defined as a disease characterized by a variable airflow limitation or AHR secondary to causes and conditions attributable to a particular working environment and not to stimuli encountered outside the workplace. Toluene diisocyanate is the most common cause of occupational asthma and is the best studied. Other causes of occupational asthma are listed in Table 23-4.

Generally, the treatment of occupational asthma is identical to treatment of other types of asthma. However, early diagnosis is important, and emphasis is placed on environmental control, in particular, cessation of exposure. Complete cessation of exposure is usually necessary because once sensitization has occurred, bronchoconstriction can be triggered by minimal subsequent exposure.[68,75]

Cough-Variant Asthma

Coughing may be the sole complaint of patients with asthma. In such patients, the cough may be relieved by a bronchodilator or the avoidance of inhaled allergens. If bronchospasm is not present at the time of examination

TABLE 23-4

Occupational Causes of Asthma

Occupation or Industry	Agent
Laboratory animal workers, veterinarians	Animals (dander, urine protein)
Food processing	Shellfish, egg proteins, pancreatic enzymes
Dairy farming	Storage mites
Poultry farming	Poultry mites, droppings, feathers
Detergent manufacturing	*Bacillus subtilis* enzymes
Baking	Flour
Sawmill workers, carpentry	Wood dust (western red cedar, oak, mahogany, zebrawood, redwood)
Nursing	Psyllium
Refining	Platinum salts
Plating	Nickel salts
Stainless steel welding	Chromium salts
Cosmetology	Persulfate
Refinery workers	Vanadium
Rubber processing	Formaldehyde, ethylenediamine
Plastics industry	Toluene diisocyanate, trimellitic anhydride

and spirometry is normal (which is often the case), the diagnosis can be confirmed by showing reversible airway obstruction by a methacholine challenge test. Ipratropium bromide may be particularly helpful in the treatment of cough-variant asthma. Otherwise, the treatment is the same as for other types of asthma.

Nocturnal Asthma

Nocturnal asthma is a characteristic problem in poorly controlled asthma and is reported by more than two-thirds of patients who receive suboptimal treatment. It probably is due to the known physiologic decrease in the airway tone during sleep, which has been attributed to variation in catecholamine and cortisol secretion. Aspiration of gastric acid also may play a role in some patients with increased symptoms at night.

After ensuring adequate antiinflammatory therapy, medications for nocturnal asthma should be focused toward the night and especially the early morning hours, when the airway tone is lowest. Sustained-release theophylline and newer long-acting beta-2 agonists such as salmeterol are particularly helpful for controlling nocturnal asthma symptoms.[68,75] Addition of a proton pump inhibitor such as esomeprazole has not been shown to enhance asthma control.[89]

Aspirin Sensitivity

At least 5% of adults with asthma experience severe and even fatal exacerbation of asthma after taking aspirin or other nonsteroidal antiinflammatory drugs (NSAIDs). Many of these patients have nasal polyps, although the relationship is not causal. The presumed mechanism is the inhibition of the cyclooxygenase pathway by aspirin and NSAIDs, with subsequent shunting of all arachidonic acid into the 5-lipoxygenase pathway, causing overproduction of bronchoconstrictor leukotrienes. Individuals with asthma should avoid aspirin and NSAIDs and instead use alternatives such as acetaminophen (e.g., Tylenol). Patients should be informed that many over-the-counter medications contain aspirin and should be avoided as well.[68,75]

Gastroesophageal Reflux

The relationship between asthma and gastroesophageal reflux is controversial, although gastroesophageal reflux is nearly three times more prevalent in patients with asthma than in persons without asthma. Presumably, acid reflux into the esophagus causes vagal stimulation, resulting in a reflex increase in bronchial tone in patients with asthma. However, addition of a proton pump inhibitor to an asthma regimen has not been shown to enhance asthma control significantly.[89]

Asthma During Pregnancy

During pregnancy, one-third of patients have worse control of their asthma, one-third have better control of asthma, and one-third have asthma that is unchanged. The potential threat of adverse effects from asthma medications is far outweighed by the danger of uncontrolled asthma to the fetus and mother. Poorly controlled asthma during pregnancy can cause increased perinatal mortality, increased prematurity, and low birth weight. Theophyllines, beta-2 agonists, inhaled or oral corticosteroids, or cromolyn can be used during pregnancy without significant risk of fetal abnormalities.[90]

Sinusitis

Acute sinusitis and chronic sinusitis have been related to exacerbations and poor control of asthma by causing postnasal drip and interfering with nasal patency. A limited CT scan of the sinuses should be obtained for patients with uncontrolled asthma. If sinusitis is present, therapy with antibiotics for 2 to 3 weeks, nasal decongestants, and nasal corticosteroid inhalers may help improve asthma control.[67,68]

Surgery

Patients with asthma are predisposed to respiratory complications after surgery, including respiratory arrest during induction of anesthesia, hypoxemia and possible hypercapnia, impaired effectiveness of cough, atelectasis, and respiratory infection. The likelihood of these complications depends on the severity of the patient's AHR, the degree of airflow obstruction, and the amount of excess airway secretions at the time of surgery. Optimizing the patient's lung function before surgery, including the administration of perioperative corticosteroids, is an important strategy for minimizing perioperative complications.[67,68]

BRONCHIECTASIS

Clinical Presentation

Bronchiectasis refers to the abnormal, irreversible dilation of the bronchi caused by destructive and inflammatory changes in the airway walls. Bronchiectasis has the following three major anatomic patterns[91]:

1. *Cylindrical bronchiectasis:* Airway wall is regularly and uniformly dilated
2. *Varicose bronchiectasis:* Irregular pattern, with alternating areas of constriction and dilation
3. *Cystic bronchiectasis:* Progressive, distal enlargement of the airways, resulting in saclike dilations

Bronchiectasis is thought to result from damage to the bronchial wall by chronic inflammation. Predisposing conditions are listed in Box 23-4.

Evaluation

The hallmark of bronchiectasis is the chronic production of large quantities of purulent sputum. Dyspnea is variable and depends on the extent of involvement and the underlying disease. Hemoptysis occurs frequently and is usually mild, but severe hemoptysis can be seen. Radiographic

Box 23-4 Causes of Bronchiectasis

LOCAL BRONCHIECTASIS
- Foreign body
- Benign airway tumor (e.g., adenoma)
- Bronchial compression by surrounding lymph nodes (e.g., middle lobe syndrome)

DIFFUSE BRONCHIECTASIS
- Cystic fibrosis
- Ciliary dyskinesia disorders (e.g., Kartagener syndrome, Young syndrome)
- Hypogammaglobulinemia
- AAT deficiency
- Allergic bronchopulmonary aspergillosis
- Rheumatoid arthritis
- Serious lung infection (e.g., from whooping cough, measles, or influenza)

studies confirm the diagnosis by showing airway dilation. A chest radiograph may show cystic spaces and tram tracks (thin parallel lines representing the airway walls). CT is the diagnostic standard; the diagnosis of bronchiectasis is established when the diameter of the bronchus exceeds the diameter of the adjacent pulmonary artery branch.[92] Because reversible airway changes consistent with bronchiectasis can follow pneumonia, CT should be deferred for 6 to 8 weeks after pneumonia resolves, when a diagnosis of bronchiectasis can be made.

Management

Antibiotics and bronchopulmonary hygiene are the mainstays of bronchiectasis management. Antibiotics can be given as needed or following a regularly scheduled regimen. Sputum cultures may be helpful in guiding antibiotic choice. Inhaled aminoglycosides may be a useful option for patients with chronic colonization by *Pseudomonas aeruginosa*. Infection by *P. aeruginosa* in bronchiectasis patients is a marker of severity but is not linked to accelerated decline in pulmonary function.[93] Secretions can be cleared by chest physiotherapy with postural drainage, cough maneuvers, and humidification. Inhaled bronchodilators may be helpful in some patients because accompanying airflow obstruction is common.[91] Inhaled hyperosmolar substances may be helpful in clearing secretion in patients with bronchiectasis. A Cochrane review concluded that dry powder mannitol improves tracheobronchial clearance in patients with bronchiectasis, patients with cystic fibrosis patients, asthmatics, and normal subjects.[94] Hypertonic saline has not been specifically tested in bronchiectasis, but it improves clearance in these other conditions and in chronic bronchitis. In cases that are complicated by massive hemoptysis, embolization of the bleeding bronchial artery may be helpful. Surgical resection should be reserved for patients with localized disease who develop massive hemoptysis or who are severely symptomatic despite appropriate medical therapy.[95-97]

ROLE OF THE RESPIRATORY THERAPIST IN OBSTRUCTIVE LUNG DISEASE

RTs play key roles in all aspects of managing patients with obstructive lung diseases; they are involved in diagnosis, acute treatment, and follow-up and monitoring. In diagnosis, RTs often perform the lung function testing that indicates the presence of airflow obstruction that is essential for diagnosis. Because of their close involvement with patients, RTs also play important roles in recognizing clinical features that may prompt physicians' appreciation of COPD variants, such as the presence of copious secretions or hemoptysis or both that might lead to suspicion of bronchiectasis or the early onset or familial clustering of COPD that might prompt suspicion of AAT deficiency.

In acute management, hospital-based RTs often administer medications and therapies to patients with acute exacerbations of asthma or COPD. Examples include the delivery of bronchodilators in small volume nebulizers, administration of chest physiotherapy in the management of bronchiectasis, and set-up of supplemental O_2. For patients with severe exacerbations, ICU management of arterial lines, blood gases, and mechanical ventilation often involves RTs in key management roles. In managing patients with bronchiectasis, RTs are pivotal in administering chest physiotherapy and instructing in the use of flutter valves and percussive vests that may be critical parts of acute management.

Finally, in longitudinal follow-up of patients with obstructive lung diseases, RTs are involved in counseling (e.g., smoking cessation, medication management), administering pulmonary rehabilitation programs, and certifying and recertifying long-term O_2 therapy. RTs working in home care may conduct home visits to patients and set up and adjust equipment in the home. This description of activities of the RT in care of the patient with obstructive lung disease suggests that RTs are indispensable caregivers for patients with asthma, COPD, and bronchiectasis and that the care of patients with obstructive lung diseases constitutes a major component of RTs' activities.

SUMMARY CHECKLIST

- Classic symptoms of asthma are episodic wheezing, shortness of breath, chest tightness, and cough.
- The goal of stable asthma management is to maintain a high quality of life for the patient, uninterrupted by asthma symptoms, side effects from medications, or limitations on the job or during exercise. This goal can be accomplished by objective measurements and monitoring lung function, pharmacologic therapy, environmental control, and patient education.
- The goals of emergency management of acute asthma are to decrease mortality and morbidity and to return

Continued

the patient to preadmission stability and function as quickly as possible. These goals are accomplished by O_2 supplementation and frequent administration of high doses of aerosolized beta-2 agonists, high-dose parenteral corticosteroids, and antibiotics if there is evidence of infection.

- The hallmark of bronchiectasis is the chronic production of large quantities of purulent sputum. Dyspnea is variable and depends on the extent of involvement and the underlying disease. Antibiotics and bronchopulmonary hygiene are the mainstays of management.

References

1. American Thoracic Society: COPD guidelines. http://www.thoracic.org/COPD. Accessed December 19, 2010.
2. The Global Initiative for Chronic Obstructive Lung Disease (GOLD): http://www.goldcopd.com. Accessed December 19, 2010.
3. World Health Organization: Global surveillance, prevention and control of chronic respiratory diseases: a comprehensive approach, Geneva, 2007, WHO Press.
4. Brown DW, Croft JB, Greenlund KJ, et al: Deaths from chronic obstructive pulmonary disease—United States, 2000-2005. MMWR Morb Mortal Wkly Rep 57:1229, 2008.
5. Centers for Disease Control and Prevention: http://www.cdc.gov/copd Accessed December 18, 2010.
6. Mannino DM, Homa DM, Akinbami LJ, et al: Chronic obstructive pulmonary disease surveillance—United States, 1971-2000. MMWR Morb Mortal Wkly Rep 51:1-16, 2002.
7. Hardie JA, Vollmer WM, Buist AS, et al: Respiratory symptoms and obstructive pulmonary disease in a population aged over 70 years. Respir Med 99:186-195, 2005.
8. Stoller JK, Aboussouan LS: Alpha-1 antitrypsin deficiency. Lancet 365:2225-2236, 2005.
9. Anthonisen SR, Connett JE, Kiley JP, et al: Effects of smoking intervention and the use of an anticholinergic bronchodilator on the rate of decline of FEV_1: the Lung Health Study. JAMA 272:1497-1504, 1994.
10. Anthonisen NR, Skeans MA, Wise RA, et al: Lung Health Study Research Group: the effects of a smoking cessation intervention on 14.5-year mortality: a randomized clinical trial. Ann Intern Med 142:233-239, 2005.
11. U.S. Department of Health and Human Services: The health consequences of smoking: chronic obstructive lung disease—a report of the Surgeon General, No. (PHS) 84-50205, Rockville, MD, 1984, U.S. Department of Health and Human Services, Public Health Service, Office on Smoking and Health.
12. Stoller JK, Smith P, Yang P, et al: Physical and social impact of alpha-1 antitrypsin deficiency: results of a survey. Cleve Clin J Med 61:461-467, 1994.
13. Stoller JK, Sandhaus RA, Turino G, et al: Delay in diagnosis of alpha-1 antitrypsin deficiency: a continuing problem. Chest 128:1989-1994, 2005.
14. American Thoracic Society/European Respiratory Society: Standards for the diagnosis and management of patients with alpha-1 antitrypsin deficiency. Am J Respir Crit Care Med 168:816-900, 2003.
15. Gadek JE, Fells GA, Zimmerman RL, et al: Antielastases of the human alveolar structures: implications for the protease-antiprotease therapy of emphysema. J Clin Invest 68:889-898, 1981.
16. Stockley RA, Mannino D, Barnes PJ: Burden and pathogenesis of chronic obstructive pulmonary disease. Proc Am Thorac Soc 6:524-526, 2009.
17. Eisner MD, Anthonisen N, Coultas D, et al: Committee on Nonsmoking COPD, Environmental and Occupational Health Assembly. An official American Thoracic Society public policy statement: novel risk factors and the global burden of chronic obstructive pulmonary disease. Am J Respir Crit Care Med 182:693-718, 2010.
18. Stoller JK, Aboussouan LS: Other causes of emphysema. In Albert RK, Spiro S, Jett J, editors: Principles of respiratory medicine, St Louis, 1999, Mosby-Year Book.
19. Anthonisen NR, Wright EC, IPPB Trial Group: Response to inhaled bronchodilators in COPD. Chest 91:36S-39S, 1987.
20. Stoller JK: Clinical practice: acute exacerbations of chronic obstructive pulmonary disease. N Engl J Med 346:988-994, 2002.
21. Sutherland ER, Cherniack RM: Management of chronic obstructive pulmonary disease. N Engl J Med 350:2689-2697, 2004.
22. Barr RG, Bourbeau J, Camargo CA, et al: Inhaled tiotropium for stable chronic obstructive pulmonary disease. Cochrane Database Syst Rev (2):CD002876, 2005.
23. Niewoehner DE, Rice K, Cote C, et al: Prevention of exacerbations of chronic obstructive pulmonary disease with tiotropium, a once-daily inhaled anticholinergic bronchodilator: a randomized trial. Ann Intern Med 143:317-326, 2005.
24. Sin DD, McAlister FA, Man SF, et al: Contemporary management of chronic obstructive pulmonary disease: scientific review. JAMA 290:2301-2312, 2003.
25. Singh S, Loke YK, Furberg CD: Inhaled anticholinergics and risk of major adverse cardiovascular events in patients with chronic obstructive pulmonary disease: a systematic review and meta-analysis. JAMA 300:1439-1450, 2008.
26. Celli B, Decramer M, Kesten S, et al: Mortality in the 4-year trial of tiotropium (UPLIFT) in patients with chronic obstructive pulmonary disease. Am J Respir Crit Care Med 180:948-955, 2009.
27. Callahan D, Dittus R, Katz B: Oral corticosteroid therapy for patients with stable chronic obstructive pulmonary disease: a meta-analysis. Ann Intern Med 114:216-223, 1991.
28. McEvoy CE, Niewohener DE: Adverse effects of corticosteroid therapy for COPD: a critical review. Chest 111:732-743, 1997.
29. Calverley PM, Anderson JA, Celli B, et al: TORCH investigators: salmeterol and fluticasone propionate and survival in chronic obstructive pulmonary disease. N Engl J Med 356:775-789, 2007.
30. Kardos P, Wencker M, Glaab T, et al: Impact of salmeterol/fluticasone propionate versus salmeterol on exacerbations in severe chronic obstructive pulmonary disease. Am J Respir Crit Care Med 175:144-149, 2007.
31. Celli BR, MacNee W: Standards for the diagnosis and treatment of patients with COPD: a summary of the ATS/ERS position paper. Eur Respir J 23:932-946, 2004.
32. Mahler D, Matthay RA, Snyder PE, et al: Sustained-release theophylline reduces dyspnea in nonreversible obstructive airway disease. Am Rev Respir Dis 131:22-25, 1985.
33. Nair S, Thomas E, Pearson SB, et al: A randomized controlled trial to assess the optimal dose and effect of nebulized albuterol in acute exacerbations of COPD. Chest 128:48-54, 2005.
34. Albert R, Martin T, Lewis S: Controlled clinical trial of methylprednisolone in patients with chronic bronchitis and acute respiratory insufficiency. Ann Intern Med 92:753-758, 1980.
35. Niewoehner DE, Erbland ML, Deupree RH, et al: Effect of systemic glucocorticoids on exacerbations of chronic

obstructive pulmonary disease. N Engl J Med 340:1941–1947, 1999.
36. Saint S, Bent S, Vittinghoff E, et al: Antibiotics in chronic obstructive pulmonary disease exacerbations: a meta-analysis. JAMA 273:957–960, 1995.
37. Anthonisen NR, Manfreda J, Warren CPW, et al: Antibiotic therapy in exacerbations of chronic obstructive pulmonary disease. Ann Intern Med 106:196–204, 1987.
38. Rice KL, Leatherman JW, Duane PG, et al: Aminophylline for acute exacerbations of chronic obstructive pulmonary disease: a controlled trial. Ann Intern Med 107:305–309, 1987.
39. Duffy N, Walker P, Diamantea F, et al: Intravenous aminophylline in patients admitted to hospital with non-acidotic exacerbations of chronic obstructive pulmonary disease: a prospective randomized controlled trial. Thorax 60:713–717, 2005.
40. Keenan SP, Sinuff T, Cook DJ, et al: Which patients with acute exacerbation of chronic obstructive pulmonary disease benefit from noninvasive positive-pressure ventilation? A systematic review of the literature. Ann Intern Med 138: 861–870, 2003.
41. Bach JR, Brougher P, Hess DR, et al: Consensus statement: non-invasive positive pressure ventilation. Respir Care 42: 365–369, 1997.
42. International Consensus Conferences in Intensive Care Medicine: Noninvasive positive pressure ventilation in acute respiratory failure. Am J Respir Crit Care Med 163:283–291, 2001.
43. Troosters T, Janssens W, Decramer M: Pulmonary rehabilitation. In Barnes PJ, Drazen JM, Rennard SI, et al, editors: Asthma and COPD: basic mechanisms and clinical management, ed 2, Waltham, MA, 2009, Academic Press.
44. Ries AL, Kaplan RM, Limberg TM, et al: Effects of pulmonary rehabilitation on physiological and psychosocial outcomes in patients with chronic obstructive pulmonary disease. Ann Intern Med 122:823–832, 1995.
45. Celli BR: Is pulmonary rehabilitation an effective treatment for chronic obstructive pulmonary disease? Am J Respir Crit Care Med 155:781–783, 1997.
46. Sillen MJ, Speksnijder CM, Eterman RM, et al: Effects of neuromuscular electrical stimulation of muscles of ambulation in patients with chronic heart failure or COPD: a systematic review of the English-language literature. Chest 136:44–61, 2009.
47. Shi Y, Warner DO: Surgery as a teachable moment for smoking cessation. Anesthesiology 112:102–107, 2010.
48. Kottke TE, Battista RN, DeFriese GH, et al: Attributes of successful cessation interventions in medical practice: a meta-analysis of 39 controlled trials. JAMA 259:2882–2889, 1988.
49. Marlow S, Stoller JK: Smoking cessation. Respir Care 48:1238–1256, 2003.
50. Nocturnal Oxygen Therapy Trial Group: Continuous or nocturnal oxygen therapy in hypoxemic chronic obstructive lung disease: a clinical trial. Ann Intern Med 93:391–398, 1980.
51. British Medical Research Council Working Party: Long-term domiciliary oxygen therapy in chronic hypoxic cor pulmonale complicating chronic bronchitis and emphysema. Lancet 1:681–685, 1981.
52. Flenley DC: Long-term oxygen therapy. Chest 87:99–103, 1985.
53. Stoller JK, Panos R, Krachman S, et al: Oxygen therapy for patients with COPD: evidence for current therapy and the Long-term Oxygen Treatment Trial (LOTT). Chest 138:179–187, 2010.
54. Guyatt GH, Nomoyama M, Lachetti C, et al: A randomized trial of strategies for assessing the eligibility for long-term domiciliary oxygen therapy. Am J Respir Crit Care Med 172:573–580, 2005.
55. Chaney JC, Jones K, Grathwohl K, et al: Implementation of an oxygen therapy clinic to manage users of long-term oxygen therapy. Chest 122:1661–1667, 2002.
56. Gardner P, Schaffner W: Immunization of adults. N Engl J Med 328:1252–1258, 1993.
57. International Society for Heart and Lung Transplantation: http://www.ishlt.org. Accessed December 27, 2010.
58. Brantigan OC, Mueller E: Surgical treatment of pulmonary emphysema. Am Surg 23:789, 1957.
59. National Emphysema Treatment Trial: Randomized trial comparing lung-volume-reduction surgery with medical therapy for severe emphysema. N Engl J Med 348:2059–2073, 2003.
60. Naunheim KS, Wood DE, Mohsenifar Z, et al: National Emphysema Treatment Trial Research Group: long term follow-up of patients receiving lung-volume-reduction surgery versus medical therapy for severe emphysema. Ann Thorac Surg 82:431–443, 2006.
61. National Emphysema Treatment Trial Research Group: Patients at high risk of death after lung-volume-reduction surgery. N Engl J Med 345:1075–1083, 2001.
62. Sciurba FC, Ernst A, Herth FJ, et al: VENT Study Research Group: A randomized study of endobronchial valves for advanced emphysema. N Engl J Med 363:1233–1244, 2010.
63. Berger RL, DeCamp MM, Criner GJ, et al: Lung volume reduction therapies for advanced emphysema: an update. Chest 138:407–417, 2010.
64. Dirksen A, Dijkman JH, Madsen F, et al: A randomized clinical trial of alpha1-antitrypsin augmentation therapy. Am J Respir Crit Care Med 160:1468–1472, 1999.
65. Dirksen A, Piitulainen E, Parr DG, et al: Exploring the role of CT densitometry: a randomised study of augmentation therapy in alpha1-antitrypsin deficiency. Eur Respir J 33: 1345–1353, 2009.
66. Abboud RT, Ford GT, Chapman KR: Standards Committee of the Canadian Thoracic Society: Alpha1-antitrypsin deficiency: a position statement of the Canadian Thoracic Society. Can Respir J 8:81–88, 2001.
67. National Asthma Education and Prevention Program: Expert Panel Report III: guidelines for the diagnosis and management of asthma, NIH Publication No. 07-4051, Bethesda, MD, 2007, National Institutes of Health, National Heart, Lung, and Blood Institute.
68. National Heart, Lung, and Blood Institute: International consensus report on diagnosis and treatment of asthma, No. 92-3091, Bethesda, MD, 1992, U.S. Department of Health and Human Services/National Institutes of Health.
69. Asthma Management and Prevention/Global Initiative for Asthma: A practical guide for public health officials and healthcare professionals, No. 96-3659A, Bethesda, MD, 1995, U.S. Department of Health and Human Services/National Institutes of Health.
70. Centers for Disease Control and Prevention, National Center for Health Statistics: Asthma prevalence, health care use and mortality, 2000-2001. http://www.cdc.gov/asthma/faststats.html. Accessed December 28, 2010.
71. McFadden ER, Jr, Gilbert IA: Asthma. N Engl J Med 327:1928–1937, 1992.
72. Barnes PJ: A new approach to the treatment of asthma. N Engl J Med 321:1517–1527, 1989.
73. Wiedemann HP, Kavuru MS: Diagnosis and management of asthma, Caddo, OK, 1994, Professional Communications.
74. Woolcock AJ: Asthma. In Murray JF, Nadel JA, editors: Textbook of respiratory medicine, Philadelphia, 2005, Saunders.
75. Fanta CH: Asthma. N Engl J Med 360:1002–1014, 2009.

76. Barnes PJ: Inhaled corticosteroids for asthma. N Engl J Med 332:868–875, 1995.
77. Zafirlukast for asthma. Med Lett Drugs Ther 38:111–112, 1996.
78. Kavuru MS, Pien L, Litwin D, et al: Asthma: current controversies and emerging therapies. Cleve Clin J Med 62:293–304, 1995.
79. Salpeter SR, Buckley NS, Ormiston TM, et al: Meta-analysis: effect of long-acting β-agonists on severe asthma exacerbations and asthma-related deaths. Ann Intern Med 144:904–912, 2006.
80. U.S. Food and Drug Administration, Center for Drug Evaluation and Research: Advair Diskus, Advair HFA, Brovana, Foradil, Serevent Diskus, and Symbicort information (long acting beta agonists. http://www.fda.gov/cder/drug/infopage/LABA/default.htm. Accessed December 28, 2010.
81. Peters SP, Kunselman SJ, Icitovic N, et al: Tiotropium bromide step-up therapy for adults with uncontrolled asthma. N Engl J Med 363:1715–1726, 2010.
82. Burrows B, Martinez FD, Halonen M, et al: Association of asthma with serum IgE levels and skin-test reactivity to allergens. N Engl J Med 320:271–277, 1989.
83. Omalizumab (Xolair): an anti-IgE antibody for asthma. Med Lett Drugs Ther 45:67, 2003.
84. Busse W, Corren J, Lanier BQ, et al: Omalizumab, anti-IgE recombinant humanized monoclonal antibody, for the treatment of severe allergic asthma. J Allergy Clin Immunol 108:184–190, 2001.
85. Bronchial thermoplasty for asthma. Med Lett Drugs Ther 52:65–66, 2010.
86. Cox G, Thomson NC, Rubin AS, et al: AIR Trial Study Group: asthma control during the year after bronchial thermoplasty. N Engl J Med 356:1327–1337, 2007.
87. Castro M, Rubin AS, Laviolette M, et al: AIR2 Trial Study Group: effectiveness and safety of bronchial thermoplasty in the treatment of severe asthma: a multicenter, randomized, double-blind, sham-controlled clinical trial. Am J Respir Crit Care Med 181:116–124, 2010.
88. Abrahamson MJ, Puy RM, Weiner JM: Injection allergen immunotherapy for asthma. Cochrane Database Syst Rev 8:6–114, 2010.
89. Kiljander TO, Junghard O, Beckman O, et al: Effect of esomeprazole 40 mg once or twice daily on asthma: a randomized, placebo-controlled study. Am J Respir Crit Care Med 181:1042–1048, 2010.
90. National Asthma Education Program Report of the Working Group on Asthma and Pregnancy: Management of asthma during pregnancy, No. 93-3279A, Bethesda, MD, 1993, U.S. Department of Health and Human Services, National Institutes of Health.
91. Barker AF: Bronchiectasis. N Engl J Med 346:1383–1393, 2002.
92. Stanford W, Galvin JR: The diagnosis of bronchiectasis. Clin Chest Med 9:691–699, 1988.
93. Davies G, Wells AU, Doffman S, et al: The effect of *Pseudomonas aeruginosa* on pulmonary function in patients with bronchiectasis. Eur Respir J 28:974–979, 2006.
94. Wills P, Greenstone M: Inhaled hyperosmolar agents for bronchiectasis. Cochrane Database Syst Rev (2):CD002996, 2006.
95. Dweik RA, Stoller JK: Role of bronchoscopy in massive hemoptysis. Clin Chest Med 20:89–105, 1999.
96. Fujimoto T, Hillejan L, Stamatis G: Current strategy for surgical management of bronchiectasis. Ann Thorac Surg 72:1711–1715, 2001.
97. Mal H, Rullon I, Mellot F, et al: Immediate and long-term results of bronchial artery embolization for life-threatening hemoptysis. Chest 115:996–1001, 1999.

Chapter 24

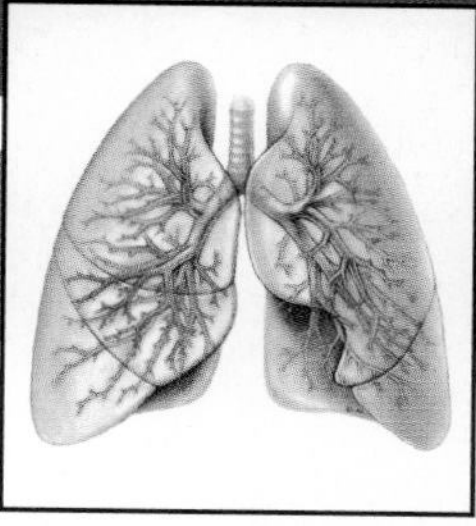

Interstitial Lung Disease

JEFFREY T. CHAPMAN

CHAPTER OBJECTIVES

After reading this chapter you will be able to:

- Organize and distinguish between the entities grouped as interstitial lung diseases (ILDs).
- Interpret symptoms, examination signs, and pulmonary function testing in ILD.
- List emerging pathophysiologic characteristics that are associated with selected ILDs.
- Describe how to manage ILD in general and how some specific ILDs can be treated.

CHAPTER OUTLINE

KEY TERMS

asbestosis
connective tissue disease
corticosteroids
hypersensitivity pneumonitis (HP)
idiopathic pulmonary fibrosis (IPF)
interstitial lung disease (ILD)
lymphangioleiomyomatosis (LAM)
occupational ILD
organizing pneumonia (OP)
pulmonary Langerhans cell histiocytosis (PLCH)
sarcoidosis
silicosis

Interstitial lung disease (ILD) comprises a broad category of lung diseases rather than a specific disease entity.[1,2] This category includes various illnesses affecting the lung parenchyma with many different causes, treatments, and prognoses. These disorders are grouped together because of similarities in their clinical presentations, appearance on plain chest radiography, and physiologic features.

With over 100 separate disorders, it is essential to group ILDs based on etiology, disease associations, or pathology. An organizational scheme is presented in Figure 24-1. When evaluating patients with an ILD, one first must consider diseases with known causes or associations, such as diseases related to specific exposures, diseases associated with systemic conditions, and diseases with a known genetic basis. Most patients do not have an ILD with a

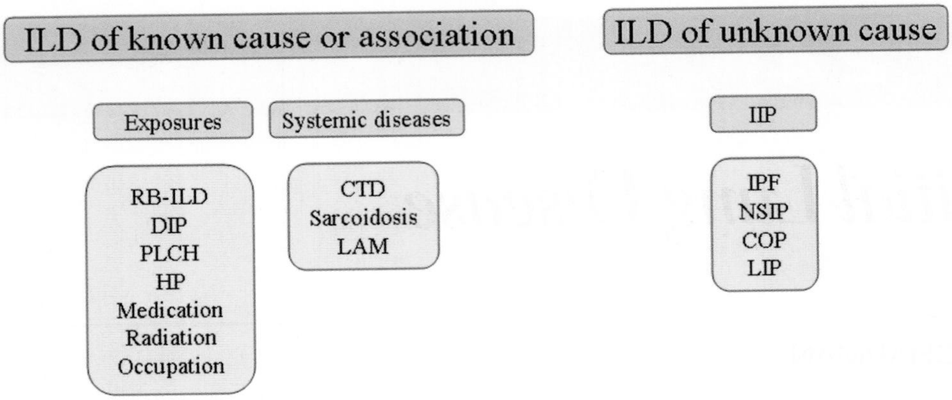

FIGURE 24-1 Current organization of ILD. *COP,* Cryptogenic organizing pneumonia; *CTD,* connective tissue disease; *IBD,* inflammatory bowel disease; *IPF,* idiopathic pulmonary fibrosis; *LAM,* lymphangioleiomyomatosis; *LIP,* lymphocytic interstitial pneumonia; *NSIP,* nonspecific interstitial pneumonitis; *PAP,* pulmonary alveolar proteinosis; *PLCH,* pulmonary Langerhans cell histiocytosis.

known cause, and their disorder is classified by pathologic pattern. These groups are divided into specific disease entities. Using this organizational scheme to guide a careful and complete history, one is able to understand the disease processes and work efficiently toward an accurate diagnosis.

As the name ILD implies, the histologic abnormalities that characterize ILD involve the pulmonary interstitium to a greater extent than the alveolar spaces or airways, although exceptions exist. Figure 24-2 illustrates the components of the normal pulmonary parenchyma. The interstitium is the area between the capillaries and the alveolar space. As Figure 24-2 shows, in the normal state, this space allows close apposition of gas and capillaries with minimal connective tissue matrix, fibroblasts, and inflammatory cells such as macrophages. The interstitium supports the delicate relationship between the alveoli and capillaries allowing for efficient gas exchange. When responding to any injury—whether from a specific exposure (e.g., asbestos, nitrofurantoin, or moldy hay), an autoimmune-mediated inflammation from a systemic **connective tissue disease** (e.g., rheumatoid arthritis), or unknown injury (e.g., idiopathic pulmonary fibrosis [IPF])—the lung must respond to the damage and repair itself. If the exposure or injury persists or if the injury repair process is imperfect, the lung may be permanently damaged with increased interstitial tissue replacing the normal capillaries, alveoli, and healthy interstitium.

These pathologic abnormalities can lead to profound impairment in lung physiology. Gas exchange is impaired owing to $\dot{V}/\dot{Q}$ mismatching, shunt, and decreased diffusion across the abnormal interstitium. Work of breathing is markedly increased because of decreased lung compliance. Together, these physiologic impairments lead to the exercise intolerance seen in all of the ILDs. If the initiating injury or abnormal repair from injury is not halted, progressive tissue damage leading to worsening physiologic impairment and death can occur.

CHARACTERISTICS OF INTERSTITIAL LUNG DISEASE

Clinical Signs and Symptoms of Interstitial Lung Disease

Many ILDs have similar clinical features and are not easily distinguished based on history or examination. Symptoms are generally limited to the respiratory tract. However, extrapulmonary symptoms should not be ignored because they may point to an ILD associated with a systemic diagnosis. Exertional breathlessness (dyspnea) and a nonproductive cough are the most common reasons patients seek medical attention. Other respiratory symptoms, such as sputum production, hemoptysis, pneumothorax, or wheezing, can occur and be suggestive of specific diseases (Table 24-1). If the patient also has prominent extrapulmonary symptoms, such as myalgia, arthralgia, sclerodactyly, gastroesophageal reflux, or Raynaud phenomenon, ILD resulting from underlying connective tissue disease may be present (Table 24-2).

Physical Examination

Most patients with ILD have bilateral fine inspiratory, crackles, which usually are most prominent at the lung bases. However, some diseases, such as sarcoidosis and lymphangioleiomyomatosis (LAM), may have only decreased breath sounds without adventitious sounds despite a markedly abnormal chest radiograph. Expiratory wheezing is uncommon, and its presence suggests either airway involvement as part of the primary disease process (LAM, sarcoidosis, respiratory bronchiolitis–associated interstitial lung disease [RB-ILD], desquamative interstitial pneumonitis [DIP], pulmonary Langerhans cell histiocytosis [PLCH]) or concomitant airways disease, such as emphysema or asthma. Signs of pulmonary arterial

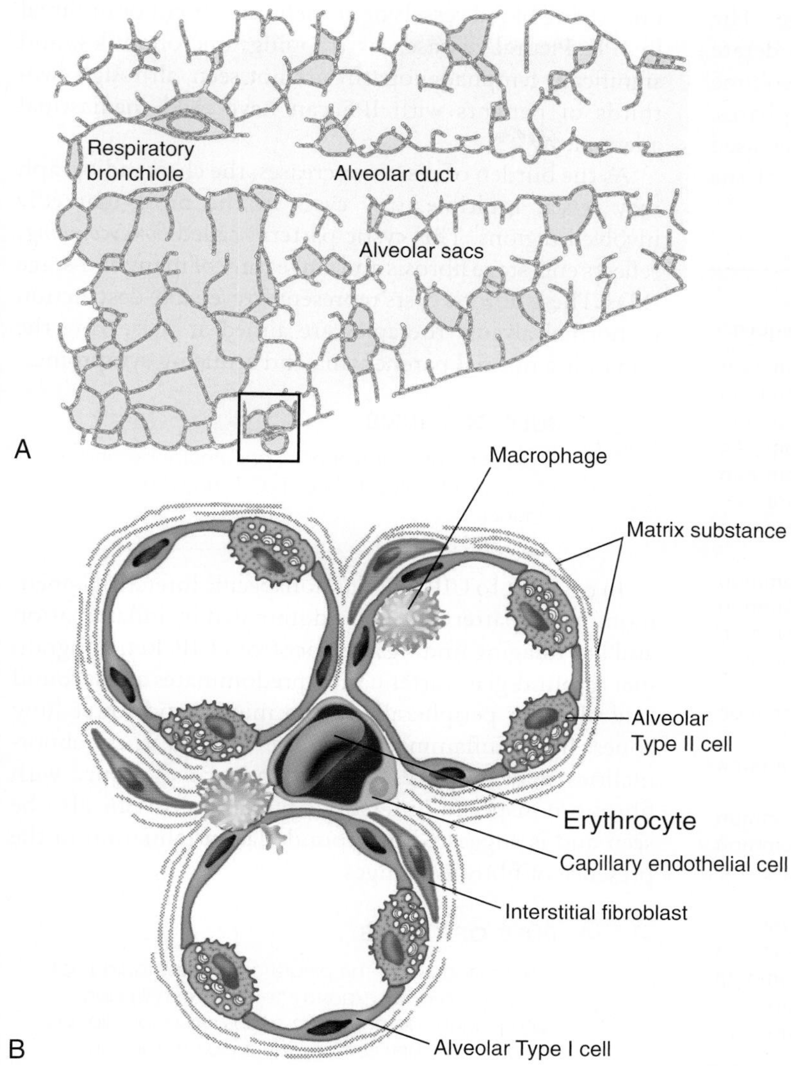

FIGURE 24-2 A, Diagram of the pulmonary parenchyma shows the respiratory bronchiole, alveolar duct, and alveolar sacs. **B,** The constituents of the interstitial space, including type I and type II alveolar epithelial cells, a capillary with vascular endothelial cells and erythrocytes in transit, resident macrophages, interstitial fibroblasts, and matrix substance.

TABLE 24-1

Unusual Pulmonary Findings and Likely Diagnosis

Pulmonary Findings	Disease	Frequency
Hemoptysis	LAM	Rare
Chyloptysis	LAM	Rare
Pneumothorax	LAM, BHD	Common
Wheeze	Sarcoidosis, LAM	Common
Chylous pleural effusion	LAM	Common
Exudative pleural effusion	RA	Common

BHD, Birt Hogg Dubé syndrome; *RA,* rheumatoid arthritis.

hypertension with right ventricular dysfunction, such as lower extremity edema or jugular venous distention, may occur late in the course of any ILD and are not helpful in the diagnosis of a specific ILD. Examination also may disclose features of underlying connective tissue disease, including synovitis, joint deformities, or skin rash.

Radiographic Features

ILDs manifest as abnormal lung parenchyma that cast abnormal radiographic shadows. For most ILDs, the chest radiograph reveals reduced lung volumes with bilateral reticular or reticulonodular opacities. However, the chest radiograph has limited value because the three-dimensional abnormalities are summed into a two-dimensional image with loss of spatial information. High-resolution cross-sectional imaging via computed tomography (CT) provides detailed images representing pulmonary pathology.[3] High-resolution CT images allow noninvasive evaluation of ILDs and are a key element in making a confident diagnosis and managing ILD.[4]

Plain chest radiographs and high-resolution CT images of usual interstitial pneumonitis (UIP) show the prototypic fibrotic injury pattern. The chest radiograph (Figure 24-3, *A*) and high-resolution CT image (Figure 24-3, *B*) in UIP typically reveal a bilateral, patchy, peripheral (subpleural), and basilar predominant disease with reticulonodular infiltrates, often with honeycomb, cystic change. The lung architecture is distorted in patients with moderate or severe disease burden, with reduced lung volume and traction bronchiectasis, especially at the lung bases. Reticulogranular (ground-glass) abnormalities, increased attenuation of the lung tissue without distortion of the underlying blood vessels or bronchi, are absent or minimal in IPF. Pleural disease, air trapping, micronodules, and significant lymphadenopathy are not seen, although two-thirds of patients with IPF can have mild mediastinal adenopathy.[5]

As the burden of disease increases, the chest radiograph may reveal multiple, tiny cysts in the most markedly involved regions. This cystic pattern, called *honeycombing*, reflects end-stage fibrosis and is a feature of many end-stage ILDs. These fibrotic cysts represent irreversible destruction of normal alveoli; therapies are aimed at preserving the remaining normal parenchyma and reducing symptoms.

TABLE 24-2

Extrapulmonary Findings and Likely Diagnosis

Extrapulmonary Findings	Disease	Frequency
Raynaud phenomenon	All CTD	Common
Arthralgia	All CTD	Common
Myalgia	Polymyositis	Common
Large muscle weakness	Polymyositis	Common
Sclerodactyly	Scleroderma	Common
Rheumatoid skin nodules	RA	Rare
Fingertip fissures	Antisynthetase syndrome	Common
Dorsal hand rash	Dermatomyositis	Common
Facial rash	Dermatomyositis	Common
Exudative pleural effusion	RA	Common
Shawl distribution skin nodules	TSC	Common
"Pencil eraser" facial skin nodules	BHD	Common
Central nervous system benign cortical tuber	TSC	Common
Abdominal angiomyolipoma	LAM	Common
Renal cancer	BHD	Common
Cardiomyopathy	Sarcoidosis, polymyositis	Rare
Cardiac conduction block	Sarcoidosis	Rare
Violaceous facial skin nodules	Sarcoidosis	Common
Subcutaneous nodules	Sarcoidosis	Common
Cranial neuropathy	Sarcoidosis	Rare
Small fiber neuropathy	Sarcoidosis	Rare

BHD, Birt Hogg Dubé syndrome; *CTD,* connective tissue disease; *RA,* rheumatoid arthritis; *TSC,* tuberous sclerosis complex.

RULE OF THUMB

In patients with spontaneous pneumothorax and interstitial infiltrates, LAM or PLCH should be considered.

In contrast to UIP, cellular nonspecific interstitial pneumonitis is a pattern of injury dominated by inflammation and has imaging findings distinct from UIP. Reticulogranular (ground-glass) attenuation predominates and is found centrally and peripherally in the middle and lower lung zones. If the inflammation can be reduced, these abnormalities may improve. A mixed pattern of injury with fibrotic nonspecific interstitial pneumonitis can also be seen and is suggested by ground-glass attenuation in the presence of fibrotic changes.

RULE OF THUMB

Calcification along the pleura on a chest radiograph suggests previous exposure to asbestos. Although such plaques do not cause symptoms or physiologic abnormality, they can provide a clue to the cause of ILD.

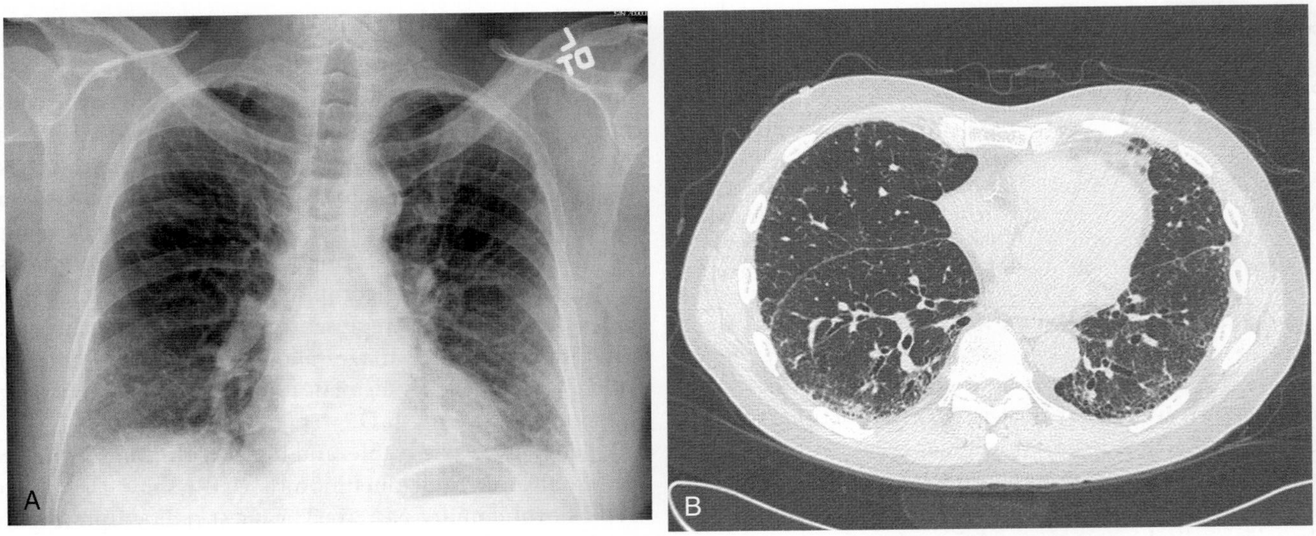

FIGURE 24-3 **A,** Posteroanterior chest radiograph showing the characteristic features of IPF, a common ILD. Notice the bilateral lower zone reticulonodular infiltrates and the loss of lung volume in the lower lobes. **B,** Chest CT image shows the peripheral nature of the fibrosis.

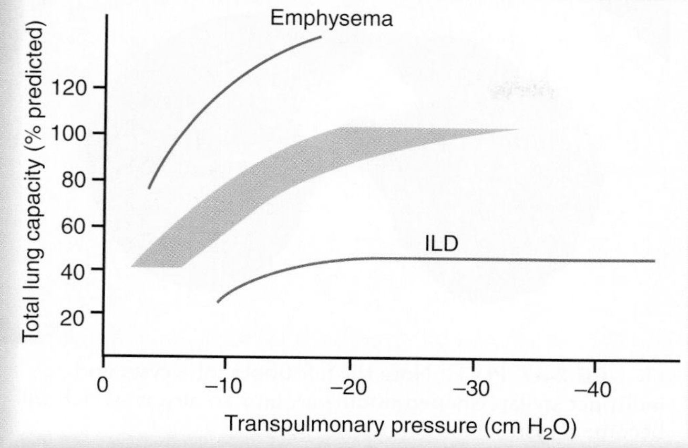

FIGURE 24-4 Static pressure-volume curve. The compliance characteristics of the lung are illustrated with a plot of lung volume against the corresponding transthoracic pressure measured during static (i.e., no flow) conditions. The *shaded area* represents the range of values expected with a normally compliant lung. The line labeled *ILD* represents an example of a patient with ILD. At any particular lung volume, the transthoracic pressure is greater than expected. For comparison, the line labeled *Emphysema* shows the compliance characteristics of patients with emphysema.

Physiologic Features

Similar to the radiographic findings, there can be considerable variability among the specific diseases in the physiologic abnormalities seen. However, a restrictive physiologic impairment is the common finding.[6] Both forced expiratory volume in 1 second (FEV_1) and forced vital capacity (FVC) are diminished, and the FEV_1/FVC ratio is preserved or even supranormal. Lung volumes are reduced, as is the diffusing capacity of the lung for carbon monoxide (DLCO). This reduction in diffusing capacity reflects a pathologic disturbance of the alveolus-capillary interface.

Although not commonly pursued, the compliance characteristics of the lungs can be evaluated with an esophageal balloon to measure intrathoracic pressure at various lung volumes. In almost all ILDs, the lungs have reduced compliance and require supranormal transpleural pressures to ventilate (Figure 24-4). This lack of compliance results in small lung volumes and increased work of breathing.

Less frequently, a pattern of physiologic obstruction may be seen. This obstruction can be the result of the primary disease process (e.g., LAM, PLCH, or sarcoidosis in some patients) or concomitant emphysema or asthma.[7] If ILD develops in a patient with significant emphysema, the opposing physiologic effects of the two diseases may result in deceptively normal spirometry and lung volume measurements and apparently normally compliant lungs. However, because both emphysema and ILD result in impaired gas exchange, DLCO is significantly decreased.

RULE OF THUMB

Among smokers with IPF, normal spirometry and lung volumes with reduced DLCO suggest the presence of coexisting emphysema.

SELECTED SPECIFIC TYPES OF INTERSTITIAL LUNG DISEASE AND THERAPIES

Exposure-Related Interstitial Lung Disease

Tobacco-Associated Interstitial Lung Disease

Although the association of first-hand tobacco smoke and obstructive lung disease is common and well known, tobacco smoke is also an avoidable cause of ILD. Although the association is rarer than with obstructive lung disease, first-hand tobacco smoke inhalation can lead to three types of ILD in susceptible individuals: RB-ILD, DIP, and PLCH. The first two disorders are related. Each disease consists of increased numbers of polyclonal activated macrophages. The diseases differ by the location of these overly abundant cells. In RB-ILD, macrophages accumulate in the respiratory bronchioles leading to bronchiolar remodeling and fibrosis of adjacent alveoli. As expected for a disease with combined airway and alveolar injury, pulmonary function testing reveals mixed restriction and obstruction with frequent air trapping. High-resolution CT images show this mixed pathologic location with indistinct centrilobular nodules (Figure 24-5). In DIP, the increased macrophages fill the alveoli, manifesting as restrictive impairment on pulmonary function testing and diffuse ground-glass attenuation on high-resolution CT imaging (Figure 24-6).

Pulmonary Langerhans cell histiocytosis (PLCH) is the third interstitial manifestation of tobacco smoke. Increased numbers of polyclonal macrophages play a prominent role. However, in PLCH, they are accompanied by fibroblasts and eosinophils in nodules concentrated around small airways. These nodules are stellate and destroy adjacent lung tissue, leading to the classic high-resolution CT image of stellate nodules associated with

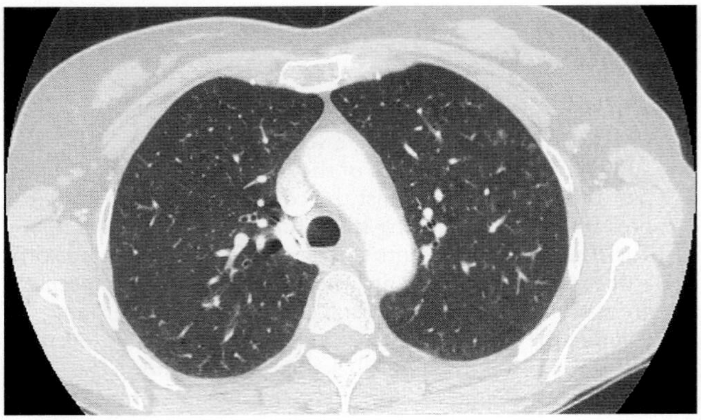

FIGURE 24-5 RB-ILD. There are numerous indistinct centrilobular nodules. Air trapping can also be seen in RB-ILD but is not present in this case.

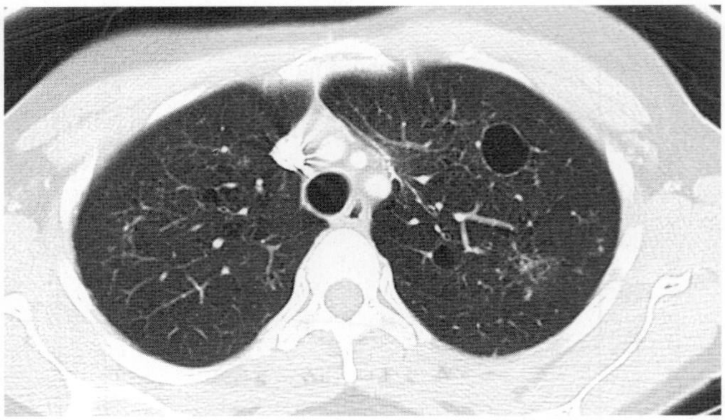

FIGURE 24-7 PLCH. Note the left upper lobe cysts and indistinct stellate-shaped nodule around an airway, which will become a cyst.

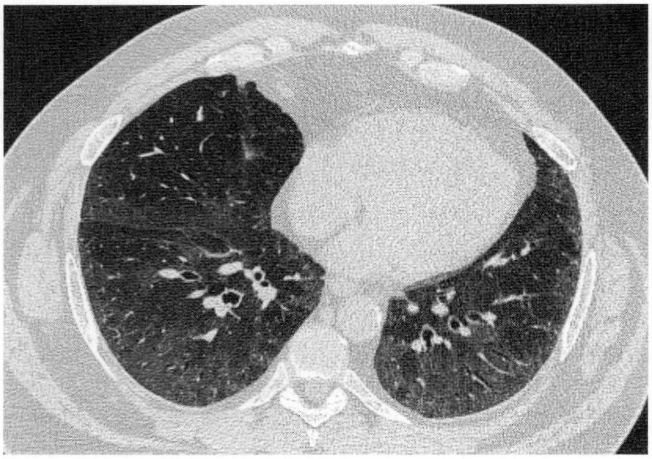

FIGURE 24-6 DIP. Note the diffuse ground-glass attenuation.

cysts as seen in Figure 24-7. Although adult smoking-associated PLCH is pathologically similar to childhood Langerhans cell histiocytosis, the adult form does not involve bone and has not proven to respond to chemotherapy as the childhood form does. The relationship of these two disorders has yet to be defined.

In each of these three diseases, the primary treatment is complete tobacco abstinence. With abstinence, most patients either minimally improve or remain stable,[8] but a few progressively worsen and may require lung transplantation. Active treatment with prednisone or other immunosuppressive medications is discouraged because few, if any, patients improve.[9]

Box 24-1 Drugs Associated With the Development of Interstitial Lung Disease

ANTIBIOTICS
Nitrofurantoin
Sulfasalazine

ANTIINFLAMMATORY AGENTS
Methotrexate
Etanercept
Infliximab

CARDIOVASCULAR AGENTS
Amiodarone
Tocainide

CHEMOTHERAPEUTIC AGENTS
Bleomycin
Mitomycin C
Busulfan
Cyclophosphamide
Chlorambucil
Melphalan
Methotrexate
Etoposide
Vinblastine
Imatinib

ILLICIT DRUGS
Heroin
Methadone
Talc as an intravenous drug contaminant

Drug-Related and Radiation-Related Interstitial Lung Disease

Many drugs have been associated with pulmonary complications of various types, including interstitial inflammation and fibrosis, bronchospasm, pulmonary edema, and pleural effusions. Drugs from many different therapeutic classes can cause ILD, most commonly chemotherapeutic agents, antibiotics, antiarrhythmic drugs, and immunosuppressive agents (Box 24-1). There are no distinct physiologic, radiographic, or pathologic patterns of drug-induced ILD, and the diagnosis is usually made when a patient is exposed to a medication known to result in lung disease, the timing of the exposure is appropriate for the development of the disease, and other causes of ILD have been eliminated. Treatment is avoidance of further exposure and systemic corticosteroids in markedly impaired or declining patients. In addition to future drug exposure, bleomycin injury is accentuated by increased

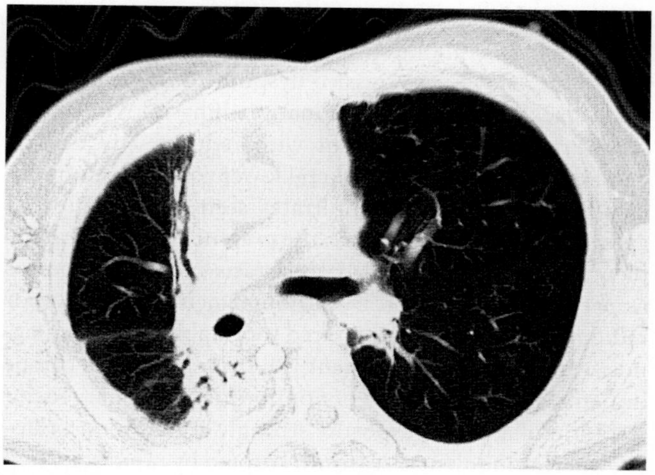

FIGURE 24-8 High-resolution CT slice shows dense fibrosis with a nonanatomic straight line boundary.

fractional inspired oxygen (FiO_2), even months after last drug exposure, and supplemental oxygen (O_2) should be used only if absolutely necessary in these patients.[10]

Exposure to therapeutic radiation in the management of cancer may result in ILD. Patients presenting within 6 months of radiation therapy generally have ground-glass abnormalities thought to represent acute inflammation. The ground-glass abnormalities can occur in both radiation-exposed tissue and unexposed tissue. Short-term systemic corticosteroid treatment can improve lung function. In contrast, radiographic abnormalities that develop more than 6 months after therapy typically appear as densely fibrotic tissue within the radiation port. On CT scan, a straight line indicating the margin of radiation is frequently evident as seen in Figure 24-8. These patients do not improve with corticosteroid therapy, and treatment is supportive.

Hypersensitivity Pneumonitis

Hypersensitivity pneumonitis (HP) is a cell-mediated immune reaction to inhaled antigens in susceptible persons.[11] Patients must be sensitized by an initial exposure, with subsequent reexposure leading to either acute HP usually after a brief but intense exposure or chronic HP from persistent exposure. Patients with acute HP present to medical attention with a history of a few days of shortness of breath, chest pain, fever, chills, malaise, and a cough that may be productive of purulent sputum. Patients who are chronically exposed to low levels of inhaled antigens may develop subtle interstitial inflammatory reactions in the lung that do not result in noticeable symptoms for months to years and can present with severe, impairing disease, which can be very difficult to distinguish from IPF.

Common organic antigens known to cause HP include bacteria and fungi, which may be found in moldy hay (farmer's lung) or in the home environment, in particular, in association with central humidification systems (humidifier lung), indoor hot tubs, and animal proteins (e.g., bird breeder's lung). Inorganic antigens from vaporized paints and plastics can also lead to HP. Numerous established antigens are listed in Table 24-3 along with the typical source of exposure and the associated syndrome.

Because the causal relationship between exposure and lung disease may not be obvious, a careful systematic occupational, environmental, and avocational history is crucial in evaluating patients with ILD. Elements that strongly suggest a diagnosis of HP are exposure to an appropriate antigen and the correct temporal relationship of symptoms to the exposure. Blood samples may be obtained to determine whether there has been an antibody response to certain antigens associated with HP (serum precipitins). However, the presence of such antibodies is insufficient to

TABLE 24-3

Etiologies of Hypersensitivity Pneumonitis

Antigen	Exposure	Syndrome
Bacteria		
Thermophilic Bacteria		
Saccharopolyspora rectivirgula	Moldy hay	Farmer's lung
Thermoactinomyces vulgaris	Moldy sugarcane	Bagassosis
Thermoactinomyces sacchari	Mushroom compost	Mushroom worker's lung
Thermoactinomyces candidus	Heated water reservoirs	Humidifier lung Air conditioner lung
Nonthermophilic Bacteria		
Bacillus subtilis, Bacillus cereus	Water, detergent	Humidifier lung Washing powder lung
Fungi		
Aspergillus species	Moldy hay	Farmer's lung
Aspergillus clavatus	Barley	Malt worker's lung
Penicillium casei, Penicillium roqueforti	Cheese	Cheese washer's lung
Alternaria species	Wood pulp	Woodworker's lung
Merulius lacrymans	Rotten wood	Dry rot lung
Penicillium frequentans	Cork dust	Suberosis
Aureobasidium pullulans	Water	Humidifier lung
Cladosporium species	Hot tub mists	Hot tub HP*
Trichosporon cutaneum	Damp wood and mats	Japanese summer-type HP*
Animal Proteins		
Avian proteins	Bird droppings, feathers	Bird-breeder's lung
Urine, serum, pelts	Rats, gerbils	Animal handler's lung
Chemicals		
Isocyanates, trimellitic anhydride	Paints, resins, plastics	Chemical worker's lung
Copper sulfate	Bordeaux mixture	Vineyard sprayer's lung
Phthalic anhydride	Heated epoxy resin	Epoxy resin lung

establish the diagnosis of HP because many individuals develop antibodies in the absence of disease. Likewise, the absence of detectable antibodies does not rule out the diagnosis of HP because the culprit may be an antigen that is not included in the blood analysis.[12]

Specific therapies for HP are strict antigen avoidance and immunosuppression with corticosteroids in patients with symptomatic or physiologically impairing disease. In acute HP, corticosteroids seem to hasten recovery but do not improve ultimate lung function.[13] In chronic HP, patients with fibrosis on CT scan have a shorter survival, and it is unknown if long-term immunosuppression is beneficial.[14]

Occupational Interstitial Lung Disease

The three most common types of **occupational ILD** are **asbestosis,** chronic **silicosis,** and coal workers' pneumoconiosis. Awareness of the associated risk and reduction in exposure has greatly reduced the incidence of these diseases in developed countries. However, they remain common in developing countries and emigrants from these countries.

Predictable clinical and radiographic abnormalities occur in susceptible patients who have been exposed to asbestos.[15] These abnormalities include pleural changes (plaques, fibrosis, effusions, atelectasis, and mesothelioma) and parenchymal scarring and lung cancer. Asbestos exposure alone increases the risk of lung cancer only minimally (1.5 to 3.0 times). However, asbestos exposure and cigarette smoking act synergistically to increase greatly the risk of cancer. Asbestos exposure also may result in benign asbestos pleural effusions or an entity known as *rounded atelectasis*. Benign asbestos pleural effusions may be asymptomatic or may be associated with acute chest pain, fever, and dyspnea. Generally, a shorter lag time exists between initial asbestos exposure and the development of benign asbestos pleural effusions (<15 years) than is seen with other manifestations of asbestos exposure. The effusions are characteristically exudative and are often bloody. In a patient with a history of asbestos exposure and a bloody pleural effusion, the major differential diagnostic concern is malignant pleural effusion from a mesothelioma. The clinical course of benign asbestos pleural effusions is characterized by spontaneous resolution, often with recurrences, and treatment is drainage to reduce symptoms. Rounded atelectasis typically manifests as a pleural-based parenchymal mass that may be mistaken for carcinoma. The characteristic CT features, such as local volume loss, pleural thickening, and the "comet tail" appearance of bronchi and vessels curving into the lesion, help distinguish rounded atelectasis from carcinoma.

The term *asbestos-related pulmonary disease* encompasses all of these entities, whereas *asbestosis* is reserved for patients who have evidence of parenchymal fibrosis. Most patients with asbestosis have had considerable airborne asbestos exposure many years before manifestation of the lung disease. Exposure frequently is associated with occupations such as shipbuilding or insulation work. Patients report very slowly progressive dyspnea on exertion[16] and have crackles on lung examination. Physiologic testing shows restrictive impairment with reduced DLCO. The chest radiograph reveals bilateral lower zone reticulonodular infiltrates similar to infiltrates seen in IPF. With an appropriate exposure history, the presence of radiographic pleural plaques or rounded atelectasis indicates asbestos as the likely cause of ILD, although neither history nor radiographic findings is required for establishing the diagnosis. Differentiating indolent IPF from asbestosis can be difficult, and the presence of nonfibrotic pulmonary manifestation of asbestos exposure strongly argues for asbestosis, whereas indolent disease interrupted by rapid stair step decline usually occurs only in IPF. Surgical lung biopsy with asbestos body determination can establish a definitive diagnosis, but this is infrequently performed owing to the age and debility of these patients. No medical therapy has been shown to improve or decrease progression of asbestosis. Severe impairment typically occurs 30 to 40 years after exposure, making almost all patients ineligible for lung transplantation because of age. Management of asbestosis is supportive.

Chronic silicosis results from chronic exposure to inhaled silica particles. Occupations that commonly entail exposure to silica include mining, tunneling, sandblasting, and foundry work. The chest radiograph commonly shows upper lung zone–predominant abnormalities characterized by multiple small nodular opacities in the central lung tissue. These nodules (simple silicosis) are asymptomatic and may never progress or cause symptoms. However, in susceptible individuals, the nodules coalesce into large midlung zone masses known as *progressive massive fibrosis*. Enlargement and eggshell calcification of the hilar lymph nodes are common in both types. Functional and physiologic impairment in chronic silicosis is quite variable. Some patients with abnormal chest radiographs report few, if any, symptoms and may have normal lung examination and pulmonary function testing. Many patients are impaired and have mixed restrictive and obstructive impairment with reduced diffusion capacity. The physiologic impairment may remain stable or, if progressive massive fibrosis occurs, may progress even in the absence of continued exposure. Symptoms are typically exertional dyspnea and variable mucus production.

It is important to recognize the association of silicosis with lung cancer and active tuberculosis.[17] Patients with silicosis are at increased risk of lung cancer, and the risk is increased when combined with exposure to tobacco smoke, diesel exhaust, or radon gas. Patients with silicosis develop active tuberculosis 2-fold to 30-fold more frequently than coworkers without silicosis. This association is especially important in societies with a high incidence of HIV infection, which markedly increases the risk of silicosis-associated active tuberculosis.

Coal workers' pneumoconiosis develops as the result of chronic inhalation of coal dust. In the past, it was assumed that silica dust was responsible for the pulmonary disease seen among coal miners because the clinical and radiographic features are quite similar to chronic silicosis. However, it is now recognized that coal workers' pneumoconiosis and silicosis are the result of distinct exposures. Simple coal workers' pneumoconiosis, characterized by multiple small nodular opacities on the chest radiograph, is asymptomatic. Cough and shortness of breath do not develop unless the disease progresses to progressive massive fibrosis similar to that seen in silicosis.

There are no proven therapies for either silicosis or coal workers' pneumoconiosis other than eliminating future exposure. In patients with significant obstructive impairment or mucus production, inhaled bronchodilators and **corticosteroids** may relieve some symptoms. Exacerbations can be frequent and are treated with antibiotics and systemic corticosteroids.

Systemic Disease–Associated Interstitial Lung Disease

Connective Tissue Disease–Associated Interstitial Lung Disease

ILD is a well-known complication of various connective tissue diseases.[18] The most commonly implicated disorders are scleroderma, rheumatoid arthritis, Sjögren syndrome, polymyositis/dermatomyositis, and systemic lupus erythematosus.

In any of these disorders, pulmonary involvement may remain undetected until significant impairment is present because these patients may be inactive owing to the underlying connective tissue disease. In addition, there is generally poor correlation between the severity of the pulmonary and nonpulmonary manifestations of these diseases. In some instances, the lung disease may overshadow or predate the other symptoms of the underlying disease. When symptoms develop, dyspnea and cough are common. On chest examination, rales, wheezing, or pleural rub may be heard because of the varied patterns of lung involvement in these disorders. Physiology is usually restrictive with decreased DLCO but may be obstructive depending on the anatomic location of the disease, especially with Sjögren syndrome because the collections of lymphocytes that define this disease are most frequent in the bronchioles.

High-resolution CT findings are variable and range from normal lung architecture to ground-glass abnormalities to reticular and fibrotic changes.[19] The pathologic pattern of injury with these diseases is as equally diverse and correlates with the high-resolution CT findings. Inflammatory injury patterns are most commonly seen, such as nonspecific interstitial pneumonitis (NSIP) and organizing pneumonia (OP). The NSIP inflammatory injury pattern appears as ground-glass abnormalities on high-resolution CT scan, whereas OP is shown by patchy consolidated lung with air bronchograms. Both of these pathologic patterns can improve with aggressive immunosuppression. At the other end of the pathologic response spectrum is fibrotic injury, which manifests as UIP, which shows reticular fibrotic opacities and honeycomb cystic changes on high-resolution CT scan and typically does not improve with immunosuppression, although long-term controlled studies are lacking.

Specific treatment of connective tissue disease–associated ILD must be individualized. Patients with evidence of extrapulmonary inflammation, an inflammatory pathologic pattern such as NSIP or OP on high-resolution CT or biopsy, or rapidly progressive symptoms are usually treated with prolonged immunosuppressive agents such as cyclophosphamide, azathioprine, mycophenolate, or tacrolimus.[20,21]

More recent studies have begun to provide evidence-based therapy for these diverse patients. The Scleroderma Lung Study showed that 1 year of oral cyclophosphamide modestly improved lung function compared with modest decline in the control group.[20] The patients with the highest degree of fibrosis on high-resolution CT improved most, and ground-glass abnormalities or an inflammatory pattern on bronchoalveolar lavage were not predictive of benefit. After 1 year off immunosuppressive therapy, the patients treated with cyclophosphamide worsened and were indistinguishable from the untreated patients in the control group.[22] Many clinicians hypothesize that to preserve any lung function gained by cyclophosphamide, continued immunosuppression may be necessary, and mycophenolate is most often used.

Polymyositis-associated ILD is being increasingly recognized as a common disease entity. Patients usually present with "mechanic's hands" consisting of thickened skin and painful fingertip fissures, and 50% have Jo-1 antibodies on antinuclear antibody testing. Lung pathology is typically fibrotic NSIP or OP. As would be expected with these inflammatory patterns of injury, patients usually benefit from immunosuppression. Classic treatment is with cyclophosphamide, but tacrolimus and rituximab are emerging as salvage agents.

Sarcoidosis

Sarcoidosis is an idiopathic multisystem inflammatory disorder that commonly involves the lung.[23] It is the most common ILD in the United States. The tissue inflammation that occurs in sarcoidosis has a characteristic pattern in which the inflammatory cells collect in microscopic nodules called *granulomas*. In contrast to IPF, sarcoidosis is more common among young adults than among older adults. Sarcoidosis often follows a benign course of inflammation without symptoms or long-term consequences that spontaneously remits.

The most common manifestation of sarcoidosis is asymptomatic hilar adenopathy. Less frequently, the chest radiograph shows parenchymal opacities in the midlung zone that may be nodular, reticulonodular, or alveolar. When symptoms occur, cough, chest pain, dyspnea, and wheezing are most common. Pulmonary physiology may be normal, restrictive, obstructive, or mixed, all with reduced DLCO. Obstructive impairment may be related to endobronchial granulomatous inflammation or scarring.[24]

Corticosteroids are commonly used in the management of sarcoidosis, but treatment usually is reserved for patients with marked symptoms or physiologic impairment attributable to the disease.[25] Although corticosteroids almost always reduce active sarcoid inflammation, long-term side effects should limit duration. For patients requiring long-term immunosuppression, alternative immunosuppressive agents such as methotrexate, azathioprine, leflunomide, or tumor necrosis factor-alpha inhibitors such as infliximab should be used.[26] Other organs that may require corticosteroid therapy include cardiac involvement, uveitis, and peripheral or central nervous system involvement with cranial nerve abnormalities. Disease activity is difficult to ascertain in many patients. Serum angiotensin-converting enzyme levels and gallium scans are not well correlated with disease activity, and their routine use is discouraged.[27]

Lymphangioleiomyomatosis

Lymphangioleiomyomatosis (LAM) is a rare disorder of abnormal smooth muscle tissue proliferating around small airways leading to severe obstruction and destruction of alveoli with resultant thin-walled cyst formation.[28] All patients are women, although both men and women with tuberous sclerosis complex can develop lung pathology identical to LAM that is called *tuberous sclerosis complex LAM*. This peculiar pathology is caused by abnormalities in the *TSC-2* gene.[29]

Dyspnea on exertion and an obstructive ventilatory impairment with reduced DLCO is almost always present except in very early disease. Disease progression is quite variable; some women having steadily worsening lung function during midlife, whereas some elderly women experience extremely slow decline over many years. Risk factors for worsening lung function include a significant bronchodilator response and possibly pregnancy. Other important disease manifestations include pneumothorax from a ruptured subpleural cyst. Unilateral or, less commonly, bilateral chylothorax is seen in about one-third of patients. This results from lymphatic obstruction by abnormal smooth muscle tissue. Treatment with a low-fat diet or blocking gut fat absorption is usually ineffective, and pleurodesis is required. Pleurodesis does not preclude subsequent lung transplantation.

Treatment is with inhaled bronchodilators and inhaled corticosteroids. Younger patients may ultimately require lung transplantation. Ongoing studies with rapamycin, which blocks the abnormal *TSC-2* gene and inhibits LAM cell proliferation, may suggest the first disease-specific therapy for an ILD.

Interstitial Lung Disease of Unknown Cause

Idiopathic Interstitial Pneumonias

Despite a careful history, physical examination, and high-resolution CT scan, most patients are not found to have an exposure or systemic illness as a cause of ILD. These patients have a disorder isolated to the lung termed *idiopathic interstitial pneumonia (IIP)*. Prognosis and potential therapies are completely dependent on the type of pathologic pattern of IIP.

Idiopathic Pulmonary Fibrosis. Idiopathic pulmonary fibrosis (IPF) is the most common IIP and is defined as a progressive fibrotic lung disease isolated to the lung.[30] Most patients are older than 60 years, and IPF is extremely unusual in persons younger than 40. Risk factors for development of IPF include exposure to smoke, metal dust, farming dust, and hairdressing chemicals. Patients present with chronic cough and exertional dyspnea, and high-resolution CT suggests a fibrotic process.

The diagnosis is made by noting a lack of exposure or systemic disease known to cause ILD and determining UIP as the pathologic pattern of injury. The diagnosis of UIP is made when high-resolution CT shows bilateral and basilar-predominant peripheral reticular fibrosis and honeycomb cystic change with absence of significant ground-glass abnormalities, micronodules, and air trapping. Without these classic findings, a surgical lung biopsy is needed for diagnosis.[31,32] Patients who do not have IPF can have UIP on surgical lung biopsy (e.g., connective tissue disease), so this pattern of injury and repair is not unique to IPF.

Most patients die as a result of progressive fibrotic lung disease within 4 years of diagnosis. Data show that approximately half of patients die with gradually progressive disease over several years.[33] The other half experience stable lung function or minimal decline for months to years and then have sudden worsening over a few weeks or months leading to death.[34] Baseline parameters that predict an increased risk of death include severity of dyspnea, severity of restrictive physiologic defect, reduced DLCO, pulmonary arterial hypertension, degree of fibrosis on high-resolution CT, and SaO_2 desaturation on exertion.[35] Serial parameters that predict poor survival include worsening dyspnea, FVC, and DLCO.

No medical therapy has proven beneficial or is recommended for IPF. Prior trials have shown no benefit with aggressive immunosuppression,[36-38] interferon gamma,[39] etanercept,[40] bosentan, ambrisentan, sildenafil,[41] or imatinib.[42] Several medications are currently under investigation, including pirfenidone, azathioprine in combination with oral corticosteroids and *N*-acetyl cysteine, and warfarin.

More recent studies have highlighted the importance of pulmonary arterial hypertension in IPF.[43] The degree of pulmonary arterial hypertension does not always correlate with the burden of fibrosis on CT scan or FVC, implying that a vascular process other than obliteration of the capillary bed from fibrosis occurs.[44] Significant pulmonary arterial hypertension is suggested in patients with markedly impaired diffusion capacity but relatively preserved FVC. At the present time, medications that benefit pulmonary arterial hypertension such as bosentan and sildenafil have not proven beneficial for IPF. Treatment with other agent used for pulmonary arterial hypertension are under investigation in IPF, but their use outside of trials is not recommended.

Nonspecific Interstitial Pneumonia. NSIP is an IIP with diffuse inflammation seen on surgical lung biopsy.[45] Patients are on average 7 to 10 years younger than patients with IPF, but considerable overlap exists. The degree of accompanying interstitial fibrosis is variable among patients. The combination of fibrosis and inflammation (fibrotic NSIP) is most common, whereas pure cellular NSIP is less common. Patients present with chronic or subacute cough and dyspnea. High-resolution CT shows predominant ground-glass abnormalities in cellular NSIP and both ground-glass abnormalities and fibrotic changes in fibrotic NSIP. Given that there is significant clinical and radiographic overlap between fibrotic NSIP and IPF, surgical lung biopsy is frequently required to distinguish these two entities, such as when elements of classic UIP are not present on high-resolution CT images.

The prognosis is much better for NSIP than IPF with most patients surviving 7 to 10 years. Immunosuppression with oral corticosteroids and cytotoxic immunosuppressive agents is the primary therapy. Type and duration of therapy are guided by disease activity and degree of inflammation on biopsy and ground-glass abnormalities on high-resolution CT. Pathologic NSIP is found frequently as an IIP and is the most common pattern of injury seen in connective tissue disease–associated ILD. Owing to this frequent association, many authors consider NSIP a connective tissue disease isolated to the lung.[46,47]

Organizing Pneumonia. Organizing pneumonia (OP) is the revised nomenclature for *bronchiolitis obliterans organizing pneumonia*. The term *cryptogenic organizing pneumonia* is used when this pattern of injury occurs as an IIP, and it is termed OP when found in the setting of connective tissue disease. Patients are younger than patients with IPF and present with acute or subacute dyspnea and cough. About one-third describe an antecedent viral illness. However, no other risk factors are known. High-resolution CT shows alveolar filling with air bronchograms mimicking acute pneumonia, and the classic OP patient presents after having failed to improve despite several courses of antibiotics. Diagnosis usually requires surgical lung biopsy, especially if the clinical and radiographic features are uncertain because small areas of OP can be seen in various inflammatory and fibrotic disorders on transbronchial lung biopsy. Surgical lung biopsy specimens show young fibroblasts within the alveoli that are presumably recovering from an injury. The alveolar basement membrane is intact, allowing for significant recovery if the inflammation or injury can be suppressed.

Most patients improve with oral corticosteroids (0.5 to 1.0 mg/kg for 6 to 12 weeks). However, many patients have recrudescence after corticosteroid withdrawal and require long-term immunosuppression with cytotoxic immunosuppressive agents. A few patients develop progressive fibrosis despite aggressive immunosuppression and can be offered lung transplantation.

Lymphocytic Interstitial Pneumonia

Lymphocytic interstitial pneumonia is a rare disorder of polyclonal lymphocyte aggregates that accumulate diffusely in the interstitium.[48] The diagnosis almost always requires surgical lung biopsy. Patients are typically younger than patients with IPF and present with subacute dyspnea and cough. Pulmonary function testing may show a mixed picture, and high-resolution CT typically shows diffuse ground-glass attenuation with variable amounts of fibrosis. Most patients respond well to oral corticosteroids with a few requiring long-term immunosuppression. Lymphocytic interstitial pneumonia is frequently associated with connective tissue diseases, especially Sjögren syndrome, and with immunodeficiency, and these possibilities should be investigated in all patients with lymphocytic interstitial pneumonia.

MINI-CLINI

Clinical Deterioration in a Patient With Interstitial Lung Disease

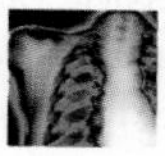

PROBLEM: A 50-year-old man with fibrotic NSIP is being treated with oral corticosteroids and cyclophosphamide. After 6 months of therapy, he begins to report progressive breathlessness. Why is this occurring?

SOLUTION: Many ILDs follow a gradually progressive course to end-stage disease and death. The available treatments may result in temporary improvement or retard progression of the disease. These treatments seldom are curative, however. Progressive symptoms (exertional dyspnea or cough) in a patient being treated for ILD often, although not always, is indicative of disease progression.

The following possibilities must be considered and separated from progression of the disease.

Superimposed Infection: Immunosuppressive agents used in the management of some ILDs increase the risk of infection in the lung and elsewhere. Common bacteria or uncommon opportunistic infections may be responsible. Pneumonia may be difficult to detect radiographically because of preexisting radiographic abnormalities, and bronchoscopy with bronchoalveolar lavage and transbronchial lung biopsy may be needed.

Continued

MINI-CLINI

Clinical Deterioration in a Patient with Interstitial Lung Disease—cont'd

Drug Reaction: Virtually all medications used to treat ILD have been reported to be capable of causing an adverse pulmonary reaction, albeit rarely. Some, such as methotrexate, have been described to result in pulmonary reactions in 5% to 10% of users. An adverse drug reaction should be considered in all patients with ILD who are being actively treated, particularly if there is a clear temporal relationship between the institution of a medication and new or progressive respiratory symptoms.

Steroid-related muscle weakness is a less common complication of corticosteroid therapy and can cause exercise intolerance indistinguishable from progression of the underlying lung disease. Steroid-related muscle weakness (steroid myopathy) is difficult to diagnose because the weakness can result in worsening of the underlying restrictive physiologic defect. When proximal muscle weakness occurs in combination with progressive respiratory symptoms, the possibility of steroid myopathy should be considered. A greater than 25% reduction of the FVC in the supine position compared with the sitting position suggests neuromuscular dysfunction.

Pulmonary Embolism: Inactivity as a result of disease-related physiologic impairment and right ventricular dysfunction may be a risk factor for thromboembolic disease. A sudden decline in respiratory status, sometimes associated with pleuritic chest pain, raises the possibility of acute pulmonary embolism.

Lung Carcinoma: Patients with pulmonary fibrosis have an increased risk of lung cancer, and its development may contribute to clinical decline.

Atherosclerotic Vascular Disease: Many patients with ILD have independent risk factors for atherosclerotic vascular disease. They may have unrelated cardiac disease, such as coronary artery disease, left ventricular dysfunction, or valvular disease, which can be mistaken for a worsening of the pulmonary process.

Each of the possible explanations for the patient's breathlessness should be considered before ascribing it to disease progression.

NONSPECIFIC THERAPIES FOR INTERSTITIAL LUNG DISEASE

Oxygen Therapy

Because hypoxemia is common in ILD, supplemental O_2 therapy is frequently prescribed, although it has not been studied as extensively as in chronic obstructive pulmonary disease (COPD). Patients with ILD should have arterial O_2 saturation determined at rest and especially during exertion because many patients with only mild disease desaturate with exertion despite normal saturation at rest. Although studies are limited, supplemental O_2 delivered via nasal cannula can prevent resting hypoxemia and allow greater exertion before desaturation. These benefits may improve quality of life and potentially ward off development of pulmonary arterial hypertension, although further studies are needed.

We favor continuous rather than pulse delivery because the desaturation with activity seen in most patients that is not rectified with pulse therapy, and pulse units vary greatly in the amount of O_2 delivered.[49] For most patients, liquid O_2 is the best source to provide adequate flow rates. In motivated patients, transtracheal delivery of supplemental O_2 increases the efficiency of delivery and improves cosmetics. However, patients must be chosen carefully because of the need for frequent care and risk of mucus dessication and rare hemorrhage.

MINI-CLINI

Tobacco Use and Interstitial Lung Disease

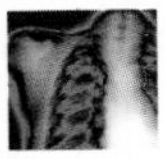

PROBLEM: A 30-year-old woman has ILD and is a current smoker. She is concerned that quitting on her own is too difficult and comments that tobacco use is associated with emphysema, not with scarring. Should she be encouraged to quit smoking? Why or why not?

SOLUTION: Yes! Although the association between tobacco use and COPD is well known, the relationship with ILD is less well appreciated. It is a risk factor for the development of IPF but not the sole cause. However, the following three types of ILD have a strong association with cigarette smoking: the IIPs of DIP, RB-ILD, and PLCH.

Approximately 90% of patients with DIP and RB-ILD are current or former tobacco smokers. More than 90% of patients with PLCH smoke, often quite heavily. As with other toxic exposures, complete avoidance of all smoke is important for these patients. In RB-ILD and PLCH, physiologic stabilization and occasionally even improvement can occur after stopping smoking. In DIP, the benefits of smoking cessation are unclear.

In addition to having concerns about these specific disease considerations, patients with ILD of any type cannot afford to risk the development of additional, smoking-related cardiorespiratory impairment. The patient should be encouraged to stop smoking.

Pulmonary Rehabilitation and Exercise Therapy

Pulmonary rehabilitation, a mainstay of treatment for obstructive lung disease, has also proven beneficial in the management of ILD. Pulmonary rehabilitation is important in building aerobic fitness, maintaining physical activity, and improving quality of life. When pulmonary rehabilitation is stopped, the benefits wane over a few months.[50] We encourage all of our patients to enroll in outpatient pulmonary rehabilitation and to continue maintenance therapy.

Vaccinations and Infection Avoidance

Because patients with ILD have increased consequences of respiratory infections, patients with ILD should receive a pneumococcal vaccine per U.S. Centers for Disease Control and Prevention guidelines and a yearly influenza virus vaccine. Additionally, we recommend that patients practice good hand hygiene (frequent handwashing). We do not recommend use of masks or special antibacterial products. Patients treated with prednisone in doses greater than 15 mg daily or with a steroid-sparing immunosuppressant should receive *Pneumocystis* prophylaxis.

Transplantation

The only therapy shown to prolong life in patients with end-stage, particularly fibrotic, ILD is lung transplantation.[51] Transplantation has been performed successfully in the management of most ILDs. Enthusiasm for the procedure is tempered by the significant risk of mortality at 1 year (10% to 25%) and 5 years (50% to 60%). Many patients with ILD are older than the upper age limit of "physiologic" age 65. Additionally, comorbidities such as gastroesophageal reflux disease, which is common in many ILDs, preclude lung transplantation owing to the increased risk of chronic rejection and death.

SUMMARY OF INTERSTITIAL LUNG DISEASES

The entities grouped as ILDs are a diverse group of illnesses of varied causation, treatment, and prognosis. These diseases generally manifest as chronic, progressive dyspnea on exertion and cough. Findings on examination are often limited to the chest in the form of fine, inspiratory crackles. The most common finding on chest radiograph is diffuse reticular or reticulonodular infiltrates with reduced lung volumes. Pulmonary function testing usually reveals restrictive physiology and decreased diffusion capacity; however, other patterns can be seen. Therapy depends on the underlying disease and may consist of immunosuppressive drugs and the avoidance of disease-inducing exposures.

ROLE OF THE RESPIRATORY THERAPIST IN INTERSTITIAL LUNG DISEASE

The respiratory therapist (RT) encounters patients with ILD in one of two settings. RTs assess and treat outpatients in several manners. In the role of pulmonary function technician, RTs assess disease burden and serial changes in lung function. At the initial evaluation, the RT needs to provide accurate spirometry, lung volume, and DLCO, along with 6-minute walk distance and saturation, because these measures have important prognostic value. At subsequent visits, serial changes in these parameters are important to assess a patient's response to therapy or disease progression. Besides having important prognostic values, changes in lung function over time help determine whether to continue therapy or refer eligible patients for lung transplantation.

RTs determine supplemental O_2 requirements at rest and with exertion and recommend the appropriate delivery amount, mode, and source of O_2. Additionally, RTs typically perform outpatient pulmonary rehabilitation, which can benefit many patients with ILD.

The needs of ILD patients change when admitted to the hospital. The RT plays a crucial role in assessing supplemental O_2 needs and delivering O_2 by the proper mode (nasal cannula, face mask, high-flow O_2 with nonrebreathing face mask, or intubation and mechanical ventilation). If obstructive impairment is suspected, the RT can recommend and deliver the appropriate bronchodilators or inhaled corticosteroids. Owing to the tenuous nature of these patients, careful monitoring of ILD patients by the RT is required to prevent hypoxemia and its acute complications.

SUMMARY CHECKLIST

- The entities grouped as ILDs are a diverse group of illnesses encompassing various etiologies, treatments, and prognoses.
- These diseases generally manifest as chronic, progressive dyspnea on exertion and cough.
- Findings on examination are often limited to the chest in the form of fine, inspiratory crackles.
- The most common chest radiograph finding is diffuse reticular or reticulonodular infiltrates with reduced lung volumes.
- Pulmonary function testing usually reveals restrictive physiology and decreased diffusion capacity; however, other patterns can be seen.
- Treatment depends on the underlying disease and may consist of immunosuppressive drugs and avoidance of disease-inducing exposures.

References

1. Raghu G, Brown KK: Interstitial lung disease: clinical evaluation and keys to an accurate diagnosis. Clin Chest Med 25:409–419, 2004.
2. King TE, Jr: Clinical advances in the diagnosis and therapy of the interstitial lung diseases. Am J Respir Crit Care Med 172:268–279, 2005.
3. Elliot TL, Lynch DA, Newell JD, Jr, et al: High-resolution computed tomography features of non-specific interstitial

pneumonia and usual interstitial pneumonia. J Comput Assist Tomogr 29:339–345, 2005.
4. Hunninghake GW, Lynch DA, Galvin JR, et al: Radiologic findings are strongly associated with a pathologic diagnosis of usual interstitial pneumonia. Chest 124:1215–1223, 2003.
5. Souza CA, Muller NL, Lee KS, et al: Idiopathic interstitial pneumonias: prevalence of mediastinal lymph node enlargement in 206 patients. AJR Am J Roentgenol 186:995–999, 2006.
6. Chetta A, Marangio E, Olivieri D: Pulmonary function testing in interstitial lung diseases. Respiration 71:209–213, 2004.
7. Cottin V, Nunes H, Brillet PY, et al: Combined pulmonary fibrosis and emphysema: a distinct underrecognised entity. Eur Respir J 26:586–593, 2005.
8. Ryu JH, Myers JL, Capizzi SA, et al: Desquamative interstitial pneumonia and respiratory bronchiolitis-associated interstitial lung disease. Chest 127:178–184, 2005.
9. Portnoy J, Veraldi KL, Schwarz MI, et al: Respiratory bronchiolitis-interstitial lung disease: long-term outcome. Chest 131:664–671, 2007.
10. Goldiner PL, Carlon GC, Cvitkovic E, et al: Factors influencing postoperative morbidity and mortality in patients treated with bleomycin. BMJ 1:1664–1667, 1978.
11. Selman M. Hypersensitivity pneumonitis: a multifaceted deceiving disorder. Clin Chest Med 25:531–547, 2004.
12. Lacasse Y, Selman M, Costabel U, et al: Clinical diagnosis of hypersensitivity pneumonitis. Am J Respir Crit Care Med 168:952–958, 2003.
13. Monkare S: Influence of corticosteroid treatment on the course of farmer's lung. Eur J Respir Dis 64:283–293, 1983.
14. Vourlekis JS, Schwarz MI, Cherniack RM, et al: The effect of pulmonary fibrosis on survival in patients with hypersensitivity pneumonitis. Am J Med 116:662–668, 2004.
15. American Thoracic Society: Diagnosis and initial management of nonmalignant diseases related to asbestos. Am J Respir Crit Care Med 170:691–715, 2004.
16. Schwartz DA, Davis CS, Merchant JA, et al: Longitudinal changes in lung function among asbestos-exposed workers. Am J Respir Crit Care Med 150:1243–1249, 1994.
17. Ross MH, Murray J: Occupational respiratory disease in mining. Occup Med (Lond) 54:304–310, 2004.
18. Strange C, Highland KB: Interstitial lung disease in the patient who has connective tissue disease. Clin Chest Med 25:549–559, 2004.
19. Tanaka N, Newell JD, Brown KK, et al: Collagen vascular disease-related lung disease: high-resolution computed tomography findings based on the pathologic classification. J Comput Assist Tomogr 28:351–360, 2004.
20. Tashkin DP, Elashoff R, Clements PJ, et al: Cyclophosphamide versus placebo in scleroderma lung disease. N Engl J Med 354:2655–2666, 2006.
21. Swigris JJ, Olson AL, Fischer A, et al: Mycophenolate mofetil is safe, well tolerated, and preserves lung function in patients with connective tissue disease-related interstitial lung disease. Chest 130:30–36, 2006.
22. Tashkin DP, Elashoff R, Clements PJ, et al: Effects of 1-year treatment with cyclophosphamide on outcomes at 2 years in scleroderma lung disease. Am J Respir Crit Care Med 176:1026–1034, 2007.
23. Baughman RP: Pulmonary sarcoidosis. Clin Chest Med 25:521–530, 2004.
24. Shorr AF, Torrington KG, Hnatiuk OW: Endobronchial involvement and airway hyperreactivity in patients with sarcoidosis. Chest 120:881–886, 2001.
25. Paramothayan NS, Lasserson TJ, Jones PW: Corticosteroids for pulmonary sarcoidosis. Cochrane Database Syst Rev (2):CD001114, 2005.
26. Rossman MD, Newman LS, Baughman RP, et al: A double-blinded, randomized, placebo-controlled trial of infliximab in subjects with active pulmonary sarcoidosis. Sarcoidosis Vasc Diffuse Lung Dis 23:201–208, 2006.
27. Keir G, Wells AU: Assessing pulmonary disease and response to therapy: which test? Semin Respir Crit Care Med 31:409–418, 2010.
28. Ryu JH, Moss J, Beck GJ, et al: The NHLBI lymphangioleiomyomatosis registry: characteristics of 230 patients at enrollment. Am J Respir Crit Care Med 173:105–111, 2006.
29. McCormack FX: Lymphangioleiomyomatosis: a clinical update. Chest 133:507–516, 2008.
30. Raghu G, Weycker D, Edelsberg J, et al: Incidence and prevalence of idiopathic pulmonary fibrosis. Am J Respir Crit Care Med 174:810–816, 2006.
31. Raghu G, Mageto YN, Lockhart D, et al: The accuracy of the clinical diagnosis of new-onset idiopathic pulmonary fibrosis and other interstitial lung disease: a prospective study. Chest 116:1168–1174, 1999.
32. Hunninghake GW, Zimmerman MB, Schwartz DA, et al: Utility of a lung biopsy for the diagnosis of idiopathic pulmonary fibrosis. Am J Respir Crit Care Med 164:193–196, 2001.
33. Martinez FJ, Safrin S, Weycker D, et al: The clinical course of patients with idiopathic pulmonary fibrosis. Ann Intern Med 142:963–967, 2005.
34. Collard HR, Moore BB, Flaherty KR, et al: Acute exacerbations of idiopathic pulmonary fibrosis. Am J Respir Crit Care Med 176:636–643, 2007.
35. Collard HR, King TE, Jr, Bartelson BB, et al: Changes in clinical and physiologic variables predict survival in idiopathic pulmonary fibrosis. Am J Respir Crit Care Med 168:538–542, 2003.
36. Richeldi L, Davies HR, Ferrara G, et al: Corticosteroids for idiopathic pulmonary fibrosis. Cochrane Database Syst Rev (3):CD002880, 2003.
37. Davies HR, Richeldi L, Walters EH: Immunomodulatory agents for idiopathic pulmonary fibrosis. Cochrane Database Syst Rev (3):CD003134, 2003.
38. Collard HR, Ryu JH, Douglas WW, et al: Combined corticosteroid and cyclophosphamide therapy does not alter survival in idiopathic pulmonary fibrosis. Chest 125:2169–2174, 2004.
39. King TE, Jr, Albera C, Bradford WZ, et al: Effect of interferon gamma-1b on survival in patients with idiopathic pulmonary fibrosis (INSPIRE): a multicentre, randomised, placebo-controlled trial. Lancet 374:222–228, 2009.
40. Raghu G, Brown KK, Costabel U, et al: Treatment of idiopathic pulmonary fibrosis with etanercept: an exploratory, placebo-controlled trial. Am J Respir Crit Care Med 178:948–955, 2008.
41. Idiopathic Pulmonary Fibrosis Clinical Research Network, Zisman DA, Schwarz M, Anstrom KJ, et al: A controlled trial of sildenafil in advanced idiopathic pulmonary fibrosis. N Engl J Med 363:620–628, 2010.
42. Daniels CE, Lasky JA, Limper AH, et al: Imatinib treatment for idiopathic pulmonary fibrosis: randomized placebo-controlled trial results. Am J Respir Crit Care Med 181:604–610, 2010.
43. Nadrous HF, Pellikka PA, Krowka MJ, et al: Pulmonary hypertension in patients with idiopathic pulmonary fibrosis. Chest 128:2393–2399, 2005.
44. Lettieri CJ, Nathan SD, Barnett SD, et al: Prevalence and outcomes of pulmonary arterial hypertension in

advanced idiopathic pulmonary fibrosis. Chest 129:746–752, 2006.
45. Martinez FJ: Idiopathic interstitial pneumonias: usual interstitial pneumonia versus non-specific interstitial pneumonia. Proc Am Thorac Soc 3:81–95, 2006.
46. Fischer A, West SG, Swigris JJ, et al: Connective tissue disease-associated interstitial lung disease: a call for clarification. Chest 138:251–256, 2010.
47. Kinder BW, Collard HR, Koth L, et al: Idiopathic non-specific interstitial pneumonia: lung manifestation of undifferentiated connective tissue disease? Am J Respir Crit Care Med 176:691–697, 2007.
48. Cha SI, Fessler MB, Cool CD, et al: Lymphoid interstitial pneumonia: clinical features, associations and prognosis. Eur Respir J 28:364–369, 2006.
49. Palwai A, Skowronski M, Coreno A, et al: Critical comparisons of the clinical performance of oxygen-conserving devices. Am J Respir Crit Care Med 181:1061–1071, 2010.
50. Holland AE, Hill CJ, Conron M, et al: Short term improvement in exercise capacity and symptoms following exercise training in interstitial lung disease. Thorax 63:549–554, 2008.
51. Orens JB, Estenne M, Arcasoy S, et al: International guidelines for the selection of lung transplant candidates: 2006 update—a consensus report from the Pulmonary Scientific Council of the International Society for Heart and Lung Transplantation. J Heart Lung Transplant 25:745–755, 2006.

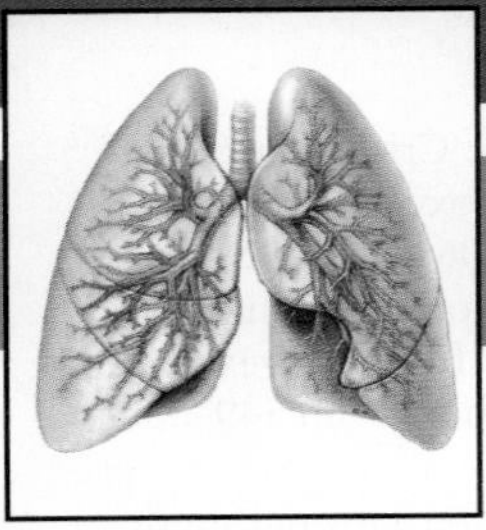

Chapter 25

Pleural Diseases

CHARLIE STRANGE

CHAPTER OBJECTIVES

After reading this chapter you will be able to:

- Describe important anatomic features and physiologic function of the visceral and parietal pleural membranes.
- Describe how pleural effusions occur and the difference between transudative and exudative effusions.
- Identify common causes of transudative and exudative pleural effusions.
- Write definitions of chylothorax, hemothorax, and pneumothorax.
- Describe the impact of moderate to large pleural effusions on lung function.
- State the role of a chest radiograph in recognizing pleural effusions.
- State the purpose of thoracentesis and the potential complications.
- Identify the definitions of spontaneous, secondary, and tension pneumothorax.
- Describe the diagnosis and treatment of pneumothorax.

CHAPTER OUTLINE

KEY TERMS

bronchopleural fistula
chyle
chylothorax
empyema
exudative pleural effusion
hemothorax
parietal pleura
pleural effusion
pleurisy
pleurodesis
pneumothorax
primary spontaneous pneumothorax
reexpansion pulmonary edema
secondary spontaneous pneumothorax
stomata
tension pneumothorax
thoracentesis
transudative pleural effusion

A spectrum of pleural diseases affects respiratory function. An understanding of pleural anatomy, physiology, and pathology is essential to delivering effective respiratory care. This chapter focuses on the two major disease processes that occur in the pleural space: pleural effusion and pneumothorax.

PLEURAL SPACE

Overview and Definitions

Each lung is covered by a thin membrane called the *visceral pleura,* which adheres closely to the subjacent alveoli of the lung. The visceral pleura dips into the fissures of the lung, allowing the surgeon easy access between the lung lobes and allowing pleural fluid to travel freely between the lobes while remaining in the pleural space.

The ribs and connective tissue of the chest wall are covered on the inner surface by a similar membrane called the **parietal pleura.** The parietal pleura can be thought of as a sac that covers not only the rib surface (costal pleura) but also the diaphragm (diaphragmatic pleura) and the mediastinum (mediastinal pleura).

The blood vessels and airways that enter the lung connect to the mediastinum at the lung hilum. At this juncture, the visceral pleura meets the mediastinal parietal pleura to form a single, continuous pleural membrane (Figure 25-1).

Because the lung usually is completely inflated, it might be thought that the pleural membranes always touch. However, freeze-fracturing has shown that there is a space between the visceral and parietal pleura that averages 10 to 20 μm in width and is filled with pleural fluid. This thin film of fluid allows the lung to slide over the ribs and allows for a gliding movement that takes little energy and produces little friction.

The average person has approximately 8 ml of pleural fluid per hemithorax.[1] The pleural fluid is estimated to have a total protein concentration similar to that of interstitial fluid elsewhere in the body: between 1.3 g/dl and 1.4.[2]

In humans, the pleural spaces surrounding each lung are completely independent, being separated by the mediastinum. This is not the case in all other mammals. The slaughter of the American buffalo could occur with a single spear or rifle shot because the pleural spaces of the buffalo lung are connected. Consequently, air in the pleural space collapses both lungs. An analogous situation can occur in any patient who has undergone median sternotomy, during which both pleural spaces were entered. Common operations resulting in this condition are lung volume reduction surgery and bilateral lung transplantation.

The pleural space is under negative pressure except during forced expiration. The intact thoracic rib cage provides elastic recoil pressure outward, whereas the intrinsic recoil pressure of the lung is inward toward the lung hilum. The diaphragm further decreases the intrapleural pressure below the atmospheric pressure to allow inspiration to occur. In an upright person, the pressure is more negative at the lung apex than at the lung base because of the weight of the lung and the effects of gravity. The net effect of the negatively pressurized pleural space is that fluid moves into the pleural space from adjacent sites when a communication is present. A patient with ascitic fluid and a diaphragmatic defect preferentially pulls fluid into the chest.

PLEURAL EFFUSIONS

Any abnormal amount of pleural fluid in the pleural space is called **pleural effusion.** The many causes of pleural effusion are categorized according to etiologic factor and the content of the fluid.[3]

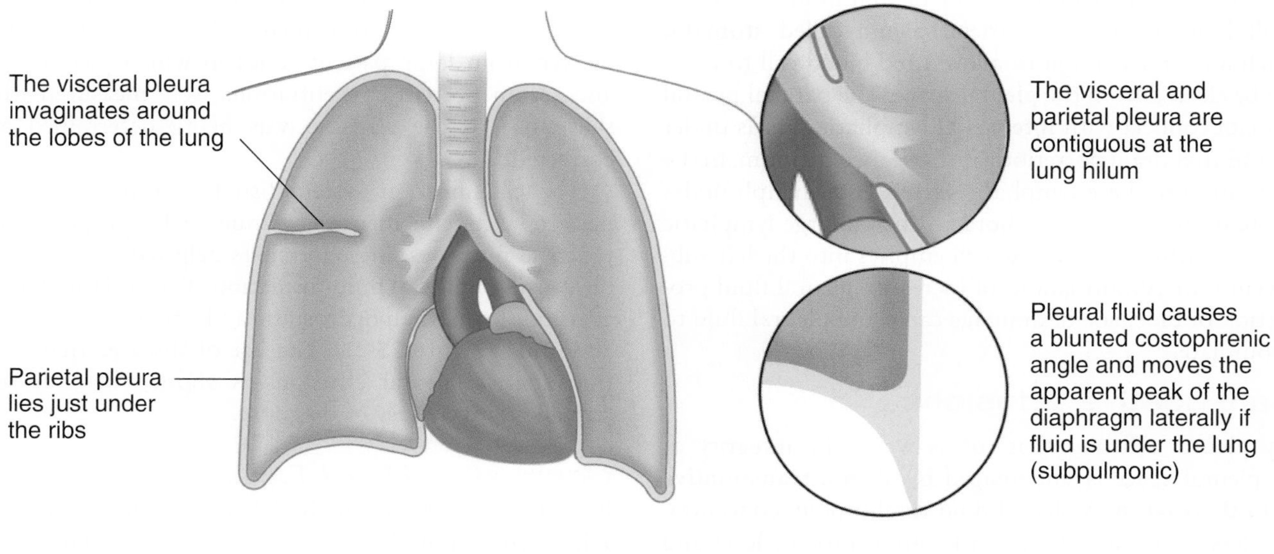
The visceral pleura invaginates around the lobes of the lung
Parietal pleura lies just under the ribs
The visceral and parietal pleura are contiguous at the lung hilum
Pleural fluid causes a blunted costophrenic angle and moves the apparent peak of the diaphragm laterally if fluid is under the lung (subpulmonic)

FIGURE 25-1 Anatomy of the pleura.

Box 25-1 Causes of Pleural Effusion

- Transudative pleural effusion
  - CHF
  - Cirrhosis
  - Nephrotic syndrome
  - Hypoalbuminemia
  - Lymphatic obstruction
  - Peritoneal dialysis
  - Atelectasis
  - Central venous catheter in pleural space
  - Urinothorax
  - Trapped lung
- Exudative pleural effusion
- Neoplastic disease
  - Carcinoma
  - Lymphoma
  - Mesothelioma
- Infectious disease
  - Bacterial infection
  - Tuberculosis
  - Fungal infection
  - Paragonimiasis
  - Viral pleurisy
- Pulmonary embolism
- Gastrointestinal disease
  - Pancreatic disease
  - Intraabdominal abscess
  - Splenic infarction
  - Esophageal perforation
  - Abdominal surgery
  - Endoscopic variceal sclerotherapy
- Collagen vascular disease
  - Rheumatoid pleurisy
  - Systemic lupus erythematosus
  - Drug-induced lupus
  - Immunoblastic lymphadenopathy
  - Sjögren syndrome
  - Familial Mediterranean fever
  - Churg-Strauss syndrome
  - Wegener granulomatosis
- Drug-induced pleural disease
  - Nitrofurantoin
  - Minoxidil
  - Dantrolene
  - Methysergide
  - Bromocriptine
  - Amiodarone
  - Procarbazine, bleomycin, mitomycin
  - Methotrexate
  - Practolol
- Miscellaneous diseases and conditions
  - Benign asbestos pleural effusion
  - Post–cardiac injury syndrome
  - Meigs syndrome
  - Yellow nail syndrome
  - Sarcoidosis
  - Pericardial disease
  - Fetal pleural effusion
  - Uremic pleural effusion
  - Lung entrapment
  - Radiation pleurisy
  - Amyloidosis
  - Electrical burns
- Hemothorax
- Chylothorax

Pleural fluid enters the pleural space across both the visceral and the parietal pleurae, particularly when the interstitial pressure within either the lung or the chest wall is increased. The main route for pleural fluid removal is small holes within the parietal pleura called **stomata,** which are large enough to allow a red blood cell to enter and be cleared from the pleural space. The parietal pleural stomata connect with intercostal lymphatic vessels under the ribs that drain posteriorly into the mediastinum. In the mediastinum, these lymphatic vessels enter lymph nodes before draining into the thoracic duct, a large lymphatic channel within the chest, which empties into the left subclavian vein. Abnormalities of increased pleural fluid production or blockade of drainage can cause pleural fluid to accumulate.

Transudative Effusions

Any pleural effusion that forms when the integrity of the pleural space is undamaged is called a **transudative pleural effusion.** A pleural fluid total protein concentration less than 50% of the serum total protein level and lactate dehydrogenase values in the pleural fluid less than 60% of the serum value indicate the presence of a transudative pleural effusion. In the absence of serum values, an absolute pleural fluid lactate dehydrogenase level less than two-thirds normal for serum suggests the presence of a transudate. These numbers were derived from large patient series in which pleural fluid and serum protein concentrations were measured while the cause of the effusion was being determined and corrected.[4]

The classification system listed in Box 25-1 is not perfect, and refinements continue to be proposed. For practical purposes, these numbers help narrow the possible causes of pleural fluid formation. Transudative pleural effusions form when hydrostatic and oncotic pressures are abnormal (Figure 25-2).[5] The list of diseases that cause transudative pleural effusions is short. These diseases remain relatively easy to diagnose.

Congestive Heart Failure

Elevation of pressure in the left atrium and pulmonary veins is the hallmark of *congestive heart failure* (CHF). Elevation of pulmonary venous pressure increases the amount

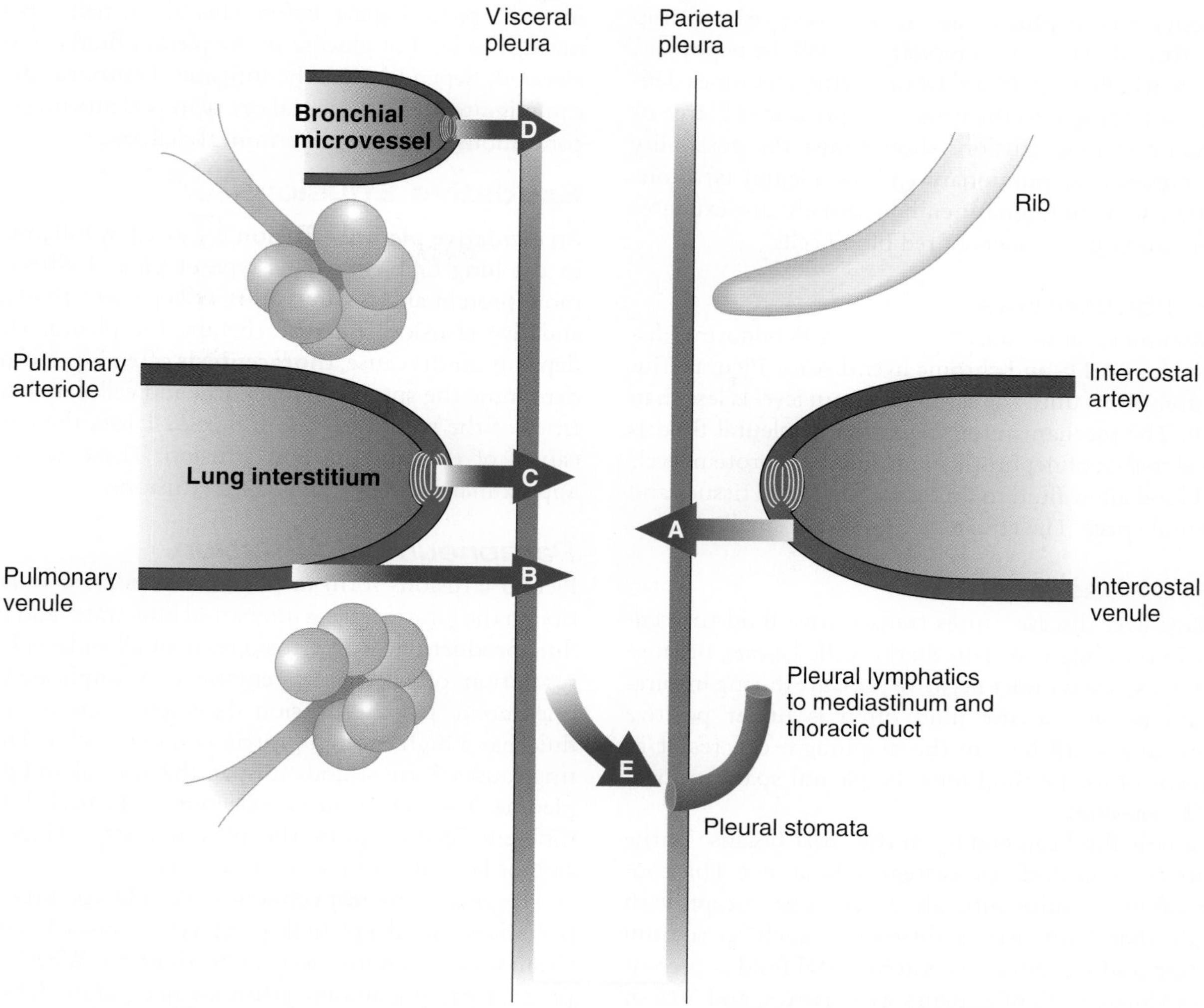

FIGURE 25-2 Pleural fluid formation requires both excess fluid formation and decreased elimination. In diseases such as pulmonary arterial hypertension, in which right-sided heart pressure is increased and systemic veins, such as the intercostal veins *(A)*, are pressurized, pleural fluid does not form because pleural fluid formation is not increased, and lymphatic drainage remains intact. However, when left ventricular failure causes pulmonary venule pressure *(B)* to increase, the addition of interstitial lung water overwhelms the drainage and produces a transudative pleural effusion. Injury to the capillaries *(C)*, as in pneumonia or ARDS, causes fluid to leak into the lung interstitium and pleural space at increased rates. Under these conditions, fibrin can occlude the pleural lymphatic vessels *(E)* and cause fluid to accumulate. The bronchial microvessels *(D)* supply the pleura with blood and likely participate to some extent in production of pleural fluid.

of interstitial fluid in the lung. In severe cases, flooding of the alveoli causes pulmonary edema, but in less severe cases, interstitial lung water increases and decompresses into the pleural space. Because systemic venous pressure also is elevated, there is limited capability to remove pleural fluid through the intercostal veins. Pleural fluid must be predominantly removed by the lymphatic vessels. Pleural effusions result when the capacity of pleural lymphatic drainage is overcome.[6]

CHF is the most common cause of clinical pleural effusions. The effusions can be massive, filling the entire hemithorax and compressing the lung. More commonly, they are small and bilateral. The effusions are rarely drained because outcome is heavily influenced by successful management of the underlying CHF, which also clears the effusions.[7]

Nephrotic Syndrome

In *nephrotic syndrome* (also known as *nephrosis*), the kidneys leak more than 3 g of protein per day into the urine. Because patients become protein depleted, there is insufficient oncotic pressure within the blood to hold appropriate amounts of fluid within the blood vessels. These patients become edematous, and fluid leaks into the lung interstitium and pleural space. Pleural effusions are common but usually are small.

Patients with nephrosis are at increased risk of deep venous thrombosis and pulmonary emboli. In nephrosis, protein S, which keeps blood from clotting, becomes deficient from leaking into the urine. The presence of large or asymmetric pleural effusions should raise the possibility of the presence of pulmonary emboli. Pleural effusions associated with pulmonary emboli usually are exudates and contain large numbers of red blood cells.

Hypoalbuminemia

Hypoalbuminemia is caused by various debilitating diseases, such as AIDS and chronic liver disease. Pleural effusions rarely form until the serum albumin level is less than 1.8 g/dl. The mechanism of formation of pleural fluid is identical to that of nephrotic syndrome. Low protein levels in the blood allow fluid to leak into interstitial tissues and the pleural space. The effusions usually are small.

Liver Disease

End-stage liver disease causes transudative fluid to accumulate in the abdomen. This fluid is called *ascites*. Because the pleural space is under negative pressure during inspiration and because ascitic fluid often is under positive pressure, any small hole in the diaphragm can result in movement of ascitic fluid into the pleural space to form *hepatic hydrothorax*.

All ascitic fluid can end up in the chest because of the pressure gradient, and true ascites can be absent. This condition often is quite difficult to manage except with methods that limit ascites formation, such as sodium restriction and diuretics. Excessive pleural fluid is present in approximately 6% of patients with ascites, and 70% of these fluid collections are on the right side.[8]

Atelectasis

When segments of the lung collapse, intrapleural pressure becomes more negative and can produce small effusions. With relief of bronchial obstruction and postoperative pain, these effusions regress.

Lymphatic Obstruction

Lymphatic obstruction within the mediastinum causes poor pleural fluid egress from the pleural space, although the pleural space is otherwise normal. The most common condition that causes this abnormality is cancer that metastasizes to the mediastinum. This condition should be differentiated from a true malignant pleural effusion, defined as cancer cells within the pleural space.

Rare Causes

There are other rare causes of transudative pleural effusions. Urinothorax occurs after rupture of the ureter causing a urine leak into the retroperitoneal space that refluxes into the chest. The pleural fluid has a low pH. A central venous line that is inappropriately placed into the pleural space can put large amounts of transudative fluid into the pleural space before this abnormality is recognized. The level of glucose in the pleural fluid can be very elevated, depending on the infusion. Peritoneal dialysate can migrate into the pleural cavity in patients undergoing continuous ambulatory peritoneal dialysis.

Exudative Effusions

An **exudative pleural effusion** is caused by inflammation in the lung or pleura. This type of pleural effusion has more protein and inflammatory cells present than a transudative effusion. Because therapy for pleural effusion depends on the cause, **thoracentesis** often is performed to determine the specific biochemical and cellular characteristics of the pleural effusion. Box 25-1 lists the common causes of exudative pleural effusion. These account for approximately 70% of all pleural effusions.

Parapneumonic Effusion

Pleural effusions form in pneumonia because inflammation in the lung increases interstitial lung water and pleural fluid production. Most effusions are small and resolve with resolution of bacterial pneumonia.[9] Complicated parapneumonic pleural effusion develops when the pleural fluid has a high enough protein content to clot. The clotting causes fibrin strands to span the visceral and parietal pleurae. The net result is collection of pleural fluid into different loculi within the pleural cavity. These often cannot be drained by a single chest tube.

Progression to **empyema** is marked by the presence of bacteria within the pleural space, seen as pus or bacteria on Gram stain. Empyema necessitates drainage. Whether complicated parapneumonic effusions necessitate drainage is controversial, although most physicians perform drainage because some of these effusions can progress to empyema.[10]

Parapneumonic effusions are common causes of persistent fever among patients with pneumonia in the intensive care unit (ICU). Sampling by thoracentesis is commonly performed to exclude empyema. Pleural fluid drainage can improve ventilation if the fluid volume is large.

Viral Pleurisy

Viral lung infections can cause pleural inflammation **(pleurisy),** small pleural effusions, and pain. The effusions may be so small they may be overlooked on a routine chest radiograph; when they can be seen, the effusions often are too small to sample. Pleural pain, which is called *pleurodynia* and which can be the result of many other pleural processes, often is difficult to manage. A typical patient with pleurodynia has shallow respirations; deeper breaths are limited by pain. The subsequent atelectasis can cause oxygenation difficulty secondary to shunting.

Tuberculous Pleurisy

In many parts of the world, any lymphocyte-predominant exudative effusion is considered tuberculosis until proven otherwise. Tuberculous pleural effusions occur when a caseous granuloma in the lung ruptures through the visceral pleural surface causing an exudative inflammatory effusion. Experiments in which purified protein derivative (PPD) is placed into the pleural space of animals have shown that such effusions result from the body's immune reaction to tuberculin proteins.

Although these patients require respiratory isolation, only 25% of them have sputum that subsequently grows *Mycobacterium tuberculosis*. The PPD skin test result is negative in 30% of patients when they come to medical attention but turns positive in 6 to 8 weeks in almost everyone.[11]

Malignant Disease

Malignant disease is the most common cause of large unilateral pleural effusions among individuals older than 60 years. Common cancers that form malignant pleural effusions include lung cancer and breast cancer, although any cancer can metastasize to the pleural surface. The effusions usually are lymphocyte predominant; malignant cells are found during cytologic examination of the pleural fluid.

Some malignant pleural effusions, such as effusions from lymphoma, respond to therapy for the malignant disease. However, most patients with symptomatic malignant pleural effusions need primary therapy with pleurodesis. In **pleurodesis,** the visceral and parietal pleural membranes are fused by talc, other chemicals, or surgery to obliterate the pleural space.

Postoperative Causes

Various operations involving the chest or upper abdomen produce pleural fluid.[12] Effusions following cardiac surgery usually are predominant on the left side and tend to be bloody. These effusions are particularly prevalent after a cutdown of the internal mammary artery for coronary artery bypass.

Small transudative pleural effusions are common when there is any atelectasis in the lung. Upper abdominal operations cause inflammation of the diaphragm and effusion that has been termed *sympathetic*. Lung surgery in which the lung is unable to fill the thoracic cavity leaves a space under negative pressure, which fills with inflammatory pleural fluid. When the lung is unable to fill the space because of small postoperative size or visceral pleural fibrosis, the resulting pleural effusion can never be completely drained because of the "trapped lung."

Chylothorax

The thoracic duct is a lymphatic channel that runs from the abdomen through the mediastinum to enter the left subclavian vein. Disruption of the thoracic duct anywhere along its course can cause leakage of **chyle** into the mediastinum, which may rupture into the pleural space and cause a **chylothorax.** The most common causes of rupture are malignancy (50%), surgery (20%), and trauma (5%).[13] The thoracic duct courses through the right side of the mediastinum in the lower thoracic cavity before crossing to the left side of the mediastinum at T4 to T6. Rupture below this level causes right-sided pleural effusion, whereas rupture above this level causes left-sided pleural effusion.

In a patient who has eaten recently, the effusions are milky white as a result of the presence of chylomicrons (microscopic fat particles) absorbed by abdominal lymphatic vessels. In a fasting patient, these effusions usually are yellow. The effusions may be bloody. A pleural fluid triglyceride concentration greater than 110 mg/dl confirms the diagnosis.[14] Computed tomography (CT) should be performed to evaluate the cause of the chylothorax.

Hemothorax

Hemothorax is the presence of blood in the pleural space. Hemothorax is arbitrarily defined as a pleural fluid hematocrit greater than 50% of the serum value. Small amounts of blood in otherwise clear fluid can turn the fluid red.

Although hemothorax is seen most commonly after blunt or penetrating chest trauma, numerous medical conditions can give rise to blood in the pleural space. These conditions should be considered in the absence of trauma. Any vein or artery in the thorax can bleed into the pleural space. A chest tube usually is inserted to monitor the rate of bleeding and determine whether the source is arterial or venous.[15]

Connective Tissue Diseases

Pleural effusions are found in various connective diseases, although the effusions usually are small. Effusions caused by inflammation of small blood vessels are the most common chest manifestation of systemic lupus erythematosus. Pleural effusions often accompany pericardial effusions in systemic lupus erythematosus and disappear with corticosteroid therapy. Rheumatoid arthritis produces a characteristic effusion with a very low glucose content and low pH. These effusions can cause visceral pleural fibrosis and a trapped lung.

Uremia

Uremic pleurisy occurs under the same conditions as uremic pericarditis. A typical patient is undergoing dialysis that is inadequate in duration or frequency. Although the cause of pleural and pericardial inflammation in kidney failure remains unknown, the inflammatory process can take weeks to resolve.

Miscellaneous Causes

Discussion of the other causes of exudative effusions is beyond the scope of this chapter. Thoracentesis that yields findings compatible with any of the systemic diseases listed in Box 25-1 can narrow the differential diagnosis.

Physiologic Importance

Mechanics of Ventilation

Pleural effusions cause lung atelectasis because the capacity of the thorax is limited, and fluid collapses the lung. Spirometry shows restriction. Studies correlating the volume of pleural fluid removed with improvement in forced vital capacity (FVC) show much variability from patient to patient.

> **RULE OF THUMB**
>
> The patient's vital capacity improves by one-third of the pleural fluid volume removed.[16] The remainder of the pleural fluid volume causes diaphragmatic compression and chest wall expansion. Some patients have a delay of 24 to 48 hours before the improvement can be seen as atelectasis resolves. Lack of any improvement suggests that lung consolidation or endobronchial obstruction is present.

Dyspnea is common with small pleural effusions, even when lung mechanics are preserved. The mechanisms are unknown but likely involve activation of stretch receptors or irritant receptors within the airways or nonadrenergic, noncholinergic C fibers in the chest wall or diaphragm. The net result is that dyspnea relief is variable after removal of pleural fluid. Some patients have symptomatic relief after removal of small pleural fluid volumes. Others can have more dyspnea if the fluid is removed in situations such as trapped lung, in which neural activation may increase with fluid withdrawal.

In rare instances, the pleurae thicken with a disease process sufficient to cause fibrothorax. Technically, fibrothorax is any process that causes fibrosis of the thoracic cage that affects pulmonary function. Fibrothorax can be caused by skin (e.g., fibrothorax that occurs rarely in scleroderma), soft tissue, bone (e.g., myositis ossificans, a disease in which muscles calcify), or pleura. Causes of pleural thickening significant enough to produce restriction include severe asbestos pleurisy, rheumatoid pleurisy, complicated trauma, cancer, and empyema.

Hypoxemia

Most patients with a pleural effusion have an increased alveolar-arterial gradient resulting from the pathologic changes in the lung that are causing the effusion. Oxygenation can worsen after thoracentesis because changes in ventilation/perfusion matching are not instantaneous. Recovery to baseline PO_2 and subsequent small improvement usually occur within 90 minutes.[16]

Diagnostic Tests

Chest Radiography

The chest radiograph is the most common method of detecting a pleural effusion. It is important that, if possible, the chest radiograph be obtained with the patient in an upright position to show a pleural fluid meniscus at the costophrenic angles. When the same patient undergoes radiography in the supine position, the effusion is distributed throughout the posterior part of the chest. The chest radiograph shows a generalized haze, which interferes with the detection of pulmonary infiltrates and quantification of pleural effusion. A lateral decubitus chest radiograph also can help define the presence or absence of pleural effusion.

Ultrasonography and Computed Tomography

Pleural fluid and loculi can be detected easily with ultrasonography of the chest. The sensitivity of ultrasonography for pleural effusions is high, although ultrasonography is an operator-dependent study. Small portable ultrasound machines with high diagnostic accuracy have become available to localize the presence of pleural effusions. Some physicians have begun to use these machines routinely to optimize thoracentesis success.

CT scanning of the chest is the most sensitive study for identification of pleural effusion. A contrast-enhanced scan is essential to delineate the pleural membrane and differentiate peripheral lung consolidation from pleural fluid formation. In addition to showing the size and location of a pleural effusion, a chest CT scan often gives information about the underlying lung parenchyma and the primary process causing the effusion.

Thoracentesis

In thoracentesis, pleural fluid is sampled percutaneously by means of insertion of a needle into the pleural space (Figure 25-3). Administration of adequate local anesthetic ensures a painless procedure if care is taken to place lidocaine at the skin insertion site, along the periosteum of the involved rib, and at the parietal pleura, which is richly innervated with sensory nerve fibers. Diagnostic sampling

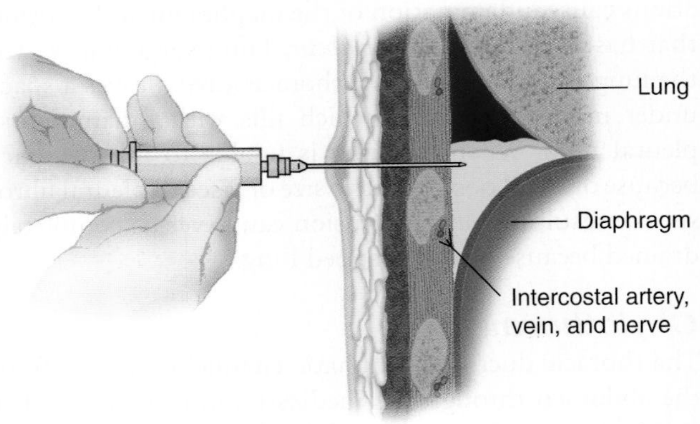

FIGURE 25-3 The technique of thoracentesis involves passage of a needle just superior to the rib. If the needle is placed too low on the chest, the diaphragm or organs below the diaphragm can be punctured. Diagnostic thoracentesis can be performed with small amounts of pleural fluid.

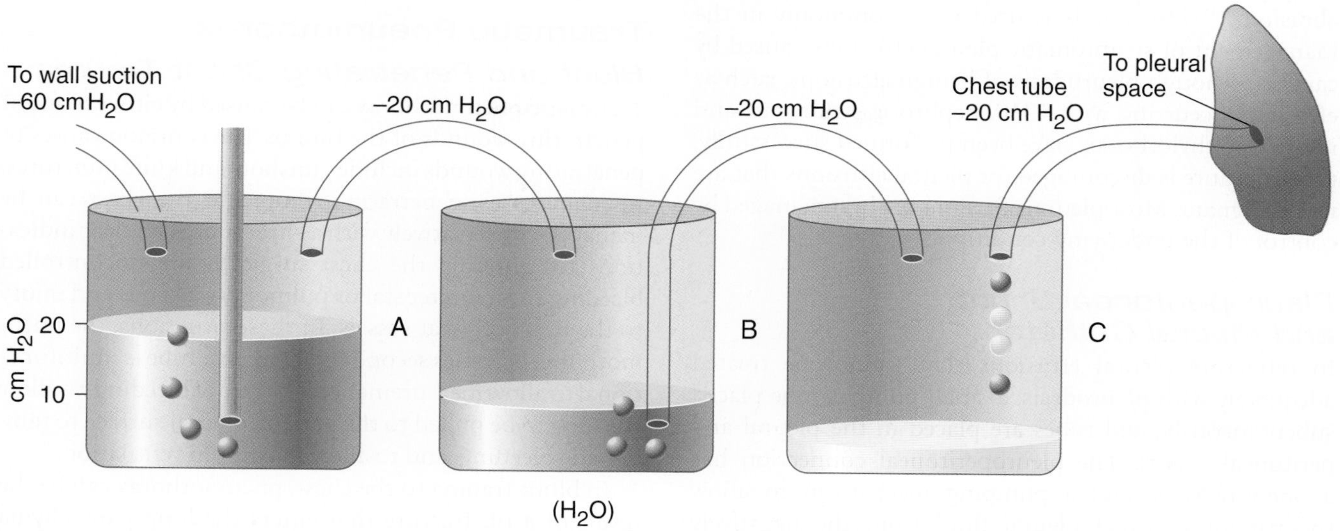

FIGURE 25-4 A-C, The standard three-bottle system is the basis for all commercial chest tube drainage systems. Pleural fluid and pleural air enter compartment **C**, which serves as a fluid collection trap so that the water-seal fluid volume does not increase (compartment **B**) and create resistance to air escaping the chest. Air cannot be inspired into the chest because of the water in compartment **B.** Open entrainment of room air through a submerged tube in compartment **A** buffers the amount of wall suction applied (−60 cm H_2O) to the height of the water column to standardize the pressure (−20 cm H_2O) transmitted to the chest.

of pleural fluid for cell counts, cultures, chemistries, and cytologic examination usually can be performed with a single syringe and a small needle. Samples for pleural pH should be kept from contact with room air. Pleural fluid drainage for lung reexpansion generously involves placing a larger catheter into the pleural space for a longer time.

Thoracentesis involves the following three major risks: (1) intercostal artery laceration, (2) infection, and (3) pneumothorax.[17] Both an artery and a vein course under every rib, and the vessels become increasingly serpiginous with aging. Ensuring needle passage just superior to the rib margin makes bleeding during thoracentesis rare. Ideally, anticoagulants should be stopped before the procedure to lessen bleeding risk.

Because infection can be introduced into the pleural space, a totally sterile procedure is necessary. In some situations, the risk of infection is so high that thoracentesis rarely should be performed. When a lung is surgically removed, the space fills with sterile fluid. An infection introduced into this space usually necessitates open surgical drainage. Any trapped lung also carries a high risk of empyema because of the inability of the visceral and parietal pleurae to meet and contain any infectious process. Needle puncture is one of the most common causes of pneumothorax (see discussion of pneumothorax later in this chapter).

Chest Thoracotomy Tubes

Chest tubes currently are manufactured in various sizes and shapes, ranging from 7 French (F) to 40F catheters. Catheter choice is frequently a matter of physician preference. Larger tubes are less likely to become obstructed and are capable of high airflow rates.

Intercostal placement is designed for the skin and soft tissue to approximate the tube and prevent air from entering the pleural space from the outside. The chest tube is connected to a water-sealed chamber, which usually is contained within a commercially marketed three-bottle system that also regulates pleural pressure and is used to measure pleural fluid volume (Figure 25-4).

Thoracoscopy

The video-assisted thoracoscope is ideally designed for diagnostic and therapeutic work in the pleural space. Diagnostic thoracoscopy often is performed in a medical procedure room with the use of local anesthesia and conscious sedation. The procedure involves placing the thoracoscope through an intercostal incision for visualization of the lung surfaces, drainage of pleural fluid, biopsy under direct visualization, and pleurodesis if needed.

Pleurodesis

Pleurodesis is the process of fusing the parietal and visceral pleurae with a fibrotic reaction that prevents further pleural fluid formation. Methods to produce pleural symphysis include surgical abrasion and the application of intrapleural chemicals such as doxycycline, minocycline, and talc. Talc has been applied as a powder suspended in sterile saline solution and injected through the chest tube (talc slurry) or dusted through a thoracoscope (talc insufflation). The success of talc pleurodesis, approximately 90%, is higher than that of all alternatives except surgical abrasion.[18,19] Pleurodesis is used most commonly in the management of symptomatic pleural effusions caused by cancer. Although pleurodesis of benign effusions, such as effusions occurring with CHF, nephrotic syndrome, and idiopathic chylothorax, have been performed successfully, the procedure is discouraged for pleural effusions that are not malignant. Most pleural effusions are best managed by control of the underlying condition.[20]

Pleuroperitoneal Shunt and Pleural Catheter

In refractory pleural effusions that cannot be treated adequately with pleurodesis, a small pump can be placed subcutaneously, and tubes are placed in the pleural and peritoneal spaces. The pleuroperitoneal connection has a one-way valve and a pumping mechanism to allow the patient to expel pleural fluid from the negatively pressurized chest to the positively pressurized peritoneum. The pleuroperitoneal shunt is placed as a last resort for refractory pleural effusions for which there is no other treatment. A Pleurx (CareFusion, San Diego, CA) catheter has an adapter for connection to vacuum bottles. It is inserted into the pleural space so that pleural fluid can be removed at home for recurrent effusions. In malignant effusions, pleural drainage lessens over time, and the Pleurx catheter can usually be removed when cancer cells have bridged the pleural space, creating a pleurodesis.

PNEUMOTHORAX

Pneumothorax refers to air in the pleural space. Although air can enter the pleural space from outside the body, as occurs in sucking chest wounds, most cases of pneumothorax occur when disruption of the visceral pleura allows air from the lung to enter the pleural space. Pneumothorax is discussed according to etiologic factor because traumatic pneumothorax is managed differently from spontaneous pneumothorax. Spontaneous pneumothorax is of two types:

1. **Primary spontaneous pneumothorax,** in which there is no underlying lung disease
2. **Secondary spontaneous pneumothorax,** in which lung disease is present

Chest pain, which is typically sharp and abrupt, occurs in nearly every patient with pneumothorax. Palpation of the chest wall does not worsen the pain, although respiratory efforts may be difficult. Dyspnea occurs in approximately two-thirds of patients when decreases in vital capacity and PO_2, probably secondary to airway closure at low lung volumes, cause ventilation/perfusion defects and shunting. When spontaneous pneumothorax is evacuated, hypoxemia may persist in some patients. The following sections describe the diseases that cause pneumothorax and the important treatment differences between them.

Traumatic Pneumothorax

Blunt and Penetrating Chest Trauma

Traumatic pneumothorax can be caused by either blunt or penetrating wounds of the thorax. The common causes of penetrating wounds include gunshots and knife punctures. In many cases, penetrating trauma to the chest can be managed conservatively with a chest tube. The clear indications for entering the chest surgically are uncontrolled bleeding from intercostal or pulmonary arteries and injury to the heart or great vessels. In these situations, the pneumothorax becomes secondary. The chest tube is multifunctional to allow measurement of the rate of bleeding, to allow the lung to be pulled to the parietal pleural surface to tamponade bleeding, and to allow maximum ventilation.

In blunt trauma to the chest, pneumothorax can be the result of a rib fracture that enters the lung parenchyma and allows air to leak into the pleural space. For this type of injury, a chest tube is placed, and the rib fractures necessitate no specific therapy. A more common injury is alveolar rupture, which breaks through the pleural membrane.

Two special injuries that produce pneumothorax are tracheal fracture and esophageal rupture. Tracheal fracture results from severe deceleration injury and often occurs in concert with fractures of the anterior aspect of the first through third ribs. In this case, urgent bronchoscopy is appropriate because tracheal fracture must be corrected surgically. Esophageal rupture produces an air-fluid level in the pleural space. Pleural fluid amylase concentration is elevated from a salivary source.

Large-caliber chest tubes are placed for trauma-related pneumothoraces to allow exit of blood and blood clots, which can be difficult to remove through small-bore catheters. Air leaks from an injured lung can be large. When bleeding is a major component of pleural injury, two chest tubes are used: a posterior chest tube to drain blood that is gravity-dependent and an anterior and apical chest tube to drain air that moves to the lung apex in the absence of pleural disease.

Iatrogenic Pneumothorax

Iatrogenic pneumothorax is the most common type of traumatic pneumothorax. Common causes are punctures of the lung from needle aspiration lung biopsy, thoracentesis, and central venous catheter placement. Unusual causes, such as feeding tube placement into the pleural space, also have been recorded. Because the pleural rupture is typically small in the absence of parenchymal lung disease, these lung punctures usually resolve within 24 hours and can be observed without chest tubes as long as serial radiographs are obtained.

Neonatal Pneumothorax

In radiographic series, spontaneous pneumothorax occurs in 1% to 2% of all infants soon after birth.[21] The cause of pneumothorax is likely high transpulmonary pressure during birth coupled with transient bronchial blockade caused by meconium, mucus, or aspiration of blood; transpulmonary pressure gradients of 100 cm H_2O can be produced.

Recognizing pneumothorax is difficult because breath sounds are transmitted widely through the chest of the neonate. A shift of the heart sounds away from the side of the pneumothorax may provide a clue. Transillumination of the chest with a high-intensity light is used in some centers. Almost all neonates with pneumothorax need a chest tube.

Spontaneous Pneumothorax

Spontaneous pneumothorax is defined as any pneumothorax caused by the escape of air into the pleural space without an obvious cause.

Primary Spontaneous Pneumothorax

Primary spontaneous pneumothorax occurs without underlying lung disease. In a way, this term is a misnomer because CT scans have shown the presence of small subpleural blebs in more than 80% of patients.[22]

Primary spontaneous pneumothorax usually occurs in patients in their late teenage years or early 20s. Patients often are tall and slender, and the lungs and pleural membrane may not have grown at the same pace; the result is airspace enlargement and a thin pleural membrane. Results of some studies suggest that cigarette smoking is a risk factor in more than 90% of cases of primary spontaneous pneumothorax.[23] The smoking history is typically short, and smoking cessation is recommended.

Secondary Spontaneous Pneumothorax

Secondary spontaneous pneumothorax occurs in patients with underlying lung disease. In most cases, the underlying lung disease is chronic obstructive pulmonary disease (COPD) with some component of emphysema. Pneumothorax also can occur with asthma and cystic fibrosis, usually during an exacerbation of disease. Interstitial lung diseases in which lung volumes are spared, such as sarcoidosis, organizing pneumonia, pulmonary Langerhans cell histiocytosis, and lymphangioleiomyomatosis, have a higher incidence than diseases without any component of obstruction, such as idiopathic pulmonary fibrosis.

Depending on the extent of parenchymal lung disease, pneumothorax can be devastating. A Veterans Affairs cooperative study included 185 patients with secondary spontaneous pneumothorax and monitored them for 5 years.[24] Although only three patients died of pneumothorax, the mortality rate was 43%.[1] Severe underlying lung disease caused most deaths. This finding suggested that most pneumothoraces occur in patients with severe lung dysfunction. The degree of dyspnea is disproportionate to the size of pneumothorax in this group of patients because pulmonary reserve is already diminished. Pneumothorax usually should be evacuated and not observed in this patient cohort.

Catamenial Pneumothorax

Catamenial pneumothorax occurs in conjunction with menstruation and usually is recurrent and right-sided. The reason for the right-sided predominance is unclear. Many patients have endometriosis on the pleural surface, although it may be impossible to see because of hormonal involution during menses. Once the diagnosis is considered, catamenial pneumothorax is not difficult to manage because most patients do not have a recurrence when ovulation is suppressed.

MINI CLINI

Subcutaneous Emphysema

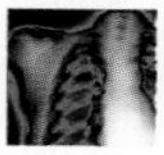

PROBLEM: A patient with ARDS experiences subcutaneous emphysema. How does the clinician determine where the air leak is occurring? Is a pneumothorax always present?

SOLUTION: Subcutaneous emphysema occurs when air enters the soft tissues. Although physical examination reveals subcutaneous bubbles, the patient's family needs to be reassured that the condition is rarely, if ever, physiologically significant. What is important to recognize, however, is that alveolar disruption has occurred, most commonly as the result of barotrauma.

Barotrauma disrupts alveoli and allows air to enter the interstitium of the lung. Rupture of the visceral pleura allows air to produce pneumothorax, or the air can travel along the low-resistance tissue planes of the bronchovascular bundles and through the hilum of the lung to enter the mediastinum. From the mediastinum, air has easy access to the retroperitoneal space, including the scrotum and the neck. The presence of subcutaneous air does not mean that pneumothorax has occurred, although the risk factors for its development are present.

Air under pressure in the pleural space can enter the subcutaneous tissues through the intercostal incision made for chest tube placement. Subcutaneous air often is seen on a chest radiograph after chest tube placement, but the air rarely spreads unless the chest tube is occluded.

In the absence of pneumothorax, there is no way to determine which lung is causing subcutaneous emphysema. For any deterioration in gas exchange, radiographs should be repeated. Because air in the mediastinum can displace the mediastinal parietal pleura, it can be difficult to tell without chest CT whether a small pneumothorax is present. Because patients often are too unstable to be moved, a chest tube sometimes is placed because the potential benefits are greater than the risks.

Complications

Tension Pneumothorax

Tension pneumothorax occurs when air in the pleural space exceeds atmospheric pressure. The radiographic appearance includes mediastinal shift to the contralateral side, diaphragmatic depression, and expansion of the ribs. The lung does not collapse completely if it is involved with a disease process such as acute respiratory distress syndrome (ARDS). Not all patients with radiographic tension have the physiologic changes commonly associated with tension pneumothorax. However, almost all pneumothoraces that occur during mechanical ventilation enlarge if not drained.

As pressure in the thorax increases and mediastinal shift places torsion on the inferior vena cava, venous return to the right side of the heart decreases. Cardiac output decreases, and hypotension with tachycardia results. Hypoxemia occurs as the lung continues to compress because of intrapulmonary shunting through the collapsed lung.

The respiratory therapist (RT) can make the diagnosis of tension pneumothorax. Treatment is emergency decompression of the chest. This procedure usually is done with an 18-gauge intravenous (e.g., Jelco) catheter inserted just over the second rib on the anterior aspect of the chest in the midclavicular line. Catheter placement should elicit a rush of air through the catheter, and this sign confirms the diagnosis. Blood pressure recovery should be rapid, although resolution of hypoxemia depends on complete lung reexpansion and can be delayed. The soft intravenous catheter can be left in place while a more conventional chest tube is inserted.

RULE OF THUMB

Tension pneumothorax is a clinical diagnosis made at the bedside in more than 50% of cases. The clinical signs are diminished breath sounds, hyperresonance to percussion, tachycardia, and hypotension.

In one case series of 74 patients with tension pneumothorax, a clinical diagnosis was made for 45 patients; the associated mortality rate was 7%. In the other cases, the diagnosis was delayed from the onset of clinical signs by 30 minutes to 8 hours, resulting in a 31% mortality rate.[25] RTS are in the perfect position to make a timely diagnosis because ventilator alarms give early warnings (e.g., high pressure, lower compliance).

Reexpansion Pulmonary Edema

Reexpansion pulmonary edema occurs in a lung that has been rapidly reinflated from low lung volumes, particularly when the pneumothorax has been long-standing or when the pressure gradient across the lung has become high, as might occur when there is endobronchial obstruction from cancer, mucus, or blood. For many years, it was believed that alveolar edema occurs because intraalveolar pressure becomes negative and pulls fluid from the vasculature. However, the lung fluid has high protein content, a finding that suggests blood vessels have been injured as well.

One proposed mechanism of vascular injury is a phenomenon of reperfusion injury caused by reactive oxygen species. Support for this hypothesis has come from experimental studies that have shown administration of antioxidants before reexpansion decreases the amount of reexpansion pulmonary edema.

Regardless of the cause, lung reexpansion in nonemergency situations should proceed slowly, and transpulmonary pressure should not become excessive. Most physicians who insert a chest tube for a large pneumothorax first place it to water seal without suction. If the lung is not completely inflated on the subsequent chest radiograph, the chest tube is placed to suction. Reexpansion pulmonary edema also occurs after drainage of pleural effusions. As a rule, thoracentesis should be limited to 1000 ml, unless pleural pressures are monitored and not allowed to become less than −20 cm H_2O.

Diagnosis

The diagnosis of pneumothorax is established with chest radiography. The diagnosis requires a high-quality film for visualization of a visceral pleural line. In the ICU, 30% of cases of pneumothorax may be missed in retrospect on a chest radiograph. Impediments to diagnosis include a low-quality radiograph, supine position of the patient, concomitant presence of mediastinal air, and subpulmonic or mediastinal position of the pneumothorax. Diagnosis is enhanced with additional upright radiographs or decubitus views.

The size of a pneumothorax is difficult to assess with a chest radiograph because a two-dimensional picture is being taken of a three-dimensional thorax. Size can be confirmed with CT if needed.

RULE OF THUMB

The size of a pneumothorax on a chest radiograph can be estimated with the knowledge that the volume of the lung and thorax is proportional to the cube of their diameters.

For example, on a chest radiograph, the chest measures 8 cm from the spine to the lateral chest wall. A pneumothorax is measured 2 cm from the chest wall:

$$\text{Volume of the lung} = (6\text{ cm})^3 \approx 216\text{ cm}^3$$
$$\text{Volume of the hemithorax} = (8\text{ cm})^3 = 512\text{ cm}^3$$
$$\text{Lung size} = 216/512 = 42\%$$
$$\text{Pneumothorax size} \approx 58\%$$

The equation shows the large volume of lung that a pneumothorax can displace despite a "small" distance from the lung to the chest wall. Use of the equation is not as accurate as chest CT because in many pneumothoraces, the lung collapses asymmetrically.

Therapy

Oxygen

Oxygen (O_2) should be administered to all patients who have a pneumothorax. Most of the air in a pneumothorax is nitrogen because O_2 is readily absorbed. If an air leak is continuing, supplemental O_2 rather than nitrogen leaks into the pleural space. After an air leak has been stopped, administration of O_2 decreases the blood and tissue partial pressure of nitrogen surrounding the pleural space. Pneumothorax resolution is normally 1.25% of the air per day. O_2 speeds recovery by increasing the gradient of nitrogen from the pleural space to the pleural tissues.

Observation

Consensus conferences have recommended observation of patients in stable condition with primary spontaneous pneumothorax and of some patients with small secondary spontaneous pneumothorax before recurrence prevention is administered.[26] Small iatrogenic pneumothorax also should be managed with observation. Primary spontaneous pneumothorax often is observed for 4 hours in the emergency department before discharge to home follow-up care as long as no pneumothorax enlargement is found on chest radiographs. Discharged patients should have ready access to emergency care facilities.

Patients with secondary spontaneous pneumothorax should be admitted to the hospital. During observation, it is important to record the respiratory rate and any signs of deteriorating respiratory function. A decrease in oxygen saturation can be an early warning of pneumothorax enlargement. Any deterioration indicates that the pneumothorax must be drained.

Simple Aspiration

Simple aspiration can be used in the emergency department when pneumothorax is first identified. A small catheter is placed into the pleural space, and air is sequentially evacuated with a three-way stopcock until no more air can be removed. If more than 4 L of air is aspirated and no resistance to further aspiration is felt, a chest tube is needed for continuing pleural air leak.

The goal of aspiration is to reexpand the lung. Many patients have a pneumothorax from air leak that subsequently heals between the time of onset and the time treatment is sought in the emergency department. Patients with primary spontaneous pneumothorax who undergo simple aspiration for lung reexpansion and who have a stable chest radiograph 4 hours after aspiration can go home without hospital admission.[26,27] Aspiration can decrease the number of patients admitted to the hospital with no increase in complications.[27]

Chest Tubes

Chest thoracostomy tubes (chest tubes) come in various sizes, ranging from 7F to 40F, and can be connected to a variety of one-way devices (e.g., Heimlich valves) that prevent entry of air into the pleural space from the outside environment. Regardless of chest tube size and the presence of a Heimlich valve or water seal, the effectiveness of chest tube placement for pneumothorax resolution depends more on lung surface healing than on the device used.

Small-Bore Catheter. One simple device is a small-bore 7F catheter with a one-way valve apparatus (Heimlich valve) that prevents air movement back into the chest. Small-bore catheters can be placed with a small skin incision, although they require a trocar for transthoracic placement, and the trocar can injure the lung.

All chest tubes used to drain pneumothorax should be directed to the apex of the lung. Small-bore catheters can be placed in the second intercostal space anteriorly in the midclavicular line or laterally in the chest from the fifth through the seventh intercostal space.

It is difficult to determine whether a Heimlich valve has an ongoing leak unless it is placed to underwater seal. This procedure can be done in the emergency department by placing the Heimlich valve into a cup of water or by placing it in line with a water-seal chamber to see whether an air leak is continuing after lung expansion. Some automated devices also are available that show ongoing air leaks.

Large-Bore Chest Tube. Large-bore chest tubes usually are connected to a commercial equivalent of a three-bottle system to collect any pleural fluid present, to determine whether an air leak is ongoing, and to measure intrapleural pressure (Figure 25-5). Insertion of large-bore catheters is accomplished with local anesthetic and blunt dissection of soft tissue down to the parietal pleura. Dissection should be wide enough to allow insertion of a finger into the pleural space to ensure that no adhesions are holding the lung close to the insertion site and to allow unobstructed entrance of the tube into the pleural space, where it can be directed to the position of choice.

Chest tubes are secured with sutures. The insertion distance should be recorded and be checked on subsequent days to ensure that the chest tube does not migrate outward. If the most proximal hole in the tube emerges from the skin, air will enter the tube, and it will appear as if the lung is persistently leaking. Another problem of apparent chest tube leak can occur when the insertion wound is large enough to allow air entry into the pleural space; this usually is accompanied by a sucking sound at the entrance, which can be occluded with petroleum gauze.

A chest radiograph is routinely obtained. However, unless a lateral radiograph also is obtained, confirmation of precise placement often is difficult. In addition, many

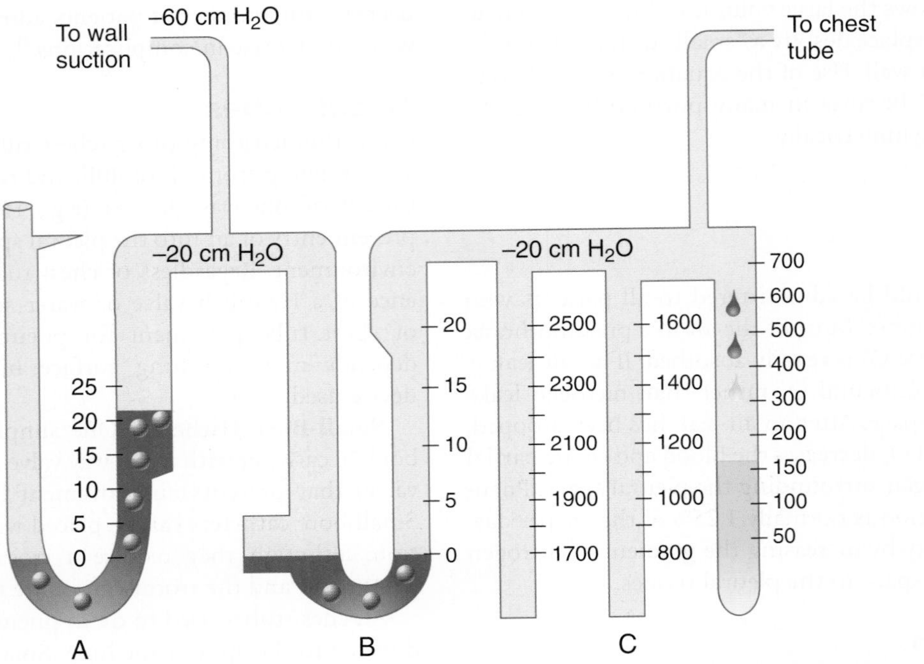

FIGURE 25-5 A-C, The Pleur-evac (Teleflex, Research Triangle Park, NC) chest tube collection system collects fluid in compartment **C** so that it does not spill into the water-seal compartment **(B).** A patent chest tube should cause respiratory variation to be seen on the scale adjacent to compartment **B,** which measures intrapleural pressure. Compartment **B** also is the place to see bubbles if an air leak is present. The water level in compartment **A** controls intrapleural pressure and should be adjusted daily.

chest tubes end up in the major fissure, where their function may be suboptimal.

Chest tube removal remains a highly variable practice. Removal of a chest tube as soon as an air leak visually ceases is associated with a 25% rate of recurrence of pneumothorax. The recurrence rate is near zero when chest tubes are removed 48 hours after the air leak no longer is seen in the water-seal chamber.[28,29] A common practice of clamping the chest tube, with chest radiographs before and after a 4-hour observation period, can be accompanied by the return of pneumothorax. If symptoms develop during chest tube clamping, the clamp should be removed immediately, and the presence of air leak should be assessed.

Bronchopleural Fistula

Air leaks from the lung through a chest tube can come in many sizes. If a large bronchus is involved in the lung injury, the large air leak is called a **bronchopleural fistula** (BPF). Many patients with a BPF are receiving mechanical ventilation, and positive airway pressures contribute to the perpetuation of pleural air.

Because a BPF can leak large quantities of air, more than one chest tube may be used to approximate the lung to the chest wall. This maneuver results in tamponade of the site of the air leak and allows pleural healing to occur. Therapy for BPF involves meticulous monitoring of tidal volume, airway pressures, and positive end-expiratory pressure (PEEP); avoidance of auto-PEEP; and consideration of bronchoscopic closure or thoracoscopic surgery.[30] Also, endobronchial valves placed by flexible bronchoscopy have shown high rates of success for patients who are not operative candidates.[31]

Pleurodesis

Patients who have had one pneumothorax are more likely than the general population to have a second. The recurrence rate is greater than 30% among patients with primary spontaneous pneumothorax and approximately 40% among patients with secondary spontaneous pneumothorax. These high recurrence rates indicate that prevention of recurrence of pneumothorax should be undertaken, in particular, for patients in whom pneumothorax may be life-threatening. Preventing recurrence involves production of adhesions between the parietal and the visceral pleura in the involved area and is termed *pleurodesis*.

The most noninvasive approaches to pleurodesis entail chemical sclerosis of the pleural space through the chest tube after the pleural air leak has ceased. The two most common preparations used at the present time in the United States include 500 mg of doxycycline or 5 g of talc mixed into a 50-ml syringe of sterile saline solution. The agent is injected through the chest tube into the pleural space. The chest tube is then clamped for 2 hours before drainage is allowed.

More invasive methods have included thoracoscopy with pleural poudrage (blowing talc onto the pleural surface under direct visualization), pleural abrasion through a thoracoscope, and thoracotomy with pleurectomy (removing the pleural surface to ensure lung adhesion). More recent recommendations are for pleurodesis to occur after the first secondary spontaneous pneumothorax with thoracoscopic bullae stapling and talc poudrage.[28]

Because the diseases that produce pneumothorax often involve both lungs, patients may experience sequential events in opposite lungs. In this situation, median sternotomy with bilateral abrasion or pleurectomy can be performed, particularly for patients at considerable risk of development of pneumothorax, such as divers and aviators.

MINI CLINI

Bronchopleural Fistula

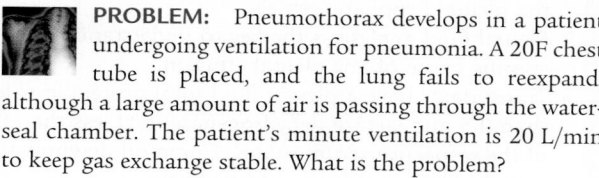

PROBLEM: Pneumothorax develops in a patient undergoing ventilation for pneumonia. A 20F chest tube is placed, and the lung fails to reexpand, although a large amount of air is passing through the water-seal chamber. The patient's minute ventilation is 20 L/min to keep gas exchange stable. What is the problem?

SOLUTION: The problem is a BPF caused by a large hole in the pleura, which is difficult to manage. The lung surface of patients with underlying emphysema can contain large bullae that do not heal readily when ruptured. Large pleural holes also can develop in patients with necrotizing pneumonia and patients who have undergone surgery on the lung.

The Fanning equation states that humidified airflow through a chest tube is proportional to the chest tube radius to the fifth power. The chest tube radius is the most important determinant of maximal airflow. Airflow through large BPFs has been measured as 16 L/min, a volume impossible to remove through a chest tube smaller than 24F, regardless of the amount of pressure applied.

This patient should receive a second, larger chest tube. The seal of the chest tube at the skin surface should be inspected to ensure that no air is entering the body from the outside. The position of both chest tubes should be confirmed either radiographically or manually to ensure the tubes are in the pleural space. When the lung is expanded, the minute ventilation should decrease because effective alveolar ventilation is improved.

Flow through stopcocks and chest tube collection devices is governed by the same considerations as chest tube size. The manufacturer of the chest tube collection device in your hospital would have the resistance figures necessary to ensure that 16 L/min of airflow can be accommodated.

MINI CLINI

Measuring a Large Air Leak

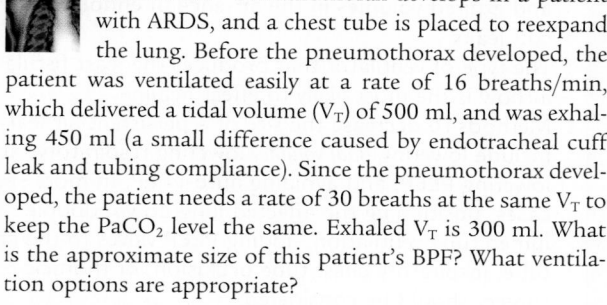

PROBLEM: Pneumothorax develops in a patient with ARDS, and a chest tube is placed to reexpand the lung. Before the pneumothorax developed, the patient was ventilated easily at a rate of 16 breaths/min, which delivered a tidal volume (V_T) of 500 ml, and was exhaling 450 ml (a small difference caused by endotracheal cuff leak and tubing compliance). Since the pneumothorax developed, the patient needs a rate of 30 breaths at the same V_T to keep the $PaCO_2$ level the same. Exhaled V_T is 300 ml. What is the approximate size of this patient's BPF? What ventilation options are appropriate?

SOLUTION: Although research laboratories can measure airflow through a chest tube with a pneumotachometer, clinical care can be provided by estimating the pleural air leak. The following simple calculations suggest that the excess difference in returned V_T (450 to 300 ml) is due to air passing through the chest tube:

30 breaths/min (150 ml differential = 4.5 L of pleural ventilation)

One other problem is that large amounts of CO_2 (up to 20%) may be removed through the chest tube.[30,32] Removal of CO_2 is beneficial because it allows lower V_T and respiratory rates for any given PCO_2. However, as the air leak closes, CO_2 has to be eliminated from the endotracheal tube, necessitating higher minute ventilation. This effect might falsely suggest that ARDS is worsening when the reality is that the air leak is closing.

Nevertheless, when the air leak is measured with every ventilatory change, the mode of ventilation that minimizes air leak is the one most likely to allow pleural healing. Breath-by-breath analysis shows the difference between delivered V_T and exhaled V_T and approximates the volume of the pleural leak.

PEEP can be a major cause of large BPF and should be turned off. Because there is no such thing as a true plateau pressure when air is exiting through the pleural space, V_T should be adjusted to produce the lowest peak airway pressure that can sustain ventilation and oxygenation. The patient should be positioned so that the lung with the air leak is in the bed.[33]

Auto-PEEP can be impossible to measure if the fistula is large and decompressing the airways. Long expiratory times are preferred. Trials of pressure-controlled and high-frequency jet ventilation are appropriate. In a practical sense, these adjustments are the same ones made to prevent barotrauma in the first place and are limited by the severity of lung injury, which requires more support than would optimally close the air leak.

MINI CLINI

Management of Bronchopleural Fistula

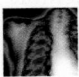

PROBLEM: A 40-year-old trauma patient with ARDS cannot be ventilated because of a large (16 L/min) BPF located entirely in the left lung. If surgery is not possible, what ventilatory options would be appropriate?

SOLUTION: Two ventilatory interventions have been attempted for large BPFs. The first is placement of a double-lumen endotracheal tube, which can carry most ventilation and PEEP on the right lung while under-ventilating the lung with the fistula to aid in its closure.[34] Long-term double-lumen ventilation is difficult for the following reasons: tenuous tube position, the need for continuous paralysis, difficulty with secretion clearance, and high airway resistance through the small endotracheal tube lumens.

The second intervention is application of positive pressure to the chest tube. This back pressure increases resistance across the BPF and allows the remainder of the lung to ventilate better. One simple way to add chest tube resistance is to connect a PEEP valve to the expiratory port of the water-seal chamber.[35] PEEP usually is placed at the same level as the ventilator. Inspiratory pressures exceed PEEP, and air flows through the chest tube. However, as expiratory pressures equilibrate, PEEP can be held within the lung, allowing the beneficial effects on oxygenation.

Pressurizing the chest tube entails synchronous closure of the chest tube during inspiration[36] and requires specialized equipment, which must be set up under controlled conditions. When used in combination with an in-line PEEP valve, BPF flow can be slowed during both inspiration and expiration.

These techniques usually increase the volume of intrapleural air. The net effect on oxygenation necessitates careful bedside observation because hypoxemia can worsen with any degree of lung collapse. Tension pneumothorax can occur and should be managed expectantly.

ROLE OF THE RESPIRATORY THERAPIST IN PLEURAL DISEASES

The RT has important roles in both the diagnosis and the management of pleural disease. Diagnostically, careful palpation and auscultation of the chest by the RT may show the dullness and decreased breath sounds that may prompt suspicion of a pleural effusion and lead the physician to order imaging studies to confirm the presence of a pleural effusion. The RT is in the most proximate position to suggest the diagnosis of pneumothorax because of changing ventilatory function in the ICU. The RT may be called on to assist in performing a thoracentesis or placing a chest tube. Therapeutically, the RT may be called on to assist in setting up the fluid collection chamber after the chest tube is placed or in performing a talc pleurodesis. This broad spectrum of potential roles for the RT makes knowledge of the diagnosis and management of pleural disease essential for the capable RT.

SUMMARY CHECKLIST

- Pleural effusions form when excess pleural fluid is produced by the lung or chest wall in sufficient quantities to overcome the resorptive capacity of the pleural lymphatic vessels.
- Pleural fluid analysis is the key to understanding the specific cause of any pleural effusion.
- Transudates have a pleural fluid total protein level less than 0.5 and lactate dehydrogenase level less than 0.6 of the respective serum values. Common diagnoses include CHF, nephrosis, and cirrhosis.
- Pleural fluid drainage returns approximately one-third of the lung volume as measured by FVC. The other two-thirds of fluid drainage allow the diaphragm to rise and the chest wall to normalize.
- Pneumothorax size is underestimated with a one-dimensional view of the chest. Measurement accuracy requires a three-dimensional perspective.
- The risk factors for pneumothorax and pneumomediastinum are the same. Air ruptures a pleural membrane in pneumothorax, and air passes through the lung hilum in pneumomediastinum.
- O_2 therapy speeds resolution of all pneumothoraces by improving nitrogen absorption.
- Chest tube flow depends on tube size, stopcock size, and collection system resistance.
- Breath-by-breath measurement of an air leak can be approximated by the difference between inspired and expired volumes in the absence of endotracheal cuff leaks.
- The type of ventilator that produces the least fistula airflow is the most likely to effect healing.
- Methods to decrease the size of a persistent air leak include lowering *tidal volume,* lowering respiratory rate, lowering PEEP, and avoiding auto-PEEP. In more severe cases, positioning the affected lung down, double-lumen tube ventilation, adding PEEP valves to the chest tube, inspiratory chest tube occlusion, or thoracic surgery should be considered.

References

1. Noppen M, De Waele M, Li R, et al: Volume and cellular content of normal pleural fluid in humans examined by pleural lavage. Am J Respir Crit Care Med 162:1023, 2000.
2. Light RW: Pleural diseases, ed 2, Philadelphia, 1990, Lea & Febiger.
3. Sahn SA: The diagnostic value of pleural fluid analysis. Semin Respir Crit Care Med 16:269, 1995.
4. Light RW, Macgregor MI, Luchsinger PC, et al: Pleural effusions: the diagnostic separation of transudates and exudates. Ann Intern Med 77:507, 1972.

5. Staub NC, Wiener-Kronish JP, et al: Transport through the pleura: physiology of normal liquid and solute exchange in the pleural space. In Chretien J, Bignon J, Hirsch A, editors: The pleura in health and disease, New York, 1985, Marcel Dekker.
6. Wiener-Kronish JP, Matthay MA, Callen PW, et al: Relationship of pleural effusions to pulmonary hemodynamics in patients with congestive heart failure. Am Rev Respir Dis 132:1253, 1985.
7. Peterman TA, Brothers SK: Pleural effusions in congestive heart failure and in pericardial disease. N Engl J Med 309:313, 1983.
8. Lieberman FL, Hidemura R, Peters RL, et al: Pathogenesis and treatment of hydrothorax complicating cirrhosis with ascites. Ann Intern Med 64:341, 1966.
9. Lieberman FL, Hidemura R, Peters RL, et al: Parapneumonic effusions. Am J Med 69:507, 1980.
10. Colice GL, Curtis A, Deslauriers J, et al: Medical and surgical treatment of parapneumonic effusions: an evidence-based guideline. Chest 118:1158, 2000.
11. Berger HW, Mejia E: Tuberculous pleurisy. Chest 63:88, 1973.
12. Light RW, George RB: Incidence and significance of pleural effusion after abdominal surgery. Chest 69:621, 1976.
13. Sahn SA: State of the art: the pleura. Am Rev Respir Dis 138:184, 1988.
14. Seriff NS, Cohen ML, Samuel P, et al: Chylothorax: diagnosis by lipoprotein electrophoresis of serum and pleural fluid. Thorax 32:98, 1977.
15. Strange C: Hemothorax. Semin Respir Crit Care Med 16:324, 1995.
16. Judson MA, Sahn SA: Pulmonary physiological abnormalities caused by pleural disease. Semin Respir Crit Care Med 16:346, 1995.
17. Collins TR, Sahn SA: Thoracocentesis: clinical value, complications, technical problems, and patient experience. Chest 91:817, 1987.
18. Walker-Renard PB, Vaughan LM, Sahn SA: Chemical pleurodesis for malignant pleural effusions. Ann Intern Med 120:56, 1994.
19. Kennedy L, Sahn SA: Talc pleurodesis for the treatment of pneumothorax and pleural effusion. Chest 106:1215, 1994.
20. Sudduth CD, Sahn SA: Pleurodesis for nonmalignant pleural effusions: recommendations. Chest 102:1855, 1992.
21. Chernick V, Reed MH: Pneumothorax and chylothorax in the neonatal period. J Pediatr 76:624, 1970.
22. Bense L, Lewander R, Eklund G, et al: Nonsmoking, non-alpha 1-antitrypsin deficiency-induced emphysema in nonsmokers with healed spontaneous pneumothorax, identified by computed tomography of the lungs. Chest 103:433, 1993.
23. Bense L, Eklund G, Wiman LG: Smoking and the increased risk of contracting spontaneous pneumothorax. Chest 92:1009, 1987.
24. Light RW, O'Hara VS, Moritz TE, et al: Intrapleural tetracycline for the prevention of recurrent spontaneous pneumothorax. Results of a Department of Veterans Affairs cooperative study. JAMA 264:2224, 1990.
25. Steier M, Ching N, Roberts EB, et al: Pneumothorax complicating continuous ventilatory support. J Thorac Cardiovasc Surg 67:17, 1979.
26. MacDuff A, Arnold A, Harvey J: BTS Pleural Disease Guideline Group (December 2010): Management of spontaneous pneumothorax: British Thoracic Society pleural disease guideline 2010. Thorax 65:18, 2010.
27. Wakai A, O'Sullivan RG, McCabe G: Simple aspiration versus intercostal tube drainage for primary spontaneous pneumothorax in adults. Cochrane Database Syst Rev (1):CD004479, 2007.
28. Baumann MH, Strange C, Heffner JE, et al: Management of spontaneous pneumothorax: an American College of Chest Physicians Delphi consensus statement. Chest 119: 590, 2001.
29. Sharma TN, Agnihotri SP, Jain NK, et al: Intercostal tube thoracostomy in pneumothorax. Indian J Chest Dis Allied Sci 30:32, 1988.
30. Baumann MH, Sahn SA: Medical management and therapy of bronchopleural fistulas in the mechanically ventilated patient. Chest 97:721, 1990.
31. Traveline JM, McKenna RJ, DeGiacomo T, et al: Endobronchial Valve for Persistent Air Leak Group: Treatment of persistent pulmonary air leaks using endobronchial valves. Chest 136:355, 2009.
32. Bishop MJ, Benson MS, Pierson DJ: Carbon dioxide excretion via bronchopleural fistulas in adult respiratory distress syndrome. Chest 91:400, 1987.
33. Lau KY: Postural management of bronchopleural fistula. Chest 94:1122, 1988.
34. Dodds CP, Hillman KM: Management of massive air leak with asynchronous independent lung ventilation. Intensive Care Med 8:287, 1982.
35. Weksler N, Ovadia L: The challenge of bilateral bronchopleural fistula. Chest 95:938, 1989.
36. Gallagher TJ, Smith RA, Kirby RR, et al: Intermittent inspiratory chest tube occlusion to limit bronchopleural cutaneous air leaks. Crit Care Med 4:328, 1976.

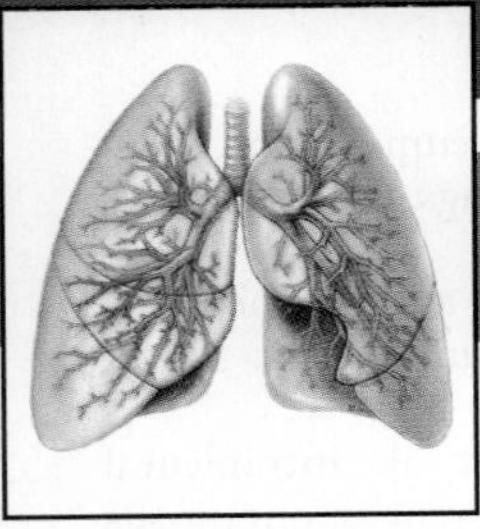

Chapter 26

Pulmonary Vascular Disease

ADRIANO R. TONELLI, ALEJANDRO C. ARROLIGA, AND RAED A. DWEIK

CHAPTER OBJECTIVES

After reading this chapter you will be able to:

- State how many patients develop venous thromboembolism each year.
- Describe how and where thromboemboli originate.
- Describe how pulmonary emboli alter lung and cardiac function.
- Identify the clinical features and electrocardiographic, chest radiograph, and arterial blood gas findings associated with pulmonary embolism.
- Describe how pulmonary embolism is diagnosed and managed.
- Describe hemodynamic findings associated with pulmonary hypertension.
- Describe the possible mechanisms believed to be responsible for the onset of idiopathic pulmonary arterial hypertension (IPAH).
- State patients who are at risk for the development of IPAH.
- Identify the clinical features associated with IPAH.
- Describe the treatment for patients with IPAH.
- Describe the pathogenesis and management of pulmonary hypertension associated with chronic obstructive pulmonary disease.

CHAPTER OUTLINE

KEY TERMS

deep venous thrombosis (DVT)
pulmonary embolism (PE)
pulmonary hypertension
venous thromboembolism

The pulmonary vasculature is affected by various diseases, ranging from obstructive airway disease to parenchymal disease such as interstitial fibrosis. Generally, the presence of **pulmonary hypertension** is determined by the severity of the underlying lung disease. Pulmonary hypertension is present in other conditions such as heart disease (congenital and acquired) and in systemic disorders, the most common of which are connective tissue diseases such as systemic sclerosis and systemic lupus erythematosus. Another systemic problem that affects the pulmonary vasculature is venous thromboembolic disease (**deep venous thrombosis [DVT]** and **pulmonary embolism [PE]**). This chapter reviews disorders associated with the pulmonary vasculature. The focus is on venous thromboembolic disease and *idiopathic pulmonary artery hypertension (IPAH),* a rare but life-threatening disease affecting young people, with a brief review of pulmonary heart disease *(cor pulmonale).*

VENOUS THROMBOEMBOLIC DISEASE

Venous thromboembolism is a major health problem in the United States. The prevalence of venous thromboembolism, which includes PE and DVT, has remained relatively constant over time and has been calculated to be 117 cases per 100,000 persons (i.e., DVT at 48 cases per 100,000 and PE at 69 cases per 100,000). It is estimated that 200,000 to 300,000 new cases occur yearly in the United States.[1]

Venous thromboembolism is treatable but requires prompt diagnosis and therapy to avert serious consequences. One-third of deaths from PE occur within 1 hour of onset of symptoms, and more than 70% of patients who die of PE are not suspected to have PE before death.[2] Although mortality from PE has decreased in recent years,[3] the death rate for the first episode of PE among hospitalized patients may be 17.4% at 3 months.[3,4] Recurrent PE is associated with a much higher mortality rate because only one-quarter of patients survive 3 months.[5] The diagnosis is not suspected in approximately two-thirds of patients who die of PE, and the frequency of recognizable emboli in routine autopsies of adult patients ranges from 1.5% to almost 30%.[6-8] In a population-based study of PE as a cause of death in New Mexico, only 34% of 812 postmortem documented cases of PE were diagnosed before death.[5] Morpurgo and Schmid[9] reported their experience with 92 postmortem cases of massive or submassive PE detected during the years 1986-1989. Only 28% of the cases were diagnosed before death, a finding that emphasizes the underdiagnosis of venous thromboembolic disease.

Two-thirds of cases of initial embolus from which patients survive remain undiagnosed. The mortality rate among these patients with undiagnosed embolism is approximately 30%,[10] which emphasizes the importance of recognizing PE. If venous thromboembolism is recognized and treated, the mortality rate decreases to less than 8%, and the long-term outcome is generally favorable.[11] The long-term survival rates after venous thromboembolism in an inception cohort of 2218 patients were 72% at 1 month and 63% at 1 year.[12]

Because the accuracy of the clinical impression (i.e., without testing) of venous thromboembolism is less than 50%,[13] objective tests are needed to confirm or exclude the diagnosis. Patients with multiple injuries, immobilization, bed rest, or intravascular catheters and elderly patients are at high risk of venous thromboembolic disease (Table 26-1) and should be considered candidates for testing when appropriate symptoms develop.

TABLE 26-1

Frequency of Venous Thrombosis in Various Hospitalized Patient Groups

Group	Frequency (%)
Orthopedic (e.g., fractured hip)	54-67
Urologic (e.g., prostatectomy)	25
Surgical patients >40 yr old	28
Gynecologic surgery	18
Cardiovascular surgery (e.g., acute myocardial infarction)	39
Obstetrics	3

From Arroliga AC, Matthay MA, Matthay RA: Pulmonary thromboembolism and other pulmonary vascular diseases. In George RB, et al, editors: Chest medicine: essentials of pulmonary and critical care medicine, ed 3, Baltimore, 1995, Williams & Wilkins.

Pathogenesis

Pulmonary emboli arise from detached portions of venous thrombi that form, in most cases, in deep veins of the lower extremities or pelvis (86%); the point of origin of pulmonary emboli is actually found in only one-half of patients.[9] A small percentage of pulmonary emboli arise from the right-sided heart chambers (3.15%) or the superior vena cava (3%).[9]

Conditions that favor thrombus formation include blood *stasis,* the presence of hypercoagulable states, and vessel wall abnormalities (factors known as Virchow's triad). Causes of blood stasis include local pressure, venous obstruction, and immobilization. Other causes of stasis include congestive heart failure, shock and dehydration, varicose veins, and enlargement of the right heart chambers. Several conditions enhance the intravascular coagulability of the blood and predispose to venous thromboembolic disease (Box 26-1).[14] The most frequent causes of an inherited hypercoagulable state are the factor V Leiden mutation and the prothrombin gene mutation, which together account for 50% to 60% of cases.[15] The major acquired risk factors for venous thromboembolism include recent major surgery, trauma, immobilization, antiphospholipid antibody syndrome, malignancy, pregnancy, oral contraceptives, and myeloproliferative disorders.[16] Vessel wall abnormalities are found most often in patients who have sustained trauma or have undergone major surgery.

Pathology

Stasis, an important factor for the formation of DVT, is rarely the only risk factor.[17] Deposition of platelets and fibrin in the venous valve cups of the lower extremities occurs as a result of stasis. The combination of diminished blood flow and the presence of trauma and toxins can worsen endothelial damage and promote the release of

Box 26-1 Conditions Predisposing to Venous Thrombosis and Pulmonary Thromboembolism

- Advanced age
- Postoperative status
- Previous venous thrombosis
- Trauma
- Oral contraceptive use
- Pregnancy
- Prolonged bed rest
- Long periods of travel
- Diagnosis of cancer
- Obesity
- Cerebrovascular accidents
- Thrombocytosis
- Erythrocytosis
- Hyperhomocysteinemia
- Mutation in gene coding for factor V (factor V Leiden)
- Mutation of prothrombin gene
- Antiphospholipid antibody
- Antithrombin deficiency
- Proteins C and S deficiency
- Abnormalities of fibrinogen
- Deficiency of plasminogen
- Sickle cell anemia
- Myeloproliferative disorder
- Paroxysmal nocturnal hemoglobinuria
- Heparin-induced thrombocytopenia

Modified from Arroliga AC, Matthay MA, Matthay RA: Pulmonary thromboembolism and other pulmonary vascular diseases. In George RB, et al, editors: Chest medicine: essentials of pulmonary and critical care medicine, ed 3, Baltimore, 1995, Williams & Wilkins.

mediators that encourage adhesion, aggregation, and degranulation of platelets. The result is activation of the coagulation cascade and production of thrombi and fibrin.

PE is a frequent complication of DVT, occurring in more than 50% of cases with DVT confirmed on phlebography.[18] PE occurs when a fragment of the thrombus in the venous system travels to the pulmonary circulation. Pulmonary emboli occur more frequently in the lower lobes and are more often found in the right lung than in the left lung, a phenomenon probably related to the flow distribution that favors the right lung and the lower lobes.[6] Embolism to the pulmonary circulation produces pulmonary hemorrhage in the ischemic or infarcted lung in less than 10% of cases of PE. Infarction, secondary to thromboembolism, is less common in the lung than in other tissues because the lung has two blood supplies: the pulmonary arterial circulation and the bronchial circulation. At a capillary level, extensive connections exist within the pulmonary and bronchial circulations that prevent serious damage to lung tissue deprived of its pulmonary artery supply.[6] Patients with underlying cardiovascular disease may have impairment of the remaining bronchial circulation with resultant lung tissue necrosis when emboli occur.

Pulmonary infarction is associated with thromboembolic obstruction of a medium-sized pulmonary artery. Generally, infarcts occur at the lung bases, are pleural-based, and may be accompanied by pleural effusion. Microscopic examination of the lung in pulmonary infarction shows necrosis of alveolar walls, alveoli filled with red blood cells, and a mild inflammatory response in the periphery.[6]

RULE OF THUMB

PE is a complication of venous thrombosis. Patients with venous thrombosis in the proximal venous system of the lower extremities and in the upper extremities are at high risk for development of PE.

Pathophysiology

The sudden obstruction of a pulmonary arterial branch causes a decrease in or total cessation of blood flow to the distal area of the lung that leads to respiratory and hemodynamic alterations.[19] In the appropriate context, massive PE should be suspected anytime there is unexplained hypotension accompanied by an elevated central venous pressure (jugular vein distention).[20] It is a catastrophic entity that frequently results in acute right ventricular failure and death. Death from massive PE is the result of cardiovascular collapse rather than of respiratory failure.

Embolic obstruction of the pulmonary artery increases the alveolar dead space, causes bronchoconstriction, and decreases the production of alveolar surfactant. Wasted or dead space areas occur when areas of the lung parenchyma are ventilated but not perfused. The response is to increase total ventilation ($\dot{V}$). The increased $\dot{V}$ contributes to the sensation of dyspnea that accompanies PE. Bronchoconstriction from diminished carbon dioxide concentration, regional hypoxia, and the production of serotonin and histamine cause further ventilation/perfusion ($\dot{V}/\dot{Q}$) mismatching.[21]

Not all patients with PE have significant arterial hypoxemia, but the presence of a widened alveolar-arterial oxygen (O_2) tension gradient and reduced PaO_2 are common. Hypoxemia develops because of $\dot{V}/\dot{Q}$ mismatch, intrapulmonary shunt, and cardiogenic shock. Shock is caused by obstruction of the pulmonary vasculature by massive emboli or by numerous small emboli in the presence of cardiopulmonary disease. Cardiac output decreases, and O_2 delivery declines. With the decrease in O_2 delivery, the peripheral tissues increase O_2 extraction causing venous O_2 desaturation. In patients with significantly increased right heart pressures, intracardiac right-to-left shunt may develop when blood flows through a patent foramen ovale.[19,21] In addition, the depletion of surfactant material as a result of embolic occlusion can lead to atelectasis and intrapulmonary shunt, which can cause hypoxemia.[19]

The main hemodynamic consequence of PE is increased resistance to blood flow caused by obstruction of the pulmonary arterial bed. The hemodynamic consequences are determined by the extent of the cross-sectional area of the pulmonary circulation involved, the underlying cardiopulmonary reserve, and the neurohumoral response to the embolism. Pulmonary hypertension occurs when 50% of the pulmonary vascular bed has been occluded.[19,21] To maintain the same flow at a higher pressure, the right ventricle must work harder. The result is an increase in right ventricular work that causes the right ventricle to become dilated and ischemic. The thin-walled right ventricle is not designed to work with acute heavy pressure loads. When the mean pulmonary artery pressure increases to greater than 40 mm Hg during an acute first PE, the right ventricle fails, and hemodynamic collapse and death occur.[22] The exact role of vasoconstriction in the pathogenesis of pulmonary hypertension is uncertain, but vasoconstrictors such as serotonin and thromboxane A_2 may also play a role in the development of pulmonary hypertension after acute PE.

Although the usual course of PE is to resolve rapidly (because the body lyses the embolism with endogenous fibrinolytic agents), permanent residual emboli do occur.[23] Massive emboli are likely to resolve within weeks, particularly in young patients. Overall, less than 10% of patients have perfusion defects after 6 weeks. Vascular patency is restored when the unresolved emboli organize or form scars against the vessel wall.

Clinical Features

A high index of suspicion for venous thromboembolism is crucial to make the diagnosis for patients at risk. No specific signs or symptoms indicate the presence of venous thromboembolic disease, and a significant proportion of patients are asymptomatic (32%).[2,24] The physical findings of DVT in the lower extremities include erythema and warm skin in one-third of patients and swelling and tenderness in three-fourths of patients. In patients who have swelling above and below the knee, fever, and a history of immobility and cancer, the likelihood of finding DVT on a venogram is only 42%.[25]

The most frequent symptoms in patients with confirmed PE are dyspnea, followed by pleuritic chest pain and cough (Table 26-2).[26] The onset of dyspnea is usually rapid, within seconds (46%) or minutes (26%).[26] Hemoptysis occurs in 13% to 20% of patients. The combination of dyspnea of sudden onset, fainting, and acute chest pain should raise suspicion of PE. In one study, this combination of symptoms was present in 96% of patients with confirmed PE compared with 59% of patients in whom PE was suspected but not confirmed.[27] In some patients, dyspnea lasts only a few minutes, and this episode may be wrongly dismissed as being trivial.[19,27-29]

There are no characteristic physical findings of PE. The most frequent physical findings include tachypnea, rales on chest examination, and tachycardia. Similar to dyspnea, these signs may be short-lived. Other common physical findings include an accentuated pulmonary component of the second heart sound (loud P_2) consistent with pulmonary hypertension. Fever may be present in 54% of patients.[27-29] Similar to what occurs in the diagnosis of DVT, less than 35% of patients in whom PE is clinically suspected actually have it.[2]

TABLE 26-2

Clinical Characteristics in Patients With Pulmonary Embolism and No Cardiopulmonary Disease

Symptoms	Frequency (%)	Signs	Frequency (%)
Dyspnea at rest or with exercise	73	Tachypnea	54
Pleuritic pain	44	Tachycardia	24
Calf or thigh pain	44	Rales	18
Cough	34	Decreased breath sounds	17
Orthopnea	28	Loud P_2	15
Wheezing	21	Jugular venous distention	14

Modified from Stein PD, Beemath A, Matta F, et al: Clinical characteristics of patients with acute pulmonary embolism: data from PIOPED II. Am J Med 120:871–879, 2007.

Because the clinical features are not specific and because treatment is anticoagulation (which carries risk of bleeding over time), confirming or excluding the diagnosis with appropriate testing is necessary, rather than committing the patient to long-term anticoagulation on the basis of clinical suspicion alone. However, unless there is a contraindication to anticoagulating the patient (e.g., recent bleeding, head trauma), anticoagulation is often begun when the diagnosis of PE is first suspected and continued until it is ruled out by tests. The rationale for this approach is that the mortality rate associated with PE is high soon after its occurrence.

Chest Radiograph

The chest radiograph cannot confirm the presence of PE but is helpful to rule out other potentially life-threatening conditions, such as pneumothorax or pneumonia, which can manifest in a similar way. In dyspneic patients, a normal chest radiograph may be a clue to the presence of PE; however, chest radiography is abnormal in more than 80% of cases. Abnormalities include enlargement of the right descending pulmonary artery (66%), elevation of the diaphragm (61%), cardiomegaly (55%), and small pleural effusion (50%). Parenchymal densities (patchy infiltrates or round nodular lesions) predominantly appearing next to the pleural surface are present in patients who have infarction or atelectasis. Other, less common findings include the *Westermark sign,* in which there is pulmonary hyperlucency caused by a marked reduction in blood flow. The so-called *Hampton hump,* an opacity in the costophrenic angle, is present in 25% to 30% of patients.[27]

Electrocardiogram

The electrocardiogram (ECG) is helpful to rule out other diagnoses, such as acute myocardial infarction and pericarditis. The ECG is frequently abnormal in patients with PE (87% of the time), but the ECG abnormalities accompanying PE are nonspecific in 70% to 75% of cases; tachycardia and ST segment depression are most common.[27] Abnormalities such as T wave inversion in right precordial leads, depression of the ST segment, and T wave inversion in V_1 and V_2 may be present. A so-called $S_1Q_3T_3$ pattern is associated with massive PE and is present in 19% of such patients.[25]

Arterial Blood Gases

Most patients with acute PE have hypoxemia and hypocapnia,[27] but a significant percentage of patients (15% to 25%) with or without previous cardiopulmonary disease have a PaO_2 exceeding 80 mm Hg.[29] Although a widened alveolar-arterial O_2 gradient is frequently present, a normal alveolar-arterial O_2 gradient may occur in approximately 20% of patients with angiographically documented PE.[27,29] Although an arterial blood gas measurement may be helpful in identifying patients with hypoxemia or hypocapnia accompanying PE, arterial blood gas measurements can never secure the diagnosis of PE.

In intubated patients or patients with chronic obstructive lung disease (COPD), a decrease in PaO_2 and an increase in $PaCO_2$ can accompany PE and should prompt suspicion. Massive PE with hypotension and respiratory collapse can result in hypercapnia and respiratory acidosis. Overall, although measurement of arterial blood gases is not helpful to confirm or exclude the diagnosis of venous thromboembolic disease, the value of arterial blood gases is to document hypoxemia, direct O_2 supplementation, or show hypercapnia in patients with limited cardiopulmonary reserve.

Diagnostic Modalities

The diagnosis of venous thromboembolic disease relies on the diagnosis of DVT or PE. The absence of one condition does not exclude the other.

By-Products of Thrombin and Plasmin

Clot formation is invariably associated with thrombin generation. Measurement of cross-linked fibrin split products (D-dimers) has been found to be sensitive for the diagnosis of acute venous thromboembolism. The specificity of D-dimer enzyme-linked immunosorbent assay (ELISA) can exclude all but 5% to 10% of patients with acute PE, so this test has been used as an important tool for early assessment.[30] The specificity of the test is only 39%, but a value less than the recommended cutoff for current quantitative ELISA assays has been shown to rule out venous thromboembolic disease in 98% of patients.[31-33] In patients in whom DVT is suspected clinically, negative results of the D-dimer assay combined with negative findings on impedance plethysmography have a negative predictive value of 98% for DVT (i.e., if the test is negative, the chance of a DVT is only 2%).[31] D-dimer results have been particularly useful in the emergency department and outpatient area for the evaluation of patients with suspected DVT[31] and PE.[33] In patients with a low pretest probability of DVT or PE and a negative D-dimer result, the negative predictive value for the strategy has been greater than 99%.[32,33]

Although there are several laboratory methods to measure D-dimer levels, tests using ELISAs are the most widely used and best performing among the D-dimer assays regarding the sensitivity and negative likelihood ratio. For excluding PE or DVT, a negative result on quantitative rapid ELISA is as diagnostically useful as a normal lung scan or negative duplex ultrasonography finding. D-dimer ELISA can be used to exclude PE in outpatients with a low to moderate suspicion without the need for further costly testing. However, inpatients should undergo an imaging study as the initial test for PE because most will already have elevated D-dimer levels because of comorbid conditions.[33]

Testing for Lower Extremity Deep Venous Thrombosis

To evaluate the clinical pretest probability of DVT, the Wells criteria are frequently used. These criteria include the following clinical parameters: presence of cancer, immobilization, localized tenderness, swelling, edema, previous DVT, collateral superficial veins, and absence of an alternative diagnosis.[34] In cases in which there is a moderate to high pretest probability, several modalities could be used for diagnosing DVT in the extremities, such as compression ultrasonography, impedance plethysmography, and venography. In patients with low pretest probability of DVT and a negative D-dimer, further testing may be unnecessary.[31,35-37]

Venography. Venography involves the injection of contrast dye into a foot vein to allow venous visualization by x-rays. It is the standard for the diagnosis of DVT. However, many problems with the test may be encountered, including inability to cannulate the vein; adverse reaction to contrast material; and, in a small percentage of patients, formation of deep venous thrombi. When results of noninvasive studies are negative, venography is recommended for the evaluation of patients at high risk in whom iliac or pelvic vein thrombus is suspected.

Impedance Plethysmography. Impedance plethysmography is a noninvasive method and measures electrical impedance to blood flow, which changes with inflation and deflation of a lower extremity cuff. The quality of the test is operator-dependent and requires that the patient be supine and lay still for at least 2 minutes. The test has a sensitivity and specificity of 91% and 96% for symptomatic proximal venous thrombi. A lower sensitivity of 65% has been reported.[38,39]

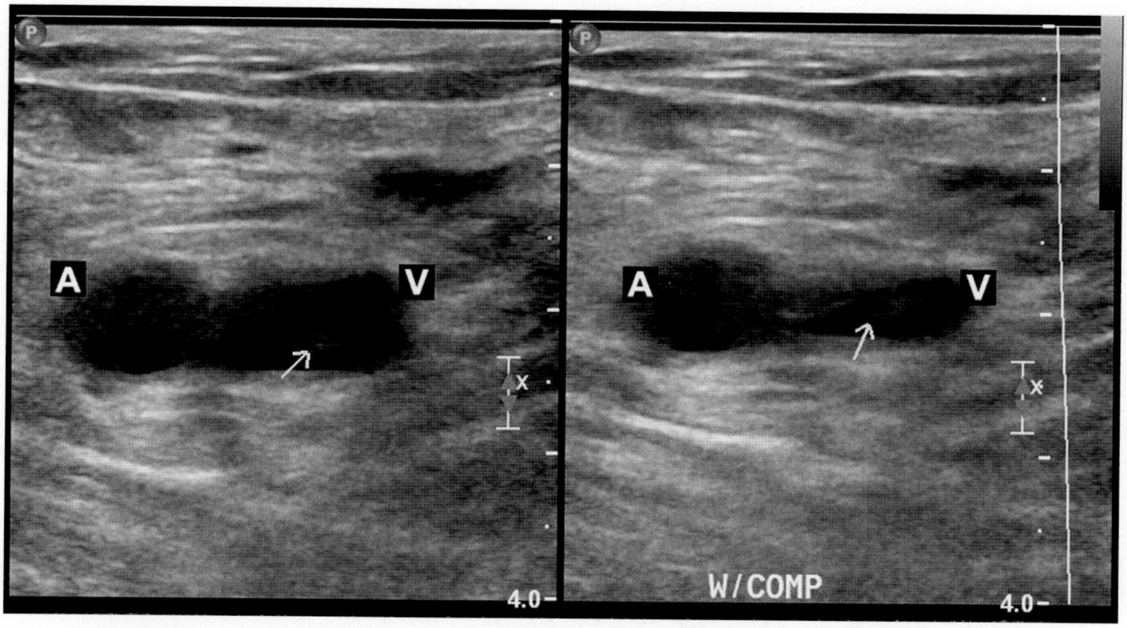

FIGURE 26-1 Deep vein thrombosis diagnosed by ultrasonography. In the *left panel,* an intraluminal thrombus is visible in the right common femoral vein *(arrow)*. The *right panel* shows incomplete collapse of the femoral vein owing to the presence of a clot. *A,* Femoral artery; *V,* femoral vein.

Compression Ultrasonography. Compression ultrasonography has proved to be sensitive and specific for the diagnosis of symptomatic proximal DVT. This test is noninvasive, portable, and accurate and is the modality of choice for the diagnosis of DVT. Compression ultrasonography combines B-mode scanning with a tightly focused pulse Doppler beam directed at the vessels of interest. DVT is diagnosed with the findings of venous noncompressibility, an echogenic filling defect, absence of Doppler flow, free-floating thrombus in the vein, and venous distention.[40] The most reliable sign of DVT is lack of compressibility of the vein, although a free-floating thrombus has the highest embolic potential (Figure 26-1). The sensitivity and specificity of compression ultrasonography in symptomatic patients vary between 95% and 100% for the detection of a proximal lower extremity thrombus.[40,41] Areas not well visualized with compression ultrasonography include the iliac veins, the superficial femoral veins in the adductor canal, and the calf veins. However, the accuracy of compression ultrasonography, even with the addition of color Doppler ultrasonography, is moderate to low for the detection of DVT in patients at high risk who do not have symptoms.[42] These results suggest that ultrasonography, although sensitive and specific for the diagnosis of DVT, is not a good screening test for patients at high risk who do not have symptoms.

The increased incidence of upper extremity DVT poses diagnostic problems. Ultrasonography still may be the initial diagnostic test of choice, although venography is more commonly used for detection of thrombi in hidden areas that cannot be assessed with ultrasonography and in the evaluation of patients without symptoms who have negative findings with noninvasive modalities but have a high risk of DVT.

Testing for Pulmonary Embolism

Noninvasive tests for the diagnosis of PE include $\dot{V}/\dot{Q}$ scan and helical or spiral computed tomography (CT) angiography scan of the chest. Either of these tests, depending on the resources available, may be the initial diagnostic examination if the presence of acute PE is clinically suspected.[43] Echocardiography can suggest the diagnosis (right ventricular dilation, dysfunction, or thrombus) and provide prognostic information.[44] In certain cases when these noninvasive tests are nondiagnostic, pulmonary angiography may be needed to confirm or exclude the diagnosis of PE.

$\dot{V}/\dot{Q}$ scanning involves the inhalation of a radiolabeled gas (usually xenon-133, xenon-127, krypton-181m, or technetium-99m) and the intravenous injection of macroaggregated albumin tagged with a gamma-emitting radioisotope. The distribution of lung ventilation ($\dot{V}$) and lung perfusion ($\dot{Q}$) is studied, and areas of mismatch where $\dot{Q}$ is less than $\dot{V}$ are sought. The presence of mismatches most often indicates embolic occlusion of the blood vessel, although other rare causes of mismatches exist, such as extrinsic compression of the vessel by a mass, intraluminal obstruction by angiosarcoma, or obliteration of a vessel by vasculitis. The addition of $\dot{V}$ scan increases the specificity of $\dot{Q}$ scan.[45] Generally, with the presence of a parenchymal abnormality, the $\dot{V}$ defect coincides with the $\dot{Q}$ defect, and matched abnormalities are found. Normal results of a $\dot{V}/\dot{Q}$ scan exclude the presence of a clinically significant PE in

TABLE 26-3

Revised PIOPED (Prospective Investigation of Pulmonary Embolism Diagnosis) Ventilation/Perfusion Scan Interpretation Criteria

High probability	Two or more large (>75% of a segment) segmental $\dot{Q}$ defects without corresponding $\dot{V}$ or abnormalities on chest radiograph
	One large segment $\dot{Q}$ defect and two or more moderate (25%-75% of a segment) segmental $\dot{Q}$ defects without corresponding $\dot{V}$ or abnormalities on chest radiograph
	Four or more moderate segmental $\dot{Q}$ defects without corresponding $\dot{V}$ or abnormalities on chest radiograph
Intermediate probability	One moderate or up to two large segment $\dot{Q}$ defects without corresponding $\dot{V}$ defect or abnormalities on chest radiograph
	Corresponding $\dot{V}/\dot{Q}$ defects and parenchymal opacity in lower lung zone on chest radiograph
	Corresponding $\dot{V}/\dot{Q}$ defects and small pleural effusion
	Single moderate matched $\dot{V}/\dot{Q}$ defects with normal findings on chest radiograph
	Findings difficult to categorize as normal, low, or high probability
Low probability	Multiple matched $\dot{V}/\dot{Q}$ defects, regardless of size, with normal findings on chest radiograph
	Corresponding $\dot{V}/\dot{Q}$ defects and parenchymal opacity in upper or middle lung zone on chest radiograph
	Corresponding $\dot{V}/\dot{Q}$ defects and large pleural effusion
	Any $\dot{Q}$ defects with substantially larger abnormality on chest radiograph
	Defects surrounded by normally perfused lung (stripe sign)
	Single or multiple small (<25% of a segment) segmental $\dot{Q}$ defects with a normal chest radiograph
	Nonsegmental $\dot{Q}$ defects (cardiomegaly, aortic impression, enlarged hila)
Normal	No $\dot{Q}$ defects; $\dot{Q}$ outlines the shape of the lung on chest radiograph

Modified from Worsley DF, Alavi A, Palevsky JH: Role of radionuclide imaging in patients with suspected pulmonary embolism. Radiol Clin North Am 31:849, 1993.

the context of a low clinical probability of PE. In these cases, anticoagulant therapy can be safely withheld.[46] Abnormal $\dot{V}/\dot{Q}$ scan results can be classified as high probability, intermediate (or indeterminate) probability, and low probability for PE, according to the size of the defect and the degree of mismatch between the $\dot{V}/\dot{Q}$ scan and chest radiographic abnormalities.[45] Diagnostic accuracy is greatest when $\dot{V}/\dot{Q}$ scan results are combined with clinical probability (Table 26-3).[47] The presence of concomitant cardiopulmonary disease (e.g., COPD), even if severe, does not diminish the diagnostic usefulness of $\dot{V}/\dot{Q}$ scans in the diagnosis of acute PE.[48-50]

For the one-third of patients who do not receive a definitive diagnosis on the basis of the results of noninvasive studies, *pulmonary angiography* is the test of choice. The mortality rate for pulmonary angiography is 0.5%, and the prevalence of major nonfatal complications is 1%. Nevertheless, patients in a medical intensive care unit are at higher risk of morbidity and mortality (approximately 4%), including respiratory failure, renal failure, and hematoma necessitating transfusion, than other patients.[47] Pulmonary angiography signs of acute PE include filling defects and cutoff of the pulmonary arteries. Other signs on angiography include absent, decreased, or delayed filling of pulmonary arteries; delayed venous emptying; pruning; and abnormal tapering. None of these findings is as specific as filling defects, in particular, in the presence of other cardiopulmonary diseases. Table 26-4 shows the probability of finding PE with angiography on the basis of results of $\dot{V}/\dot{Q}$ scan and clinical probability.[47] A definite diagnosis can be established with noninvasive diagnostic tools in two-thirds of cases.[51]

TABLE 26-4

Likelihood of Identifying Pulmonary Embolism on Pulmonary Angiogram on the Basis of Results of Ventilation/Perfusion Lung Scan and Clinical Probability

Scan Interpretation	High Clinical Probability (%)	Intermediate Clinical Probability (%)	Low Clinical Probability (%)
High probability	96	88	56
Intermediate probability	66	28	16
Low probability	40	16	4
Near-normal/normal	0	6	2

From Arroliga AC, Matthay MA, Matthay RA: Pulmonary thromboembolism and other pulmonary vascular diseases. In George RB, et al, editors: Chest medicine: essentials of pulmonary and critical care medicine, ed 3, Baltimore, 1995, Williams & Wilkins.

Helical CT angiography has been used extensively in the diagnostic evaluation of PE and has become the principal diagnostic imaging method to evaluate suspected PE (Figure 26-2).[52,53] The reported sensitivity of helical CT angiography ranges from 53% to 100%, and the specificity ranges from 81% to 100%.[53] The variability is probably due to the experience of the radiologists and image quality.[54] Studies indicate that helical CT scanning detects large pulmonary emboli involving main and lobar emboli. However, this test is generally unable to detect smaller pulmonary emboli. One potential advantage of helical CT angiography is its ability to identify alternative diagnoses in cases

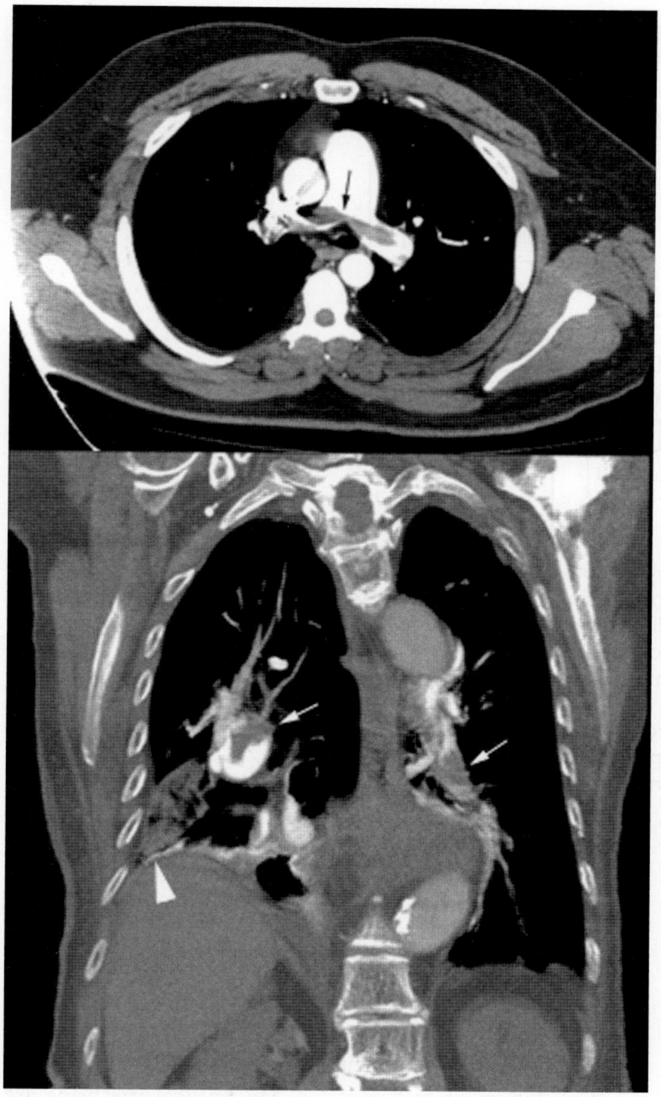

FIGURE 26-2 Pulmonary embolism diagnosed by CT angiography. Axial (at the level of the pulmonary artery bifurcation, *upper panel*) and coronal cuts (just anterior to the thoracic spine, *lower panel*) show the presence of pulmonary embolism involving the right and left pulmonary arteries, also known as *saddle embolism (arrows)*. On the coronal cut, there is a wedge-shaped area in the right lower lobe that represents lung infarction *(arrowhead)*.

in which PE is not present (e.g., pneumonia, pleural disease). Helical CT angiography scanning can be as cost-effective as $\dot{V}/\dot{Q}$ scanning and duplex ultrasound examination of the lower extremity but only when combined with D-dimer testing.

Multicenter trials suggest that helical CT scanning is safe to use for ruling out PE, at least in patients with a low or intermediate clinical probability of embolism. The PIOPED (Prospective Investigation of Pulmonary Embolism Diagnosis) II trial evaluated the accuracy of multidetector CT angiography alone and combined with venous phase imaging (CT angiography–CT venography) for the diagnosis of acute PE. Among 824 patients with a reference diagnosis and a completed CT study, CT angiography was inconclusive in 51 because of poor image quality. Excluding such inconclusive studies, the sensitivity of CT angiography was 83%, and the specificity was 96%. CT angiography–CT venography was inconclusive in 87 of 824 patients because the image quality of either CT angiography or CT venography was poor. The sensitivity of CT angiography–CT venography for PE was 90%, and specificity was 95%. The predictive value of either CT angiography or CT angiography–CT venography is high with a concordant clinical assessment, but additional testing is necessary when the clinical probability is inconsistent with the imaging results.[53,55] Several algorithms for the diagnosis of PE are available, but no approach has proven superior to others.[56-58] Figure 26-3 summarizes the diagnostic approach to PE using CT angiography.

MINI CLINI

Respiratory Distress After Hip Replacement

PROBLEM: The RT is told to evaluate a 65-year-old man who has undergone right hip replacement. On the third day after surgery, the patient experienced dyspnea and pleuritic chest pain in the right hemithorax. On physical examination, his heart rate is 120 beats/min, respiratory rate is 25 breaths/min, and blood pressure is 120/85 mm Hg. The lungs are clear, and the heart examination does not show any gallops or murmurs. Arterial blood gas measurements on room air reveal a pH of 7.49, $PaCO_2$ 30 mm Hg, and PO_2 85 mm Hg. The chest radiograph is unremarkable. What is the differential diagnosis, and how should the RT treat this patient?

DISCUSSION: The differential diagnosis is extensive and should include an ischemic cardiac event such as myocardial infarction and bacterial pneumonia. The type of chest pain is not typical of myocardial infarction. An ECG may be valuable because in patients with myocardial infarction, elevation of the ST segments is prominent in the acute phase. Other laboratory data include elevation of the creatinine kinase and troponin levels, although these test results may become abnormal after several hours. The normal chest radiograph decreases the likelihood of the presence of pneumonia.

Because of the history of surgery on the right hip, DVT and PE are the most likely diagnoses. The next examinations are duplex ultrasonography of the lower extremities followed by a $\dot{V}/\dot{Q}$ radionuclide study or a CT angiography scan of the chest. DVT should be sought in patients diagnosed with PE to investigate the origin of the thrombus and because patients with PE found to have a coexisting DVT are at increased risk for mortality.[59] The presence of a "normal" PaO_2 of 85 mm Hg in this patient may be misleading. The wide alveolar-arterial gradient probably is caused by the presence of a pulmonary embolus. The patient needs to be anticoagulated (e.g., with heparin, continuous intravenous drip) followed by warfarin.

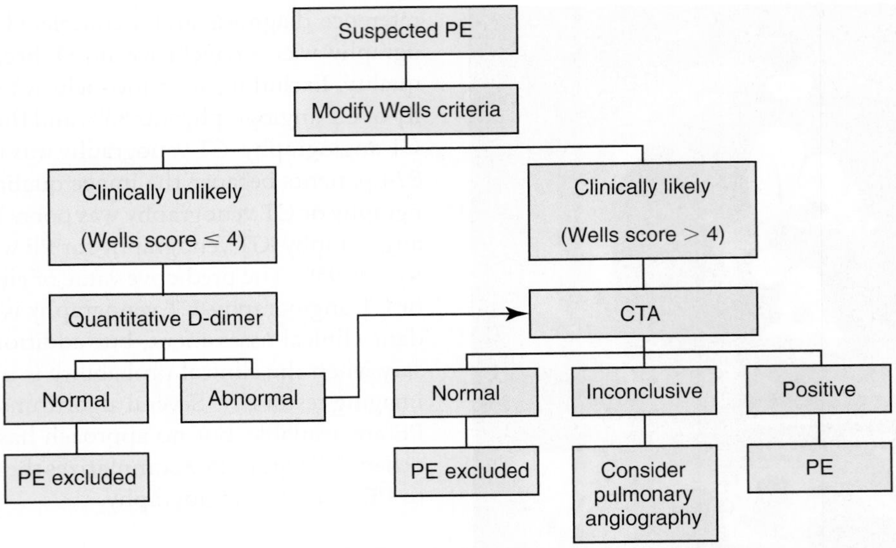

FIGURE 26-3 Strategy for diagnosis of pulmonary embolism using D-dimer and CT angiography. Diagnosis is based on clinical suspicion (using Wells modified criteria) and the results of CT angiography scan. The modified Wells criteria include the following: clinical symptoms of DVT (3 points), other diagnoses less likely than PE (3 points), heart rate greater than 100 beats/min (1.5 points), immobilization lasting 3 days or more or surgery in previous 4 weeks (1.5 points), previous DVT or PE (1.5 points), hemoptysis (1 point), and malignancy (1 point). (Modified from van Belle A, Buller HR, Huisman MV, et al: Effectiveness of managing suspected pulmonary embolism using an algorithm combining clinical probability, D-dimer testing, and computed tomography. JAMA 295:172–179, 2006.)

Other diagnostic modalities have been used to make the diagnosis of PE. Magnetic resonance imaging (MRI) has been suggested as an alternative noninvasive method for confirming the presence or absence of DVT. The sensitivity, specificity, and accuracy of MRI all are approximately 97%.[60] MRI with radial pulse acquisition seems accurate in the diagnosis of acute DVT. Because of respiratory and cardiac motion artifacts and suboptimal resolution from the adjacent air-containing lung, MRI may not be useful in the acute setting.[61]

Treatment

Prophylaxis

Prophylactic therapy reduces the risk of venous thromboembolism in patients at risk. The frequency of proximal DVT ranges from 2% to 4% among general surgical patients undergoing minor surgery to 40% to 80% among patients at the highest risk, such as patients who have undergone hip or knee surgery.[62] Patients at moderate to high risk include patients with acute spinal cord injury, myocardial infarction, ischemic stroke, or other medical conditions such as heart failure and pneumonia.[62] Patients admitted to medical intensive care units are another group at risk for DVT; 33% of these patients have been found to have DVT.[63] Compliance in the use of prophylaxis varies between 28% and 100%.[62]

Pharmacologic choices for prophylaxis include low-dose subcutaneous heparin, low-molecular-weight heparin, and fondaparinux.[64-66] Mechanical measures to reduce venous stasis include early ambulation, wearing elastic stockings, pneumatic calf compression, and electrical stimulation of calf muscles. Mechanical methods are reserved for patients with contraindications to anticoagulant thromboprophylaxis.[67] Current prophylactic strategies for DVT and PE are summarized in Table 26-5. Most hospitalized patients who are immobile need prophylaxis for venous thromboembolism.

RULE OF THUMB

Most hospitalized patients who are immobile need prophylaxis for venous thromboembolism.

Management of Venous Thromboembolism

Anticoagulation. Heparin is the standard therapy for venous thromboembolic disease. Unfractionated heparin is the time-honored drug treatment, but low-molecular-weight heparin (e.g., enoxaparin) is widely used and has been endorsed in some guidelines as first-line therapy.[68] Heparin has an immediate action and is relatively safe.

TABLE 26-5

Thromboembolism Risk and Recommended Thromboprophylaxis in Hospitalized Patients

Risk		DVT Risk Without Prophylaxis	Suggested Option
Low	(a) Minor surgery in mobile patient	<10%	(a) No specific prophylaxis
	(b) Medical patients fully mobile		(b) Early and aggressive ambulation
Moderate	(a) Most general, open gynecologic or urologic surgery	10%-40%	(a) LMWH, UF heparin, or fondaparinux
	(b) Medical patients, bed rest or sick		(b) LMWH, UF heparin, or fondaparinux
	(c) High bleeding risk		(c) Mechanical prophylaxis
High	(a) Hip or knee arthroplasty, major trauma, hip fracture, and spinal cord injury	40%-80%	(a) LMWH, fondaparinux, warfarin (INR 2-3)
	(b) High bleeding risk		(b) Mechanical prophylaxis

Modified from Geerts WH, Bergqvist D, Pineo GF, et al: Prevention of venous thromboembolism. American College of Chest Physicians Evidence-Based Clinical Practice Guidelines (8th Edition). Chest 133:381S-453S, 2008.
INR, International normalized ratio; *LMWH,* low molecular weight heparin; *UF,* unfractionated.

It potentiates the action of antithrombin and heparin cofactor 2 and in this way inactivates thrombin, factor IXa, and factor Xa. Heparin does not lyse existing clots but prevents formation and propagation of new clots. Unfractionated heparin should be administered as a bolus followed by a continuous infusion.[62] Low-molecular-weight heparin is administered subcutaneously, once or twice a day, and does not characteristically require blood test monitoring to ensure therapeutic benefit.[68]

The heparin regimen should be selected to maximize its antithrombotic effect without increasing the risk of bleeding. It is very important to achieve a therapeutic effect in the first 24 to 48 hours of starting therapy. The goal of unfractionated heparin therapy is to maintain an activated partial thromboplastin time greater than 1.5 times the control value.[69] Clinical recurrence of DVT and PE is rare when heparin is infused at doses of at least 1250 units/hr.[69] The fastest way to achieve a therapeutic heparin effect is to follow an established nomogram. Several nomograms are available, and one is shown in Table 26-6.[69-71] These nomograms have been well accepted by clinicians and have led to aggressive heparin dosing and improvement in intermediate outcome. The use of nomograms has been associated with decreasing time to achieve therapeutic activated partial thromboplastin time (85% to 90% of patients achieve a therapeutic level within 24 hours) and a decrease in the variance of these parameters without any changes in bleeding rate.[71] The complications of intravenous heparin administration include major bleeding (3.8%) and thrombocytopenia caused by IgG antiheparin antibodies (2.5% to 3% of patients to whom heparin is given therapeutically, <0.5% of patients to whom it is given prophylactically). If thrombocytopenia or bleeding occurs, heparin should be discontinued promptly.

Heparin should be given for a minimum of 5 to 7 days.[69] Oral anticoagulation can be started at the same time, not before, as the initiation of heparin.[72] Coumarin derivatives are drugs that inhibit the formation of vitamin K–dependent factors II, VII, IX, and X. The coumarin derivative warfarin sodium is the most commonly used oral anticoagulant. Warfarin should be overlapped with heparin for a minimum of 5 days and until the international normalized ratio has been therapeutic for at least 24 hours to achieve a full antithrombotic effect.[72] Warfarin should not be used solely for the initial management of venous thromboembolism because the peak effect is delayed for at least 72 to 96 hours. Because warfarin also decreases production of proteins C and S, a relative hypercoagulable state may occur in the first 24 hours as a result of the depletion of these proteins. The loading dose of warfarin varies between 5 mg/day and 10 mg/day. The 5-mg/day dose produces a lesser degree of anticoagulation and avoids the development of a potential hypercoagulable state caused by the decrease in the level of protein C during the first 36 hours of therapy.[73]

TABLE 26-6

Weight-Based Nomogram for Administration of Heparin

Initial dose	80 U/kg bolus, then 18 U/kg/hr
aPTT < 35 sec (<1.2× control value)	80 U/kg bolus, then 4 U/kg/hr
aPTT 35-45 sec (1.2-1.5× control value)	40 U/kg bolus, then 2 U/kg/hr
aPTT 46-70 sec (1.5-2.3× control value)	No change
aPTT 71-90 sec (2.3-3× control value)	Decrease infusion rate by 2 U/kg/hr
aPTT > 90 sec (>3× control value)	Hold infusion 1 hr, then decrease infusion rate by 3 U/kg/hr

Modified from Raschke RA, Gollihake B, Pierce JC: The effectiveness of implementing the weight-based heparin nomogram as a practice guideline. Arch Intern Med 156:1645, 1996.
aPTT, Activated partial thromboplastin time.
Note: Doses are calculated on actual body weight.

Management of Deep Venous Thrombosis

Patients generally need treatment with oral anticoagulants for 6 months, although in patients with transient risk of DVT (postoperative period), a 4- to 6-week course of anticoagulation may be adequate.[69,74] Patients who need therapy for more than 6 months include patients with idiopathic venous thromboembolism. Patients who need therapy for more than 1 year or for life are patients with a history of cancer, anticardiolipin antibody, or antithrombin deficiency.[69]

Low-molecular-weight heparin, as a single dose or twice a day given via the subcutaneous route, is the suggested therapy for proximal DVT if no contraindication exists.[72] This agent has been shown to be as effective and as safe as, and less expensive than, intravenous heparin therapy. In selected patients, low-molecular-weight heparin can be administered at home in an efficacious and safe way that can potentially decrease the number of days of hospital admission for acute DVT.[69] It has been suggested that $250 million could be saved annually in the United States if patients were treated in the outpatient setting. Patients chosen for outpatient therapy should be in stable condition, should have a low risk of bleeding, and should not have renal insufficiency. At-home administration of low-molecular-weight heparin should be closely supervised.

The role of thrombolytic therapy with streptokinase, urokinase, or tissue plasminogen activator is not well defined in the management of acute DVT. Administration of early thrombolytic therapy decreases the pain and the incidence of postphlebitic syndrome, but the risks and benefits of this therapy are not well established.[69] A systematic review of the efficacy and the safety of the use of recombinant tissue plasminogen activator in the management of lower extremity DVT did not support the routine use of this medication.[75] It may be indicated in patients with massive proximal DVT and high risk of limb gangrene.[72] Knowledge of the patient's values and preferences must be used to guide the best decision.[76]

Management of Pulmonary Embolism

The management of PE depends on the extent of PE and the status of the cardiopulmonary system. Therapy with unfractionated or low-molecular-weight heparin followed by oral coumarin in a regimen similar to that for acute DVT is the treatment of choice. When the heparin effect is therapeutic within the first 24 hours, the risk of recurrent PE, which is associated with higher mortality, is decreased.[77]

Patients with an acute pulmonary embolus need additional supportive measures. Supplemental O_2 should be administered to patients who have hypoxemia, and adequate analgesia should be prescribed for patients who have pain and anxiety. Resuscitation with fluids and vasopressor agents is necessary for patients who develop hypotension and shock. The vasopressors of choice include agents that may reduce pulmonary vascular resistance and increase cardiac output, such as norepinephrine and dopamine.[78,79] Anticoagulation prevents further clot formation but does not lyse existing thromboemboli or decrease thrombus size. In the care of patients with severe hypoxemia, acute right heart failure, or shock, thrombolytic therapy may be administered for lysis of the emboli. Persistent hypotension secondary to massive PE is the most commonly accepted indication for thrombolytic therapy; however, no major trial has conclusively shown a mortality benefit of this intervention.[72] When thrombolytic therapy with streptokinase and urokinase is used, heparin should not be infused concurrently. However, the use of heparin is optional in the treatment of patients receiving tissue plasminogen activator or reteplase.[69]

Other options in the care of a patient with confirmed massive PE, in whom thrombolysis is either contraindicated or unsuccessful, include pulmonary embolectomy, catheter tip embolectomy (physical removal of the embolism), and catheter tip fragmentation. Because of associated risks, these techniques should be used in centers with appropriate experience.[43] Patients who have undergone attempts at embolectomy and catheter extraction have had massive embolism and shock.[69]

For patients in whom anticoagulation is contraindicated (e.g., because of bleeding risk), placement of a filter into the inferior vena cava to prevent movement of clot from the lower extremities to the pulmonary arteries is a treatment option. Another reason for placing an inferior vena cava filter is that a recurrent embolism has occurred despite adequate anticoagulation or that the patient has experienced multiple past emboli and is considered to be unable to tolerate another pulmonary embolus. Filter placement reduces the risk of PE in the period immediately after insertion but is associated over the longer term with a higher incidence of recurrent DVT.[69,80]

PULMONARY HYPERTENSION

Pulmonary hypertension is defined by an elevation in mean pulmonary artery pressure greater than 25 mm Hg at rest.[81] Pulmonary hypertension is grouped in five categories; this classification that was updated in 2008 by the Fourth World Symposium on Pulmonary Hypertension in Dana Point, California (Box 26-2).[82] The importance of the clinical system, outside of allowing a better understanding of pathophysiology, is to give a framework for understanding important branch-points in the management and treatment of different conditions known to cause pulmonary hypertension. The first category, *pulmonary artery hypertension (PAH)*, is characterized by an elevation in pulmonary artery pressure associated with high pulmonary vascular resistance (≥3 Wood units) and normal left ventricular filling pressures (pulmonary artery occlusion pressure ≤15 mm Hg). PAH may be associated with several conditions, including congenital heart disease, collagen vascular disease, cirrhosis of the liver, viral infections (e.g., HIV), and drugs and toxins (diet pills or anorexiants).[82] In

Box 26-2	Clinical Classification of Pulmonary Hypertension (Dana Point, 2008)

1. PAH
2. Pulmonary hypertension owing to left heart disease
3. Pulmonary hypertension owing to lung diseases or hypoxia or both
4. Chronic thromboembolic pulmonary hypertension
5. Pulmonary hypertension with unclear multifactorial mechanisms

Modified from Simonneau G, Robbins IM, Beghetti M, et al: Updated clinical classification of pulmonary hypertension. J Am Coll Cardiol 54:S43–S54, 2009.

patients in whom no underlying etiology of pulmonary hypertension can be identified, the disease is referred to as *idiopathic pulmonary arterial hypertension (IPAH)*, previously known as *primary pulmonary hypertension*.[83-86] Pulmonary hypertension can also develop as a consequence of PE, and this entity is known as *chronic thromboembolic pulmonary hypertension*.[87]

Pathogenesis

The initial event of IPAH is probably an insult to the pulmonary endothelium (the cells that line the blood vessel). A genetic predisposition is probably necessary. The damage to the endothelium alters the balance between vasoconstrictive mediators such as thromboxane and endothelin I and vasodilators such as nitric oxide and prostacyclin, and vasoconstriction results. Vasoconstriction may not be the primary event, but it is an important component in the pathogenesis of IPAH.[88-90] In addition to vasoconstriction, inflammation, thrombosis, cell proliferation, apoptosis, and fibrosis lead to pulmonary vascular remodeling and irreversible PAH.[91] More recent research suggests the presence of other potential pathways involved in the pathogenesis of PAH, including downregulation of potassium channels,[92] increased matrix metalloproteinases,[93] decreased vasoactive intestinal peptide,[94] elevated serotonin,[95] transforming growth factor beta,[96] and others.[97] Potential new biomarkers and lines of therapies could result from these discoveries.[83-86,88-90,98]

Epidemiology and Clinical Findings

IPAH is more common among women than among men, with a ratio of 3:1. Approximately 7% of all cases are heritable. IPAH can occur at any age, although it is more common from ages 20 to 50 years. On average, the diagnosis of IPAH is delayed for 2 years after the onset of IPAH. The condition frequently is misdiagnosed as anxiety or depression because it is characterized by onset of vague symptoms and hyperventilation. The most common initial symptom is dyspnea (60% of patients). Angina, probably caused by underperfusion of the right ventricle or stretching of the large pulmonary arteries, is present in approximately 50% of patients. Syncope (passing out) is present in 8% of patients as an early symptom. Other symptoms include cough, hemoptysis, hoarseness, and Raynaud phenomenon (blanching of the fingers on exposure to cold) in approximately 10% of patients. Physical findings associated with IPAH include a loud second heart sound and a right-sided third or fourth heart sound. Other common signs are a palpable right ventricular heave and impulse of the pulmonary artery and both pulmonary ejection and pulmonary tricuspid regurgitation murmurs. Signs of right ventricular failure are common. Cyanosis often is present as a result of low cardiac output or the presence of an intracardiac right-to-left shunt that occurs as cor pulmonale develops. Clubbing does not occur in IPAH. Findings on chest radiograph include enlargement of the main and hilar pulmonary arteries, "pruning" (or narrowing) of the peripheral arteries, enlargement of the right ventricle and atrium, and pleural effusion, although the chest radiograph may remain normal in 6% of patients. In pulmonary venoocclusive disease, a histopathologic type of IPAH, there is an increase in vascular markings, and so-called Kerley B lines may be present on the chest radiograph (thin lines that represent congested pulmonary lymphatics that extend from the pleural surface into the lung).[83-86]

Diagnosis

Before the diagnosis of IPAH can be made, other underlying diseases that can be associated with PAH must be excluded. Tests commonly ordered to establish the diagnosis include blood tests, ECG, pulmonary function testing, echocardiogram, $\dot{V}/\dot{Q}$ scan, CT angiography, and pulmonary artery catheterization.

Laboratory tests include complete blood count, HIV, rheumatologic panel, and liver function testing. These tests help identify conditions associated with PAH. ECG findings usually include right-axis deviation, right ventricular hypertrophy, and strain. Pulmonary function tests are useful to rule out the presence of significant restrictive or obstructive airway disease. The most common abnormality on pulmonary function testing of patients with IPAH is a low carbon monoxide diffusing capacity (DLCO), associated with normal pulmonary mechanics. The echocardiogram may show dilation of the right ventricle and right atrium and tricuspid regurgitation (Figure 26-4).

One of the most important noninvasive tests for IPAH is the $\dot{V}/\dot{Q}$ lung scan, which helps to rule out the possibility of chronic thromboembolic pulmonary hypertension, a mimic of IPAH that has different treatment. In patients with IPAH, the $\dot{V}/\dot{Q}$ scan may be normal or show only patchy subsegmental defects. In patients with chronic thromboembolic pulmonary hypertension, the $\dot{V}/\dot{Q}$ scan shows segmental defects; in these cases, confirmation of chronic thromboembolic pulmonary hypertension requires pulmonary angiography. High-resolution CT is helpful to rule out associated etiologies and may be useful in evaluating the small group of patients with chronic interstitial disease and normal chest radiographs.

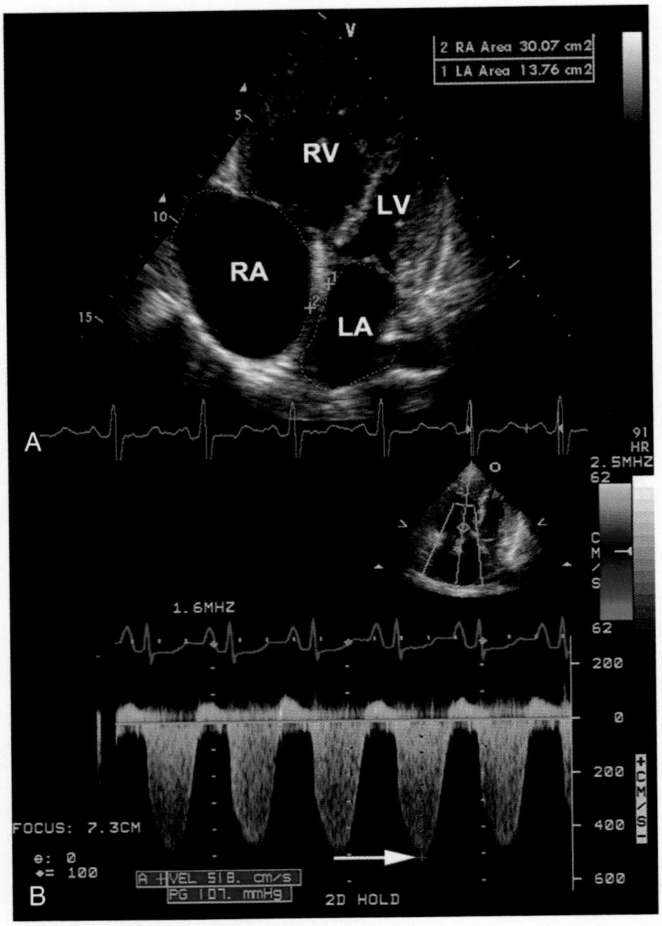

FIGURE 26-4 Echocardiography in pulmonary hypertension. **A,** Apical four-chamber view of the heart reveals enlarged right atrium and ventricle compressing the left cardiac chambers. **B,** Doppler echocardiography shows tricuspid insufficiency jet *(arrow)* used to estimate the right ventricular systolic pressure, in this case 107 mm Hg. *LA,* Left atrium; *LV,* left ventricle; *RA,* right atrium; *RV,* right ventricle.

Right heart catheterization is required to confirm the diagnosis and determine the degree of hemodynamic impairment, the presence of vasoreactivity, and the prognosis of patients with PAH (Figure 26-5). Patients with severe degrees of pulmonary hypertension, high right atrial pressure, and low cardiac output have a very poor prognosis.[14,83-86]

Systemic lupus erythematosus, systemic sclerosis, and mixed connective tissue disease may be ruled out by the appropriate clinical examinations and laboratory tests. Schistosomiasis, a parasitic disease and the most common cause of pulmonary hypertension worldwide, must be ruled out in the appropriate setting.

Management of Pulmonary Hypertension

IPAH can be life-threatening and is associated with a poor prognosis. Without therapy, only 33% of patients are alive 5 years after the onset of the disorder. During the past decade, treatment has improved considerably.[99-104] Current treatment options include using calcium channel blockers, prostanoids, endothelin receptor antagonists, and phosphodiesterase 5 (PDE5) inhibitors (discussed later).

General Measures

Oral anticoagulation improves survival in IPAH and is recommended in all patients with IPAH unless there is a contraindication to anticoagulation.[105] The recommended target international normalized ratio is approximately 2. The role of anticoagulation in other forms of PAH is less clear. Supplemental O_2 should be used to maintain O_2 saturation greater than 90%, especially because hypoxemia is a major cause of pulmonary vasoconstriction. Diuretics are indicated for right ventricular volume overload, and digoxin is reserved for patients with refractory right ventricular failure and for rate control in atrial flutter or fibrillation.[103,104]

Calcium Channel Blockers

Patients with IPAH who respond to vasodilators in the short-term have improved survival with long-term use of calcium channel blockers. These agents should be considered in all patients who have significant and definite response to a short-acting vasodilator such as nitric oxide. Nitric oxide is the preferred agent for pulmonary vasodilator testing because its half-life is very short, it does not affect cardiac output, and it enhances $\dot{V}/\dot{Q}$ matching.[106] It is usually administered by mask at 10 to 40 parts per million for 2 to 5 minutes.[106] Only a small fraction of patients with IPAH qualify for and benefit from long-term therapy with oral calcium channel blockers.[103,104]

Prostanoids

Prostanoids available for treating patients with pulmonary hypertension, especially IPAH, include epoprostenol, treprostinil, and iloprost. Epoprostenol, delivered via continuous intravenous infusion, improves exercise capacity, hemodynamic variables, and survival in patients with IPAH and is the treatment of choice for severely ill patients.[107] Epoprostenol therapy is complicated, however, by the instability of the drug at room temperature and the need for continuous intravenous infusion because of the short half-life of the drug. Common side effects include headache, flushing, jaw pain, diarrhea, nausea, skin rash, and musculoskeletal pain. Catheter-related complications include infection, sometimes serious (e.g., bacteremia), and thrombosis. By changing the buffer, a thermostable epoprostenol was developed and has been approved for clinical use by the U.S. Food and Drug Administration (FDA).

Another prostanoid, treprostinil, is a stable prostacyclin analogue with a longer half-life, allowing for subcutaneous,[108] intravenous,[109] or inhaled delivery.[110] In addition to side effects seen with epoprostenol, patients receiving treprostinil subcutaneously may experience pain at the infusion site. Inhaled treprostinil is administered by using

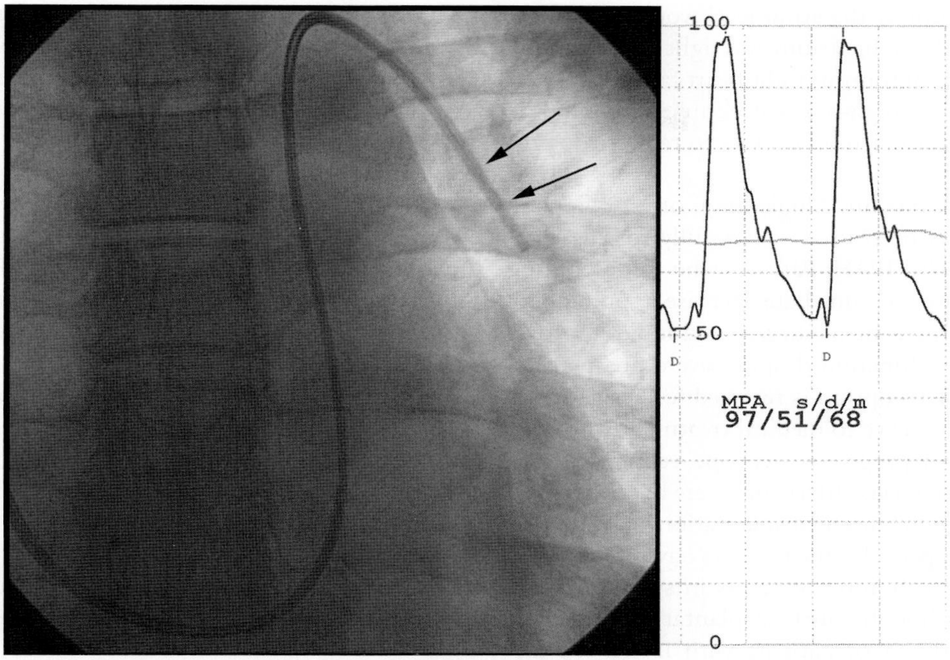

FIGURE 26-5 Right heart catheterization in pulmonary hypertension. In the *left panel,* a pulmonary artery catheter is observed in the left pulmonary artery *(arrows)*. In the *right panel,* the corresponding pulmonary artery pressure tracing is shown, confirming the diagnosis of pulmonary hypertension. In this case, the pulmonary artery systolic, diastolic, and mean pressures were 97 mm Hg, 51 mm Hg, and 68 mm Hg.

the Tyvaso Inhalation System (ultrasonic, pulsed-delivery device). It is initially dosed at 3 inhalations four times a day. If this dose is tolerated, it may be increased up to 9 inhalations four times a day.

Iloprost is a stable prostacyclin analogue that can be delivered via inhalation and is an effective therapy for PAH.[111] Because of the relatively short duration of action of inhaled iloprost, it needs to be administered as 1 to 2 inhalations six to nine times a day. For its administration, the I-neb adaptive aerosol delivery (AAD) or Prodose AAD system should be used. Common side effects include cough, flushing, and headache. Inhaled iloprost may be useful as an adjunct to oral therapy. The main impediment to the use of prostanoids has been the route of delivery. The development of orally administered prostanoids is under way.[99,100,103,104]

Endothelin Receptor Antagonists

Endothelin antagonists represent another class of medications available for treating pulmonary hypertension. Bosentan, an orally administered nonselective endothelin-1 receptor antagonist, improves walking distance, hemodynamic variables, and functional class in patients with PAH.[112] The main side effect is the asymptomatic increase in hepatic aminotransferase levels, which necessitates monitoring liver function at least monthly in all patients receiving the medication. Ambrisentan is a selective type A endothelin-1 receptor antagonist that is also beneficial in patients with PAH. Its main side effect is peripheral edema.[113,114] All endothelin receptor antagonists are potent teratogens, and meticulous contraception must be observed by patients receiving these medications.

Phosphodiesterase 5 Inhibitors

Sildenafil, a PDE5 inhibitor, reduces pulmonary artery pressure and is effective in the treatment of pulmonary hypertension.[101] By inhibiting PDE5, sildenafil stabilizes cyclic guanosine monophosphate (cGMP), the second messenger of nitric oxide, allowing a more sustained effect of endogenous nitric oxide, an indirect but effective and practical way of using the nitric oxide–cGMP pathway. Tadalafil, a long-acting PDE5 inhibitor, also improves outcomes in PAH and has some differences in the acute effects compared with sildenafil.[115,116] These medications are usually well-tolerated; rarely, patients can have vision or hearing loss, priapism, and hypotension.

Surgical Therapy

Atrial Septostomy. The role of balloon atrial septostomy in the treatment of patients with PAH is uncertain. Septostomy might be beneficial in the setting of severe disease with recurrent syncope or right heart failure despite maximal medical therapy. The procedure can also be used as a palliative bridge to lung transplantation. The rationale for its use is that the controlled creation of an atrial septal defect would allow right-to-left shunting, leading to increased systemic output and systemic O_2 transport despite the accompanying decrease in systemic arterial O_2

saturation. The shunt at the atrial level would also allow decompression of the right atrium and right ventricle, alleviating signs and symptoms of right heart failure. Balloon atrial septostomy is a high-risk procedure and should be performed only in experienced centers to reduce the procedural risks.[103]

Lung Transplantation. Single-lung or double-lung transplantation has been used successfully in the treatment of patients with IPAH. Patients who undergo lung transplantation have an immediate decrease in pulmonary artery pressure at the time of surgery and rapid improvement in right heart function despite severe preoperative cor pulmonale.[103] This option is reserved for special cases of patients not responsive to medical treatment who have an indicator of poor prognosis (syncope, refractory right heart failure, function class III/IV, or severe hypoxemia).[117] Perioperative mortality for transplantation is higher in PAH, but after this period some patients have an excellent response with dramatic improvements in symptoms and quality of life.[118] Although lung transplantation is an alternative in the treatment of patients with IPAH, the disadvantages of transplantation are the need for lifelong immunosuppression and the morbidity and mortality of lung transplantation, which increase over time. The survival rate 3 years after lung transplantation is approximately 60%. By the time patients with PAH and CHD are considered for transplantation, they are usually poor candidates because of multiple organ system failures.

RULE OF THUMB

In patients with shortness of breath who have unremarkable results at physical examination, the presence of low DLCO and normal pulmonary mechanics suggests a pulmonary vascular cause (e.g., pulmonary hypertension) as a cause of the symptoms.

Pulmonary Hypertension in Chronic Lung Disease

Pulmonary hypertension is a frequent complication of chronic pulmonary disease (see Chapter 23). Approximately 50% of elderly patients with COPD have pulmonary hypertension with significant reduction in survival and quality of life. The pulmonary hypertension associated with COPD is multifactorial. Loss of vascular surface caused by destruction of lung parenchyma, compression of the vascular bed as a result of hyperinflation, hyperviscosity of the blood as a result of polycythemia, and left ventricular dysfunction are important contributory factors. Alveolar hypoxia, because of its potent pulmonary vasoconstrictive effect, is probably the most important factor contributing to pulmonary hypertension in patients with COPD. Sustained alveolar hypoxia causes pulmonary vasoconstriction and eventually medial hypertrophy, fibrosis of the intima, and narrowing of the lumen of the pulmonary blood vessels. The increases in pulmonary artery pressure and vascular resistance lead to an increase in the afterload of the right ventricle with dilation and hypertrophy in an effort to maintain the cardiac output.

Patients with COPD may have worsening of dyspnea and a decrease in exercise tolerance without a change in the degree of airway obstruction. The presence of pulmonary hypertension in patients with COPD correlates with the severity of the disease. Patients with severe hypoxemia (PaO_2 < 55 mm Hg) may have more elevated pulmonary artery pressures, although the mean pulmonary artery pressure owing to COPD alone rarely exceeds 35 to 40 mm Hg.[119-122] Patients with mean pulmonary artery pressure higher than this have a poor prognosis.[123]

MINI CLINI

Dyspnea and Near-Syncope

PROBLEM: A 35-year-old woman has shortness of breath. She had an episode of near-syncope approximately 6 months ago; a diagnostic evaluation was done, and the results were negative. The physical examination shows a loud second heart sound. A chest radiograph shows questionable cardiomegaly. Values for forced vital capacity and forced expiratory volume in 1 second are normal, but DLCO is only 40% of the predicted value. What is the cause of the dyspnea and the low DLCO?

DISCUSSION: This patient could have pulmonary hypertension of unknown cause—IPAH. She has physical findings consistent with high pressure in the right side of the heart (a loud second heart sound), and she has symptoms that are common in this disorder, such as dyspnea and near-syncope or syncope. The diagnosis is difficult, but low DLCO in the presence of normal lung mechanics could indicate an abnormality of the pulmonary vasculature.

An echocardiogram is usually the first test of choice to assess for the presence of pulmonary hypertension. If the echocardiogram is consistent with the diagnosis, pulmonary artery (also known as right heart) catheterization is usually needed to confirm the diagnosis, determine the severity, and exclude left heart disease. For the diagnosis of IPAH, other underlying diseases that can be associated with pulmonary artery hypertension must be excluded. A $\dot{V}/\dot{Q}$ scan or pulmonary angiogram can exclude chronic thromboembolic disease, a CT scan of the chest and pulmonary function tests can help determine the presence of parenchymal lung disease, and blood serologic tests can be used to evaluate for connective tissue disease. A 6-minute walk test may help in determining the functional capacity of the patient and assess the patient's response to treatment. Several treatment options are currently available for patients with pulmonary hypertension. The best option depends on the underlying diagnosis (if any) and the severity of the disease.

O_2 therapy is the main treatment that improves survival among patients with COPD and pulmonary hypertension, although smoking cessation and lung volume reduction (in selected individuals) may also confer survival benefits in patients with COPD. Vasodilator agents used for IPAH could potentially be used in these patients, but the results of large clinical trials are not yet available.[121,123]

ROLE OF RESPIRATORY THERAPISTS IN PULMONARY VASCULAR DISEASE

Respiratory therapists (RTs) can play a key role in the diagnosis and management of patients with pulmonary vascular disease. An astute RT may help in diagnosing venous thromboembolism and pulmonary hypertension by recognizing the signs and symptoms of DVT and PE and pulmonary hypertension (e.g., acute onset of dyspnea, pleuritic pain, pedal edema). Communication with the managing physician to point out these findings and to suggest a work-up may prove lifesaving.

RTs may also play an important role in preventing and managing pulmonary vascular disease. Ensuring patients' compliance with vascular compression stockings can help prevent PE. RTs may also be members of teams that care for patients with pulmonary hypertension, as in performing right heart catheterization and in managing therapy (e.g., inhaled iloprost and treprostinil).

SUMMARY CHECKLIST

- Venous thromboembolism (DVT and PE) is an important cause of morbidity and mortality among hospitalized patients.
- Early recognition and treatment are essential and lifesaving. One-third of deaths caused by PE occur within 1 hour of symptom onset. The mortality rate in patients with PE that goes undiagnosed is 30%; if venous thrombosis is recognized and managed, the mortality rate is less than 8%.
- The point of origin of PE is DVT of the lower extremities or pelvis in 86% of cases.
- Most of the time, the clinical presentation of PE and DVT is nonspecific. A high index of suspicion is important to make the diagnosis in patients at risk.
- Prophylactic therapy reduces the risk of venous thromboembolism in patients who are at risk, but prophylactic therapy is underused.
- Pharmacologic choices for prophylaxis include low-dose subcutaneous heparin, warfarin, low-molecular-weight heparin, and dextran. Mechanical measures include early ambulation, wearing elastic stockings, pneumatic calf compression, and electrical stimulation of calf muscles.
- Management of venous thromboembolism includes anticoagulation therapy (heparin and warfarin).
- IPAH is a rare disease that mainly affects young adults. In IPAH, damage to the endothelium of the pulmonary artery alters the balance between vasoconstrictors and vasodilators, favoring vasoconstriction. Thrombosis and cellular proliferation are additional components in the pathogenesis of pulmonary hypertension.
- Management of IPAH includes anticoagulation and administration of vasodilators (calcium channel blockers, prostanoids, endothelin receptor antagonists, and PDE5 inhibitors). Lung transplantation is an option.

References

1. Silverstein MD, Heit JA, Mohr DN, et al: Trends in the incidence of deep vein thrombosis and pulmonary embolism: a 25-year population-based study. Arch Intern Med 158:585–593, 1998.
2. Rosenow EC, 3rd: Venous and pulmonary thromboembolism: an algorithmic approach to diagnosis and management. Mayo Clin Proc 70:45–49, 1995.
3. Horlander KT, Mannino DM, Leeper KV: Pulmonary embolism mortality in the United States, 1979-1998: an analysis using multiple-cause mortality data. Arch Intern Med 163:1711–1717, 2003.
4. Goldhaber SZ, Visani L, De Rosa M: Acute pulmonary embolism: clinical outcomes in the International Cooperative Pulmonary Embolism Registry (ICOPER). Lancet 353:1386–1389, 1999.
5. Nijkeuter M, Sohne M, Tick LW, et al: The natural course of hemodynamically stable pulmonary embolism: clinical outcome and risk factors in a large prospective cohort study. Chest 131:517–523, 2007.
6. Wagenvoort CA: Pathology of pulmonary thromboembolism. Chest 107(1 Suppl):10S–17S, 1995.
7. Sperry KL, Key CR, Anderson RE: Toward a population-based assessment of death due to pulmonary embolism in New Mexico. Hum Pathol 21:159–165, 1990.
8. Sandler DA, Martin JF: Autopsy proven pulmonary embolism in hospital patients: are we detecting enough deep vein thrombosis? J R Soc Med 82:203–205, 1989.
9. Morpurgo M, Schmid C: The spectrum of pulmonary embolism: clinicopathologic correlations. Chest 107(1 Suppl):18S–20S, 1995.
10. Dalen JE, Alpert JS: Natural history of pulmonary embolism. Prog Cardiovasc Dis 17:259–270, 1975.
11. Carson JL, Kelley MA, Duff A, et al: The clinical course of pulmonary embolism. N Engl J Med 326:1240–1245, 1992.
12. Heit JA, Silverstein MD, Mohr DN, et al: Predictors of survival after deep vein thrombosis and pulmonary embolism: a population-based, cohort study. Arch Intern Med 159:445–453, 1999.
13. Dalen JE: When can treatment be withheld in patients with suspected pulmonary embolism? Arch Intern Med 153:1415–1418, 1993.
14. Arroliga AC, Matthay M, Matthay R: Pulmonary thromboembolism and other pulmonary vascular diseases. In George RB, editor: Chest medicine: essentials of pulmonary and critical care medicine, ed 4, Philadelphia, 2000, Lippincott Williams & Wilkins.
15. Crowther MA, Kelton JG: Congenital thrombophilic states associated with venous thrombosis: a qualitative overview and proposed classification system. Ann Intern Med 138:128–134, 2003.

16. Goldhaber SZ: Risk factors for venous thromboembolism. J Am Coll Cardiol 56:1–7, 2010.
17. Haemostasis and Thrombosis Task Force, British Committee for Standards in Haematology: Investigation and management of heritable thrombophilia. Br J Haematol 114:512–528, 2001.
18. Girard P, Decousus M, Laporte S, et al: Diagnosis of pulmonary embolism in patients with proximal deep vein thrombosis: specificity of symptoms and perfusion defects at baseline and during anticoagulant therapy. Am J Respir Crit Care Med 164:1033–1037, 2001.
19. Riedel M: Acute pulmonary embolism, 1: pathophysiology, clinical presentation, and diagnosis. Heart 85:229–240, 2001.
20. Kucher N, Goldhaber SZ: Management of massive pulmonary embolism. Circulation 112:e28–e32, 2005.
21. Elliott CG: Pulmonary physiology during pulmonary embolism. Chest 101(4 Suppl):163S–171S, 1992.
22. Benotti JR, Dalen JE: The natural history of pulmonary embolism. Clin Chest Med 5:403–410, 1984.
23. Thomas D, Stein M, Tanabe G, et al: Mechanism of bronchoconstriction produced by thromboemboli in dogs. Am J Physiol 206:1207–1212, 1964.
24. Stein PD, Matta F, Musani MH, et al: Silent pulmonary embolism in patients with deep venous thrombosis: a systematic review. Am J Med 123:426–431, 2010.
25. Landefeld CS, McGuire E, Cohen AM: Clinical findings associated with acute proximal deep vein thrombosis: a basis for quantifying clinical judgment. Am J Med 88:382–388, 1990.
26. Stein PD, Beemath A, Matta F, et al: Clinical characteristics of patients with acute pulmonary embolism: data from PIOPED II. Am J Med 120:871–879, 2007.
27. Miniati M, Prediletto R, Formichi B, et al: Accuracy of clinical assessment in the diagnosis of pulmonary embolism. Am J Respir Crit Care Med 159:864–871, 1999.
28. Manganelli D, Palla A, Donnamaria V, et al: Clinical features of pulmonary embolism: doubts and certainties. Chest 107(1 Suppl):25S–32S, 1995.
29. Stein PD, Terrin ML, Hales CA, et al: Clinical, laboratory, roentgenographic, and electrocardiographic findings in patients with acute pulmonary embolism and no pre-existing cardiac or pulmonary disease. Chest 100:598–603, 1991.
30. Bates SM, Kearon C, Crowther M, et al: A diagnostic strategy involving a quantitative latex D-dimer assay reliably excludes deep venous thrombosis. Ann Intern Med 138:787–794, 2003.
31. Wells PS, Anderson DR, Rodger M, et al: Evaluation of D-dimer in the diagnosis of suspected deep-vein thrombosis. N Engl J Med 349:1227–1235, 2003.
32. Kearon C, Ginsberg JS, Douketis J, et al: A randomized trial of diagnostic strategies after normal proximal vein ultrasonography for suspected deep venous thrombosis: D-dimer testing compared with repeated ultrasonography. Ann Intern Med 142:490–496, 2005.
33. Stein PD, Hull RD, Patel KC, et al: D-dimer for the exclusion of acute venous thrombosis and pulmonary embolism: a systematic review. Ann Intern Med 140:589–602, 2004.
34. Tamariz LJ, Eng J, Segal JB, et al: Usefulness of clinical prediction rules for the diagnosis of venous thromboembolism: a systematic review. Am J Med 117:676–684, 2004.
35. Carrier M, Le Gal G, Bates SM, et al: D-dimer testing is useful to exclude deep vein thrombosis in elderly outpatients. J Thromb Haemost 6:1072–1076, 2008.
36. Stender MT, Frokjaer JB, Hagedorn Nielsen TS, et al: Combined use of clinical pre-test probability and D-dimer test in the diagnosis of preoperative deep venous thrombosis in colorectal cancer patients. Thromb Haemost 99:396–400, 2008.
37. Qaseem A, Snow V, Barry P, et al: Current diagnosis of venous thromboembolism in primary care: a clinical practice guideline from the American Academy of Family Physicians and the American College of Physicians. Ann Fam Med 5:57–62, 2007.
38. Hull R, Taylor DW, Hirsh J, et al: Impedance plethysmography: the relationship between venous filling and sensitivity and specificity for proximal vein thrombosis. Circulation 58:898–902, 1978.
39. Ginsberg JS, Wells PS, Hirsh J, et al: Reevaluation of the sensitivity of impedance plethysmography for the detection of proximal deep vein thrombosis. Arch Intern Med 154:1930–1933, 1994.
40. Cronan JJ: Venous thromboembolic disease: the role of US. Radiology 186:619–630, 1993.
41. Lensing AW, Prandoni P, Brandjes D, et al: Detection of deep-vein thrombosis by real-time B-mode ultrasonography. N Engl J Med 320:342–345, 1989.
42. Lensing AW, Doris CI, McGrath FP, et al: A comparison of compression ultrasound with color Doppler ultrasound for the diagnosis of symptomless postoperative deep vein thrombosis. Arch Intern Med 157:765–768, 1997.
43. Opinions regarding the diagnosis and management of venous thromboembolic disease. ACCP Consensus Committee on Pulmonary Embolism. American College of Chest Physicians. Chest 113:499–504, 1998.
44. ten Wolde M, Sohne M, Quak E, et al: Prognostic value of echocardiographically assessed right ventricular dysfunction in patients with pulmonary embolism. Arch Intern Med 164:1685–1689, 2004.
45. Worsley DF, Alavi A, Palevsky HI: Role of radionuclide imaging in patients with suspected pulmonary embolism. Radiol Clin North Am 31:849–858, 1993.
46. van Beek EJ, Kuyer PM, Schenk BE, et al: A normal perfusion lung scan in patients with clinically suspected pulmonary embolism: frequency and clinical validity. Chest 108:170–173, 1995.
47. Value of the ventilation/perfusion scan in acute pulmonary embolism. Results of the prospective investigation of pulmonary embolism diagnosis (PIOPED). The PIOPED Investigators. JAMA 263:2753–2759, 1990.
48. Stein PD, Coleman RE, Gottschalk A, et al: Diagnostic utility of ventilation/perfusion lung scans in acute pulmonary embolism is not diminished by pre-existing cardiac or pulmonary disease. Chest 100:604–606, 1991.
49. Henry JW, Stein PD, Gottschalk A, et al: Scintigraphic lung scans and clinical assessment in critically ill patients with suspected acute pulmonary embolism. Chest 109:462–466, 1996.
50. Hartmann IJ, Hagen PJ, Melissant CF, et al: Diagnosing acute pulmonary embolism: effect of chronic obstructive pulmonary disease on the performance of D-dimer testing, ventilation/perfusion scintigraphy, spiral computed tomographic angiography, and conventional angiography. ANTELOPE Study Group. Advances in New Technologies Evaluating the Localization of Pulmonary Embolism. Am J Respir Crit Care Med 162:2232–2237, 2000.
51. Stein PD, Woodard PK, Weg JG, et al: Diagnostic pathways in acute pulmonary embolism: recommendations of the PIOPED II investigators. Am J Med 119:1048–1055, 2006.
52. Perrier A, Nendaz MR, Sarasin FP, et al: Cost-effectiveness analysis of diagnostic strategies for suspected pulmonary embolism including helical computed tomography. Am J Respir Crit Care Med 167:39–44, 2003.

53. Perrier A, Roy PM, Sanchez O, et al: Multidetector-row computed tomography in suspected pulmonary embolism. N Engl J Med 352:1760–1768, 2005.
54. Rathbun SW, Raskob GE, Whitsett TL: Sensitivity and specificity of helical computed tomography in the diagnosis of pulmonary embolism: a systematic review. Ann Intern Med 132:227–232, 2000.
55. Stein PD, Fowler SE, Goodman LR, et al: Multidetector computed tomography for acute pulmonary embolism. N Engl J Med 354:2317–2327, 2006.
56. Wells PS, Ginsberg JS, Anderson DR, et al: Use of a clinical model for safe management of patients with suspected pulmonary embolism. Ann Intern Med 129:997–1005, 1998.
57. van Belle A, Buller HR, Huisman MV, et al: Effectiveness of managing suspected pulmonary embolism using an algorithm combining clinical probability, D-dimer testing, and computed tomography. JAMA 295:172–179, 2006.
58. Wells PS, Anderson DR, Rodger M, et al: Excluding pulmonary embolism at the bedside without diagnostic imaging: management of patients with suspected pulmonary embolism presenting to the emergency department by using a simple clinical model and D-dimer. Ann Intern Med 135: 98–107, 2001.
59. Jimenez D, Aujesky D, Diaz G, et al: Prognostic significance of deep vein thrombosis in patients presenting with acute symptomatic pulmonary embolism. Am J Respir Crit Care Med 181:983–991, 2010.
60. Kluge A, Luboldt W, Bachmann G: Acute pulmonary embolism to the subsegmental level: diagnostic accuracy of three MRI techniques compared with 16-MDCT. AJR Am J Roentgenol 187:W7–W14, 2006.
61. Tapson VF: Pulmonary embolism—new diagnostic approaches. N Engl J Med 336:1449–1451, 1997.
62. Geerts WH, Heit JA, Clagett GP, et al: Prevention of venous thromboembolism. Chest 119(1 Suppl):132S–175S, 2001.
63. Hirsch DR, Ingenito EP, Goldhaber SZ: Prevalence of deep venous thrombosis among patients in medical intensive care. JAMA 274:335–337, 1995.
64. Alikhan R, Cohen AT: Heparin for the prevention of venous thromboembolism in general medical patients (excluding stroke and myocardial infarction). Cochrane Database Syst Rev (3):CD003747, 2009.
65. King CS, Holley AB, Jackson JL, et al: Twice vs three times daily heparin dosing for thromboembolism prophylaxis in the general medical population: a metaanalysis. Chest 131:507–516, 2007.
66. Cohen AT, Davidson BL, Gallus AS, et al: Efficacy and safety of fondaparinux for the prevention of venous thromboembolism in older acute medical patients: randomised placebo controlled trial. BMJ 332:325–329, 2006.
67. Geerts WH, Bergqvist D, Pineo GF, et al: Prevention of venous thromboembolism. American College of Chest Physicians Evidence-Based Clinical Practice Guidelines (8th Edition). Chest 133(6 Suppl):381S–453S, 2008.
68. Snow V, Qaseem A, Barry P, et al: Management of venous thromboembolism: a clinical practice guideline from the American College of Physicians and the American Academy of Family Physicians. Ann Intern Med 146:204–210, 2007.
69. Hyers TM, Agnelli G, Hull RD, et al: Antithrombotic therapy for venous thromboembolic disease. Chest 119(1 Suppl): 176S–193S, 2001.
70. Raschke RA, Reilly BM, Guidry JR, et al: The weight-based heparin dosing nomogram compared with a "standard care" nomogram: a randomized controlled trial. Ann Intern Med 119:874–881, 1993.
71. Raschke RA, Gollihare B, Peirce JC: The effectiveness of implementing the weight-based heparin nomogram as a practice guideline. Arch Intern Med 156:1645–1649, 1996.
72. Kearon C, Kahn SR, Agnelli G, et al: Antithrombotic therapy for venous thromboembolic disease. American College of Chest Physicians Evidence-Based Clinical Practice Guidelines (8th Edition). Chest 133(6 Suppl):454S–545S, 2008.
73. Harrison L, Johnston M, Massicotte MP, et al: Comparison of 5-mg and 10-mg loading doses in initiation of warfarin therapy. Ann Intern Med 126:133–136, 1997.
74. Pinede L, Ninet J, Duhaut P, et al: Comparison of 3 and 6 months of oral anticoagulant therapy after a first episode of proximal deep vein thrombosis or pulmonary embolism and comparison of 6 and 12 weeks of therapy after isolated calf deep vein thrombosis. Circulation 103:2453–2460, 2001.
75. Watson LI, Armon MP: Thrombolysis for acute deep vein thrombosis. Cochrane Database Syst Rev (4):CD002783, 2004.
76. O'Meara JJ, 3rd, McNutt RA, Evans AT, et al: A decision analysis of streptokinase plus heparin as compared with heparin alone for deep-vein thrombosis. N Engl J Med 330:1864–1869, 1994.
77. Hull RD, Raskob GE, Brant RF, et al: Relation between the time to achieve the lower limit of the APTT therapeutic range and recurrent venous thromboembolism during heparin treatment for deep vein thrombosis. Arch Intern Med 157:2562–2568, 1997.
78. Tapson VF, Witty LA: Massive pulmonary embolism: diagnostic and therapeutic strategies. Clin Chest Med 16:329–340, 1995.
79. Goldhaber SZ: Contemporary pulmonary embolism thrombolysis. Chest 107(1 Suppl):45S–51S, 1995.
80. Decousus H, Leizorovicz A, Parent F, et al: A clinical trial of vena caval filters in the prevention of pulmonary embolism in patients with proximal deep-vein thrombosis. Prevention du Risque d'Embolie Pulmonaire par Interruption Cave Study Group. N Engl J Med 338:409–415, 1998.
81. Badesch DB, Champion HC, Sanchez MA, et al: Diagnosis and assessment of pulmonary arterial hypertension. J Am Coll Cardiol 54(1 Suppl):S55–S66, 2009.
82. Simonneau G, Robbins IM, Beghetti M, et al: Updated clinical classification of pulmonary hypertension. J Am Coll Cardiol 54(1 Suppl):S43–S54, 2009.
83. Farber HW, Loscalzo J: Pulmonary arterial hypertension. N Engl J Med 351:1655–1665, 2004.
84. Ghamra ZW, Dweik RA: Primary pulmonary hypertension: an overview of epidemiology and pathogenesis. Cleve Clin J Med 70(Suppl 1):S2–S8, 2003.
85. Fishman AP: Primary pulmonary arterial hypertension: a look back. J Am Coll Cardiol 43(12 Suppl S):2S–4S, 2004.
86. Arroliga AC, Dweik RA, Kaneko FJ, et al: Primary pulmonary hypertension: update on pathogenesis and novel therapies. Cleve Clin J Med 67:175–178, 2000.
87. Kline JA, Steuerwald MT, Marchick MR, et al: Prospective evaluation of right ventricular function and functional status 6 months after acute submassive pulmonary embolism: frequency of persistent or subsequent elevation in estimated pulmonary artery pressure. Chest 136:1202–1210, 2009.
88. Christman BW, McPherson CD, Newman JH, et al: An imbalance between the excretion of thromboxane and prostacyclin metabolites in pulmonary hypertension. N Engl J Med 327:70–75, 1992.
89. Giaid A, Yanagisawa M, Langleben D, et al: Expression of endothelin-1 in the lungs of patients with pulmonary hypertension. N Engl J Med 328:1732–1739, 1993.

90. Kaneko FT, Arroliga AC, Dweik RA, et al: Biochemical reaction products of nitric oxide as quantitative markers of primary pulmonary hypertension. Am J Respir Crit Care Med 158:917–923, 1998.
91. Rabinovitch M: Pulmonary hypertension: pathophysiology as a basis for clinical decision making. J Heart Lung Transplant 18:1041–1053, 1999.
92. Newman JH, Fanburg BL, Archer SL, et al: Pulmonary arterial hypertension: future directions: report of a National Heart, Lung and Blood Institute/Office of Rare Diseases workshop. Circulation 109:2947–2952, 2004.
93. Lepetit H, Eddahibi S, Fadel E, et al: Smooth muscle cell matrix metalloproteinases in idiopathic pulmonary arterial hypertension. Eur Respir J 25:834–842, 2005.
94. Petkov V, Mosgoeller W, Ziesche R, et al: Vasoactive intestinal peptide as a new drug for treatment of primary pulmonary hypertension. J Clin Invest 111:1339–1346, 2003.
95. Guignabert C, Izikki M, Tu LI, et al: Transgenic mice overexpressing the 5-hydroxytryptamine transporter gene in smooth muscle develop pulmonary hypertension. Circ Res 98:1323–1330, 2006.
96. Zaiman AL, Podowski M, Medicherla S, et al: Role of the TGF-beta/Alk5 signaling pathway in monocrotaline-induced pulmonary hypertension. Am J Respir Crit Care Med 177:896–905, 2008.
97. Morrell NW, Adnot S, Archer SL, et al: Cellular and molecular basis of pulmonary arterial hypertension. J Am Coll Cardiol 54(1 Suppl):S20–S31, 2009.
98. Erzurum S, Rounds SI, Stevens T, et al: Strategic plan for lung vascular research: An NHLBI-ORDR Workshop Report. Am J Respir Crit Care Med 182:1554–1562, 2010.
99. Kuhn KP, Byrne DW, Arbogast PG, et al: Outcome in 91 consecutive patients with pulmonary arterial hypertension receiving epoprostenol. Am J Respir Crit Care Med 167:580–586, 2003.
100. McLaughlin VV, Gaine SP, Barst RJ, et al: Efficacy and safety of treprostinil: an epoprostenol analog for primary pulmonary hypertension. J Cardiovasc Pharmacol 41:293–299, 2003.
101. Galie N, Ghofrani HA, Torbicki A, et al: Sildenafil citrate therapy for pulmonary arterial hypertension. N Engl J Med 353:2148–2157, 2005.
102. Channick RN, Simonneau G, Sitbon O, et al: Effects of the dual endothelin-receptor antagonist bosentan in patients with pulmonary hypertension: a randomised placebo-controlled study. Lancet 358:1119–1123, 2001.
103. Rubin LJ, Badesch DB: Evaluation and management of the patient with pulmonary arterial hypertension. Ann Intern Med 143:282–292, 2005.
104. Humbert M, Sitbon O, Simonneau G: Treatment of pulmonary arterial hypertension. N Engl J Med 351:1425–1436, 2004.
105. Johnson SR, Mehta S, Granton JT: Anticoagulation in pulmonary arterial hypertension: a qualitative systematic review. Eur Respir J 28:999–1004, 2006.
106. Tonelli AR, Alnuaimat H, Mubarak K: Pulmonary vasodilator testing and use of calcium channel blockers in pulmonary arterial hypertension. Respir Med 104:481–496, 2010.
107. Barst RJ, Rubin LJ, Long WA, et al: A comparison of continuous intravenous epoprostenol (prostacyclin) with conventional therapy for primary pulmonary hypertension. The Primary Pulmonary Hypertension Study Group. N Engl J Med 334:296–302, 1996.
108. Simonneau G, Barst RJ, Galie N, et al: Continuous subcutaneous infusion of treprostinil, a prostacyclin analogue, in patients with pulmonary arterial hypertension: a double-blind, randomized, placebo-controlled trial. Am J Respir Crit Care Med 165:800–804, 2002.
109. Tapson VF, Gomberg-Maitland M, McLaughlin VV, et al: Safety and efficacy of IV treprostinil for pulmonary arterial hypertension: a prospective, multicenter, open-label, 12-week trial. Chest 129:683–688, 2006.
110. Channick RN, Olschewski H, Seeger W, et al: Safety and efficacy of inhaled treprostinil as add-on therapy to bosentan in pulmonary arterial hypertension. J Am Coll Cardiol 48:1433–1437, 2006.
111. Olschewski H, Simonneau G, Galie N, et al: Inhaled iloprost for severe pulmonary hypertension. N Engl J Med 347:322–329, 2002.
112. Rubin LJ, Badesch DB, Barst RJ, et al: Bosentan therapy for pulmonary arterial hypertension. N Engl J Med 346:896–903, 2002.
113. Galie N, Olschewski H, Oudiz RJ, et al: Ambrisentan for the treatment of pulmonary arterial hypertension: results of the ambrisentan in pulmonary arterial hypertension, randomized, double-blind, placebo-controlled, multicenter, efficacy (ARIES) study 1 and 2. Circulation 117:3010–3019, 2008.
114. Oudiz RJ, Galie N, Olschewski H, et al: Long-term ambrisentan therapy for the treatment of pulmonary arterial hypertension. J Am Coll Cardiol 54:1971–1981, 2009.
115. Galie N, Brundage BH, Ghofrani HA, et al: Tadalafil therapy for pulmonary arterial hypertension. Circulation 119:2894–2903, 2009.
116. Ghofrani HA, Voswinckel R, Reichenberger F, et al: Differences in hemodynamic and oxygenation responses to three different phosphodiesterase-5 inhibitors in patients with pulmonary arterial hypertension: a randomized prospective study. J Am Coll Cardiol 44:1488–1496, 2004.
117. Klepetko W, Mayer E, Sandoval J, et al: Interventional and surgical modalities of treatment for pulmonary arterial hypertension. J Am Coll Cardiol 43(12 Suppl S):73S–80S, 2004.
118. Trulock EP: Lung and heart-lung transplantation: overview of results. Semin Respir Crit Care Med 22:479–488, 2001.
119. Matthay RA, Arroliga AC, Wiedemann HP, et al: Right ventricular function at rest and during exercise in chronic obstructive pulmonary disease. Chest 101(5 Suppl):255S–262S, 1992.
120. Weitzenblum E, Kessler R, Oswald M, et al: Medical treatment of pulmonary hypertension in chronic lung disease. Eur Respir J 7:148–152, 1994.
121. Higenbottam T: Pulmonary hypertension and chronic obstructive pulmonary disease: a case for treatment. Proc Am Thorac Soc 2:12–19, 2005.
122. Standards for the diagnosis and care of patients with chronic obstructive pulmonary disease. American Thoracic Society. Am J Respir Crit Care Med 152(5 Pt 2):S77–S121, 1995.
123. Weitzenblum E, Chaouat A, Canuet M, et al: Pulmonary hypertension in chronic obstructive pulmonary disease and interstitial lung diseases. Semin Respir Crit Care Med 30:458–470, 2009.

Chapter 27

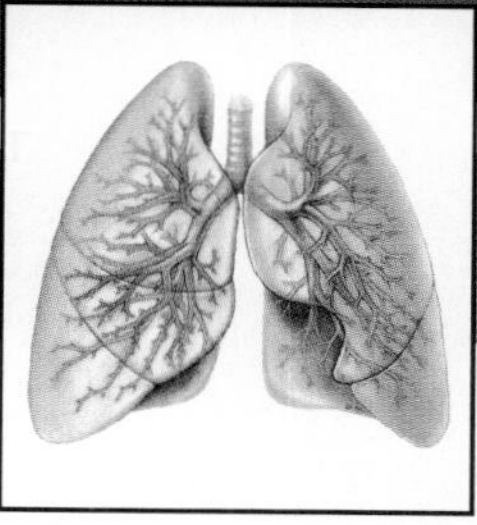

Acute Lung Injury, Pulmonary Edema, and Multiple System Organ Failure

ELLIOTT D. CROUSER, MATTHEW C. EXLINE, AND RUAIRI J. FAHY

CHAPTER OBJECTIVES

After reading this chapter you will be able to:

- Identify the approximate incidence rate of acute respiratory distress syndrome (ARDS) and how the mortality rate has changed over the past several decades.
- State the risk factors associated with the onset of ARDS.
- Describe how the normal lung prevents fluid from collecting in the parenchyma and how these mechanisms can fail and cause pulmonary edema.
- Describe the effect pulmonary edema has on lung function, including gas exchange and lung compliance.
- Describe the relationship between multiple organ dysfunction syndrome (MODS) and ARDS.
- Identify the histopathology associated with the exudative phase and the fibroproliferative phase of ARDS.
- Differentiate hydrostatic and nonhydrostatic pulmonary edema based on clinical setting.
- Describe the principles of supportive care followed for patients with ARDS.
- Describe how ventilator settings (e.g., tidal volume, positive end expiratory pressure, respiratory rate) are adjusted for patients with ARDS and MODS.
- Describe how mechanical ventilation can cause lung injury and how ventilator-induced lung injury can be avoided.
- State the approaches to the management of ARDS and MODS.
- Describe the use of innovative mechanical ventilation strategies in the support of patients with ARDS.
- State the effect of prone positioning on oxygenation and mortality in a patient with ARDS.
- Describe the value of pharmacologic therapies such as nitric oxide and corticosteroids in the treatment of patients with ARDS.

CHAPTER OUTLINE

KEY TERMS

acute lung injury (ALI)
acute respiratory distress syndrome (ARDS)
airway pressure release ventilation (APRV)
barotrauma
compliance
congestive heart failure (CHF)
extracorporeal carbon dioxide removal ($ECCO_2R$)
extracorporeal membrane oxygenation (ECMO)
high-frequency ventilation (HFV)
hydrostatic
hydrostatic pulmonary edema
lymphatic drainage system
multiple organ dysfunction syndrome (MODS)
nonhydrostatic pulmonary edema
positive end expiratory pressure (PEEP)
pulmonary edema
volume-controlled ventilation

Acute hypoxemic respiratory failure may develop in many clinical settings and is a common reason for admission to the intensive care unit (ICU). Most cases of acute hypoxemic respiratory failure develop as a result of abnormal accumulations of fluid within the lung parenchyma and alveoli. These accumulations are collectively referred to as **pulmonary edema.** Pulmonary edema may arise from acute illnesses associated with increased pulmonary venous pressure (hydrostatic pulmonary edema or **congestive heart failure [CHF]**) or may result from conditions associated with **acute lung injury (ALI),** in which the normal barriers to fluid movement within the lungs are disrupted (nonhydrostatic pulmonary edema). ALI of sufficient severity to cause acute hypoxemic respiratory failure is commonly referred to as **acute respiratory distress syndrome (ARDS).** ALI and ARDS represent a spectrum of lung injury with many patients initially presenting with *ALI* and progressing to *ARDS* with more severe gas exchange abnormalities (Table 27-1).[1,2]

The arbitrary dividing line between ALI and ARDS may have clinical relevance because patients with more severe lung injury often have simultaneous injury to other systemic organs. Acute illnesses associated with widespread systemic organ injury are referred to as **multiple organ dysfunction syndrome (MODS),** which is the most common cause of death in ICUs. ARDS is the pulmonary manifestation of MODS.

CHF and ARDS are distinct disease processes that require different management strategies. Failure to differentiate these two forms of pulmonary edema may delay appropriate therapy for the underlying disease, resulting in prolonged hospitalization and worse outcome. Because of similarities in clinical presentations, differentiating **hydrostatic** and nonhydrostatic pulmonary edema is often difficult for even the most skilled clinician.

This chapter initially focuses on the unique mechanisms responsible for acute respiratory failure caused by hydrostatic or nonhydrostatic (sometimes called *cardiogenic* and *noncardiogenic*) pulmonary edema. Emphasis is on identifying key clinical features that differentiate these two forms of respiratory failure. This discussion sets the stage for a better understanding of the established principles of supportive care and of the rationale behind innovative treatments of patients with ARDS and MODS.

EPIDEMIOLOGY

ARDS is a common cause of respiratory failure. It can occur as a consequence of critical illnesses of diverse causes. The exact incidence of ARDS varies depending on the population being studied, but in the United States it is thought to range from 13.5 to 64 cases per 100,000 person-years.[3,4] ARDS may be present in 16% of mechanically ventilated patients on admission to the ICU.[2] Despite uncertainties regarding the incidence of ARDS, the mortality rate associated with ARDS has seemed to decline over the past 3 decades from more than 90% to the present level of 30% to 40%.[5,6]

The explanation for this favorable trend is likely multifactorial and includes advances in supportive care, early detection, effective management of comorbid diseases such as nosocomial infection, and the broad application

TABLE 27-1

Recommended Criteria for Acute Lung Injury (ALI) and Acute Respiratory Distress Syndrome (ARDS)

Criteria Pressure	Timing	Oxygenation	Chest Radiograph	Pulmonary Artery Wedge
ALI	Acute onset	$PaO_2/FiO_2 \leq 300$ mm Hg (regardless of PEEP level)	Bilateral infiltrates seen on frontal chest radiograph	≤18 mm Hg when measured or no clinical evidence of left atrial hypertension
ARDS	Acute onset	$PaO_2/FiO_2 \leq 200$ mm Hg (regardless of PEEP level)	Bilateral infiltrates seen on frontal chest radiograph	≤18 mm Hg when measured or no clinical evidence of left atrial hypertension

Modified from Bernard GR, Artigas A, Brigham KL, et al: The American-European Consensus Conference on ARDS. Definitions, mechanisms, relevant outcomes, and clinical trial coordination. Am J Respir Crit Care Med 49(3 Pt 1):818-824, 1994.

Box 27-1 Risk Factors for Acute Lung Injury and Acute Respiratory Distress Syndrome

DIRECT INJURY
- Pneumonia (viral, bacterial, fungal)
- Gastric aspiration
- Toxic inhalation (phosgene, cocaine, smoke, high concentration of O_2)
- Near-drowning
- Lung contusion

INDIRECT INJURY
- Sepsis
- Burn injury (chemical or heat-induced)
- Prolonged systemic hypotension and shock
- Multiple trauma
- Pancreatitis
- Gynecologic (abruptio placentae, amniotic embolism, eclampsia)
- Drug effect (salicylates, thiazides, others)
- Fulminant hepatic failure
- Sickle cell crisis
- Multiple drug transfusions

of innovative mechanical ventilation techniques. However, the cumulative cost of ARDS and MODS in terms of both human lives and medical resource use remains unacceptably high. The medical community awaits the results of ongoing investigations that may provide insight into the pathogenesis and management of ARDS.

RISK FACTORS FOR ACUTE RESPIRATORY DISTRESS SYNDROME

It has been proposed that ARDS can develop via different mechanisms and that the risk factors for ARDS should be categorized as either direct injury via damage directly to the alveolar space or indirect injury initiated by systemic disease (Box 27-1).[1] However, all of these risk factors share the common ability to initiate a systemic inflammatory reaction, which, if sufficiently vigorous, may lead to diffuse lung injury (ARDS). In this regard, the probability of developing ARDS may depend in part on the severity and characteristics of the initial injury. Gastric aspiration and septic shock (sepsis with refractory hypotension) are associated with a greater than 25% risk of ARDS, whereas the administration of multiple blood transfusions is associated with an ARDS risk of less than 5%.[7] The risk of ARDS seems to be additive when multiple risk factors are present.[8]

PATHOPHYSIOLOGY

Normal Physiology

The lung structure is optimally designed to fulfill its physiologic functions. These are as follows:
- To deliver inhaled oxygen (O_2) to the site of gas exchange—the alveoli
- To diffuse gases, mainly O_2 and carbon dioxide (CO_2), between the alveolar capillary membrane and the lumen of the alveolus
- To match alveolar ventilation with pulmonary capillary blood flow so that gas exchange is optimized
- To maintain a net flux of fluid through the lung parenchyma without inducing lung edema or alveolar consolidation
- To provide a barrier against toxic environmental exposures, including infectious agents, dusts, and fumes

For optimization of gas exchange, the entire cardiac output passes through the vascular system of the lungs. Gas exchange primarily occurs through the extensive capillary network surrounding the alveolar airspaces. The entire surface of alveolar walls is in close approximation to pulmonary capillaries. The diffusion distances between inspired gases and capillary blood are very small (<0.5 μ). Diffusion of gases at the alveolar-capillary interface depends on the relative concentrations of gases in the inspired air and in the blood. There is net diffusion of O_2 from the alveolus into the blood, whereas CO_2 diffuses from the blood to the alveolus. These diffusion gradients are constantly renewed by provision of deoxygenated and CO_2-rich blood from the systemic circulation to the lungs and by ventilation of the lungs with oxygenated, CO_2-depleted air. In this way, the heart and lungs are vitally linked.

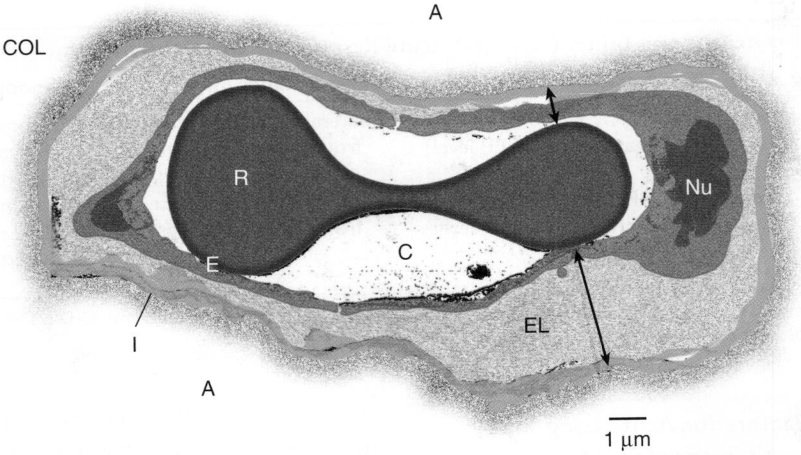

FIGURE 27-1 Cross section of an alveolar wall shows the path for O_2 and CO_2 diffusion. The thin side of the alveolar wall barrier *(short double arrow)* consists of type I epithelium *(I)*, interstitium formed by the fused basal laminae of the epithelial and endothelial cells, capillary endothelium *(E)*, plasma in the alveolar capillary *(C)*, and the cytoplasm of the red blood cell *(R)*. The thick side of the gas exchange barrier *(long double arrow)* has an accumulation of elastin *(EL)*, collagen *(COL)*, and matrix that separates the alveolar epithelium from the alveolar capillary endothelium. As long as the red blood cells are flowing, O_2 and CO_2 diffusion probably occur across both sides of the air-blood barrier. *A,* Alveolus; *Nu,* nucleus of the capillary endothelial cell. (Human lung surgical specimen, transmission electron photomicrograph.)

Pulmonary Blood Flow

The intricate design of the pulmonary circulation provides for the efficient transfer of gases between the alveoli and the blood. On average, the entire blood volume of the body circulates through the lungs in 1 minute or less. This incredible feat is achieved through an ingenious design. Starting at the outflow tract of the right ventricle (pulmonary valve), the relatively thick-walled, smooth muscle–lined pulmonary artery branches successively and follows the divisions of the bronchi as far as the terminal bronchioles. Beyond the terminal bronchioles, the pulmonary vasculature divides further to form a fine capillary meshwork surrounding the alveoli. The large surface area of the capillary network provides for a low-pressure (5 to 12 mm Hg), high-volume system wherein large volumes of blood come into immediate contact with alveolar gases. At a capillary level, the vessel walls are composed solely of endothelial cells bound to a basal lamina. Because of the delicate nature of the alveolar-capillary interface, injury to the alveolar-capillary interface and high capillary blood pressure result in disruption of pulmonary gas exchange (see later section on Pulmonary Edema).

Lung Interstitium

The interstitial space of the lung is the space between the alveolar epithelium and the capillaries. The interstitium is composed of several structural proteins (types I, III, and IV collagen and elastin) and proteoglycans. The proteoglycans make up the ground substance of the interstitium and are composed of 20% protein and 80% glycosaminoglycans. The alveolar-capillary interstitial space is composed of endothelial and epithelial cell membranes bound to a common basement membrane with a very thin (<0.5 μ) interstitial space. In contrast, the interstitium on the nonalveolar side of the capillaries contains separate basement membranes for both epithelial cells and endothelial cells and fibroblasts, structural collagen, elastin proteins, and mucopolysaccharides in a hyaluronic acid gel (Figure 27-1).

The physical properties of the matrix allow absorption of water into the interstitial space without an increase in hydrostatic pressure and without an effect on pulmonary gas exchange. The interstitium is highly compliant under normal circumstances (large increases in fluid volume produce little change in interstitial pressure). However, the **compliance** of the interstitium dramatically decreases when the interstitial space becomes saturated. This phenomenon has important implications with respect to protecting against pulmonary edema.

Liquid and Solute Transport in the Lungs

The alveolar capillaries are selectively permeable to protein and are consequently "leaky." This capillary porosity allows movement of solutes between the intravascular space and the interstitium of the lungs. The net exchange of fluids between the intravascular space and the interstitium of the lungs is determined by the combined influences of hydrostatic and osmotic forces. The relationship between these two forces is described by the Starling equation:

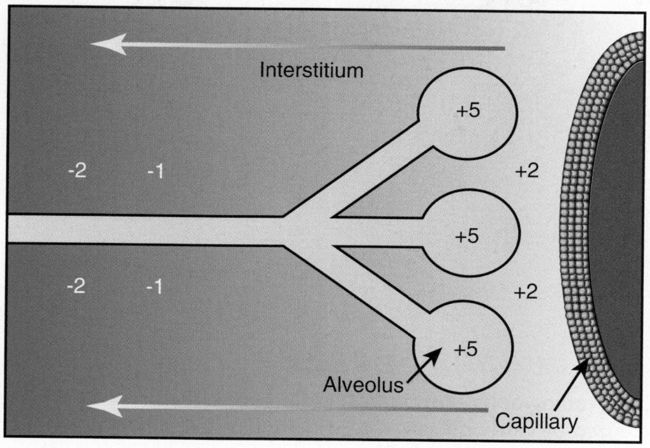

FIGURE 27-2 Relative hydrostatic pressures (in cm H_2O) that typically exist within the various compartments of the lung. Hydrostatic forces favor the movement of fluid along the pressure gradient *(arrows)* between the alveolar and pericapillary spaces and pulmonary lymphatic vessels. This hydrostatic pressure gradient favors the movement of fluid away from the alveolar capillary interface and protects against alveolar and interstitial edema formation.

$$Q_f = K_{fc}[(P_{mv} - P_i) - (s_d)(TT_{mv} - TT_i)]$$

where Q_f is net fluid filtration, K_{fc} is the capillary filtration coefficient (permeability constant) of the microvascular endothelium, P_{mv} is microvascular hydrostatic pressure, P_i is interstitial hydrostatic pressure, s_d is average osmotic reflection coefficient, TT_{mv} is microvascular osmotic pressure, and TT_i is interstitial osmotic pressure.

Under normal conditions, forces influencing the movement of fluid from the bloodstream to the interstitium of the lungs ($P_{mv} + TT_i$) are slightly greater than forces opposing this movement ($TT_{mv} + P_i$). Consequently, as fluid and proteins move from the vascular space into the interstitium, a small fraction of the cardiac output (approximately 0.01%) normally filters through the interstitium of the lungs. This filtration process plays a role in the immune defenses of the lung and is a major determinant of total lung fluid content.

The lung protects itself from the devastating consequences of excessive fluid accumulation by several mechanisms. The lung **lymphatic drainage system** is the primary operant system under nonpathologic conditions. The lymphatic drainage system is the main conduit for the removal of filtered fluid and protein from the lungs. Fluid and solutes enter the lymphatic drainage channels from small lymphatic capillaries located around the respiratory bronchioles. This process is assisted by the presence of a modest pressure gradient within the lungs. That is, pressure is greatest within the dense alveolar interstitium and gradually decreases in the nonalveolar interstitium and terminal lymphatic vessels (Figure 27-2). Drainage is enhanced further by intrathoracic pressure alterations that occur with respiration, and retrograde flow is prevented by the presence of one-way lymphatic valves. Ultimately, lymphatic fluid drains into the superior vena cava through the thoracic duct.[9]

When fluid filtration exceeds the capacity for drainage through pulmonary lymphatic vessels, several "backup" systems exist for storing additional fluid and for protection against alveolar flooding. Loose connective tissue located along the peribronchovascular space and extending to the level of the bronchiole is capable of storing twice the normal fluid content of the lungs.[9] Filling of these spaces or cuffs manifests radiographically as increased interstitial infiltrates (Figure 27-3), or Kerley's lines, which are caused by increased fluid in interlobular septal spaces. The peribronchovascular spaces drain into the local blood vessels or follow the intrinsic pressure gradient in the lung and empty into pulmonary lymphatic vessels. As total lung fluid accumulation increases further, the gel-like matrix of the lung is capable of absorbing additional fluid without affecting interstitial pressure. The latter property is important because fluid is allowed to accumulate in the lungs without transmitting additional hydrostatic pressure to

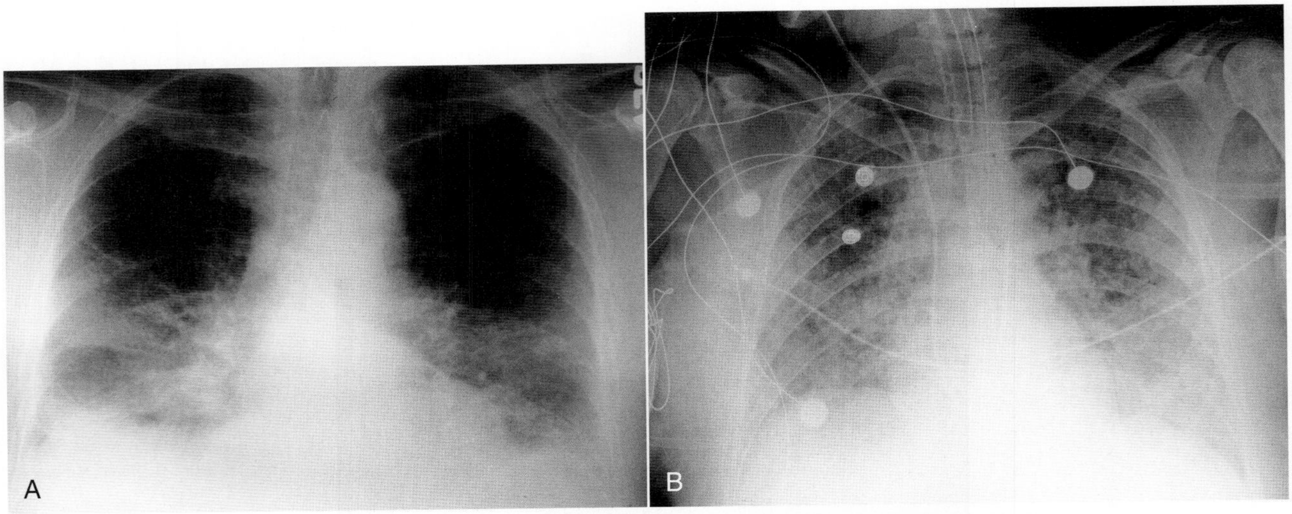

FIGURE 27-3 Chest radiographs show typical radiographic features of CHF and ARDS. **A,** CHF is characterized by cardiomegaly, interstitial infiltrates, bilateral perihilar and basilar alveolar infiltrates, and bilateral pleural effusions, which cause blunting of the costophrenic angles. **B,** ARDS is commonly associated with normal cardiac size, diffuse peripheral alveolar infiltrates, and minimal or absent pleural effusions.

the alveolar barrier. Additional fluid movement into the lungs is avoided. The dense connective tissue making up the alveolar matrix resists edema formation in response to elevated hydrostatic or oncotic pressure.

Pulmonary Edema

Despite these protective mechanisms, in certain disease states, fluid flux into the lungs exceeds the capacity of the lung to remove or store the fluid. Under such circumstances, small increases in lung fluid content produce large increases in interstitial hydrostatic pressure. The result is *alveolar flooding (pulmonary edema).* This pulmonary edema can be due to increased vascular hydrostatic pressure—**hydrostatic pulmonary edema**—or loss of the endothelial membrane integrity—**nonhydrostatic pulmonary edema.** Impaired gas exchange in the setting of pulmonary edema is complicated further by an increase in the work of breathing caused by dramatic reductions in lung compliance resulting from alveolar collapse and interstitial fluid accumulation. This scenario commonly results in acute respiratory failure.

Hydrostatic Pulmonary Edema

Hydrostatic pulmonary edema, also called *cardiogenic pulmonary edema,* is the result of increased venous hydrostatic pressure leading to fluid accumulation and alveolar flooding. The alveolar barrier is composed of the dense alveolar matrix (described earlier), the epithelial basement membrane, and the lining epithelial cells. The alveolar basement membrane is selectively permeable to only very small solutes such that osmotic forces favor the retention of fluid in the intravascular space. Alveolar pressure generally is slightly higher than interstitial pressure, and this difference provides further protection against alveolar fluid accumulation (see Figure 27-2). Under normal circumstances, there is little fluid movement into the alveoli across the alveolar barrier. Fluid that does form is composed of low-molecular-weight proteins and is actively transported back into the interstitium by type II pneumocytes.[10] In contrast, when the vascular hydrostatic pressure increases and overwhelms the defense mechanisms against fluid accumulation in the lung, hydrostatic pressure increases sharply within the interstitium of the lung, and alveolar flooding ensues. The precise mechanism of alveolar flooding in hydrostatic pulmonary edema is unknown. It has been shown, however, that alveolar flooding occurs in an "all-or-none" manner. The alveolar fluid formed in the setting of increased hydrostatic pressure has characteristics identical to interstitial fluid even though the alveolar epithelium is normally impermeable to large proteins and molecules.[9] This observation lends support to the findings of Conhaim,[11] who showed experimentally that high interstitial fluid pressure leads to alveolar flooding through leakage of fluid from the epithelium of respiratory bronchioles, alveolar ducts, and their associated alveoli. The epithelium of the respiratory bronchioles and alveolar ducts may be particularly prone to hydrostatic injury because these locations represent the transition zone between respiratory and alveolar epithelium.

Nonhydrostatic Pulmonary Edema

Nonhydrostatic pulmonary edema, also called *noncardiogenic pulmonary edema,* is the result of the loss of microvascular membrane integrity. In contrast to hydrostatic pulmonary edema, nonhydrostatic pulmonary edema is associated with increased total lung water despite normal microvascular hydrostatic pressure. The mechanisms of nonhydrostatic pulmonary edema that ultimately lead to

ARDS are more complex than the mechanisms responsible for hydrostatic pulmonary edema. Although many seemingly unrelated risk factors for ARDS have been identified, all causes of ARDS evoke disruption of endothelial and epithelial barriers and typically occur under conditions associated with widespread microvascular injury to the lungs. Vascular endothelial injury in the lungs results in increased microvascular permeability and fluid filtration, such that there is uninhibited entry of protein-rich fluid into the pulmonary interstitium. Alveolar flooding develops when the osmotic gradient between the capillary and the lung becomes essentially zero and no longer opposes the hydrostatic forces favoring fluid movement from the capillary into the lung: $K_{fc}(P_{mv} - P_i) >> (s_d)(TT_{mv} - T_{ti})$ (see earlier equation). This process is likely facilitated both by damage to the normally impermeable alveolar epithelial barrier, which is a key feature of ARDS,[12] and by impaired alveolar fluid clearance in ALI and ARDS.[13] Investigations support a role for both necrotic epithelial cell death and programmed cell death (apoptosis) in the pathogenesis of alveolar wall damage.[14,15] In addition, therapies aimed at improving the vascular barrier to fluid movement have shown protection against ALI animal models.

Nonhydrostatic pulmonary edema is caused by the loss of the normal osmotic gradient that normally opposes fluid movement into the lungs. Fluid accumulation in the lung is further amplified by impaired pulmonary fluid clearance and in the presence of higher hydrostatic pressures (i.e., pulmonary capillary pressure).

A common mechanism to explain how different acute illnesses (e.g., sepsis, gastric acid aspiration, pancreatitis) can lead to the development of ARDS was proposed by Weiland and colleagues.[16] These investigators showed that ARDS, regardless of the cause, is associated with an influx of polymorphonuclear neutrophils (PMNs) and PMN-derived inflammatory by-products, such as neutrophil elastase and myeloperoxidase, into the lung. The PMN-activating cytokine interleukin (IL)-8 has been shown to be increased in the lungs of patients with ARDS, whereas a reduction in IL-8 and PMNs has been shown to correlate with recovery from ARDS.[17] Taken together, the results of these studies suggest that the common mechanism for the development of ARDS is induction of lung inflammation leading to loss of membrane integrity, as a result of either local lung injury (direct injury) or systemic inflammation (indirect injury).

Although PMNs play a central role in the development of ARDS, other chemical (e.g., gastric aspiration) and immunologic pathways participate in the initiation and development of the systemic inflammatory response to critical illnesses associated with ARDS. Sepsis is associated with intense activation of systemic inflammatory pathways such that cytokines (e.g., tumor necrosis factor [TNF]-alpha, IL-1beta, IL-6, and IL-8), arachidonic acid metabolites (e.g., platelet-activating factor, leukotrienes), and nitric oxide (NO) all contribute to the hemodynamic and inflammatory events characteristic of this syndrome.[18] The relative contributions and exact roles of these proinflammatory mediators in the pathogenesis of ARDS and MODS remain a topic of intense investigation and controversy.[19,20] It is likely that there is no single dominant pathway in the development of ARDS because attempts to control the inflammatory response in sepsis by blocking specific mediators, such as anti-TNF antibodies, have not proved beneficial and may worsen outcome.

Gas Exchange and Lung Mechanics in Acute Respiratory Distress Syndrome

ARDS is associated with restrictive physiology and refractory hypoxemia, which are largely a result of pulmonary microvascular injury. Specifically, increased pulmonary capillary permeability facilitates the influx of inflammatory fluid into the lung interstitium and alveolar spaces and causes decreased lung compliance and alveolar consolidation. The presence of intraalveolar inflammatory fluid impairs surfactant synthesis and function so that pulmonary gas exchange (i.e., related to atelectasis) and compliance are further impaired. The negative effects of alveolar consolidation and atelectasis on pulmonary gas exchange are exacerbated by a loss of the normal vascular response to alveolar hypoxemia. The body is unable to shunt blood away from the diseased alveoli, and these unaerated alveoli receive excessive blood flow, which contributes to severe ventilation/perfusion mismatching and an effective intrapulmonary right-to-left shunting of blood flow in ARDS. The pulmonary manifestations of ARDS and CHF are summarized in Box 27-2.

Role of Organ-Organ Interactions in the Pathogenesis of Acute Respiratory Distress Syndrome and Multiple Organ Dysfunction Syndrome

The notion that factors operating outside the lungs may participate in the initiation and progression of ARDS has generated interest in the role of organ system interactions in the pathogenesis of ARDS and MODS. For example, injury to remote systemic organs is known to occur after ALI,[21] apparently related to PMN-mediated mechanisms.[22] In this way, ALI may perpetuate the systemic inflammatory response and lead to further lung and systemic organ injury. The gut-liver-lung axis may be most influential in causing the systemic inflammatory response associated with ARDS and MODS. The gastrointestinal (GI) tract contains large quantities of potentially pathogenic bacteria against which the host is normally protected by intact mucosal barriers and the reticuloendothelial system. However, the function of the GI tract and the liver is frequently compromised in critical illness. The widespread use of broad-spectrum antibiotics in the care of critically ill patients often leads to overgrowth of antibiotic-resistant

Box 27-2 Clinical Features of Congestive Heart Failure and Acute Respiratory Distress Syndrome

FEATURES COMMON TO CHF AND ARDS
- Symptoms of anxiety, dyspnea, tachypnea
- Reduced lung volumes and decreased compliance
- Arterial blood gases initially show respiratory alkalosis and arterial hypoxemia
- Chest radiograph shows diffuse alveolar and interstitial infiltrates

FEATURES FAVORING CHF
- Clinical history suggestive of CHF (see Box 27-1)
- Cardiomegaly or pleural effusions on chest radiograph (see Figure 27-3)
- PCWP > 18 mm Hg
- BALF nonproteinaceous and noninflammatory

FEATURES FAVORING ARDS
- Clinical history of risk factors for ARDS (see Table 27-1)
- Peripheral infiltrates on chest radiograph (see Figure 27-3)
- PCWP > 18 mm Hg
- BALF proteinaceous and inflammatory
- Pathologic examination shows diffuse alveolar damage, type II pneumocyte hyperplasia with or without fibrosis
- Ratio of $PaO_2/FiO_2 < 200$*

BALF, Bronchoalveolar lavage fluid.
*Impaired oxygenation is characteristic of ARDS. By definition, ARDS and ALI are distinguished by the ratio of PaO_2 to FiO_2. In ARDS, this ratio is <200, and in ALI, the ratio is <300.

bacteria within the GI tract. These bacteria and their toxic by-products (e.g., endotoxin) escape from the GI tract and are taken up by the reticuloendothelial cells of the liver, spleen, and regional lymph nodes. The resultant activation of the reticuloendothelial system may initiate and perpetuate a systemic inflammatory response that leads to systemic organ injury (i.e., ARDS and MODS).[23] This sequence of events forms the basis for strategies designed to reduce the release of proinflammatory mediators from the GI tract, including selective decontamination, early enteral feeding, and other approaches designed to moderate the systemic inflammatory response in ARDS and MODS (see later section on Therapeutic Approach to Acute Respiratory Distress Syndrome).

Why ARDS and MODS develop in some patients with ALI and not in others is unknown. The determinants of ARDS may relate to the balance between proinflammatory and antiinflammatory factors within the body. In this regard, the liver plays a major role in both induction and *modulation* of the systemic inflammatory response to all kinds of initiating events and is primarily responsible for the breakdown of endogenous proinflammatory mediators, including TNF-alpha, leukotrienes, and others.[24] Patients with liver disease have higher levels of circulating proinflammatory mediators, are more prone to bacteremia, and have a high incidence of ARDS compared with patients without liver disease.[25]

The liver is not the sole determinant of ARDS and MODS in critically ill patients. Other factors, such as the severity of the primary illness and comorbid diseases (e.g., cardiac disease, advanced age, renal failure, malignant disease) and perhaps the genetic profile of the patient, also seem to predispose patients to ARDS and MODS.[23,26]

HISTOPATHOLOGY AND CLINICAL CORRELATES OF ACUTE RESPIRATORY DISTRESS SYNDROME

Exudative Phase (1 to 3 Days)

The exudative phase is characterized by diffuse damage to alveoli and blood vessels and the influx of inflammatory cells into the interstitium. Many of the alveolar spaces become filled with a proteinaceous, eosinophilic (on hematoxylin and eosin stain) material called *hyaline membranes,* which are composed of cellular debris and condensed plasma proteins. Pathologically, there is destruction of type I pneumocytes, which are normally the predominant cells lining the alveoli; type II pneumocytes are relatively resistant to injury.[27,28] Patients with ARDS have profound dyspnea, tachypnea, and refractory hypoxemia. This phase of ARDS often is difficult to differentiate from respiratory failure related to hydrostatic pulmonary edema (CHF). The clinical presentations of these two forms of acute respiratory failure are discussed later (see the section on Differentiating Hydrostatic from Nonhydrostatic Pulmonary Edema in the Clinical Setting). The exudative phase may be self-limited or may progress to a fibroproliferative phase.

RULE OF THUMB

A careful history and physical examination often are the most useful means by which CHF and ARDS can be initially differentiated in a patient who has refractory hypoxemia and bilateral infiltrates on chest radiographs. A history consistent with one of the common causes of CHF (Box 27-3) combined with physical examination findings of jugular venous distention, cardiac murmurs or gallops, bibasilar crackles, or peripheral edema suggests a diagnosis of CHF. ARDS is more likely when the history is positive for one of the established risk factors (see Box 27-1) and there is no clinical evidence in support of CHF.

Fibroproliferative Phase (3 to 7 Days)

After inflammatory injury to the lung is established and the initiating events are controlled, a process of lung repair begins. Pathologically, there is hyperplasia of alveolar type

II pneumocytes and proliferation of fibroblasts within the alveolar basement membrane and intraalveolar spaces. Fibroblasts mediate the formation of intraalveolar and interstitial fibrosis.[27] The extent of fibrosis determines the degree of pulmonary disability in patients who survive ARDS.

The exact mechanisms controlling lung remodeling in ALI are not well established but very likely involve by-products of inflammatory cells (e.g., proteases, antiproteases, IL-6) and various growth factors (transforming growth factor [TGF]-alpha, TGF-beta).[29,30] However, the remodeling process after ARDS is quite variable. In some cases, patients have nearly complete normalization of lung compliance and oxygenation for 6 to 12 months after the illness. In other cases, the architecture of the lung never returns to normal, and patients experience severe respiratory disability related to extensive pulmonary fibrosis and obliteration of the pulmonary vasculature. The pattern of fibrosis after ALI suggests that, as in repair of the skin, an intact basement membrane is necessary for normal repair of the epithelium of the alveoli. It follows that disruption of the alveolar basement membrane is a prerequisite to the development of fibrosis after ALI. This line of reasoning is supported by the observation that the extent of recovery depends on the severity of the initial lung injury and on the influence of secondary forms of injury. Secondary forms of lung injury include nosocomial infection, O_2 toxicity, and **barotrauma** (see later section on Therapeutic Approach to Acute Respiratory Distress Syndrome).

Differentiating Hydrostatic from Nonhydrostatic Pulmonary Edema in the Clinical Setting

The diagnostic criteria for ARDS are shown in Table 27-1. However, despite the existence of distinct pathophysiologic mechanisms of hydrostatic and nonhydrostatic pulmonary edema, differentiating these two forms of acute respiratory failure may be difficult because of similarities in their early clinical presentations. CHF is more common than ARDS and should be considered when any patient has pulmonary edema, in particular, when the history and physical examination findings suggest one of the causes of CHF listed in Box 27-3. Alveolar flooding by either hydrostatic or nonhydrostatic mechanisms results in diffuse radiographic infiltrates, altered gas exchange, and abnormal mechanical properties of the lung (see Box 27-2). A clinical history of infection, recent trauma, or risk factors for aspiration may be present in either patient group. Likewise, many patients with ARDS are older and have preexisting illnesses that place them at risk of CHF. In patients with acute hypoxemic respiratory failure, CHF must always be considered, even when the patient has obvious risk factors for ARDS.

Box 27-3 Common Causes of Hydrostatic Pulmonary Edema

CARDIAC
- Left ventricular failure (e.g., myocardial infarction, myocarditis)
- Cardiac valvular disease (aortic, mitral)

VASCULAR
- Systemic hypertension
- Pulmonary embolism

VOLUME OVERLOAD
- Excessive fluid administration
- Renal failure

The ability to discern CHF and ARDS solely on the basis of radiographic findings is difficult and is complicated by technical limitations associated with obtaining chest radiographs in the ICU. Both CHF and ARDS are characterized by diffuse alveolar infiltrates prevalent in dependent lung zones. CHF is more often associated with cardiomegaly and the presence of perihilar infiltrates and pleural effusions. ARDS is more often associated with the presence of peripheral alveolar infiltrates, air bronchograms, sparing of the costophrenic angles, and normal cardiac size. However, cardiac size may be difficult to interpret on an anteroposterior chest x-ray, and when images are obtained with the patient in the supine position, pleural effusions may be obscured. Consequently, the hallmark radiographic distinctions between CHF and ARDS are often invisible to the clinician, a situation further complicated by the occasional coexistence of both hydrostatic and nonhydrostatic pulmonary edema.

Alveolar flooding of any cause (i.e., hydrostatic or nonhydrostatic) is associated with impaired gas exchange and abnormal lung mechanics. Both CHF and early ARDS (exudative phase) are associated with interstitial and alveolar accumulation of fluid. As a result of ventilation/perfusion mismatching and shunt accompanying this fluid accumulation, arterial hypoxemia develops. Patients with interstitial and alveolar edema of any cause use a higher fraction (25% to 50%) of their total metabolic output to support the increased work of breathing attendant to reduced lung compliance and higher ventilatory rates. However, on the basis of gas exchange and lung mechanics alone, alveolar flooding related to hydrostatic causes may be indistinguishable from alveolar flooding related to nonhydrostatic causes.

In many cases, measurement of hemodynamic variables is necessary to determine whether hydrostatic or nonhydrostatic forces underlie the development of acute hypoxemic respiratory failure. To this end, a pulmonary artery (Swan-Ganz) catheter is a useful clinical tool because it allows estimation of clinically relevant data, such as cardiac output and pulmonary capillary wedge pressure

(PCWP), also called *pulmonary artery occlusion pressure.* Under ideal circumstances, PCWP closely corresponds to left ventricular end-diastolic pressure and is a reflection of the hydrostatic forces applied to the pulmonary capillary system. In this regard, PCWP greater than 18 mm Hg is necessary for the development of hydrostatic pulmonary edema. Conversely, alveolar flooding resulting from nonhydrostatic pulmonary edema can occur at any PCWP and is the exclusive cause of pulmonary edema at PCWP less than 18 mm Hg.

Invasive hemodynamic monitoring may be unreliable in patients with high airway pressure. In particular, high levels of **positive end expiratory pressure (PEEP)** lead to expansion of non-zone 3 lung areas in which alveolar pressure exceeds venous pressure. PCWP measured in non-zone 3 lung reflects alveolar pressure and not left ventricular pressure.[31] Hydrostatic forces may be overestimated or misdiagnosed in ARDS as hydrostatic pulmonary edema. These confounding variables may lead to misinterpretation of the hemodynamic status of the patient, resulting in mismanagement of his or her condition, and could explain why the routine use of pulmonary artery catheters in patients with ARDS is not beneficial.[32] A similar estimate of pulmonary capillary hydrostatic pressure may be obtained via central venous pressure (CVP) obtained from a central line placed in the superior vena cava. CVP is less technically difficult to obtain and interpret compared with PCWP; in a large clinical trial, therapy guided by CVP estimation of the patient's volume status was equivalent to therapy guided by PCWP.[33]

Another useful method of separating nonhydrostatic from hydrostatic pulmonary edema is based on differences in the characteristics of the edema fluid. As previously discussed (see the section on Pathophysiology), ARDS is associated with inflammatory injury to the pulmonary microvasculature, which allows the influx of inflammatory cells and proteinaceous fluid into the interstitium and alveolar spaces. The inflammatory nature of this exudative fluid is reflected by the presence of large quantities of inflammatory cells (predominantly neutrophils) in bronchoalveolar lavage fluid (BALF). The BALF findings provide diagnostic insights if infectious agents or signs of aspiration (e.g., food particles) are present. In contrast, although hydrostatic pulmonary edema is associated with alveolar flooding, the edema fluid typically is noninflammatory, and the protein content is much lower than the protein content of BALF.[34] BALF often provides useful insight into the underlying cause of hypoxemic respiratory failure, but the role of BALF in the clinical management of patients with acute respiratory failure caused by pulmonary edema is not well established. The clinical characteristics that differentiate acute hypoxemic failure caused by hydrostatic pulmonary edema from acute hypoxemic failure caused by nonhydrostatic pulmonary edema are summarized in Box 27-2.

MINI CLINI

Determination of "Optimal" PEEP

PROBLEM: Although PEEP is capable of recruiting collapsed alveolar units in patients with ARDS, it adversely affects cardiac output and increases ventilatory pressure. The clinician must approach PEEP as a therapy that has risks and benefits.

DISCUSSION: In patients with ARDS, increasing levels of PEEP are associated with improved oxygenation and a reduction in the measured shunt fraction (PaO_2/FiO_2 ratio) (see Figure 27-5). Routine use of high levels of PEEP has not been shown to be beneficial for all patients. However, patients with severe ARDS may benefit from higher PEEP levels to maintain oxygenation.[35] Despite initial increases in oxygenation above the level of PEEP designated the "optimal level" in Figure 27-5, there is a net decrease in systemic O_2 delivery. Lung compliance may begin to decline at higher levels of PEEP, and the risk of volutrauma increases. Also, healthy alveoli may become overdistended, resulting in decreased perfusion and stretch-induced injury of the "good lung." The pressure-volume relationships of the lungs may be used to adjust PEEP such that end expiratory alveolar collapse and end inspiratory overinflation are minimized (see Figure 27-6).

Although the optimal PEEP must be determined for each patient, optimal levels of PEEP usually are in the range of 8 to 20 cm H_2O. The tidal volume may have to be decreased whenever PEEP is increased to avoid alveolar overdistention.

THERAPEUTIC APPROACH TO ACUTE RESPIRATORY DISTRESS SYNDROME

The management of critical illness associated with ARDS previously was confined to supportive therapy (Box 27-4) designed to preserve systemic organ function and allow recovery from the underlying illness. Strategies have evolved for controlling the systemic inflammatory response that leads to lung and other organ injury. This section presents an overview of the current approach to supportive care and new potential therapies for ARDS and MODS (Figure 27-4).

Supportive Care of Patients With Acute Respiratory Distress Syndrome and Multiple Organ Dysfunction Syndrome

The fundamental principles of supportive care of patients with ARDS and MODS are outlined in Box 27-4.

Hemodynamics and Fluid Management in Acute Respiratory Distress Syndrome

Preservation of vital organ integrity through the optimization of systemic O_2 delivery is a principal goal of supportive management in all causes of respiratory failure. Ventilator strategies designed to improve arterial oxygenation must be weighed against any potential changes in hemodynamic values incurred as a result of these strategies. In view of the deleterious cardiopulmonary effects of high-pressure mechanical ventilation (e.g., PEEP) in ARDS, it is logical to imagine that invasive monitoring of both cardiac output and systemic O_2 delivery (DO_2) would be beneficial. As previously mentioned, the role of invasive hemodynamic monitoring (e.g., pulmonary artery catheters) in the management of ARDS was historically controversial. However, clarity was provided by the National Institutes of Health National Heart, Lung and Blood Institute–sponsored ARDS Clinical Trials Network, which evaluated the benefits and risks of the use of pulmonary artery catheters to guide treatment in the setting of ALI. The study involved 1000 participants and showed no benefit in terms of mortality, ventilator-free days, and duration of ICU admission and no difference in terms of overall fluid balance. The authors of the study concluded that pulmonary artery catheters "should not be routinely used for the management of ALI."[33]

Gas exchange is highly dependent on total lung fluid during the exudative phase of ARDS, and small increases in hydrostatic forces (PCWP) lead to significant decreases in oxygenation consequent to alveolar flooding and associated right-to-left shunting. Measures that restrict intravascular volume are associated with improved oxygenation. However, as with increasing PEEP, improvements in arterial oxygenation attendant to reducing PCWP must be weighed against reduced cardiac output, as reflected by the measured DO_2 or other measures of systemic tissue oxygenation. In this context, a randomized, multicenter study conducted by the ARDS Clinical Trials Network compared conservative and liberal fluid management strategies for the first 7 days of treatment of 1000 patients with ALI. In keeping with the concept of "leaky" pulmonary capillaries in the setting of ALI resulting in increased susceptibility to lung fluid accumulation in response to increased hydrostatic forces, conservative fluid management was associated with improved arterial oxygenation, increased ventilator-free days, and shorter stays in the ICU. There was no statistical improvement in 60-day mortality, and

Box 27-4 Supportive Care of Patients With Acute Respiratory Distress Syndrome

1. Identify and manage underlying cause of ARDS.
2. Avoid secondary (iatrogenic or nosocomial) lung injury:
   a. Avoid O_2 toxicity.
   b. Avoid aspiration.
   c. Avoid barotrauma and volutrauma.
   d. Identify and manage nosocomial infection and pneumonia.
   e. Extubate as soon as is feasible.
3. Maintain adequate DO_2 to systemic organs.
   a. Minimize demand by reducing metabolic rate:
      Control fever.
      Control anxiety and pain.
   b. Support cardiovascular system with intravenous fluids and vasopressor agents, as necessary, to
      Prevent hypotension (systolic blood pressure >90 mm Hg and mean arterial pressure >60-70 mm Hg).
      Reverse lactic acidosis.
      Maintain adequate urine output.
4. Provide nutritional support.
5. Optimize gas exchange by avoiding excessive fluid administration.

Lung Injury Severity	Clinical Manifestation	Interventions
↓	Acute lung injury	• Low tidal volume ventilation (6 ml/kg) • Conservative fluid management • Daily spontaneous breathing trials
	Acute respiratory distress	• Adjust PEEP and FiO_2 to maintain $PaO_2 > 55$ mm Hg • Consider transfer to tertiary care center
	Refractory hypoxemia	• Prone ventilation • Continuous paralytics • Inhaled vasodilators (nitric oxide/epoprostenol) • High-frequency ventilation • Extracorporeal membrane oxygenation (ECMO) • Extracorporeal carbon dioxide removal ($ECCO_2R$)

FIGURE 27-4 As the severity of lung injury worsens, clinical teams should provide the best evidence-based supportive care including low tidal volume ventilation, conservative fluid management, and daily attempts at ventilator liberation. In patients with significant ARDS and refractory hypoxemia (arbitrarily defined as a PaO_2/FiO_2 ratio <100), transfer to a center with one or more rescue therapies should be considered.

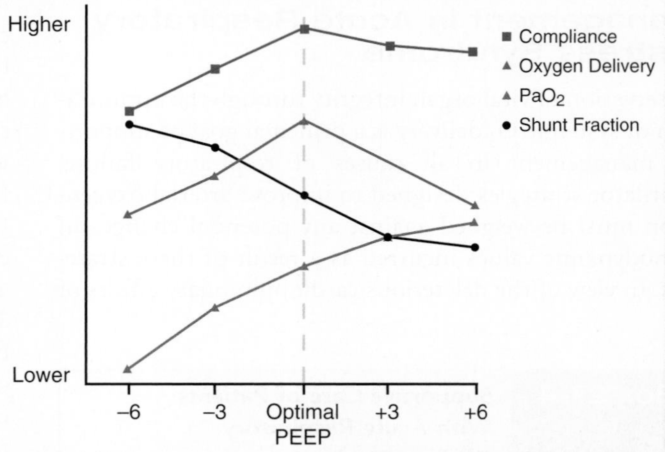

FIGURE 27-5 Determination of "optimal PEEP" from simultaneous measurements of hemodynamic (DO_2), gas exchange (shunt fraction and arterial oxygenation [PaO_2]), and physiologic values. Optimal PEEP does not correspond to PEEP associated with optimal pulmonary gas exchange. When adjusting PEEP, the clinician should consider its effects on systemic DO_2 and lung compliance such that systemic organ injury and lung injury are minimized.

there was no difference between the groups in terms of vital organ failures. Nonetheless, the results of this study strongly favor the routine use of a conservative fluid management strategy in patients with ARDS.[36]

RULE OF THUMB

The beneficial effects of PEEP are optimal at a pressure of 20 cm H_2O or less in most patients with ARDS. Levels of PEEP greater than 20 cm H_2O should not be routinely used unless the benefits of higher levels of PEEP are supported by objective end points, such as improved lung compliance (Figure 27-5) or optimal alveolar recruitment (see Figure 27-6).

With regard to tissue oxygenation in critical illness, various investigations have shown that an abnormal dependence of O_2 consumption ($\dot{V}O_2$) on DO_2 exists throughout the physiologic range of DO_2 in many critically ill patients.[37] This abnormal dependence of $\dot{V}O_2$ on DO_2 is associated with impaired O_2 extraction. These observations have been interpreted to imply that tissue hypoxia may exist and is contributing to organ failure (MODS) in these patients. This notion formed the basis for studies in which DO_2 was increased to "supranormal" levels in patients at risk of sepsis and ARDS.[7] The encouraging results of early trials using this strategy[38,39] were not supported by larger, well-designed clinical trials in cohorts of patients with established sepsis.[40,41] One study showed a higher mortality associated with the use of this strategy.[40] Because of these findings, efforts to increase DO_2 beyond normal values (3.5 L/min/kg) are not currently recommended. The "optimal DO_2" for critically ill patients may never be established because the needs of individual patients must be factored into the decision to augment DO_2. New techniques for detecting tissue hypoxia are needed for guiding the hemodynamic management of these patients. Until such tools become available, it seems prudent to prevent hypotension (systolic arterial blood pressure >90 mm Hg, mean arterial blood pressure >60 mm Hg), consider augmentation of DO_2 in the setting of hyperlactatemia, optimize hemoglobin saturation (>90%), and ensure adequate organ function (e.g., urine output).

Mechanical Ventilation in Acute Respiratory Distress Syndrome

Despite the presence of widespread pulmonary injury and altered gas exchange in ARDS, more recent investigation has shown that aerated portions of the lung have near-normal mechanical characteristics. Gattinoni and Pesenti[42] suggested that three distinct zones exist in the lungs of patients with ARDS. The most dependent lung zones are characterized by dense pulmonary infiltrates corresponding to nonventilated lung units. A second lung zone also has dense pulmonary infiltrates and nonventilated alveolar units but is distinct from the more dependent lung zones in that these areas may be made available for gas exchange through changes in the mode of mechanical ventilation. Finally, nondependent lung zones are fully inflated and receive most of the ventilation. The aerated lung zones have been shown to retain normal mechanical characteristics as reflected by the measured specific compliance (static compliance adjusted for the volume of ventilated lung). In ARDS, the lungs are effectively diminished in size to 20% to 30% of normal, but the aerated portions of the lungs retain near-normal physiologic properties.

Setting Tidal Volume

Because of the heterogeneous properties of the lungs in ARDS, mechanical ventilation with large tidal volumes is inappropriate for these patients. Tidal volumes of 10 to 15 ml/kg, when distributed primarily to the relatively small aerated lung zones, lead to hyperinflation and overdistention of the alveoli in these areas. In animal models, alveolar hyperinflation has been shown to result in altered alveolar capillary permeability identical to that associated with ARDS. The excessive volume, not high pressure, is responsible for lung injury.[43] Lung tissue injury induced by alveolar hyperinflation has been termed *volume trauma* or *volutrauma* and can be avoided with the use of lower tidal volumes. In the original ARDSNet trial, patients with ARDS ventilated with an initial tidal volume of 6 ml/kg and a targeted plateau pressure of 30 cm H_2O had a significantly reduced mortality compared with patients ventilated with 12 ml/kg.[44]

Tidal volume ideally would be selected on the basis of the patient's individual pressure-volume relationships. Pressure-volume relationships can be established for each patient by measuring airway pressure changes over a wide range of tidal volumes. These measurements are used to describe the lower inflection point (LIP) and upper inflection point (UIP) (Figure 27-6). The UIP corresponds to the development of regional lung overdistention. Ventilatory pressure exceeding the pressure associated with the UIP is likely to cause lung injury. In contrast, the LIP represents the point in the pressure-volume curve at which dynamic collapse of alveolar units begins to occur. At ventilator pressures associated with lung volumes below the LIP, alveoli begin to collapse, and oxygenation is impaired. As airway pressure decreases to less than the LIP at end-expiration and increases to more than the LIP during the ventilatory cycle, the alveoli undergo repeated collapse and reexpansion. The shear stress induced by this cyclic opening and closing of the alveoli, particularly relating to forces generated when an alveolus opens adjacent to closed alveolar units creating tremendous distortion of the alveolar walls, represents another possible mechanism of ventilator-associated lung injury.[45]

Ventilator strategies designed to optimize pressure-volume relationships and minimize ventilator-associated lung injury were initially described by Amato and colleagues[46] and were subsequently evaluated by the ARDS Clinical Trials Network. These strategies, termed **volume-controlled ventilation** (see later section on Innovative Ventilation Strategies for Acute Respiratory Distress Syndrome), have been an encouraging finding in an otherwise disappointing quest to discover effective treatments for patients with ARDS.

MINI CLINI

Managing Hydrostatic Pressure in Patients With ARDS

PROBLEM: Critically ill patients requiring mechanical ventilation for acute respiratory failure often receive large volumes of fluid in the form of intravenous medications, maintenance fluids, and enteral or parenteral feedings. These patients consequently are at very high risk for the development of iatrogenic pulmonary edema secondary to increased pulmonary vascular hydrostatic pressure (increased intravascular volume). Excessive fluid administration is of particular concern in patients with ARDS who have "leaky capillaries," particularly in the early phases of the disease, and are remarkably sensitive to changes in pulmonary vascular hydrostatic pressure. How can iatrogenic pulmonary edema be avoided in these patients so that liberation from the ventilator can be expedited?

DISCUSSION: Patients with respiratory insufficiency of any cause may not tolerate additional demands on the cardiorespiratory system, including the demands associated with pulmonary edema owing to intravascular volume overload. The patient's volume status must be monitored closely by noninvasive and, in the case of more severely ill patients, invasive means. Noninvasive estimates of total body water, such as daily weights and total fluid intake and total fluid output measurements, are prone to error related to confounding variables. For example, limited patient mobility interferes with the ability to obtain exact measurements of the patient's weight. Likewise, total fluid intake and output measurements are limited by the loss of information related to insensible fluid losses (e.g., perspiration and respiration-related fluid loss).

Inaccuracies related to noninvasive estimates of total body fluid content are tolerable as long as the patient's overall clinical status is improving and the hemodynamic status remains stable. However, in the setting of worsening pulmonary gas exchange or inadequate systemic DO_2 despite appropriate supportive therapy, invasive measurement of intravascular volume status (e.g., CVP) often is necessary to optimize pulmonary and systemic gas exchange. In this regard, the goals of invasive monitoring should be to guide therapy so that the minimum intravascular volume associated with safe levels of inspired O_2 ($FiO_2 < 0.6$) and signs of effective circulation (e.g., urine output >0.5 ml/kg/hr, capillary refill <2 seconds) are attained. Invasive monitoring is particularly useful in the care of patients with ARDS, who have increased pulmonary capillary permeability and are consequently very sensitive to increases in pulmonary hydrostatic pressure. According to the protocol used by the National Institutes of Health National Heart, Lung and Blood Institute–sponsored ARDS Clinical Trials Network, in patients with signs of effective circulation, as described previously, a conservative fluid management strategy (i.e., CVP < 13 mm Hg) was associated with improved oxygenation and shorter duration of mechanical ventilation relative to a more liberal fluid management approach (i.e., CVP < 18 mm Hg).[36]

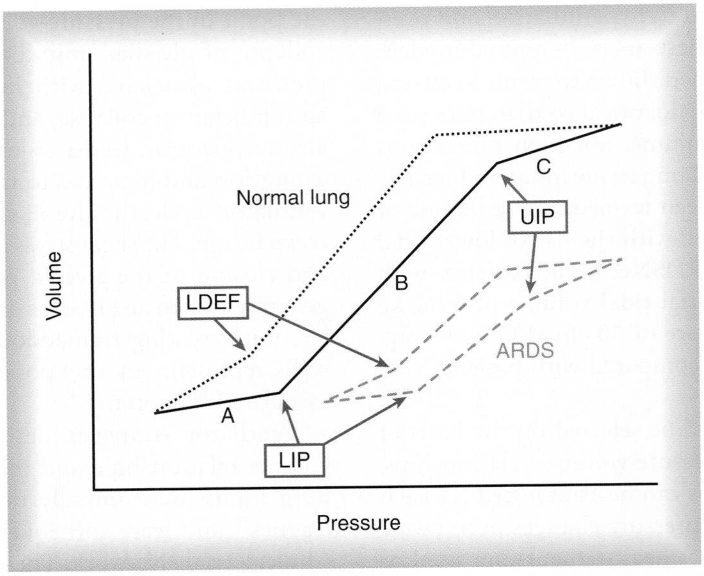

FIGURE 27-6 Typical pressure-volume relationships during normal conditions and during ARDS. At low lung volume, inspiratory pressure increases faster than lung volume *(line A)* owing to high alveolar surface tension. As alveoli open, surface tension decreases, and the pressure required to increase lung volume further decreases *(line B)*. The lower inflection point *(LIP)* occurs between *lines A* and *B* and represents the volume above which most alveolar units are open. The upper inflection point *(UIP)* occurs at near-maximal lung volume and corresponds to the point at which further increases in pressure result in minimal increases in lung volume *(line C)*. Pressure applied above the *UIP* is associated with alveolar distention. During the expiratory phase of the respiratory cycle *(dotted line)*, the lower deflection point *(LDEF)* is the point below which lung volumes slowly decrease (alveolar units collapse). During ARDS *(gray dashed curve)*, pressure-volume relationships change such that higher pressure is needed to maintain alveolar patency, and alveolar distention occurs at lower tidal volumes. Near-maximal lung volumes are typically achieved at an inspiratory pressure of approximately 35 cm H_2O in normal conditions and during *ARDS*. Attempts to increase inspiratory pressure to more than 35 cm H_2O provide little additional ventilation and substantially increase the risk of volume trauma to the lungs. The *LIP* corresponds to pressure below which alveolar collapse occurs *(line A)*. Under normal conditions, the *LIP* may not be evident (i.e., minimal alveolar collapse occurs at end-inspiration under normal conditions). In contrast, during *ARDS*, the *LIP* often is evident during measurements of pressure-volume relationships and frequently occurs at a pressure of 5 to 15 cm H_2O. PEEP at levels greater than *LIP* may prevent end expiratory alveolar collapse and reduce lung injury secondary to alveolar shear stress.

Adjusting Positive End Expiratory Pressure

The rationale behind the use of PEEP in the care of patients with ARDS is not directly related to its effect on lung injury. PEEP may contribute to further pulmonary injury (volutrauma) in these patients. The benefits of PEEP relate to recruitment of additional alveoli, which results in an increase in functional residual capacity (FRC) and improved oxygenation. By improving arterial oxygenation, PEEP may enable reduction of the fraction of inspired O_2 (FiO_2) and diminish the risk of O_2 toxicity to the lungs. When patency of alveolar units is maintained throughout the ventilatory cycle, the damaging effects of opening and closing alveoli with each ventilatory cycle can be avoided. The form of lung injury occurring at lower lung volumes has been termed *airway shear trauma*, and the point at which it occurs is reflected by the LIP of the pressure-volume curve (see Figure 27-6).

The beneficial effects of PEEP must be balanced against the negative effects. Because the primary goal of mechanical ventilation is to provide adequate oxygenation at safe levels of FiO_2 while maintaining adequate DO_2 to the body, the inverse relationship between PEEP and cardiac output must be considered. One common clinical scenario involves increasing PEEP to improve arterial oxygenation at the expense of a reduction in the overall DO_2. For this reason, patients who present with ARDS necessitating the use of PEEP may benefit from invasive hemodynamic monitoring. The more recent ARDS Clinical Trials Network study that evaluated low tidal volume with either high or low PEEP failed to show a survival advantage or shorter ventilator time with either measure.[47] It is reasonable to use the lowest level of PEEP that maintains adequate oxygenation.

As with tidal volume adjustments, the optimal level of PEEP is different for each patient. On the basis of the previous discussion, the goals of PEEP therapy are as follows:

- Provide adequate oxygenation ($PaO_2 > 55$ mm Hg) at a safe FiO_2 (<0.6).
- Ensure adequate tissue oxygenation.
- Maintain the patency of alveolar units throughout the ventilatory cycle (see Figure 27-6).
- Avoid barotrauma by maintaining mean airway pressure less than 35 cm H_2O or less than the pressure that corresponds to the UIP of the pressure-volume curve (see Figure 27-6).

RULE OF THUMB

Administration of high levels of supplemental O_2 ($FiO_2 > 0.6$) for longer than 24 hours can cause lung injury as a result of O_2 toxicity (oxidative stress), which advances ARDS and lung fibrosis. As the FiO_2 becomes greater than 0.6, the time required to cause lung injury decreases. The FiO_2 should be decreased to 0.6 as soon as possible via supportive therapy, such as positive pressure ventilation, PEEP, manipulations of pulmonary vascular pressure, or another recommended therapy (Tables 27-2 and 27-3).

Adjusting the Ventilatory Rate

ARDS is associated with alveolar consolidation and ventilation/perfusion mismatching, which results in a decrease in the number of normally functioning alveoli. Critically ill patients often have elevated metabolic rates so that CO_2 production is increased. Compared with individuals with normal lungs, patients with ARDS require much higher minute ventilation to maintain $PaCO_2$ in the normal range. In patients with ARDS, it is desirable to maintain lower tidal volumes and avoid volutrauma. The goal of reducing tidal volume and controlling ventilatory rate is achieved at the expense of considerable CO_2 retention in patients with ARDS. In most cases, the $PaCO_2$ increases to 60 to 80 mm Hg, and the arterial pH decreases to approximately 7.25. Subsequent metabolic compensation tends to correct the acidosis over several days.[48] In some cases, the acidosis is more severe but appears to be well tolerated as long as tissue oxygenation is maintained. This ventilatory strategy has been designated *permissive hypercapnia* or *controlled hypoventilation* and often requires increased levels of sedation and, in some cases, paralysis to avoid patient discomfort owing to air hunger and a high respiratory rate.[48]

Animal models and human studies have confirmed the safety of controlled hypoventilation.[49] Several investigations have shown a survival benefit of low-volume

TABLE 27-2

Criteria for Evidence-Based Recommendations for Management of Acute Respiratory Distress Syndrome (ARDS)

Quality of Evidence	
Level 1	Randomized, prospective, controlled investigations of ARDS
Level 2	Nonrandomized concurrent cohort investigations, historical cohort investigations, and case series of patients with ARDS
Level 3	Randomized, prospective, controlled investigations of sepsis or other relevant conditions that have potential application to ARDS
Level 4	Case reports of ARDS
Grading of Recommendations	
A	Supported by at least two Level 1 investigations
B	Supported by only one Level 1 investigation
C	Supported by Level 2 investigations only
D	Supported by at least one Level 3 investigation
Ungraded	No available clinical investigations

Modified from Kollef MH, Schuster D: Acute respiratory distress syndrome. Dis Mon 42:270–326, 1996.

TABLE 27-3

Recommendations for Nonpharmacologic Management of Acute Respiratory Distress Syndrome

Treatment	Recommendation	Grade
Mechanical ventilation		Ungraded
Initial settings: assist control mode; FiO_2 1.0; PEEP ≤5 cm H_2O; inspiratory flow, 60 L/min	Yes	
Tidal volume, 6-10 ml/kg	Yes	C
Prophylactic PEEP (≤5 cm H_2O)	No	B
Least PEEP with $SaO_2 \geq 0.9$ and $FiO_2 \leq 0.6$	Yes	Ungraded
Permissive hypercapnia to maintain peak airway pressure <40-45 cm H_2O and plateau pressure <35 cm H_2O	Yes	C
Routine use of IRV	No	C
IRV for persistent hypoxemia or elevated airway pressure	Yes	C
APRV	No*	
HFV	No	B
Tracheal gas insufflation	*	
Partial liquid ventilation	*	
ECMO	No	B
$ECCO_2R$	No	B
Patient repositioning (including prone position)	Yes	C
Early fluid restriction or diuresis	Yes	B
Supranormal DO_2 goals	No	D

Modified from Kollef MH, Schuster D: Acute respiratory distress syndrome. Dis Mon 42:270–326, 1996.
IRV, Inverse ratio ventilation; *APRV;* airway pressure release ventilation; *HSV,* high frequency ventilation; *ECMO,* extracorporeal membrane oxygenation; *$ECCO_2R$,* extracorporeal carbon dioxide removal.
*Pending results of ongoing clinical trials.

ventilation and permissive hypercapnia in patients with ARDS. This strategy is contraindicated in the care of patients with elevated intracranial pressure because this condition may be negatively affected by elevated $PaCO_2$. Respiratory acidosis secondary to permissive hypercapnia may result in a further decrease in systolic blood pressure in patients with shock, especially patients receiving vasoactive medications; this generally occurs at an arterial pH less than 7.20. In these patients, parenteral replacement of bicarbonate may be considered to maintain an arterial pH of greater than 7.20 while still achieving the goal of low tidal volume ventilation.

Innovative Ventilation Strategies for Acute Respiratory Distress Syndrome

The mainstay of therapy for patients with ALI and ARDS is generally supportive care aimed at avoiding complications associated with mechanical ventilation, volutrauma, and nosocomial pneumonia. No specific ventilator modality has been shown to be consistently superior in improving outcomes in patients with ARDS. However, some ventilator strategies and pharmacotherapies have been shown to improve patients' oxygenation acutely. Patients with ARDS requiring high levels of inspired O_2 ($FiO_2 > 0.6$) despite conventional supportive therapy may benefit from one or more of these ventilatory strategies. The choice of which strategy to use depends on the patient's clinical condition; patient comfort; and the familiarity, comfort, and availability of these modalities to the clinical team.

Volume-Controlled Mechanical Ventilation

Volume-controlled mechanical ventilation represents an exciting new area of ARDS research. A large, well-designed clinical trial sponsored by the National Institutes of Health ARDS Clinical Trials Network showed a significant reduction in mortality (approximately 20%) when lower tidal volumes were used in patients with ALI and ARDS.[44] Volume-controlled ventilation is now considered a preferred ventilation strategy for patients with ARDS. This ventilation technique is typically adjusted to the specific pressure-volume relationships of each patient; however, a range of optimal initial ventilator settings can be derived from more recent experimental observations. A tidal volume of 10 ml/kg exceeds the volume at which the UIP is reached in more than 80% of patients with ARDS, and most patients need only 5 to 7 ml/kg tidal volume to reach this inflection point.[50]

On the basis of these observations, it is now recommended that the tidal volume for patients with ARDS be initiated at 5 to 7 ml/kg. Subsequent tidal volume adjustments should be made on the basis of each patient's pressure-volume relationships (see Figure 27-6). Ideal PEEP should be determined as previously described (see Figure 27-5 and Mini Clini, "Determination of 'Optimal' PEEP"). Despite the convincing evidence that low-volume ventilation decreases mortality, institutional practices vary considerably, and overall compliance with this recommended approach to the management of patients with ALI is currently quite poor.[51]

High-Frequency Ventilation

High-frequency ventilation (HFV) was designed to maintain adequate ventilation and reduce alveolar collapse simultaneously through ventilation with high expiratory lung volumes and rapid (up to 300 breaths/min), small tidal volumes (3 to 5 ml/kg). This technique has been successfully applied to the ventilation of neonates with respiratory distress related to insufficient surfactant production.[52] However, despite anecdotal evidence suggesting that HFV may be beneficial to adults with ARDS,[53,54] larger clinical trials do not support the routine use of HFV in this patient population.[55]

Experience with the H1N1 influenza epidemic of 2009 has resulted in renewed interest in HFV. In many centers, high-frequency oscillatory ventilation (HFOV) is a rescue therapy applied to patients with inadequate response to conventional ARDS ventilator strategies.[56] Although smaller trials seem to show equivalence with conventional ventilation,[57] a more recent meta-analysis suggested that HFOV may provide a survival advantage relative to conventional modes of ventilation.[58] Additionally, the combination of HFOV with pumpless interventional lung assist devices to remove CO_2 has proven useful in small trials.[59] Patients on HFOV usually have high mean airway pressures (≥30 cm H_2O), and as with the use of high levels of PEEP, care must be taken that these elevated airway pressures do not overly reduce the cardiac output and the overall O_2 delivery despite elevated arterial oxygenation.

Inverse-Ratio Ventilation

Inverse-ratio ventilation (IRV) is designed to recruit alveolar units through prolongation of the inspiratory phase of the ventilatory cycle and improve oxygenation. In conventional modes of mechanical ventilation, the respiratory cycle is characterized by *inspiratory-to-expiratory (I:E) ratios* exceeding 1:2. During IRV, the inspiratory time on the ventilator is prolonged so that the I:E ratio is reversed and may exceed 4:1. Initial reports of the use of this strategy showed significant improvement in oxygenation in patients with ARDS.[60] However, these studies did not take into account other variables, such as the level of PEEP. After controlling for the level of PEEP, no change in oxygenation was observed in patients with ARDS who received IRV.[61] No study has shown a significant survival benefit with this ventilator mode. Because of the discomfort associated with this mode of ventilation and the risk of asynchronous spontaneous ventilatory efforts, patients often demand heavy sedation or paralysis during IRV. The routine use of IRV in ARDS cannot be advocated at this time.

MINI CLINI

Avoiding Ventilator-Induced Lung Injury

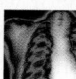

PROBLEM: How can ventilator-induced lung injury be minimized in patients with ARDS through adjustments of PEEP and tidal volume?

DISCUSSION: Alveolar shear stress occurs when alveoli collapse during expiration and are reopened as the next tidal volume is delivered. Patients with ARDS are prone to development of this form of lung injury because surface tension increases as a result of impaired surfactant synthesis and function and decreased lung compliance. Alveolar collapse at end-expiration (the LIP of the pressure-volume curve) can be avoided with PEEP, which reduces alveolar shear stress by preventing the cyclic opening and closing of the alveoli during each ventilatory cycle. Because partially patent alveoli require less pressure to inflate than collapsed alveoli, PEEP also improves lung compliance. Improved compliance is reflected by an increase in the slope of the pressure-volume curve (see Figure 27-6).

Many newer ventilators can provide pressure-volume relationships. This information allows the clinician to estimate the PEEP needed to maintain alveolar patency (see Figure 27-6). Alternatively, the clinician can gauge the effects of PEEP on the basis of calculated changes in lung compliance (see Figure 27-5). In the clinical setting, changes in lung compliance are estimated from the compliance of the entire respiratory system, which includes the combined influences of lung compliance, chest wall compliance, and abdominal pressure:

$$\text{Compliance of the respiratory system} = \text{Tidal volume} \div (\text{Plateau pressure} - \text{Total PEEP})$$

As PEEP increases, so do airway pressure and the risk of lung injury owing to volutrauma. Volutrauma occurs when alveoli are exposed to pressure greater than that necessary to provide optimal ventilation. Volutrauma is particularly problematic in the care of patients with ARDS because the tidal volume necessary for complete inflation of the lungs is reduced. It becomes critical during ARDS to avoid lung injury related to alveolar overinflation by reducing plateau airway pressures to less than approximately 30 cm H_2O.

Just as alveolar collapse during end-expiration is associated with decreased lung compliance, alveolar overinflation during end-inspiration is reflected by decreasing compliance and corresponds to the UIP of the pressure-volume curve (see Figure 27-6). Tidal volumes should be adjusted so that maximal inspiratory pressure does not exceed the pressure corresponding to the UIP of the pressure-volume curve. In most patients, the UIP is attained at tidal volumes less than 10 ml/kg and plateau pressure less than 35 cm H_2O.[61]

Pressure Control Ventilation

Pressure control ventilation (PCV) is designed to prevent ventilator-associated lung injury. The clinician sets the maximal inspiratory airway pressure. A maximal inspiratory pressure (30 to 35 cm H_2O) is chosen that is likely to avert alveolar overdistention and prevent volume-associated lung injury. Minute ventilation is maintained by setting the respiratory rate. Tidal volume becomes a dynamic variable during PCV. That is, tidal volume primarily depends on the driving pressure (maximum inspiratory pressure—PEEP), airway resistance, inspiratory time, and lung compliance. Changes in intrathoracic pressure (e.g., owing to spontaneous inspiratory efforts) or airway resistance or changes in lung compliance influence tidal volume. Large swings in ventilation (increases or decreases in $PaCO_2$) may be observed during PCV. Close monitoring of the ventilatory status of the patient must be maintained while the PCV mode is in use. Despite its theoretic benefits, PCV has not been shown to be superior to volume-controlled ventilation in clinical trials.[62,63]

Many modern ventilators now have hybrid modes that combine the benefit of pressure control ventilation, a set maximal inspiratory pressure, with a targeted tidal volume that allows the ventilator to reduce the drive pressure as the lung compliance improves and avoid overdistention. These modes rely on algorithms to adjust the drive pressure that are often proprietary to the ventilator manufacturer. To date, data showing that these hybrid modes improve outcomes in ARDS are insufficient, but they may improve patient comfort.

Airway Pressure Release Ventilation

Airway pressure release ventilation (APRV) is designed to optimize ventilation by recruiting collapsed alveolar units while minimizing ventilator-induced barotrauma in patients with ARDS. APRV generally features two levels of PEEP: a high PEEP often set to approximately 25 to 30 cm H_2O and a low PEEP that is usually set to zero. Similar to IRV, APRV prolongs the inspiratory phase of the ventilatory cycle with inspiratory times often of 4 to 6 seconds at the high PEEP level. During APRV, patients may spontaneously breathe while on this high PEEP, making it more comfortable than traditional IRV. After a period at the high PEEP level, there are brief, approximately 0.5 second, decreases in airway pressure to the low PEEP level, which may be triggered by the patient, allowing volume release and generating a "tidal volume" for this mode. Owing to the prolonged inspiratory times, APRV is associated with an increase in mean airway pressure and a tendency to stack breaths (increased intrinsic PEEP). Increased intrinsic PEEP is the likely mechanism by which APRV improves arterial oxygenation.

Comparisons of APRV with other forms of mechanical ventilation, including pressure support and synchronized intermittent mandatory ventilation, have shown APRV to be effective and well tolerated. In a study by Sydow and associates[64] in which APRV was compared with IRV in patients with ARDS, APRV was better tolerated and was associated with lower peak airway pressures. Alveolar recruitment improved over time with APRV but not with IRV. Despite these potential advantages, APRV has not proved to be superior to conventional mechanical ventilation in large clinical trials in patients with ARDS.[65]

Adjunctive Strategies for Acute Respiratory Distress Syndrome

Patient Positioning

In view of the heterogeneous distribution of lung injury in patients with ARDS, it has been proposed that changing the position of the patient could result in improved ventilation/perfusion matching within the lungs. In this regard, it is known that alveolar consolidation tends to be most pronounced in the dependent lung zones in patients with ARDS where blood flow is greatest.[66] These observations led investigators to experiment with positioning the patient so that aerated lung fields (nondependent lung zones) become dependent (by positioning of the patient in the prone position). Douglas and colleagues[67] were the first to describe improved oxygenation with prone positioning of patients with ARDS. For unclear reasons, this ventilation strategy was not popularized until more recently, when other investigators showed similar beneficial effects in patients with ARDS.[68]

The mechanisms by which prone positioning improves oxygenation is the subject of ongoing debate. Some proposed mechanisms include improved matching of ventilation with perfusion, increased FRC, increased cardiac output, more effective drainage of upper and lower airway secretions, and improved diaphragmatic excursion. Investigations using animal models of ALI have shown that ventilation in the supine position causes compressive forces on the dorsal airspaces resulting in derecruitment of lung units. This phenomenon is reversed by ventilation in the prone position.[69,70]

A large multicenter, randomized clinical trial failed to show a survival benefit when ventilation in the prone position was used for at least 6 hours a day in the care of patients with ALI or ARDS, even though oxygenation was significantly improved in the prone position.[69] A more recent trial that evaluated the implementation of prone ventilation very early in the course of ARDS and for prolonged periods appeared to show a survival benefit.[71] It is also encouraging that a more recent meta-analysis suggested a survival advantage for prone ventilation, which was evident in patients with more severe hypoxemia, defined as a PaO_2/FiO_2 ratio less than 100 mm Hg.[72]

The advantages of prone ventilation are the improvement in oxygenation and potentially a survival advantage over supine ventilation without the need for expensive pharmacologic interventions or new ventilator modalities. Despite these advantages, there is a significant downside to this intervention. Some patients do not tolerate prone positioning because of hemodynamic instability or worsening gas exchange, and all patients treated in this way require specialized nursing care. Prone positioning of a patient with ARDS requires experienced and committed nursing staff and may require special equipment to facilitate turning, especially obese patients. The improvements in gas exchange related to repositioning the patient tend to be transient necessitating subsequent repositioning. At this point, it is difficult to offer definitive guidance for the use of prone ventilation, but centers experienced with prone ventilation may use it in patients who fail to respond to usual interventions.

Extracorporeal Membrane Oxygenation and Extracorporeal Carbon Dioxide Removal

Extracorporeal membrane oxygenation (ECMO) was first introduced in 1972 as a form of respiratory support for patients with severe, acute hypoxemic respiratory failure. This modality involves the establishment of an arteriovenous circuit for diverting a large proportion of the cardiac output through an artificial gas exchange device, or "artificial lung," to facilitate the exchange of CO_2 and O_2. Following an initial flurry of interest during the 1970s, a trial comparing ECMO plus conventional mechanical ventilation with conventional mechanical ventilation alone in ARDS showed no survival benefit with ECMO.[73]

Several more recent studies reported a significant improvement in survival[74,75] and less severe disability at 6 months in patients who were managed with ECMO compared with patients who received conventional therapy.[75] These promising results, along with others not mentioned here, have led many institutions to use ECMO as rescue therapy for patients with H1N1-induced ARDS who cannot be managed with conventional ventilatory modes or HFOV.[74] The merits of ECMO for routine management of all patients with ARDS is an area of intense debate and conflicting opinions, but ECMO is currently a reasonable alternative to conventional ventilation strategies in the setting of refractory hypoxemia in patients with ARDS.[76]

Similar to ECMO, **extracorporeal carbon dioxide removal ($ECCO_2R$)** entails the use of artificial membranes to supplement the gas exchange deficiencies of damaged lungs. In contrast to ECMO, $ECCO_2R$ has a venovenous circuit that diverts a fraction of the cardiac output (approximately 20%) through the membrane lung, is primarily designed to remove CO_2, and does not directly influence oxygenation. Oxygenation is indirectly facilitated through the removal of CO_2, which would otherwise compete with O_2 exchange within the alveoli. By this mechanism, $ECCO_2R$ allows the clinician to maintain the same level of oxygenation at lower ventilatory rates and reduce the risk of lung injury related to mechanical ventilation.

Clinical trials comparing $ECCO_2R$ with conventional mechanical ventilation in the care of adults with ARDS have shown improved gas exchange, lower peak airway pressure, lower ventilatory rate, and reduced thoracic volume (less overinflation of the lungs) in patients treated with $ECCO_2R$ ventilation.[77] This trial failed to show a survival benefit with $ECCO_2R$ at 30 days in 40 patients.

The H1N1 influenza outbreak of 2009 generated many reports supporting the use of $ECCO_2R$ employing technology, such as the Novalung (Heilbronn, Germany), in patients with ARDS failing to respond to conventional therapy.[78] As experience grows in its use in specialized centers around the world, $ECCO_2R$ has become a therapy of last resort especially for viral-induced ARDS. Most hospitals have put in place contingency plans to move patients to these centers when deemed appropriate by critical care clinicians.

Pharmacologic Therapies for Acute Respiratory Distress Syndrome

Exogenous Surfactant Administration

The assumed role of surfactant deficiency in the pathogenesis of infant respiratory distress is well established. Exogenous surfactant administration is a cornerstone of therapy for infant respiratory distress syndrome. The pathogenesis of ARDS is more complex, however (see earlier section on Pathophysiology). Although surfactant is known to be qualitatively and quantitatively altered during ARDS, other factors, such as the severity of pulmonary microvascular injury, contribute to the gas exchange abnormalities associated with this condition. Nonetheless, surfactant has been shown to have immunomodulating (i.e., affecting immune function) properties that may reduce microvascular injury in the lungs. Surfactant dysfunction may contribute to the development of ARDS by promoting instability of the alveolar units (airway shear trauma, atelectasis, and right-to-left shunt) and by allowing inflammatory injury to alveoli to continue unchecked. This rationale explains the observed correlation between the degree of surfactant dysfunction and the severity of gas exchange abnormalities during adult ARDS and forms the basis for clinical trials of exogenous surfactant administration during ARDS.

Exogenous surfactant replacement is of greatest benefit in models of pure surfactant deficiency, such as infant respiratory distress or the aftermath of saline lavage. However, in adult ARDS, in which deactivation of surfactant relates to the influx of inflammatory cells and mediators into the alveolar space, the effects of exogenous surfactant are less apparent. Although initial studies showed a benefit in oxygenation with surfactant administration, either synthetic (Alveofact [Lyomark Pharma, Oberhaching, Germany])[79] or a modified bovine lung surfactant (beractant [Survanta, Abbott Nutrition, Chicago, IL]),[80] subsequent trials failed to show a survival benefit, and one trial showed a trend toward increasing mortality.[81,82] Surfactant replacement therapy cannot be recommended for the routine management of patients with ARDS.

Neuromuscular Blockade

Neuromuscular blocking agents have been used for decades to enhance compliance with mechanical ventilation in patients with ARDS, especially when the ventilatory mode has involved low-volume ventilation, or inverse ratio ventilation. Although earlier studies showed improved oxygenation with neuromuscular blockade for the first 48 hours, they did not address any survival advantage gained from this intervention. A multicenter randomized trial considered 90-day in-hospital mortality as the outcome measure after therapeutic intervention with a bolus of the paralytic drug cisatracurium followed by a 48-hour infusion. The cisatracurium group showed an improvement in the adjusted 90-day survival, days off the ventilator, and incidence of barotrauma complications. In post hoc analysis of the study, the benefit seemed to be most evident in more severe disease as defined by a PaO_2/FiO_2 ratio less than 120. Although problems with muscle weakness related to neuromuscular blocker use were thought to be more likely in the intervention arm, this was not seen in practice in the study and may reflect the short duration of paralysis.[83] At this time, it is difficult to make firm conclusions about the routine use of neuromuscular blockade, and further trials are needed to clarify this area.

Inhaled Nitric Oxide

NO is a potent vasodilator that plays a critical role in the regulation of blood flow within the lungs. NO is soluble in liquids and gases and diffuses readily through various tissues. In vitro, the vasodilatory effects of NO are short-lived because NO is quickly bound and neutralized by hemoglobin and competes with O_2 for mitochondrial oxidization. Consequently, the effects of NO are localized and temporally self-limited.

The potential role of inhaled NO in ARDS is based on the idea that NO is preferentially distributed to well-ventilated portions of the lung, where it causes local vasodilation. In this way, well-ventilated areas of the lung receive a greater portion of the total pulmonary blood flow, which results in improved oxygenation by reducing ventilation/perfusion mismatch (Figure 27-7). In practice, the effects of inhaled NO in patients with ARDS have been variable. Generally, patients with high pulmonary vascular resistance, who presumably have more severe alterations in pulmonary vascular regulation, seem to benefit the most. The beneficial effects of NO can be achieved at low concentrations of inhaled NO, which explains the low incidence of systemic hypotension associated with its use. However, sudden discontinuation of inhaled NO may be associated with severe pulmonary vasoconstriction; slow weaning is necessary.

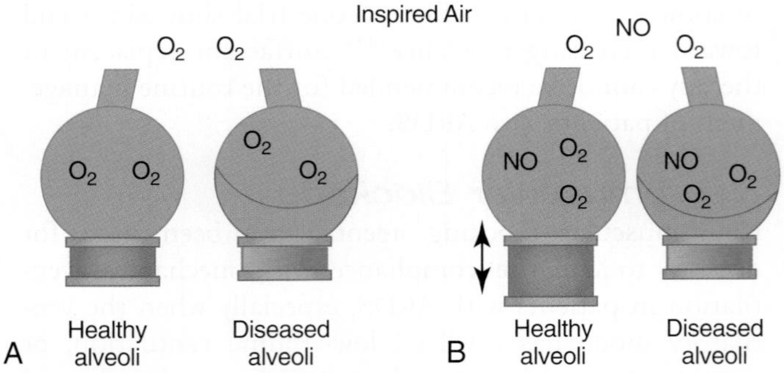

FIGURE 27-7 The damage of ALI and ARDS is heterogeneous. **A,** Despite autoregulatory changes that favor vasodilation of well-oxygenated alveoli, perfusion goes to both the healthy, unaffected alveoli and the diseased alveoli that are unable to oxygenate blood. This results in ventilation/perfusion mismatch or a shuntlike state resulting in deoxygenated blood returning from the lung and hypoxemia. **B,** The addition of inhaled NO to the inspired gas results in vasodilation of the capillaries adjacent to healthy alveoli promoting increased blood flow to the "good" alveoli and diminishing the percentage of blood going to diseased alveoli, resulting in improved ventilation/perfusion match and improved oxygenation.

Despite encouraging results of animal studies showing tolerance of low doses of inhaled NO for 6 months, the safety and effectiveness of inhaled NO therapy for ARDS have not been established. The breakdown products of NO are potentially toxic and include highly reactive free radicals (e.g., peroxynitrite) and methemoglobin, potentially contributing to further lung injury in patients with ARDS or in individuals with normal lung function. The use of inhaled NO during mechanical ventilation involves close monitoring and special exhaust systems to prevent exposure of health care personnel to NO and its potentially toxic by-products. Many phase II and phase III studies have been completed with NO. No study has shown that NO improves outcome or mortality. Most recently, a large multicenter randomized trial involving more than 300 patients reported that NO at a dose of 5 ppm was ineffective in altering mortality, or duration of ventilator support, although there was a short-term benefit on oxygenation.[84] Because of these uncertainties, inhaled NO, although promising, remains an experimental therapy for ARDS.

Inhaled Epoprostenol

Similar to NO, epoprostenol (Flolan) is a potent vasodilator with a short half-life. Epoprostenol is generally given intravenously to patients with pulmonary hypertension; however, because of the significantly lower costs compared with NO, there is interest in the use of inhaled epoprostenol in a nebulized form for refractory hypoxemia associated with ARDS. In patients with ARDS, nebulized epoprostenol is associated with improved oxygenation presumably secondary to preferential vasodilation of the good lung, as discussed earlier, leading to improvement in ventilation/perfusion matching.[85] To date, there is no evidence of a mortality benefit with the use of inhaled epoprostenol to recommend its routine use in ARDS.[86] Epoprostenol should be viewed as salvage therapy for refractory hypoxemia.

Corticosteroids for Late, Uncomplicated Acute Respiratory Distress Syndrome

Although most patients who survive ARDS have minimal residual pulmonary impairment, a small but significant number of patients cannot be weaned from mechanical ventilatory support because of abundant fibroproliferation during recovery from ARDS. The high mortality among these patients seems to relate to the extent and severity of pulmonary fibrosis.[87] High-dose corticosteroids have been used to manage uncomplicated pulmonary fibrosis following ARDS. In a well-publicized but uncontrolled study by Meduri and coworkers,[88] patients treated with corticosteroids for ARDS-related pulmonary fibrosis had improved gas exchange and low mortality (24%). Subsequently, the same investigators performed a randomized double-blind, placebo-controlled trial to determine the effect of prolonged methylprednisolone therapy for unresolving ARDS. The results were encouraging, showing improvement in lung injury scores and reduced mortality.[89] The ARDS Clinical Trials Network conducted a large multicenter trial of corticosteroids for the treatment of patients with late, fibroproliferative ARDS (>7 days' duration). The results showed no survival benefit with steroid use at 60 days and 180 days, and patients given steroids after 14 days from ARDS onset experienced a higher mortality. At this time, the routine use of corticosteroids for the treatment of established ARDS cannot be advocated and should be strictly avoided after 14 days from onset.[90]

Beta-2 Agonists

Although beta-2 agonists were first shown to decrease alveolar permeability to fluid in humans more than 20 years ago, the therapeutic implications of this class of drug were assessed in humans with ARDS only more recently. A cohort of patients with ALI or ARDS were randomly assigned to treatment with intravenous salbutamol (15 μg/kg/hr) or placebo for 7 days and assessed for the degree of extravascular lung water, measured by thermodilution (PiCCO) at day 7. Patients treated with salbutamol exhibited significantly lower lung water and lower plateau pressures, although there was no difference in the PaO_2/FiO_2 ratio at day 7, ventilator days, or 28-day mortality.[91] It is not yet determined whether beta-2 agonists provide a mortality benefit or if this promising therapy will join the ever-increasing list of ineffective ARDS treatments.

ROLE OF THE RESPIRATORY THERAPIST IN ACUTE LUNG INJURY AND ACUTE RESPIRATORY DISTRESS SYNDROME

Patients with ALI and ARDS represent some of the most challenging patients to manage on the ventilator. Respiratory therapists (RTs) play a pivotal role in caring for patients with ALI and ARDS. RTs participate in the close monitoring that these patients require, for example, in drawing arterial blood gases, sometimes placing arterial lines or performing hemodynamic assessments, and monitoring pulse oximeter data.

In treating patients with ARDS and ALI, RTs are key members of the ICU team. In multiple randomized trials, RT-driven ventilator management protocols have outperformed usual care protocols in ventilator liberation.[92] RT assistance in ventilator management, with regard to offering advice concerning ventilatory strategies; reinforcing the value of "low stretch" approaches to all members of the team; and performing the ventilator setups, adjustments, and checks, is essential to the care of patients with ALI and ARDS.

SUMMARY CHECKLIST

- CHF and ARDS are common causes of acute respiratory failure that often are difficult to differentiate on the initial clinical evaluation.
- Although CHF and ARDS both cause pulmonary edema, CHF-associated pulmonary edema is caused by elevated hydrostatic pressure in the pulmonary vasculature. Pulmonary edema associated with ARDS results from inflammatory injury to the lungs and occurs at normal hydrostatic pressure.
- ARDS is the likely diagnosis in a patient who has an established risk factor for ARDS (see Box 27-1), in the presence of diagnostic criteria, and whose history is not suggestive of one of the causes of CHF (see Box 27-3).
- When the clinical history, physical examination, and chest radiograph do not provide sufficient information for a diagnosis, alternative diagnostic techniques, such as bronchoscopy or pulmonary artery catheterization, may be necessary to differentiate CHF and ARDS.
- No drug therapy is effective in preventing or reversing ARDS or MODS in critically ill patients. Recommendations regarding the management of ARDS have focused on supportive care, including optimization of gas exchange and support of systemic organ function (e.g., mechanical ventilation), until the patient recovers from the underlying illness.
- A consensus is beginning to emerge regarding supportive care of patients with ARDS. Currently recommended ventilatory strategies for patients with ARDS are designed to minimize ventilator-induced lung injury by use of PEEP, low tidal volumes, reduced airway pressures, and nontoxic levels of inspired O_2. Gas exchange and duration of mechanical ventilation are improved when conservative fluid management strategies are used.
- Innovative ventilatory strategies and therapies for ARDS that does not resolve with conventional supportive therapy are under active investigation.
- Ambiguity surrounds the treatment of patients with ARDS because of the heterogeneous nature of the patient population, the complex pathophysiologic determinants of ARDS and MODS, and the limitations of the studies designed to evaluate each form of therapy.
- An evidence-based approach to the development of a rational therapeutic plan for treatment of patients with ARDS is needed to standardize the care of these patients (see Tables 27-2 and 27-3).

References

1. Bernard GR, Artigas A, Brigham KL, et al: The American-European Consensus Conference on ARDS. Definitions, mechanisms, relevant outcomes, and clinical trial coordination. Am J Respir Crit Care Med 49(3 Pt 1):818–824, 1994.
2. Brun-Buisson C, Minelli C, Bertolini G, et al: Epidemiology and outcome of acute lung injury in European intensive care units: results from the ALIVE study. Intensive Care Med 30:51–61, 2004.
3. Luhr OR, Antonsen K, Karlsson M, et al: Incidence and mortality after acute respiratory failure and acute respiratory distress syndrome in Sweden, Denmark, and Iceland. The ARF Study Group. Am J Respir Crit Care Med 159:1849–1861, 1999.
4. Rubenfeld GD, Caldwell E, Peabody E, et al: Incidence and outcomes of acute lung injury. N Engl J Med 353:1685–1693, 2005.
5. Milberg JA, Davis DR, Steinberg KP, et al: Improved survival of patients with acute respiratory distress syndrome (ARDS): 1983–1993. JAMA 273:306–309, 1995.
6. Sheu CC, Gong MN, Zhai R, et al: Clinical characteristics and outcomes of sepsis-related vs non-sepsis-related ARDS. Chest 138:559–567, 2010.
7. Fowler AA, Hamman RF, Good JT, et al: Adult respiratory distress syndrome: risk with common predispositions. Ann Intern Med 98(5 Pt 1):593–597, 1983.
8. Sloane PJ, Gee MH, Gottlieb JE, et al: A multicenter registry of patients with acute respiratory distress syndrome: physiology and outcome. Am Rev Respir Dis 146:419–426, 1992.
9. Flick M, Matthay M: Pulmonary edema and acute lung injury, Philadelphia, 1994, Saunders.
10. Matthay MA, Zimmerman GA: Acute lung injury and the acute respiratory distress syndrome: four decades of inquiry into pathogenesis and rational management. Am J Respir Cell Mol Biol 33:319–327, 2005.
11. Conhaim RL: Airway level at which edema liquid enters the air space of isolated dog lungs. J Appl Physiol 67:2234–2242, 1989.
12. Pugin J, Verghese G, Widmer MC, et al: The alveolar space is the site of intense inflammatory and profibrotic reactions in

the early phase of acute respiratory distress syndrome. Crit Care Med 27:304–312, 1999.
13. Ware LB, Matthay MA: Alveolar fluid clearance is impaired in the majority of patients with acute lung injury and the acute respiratory distress syndrome. Am J Respir Crit Care Med 163:1376–1383, 2001.
14. Katzenstein AL, Bloor CM, Leibow AA: Diffuse alveolar damage—the role of oxygen, shock, and related factors: a review. Am J Pathol 85:209–228, 1976.
15. Matute-Bello G, Liles WC, Steinberg KP, et al: Soluble Fas ligand induces epithelial cell apoptosis in humans with acute lung injury (ARDS). J Immunol 163:2217–2225, 1999.
16. Weiland JE, Davis WB, Holter JF, et al: Lung neutrophils in the adult respiratory distress syndrome: clinical and pathophysiologic significance. Am Rev Respir Dis 133:218–225, 1986.
17. Baughman RP, Gunther KL, Rashkin MC, et al: Changes in the inflammatory response of the lung during acute respiratory distress syndrome: prognostic indicators. Am J Respir Crit Care Med 154:76–81, 1996.
18. Marsh CB, Wewers MD: The pathogenesis of sepsis: factors that modulate the response to gram-negative bacterial infection. Clin Chest Med 17:183–197, 1996.
19. Parsons PE: Mediators and mechanisms of acute lung injury. Clin Chest Med 21:467–476, 2000.
20. Ware LB, Matthay MA: The acute respiratory distress syndrome. N Engl J Med 342:1334–1349, 2000.
21. Crouser ED, Julian MW, Weisbrode SE, et al: Acid aspiration results in ileal injury without altering ileal V(O2)-D(O2) relationships. Am J Respir Crit Care Med 153(6 Pt 1):1965–1971, 1996.
22. St John RC, Mizer LA, Kindt GC, et al: Acid aspiration-induced acute lung injury causes leukocyte-dependent systemic organ injury. J Appl Physiol 74:1994–2003, 1993.
23. Crouser ED, Dorinsky PM: Gastrointestinal tract dysfunction in critical illness: pathophysiology and interaction with acute lung injury in adult respiratory distress syndrome/multiple organ dysfunction syndrome. New Horiz 2:476–487, 1994.
24. Matuschak GM, Mattingly ME, Tredway TL, et al: Liver-lung interactions during E. coli endotoxemia: TNF-alpha: leukotriene axis. Am J Respir Crit Care Med 149:41–49, 1994.
25. Wiklund RA: Preoperative preparation of patients with advanced liver disease. Crit Care Med 32(4 Suppl):S106–S115, 2004.
26. Barnes KC: Genetic determinants and ethnic disparities in sepsis-associated acute lung injury. Proc Am Thorac Soc 2:195–201, 2005.
27. Tomashefski JF, Jr: Pulmonary pathology of acute respiratory distress syndrome. Clin Chest Med 21:435–466, 2000.
28. Matthay MA, Robriquet L, Fang X: Alveolar epithelium: role in lung fluid balance and acute lung injury. Proc Am Thorac Soc 2:206–213, 2005.
29. Fahy RJ, Lichtenberger F, McKeegan CB, et al: The acute respiratory distress syndrome: a role for transforming growth factor-beta 1. Am J Respir Cell Mol Biol 28:499–503, 2003.
30. Marinelli WA, Henke CA, Harmon KR, et al: Mechanisms of alveolar fibrosis after acute lung injury. Clin Chest Med 11:657–672, 1990.
31. O'Quin R, Marini JJ: Pulmonary artery occlusion pressure: clinical physiology, measurement, and interpretation. Am Rev Respir Dis 128:319–326, 1983.
32. Richard C, Warszawski J, Anguel N, et al: Early use of the pulmonary artery catheter and outcomes in patients with shock and acute respiratory distress syndrome: a randomized controlled trial. JAMA 290:2713–2720, 2003.
33. Wheeler AP, Bernard GR, Thompson BT, et al: Pulmonary-artery versus central venous catheter to guide treatment of acute lung injury. N Engl J Med 354:2213–2224, 2006.
34. Idell S, Cohen AB: Bronchoalveolar lavage in patients with the adult respiratory distress syndrome. Clin Chest Med 6:459–471, 1985.
35. Briel M, Meade M, Mercat A, et al: Higher vs. lower positive end-expiratory pressure in patients with acute lung injury and acute respiratory distress syndrome: systematic review and meta-analysis. JAMA 303:865–873, 2010.
36. Wiedemann HP, Wheeler AP, Bernard GR, et al: Comparison of two fluid-management strategies in acute lung injury. N Engl J Med 354:2564–2575, 2006.
37. Schumacker PT: Oxygen supply dependency in critical illness: an evolving understanding. Intensive Care Med 24:97–99, 1998.
38. Shoemaker WC, Appel PL, Kram HB, et al: Prospective trial of supranormal values of survivors as therapeutic goals in high-risk surgical patients. Chest 94:1176–1186, 1988.
39. Tuchschmidt J, Fried J, Astiz M, et al: Elevation of cardiac output and oxygen delivery improves outcome in septic shock. Chest 102:216–220, 1992.
40. Gattinoni L, Brazzi L, Pelosi P, et al: A trial of goal-oriented hemodynamic therapy in critically ill patients. SvO2 Collaborative Group. N Engl J Med 333:1025–1032, 1995.
41. Hayes MA, Timmins AC, Yau EH, et al: Elevation of systemic oxygen delivery in the treatment of critically ill patients. N Engl J Med 330:1717–1722, 1994.
42. Gattinoni L, Pesenti A: Computerized tomography scanning in acute respiratory failure, New York, 1991, Marcel Dekker.
43. Dreyfuss D, Soler P, Basset G, et al: High inflation pressure pulmonary edema: respective effects of high airway pressure, high tidal volume, and positive end-expiratory pressure. Am Rev Respir Dis 137:1159–1164, 1988.
44. Ventilation with lower tidal volumes as compared with traditional tidal volumes for acute lung injury and the acute respiratory distress syndrome. The Acute Respiratory Distress Syndrome Network. N Engl J Med 342:1301–1308, 2000.
45. Gattinoni L, Protti A, Caironi P, et al: Ventilator-induced lung injury: the anatomical and physiological framework. Crit Care Med 38(10 Suppl):S539–S548, 2010.
46. Amato MB, Barbas CS, Medeiros DM, et al: Beneficial effects of the "open lung approach" with low distending pressures in acute respiratory distress syndrome: a prospective randomized study on mechanical ventilation. Am J Respir Crit Care Med 152(6 Pt 1):1835–1846, 1995.
47. Brower RG, Lanken PN, MacIntyre N, et al: Higher versus lower positive end-expiratory pressures in patients with the acute respiratory distress syndrome. N Engl J Med 351:327–336, 2004.
48. O'Croinin D, Ni Chonghaile M, Higgins B, et al: Bench-to-bedside review: permissive hypercapnia. Crit Care 9:51–59, 2005.
49. Kregenow DA, Rubenfeld GD, Hudson LD, et al: Hypercapnic acidosis and mortality in acute lung injury. Crit Care Med 34:1–7, 2006.
50. Roupie E, Dambrosio M, Servillo G, et al: Titration of tidal volume and induced hypercapnia in acute respiratory distress syndrome. Am J Respir Crit Care Med 152:121–128, 1995.
51. Young MP, Manning HL, Wilson DL, et al: Ventilation of patients with acute lung injury and acute respiratory distress syndrome: has new evidence changed clinical practice? Crit Care Med 32:1260–1265, 2004.

52. Paulson TE, Spear RM, Silva PD, et al: High-frequency pressure-control ventilation with high positive end-expiratory pressure in children with acute respiratory distress syndrome. J Pediatr 129:566–573, 1996.
53. Fort P, Farmer C, Westerman J, et al: High-frequency oscillatory ventilation for adult respiratory distress syndrome—a pilot study. Crit Care Med 25:937–947, 1997.
54. Gluck E, Heard S, Patel C, et al: Use of ultrahigh frequency ventilation in patients with ARDS: a preliminary report. Chest 103:1413–1420, 1993.
55. Derdak S, Mehta S, Stewart TE, et al: High-frequency oscillatory ventilation for acute respiratory distress syndrome in adults: a randomized, controlled trial. Am J Respir Crit Care Med 166:801–808, 2002.
56. Pipeling MR, Fan E: Therapies for refractory hypoxemia in acute respiratory distress syndrome. JAMA 304:2521–2527, 2010.
57. Bollen CW, van Well GT, Sherry T, et al: High frequency oscillatory ventilation compared with conventional mechanical ventilation in adult respiratory distress syndrome: a randomized controlled trial [ISRCTN24242669]. Crit Care 9:R430–R439, 2005.
58. Sud S, Sud M, Friedrich JO, et al: High frequency oscillation in patients with acute lung injury and acute respiratory distress syndrome (ARDS): systematic review and meta-analysis. BMJ 340:c2327, 2010.
59. Lubnow M, Luchner A, Philipp A, et al: Combination of high frequency oscillatory ventilation and interventional lung assist in severe acute respiratory distress syndrome. J Crit Care 25:436–444, 2010.
60. Tharratt RS, Allen RP, Albertson TE: Pressure controlled inverse ratio ventilation in severe adult respiratory failure. Chest 94:755–762, 1988.
61. Mercat A, Graini L, Teboul JL, et al: Cardiorespiratory effects of pressure-controlled ventilation with and without inverse ratio in the adult respiratory distress syndrome. Chest 104:871–875, 1993.
62. Esteban A, Alia I, Gordo F, et al: Prospective randomized trial comparing pressure-controlled ventilation and volume-controlled ventilation in ARDS. For the Spanish Lung Failure Collaborative Group. Chest 117:1690–1696, 2000.
63. Lessard MR, Guerot E, Lorino H, et al: Effects of pressure-controlled with different I:E ratios versus volume-controlled ventilation on respiratory mechanics, gas exchange, and hemodynamics in patients with adult respiratory distress syndrome. Anesthesiology 80:983–991, 1994.
64. Sydow M, Burchardi H, Ephraim E, et al: Long-term effects of two different ventilatory modes on oxygenation in acute lung injury: comparison of airway pressure release ventilation and volume-controlled inverse ratio ventilation. Am J Respir Crit Care Med 149:1550–1556, 1994.
65. Varpula T, Pettila V, Nieminen H, et al: Airway pressure release ventilation and prone positioning in severe acute respiratory distress syndrome. Acta Anaesthesiol Scand 45:340–344, 2001.
66. Boonyapisit K, Katirji B: Multifocal motor neuropathy presenting with respiratory failure. Muscle Nerve 23:1887–1890, 2000.
67. Douglas WW, Rehder K, Beynen FM, et al: Improved oxygenation in patients with acute respiratory failure: the prone position. Am Rev Respir Dis 115:559–566, 1977.
68. Chatte G, Sab JM, Dubois JM, et al: Prone position in mechanically ventilated patients with severe acute respiratory failure. Am J Respir Crit Care Med 155:473–478, 1997.
69. Gattinoni L, Tognoni G, Pesenti A, et al: Effect of prone positioning on the survival of patients with acute respiratory failure. N Engl J Med 345:568–573, 2001.
70. Mutoh T, Guest RJ, Lamm WJ, et al: Prone position alters the effect of volume overload on regional pleural pressures and improves hypoxemia in pigs in vivo. Am Rev Respir Dis 146:300–306, 1992.
71. Mancebo J, Fernandez R, Blanch L, et al: A multicenter trial of prolonged prone ventilation in severe acute respiratory distress syndrome. Am J Respir Crit Care Med 173:1233–1239, 2006.
72. Sud S, Friedrich JO, Taccone P, et al: Prone ventilation reduces mortality in patients with acute respiratory failure and severe hypoxemia: systematic review and meta-analysis. Intensive Care Med 36:585–599, 2010.
73. Zapol WM, Snider MT, Schneider RC: Extracorporeal membrane oxygenation for acute respiratory failure. Anesthesiology 46:272–285, 1977.
74. Davies A, Jones D, Bailey M, et al: Extracorporeal membrane oxygenation for 2009 influenza A(H1N1) acute respiratory distress syndrome. JAMA 302:1888–1895, 2009.
75. Peek GJ, Mugford M, Tiruvoipati R, et al: Efficacy and economic assessment of conventional ventilatory support versus extracorporeal membrane oxygenation for severe adult respiratory failure (CESAR): a multicentre randomised controlled trial. Lancet 374:1351–1363, 2009.
76. Park PK, Dalton HJ, Bartlett RH: Point: efficacy of extracorporeal membrane oxygenation in 2009 influenza A(H1N1): sufficient evidence? Chest 138:776–778, 2010.
77. Brunet F, Mira JP, Belghith M, et al: Extracorporeal carbon dioxide removal technique improves oxygenation without causing overinflation. Am J Respir Crit Care Med 149:1557–1562, 1994.
78. Freed DH, Henzler D, White CW, et al: Extracorporeal lung support for patients who had severe respiratory failure secondary to influenza A (H1N1) 2009 infection in Canada. Can J Anaesth 57:240–247, 2010.
79. Walmrath D, Grimminger F, Pappert D, et al: Bronchoscopic administration of bovine natural surfactant in ARDS and septic shock: impact on gas exchange and haemodynamics. Eur Respir J 19:805–810, 2002.
80. Gregory TJ, Steinberg KP, Spragg R, et al: Bovine surfactant therapy for patients with acute respiratory distress syndrome. Am J Respir Crit Care Med 155:1309–1315, 1997.
81. Spragg RG, Lewis JF, Walmrath HD, et al: Effect of recombinant surfactant protein C-based surfactant on the acute respiratory distress syndrome. N Engl J Med 351:884–892, 2004.
82. Kesecioglu J, Beale R, Stewart TE, et al: Exogenous natural surfactant for treatment of acute lung injury and the acute respiratory distress syndrome. Am J Respir Crit Care Med 180:989–994, 2009.
83. Papazian L, Forel JM, Gacouin A, et al: Neuromuscular blockers in early acute respiratory distress syndrome. N Engl J Med 363:1107–1116, 2010.
84. Taylor RW, Zimmerman JL, Dellinger RP, et al: Low-dose inhaled nitric oxide in patients with acute lung injury: a randomized controlled trial. JAMA 291:1603–1609, 2004.
85. van Heerden PV, Barden A, Michalopoulos N, et al: Dose-response to inhaled aerosolized prostacyclin for hypoxemia due to ARDS. Chest 117:819–827, 2000.
86. Afshari A, Brok J, Moller AM, et al. Inhaled nitric oxide for acute respiratory distress syndrome (ARDS) and acute lung injury in children and adults. Cochrane Database Syst Rev (7):CD002787, 2010.
87. Martin C, Papazian L, Payan MJ, et al: Pulmonary fibrosis correlates with outcome in adult respiratory distress syndrome: a study in mechanically ventilated patients. Chest 107:196–200, 1995.

88. Meduri GU, Chinn AJ, Leeper KV, et al: Corticosteroid rescue treatment of progressive fibroproliferation in late ARDS: patterns of response and predictors of outcome. Chest 105:1516–1527, 1994.
89. Meduri GU, Headley AS, Golden E, et al: Effect of prolonged methylprednisolone therapy in unresolving acute respiratory distress syndrome: a randomized controlled trial. JAMA 280:159–165, 1998.
90. Steinberg KP, Hudson LD, Goodman RB, et al: Efficacy and safety of corticosteroids for persistent acute respiratory distress syndrome. N Engl J Med 354:1671–1684, 2006.
91. Perkins GD, McAuley DF, Thickett DR, et al: The beta-agonist lung injury trial (BALTI): a randomized placebo-controlled clinical trial. Am J Respir Crit Care Med 173:281–287, 2006.
92. Girard TD, Kress JP, Fuchs BD, et al: Efficacy and safety of a paired sedation and ventilator weaning protocol for mechanically ventilated patients in intensive care (Awakening and Breathing Controlled trial): a randomised controlled trial. Lancet 371:126–134, 2008.

Chapter 28

Lung Cancer

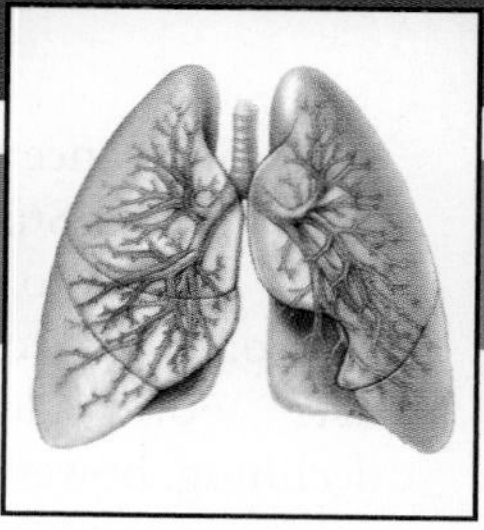

PETER MAZZONE AND HILARY PETERSEN

CHAPTER OBJECTIVES

After reading this chapter you will be able to:

- Describe the epidemiology of lung cancer in the United States, particularly current trends.
- Identify risk factors for lung cancer.
- State the classification of lung cancer types and the cellular features of the four common types of lung cancer.
- Describe current understanding of the pathophysiology of lung cancer.
- Identify the clinical features of the common types of lung cancer.
- Describe the diagnostic approach to lung cancer.
- State the staging system for lung cancer.
- Describe the treatment and outcomes for the common types of lung cancer by stage.
- State the role of the respiratory therapist in managing patients with lung cancer.

CHAPTER OUTLINE

KEY TERMS

adenocarcinoma
chemotherapy
computed tomography (CT)
flexible bronchoscopy
large cell carcinoma
magnetic resonance imaging (MRI)
mass
nodule
non-small cell carcinoma
Pancoast syndrome
paraneoplastic syndrome
positron emission tomography (PET)
radiotherapy
screening
small cell carcinoma
squamous cell carcinoma
staging system
surgical resection
TNM staging
transbronchial needle aspiration
transthoracic needle biopsy

Lung cancer is a major public health problem. In the United States, approximately 28% of cancer deaths are due to lung cancer.[1] Most of these deaths could be avoided if people did not smoke tobacco-related products. Worldwide tobacco consumption has not been declining, however, suggesting lung cancer will remain an epidemic for years to come. Advances in early detection and treatment have been slow, leaving the overall prognosis very poor when lung cancer has been detected. Just over one in eight lung cancer patients is still living 5 years after diagnosis. This chapter provides an overview of lung cancer for the respiratory therapist (RT).

EPIDEMIOLOGY

New Cases

In 2010, an estimated 222,520 new cases of lung cancer were diagnosed in the United States.[1] Lung cancer is the second most frequently diagnosed cancer in men and women (prostate and breast cancers are most frequent in men and women) (Figure 28-1). The incidence of lung cancer peaked in men in 1984 (86.5 per 100,000 men) and has since been declining (69.1 per 100,000 in 1997). In women, the incidence increased during the 1990s, with a leveling off toward the end of the decade (43.1 per 100,000 women). These trends parallel the smoking patterns of men and women.[1] The World Health Organization estimates that there are 2 million cases of lung cancer worldwide each year.

Deaths

Lung cancer is the leading cause of cancer-related mortality in men and women; it surpassed colon cancer in the early 1950s in men and breast cancer in the late 1980s in women. Mortality rates in men declined significantly in the 1990s, whereas a slow increase occurred in women. These rates parallel the smoking patterns of men and women (Figures 28-2 and 28-3). In 2010 in the United States, an estimated 157,300 deaths were due to lung cancer. In men, lung cancer is the leading cause of cancer-related mortality from age 40 on. In women, lung cancer surpasses breast cancer in the age group of 60 and older.[1]

Risk Factors

Tobacco-Related Products

Direct exposure to tobacco has occurred in 85% to 90% of individuals with lung cancer. Many tobacco-related carcinogens have been identified. The two major classes are

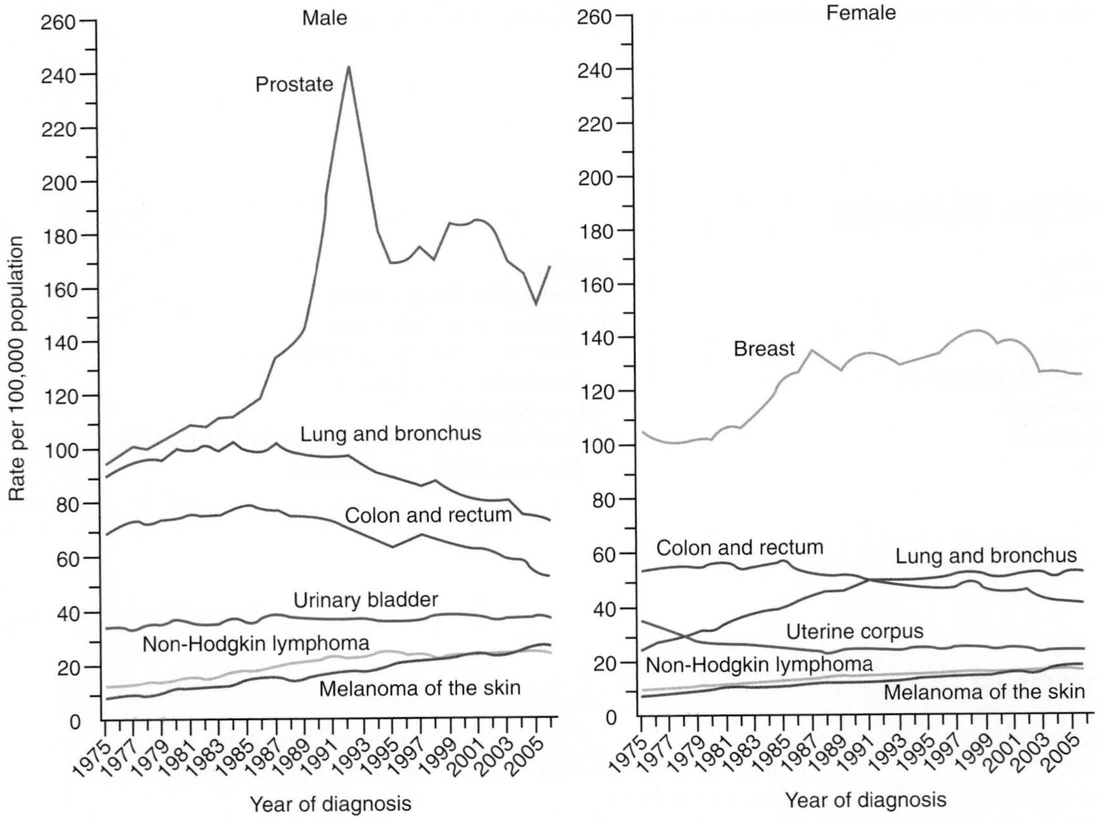

FIGURE 28-1 Age-adjusted cancer incidence rates for women and men, United States, 1975-2006. Rates are per 100,000 female population, adjusted to the 2000 U.S. standard population. The incidence of lung cancer in men and women has paralleled smoking habits. (Modified from Jemal A, Siegal R, Xu J, et al: Cancer statistics, 2010. CA Cancer J Clin 60:277-300, 2010.)

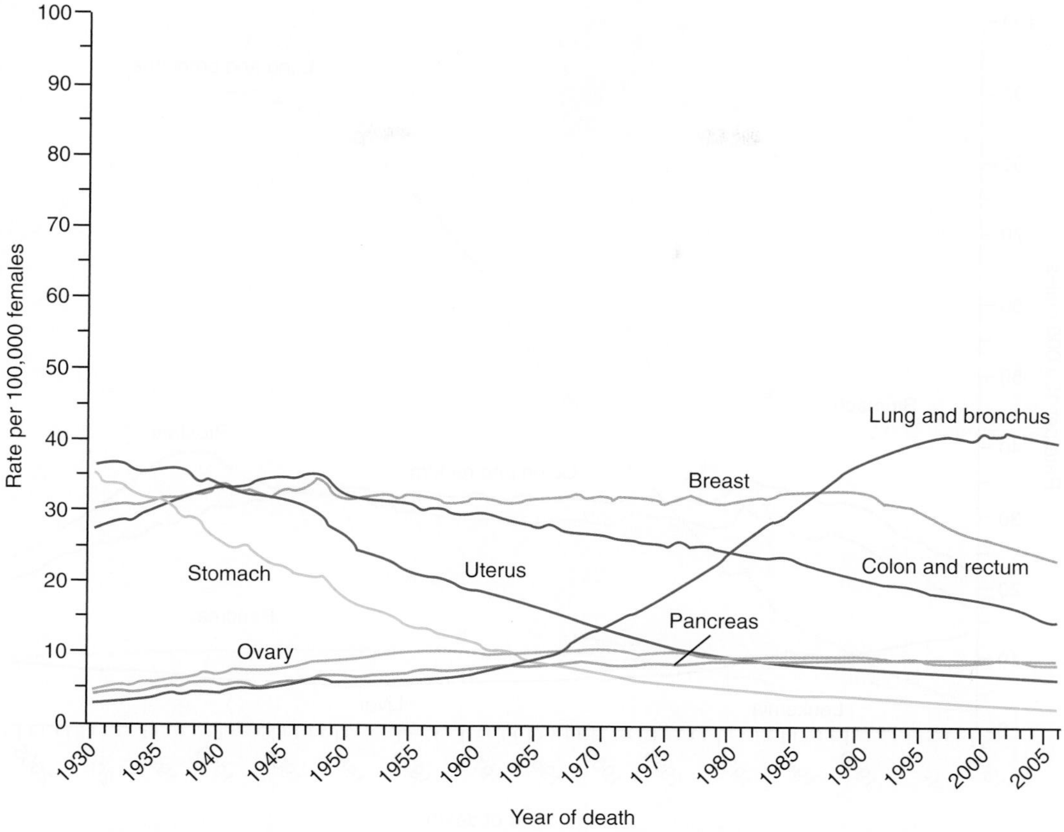

FIGURE 28-2 Age-adjusted cancer death rates for women, United States, 1930-2006. Rates are per 100,000, adjusted to the 2000 U.S. standard population. Lung cancer surpassed breast cancer as the leading cause of cancer-related mortality in women in the late 1980s. (Modified from Jemal A, Siegal R, Xu J, et al: Cancer statistics, 2010. CA Cancer J Clin 60:277-300, 2010.)

the *N-nitrosamines* and *polycyclic aromatic hydrocarbons.* A dose-response relationship exists between the degree of exposure to cigarette smoke and the development of lung cancer. The age at which smoking began, the number of cigarettes smoked per day, and the duration of smoking all influence the likelihood of developing lung cancer. Also, the intensity of smoking, the depth of inhalation, and the composition of the cigarette influence the risk. All types (see later) of lung cancer are associated with smoking. The strongest associations are with two of the cell types: *small cell* and *squamous cell carcinoma*. The risk of developing lung cancer decreases over time after smoking cessation, although it never reaches that of a lifelong nonsmoker.

There is evidence that *nicotine,* a chemical in tobacco, is highly addictive.[2] Approximately one-fifth of all adults in the United States smoke cigarettes. Progress had been made in the fight against cigarette use; in the decades from 1970-1990, the percentage of women who smoked declined from 33% to 25%, and the rate of smoking among men decreased from 43% to 28%. The annual decline that had occurred since the early 1970s began to slow through the 1990s despite mounting evidence associating smoking with disease and death.[3] In addition, a decrease in smoking has not been observed among adults 18 to 24 years old. Cigarette smoking among young people remains a major public health concern. Of young adults (18 to 24 years old), 33% have been reported to be current users of tobacco,[4] and 3000 teenagers begin smoking each day.[5] Approximately 13% of middle school children and 28% of high school students use tobacco products. In the context that a person who has not started smoking as a teenager is unlikely ever to become a smoker, the tobacco industry has focused on young people and developing countries as the primary sources of new customers.[6,7]

Other forms of exposure to tobacco-related products also pose risk of promoting lung cancer. Cigar smoking, which has increased considerably over the past several years, is known to be an independent risk factor for developing lung cancer.[8]

Exposure to *sidestream smoke,* or *passive smoking,* may also lead to an increased risk of lung cancer. The risk is generally much lower than active smoking but varies with the intensity of exposure.[7] The risk of developing lung cancer has been reported to be 30% higher in individuals exposed to sidestream smoke. It has been estimated that 3000 to 5000 deaths in the United States and 21,400 deaths worldwide from lung cancer occur each year because of secondhand smoke exposure.[9,10]

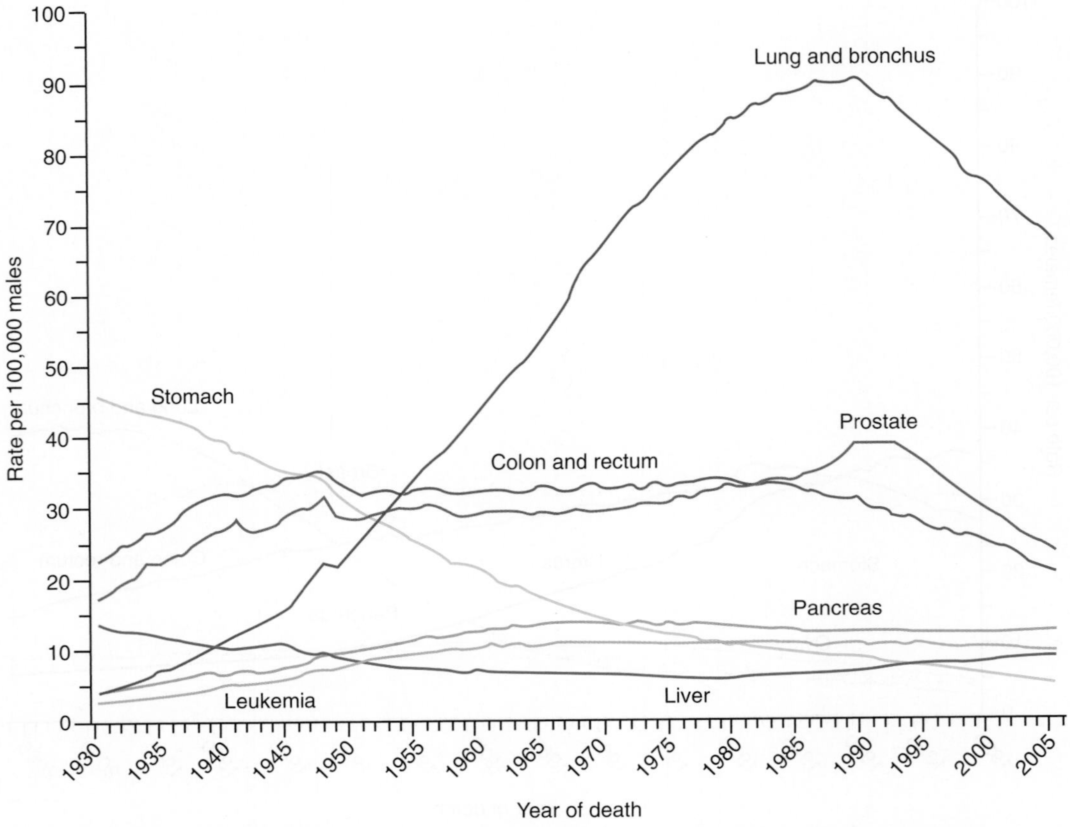

FIGURE 28-3 Age-adjusted cancer death rates for men, United States, 1930-2006. Rates are per 100,000, adjusted to the 2000 U.S. standard population. Lung cancer has been the leading cause of cancer-related mortality in men since the early 1950s. Mortality rates have declined more recently. (Modified from Jemal A, Siegal R, Xu J, et al: Cancer statistics, 2010. CA Cancer J Clin 60:277-300, 2010.)

Occupational Agents and Other Risks

Many other risk factors have been identified (Box 28-1). Occupational agents are known to act as lung cancer carcinogens. Arsenic, asbestos, and chromium confer the highest risk. Of lung cancers, 2% to 9% have been estimated to be related to occupational exposures. This risk is increased when there is concomitant exposure to tobacco products. Indoor radon exposure is also a risk factor for developing lung cancer.[11] Radon is a product generated by the breakdown of uranium. Particulates in the atmosphere (i.e., pollution) can increase the risk of lung diseases including lung cancer.

An inherited genetic predisposition has epidemiologic support as a risk factor, but the mechanisms are not proven. Family members of people who develop lung cancer have an increased risk.[12,13] Women seem to have a higher baseline risk of developing lung cancer and a greater susceptibility to the effects of smoking. Differences in the metabolism of tobacco-related carcinogens and their metabolites, an effect of hormone differences, or both are thought to account for the increased susceptibility.[14] Dietary factors can also modify risks. Higher

Box 28-1 Lung Cancer Risk Factors

- Tobacco smoke exposure
  - Active (mainstream)—cigarette, cigar
  - Passive (sidestream)
- Occupational and environmental exposures
  - Arsenic
  - Chromium
  - Asbestos
  - Nickel
  - Beryllium
  - Polycyclic aromatic hydrocarbons
  - Bis(chloromethyl)ether
  - Radon
  - Cadmium
  - Vinyl chloride
- Genetic predisposition
- Gender
- Dietary factors
- COPD
- Air pollution

Courtesy The Cleveland Clinic, Cleveland, Ohio.

consumption of fruits and vegetables is associated with a reduced lung cancer risk, and increased dietary fat intake may lead to a higher risk.[15,16] Supplementation with vitamin A, vitamin E, or beta-carotene has not positively influenced risk.[15] The presence of chronic obstructive pulmonary disease (COPD) is an independent risk factor.[17] This risk increases as the forced expiratory volume in 1 second (FEV_1) decreases.[18,19]

LUNG CANCER CLASSIFICATION

Lung cancers are divided into two major groups—**small cell carcinoma** and **non-small cell carcinoma**—based on pathologic features that are visible under light microscopy. The evaluation and management of a patient are guided by the category and stage (see later) of lung cancer. The non-small cell cancer category consists of **adenocarcinoma, squamous cell carcinoma, large cell carcinoma,** and variants (Figure 28-4). Table 28-1 presents the pathologic and epidemiologic features of the four most common types of lung cancer: adenocarcinoma, squamous cell carcinoma, large cell carcinoma, and small cell carcinoma.

PATHOPHYSIOLOGY

The pathophysiology of lung cancer development is complex and incompletely understood. Damage to genetic material in lung cells is the result of exposure to chemical carcinogens such as the carcinogens contained in tobacco smoke.[20] People who develop lung cancer may have a genetic predisposition to the effects of these carcinogens. The genes influenced in the pathogenesis of lung cancer produce proteins involved in cell growth and differentiation, cell cycle processes, *apoptosis* (programmed cell death), *angiogenesis* (production of new blood vessels), tumor progression, and immune regulation. If enough of these pathways have been affected, the uncontrolled growth of cells that defines cancer occurs. If the mechanisms that lead to

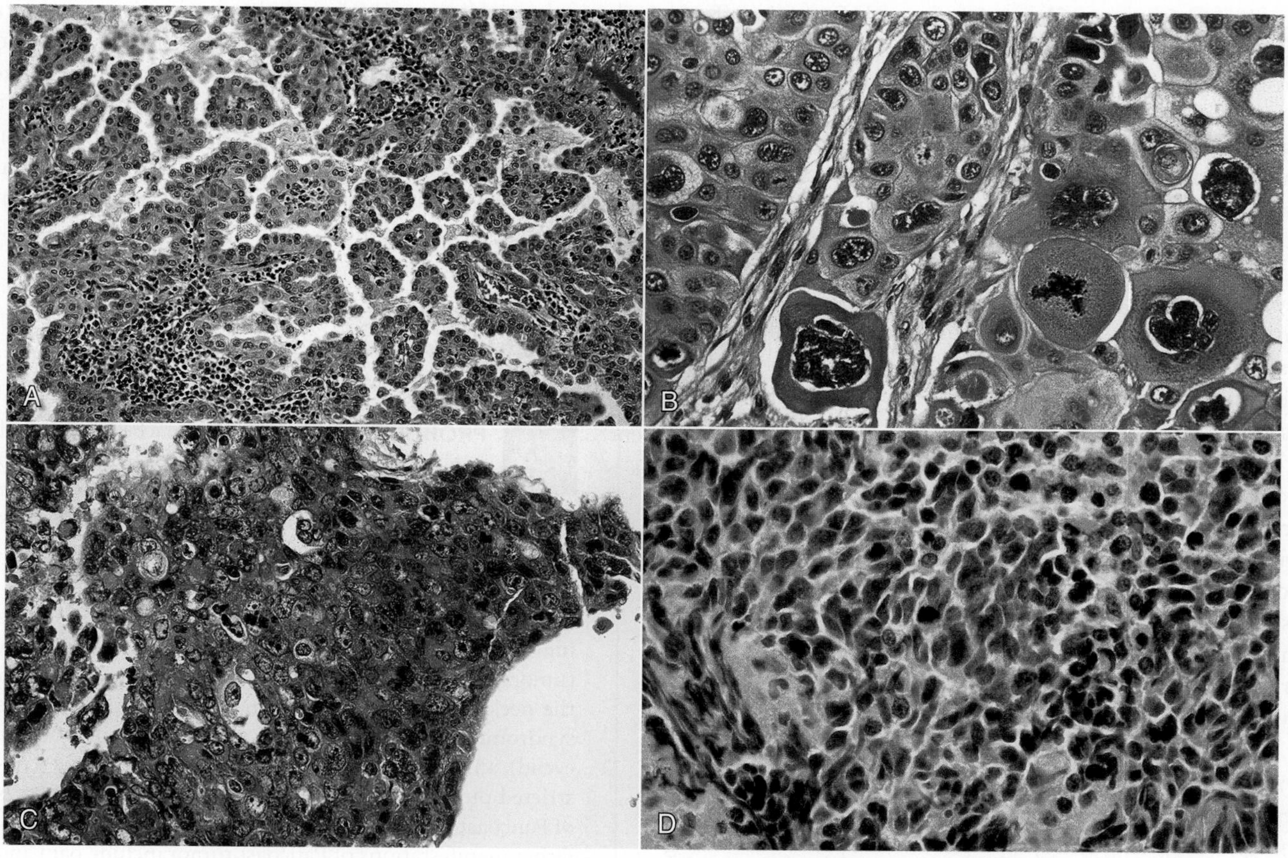

FIGURE 28-4 Lung cancer histology. **A,** Adenocarcinoma, characterized by heterogeneous differentiation in the same tumor. **B,** Squamous cell carcinoma, characterized by the presence of cytokeratin differentiation with keratinization and intercellular bridges. **C,** Large cell carcinoma, characterized by sheets and nest with extensive necrosis, large nuclei with prominent nucleoli, and lack of definitive evidence of squamous or glandular differentiation. **D,** Small cell carcinoma, characterized by round to fusiform nuclei, nuclear molding, faint or absent nucleoli, and scant cytoplasm. (Courtesy The Cleveland Clinic, Cleveland, Ohio.)

TABLE 28-1

Classification of Most Common Types of Lung Cancer

Category	Cell Type	Pathologic Features (Light Microscopy)	Epidemiology
Non–small cell carcinoma	Adenocarcinoma	Formation of glandular structures; heterogeneous differentiation	Accounts for >40% of lung cancers in North America; increasing frequency in women
	Squamous cell carcinoma	Cytokeratin and intercellular bridges	Second most frequent type of lung cancer in United States
	Large cell carcinoma	Sheets and nests of cells, necrosis, lack of squamous cell or glandular features	Less common than adenocarcinoma or squamous cell carcinoma
Small cell carcinoma	Small cell carcinoma	Round to fusiform nuclei; faint to absent nucleoli; scant cytoplasm	Accounts for 13% of lung cancers

genetic damage can be identified and the means by which the pathways involved are controlled, novel means of risk stratification, prevention, early detection, and therapy should be able to be developed.

CLINICAL FEATURES

The clinical features of lung cancer result from the effects of local growth of the tumor, regional growth or spread through the lymphatic system, hematogenous (blood-borne) distant metastatic spread, and remote paraneoplastic effects from tumor products or immune cross reaction with tumor antigens (Box 28-2). Some manifestations occur more commonly with a particular cell type. Despite modern imaging advances, only approximately 15% of patients with a diagnosis of lung cancer do not have symptoms at the time of presentation. Some of the initial symptoms may be related to accompanying illnesses because these patients are at risk for other medical problems in addition to lung cancer (e.g., COPD, heart disease).

Local growth in a central location (e.g., in a main stem bronchus) can cause cough, hemoptysis, or features of large airway obstruction. Squamous cell carcinoma and small cell carcinoma are more likely to grow in a central location than other cell types. Peripheral growth may also cause cough and dyspnea. If the pleura or chest wall is involved, pain may occur. Adenocarcinoma and large cell carcinoma occur more commonly in the periphery of the lung.

Regional growth may lead to esophageal compression *(dysphagia),* recurrent laryngeal nerve paralysis (hoarseness), phrenic nerve paralysis with an elevated hemidiaphragm (dyspnea), and sympathetic nerve paralysis leading to Horner syndrome (ptosis [droopy eyelid], miosis [small pupils], anhidrosis [lack of facial sweating], and enophthalmos [sunken eye]). Apical growth may lead to **Pancoast syndrome,** with shoulder pain radiating in an ulnar distribution as a result of involvement of the brachial plexus. The superior vena cava can become obstructed, resulting in swelling of the face, neck, and upper chest; plethora; and dilation of superficial veins over these areas; this is called the *superior vena cava syndrome.* Lung cancer can grow to involve the heart and pericardium. Lymphatic obstruction and spread can lead to dyspnea, hypoxemia, and pleural effusions.

Distant metastatic disease can affect most organs; the brain, bones, liver, and adrenal glands are most commonly involved. Neurologic symptoms such as headaches, vision changes, and seizures may suggest brain metastases. Back pain and changes in strength or sensation in an extremity may indicate spinal cord compression. Bone pain could indicate bone metastases. Laboratory abnormalities may point to bone marrow or liver involvement. Imaging may detect adrenal involvement.

MINI CLINI

Pancoast Tumor

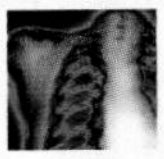

PROBLEM: A 65-year-old man who has smoked two packs of cigarettes per day for the past 40 years has had drooping of the left eyelid for the past 3 weeks. A chest radiograph reveals a mass in the apex of the left lung. Is there a link between the drooping of the eyelid and the lung mass?

DISCUSSION: Lung tumors involving the apex of the lung (superior sulcus tumors) are also known as Pancoast tumors. If they involve the cervical sympathetic nerves in the neck, these tumors result in Horner syndrome. This syndrome is characterized by ptosis (drooping of the eyelid), anhidrosis (absence of sweating), and miosis (constricted pupil) on the same side as the tumor. Most cases of Pancoast tumor are caused by squamous cell carcinoma. Other manifestations of Pancoast tumor include pain and weakness in the upper extremity (owing to involvement of the brachial plexus), rib destruction, and destruction of vertebral bodies. This condition usually reflects the presence of advanced disease that may not be amenable to surgical resection.

MINI CLINI

Hilar Adenopathy

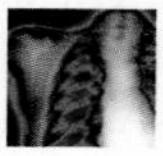

PROBLEM: A 60-year-old man has been found to have small cell lung cancer on the basis of results of bronchoscopic biopsy. CT scan of the chest shows extensive hilar adenopathy. The patient has been admitted to the oncology floor for chemotherapy. You are called to assess him because he cannot lie down owing to shortness of breath (orthopnea). When you arrive, the patient is sitting on the edge of the bed. You notice that his face and neck are swollen. He also has dilated veins over the face, neck, chest, and arms. How do you explain these findings?

DISCUSSION: This patient has superior vena cava obstruction caused by compression by the mediastinal tumor. The swelling of the face, neck, and arms is caused by impairment of the venous drainage from the upper body (the superior vena cava distribution). The dilated chest and arm veins are collateral vessels (or alternative pathway vessels) that compensate for the superior vena cava obstruction. Superior vena cava obstruction can be caused by various benign or malignant conditions that involve the mediastinum or the right upper lung. Treatment usually is therapy for the underlying problem. For this patient, the preferred treatment is chemotherapy because small cell lung cancer is highly responsive to this modality. Other cancers may be more responsive to radiation. Good responses occur in 75% of patients within 2 weeks of initiation of therapy. Surgical resection rarely is needed.

When symptoms develop that are the result of the presence of cancer but are not related to the growth or spread of the cancer, these symptoms constitute a **paraneoplastic syndrome.** Paraneoplastic syndromes can result from the effects of proteins produced by the tumor that circulate through the body to have their effects on distant organs or result from the immune response of the body to a tumor antigen that is similar to antigens in other parts of the body, causing immune injury to the distant organ. Paraneoplastic syndromes may occur before the primary tumor appears and be the first sign of disease or an indication of tumor recurrence. Examples include production of excess glucocorticoids (ectopic Cushing syndrome), parathyroid hormone (hypercalcemia of malignancy), and antidiuretic hormone (syndrome of inappropriate antidiuretic hormone [SIADH]). Paraneoplastic neurologic syndromes can affect all parts of the neurologic system resulting in emotional lability (limbic encephalitis), loss of balance (cerebellar degeneration), and muscle weakness with a characteristic recruitment of strength on electrical stimulation (Lambert-Eaton syndrome). Other paraneoplastic syndromes include skeletal and connective tissue syndromes (clubbing, hypertrophic pulmonary

Box 28-2 Lung Cancer Manifestations

- Local growth
  - Cough
  - Dyspnea
  - Hemoptysis
  - Pain
- Regional growth
  - Dysphagia
  - Dyspnea
  - Hoarseness
  - Horner syndrome
  - Hypoxia
  - Pancoast syndrome
- Pericardial and pleural effusions
  - Superior vena cava syndrome
- Metastatic disease
  - Headache
  - Hepatomegaly
  - Mental status change
  - Pain
  - Papilledema
  - Seizures
  - Skin or soft tissue mass
  - Syncope
  - Weakness
- Paraneoplastic
  - Cutaneous or skeletal
  - Acanthosis nigricans
  - Clubbing
  - Dermatomyositis
  - Hypertrophic osteoarthropathy
- Endocrine
  - Cushing syndrome
  - Humoral hypercalcemia
  - SIADH
  - Tumor necrosis factor (cachexia)
- Hematologic
  - Anemia or polycythemia
- Disseminated intravascular coagulation
- Eosinophilia
  - Granulocytosis
  - Thrombophlebitis
- Neurologic
- Cancer-associated retinopathy
- Encephalomyelitis
  - Lambert-Eaton syndrome
  - Neuropathies
  - Cerebellar degeneration
- Renal
  - Glomerulonephritis
  - Nephrotic syndrome

Courtesy The Cleveland Clinic, Cleveland, Ohio.

osteoarthropathy), coagulation and hematologic disorders, cutaneous and renal manifestations, and systemic symptoms (anorexia, cachexia, and weight loss).[21]

MINI CLINI

Paraneoplastic Syndrome

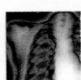

PROBLEM: A 55-year-old man is brought to the emergency department by family members because of confusion and progressive generalized weakness. Examination in the emergency department shows the patient is dehydrated, lethargic, and confused. Chest radiograph reveals a cavitary lesion in the right upper lobe. Results of arterial blood gas analysis are normal. Results of chemical analysis urgently performed with the blood gas analysis reveal a sodium level of 150 mEq/L (normal 135 to 145 mEq/L) and a calcium level of 17 mg/dl (normal 9 to 10.5 mg/dl). How is the lung mass related to this patient's presentation and biochemical abnormalities?

DISCUSSION: This patient's confusion and weakness are due to hypercalcemia, which is a paraneoplastic presentation of lung cancer, especially squamous cell carcinoma (the cavitating mass on the chest radiograph). Paraneoplastic syndromes are systemic manifestations of lung cancer that are not caused by metastasis. Most paraneoplastic syndromes are associated with small cell lung cancer. However, hypercalcemia is more common with squamous cell carcinoma and is caused by secretion by the tumor of parathyroid hormone–related peptide. Treatment consists of hydration, diuresis, and use of medications that can reduce the levels of calcium.

DIAGNOSIS

Approximately 85% of patients with lung cancer present with one or more of the previously described symptoms. In the remainder, lung cancer is detected by radiographic evaluation performed for an unrelated problem. This proportion may change in the future if **computed tomography (CT)** screening programs become widespread. Most patients have a chest radiograph and CT scan of the chest performed in their initial evaluation. These studies show a small spot (<3 cm in diameter) termed a **nodule** in the lungs or a larger spot (>3 cm in diameter) termed a **mass.** Other findings on imaging include enlarged lymph nodes in the hila (where the bronchi and central blood vessels emerge from the mediastinum into the lung) or mediastinum or a pleural effusion. An individual patient's clinical and radiographic presentation dictates further evaluation.

The symptoms of lung cancer are nonspecific. There are many reasons that someone could have a cough or be short of breath. Similarly, an abnormality such as a lung nodule can be present on chest imaging for various reasons. Certain clinical and radiographic features make it more likely that the presentation represents lung cancer. Clinical features to consider include age, smoking history, history of other cancers, and presence of key symptoms. The older the patient is and the more he or she has smoked over time, the more likely the chest finding is lung cancer. Also, individuals with prior cancers are more likely to have lung cancer. Hemoptysis increases concern about cancer.

Radiographic features are also used to determine the probability of cancer. The larger the lung abnormality, the more likely it is to be cancer. When the abnormality has reached the size of a mass (3 cm), it needs to be considered a cancer until proven otherwise. The rate of growth of the lesion is also helpful. If a nodule grows rapidly (doubles in size in <1 month) or grows very slowly or not at all over a couple of years, it is unlikely to be due to cancer. If the nodule appears to be heavily calcified on imaging, it has likely been present for quite some time and is unlikely to represent cancer. If the abnormality has an irregular border, is lobulated, or is spiculated, it is more likely to be a cancer than if the border is smooth and rounded. Finally, if the lesion is cavitary, the thickness of the wall of the cavity can suggest cancer. A wall thickness of 14 mm or greater is likely to represent a cancer.[22]

RULE OF THUMB

A solitary pulmonary nodule that has not grown in 24 months is unlikely to be malignant.

MINI CLINI

No Response to Antibiotics

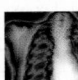

PROBLEM: A 55-year-old woman who does not smoke has a 3-month history of dyspnea on exertion, weight loss, and cough productive of copious amounts of clear, frothy sputum. She has no fever or chills. She has been treated for 2 weeks for "double pneumonia" without relief of the symptoms. Examination reveals finger clubbing and decreased air entry in both lung bases with dullness to percussion. A chest radiograph shows bilateral alveolar infiltrates. What should be done next?

DISCUSSION: The patient has a variant of adenocarcinoma of the lung. Cough productive of copious amounts of clear, frothy sputum is characteristic of this type of lung cancer. The radiographic appearance may be indistinguishable from pneumonia, especially when there is sputum production. The absence of fever, the chronic presence of infiltrates, and the lack of response to antibiotic therapy should raise suspicion for this type of lung cancer. Bronchoscopy with transbronchial biopsy would be a reasonable next step to confirm the diagnosis.

After the clinical and standard imaging features are reviewed, a probability of malignancy can be determined. If the probability is very high, the potential cancer does not seem to have spread, and the individual is fit, proceeding directly to surgery would be reasonable. If the previously mentioned features suggest a very low probability of malignancy, the clinician and patient might choose to follow along with serial chest imaging over time to assess for further growth. When the probability falls between these extremes, adjunctive imaging and invasive procedures can be used to help alter the probability. The most commonly used additional imaging technique is **positron emission tomography (PET)** with fluorodeoxyglucose (FDG-PET). Because malignant cells are metabolically very active, they take up the glucose analogue more avidly than nonmalignant cells. The attached radioactive tracer becomes trapped in the cells, allowing it to be imaged. When this test is used to help predict the presence of lung cancer, it has a sensitivity of 97% and a specificity of 78%.[23] PET imaging can produce false-positive results in other metabolically active conditions such as infections. It can be falsely negative if the lesion is too small (<10 mm) or if the tumor is slow growing and not very metabolically active (e.g., some adenocarcinomas, carcinoid tumor). Single photon emission computed tomography (SPECT) and lung nodule enhancement with contrast-enhanced CT are other imaging techniques that have been studied but are not being used clinically.[22]

Ultimately, tissue is obtained to confirm the diagnosis of lung cancer. **Flexible bronchoscopy** and **transthoracic needle biopsy** are invasive, nonsurgical approaches used to obtain tissue. If these procedures fail or are deemed unnecessary, a surgical approach is used.

Flexible bronchoscopy is a procedure in which a long, thin, flexible camera is passed through a patient's nostril or mouth into the lungs. The camera can be extended into the branches of the lung as far as the branches are large enough to admit it. The camera has a small channel through which very thin biopsy instruments can be passed out deeper into the lung to take samples from concerning areas. Flexible bronchoscopy has a high diagnostic yield for lesions that are endoscopically visible within the larger airways. Samples are collected by washing saline over the lesion, sending a small brush through the camera to collect cells on its bristles, and taking biopsy samples with a forceps or needle.

Addition of needle aspiration to the conventional sampling techniques (washing, brushing, and forceps biopsy) improves the yield. The diagnostic yield from lesions in the periphery of the lung, beyond where the camera is able to see, is lower. Conventional sampling techniques and peripheral **transbronchial needle aspiration** complement each other. Factors that influence the diagnostic yield of flexible bronchoscopy for peripheral lesions include the size of the lesion, its location, and the presence of a "bronchus sign" on CT (an airway leading directly into the lesion). Smaller, more peripheral lesions, without a visible bronchus within or leading directly to them, are unlikely to be diagnosed by flexible bronchoscopy.[22] More recent technologic advances, such as multiplanar imaging, electromagnetic navigation of the bronchoscopy instruments, and peripheral endobronchial ultrasound, have been able to improve the yield of flexible bronchoscopy for these small peripheral lesions.[24] Endobronchial ultrasound can also be used to guide biopsies of hilar and mediastinal lymph nodes.[25-26]

Transthoracic needle biopsy, using fluoroscopic or CT guidance, can also be used to obtain tissue. With this procedure, an aspirating needle is passed through the skin into the lung lesion under the guidance of chest imaging. The positive predictive value of this procedure is high, the negative predictive value is modest, and the rate of establishing a specific benign diagnosis is low. Smaller nodules in central locations have lower diagnostic rates. A higher rate of pneumothorax occurs with transthoracic needle biopsy.[24] The choice of which procedure to use is guided by the size and location of the lesion and by the local expertise with each technique.

STAGING

A major factor that determines the prognosis of lung cancer and guides the selection of appropriate treatment is the extent to which the cancer has spread in the lungs and throughout the body. The extent of cancer spread is termed the *stage* of the cancer. Non-small cell lung cancer is staged using the **TNM staging** system (*T* for extent of primary tumor, *N* for regional lymph node involvement, and *M* for metastases).

The T component of the **staging system** is divided into T1 through T4 lesions, as follows:

- A *T1 tumor* is a small tumor confined to the lung. It must be less than 3 cm in diameter and be surrounded by lung or visceral pleura and cannot extend into a main bronchus. T1a tumors are less than 2 cm in diameter, and T1b tumors are 2 to 3 cm.
- A *T2 tumor* is larger than a T1 lesion, but its local growth remains minimally invasive. It is greater than 3 cm in diameter (3 to 5 cm for T2a, 5 to 7 cm for T2b), may invade the visceral pleura, or may extend into the main bronchus, but it remains greater than 2 cm from the main carina. It may cause segmental or lobar atelectasis.
- A *T3 tumor* is locally advanced or invasive up to but not including the major intrathoracic structures. It can be any size, and it may involve the chest wall, diaphragm, mediastinal pleura, parietal pericardium, or main bronchus within 2 cm of the main carina (but not involving the main carina). It may cause atelectasis of an entire lung. There may be separate tumor nodules in the same lobe as the primary tumor. A tumor larger than 7 cm in diameter is considered T3 even if unaccompanied by local invasion.

- A *T4 tumor* is a tumor of any size that has invaded one of the major intrathoracic structures, such as the mediastinum, heart, great vessels, trachea, esophagus, vertebral body, or main carina. The tumor is also classified T4 if there are tumor nodules in a different ipsilateral lobe of the lung.

The N component of the staging system is determined by which lymph nodes, if any, are involved with tumor, as follows:

- *N0 spread* does not involve any lymph nodes.
- *N1 spread* indicates the presence of cancer in nodes within the ipsilateral lung (the same side as the tumor).
- *N2 spread* signifies cancer in nodes in the mediastinum ipsilateral to the primary tumor.
- *N3 spread* signifies cancer in nodes distant to the nodes included in N2 such as *contralateral* ("opposite side") mediastinal or hilar nodes, *ipsilateral* ("same side") or contralateral scalene, or supraclavicular nodes.[27-29]

The M part of the staging system represents the absence *(M0)* or presence *(M1)* of metastases outside of the chest. *M1a* refers to metastasis of separate tumor nodules in the contralateral lung or malignant pleural involvement (including a malignant pleural or pericardial effusion). *M1b* refers to distant metastatic spread, such as liver, bone, or brain lesions.

The most recent revision[27] to this staging system occurred in 2009 (Table 28-2 and Figure 28-5). The stages are labeled from stage IA to stage IV based on the combination of T, N, and M features.

For patients with small cell lung cancer, the TNM staging system was previously thought to be less useful. Instead, small cell lung cancer has been staged as limited or extensive disease. *Limited stage* disease is present when the tumor is confined to a hemithorax (including ipsilateral mediastinal and supraclavicular lymph nodes) and can be contained within a radiotherapy port. *Extensive stage* disease is present when the tumor extends beyond these boundaries. The recent lung cancer staging revision recognized a benefit to applying the TNM staging system used for non–small cell cancer to small cell cancer as well.[27,29]

The proper use of testing to stage a patient with lung cancer is addressed in a more recent set of guidelines.[30] The history and physical examination are important in guiding testing. The extent of spread is best evaluated using CT of the chest extending to the upper abdomen to include the liver and adrenal glands; this should be ordered in all patients. **Magnetic resonance imaging (MRI)** has not proved to be more accurate except in the setting of a Pancoast tumor. The sensitivity and specificity of CT for the evaluation of regional lymph node involvement are modest, commonly noted to be 60% and rarely greater than 75%. Imaging with FDG-PET scanning seems to have better test characteristics for staging mediastinal nodes, with sensitivity and specificity greater than 90%.[31] Integrated PET/CT scanning seems to have better test characteristics than PET and CT used alone or together.[32]

Because noninvasive tests can have false-positive results, tissue confirmation is necessary. Bronchoscopy with transbronchial needle aspiration is useful to stage the mediastinum. The addition of endobronchial and endoscopic ultrasound has increased the yield of nonsurgical mediastinal staging.[26,33] If such staging is negative, mediastinoscopy, mediastinotomy, or thoracoscopy can confirm the nodal status. Despite the advances in imaging technology and sampling techniques, definitive staging with **surgical resection** and mediastinal dissection remains the "gold standard" in a patient with resectable disease. The assigned clinical stage (determined by the previously listed testing, including mediastinoscopy) can be lower than the pathologic staging (assigned after surgery).

The evaluation of metastatic disease also takes into consideration the history, physical examination, laboratory results (electrolytes, calcium, alkaline phosphatase, liver profile, and creatinine), and pathology results. All patients should have the chest CT scan extended through the adrenal glands because metastatic disease to the adrenal glands is usually asymptomatic, and frequently no alterations are seen in routine laboratory tests. Contrast-enhanced CT, ultrasound, or MRI of the liver should be performed if the chest CT scan, laboratory results, or clinical evaluation suggests metastatic liver disease.

Per guidelines, a head CT or MRI scan should be performed if symptoms or signs of metastatic disease are present or when evaluating what appears to be stage IIIA through IV disease. Although there is no proven survival benefit from CT versus MRI, many clinicians prefer to use MRI of the brain because it has greater sensitivity to detect metastatic disease.[30,34] Bone scanning was previously performed if symptoms or signs suggest bone involvement, if the patient has an elevated calcium or alkaline phosphatase level, or if the patient is in stage IIIA/B disease. This scan has been largely replaced by PET. PET has been used to stage all but brain metastases. The rate of detecting distant metastases using PET appears to be higher than using non-PET approaches.[35]

Along with evaluating the anatomic extent of disease, a patient's performance status is important in determining his or her prognosis and ability to tolerate any proposed treatment. The two most commonly used scales of performance status are the *Zubrod scale* and the *Karnofsky scale.*

TABLE 28-2
Staging

Stage	
IA	T1a,bN0M0
IB	T2aN0M0
IIA	T1a,bN1M0, T2aN1M0, T2bN0M0
IIB	T2bN1M0, T3N0M0
IIIA	T3N1M0, T(1-3)N2M0, T4N0-1
IIIB	T4N2M0, T(1-4)N3M0
IV	T(any)N(any)M1a,b

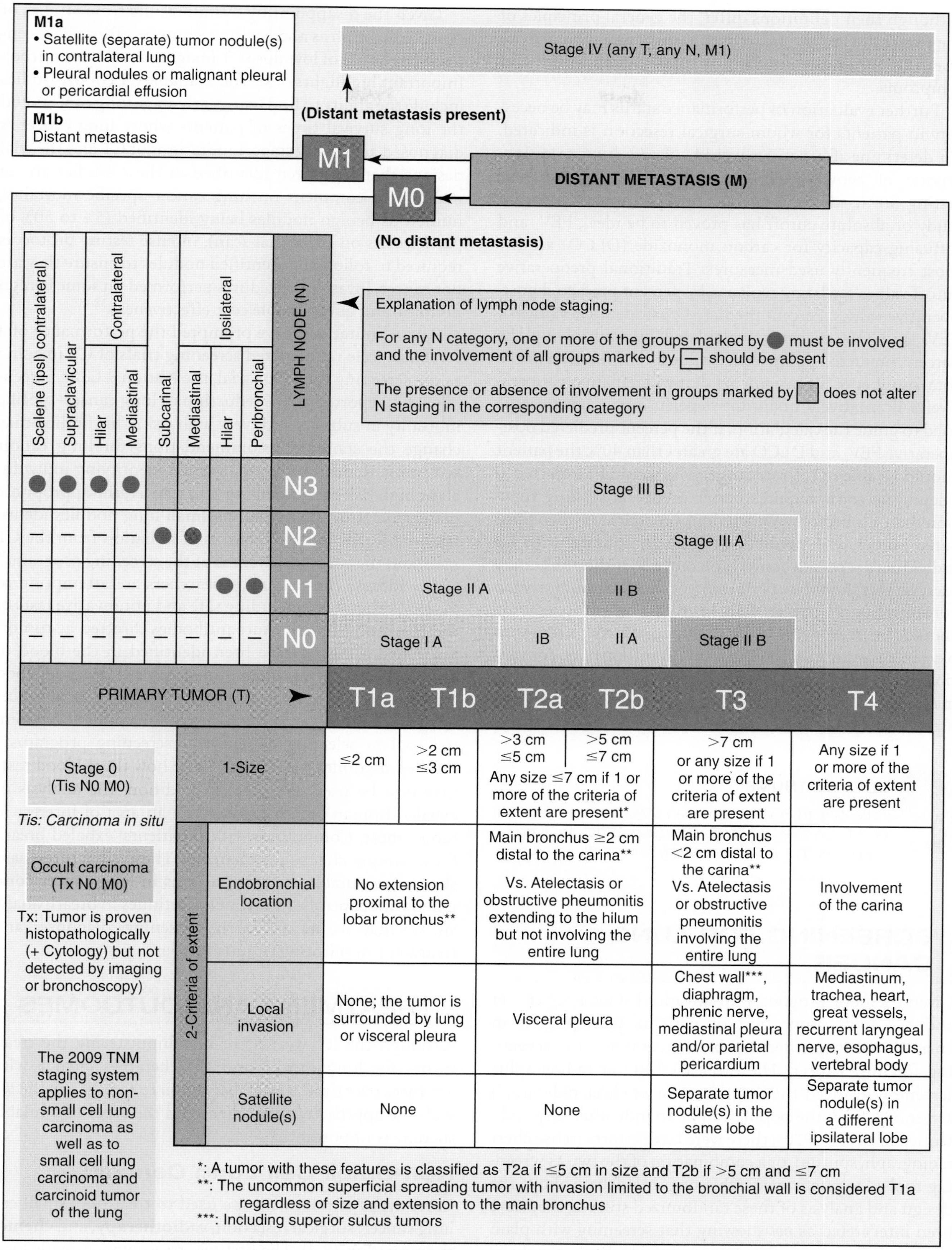

FIGURE 28-5 Reference chart for TNM staging of lung cancer. (Modified from Lababede O, Meziane M, Rice T: Seventh edition of the cancer staging manual and stage grouping of lung cancer: quick reference chart and diagrams. Chest 139:183–189, 2011.)

Although their definitions differ, the general principles of the two scales are the same, with ratings based on activity level, independence in daily activities, and severity of symptoms.

Further evaluation of performance status may be necessary in patients for whom surgical resection is indicated. To determine if a patient would tolerate lung resection, reports of activity tolerance and pulmonary function testing are used. Although no one pulmonary function study or absolute cutoff has proved to be ideal, FEV_1 and diffusing capacity for carbon monoxide (DLCO) are the most frequently used measures. Traditional preoperative cutoff values are being replaced by percent predicted postoperative values. Percent predicted postoperative values of FEV_1 and DLCO can be calculated by multiplying the percent predicted preoperative value by the fraction of the total number of lung segments that will remain postoperatively. Alternatively, quantitative perfusion imaging can be used to guide the calculation. If the percent predicted postoperative FEV_1 and DLCO are greater than 40%, the patient should be able to tolerate surgery. As would be expected, a pneumonectomy requires better preoperative lung function than a lobectomy. When doubt remains or when measured values and predictions seem discordant with an individual's reported activity tolerance, a cardiopulmonary exercise test should be performed. If the maximum oxygen consumption is greater than 15 ml/kg/min, a lobectomy should be reasonably well tolerated. If the maximum oxygen consumption is less than 10 ml/kg/min, conventional surgery should not be performed. Patients with a maximum oxygen consumption value between these two limits should be considered on a case-by-case basis.[36]

RULE OF THUMB

Patients with FEV_1 greater than 80% predicted value or 2 L can safely undergo surgical resection for lung cancer, even if pneumonectomy is needed.

SCREENING FOR LUNG CANCER

Given the poor prognosis for advanced stage lung cancer and the high proportion of patients who present in an advanced stage, there has been great interest in **screening** for lung cancer. The earliest efforts at radiographic screening involved the analysis of mass chest radiograph screenings from the population of an individual city. Subsequently in the 1970s, there were large efforts to use chest radiograph, sputum, or a combination of the two as screening tools. Despite considerable ongoing debate about the design and analysis of these randomized studies, they have been interpreted as *not* showing that screening with plain chest radiograph or sputum examination has a beneficial effect on mortality from lung cancer.[37]

Given the disappointing overall results from studies of chest radiograph as a screening technique, efforts have centered on the use of low-dose CT imaging as a screening tool. Important highlights of several available CT cohort studies include the ability to find many early stage lung cancers and the long survival times of patients whose lung cancer is diagnosed at an early stage. Limitations of CT and the trial designs that have been identified in these studies are an inability to comment on lung cancer–specific mortality, numerous benign nodules being identified (5% to 50% of participants on the initial scan), intense testing protocols required to follow the identified nodules to ensure they are not cancer, invasive procedures performed on some benign nodules, and questionable cost-effectiveness.[38-45]

These limitations have prompted the performance of a few large-scale randomized screening trials of CT imaging as the screening tool. One trial, the National Lung Screening Trial, reported a 20% reduction in lung cancer–specific mortality in subjects with very high risk. This finding may change the standard recommendations for lung cancer screening. Remaining issues include identifying individuals at high risk for developing lung cancer, the appropriate management of the numerous small lung nodules identified on CT, the potential harms of radiation from the CT scan, and the cost-effectiveness of the screening program.[46]

To address these issues, researchers are attempting to develop other tests, including safe and noninvasive tests of the blood and breath. Autoantibodies directed at tumor-associated antigens have been identified in the blood of some patients with primary lung cancer. A positive blood test such as this may be an early indicator of lung cancer before a tumor appears in the lungs and could be a potential tool in selecting patients for screening programs.[47] Studies are under way to determine how these blood tests may best be used clinically. In addition, the analysis of exhaled human breath has become an area of interest in lung cancer. Compounds within patients' exhaled breath form unique chemical signatures. These signatures have shown measurable, specific patterns in lung cancer compared with controls. As research continues in breath analysis, we may see its use in the screening, diagnosis, and treatment monitoring of lung cancer.[48]

TREATMENT AND OUTCOMES

Although the RT would not be administering the treatments for lung cancer, and the therapies change with advances over time, a brief discussion to familiarize the RT with the approach to treatment and the types of available therapy is important.

Non–Small Cell Lung Cancer

Three types of treatment are used to treat non–small cell lung cancer: surgical resection, **radiotherapy,** and **chemotherapy** (Box 28-3). The first two treatments provide local control of the cancer, and the last is used to treat systemic

Box 28-3 Options for Treatment of Lung Cancer

NON–SMALL CELL

Stages IA, IB, IIA, IIB

- Surgical resection standard of care if patient deemed able to tolerate resection
- Limited resection if patient is unable to tolerate larger resection
- Radiotherapy, particularly stereotactic body radiotherapy in N0 disease, if patient is unable to tolerate or chooses not to undergo resection
- Adjuvant radiotherapy possibly of use if incomplete resection has occurred
- Adjuvant chemotherapy in patient with stage II disease who can tolerate it; consider in stage IB

Stage IIIA

- Concurrent chemoradiotherapy using platinum-based regimen if performance status is reasonable
- Induction chemoradiotherapy followed by resection and adjuvant chemotherapy in selected patients, ideally as part of a study protocol

Stage IIIB

- Concurrent chemoradiotherapy using platinum-based regimen if performance status is reasonable
- Induction chemoradiotherapy followed by resection in highly selected patients, only as part of a study protocol

Stage IV

- Platinum-based chemotherapy regimen in patients with adequate performance status
- Targeted therapies (EGFR and VEGF inhibitors) in appropriate subgroups

SMALL CELL

Limited Stage

- Combination chemotherapy with concurrent hyperfractionated radiotherapy if performance status is adequate
- Prophylactic cranial radiation for patients with complete response to chemoradiotherapy

Extensive Stage

- Combination chemotherapy if performance status is adequate

Courtesy The Cleveland Clinic, Cleveland, Ohio.
EGFR, Epithelial growth factor receptor; *NEGF,* vascular endothelial growth factor.

disease. Which therapy or combination of therapies is recommended depends on the stage of the cancer, the patient's ability to tolerate treatment, and the type of cancer (or its histology). Molecular changes within the tumor are beginning to influence treatment choices as well.

Early Stage Non–Small Cell Carcinoma

Surgical resection offers the best chance of cure for early stage non–small cell lung cancer (stages I and II) (Table 28-3). Survival after resection in pathologic stage IA approaches 70% at 5 years; in pathologic stage IB, 5-year survival is closer to 55%. The surgery of choice is a *lobectomy,* in which the entire lobe of the lung containing the cancer is removed. If the tumor is very central, a pneumonectomy may be required. Lesser resections, such as *segmentectomy,* or *wedge resection,* can be performed in patients with modest lung function to spare as much lung tissue as possible. In most patients, limited resection leads to a slightly lower survival rate and a higher rate of local recurrence of cancer.[49,50] In elderly patients and in patients with the poorest lung function, much of the decrease in survival is due to mortality not related to lung cancer.[51] In the smallest cancers and in patients who are older than 70 years, a limited resection may be as effective as a lobectomy.[51,52] Vascular invasion and tumor differentiation may be prognostic factors. There does not seem to be a difference in survival between patients who have adenocarcinoma and patients who have squamous cell carcinoma. Recurrence usually involves distant metastases.

Survival after resection in pathologic stage IIA is 50% to 55% at 5 years and in pathologic stage IIB is approximately 40% (see Table 28-3). Limited resections are not typically an option in stage II cancers. Patients with adenocarcinoma may have poorer survival than patients with squamous cell carcinoma. Most recurrences involve distant metastases.

Radiotherapy has been used with curative intent in early stage non–small cell lung cancer in patients who cannot tolerate surgery or in patients who elect not to undergo surgery. The 5-year survival rate in stage I and II disease approaches 15% with standard radiotherapy alone. There is a high rate of local recurrence, and most deaths are due to lung cancer. Stereotactic body radiotherapy is a novel radiation therapy technique in which multiple convergent beams of radiation are precisely targeted on the tumor. This targeting allows very high doses of radiation to be delivered to the tumor while sparing the normal lung tissue. Rates of local control and survival are impressive in

TABLE 28-3

Non–Small Cell Lung Cancer: 5-Year Survival by Stage

Stage	Clinical	Pathologic
IA	50%	73%
IB	43%	58%
IIA	36%	46%
IIB	25%	36%
IIIA	19%	24%
IIIB	7%	9%
IV	2%	13%

Adapted from Goldstraw P, Crowley J, Chansky K, et al; International Association for the Study of Lung Cancer International Staging Committee; Participating Institutions: The IASLC Lung Cancer Staging Project: proposals for the revision of the TNM stage groupings in the forthcoming (seventh) edition of the TNM Classification of malignant tumours. J Thorac Oncol 2:706–714, 2007.

selected groups reported in many case series, approaching the rates of lung resection.[53] Lung resection and stereotactic body radiotherapy have not been compared head to head. Lung resection remains the standard of care in patients able to tolerate it. *Adjuvant* ("applied after initial treatment") radiotherapy in patients who have undergone surgical resection may improve local control but does not improve survival (with the possible exception of patients who have undergone incomplete resection).

Adjuvant platinum-based chemotherapy leads to a significant survival benefit in selected patients with completely resected stage II lung cancers.[54] The potential benefit of adjuvant chemotherapy in patients with stage IB disease is debated.

Locally and Regionally Advanced Non–Small Cell Carcinoma

Locally advanced tumors (T3) frequently can be completely resected, although central T3 tumors are less resectable than tumors involving the chest wall. The survival in patients with T3 tumors and chest wall involvement and negative nodes approximates the survival of other stage IIB patients. The best results occur when complete resection is possible. With nodal involvement at any level, survival decreases dramatically, and the tumor is classified in a higher stage. T3 involvement of the mediastinum or main stem bronchus portends a poorer prognosis, with 5-year survival rates less than 30%.

When a *Pancoast tumor* is present, chemoradiotherapy followed by surgical resection (lobectomy and chest wall resection) is performed if possible. The invasion of local structures (rib, vertebral body, subclavian artery, or sympathetic chain) is a poor prognostic sign. Two-thirds of patients have a recurrence, and two-thirds of these recurrences are local.

The approach to N2 (stage IIIA) disease varies among institutions. Unselected patients have a low rate of complete resection with primary surgery, and patients with incomplete resection do poorly. Patients without radiographic evidence of N2 disease but who are found at surgery to have N2 disease do better than patients with preoperative evidence of N2 disease. Adjuvant chemotherapy should be offered to this group. Generally, the more advanced the node involvement (number, extension, or location), the poorer the prognosis; protocols using multimodal therapy are being investigated. Induction with chemotherapy with or without radiotherapy leads to objective responses in most patients, some of whom go to a more favorable stage and become candidates for surgical resection. Patients who have bulky nodes or who require a pneumonectomy are less likely to benefit from resection after induction therapy. At the present time, concurrent chemoradiotherapy should be considered the standard of care, with resection included in specialized centers, often in the setting of a study. Survival rates are 5% to 13% at 5 years. It is suggested that newer agents may be as effective with less toxicity. With advances in each of the modes of therapy, treatment will evolve over time.[55-58]

T4 disease without advanced nodal status (stage IIIB) may be considered for surgical treatment in only a few settings. T4 disease involving the main carina may be considered for resection at centers with expertise. The role of induction therapy in this setting has not yet been defined. Disease at the N3 level (stage IIIB) is generally considered nonsurgical. Advances in induction therapy may alter this notion in time, and trials of multimodality therapy are ongoing.[57,58]

Metastatic Non–Small Cell Carcinoma

In stage IV lung cancer, platinum-based chemotherapy regimens have been shown to improve survival and enhance quality of life. They are also cost-effective. This treatment is most appropriate for individuals with a good performance status. Resection of an isolated brain metastasis in patients with a good performance status can improve survival. Standard chemotherapy typically involves two agents administered in cycles, each approximately 3 weeks apart, for a total of four to six cycles. The addition of a third agent or additional cycles has traditionally added risk without benefit. More recently, agents with improved tolerance have been shown to benefit patients who have shown a good response to treatment when administered as maintenance treatment, until progression is noted.[59]

Standard chemotherapy targets all growing cells, not just cancer cells (hence the common side effects seen). Targeted therapies have been developed where the mechanism of action is more specific to the cancer cell. In lung cancer, inhibitors of epidermal growth factor receptors (EGFRs), known to be highly expressed on lung cancer cells, and vascular endothelial growth factor (VEGF) have been studied. EGFR inhibitors have been most successful in patients with EGFR activating mutations in their cancer tissue. The patients most likely to have EGFR mutations include female never-smokers with adenocarcinoma, in particular, patients of Asian origin. This subgroup has been found to have an improved survival overall, which is improved further by the use of an EGFR inhibitor. The VEGF receptor inhibitor has been shown to improve survival when added to standard chemotherapy in patients with nonsquamous cell histology.[59,60] These treatments can be continued until progression is noted. Other promising agents in late phase development include inhibitors of insulin-like growth factor receptor and the EML4-anaplastic lymphoma kinase *(ALK)* gene rearrangement.[59-62] Further successes with targeted therapy are expected in the future.

Small Cell Lung Cancer

Treatment of small cell lung cancer is based on its staging (see Box 28-3). In limited stage disease, combination chemotherapy with concurrent hyperfractionated radiotherapy is recommended. The drug etoposide and a platinum agent are standard, but trials with newer agents are ongoing. Prophylactic cranial radiation is generally recommended for patients who have a complete response to chemoradiotherapy. Surgery is limited to cases in which the diagnosis is in doubt or in cases that have not responded to chemoradiotherapy but remain resectable. In patients with extensive stage disease, combination chemotherapy improves the quality of life and median survival. A poor performance status and an elevated lactate dehydrogenase level portend a poor prognosis. Radiotherapy to the chest may be used in patients who have a complete response to chemotherapy in disease outside the chest.[59,63]

RULE OF THUMB

Surgery is the treatment of choice for early stage non–small cell lung cancer. Chemotherapy is the modality of choice for advanced non–small cell lung cancer. Chemotherapy with or without radiation therapy is used to treat small cell lung cancer.

Palliation of symptoms related to lung cancer is an important aspect of overall management. The judicious use of analgesic agents for pain, antiemetics for nausea, and antidepressants can improve quality of life. Radiotherapy can be used to palliate bone pain related to metastatic disease, hemoptysis, or symptoms of airway obstruction. Invasive bronchoscopic procedures (e.g., laser ablation, electrocautery, stent placement) may be palliative in patients with airway obstruction.

FUTURE SCENARIO

The prospect of major advances in the prevention, detection, and treatment of lung cancer is strong. An attainable vision for 2031 could be as follows: Primary prevention campaigns have successfully minimized the number of individuals who are smoking, legislation has passed broadly to prevent exposure to tobacco smoke in public places, progress has been made in occupational exposure avoidance, and successful measures have been enacted to clean the air. Individuals are now identified who have changes in lung cells that suggest lung cancer could develop and are being treated with medication to prevent it from developing. Individuals at risk for developing lung cancer are part of a screening program that detects early stage lung cancer with a test that is inexpensive and acceptable to all. Technology has improved diagnostic abilities by making imaging more specific and biopsies more accurate. Noninvasive diagnostics have expanded with advances in blood and breath testing.[47,48,64,65] In addition to tumor appearance, researchers are identifying characteristics of tumor biology that allow more selection in choosing treatments.[66,67] The best form of local control for a given tumor (resection, radiation) is known, and means have been developed to minimize the effect of these interventions on the quality of life. Novel agents have been developed that can reach and kill tumor cells, while avoiding injury to healthy tissue. As evidence of successes to date, lung cancer is no longer the leading cause of cancer-related mortality in the United States.

MINI CLINI

Evaluating Surgical Risk

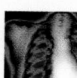

PROBLEM: A 62-year-old man with a long history of smoking has a chronic, productive cough. A chest radiograph obtained because of a recent episode of hemoptysis reveals a right lung mass. Results of transbronchial biopsy suggest the presence of large cell carcinoma. There is no evidence of metastasis. As part of the patient's evaluation for surgery, he has the following spirometry results:

Forced vital capacity (FVC) 4.2 L (80% of predicted value)

FEV_1 1.6 L (60% of predicted value)

FEV_1/FVC 0.4

Can he undergo surgery?

DISCUSSION: Assessment of lung reserve is an important step in the preoperative evaluation of patients with lung cancer being considered for surgical resection. A preoperative FEV_1 of more than 2 L (or >80% of predicted value) indicates good lung reserve with low surgical risk even if pneumonectomy is needed. FEV_1 less than 35% to 40% of predicted value is a contraindication to surgery because of the high risk of postoperative mortality and morbidity. Other options, such as radiation therapy or chemotherapy, must be considered for these patients. This patient, similar to most patients with lung cancer, has FEV_1 between 35% and 80% because of underlying COPD. He needs reevaluation after appropriate management of the underlying COPD. If the patient's lung function does not improve to the low-risk level with treatment, a quantitative lung perfusion scan may be necessary for assessment of the percentage of functional contribution by each lung and for prediction of residual lung function after surgical resection.

ROLE OF THE RESPIRATORY THERAPIST IN MANAGING PATIENTS WITH LUNG CANCER

RTs perform many important roles in the evaluation and management of patients with lung cancer. Many patients in the care of the RT are smokers, and the RT has the opportunity to educate these individuals on the dangers of smoking and on the means available to help one quit.

Because many of these patients also have smoking-related lung disorders (e.g., COPD), RTs can offer guidance on the proper use of inhaled medications, the use of supplemental oxygen, and the role of pulmonary rehabilitation before and after treatment. Also, many RTs assist with diagnostic tests such as bronchoscopy and the measurement of pulmonary function. Finally, in the context that the RT may spend substantial time with the patient with lung cancer, the RT may be an important source of psychologic support and help. Taken together, these various diagnostic and treatment roles establish that the RT plays a crucial role in helping to manage patients with lung cancer.

SUMMARY CHECKLIST

- Approximately 222,520 cases of bronchogenic carcinoma were newly diagnosed in the United States in 2010, making bronchogenic carcinoma a major health hazard. It is the leading cause of cancer-related mortality in the United States.
- Approximately 85% of all cases of bronchogenic carcinoma are linked to smoking.
- The major histopathologic types of bronchogenic carcinoma include adenocarcinoma, squamous cell carcinoma, small cell carcinoma, and large cell carcinoma. Adenocarcinoma is the most common type, representing more than 40% of all cases.
- The clinical manifestations of bronchogenic carcinoma result from local growth of the tumor, regional spread, metastases to extrathoracic and intrathoracic organs, and paraneoplastic syndromes.
- The staging system most commonly used for non-small cell bronchogenic carcinoma is based on status of the primary tumor (T), local and regional lymph node involvement (N), and the presence of metastasis (M). The TNM classification groups patients in stages or categories that correlate with survival. Small cell lung cancer is classified in two stages, limited and extensive, although the TNM system can be used as well.
- The most commonly used treatments for patients with non-small cell lung cancer are surgical resection, radiation therapy, and chemotherapy. Treatment of most patients with small cell carcinoma includes chemotherapy and possibly radiation therapy.
- The most effective way to prevent lung cancer is to prevent smoking.

References

1. Jemal A, Siegal R, Xu J, et al: Cancer statistics, 2010. CA Cancer J Clin 60:277–300, 2010.
2. Fontham ET, Correa P, Reynolds P, et al: Environmental tobacco smoke and lung cancer in nonsmoking women: a multi-center study. JAMA 271:1752–1759, 1994.
3. Bartecchi CE, MacKenzie TD, Schrien RW: The human cost of tobacco use. N Engl J Med 330:907–912, 1994.
4. Rigotti NA, Lee JE, Wechsler H: U.S. college students' use of tobacco products: results of a national survey. JAMA 284:699–705, 2000.
5. Kessler DA: Nicotine addiction in young people. N Engl J Med 333:186–189, 1995.
6. Marshall L, Schooley M, Ryan H, et al: Youth tobacco surveillance–US, 2001-2002. MMWR Surveill Summ 55:1–56, 2006.
7. Iribarren C, Tekawa IS, Sidney S, et al: Effect of cigar smoking on the risk of cardiovascular disease, chronic obstructive pulmonary disease, and cancer in men. N Engl J Med 340:1773–1780, 1999.
8. Vineis P, Airoldi L, Veglia F, et al: Environmental tobacco smoke and risk of respiratory cancer and chronic obstructive pulmonary disease in former smokers and never smokers in the EPIC prospective study. BMJ 330:277–281, 2005.
9. Oberg M, Jaakkola MS, Woodward A, et al: Worldwide burden of disease from exposure to second hand smoke: a retrospective analysis of data from 193 countries. Lancet 377:139–146, 2011.
10. Darby S, Hill D, Auvinen A, et al: Radon in homes and risk of lung cancer: collaborative analysis of individual data from 13 European case-control studies. BMJ 330:223–228, 2005.
11. Cote ML, Kardia SLR, Wenzlaff AS, et al: Risk of lung cancer among white and black relatives of individuals with early-onset lung cancer. JAMA 293:3036–3042, 2005.
12. Nitadori J, Inoue M, Iwasaki M, et al: Association between lung cancer incidence and family history of lung cancer: data from a large-scale population-based cohort study, the JPHC study. Chest 130:968–975, 2006.
13. Dresler CM, Fratelli C, Babb J, et al: Gender differences in genetic susceptibility for lung cancer. Lung Cancer 30:153–160, 2000.
14. Schabath MD, Hernandez LM, Wu X, et al: Dietary phytoestrogens and lung cancer risk. JAMA 294:1493–1504, 2005.
15. Brennan P, Hsu C, Moullan N, et al: Effect of cruciferous vegetables on lung cancer in patients stratified by genetic status: a mendelian randomization approach. Lancet 366: 1558–1560, 2005.
16. Virtamo J, Pietinen P, Huttunen JK, et al; ATBC Study Group: Incidence of cancer and mortality following alpha-tocopherol and beta-carotene supplementation: a postintervention follow-up. JAMA 290:476–485, 2003.
17. Mannino DM, Aguayo SM, Petty TL, et al: Low lung function and incident lung cancer in the United States: data from the first National Health and Nutrition Examination Survey follow-up. Arch Intern Med 163:1475–1480, 2003.
18. Wasswa-Kintu S, Gan WQ, Man SF, et al: Relationship between reduced forced expiratory volume in one second and the risk of lung cancer: a systematic review and meta-analysis. Thorax 60:570–575, 2005.
19. Christiani DC: Smoking and the molecular epidemiology of lung cancer. Clin Chest Med 21:87, 2000.
20. Gerber RB, Mazzone PJ, Arroliga AC: Paraneoplastic syndromes associated with bronchogenic carcinoma. Clin Chest Med 23:257–264, 2002.
21. Mazzone P, Stoller JK: The pulmonologist's perspective regarding the solitary pulmonary nodule. Semin Thorac Cardiovasc Surg 14:250–260, 2002.
22. Gould MK, Maclean CC, Kuschner WG, et al: Accuracy of positron emission tomography for diagnosis of pulmonary nodules and mass lesions: a meta-analysis. JAMA 285:914–924, 2001.
23. Mazzone PJ, Jain P, Arroliga AC, et al: Bronchoscopy and needle biopsy techniques for the diagnosis and staging of lung cancer. Clin Chest Med 23:137–158, 2002.

24. Gildea T, Mazzone PJ, Karnak D, et al: Electromagnetic navigation bronchoscopy: a prospective study. Am J Respir Crit Care Med 174:982–989, 2006.
25. Wallace MB, Pascaul JM, Raimondo M, et al: Minimally invasive endoscopic staging of lung cancer. JAMA 299:540–546, 2008.
26. Detterbeck FC, Boffa DJ, Tanour LT: The new lung cancer staging system. Chest 126:260–271, 2009.
27. Lababede O, Meziane M, Rice T: Seventh edition of the cancer staging manual and stage grouping of lung cancer: quick reference chart and diagrams. Chest 139:183–189, 2011.
28. Goldstraw P, Crowley J, Chansky K, et al: The IASLC lung cancer staging project: proposals for the revision of the TNM stage groupings in the forthcoming (seventh) edition of the TNM classification of malignant tumours. J Thorac Oncol 2:706–714, 2007.
29. Silvestri GA, Tanoue LT, Margolis ML, et al: The noninvasive staging of non-small cell lung cancer: the guidelines. Chest 123:147S–156S, 2007.
30. Vansteenkiste JF, Stroobants SG, De Leyn PR, et al: Mediastinal lymph node staging with FDG-PET scan in patients with potentially operable non-small-cell lung cancer: a prospective analysis of 50 cases. Leuven Lung Cancer Group. Chest 112:1480–1486, 1997.
31. Lardinois D, Weder W, Hany TF, et al: Staging of non-small-cell lung cancer with integrated positron-emission tomography and computed tomography. N Engl J Med 348:2500–2507, 2003.
32. Annema JT, Versteegh MI, Veselic M, et al: Endoscopic ultrasound-guided fine-needle aspiration in the diagnosis and staging of lung cancer and its impact on surgical staging. J Clin Oncol 23:8357–8361, 2005.
33. Yokoi K, Kamiya N, Matsuguma H, et al: Detection of brain metastasis in potentially operable non-small cell lung cancer: a comparison of CT and MRI. Chest 114:714–719, 1999.
34. Pieterman RM, van Putten JW, Meuzelaar JJ, et al: Preoperative staging of non-small-cell lung cancer with positron-emission tomography. N Engl J Med 343:254–261, 2000.
35. Mazzone PJ, Arroliga AC: Lung cancer: preoperative pulmonary evaluation of the lung resection candidate. Am J Med 118:578–583, 2005.
36. Manser RL, Irving LB, Byrnes G, et al: Screening for lung cancer: a systematic review and meta-analysis of controlled trials. Thorax 58:784–789, 2003.
37. Henschke CI, Naidich DP, Yankelevitz DF, et al: Early Lung Cancer Action Project: initial findings on repeat screening. Cancer 92:153–159, 2001.
38. Nawa T, Nakagawa T, Kusano S, et al: Lung cancer screening using low-dose spiral CT: results of baseline and 1-year follow-up studies. Chest 122:15–20, 2002.
39. Swensen SJ, Jett JR, Sloan JA, et al: Screening for lung cancer with low-dose spiral computed tomography. Am J Respir Crit Care Med 165:508–513, 2002.
40. Swensen SJ, Jett JR, Hartman TE, et al: Lung cancer screening with CT: Mayo Clinic experience. Radiology 226:756–761, 2003.
41. Swensen SJ, Jett JR, Hartman TE, et al: CT screening for lung cancer: five-year prospective experience. Radiology 235:259–265, 2005.
42. Pastorino U, Bellomi M, Landoni C, et al: Early lung-cancer detection with spiral CT and positron emission tomography in heavy smokers: 2-year results. Lancet 362: 593–597, 2003.
43. Mahadevia PJ, Fleisher LA, Frick KD, et al: Lung cancer screening with helical computed tomography in older adult smokers: a decision and cost-effectiveness analysis. JAMA 289:313–322, 2003.
44. International Early Lung Cancer Action Program Investigators, Henschke CI, Yankelevitz DF, Libby DM, et al: Survival of patients with stage I lung cancer detected on CT screening. N Engl J Med 355:1763–1771, 2006.
45. National Lung Cancer Screening Research Team, Aberle DR, Berg CD, Black WC, et al: The National Lung Cancer Screening Trial: overview and study design. Radiology 258: 243–253, 2011.
46. Murray A, Chapman CJ, Healey G, et al: The technical validation of an autoantibody test for lung cancer. Ann Oncol 21:1687–1693, 2010.
47. Mazzone P: Analysis of volatile organic compounds in the exhaled breath for the diagnosis of lung cancer. J Thorac Oncol 7:774–780, 2008.
48. Ginsberg RJ, Rubenstein LV: Randomized trial of lobectomy versus limited resection for T1N0 non-small cell lung cancer. Lung Cancer Study Group. Ann Thorac Surg 60:615–622, 1995.
49. Landreneau RJ, Sugarbaker DJ, Mack MJ, et al: Wedge resection versus lobectomy for stage I (T1N0M0) non-small-cell lung cancer. J Thorac Cardiovasc Surg 113:691–700, 1997.
50. Mery CM, Pappas AN, Bueno R, et al: Similar long-term survival of elderly patients with non-small cell lung cancer treated with lobectomy or wedge resection within the Surveillance, Epidemiology, and End Results database. Chest 128:237–245, 2005.
51. Okada M, Nishio W, Sakamoto T, et al: Effect of tumor size on prognosis in patients with non-small cell lung cancer: the role of segmentectomy as a type of lesser resection. J Thorac Cardiovasc Surg 129:87–93, 2005.
52. Timmerman R, Paulus R, Galvin J, et al: Stereotactic body radiation therapy for inoperable early stage lung cancer. JAMA 303:1070–1076, 2010.
53. Arriagada R, Bergman B, Dunant A, et al; International Adjuvant Lung Cancer Trial Collaborative Group: Cisplatin-based adjuvant chemotherapy in patients with completely resected non-small-cell lung cancer. N Engl J Med 350:351–360, 2004.
54. Spira A, Ettinger DS: Multidisciplinary management of lung cancer. N Engl J Med 350:379–392, 2004.
55. Georgoulias V, Papadakis E, Alexopoulos A, et al: Platinum-based and non-platinum-based chemotherapy in advanced non-small-cell lung cancer: a randomised multicentre trial. Lancet 357:1478–1484, 2001.
56. Albain KS, Swann RS, Rusch VW, et al: Radiotherapy plus chemotherapy with or without surgical resection for stage III non-small-cell lung cancer: a phase III randomised controlled trial. Lancet 374:379–386, 2009.
57. van Meerbeeck JP, Kramer GW, Van Schil PE, et al: Randomized controlled trial of resection versus radiotherapy after induction chemotherapy in stage IIIA-N2 non-small-cell lung cancer. J Natl Cancer Inst 99:442–450, 2007.
58. Azzoli CG, Baker S Jr, Temin S, et al: American Society of Clinical Oncology Clinical Practice Guideline update on chemotherapy for stage IV non-small-cell lung cancer. J Clin Oncol 27:6251–6266, 2009.
59. Sharma SV, Bell DW, Settleman J, et al: Epidermal growth factor receptor mutations in lung cancer. Nat Rev Cancer 7:169–181, 2007.
60. Silvestri GA, Rivera P: Targeted therapy for the treatment of advanced non-small cell lung cancer: a review of the epidermal growth factor receptor antagonists. Chest 128: 3975–3984, 2005.

61. Kwak EL, Bang Y, Camidge R, et al: Anaplastic lymphoma kinase inhibition in non-small cell lung cancer. N Engl J Med 363:1693–1703, 2010.
62. Jackman DM, Johnson BE: Small-cell lung cancer. Lancet 366:1385–1396, 2005.
63. Zhong L, Hidalgo GE, Stromberg AJ, et al: Using protein microarray as a diagnostic assay for non-small cell lung cancer. Am J Respir Crit Care Med 172:1308–1314, 2005.
64. Machado RF, Laskowski D, Deffenderfer O, et al: Detection of lung cancer by sensor array analyses of exhaled breath. Am J Respir Crit Care Med 171:1286–1291, 2005.
65. Potti A, Mukherjee S, Petersen R, et al: A genomic strategy to refine prognosis in early-stage non-small-cell lung cancer. N Engl J Med 355:570–580, 2006.
66. Olaussen KA, Dunant A, Fouret P, et al: DNA repair by ERCC1 in non-small cell lung cancer and cisplatin-based adjuvant chemotherapy. N Engl J Med 355:983–991, 2006.
67. Yanagisawa K, Shyr Y, Xu BJ, et al: Proteomic patterns of tumor subsets in non-small-cell lung cancer. Lancet 362:433–439, 2003.

Chapter 29

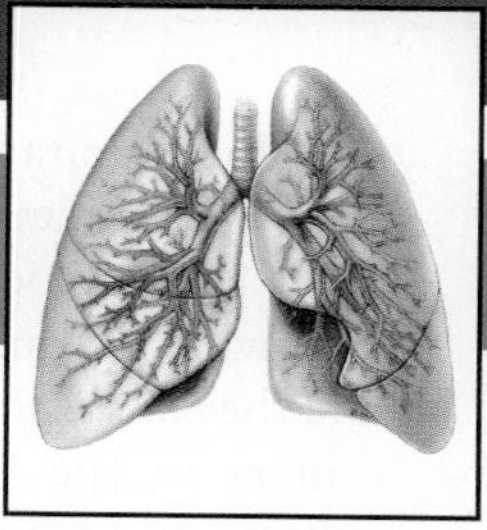

Neuromuscular and Other Diseases of the Chest Wall

RENDELL W. ASHTON

CHAPTER OBJECTIVES

- Identify pulmonary function test results seen in patients with neuromuscular disease.
- List the potential respiratory complications associated with neuromuscular disease.
- Identify the clinical signs and symptoms associated with respiratory muscle weakness.
- Describe techniques for monitoring patients with respiratory muscle weakness.
- Describe general respiratory care management of patients with respiratory muscle weakness.
- Describe the clinical findings and treatment for each of the following neuromuscular disorders: Duchenne muscular dystrophy, myotonic dystrophy, polymyositis, myasthenia gravis, Lambert-Eaton syndrome, Guillain-Barré syndrome, unilateral diaphragmatic paralysis, amyotrophic lateral sclerosis, critical illness myopathy and polyneuropathy, spinal cord injury, stroke, traumatic brain injury, kyphoscoliosis, and flail chest.

CHAPTER OUTLINE

KEY TERMS

amyotrophic lateral sclerosis (ALS)
ankylosing spondylitis
apneustic breathing
ataxic breathing
Becker muscular dystrophy
central neurogenic hyperinflation
Cheyne-Stokes respirations
critical illness myopathy
critical illness polyneuropathy
dermatomyositis
Duchenne muscular dystrophy (DMD)
flail chest
gasping
Guillain-Barré syndrome (GBS)
inclusion body myositis
kyphoscoliosis
Lambert-Eaton syndrome (LES)
Lou Gehrig disease
myasthenia gravis (MG)
myopathy
myositis
myotonic dystrophy
neuropathy
Ondine curse
paradoxical motion
periodic breathing
polymyositis
stroke
traumatic brain injury

The respiratory system comprises the *lungs,* which provide an interface between inhaled air and circulating blood, mediating gas exchange; the *thoracic cage,* which forms the structure of the ventilatory pump; and the *muscles of respiration,* which are linked to respiratory centers in the brainstem by nerves exiting the spinal column and whose action on the thoracic cage produces movement of air into and out of the lungs. Understanding the interactions between these components is essential to understanding how their dysfunction leads to disease. The neuromuscular organization of the components of the respiratory system is shown in Figure 29-1. Maintenance of normal ventilation depends critically on intact, functional components of the neuromuscular system, which contribute to breathing in three principal ways: (1) regulation of respiratory drive and rate, (2) control of the mechanics of ventilation, and (3) cough and other airway protection. Diseases that affect the brain, nerves, muscles, or thoracic cage can lead to respiratory failure or hypoxemia even if the lungs are normal. The pulmonary consequences of neuromuscular disease include the following:

1. Dysregulation of respiratory drive or rate
   - Hyperventilation
   - Hypoventilation
   - Central apnea
   - Other pathologic breathing patterns (listed in Table 29-6)
2. Loss of strength or control of the mechanics of breathing
   - Respiratory failure owing to excessive work of breathing
   - Atelectasis leading to hypoxemia
   - Secondary effects of chronic hypoxemia (e.g., cor pulmonale, pulmonary hypertension)
3. Loss of strength or control of the muscles that produce cough and protect the airway
   - Aspiration
   - Obstructive apnea
   - Mucous plugging
   - Pneumonia

Some systemic diseases that affect the neuromuscular system also cause interstitial lung disease, which can lead to considerable respiratory dysfunction (see Chapter 24). Respiratory failure, often associated with pulmonary infection, is a frequent cause of death in patients with neuromuscular disorders.

A thorough understanding of the physiology of ventilation and chest wall mechanics (see Chapters 10 and 18) is needed to help the reader understand how abnormalities of the upper airway, chest wall, diaphragm, and abdominal muscles cause disease. This chapter reviews major disorders of the neuromuscular and skeletal systems that affect breathing. Disorders are grouped according to which functional unit of the neuromuscular system is affected, focusing on pulmonary manifestations of these disease processes (Table 29-1).

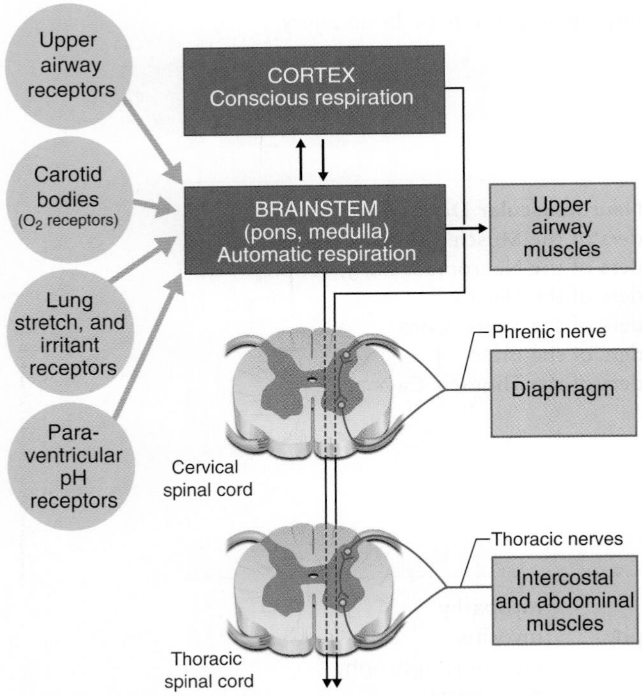

FIGURE 29-1 The neuromuscular components of the respiratory system include elements of the cortex (which allow conscious alteration of breathing) and motor centers (which maintain upper airway tone). Brainstem structures receive input from peripheral oxygen, pH, and stretch receptors and generate automatic respiration. Efferent nerves carry central nervous impulses to the muscles of respiration through the phrenic and spinal nerves, which drive the muscles of respiration.

TABLE 29-1

Locations at Which Several Neuromuscular Diseases Affect the Respiratory System

Location	Disease
Cortex and upper motor neurons	Stroke, traumatic brain injury
Spinal cord	Trauma, transverse myelitis, multiple sclerosis
Anterior horn cells (lower motor neurons)	ALS, spinal muscular atrophy, poliomyelitis and postpoliomyelitis
Peripheral nerves	GBS, critical illness polyneuropathy, Lyme disease
Neuromuscular junction	MG, LES, botulism
Muscle	DMD, polymyositis, acid maltase deficiency
Interstitial lung disease*	Polymyositis, dermatomyositis, tuberous sclerosis, neurofibromatosis

*A category of systemic diseases that can affect neuromuscular function.

TABLE 29-2

Pulmonary Function Testing Results from a Patient With Profound Diaphragm Weakness

	Predicted Value	Lower Limit of Normal	Sitting Position	% of Predicted	Supine Position	% Change from Sitting
FVC	4.42	3.55	1.85	42	0.89	−52
FEV_1	3.36	2.62	1.51	45	0.68	−55
FEV_1/FVC	75.88	66.20	81.75	108	75.76	−7
TLC	6.53	4.92	4.21	64		
RV	2.10	1.34	2.39	114		
DLCO	24.93	16.67	17.16	69		
DLCO/VA	3.88	2.38	5.57	144		
PImax	110.58	75.02	18.46	17		
PEmax	207.29	140.04	26.52	13		

GENERAL PRINCIPLES RELATING TO NEUROMUSCULAR WEAKNESS OF THE VENTILATORY MUSCLES

This section describes the evaluation and testing of patients with suspected neuromuscular weakness of the respiratory muscles, regardless of the disease causing the weakness.

Pathophysiology and Pulmonary Function Testing

Weakness of the respiratory muscles leads to the inability to generate or maintain normal respiratory pressures. Pulmonary function testing in patients with neuromuscular weakness typically reveals a restrictive ventilatory defect even if the lungs are normal. Vital capacity (VC), forced expiratory volume in 1 second (FEV_1), and total lung capacity (TLC) are decreased. Residual volume (RV) is normal or decreased, and diffusing capacity corrected for alveolar volume is normal or near-normal but has been reported to be decreased.[1] Comparison of spirometric results obtained with the patient in seated and supine positions can be useful in showing that orthopnea is caused by neuromuscular weakness. A decrease in VC or FEV_1 of greater than 20% when a patient moves from the seated to the supine position suggests diaphragmatic weakness (Table 29-2 and Figure 29-2). The inability to generate normal respiratory pressures is reflected in a decreased maximal inspiratory pressure (PImax). Expiratory muscle weakness is characterized by a decreased maximal expiratory pressure (PEmax).

Arterial blood gases in the setting of a rapid, shallow breathing pattern may show a decreased $PaCO_2$, although progressive inspiratory muscle weakness leads to hypoventilation and hypercapnia. Hypoxemia can occur in patients unable to take deep breaths and may be caused by microatelectasis, which leads to ventilation/perfusion mismatching within the lung and a resulting decrease in PaO_2 (Figure 29-3). Chronic hypoxemia in this situation may be protective against acute respiratory muscle failure. Experimental data suggest that when hypoxemia is chronic, it may increase diaphragm muscle endurance.[2] Hypoventilation that occurs with progressive neuromuscular disease may be a protective mechanism that avoids acute respiratory muscle fatigue. However, when hypoxemia is acute, it potentiates respiratory muscle fatigue, hastening respiratory failure.[3]

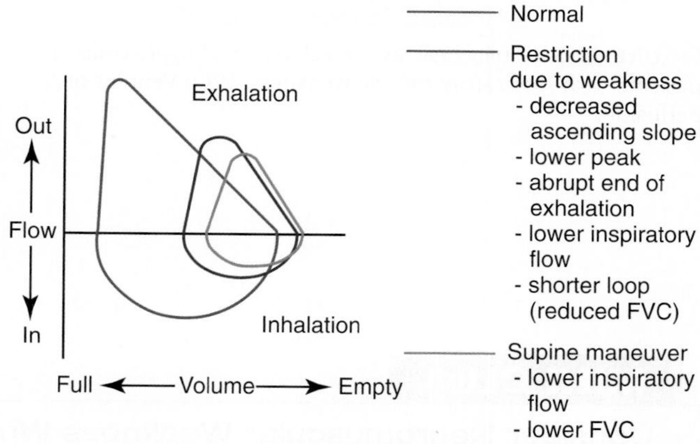

FIGURE 29-2 Normal flow-volume loop compared with loops from a patient with neuromuscular weakness, showing characteristic ventilatory restriction, which worsens when the patient is placed in the supine position.

RULE OF THUMB

Neuromuscular weakness of the respiratory muscles may be present before any substantial decrease in VC or FEV_1 is noticed. Values of PEmax may be decreased by 50% or more before any decrement in VC or FEV_1 is noticed.

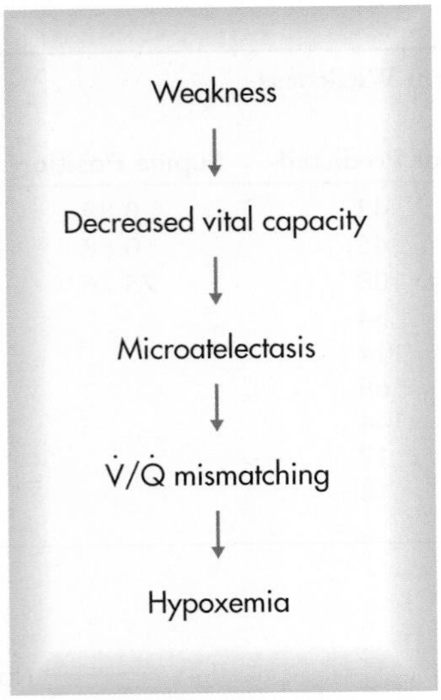

FIGURE 29-3 Atelectasis as a mechanism of hypoxemia in patients with respiratory muscle weakness. $\dot{V}/\dot{Q}$, Ventilation/perfusion.

Clinical Signs and Symptoms

In the early stages of neuromuscular disease, patients with respiratory muscle weakness initially report exertional dyspnea and fatigue. As the disease process progresses, patients may complain of orthopnea or symptoms of cor pulmonale. These symptoms occur because the muscles involved with respiration can no longer generate or maintain normal ventilation. The response to hypoxemia and respiratory drive, measured with airway occlusion pressure (P0.1), is preserved in most patients with neuromuscular weakness.[4] Because these patients do not have the strength to take deep breaths, they increase minute ventilation by increasing respiratory rate and adopting a rapid, shallow breathing pattern, which uses less respiratory muscle strength but provides less efficient ventilation. Patients with poor inspiratory muscle function (especially diaphragm weakness) may have marked orthopnea and prefer to sleep in a seated position. They may also experience a decline in the volume and power of voice or voice quality. Progressive muscle weakness can progress to the point where adequate ventilation is no longer maintained, and hypercapnia occurs.

MINI CLINI

Consider Neuromuscular Weakness When a Patient Complains of Dyspnea

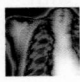

PROBLEM: A 27-year-old woman was referred to the pulmonary clinic for persistent shortness of breath for 2 months, along with a sore throat and a hoarse voice. The symptoms had begun with a viral syndrome including sore throat, myalgias, and fever, progressing to cough and chest discomfort. All symptoms except her shortness of breath and hoarseness had resolved. She complained of being particularly short of breath while lying down and not being able to lie down on her left side at all because she felt she could not breathe in that position. She also described running out of breath in the middle of sentences and of her voice having a hoarse, "airy" quality. She had been evaluated previously, including a normal chest x-ray and spirometry, and had been told her dyspnea was due to anxiety. No other diagnosis was made. What clues in her history might suggest a pulmonary disease, and what additional testing could help identify it?

DISCUSSION: This patient had already been evaluated and had been told that her dyspnea was psychologic in nature because her chest x-ray and standard pulmonary function testing were normal. Spirometry was within the normal range of values, but when repeated in the supine position, FEV_1 decreased by 41%. Lung volumes were normal except for a slight elevation of residual volume. Diffusing capacity was also normal. A fluoroscopic sniff test, in which her diaphragms were visualized in real time as she performed a simple sniff maneuver, showed paradoxical motion of the right hemidiaphragm. She was diagnosed with neuralgic amyotrophy, a rare neuromuscular condition affecting the phrenic nerve, which is often triggered by a viral syndrome and which usually improves gradually with time.

The important clue that led to the diagnosis of neuromuscular weakness was her complaint of orthopnea, especially the inability to breathe comfortably on one side or the other. When one diaphragm is weak or paralyzed, a patient often cannot breathe when lying on the opposite side because this prevents the good side from compensating for the weak side. When the details of her history were recognized as classic symptoms of diaphragm weakness, testing to establish the diagnosis was straightforward.

PROBLEM: What physical findings may suggest respiratory distress in a patient with diaphragmatic weakness?

DISCUSSION: Patients whose diaphragmatic strength is inadequate to meet their ventilatory needs may use *accessory* muscles of inspiration. The sternocleidomastoid, intercostal, and scalene muscles all may be found active in the setting of respiratory distress. Use of these muscles in the setting of a weak or paralyzed diaphragm can lead to cephalad movement of the diaphragm during inspiration that is accompanied by paradoxical inward movement of the abdomen during inspiration (which is called *paradoxical breathing*). The presence of these signs in this patient should prompt evaluation of ventilatory adequacy and the need for ventilatory support.

RULE OF THUMB

When a patient complains of immediate shortness of breath on lying down, especially if one side is worse than the other, the problem is diaphragm weakness until proved otherwise.

Monitoring and Assessing Patients With Muscle Weakness for Respiratory Insufficiency

If respiratory muscle weakness progresses and cannot be stopped, the eventual result is respiratory failure. The onset of respiratory failure is acute or chronic depending on the time course of the disease process and the circumstances of the patient. When this progression toward respiratory failure is noted, careful follow-up and monitoring of symptoms and pulmonary function are necessary for assessment of the need for mechanical ventilation.

Monitoring the ventilatory function of a patient with neuromuscular weakness can involve repeated measurement of inspiratory pressure, VC, and arterial blood gas values. Depending on the condition, the need for mechanical support can be signaled by reaching either a critical value on testing or an overall clinical condition that does not allow unassisted ventilation to continue. Additional measurements that have been suggested to be more indicative of early respiratory insufficiency, at least in amyotrophic lateral sclerosis (ALS), include maximal sniff nasal inspiratory force[5] and nocturnal oximetry.[6]

At least two caveats to this general approach should be mentioned. First, patients with myasthenia gravis having an acute myasthenic crisis may have normal test results within minutes of acute ventilatory failure because of the nature of the disorder.[7] Second, the need to protect the upper airway from secretions and aspiration may not be clearly reflected in results of pulmonary function tests, which evaluate only the mechanical function of the ventilatory pump. Neuromuscular weakness may not manifest uniformly in all muscle groups. Ventilation may be only moderately reduced in patients with gross oropharyngeal dysfunction leading to aspiration. Patients with ventilatory weakness can have a high risk of acute respiratory failure if upper respiratory tract infection or pneumonia develops. In these patients, inability to clear secretions can increase the work of breathing; the results are muscle fatigue, hypoventilation, and acute respiratory failure.

Patients with significant weakness of the respiratory muscles can have a high risk of respiratory failure when any pulmonary process increases the work of breathing. Pulmonary edema, pneumonia, and mucous plugging are examples of clinical conditions that can precipitate respiratory failure rapidly in patients with significant neuromuscular weakness. Such patients may need observation of their respiratory status when they are in the hospital with these conditions. Although the underlying disease may not have progressed to the point that these patients need continual or routine ventilatory support, that support may be critical in the setting of acute, exacerbating illness.

Nocturnal oximetry or formal sleep testing with polysomnography may be suggested in some clinical settings when patients have cor pulmonale, sleep disturbance, or excessive daytime somnolence that is otherwise unexplained.

MINI CLINI

Assessment of a Patient With Neuromuscular Weakness

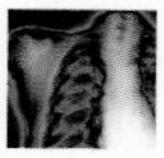

PROBLEM: A 50-year-old man with ALS is admitted to the hospital because of right lower lobe pneumonia. The patient is moderately hypoxemic, with PO_2 of 68 mm Hg on room air. ALS was diagnosed 3 years previously, and he has had progressive worsening of dyspnea since then. These symptoms first occurred with mild exertion and then with supine position, which the patient has noticed in the last 1 or 2 months. A recent measurement of VC at the physician's office was 35 ml/kg. The patient has noticed recent difficulty with swallowing and frequent coughing at meals. What features in the patient's history may be relevant with regard to management?

DISCUSSION: This patient has a disease that is associated with respiratory compromise, which progresses slowly in most cases, in contrast the acute case described here. All patients with ALS ultimately have respiratory insufficiency. The earliest symptom of neuromuscular weakness in the respiratory muscles is exertional dyspnea, which this patient has had for some time. A more significant finding is orthopnea, which is highly suggestive of diaphragmatic weakness. Patients with significant diaphragmatic weakness prefer the upright seated position, which allows the abdominal contents to shift toward the feet and allows unimpeded diaphragmatic descent. Although the patient may not have had a critically low VC recently, this value is low. Additional loading of already compromised ventilatory machinery can lead to fatigue and frank respiratory failure. It is important to recognize that the underlying neuromuscular weakness coupled with pneumonia may predispose this patient to respiratory fatigue and subsequent respiratory failure. The history of difficulty with feeding may suggest that the pneumonia is related to aspiration. The location of pneumonia in the lower lobe also favors the diagnosis if the aspiration occurs when the patient is seated.

Management of Respiratory Muscle Weakness

Respiratory insufficiency and failure to clear secretions are the major consequences of inspiratory and expiratory muscle weakness. Treatment of these patients involves consideration of mechanical ventilation via face mask or other noninvasive interfaces or via tracheostomy. Although often overlooked, therapies to augment secretion clearance and assist with cough are important in these patients (see Chapters 39 and 40). Used together, these interventions can decrease hospitalizations secondary to respiratory complications in patients with neuromuscular disease.[8] These measures may also be useful in delaying or preventing the need for intubation or tracheostomy, although severe bulbar muscle weakness may limit a patient's ability to avoid invasive ventilatory support.[9] In addition to these interventions, general rehabilitation focusing on aerobic conditioning, muscle strengthening, and respiratory muscle training can often delay the need for ventilatory support and improve the overall quality of life for patients with muscle weakness.[10]

Noninvasive ventilation is being used increasingly for short-term and intermittent ventilatory support of patients with neuromuscular disease.[11] Acute deterioration, such as during a pneumonia, and surgical procedures such as gastrostomy tube insertion are situations where noninvasive ventilation is safe and effective if used carefully.[9,12] If a patient needs long-term ventilatory support on an intermittent basis, such as at night only, noninvasive ventilation may be appropriate.[13] Decisions to begin mechanical ventilation in some patients with neuromuscular weakness have varied greatly among physicians[14] and may be motivated by many different patient factors.[15] No uniform guidelines exist for the use of long-term mechanical ventilation for patients with neuromuscular weakness. However, it is considered a standard option for patients who have reached the point of respiratory failure. Starting a patient on long-term mechanical ventilation requires careful planning and consideration of various issues related to respiratory care in alternative settings. These issues have been addressed in consensus statements[16,17] and are discussed in Chapter 51.

Diaphragm pacing in patients with spinal cord injury has been described for some time using direct stimulation of an intact phrenic nerve to contract the diaphragm and produce negative intrathoracic pressure and inspiration.[18] This technique usually requires a thoracotomy, with its associated risks and high cost, and carries some risk of phrenic nerve injury. These objections have led to the development of an alternative system for diaphragm pacing using direct pacing of the diaphragm employing intramuscular electrodes implanted laparoscopically.[19] When the electrodes can be placed in the diaphragm muscle at an electrophysiologically mapped *motor point,* the result is often elimination of the need for mechanical ventilation in patients with spinal cord injury and delay in the need to start mechanical ventilation in patients with ALS and other neuromuscular diseases.[20]

MINI CLINI

Care of a Patient With Neuromuscular Weakness

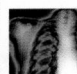

PROBLEM: A 45-year-old man has myotonic dystrophy. He has progressive dyspnea that has increased particularly in the last year. PCO_2 determined from arterial blood gas analysis is 55 mm Hg. VC is 45% of the predicted value. The patient has no underlying pulmonary disease. Cough is decreased, but the patient maintains adequate control of secretions. The patient sleeps in a seated to semirecumbent position. What interventions are indicated for this patient?

DISCUSSION: The patient has a disease that can result in respiratory insufficiency. VC is decreased, and arterial carbon dioxide levels are increased. These factors are consistent with hypoventilation secondary to neuromuscular weakness. The patient has dyspnea on exertion and orthopnea. All these factors suggest that mechanical ventilation should be considered.

Noninvasive positive pressure ventilation (NIPPV) may be a reasonable first choice in the care of this patient. The patient's mental status and bulbar function are intact. He has no significant problems with secretions. (Important factors for successful application of NIPPV are discussed in Chapter 45.) Use of a nasal mask with a biphasic positive airway pressure unit may be instituted and titrated to patient tolerance. (Most pressure or volume-cycled ventilators can be used to deliver NIPPV and invasive ventilation.) A time-cycled backup rate can be set on some ventilators to facilitate ventilation of patients who may inadequately trigger the ventilator. If the ability to clear secretions becomes compromised, cough augmentation strategies should be implemented. As long as bulbar function—swallowing and secretion management—are maintained, noninvasive ventilation is a reasonable choice for ventilatory support.

RULE OF THUMB

Patients with neuromuscular weakness who require noninvasive ventilation generally prefer a low expiratory pressure (2 to 3 cm H_2O) with a significantly higher inspiratory pressure (7 to 15 cm H_2O).

SPECIFIC NEUROMUSCULAR DISEASES

Disorders of the Muscle (Myopathic Disease)

Primary muscle disease can decrease the ability of a normal neural impulse to generate effective muscle contraction. Some commonly recognized myopathies include

TABLE 29-3

Myopathic Diseases With Associated Respiratory Dysfunction

Muscular Dystrophies	Myopathies
DMD	Congenital myopathies
Myotonic dystrophy	Nemaline rod myopathy
Facioscapulohumeral muscular dystrophy	Centronuclear myopathy
Limb-girdle dystrophy	Metabolic myopathies
Oculopharyngeal dystrophy	Acid maltase deficiency
	Mitochondrial myopathies (Kearns-Sayre syndrome)
	Inflammatory myopathies
	Polymyositis
	Dermatomyositis
	Hypothyroid-related and hyperthyroid-related myopathies
	Endocrine myopathies
	Steroid-induced myopathies (including critical illness myopathy)
	Miscellaneous myopathies
	Electrolyte disorders (e.g., hypophosphatemia, hypokalemia)
	Rhabdomyolysis
	Periodic paralysis
	Postneuromuscular blockade myopathy

Duchenne muscular dystrophy (DMD), myotonic dystrophy, and polymyositis. Table 29-3 presents a more complete list of myopathic diseases associated with ventilatory dysfunction.

Duchenne Muscular Dystrophy and Becker Muscular Dystrophy

Duchenne muscular dystrophy (DMD) is a genetic muscle-wasting disorder caused by mutations in the dystrophin gene.[21] Because it is an X-linked recessive disorder, it affects mostly males. The diagnosis is made when a dystrophin mutation is found in DNA from peripheral white blood cells or when dystrophin is found to be absent or abnormal in muscle biopsy tissue.

DMD manifests early in life with proximal muscle weakness that leads to a waddling gait, exaggerated lumbar curvature (lordosis), and frequent falls. Most affected children need a wheelchair by 12 years of age. Death generally occurs by 20 years of age, usually as a result of declining respiratory muscle strength and subsequent infection. **Becker muscular dystrophy,** a milder form of DMD, also is associated with dysregulation of the dystrophin gene and manifests later in life.

Other systemic effects of DMD include scarring of the left ventricle and decreased bowel motility (intestinal pseudoobstruction). The progressive decline in respiratory function in patients with DMD parallels limb weakness and typically occurs at the point of wheelchair dependence. Respiratory weakness is primarily due to loss of muscle strength and leads to a lower PImax at all lung volumes than is present in healthy persons.

Progressive scoliosis is associated with DMD and can contribute further to respiratory insufficiency. Many patients undergo spine fusion surgery, and often the procedure allows greater comfort and ease in maintaining an upright posture. Although no randomized trials have proven any benefit of surgery on pulmonary function,[22] observational data suggest that the rate of respiratory decline is slower after fusion surgery.[23]

Obstructive sleep apnea has been described in a significant proportion of patients with DMD, prompting some authors to recommend formal polysomnography in patients with symptoms of obstructive sleep apnea or at the stage of becoming wheelchair-bound.[24] Institution of positive pressure ventilation (PPV) is a decision most patients face at some point in the disease. The point at which to begin different stages of ventilatory support depends on both test results and clinical condition. Nocturnal PPV is usually indicated when FVC reaches 30% of predicted with signs of hypoventilation.[25,26] It can be instituted in response to oxygen desaturation during sleep, which is common in patients with increased disability and scoliosis. Nocturnal ventilation seems to improve daytime ventilatory function in patients with DMD,[27] presumably through the prevention of fatigue of the affected respiratory muscles. Despite this improvement, results of studies of early "prophylactic" institution of PPV in the care of patients with DMD have shown that early PPV failed to delay the need for formal ventilatory support.[28] However, long-term inspiratory muscle training using resistive loading was shown in at least one study to improve PImax in patients with DMD and VC values greater than 27%,[29] theoretically delaying the need for ventilatory support. Although there are concerns that pulmonary rehabilitation could produce deleterious effects through overloading weak respiratory muscles, such concerns have not been confirmed in studies in Becker muscular dystrophy.[30]

Myotonic Dystrophy

Myotonic dystrophy is the most common form of muscular dystrophy in adults, with an estimated frequency of 1 in 8000 persons.[31] *Myotonia,* or delayed muscle relaxation, is the hallmark of this neuromuscular disorder but does not clearly occur in respiratory muscles or directly cause respiratory insufficiency.[32] This autosomal dominant disorder causes progressive muscle weakness, abnormalities of the cardiac conduction system, endocrine dysfunction, and cataracts. There are two main types of myotonic dystrophy, both caused by an expansion of a repeated DNA sequence on chromosome 19.[33]

Respiratory dysfunction in myotonic dystrophy is common, usually occurring late in the course of disease, and can include respiratory muscle weakness, obstructive sleep apnea, central sleep apnea, and bulbar muscle dysfunction leading to aspiration. Sleep-related disorders are particularly common, even at an early age.[34]

Patients with myotonic dystrophy can be very sensitive to anesthesia and respiratory depressants. Both respiratory failure and prolonged neuromuscular blockade have been reported in patients with myotonic dystrophy given usual doses of these agents. For this reason, prolonged perioperative monitoring after surgery is important.[35,36]

Nocturnal ventilation by nasal mask often is effective for these patients and should be considered if the patient has declining oxygen saturation or hypercapnia. If present, central hypoventilation may necessitate tracheostomy and mechanical ventilation.

Polymyositis

Polymyositis, dermatomyositis, and **inclusion body myositis** are inflammatory myopathies of unknown cause. Respiratory compromise is rare in inclusion body **myositis** but can be seen in both polymyositis and dermatomyositis. Clinical respiratory muscle weakness is uncommon but can lead to respiratory weakness or failure within weeks to months in the setting of rapidly progressing disease. Diagnosis of these diseases is based on clinical findings of myalgia, elevated muscle enzyme levels (creatine phosphokinase or aldolase), and compatible electromyographic or muscle biopsy results. Diagnostic criteria may apply to any inflammatory **myopathy,** and specific findings or antibody identification may be needed to differentiate the various diseases (Table 29-4).[37,38]

Ventilatory insufficiency and failure caused by these inflammatory myopathies are unusual but tend to parallel the development of limb muscle weakness when they occur. In rare reported instances, diaphragmatic function is decreased disproportionately to the degree of limb weakness.[39]

Corticosteroids are the mainstay of initial management of polymyositis and dermatomyositis, although other immunosuppressive and cytotoxic regimens are used to limit long-term steroid exposure; 35% to 40% of patients with inflammatory myopathy have interstitial lung disease associated with myopathy. This lung disease appears as diffuse interstitial infiltrates that may be caused by various lung processes, but the most common (56%) is nonspecific interstitial pneumonia.[40] Various antisynthetase antibodies (e.g., Jo-1) have been identified that are associated with polymyositis and dermatomyositis,[41-43] although the role of these antibodies in the pathogenesis of these diseases is unclear. Pulmonary vasculitis can occur with polymyositis and dermatomyositis and can lead to oxygen exchange abnormalities and pulmonary hypertension.

Critical Illness Myopathy

Critical illness myopathy is a heterogeneous entity that occurs commonly in intensive care units (ICUs) and in which patients develop flaccid weakness of proximal muscles. Patients are often very difficult to wean from mechanical ventilation. Risk factors for developing this myopathy include use of corticosteroids (likely dose-dependent); use of paralytic agents; hyperglycemia; hyperthyroidism; and possibly systemic inflammatory response syndrome, with or without sepsis.[44,45] Weakness improves on its own in most cases but may take weeks or months to resolve. There is no specific therapy, and prevention by avoiding the aforementioned risk factors is the best approach.

TABLE 29-4

Diagnostic Criteria for Inflammatory Myopathies

Criterion	Polymyositis	Dermatomyositis	Inclusion Body Myositis
Symmetric proximal muscle weakness on physical examination	Yes	Yes	May be asymmetric and more distal weakness
Elevation of serum muscle enzymes (creatine kinase, aldolase, glutamate oxaloacetate, pyruvate transaminases, and lactate dehydrogenase)	Yes	Yes	Yes, lower levels than in polymyositis or dermatomyositis
Electromyographic triad of (1) short, small polyphasic potentials, (2) fibrillations, (3) high-frequency repetitive discharges	Yes	Yes	Yes
Muscle biopsy showing mononuclear inflammation, phagocytosis, necrosis, degeneration, and regeneration	Yes	Yes	Yes, may have fatty infiltration
Skin findings: Gottron sign and papules; heliotrope rash	No	Common	No
Anti–Jo-1 antibody (or other antisynthetase antibodies)	30%-50%, may indicate antisynthetase syndrome		No
Interstitial lung disease	86% in patients with antisynthetase syndrome		No

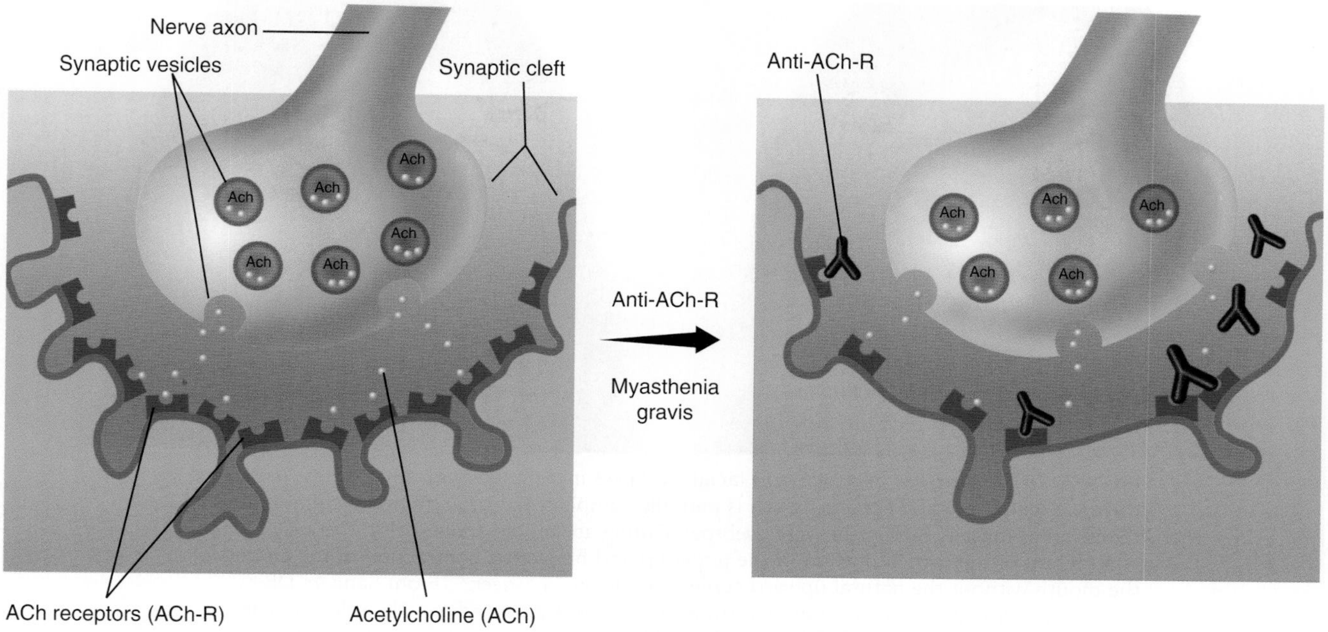

FIGURE 29-4 The neuromuscular junction with acetylcholine (ACh) stored in presynaptic vesicles. ACh is released by exocytosis into the synaptic cleft in response to a presynaptic nerve impulse. ACh binds to its cognate ACh-R on the postsynaptic membrane. This process depolarizes the nerve, propagates the impulse, and causes muscle contraction. Binding of anti-ACh-R antibodies to ACh-R mediates autoimmune destruction of the receptors. This process leads to abnormal muscle activation and the weakness that occurs in patients with MG.

Disorders of the Neuromuscular Junction

Disorders of the neuromuscular junction decrease conduction of nervous system impulses to the peripheral muscles, resulting in muscle weakness. Different clinical syndromes are caused by defects in different molecules or components of the neuromuscular junction, which is represented schematically in Figure 29-4. Disorders of the neuromuscular junction include the following:

1. Myasthenia gravis (MG)
2. Lambert-Eaton syndrome (LES)
3. Poisoning (organophosphate, tetanus, botulism)

Myasthenia Gravis

Myasthenia gravis (MG) is characterized by intermittent muscular weakness, which worsens on repetitive stimulation and improves with administration of anticholinesterase medications, such as edrophonium (Tensilon) or neostigmine. Most cases of MG arise from production of antibodies directed against the acetylcholine receptor (ACh-R). The antibodies inactivate the ACh-R and block transmission of electrical impulses from the nerve to the muscle.[46]

Approximately 20% of patients with MG do not exhibit such antibodies but may have antibodies to alternative targets, such as muscle-specific kinase.[47] Abnormalities of the thymus gland are common in MG. Approximately 10% of patients with MG have a neoplastic growth within the thymus called *thymoma,* which can be malignant but usually is not. Patients without thymoma typically have some degree of thymic hyperplasia. Congenital or fetal myasthenic syndromes are caused by either autoantibodies or inherited defects in the ACh-R.

MG typically occurs earlier in life in women and later in men. As the population has aged, more patients are diagnosed with MG later in life, and now there are more men affected than women.[48] This disorder may be associated with other autoimmune diseases, such as endocrinopathies, rheumatoid arthritis, ulcerative colitis, sarcoidosis, and pernicious anemia.

MG is characterized by progressive loss of muscular function, which may affect only the eye muscles (ocular myasthenia) or may be more widespread. The initial symptom is diplopia (double vision) or ptosis (a drooping eyelid) in greater than 65% of patients (Figure 29-5).[49] The patient typically reports weakness of the affected muscles that may vary through the day or progress, especially with repetitive use. The diagnosis of MG is supported by the detection of anti-ACh-R antibodies in the blood, a characteristic fading of nerve impulses with repeated nerve stimulation testing during electromyography, and improvement of strength or symptoms in response to an anticholinesterase inhibitor drug (edrophonium) (Figure 29-6).

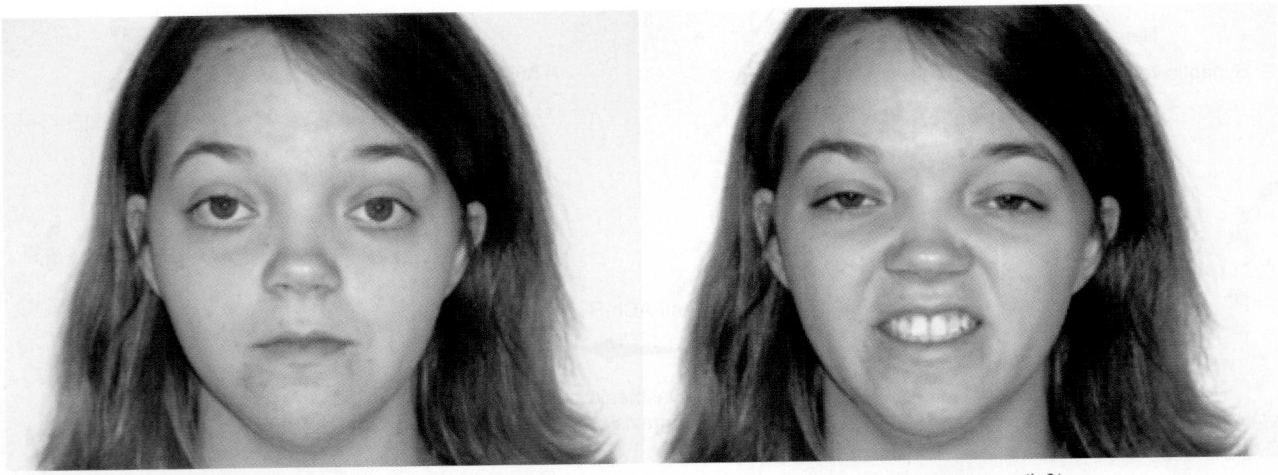

FIGURE 29-5 Features of ocular and facial weakness in a patient with MG. At rest *(left)*, there is slight bilateral lid ptosis, which is partially compensated by asymmetric contraction of the frontalis muscle, raising the right eyebrow. During attempted smile *(right)*, there is contraction of the medial portion of the upper lip and horizontal contraction of the corners of the mouth without the natural upward curling, producing a "sneer." (From Sanders DB, Howard JF: Disorders of neuromuscular transmission. In Bradley, editor: Neurology in clinical practice, ed 5, Philadelphia, 2008, Butterworth Heinemann.)

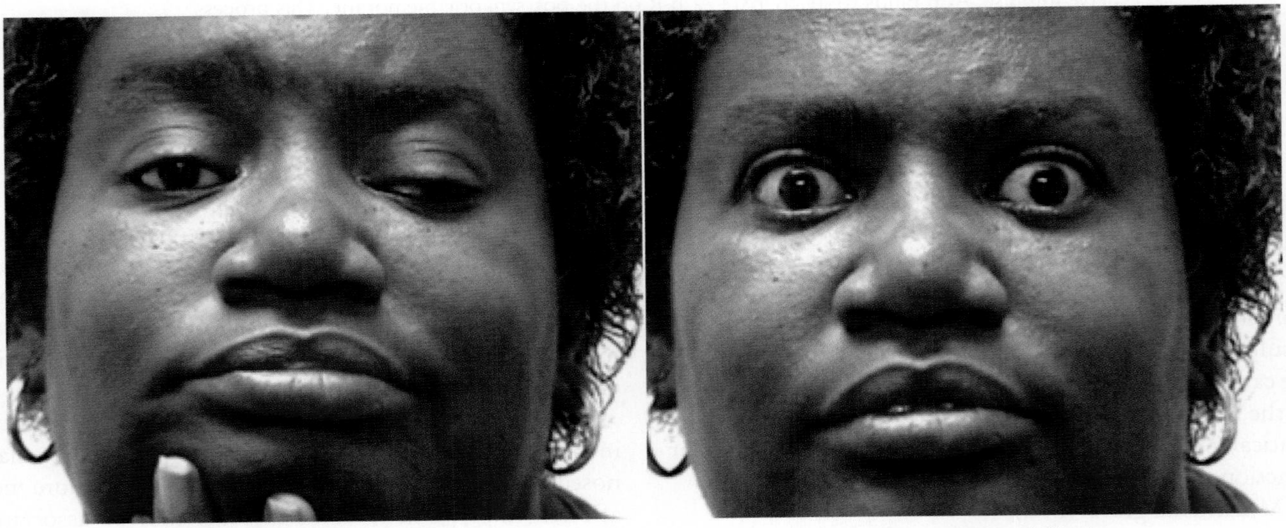

FIGURE 29-6 Clinical effect of edrophonium on a patient with MG. Before testing *(left)*, the patient has ptosis of the left eyelid and lateral deviation of the left eye, and she must support her jaw. At 5 seconds after injection of 0.1 mg of edrophonium *(right)*, ptosis and lateral deviation are resolved, and her jaw no longer requires support. (From Sanders DB, Massey JM: Clinical features of myasthenia gravis. In Engel AG, editor: Neuromuscular junction disorders, New York, Elsevier.)

Treatment of MG is generally effective, although it is largely empiric because clinical trials are rare. Long-term management includes thymectomy[50] and administration of anticholinesterases (edrophonium, neostigmine, pyridostigmine) with or without corticosteroids or other immunosuppressants, such as azathioprine or cyclosporine.[49] For patients in acute myasthenic crisis, who often are in respiratory failure on mechanical ventilation, circulating antibodies can be removed by plasmapheresis, which results in clinical improvement[51,52] usually after five or six treatments and has been used to facilitate weaning from mechanical ventilation in the care of patients with myasthenic crisis.[53] Intravenous IgG has also been used and can improve muscle strength and hasten recovery from respiratory failure. Neither apheresis nor intravenous IgG is generally used for long-term management of MG. The effect of both treatments is temporary but may last several months.[49] Clinical trials comparing these treatments have shown a slight efficacy advantage of plasmapheresis but at the cost of a higher complication rate.[54,55]

The pulmonary complications of MG depend on the magnitude and location of the affected muscle groups and tend to occur in patients most severely disabled with the disease. Upper airway obstruction, exertional dyspnea, and overt ventilatory failure all are reported in MG. Pulmonary function testing of MG patients who have respiratory muscle weakness shows decreased TLC, VC, PImax, and PEmax similar to other neuromuscular disorders, with PImax and PEmax being more sensitive markers of early respiratory muscle weakness.[56]

Myasthenic crisis is an acute event in MG and is characterized either by respiratory failure or by inability to maintain a patent airway. Myasthenic crisis can occur acutely in response to worsening of disease, intercurrent infection, or surgery or when excess anticholinesterase inhibitors have been given. Endotracheal intubation and mechanical ventilation are required immediately and may be prolonged.[57]

Lambert-Eaton Syndrome

Another syndrome of neuromuscular weakness arising from a disorder at the neuromuscular junction is **Lambert-Eaton syndrome (LES).** More than 50% of cases of LES are associated with cancer. Of these cancer-related cases, greater than 80% are associated with small cell carcinoma of the lung.[58] The mean age at presentation is approximately 60 years, although LES can occur in all age groups. Autoantibodies against voltage-gated calcium channels at the nerve terminals impair the release of acetylcholine and can lead to both muscular weakness and autonomic insufficiency.[59] These autoantibodies can be detected in a patient's serum, which confirms the diagnosis.[60] The clinical diagnosis of LES is supported by results of nerve conduction studies. Increasing muscle strength with repetitive stimuli is a characteristic feature of LES, which differentiates it from MG. In contrast, MG is characterized by progressive fatigue of muscular contraction with repetitive stimulation.

Patients with LES usually present with tiredness or weakness of proximal muscle groups out of proportion to findings on clinical examination. Although patients are subject to respiratory complications because of their increased sensitivity to the effects of anesthesia, respiratory failure is rare. The clinical course of LES tends to be one of relative stability with less fluctuation than MG. Management of LES includes treatment of the underlying malignancy when present. If no malignancy is found, surveillance for lung cancer is recommended every 6 months, and LES is managed symptomatically with immunosuppressive medication or acetylcholinesterase inhibitors.[60]

Disorders of the Nerves

The peripheral nerves may be affected by toxic agents, inflammatory processes, vascular disorders, malignant diseases, and metabolic or nutritional imbalances. Hundreds of conditions have been associated with neuropathies leading to respiratory muscle dysfunction. Representative conditions are listed in Box 29-1.

Box 29-1 Causes of Phrenic Nerve Dysfunction Leading to Respiratory Dysfunction

- Cardiac surgery (cold cardioplegia to arrest the heart can cause "frostbitten" phrenic nerves; ischemic injury to nerves can also complicate cardiac surgery)
- Diabetes
- Trauma
- Thoracic aneurysm

Guillain-Barré Syndrome

Guillain-Barré syndrome (GBS) is acute inflammatory demyelinating polyneuropathy and is the most common peripheral **neuropathy** causing respiratory insufficiency. GBS is characterized by paralysis and hyporeflexia with or without sensory symptoms. GBS is typically a self-limited disease, but overall mortality ranges from 3% to 6%.[61] Before modern mechanical ventilation techniques, mortality in this condition was greater than 33%.[62] Most patients recover their respiratory muscle strength completely, but the proportion of patients with significant disability 1 year after onset of the disease can be 20%.[63] Autonomic nervous system problems, such as hypotension, flushing, bronchorrhea, dermatographia, and bradycardia, are common. Two-thirds of patients with GBS report a triggering event, such as respiratory or gastrointestinal infection, immunization, or surgery, 1 to 4 weeks before the onset of symptoms. Other reported triggers include pregnancy and malignancy.[62]

GBS is a demyelinating process widely believed to be caused by autoantibodies directed against the myelin constituting the nerve sheath. The diagnosis of GBS is based on a combination of clinical, laboratory, and electrophysiologic data (Table 29-5).[64] Cerebrospinal fluid protein levels are elevated with minimal cellularity after approximately 1 week of illness. Nerve conduction studies show slowing of conduction with preserved amplitude, which is typical of demyelination. Approximately one-third of all patients with GBS have respiratory muscle compromise. Although the diaphragm is typically affected later in the course of GBS, cases of respiratory failure in the absence of substantial peripheral weakness have been reported. The need for mechanical ventilatory support for patients with GBS increases with age.[62]

Treatment strategies that have improved outcome in GBS include intravenous immunoglobulin infusions and plasmapheresis. Both treatments are equally effective in hastening recovery of muscle strength. The benefit is greatest when treatment is started within 2 weeks of symptom onset. There is no additional benefit of combining the two therapies. Corticosteroids have no beneficial role in GBS.[65]

TABLE 29-5

Diagnostic Criteria for Guillain-Barré Syndrome

Required for Diagnosis	Supportive of Diagnosis
Progressive weakness of both legs and arms	Symptoms progress over days to weeks
Areflexia	Symmetry of weakness
	Cranial nerve involvement (facial palsies)
	Improvement begins 2-4 wk after progression stops
	Absence of fever at onset of symptoms
	Laboratory features not suggestive of alternate diagnosis
	Cerebrospinal fluid with high protein, low cell count
	Nerve conduction slowing or block with normal amplitude

Patients with dyspnea, orthopnea, or impaired ability to maintain a patent airway should receive spirometry every 4 to 6 hours for documentation of function and assessment of the need for endotracheal intubation. Patients with poor upper airway control, weak cough, or large amounts of secretions should be considered for endotracheal intubation even though their VC is greater than 20 ml/kg. The increased work of breathing imposed by mucous plugging or atelectasis can hasten decompensation. A small subgroup may need mechanical ventilation for 1 year or more. Weaning of patients with GBS from mechanical ventilation is predicted by VC greater than 18 ml/kg,[68] transdiaphragmatic pressure greater than 31 cm H_2O, or a PImax stronger than −30 cm H_2O.[69]

RULE OF THUMB

Patients with GBS whose VC becomes less than 20 ml/kg or declines more than 30% from baseline or whose maximal inspiratory pressure is less than −30 cm H_2O and maximal expiratory pressure is less than 40 cm H_2O are at risk of respiratory failure and may need ventilatory support. Patients who meet the criteria of this "20-30-40 rule" should be observed in an ICU.[66]

RULE OF THUMB

Patients with GBS should be intubated for mechanical ventilatory support when VC decreases to 12 to 15 ml/kg or sooner if they have bulbar dysfunction with difficulty managing oral secretions or when PaO_2 values are less than 70 mm Hg while breathing room air.[62] As with all patients requiring intubation, as soon as it is clear that intubation will exceed 2 weeks' duration, a tracheostomy should be considered.[67]

Phrenic Nerve Damage and Diaphragmatic Paralysis

Each hemidiaphragm is supplied by its own phrenic nerve. The phrenic nerves emerge from the spinal cord at level C3-5 and descend through the mediastinum along the great vessels of the chest and pericardium. Damage to or interruption of either phrenic nerve leads to paralysis of the ipsilateral hemidiaphragm. Bilateral interruption is seen in high spinal cord injury and causes complete diaphragmatic paralysis. Unilateral diaphragmatic paralysis can be seen in various disease processes. Reversible unilateral diaphragmatic paralysis is a rare complication of acute pneumonia, but it can occur in 10% of patients who undergo cardiac surgery with cardiopulmonary bypass, usually secondary to cold cardioplegia or traction on the nerve during surgery or ischemic nerve injury.[70]

Patients with unilateral diaphragmatic paralysis may have a 15% to 20% reduction in VC and TLC in the upright position and a further reduction while supine. If they have no other diseases, patients with unilateral diaphragmatic paralysis may have no symptoms. Athletes, musicians, and others who use their lungs more fully are more likely to notice the decreased ventilatory capacity caused by unilateral diaphragm weakness. Diaphragmatic paralysis is diagnosed most often with chest radiography. The paralyzed side retains its contour but is displaced upward (Figure 29-7, *A*). At fluoroscopy, the paralyzed hemidiaphragm paradoxically rises into the thorax during a sudden forceful inspiration (sniff test). This paradoxical motion dampens the effect of the normal diaphragm on the opposite side.

For patients with unilateral diaphragm paralysis, surgical plication of the weak side can move the diaphragm downward to a more normal position (Figure 29-7, *B*) and minimize paradoxical motion and improve overall lung function.[71,72] Historically, results of diaphragm plication procedures have been disappointing, but newer laparoscopic techniques are more promising.[73] Appropriate patient selection is crucial to avoid operating on patients whose diaphragms would recover their strength in time and patients whose weakness is due to primary neuromuscular disorders, which would not be improved by plication.

RULE OF THUMB

Diaphragm weakness resulting from phrenic nerve injury (not transection) often improves very slowly, sometimes over years, so plication should be delayed until serial testing shows that no further improvement is occurring, usually at least 1 to 2 years from the onset of weakness.

Critical Illness Polyneuropathy

In contrast to critical illness myopathy, discussed previously, **critical illness polyneuropathy** is associated almost entirely with severe sepsis in the ICU. Patients

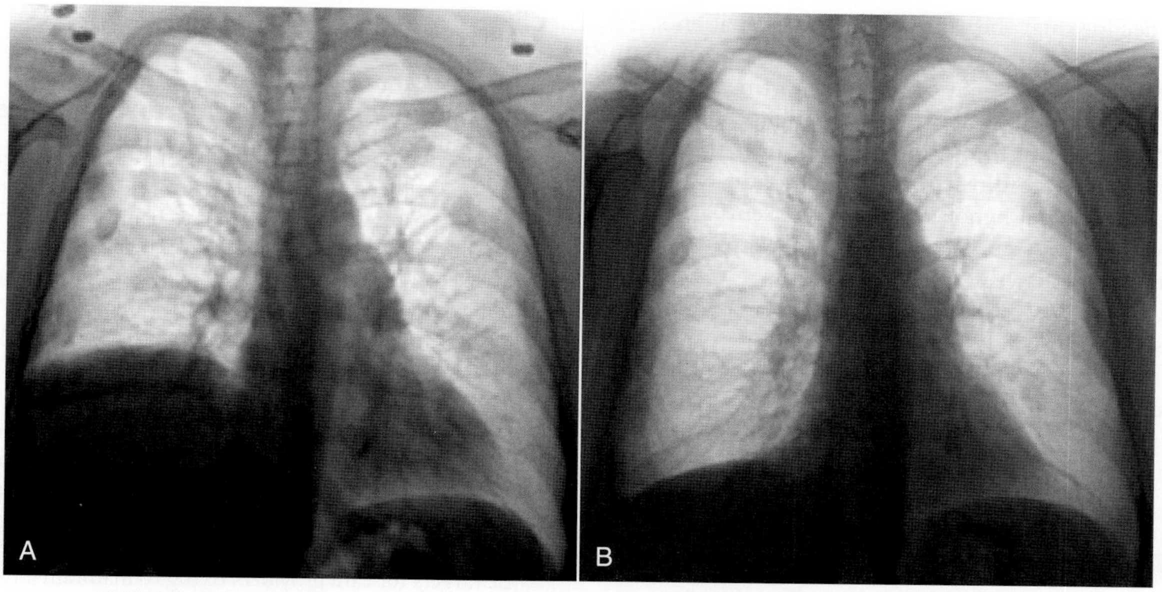

FIGURE 29-7 **A,** Chest x-ray showing elevation of a right hemidiaphragm. **B,** Chest x-ray in the same patient 1 year after laparoscopic diaphragm plication. (From Groth SS, Andrade RS: Diaphragm plication for eventration or paralysis: a review of the literature. Ann Thorac Surg 89:S2146–S2150, 2010.)

develop muscle weakness and atrophy, loss of deep tendon reflexes, and loss of peripheral sensation to pinprick and touch. Cranial nerve function is usually spared. The mechanism of nerve damage is unknown but, similar to other complications of sepsis, may be related to ischemia caused by thrombosis or underperfusion of the microcirculation, or both, in this case of the affected nerves.[45]

Effects of critical illness polyneuropathy may persist for years, or permanently, but often improve with time and rehabilitation. As in critical illness myopathy, there is no specific treatment; optimal management of the patient's severe sepsis following protocols to restore adequate circulation and limit the length of organ system failure is thought to be beneficial.

Disorders of the Spinal Cord

Upper motor neurons arise from cell bodies in the motor areas of the brain and terminate at the anterior horn cells in the spinal cord, which constitute the lower motor neurons because it is axons from these cells that extend out of the central nervous system to the skeletal muscles. Disorders in this group (e.g., ALS) can affect specific parts of this chain or nonspecifically disrupt these tracts (e.g., spinal cord injury). Other examples of lesions in this anatomic location include transverse myelitis, syringomyelia, poliomyelitis, and spinal cord tumors.

Amyotrophic Lateral Sclerosis

Amyotrophic lateral sclerosis (ALS), or **Lou Gehrig disease,** is a neuromuscular disease characterized by progressive degeneration of both upper and lower motor neurons; early in the disease, degeneration of either upper or lower motor neurons may predominate. Approximately 5% to 10% of cases are familial; others are sporadic. The male-to-female ratio for ALS is approximately 1.2 : 1, and the peak incidence is between 65 years old and 75 years old, although cases have been reported in patients younger than 30 years old. The prognosis of ALS is poor, with a mean survival from diagnosis of 3 years. By 5 years, 80% of patients have died, and 90% have died by 10 years.[74] Medical treatment of ALS is disappointing. There is no cure, and therapies to halt or slow progression of the disease are few and ineffective. One approved therapy for ALS is riluzole, an antiglutamate agent. Randomized trials have shown modest improvements in median survival of 4.2 months.[75] The cost of the medication is prohibitive for many patients, especially in light of the modest results usually seen.

Muscle weakness secondary to ALS usually begins in a localized muscle group and spreads out geographically from there. It most often begins in the arms but may originate in the bulbar muscles (i.e., muscles supplied by nerves in the upper spinal cord, such as the nerves controlling swallowing and speaking) 25% of the time. In 1% to 2% of cases, ALS manifests initially as isolated respiratory muscle dysfunction in an otherwise relatively intact patient. Respiratory involvement eventually occurs in all patients with ALS, and pulmonary complications are the most frequent cause of death. Muscle weakness is associated with fasciculations, or involuntary quivering of the affected muscles. If muscle fasciculation does not develop in a patient with presumed ALS soon after weakness, another diagnosis should be considered.[76]

Inspiratory muscle decline, measured by FVC, tends to be linear with time in any one patient, although the rate of decline may be different between patients. As respiratory muscle strength gradually declines, acute respiratory decompensation may occur in the setting of respiratory infection or aspiration. ALS patients may have respiratory difficulty for various disease-related reasons, not all of which are direct results of respiratory muscle weakness. Nocturnal hypoxemia and hypoventilation can lead to disrupted sleep, frequent arousal, daytime headaches, and somnolence.

Monitoring FVC, PImax, and PEmax or maximal sniff nasal inspiratory force is helpful in these patients and can provide important information regarding the ability to clear secretions and maintain gas exchange. Ineffective cough can lead to atelectasis, pneumonia, and worsening gas exchange and hypoxemia.

RULE OF THUMB

Effective cough typically requires a PEmax greater than 40 cm H_2O to compress airways and generate sufficient flow velocities within the tracheobronchial tree to clear obstructing secretions or aspirated material.

The prevention of respiratory complications and assessment of the need for ventilatory assistance are central in caring for patients with advancing ALS. Helpful therapeutic interventions include (1) modification of food consistency or placement of feeding tubes in patients with marked bulbar dysfunction, (2) clearing of secretions with assisted cough techniques or postural drainage, and (3) ventilatory assistance with positive or negative pressure devices. Noninvasive techniques are a viable option for many patients and have been shown to slow the rate of pulmonary decline, improve symptoms, and prolong survival.[77] When these techniques no longer suffice, many patients with ALS choose not to receive invasive mechanical ventilation and opt for palliative management at that point. However, many patients do desire invasive ventilatory support, and 90% of such patients in one study reported satisfaction with their decision and would choose tracheostomy and ventilation again in the same situation.[78] Although overall survival with ALS is poor, prolonged survival of ventilated patients has been reported.

RULE OF THUMB

The timing and type of ventilatory intervention (noninvasive or invasive) in the care of patients with ALS are the subject of much discussion. General guidelines for considering ventilatory assistance[79] include the following: VC less than 50% predicted, orthopnea, maximal sniff nasal inspiratory force less than −40 cm H_2O, PImax less than (i.e., more negative than) −60 cm H_2O, and abnormal nocturnal oximetry.

MINI CLINI

Respiratory Care of a Patient with Amyotrophic Lateral Sclerosis

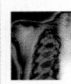

PROBLEM: A 57-year-old practicing attorney with a diagnosis of ALS for 2 years has a tracheostomy for nocturnal mechanical ventilation. He is still able to function and practice law in a specialized wheelchair and wants to maintain his independence and professional practice as long as possible. What measures can be offered to help him maintain his respiratory function, avoid exacerbations that could lead to acute respiratory failure, and preserve his quality of life?

DISCUSSION: Respiratory muscle failure can be influenced by many factors in addition to the primary neuromuscular disease. These additional factors can be significant contributors to a patient's quality of life or progressive decline in function, and they provide additional therapeutic targets for care providers trying to maintain a patient's function and comfort.

Reduced lung compliance owing to atelectasis or retained secretions can greatly increase the work of breathing for weakened muscles and worsen gas exchange. Maneuvers to recruit collapsed alveoli and augment his cough to clear secretions can counteract these factors. These maneuvers include chest physiotherapy and mechanical insufflation and exsufflation devices. Increased secretion production is another factor in many patients' illness, which can be managed with medications such as atropine or amitriptyline. In some cases, salivary glands are treated with low-dose radiation. Patients with bulbar dysfunction may lose additional respiratory muscle strength as a result of poor nutrition; placement of a percutaneous endoscopic gastrostomy tube for nutrition may avoid this as eating becomes more difficult. Keeping these additional aspects in mind allows a care provider to address them along with the primary weakness, and it is this care in many cases that prolongs a patient's ability to breathe independently and function as he or she would like.[80]

RULE OF THUMB

ALS is a complex and devastating disease and often requires a multidisciplinary approach, with input and active participation from numerous clinical specialties, including pulmonary, neurology, critical care, gastroenterology, palliative medicine, physical therapy, occupational therapy, social work, home nursing, psychiatry, and spiritual care.

Spinal Cord Trauma

Approximately 12,000 new spinal cord injuries occur in the United States each year, and 55% involve the cervical spine. The causes are varied, but the most common causes are motor vehicle accidents, falls, violence, and sports. Many patients with a spine injury have other injuries associated with their trauma, including 25% to 50% with traumatic

RULE OF THUMB

Patients with ALS typically need psychologic support because of the progressive, incurable nature of their disease. Care providers must address issues such as depression, social and family support and education, and end-of-life planning. Because end-of-life discussions with patients can be uncomfortable for care providers, many avoid them and assume someone else will address this difficult topic, but that is a disservice to patients who need to understand and confront issues of eventual respiratory failure and death from their disease.

head injury[81]; 5% to 10% of these spinal cord injuries cause quadriplegia. Complete cord injury is associated with absent motor and sensory function below the level of injury, and the patient's condition rarely improves. Patients with incomplete injury have residual function and tend to improve to varying degrees.

The respiratory manifestations of spinal cord injury depend on the level of injury and extent of damage. The injuries can be functionally divided into two classes: high cervical cord lesions (C1-2) and middle to low cervical cord lesions (C3-8). The diaphragm receives innervation from nerve roots exiting the spinal cord at levels C3-5. Complete injury above this level results in total respiratory muscle paralysis and death, unless urgent intubation and ventilation are performed. Injury to the cord at C3-5 can severely reduce respiratory strength as manifested by reductions in PEmax, PImax, FVC, and FEV_1, consistent with a restrictive ventilatory defect. Patients adopt a rapid, shallow breathing pattern and use accessory inspiratory muscles (scalene and sternocleidomastoid muscles). *Abdominal paradox* (inward movement of the abdomen while the thorax expands) is the hallmark of significant bilateral diaphragmatic weakness. Despite the serious nature of injury between C3 and C5, 80% of intubated patients with this lesion can ultimately be liberated from mechanical ventilation. The muscles of expiration receive neural input from spinal levels T1-L1 and are predominantly affected by middle to low cervical cord lesions. This condition manifests as a marked reduction in PEmax compared with PImax and a diminished or absent effective cough.

The differential weakness of respective muscle groups in patients with neuromuscular weakness affects ventilatory capacity in the supine and seated positions. Patients with predominantly diaphragmatic weakness have orthopnea and are most comfortable in the upright seated position. The upright seated position favors gravity-assisted descent of the diaphragm, which is less affected by the abdominal contents that shift caudally (toward the bottom of the patient's spine) in the seated patient.

Recumbent patients with bilateral diaphragmatic weakness accompanying spinal cord injury may display paradoxical breathing, or abdominal paradox. Observation of the chest and abdomen of patients reveals paradoxic inward movement of the abdomen during inspiration. Conversely, patients with expiratory muscle weakness similar to that produced by low cervical cord injury prefer the supine position, in which the tendency of the abdominal contents to move toward the head assists expiration in the absence of marked expiratory muscle tone. These physiologic principles form the basis for the use of "rocking beds" and pneumatic belt devices as ventilatory adjuncts in the care of patients with considerable respiratory muscle weakness.

MINI CLINI

Respiratory Dysfunction in Spinal Cord Injury

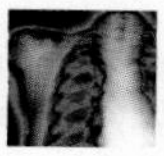

PROBLEM: A young man who is otherwise healthy falls from a ladder and transects the spinal cord at the level of C6. Which muscles of the respiratory system will be affected, and what will be the effect?

DISCUSSION: Transection of the spinal cord at the level of the sixth cervical vertebra paralyzes any muscle group that receives its innervation from nerve roots that exit the spinal vertebral canal below C6. A review of the innervation of the major muscles of inspiration and expiration is important:

Upper airway, tongue, palate: Cranial nerves IX, X, XI, and XII
C3-5: Diaphragm
C4-8: Shoulder girdle muscle (scalenes)
T1-12: Intercostal muscles
T7-L1: Abdominal muscles

The upper airway, tongue, shoulder girdle muscles, and diaphragm should be intact in this patient's injury. Maintenance of intrathoracic volume depends partly on continuous activation of intercostal muscles, which stabilize and expand the thoracic cage. With these muscles paralyzed, expiratory reserve volume decreases, and normal activation of the diaphragm results in a tendency toward inward excursion of the chest wall and loss of effective volume. Forceful exhalation and the development of cough depend on activation of abdominal and intercostal muscle groups, both of which are paralyzed in this injury. Although he has an intact diaphragm, this patient has a poor cough, which is a predisposing factor for atelectasis, pooling of secretions, and pneumonia. Successful management of spinal cord injury at this level includes aggressive postural drainage and percussion (when the injury has been stabilized) and possibly assisted cough in the respiratory care regimen.

Disorders of the Brain

Traumatic brain injury, stroke, hemorrhage, and infection can lead to abnormality of respiration through various mechanisms. The motor cortex contains voluntary centers

TABLE 29-6

Abnormal Respiratory Patterns Associated With Stroke

Cheyne-Stokes respiration	Common abnormal pattern characterized by crescendo-decrescendo breathing force and tidal volume; it is not specific for stroke and is more commonly due to cardiopulmonary disease
Periodic breathing	Similar to Cheyne-Stokes but with complete central apneas in between periods of crescendo-decrescendo breathing; it is seen in 25% of acute strokes, especially in patients with subarachnoid hemorrhage
Gasping	Very short inspiration, often involving contraction of accessory muscles, with long expiratory phase; it often heralds impending respiratory failure
Ataxic breathing	Irregularly irregular respiratory rate and tidal volumes; it nearly always means a medullary stroke or lesion; it is not the sign of a poor prognosis
Apneustic breathing	Very long inspiratory phase (several seconds), then brief, rapid exhalation followed by a respiratory pause; it is usually associated with bulbar dysfunction with difficulty protecting airway from secretions, so usually requires intubation, and may be difficult to wean from ventilator
Central neurogenic hyperventilation	Rapid deep breaths resulting in hypocapnia; other causes of hyperventilation must be ruled out, but if so, this pattern signifies a poor prognosis
Apnea	Unusual in strokes except in brain death; prognosis is generally poor
Ondine curse	Apnea during sleep with normal respiration while awake; it is treated with mechanical ventilation during sleep only; some patients improve and no longer need ventilatory support

Data from references 82-84.

for control of the upper airway and pharynx (see Chapter 14). The pons and medulla, located in the brainstem, contain (1) chemoreceptors for automatic control of ventilation in response to increasing pH and hypercapnia and (2) centers that generate and modify patterns of automatic ventilation in response to visceral and chemical afferent information (see Figure 29-1). Both stroke and traumatic brain injury can lead to disordered patterns of breathing, which are listed in Table 29-6, and abnormalities in the lungs themselves, such as neurogenic pulmonary edema. This section describes the clinical entities of stroke and traumatic brain injury and their effects on the respiratory system.

Stroke

Stroke is a clinical syndrome produced by acute interruption of the normal blood flow to an area of the brain. The result is persistent dysfunction related to the affected structures. Stroke can be thrombotic (related to local formation of a clot), embolic (related to a clot traveling from a remote place in the body), or hemorrhagic. The effect of a stroke on respiration depends on which of the control elements of ventilation are damaged.

Strokes in the cerebral cortex can produce decreased chest wall and diaphragmatic movement. Infarction in this area usually does not lead to significant alteration of ventilation. However, the patient may have significant impairment of speech and movement, including impairment of muscles that affect upper airway tone and control secretions. Swallowing is also frequently a problem, leading to aspiration or poor nutrition. Chronic changes in pharyngeal muscle tone can also lead to obstructive sleep apnea. Rarely, localized strokes lead to profound alterations of the respiratory system. These alterations often result from strokes in the midbrain and brainstem or from subarachnoid hemorrhage. They often resolve or improve after the acute time frame of the stroke (see Table 29-6).

Therapy for stroke has evolved considerably. Previous therapy for thrombotic stroke was largely supportive. At the present time, early use of thrombolytic therapy to dissolve the clot and restore circulation and function has been shown to improve function and survival, particularly if the thrombolytic agent is given less than 3 hours after the onset of symptoms.[85,86] More recent trials have also shown benefit in a more restricted patient population when thrombolytic therapy was given in the 3- to 4.5-hour time frame.[87,88] Physical therapy and occupational therapy continue to be important components for optimizing function in the setting of residual deficit after stroke. Patients with substantial impairment of speech and swallowing may be at risk of aspiration pneumonia. As in many catastrophic illnesses, stroke presents a complex set of problems, and patients do best when managed using a multidisciplinary approach in a center with high volumes of similar patients and well-developed expertise.[89]

Traumatic Brain Injury

Traumatic brain injury is a general term referring to numerous focal or diffuse lesions of the brain resulting from blunt or penetrating force. In some patients, direct trauma to the respiratory centers in the brain may cause the same derangements of ventilation as strokes (mentioned previously); traumatic brain injury can also lead to secondary effects on the respiratory system, such as neurogenic pulmonary edema and hypersecretion of mucus, leading to hypoxemia and respiratory insufficiency through mechanisms other than muscular weakness. There may be other injuries in patients with traumatic brain injury that affect the respiratory system, such as spinal cord injury or rib fractures, or there may be factors that helped lead to

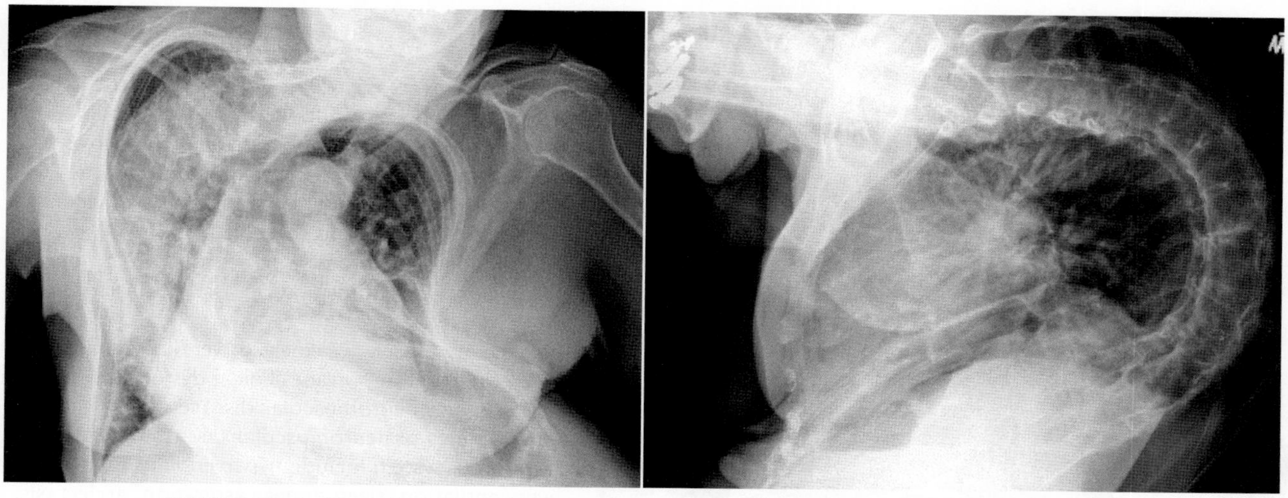

FIGURE 29-8 Frontal and lateral chest x-ray views of the same patient, showing severe scoliosis and kyphosis.

the injury, which may independently affect breathing, such as intoxication or underlying illness.

Disorders of the Thoracic Cage

The thoracic cage contains the lungs and supports the muscles of respiration. Normal ventilatory mechanics depend on a compliant thoracic cage with free excursion throughout the respiratory cycle.

Kyphoscoliosis

Kyphosis is posterior angulation of the thoracic cage. *Scoliosis* is lateral curvature of the spine (Figure 29-8). These two deformities often occur together (called **kyphoscoliosis**) as a result of the compensatory effects of the spine in response to the primary lateral curve in scoliosis.

Scoliosis is typically noticed during childhood and progresses during adolescence, although idiopathic adult kyphoscoliosis has been reported. The degree of scoliosis is measured by the *Cobb angle,* which is determined by the intersection of lines drawn between the upper and lower limbs of the primary curve in scoliosis (Figure 29-9). Severe kyphoscoliosis (Cobb angle >90 to 100 degrees) can lead to hypoventilation, hypercapnia, and, if untreated, complications of pulmonary hypertension. However, the degree of pulmonary dysfunction cannot be predicted from the Cobb angle alone.[90,91] Respiratory dysfunction is probably multifactorial in most patients. Compliance of the chest wall and lung is decreased in patients with significant kyphoscoliosis. The result is a restrictive ventilatory defect with decreased TLC and VC in pulmonary function testing. Maximal transdiaphragmatic pressure also is decreased, a sign of impaired diaphragmatic function in the pathogenesis of respiratory dysfunction in severe kyphoscoliosis.

Anterior or posterior spinal fixation can stabilize kyphoscoliosis and restore the thoracic curvature to a condition close to normal. Fixation prevents complications secondary to progressive curvature, loss of compliance, and subsequent ventilatory dysfunction. Few options are available to restore pulmonary function to older patients with established kyphoscoliosis. Surgery to correct the deformity can be undertaken, but this treatment generally does not improve pulmonary function.[92] Better long-term results are seen when surgery or brace therapy to correct the angulation are undertaken in adolescence.[93]

Both noninvasive and invasive ventilation are used in some patients with severe kyphoscoliosis, with improvement in blood gas values, respiratory muscle strength, symptoms of dyspnea,[94] and exercise capacity.[95] Both negative pressure[96] and positive pressure[97] ventilation have been reported to stabilize respiratory function in patients with severe kyphoscoliosis.

Flail Chest

Flail chest is defined in different ways but occurs as a result of multiple rib fractures that cause a portion of the chest wall to become free-floating. The destabilized segment of the thoracic cage exhibits **paradoxical motion** during the respiratory cycle, bowing out with expiration and collapsing inward during a spontaneous breath. The movement is associated with a decreased pressure gradient to drive inspiration and expiration and can result in respiratory failure. Flail chest frequently is accompanied by other pulmonary injuries as a result of the mechanism of injury and the force required to fracture multiple ribs. Pulmonary contusion, hemothorax, and pneumothorax are frequently associated with flail chest and often necessitate urgent or emergency treatment in the trauma patient.[98] Flail chest is managed with analgesia and positive pressure ventilation.

Ankylosing Spondylitis

Ankylosing spondylitis is a rheumatologic disease that affects the spine and thoracic cage. Chronic joint inflammation ultimately leads to fusion of the vertebral bodies

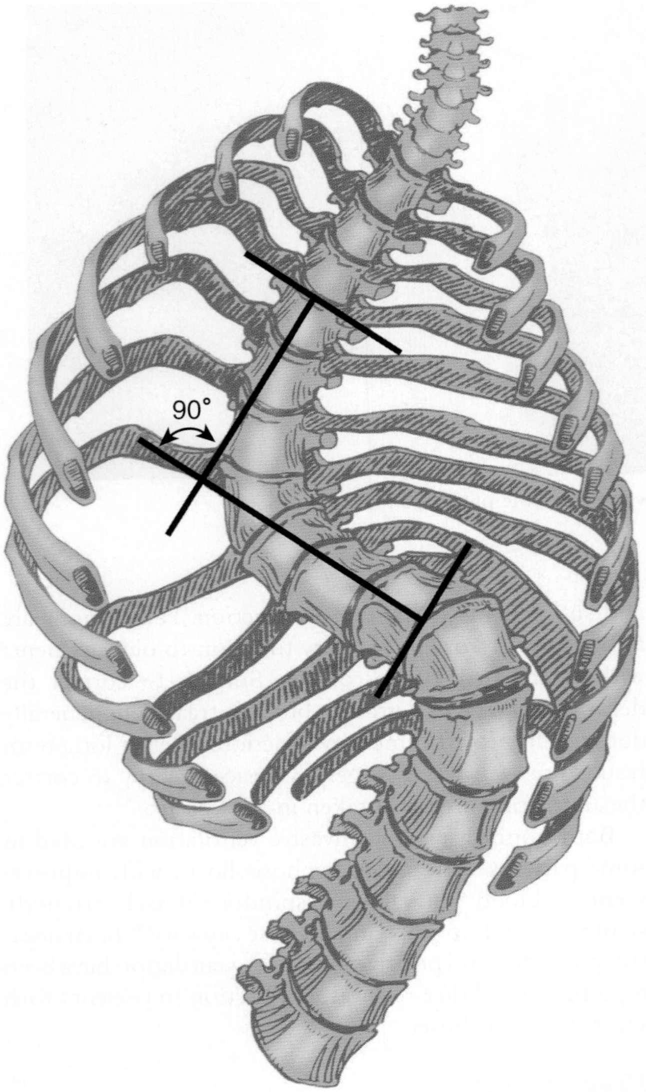

FIGURE 29-9 Scoliosis is lateral curvature of the spine. The degree of scoliosis is measured by the Cobb angle, which is determined by the intersection of lines drawn between the upper and lower limbs of the primary curve in scoliosis. Respiratory insufficiency rarely occurs until the Cobb angle exceeds 90 to 100 degrees. (Modified from Fishman AP: Acute respiratory failure. In Fishman AP, editor: Pulmonary disease, New York, 1992, McGraw-Hill, p 2300.)

and the costovertebral joints, typically leading to severe kyphosis and a dramatic decrease in thoracic cage compliance. Because diaphragmatic movement is retained, TLC and VC are only slightly reduced. The most severe respiratory consequence is parenchymal lung disease, which occurs in about 10% of patients with ankylosing spondylitis, in the form of apical fibrocystic changes that can decrease gas exchange and often provide a location for superinfection, especially fungal infection.[99]

SUMMARY CHECKLIST

- The components of the neuromuscular system that affect respiration include the brain (especially respiratory centers in the brainstem); the nerves (the phrenic nerve supplying the diaphragm and the intercostal nerves supplying many of the other respiratory muscles and the bulbar muscles coordinating the throat); the neuromuscular junction; and the muscles of inspiration, expiration, and upper airway control.
- Respiratory muscle weakness or ventilatory failure is often the most important clinical dysfunction for many patients with neuromuscular diseases.
- Other effects of neuromuscular disease on the respiratory system include hyperventilation or hypoventilation, sleep apnea, aspiration, atelectasis, pulmonary hypertension, and cor pulmonale.
- Signs and symptoms that may indicate weakness of the respiratory muscles include exertional dyspnea, orthopnea, decreased volume of voice, weak or ineffective cough, accessory muscle use, and paradoxical breathing pattern (abdominal paradox).
- Pulmonary function abnormalities in patients with inspiratory muscle weakness typically include decreases in PImax, TLC, VC, and FEV_1. Residual volume can be increased. There often is an abnormally large decrease in FVC and FEV_1 (30% to 50%) when patients undergo testing in the seated and supine positions. Diffusing capacity corrected for alveolar volume typically is normal.
- Common neuromuscular disorders that cause respiratory compromise include amyotrophic lateral sclerosis, myotonic dystrophy, spinal cord injury, Guillain-Barré syndrome, Duchenne muscular dystrophy, and myasthenia gravis.
- Cervical spine injury above the C3 level results in complete paralysis of the respiratory muscles and necessitates emergency mechanical ventilation. Cervical spine injury below C5 leads to weakness of the expiratory muscles with decreased ability to cough and clear secretions.
- Unilateral diaphragmatic paralysis resulting from phrenic nerve damage usually is asymptomatic and is associated with minor reductions in respiratory function in an otherwise healthy patient.
- Scoliosis is abnormal lateral curvature of the spine. Respiratory insufficiency can occur if the curve is severe.
- Flail chest typically results from trauma to the chest. Multiple fractures of adjacent ribs produce a free-floating segment of the thoracic cage, which displays paradoxical excursion during the respiratory cycle. Flail chest often is associated with serious damage to the lungs, heart, or great vessels. Respiratory insufficiency in patients with flail chest can occur through numerous mechanisms.

References

1. American Thoracic Society/European Respiratory Society ATS/ERS Statement on respiratory muscle testing. Am J Respir Crit Care Med 166:518–624, 2002.
2. McMorrow C, Fredsted A, Carberry J, et al: Chronic hypoxia increases rat diaphragm muscle endurance and Na+-K+ ATPase pump content. Eur Respir J 37:1474–1481, 2010.
3. Verges S, Bachasson D, Wuyam B: Effect of acute hypoxia on respiratory muscle fatigue in healthy humans. Respir Res 11:109, 2010.
4. Begin R, Bureau MA, Lupien L, et al: Control of breathing in Duchenne's muscular dystrophy. Am J Med 69:227–234, 1980.
5. Morgan RK, McNally S, Alexander M, et al: Use of sniff nasal-inspiratory force to predict survival in amyotrophic lateral sclerosis. Am J Respir Crit Care Med 171:269, 2005.
6. Elman LB, Siderowf AD, McCluskey LF: Nocturnal oximetry: utility in the respiratory management of amyotrophic lateral sclerosis. Am J Phys Med Rehabil 82:866, 2003.
7. Yavagal DR, Mayer SA: Respiratory complications of rapidly progressive neuromuscular syndromes: Guillain-Barré syndrome and myasthenia gravis. Semin Respir Crit Care Med 23:221–229, 2002.
8. Tzeng AC, Bach JR: Prevention of pulmonary morbidity for patients with neuromuscular disease. Chest 118:1390, 2000.
9. Servera E, Sancho J, Zafra MJ, et al: Alternatives to endotracheal intubation for patients with neuromuscular diseases. Am J Phys Med Rehabil 84:851–857, 2005.
10. Aboussouan LS: Mechanisms of exercise limitation and pulmonary rehabilitation for patients with neuromuscular disease. Chron Respir Dis 6:231–249, 2009.
11. Vianello A, Bevilacqua M, Arcaro G, et al: Non-invasive ventilatory approach to treatment of acute respiratory failure in neuromuscular disorders: a comparison with endotracheal intubation. Intensive Care Med 26:384, 2000.
12. Boitano LJ, Jordan T, Benditt JO: Noninvasive ventilation allows gastrostomy tube placement in patients with advanced ALS. Neurology 56:413, 2001.
13. Robert D, Argaud L: Clinical review: long-term noninvasive ventilation. Crit Care 11:210, 2007.
14. Melo J, Homma A, Iturriaga E, et al: Pulmonary evaluation and prevalence of non-invasive ventilation in patients with amyotrophic lateral sclerosis: a multicenter survey and proposal of a pulmonary protocol. J Neurol Sci 169:114, 1999.
15. Laub M, Berg S, Midgren B: Symptoms, clinical and physiological finding motivating home mechanical ventilation in patients with neuromuscular diseases. J Rehabil Med 38:250, 2006.
16. Make BJ, Hill NS, Goldberg AI, et al: Mechanical ventilation beyond the intensive care unit: report of a consensus conference of the American College of Chest Physicians. Chest 113(Suppl):289S, 1998.
17. MacIntyre NR, Epstein SK, Carson S, et al: Management of patients requiring prolonged mechanical ventilation: report of a NAMDRC consensus conference. Chest 128:3937–3954, 2005.
18. Elefteriades JA, Quin JA, Hogan JF, et al: Long-term follow-up of pacing of the conditioned diaphragm in quadriplegia. Pacing Clin Electrophysiol 25:897, 2002.
19. DiMarco AF, Onders RP, Ignagni A, et al: Phrenic nerve pacing via intramuscular diaphragm electrodes in tetraplegic subjects. Chest 127:671, 2005.
20. Onders RP, Elmo M, Khansarinia S, et al: Complete worldwide operative experience in laparoscopic diaphragm pacing: results and differences in spinal cord injured patients and amyotrophic lateral sclerosis patients. Surg Endosc 23:1433–1440, 2009.
21. Hoffman E, Brown R, Kunkel L: Dystrophin: the product of the Duchenne muscular dystrophy locus. Cell 51:919, 1987.
22. Cheuk DK, Wong V, Wraige E, et al: Surgery for scoliosis in Duchenne muscular dystrophy, Cochrane Database Syst Rev 24:CD005375, 2007.
23. Velasco MV, Colin AA, Zurakowski D, et al: Posterior spinal fusion for scoliosis in Duchenne muscular dystrophy diminishes the rate of respiratory decline. Spine (Phila Pa 1976) 32:459–465, 2007.
24. Suresh S, Wales P, Harris M, et al: Sleep-related breathing disorder in Duchenne muscular dystrophy: disease spectrum in the paediatric population. J Paediatr Child Health 41:500, 2005.
25. Bushby K, Finkel R, Birnkrant DJ, et al; Care Considerations Working Group: Diagnosis and management of Duchenne muscular dystrophy, part 2: implementation of multidisciplinary care. Lancet Neurol 9:177–189, 2010.
26. Birnkrant DJ, Bushby KM, Amin RS, et al: The respiratory management of patients with Duchenne muscular dystrophy: a DMD care considerations working group specialty article. Pediatr Pulmonol 45:739–748, 2010.
27. Mohr C, Hill N: Long-term follow-up of nocturnal ventilatory assistance in patients with respiratory failure due to Duchenne-type muscular dystrophy. Chest 97:91, 1990.
28. Raphael JC, Chevret S, Chastang C, et al: Randomized trial of preventive nasal ventilation in Duchenne muscular dystrophy: French Multicentre Cooperative Group on Home Mechanical Ventilation Assistance in Duchenne de Boulogne Muscular Dystrophy. Lancet 343:1600–1604, 1994.
29. Kessler W, Wanke T, Winkler G, et al: 2 Years experience with inspiratory muscle training in patients with neuromuscular disorders. Chest 120:765, 2001.
30. Sveen ML, Jeppesen TD, Hauerslev S, et al: Endurance training improves fitness and strength in patients with Becker muscular dystrophy. Brain 131:2824–2831, 2008.
31. Harper P: Myotonic dystrophy: major problems in neurology, vol 21, Philadelphia, 1989, Saunders.
32. Rimmer K, Golar SD, Lee MA, et al: Myotonia of the respiratory muscles in myotonic dystrophy. Am Rev Respir Dis 148:1018–1022, 1993.
33. Pizzuti A, Friedman D, Caskey C: The myotonic dystrophy gene. Arch Neurol 50:1173, 1993.
34. Culebras A: Sleep and neuromuscular disorders. Neurol Clin 23:1209–1223, 2005.
35. Mathieu J, Allard P, Gobeil G, et al: Anesthetic and surgical complications in 219 cases of myotonic dystrophy. Neurology 49:1646–1650, 1997.
36. Gupta N, Saxena K, Kumar PA, et al: Myotonic dystrophy: an anaesthetic dilemma. Indian J Anaesth 53:688–691, 2009.
37. Bohan A, Peter JB: Polymyositis and dermatomyositis (first of two parts). N Engl J Med 292:344–347, 1975.
38. Bohan A, Peter JB: Polymyositis and dermatomyositis (second of two parts). N Engl J Med 292:403–407, 1975.
39. Blumbergs P, Byrne E, Kakulas B: Polymyositis presenting with respiratory failure. J Neurol Sci 65:221, 1984.
40. Connors GR, Christopher-Stine L, Oddis CV, et al: Interstitial lung disease associated with the idiopathic inflammatory myopathies: what progress has been made in the past 35 years? Chest 138:1464–1474, 2010.
41. Arnett F, Hirsch TJ, Bias WB, et al: The Jo-1 antibody system in myositis: relationships to clinical features and HLA. J Rheumatol 8:925, 1981.

42. Targoff IN: Myositis specific autoantibodies. Curr Rheumatol Rep 8:196–203, 2006.
43. Betteridge Z, Gunawardena H, North J, et al: Anti-synthetase syndrome: a new autoantibody to phenylalanyl transfer RNA synthetase (anti-Zo) associated with polymyositis and interstitial pneumonia. Rheumatology (Oxford) 46:1005–1008, 2007.
44. Lacomis D, Giuliani MJ, Van Cott A, et al: Acute myopathy of intensive care: clinical, electromyographic, and pathological aspects. Ann Neurol 40:645–654, 1996.
45. Latronico N, Shehu I, Seghelini E: Neuromuscular sequelae of critical illness. Curr Opin Crit Care 11:381–390, 2005.
46. Vincent A: Unravelling the pathogenesis of myasthenia gravis. Nat Rev Immunol 2:797–804, 2002.
47. Hoch W, McConville J, Helms S, et al: Auto-antibodies to the receptor tyrosine kinase MuSK in patients with myasthenia gravis without acetylcholine receptor antibodies. Nat Med 7:365, 2001.
48. Phillips LH: The epidemiology of myasthenia gravis. Semin Neurol 24:17–20, 2004.
49. Sanders DB, Howard JF: Disorders of neuromuscular transmission. In Bradley WG, Davoff RB, Fenichel GM, et al, editors: Neurology in Clinical Practice, ed 5, Philadelphia, 2008, Butterworth Heinemann.
50. Gronseth GS, Barohn RJ: Practice parameter: thymectomy for autoimmune myasthenia gravis (an evidence-based review). Neurology 55:5–15, 2000.
51. Norris FH Jr, Denys EH, Mielke CH Jr: Plasmapheresis (plasma exchange) in neurologic disorders. Clin Neuropharmacol 5:93, 1982.
52. Batocchi AP, Evoli A, Di Schino C, et al: Therapeutic apheresis in myasthenia gravis. Ther Apher 4:275, 2000.
53. Gracey DR, Howard FM Jr, Divertie MB: Plasmapheresis in the treatment of ventilator-dependent myasthenia gravis patients: report of four cases. Chest 85:739, 1984.
54. Gajdos P, Chevret S, Clair B, et al: Clinical trial of plasma exchange and high-dose intravenous immunoglobulin in myasthenia gravis. Myasthenia Gravis Clinical Study Group. Ann Neurol 41:789–796, 1997.
55. Qureshi AI, Choudhry MA, Akbar MS, et al: Plasma exchange versus intravenous immunoglobulin treatment in myasthenic crisis. Neurology 52:629–632, 1999.
56. Mier-Jedzejowicz A, Brophy C, Green M: Respiratory muscle function in myasthenia gravis. Am Rev Respir Dis 138:867, 1988.
57. Gracey D, Divertie M, Howard FJ: Mechanical ventilation for respiratory failure in myasthenia gravis: two year experience with 22 patients. Mayo Clin Proc 58:597, 1983.
58. O'Neill JH, Murray NM, Newsom-Davis J: The Lambert-Eaton myasthenic syndrome: a review of 50 cases. Brain 111(Pt 3):577–596, 1988.
59. Lennon VA, Lambert EH: Autoantibodies bind solubilized calcium channel-omega-conotoxin complexes from small cell carcinoma: a diagnostic aid for Lambert-Eaton myasthenic syndrome. Mayo Clin Proc 64:1498, 1989.
60. Mareska M, Gutmann L: Lambert-Eaton myasthenic syndrome. Semin Neurol 24:149–153, 2004.
61. Ropper AH, Kehne S: Guillain-Barré syndrome: management of respiratory failure. Neurology 35:1662, 1985.
62. Harati Y, Bosch EP: Disorders of peripheral nerves. In Bradley WG, Davoff RB, Fenichel GM, et al, editors: Neurology in Clinical Practice, ed 5, Philadelphia, 2008, Butterworth Heinemann.
63. Winer J, Hughes R, Osmond C: A prospective study of acute idiopathic neuropathy, I: clinical features and their prognostic value. J Neurol Neurosurg Psychiatry 51:605, 1988.
64. Ashbury AK, Cornblath DR: Assessment of current diagnostic criteria for Guillain-Barré syndrome. Ann Neurol 27(Suppl):S21–S24, 1990.
65. Lehmann HC, Hartung HP, Hetzel GR, et al: Plasma exchange in neuroimmunological disorders, part 2: treatment of neuromuscular disorders. Arch Neurol 63:1066–1071, 2006.
66. Lawn ND, Fletcher DD, Henderson RD, et al: Anticipating mechanical ventilation in Guillain-Barré syndrome. Arch Neurol 58:893–898, 2001.
67. Marsh M, Gillespie D, Baumgartner A: Timing of tracheostomy in critically ill patients. Chest 96:190, 1989.
68. Chevrolet JC, Deleamont P: Repeated vital capacity measurements as predictive parameters for mechanical ventilation need and weaning success in Guillain-Barré syndrome. Am Rev Respir Dis 144:814, 1991.
69. Borel CO, Teitelbaum J, Hanley D: Ventilatory drive and CO2-response in ventilatory failure due to myasthenia gravis and Guillain-Barré. Crit Care Med 21:1717, 1993.
70. Canbaz S, Turgut N, Halici U, et al: Electrophysiological evaluation of phrenic nerve injury during cardiac surgery—a prospective, controlled, clinical study. BMC Surg 4:2, 2004.
71. Celik S, Celik M, Aydemir B, et al: Long-term results of diaphragmatic plication in adults with unilateral diaphragm paralysis. J Cardiothorac Surg 15:111, 2010.
72. Groth SS, Andrade RS: Diaphragm plication for eventration or paralysis: a review of the literature. Ann Thorac Surg 89:S2146–S2150, 2010.
73. Groth SS, Rueth NM, Kast T, et al: Laparoscopic diaphragmatic plication for diaphragmatic paralysis and eventration: an objective evaluation of short-term and midterm results. J Thorac Cardiovasc Surg 139:1452–1456, 2010.
74. Murray B: Natural history and prognosis in amyotrophic lateral sclerosis. In Mitsumoto H, Przedborski S, Gordon PH, editors: Amyotrophic lateral sclerosis, New York, 2006, Taylor & Francis Group, pp 227–255.
75. Traynor BJ, Alexander M, Corr B, et al: An outcome study of riluzole in amyotrophic lateral sclerosis: a population based study in Ireland, 1996–2000. J Neurol 250:473, 2003.
76. Murray B, Mitsumoto H: Disorders of upper and lower motor neurons. In Bradley WG, Davoff RB, Fenichel GM, et al: Neurology in Clinical Practice, ed 5, Philadelphia, 2008, Butterworth Heinemann.
77. Aboussouan LS, Khan SU, Arroliga AC, et al: Effect of noninvasive positive-pressure ventilation on pulmonary function, respiratory muscle strength and arterial blood gases in amyotrophic lateral sclerosis. Muscle Nerve 24:403–409, 2001.
78. Moss AH, Casey P: Home ventilation for amyotrophic lateral sclerosis patients: outcomes, costs and patient, family and physician attitudes. Neurology 43:438, 1993.
79. Miller RG, Jackson CE, Kasarskis EJ, et al: Practice parameter update: the care of the patient with amyotrophic lateral sclerosis: drug, nutritional, and respiratory therapies (an evidence-based review). Report of the Quality Standards Subcommittee of the American Academy of Neurology. Neurology 73:1218–1226, 2009.
80. Hardiman O: Management of respiratory symptoms in ALS. J Neurol 258:359–365, 2011.
81. Gala VC, Vovadzis JM, Kim DH, et al: Trauma of the nervous system: spinal cord trauma. In Bradley WG, Davoff RB, Fenichel GM, et al, editors: Neurology in Clinical Practice, ed 5, Philadelphia, 2008, Butterworth Heinemann.
82. North JB, Jennett S: Abnormal breathing patterns associated with acute brain damage. Arch Neurol 31:338–344, 1974.
83. Lee MC, Klassen AC, Resch JA: Respiratory pattern disturbances in ischemic cerebral vascular disease. Stroke 5:612–616, 1974.

84. Frank JI: Abnormal breathing patterns. In: Hanley DC, Einhaupl KM, Bleck TP, et al, editors: Neurocritical care, Heidelberg, 1994, Springer-Verlag.
85. Adams HP Jr, Brott TG, Furlan AJ, et al: Guidelines for thrombolytic therapy for acute stroke: a supplement to the guidelines for the management of patients with acute ischemic stroke: a statement for healthcare professionals from a Special Writing Group of the Stroke Council, American Heart Association. Circulation 94:1167, 1996.
86. Pereira AC, Martin PJ, Warburton EA: Thrombolysis in acute ischaemic stroke. Postgrad Med J 77:166, 2001.
87. Hacke W, Kaste M, Bluhmki E, et al; ECASS Investigators: Thrombolysis with alteplase 3 to 4.5 hours after acute ischemic stroke. N Engl J Med 359:1317–1329, 2008.
88. Bluhmki E, Chamorro A, Davalos A, et al: Stroke treatment with alteplase given 3.0–4.5 h after onset of acute ischaemic stroke (ECASS III): additional outcomes and subgroup analysis of a randomised controlled trial. Lancet Neurol 8:1095–1102, 2009.
89. Adams HP Jr, del Zoppo G, Alberts MJ, et al; American Heart Association/American Stroke Association Stroke Council; American Heart Association/American Stroke Association Clinical Cardiology Council; American Heart Association/American Stroke Association Cardiovascular Radiology and Intervention Council; Atherosclerotic Peripheral Vascular Disease Working Group; Quality of Care Outcomes in Research Interdisciplinary Working Group: Guidelines for the early management of adults with ischemic stroke: a guideline from the American Heart Association/American Stroke Association Stroke Council, Clinical Cardiology Council, Cardiovascular Radiology and Intervention Council, and the Atherosclerotic Peripheral Vascular Disease and Quality of Care Outcomes in Research Interdisciplinary Working Groups. Circulation 115:e478–e534, 2007.
90. Upadhyay SS, Mullaji AB, Luk KD, et al: Evaluation of deformities and pulmonary function in adolescent idiopathic thoracic scoliosis. Eur Spine J 4:274, 1995.
91. Kearon C, Viviani GR, Kirkley A, et al: Factors determining pulmonary function in adolescent idiopathic thoracic scoliosis. Am Rev Respir Dis 148:288, 1993.
92. Wong CA, Cole AA, Watson L, et al: Pulmonary function before and after anterior spinal surgery in adult idiopathic scoliosis. Thorax 51:534, 1996.
93. Pehrsson K, Danielsson A, Nachemson A: Pulmonary function in adolescent idiopathic scoliosis: a 25 year follow up after surgery or start of brace treatment. Thorax 56:388–393, 2001.
94. Gonzalez C, Ferris G, Diaz J, et al: Kyphoscoliotic ventilatory insufficiency: effects of long-term intermittent positive-pressure ventilation. Chest 124:857–862, 2003.
95. Fuschillo S, De Felice A, Gaudiosi C, et al: Nocturnal mechanical ventilation improves exercise capacity in kyphoscoliotic patients with respiratory impairment. Monaldi Arch Chest Dis 59:281–286, 2003.
96. Jackson M, Kinnear W, King M, et al: The effects of five years of nocturnal cuirass-assisted ventilation in chest wall disease. Eur Respir J 6:630, 1993.
97. Hoeppner V, Cockcroft DW, Dosman JA, et al: Nighttime ventilation improves respiratory failure in secondary kyphoscoliosis. Am Rev Respir Dis 129:240, 1984.
98. Ciraulo D, Elliott D, Mitchell KA, et al: Flail chest as a marker for significant injuries. J Am Coll Surg 178:466, 1994.
99. Kanathur N, Lee-Chiong T: Pulmonary manifestations of ankylosing spondylitis. Clin Chest Med 31:547–554, 2010.

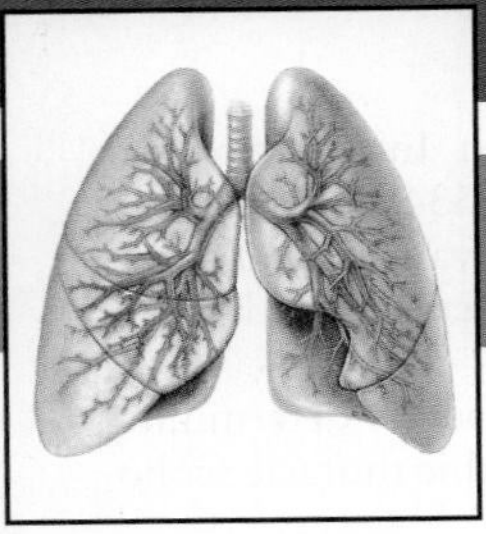

Chapter 30

Disorders of Sleep

EUHAN JOHN LEE AND PATRICK J. STROLLO, JR.

CHAPTER OBJECTIVES

After reading this chapter you will be able to:

- Define obstructive sleep apnea (OSA).
- Identify why airway closure occurs only during sleep.
- State the long-term consequences of uncontrolled OSA.
- State how a diagnosis of OSA is made.
- Identify what groups of patients are at particular risk of OSA.
- State what treatments are available for patients with OSA.
- Describe how continuous positive airway pressure (CPAP) works.
- Identify problems associated with CPAP.
- Determine when bilevel pressure is useful in the treatment of OSA.
- Define "auto-titrating" CPAP.
- Identify the surgical alternatives for patients with severe OSA.

CHAPTER OUTLINE

KEY TERMS

bilevel positive airway pressure (bilevel PAP)
central sleep apnea (CSA)
continuous positive airway pressure (CPAP)
obesity hypoventilation
obstructive sleep apnea (OSA)
sleep-disordered breathing
uvulopalatopharyngoplasty (UPPP)

Obstructive sleep apnea (OSA) syndrome is a common clinical problem that is underdiagnosed.[1] It is estimated that approximately 2% to 4% of adults have OSA.[2] This prevalence is equivalent to asthma and diabetes in the general population. The spectrum of disease ranges from sleep disruption related to increased airway resistance to profound daytime sleepiness in conjunction with severe oxyhemoglobin desaturation, pulmonary hypertension, and right heart failure. The common feature in all variants of OSA syndrome is sleep disruption secondary to increased ventilatory effort that results in daytime hypersomnolence (Figure 30-1).[3] Treatment decreases morbidity and mortality.

Sleep apnea is defined as repeated episodes of complete cessation of airflow for 10 seconds or longer. The events can be obstructive (caused by upper airway closure) or central (caused by lack of ventilatory effort). Primary central nervous system lesions, stroke, congestive heart

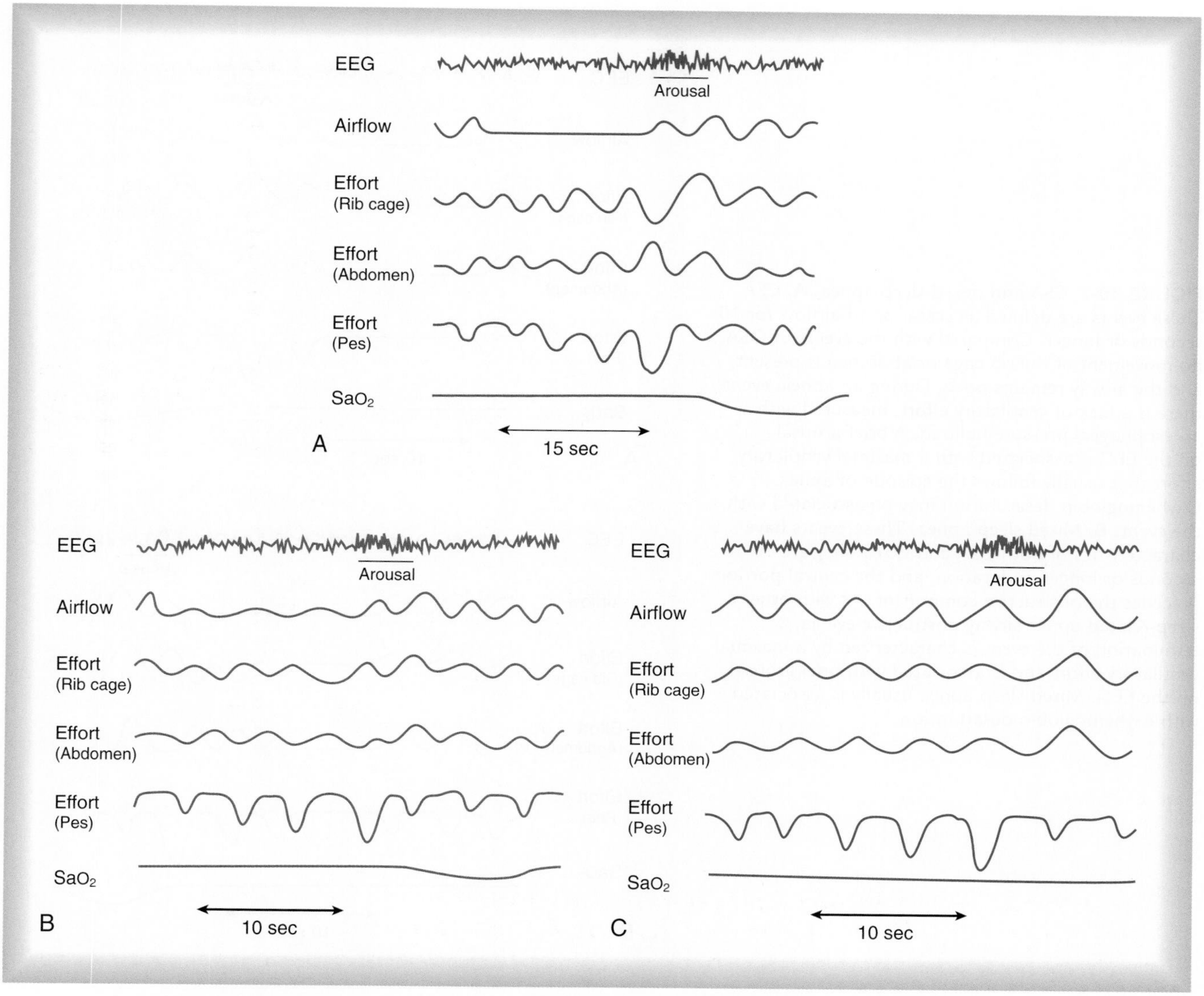

FIGURE 30-1 Spectrum of sleep-related upper airway obstruction. **A,** OSA. These events are defined as cessation of airflow for 10 seconds or longer. Paradoxical movement of the rib cage and abdomen in response to the closed airway occurs. Ventilatory effort, measured with an esophageal pressure balloon, usually increases until a threshold is reached that triggers a brief arousal seen on the EEG, and airway opening occurs. Oxyhemoglobin desaturation usually accompanies the event. **B,** Obstructive hypopnea. These events have been defined as a reduction of airflow by 30% to 50% for 10 seconds or longer. Paradoxical movement of the rib cage and abdomen in response to the narrowed airway occurs. Ventilatory effort, measured with an esophageal pressure balloon, usually increases until a threshold is reached that triggers a brief arousal seen on the EEG, and complete airway opening occurs. Oxyhemoglobin desaturation usually accompanies the event and usually is of a lesser degree than occurs with apnea. **C,** Respiratory effort-related arousals. These events are characterized by no discernible reduction in airflow. Subtle paradoxical movement of the rib cage and abdomen in response to narrowing of the airway may occur. As in apnea and hypopnea, ventilatory effort, measured with an esophageal pressure balloon, usually increases until a threshold is reached that triggers a brief arousal seen on the EEG, and complete airway opening occurs. By definition, no oxyhemoglobin desaturation is associated with the event.

failure, and high-altitude hypoxemia can diminish respiratory control and cause central apnea events.[3] **Central sleep apnea (CSA)** is not as common as OSA. Only 10% to 15% of patients with sleep-disordered breathing are classified as having CSA.[4] Mixed sleep apnea has an initial central component followed by an obstructive component (Figure 30-2).

Hypopnea is a significant decrease in breathing without complete cessation of airflow.[5] Hypopnea is defined as a 30% decrease in airflow in conjunction with 4% oxygen (O_2)

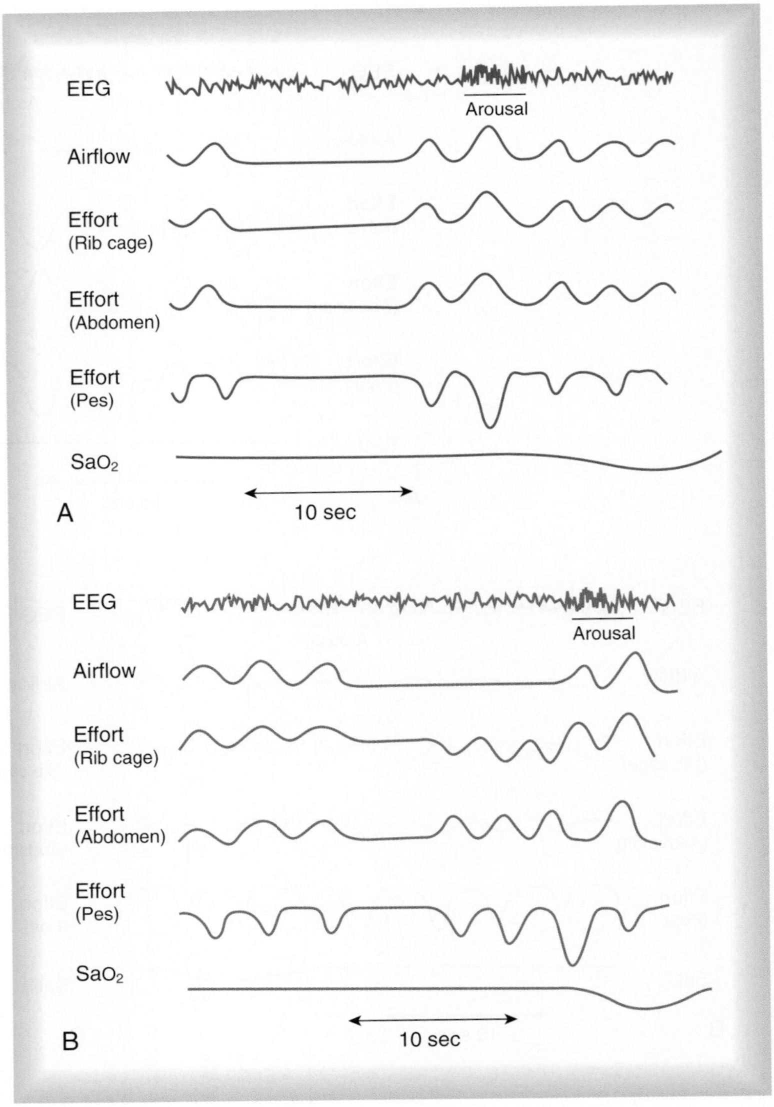

FIGURE 30-2 CSA and mixed sleep apnea. **A,** CSA. These events are defined as cessation of airflow for 10 seconds or longer. Compared with the events of OSA, no movement of the rib cage or abdomen is present, and the airway remains open. During an apneic event, there is a lack of ventilatory effort, measured with an esophageal pressure balloon. A brief arousal on the EEG is associated with a maximal ventilatory effort that usually follows the episode of apnea. Oxyhemoglobin desaturation may be associated with the event. **B,** Mixed sleep apnea. These events have characteristics of both CSA and OSA. They are 10 seconds or longer in duration, and the central portion precedes the obstructive component. As with other sleep-related upper airway obstructive events, termination of the event is characterized by a maximal ventilatory effort and is associated with brief arousal on the EEG. Mixed sleep apnea usually is associated with oxyhemoglobin desaturation.

desaturation.[6] Most investigators agree that physiologically significant hypopnea is associated with a decrease in O_2 saturation or arousal from sleep.[7]

Respiratory therapists (RTs) are likely to encounter both OSA and CSA when treating patients. Because OSA is the most commonly encountered type of sleep apnea and is underdiagnosed by health professionals, the focus of this chapter is on the pathophysiology and management of the variants of OSA.

PATHOPHYSIOLOGY

Obstructive Sleep Apnea

The primary cause of OSA is a small or unstable pharyngeal airway. This condition can be caused by soft tissue factors, such as upper body obesity or tonsillar hypertrophy (rare in adults), and skeletal factors, such as a small or recessed chin.[8] During the waking state, pharyngeal patency is maintained by increased activity of the upper airway dilator muscles. Sleep onset is associated with a decrease in the activity of these muscles. The result is airway narrowing or closure of airways that are at risk.[9] In an unstable upper airway, narrowing and closure during sleep may involve multiple sites.[10]

Partial or complete closure of the upper airway during sleep has many serious neurobehavioral, metabolic, and cardiopulmonary consequences (Box 30-1). Compared with the general population, patients with untreated OSA have an increased risk of systemic and pulmonary hypertension, stroke, nocturnal arrhythmia, heart failure, and myocardial infarction.[11,12] The repetitive cycle of upper airway closure and opening during sleep is believed to have effects on the autonomic nervous system, specifically, an increase in sympathetic tone.[13] These effects are caused in part by episodes of hypoxemia and hypercapnia that are due to airway closure and hypoventilation that can occur throughout the night in patients with OSA. The arousals and microarousals during sleep also play an important role in the increase in sympathetic tone.[13] Over time, increased sympathetic tone may result in systemic and modest pulmonary hypertension.[14] Patients with OSA may have right ventricular hypertrophy and right heart failure if they are not treated.[15,16]

Obesity, especially of the upper body, has been found to correlate positively with the presence of OSA. In most instances, patients with OSA are obese with a large amount of peripharyngeal tissue and adipose tissue in the neck.[17] A body mass index greater than 28 (>120% of ideal body weight normalized for height) should alert the practitioner to the possibility of OSA, particularly if the patient has excessive daytime sleepiness (EDS).[2]

Patients who are of normal body weight can be predisposed to OSA if they have an abnormal craniofacial configuration. Men often grow a beard to disguise such a craniofacial abnormality. If the chin is recessed (retrognathic) or small (micrognathic), the upper airway space may be narrow, and the risk of airway closure during sleep increases.[2,8,14] Patients with a deviated nasal septum or trauma to the nasal passages may be predisposed to upper airway closure during sleep as a result of the increased resistive load to the upper airway. An isolated nasal abnormality is an unusual cause of OSA.

OSA may have a genetic predisposition.[18] There have been reports of families in which obesity alone does not explain the increased prevalence of OSA.[19] It has been postulated that craniofacial abnormalities and defects in ventilatory control explain the increased frequency of OSA in these families.

Central Sleep Apnea

Although a detailed discussion of the pathophysiology of CSA is beyond the scope of this chapter, several concepts are important to RTs. In contrast to OSA, which represents a spectrum of the same disease, CSA is a heterogeneous group of disorders. Patients have a ventilatory pattern known as *periodic breathing*, in which there is a waxing and waning of respiratory drive, which is reflected clinically as an increase and then a decrease in respiratory rate and tidal volume (V_T). Cheyne-Stokes respiration, which often occurs in patients with congestive heart failure or stroke, is a severe type of periodic breathing characterized by a crescendo-decrescendo pattern of hyperpnea alternating with apnea. After apnea occurs, there may be an increase in central ventilatory drive and an increase in V_T.[3]

Overlap Syndrome

Some patients with chronic obstructive pulmonary disease (COPD) have coexisting OSA. This combination is referred to as *overlap syndrome*.[20] Patients are usually obese and have a history of smoking. They have moderate to severe nocturnal oxyhemoglobin desaturation secondary to both OSA and COPD. The worst desaturation values occur during rapid eye movement (REM) sleep and are related to the loss of accessory muscle use encountered in this physiologic state. Patients with overlap syndrome tend to have a worse prognosis and more severe blood gas abnormalities than patients with the same degree of OSA but without COPD.[20] They may arrive in the intensive care unit with a "COPD exacerbation" and decompensated right heart failure. Undiagnosed OSA complicates the course at night with arousals, increased dyspnea, and O_2 desaturation values resistant to supplemental O_2.[20]

CLINICAL FEATURES

Patients with sleep apnea are more commonly men (three times greater frequency than among women), are older than 40 years, and have hypertension (Box 30-2). Most patients with sleep apnea report habitual snoring that has become progressively worse.[2,21] Sensations of nocturnal choking, gasping, or resuscitative snorting are frequently reported. If a bed partner observes periods of apnea, the diagnosis of OSA is highly likely.

The presence of EDS may be underestimated because OSA manifests in a subacute manner. As a result, patients with OSA may report symptoms of fatigue alone. These

Box 30-1 Adverse Consequences of Obstructive Sleep Apnea

CARDIOPULMONARY
- Nocturnal arrhythmia
- Diurnal hypertension
- Pulmonary hypertension
- Right or left ventricular failure
- Myocardial infarction
- Stroke

NEUROBEHAVIORAL
- Excessive daytime sleepiness
- Diminished quality of life
- Adverse personality change
- Motor vehicle accidents

METABOLIC
- Insulin resistance
- Altered lipid metabolism

Box 30-2 Common Clinical Features of Obstructive Sleep Apnea

- Male
- Age >40 years
- Upper body obesity (neck >16.5 in)
- Habitual snoring
- Fatigue or daytime sleepiness
- Diurnal hypertension

patients also frequently report nocturnal reflux, nocturia, chronic nasal obstruction, morning headaches, and symptoms of depression.

Patients with OSA have arousals from sleep and sleep fragmentation, which can lead to fatigue, EDS, and irritability.[22] Patients who have an increased frequency of awakenings and microarousals have more daytime sleepiness and greater difficulty with daytime functioning than the general population.[23] Patients with OSA may have neuropsychologic deficits and impairment in vigilance.[24] Compared with the general population, untreated OSA patients are at increased risk of motor vehicle accidents because of EDS.[25-27]

The physical examination of most patients reveals evidence of obesity, particularly in the upper body. Upper body obesity can be quantitated with neck size. A neck circumference of 42 cm (16.5 in) increases the likelihood of the diagnosis of sleep apnea.[14] Examination of the oropharynx frequently reveals a long soft palate. Although tonsillar hypertrophy is common in children with sleep apnea, it is seldom found in adults. Large palatine tonsils may increase the risk of airway closure during sleep. A retrognathic or micrognathic mandible can narrow the pharyngeal airway, placing a patient of normal weight at risk of airway closure during sleep.[8]

The cardiovascular examination may reveal evidence of pulmonary hypertension or right heart failure (lower extremity edema).[28,29] These findings are determined primarily by the hypoxic burden experienced by the patient. Pulmonary hypertension or right heart failure is more commonly encountered in patients with concomitant daytime hypoxemia. Patients with OSA and COPD or severe obesity (body mass index greater than 40) appear to be at particular risk of this complication.[30] Recurrent moderate to severe oxyhemoglobin desaturation and resaturation secondary to OSA can be associated with an increased incidence of cardiac arrhythmia.[31,32] Repeated nocturnal desaturation can be a cause of secondary polycythemia.[14,33]

RULE OF THUMB

Uncontrolled OSA can cause daytime hypoxemia. The diagnosis of OSA should be considered when the degree of hypoxemia is out of proportion to the defect on pulmonary spirometry. When the arterial partial pressure of O_2 is less than 60 mm Hg and the FEV_1 is greater than 30% of predicted, COPD alone is inadequate to explain the hypoxemia, and coexisting OSA should be considered. OSA in this setting is frequently associated with pulmonary hypertension and evidence of right heart failure on physical examination. Hypoxemia, pulmonary hypertension, and right heart failure can be substantially improved with management of OSA. If the patient adheres to therapy, the need for supplemental O_2 may be reduced or eliminated.

OSA and poor sleep quality are also associated with metabolic syndrome independent of obesity.[34,35] Metabolic syndrome includes three of the following: waist circumference 102 cm or greater in men or 88 cm or greater in women, hypertension, impaired glucose tolerance, insulin resistance, and elevated triglycerides.[36,37] These interactions can also increase the patient's cardiac risks and increased morbidity and mortality from cardiovascular disease.[12,38]

In the acute care setting, patients frequently present with previously undiagnosed OSA and can pose a particular challenge for diagnosis and management.[39-41] A high clinical suspicion for OSA in the hospital setting is necessary because untreated or unrecognized OSA can complicate recovery from acute illness, trauma, heart failure, and recent surgery.[42-45] Patients with known OSA are frequently not placed on continuous positive airway pressure (CPAP) while in the hospital or may require a temporary adjustment in pressure settings.[46] Patients who are unstable for testing in a sleep laboratory can undergo portable bedside testing or empiric treatment with positive pressure if the diagnosis cannot be confirmed.[47] Outpatient follow-up with confirmatory sleep evaluation is important for long-term treatment and compliance.

LABORATORY TESTING

When sleep apnea is suspected, an overnight polysomnogram (PSG) should be obtained for confirmation of the clinical diagnosis. A full-night PSG in the sleep laboratory monitored by a sleep technologist is considered the standard method of diagnosing OSA.

RTs play a vital role in the diagnosis and treatment of OSA. As part of the multidisciplinary team, RTs prepare patients for the overnight PSG and obtain key information relating to their sleep history. During the study, RTs assess for **sleep-disordered breathing** and apply and titrate positive pressure. They are also involved with education, which is important in assisting with the patient's understanding and compliance with positive pressure therapy.

In a laboratory sleep study, several physiologic signals are recorded to determine whether airway closure occurs during sleep and to what extent the events disturb sleep continuity and cardiopulmonary function. An electroencephalogram (EEG), electrooculogram (EOG), and chin electromyogram (EMG) are obtained for assessment of sleep stage and documentation of sleep disruption secondary to sleep-related breathing disturbance. Airflow (measured at the nose and mouth), ventilatory effort (using inductive plethysmography or piezoelectric belts), cardiac rhythm (with a modified lead II electrocardiogram [ECG]), and O_2 saturation (measured with pulse oximetry) are included in the standard testing montage.

In obstructive apnea or hypopnea, airflow is absent or decreased in the presence of continued ventilatory effort. Asynchronous (paradoxical) movement of the abdomen and rib cage can be observed. O_2 desaturation may or may not occur. The degree of the O_2 desaturation depends on the length of the apneic event or the patient's baseline saturation (see Figure 30-1). Respiratory effort-related arousals are characterized by increased respiratory effort, leading to arousal from sleep that does not meet the criteria of an apneic or a hypopneic event (see Figure 30-1).[48,49]

Measuring devices that are adequate for assessing hypopnea also are adequate for assessing apnea; however, devices used for measuring apnea cannot always detect hypopnea. The diagnosis of hypopnea may be affected by the measurement technique used. In 1999, an American Academy of Sleep Medicine (AASM) task force conducted an evidence-based review of measurement techniques for detection of hypopnea.[50] The scoring system was as follows: *A,* good to excellent agreement with a reference standard (face mask pneumotachygraph); *B,* limited data, but good theoretical framework and clinical experience suggest the method is valid; *C,* no data, weak theoretical framework or clinical experience; and *D,* research or clinical experience suggests the method is invalid.

The measuring techniques were scored as follows: nasal pressure, B; respiratory inductance plethysmography (RIP) with sum of chest and abdominal signals, B; dual-channel RIP, C; single-channel RIP, C; piezoelectricity sensors, strain gauges, and thoracic impedance, D; breathing measurement signal with a desaturation or arousal, B; expired carbon dioxide (CO_2), D; and thermal sensors, D. A face mask pneumotachygraph allows the greatest precision in measuring airflow, but it is poorly tolerated. Nasal pressure is a reliable way to detect hypopnea and is well tolerated by patients undergoing a diagnostic PSG.[5,50]

After the sleep study is completed, the sleep technologist scores it. The number of apneas and of hypopneas per hour of sleep are reported as an apnea-hypopnea index (AHI) or respiratory disturbance index (RDI). The AASM has operationally defined the severity of OSA as follows: mild, AHI 5 to 15; moderate, AHI 15 to 30; severe, AHI greater than 30. AHI less than 5 is considered within the normal range for adults. The number of arousals per hour (arousal index), percentage of each sleep stage, frequency of O_2 desaturation, mean O_2 saturation, and nadir of O_2 saturation also are reported (Box 30-3).

RULE OF THUMB

Intermittent checks of O_2 saturation cannot reliably exclude sleep-related desaturation secondary to OSA. Placing the oximetry probe on the patient frequently awakens the patient. In addition, isolated readings may not allow sampling of all sleep stages, especially REM sleep, during which sleep-disordered breathing and nocturnal desaturation tend to be prominent. Continuous overnight oximetry is a better assessment of the degree of oxyhemoglobin desaturation with sleep.

Box 30-3 Key Features of Sleep Studies to Be Analyzed and Reported for Obstructive Sleep Apnea

- AHI
- Arousal index
- Sleep stage distribution
- Frequency of oxyhemoglobin desaturations
- Mean oxyhemoglobin saturation
- Nadir of oxyhemoglobin saturation

Box 30-4 Goals of Treatment for Obstructive Sleep Apnea

- Eliminate apnea, hypopnea, and snoring
- Normalize O_2 saturation and ventilation
- Improve sleep architecture and continuity

Abbreviated (portable) cardiopulmonary testing has been used to confirm a diagnosis of OSA. These studies do not record the electrophysiologic signals (EEG, EOG, and EMG) required to stage and score sleep. The portable studies vary in the type and number of cardiopulmonary values recorded. Controversy exists whether portable systems are sufficient to diagnose OSA. Many variables, such as airflow, ventilatory effort, sleep stage, and O_2 saturation values, may be less precise or may not be measured at all with these devices. Currently, portable monitoring for the diagnosis of OSA is acceptable in patients with high pretest probability but without significant comorbidities that may affect the accuracy of testing.[51] Excerpts of American Association for Respiratory Care (AARC) Clinical Practice Guidelines for a PSG are provided in Clinical Practice Guideline 30-1.

TREATMENT

Management of OSA should be individualized but generally can be classified into three options: behavioral, medical, and surgical interventions.[52] Behavioral therapy should be pursued in the care of all patients. Medical therapy and surgical therapy must be tailored to the individual patient. The likelihood of acceptance of and adherence to the prescribed therapeutic intervention must be considered. The goals of treatment are to normalize O_2 saturation and ventilation; eliminate apnea, hypopnea, and snoring; and improve sleep architecture and continuity (Box 30-4).

Behavioral Interventions and Risk Counseling

Patients need to be informed of the risks of uncontrolled sleep apnea. Several behavioral interventions can be beneficial, including weight loss in obese patients; avoidance of alcohol, sedatives, and hypnotics; and avoidance of sleep

30-1 Polysomnography

AARC Clinical Practice Guideline (Excerpts)*

INDICATIONS

Polysomnography may be indicated in patients with:

- COPD whose awake PaO_2 is >55 mm Hg but whose illness is complicated by pulmonary hypertension, right heart failure, polycythemia, or excessive daytime sleepiness
- Restrictive ventilatory impairment secondary to chest wall and neuromuscular disturbances whose illness is complicated by chronic hypoventilation, polycythemia, pulmonary hypertension, disturbed sleep, morning headaches, or daytime somnolence or fatigue
- Disturbances in respiratory control whose awake $PaCO_2$ is >45 mm Hg or whose illness is complicated by pulmonary hypertension, polycythemia, disturbed sleep, morning headaches, or daytime somnolence or fatigue
- Nocturnal cyclic bradyarrhythmia or tachyarrhythmia, nocturnal abnormalities of atrioventricular conduction, or ventricular ectopy that seems to increase in frequency during sleep
- Excessive daytime sleepiness or insomnia
- Snoring associated with observed apneas or excessive daytime sleepiness or both
- Other symptoms of sleep-disordered breathing as described in *The International Classification of Sleep Disorders, Diagnostic and Coding Manual*

CONTRAINDICATIONS

There are no absolute contraindications to polysomnography when indications are clearly established. However, risk-benefit ratios should be assessed if transferring medically unstable inpatients.

PRECAUTIONS AND COMPLICATIONS

- Skin irritation may occur as a result of the adhesive used to attach electrodes to the patient.
- At the conclusion of the study, adhesive remover is used to dissolve adhesive on the patient's skin. Adhesive removers (e.g., acetone) should be used only in well-ventilated areas.
- The integrity of the electrical isolation of polysomnographic equipment must be certified by engineering or biomedical personnel qualified to make such assessment.
- The adhesive used to attach EEG electrodes should not be used to attach electrodes near the patient's eyes and should always be used in well-ventilated areas.
- Because of the high flammability of adhesives and acetone, these substances should be used with caution, especially in patients who require supplemental O_2.
- Adhesives should be used with caution in patients with reactive airways disease and in small infants.
- Patients with parasomnias or seizures may be at risk of injury related to movements during sleep.
- Institution-specific policies and guidelines describing personnel responsibilities and appropriate responses should be developed.

ASSESSMENT OF NEED

Polysomnography is indicated for patients suspected to have sleep-related respiratory disturbances described in *The International Classification of Sleep Disorders, Diagnostic and Coding Manual*.

ASSESSMENT OF TEST QUALITY

- Polysomnography should either confirm or eliminate a sleep-related diagnosis.
- Documentation of findings, suggested therapeutic intervention, and other clinical decisions resulting from polysomnography should be noted in the patient's chart.
- Each laboratory should implement a quality assurance program that addresses equipment calibration and maintenance, patient preparation and monitoring, scoring methodology, and intertechnician scoring variances.

MONITORING

- Patient variables to be monitored include EEG, EOG, EMG, ECG, respiratory effort, nasal or oral airflow, SpO_2, body position, and limb movement; intervention should occur if the physiologic signals are lost.
- Infrared or low-light video cameras and recording equipment should permit visualization of the patient by the technician throughout the procedure.
- The technician should intervene if an acute change in physiologic status occurs and communicate that change to appropriate medical personnel.

For complete guidelines, see AARC-APT (American Association for Respiratory Care-Association of Polysomnography Technologists) clinical practice guideline. Polysomnography. Respir Care 40:1336–1343, 1995.

deprivation. Although weight loss clearly influences the severity of sleep apnea, it is a difficult behavioral strategy to implement. Involvement of the patient with a dietitian or nutritionist can be helpful. Alcohol decreases the arousal threshold and as a result can increase the duration of apnea. Alcohol also reduces upper airway muscle tone, causing the airway to be more compliant and more prone to complete or partial closure.[53] For these reasons, alcohol should be avoided by patients believed to have sleep apnea. Sedatives and hypnotics can decrease the stability of the upper airway and suppress certain stages of sleep.[54]

Positional Therapy

When a sleep study indicates that apnea and snoring occur only in the supine position, instruction on sleeping in the lateral position or head of bed elevation can be beneficial.[55,56] Use of the "tennis ball" technique, in which a ball is sewn onto the back of the patient's sleeping garment, or other positional devices that discourage the patient from rolling into the supine position can be effective in treating positional OSA.[57] However, the long-term effects of positional therapy are unknown. Positional therapy is generally recommended for milder cases of positional OSA.

Medical Interventions

Positive Pressure Therapy

Continuous Positive Airway Pressure Therapy. Continuous positive airway pressure (CPAP) therapy was introduced for management of OSA in 1981.[58] CPAP has become the first-line medical therapy for OSA. Numerous studies have documented the effectiveness of CPAP in decreasing the morbidity and mortality associated with OSA.[9,11,59,60] For most patients, obstruction of the upper airway is abolished by CPAP pressures between 7.5 cm H_2O and 12.5 cm H_2O.[61] The level of CPAP required for optimal management of OSA is best determined with a titration performed in the sleep laboratory.[60] Attempts to use an algorithm or a prediction equation as a replacement for in-laboratory titration have not been uniformly successful.[62]

CPAP therapy has been shown to decrease daytime sleepiness and improve neurocognitive testing, vigilance scores, insulin sensitivity, and lipid profiles. CPAP decreases the incidence of pulmonary hypertension and right heart failure and decreases the number of ventilation-related arousals and nocturnal cardiac events. Reductions in daytime hypoxemia and hypercapnia also have been attributed to CPAP therapy.[61,63-67]

RULE OF THUMB

Retrognathia can be the cause of OSA in young patients who are at or close to ideal body weight. CPAP therapy is highly effective for these patients, but upper airway reconstruction (phases I and II surgery) can be curative.

MINI CLINI

Nocturnal Angina in an Obese Middle-Aged Man

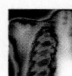

HISTORY: A 45-year-old, morbidly obese nonsmoker is admitted to the coronary care unit after awakening at 4 AM with chest pain typical of angina pectoris. The pain has resolved by the time he reaches the emergency department. The patient is unsure of the duration of the pain before he called for his wife, who sleeps in a separate bedroom because of his very loud habitual snoring. The patient reports exertional shortness of breath but no chest pain before this event. He states that he frequently gets "indigestion" that sometimes is worse at night, but that this pain was different.

MEDICATIONS
- Captopril, 25 mg by mouth twice a day
- Furosemide (Lasix), 20 mg by mouth every day
- Cimetidine (Tagamet), 300 mg by mouth at bedtime

MEDICAL HISTORY
- Hypertension and gastroesophageal reflux
- No significant cardiac disease
- Cardiac catheterization 1 year ago showed normal left ventricular function and minimal coronary artery occlusion

PHYSICAL EXAMINATION
- *Vital signs:* Blood pressure 160/98 mm Hg, heart rate 100 beats/min, temperature 98.6° F (37° C), respiration 18 breaths/min
- *General:* Mildly diaphoretic obese white man
- *Neck:* 52 cm (20.5 in) in circumference
- *Lungs:* Clear breath sounds bilaterally
- *Heart:* Regular rate and rhythm
- *Abdomen:* Obese, soft, normal bowel sounds
- *Extremities:* 4 mm pretibial pitting edema

LABORATORY DATA
- *Room air arterial blood gases:* pH 7.36, PCO_2 37 mm Hg, PO_2 62 mm Hg, SaO_2 92%
- *Chest radiograph:* Pulmonary congestion, otherwise normal
- *ECG:* Sinus tachycardia without acute changes

PROBLEM: Why did this patient experience angina during sleep?

DISCUSSION: Serial cardiac enzyme values show no myocardial infarction. A stress test result is negative, but a submaximal effort is obtained. The patient's weight precludes an adenosine thallium stress test. A repeat cardiac catheterization shows no change in the minimal coronary artery occlusion reported previously. The pulmonary consultant called to evaluate the patient's shortness of breath recommends a nocturnal PSG to rule out sleep apnea. The sleep study result is positive for severe sleep apnea (AHI 110; lowest SaO_2 70% on the oximeter during REM sleep). A CPAP titration test is performed. The patient is discharged home on CPAP 17.5 cm H_2O via a nasal mask. He returns to the pulmonary clinic 1 month after discharge. He reported no further episodes of nocturnal angina. Reflux and shortness of breath have been relieved. The patient has lost 10 lb (4.5 kg) without dieting. Lower extremity edema is markedly relieved.

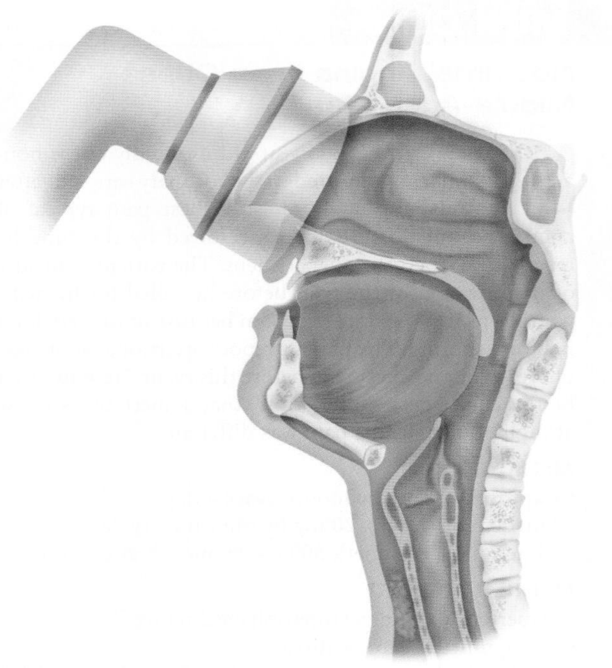

FIGURE 30-3 Nasal CPAP. Positive airway pressure is applied with a nasal mask. The soft palate falls against the base of the tongue so that the upper airway is pneumatically splinted open.

CPAP therapy primarily works by splinting the upper airway open, increasing the intraluminal pressure of the upper airway above a critical transmural pressure of the pharynx and hypopharynx that is associated with airway closure. The soft palate is effectively moved anteriorly up against the tongue, "pressurizing" the upper airway (Figure 30-3).[68] CPAP allows the upper airway to be splinted open whether there is a single site (uncommon) or multiple sites (more common) of airway narrowing or closure. Investigators have found that when nasal CPAP is applied, EMG activity of the upper airway dilator muscles is decreased.[69]

To be successful, CPAP titration should obliterate all apneic episodes and reduce the number of hypopneic episodes for prevention of arterial O_2 desaturation. Paradoxical thoracoabdominal movement and snoring should be eliminated.[70] For improvement of sleep continuity, respiration-related EEG arousals and microarousals must be abolished. There is no evidence to support the misconception that a higher level of CPAP always is necessary in patients with severe sleep apnea. There is variability in the CPAP requirement to treat OSA effectively. Some patients with relatively mild elevation of the AHI need higher levels of CPAP than patients with a substantially higher AHI.[71]

Patients who report EDS without an increase in AHI may have repetitive 2- to 3-second transient EEG arousals during episodes of snoring. These short arousals occur during episodes of increased upper airway resistance, and although not associated with any significant arterial O_2 desaturation, they may cause EDS and fatigue.[72,73] This pattern is known as *upper airway resistance syndrome,* generally occurs in younger patients, and is characterized by respiratory effort–related arousals (see Figure 30-1). With the emergence of upper airway resistance syndrome as a clinical entity, some researchers have suggested that CPAP titrations may be suboptimal without measurement of esophageal pressure.[71,74,75] Many sleep laboratories do not measure esophageal pressure. In addition, many patients refuse this type of monitoring because of perceived or real discomfort.

The contour of the inspiratory flow signal, when measured by a pressure transducer, correlates with ventilatory effort as reflected by esophageal pressure.[48] When esophageal pressure is not used, nasal pressure can be useful in facilitating CPAP titrations.[75] Condos and colleagues[48] hypothesized that during CPAP titration, there is a period during the transition to deeper stages of sleep when there is flow limitation and increased intrathoracic pressure without EEG arousals. These investigators suggested that if this condition is not corrected, patients may have incomplete and suboptimal titrations. The clinical significance of flow limitation without EEG arousals is uncertain at the present time.

Despite numerous studies documenting the efficacy of CPAP in the treatment of patients in the sleep laboratory, clinicians have encountered difficulty with adherence of patients to CPAP therapy. Approximately 80% of patients accept CPAP, although long-term objective compliance is frequently suboptimal. *Objective compliance*—defined as use of the machine for more than 4 hours per night for more than 70% of observed nights—has been measured to be 46%.[76,77] Severity of the AHI does not always correlate with compliance, and the benefit perceived by the patient is a better predictor. Data reported by McArdle and associates[78] indicate that patients who are subjectively sleepy and have an AHI 30 or greater are likely to accept and comply with CPAP therapy. Clinic follow-up with objective compliance monitoring is essential. Compliance 1 month after the initiation of therapy is reported to be a good predictor of CPAP use at 3 months.

It is unclear whether higher levels of CPAP cause a decrease in compliance. Some patients report breathing against a continuous pressure to be uncomfortable. Discomfort with the interface and the device may also reduce acceptance and compliance.[79-81] Since the introduction of CPAP, various interfaces have been designed to improve comfort and have a favorable impact on compliance. Nasal pillows or prongs, nasal masks with comfort flaps or bubbles, oronasal masks, and full-face masks are available.[82-86] No studies have been conducted for direct comparison of efficacy, subjective patient comfort, or objective patient compliance with these interfaces.[82] In clinical practice, some patients tolerate one interface better than another. Technician bias may affect the choice of an interface, and this may have a positive or negative impact.

MINI CLINI

Young Man Hospitalized for Observation after a Single-Vehicle Accident in the Midafternoon

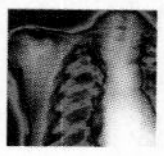

HISTORY: A 27-year-old nonsmoker is admitted to the coronary care unit for monitoring so that the diagnosis of cardiac contusion can be ruled out. The patient has been involved in a single-vehicle automobile accident. The accident occurred at 3:30 PM on a clear day. The patient felt drowsy immediately before the event. He became conscious after hitting the guardrail. The patient's chest hit the steering wheel. The patient reports anterior chest wall pain and denies having angina or presyncope.

MEDICATIONS

- None

MEDICAL HISTORY

- Negative

PHYSICAL EXAMINATION

- *Vital signs:* Blood pressure 140/88 mm Hg, heart rate 100 beats/min, temperature 98.6° F (37° C), respirations 16 breaths/min
- *General:* Well-developed, well-nourished white man
- *Head, eyes, ears, nose throat:* Elongated soft palate, mild crowding of tonsillar pillars, retrognathic chin
- *Neck:* 40 cm (16 in) in circumference
- *Chest:* Contusion on anterior portion of the chest
- *Lungs:* Clear breath sounds bilaterally
- *Heart:* Regular rate and rhythm
- *Abdomen:* Soft with normal bowel sounds
- *Extremities:* No clubbing, cyanosis, or edema
- *Skin:* Multiple small lacerations

LABORATORY DATA

- *Chest radiograph:* No cardiomegaly, mass, infiltrate, or effusion
- *ECG:* Sinus tachycardia
- *Creatine kinase:* 350 IU/L (no MB fraction)

PROBLEM: What caused the patient to fall asleep at the wheel?

DISCUSSION: The patient is found to have bradycardia during sleep on the night of admission. This sign is associated with snoring and oxyhemoglobin desaturation on O_2 at 2 L/min through a nasal cannula. The cardiology consultant recommends a diagnostic nocturnal PSG to rule out sleep apnea. The study shows severe sleep apnea (AHI 85 with a low SaO_2 of 60%). A CPAP titration study reveals that the patient requires 10 cm H_2O of CPAP via nasal pillows. At follow-up 1 month later, the patient states he no longer experiences the fatigue he had previously. In retrospect, the patient believes that before treatment with CPAP, he was quite sleepy during the day. Despite this improvement, he wants to explore other treatment options. A surgical consultation is obtained.

Bilevel Pressure Therapy. Another form of positive pressure therapy is **bilevel positive airway pressure (bilevel PAP).** Bilevel PAP therapy was developed to take advantage of the fact that some patients may have different pressure requirements between inspiration and expiration.[81] It was hypothesized that because a patient may have a lower expiratory pressure requirement to splint the airway open, patient acceptance and compliance would be favorably affected. Bilevel units operate on household electricity and are similar in size and appearance to conventional CPAP units. There is a difference in cost, however, with bilevel devices generally more expensive than CPAP devices.

Although patient acceptance may be slightly better with bilevel PAP, published data have shown no difference in compliance between conventional CPAP and bilevel PAP in patients who have not previously received CPAP therapy.[87] However, bilevel PAP may be better tolerated by the subgroup of patients who need higher CPAP settings or who are uncomfortable exhaling against a continuous pressure.

In contrast to conventional CPAP, bilevel PAP is titrated by increasing inspiratory positive airway pressure and expiratory positive airway pressure separately in response to apnea, hypopnea, and desaturation. The specific titration algorithm may vary from laboratory to laboratory. Generally, inspiratory positive airway pressure and expiratory positive airway pressure are titrated upward together (as CPAP) until apnea is eliminated. Inspiratory positive airway pressure is then increased independently to eliminate hypopnea, snoring, and arousals.

Autotitrating Devices. A new generation of self-titrating CPAP devices has been developed to address issues of patient compliance, patient comfort, and variability of the CPAP requirement throughout the night.[88-91] These devices are referred to as *auto-CPAP, intelligent CPAP,* or *smart CPAP.* These devices use a computer algorithm for adjusting the level of CPAP in response to dynamic changes in airflow or vibration secondary to snoring or both. Abnormal function manifests as snoring, hypopnea, and apnea. The average overnight pressure required to treat OSA effectively may be decreased, which may have a favorable impact on interface-related leaks. It is unknown whether these devices are capable of eliminating the need for standard CPAP titration in a sleep laboratory. Self-titrating devices may be useful in facilitating therapeutic CPAP titrations by technologists in the sleep laboratory but cannot be used as a surrogate for proper diagnostic testing.[47] Further studies are needed to determine whether self-titrating CPAP devices provide any improvement over conventional CPAP units in the areas of compliance and EDS, in particular, in patients who have not previously received CPAP therapy.

Side Effects and Troubleshooting Strategies. Side effects of positive pressure therapy are related to the interface and to the pressure prescribed. These effects include

MINI CLINI

Middle-Aged Woman With Primary Pulmonary Hypertension

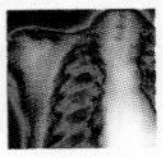

HISTORY: A 59-year-old former smoker is admitted to the hospital for right and left heart catheterization. A previous ECG showed pulmonary hypertension. The patient denies having angina or exertional chest discomfort. She admits to dyspnea on exertion that has been increasing over the past few months and to a chronic nonproductive cough. She denies taking "diet pills."

MEDICATIONS
- Nifedipine, 10 mg by mouth three times a day
- Furosemide (Lasix), 20 mg by mouth daily
- Potassium chloride, 20 mEq by mouth twice a day

MEDICAL HISTORY
- Hypertension and allergic rhinitis
- No cardiac disease

PHYSICAL EXAMINATION
- *Vital signs:* Blood pressure 140/88 mm Hg, heart rate 90 beats/min, temperature 98.6° F (37° C), respirations 12 breaths/min
- *General:* Obese white woman in no acute distress
- *Neck:* 40 cm (16 in) in circumference
- *Lungs:* Clear breath sounds bilaterally
- *Heart:* Regular rate and rhythm, increased second heart sound (P_2)
- *Abdomen:* Obese, soft, normal bowel sounds
- *Extremities:* 2-mm pretibial pitting edema

LABORATORY DATA
- *Chest radiograph:* Mildly enlarged heart, no mass, infiltrate, or effusion
- *ECG:* Normal sinus rhythm with P pulmonale
- *Left heart catheterization:* No significant coronary artery disease, normal left ventricular function
- *Right heart catheterization:* Pulmonary hypertension (75/25 mm Hg), pulmonary artery wedge pressure 23 mm Hg
- *Room air arterial blood gases:* pH 7.45, PCO_2 41 mm Hg, PO_2 54 mm Hg, SaO_2 84%
- *Spirometry:* FVC 1.69 L (55% of predicted value), FEV_1 1.27 L (55% of predicted value), FEV_1/FVC 75, forced expiratory flow midexpiratory phase ($FEF_{25\%-75\%}$) 0.96 L/sec (37% of predicted value); no significant improvement with single-dose bronchodilator

PROBLEM: What is the cause of the pulmonary hypertension?

DISCUSSION: The pulmonary service is consulted for evaluation for pulmonary hypertension in association with abnormal spirometric results. Results of bilateral lower extremity Doppler examinations and a ventilation/perfusion scan are normal. Because of a history of snoring, an overnight portable cardiopulmonary sleep study is performed. The study reveals evidence of snoring, nonpositional apnea and hypopnea, and desaturation to less than 60% on the oximeter for most of the monitoring period. Results of a PSG performed in the sleep laboratory verify the presence of moderate to severe OSA, which responds well to the application of CPAP. Follow-up examinations show the dyspnea is relieved, and arterial blood gas values have improved. The patient no longer needs portable liquid O_2 to maintain O_2 saturation greater than 90% at rest or with exercise.

It is unlikely this patient has primary pulmonary hypertension, which generally affects younger women. Chronic thromboembolic disease should be excluded, as it was in this case. Chronic right heart failure secondary to sleep apnea is relieved with proper treatment.

feelings of claustrophobia, nasal congestion, rhinorrhea, skin irritation, and nasal dryness (Figure 30-4). Claustrophobia and skin irritation can be managed by changing the interface to one that is more easily tolerated by the patient. Nasal congestion, rhinorrhea, skin irritation, and nasal dryness can be managed by use of combinations of topical nasal steroids, antihistamines, nasal saline sprays, and lotions. A humidifier can be used in-line with the machine. Heated humidification has been shown to improve compliance.[92] If the patient has a sensation of too much pressure in the nose, adding a system equipped with a ramp may be beneficial.[62] The ramp allows a gradual increase in pressure over 5 to 45 minutes. The ramp time is empirically determined by the prescribing physician. There is no objective evidence that a ramp feature improves patient acceptance or compliance.[76]

Pressure leaks are another problem RTs encounter. Most interfaces are of the nasal variety. Some patients tend to breathe partially or mainly through the mouth. The addition of a chin strap may not resolve the problem. Changing the interface to an oronasal mask may be required for effective "pressurization" of the upper airway in these patients.[82]

Oral Appliances

Oral appliances are devices that enlarge the airway by moving the mandible forward or by keeping the tongue in an anterior position (Figure 30-5). Patients who have mild sleep apnea and are unwilling to use CPAP may benefit from these devices. Oral appliances are worn only during sleep and come in various forms. The appliances are custom-fitted by dentists and are generally well tolerated by patients. They are overall less effective than CPAP therapy and are regarded as a second-line intervention, particularly for severe OSA.[93,94]

Medications

Medications have proved ineffective for most patients with sleep apnea. Benzodiazepines and other sedative-hypnotics should be avoided because they can potentiate upper

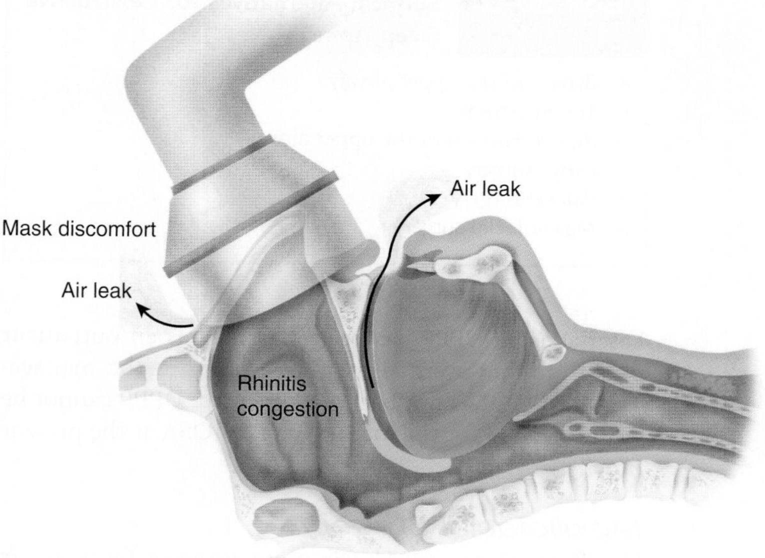

FIGURE 30-4 Positive airway pressure problems. Various problems can be encountered with CPAP.

MINI CLINI

Worsening Right-Sided Heart Failure in a Patient With Chronic Obstructive Pulmonary Disease Who Is Using Oxygen

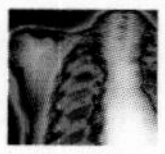

HISTORY: A 50-year-old former smoker previously found to have severe COPD, with FEV_1 of 0.9 L (30% of predicted value), is admitted to the hospital for evaluation and management of worsening shortness of breath and persistent bilateral leg swelling. He has been using O_2 at 2 L/min 24 hours per day for the last 3 months. A chronic productive cough of clear sputum has been unchanged. He denies having chest pain.

MEDICATIONS

- Ipratropium bromide by metered dose inhaler, 2 puffs four times a day
- O_2, 2 L/min 24 hours per day
- Hydrochlorothiazide, 50 mg by mouth daily
- Theophylline, 300 mg by mouth twice a day

MEDICAL HISTORY

- Hypertension and chronic bronchitis
- No cardiac disease

PHYSICAL EXAMINATION

- *Vital signs:* Blood pressure 150/90 mm Hg, heart rate 100 beats/min, temperature 98.6° F (37° C), respirations 18 breaths/min
- *General:* Obese white man who appears short of breath
- *Neck:* 46 cm (18 in) in circumference
- *Lungs:* Decreased breath sounds bilaterally
- *Heart:* Faint sounds but regular rate and rhythm
- *Abdomen:* Obese, soft, normal bowel sounds
- *Extremities:* "Dusky" lower extremities with 4 mm pitting edema to the knees

LABORATORY DATA

- *Theophylline level:* 12 mcg/ml
- *Arterial blood gases:* pH 7.36, PCO_2 44 mm Hg, PO_2 56 mm Hg, SaO_2 89% (on 2 L/min O_2)
- *Chest radiograph:* "Pulmonary congestion"; otherwise normal
- *ECG:* Sinus tachycardia without acute changes
- *Echocardiogram:* "Technically limited" but reported to be without segmental wall abnormalities or to show normal left ventricular function
- *Bilateral lower extremity Doppler examination:* Negative for deep venous thrombosis

PROBLEM: What could be the cause of this patient's continued signs of right heart failure?

DISCUSSION: The patient has overlap syndrome (COPD and OSA). He has been appropriately treated for COPD (bronchodilators and O_2) but has not been treated for OSA. His physician never asked and the patient never volunteered a history of nightly loud snoring with observed apnea and daytime fatigue. Subsequent evaluation with a nocturnal PSG reveals severe nocturnal desaturation to 40% on the oximeter despite treatment with O_2 at 2 L/min. A CPAP titration study is performed. The patient is discharged with CPAP set at 15 cm H_2O via a nasal mask. He returns to the outpatient clinic 3 months later and reports "feeling great." He reports that the shortness of breath has decreased and that he has much more energy during the day. Physical examination shows trace pedal edema. Arterial blood gas studies on 2 L/min of O_2 reveal pH 7.40, PCO_2 40 mm Hg, PO_2 75 mm Hg, and SaO_2 93%.

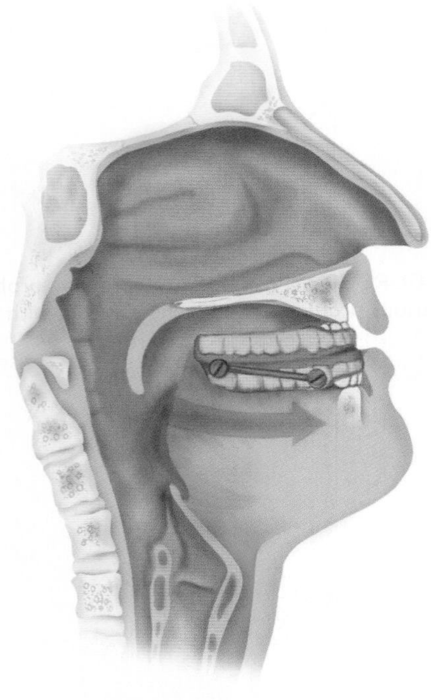

FIGURE 30-5 Oral appliance. The oral appliance covers the teeth of the upper and lower jaws and is adjusted to move the mandible (lower jaw) forward mechanically to open the airway.

airway collapse. The antidepressants protriptyline and fluoxetine have been used to manage mild sleep apnea but are ineffective in most patients.[14] O_2 therapy is useful for patients with oxyhemoglobin desaturation who refuse positive pressure therapy. O_2 therapy can improve nocturnal desaturation but has no significant effect on ventilatory arousals and daytime sleepiness.[95] O_2 therapy should be used with caution by patients with concomitant severe COPD, who may retain CO_2.

Surgical Interventions

Surgical alternatives can be divided into two broad categories: (1) procedures that bypass the upper airway and (2) procedures that reconstruct the upper airway (Box 30-5). Before the advent of CPAP therapy, tracheostomy was the primary therapy for severe OSA. Because of the psychosocial and medical morbidity associated with the procedure, use of tracheostomy today is limited to management of severe OSA when all other therapies have been exhausted.[96,97]

Palatal Surgery

Uvulopalatopharyngoplasty (UPPP) is palatal surgery performed with a standard "cold knife" technique or a laser. Portions of the soft palate, the uvula, and additional redundant tissue are removed in these procedures. The success rate of UPPP is reported to be less than 50% overall.[98] The site of the physiologic obstruction cannot be predicted correctly with preoperative imaging.

Box 30-5 Surgical Alternatives for Obstructive Sleep Apnea

- Bypass of the upper airway
- Tracheostomy
- Reconstruction of the upper airway
- Nasal surgery
- Palatal surgery
- Maxillofacial surgery

Laser-assisted UPPP has been marketed as an outpatient procedure; however, substantial efficacy in the management of OSA has not been documented. UPPP cannot be recommended for the management of OSA at the present time.[99,100]

Maxillofacial Surgery

Maxillofacial surgery shows more promise for patients with OSA (Figure 30-6). Phase I surgical procedures combine UPPP with genioglossal advancement. Patients are identified preoperatively with a combination of radiologic imaging and direct visualization of the upper airway. It is beneficial to have these patients use CPAP therapy perioperatively to reduce the chronic upper airway swelling and edema present before surgery and to reduce postoperative airway edema.[101] When phase I surgery is unsuccessful, phase II surgery involves advancement of the maxilla and the mandible.[102] These surgical procedures are performed at only a few specialized centers. A coordinated effort by a dedicated team of otolaryngologists, oral surgeons, and sleep specialists is essential. Regardless of the surgical option chosen, a postoperative PSG should be obtained to document improvement objectively.[103]

ROLE OF THE RESPIRATORY THERAPIST IN DISORDERS OF SLEEP

RTs play a key role in the management of patients with sleep disorders. RTs may see patients with sleep disorder–related symptoms in the course of their clinical practice and can prompt diagnostic testing by discussion with the patient or the managing physician or both. In the acute care setting, RTs and nursing staff are in a unique position to observe directly evidence of abnormal breathing during sleep or other clinical clues that may prompt further clinical action. RTs may also be members of the sleep laboratory team, where they may assist with titrations of CPAP and interface fitting and management. Some RTs pursue special certification in Sleep Technology.

Therapeutically, RTs may see patients in their home and assist with managing the CPAP or bilevel PAP machines, interfaces, and supplemental O_2. In the context of rehabilitation or bariatric surgery, RTs may help care for patients recovering from surgery or participating in

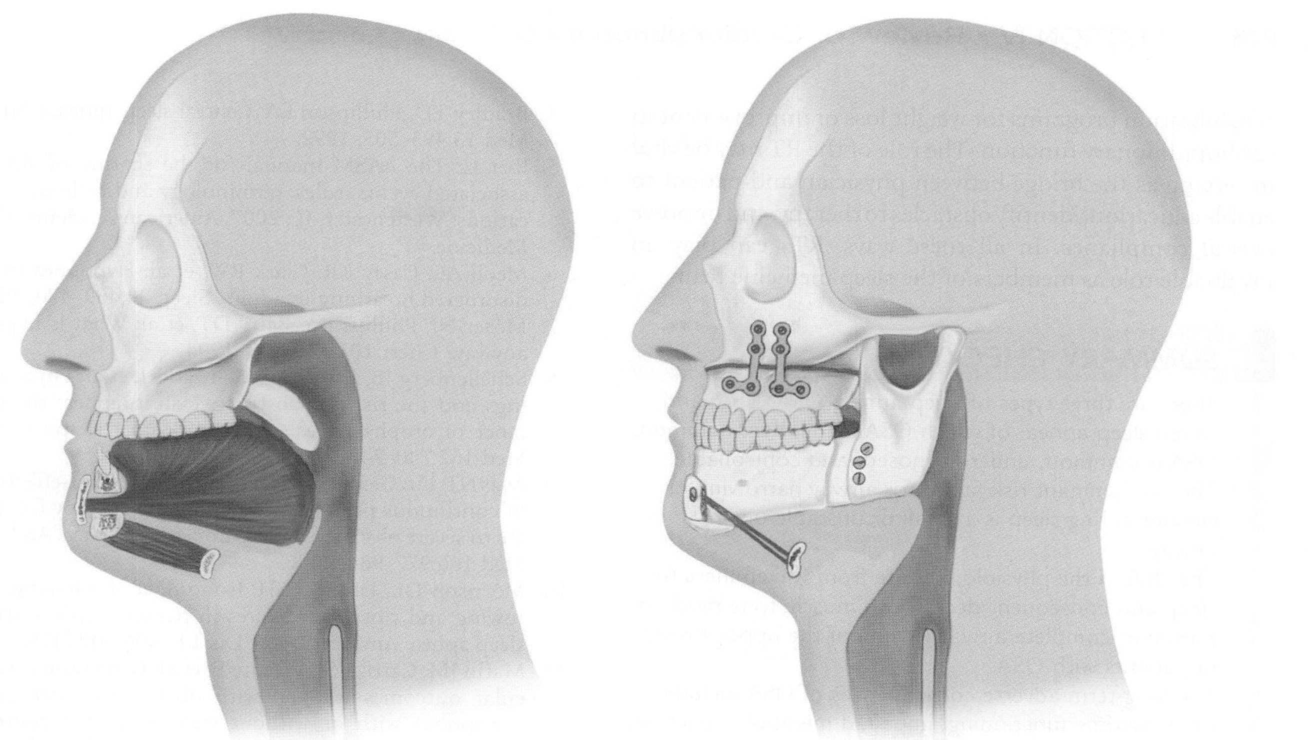

A B

FIGURE 30-6 Phase I and phase II upper airway reconstruction. **A,** Phase I surgery. Lateral cutaway view of the skull shows tongue (genioglossal) and hyoid bone advancement in conjunction with UPPP. **B,** Phase II surgery. Lateral cutaway view of the skull shows advancement of the maxilla (upper jaw) and mandible (lower jaw) in a patient who has undergone a phase I procedure.

MINI CLINI

Young Woman With Mental Status Changes After Orthopedic Surgery

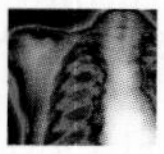

HISTORY: A 37-year-old obese smoker is admitted to the hospital after elective surgical repair of a biceps tendon and ulnar collateral ligament. She initially sustained the injury after a fall when riding a bicycle. After outpatient orthopedic evaluation and preoperative cardiac clearance, an elective repair of the tendon and ligament was scheduled. She was intubated electively for the procedure, and her operative course was unremarkable. Postoperatively, she was extubated and noted to be slightly lethargic but easily arousable and in pain while in postoperative recovery. On transfer to the floor, she became increasingly lethargic and hypoxemic despite the addition of up to 6 L/min of supplemental O_2 via nasal cannula. An emergency code is called. She is transferred to a step-down bed, and further testing is obtained.

MEDICATIONS AT HOME

- None

MEDICAL HISTORY

- Hypertension, not on medications

PHYSICAL EXAMINATION

- *Vital signs:* Blood pressure 158/74 mm Hg, heart rate 68 beats/min, temperature 98.6° F (38.6° C), respirations 12 breaths/min
- *General:* Obese woman, lethargic and arousable
- *Neck:* 46 cm (18 in) in circumference
- *Lungs:* Diminished breath sounds bilaterally
- *Heart:* Faint sounds but regular rate and rhythm
- *Abdomen:* Obese, soft, normal bowel sounds
- *Extremities:* Right arm wound intact with bandages in place, pulses equal

LABORATORY DATA

- *Arterial blood gases on 6 L/min O_2 via nasal cannula:* pH 7.11, PCO_2 109 mm Hg, PO_2 110 mm Hg, SaO_2 87%
- *Chest x-ray:* No mass, infiltrate, or effusion
- *ECG:* Normal sinus rhythm
- *CT scan of the head without contrast agent:* No mass, hemorrhage, or midline shift
- *CT scan of the chest with contrast agent:* No evidence of pulmonary embolism or parenchymal abnormality
- *EEG:* No seizure activity
- *PROBLEM:* How should this patient be managed?

DISCUSSION: The patient requires bilevel noninvasive ventilator support intermittently for the next several days. After her work-up reveals nothing remarkable, a pulmonary and sleep consultation is obtained. Review of the medical records reveals the patient has been receiving hydromorphone (Dilaudid) frequently for pain control. After cessation of opioid medication, the patient's mental status gradually returns to baseline. Repeat arterial blood gases on room air show pH 7.39, PCO_2 62 mm Hg, PO_2 110 mm Hg, and SaO_2 93%. A diagnostic nocturnal PSG is performed, which reveals severe OSA with AHI of 55 and low SaO_2 of 72% and evidence of chronic **obesity hypoventilation.** Positive pressure titration is performed successfully with average volume assisted pressure support with goal V_T of 8 ml/kg. The patient is discharged home with a follow-up appointment in the sleep clinic.

rehabilitation programs for weight loss or improvement in cardiopulmonary function. The role of the RT may be vital in serving as the bridge between physician and patient to enable education, identify obstacles to therapy, and improve overall compliance. In all these ways, RTs can play an invaluable role as members of the sleep medicine team.

SUMMARY CHECKLIST

- There are three types of sleep apnea: OSA, CSA, and mixed sleep apnea, of which OSA is the most common.
- OSA is common, underdiagnosed, and controllable.
- The predominant risk factor for airway narrowing or closure during sleep is a small or unstable upper airway.
- The shift in the physiologic state from wakefulness to sleep and consequent decrease in muscle tone result in partial or complete airway closure of the upper airway in patients with OSA.
- The long-term adverse consequences of OSA include poor daytime functioning, impaired metabolic function, and increased risk of cardiovascular morbidity and mortality.
- Risk factors for OSA include male sex, age older than 40 years, upper body obesity (neck size >16.5 in), habitual snoring, and diurnal hypertension.
- PSG is the most accurate way to make the diagnosis of OSA. The PSG measures several physiologic variables and allows for the staging of sleep and measurement of airflow, ventilatory effort, ECG, and O_2 saturation.
- First-line medical therapy for OSA is CPAP. This modality is almost always effective in the laboratory, although long-term compliance with CPAP therapy may be suboptimal.
- Bilevel PAP therapy may be useful in salvaging selected patients who have difficulty accepting or complying with CPAP.
- The role of autotitrating positive airway pressure devices (auto-CPAP or auto-bilevel PAP) in the management of OSA remains to be defined.
- Oral appliances can be effective, in particular, in patients with mild to moderate OSA.
- Surgical therapy may be an option for a select group of patients who have undergone an extensive preoperative analysis of the upper airway and do not accept or comply poorly with medical therapy. Optimal management of OSA, regardless of the modality, requires patient education, continued monitoring, and reassessment.

References

1. Kapur V, Strohl KP, Redline S, et al: Underdiagnosis of sleep apnea syndrome in U.S. communities. Sleep Breath 6:49-54, 2002.
2. Young T, Peppard PE, Gottlieb DJ: Epidemiology of obstructive sleep apnea: a population health perspective. Am J Respir Crit Care Med 165:1217-1239, 2002.
3. White DP: Pathogenesis of obstructive and central sleep apnea. Am J Respir Crit Care Med 172:1363-1370, 2005.
4. Bradley TD, Phillipson EA: Central sleep apnea. Clin Chest Med 13:493-505, 1992.
5. Iber C: The AASM manual for the scoring of sleep and associated events: rules, terminology and technical specifications. Westchester, IL, 2007, American Academy of Sleep Medicine.
6. Meoli AL, Casey KR, Clark RW, et al: Hypopnea in sleep-disordered breathing in adults. Sleep 24:469-470, 2001.
7. Moser NJ, Phillips BA, Berry DT, et al: What is hypopnea, anyway? Chest 105:426-428, 1994.
8. Schellenberg JB, Maislin G, Schwab RJ, et al: Physical findings and the risk for obstructive sleep apnea: the importance of oropharyngeal structures. Am J Respir Crit Care Med 162:740-748, 2000.
9. Ayas NT, FitzGerald JM, Fleetham JA, et al: Cost-effectiveness of continuous positive airway pressure therapy for moderate to severe obstructive sleep apnea/hypopnea. Arch Intern Med 166:977-984, 2006.
10. Morrison DL, Launois SH, Isono S, et al: Pharyngeal narrowing and closing pressures in patients with obstructive sleep apnea. Am Rev Respir Dis 148:606-611, 1993.
11. Marin JM, Carrizo SJ, Vicente E, et al: Long-term cardiovascular outcomes in men with obstructive sleep apnoea-hypopnoea with or without treatment with continuous positive airway pressure: an observational study. Lancet 365:1046-1053, 2005.
12. Shahar E, Whitney CW, Redline S, et al: Sleep-disordered breathing and cardiovascular disease: cross-sectional results of the Sleep Heart Health Study. Am J Respir Crit Care Med 163:19-25, 2001.
13. Shamsuzzaman AS, Gersh BJ, Somers VK: Obstructive sleep apnea: implications for cardiac and vascular disease. JAMA 290:1906-1914, 2003.
14. Strollo PJ, Jr, Rogers RM: Obstructive sleep apnea. N Engl J Med 334:99-104, 1996.
15. Guidry UC, Mendes LA, Evans JC, et al: Echocardiographic features of the right heart in sleep-disordered breathing: the Framingham Heart Study. Am J Respir Crit Care Med 164:933-938, 2001.
16. Shivalkar B, Van de Heyning C, Kerremans M, et al: Obstructive sleep apnea syndrome: more insights on structural and functional cardiac alterations, and the effects of treatment with continuous positive airway pressure. J Am Coll Cardiol 47:1433-1439, 2006.
17. Schwab RJ, Gupta KB, Gefter WB, et al: Upper airway and soft tissue anatomy in normal subjects and patients with sleep-disordered breathing: significance of the lateral pharyngeal walls. Am J Respir Crit Care Med 152:1673-1689, 1995.
18. Palmer LJ, Buxbaum SG, Larkin E, et al: A whole-genome scan for obstructive sleep apnea and obesity. Am J Hum Genet 72:340-350, 2003.
19. Mathur R, Douglas NJ: Family studies in patients with the sleep apnea-hypopnea syndrome. Ann Intern Med 122:174-178, 1995.
20. Gay PC: Chronic obstructive pulmonary disease and sleep. Respir Care 49:39-51, 2004.
21. Malhotra A, White DP: Obstructive sleep apnoea. Lancet 360:237-245, 2002.
22. Seneviratne U, Puvanendran K: Excessive daytime sleepiness in obstructive sleep apnea: prevalence, severity, and predictors. Sleep Med 5:339-343, 2004.
23. Gottlieb DJ, Whitney CW, Bonekat WH, et al: Relation of sleepiness to respiratory disturbance index: the Sleep Heart Health Study. Am J Respir Crit Care Med 159:502-507, 1999.
24. Adams N, Strauss M, Schluchter M, et al: Relation of measures of sleep-disordered breathing to neuropsychological

functioning. Am J Respir Crit Care Med 163:1626–1631, 2001.
25. George CF, George CFP: Sleep. 5: driving and automobile crashes in patients with obstructive sleep apnoea/hypopnoea syndrome. Thorax 59:804–807, 2004.
26. Hartenbaum N, Collop N, Rosen IM, et al: Sleep apnea and commercial motor vehicle operators: statement from the joint task force of the American College of Chest Physicians, the American College of Occupational and Environmental Medicine, and the National Sleep Foundation. Chest 130:902–905, 2006.
27. Teran-Santos J, Jimenez-Gomez A, Cordero-Guevara J: The association between sleep apnea and the risk of traffic accidents. Cooperative Group Burgos-Santander. N Engl J Med 340:847–851, 1999.
28. Blankfield RP, Hudgel DW, Tapolyai AA, et al: Bilateral leg edema, obesity, pulmonary hypertension, and obstructive sleep apnea. Arch Intern Med 160:2357–2362, 2000. [erratum in Arch Intern Med 2000;160(17):2650].
29. Badesch DB, Raskob GE, Elliott CG, et al: Pulmonary arterial hypertension: baseline characteristics from the REVEAL Registry. Chest 137:376–387, 2010.
30. Kessler R, Chaouat A, Schinkewitch P, et al: The obesity-hypoventilation syndrome revisited: a prospective study of 34 consecutive cases. Chest 120:369–376, 2001.
31. Mehra R, Benjamin EJ, Shahar E, et al: Association of nocturnal arrhythmias with sleep-disordered breathing: the Sleep Heart Health Study. Am J Respir Crit Care Med 173: 910–916, 2006.
32. Monahan K, Storfer-Isser A, Mehra R, et al: Triggering of nocturnal arrhythmias by sleep-disordered breathing events. J Am Coll Cardiol 54:1797–1804, 2009.
33. Yamashiro Y, Kryger M: Why should sleep apnea be diagnosed and treated? Clin Pulm Med 1:250, 1994.
34. Coughlin SR, Mawdsley L, Mugarza JA, et al: Obstructive sleep apnoea is independently associated with an increased prevalence of metabolic syndrome. Eur Heart J 25:735–741, 2004.
35. Troxel WM, Buysse DJ, Matthews KA, et al: Sleep symptoms predict the development of the metabolic syndrome. Sleep 33:1633–1640, 2010.
36. Reaven GM: Banting Lecture 1988. Role of insulin resistance in human disease. Nutrition 13:65, 1997.
37. Punjabi NM, Beamer BA: Alterations in glucose disposal in sleep-disordered breathing. Am J Respir Crit Care Med 179:235–240, 2009.
38. Gottlieb DJ, Yenokyan G, Newman AB, et al: Prospective study of obstructive sleep apnea and incident coronary heart disease and heart failure: the Sleep Heart Health Study. Circulation 122:352–360, 2010.
39. Gay PC: Sleep and sleep-disordered breathing in the hospitalized patient. Respir Care 55:1240–1254, 2010.
40. Gross JB, Bachenberg KL, Benumof JL, et al: Practice guidelines for the perioperative management of patients with obstructive sleep apnea: a report by the American Society of Anesthesiologists Task Force on Perioperative Management of patients with obstructive sleep apnea. Anesthesiology 104:1081–1093, 2006.
41. Meoli AL, Rosen CL, Kristo D, et al: Upper airway management of the adult patient with obstructive sleep apnea in the perioperative period—avoiding complications. Sleep 26:1060–1065, 2003.
42. Khayat RN, Jarjoura D, Patt B, et al: In-hospital testing for sleep-disordered breathing in hospitalized patients with decompensated heart failure: report of prevalence and patient characteristics. J Card Fail 15:739–746, 2009.
43. Memtsoudis S, Liu SS, Ma Y, et al: Perioperative pulmonary outcomes in patients with sleep apnea after noncardiac surgery. Anesth Analg 112:113–121, 2011.
44. Weingarten TN, Flores AS, McKenzie JA, et al: Obstructive sleep apnoea and perioperative complications in bariatric patients. Br J Anaesth 106:131–139, 2011.
45. Adesanya AO, Lee W, Greilich NB, et al: Perioperative management of obstructive sleep apnea. Chest 138:1489–1498, 2010.
46. Spurr KF, Graven MA, Gilbert RW: Prevalence of unspecified sleep apnea and the use of continuous positive airway pressure in hospitalized patients, 2004 National Hospital Discharge Survey. Sleep Breath 12:229–234, 2008.
47. Morgenthaler TI, Aurora RN, Brown T, et al: Practice parameters for the use of autotitrating continuous positive airway pressure devices for titrating pressures and treating adult patients with obstructive sleep apnea syndrome: an update for 2007. An American Academy of Sleep Medicine report. Sleep 31:141–147, 2008.
48. Condos R, Norman RG, Krishnasamy I, et al: Flow limitation as a noninvasive assessment of residual upper-airway resistance during continuous positive airway pressure therapy of obstructive sleep apnea. Am J Respir Crit Care Med 150:475–480, 1994.
49. Cracowski C, Pepin JL, Wuyam B, et al: Characterization of obstructive nonapneic respiratory events in moderate sleep apnea syndrome. Am J Respir Crit Care Med 164:944–948, 2001.
50. Sleep-related breathing disorders in adults: recommendations for syndrome definition and measurement techniques in clinical research. Report of an American Academy of Sleep Medicine Task Force. Sleep 22:667–689, 1999.
51. Collop NA, Anderson WM, Boehlecke B, et al: Clinical guidelines for the use of unattended portable monitors in the diagnosis of obstructive sleep apnea in adult patients. Portable Monitoring Task Force of the American Academy of Sleep Medicine. J Clin Sleep Med 3:737–747, 2007.
52. Epstein LJ, Kristo D, Strollo PJ, Jr, et al: Clinical guideline for the evaluation, management and long-term care of obstructive sleep apnea in adults. J Clin Sleep Med 5:263–276, 2009.
53. Herzog M, Riemann R, Herzog M, et al: Alcohol ingestion influences the nocturnal cardio-respiratory activity in snoring and non-snoring males. Eur Arch Otorhinolaryngol 261:459–462, 2004.
54. Guilleminault C, Guilleminault C: Benzodiazepines, breathing, and sleep. Am J Med 88:25S–28S, 1990.
55. Skinner MA, Kingshott RN, Jones DR, et al: Elevated posture for the management of obstructive sleep apnea. Sleep Breath 8:193–200, 2004.
56. Mador MJ, Kufel TJ, Magalang UJ, et al: Prevalence of positional sleep apnea in patients undergoing polysomnography. Chest 128:2130–2137, 2005.
57. Permut I, Diaz-Abad M, Chatila W, et al: Comparison of positional therapy to CPAP in patients with positional obstructive sleep apnea. J Clin Sleep Med 6:238–243, 2010.
58. Sullivan CE, Issa FG, Berthon-Jones M, et al: Reversal of obstructive sleep apnoea by continuous positive airway pressure applied through the nares. Lancet 1:862–865, 1981.
59. Kushida CA, Littner MR, Hirshkowitz M, et al: Practice parameters for the use of continuous and bilevel positive airway pressure devices to treat adult patients with sleep-related breathing disorders. Sleep 29:375–380, 2006.
60. Kushida CA, Chediak A, Berry RB, et al: Clinical guidelines for the manual titration of positive airway pressure in

patients with obstructive sleep apnea. J Clin Sleep Med 4:157–171, 2008.
61. Hoffstein V, Viner S, Mateika S, et al: Treatment of obstructive sleep apnea with nasal continuous positive airway pressure: patient compliance, perception of benefits, and side effects. Am Rev Respir Dis 145:841–845, 1992.
62. Miljeteig H, Hoffstein V: Determinants of continuous positive airway pressure level for treatment of obstructive sleep apnea. Am Rev Respir Dis 147:1526–1530, 1993.
63. Engleman HM, Martin SE, Deary IJ, et al: Effect of continuous positive airway pressure treatment on daytime function in sleep apnoea/hypopnoea syndrome. Lancet 343:572–575, 1994.
64. Sforza E, Lugaresi E: Daytime sleepiness and nasal continuous positive airway pressure therapy in obstructive sleep apnea syndrome patients: effects of chronic treatment and 1-night therapy withdrawal. Sleep 18:195–201, 1995.
65. Montplaisir J, Bedard MA, Richer F, et al: Neurobehavioral manifestations in obstructive sleep apnea syndrome before and after treatment with continuous positive airway pressure. Sleep 15:S17–S19, 1992.
66. Lamphere J, Roehrs T, Wittig R, et al: Recovery of alertness after CPAP in apnea. Chest 96:1364–1367, 1989.
67. Leech JA, Onal E, Lopata M: Nasal CPAP continues to improve sleep-disordered breathing and daytime oxygenation over long-term follow-up of occlusive sleep apnea syndrome. Chest 102:1651–1655, 1992.
68. Strollo PJ, Sanders MH, Striller RA: Continuous and bilevel positive airway pressure therapy in sleep disordered breathing. Oral Maxillofac Surg Clin N Am 7:221, 1995.
69. Strohl KP, Redline S: Nasal CPAP therapy, upper airway muscle activation, and obstructive sleep apnea. Am Rev Respir Dis 134:555–558, 1986.
70. Grunstein RR: Sleep-related breathing disorders. 5. Nasal continuous positive airway pressure treatment for obstructive sleep apnoea. Thorax 50:1106–1113, 1995.
71. Sforza E, Krieger J, Bacon W, et al: Determinants of effective continuous positive airway pressure in obstructive sleep apnea: role of respiratory effort. Am J Respir Crit Care Med 151:1852–1856, 1995.
72. Guilleminault C, Stoohs R, Clerk A, et al: From obstructive sleep apnea syndrome to upper airway resistance syndrome: consistency of daytime sleepiness. Sleep 15:S13–S16, 1992.
73. Guilleminault C, Stoohs R, Clerk A, et al: A cause of excessive daytime sleepiness: the upper airway resistance syndrome. Chest 104:781–787, 1993.
74. Guilleminault C, Stoohs R, Duncan S: Snoring, I: daytime sleepiness in regular heavy snorers. Chest 99:40–48, 1991.
75. Montserrat JM, Ballester E, Olivi H, et al: Time-course of stepwise CPAP titration: behavior of respiratory and neurological variables. Am J Respir Crit Care Med 152:1854–1859, 1995.
76. Zozula R, Rosen R: Compliance with continuous positive airway pressure therapy: assessing and improving treatment outcomes. Curr Opin Pulm Med 7:391–398, 2001.
77. Sin DD, Mayers I, Man GC, et al: Long-term compliance rates to continuous positive airway pressure in obstructive sleep apnea: a population-based study. Chest 121:430–435, 2002.
78. McArdle N, Devereux G, Heidarnejad H, et al: Long-term use of CPAP therapy for sleep apnea/hypopnea syndrome. Am J Respir Crit Care Med 159:1108–1114, 1999.
79. Sanders MH, Gruendl CA, Rogers RM: Patient compliance with nasal CPAP therapy for sleep apnea. Chest 90:330–333, 1986.
80. Kribbs NB, Pack AI, Kline LR, et al: Objective measurement of patterns of nasal CPAP use by patients with obstructive sleep apnea. Am Rev Respir Dis 147:887–895, 1993.
81. Sanders MH, Kern N: Obstructive sleep apnea treated by independently adjusted inspiratory and expiratory positive airway pressures via nasal mask: physiologic and clinical implications. Chest 98:317–324, 1990.
82. Sanders MH, Kern NB, Stiller RA, et al: CPAP therapy via oronasal mask for obstructive sleep apnea. Chest 106:774–779,1994.
83. Prosise GL, Berry RB: Oral-nasal continuous positive airway pressure as a treatment for obstructive sleep apnea. Chest 106:180–186, 1994.
84. Criner GJ, Travaline JM, Brennan KJ, et al: Efficacy of a new full face mask for noninvasive positive pressure ventilation. Chest 106:1109–1115, 1994.
85. Mayer LS, Kerby GR, Whitman RA: Evaluation of a new nasal device for administration of continuous positive airway pressure for treatment of obstructive sleep apnea. Am Rev Respir Dis 139:A114, 1989.
86. Harris C, Daniels B, Herold D, et al: Comparison of cannula and mask systems for administration of nasal continuous positive airway pressure for treatment of obstructive sleep apnea. Sleep Res 19:233, 1990.
87. Reeves-Hoche MK, Hudgel DW, Meck R, et al: Continuous versus bilevel positive airway pressure for obstructive sleep apnea. Am J Respir Crit Care Med 151:443–449, 1995.
88. Littner M, Hirshkowitz M, Davila D, et al: Practice parameters for the use of auto-titrating continuous positive airway pressure devices for titrating pressures and treating adult patients with obstructive sleep apnea syndrome. An American Academy of Sleep Medicine report. Sleep 25:143–147, 2002.
89. d'Ortho MP, d'Ortho MP: Auto-titrating continuous positive airway pressure for treating adult patients with sleep apnea syndrome. Curr Opin Pulm Med 10:495–499, 2004.
90. Berry RB, Parish JM, Hartse KM, et al: The use of auto-titrating continuous positive airway pressure for treatment of adult obstructive sleep apnea. An American Academy of Sleep Medicine review. Sleep 25:148–173, 2002.
91. Ayas NT, Patel SR, Malhotra A, et al: Auto-titrating versus standard continuous positive airway pressure for the treatment of obstructive sleep apnea: results of a meta-analysis. Sleep 27:249–253, 2004.
92. Rakotonanahary D, Pelletier-Fleury N, Gagnadoux F, et al: Predictive factors for the need for additional humidification during nasal continuous positive airway pressure therapy. Chest 119:460–465, 2001.
93. Kushida CA, Morgenthaler TI, Littner MR, et al: Practice parameters for the treatment of snoring and obstructive sleep apnea with oral appliances: an update for 2005. Sleep 29:240–243, 2006.
94. Ferguson KA, Cartwright R, Rogers R, et al: Oral appliances for snoring and obstructive sleep apnea: a review. Sleep 29:244–262, 2006.
95. Fletcher EC, Munafo DA: Role of nocturnal oxygen therapy in obstructive sleep apnea: when should it be used? Chest 98:1497–1504, 1990.
96. Guilleminault C, Simmons FB, Motta J, et al: Obstructive sleep apnea syndrome and tracheostomy: long-term follow-up experience. Arch Intern Med 141:985–988, 1981.
97. Conway WA, Victor LD, Magilligan DJ, Jr, et al: Adverse effects of tracheostomy for sleep apnea. JAMA 246:347–350, 1981.
98. Sher AE, Schechtman KB, Piccirillo JF: The efficacy of surgical modifications of the upper airway in adults with obstructive sleep apnea syndrome. Sleep 19:156–177, 1996.

99. Sundaram S, Bridgman SA, Lim J, et al: Surgery for obstructive sleep apnoea. Cochrane Database Syst Rev (4): CD001004, 2005.
100. Littner M, Kushida CA, Hartse K, et al: Practice parameters for the use of laser-assisted uvulopalatoplasty: an update for 2000. Sleep 24:603–619, 2001.
101. Johnson NT, Chinn J: Uvulopalatopharyngoplasty and inferior sagittal mandibular osteotomy with genioglossus advancement for treatment of obstructive sleep apnea. Chest 105:278–283, 1994.
102. Dattilo DJ, Drooger SA: Outcome assessment of patients undergoing maxillofacial procedures for the treatment of sleep apnea: comparison of subjective and objective results. J Oral Maxillofac Surg 62:164–168, 2004.
103. Kushida CA, Littner MR, Morgenthaler T, et al: Practice parameters for the indications for polysomnography and related procedures: an update for 2005. Sleep 28:499–521, 2005.

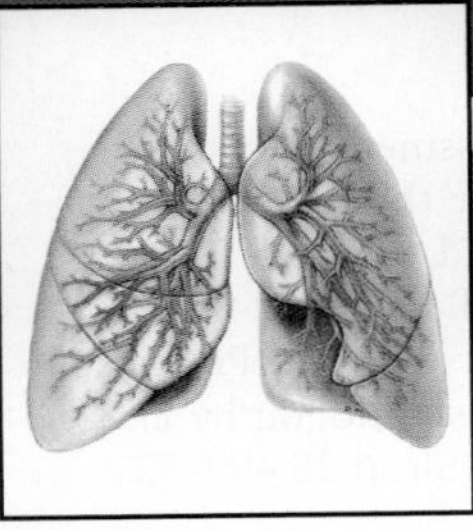

Chapter 31

Neonatal and Pediatric Respiratory Disorders

DOUGLAS D. DEMING AND N. LENNARD SPECHT

CHAPTER OBJECTIVES

After reading this chapter you will be able to:

- Discuss the clinical findings, radiographic abnormalities, and treatment of patients with respiratory distress syndrome.
- Describe the clinical manifestations and treatment of patients with transient tachypnea of the newborn.
- Describe the pathophysiology, presentation, and treatment of meconium aspiration syndrome.
- Identify the clinical signs and symptoms associated with bronchopulmonary dysplasia and the approaches used to manage these infants.
- State the etiology and treatment of apnea of prematurity.
- Describe the pathophysiology, diagnosis, and treatment of persistent pulmonary hypertension of the newborn.
- Discuss the pathophysiology, diagnosis, and treatment of congenital diaphragmatic hernia.
- Identify the anatomic defects associated with tetralogy of Fallot.
- Describe the clinical presentation of a ventricular septal defect.
- Define the epidemiologic factors associated with increased risk of sudden infant death syndrome.
- Identify the respiratory problems associated with gastroesophageal reflux disease.
- State the clinical findings commonly observed in patients with bronchiolitis.
- Describe the clinical features and treatment of children with epiglottitis.
- Describe the clinical manifestations and treatment of cystic fibrosis.

CHAPTER OUTLINE

Neonatal Respiratory Disorders
- Lung Parenchymal Disease
- Control of Breathing
- Pulmonary Vascular Disease
- Congenital Abnormalities Affecting Respiration
- Congenital Heart Disease

Neonatal Resuscitation

Pediatric Respiratory Disorders
- Sudden Infant Death Syndrome
- Gastroesophageal Reflux Disease
- Bronchiolitis
- Croup
- Epiglottitis
- Cystic Fibrosis

Role of the Respiratory Therapist in Neonatal and Pediatric Respiratory Disorders

KEY TERMS

apnea of prematurity
bronchiolitis
bronchopulmonary dysplasia (BPD)
croup
cystic fibrosis (CF)
ductus arteriosus
epiglottitis
gastroesophageal reflux disease (GERD)
meconium aspiration syndrome (MAS)
nasal flaring
persistent pulmonary hypertension of the newborn (PPHN)
respiratory distress syndrome (RDS)

sudden infant death syndrome (SIDS)
tetralogy of Fallot
transient tachypnea of the newborn (TTN)
transposition of the great arteries

Many perinatal disorders affect the respiratory system. Some disorders are developmental abnormalities of the heart, lungs, or airways; some are caused by prematurity; some are caused by problems during labor and delivery; and some are caused by treatments. Common disorders in the neonatal period with which respiratory therapists (RTs) should be familiar are respiratory distress syndrome (RDS), transient tachypnea of the newborn (TTN), meconium aspiration syndrome (MAS), apnea of prematurity, bronchopulmonary dysplasia (BPD), persistent pulmonary hypertension of the newborn (PPHN), and congenital cardiopulmonary abnormalities.

NEONATAL RESPIRATORY DISORDERS

Lung Parenchymal Disease

Respiratory Distress Syndrome

Background. Neonatal **respiratory distress syndrome (RDS)** affects 60,000 to 70,000 infants each year in the United States. Although the death rate has decreased dramatically over the past 3 decades, many infants still die or have chronic effects of the syndrome. RDS, also known as *hyaline membrane disease,* is a disease of prematurity. The incidence increases with decreasing gestational age. The major factors in the pathophysiology of RDS are qualitative surfactant deficiency, decreased alveolar surface area, increased small airways compliance, and presence of a **ductus arteriosus.**

> **RULE OF THUMB**
> The incidence of RDS increases with decreasing gestational age.

Surfactant production depends on both the relative maturity of the lung and the adequacy of fetal perfusion. Maternal factors that impair fetal blood flow, such as abruptio placentae and maternal diabetes, also may lead to RDS.

Pathophysiology. In preterm infants, adequate amounts of surfactant are present in the lung; however, the surfactant is trapped inside type II cells. In infants with RDS, type II cells do not release adequate amounts of surfactant. The surfactant that is released is incompletely formed, so it does not make tubular myelin and does not cause a decrease in alveolar surface tension. Because the surfactant molecule in the alveolus is structurally abnormal, the type II cells and alveolar macrophages have more rapid uptake for recycling. There is a qualitative deficiency of alveolar surfactant.

Figure 31-1 outlines the pathophysiologic events associated with RDS. A qualitative decrease in surfactant increases alveolar surface tension forces. This process causes alveoli to become unstable and collapse and leads to atelectasis and increased work of breathing. At the same time, the increased surface tension draws fluid from the pulmonary capillaries into the alveoli. In combination, these factors impair oxygen (O_2) exchange and cause severe hypoxemia. The severe hypoxemia and acidosis increase *pulmonary vascular resistance (PVR)*. As pulmonary arterial pressure increases, extrapulmonary right-to-left shunting increases, and hypoxemia worsens. Hypoxia and acidosis also impair further surfactant production. Antenatal steroids have been shown to mature surfactant function.

Clinical Manifestations. The first signs of respiratory distress in infants with RDS usually appear soon after birth. Tachypnea usually occurs first. After tachypnea, worsening retractions, paradoxical breathing, and audible grunting are observed. **Nasal flaring** also may be seen. Chest auscultation often reveals fine inspiratory crackles. Cyanosis may or may not be present. If central cyanosis is observed, it is likely that the infant has severe hypoxemia. Certain other conditions, such as systemic hypotension, hypothermia, and poor perfusion, can mimic this aspect of RDS.

A definitive diagnosis of RDS usually is made with chest radiography (Figure 31-2). Diffuse, hazy, reticulogranular densities with the presence of air bronchograms with low lung volumes are typical of RDS. The reticulogranular pattern is caused by aeration of respiratory bronchioles and collapse of the alveoli. Air bronchograms appear as aerated, dark, major bronchi surrounded by the collapsed or consolidated lung tissue.

Treatment. *Continuous positive airway pressure (CPAP)* and *positive end expiratory pressure (PEEP)* are the traditional support modes used to manage RDS. Surfactant replacement therapy and *high-frequency ventilation (HFV)* have been added to these traditional approaches.[1-5] Unless the infant's condition is severe, a trial of nasal CPAP is indicated (4 to 6 cm H_2O).[6,7] Because of the hazards of endotracheal tubes, nasal prongs are preferred. If the infant's clinical condition deteriorates rapidly, a more aggressive approach is required. Endotracheal intubation should be performed under controlled conditions as an elective procedure. Mechanical ventilation with PEEP should be initiated if oxygenation

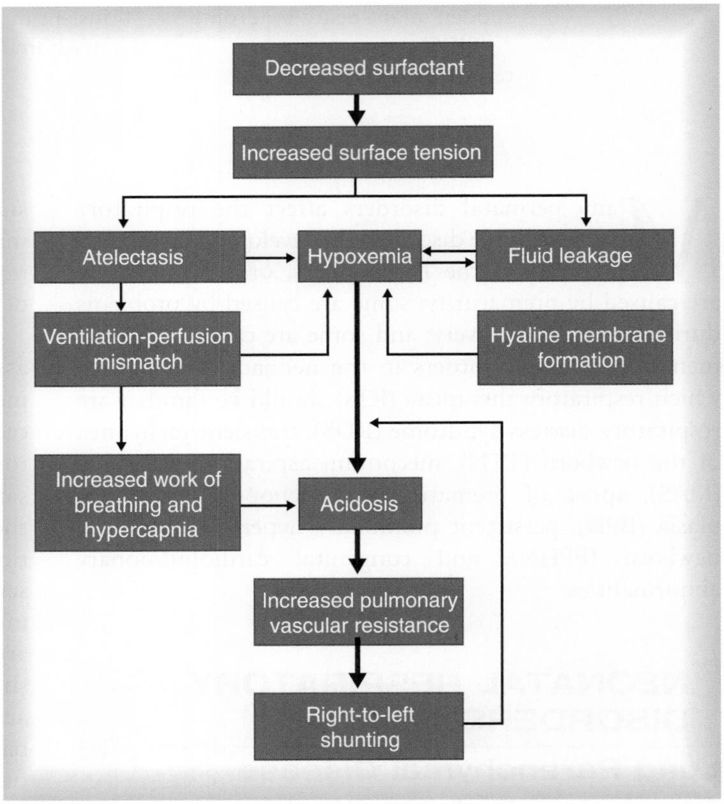

FIGURE 31-1 Pathophysiology of RDS.

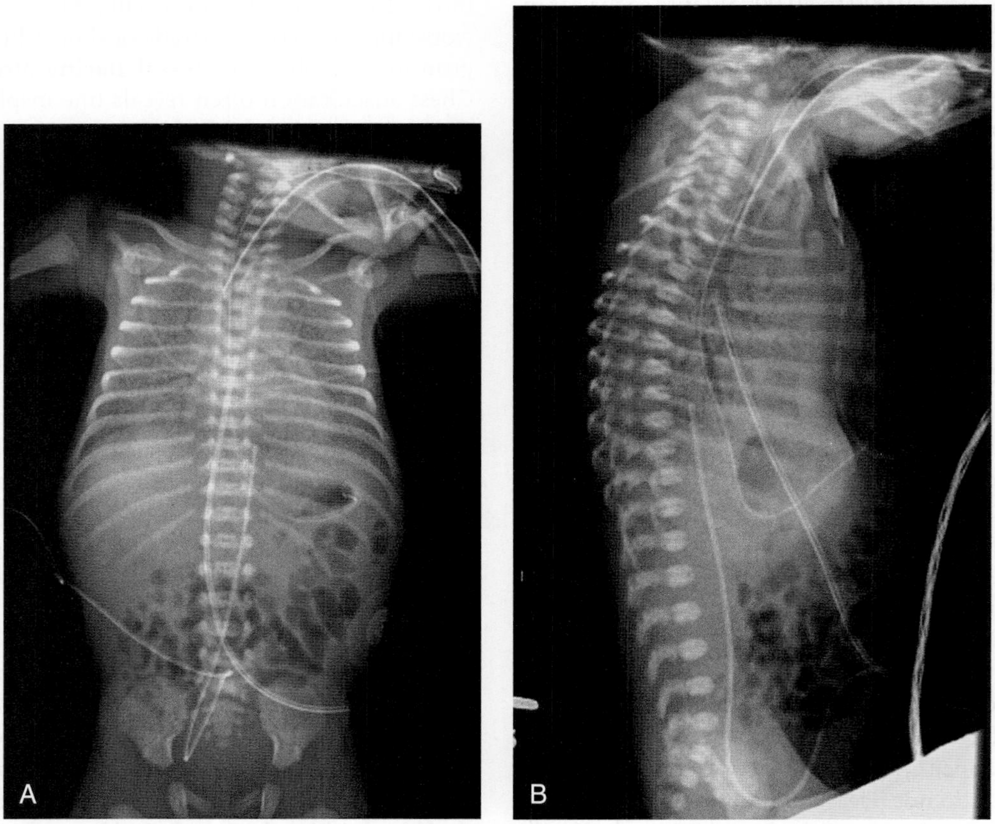

FIGURE 31-2 Radiopaque appearance of severe RDS. Anteroposterior **(A)** and lateral **(B)** radiographs show diffuse hazy appearance with low lung volumes and air bronchograms that extend into the periphery.

TABLE 31-1
Surfactant Dosing

	Beractant (Survanta)	Calfactant (Infasurf)	Poractant alfa (Curosurf)
Dose mg/kg of phospholipid	100	100	100-200
ml/kg	4	3	1.25-2.5
Administration	¼ dose quickly in each of four positions	½ dose slowly supine then rotated	Whole or ½ dose supine
Dosing interval	Every 6 hr or more often	Every 12 hr or more often	Every 12 hr or more often

does not improve with CPAP or if the patient is apneic or acidotic. There is significant interest in an approach comprising intubation, delivery of surfactant, extubation, and then nasal CPAP.[8] However, more research is needed to understand the risks and benefits of this approach.

The aim of mechanical ventilation for RDS is to prevent lung collapse and maintain alveolar inflation. In severe RDS, collapse of alveoli with every breath necessitates very high reinflation pressure. To prevent the need for this high reinflation pressure, use of end-tidal pressure is desirable.

Because of the relationship between arterial partial pressure of carbon dioxide ($PaCO_2$) and functional residual capacity (FRC), $PaCO_2$ is lowest when PEEP is used to optimize FRC. The time constant of the lungs in RDS is short, so the lung empties very quickly with each ventilator cycle. If alveolar ventilation is inadequate, either peak inspiratory pressure or rate should be increased. For minimization of the potential for volutrauma, the peak inspiratory pressure should be kept less than 30 cm H_2O for larger premature infants, and even lower peak inspiratory pressure is indicated for more immature infants.

Three surfactant preparations are used in the United States for management of neonatal RDS: beractant (Survanta; Abbott Laboratories, North Chicago, IL), calfactant (Infasurf; ONY, Inc, Amherst, NY), and poractant alfa (Curosurf; Chiesi, Cheadle, United Kingdom).[4,5,7-9] Beractant and calfactant are natural bovine surfactant extracts. Poractant alfa is a natural porcine surfactant extract. Each of these three natural surfactants has surfactant proteins B and C as part of the formulation. These surfactant proteins are important for decreasing alveolar surface tension. All of these preparations are liquid suspensions that are instilled directly into the trachea. The current standard of care is to deliver replacement surfactant to all infants with RDS. An additional artificial surfactant, lucinactant, is being actively studied.[9] The ability to nebulize with this new surfactant is an exciting possibility. At the present time, no evidence supports the use of a particular brand of surfactant.

Surfactant replacement therapy also is used as both a rescue treatment (of infants who already have RDS) and a prophylactic therapy (in the care of infants delivered prematurely).[10-13] Some centers use prophylactic surfactant replacement therapy in the care of all very small infants (<1500 g). Therapies aimed at decreasing pulmonary edema, improving cardiac output, and weaning from O_2 and high ventilator pressures are essential in the successful treatment of infants receiving surfactant.

All surfactants are delivered via the endotracheal tube. Animal studies suggest that surfactant is rapidly distributed throughout the lung.[14] Each specific surfactant has different dosing volumes and intervals (Table 31-1). The surfactant product insert describes the positioning of the infant for surfactant delivery. Basically, the infant is positioned with different sections of the lung dependent so that the surfactant enters that section of the lung with gravity flow. If the infant is very sick and cannot be repositioned, surfactant can be administered with the infant in a supine position.

MINI CLINI

Respiratory Distress Syndrome

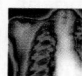

PROBLEM: A woman is about to deliver at 26 weeks' gestational age. What should the RT have available for the resuscitation of the infant?

DISCUSSION: An infant at 26 weeks' gestational age is most likely going to have RDS—ranging from mild to severe disease. The RT should have equipment, supplies, and drugs necessary to support the infant. Many infants require mask-bag ventilation. It is crucial that the RT be acutely attuned to using the lowest pressures necessary to move the chest. It is very easy to injure the lung with high V_T. Most authorities recommend the use of a T-piece resuscitator that delivers manual breaths at fixed pressures, decreasing the risk of traumatic injury from high V_T.

Some infants have severe disease that requires intubation and immediate administration of surfactant. Some infants have only mild disease. These less sick infants may require only nasal CPAP. For infants who have intermediate disease, at some centers clinicians intubate the infant, administer surfactant, and then extubate the infant back to nasal CPAP.

Transient Tachypnea of the Newborn

Background. Transient tachypnea of the newborn (TTN), often called *type II RDS,* is probably the most common respiratory disorder of newborns. The cause of

TTN is unclear, but it is most likely related to delayed clearance of fetal lung liquid.[15-29] During most births, approximately two-thirds of this fluid is expelled by thoracic squeeze in the birth canal; the rest is reabsorbed through the lymphatic vessels during initial breathing. These mechanisms are impaired in infants born by cesarean section or infants with incomplete development of the lymphatic vessels (preterm or small-for-gestational-age infants). The residual lung fluid causes an increase in airway resistance and an overall decrease in lung compliance. Because compliance is low, the infant must generate more negative pleural pressure to breathe. This process can result in hyperinflation of some areas and air trapping in others. Most infants with TTN are born at term without any specific predisposing factors in common. Mothers of neonates who have TTN tend to have longer labor intervals and a higher incidence of failure to progress in labor, which leads to cesarean delivery. In many cases, however, maternal history and labor and delivery are normal.

Clinical Manifestations. During the first few hours of life, infants with TTN breathe rapidly. Alveolar ventilation, as measured by arterial pH and$PaCO_2$, usually is normal. The chest radiographic findings, which may initially be indistinguishable from pneumonia, are hyperinflation, which is secondary to air trapping, and perihilar streaking. The perihilar streaking probably represents lymphatic engorgement. Pleural effusions may be evident in the costophrenic angles and interlobar fissures.

Treatment. Infants with TTN usually respond readily to a low FiO_2 by infant O_2 hood or nasal cannula. Infants requiring a higher FiO_2 may benefit from CPAP. Because the retention of lung fluid may be gravity-dependent, frequent changes in the infant's position may help speed lung fluid clearance. Because TTN and neonatal pneumonia have similar clinical signs, intravenous administration of antibiotics should be considered for at least 3 days after appropriate culture samples are obtained. Mechanical ventilation is rarely needed, and when it is, this probably indicates a complication. Clearing of the lungs evident on a chest radiograph and with clinical improvement usually occurs within 24 to 48 hours. A few infants with TTN eventually have persistent pulmonary hypertension.

Meconium Aspiration Syndrome

Background. Meconium aspiration syndrome (MAS) is a disease of term and near-term infants. It involves aspiration of meconium into the central airways of the lung. It usually is associated with perinatal depression and asphyxia.

Pathophysiology. Amniotic fluid consists mainly of fetal lung fluid, fetal urine, and transudate from the uterine wall. *Meconium,* the contents of the fetal intestine, occasionally is expelled from the fetus into the surrounding amniotic fluid. Meconium consists of mucopolysaccharides, cholesterol, bile acids and salts, intestinal enzymes, and other substances. Meconium normally is not passed until after delivery.[30] Infants who have marked perinatal depression or perinatal asphyxia may pass meconium in utero. The pathophysiologic control mechanisms for the passage of meconium in utero are not completely understood. It is widely accepted that infants can have meconium aspiration in utero. Amniotic fluid stained with meconium is found in approximately 12% of all births.[30] Meconium-stained amniotic fluid is rare among infants of less than 37 weeks' gestational age. The clinical syndrome develops in 2 of every 1000 infants. Of infants with inhaled meconium, 95% clear their lungs spontaneously.[30]Amniotic fluid infusion into the uterus before the delivery of infants with meconium-stained fluid has been shown to improve neonatal outcomes.[31,32]

For many years, the aspirated meconium itself was considered the primary cause of MAS. More recent evidence suggests that the real causative agent is fetal asphyxia that precedes aspiration.[23] Fetal asphyxia causes pulmonary vasospasm and hyperreactivity of the vasculature, which lead to persistent pulmonary hypertension.

MAS involves three primary problems: pulmonary obstruction, lung tissue damage, and pulmonary hypertension.[33] Obstruction occurs because of plugging of the airways with particulate meconium. This obstruction often is of the ball-valve type, which allows gas entry but prevents gas exit. Ball-valve obstruction causes air trapping and can lead to volutrauma (Figure 31-3). The lung tissue injury caused by MAS is chemical pneumonitis. Additionally, there are various chemical effects, inflammatory responses, cytokine and chemokine activations, complement activation, and phospholipase A_2 activation.[33-37] Persistent pulmonary hypertension with intracardiac and extracardiac right-to-left shunting frequently complicates MAS.[30]

Clinical Manifestations. Before birth, thick meconium, fetal tachycardia, and absent fetal cardiac accelerations during labor are evidence that the fetus is at high risk of MAS.[38] After delivery, if the infant has a low umbilical artery pH, an Apgar score less than 5, and meconium aspirated from the trachea, intensive care and close observation for MAS are warranted. Infants with MAS typically have gasping respirations, tachypnea, grunting, and retractions. The chest radiograph usually shows irregular pulmonary densities, which represent areas of atelectasis, and hyperlucent areas, which represent hyperinflation secondary to air trapping (Figure 31-4). Arterial blood gases typically show hypoxemia with mixed respiratory and metabolic acidosis. In the most severe cases, there is right-to-left shunting and persistent pulmonary hypertension.[30]

Treatment. It is no longer recommended that vigorous infants with meconium-stained fluid be intubated and suctioned.[31,39-41] However, it is important that an endotracheal tube be inserted immediately in severely depressed infants with thick meconium, and suction should be applied directly to the endotracheal tube.[40] The endotracheal tube is removed and inspected for meconium. If meconium is

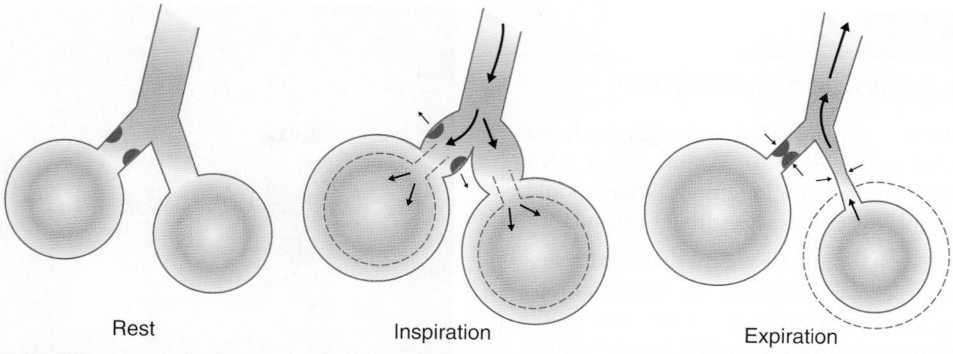

FIGURE 31-3 Ball-valve effect. At rest, the airway lumen is partially obstructed. With inspiration, negative intrathoracic pressure opens the airway and relieves obstruction. Gas enters and expands the alveoli. With expiration, intrathoracic pressure changes to positive force, which narrows the airway and causes total occlusion. Gas cannot be expelled and is trapped within the alveoli. (Modified from Koff PB, Eitzman DV, Neu J: Neonatal and pediatric care, ed 2, St Louis, 1993, Mosby.)

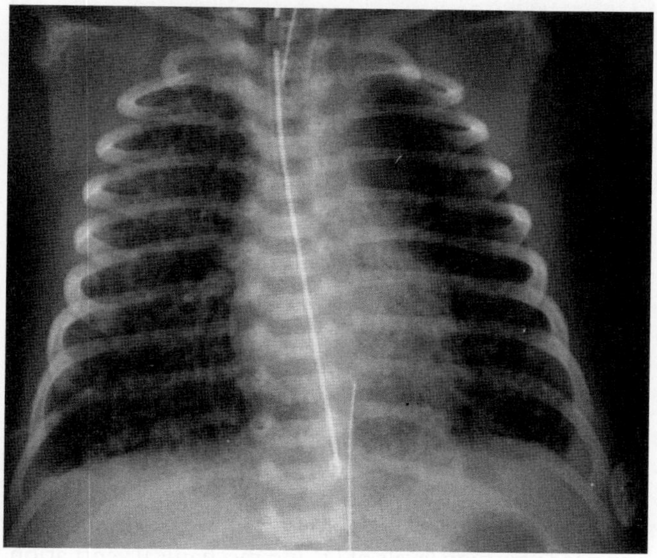

FIGURE 31-4 Radiograph of a patient with MAS. Anteroposterior radiograph shows diffuse patchy areas of atelectasis and emphysema.

present, the procedure is repeated with a new endotracheal tube until no further meconium is aspirated or until two to four aspirations have been performed. The endotracheal tube should be left in place, and mechanical ventilation should be started. For prevention of hypoxemia, a flow of warmed 100% O_2 should be blown across the infant's face during the aspiration efforts. No evidence suggests an improved outcome because of endotracheal suctioning in the care of infants who have meconium and are vigorous and would not otherwise require intubation.[42,43] There is evidence that tracheal lavage with dilute surfactant improves the clinical course and outcome of infants with MAS.[44-46]

If the infant's condition worsens, CPAP or mechanical ventilation may be indicated. CPAP is indicated if the primary problem is hypoxemia. By distending the small airways, CPAP can sometimes overcome the ball-valve obstruction and improve both oxygenation and ventilation. If respiratory acidosis is severe or clinical assessment indicates excessive work in breathing, mechanical ventilation should be started. Figure 31-3 shows the ball-valve effect. At rest, the airway lumen is partially obstructed. With inspiration, negative intrathoracic pressure opens the airway and relieves the obstruction. Gas enters and expands the alveoli. With expiration, intrathoracic pressure changes to a positive force, which narrows the airway and causes total occlusion. Gas cannot be expelled and is trapped within the alveoli. It is difficult to provide ventilation to infants with severe MAS. These infants often retain CO_2 and need increased ventilator support. Because of high airways resistance, the lungs have a long time constant. High ventilator rates and pressures increase the risk of air trapping and volutrauma.

Evidence suggests that both HFV and synchronous intermittent mechanical ventilation decrease the risk of air leak.[47] Various studies have shown improvement in MAS with the use of HFV and surfactant.[48] Nitric oxide has become a major adjunct in the management of persistent pulmonary hypertension.[49] Corticosteroids have not yet been shown to improve outcomes for infants with MAS.[50] High mean airway pressures may worsen pulmonary hypertension and aggravate right-to-left cardiac shunting.[38]

Bronchopulmonary Dysplasia

Background. Infants, especially preterm infants, with severe respiratory failure in the first few weeks of life may develop a chronic pulmonary condition called **bronchopulmonary dysplasia (BPD).** BPD is a complex disease that is poorly defined.[51-54] Historical definitions have included radiographic patterns and the requirement for supplemental O_2 at fixed time points in the infant's life. Immaturity, genetics, malnutrition, O_2 toxicity, and mechanical ventilation all have been implicated in the origin of BPD.[51,55-62]

MINI CLINI

Meconium Aspiration Syndrome

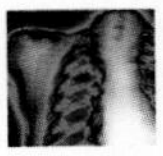

PROBLEM: You are called to the delivery room to attend the delivery of a term infant with meconium-stained amniotic fluid. What should the RT have available for the resuscitation of this infant?

DISCUSSION: The RT should have the standard resuscitation equipment available. Current recommendations for resuscitating a newborn with meconium staining do not include immediate intubation and tracheal suctioning for a vigorous infant. If the infant is depressed and not breathing, the infant should be resuscitated similar to any other depressed and apneic infant, which includes intubation. However, there is no evidence for whether the depressed infant would benefit from intubation and tracheal suctioning.[43]

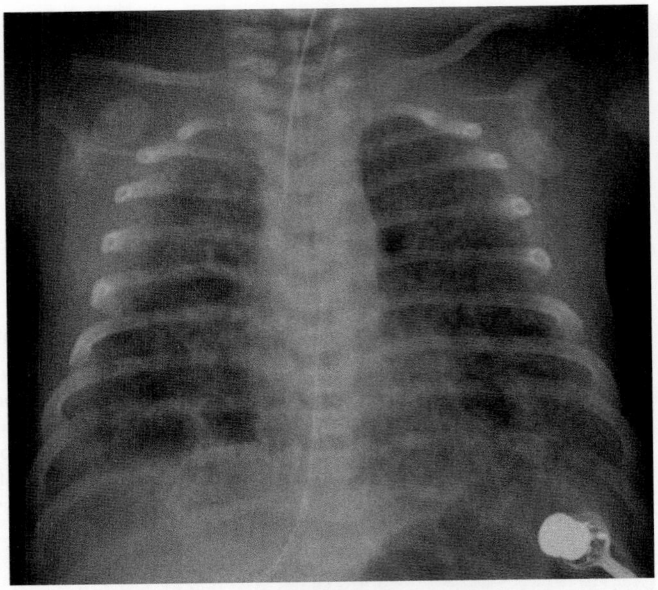

FIGURE 31-5 Radiograph of a patient with BPD. Anteroposterior radiograph shows areas of scarring, atelectasis, emphysema, and cysts. This film is consistent with severe BPD.

Pathophysiology. The development of BPD is complex and involves many pathways. The initiating factors are related to *atelectrauma* (lung collapse) and *volutrauma* (large tidal volume [V_T]). Factors such as hyperoxia and hypoxia, mechanical forces, vascular maldevelopment, inflammation, nutrition, and genetics contribute to the abnormal development of the lung and lead to BPD.[56,59,63-67] *Atelectrauma* is a term coined to describe loss of alveolar volume that is both a consequence and a cause of lung injury. *Volutrauma* is the term used to describe local overinflation (and stretch) of airways and alveoli. Atelectrauma leads to derecuitment (e.g., areas of alveolar collapse) of the lung. Volutrauma leads to damage to airways, pulmonary capillary endothelium, alveolar and airway epithelium, and basement membranes. The combination of atelectrauma and volutrauma synergistically increases lung injury.

Both atelectrauma and volutrauma cause a need for increased supplemental O_2 concentrations. This use of supplemental O_2 leads to overproduction of superoxide, hydrogen peroxide, and perhydroxyl radicals. Preterm infants are particularly susceptible to O_2 radicals because the antioxidant systems develop in the last trimester of pregnancy. Prolonged hyperoxia begins a sequence of lung injury that leads to inflammation, diffuse alveolar damage, pulmonary dysfunction, and death.

The response of the lungs to the combination of trauma and O_2 toxicity is the production and release of soluble mediators. These mediators probably are released from granulocytes residing in the lung. The release of these mediators can injure the alveolar-capillary barrier and induce an inflammatory response.[62] A "new" BPD is being described that shows decreased alveolarization rather than the prominent airway damage of the "old" BPD. This change in the pathologic characteristics of BPD is thought to be related to improvements in ventilator management, the use of surfactant, and processes that interrupt alveolar development (e.g., postnatal steroid therapy).[54,68-70] Some authors speculate that the "new" BPD and "old" BPD are the same disease. The difference is that clinicians are better at performing mechanical ventilation in infants and do less damage to the airway compared with 20 years ago.[71]

Clinical Manifestations. BPD has various clinical manifestations. Some very immature infants may start with little or no O_2 requirement and little or no mechanical ventilation requirement. Progressive respiratory distress develops at approximately 2 to 3 weeks of life, and then the infant needs O_2 and mechanical ventilation. Other immature infants may begin with pneumonia or sepsis and need very high levels of O_2 and mechanical ventilation. In either of these scenarios, progressive vascular leakage and areas of atelectasis and emphysema develop in the lungs, and progressive pulmonary damage occurs. The chest radiograph in severe disease shows areas of atelectasis, emphysema, and fibrosis diffusely intermixed throughout the lung (Figure 31-5).[67,72] Arterial blood gas measurements reveal varying degrees of hypoxemia and hypercapnia secondary to airway obstruction, air trapping, pulmonary fibrosis, and atelectasis. There is a marked increase in airway resistance with an overall decrease in lung compliance.

Treatment. The best management of BPD is prevention. Prevention of atelectrauma and volutrauma begins in the delivery room. Establishment of an optimal FRC without overstretching the lung requires careful attention to detail in providing end-tidal pressure and avoiding large V_T. Surfactant should be delivered early in the course of treatment.

Treatment of infants with BPD involves steps to minimize additional lung damage and prevent pulmonary hypertension and cor pulmonale. Infants with severe

TABLE 31-2

Evaluation of an Infant With Apnea

Possible Cause	Associated Signs	Investigation
Infection	Lethargy, respiratory distress, temperature instability	Complete blood count, sepsis evaluation
Metabolic disorder	Poor feeding, lethargy, jitteriness	Glucose, calcium, electrolyte levels
Impaired oxygenation	Respiratory distress, tachypnea, cyanosis	O_2 monitoring, arterial blood gases, chest radiograph
Maternal drugs	Maternal history, hypotonia, central nervous system depression	Magnesium level, urine drug screen
Intracranial lesion	Abnormal neurologic findings, seizures	Cranial ultrasonography
Environmental	Lethargy	Monitor temperature (infant and environment)
Gastroesophageal reflux	Feeding difficulty	Specific observation, radiographic barium swallow examination

From Stark AR: Disorders of respiratory control in infants. Respir Care 36:673, 1991.

disease may be dependent on supplemental O_2 or mechanical ventilation for months and have symptoms of airway obstruction for years. Therapy usually is supportive throughout the course of the disease. An infant with BPD is given respiratory support as needed. Supplemental O_2 can help decrease the pulmonary hypertension that is common with BPD.

Multiple pharmacologic treatments have been advocated for infants with BPD.[73] Diuretics are given as needed to decrease pulmonary edema; antibiotics are given to manage existing pulmonary infection.[74] Chest physical therapy may help mobilize secretions and prevent further atelectasis. Bronchodilator therapy may be useful in decreasing airway resistance.[75] Steroid therapy with dexamethasone can produce substantial short-term improvement in lung function, often allowing rapid weaning from ventilatory support. However, steroid therapy has little effect on long-term outcome such as mortality and duration of O_2 therapy.[76,77] Steroid therapy also has been implicated in decreased alveolarization and increased developmental delay.[78] Although steroids are still given in clinical practice, they should be used cautiously and only after the risks have been thoroughly explained to the parents.

Control of Breathing

Apnea of Prematurity

Background. Apnea of prematurity is a common, controllable disorder among premature infants. It usually resolves over time.[79-84] Premature infants frequently have periodic respiration, which comprises sequential short apneic episodes of 5 to 10 seconds followed by 10 to 15 seconds of rapid respiration. Apneic spells are abnormal if (1) they last longer than 15 seconds; or (2) they are associated with cyanosis, pallor, hypotonia, or bradycardia.

If no effort to breathe occurs during a spell, the apnea is called *central* apnea. If breathing efforts occur, but obstruction prevents airflow, the apnea is termed *obstructive*. *Mixed* apnea is a combination of the central and obstructive types that starts as obstructive apnea and then develops into central apnea.[79-83,85]

Etiology. Premature infants have immature control of respiratory drive in response to oxygen and carbon dioxide. In mature animals, an increase in alveolar $PaCO_2$ elicits an increase in V_T and respiratory rate. A decrease in FiO_2 below room air also triggers an increase in V_T. Conversely, in premature animals, an increase in $PaCO_2$ temporarily increases V_T but does not increase respiratory rate. A decrease in FiO_2 below room air decreases V_T and respiratory rate. This effect can lead to apnea in a premature infant. Several factors in addition to prematurity can cause apnea in infants. Table 31-2 summarizes the potential causes, associated signs, and diagnostic indicators.[86]

Treatment. Infants with apnea need continuous monitoring of heart and respiratory rates. Continuous noninvasive monitoring of oxygenation by transcutaneous electrode or pulse oximetry is recommended. Most apneic incidents can be quickly terminated with gentle mechanical stimulation, such as picking the infant up, flicking the sole of the foot, or rubbing the skin.[79,81,82,85,87] If the cause of apnea is not prematurity, treatment must be directed at resolving the underlying condition. Table 31-3 outlines current treatment strategies for infants with apnea.[86] Apnea secondary to prematurity responds well to methylxanthines, especially theophylline and caffeine.[82,85,87] These agents stimulate the central nervous system and increase the infant's responsiveness to CO_2. For infants with apnea that is refractory to treatment with theophylline, doxapram can be used.[88-90] However, doxapram is delivered by continuous infusion and has multiple toxicities.

CPAP can also be used to manage infant apnea.[91] Although the mechanism of action is not established, CPAP probably increases FRC and improves arterial partial pressure of oxygen (PaO_2) and $PaCO_2$. CPAP may also stimulate vagal receptors in the lung, increasing the output of the brainstem respiratory centers. Severe or recurrent apnea that is unresponsive to these interventions may necessitate mechanical ventilatory support.

As the respiratory control mechanisms mature, apnea of prematurity normally resolves without intervention.

TABLE 31-3

Treatment Strategies for Infants With Apnea

Treatment	Rationale
Manage underlying cause if identified	Removes precipitating factor
Tactile stimulation	Increases respiratory drive by sensory stimulation
CPAP	Reduces mixed and obstructive apnea by splinting the upper airway
Theophylline or caffeine	Increases respiratory center output and CO_2 response, enhances diaphragm strength, adenosine antagonist
Doxapram	Stimulates respiratory center and peripheral chemoreceptors
Transfusion	Decreases hypoxic depression by increasing O_2-carrying capacity
Mechanical ventilation	Provides support when respiratory effort is inadequate

From Stark AR: Disorders of respiratory control in infants. Respir Care 36:673, 1991.

Apneic spells begin to disappear by week 37 to 44 of postmenstrual age with no apparent long-term effects. Infants who have apnea of prematurity are not at higher risk of sudden infant death syndrome (SIDS) than other infants.

Apnea monitoring can allow infants who are otherwise ready for discharge but still having occasional episodes of apnea to go home.[79,81,85,92-95] However, the presence of a home apnea monitor is a significant inconvenience to the family. Home monitors lack the sophisticated filtering systems of hospital monitors, and they have very frequent false alarms.

Pulmonary Vascular Disease

Persistent Pulmonary Hypertension of the Newborn

Background. **Persistent pulmonary hypertension of the newborn (PPHN)** is a complex syndrome with many causes.[96] The common denominator in PPHN is a return to fetal circulatory pathways, usually because of elevated PVR. This condition results in further right-to-left shunting, severe hypoxemia, and metabolic and respiratory acidosis.

Pathophysiology. In the uterus, the fetus does not use the lungs as a gas exchange organ. PVR is high, and *systemic vascular resistance (SVR)* is low. This condition produces a PVR/SVR ratio greater than 1. A fetus has two anatomic shunts that are not present in older infants, children, or adults: *foramen ovale* and *ductus arteriosus*. With a PVR/SVR ratio greater than 1 and the anatomic shunts, blood flow bypasses the lung either at the atrial level (foramen ovale) or at the pulmonary artery (ductus arteriosus). Intrauterine total pulmonary blood flow and systemic arterial O_2 saturation are low.

In the transition to extrauterine life, PVR decreases owing to gas filling of the lung and increasing PaO_2 in the pulmonary venous circulation. SVR increases with the removal of the placenta from the circulation, and this makes the PVR/SVR ratio less than 1. If PVR does not decrease to allow the PVR/SVR ratio to become less than 1, the infant has PPHN.

There are three fundamental types of PPHN: vascular spasm, increased muscle wall thickness, and decreased cross-sectional area of pulmonary vessels.[97] *Vascular spasm* is an acute event that can be triggered by many different conditions, including hypoxemia, hypoglycemia, hypotension, and pain. *Increased muscle wall thickness* is a chronic condition that develops in utero in response to several different etiologic factors, including chronic fetal hypoxia, increased pulmonary blood flow (e.g., intrauterine closure of the ductus arteriosus), and pulmonary venous obstruction (e.g., total anomalous pulmonary venous return with obstructed below-diaphragm return). *Decreased cross-sectional area* is related to hypoplasia of the lungs and occurs with congenital diaphragmatic hernia, Potter sequence (absent kidneys), and oligohydramnios syndromes (decreased amniotic fluid).

Clinical Manifestations. PPHN should be suspected when an infant has rapidly changing O_2 saturation without changes in FiO_2 or has hypoxemia out of proportion to the lung disease detected with chest radiography or $PaCO_2$ measurement. In infants with a significant shunt through the ductus arteriosus, there usually is a substantial gradient (>5%) between preductal and postductal O_2 saturation. This gradient can be found easily if two pulse oximeters are placed on the infant, one on the right arm and the other on either leg.

Treatment. Initial therapy for PPHN is removal of the underlying cause, such as administration of O_2 for hypoxemia, surfactant for RDS, glucose for hypoglycemia, and inotropic agents for low cardiac output and systemic hypotension. If correction of the underlying problem does not correct hypoxemia, the infant needs intubation and mechanical ventilation. Because pain and anxiety may contribute to PPHN, the infant may need sedation and, frequently, paralysis. If these measures do not improve oxygenation, the next step is HFV. This mode of ventilation allows a higher FRC without a large V_T. Inhaled nitric oxide is considered the next intervention.[98-100] If all of these modalities fail to improve oxygenation, the infant may be a candidate for extracorporeal membrane oxygenation (ECMO).[99,101-103] Even with all of these therapeutic modalities, PPHN remains a complex disease with high morbidity.

Congenital Abnormalities Affecting Respiration

Congenital abnormalities that affect respiration can be divided into several groups: airway diseases, lung malformations, chest wall abnormalities, abdominal wall abnormalities, and diseases of neuromuscular control.

Airway Diseases

Airway abnormalities have three fundamental mechanisms: internal obstruction, external obstruction, and disruption. Internal obstruction includes common problems, such as laryngomalacia, that cause obstructive apnea. Less common problems caused by internal obstruction are tracheomalacia, laryngeal webs, tracheal stenosis, and hemangiomas. All of these diseases usually manifest as a combination of inspiratory stridor, gas trapping, expiratory wheezing, and accessory respiratory muscle activity.

External compression can be caused by hemangiomas, neck or thoracic masses, and vascular rings. These lesions are far less common than diseases caused by internal obstruction, but they are not rare. The symptoms are similar to symptoms of internal obstruction. Neck masses usually are obvious at visual inspection. Intrathoracic masses and vascular rings must be suspected on the basis of the clinical manifestations: noise during the respiratory cycle that worsens with exertion. The infant may have difficulty with swallowing.

Airway disruptions usually are related to *tracheoesophageal fistula (TEF)* in a newborn. This malformation usually is associated with esophageal atresia. There are five types of TEF: esophageal atresia with a proximal fistula, esophageal atresia with a distal fistula, esophageal atresia with both a proximal and a distal fistula, esophageal atresia without either fistula, and an intact esophagus with a so-called H fistula.[104] The most common of these malformations is esophageal atresia with a distal fistula, which accounts for 85% to 90% of all TEFs. The least common is the H fistula. All of these malformations manifest as difficulty swallowing, bubbling and frothing at the mouth, and choking, in particular, during attempts at feeding. These anomalies can occur in isolation or as part of an association of defects. The most common is the *VATER* or *VACTERL* association of *v*ertebral anomalies, imperforate *a*nus, *t*racheo*e*sophageal fistula, and *r*enal or *r*adial anomalies. In *VACTERL*, *c*ardiac anomalies are added, and *r*enal and *l*imb anomalies replace renal or radial anomalies in the acronym. These associated anomalies must be sought in any infant with TEF. TEF is managed with surgical ligation of the fistula and reconnection of the interrupted esophagus.[105] Most infants with TEF have a good outcome; however, some infants have severe malformations that can cause chronic problems. Infants with TEF usually need only supportive respiratory care. They usually do not have lung disease. However, some infants need HFV because the air leak through the fistula can become larger than the airflow to the alveoli.

Lung Malformations

There is a broad spectrum of rare lung malformations that occur in the newborn period.[106-108] These lesions are thought to be part of a continual spectrum of diseases that originate as defects in lung segmentation. The most common is *congenital pulmonary adenomatoid malformation (CPAM)*; this was previously known as *cystic adenomatoid malformation of the lung*. CPAM is classified into five types on the basis of the type and size of the cyst.[109,110] The disease may affect entire lobes of the lung. The affected parts of the lung do not exchange gas and can become infected. The usual treatment is surgical removal of the affected lobe. There is also the potential for malignant transformation.

Some affected fetuses can develop hydrops in utero. Most infants with CPAM have symptoms of lung volume loss. As the mass expands, the normal surrounding lung is compressed. Some CPAMs resolve spontaneously. A few infants have severe cardiorespiratory compromise and need respiratory support and emergency surgery. However, better results are seen when surgery can be performed electively.

Other, less common lung malformations include pulmonary sequestration and lobar emphysema. Both of these diseases involve maldevelopment of lobes of the lung. Sequestration is a primitive, frequently cystic, lung lobe that is not in communication with the tracheobronchial tree and frequently receives no pulmonary vascular blood flow.

Lobar emphysema is an airway malformation that causes gas trapping in a lobe of the lung. These malformations manifest as space-occupying masses within the thorax. They usually are managed with surgical resection.

Congenital Diaphragmatic Hernia

Congenital diaphragmatic hernia is a severe disease that usually manifests in newborns as severe respiratory distress. The pathophysiologic mechanism is a complex combination of lung hypoplasia, including decreased alveolar count and decreased pulmonary vasculature; pulmonary hypertension; and unusual anatomy of the inferior vena cava.[111] This disorder varies between asymptomatic (rare) and severe life-threatening disease (frequent). There are two types of hernia: Bochdalek hernia (lateral and posterior defect, usually on the left) and Morgagni hernia (medial and anterior, may be on either side). Hernias that occur in the right hemidiaphragm may be less severe because the liver can block the defect and decrease the volume of abdominal contents that can enter the thorax.[112]

Some authors speculate that the diaphragmatic hernia complex is a developmental field defect and not just a simple cascade of events related to a hole in the diaphragm. This theory is partly based on long-term outcomes of survivors with diaphragmatic hernias. These survivors frequently have severe scoliosis in the direction of the diaphragm defect. They also frequently have severe esophageal reflux disease.

Most cases of congenital diaphragmatic hernia can be diagnosed in utero with ultrasonography. Physical examination may yield the following findings: scaphoid abdomen (because the abdominal contents are in the thorax), decreased breath sounds, displaced heart sounds (because the heart is pushed away from the hernia), and severe cyanosis (from lung hypoplasia and pulmonary hypertension). The diagnosis is established with chest radiography.

The general treatment of infants with congenital diaphragmatic hernia involves neonatologists and pediatric surgeons. Initial treatment is insertion of an endotracheal tube, paralysis, and mechanical ventilation. A large sump tube is placed in the stomach and connected to continuous suction. These therapies allow adequate ventilation and oxygenation and prevent gas insufflation of the intestine. Most centers delay surgical repair for several days to allow the natural decrease in PVR. On day 7 to 10 of life, a surgeon closes the defect. This scenario occurs only for infants with easily correctable pulmonary hypertension. Infants with severe pulmonary hypertension may need HFV and ECMO. At some centers, the diaphragm is repaired during ECMO. Most centers try to wean the infant from ECMO and then perform the repair. Despite all these advanced therapies, the mortality for this disease is high.[113] Survival depends on many complex variables (e.g., liver herniation into the thorax, fetal head-to-lung ratio, initial PaO_2 and $PaCO_2$).[113,114]

Abdominal Wall Abnormalities

Because all newborns are primarily abdominal breathers, the abdominal wall is an intrinsic part of the respiratory system. Large defects in the abdominal wall can cause severe respiratory compromise.[115] One of the most common of these defects is *omphalocele*. An omphalocele is an abdominal wall defect that involves the insertion of the umbilical cord. The umbilical cord goes into the omphalocele. The bowel of an infant with an omphalocele is usually covered by a membrane that looks like the surface of the umbilical cord. Occasionally, the omphalocele membrane ruptures and exposes the bowel of the infant. Omphaloceles must be distinguished from gastroschisis. Gastroschisis is an abdominal wall defect that is completely separate from the insertion of the umbilical cord. The bowel of an infant with a gastroschisis is not covered by a membrane. Usually only large omphaloceles cause respiratory distress. When they are greater than 10 cm in diameter, these defects can cause severe respiratory distress and frequently necessitate prolonged mechanical ventilation.

Neuromuscular Control

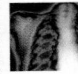

Many diseases of poor neuromuscular control affect newborns,[116-119] including spinal muscular atrophy, congenital myasthenia gravis, and myotonic dystrophy. These diseases frequently necessitate respiratory support in the newborn and pediatric periods. The morbidity and mortality of these diseases are extremely variable. New technologies may allow noninvasive respiratory support of some patients.[120] Some diseases can be quite severe in the newborn period and be relieved with age. It is important to make an accurate diagnosis to be able to estimate prognosis and to provide genetic counseling. Many of these diseases are inherited with known inheritance patterns.

> **MINI CLINI**
>
> **Delivery of an Infant With an Abdominal Wall Defect**
>
> **PROBLEM:** The RT is called to the delivery room to assist in the delivery of a term infant with an abdominal wall defect. What should the RT consider for assisting this infant?
>
> **DISCUSSION:** There are many types of abdominal wall defects. The two most common are gastroschisis and omphalocele. These anomalies can be differentiated by whether the insertion of the umbilical cord into the abdomen is involved in the defect. In a gastroschisis, the umbilical cord inserts directly into the abdomen and is separate from the defect. In an omphalocele, the umbilical cord inserts directly into the defect. Although there is usually a membrane covering the bowel in an omphalocele, if the membrane has ruptured, the only means of distinguishing an omphalocele is by the umbilical cord insertion.
>
> Most infants with these abdominal wall defects are term. Most do not have significant lung disease. An abdominal wall defect increases the intraabdominal pressure. It pushes the diaphragm up into the thorax decreasing FRC. The RT should be aware that these patients will need support of their FRC. Typically, if the FRC can be supported with CPAP or PEEP, the infant will not need high rates or a high V_T to achieve adequate gas exchange.

Congenital Heart Disease

A full discussion of congenital heart disease is beyond the scope of this chapter. However, basic knowledge of the common defects is essential to good practice in pediatric and neonatal respiratory care. Congenital heart diseases usually are divided into two large categories: cyanotic and acyanotic heart disease. *Cyanotic* heart diseases are diseases in which blood shunts from right to left, bypassing the lungs, and is deoxygenated. *Acyanotic* heart diseases are diseases in which blood shunts from left to right causing congestive heart failure. Figure 31-6 compares normal cardiac anatomy with the features of the five most common congenital defects.

Cyanotic Heart Diseases

The two most common cyanotic heart diseases are tetralogy of Fallot and transposition of the great arteries.

Tetralogy of Fallot. Tetralogy of Fallot is a defect that includes (1) obstruction of right ventricular outflow (pulmonary stenosis), (2) ventricular septal defect (a hole between the right and left ventricles), (3) dextroposition of

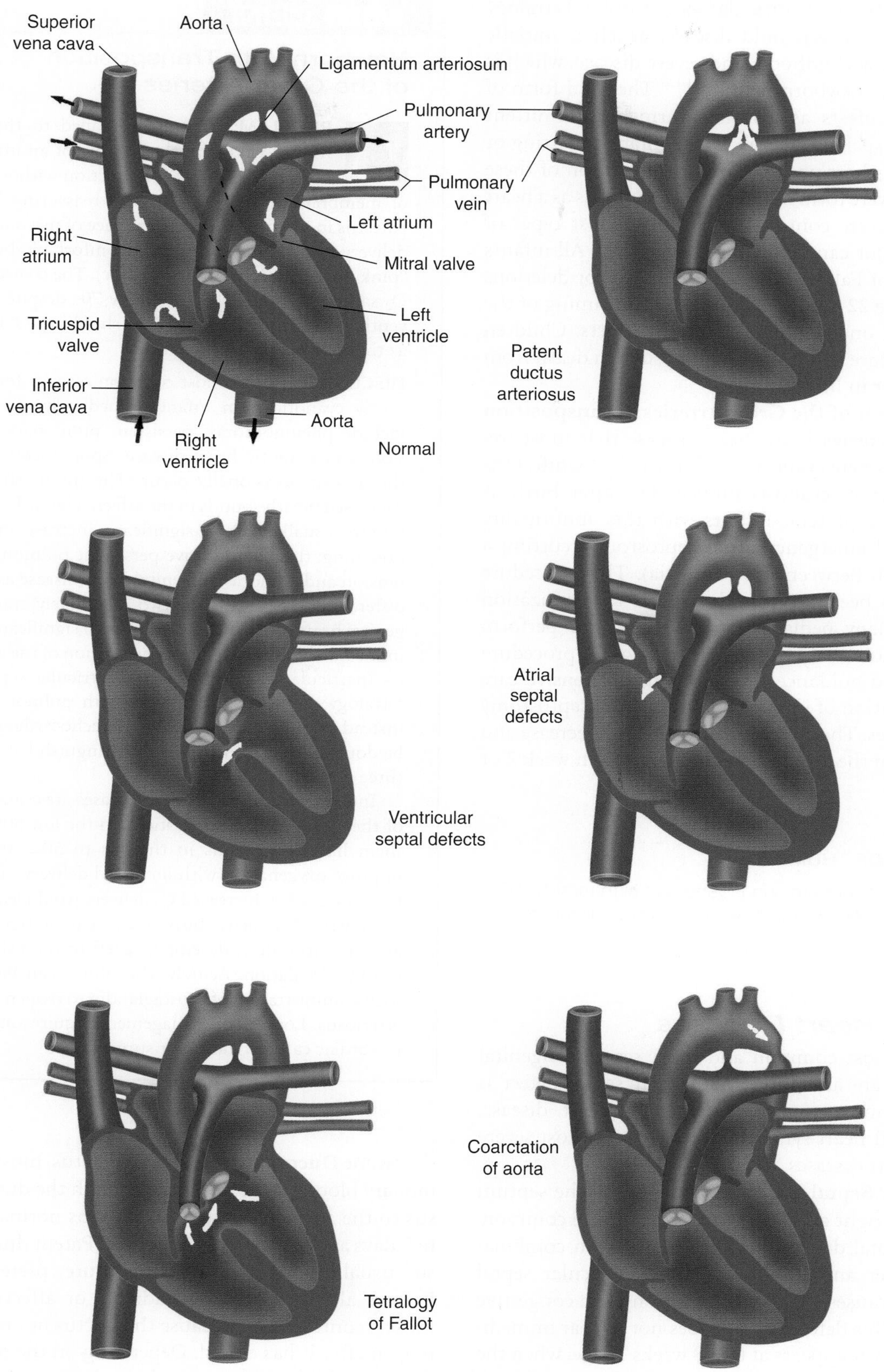

FIGURE 31-6 Normal flow of blood through the heart and some congenital defects that cause abnormal flow. (Modified from Jacob S, Francone C, Lossow WJ: Structure and function in man, ed 5, Philadelphia, 1982, Saunders.)

the aorta, and (4) right ventricular hypertrophy. Tetralogy of Fallot varies between mild disease, which is initially diagnosed in early childhood, and severe disease, which is diagnosed in the newborn period.[121-123] The mild form of the disease manifests as a heart murmur, intermittent severe cyanotic spells, a history of the infant squatting or entering a knee-chest position, or a combination of these features. The severe form of the disease manifests as a heart murmur and severe continuous cyanosis. Most types of tetralogy of Fallot can be managed surgically. All infants with tetralogy of Fallot should be evaluated for deletions on chromosome 22 (22q11).[124] The type and timing of the surgery depend on the anatomy of the defects. Children with this defect are at increased risk of sudden death from arrhythmia later in life.

Transposition of the Great Arteries. **Transposition of the great arteries** is the heart disease that most frequently causes severe cyanosis.[125-128] It usually manifests as moderate to severe cyanosis immediately after birth. A murmur may be present. Infants with this abnormality frequently need emergency atrial septostomy (cutting a hole in the wall between the two atria). This procedure historically has been performed in heart catheterization laboratories. Many pediatric cardiologists who perform invasive procedures have begun performing this procedure with ultrasound guidance in the neonatal intensive care unit. The condition of infants who need atrial septostomy usually stabilizes. The goal is to allow PVR to decrease and then to perform the arterial switch operation in week 2 or 3 of life.

RULE OF THUMB

An infant with profound cyanosis at birth most likely has cyanotic heart disease or persistent pulmonary hypertension.

Acyanotic Heart Diseases

Some of the most common and most severe congenital heart diseases are acyanotic. Ventricular septal defect is probably the most common congenital heart disease. Hypoplastic left heart syndrome is one of the most severe congenital heart diseases.

Ventricular Septal Defect. Defects along the septum separating the right and left ventricles are quite common. Ventricular septal defect can occur alone or in combination with other anomalies. A simple ventricular septal defect usually causes left-to-right shunting and congestive heart failure. This defect usually does not appear immediately after birth. It appears at 6 to 8 weeks of age, when the PVR has decreased enough that the shunt becomes large.

Atrial Septal Defect. The most common type of atrial septal defect is a small, slitlike opening that persists after closure of the foramen ovale. An isolated atrial septal defect is of little clinical importance.

MINI CLINI

Newborn With Transposition of the Great Arteries

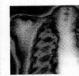

PROBLEM: The RT is called to the delivery room to assist in the delivery of an infant to be born by repeat cesarean section without rupture of membranes. The fetus has had reassuring heart rate patterns in utero. There is no evidence of meconium. After delivery, the infant is breathing comfortably but fails to "pink up" (i.e., the infant is cyanotic). The transcutaneous O_2 saturation stabilizes in the low 70s despite mask-bag ventilation with FiO_2 of 1. What should the RT consider as the source of this problem?

DISCUSSION: The most common reasons for a significantly cyanotic term infant immediately after delivery include pneumothorax, persistent pulmonary hypertension, and cyanotic heart disease. Spontaneous pneumothorax can occasionally occur. The infant should have decreased breath sounds in the affected hemithorax. These infants usually have a significant increase in work of breathing; this should leave persistent pulmonary hypertension and cyanotic congenital heart disease as the main differential diagnoses. The two most likely cyanotic congenital heart diseases to manifest with significant cyanosis immediately after birth are transposition of the great arteries (particularly with an intact ventricular septum) and tetralogy of Fallot (particularly with pulmonary atresia instead of pulmonary stenosis). An echocardiogram must be done as soon as possible to distinguish between these three possibilities.

Infants with cyanotic heart diseases are cyanotic. Some of these infants have saturations in the low 80s. Some of them have saturations in the 40s to 50s. Attempts to improve oxygenation with increased delivery of O_2 would be unsuccessful. Increased O_2 delivery would lead to problems with O_2 toxicity. Improvement in systemic oxygenation occurs only by developing a left-to-right shunt in the central circulation. Acutely, this shunt can be managed with administration of prostaglandin to reopen the ductus arteriosus. Long-term management requires intervention by cardiac catheterization or surgery.

Patent Ductus Arteriosus. In a fetus, most of the pulmonary blood flow is shunted through the ductus arteriosus to the aorta. Closure of the ductus normally occurs 5 to 7 days after birth of a term infant. Patent ductus arteriosus usually is a disease of immature, preterm infants. Factors altering pressure gradients or affecting smooth muscle contraction can cause the ductus not to close or to reopen after it has closed. Depending on the pressure gradients established, shunting through an open ductus may be either right to left (pulmonary pressure greater than aortic) or left to right (aortic pressure greater than pulmonary). Treatment is either pharmacologic (indomethacin) or surgical (ligation). In recent years, the best timing of

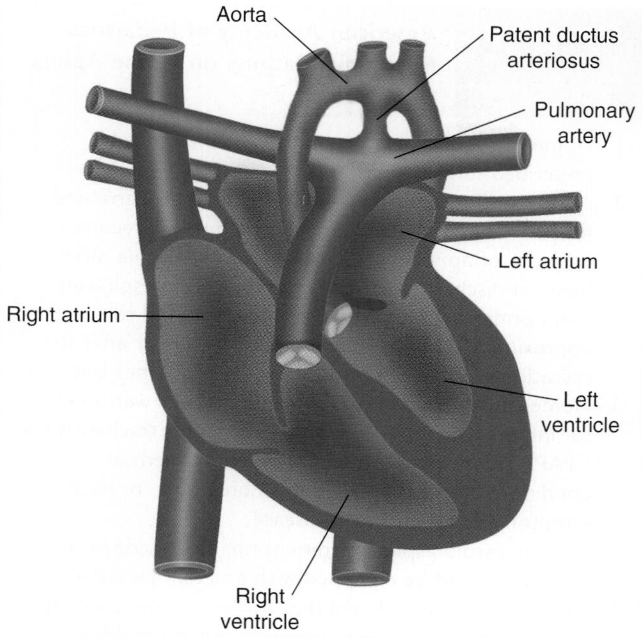

FIGURE 31-7 Hypoplastic left heart syndrome.

Box 31-1	Factors Associated With Increased Frequency of Sudden Infant Death Syndrome

MATERNAL CHARACTERISTICS

- Younger than 20 years
- Poor
- African-American, Native American, or Alaskan Native
- Previous fetal loss
- Cigarette smoking
- Narcotic abuse
- Illness during pregnancy
- Inadequate prenatal care

INFANT CHARACTERISTICS AT BIRTH

- Male gender
- Premature birth
- Small for gestational age
- Low Apgar score
- Resuscitation with O_2 and ventilation at birth
- Second or third in birth order or of a multiple birth
- Sibling death from SIDS

From Koff PB, Eitzman DV, Neu J: Neonatal and pediatric respiratory care, ed 2, St Louis, 1993, Mosby.

treatment and the treatment mechanism have become quite controversial.[129]

Left Ventricular Outflow Obstructions. Hypoplastic left heart syndrome (Figure 31-7), interrupted aortic arch, and coarctation of the aorta have in common obstruction of left ventricular outflow.[130-132] They all manifest in the newborn period with symptoms of acute heart failure. Systemic blood flow depends on patency of the ductus arteriosus. When the ductus spontaneously closes (usually at 5 to 7 days of age), severe congestive heart failure develops. The symptoms range from moderate respiratory distress to complete cardiovascular collapse. Initial treatment is intravenous administration of prostaglandin E_1. Most infants with these defects need support with mechanical ventilation. These infants do not have lung disease. The pressures and rates used should be set appropriately.

There are standard surgical repairs for both interrupted aortic arch and coarctation of the aorta. Hypoplastic left heart syndrome has several accepted treatments, including a palliative surgical procedure (Norwood) and transplantation.[130-132] Neither the Norwood procedure nor transplantation is ideal, and each option has significant associated problems. The decision must be made in consultation with the family.

NEONATAL RESUSCITATION

Resuscitation of a newborn is a subset of resuscitation techniques. Most infant resuscitations occur in the delivery room. Although these resuscitations can range from minimal intervention to full resuscitation, more than 90% of them can be successfully dealt with by stimulation, ensuring the presence of an airway, and providing breathing support.[133-135] RTs are a vital part of any resuscitation team. Their expertise in establishing and supporting an airway and initiating respiratory support is essential. It is beyond the scope of this chapter to delineate the guidelines of neonatal resuscitation. The reader should refer to the neonatal resuscitation guidelines published by the American Academy of Pediatrics (AAP).[133-139]

PEDIATRIC RESPIRATORY DISORDERS

Compared with the common cardiopulmonary diseases in the neonatal period, the pulmonary conditions that occur among older infants and children commonly result from airway obstruction caused by bacterial or viral infections. Other entities discussed in this section include asthma, SIDS, gastroesophageal reflux disease (GERD), and CF.

Sudden Infant Death Syndrome

Sudden infant death syndrome (SIDS) is the leading cause of death (40%) among infants younger than 1 year in the United States. Approximately 7000 infants die of SIDS each year in the United States.[83,92,140] A presumptive diagnosis is based on the conditions of death in which a previously healthy infant dies unexpectedly, usually during sleep. Autopsy shows that many infants who die of SIDS have evidence of repeated episodes of hypoxemia or ischemia. Factors associated with increased frequency of SIDS are presented in Box 31-1. If the infant is found and resuscitation is successful, the diagnosis would be *apparent life-threatening event.*

Box 31-2 Infant Characteristics Near the Time of Death from Sudden Infant Death Syndrome

- Age <6 months (peak between 1 month and 3 months)
- Winter season
- Asleep at night
- Mild illness in week before death
- History of apparent life-threatening event
- Prone sleep position

Etiology

The cause of SIDS is unknown. Apnea of prematurity is not a predisposing factor, and there is no evidence that immaturity of the respiratory centers is a cause. Although infants in families in which two or more SIDS deaths have occurred are at slightly higher risk, there is no evidence of a genetic link. The best knowledge of SIDS comes from population or epidemiologic studies and is summarized in Box 31-2. An infant who dies of SIDS typically is a preterm African-American boy born to a poor mother younger than 20 years who received inadequate prenatal care. Infants 1 to 3 months old are most susceptible, and death is most likely to occur at night during the winter. The risk of SIDS also is high among infants who previously experienced an apparent life-threatening event. Such an event occurs when an infant becomes apneic, cyanotic, or limp enough to frighten the parent or caregiver. The prone sleeping position has been strongly associated with increased risk of SIDS. It is difficult to differentiate death of SIDS from death of intentional suffocation. The possibility of intentional suffocation must be investigated but with great sensitivity.[141]

Prevention

Because of the unknown causation and unexpected occurrence, there is no therapy for SIDS. Prevention is the goal. Successful prevention requires that infants at high risk be identified through a history of risk factors and documented monitoring or event recording. After identification that an infant is at risk, the family is trained in apnea monitoring and *cardiopulmonary resuscitation (CPR)*. The AAP recommends placing infants in either the supine or the side-lying position for the first 6 months of life and reducing soft objects in the infant's sleeping environment.[92,140-142] To define the need and appropriate approach for home monitoring of infants, the AAP has developed a policy statement on infantile apnea and home monitoring.[92] The AAP recommendations for the need for and use of home monitoring are summarized in Box 31-3.

Box 31-3 American Academy of Pediatrics Recommendations on Home Apnea Monitoring

1. Home cardiorespiratory monitoring should not be prescribed to prevent SIDS.
2. Home cardiorespiratory monitoring may be warranted for premature infants who are at high risk of recurrent episodes of apnea, bradycardia, and hypoxemia after hospital discharge. The use of home cardiorespiratory monitoring in these infants should be limited to approximately 43 weeks postmenstrual age or after the cessation of extreme episodes, whichever comes last.
3. Home cardiorespiratory monitoring may be warranted for infants who are technology-dependent (tracheostomy, CPAP), have unstable airways, have rare medical conditions affecting regulation of breathing, or have symptomatic chronic lung disease.
4. If home cardiorespiratory monitoring is prescribed, the monitor should be equipped with an event recorder.
5. Parents should be advised that home cardiorespiratory monitoring has not been proven to prevent sudden unexpected deaths in infants.
6. Pediatricians should continue to promote proven practices that decrease the risk of SIDS, including supine sleep position, safe sleeping environments, and elimination of prenatal and postnatal exposure to tobacco smoke.

From Committee on Fetus and Newborn: American Academy of Pediatrics: Apnea, sudden infant death syndrome, and home monitoring. Pediatrics 111(4 Pt 1):914–917, 2003.

Gastroesophageal Reflux Disease

Gastroesophageal reflux disease (GERD) is the regurgitation of stomach contents into the esophagus and is common in childhood. Some causes of GERD are not pathologic. There is general agreement that there are important interactions between GERD and various disorders of the respiratory system.[143] Respiratory problems caused by gastroesophageal reflux include reactive airways disease, aspiration pneumonia, laryngospasm, stridor, chronic cough, choking spells, and apnea.[143-147] GERD should be considered when an infant has faced a sudden life-threatening event and when an older child has unexplained chronic head and neck problems. GERD can be diagnosed with esophageal pH testing, upper gastrointestinal contrast studies, and gastric scintiscan. When GERD has been diagnosed, medical therapy can begin.[148-150] Occasional cases that do not respond to medical management may require surgical intervention.

Bronchiolitis

Bronchiolitis is an acute infection of the lower respiratory tract, usually caused by *respiratory syncytial virus (RSV)*. Nearly 1 in 10 infants younger than 2 years acquires a bronchiolitis infection. The outcome is generally good, although approximately 1% of infants hospitalized for bronchiolitis die of respiratory failure. Infants most prone to respiratory failure as a consequence of bronchiolitis are very young and immunodeficient and have comorbidity, such as congenital heart disease, BPD, CF, or childhood asthma.[151-155]

Clinical Manifestations

The clinical manifestations of bronchiolitis are inflammation and obstruction of the small bronchi and bronchioles. Bronchiolitis commonly occurs soon after a viral upper respiratory infection. The infant may have a slight fever with an intermittent cough. After a few days, signs of respiratory distress develop, in particular, dyspnea and tachypnea. Progressive inflammation and narrowing of the airways cause inspiratory and expiratory wheezing and increase airway resistance. A chest radiograph shows signs of hyperinflation with areas of consolidation. The diagnosis of RSV infection can be established by immunofluorescent assay the same day and assists in the implementation of a treatment plan.

Prophylaxis. In recent years, passive immunization for RSV has become available.[156-158] Initially, passive immunization was recommended only for preterm infants with BPD. However, passive immunization is now recommended for infants younger than 2 years who require medical therapy for chronic lung disease, infants born at less than 32 weeks' gestational age, and infants with congenital heart disease who have cardiovascular compromise (Box 31-4).[156-160]

Treatment. Treatment of a patient with bronchiolitis varies with the severity of the infection and the clinical signs and symptoms. Many patients can be treated at home with humidification and oral decongestants. Patients with more severe symptoms (apnea) and comorbidity usually are hospitalized, and treatment is directed at relieving the airway obstruction and associated hypoxemia. Hospitalized children frequently are treated with systemic hydration and O_2 hood, croup tent, or nasal cannula and assisted with airway clearance.[154,155,161-163]

Box 31-4 American Academy of Pediatrics Recommendations for Respiratory Syncytial Virus Prophylaxis

INDICATIONS FOR RSV PROPHYLAXIS

Infants with chronic lung disease
Infants born at <32 weeks' gestational age
Infants born at 32 to 35 weeks' gestational age who are at high risk of severe infection and <90 days of age
If two or more of following risks are present
- Child care attendance
- School-age siblings
- Exposure to environmental air pollutants
- Congenital abnormalities of the airways
- Severe neuromuscular disease

Infants with hemodynamically significant congenital heart disease (cyanotic and acyanotic)
Following cardiopulmonary bypass

Antibiotics may be administered to control secondary bacterial infections. If bronchiolitis progresses to acute respiratory failure, mechanical ventilation is required. Because of the obstructive nature of this disorder, low respiratory rates and long expiratory times may be needed to prevent air trapping. Heliox has been used for severe airways disease requiring mechanical ventilation.[164] Vigorous bronchial hygiene, occasionally including tracheobronchial aspiration, usually is needed to maintain a patent airway.

Croup

Croup is a viral disorder of the upper airway that normally results in subglottic swelling and obstruction. Termed *laryngotracheobronchitis,* viral croup is usually caused by the parainfluenza virus and is the most common form of airway obstruction in children 6 months to 6 years old. RSV and influenza virus are less common as causative agents. Bacterial superinfection with *Staphylococcus aureus,* group A *Streptococcus pyogenes,* or *Haemophilus influenzae* may worsen croup.

Clinical Manifestations

Symptoms become evident after 2 or 3 days of nasal congestion, fever, and coughing. A child typically has slow, progressive inspiratory and expiratory stridor and a barking cough. As the disease progresses, dyspnea, cyanosis, exhaustion, and agitation occur. A radiograph of the upper airway is helpful in confirming the diagnosis and ruling out epiglottitis but is usually not needed in most cases of croup.[84] Classic croup is seen on an anteroposterior radiograph as characteristic subglottic narrowing of the trachea, called the *steeple sign* (Figure 31-8).

Treatment

The evaluation and treatment of a child with croup must focus on the degree of respiratory distress and associated clinical findings. If stridor is mild or occurs only on exertion and cyanosis is not present, hospitalization is generally not required, and the child is treated at home. If there is stridor at rest (accompanied by harsh breath sounds, suprasternal retractions, and cyanosis with breathing of room air), hospitalization is indicated. The traditional treatment of a child with mild to moderate croup has involved cool mist therapy with or without supplemental O_2. However, there is no evidence that this practice is beneficial.[165] Corticosteroids and epinephrine have been shown to have the greatest benefit for decreasing the length and severity of respiratory symptoms associated with viral croup.[166,167] The addition of budesonide has been shown to reduce the severity of symptoms in mild to moderate cases of croup.[166,167] Progressive worsening of the clinical signs despite treatment indicates the need for intubation and mechanical ventilation. Heliox has been used for infants and children with severe disease. However, there is insufficient evidence to show whether this is beneficial.[168]

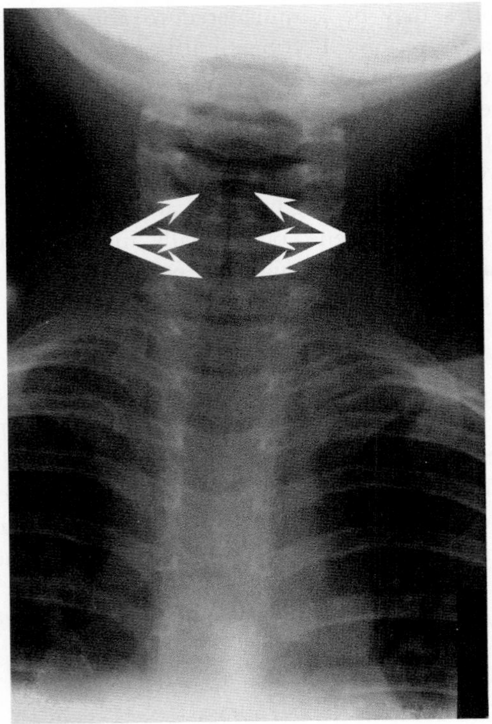

FIGURE 31-8 Anteroposterior chest radiograph of a patient with croup. Subglottic narrowing typical of croup is evident *(arrows)*.

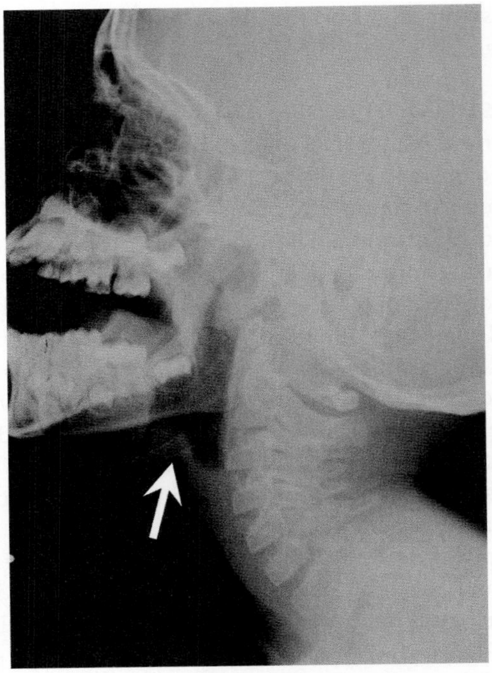

FIGURE 31-9 Lateral radiograph of the neck of a patient with epiglottitis. The thumb sign is prominent *(arrow)*.

Epiglottitis

Epiglottitis is an acute and often life-threatening infection of the upper airway that causes severe obstruction secondary to supraglottic swelling. Evidence suggests that the incidence of epiglottitis is decreasing among children and increasing in adults,[169] probably because of the use of vaccines. The most common cause is *H. influenzae* type B infection. Other organisms that are increasingly found to be causes of acute epiglottitis include group A *S. pneumoniae, S. aureus, Klebsiella pneumoniae, Haemophilus parainfluenzae,* and beta-hemolytic streptococci (groups A, B, C, and F).[170]

Clinical Manifestations

A child with epiglottitis usually has a high fever, sore throat, stridor, and labored breathing.[170-172] The patient does not have a croupy bark but instead has a muffled voice. Older children may report a sore throat and difficulty swallowing. Difficulty swallowing may cause drooling. Lateral radiographs of the neck (Figure 31-9) show the epiglottis is markedly thickened and flattened (thumb sign) and the aryepiglottic folds are swollen; the vallecula may not be visualized. Visual examination of the upper airway is dangerous in these children and always should be performed in a controlled setting by personnel expert in emergency intubation. Inadvertent traction of the tongue can cause further and immediate swelling of the epiglottis and abrupt and total upper airway obstruction. Children with suspected epiglottitis should be accompanied by personnel expert in emergency intubation during any transport for diagnostic procedures.

MINI CLINI

Extubation

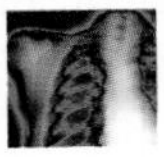

PROBLEM: A 3-year-old child underwent emergency intubation 5 days earlier for epiglottitis. The physician asks the RT to evaluate the patient for extubation. What would the RT evaluate before making the decision for extubation? What equipment would the RT want to have at the bedside during extubation?

DISCUSSION: Clinical examination of vital signs (e.g., body temperature), breath sounds, sensorium, and degree of airway leak should be considered. Equipment for rapid reintubation must be at the bedside, including racemic epinephrine for aerosolization.

Extubation of any patient should take into consideration the pathophysiologic condition that led to intubation. In this case, the RT should look for evidence that the infection is resolving and that the upper airway is no longer inflamed. A lack of fever for at least 12 hours and visual inspection of the throat that reveals minimal inflammation would be most helpful. After extubation, close monitoring must be performed for evidence of airway compromise. Cool mist may be helpful to minimize inflammation after extubation.

Treatment

Children with epiglottitis need elective intubation under general anesthesia in the operating room. Tracheostomy may be needed if the patient's condition warrants it; however, this procedure is rarely used. There should be no attempt to lie the child down or attempts to intubate until the child is sedated. Premature attempts at intubation can precipitate acute airway obstruction and respiratory arrest. After an airway is secured, a sample for bacterial culture should be obtained, and antibiotic therapy should be started. Corticosteroids may decrease the swelling.[170] Children with an endotracheal tube should be sedated and restrained to prevent inadvertent extubation. Extubation should not be attempted until an upper airway leak is readily detected.

Cystic Fibrosis

Cystic fibrosis (CF) is the most common lethal genetic disease among whites in the United States. It is inherited as an autosomal recessive trait that affects approximately 30,000 persons in the United States.[173] The disease is caused by a genetic mutation of the gene coding for a large protein that controls the movement of chloride ions through the cell membrane.[174] This protein is called the *cystic fibrosis transmembrane conductance regulator (CFTR)*. Movement of chloride ions is vital to the proper production and regulation of secretions. CFTR can be mutated in more than 1000 different ways to cause CF.[175] Some CF mutations cause more severe CFTR dysfunction than others. The variety of mutations that can be inherited explains some of the variability in the severity of clinical CF. In CF, abnormalities of chloride movement through the surface of exocrine glands cause most of the clinical manifestations.

RULE OF THUMB

Both parents must be carriers of the CF gene for any child to be born with CF. If both parents carry the CF gene, the chance that CF will develop in offspring is 1 : 4.

Clinical Manifestations

Patients with CF experience abnormalities in nearly all organs with exocrine function. The most severely affected organs are the sweat glands, pancreas, and lungs. Normal sweat is produced as a saline solution that has much of the salt removed on its way to the surface of the skin. Sweat glands of patients with CF are unable to remove salt from sweat properly.[176] As a result, the skin of patients with CF develops a salty taste, and they are prone to dehydration during hot weather.[177] The sweat chloride test used for diagnosis of the disease is based on the high salt concentration in the sweat of patients with CF.[178] Most patients with CF also have exocrine pancreatic insufficiency, which usually starts in infancy. Exocrine pancreatic insufficiency dramatically reduces the number of digestive enzymes, and patients lacking digestive enzymes do not break down large proteins, carbohydrates, and fats for absorption, causing malnutrition and diarrhea. Digestion of fats is particularly compromised in patients with CF. These patients often have deficiencies of the fat-soluble vitamins A, D, E, and K and have large amounts of undigested fat in the stool (steatorrhea).

Complications of lung disease are the leading cause of death in patients with CF. Patients have recurring pulmonary infections, often beginning during the first few years of life. The organisms associated with these infections frequently include *S. aureus, H. influenzae,* and *Pseudomonas aeruginosa.* Patients with CF have bronchiolitis and bronchiectasis and produce copious amounts of thick, mucoid secretions. Mucus sometimes obstructs the airways and causes atelectasis, pneumonia, or lung abscesses. As the disease progresses, the lungs become hyperinflated, and bronchiectatic exacerbations increase in frequency. Patients with end-stage CF have severe debility with marked hypoxemia and may develop pulmonary hypertension and cor pulmonale.

Diagnosis

The diagnosis of CF is suspected when a patient has clinical manifestations of the disease or has close family members with CF. Findings of recurrent pulmonary infections or failure to grow as rapidly as expected are clinical clues that often prompt physicians to initiate testing for CF. The diagnosis usually is confirmed with the sweat chloride test, which is done with electrical stimulation of the skin to produce sweat (iontophoresis). In a child, a sweat chloride level greater than 60 mEq/L confirms the diagnosis of CF.[179]

Monitoring

The lung disease of CF is progressive. Careful monitoring of progression and response to treatment is routinely accomplished with spirometry and chest films. Cultures of sputum are often used to monitor for airway flora and resistance.

Treatment

The deficiency of pancreatic enzymes that occurs in patients with CF is managed with pancreatic enzyme supplementation. Several important steps are taken to help patients with CF maintain lung function. Regular chest physical therapy improves lung function and clearance of secretions.[180] When patients with CF become teenagers or young adults, they may have no partner to assist with chest physiotherapy. For these patients, strenuous exercise, external pneumatic vests,[181] PEEP devices, or autogenic drainage may substitute for regular chest physiotherapy. Another mucus clearance adjunct is inhaled recombinant deoxyribonuclease (DNase or DNAase). The routine daily use of inhaled DNase reduces the frequency of respiratory infections.[182,183] The daily use of nebulized 7% saline both preserves lung function and decreases the likelihood of bronchiectatic flare-ups.[184]

Antibiotics directed against the usual infectious organisms are required with each bronchiectatic exacerbation. As CF progresses, the bacteria causing exacerbations can become progressively more resistant to antibiotic treatments. Intravenous antibiotics are often required if a bronchiectatic exacerbation is caused by resistant bacteria. A nebulized form of the antibiotic tobramycin is used to prevent infection. When inhaled tobramycin is used twice daily every other month, there is a marked reduction in the number of bronchiectatic exacerbations.[185] The regular use of azithromycin helps preserve lung function and decreases the frequency of pulmonary flare-ups.[186]

High doses of the antiinflammatory drug ibuprofen reduce the rate of lung function loss in patients younger than 13 years old.[187] Many patients with CF have asthma symptoms. These patients benefit from bronchodilators.

Lung transplantation is commonly performed in patients with advanced CF lung disease. Double-lung transplantation is the most commonly used form of lung transplantation in the treatment of patients with CF. New therapies for CF focus on improving the function of specific CFTR mutations.[188]

Prognosis

When CF was first described more than 60 years ago, children with the disease rarely lived more than a few years. Today, median survival of patients with CF is nearly 38 years.[173]

ROLE OF THE RESPIRATORY THERAPIST IN NEONATAL AND PEDIATRIC RESPIRATORY DISORDERS

As with any clinical situation, the role of the RT in the special environment of neonatal and pediatric care is to use his or her expertise and knowledge to improve the outcome of the patients. Because there are significant differences in the diseases, pathophysiologies, and function of respiratory support equipment between adult and pediatric patients, the RT must be thoroughly familiar with all aspects of pediatric care. The old adage "children are not little adults" is very true. Equally, newborns are not little children. Each of these age groups has unique characteristics that require specialized knowledge and experience. The role of the RT should be part of a team that is dedicated to the health and well-being of these fragile patients.

Additionally, the RT has an important role in the education and emotional support not only of the pediatric patient but also of the families and caregivers. Frequently, the RT is at the bedside of patients when the parents or caregivers are present. The RT is invaluable in helping patients and parents understand the respiratory goals of each individual patient.

SUMMARY CHECKLIST

- The incidence of RDS increases with decreasing gestational age.
- A qualitative decrease in surfactant increases alveolar surface tension forces in RDS patients. This process causes alveoli to become unstable and collapse and leads to atelectasis and increased work of breathing.
- The definitive diagnosis of RDS usually is made with chest radiography. Diffuse, hazy, reticulogranular densities with the presence of air bronchograms and low lung volumes are typical of RDS.
- TTN, often referred to as type II RDS, is probably the most common respiratory disorder of the newborn. The cause of TTN is unclear but is most likely related to delayed clearance of fetal lung liquid. Infants with TTN usually respond readily to low FiO_2 by O_2 hood or nasal cannula. Infants who need higher FiO_2 levels may benefit from CPAP.
- MAS is a disease of term and near-term infants. It involves aspiration of meconium into the central airways of the lung. This disorder usually is associated with perinatal depression and asphyxia.
- The best management of BPD is prevention. Prevention of atelectrauma and volutrauma begins in the delivery room.
- PPHN should be suspected when an infant has rapidly changing O_2 saturation without changes in FiO_2 or has hypoxemia out of proportion to the lung disease detected with a chest radiograph or on the basis of $PaCO_2$.
- Congenital diaphragmatic hernia is a severe disease that usually manifests as severe respiratory distress in the newborn period. The pathophysiologic mechanism is a complex combination of lung hypoplasia, including decreased alveolar count and decreased pulmonary vasculature; pulmonary hypertension; and unusual anatomy of the inferior vena cava.
- The cause of SIDS is unknown. Apnea of prematurity is not a predisposing factor, and there is no evidence that immaturity of the respiratory centers is a cause.
- Bronchiolitis is an acute infection of the lower respiratory tract usually caused by RSV.
- Croup is a viral disorder of the upper airway that normally results in subglottic swelling and obstruction. Termed *laryngotracheobronchitis,* viral croup is caused by the parainfluenza virus and is the most common form of airway obstruction in children 6 months to 6 years old.
- Epiglottitis is an acute, often life-threatening infection of the upper airway that causes severe obstruction secondary to supraglottic swelling. Evidence suggests that the incidence of epiglottitis is decreasing among children, probably because of the use of vaccines. A child with epiglottitis usually has a high fever, sore throat, stridor, and labored breathing.

- CF is the most common lethal genetic disorder among whites. It is inherited as an autosomal recessive trait that affects approximately 30,000 people in the United States. Treatment of CF lung disease requires aggressive efforts to control pulmonary infections and clear pulmonary secretions. RTs often play a key role in treating patients with CF.

References

1. Sweet DG, Halliday HL: The use of surfactants in 2009. Arch Dis Child Educ Pract Ed 94:78–83, 2009.
2. Sweet DG, Carnielli V, Greisen G, et al: European Consensus Guidelines on the Management of Neonatal Respiratory Distress Syndrome in Preterm Infants—2010 Update. Neonatology 97:402–417, 2010.
3. Soll R, Ozek E: Multiple versus single doses of exogenous surfactant for the prevention or treatment of neonatal respiratory distress syndrome. Cochr Database Syst Rev (1):CD000141, 2009.
4. Soll RF: Current trials in the treatment of respiratory failure in preterm infants. Neonatology 95:368–372, 2009.
5. Wirbelauer J, Speer CP: The role of surfactant treatment in preterm infants and term newborns with acute respiratory distress syndrome. J Perinatol 29:S18–S22, 2009.
6. Sekar KC, Corff KE: To tube or not to tube babies with respiratory distress syndrome. J Perinatol 29:S68–S72, 2009.
7. Verder H, Bohlin K, Kamper J, et al: Nasal CPAP and surfactant for treatment of respiratory distress syndrome and prevention of bronchopulmonary dysplasia. Acta Paediatr 98:1400–1408, 2009.
8. Dani C, Corsini I, Bertini G, et al: The INSURE method in preterm infants of less than 30 weeks' gestation. J Matern Fetal Neonatal Med 23:1024–1029, 2010.
9. Lal MK, Sinha SK: Review: Surfactant respiratory therapy using Surfaxin/sinapultide. Ther Adv Respir Dis 2:339–344, 2008.
10. Soll RF: Synthetic surfactant for respiratory distress syndrome in preterm infants. Cochrane Database Syst Rev (2):CD001149, 2000.
11. Soll RF: Prophylactic synthetic surfactant for preventing morbidity and mortality in preterm infants. Cochrane Database Syst Rev (2):CD001079, 2000.
12. Soll RF: Prophylactic natural surfactant extract for preventing morbidity and mortality in preterm infants. Cochrane Database Syst Rev (2):CD000511, 2000.
13. Soll RF: Natural surfactant extract versus synthetic surfactant for neonatal respiratory distress syndrome. Cochrane Database Syst Rev (2):CD000144, 2000.
14. Davis JM, Russ GA, Metlay L, et al: Short-term distribution kinetics of intratracheally administered exogenous lung surfactant. Pediatr Res 31:445–450, 1992.
15. Eaton DC, Chen J, Ramosevac S, et al: Regulation of Na+ channels in lung alveolar type II epithelial cells. Proc Am Thorac Soc 1:10–16, 2004.
16. Eaton DC, Helms MN, Koval M, et al: The contribution of epithelial sodium channels to alveolar function in health and disease. Annu Rev Physiol 71:403–423, 2009.
17. Eaton DC, Malik B, Bao HF, et al: Regulation of epithelial sodium channel trafficking by ubiquitination. Proc Am Thorac Soc 7:54–64, 2010.
18. Jain L: Respiratory morbidity in late-preterm infants: prevention is better than cure! Am J Perinatol 25:75–78, 2008.
19. Jain L: Morbidity and mortality in late-preterm infants: more than just transient tachypnea! J Pediatr 151 :445–446, 2007.
20. Jain L: Alveolar fluid clearance in developing lungs and its role in neonatal transition. Clin Perinatol 26:585–599, 1999.
21. Jain L, Eaton DC: Physiology of fetal lung fluid clearance and the effect of labor. Semin Perinatol 30:34–43, 2006.
22. Jain L, Eaton DC: Alveolar fluid transport: a changing paradigm. Am J Physiol Lung Cell Mol Physiol 290:L646–L648, 2006.
23. Jain L, Ferre C, Vidyasagar D: Cesarean delivery of the breech very-low-birth-weight infant: does it make a difference? J Matern Fetal Med 7:28–31, 1998.
24. Jain L, Wapner R: Cesarean delivery: its impact on the mother and newborn, part I. Preface. Clin Perinatol 35:xi–xii, 2008.
25. Jain L, Wapner RJ: Cesarean delivery: its impact on the mother and newborn, part II. Preface. Clin Perinatol 35:xv–xvi, 2008.
26. Beall MH, van den Wijngaard JPHM, van Gemert MJC, et al: Regulation of amniotic fluid volume. Placenta 28:824–832, 2007.
27. Beall MH, Wang S, Yang B, et al: Placental and membrane aquaporin water channels: correlation with amniotic fluid volume and composition. Placenta 28:421–428, 2007.
28. Ross MG, Beall MH: Cesarean section and transient tachypnea of the newborn. Am J Obstet Gynecol 195:1496–1497, 2006.
29. Ross MG, Beall MH, Christenson PD: Amniotic fluid volume and perinatal outcome. Am J Obstet Gynecol 196:e17, 2007.
30. Katz VL, Bowes WA, Jr: Meconium aspiration syndrome: reflections on a murky subject. Am J Obstet Gynecol 166 (1 Pt 1):171–183, 1992.
31. de Beaufort AJ: Early human development at the perinatal interface: meconium stained amniotic fluid (MSAF) and meconium aspiration syndrome (MAS). Early Hum Dev 85: 605, 2009.
32. Hofmeyr GJ, Xu H: Amnioinfusion for meconium-stained liquor in labour. Cochrane Database Syst Rev (1):CD000014, 2010.
33. Ivanov VA, Gewolb IH, Uhal BD: A new look at the pathogenesis of the meconium aspiration syndrome: a role for fetal pancreatic proteolytic enzymes in epithelial cell detachment. Pediatr Res 68:221–224, 2010.
34. Kaapa P, Soukka H: Phospholipase A2 in meconium-induced lung injury. J Perinatol 28(Suppl 3):S120–S122, 2008.
35. Saugstad OD, Tollofsrud PA, Lindenskov P, et al: Toxic effects of different meconium fractions on lung function: new therapeutic strategies for meconium aspiration syndrome. J Perinatol 28(Suppl 3):S113–S115, 2008.
36. Vidyasagar D, Zagariya A: Studies of meconium-induced lung injury: inflammatory cytokine expression and apoptosis. J Perinatol 28(Suppl 3):S102–S107, 2008.
37. Wang PW, Jeng MJ, Wang LS, et al: Surfactant lavage decreases systemic interleukin-1beta production in meconium aspiration syndrome. Pediatr Int 52:432–437, 2010.
38. Rossi EM, Philipson EH, Williams TG, et al: Meconium aspiration syndrome: intrapartum and neonatal attributes. Am J Obstet Gynecol 161:1106–1110, 1998.
39. Jain L, Vidyasagar D: Controversies in neonatal resuscitation. Pediatr Ann 24:540–545, 1995.
40. Vain NE, Szyld EG, Prudent LM, et al: What (not) to do at and after delivery? Prevention and management of meconium aspiration syndrome. Early Hum Dev 85:621–626, 2009.

41. van Ierland Y, de Boer M, de Beaufort AJ: Meconium-stained amniotic fluid: discharge vigorous newborns. Arch Dis Child Fetal Neonatal Ed 95:F69–F71, 2010.
42. Halliday HL: Endotracheal intubation at birth for preventing morbidity and mortality in vigorous, meconium-stained infants born at term. Cochrane Database Syst Rev (1): CD000500, 2001.
43. Wiswell TE: Delivery room management of the meconium-stained newborn. J Perinatol 28(Suppl 3):S19–S26, 2008.
44. Dargaville PA, Copnell B, Mills JF, et al: Randomized controlled trial of lung lavage with dilute surfactant for meconium aspiration syndrome. J Pediatr 158:383–389.e2, 2011.
45. Halliday HL, Speer CP, Robertson B: Treatment of severe meconium aspiration syndrome with porcine surfactant. Collaborative Surfactant Study Group. Eur J Pediatr 155: 1047–1051, 1996.
46. Jeng MJ, Soong WJ, Lee YS: Effective lavage volume of diluted surfactant improves the outcome of meconium aspiration syndrome in newborn piglets. Pediatr Res 66: 107–112, 2009.
47. Greenough A, Dimitriou G, Prendergast M, et al: Synchronized mechanical ventilation for respiratory support in newborn infants. Cochrane Database Syst Rev (1): CD000456, 2008.
48. Soll RF, Dargaville P: Surfactant for meconium aspiration syndrome in full term infants. Cochrane Database Syst Rev (2):CD002054, 2000.
49. Finer N, Barrington K: Nitric oxide for respiratory failure in infants born at or near term. Cochrane Database Syst Rev (4):CD000399, 2006.
50. Ward M, Sinn J: Steroid therapy for meconium aspiration syndrome in newborn infants. Cochrane Database Syst Rev (4):CD003485, 2003.
51. Bancalari E, Claure N: Definitions and diagnostic criteria for bronchopulmonary dysplasia. Semin Perinatol 30:164–170, 2006.
52. Northway WH, Jr: Bronchopulmonary dysplasia: twenty-five years later. Pediatrics 89(5 Pt 1):969–973, 1992.
53. Northway WH, Jr, Rosan RC, Porter DY: Pulmonary disease following respiratory therapy of hyaline-membrane disease: bronchopulmonary dysplasia. N Engl J Med 276:357–368, 1967.
54. Merritt TA, Deming DD, Boynton BR: The "new" bronchopulmonary dysplasia: challenges and commentary. Semin Fetal Neonatal Med 14:345–357, 2009.
55. Bancalari E, Gerhardt T: Bronchopulmonary dysplasia. Pediatr Clin North Am 33:1–23, 1986.
56. Bhandari A, Bhandari V: Bronchopulmonary dysplasia: an update. Indian J Pediatr 74:73–77, 2007.
57. Bhandari V, Gruen JR: The genetics of bronchopulmonary dysplasia. Semin Perinatol 30:185–191, 2006.
58. Biniwale MA, Ehrenkranz RA: The role of nutrition in the prevention and management of bronchopulmonary dysplasia. Semin Perinatol 30:200–208, 2006.
59. Chess PR, D'Angio CT, Pryhuber GS, et al: Pathogenesis of bronchopulmonary dysplasia. Semin Perinatol 30:171–178, 2006.
60. Frank L, Sosenko IR: Undernutrition as a major contributing factor in the pathogenesis of bronchopulmonary dysplasia. Am Rev Respir Dis 138:725–729, 1988.
61. Chambers HM, van Velzen D: Ventilator-related pathology in the extremely immature lung. Pathology 21:79–83, 1989.
62. Nickerson BG: Bronchopulmonary dysplasia: chronic pulmonary disease following neonatal respiratory failure. Chest 87:528–535, 1985.
63. Abman SH, Wolfe RR, Accurso FJ, et al: Pulmonary vascular response to oxygen in infants with severe bronchopulmonary dysplasia. Pediatrics 75:80–84, 1985.
64. Aghai ZH, Faqiri S, Saslow JG, et al: Angiopoietin 2 concentrations in infants developing bronchopulmonary dysplasia: attenuation by dexamethasone. J Perinatol 28:149–155, 2008.
65. Aghai ZH, Saslow JG, Meniru C, et al: High-mobility group box-1 protein in tracheal aspirates from premature infants: relationship with bronchopulmonary dysplasia and steroid therapy. J Perinatol 30:610–615, 2010.
66. Bose CL, Dammann CE, Laughon MM: Bronchopulmonary dysplasia and inflammatory biomarkers in the premature neonate. Arch Dis Child Fetal Neonatal Ed 93:F455–F461, 2008.
67. Coalson JJ: Pathology of new bronchopulmonary dysplasia. Semin Neonatol 8:73–81, 2003.
68. Nadeau K, Jankov RP, Tanswell AK, et al: Lgl1 is suppressed in oxygen toxicity animal models of bronchopulmonary dysplasia and normalizes during recovery in air. Pediatr Res 59:389–395, 2006.
69. Nakanishi H, Sugiura T, Streisand JB, et al: TGF-beta-neutralizing antibodies improve pulmonary alveologenesis and vasculogenesis in the injured newborn lung. Am J Physiol Lung Cell Mol Physiol 293:L151–L161, 2007.
70. Stenmark KR, Abman SH: Lung vascular development: implications for the pathogenesis of bronchopulmonary dysplasia. Annu Rev Physiol 67:623–661, 2005.
71. Ambalavanan N, Carlo WA: Ventilatory strategies in the prevention and management of bronchopulmonary dysplasia. Semin Perinatol 30:192–199, 2006.
72. Coalson JJ: Pathology of bronchopulmonary dysplasia. Semin Perinatol 30:179–184, 2006.
73. Baveja R, Christou H: Pharmacological strategies in the prevention and management of bronchopulmonary dysplasia. Semin Perinatol 30:209–218, 2006.
74. Blanchard PW, Brown TM, Coates AL: Pharmacotherapy in bronchopulmonary dysplasia. Clin Perinatol 14:881–910, 1987.
75. Wilkie RA, Bryan MH: Effect of bronchodilators on airway resistance in ventilator-dependent neonates with chronic lung disease. J Pediatr 111:278–282, 1987.
76. Benini F, Rubaltelli FF, Griffith P, et al: Dexamethasone in the treatment of bronchopulmonary dysplasia. Acta Paediatr Scand Suppl 360:108–112, 1987.
77. Harkavy KL, Scanlon JW, Chowdhry PK, et al: Dexamethasone therapy for chronic lung disease in ventilator- and oxygen-dependent infants: a controlled trial. J Pediatr 115: 979–983, 1989.
78. Grier DG, Halliday HL: Corticosteroids in the prevention and management of bronchopulmonary dysplasia. Semin Neonatol 8:83–91, 2003.
79. Silvestri JM, Lister G, Corwin MJ, et al: Factors that influence use of a home cardiorespiratory monitor for infants: the collaborative home infant monitoring evaluation. Arch Pediatr Adolesc Med 159:18–24, 2005.
80. Hunt CE: Small for gestational age infants and sudden infant death syndrome: a confluence of complex conditions. Arch Dis Child Fetal Neonatal Ed 92:F428–F429, 2007.
81. Hunt CE: Ontogeny of autonomic regulation in late preterm infants born at 34-37 weeks postmenstrual age. Semin Perinatol 30:73–76, 2006.
82. Hunt CE: Sudden infant death syndrome and other causes of infant mortality: diagnosis, mechanisms, and risk for recurrence in siblings. Am J Respir Crit Care Med 164:346–357, 2001.

83. Hunt CE, Brouillette RT: Sudden infant death syndrome: 1987 perspective. J Pediatr 110:669–678, 1987.
84. Hunt CE, Corwin MJ, Lister G, et al: Precursors of cardiorespiratory events in infants detected by home memory monitor. Pediatr Pulmonol 43:87–98, 2008.
85. Hunt CE, Corwin MJ, Baird T, et al: Cardiorespiratory events detected by home memory monitoring and one-year neurodevelopmental outcome. J Pediatr 145:465–471, 2004.
86. Stark A: Disorders of respiratory control in infants. Respir Care 36:673, 1991.
87. Hunt CE, Lesko SM, Vezina RM, et al: Infant sleep position and associated health outcomes. Arch Pediatr Adolesc Med 157:469–474, 2003.
88. Henderson-Smart D, Steer P: Doxapram treatment for apnea in preterm infants. Cochrane Database Syst Rev (4):CD000074, 2004.
89. Henderson-Smart DJ, Davis PG: Prophylactic doxapram for the prevention of morbidity and mortality in preterm infants undergoing endotracheal extubation. Cochrane Database Syst Rev (3):CD001966, 2000.
90. Henderson-Smart DJ, Steer P: Doxapram versus methylxanthine for apnea in preterm infants. Cochrane Database Syst Rev (4):CD000075, 2000.
91. Abu-Shaweesh JM, Martin RJ: Neonatal apnea: what's new? Pediatr Pulmonol 43:937–944, 2008.
92. Committee on Fetus and Newborn: American Academy of Pediatrics: Apnea, sudden infant death syndrome, and home monitoring. Pediatrics 111(4 Pt 1):914–917, 2003.
93. Kelly MM: The medically complex premature infant in primary care. J Pediatr Health Care 20:367–373, 2006.
94. Kelly MM: Primary care issues for the healthy premature infant. J Pediatr Health Care 20:293–299, 2006.
95. Hall KL, Zalman B: Evaluation and management of apparent life-threatening events in children. Am Fam Physician 71:2301–2308, 2005.
96. Steinhorn RH: Neonatal pulmonary hypertension. Pediatr Crit Care Med 11(2 Suppl):S79–S84, 2010.
97. Gao Y, Raj JU: Regulation of the pulmonary circulation in the fetus and newborn. Physiol Rev 90:1291–1335, 2010.
98. Golombek SG: The use of inhaled nitric oxide in newborn medicine. Heart Dis 2:342–347, 2000.
99. Walsh MC, Stork EK: Persistent pulmonary hypertension of the newborn: rational therapy based on pathophysiology. Clin Perinatol 28:609–627, 2001.
100. Weinberger B, Weiss K, Heck DE, et al: Pharmacologic therapy of persistent pulmonary hypertension of the newborn. Pharmacol Ther 89:67–79, 2001.
101. Kinsella JP, Abman SH: Inhaled nitric oxide: current and future uses in neonates. Semin Perinatol 24:387–395, 2000.
102. Kinsella JP, Abman SH: Clinical approach to inhaled nitric oxide therapy in the newborn with hypoxemia. J Pediatr 136:717–726, 2000.
103. Somme S, Liu DC: New trends in extracorporeal membrane oxygenation in newborn pulmonary diseases. Artif Organs 25:633–637, 2001.
104. El-Gohary Y, Gittes GK, Tovar JA: Congenital anomalies of the esophagus. Semin Pediatr Surg 19:186–193, 2010.
105. Holland AJA, Fitzgerald DA: Oesophageal atresia and tracheo-oesophageal fistula: current management strategies and complications. Paediatr Respir Rev 11:100–107, 2010.
106. Azizkhan R, Crombleholme T: Congenital cystic lung disease: contemporary antenatal and postnatal management. Pediatr Surg Int 24:643–657, 2008.
107. Bush A: Prenatal presentation and postnatal management of congenital thoracic malformations. Early Hum Dev 85:679–684, 2009.
108. Correia-Pinto J, Gonzaga S, Huang Y, et al: Congenital lung lesions—underlying molecular mechanisms. Semin Pediatr Surg 19:171–179, 2010.
109. Stocker JT: Cystic lung disease in infants and children. Fetal Pediatr Pathol 28:155–184, 2009.
110. Stocker JT: Congenital pulmonary airway malformation—a new name for and an expanded classification of congenital cystic adenomatoid malformation of the lung. Histopathology 41(Suppl 2):424–430, 2002.
111. Cullen ML, Klein MD, Philippart AI: Congenital diaphragmatic hernia. Surg Clin North Am 65:1115–1138, 1985.
112. Keijzer R, Puri P: Congenital diaphragmatic hernia. Semin Pediatr Surg 19:180–185, 2010.
113. Hoffman SB, Massaro AN, Gingalewski C, et al: Predictors of survival in congenital diaphragmatic hernia patients requiring extracorporeal membrane oxygenation: CNMC 15-year experience. J Perinatol 30:546–552, 2010.
114. de Buys Roessingh A, Dinh-Xuan A: Congenital diaphragmatic hernia: current status and review of the literature. Eur J Pediatr 168:393–406, 2009.
115. Islam S: Clinical care outcomes in abdominal wall defects. Curr Opin Pediatr 20:305–310, 2008.
116. Kennedy JD, Martin AJ: Chronic respiratory failure and neuromuscular disease. Pediatr Clin North Am 56:261–273, 2009.
117. Panitch HB: The pathophysiology of respiratory impairment in pediatric neuromuscular diseases. Pediatrics 123(Suppl 4):S215–S218, 2009.
118. Schroth MK: Special considerations in the respiratory management of spinal muscular atrophy. Pediatrics 123 (Suppl 4):S245–S249, 2009.
119. Yang ML, Finkel RS: Overview of paediatric neuromuscular disorders and related pulmonary issues: diagnostic and therapeutic considerations. Paediatr Respir Rev 11:9–17, 2007.
120. Benditt JO: Initiating noninvasive management of respiratory insufficiency in neuromuscular disease. Pediatrics 123(Suppl 4):S236–S238, 2009.
121. Duro RP, Moura C, Leite-Moreira A: Anatomophysiologic basis of tetralogy of Fallot and its clinical implications. Rev Port Cardiol 29:591–630, 2010.
122. Naguib MA, Dob DP, Gatzoulis MA: A functional understanding of moderate to complex congenital heart disease and the impact of pregnancy. Part II: tetralogy of Fallot, Eisenmenger's syndrome and the Fontan operation. Int J Obstet Anesth 19:306–312, 2010.
123. Starr J: Tetralogy of Fallot: yesterday and today. World J Surg 34:658–668, 2010.
124. Momma K: Cardiovascular anomalies associated with chromosome 22q11.2 deletion syndrome. Am J Cardiol 105:1617–1624, 2010.
125. Dob DP, Naguib MA, Gatzoulis MA: A functional understanding of moderate to complex congenital heart disease and the impact of pregnancy. Part I: the transposition complexes. Int J Obstet Anesth 19:298–305, 2010.
126. Martins P, Castela E: Transposition of the great arteries. Orphanet J Rare Dis 3:27, 2008.
127. Martins P, Tran V, Price G, et al: Extending the surgical boundaries in the management of the left ventricular outflow tract obstruction in discordant ventriculo-arterial connections—a surgical and morphological study. Cardiol Young 18:124–134, 2008.
128. Skinner J, Hornung T, Rumball E: Transposition of the great arteries: from fetus to adult. Heart 94:1227–1235, 2008.
129. Benitz WE: Treatment of persistent patent ductus arteriosus in preterm infants: time to accept the null hypothesis? J Perinatol 30:241–252, 2010.

130. Barron DJ, Kilby MD, Davies B, et al: Hypoplastic left heart syndrome. Lancet 374:551–564, 2009.
131. Stumper O: Hypoplastic left heart syndrome. Postgrad Med J 86:183–188, 2010.
132. Wernovsky G, Ghanayem N, Ohye RG, et al: Hypoplastic left heart syndrome: consensus and controversies in 2007. Cardiol Young 17(Suppl 2):75–86, 2010.
133. Kattwinkel J, Perlman JM, Aziz K, et al: Part 15: Neonatal resuscitation: 2010 American Heart Association Guidelines for Cardiopulmonary Resuscitation and Emergency Cardiovascular Care. Circulation 122(18 Suppl 3):S909–S919, 2010.
134. Kattwinkel J, Perlman JM, Aziz K, et al: Neonatal resuscitation: 2010 American Heart Association Guidelines for Cardiopulmonary Resuscitation and Emergency Cardiovascular Care. Pediatrics 126:e1400–e1413, 2010.
135. Perlman JM, Wyllie J, Kattwinkel J, et al: Part 11: Neonatal resuscitation: 2010 International Consensus on Cardiopulmonary Resuscitation and Emergency Cardiovascular Care Science with Treatment Recommendations. Circulation 122(16 Suppl 2):S516–S538, 2010.
136. Berg MD, Schexnayder SM, Chameides L, et al: Pediatric basic life support: 2010 American Heart Association Guidelines for Cardiopulmonary Resuscitation and Emergency Cardiovascular Care. Pediatrics 126:e1345–e1360, 2010.
137. Kleinman ME, Chameides L, Schexnayder SM, et al: Pediatric advanced life support: 2010 American Heart Association Guidelines for Cardiopulmonary Resuscitation and Emergency Cardiovascular Care. Pediatrics 126:e1361–e1399, 2010.
138. Kleinman ME, de Caen AR, Chameides L, et al: Part 10: Pediatric Basic and Advanced Life Support: 2010 International Consensus on Cardiopulmonary Resuscitation and Emergency Cardiovascular Care Science with Treatment Recommendations. Circulation 122(16 Suppl 2):S466–S515, 2010.
139. Perlman JM, Wyllie J, Kattwinkel J, et al: Neonatal resuscitation: 2010 International Consensus on Cardiopulmonary Resuscitation and Emergency Cardiovascular Care Science with Treatment Recommendations. Pediatrics 126:e1319–e1344, 2010.
140. Hunt CE, Hauck FR: Sudden infant death syndrome. Can Med Assoc J 174:1861–1869, 2006.
141. American Academy of Pediatrics Task Force on Sudden Infant Death Syndrome: The changing concept of sudden infant death syndrome: diagnostic coding shifts, controversies regarding the sleeping environment, and new variables to consider in reducing risk. Pediatrics 116:1245–1255, 2005.
142. Grazel R, Phalen AG, Polomano RC: Implementation of the American Academy of Pediatrics recommendations to reduce sudden infant death syndrome risk in neonatal intensive care units: an evaluation of nursing knowledge and practice. Adv Neonatal Care 10:332–342, 2010.
143. Tolia V, Vandenplas Y: Systematic review: the extra-oesophageal symptoms of gastro-oesophageal reflux disease in children. Aliment Pharmacol Ther 29:258–272, 2009.
144. Bhatia J, Parish A: GERD or not GERD: the fussy infant. J Perinatol 29(Suppl 2):S7–S11, 2009.
145. Golski CA, Rome ES, Martin RJ, et al: Pediatric specialists' beliefs about gastroesophageal reflux disease in premature infants. Pediatrics 125:96–104, 2010.
146. Sherman PM, Hassall E, Fagundes-Neto U, et al: A global, evidence-based consensus on the definition of gastroesophageal reflux disease in the pediatric population. Am J Gastroenterol 104:1278–1295, 2009.
147. Thakkar K, Boatright RO, Gilger MA, et al: Gastroesophageal reflux and asthma in children: a systematic review. Pediatrics 125:e925–e930, 2010.
148. Higginbotham TW: Effectiveness and safety of proton pump inhibitors in infantile gastroesophageal reflux disease. Ann Pharmacother 44:572–576, 2010.
149. Horvath A, Dziechciarz P, Szajewska H: The effect of thickened-feed interventions on gastroesophageal reflux in infants: systematic review and meta-analysis of randomized, controlled trials. Pediatrics 122:e1268–e1277, 2008.
150. Sopo SM, Radzik D, Calvani M: Does treatment with proton pump inhibitors for gastroesophageal reflux disease (GERD) improve asthma symptoms in children with asthma and GERD? A systematic review. J Invest Allergol Clin Immunol 19:1–5, 2009.
151. Anne BC, Christina CC, Grady KO, et al: Lower respiratory tract infections. Pediatr Clin North Am 56:1303–1321, 2009.
152. Ralston S, Hill V: Incidence of apnea in infants hospitalized with respiratory syncytial virus bronchiolitis: a systematic review. J Pediatr 155:728–733, 2009.
153. Vicencio AG: Susceptibility to bronchiolitis in infants. Curr Opin Pediatr 22:302–306, 2010.
154. Wainwright C: Acute viral bronchiolitis in children—a very common condition with few therapeutic options. Paediatr Respir Rev 11:39–45, 2010.
155. Zorc JJ, Hall CB: Bronchiolitis: recent evidence on diagnosis and management. Pediatrics 125:342–349, 2010.
156. Fitzgerald DA: Preventing RSV bronchiolitis in vulnerable infants: the role of palivizumab. Paediatr Respir Rev 10:143–147, 2009.
157. Wang D, Cummins C, Bayliss S, et al: Immunoprophylaxis against respiratory syncytial virus (RSV) with palivizumab in children: a systematic review and economic evaluation. Health Technol Assess 12:1–86, 2008.
158. Vogel AM, Lennon DR, Broadbent R, et al: Palivizumab prophylaxis of respiratory syncytial virus infection in high-risk infants. J Paediatr Child Health 38:550–554, 2002.
159. Carbonell-Estrany X, Bont L, Doering G, et al: Clinical relevance of prevention of respiratory syncytial virus lower respiratory tract infection in preterm infants born between 33 and 35 weeks gestational age. Eur J Clin Microbiol Infect Dis 27:891–899, 2008.
160. Nokes JD, Cane PA: New strategies for control of respiratory syncytial virus infection. Curr Opin Infect Dis 21:639–643, 2008.
161. Wacogne I: Nebulised hypertonic saline reduced the severity of illness in infants with bronchiolitis. Arch Dis Child Educ Pract Ed 95:168, 2010.
162. Fernandes RM, Bialy LM, Vandermeer B, et al: Glucocorticoids for acute viral bronchiolitis in infants and young children. Cochrane Database Syst Rev (10):CD004878, 2010.
163. Mitchell I: Treatment of RSV bronchiolitis: drugs, antibiotics. Paediatr Respir Rev 10(Suppl 1):14–15, 2009.
164. Liet JM, Ducruet T, Gupta V, et al: Heliox inhalation therapy for bronchiolitis in infants. Cochrane Database Syst Rev (4):CD006915, 2010.
165. Moore M, Little P: Humidified air inhalation for treating croup: a systematic review and meta-analysis. Fam Pract 24:295–301, 2007.
166. Bjornson CL, Johnson DW: Croup. Lancet 371:329–339, 2008.
167. Cherry JD: Croup. N Engl J Med 358:384–391, 2008.
168. Vorwerk C, Coats T: Heliox for croup in children. Cochrane Database Syst Rev (2):CD006822, 2010.
169. Berger G, Landau T, Berger S, et al: The rising incidence of adult acute epiglottitis and epiglottic abscess. Am J Otolaryngol 24:374–383, 2003.

170. Sobol SE, Zapata S: Epiglottitis and croup. Otolaryngol Clin North Am 41:551–566, 2008.
171. Rotta AT, Wiryawan B: Respiratory emergencies in children. Respir Care 48:248–258, 2003.
172. Shah S, Sharieff GQ: Pediatric respiratory infections. Emerg Med Clin North Am 25:961–979, 2007.
173. Cystic Fibrosis Foundation: www.cff.org. Accessed February 14, 2011.
174. Anderson MP, Gregory RJ, Thompson S, et al: Demonstration that CFTR is a chloride channel by alteration of its anion selectivity. Science 253:202–205, 1991.
175. Cystic fibrosis mutation database: www.genet.sickkids.on.ca/cftr. Accessed February 12, 2011.
176. Quinton PM, Bijman J: Higher bioelectric potentials due to decreased chloride absorption in the sweat glands of patients with cystic fibrosis. N Engl J Med 308:1185–1189, 1983.
177. Di Sant'Agnese PA: Abnormal electrolyte composition of sweat in cystic fibrosis of the pancreas. Pediatrics 23:549, 1953.
178. Gibson LE, Cooke RE: A test for concentration of electrolytes in sweat in cystic fibrosis of the pancreas utilizing pilocarpine by iontophoresis. Pediatrics 23:545–549, 1959.
179. Stern RC: The diagnosis of cystic fibrosis. N Engl J Med 336:487–491, 1997.
180. Thomas J, Cook DJ, Brooks D: Chest physical therapy management of patients with cystic fibrosis: a meta-analysis. Am J Respir Crit Care Med 151(3 Pt 1):846–850, 1995.
181. Arens R, Gozal D, Omlin KJ, et al: Comparison of high frequency chest compression and conventional chest physiotherapy in hospitalized patients with cystic fibrosis. Am J Respir Crit Care Med 150:1154–1157, 1994.
182. Fuchs HJ, Borowitz DS, Christiansen DH, et al: Effect of aerosolized recombinant human DNase on exacerbations of respiratory symptoms and on pulmonary function in patients with cystic fibrosis. The Pulmozyme Study Group. N Engl J Med 331:637–642, 1994.
183. Jones AP, Wallis C: Dornase alfa for cystic fibrosis. Cochrane Database Syst Rev (3):CD001127, 2010.
184. Elkins MR, Robinson M, Rose BR, et al: A controlled trial of long-term inhaled hypertonic saline in patients with cystic fibrosis. N Engl J Med 354:229–240, 2006.
185. Ramsey BW, Pepe MS, Quan JM, et al: Intermittent administration of inhaled tobramycin in patients with cystic fibrosis. Cystic Fibrosis Inhaled Tobramycin Study Group. N Engl J Med 340:23–30, 1999.
186. Wolter J, Seeney S, Bell S, et al: Effect of long term treatment with azithromycin on disease parameters in cystic fibrosis: a randomised trial. Thorax 57:212–216, 2002.
187. Konstan MW, Byard PJ, Hoppel CL, et al: Effect of high-dose ibuprofen in patients with cystic fibrosis. N Engl J Med 332:848–854, 1995.
188. Accurso FJ, Rowe SM, Clancy JP, et al: Effect of VX-770 in persons with cystic fibrosis and the G551D-CFTR mutation. N Engl J Med 363:1991–2003, 2010.

SECTION V

BASIC THERAPEUTICS

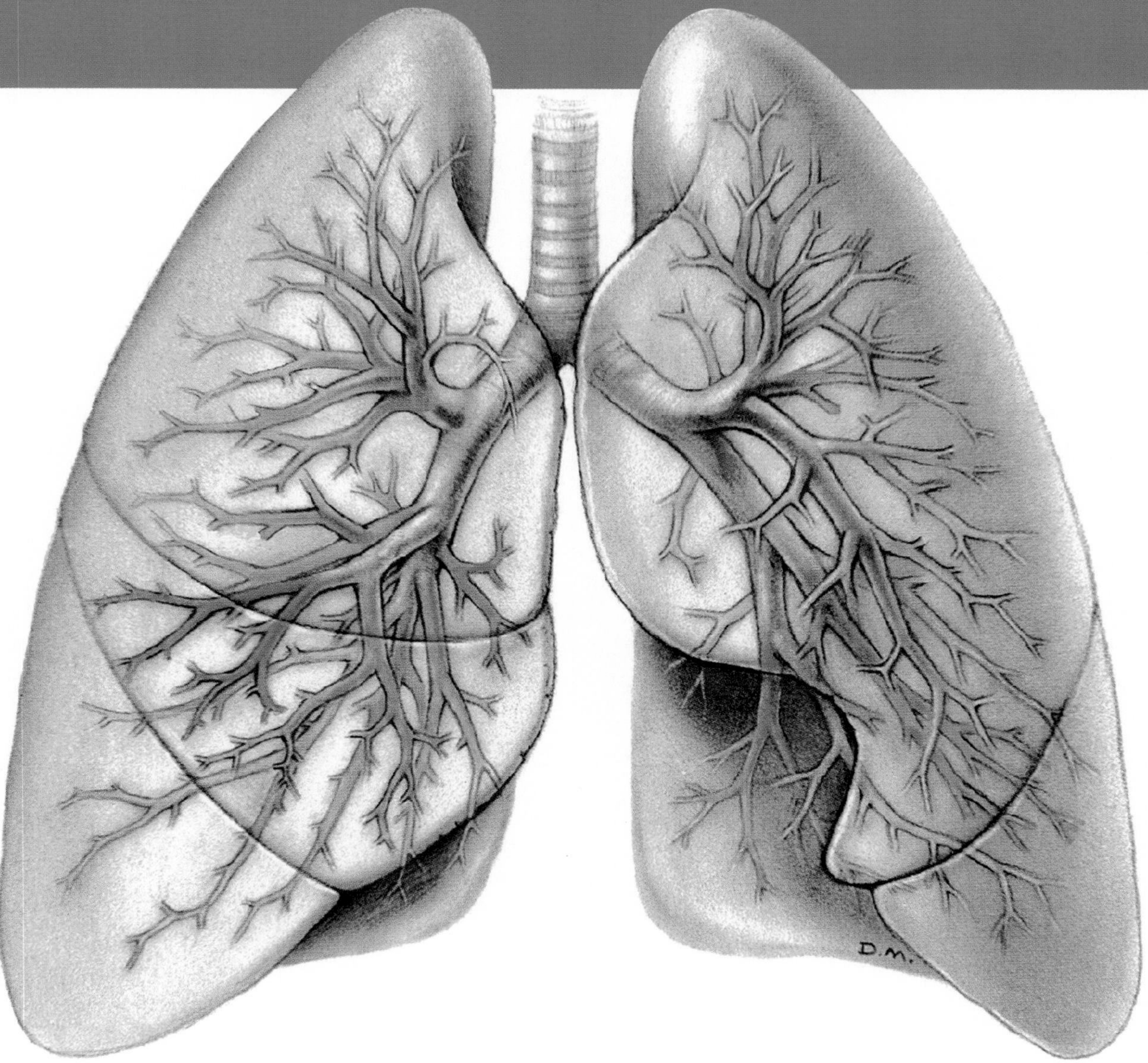

Chapter 32

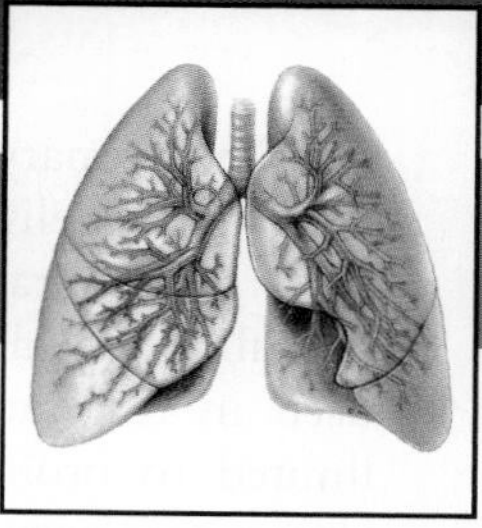

Airway Pharmacology

DOUGLAS S. GARDENHIRE

CHAPTER OBJECTIVES

After reading this chapter you will be able to:

- Analyze three phases that constitute the course of drug action from dose to effect.
- Describe classes of drugs that are delivered via the aerosol route.
- Compare mode of action, indications, and adverse effects that characterize each major class of aerosolized drug.
- Compare available aerosol formulations, brand names, and dosages for each specific drug class.
- Select the appropriate drug class for a specific patient or clinical situation.
- Assess the outcomes for each class of aerosol drug therapy.

CHAPTER OUTLINE

Principles of Pharmacology
- Drug Administration Phase
- Pharmacokinetic Phase
- Pharmacodynamic Phase
- Airway Receptors and Neural Control of the Lung

Adrenergic Bronchodilators
- Indications for Use
- Mode of Action and Effects
- Adrenergic Bronchodilator Agents
- Adverse Effects
- Assessment of Bronchodilator Therapy

Anticholinergic Bronchodilators
- Indications for Use
- Mode of Action
- Adverse Effects
- Assessment

Mucus-Controlling Agents
- *N*-Acetyl Cysteine
- Dornase Alfa
- Other Mucoactive Agents
- Assessment of Mucoactive Drug Therapy

Inhaled Corticosteroids
- Indications and Purposes
- Mode of Action
- Adverse Effects
- Special Considerations
- Assessment of Drug Therapy

Nonsteroidal Antiasthma Drugs
- Indication for Use
- Mode of Action
- Adverse Effects
- Assessment of Drug Therapy

Aerosolized Antiinfective Agents
- Pentamidine Isethionate
- Ribavirin
- Inhaled Tobramycin
- Inhaled Aztreonam
- Colistimethate Sodium
- Inhaled Zanamivir

Inhaled Pulmonary Vasodilators
- Nitric Oxide
- Iloprost
- Treprostinil

KEY TERMS

adrenergic
agonists
antagonists
antiadrenergic
anticholinergic
catecholamine
cholinergic
drug signaling
L/T ratio
leukotriene
muscarinic
mydriasis
neutropenia
pharmacodynamic phase
pharmacokinetic phase
prodrug
tachyphylaxis
vasopressor

The primary focus of respiratory care pharmacology is the delivery of bronchoactive inhaled aerosols to the respiratory tract for the diagnosis and treatment of pulmonary diseases. Although other drug classes are used in respiratory care, discussion in this chapter is limited to bronchoactive inhaled aerosols. Other drug classes are reviewed in pharmacology texts.[1,2]

PRINCIPLES OF PHARMACOLOGY

The course of drug action from dose to effect comprises three phases: *drug administration, pharmacokinetic,* and *pharmacodynamic phases.* These three phases of drug action can be applied to drug treatment of the respiratory tract with bronchoactive inhaled agents.

Drug Administration Phase

The drug administration phase describes the method by which a drug dose is made available to the body. Administering drugs directly to the respiratory tract uses the inhalation route, and the dose form is an aerosol of liquid solutions, suspensions, or dry powders. The most commonly used devices to administer orally or nasally inhaled aerosols are the metered dose inhaler (MDI), the small volume nebulizer (SVN), and the dry powder inhaler (DPI). Reservoir devices, including holding chambers with one-way inspiratory valves and simple, nonvalved spacer devices, are often added to MDIs to reduce the need for complex hand-breathing coordination and to reduce oropharyngeal impaction of the aerosol drug (see Chapter 36).

The advantages of treatment of the respiratory tract with inhaled aerosols are as follows:

- Aerosol doses are usually smaller than doses for systemic administration.
- Onset of drug action is rapid.
- Delivery is targeted to the organ requiring treatment.
- Systemic side effects are often fewer and less severe.

Disadvantages of the delivery of inhaled aerosols in treating respiratory disease include the number of variables affecting the delivered dose and lack of adequate knowledge of device performance and use among patients and caregivers.[3]

Pharmacokinetic Phase

The **pharmacokinetic phase** of drug action describes the time course and disposition of a drug in the body based on its absorption, distribution, metabolism, and elimination. Inhaled bronchoactive aerosols are intended for local effects in the airway. Undesired systemic effects result from absorption and distribution throughout the body. One method of limiting distribution of inhaled aerosols is use of a fully ionized drug rather than a nonionized agent. A fully ionized drug is not absorbed across lipid membranes, whereas a nonionized drug is lipid-soluble and diffuses across cell membranes and into the bloodstream. Examples are ipratropium and atropine sulfate. Ipratropium is a fully ionized quaternary ammonium compound that diffuses poorly across lipid membranes. Atropine is poorly ionized and diffuses well, distributing throughout the body. As a result, atropine produces systemic side effects such as **mydriasis** (dilation of the pupils) and blurring of vision. The effects of ipratropium are largely local to the airway, and systemic effects are nonexistent or minimal.

An inhaled aerosol distributes to the lung by inhalation and the stomach through swallowing of drug that deposits in the oropharynx. The therapeutic effect of the aerosol drug is caused by the portion in the airway. Systemic effects are due to absorption of the drug from the airway and gastrointestinal (GI) tract. The ideal aerosol would distribute only to the airway with none reaching the stomach. The lung availability-to-total systemic availability ratio **(L/T ratio)** quantifies the efficiency of aerosol delivery to the lung:

$$\text{L/T ratio} = \text{Lung availability}/(\text{Lung} + \text{GI availability})$$

This concept, proposed by Borgström[4] and elaborated by Thorsson,[5] is illustrated in Figure 32-1, showing delivery of albuterol by inhalation using an MDI and a DPI.

Pharmacodynamic Phase

The **pharmacodynamic phase** describes the mechanisms of drug action by which a drug molecule causes its effects in the body. Drug effects are caused by the combination of a drug with a matching receptor. **Drug signaling** mechanisms include the following:

Signaling Mechanism	Example
Mediation by G protein (guanine nucleotide)–linked receptors	Beta-adrenergic agonists, antimuscarinic agents
Attachment to intracellular receptors by lipid-soluble drugs	Corticosteroids

The mechanisms of drug action are briefly described for each class of bronchoactive drug.

Airway Receptors and Neural Control of the Lung

Pharmacologic control of the airway is mediated by receptors found on airway smooth muscle, secretory cells, bronchial epithelium, and pulmonary and bronchial blood vessels. There are *sympathetic (adrenergic)* and *parasympathetic (cholinergic)* receptors in the lung. The terminology for drugs acting on these receptors is based on the usual neurotransmitter that acts on the receptor. The usual

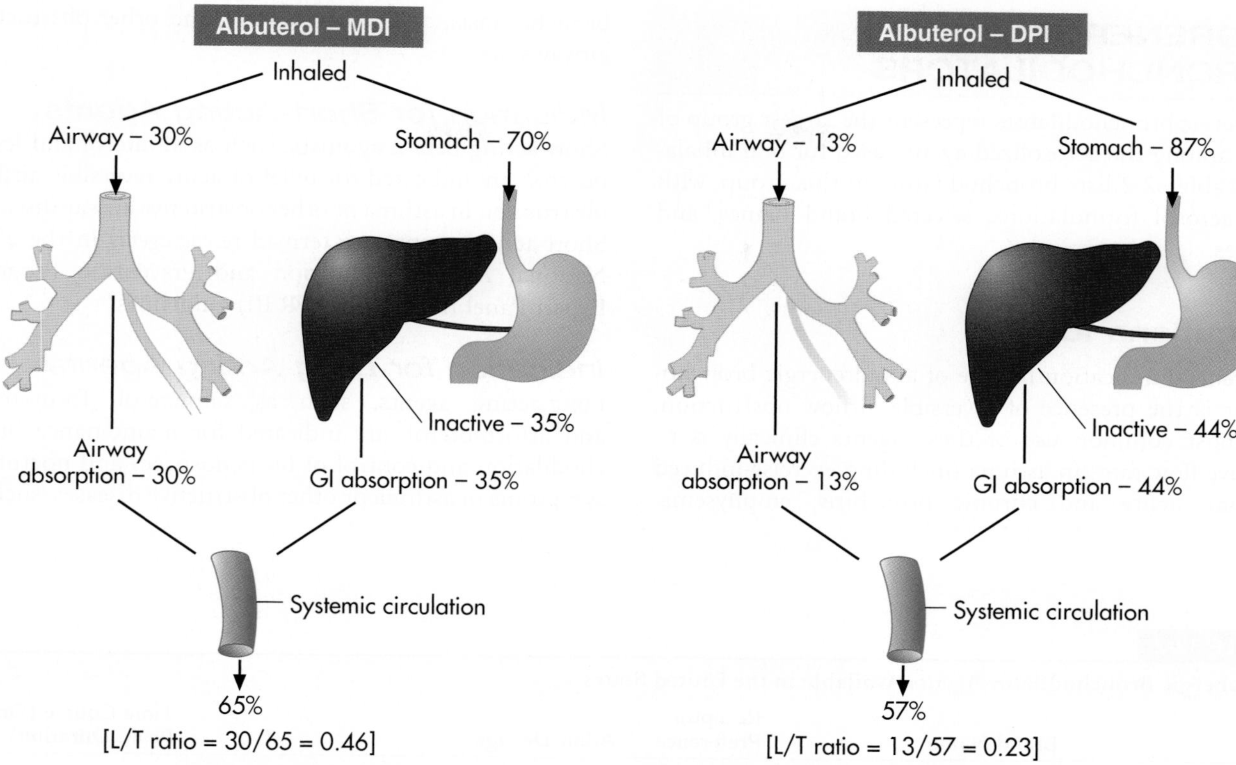

FIGURE 32-1 Comparison of efficiency of aerosol delivery with MDI and DPI using the L/T availability ratio. (From Gardenhire DS: Rau's respiratory care pharmacology, ed 8, St. Louis, 2012, Elsevier.)

neurotransmitter in the sympathetic system is norepinephrine, which is similar to epinephrine, also known as adrenaline (Adrenalin). The usual neurotransmitter in the parasympathetic system is acetylcholine. The receptors responding to these neurotransmitters are termed *adrenergic* and *cholinergic*. **Agonists** (stimulating agents) and **antagonists** (blocking agents) that act on these receptors are given the following classifications:

- **Adrenergic** (adrenomimetic): Drug that stimulates a receptor responding to norepinephrine or epinephrine
- **Antiadrenergic:** Drug that blocks a receptor for norepinephrine or epinephrine
- **Cholinergic** (cholinomimetic): Drug that stimulates a receptor for acetylcholine
- **Anticholinergic:** Drug that blocks a receptor for acetylcholine
- **Muscarinic:** Drug that stimulates acetylcholine receptors specifically at parasympathetic nerve-ending sites

Because cholinergic receptors exist at autonomic ganglia and at the myoneural junction in skeletal muscle, the terms *muscarinic* and *antimuscarinic* distinguish cholinergic agents whose action is limited to parasympathetic sites. Neostigmine is a cholinergic (indirect-acting) drug that increases receptor stimulation at both the myoneural junction and the parasympathetic sites. By contrast, atropine is an antimuscarinic agent, which blocks the action of acetylcholine only at the parasympathetic sites. Table 32-1 summarizes receptors and their effects for the cardiopulmonary system. A more detailed description of the autonomic nervous system and receptor subtypes is provided by Katzung and colleagues.[2]

TABLE 32-1
Airway Receptors and Their Effects in the Cardiopulmonary System*

Location	Receptor	Effect
Heart	Beta-1-adrenergic	Increased rate, force
	M_2-cholinergic	Decreased rate
Bronchiolar smooth muscle	Beta-2-adrenergic	Bronchodilation
	M_3-cholinergic	Bronchoconstriction
Pulmonary blood vessels	Alpha-1-adrenergic	Vasoconstriction
	Beta-2-adrenergic	Vasodilation
	M_3-cholinergic	Vasodilation
Bronchial blood vessels	Alpha-1-adrenergic	Vasoconstriction
	Beta-2-adrenergic	Vasodilation
Submucosal glands	Alpha-1-adrenergic	Increased fluid, mucin
	Beta-2-adrenergic	Increased fluid, mucin
	M_3-cholinergic	Exocytosis, secretion

M_2, M_3, Subtypes of muscarinic *(M)* cholinergic receptors.
*Adrenergic and muscarinic cholinergic receptor subtypes are indicated.

ADRENERGIC BRONCHODILATORS

Adrenergic bronchodilators represent the largest group of drugs among the aerosolized agents used for oral inhalation. Table 32-2 lists bronchodilators in this group, with their aerosol formulations, selected brand names, and dosages.

Indications for Use

The general indication for use of an adrenergic bronchodilator is the presence of reversible airflow obstruction. The most common use of these agents clinically is to improve flow rates in asthma (including exercise-induced asthma), acute and chronic bronchitis, emphysema, bronchiectasis, cystic fibrosis (CF), and other obstructive airway states.

Indication for Short-Acting Agents

Short-acting beta-2 agonists, such as albuterol and levalbuterol, are indicated for relief of acute reversible airflow obstruction in asthma or other obstructive airway diseases. Short-acting agents are termed *rescue agents* in the 2007 National Asthma Education and Prevention Program Expert Panel III (NAEPP EPR III) guidelines.[6]

Indication for Long-Acting Agents

Long-acting agents, such as salmeterol, formoterol, and arformoterol, are indicated for maintenance bronchodilation and control of bronchospasm and nocturnal symptoms in asthma or other obstructive diseases, such as

TABLE 32-2

Adrenergic Bronchodilator Agents Available in the United States

Drug	Brand Name	Receptor Preference	Adult Dosage	Time Course (Onset, Peak, Duration)
Ultra-Short-Acting Adrenergic Bronchodilator Agents				
Epinephrine	Adrenalin Chloride	Alpha, beta	SVN: 1% solution (1 : 100), 0.25-0.5 ml (2.5-5.0 mg) 4 times daily	*Onset:* 3-5 min *Peak:* 5-20 min *Duration:* 1-3 hr
	Primatene Mist		MDI: 0.22 mg/puff, puffs as ordered or needed	
Racemic epinephrine	microNefrin, Nephron, S-2	Alpha, beta	SVN: 2.25% solution, 0.25-0.5 ml (5.63-11.25 mg) 4 times daily	*Onset:* 3-5 min *Peak:* 5-20 min *Duration:* 0.5-2 hr
Short-Acting Adrenergic Bronchodilator Agents				
Metaproterenol	Alupent	Beta-2	SVN: 0.4%, 0.6% solution, tid, qid Tab: 10 mg and 20 mg, tid, qid Syrup: 10 mg per 5 ml	*Onset:* 1-5 min *Peak:* 60 min *Duration:* 2-6 hr
Albuterol	Proventil HFA, Ventolin HFA, ProAir HFA, AccuNeb, VoSpire ER	Beta-2	SVN: 0.5% solution, 0.5 ml (2.5 mg), 0.63 mg, 1.25 mg and 2.5 mg unit dose, tid, qid MDI: 90 μg/puff, 2 puffs tid, qid Tab: 2 mg, 4 mg, and 8 mg, bid, tid, qid Syrup: 2 mg/5 ml, 1-2 tsp tid, qid	*Onset:* 15 min *Peak:* 30-60 min *Duration:* 5-8 hr
Pirbuterol	Maxair Autohaler	Beta-2	MDI: 200 μg/puff, 2 puffs every 4-6 hr	*Onset:* 5 min *Peak:* 30 min *Duration:* 5 hr
Levalbuterol	Xopenex, Xopenex HFA	Beta-2	SVN: 0.31 mg/3 ml 3 times daily, 0.63 mg/3 ml 3 times daily, or 1.25 mg/3 ml 3 times daily, concentrate 1.25 mg/0.5 ml, 3 times daily MDI: 45 μg/puff, 2 puffs every 4-6 hr	*Onset:* 15 min *Peak:* 30-60 min *Duration:* 5-8 hr
Long-Acting Adrenergic Bronchodilator Agents				
Salmeterol	Serevent Diskus	Beta-2	DPI: 50 μg/blister twice daily	*Onset:* 20 min *Peak:* 3-5 hr *Duration:* 12 hr
Formoterol	Perforomist, Foradil	Beta-2	SVN: 20 μg/2 ml unit dose, bid DPI: 12 μg/inhalation, bid	*Onset:* 15 min *Peak:* 30-60 min *Duration:* 12 hr
	Foradil Certihaler	Beta-2	DPI: 8.5 μg/inhalation, bid	
Arformoterol	Brovana	Beta-2	SVN: 15 μg/2 ml unit dose, twice daily	*Onset:* 15 min *Peak:* 30-60 min *Duration:* 12 hr

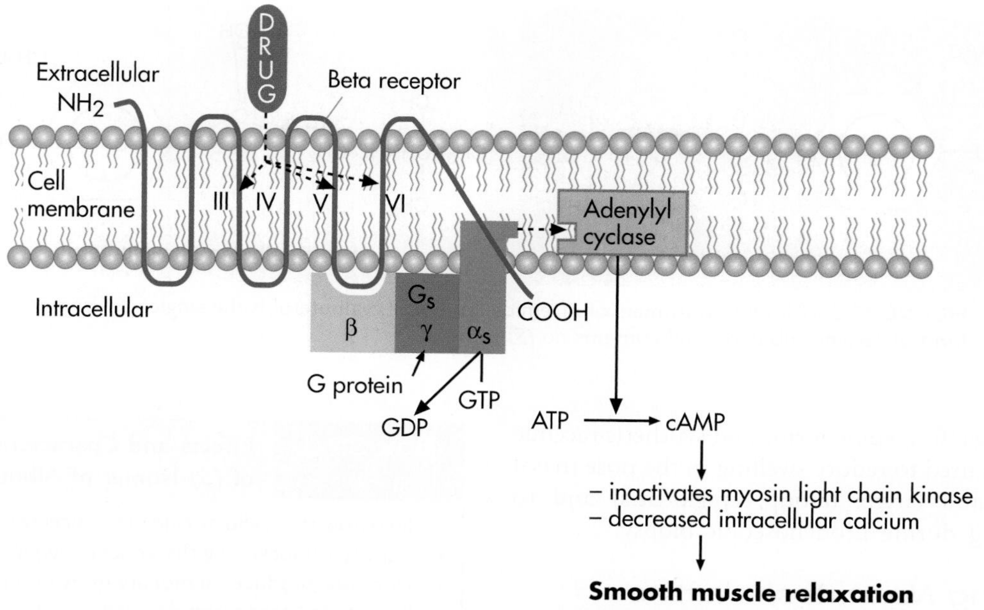

FIGURE 32-2 Mode of action by which a beta agonist stimulates the G protein–linked beta receptor to cause smooth muscle relaxation. Adrenergic agonists, such as albuterol or epinephrine, attach to beta receptors, which are polypeptide chains traversing the cell membrane seven times. This causes activation of the stimulatory G protein, designated G_S, linked to the receptor. When stimulated, the receptor undergoes a conformational change, and the alpha subunit of the G protein attaches to adenyl cyclase. Activation of adenyl cyclase by the G_S protein causes an increased synthesis of the second messenger, cyclic adenosine monophosphate (cAMP). This ultimately causes smooth muscle relaxation and bronchodilation. *ATP,* Adenosine triphosphate; *COOH,* carboxy terminus; *GDP,* guanosine diphosphate; *GTP,* guanosine triphosphate. (From Gardenhire DS: Rau's respiratory care pharmacology, ed 8, St. Louis, 2012, Elsevier.)

chronic obstructive pulmonary disease (COPD). NAEPP EPR III guidelines consider salmeterol a *controller;* its slow time to peak effect makes it a poor rescue drug. In asthma, a long-acting bronchodilator is usually combined with antiinflammatory medication for control of airway inflammation and bronchospasm. Although formoterol has a rapid onset and peak effect similar to albuterol, its prolonged activity makes it a better maintenance drug compared with an acute reliever or rescue agent.

Indication for Racemic Epinephrine

Racemic epinephrine is often used either by inhaled aerosol or by direct lung instillation for its strong beta-adrenergic vasoconstricting effect to reduce airway swelling after extubation or during epiglottitis, croup, or bronchiolitis or to control airway bleeding during endoscopy.

Mode of Action and Effects

Adrenergic bronchodilators can stimulate one or more of the following receptors, with the effects described:

- *Alpha-receptor stimulation:* Causes vasoconstriction and a **vasopressor** effect (increased blood pressure)
- *Beta-1-receptor stimulation:* Causes increased heart rate and myocardial contractility
- *Beta-2-receptor stimulation:* Relaxes bronchial smooth muscle, stimulates mucociliary activity, and has some inhibitory action on inflammatory mediator release

Bronchodilation, through stimulation of beta-2 receptors, is the desired therapeutic effect. Both alpha-adrenergic and beta-adrenergic receptors are G protein–linked receptors. Figure 32-2 illustrates the mode of action for relaxation of airway smooth muscle when a beta-2 receptor is stimulated. The nature of the beta receptor and its activity is presented in detail in a review by Barnes.[7]

Adrenergic Bronchodilator Agents

Adrenergic bronchodilator agents represent the evolution of a drug class. Although all of these agents are adrenergic agonists, the differences among individual agents are due to their receptor preference (alpha-adrenergic, beta-1-adrenergic, beta-2-adrenergic) and their different pharmacokinetics as listed in Table 32-2. These differences determine the optimal clinical application of individual agents, as discussed subsequently. The adrenergic bronchodilators form three subgroups.

Ultra-Short-Acting Catecholamines

The older agents, epinephrine and isoproterenol, are both **catecholamines.** These agents lack beta-2 specificity. As a result, cardiac effects, especially tachycardia and increased blood pressure, are common. As catecholamines, they are metabolized rapidly by the enzyme catechol *O*-methyltransferase, which causes a short duration of action. Because of their strong alpha-1 activity and

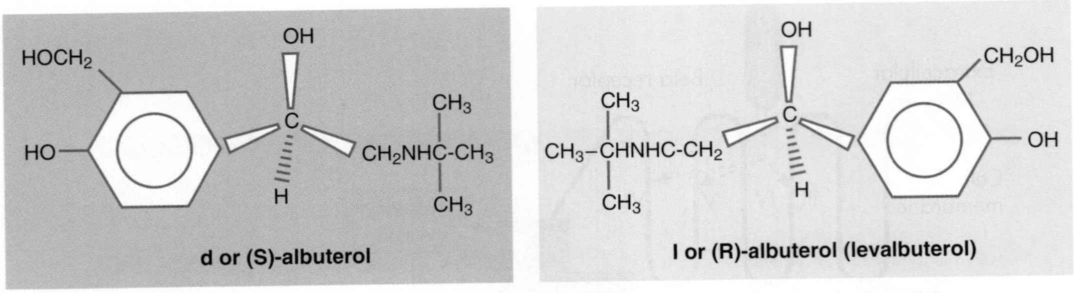

FIGURE 32-3 *(R)*- and *(S)*-isomers of racemic albuterol. Levalbuterol is the single, *(R)*-isomer form of racemic albuterol and contains no *(S)*-isomer.

vasoconstricting effect, epinephrine and synthetic racemic epinephrine are used to reduce swelling in the nose (nasal decongestant) and larynx (croup, epiglottitis) and to control bleeding during bronchoscopic biopsy.

Short-Acting Noncatecholamine Agents

Because of their short duration of action and lack of beta-2 specificity, catecholamines were replaced with longer acting, beta-2-specific agents, including metaproterenol, pirbuterol, albuterol, and levalbuterol. Because their duration of action is approximately 4 to 6 hours, these drugs are more suited to maintenance therapy than catecholamines and can be taken on a four-times-daily schedule. However, their modest duration of action results in loss of bronchodilating effect overnight.

Single-Isomer Beta Agonists. Levalbuterol is approved as a single-isomer beta-2-selective agonist. Previous inhaled formulations of adrenergic bronchodilators all were synthetic racemic mixtures, containing both the *(R)*-isomer and the *(S)*-isomer in equal amounts. Levalbuterol is the pure *(R)*-isomer of racemic albuterol. Both stereoisomers of albuterol are shown in Figure 32-3 with the single-isomer (*R*-isomer) form of levalbuterol. Although the *(S)*-isomer is physiologically inactive on adrenergic receptors, there is accumulating evidence that the *(S)*-isomer is not completely inactive. Box 32-1 lists some of the physiologic effects of *(S)*-albuterol noted in the literature.[8-14] The effects noted antagonize the bronchodilating effects of the *(R)*-isomer and promote bronchoconstriction. In addition, the *(S)*-isomer is more slowly metabolized than the *(R)*-isomer.

Levalbuterol is available as a nebulization solution in three strengths: 0.31 mg/3 ml, 0.63 mg/3 ml, and 1.25 mg/3 ml. As a result of mixing of other inhaled agents, levalbuterol is also available as a concentrate of 1.25 mg/0.5 ml and an MDI. In a study by Nelson and associates,[15] the 0.63-mg dose was found to be comparable to the 2.5-mg racemic albuterol dose in onset and duration. Side effects of tremor and heart rate changes were less with the single-isomer formulation. The 1.25-mg dose showed a higher peak effect on forced expiratory volume in 1 second (FEV_1) with an 8-hour duration compared with racemic albuterol.

Box 32-1 Effects and Characteristics of *(S)*-Isomer of Albuterol

- Increases intracellular calcium concentration in vitro[8]
- Activity is blocked by the anticholinergic atropine[8]
- Does not produce pulmonary or extrapulmonary beta-2-mediated effects[9]
- Enhances experimental airway responsiveness in vitro[10]
- Increases contractile response of bronchial tissue to histamine or leukotriene C_4 in vitro[11]
- Enhances eosinophil superoxide production with interleukin-5 stimulation[12]
- Slower metabolism than *(R)*-albuterol in vivo[13]
- Preferential retention in the lung when inhaled by MDI (in vivo)[14]

Side effects with this dose were equivalent to the side effects seen with racemic albuterol. An equivalent clinical response was seen with one-fourth of the racemic dose (0.63 mg) using the pure isomer, although the racemic mixture contains 1.25 mg of the *(R)*-isomer (half of the total 2.5-mg dose). A detailed review is available of levalbuterol and differences between the *(R)*-isomer and *(S)*-isomer of albuterol.[16]

Long-Acting Adrenergic Bronchodilators

The release of salmeterol offered the first long-acting adrenergic bronchodilator in the United States. In contrast to previous agents, the duration of action of salmeterol is about 12 hours. The pharmacokinetics of salmeterol makes it suitable for maintenance therapy, in particular, with nocturnal asthma. However, it is not well suited for relief of acute airflow obstruction or bronchospasm because its onset is longer than 20 minutes, with a peak effect occurring by 3 to 5 hours. Although this agent is a beta-2 agonist, its exact mode of action differs from previous beta-2 agonists, allowing persistent receptor stimulation over a prolonged period of hours. A more detailed discussion of the action of salmeterol can be found in a review by Johnson and colleagues.[17]

Formoterol is a second long-acting, beta-2-specific agent and is approved for general clinical use in the United States. The duration of effect is approximately 12 hours, but in contrast to salmeterol, the onset of action and peak effect of formoterol are rapid and similar to albuterol.[18] Nonetheless, patients should be cautioned about the risk of accumulation and toxicity if formoterol is used as a rescue agent in the same way that shorter acting beta agonists, such as albuterol, are used. As with salmeterol, the extensive side chain or tail makes formoterol more lipophilic than shorter acting bronchodilators and is the basis for its longer duration of effect.

Arformoterol (Brovana), the single *(R)*-isomer of formoterol, is the newest long-acting beta agonist on the market. Arformoterol is available as a 2-ml unit dose vial inhalation solution delivering 15 mcg per dose. The recommended dosage is one unit dose twice daily. Arformoterol is indicated for the maintenance of bronchospasm in COPD, including chronic bronchitis and emphysema. In phase III trials, the manufacturer reported an increase in bronchodilation compared with placebo.

A new novel once-daily, long-acting beta-agonist, indacaterol, was approved in the United States in 2011 under the brand name of Arcapta Neohaler. It has been used mainly to treat asthma, and additional indications for COPD are being examined. Indacaterol is also being studied in combination with tiotropium bromide with successful preliminary outcomes.[1]

Adverse Effects

Older adrenergic agents, such as isoproterenol, commonly caused tachycardia, palpitations, and an "adrenaline effect" of shakiness and nervousness. The newer, more beta-2-selective agents are safer and typically cause tremor as the main side effect. Other common side effects with the inhaled agents include headache, insomnia, and nervousness. Patients should be reassured that some tolerance to these effects does occur. Potential adverse effects with use of adrenergic bronchodilators include the following:

- Dizziness
- Hypokalemia
- Loss of bronchoprotection
- Nausea
- Tolerance **(tachyphylaxis)**
- Worsening ventilation/perfusion ($\dot{V}/\dot{Q}$) ratio (decrease in PaO_2/SpO_2)

Inhalation results in fewer and less severe side effects than oral administration. Although tolerance develops to the bronchodilating effect, this is not a contraindication to use of the drugs, and relaxation of airway smooth muscle still occurs. Desaturation resulting from mismatching of $\dot{V}/\dot{Q}$ with inhalation of the aerosol is not clinically significant and reverses quickly. Bronchospasm resulting from chlorofluorocarbon propellants can be prevented by changing to newer hydrofluoroalkane-propelled MDIs or a different aerosol delivery form.

The implication of beta-2-adrenergic agonists in deaths from asthma—termed the *asthma paradox* or the *beta agonist controversy*—remains debated.[19] There is evidence of loss of a bronchoprotective effect with use of beta agonists, and patients should be cautioned to avoid asthma triggers.[20] The increased prevalence of asthma in general remains a troublesome and unresolved issue.

Assessment of Bronchodilator Therapy

Assessment of therapy with adrenergic bronchodilators should be based on the indication for the aerosol agent (presence of reversible airflow obstruction owing to primary bronchospasm or other obstruction secondary to an inflammatory response or secretions, either acute or chronic). With all aerosol drug therapy, basic vital signs (respiratory rate and pattern, pulse, breath sounds) should be assessed before and after treatment, especially for initial drug use, and the patient's subjective reaction (complaints of breathing difficulty) should be assessed. Patients should be instructed in the correct use of the aerosol device used, with verification of correct use. Finally, the patient's subjective reaction to the treatment should be monitored for any change in breathing effort. This assessment applies to all subsequent drug groups by aerosol and is not repeated for each class. The following specific actions are suggested to evaluate patient response to this class of drugs:

- Monitor flow rates using bedside peak flowmeters, portable spirometry, or laboratory reports of pulmonary function before and after bronchodilator studies to assess reversibility of airflow obstruction.
- Assess arterial blood gases or pulse oximetry saturation, as needed, for acute states with asthma or COPD to monitor changes in ventilation and gas exchange (oxygenation).
- Note the effect of beta agonists on blood glucose (increase) and K^+ (decrease) laboratory values, if using high doses, such as with continuous nebulization or emergency department treatments.
- In the long-term, monitor pulmonary function studies of lung volumes, capacities, and flows.
- Instruct asthmatic patients in the use and interpretation of disposable peak flowmeters to assess severity of asthmatic episodes and provide an action plan for treatment modification.
- Emphasize in patient education that beta agonists do not treat underlying inflammation and do not prevent progression of asthma, and additional antiinflammatory treatment or more aggressive medical therapy may be needed if there is a poor response to the rescue beta agonist.
- Instruct and then verify correct use of aerosol delivery device (SVN, MDI, reservoir, DPI).

- Instruct patients in use, assembly, and especially cleaning of aerosol inhalation devices.

The following actions are suggested to evaluate patient response to long-acting beta agonists:

- Assess ongoing lung function, including predose FEV_1 over time and variability in peak expiratory flows.
- Assess amount of rescue beta agonist use and nocturnal symptoms.
- Assess number of exacerbations, unscheduled clinic visits, and hospitalizations.
- Assess days of absence from school or work because of symptoms.
- Assess ability to reduce the dose of concomitant inhaled corticosteroids.

Note: Death has been associated with excessive use of inhaled adrenergic agents in severe acute asthma crises. Individuals using such drugs should be instructed to contact a physician or an emergency department if there is no response to the usual dose of the inhaled agent.

Because of the ongoing safety concerns of long-acting beta-2 agonists, the FDA is requiring changes on how long-acting beta-2 agonists are used in the treatment of asthma. As of June 2, 2010, the FDA suggests the following:

- Long-acting beta-2 agonists are not to be used without a controller medication (i.e., corticosteroid).
- Long-acting beta-2 agonists should not be used by patients who are controlled on low-dose or medium-dose inhaled corticosteroids.
- Long-acting beta-2 agonists should be used only if patients are not controlled with agents such as inhaled corticosteroids.
- Long-acting beta-2 agonists should be for short-term use only. A long-acting beta-2 agonist should be discontinued when asthma is controlled.
- Children should use a long-acting beta-2 agonist only in conjunction with a corticosteroid. The use of a combination product is needed to increase adherence.

ANTICHOLINERGIC BRONCHODILATORS

A second method of producing airway relaxation is through blockade of cholinergic-induced bronchoconstriction. An important difference between beta agonists and anticholinergic bronchodilators is the active stimulatory action of the former versus the passive blockade of the latter. A cholinergic blocking agent is effective only if bronchoconstriction exists secondary to cholinergic activity.

Indications for Use

Ipratropium bromide and tiotropium bromide are the only inhaled anticholinergic bronchodilators available in the United States. Table 32-3 lists the dosage forms and pharmacokinetics of ipratropium and tiotropium. Generally, anticholinergic agents have been found to be as effective as beta agonists in airflow improvement in COPD but

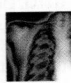

MINI CLINI

Assessing Beta Agonist Side Effects

PROBLEM: The respiratory therapist (RT) has administered an aerosol treatment of albuterol using an MDI with a holding chamber to a 67-year-old patient with newly diagnosed COPD who was admitted for an acute exacerbation and shortness of breath. When the RT returns for the second treatment that day, the patient informs the RT that he began to feel very shaky and nervous, beginning about 30 minutes after the previous treatment. He also noticed a tremor when he held his water cup and took a drink. His pulse during the earlier treatment was 84 beats/min. Clinical assessment shows that he is coherent, has good color, is not diaphoretic, and is in no respiratory distress. His respiratory rate is 16 breaths/min and regular, and his pulse is 82 beats/min and regular. Auscultation reveals mild wheezing and scattered rhonchi, with little change from earlier breath sounds. A mild tremor is apparent when he holds his hand out. On questioning, he states that he is now feeling better, and the "shakiness" has subsided a bit.

DISCUSSION: This patient's situation exemplifies a common reaction to inhaled adrenergic bronchodilators. Although albuterol is beta-2 preferential, it is still an epinephrine-like drug and can produce side effects secondary to sympathetic stimulation. The description of the symptoms is suggestive of common adrenergic side effects (tremor, shakiness). The timing of the symptoms coincides with the pharmacokinetics of albuterol (peak effect in 30 to 60 minutes). As presented in the case description, it is important to rule out other complications. The physical examination shows no changes from the earlier treatment in his vital signs.

It is important to caution patients about "normal" expected side effects and to reassure them that the side effects decrease with tolerance to the medication. In addition, the RT needs to be alert to the possibility that patients may have deteriorated or changed in their respiratory status.

RULE OF THUMB

Choosing an Aerosol Agent

An aerosol agent to treat the respiratory tract is chosen based on the indication for the agent or class of drugs and a corresponding presence of the indication in the patient.

- *Example: Adrenergic bronchodilator.* The indication is presence of reversible airflow obstruction. The patient shows a 20% improvement in FEV_1 on spirometry with use of inhaled albuterol. Choose an adrenergic bronchodilator.
- *Example: Inhaled corticosteroid.* The indication is mild, moderate, or persistent asthma. The patient with asthma reports a need to use a beta-agonist inhaler more than a few days each week and complains of waking up at night with shortness of breath. Choose an inhaled corticosteroid.

TABLE 32-3

Inhaled Anticholinergic Bronchodilator Agents*

Drug	Brand Name	Adult Dosage	Time Course (Onset, Peak, Duration)
Ipratropium bromide	Atrovent HFA	HFA MDI: 17 μg/puff, 2 puffs 4 times daily SVN: 0.02% solution (0.2 mg/ml), 500 μg 3-4 times daily Nasal spray: 21 μg or 40 μg, 2 sprays per nostril 2-4 times daily (dosage varies)	*Onset:* 15 min *Peak:* 1-2 hr *Duration:* 4-6 hr
Ipratropium bromide and albuterol	Combivent	MDI: Ipratropium 18 μg/puff and albuterol 90 μg/puff, 2 puffs 4 times daily	*Onset:* 15 min *Peak:* 1-2 hr *Duration:* 4-6 hr
	DuoNeb	SVN: Ipratropium 0.5 mg and albuterol 2.5 mg	
Tiotropium bromide	Spiriva	DPI: 18 μg/inhalation, 1 inhalation daily (1 capsule)	*Onset:* 30 min *Peak:* 3 hr *Duration:* 24 hr

HFA, Hydrofluoroalkane.
*A holding chamber is recommended with MDI administration to prevent accidental eye exposure.

less so in asthma. A nasal formulation of ipratropium is also available for relief of allergic and nonallergic perennial rhinitis, including the common cold.[21]

Indication for Anticholinergic Bronchodilators

Ipratropium and tiotropium are indicated as bronchodilators for maintenance treatment in COPD, including chronic bronchitis and emphysema.

Indication for Combined Anticholinergic and Beta-Agonist Bronchodilators

A combination anticholinergic and beta agonist, such as ipratropium bromide and albuterol (Combivent; DuoNeb), is indicated for use in patients with COPD receiving regular treatment who require additional bronchodilation for relief of airflow obstruction. Ipratropium bromide is also commonly used in severe asthma in addition to beta agonists, especially in acute bronchoconstriction that does not respond well to beta agonist therapy.

Mode of Action

As antimuscarinic agents, ipratropium and tiotropium act as competitive antagonists for acetylcholine at muscarinic receptors on airway smooth muscle. Part of the airflow obstruction in COPD may be due to vagally mediated, reflex cholinergic stimulation. Airway irritation and inflammation stimulate afferent sensory C-fibers in the airway, which synapse with efferent vagal (cholinergic) fibers to the airway and mucous glands. The muscarinic receptor subtype on smooth muscle and submucosal mucous glands is the M_3 receptor, which is a G protein–linked receptor. The effect of acetylcholine, the usual neurotransmitter, on the muscarinic (M_3) receptors on airway smooth muscle is bronchoconstriction. The M_1 receptor at the ganglionic junction enhances cholinergic nerve transmission. The M_2 receptor is an autoreceptor inhibiting further release of acetylcholine so that blockade can increase acetylcholine release and may offset the bronchodilating effect of antimuscarinics.[22]

Ipratropium and tiotropium block the action of acetylcholine at the M_3 receptor in the airway, reversing bronchoconstriction secondary to cholinergic activity. Ipratropium is a nonselective muscarinic receptor blocker and has affinity for M_1, M_2, and M_3 receptors. Blockade of the M_2 receptor can theoretically reverse the bronchodilating effect of ipratropium or other nonselective muscarinic receptor antagonists because the autoinhibitory action of the M_2 receptor is blocked. Both ipratropium and tiotropium are quaternary ammonium compounds and are poorly absorbed after inhalation.

Tiotropium exhibits receptor subtype selectivity for M_1 and M_3 receptors. The drug binds to all three muscarinic receptors (M_1, M_2, and M_3) but dissociates much more slowly than ipratropium from the M_1 and M_3 receptors; this results in a selectivity of action on M_1 and M_3 receptors. In patients with COPD, tiotropium provides a bronchodilating effect for 24 hours with an adequate dose.[22] Inhalation of a single dose gives a peak plasma level within 5 minutes, with a rapid decline to very low levels within 1 hour. The site of action of anticholinergic agents in reversing cholinergic-induced airflow obstruction is shown in Figure 32-4.

Adverse Effects

Ipratropium bromide and tiotropium bromide are fully ionized compounds that are not well absorbed and distributed throughout the body, whereas atropine sulfate is a tertiary ammonium compound that is easily absorbed into the bloodstream. As a result, atropine produces many systemic side effects when inhaled, even though it is delivered

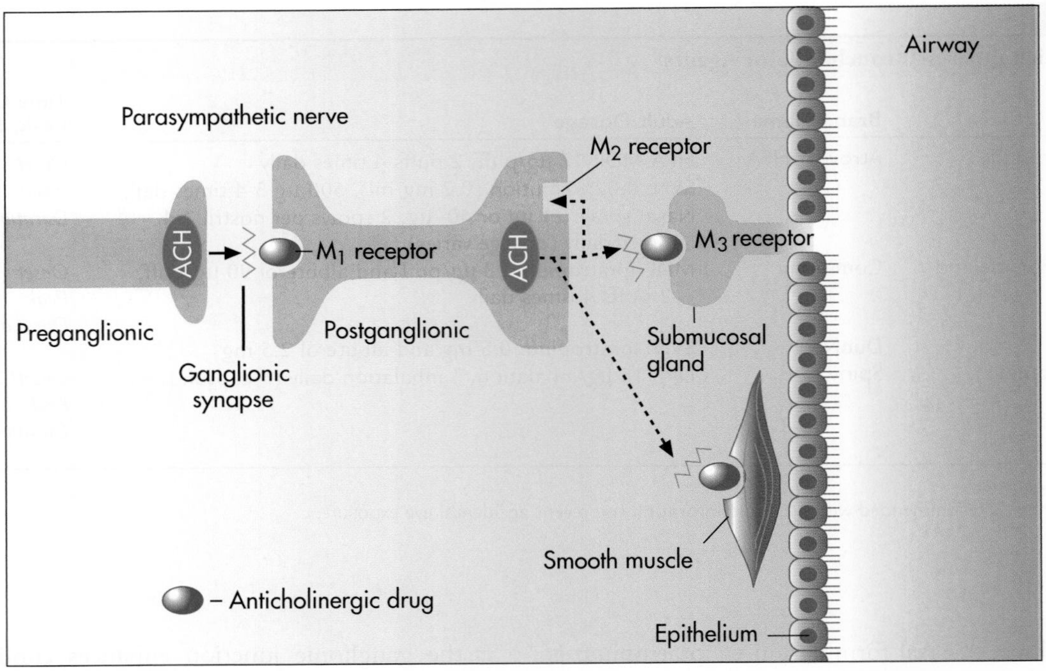

FIGURE 32-4 Mode of action of anticholinergic agents in blocking muscarinic receptors in the airway to inhibit cholinergic-induced bronchoconstriction. *ACH,* Acetylcholine. (From Gardenhire DS: Rau's respiratory care pharmacology, ed 8, St. Louis, 2012, Elsevier.)

locally to the lung. Side effects include the local topical effect of dry mouth, pupillary dilation, lens paralysis, increased intraocular pressure, increased heart rate, urinary retention, and altered mental state. Because of its many side effects and the availability of ionized compounds such as ipratropium, the use of atropine sulfate by nebulization is not recommended. In contrast, the side effects of inhaled anticholinergics are largely limited to its local site of action (Box 32-2).

The amount of drug in the nebulizer dose of ipratropium is more than 10 times greater than the MDI dose (500 mcg vs. 34 mcg). If a patient receives approximately 10% of an inhaled aerosol to the lung, a much larger dose is given with an SVN. Although ipratropium is not contraindicated in subjects with prostatic hypertrophy, urinary retention, or glaucoma, the drug should be used with precaution and adequate evaluation for possible systemic side effects in these subjects. The eye must be protected from drug exposure with aerosol use owing to accidental spraying from an MDI or with nebulizer-mask delivery. There is less chance of eye exposure with the MDI formulation than the SVN solution; a holding chamber is recommended with MDI use.

Assessment

The assessment of bronchodilator therapy with an anticholinergic agent is the same as assessment for adrenergic agents. In addition, preexisting conditions of narrow-angle glaucoma, prostatic hypertrophy, or urinary retention warrant caution with continued evaluation.

Box 32-2 Side Effects Seen With Anticholinergic Aerosol Agents*

SVN, MDI, AND DPI (COMMON)
- Cough, dry mouth

MDI (OCCASIONAL)
- Nervousness, irritation, dizziness, headache, palpitation, rash

SVN AND DPI
- Pharyngitis, dyspnea, flulike symptoms, bronchitis, upper respiratory infections, nausea, occasional bronchoconstriction, eye pain, urinary retention

Precautions: Use with caution in patients with narrow-angle glaucoma, prostatic hypertrophy, bladder neck obstruction, constipation, bowel obstruction, or tachycardia.
*Side effects were reported in a small percentage (1% to 5%) of patients.

MUCUS-CONTROLLING AGENTS

The two agents approved in the United States for oral inhalation with an effect on mucus are *N*-acetyl-cysteine (NAC) and dornase alfa. Both agents are mucolytic, although their modes of action differ. Table 32-4 lists these agents, their formulations, dosages, and bland aqueous aerosols. A review by Rubin[23] provides additional detail.

TABLE 32-4

Mucoactive Agents Available for Aerosol Administration

Drug	Brand Name	Adult Dosage	Use
N-Acetylcysteine 10%	Mucomyst	SVN: 3-5 ml	Bronchitis, efficacy not proven
N-Acetylcysteine 20%	Mucomyst	SVN: 3-5 ml	Bronchitis, efficacy not proven
Dornase alfa	Pulmozyme	SVN: 2.5 mg/ampule, 1 ampule daily*	CF
Aqueous aerosols: water, saline (0.45%, 0.9%, 5%-10%)	NA	SVN: 3-5 ml, as ordered USN: 3-5 ml, as ordered	Sputum induction, secretion mobilization

NA, Not applicable.
*Use recommended nebulizer system (see package insert). Approved nebulizers include Hudson T Updraft II, Marquest II with Pulmo-Aide compressor, or PARI LC Jet Plus with PARI Inhaler Boy compressor.

N-Acetyl Cysteine

NAC is the *N*-acetyl derivative of the amino acid L-cysteine and is given either by nebulization or by direct tracheal instillation.

MINI CLINI

Calculating Drug Doses

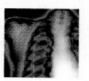

PROBLEM: The dose of ipratropium bromide (Atrovent) released from the valve of the MDI is 17 µg. With a usual dose of two actuations, this would release 34 µg total. The SVN solution is a vial of 2.5 ml of a 0.02% strength concentration, all of which is placed in the nebulizer. Does the nebulizer dose contain the same amount of drug as the two actuations from the MDI?

DISCUSSION: The amount of drug in milligrams or micrograms can be calculated for the nebulizer solution, using the following formula for percentage strength:

$$\%\ (\text{as decimal}) = \frac{\text{Drug solute (in g)}}{\text{Total solution (in ml)}}$$

$$0.0002 = \frac{x\ \text{g}}{2.5\ \text{ml}}$$

$$x\ \text{g} = 0.0002 \times 2.5\ \text{ml} = 0.0005\ \text{g}$$

Converting 0.0005 g to milligrams gives 0.5 mg, or 500 µg. Two actuations of the MDI release 34 µg, whereas the dose contained in the SVN is 500 µg (or >10 times more). The lower dose MDI is the reason that additional actuations of four or six are needed if a patient does not obtain relief. The SVN solution may also provide relief by giving a higher dose of the drug.

Indications for Use

NAC is indicated to reduce accumulation of airway secretions, with concomitant improvement in pulmonary function and gas exchange and prevention of recurrent respiratory infection and airway damage. Diseases of excessive viscous mucus secretions and poor airway clearance include COPD, acute tracheobronchitis, and bronchiectasis. NAC also is used to treat or prevent liver damage that can occur when a patient takes an overdose of acetaminophen.[24] Despite excellent in vitro mucolytic activity and a long history of use, no data clearly show that oral or aerosolized NAC is effective therapy for treating any lung disease.[25] This situation may be partially due to NAC selectively depolymerizing the essential mucin polymer structure and leaving the pathologic polymers of DNA and F-actin intact in respiratory secretions.

Mode of Action

The mucus macromolecule consists of a polypeptide (protein) chain of amino acids, to which carbohydrate side chains are attached. There is internal cross-linking between strands with disulfide (–S–S–) bonds and hydrogen bonds.[26] NAC acts as a classic mucolytic to reduce the viscosity of mucus by substituting its own sulfhydryl group for the disulfide group in mucus, breaking a portion of the bond forming the gel structure. The drug is effective in reducing viscosity and can be helpful by direct bronchial instillation during bronchoscopy to remove mucus plugs.

Side Effects

Several side effects to NAC have led to less use in patients with hypersecretory states. The drug is irritating to the airway and can produce bronchospasm, especially in subjects with asthma and hyperreactive airways. The general effect of airway irritation is counterproductive to reduction of mucus hypersecretion. To reduce the occurrence of bronchospasm, use of the 10% solution, which is less hypertonic than the 20% solution, is recommended. Pretreatment with an adrenergic bronchodilator, allowing adequate time for production of a bronchodilatory effect, can prevent or reduce airway resistance with NAC.

Other side effects that can occur include the following:

- Airway obstruction secondary to rapid liquefaction of secretions
- Disagreeable odor secondary to hydrogen sulfide
- Incompatibility with certain antibiotics (sodium ampicillin, amphotericin B, erythromycin, tetracyclines, and aminoglycosides) if mixed in solution

Reduction in Viscosity: (Pourability)

	0 min	15 min	30 min
Saline	0	+1	+1
rhDNase, 50 μg/ml	0	+3	+4
Bovine DNase, 50 μg/ml	0	+2	+4

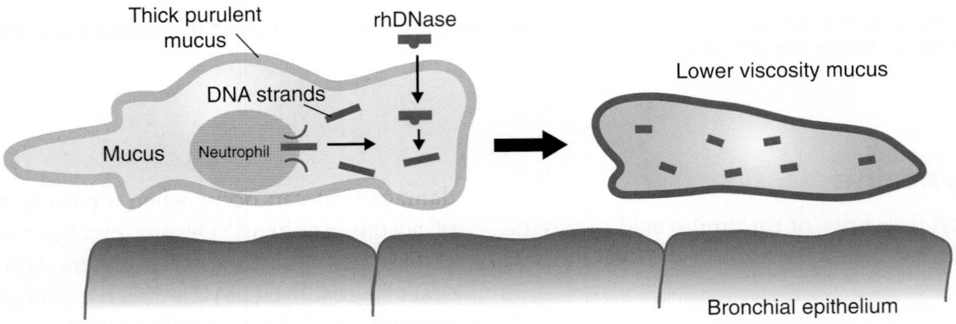

FIGURE 32-5 Mode of action of dornase alfa (rhDNase) in reducing viscosity of infected sputum. (Based on data from Shak S, Capon DJ, Hellmiss R, et al: Recombinant human DNase I reduces the viscosity of cystic fibrosis sputum. Proc Natl Acad Sci U S A 87:9188, 1990; modified from Rau JL: Respiratory care pharmacology, ed 5, St. Louis, 1998, Mosby.)

- Increased concentration and toxicity of nebulizer solution toward end of treatment
- Nausea and rhinorrhea
- Stomatitis
- Reactivity of acetylcysteine with rubber, copper, iron, and cork

If NAC is administered by direct tracheal instillation, tracheobronchial suction should be immediately available to maintain the airway. To prevent concentration of solution in the nebulizer during treatment, it is suggested that the last fourth of the solution in the nebulizer be diluted with an equal volume of sterile water to prevent concentrated residue, possibly leading to airway irritation. Aerosolizing NAC may leave a sticky film on surfaces, including hands and face.

Dornase Alfa

Dornase alfa (Pulmozyme) is a genetically engineered clone of the natural human pancreatic DNase enzyme, which can digest extracellular DNA material. It is a peptide mucolytic and can reduce extracellular DNA and F-actin polymers. It is occasionally referred to as *rhDNase* (recombinant human DNase). It is designated as an orphan drug. Administration and dosage are given in Table 32-4.

Indication for Use

Dornase alfa is indicated in the management of CF to reduce the frequency of respiratory infections requiring parenteral antibiotics and to improve pulmonary function of these patients.[27]

Mode of Action

Dornase alfa is a proteolytic enzyme that can break down the DNA material from neutrophils found in purulent secretions (Figure 32-5). This agent has been shown to be more effective than acetylcysteine in reducing the viscosity of infected sputum in CF.[28]

Side Effects

In contrast to its predecessor, pancreatic dornase (Dornavac), a natural enzyme obtained from animal preparations, dornase alfa has not been shown to produce antibodies that might cause allergic reactions, including bronchospasm. Common side effects associated with the drug include pharyngitis and voice alteration, laryngitis, rash, chest pain, and conjunctivitis. Other effects are less common but are reported as various respiratory symptoms (cough, dyspnea, pneumothorax, hemoptysis, rhinitis, sinusitis), flu syndrome, GI obstruction, hypoxia, malaise, and weight loss. Contraindications to the drug include hypersensitivity to dornase, Chinese hamster ovary (CHO) cell products, or other components of the drug preparation.

Other Mucoactive Agents

Bland aerosols of water, including distilled water and normotonic, hypertonic, and hypotonic saline, have traditionally been nebulized to improve mobilization of secretions in respiratory disease states. The mucus gel layer is relatively resistant to the addition or removal of water after it is formed. Bland aerosols have been found to increase secretion clearance and sputum production and cause productive coughing.[29] The effect is probably a vagally mediated reflex production of cough and mucus secretion. Bland aerosols are more properly considered expectorants rather than mucolytic agents. Clinicians must be alert to the possibility of bronchospasm with nonisotonic solutions, in particular, in patients with hyperreactive airways.

Sodium bicarbonate has been aerosolized and directly instilled into the airway in intubated subjects to reduce the viscosity of airway secretions. This agent is not approved for such use. The reduction in secretion viscosity is thought to be caused by the increase in topical airway pH, with degradation of bonding in the mucin polysaccharide.

Expectorants are mucoactive but stimulate the production and clearance of airway secretions rather than cause mucolysis. Examples of such agents include guaifenesin (also known as glyceryl guaiacolate), iodinated glycerol, and saturated solution of potassium iodide (SSKI). Guaifenesin is found in many over-the-counter cough and cold products.

Assessment of Mucoactive Drug Therapy

Assessment of drug therapy for respiratory secretions is difficult. FEV_1 is relatively insensitive to changes in mucociliary clearance. The rate of change in lung function over time is a better marker. In addition, during maintenance therapy, the volume of sputum expectorated varies from day to day and does not reflect effective therapy. The following assessments should be performed.

Before Treatment

- Assess the patient's adequacy of cough and level of consciousness to determine need for treatment with mechanical suctioning or adjunct bronchial hygiene (postural drainage or percussion, positive expiratory pressure therapy) to clear the airway or if treatment is contraindicated.

During Treatment and Short-Term

- Teach and then verify correct use of aerosol nebulization system, including cleaning.
- Assess therapy based on indication for drug: mucolysis and improved clearance of secretions.
- Monitor airflow changes or adverse effects such as a decrease in FEV_1.
- Assess the patient's breathing pattern and rate.
- Assess the patient's subjective reaction to treatment (changes in breathing effort or pattern).
- Discontinue therapy if the patient experiences adverse reactions.

Long-Term

- Discontinue therapy if the patient experiences adverse reactions.
- Monitor number and severity of respiratory tract infections and need for antibiotic therapy, emergency visits, and hospitalizations.
- Monitor pulmonary function for improvement or slowing in the rate of deterioration.

General Contraindications

Mucoactive therapy should be used with caution in patients with severely compromised vital capacity and expiratory flow, such as in the presence of end-stage pulmonary disease or neuromuscular disorders. Generally, if FEV_1 is less than 25% of predicted, it becomes difficult to mobilize and expectorate secretions. Theoretically, with profound airflow compromise, secretion clearance could decline.

Gastroesophageal reflux and inability of the patient to protect the airway are risk factors for postural drainage that should be considered if postural drainage is necessary with mucoactive therapy. Mucoactive agents should be discontinued if there is evidence of clinical deterioration. Patients with acute bronchitis or exacerbation of chronic disease (CF, COPD) may be less responsive to mucoactive therapy, possibly secondary to infection and muscular weakness, which can reduce airflow-dependent mechanisms further.[26]

INHALED CORTICOSTEROIDS

Corticosteroids are endogenous hormones produced in the adrenal cortex, which regulate basic metabolic functions in the body and exert an antiinflammatory effect.[30] The use of aerosolized corticosteroids is reviewed in this section. All corticosteroids used to treat asthma and COPD are glucocorticoids.

Indications and Purposes

The two general formulations of aerosolized glucocorticoids are orally inhaled and intranasal aerosol preparations. Orally inhaled preparations are listed in Table 32-5. The primary use of orally inhaled corticosteroids is for antiinflammatory maintenance therapy of persistent asthma[6] and severe COPD.[31] The use of intranasal steroids is for control of seasonal allergic or nonallergic rhinitis. Most agents in Table 32-5 are available as intranasal preparations, with the exception of the combination drugs.

Mode of Action

Glucocorticoids are lipid-soluble drugs that act on intracellular receptors. The complex action of steroids is illustrated in Figure 32-6.[32-34] Because steroid action involves modification of cell transcription, full antiinflammatory effects require hours to days. It is important for patients to understand that inhalation of an aerosolized steroid does not provide immediate relief as with an adrenergic bronchodilator. However, daily compliance with the inhaled medication is essential to controlling the inflammation of asthma. Oral corticosteroids may be needed initially to clear the airway or as "burst" therapy to control asthma exacerbations.

TABLE 32-5

Corticosteroids and Combination Products Available by Aerosol for Oral Inhalation*

Drug	Brand Name	Formulation and Dosage
Beclomethasone dipropionate HFA	QVAR	MDI: 40 and 80 μg/puff Adults and children ≥12 yr: 40-80 μg twice daily† or 40-160 μg twice daily‡ Children ≥5 yr: 40-80 μg twice daily
Ciclesonide	Alvesco	MDI: 40 μg/puff and 80 μg/puff Adults and children ≥12 yr: 80-160 μg twice daily† or 80-320 μg twice daily‡
Flunisolide hemihydrate HFA	AeroSpan	MDI: 80 μg/puff Adults and children ≥12 yr: 2 puffs twice daily, adults no more than 4 puffs daily§ Children 6-11 yr: 1 puff daily, no more than 2 puffs daily
Fluticasone propionate	Flovent HFA	MDI: 44, 110, and 220 μg/puff Adults and children ≥12 yr: 88 μg twice daily†, 88-220 μg twice daily‡, or 880 μg twice daily§ Children 4-11 yr: 88 μg twice daily¶
	Flovent Diskus	DPI: 50, 100, and 250 μg Adults and children ≥12 yr: 100 μg twice daily†, 100-250 μg twice daily‡, 1000 μg twice daily§ Children 4-11 yr: 50 μg twice daily
Budesonide	Pulmicort Flexhaler	DPI: 90 μg/actuation and 180 μg/actuation Adults and children ≥12 yr: 180-360 μg bid†, 180-360 μg bid‡, 360-720 μg bid§ Children ≥6 yr: 180-360 μg bid
	Pulmicort Respules	SVN: 0.25 mg/2 ml, 0.5 mg/2 ml, 1 mg/2 ml Children 1-8 yr: 0.5-mg total dose given once daily or twice daily in divided doses†,‡ 1 mg given as 0.5 mg twice daily or once daily§
Mometasone furoate	Asmanex Twisthaler	DPI: 220 μg/actuation; or 110 μg actuation Adults and children ≥12 yr: 220-440 μg daily†, 220-440 μg daily‡, 440-880 μg daily§; children 4-11 yrs: 110-220 μg daily
Fluticasone propionate/salmeterol	Advair Diskus	DPI: 100 μg fluticasone/50 μg salmeterol, 250 μg fluticasone/50 μg salmeterol, or 500 μg fluticasone/50 μg salmeterol
	Advair HFA	Adults and children ≥12 yr: 100 μg fluticasone/50 μg salmeterol, 1 inhalation twice daily, about 12 hr apart (starting dose if not currently taking inhaled corticosteroids) Maximal recommended dose 500 μg fluticasone/50 μg salmeterol twice daily Children ≥4 yr: 100 μg fluticasone/50 μg salmeterol, 1 inhalation twice daily, about 12 hr apart (for patients who are symptomatic while taking an inhaled corticosteroid)§ MDI: 45 μg fluticasone/21 μg salmeterol, 115 μg fluticasone/21 μg salmeterol, or 230 μg fluticasone/21 μg salmeterol§ Adults and children ≥12 yr: 2 inhalations twice daily, about 12 hr apart
Budesonide/formoterol fumarate HFA	Symbicort	MDI: 80 μg budesonide/4.5 μg formoterol and 160 μg budesonide/4.5 μg formoterol twice daily Adults and children ≥12yr: 320 μg budesonide/9 μg formoterol; or 160 μg budesonide/9 μg formoterol twice daily
Mometasone furoate/formoterol fumarate HFA	Dulera	MDI: 100 μg mometasone/5 μg formoterol and 200 μg mometasone/5 μg formoterol Adults and children ≥12 yr: If previously on medium dose of corticosteroids, ≤400 μg mometasone/20 μg formoterol daily; if previously on high dose of corticosteroid, ≤800 μg mometasone/20 μg formoterol daily

HFA, Hydrofluoroalkane.
*Individual agents are discussed in the text. Detailed information about each agent should be obtained from the manufacturer's drug insert.
†Recommended starting dose if taking only bronchodilators.
‡Recommended starting dose if previously taking inhaled corticosteroids.
§Recommended starting dose if previously taking oral corticosteroids.
¶This dose should be used regardless of previous therapy.

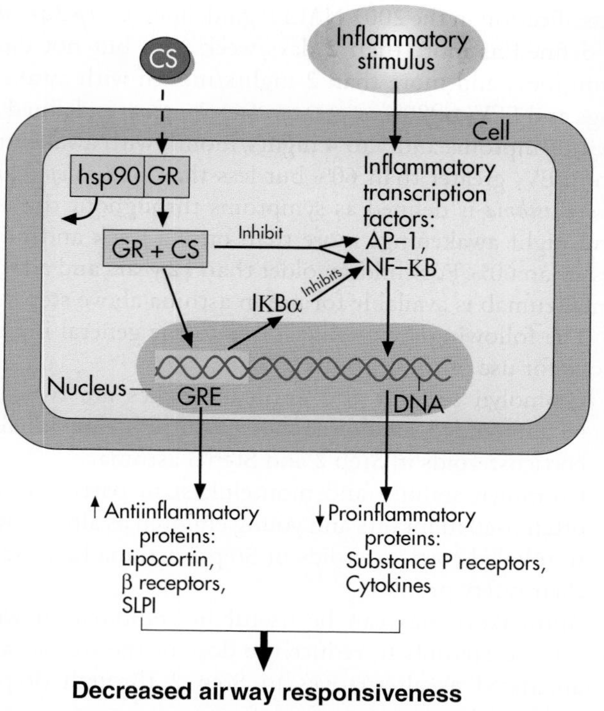

FIGURE 32-6 Mode of action by which corticosteroids modify cell response to inhibit inflammatory response in the airway. Corticosteroids (CS) diffuse into the cell and bind to a glucocorticoid receptor (GR). When the steroid binds to the GR, a protein, hsp 90, dissociates from the GR, and the steroid-GR complex moves into the cell nucleus. The drug-receptor complex binds to glucocorticoid response elements (GRE) of the nuclear DNA to upregulate transcription of antiinflammatory substances such as lipocortin, a protein that inhibits the generation of the arachidonic acid cascade by phospholipase A_2.There is evidence that steroids also upregulate inhibitors of factors in the cell, such as nuclear factor-κB (NF-κB), which can cause transcription of inflammatory substances. There may be direct inhibition of factors such as NF-κB to limit the inflammatory process further. (From Gardenhire DS: Rau's respiratory care pharmacology, ed 8, St. Louis, 2012, Elsevier.)

Adverse Effects

The type and severity of side effects seen with inhaled aerosolized corticosteroids are much less than with systemic use, as with other classes of aerosolized drugs. Box 32-3 lists systemic and local effects that can occur with inhaled steroids. The systemic effect of adrenal suppression is not usually seen with inhaled doses less than 800 mcg/day in adults or less than 400 mcg/day in children. Use of a reservoir device should be routine with inhaled steroids to prevent a swallowed portion adding to the systemic effect and to prevent the local effects of oral candidiasis and dysphonia. Growth retardation with use of inhaled steroids in asthma is controversial. Some investigators found no growth suppression even with high-dose inhaled steroids. Allen and colleagues[35] published a comprehensive review of inhaled steroids.

Box 32-3 Potential Hazards and Side Effects of Aerosolized Corticosteroids

SYSTEMIC
- Adrenal insufficiency*
- Extrapulmonary allergy*
- Acute asthma*
- HPA suppression (minimal, dose-dependent)
- Growth retardation†
- Osteoporosis†

LOCAL (TOPICAL)
- Oropharyngeal fungal infections
- Dysphonia
- Cough, bronchoconstriction
- Incorrect use of MDI

HPA, Hypothalamo-pituitary-adrenocortical.
*Following substitution for systemic corticosteroid therapy.
†Effect with inhaled corticosteroids alone is unclear.

Special Considerations

The modes of action of all inhaled glucocorticoids are the same with one exception. Ciclesonide, a **prodrug,** is given as an inactive compound and is converted to an active metabolite, desisobutyryl-ciclesonide, by intracellular enzymes. Ciclesonide is available as an intranasal formulation (Omnaris) and a pressurized MDI (Alvesco).

Assessment of Drug Therapy

The basic actions to evaluate an aerosol drug treatment should be followed (see section on Assessment of Bronchodilator Therapy). As with other drug therapy, the indications for this class of drug should be present. The 2007 NAEPP and 2010 Global Initiative on Obstructive Lung Disease (GOLD) COPD guidelines are recommended for guidance.[6,31] In addition, with inhaled corticosteroids, the following actions are suggested:

- Verify that the patient understands that a corticosteroid is a controller agent and is different from a rescue bronchodilator (relieving agent); assess the patient's understanding of the need for consistent use of an inhaled corticosteroid (compliance with therapy).
- Instruct the patient in the use of a peak flowmeter to monitor baseline peak expiratory flow (PEF) and changes. Verify that there is a specific action plan, based on symptoms and PEF results. The patient should understand when to contact a physician with deterioration in PEF or exacerbation of symptoms.

Long-Term

- Assess severity of symptoms (coughing, wheezing, nocturnal awakenings, symptoms during exertion; use of rescue bronchodilator; number of exacerbations; missed work or school days; and pulmonary function), and modify level or dosage as recommended by NAEPP and GOLD guidelines.[6,31]

- Assess for the presence of side effects with inhaled steroid therapy (oral thrush, hoarseness or voice changes, cough or wheezing with MDI use); use a reservoir (preferably a holding chamber) with MDI use, and verify correct technique.

MINI CLINI

Patient Education

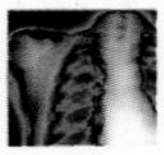

PROBLEM: A 24-year-old patient with asthma has complained of waking up at night and being short of breath. She also reports feeling tight in her chest and needs to use her albuterol inhaler 5 to 6 days a week to get relief. She is not currently on other inhaled medications. Her allergist prescribes an inhaled MDI corticosteroid and salmeterol to be taken on a daily basis. What instructions should she be given in using these agents by inhalation?

DISCUSSION: The key points with corticosteroid inhalation should be reviewed. These are small doses and safe to take. However, it is important to take the prescribed corticosteroid dose regularly every day if the drug is to have an antiinflammatory effect in the lung. She should also use a reservoir device with the MDI. Rinsing her mouth with water after a treatment can reduce further the chance of oral candidiasis or dysphonia. With salmeterol, she should also be instructed to follow her prescribed dose, which is usually two inhalations, twice daily. Because of its pharmacokinetics, salmeterol is considered a long-term controller and not a quick reliever. It is not helpful in relieving bronchospasm if she experiences acute difficulty in breathing. For acute respiratory problems, she should have a quick-acting adrenergic agent such as albuterol or levalbuterol. If she experiences wheezing or chest tightness, one or two actuations of one of these agents would help. Salmeterol should be taken at the regularly prescribed time, usually every 12 hours.

NONSTEROIDAL ANTIASTHMA DRUGS

Nonsteroidal antiinflammatory drugs constitute a growing class of drugs in the treatment of asthma. These include mast cell stabilizers (cromolyn sodium); antileukotrienes, also termed **leukotriene** modifiers (zafirlukast, zileuton, montelukast); and a new class, monoclonal antibodies or anti-IgE agents (omalizumab). Antileukotrienes are administered orally, and the monoclonal antibody agent omalizumab is given parenterally, but these are included as bronchoactive drugs. Table 32-6 lists pharmaceutical details for each agent.

Indication for Use

The general indication for clinical use of nonsteroidal antiasthma agents is prophylactic management (control) of persistent asthma (Step 2 or greater asthma, using the classification in the 2007 NAEPP guidelines[6]). *Step 2 asthma* is defined as more than 2 days/week with but not daily symptoms and more than 2 nights/month with awakenings and FEV_1 of 80% or greater. *Step 3 asthma* is defined as daily symptoms and 3 to 4 nights/month with awakening and FEV_1 greater than 60% but less than 80%. *Step 4 and above asthma* is defined as symptoms throughout the day and night awakenings more than once a week and FEV_1 less than 60%. For children older than 12 years and adults, omalizumab is available for use in asthma above step 4.[36]

The following are qualifications to the general indications for use of these agents:

- Cromolyn sodium and antileukotrienes are typically recommended as alternatives to introducing inhaled corticosteroids in Step 2 and Step 3 asthma.
- Cromolyn sodium and montelukast in particular are often used in infants and young children as alternatives to inhaled corticosteroids in Step 2 asthma because of their safety profiles.
- Antileukotrienes can be useful in combination with inhaled steroids to reduce the dose of the steroid and are listed as alternatives in Step 2 through Step 4 asthma.
- The monoclonal antibody omalizumab is available for consideration in the appropriate population.[37]

All of the nonsteroidal antiasthma drugs described in this chapter are controllers, not relievers, and are used in asthma requiring antiinflammatory drug therapy (Box 32-4).

Mode of Action

Cromolyn sodium acts by inhibiting the degranulation of mast cells in response to allergic and nonallergic stimuli. This inhibition prevents release of histamine and other mediators of inflammation. These mediators cause

Box 32-4 Bronchoactive Agents Distinguished as Controllers or Relievers in Treating Asthma

LONG-TERM CONTROL

Inhaled corticosteroids
Cromolyn sodium
Long-acting beta-2 agonists
  Inhaled: salmeterol, formoterol
  Oral: sustained-release albuterol
Leukotriene modifiers
Systemic corticosteroids
Methylxanthines (theophylline)

QUICK RELIEF

Short-acting inhaled beta-2 agonists: albuterol, levalbuterol
Anticholinergic (antimuscarinic): ipratropium
Systemic corticosteroids (oral burst therapy, IV)

From National Asthma Education and Prevention Program, National Heart, Lung and Blood Institute, National Institutes of Health: Expert Panel Report 3: Guidelines for the diagnosis and management of asthma, NIH Publication No. 08-4051. Bethesda, MD, 2007, NIH.

TABLE 32-6

Nonsteroidal Antiasthma Medications*

Generic Drug	Brand Name	Formulation and Dosage
Mast Cell Stabilizer		
Cromolyn sodium		SVN: 20 mg/ampule or 20 mg/2 ml Adults and children ≥2 yr: 20 mg inhaled 4 times daily
	NasalCrom	Spray: 40 mg/ml (4%) (5.2 mg per actuation) Adults and children ≥2 yr: 1 spray each nostril, 3-6 times daily every 4-6 hr
	Gastrocrom	Oral concentrate: 100 mg/5 ml Adults and children ≥13 yr: 2 ampules 4 times daily, 30 min before meals and at bedtime Children 2-12 yr: 1 ampule 4 time daily, 30 min before meals and at bedtime
Antileukotrienes		
Zafirlukast	Accolate	Tablets: 10 and 20 mg Adults and children ≥12 yr: 20 mg twice daily, without food Children 5-11 yr: 10 mg twice daily
Montelukast	Singulair	Tablets: 10 mg and 4-mg and 5-mg cherry-flavored chewable; 4-mg packet of granules Adults and children ≥15 yr: 1 10-mg tablet daily Children 6-14 yr: 1 5-mg chewable tablet daily Children 2-5 yr: 1 4-mg chewable tablet or 1 4-mg packet of granules daily 6-23 mo: 1 4-mg packet of granules daily
Zileuton	Zyflo; Zyflo CR	Tablets: 600 mg Adults and children ≥12 yr: 1 600-mg tablet 4 times per day; CR, 2 tablets twice daily, within 1 hr of morning and evening meals
Monoclonal Antibody		
Omalizumab	Xolair	Adults and children ≥12 yr: subcutaneous injection every 4 wk; dose dependent on weight and serum IgE level

*Detailed prescribing information should be obtained from the manufacturer's package insert.

bronchospasm and trigger an increasing cascade of further mediator release and inflammatory cell activity in the airway.[38]

Zafirlukast and montelukast act as leukotriene receptor antagonists and are selective competitive antagonists of leukotriene receptors LTD_4 and LTE_4. Leukotrienes such as LTC_4, LTD_4, and LTE_4 (previously known as SRS-A) stimulate leukotriene receptors termed $CysLT_1$ to cause bronchoconstriction, mucus secretion, vascular permeability, and plasma exudation into the airway. The mode of action is shown in Figure 32-7. The drug inhibits asthma reactions induced by exercise, cold air, allergens, and aspirin.[39]

Zileuton inhibits the 5-lipoxygenase enzyme that catalyzes the formation of leukotrienes from arachidonic acid (see Figure 32-7).[40] Omalizumab is a recombinant DNA-derived humanized antibody that binds to IgE. The agent inhibits the attachment of IgE to mast cells and basophils, reducing the release of chemical mediators of the allergic response.[41]

Adverse Effects

A potential adverse effect with any nonsteroidal antiasthma drug is inappropriate use. These agents are not bronchodilators and offer no benefit for acute airway obstruction in asthma. Using the NAEPP terminology, all of these agents are controllers rather than relievers.[6]

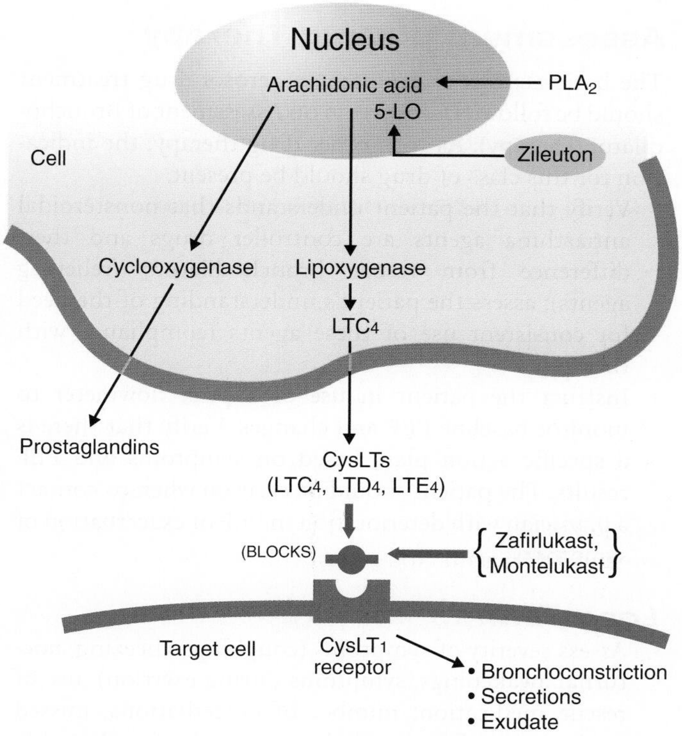

FIGURE 32-7 Modes and sites of action for leukotriene modifiers zileuton, zafirlukast, and montelukast. Zileuton inhibits the 5-LO enzyme, whereas zafirlukast and montelukast block the leukotriene receptor ($CysLT_1$).

TABLE 32-7
Summary of Comparative Features of Three Available Antileukotriene Agents

	Zileuton	Zafirlukast	Montelukast
Brand name	Zyflo; Zyflo CR	Accolate	Singulair
Action	5-LO inhibitor	$CysLT_1$ receptor block	$CysLT_1$ receptor block
Age range	≥12 yr	≥5 yr	≥6 mos
Dosage	600-mg tab, qid; CR: 2 600-mg tab bid; 1 hr within morning and evening meal	Adult: 20-mg tab bid Children 5-11 yr: 10-mg tab bid	Adult: 10-mg tab q evening 6-14 yr: 5-mg tab q evening 2-5 yr: 4-mg tab q evening 6-23 mo: 4-mg oral granules q evening
Administration	Can be taken with food	1 hr before or 2 hr after meal	Taken with or without food
Drug interaction	Yes (theophylline, warfarin, propranolol)	Yes (warfarin, theophylline, aspirin)	No
Side effects (common)	Headache, dyspepsia, unspecified pain, liver enzyme elevations	Headache, infection, nausea, possible liver enzyme changes	Headache, influenza, abdominal pain
Contraindications	Active liver disease or elevated liver enzyme levels, hypersensitivity to components	Hypersensitivity to components	Hypersensitivity to components

Table 32-7 summarizes information and comparative features of the three antileukotriene agents, including drug interactions, common side effects, and contraindications. The most common adverse reactions seen with omalizumab include injection site reaction, viral infections, respiratory tract infections, headache, sinusitis, and pharyngitis.

Assessment of Drug Therapy

The basic actions to evaluate an aerosol drug treatment should be followed (see section on Assessment of Bronchodilator Therapy). As with other drug therapy, the indication for this class of drug should be present.

- Verify that the patient understands that nonsteroidal antiasthma agents are controller drugs and their difference from rescue bronchodilators (relieving agents); assess the patient's understanding of the need for consistent use of these agents (compliance with therapy).
- Instruct the patient in use of a peak flowmeter to monitor baseline PEF and changes. Verify that there is a specific action plan, based on symptoms and PEF results. The patient should be clear on when to contact a physician with deterioration in PEF or exacerbation of symptoms.

Long-Term

- Assess severity of symptoms (coughing, wheezing, nocturnal awakenings, symptoms during exertion); use of rescue medication; number of exacerbations; missed work or school days; pulmonary function), and modify level of asthma therapy (up or down, as described in the 2007 NAEPP EPR III guidelines for step therapy).
- Assess for the presence of side effects with nonsteroidal antiasthma agents; refer to the particular agent and its side effects (listed previously).

AEROSOLIZED ANTIINFECTIVE AGENTS

Multiple aerosolized antiinfective agents are available. Some agents may be used less often than others in respiratory therapy. The antiinfective agents pentamidine, ribavirin, inhaled tobramycin, and zanamivir are briefly outlined here. Drug formulations and dosages are given in Table 32-8.

Pentamidine Isethionate

Pentamidine isethionate (NebuPent) is an antiprotozoal agent that has been used in the treatment of opportunistic pneumonia caused by *Pneumocystis jiroveci,* which is the causative agent of pneumocystis pneumonia (PCP). PCP is seen in immunocompromised patients, especially patients with AIDS.

Indication for Use

Comparisons of the efficacy of aerosolized pentamidine with oral trimethoprim-sulfamethoxazole (TMP-SMX), together with reports of serious adverse effects with aerosolized pentamidine, led to a reevaluation of aerosol therapy with pentamidine for prophylaxis of PCP. General recommendations for prophylaxis of PCP were published by the U.S. Centers for Disease Control and Prevention (CDC) in for HIV-positive children[42] and adults.[43] In the 2009 CDC recommendations, oral TMP-SMX was preferred for prophylaxis of PCP as long as adverse side effects

TABLE 32-8

Inhaled Antiinfective Agents*

Drug	Brand Name	Formulation and Dosage	Clinical Use
Pentamidine isethionate	NebuPent	300 mg powder in 6 ml sterile water; 300 mg once every 4 wk	PCP prophylaxis
Ribavirin	Virazole	6 g powder in 300 ml sterile water (20-mg/ml solution); given every 12-18 hr/day for 3-7 days by SPAG nebulizer	RSV
Tobramycin	TOBI	300-mg/5-ml ampule; adults and children ≥6 years: 300 mg bid, 28 days on/28 days off drug	*P. aeruginosa* infection in CF
Aztreonam	Cayston	75 mg/1 ml; adults and children ≥7 yr: 75 mg tid, 28 days on/28 days off drug	*P. aeruginosa* infection in CF
Zanamivir	Relenza	DPI: 5 mg/inhalation; adults ≥5 years: 2 inhalations (1 5-mg blister per inhalation) bid, 12 hr apart for 5 days	Influenza

*Details on use and administration should be obtained from manufacturer's drug insert material before use.

from TMP-SMX were absent or acceptable.[43] Aerosolized pentamidine is recommended as an alternative therapy for prophylaxis of PCP if TMP-SMX cannot be tolerated.

Adverse Effects

Possible side effects with aerosolized pentamidine include cough, bronchial irritation, bronchospasm and wheezing, shortness of breath, fatigue, bad or metallic taste, pharyngitis, conjunctivitis, rash, and chest pain. Systemic effects have also been noted with inhaled pentamidine, including decreased appetite, dizziness, rash, nausea, night sweats, chills, spontaneous pneumothoraces, **neutropenia,** pancreatitis, renal insufficiency, and hypoglycemia. It is difficult to distinguish systemic effects caused by the drug versus the disease. Extrapulmonary infection with *P. jiroveci* can occur with prophylactic inhaled pentamidine.

Assessment

When administering aerosolized pentamidine, isolation, an environmental containment system (e.g., a booth or negative pressure room), and personnel barrier protection should be provided. Patients should be screened for tuberculosis. The drug is given using a nebulizer system with one-way valves and scavenging expiratory filters (e.g., Respirgard); this reduces environmental contamination. Nebulizer systems capable of producing a mass median astrodynamic diameter of 1 to 2 μm for peripheral lung deposition may reduce coughing. The patient should be monitored for onset of any of the previously described adverse reactions. In addition, the following actions are recommended:

- If coughing and bronchospasm are present, provide a short-acting beta agonist or an anticholinergic bronchodilator such as ipratropium if present with inhaled pentamidine.
- Monitor for occurrence rate of PCP and rate of long-term hospitalizations.
- Monitor for presence of side effects (shortness of breath, possible pneumothorax, conjunctivitis, rash, neutropenia, dysglycemia) or appearance of extrapulmonary *P. jiroveci* infection.
- Evaluate need for prior use of a bronchodilator if symptoms of bronchospasm or coughing occur after inhalation of pentamidine.

Long-Term

- Monitor efficacy of pentamidine prophylaxis in preventing episodes of PCP.

Ribavirin

Ribavirin (Virazole) is an antiviral agent used in the treatment of severe lower respiratory tract infections caused by respiratory syncytial virus (RSV). RSV is a common seasonal respiratory infection in infants and young children, which is usually self-limiting. The cost-effectiveness of ribavirin continues to be debated. Recommendations for use of the drug were published in a statement by the American Academy of Pediatrics.[44] Administration of the aerosol requires use of a special large-reservoir nebulizer called a *small particle aerosol generator (SPAG).* The mode of action of ribavirin is ascribed to the similarity of the drug to guanosine, a natural nucleoside. Substitution of ribavirin for the natural nucleoside interrupts the viral replication process in the host cell.

Adverse Effects

Skin rash, eyelid erythema, and conjunctivitis have been noted with aerosol administration. Important equipment-related effects during mechanical ventilation include endotracheal tube occlusion and occlusion of ventilator expiratory valves or sensors. Deterioration of pulmonary function can occur. Patients or practitioners who are pregnant should not have exposure to ribavirin.

Assessment

- Monitor signs of improvement in RSV infection severity, including vital signs, respiratory pattern and work of breathing (clinically), level of fractional inspired oxygen (FiO_2) needed, level of ventilatory support,

arterial blood gases, body temperature, and other indicators of pulmonary gas exchange.
- Monitor the patient for evidence of side effects, such as deterioration in lung function, bronchospasm, occlusion of endotracheal tube (if present), cardiovascular instability, skin irritation from the aerosol drug, and equipment malfunction related to drug residue.

Inhaled Tobramycin

Patients with CF have chronic respiratory infection with *Pseudomonas aeruginosa* and other microorganisms. Such chronic infection causes recurrent acute respiratory infections and deterioration of lung function. With the exception of the quinoline derivatives such as ciprofloxacin, antibiotics such as the aminoglycosides (e.g., tobramycin), which are effective against *Pseudomonas* organisms, have poor lung bioavailability when taken orally. Consequently, these antibiotics must be given either intravenously or by inhalation. The aminoglycoside tobramycin has been approved for inhaled administration (TOBI) and is intended to manage chronic infection with *P. aeruginosa* in patients with CF. Goals of therapy are to treat or prevent early colonization with *P. aeruginosa* and maintain present lung function or reduce the rate of deterioration. The emergence of bacterial resistance was not seen in clinical trials with inhaled tobramycin.[45]

Adverse Effects

Side effects with parenteral aminoglycosides include possible auditory and vestibular damage with potential for deafness and nephrotoxicity. Other possible effects are listed in Box 32-5. Side effects observed since the introduction of inhaled tobramycin have been minimal and include voice alteration and tinnitus in a small percentage of patients. Risk for more serious side effects with tobramycin, whether by inhaled or parenteral routes, increases with the use of other aminoglycosides, in the presence of poor renal function and dehydration, with preexisting neuromuscular impairment, or with use of other ototoxic drugs.

Box 32-5 Side Effects With Aminoglycosides and Tobramycin

PARENTERAL ADMINISTRATION
- Ototoxicity (auditory and vestibular)
- Nephrotoxicity
- Neuromuscular blockade
- Hypomagnesemia
- Cross-allergenicity
- Fetal harm (deafness)

INHALED NEBULIZED TOBRAMYCIN
- Voice alteration
- Tinnitus
- Nonsignificant increase in bacterial resistance

The following precautions are suggested with use of inhaled tobramycin:
- Inhaled tobramycin should be used with caution in patients with preexisting renal, auditory, vestibular, or neuromuscular dysfunction.
- Tobramycin solution should not be mixed with beta-lactam antibiotics (penicillins, cephalosporins) because of admixture incompatibility, and mixing with other drugs in general is discouraged.
- Nebulization of antibiotics during hospitalization should be performed under conditions of containment, as previously described for pentamidine and ribavirin, to prevent environmental saturation and development of resistant organisms in the hospital.
- Aminoglycosides can cause fetal harm if administered to pregnant women; exposure to ambient aerosol drug should be avoided by women who are pregnant or trying to become pregnant.
- Local airway irritation resulting in cough and bronchospasm with decreased ventilatory flow rates is possible with inhaled antibiotics and seems to be related to the osmolality of the solution.[46,47] Peak flow rates and chest auscultation should be used before and after treatments to evaluate airway changes. Pretreatment with a beta agonist may be needed.
- Allergic reactions in the patient, staff, or family should be considered if exposure to the aerosolized drug is not controlled. The use of a nebulizing system with a scavenging filter, one-way valves, and thumb control could reduce ambient contamination with the drug, as previously described.

In clinical trials, inhaled tobramycin was administered using the PARI LC Plus nebulizer with a DeVilbiss Pulmo-Aide compressor. Other nebulizer systems must be tested to ensure adequate drug output and particle size because antibiotic solutions differ in viscosity from the aqueous bronchodilator solutions used in common disposable nebulizers. Studies have reported that not all nebulizer-compressor systems perform adequately with antibiotic solutions, and higher flow rates of 10 to 12 L/min may be needed with nebulizers.[48,49]

Assessment

- Verify that the patient understands that nebulized tobramycin should be given after other CF therapies, including other inhaled drugs.
- Check whether the patient has renal, auditory, vestibular, or neuromuscular problems or is taking other aminoglycosides or ototoxic drugs. Consider whether tobramycin should be used for the patient based on severity of preexisting or concomitant risk factors.
- Monitor lung function to note improvement in FEV_1.
- Assess rate of hospitalization before and after institution of inhaled tobramycin.
- Assess need for IV antipseudomonal therapy.
- Assess improvement in weight.

- Monitor for occurrence of side effects, such as tinnitus or voice alteration; have the patient rinse and expectorate after aerosol treatments.
- Evaluate for changes in hearing or renal function during use of inhaled tobramycin.

Inhaled Aztreonam

Aztreonam was approved in December 1986 by the FDA as a monobactam, a synthetic bactericidal antibiotic; it is given as an IV solution. Inhaled aztreonam (Cayston) was approved in 2010 to improve pulmonary symptoms in patients with CF colonized with *P. aeruginosa.*[50] Inhaled aztreonam is not indicated for patients younger than 7 years old or patients with *Burkholderia cepacia* infection. This agent has been studied only in patients with FEV_1 greater than 25% or less than 75% of predicted. The agent is delivered by itself using the Altera Nebulizer System.

Adverse Effects

Inhaled aztreonam can cause bronchospasm and decrease FEV_1. All patients should be screened for baseline pulmonary function results and be treated with a bronchodilator before administering inhaled aztreonam.

Patients have been reported to experience severe allergic reactions with injectable aztreonam. Careful observation is warranted when first using inhaled aztreonam because it could cause an allergic reaction. If any signs occur during the delivery of inhaled aztreonam, the treatment should be stopped immediately, and the health care team should be informed.

The use of antibiotics in the absence of infection may lead to the development of drug-resistant bacteria. Inhaled aztreonam should not be used in patients with CF not infected with *P. aeruginosa.*

Colistimethate Sodium

Colistimethate sodium (colistin) is an antibiotic used to treat sensitive strains of gram-negative bacilli, particularly *P. aeruginosa.* Colistimethate sodium is available as an inhaled formulation in Europe as Promixin; this agent is not approved for inhalation by the FDA. However, nebulization of the parenteral formulation is commonly used in patients with CF. Falagas and colleagues[51] published a review of IV and aerosolized colistimethate sodium.

Adverse Effects

Side effects seen with parenteral administration include neurotoxic events and nephrotoxicity. Because colistimethate sodium is mainly eliminated by the renal system, renal insufficiency should be considered. Neurotoxic events associated with colistimethate sodium include dizziness, confusion, muscle weakness, and possible neuromuscular blockade, leading to respiratory arrest. When using aerosolized colistimethate sodium, the most common complication seen is bronchospasm. Pretreatment with a beta agonist can decrease the potential for this complication.

Inhaled Zanamivir

Zanamivir is an inhaled powder aerosol (DPI). Despite the availability of zanamivir and the oral antiinfluenza agent oseltamivir (Tamiflu), prophylactic vaccination against influenza is still recommended, especially in high-risk individuals with cardiovascular or pulmonary disease. Zanamivir and oseltamivir represent a new class of antiviral agents termed *neuraminidase inhibitors.*

Indication for Use

Inhaled zanamivir is indicated for the treatment of uncomplicated acute illness caused by influenza virus in adults and children 5 years or older who have been symptomatic for no longer than 2 days. The agents have an off-label use for treatment and prophylaxis of H1N1 influenza A.

Mode of Action

The influenza virus attaches to respiratory tract cells by binding of viral surface hemagglutinin to the cell's surface molecule of sialic acid (Figure 32-8). The viral particle also has an enzyme, neuraminidase, on its surface. When replicated viral particles are released from the host cell after

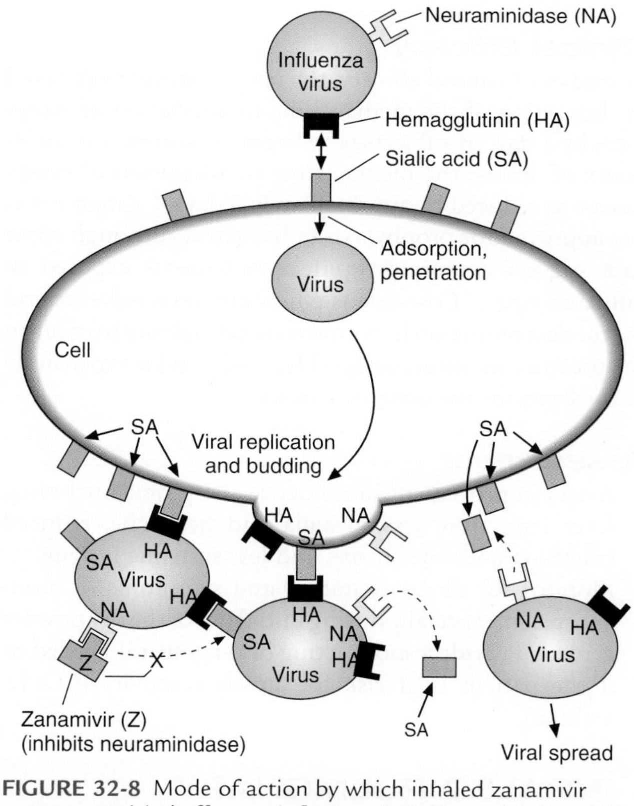

FIGURE 32-8 Mode of action by which inhaled zanamivir exerts an antiviral effect on influenza virus. Zanamivir is a sialic acid analogue and binds to neuraminidase, the enzyme responsible for cleaving sialic acid and preventing viral binding to sialic acid. This causes viral aggregation, with binding of viral particles to each other and to the host cell, preventing viral spread. (From Gardenhire DS: Rau's respiratory care pharmacology, ed 8, St. Louis, 2012, Elsevier.)

infection, the viral neuraminidase cleaves the sialic acid on both the host cell surface and other viral particle surfaces so that mature virus can be released and spread. Without neuraminidase, influenza virus would clump together and to the host cell, preventing spread. Zanamivir and oseltamivir combine with the surface neuraminidase, preventing its action and the spread of viral particles.

Adverse Effects

Several adverse effects can occur with inhaled zanamivir:

- Bronchospasm and deterioration in lung function, especially in patients with COPD or asthma
- Possible undertreatment of bacterial infection masquerading as a viral infection or a secondary bacterial infection in the presence of influenza
- Allergic reactions, as may occur with any drug
- Adverse reactions, such as diarrhea, nausea, vomiting, bronchitis, cough, sinusitis, dizziness, and headaches

Because of the effect on lung function in patients with respiratory disease and reports of adverse reactions, revised labeling for the drug carries a warning that zanamivir is not generally recommended for patients with underlying airways disease.[52] However, other studies have determined that high-risk patients such as patients with asthma and COPD were not affected by the use of zanamivir.[53]

Clinical Efficacy

In studies of clinical efficacy, the use of zanamivir resulted in shortening of the median time to alleviation of symptoms by 1 day. In subjects who began treatment within 30 hours of illness, the median time to alleviation of symptoms was reduced by approximately 3 days.[54] Zanamivir is not approved for prophylaxis of influenza, although some data suggest a preventive effect in patients exposed to influenza virus.[53] Cost-versus-efficacy issues revolve around the modest reduction in symptoms and inability to confirm the presence of influenza quickly, easily, and inexpensively as the basis for the drug treatment.

Assessment

- Assess improvement in influenza symptoms, including fever reduction, less myalgia and headache, reduced coughing and sore throat, and less systemic fatigue.
- Monitor for airway irritation and symptoms of bronchospasm, especially during initial use of the dry powder aerosol. Provide a short-acting beta agonist if needed or if the patient is at risk for airway reactivity (COPD, asthma).

INHALED PULMONARY VASODILATORS

The use of nitric oxide gas to treat neonates with persistent pulmonary hypertension is approved by the FDA and is discussed in detail in Chapter 38. In addition to this medical gas, inhaled medications are being tested and used to treat pulmonary hypertension. Several such agents are being studied, including epoprostenol (Flolan) and alprostadil (Prostin VR Pediatric); however, only two, iloprost, and treprostenil, are approved by the FDA for widespread use. Siobal[55] published a review of aerosolized prostacyclins and nitric oxide.

Nitric Oxide

Indications for Use

As described in more detail in Chapter 38, nitric oxide (INOmax) is indicated in the treatment of neonates (>34 weeks' gestational age) with hypoxic respiratory failure.[56] The patient should have evidence of pulmonary hypertension in which nitric oxide would improve oxygenation and decrease the need for extracorporeal membrane oxygenation. Off-label uses include reducing pulmonary artery pressure in the neonate.[57]

Mode of Action

Nitric oxide is produced by cells in the body. It relaxes vascular smooth muscle by binding to the heme group of cytosolic guanylate cyclase, activating guanylate cyclase, and increasing cyclic guanosine monophosphate. When inhaled, nitric oxide produces pulmonary vasodilation, reducing pulmonary artery pressure and improving $\dot{V}/\dot{Q}$ mismatching.

Adverse Effects

Nitric oxide is contraindicated in neonates with dependent right-to-left shunts. Precautions include methemoglobinemia and nitric dioxide formation. The most common adverse events are hypotension and withdrawal.[58]

Iloprost

Indications for Use

Iloprost (Ventavis) inhalation is indicated for the treatment of pulmonary hypertension.[59] Iloprost inhalation is administered with the I-neb nebulizer.

Mode of Action

Iloprost is a synthetic analogue of prostacyclin (PGI_2). This agent dilates pulmonary arterial vascular beds and affects platelet aggregation. It is unknown whether platelet aggregation plays a role in the treatment of pulmonary hypertension.

Adverse Effects

Syncope and pulmonary edema may occur secondary to the vasodilatory properties of iloprost. During the 12-week clinical trial, headache and increased cough were the most noted adverse reactions.

Treprostinil

Indication for Use

Treprostinil (Tyvaso) is indicated for the treatment of pulmonary arterial hypertension to increase walking distance in patients with New York Heart Association class III symptoms.[60] It is administered using the Tyvaso

Inhalation System, which is an ultrasonic, pulsed-delivery device.

Mode of Action

Treprostinil is a prostacyclin analogue that causes vasodilation of the pulmonary and systemic arterial vascular beds and inhibits platelet aggregation. Treprostinil is available in a 2.9-mL ampule, which contains 1.74 mg of treprostinil (0.6 mg/mL). It is provided as a nebulization in the Tyvaso Inhalation System. The ampule is dumped into the medication cup of the nebulizer and is used for the entire day.

The patient receives the prescribed amount of drug as a nebulization in four separate, equally spaced treatment sessions per day during waking hours. Each breath delivers 6 mcg of treprostinil. The initial dose is 3 breaths (18 mcg) per treatment session. If not tolerated, the dose may be reduced to 1 to 2 breaths per session and then increased to 3 breaths. Treprostinil should be increased by 3 breaths every 1 to 2 weeks until a dose of 9 breaths (54 mcg) per treatment session is reached.

Adverse Effects

Treprostinil has not been studied in patients with underlying lung disease (e.g., asthma, COPD). Treprostinil may cause bronchospasm. This agent should not be mixed with any other agents.

SUMMARY CHECKLIST

- Orally inhaled aerosol drug classes include beta-agonist bronchodilators, anticholinergic (antimuscarinic) bronchodilators, mucolytics, corticosteroids, nonsteroidal antiasthma drugs, and antiinfective agents.
- Beta-agonist and anticholinergic bronchodilators are used to reverse or improve airflow obstruction; mucolytics are used to reduce mucus viscosity and improve mucociliary clearance; corticosteroids and nonsteroidal antiasthma agents are used to reduce or prevent airway inflammation in asthma; the antiinfective agent pentamidine is used to treat PCP, especially in patients with AIDS; ribavirin is used to treat RSV infection in at-risk infants and children; inhaled tobramycin is used in patients with CF to prevent or manage gram-negative *Pseudomonas* infections; and inhaled zanamivir is used to treat acute influenza.
- Selection of an appropriate aerosol class of drug is based on matching the indication for the drug class to the presence of the indication in the patient. For example, the presence of repeated respiratory infections requiring IV antibiotics and hospitalizations and causing declining lung function in a patient with CF matches the indication for use of dornase alfa or inhaled tobramycin or both agents.
- All aerosol treatments are assessed immediately by monitoring respiratory "vital signs," which include respiratory rate and pattern, pulse, breath sounds on auscultation, general patient appearance (e.g., color, diaphoresis), and patient report of subjective reaction (e.g., "chest tightness"). Additional assessment should be related to the indication for the drug (e.g., monitoring of peak flow rates or bedside spirometry with bronchodilator use; frequency of exacerbation or beta agonist use with inhaled corticosteroids in asthma).
- Each class of aerosol drug has its own mode of action. Beta agonists stimulate G protein–linked beta receptors to increase cyclic adenosine monophosphate and relax smooth muscle; anticholinergic agents block cholinergic (muscarinic) receptors in the airway to prevent bronchoconstriction; mucolytics lyse mucus; corticosteroids modify cell nuclear transcription to cause an antiinflammatory effect; cromolyn-like agents inhibit inflammatory mediator release or action; leukotriene modifiers competitively block leukotriene receptors (montelukast, zafirlukast) or 5-LO enzyme (zileuton); and antiinfectives inhibit particular infecting organisms (*P. jiroveci,* RSV, *Pseudomonas,* influenza).
- Common side effects with each class of drug include tremor and shakiness with beta agonists; dry mouth with anticholinergic agents; bronchial irritation with acetylcysteine; dysphonia and voice changes with dornase alfa; and oral fungal infections with corticosteroids. Miscellaneous reactions include cough, unpleasant taste, headache, and liver enzyme changes (zileuton) with nonsteroidal antiasthma agents, depending on the specific agent; bronchial irritation and bronchospasm (pentamidine); and skin rash, conjunctivitis, bronchial irritation, and equipment or endotracheal tube occlusion by drug precipitate (ribavirin). Nebulized antibiotics and zanamivir may cause bronchospasm and require higher than normal power gas flow rates (10 to 12 L/min).
- Agents used in asthma that provide quick relief include short-acting beta agonists (albuterol, levalbuterol, pirbuterol) and anticholinergic bronchodilators. Agents that provide long-term control include long-acting beta agonists (salmeterol, formoterol, arformoterol); inhaled corticosteroids; and nonsteroidal antiasthma drugs (cromolyn, nedocromil, montelukast, and other leukotriene antagonists). Systemic corticosteroids are used for both quick relief (intravenously) and long-term control (orally).
- Newer inhaled medications within a class known as aerosolized prostacyclins are being introduced to help treat pulmonary hypertension. Several agents are being studied, including epoprostenol (Flolan) and alprostadil (Prostin VR Pediatric); however, only treprostinil (Tyvaso) and iloprost (Ventavis) are being used on a widespread basis.

References

1. Gardenhire DS: Rau's respiratory care pharmacology, ed 8, St. Louis, 2012, Elsevier.
2. Katzung BG, Masters, SB, Trevor AJ: Basic and clinical pharmacology, ed 11, New York, 2009, McGraw-Hill.

3. Rau JL: The inhalation of drugs: advantages and problems. Respir Care 50:367, 2005.
4. Borgström L: A possible new approach of comparing different inhalers and inhaled substances. J Aerosol Med 4:A13, 1991.
5. Thorsson L: Influence of inhaler systems on systemic availability, with focus on inhaled corticosteroids. J Aerosol Med 8(Suppl 3):S29, 1995.
6. National Asthma Education and Prevention Program, National Heart, Lung and Blood Institute, National Institutes of Health: Expert Panel Report 3: Guidelines for the diagnosis and management of asthma, NIH Publication No. 08-4051, Bethesda, MD, 2007, NIH.
7. Barnes PJ: Beta-adrenergic receptors and their regulation. Am J Respir Crit Care Med 152:838, 1995.
8. Mitra S, Ugur M, Ugur O, et al: (S)-Albuterol increases intracellular free calcium by muscarinic receptor activation and a phospholipase C-dependent mechanism in airway smooth muscle. Mol Pharmacol 53:347, 1998.
9. Lipworth BJ, Clark DJ, Koch P, et al: Pharmacokinetics and extrapulmonary β_2 adrenoceptor activity of nebulised racemic salbutamol and its R- and S-isomers in healthy volunteers. Thorax 52:849, 1997.
10. Johansson FJ, Rydberg I, Aberg G, et al: Effects of albuterol enantiomers on in vitro bronchial reactivity. Clin Rev Allergy Immunol 14:57, 1996.
11. Templeton AG, Chapman ID, Chilvers ER, et al: Effects of S-salbutamol on human isolated bronchus. Pulm Pharmacol Ther 11:1, 1998.
12. Volcheck GW, Gleich GJ, Kita H: Pro- and anti-inflammatory effects of β-adrenergic agonists on eosinophil response to IL-5. J Allergy Clin Immunol 101:S35, 1998.
13. Schmekel B, Rydberg I, Norlander B, et al: Stereoselective pharmacokinetics of S-salbutamol after administration of the racemate in healthy volunteers. Eur Respir J 13:1230, 1999.
14. Dhand R, Goode M, Reid R, et al: Preferential pulmonary retention of (S)-albuterol after inhalation of racemic albuterol. Am J Respir Crit Care Med 160:1136, 1999.
15. Nelson HS, Bensch G, Pleskow WW, et al: Improved bronchodilation with levalbuterol compared with racemic albuterol in patients with asthma. J Allergy Clin Immunol 102:943, 1998.
16. Rau JL: Introduction of a single isomer β-agonist. Respir Care 45:962, 2000.
17. Johnson M, Butchers PR, Coleman RA, et al: The pharmacology of salmeterol. Life Sci 52:2131, 1993.
18. Bartow RA, Brogden RN: Formoterol: an update of its pharmacological properties and therapeutic efficacy in the management of asthma. Drugs 56:303, 1998.
19. McFadden ER, Jr: The β_2-agonist controversy revisited. Ann Allergy Asthma Immunol 75:173, 1995.
20. Jenne JW: Adverse effects of β-adrenergic agonists. In Leff AR, editor: Pulmonary and critical care pharmacology and therapeutics, New York, 1996, McGraw-Hill.
21. Meltzer EO: Intranasal anticholinergic therapy of rhinorrhea. J Allergy Clin Immunol 90:1055, 1992.
22. Barr RG, Bourbeau J, Camargo CA, Jr, et al. Tiotropium for stable chronic obstructive pulmonary disease: a meta-analysis. Thorax 61:854, 2006.
23. Rubin BK: The pharmacologic approach to airway clearance: mucoactive agents. Paediatr Respir Rev 7:S215, 2006.
24. Macy AM: Preventing hepatotoxicity in acetaminophen overdose. Am J Nurs 79:301, 1979.
25. Decramer M, Rutten-van Molken M, Dekhuijzen PN, et al: Effects of N-acetylcysteine on outcomes in chronic obstructive pulmonary disease (Bronchitis Randomized on NAC Cost-Utility Study, BRONCUS): a randomised placebo-controlled trial. Lancet 365:1552, 2005.
26. King M, Rubin BK: Mucus-controlling agents: past and present. Respir Care Clin N Am 5:575, 1999.
27. Consensus Conference: Practical applications of Pulmozyme. Pediatr Pulmonol 17:404, 1994.
28. Shak S, Capon DJ, Hellmiss R, et al: Recombinant human DNase I reduces the viscosity of cystic fibrosis sputum. Proc Natl Acad Sci U S A 87:9188, 1990.
29. Robinson M, Regnis JA, Bailey DL, et al: Effect of hypertonic saline, amiloride, and cough on mucociliary clearance in patients with cystic fibrosis. Am J Respir Crit Care Med 153:1503, 1996.
30. Johnson M: Pharmacodynamics and pharmacokinetics of inhaled glucocorticoids. J Allergy Clin Immunol 97:169, 1996.
31. Global Initiative for Chronic Obstructive Lung Disease: Executive Summary: December 2010, Global Strategy for the Diagnosis, Management, and Prevention of COPD, National Heart, Lung, and Blood Institute (Bethesda, Md) and World Health Organization (Geneva, Switzerland), 2010.
32. Baraniuk JN: Molecular actions of glucocorticoids: an introduction. J Allergy Clin Immunol 97:141, 1996.
33. Anderson GP: Interactions between corticosteroids and β-adrenergic agonists in asthma disease induction, progression, and exacerbation. Am J Respir Crit Care Med 161:S188, 2000.
34. Barnes PJ: Inhaled glucocorticoids for asthma. N Engl J Med 332:868, 1995.
35. Allen DB, Bielory L, Derendorf H, et al: Inhaled corticosteroids, past lessons and future issues. J Allergy Clin Immunol 112(Suppl 3):S1, 2003.
36. Ayres JG, Higgins B, Chilvers ER, et al: Efficacy and tolerability of anti-immunoglobulin E therapy with omalizumab in patients with poorly controlled (moderate-to-severe) allergic asthma. Allergy 59:701, 2004.
37. Lanier BQ, Corren J, Lumry W, et al: Omalizumab is effective in the long-term control of severe allergic asthma. Ann Allergy Asthma Immunol 91:154, 2003.
38. Holgate ST: Inhaled sodium cromoglycate. Respir Med 90:387, 1996.
39. Bisgaard H: Role of leukotrienes in asthma pathophysiology. Pediatr Pulmonol 30:166, 2000.
40. Drazen JM, Israel E, O'Byrne PM: Treatment of asthma with drugs modifying the leukotriene pathway. N Engl J Med 340:197, 1999.
41. Holgate ST, Djukanovic R, Casale T, et al: Anti-immunoglobulin E treatment with omalizumab in allergic diseases: an update on anti-inflammatory activity and clinical efficacy. Clin Exp Allergy 35:408, 2005.
42. Mofenson LM, Brady MT, Danner SP, et al: Guidelines for the prevention and treatment of opportunistic infections among HIV-exposed and HIV-infected children: recommendations from CDC, the National Institutes of Health, the HIV Medicine Association of the Infectious Diseases Society of America, the Pediatric Infectious Diseases Society, and the American Academy of Pediatrics. MMWR Recomm Rep 58(RR-11):1–166, 2009.
43. Kaplan JE, Benson C, Holmes KH, et al: Guidelines for prevention and treatment of opportunistic infections in HIV-infected adults and adolescents: recommendations from CDC, the National Institutes of Health, and the HIV Medicine Association of the Infectious Diseases Society of America. MMWR Recomm Rep 58(RR-4):1–198, 2009.
44. American Academy of Pediatrics Committee on Infectious Diseases: Respiratory syncytial virus. In Pickering LK, editor:

Red Book: 2009 report of the Committee on Infectious Diseases, ed 28, Elk Grove Village, IL, 2009, AAP.
45. Ramsey BW, Pepe MS, Quan JM, et al: Intermittent administration of inhaled tobramycin in patients with cystic fibrosis. N Engl J Med 340:23, 1999.
46. Littlewood JM, Smye SW, Cunliffe H: Aerosol antibiotic treatment in cystic fibrosis. Arch Dis Child 68:788, 1993.
47. Dally MB, Kurrle S, Breslin AB: Ventilatory effects of aerosol gentamicin. Thorax 33:54, 1978.
48. Hurley PK, Smye SW, Cunliffe H: Assessment of antibiotic aerosol generation using commercial jet nebulizers. J Aerosol Med 7:217, 1994.
49. Newman SP, Pellow PG, Clay MM, et al: Evaluation of jet nebulizers for use with gentamicin solution. Thorax 40:671, 1985.
50. Anderson P: Emerging therapies in cystic fibrosis. Ther Adv Respir Dis 4:177, 2010.
51. Falagas ME, Kasiakou SK, Tsiodras S, et al: The use of intravenous and aerosolized polymyxins for the treatment of infections in critically ill patients: a review of the recent literature. Clin Med Res 4:138, 2006.
52. Food and Drug Administration: Revised labeling for zanamivir. JAMA 284:1234, 2000.
53. Gubareva LV, Kaiser L, Hayden FG: Influenza virus neuraminidase inhibitors. Lancet 355:827, 2000.
54. Hayden FG, Gubareva LV, Monto AS, et al: Inhaled zanamivir for the prevention of influenza in families. N Engl J Med 343:1282, 2000.
55. Siobal M: Aerosolized prostacyclins. Respir Care 49:640, 2004.
56. Taylor RW, Zimmerman JL, Dellinger RP, et al; Inhaled Nitric Oxide in ARDS Study Group: Low dose inhaled nitric oxide in patients with acute lung injury. JAMA 291:1603, 2004.
57. Palevsky HI: Treatment of pulmonary hypertension. In Leff AR, editor: Pulmonary and critical care pharmacology and therapeutics, New York, 2000, McGraw-Hill.
58. Martin WJ, Rehm S: Toxic injury of the lung parenchyma. In Leff AR, editor: Pulmonary and critical care pharmacology and therapeutics, New York, 2000, McGraw-Hill.
59. Olschewski H, Simonneau G, Galie N, et al; Aerosolized Iloprost Randomized Study Group. Inhaled iloprost for severe pulmonary hypertension. N Engl J Med 347:322, 2002.
60. Channick RN, Olschewski H, Seeger W, et al: Safety and efficacy of inhaled treprostinil as add-on therapy to bosentan in pulmonary arterial hypertension. J Am Coll Cardiol 48:1433, 2006.

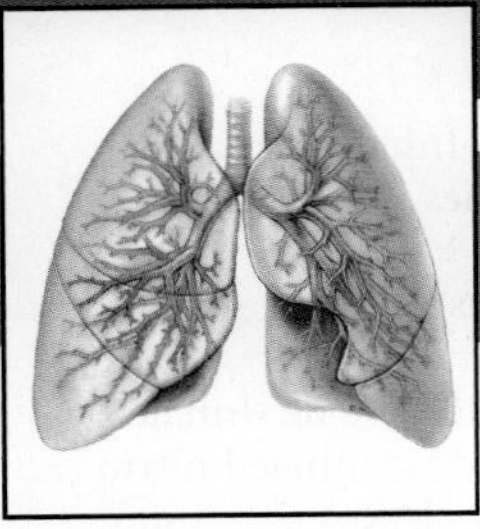

Chapter 33

Airway Management

NEILA ALTOBELLI

CHAPTER OBJECTIVES

After reading this chapter you will be able to:

- Describe how to perform endotracheal and nasotracheal suctioning safely.
- Describe how to obtain sputum samples properly.
- Assess the need for and select an artificial airway.
- Identify the complications and hazards associated with insertion of artificial airways.
- Describe how to perform orotracheal and nasotracheal intubation of an adult.
- Assess and confirm proper endotracheal tube placement.
- Describe the rationale and the methods for performing a tracheotomy.
- Identify the types of damage that artificial airways can cause.
- Describe how to maintain and troubleshoot artificial airways properly.
- Describe techniques for measuring and adjusting tracheal tube cuff pressures.
- Identify when and how to extubate or decannulate a patient.
- Describe how to use alternative airway devices.
- Describe how to assist a physician in setting up and performing bronchoscopy.

CHAPTER OUTLINE

KEY TERMS

American Society for Testing and Materials (ASTM)
bronchoscopy
decannulation
endotracheal tubes
extubation
fenestrated
intubation
obturator
pharyngeal airways
radiopaque
stenosis
suctioning
tracheoesophageal fistula
tracheoinnominate artery fistula
tracheomalacia
tracheostomy
tracheostomy tubes
tracheotomy

Respiratory therapists (RTs) are an important part of the health care team who aim to optimize patient ventilation and gas exchange. Because adequate ventilation and gas exchange are impossible without a patent airway, RTs often assume responsibility for airway management of patients in both the acute care and the postacute care settings. RTs must develop skills in three broad areas of airway care. First, the RT must be proficient in airway clearance techniques, including methods designed to ensure the patency of the patient's natural or artificial airway. Second, the RT must be able to insert and maintain artificial airways designed to support patients whose own natural airways are inadequate. Third, the RT must be able to assist physicians in performing special procedures related to airway management. This chapter explores each of these areas.

SUCTIONING

Airway obstruction can be caused by retained secretions, foreign bodies, and structural changes such as edema, tumors, or trauma. Retained secretions increase airway resistance and the work of breathing and can cause hypoxemia, hypercapnia, atelectasis, and infection. Difficulty in clearing secretions may be due to the thickness or amount of the secretions or to the patient's inability to generate an effective cough.

RTs can remove retained secretions or other semiliquid fluids from the airways by suctioning. **Suctioning** is the application of negative pressure (vacuum) to the airways through a collecting tube (flexible catheter or suction tip). Removal of foreign bodies, secretions, or tissue masses beyond the main stem bronchi requires bronchoscopy, which is performed by a physician. RTs often assist physicians in performing bronchoscopy, which is discussed at the end of the chapter.

Suction can be performed in either the upper airway (oropharynx) or the lower airway (trachea and bronchi). Secretions or fluids can also be removed from the oropharynx by using a rigid tonsillar, or Yankauer, suction tip (Figure 33-1). Access to the lower airway is via introduction of a flexible suction catheter (Figure 33-2) through the nose (nasotracheal suctioning) or artificial airway (endotracheal suctioning). Tracheal suctioning through the mouth should be avoided because it causes gagging.

Endotracheal Suctioning

Clinical Practice Guideline

To guide practitioners in safe and effective application of this procedure, the American Association for Respiratory Care (AARC) has developed a clinical practice guideline on endotracheal suctioning of mechanically ventilated patients with artificial airways. Excerpts from the AARC guideline, including indications, contraindications, hazards and complications, assessment of need, assessment of outcome, and monitoring, appear in Clinical Practice Guideline 33-1.[1]

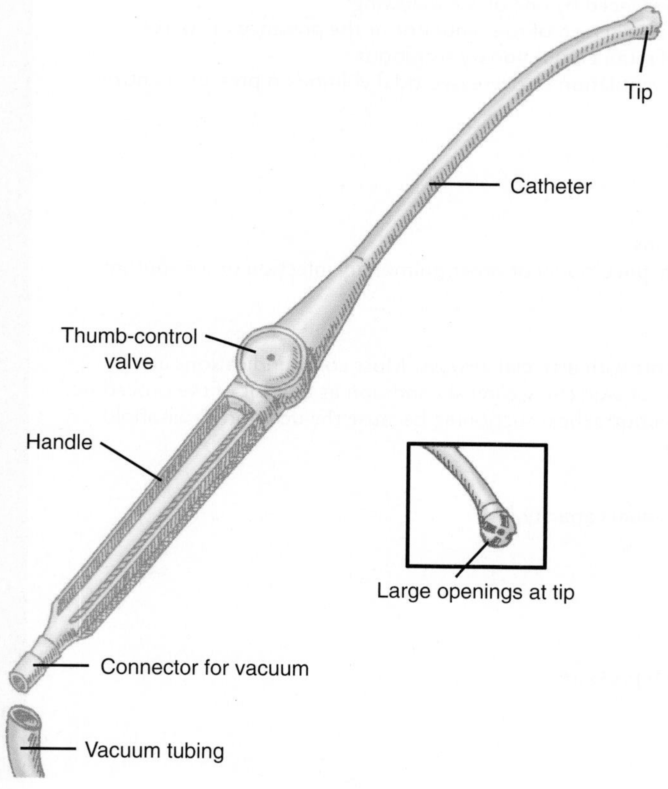

FIGURE 33-1 Rigid tonsillar, or Yankauer, suction tip. (Modified from Sills JR: The comprehensive respiratory therapist exam review, entry and advanced levels, ed 5, St. Louis, 2010, Mosby.)

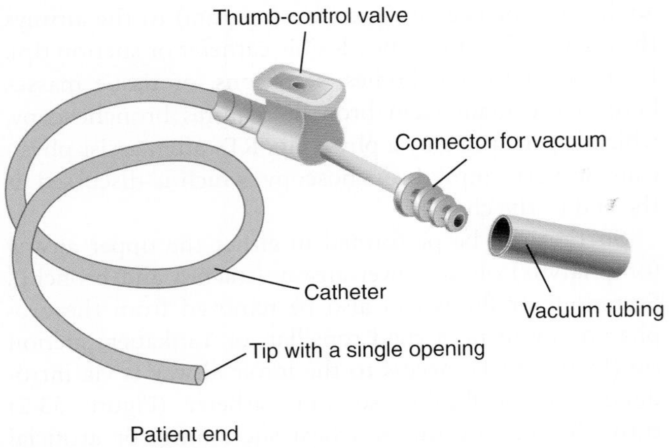

FIGURE 33-2 Flexible suction catheter for lower airway suctioning.

Equipment and Procedure

The procedure described here is for endotracheal suctioning of adults or children. Nasotracheal suctioning is described separately later in this chapter. There are two techniques for endotracheal suctioning: open and closed. The open, sterile technique requires disconnecting the patient from the ventilator. The closed technique uses a sterile, closed, in-line suction catheter later is attached to the ventilator circuit so that the suction catheter can be advanced into the patient's endotracheal airway without disconnecting the patient from the ventilator.

There are also two methods of suctioning based on how deep the suction catheter is inserted in the artificial airway: deep suctioning and shallow suctioning. Deep suctioning is when the catheter is inserted until resistance is met and then withdrawn approximately 1 cm before applying suction. Shallow suctioning is when the catheter

33-1 Endotracheal Suctioning of Mechanically Ventilated Patients With Artificial Airways

AARC Clinical Practice Guideline (Excerpts)*

INDICATIONS

- Need to maintain patency and integrity of the artificial airway
- Need to remove accumulated pulmonary secretions as evidenced by one of the following:
  - Sawtooth pattern on the flow-volume loop on the monitor screen of the ventilator or the presence of coarse crackles over the trachea—both are strong indicators of retained pulmonary secretions
  - Increased peak inspiratory pressure on volume-control ventilation or decreased tidal volume on pressure control ventilation
  - Deterioration of O_2 saturation or blood gas values
  - Visible secretions in the airway
  - Inability of patient to generate an effective cough
  - Acute respiratory distress
  - Suspected aspiration of gastric or upper airway secretions
- Need to obtain a sputum specimen to rule out or identify pneumonia or other pulmonary infection or for sputum cytology

CONTRAINDICATIONS

Endotracheal suctioning is a necessary procedure for patients with artificial airways. Most contraindications are relative to the patient's risk of developing adverse reactions or worsening clinical condition as a result of the procedure. When indicated, there is no absolute contraindication to endotracheal suctioning because the decision to withhold suctioning to avoid possible adverse reaction may be lethal.

HAZARDS AND COMPLICATIONS

- Decrease in dynamic lung compliance and functional residual capacity
- Atelectasis
- Hypoxia or hypoxemia
- Tissue trauma to the tracheal or bronchial mucosa
- Bronchoconstriction or bronchospasm
- Increased microbial colonization of lower airway
- Changes in cerebral blood flow and increased intracranial pressure
- Hypertension
- Hypotension
- Cardiac dysrhythmias

33-1 Endotracheal Suctioning of Mechanically Ventilated Patients With Artificial Airways—cont'd

AARC Clinical Practice Guideline (Excerpts)*

Routine use of normal saline instillation may be associated with the following adverse events:
- Excessive coughing
- Decreased O_2 saturation
- Bronchospasm
- Dislodgment of the bacterial biofilm that colonizes the endotracheal tube into the lower airway
- Pain, anxiety, dyspnea
- Tachycardia
- Increased intracranial pressure

ASSESSMENT OF NEED

Qualified personnel should assess the need for endotracheal suctioning as a routine part of a patient and ventilator system assessment as detailed under Indications.

ASSESSMENT OF OUTCOME

- Improvement in appearance of ventilator graphics and breath sounds
- Decreased peak inspiratory pressure with narrowing of peak inspiratory pressure to plateau pressure difference; decreased airway resistance or increased dynamic compliance; increased tidal volume delivery during pressure-limited ventilation
- Improvement in arterial blood gas values or saturation as reflected by pulse oximetry (SpO_2)
- Removal of pulmonary secretions

MONITORING

The following should be monitored before, during, and after the procedure:
- Breath sounds
- O_2 saturation
- Skin color
- Pulse oximeter
- Respiratory rate and pattern
- Hemodynamic parameters
- Pulse rate
- Blood pressure, if indicated and available
- Electrocardiogram, if indicated and available
- Sputum characteristics—color, volume, consistency, odor
- Cough characteristics
- Intracranial pressure, if indicated and available
- Ventilator parameters
- Peak inspiratory pressure and plateau pressure
- Tidal volume
- Pressure, flow, and volume graphics, if available
- FiO_2

**For complete guidelines, see American Association for Respiratory Care: Clinical practice guideline. Endotracheal suctioning of mechanically ventilated patients with artificial airways, Respir Care 55:758, 2010.*

is advanced to a predetermined depth, which is usually the length of the airway plus the adapter.[2] Using shallow suctioning rather than deep suctioning is recommended in infants and children.[3]

Step 1: Assess Patient for Indications. Generally, a patient should never be suctioned according to a preset schedule. Although very thick secretions may not move with airflow and may not create any adventitious sounds, the patient should be assessed for clinical indicators, such as rhonchi heard on auscultation, which suggest the need for suctioning (see Clinical Practice Guideline 33-1).

Step 2: Assemble and Check Equipment. The equipment needed for endotracheal suctioning is listed in Box 33-1. The suction catheter, gloves, and cup are often prepackaged together in disposable sterile kits for use during the open suctioning technique. The AARC Clinical Practice Guideline suggests the closed suctioning technique to avoid disconnecting the patient from the ventilator, which interrupts ventilation and exposes the patient to infection risk. Suction pressure should always be checked by occluding the end of the suction tubing before attaching the suction catheter. The suction pressure should be set at the lowest effective level. Negative pressures of 80 to 100 mm Hg in neonates and less than 150 mm Hg in adults are generally recommended.[4]

Suction catheters are available in various designs, most with side ports to minimize mucosal damage. Most suction catheters for general purposes are 22 inches long (sufficient to reach the main stem bronchi) and sized in French units (external circumference). A curved-tip catheter, or catheter coudé, is available to help direct access to the left main stem bronchus. The size of the catheter may be more important than its design. A catheter that is too large can obstruct part or all of the airway by occupying too much of its opening. Too large a suction catheter combined with negative pressure quickly evacuates lung volume and can cause atelectasis and hypoxemia. To avoid this problem, the diameter of the catheter should be less than 50% of the internal diameter of the artificial airway in adults.[5,6] In infants and small children, the diameter of the suction catheter should be less than 70% of the internal diameter of the artificial airway.[7]

Box 33-1 Equipment Needed for Suctioning

- Vacuum source
- Calibrated, adjustable regulator
- Collection bottle and connecting tubing
- Disposable gloves: sterile (open suction) or clean (closed suction)
- Sterile suction catheter
- Sterile water and cup (open suction)
- Goggles, mask, and other appropriate equipment for standard precautions
- O_2 source with a calibrated flowmeter (open suction) or ventilator (closed suction)
- Pulse oximeter
- Manual resuscitation bag equipped with O_2-enrichment device for emergency backup use
- Stethoscope

OPTIONAL EQUIPMENT

- Electrocardiograph
- Sterile sputum trap for culture specimen

RULE OF THUMB

To estimate quickly the proper size of suction catheter to use with a given tracheal tube, first multiply the tube's inner diameter by 2. Then use the next smallest size catheter.

Example: 6-mm endotracheal tube: 2 × 6 = 12; next smallest catheter is 10F

Example: 8-mm endotracheal tube: 2 × 8 = 16; next smallest catheter is 14F

An in-line suction catheter can be used for patients receiving ventilatory support (Figure 33-3). These systems are incorporated directly into the ventilator circuit and used repeatedly. Because this system allows suctioning without disconnecting the patient from the ventilator, it is recommended for suctioning patients who require

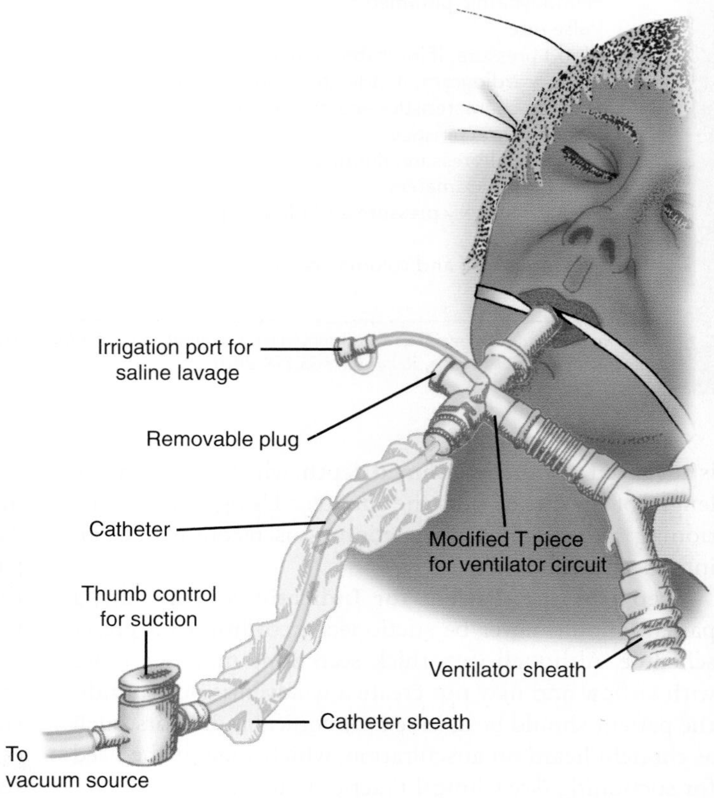

FIGURE 33-3 In-line, closed-system multiuse suction catheter. (Modified from Sills JR: The comprehensive respiratory therapist exam review, entry and advanced levels, ed 5, St. Louis, 2010, Mosby.)

high fractional inspired oxygen (FiO_2) and positive end-expiratory pressure (PEEP), who are at risk for lung derecruitment, and for neonates.[8-10] In addition, cross contamination is less likely with such systems. The use of in-line suction catheters has been shown to be cost-effective because they need to be changed only if soiled or malfunctioning and not on a daily basis.[11] However, in-line suction catheters have not been shown either to increase or to decrease the risk of ventilator-associated pneumonia.[12] The extra weight an in-line catheter adds to a ventilator circuit may increase tension on the endotracheal tube, so care should be taken to support the ventilator tubing appropriately.

Basic indications for the use of closed suction catheters are listed in Box 33-2.[13] Routine instillation of sterile normal saline to aid secretion removal before suctioning is not recommended because there is insufficient evidence that this practice is beneficial, and it may increase infection risk (see Hazards and Complications in Clinical Practice Guideline 33-1). If the secretions are extremely tenacious, instillation of acetylcysteine or sodium bicarbonate (2%) may be more effective than normal saline; this generally requires a physician's order. The use of these medications is discussed in more detail in Chapter 32.

After connecting the catheter to the suction source, the level of suction pressure should be checked by closing the catheter thumb port and aspirating some sterile water or saline from the basin. If no vacuum is generated, it is necessary to check for leaks in the tubing, at the collection container, or at the suction regulator. In addition, if the collecting bottle is full, the float-valve closes and prevents vacuum transmission.

RULE OF THUMB

Set suction pressure to −120 to −150 mm Hg for adults, 100 to 120 mm Hg for children, and 80 to 100 mm Hg for infants.

Box 33-2 Indications for Use of Closed Suctioning Technique

Mechanically ventilated patients, especially neonates and patients with:

- PEEP ≥ 10 cm H_2O
- Mean airway pressure ≥20 cm H_2O
- Inspiratory time ≥1.5 seconds
- FiO_2 ≥ 0.60
- Frequent suctioning (≥6 times/day)
- Hemodynamic instability associated with ventilator disconnection
- Respiratory infections requiring airborne or droplet precautions (see Chapter 4)
- Inhaled agents that cannot be interrupted by ventilator disconnection (e.g., nitric oxide, helium/O_2 mixture)

Step 3: Hyperoxygenate Patient. Before suctioning, delivery of 100% oxygen (O_2) for 30 to 60 seconds to pediatric and adult patients is suggested, especially to patients who are at risk for hypoxemia. Also, the O_2 concentration should be increased by 10% in neonates before suctioning[14]; this may be done by increasing the set FiO_2 or activating the temporary 100% setting on microprocessor ventilators. Manual ventilation is not recommended because it is sometimes difficult to deliver 100% O_2 this way.[15] However, if there is no other alternative to hyperoxygenate the patient, PEEP should be maintained during the manual ventilation with 100% O_2.

Step 4: Insert Catheter. To prevent tracheal mucosal trauma, especially in infants, the shallow suction method should be used advancing the catheter just to the end of the artificial airway as recommended in the AARC guidelines.

Step 5: Apply Suction and Clear Catheter. Suction is applied while withdrawing the catheter. Total suction time should be kept to less than 15 seconds.[16,17] After removing the catheter, it should be cleared using the sterile cup filled with sterile water or saline. The closed suction catheter has an adapter for saline vials to be placed in line with the device. The catheter is cleared by squeezing the saline vial and applying suction at the same time. Caution must be used to ensure saline is being drawn into the catheter and not down the airway. If any untoward response occurs during suctioning, the catheter should be immediately removed, and the patient should be oxygenated.

Step 6: Reoxygenate Patient. The patient should be hyperoxygenated by the same method used in Step 3 for at least 1 minute. Routine hyperventilation is not recommended. If there are indications of derecruitment, lung recruitment maneuvers may be used.

Step 7: Monitor Patient and Assess Outcomes. Steps 3 through 7 are repeated as needed until improvement is seen or an adverse response is observed. Any necessary corrective steps should be taken.

Minimizing Complications and Adverse Responses

Careful adherence to procedure is the best way to avoid or minimize complications of endotracheal suctioning. First, preoxygenation helps minimize the incidence of hypoxemia during suctioning. Also, it is recommended to preoxygenate and suction without disconnecting the patient from the ventilator, rather than disconnecting the patient and manually ventilating.[18] A manual resuscitator cannot always provide 100% O_2 or deliver a consistent tidal volume, and maintaining sterile technique and PEEP levels can be difficult. As previously described, use of the closed suction technique on ventilator patients can decrease the likelihood of hypoxemia, especially in neonates and adults requiring high FiO_2 or PEEP, or both, or at risk for lung derecruitment.

Cardiac dysrhythmias occur mainly as a result of hypoxemia. Mechanical stimulation of the airway also can cause dysrhythmias. If the patient is connected to a cardiac monitor, it should be checked often for gross dysrhythmias. Vagal stimulation can cause transient bradycardia or asystole. Tachycardia may result from patient agitation and hypoxemia. If any major change is seen in the heart rate or rhythm, the RT should immediately stop suctioning, administer O_2 to the patient, provide ventilation as needed, and notify the nurse and physician.

Hypotension during suctioning may be due to cardiac dysrhythmias or severe coughing episodes that decrease venous return. As with dysrhythmias, if the patient becomes hypotensive, the procedure should be stopped, and oxygenation and ventilation should be restored. Hypertension may be caused by hypoxemia or increased sympathetic tone secondary to stress, anxiety, pain, or changes in hemodynamics.

Atelectasis can be caused by removal of too much air from the lungs in a short time. This complication can be avoided by (1) limiting the amount of negative pressure used, (2) keeping the duration of suctioning as short as possible, (3) using the appropriate size suction catheter, and (4) avoiding disconnection from the ventilator.

Mucosal trauma can also occur when the catheter comes in contact with the wall of the airway during suctioning. To avoid this problem, the amount of negative pressure used should be limited, and the shallow suctioning method as described previously should be used.

Increased intracranial pressure (ICP) has been reported during suctioning. These changes are transient, with values normally returning to baseline within 1 minute. However, in patients who already have an elevated ICP, these changes may be clinically significant. Should this problem occur, an aerosolized topical anesthetic given 15 minutes before suctioning may help reduce coughing and discomfort and any increase in ICP.[19]

Also, steps should be taken to minimize bacterial colonization of the lower airway. Sterile technique should be used during suctioning, and care must be taken when manually ventilating the patient not to contaminate the airway. Also, sterile normal saline should not be instilled routinely into the artificial airway before suctioning unless it is necessary to help mobilize very thick secretions.

RULE OF THUMB

To minimize hypoxemia and lung derecruitment when suctioning a mechanically ventilated patient, preoxygenate and suction the artificial airway with a closed-system in-line catheter to avoid disconnecting the patient from the ventilator.

Nasotracheal Suctioning

Nasotracheal suctioning is indicated for patients who have retained secretions but do not have an artificial tracheal airway.

Clinical Practice Guideline

The AARC has developed and published a clinical practice guideline on nasotracheal suctioning to guide practitioners in safe and effective application of this procedure. Excerpts from the AARC guideline, including indications, contraindications, hazards and complications, assessment of need, assessment of outcome, and monitoring, appear in Clinical Practice Guideline 33-2.[20]

Equipment and Procedure

The equipment and procedure for nasotracheal suctioning are similar to the equipment and procedure for endotracheal suctioning. Only the key differences are highlighted here. In addition to the equipment and supplies used for endotracheal suctioning (see Box 33-1), sterile water-soluble lubricating jelly is needed to aid catheter passage through the nose. Use of a nasopharyngeal airway should be considered to help reduce mucosal trauma in the nose of patients who require repeated, long-term nasotracheal suctioning.

The key aspect of the nasotracheal suctioning procedure is catheter insertion. After lubricating the catheter, the RT inserts it gently through the nostril, directing it toward the septum and floor of the nasal cavity, without applying negative pressure. The catheter is gently twisted if any resistance in the nose is felt. If twisting does not help, the catheter is withdrawn and inserted through the other nostril.

As the catheter enters the lower pharynx, the patient should assume a "sniffing" position (Figure 33-4). This position helps align the opening of the larynx with the lower pharynx, making catheter passage through the larynx more likely. The catheter is continually advanced until the patient coughs or a resistance is felt.

Minimizing Complications and Adverse Responses

Advancing the catheter into the oropharynx or esophagus may cause gagging or regurgitation. The RT must always be ready to reposition the patient and suction the oropharynx if this occurs. The risk of regurgitation can also be minimized by avoiding suctioning too soon after a meal or tube feeding; this can be accomplished by close coordination with nursing personnel.

Airway trauma can occur as the catheter is passed through the upper airway. The presence of blood in the catheter or patient's nose or mouth suggests tissue damage. Trauma can range from simple mucosal bleeding to laceration of nasal turbinates and pharyngeal perforation. To minimize airway trauma, excessive force should be avoided when advancing the catheter. Lubrication of the catheter also eases its passage. As previously indicated, placement of a nasopharyngeal airway can help minimize nasal trauma when repeated access is needed.

Contamination of the lungs with bacteria from the upper airway is another complication of nasotracheal

33-2 Nasotracheal Suctioning

AARC Clinical Practice Guideline (Excerpts)*

INDICATIONS

- Need to maintain a patent airway and remove saliva, pulmonary secretions, blood, vomitus, or foreign material from the trachea in the presence of inability to clear secretions when audible or visible evidence of secretions in the large or central airways that persist despite patient's best cough effort, as evidenced by one or more of the following:
  - Visible secretions in airway
  - Chest auscultation of coarse, gurgling breath sounds, rhonchi, or diminished breath sounds
  - Feeling of secretions in the chest (increased tactile fremitus)
  - Suspected aspiration of gastric or upper airway secretions
  - Clinically apparent increased work of breathing
  - Deterioration of arterial blood gas values suggesting hypoxemia or hypercarbia
  - Chest radiographic evidence of retained secretions resulting in atelectasis or consolidation
  - Restlessness
- Stimulate cough or for unrelieved coughing
- Obtain a sputum sample for microbiologic or cytologic analysis

CONTRAINDICATIONS

Listed contraindications are relative unless noted to be absolute.

- Occluded nasal passages
- Nasal bleeding
- Epiglottis or croup—absolute
- Acute head, facial, or neck injury
- Coagulopathy or bleeding disorder
- Laryngospasm
- Irritable airway
- Upper respiratory tract infection
- Tracheal surgery
- Gastric surgery with high anastomosis
- Myocardial infarction
- Bronchospasm

HAZARDS AND COMPLICATIONS

- Mechanical trauma
- Laceration of nasal turbinates
- Perforation of pharynx
- Nasal irritation or bleeding
- Tracheitis
- Mucosal hemorrhage
- Edema of uvula
- Hypoxia or hypoxemia
- Cardiac dysrhythmias or arrest
- Bradycardia
- Increased blood pressure
- Hypotension
- Respiratory arrest
- Uncontrolled coughing
- Gagging or vomiting
- Laryngospasm
- Bronchoconstriction or bronchospasm
- Discomfort and pain
- Nosocomial infection
- Atelectasis
- Misdirection of the catheter
- Increased intracranial pressure
- Intraventricular hemorrhage
- Exacerbation of cerebral edema
- Pneumothorax

Continued

33-2 Nasotracheal Suctioning—cont'd

AARC Clinical Practice Guideline (Excerpts)*

■ ASSESSMENT OF NEED

Personnel should perform a baseline assessment for indications of respiratory distress and the need, as recognized by above-listed presenting indications. This assessment should include but not be limited to the following:

- Auscultation of the chest
- Monitoring of heart rate
- Assessment of respiratory rate
- Assessment of cardiac rhythm
- Assessment of O_2 saturation
- Assessment of skin color and perfusion
- Assessment of effectiveness of cough

Prepare the patient for the procedure by providing an appropriate explanation along with adequate sedation and pain relief as needed.

■ ASSESSMENT OF OUTCOME

Assess the patient after suction for the following:

- Improved breath sounds
- Removal of secretions
- Improved blood gas data or pulse oximetry
- Decreased work of breathing (decreased respiratory rate or dyspnea)

■ MONITORING

The following should be monitored before, during, and after the procedure:

- Breath sounds
- Skin color
- Breathing pattern and rate
- Pulse rate, dysrhythmia, electrocardiogram if available
- Color, consistency, and volume of secretions
- Presence of bleeding or evidence of physical trauma
- Subjective response, including pain
- Oxygenation (pulse oximeter)
- Intracranial pressure, if equipment is available
- Arterial blood pressure, if available
- Laryngospasm

**For complete guidelines, see American Association for Respiratory Care: Clinical practice guideline. Nasotracheal suctioning—2004 revision and update, Respir Care 49:1080, 2004.*

suctioning. Immunosuppressed patients are likely to develop more serious complications. Sterile technique and gentle insertion help minimize this complication.

The presence of the catheter in the lower airway may stimulate normal protective mechanisms, resulting in coughing, laryngospasm, or bronchospasm. The bronchospastic response may be particularly strong in patients with hyperactive airway disease. These patients should be assessed for the development of wheezes associated with suctioning.

Sputum Sampling

Sputum samples are often collected to identify organisms infecting the airway. To obtain the samples, the suctioning procedures described previously should be followed. In addition to the usual equipment, a sterile specimen container is needed. This device consists of a plastic tube or cup with flexible tubing on one end to attach to the suction catheter. The other outlet is a stiff plastic nozzle that connects to the suction tubing from the wall vacuum unit (Figure 33-5).

It is important to maintain sterile technique when touching the connection points on the trap. If a closed suction system is being used, a new catheter should be placed just before suctioning the patient for the sample. When an adequate sample is obtained, the container is removed from the suction catheter and suction tubing. The flexible tubing on the container is attached to the open nozzle; this creates a closed container. The container and process should be labeled according to hospital or facility policy. The suctioning procedure is completed as previously described.

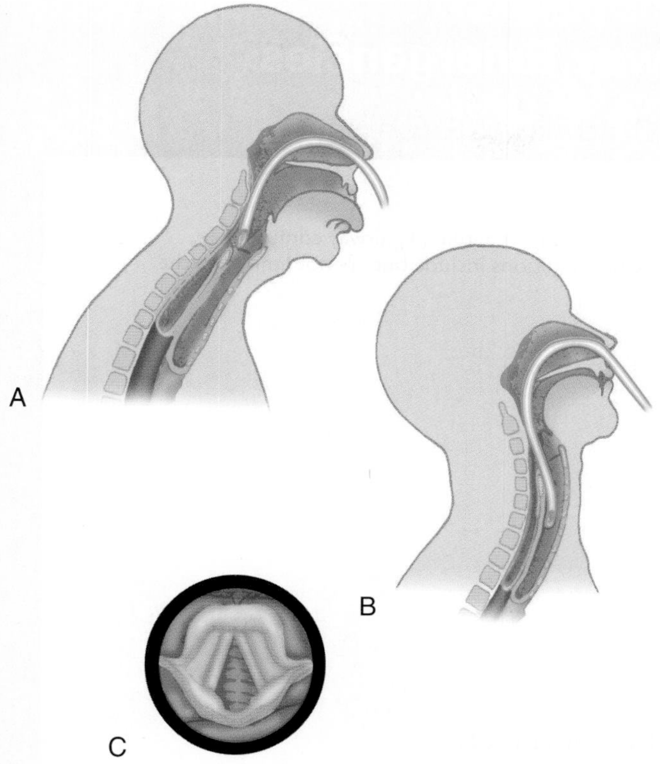

FIGURE 33-4 Nasotracheal suctioning technique. **A,** Optimal position of the head to insert catheter into the trachea. The neck is flexed, and the head is extended. The tongue is protruded (and held by a 4 × 4 gauze pad). **B,** After catheter has advanced into the trachea, the tongue is released, and the patient's head is allowed to assume a comfortable position. **C,** View of vocal cords from above. The cords are most widely separated during inspiration. (Modified from Sanderson RG: The cardiac patient: a comprehensive approach, Philadelphia, 1972, Saunders.)

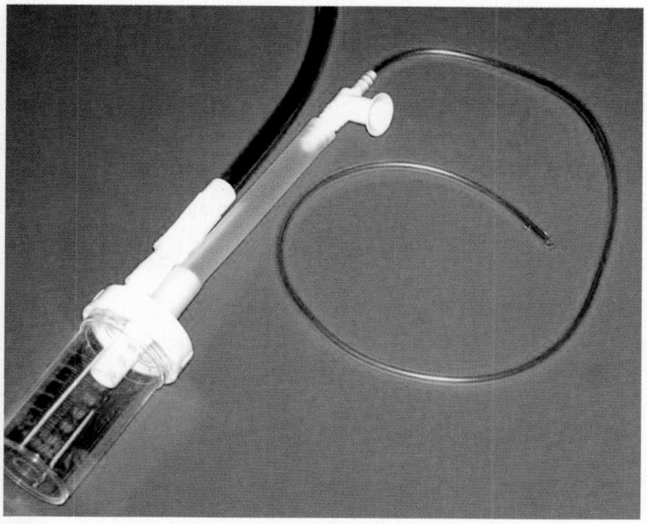

FIGURE 33-5 Specimen container placement between the suction catheter and wall suction source.

ESTABLISHING AN ARTIFICIAL AIRWAY

Clinical Practice Guideline

An artificial airway is required when the patient's natural airway can no longer perform its proper functions. To guide practitioners in the identification, assessment, and treatment of patients requiring artificial airways, the AARC has developed a clinical practice guideline on management of airway emergencies. Excerpts from the AARC guideline, including indications; contraindications; precautions, hazards, and possible complications; assessment of need and outcome; and monitoring, appear in Clinical Practice Guideline 33-3.[21]

Routes

Artificial airways are inserted for various reasons and involve varying degrees of invasion into the upper airway. **Pharyngeal airways** extend only into the pharynx. Artificial airways that are placed through the mouth or nose into the trachea are called **endotracheal tubes.** The process of placing an artificial airway into the trachea is referred to as **intubation.** Clinically, the term *intubation* is most often used to refer to the process of passing a tube through the nose or mouth into the larynx and trachea. When the endotracheal tube is passed through the nose first, the procedure is referred to as *nasotracheal intubation*. When the tube is passed through the mouth on its way into the trachea, the procedure is called *orotracheal intubation*.

Pharyngeal Airways

Pharyngeal airways prevent airway obstruction by keeping the tongue pulled forward and away from the posterior pharynx. This type of obstruction is common in an unconscious patient as a result of a loss of muscle tone.

A *nasopharyngeal airway* (Figure 33-6) is most often placed in a patient who requires frequent nasotracheal suctioning. Although it does not ensure entry into the trachea, it minimizes damage to the nasal mucosa that can be caused by the suction catheter. A nasopharyngeal airway may also be placed in a patient who was recently extubated after facial surgery. The nasopharyngeal airway helps to maintain the patency of the upper airway despite swelling.

Oropharyngeal airways (see Figure 33-6) are inserted into the mouth and over the tongue. Use of oropharyngeal airways should be restricted to unconscious patients to avoid gagging and regurgitation. These airways maintain a patent airway when the tongue would otherwise obstruct the oropharynx. The airway can also be used as a bite-block for patients with oral tubes.

Pharyngeal airways are used mainly in emergency life support. Further details on their use, insertion techniques, and size selection are provided in Chapter 34.

33-3 Management of Airway Emergencies

AARC Clinical Practice Guideline (Excerpts)*

■ INDICATIONS

In general, conditions requiring management of the airway are impending or actual (1) airway compromise, (2) respiratory failure, and (3) need to protect the airway. Specific conditions include but are not limited to the following:

- Airway emergency before endotracheal intubation
- Obstruction of the artificial airway
- Apnea
- Acute traumatic coma
- Penetrating neck trauma
- Cardiopulmonary arrest and unstable dysrhythmias
- Severe bronchospasm
- Severe allergic reactions with cardiopulmonary compromise
- Pulmonary edema
- Sedative/narcotic drug effect
- Foreign body obstruction
- Choanal atresia in neonates
- Aspiration
- Risk of aspiration
- Severe laryngospasm
- Self-extubation

Conditions requiring emergency tracheal intubation include but are not limited to:

- Persistent apnea
- Traumatic upper airway obstruction
- Accidental extubation of a patient unable to maintain adequate spontaneous ventilation
- Obstructive angioedema
- Massive uncontrolled upper airway bleeding
- Infection-related upper airway obstruction (partial or complete)
  - Epiglottitis in children or adults
  - Acute uvular edema
  - Tonsillopharyngitis or retropharyngeal abscess
  - Suppurative parotitis
- Coma with potential for increased intracranial pressure
- Neonatal- or pediatric-specific conditions
  - Perinatal asphyxia
  - Severe adenotonsillar hypertrophy
  - Severe laryngomalacia
  - Bacterial tracheitis
  - Neonatal epignathus
  - Obstruction from abnormal laryngeal closure owing to arytenoid masses
  - Mediastinal tumors
  - Congenital diaphragmatic hernia
  - Presence of thick or particulate meconium in amniotic fluid
  - Absence of airway protective reflexes
  - Cardiopulmonary arrest
  - Massive hemoptysis

A patient in whom airway control is not possible by other methods may require surgical placement of an airway (needle or surgical cricothyrotomy).

Conditions in which endotracheal intubation may be impossible and in which alternative techniques may be used include but are not limited to the following:

- Restriction of endotracheal intubation by policy or statute
- Difficult or failed intubation in the presence of risk factors associated with difficult tracheal intubations such as
  - Short neck or bull neck
  - Protruding maxillary incisors
  - Receding mandible
  - Reduced mobility of atlantooccipital joint
  - Temporomandibular ankylosis
  - Congenital oropharyngeal wall stenosis
  - Anterior osteophytes of the cervical vertebrae, associated with diffuse idiopathic skeletal hyperostosis

33-3 Management of Airway Emergencies—cont'd

AARC Clinical Practice Guideline (Excerpts)*

- Large substernal or cancerous goiters
- Treacher Collins syndrome
- Morquio-Brailsford syndrome
- Endolaryngeal tumors
- When endotracheal intubation is not immediately possible

CONTRAINDICATIONS

Aggressive airway management (intubation or establishment of a surgical airway) may be contraindicated when the patient's desire not to be resuscitated has been clearly expressed and documented in the patient's medical record or other valid legal document.

PRECAUTIONS, HAZARDS, AND COMPLICATIONS

Possible hazards or complications related to the major facets of management of airway emergencies include the following:

- Failure to establish a patent airway
- Failure to intubate the trachea
- Failure to recognize intubation of esophagus
- Upper airway trauma, laryngeal, and esophageal damage
- Aspiration
- Cervical spine trauma
- Unrecognized bronchial intubation
- Eye injury
- Vocal cord paralysis
- Problems with endotracheal tubes
  - Cuff perforation
  - Cuff herniation
  - Pilot-tube-valve incompetence
  - Tube kinking during biting
  - Inadvertent extubation
  - Tube occlusion
  - Bronchospasm
  - Laryngospasm
  - Dental accidents
  - Dysrhythmias
  - Hypotension and bradycardia secondary to vagal stimulation
  - Hypertension and tachycardia
  - Inappropriate tube size
  - Bleeding
  - Mouth ulceration
- Nasal intubation specific
  - Nasal damage including epistaxis
  - Tube kinking in pharynx
  - Sinusitis and otitis media
  - Tongue ulceration
  - Tracheal damage including tracheoesophageal fistula, tracheal innominate fistula, tracheal stenosis, and tracheomalacia
  - Pneumonia
  - Laryngeal damage with consequent laryngeal stenosis, laryngeal ulcer, granuloma, polyps, synechiae
- Surgical cricothyrotomy or tracheostomy specific
  - Stomal stenosis
  - Innominate erosion
- Needle cricothyrotomy specific
  - Bleeding at insertion site with hematoma formation
  - Subcutaneous and mediastinal emphysema
  - Esophageal perforation
  - Emergency ventilation
  - Inadequate O_2 delivery
  - Hypoventilation or hyperventilation
  - Gastric insufflation or rupture

Continued

33-3 Management of Airway Emergencies—cont'd

AARC Clinical Practice Guideline (Excerpts)*

- Barotrauma
- Hypotension owing to reduced venous return secondary to high mean intrathoracic pressure
- Vomiting and aspiration
- Prolonged interruption of ventilation for intubation
- Failure to establish adequate functional residual capacity in a newborn
- Movement of unstable cervical spine (more than by any commonly used method of endotracheal intubation)
- Failure to exhale owing to upper airway obstruction during percutaneous transtracheal ventilation

ASSESSMENT OF NEED

The need for airway management is dictated by the clinical condition of the patient. Careful observation, implementation of basic airway management techniques, and laboratory and clinical data should help determine the need for more aggressive measures. Specific conditions requiring intervention include the following:

- Inability to protect airway adequately (e.g., coma, lack of gag reflex, inability to cough) with or without other signs of respiratory distress
- Partially obstructed airway. Signs of a partially obstructed upper airway include ineffective patient efforts to ventilate, paradoxical respiration, stridor, use of accessory muscles, patient pointing to neck, choking motions, cyanosis, and distress. Signs of lower airway obstruction may include the above-mentioned signs and wheezing
- Complete airway obstruction. Respiratory efforts with no breath sounds or suggestion of air movement are indicative of complete obstruction
- Apnea. No respiratory efforts are seen; may be associated with cardiac arrest
- Hypoxemia, hypercarbia, or acidemia seen on arterial blood gas analysis, oximetry, or exhaled gas analysis
- Respiratory distress. Elevated respiratory rate, high or low ventilatory volumes, and signs of sympathetic nervous system hyperactivity may be associated with respiratory distress

ASSESSMENT OF PROCESS AND OUTCOME

Timely intervention to maintain the patient's airway can improve outcomes. Under rare circumstances, maintenance of an airway by nonsurgical means may be impossible. Despite optimal airway maintenance, outcomes are affected by patient-specific factors. Lack of appropriate equipment and personnel may adversely affect outcomes. Monitoring and recording can help improve emergency airway management. Some aspects (e.g., frequency of complications of tracheal intubations or time to establishment of a definitive airway) are easy to quantify and can help improve hospital-wide systems. The patient's condition after the emergency should be evaluated from this perspective.

MONITORING

Clinical Signs

Continuous patient observation and repeated clinical assessment by a trained observer provide optimal monitoring of the airway. Special consideration should be given to the following:

- Level of consciousness
- Presence and character of breath sounds
- Ease of ventilation
- Symmetry and amount of chest movement
- Skin color and character (temperature and presence or absence of diaphoresis)
- Presence of upper airway sounds (crowing, snoring, stridor)
- Presence of excessive secretions, blood, vomitus, or foreign objects in the airway
- Presence of epigastric sounds
- Presence of retractions
- Presence of nasal flaring

Physiologic Variables

Repeated assessment of physiologic data by trained professionals supplements clinical assessment in managing patients with airway difficulties. Monitoring devices should be available, accessible, functional, and periodically evaluated for function. These data include but are not limited to:

- Ventilatory frequency, tidal volume, and airway pressure
- Presence of CO_2 in exhaled gas
- Heart rate and rhythm
- Pulse oximetry
- Arterial blood gas values
- Chest radiograph

33-3 Management of Airway Emergencies—cont'd

AARC Clinical Practice Guideline (Excerpts)*

Endotracheal Tube Position

Regardless of the method of ventilation used, the most important consideration is detection of esophageal intubation.

- Tracheal intubation is suggested but may not be confirmed by
  - Bilateral breath sounds over the chest
  - Symmetric chest movement
  - Absence of ventilation sounds over the epigastrium
  - Presence of condensate inside the tube, corresponding with exhalation
  - Visualization of the tip of the tube passing through the vocal cords
  - Esophageal detector devices may be useful in differentiating esophageal from tracheal intubation
- Tracheal intubation is confirmed by detection of CO_2 in the exhaled gas, although cases of transient CO_2 excretion from the stomach have been reported
- Tracheal intubation is confirmed by endoscopic visualization of the carina or tracheal rings through the tube
- Position of the endotracheal tube (i.e., depth of insertion) should be appropriate on chest radiograph

AIRWAY MANAGEMENT PROCESS

A properly managed airway may improve patient outcome. Continuous evaluation of the process identifies components needing improvement. These include response time, equipment function, equipment availability, practitioner performance, complication rate, and patient survival and functional status.

For complete guidelines, see American Association for Respiratory Care: Clinical practice guideline. Management of airway emergencies, Respir Care 40:749, 1995.

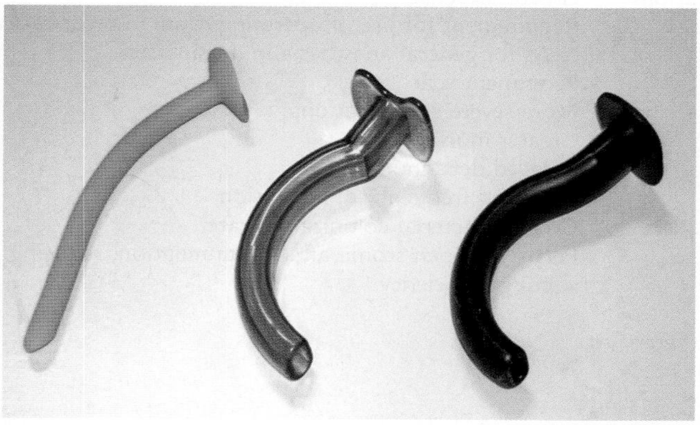

FIGURE 33-6 Pharyngeal airways. **A,** Nasopharyngeal airway. **B** and **C,** Oropharyngeal airways.

Tracheal Airways

Tracheal airways extend beyond the pharynx into the trachea. The two basic types of tracheal airways are *endotracheal (translaryngeal) tubes* and *tracheostomy tubes*. Endotracheal tubes are inserted through either the mouth or the nose (orotracheal or nasotracheal), through the larynx, and into the trachea. **Tracheostomy tubes** are inserted through a surgically created opening in the neck directly into the trachea. Table 33-1 summarizes the advantages and disadvantages of each of these three approaches.

Airway Tubes

Endotracheal Tubes

Endotracheal tubes are semirigid tubes most often composed of polyvinyl chloride or related plastic polymers.[22] Specifications covering the sizing, labeling, performance requirements, and test methods for endotracheal tubes are established by the **American Society for Testing and Materials (ASTM).**[23] Figure 33-7 shows a typical endotracheal tube, its key components, and a stylet used for insertion. The proximal end of the tube is attached to a standard adapter with a 15-mm external diameter. The curved body of the tube usually has length markings, indicating the distance (in centimeters) from the beveled tube tip. In addition to the beveled opening at the tip, there is a side port, or "Murphy eye," which ensures gas flow if the main port should become obstructed. The angle of the bevel minimizes mucosal trauma during insertion. The tube cuff is permanently bonded to the tube body. Inflation of the cuff seals off the lower airway, either for protection from gross aspiration or to provide positive pressure ventilation. A small filling tube leads from the cuff to a pilot balloon, used to monitor cuff status and pressure when the tube is in place. Finally, a spring-loaded valve with a standard connector for a syringe allows inflation and deflation of the cuff. Although not shown in Figure 33-7, included with most modern endotracheal tubes is a **radiopaque** indicator that is embedded in the distal end of the tube body.

TABLE 33-1

Advantages and Disadvantages of Tracheal Airway Routes

Route	Advantages	Disadvantages
Oral intubation	Insertion is faster, easier, less traumatic, and more comfortable Larger tube is tolerated Easier suctioning Less airflow resistance Decreased work of breathing Easier passage of bronchoscope Reduced risk of tube kinking Avoidance of nasal and paranasal complications, including epistaxis and sinusitis	Esthetically displeasing, especially long-term Greater risk of self-extubation or inadvertent extubation Greater risk of main stem intubation Risk of tube occlusion by biting or trismus Risk of injury to lips, teeth, tongue, palate, and oral soft tissues May require additional use of oral airway Great risk of retching, vomiting, and aspiration Pain and discomfort, especially with inadequate preparation
Nasal intubation	Less retching and gagging Greater comfort in long-term use Less salivation Improved ability to swallow oral secretions Improved communication Improved mouth care and oral hygiene Avoidance of occlusion by biting or trismus Easier nursing care Avoidance of oral route complications Less posterior laryngeal ulceration Better tube anchoring, less chance of inadvertent extubation Reduced risk of main stem intubation Some patients can swallow liquids, providing a means of nutritional support Blind nasal intubation does not require muscle relaxants or sedatives May avert "crash" oral intubation	Nasal and paranasal complications, including epistaxis, sinusitis, otitis More difficult to perform Spontaneous breathing required for blind nasal intubation Smaller tube is necessary Greater suctioning difficulty Increased airflow resistance Increased work of breathing Difficulty passing bronchoscope Smaller risk of transient bacteremia
Tracheotomy	Avoidance of laryngeal and upper airway complications of translaryngeal intubation Greater comfort Aids feeding, oral care, suctioning, speech Psychologic benefit (improved motivation) Easier passage of fiberoptic bronchoscope Easier reinsertion Esthetically less objectionable Facilitation of weaning from ventilator Elimination of risk of main stem intubation Reduced work of breathing Better anchoring (reduced risk of decannulation) Improved ability to place curve-tipped suction catheter in left bronchus Improved mobility (transfer out of ICU to ward or extended-care facility)	Greater expense Requirement for use of operating room in most cases Need for general anesthesia in most cases Permanent scar More severe complications Greater mortality rate Delayed decannulation Increased frequency of aspiration Greater bacterial colonization rate Persistent open stoma after decannulation, reducing cough efficiency

From Stauffer JL, Silvestri RC: Complications and consequences of endotrachial intubation and tracheostomy, Respir Care 27:417, 1982.

This indicator allows for easy identification of tube position on the radiograph.

Specialized Endotracheal Tubes. The standard endotracheal tube has been modified for specific uses, including special ventilation methods, lung pathology, and surgical procedures. A detailed description of the various tubes is beyond the scope of this chapter but is provided elsewhere in this text. Some more common tubes, including double-lumen tubes, tubes with special adapters for jet ventilation, and tubes with subglottic suction ports, are discussed.[24]

Special mechanical ventilation techniques may require unique types of endotracheal tubes. When unilateral lung disease occurs, independent lung ventilation may be needed. This ventilation requires the use of a double-lumen endotracheal tube (Figure 33-8). This tube has two proximal ventilator connectors (15-mm adapter), two inner lumens for gas flow, two cuffs, and two distal openings. The larger cuff seals the tracheal lumen and allows gas to flow into one bronchus. The smaller cuff seals the opposite bronchial lumen (Figure 33-9).

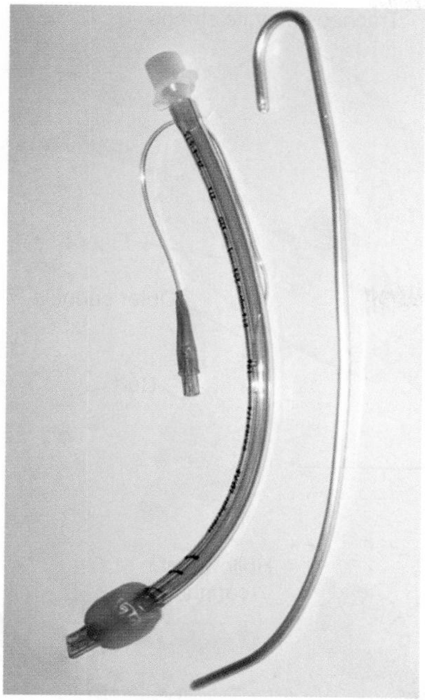

FIGURE 33-7 Typical endotracheal tube and stylet.

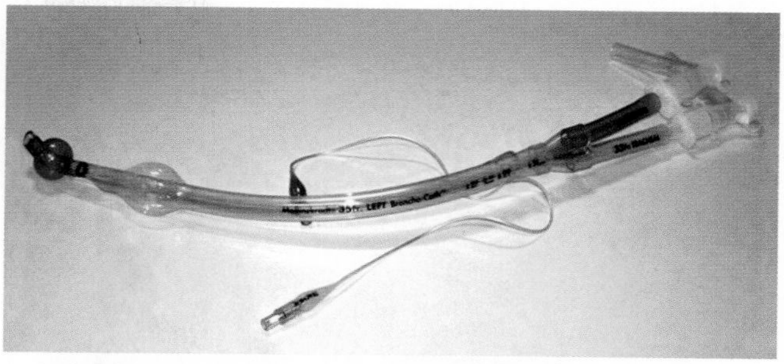

FIGURE 33-8 Double-lumen endotracheal tube for independent lung ventilation.

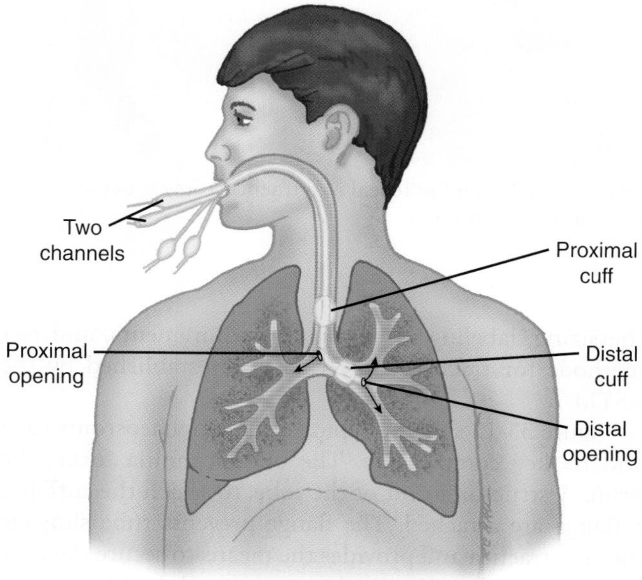

FIGURE 33-9 Correct positioning of double-lumen endotracheal tube.

There are important points to consider when using double-lumen endotracheal tubes. These tubes are stiffer and bulkier to insert than standard tubes and must be rotated during insertion to align with the proper bronchus. Fiberoptic bronchoscopy should be performed to ensure proper placement. The resistance to flow through each tube is increased because each lumen is smaller than the same-size single-lumen tubes.

High-frequency jet ventilation uses a special endotracheal tube adapter (Figure 33-10). This adapter replaces the standard endotracheal tube adapter. There is a jet port allows for the injection of high flow pulses from the jet ventilator and a 15 minute connection for conventional ventilation. A pressure monitoring tube is also available for monitoring airway pressures.

A specialized endotracheal tube with an attached subglottic suction port has been designed to allow for removal of secretions that often accumulate above the cuff (Figure 33-11). This tube has a separate channel in the wall of the tube that attaches to a wall suction source. The suction source is run continuously at negative pressures of 20 to 30 cm H_2O. The aspirated material is collected in a small container, which is emptied on a regular basis. Every 4 hours, a small amount of air should be injected into the suction port to ensure the port and tubing are not clogged. Use of this tube has been reported to decrease the incidence of ventilator-associated pneumonia.[25,26]

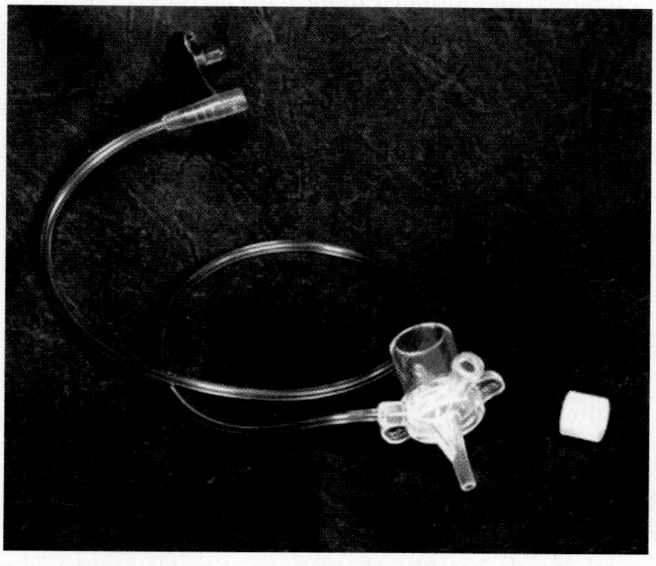

FIGURE 33-10 Endotracheal tube adapter for jet ventilation. LifePort Adapter. (Courtesy Bunnell Incorporated, Salt Lake City, Utah.)

Tracheostomy Tubes

Tracheostomy tubes are generally made from plastic polymers such as polyvinyl chloride or silicone, although some are still made from metal. Specifications covering

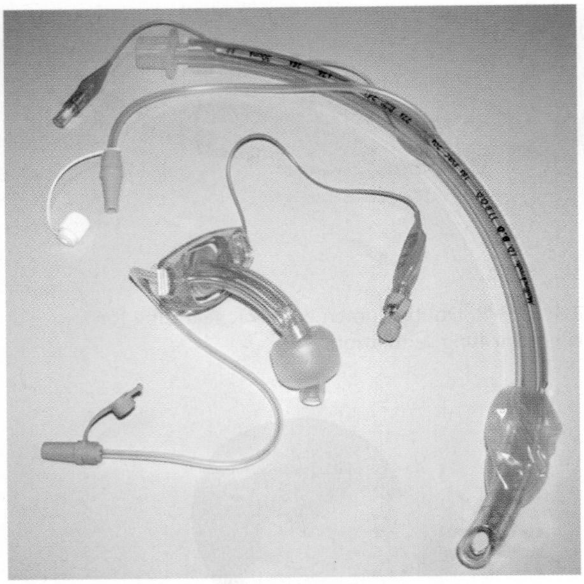

FIGURE 33-11 Endotracheal and tracheostomy tubes with subglottic suction ports.

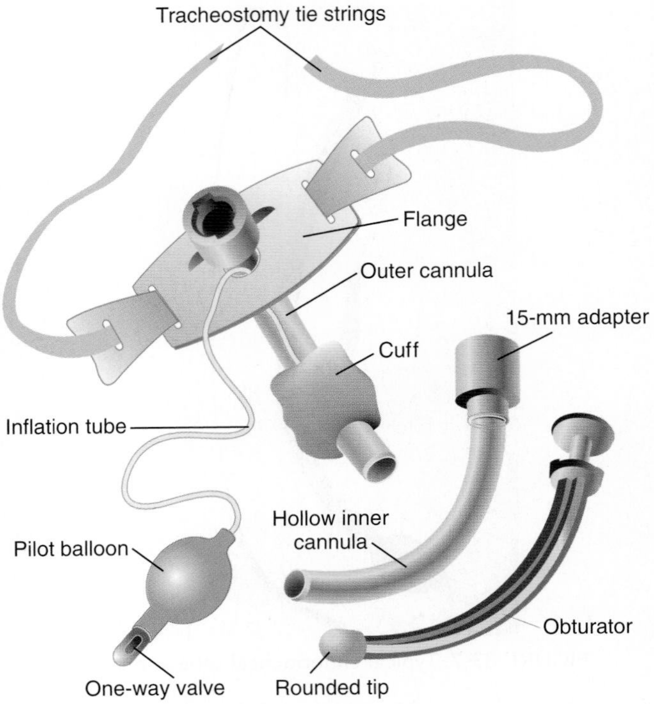

FIGURE 33-12 Parts of a tracheostomy tube.

the sizing, labeling, performance requirements, and test methods for tracheostomy tubes are established by the ASTM.[27]

Figure 33-12 shows a typical plastic tracheostomy tube and its key components. The outer cannula forms the primary structural unit of the tube, to which the cuff and a flange are attached. The flange prevents tube slippage into the trachea and provides the means to secure the tube to the neck. There are single-cannula and double-cannula tracheostomy tubes. The double-cannula tube has a removable inner cannula with a standard 15-mm adapter. It is normally kept in place within the outer cannula but can be removed for routine cleaning or if it becomes obstructed. To prevent accidental removal, the inner cannula can be locked in place at the proximal end of the outer cannula. As with an endotracheal tube, an inflation tube leads from the cuff to a pilot balloon and spring-loaded valve. The tube is stabilized at the stoma site with cotton tape, which attaches to the flange and is tied around the neck, or a soft tracheostomy tube holder with Velcro fasteners. An **obturator** with a rounded tip is used for tube insertion. Before insertion, the obturator is placed within the outer cannula, with its tip extending just beyond the far end of the tube; this minimizes mucosal trauma during insertion. Finally, as with endotracheal tubes, a radiopaque indicator in the distal end of the tube helps confirm tube position on a radiograph.

As with endotracheal tubes, various modified tracheostomy tubes are available. Extra-long tracheostomy tubes may be used in patients who require extra proximal or distal length because of anatomic considerations. The metal Jackson tracheostomy tube is made of stainless steel

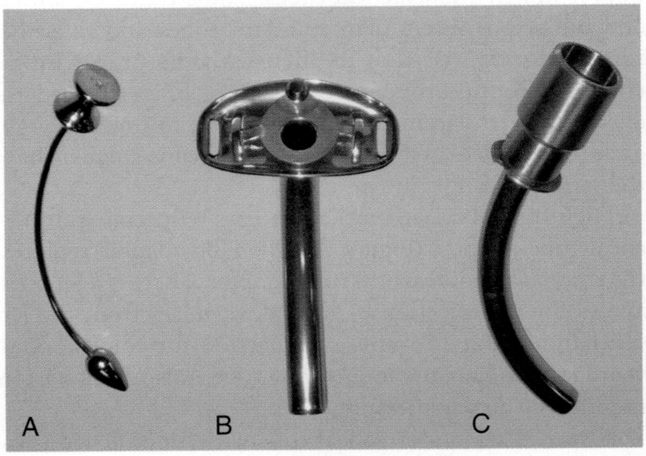

FIGURE 33-13 Jackson tracheostomy tube made from stainless steel. It has no cuff and no 15-mm adapter. **A,** Obturator. **B,** Outer cannula. **C,** Inner cannula.

with an inner and outer cannula (Figure 33-13). There is no cuff at the distal end or 15-mm adapter at the proximal end. This tracheostomy tube is generally used in patients with a long-term need for an airway but who do not require a seal to protect the airway from aspiration or to facilitate positive pressure ventilation. If the patient requires manual ventilation, a 15-mm adapter should be inserted into the proximal opening. If the patient requires a sealed airway, the tube needs to be changed to the standard cuffed tube described earlier.

Procedures

Orotracheal Intubation

Orotracheal intubation is the preferred route for establishing an emergency tracheal airway because the oral passage is the quickest and easiest route in most cases. Orotracheal intubation can be safely performed by an appropriately trained physician, RT, nurse, or paramedic.[28] Typically, this training involves manikin practice and application on anesthetized patients under the guidance of an anesthesiologist or other appropriately skilled individual. The basic steps in orotracheal intubation are described here.[29] Proficiency in this technique can be developed only with extensive training and experience.

Step 1: Assemble and Check Equipment. Box 33-3 lists the equipment necessary for intubation. All suction equipment is assembled, and the vacuum pressure is checked before intubation because vomitus or secretions may obscure the pharynx or glottis. The appropriate-size laryngoscope blade (see Box 33-3) is attached to its handle, and the light source is checked for secure attachment and brightness. If the light does not function, the bulb first should be checked to see if it is tight. If the scope still does not light, the batteries should be checked, or the bulb should be replaced.

A tube that is the right size for the patient should be selected, but one should be sure to have available tubes that are at least one size larger and one size smaller. Table 33-2 lists recommended orotracheal tube sizes according to patient weight or age. Endotracheal tubes are sized by their internal diameter (in millimeters). Tube lengths given in Table 33-2 are averages after insertion, confirmed placement, and fixation (teeth to tube tip).

Box 33-3 Equipment Needed for Endotracheal Intubation

- O_2 flowmeter and tubing
- Suction apparatus
- Flexible sterile suction catheters
- Sterile gloves for endotracheal suctioning
- Yankauer (tonsillar) tip suction
- Manual resuscitation bag and mask
- Colorimetric CO_2 detector
- Oropharyngeal airways
- Laryngoscope (2) with assorted blades (size 2-3 for adults, size 1-2 for children, size 0-1 for infants)
- Endotracheal tubes (3 appropriate sizes)
- Tongue depressor
- Stylet
- Stethoscope
- Tape or endotracheal tube holder
- 10-ml or 12-ml syringe
- Water-soluble lubricating gel
- Magill forceps
- Local anesthetic (spray)
- Towels (for positioning)
- CDC barrier precautions (gloves, gowns, masks, goggles, or face shields)

CDC, U.S. Centers for Disease Control and Prevention.

RULE OF THUMB

Generally, a woman is intubated with a No. 7 or No. 7.5 orotracheal tube, and a man is intubated with a No. 8.0 or No. 8.5 orotracheal tube.

After selecting the correct size of tube, the RT inflates the tube cuff and checks for leaks. The RT must be sure to deflate the cuff before insertion. To ease insertion, the outer surface of the tube should be lubricated with a water-soluble gel. Last, many clinicians insert a stylet into the tube to add rigidity and maintain shape during insertion. The tip of the stylet must never extend beyond the endotracheal tube tip.

Step 2: Position Patient. To visualize the glottis and insert the tube, the RT aligns the patient's mouth, pharynx, and larynx. This alignment is achieved by combining moderate cervical flexion with extension of the atlantooccipital joint. Placement of one or more rolled towels under the patient's shoulders helps. Next the RT flexes the patient's neck and tilts the head backward with his or her hand (Figure 33-14).

TABLE 33-2

Guideline for Infant, Pediatric, and Adult Oral Endotracheal Tube Sizes

Age	Tube Size (mm Internal Diameter)	Distance (in cm) from Incisors (Lip in Infants) to Tip of Tube
Infant, <1 kg	2.5	6.5-8
Infant, 1-2 kg	3.0	7-8
Infant, 2-3 kg	3.5	8-9
Infant, 4 kg	3.5-4.0	9-10
6 mo	3.5-4.0	10-11
18 mo	3.5-4.5	11-13
3 yr	4.5-5.0	12-14
5 yr	4.5-5.0	13-15
6 yr	5.5-6.0	14-16
8 yr	6.0-6.5	15-17
12 yr	6.0-7.0	17-19
16 yr/small women	6.5-7.0	18-20
Women (average)	7.5-8.0	19-21
Men	8.0-9.0	21-23

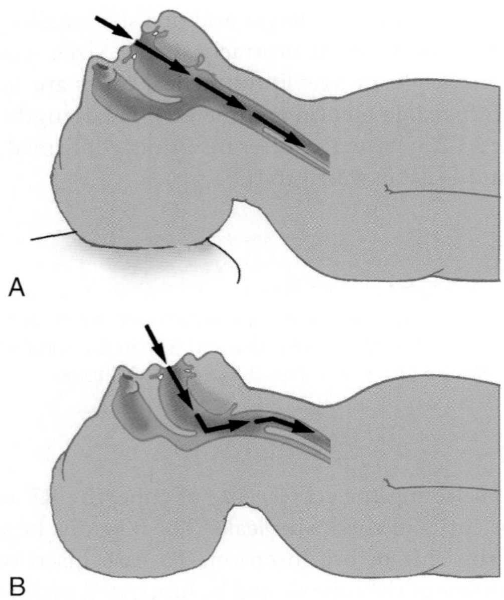

FIGURE 33-14 **A,** Correct head position before intubation. **B,** Incorrect head position before intubation.

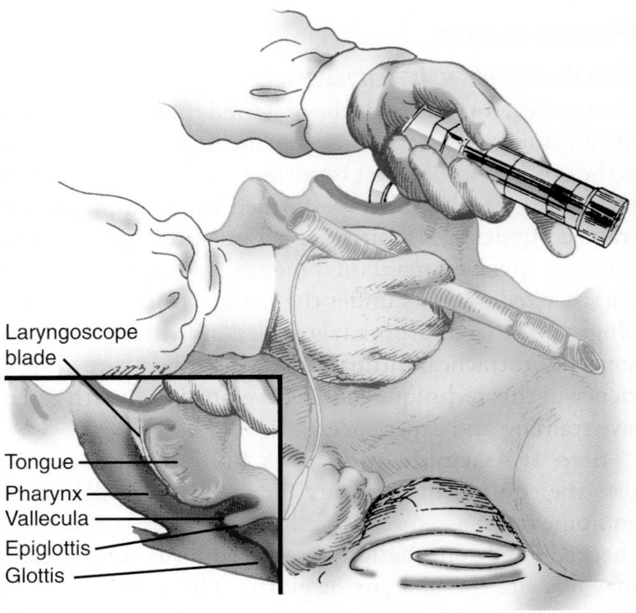

FIGURE 33-15 To achieve orotracheal intubation, the RT holds the laryngoscope in the left hand, introduces the blade into the right side of mouth, and displaces the tongue to the left. (Modified from Ellis PD, Billings DM: Cardiopulmonary resuscitation: procedures for basic and advanced life support, St. Louis, 1980, Mosby.)

MINI CLINI

Indications for Artificial Airway Management

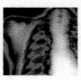

PROBLEM: A woman is admitted to the emergency department after sustaining chest trauma during a motor vehicle accident. The patient is unconscious, cyanotic, and tachypneic and has blood in the mouth and pharynx. Breath sounds are diminished on both sides. The physician requests that the RT immediately perform orotracheal intubation. Why?

DISCUSSION: This patient exhibits several indications for insertion of an artificial airway. First, being unconscious, the patient is probably unable to protect her lower airway adequately. With blood in the mouth and pharynx, there should be increased concern for protecting her lungs from aspiration. The blood also may indicate partial airway obstruction; the breath sounds, cyanosis, and respiratory distress contribute to that conclusion. Finally, the cyanosis and chest trauma indicate potential hypoxemic respiratory failure, which may require positive pressure ventilatory support via a cuffed endotracheal tube.

Step 3: Preoxygenate and Ventilate Patient. A patient in need of intubation is often apneic or in respiratory distress. Providing ventilation and oxygenation by manual resuscitator bag and mask with 100% O_2 before intubation helps ensure the patient tolerates the intubation procedure. No more than 30 seconds should be devoted to any intubation attempt. If intubation fails, immediate ventilation and oxygenation of the patient for 3 to 5 minutes before the next attempt should occur.

Step 4: Insert Laryngoscope. The RT should use the left hand to hold the laryngoscope and the right hand to open the mouth (Figure 33-15). The laryngoscope is inserted into the right side of the mouth and moved toward the center, displacing the tongue to the left. The tip of the blade is advanced along the curve of the tongue until the epiglottis is visualized.

RULE OF THUMB

A No. 3 curved Macintosh or straight Miller laryngoscope blade is commonly used to intubate adults.

Step 5: Visualize Glottis. As the laryngoscope blade reaches the base of the tongue, the RT looks for the arytenoid cartilage and epiglottis (Figure 33-16). If these structures are not visible, the blade is probably advanced too far and may be in the esophagus. If this is the case, the RT should maintain upward force on the laryngoscope and slowly withdraw the blade until the larynx is seen.

Step 6: Displace Epiglottis. The technique used to displace the epiglottis depends on the type of blade chosen (Figure 33-17). With the curved or MacIntosh blade, the epiglottis is displaced indirectly by advancing the tip of the blade into the vallecula (at the base of the tongue), and the laryngoscope is lifted up and forward (see Figure 33-17, *A*). With the straight or Miller blade, the epiglottis is

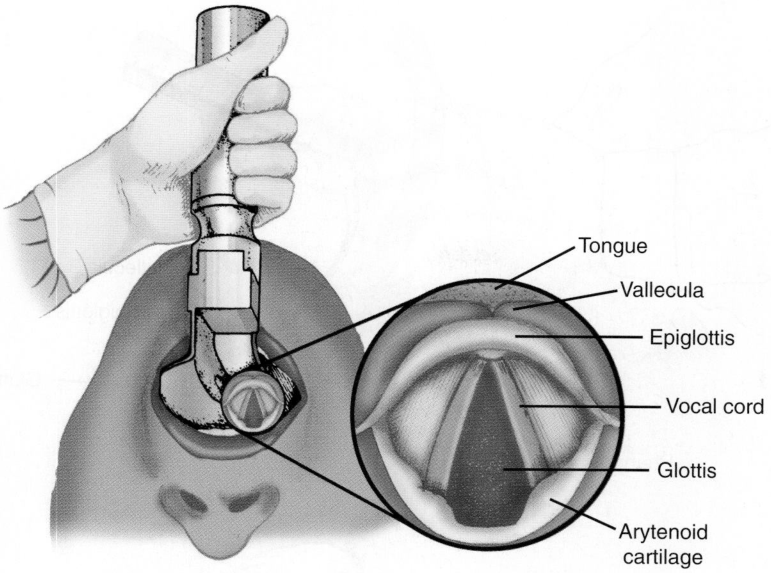

FIGURE 33-16 Visualization of vocal cords is achieved with a laryngoscope. (Modified from Ellis PD, Billings DM: Cardiopulmonary resuscitation: procedures for basic and advanced life support, St. Louis, 1980, Mosby.)

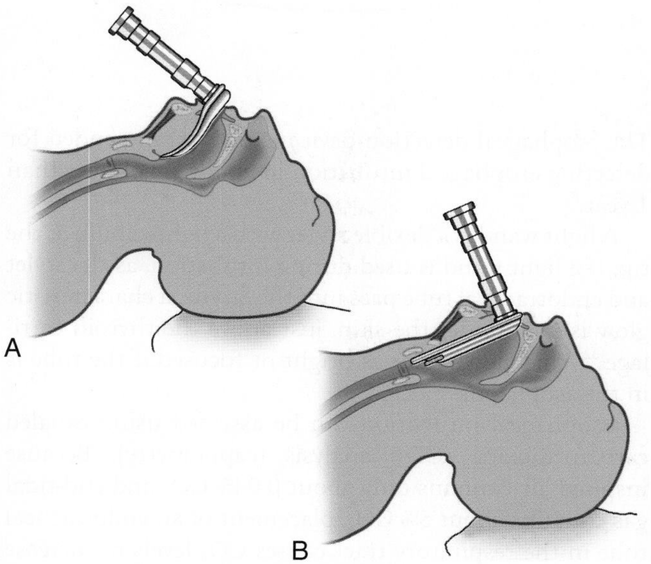

FIGURE 33-17 Placement of curved **(A)** versus straight **(B)** laryngoscope blade.

displaced directly by advancing the tip of the blade over its posterior surface, and the laryngoscope is lifted up and forward (see Figure 33-17, *B*).

One should avoid levering the laryngoscope against the teeth while lifting the tip of the blade because this can damage the teeth and gums. This problem can be avoided by keeping one's wrist fixed and moving the handle of the laryngoscope in the direction it is pointing when visualizing the epiglottis.

Step 7: Insert Tube. When the epiglottis is displaced and the glottis is visualized, the tube is inserted from the right side of the mouth and advanced without obscuring the glottic opening (Figure 33-18). When the tube tip is seen passing through the glottis, it is advanced until the cuff has passed the vocal cords. When the tube is in place, the RT stabilizes it with the right hand and uses the left hand to remove the laryngoscope and stylet. The cuff is inflated to seal the airway, and ventilation and oxygenation are immediately provided.

Step 8: Assess Tube Position. Ideally, the tip of an endotracheal tube should be positioned in the trachea about 3 to 6 cm above the carina.[30] One or more of several bedside methods can be used to assess positioning of the endotracheal tube before stabilization (Box 33-4). With the exception of fiberoptic laryngoscopy or bronchoscopy and videolaryngoscopy, none of these methods can absolutely confirm proper tube placement.

After tube passage and cuff inflation, the RT listens for equal and bilateral breath sounds as the patient is being ventilated. Air movement or gurgling sounds over the epigastrium indicate possible esophageal intubation. In addition, the chest wall is observed for adequate and equal chest expansion. These movements, combined with good breath sounds, are reinforcing. The combination of decreased breath sounds and decreased chest wall movement on the left side may indicate right main stem intubation. Right main stem intubation is corrected by slowly withdrawing the tube, while listening for the return of left-side breath sounds. Other conditions may cause decreased breath sounds in the left lung (e.g., atelectasis, pleural effusion).

The depth of tube insertion (length from teeth to tip) is useful to help determine tube position. As indicated in Table 33-2, the average length from the teeth (incisors) to the tip of a properly positioned oral endotracheal tube in men is 21 to 23 cm. For women, this distance is about 2 cm less. Tube length alone cannot confirm proper placement; a tube with the 23-cm mark positioned at the teeth could just as well be in the esophagus as in the trachea.

An esophageal detection device may be used to determine whether the tube is in the esophagus or trachea.[31]

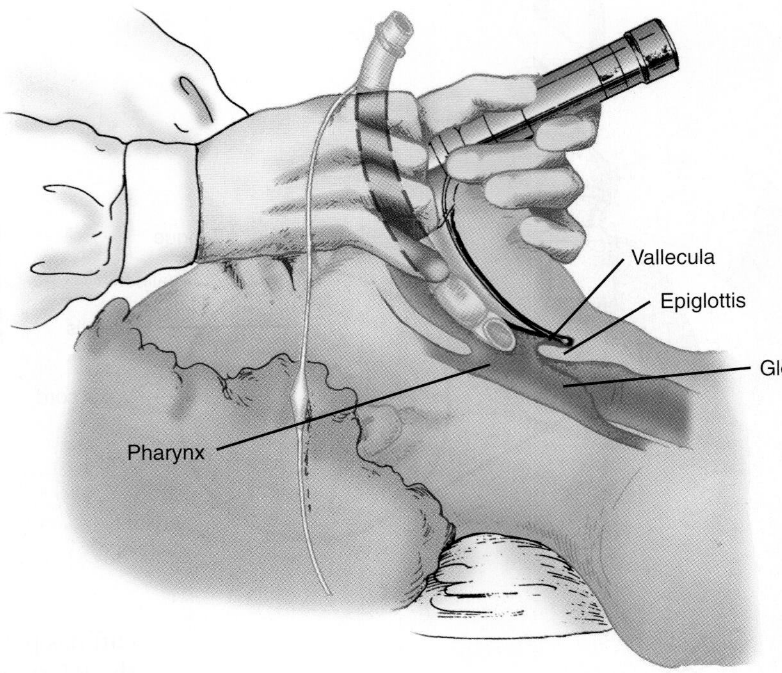

FIGURE 33-18 Insertion of endotracheal tube. (Modified from Ellis PD, Billings DM: Cardiopulmonary resuscitation: procedures for basic and advanced life support, St. Louis, 1980, Mosby.)

Box 33-4 Bedside Methods to Assess Endotracheal Tube Position

- Auscultation of chest and abdomen
- Observation of chest movement
- Tube length (cm to teeth)
- Esophageal detection device
- Light wand
- Capnometry
- Colorimetry
- Fiberoptic laryngoscopy or bronchoscopy
- Videolaryngoscopy

This device is more commonly used outside the hospital setting. The original device consists of a squeeze-bulb aspirator attached to a standard 15-mm adapter. After creating a negative pressure (−80 to −90 mm Hg) by squeezing the bulb, one attaches it to the positioned endotracheal tube. If the tube is placed correctly, the bulb quickly reexpands on release because the tracheal lumen is held open by cartilaginous rings. If the tube is in the esophagus, it does not reinflate because the more pliable esophagus collapses around the tip of the endotracheal tube preventing the bulb from reinflating. Instead of a squeeze-bulb, a large syringe with a 15-mm adapter can be used. If the endotracheal tube is in the esophagus, strong resistance is noticed when aspirating air (the barrel tends to recoil if released); if the tube is in the trachea, aspirating air into the syringe is easy. In patients with copious secretions, the esophageal detection device may become occluded and not reexpand. The esophageal detection device is not recommended for detecting esophageal intubation in children younger than 1 year.[31]

A light wand is a flexible stylet with a lighted bulb at the tip. If a light wand is used during intubation, as the stylet and endotracheal tube pass into the larynx, a characteristic glow is seen under the skin, just above the thyroid cartilage.[32] This glow is not as bright or focused if the tube is in the esophagus.

Esophageal intubation can be assessed using exhaled carbon dioxide (CO_2) analysis (capnometry). Because inspired air contains only about 0.04% CO_2 and end-tidal gas contains about 5% CO_2, placement of an endotracheal tube in the respiratory tract causes CO_2 levels to increase abruptly during expiration. This increase is evident on a capnographic display (Figure 33-19). If the tube is in the esophagus, CO_2 levels remain near zero.[33]

Colorimetric CO_2 analysis is an inexpensive alternative to capnometry. Functioning similar to pH paper, a colorimetric system has an indicator that changes color when exposed to different CO_2 levels.[34] Figure 33-20 shows a disposable colorimetric system designed specifically to confirm tube placement during intubation. Colorimetric devices are portable and disposable and are commonly used in hospitals.

Both devices are effective in detecting most esophageal intubations. However, in patients with cardiac arrest, expired CO_2 levels may be near zero because of poor pulmonary blood flow, yielding a false-negative result.[32-34] Generally, expired CO_2 levels increase with the return of spontaneous circulation. CO_2 analysis is an unreliable indicator of main stem bronchial intubation.

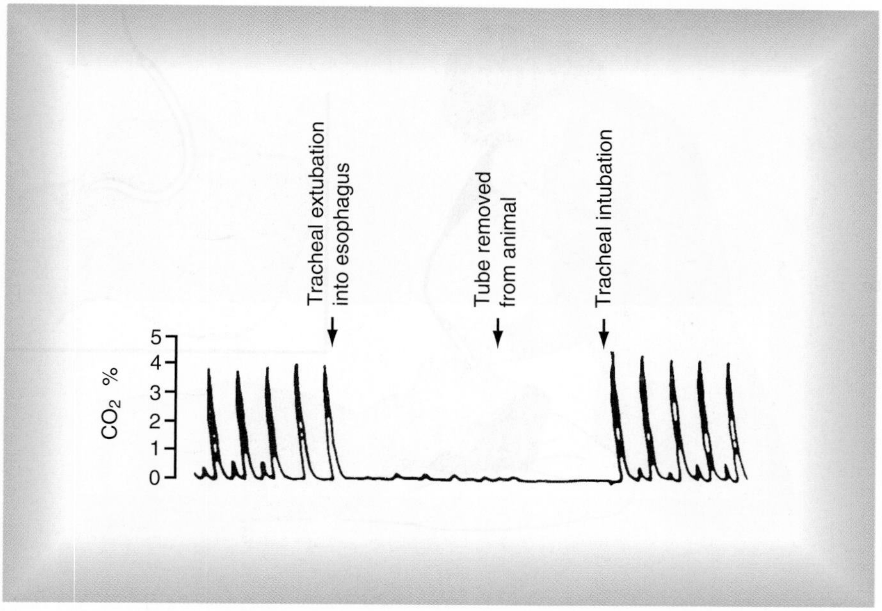

FIGURE 33-19 Capnogram tracing showing changes in expired percent CO_2 with proper and improper placement of endotracheal tube in test animals.

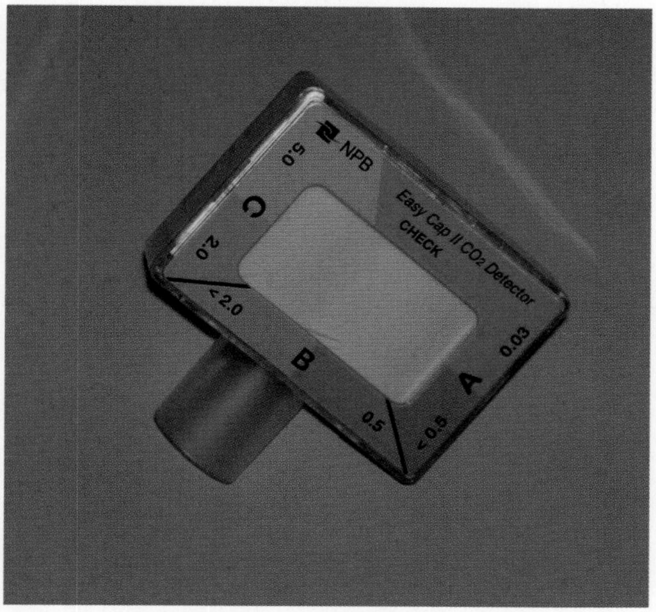

FIGURE 33-20 Disposable colorimetric CO_2 detector for confirming tracheal intubation. (Used by permission from Nellcor Puritan Bennett LLC, Boulder, Colorado, doing business as Covidien.)

RULE OF THUMB

Generally, an orotracheal tube should initially be inserted to the 21- to 23-cm mark at the teeth in men and to the 19- to 21-cm mark at the teeth in women and adjusted based on the results of the patient assessment (bilateral breath sounds) and chest x-ray findings after intubation.

Proper tube placement in the trachea can be confirmed without a chest radiograph by using a fiberoptic laryngoscope or bronchoscope.[35] After ensuring patient reoxygenation, a fiberoptic laryngoscope or bronchoscope can be inserted directly into the endotracheal tube (Figure 33-21). Visualization of the carina distal to the tip of the endotracheal tube ensures proper placement in the trachea. More

MINI CLINI

Capnometry and Endotracheal Tube Placement

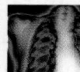

PROBLEM: At a Code Blue in the emergency department, a patient is intubated by the RT. A capnometer is attached to the endotracheal tube to confirm placement in the trachea. The end-expired CO_2 reads 0% as the patient is ventilated with a manual resuscitator. At this time, no one is performing cardiac compressions. Should the RT conclude that the endotracheal tube is not in the trachea?

DISCUSSION: No. If the patient is in cardiac arrest, no blood is perfusing the alveoli, and no CO_2 is entering the alveoli. The result is an end-tidal CO_2 of 0%. When cardiac compressions begin (and they should begin immediately in confirmed cardiac arrest) and if compressions are effective, one should see an increase in end-tidal CO_2 as blood begins to perfuse the alveoli, and CO_2 diffuses the blood.

There are other simple ways to assess endotracheal tube placement in the trachea, such as bilateral breath sounds on auscultation and chest excursions. However, an increase in end-tidal CO_2 is a sure indication that the endotracheal tube is in the lungs because the only source of CO_2 is in the alveoli.

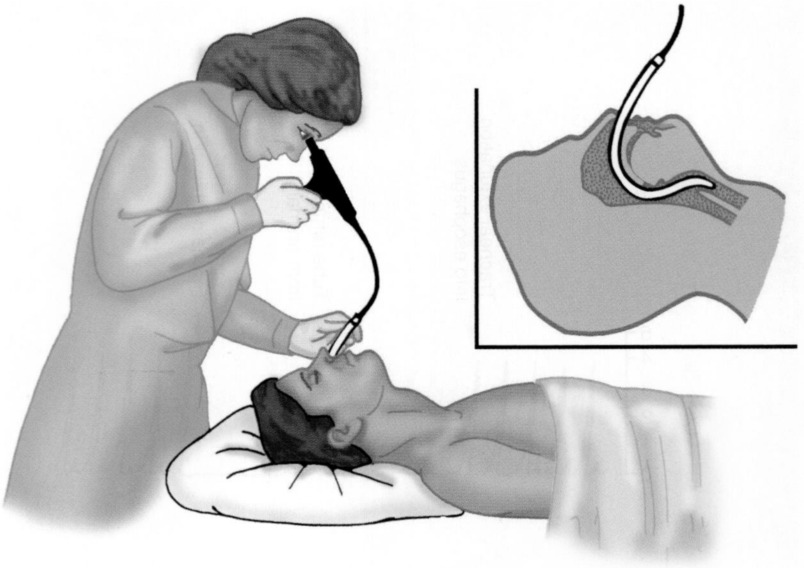

FIGURE 33-21 Fiberoptic laryngoscopy used to confirm endotracheal tube placement.

precise placement is possible by moving the laryngoscope from the tube tip to the carina, while measuring this distance. Also, a videolaryngoscope can be used to ensure proper placement of the endotracheal tube, especially in anticipated difficult intubations. It provides a better view of the airway, especially when there is limited mobility of the patient's neck or mouth. Also, other clinicians can see the airway and help if needed.[36]

Step 9: Stabilize Tube and Confirm Placement. The tube should not be secured until correct placement has been assessed by using one or more of the above-mentioned methods. After assessing placement and while holding the tube in position, the RT secures the tube to the skin above the lip and on the cheeks using tape or an endotracheal tube holder. A bite-block, oropharyngeal airway, or similar device may be needed to prevent the patient from biting down on the tube (Figure 33-22). After the tube is stabilized, a chest radiograph should be taken to confirm its position.

The most common complication of emergency airway management is tissue trauma. The most serious complications are acute hypoxemia, hypercapnia, bradycardia, and cardiac arrest.[37] These problems can be minimized by using proper technique, providing the patient with adequate ventilation and oxygenation (before, during, and after), and strictly adhering to intubation time limits. In addition, sedation and anesthesia can reduce complications and facilitate intubation in a semicomatose or combative patient.[28] Muscle relaxing or paralyzing agents can be used in a combative patient who cannot be controlled by sedation. A paralyzed patient has no ability to compensate for hypoxemia or hypercapnia. It is imperative that the patient can be adequately ventilated by bag and mask. Rapid-sequence induction is used with the administration of a sedative-hypnotic medication and a muscle relaxing or paralyzing agent.

Difficult intubations occur because of inability to open the patient's mouth, inability to position the patient, or unusual airway anatomy. Special intubation equipment (e.g., laryngoscope blades, videolaryngoscopy, or specialized stylets) or alternative techniques can be employed.[28,37] Additional details of these techniques are beyond the scope of this chapter.

Nasotracheal Intubation

Although nasotracheal intubation is more difficult than orotracheal intubation, it is the route of choice in certain clinical situations. Examples include intubation of patients when the oral route is unavailable, such as patients with maxillofacial injuries or undergoing oral surgery.

Nasotracheal intubation is performed either blindly or by direct visualization.[38] The direct visualization approach requires either a standard or a fiberoptic laryngoscope. For the blind technique to work, the patient must be breathing spontaneously. Equipment assembly, patient positioning, and preoxygenation are essentially the same as with oral intubation. A mixture of 0.25% phenylephrine and 3% lidocaine may be applied to the nasal mucosa with a long cotton-tipped swab to provide local anesthesia and vasoconstriction of the nasal passage.

Direct Visualization. The equipment needed for nasal intubation by direct visualization is the same as for oral intubation, with the addition of Magill forceps. A smaller size endotracheal tube may also be needed. The tube should be prelubricated with water-soluble gel to aid passage. To insert the tube, the bevel is positioned toward the septum and advanced along the floor of the meatus (inferiorly). When the tip of the tube is in the patient's oropharynx, the RT opens the patient's mouth, inserts the laryngoscope (with the left hand), and visualizes the glottis. The RT uses the Magill forceps with the right hand to grasp the tube just above the cuff and direct it between the

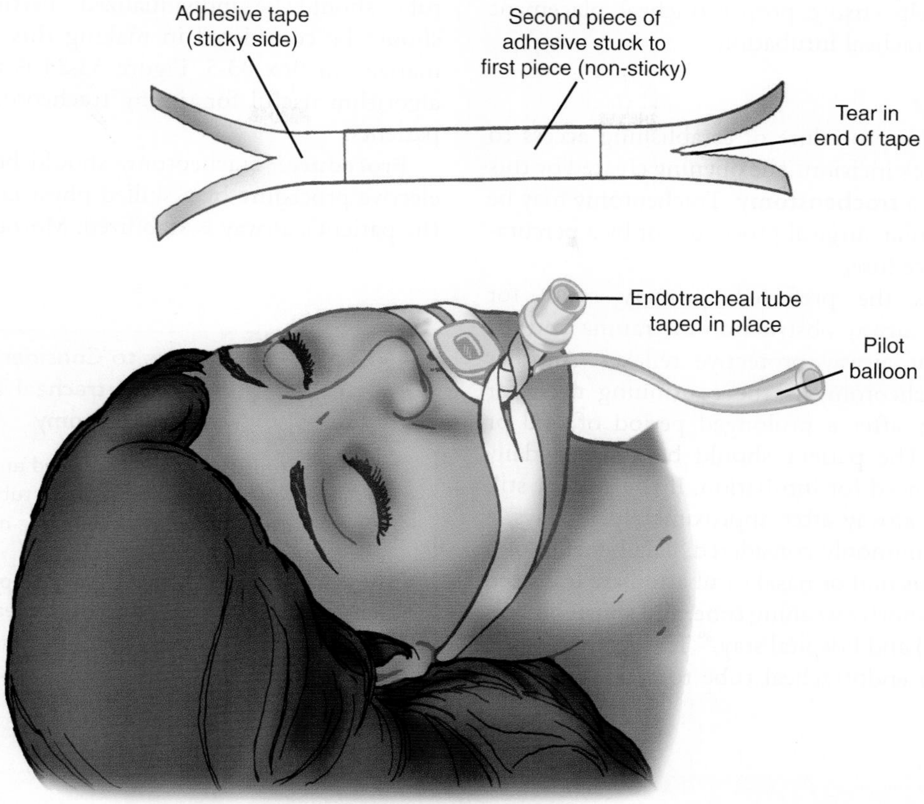

FIGURE 33-22 Securing the endotracheal tube.

vocal cords (Figure 33-23). To help advance the tube past the vocal cords, the neck may need to be flexed. Confirmation of position and stabilization follows, as with the oral route.

Alternatively, a fiberoptic bronchoscope or laryngoscope can be used to guide tube passage.[35] With the bronchoscopic method, the distal end of the scope is passed through the endotracheal tube and directly into the trachea. When placement is ensured, the RT slides the endotracheal tube down over the scope into proper position. The procedure is similar with a fiberoptic laryngoscope. However, because directional control of the scope is limited, the RT may have to reposition the patient's head and neck to help guide the tube.

Blind Passage. For blind nasal intubation, the patient is placed in either the supine or the sitting position. As with direct visualization, the tube is inserted through the nose. As the tube approaches the larynx, one can listen through the tube for air movement. The breath sounds become louder and more tubular when the tube passes through the larynx. Successful passage of the tube through the larynx usually is indicated by a harsh cough, followed by vocal silence. If the sounds disappear, the tube is moving toward the esophagus. A malpositioned tube can be corrected by manipulating the tube and repositioning the patient's head and neck. Confirmation of tube placement and stabilization should follow. As previously indicated, a

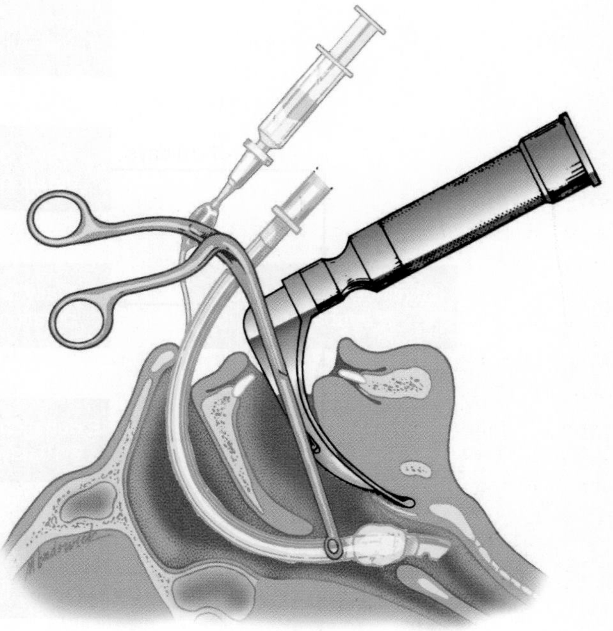

FIGURE 33-23 Nasal intubation using Magill forceps. (Modified from Finucane BT, Santora AH: Principles of airway management, Philadelphia, 1988, FA Davis.)

light wand can help ensure proper tracheal placement during blind nasotracheal intubation.

Tracheotomy

Tracheotomy is the procedure of establishing access to the trachea via a neck incision. The opening created by this procedure is called a **tracheostomy.** Tracheotomy may be performed as a regular surgical procedure or by a percutaneous dilation procedure.

Tracheotomy is the preferred, primary route for overcoming upper airway obstruction or trauma and for patients with poor airway protective reflexes. Another indication for tracheotomy is the continuing need for an artificial airway after a prolonged period of oral or nasal intubation. The patient should be assessed daily for the continued need for intubation. If the patient still needs an artificial airway after approximately 14 days, a tracheostomy is commonly considered. The benefits of a tracheostomy versus oral or nasal intubation are less need for deep sedation, shorter weaning time, and shorter intensive care unit (ICU) and hospital stay.[39] The decision when to switch from an endotracheal tube to a tracheostomy tube should be individualized. Pertinent factors that should be considered in making this decision are summarized in Box 33-5. Figure 33-24 is a decision-making algorithm useful for timing tracheotomy in critically ill patients.

Procedure. Tracheotomy should be performed as an elective procedure by a skilled physician or surgeon after the patient's airway is stabilized. Mortality and morbidity

Box 33-5 Factors to Consider in Switching from Endotracheal Tube to Tracheostomy

- Projected time the patient will need an artificial airway
- Patient's tolerance of endotracheal tube
- Patient's overall condition (including nutritional, cardiovascular, and infection status)
- Patient's ability to tolerate a surgical procedure
- Relative risks of continued endotracheal intubation vs. tracheostomy

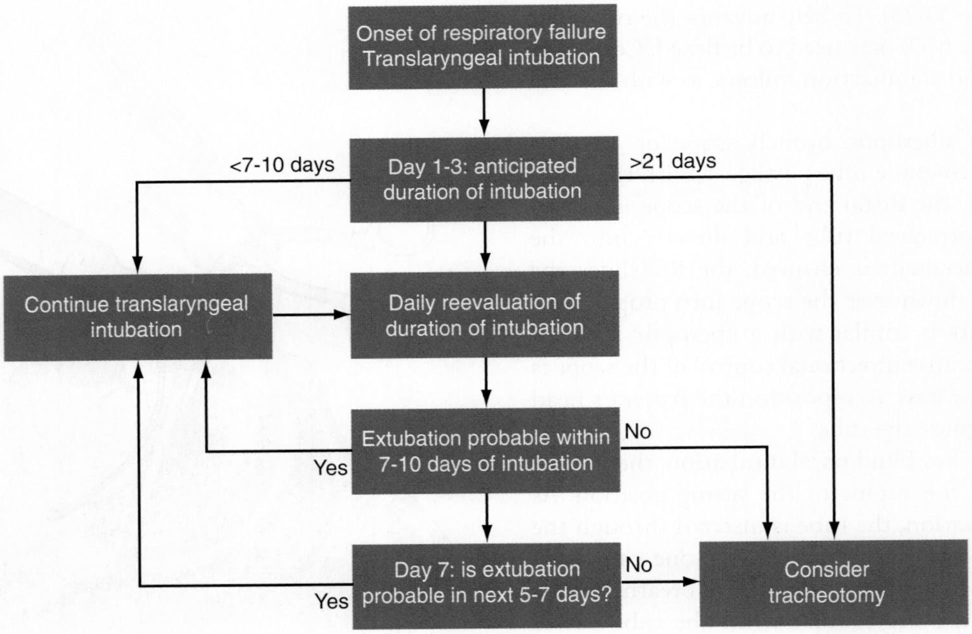

FIGURE 33-24 Approach to timing tracheotomy in patients intubated and mechanically ventilated for respiratory failure. (From Heffner JE: Timing of trachiostomy in ventilator-dependant patients, Clin Chest Med 12:611, 1991.)

are greater when the procedure is performed on an emergency basis. The RT may be asked to assist in tracheotomy, especially if performed at the bedside. For this reason, we briefly describe both the traditional surgical procedure and the percutaneous dilation method.[39]

A local anesthetic is used, and the patient is mildly sedated if conditions permit. If an endotracheal tube is in place, it should not be removed until just before the insertion of the tracheostomy tube. Keeping the endotracheal tube in place this way ensures a patent airway and provides additional stability to the trachea during the procedure.

In traditional surgical tracheotomy, the surgeon makes an incision in the neck over the second or third tracheal ring. After the skin and subcutaneous tissue have been incised, the surgeon divides the platysma muscles and locates the underlying thyroid gland. The surgeon divides and ligates the thyroid isthmus, which overlies the second and third tracheal rings. The surgeon then enters the trachea through either a horizontal incision between rings or a vertical incision through the second and third rings. As little cartilage as possible should be removed to promote better closure after extubation.

In percutaneous dilation tracheotomy, the initial steps to prepare the patient are similar to the steps in the traditional tracheotomy procedure. After dissection to the anterior tracheal wall, the endotracheal tube is retracted to keep the tip of the tube inside the larynx. A bronchoscope can be used to reassess placement for the endotracheal tube for the duration of the procedure. A large leak around the endotracheal tube develops for patients on mechanical ventilation. If the patient is unable to tolerate the large leak, and adjustments to ventilatory support cannot be used to compensate for the leak, a surgical procedure may be indicated for that patient.

The physician inserts a needle and sheath into the trachea between the cricoid and first tracheal ring or between the first and second rings. The physician then inserts a guidewire through the sheath, the sheath is removed, and a dilator is passed over the guidewire. Larger and larger dilators are introduced until the stoma is large enough for a standard tracheostomy tube. The physician slips the tracheostomy tube over the last dilator used. An alternative to the use of multiple dilators is to use a single dilator with increasing diameter from the proximal to the distal end.

The procedure may be performed under direct vision with a bronchoscope passed through the endotracheal tube or a laryngeal mask airway (LMA). Compared with the traditional surgical procedure, a percutaneous dilation tracheotomy is rapid with fewer complications from the surgical site and has a better cosmetic appearance after decannulation. Contraindications for percutaneous tracheotomy are listed in Box 33-6.

Insertion of the tube, inflation of the cuff, and securing the tube follow both methods. Tracheostomy tube ties should be secure enough to prevent movement of the tube but not so tight as to cause skin ulceration. The role of the RT in the procedure may include managing the endotracheal tube, making ventilator changes as needed, assisting with the bronchoscope, and monitoring the patient.

Box 33-6 Contraindications for Percutaneous Dilation Tracheostomy

ABSOLUTE
- Need for emergent surgical airway

RELATIVE
- Children <12 years old
- Poor landmarks secondary to body habitus, abnormal anatomy, or occluding thyroid mass
- PEEP > 15 cm H_2O
- Coagulopathy
- Pulsating blood vessel over tracheotomy site
- Limited ability to extend cervical spine
- History of difficult intubation
- Infection, burn, or malignancy at tracheotomy site

From Park S, Goldenberg D: Percutaneous tracheotomy: Griggs technique. Op Tech Otolaryngol 18:95, 2007.

Generally, the tube size is correct if it occupies two-thirds to three-quarters of the internal tracheal diameter. Tracheostomy tubes come in various sizes, lengths, and shapes depending on the manufacturer. The size marked on the flange usually indicates the internal diameter, but some tracheostomy tubes with inner cannulas use Jackson sizing. Table 33-3 lists the sizes, internal diameter, external diameter, and length of commonly used brands and styles of adult tracheostomy tubes. Table 33-4 provides guidelines for selecting a tracheostomy tube according to a patient's age. Within an age category, the exact size of tube chosen depends on the patient's height, weight, and airway anatomy. To choose a tracheostomy tube that fits a patient properly, it is important to consider not only the internal and external diameter of the tube but also the length and shape of the tube.

AIRWAY TRAUMA ASSOCIATED WITH TRACHEAL TUBES

Artificial airways do not conform exactly to patients' anatomy, which may result in pressure on soft tissues that can result in ischemia and ulceration.[40] In addition, artificial airways tend to shift position as the patient's head and neck move or as the tube is manipulated. This shifting can result in friction-like injuries. Occasional reaction to the materials composing the tube may also cause problems.

Depending on the type of tube, damage to the patient's airway can occur anywhere from the nose down into the lower trachea. Because tracheostomy tubes do not pass through the larynx, structural injury resulting from these airways is limited to tracheal sites. Laryngeal dysfunction

TABLE 33-3

Comparison of Commonly Used Brands of Adult Tracheostomy Tubes

Portex Flex DIC—Sized by ID; Also Available Cuffless or Fenestrated

ID (mm)	OD (mm)	Length (mm)*
6.0	8.2	64
7.0	9.6	70
8.0	10.9	74

Shiley SCT—Sized by ID; Also Available Cuffless

ID (mm)	OD (mm)	Length (mm)*
6.0	8.3	67
7.0	9.6	80
8.0	10.9	89

Shiley Double Cannula (LPC, DC, CFS, CFN, FEN, PERC) With Disposable or Nondisposable Inner Cannula—Sized by Jackson Scale; Also Available Cuffless or Fenestrated

Size (Jackson)	ID (mm)	OD (mm)	Length (mm)
4	5.0	9.4	65
6	6.4	10.8	76 (PERC 74)
8	7.6	12.2	81 (PERC 79)

Jackson Double Cannula Stainless Steel Tube; Available Cuffless Only; Available Fenestrated

Size (Jackson)	ID (mm)	OD (mm)	Length (mm)
4	5.3	8.0	62
6	7.2	10.0	69
8	9.2	12.0	69

Extra Length Tubes: Shiley TracheoSoft XLT Proximal or Distal Extension With DIC—Sized by ID

ID (mm)	OD (mm)	Length (mm)
6.0	11	95
7.0	12.3	100
8.0	13.3	105

Bivona Mid-Range Aire-Cuf Extra Length Fixed or Adjustable Neck Flange—Sized by ID

ID (mm)	OD (mm)	Length (mm)
6.0	8.7	100 (adjustable 110)
7.0	10.0	110 (adjustable 120)
8.0	11.0	120 (adjustable 130)

Bivona TTS—Sized by ID; Cuff Inflated With Sterile Water Not Air

ID (mm)	OD (mm)	Length (mm)
6.0	8.7	70
7.0	10.0	80
8.0	11.0	88

DIC, Disposable inner cannula; *ID,* inner diameter; *OD,* outer diameter; *SCT,* single cannula tracheostomy.
*The main difference between these tubes is the length.

TABLE 33-4

Guideline for Infant, Pediatric, and Adult Tracheostomy Tube Sizes

Age/Weight*	ID (mm)
Premature <2 kg	2.5 cuffless neonatal
Infant	3.0-3.5 cuffless neonatal
6-18 mo	3.5-4.0 neonatal or pediatric
18 mo to 4-5 yr	4.0-4.5 pediatric
4-5 yr to 10 yr	4.5-6.0 pediatric
10-14 yr	5.0-6.5 pediatric or adult
14 years to adult	6.0-9.0 adult

ID, Inner diameter.
Note: The difference between the same size (ID) neonatal and pediatric tube or pediatric and adult tube is the length; that is, the adult tube is longer than the pediatric tube, and the pediatric tube is longer than the neonatal tube.
*Typical pediatric size = (16 + age)/4 or (age/4) + 4

may occur secondary to a lack of stimulation from airflow or restricted movement secondary to equipment.[41]

Because injury often cannot be assessed while an artificial airway is in place, the patient's airway should always be evaluated carefully after extubation. Techniques commonly used to diagnose airway damage include physical examination, air tomography, fluoroscopy, laryngoscopy, bronchoscopy, magnetic resonance imaging, and pulmonary function studies.[40]

Laryngeal Lesions

The most common laryngeal injuries associated with endotracheal intubation are glottic edema, vocal cord inflammation, laryngeal or vocal cord ulcerations, and vocal cord polyps or granulomas. Less common and more serious injuries are vocal cord paralysis and laryngeal stenosis.[29,40]

Glottic edema and vocal cord inflammation are transient changes that occur as a result of pressure from the endotracheal tube or trauma during intubation.[40] The primary concern with glottic edema and vocal cord inflammation occurs after extubation. Because swelling can worsen over 24 hours after extubation, patients should be evaluated periodically for delayed development of glottic edema.

The primary symptoms of glottic edema and vocal cord inflammation are hoarseness and stridor. Hoarseness occurs in most extubated patients and usually resolves quickly. Stridor is a more serious symptom than hoarseness, indicating a significant decrease in diameter of the airway. Stridor is often treated with epinephrine (2.25%

racemic solution or levoepinephrine 1 : 1000) via aerosol.[40] The goal of treatment is to reduce glottic or airway edema by mucosal vasoconstriction. A steroid may also be added to the aerosol to reduce inflammation further. Both of these techniques are more commonly used in children than in adults.

To reduce laryngeal edema in patients who have had prolonged intubation or patients who have failed prior extubation because of glottic edema, intravenous steroids may be given 24 hours before extubation.[9,40] If stridor continues and is unresponsive to treatment, structural changes that narrow the airway should be suspected.

Laryngeal and vocal cord ulcerations may also cause hoarseness soon after extubation. Symptoms usually resolve spontaneously, and no treatment is indicated. Vocal cord polyps and granulomas develop more slowly, taking weeks or months to form.[41] Symptoms include difficulty in swallowing, hoarseness, and stridor. If symptoms are severe or persistent, the polyps or granulomas may have to be removed surgically.

Vocal cord paralysis is likely in extubated patients with hoarseness and stridor that does not resolve with treatment or time. In some patients, symptoms may resolve within 24 hours, and full movement of the vocal cords can return over several days. If the obstructive symptoms continue, tracheotomy may be indicated.

Laryngeal **stenosis** occurs when the normal tissue of the larynx is replaced by scar tissue, which causes stricture and decreased mobility. The symptoms of laryngeal stenosis are similar to symptoms of vocal cord paralysis—stridor and hoarseness. Because laryngeal stenosis does not resolve spontaneously, surgical correction is usually required. Some patients require a permanent tracheostomy.

Tracheal Lesions

Although laryngeal lesions occur only with oral or nasal endotracheal tubes, tracheal lesions can occur with any tracheal airway. These tracheal lesions include granulomas, **tracheomalacia,** and tracheal stenosis.[40,41] Less common, but more serious complications are tracheoesophageal and tracheoinnominate artery fistulas.

Tracheomalacia and tracheal stenosis can occur either separately or together. *Tracheomalacia* is the softening of the cartilaginous rings, which causes collapse of the trachea during inspiration. *Tracheal stenosis* is a narrowing of the lumen of the trachea, which can occur as fibrous scarring causes the airway to narrow. In patients with endotracheal tubes, this type of damage most often occurs at the cuff site. In patients with tracheostomy tubes, stenosis may occur at the cuff, tube tip, or stoma sites; the stoma site is the most common. Stenosis at the stoma site is associated with too large a stoma, infection of the stoma, movement of the tube, frequent tube changes, and advanced age.[41]

Signs of possible tracheal damage before extubation include difficulty in sealing the trachea with the cuff and evidence of tracheal dilation on chest radiograph.[40] Signs and symptoms of postextubation problems include difficulty with expectoration, dyspnea, and stridor. Although these findings may appear acutely, they may develop over several months and may not be present until the radius is reduced by 50% to 75%. Dyspnea at rest may not be seen until the diameter of the trachea is less than 5 mm. Symptoms are often incorrectly attributed to the development of asthma or chronic lung disease.[41]

Tomography, fluoroscopy, and pulmonary function studies (especially flow-volume loops) may be helpful in quantifying the severity of the damage. Flow-volume loops are also helpful in distinguishing between tracheomalacia and tracheal stenosis. Tracheomalacia appears as a variable obstruction with different inspiratory and expiratory patterns. Tracheal stenosis appears as a fixed obstructive pattern, with flattening of both the inspiratory and the expiratory limbs of the flow-volume loop (Figure 33-25).

Treatment depends on the severity of the lesion, especially the length and circumference of the damage.[41] Laser therapy may be useful if the lesion is small. Resection and end-to-end anastomosis may be indicated when the damage involves fewer than three tracheal rings. More involved damage may require staged repair. Stents may also be placed to maintain the patency of the airway.

A **tracheoesophageal fistula** is a direct communication between the trachea and the esophagus. Tracheoesophageal fistula is a rare complication of both tracheotomy and endotracheal intubation. If it occurs soon after a tracheotomy, incorrect surgical technique may be the cause. Later development is related to sepsis, malnutrition, tracheal erosion from the cuff and tube, and esophageal erosion from nasogastric tubes.[40] The diagnosis can be made based on a history of recurrent aspiration and abdominal distention as air is forced into the esophagus during positive pressure ventilation. Diagnosis is also made by direct endoscopic examination of the trachea and esophagus. Treatment involves surgical closure of the defect.

A **tracheoinnominate artery fistula** can occur when a tracheostomy tube causes tissue erosion through the innominate artery. The result is massive hemorrhage and, in most cases, death. Tracheoinnominate artery fistula is a rare complication, probably caused by improper low positioning of the stoma or excessive movement of the tube.[41] Pulsation of the tracheostomy tube may be the only clue before actual hemorrhage. When hemorrhage begins, hyperinflation of the cuff may slow the bleeding, but the patient still needs surgical intervention.[41] Even with proper corrective action, only 25% of patients who develop this serious complication survive.

Prevention

Several actions can minimize the trauma caused by tracheal airways. Many studies suggest that tube movement is a primary cause of injury.[40,41] Several methods can be used to limit tube movement. Sedation can help keep patients comfortable and decrease the likelihood of

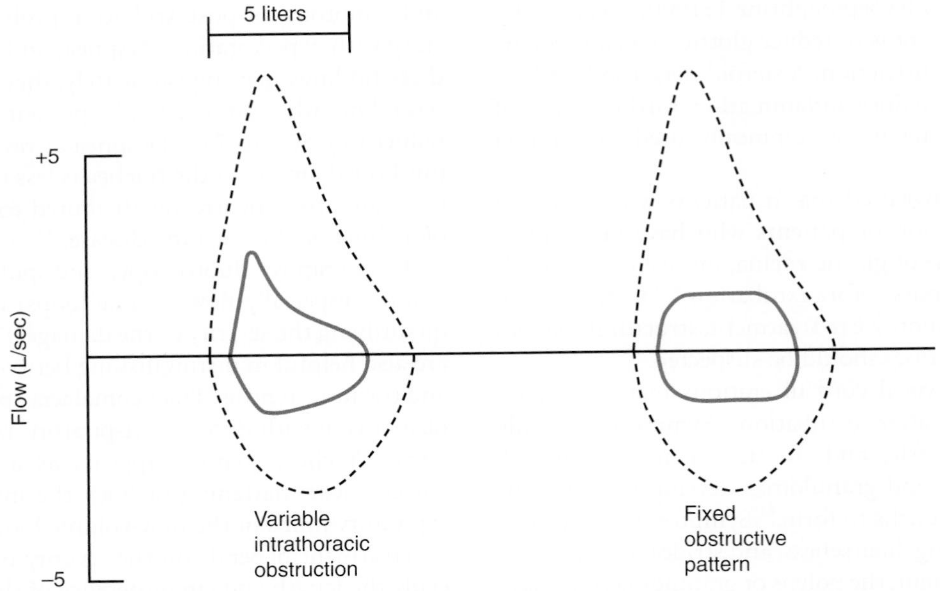

FIGURE 33-25 Variable intrathoracic *(left)* versus fixed obstructive pattern *(right)* flow-volume loops. *Dotted lines* are normal values for comparison. Tracheomalacia is typically seen as a variable obstruction, whereas tracheal stenosis most often manifests with a fixed pattern.

self-extubation. Nasotracheal tubes are easier to stabilize and may move less than orotracheal tubes. Swivel adapters can be used to minimize tube traction whenever respiratory therapy equipment is attached to patients with tracheostomies. If a patient with a tracheostomy requires O_2 therapy, tracheostomy collars are preferred to T-tubes or Briggs adapters.

Selection of the correct airway size is also important. Once in place, endotracheal and tracheostomy tubes should not be changed unless necessary. To minimize vocal cord closure around endotracheal tubes, patients should be discouraged from unnecessary coughing or efforts to talk. Tracheal wall injury from the endotracheal or tracheostomy tube cuff can be reduced by maintaining pressures of 25 to 35 cm H_2O.[13,42] If the airway is in place solely for suctioning or to bypass an obstruction, a cuff may not be needed.

Infected secretions have been implicated in the development of tracheitis and mucosal destruction, and infection of the tracheotomy stoma has been linked to tracheal stenosis.[41] Sterile techniques should be used when cleaning or suctioning tracheostomy tubes. Good tracheostomy care, including aseptic cleaning of the stoma with sterile normal saline or half-strength hydrogen peroxide, should be carried out routinely. Also, soiled tracheostomy dressings should be changed as needed.

RULE OF THUMB

In adults, tracheal tube cuff pressure should be maintained at 25 to 35 cm H_2O to minimize tracheal mucosal injury and aspiration of oral secretions.

AIRWAY MAINTENANCE

The RT must attend to several aspects of airway maintenance when a tracheal airway is in place. Critical responsibilities in this area include (1) securing the tube and maintaining its proper placement, (2) providing for patient communication, (3) ensuring adequate humidification, (4) minimizing the possibility of infection, (5) aiding in secretion clearance, (6) providing appropriate cuff care, and (7) troubleshooting airway-related problems.

Securing the Airway and Confirming Placement

The most common way to secure endotracheal tubes is with tape. The tape is secured to one side of the face and then wound around the tube and airway once or twice before the end is secured to the skin again (see Figure 33-22). Silk tape is adequate if the period of intubation is short, such as during surgery; however, silk tape is easily loosened by oral secretions. Cloth tape seems to be better for longer use and may adhere better if the skin is prepared with tincture of benzoin. Instead of using tape to secure the tube, practitioners can choose among several commercial endotracheal tube holders or stabilizers. Case reports indicate that use of these stabilizers can result in less skin damage, tube movement, and self-extubations than with traditional taping. However, of and by themselves, these stabilizing devices cannot prevent airway trauma.

A tracheostomy tube can be secured by threading cloth ties through the tube flange and tying them together on the side of the patient's neck. Alternatively, a commercial tracheostomy tube holder made of soft foam with Velcro attachments threaded through the tube flange can be used.

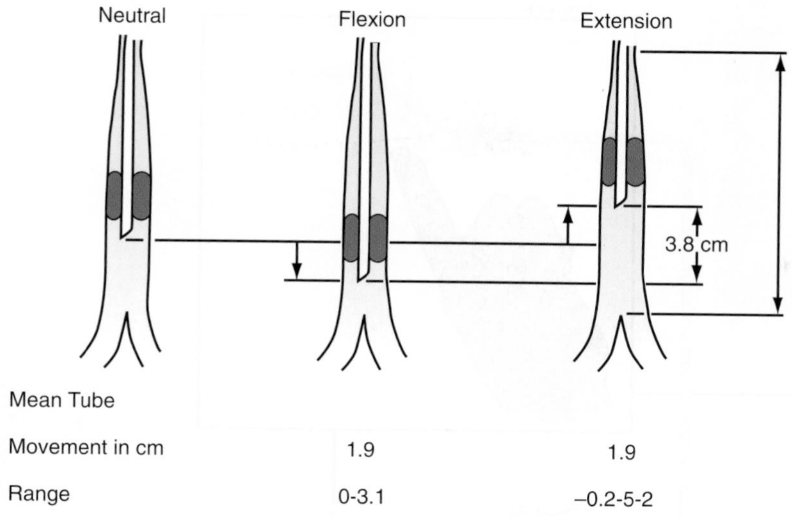

FIGURE 33-26 Effect of neck flexion and extension on endotracheal tube position. (Modified from Conrardy PA, Goodman L, Lainge F, et al: Alteration of endotracheal tube position: flexion and extension of the neck. Crit Care Med 4:8, 1976.)

This soft tracheostomy tube holder is easier to change and does not cause skin ulceration as often as cloth ties. Whichever tube holder is used, skin damage can be minimized by keeping the ties loose enough to slip one finger underneath easily.

Proper placement of an endotracheal or tracheostomy tube normally is confirmed by radiograph. The tube tip should be about 3 to 6 cm above the carina in adults, or between the second and fourth tracheal rings.[30,43] Keeping the tube position in this range minimizes the chance of the tube moving down into the main stem bronchi or up into the larynx. Even so, the endotracheal tube position changes with movement of the head and neck (Figure 33-26).[44] Flexion of the neck moves the tube toward the carina, whereas extension pulls the tube toward the larynx. When reviewing a radiograph for tube placement, the clinician should also check the position of the head and neck. If the tube is malpositioned, the old tape should be removed and the tube should be repositioned, using the centimeter markings as a guide. This maneuver usually requires two people to prevent extubation.

As an alternative to using chest films to confirm tube placement, a practitioner trained in fiberoptic laryngoscopy or bronchoscopy may confirm the position of the tube visually.[45] With this method, the fiberoptic scope is inserted into the tube, and the carina is directly visualized. By moving the scope from the tube tip to the carina and measuring the distance of laryngoscope displacement, the exact distance of insertion can be determined.

Providing for Patient Communication

One of the most frustrating aspects of caring for a patient with a tracheal tube is his or her inability to talk. Phonation requires moving vocal cords, resulting in airflow between them. Endotracheal tubes prevent vocal cord movement and airflow through the cords. Standard tracheostomy tubes allow vocal cord movement but prevent airflow. Without the ability to speak, the patient cannot easily inform the health care providers of changes in symptoms or make basic requests. This situation may lead to agitation and stress in the patient. If that agitation is treated with sedatives, a patient on a ventilator may wean more slowly.[46]

An experienced practitioner may use lip reading, but this technique is very difficult in patients with orotracheal tubes. Alternatively, an alert patient may write messages on paper or some other writing surface. For many patients, however, restricted hand movement because of restraints or vascular catheters makes writing impossible. Some critically ill patients simply cannot hold up their heads. A better solution is a letter, phrase, or picture board.[46] These devices allow patients to communicate by simple pointing. Large and simple drawings are particularly important for patients who cannot see print clearly.

For conscious patients with a long-term tracheostomy who are ventilator-dependent, communication can be enhanced with a "talking" tracheostomy tube (Figure 33-27).[47] These special airways provide a separate inlet for compressed gas, which escapes above the tube, allowing phonation. There are some problems associated with these tubes, however. The continuous gas flow through a new tracheostomy may cause air leaks. High flow rates may cause mucosal drying and irritation. Finally, secretions may occlude the speaking gas outlets. Although not life-threatening, these problems can be frustrating for both the patient and the practitioner.

An alternative to a speaking tracheostomy tube is to place a one-way valve (speaking valve) on the external opening of the tracheostomy tube.[47] With this device in place and the tracheostomy tube cuff deflated, the patient inhales around and through the tube and exhales only around the tube through the larynx. Speech is coordinated with exhalation through the larynx. A patient who is a good candidate for a speaking valve is one who is medically stable, is able to communicate, and has a low risk of

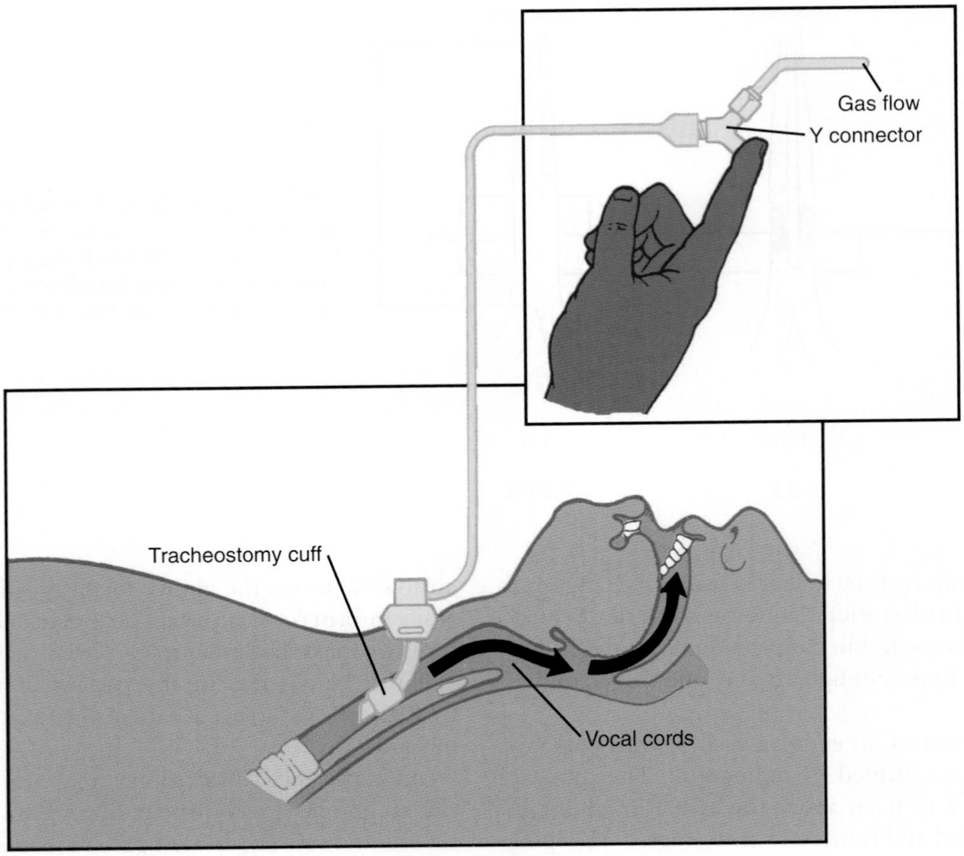

FIGURE 33-27 "Talking" tracheostomy tube.

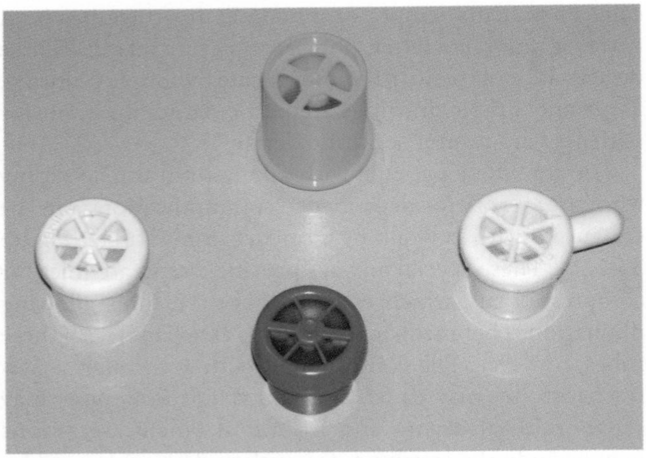

FIGURE 33-28 Speaking valves.

aspiration. Several types of speaking valves are available, as shown in Figure 33-28. They can be used with spontaneously breathing or ventilator-dependent patients. When using the speaking valve, the cuff on the tube must be deflated to allow airflow around the tube. This deflation of the cuff causes a leak on inspiration and a decrease in tidal volume delivery during mechanical ventilation. However, an increase in the set tidal volume on the ventilator during initial trials of the valve should compensate for this.

During the initial placement of the speaking valve, the patient's ability to exhale around the tracheostomy tube should be assessed by measuring the tracheal pressure during exhalation with the valve in place as shown in Figure 33-29. If the tracheal pressure is greater than 5 cm H_2O, it may indicate that there is increased resistance during exhalation. The most common causes of this problem are the size of the tracheostomy tube relative to the size of the trachea, tube position, inadequate cuff deflation, or an upper airway abnormality.[47] The tube may need to be changed to a smaller size, to a cuffless tube, or to a tube with a tight-to-shaft (TTS) cuff. The speaking valve then can be placed and the tracheal pressure measured again. If an upper airway abnormality is suspected, an otolaryngologist should be consulted. A speech-language pathologist may be consulted to assist in the assessment of the patient's risk of aspiration and tolerance of the speaking valve.

Assessment of heart rate, respiratory rate, and saturation should follow initial placement of the valve for all patients.[48] In addition to facilitating communication, other benefits of airflow over the upper airway include better function of the vocal cords, better sense of smell, and fewer secretion problems. Improved swallowing function and less aspiration have been reported with the speaking valve.[47,48]

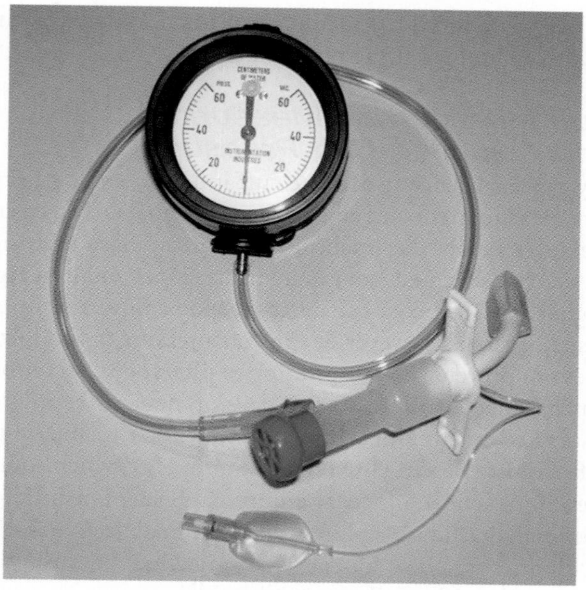

FIGURE 33-29 Setup to measure transtracheal pressures with speaking valve on tracheostomy tube.

RULE OF THUMB

The tracheostomy tube cuff must always be deflated before a speaking valve is placed on the tracheostomy tube.

Ensuring Adequate Humidification

Although tracheal tubes provide an artificial airway to conduct gas to and from the lungs, they do not function as well as natural airways. Specifically, artificial tracheal airways bypass the normal humidification, filtration, and heating functions of the upper airway. The decreased humidity in the inspired air can cause secretions to thicken. Cool air also can decrease ciliary function. These conditions may impair mucociliary clearance and cause retention of secretions. If a patient is intubated to help clear secretions, failure to provide adequate humidification only worsens the problem. In the worst case, thick secretions can obstruct a tracheal tube and cause asphyxiation.

Either a heated humidifier or a large volume jet nebulizer should be used to deliver heated humidity to nonventilated patients with a tracheostomy. However, some patients may have increased airway resistance or bronchospasm from the aerosol produced by a large volume jet nebulizer. A heat and moisture exchanger may be used to provide humidity to patients who do not require O_2 and do not have thick secretions. For ventilated patients, a heated humidifier or heat and moisture exchanger can be used. These devices can provide saturated gas to the airway at temperatures between 32° C and 35° C.[49] The selection of a humidification device ultimately should be based on patient needs and assessment of the airway and include the volume and thickness of secretions and the history of mucous plugging or tube occlusions. More details are provided in the AARC Clinical Practice Guideline for humidification during mechanical ventilation, which is included in Chapter 35.[50]

Box 33-7 Why Tracheal Airways Increase the Incidence of Pulmonary Infection

- Bypassed upper airway filtration
- Increased aspiration of pharyngeal secretions
- Contaminated equipment or solutions
- Impaired mucociliary clearance in trachea
- Increased mucosal damage owing to tube or suctioning
- Ineffective clearance via cough

Minimizing Nosocomial Infections

Patients with tracheal airways are very susceptible to bacterial colonization and infection of the lower respiratory tract. The presence of infection is suggested by changes in the patient's sputum (color, consistency, or amount), breath sounds (wheezes, crackles, or rhonchi), or chest radiograph (infiltrates or atelectasis).[51] Additional changes associated with bacterial infection include fever, increased heart rate, and leukocytosis.

There are several reasons why tracheal tubes increase the incidence of pulmonary infection (Box 33-7).[51,52] To guard against infection, the clinician first should avoid introducing organisms into the airway. The clinician does this by (1) adhering to sterile technique during suctioning, (2) ensuring that only aseptically clean or sterile respiratory equipment is used for each patient, and (3) consistently performing hand hygiene between patient contacts (see Chapter 4).[53]

In addition, efforts should be made to prevent retention of secretions. Suctioning, chest physiotherapy, and adequate humidification are useful to this end. Closed suction systems may be preferred to open suction systems in the prevention of infection.[53] Routinely changing the inner cannula on tracheostomy tubes may also help minimize bacterial contamination and infection. Techniques to decrease the consequences of pharyngeal aspiration include (1) use of medications for stress ulcer prophylaxis, such as sucralfate, that maintain normal gastric pH; (2) positioning of patients with the head of the bed elevated 30 degrees or more to decrease reflux; and (3) continuous aspiration of subglottic secretions.[54]

Facilitating Secretion Clearance

The most common cause of airway obstruction in critically ill patients is retained secretions. To remove retained secretions, blood, or other semiliquid fluids from the large airways, the patient is suctioned as described previously in this chapter. Suctioning involves application of negative pressure to the large airways through a catheter. This method may be used alone or in combination with noninvasive techniques described in Chapter 40.

One noninvasive technique is the mechanical insufflator-exsufflator (Cough Assist). It has been shown to facilitate secretion clearance in patients with an ineffective cough, especially secondary to neuromuscular disease, such as amyotrophic lateral sclerosis and muscular dystrophy.[55,56] These patients have decreased vital capacities and expiratory flows. During inspiration, the mechanical insufflator-exsufflator delivers positive pressure usually set between 30 cm H_2O and 40 cm H_2O for 1 to 3 seconds to inflate the lungs. During expiration, it delivers negative pressure usually set between 30 cm H_2O and 40 cm H_2O for 2 to 3 seconds, which increases the expiratory flow rates mobilizing secretions upward into the larger airways.

The mechanical insufflator-exsufflator can be used with a face mask, mouthpiece, or artificial airway. The patient's oropharynx may need to be suctioned after using the mechanical insufflator-exsufflator with a face mask or mouthpiece if the patient is unable to expectorate the secretions. A patient with a tracheostomy tube may also require suctioning to clear the tube of secretions after using the mechanical insufflator-exsufflator. The mechanical insufflator-exsufflator may also be used to improve secretion clearance in patients with chronic obstructive pulmonary disease (COPD) and in pediatric patients, but the evidence is unclear as to how beneficial it is in these patients.[57]

Providing Cuff Care

Tracheal tube cuffs are used to seal the airway for mechanical ventilation or to prevent or minimize aspiration. As previously mentioned, tracheal stenosis and tracheomalacia are associated with cuff use. The pathogenesis of these problems is related to the amount of cuff pressure transmitted to the tracheal wall, impeding the flow of blood and lymphatic fluid. If cuff pressure exceeds the mucosal perfusion pressure, ischemia, ulceration, necrosis, and exposure of the cartilage may result (Figure 33-30).

Importance of Cuff Pressure

In the past, high-pressure tracheal tube cuffs were a major cause of airway damage. Since the 1970s, high-residual-volume, low-pressure cuffs have become the norm (Figure 33-31). The fully inflated diameter of these cuffs is greater than the diameter of the trachea. This means that the cuff does not have to be fully inflated to seal the airway, and less internal cuff pressure is needed. When properly used, these cuffs transmit less pressure to the tracheal wall than the older high-pressure designs. Although low-pressure cuffs have reduced the incidence of tracheal damage, they have not eliminated the problem entirely.

Cuff Inflation and Measuring and Adjusting Cuff Pressure

Key aspects of airway care are cuff inflation and cuff pressure measurement and adjustment. The goal is to keep cuff pressures below the tracheal mucosal capillary perfusion pressure, estimated to range from 25 to 30 mm Hg.[42] Higher pressure cuts off mucosal blood flow and causes tissue damage. However, if the cuff pressure is too low, it does not prevent silent aspiration of pharyngeal secretions, which can contribute to the development of ventilator-associated pneumonia. It is recommended to inflate the cuff to 25 to 35 cm H_2O (20 to 25 mm Hg), which should prevent tracheal mucosal injury and silent aspiration. Minimal occluding volume and minimal leak inflation techniques are no longer recommended because they increase the risk of silent aspiration.[42]

Cuff pressure can be measured with various devices designed for this purpose. These devices have the ability to measure the pressure and allow air to be added or withdrawn from the cuff. There are two key considerations when making these adjustments. First, most manometers are calibrated in cm H_2O and not mm Hg. The "acceptable range" of 20 to 25 mm Hg equates to 25 to 35 cm H_2O.[42] Second, attaching the measurement system to the pilot tube evacuates some volume from the cuff (and decreases its pressure). For this reason, the clinician should always adjust the pressure to the desired level and never just measure it.

High cuff pressures may be caused by the need to overinflate the cuff to seal the airway. This problem is common if the tube chosen is too small for the patient's trachea or positioned too high in the trachea, or if the patient has developed tracheomalacia, which is a softening of the tracheal tissue. Another cause of high cuff pressures is high airway pressures generated by mechanical ventilation, which may require adding air to the cuff to maintain an adequate tracheal seal. Intracuff pressure measurements should be done regularly to maintain the cuff pressure in the safe range to avoid tracheal wall injury and minimize risk of aspiration of oral secretions.

Alternative Cuff Designs

Several different types of cuffs have been designed to minimize mucosal trauma.[24] The Lanz tube incorporates an external pressure regulating valve and control reservoir designed to limit the cuff pressure to 16 to 18 mm Hg. The foam cuff is another alternative, which is designed to seal the trachea with atmospheric pressure in the cuff (Figure 33-32). Before insertion, the foam cuff must be deflated by actively withdrawing air from the cuff with a cuff pressure device or syringe. When in position, the pilot tube is opened to the atmosphere, and the foam is

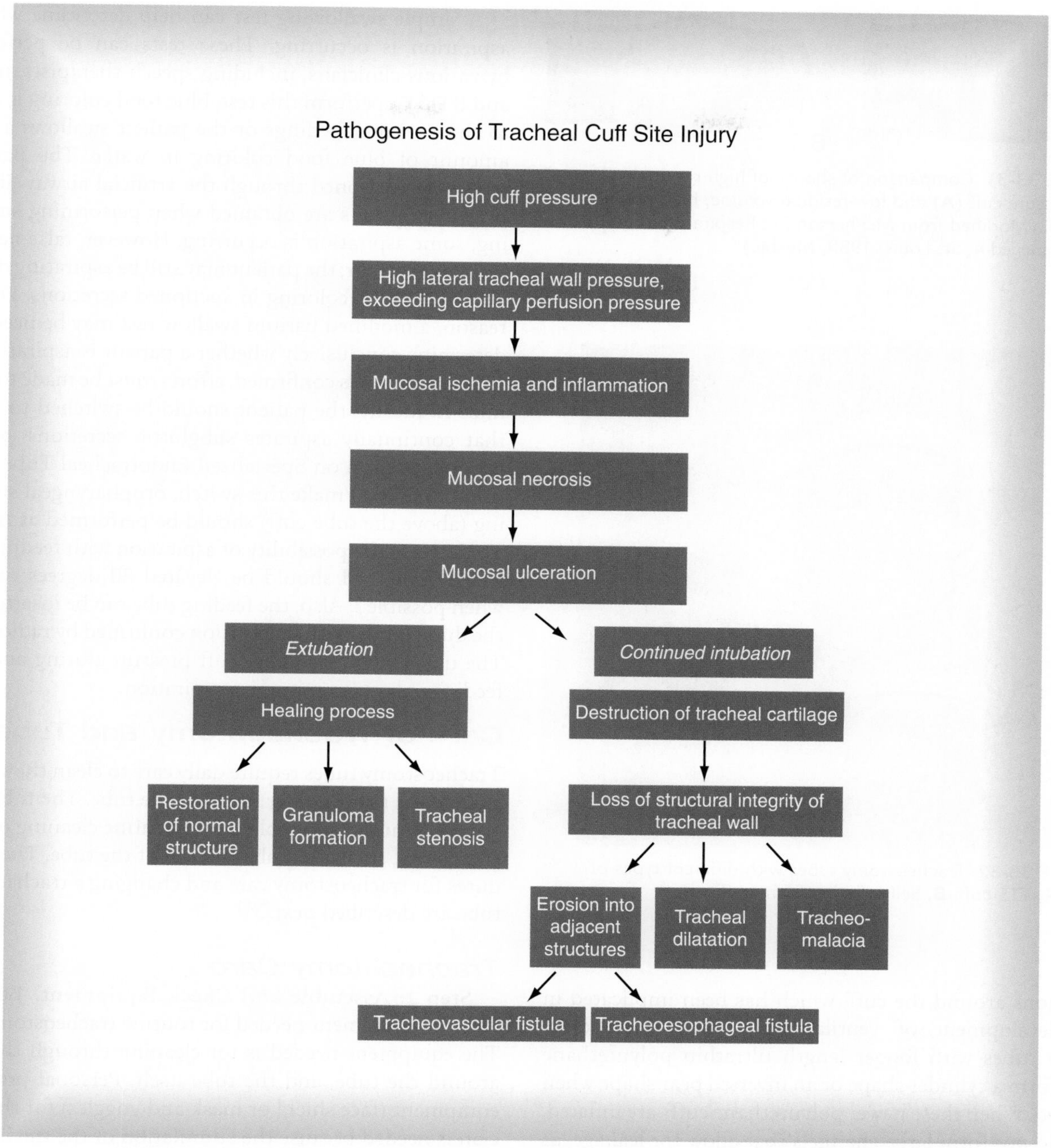

FIGURE 33-30 Tracheal injury may occur secondary to trauma from the cuff. (Modified from Stauffer JL: Complications of endotracheal intubation and tracheostomy. Respir Care 44:828, 1999.)

allowed to expand against the tracheal wall. Expansion of the cuff stops when the tracheal wall is encountered. If too much air leak and volume loss occur around the tube, the pilot tube can be placed in line with the endotracheal tube. Foam cuff tubes are not commonly used except in patients who have already developed tracheal injury. Both of these cuffs can minimize tracheal mucosal trauma but may not minimize the risk of aspiration of oral secretions.

Another cuff design is the TTS cuff on some tracheostomy tubes (see Figure 33-32). This is a low-volume, high-pressure cuff designed to maximize airflow around the tube when it is deflated. It should be inflated only intermittently as recommended by the manufacturer. Because the cuff is made of a porous silicone material, it can be inflated only with sterile water and not air.

More recent data suggest the shape and material of the cuff can help to minimize microaspiration of oral

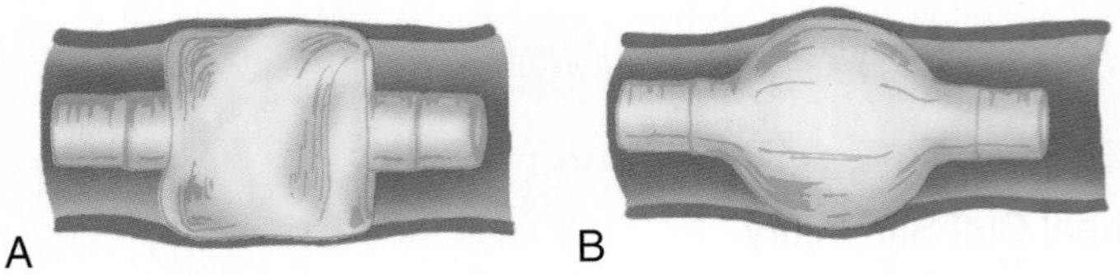

FIGURE 33-31 Comparison of shapes of high-residual-volume, low-pressure cuff **(A)** and low-residual-volume, high-pressure cuff **(B).** (Modified from McPherson SP: Respiratory therapy equipment, ed 4, St. Louis, 1989, Mosby.)

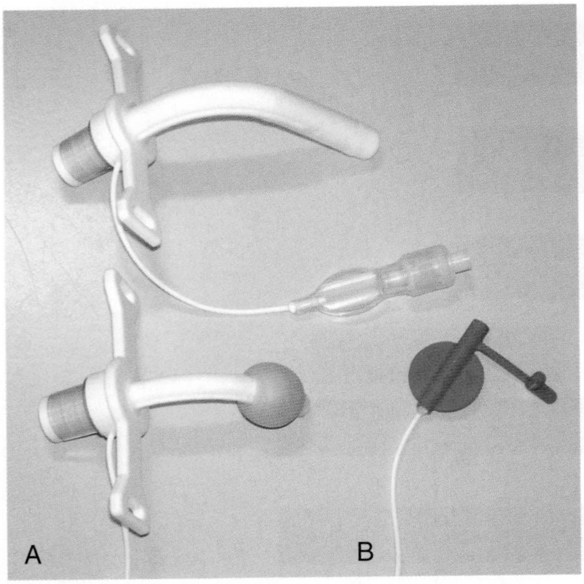

FIGURE 33-32 Tracheostomy tubes with different types of cuffs: **A,** TTS cuff. **B,** Self-inflating foam cuff.

secretions around the cuff, which has been implicated in the development of ventilator-associated pneumonia. Newer tubes with longer length ultrathin polyurethane cuffs form a cylinder shape or an inverted pear shape when inflated. When these newer polyurethane cuffs are inflated, they do not form large channels that allow for leakage, as occurs around the standard length and rounder shaped polyvinyl chloride cuffs.[57,58] Using these newer tubes may help to reduce the incidence of microaspiration.

Minimizing Likelihood of Aspiration

When judging the adequacy of a tracheal seal, the potential for aspiration should also be taken into account. Keeping the cuff pressure between 25 cm H_2O and 35 cm H_2O (20 mm Hg and 25 mm Hg) helps minimize aspiration and injury. Also, aspiration is reported to be more common in spontaneously breathing patients than in patients receiving positive pressure ventilation; this may be due to the movement of pharyngeal secretions around the cuff during the negative pressure phase of a spontaneous inspiration.

A simple swallowing test can help determine whether aspiration is occurring. These tests can be performed by various clinicians, including speech therapists, nurses, and RTs. To perform this test, blue food coloring is added to the patient's feedings or the patient swallows a small amount of blue food coloring in water. The patient's trachea is suctioned through the artificial airway. If blue-tinged secretions are obtained when performing suctioning, some aspiration is occurring. However, false-negative results can occur; the patient may still be aspirating despite no sign of blue coloring in suctioned secretions. For this reason, a modified barium swallow test may be needed to determine conclusively whether a patient is aspirating.[59]

If aspiration is confirmed, efforts must be made to minimize it. Ideally, the patient should be switched to a tube that continually aspirates subglottic secretions (see the previous section on Specialized Endotracheal Tubes). If it is impossible to make this switch, oropharyngeal suctioning (above the tube cuff) should be performed as needed. To decrease the possibility of aspiration with feedings, the head of the bed should be elevated 30 degrees or more when possible.[54] Also, the feeding tube can be inserted into the duodenum, with its position confirmed by radiograph. The use of slightly higher cuff pressure during and after feedings may also minimize aspiration.

Care of Tracheostomy and Tube

Tracheostomy tubes require daily care to clean the site and change the tie or holder securing the tube. The tubes may also be removed and replaced for routine cleaning or in an emergency, such as an obstruction of the tube. The procedures for tracheostomy care and changing a tracheostomy tube are described next.[60,61]

Tracheostomy Care

Step 1: Assemble and Check Equipment. Box 33-8 lists the equipment needed for routine tracheostomy care. The equipment needed is for cleaning through the tube, around the tube, and the tube itself. Personal protective equipment (face shield or mask and goggles) for the clinician is needed because the stimulation of the trachea may result in coughing and expectorated secretions. Use of suction equipment to remove secretions from the tube before the procedure can decrease the possibility of secretions contaminating the environment. O_2 and a manual resuscitator are needed for the suctioning procedure and in case any problems such as desaturation occur. To clean around the tube, hydrogen peroxide (diluted to half-strength with sterile water or saline), sterile water, cotton-tipped applicators, and tracheostomy sponges are needed along with a new tie or tracheostomy tube holder to secure the tube. A tracheostomy tube kit includes a basin and brush to clean the inner cannula of the tube. Alternatively, a disposable inner cannula may be used. The function of the manual resuscitator, O_2 flow, and suction control must be checked before starting.

Box 33-8 Equipment for Tracheostomy Care

Personal protective equipment: goggles and mask or face shield
Sterile gloves
Suction equipment
Resuscitation bag
O_2
Tracheostomy care kit (basin and brush)
- Spare inner cannula
- Disposable inner cannula (if appropriate)
- Hydrogen peroxide and sterile water
- Cotton-tipped applicators
- Precut gauze pad or precut foam dressing (to absorb excessive drainage)
- New tracheostomy tube tie or Velcro tracheostomy tube holder
- Another tracheostomy tube of the same size as backup

Additional equipment needed if changing tracheostomy tube
- New tracheostomy tube with component parts and another tube one size smaller
- Water-soluble lubricant
- 10-ml or 12-ml syringe

Step 2: Explain Procedure to Patient

Step 3: Suction Patient. The procedures previously described for endotracheal suctioning are appropriate for this situation. A tracheostomy tube is much shorter than an endotracheal tube. The catheter is inserted just to the end of the tracheostomy tube to avoid causing mucosal injury to the carina.

Step 4: Clean Inner Cannula (If Present and Nondisposable). The inner cannula is removed and placed in the basin. If appropriate, such as in the case of a ventilator-dependent patient, the spare inner cannula is inserted. Patients with certain types of tracheostomy tubes (Portex, Smith Medical International, Ltd., Kent, United Kingdom) can be mechanically ventilated without an inner cannula in place. If the patient is not mechanically ventilated, the O_2 therapy device is reapplied as necessary. Sterile water and hydrogen peroxide are added to the basin, and the cannula is left to soak. The brush is used to remove any dried secretions from the inner lumen or the outside of the cannula. The cannula is rinsed with sterile water and allowed to air dry on sterile gauze.

Step 5: Clean and Examine Stoma Site. The dressing (if present) is removed and disposed of in a biohazard container. Applicators that have been dipped in the hydrogen peroxide and water solution are used to clean around the stoma site. A clean dressing, if needed, is placed under the flange of the tube. Gauze should not be cut for this purpose because fibers may loosen and become caught in the stoma. Either precut gauze or an absorbent foam dressing, especially if there is excessive drainage around stoma, should be used. If the stoma site appears red or swollen, has pus around it, or is emitting a foul smell, the physician and nurse should be notified.

Step 6: Change Tie or Holder. The clinician cuts the old tie or loosens the Velcro holder. One hand is kept on the flange of the tracheostomy tube to keep it secure. The old tie or holder is removed and discarded. The clinician replaces the tie or holder, keeping one finger-width of space between the neck and tie or holder.

Step 7: Replace Clean Inner Cannula (If Present). If the inner cannula is marked disposable and is not to be reused, a new one is inserted.

Step 8: Reassess Patient. The clinician checks for adequate breath sounds, checks vital signs and oxygenation, and confirms no adverse effects.

RULE OF THUMB

An extra tracheostomy tube of the same size and another, one size smaller, should be kept readily available in or nearby the patient's room in case of an accidental decannulation.

Changing a Tracheostomy Tube

A tracheostomy tube may need to be replaced according to schedule in the case of long-term mechanical ventilation; if the current tube develops a problem, such as a mucous plug or damage to the cuff; or if a different size or type of tube is needed.[61] If a tube needs to be replaced before the stoma heals (7 to 10 days), it is best done by a physician. Intubation equipment should also be available. Because a single cannula tube has no inner cannula to remove for cleaning, it may need to be replaced periodically.

Step 1: Assemble and Prepare Equipment. In addition to the equipment described previously, the new tube, an extra tube one size smaller, and water-soluble lubricant are necessary.

Step 2: Explain Procedure to Patient

Step 3: Prepare Equipment. Sterile technique must always be maintained for the distal portion of the cannula, which goes into the trachea. The inner cannula is removed and placed on a sterile surface. The obturator is inserted. The tie or tracheostomy tube holder is attached to one side of the flange of the tube. The clinician inflates the cuff, checks for leaks, and deflates the cuff. Lubricant is applied to the distal portion of the cannula.

Step 4: Prepare Patient. The patient should be placed with the neck extended so that the tracheal stoma is accessible. The patient is suctioned and hyperoxygenated.

Step 5: Remove Old Tube. The tie is cut, or the Velcro tracheostomy tube holder is opened. The cuff is deflated. The clinician removes the tube by following the curve of the tube. The clinician grasps the outer portion of the tracheostomy tube with one hand and rotates

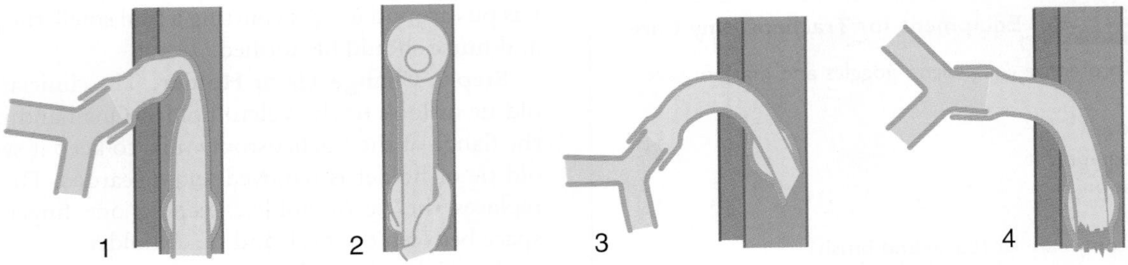

FIGURE 33-33 Causes of tube obstruction. (See text for details.) (Modified from Sykes MK, McNichol MW, Campbell EJM: Respiratory failure, Philadelphia, 1969, FA Davis.)

the wrist toward the chest. The stoma is inspected for any bleeding or other problems, such as granuloma or ulceration.

Step 6: Insert New Tube and Assess Patient. The new tube is picked up by the proximal portion. The surface that enters the trachea should not be touched. The tip of the obturator is inserted into the stoma, and the tube is advanced following the curve of the tube. While holding the flange of the tube against the neck, the clinician immediately removes the obturator. The clinician assesses for airflow through the tube. Coughing may reflect pressure on the outside of the trachea. The patient is assessed for proper tube placement and tolerance of the procedure. If extreme difficulty is encountered inserting the new tube, insertion of the "stand-by" tube, which is one size smaller, is attempted.

Step 7: Secure Tube. While still holding onto the flange, the clinician secures the tracheostomy tube tie or holder without overtightening. The inner cannula, if present, is inserted. The clinician reassesses for airflow and reapplies the O_2 therapy device or ventilator.

Step 8: Reassess Patient. Suctioning may be required again. The clinician checks vital signs and O_2 saturation and assesses the patient's overall tolerance of the procedure.

Troubleshooting Airway Emergencies

The areas discussed so far are routine aspects of airway care. Three emergency situations that may occur are tube obstruction, cuff leaks, and accidental extubation. Clinical signs frequently encountered under these circumstances include various degrees of respiratory distress; changes in breath sounds; air movement through the mouth; or, if the patient is mechanically ventilated, changes in pressures.

Decreased breath sounds are a common finding in airway emergencies. The RT must try to identify specific indications of decreased breath sounds, such as the inability to pass a suction catheter (obstruction, occluded tube) or airflow around the tube (leaking cuff). Replacement airways, a manual resuscitator, mask, and gauze pads (for patients with tracheostomies) should be kept at the bedside.

Tube Obstruction

Obstruction of the tube is one of the most common causes of airway emergencies. Tube obstruction can be caused by (1) the kinking of the tube or the patient biting on the tube, (2) herniation of the cuff over the tube tip,[62] (3) obstruction of the tube orifice against the tracheal wall, and (4) mucus plugging (Figure 33-33).

Different clinical signs are present depending on whether the tube obstruction is partial or complete.[40] A spontaneously breathing patient with partial airway obstruction exhibits decreased breath sounds and decreased airflow through the tube. If the patient is receiving volume-controlled ventilation, peak inspiratory pressures increase, often causing the high-pressure alarm to sound; during pressure-controlled ventilation, delivered tidal volumes decrease. With complete tube obstruction, the patient exhibits severe distress, no breath sounds are heard, and there is no gas flow through the tube.

If the tube is kinked or positioned against the tracheal wall, the obstruction can be reversed by moving the patient's head and neck or repositioning the tube.[40] If this action does not relieve the obstruction, a herniated cuff may be blocking the airway. Deflating the cuff relieves the obstruction in such cases. If these steps fail to overcome the obstruction, the clinician can try to pass a suction catheter through the tube. The distance the catheter inserts before stopping helps determine the site of obstruction. If the catheter does not travel much beyond the tube tip and insertion does not cause coughing, the likely problem is a herniated cuff or a mucous plug. In the case of mucous plugging, the clinician can attempt to remove the plug by suctioning the tube before considering more drastic action. Although instillation of sterile normal saline into the tube is not routinely needed during suctioning, it may facilitate mobilizing the mucous plug so that it can be more easily removed by suctioning.

When the patient has a tracheostomy tube with an inner cannula, it should be removed and checked to see if the plug is lodged in the tube. O_2 should be provided to the patient through the outer cannula, or the inner cannula should be replaced with a spare one to facilitate manual ventilation.

If the obstruction cannot be cleared by using these techniques, the airway should be removed and replaced. In patients who have undergone recent tracheotomy (4 or 5 days earlier), the stoma may not be well established and may close when the tube is removed. If suture ties were left in place by the surgeon, they can be used to pull open the stoma.

After the obstructed airway is removed, the clinician should immediately try to restore adequate ventilation and oxygenation. For a patient with a tracheotomy stoma, the stoma may need to be covered with a gauze pad and the patient may need to be manually ventilated with a mask. Airway reinsertion by a properly trained RT or physician should be undertaken only after adequate ventilation and oxygenation are restored.

Cuff Leaks

A leak in the cuff, pilot tube, or one-way valve is a problem mostly for patients receiving mechanical ventilation. This leak causes a system leak, with a resultant loss of delivered volume or decreased inspiratory pressure or both.

A small cuff leak can be detected by noting decreasing cuff pressures over time. A large leak, such as occurs with a ruptured cuff, generally has a more rapid onset. Breath sounds are decreased, but a spontaneously breathing patient has air movement through the tube. With positive pressure breaths, airflow often is felt at the mouth. Under such circumstances, the RT should try to reinflate the cuff, while checking the pilot tube and valve for leaks.[13] If the pilot tube or valve is leaking, the tube needs to be changed as soon as possible. However, a pilot valve (pilot balloon) repair kit, which permits the insertion of a replacement valve into the pilot tubing, can offer a safe and effective alternative until a replacement tube can be inserted.

A ruptured cuff requires extubation and reintubation emergently if the patient is being mechanically ventilated. This procedure can be done via the standard reintubation procedure or by using an endotracheal tube exchanger, which is a semirigid guide over which the damaged tube can be removed and the new tube promptly inserted. An endotracheal tube exchanger should be used only by an individual trained in its use, and all necessary intubation equipment and personnel should be available to perform a standard intubation if problems occur. An endotracheal tube that is positioned too high in the trachea and near the glottic opening can mimic a cuff leak. Before presuming a cuff leak, the RT should check the tube depth by noting the markings, and if the tube appears shallow, the RT should attempt to advance the tube slightly and reassess the leak. A leak around a tracheal tube can occur from a tube or cuff problem. Figure 33-34 is a diagram of the process to investigate the source of a leak around a tube.[13]

MINI CLINI

Airway Cuff Problems

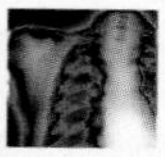

PROBLEM: The RT is called to assist with a 220-lb, 6 ft 2 in male patient who is intubated with a 7-mm endotracheal tube and receiving positive pressure ventilation. The patient's nurse reports to the RT that over the last week it has been increasingly difficult to get a good seal with the tube cuff and that she has had to add "more and more air" to prevent gross leakage. When asked if the cuff pressures have been monitored, she says no. What is the likely problem and solution?

DISCUSSION: "Low-pressure" cuffs can exert high pressure at high inflation volumes. The need for high volumes to get a good seal usually indicates that the endotracheal or tracheostomy tube is too small for the patient. This large man probably should have been intubated with at least an 8-mm tube. In addition, because cuff pressures were not monitored, it is possible that tracheal damage has already occurred. The fact that the nurse reports having to add "more and more air" to get a seal suggests tracheomalacia, which could be confirmed by radiographic or bronchoscopic examination.

Tracheomalacia can cause a vicious cycle in which high pressure causes more tracheal dilation, which requires higher pressures to seal the cuff, and so on. If tracheomalacia is confirmed, and the patient still needs an artificial airway, the smaller tube should be replaced with a larger one that allows a good seal at acceptable cuff pressures. It may also be necessary to reposition the tube so that the cuff is not proximal to the original site of damage.

Accidental Extubation

Partial displacement of an airway out of the trachea can be detected by noting decreased breath sounds, decreased airflow through the tube, and the ability to pass a catheter to its full length without meeting an obstruction or eliciting a cough. With positive pressure ventilation, airflow through the mouth or into the stomach may be heard, and a decrease in delivered volumes or pressures occurs. In these cases, the tube should be completely removed, and ventilatory support should be provided by manual resuscitator and mask as needed until the patient can be reintubated or the tracheostomy tube reinserted. To monitor trends and optimize quality outcomes associated with unplanned extubations, hospitals often require certain details of such incidents to be recorded.

EXTUBATION OR DECANNULATION

For most patients, tracheal intubation is a temporary measure. The artificial airway should be removed when it is no longer needed. The process of removing an artificial

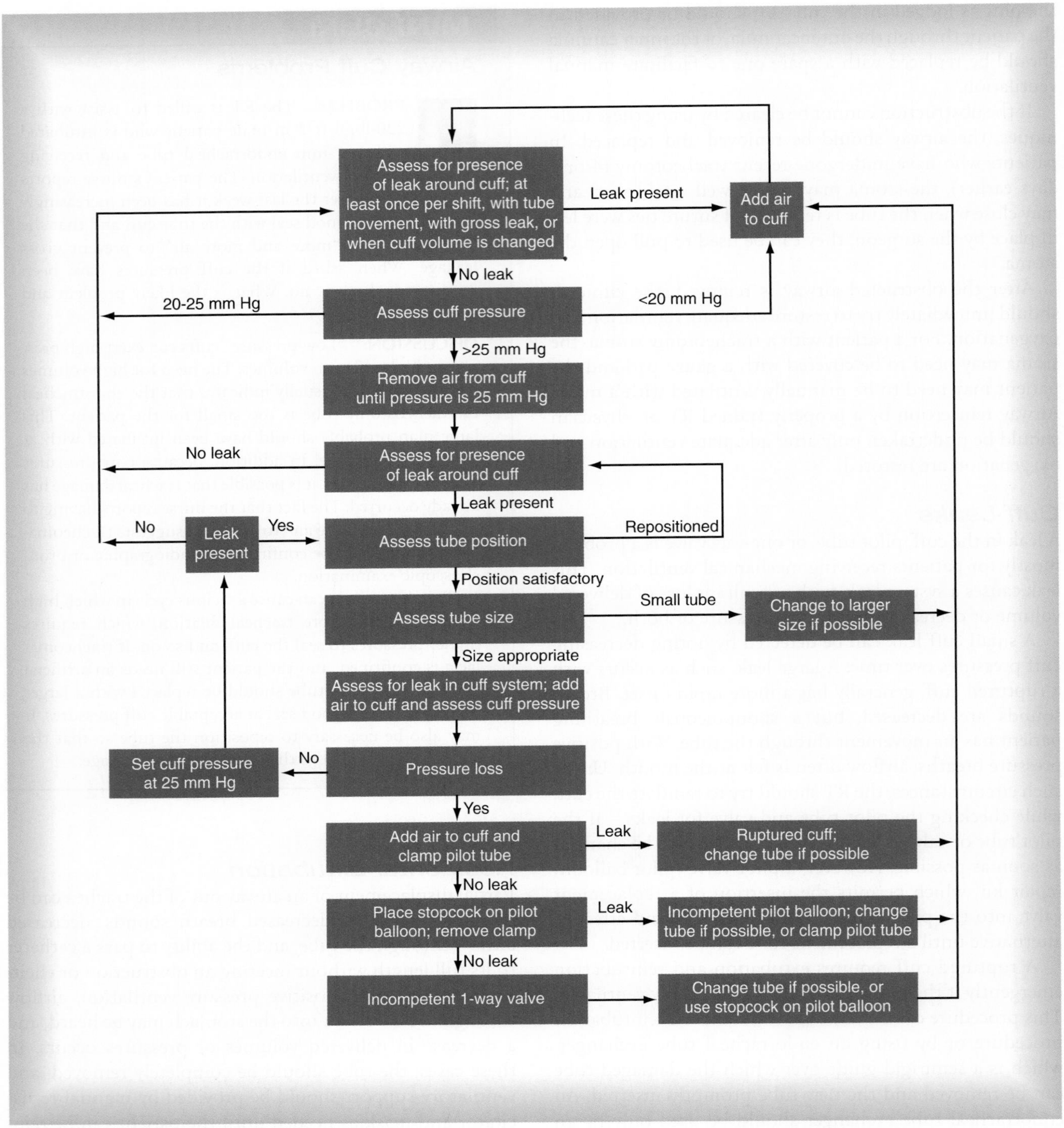

FIGURE 33-34 Algorithm for solving leaking cuff problems. (From Hess D: Managing the artificial airway. Respir Care 44:759, 1999.)

tracheal airway is called **extubation** (endotracheal tube) or **decannulation** (tracheostomy tube). Although most patients eventually undergo extubation, a few need to maintain a permanent artificial route, usually by tracheostomy. Permanent tracheostomies are common among patients with surgically treated throat or laryngeal cancer and patients requiring long-term positive pressure ventilation. Advances in noninvasive mechanical ventilation have reduced the need for permanent tracheostomies in the latter group.

Assessing Patient Readiness for Extubation

A patient is ready to be extubated when the original need for the artificial airway no longer exists. Because artificial airways are inserted for many different reasons, several different criteria to establish readiness for extubation need to be considered.[63] Some basic assessments include the ability of the patient to protect the airway by the presence of a gag reflex, the ability to manage secretions based on cough strength, the quantity and thickness of secretions, and the patency of the upper airway.

MINI CLINI

Extubation Assessment

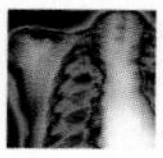

PROBLEM: A physician informs the RT that a patient recently removed from a ventilator is maintaining adequate oxygenation and ventilation via spontaneous breathing through an oral endotracheal tube. She requests that the RT evaluate the patient for extubation. What would the RT assess and why?

DISCUSSION: Because the patient is maintaining adequate oxygenation and ventilation off the ventilator, two key criteria for extubation have already been met. Further assessment is needed to determine (1) the risk for upper airway obstruction after extubation, (2) the level of protection against aspiration, and (3) the ability of the patient to clear secretions after extubation. First, the RT should perform a leak test to assess for upper airway edema. Second, the RT should determine the patient's level of consciousness and neuromuscular function by assessing the gag reflex or having the patient try to raise and hold his or her head off the bed. Third, the RT should determine the patient's ability to cough, using either subjective assessment (on suctioning) or measurement of maximum expiratory pressure or peak cough flow. Extubation should be recommended only if all three areas yield positive results.

The decision to remove the airway may not be the same as the decision to discontinue mechanical ventilation. The ventilator and airway may be removed simultaneously in the case of patients with normal lungs intubated for surgery. If a patient was intubated because of respiratory failure and has improved, but the upper airway problems remain (e.g., no gag reflex), the ventilator may be discontinued before extubation.

The cuff-leak test is designed to help predict the occurrence of glottic edema or stridor after extubation.[63,64] The clinician totally deflates the tube cuff and assesses the leak around the tube during positive pressure ventilation in a volume-controlled mode. The percent of the cuff leak should be approximately 15% or greater, as determined by the difference between the measured expiratory tidal volume with the cuff inflated and then deflated.[63] If the exhaled volume is 500 ml with the cuff inflated and 400 ml with the cuff deflated, the difference is 100 ml. The percent cuff leak is 20% (100 ml divided by 500 ml), which suggests that there is no significant upper airway edema or obstruction. However, some data suggest that this test may not always be predictive of the presence of upper airway obstruction or edema. This test may be most useful in patients who are at greatest risk for postextubation stridor, such as children, women, and patients intubated for more than 6 days.[65] Some patients who fail the test or who have questionable results may still be extubated, but they must be closely monitored with the appropriate personnel and equipment available to reestablish the airway if needed.

Clinical Practice Guideline

To guide practitioners in safe and effective application of this procedure, the AARC has developed a clinical practice guideline on removal of the endotracheal tube. Excerpts from the AARC guideline, including indications, contraindications, hazards and complications, assessment of need, assessment of outcome, and monitoring, appear in Clinical Practice Guideline 33-4.[63]

Procedures

Because RTs play a key role in extubation and decannulation and the techniques differ, the procedures for removing orotracheal or nasotracheal (extubation) and tracheostomy tubes (decannulation) are reviewed separately.

Orotracheal or Nasotracheal Tubes

The procedure for orotracheal or nasotracheal extubation is as follows.

Step 1: Assemble Needed Equipment. Needed equipment includes suctioning apparatus; two age-appropriate suction kits with sterile suction catheters and gloves; tonsillar suction tip (Yankauer); 10-ml or 12-ml syringe; O_2 and aerosol therapy equipment; manual resuscitator and mask; aerosol nebulizer with racemic epinephrine and normal saline (if ordered); and intubation equipment (laryngoscope blades, handle, endotracheal tubes, stylets, water-soluble lubricant, syringe to inflate cuff, tape or holder to secure tube).

Step 2: Suction Endotracheal Tube and Pharynx to Above Cuff. Suctioning before extubation helps prevent aspiration of secretions after cuff deflation. After use, the first suction kit should be discarded, and another should be prepared for use, or a rigid tonsillar (Yankauer) suction tip should be prepared to suction the oropharynx.

Step 3: Oxygenate Patient Well After Suctioning. Extubation is a stressful procedure that can cause hypoxemia and unwanted cardiovascular side effects. To help avoid these problems, 100% O_2 should be administered for 1 to 2 minutes.

Step 4: Deflate Cuff. The 10-ml or 12-ml syringe is attached to the pilot tubing. All the air is withdrawn from the cuff while applying positive pressure to direct any pooled secretions above the cuff up into the oropharynx, where they can immediately be suctioned with the tonsillar suction tip. The RT should listen for an audible leak around the tube. If no audible leak is present, the RT

33-4 Removal of the Endotracheal Tube

AARC Clinical Practice Guideline (Excerpts)*

ENVIRONMENT

The endotracheal tube should be removed in an environment in which the patient can be physiologically monitored and in which emergency equipment and appropriately trained health care providers with airway management skills are immediately available.

INDICATIONS

- The airway control afforded by the endotracheal tube is deemed to be no longer necessary for the continued care of the patient.
- Subjective or objective determination of improvement of the underlying condition impairing pulmonary function or gas exchange capacity, or both, is made before extubation. To maximize the likelihood for successful extubation, the patient should be capable of maintaining a patent airway and generating adequate spontaneous ventilation. Generally, the patient needs to possess adequate central inspiratory drive, respiratory muscle strength, cough strength to clear secretions, laryngeal function, nutritional status, and clearance of sedative and neuromuscular blocking effects.
- Occasionally, acute airway obstruction of the artificial airway caused by mucus or mechanical deformation mandates immediate removal of the artificial airway. Reintubation or other appropriate techniques for reestablishing the airway (i.e., surgical airway management) must be used to maintain effective gas exchange.
- Patients in whom an explicit declaration of the futility of further medical care is documented may have the endotracheal tube removed despite failure to meet the above-listed indications.

CONTRAINDICATIONS

There are no absolute contraindications to extubation. However, some patients may require one or more of the following to maintain acceptable gas exchange after extubation: noninvasive ventilation, continuous positive airway pressure (CPAP), high inspired O_2 fraction, or reintubation. Airway protective reflexes may be depressed immediately after as well as for some time after extubation. Measures to prevent aspiration should be considered.

HAZARDS AND COMPLICATIONS

- Hypoxemia after extubation may result from but is not limited to
  - Failure to deliver adequate FiO_2 through the natural upper airway
  - Acute upper airway obstruction secondary to laryngospasm
  - Development of postobstruction pulmonary edema
  - Bronchospasm
  - Development of atelectasis, or lung collapse
  - Pulmonary aspiration
  - Hypoventilation
- Hypercapnia after extubation may be caused by but is not limited to
  - Upper airway obstruction resulting from edema of the trachea, vocal cords, or larynx
  - Respiratory muscle weakness
  - Excessive work of breathing
  - Bronchospasm
- Death may occur when medical futility is the reason for removing the endotracheal tube

ASSESSMENT OF EXTUBATION READINESS

The endotracheal tube should be removed as soon as the patient no longer requires an artificial airway. Patients should show some evidence for the reversal of the underlying cause of respiratory failure and should be capable of maintaining adequate spontaneous ventilation and gas exchange. The determination of extubation readiness may be individualized using the following guidelines:

- Patients with an artificial airway to facilitate treatment of respiratory failure should be considered for extubation when they have met established extubation readiness criteria; examples of these criteria include but are not limited to
  - The capacity to maintain adequate arterial partial pressure of O_2 (PaO_2/FiO_2 ratio >150 to 200) on inspired O_2 fractions provided with simple O_2 devices ($FiO_2 \leq 0.4$ to 0.5) and with low levels of PEEP (≤5 to 8 cm H_2O)
  - The capacity to maintain appropriate pH (pH ≥ 7.25) and arterial partial pressure of CO_2 during spontaneous ventilation
  - Successful completion of 30- to 120-minute spontaneous breathing trial performed with a low level of CPAP (e.g., 5 cm H_2O) or low level of pressure support (e.g., 5 to 7 cm H_2O) showing adequate respiratory pattern and gas exchange, hemodynamic stability, and subjective comfort
  - In adults, respiratory rate less than 35 breaths/min during spontaneous breathing; in infants and children, acceptable respiratory rate decreases inversely with age and can be measured with good repeatability with a stethoscope
  - Adequate respiratory muscle strength

33-4 Removal of the Endotracheal Tube—cont'd

AARC Clinical Practice Guideline (Excerpts)*

- Maximum negative inspiratory pressure greater than −30 cm H_2O, although current clinical practice may accept greater than −20 cm H_2O
- Vital capacity greater than 10 ml/kg ideal body weight or in neonates greater than 150 ml/m^2
- Pressure measured across the diaphragm during spontaneous ventilation less than 15% of maximum
- In adults, spontaneous exhaled minute ventilation less than 10 L/min
- In adults, a rapid shallow breathing index (respiratory rate-to-tidal volume ratio of ≤105); in infants and children, variables standardized by age or weight prove more useful
- Thoracic compliance greater than 25 ml/cm H_2O
- Work of breathing less than 0.8 J/L
- O_2 cost of breathing less than 15% total, especially for patients with chronic respiratory insufficiency requiring long-term mechanical ventilation
- Dead space-to-tidal volume ratio (V_D/V_T) less than 0.6; in children, V_D/V_T less than or equal to 0.5 equates to 96% successful extubation, 0.51 to 0.64 equates to 60% successful extubation, 0.65 equates to 20% successful extubation
- Airway occlusion pressure at 0.1 second (P0.1) less than 6 cm H_2O and when normalized for maximal inspiratory pressure (MIP), as indicated by P0.1/MIP (107-109) (this measurement is primarily a research tool)
- Maximum voluntary ventilation more than twice the resting minute ventilation
- In preterm infants, minute ventilation testing vs. standard clinical evaluation resulted in shorter time to extubation
- Peak expiratory flow greater than or equal to 60 L/min after three cough attempts measured with an in-line spirometer
- Time to recovery of minute ventilation to pre-spontaneous breathing trial baseline levels
- Sustained maximal inspiratory pressures greater than 57.5 pressure time units predicted extubation outcome
- In neonates, total respiratory compliance (derived from V_T/PIP − PEEP) less than or equal to 0.9 ml/cm H_2O was associated with extubation failure, whereas a value greater than or equal to 1.3 ml/cm H_2O was associated with extubation success
- Preterm infants extubated directly from low-rate ventilation without a trial of endotracheal tube CPAP showed a trend toward increased chance of successful extubation
- Integrated indices of measured vital capacity (threshold value 635 ml), respiratory frequency-to-tidal volume ratio (threshold value 88 breaths/min/L), and maximal expiratory pressure (threshold value 28 cm H_2O)

- In addition to treatment of respiratory failure, artificial airways are sometimes placed for airway protection. Resolution of the need for airway protection may be assessed by but is not limited to
  - Appropriate level of consciousness
  - Adequate airway protective reflexes
  - Reduced cough strength (grade 0 to 2) measured by the white card test and increased secretion burden predicted unsuccessful extubation
  - Easily managed secretions
- In addition to resolution of the processes requiring the insertion of an artificial airway, issues that should be considered in all patients before extubation include the following:
  - No immediate need for reintubation
  - Known risk factors for extubation failure
  - Patient features of high risk for extubation failure include admission to medical ICU, age older than 70 years or younger than 24 months, higher severity of illness on weaning, hemoglobin less than 10 mg/dl, use of continuous intravenous sedation, longer duration of mechanical ventilation, presence of a syndromic or chronic medical condition, known medical or surgical airway condition, frequent pulmonary toilet, and loss of airway protective reflexes
  - Risk factors for a known history of a difficult airway include syndromic or congenital conditions associated with cervical instability (i.e., Klippel-Feil syndrome or trisomy 21); limited physical access to the airway (i.e., halo-vest or anatomic hindrances); and multiple failed direct laryngoscopy attempts by an experienced laryngoscopist or a failed laryngoscopy attempt followed by tracheal intubation using fiberoptic bronchoscopy or a nasal light wand or requiring placement of a LMA
  - In the pediatric patients undergoing cardiothoracic surgery, presence of one or more of these variables increases the likelihood of failed extubation: age younger than 6 months, history of prematurity, congestive heart failure, and pulmonary hypertension
  - For pediatric patients, validated bedside measures of respiratory function identifying low-risk (<10%) and high-risk (>25%) threshold values of extubation failure may be useful in generating discussion but do not apply to individual risk
  - Presence of upper airway obstruction or laryngeal edema as detected by diminished gas leak around the endotracheal tube with positive pressure breaths

Continued

33-4 Removal of the Endotracheal Tube—cont'd

AARC Clinical Practice Guideline (Excerpts)*

- Percent cuff leak or the difference between expiratory tidal volume measured with the cuff inflated and then deflated in a volume-controlled mode of 15.5% or greater; this test was found not to be predictive in a study of patients undergoing cardiothoracic surgery
- Air leak may be an age-dependent predictor of postextubation stridor in children. An air leak greater than 20 cm H_2O was predictive of postextubation stridor in children 7 years old or older but was not predictive in children younger than 7 years
- Air leak test has been predictive of postextubation stridor or extubation failure for children with upper airway pathology, including trauma patients, patients with croup, and patients after tracheal surgery
- Evidence of stable, adequate hemodynamic function
- Evidence of stable nonrespiratory functions
- Electrolyte values within normal range
- Evidence of malnutrition decreasing respiratory muscle function and ventilatory drive
- Anesthesia literature indicates the patient must have no intake of food or liquid by mouth for a period of time before airway manipulation; continuation of transpyloric feedings during an extubation procedure is controversial

- Prophylactic medication before extubation to avoid or reduce the severity of postextubation complications
  - Consider use of lidocaine to prevent cough or laryngospasm in patients at risk
  - Prophylactic administration of steroids may be helpful to prevent reintubation rates in high-risk neonates but not in children
  - Prophylactic administration of steroids may help reduce the incidence of postextubation stridor in children but not in neonates or adults
  - Prophylactic administration of steroids for patients with laryngotracheobronchitis (croup) correlates with reduced rates of reintubation
  - Caffeine citrate reduced the risk of apnea for infants but did not reduce the risk of extubation failure
  - Methylxanthine treatment stimulates breathing and reduces the rate of apnea for neonates with poor respiratory drive, especially low-birth-weight infants

ASSESSMENT OF OUTCOME

- Removal of the endotracheal tube should be followed by adequate spontaneous ventilation through the natural airway, adequate oxygenation, and no need for reintubation.
- Clinical outcome may be assessed by physical examination, auscultation, invasive and noninvasive measurements of gas exchange, and chest radiography.
- When a patient experiences an unplanned self-extubation and does not require reintubation, this suggests that planned extubation should have been considered earlier.
- Some patients may require support after extubation or intervention to maintain adequate gas exchange independent of controlled mechanical ventilation.

Noninvasive Respiratory Support

- Nasal CPAP is used in infants.
- Routine use of noninvasive positive pressure ventilation in adults is not supported.
- In patients with COPD, CPAP of 5 cm H_2O and pressure support ventilation of 15 cm H_2O have improved pulmonary gas exchange, decreased intrapulmonary shunt fraction, and reduced patient work of breathing.

Postextubation Medical Therapy

- Aerosolized levoepinephrine is as effective as aerosolized racemic epinephrine in the treatment of postextubation laryngeal edema in children.
- Heliox may alleviate symptoms of partial airway obstruction and resultant stridor, improve patient comfort, decrease work of breathing, and prevent reintubation.

Diagnostic Therapy

- For patients with postextubation complications such as stridor or obstruction, fiberoptic bronchoscopy may provide direct airway inspection and therapeutic interventions (secretion clearance, instillation of drugs, removal of aspirated foreign objects).

**For complete guidelines, see American Association for Respiratory Care: Clinical practice guideline. Removal of the endotracheal tube—2007 revision and update, Respir Care 52:81, 2007.*

should reinflate the cuff and discuss with the physician how to proceed.

Step 5: Remove Tube. The tape or holder that is securing the tube is removed. The technique used to remove the tube should help avoid aspiration of pharyngeal secretions and maximally abduct the vocal cords. Clinicians use one of two different techniques to accomplish these goals. In the first method, a large breath is given with the manual resuscitator, and the tube is removed at peak inspiration (when the vocal cords are maximally abducted). In the second method, the patient coughs, and the tube is pulled during the expulsive expiratory phase. This technique also results in maximal abduction of the vocal cords.

Step 6: Apply Appropriate Oxygen and Humidity Therapy. Patients who have been receiving mechanical ventilation may still require O_2 therapy, usually at a higher FiO_2. Other patients may require some O_2 because this is a stressful procedure. If humidity or aerosol therapy is indicated, most clinicians suggest a cool mist immediately after extubation.

Step 7: Assess or Reassess Patient. After extubation, auscultation is performed to check for good air movement. Stridor or decreased air movement after extubation indicates upper airway problems. Next, the patient's respiratory rate, breathing pattern, heart rate, blood pressure, and O_2 saturation are checked. Mild hypertension and tachycardia immediately after extubation are common and resolve spontaneously in most cases. The patient should be monitored for nosebleeding after nasotracheal extubation. The patient is encouraged to cough, with assistance as needed. Because laryngeal edema may worsen with time and stridor may develop, racemic epinephrine for nebulization should be available. Arterial blood gas values should be sampled and analyzed as needed.

The most common problems that occur after extubation are hoarseness, sore throat, and cough.[40] These problems are benign and improve with time. A rare, but serious complication associated with extubation is laryngospasm. Postextubation laryngospasm is usually a transient event, lasting several seconds. If laryngospasm occurs, oxygenation can be maintained with a high FiO_2 and the application of positive pressure. If laryngospasm persists, a neuromuscular blocking agent may need to be given, which necessitates manual ventilation or reintubation.

Because the vocal cords have had limited function during the intubation period, they may not close fully as needed when the airway has been removed. To avoid aspiration, oral feedings, especially liquids, should be withheld for 24 hours after extubation. Patients may aspirate liquids even with an intact gag reflex.[48]

Extubation failure, defined as the sudden need for reinsertion of the airway because of airway problems, often occurs within 8 hours of extubation. Aspiration and edema are the most common problems. If the patient was also mechanically ventilated, reintubation may be required for work of breathing issues unrelated to the airway.

Tracheostomy Tube Removal (Decannulation)

Decannulation refers to removal of the tracheostomy tube. Several approaches exist to remove tracheostomy tubes. Patients who received a tracheostomy as a result of upper airway obstruction that has been resolved may have their tube removed in one step. Patients who have been on mechanical ventilation for an extended time may have problems with muscle weakness, problems adjusting to the increase in anatomic dead space, and upper airway problems with secretions and glottic closure. For these patients, a weaning process is used rather than abrupt removal of the tube. Weaning is accomplished by using fenestrated tubes, progressively smaller tubes, or tracheostomy buttons.[66]

Before decannulation, a comprehensive patient assessment is required. The patient should have sufficient muscle strength (peak expiratory pressure >40 cm H_2O) to generate an effective cough. Ideally, there should be no active pulmonary infection, and the volume and thickness of secretions should be acceptable. Patency of the upper airway can be assessed via bronchoscopy.[67] An adequate swallow must be present to decrease the risk of aspiration. After removal of the tube, the stoma closes on its own in a few days. After cleaning around the stoma, a sterile occlusive dressing should be applied over the stoma until it closes. The particular decannulation technique used depends on the patient's needs and the experience and preferences of the attending physician.

Fenestrated Tracheostomy Tubes

A **fenestrated** tracheostomy tube is a double cannulated tube that has an opening in the posterior wall of the outer cannula above the cuff (Figure 33-35). Removal of the inner cannula opens the fenestration allowing air to pass into the upper airway. Capping or placing a speaking valve on the proximal opening of the tube's outer cannula, accompanied by deflation of the cuff, allows for assessment of upper airway function. Removal of the cap or speaking valve allows access for suctioning. If mechanical ventilation is needed, the inner cannula can be reinserted, and the cuff can be reinflated.

One problem associated with this type of tracheostomy tube is malposition of the fenestration, such as between the skin and stoma, or against the posterior wall of the larynx.[42] Customizing the fenestration or trying a fenestrated tube of a different size or by a different manufacturer can help avoid this problem. Proper placement can be confirmed by using fiberoptic bronchoscopy.

Case reports have shown granular tissue formation in some patients using a fenestrated tracheostomy tube. Granular tissue tends to form on the posterior tracheal wall, above the tube fenestration. This granular tissue may occlude the fenestration, cause bleeding (especially with tube changes), or result in airway obstruction on decannulation. Given the location of this granular tissue, these problems may be due to poor positioning of the fenestration within the airway.

Progressively Smaller Tubes

A second airway weaning technique is to use progressively smaller tracheostomy tubes. Similar to fenestrated tubes, this approach maintains the airway, but it allows for increasing use of the upper airway. This technique is also indicated in patients whose airway is too small for the available fenestrated tubes. The use of progressively smaller tubes may also allow for better healing of the stoma.

The problem with these techniques is the continued presence of a tube within the lumen of the airway.[66] The presence of the tube (cuffed or uncuffed) increases airway resistance. In patients with preexisting obstructive disorders, this added airway resistance may be too much to bear, resulting in failed decannulation. These tubes can also impair coughing by preventing full compression of the inspired thoracic volume. The last factor to consider when using smaller tubes is the fit of the tube within the trachea. Smaller tubes not only have a smaller diameter but also a different length; this may result in the curve of the tube impacting the posterior tracheal wall.

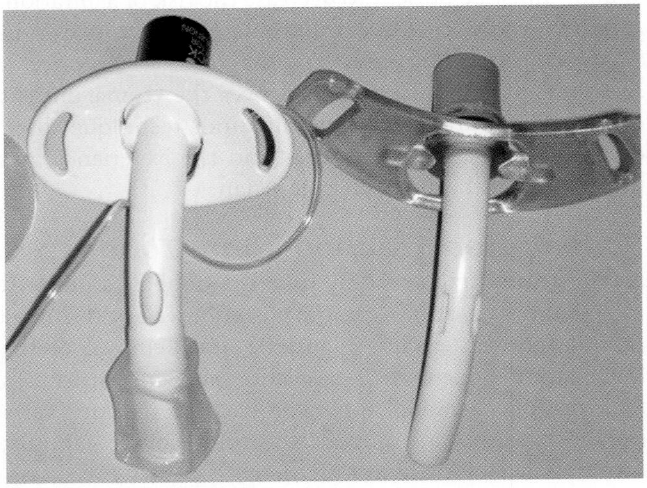

FIGURE 33-35 Fenestrated tracheostomy tubes.

Tracheal Buttons

The tracheal button also may be used to maintain a tracheal stoma.[42] In contrast to the fenestrated tube, the tracheal button fits through the skin to just inside the anterior wall of the trachea (Figure 33-36), which avoids the problem of added resistance. Because the tracheal button has no cuff, its use is limited to relieving airway obstruction and aiding the removal of secretions. When the inner cannula is removed, the clinician can suction through the outer cannula. However, when the inner cannula is removed, the clinician needs to hold the outer cannula in place to prevent it from being coughed out during suctioning.

Assessment After Tracheostomy Decannulation

After tracheostomy decannulation, the patient should be assessed for vocal cord responses.[47,67] Vocal cord abnormalities can result in either aspiration or acute airway obstruction. Symptoms such as stridor, retractions, and inability to feel airflow through the upper airway indicate upper airway obstruction. A replacement tracheostomy tube and suctioning equipment should be available in case the patient develops any of these symptoms of obstruction.

ALTERNATIVE AIRWAY DEVICES

Placement of an endotracheal tube is a complex skill and is not always accomplished easily, even in experienced hands. Emergency medical services personnel are not always in the best situation to intubate. A patient's particular anatomy may make intubation difficult. Several alternative devices and techniques can be used in such circumstances. An algorithm for difficult intubations created by the American Society of Anesthesiologists

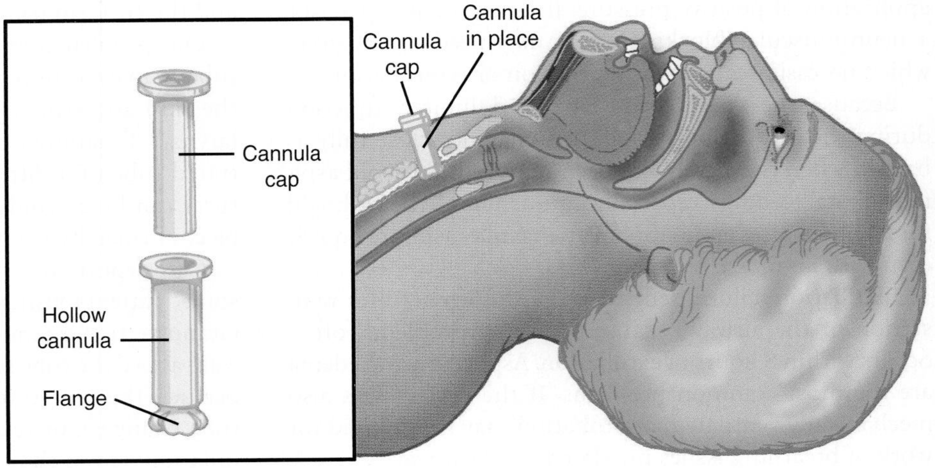

FIGURE 33-36 Tracheostomy button.

TABLE 33-5

Advantages and Disadvantages of Alternatives to Endotracheal Intubation for Maintaining Upper Airway Patency

	Advantages	Disadvantages
Oral and nasal airways	Little training required No special equipment necessary Inexpensive Can be quickly placed	Does not guarantee airway patency May worsen obstruction Poorly tolerated by awake patient Does not prevent aspiration Short-term use Does not facilitate positive pressure ventilation
Double-lumen airway (Combitube) placement	Less skill than bag-valve-mask or intubation No special equipment necessary Protection against aspiration Facilitates positive pressure ventilation	Difficulty distinguishing tracheal vs. esophageal Short-term use Aspiration during removal Cannot suction in esophageal position Only 1 size (adult) Potential for esophageal injury
LMA	Easy to insert No special equipment necessary Can intubate without removing LMA Avoids laryngeal and tracheal trauma	Short-term use Aspiration not avoided Cannot provide high ventilation pressures if needed

provides extensive options.[68] Two devices, the *LMA* and the *double-lumen airway* (Combitube), are referred to as *nonintermediate airways*. They can be used to ventilate a patient, but an endotracheal tube or tracheostomy tube may be needed eventually. These two devices may be inserted by respiratory care practitioners and are discussed subsequently. The advantages and disadvantages of each device are summarized in Table 33-5.

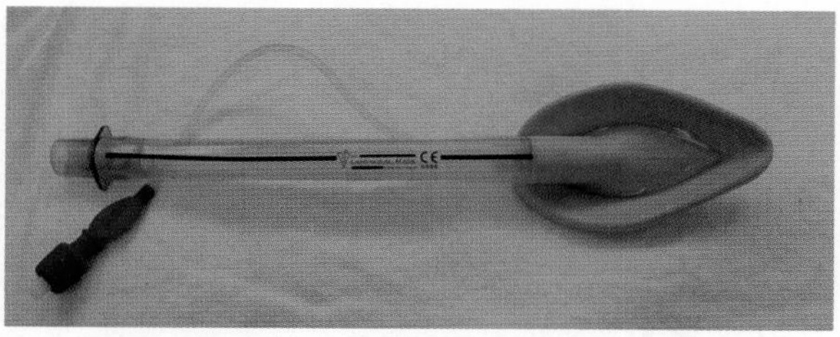

FIGURE 33-37 LMA. (From Gartsman G: Shoulder arthroscopy, ed 2, Philadelphia, 2009, Saunders.)

Laryngeal Mask Airway

The algorithm for the management of a difficult airway has been modified to show the various uses of the LMA. The LMA consists of a short tube and a small mask that is inserted deep into the oropharynx (Figure 33-37).[28,69] The open surface of the mask faces the laryngeal opening and the tip of the mask is just above the esophageal sphincter. The short tube has a 15-mm adapter that can be connected to a manual resuscitator bag. A small tube is used to inflate a cuff when the device is in place. LMAs range in size from size 5 for adults to size 1 for infants.

Compared with bag and mask ventilation, a greater amount of ventilation is directed to the lungs by the LMA. The ease and speed of insertion offer an advantage over intubation when the intubator is inexperienced, the patient cannot be positioned for intubation, or the intubation is difficult.

The insertion of the LMA does not require any equipment (Figure 33-38).[69] Before insertion, the posterior surface of the mask must be lubricated, and the cuff must be fully deflated. The index finger is used to guide insertion of the mask along the palate and down into the oropharynx. When the cuff is in place, it is inflated to a maximum of 60 cm H_2O. Inflation causes the mask to rise slightly out of the mouth.

Use of the LMA has two major limitations.[69] First, it cannot be used in a conscious or semicomatose patient because of stimulation of the gag reflex. Second, if ventilating pressures greater than 20 cm H_2O are needed, gastric distention may occur. This device does not protect against aspiration should regurgitation occur.

The classic LMA can be used to facilitate intubation because the opening faces the glottis. However, because of the small size of the ventilating tube on the mask, a small endotracheal tube is needed. A specially designed LMA with a small handle facilitates intubation (Figure 33-39).

Double-Lumen Airway

The double-lumen airway (Combitube) is designed to be inserted blindly through the oropharynx and into the trachea or the esophagus (Figure 33-40).[69] Its external design is similar to a double-lumen endotracheal tube with two external openings, two 15-mm adapters, two lumens, and two cuffs. One cuff seals the oropharynx. The second seals the trachea or the esophagus.

If the tube is placed into the esophagus and the cuffs are inflated, ventilation is accomplished by air passing

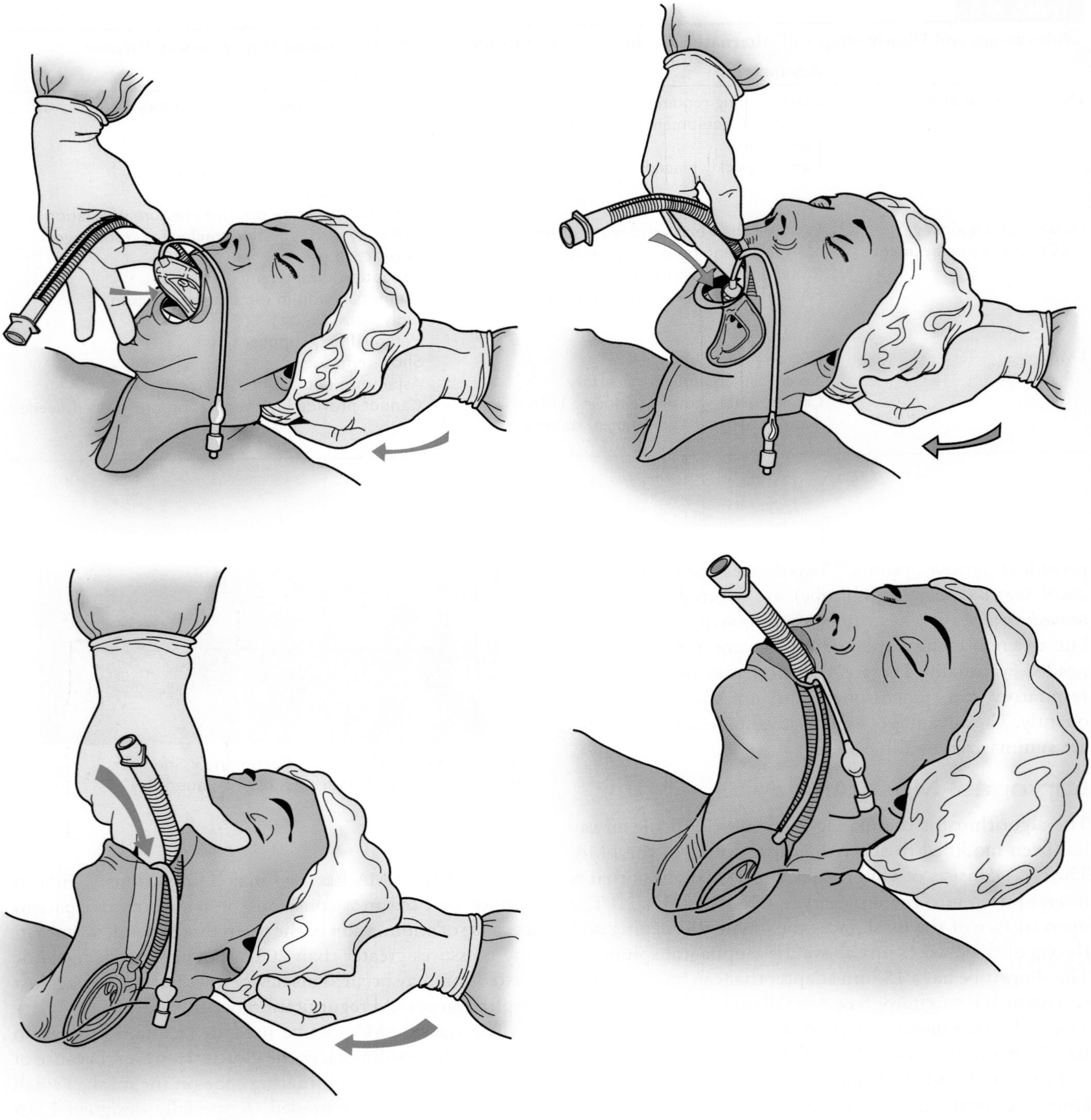

FIGURE 33-38 Insertion of LMA. (Modified from Cairo JM, Pilbeam SP: Mosby's respiratory care equipment, ed 8, St. Louis, 2010, Mosby.)

through a series of holes in the area of the hypopharynx and into the trachea. The pharyngeal cuff prevents air from leaving through the mouth. The distal cuff in the esophagus helps to decrease regurgitation. If the tube is placed in the trachea, it functions like an endotracheal tube. To assess placement, the RT can manually ventilate through the external adapters and determine which gives the best breath sounds.

Surgical Emergency Airways

Despite various alternatives to establish ventilation, occasionally the problem of "cannot intubate/cannot ventilate" occurs.[28] In these situations, a surgical transtracheal airway must be established. Cricothyroidotomy and percutaneous transtracheal ventilation are options. Commercial kits are available, or a series of available supplies can be used (Figures 33-41 and 33-42).[70]

Complications include bleeding, subcutaneous emphysema secondary to inspiratory airway resistance through a small lumen, and air trapping secondary to expiratory flow resistance. Nevertheless, cricothyroidotomy and percutaneous transtracheal ventilation are the preferred routes over emergent tracheotomy until a more definitive airway can be placed after the emergency has passed. A surgical transtracheal airway should be accomplished in 48 to 72 hours.[40,70]

BRONCHOSCOPY

Bronchoscopy is the general term used to describe the insertion of a visualization instrument (endoscope) into the bronchi. The purposes of bronchoscopy are to inspect the airway, remove objects from the airway, collect samples from the airway, and place devices into the airway.[35] Two different bronchoscopic techniques are in use: rigid tube bronchoscopy and flexible bronchoscopy. Although RTs most often assist in flexible fiberoptic bronchoscopy, they should understand the differences between these two approaches.

Rigid Tube Bronchoscopy

A *rigid bronchoscope* is an open metal tube with a distal light source and a port for attaching O_2 or ventilating equipment. A rigid bronchoscope is used most often by otorhinolaryngologists or thoracic surgeons. The tube is passed through the mouth, down into the trachea, and as far as the bronchi. A telescoping tube with mirrors is used to advance to and view segmental bronchi. Suctioning is accomplished via a metal tube passed through the

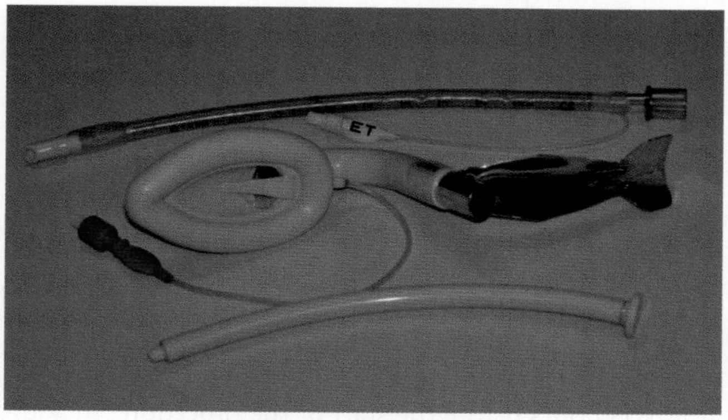

FIGURE 33-39 Intubating LMA.

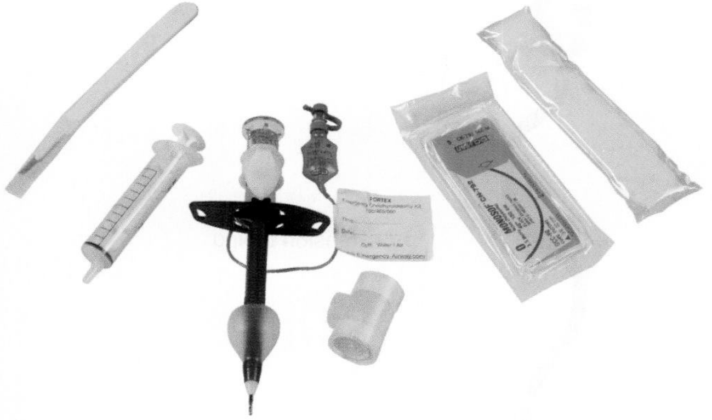

FIGURE 33-41 Commercially available cricothyroidotomy kit. (Courtesy Smith's Medical International, Ltd., Kent, United Kingdom.)

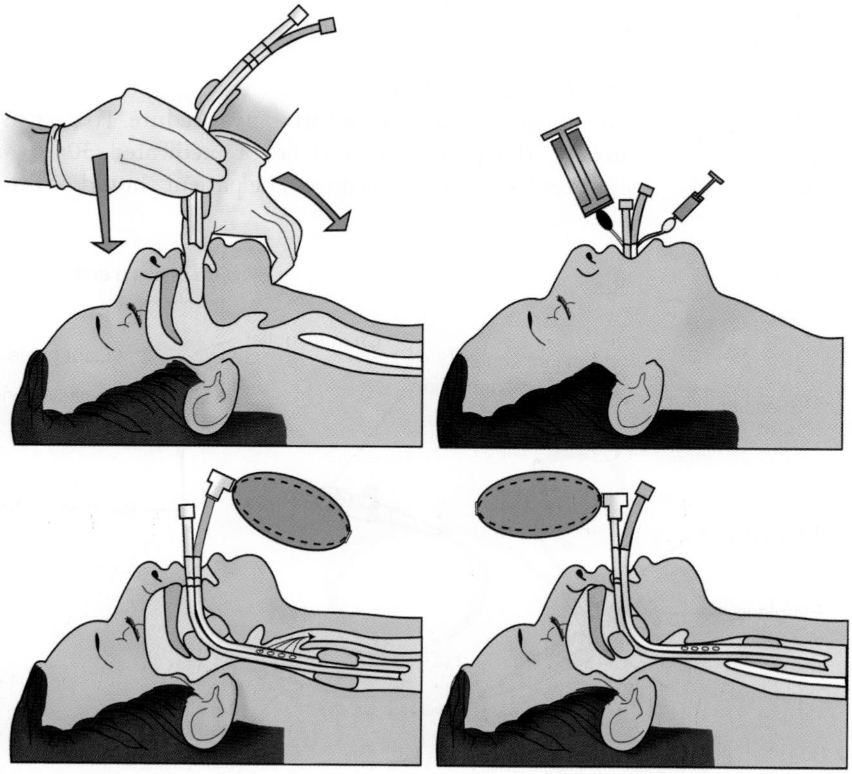

FIGURE 33-40 Insertion of a double-lumen airway (Combitube). (Modified from Cairo JM, Pilbeam SP: Mosby's respiratory care equipment, ed 8, St. Louis, 2010, Mosby.)

bronchoscope. The large internal diameter of this suction tube allows for aspiration of thick inspissated secretions and large mucous plugs. Grasping forceps passed through the device allow removal of foreign bodies and biopsies of airway tumors.

Rigid bronchoscopy has several disadvantages. First, it is very uncomfortable for conscious patients. It usually requires the assistance of an anesthesiologist and the use of an operating room. Last, and most important, rigid bronchoscopy cannot access the smaller airways.

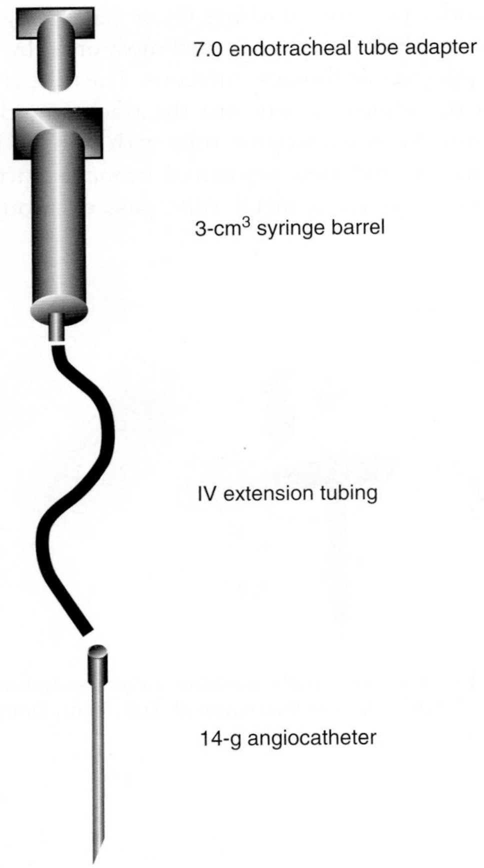

FIGURE 33-42 Percutaneous tracheal ventilation supplies. (Modified from Rodrick MB, Deutschman CS: Emergent airway management: indications and methods in the face of confounding conditions. Crit Care Clin 16:396, 2000.)

Flexible Fiberoptic Bronchoscopy

Flexible fiberoptic bronchoscopy has gained popularity over the years as a result of both its versatility and its ability to access very small airways. A typical fiberoptic bronchoscope has a light transmission channel, a visualizing channel, and a multipurpose open channel (Figure 33-43). The open channel can be used for aspiration, tissue sampling, or O_2 administration. After insertion, the physician can direct the tip of the scope via the control section to the location desired. This type of bronchoscope is most often used by the pulmonologist, often with the assistance of the RT.[71]

To guide practitioners in assisting physicians performing this procedure, the AARC has developed and published a clinical practice guideline on fiberoptic bronchoscopy assisting. Excerpts from the AARC guideline, including indications, contraindications, precautions and possible complications, assessment of need, assessment of outcome, and monitoring, appear in Clinical Practice Guideline 33-5.[72]

Fiberoptic Bronchoscopy Procedure

Key factors in planning and conducting fiberoptic bronchoscopy include premedication, equipment preparation, airway preparation, and monitoring.[72,73] To reduce the risk of aspiration secondary to gagging and loss of airway reflexes, the patient should refrain from food or drink for at least 8 hours before the start of the procedure. In addition, if the intravenous route is not already available, vascular access should be obtained before the start of the procedure.

Premedication

Bronchoscopy is an uncomfortable procedure. To decrease anxiety, the patient should be premedicated 30 to 45 minutes before the procedure. The patient should be calm

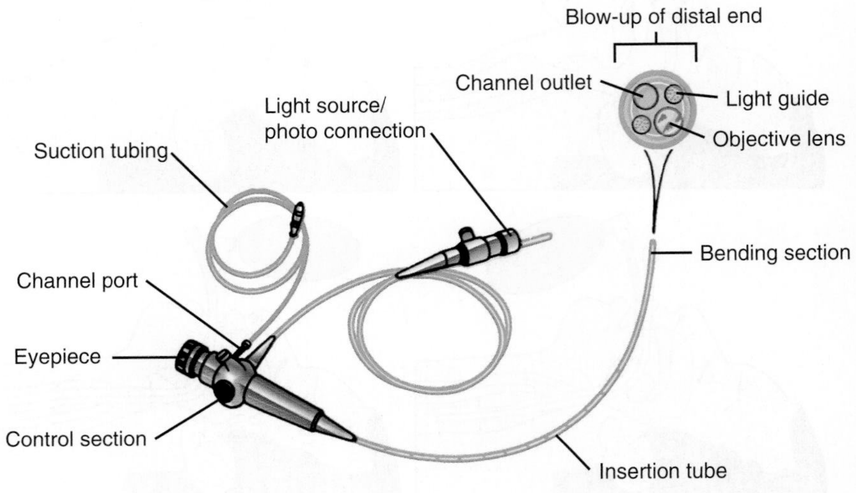

FIGURE 33-43 Flexible fiberoptic bronchoscope.

33-5 Bronchoscopy Assisting

AARC Clinical Practice Guideline (Excerpts)*

INDICATIONS

- Presence of lesions of unknown etiology on the chest radiograph or need to evaluate recurrent pneumonia, persistent atelectasis, or pulmonary infiltrates
- Need to assess patency or mechanical properties of the upper airway
- Need to investigate hemoptysis, unexplained cough, wheeze, or stridor
- Suspicious or positive sputum cytology results
- Suspicion that secretions or mucous plugs are causing atelectasis
- Need to obtain lower respiratory tract secretions, cell washings, and biopsy specimens for cytologic, histologic, and microbiologic evaluation
- Need to determine location and extent of injury from toxic inhalation or aspiration
- Need to evaluate problems associated with endotracheal or tracheostomy tubes (tracheal damage, airway obstruction, or tube placement)
- Need for aid in performing difficult intubations or percutaneous tracheostomies
- Suspicion that secretions or mucous plugs are responsible for lobar or segmental atelectasis
- Need to remove abnormal endobronchial tissue or foreign material by forceps, basket, or laser
- Need to retrieve a foreign body (although rigid bronchoscopy is preferred under most circumstances)
- Therapeutic management of endobronchial toilet in ventilator-associated pneumonia
- Selective intubation of a main stem bronchus
- Need to place or assess airway stent function
- Need for airway balloon dilation in treatment of tracheobronchial stenosis

CONTRAINDICATIONS

Flexible bronchoscopy should be performed only when the relative benefits outweigh the risks. Absolute contraindications include the following:

- Absence of consent from the patient or his or her representative unless a medical emergency exists and patient is not competent to give permission
- Absence of an experienced bronchoscopist to perform or supervise closely and directly the procedure
- Lack of adequate facilities and personnel to care for emergencies such as cardiopulmonary arrest, pneumothorax, or bleeding
- Inability to oxygenate the patient adequately during the procedure
- Danger of a serious complication from bronchoscopy is especially great in patients with the following disorders, and these conditions are usually considered absolute contraindications unless the risk-benefit assessment warrants the procedure:
  - Coagulopathy or bleeding diathesis that cannot be corrected
  - Severe refractory hypoxemia
  - Unstable hemodynamic status including dysrhythmias

  Relative contraindications (or conditions involving increased risk), according to the American Thoracic Society guidelines for fiberoptic bronchoscopy in adults, include the following:
  - Lack of patient cooperation
  - Recent (within 6 weeks) myocardial infarction or unstable angina
  - Partial tracheal obstruction
  - Moderate to severe hypoxemia or any degree of hypercarbia
  - Uremia and pulmonary hypertension (possible serious hemorrhage after biopsy)
  - Lung abscess (danger of flooding airway with purulent material)
  - Obstruction of superior vena cava (possibility of bleeding and laryngeal edema)
  - Debility and malnutrition
  - Disorders requiring laser therapy, biopsy of lesions obstructing large airways, or multiple transbronchial lung biopsies
  - Known or suspected pregnancy (safety concern of possible radiation exposure)
  - Safety of bronchoscopic procedures in asthmatic patients is a concern, but the presence of asthma does not preclude use of these procedures
  - Patients with recent head injury are susceptible to increased intracranial pressures
  - Inability to sedate (including time constraints of oral ingestion of solids or liquids)

HAZARDS AND COMPLICATIONS

- Adverse effects of medication used before and during bronchoscopic procedure
- Hypoxemia
- Hypercarbia
- Bronchospasm
- Hypotension

Continued

33-5 Bronchoscopy Assisting—cont'd

AARC Clinical Practice Guideline (Excerpts)*

- Laryngospasm, bradycardia, or other vagally mediated phenomena
- Mechanical complications such as epistaxis, pneumothorax, and hemoptysis
- Increased airway resistance
- Cross-contamination of specimens or bronchoscopes
- Nausea, vomiting
- Fever and chills
- Cardiac dysrhythmias
- Death
- Infection hazard for health care workers or other patients

ASSESSMENT OF NEED

Need is determined by bronchoscopist assessment of the patient and treatment plan in addition to the presence of clinical indications and the absence of contraindications, as described previously.

ASSESSMENT OF OUTCOME

Patient outcome is determined by clinical, physiologic, and pathologic assessment. Procedural outcome is determined by the accomplishment of the procedural goals as indicated and by appropriate quality assessment indicators.

MONITORING

The following should be monitored continuously before, during, and after bronchoscopy, until the patient returns to presedation level of consciousness.

Patient

- Level of consciousness
- Medications administered, dosage, route, and time of delivery
- Subjective response to procedure (e.g., pain, discomfort, dyspnea)
- Blood pressure, breath sounds, heart rate, rhythm, and changes in cardiac status
- SpO_2, FiO_2, and end-tidal CO_2
- Tidal volume, peak inspiratory pressure, adequacy of inspiratory flow, and other ventilator parameters if patient is mechanically ventilated
- Lavage volumes (delivered and retrieved)
- Monitor and document site of biopsies and washings; record which laboratory tests were requested on each sample
- Periodic follow-up monitoring of patient condition after the procedure is advisable for 24 to 48 hours for inpatients. Outpatients should be instructed to contact the bronchoscopist regarding fever, chest pain or discomfort, dyspnea, wheezing, hemoptysis, or any new findings manifesting after procedure has been completed. Oral instructions should be reinforced by written instructions that include names and phone numbers of persons to be contacted in emergency.
- Chest radiograph 1 hour after transbronchial biopsy to exclude pneumothorax

Technical Devices

- Bronchoscope integrity (fiberoptic or channel damage, passage of leak test)
- Strict adherence to the manufacturer's and institutional recommended procedures for cleaning, disinfection, and sterilization of the devices and integrity of disinfection or sterilization packaging
- Smooth, unhampered operation of biopsy devices (forceps, needles, brushes)

Recordkeeping

- Quality assessment indicators are determined appropriate by the institution's quality assessment committee
- Documentation of patient and device monitoring
- Identification of bronchoscope used for each patient
- Annual assessment of the institutional or departmental bronchoscopy procedure, including (1) evaluation of the adequacy of bronchoscopic specimens; (2) review of infection control procedures and compliance with current guidelines for semicritical patient care objects; (3) synopsis of complications; (d) control washings to ensure that infection control and disinfection and sterilization procedures are adequate, and that cross contamination of specimens does not occur; and (e) annual review of the bronchoscopy service and all of the above-listed records with physician bronchoscopists

**For complete guidelines, see American Association for Respiratory Care: Clinical practice guideline. Bronchoscopy assisting–2007 revision and update, Respir Care 52:74, 2007.*

but alert enough to follow commands, such as taking a deep breath. Sedative agents, such as benzodiazepines (e.g., midazolam, diazepam), are frequently used for this purpose; this is known as moderate or conscious sedation.

Another goal of premedication is to dry the patient's airway. A dry airway promotes anesthetic deposition, aids visibility, and can reduce procedure time. An anticholinergic agent, such as atropine, given before the procedure is used for this purpose. Atropine may also help decrease vagal responses (e.g., bradycardia and hypotension) that can occur during bronchoscopy.

Narcotic analgesics such as morphine or fentanyl may also be given. In addition to reducing pain, these agents help diminish laryngeal reflexes. However, narcotics should be withheld until procedures requiring patient cooperation are completed. Caution must be exercised to avoid respiratory depression. Naloxone (Narcan) must be available in the event of respiratory depression.

Additional narcotics and sedatives (e.g., propofol) may be needed for patient comfort and should be available. The need for antiarrhythmics, resuscitative drugs, narcotic antagonists, and intravenous fluids is harder to predict. Advance preparation results in a more efficient and rapid response.

Equipment Preparation

The RT is often responsible for preparing the equipment needed for bronchoscopy. Box 33-9 lists needed equipment. Special procedure rooms are often used for bronchoscopy and usually have most of the ancillary equipment already in place. All equipment must be thoroughly checked for function, tight connections, and integrity. This check is especially important for small parts and connectors, which can be aspirated if they loosen and disconnect.

Airway Preparation

The goals of airway preparation are to prevent bleeding, decrease cough and gagging, and decrease pain. Topical vasoconstrictors such as pseudoephedrine or dilute epinephrine (usually 1:10,000) may be used to prevent or treat bleeding.

Box 33-9 Equipment Needed for Bronchoscopy

EQUIPMENT FOR BRONCHOSCOPIST AND ASSISTANT
- Masks
- Gloves (sterile for bronchoscopist)
- Gown

BRONCHOSCOPIC DEVICES

Appropriate size bronchoscope, as determined by bronchoscopist
Bronchoscopic light source
Bronchoscope adapter for endotracheal tube
Cytology brushes, flexible forceps, transbronchial aspiration needles, retrieval baskets, as determined by the bronchoscopist
Syringes for medication delivery, normal saline lavage, and needle aspiration
Sterile normal saline
Specimen collection devices and fixatives as determined by institutional policies
Bite-block
Sterile gauze pads for cleaning tip of bronchoscope, as needed
Water-soluble lubricant
Venous access equipment
In case intubation is required
  Endotracheal tubes (various sizes, laryngoscope, LMAs, thoracostomy set/tray)
  Appropriate procedure documentation paperwork, including laboratory requisitions

FOR PATIENT SUPPORT AND MONITORING
- Pulse oximeter
- O_2 and related delivery equipment
- Electrocardiographic monitoring equipment
- Sphygmomanometer
- Suction system with suction supplies for mouth and scope
- Resuscitation equipment, in case needed

MEDICATIONS*
- Topical anesthetics—lidocaine 1%, 2%, 4%; benzocaine 14%, lidocaine 3% with phenylephrine (for nares)
- Sedatives—codeine, midazolam, morphine, diazepam, fentanyl, propofol
- Benzodiazepine antagonist (flumazenil), narcotic antagonist (naloxone)
- Anticholinergic agent (atropine, glycopyrrolate) to reduce secretions and minimize vasovagal reflexes
- Sterile nonbacteriostatic 0.9% sodium chloride solution for bronchial washings or lavage
- Dilute epinephrine (usually 1 : 10,000) for bleeding control
- Inhaled beta agonist (albuterol, levalbuterol)
- Nasal decongestants (pseudoephedrine)
- Water-soluble lubricant or combined lubricant and anesthetic (viscous lidocaine)
- Mucolytics or mucokinetics (10% or 20% acetylcysteine, 7.5% sodium bicarbonate, rhDNAse)
- Emergency and resuscitation drugs as deemed appropriate

From American Association for Respiratory Care: Clinical practice guideline. Bronchoscopy assisting—2007 revision and update. Respir Care 52:74, 2007.
*Depend on institutional policy and bronchoscopist preference. Aerosolized, atomized, or instilled drugs may be administered by an appropriately trained RT. Intravenous medications must be administered by a physician or nurse.

Airway anesthesia is achieved by topical anesthetics or nerve block. Topical anesthetics are more common. The particular anesthetic and route of administration vary depending on experience and locale. Lidocaine (1%, 2%, or 4%) and benzocaine (14%) are often used. Lidocaine is commonly delivered via an atomizer to the nose, via mouthwash to the oropharynx, and via nebulizer or instillation through the bronchoscope to the lower airways. If lidocaine given by nebulizer, the RT usually performs this function. The use of lidocaine by nebulizer before bronchoscopy may limit the need for lidocaine instillations into the lower airways and can make the procedure less unpleasant for the patient. Superior laryngeal nerve block provides anesthesia in the upper larynx, but it does not affect the vocal cords. Transtracheal block through the cricoid membrane anesthetizes both the vocal cords and the trachea.

Monitoring

The RT has an active role in monitoring the patient and should communicate any changes to the physician. Oxygenation should be monitored continuously via pulse oximetry. If desaturation occurs, FiO_2 is increased with an O_2 therapy device. Alternatively, the procedure can be temporarily halted, and O_2 can be given through the scope's open channel. The latter technique has the advantage of defogging the scope.

Respiratory rate and depth are also observed. Decreases in rate or depth may indicate oversedation. Continuous electrocardiogram and periodic blood pressure monitoring should also be routine. Arrhythmias and changes in blood pressure that occur are usually due to hypoxemia, vagal stimulation, pain, or anxiety. Prompt recognition of a problem and appropriate response aid recovery.

Assisting With the Procedure

The physician inserts the bronchoscope into the airway and guides it by directing the tip with the thumb lever. While monitoring the patient, the RT may also assist the physician by supplying syringes filled with anesthetic, vasoconstrictor, mucolytic agents, or lavage solutions. Forceps or brushes are often inserted into the bronchoscope by the RT. The physician guides these devices to the desired area. In addition, sputum or tissue samples obtained by the physician may be collected by the RT and prepared for laboratory analysis. When the goals of the procedure have been achieved, the bronchoscope is removed, and the patient's recovery period begins.

Recovery

Hypoxemia that occurs during the procedure may persist after completion. O_2 therapy should be maintained for up to 4 hours. Adequate oxygenation, via pulse oximetry, should be confirmed before therapy is discontinued.

The risk of aspiration persists as long as the airway is anesthetized. Patients should remain in a sitting position and refrain from eating or drinking until sensation returns. Patients are assessed for the development of stridor or wheezes. The physician is notified, and appropriate aerosol therapy with nebulized racemic epinephrine or bronchodilators is given in such cases.

Complications

The complications of bronchoscopy are similar to the complications associated with suctioning. However, the greater patient discomfort, longer duration, and the extent of airway penetration make bronchoscopy a more hazardous and complex procedure.

Hypoxemia is most severe in patients with underlying lung disease. To minimize this problem, all patients should receive O_2 before and during the procedure. When the nasal route is used to insert the bronchoscope, O_2 can be administered by a nasal catheter (in the opposite naris) or by a mask adapted to allow passage of the bronchoscope.

Hemodynamic changes (heart rate, blood pressure, and cardiac output) vary and may be related to differences in techniques or medications. Bronchospasm also has been reported and is most severe in patients with asthma. Premedication with albuterol and ipratropium bromide may help relieve this problem; the use of sedatives or narcotic analgesics, which do not release histamine, would also be helpful. Meperidine (Demerol) and fentanyl are better for patients with asthma.[35]

In patients with artificial airways, placing a bronchoscope through an endotracheal tube or tracheostomy tube may decrease the radius by 50%. If the patient is on a ventilator, peak inspiratory pressure may increase, or tidal volumes may decrease. Inadvertent PEEP also may increase. An RT should be present during the procedure to adjust the ventilator and monitor O_2 saturation and exhaled volumes.

SUMMARY CHECKLIST

- Retained secretions, or other semiliquid fluids, are removed from the large airways via suctioning. Removal of foreign bodies or tissue masses beyond the main stem bronchi requires bronchoscopy.
- To avoid or minimize the complications of suctioning, the RT needs to (1) preoxygenate, (2) limit negative pressure and suction time, and (3) use sterile technique.
- The primary indications for an artificial tracheal airway are (1) to relieve airway obstruction, (2) to facilitate secretion removal, (3) to protect against aspiration, and (4) to provide positive pressure ventilation.
- There are two basic types of tracheal airways: endotracheal (translaryngeal) tubes and tracheostomy tubes.
- Orotracheal intubation is the preferred route for establishing an emergency tracheal airway.
- Before intubation, adequate ventilation and 100% O_2 by manual resuscitator and mask should be provided.
- No more than 30 seconds should be devoted to any intubation attempt.

- There are many ways to assess endotracheal tube position; only laryngoscopy or bronchoscopy can confirm correct positioning.
- Serious complications of emergency airway management include acute hypoxemia, hypercapnia, bradycardia, and cardiac arrest.
- Nasotracheal intubation is the preferred route for intubation of patients with maxillofacial injuries.
- The primary indication for tracheotomy is the continuing need for an artificial airway after a prolonged period of oral or nasal intubation; the decision when to switch from endotracheal tube to tracheostomy tube should be individualized.
- The most common laryngeal injuries associated with endotracheal intubation are glottic edema, vocal cord inflammation, laryngeal or vocal cord ulcerations, and vocal cord polyps or granulomas.
- Although laryngeal lesions occur only with oral or nasal endotracheal tubes, tracheal lesions can occur with any tracheal airway. The most common tracheal lesions are granulomas, tracheomalacia, and tracheal stenosis.
- To minimize or prevent trauma secondary to tracheal airways, the RT needs to (1) select the correct size of airway, (2) avoid tube movement or traction, (3) limit cuff pressures, and (4) use sterile techniques.
- To minimize the risk of infection, the RT needs to (1) use closed suction devices, (2) use passive humidification, (3) monitor cuff pressure carefully, (4) use subglottic suction, and (5) keep the head of the bed elevated.
- Endotracheal tube obstruction can be caused by (1) kinking of or biting on the tube, (2) herniation of the cuff over the tube tip, (3) obstruction of the tube orifice against the tracheal wall, and (4) mucous plugging.
- If a tracheal airway appears to be completely obstructed, the RT needs to perform the following steps in order until the obstruction is relieved: (1) reposition the patient's head and neck, (2) deflate the tube cuff, (3) try passing a suction catheter, (4) try removing the inner cannula of the tracheostomy tube, (5) remove the airway and provide bag-valve-mask ventilation or oxygenation.
- A patient is ready for extubation if the patient (1) can maintain adequate spontaneous oxygenation and ventilation, (2) is at minimal risk for upper airway obstruction, (3) has adequate airway protective reflexes, and (4) can adequately clear secretions.
- Tracheostomy decannulation can be accomplished by using fenestrated tubes, progressively smaller tubes, or tracheostomy buttons. An LMA or a double-lumen airway (Combitube) can be used in a difficult intubation.
- Cricothyroidotomy is performed when a patient cannot be intubated or ventilated.
- Key factors in planning and conducting fiberoptic bronchoscopy include premedication, equipment preparation, airway preparation, and monitoring.

References

1. American Association for Respiratory Care: Clinical practice guideline. Endotracheal suctioning of mechanically ventilated patients with artificial airways. Respir Care 55:758, 2010.
2. Koeppel R: Endotracheal tube suctioning in the newborn: a review of the literature. Newborn Infant Nurs Rev 6:94, 2006.
3. Spence K, Gillies D, Waterworth L: Deep versus shallow suction of endotracheal tubes in ventilated neonates and young infants. Cochrane Database Syst Rev (3):CD003309, 2003.
4. Plevak D, Ward J: Airway management. In: Burton G, Hodgkin J, editors: Respiratory care: a guideline to clinical practice, New York, 1997, Lippincott Williams & Wilkins.
5. Tiffin NH, Keim MR, Trewen TC: The effects of variations in flow through an insufflating catheter and endotracheal tube and suction catheter size on test lung pressures. Respir Care 35:889, 1990.
6. Vanner R, Bick E: Tracheal pressures during open suctioning. Anaesthesia 63:313, 2008.
7. Singh NC, Kissoon N, Frewen T, et al: Physiological responses to endotracheal and oral suctioning in pediatric patients: the influence of endotracheal tube sizes and suction pressures. Clin Intensive Care 2:345, 1991.
8. Maggiore S, Lellouche F, Pigeot J, et al: Prevention of endotracheal suctioning-induced alveolar derecruitment in acute lung injury. Am J Respir Crit Care Med 1:1215, 2003.
9. Kalyn A, Blatz S, Feuerstake S, et al: Closed suctioning of intubated neonates maintains better physiologic stability: a randomized trial. J Perinatol 23:218, 2003.
10. Caramez M, Schettino G, Suchodolski K, et al: The impact of endotracheal suctioning on gas exchange and hemodynamics during lung-protective ventilation in acute respiratory distress syndrome. Respir Care 51:497, 2006.
11. Stoller J, Orens D, Fotica C, et al: Weekly versus daily changes of in-line suction catheters: impact on rates of ventilator-associated pneumonia and associated costs. Respir Care 48:494, 2003.
12. Topeli A, Harmanci A, Cetinkaya Y, et al: Comparison of the effect of closed versus open endotracheal suction systems on the development of ventilator-associated pneumonia. J Hosp Infect 58:14, 2004.
13. Hess DR: Managing the artificial airway. Respir Care 44:759, 1999.
14. Pritchard MA, Flenady V, Woodgate P: Systematic review of the role of pre-oxygenation for tracheal suctioning in ventilated newborn infants. J Paediatr Child Health 39:163, 2003.
15. Barnes TA, McGarry WP: Evaluation of ten disposable manual resuscitators. Respir Care 35:960, 1990.
16. Woodgate PG, Flenady V: Tracheal suctioning without disconnection in intubated ventilated neonates. Cochrane Database Syst Rev (2):CD003065, 2001.
17. Pedersen C, Rosendahl-Nielsen M, Hjermind J, et al: Endotracheal suctioning of the adult intubated patient—what is the evidence? Intensive Crit Care Nurs 25:21, 2009.
18. Morrow BM, Argent AC: A comprehensive review of pediatric endotracheal suctioning: effects, indications, and clinical practice. Pediatr Crit Care Med 9:465, 2008.
19. Oh H, Seo W: A meta-analysis of the effects of various interventions in preventing endotracheal suction-induced hypoxemia. J Clin Nurs 12:912, 2003.
20. American Association for Respiratory Care: Clinical practice guideline. Nasotracheal suctioning—2004 revision and update. Respir Care 49:1080, 2004.
21. American Association for Respiratory Care: Clinical practice guideline. Management of airway emergencies. Respir Care 40:749, 1995.

22. Colice GL: Technical standards for tracheal tubes. Clin Chest Med 12:433, 1991.
23. American Society for Testing and Materials: Standard specification for cuffed and uncuffed tracheal tubes (F1242-96), Conshohocken, PA, 1996, ASTM.
24. Jaeger JM, Durbin CG: Special purpose endotracheal tubes. Respir Care 44:661, 1999.
25. Diaz E, Rodriquez A, Rello J: Ventilator-associated pneumonia: issues related to the artificial airway. Respir Care 50:900, 2005.
26. Deem S, Treggiari M: New endotracheal tubes designed to prevent ventilator-associated pneumonia: do they make a difference? Respir Care 55:1046, 2010.
27. American Society for Testing and Materials: Standard specification for adult tracheostomy tubes (F1666-95), Conshohocken, PA, 1996, ASTM.
28. Gudzenko V, Bittner E, Schmidt U: Emergency airway management. Respir Care 55:1026, 2010.
29. Levitan R, Ochroch EA: Airway management and direct laryngoscopy: a review and update. Crit Care Clin 16:373, 2000.
30. Reed D, Clinton J: Proper depth of placement of nasotracheal tubes in adults prior to radiographic confirmation. Acad Emerg Med 4:1111, 1997.
31. American Heart Association: 2010 American Heart Association Guidelines for Cardiopulmonary Resuscitation and Emergency Cardiovascular Care. Circulation 122:S729, 2010.
32. Salem MR: Verification of endotracheal tube position. Anesthesiol Clin N Am 19:813, 2001.
33. Li J: Capnography alone is imperfect for endotracheal tube placement confirmation during emergency intubation. J Emerg Med 20:223, 2001.
34. Hogg K, Teece S: Colourimetric CO_2 detector compared with capnography for confirming ET tube placement. Emerg Med J 20:265, 2003.
35. Leibler JM, Markin CJ: Fiberoptic bronchoscopy for diagnosis and treatment. Crit Care Clin 16:83, 2000.
36. Hurford WE: Video revolution: a new view of laryngoscopy. Respir Care 55:1036, 2010.
37. Jaber S, Amraoui J, Lefrant JY, et al: Clinical practice and risk factors for immediate complications of endotracheal intubation in the intensive care unit: a prospective, multiple-center study. Crit Care Med 34:2355, 2006.
38. Hurford WE: Nasotracheal intubation. Respir Care 44:643, 1999.
39. Durbin CG: Tracheostomy: why, when, and how? Respir Care 55:1056, 2010.
40. Stauffer JL: Complications of endotracheal intubation and tracheostomy. Respir Care 44:828, 1999.
41. Epstein SK: Late complications of tracheostomy. Respir Care 50:542, 2005.
42. Hess, DR: Tracheostomy tubes and related appliances. Respir Care 50:495, 2005.
43. Lotano R, Gerber D, Aseron C, et al: Utility of postintubation chest radiographs in the intensive care unit. Crit Care 4:50, 2000.
44. Olufolab AJ, Charlto GA, Sparg PM: Effect of head posture on tracheal tube position in children. Anesthesia 59:1069, 2004.
45. Reyes G, Ramilo J, Horowitz I, et al: Use of an optical fiber scope to confirm endotracheal tube placement in pediatric patients. Crit Care Med 24:175, 2001.
46. Williams ML: An algorithm for selecting a communication technique with intubated patients. Dimens Crit Care Nurs 11:222, 1992.
47. Hess DR: Facilitating speech in the patient with a tracheostomy. Respir Care 50:519, 2005.
48. Orringer MK: Tracheostomy: communication and swallowing. Respir Care 44:845, 1999.
49. Branson RD: Humdification for patients with artificial airways. Respir Care 44:630, 1999.
50. American Association for Respiratory Care: Clinical practice guideline. Humidification during mechanical ventilation. Respir Care 37:887, 1992.
51. Levine SA, Neederman MS: The impact of tracheal intubation on host defenses and risks for nosocomial pneumonia. Clin Chest Med 12:523, 1991.
52. Safdar N, Crinch CJ, Maki DG: The pathogenesis of ventilator-associated pneumonia: its relevance to developing effective strategies for prevention. Respir Care 50:725, 2005.
53. Hess DR, Kallstrom T, Mottram CD, et al: Care of the ventilator circuit and its relation to ventilator-associated pneumonia. Respir Care 48:869, 2003.
54. Hijazi M, Al-Ansari M: Therapy for ventilator associated pneumonia: what works and what doesn't. Respir Care Clin North Am 10:341, 2004.
55. Boitano LJ: Management of airway clearance in neuromuscular disease. Respir Care 51:913, 2006.
56. Panitch HB: Respiratory issues in the management of children with neuromuscular disease. Respir Care 51:885, 2006.
57. Homnick DN: Mechanical insufflation-exsufflation for airway mucus clearance. Respir Care 52:1296, 2007.
58. Pitts R, Fisher D, Sulemanji D, et al: Variables affecting leakage past endotracheal tube cuffs: a bench study. Intensive Care Med 36:2066, 2010.
59. Kacmarek R, Dimas S, Mack C: Airway care. In: The essentials of respiratory care, St. Louis, 2005, Mosby.
60. Dhand R, Johnson J: Care of chronic tracheostomy. Respir Care 51:984, 2006.
61. White AC, Kher S, O'Connor HH: When to change a tracheostomy tube. Respir Care 55:1069, 2010.
62. Saini S, Taxak S, Singh MR: Tracheostomy tube obstruction caused by an overinflated cuff. Otolaryngol Head Neck Surg 122:768, 2000.
63. American Association for Respiratory Care: Clinical practice guideline. Removal of the endotracheal tube—2007 revision and update. Respir Care 52:81, 2007.
64. Kriner EJ, Shafazand S, Coilice GL: The endotracheal tube cuff-leak test as a predictor of postextubation stridor: a prospective study. Respir Care 50:1632, 2005.
65. Deem S: Limited value of the cuff leak test. Respir Care 50:1627, 2005.
66. Christopher KL: Tracheostomy decannulation. Respir Care 50:538, 2005.
67. O'Connor H, White A: Tracheostomy decannulation. Respir Care 55:1076, 2010.
68. American Society of Anesthesiologists: Practice guidelines for management of the difficult airway. Clin Anesth 18:531, 2004.
69. Foley LJ, Ochroch EA: Bridges to establish an emergency airway and alternate intubating techniques. Crit Care Clin 16:429, 2000.
70. Roderick MB, Duetschman CS: Emergent airway management: indications and methods in the face of confounding conditions. Crit Care Med 16:389, 2000.
71. Treanor S, Benitez WD, Raffin TA: Respiratory therapists as fiberoptic bronchoscopy assistants. Respir Care 30:321, 1985.
72. American Association for Respiratory Care: Clinical practice guideline. Bronchoscopy assisting—2007 revision and update. Respir Care 52:74, 2007.
73. Ernst A, Silvestri GA, Johnstone D: Interventional pulmonary procedures: guidelines from the American College of Chest Physicians. Chest 123:1693, 2003.

Chapter 34

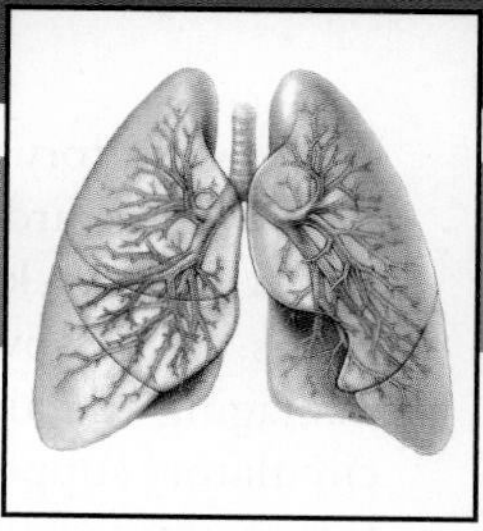

Emergency Cardiovascular Life Support

THOMAS A. BARNES

CHAPTER OBJECTIVES

After reading this chapter you will be able to:

- List the causes of sudden cardiac arrest (SCA).
- List the signs of SCA, heart attack, stroke, and foreign body airway obstruction.
- Describe how to perform cardiopulmonary resuscitation (CPR) on adults, children, and infants.
- Describe how to perform defibrillation with automated external defibrillators and manual defibrillators.
- State how to administer synchronized cardioversion.
- Describe how to evaluate quality and effectiveness of CPR.
- List the complications that can occur as a result of resuscitation of SCA.
- State when not to initiate CPR.
- Describe how to apply key adjunct equipment during advanced cardiovascular life support (ACLS).
- State common drugs and drug routes used during ACLS.
- Describe how to monitor patients before cardiac arrest, during CPR, and after cardiac arrest.

CHAPTER OUTLINE

KEY TERMS

abdominal thrust
advanced cardiovascular life support (ACLS)
automated external defibrillators (AEDs)
basic life support (BLS)
cardiopulmonary resuscitation (CPR)
cardioversion
defibrillation
gastric inflation
synchronized cardioversion

Respiratory therapists (RTs) play a vital role in emergency cardiovascular life support. In hospitals, RTs serve as key members of the medical emergency teams, also known as *rapid response teams*. In addition to managing the airway, RTs often provide ventilatory and circulatory support; drug and electrical therapy; and monitoring immediately before, during, and after a cardiac arrest.

In the community, RTs may also be certified **cardiopulmonary resuscitation (CPR)** instructors, extending their knowledge to laypeople through organizations such as the American Heart Association (AHA) or the American Red Cross. Mastery of an extensive knowledge base and the development of various, sometimes difficult manual skills are required for teaching and performing CPR. The practitioner is encouraged to obtain further competencies by completion of formal courses in CPR, **advanced cardiovascular life support (ACLS),** pediatric advanced life support, and neonatal resuscitation program.

CAUSES AND PREVENTION OF SUDDEN DEATH

Sudden cardiac arrest (SCA) is a leading cause of death in many parts of the world.[1] In the United States and Canada, approximately 350,000 people per year experience SCA and receive an attempted resuscitation.[2] The incidence of out-of-hospital SCA is 50 to 55 per 100,000 persons per year.[2] The incidence of in-hospital cardiac arrest is 3 to 6 per 1000 admissions. Pulseless ventricular rhythms are the first manifestation of cardiac arrest in 25% of cases.[2,3] Successful resuscitation depends on immediate CPR and delivery of a shock before pulseless ventricular rhythms deteriorate into asystole. In cases of SCA related to asphyxia secondary to trauma, drug overdose, or upper airway obstruction, CPR with chest compressions and ventilation before the shock is critical.

BASIC LIFE SUPPORT

The goal of **basic life support (BLS)** is to restore ventilation and circulation to victims of airway obstruction and respiratory or cardiac arrest. These skills can be used by a single practitioner to restore ventilation and circulation until the victim is revived or until ACLS equipment and personnel are available. The steps for administering BLS by a single health care practitioner are as follows:

1. Check for lack of movement or response and no normal breathing or only gasping.
2. If no response and no breathing or only gasping, check pulse within 10 seconds (health care providers only).
3. Activate emergency response system (get automated external defibrillator [AED] if close to your location).
4. If no AED is available, start chest compressions and rescue breathing for adult cardiac arrest (use cycles of 30 compressions to two ventilations).
5. Open airway and check breathing.
6. If not breathing, give two breaths that produce chest rise and immediately resume chest compressions (push hard and deep).
7. AED arrives with response team.

Steps 4 through 7 are referred to as the *CABDs* of resuscitation—*c*irculation, *a*irway, *b*reathing, and *d*efibrillation. Table 34-1 summarizes the CABDs of CPR for adults, children (1 year old to puberty), and infants (<1 year old).

Determining Unresponsiveness

BLS begins when a victim is found unresponsive and not moving. Because many hospitalized patients exhibit decreased levels of consciousness, health care personnel should avoid needless intervention by careful assessment of the patient.

When a person encounters a collapsed victim outside the hospital setting who appears to be unconscious, he or she should first look for any obvious head or neck injuries. If such injuries are apparent, great care should be taken in subsequent manipulation of the neck and in any effort to move the individual.

Whatever the location, the victim's level of consciousness should be assessed quickly by checking for signs of life (e.g., movement and normal breathing). The rescuer should call for help and activate the emergency medical services (EMS) system if the patient is not moving or breathing or only gasping. Outside the hospital, someone may need to call 911 or the emergency number for the local EMS system. Within the hospital, specific protocols exist for "calling a code." All RTs must be familiar with the protocols of their institution for handling these emergency situations.

Restoring Circulation

Determining Pulselessness

For ease of training, the lay rescuer should be taught to assume that a cardiac arrest is present if the unresponsive victim is not breathing or gasping. Health care workers may also take too long for a pulse check and have difficulty determining if a pulse is present. For this reason, rescuers should proceed with chest compressions if no pulse is found within 10 seconds.

RULE OF THUMB

Assessment of the pulse of an unresponsive patient by health care providers should be limited to 5 to 10 seconds to avoid delaying chest compressions. Pulse checks are difficult to accomplish with any fidelity. Pulse and rhythm checks should not be done after a shock until five cycles of CPR have been completed. Pulse checks should not be done by lay rescuers.[4]

Pulselessness is evaluated by palpating a major artery. In adults and children older than 1 year, the carotid artery in the neck or femoral artery should be palpated. To locate

TABLE 34-1

Steps for Cardiopulmonary Resuscitation (CPR) in Adults, Children, and Infants

Procedure	Adult	Child	Infant
Compressions			
Where to check pulse (limit pulse check to <10 sec)	Carotid artery	Carotid or femoral artery	Brachial artery
Hand placement	Heel of one hand on sternum in center of chest, between nipples. Second hand on top of first with hands overlapped and parallel	Lower half of sternum with heel of one hand or with two hands (for larger children). Do not compress over xiphoid	Sternum with two fingers placed just below nipple line in center of chest
Compression-to-ventilation ratio	One or two rescuers 30 : 2	One rescuer 30 : 2; two rescuers 15 : 2	One rescuer 30 : 2; two rescuers 15 : 2
Cycles of compression-to-ventilation	5	5	5
Depth of compressions (push in hard and fast, allow chest to recoil fully)	2 in	At least one-third anteroposterior diameter of chest or 2 in (5 cm)	At least one-third anteroposterior diameter of chest or 1½ in (4 cm)
Compression rate	100/min	100/min	100/min
Breathing			
Obstructive procedure	*Responsive:* If mild, allow victim to clear the airway by coughing. If severe, repeat abdominal thrusts until foreign body is expelled, or the choking victim becomes unresponsive. Consider chest thrusts if abdominal thrusts are ineffective, if rescuer is unable to encircle victim's abdomen, or if victim is in the late stages of pregnancy *Unresponsive:* Carefully move victim to the ground, immediately activate EMS system, and begin CPR, but look into the mouth before giving breaths. If a foreign body is seen, it should be removed. Follow ventilation with chest compressions	Same as for adult	*Responsive:* If mild, allow infant to clear the airway by coughing. If infant is unable to make a sound (severe obstruction), deliver five back blows (slaps) followed by chest thrusts repeatedly until object is expelled or infant becomes unresponsive. Abdominal thrusts should not be done on infants because they may damage the largely unprotected liver *Unresponsive:* Activate EMS system and begin CPR, but look into the mouth before giving breaths. If a foreign body is seen, it should be removed. Follow ventilation with chest compressions
Rescue Breathing			
Palpable pulse, but no spontaneous breaths or inadequate breathing	10-12/min, 1 breath every 5-6 sec	12-20/min, 1 breath every 3-5 sec, if palpable pulse ≥60/min	20/min, 1 breath every 3 sec, if palpable pulse ≥60/min

the carotid artery, the rescuer should maintain the head-tilt with one hand while sliding the fingers of the other hand into the groove created by the trachea and the large neck muscles (Figure 34-1). The carotid artery area must be palpated gently to avoid compressing the artery or pushing on the carotid sinus. Because the pulse may be slow, weak, or irregular, the artery may need to be assessed for approximately 10 seconds for the presence or absence of a pulse to be confirmed.

For infants, the brachial artery is preferred for assessing pulselessness. To palpate the brachial artery, the rescuer must grasp the infant's arm with his or her thumb outward, slide his or her fingers down toward the antecubital fossa, and press gently to feel for a pulse. The femoral artery also can be palpated, which may be done for an adult, a child, or an infant.

In hospital critical care settings, bedside monitoring equipment may provide supporting or confirming information regarding the respiratory or circulatory status of a patient. However, information obtained from these devices should never be a substitute for careful clinical assessment.

If the patient has a pulse but is not breathing, ventilation must be started immediately, at the appropriate rate

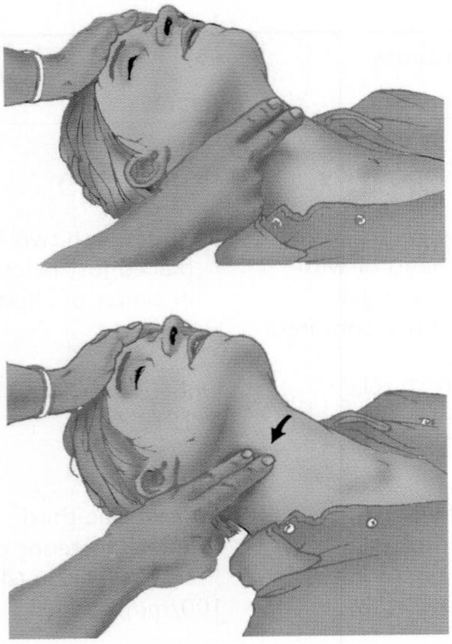

FIGURE 34-1 Determining pulselessness.

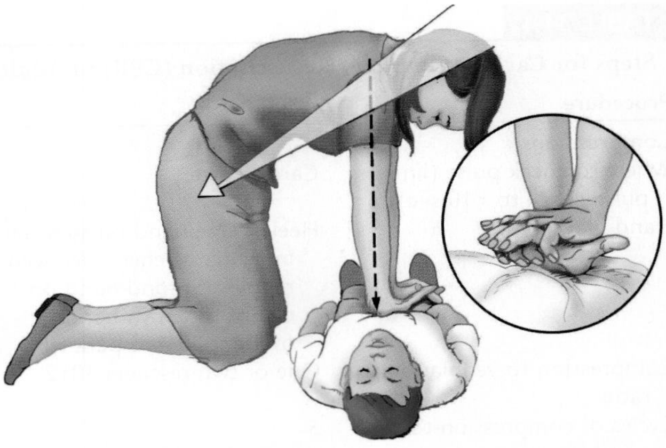

FIGURE 34-2 Position of practitioner for external cardiac compression. Note interlocked fingers to prevent pressure on rib cage.

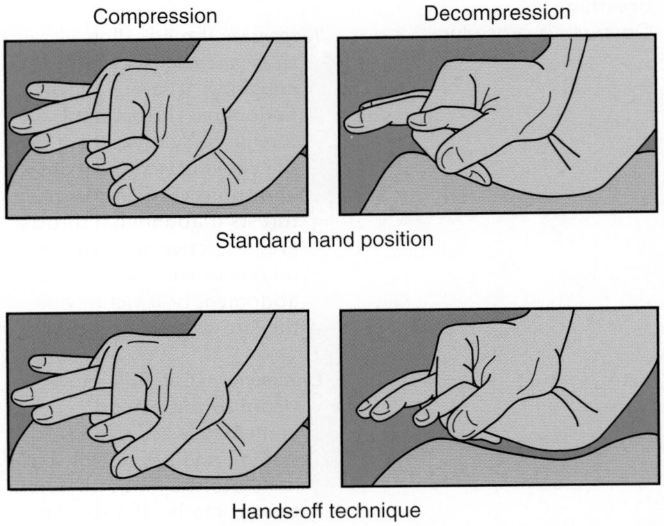

FIGURE 34-3 Techniques for hand position.

of 8 to 10 breaths/min (every 6 to 8 seconds). If no pulse is palpable, external chest compressions must be interposed with ventilatory support (see Table 34-1).

Providing Chest Compressions

Adequate circulation can be restored in a pulseless victim using external chest compressions. The rescuer manually compresses the lower half of the sternum (for an adult patient) at a rate of 100 compressions/min. The duty cycle for downstroke and upstroke (release) is 600 msec with a 1:1 downstroke-to-upstroke ratio. It is very important to have a complete upstroke so as not to increase intrathoracic pressure during the diastolic phase. The best way to ensure that the upstroke is complete is for the rescuer to take his or her hand slightly off the chest between compressions.[5] Cardiac output produced by external chest compressions is approximately one-fourth of normal cardiac output, with arterial systolic blood pressures between 60 mm Hg and 80 mm Hg. Blood flow during chest compression probably results from changes in the intrathoracic pressure.

Adults. The procedure for providing chest compressions to adults is as follows (Figures 34-2 and 34-3):

1. Place the victim in a supine position on a firm surface, such as the ground or the floor, because chest compressions are more effective when the victim is on a firm surface. When victims are in bed or on a stretcher, place a board or tray under them. A cardiac arrest board is ideal, but a removable bed piece or food tray may have to be used.
2. Expose the patient's chest to identify landmarks for correct hand position. If the victim is fully clothed, quickly remove or cut off any clothing or underwear.
3. Choose a position close to the patient's upper chest so that the weight of your upper body can be used for compression. If the patient is on a bed or stretcher, stand next to it with the patient close to that side. If the bed is high or you are short, you may need to lower the bed, stand on a stool or chair, or kneel on the bed next to the victim. If the patient is on the ground, kneel at his or her side.
4. Identify the lower half of the victim's sternum, in the center of the chest between the nipples, and place the heel of your hand on the sternum with your other hand on top, and lock your elbows.[6]
5. Perform compression with the weight of your body exerting force on your outstretched arms, elbows held straight. Your shoulders should be positioned above the patient so that the thrust of each compression goes straight down onto the sternum, using your upper body weight and the hip joints as a fulcrum (see Figure 34-2). It is acceptable to let your hands leave the victim's chest ever so slightly to ensure a complete upstroke (see Figure 34-3).

6. Compress the sternum 2 in (5 cm) at a rate of 100 compressions/min. The compression phase of the cycle should be equal in duration to the upstroke phase.
7. If CPR must be interrupted for transportation or advanced life support measures, resume chest compressions as quickly as possible. Compressions should not cease for more than 5 seconds (30 seconds if the victim is being intubated).

Children. Children who have reached puberty should receive chest compressions as outlined for adults. The procedure for younger children (1 year old to puberty) is as follows:

1. Place the victim in the supine position on a firm surface. Small children may require additional support under the upper body; this is particularly true when chest compressions are given with mouth-to-mouth ventilation because extension of the neck raises the shoulders. The head should be no higher than the body.
2. As with an adult, identify the lower half of the sternum. Because the liver and spleen of younger children lie higher in the abdominal cavity, take special care to ensure proper positioning as described previously. However, use only one hand to compress. Use the other hand to maintain head position and maintain an airway.
3. Compress the chest approximately 2 in (5 cm) at a rate of 100 compressions/min. Generally, the heel of one hand is sufficient to achieve compression. As with adults, compression and relaxation times should be equal in length and delivered smoothly.

Infants. The procedure for infants (≤1 year of age) is as follows (Figure 34-4):

1. Use the lower half of the sternum for compression in an infant. Proper placement is determined by imagining a line across the chest connecting the nipples. Place your index finger along this line on the sternum. Then place your middle and ring fingers next to the index finger. Raise your index finger and perform compressions with the middle and ring fingers. Use the other hand to maintain the infant's head position and airway.
2. Compress the sternum approximately 1.5 in (4 cm) at a rate of at least 100 compressions/min. Compression and upstroke phases should be equal in length and delivered smoothly. Your fingers should remain on the chest at all times.

Neonates. Chest compressions are indicated if the neonate's heart rate decreases to less than 60 beats/min despite adequate ventilation with 100% oxygen (O_2) for 30 seconds. Before starting chest compressions, the rescuer should ensure that the neonate is being ventilated optimally.[7] Neonatal chest compressions are delivered on the lower third of the sternum to a depth of approximately one-third of the anteroposterior diameter of the chest to achieve an approximate rate of 100 compressions/min.[7-10] Two methods have been described. The first method uses a "wraparound" technique (Figure 34-5). To use this method, the rescuer encircles the neonate's chest with both hands and compresses the sternum with two thumbs, using the other fingers of both hands to support the neonate's back. The rescuer should position the thumbs just below the victim's intermammary line, taking care not to compress the xiphoid process. Compression should be performed smoothly, with downstroke and upstroke times approximately equal. Delivering a slightly shorter compression than relaxation phase may allow for more blood flow in a very young infant.[11] In all infants, the chest should be allowed to expand fully after a compression. After every third compression, the neonate should receive a breath of 100% O_2, coordinated with compressions to avoid simultaneous delivery. The second method, the two-finger technique (see Figure 34-4), may have advantages when access to the umbilicus is required.

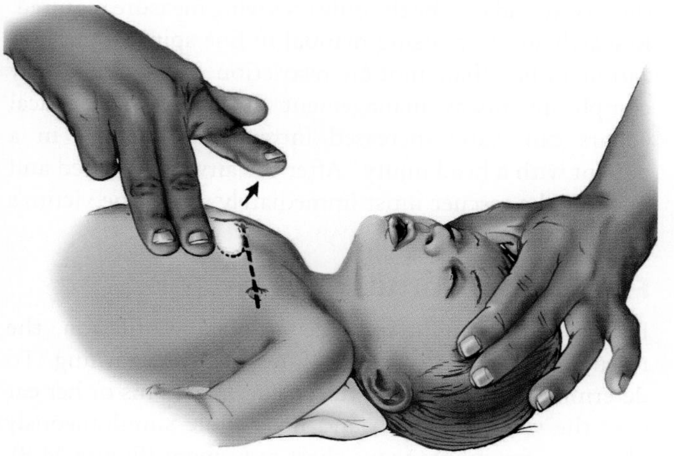

FIGURE 34-4 Position for chest compression in infants.

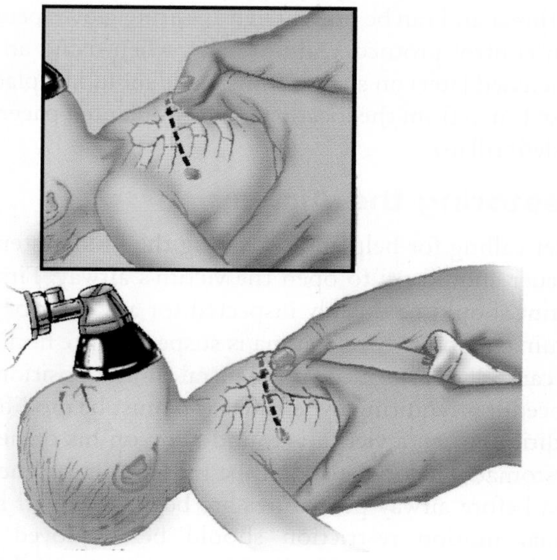

FIGURE 34-5 Neonatal chest compression using the wraparound technique.

Chest Compressions Under Special Circumstances

The following unique circumstances require modification of the normal procedures for applying cardiac compressions: near drowning, electrical shock, and patients with implanted pacemakers or defibrillators.

Near Drowning. When cardiac arrest occurs as a result of drowning, the victim must be moved as quickly as possible to a firm surface. Cardiac compressions are difficult to perform while a victim is in the water and may be ineffective. Mouth-to-mouth ventilation in the water may be helpful when administered properly. Stabilization of the cervical spine is unnecessary unless circumstances leading to the incident indicate that trauma is likely. Manual cervical spine and spine immobilization equipment may restrict adequate opening of the airway and may delay the delivery of adequate ventilation.

Electrical Shock. Electrical shock can cause either cardiac or respiratory arrest. Cardiac arrest is caused by ventricular fibrillation (VF). Respiratory arrest may occur secondary to paralysis of ventilatory muscles. Initially, the victim must be removed from contact with the source of electricity and evaluated. The rescuers must pay special attention to their own safety. A victim who is still connected to an electrical source must not be touched. The power must be turned off. If cardiac arrest has occurred, airway control, CPR, and attempts at defibrillation should be administered immediately.

Implanted Pacemakers and Defibrillators. Compressions should be done on a victim with an implanted pacemaker or defibrillator in essentially the same way they are done on other victims. These devices are generally located in the upper left chest or occasionally in the abdomen. They generally do not interfere with the administration of compressions. However, if the implanted defibrillator administers a shock during compressions, the rescuer may feel a tingling sensation; this sensation poses no threat and can be prevented by wearing gloves per infection control protocol. Additionally, when using an AED (discussed later) on such victims, pads should be placed at least 1 inch from the location of the implanted pacemaker or defibrillator.

Restoring the Airway

After calling for help and activating the EMS system, the rescuer should try to open the victim's airway. First, the victim should be quickly inspected for any neck or facial trauma. If spinal cord trauma is suspected, the neck must be carefully positioned in a neutral in-line position, and procedures requiring hyperextension must be modified. In addition, when a victim is found lying on his or her side or stomach, he or she should be moved to a supine position before airway procedures are begun. Manual in-line spinal motion restriction should be employed when moving the patient. The rescuer must ensure that the victim is positioned on a hard, flat surface.

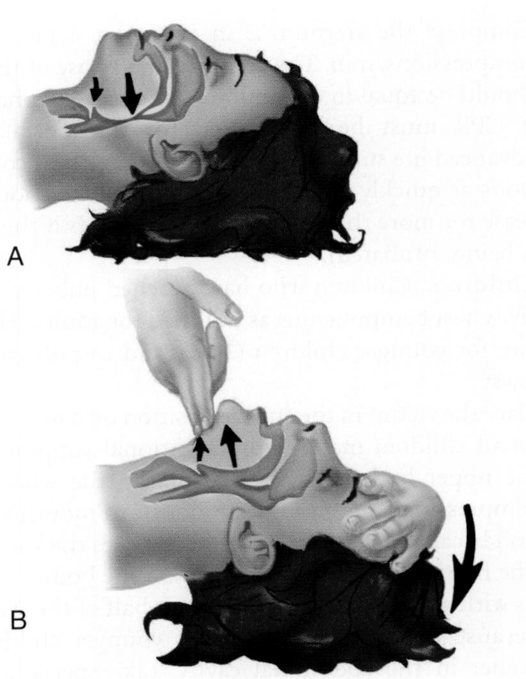

FIGURE 34-6 Opening the airway. **A,** Airway obstruction produced by tongue and epiglottis. **B,** Relief by head-tilt/chin-lift method.

The most common cause of airway obstruction is loss of muscle tone, which causes the tongue to fall back into the pharynx, blocking airflow. Movement of the lower jaw and extension of the neck pulls the tongue from the posterior pharyngeal wall and opens the airway. One of two procedures can be used: (1) The head-tilt/chin-lift method is the primary procedure recommended for a layperson when spinal trauma is not suspected (Figures 34-6 and 34-7). (2) The jaw thrust is used mainly by trained clinicians when spinal neck injuries are suspected and is no longer recommended by the AHA for lay rescuers (see Figure 34-7). Health care providers should use a head-tilt/chin-lift procedure if the jaw thrust maneuver does not open the airway.[4] One of these maneuvers usually can open the airway and may be the only lifesaving measure required. Research supports using manual in-line spinal immobilization rather than motion restriction devices that may complicate airway management during CPR.[8] Cervical collars can cause increased intracranial pressure in a patient with a head injury.[9] After the airway is cleared and opened, the rescuer must immediately assess the victim's ventilation.

Restoring Ventilation

Before attempting to provide artificial ventilation, the rescuer should assess for the presence of breathing. To determine breathlessness, the rescuer places his or her ear over the victim's mouth and nose while simultaneously observing for spontaneous chest movement (Figure 34-8). Breathlessness exists if no chest movement or breath

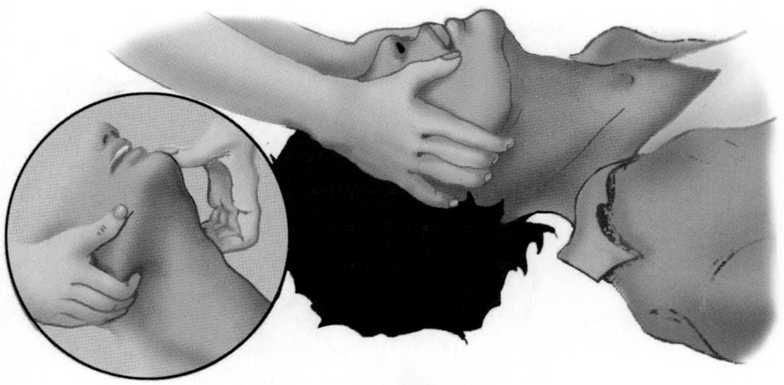

FIGURE 34-7 Jaw-thrust maneuver.

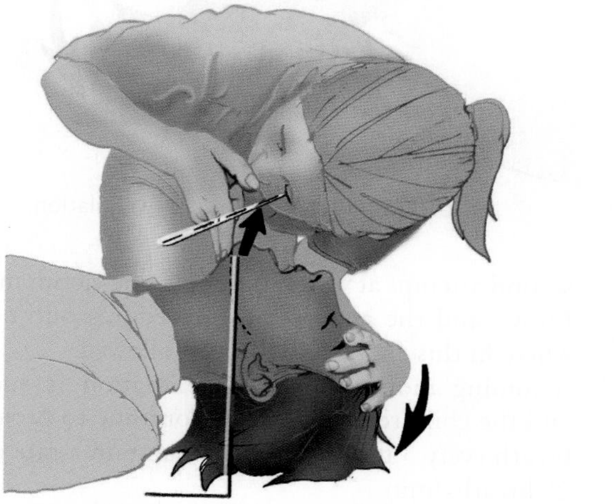

FIGURE 34-8 Determining breathlessness.

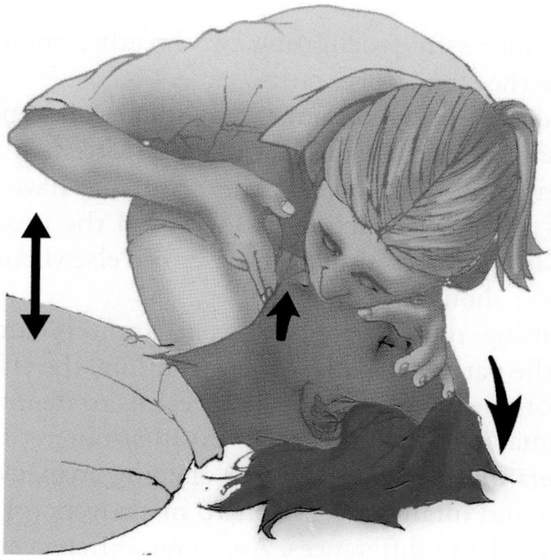

FIGURE 34-9 Adult mouth-to-mouth ventilation.

sounds are present or only gasping is present. This evaluation should take no longer than 3 to 5 seconds to complete.

Providing Artificial Ventilation

During respiratory arrest, the victim must be provided with O_2 within 4 to 6 minutes, or biologic death follows. The rescuer can restore O_2 supply to the victim's lungs by exhaling into the victim's mouth, nose, or tracheal stoma. These procedures can be used for any victim, with appropriate modification for the patient's age.

Mouth-to-Mouth Ventilation. Adequate oxygenation can be restored through mouth-to-mouth ventilation. To do this, the rescuer must take a slightly deeper than normal breath (700 to 1000 ml) and exhale directly into the victim's mouth over 1 second to produce visible chest rise. Exhaled air provides approximately 16% O_2, which is sufficient to achieve an arterial oxygen tension (PaO_2) of 50 to 60 mm Hg. A tidal volume (V_T) between 700 ml and 1000 ml is ideal for most adults. A V_T of 500 ml should be delivered when chest compressions are being administered. Children require proportionally smaller volumes.

During resuscitation of a victim of cardiac arrest, two breaths should be given over a period of 1 second each. Excessive volumes (>500 ml) or an inspiratory rate that is too fast (>8 to 10 breaths/min) must be avoided because this can push air into the stomach causing **gastric inflation** and increase intrathoracic pressure. Increased intrathoracic pressure can decrease coronary and cerebral perfusion. Visible chest rise should be used to gauge the V_T needed in children and adults.

Adults. The procedure for adults is as follows (Figure 34-9):

1. Place the victim on his or her back on a hard, flat surface.
2. Kneel at the patient's side, and open and clear the airway as previously described. Pinch the victim's nose with your thumb and index finger close to the nares to prevent air from escaping during ventilation.
3. Take a slightly deeper than normal breath and deliver 500 ml over 1 second, while making a seal over the victim's mouth. A good seal over the patient's mouth is essential. If a good seal cannot be obtained using this method, attempt mouth-to-nose ventilation.
4. Remove your mouth from the patient's mouth, and allow the victim to exhale passively. Provide a second breath after exhalation is complete.

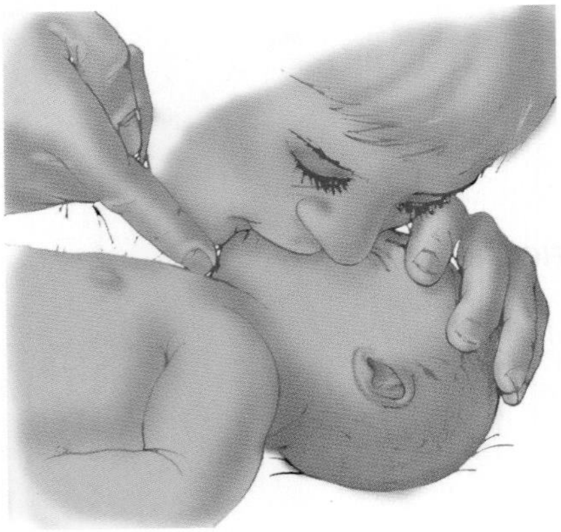

FIGURE 34-10 Mouth-to-mouth and nose seal for infants.

5. After successfully delivering two breaths, immediately assess the circulatory status.
6. Should the initial attempt to ventilate fail, reposition the victim's head and repeat the effort. If a second attempt at ventilation fails, the victim may have foreign body airway obstruction (FBAO), and the procedures for handling such situations described elsewhere in this chapter should be followed.
7. Assuming mouth-to-mouth ventilation is successful and the patient remains apneic, continue the effort at a rate of one breath every 6 to 7 seconds to maintain the minimal adult rate of 8 to 10 breaths/min.

Infants and Children. Airway opening maneuvers for children and infants are similar to maneuvers for adults, with several key differences. Anatomic differences in the infant's airway make it especially susceptible to occlusion by the tongue. The infant's head should be extended only slightly, or it should be tilted back gently into a neutral position when the head-tilt/chin-lift maneuver is used. The procedure for children and infants is as follows (Figure 34-10):

1. If the patient is an infant (<1 year old), create an airtight seal by placing your mouth over the infant's nose and mouth (see Figure 34-10).
2. If the patient is a child between 1 year old and puberty, ventilate the victim's lungs using the same technique as would be used for an adult (see Figure 34-9).
3. Provide an initial breath (over 1 second) sufficient to cause a visible rise in the chest. In infants, small puffs of air from the rescuer's cheeks are usually sufficient to achieve adequate ventilation.
4. Remove your mouth, and allow the victim to exhale passively. Provide a second breath after this deflation pause.
5. After successfully delivering two breaths, immediately assess the pulse (<10 seconds).
6. If the initial attempt to ventilate fails, reposition the victim's head and repeat the effort. A child's head may need to be moved through a wide range of positions to secure an open airway. Hyperextension of a child's neck can cause obstruction and should be avoided. If a second attempt at ventilation fails, the victim may have FBAO, and the appropriate procedures outlined elsewhere in this chapter should be followed.
7. Assuming mouth-to-mouth ventilation is successful and the child remains apneic, continue to provide one breath every 3 to 5 seconds to maintain a rate of 12 to 20 breaths/min.

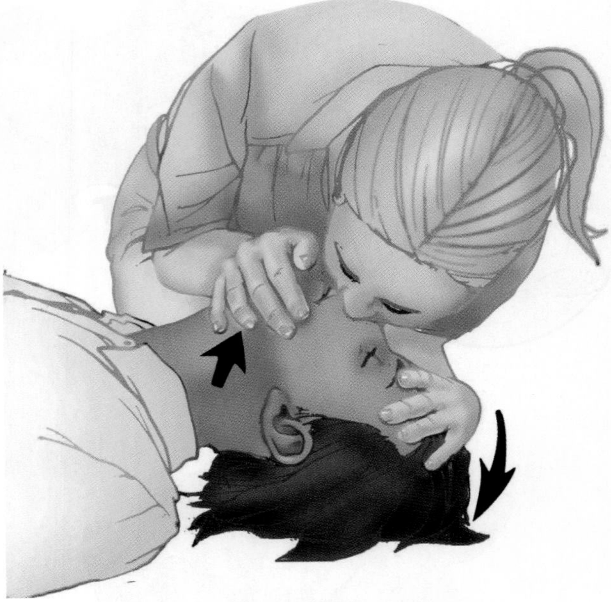

FIGURE 34-11 Mouth-to-nose ventilation.

Mouth-to-Nose Ventilation. Mouth-to-mouth ventilation cannot be performed in some situations; these include trismus (involuntary contraction of the jaw muscles, also known as *lockjaw*) and traumatic jaw or mouth injury. Also, sometimes it is difficult to maintain a tight seal with the lips using the mouth-to-mouth method. In these situations, mouth-to-nose ventilation should be used. The procedure is as follows (Figure 34-11):

1. Place the victim on his or her back.
2. Use the head-tilt/chin-lift maneuver to establish the airway, taking care to close the mouth completely.
3. Inhale slightly deeper than normal and exhale into the patient's nose. Greater force may need to be applied than would be used with mouth-to-mouth ventilation because the nasal passageways are smaller.
4. Remove your mouth from the victim's nose to allow the patient to exhale passively. If the patient does not exhale through the nose (because of nasopharyngeal obstruction from the soft palate), open the victim's mouth or separate his or her lips to facilitate exhalation.
5. After successfully delivering two slow breaths, immediately assess the circulatory status.
6. If the victim remains apneic, maintain ventilation at the rate appropriate for his or her age.

Mouth-to-Stoma Ventilation. Patients with tracheostomies or laryngectomies can be ventilated directly through the stoma or tube. These patients can be identified by an obvious stoma or a tracheostomy or laryngectomy tube in place. Some patients wear a medical alert tag or bracelet indicating that a stoma is present. The procedure for mouth-to-stoma ventilation is as follows:

1. Place the victim on his or her back with the neck in vertical alignment. Usually, the neck does not need to be extended and the nose or mouth does not need to be sealed because oropharyngeal structures are bypassed by the stoma.
2. Ensure that the stoma is clear of any obstructing matter and breathe directly into the stoma (or tube). If the victim has a cuffed tracheostomy tube in place, inflate the cuff to prevent air from escaping around the tube. If the tube is uncuffed, the mouth and nose may need to be sealed off with your hand or a tight-fitting face mask, using a pediatric face mask to create an adequate peristomal seal for bag-mask ventilation.
3. After delivering two breaths, immediately assess the circulatory status.
4. If the victim remains apneic, maintain ventilation at the rate appropriate for his or her age.

One-Rescuer versus Two-Rescuer Adult Cardiopulmonary Resuscitation

Outside the hospital, one-rescuer CPR is common. In such cases, the rescuer must assess the victim, call for help, and begin CPR without assistance from others. The rescuer must remain calm and remember the steps of one-rescuer CPR. The technique for performing chest compressions, opening the airway, and giving mouth-to-mouth breaths is the same, regardless of the number of rescuers.

When performing CPR alone, the lay rescuer must remember to give only compressions for adults, children, and infants until an AED arrives. When two rescuers are available, the second rescuer ventilates and evaluates the effectiveness of CPR. The other rescuer administers cardiac compressions. To facilitate movement, each rescuer should assume the appropriate rescue position on opposite sides of the victim. For an adult and child, the compression-to-ventilation ratio is the same as for a single rescuer (30:2), and the timing for compressions is "one and two and three and four and five" (a rate of 100 times/min). In infants, two rescuers should use a compression-to-ventilation ratio of 3:1 with 90 compressions and 30 breaths delivered per minute (120 events/min). Each breath is delivered over half second with exhalation occurring on the next compression.

RULE OF THUMB

Lay rescuers should be taught to do 100 compressions/min until the AED arrives for all age groups because it is easier to remember.[4] Emphasis should be placed on teaching lay rescuers to "push hard and fast" on the sternum.

RULE OF THUMB

Health care providers should use a 30:2 compression-to-ventilation ratio on adults and children. A 3:1 compression-to-ventilation ratio for infants (≤1 year of age) should be used when there are two rescuers.[4,10,11]

When two health care providers resuscitate a patient, the individual providing compressions briefly pauses after 30 compressions so that the other person can administer two ventilations. The cycle is repeated without interruption of compressions to check for signs of circulation or response until an AED arrives or until the hospital code team take over CPR. Health care providers should limit interruptions in chest compressions to no longer than 10 seconds except for interventions such as insertion of an advanced airway or defibrillation.

To provide rest for the individual delivering cardiac compressions, the rescuers should change positions every five cycles (approximately 2 minutes). The individual doing cardiac compressions calls for the change, saying "we will change next time" in sequence with compressions. The switch should be accomplished in less than 5 seconds. The cycle continues with the two rescuers in their new positions. Alternatively, to avoid fatigue, teams of three health care providers can be assigned to do chest compression, switching every five cycles of 30:2 compression-to-ventilation ratio. The goal is to push "hard and fast" at a rate of 100/min without fatigue diminishing that goal.

RULE OF THUMB

The person doing chest compressions should be changed every 2 minutes. Doing chest compressions is tiring, and fatigue occurs within a few minutes leading to a compression rate less than 100 compressions/min, shallow chest compressions, and incomplete chest recoil.[4]

Rescue attempts continue until advanced life support is available, the rescuers note spontaneous pulse and breathing, or a physician pronounces the victim dead. A cardiopulmonary emergency is a crisis for the victim and his or her family, and appropriate support and intervention should be provided all individuals affected. Victims who survive CPR should be transported quickly to tertiary care facilities, ideally only after advanced life support is instituted.

Automated External Defibrillation

Early Defibrillation

Since 1990, the AHA has recommended adding a fourth step to the treatment of cardiac arrest. This step involves early **defibrillation** after CPR has been initiated. The rationale is as follows:

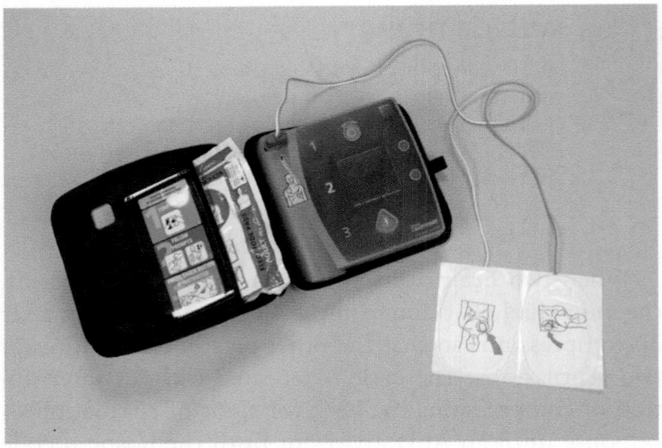

FIGURE 34-12 AED with pads attached. (From Chapleau W: Emergency First Responder, Making the Difference, Revised 2nd edition, 2011, St. Louis, Mosby JEMS.)

1. The most common initial rhythm in witnessed sudden cardiac arrest is VF.
2. The treatment for VF is electrical defibrillation.
3. The probability of successful defibrillation diminishes rapidly over time.
4. VF tends to convert to asystole within a few minutes.

Studies have shown that survival rates are highest when immediate bystander CPR is provided and defibrillation occurs within 5 minutes after SCA.[12]

The AHA recommendation is that **automated external defibrillators (AEDs)** be made available to individuals expected to respond to emergencies, such as police, security personnel, ski patrol personnel, flight attendants, and first-aid volunteers (Figure 34-12). Early defibrillation has already proven to be effective in saving lives of people who otherwise may have not been successfully resuscitated.[12] After appropriate training and implementation of the *CABs,* this step is inserted as the letter *D,* for defibrillation. This step should be initiated within 2 minutes of when CPR is begun. EMS providers arriving at the scene of a cardiac arrest should give a period of CPR (five cycles, or about 2 minutes) before checking a rhythm and attempting defibrillation. If the EMS provider witnesses the collapse or for in-hospital situations, the rescuer should use the defibrillator as soon as it is available. In an adult drowning victim or a victim of FBAO who becomes unconscious, a health care provider working alone may give about five cycles (approximately 2 minutes) of CPR before activating the emergency response system.[4]

Personnel employed at high-acuity hospitals may not be equipped with AEDs because access to ACLS is readily available, usually within minutes of the code being called. However, low-acuity hospitals, skilled nursing facilities, and other medical facilities that do not have a code team on the premises would benefit from AEDs. RTs working at such facilities should inquire whether one is on the premises and, if so, where it is located and how it functions. If an AED is not present, a recommendation should be made to the administration of the facility to purchase one. The AHA recommends that an AED be available wherever CPR is likely to be performed.

VF cardiac arrest is less common in children than adults and accounts for 5% to 15% of pediatric and adolescent arrests.[13,14] The AHA recommends use of an AED for children older than 1 year who are in cardiac arrest and encourages the use of a pediatric dose-attenuator system if one is available. If such a system is unavailable, a standard AED is recommended. The standard doses recommended by the AHA for manual defibrillation of children are 2 J/kg for the first attempt and 4 J/kg for subsequent attempts.[15] Research has shown that lower energy (120 to 200 J) biphasic waveform shocks have equivalent or higher success in terminating VF than three stacked monophasic waveform shocks delivering escalating energy of 200 J, 300 J, and 360 J.[16] AEDs should be deployed in locations where there is a high incidence of witnessed SCA, such as airports, casinos, and sports facilities.

Automated External Defibrillators

AEDs function more in a semiautomated fashion; the device only recommends that a shock be delivered, rather than initiating one automatically. Fully automatic defibrillators are available but are used only in special circumstances. Adhesive electrodes from the AED are attached to the patient. When all of the equipment is hooked up, the "Analyze" button should be pressed to begin. A rhythm recognition program analyzes the patient's rhythm. If it detects ventricular tachycardia (VT) or VF, it advises the rescuer through voice and visual prompts that a shock be delivered. If a shock is indicated, the rescuer should "Clear" the patient and press the "Shock" button. After pressing the shock button, the rescuer should deliver five cycles of CPR beginning with chest compression using a 30:2 compression-to-ventilation ratio.

The rescuer should not delay chest compressions by stopping to recheck the rhythm or pulse. The rhythm is checked by the AED after five cycles (approximately 2 minutes) of CPR have been completed. The rescuers should be prepared to initiate another five cycles of CPR immediately after a second shock has been delivered. The rescuer administering chest compressions should be changed every 2 minutes. The rescuer providing 2 minutes of chest compressions should be prepared to deliver a shock as soon as he or she removes the hands from the victim's chest. The second rescuer should be in position to start chest compressions as soon as the shock is delivered. If no shock is advised by the AED, the AED voice prompt should instruct the rescuer to resume CPR immediately starting with chest compressions. If the message reads "No shock indicated," CPR should be performed for 1 to 2 minutes, and then the rhythm analysis should be repeated. A 1- to 2-minute period of CPR after a no-shock prompt from the AED delivers O_2 and metabolic substrates to the myocardium, increasing the probability that a perfusing

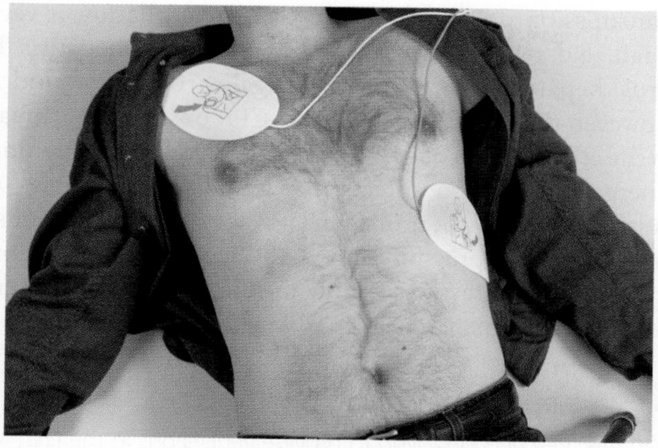

FIGURE 34-13 Positioning of rescuer and placement of pads when using AED. (From Chapleau W: Emergency First Responder, Making the Difference, Revised 2nd edition, 2011, St. Louis, Mosby JEMS.)

rhythm will occur. The rescuer should not be concerned that chest compressions might trigger the return of VF in the presence of a postshock organized rhythm.[17] Figure 34-13 indicates how the AED is used by the rescuer.

RULE OF THUMB

Patients in VF or pulseless VT cardiac arrest should receive only one shock followed immediately by five cycles of CPR before the pulse and rhythm are rechecked.[15]

Evaluating Effectiveness of Cardiopulmonary Resuscitation

CPR providers need to judge continuously both the effectiveness of CPR and the victim's response. Ventilation can be evaluated by observing visible rise and fall of the victim's chest during mouth-to-mouth resuscitation. Air that is escaping can be heard and felt during exhalation. Researchers at the AHA 2005 CPR and emergency cardiovascular care consensus conference reached the following conclusions regarding the effectiveness of chest compressions:[18]

1. "Effective" chest compressions are essential for providing blood flow during CPR.
2. To give "effective" chest compressions, "push hard and push fast." Compress the adult chest at a rate of about 100 compressions/min, with a depth of 2 inches (for adults). Allow the chest to recoil completely after each compression, and allow approximately equal compression and relaxation times.
3. Minimize interruptions in chest compressions.

The cycle time is 600 msec if the chest is compressed at a rate of 100 compressions/min. The time to deliver 30 compressions is 18 seconds if the compression rate is held constant at 100 compressions/min. It takes a rescuer 4 seconds to deliver two breaths with a 1-second inspiratory time and a 1-second expiratory time. Assuming 2 seconds are lost switching from compressions to ventilations, the total ventilation time is 6 seconds. The CPR cycle time is 24 seconds; 2.5 cycles/min would optimally deliver 75 compressions and five breaths. The AHA has encouraged the use of CPR prompts after studies showing compression and ventilation rates are frequently too fast or slow.[19,20] Every effort possible must be made to decrease the number of interruptions in chest compressions.

Hazards and Complications

The most common complications that occur with CPR are worsening of existing neck or spine injuries, gastric inflation and vomiting, trauma to internal structures during chest compressions, and problems associated with the removal of foreign objects to clear an obstructed airway.

Neck and Spine Injuries

Health care providers can aggravate neck or spine injuries by inappropriately moving the victim's head. However, only approximately 2% of victims with blunt trauma have a spinal injury. Spinal injury risk is greatest if the victim has craniofacial injury or a Glasgow Coma Scale score of less than 8.[21] The victim should be carefully assessed for head, neck, or spine injuries. If this type of injury is apparent, the head should be carefully supported, and side-to-side motion must be avoided. In such situations, using the jaw thrust maneuver rather than the head-tilt/chin-lift method to open the airway is recommended by the AHA.[4] If jaw thrust is unsuccessful in establishing an airway, the rescuer should try a slight head-tilt.[4]

Gastric Inflation

During prolonged mouth-to-mouth ventilation, air enters the esophagus and stomach. Some gastric inflation is not unusual, particularly in children, and occurs in approximately 17% of cases.[22] Severe gastric inflation puts pressure on the diaphragm, restricting lung expansion. Gastric inflation also can increase vagal tone and cause reflex bradycardia and hypotension.

RULE OF THUMB

The best way to avoid gastric inflation during bag-mask ventilation is to deliver breaths with low to moderate flow (<30 L/min) over 1 second.[23] V_T size should be only large enough to cause visible chest rise. The health care provider should not ventilate and compress the chest simultaneously with a bag-mask device.

However, most important is the fact that severe gastric inflation prompts regurgitation. Because an unconscious patient lacks normal upper airway reflexes, regurgitated stomach contents can be aspirated easily into the lungs. Aspiration of stomach contents into the lungs may cause death by making ventilation virtually impossible or lead to severe lung injury such as aspiration pneumonia that may cause death days or weeks later.

Vomiting

Vomiting is another complication associated with **abdominal thrusts,** and it is impossible to avoid in some victims. Vomiting itself is a minor problem. The hazard is the aspiration of vomitus into the lung. Aspiration can be prevented only by using advanced airway devices such as an endotracheal tube, laryngeal mask airway, or esophageal-tracheal double-lumen airway (Combitube).

Internal Trauma

External cardiac compression is hazardous, and every attempt should be made to minimize trauma by using the correct technique. Complications associated with chest compression include gastric perforation, laceration of the liver, contusion of the lung, fractured ribs or sternum, pneumothorax, hemothorax, cardiac tamponade, and soft tissue emphysema.[24,25] These complications most often are linked to improper hand position. Placement of the hands too far to either the left or the right can cause fractured ribs or lacerated lung. Incorrect placement on the left can injure the heart. Placing the hands too high on the sternum can fracture the sternum; placing the hands too low can cause a fractured xiphoid process or a lacerated liver. Correct identification of landmarks and proper hand placement minimize the likelihood of these complications.

Foreign Body Airway Obstruction

Manual removal of FBAO from the upper airway also can be hazardous because of the possibility of forcing the object deeper into the airway or traumatizing the airway. This hazard can be minimized by attempting to remove FBAO only when the provider can see solid material obstructing the airway in an unresponsive patient and using extreme care in removing it.[4]

Contraindications to Cardiopulmonary Resuscitation

A pulseless, apneic patient dies within 4 to 6 minutes without intervention. Fear of further harm should never influence the decision to begin CPR. CPR is contraindicated only when the patient is obviously biologically dead (as noted by such findings as rigor mortis). In the hospital, CPR is contraindicated when a valid "do not resuscitate" order is in effect or when a properly executed living will (advance directive) specifically requests that CPR not be initiated.

Health Concerns and Cardiopulmonary Resuscitation

Laypeople and health care professionals are concerned regarding possible transmission of infectious diseases, such as AIDS, during CPR.[26] In one survey, 45% of the physicians and 80% of the nurses who responded indicated that they would refuse to provide mouth-to-mouth ventilation for a stranger.[27] The actual risk of disease transmission during mouth-to-mouth ventilation is very small. No reports on transmission of HIV, hepatitis B virus, hepatitis C virus, or cytomegalovirus were found.[28] However, the reluctance to initiate CPR poses a clear threat to the effectiveness of early intervention in life-threatening emergencies, which affects the public as a whole. A bystander who is not trained in CPR should provide hands-only (chest compression only) CPR, with an emphasis on "push hard and fast," or follow the directions of the emergency medical dispatcher.[4]

RULE OF THUMB

Rescuers unwilling to provide ventilations in the first few minutes of adult VF cardiac arrest should provide chest compressions at a rate of 100 compressions/min, with an emphasis on "push hard and fast." Periodic gasps and chest recoil in adult cardiac arrest may provide some ventilation if the airway is open. Most children and infants with cardiac arrest require both prompt ventilations and chest compressions.

Health care providers with a duty to provide CPR should follow the guidelines established by the U.S. Centers for Disease Control and Prevention (CDC) and the Occupational Safety and Health Administration. These recommendations include the use of latex gloves, masks, and goggles. Mechanical barrier aids to ventilation (e.g., masks, filters, valves) also have been suggested to allay fear and to protect the rescuer. However, these devices require training to be used properly, are not universally available, and may not be as effective as mouth-to-mouth ventilation.

Although technically blood or body fluids can be exchanged through mouth-to-mouth ventilation, CDC surveillance of job-related contraction of AIDS has never discovered such an incident.[28] Other infectious diseases, such as herpes simplex and tuberculosis, may present a higher risk to the rescuer, but few cases have been reported. Although the risk of transmission is believed to be low, health care providers who perform mouth-to-mouth ventilation on someone suspected to have tuberculosis should obtain a follow-up evaluation using standard approaches. In addition, any health care provider who might hesitate to provide mouth-to-mouth ventilation to a victim in need should always carry (and know how to use) an appropriate barrier device for this purpose. Equipment contaminated with blood or other body fluids during a resuscitation effort should always be discarded in appropriate receptacles or thoroughly cleaned and disinfected according to hospital protocols.

Treating Foreign Body Airway Obstruction

Early recognition of FBAO is critical. Foreign bodies may cause partial or complete obstruction. Partial obstruction may allow nearly adequate air exchange, in which case the patient remains conscious and coughing. As long as air exchange is present, the patient should be reassured and allowed to clear his or her own airway by coughing. If partial obstruction persists, or air exchange worsens, the EMS system should be activated. Poor air exchange exists when the patient has a weak or ineffective cough, increased inspiratory difficulty, or cyanosis.

With a completely obstructed airway, the patient commonly clutches at his or her throat. This is known as the *universal distress signal for foreign body obstruction.* A person with a complete obstruction cannot talk, cough, or breathe and is in dire need of emergency intervention using abdominal thrusts, chest thrusts, back blows, or a combination of two or more maneuvers.

Several procedures can be used to obtain a clear passageway if attempts to open a victim's airway are unsuccessful or if a foreign body is observed but cannot be removed from the mouth or pharynx. For adults and children, the procedure for health care providers for clearing a foreign body is the *abdominal thrust.* The rescuer should attempt back blows first for infants with an obstructed airway; if these are unsuccessful, the rescuer should try chest thrusts. *Chest thrusts* may be used in place of abdominal thrusts on women in advanced stages of pregnancy and on markedly obese individuals. Both abdominal thrusts and chest thrusts normally are followed by a visual check and manual removal of any observed obstructing foreign material.

Abdominal Thrusts (Heimlich Maneuver)

Forceful thrusts applied to the epigastrium can dislodge an obstruction caused by a food bolus, vomitus, or other foreign body. Quick thrusts to the abdomen rapidly displace the diaphragm upward, increasing intrathoracic pressure and creating expulsive expiratory airflow. As with a normal cough, this expulsive airflow may be sufficient to expel the foreign body from the airway. The procedure for performing abdominal thrusts on adults and children is as follows (Figure 34-14):

1. If the victim is sitting or standing, stand behind the victim and wrap your arms around his or her waist. Make a fist with one hand and place the thumb side midline on the abdomen slightly above the navel and well below the tip of the xiphoid process (see Figure 34-14). Grasp the fist with the other hand and deliver a quick upward and inward thrust. Each thrust should be a separate and distinct movement. Repeat the process until the obstruction is removed or the victim loses consciousness.
2. If an adult victim with FBAO becomes unresponsive, the rescuer should move the patient to the ground, activate the EMS system, and begin CPR. Each time the mouth is opened during cycles of compressions and ventilation, the rescuer should look into the victim's mouth for FBAO and remove it; this should be done without increasing the time to deliver two breaths (approximately 6 seconds). The routine use of blind finger sweeps to remove FBAO in adults, children, and infants is not recommended by the AHA.[4,11]
3. A conscious victim who is alone can attempt to dislodge the foreign body with self-administered abdominal thrusts, performed by pressing his or her fist into the abdomen or pushing the abdomen against a firm surface such as a counter top, sink, chair back, railing, or tabletop.

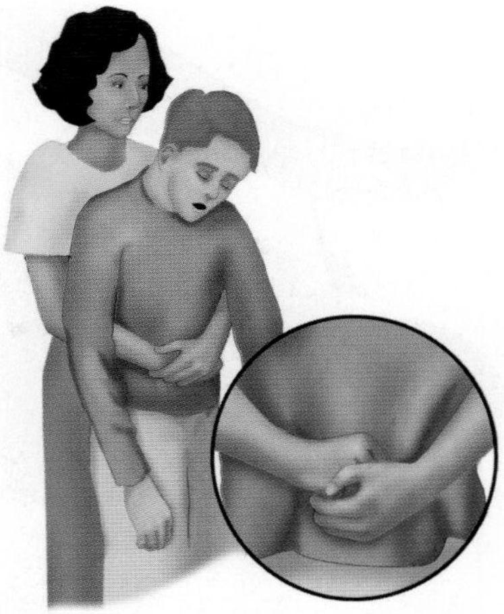

FIGURE 34-14 Abdominal thrusts, adult victim standing. (From Chapleau W: Emergency First Responder, Making the Difference, Revised 2nd edition, 2011, St. Louis, Mosby JEMS.)

Internal Organ Damage. The major hazard associated with abdominal thrusts that are performed when an individual has choked and lost consciousness is possible damage to internal organs, such as laceration or rupture of abdominal or thoracic viscera.[29] The body of clinical data regarding choking is largely retrospective and anecdotal. Abdominal thrusts have been recommended for relief of FBAO in adults and children since 1975 based mostly on early anecdotal case reports. Abdominal thrusts are recommended by the AHA and several other resuscitation councils for use for *unresponsive* adult and child (but not infant) victims. Abdominal thrusts are not recommended for infants younger than 1 year because of their relatively unprotected abdomens and large livers. Rational conjecture and common practices suggest that back blows may loosen obstruction so that subsequent abdominal or chest thrusts may relieve obstruction. The risk of internal organ damage from abdominal thrusts in a conscious patient can be minimized by the rescuer placing his or her arms and fist below the victim's xiphoid process and lower margin of the ribs.

Back Blows and Chest Thrusts

Because abdominal maneuver can easily cause abdominal injury when applied to infants, a combination of back blows and chest thrusts should be used to clear foreign bodies from the upper airway. Back blows alone may create sufficient force to dislodge trapped objects, but if this is ineffective, the back blows should be followed with five

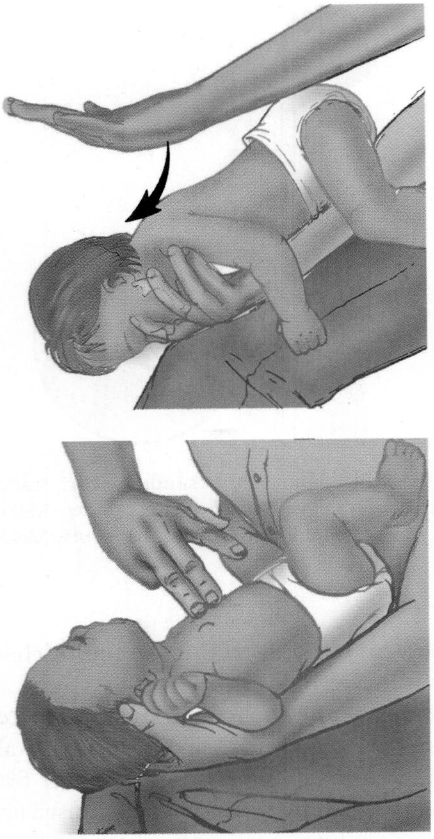

FIGURE 34-15 Use of back blows and chest thrusts to clear foreign bodies from infant airway.

chest thrusts. The rescuer should continue inspecting the airway until the airway is restored. This procedure is as follows (Figure 34-15):

1. Back blows can be administered to infants more efficiently if the child is held straddled over one arm with the head lower than the body.
2. Use the flat portion of your hand to deliver gently, but quickly, five back blows between the shoulder blades.
3. If the back blows do not clear the infant's airway, turn the infant over and institute a series of five chest thrusts. Similar to abdominal thrust, chest thrust creates a rapid increase in intrathoracic pressure, aiding expulsion of the foreign body. Chest thrusts for infants are performed in the same manner and at the same location as cardiac compressions but at a slower rate.
4. Try to clear the airway between attempts to expel the foreign body. First, visually inspect the oral cavity and remove any foreign matter that can be seen. Deep blind finger sweeps of the mouth of an infant, child, or adult are not recommended.

Evaluating Effectiveness of Foreign Body Removal

After each airway restoration maneuver, the rescuer must determine whether the foreign body has been expelled and the obstructed airway cleared. If the foreign body has not been dislodged, the appropriate sequence (abdominal thrusts or chest thrusts for adults and children, back blows and chest thrusts for infants) should be repeated until successful. Successful removal of an obstructing body is indicated by the following:

- Confirmed expulsion of foreign body
- Clear breathing and ability to speak
- Return of consciousness
- Return of normal color

If successive attempts to clear the airway fail, more aggressive techniques are indicated, if available. These include direct laryngoscopy and foreign body removal with Magill forceps, transtracheal catheterization, cricothyrotomy, and tracheotomy. These methods require specially trained health care professionals and equipment, and they are aptly categorized as advanced life support techniques. Transtracheal catheterization and cricothyrotomy are discussed later in this chapter, and laryngoscopy, bronchoscopy, and tracheotomy were described in Chapter 33.

ADVANCED CARDIOVASCULAR LIFE SUPPORT

ACLS extends BLS capabilities by providing additional measures beyond immediate ventilatory and circulatory assistance. These measures include using accessory equipment to support ventilation and oxygenation, monitoring the electrocardiogram (ECG), establishing an intravenous (IV) route for drug administration, and applying selected pharmacologic agents and electrical therapies (Figure 34-16). The AHA claims that "the foundation of ACLS is good BLS care, beginning with prompt high-quality bystander CPR and, for pulseless ventricular rhythms, attempted defibrillation within minutes of collapse."[28]

During ACLS in the hospital, the RT assumes primary responsibility for supporting oxygenation, establishing and maintaining the airway, and providing ventilation. RTs must demonstrate high levels of proficiency in these advanced life support skills and other ACLS skills that may be assigned by the resuscitation team leader.

Support for Oxygenation

Although expired air ventilation provides an acceptable level of oxygenation, low cardiac output, pulmonary shunting, and abnormalities during CPR lead to hypoxia. Hypoxia results in anaerobic metabolism and metabolic acidosis. Metabolic acidosis impedes the action of certain drugs and can diminish the effectiveness of electrical therapies. For these reasons, the highest possible concentration of O_2 should be administered as soon as possible. Concerns about O_2 toxicity are not valid during this period of resuscitation.

During ACLS, supplemental O_2 is normally given through accessory devices designed to support ventilation. The ability of these devices to provide high fractional

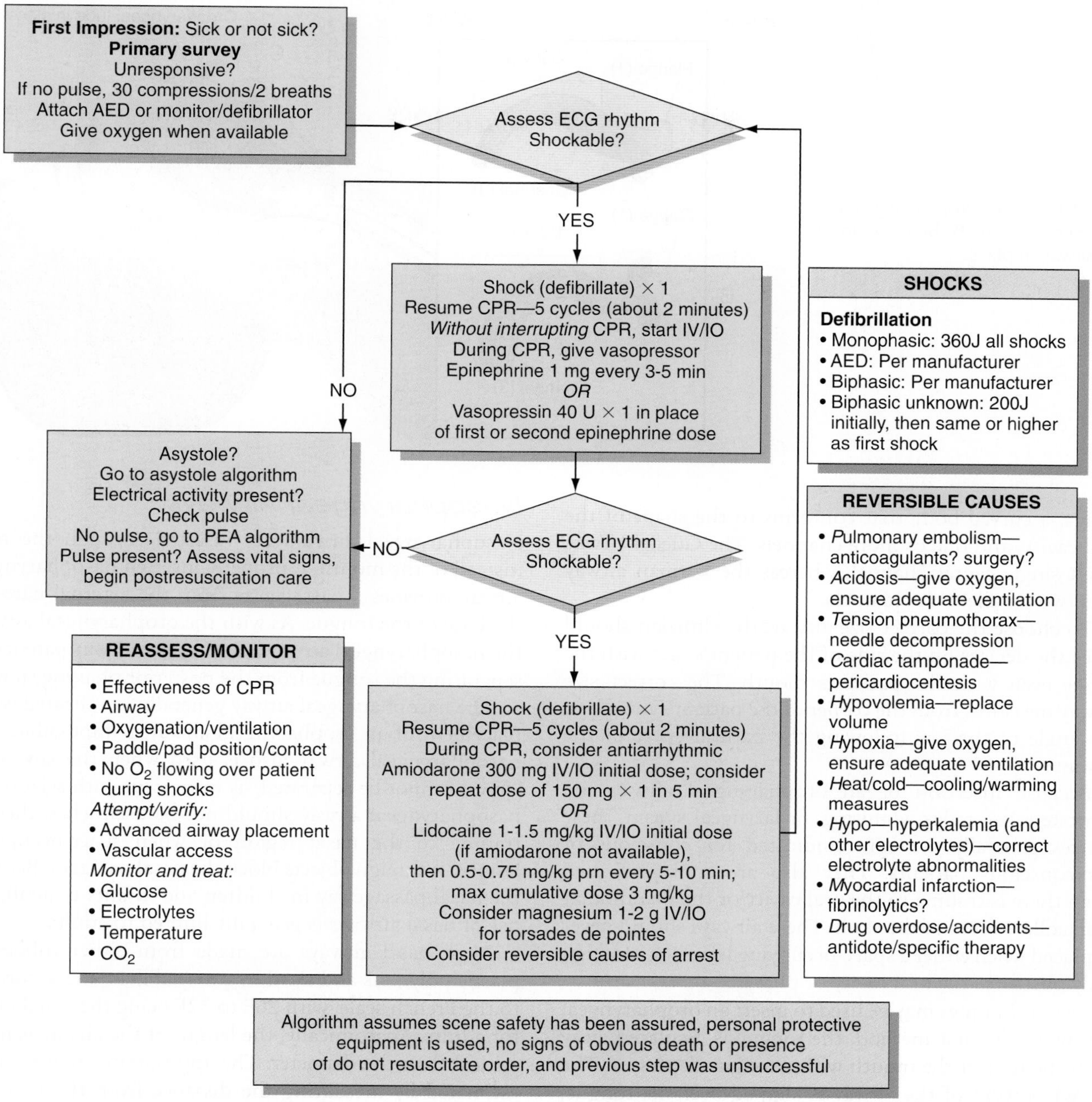

First Impression: Sick or not sick?
Primary survey
Unresponsive?
If no pulse, 30 compressions/2 breaths
Attach AED or monitor/defibrillator
Give oxygen when available
Assess ECG rhythm
Shockable?
YES
NO
Shock (defibrillate) × 1
Resume CPR—5 cycles (about 2 minutes)
Without interrupting CPR, start IV/IO
During CPR, give vasopressor
Epinephrine 1 mg every 3-5 min
OR
Vasopressin 40 U × 1 in place
of first or second epinephrine dose
SHOCKS
Defibrillation
• Monophasic: 360J all shocks
• AED: Per manufacturer
• Biphasic: Per manufacturer
• Biphasic unknown: 200J initially, then same or higher as first shock
Asystole?
Go to asystole algorithm
Electrical activity present?
Check pulse
No pulse, go to PEA algorithm
Pulse present? Assess vital signs,
begin postresuscitation care
NO
Assess ECG rhythm
Shockable?
YES
REVERSIBLE CAUSES
• Pulmonary embolism—anticoagulants? surgery?
• Acidosis—give oxygen, ensure adequate ventilation
• Tension pneumothorax—needle decompression
• Cardiac tamponade—pericardiocentesis
• Hypovolemia—replace volume
• Hypoxia—give oxygen, ensure adequate ventilation
• Heat/cold—cooling/warming measures
• Hypo—hyperkalemia (and other electrolytes)—correct electrolyte abnormalities
• Myocardial infarction—fibrinolytics?
• Drug overdose/accidents—antidote/specific therapy
REASSESS/MONITOR
• Effectiveness of CPR
• Airway
• Oxygenation/ventilation
• Paddle/pad position/contact
• No O_2 flowing over patient during shocks
Attempt/verify:
• Advanced airway placement
• Vascular access
Monitor and treat:
• Glucose
• Electrolytes
• Temperature
• CO_2
Shock (defibrillate) × 1
Resume CPR—5 cycles (about 2 minutes)
During CPR, consider antiarrhythmic
Amiodarone 300 mg IV/IO initial dose; consider
repeat dose of 150 mg × 1 in 5 min
OR
Lidocaine 1-1.5 mg/kg IV/IO initial dose
(if amiodarone not available),
then 0.5-0.75 mg/kg prn every 5-10 min;
max cumulative dose 3 mg/kg
Consider magnesium 1-2 g IV/IO
for torsades de pointes
Consider reversible causes of arrest
Algorithm assumes scene safety has been assured, personal protective
equipment is used, no signs of obvious death or presence
of do not resuscitate order, and previous step was unsuccessful

FIGURE 34-16 Pulseless VT/VF algorithm. (From Aehlert B: ACLS study guide, ed 4, St. Louis, 2012, Mosby.)

inspired oxygen (FiO_2) is a key factor in judging their performance.

Airway Management

Accessory equipment designed to provide airway management during ACLS includes a variety of masks and artificial airways.

Pharyngeal Airways

Pharyngeal airways can help restore airway patency and maintain adequate ventilation, in particular, when using a bag-mask device. A properly placed pharyngeal airway also may help provide access for suctioning. Pharyngeal airways should be used only after BLS methods have successfully opened and cleared the airway.

Pharyngeal airways restore airway patency by separating the tongue from the posterior pharyngeal wall. Two types of pharyngeal airways are used in clinical practice: (1) oropharyngeal airway and (2) nasopharyngeal airway.

Oropharyngeal airways come in many different sizes to fit adults, children, and infants. Figure 34-17 shows the two most common oropharyngeal airway designs: (1) the Guedel airway (see Figure 34-17, *A*) and (2) the Berman airway (see Figure 34-17, *B*). Both types have an external

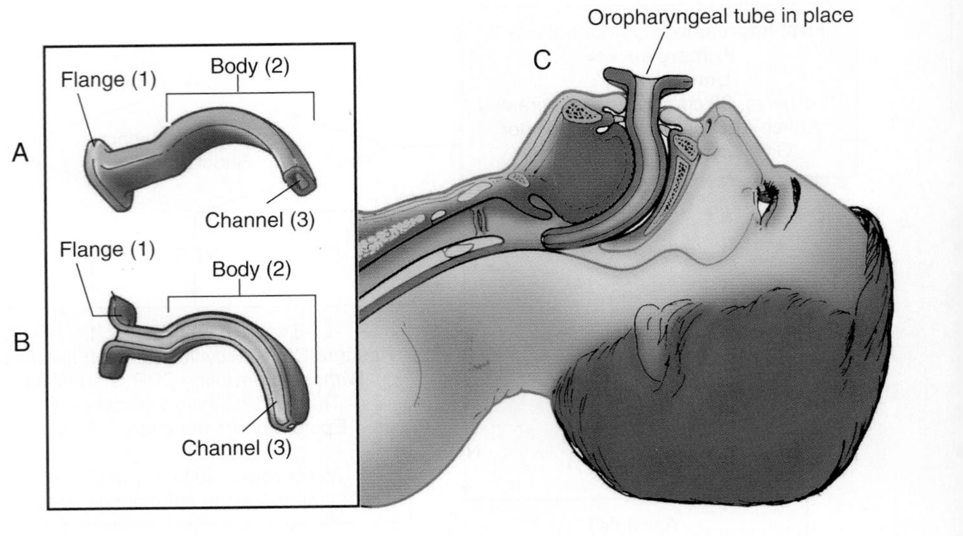

FIGURE 34-17 Oropharyngeal airways. **A,** Guedel airway. **B,** Berman airway. **C,** Airway in place.

flange, a curved body that conforms to the shape of the oral cavity, and one or more channels. The Guedel airway has a single center channel, whereas the Berman airway uses two parallel side channels.

To choose the correct size airway, the clinician should place the devices on the side of the patient's face with the flange even with the patient's mouth. The correct size airway measures from the corner of the patient's mouth to the angle of the jaw following the natural curve of the airway.

Because insertion of an oropharyngeal airway can provoke a gag reflex, vomiting, or laryngeal spasm, these devices generally are contraindicated for conscious or semiconscious patients. They also are contraindicated when there is trauma to the oral cavity or the mandibular or maxillary areas of the skull. These airways should never be placed when either a space-occupying lesion or a foreign body obstructs the oral cavity or pharynx.

Two techniques may be used to insert an oropharyngeal airway. In the first method, the tongue is displaced away from the roof of the mouth with a tongue depressor. The curved portion of the airway is slipped over the tongue, following the curve of the oral cavity.

In the second approach, the jaw-lift technique is used to help displace the tongue. The oropharyngeal airway is rotated 180 degrees before insertion. In this manner, the airway itself helps separate the tongue from the posterior wall of the pharynx. As the tip of the airway reaches the hard palate, it is rotated 180 degrees, aligning it in the pharynx.

In either approach, incorrect placement can displace the tongue, pushing it farther back into the pharynx and worsening the obstruction. Oropharyngeal airways must be inserted carefully and by trained personnel only. As shown in Figure 34-17, *C,* when properly inserted, the tip of an oropharyngeal airway lies at the base of the tongue above the epiglottis, with the flange portion extending outside the teeth. Only in this position can the device properly maintain airway patency.

Nasopharyngeal Airways

Nasopharyngeal airways are inserted through the nose instead of the mouth. A properly inserted nasopharyngeal airway provides a passageway from the external nares to the base of the tongue. As with the oropharyngeal airway, the nasopharyngeal airway helps restore airway patency by separating the tongue from the posterior pharyngeal wall.

The nasopharyngeal airway generally is indicated when placement of an oropharyngeal airway is impossible. The nasopharyngeal airway also is used when the jaws of a victim cannot be separated, as may occur with seizures. A nasopharyngeal airway should not be used when there is trauma to the nasal region or when space-occupying lesions or foreign objects block the nasal passages. Because the nasal passageway in children and infants is small, the use of nasal airways is generally limited to adults.

Most nasal airways are made from either rubber or plastic polymers and sized by external diameter according to the French scale, with 26F to 32F being the usual range for adults. Anatomically, the length of the airway is more critical than the diameter. The appropriate length can be estimated by measuring the distance from the patient's earlobe to the tip of the nose.

To insert a nasopharyngeal airway, the victim's head is tilted slightly backward. The airway is lubricated with a water-soluble agent to ease insertion, and it is positioned perpendicular to the frontal plane of the victim's face. The airway is advanced slowly through the inferior meatus of either the right or the left nasal cavity, with the bevel edge facing the septum. If an obstruction is felt during insertion, gentle twisting may facilitate placement. If the resistance continues, the most likely cause is a deviated nasal septum. In this case, one should attempt to insert the airway through the other naris or try a smaller diameter tube.

After the airway is inserted, one should try to visualize and confirm its correct position quickly, using a tongue depressor if necessary. When properly positioned, a nasopharyngeal airway is usually stabilized by its own flange.

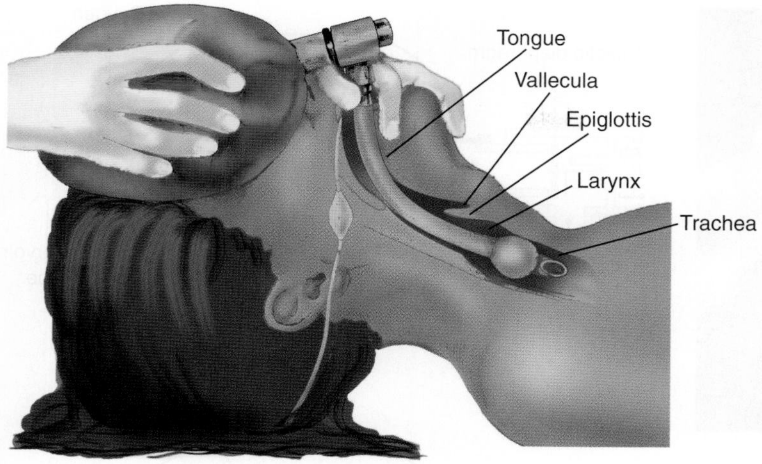

FIGURE 34-18 Orotracheal tube in place, being used with a bag-valve resuscitator.

Masks

A mask that fits the patient is a useful tool for the application of artificial ventilation by appropriately trained rescuers. An ideal mask should be made of transparent material, be capable of sealing tightly against the face, provide an inlet for supplemental O_2, and have a standard 22-mm port for connection to a bag-mask device. The mask should be available in various sizes to accommodate adults, children, and infants. Infant masks often have a 15-mm male connector instead of a 22-mm port. The use of masks to support ventilation presumes that the airway can be maintained by conventional BLS techniques. Which mask should be used in a given situation depends on careful assessment of the status of the victim and an in-depth knowledge of the capabilities and limitations of the equipment at hand.

Endotracheal Intubation

An advanced airway allows the rescuer to achieve one or more of the following goals:

1. Deliver ventilations that are not synchronous with chest compressions
2. Restore airway patency
3. Maintain adequate ventilation
4. Isolate and protect the airway from aspiration
5. Provide access for clearance of secretions
6. Provide an alternative route for administration of selected drugs

Endotracheal intubation is the preferred method for securing the airway during CPR. When positioned properly, an endotracheal tube can maintain a patent airway, prevent aspiration of stomach contents, permit suctioning of the trachea and main stem bronchi, facilitate ventilation and oxygenation, and provide a route for drug administration.

Attempts to intubate the trachea must never interfere with providing adequate ventilation and oxygenation by other means. Only highly trained personnel should perform endotracheal intubation, and each attempt should not exceed 30 seconds because ventilation is absent during the procedure. Adequate ventilation and oxygenation must be provided between attempts. Figure 34-18 shows a cuffed orotracheal tube properly positioned in the trachea. It is being used with a manual bag-mask device to provide ventilation and oxygenation. Adequate ventilation and oxygenation can be provided with 10 to 12 breaths/min.

RTs should be trained in endotracheal intubation techniques, as applied in both emergency life support and mechanical ventilation situations. Details about the necessary equipment, procedures, and short-term and long-term complications of endotracheal intubation are provided in Chapter 33.

Ventilation

Accessory equipment used to support ventilation in advanced life support includes manual and O_2-powered resuscitators. Manual resuscitators, also called *bag-mask devices,* are available for adults, children, and infants. Conversely, O_2-powered resuscitators are strictly limited to adult application and are not discussed in this chapter.

Bag-Mask Devices

One-way valves on bag-mask devices should be simple, dependable, and jam-free. All health care professionals responding to a cardiac arrest call should be familiar and skilled in the use of such a device for support of ventilation and oxygenation. Application of the bag-mask device is best performed with the practitioner positioned at the head of the victim, using the head-tilt maneuver to maintain the airway (Figure 34-19). The rescuer delivers V_T adequate to produce visible chest rise (6 to 7 ml/kg or 500 to 600 ml) over 1 second. Using this smaller V_T decreases airway pressure and minimizes risk of gastric inflation.

It is important to deliver the two breaths during CPR over only 3 to 4 seconds so that the optimal number of chest compressions per minute can be delivered (75 compressions/min, rate of delivery 100 compressions/min). The 30 : 2 compression-to-ventilation ratio allows for only five breaths to be delivered per minute. It is critical

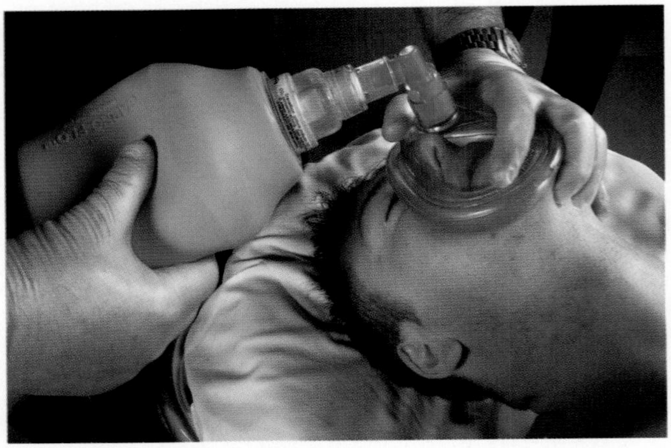

FIGURE 34-19 Ventilation using a bag-mask device and head-tilt/chin-lift method to open the airway. (From Henry MC, Stapleton ER: EMT prehospital care, revised ed 4, St. Louis, 2009, Mosby.)

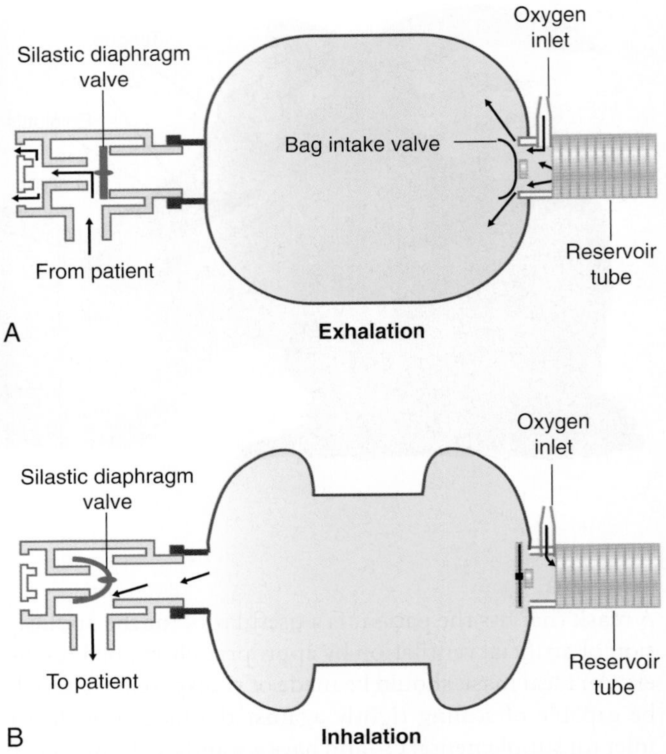

FIGURE 34-20 Components of bag-mask device.

that all five breaths be delivered with visible chest rise. After an advanced airway replaces the face mask, the ventilatory rate should be 8 to 10 breaths/min during CPR. Slower rates of 6 to 8 breaths/min might be needed for patients with chronic obstructive pulmonary disease (COPD) to prevent air trapping and the development of auto-positive end expiratory pressure (PEEP). Ventilatory rates greater than 12 breaths/min are not recommended during CPR because they lead to increased intrathoracic pressure, impeding venous return to the heart during chest compressions,[30] and hyperventilation.

The rescuer delivers each breath over 1 second and should not attempt to synchronize ventilations with the chest compressions. Nonsynchronized delivery of ventilation and compressions allows the number of chest compressions delivered per minute to increase from 75 to 100 (33% increase) and breaths delivered per minute increase from 5 to 10 (100% increase). After restoration of a perfusing rhythm, the ventilation rate should be 10 to 12 breaths/min delivered over 1 second.

RULE OF THUMB

Rescuers should not hyperventilate victims of cardiac arrest. Once an advanced airway is placed, ventilations should be delivered over 1 second at a rate of 8 to 10 breaths/min (every 6 to 8 seconds). One should not attempt to synchronize ventilations with chest compressions. Ventilation for patients with a perfusing rhythm should be at a rate of 10 to 12 breaths/min (one breath every 5 to 6 seconds). Patients with COPD may need ventilation rates of 6 to 8 breaths/min to prevent auto-PEEP.

Bag-mask devices combine a mask with a self-inflating bag and a nonrebreathing valve mechanism. These devices may be used to ventilate patients by applying the mask over the patient's mouth and nose or by attaching the self-inflating bag directly to an endotracheal tube or other advanced airways. All devices are capable of providing ventilation with air or with supplemental O_2. Bag-mask devices can provide 100% O_2 when properly applied. Although initially designed as adjuncts for emergency life support, they are used extensively in other respiratory care settings, in particular, in the areas of airway management and continuous mechanical ventilation.

Design

Figure 34-20 is a schematic of a typical bag-mask device, showing gas movement and valve action during both the inhalation-compression and exhalation-relaxation phases. The key components shown in this schematic are the nonrebreathing valve *(left)*, the bag itself, the O_2 inlet and bag inlet valve *(to the right of the bag)*, and the O_2 reservoir tube *(far right)*.

During exhalation (see Figure 34-20, *A*), gas flows out from the patient's lungs through the nonrebreathing valve into the atmosphere. At the same time (while the bag expands), the intake valve opens, and 100% O_2 flows into the bag from both the reservoir and the O_2 inlet.

During the inhalation phase (see Figure 34-20, *B*), the bag is compressed manually, causing bag pressure to increase. This increase in bag pressure simultaneously closes the inlet valve and opens the nonrebreathing valve, forcing gas into the patient. While the bag inlet valve is closed, O_2 coming in through the O_2 inlet goes into the reservoir tube, where it is stored for the next breath.

Use

To use a bag-mask device, the health care provider is positioned at the head of the patient's bed. Ideally, an oral airway is inserted, and the head-tilt method is used to keep the airway open (assuming there are no neck injuries). While using one hand to keep the patient's head extended and the mask tightly sealed to the patient's face, the health care provider uses the other hand to compress the bag (see Figure 34-19).

In addition to providing adequate ventilation, bag-mask devices can provide high FiO_2. Theoretically, all such devices on the market can deliver 100% O_2; however, the actual FiO_2 provided at the bedside depends on several factors, including O_2 input flow, reservoir volume, delivered volume and rate, and bag refill time. As a guideline to achieve the highest possible FiO_2 with a bag-mask device, the following should always be done:

1. Use an O_2 reservoir of adequate size
2. Set O_2 input flow at 10 to 15 L/min
3. Deliver appropriate V_T for a 1-second period (when using a mask)
4. Ensure the longest possible bag refill time

Hazards and Troubleshooting

Bag-mask devices are simple and safe advanced life support devices. However, several major hazards are associated with their use. The first and most common problem is unrecognized equipment failure. Knowledge of how such devices operate can help clinicians understand the operational testing of and troubleshooting for these devices.

Gastric inflation is another common hazard encountered when using a bag-valve device with a face mask. Gastric inflation can be minimized by providing low to moderate inspiratory flows (<30 L/min).[23] For an adult, a full 1 second should be used to deliver V_T of 500 ml.

Barotrauma has long been recognized as a potential hazard of bag-mask device use. However, with the full-bag volume of adult-size devices (generally ≤2000 ml), the potential for barotrauma is small if the nonrebreathing valve is working properly, and a bronchial intubation has not occurred. The average mask leak with bag-mask devices ranges from 20% to 40% of stroke volume and substantially reduces the risk of barotrauma, especially if visible chest rise is used to determine adequate V_T. Some pediatric bag-mask devices have bag volumes of more than 500 ml, and rescuers may cause barotrauma to small children or infants if they do not adjust stroke volume by squeezing the bag so that only one-half to one-third of the volume is delivered to the mask.

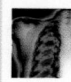

Hyperventilation during resuscitation of a cardiac arrest victim markedly decreases coronary perfusion pressure and survival rates.[30] Overzealous ventilation with high rates (>12 breaths/min) during resuscitation of cardiac arrest increases intrathoracic pressure, impedes venous return, decreases cardiac output, decreases coronary artery perfusion pressure, increases gastric inflation, and provides more ventilation than is needed.

MINI CLINI

Ventilation During Cardiopulmonary Resuscitation

PROBLEM: A student is observing a Code Blue in progress in the intensive care unit. The patient has had a cardiac arrest, and CPR is being administered. The student notices that the RT is ventilating the patient's lungs with a bag-valve device through an endotracheal tube at a considerably higher rate and minute ventilation than one would normally establish on a mechanical ventilator for a patient of this size. Is this increased minute ventilation needed?

SOLUTION: No, it is not. The ventilation rate should be 8 to 10 breaths/min, and V_T should be limited to achieve chest rise to avoid excessive ventilation.[30] Ventilation rates greater than 12 breaths/min and large V_T (>6 to 7 ml/kg) increase intrathoracic pressure and impede venous return to the heart during chest compressions.[30] During CPR, hyperventilation reduces cardiac output and decreases coronary and cerebral perfusion. Increases in central venous pressure, as a result of increased intrathoracic pressure, can decrease cerebral blood flow. Increased airway pressures and auto-PEEP generated by hyperventilation should be avoided. The AHA 2010 guidelines for CPR and emergency cardiovascular care state that "routine hyperventilation during and after cardiac arrest is detrimental and it is considered a Class III procedure" (i.e., the risk is greater than the benefit).[4] Ventilation with V_T of 500 to 600 ml at rates of one breath every 6 to 8 seconds is all that is needed to maintain a normocarbic level during CPR.

Restoring Cardiac Function

Perfusion support techniques, such as chest compressions, can restore circulation only temporarily. ACLS must go beyond simple perfusion support to identify and remove, or relieve the underlying cause of cardiac failure; this is done by combining ECG monitoring with pharmacologic and electrical therapies.

Electrocardiogram Monitoring

Because most cases of cardiac arrest are caused by arrhythmias, ECG monitoring should be started as soon as the necessary equipment and personnel arrive. Monitoring may be done with either standard electrocardiographic equipment or the quick-look paddles now available on most defibrillators.

Given their important role in ACLS, RTs must be skilled in recognizing arrhythmias. Although an experienced RT may be able to interpret quickly gross arrhythmias appearing on electrocardiographic monitors at the bedside, these skills develop only after much practice with actual rhythm strips. Chapter 17 presents a review of ECG interpretation. The reader should focus on the following arrhythmias:

- VT
- VF
- Sinus tachycardia
- Sinus bradycardia
- Sinus arrest
- Premature atrial contractions
- Supraventricular tachycardia (SVT)—a classification of arrhythmias, including but not limited to:
  - Sinus tachycardia
  - Atrial flutter
  - Atrial fibrillation
- Atrioventricular blocks—first degree, second degree types I and II, and third degree
- Premature ventricular contractions
- Pulseless electrical activity (PEA)
- Systole

This section briefly discusses the arrhythmias closely associated with CPR conditions, including SVT, VT, VF, and PEA.

Supraventricular Tachycardia. The term *supraventricular tachycardia* is commonly used to describe any tachycardia not of ventricular origin. This grouping can include sinus tachycardia, atrial tachycardia, junctional tachycardia, atrial flutter, and atrial fibrillation (with rates >100 beats/min). These individual supraventricular arrhythmias are identified by ECG and treated accordingly (Figure 34-21).

A more specific form of SVT involves rapid impulse formation caused by a reentry mechanism that develops in the atria or atrioventricular junction. Normally, a single impulse from the sinoatrial node traverses the atria and continues down into the ventricles, causing depolarization and contraction. In reentry, an ectopic focus disrupts this normal conduction. The impulse not only moves down to the ventricles but also returns to the atria. This pattern repeats in a self-perpetuating, or circular, manner.

Typically, this form of SVT results in heart rates between 160 beats/min and 220 beats/min. The rhythm is regular, which distinguishes it from rapid atrial fibrillation. However, because of its rapid rate, P waves may not be seen. If identifiable, the P waves appear abnormal. In addition to the rate and regular rhythm, SVT is characterized by a normal QRS complex. At very high rates, the ventricles may not have enough time to fill completely. Incomplete ventricular filling can result in decreased cardiac output, congestive heart failure, and tissue hypoxia. SVT may deteriorate to VT if it is not recognized and treated in a timely manner.

The treatment of SVT varies according to the clinical situation (Figure 34-22). If a patient with SVT is ill or unstable, the treatment of choice is immediate synchronized electrical cardioversion as described elsewhere in this chapter. If the patient is stable, other interventions are tried before cardioversion is considered. The most common nonelectrical treatment for SVT is vagal stimulation by carotid artery massage or Valsalva maneuver. If these attempts are ineffective and the patient remains stable, drugs such as adenosine, diltiazem, verapamil, or beta blockers (as a second-line agent) may halt SVT. These drugs work primarily on the nodal tissue by slowing ventricular response to atrial arrhythmias, or they block the reentry SVT that travels through the atrioventricular node.

Ventricular Tachycardia. VT occurs when one or more irritable foci within the ventricle discharge at rapid rates, creating the appearance of a prolonged chain of premature ventricular contractions. Rates typically range from 140 to 220 beats/min and usually are regular (Figure 34-23).

Although VT may come and go in brief episodes, or *paroxysms,* it is always a sign of a serious underlying pathologic condition and should be treated immediately. In stable patients, VT is managed with amiodarone.[31] Alternative drugs for wide-complex regular tachycardias are procainamide and sotalol.[32] For patients with sustained VT who exhibit hypotension, ischemic chest pain, shortness of breath, decreased consciousness, or signs of pulmonary edema, immediate **synchronized cardioversion** is indicated (Figure 34-24). Patients with sustained VT in full cardiac arrest are treated similarly to patients with VF.

Ventricular Fibrillation. VF is a rapid, sustained, and uncontrolled depolarization of the ventricles. During VF, the ECG is characterized by irregular, widened, and poorly defined QRS complexes, known as *coarse* VF (Figure 34-25, *A*). These complexes widen farther and lose amplitude, resembling a coarse asystole, which now is defined as *fine* VF (Figure 34-25, *B*). Rather than exhibiting coordinated contractions, the ventricles quiver in a totally disorganized manner. Cardiac output during VF is zero. The rapid

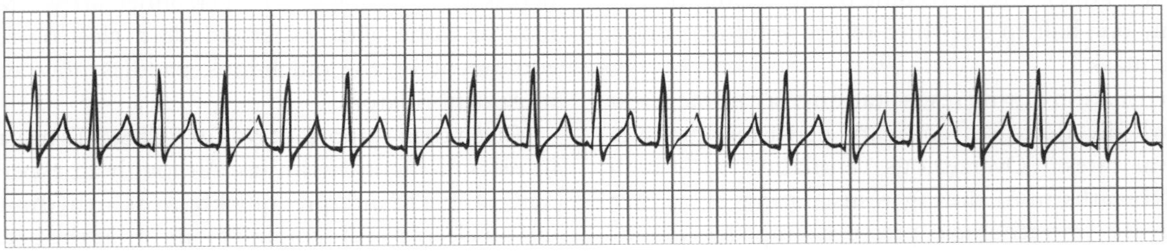

FIGURE 34-21 SVT, lead II.

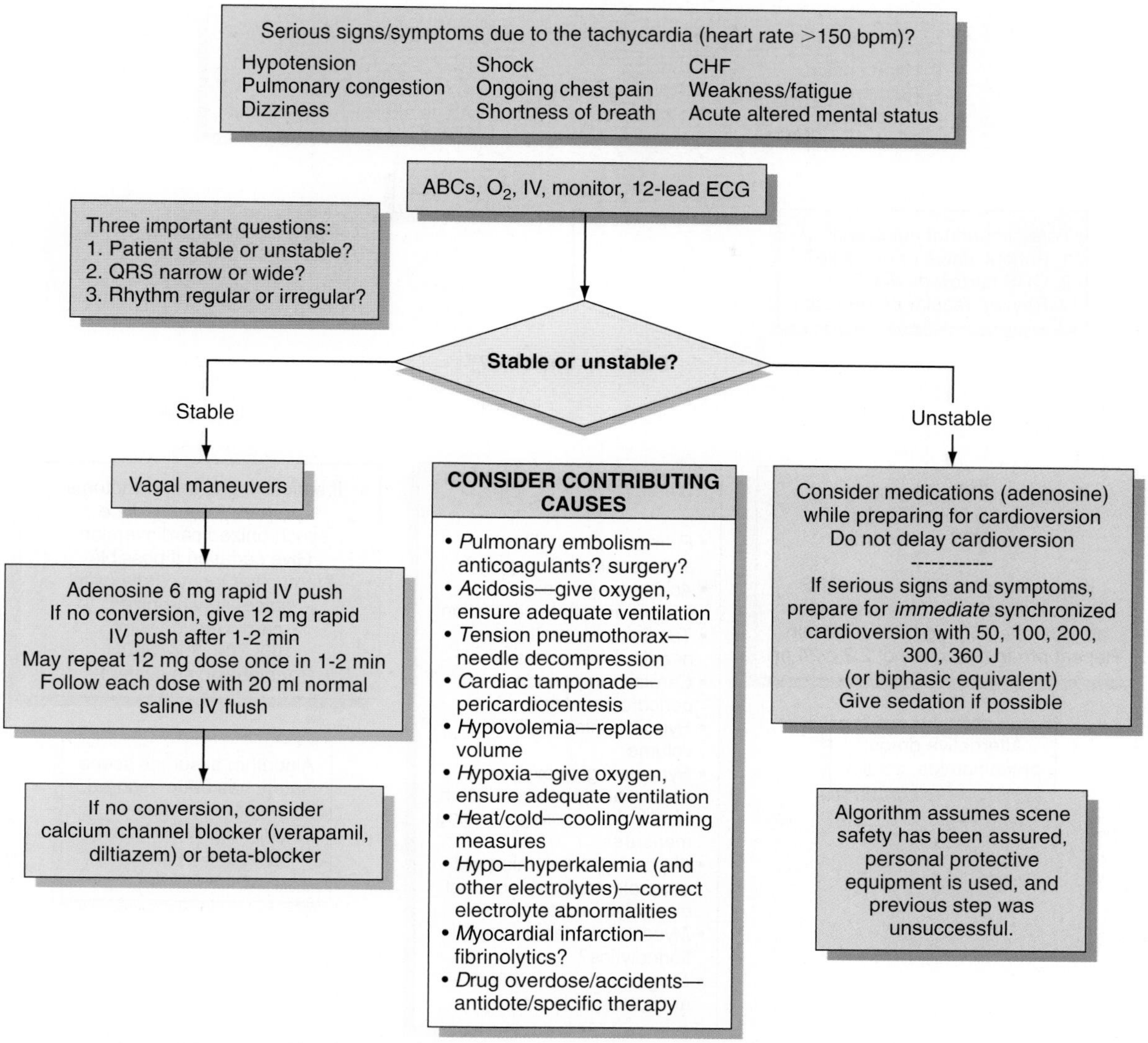
Serious signs/symptoms due to the tachycardia (heart rate >150 bpm)?
Hypotension
Pulmonary congestion
Dizziness
Shock
Ongoing chest pain
Shortness of breath
CHF
Weakness/fatigue
Acute altered mental status
ABCs, O_2, IV, monitor, 12-lead ECG
Three important questions:
1. Patient stable or unstable?
2. QRS narrow or wide?
3. Rhythm regular or irregular?
Stable or unstable?
Stable
Unstable
Vagal maneuvers
Adenosine 6 mg rapid IV push
If no conversion, give 12 mg rapid IV push after 1-2 min
May repeat 12 mg dose once in 1-2 min
Follow each dose with 20 ml normal saline IV flush
If no conversion, consider calcium channel blocker (verapamil, diltiazem) or beta-blocker
CONSIDER CONTRIBUTING CAUSES
• Pulmonary embolism—anticoagulants? surgery?
• Acidosis—give oxygen, ensure adequate ventilation
• Tension pneumothorax—needle decompression
• Cardiac tamponade—pericardiocentesis
• Hypovolemia—replace volume
• Hypoxia—give oxygen, ensure adequate ventilation
• Heat/cold—cooling/warming measures
• Hypo—hyperkalemia (and other electrolytes)—correct electrolyte abnormalities
• Myocardial infarction—fibrinolytics?
• Drug overdose/accidents—antidote/specific therapy
Consider medications (adenosine) while preparing for cardioversion
Do not delay cardioversion

If serious signs and symptoms, prepare for immediate synchronized cardioversion with 50, 100, 200, 300, 360 J
(or biphasic equivalent)
Give sedation if possible
Algorithm assumes scene safety has been assured, personal protective equipment is used, and previous step was unsuccessful.

FIGURE 34-22 Narrow-complex QRS tachycardia. (From Aehlert B: ACLS study guide, ed 4, St. Louis, 2012, Mosby.)

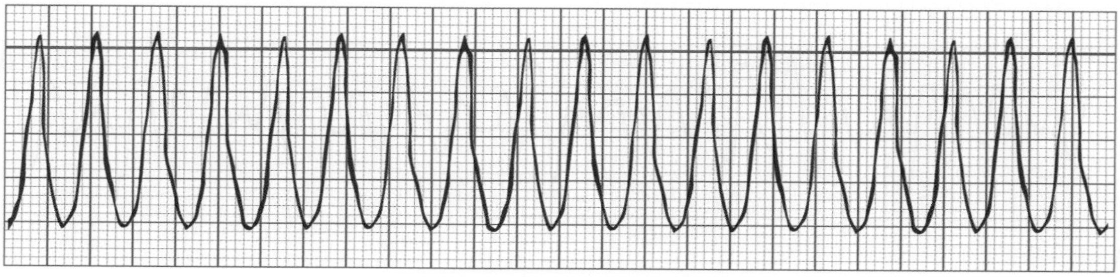

FIGURE 34-23 VT, lead II.

decrease in cardiac output produces an acute cerebral hypoxia, often manifested by convulsions. VF is uniformly fatal if not corrected immediately.

Many conditions cause VF. The most common causes include electrical shock, anesthesia, mechanical irritation of the heart, severe hypoxia, myocardial infarction, and large doses of digitalis or epinephrine. Regardless of the cause, VF constitutes a true emergency. Patient survival depends on immediate provision of ACLS, especially electrical defibrillation. Early defibrillation is the major determinant of survival in cardiac arrest caused by VF.

Pulseless Electrical Activity. PEA that is not shockable can result from several reversible causes (Figure 34-26). The immediate primary treatment is uninterrupted CPR

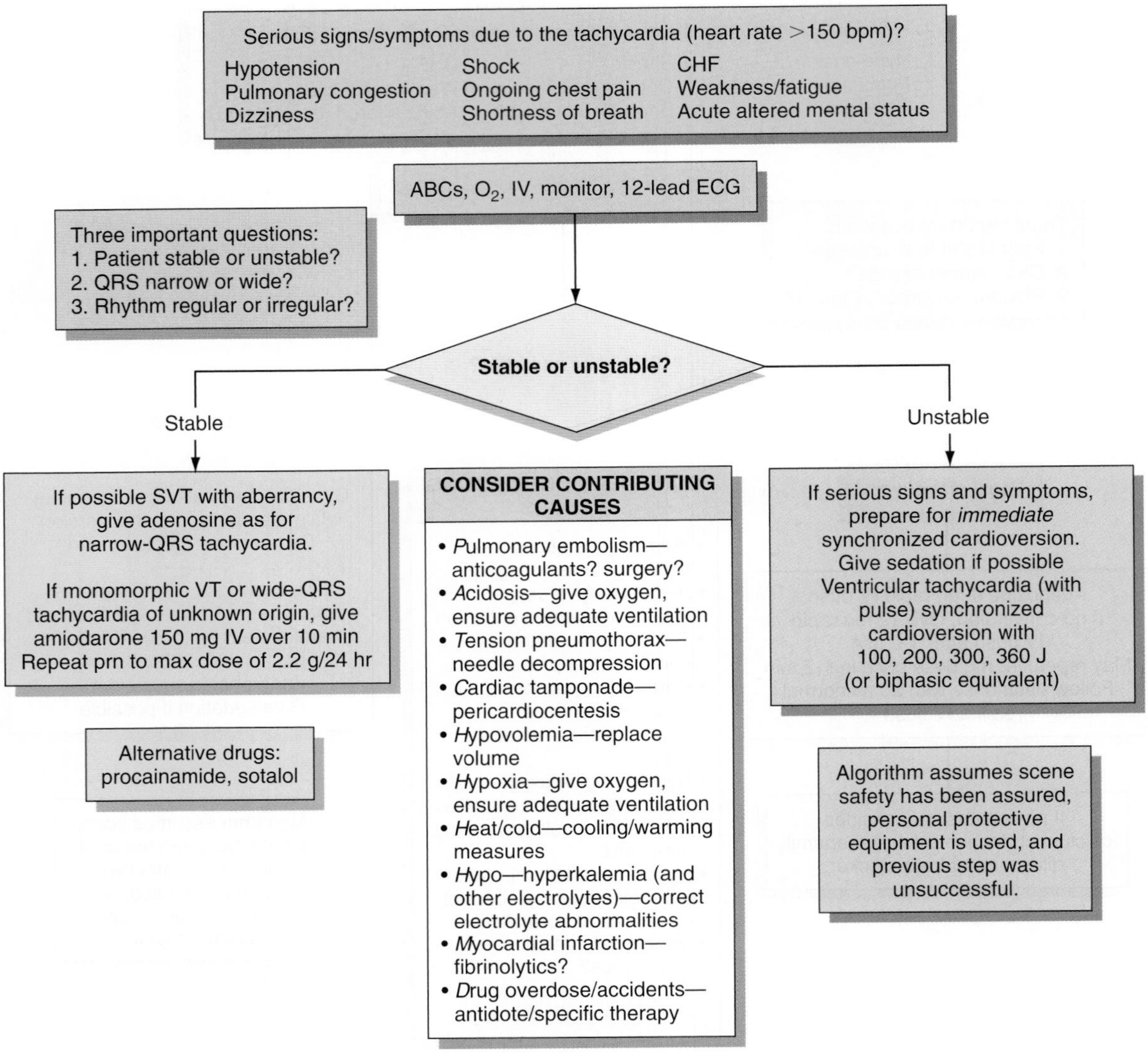

Serious signs/symptoms due to the tachycardia (heart rate >150 bpm)?
Hypotension
Pulmonary congestion
Dizziness
Shock
Ongoing chest pain
Shortness of breath
CHF
Weakness/fatigue
Acute altered mental status
ABCs, O_2, IV, monitor, 12-lead ECG
Three important questions:
1. Patient stable or unstable?
2. QRS narrow or wide?
3. Rhythm regular or irregular?
Stable or unstable?
Stable
Unstable
If possible SVT with aberrancy, give adenosine as for narrow-QRS tachycardia.
If monomorphic VT or wide-QRS tachycardia of unknown origin, give amiodarone 150 mg IV over 10 min Repeat prn to max dose of 2.2 g/24 hr
Alternative drugs: procainamide, sotalol
CONSIDER CONTRIBUTING CAUSES
• Pulmonary embolism—anticoagulants? surgery?
• Acidosis—give oxygen, ensure adequate ventilation
• Tension pneumothorax—needle decompression
• Cardiac tamponade—pericardiocentesis
• Hypovolemia—replace volume
• Hypoxia—give oxygen, ensure adequate ventilation
• Heat/cold—cooling/warming measures
• Hypo—hyperkalemia (and other electrolytes)—correct electrolyte abnormalities
• Myocardial infarction—fibrinolytics?
• Drug overdose/accidents—antidote/specific therapy
If serious signs and symptoms, prepare for *immediate* synchronized cardioversion. Give sedation if possible Ventricular tachycardia (with pulse) synchronized cardioversion with 100, 200, 300, 360 J (or biphasic equivalent)
Algorithm assumes scene safety has been assured, personal protective equipment is used, and previous step was unsuccessful.

FIGURE 34-24 Wide-complex QRS tachycardia. (From Aehlert B: ACLS study guide, ed 4, St. Louis, 2012, Mosby.)

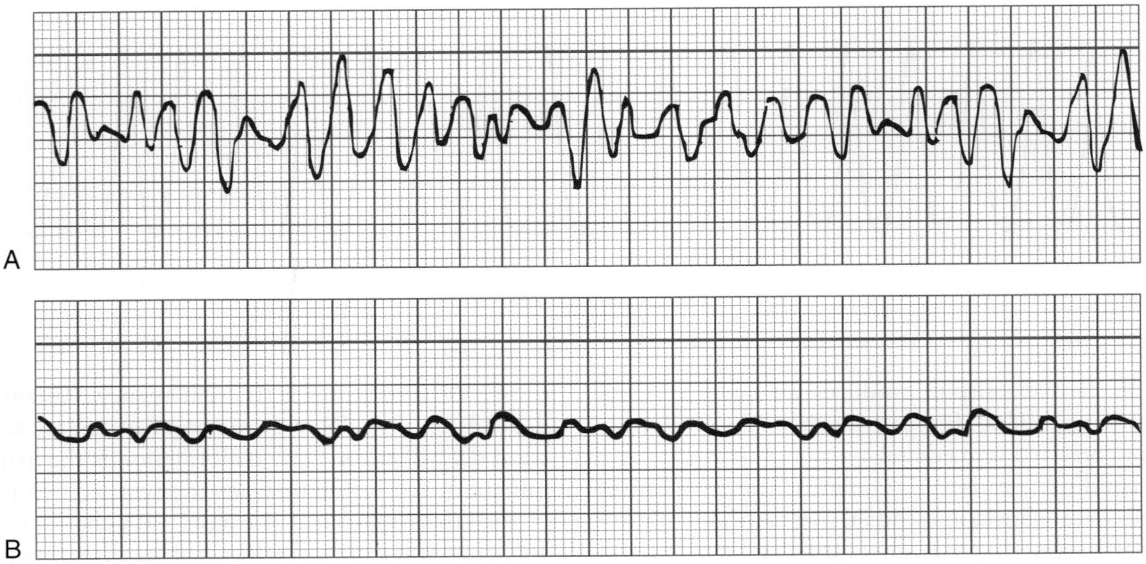

FIGURE 34-25 VF. **A,** Coarse VF. **B,** Fine VF, lead II.

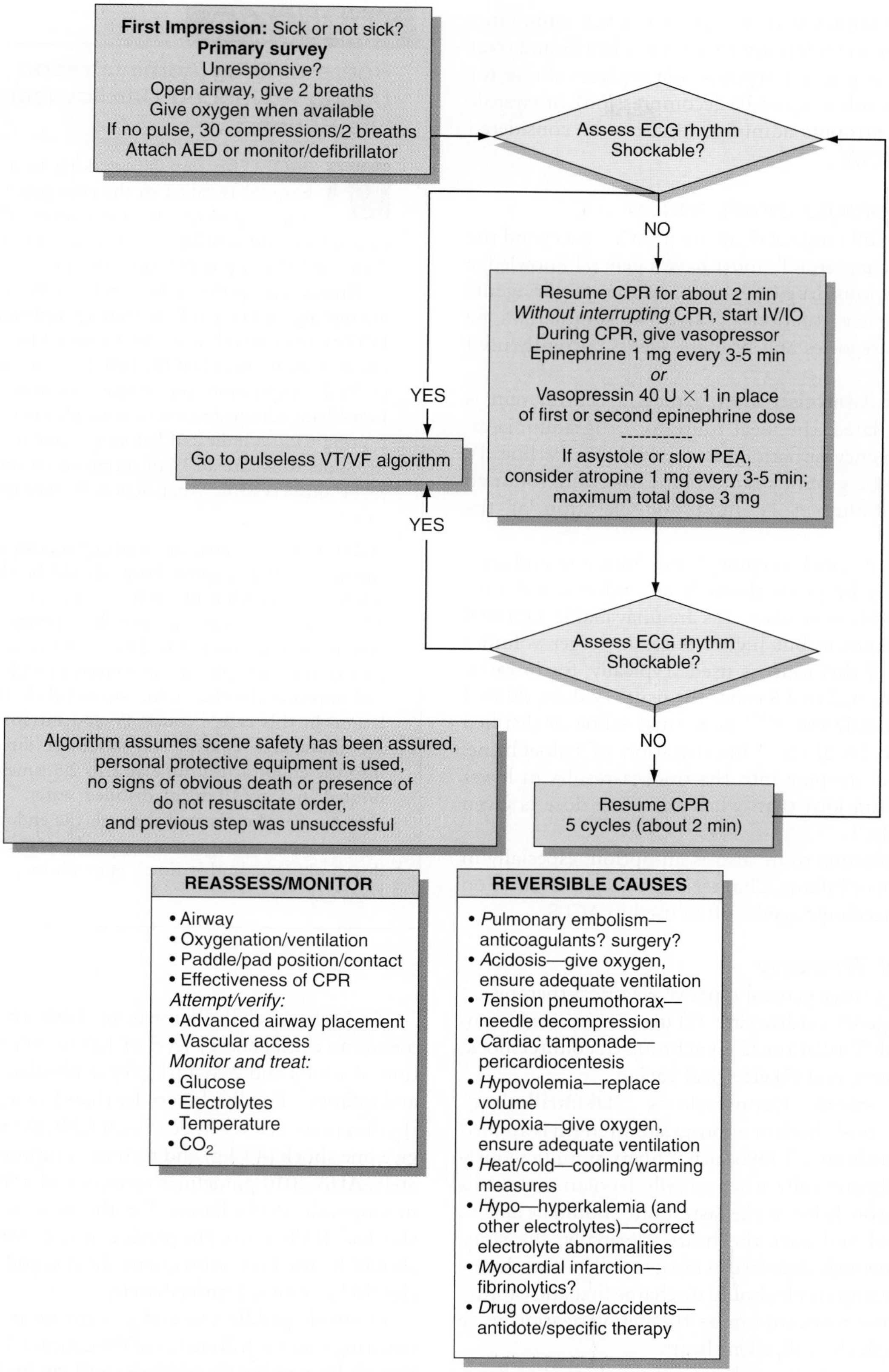
First Impression: Sick or not sick?
Primary survey
Unresponsive?
Open airway, give 2 breaths
Give oxygen when available
If no pulse, 30 compressions/2 breaths
Attach AED or monitor/defibrillator
Assess ECG rhythm
Shockable?
NO
YES
Resume CPR for about 2 min
Without interrupting CPR, start IV/IO
During CPR, give vasopressor
Epinephrine 1 mg every 3-5 min
or
Vasopressin 40 U × 1 in place
of first or second epinephrine dose
If asystole or slow PEA,
consider atropine 1 mg every 3-5 min;
maximum total dose 3 mg
Go to pulseless VT/VF algorithm
YES
Assess ECG rhythm
Shockable?
NO
Algorithm assumes scene safety has been assured,
personal protective equipment is used,
no signs of obvious death or presence of
do not resuscitate order,
and previous step was unsuccessful
Resume CPR
5 cycles (about 2 min)
REASSESS/MONITOR
• Airway
• Oxygenation/ventilation
• Paddle/pad position/contact
• Effectiveness of CPR
Attempt/verify:
• Advanced airway placement
• Vascular access
Monitor and treat:
• Glucose
• Electrolytes
• Temperature
• CO2
REVERSIBLE CAUSES
• Pulmonary embolism—
anticoagulants? surgery?
• Acidosis—give oxygen,
ensure adequate ventilation
• Tension pneumothorax—
needle decompression
• Cardiac tamponade—
pericardiocentesis
• Hypovolemia—replace
volume
• Hypoxia—give oxygen,
ensure adequate ventilation
• Heat/cold—cooling/warming
measures
• Hypo—hyperkalemia (and
other electrolytes)—correct
electrolyte abnormalities
• Myocardial infarction—
fibrinolytics?
• Drug overdose/accidents—
antidote/specific therapy

FIGURE 34-26 Asystole or PEA algorithm. (From Aehlert B: ACLS study guide, ed 4, St. Louis, 2012, Mosby.)

for about 2 minutes with vasopressor given simultaneously. The best secondary approach is to identify and treat reversible causes (e.g., for hypovolemia, replace volume; for tension pneumothorax, needle decompression). In asystole or slow PEA, atropine administration can be considered (see Figure 34-26).

Pharmacologic Intervention

Although the full range of drug use in ACLS is beyond the scope of this chapter, RTs must have a general knowledge of both the various drug categories and the specific agents used in emergency situations.[33] Table 34-2 summarizes the major drug categories and primary agents currently used in ACLS.

Routes of Administration. Unless a central vein is already cannulated, the ideal route for drug administration in emergency situations is a peripheral IV line. IV drugs should be given by rapid bolus injection, followed by a 20-ml bolus of IV fluid and elevation of the extremity.

Selected drugs, such as epinephrine, lidocaine, and atropine, also may be given through an endotracheal tube when IV and intraosseous access are unavailable. Optimal doses are unknown, but higher doses in larger volumes are necessary if this route is used. Typically, for intratracheal instillation, 2 to 2.5 times the usual IV dose, diluted in 10 ml of sterile water[34,35] or normal saline or distilled water, should be given. Administration of epinephrine, lidocaine, and atropine into the trachea results in lower blood concentrations than when the same dose is given intravascularly.[32]

The intraosseous route also is an option, especially in small children or infants. Chapter 32 provides information about pharmacologic agents often used in ACLS.

MINI CLINI

Route of Drug Administration During Advanced Cardiovascular Life Support

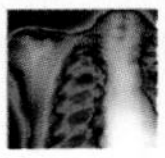

PROBLEM: An RT working in a small, rural hospital is called to the emergency department where a patient is in cardiac arrest. The RT is able to intubate and ventilate the patient, using a bag-valve device at 100% inspired O_2 concentration.

Nurses are performing cardiac compressions and attempting unsuccessfully to start a peripheral IV line. The ECG monitor reveals a fine VF pattern. Electrical defibrillation is unsuccessful on the first attempt, and five cycles of 30 : 2 compression-to-ventilation ratio are in progress. Immediate administration of epinephrine without interrupting CPR is indicated before or after the next shock. Attempts to secure an IV or intraosseous route continue to be unsuccessful. What action is appropriate at this time?

SOLUTION: Because of its strong inotropic and alpha-adrenergic effects, epinephrine should be the first drug during resuscitation of cardiac arrest, and it should be administered as soon as possible. Drugs given via a peripheral vein require 1 to 2 minutes to reach the central circulation. Epinephrine can convert fine VF to coarse VF and improves the chance for successful electrical defibrillation. In this case, because IV and intraosseous routes are unavailable, epinephrine should be directly instilled into the endotracheal tube at 2 to 2.5 times the IV dose diluted in 5 to 10 ml of distilled water.[32] Other drugs that can be administered through the endotracheal tube are naloxone, atropine, vasopressin (direct instillation dose unknown at this time), epinephrine, and lidocaine *(NAVEL)*.

Electrical Therapy

The following three general types of electrical therapy are used in emergency cardiac care: (1) unsynchronized countershock, or defibrillation; (2) synchronized countershock, or cardioversion; and (3) electrical pacing.

Unsynchronized Countershock (Defibrillation). When an electrical shock of appropriate strength is applied to the myocardium, all myocardial fibers simultaneously depolarize. Theoretically, when all cells depolarize, the cells that spontaneously fire at the fastest rate should be able to regain control and pace the heart. Normally, the sinus node spontaneously depolarizes most rapidly. After electrical shock, the sinus node should discharge first and capture all parts of the myocardium as the depolarization wave travels through the still, silent heart.

Defibrillation is an unsynchronized shock used to depolarize the myocardial fibers simultaneously. It is the definitive treatment for both VF and pulseless VT. If one of these arrhythmias is present, and the proper equipment and trained personnel are available, defibrillation of the patient should be performed immediately.

If a biphasic defibrillator is available, the AHA recommends an initial energy level of 120 to 200 J for defibrillation of adults and 2 to 4 J/kg for defibrillation of children and infants.[15] For children older than 1 year, if a shockable rhythm persists after five cycles of CPR, the rescuer should give one shock (4 J/kg) and resume compressions immediately. AHA 2010 guidelines recommend a 360-J shock for monophasic defibrillators for the first and subsequent shocks.[15] If VF recurs, the previously successful energy level should be used for subsequent shocks, and compressions should be resumed immediately.

Electrode paddle size and placement are important in ensuring that the full energy of the countershock is applied. For adults, paddles should be 8 to 12 cm in diameter; adult paddles are adequate size for children older than 1 year. Normally, one paddle is placed below the clavicle and just to the right of the upper portion of the sternum, with the other positioned on the midaxillary line to the left of the left nipple. Alternatively, one paddle may be placed on

TABLE 34-2

Drugs Used in Advanced Cardiovascular Life Support

Drug	Indications	Contraindications	Route	Dosage	Pharmacologic Effects
Adenosine	PSVT	Use with caution if patient has asthma; poison-induced or drug-induced tachycardia; second-degree or third-degree heart block	IV bolus	6 mg IV for 1-2 sec followed by 20-ml saline bolus; repeat twice with 12 mg in 1-2 min if needed	Decrease in AV node conduction
Amiodarone	Atrial and ventricular tachyarrhythmias	Prolonged QT interval	IV; IO	150-300 mg IV over 10 min; may repeat every 10 min to maximum of 2.2 g in 24 hr	Increased PR and QT intervals; decreased sinus node function; inhibited alpha- and beta-adrenergic responses
Atropine sulfate	Sinus bradycardia; asystole; PEA; organophosphate poisoning	Sinus, atrial, and ventricular tachycardia; hypothermic bradycardia; infranodal (type II) AV block; new third-degree with wide QRS complexes	IV bolus; IO; endotracheal*	0.5-1.0 mg IV repeated every 3-5 min to total dose of 3 mg	Increased heart rate; increased force of atrial contractions
Calcium chloride	Hypokalemia; hyperkalemia; calcium channel blocker toxicity	Do not use routinely in cardiac arrest	IV (not to be mixed with other drugs)	500-1000 mg for hyperkalemia and channel blocker overdose	Increased force of contractions; increased ventricular excitability
Diuretics: furosemide (Lasix)	CHF; pulmonary edema	Hypovolemia	IV infusion	0.5-1.0 mg/kg bolus over 1-2 min; slowly increase to 2.0 mg/kg over 1-2 min if no response	Diuresis or venodilation
Dobutamine	Depressed myocardial contractility	Systolic blood pressure <100 mm Hg and signs of shock; suspected poison-induced or drug-induced shock	IV infusion	2.0-20 μg/kg/min, titrate so heart rate does not increase by >10% of baseline	Increased force of contractions; enhanced AV conduction
Dopamine	Hypotension with signs and symptoms of shock; second-line drug for symptomatic bradycardia	Use with caution in cardiogenic shock with accompanying CHF	IV infusion	2.0-20 μg/kg/min	Increased renal and splenic flow at low doses (1-5 μg/kg/min); beta-adrenergic effects at moderate doses (5-10 μg/kg/min); alpha-adrenergic effects at high doses (>10 μg/kg/min)

Continued

TABLE 34-2

Drugs Used in Advanced Cardiovascular Life Support—cont'd

Drug	Indications	Contraindications	Route	Dosage	Pharmacologic Effects
Epinephrine	Cardiac arrest; VF; pulseless tachycardia; asystole; PEA; symptomatic bradycardia; severe hypotension; anaphylaxis; severe allergic reaction	VT and frequent PVCs	IV bolus; IO; endotracheal*; IV infusion	1 mg every 3-5 min in cardiac arrest, up to 0.2 mg/kg; 2-10 μg/min infusion, titrate to patient response	Increased heart rate; increased force of contractions; vasoconstriction; increased coronary perfusion pressure; increased myocardial irritability; increased myocardial O_2 consumption
Isoproterenol	Refractory torsades de pointes unresponsive to magnesium sulfate; temporary control of bradycardia in heart transplant patients; poisoning from beta blockers	Cardiac arrest; VT; frequent PVCs	IV infusion	2-10 μg/min, titrate to adequate heart rate	Increased heart rate; increased force of contractions; vasodilation
Lidocaine	Alternative to amiodarone in cardiac arrest from VF/VT; stable monomorphic VT with preserved ventricular function; stable polymorphic VT with normal baseline QT interval and preserved left ventricular function when ischemia is treated and electrolyte balance is corrected; stable polymorphic VT with baseline QT prolongation if torsades suspected	Signs of lidocaine toxicity; prophylactic use in acute MI	IV bolus; IV infusion; IO; endotracheal†	1-1.5 mg/kg bolus every 5-10 min up to 3 mg/kg	Increased electrical stimulation threshold; depressed ventricular electrical activity
Magnesium sulfate	Cardiac arrest only if torsades de pointes or hypomagnesemia is present; life-threatening arrhythmias caused by digitalis toxicity	Routine administration in hospitalized patients with acute MI; use with caution in renal failure	IV infusion; IO infusion	Cardiac arrest: 1-2 g (2-4 mL of 50% solution) diluted in 10 mL of 5% dextrose in water over 20 min	Hypomagnesemia hinders replenishment of intracellular potassium
Norepinephrine	Cardiogenic or vasogenic shock	Hypovolemia; use with caution in patients with acute ischemia	IV infusion	0.5-1.0 μg/min, titrate to effect up to 30 μg/min	Alpha-adrenergic stimulation

Procainamide	Stable monomorphic VT with normal QT interval and preserved left ventricular function; treatment of PSVT uncontrolled by adenosine and vagal maneuvers if blood pressure is stable; stable wide-complex tachycardia of unknown origin; AF with Wolff-Parkinson-White syndrome	Heart block, asystole, PEA, proarrhythmic especially in setting of acute MI, hypokalemia, or hypomagnesemia	IV bolus; IV infusion	20 mg/min, 50 mg/min in urgent situations up to maximum dose of 17 mg/kg; 1-4 mg/min	Raised electrical stimulation threshold; depressed ventricular electrical activity; may cause hypotension
Propranolol	Suspected MI and unstable angina; SVTs	Bronchospastic disease; severe bradycardia; hypotension; second-degree or third-degree heart block; cocaine-induced acute coronary syndrome	IV	Total dose: 0.1 mg/kg by slow IV push, divided into 3 equal doses at 2- to 3-min intervals. Do not exceed 1 mg/min, repeat in 2 min up to a total dose of 0.1 mg/kg if required	Decreased heart rate; decreased stroke volume; decreased myocardial O_2 consumption; increased LVEDP
Sodium nitroprusside	Hypertension	Hypotension; CHF; reactive airway disease	IV infusion	0.1-5.0 μg/kg/min	Direct peripheral vasodilation
Vasopressin	Alternative pressor to epinephrine in treatment of adult shock-refractory VF; alternative to epinephrine in asystole and PEA, hemodynamic support in vasodilatory shock	Responsive patients with coronary artery disease	IV bolus; IO bolus	40-unit push may replace either first or second dose of epinephrine	Potent peripheral vasoconstrictor
Verapamil	Alternative drug (after adenosine) to terminate PSVT with narrow QRS complex and adequate blood pressure and preserved left ventricular function	Wide-complex QRS tachycardias of uncertain origin, Wolff-Parkinson-White syndrome and AF, sick sinus syndrome, second-degree or third-degree block without pacemaker, concurrent IV administration with IV beta blockers	IV bolus	First dose: 2.5- to 5-mg IV bolus over 2 min (over 3 min in older patients). Second dose: 5-10 mg, if needed, every 15-30 min; maximum dose 20 mg. Alternative: 5-mg bolus every 15 min to a total dose of 30 mg	Decreased sinoatrial node automaticity; slowed AV node conduction

AF, Atrial fibrillation; *AV,* atrioventricular; *CHF,* congestive heart failure; *IO,* intraosseous; *LVEDP,* left ventricular end-diastolic pressure; *MI,* myocardial infarction; *PSVT,* paroxysmal supraventricular tachycardia; *PVC,* premature ventricular contraction.

*Endotracheal tube dosage is usually double IV dosage.

†Dose of lidocaine via an endotracheal tube is 2.0-2.5 times the normal IV dose diluted in 10 mL of normal saline or sterile water to be used only when IV and IO access is unavailable.

the left precordium, with the other positioned posteriorly under the patient, behind the heart. Paddles should be prepared with conducting gel and applied with firm pressure (approximately 25 lb).

Synchronized Countershock (Cardioversion). Cardioversion is similar to defibrillation, with two major exceptions. First, the countershock is synchronized with the heart's electrical activity (the R wave). Synchronization is necessary because electrical stimulation during the refractory phase (part of the T wave) can cause VF or VT. Second, the energy used during cardioversion usually is less than the energy applied during defibrillation.

Cardioversion is considered when a patient with an organized arrhythmia producing a high ventricular rate exhibits signs or symptoms of cardiac decompensation. These so-called tachyarrhythmias include SVT, atrial flutter, atrial fibrillation, and monomorphic VT with pulses. Cardioversion is ineffective for treatment of junctional tachycardia or multifocal atrial tachycardia.[15]

If the arrhythmia is not causing serious signs or symptoms, drug therapy is used first. However, if the patient is hypotensive, exhibits signs of decreased consciousness or pulmonary congestion, or complains of chest pain, cardioversion is indicated.

Electrical Pacing. Another application of electrical therapy uses intermittently timed, low-energy discharges to replace or supplement the natural pacemaker of the heart. There are two primary types of electrical pacing. First, the electrical discharge can be delivered from an external power pack through wires inserted into the patient's chest wall (transcutaneous, or transthoracic, pacing). Alternatively, wire electrodes may be floated through the large veins and implanted directly inside the heart (transvenous pacing). Because it can be started quickly, transcutaneous pacing is the method used most often in emergency cardiac care.

Pacemaker therapy is used to treat sinus bradycardias that produce serious signs and symptoms and that do not respond to atropine (Figure 34-27). Electrical pacing also is used to manage second-degree type II and third-degree heart block. Electrical pacing also can be used to treat some tachyarrhythmias. In these cases, the pacemaker is set to discharge faster than the underlying rate. After a few seconds, the pacemaker is stopped to allow the heart's intrinsic rate to return. This is called *overdrive pacing*. Although overdrive pacing has shown promise in treating certain types of SVT and VT, pharmacologic intervention (when the patient is stable) and cardioversion (when the patient is unstable) remain the treatments of choice.

Because defibrillation can cause damage to permanent pacemakers, care should be taken not to place the electrode paddles near these devices. After a patient with a permanent pacemaker undergoes either cardioversion or defibrillation, the device should be checked for proper functioning. Pacing is not recommended by the AHA for patients in asystolic cardiac arrest because it is ineffective and may delay or interrupt the delivery of chest compressions.[15]

Monitoring During Advanced Cardiac Life Support

Although extensive monitoring is used in most critical care settings, monitoring during emergency life support is usually limited to ECG, pulse, blood pressure, and intermittent arterial blood gas (ABG) sampling. Several approaches designed to enhance knowledge of patient status during CPR have been proposed more recently. These include methods to monitor ventilation, oxygenation, and airway status better.

The ECG is the most common and one of the most useful types of monitoring used during ACLS. The ECG provides the basis for selecting various drug and electrical therapies during CPR and helps indicate patient response to these interventions. However, an acceptable ECG rhythm does not mean that cardiac output is adequate. Other indices of perfusion, such as pulse, blood pressure, and skin temperature, are needed to confirm adequate cardiac output.

Patient Care Following Resuscitation

Following cardiac arrest, a patient may exhibit an optimal response, in which case the patient regains consciousness, is responsive, and breathes spontaneously. More often, however, the patient requires support of one or more organ systems. Acidemia associated with cardiac arrest usually improves when normal ventilation and perfusion are restored.

If the patient is conscious and breathing spontaneously after resuscitation, supplemental O_2, maintenance of an IV infusion, and continuous cardiac and hemodynamic monitoring may be all that is necessary. A 12-lead ECG, chest x-ray, ABG analysis, and clinical chemistry profile should be obtained as soon as possible. The 2010 AHA guidelines recommend that providers of care after cardiac arrest should "(1) control body temperature to optimize survival and neurological recovery; (2) identify and treat acute coronary syndromes; (3) optimize mechanical ventilation to minimize lung injury; (4) reduce the risk of multiorgan injury and support organ function if required; (5) objectively assess prognosis for recovery; and (6) assist survivors with rehabilitation services when required."[36] The patient should be closely supervised in an intensive care or coronary care unit, especially during the first 24 hours after a cardiac arrest.[37]

Only in this setting can underlying organ system insufficiency or failure be properly identified and managed.[37] The organs most likely to exhibit failure after resuscitation are the lung, heart and vasculature, and kidneys. Central nervous system failure is an ominous sign and generally indicates a failed resuscitation attempt.

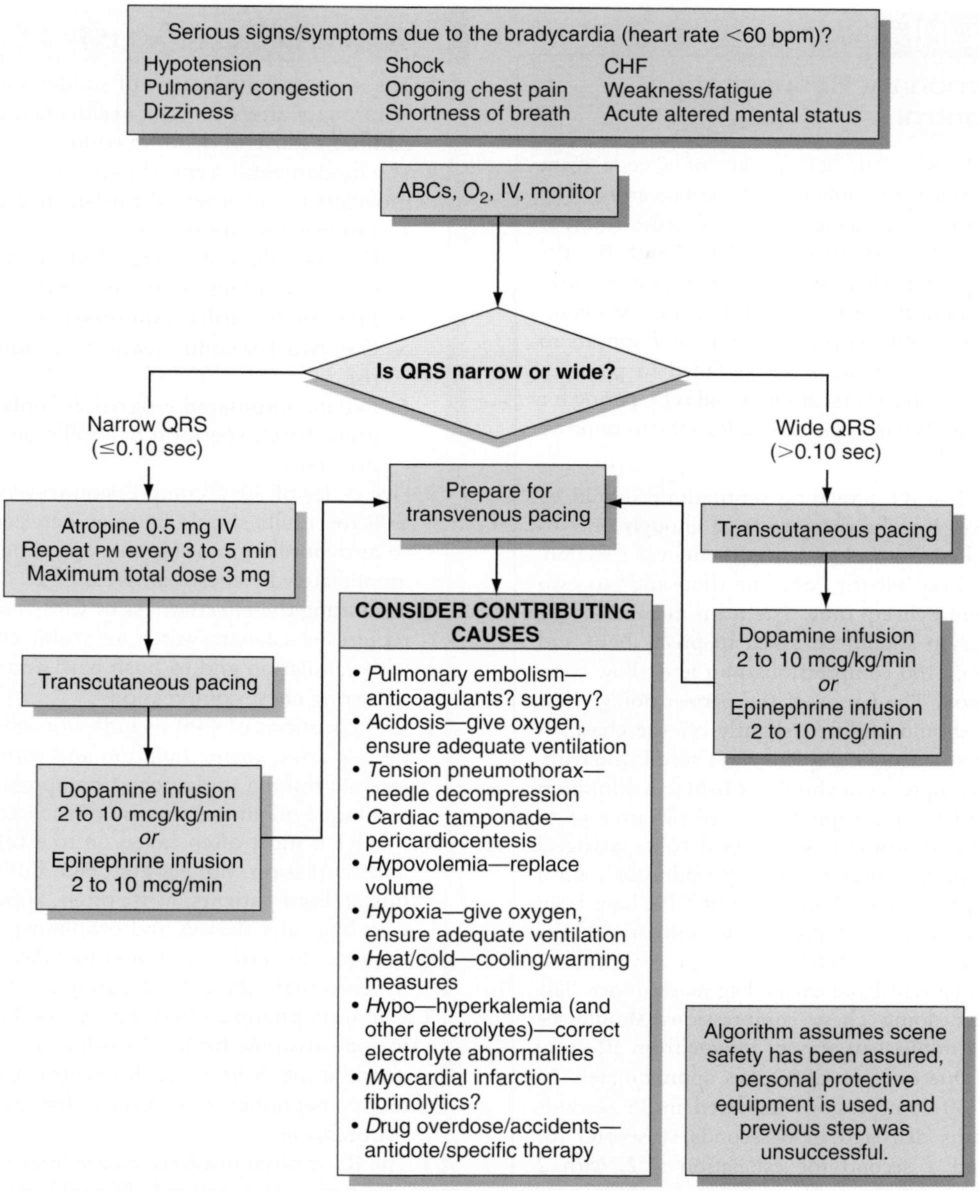
Serious signs/symptoms due to the bradycardia (heart rate <60 bpm)?
Hypotension
Pulmonary congestion
Dizziness
Shock
Ongoing chest pain
Shortness of breath
CHF
Weakness/fatigue
Acute altered mental status
ABCs, O2, IV, monitor
Is QRS narrow or wide?
Narrow QRS (≤0.10 sec)
Wide QRS (>0.10 sec)
Atropine 0.5 mg IV
Repeat PM every 3 to 5 min
Maximum total dose 3 mg
Transcutaneous pacing
Dopamine infusion
2 to 10 mcg/kg/min
or
Epinephrine infusion
2 to 10 mcg/min
Prepare for transvenous pacing
Transcutaneous pacing
Dopamine infusion
2 to 10 mcg/kg/min
or
Epinephrine infusion
2 to 10 mcg/min
CONSIDER CONTRIBUTING CAUSES
• Pulmonary embolism—anticoagulants? surgery?
• Acidosis—give oxygen, ensure adequate ventilation
• Tension pneumothorax—needle decompression
• Cardiac tamponade—pericardiocentesis
• Hypovolemia—replace volume
• Hypoxia—give oxygen, ensure adequate ventilation
• Heat/cold—cooling/warming measures
• Hypo—hyperkalemia (and other electrolytes)—correct electrolyte abnormalities
• Myocardial infarction—fibrinolytics?
• Drug overdose/accidents—antidote/specific therapy
Algorithm assumes scene safety has been assured, personal protective equipment is used, and previous step was unsuccessful.

FIGURE 34-27 Symptomatic bradycardia algorithm. (From Aehlert B: ACLS study guide, ed 4, St. Louis, 2012, Mosby.)

Respiratory Management

If the patient remains apneic or exhibits irregular breathing after resuscitation, mechanical ventilation is instituted through a properly positioned endotracheal tube, with an initial O_2 concentration of 100%. ABGs, preferably obtained through an arterial line, are analyzed as needed until the oxygenation and acid-base status of the patient stabilize. ABG analysis also helps differentiate between pulmonary and nonpulmonary (or cardiac) causes of hypoxemia and tissue hypoxia. Mechanical ventilation is adjusted to maintain a normal $PaCO_2$ level. Hyperventilation is detrimental and should be avoided. Higher ventilatory rates and larger V_T may cause hyperventilation. This hyperventilation may generate increased airway pressures and auto-PEEP, leading to an increase in cerebral venous and intracranial pressures and a decrease in coronary artery and cerebral arterial pressures.[38] Cerebral blood flow may decrease, causing increased brain ischemia, if hyperventilation results in increased intrathoracic pressure. For details of the selection and use of mechanical ventilators and appropriate patient monitoring procedures, see Chapters 41 to 46.

Cardiovascular Management

The 12-lead ECG, chest x-ray, clinical chemistry profile, cardiac enzyme results, and current and past drug histories should be reviewed. Invasive hemodynamic monitoring

MINI CLINI

Cardiopulmonary Resuscitation Quality Control

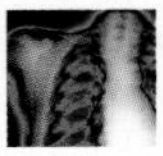

PROBLEM: The RT is part of a code team resuscitating a patient in VF cardiac arrest. The RT notices several quality control issues: Another therapist is providing bag-mask ventilation with breaths that are too large and delivered with a fast inspiratory flow. Another member of the team is administering chest compressions at rate of 80 compressions/min and appears to be tiring. A house-staff member has failed to place an endotracheal tube on the first attempt and is preparing for a second attempt. What steps can the RT take to improve the quality of CPR?

SOLUTION: The RT providing ventilations should be asked to deliver breaths that are large enough only to create visible chest rise and to deliver them over 1 second. The RT should say silently "one-one thousand" to estimate a 1-second delivery time. The team member doing chest compression should be asked to push "hard and fast" at a rate of 100 compressions/min and allow complete chest recoil. The hands of the person doing chest compressions should be lifted slightly off the chest on each upstroke to ensure complete chest recoil. Interruptions in chest compressions should be held to a minimum and should not be interrupted by a second attempt to place an advanced airway (endotracheal tube, laryngeal mask airway, double-lumen airway [Combitube]) until five cycles (approximately 2 minutes) of CPR have been completed using a 30:2 compression-to-ventilation ratio. Postponing the second intubation attempt assumes that the victim can be ventilated with a bag-mask device. The team members doing chest compressions should be rotated every 2 minutes to prevent fatigue from affecting performance. One cycle of CPR takes approximately 24 seconds with 30 compressions delivered in 18 seconds and two breaths delivered in 6 seconds (1 second for inspiration and 1 second for exhalation × 2, with 2 seconds lost to transitioning between compressions and ventilation). Perfect CPR would result in 75 compressions and five breaths being delivered each minute. Code team members should not stop CPR to check the rhythm or a pulse immediately after shock delivery. After the shock, they should immediately administer five cycles of uninterrupted CPR beginning with chest compressions and should check the rhythm and pulse after about 2 minutes.

may be needed to monitor blood pressure and cardiac output. This monitoring provides needed data on the adequacy of vascular volumes, left ventricular performance, and overall tissue perfusion. Based on these data, judgments can be made regarding the need for fluid therapy and the selection and use of appropriate drugs.

SUMMARY CHECKLIST

- The most common cause of sudden death in adults is coronary artery disease; accidents are the most common cause of death in young people.
- The fundamental steps of basic CPR of health care providers for a witnessed cardiac arrest are as follows:
  1. Confirm unresponsiveness.
  2. Call for help and activate EMS system.
  3. Check for a pulse (<10 seconds).
  4. Perform 30 cardiac compressions
  5. Give two 1-second breaths to produce visible chest rise.
  6. Initiate automated external defibrillation immediately (perform defibrillation as soon as possible).
- Five cycles of 30:2 compression-to-ventilation ratio CPR for adults should be given between attempts to at defibrillation using only one shock followed immediately by chest compressions.
- Evaluating the effectiveness of CPR is important and requires rescuers to watch for visible chest rise and fall with ventilation and to push hard and fast when delivering chest compression.
- Complications of CPR include worsening of potential neck injuries, gastric inflation and vomiting, and internal trauma during chest compressions. Correct technique minimizes the risk of such complications.
- The RT is most often called on to establish an airway and ventilation with elevated FiO_2 during ACLS of hospitalized patients. Most often, knowledge and skill with bag-valve devices and oropharyngeal airways are required. Special care should be taken not to hyperventilate the patient during or after cardiac arrest.
- Common pharmacologic agents used during ACLS include atropine for bradycardia, epinephrine and amiodarone or lidocaine for ventricular arrhythmias, and epinephrine or vasopressin for cardiac arrest and hypotension.
- The RT is often involved in care after cardiac arrest of a victim who responds favorably to CPR. In the postresuscitative phase, the RT may need to maintain normal ventilation and oxygenation and assist the physician and nurses in monitoring the patient's condition.

References

1. Lloyd-Jones D, Adams RJ, Brown TM, et al: American Heart Association Statistics Committee and Stroke Statistics Subcommittee: Heart disease and stroke statistics—2010 update: a report from the American Heart Association. Circulation 121:e46, 2010.
2. Nichol G, Thomas E, Callaway CW, et al: Regional variation in out-of-hospital cardiac arrest incidence and outcome. JAMA 300:1423, 2008.
3. Nadkarni VM, Larkin GL, Peberdy MA, et al: First documented rhythm and clinical outcome from in-hospital cardiac arrest among children and adults. JAMA 295:50, 2006.

4. American Heart Association 2010 Guidelines for cardiopulmonary resuscitation and emergency cardiovascular care. Part 5. Adult basic life support. Circulation 122:S639, 2010.
5. Aufderheide TP, Pirrallo RG, Yannopoulos D, et al: Incomplete chest wall decompression: a clinical evaluation of CPR performance by EMS personnel and assessment of alternative manual chest-decompression techniques. Resuscitation 64:353, 2005.
6. Handley AJ: Teaching hand placement for chest compression—a simpler technique. Resuscitation 53:29, 2002.
7. American Heart Association 2010 guidelines for cardiopulmonary resuscitation and emergency cardiovascular care. Part 15: Neonatal resuscitation guidelines. Circulation 122:S639, 2010.
8. Hastings RH, Wood PR: Head extension and laryngeal view during laryngoscopy with cervical spine stabilization maneuvers. Anesthesiology 80:825, 1994.
9. Mobbs RJ, Stoodley MA, Fuller J: Effect of cervical hard collar on intracranial pressure after head injury. Aust N Z J Surg 72:389, 2002.
10. American Heart Association 2010 guidelines for cardiopulmonary resuscitation and emergency cardiovascular care. Part 13. Pediatric life support guidelines. Circulation 122:S639, November 10, 2010.
11. American Heart Association 2010 guidelines for cardiopulmonary resuscitation and emergency cardiovascular care. Part 15. Neonatal resuscitation. Circulation 122:S639, 2010.
12. White RD, Bunch TJ, Hankins DG: Evolution of a community-wide early defibrillation program experience over 13 years using police/fire personnel and paramedics as responders. Resuscitation 65:279, 2005.
13. Hickey RW, et al: Pediatric patients requiring CPR in the prehospital setting. Ann Emerg Med 25:495, 1995.
14. Atkins DL, Everson-Stewart S, Sears GK, et al: Epidemiology and outcomes from out-of-hospital cardiac arrest in children: the Resuscitation Outcomes Consortium Epistry-Cardiac Arrest. Circulation 119:1484, 2009.
15. American Heart Association 2010 guidelines for cardiopulmonary resuscitation and emergency cardiovascular care. Part 6. Electrical therapies. Circulation 122:S639, 2010.
16. Faddy SC, Powell J, Craig J: Biphasic and monophasic shocks for transthoracic defibrillation: a metaanalysis of randomized controlled trials. Resuscitation 58:9, 2000.
17. Hess EP, White RD: Ventricular fibrillation is not provoked by chest compression during post-shock organized rhythms in out-of-hospital cardiac arrest. Resuscitation 66:7, 2005.
18. Berg RA, Hilwig RW, Berg MD, et al: Immediate post-shock chest compressions improve outcome from prolonged ventricular fibrillation. Resuscitation 78:71, 2008.
19. Wik L, Kramer-Johansen J, Myklebust H, et al: Quality of cardiopulmonary resuscitation during out-of-hospital cardiac arrest. JAMA 293:299, 2005.
20. Abella BS, Alvarado JP, Myklebust H, et al: Quality of cardiopulmonary resuscitation during in-hospital cardiac arrest. JAMA 293:305, 2005.
21. Demetriades D, Charalambides K, Chahwan S, et al: Nonskeletal cervical spine incidence, epidemiology and diagnostic pitfalls. J Trauma 48:724, 2000.
22. Berg MD, Idris AH, Berg RA: Severe ventilatory compromise due to gastric distention during pediatric cardiopulmonary resuscitation. Resuscitation 36:71, 1998.
23. Barnes TA, Catino ME, Burns EC, et al: Comparison of an oxygen-powered flow-limited resuscitator to manual ventilation with an adult 1,000 mL self-inflating bag. Respir Care 50:1445, 2005.
24. Oschatz E, Wunderbaldinger P, Sterz F, et al: Cardiopulmonary resuscitation performed by bystanders does not increase adverse effects as assessed by chest radiographs. Anesth Analg 93:128, 2001.
25. Sullivan F, Avstreih D: Pneumothorax during CPR training: a case report and review of the CPR literature. Prehosp Disaster Med 15:64, 2000.
26. Hew P, Brenner B, Kaufman J: Reluctance of paramedics and emergency medical technicians to perform mouth-to-mouth resuscitation. J Emerg Med 15:279, 1997.
27. Brenner BE, Kaufman J: Reluctance of internists and medical nurses to perform mouth-to-mouth resuscitation. Arch Intern Med 153:1763, 1993.
28. Mejicano GC, Maki DG: Infections acquired during cardiopulmonary resuscitation: estimating the risk and defining strategies for prevention. Ann Intern Med 129:813, 1998.
29. van der Ham AC, Lange JF: Traumatic rupture of the stomach after Heimlich maneuver. Emerg Med 8:713, 1990.
30. Aufderheide TP, Sigurdsson G, Pirrallo RG, et al: Hyperventilation-induced hypotension during cardiopulmonary resuscitation. Circulation 109:1960, 2004.
31. Somerberg JC, Bailin SJ, Haffajee CI, et al: Intravenous lidocaine versus intravenous amiodarone (in a new aqueous formulation) for incessant ventricular tachycardia. Am J Cardiol 90:853, 2002.
32. American Heart Association 2010 guidelines for cardiopulmonary resuscitation and emergency cardiovascular care. Part 8. Advanced cardiovascular life support. Circulation 122:S639, 2010.
33. Barnes TA, Gale DD, Kacmarek RM, et al: Competencies needed by graduate respiratory therapists in 2015 and beyond. Respir Care 55:601, 2010.
34. Hahnel JH, Lindner KH, Schurmann C, et al: Plasma lidocaine levels and PaO_2 with endobronchial administration: dilution with normal saline or distilled water? Ann Emerg Med 19:1314, 1990.
35. Naganobu K, Hasebe Y, Uchiyama Y, et al: A comparison of distilled water and normal saline as diluents for endobronchial administration of epinephrine in the dog. Anesth Analg 91:317, 2000.
36. American Heart Association 2010 guidelines for cardiopulmonary resuscitation and emergency cardiovascular care. Part 9. Post cardiac-arrest care. Circulation 122:S639, 2010.
37. Sunde K, Pytte M, Jacobsen D, et al: Implementation of a standardised treatment protocol for post resuscitation care after out-of-hospital cardiac arrest. Resuscitation 73:29, 2007.
38. Herff H, Paal P, von Goedecke A, et al: Influence of ventilation strategies on survival in severe controlled hemorrhagic shock. Crit Care Med 36:2613, 2008.

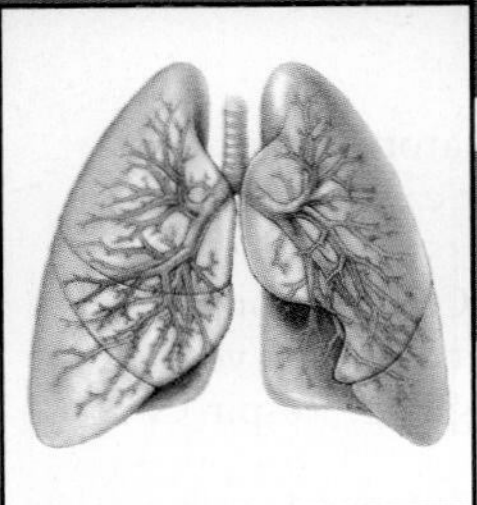

Chapter 35

Humidity and Bland Aerosol Therapy

JIM FINK AND ARZU ARI

CHAPTER OBJECTIVES

After reading this chapter you will be able to:

- Describe how airway heat and moisture exchange normally occurs.
- State the effect dry gases have on the respiratory tract.
- State when to humidify and warm inspired gas.
- Describe how various types of humidifiers work.
- Describe how to enhance humidifier performance.
- State how to select and use humidifier heating and feed systems safely.
- Identify the indications, contraindications, and hazards that pertain to humidification during mechanical ventilation.
- Describe how to monitor patients receiving humidity therapy.
- Describe how to identify and resolve common problems with humidification systems.
- State when to apply bland aerosol therapy.
- Describe how large volume aerosol generators work.
- Identify the delivery systems used for bland aerosol therapy.
- Describe how to identify and resolve common problems with aerosol delivery systems.
- Describe how to perform sputum induction.
- State how to select the appropriate therapy to condition a patient's inspired gas.

CHAPTER OUTLINE

KEY TERMS

American Society for Testing and Materials (ASTM)
baffling
body humidity
heat and moisture exchangers (HMEs)
humidifier
hydrophobic
hygrometer
hygroscopic
hypothermia
inspissated
International Organization for Standardization (ISO)
isothermic saturation boundary (ISB)
nebulizer
piezoelectric crystal
servo-controlled heating system
ultrasonic nebulizer (USN)

Vapors and mists have been used for thousands of years to treat respiratory disease. Modern respiratory care still uses these treatments at the bedside, in the form of water vapor (humidity) and bland water aerosols. Concepts of absolute and relative humidity are essential for understanding humidity therapy; these concepts are covered in Chapter 6. This chapter reviews the principles, methods, equipment, and procedures for using these concepts appropriately.

HUMIDITY THERAPY

Humidity therapy involves adding water vapor and (sometimes) heat to the inspired gas. To understand the need for humidity therapy, clinicians first must understand the normal control of heat and moisture exchange.

Physiologic Control of Heat and Moisture Exchange

Heat and moisture exchange is a primary function of the upper respiratory tract, mainly the nose.[1] The nose heats and humidifies gas on inspiration and cools and reclaims water from gas that is exhaled. The nasal mucosal lining is kept moist by secretions from mucous glands, goblet cells, transudation of fluid through cell walls, and condensation of exhaled humidity. The nasal mucosa is very vascular, actively regulating temperature changes in the nose and serving as an active element in promoting effective heat transfer. Similarly, the mucosa lining the sinuses, trachea, and bronchi aid in heating and humidifying inspired gases.

During inspiration through the nose, the tortuous path of gas through the turbinates increases contact between the inspired air and the mucosa. As the inspired air enters the nose, it warms *(convection)* and picks up water vapor from the moist mucosal lining *(evaporation)*, cooling the mucosal surface.

During exhalation, the expired gas transfers heat back to the cooler tracheal and nasal mucosa by convection. As the saturated gas cools, it holds less water vapor. Condensation occurs on the mucosal surfaces during exhalation, and water is reabsorbed by the mucus *(rehydration)*. In cold environments, the formation of condensate may exceed the ability of the mucus to reabsorb water (resulting in a "runny nose").

The mouth is less effective at heat and moisture exchange than the nose because of the low ratio of gas volume to moist and warm surface area and the less vascular squamous epithelium lining the oropharynx and hypopharynx. When a person inhales through the mouth at normal room temperature, pharyngeal temperatures are approximately 3° C less than when the person breathes through the nose, with 20% less relative humidity. During exhalation, the relative humidity of expired gas varies little between mouth breathing and nose breathing, but the mouth is much less efficient in reclaiming heat and water.[2]

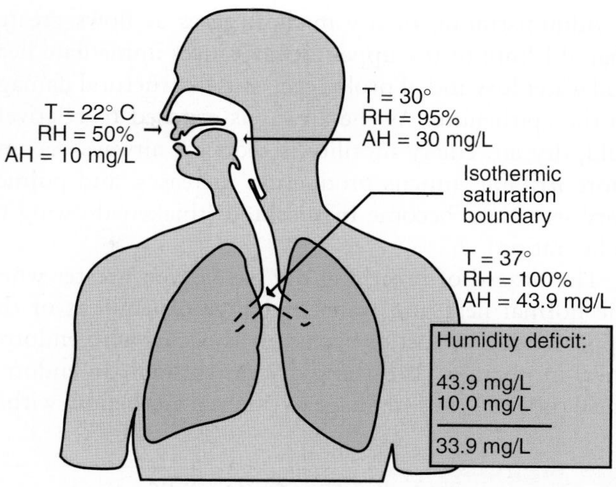

FIGURE 35-1 As a person breathes typical ambient air, the upper airway adds 20 mg/L of water vapor, and the lower airway adds 13.9 mg/L. If all of that humidity were exhaled, this would represent a 33.9 mg/L humidity deficit. (From Fink J: Humidity and aerosol therapy. In Cairo J, Pilbeam S, editors: Mosby's respiratory equipment, ed 8, St. Louis, 2010, Mosby.)

As inspired gas moves into the lungs, it achieves BTPS conditions (body temperature, 37° C; barometric pressure; saturated with water vapor [100% relative humidity at 37° C]) (Figure 35-1). This point, normally approximately 5 cm below the carina, is called the **isothermic saturation boundary (ISB).**[3] Above the ISB, temperature and humidity decrease during inspiration and increase during exhalation. Below the ISB, temperature and relative humidity remain constant (BTPS).

Numerous factors can shift the ISB deeper into the lungs. The ISB shifts distally when a person breathes through the mouth rather than the nose; when the person breathes cold, dry air; when the upper airway is bypassed (breathing through an artificial tracheal airway); or when the minute ventilation is higher than normal. When this shift of ISB occurs, additional surfaces of the airway are recruited to meet the heat and humidity requirements of the lung. This recruitment of airways that do not typically provide this level of heat and humidity can have a negative impact on epithelial integrity. These shifts of the ISB can compromise the body's normal heat and moisture exchange mechanisms, and humidity therapy is indicated.

Indications for Humidification and Warming of Inspired Gases

The primary goal of humidification is to maintain normal physiologic conditions in the lower airways. Proper levels of heat and humidity help ensure normal function of the mucociliary transport system. Humidity therapy is also used to treat abnormal conditions. Box 35-1 summarizes the primary and secondary indications for humidity therapy.

Administration of dry medical gases at flows greater than 4 L/min to the upper airway causes immediate heat and water loss and, if prolonged, causes structural damage to the epithelium. As the airway is exposed to relatively cold, dry air, ciliary motility is reduced, airways become more irritable, mucus production increases, and pulmonary secretions become **inspissated** (thickened owing to dehydration).

The hazard of breathing dry gas is even greater when the normal heat and water exchange capabilities of the upper airway are lost or bypassed, as occurs with endotracheal intubation.[4] Breathing dry gas through an endotracheal tube can cause damage to tracheal epithelium within minutes. However, as long as the inspired humidity is at least 60% of BTPS conditions, no injury occurs in normal lungs.[5,6] Prolonged breathing of improperly conditioned gases through a tracheal airway can result in **hypothermia** (reduced body temperature), inspissation of airway secretions, mucociliary dysfunction, destruction of airway epithelium, and atelectasis.[7] Box 35-2 summarizes the signs and symptoms associated with breathing cold, dry gases.

Figure 35-2 illustrates the level of dysfunction in the airway caused by changes in absolute humidity below BTPS and over hours of exposure. A reduction of 20 mg/L

Box 35-1 Indications for Humidification Therapy

PRIMARY
- Humidifying dry medical gases
- Overcoming humidity deficit created when upper airway is bypassed

SECONDARY
- Managing hypothermia
- Treating bronchospasm caused by cold air

Box 35-2 Clinical Signs and Symptoms of Inadequate Airway Humidification

- Atelectasis
- Dry, nonproductive cough
- Increased airway resistance
- Increased incidence of infection
- Increased work of breathing
- Patient complaint of substernal pain and airway dryness
- Thick, dehydrated secretions

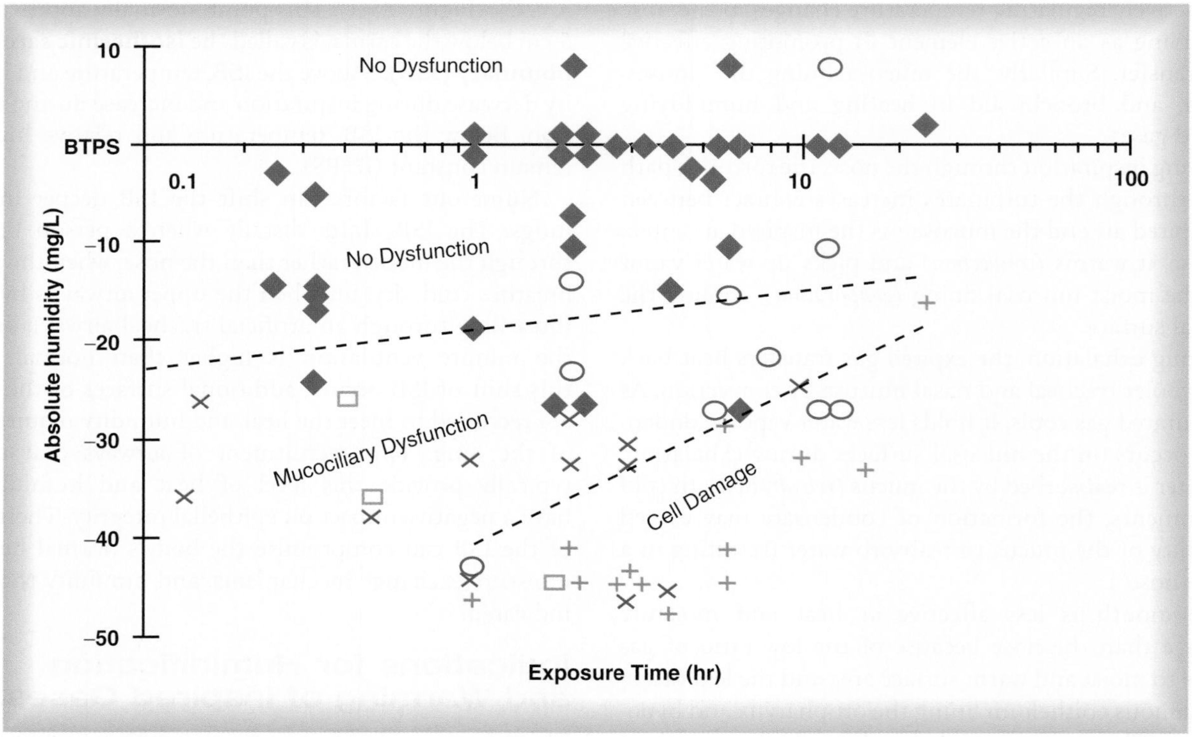

FIGURE 35-2 Diagram of published data describing the effects of humidity versus exposure time on airway dysfunction. Each point represents a single measurement coded as no dysfunction *(diamond)*, mucus thick or thin *(circle)*, mucociliary transport stopped *(square)*, cilia stopped *(X)*, or cell damage *(+)*. Data are grouped in categories of no dysfunction, mucociliary dysfunction, or cell damage. (Redrawn from Williams R, Rankin N, Smith T, et al: Relationship between the humidity and temperature of inspired gas and the function of the airway mucosa. Crit Care Med 24:1920, 1996.)

TABLE 35-1

Recommended Heat and Humidity Levels

Delivery Site	Temperature Range (° C)	Relative Humidity (%)	Absolute Humidity (mg/L)
Nose/mouth	20-22	50	10
Hypopharynx	29-32	95	28-34
Trachea	32-35	100	36-40

From Chatburn R, Primiano F: A rational basis for humidity therapy. Respir Care 32:249, 1987.

below BTPS (44 mg/L) is less than 60% relative humidity at BTPS.

The amount of heat and humidity that a patient needs depends on the site of gas delivery (e.g., nose or mouth, hypopharynx, trachea). Table 35-1 summarizes the recommended levels based on current standards.[8]

Warmed, humidified gases are used to prevent or treat various abnormal conditions. For treatment of a patient with hypothermia, heating and humidifying the inspired gas is one of several techniques used to raise core temperatures back to normal.[9,10] Heated humidification is also used to prevent intraoperative hypothermia.[11] Of possibly greater clinical significance, warming and humidifying the inspired gas can help alleviate bronchospasm in patients who develop airway narrowing after exercise or when they breathe cold air. Although the cause of this condition is not known for certain, the primary stimulus is probably a combination of airway cooling and drying, which leads to hypertonicity of airway lining fluid and the release of chemical mediators.[12] Patients may reduce the incidence of cold air–induced bronchospasm by simply wearing a scarf over the nose and mouth when outside in cold weather; the scarf serves as a crude passive heat and moisture exchanger (HME).

The delivery of cool humidified gas is used to treat upper airway inflammation resulting from croup, epiglottitis, and postextubation edema. This technique is used most often in conjunction with bland aerosol delivery (see the section on Bland Aerosol Delivery).

Equipment

A **humidifier** is a device that adds molecular water to gas. This process occurs by evaporation of water from a surface (see Chapter 6), whether the water is in a reservoir, a wick, or a sphere of water in suspension (aerosol).

Physical Principles Governing Humidifier Function

The following four variables or principles affect the quality of performance of a humidifier: (1) temperature, (2) surface area, (3) time of contact, and (4) thermal mass. These factors are exploited to various degrees in the design of humidification devices (Box 35-3).

Box 35-3 Physical Principles Governing Humidifier Function

Temperature: The higher the temperature of a gas, the more water vapor it can hold (increased capacity) or vice versa

Surface area: The greater the surface area of contact between water and gas, the more opportunity for evaporation to occur

Contact time: The longer a gas remains in contact with water, the greater the opportunity for evaporation to occur

Thermal mass: The greater the mass of water or the core element of a humidifier, the greater its capacity to hold and transfer heat

Temperature. Temperature is an important factor affecting humidifier performance. The greater the temperature of a gas, the more water vapor it can hold (increased capacity). As gas expansion and evaporation cool water in unheated humidifiers to 10° C below ambient temperature, the humidifiers become less efficient.

Figure 35-3 shows this concept, where, owing to evaporative cooling, the unheated humidifier on the left is operating at 10° C. Although the humidifier fully saturates the gas, the low operating temperature limits total water vapor capacity to approximately 9.4 mg/L water vapor, equivalent to approximately 21% of **body humidity.** Simply heating the humidifier to 40° C (see Figure 35-3, right) increases its output to 51 mg/L, which is sufficient to meet BTPS conditions.

Surface Area. The greater the area of contact between water and gas, the more opportunity there is for evaporation to occur. Passover humidifiers pass gas over a large surface area of water. More space-efficient ways to increase the water/gas surface-area ratio include bubble diffusion, aerosol, and wick technologies.

The *bubble-diffusion* technique directs a stream of gas underwater, where it is broken up into small bubbles. As the gas bubbles rise to the surface, evaporation increases the water vapor content within the bubble. The smaller the bubble, the greater the water/air surface-area ratio.

An alternative to dispersing gas bubbles in water is spraying water particles into the gas. This is accomplished by generating an *aerosol* (suspension of water droplets) in the gas stream. The higher the aerosol density (number of particles per volume of gas), the greater the gas/water surface area available for evaporation.

Wick technologies use porous water-absorbent materials to increase surface area. A wick draws water (similar to a sponge) into its fine honeycombed structure by means of capillary action. The surfaces of the wick increase the area of contact between the water and gas, which aids evaporation.

Contact Time. The longer a gas remains in contact with water, the greater the opportunity for evaporation to occur. For bubble humidifiers, contact time depends on

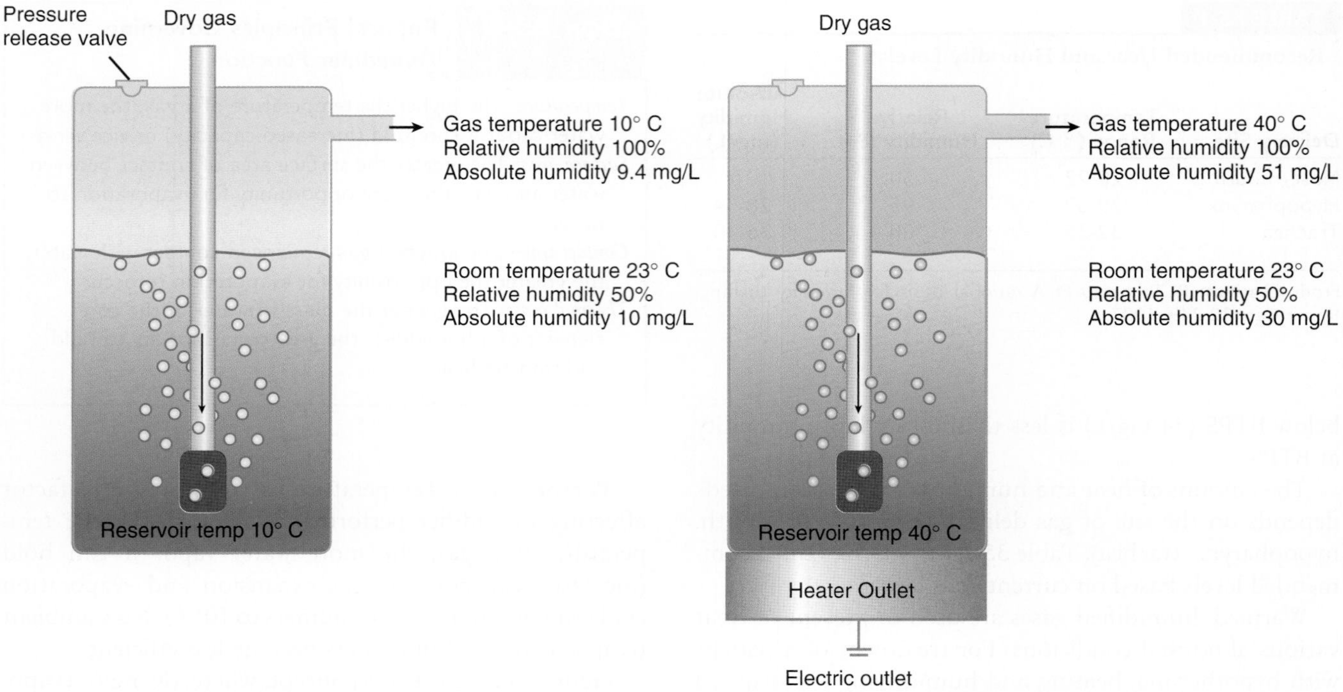

FIGURE 35-3 Effects of reservoir temperature on humidity output with unheated *(left)* and heated *(right)* bubble-type humidifiers. (Modified from Fink J, Cohen N: Humidity and aerosols. In Eubank D, Bone R, editors: Principles and applications of cardiorespiratory care equipment, St. Louis, 1994, Mosby.)

the depth of the water column; the deeper the column, the greater the time of contact as the bubbles rise to the surface. In passover and wick-type humidifiers, the flow rate of gas through the humidifier is inversely related to contact time, with high flow rates reducing the time available for evaporation to occur. Aerosols suspended in a gas stream have extended contact time (and opportunity for evaporation) as the aerosol and gas travel to the patient.

Thermal Mass. The greater the amount of water in a humidifier, the greater the thermal mass. Increased thermal mass within a humidifier equates to increased capacity to hold and transfer heat to therapeutic gases. Larger reservoir humidifiers can provide more consistent heat and humidification with a broader range of gas flow.

Types of Humidifiers

Humidifiers are either *active* (actively adding heat or water or both to the device-patient interface) or *passive* (recycling exhaled heat and humidity from the patient). Active humidifiers typically include (1) bubble humidifiers, (2) passover humidifiers, (3) nebulizers of bland aerosols, and (4) vaporizers. Passive humidifiers refer to typical **heat and moisture exchangers (HMEs).** Specifications covering the design and performance requirements for medical humidifiers are established by the **American Society for Testing and Materials (ASTM).**[13]

Active Humidifiers

Bubble. A bubble humidifier breaks (diffuses) an underwater gas stream into small bubbles (Figure 35-4). Use of a foam or mesh diffuser produces smaller bubbles than an open lumen, allowing greater surface area for gas/water interaction. Unheated bubble humidifiers are commonly used with oxygen (O_2) delivery systems (see Chapter 38) to raise the water vapor content of the gas to ambient levels.

As indicated in Table 35-2, unheated bubble humidifiers can provide absolute humidity levels between approximately 15 mg/L and 20 mg/L.[14-16] At room temperature, 10 mg/L absolute humidity corresponds to approximately 80% relative humidity but only approximately 25% body humidity (see Chapter 6). As gas flow increases, these devices become less efficient as the reservoir cools and contact time is reduced, limiting their effectiveness at flow rates greater than 10 L/min. Heating the reservoirs of these units can increase humidity content, but this is not

TABLE 35-2

Absolute Humidity (mg/L) Provided by Unheated Bubble Humidifiers

L/min	Aquapak 301 (Hudson RCI, Corp, Dunham, NC)	Traveral 500 (Baxter-Travenol, Corp, Deerfield, IL)
2	17.6	20.4
4	17.7	19.5
6	16.9	16.2
8	14.9	15.7

Modified from Darin J, Broadwell J, MacDonell R: An evaluation of water-vapor output from four brands of unheated, prefilled bubble humidifiers. Respir Care 27:41, 1982.

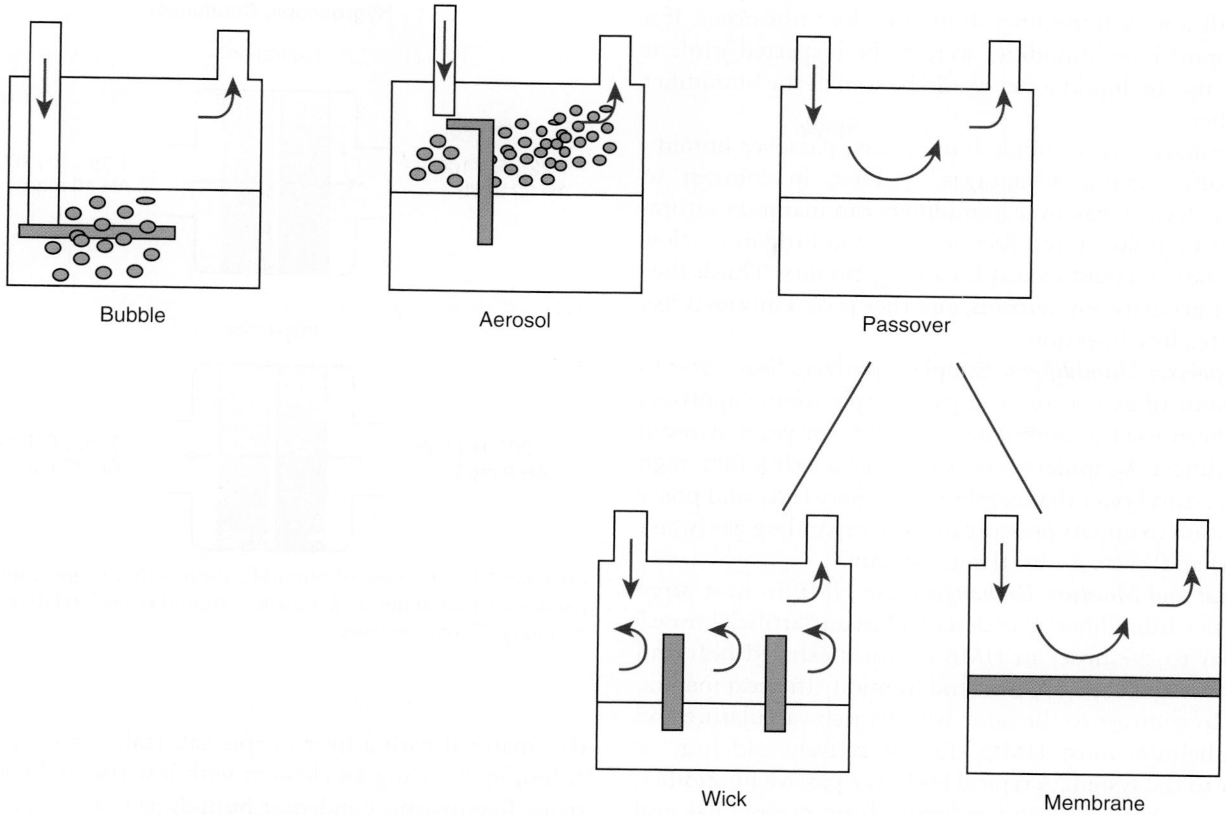

FIGURE 35-4 Primary types of active humidifiers. Gas passes through the water (bubble), around drops of water (aerosol) or over the surface of water (Passover), a saturated material (wick) or a semipermeable membrane (membrane). (From Fink J: Humidity and aerosol therapy. In Cairo J, Pilbeam S, editors; Mosby's respiratory equipment, ed 8, St. Louis, 2010, Mosby.)

recommended because the resulting condensate tends to obstruct the small bore delivery tubing to which these units connect.

To warn of flow-path obstruction and to prevent bursting of the humidifier bottle, bubble humidifiers incorporate a simple pressure-relief valve, or *pop-off*. Typically, the pop-off is either a gravity or spring-loaded valve that releases pressures greater than 2 psi. Humidifier pop-offs should provide both an audible and a visible alarm and should automatically resume normal position when pressures return to normal.[13] The pop-off also can be used to test an O_2 delivery system for leaks. If the system is obstructed at or near the patient interface and the pop-off sounds, the system is leak-free; failure of the pop-off to sound may indicate a leak (or a faulty pop-off valve).

At high flow rates, bubble humidifiers can produce aerosols. Although invisible to the naked eye, these water droplet suspensions can transmit pathogenic bacteria from the humidifier reservoir to the patient.[17] Because any device that generates an aerosol poses a high risk of spreading infection, strict infection control procedures must be followed when using these systems (see Chapter 4).

Passover. Passover humidifiers direct gas over a surface containing water. There are three common types of passover humidifiers: (1) simple reservoir type, (2) wick type, and (3) membrane type (see Figure 35-4).

The simple reservoir device directs gas over the surface of a volume of water (or fluid). The surface for gas-fluid interface is limited. These systems are typically used with heated fluids for use with mechanical ventilation, but they may also be used with room temperature fluids with noninvasive ventilatory support (nasal continuous positive airway pressure or bilevel ventilation).

A wick humidifier uses an absorbent material to increase the surface area for dry air to interface with heated water. Typically, a wick is placed upright with the gravity-dependent end in a heated water reservoir. Heating elements might be below or surrounding the wick. Capillary action continually draws water up from the reservoir and keeps the wick saturated. As dry gas enters the chamber, it flows around the wick, quickly picking up heat and moisture and leaving the chamber fully saturated with water vapor. No bubbling occurs, so no aerosol is produced.

A membrane-type humidifier separates the water from the gas stream by means of a **hydrophobic** membrane (see Figure 35-4). Water vapor molecules can easily pass through this membrane, but liquid water (and pathogens) cannot.

As with a wick humidifier, bubbling does not occur. If a membrane-type humidifier were to be inspected while it was in use, no liquid water would be seen in the humidifier chamber.

Compared with bubble humidifiers, passover humidifiers offer several advantages.[17,18] First, in contrast to bubble devices, passover humidifiers can maintain saturation at high flow rates. Second, they add little or no flow resistance to spontaneous breathing circuits. Third, they do not generate any aerosols, and they pose a minimal risk for spreading infection.

Vaporizer Humidifiers. Simple vaporizers heat water to the point of expansion as a gas. Simple room vaporizers have been used in ambulatory settings for years as room humidifiers. A capillary force vaporizer is a thin-film, high surface area boiler that combines capillary force and phase transition to impart pressure onto an expanding gas (water vapor) and ejects it into the gas stream.

Heat and Moisture Exchangers. An HME is most often a passive humidifier, also described as an "artificial nose." Similar to the nose, an HME captures exhaled heat and moisture and uses it to heat and humidify the next inspiration. In contrast to the nose, with its rich vasculature and endothelium, most HMEs do not actively add heat or water to the system. A typical HME is a passive humidifier, capturing both heat and moisture from expired gas and returning up to 70% of both to the patient during the next inspiration.

Traditionally, use of HMEs has been limited to providing humidification to patients receiving invasive ventilatory support via endotracheal or tracheostomy tubes. More recently, HMEs have been used successfully in meeting the short-term humidification needs of spontaneously breathing patients with tracheostomy tubes.[19] Kapadia[20] reviewed airway accidents in the intensive care unit for a 4-year period and noted an increasing trend in the incidence of blocked tracheal tubes, which was associated with an increased duration of HME filter use. More recent evidence supports long-term use of HMEs for spontaneously breathing patients.[21]

The three basic types of HMEs are (1) simple condenser humidifiers, (2) **hygroscopic** condenser humidifiers, and (3) hydrophobic condenser humidifiers. Simple condenser humidifiers contain a condenser element with high thermal conductivity, usually consisting of metallic gauze, corrugated metal, or parallel metal tubes. On inspiration, inspired air cools the condenser element. On exhalation, expired water vapor condenses directly on its surface and rewarms it. On the next inspiration, cool, dry air is warmed and humidified as its passes over the condenser element. Simple condenser humidifiers are able to recapture only approximately 50% of a patient's exhaled moisture (50% efficiency).

Hygroscopic condenser humidifiers provide higher efficiency by (1) using a condensing element of low thermal conductivity (e.g., paper, wool, foam) and (2) impregnating

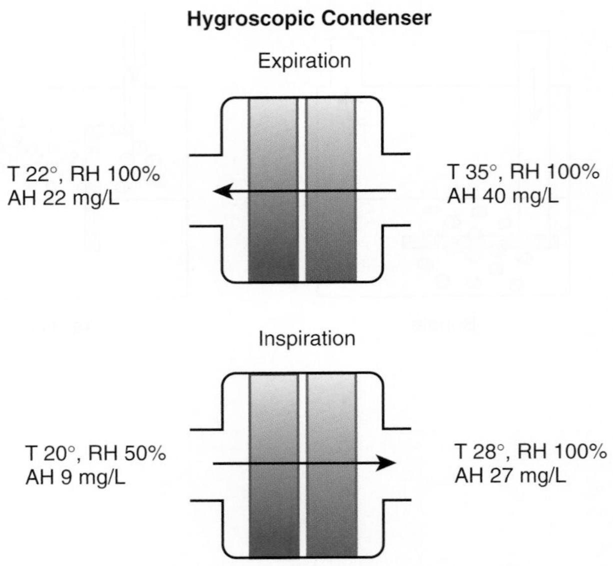

FIGURE 35-5 Process of humidification with a hygroscopic condenser humidifier. *AH,* Absolute humidity; *RH,* relative humidity; *T,* temperature.

this material with a hygroscopic salt (calcium or lithium chloride). By using an element with low thermal conductivity, hygroscopic condenser humidifiers can retain more heat than simple condenser systems. In addition, the hygroscopic salt helps capture extra moisture from the exhaled gas. During exhalation, some water vapor condenses on the cool condenser element, whereas other water molecules bind directly to the hygroscopic salt. During inspiration, the lower water vapor pressure in the inspired gas liberates water molecules directly from the hygroscopic salt, without cooling. Figure 35-5 depicts the overall process of humidification with a hygroscopic condenser humidifier, showing the changes in temperature and the relative and absolute humidity occurring during the cycle of breathing. As shown, these devices typically achieve approximately 70% efficiency (40 mg/L exhaled, 27 mg/L returned).

Hydrophobic condenser humidifiers use a water-repellent element with a large surface area and low thermal conductivity (Figure 35-6). During exhalation, the condenser temperature increases to approximately 25° C because of conduction and latent heat of condensation. On inspiration, cool gas and evaporation cools the condenser down to 10° C. This large temperature change results in the conservation of more water to be used in humidifying the next breath. The efficiency of these devices is comparable to hygroscopic condenser humidifiers (approximately 70%). However, some hydrophobic humidifiers that provide bacterial filtration may reduce the risk of pneumonia but be unsuitable for patients with limited respiratory reserve or who are prone to airway blockage because they may increase artificial airway occlusion.[22,23]

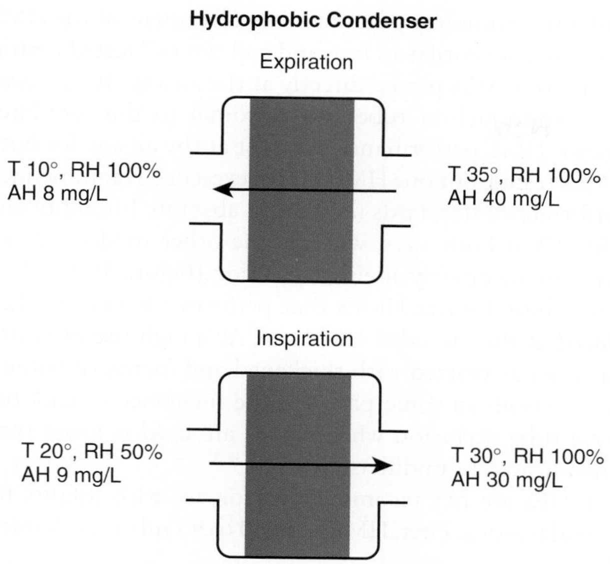

FIGURE 35-6 Process of humidification with a hydrophobic condenser humidifier. *AH,* Absolute humidity; *RH,* relative humidity; *T,* temperature.

Design and performance standards for HMEs are set by the **International Organization for Standardization (ISO).**[24] The ideal HME should operate at 70% efficiency or better (providing at least 30 mg/L water vapor); use standard connections; have a low compliance; and add minimal weight, dead space, and flow resistance to a breathing circuit.[25] According to Lellouche and colleagues,[26] HME performance varies from brand to brand, and only 37.5% of 32 HMEs tested in the study performed well. Table 35-3 compares performance of several commercially available HMEs according to their moisture output, flow resistance, and dead space.[26]

As shown in Table 35-3, the moisture output of HMEs tends to decrease at high volumes and rates of breathing. In addition, high inspiratory flows and high FiO_2 levels can decrease HME efficiency.[25] Flow resistance through the HME also is important. When an HME is dry, resistance across most devices is minimal. However, because of water absorption, HME flow resistance increases after several hours of use.[27,28] For some patients, the increased resistance imposed by the HME may not be well tolerated, in particular, if the underlying lung disease already causes increased work of breathing.

TABLE 35-3

Comparison of 25 Heat and Moisture Exchangers

Device	Manufacturer	Measured AH (mg H_2O/L)	AH/ml of Dead Space	Measured Resistance at 60 L/min cm H_2O
Hygrovent	Peters	31.9 ± 0.6	0.34	1.8
Hygrobac	Mallinckrodt	31.7 ± 0.7	0.33	2.1
Hygrovent S	Peters	31.7 ± 0.5	0.58	2.8
Hygrobac S	Mallinckrodt	31.2 ± 0.2	0.69	2.3
9000/100	Allégiance	31.2 ± 1.4	0.35	2.7
Servo Humidifier 172	Siemens	30.9 ± 0.3	0.56	NA
Humid Vent Filter	Hudson	30.8 ± 0.3	0.88	2.3
Hygroster	Mallinckrodt	30.7 ± 0.6	0.32	2.3
Humid Vent 2	Hudson	29.7 ± 0.4	1.03	NA
Servo Humidifier 162	Siemens	29.7 ± 0.8	0.78	NA
Humid Vent 2S	Hudson	29.2 ± 0.4	1.01	NA
9040/01	Allégiance	28.6 ± 1.1	0.61	2.4
9000/01	Allégiance	28.5 ± 0.8	0.32	3.9
BB100E	Pall	27.2 ± 0.7	0.32	1.4
BB100	Pall	26.8 ± 0.5	0.30	2.0
Stérivent	Mallinckrodt	23.8 ± 0.9	0.26	1.9
Iso Gard Hepa Light	Hudson	23.6 ± 0.3	0.47	2.4
Stérivent S	Mallinckrodt	22.2 ± 0.2	0.36	1.7
BB25	Pall	19.6 ± 1.4	0.56	2.6
BB2000AP	Pall	18.9 ± 0.4	0.54	3.1
Stérivent Mini	Mallinckrodt	16.6 ± 1.0	0.47	2.2
4444/66	Allégiance	16.4 ± 0.6	0.35	3.4
4000/01	Allégiance	15.1 ± 0.9	0.40	2.2
Barrierbac S	Mallinckrodt	13.2 ± 0.2	0.38	2.1

Modified from Lellouche F, Taille S, Lefrancois F, et al: Humidification performance of 48 passive airway humidifiers: comparison with manufacturer data. Chest 135:276, 2009.
AH, Absolute humidity; *NA,* not available.

Because HMEs eliminate the problem of breathing circuit condensation, many clinicians consider these devices (especially hydrophobic filter HMEs) to be helpful in preventing nosocomial infections and ventilator-associated pneumonia.[29] Compared with active humidification systems, HMEs do reduce bacterial colonization of ventilator circuits.[30] However, circuit colonization plays a minor role in the development of nosocomial infections, provided that usual maintenance precautions are applied.[31] Evidence indicates no difference in incidence of ventilator-associated pneumonia, mortality, morbidity, and respiratory complications among patients managed with HMEs and heated humidifiers.[23,26,30,32,33]

The position of the HME relative to the patient's airway can affect its ability both to heat and to humidify inhaled gas. Secretions can foul HMEs attached directly to the airway. The use of devices such as closed suction catheters and airway monitor ports requires placement of the HME closer to the ventilator. Inui and colleagues[34] tested performance of HMEs placed directly at the airway, 10 cm away from endotracheal tube and proximal to the ventilator circuit. HME performance was best at the airway for both HMEs tested, but one HME model exceeded recommended performance standards (≥30 mg/L absolute humidity and ≥30° C) at both sites, whereas the other model did not perform adequately at either position (Figure 35-7). Clinicians should select HMEs that perform adequately when placed at the intended HME site. Although use of HMEs has been associated with thickened and increased volume of secretions in some patients, the incidence of endotracheal tube occlusion when HMEs are used is lower than when heated humidifiers are used.[35,36]

HMEs are not recommended for use with infants for several reasons. First, HMEs add 30 to 90 ml of mechanical

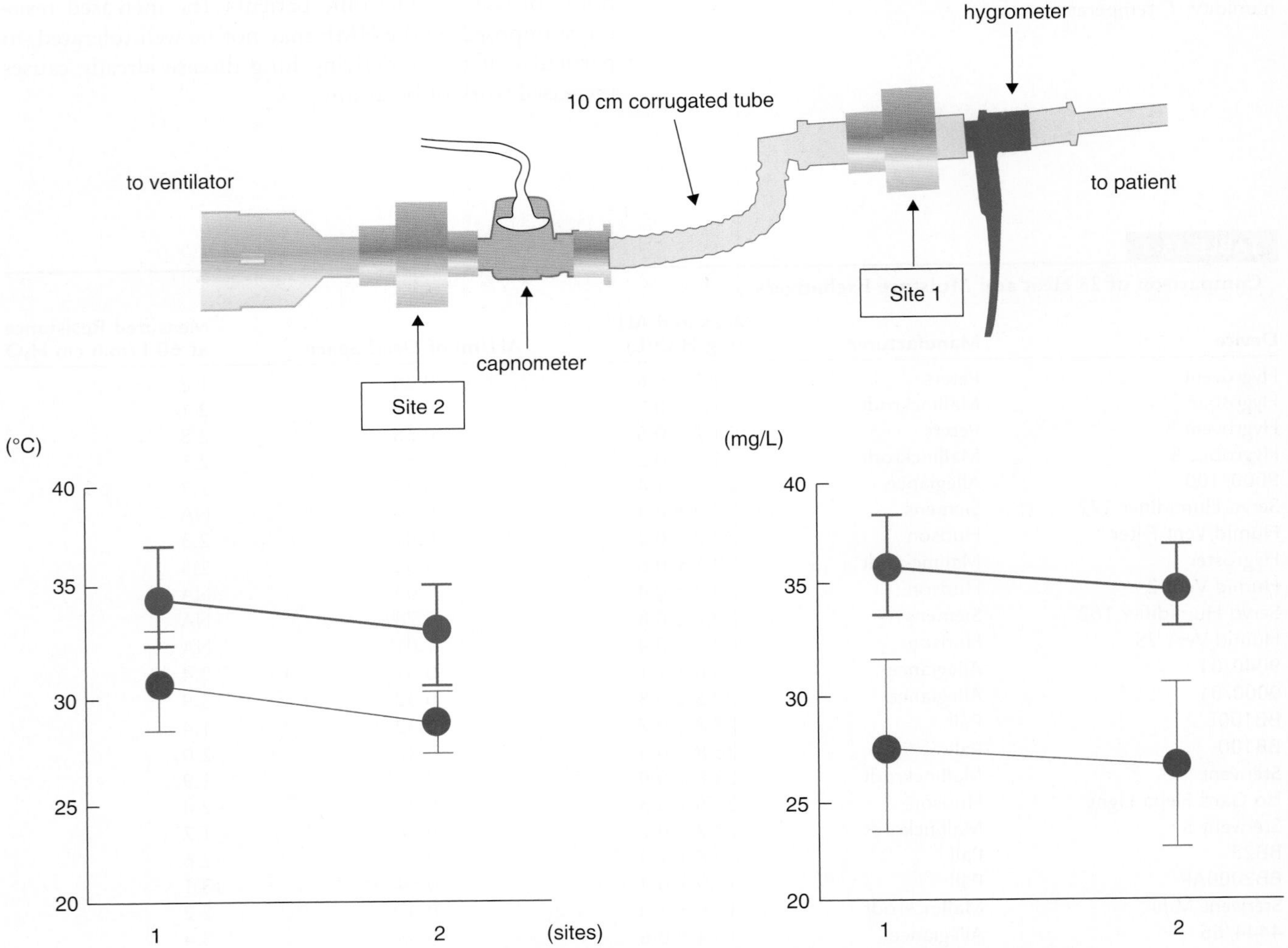

FIGURE 35-7 Placement of HMEs (Hygrobac S [Mallinckrodt-Dar, Mirandola, Italy, *blue circle*] or Thermovent HEPA [Smiths Medical International, Ltd, Kent, United Kingdom, *red circle*]) at the airway *(site 1)* or proximal to the ventilator circuit *(site 2)*. Temperature mean ± SD (TEMP; *left*) and absolute humidity were significantly higher with both HMEs. $P < .05$ placed at *site 1* compared with *site 2*. (Modified from Inui D, Oto J, Nishimura M: Effect of heat and moisture exchanger (HME) positioning on inspiratory gas humidification. BMC Pulm Med 6:19, 2006.)

dead space, exceeding the tidal volume of the infant. In addition, infants are commonly ventilated through uncuffed endotracheal tubes, which allow exhaled gas to leak around the tube and bypass the HME reducing recovered heat and humidity.

Active Heat Moisture Exchangers. Active HMEs add humidity or heat or both to inspired gas by chemical or electrical means.[37] The Humid-Heat (Louis Gibeck AB, Upplands Väsby, Sweden) consists of a supply unit with a microprocessor, water pump, and humidification device, which is placed between the Y-piece and the endotracheal tube. The humidification device is based on a hygroscopic HME, which absorbs the expired heat and moisture and releases it into the inspired gas. External heat and water are added to the patient side of the HME, so the inspired gas should reach 100% humidity at 37° C (44 mg H_2O/L air). The external water is delivered to the humidification device via a pump onto a wick and evaporated into the inspired air by an electrical heater. The microprocessor controls the water pump and the heater by an algorithm using the minute ventilation (which is fed into the microprocessor) and the airway temperature measured by a sensor mounted in the flex-tube on the patient side of the humidification device. The HME Booster (King Systems, Noblesville, IN) has a T-piece containing an electrically heated element that was designed for use as an adjunct to a passive HME. The heating element heats water so that water vapor passes into the airway between the artificial airway and the endotracheal tube, via a Gore-Tex membrane and aluminum. Using a gravity feedbag via a flow regulator that limits flow to 10 mL/hr, water is fed to the heater, which operates at 110° C and adds 3 to 5.5 mg/L of humidity and 3° C to 4° C to inspired gas compared with HME alone. The Humid-Booster was designed for patients with minute volumes of 4 to 20 L, and it is not appropriate for use with pediatric patients or infants. Active HMEs add weight and complexity at the patient airway.

Heating Systems

Heat improves the water output of humidifiers. Heated humidifiers are used mainly for patients with bypassed upper airways and patients receiving mechanical ventilatory support. Although heating a humidifier provides benefits, it also presents additional risks. Humidifier heating systems generally have a controller that regulates the power to the heating element by monitoring the heating element, which matches a preset or an adjustable temperature. They may also use a thermistor placed at the outlet of the humidifier, with a heater set to control output temperature. Servo-controlled heating systems monitor the temperature at the humidifier's outlet and at the patient's airway using a thermistor probe. The controller adjusts the heater power to reach the desired airway temperature and incorporates alarms and an alarm-activated heater shutdown function.

An electrical heating element provides the needed energy. Five types of heating elements are common: (1) a hot plate element at the base of the humidifier; (2) a wraparound type that surrounds the humidifier chamber; (3) a yolk, or collar, element that sits between the water reservoir and the gas outlet; (4) an immersion-type heater, with the element placed in the water reservoir; (5) a heated wire in the inspiratory limb warming a saturated wick or hollow fiber; and (6) a thin-film, high surface area broiler.

Humidifier heating systems have a controller that regulates the element's electrical power. In the simplest systems, the controller monitors the heating element, varying the delivered current to match either a preset or an adjustable temperature. In these systems, the temperature of the patient's airway has no effect on the controller. Conversely, a **servo-controlled heating system** monitors temperature at or near the patient's airway using a thermistor probe. The controller adjusts heater power to achieve the desired airway temperature. Both types of controller units usually incorporate alarms and alarm-activated heater shutdown. Box 35-4 outlines key features of modern heated humidification systems.[38]

RULE OF THUMB

Place heated humidifier thermistor probes in the inspiratory limb of a ventilator circuit far away from the patient "wye" to ensure that warm exhaled gas does not fool the controller system. Similarly, never place a thermistor probe in an isolette or a radiant warmer, where the probe is warmed externally and the humidifier is fooled into shutting down, reducing the humidity available to the patient.

Reservoir and Feed Systems

Heated humidifiers operating continuously in breathing circuits can evaporate more than 1 L of water per day. To avoid constant refilling, these devices either incorporate a large water reservoir or use a gravity feed system. An ideal reservoir or feed system should be safe, dependable, and easy to set up and use and should allow for continuity of therapy, even when the reservoir is being replenished.

Manual Systems. Simple large reservoir systems are manually refilled (with sterile or distilled water). If a manual system is used, momentary interruption of humidifier operation and mechanical ventilation is required for refilling. Because the system must be "opened" for refilling, cross contamination can occur. Water levels in manually filled systems are constantly changing, and changes in the humidifier fill volume alter the gas compression factor and the delivered volume during mechanical ventilation.

A small inlet that can be attached to a gravity-fed intravenous bag and line allows refilling without interruption of ventilation. Such systems still require constant checking and manual replenishment by opening the line valve or

Box 35-4 Key Features for Heated Humidification Systems

Gas temperature delivered to the patient should not be greater than 40° C. When temperatures greater than 40° C are reached, audible and visual alarms should indicate an over-temperature condition and interrupt power to the heater.

Audible and visual alarms should indicate when remote temperature sensors are disconnected, absent, or defective, and power to the heater should be interrupted to prevent overheating.

Temperature overshoot should be minimized. Overshoot can occur when servo-controlled units warm up without flow through the circuit, when the temperature probe is not inserted in the circuit (or becomes dislodged), or when flow changes during normal operation. Non–servo-controlled units can overshoot when temperature controls are set too high or when gas flow is abruptly reduced.

Indicators for delivered gas temperature should be accurate to ±3° C of the indicated value.

Humidifier temperature output should not vary more than 2° C from the set value (proximal to the patient).

Warm-up time should not exceed 15 minutes.

The water level should be readily visible in either the humidifier or the remote reservoir.

Humidifiers should be able to withstand ventilation pressures greater than 100 cm H_2O.

Internal compliance should be low and stable so that changes in the water level do not significantly alter the delivered tidal volume.

The exposed surface of a humidifier should not be too hot to touch during operation. Readily accessible surfaces should not be greater than 37.5° C. A warning label is needed for hotter surfaces.

Operator, or feed, systems must not be able to overfill the humidifier to the point that water can block gas flow through the humidifier or ventilator circuit. Humidifiers should not be damaged by spilled fluids.

Electromagnetic interference from other devices should not affect humidifier performance. The unit should not be damaged by 95 to 135 V rms.

Fuses or circuit breakers should be clearly labeled and easily reset or replaced. The unit should have adequate overcurrent protection to prevent ventilator shutdown or loss of power to other equipment on the same branch circuit because of internal equipment failures.

It should be impossible to assemble the unit in a way that would be hazardous to the patient. The direction of gas flow should be indicated on interchangeable components, for which proper direction is essential.

The humidifier should be assembled and filled in a manner that minimizes the introduction of infectious materials or foreign objects.

Service and operation manuals should be provided with the humidifier and should cover all aspects of its use and service.

Modified from Emergency Care Research Institute: Heated humidifiers, Health Devices. 1987. http://www.fda.gov/oc/po/firmrecalls/Vapotherm2000i_01_06.html. Accessed March 2, 2011.

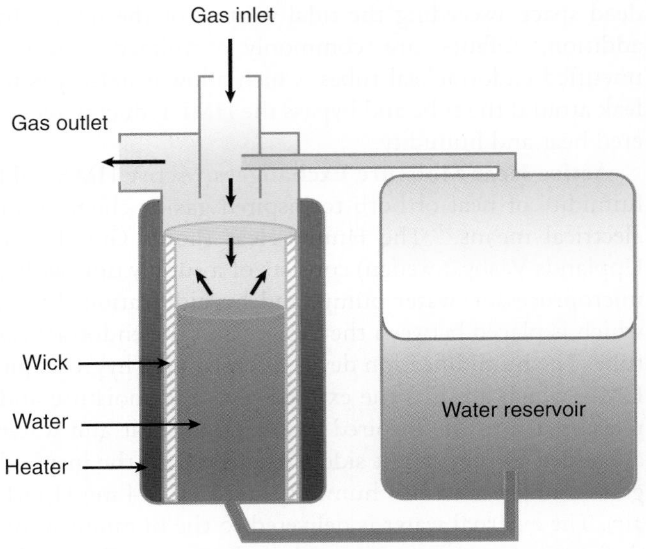

FIGURE 35-8 Schematic of the Concha-Column wick-type humidifier with level-compensated reservoir feed system (Hudson RCI, Temecula, CA). (Modified from Fink J, Cohen N: Humidity and aerosols. In Eubank D, Bone R, editors: Principles and applications of cardiorespiratory care equipment, St. Louis, 1994, Mosby.)

clamp. If not checked regularly, the reservoir in these systems can go dry, placing the patient at considerable risk.

Automatic Systems. Automatic feed systems avoid the need for constant checking and manual refilling of humidifiers. The simplest type of automatic feed system is the level-compensated reservoir (Figure 35-8). In these systems, an external reservoir is aligned horizontally with the humidifier, maintaining relatively consistent water levels between the reservoir and the humidifier chamber.

Flotation valve controls can be used to maintain humidifier reservoir fluid volume. In flotation-type systems, a float rises and falls with the water level. As the water level falls below a preset value, the float opens the feed valve; as the water rises back to the set fill level, the float closes the feed valve. An optical sensor can also be used to sense water level, driving a solenoid valve to allow refilling of the humidifier reservoir.

Membrane-type humidifiers do not require a flow control system. Because the liquid water chamber underlying the membrane cannot overfill, these devices require only an open gravity feed system to ensure proper function. Two examples are the Vapotherm (Vapotherm Inc, Stevensville, MD) membrane cartridge system and the Hummax II (Metran Medical Instruments Mfg Co, Ltd, Saitama, Japan), which uses a heated wire to warm the polyethylene microporous hollow fiber placed in the inspiratory circuit.

The Hydrate (Pari Respiratory Equipment, Midlothian, VA) capillary force vaporizer is driven by software that controls a heater element and water flow. The 19-mm diameter disc can deliver 2.2 mg of water vapor/min at 37° C. Data

MINI CLINI

Selecting the Appropriate Therapy to Condition a Patient's Inspired Gas

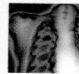

PROBLEM: A survivor of near drowning has just been intubated and placed on mechanical ventilatory support. Her body temperature is 31° C, and her minute ventilation is high. What would be the appropriate humidification system to recommend for this patient?

SOLUTION: Normally, patients supported by mechanical ventilation can be started with an HME, unless its use is contraindicated. According to AARC Clinical Practice Guideline 35-1, using an HME with this patient is contraindicated because (1) she is hypothermic, and (2) she has a high minute ventilation. Based on this assessment, the best choice is a heated humidifier, preferably with servo-controlled airway temperature.

from prototypes suggest temperature control from 33° C to 41° C for flows 2 to 40 L/min (Figure 35-9).[39]

To guide practitioners in applying humidity therapy during ventilatory support, the American Association for Respiratory Care (AARC) has published Clinical Practice Guideline: Humidification During Mechanical Ventilation; excerpts from the AARC guideline appear in Clinical Practice Guideline 35-1.[7]

Setting Humidification Levels

Although the American National Standards Institute (ANSI) recommends minimum levels of humidity for intubated patients (>30 mg/L), there is less guidance regarding appropriate settings for optimal humidification. One suggestion is to target the temperature and level of humidity for normal conditions at the point that the gas is entering the airway. For example, the humidity of air entering the carina is typically 35 to 40 mg/L. When humidifiers run too cold (<32° C), humidity can be reduced to the point of increased airway plugging. Not all active heated

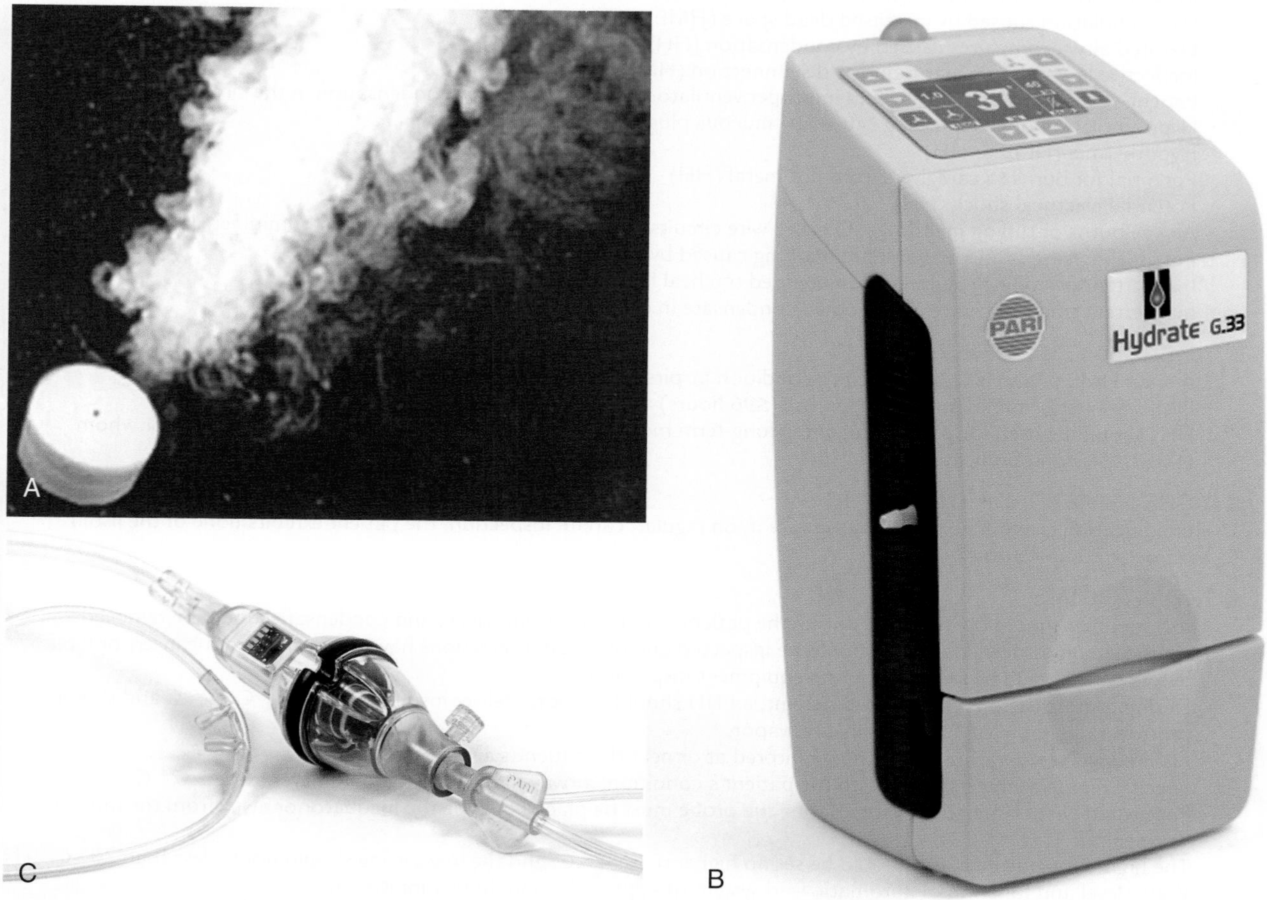

FIGURE 35-9 The capillary force vaporizer (CFV) is a thin-film, high surface area boiler that combines capillary force and phase transition. **A,** Inducing phase transition in a capillary environment, the CFV imparts pressure onto the expanding gas and ejects it. **B,** The CFV is incorporated to provide controlled heated humidity in the Hydrate (Pari, MidLothian, VA). **C,** Temperature probe. (Courtesy Pari.)

35-1 Humidification During Mechanical Ventilation

AARC Clinical Practice Guideline (Excerpts)*

INDICATIONS

Humidification of inspired gas during mechanical ventilation is mandatory when an endotracheal or a tracheostomy tube is present.

CONTRAINDICATIONS

There are no contraindications to providing physiologic conditioning of inspired gas during mechanical ventilation. However, an HME is contraindicated in the following circumstances:

- For patients with thick, copious, or bloody secretions
- For patients with an expired tidal volume less than 70% of the delivered tidal volume (e.g., patients with large bronchopleural fistulas or incompetent or absent endotracheal tube cuffs)
- For patients whose body temperature is less than 32° C
- For patients with high spontaneous minute volumes (>10 L/min)
- For patients receiving in-line aerosol drug treatments (an HME must be removed from the patient circuit during treatments)

HAZARDS AND COMPLICATIONS

Hazards and complications associated with the use of heated humidifier (HH) and HME devices during mechanical ventilation include the following:

- High flow rates during disconnect may aerosolize contaminated condensate (HH)
- Underhydration and mucous impaction (HME or HH)
- Increased work of breathing (HME or HH)
- Hypoventilation caused by increased dead space (HME)
- Elevated airway pressures caused by condensation (HH)
- Ineffective low-pressure alarm during disconnection (HME)
- Patient-ventilator dyssynchrony and improper ventilator function caused by condensation in the circuit (HH)
- Hypoventilation or gas trapping caused by mucous plugging (HME or HH)
- Hypothermia (HME or HH)
- Potential for burns to caregivers from hot metal (HH)
- Potential electrical shock (HH)
- Airway burns or tubing meltdown if heated wire circuits are covered or incompatible with humidifier (HH)
- Possible increased resistive work of breathing caused by mucous plugging (HME or HH)
- Inadvertent overfilling resulting in unintended tracheal lavage (HH)
- Inadvertent tracheal lavage from pooled condensate in circuit (HH)

ASSESSMENT OF NEED

Either an HME or an HH can be used to condition inspired gases:

- HMEs are better suited for short-term use (≤96 hours) and during transport.
- HHs should be used for patients requiring long-term mechanical ventilation (>96 hours) or for patients for whom HME use is contraindicated.

ASSESSMENT OF OUTCOME

Humidification is assumed to be appropriate if, on regular, careful inspection, the patient exhibits none of the listed hazards or complications.

MONITORING

The humidifier should be inspected during the patient-ventilator system check, and condensate should be removed from the circuit as needed. HMEs should be inspected and replaced if secretions have contaminated the insert or filter. The following should be recorded during equipment inspection:

- During routine use on an intubated patient, an HH should be set to deliver inspired gas at 33° C ± 2° C and should provide a minimum of 30 mg/L of water vapor.
- Inspired gas temperature should be monitored at or near the patient's airway opening (HH).
- Specific temperatures may vary with the patient's condition; airway temperature should never exceed 37° C.
- For heated wire circuits used with infants, the probe must be placed outside the incubator or away from the radiant warmer.
- The high-temperature alarm should be set no higher than 37° C, and the low setting should not be less than 30° C.
- Water level and function of automatic feed system (if applicable) should be monitored.
- Quantity, consistency, and other characteristics of secretions should be noted and recorded. When using an HME, if secretions become copious or appear increasingly tenacious, an HH should replace the HME.

For the complete guideline, see American Association for Respiratory Care: Clinical practice guideline: humidification during mechanical ventilation, Respir Care 37:887, 1992.

humidifiers perform the same under all conditions. Nishida[40] compared the performance of four active humidifiers (MR290 with MR730 [Fisher & Paykel Healthcare Inc, Laguna Hills, CA], MR310 with MR730 [Fisher & Paykel Healthcare Inc], ConchaTherm IV [Hudson RCI, Temecula, CA], and Hummax II), which were set to maintain the temperature of the airway opening at 32° C and 37° C under various ventilator parameters. The greater the minute ventilation, the lower the humidity delivered with all devices except the Hummax II. When the airway temperature control of the devices was set at 32° C, the ConchaTherm IV, the MR 310, and the MR 730 all failed to deliver 30 mg/L of vapor, which is the value recommended by ANSI. This study emphasizes the need to set humidifiers to maintain airway temperatures between 35° C and 37° C.

Controversy exists regarding the appropriate temperature and humidity of inspired gas delivered to mechanically ventilated patients with artificial airways. The current AARC Clinical Practice Guideline recommends 33° C, within 2° C, with a minimum of 30 mg/L of water vapor. In a comprehensive review, Williams[41] suggested that inspired humidity be maintained at an optimal level, 37° C with 100% relative humidity and 44 mg/L, to minimize mucosal dysfunction. Theoretically, optimal humidity offers improved mucociliary clearance. The benefits of this strategy are theory based but have yet to be shown conclusively in the clinical setting. Further controlled studies are needed to support better the need for optimal humidity.

Problem Solving and Troubleshooting

Common problems with humidification systems include dealing with condensation, avoiding cross contamination, and ensuring proper conditioning of the inspired gas.

Condensation

In all standard heated humidifier systems, saturated gas cools as it leaves the point of humidification and passes through the delivery tubing en route to the patient. As the gas cools, its water vapor capacity decreases, resulting in condensation or "rain out." Factors influencing the amount of condensation include (1) the temperature difference across the system (humidifier to airway); (2) the ambient temperature; (3) the gas flow; (4) the set airway temperature; and (5) the length, diameter, and thermal mass of the breathing circuit.

Figure 35-10 provides an example of the condensation process. In this case, because of cooling along the circuit, the humidifier temperature has to be set to a higher level (50° C) than desired at the airway. At 50° C, the humidifier fully saturates the gas to an absolute humidity level of 84 mg/L of water. As cooling occurs along the tubing, the capacity of the gas to hold water vapor decreases. By the time the gas reaches the patient, the temperature of the gas has decreased to 37° C, and it is holding only 44 mg/L of water vapor. Although BTPS conditions have been achieved, 40 mg/L, half the total output of the humidifier (84 mg/L − 44 mg/L = 40 mg/L), has condensed in the inspiratory limb of the circuit.

The condensation process poses risks to patients and caregivers and can waste a lot of water. First, condensation can disrupt or occlude gas flow through the circuit, potentially altering fractional inspired oxygen (FiO_2) or ventilator function or both. Condensate can work its way toward the patient and be aspirated. For these reasons, circuits must be positioned to drain condensate away from the patient and must be checked often, and excess condensate must be drained from heated humidifier breathing circuits on a regular basis.

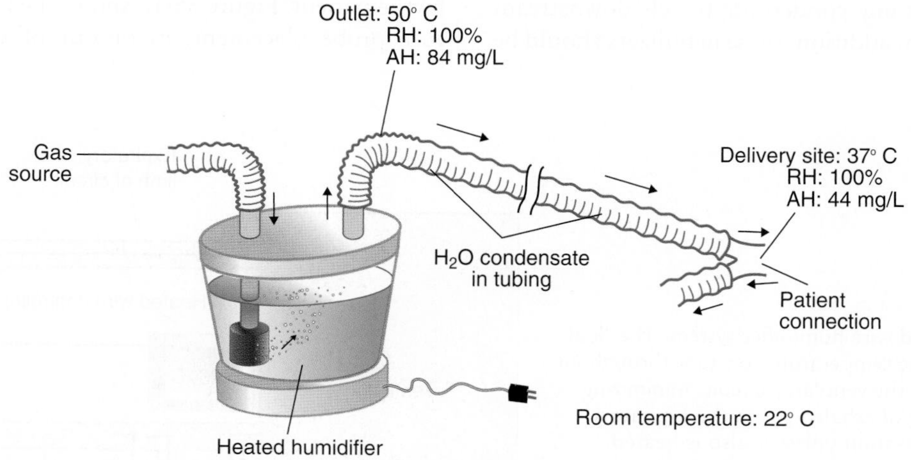

FIGURE 35-10 Gases leaving a standard heated humidifier are cooled en route to the patient. Although the gas remains saturated (100% relative humidity *[RH]*), cooling reduces its water vapor capacity, and condensation forms. Almost half of the original water (500 ml/day) is lost to condensation. The temperature at the patient connection (37° C) shown here is for illustrative purposes only. Heated humidifiers should be set to deliver inspired gas at 33° C ± 2° C. *AH,* Absolute humidity.

Typically, patients contaminate ventilator circuits within hours, and condensate is colonized with bacteria and poses an infection risk.[42] To avoid problems in this area, health care personnel should treat all breathing circuit condensate as infectious waste. See Chapters 4 and 43 for more detail on control procedures used with breathing circuits, including the AARC Clinical Practice Guideline on changing ventilator circuits (see Clinical Practice Guideline 4-1).

RULE OF THUMB

Always treat breathing circuit condensate as infectious waste. Use standard precautions, including wearing gloves and goggles. Always drain the tubing away from the patient's airway into an infectious waste container, and dispose of the waste according to the policies and procedures of the institution.

Several techniques are used to minimize problems with breathing circuit condensate. One common method is to place water traps at low points in the circuit (both the inspiratory and the expiratory limbs of ventilator circuits). This method aids drainage of condensate and reduces the likelihood of gas flow obstruction. When used in ventilator circuits, water traps should have little effect on circuit compliance, allow emptying without disrupting ventilation, and not be prone to leakage.

Nebulizers, with medication reservoirs below the aerosol generator and placed in the ventilator circuit, can act as a "water trap," collecting contaminated condensate. There is a tremendous risk that contaminated aerosols can be generated and pathogens delivered to the deep lung. To minimize this risk, nebulizers should be placed in a superior position so that any condensate travels downstream from the nebulizer. In addition, these nebulizers should be removed from the ventilator circuit between treatments, rinsed and air dried, washed, and sterilized or disposed of and replaced.

One way to avoid condensation problems is to prevent condensation from forming. Because the decrease in temperature in gas traveling from the humidifier to the airway causes condensation, maintaining an appropriate temperature in the circuit can prevent formation of condensate. Several methods, such as insulation or increasing the thermal mass of the circuit, can reduce circuit cooling by keeping the circuit at a constant temperature. The most common approach uses wire heating elements inserted into the ventilator circuit.

Most heated wire circuits use dual controllers with two temperature sensors: one monitoring the temperature of gas leaving the humidifier and the other placed at or near the patient's airway (Figure 35-11). The controller regulates the temperature difference between humidifier output and patient airway. When heated wire circuits are used, the humidifier heats gas to a lower temperature (32° C to 40° C) than with conventional circuits (45° C to 50° C). The reduction in condensate in the tubing results in less water use, reduced need for drainage, and less infection risk for patients and health care workers.

Even heated wire circuits can produce unwanted levels of condensate. One strategy is to provide absorptive material in the inspiratory limb of the ventilator circuit, which acts as a wick warmed by the heated wire system (Fisher & Paykel Healthcare Inc).

Use of heated wire circuits in neonates is complicated by the use of incubators and radiant warmers. Incubators provide a warm environment surrounding the infant and radiant warmers use radiant energy to warm objects that intercept radiant light. In both cases, a temperature probe placed in the heated environment would affect humidifier performance, resulting in reduced humidity received by the patient. Figure 35-12 shows the impact of temperature probe placement, in or out of the incubator, on

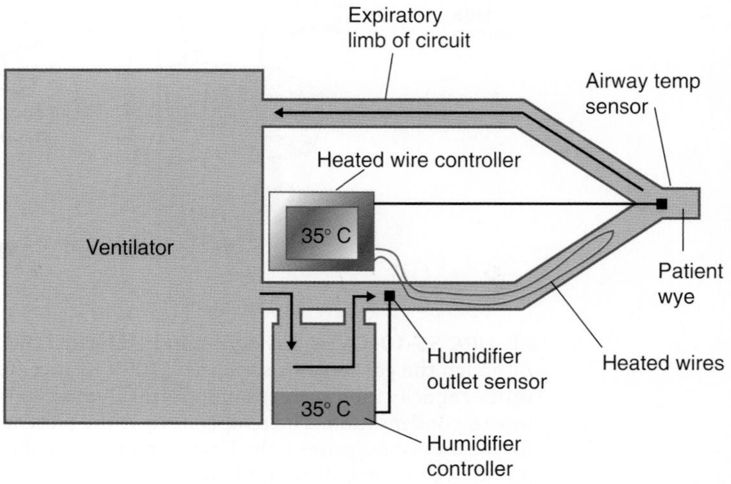

FIGURE 35-11 Heated wire humidifier system. The dual sensor system keeps the temperature constant throughout the inspiratory limb of the ventilator circuit, minimizing condensation. Cooling of exhaled gas in the expiratory limb can cause condensation unless it also is heated.

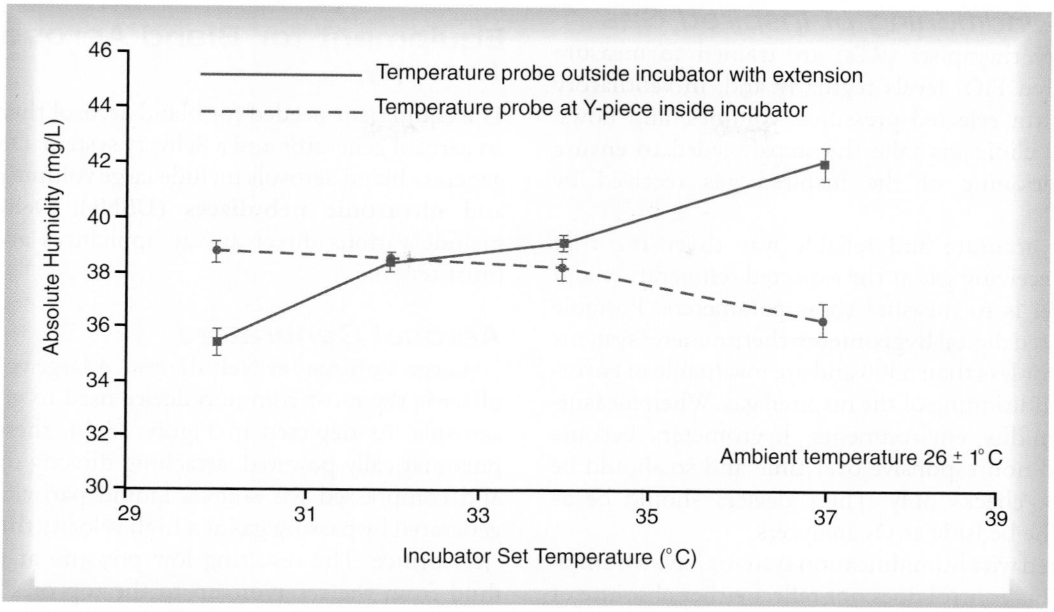

FIGURE 35-12 Humidity achieved at the Y-piece of a neonatal humidification system when used inside an incubator *(dotted line)* and outside or under an incubator *(solid line)*.

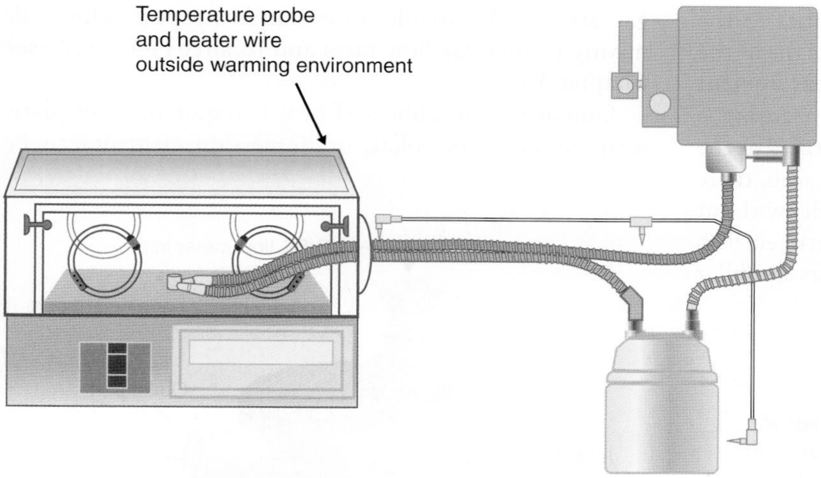

FIGURE 35-13 Neonatal breathing circuit configuration used with an incubator, with the temperature probe placed outside of the warming environment and an unheated portion of the inspiratory circuit delivering the gases to the Y-piece.

absolute humidity delivered to the neonate. Consequently, temperature probes should always be placed outside of the radiant field or incubator (Figure 35-13).

Cross Contamination

Aerosol and condensate from ventilator circuits are known sources of bacterial colonization.[42] However, advances in both circuit and humidifier technology have reduced the risk of nosocomial infection when these systems are used. Wick-type or membrane-type passover humidifiers prevent formation of bacteria-carrying aerosols. Heated wire circuits reduce production and pooling of condensate within the circuit. In addition, the high reservoir temperatures in humidifiers are bactericidal.[43] In ventilator circuits using wick-type humidifiers with heated wire systems, circuit contamination usually occurs from the patient to the circuit, rather than vice versa.

For decades, the traditional way to minimize the risk of circuit-related nosocomial infection in critically ill patients receiving ventilatory support was to change the ventilator tubing and its attached components every 24 hours.[44] It is now known that frequent ventilator circuit changes increase the risk of nosocomial pneumonia.[45] Current research indicates that there is minimal risk of ventilator-associated pneumonia with weekly circuit changes and that there may be no need to change circuits at all.[30,31,46,47] In addition, substantial cost savings can accrue with decreased frequency of circuit changes.

Proper Conditioning of Inspired Gas

All respiratory therapists (RTs) are trained to measure patient inspired FiO_2 levels regularly and, in ventilatory care, to monitor selected pressures, volumes, and flows. However, few clinicians take the steps needed to ensure proper conditioning of the inspired gas received by patients.

The most accurate and reliable way to ensure that patients are receiving gas at the expected temperature and humidity level is to measure these parameters. Portable battery-operated digital **hygrometer**-thermometer systems are available for less than $300 and are invaluable in ensuring proper conditioning of the inspired gas. When measuring high-humidity environments, hygrometers become saturated and nonresponsive over time and so should be used for spot checks only. These devices should be as common at the bedside as O_2 analyzers.

Many heated wire humidification systems have a humidity control. This control does not reflect either absolute or relative humidity but only the temperature differential between the humidifier and the airway sensor. If the heated wires are set warmer than the humidifier, less relative humidity is delivered to the patient. To ensure that the inspired gas is being properly conditioned, clinicians should always adjust the temperature differential to the point that a few drops of condensation form near the patient connection, or "wye." Lacking direct measurement of humidity, observation of this minimal condensate is the most reliable indicator that the gas is fully saturated at the specified temperature. If condensate cannot be seen, there is no way of knowing the level of relative humidity without direct measurement–it could be anywhere between 99% and 0%. HME performance can be evaluated in a similar manner.[48]

> **RULE OF THUMB**
>
> You can estimate if an HME is performing well at the bedside by visually confirming condensation in the flex tube between the airway and HME. Lack of condensate may be a clue that humidification is inadequate and that alternative systems may be appropriate for use with the patient.

BLAND AEROSOL THERAPY

Humidity is simply water in the gas phase, whereas a bland aerosol consists of liquid particles suspended in a gas (see Chapter 36 for details on aerosol physics). Bland aerosol therapy involves the delivery of sterile water or hypotonic, isotonic, or hypertonic saline aerosols. Bland aerosol administration may be accompanied by O_2 therapy. To guide practitioners in applying this therapy, the AARC has published Clinical Practice Guideline: Bland Aerosol Administration; excerpts appear in Clinical Practice Guideline 35-2.[49]

Equipment for Bland Aerosol Therapy

The equipment needed for bland aerosol therapy includes an aerosol generator and a delivery system. Devices used to generate bland aerosols include large volume jet nebulizers and **ultrasonic nebulizers (USNs).** Delivery systems include various direct airway appliances and enclosures (mist tents).

Aerosol Generators

Large Volume Jet Nebulizers. A large volume jet nebulizer is the most common device used to generate bland aerosols. As depicted in Figure 35-14, these devices are pneumatically powered, attaching directly to a flowmeter and compressed gas source. Liquid particle aerosols are generated by passing gas at a high velocity through a small "jet" orifice. The resulting low pressure at the jet draws fluid from the reservoir up to the top of a siphon tube, where it is sheared off and shattered into liquid particles. The large, unstable particles fall out of suspension or impact on the internal surfaces of the device, including the fluid surface **(baffling).** The remaining small particles leave the nebulizer through the outlet port, carried in the gas stream. A variable air-entrainment port allows air mixing to increase flow rates and to alter FiO_2 levels (see Chapter 38).

Similar to humidifiers, if heat is required, a hot plate, wraparound, yolk collar, or immersion element can be

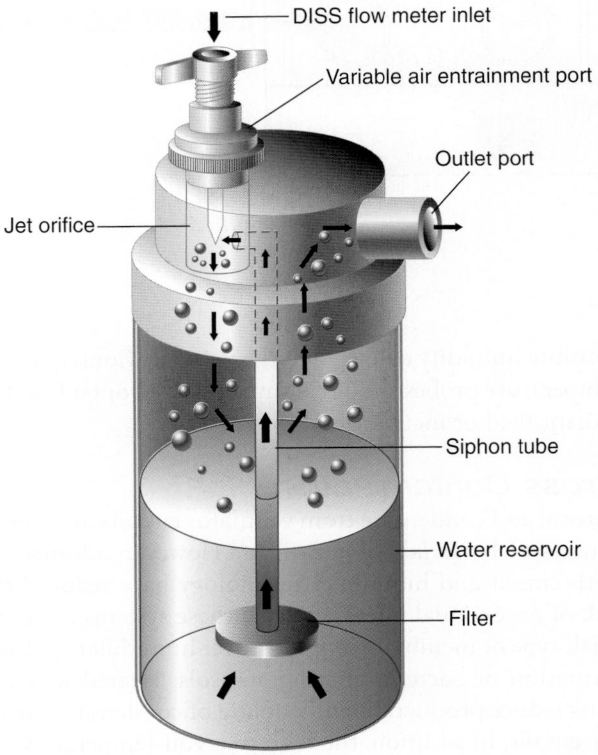

FIGURE 35-14 All-purpose large volume jet nebulizer.

35-2 Bland Aerosol Administration

AARC Clinical Practice Guideline (Excerpts)*

INDICATIONS
- Presence of upper airway edema—cool, bland aerosol
- Laryngotracheobronchitis
- Subglottic edema
- Postextubation edema
- Postoperative management of the upper airway
- Presence of a bypassed upper airway
- Need for sputum specimens or mobilization of secretions

CONTRAINDICATIONS
- Bronchoconstriction
- History of airway hyperresponsiveness

HAZARDS AND COMPLICATIONS
- Wheezing or bronchospasm
- Bronchoconstriction when artificial airway is used
- Infection
- Overhydration
- Patient discomfort
- Caregiver exposure to airborne contagions produced during coughing or sputum induction
- Edema of the airway wall
- Edema associated with decreased compliance and gas exchange and with increased airway resistance
- Sputum induction by hypertonic saline inhalation can cause bronchoconstriction in patients with chronic obstructive pulmonary disease, asthma, cystic fibrosis, or other pulmonary diseases.

ASSESSMENT OF NEED
The presence of one or more of the following may be an indication for administration of a water or isotonic or hypotonic saline aerosol:
- Stridor
- Brassy, crouplike cough
- Hoarseness after extubation
- Diagnosis of laryngotracheobronchitis or croup
- History of upper airway irritation and increased work of breathing (e.g., smoke inhalation)
- Patient discomfort associated with airway instrumentation or insult
- Bypassed upper airway

Need for sputum induction (e.g., pneumocystis pneumonia or tuberculosis) is an indication for administration of hypertonic saline aerosol.

ASSESSMENT OF OUTCOME
With administration of water or hypotonic or isotonic saline, the desired outcome is one or more of the following:
- Decreased work of breathing
- Improved vital signs
- Decreased stridor
- Decreased dyspnea
- Improved arterial blood gas values
- Improved O_2 saturation, as indicated by pulse oximetry

With administration of hypertonic saline, the desired outcome is a sputum sample that is adequate for analysis.

MONITORING
The extent of patient monitoring should be determined based on the stability and severity of the patient's condition:
- Patient subjective response—pain, discomfort, dyspnea, restlessness
- Heart rate and rhythm; blood pressure
- Respiratory rate, pattern, mechanics; accessory muscle use
- Sputum production—quantity, color, consistency, odor
- Skin color
- Breath sounds
- Pulse oximetry (if hypoxemia is suspected)
- Spirometry equipment (if adverse reaction is a concern)

**For the complete guideline, see Kallstrom T: American Association for Respiratory Care: AARC clinical practice guideline. Bland aerosol administration—2003 revision and update, Respir Care 48:529, 2003.*

added. However, in contrast to heated humidifiers, these devices rarely have sophisticated servo-controlled systems to control delivery temperature. Many systems do not shut down when the reservoir empties, resulting in the delivery of hot, dry gas to the patient. Failure of the element can also cause a loss of heating capacity, without warning to the clinician.

Depending on the design, input flow, and air-entrainment setting, the total water output of unheated large volume jet nebulizers varies between 26 mg H_2O/L and 35 mg H_2O/L. When heated, output increases to between 33 mg H_2O/L and 55 mg H_2O/L, mainly because of increased vapor capacity.[49,50] Larger versions of these devices (with 2-L to 3-L reservoirs) are used to deliver bland aerosols into mist tents. These enclosure systems can generate flow rates faster than 20 L/min, with water outputs of 5 ml/min (300 ml/hr). Because heat buildup in enclosures is a problem, these systems are always run unheated.

Ultrasonic Nebulizers. A USN is an electrically powered device that uses a **piezoelectric crystal** to generate aerosol. This crystal transducer converts radio waves into high-frequency mechanical vibrations (sound). These vibrations are transmitted to a liquid surface, where the intense mechanical energy creates a cavitation in the liquid, forming a standing wave, or "geyser," which sheds aerosol droplets. Figure 35-15 provides a schematic of a large volume USN. Output from a radiofrequency generator is transmitted over a shielded cable to the piezoelectric crystal. Vibrational energy is transmitted either indirectly through a water-filled couplant reservoir or directly to a solution chamber. Gas entering the chamber inlet picks up the aerosol particles and exits through the chamber outlet.

The properties of the ultrasonic signal determine the characteristics of the aerosol generated by these nebulizers. The frequency at which the crystal vibrates, preset by the manufacturer, determines aerosol particle size. Particle size is inversely proportional to signal frequency. A USN operating at a frequency of 2.25 MHz may produce an aerosol with a mass median aerodynamic diameter (MMAD) of approximately 2.5 μm, whereas another nebulizer operating at 1.25 MHz produces an aerosol with MMAD between 4 μm and 6 μm. Signal amplitude directly affects the amount of aerosol produced; the greater the amplitude, the greater the volume of aerosol output. In contrast to frequency, signal amplitude may be adjusted by the clinician.

Particle size and aerosol density delivered to the patient are also affected by the source and flow of gas through the aerosol-generating chamber. Some large volume USNs have built-in fans that direct room air through the solution chamber conducting the aerosol to the patient. The airflow may be adjusted by changing the fan speed or use of a simple damper valve. Alternatively, compressed anhydrous gases can be delivered to the chamber inlet through a flowmeter. For precise control over delivered O_2 concentrations, clinicians can attach a flowmeter with an O_2 blender or air-entrainment system to the chamber inlet.

The flow and amplitude settings interact to determine aerosol density (mg/L) and total water output (ml/min). Amplitude affects water output. At a given amplitude setting, the greater the flow through the chamber, the less

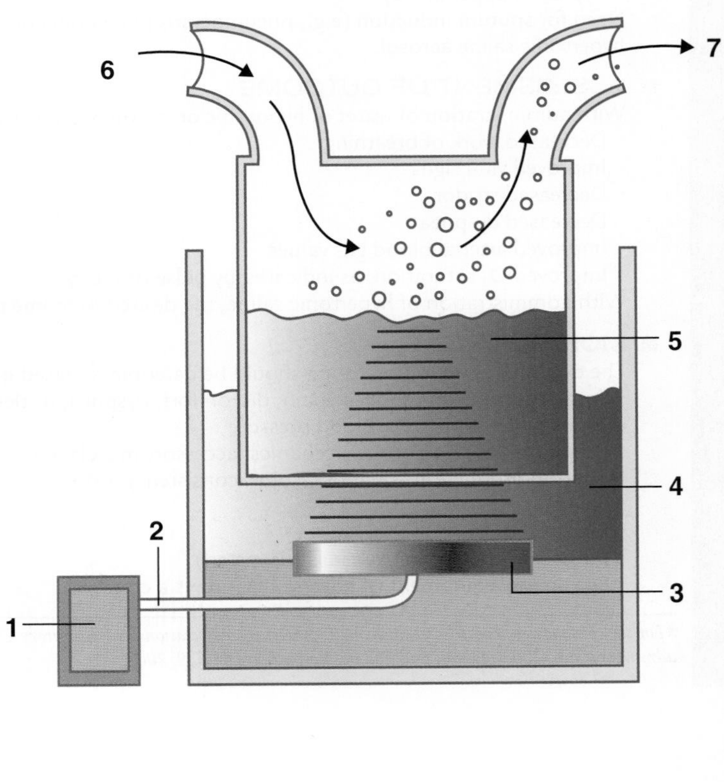

FIGURE 35-15 Functional schematic of a typical large volume USN. *1,* Radiofrequency generator; *2,* shielded cable; *3,* piezoelectric crystal transducer; *4,* water-filled couplant reservoir; *5,* solution chamber; *6,* chamber inlet; and *7,* chamber outlet. (Modified from Barnes TA: Core textbook for respiratory care practice, ed 2, St. Louis, 1994, Mosby.)

the density of the aerosol. Conversely, low flows result in aerosols of higher density. Total aerosol output (ml/min) is greatest when both flow and amplitude are set at the maximum. Using these settings, some units can achieve total water outputs of 7 ml/min.

Particle size, aerosol density, and output are also affected by the relative humidity of the carrier gas (see Chapter 36). In contrast to jet nebulizers, the temperature of the solution placed in a USN increases during use. Although this increase in temperature affects water vapor capacity, its impact on aerosol output is minimal.

RULE OF THUMB

To produce a high-density aerosol using a USN (useful for sputum induction), set the amplitude high and the flow rate low. To maximize aerosol delivery per minute (when trying to help mobilize secretions), set the flow rate to match and slightly exceed patient inspiratory flow rate, and set the amplitude at the maximum.

Although USNs have some unique capabilities, in most cases of bland aerosol administration, their relative advantages over jet nebulizers are outweighed by their high cost and erratic reliability. Exceptions include the use of a USN for sputum induction, where the high output (1 to 5 ml/min) and aerosol density seem to yield higher quantity and quality of sputum specimens for analysis, although at some cost in increased airway reactivity.[51] Although a major manufacturer of USNs (DeVilbiss) discontinued their product line, other manufacturers in both the United States and Europe still manufacture units for clinical use.

Commercially available USNs (usually marketed as "cool" mist devices) have found a place in the home, being used as room humidifiers. As with any nebulizer, the reservoirs of these devices can easily become contaminated, resulting in airborne transmission of pathogens. Care should be taken to ensure that these units are cleaned according to the manufacturer's recommendations and that water is discarded from the reservoir periodically between cleanings. In the absence of a manufacturer's recommendation, these units should undergo appropriate disinfection at least every 6 days.[52] Generally, passover and wick-type humidifiers present less risk than the USN as a room humidifier.

Airway Appliances

Airway appliances used to deliver bland aerosol therapy include aerosol mask, face tent, T-tube, and tracheostomy mask (Figure 35-16). The aerosol mask and face tent are used for patients with intact upper airways. The T-tube is used for patients who are orally or nasally intubated or who have a tracheostomy. The tracheostomy mask is used only for patients who have a tracheostomy. In all cases, large bore tubing is required to minimize flow resistance and prevent occlusion by condensate.

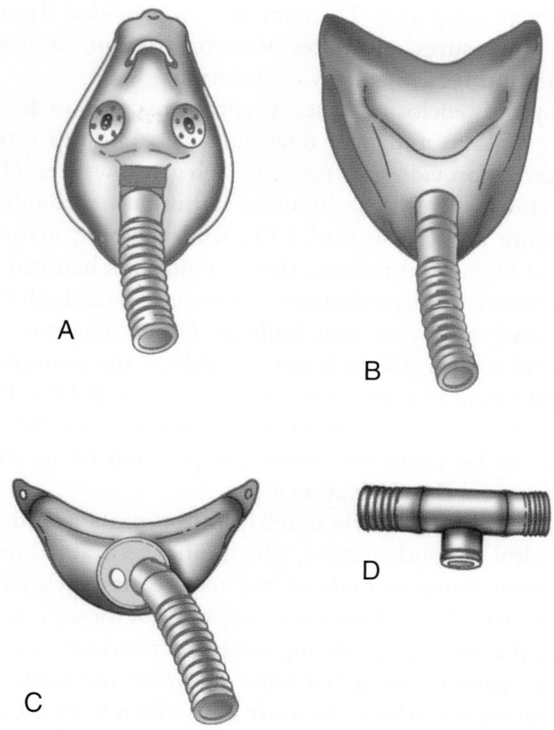

FIGURE 35-16 Airway appliances used to deliver bland aerosol therapy. **A,** Aerosol mask. **B,** Face tent. **C,** Tracheostomy mask. **D,** T-tube.

For short-term therapy to patients with intact upper airways, the aerosol mask is the device of choice. However, some patients cannot tolerate masks and may do better with a face tent. No data support preferential use of an open aerosol mask versus a face tent.

Although the T-tube is the most common application for tracheostomy patients, unless moderate to high FiO_2 levels are needed, a tracheostomy mask is a better choice. In contrast to T-tubes, tracheostomy masks exert no traction on the airway, and they allow secretions and condensate to escape from the airway, reducing airway resistance.

Enclosures (Mist Tents and Hoods)

Infants and small children may not readily tolerate direct airway appliances such as masks, so enclosures such as mist tents and aerosol hoods are used to deliver bland aerosol therapy to these patients. More recent studies have shown that aerosol hoods can provide aerosol delivery with similar efficiency to a properly fitted aerosol mask in infants, with less discomfort for the patient.[53]

Because mist tents were used for more than 40 years mainly to treat croup, clinicians may still refer to these devices as *croup tents*. The cool aerosol provided through these enclosures promotes vasoconstriction, decreases edema, and reduces airway obstruction.

Any body enclosure poses two problems: carbon dioxide (CO_2) buildup and heat retention. CO_2 buildup can be reduced by providing sufficiently high gas flow rates. These high flows of fresh gas circulate continually through the enclosure and "wash out" CO_2, while helping maintain desired O_2 concentrations. Heat retention is handled differently by each manufacturer. Some devices use high fresh gas flows to prevent heat buildup. Others incorporate a separate cooling device. Some tent devices use a simple ice compartment to cool the aerosol. The Ohmeda Ohio Pediatric Aerosol Tent (Ohmeda Ohio Corp., Gurnee, IL) and other similar units use electrically powered refrigeration units to cool the circulating air.

The cooling from these refrigeration units produces a great deal of condensation, which must be drained into a collection bottle outside of the tent. Units such as the Mistogen CAM-3M have overcome some of these problems with a thermoelectric cooling system, in which an electrical current passing through a semiconductor augments heat absorption and release. As warm air is taken from the tent, heat is transferred and released in the room, and cool air is returned to the tent.

Sputum Induction

As a diagnostic procedure, sputum induction (Box 35-5) warrants separate attention from other modes of bland aerosol therapy. Over the years, sputum induction has proved a useful, cost-effective, and safe method for diagnosing tuberculosis, pneumocystis pneumonia (caused by *Pneumocystis jiroveci* [formerly *Pneumocystis carinii*]), and lung cancer.[54-56]

Sputum induction involves short-term application of high-density hypertonic saline (3% to 10%) aerosols to the airway to assist in mobilizing pulmonary secretions for evacuation and recovery. These high-density aerosols are most easily generated using ultrasonic nebulization. The exact mechanism by which high-density hypertonic aerosols aid mucociliary clearance is unknown. However, an increased volume of surface fluid delivered to the airways, combined with stimulation of the irritant (cough) reflex, is a likely mechanism.

Box 35-5 outlines a procedure for sputum induction using a 3% saline solution.[57] To ensure a good sputum sample, every effort must be made to separate saliva from true respiratory tract secretions.[56] In some cases, protocols include having patients brush their teeth and tongue surface thoroughly and rinse their mouths before sputum induction. Although the distinction between saliva and sputum can be made in the diagnostic laboratory, care during the collection procedure eliminates the need for repeat inductions.

Box 35-5 Sputum-Induction Procedure

- Gather the necessary equipment: USN, aerosol mask, large bore tubing, specimen container, 3% sterile saline, and stethoscope.
- Check the chart for order or protocol, diagnosis, history, and other pertinent information.
- Wash your hands and follow applicable standard, airborne, and tuberculosis precautions.
- Introduce yourself and identify your department; verify the patient's identity; and explain the procedure and verify that the patient understands it.
- Have the patient assume an upright, seated position if possible.
- Have the patient rinse his or her mouth with water, blow his or her nose, and clear any excess saliva.
- Perform pretreatment assessment, including vital signs, muscle tone, ability to cough, and auscultation.
- Assemble the nebulizer; fill the couplant chamber with tap water; plug the unit into a grounded electrical outlet; and attach the delivery tubing and mask.
- Aseptically fill the medication chamber of the nebulizer with 3% sterile saline.
- Turn the unit on, and adjust the output control to achieve adequate flow and high density.
- Place the mask comfortably on the patient's face, and instruct the patient to take slow, deep breaths, with occasional inspiratory hold as tolerated.
- Periodically reassess the patient's condition (including breath sounds) throughout the application.
- Modify the technique and reinstruct the patient as needed, based on his or her response.
- Terminate the treatment after 15 to 30 minutes, if significant adverse reactions occur, or when sputum specimen has been obtained.
- Encourage the patient to cough and expectorate sputum into specimen cup; observe for volume, color, consistency, odor, and presence or absence of blood.
- Label the specimen container with patient identification and required information, and deliver to the appropriate personnel.
- Chart the therapy according to departmental and institutional protocol.
- Notify the appropriate personnel of any adverse reactions or other concerns.

Modified from Butler TJ: Laboratory exercises for competency in respiratory care, ed 2, Philadelphia, 2009, FA Davis.

Problem Solving and Troubleshooting

The most common problems with bland aerosol delivery systems are cross contamination and infection, environmental safety, inadequate mist production, overhydration, bronchospasm, and noise.

Cross Contamination

Rigorous adherence to the infection control guidelines detailed in Chapter 4, especially guidelines covering solutions and equipment processing, should help minimize the cross contamination and infection risks involved in using these systems. In addition, the water should be changed regularly, and the couplant compartments and nebulizer chambers of USNs should be disinfected or replaced regularly.

Environmental Exposure

Environmental safety issues from secondhand and exhaled aerosol arise mainly when aerosol therapy is prescribed for immunosuppressed patients or for patients with tuberculosis. A survey suggested that RTs may be at increased risk for developing asthma-like symptoms, attributed partly to secondhand exposure to aerosols such as ribavirin or albuterol.[58] To minimize problems in this area, all clinicians should strictly follow U.S. Centers for Disease Control and Prevention standards and airborne precautions, including precautions specified for control of exposure to tuberculosis (see Chapter 4). Additional methods for dealing with environmental control of drug aerosols are described in Chapter 36.

Inadequate Aerosol Output

Inadequate mist production is a common problem with all nebulizer systems. With pneumatically powered jet nebulizers, poor mist production can be caused by inadequate input flow of driving gas, siphon tube obstruction, or jet orifice misalignment. With the exception of inadequate driving gas flow, these problems require unit repair or replacement. If a USN is not functioning properly, the electrical power supply (cord, plug, and fuse or circuit breakers) should be checked first. The clinician next should check to confirm that (1) carrier gas is flowing through the device and (2) the amplitude, or output, control is set above minimum. If there is still no visible mist output, the clinician should inspect the couplant chamber to confirm proper fill level and the absence of any visible dirt or debris. Finally, the clinician must ensure that the couplant chamber solution meets the manufacturer's specifications (most units do not function properly with distilled water).

Overhydration

Overhydration is a problem with continuous use of heated jet nebulizers and USNs. With USNs capable of such extraordinarily high water outputs, they should never be used for continuous therapy. The risk of overhydration is highest for infants, small children, and patients with preexisting fluid or electrolyte imbalances. Even if used only to meet BTPS conditions, bland aerosol therapy effectively eliminates insensible water loss through the lungs and should be equated to a daily water gain (approximately 200 ml/day for an average adult). In addition to overhydration of the patient, inspissated pulmonary secretions can swell after high-density aerosol therapy, worsening airway obstruction. Careful patient selection and monitoring can prevent most potential problems with overhydration.

Bronchospasm

Even bland water aerosols can cause bronchospasm in some patients. Ultrasonic nebulization of distilled water is used in some pulmonary function laboratories to provoke bronchospasm and to assess bronchial hyperactivity.[57] To avoid this problem at the bedside, the clinician should always carefully review the patient's history and diagnosis before administering any bland aerosol, especially a hypotonic water solution. As indicated in the AARC practice guideline (see Clinical Practice Guideline 35-2), patients receiving continuous bland aerosol therapy should be initially monitored carefully (including breath sounds and subjective response) and reevaluated every 8 hours or with any change in clinical condition.[49] If bronchospasm occurs during therapy, treatment must be stopped immediately, O_2 must be provided, and appropriate bronchodilator therapy should be initiated as soon as possible. If the physician still requests bland aerosol therapy for such a patient, pretreatment with a bronchodilator may be needed. In addition, isotonic solutions (0.9% saline) may be better tolerated by these patients than water.

A problem unique to large volume, air entrainment jet nebulizers is the noise they generate, especially at high flows. The American Academy of Pediatrics recommends that sound levels remain less than 58 dB to avoid hearing loss for infants being cared for in incubators and O_2 hoods. Because many commercial nebulizers exceed this noise level when in operation, careful selection of equipment is necessary. However, the best way to avoid this problem and minimize infection risks further is to use heated passover humidification instead of nebulization.

SELECTING THE APPROPRIATE THERAPY

Figure 35-17 provides a basic algorithm for selecting or recommending the appropriate therapy to condition a patient's inspired gas. Key considerations include (1) gas flow, (2) presence or absence of an artificial tracheal airway, (3) character of the pulmonary secretions, (4) need for and expected duration of mechanical ventilation, and (5) contraindications to using an HME.

Regarding delivery of O_2 to the upper airway, the American College of Chest Physicians advises against using a bubble humidifier at flow O_2 rates of 4 L/min or less.[59] For the occasional patient who complains of nasal dryness or

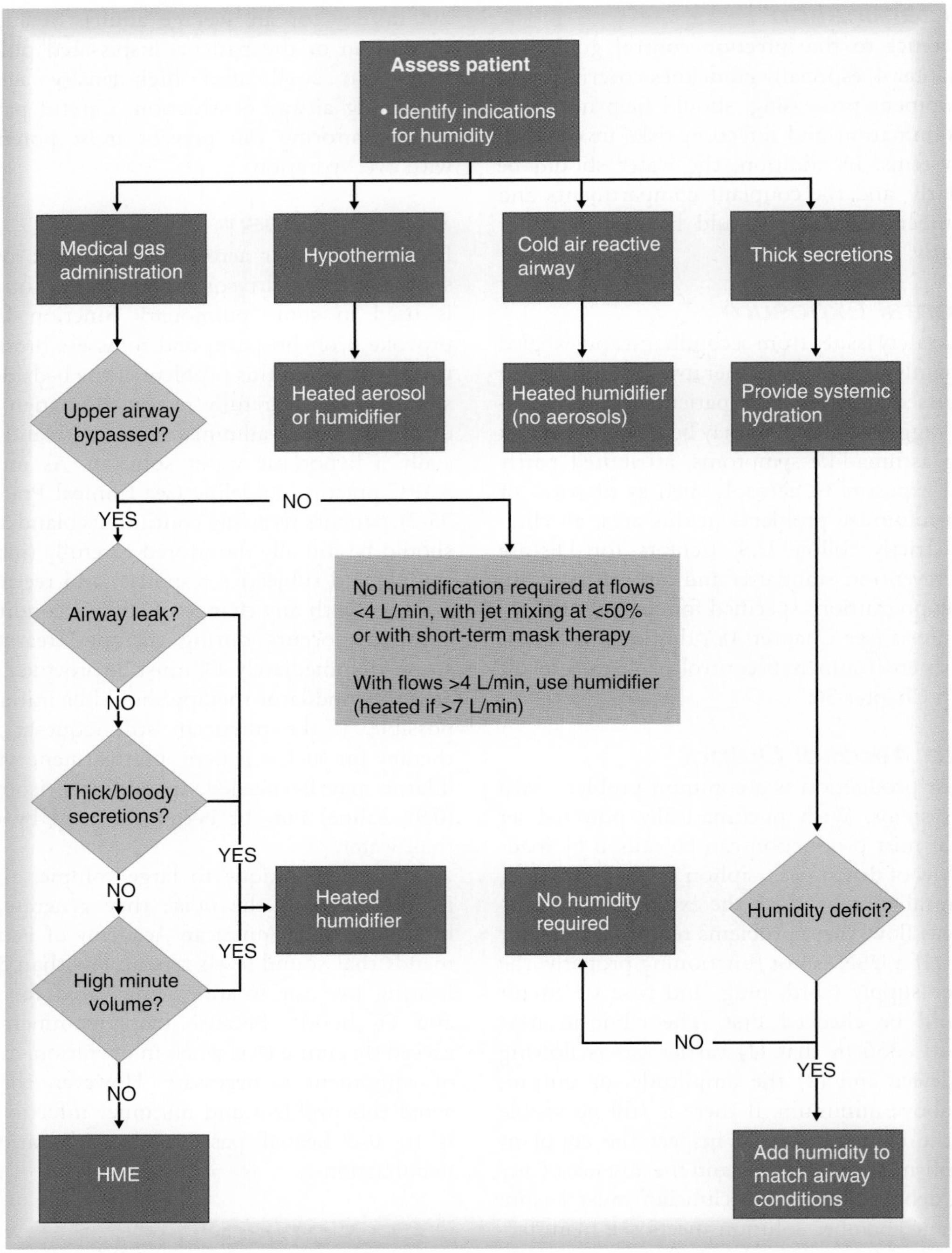

FIGURE 35-17 Selection algorithm for humidity and bland aerosol therapy.

irritation when receiving low-flow O_2, a humidifier should be added to the delivery system. Conversely, the relative inefficiency of unheated bubble humidifiers means that the clinician may need to consider heated humidification for patients receiving long-term O_2 at high flow rates (>10 L/min without air entrainment).

HMEs provide an inexpensive alternative to heated humidifiers when used for ventilation of patients who do not have complex humidification needs. However, passive HMEs may not provide sufficient heat or humidification for long-term management of certain patients. When an HME is to be used, it should be selected based on individual patient need and ventilatory pattern and the unit's performance, efficiency, and size. All patients using HMEs should be reevaluated regularly to confirm the appropriateness of continued use.[60]

MINI CLINI

Cost-Effectiveness of Humidification Systems

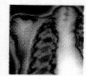

PROBLEM: There is a lot of controversy over which is more cost-effective—heated water humidifiers or HMEs. How can the cost of passover humidifiers, with standard circuit and heated wire circuits, be compared with the cost of HMEs?

SOLUTION: First, determine the frequency of circuit setup and component changes for each type of humidification system. Second, determine supplies and time required to set up the system and to operate the system on a daily basis.

The following table compares the costs associated with three humidification strategies in terms of circuit setup costs, water usage, and labor for a typical patient requiring 12 days of mechanical ventilation at a large, comprehensive acute care hospital. Labor costs were calculated as the time required to perform setup or maintenance multiplied by the average salary. This example assumes no circuit changes for a patient over 14 days and that the HME is changed daily.

Components of Circuit Setup and Operating Costs	Heated Humidifier With Standard Circuit	Heated Humidifier With Heated Wire Circuit	Heat Moisture Exchanger
Vent circuit	$3.00	$11.00	$3.00
Humidifier/ water feed system	$12.00	$12.00	—
HME filter	—	—	$5.00
Setup cost (labor)	$18.00	$23.00	$8.00
Daily cost (labor)	$11.00	$1.50	$5.00
Total costs (5 days)	$62.00	$29.00	$28.00
Total costs (12 days)	$139.00	$39.50	$63.00

In this example, the standard circuit costs less than the heated wire circuit but has twice the daily water usage, with an additional labor cost of $9.50 per day for adding and removing water from the system. The HME has the lowest setup cost, but after ventilator day 5, total costs of daily filter replacement exceed the cost associated with operation of the heated wire circuit. Although different component costs may shift the analysis, this example shows that use of active humidity employing heated wire circuits is more cost-effective than standard circuits and possibly even HMEs.

SUMMARY CHECKLIST

- Conditioning of inhaled and exhaled gas is accomplished primarily by the nose and upper airway. Bypassing the upper airway without providing similar levels of heat and humidity to inhaled gas can cause damage to the respiratory tract.
- The primary goal of humidification is to maintain normal physiologic conditions in the lower airways.
- Gases delivered to the nose and mouth should be conditioned to 20° C to 22° C with 10 mg/L water vapor (50% relative humidity).
- When being delivered to the trachea, gases should be warmed and humidified to 32° C to 40° C with 36 to 40 mg/L water vapor (>90% relative humidity).
- A humidifier is a device that adds invisible molecular water to gas.
- A nebulizer generates and disperses liquid particles in a gas stream.
- Water vapor cannot carry pathogens, but aerosols and condensate can carry pathogens.
- Temperature is the most important factor affecting humidifier output. The higher the temperature, the greater the water vapor content of the delivered gas.
- Bubble humidifiers, passover humidifiers, wick humidifiers, and HMEs are the major types of humidifiers. Active humidifiers incorporate heating devices and reservoir and feed systems.
- At high flow rates, some bubble humidifiers can produce microaerosol particles, which can carry infectious bacteria.
- Most HMEs are passive, capturing both heat and moisture from expired gas and returning it to the patient, at about 70% efficiency. HMEs are not recommended for use with infants because of the increased mechanical dead space and use of uncuffed endotracheal tubes, which allow some exhaled gas to bypass the HME.
- Common problems with humidification systems include condensation, cross contamination, and ensuring proper conditioning of the inspired gas.
- Breathing circuit condensate must always be treated as infectious waste.
- Bland aerosol therapy with sterile water or saline is used to (1) treat upper airway edema, (2) overcome heat and humidity deficits in patients with tracheal airways, and (3) help obtain sputum specimens.
- Large volume jet nebulizers and USNs are used to generate bland aerosols. Delivery systems include various direct airway appliances and mist tents.
- Common problems with bland aerosol therapy are cross contamination and infection, environmental safety, inadequate mist production, overhydration, bronchospasm, and noise.

References

1. Kapadia F, Shelley M: Normal mechanisms of humidification. Probl Respir Care 4:395, 1991.
2. Primiano F, Montague F, Saidel G: Measurement system for water vapor and temperature dynamics. J Appl Physiol 56:1679, 1984.
3. Shelley M, Lloyd G, Park G: A review of the mechanisms and the methods of humidification of inspired gas. Intensive Care Med 14:1, 1998.
4. Ingelstedt S: Studies on the conditioning of air in the respiratory tract. Acta Otolaryngol 131(Suppl):1, 1956.
5. Chalon J, Loew D, Malbranche J: Effects of dry air and subsequent humidification on tracheobronchial ciliated epithelium. Anesthesiology 37:338, 1972.
6. Marfatia S, Donahoe P, Henderson W: Effect of dry and humidified gases on the respiratory epithelium in rabbits. J Pediatr Surg 10:583, 1975.
7. American Association for Respiratory Care: Clinical practice guideline: humidification during mechanical ventilation. Respir Care 37:887, 1992.
8. Chatburn R, Primiano F: A rational basis for humidity therapy. Respir Care 32:249, 1987.
9. Anderson S, Herbring B, Widman B: Accidental profound hypothermia. Br J Anaesth 42:653, 1970.
10. Weinberg A: Hypothermia. Ann Emerg Med 22:370, 1993.
11. Chen T: The effect of heated humidifier in the prevention of intra-operative hypothermia. Acta Anaesthesiol Sin 32:27, 1994.
12. Giesbrecht G, Younes M: Exercise and cold-induced asthma. Can J Appl Physiol 20:300, 1995.
13. American Society for Testing and Materials (ASTM): Standard specification for humidifiers for medical use (F1690), Conshohocken, PA, 1996, ASTM.
14. Gray H: Humidifiers. Probl Respir Care 4:423, 1992.
15. Klein E: Performance characteristics of conventional prototype humidifiers and nebulizers. Chest 64:690, 1993.
16. Darin J, Broadwell J, MacDonell R: An evaluation of water-vapor output from four brands of unheated, prefilled bubble humidifiers. Respir Care 27:41, 1992.
17. Rhame F, Streifel A, McComb C: Bubbling humidifiers produce microaerosols which can carry bacteria. Infection Control 7:403, 1986.
18. Cairo JM, Pilbeam SP: Mosby's respiratory care equipment, ed 8, St. Louis, 2010, Mosby.
19. Vitacca M: Hygroscopic condenser humidifiers in chronically tracheostomized patients who breathe spontaneously. Eur Respir J 7:2026, 1994.
20. Kapadia F: Changing patterns of airway accidents in intubated ICU patients. Intensive Care Med 27:296, 2001.
21. Bien S, Okla S, van As-Brooks CJ, et al: The effect of a Heat and Moisture Exchanger (Provox HME) on pulmonary protection after total laryngectomy: a randomized controlled study. Eur Arch Otorhinolaryngol 267:429, 2010.
22. Hedley R, Allt-Graham J: A comparison of the filtration properties of heat and moisture exchangers. Anaesthesia 47:414, 1992.
23. Kelly M, Gillies D, Todd DA, et al: Heated humidification versus heat and moisture exchangers for ventilated adults and children. Cochrane Database Syst Rev (4):CD004711, 2010.
24. International Organization for Standardization: Heat and moisture exchangers for use in humidifying respired gases in humans (ISO 9360), Geneva, 1992, International Organization for Standardization.
25. Shelly M: Inspired gas conditioning. Respir Care 37:1070, 1992.
26. Lellouche F, Taille S, Lefrancois F, et al: Humidification performance of 48 passive airway humidifiers: comparison with manufacturer data. Chest 135:276, 2009.
27. Branson R, Davis K: Evaluation of 21 passive humidifiers according to the ISO 9360 standard: moisture output, deadspace, and flow resistance. Respir Care 41:736, 1996.
28. Ploysongsang Y: Effect of flowrate and duration of use on the pressure drop across six artificial noses. Respir Care 34:902, 1989.
29. Kola A, Eckmanns T, Gastmeier P: Efficacy of heat and moisture exchangers in preventing ventilator-associated pneumonia: meta-analysis of randomized controlled trials. Intensive Care Med 31:5, 2005.
30. Ricard JD, Boyer A, Dreyfuss D: The effect of humidification on the incidence of ventilator-associated pneumonia. Respir Care 12:263, 2006.
31. Dreyfuss D: Mechanical ventilation with heated humidifiers or heat and moisture exchangers: effect on patient colonization and incidence of nosocomial pneumonia. Am J Respir Crit Care Med 151:986, 1995.
32. Siempos I, Vardakas KZ, Kopterides P, et al: Impact of passive humidification on clinical outcomes of mechanically ventilated patients: a meta-analysis of randomized controlled trials. Crit Care Med 35:2843, 2007.
33. Lacherade J, Auburtin M, Cerf C, et al: Impact of humidification systems on ventilator-associated pneumonia: a randomized multicenter trial. Am J Respir Crit Care Med 172:1276, 2005.
34. Inui D, Oto J, Nishimura M: Effect of heat and moisture exchanger (HME) positioning on inspiratory gas humidification. BMC Pulm Med 6:19, 2006.
35. Solomita M, Palmer B, Daroowalla F, et al: Humidification and secretion volume in mechanically ventilated patients. Respir Care 54:1329, 2009.
36. Jean-Claude L: Impact of humidification systems on ventilator-associated pneumonia. Am J Respir Crit Care Med 17:1276, 2005.
37. Larsson A, Gustafsson A, Svanborg L: A new device for 100 per cent humidification of inspired air. Crit Care Med 4:54, 2000.
38. Emergency Care Research Institute: Heated humidifiers, Health Devices. 1987. http://www.fda.gov/oc/po/firmrecalls/Vapotherm2000i_01_06.html. Accessed March 2, 2011.
39. Tiffin N, Weinstein L, Sunstein D: The performance of a novel humidification device for mechanical ventilation. Presented at European Respiratory Society 16th Annual Congress, Munich, Germany, 2006.
40. Nishida T: Performance of heated humidifiers with a heated wire according to ventilatory settings. J Aerosol Med 14:43, 2001.
41. Williams R: Relationship between the humidity and temperature of inspired gas and the function of the airway mucosa. Crit Care Med 24:1920, 1996.
42. Craven D, Goularte T, Make B: Contaminated condensate in mechanical ventilator circuits: a risk factor for nosocomial pneumonia. Am Rev Respir Dis 129:625, 1984.
43. Gilmour I, Boyle M, Streifel A: Humidifiers kill bacteria. Anesthesiology 75:498, 1991.
44. Craven D: Risk factors for pneumonia and fatality in patients receiving continuous mechanical ventilation. Am Rev Respir Dis 33:792, 1986.
45. Hess D: Weekly ventilator circuit changes: a strategy to reduce costs without affecting pneumonia rates. Anesthesiology 82:903, 1995.

46. Kollef M: Mechanical ventilation with or without 7-day circuit changes: a randomized controlled study. Ann Intern Med 123:168, 1995.
47. Fink J: Extending ventilator circuit change interval beyond two days reduces the likelihood of ventilator associated pneumonia (VAP). Chest 113:405, 1998.
48. Beydon L: Correlation between simple clinical parameters and the in vitro humidification characteristics of filter heat and moisture exchangers. Chest 112:739, 1997.
49. Kallstrom T; American Association for Respiratory Care: AARC clinical practice guideline. Bland aerosol administration—2003 revision and update. Respir Care 48:529, 2003.
50. Hill T, Sorbello J: Humidity outputs of large-reservoir nebulizers. Respir Care 32:225, 1987.
51. Loh L, Eg K, Puspanathan P: A comparison of sputum induction methods: ultrasonic vs compressed-air nebulizer and hypertonic vs isotonic saline inhalation. Asian Pac J Allergy Immunol 1:11, 2004.
52. Chatburn R, Lough M, Klinger J: An in-hospital evaluation of the sonic mist ultrasonic room humidifier. Respir Care 29:893, 1994.
53. Kugelman A, Amirav I, Mor F, et al: Hood versus mask nebulization in infants with evolving bronchopulmonary dysplasia in the neonatal intensive care unit. J Perinatol 26:31, 2006.
54. Khajotia R: Induced sputum and cytological diagnosis of lung cancer. Lancet 338:976, 1991.
55. Anderson C, Inhaber N, Menzies D: Comparison of sputum induction with fiberoptic bronchoscopy in the diagnosis of tuberculosis. Am J Respir Crit Care Med 152:1570, 1995.
56. Godwin C, Brown D, Masur H: Sputum induction: a quick and sensitive technique for diagnosing *Pneumocystis carinii* pneumonia in immunosuppressed patients. Respir Care 36:33, 1991.
57. Gershman N: Comparison of two methods of collecting induced sputum in asthmatic subjects. Eur Respir J 9:2448, 1996.
58. Dimich-Ward H, Wymer ML, Chan-Yeung M: Respiratory health survey of respiratory therapists. Chest 126:1048, 2004.
59. American College of Chest Physicians and NHLBI: National Conference on Oxygen Therapy. Respir Care 29:922, 1984.
60. Branson R, Chatburn R: Humidification during mechanical ventilation (editorial). Respir Care 38:461, 1993.

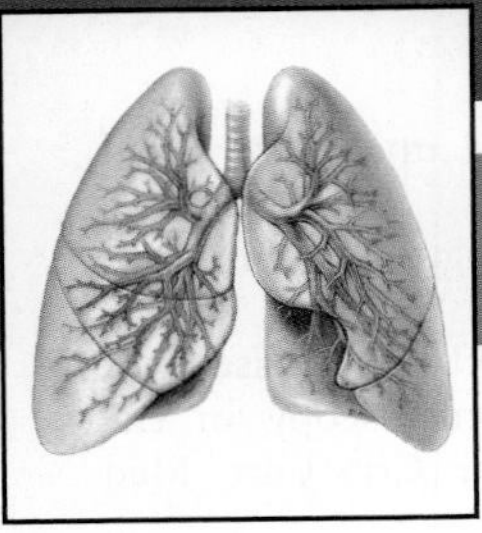

Chapter 36

Aerosol Drug Therapy

JIM FINK

CHAPTER OBJECTIVES

After reading this chapter you will be able to:

- Define the term *aerosol*.
- Describe how particle size, motion, and airway characteristics affect aerosol deposition.
- Describe how aerosols are generated.
- List the hazards associated with aerosol drug therapy.
- Describe how to select the best aerosol drug delivery system for a patient.
- Describe how to initiate and modify aerosol drug therapy.
- State the information patients need to know to self-administer drug aerosol therapy properly.
- Describe how to assess patient response to bronchodilator therapy at the point of care.
- Describe how to apply aerosol therapy in special circumstances.
- Describe how to protect patients and caregivers from exposure to aerosolized drugs.

CHAPTER OUTLINE

Characteristics of Therapeutic Aerosols
- Aerosol Output
- Particle Size
- Deposition
- Aging
- Quantifying Aerosol Delivery

Hazards of Aerosol Therapy
- Infection
- Airway Reactivity
- Pulmonary and Systemic Effects
- Drug Concentration
- Eye Irritation
- Secondhand Exposure to Aerosol Drugs

Aerosol Drug Delivery Systems
- Metered Dose Inhalers
- Dry Powder Inhalers
- Nebulizers
- Advantages and Disadvantages of Aerosol Systems
- Special Medication Delivery Issues for Infants and Children
- Selecting an Aerosol Drug Delivery System

Assessment-Based Bronchodilator Therapy Protocols
- Sample Protocol
- Assessing Patient Response
- Patient Education

Special Considerations
- Acute Care and Off-Label Use
- Aerosol Administration to Mechanically Ventilated Patients
- Aerosol Generator Placement

Controlling Environmental Contamination
- Negative Pressure Rooms
- Booths and Stations
- Personal Protective Equipment

KEY TERMS

aerosol
aerosol output
aging
atomizer
baffle
breath-actuated nebulizer
breath-enhanced nebulizer
chlorofluorocarbons (CFCs)
deposition
emitted dose
fine-particle fraction
geometric standard deviation (GSD)
heterodisperse
hydrofluoroalkane (HFA)
hygroscopic
inertial impaction
inhaled mass
mass median aerodynamic diameter (MMAD)
monodisperse

nebulizer
propellant
residual drug volume
respirable mass
scintigraphy
sedimentation
therapeutic index
volume median diameter (VMD)

An **aerosol** is a suspension of solid or liquid particles in gas. Aerosols occur in nature as pollens, spores, dust, smoke, smog, fog, and mist.[1] A primary function of the upper airway and respiratory tract is to protect the lungs from invasion by these aerosols. In the clinical setting, medical aerosols are generated with **atomizers, nebulizers,** and inhalers—devices that physically disperse matter into small particles and suspend them into a gas. Aerosols can be used to deliver bland water solutions to the respiratory tract (see Chapter 35) or to administer drugs to the lungs, throat, or nose for local and systemic effect. This chapter focuses on the principles of aerosol drug therapy.

The aim of medical aerosol therapy is to deliver a therapeutic dose of the selected agent (drug) to the desired site of action. The indication for any specific aerosol is based on the need for the specific drug and the targeted site of delivery.[1] For patients with pulmonary disorders, administration of drugs by aerosol offers higher local drug concentrations in the lung with lower systemic levels compared with other forms of administration. Improved therapeutic action with fewer systemic side effects provides a higher **therapeutic index.**[2]

CHARACTERISTICS OF THERAPEUTIC AEROSOLS

Effective use of medical aerosols requires an understanding of the characteristics of aerosols and their effect on drug delivery to the desired site of action. Key concepts include aerosol output, particle size, deposition, and a phenomenon known as *aging.*

Aerosol Output

The rate that aerosol is generated is a key parameter in aerosol administration. **Aerosol output** is defined as the mass of fluid or drug contained in aerosol produced by a nebulizer. Output is expressed as either a unit of mass leaving the nebulizer or as a proportion of the dose placed in the nebulizer. Output rate is the mass of aerosol generated per unit of time. Output varies greatly among different nebulizers and inhalers. For drug delivery systems, **emitted dose** describes the mass of drug leaving the mouthpiece of a nebulizer or inhaler as aerosol.

Aerosol output can be measured by collecting the aerosol that leaves the nebulizer on filters and measuring either their weight (gravimetric analysis) or quantity of drug (assay). Gravimetric measurements of aerosols are less reliable than drug assay techniques because weight changes resulting from water evaporation cannot be differentiated from changes in drug mass. A drug assay provides the most reliable measure of aerosol output.

A substantial proportion of particles that leave a nebulizer never reach the lungs. The ability of aerosols to travel through the air, enter the airways, and become deposited in the lungs is based on numerous variables ranging from particle size to breathing pattern. Understanding and skillful manipulation of these variables can greatly improve pulmonary delivery of aerosols.

Particle Size

Aerosol particle size depends on the substance for nebulization, the method used to generate the aerosol, and the environmental conditions surrounding the particle.[3] It is impossible to determine visually whether a nebulizer is producing an optimal particle size. The unaided human eye cannot see particles less than 50 to 100 μm in diameter (equivalent to a small grain of sand). The only reliable way to determine the characteristics of an aerosol suspension is laboratory measurement. The two most common laboratory methods used to measure medical aerosol particle size distribution are cascade impaction and laser diffraction. *Cascade impactors* are designed to collect aerosols of different size ranges on a series of stages or plates. The mass of aerosol deposited on each plate is quantified by drug assay, and a distribution of drug mass across particle sizes is calculated. In *laser diffraction,* a computer is used to estimate the range and frequency of droplet volumes crossing the laser beam.

Because medical aerosols contain particles of many different sizes **(heterodisperse),** the average particle size is expressed with a measure of central tendency, such as **mass median aerodynamic diameter (MMAD)** for cascade impaction or **volume median diameter (VMD)** for laser diffraction. These measurement techniques of the same aerosol may report different sizes, so it is important to know which measurement is used. The MMAD and VMD both describe the particle diameter in micrometers (μm). In an aerosol distribution with a specific MMAD, 50% of the particles are smaller and have less mass, and 50% are larger and have greater mass.

The **geometric standard deviation (GSD)** describes the variability of particle sizes in an aerosol distribution set at 1 standard deviation above or below the median (15.8% and 84.13%). Most aerosols found in nature and used in respiratory care are composed of particles of different sizes, described as heterodisperse. The greater the GSD, the wider the range of particle sizes, and the more heterodisperse the aerosol. Aerosols consisting of particles of similar size (GSD ≤ 1.2) are referred to as **monodisperse.** Nebulizers that produce monodisperse aerosols are used mainly in laboratory research and in nonmedical industries.

Deposition

When aerosol particles leave suspension in gas, they deposit on (attach to) a surface. Only a portion of the aerosol generated and emitted from a nebulizer (emitted dose) may be inhaled (inhaled dose). A fraction of the inhaled dose is deposited in the lungs (respirable dose). **Inhaled mass** is the amount of drug inhaled. The proportion of the drug mass in particles that are small enough **(fine-particle fraction)** to reach the lower respiratory tract is the **respirable mass.** Not all aerosol delivered to the lung is retained, or deposited. A small percentage (1% to 5%) of inhaled drug may be exhaled. Whether aerosol particles that are inhaled into the lung are deposited in the respiratory tract depends on the size, shape, and motion of the particles and on the physical characteristics of the airways and breathing pattern. Key mechanisms of aerosol **deposition** include inertial impaction, gravimetric sedimentation, and brownian diffusion.[1,3]

Inertial Impaction

Inertial impaction occurs when suspended particles in motion collide with and are deposited on a surface; this is the primary deposition mechanism for particles larger than 5 μm. The greater the mass and velocity of a moving object, the greater its inertia, and the greater the tendency of that object to continue moving along its set path (Figure 36-1). When a particle of sufficient (large) mass is moving in a gas stream and that stream changes direction, the particle tends to remain on its initial path and collide with the airway surface.

Because inertia involves both mass and velocity, the higher the flow of a gas stream, the greater the tendency for particles to impact and be deposited in the airways. Turbulent flow patterns, obstructed or tortuous pathways, and inspiratory flow rates greater than 30 L/min are associated with increased inertial impaction. Turbulent flow and convoluted passageways in the nose cause most particles larger than 10 μm to impact and become deposited. This process produces an effective filter that protects the lower airway from particulates such as dust and pollen. However, particles 5 to 10 μm tend to become deposited in the oropharynx and hypopharynx, especially with the turbulence created by the transition of air as it passes around the tongue and into the larynx.

Sedimentation

Sedimentation occurs when aerosol particles settle out of suspension and are deposited owing to gravity. The greater the mass of the particle, the faster it settles (Figure 36-2). During normal breathing, sedimentation is the primary mechanism for deposition of particles 1 to 5 μm. Sedimentation occurs mostly in the central airways and increases with time, affecting particles 1 μm in diameter. Breath holding after inhalation of an aerosol increases the residence time for the particles in the lung and enhances distribution across the lungs and sedimentation. A 10-second breath hold can increase aerosol deposition 10% and increase the ratio of aerosol deposited in lung parenchyma to central airway by fourfold.[4]

Diffusion

Brownian diffusion is the primary mechanism for deposition of small particles (<3 μm), mainly in the respiratory region where bulk gas flow ceases and most aerosol particles reach the alveoli by diffusion. These aerosol particles have very low mass and are easily bounced around by collisions with carrier gas molecules. These random molecular collisions cause some particles to contact and become deposited on surrounding surfaces. Particles 1 to 0.5 μm are so stable

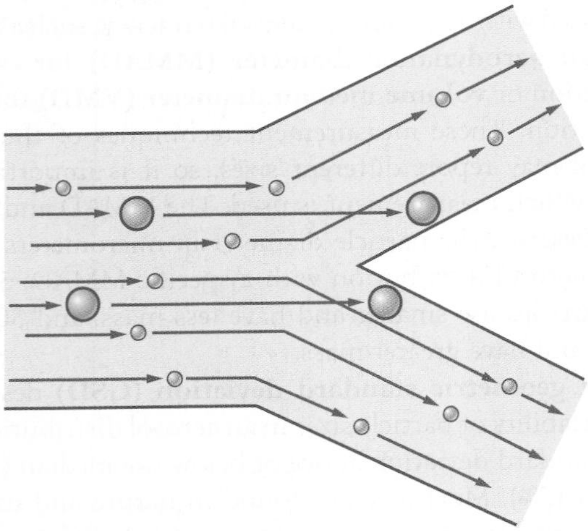

FIGURE 36-1 Inertial impaction of large particles, the masses of which tend to maintain their motion in straight lines. As airway direction changes, the particles are deposited on nearby walls. Smaller particles are carried around corners by the airstream and fall out less readily.

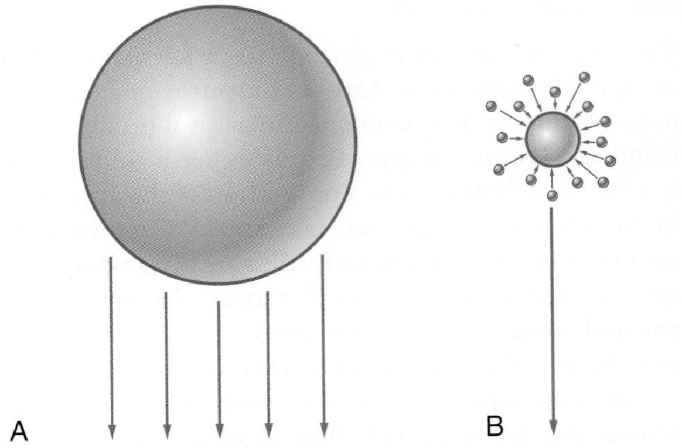

FIGURE 36-2 Effect of mass on particle size. Large particles **(A)** are more susceptible to the force of gravity than smaller particles **(B),** which are more affected by the bombardment of molecules deposited by diffusion.

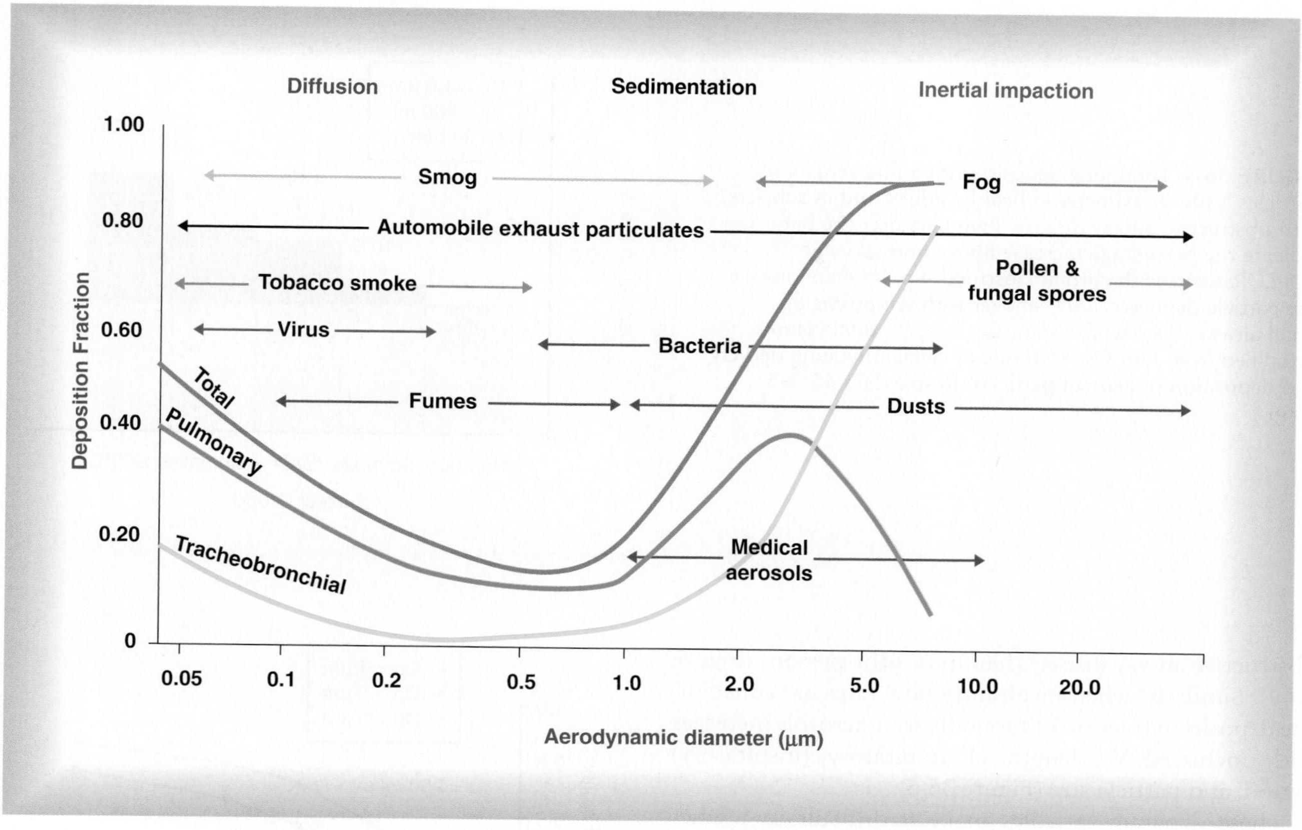

FIGURE 36-3 Range of particle size for common aerosols in the environment and the influence of inertial impactions, sedimentation, and diffusion. (Modified from Yu CP, Nicolaides P, Soong TT, et al: Effect of random airway sizes on aerosol deposition. Am Ind Hyg Assoc J 40:999, 1979.)

that most remain in suspension and are cleared with the exhaled gas, whereas particles smaller than 0.5 μm have a greater retention rate in the lungs.

Figure 36-3 summarizes the relationships between particle size and aerosol deposition in the respiratory tract. The depth of penetration and deposition of a particle in the respiratory tract tend to vary with size and tidal volume (V_T).[5] With this knowledge, it may be possible to target aerosol deposition to specific areas of the lung by using the proper particle size and breathing pattern.

RULE OF THUMB

The site of deposition in the respiratory tract varies with the size of the particle. Use of nebulizers that produce particles in a specific size range improves the targeting of aerosols for deposition to a desired site in the respiratory tract, as follows:

Desired Location	Recommended MMAD
Upper airway: nose, larynx, trachea	5 to >50 μm
Lower airways	2 to 5 μm
Parenchyma: alveolar region	1 to 3 μm
Parenchyma	<0.1 μm

Aging

Aerosols are dynamic suspensions. Individual particles constantly grow, shrink, coalesce, and fall out of suspension. The process by which an aerosol suspension changes over time is called **aging.** How an aerosol ages depends on the composition of the aerosol, the initial size of its particles, the time in suspension, and the ambient conditions to which it is exposed.

Aerosol particles can change size as a result of either evaporation or **hygroscopic** water absorption. The relative rate of particle size change is inversely proportional to the size of a particle, so small particles grow or shrink faster than large particles. Small water-based particles shrink when exposed to relatively dry gas. Aerosols of water-soluble materials, especially salts, tend to be hygroscopic, absorbing water and growing when introduced into a high-humidity environment.[5]

Particle size is not the only determinant of deposition. Inspiratory flow rate, flow pattern, respiratory rate, inhaled volume, ratio of inspiratory time to expiratory time (I:E ratio), and breath holding all influence where a particle of any specific size is deposited. The presence of airway obstruction is one of the greatest factors influencing aerosol deposition. It has been shown that total pulmonary deposition is greater in smokers and patients with

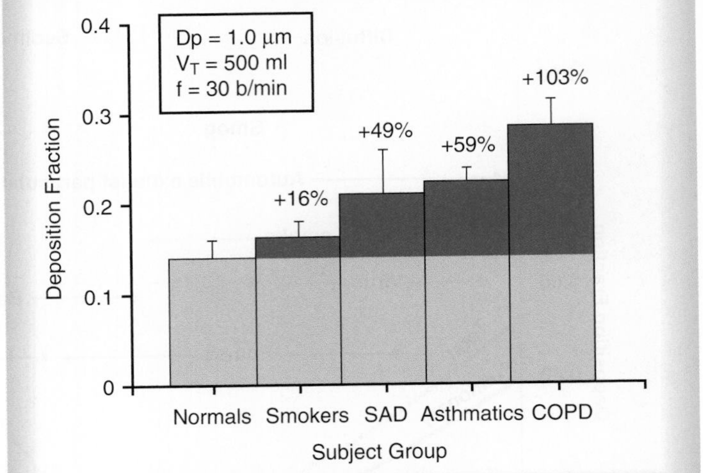

FIGURE 36-4 Total lung deposition of a fine aerosol of particles 1 μm in diameter in healthy adults and in subjects with obstructive airway disease. Numbers over the bar indicate the percentage increase above normal value. *COPD,* Patients with chronic obstructive pulmonary disease; *Dp,* particle diameter; *SAD,* smoker with symptoms of small airways disease; *f,* respiratory rate; *V_T,* tidal volume. (Modified from Kim CS: Methods of calculating lung delivery and deposition of aerosol particles. Respir Care 45:695, 2000.)

obstructive airway disease than in healthy persons (Figure 36-4). Similarly, when inspiratory flow rates are constant, the deposition fraction of monodisperse aerosols increases with increased V_T, length of respiratory (inspiratory) period, and particle size (Figure 36-5).

These dynamic variables make it difficult to predict exactly what occurs to aerosol particles when they enter a gas stream and are inhaled. For this reason, prediction of actual aerosol deposition for an individual patient is difficult.

Quantifying Aerosol Delivery

As mentioned in the preceding sections, many characteristics of aerosols can account for the variances in quantity of aerosolized medication delivered to the patient. Although the precise amount of drug delivered to the patient's airways can be difficult to determine, it can be measured in terms of the patient's clinical response to aerosol drug therapy, including the desired therapeutic effects and any unwanted adverse effects. The amount of aerosol deposited to a patient's airways can be quantified using specialized equipment and tests.

One approach used to quantify aerosol deposition to the human body (in vivo) involves **scintigraphy,** in which a drug is "tagged" with a radioactive substance (e.g., technetium), aerosolized, and inhaled. A scanner (similar to scanners used in nuclear medicine) measures the distribution and intensity of radiation across the device and the patient's head and thorax. The result is a radiation map of aerosol deposition in the upper airway, the lungs (central and peripheral airways), and the stomach. This information is used to calculate the percentage of drug retained by the device and delivered to various areas in the patient.[6]

A less direct approach relates the systemic pharmacokinetic profile of a drug delivered by aerosol to an assay of the drug in a patient's blood or urine over time. This method does not estimate actual lung delivery, but it

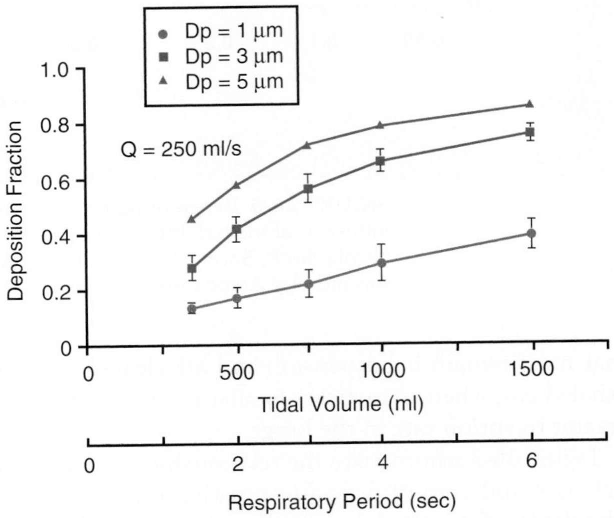

FIGURE 36-5 Total lung deposition versus V_T and respiratory time at a fixed flow: respiratory flow (Q) = 250 ml/sec. *Dp,* Particle diameter. (Modified from Kim CS: Methods of calculating lung delivery and deposition of aerosol particles. Respir Care 45:695, 2000.)

provides insight into systemic drug levels achieved after aerosol administration. Care must be taken to differentiate drug absorbed through the lungs from drug absorbed through the gastrointestinal tract. Simple laboratory, or in vitro, models, which simulate a range of V_T values, inspiratory flow rates, I:E ratios, and respiratory rates, have been useful in predicting inhaled mass of drug and relative performance of nebulizers.[7]

HAZARDS OF AEROSOL THERAPY

The primary hazard of aerosol drug therapy is an adverse reaction to the medication being administered (see Chapter 32). Other hazards to the patient include infection, airway reactivity, systemic effects of bland aerosols, drug concentration, and eye irritation. Care providers and bystanders risk these hazards as a result of exposure to secondhand aerosol drugs.

Infection

Aerosol generators can contribute to nosocomial infections by spreading bacteria by the airborne route.[8] The most common sources of bacteria are patient secretions, contaminated solutions (i.e., multiple-dose drug vials), and caregivers' hands. Offending organisms are primarily gram-negative bacilli, in particular, *Pseudomonas aeruginosa* and *Legionella pneumophila* (the cause of the highly virulent legionnaires' disease).[9]

Various procedures can help reduce contamination and infection associated with respiratory care equipment. Guidelines from the U.S. Centers for Disease Control and Prevention (CDC) state that nebulizers should be sterilized between patients, frequently replaced with disinfected or sterile units, or rinsed with sterile water (not tap water) and air dried every 24 hours (see Chapter 4).

Airway Reactivity

Cold air and high-density aerosols can cause reactive bronchospasm and increased airway resistance, especially in patients with preexisting respiratory disease.[10] Medications such as acetylcysteine, antibiotics, steroids, cromolyn sodium, ribavirin, and distilled water have been associated with increased airway resistance and wheezing during aerosol therapy. Administration of bronchodilators before or with administration of these agents may reduce the risk or duration of increased airway resistance.

The risk of inducing bronchospasm always should be considered when aerosols are administered. Monitoring for reactive bronchospasm should include peak flow measurements or percentage forced expiratory volume in 1 second (%FEV_1) before and after therapy; auscultation for adventitious breath sounds; observation of the patient's breathing pattern and overall appearance; and, most essential, communicating with the patient during therapy to determine the perceived work of breathing.[11]

Pulmonary and Systemic Effects

Pulmonary and systemic effects are associated with the site of delivery and the drug being administered. However, even bland aerosols present risk. Excess water can cause overhydration, and excess saline solution can cause hypernatremia. Animal data indicate that long-term, continuous administration of bland aerosols can cause localized inflammation and tissue damage, atelectasis, and pulmonary edema.

Preliminary assessment should balance the need versus the risk of aerosol therapy, especially among patients at high risk, such as infants, patients who are prone to fluid and electrolyte imbalances, and patients with atelectasis or pulmonary edema. For patients unable to clear their own secretions, suctioning or other airway clearance techniques may be indicated as an adjunct to aerosol therapy. Care must be taken to ensure that patients are capable of clearing secretions when the secretions are mobilized by aerosol therapy. Appropriate airway clearance techniques should accompany any aerosol therapy designed to help mobilize secretions (see Chapter 40).

Drug Concentration

During nebulization, the evaporation, heating, baffling, and recycling of drug solutions undergoing jet or ultrasonic nebulization increase solute concentrations.[12] This process can expose the patient to increasingly higher concentrations of the drug over the course of therapy and result in a larger concentration of drug remaining in the nebulizer at the end of therapy. This increase in concentration usually is time-dependent; the greatest effect occurs when nebulization of medications occurs over extended periods, as in continuous aerosol drug delivery.

Eye Irritation

Aerosol administration via a face mask may deposit drug in the eyes and cause eye irritation. In very rare cases, anticholinergic medications (see Chapter 32) have been suspected to worsen preexisting eye conditions, such as forms of glaucoma. Caution should be exercised when a face mask is used during aerosol drug therapy. In addition, special mask designs that have been shown to reduce drug deposition in the eyes or mouthpieces should be considered for at-risk patients.[13,14]

Secondhand Exposure to Aerosol Drugs

Workplace exposure to aerosol may be detectable in the plasma of bystanders and health care providers. Repeated secondhand exposure to bronchodilators is associated with increased risk of occupational asthma. Institutions should develop and implement an occupational health and safety policy to minimize the risk of secondhand aerosol exposure for care providers and bystanders.[15-17] Unless filters are placed in the expiratory limb, 40% of aerosol produced during mechanical ventilation is exhausted to the air of the intensive care unit.[18] Implementation of an occupational health and safety policy could include using systems that introduce less aerosol to the atmosphere (pressurized metered dose inhalers [pMDIs], dry powder inhalers [DPIs], and breath-actuated nebulizers), filtering exhalation to contain aerosol, and using environmental controls.

AEROSOL DRUG DELIVERY SYSTEMS

Effective aerosol therapy requires a device that quickly delivers sufficient drug to the desired site of action with minimal waste and at a low cost.[19] Aerosol generators in use include pMDIs with or without spacers or holding chambers, DPIs, small and large volume (jet) nebulizers, hand-bulb atomizers (including nasal spray pumps), ultrasonic nebulizers (USNs), and vibrating mesh (VM) nebulizers as well as numerous emerging technologies.[2]

Clinicians are often exposed to competing and sometimes conflicting claims about the different delivery systems and may not be provided the information they need to select the correct system for a given situation. Because device selection can make the difference between successful and unsuccessful therapy, clinicians must have in-depth knowledge of the operating principles and performance characteristics of these various systems and how best to select and apply them.[20]

Metered Dose Inhalers

The pMDI is the most commonly prescribed method of aerosol delivery in the United States. The pMDI is portable, compact, and easy to use and provides multidose convenience. A uniform dose of drug is dispensed within a fraction of a second after actuation and is reproducible throughout the canister life. The pMDI and actuator are designed for the specific drug formulation and dose volume to be delivered. Although the pMDI appears to be a simple device, it represents sophisticated technology and engineering. Although relatively easy to use, it is commonly misused by patients.

The pMDI is used to administer bronchodilators, anticholinergics, and steroids. More formulations of these drugs are available for use by pMDIs than for use with nebulizers. Properly used, pMDIs are at least as effective as other nebulizers for drug delivery. For this reason, pMDIs often are the preferred method for delivering bronchodilators to spontaneously breathing patients and patients who are intubated and undergoing mechanical ventilation.[21]

Most pMDIs are "press and breathe," but there is increasing presence of a variation known as breath-actuated pMDIs. The basic components of pMDI are similar regardless of type, manufacturer, or active ingredient; commonly used pMDIs are shown in Figure 36-6.

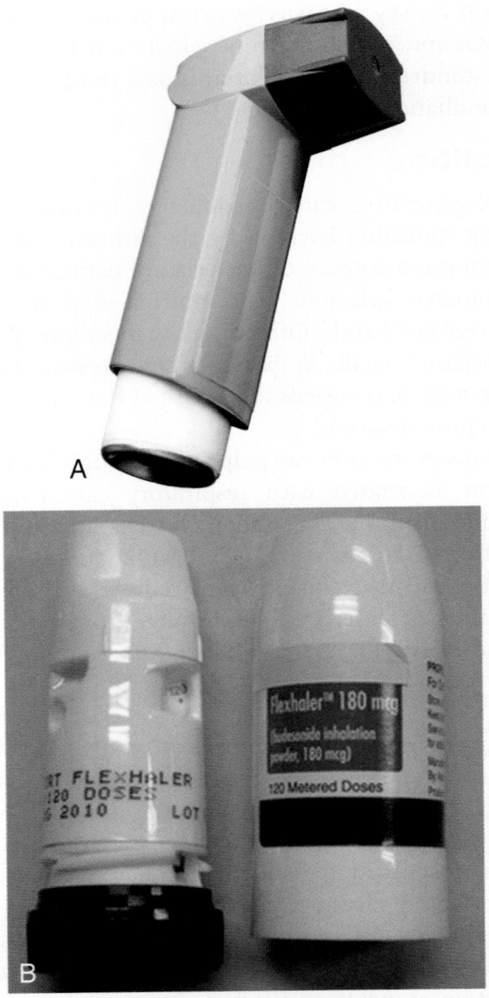

FIGURE 36-6 Examples of commonly used pMDIs. **A,** Albuterol inhaler **B,** The ASMANEX TWISTHALER. (**A,** Courtesy Hemera, Thinkstock. **B,** Reproduced with permission of Schering Corporation, subsidiary of Merck & Co. All rights reserved. ASMANEX and TWISTHALER are registered trademarks of Schering Corporation.)

A pMDI is a pressurized canister that contains the prescribed drug (a micronized powder or aqueous solution) in a volatile **propellant** combined with a surfactant and dispersing agent (Figure 36-7). When the canister is inverted (nozzle down) and placed in its actuator, or "boot," the volatile suspension fills a metering chamber that controls the amount of drug delivered. Pressing down on the canister aligns a hole in the metering valve with the metering chamber. The high propellant vapor pressure quickly forces the metered dose out through this hole and through the actuator nozzle.

Aerosol production takes approximately 20 msec. As the liquid suspension is forced out of the pMDI, it forms a plume, within which the propellants vaporize, or "flash." Initially, the velocity of this plume is high (approximately 15 m/sec). However, within 0.1 second, the plume velocity decreases to less than half its maximum as the plume moves away from the actuator nozzle. At the same time, propellant evaporation causes the initially large particles (35 μm) generated at the actuator orifice to decrease rapidly in size.

The output volume of pMDIs ranges from 30 to 100 mcl. Approximately 60% to 80% by weight of this spray consists of the propellant, with only approximately 1% being active drug (50 mcg to 5 mg, depending on the drug formulation). For a chlorofluorocarbon (CFC) pMDI used in a standard actuator, loss of drug in the valve stem housing and on the actuator mouthpiece amounts to 10% to 15% of the nominal dose from the metering valve.

From their inception in the mid-1950s to the beginning of the twenty-first century, **chlorofluorocarbons (CFCs)** such as Freon were the propellants used in pMDIs. Manufacture of CFCs for most applications was prohibited because of the effect of these compounds on

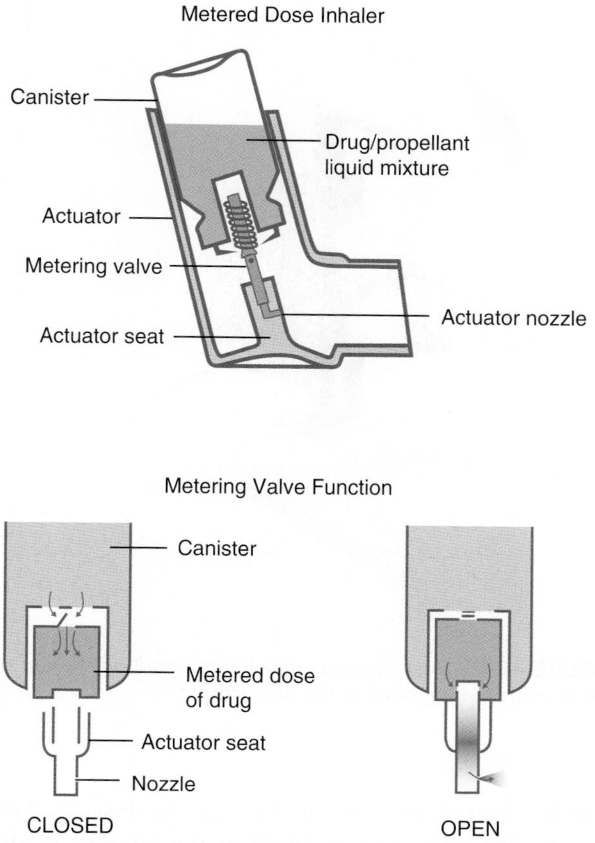

FIGURE 36-7 Components of a pMDI, including function of the metering valve. (From Gardenhire DS: Rau's respiratory care pharmacology, ed 8, St. Louis, 2012, Mosby.)

global warming, with a period of transition provided for pMDIs. A consortium of eight pharmaceutical companies developed **hydrofluoroalkane (HFA)**-134a to be more environment-friendly and possibly clinically safer than CFCs.[22] Redesign of key components of the pMDI has resulted in improved performance.[23]

In addition to the propellant, pMDIs use dispersal agents to improve drug delivery by keeping the drug in suspension. The most common dispersal agents are surfactants, such as soy lecithin, sorbitan trioleate, and oleic acid. These agents help keep the drug suspended in the propellant and lubricate the valve mechanism but may also cause adverse responses (coughing or wheezing) in some patients.

Before initial use and after storage, every pMDI should be primed by shaking and actuating the device to atmosphere one to four times (see label for the specific device). Without priming, the initial dose actuated from a new pMDI canister contains less active substance than subsequent actuations.[20] This "loss of dose" from a pMDI occurs when drug particles rise to the top of the canister over time ("cream"). A reduction in emitted dose with the first actuation commonly occurs with a pMDI after storage, particularly with the valve pointed in the downward position. Loss of prime is related to valve design and occurs when propellant leaks out of the metering chamber during periods of nonuse (e.g., 4 hours). The result is reduced pressure and drug released with the next actuation.[20] Improved designs of metering valves developed for use with HFA propellants reduce these losses. It is recommended that a single dose be wasted before the next dose is inhaled when a CFC pMDI has not been used for 4 to 6 hours. An HFA pMDI requires no wasting of dose for periods exceeding 2 days.

Breath-Actuated Pressurized Metered Dose Inhaler

A variation of a pMDI is a breath-actuated model, which incorporates a trigger that is activated during inhalation. This trigger theoretically reduces the need for the patient or caregiver to coordinate MDI actuation with inhalation.[24] However, patients may stop breathing when the MDI is actuated ("cold Freon effect") or have suboptimal inspiration. Evaluation of the efficacy of breath-actuated pMDIs in children younger than 6 years is limited, and their use should be restricted to older children and adults. Oropharyngeal deposition of steroids using these devices is still very high.

The Aerocount Autohaler is a flow-triggered pMDI developed and marketed by the 3M Corporation (St. Paul, MN) (Figure 36-8). The device is designed to eliminate the need for hand-breath coordination by automatically triggering in response to the patient's inspiratory effort.[24] To use the Autohaler, the patient cocks a lever on the top of the unit, which sets in motion a downward spring force. Using the closed-mouth technique, the patient draws through the mouthpiece. When the patient's flow rate exceeds 30 L/min, a vane releases the spring, which forces the canister down and triggers the pMDI. In the United States, the Autohaler is available only with pirbuterol, a bronchodilator similar to albuterol. Current data indicate that the device reduces pharyngeal impaction and enhances lung deposition. A possible limitation of the device is that it can be breath actuated only. Patients experiencing an acute exacerbation of bronchospasm may be unable to generate sufficient flows to trigger the Autohaler. This theoretical concern has not been widely observed in clinical studies of patients with severe exacerbation of asthma receiving treatment in emergency departments. Nevertheless, caution may be appropriate in ordering breath-triggered pMDIs for small children and patients prone to severe levels of airway obstruction.

The Easihaler (GlaxoSmithKline, Philadelphia) is a breath-actuated pMDI that has been developed with a range of medications and is currently available in Europe and Canada. Release in the United States is anticipated in the near future. A new generation of pMDIs such as the Tempo (MAP Pharmaceuticals, Mountain View, CA) have been designed to be breath actuated with lower force of the plume exiting the mouthpiece, reducing oropharyngeal deposition and increasing lung dose (Figure 36-9).

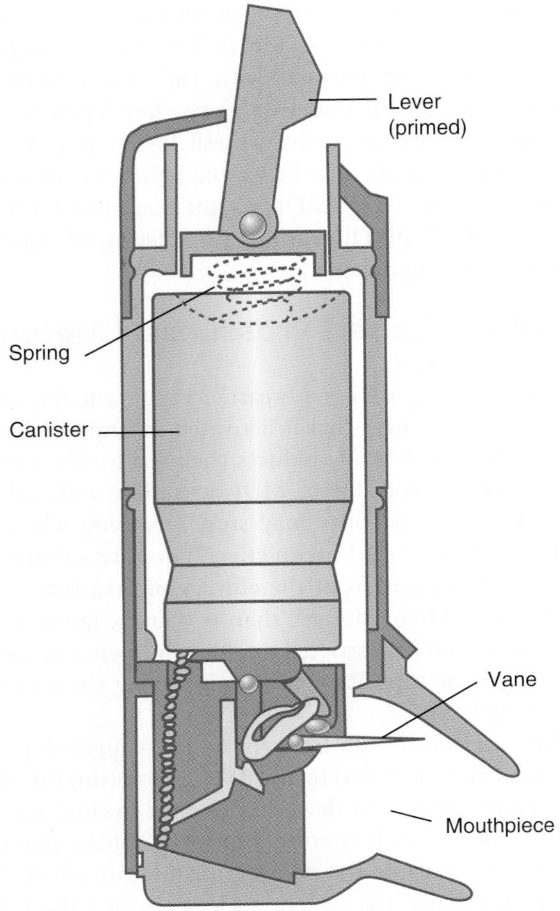

FIGURE 36-8 Autohaler (3M, St Paul, MN) flow-triggered pMDI. (Modified from Gardenhire DS: Rau's respiratory care pharmacology, ed 8, St. Louis, 2012, Mosby.)

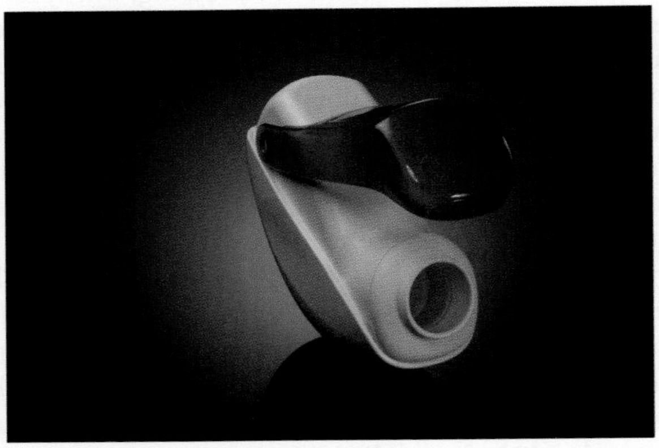

FIGURE 36-9 Tempo® Inhaler is a breath actuated pMDI with synchronous trigger for breath actuation and flow control chamber to reduce plume velocity. (Courtesy of MAP Pharmaceuticals. The TEMPO® inhaler is a registered trademark of MAP Pharmaceuticals, Inc. Mountain View, Calif.)

Dose Counters

A serious limitation of pMDIs is the lack of a "counter" to indicate the number of doses remaining in the canister. After the number of label doses have been administered, the pMDI may seem to give another 20 to 60 doses, which may deliver little or no medications as the doses "tail-off." *Tail-off effect* refers to variability in the amount of drug dispensed toward the end of the life of the canister. The result of tail-off is swings from normal to almost no dose emitted from one breath to the next with no reliable indicator to the user. Without a dose counter, there is no viable method to determine remaining drug in a pMDI other than manually keeping a log of every dose taken. The U.S. Food and Drug Administration (FDA) is requiring all new pMDIs to have a counter technology to track pMDI actuations remaining. Third-party dose counters may be added to older pMDI models but may not have the accuracy of built-in technology (Figure 36-10).

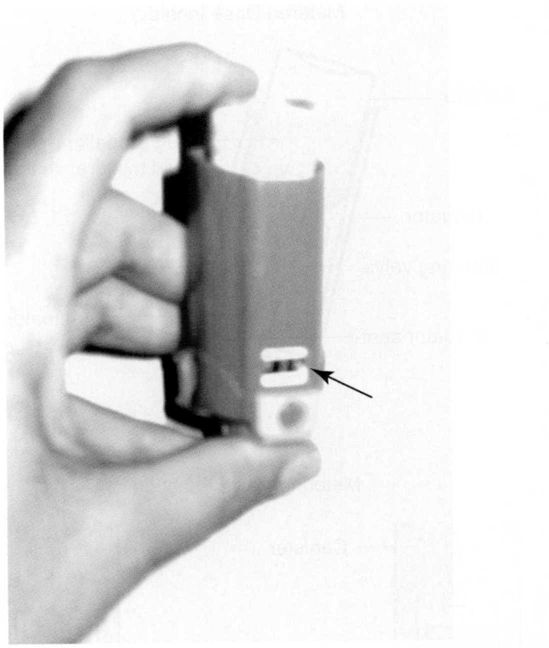

FIGURE 36-10 Dose counters may be mounted on the top of a pMDI canister integrated in the actuator boot.

Factors Affecting Pressurized Metered Dose Inhaler Performance and Drug Delivery

Temperature. Decreased temperature (<10° C) has been shown to decrease the output of CFC pMDIs. Patients with cold air–induced bronchospasm who keep their pMDIs in outer coat pockets when outside in cold winter weather may receive only a small percentage of drug compared with that administered with the same pMDI at 25° C. This problem has been less serious with the newer HFA pMDIs.[20]

Nozzle Size and Cleanliness. Aerosol drug delivery is influenced by nozzle size and cleanliness. Nozzle size is pMDI-specific. As debris builds up on the nozzle or actuator orifice, the emitted dose is reduced. Manufacturer recommendations should be followed for cleaning. pMDI canisters should never be placed under water.

MINI CLINI

Using Universal Pressurized Metered Dose Inhaler Actuator or Boot

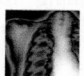

PROBLEM: The association of CFCs with degradation of the earth's atmosphere and the ozone layer has resulted in an international treaty banning use of these compounds. As HFAs become the propellants of choice, a problem arises. If the CFC and HFA drug formulations are bioequivalent, can these compounds be used with the same (universal) pMDI actuator, or boot?

SOLUTION: In the case of HFA-based albuterol (e.g., Proventil HFA), the operating pressure and stem orifice differ from those used for the CFC formulation. The result is different plume geometries. When HFA albuterol is used in a universal adapter designed for CFC albuterol, the MMAD and GSD are greatly increased. The result is that significantly less drug is available to the patient. When possible, accessory devices that are used in the manufacturer's boot with the pMDI should be selected. If these devices are unavailable, the universal adapter device that is available should be evaluated to determine how much additional dose may be required to provide an equivalent dose through a third-party adapter.

Priming. Priming is defined as shaking the device and releasing one or more sprays into the air when the pMDI is new or has not been used for awhile. It is done to mix the drug and the propellant, which can separate in the canister over time. Priming is required to provide an adequate dose, according to the manufacturer's guidelines.

Timing of Actuation Intervals. Manufacturers recommend 30 seconds to 1 minute between actuations. When propellants are released, the device cools, changing aerosol output. The pause allows the device to return to room temperature and recover normal output. However, Fink and colleagues[25] showed that pMDI output is similar at 15-second intervals. Very rapid actuation of multiple puffs per breath reduces inhaled drug per puff.

Aerosol Delivery Characteristics

Although pMDIs can produce particles in the respirable range (MMAD 2 to 6 μm),[20] the initial velocity and dispersion of the aerosol plume generate larger particles that decrease in size as they leave the pMDI, resulting in approximately 80% of the dose leaving the actuator to impact and become deposited in the oropharynx. A significant proportion of this oropharyngeal deposition is swallowed and may be a factor in systemic absorption of some drugs. Pulmonary deposition ranges from 10% to 20% in adults and larger children (less in infants).[26] The exact amount of drug delivered to an individual patient is unpredictable because of high variability between patients and because pMDI drug administration is technique-dependent.

Box 36-1 Optimal Technique for Use of a Pressurized Metered Dose Inhaler

1. Warm the pMDI canister to hand or body temperature, and shake it vigorously.
2. Before first use of a new pMDI and when the pMDI has not been used for several days, prime the pMDI by pointing it into the air (away from people) and actuating.
3. Assemble the apparatus and uncap the mouthpiece, ensuring there are no loose objects in the device.
4. Open mouth technique*: Open your mouth wide, keeping tongue down. Hold the pMDI with the canister oriented downward and the outlet aimed at your mouth. Position the pMDI approximately 4 cm (two fingerbreadths) away from your mouth.
5. Closed mouth technique†: Place mouthpiece between lips, with tongue out of the path of the outlet.
6. Breathe out normally.
7. As you slowly begin to breathe in (<0.5 L/sec), actuate the pMDI.
8. Continue inspiration to total lung capacity.
9. Hold your breath for up to 10 seconds. Then relax and breathe normally.
10. Wait 1 minute between puffs.
11. Disassemble the apparatus, and recap the mouthpiece.

*Technique is based on research with beta agonists and has been shown to reduce oropharyngeal deposition. It is not advised for use with anticholinergics because of possible eye exposure.
†Label technique recommended by pMDI manufacturers.

Technique

The successful administration of aerosol drugs by pMDI is highly technique-dependent. Two-thirds of patients and health care professionals who should teach pMDI use do not perform the procedure properly.[27] Box 36-1 outlines the recommended steps for self-administering a bronchodilator by simple pMDI. Thorough preliminary patient instruction can last 10 to 30 minutes and should include demonstration, practice, and confirmation of patient performance (demonstration pMDIs with placebo are available from manufacturers for this purpose). Repeated instruction improves performance; repeat instruction is done most appropriately with follow-up clinic or home visits. Demonstration and return demonstration must occur several times for best patient adherence to device use.

For best effect, the pMDI should be actuated once at the beginning of inspiration. Common hand-breath coordination problems include actuating the pMDI before or after the breath. Some patients, especially infants, young children, elderly adults, and patients in acute distress, may be unable to coordinate actuation of the pMDI with inspiration. Some patients exhibit a "cold Freon effect," which occurs when the cold aerosol plume reaches the back of the mouth and the patient stops inhaling. All of these problems reduce aerosol delivery to the lung to the point that the patient does not benefit from the medication, but they can be corrected entirely or in part by use of the proper pMDI accessory device.

Most pMDI labels call for placing the mouthpiece between the lips. However, research has shown that positioning the outlet of the pMDI approximately 4 cm (two fingerbreadths) in front of the mouth improves lung deposition by decreasing oropharyngeal impaction.[28] Holding the canister outside the open mouth (at two fingerbreadths) provides a space for the particles to decelerate while evaporating, allowing particle size to reduce to respirable size. Use of the open-mouth technique with a low inspiratory flow rate can result in a doubling of the dose delivered to the lower respiratory tract of an adult from approximately 7% to 10% to 14% to 20%. However, this technique is more difficult for patients to perform reliably than the closed-mouth technique. Although it may reduce oropharyngeal deposition, the technique has not been shown to improve the clinical response to pMDI bronchodilators.

Concerns have been raised about use of the open-mouth technique with ipratropium bromide because poor coordination can result in drug being sprayed into the eyes. Use of anticholinergic agents has been associated with increased ocular pressure, which could be dangerous for patients with glaucoma. For avoidance of ocular exposure, the drug manufacturer recommends patients use the closed-mouth technique with ipratropium.

The high percentage of oropharyngeal drug deposition with use of steroid pMDIs can increase the incidence of opportunistic oral yeast infection (thrush) and changes in the voice (dysphonia). Rinsing the mouth after steroid use can help avoid this problem, but most pMDI steroid aerosol impaction occurs deep in the hypopharynx, which cannot be easily rinsed with gargling. For this reason, steroid pMDIs should not be used alone but always in combination with a spacer or valved holding chamber. See Box 36-2 for instructions for determining dosage left in the pMDI.

Box 36-2 Determining Dose Left in Pressurized Metered Dose Inhaler

Tracking the number of actuations (puffs) remaining in a pMDI can be done with or without dose counters (see Figure 36-10).

WITH DOSE COUNTERS

The user should[29]:

1. Determine how many puffs of drug the pMDI has when full.
2. Learn to read the counter display because each dose counter has a different way of displaying doses left in the canister.
3. Check the counter display to track the pMDI actuations remaining in the canister.
4. Reorder the pMDI when there are a few days of drug remaining.
5. Dispose of the pMDI properly, after the last dose is dispensed.

WITHOUT DOSE COUNTERS

The user should[29]:

1. Read the label to determine how many puffs of drug the pMDI has when full.
2. Calculate how long the pMDI will last by dividing the total number of puffs in the pMDI by the total puffs used per day. If the pMDI is used more often than planned, it will run out sooner.
3. Identify the date that the medication will run out, and mark it on the canister or on a calendar.
4. For drugs that are prescribed to be taken as needed, track the number of puffs of drug administered on a daily log sheet and subtract them from the remaining puffs to determine the amount of medication left in the pMDI.
5. Keep the daily log sheet in a convenient place, such as taped to the bathroom mirror.
6. Refill the pMDI prescription when there are a few days of use remaining in the pMDI.
7. Dispose of the pMDI properly when the last dose is dispensed.

Pressurized Metered Dose Inhaler Accessory Devices

Various pMDI accessory devices have been developed to overcome the two primary limitations of these systems: hand-breath coordination problems and high oropharyngeal deposition. Accessory devices include breath-actuated pMDIs, spacers, and holding chambers.

Spacers and Holding Chambers. Spacers and valved holding chambers are pMDI accessory devices designed to reduce both oropharyngeal deposition and the need for hand-breath coordination. Despite differences in design, all spacers add distance between the pMDI and the mouth, reducing the initial forward velocity of the pMDI droplets, which occurs with partial evaporation of propellant in the time the aerosol traverses the length of the spacer. The reduction in initial forward velocity decreases the number of nonrespirable particles reaching the airway. With retention of the larger droplets in the spacer or holding chamber and evaporation of propellants before entering the airway, the “cold Freon effect,” which causes many children to stop inhaling, is reduced, as is the foul taste associated with some of the drug aerosols. The same drug used with different accessory devices may produce differences in MMAD, GSD, and fine-particle fraction. The quantity of respirable drug available at the spacer or valved holding chamber exit depends on spacer volume and design and on formulation factors. The placement of a valve between the pMDI and the chamber and the mouthpiece works like a baffle reducing the size of particles inhaled. A simple tube spacer may reduce oral deposition by 90%, whereas a valved holding chamber can reduce oral deposition by 99%.

Valved holding chambers protect the patient from poor hand-breath coordination, with exhaled gas venting to the atmosphere, allowing aerosol to remain in the chamber available to be inhaled with the next breath. Valved holding chambers allow infants, small children, and adults who cannot control their breathing pattern to be treated effectively with pMDIs.

It is increasingly common practice to provide asthmatic patients an accessory device to use with the pMDI and to teach them to use the pMDI with and without the accessory device. The patients are instructed to use the device with the pMDI whenever they feel short of breath. Many of these patients find that they get much better relief from the pMDI with an accessory device than with the pMDI alone.

Basic concepts for spacer devices include (1) small volume adapters, (2) open tube designs, (3) bag reservoirs, and (4) valved holding chambers (Figure 36-11). More

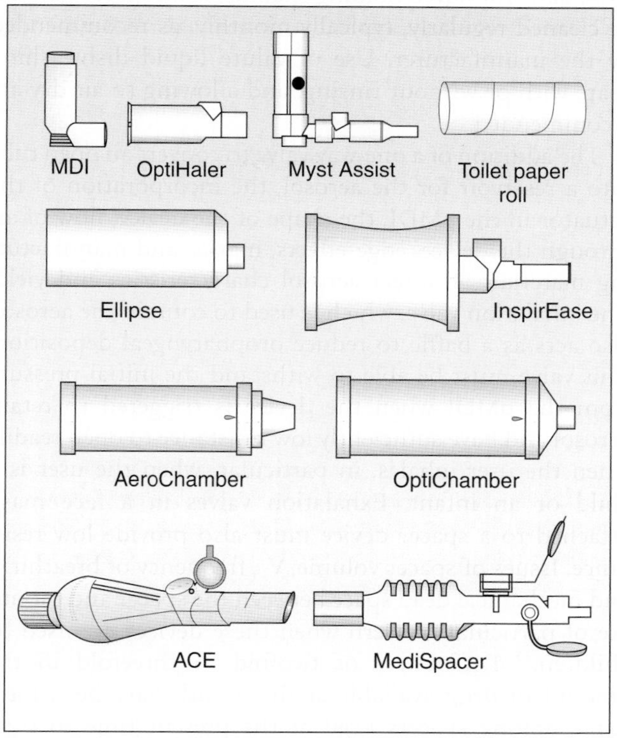

FIGURE 36-11 pMDI and accessory devices consisting of spacer and holding chambers. All of the accessory devices reduce oropharyngeal deposition. Small volume spacers (e.g., Optihaler [Philips Respironics, Murrysville, PA] and Myst Assist [Philips Respironics, Murrysville, PA]) offer no additional advantage, but large volume spacers (e.g., toilet paper roll and Ellipse [Ellipse Technologies, Irving, CA]) improve inhaled aerosol with delay between actuation and inspiration. Only the bag (e.g., Inspirease [Schering Plough, Kenilworth, NJ]) and valved holding chambers (e.g., Aerochamber [Invicare, Elyria, OH], Optichamber [Philips Respironics, Murrysville, PA], Ace [Smiths Medical, Kent, UK], and Medispacer [Cardinal Health, Dublin, OH]) protect the patient from blowing the dose away when the pMDI is actuated during expiration. (Modified from Wilkes W, Fink J, Dhand R: Selecting an accessory device with a metered-dose inhaler: variable influence of accessory devices on fine particle dose, throat deposition, and drug delivery with asynchronous actuation from a metered-dose inhaler. J Aerosol Med 14:351, 2001.)

than a dozen different devices with volumes ranging from 15 to 750 ml have been developed over the past 30 years.

A spacer is a simple valveless extension device that adds distance between the pMDI outlet and the patient's mouth. This distance allows the aerosol plume to expand and the propellants to evaporate before the medication reaches the oropharynx. Larger particles leaving the pMDI tend to impact on the spacer walls. In combination, this phenomenon reduces oropharyngeal impaction and increases pulmonary deposition. Proper use of a simple open-tube spacer still requires some hand-breath coordination because a momentary delay between triggering and inhaling the discharged spray results in a substantial loss of drug and reduced lung delivery. Exhalation into a simple spacer after pMDI actuation clears the aerosol from the device and wastes most of the dose to the atmosphere. This reduction in dose also occurs with small volume reverse-flow design spacers if there is no provision for "holding" the aerosol in the device.[30]

Similar to spacers, holding chambers allow the aerosol plume to develop and reduce oropharyngeal deposition. A holding chamber also incorporates one or more valves that prevent aerosol in the chamber from being cleared on exhalation. This allows patients with a small V_T to empty the aerosol from the chamber over two or more successive breaths. Generally, holding chambers provide less oropharyngeal deposition, higher respirable drug dosages, and better protection from poor hand-breath coordination than simple spacers.

The MMAD of the aerosol emitted from the pMDI exiting a spacer decreases approximately 25%, whereas the fraction containing particles less than 5 μm in diameter increases. This change is largely due to rapid evaporation of propellant in the spacer. With valved holding chambers, in addition to evaporation of the plume, the valves act as baffles of larger particles, increasing the respirable fraction further.

Holding chambers produce a finer, slower moving, more "respirable" aerosol with less impaction of drug in the oropharyngeal area (1% of dose) than simple spacers (10%) or a pMDI alone (80% of dose). Deposition after inhalation of a radiolabeled pMDI solution aerosol from the AeroChamber, compared with deposition from the same pMDI inhaled with the open-mouth technique, showed a 10-fold to 17-fold decrease in the amount of radioactivity deposited in the oropharyngeal-laryngeal area while a similar lung dose was maintained. This finding was true for both healthy subjects and patients with chronic obstructive pulmonary disease (COPD).[31] The advantage of reduced oropharyngeal deposition is fewer side effects from steroid aerosols, as shown in numerous published clinical trials. If multiple actuations of one or more drugs are placed into a spacer, both the total dose and the respirable dose of drug available for inhalation are reduced. The extent of these losses may vary for different drugs and spacer designs.[20]

Box 36-3 Optimal Technique for Use of a Metered Dose Inhaler With a Valved Holding Chamber

1. Warm the pMDI to hand or body temperature.
2. Assemble the apparatus, ensuring there are no objects or coins in the chamber that could be aspirated or obstruct outflow.
3. Hold the canister vertically, and shake it vigorously. Prime if necessary.
4. Place the pMDI in the holding chamber inlet, position chamber outlet in the mouth (or place the mask over nose and mouth), and encourage the patient to breathe through the mouth. Visually inspect for proper valve function.
5. With normal breathing, actuate the pMDI once and have the patient breathe through the device for three to seven breaths (three breaths for adults and seven breaths for infants).*
6. Allow 30 to 60 seconds between actuations.

*For a cooperative patient, synchronizing actuation at the beginning of larger breaths with breath holding may be encouraged. However, this maneuver has not been shown to increase clinical response to inhaled bronchodilators.

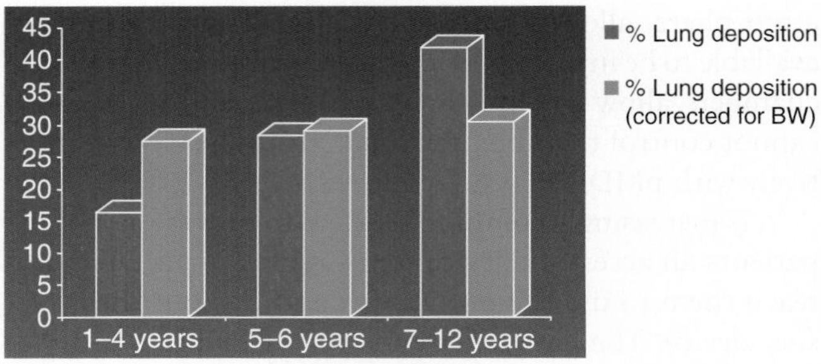

FIGURE 36-12 Although the percentage of drug deposited in the lung varies with age *(red bars)*, the percentage of lung deposition corrected for body weights is consistent across age groups. (Modified from Wildhaber JH, Janssens HM, Piérart F, et al: High percentage lung delivery in children from detergent-treated spacers, Pediatr Pulmonol 29:389-393, 2000.)

Holding chambers with masks are available for use in the care of infants, children, and adults. These units allow effective administration of aerosol from a pMDI to patients who are unable to use a mouthpiece device (because of their size, age, coordination, or mentation). Holding chambers are helpful in administration of pMDI steroids because deposition of the drug in the mouth is largely eliminated, and systemic side effects can be minimized.

Even with a holding chamber, respirable particles containing drug settle out and become deposited within the device, causing a whitish buildup on the inner chamber walls. This residual drug poses no risk to the patient but may be rinsed out periodically. Drug output from plastic spacers has been shown to decrease owing to the presence of an electrostatic charge. With these devices, a buildup of material can be seen on the walls of the chamber. As more material builds up on the wall of the chamber, the charge is dissipated, and more drug is inhaled by the patient. Washing the chamber with water (without soap) causes the electrostatic charge to be reestablished, making the device less effective for the next few puffs, until the static charge in the chamber (which attracts small particles) is again reduced.[32] Optimal technique is outlined in Box 36-3.

Use of conductive metal or nonelectrostatic plastic chambers or washing the plastic chamber periodically with deionizing detergent (liquid dishwashing soap) can overcome the loss of fine-particle mass owing to electrostatic charge and increase the inhaled mass from 20% to 50% of the emitted dose of the pMDI, even in children (Figure 36-12).[32] The effect of washing the chamber with conventional dishwashing soap reduces this static charge for up to 30 days. All valved holding chambers and spacers should be cleaned regularly, typically monthly, as recommended by the manufacturer. Use of dilute liquid dishwashing soap, with or without rinsing, and allowing to air dry are recommended.

The addition of a one-way valve to convert an open tube into a reservoir for the aerosol, the incorporation of the actuator in the pMDI, the shape of the device, flow of air through the device, edge effects, masks, and manufacturing materials all affect aerosol characteristics and yield. The inhalation valve, which is used to contain the aerosol, also acts as a baffle to reduce oropharyngeal deposition. This valve must be able to withstand the initial pressure from the pMDI when the device is triggered to retain aerosol and have sufficiently low resistance to open readily when the user inhales, in particular, when the user is a child or an infant. Exhalation valves in a face mask attached to a spacer device must also provide low resistance. Issues of spacer volume, V_T, frequency of breathing, and mechanical dead space between the spacer and mouth are of particular concern when these devices are used by children.[33] Differences of twofold to threefold in the amount of drug available at the mouth have been measured among spacers used at the present time to treat infants. Clinicians should determine the delivery efficiencies of spacer devices before using the devices in the care of a particular population.

Accessory devices are used with either the manufacturer-designed boot that comes with the pMDI or with a "universal adapter" that triggers the pMDI canister. Different formulations of pMDI drugs operate at different pressures and have a different-sized orifice in the boot that is specifically designed by the manufacturer for use exclusively with that pMDI. The output characteristics of a pMDI change when an adapter with a different-sized orifice is used. With HFA pMDIs, the diameter of the actuator orifice is smaller, and the spray is predictably finer. When the HFA pMDI is used in an actuator designed for use with CFC pMDIs, output is reduced. When these HFA formulations are used

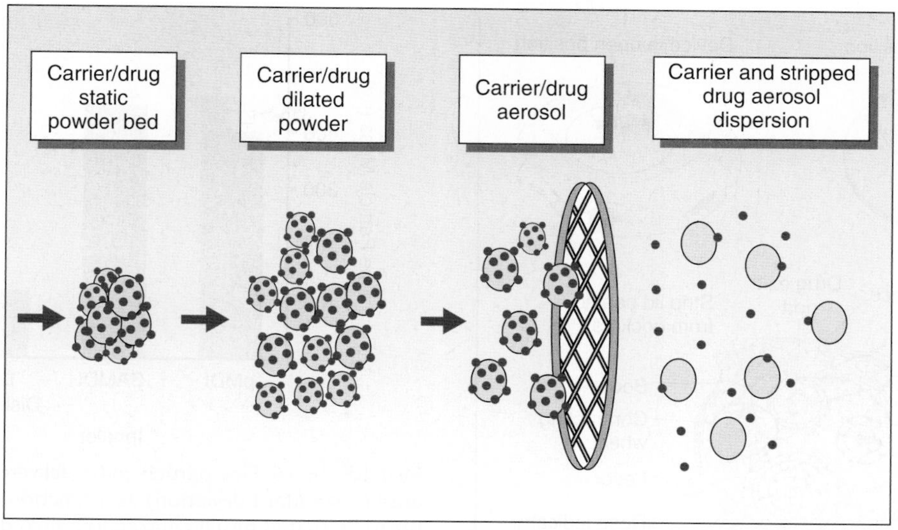

FIGURE 36-13 Aerosolization of dry powder. (Modified from Dhand R, Fink J: Dry powder inhalers. Respir Care 44:940, 1999.)

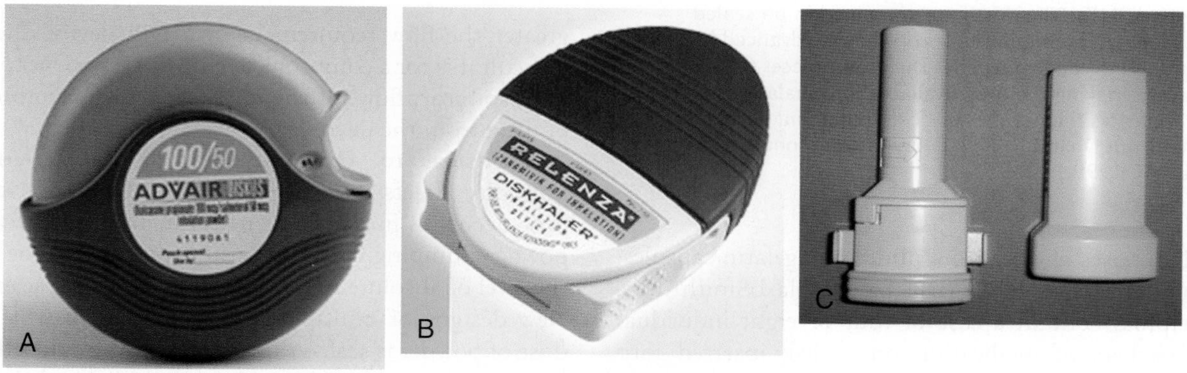

FIGURE 36-14 Some currently available DPIs: **A** and **B,** Multiple-dose dpi: diskus inhaler **C,** Unit-dose dpi: aerolizer. (**A,** GlaxoSmithKline, used with permission. **B** and **C,** Merck & Co. Inc. Whitehouse Station, NJ.)

with any particular spacer, it is important to know how comparable the available dose and particle size distribution are to the dose and particle size from an existing CFC pMDI.[20]

Dry Powder Inhalers

A DPI is typically a breath-actuated dosing system. With a DPI, the patient creates the aerosol by drawing air though a dose of finely milled drug powder with sufficient force to disperse and suspend the powder in the air. DPIs are inexpensive, do not need propellants, and do not require the hand-breath coordination needed for pMDIs. However, dispersion of the powder into respirable particles depends on the creation of turbulent flow in the inhaler. Turbulent flow is a function of the ability of the patient to inhale the powder with a sufficiently high inspiratory flow rate (Figure 36-13). In terms of both lung deposition and drug response, DPIs are as effective as pMDIs.[34]

Equipment Design and Function

Most passive dry powder–dispensing systems require the use of a carrier substance (lactose or glucose) mixed into the drug to enable the drug powder to deaggregate more readily and flow out of the device. Reactions to lactose or glucose seem to be fewer than reactions to the surfactants and propellants used in pMDIs, even though the amount of these substances is substantially greater than the amount of the drug and can represent 98% or more of the weight per inhaled dose in some formulations.

As shown in Figure 36-14, there are numerous DPIs on the market, which can be divided into three categories based on the design of their dose containers: (1) unit-dose DPI, (2) multiple unit-dose DPI, and (3) multiple dose drug reservoir DPI.

Unit-dose DPIs, such as the Aerolizer (Schering-Plough, Kenilworth, NJ) and the HandiHaler (Boehringer Ingleheim, Ingelheim am Rhein, Germany), dispense

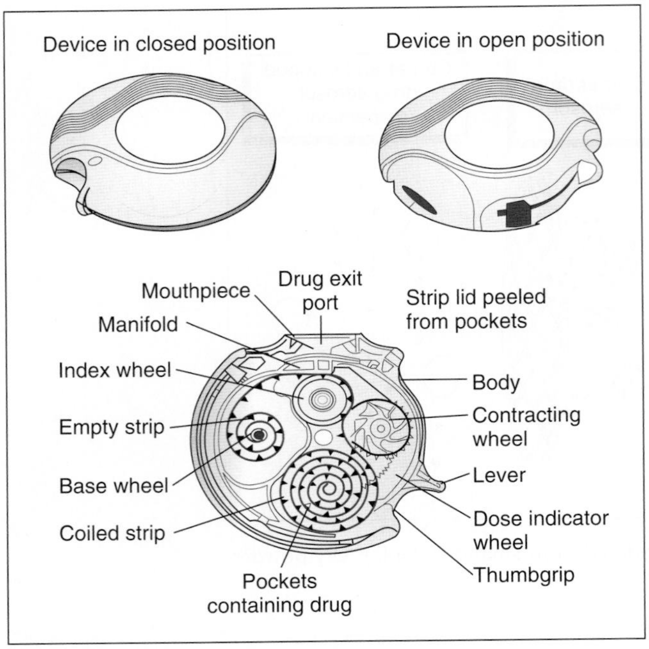

FIGURE 36-15 Diskus DPI (Glaxo Wellcome, Research Triangle Park, NC). The doses are contained in 60 sealed pockets along an aluminum-foil strip that is advanced by the lever. As the drug pocket reaches the mouthpiece, the cover is peeled away, making the drug available for inhalation. A dose counter indicates the number of doses remaining in the device. (Modified from Dhand R, Fink J: Dry powder inhalers. Respir Care 44:940, 1999.)

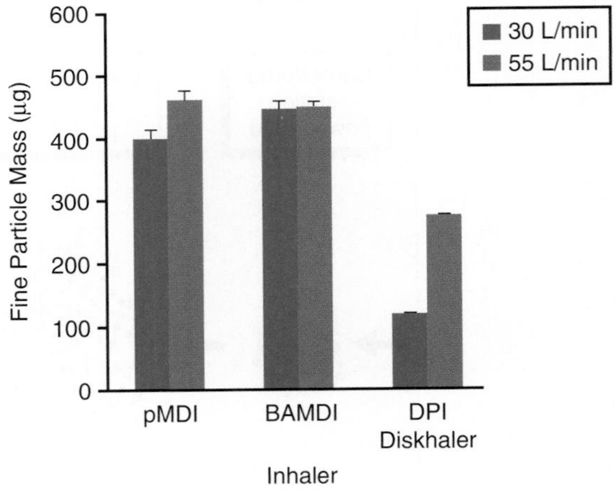

FIGURE 36-16 Fine particle mass delivered from a 1000-mg dose (± standard deviation) as a function of flow. *BAMDI,* Breath-actuated pMDI (Autohaler); *DPI,* dry powder inhaler (Diskhaler); *pMDI,* pressurized metered dose inhaler. (Modified from Smith KJ, Chan HK, Brown KF: Influence of flow rate on aerosol particle size distributions from pressurized and breath-actuated inhalers. J Aerosol Med 11:231, 1998.)

individual doses of drug from punctured gelatin capsules. Multiple unit-dose DPIs (Diskhaler; GlaxoSmithKline, Philadelphia) contain a case of four or eight individual blister packets of medication on a disk inserted into the inhaler. Multiple dose DPIs include the Twisthaler (Schering-Plough), Flexhaler (AstraZeneka, London), and the Diskus (GlaxoSmithKline). The Twisthaler and Flexhaler have a multidose reservoir powder system preloaded with a quantity of pure drug sufficient for dispensing 120 doses of medication, and the Diskus incorporates a tape system that contains up to 60 sealed single doses (Figure 36-15).

The particle size of the dry powder particles of drug ranges from 1 to 3 μm. However, the size of the lactose or glucose particles can range from approximately 20 to 65 μm, so most of the carrier (≤80%) is deposited in the oropharynx.

Factors Affecting Dry Powder Inhaler Performance and Drug Delivery

Performance of DPIs can be affected by the materials used in production and manufacturing.

Intrinsic Resistance and Inspiratory Flow Rate. Optimal performance for each DPI design occurs at a specific inspiratory flow rate. The fine-particle fraction of respirable drug from existing DPIs ranges from 10% to 60% of the nominal dose. The amount varies with inspiratory flow and device design. The higher the resistance or the greater the flow requirement of a DPI device, the more difficult it is for a compromised or young patient to generate inspiratory flow sufficient to obtain the maximum dose of drug from the device.

Exposure to Humidity and Moisture. Ambient humidity affects drug delivered from DPIs. The emitted dose decreases in a humid environment, likely because of powder clumping. The longer the exposure and the greater the level of absolute humidity, the lower the dose emitted. New designs of multiple unit-dose DPIs in which each dose of powder is sealed until used minimize the effects of moisture on the powder as long as individual doses are inhaled as soon as the seal is broken.

Patient's Inspiratory Flow Ability. The high peak inspiratory flow rates (>60 L/min) required to dispense the drug powder from most current DPI designs result in a pharyngeal dose comparable to the dose received from a typical pMDI without an add-on device. If inhalation is not performed at the optimal inspiratory flow rate for a particular device, delivery to the lung decreases as the dose of drug dispensed decreases and the particle size of the powder aerosol increases (Figure 36-16).[34]

Despite the foregoing issues, DPIs generally are convenient and easy to use. Newer designs are being developed that provide aerosols with higher fine-particle fractions and more reproducible dosing, independent of inspiratory flow rate.

Passive, or patient-driven, DPIs rely on the patient's inspiratory effort to dispense the dose. The result is differences in lung delivery and clinical response. Active or powered DPI devices, which deaggregate the powder before inhalation, are independent of patient effort. Active DPIs use an energy source to deaggregate the powder and suspend the powder into an aerosol, allowing the dose to be suspended independent of patient inspiratory flow rates. One example of an active DPI is the Exubera powder insulin delivery system (Pfizer, New York). This device is manually powered using pneumatic pressure to disperse the powder into a reservoir chamber from which the aerosol is inhaled.

Technique. As with pMDIs, to derive the maximum benefit from a DPI, proper technique is essential. Box 36-4 outlines the basic steps for ensuring optimal drug delivery. The most critical factor in using a passive DPI is the need for high inspiratory flow. Patients must generate an inspiratory flow rate of at least 40 to 60 L/min to produce a respirable powder aerosol. Because infants, small children (<5 years old) (Figure 36-17), and patients who are unable to follow instructions cannot develop flow this high, these patients cannot use DPIs. Also, patients with severe airway obstruction may be unable to achieve the required flow; DPIs should not be used in the management of acute bronchospasm.

Although hand-breath coordination is not as important with DPIs as it is with pMDIs, exhalation into the device before inspiration can result in loss of drug delivery to the lung. Some devices also require assembly, which can be cumbersome or difficult for some patients, especially in an emergency. It is important that patients receive demonstrations with their inhalers and have the opportunity to assemble and use the DPI (return demonstration) before self-administration. Although the DPI may require cleaning in accordance with the product label, the device should never be submerged in water. Moisture in the device dramatically reduces available dose. Based on the different types of DPIs and the various drug container closure systems, Table 36-1 provides methods to determine the dose in the DPI.

Box 36-4 Optimal Technique for Use of a Dry Powder Inhaler

1. Assemble the apparatus.
2. Load dose, keeping device upright.
3. Exhale slowly to functional residual capacity.
4. Seal lips around the mouthpiece.
5. Inhale deeply and forcefully (>60 L/min). A breath hold should be encouraged but is not essential.
6. Repeat the process until dose is completed.
7. Monitor adverse reactions.
8. Assess beneficial effects.

Modified from Pedersen S: How to use a Rotahaler. Arch Dis Child 61:11, 1986; and Hansen OR, Pedersen S: Optimal inhalation technique with terbutaline. Turbuhaler Eur Respir J 2:637, 1989.

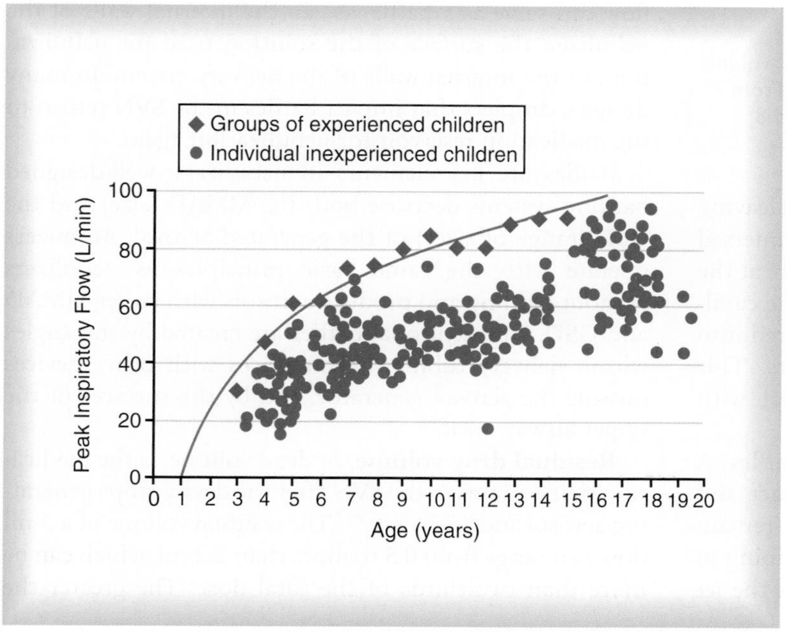

FIGURE 36-17 Peak inspiratory flows in individual inexperienced children (Pedersen et al, 1990) and groups of experienced children (Agertoft et al, 1995). (Modified from Pedersen S: Delivery options for inhaled therapy in children over the age of 6 years. J Aerosol Med 10[Suppl 1]:S41, 1997.)

Nebulizers

Nebulizers generate aerosols from solutions and suspensions. The three categories of nebulizers include (1) pneumatic jet nebulizers, (2) USNs, and (3) VM nebulizers. Nebulizers are also described in terms of their reservoir size. Small volume nebulizers (SVNs) most commonly used for medical aerosol therapy hold 5 to 20 ml of medication. Large volume nebulizers, also known as jet nebulizers, hold up to 200 ml and may be used for either bland aerosol therapy (see Chapter 35) or continuous drug administration.

Pneumatic (Jet) Nebulizers

Gas-powered jet nebulizers (Figure 36-18, *A*) have been in clinical use for longer than 100 years. Most modern jet nebulizers are powered by high-pressure air or oxygen (O_2) provided by a portable compressor, compressed gas cylinder, or 50-psi wall outlet.

Factors Affecting Nebulizer Performance. Nebulizer design, gas pressure, gas density, and medication characteristics affect SVN performance (Box 36-5).

Nebulizer Design. As shown in Figure 36-18, *B*, a typical SVN is powered by a high-pressure stream of gas directed

TABLE 36-1

Determining Doses Left in the Dry Powder Inhaler

		Drug Container	Doses	Type Indicator	Meaning of Dose Indicator
Unit-Dose DPI	Aerolizer or HandiHaler	Single capsule	1	None	Check capsule to ensure full dose was inhaled. Repeat to empty capsule
Multiple Unit-Dose DPI	Diskhaler	Dose blisters	4 or 8	None	Inspect visually to confirm use of all blisters
	Diskus	Blister strip	60	Red numbers	Red numbers indicate that ≤5 doses are left in DPI
Multiple Dose DPI	Flexhaler	Reservoir	60 or 120	"0"	Marked in intervals of 10 doses; "0" indicates empty
	Twisthaler	Reservoir	30	"01"	"01" indicates last dose

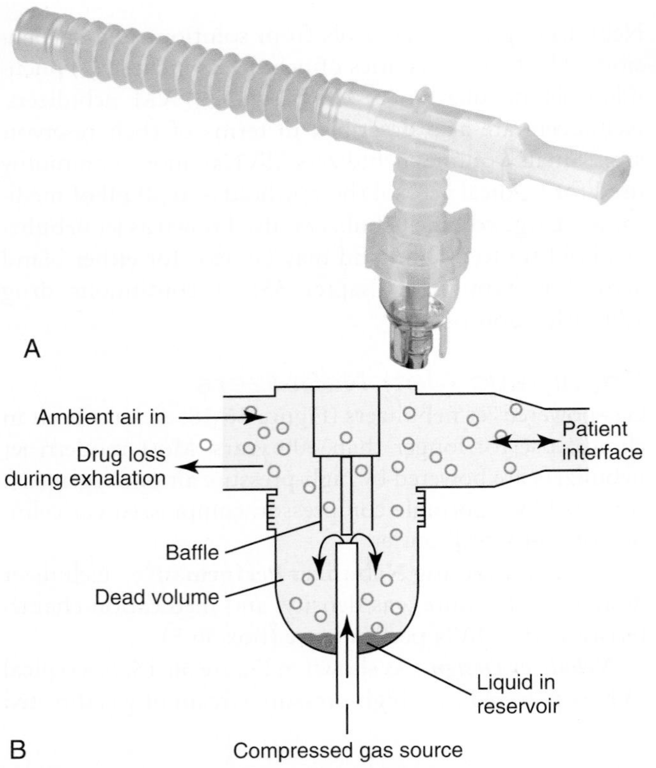

FIGURE 36-18 **A,** Small-volume jet nebulizer with tube reservoir for liquid drug delivery. **B,** Schematic of a small-volume jet nebulizer. (**A,** DeVilbiss Healthcare, Somerset PA. **B,** From Gardenhire, D: Rau's Respiratory Care Pharmacology, ed 8, St. Louis, 2012, Mosby.)

through a restricted orifice (the jet). The gas stream leaving the jet passes by the opening of a capillary tube immersed in solution. Because it produces low lateral pressure at the outlet, the high jet velocity draws the liquid up the capillary tube and into the gas stream, where it is sheared into filaments of liquid that break up into droplets. This primary spray produces a heterodisperse aerosol with droplets ranging from 0.1 to 500 μm.[35]

This spray is directed against one or more baffles. A **baffle** is a surface on which large particles impact and fall out of suspension, whereas smaller particles remain in suspension, reducing the size of particles remaining in the aerosol. A sphere or plate placed in line with the jet

Box 36-5 Factors Affecting Performance of Small Volume Nebulizers

NEBULIZER DESIGN
- Baffles
- Fill volume
- Residual drug volume
- Nebulizer position
- Continuous vs. intermittent nebulization
- Reservoirs and extensions
- Vents, valves, and gas entrainment
- Tolerances in manufacturing within lots

GAS SOURCE: WALL, CYLINDER, COMPRESSOR
- Pressure
- Flow through nebulizer
- Gas density
- Humidity
- Temperature

CHARACTERISTICS OF DRUG FORMULATION
- Viscosity
- Surface tension
- Homogeneity

flow can serve as a baffle, as can the internal walls of the nebulizer, the surface of the solution used for nebulization, or the internal walls of the delivery system. In many designs, droplets that impact baffles in the SVN return to the medication reservoir for nebulization again.

Baffles are key elements in nebulizers; well-designed baffling systems decrease both the MMAD (size) and the GSD (range of sizes) of the generated aerosol. Atomizers operate with the same basic principles as nebulizers without baffling and produce aerosols with larger MMAD and GSD. Unintentional baffles are created by the angles within delivery tubing, by interfaces with other devices outside the aerosol generator, and by the surfaces of the upper airway itself.[36]

Residual drug volume, or dead volume, is the medication that remains in the SVN after the device stops generating aerosol and "runs dry."[37] The residual volume of a 3-ml dose can range from 0.5 to more than 2.2 ml, which can be more than two-thirds of the total dose. The greater the residual drug volume, the more drug that is unavailable as aerosol, and the less efficient the delivery system. Residual volume also depends on the position of the SVN. Some SVNs stop producing aerosol when tilted 30 degrees from vertical. Increasing the fill volume allows a greater proportion of active medication to be used for nebulization. In a nebulizer with a residual volume of 1.5 ml, a fill of 3 ml would leave only 50% of the nebulizer charge (nominal dose) available for nebulization. In contrast, a fill of 5 ml would make 3.5 ml, or more than 70% of the medication, available to be inhaled. The unit-dose volumes of drugs were based on clinical response of patients using nebulizers with substantial residual drug volumes. Although increasing dose volume may increase available dose, it should be considered off-label administration, and no significant difference in clinical response has been shown to date with varying diluent volumes and flow rates.

Flow. Droplet size and nebulization time are inversely proportional to gas flow through the jet. The higher the flow of gas to the nebulizer, the smaller the particle size generated, and the shorter is the time required for nebulization of the full dose. Within the limits of the design of the nebulizer, the higher the gas pressure and flow to the nebulizer, the smaller the particle generated. Nebulizers that produce smaller particle sizes by use of baffles, such as one-way valves, may reduce total drug output per minute compared with the same nebulizer without baffling and require more time or nominal dose to deliver a standard dose of medication to the lungs.

Gas Source (Hospital versus Home). Gas pressure and flow through the nebulizer affect particle size distribution and output. Within operating limits, the higher the pressure or flow, the smaller the particle size, the greater the output, and the shorter the treatment time. A nebulizer that produces an MMAD of 2.5 μm when driven by a gas source of 50 psi at 6 to 10 L/min may produce an MMAD of more than 5 μm when operated on a home compressor (or ventilator) developing 10 psi. Too low a gas pressure or flow can result in negligible nebulizer output. Consequently, nebulizers used for home care should be matched to the compressor according to data supplied by the manufacturer so that the combination of specific equipment performs efficient nebulization of the desired medications prescribed for the patient. In Europe, equipment manufacturers are required to characterize the performance of their nebulizer and compressor combinations using standardized methods so that consumers can compare performance. Until such time that similar standards are required in the United States, clinicians should ascertain whether the system prescribed meets these criteria.

Other concerns in the use of disposable nebulizers with compressors at home involve possible degradation of performance of the plastic device over multiple uses. One study showed that repeated use did not alter MMAD or output as long as the nebulizer was cleaned properly. Failure to clean the nebulizer properly resulted in degradation of performance because of clogging of the Venturi orifice, reducing the output flow, and buildup of electrostatic charge in the device.

Density. Gas density affects both aerosol generation and delivery to the lungs. The lower the density of a carrier gas, the less turbulent the flow (i.e., the lower the Reynolds number), resulting in less aerosol impaction. This phenomenon has been shown with low-density helium-O_2 mixtures (heliox). The lower the density of a carrier gas, the less aerosol impaction occurs as gas passes through the airways, and the greater the deposition of aerosol in the lungs.[38] However, when heliox is used to drive a jet nebulizer at standard flow rates, aerosol output is substantially less than with air or O_2, and aerosol particles are considerably smaller. When driving a nebulizer with heliox, twofold to threefold greater flow is required to produce a comparable aerosol output. Heliox concentrations of 40% or greater have been shown to improve aerosol deposition.[39]

Humidity and Temperature. Humidity and temperature can affect particle size and the concentration of drug remaining in the nebulizer. Evaporation of water and adiabatic expansion of gas can reduce the temperature of the aerosol to 10° C less than ambient temperature. This cooling may increase solution viscosity and reduce the nebulizer output, while decreasing particle MMAD.[40] Aerosol particles entrained into a warm and fully saturated gas stream increase in size. These particles also can coalesce (stick together), increasing the MMAD further and, in the case of a DPI, can severely compromise the output of respirable particles. How much these particles enlarge depends primarily on the tonicity of the solution. Aerosols generated from isotonic solutions probably maintain their size as they enter the respiratory tract. Hypertonic solutions tend to enlarge, whereas evaporation can cause hypotonic droplets to evaporate and shrink.

Characteristics of Drug Formulation. The viscosity and density of a drug formulation affect both output and particle size. Some drugs, such as antibiotics, are so viscous they cannot be used effectively for nebulization in some standard SVNs. Also, in some suspensions, some aerosolized particles contain no active drug, whereas other particles, generally larger, carry the active medication.

Small Volume Nebulizers

Four categories of jet SVNs include (1) continuous nebulizer with simple reservoir, (2) continuous nebulizer with collection reservoir bag, (3) breath-enhanced nebulizer, and (4) breath-actuated nebulizer (Figure 36-19). The most commonly used SVN is the constant output design. Supplemental air is entrained across the top of the device and dilutes the aerosol produced within the nebulizer as it exits toward the patient. Aerosol is generated continuously, with 30% to 60% of the nominal dose being trapped as residual volume in the nebulizer, and more than 60% of the emitted dose is wasted to the atmosphere. Continuous nebulization wastes medication because the aerosol is

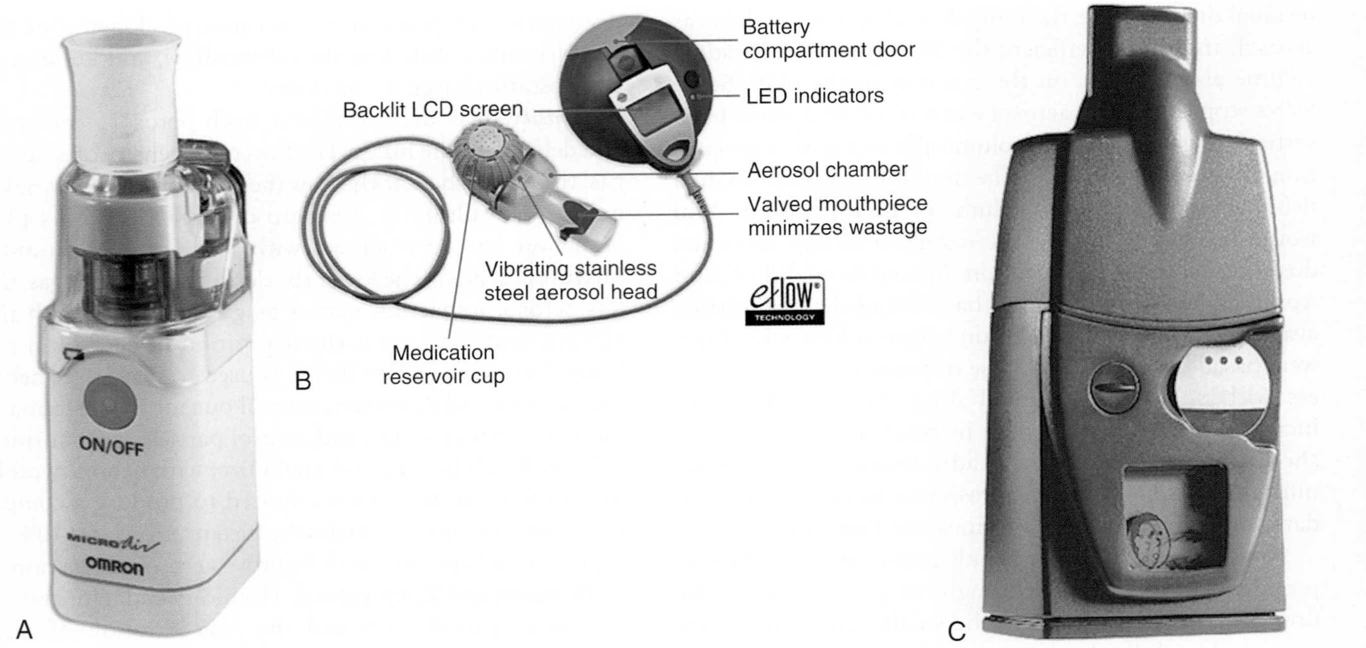

FIGURE 36-19 Variety of available aerosol devices. **A** and **C,** Passive mesh **B,** Active vibrating mesh. (**A** and **C,** Courtesy Omron Healthcare, Inc. Bannockburn, IL. **B,** Courtesy PARI Respiratory Equipment, Inc. Midloathian VA.)

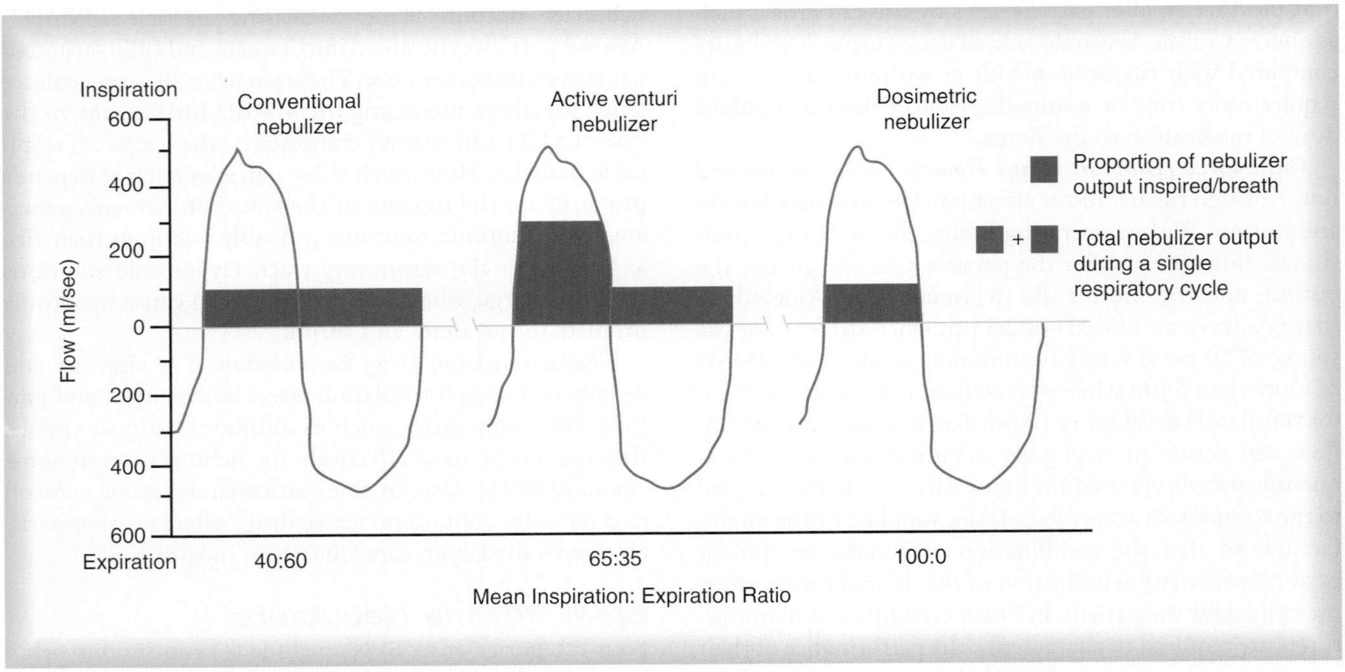

FIGURE 36-20 Proportions of nebulizer output inhaled with continuous standard jet nebulizer, vented nebulizer, and dosimetric (breath-actuated) nebulizer. (Modified from Nikander K: Drug delivery systems. Aerosol Med 7[Suppl 1]:S19, 1994.)

produced throughout the respiratory cycle and is largely lost to the atmosphere, as shown in Figure 36-20. Patients with an I:E ratio of 40:60 (or 1:1.5) lose 60% of the aerosol generated to the atmosphere. If 50% of the total dose is emitted from the nebulizer, and 50% of that aerosol is in the respiratory range and 40% of that is inhaled by the patient, less than 10% deposition is commonly measured in adults receiving continuous nebulizer therapy. In neonates and infants, given the small minute volumes and small airways with increased impaction and reduced sedimentation, deposition can be only 0.5%.

Aerosolized medication can also be conserved with reservoirs.[41] A reservoir on the expiratory limb of the nebulizer conserves drug aerosol.

Small Volume Nebulizer With a Reservoir. Many types of disposable SVNs are packaged with a 6-inch (15-cm) piece of aerosol tubing to be used as a reservoir (see Figure 36-18, *A*). This may increase inhaled dose by 5% to 10% or increase the inhaled dose from 10% to approximately 11% with the reservoir tube.

Continuous Small Volume Nebulizer With Collection Bag. Bag reservoirs hold the aerosol generated during exhalation and allow the small particles to remain in suspension for inhalation with the next breath, while larger particles rain out, attributed to a 30% to 50% increase in inhaled dose.[41] A collection bag is attached on the expiratory side of the nebulizer "T," which collects aerosol leaving the SVN when the patient is not actively inhaling. Some of the aerosol in the bag is inhaled with the next inspiration, increasing total dose efficiency. The patient inhales aerosol from the SVN and reservoir through a one-way valve with exhalation through a second valve to the atmosphere.

Breath-Enhanced Nebulizers. Breath-enhanced nebulizers generate aerosol continuously, using a system of vents and one-way valves to minimize aerosol waste.[42] In the Pari LC Sprint (Pari, Midlothian, VA) breath-enhanced nebulizer (Figure 36-21), an inspiratory vent allows the patient to draw in air through the nebulization chamber generating and containing aerosolized drug. On exhalation, the inlet vent closes, and aerosol exits by a one-way valve near the mouthpiece; this process can increase inhaled mass by 50% over standard continuous nebulizers and reduces aerosol waste to the atmosphere.

MINI CLINI

Home Nebulizer Therapy

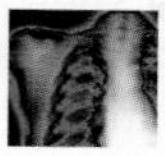

PROBLEM: Many patients are sent home with a prescription for home nebulizer therapy prescribed with the intention of giving the patient the same quality of aerosol therapy he or she received in the hospital. However, the patient often is given the same type of nebulizer used in the hospital because it is inexpensive. These nebulizers provide an aerosol that is too large for optimal deposition in the lungs. What should be done instead?

SOLUTION: Home nebulizers designed for use with compressors should be matched to ensure an MMAD of 1 to 5 μm with the medication being administered. Nebulizer manufacturers such as Pari and Medic-Aid offer matched nebulizer-compressor systems for home use. Although these devices cost a little more, they are more likely to meet therapeutic objectives.

Breath-Actuated Nebulizers. Breath-actuated nebulization can increase inhaled aerosol mass by threefold to fourfold over conventional continuous nebulization. Historically, this increase was accomplished with a patient-controlled finger port that directed gas to the nebulizer only during inspiration. Although this system wastes less aerosol, it can increase treatment time fourfold. This

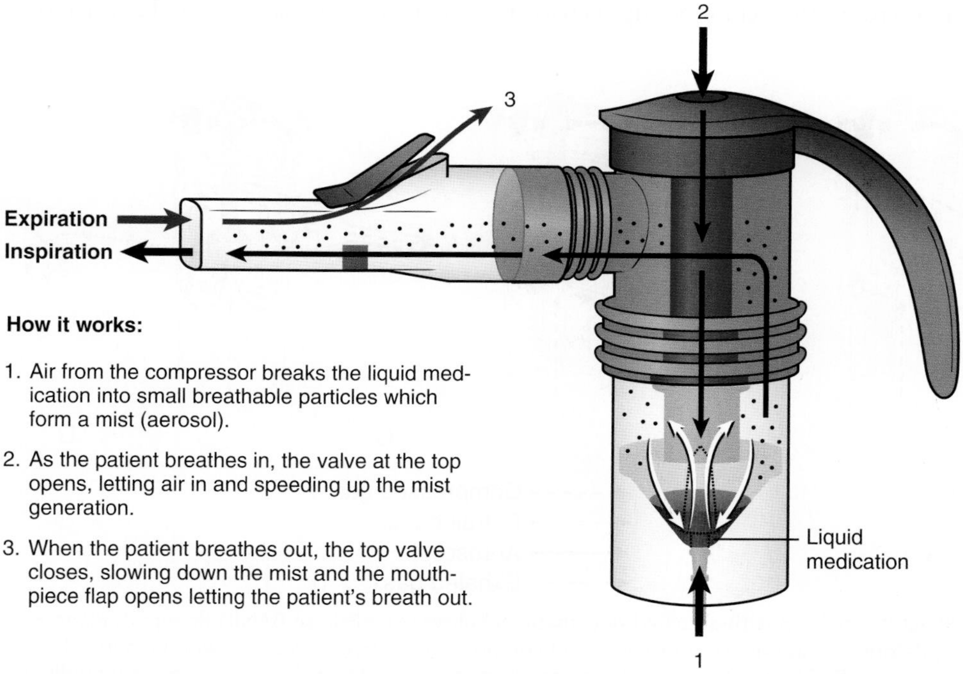

2
3
Expiration
Inspiration
How it works:
1. Air from the compressor breaks the liquid medication into small breathable particles which form a mist (aerosol).
2. As the patient breathes in, the valve at the top opens, letting air in and speeding up the mist generation.
3. When the patient breathes out, the top valve closes, slowing down the mist and the mouthpiece flap opens letting the patient's breath out.
Liquid medication
1

FIGURE 36-21 Operating principles of the Sprint (Pari, Midlothian, VA) breath-enhanced nebulizer. (From Cairo JM, Pilbeam SP: Mosby's respiratory care equipment, ed 8, St. Louis, 2009, Mosby.)

approach requires good hand-breath coordination, something not all patients possess, especially when they are distressed.

Breath-actuated SVNs have been introduced that synchronize aerosol generation based on the patient's breathing pattern. **Breath-actuated nebulizers** generate aerosol only during inspiration. This feature eliminates waste of aerosol during exhalation and increases the delivered dose threefold or more over continuous and breath-enhanced nebulizers. Dosimeters, used in pulmonary function laboratories, sense inspiration and pulse airflow to the jet orifice and transform a conventional nebulizer into a breath-actuated system.

AeroEclipse (Trudell Medical International, London, Ontario, Canada) is a breath-actuated SVN. A unique, spring-loaded, one-way valve design draws the jet to the capillary tube during inspiration and causes nebulization to cease when the patient's inspiratory flow decreases below the threshold or the patient exhales into the device (Figure 36-22). Expiratory pressure on the valve at the initiation of exhalation moves the nebulizer baffle away from its position directly above the jet orifice, reduces the pressure, and stops aerosolization. Because aerosol is generated only during inhalation, exhaled aerosol and contamination of the environment during the expiratory phase of the breathing cycle are largely eliminated.

It can be difficult to determine when a nebulizer treatment is complete. Malone and colleagues[43] found that with three different fill volumes, albuterol delivery from the nebulizer ceased after the onset of inconsistent nebulization (sputtering) (Figure 36-23). Aerosol output declined one-half within 20 seconds of the onset of sputtering. The concentration of albuterol in the nebulizer cup increased significantly when the aerosol output declined, and further weight loss in the nebulizer was caused primarily by evaporation. The authors concluded that aerosolization past the point of initial nebulizer sputter is ineffective.

Table 36-2 summarizes some of these key factors for many commercially available SVNs.[44] Numerous SVNs are on the market, and they vary widely in design and performance. SVNs of the same design and lot number can exhibit variable performance, even to the point that some nebulizers of the same model number do not work at all.[45] Managers and clinicians always must evaluate SVNs carefully before purchasing or using them. Manufacturers should provide data on the performance of their nebulizers under common use conditions.

Technique. Box 36-6 outlines the optimal technique for using an SVN for aerosol drug delivery. Use of an SVN is less technique-dependent and device-dependent than use of a pMDI or DPI delivery system. Slow inspiratory flow optimizes SVN aerosol deposition. However, deep breathing and breath holding during SVN therapy do little to enhance deposition over normal tidal breathing.[46] Because the nose is an efficient filter of particles larger than 5 mm, many clinicians prefer not to use a mask for SVN therapy. As long as the patient is mouth breathing, there is little difference in clinical response between therapy given by mouthpiece and therapy given by mask. The selection of delivery method (mask or mouthpiece) should be based on patient ability, preference, and comfort.

Infection Control Issues. The CDC recommends that nebulizers be cleaned and disinfected, or rinsed with sterile water, and air dried between uses. Oie and Kamiya,[47] studying microbial contamination of antibiotic aerosol solutions, found that after 7 days, five of six solutions were

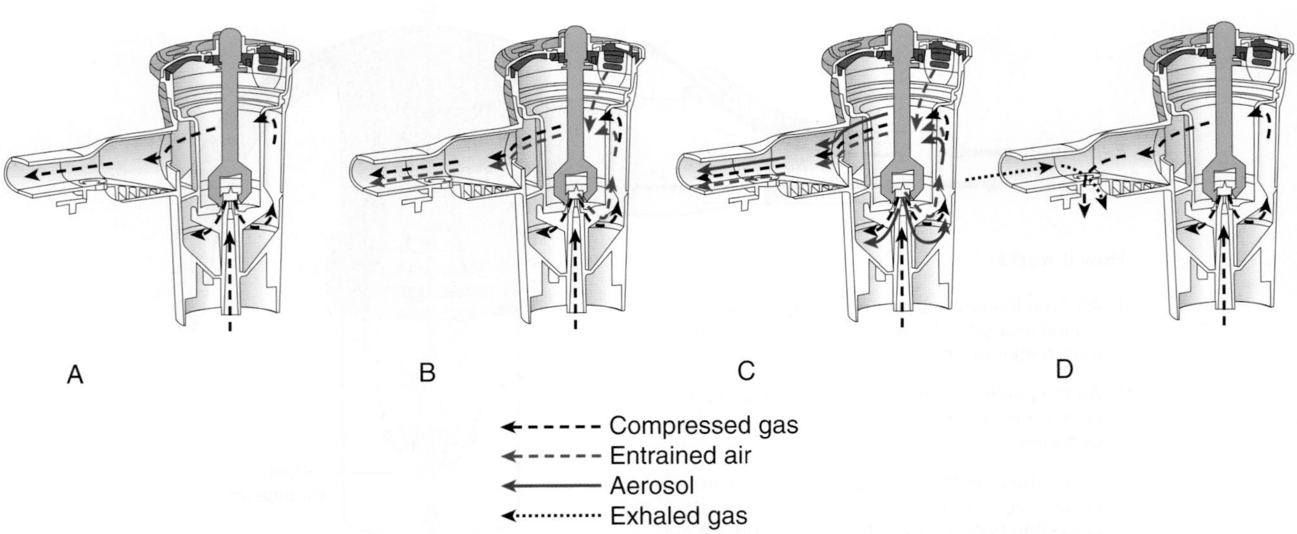

FIGURE 36-22 Breath-actuated pneumatic nebulizer (AeroEclipse BANII) flow path diagram. **A,** Before inhalation, actuator is up, and compressed gas freely circulates with no aerosol produced. **B,** Patient inhales, and actuator starts to move down. **C,** Negative pressure pulls the diaphragm down (with actuator moved down sealing around the nozzle cover), producing aerosol. **D,** Patient exhales through valve in mouthpiece; as pressure increases, the diaphragm and actuator move up, stopping aerosol production. (Courtesy Trudell Medical International, London, Ontario, Canada.)

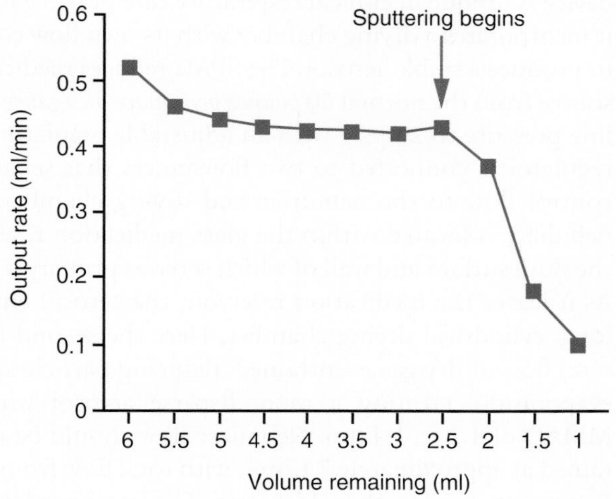

FIGURE 36-23 Output rate for jet nebulizers is substantially reduced as the nebulizer begins to sputter. The decrease in output rate correlates with reduced drug output. This finding supports a recommendation to end treatment when sputtering begins. (Modified from Malone RA, Hollie MC, Glynn-Barnhart A, et al: Optimal duration of nebulized albuterol therapy. Chest 104:1114, 1993.)

TABLE 36-2

Comparison of Different Nebulizers

	Jet	Ultrasonic	Vibrating Mesh
Features			
Power source	Compressed gas or electrical mains	Electrical mains	Batteries or electrical mains
Portability	Restricted	Restricted	Portable
Treatment time	Long	Intermediate	Short
Output rate	Low	Higher	Highest
Residual volume	0.8-2.0 ml	Variable but low	≤0.2 ml
Environmental Contamination			
Continuous use	High	High	High
Breath-activated	Low	Low	Low
Performance variability	High	Intermediate	Low
Formulation Characteristics			
Temperature	Decreases*	Increases†	Minimum change
Concentration	Increases	Variable	Minimum change
Suspensions	Low efficiency	Poor efficiency	Variable efficiency
Denaturation	Possible‡	Probable‡	Possible‡
Cleaning	Required, after single use	Required, after multiple use	Required after single use
Cost	Very low	High	High

Modified from Dolovich MB, Dhand R: Aerosol drug delivery: developments in device design and clinical use. Lancet 377:1032, 2011.
*For jet nebulizers, the temperature of the reservoir fluid decreases about 15° C during nebulization because of evaporation.
†For ultrasonic nebulizers, vibration of the reservoir fluid causes a temperature increase during aerosol generation, which can be 10° C to 15° C.
‡Denaturation of DNA occurs with all the nebulizers.

contaminated. The contamination appeared to have been caused by storage of multiple dose solutions at room temperature instead of in a refrigerator and reuse of syringes for measuring the solution. Refrigerating solutions and discarding syringes every 24 hours eliminated bacterial contamination.

Large Volume Jet Nebulizers

Large volume jet nebulizers are also used to deliver aerosolized drugs to the lung. A large volume nebulizer is particularly useful when traditional dosing strategies are ineffective in the management of severe bronchospasm. When a patient with airway obstruction does not respond to a standard dosage of bronchodilator, it is common to repeat the treatment every 15 minutes. An alternative approach is to provide continuous nebulization with a specialized large volume nebulizer.

The high-output extended aerosol respiratory therapy nebulizers HEART (Cardinal Health, Dublin, OH), and HOPE (B & B Medical Technologies, Carlsbad, CA) are examples of devices designed for this purpose. These nebulizers have a reservoir greater than 200 ml that produces an aerosol with an MMAD of 2.2 to 3.5 μm. Actual output and particle size vary with the pressure and flow at which the nebulizer operates. A potential problem with continuous bronchodilator therapy (CBT) is increase in drug concentration. Patients receiving CBT need close monitoring for signs of drug toxicity (e.g., tachycardia and tremor). An additional strategy is to use an intravenous infusion pump to drip premixed bronchodilator solution into a standard SVN. Although an equipment-intensive approach, this technique can provide dosing equivalent to every 15 minutes.[48]

Another special-purpose large volume nebulizer is a *small particle aerosol generator (SPAG)* (Figure 36-24). The SPAG was manufactured by ICN Pharmaceuticals specifically for administration of ribavirin (Virazole) to infants with respiratory syncytial virus infection. The device is unique in clinical respiratory care practice in that it incorporates a drying chamber with its own flow control to produce a stable aerosol. The SPAG reduces medical gas source from the normal 50 *pounds per square inch gauge (psig)* line pressure to 26 psig with an adjustable regulator. The regulator is connected to two flowmeters that separately control flow to the nebulizer and drying chamber. The nebulizer is located within the glass medication reservoir, the fluid surface and wall of which serve as primary baffles. As it leaves the medication reservoir, the aerosol enters a long, cylindrical drying chamber. Here the second (separate) flow of dry gas is entrained, reducing particle size by evaporation, creating a monodisperse aerosol with an MMAD of 1.2 to 1.4 μm. Nebulizer flow should be maintained at approximately 7 L/min with total flow from both flowmeters not less than 15 L/min. The latest model operates consistently even with back pressure and can be used with masks, hoods, tents, or ventilator circuits.

Two specific problems are associated with SPAG use to deliver ribavirin. The first is caregiver exposure to the drug aerosol. Approaches to limit caregiver exposure are discussed later (see the section on Controlling Environmental Contamination). The other problem occurs only when the SPAG is used to deliver ribavirin through a mechanical ventilator circuit. Drug precipitation can jam breathing valves or occlude the ventilator circuit. This problem can be overcome by (1) placing a one-way valve between the SPAG and the circuit and (2) filtering out the excess aerosol particles before they reach the exhalation valve, changing filters frequently to avoid increasing expiratory resistance.[46]

Box 36-6 Optimal Technique for Using a Small Volume Nebulizer

1. Assess the patient for need (clinical signs and symptoms, breath sounds, peak flow, $\%FEV_1$)
2. Select mask or mouthpiece delivery (nose clips may be needed with mouthpiece).
3. Use conserving system (thumb port, breath actuator or reservoir) if indicated.
4. Place drug in the nebulizer. If using a multidose vial, add saline to approved dose volume (per drug label).
5. Set gas flow to nebulizer at 6 to 10 L/min (per manufacturer label).
6. Coach patient to breathe slowly through the mouth at normal V_T.
7. Continue treatment until nebulizer begins to sputter.
8. Rinse the nebulizer with sterile water and air dry, or discard, between treatments.
9. Monitor patient for adverse response.
10. Assess outcome (change in peak flow, $\%FEV_1$).

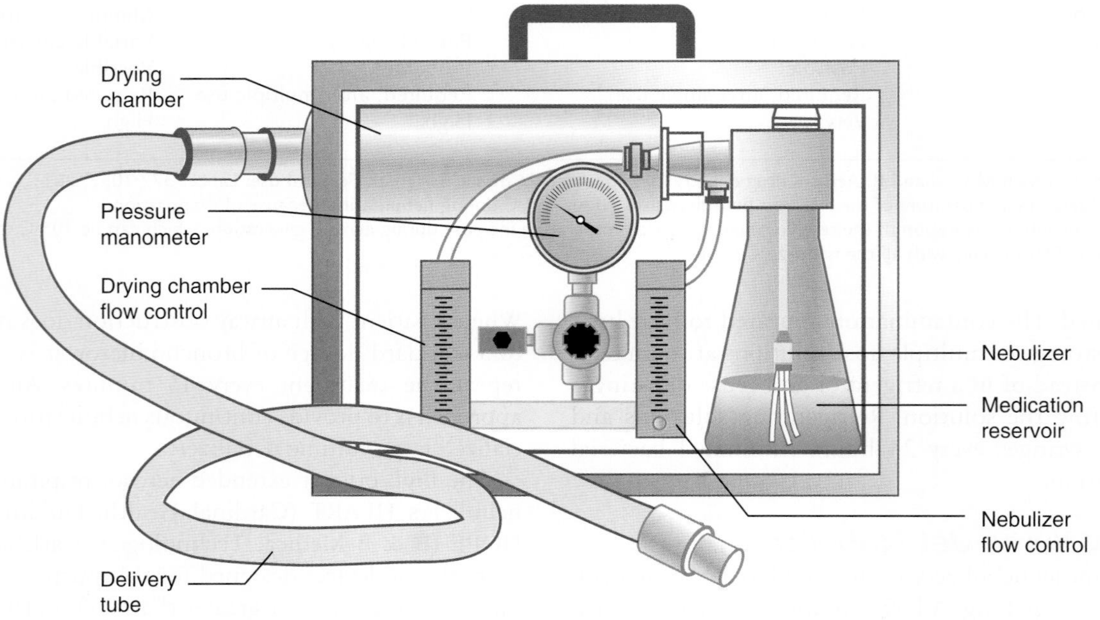

FIGURE 36-24 Small particle aerosol generator (SPAG).

Hand-Bulb Atomizers and Spray Pumps

Hand-bulb atomizers and nasal spray pumps are used to administer sympathomimetic, anticholinergic, antiinflammatory, and anesthetic aerosols to the upper airway, including nasal passages, pharynx, and larynx (see also Chapter 32). These agents are used to manage upper airway inflammation and rhinitis, to provide local anesthesia, and to achieve systemic effects. Guidelines for the delivery of drugs to the upper airway have been developed by the American Association for Respiratory Care (AARC).[49]

Because the spray pump generates relatively low pressure and does not have baffles, it produces an aerosol suspension with large particle size (high MMAD and GSD), which are ideal for upper airway deposition. (Nasopharyngeal deposition is greatest for particles 5 to 20 μm.) Deposition with the hand-bulb atomizer applied to the nose occurs mostly in the anterior nasal passages with clearance to the nasopharynx. The 100-mcl puffs appear to deposit more medication than 50-mcl puffs, and deposition to a greater surface area occurs with a 35-degree spray angle than with a 60-degree angle.

Ultrasonic Nebulizers

The USN uses a piezoelectric crystal to generate an aerosol. The crystal transducer converts an electrical signal into high-frequency (1.2- to 2.4-MHz) acoustic vibrations. These vibrations are focused in the liquid above the transducer, where they disrupt the surface and create oscillation waves (Figure 36-25). If the frequency of the signal is high enough and its amplitude strong enough, the oscillation waves form a standing wave that generates a geyser of droplets that break free as fine aerosol particles.

USNs are capable of higher aerosol outputs (0.2 to 1.0 ml/min) and higher aerosol densities than conventional jet nebulizers. Output is determined by the amplitude setting (sometimes user-selected); the greater the signal amplitude, the greater the nebulizer output. Particle size is inversely proportional to the frequency of vibrations. Frequency is device-specific and is not user-adjustable. For example, the DeVilbiss (Somerset, PA) Portasonic nebulizer operating at a frequency of 2.25 MHz produces particles with an MMAD of 2.5 μm, whereas the DeVilbiss Pulmosonic nebulizer operating at 1.25 MHz produces particles in the 4- to 6-μm range. Particle size and aerosol density also depend on the source and flow of gas conducting the aerosol to the patient.

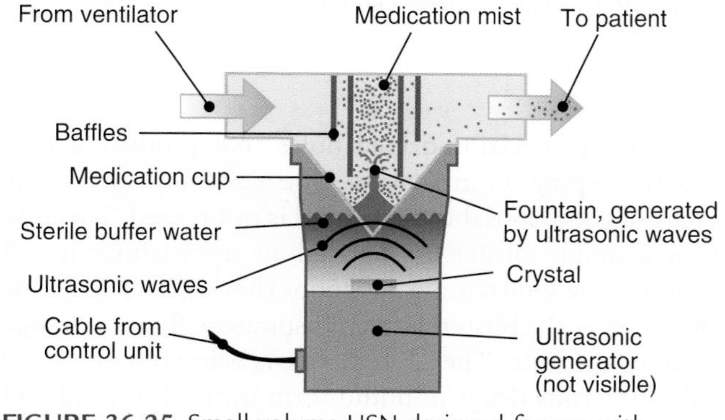

FIGURE 36-25 Small volume USN designed for use with mechanical ventilation. A vibrating piezoceramic crystal generates ultrasonic waves that pass through couplant (sterile buffer water) and the medication cup to generate a fountain (or standing wave) of medication that produces aerosol particles. (Courtesy Siemens, Tarrytown, New York.)

Large Volume Ultrasonic Nebulizers. Large volume USNs (used mainly for bland aerosol therapy or sputum induction) incorporate air blowers to carry the mist to the patient (see Chapter 35). Low flow through the USN is associated with smaller particles and higher mist density. High flow yields larger particles and less density. In contrast to jet nebulizers, the temperature of the solution placed in a USN increases during use. As the temperature increases, the drug concentration increases, as does the likelihood of undesired side effects.

Small Volume Ultrasonic Nebulizers. Many small volume USNs have been marketed for aerosol drug delivery (see Figure 36-25). In contrast to the larger units, some of these systems do not use a couplant compartment; the medication is placed directly into the manifold on top of the transducer. The transducer is connected by a cable to a power source, often battery-powered to increase portability. These devices have no blower; the patient's inspiratory flow draws the aerosol from the nebulizer into the lung.

Small volume USNs have been promoted for administration of a wide variety of formulations ranging from bronchodilators to antiinflammatory agents and antibiotics.[50] Use of a small volume USN may increase available respirable mass for designs with less residual drug volume than SVNs; this may reduce the need for a large quantity of diluent to ensure delivery of the drugs. The contained portable power source adds a great deal of convenience in mobility. Both theoretical advantages of the ultrasonic devices are outweighed by relatively high purchase costs and poor reliability.

Small volume USNs have been used to administer undiluted bronchodilators to patients with severe bronchospasm.[50] Because the nebulizers have minimal residual drug volume, the treatment time is reduced with smaller volumes; however, it may be increased with standard dosing volumes. Use of undiluted bronchodilators has been described in the literature, but this is not included at the present time in the manufacturer's label on product dosing information. Some ventilator manufacturers (e.g., Maquet, Rastatt, Germany) have promoted the use of USNs for administration of aerosols during mechanical ventilation. In contrast to SVNs, USNs do not add extra gas flow to the ventilator circuit during use. This feature reduces the need to change and reset ventilator and alarm settings during aerosol administration.[51]

Vibrating Mesh Nebulizers

Two types of VM nebulizers, active and passive, are available commercially.[52] Active VM nebulizers use a dome-shaped aperture plate, containing more than 1000 funnel-shaped apertures. This dome is attached to a plate that is also attached to a piezoceramic element that surrounds the aperture plate. Electricity applied to the piezoceramic element causes the aperture plate to be vibrated at a frequency of approximately 130 kHz (or one-tenth that of a USN), moving the aperture plate up and down by 1 μm or 2 μm, creating an electronic micropump. The plate actively pumps the liquid through the apertures, where it is broken into fine droplets. The exit velocity of the aerosol is low (<4 m/sec), and the particle size can range from 2 to 3 μm (MMAD), varying with the exit diameter of the apertures (Figure 36-26). Examples of an active VM nebulizer include the Aeroneb Go, Pro, and Solo nebulizers (Aerogen, Inc, Galway, Ireland) and the eFlow (Pari, Midlothian, VA). An active VM nebulizer can provide nebulization with single drops 15 mcl of formulations containing small and large molecules, suspensions, microsuspensions, and liposomes.

Passive VM nebulizers use a mesh separated from an ultrasonic horn by the liquid for nebulization. A piezoelectric transducer vibrates the ultrasonic horn, which pushes fluid through the mesh. Passive VM nebulizers include the NEU-22 (Omron, Kyoto, Japan) and the I-Neb (Philips Respironics, Murraysville, PA).

The residual drug volumes with either type of VM nebulizer range from 0.1 to 0.4 ml, in contrast to other types of liquid aerosol generators with residual drug volumes of 0.8 to 1.5 ml. Because a greater percentage of standard unit doses are emitted as aerosol, care should be exercised when transitioning to these devices to ensure that the higher dose does not create adverse effects.

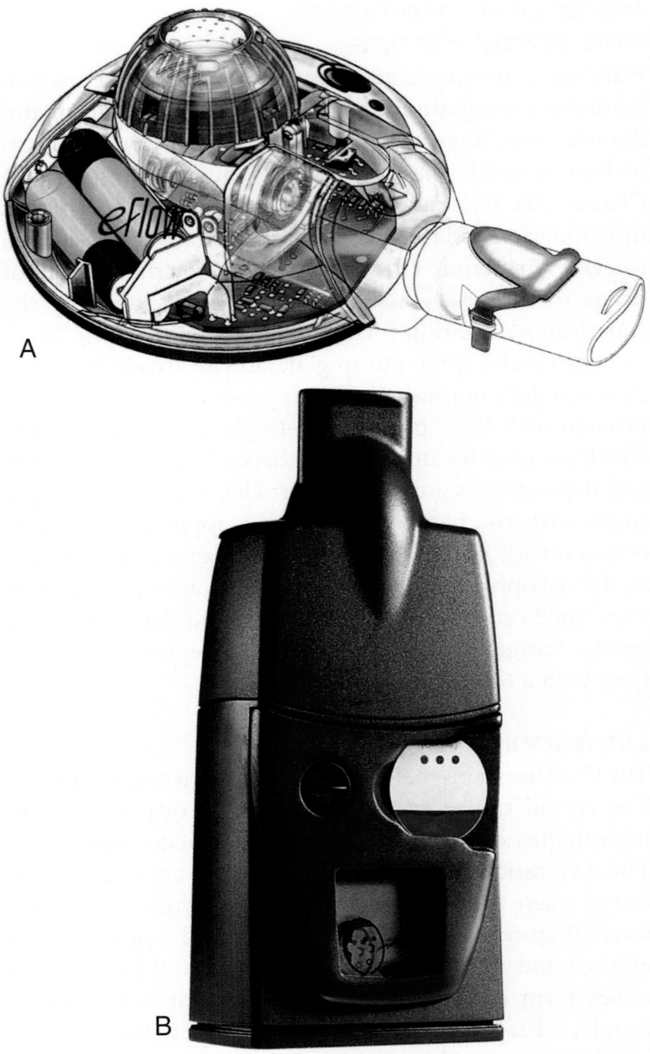

A

B

FIGURE 36-26 VM nebulizers use two basic configurations. Active VM nebulizer **(A)** has an aperture plate with funnel-shaped holes vibrated by a piezoelectric transducer surrounding the aperture plate found in the Aeroneb Solo (Aerogen, Galway, Ireland) and eFlow (Pari, Midlothian, VA; **A**). Passive VM nebulizer **(B)** uses an ultrasonic horn to push fluid through a stationary mesh found in the NEU-22 (Omron; **B**) and iNeb (Phillips/Respironics, Murrysville, PA).

New-Generation Nebulizers

Low-velocity (soft mist) aerosol, smaller particle size distribution, and systems that minimize residual volume of medication left in the nebulizer substantially improve aerosol device efficiency. Along with improved performance, some "smart" nebulizers have the capability to monitor patient compliance and aid in managing the patient's treatment schedule.

With pulmonary deposition increased from the old standard of approximately 10% to more than 60% of the nominal dose, these recent device improvements may be accompanied by greater systemic side effects, unless the delivered dose is reduced. The key is to be able to target an effective delivered dose to the lungs.

New Nebulizer Designs for Liquids. New nebulizer designs are available for delivery of liquids.[53]

AERx. The AERx device (Aradigm Corp, Hayward, CA) uses a drug solution in a unit-dose, sterile, preservative-free blister pack containing 25 to 50 mcl of fluid. The drug is extruded under pressure through a nozzle containing many small, precision-drilled holes that produce a fine, respirable spray on inhalation. The aerosolization nozzle is part of the disposable blister and is not reused. The dose from a single blister is metered in approximately 1.5 seconds. The emitted dose is more than 70% of the dose contained in the blister with an inspiratory flow rate range of 30 to 85 L/min. The AERx device is being tested for use with numerous drugs in liquid form for both topical and systemic therapy. The AERx device has built-in electronic monitoring capabilities for measuring *inspiratory flow rate (IFR)* during dosing and for triggering and dispensing the dose at the appropriate inspiratory flow rate for optimal delivery. The dose administered is logged to provide a

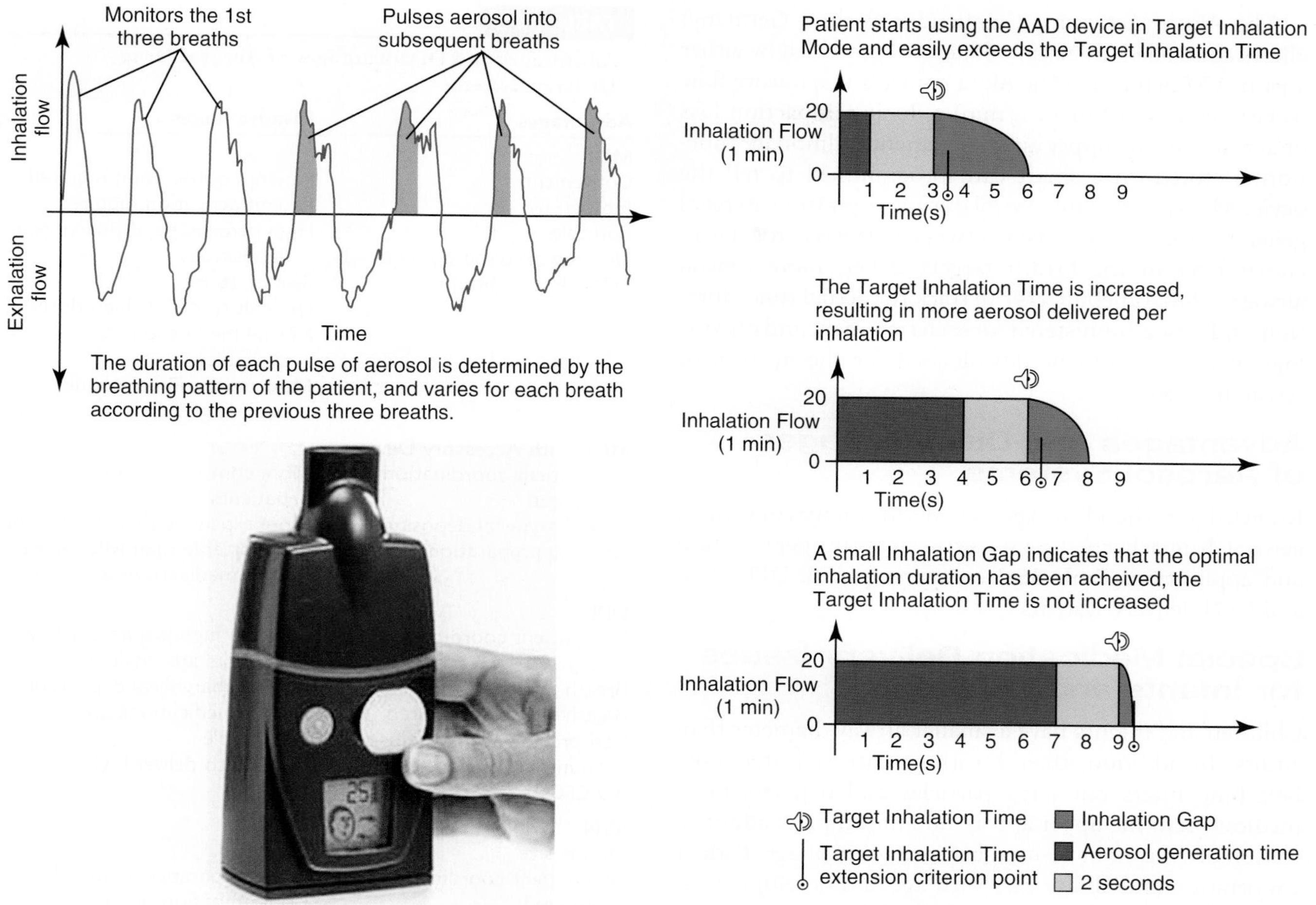

FIGURE 36-27 The iNeb *(bottom left)* is a smart nebulizer with adaptive aerosol delivery (AAD) and targeted inhalation mode (TIM). AAD delivers a precise preset dose with variation between patients. A microprocessor tracks the patient's breathing pattern on a running average of the previous three breaths, generating aerosol for 50% of the predicted inspiration *(upper left)*. TIM progressively guides the patient to take longer inspirations, increasing to achieve optimal inhalation duration *(right)*.

record of treatments and an indication of patient compliance with therapy. The AERx device is in clinical trials in the United States.

Respimat. The Respimat soft mist inhaler (Boehringer, Ingelheim am Rhein, Germany) is a small hand-held inhaler that uses mechanical energy to create an aerosol from liquid solutions to produce a low-velocity spray (10 mm/sec) that delivers a unit dose of drug in a single actuation. To operate the device, patients twist the body of the device to load an internal spring, place the mouthpiece of the Respimat between the lips, and press a button to release the drug through a uniblock to create spray, which is released over 1.1 to 1.4 seconds, depending on the formulation configuration. The Respimat device requires hand-breath coordination on the part of the patient, as does a pMDI, but because of the longer spray time, it seems more likely to get a greater percent of emitted dose despite coordination issues. Because of the small particle size and low-velocity spray, pulmonary deposition of 40% is independent of inspiratory flows with oral deposition (40%) half the oral dose used with most pMDIs and DPIs (80%). The Respimat is currently available with several drugs in Europe and is slated for introduction with tiotropium in the United States.[54]

Smart Nebulizers. The I-Neb (Phillips Respironics, Murrysville, PA) is a breath-actuated passive VM nebulizer with *adaptive aerosol delivery* that monitors pressure changes and inspiratory time for the patient's first three consecutive breaths (Figure 36-27).[55] Drug is then aerosolized over 50% of the inspiratory maneuver during the fourth and all subsequent breaths. *Targeted inhalation mode* guides the patient to take serially longer inspirations to achieve optimal inhalation duration, reducing the time for administration. When the prescribed emitted dose has been aerosolized, the system provides an audible signal indicating the treatment should be stopped and the remaining medication discarded. Built-in electronics monitor patient treatment schedules and delivered doses with the goal to improve compliance with therapy. The I-Neb has been released for delivery of prostacyclin.

The Akita (Activaero, Gemuenden/Wohra, Germany) allows controlled inhalation of aerosol produced by either a jet or VM nebulizer. The Akita controls inspiratory flow to keep it slow (12 to 15 L/min) reducing impaction loss of aerosols in the upper airways. Patient pulmonary function is stored on a smart card programmed to tell the device when to generate aerosol during inspiration. Aerosol generated early targets distal airways, whereas aerosol generated later in the breath targets larger, more central airways.[56] Smart nebulizers can track the actual time, duration, and dose administered for each treatment and provide logs of use that can be downloaded for the medical or research record.

Advantages and Disadvantages of Aerosol Systems

Knowledge of the advantages and disadvantages of various aerosol drug delivery systems is crucial for proper selection and application. Table 36-3 compares pMDI, DPI, SVN, and USN delivery systems.

Special Medication Delivery Issues for Infants and Children

Children and infants have a smaller airway diameter than adults. In addition, their breathing rate is faster, nose breathing filters out large particles and deposits more medication in the upper airway, and mouthpiece administration often cannot be used before 3 years of age. Patient cooperation and ability vary with age and developmental ability. Finally, infants and small children have lower minute volumes than adults and so inhale a smaller proportion of the output of a continuous nebulizer than adults.[7]

Normal tidal breathing is the most effective method for administering aerosols to an infant. Mouth breathing enhances medication delivery to the airways of adults, but there is little evidence to show that this is true for infants, who are preferential nose breathers up to 1 year of age. Aerosols should never be administered to a crying child. Crying greatly reduces lower airway deposition of aerosol medication (Figure 36-28).

For infants and children who can tolerate a mask, a medication nebulizer can be fitted to an appropriately sized aerosol mask. There is no difference in clinical response between mouthpiece and close-fitting mask treatment, so patient tolerance, compliance, and preference should guide selection of the device. There is evidence that the aerosol available to the patient is substantially less when a loosely fitting mask (>1-cm leak) is used rather than a snug mask or mouthpiece with either a nebulizer or a pMDI with a holder chamber.[57,58] If a patient cannot tolerate mask treatment (e.g., will not wear a close-fitting mask), a commonly used strategy is "blow-by" technique, in which the practitioner directs the aerosol from the nebulizer toward the patient's nose and mouth from a distance of several inches from the face. There are no peer-reviewed published data supporting the use of the blow-by technique. Studies suggest that almost no drug enters the airway with this method. Rather than "blow-by," it may be more efficient to take the time to condition the infant or child to tolerate the mask without crying or to deliver medication with a close-fitting mask when the patient is asleep.[59]

TABLE 36-3

Advantages and Disadvantages of Aerosol Drug Delivery Systems

Advantages	Disadvantages
MDI	
Convenient	Patient coordination required
Inexpensive	Patient activation required
Portable	High percentage of pharyngeal deposition
No drug preparation required	Risk of abuse
Difficult to contaminate	Difficult to deliver high doses
	Not all medications are available
	Most units still use ozone-depleting CFCs
MDI With Accessory Device	
Less patient coordination required	More complex for some patients
Less pharyngeal deposition	More expensive than MDI alone
No drug preparation required	Less portable than MDI alone
	Not all medications available
DPI	
Less patient coordination required	Requires high inspiratory flow
Breath-activated	Most units are single dose
Breath hold not required	Risk of pharyngeal deposition
Can provide accurate dose counts	Not all medications are available
No CFCs	Difficult to deliver high doses
SVN	
Inexpensive	Wasteful
Less patient coordination required	Drug preparation required
High doses possible (even continuous)	Contamination possible if device not cleaned carefully
No CFC release	Not all medications available
	Pressurized gas source required
	Long treatment times
USN	
Moderate residual volume	Expensive
Quiet	Prone to electrical or mechanical breakdown
Smaller residual drug volume than SVN	Not all medications available
Aerosol accumulates during exhalation	Drug preparation required
VM Nebulizer	
Low residual volume	Expensive
Quiet	Not all medications available
Does not require gas or propellant	Drug preparation required
Flow-independent delivery	
Shorter treatment times	

Modified from Hess D: Aerosol delivery. Respir Care Clin N Am 1:235, 1995.

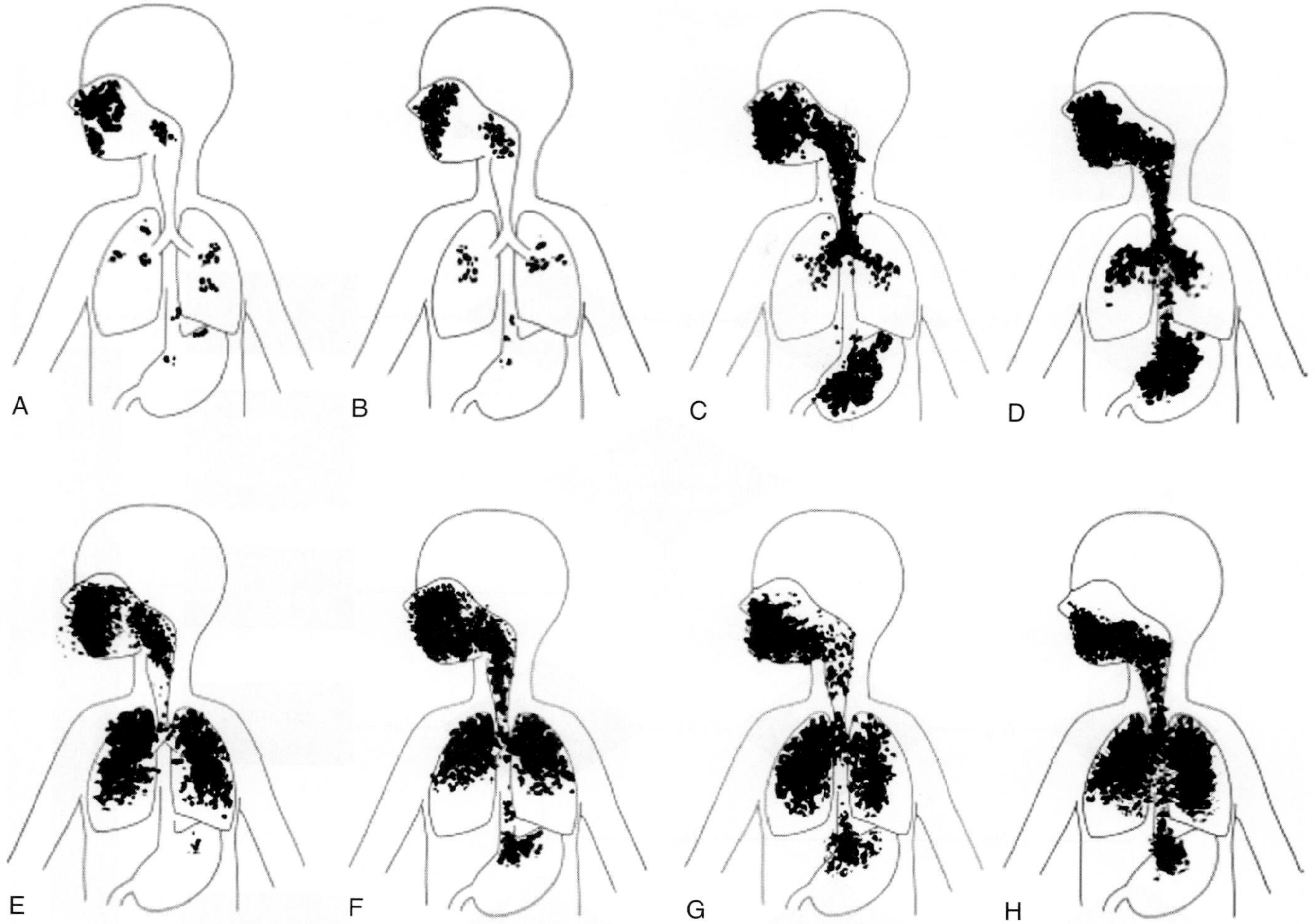

FIGURE 36-28 Drug deposition of radiolabeled albuterol in a young child **(A)** inhaling with a pMDI/space through a non-tightly fitted facemask; **(B)** inhaling with a nebulizer through a non-tightly fitted facemask; **(C)** inhaling with a pMDI/spacer through a tightly fitted facemask, screaming during inhalation; **(E, F)** inhaling with a pMDI/spacer through a tightly fitted facemask, quietly inhaling; and **(G, H)** inhaling from a nebulizer through a tightly fitted facemask, quietly inhaling. (Redrawn from Erzinger, S, Schueepp, KG, Brooks-Wildhaber, J, et al: Facemasks and aerosol delivery in vivo. J Aerosol Med 2007;20(suppl 1.):S78-S84.)

Given the cognitive and functional limitations of very young patients, not all delivery devices are suitable for these patients. To help guide clinicians, the accompanying Rule of Thumb outlines age-specific guidelines for using aerosol devices in pediatric and neonatal patients.

RULE OF THUMB

Guidelines for Use of Aerosol Devices in the Care of Infants and Children

Device	Age Group
SVN	Neonate to all ages
Valved chamber with mask	Neonate/infant/toddler
Valved chamber with mouthpiece	>3 years
pMDI alone	>4 years
Breath-actuated Neb	>4 years
DPI	≥4 years

Spontaneous breathing in all patients, including pediatric and neonatal patients, results in greater deposition of aerosol from an SVN than occurs with positive pressure breaths (e.g., intermittent positive pressure ventilation). This mode of ventilation reduces aerosol deposition more than 30% compared with the effect of spontaneously inhaled aerosols.[60]

Selecting an Aerosol Drug Delivery System

The American College of Chest Physicians commissioned an extensive evidence-based review of the literature to determine which type of aerosol delivery system is superior. It was concluded that pMDIs, DPIs, and nebulizers all work with comparable clinical results, as long as they are prescribed for the appropriate patients and are used properly.[61] Consequently, clinicians need to know the strengths and limitations of each type of device, match the device to

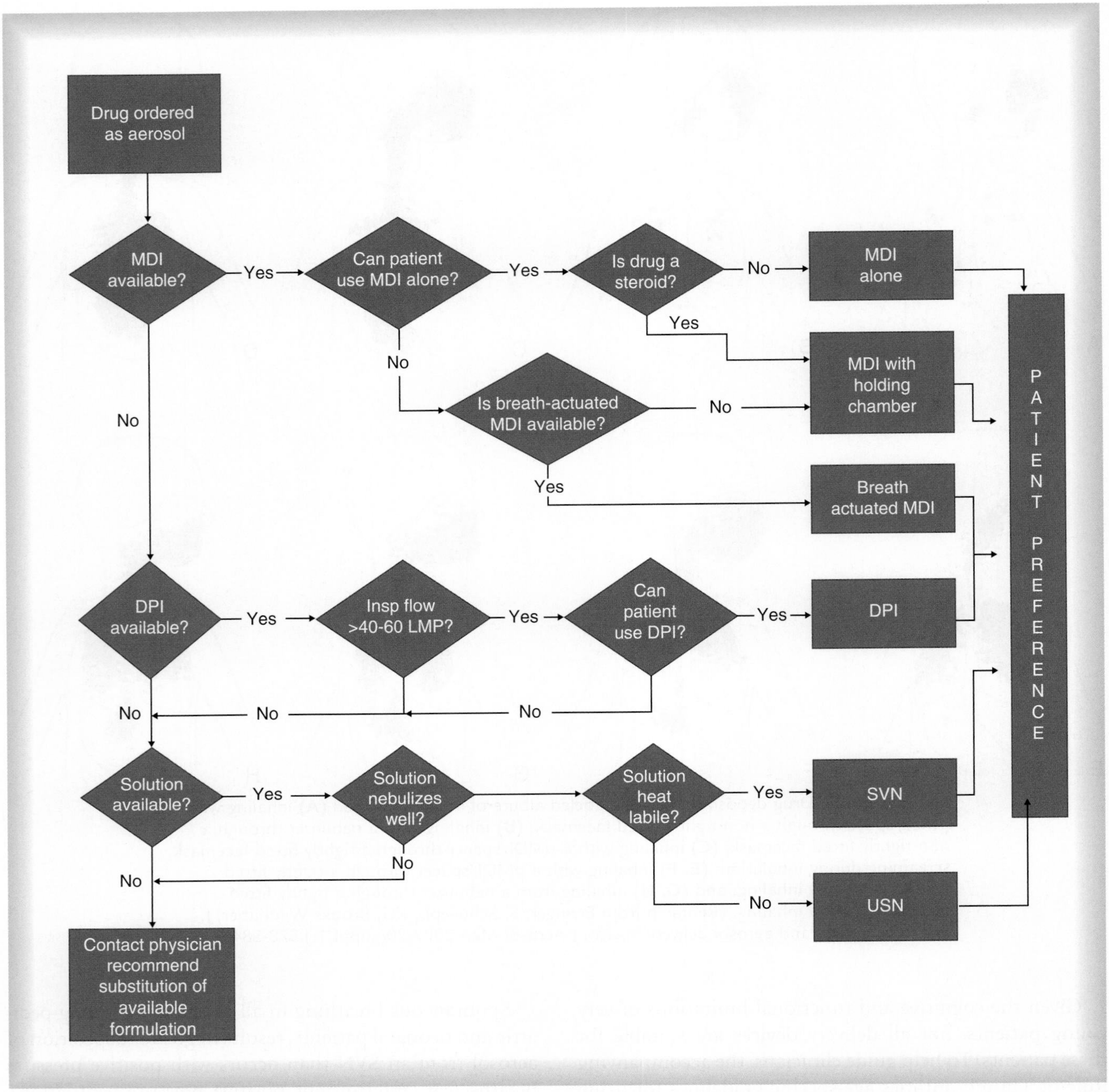

FIGURE 36-29 Selecting an aerosol drug delivery system. When the need is established for aerosol drug delivery, the formulations available for the prescribed medication should be determined. If a pMDI is available, it is the first choice for cost and convenience. The patient's ability to coordinate actuation with inspiration and the need to reduce oropharyngeal deposition (e.g., steroids) determine need for a holding chamber or a breath-actuated unit. Nebulizers are the first choice when the formulation is available only as a solution. When the ordered medication is unavailable for inhalation use, the RT should recommend a substitution to the ordering physician.

each patient, and ensure that the patient or caregiver is trained to use the device properly.[62]

To guide practitioners in selecting the best aerosol delivery system for a given clinical situation, the AARC has published relevant clinical practice guidelines for aerosol delivery to the upper airway,[49] to the lung parenchyma,[63] and to neonatal and pediatric patients.[64] Figure 36-29 is a selection algorithm that provides guidance regarding device selection.

Regardless of the device used, the clinician must be aware of the limitations of aerosol drug therapy. First, depending on the device and patient, 10% or less of drug

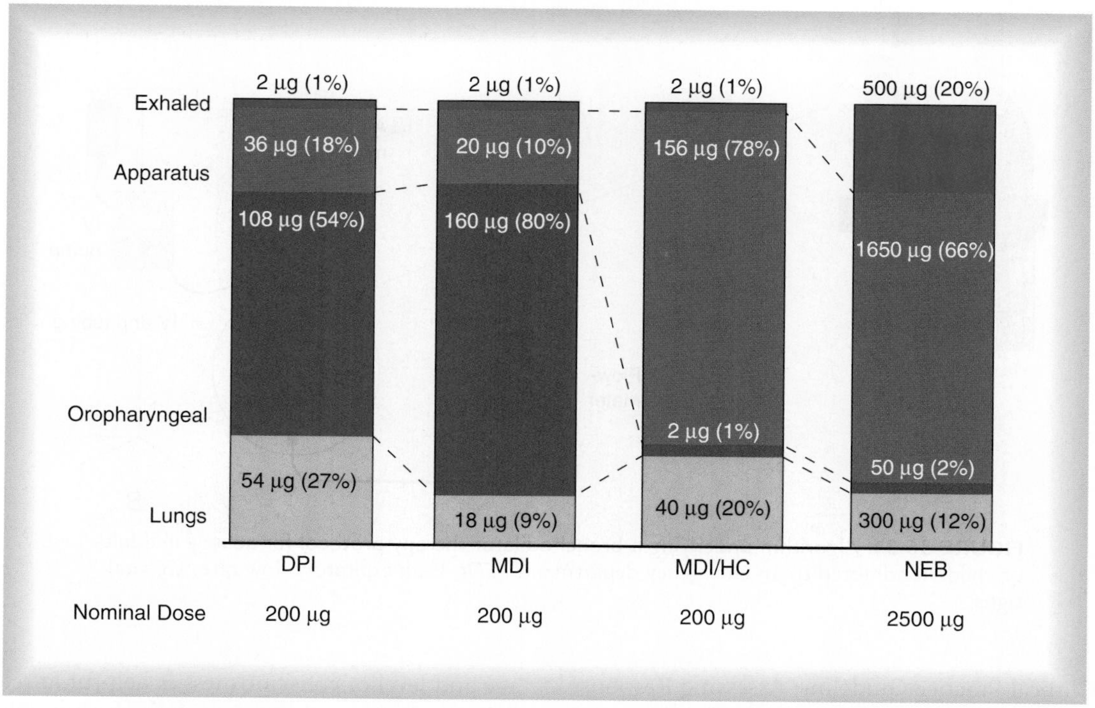

FIGURE 36-30 Distribution of albuterol via nebulizer, pMDI, pMDI with a holding chamber, and DPI. (Modified from Fink J: Metered-dose inhalers, dry powder inhalers and transitions. Respir Care 45:623, 2000.)

Box 36-7 Factors Associated With Reduced Aerosol Drug Deposition in the Lung

- Mechanical ventilation
- Artificial airways
- Reduced airway caliber (e.g., infants and children)
- Severe airway obstruction
- High gas flows
- Low minute volumes
- Poor patient compliance or technique
- Limitation of specific delivery device

emitted from an aerosol device may be deposited in the lungs (Figure 36-30). As indicated in Box 36-7, additional reductions in lung deposition can occur in many clinical situations that sometimes necessitate the use of higher dosages. Clinical efficacy varies according to both patient technique and device design. For these reasons, the best approach to aerosol drug therapy is to use an assessment-based protocol that emphasizes individually tailored therapy modified according to patient response.

ASSESSMENT-BASED BRONCHODILATOR THERAPY PROTOCOLS

Although the choice of delivery system affects how well an aerosolized drug works, it is ultimately the patient's response that determines the therapeutic outcome. Because patients vary markedly in response to the dose and route of drug administration, it makes sense to tailor aerosol drug therapy to each patient. This approach is best determined with an assessment-based protocol.

Sample Protocol

Figure 36-31 is an algorithm underlying a bronchodilator therapy protocol for acutely ill adults or children admitted to an emergency department.[65] The protocol relies heavily on bedside assessment of the severity of airway obstruction based on the patient's response to varying drug dosages.

According to the algorithm, a patient with acute airway obstruction (wheezing, cough, dyspnea, and peak expiratory flow rate [PEFR] <60% of predicted value) would receive up to three SVN treatments with a standard dose of albuterol, repeated at 20-minute intervals, or 4 puffs of pMDI albuterol with a holding chamber (up to 12 puffs). Each treatment is followed by a dose-response assessment to determine the "best" dose. Once determined, this best dose, with the pMDI or SVN, is repeated 1 hour later, then every 4 hours as needed, supplemented with patient education. If use of the SVN or pMDI with holding chamber fails to relieve the symptoms, CBT with 15 mg/hr albuterol is generally started.

Assessing Patient Response

Careful, ongoing patient assessment is key to an effective bronchodilator therapy protocol. To guide practitioners in implementing effective bedside assessment, the AARC has

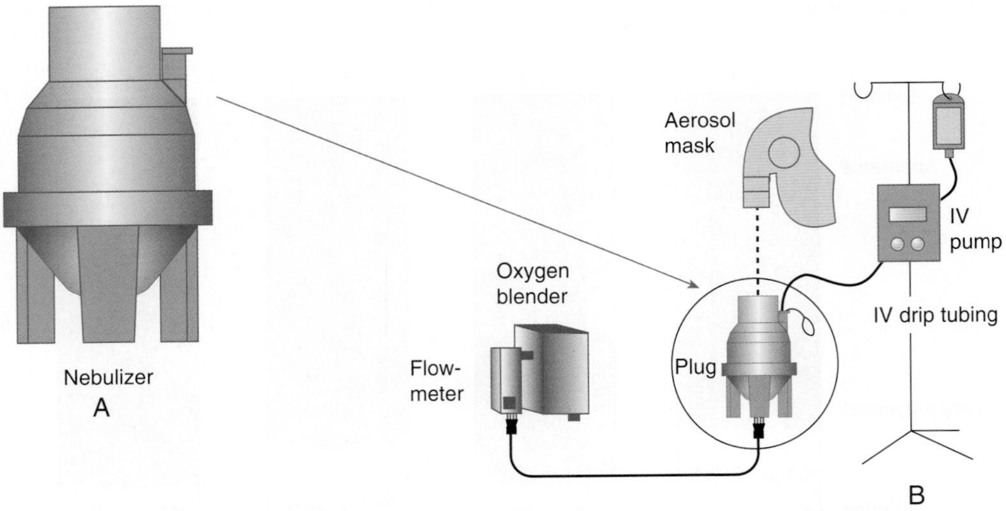

FIGURE 36-31 Algorithm underlying a bronchodilator therapy protocol for acutely ill adults or children admitted to an emergency department. *PEFR,* Peak expiratory flow rate; *VS,* vital signs.

published Clinical Practice Guideline: Assessing Response to Bronchodilator Therapy at Point of Care.[66]

Use and Limitations of Peak Flow Monitoring

Because the peak flow measurement is effort-dependent and volume-dependent, evaluation of patient performance is subjective, and there are no good acceptability criteria. In addition, agreement between conventional spirometry values, such as forced vital capacity (FVC) and FEV_1, and bedside PEFR values may be poor for individual patients. Although peak flow measurement can be used at the bedside to assess treatment effectiveness and to monitor trends, conventional spirometry remains the standard for determining bronchodilator response.[66]

Some peak flowmeters are more accurate and reliable than others. Even different units of the same model may give variable results. For this reason, the AARC recommends that when monitoring trends, the same unit be used for a given patient and that the patient's range be reestablished if a different flowmeter is used.[66]

Other Components of Patient Assessment

Sole dependence on tests of expiratory airflow for assessing patient response to therapy is unwise because not all patients can perform these maneuvers. Other components of patient assessment useful in evaluating bronchodilator therapy include patient interviewing and observation, measurement of vital signs, auscultation, blood gas analysis, and oximetry.

When possible, the patient should be interviewed to determine the pertinent respiratory history and current level of dyspnea. A validated dyspnea rating scale may be useful for this purpose. Initial determination of patient age and level of consciousness is helpful in selecting both delivery device and starting drug dosage. Observing the patient for signs of increased work of breathing (e.g., tachypnea, accessory muscle use) provides a baseline for assessing status as therapy progresses. Restlessness, diaphoresis, and tachycardia also may indicate severity of airway obstruction but must not be confused with bronchodilator overdose.

Increased cough has been associated with the onset of asthma. The frequency, severity, and effectiveness of cough should be assessed before and after therapy.

In terms of breath sounds, a decrease in wheezing accompanied by an overall decrease in the intensity of breath sounds indicates worsening airway obstruction or patient fatigue. Improvement is indicated when wheezing decreases and the overall intensity of breath sounds increases.

All patients with acute airway obstruction should be monitored for oxygenation status with pulse oximetry. This value can be used in conjunction with observational assessment to titrate the level of inspired O_2 given to the patient (see Chapter 35). Arterial blood gases are not essential for determining patient response to bronchodilator therapy but may be needed for patients in severe distress to assess for hypercapnic respiratory failure.

Dose-Response Assessment

Poor patient response to bronchodilator therapy often occurs because an inadequate amount of drug reaches the airway. To determine the "best" dose for patients with moderate obstruction, the respiratory therapist (RT) should conduct a dose-response titration.

A simple albuterol dose-response titration involves giving an initial 4 puffs (90 mcg/puff) at 1-minute intervals through a pMDI with a holding chamber. After 5 minutes, if airway obstruction is not relieved, the RT gives

1 puff per minute until symptoms are relieved, heart rate increases to more than 20 beats/min, tremors increase, or 12 puffs are delivered. The best dose is the dose that provides maximum relief of symptoms and the highest PEFR without side effects.

Frequency of Patient Assessment

How frequently patients should undergo assessment for bronchodilator therapy depends primarily on the acuity of the condition. A patient in unstable condition and in acute distress should undergo closer and more frequent scrutiny than a patient in stable condition. Box 36-8 provides guidance regarding the frequency of assessment according to acuity.

Patient Education

The desired outcome of all bronchodilator protocols is restoration of normal airflow and cessation of therapy. For patients who need ongoing maintenance therapy after the acute phase of illness, the goal should be effective self-administration. An effective program of aerosol drug self-administration depends on thorough patient education.

The patient's ability to understand the therapy and its goals significantly affects the therapeutic efficacy of any treatment. Whenever possible, patients should be taught to understand the basic administration techniques, to keep track of dosing requirements, to recognize undesirable side effects, and to understand the options and actions required to reduce or eliminate these effects. In addition, patients should be able to demonstrate good technique regarding the use of each aerosol device that they are expected to use in self-care. Practitioner demonstration followed by repeated patient return demonstration is a must and should be done frequently, such as with each office or clinic visit.

Box 36-8 Frequency of Assessment of Bronchodilator Therapy

FOR PATIENT WITH AN ACUTE DISORDER WHO IS IN UNSTABLE CONDITION

- Whenever possible, perform a full assessment and obtain a pretreatment baseline.
- Assess and document all appropriate variables before and after each treatment (breath sounds, vital signs, side effects during therapy, and PEFR or FEV_1).
- The frequency with which physical examination and PEFR or FEV_1 are repeated should be based on the acuteness of the disorder and the severity of the patient's condition.
- SpO_2 should be monitored continuously, if possible.
- Assessment should continue as dosages are changed to optimize patient response (e.g., if an asthmatic patient achieves 70% to 90% of predicted or "personal best" or becomes symptom-free).

FOR STABLE PATIENT

- In the hospital, PEFR should be measured initially before and after each bronchodilator administration. Thereafter, twice-daily determinations may be adequate.
- In the home, PEFR ideally should be measured three or four times a day: on rising, at noon, between 4 PM and 7 PM, and at bedtime.
- For a stable COPD patient at home, measuring PEFR twice a day may be adequate.
- Patients with asthma should adjust the frequency of PEFR measurement according to the severity of symptoms.
- PEFR levels before and after bronchodilator use, medication dose, date and time, and dyspnea score should be documented.
- The patient should be reevaluated periodically for response to therapy.

SPECIAL CONSIDERATIONS

Acute Care and Off-Label Use

Every drug approved for inhalation to date has been designed for and tested in populations of ambulatory patients with moderate disease. As patients with lung disease become acutely and critically ill, the approved label doses, frequency of administration, and devices may not be practical or effective, especially for treatment of patients requiring ventilatory support. In such cases, clinicians may explore and consider nonstandard methods (doses, frequency, and devices) for administration of approved inhaled drugs to patients in the acute care environment, known as *off-label use*. Another type of off-label use involves drugs that have not been approved for inhalation, ranging from heparin to certain antibiotics. Although physicians may order such drugs via inhalation, the risk to the patient and institution is greater when the administration of such drugs via inhalation has not been thoroughly studied. All forms of off-label use should be avoided when approved and viable alternatives exist. Likewise, off-label administration should always be backed by appropriate departmental or institutional policies and procedures.

Continuous Nebulization for Refractory Bronchospasm

Patients in the emergency department with severe exacerbation of asthma or acute bronchospasm often have been taking standard doses of their bronchodilators for 24 to 36 hours before admission without response. Giving nebulizer treatments with standard bronchodilator doses and repeating the treatments until the symptoms are relieved can require hours of staff time. Administering higher doses of albuterol in short time frames can be accomplished by nebulization of undiluted albuterol (8 to 20 breaths) or by protocol titration with a pMDI and holding chamber (up to 12 puffs). If these strategies fail to provide relief, CBT with albuterol nebulization doses ranging from 5 to

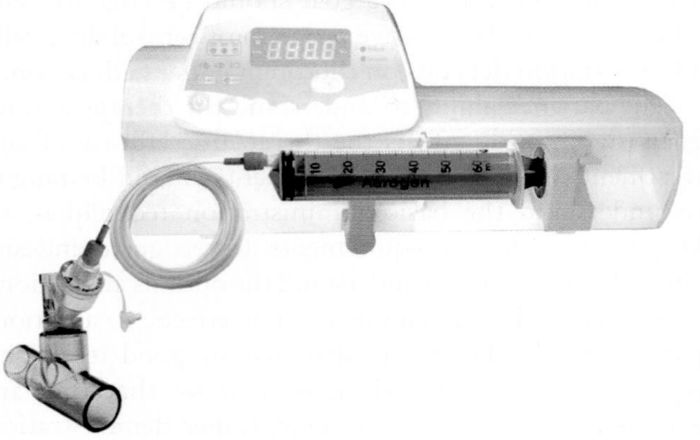

FIGURE 36-32 Continuous line from a syringe pump attached to a nebulizer.

20 mg/hr have proved safe and effective for adult and pediatric patients (Figure 36-32).

Figure 36-33 is a treatment algorithm for high-dose therapy and CBT for pediatric patients with status asthmaticus who are unable to perform peak flow maneuvers.[67] Candidates for this protocol are children who, despite frequent beta agonist treatments, remain in extremis with bronchospasm, dyspnea, cough, chest tightness, and diminished breath sounds.

According to this protocol, children older than 6 years with tachypnea, hypoxemia, increased work of breathing, and restlessness who do not respond to standard therapy are given CBT with a large volume nebulizer or SVN at a dose rate of 15 mg/hr (see the accompanying Mini Clini "CBT Dosage Computations" for dosage computations). A

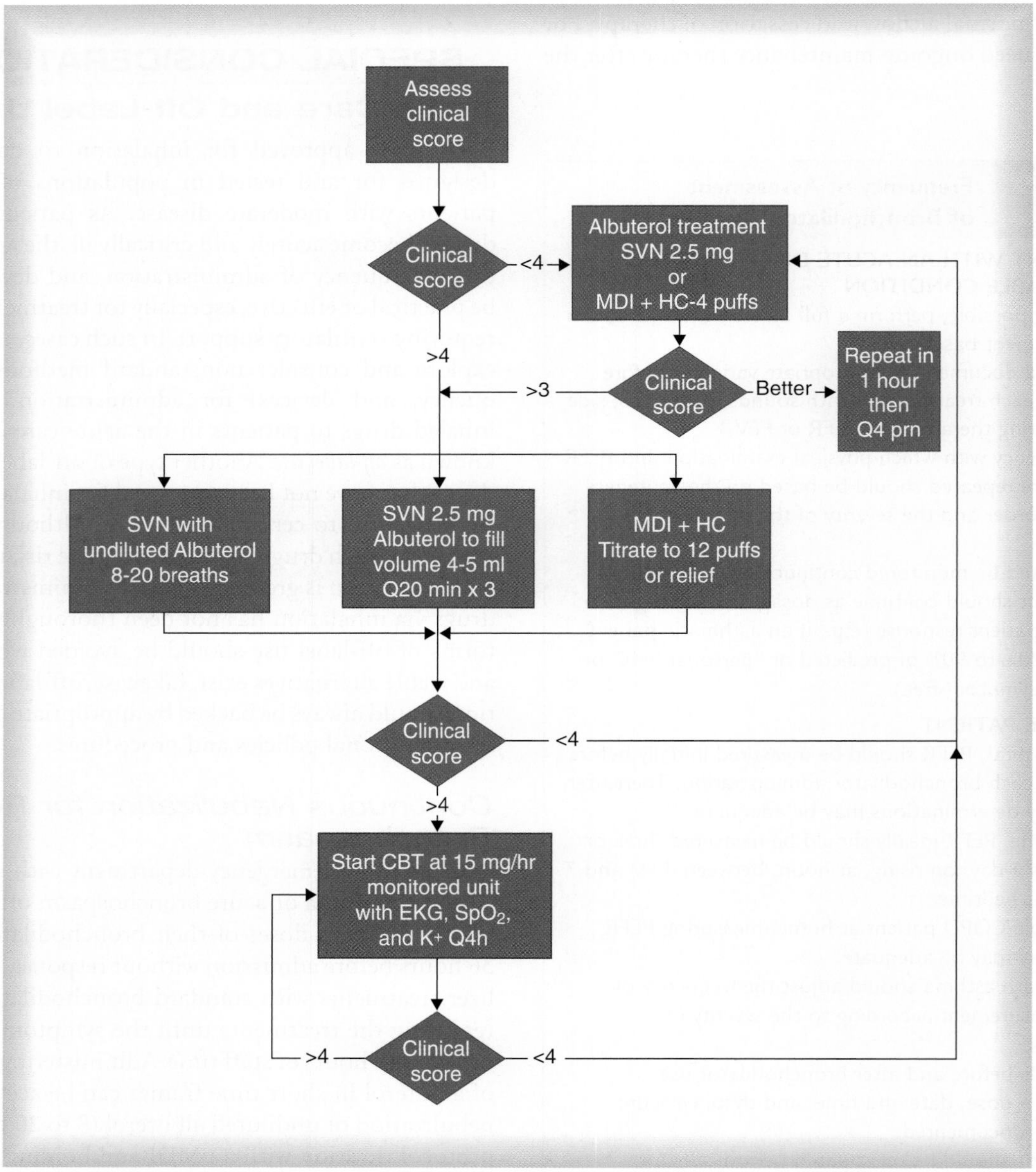

FIGURE 36-33 Algorithm for CBT for patients younger than 5 years with pediatric asthma in extremis.

TABLE 36-4

Pediatric Asthma Score

Indicator	Score: 0	Score: 1	Score: 2
PaO_2	>70 mm Hg (air)	<70 mm Hg (air)	<70 mm Hg (40% O_2)
SpO_2	>94% (air)	<94% (air)	<94% (40% O_2)
Cyanosis	No	Yes	Yes
Breath sounds	Equal	Unequal	Absent
Wheezing	None	Moderate	Marked
Accessory muscle use	None	Moderate	Marked
Level of consciousness	Alert	Agitated or depressed	Comatose

Modified from Volpe J: Therapist-driven protocols for pediatric patients. Respir Care Clin N Am 2:117, 1996.

standardized asthma score is used to evaluate children younger than 6 years for the severity of the condition (Table 36-4). Patients with an asthma score of 4 or higher are given CBT.

After CBT is started, the patient is carefully assessed every 30 minutes for the first 2 hours and thereafter every hour. A positive response is indicated by an increase in PEFR of at least 10% after the first hour of therapy. The goal is at least 50% of the predicted value. For small children, improved oxygenation (oxygen saturation by pulse oximeter [SpO_2] >92% on room air) with evidence of decreased work of breathing indicates a favorable response. Once the patient "opens up," intermittent SVN administration is resumed, or a pMDI dose-response assessment is conducted.

The patient has responded poorly to CBT if any of the indicators listed in Table 36-4 worsens. The patient must be observed for adverse drug responses, including worsening tachycardia, palpitations, and vomiting. In these situations, the attending physician must be contacted immediately.

As an alternative to large volume drug nebulizers, some protocols are based on high-dose pMDI therapy (12 to 24 puffs per hour).[68] To provide an extra margin of safety, some clinicians recommend that patients receiving CBT undergo continuous electrocardiogram monitoring and measurement of serum potassium level every 4 hours.

MINI CLINI

Continuous Bronchodilator Therapy Dosage Computations

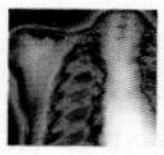

PROBLEM: Dosages for CBT are ordered in milligrams per hour, and delivery depends on both drug concentration and nebulizer output. Compute the volume of 1:200 (0.5%) albuterol and the volume of diluent (normal saline solution) needed to provide 4 hours of CBT with 15 mg/hr of albuterol in a nebulizer with an output of 25 ml/hr.

SOLUTION:

Step 1: Compute the volume of albuterol given per hour (mg/hr × ml/mg).

15.0 mg/hr × 0.2 ml/mg = 3.0 ml/hr albuterol

Step 2: Compute the volume of albuterol for the treatment period (hours × ml/hr).

4 hours × 3.0 ml/hr = 12 ml/4 hr albuterol

Step 3: Compute the volume of nebulization solution (ml/hr nebulizer output × hours).

25 ml/hr × 4 hours = 100 ml

Step 4: Compute the volume of diluent required.

100 ml − 12 ml = 88 ml normal saline solution

To prepare this dosage, mix 12 ml of 0.5% albuterol with 88 ml of normal saline solution, for a total nebulizer solution volume of 100 ml. In this example, residual volume of the nebulizer decreases total treatment time and dose.

Aerosol Administration to Mechanically Ventilated Patients

Since the advent of modern mechanical ventilation, clinicians have administered aerosols to patients with the sickest of lungs. Four primary forms of aerosol generator are used to deliver aerosols during mechanical ventilation: SVN, USN, VM nebulizer, and pMDI with third-party adapter. Table 36-5 summarizes the factors affecting aerosol drug delivery to mechanically ventilated patients. Techniques to optimize delivery to patients receiving ventilatory support are described.[69]

Regarding doses, the amount of drug required to achieve the same therapeutic end point is substantially similar for medications delivered by pMDI to intubated patients (8%) and patients who are not intubated (8% to 10%). In stable patients with COPD receiving ventilatory support, 4 puffs of albuterol via pMDI with chamber and 2.5 mg via SVN were shown to produce maximum bronchodilation with effects lasting for 4 hours. However, some differences in response were noted that may have been due to the level of airway obstruction and the techniques used for assessing response.

TABLE 36-5

Factors Affecting Aerosol Drug Delivery During Mechanical Ventilation

Category	Factor
Ventilator-related	Mode of ventilation
	V_T
	Respiratory rate
	Duty cycle
	Inspiratory waveform
	Breath-triggering mechanism
Circuit-related	Size of endotracheal tube
	Type of humidifier
	Relative humidity
	Density and viscosity of inhaled gas
Device-related MDI	Type of spacer or adapter used
	Position of spacer in circuit
	Timing of MDI actuation
SVN	Type of nebulizer used
	Fill volume
	Gas flow
	Cycling: inspiration vs. continuous
	Duration of nebulization
	Position in circuit
Patient-related	Severity of airway obstruction
	Mechanism of airway obstruction
	Presence of dynamic hyperinflation
	Spontaneous ventilation
	Disease process
Drug-related	Dose
	Aerosol particle size
	Targeted site for delivery
	Duration of action

Techniques for assessing the response to a bronchodilator in intubated patients undergoing mechanical ventilation differ from techniques used in the care of spontaneously breathing patients because expiration is passive during mechanical ventilation, and forced expiratory values (PEFR, FVC, FEV_1) cannot normally be obtained. Additional techniques can be used for mechanically ventilated patients because (1) a change in the differences between peak and plateau pressures (the most reliable indicator of a change in airway resistance during continuous mechanical ventilation) can be measured, (2) automatic positive end expiratory pressure levels may decrease in response to bronchodilators (see Chapter 41), and (3) breath-to-breath variations make measurements more reliable when the patient is not actively breathing with the ventilator.[70]

Techniques for aerosol administration vary by type of aerosol generator and device used. The optimal technique for drug delivery to mechanically ventilated patients with each type of aerosol generator is described in Box 36-9.

Box 36-9 Optimal Technique for Aerosolized Drug Delivery to Mechanically Ventilated Patients

1. Review order, identify the patient, gather equipment, and assess the need for bronchodilators.
2. Clear the airways as needed, by suctioning the patient as needed.
3. If using a circuit with heat and moisture exchanger (HME), remove HME from between the aerosol generator and the patient.
4. If using heated humidifier, do not turn off or disconnect before or during treatment.
5. Assemble equipment (tubing, nebulizer, circuit adapter).
6. Fill the nebulizer with recommended volume and medication per physician order and label.
7. Place adapter in the inspiratory limb, 6 inches from the "wye," and connect aerosol generator.
8. Turn off or minimize bias flow during treatment.
9. Connect the nebulizer to a gas or power source, as appropriate.

10a. For jet nebulizer (including SVN): Use gas source on ventilator to synchronize nebulization with inspiration, if available; otherwise, set gas flow 2 to 10 L/min as recommended on nebulizer label, and adjust ventilator volume or pressure limit and alarms to compensate for added flow and volume.

10b. For USN and VM nebulizer: Attach power source and cable from controller.

10c. For pMDI: Shake canister and connect to spacer or adapter; actuate at beginning of inspiration.

11. Observe aerosol cloud for adequate aerosol generation during nebulization.
12. After appropriate dose is administered, remove aerosol generator from the ventilator circuit.
13. Reconnect HME, as appropriate.
14. Return ventilator settings and alarms to previous values.
15. Ensure there is no leak in the ventilator circuit.
16. Rinse the nebulizer with sterile or distilled water, shake off excess water, and allow to air dry.
17. Store aerosol device in a clean, dry place.
18. Monitor heart rate, SpO_2, blood pressure, and patient-ventilator synchronization.
19. Monitor the patient for adverse response.
20. Assess the airway, and suction as needed; document findings.

Use of a Small Volume Nebulizer During Mechanical Ventilation

The aerosol administered by SVN to intubated patients receiving mechanical ventilation tends to be deposited mainly in the tubing of the ventilator circuit and expiratory filter. Under normal conditions with heated humidification and standard jet nebulizers, pulmonary deposition ranges from 1.5% to 3.0%.[70,71] When nebulizer output, humidity level, V_T, flow, and I:E ratio are optimized, deposition can increase to 15%.

There are several disadvantages with SVN use during mechanical ventilation. Although in vitro models showed 40% higher aerosol delivery compared with heated humidity, these effects have not been shown in patients, whereas the risks associated with administering cold and dry gas through an endotracheal tube have. A heat and moisture exchanger should be considered a barrier to aerosol administration and should always be removed if placed between the nebulizer and the patient airway. When available with the specific ventilator being used, breath actuation can increase aerosol delivery by 30%, but it may extend administration time by more than threefold. Introducing additional flow into the ventilator circuit may change parameters of flow and delivered volumes and require changes to alarm settings during and after nebulization. The smaller the patient, the greater the impact of added flow into the ventilator circuit, where 6 L/min of additional gas flow can more than double V_T and inspiratory pressure, placing the patient at risk. Risk is high for not changing ventilator parameters and not returning parameters to pretreatment levels after administration. There is also a tendency for condensate and secretions to drain into the nebulizer reservoir, contaminating medication being delivered to the lungs.

MINI CLINI

Never Emptying Nebulizer

PROBLEM: Jet nebulizers and USNs are commonly used to administer aerosol to patients during mechanical ventilation. Commonly, a nebulizer is filled with a standard unit dose of 3 ml of medication at the beginning of the aerosol treatment, and the RT finds as much or more fluid in the medication reservoir 20 to 30 minutes later. The additional fluid is usually condensate (often contaminated from patient secretions), which drains from the inspiratory limb into the gravity-dependent reservoir of the nebulizer. Even heated wire circuits may have condensate. Although pathogens in a dry circuit have minimal chance of contaminating the patient's airway, aerosolizing the pathogens provides a vehicle for infectious material to enter the airway and the lung parenchyma.

SOLUTION: The nebulizer should be positioned so that the upper end of the reservoir is superior to (higher than) the ventilator tubing attached to both ends of the nebulizer. This position allows the condensate and secretions to drain away from the nebulizer. Alternatively, nebulizers with physical barriers between the ventilator circuit tubing and the medication reservoir can be used. These options include use of a pMDI with spacer or a VM nebulizer.

Use of a Vibrating Mesh Nebulizer During Mechanical Ventilation

Aerosol administration by a VM nebulizer has been estimated to deliver greater than 10% deposition in adults and infants without the addition of gas into the ventilator circuit. The low residual drug volume and small particle size are associated with higher efficiency. Similar to the USN, the VM nebulizer does not add gas flow into the ventilator circuit, so ventilator parameters and alarms do not need to be adjusted before, during, or after nebulization. In contrast to jet SVNs and USNs, the medication reservoir of the VM nebulizer is above the circuit and separated from the ventilator tubing by the mesh, reducing the risk of retrograde contamination of medication in the reservoir from the ventilator circuit. Because of the nature of the mesh, the reservoir can be opened and medication can be added to the nebulizer without creating a perceptible leak during ventilation.

Use of a Pressurized Metered Dose Inhaler During Mechanical Ventilation

Results of in vitro studies show that effective aerosol delivery by pMDIs during mechanical ventilation can range from 2% to 30%. Direct pMDI actuation by simple elbow adapters typically results in the least pulmonary deposition, with most of the aerosol impacting in either the ventilator circuit or the tracheal airway. Higher aerosol delivery percentages occur only when an actuator or spacer is placed in-line in the ventilator circuit. These spacers allow an aerosol "plume" to develop before the bulk of the particles impact on the surface of the circuit or endotracheal tube. The result is a more stable aerosol mass that can penetrate beyond the artificial airway and be deposited mainly in the lung. This situation leads to a better clinical response at lower doses.[52]

Aerosol Generator Placement

Placement of aerosol generators in the ventilator circuit can have a substantial impact on the available lung dose of drug. During adult ventilation without bias flow, placement of aerosol generators distal to the patient in the inspiratory limb may increase inhaled dose for jet nebulizers, where continuous gas flow acts to charge the inspiratory limb of the ventilator circuit with aerosol increasing the inhaled dose. In contrast, pMDI, USN, and VM nebulizer devices were more efficient when placed proximal to the patient.[72] With continuous or bias flow through the ventilator circuit, the delivery is reduced as flow increases, whereas placement of a VM nebulizer near the ventilator increases delivery (Figure 36-34).[73]

Placement During Noninvasive Ventilation

Noninvasive ventilation may be administered with standard and bilevel ventilators. Bilevel ventilators often use a flow turbine, with a fixed valve or leak in the circuit that permits excess flow to vent to atmosphere. Placement of the aerosol generator between the leak and the patient's airway seems to provide the highest aerosol delivery efficiency.[74] A VM nebulizer delivers a greater fine-particle dose than an SVN during noninvasive ventilation presumably because of the lower residual drug volume and lower total flow in the circuit.[75]

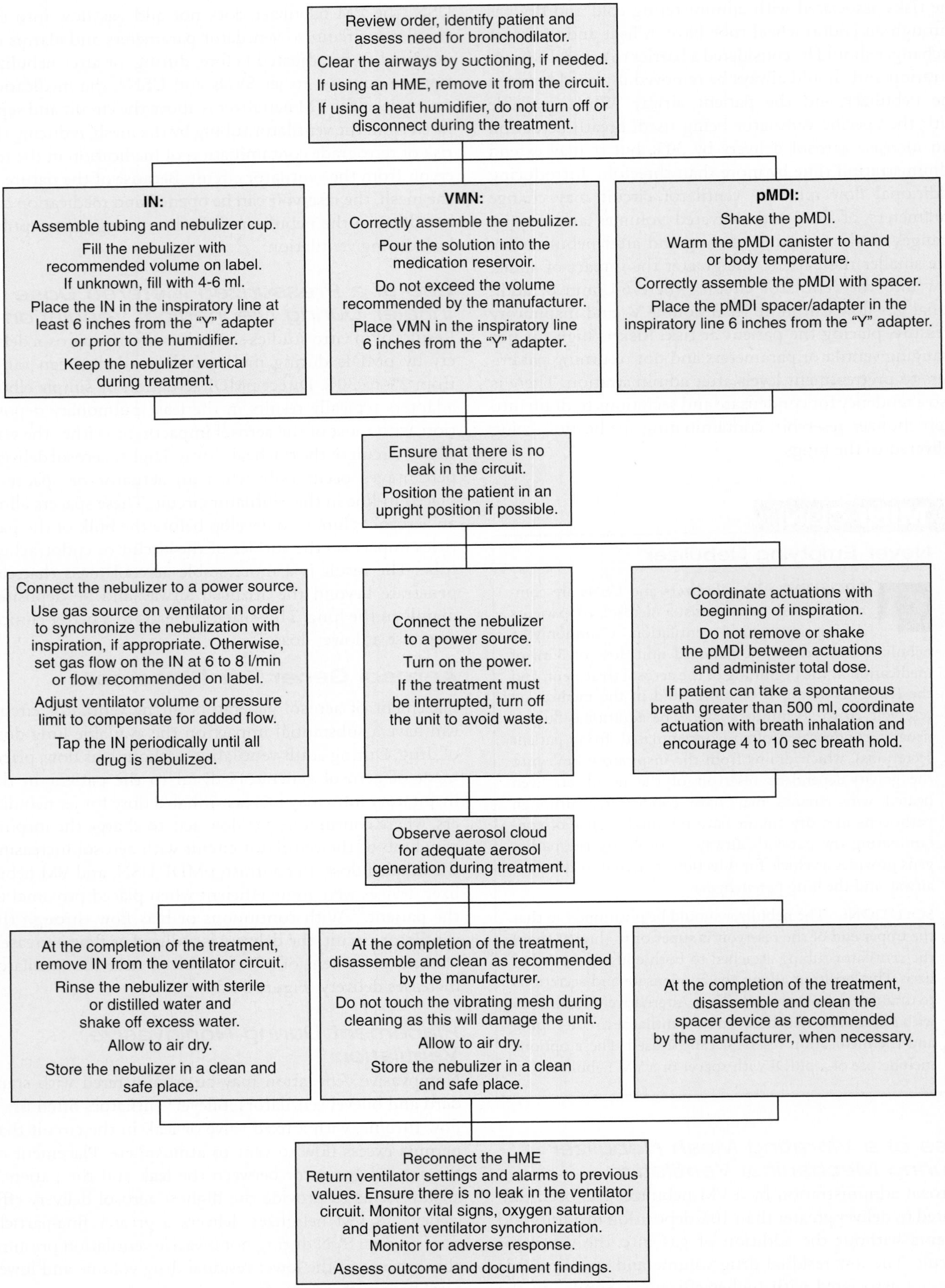

FIGURE 36-34 Frequency of assessment according to acuity. (From Ari A, Fink TB: Factors affecting bronchodilator delivery in mechanically ventilated adults. Nurs Crit Care 15:192, 2010.)

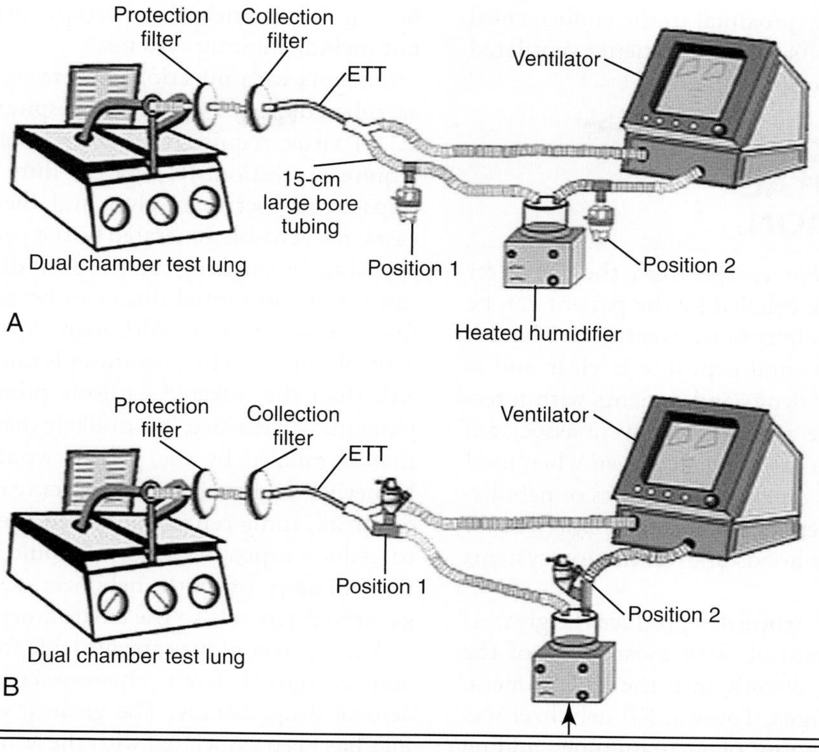

	Percent of nominal or emitted dose (mean ± SD %)							
	Adult lung model				Pediatric lung model			
	Position 1		Position 2		Position 1		Position 2	
	Bias flow 2 L/min	Bias flow 5 L/min	Bias flow 2 L/min	Bias flow 5 L/min	Bias flow 2 L/min	Bias flow 5 L/min	Bias flow 2 L/min	Bias flow 5 L/min
Jet nebulizer	4.7 ± 0.1*	4.0 ± 0.1*	5.2 ± 0.2*	4.7 ± 0.4*	4.2 ± 0.2*	3.8 ± 0.3*	5.2 ± 0.3*	4.1 ± 0.4*
Vibrating-mesh nubulizer	13.4 ± 1.1	9.7 ± 0.6	23.8 ± 1.0	21.4 ± 0.4	11.4 ± 0.7	8.4 ± 0.2	13.6 ± 1.3	10.6 ± 0.3

*Significant difference between jet nebulizer and vibrating-mesh nebulizer (p< 05).

FIGURE 36-35 Placement of SVN and VM nebulizer aerosol generators in two positions in the ventilator circuit with 2 L/min and 5 L/min of bias flow results in different deposition efficiency.

Placement During High-Flow Nasal Oxygen

Researchers used a VM nebulizer to simulate the delivery of aerosol via a high-flow nasal O_2 setup using infant, pediatric, and adult cannulas, with inhaled dose ranging from 8% to 28%.[76] Figure 36-35 shows such a setup, including the location of the VM nebulizer. In addition to the type and location of the nebulizer used with high-flow nasal O_2, the inhaled dose seems to vary based on cannula size, respiratory pattern, and O_2 flow. Heliox (80:20) appears to improve aerosol delivery at higher flow rates with these setups.[77]

Placement During Intrapulmonary Percussive Ventilation

Intrapulmonary percussive ventilation provides high-frequency oscillation of the airway while administering aerosol particles. During intrapulmonary percussive ventilation, the aerosol generator should be placed in the circuit as close to the patient's airway as practical. Aerosol administration during intrapulmonary percussive ventilation has been compared with a standard jet nebulizer. The MMAD was smaller with intrapulmonary percussive ventilation than with the jet (0.2 μm vs. 1.89 μm), and the fine-particle fraction was lower (16.2% vs. 67.5%). However, lung dose was similar (2.49% with intrapulmonary percussive ventilation vs. 4.2% with the jet nebulizer). It was concluded that intrapulmonary percussive ventilation was too variable and too unpredictable to recommend for drug delivery to the lung.[78]

Placement During High-Frequency Oscillatory Ventilation

When used in conjunction with high-frequency oscillatory ventilation, administration of albuterol sulfate via a VM nebulizer placed between the ventilator circuit and the patient airway has been reported to deliver greater than 10% of dose to both infants and adults.[79,80] A pMDI with adapter placed immediately proximal to the endotracheal tube achieved similar results in adult patients ventilated via high-frequency oscillatory ventilation.[81]

CONTROLLING ENVIRONMENTAL CONTAMINATION

Drugs for nebulization that escape from the nebulizer into the atmosphere or are exhaled by the patient can be inhaled by anyone in the vicinity of the treatment. The risk imposed by this environmental exposure is clear and is associated with a range of drugs and patients with infectious disease. Pentamidine and ribavirin were associated with health risks to health care providers even when used in conjunction with filters on exhalation ports of nebulizers, containment and scavenger systems, and *high-efficiency particulate air (HEPA)* filter hoods and ventilation systems (Figure 36-36).

Continuous pneumatic nebulizers produce the greatest amount of secondhand aerosol, with most (60%) of the aerosol produced passing directly into the environment. The Respirgard II (Vital Signs, Totowa, NJ) nebulizer was developed for administration of pentamidine, adding one-way valves and an expiratory filter to contain aerosol that is exhaled and not inhaled. Breath-actuated nebulizers, DPIs, and pMDIs tend to generate less secondhand aerosol.

A survey found that RTs were more than twice as likely as physical therapists to develop asthma-like symptoms during the course of their careers. The authors associated this with administration of ribavirin and exposure to gluteraldehyde.[17] There have been anecdotal reports of respiratory care clinicians who have developed a sensitivity to secondhand aerosol from bronchodilators. Further research is required to understand more thoroughly the hazards of secondhand exposure to aerosols in the clinical setting. Most of nebulizer therapy currently delivered does not include filtering systems.

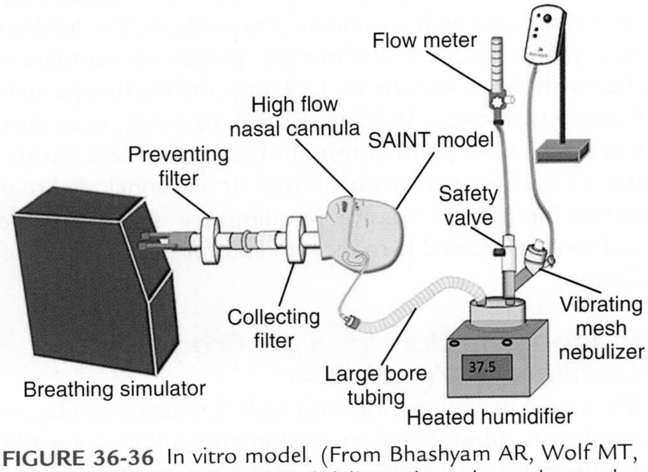

FIGURE 36-36 In vitro model. (From Bhashyam AR, Wolf MT, Marcinkowski AL, et al: Aerosol delivery through nasal cannulas: an in vitro study. J Aerosol Med Pulm Drug Deliv 21:181, 2008.)

Patients with infectious and resistant organisms, such as tuberculosis, severe acute respiratory syndrome, and H1N1 virus, require respiratory isolation, and caregivers require protection. RTs have a duty to take appropriate steps to protect themselves and their patients. In these cases, the aerosols generated by the patient from coughing, speaking, or laughing can transmit disease. These aerosols can travel substantial distances between rooms and even floors in institutions. Although exposure to secondhand aerosol generated by a nebulizer is undesirable, it poses less risk than the infected aerosols produced by mucosa of patients.[82] In essence, it is unlikely that any medical aerosol that is inhaled by the patient would be contaminated. Nonetheless, during the severe acute respiratory syndrome outbreak, some centers outlawed use of medical aerosols to reduce exposure. Efforts should be taken to reduce transmission of both nebulizer aerosols and patient-generated aerosols to the environment.

Various techniques are available for protecting patients and caregivers from environmental exposure during aerosol drug therapy. The greatest occupational risk for RTs has been associated with the administration of ribavirin and pentamidine. Conjunctivitis, headaches, bronchospasm, shortness of breath, and rashes have been reported among individuals administering these drugs.[83] Patients given aerosolized ribavirin or pentamidine must be treated in a private room, booth, or tent or at a special station designed to minimize environmental contamination.

Negative Pressure Rooms

When ribavirin or pentamidine is given, the treatment is provided in a private room. The room should be equipped for negative pressure ventilation with adequate air exchanges (at least six per hour) to clear the room of residual aerosols before the next treatment. HEPA filters should be used to filter room or tent exhaust, or the aerosol should be scavenged to the outside.

Booths and Stations

Booths or stations should be used for sputum induction and aerosolized medication treatments given in any area where more than one patient is treated. The area should be designed to provide adequate airflow to draw aerosol and droplet nuclei from the patient into an appropriate filtration system or an exhaust system directly to the outside. Booths and stations should be adequately cleaned between patients.

A variety of booths and specially designed stations are available for delivery of pentamidine or ribavirin. The Emerson containment booth (Figure 36-37) is an example of a system that completely isolates the patient during aerosol administration. The AeroStar Aerosol Protection Cart (Respiratory Safety Systems, San Diego, CA) is a portable patient isolation station for administration of

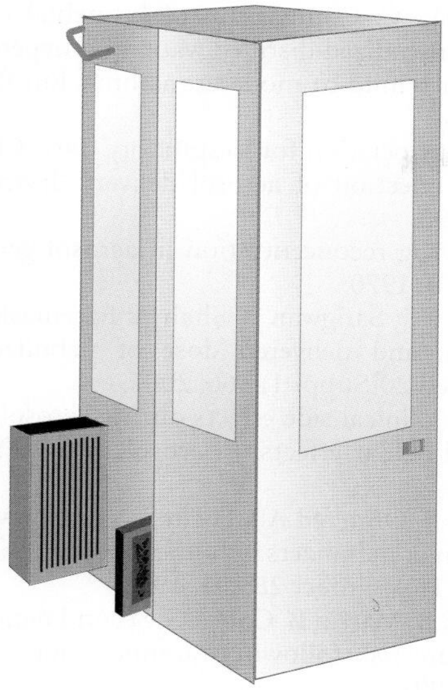

FIGURE 36-37 Emerson treatment booth provides containment of aerosol during therapy.

hazardous aerosolized medication. It has been used during sputum induction and for pentamidine treatment. The patient compartment is collapsible with a swing-out counter and three polycarbonate walls. Captured aerosols are removed with a HEPA filter. A prefilter is used to retain larger dust particles and to prevent early loading of the more expensive HEPA filter.

Filters and nebulizers used in treatments with pentamidine and ribavirin should be treated as hazardous wastes and disposed of accordingly. Goggles, gloves, and gowns should be used as splatter shields and to reduce exposure to medication residues and body substances. Staff members should be screened for adverse effects of exposure to the aerosol medication. The risks and safety procedures should be reviewed regularly.

In addition to the risks associated with administration of aerosol medication, risk of tuberculosis transmission has become a great concern because of an increase in case numbers and the development of multidrug-resistant strains of the organism. Tuberculosis is transmitted in the form of droplet nuclei (0.3 to 0.6 µm) that carry tuberculosis bacilli. Patients with known or suspected tuberculosis need private rooms with negative pressure ventilation that exhausts to the outside. If environmental isolation is impossible or the health care worker must enter the patient's room, personal protective equipment should be used.

Personal Protective Equipment

Personal protective equipment is recommended when caring for any patient with a disease that can be spread by the airborne route.[84] The greatest risk is communication of tuberculosis or chickenpox. Although environmental controls should be instituted in the care of these patients, standard and airborne precautions should also be implemented. Various masks and respirators have been recommended for use when caring for a patient with tuberculosis or other respiration-transmitted diseases. Traditional surgical masks, particulate respirators, disposable and reusable HEPA filters, and powered air-purifying respirators have been used. No data are available for determining the most effective and most clinically useful device to protect health care workers and others, although the U.S. Occupational Safety and Health Administration requires specific levels of protection (HEPA filters and powered air-purifying respirators). Guidelines from the World Health Organization recommend surgical masks for all patient care with the exception of N95 masks for aerosol-generating procedures such as sputum induction. Evidence from laboratory studies of potential airborne spread of influenza from contagious patients indicates that guidelines related to the current 1-m respiratory zone may need to be extended to a larger respiratory zone and include eye protection.[85]

SUMMARY CHECKLIST

- An aerosol is a suspension of solid or liquid particles in gas. In the clinical setting, therapeutic aerosols are made with atomizers or nebulizers.
- The general aim of aerosol drug therapy is delivery of a therapeutic dose of the selected agent to the desired site of action.
- Where aerosol particles are deposited in the respiratory tract depends on their size, shape, and motion and on the physical characteristics of the airways. Key mechanisms causing aerosol deposition include inertial impaction, sedimentation, and brownian diffusion.
- For targeting aerosols for delivery to the upper airway (nose, larynx, trachea), particles in the 5- to 20-µm MMAD range are used; for the lower airways, 2- to 5-µm particles are used; and for the lung parenchyma (alveolar region), 1- to 3-µm particles are used.
- The primary hazard of aerosol drug therapy is an adverse reaction to the medication being administered. Other hazards include infection, airway reactivity, systemic effects of bland aerosols, and drug reconcentration.
- Drug aerosol delivery systems include pMDIs, DPIs, SVNs, large volume jet nebulizers, hand-bulb atomizers (nasal spray pumps), USNs, and VM nebulizers.
- MDIs are the preferred method for maintenance delivery of bronchodilators and steroids to spontaneously breathing patients. The effectiveness of this therapy is highly technique-dependent.
- Accessory devices, spacers, and holding chambers are used with pMDIs to reduce oropharyngeal deposition of a drug and to overcome problems with poor hand-breath coordination.
- Effective use of DPIs does not require hand-breath coordination, but it does require high inspiratory flows. Some patients in stable condition prefer DPI delivery systems.

Continued

- Compared with pMDI and DPI delivery systems, use of an SVN is less technique-dependent and is more commonly used in acute care.
- Large volume drug nebulizers can be used to provide continuous aerosol delivery when traditional dosing strategies are ineffective in controlling severe bronchospasm.
- Small volume USNs can be used to administer bronchodilators, antiinflammatory agents, and antibiotics.
- Because patients vary greatly in their response to a particular drug dose and route of administration, aerosol drug therapy should be tailored to each patient with an assessment-based protocol.
- Careful, ongoing patient assessment is the key to an effective bronchodilator therapy protocol. Components of the assessment include a patient interview, observation, expiratory airflow tests, vital sign measurements, auscultation, blood gas analysis, and oximetry.
- Protocols for CBT have proved safe and effective in the management of refractory bronchospasm in both adults and children.
- Many factors affect the efficiency of aerosol drug delivery during mechanical ventilation. Proper selection of aerosol generator type, position in the circuit, dose, and accessory equipment is needed to optimize deposition and achieve the desired clinical outcome.
- Various techniques are available to protect patients and caregivers from environmental exposure during aerosol drug therapy.

References

1. Dolovich MA, MacIntyre NR, Anderson PJ, et al: Consensus statement: aerosols and delivery devices. American Association for Respiratory Care. Respir Care 45:589, 2000.
2. Dolovich MA: Aerosols and aerosol drug delivery system. In Adkinson N, Busse W, Bochner B, et al, editors: Middleton's allergy: principles and practice, Philadelphia, 2009, Mosby.
3. O'Callaghan C, Barry PW: The science of nebulised drug delivery. Thorax 52(Suppl 2):31, 1997.
4. Newhouse M, Dolovich M: Aerosol therapy in children. In Chermick V, Mellins RB, editors. Basic mechanisms of pediatric respiratory disease: cellular and integrative, Toronto, 1991, BC Decker.
5. Lange C, Finlay W: Overcoming the adverse effect of humidity in aerosol delivery via pressurized metered-dose inhalers during mechanical ventilation. Am J Respir Crit Care Med 161:1614, 2000.
6. Dolovich M, Labiris NR: Imaging drug delivery and drug responses in the lung. Proc Am Thorac Soc 1:329, 2004.
7. Dolovich MA: Assessing nebulizer performance. Respir Care 47:1290, 2002.
8. Pierce A, Sanford J, Thomas G: Long-term evaluation of inhalation therapy equipment and the occurrence of necrotizing pneumonia. N Engl J Med 282:528, 1970.
9. Hamill R, Houston E, Georghiou P: An outbreak of *Burkholderia cepacia* respiratory tract colonization and infection associated with nebulized albuterol therapy. Ann Intern Med 122: 762, 1995.
10. Wojnarowski C: Comparison of bronchial challenge with ultrasonic nebulized distilled water and hypertonic saline in children with mild-to-moderate asthma. Eur Respir J 9:1896, 1996.
11. American Association for Respiratory Care: Clinical practice guideline: selection of aerosol delivery device. Respir Care 37:891, 1992.
12. Glick R: Drug reconcentration in aerosol generators. Inhal Ther 15:179, 1970.
13. Smaldone GC, Sangwan S, Shah A: Facemask design, facial deposition, and delivered dose of nebulized aerosols. J Aerosol Med 20(Suppl 1):S66, 2007.
14. Geller DE: Clinical side effects during aerosol therapy: cutaneous and ocular effects. J Aerosol Med 20(Suppl 1):S100, 2007.
15. Jakobsson B, Onnered AB, Hjelte L, et al: Low bacterial contamination of nebulizers in home treatment of cystic fibrosis patients. J Hosp Infect 28:201, 1997.
16. Carnathan B, Martin B, Colice G: Second hand (S)-albuterol: RT exposure risk following racemic albuterol. Respir Care 46:1084, 2001.
17. Dimich-Ward H, Wymer ML, Chan-Yeung M: Respiratory health survey of respiratory therapists. Chest 126:1048, 2004.
18. Ari A, Fink JB, Harwood R, et al: Secondhand aerosol exposure during mechanical ventilation with and without expiratory filters: an in-vitro study. Respir Care 55:1566, 2010.
19. The Nebuliser Project Group of the British Thoracic Society Standards of Care Committee: Current best practice for nebuliser treatment. Thorax 52:S4, 1997.
20. Fink J: Metered-dose inhalers, dry powder inhalers and transitions. Respir Care 45:623, 2000.
21. American Association for Respiratory Care: Aerosol consensus conference statement—1991. Respir Care 36:916, 1991.
22. Leach CL: Safety assessment of the HFA propellant and the new inhaler. Eur Respir Rev 7:41, 1997.
23. Leach CL: The CFC to HFA transition and its impact on pulmonary drug development. Respir Care 50:1201, 2005.
24. Hampson N, Mueller M: Reduction in patient timing errors using a breath-activated metered dose inhaler. Chest 106:462, 1994.
25. Fink JB, Dhand R, Grychowski J, et al: Reconciling in vitro and in vivo measurements of aerosol delivery from a metered-dose inhaler during mechanical ventilation and defining efficiency-enhancing factors. Am J Respir Crit Care Med 159:63, 1999.
26. Newman S: Aerosol generators and delivery systems. Respir Care 36:939, 1991.
27. Fink JB, Rubin BK: Problems with inhaler use: a call for improved clinician and patient education. Respir Care 50:1360, 2005.
28. Chhabra SK: A comparison of "closed" and "open" mouth techniques of inhalation of a salbutamol metered-dose inhaler. J Asthma 31:123, 1994.
29. Ari A: A guide to aerosol delivery devices for respiratory therapists, San Antonio, Texas, 2009, American Association for Respiratory Care.
30. Wilkes W, Fink J, Dhand R: Selecting an accessory device with a metered-dose inhaler: variable influence of accessory devices on fine particle dose, throat deposition, and drug delivery with asynchronous actuation from a metered-dose inhaler. J Aerosol Med 14:351, 2001.
31. Dolovich M, Ruffin R, Corr D: Clinical evaluation of a simple demand inhalation MDI aerosol delivery device. Chest 84:36, 1983.
32. Wildhaber JH, Janssens HM, Piérart F, et al: High-percentage lung delivery in children from detergent-treated spacers. Pediatr Pulmonol 29:389, 2000.

33. Rubin D, Fink JB: Optimizing aerosol delivery by pressurized metered-dose inhalers. Respir Care 50:1191, 2005.
34. Dhand R, Fink J: Dry powder inhalers. Respir Care 44:940, 1999.
35. Nerbrink O, Dahlback M, Hansson H: Why do medical nebulizers differ in their output and particle characteristics? J Aerosol Med 7:259, 1994.
36. Dennis J, Hendrick D: Design characteristics for drug nebulizers. J Med Eng Technol 16:63, 1992.
37. Hess D, Fisher D, Williams P, et al: Medication nebulizer performance: effects of diluent volume, nebulizer flow, and nebulizer brand. Chest 110:498, 1996.
38. Goode ML, Fink JB, Dhand R, et al: Improvement in aerosol delivery with helium-oxygen mixtures during mechanical ventilation. Am J Respir Crit Care Med 163:109, 2001.
39. Hess DR, Fink JB, Venkataraman ST, et al: The history and physics of heliox. Respir Care 51:608, 2006.
40. Phipps P, Gonda I: Droplets produced by medical nebulizers: some factors affecting their size and solute concentration. Chest 97:1327, 1990.
41. Thomas S, Lanford J, George R: Improving the efficiency of drug administration with jet nebulisers. Lancet 1:126, 1988.
42. Rau JL, Ari A, Restrepo RD: Performance comparison of nebulizer designs: constant-output, breath-enhanced, and dosimetric. Respir Care 49:174, 2004.
43. Malone RA, Hollie MC, Glynn-Barnhart A, et al: Optimal duration of nebulized albuterol therapy. Chest 104:1114, 1993.
44. Kendrick A, Smith E, Wilson R: Selecting and using nebulizer equipment. Thorax 52:92, 1997.
45. Alvine GF, Rodgers P, Fitzsimmons KM, et al: Disposable jet nebulizers. How reliable are they? Chest 101:316, 1992.
46. Kacmarek R, Kratohvil J: Evaluation of a double-enclosure double-vacuum unit scavenging system for ribavirin administration. Respir Care 37:37, 1992.
47. Oie S, Kamiya A: Bacterial contamination of aerosol solutions containing antibiotics. Microbios 82:109, 1995.
48. Colacone A, Wolkove N, Stern E: Continuous nebulization of albuterol (salbutamol) in acute asthma. Chest 97:693, 1990.
49. American Association for Respiratory Care: Clinical practice guideline: delivery of aerosols to the upper airway. Respir Care 39:803, 1994.
50. Phillips G, Millard F: The therapeutic use of ultrasonic nebulizers in acute asthma. Respir Med 88:387, 1994.
51. Thomas SH, O'Doherty MJ, Page CJ, et al: Delivery of ultrasonic nebulized aerosols to a lung model during mechanical ventilation. Am Rev Respir Dis 148:872, 1993.
52. Dhand R: Nebulizers that use a vibrating mesh or plate with multiple apertures to generate aerosol. Respir Care 47:1406, 2002.
53. Dolovich MA, Fink J: Aerosols and devices. Respir Care Clin N Am 7:131, 2001.
54. Henriet AC, Marchand-Adam S, Mankikian J, et al: [Respimat, first Soft Mist inhaler: new perspectives in the management of COPD.] Rev Mal Respir 27:1141, 2010 [in French].
55. Denyer J, Nikander K, Smith N: Adaptive aerosol delivery (AAD) technology. Expert Opin Drug Deliv 1:165, 2004.
56. Kesser KC, Geller DE: New aerosol delivery devices for cystic fibrosis. Respir Care 54:754, 2009.
57. Erzinger S, Schueepp KG, Brooks-Wildhaber J, et al: Facemasks and aerosol delivery in vivo. J Aerosol Med 20 (Suppl 1):S78, 2007.
58. Rubin B, Fink J: Aerosol therapy for children. Respir Care Clin N Am 7:100, 2001.
59. Janssens H, Tiddens H: Aerosol therapy: the special needs of young children. Pediatr Respir Rev 7:S83, 2006.
60. Dolovich MA, Killian D, Wolff RK, et al: Pulmonary aerosol deposition in chronic bronchitis: intermittent positive pressure breathing versus quiet breathing. Am Rev Respir Dis 115:397, 1977.
61. Dolovich MB, Ahrens RC, Hess DR, et al; American College of Chest Physicians; American College of Asthma, Allergy, and Immunology: Device selection and outcomes of aerosol therapy: evidence-based guidelines. American College of Chest Physicians/American College of Asthma, Allergy, and Immunology. Chest 127:335, 2005.
62. Dolovich MB, Dhand R: Aerosol drug delivery: developments in device design and clinical use. Lancet 377:1032, 2011.
63. American Association for Respiratory Care: Clinical practice guideline: selection of a device for delivery of aerosol to the lung parenchyma. Respir Care 41:647, 1996.
64. AARC (American Association of Respiratory Care) clinical practice guideline: Selection of an aerosol delivery device for neonatal and pediatric patients. Respir Care 40:1325, 1995.
65. Volpe J: Therapist-driven protocols for pediatric patients. Respir Care Clin N Am 2:117, 1996.
66. AARC (American Association of Respiratory Care) clinical practice guideline: Assessing response to bronchodilator therapy at point of care. Respir Care 40:1300, 1995.
67. Papo MC, Frank J, Thompson AE: A prospective, randomized study of continuous versus intermittent nebulized albuterol for severe status asthmaticus in children. Crit Care Med 21:1479, 1993.
68. Fink J, Dhand R: Bronchodilator resuscitation in the emergency department, part 2: dosing. Respir Care 45:497, 2000.
69. Dhand R, Guntur VP: How best to deliver aerosol medications to mechanically ventilated patients. Clin Chest Med 29:277, 2008.
70. Duarte AG, Fink JB, Dhand R: Inhalation therapy during mechanical ventilation. Respir Care Clin N Am 7:233, 2001.
71. Ari A, Fink JB: Factors affecting bronchodilator delivery in mechanically ventilated adults. Nurs Crit Care 15:192, 2010.
72. Ari A, Areabi H, Fink JB: Evaluation of position of aerosol device in two different ventilator circuits during mechanical ventilation. Respir Care 55:837, 2010.
73. Ari A, Atalay OT, Harwood R, et al: Influence of nebulizer type, position, and bias flow on aerosol drug delivery in simulated pediatric and adult lung models during mechanical ventilation. Respir Care 55:845, 2010.
74. Hess DR: The mask for noninvasive ventilation: principles of design and effects on aerosol delivery. J Aerosol Med 20 (Suppl 1): S85, 2007.
75. Abdelrahim ME, Plant P, Chrystyn H: In-vitro characterisation of the nebulised dose during non-invasive ventilation. J Pharm Pharmacol 62:966, 2010.
76. Bhashyam AR, Wolf MT, Marcinkowski AL, et al: Aerosol delivery through nasal cannulas: an in vitro study. J Aerosol Med Pulm Drug Deliv 21:181, 2008.
77. Ari A, Harwood R, Sheard M, et al: In-vitro comparison of heliox and oxygen in aerosol delivery using pediatric high flow nasal cannula. Pediatr Pulmonol 46:795, 2011.
78. Reychler G: Comparison of lung deposition in two types of nebulization: intrapulmonary percussive ventilation vs jet nebulization. Chest 125:502, 2004.
79. Demers B, Gilley D, Fink J: Nebulized medications. American Thoracic Society (ATS) International Conference, San Diego, 2005.
80. Siobal M, Ari A, Fink J: Aerosol lung deposition using a vibrating mesh nebulizer during high frequency oscillatory ventilation in the adult lung model. Respir Care 55:1565, 2010.
81. Alzahrani W, Harwood R, Fink JB, et al: Comparison of albuterol delivery during high frequency oscillatory ventilation

and conventional mechanical ventilation of a simulated adult. Respir Care 55:1576, 2010.
82. Lindsley WG, Blachere FM, Thewlis RE, et al: Measurements of airborne influenza virus in aerosol particles from human coughs. PLoS One 5:e15100, 2010.
83. Harrison R: Reproductive risk assessment with occupational exposure to ribavirin aerosol. Pediatr Infect Dis J 9:S1025, 1990.
84. Garner J: Guideline for isolation precautions in hospitals. Infect Control Hosp Epidemiol 17:53, 1996.
85. Gralton J, McLaws ML: Protecting healthcare workers from pandemic influenza: N95 or surgical masks? Crit Care Med 38:657, 2010.

Chapter 37

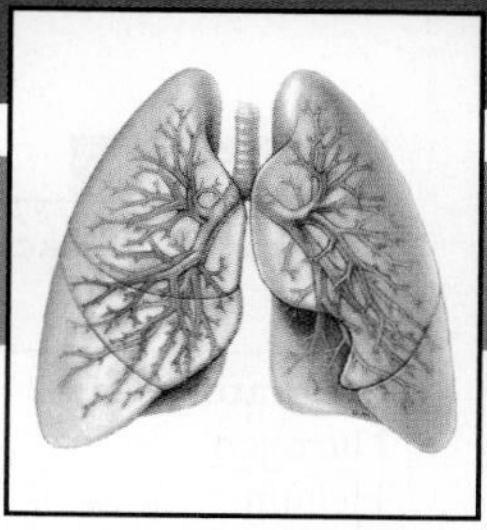

Storage and Delivery of Medical Gases

DAVID L. VINES

CHAPTER OBJECTIVES

After reading this chapter you will be able to:

- Describe how medical gases and gas mixtures are produced.
- Discuss the clinical applications for medical gases and gas mixtures.
- Distinguish between gaseous and liquid storage methods.
- Calculate the duration of remaining contents of a compressed oxygen cylinder.
- Calculate the duration of remaining contents of a liquid oxygen cylinder.
- Describe how to store, transport, and use compressed gas cylinders properly.
- Distinguish between gas supply systems.
- Describe what to do if a bulk oxygen supply system fails.
- Differentiate among safety systems that apply to various equipment connections.
- Select the appropriate devices to regulate gas pressure or control flow in various clinical settings.
- Describe how to assemble, check for proper function, and identify malfunctions in gas delivery equipment.
- Identify and correct common malfunctions of gas delivery equipment.

CHAPTER OUTLINE

Characteristics of Medical Gases
- Oxygen
- Air
- Carbon Dioxide
- Helium
- Nitric Oxide
- Nitrous Oxide

Storage of Medical Gases
- Gas Cylinders
- Bulk Oxygen

Distribution and Regulation of Medical Gases
- Central Piping Systems
- Safety Indexed Connector Systems
- Regulating Gas Pressure and Flow

KEY TERMS

American standard safety system (ASSS)
Bourdon gauge
cryogenic
diameter-index safety system (DISS)
downstream
filling density
flammable
flowmeter
fractional distillation
heliox
manifold
nonflammable
oxidizing
pin-index safety system (PISS)
psig
reducing valve
regulator
Thorpe tube
upstream
zone valves

TABLE 37-1

Physical Characteristics of Medical Gases

Gas	Chemical Symbol	Color	Taste	Odor	Can Support Life	Flammability
Laboratory Gases						
Nitrogen	N	Colorless	Tasteless	Odorless	No	Nonflammable
Helium	He	Colorless	Tasteless	Odorless	No	Nonflammable
Carbon dioxide	CO_2	Colorless	Slightly acidic	Odorless	No	Nonflammable
Therapeutic Gases						
Air	AIR	Colorless	Tasteless	Odorless	Yes	Supports combustion
Oxygen	O_2	Colorless	Tasteless	Odorless	Yes	Supports combustion
Helium/oxygen (heliox)	He/O_2	Colorless	Tasteless	Odorless	Yes	Supports combustion
Carbon dioxide/oxygen	CO_2/O_2	Colorless	Slightly acidic	Odorless	No	Supports combustion
Nitric oxide	NO	Colorless	Tasteless	Metallic	No	Supports combustion
Anesthetic Gas						
Nitrous oxide	N_2O	Colorless	Slightly sweet	Slightly sweet	No	Supports combustion

The hospital "oxygen service" is the origin from which the current technology-laden field of respiratory care evolved. Although respiratory therapists (RTs) have assumed many more challenging duties, ensuring the safe and uninterrupted supply of medical gases is still a key responsibility.

There are many commercially produced gases, but only a few are used medically (Table 37-1). Medical gases are classified as laboratory gases, therapeutic gases, or anesthetic gases. *Laboratory gases* are used for equipment calibration and diagnostic testing. *Therapeutic gases* are used to relieve symptoms and improve oxygenation of patients with hypoxemia. *Anesthetic gases* are combined with oxygen (O_2) to provide anesthesia during surgery. It is important for RTs to be familiar with all aspects of gases used in the clinical setting, especially the chemical symbols, physical characteristics, ability to support life, and fire risk. In regard to fire risk, medical compressed gases are classified as either **nonflammable** (do not burn), nonflammable but supportive of combustion (also termed **oxidizing**), or **flammable** (burns readily, potentially explosive).[1] Of the gases listed in Table 37-1, the focus of this chapter is on the therapeutic gases.

CHARACTERISTICS OF MEDICAL GASES

Oxygen

Characteristics

O_2 is a colorless, odorless, transparent, and tasteless gas.[1] It exists naturally as free molecular O_2 and as a component of a host of chemical compounds. O_2 constitutes almost 50% by weight of the earth's crust and occurs in all living matter in combination with hydrogen as water. At *standard temperature, pressure, and dry (STPD)*, O_2 has a density of 1.429 g/L, being slightly heavier than air (1.29 g/L). O_2 is not very soluble in water. At room temperature and 1 atm pressure, only 3.3 ml of O_2 dissolves in 100 ml of water.

O_2 is nonflammable, but it greatly accelerates combustion. Burning speed increases with either (1) an increase in O_2 percentage at a fixed total pressure or (2) an increase in total pressure of O_2 at a constant gas concentration. Both O_2 concentration and partial pressure influence the rate of burning.[2]

Production

O_2 is produced through one of several methods. Chemical methods for producing small quantities of O_2 include *electrolysis of water* and *decomposition of sodium chlorate* ($NaClO_3$). Most large quantities of medical O_2 are produced by fractional distillation of atmospheric air.[1] Small quantities of concentrated O_2 are produced by physical separation of O_2 from air.

Fractional Distillation. Fractional distillation is the most common and least expensive method for producing O_2. The process involves several related steps. First, atmospheric air is filtered to remove pollutants, water, and carbon dioxide (CO_2). The purified air is liquefied by compression and cooled by rapid expansion *(Joule-Thompson effect)*.

The resulting mixture of liquid O_2 and nitrogen (N, N_2) is heated slowly in a distillation tower. N_2, with its boiling point of 195.8° C (320.5° F), escapes first, followed by the trace gases of argon, krypton, and xenon. The remaining liquid O_2 is transferred to specially insulated **cryogenic** (low-temperature) storage cylinders. An alternative procedure is to convert O_2 directly to gas for storage in high-pressure metal cylinders. These methods produce O_2 that is approximately 99.5% pure. The remaining 0.5% is mostly N_2 and trace argon. U.S. Food and Drug Administration (FDA) standards require an O_2 purity of at least 99.0%.[3]

Physical Separation. Two methods are used to separate O_2 from air.[4] The first method entails use of molecular "sieves" composed of inorganic sodium aluminum silicate pellets. These pellets absorb N_2, "trace" gases, and water vapor from the air, providing a concentrated mixture of more than 90% O_2 for patient use. The second method

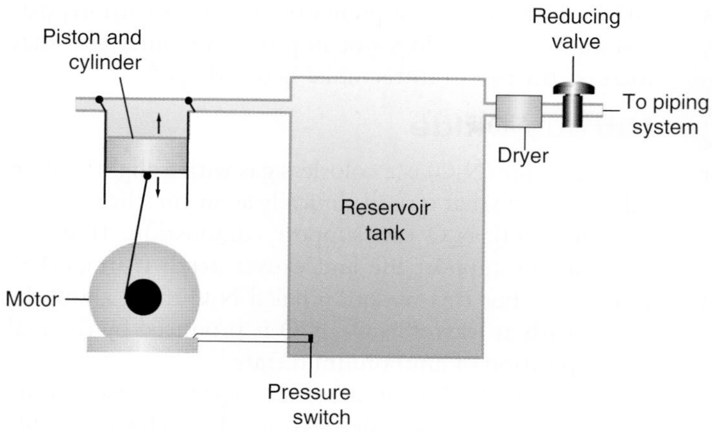

FIGURE 37-1 Large medical air compressor. The compressor sends gas to the reservoir at higher than line pressure. When the preset pressure level is reached, the pressure switch shuts off the compressor. Gas leaves the reservoir and passes through the dryer to remove moisture, and the reducing valve reduces gas to the desired line pressure. When reservoir pressure has decreased to near line pressure, the pressure switch turns the compressor back on. (Modified from McPherson SP, Spearman CB: Respiratory therapy equipment, ed 5, St Louis, 1995, Mosby.)

entails use of a vacuum to pull ambient air through a semipermeable plastic membrane. The membrane allows O_2 and water vapor to pass through at a faster rate than N_2 from ambient air. This system can produce an O_2 mixture of approximately 40%. These devices, called *oxygen concentrators,* are used primarily for supplying low-flow O_2 in the home care setting. For this reason, details about the principles of operation and appropriate use are discussed in Chapter 51.

Air

Atmospheric air is a colorless, odorless, naturally occurring gas mixture that consists of 20.95% O_2, 78.1% N_2, and approximately 1% "trace" gases, mainly argon. At STPD, the density of air is 1.29 g/L, which is used as the standard for measuring specific gravity of other gases. O_2 and N_2 can be mixed to produce a gas with an O_2 concentration equivalent to that of air. Medical-grade air usually is produced by filtering and compressing atmospheric air.[1,5]

Figure 37-1 shows a typical large medical *air compressor system.* In these systems, an electrical motor is used to power a piston in a compression cylinder. On its downstroke, the piston draws air through a filter system with an inlet valve. On its upstroke, the piston compresses the air in the cylinder (closing the inlet valve) and delivers it through an outlet valve to a reservoir tank. Air from the reservoir tank is reduced to the desired working pressure by a pressure-reducing valve before being delivered to the piping system.

For medical gas use, air must be dry and free of oil or particulate contamination.[5] The most common method used for drying air is cooling to produce condensation. For avoidance of oil or particulate contamination, medical air compressors have air inlet filters and polytetrafluoroethylene (Teflon) piston rings as opposed to oil lubrication. Large medical air compressors must provide high flow (at least 100 L/min) at the standard working pressure of 50 *pounds per square inch gauge* **(psig)** for all equipment in use.

Smaller compressors (Figure 37-2) are available for bedside or home use. These compressors have a diaphragm or turbine that compresses the air and generally do not have a reservoir. This design limits the pressure and flow capabilities of these devices. For this reason, small compressors must never be used to power equipment that needs unrestricted flow at 50 psig, such as pneumatically powered ventilators (see Chapter 42). However, small diaphragm or turbine compressors are ideal for powering devices such as small-volume medication nebulizers (see Chapter 36).

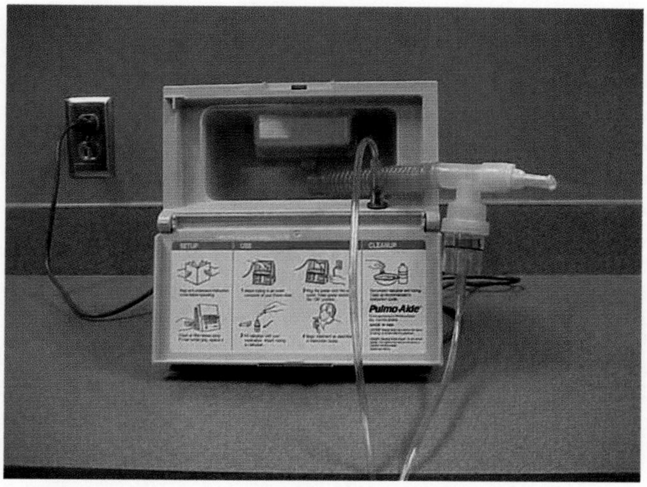

FIGURE 37-2 Small portable compressor used with a hand-held nebulizer to aerosolize medication.

Carbon Dioxide

At STPD, CO_2 is a colorless and odorless gas with a specific gravity of 1.52 (approximately 1.5 times heavier than air).[1] CO_2 does not support combustion or maintain animal life. For medical use, CO_2 usually is produced by heating limestone in contact with water. The gas is recovered from this process and liquefied by compression and cooling. The FDA purity standard for CO_2 is 99%.[3]

Mixtures of O_2 and 5% to 10% CO_2 are occasionally used for therapeutic purposes as noted in Chapter 38.

Therapeutic uses include the management of singultus (hiccups), prevention of the complete washout of CO_2 during cardiopulmonary bypass, and regulation of pulmonary vascular pressures in some congenital heart disorders. However, CO_2 mixtures are more commonly used for the calibration of blood gas analyzers (see Chapter 18) and for diagnostic purposes in the clinical laboratory.

Helium

Helium (He) is second only to hydrogen as the lightest of all gases; it has a density at STPD of 0.1785 g/L. He is odorless, tasteless, nonflammable, and chemically and physiologically inert. It is a good conductor of heat, sound, and electricity but is poorly soluble in water. Although He is present in small quantities in the atmosphere, it is commercially produced from natural gas through liquefaction to purity standards of at least 99%.[3]

He cannot support life, so breathing 100% He would cause suffocation and death. For therapeutic use, He must always be mixed with at least 20% O_2. **Heliox** (a gas mixture of O_2 and He) may be used clinically to manage severe cases of airway obstruction. Its low density decreases the work of breathing by making gas flow more laminar. He is discussed in more detail in Chapter 38.

> **RULE OF THUMB**
>
> He must always be combined with at least 20% O_2. The higher the concentration of O_2 used in a heliox mixture, the less likely it is that heliox would be beneficial. Heliox mixtures of less than 60% He are rarely used clinically.

Nitric Oxide

Nitric oxide (NO) is a colorless, nonflammable, toxic gas that supports combustion. It is produced by oxidation of ammonia at high temperatures in the presence of a catalyst. In combination with air, NO forms brown fumes of nitrogen dioxide (NO_2). Together, NO and NO_2 are strong respiratory irritants that can cause chemical pneumonitis and a fatal form of pulmonary edema. Exposure to high concentrations of NO alone can cause methemoglobinemia (see Chapter 11). High levels of methemoglobin can cause tissue hypoxia.

As discussed in Chapter 38, NO is approved by the FDA for use in the treatment of term and near-term infants for hypoxic respiratory failure. The American Academy of Pediatrics (AAP) has published a policy statement recommending the use of NO in the care of term and near-term infants when mechanical ventilation is failing because of hypoxic respiratory failure. The AAP suggests that NO be used before extracorporeal membrane oxygenation.[6] A systemic review from the Cochrane database supports the recommendation that inhaled NO at 20 ppm may be beneficial in term and near-term infants who do not have a diaphragmatic hernia (see Chapter 31).[7] The use of inhaled NO in the treatment of premature neonates with hypoxic respiratory failure does not improve outcomes and may increase the risk of intracranial hemorrhage.[8]

Nitrous Oxide

Nitrous oxide (N_2O) is a colorless gas with a slightly sweet odor and taste that is used clinically as an anesthetic agent. Similar to O_2, N_2O can support combustion. However, N_2O cannot support life and causes death if inhaled in pure form. For this reason, inhaled N_2O must always be mixed with at least 20% O_2. N_2O is produced by thermal decomposition of ammonium nitrate.[1]

The use of N_2O as an anesthetic agent is based on its central nervous system depressant effect. However, only dangerously high levels of N_2O provide true anesthesia. N_2O/O_2 mixtures are almost always used in combination with other anesthetic agents.

Long-term human exposure to N_2O has been associated with a form of neuropathy. In addition, epidemiologic studies have linked chronic N_2O exposure with an increased risk of fetal disorders and spontaneous abortion.[1] On the basis of this knowledge, the National Institute for Occupational Safety and Health (a division of the Occupational Safety and Health Administration) has set an upper exposure limit for hospital operating rooms of 25 ppm N_2O.[1]

STORAGE OF MEDICAL GASES

Medical gases are stored either in portable high-pressure cylinders or in large bulk reservoirs. Bulk reservoirs require a separate distribution system to deliver the gas to the patient.

Gas Cylinders

The containers used to store and ship compressed or liquid medical gases are high-pressure cylinders. The design, manufacture, transport, and use of these cylinders are carefully controlled by both industrial standards and federal regulations. Gas cylinders are made of seamless steel and are classified by the U.S. Department of Transportation (DOT) according to their fabrication method. DOT type 3A cylinders are made from carbon steel, and DOT type 3AA containers are manufactured with a steel alloy tempered for higher strength.[1]

Markings and Identification

Medical gas cylinders are marked with metal stamping on the shoulders that supplies specific information (Figure 37-3).[1,9] Although the exact location and order of these markings vary, the practitioner should be able to identify several key items of information.

The letters *DOT* or *ICC* (Interstate Commerce Commission) are followed by the cylinder classification (*3A* or *3AA*) and the normal filling pressure in pounds per square inch (psi). Below this information usually is the letter size of the

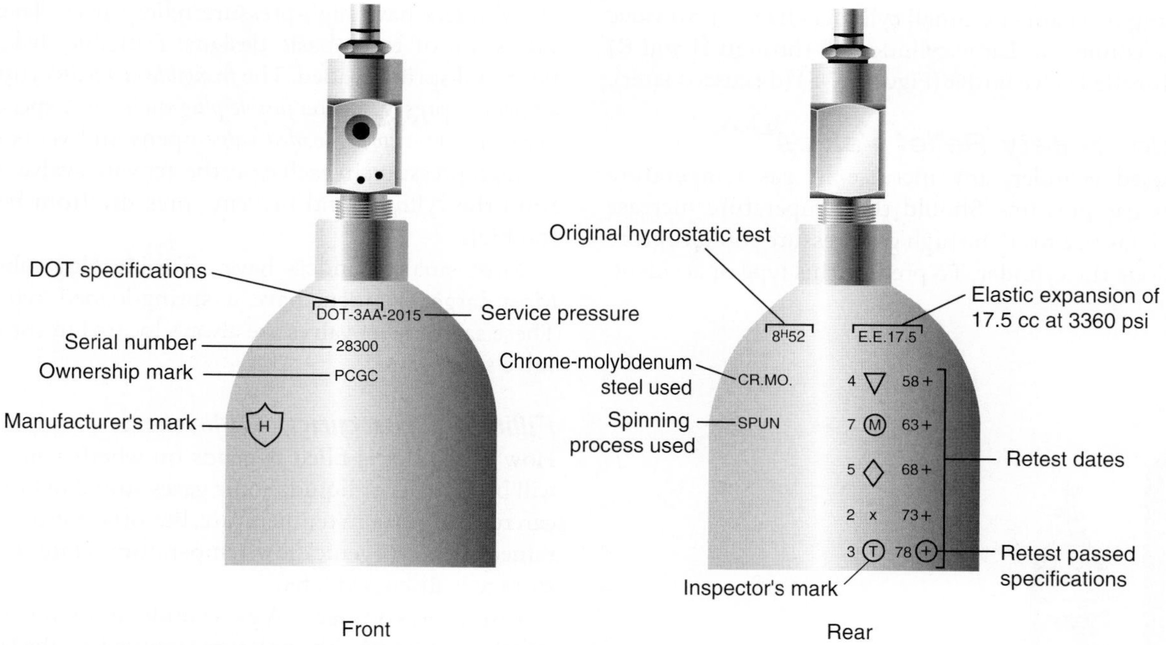

FIGURE 37-3 Typical markings of cylinders containing medical gases. Front and back views are for illustration purposes only; exact location and order of markings vary. *DOT,* Department of Transportation.

cylinder (*E, G,* and so on) followed by the cylinder serial number. A third line provides a mark of ownership, often followed by the manufacturer's stamp or a mark identifying the inspecting authority. An abbreviation indicating the method of cylinder manufacturer is usually on the opposite side of the cylinder. Also in this area is information about the original safety test and dates of all subsequent tests.

Safety tests are conducted on each cylinder every 5 or 10 years, as specified in DOT regulations.[1,9] During these tests, cylinders are pressurized to five thirds of their service pressure. While the cylinder is under pressure, technicians measure cylinder leakage, expansion, and wall stress. The notation *EE* followed by a number indicates the elastic expansion of the cylinder in cubic centimeters under the test conditions. An asterisk (*) next to the test date indicates DOT approval for 10-year testing. A plus sign (+) means the cylinder is approved for filling to 10% greater than its service pressure. An approved cylinder with a service pressure of 2015 psi can be filled to approximately 2200 psi. After hydrostatic testing, cylinders are subjected to internal inspection and cleaning.

In addition to these permanent marks, all cylinders are color-coded and labeled for identification of their contents.[1,10] Table 37-2 lists the color codes for medical gases as adopted by the Bureau of Standards of the U.S. Department of Commerce.[11] For comparison, the color codes adopted by the Canadian Standards Association also are included. Color codes are not standardized internationally. For this reason, cylinder color should be used only as a guide. As with any drug agent, the cylinder contents always must be identified through careful inspection of the label. To be absolutely sure about the O_2 concentration provided by a cylinder, the user must analyze the gas before administering it (see Chapter 18).[12]

TABLE 37-2

Color Codes for Medical Gas Cylinders

Gas	United States	Canada
O_2	Green	White*
CO_2	Gray	Gray
N_2O	Blue	Blue
Cyclopropane	Orange	Orange
He	Brown	Brown
C_2H_4	Red	Red
CO_2-O_2	Gray/green	Gray/white
He-O_2	Brown/green	Brown/white
N_2	Black	Black
Air	Yellow*	Black/white
N_2-O_2	Black/green	Pink

C_2H_4, Ethylene.

*Vacuum systems historically are identified as white in the United States and yellow in Canada. For this reason, the CGA recommends that white not be used for any cylinders in the United States and that yellow not be used in Canada.

Cylinder Sizes and Contents

Letter designations are used for different sizes of cylinders (Figure 37-4). Sizes E through AA are referred to as "small cylinders" and are used most often for transporting patients and anesthetic gases. These small cylinders are easily identified because of their unique valves and connecting mechanisms. Small cylinders have a post valve and yoke connector. Large cylinders (F through H and K) have a threaded valve outlet (Figure 37-5) (discussed later).

Cylinder Safety Relief Valves

In a closed cylinder, any increase in gas temperature increases gas pressure. Should the temperature increase too much (as in a fire), the high gas pressure could rupture and explode the cylinder. To prevent this type of accident, all cylinders have high-pressure relief valves. These relief valves are of three basic designs: frangible disk, fusible plug, and spring-loaded. The *frangible metal disk* ruptures at a specific pressure. The *fusible plug* melts at a specific temperature. The *spring-loaded valve* opens and vents gas at a set high pressure. In each case, the activated valve vents gas from the cylinder and prevents pressure from becoming too high.

Most small cylinders have a fusible plug relief valve. Most large cylinders have a spring-loaded relief valve. These safety relief valves are always located in the cylinder valve stems.

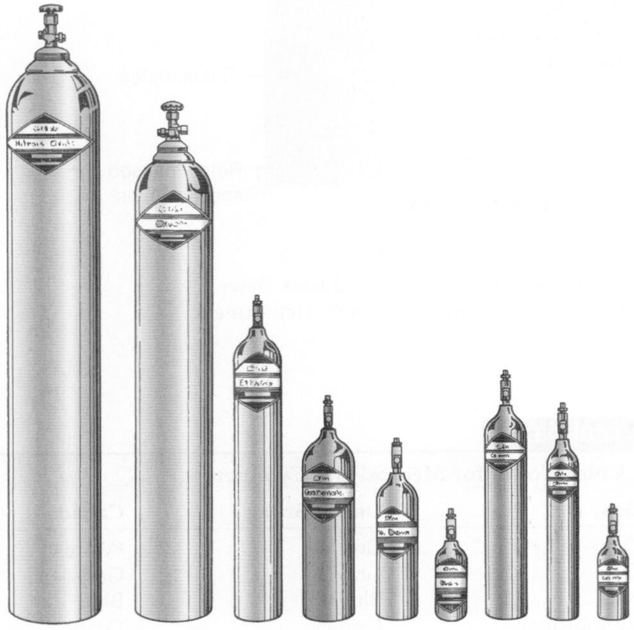

FIGURE 37-4 Cylinder sizes are identified by letter designations.

Filling (Charging) Cylinders

How a cylinder is filled depends on whether its contents will be gaseous or liquid. Some gases stored in liquid form can remain at room temperature, but others must be maintained in a cryogenic (low-temperature) state. Cryogenic storage is discussed later.

Compressed Gases. A gas cylinder normally is filled to its service pressure (the pressure stamped on the shoulder) at 21.1° C (70° F). However, approved cylinders can be filled to 10% greater than service pressure.

Liquefied Gases. Gases with critical temperatures greater than room temperature can be stored as liquids at room temperature (see Chapter 6). These gases include CO_2 and N_2O. Rather than being filled to filling pressure, cylinders of these gases are filled according to a specified filling density. The **filling density** is the ratio between the weight of liquid gas put into the cylinder and the weight of water the cylinder could contain if full. The filling density for CO_2 is 68%. This system allows the manufacturer to fill a cylinder with liquid CO_2 up to 68% of the weight of water that a full cylinder could hold. The filling density of N_2O is 55%.

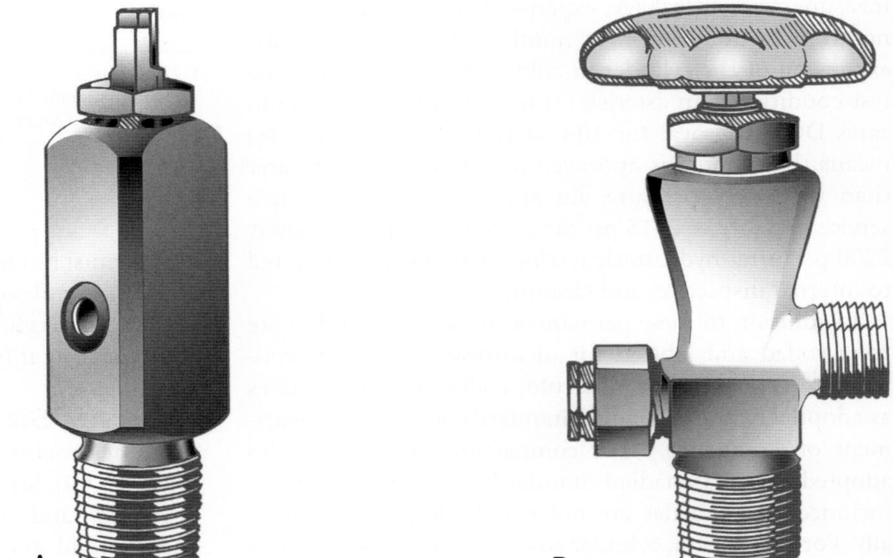

FIGURE 37-5 **A,** Post valve for yoke connector used with small cylinders (E through AA). **B,** Large, threaded valve outlet used with large cylinders (H/K, G, and M).

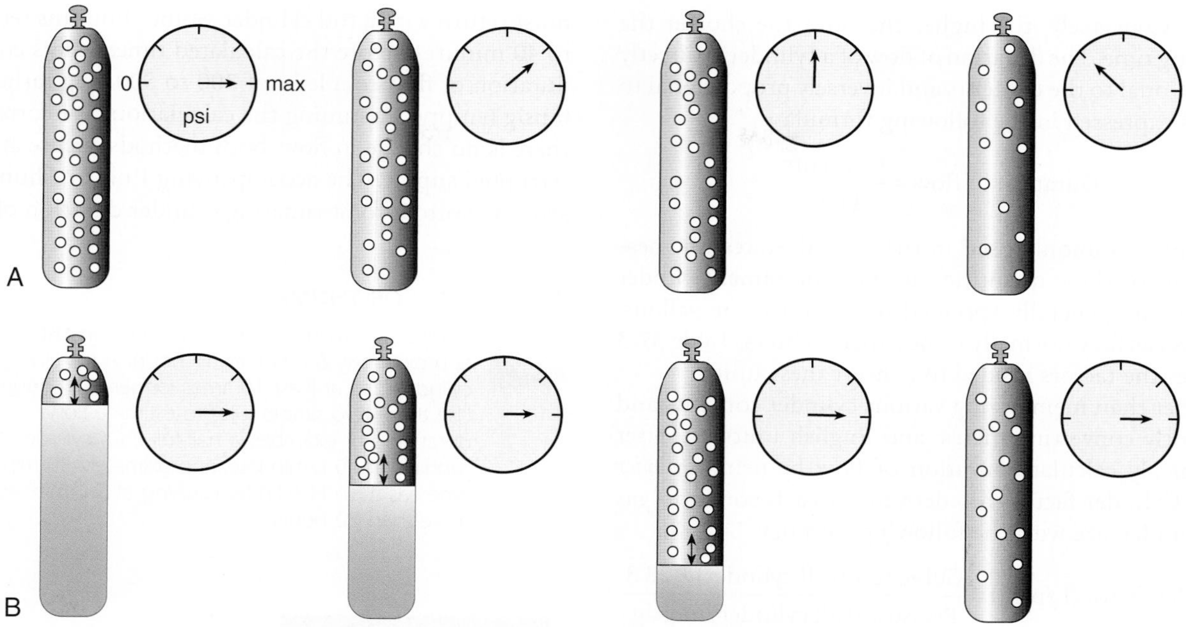

FIGURE 37-6 The content of a gas-filled cylinder **(A)** is directly proportional to the gas pressure. A pressure decrease of 50% indicates a loss of 50% of the contained gas. In a liquid-gas cylinder **(B),** gauge pressure is a measure of only the vapor pressure of gas in equilibrium with the liquid phase. This value remains constant at a given temperature as long as liquid is present. Only when all the liquid has vaporized, as the cylinder nears depletion, does the gauge pressure decrease proportionately to the terminal volume of remaining gas.

Cylinder pressures for gases stored in the liquid phase are much lower than for gases stored in the gas phase. Because the liquid does not fill the entire volume of a cylinder, the space above the liquid surface contains gas in equilibrium with the liquid. The pressure in a liquid-filled cylinder equals the pressure of the vapor at any given temperature.

Pressure in a cylinder depends on the state of its contents. In a gas-filled cylinder, the pressure represents the force required to compress the gas into its smaller volume. In contrast, the pressure in a liquid-filled cylinder is the vapor pressure needed to keep the gas liquefied at the current temperature.

Measuring Cylinder Contents

Because of the previously described differences in the physical state of matter of compressed and liquid gases, different methods are needed to measure the contents of the cylinder.

Compressed Gas Cylinders. For gas-filled cylinders, the volume of gas in the cylinder is directly proportional to its pressure at a constant temperature. If a cylinder is full at 2200 psig, it will be half full when the pressure decreases to 1100 psig. To know how much gas is contained in a compressed gas cylinder, one needs only to measure its pressure.

Liquid Gas Cylinders. In a liquid gas cylinder or container, the measured pressure is the vapor pressure above the liquid. This pressure bears no relationship to the amount of liquid remaining in the cylinder. As long as some liquid remains (and the temperature remains constant), the vapor pressure and the gauge pressure remain constant. When all the liquid is gone and the cylinder contains only gas, the pressure decreases in proportion to a reduction in volume. Monitoring the gauge pressure of liquid gas cylinders is useful only after all the liquid vaporizes. Weighing a liquid-filled cylinder is the only accurate method for determining the contents.

Figure 37-6 compares the behavior of compressed gas and liquid gas cylinders during use. The vapor pressure of liquid gas cylinders varies with the temperature of the contents. The pressure in an N_2O cylinder at 21.1° C (70° F) is 745 psig; at 15.6° C (60° F), the pressure decreases to 660 psig. As the temperature increases toward the critical point, more liquid vaporizes, and the cylinder pressure increases. If a cylinder of N_2O warms to 36.4° C (97.5° F) (its critical temperature), all the contents convert to gas. Only at this temperature and higher does the cylinder gauge pressure accurately reflect cylinder contents.

Estimating Duration of Cylinder Gas Flow

When a cylinder of therapeutic gas is used, it often is necessary to predict how long the contents will last at a given flow. The duration of flow of a cylinder can be estimated if the following are known: (1) the gas flow, (2) the cylinder size, and (3) the cylinder pressure at the start of therapy. For a given flow, the more gas a cylinder holds, the longer it lasts. Conversely, the higher the flow, the shorter the emptying time. The duration of flow of a cylinder is directly proportional to the contents and inversely proportional to flow, as expressed in the following formula:

$$\text{Duration of flow} = \frac{\text{Contents}}{\text{Flow}}$$

The units commonly used in the United States for measurement of these quantities are not the same. Cylinder contents are generally specified in cubic feet or gallons, whereas gas flow normally is measured in liters. Table 37-3 provides the factors needed to convert these units.

Rather than memorizing various cylinder contents and constantly converting metric and English units, the user can quickly calculate duration of flow by using *cylinder factors*. Cylinder factors are derived for each common gas and cylinder size with the following formula:

$$\text{Cylinder factor (L/psig)} = \frac{\text{Cubic feet (full cylinder)} \times 28.3}{\text{Pressure (full cylinder) in psig}}$$

In the numerator of the previous equation, the English-metric conversion constant (28.3) is used to convert cubic feet to liters. Dividing the resulting volume by the pressure in a full cylinder yields the cylinder factor. The derived factor represents the volume of gas leaving a given cylinder for every 1-psig decrease in pressure. Table 37-4 provides cylinder factors for the therapeutic medical gases and common cylinder sizes.

When the factor for a given gas and cylinder is known, calculating the duration of flow is a simple matter of applying the following equation:

$$\text{Duration of flow (min)} = \frac{\text{Pressure (psig)} \times \text{Cylinder factor}}{\text{Flow (L/min)}}$$

A wide margin of safety must be allowed in estimation of cylinder duration of flow. This principle is especially important if the RT cannot be present during use and must return with a full cylinder. Some clinicians return 30 to 40 minutes before the calculated time; others compute duration of flow to a level of 300 to 500 psig rather than 0 psig (empty). Assuming the calculations are correct and there is no change in flow, both methods ensure an uninterrupted supply. The accompanying Rule of Thumb presents a shortcut for estimating cylinder duration of flow.

TABLE 37-3

Gas Volume Conversion Factors

Liters	Cubic Feet	Gallons
28.316	1	7.481
1	0.03531	0.2642
3.785	0.1337	1

TABLE 37-4

Factors for Calculation of Cylinder Duration of Flow (Minutes)

	Cylinder Size			
Gas	D	E	G	H and K
O_2, O_2/N_2, air	0.16	0.28	2.41	3.14
O_2/CO_2	0.20	0.35	2.94	3.84
He/O_2	0.14	0.23	1.93	2.50

RULE OF THUMB

A full E O_2 cylinder running at 10 L/min lasts approximately 60 minutes (1 hour). A full H/K cylinder lasts at least 10 times longer (>10 hours). Use these two simple rules to estimate flow duration. For example, a half-full E O_2 cylinder running at 10 L/min lasts approximately 30 minutes, whereas a full H cylinder running at 5 L/min lasts more than 20 hours.

MINI CLINI

Computing Cylinder Duration of Flow

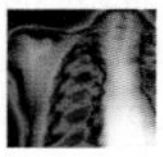

PROBLEM: The RT needs to determine how long a G cylinder of O_2 with a gauge pressure of 800 psi set to deliver 8 L/min will last until empty.

SOLUTION

Step 1: Determine the cylinder factor for an O_2 G cylinder (see Table 37-4), in this case 2.41.

Step 2: Apply the duration of flow equation:

$$\text{Duration of flow (min)} = \frac{\text{Pressure (psig)} \times \text{Cylinder factor}}{\text{Flow (L/min)}}$$

$$\text{Duration of flow (min)} = \frac{800 \times 2.41}{8} = 241 \text{ minutes}$$

(approximately 4 hours)

Estimating Duration of Liquid Oxygen Cylinder Gas Flow

The only accurate method for determining the volume of gas in a liquid-filled cylinder is by weight. Because 1 L of liquid O_2 weighs 2.5 lb and produces 860 L of O_2 in its gaseous state, the amount of gas in a liquid O_2 cylinder can be calculated with the following formula:

$$\text{Amount of gas in cylinder} = \frac{\text{Liquid } O_2 \text{ weight (lb)} \times 860}{2.5 \text{ lb/L}}$$

After the amount of O_2 remaining in the cylinder is determined, the duration of the gas in minutes can be calculated with the following formula:

$$\text{Duration of gas (min)} = \frac{\text{Amount of gas in cylinder (L)}}{\text{Flow (L/min)}}$$

As with gaseous O_2 cylinders, a wide margin of safety is needed for estimation of cylinder duration. This margin of safety varies with the size of the portable O_2 unit or large storage container.

MINI CLINI

Computing the Duration of a Liquid Oxygen Container

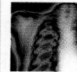

PROBLEM: The RT needs to estimate how long Mrs. Jones' portable liquid O_2 container will last if it contains 3 lb of liquid O_2 that supplies an O_2 delivery device running at 2 L/min.

SOLUTION:

Step 1: Determine the amount of O_2 in the cylinder.

$$\text{Amount of gas in cylinder} = \frac{\text{Liquid } O_2 \text{ weight (lb)} \times 860}{2.5 \text{ lb/L}} = \frac{3 \times 860}{2.5} = 1032 \text{ L}$$

Step 2: Calculate the duration of the gas in the container.

$$\text{Duration of gas} = \frac{\text{Amount of gas in the cylinder (L)}}{\text{Flow (L/min)}} = \frac{1032 \text{ L}}{2} = \frac{516 \text{ minutes}}{60 \text{ (min/hr)}} = 8 \text{ hours } 36 \text{ minutes}$$

Gas Cylinder Safety

The following guidelines for cylinder safety are from the recommendations of the National Fire Protection Agency (NFPA)[2] and the Compressed Gas Association (CGA).[1] For ease of use, these safety guidelines are divided into cylinder storage, transport, and use.

Cylinder Storage. The following guidelines apply to cylinder storage:

- Store gas cylinders in racks or chain cylinders to the wall to prevent them from falling or becoming damaged.
- Other than the wooden racks used to store the cylinders, store no other combustible material in the vicinity of cylinders or gas supply systems.
- Store gas cylinders away from sources of heat. Keep the cylinder temperature less than 125° F (<51.7° C).
- Store flammable gases separately from gases that support combustion, such as air, O_2, and N_2O.
- If a cylinder is not in use, keep the protective cylinder cap in place.
- Do not store air compressors and gas cylinders together. A fire involving one or the other can damage both gas delivery systems.
- Contain and store cylinder supply systems in an enclosure constructed of a material with at least a 1-hour fire resistive rating that is well ventilated and well drained.
- Segregate full and empty cylinders; store them separately if possible.
- Place on each door or gate of the enclosure a sign that cautions the presence of an oxidizing gas and alerts against smoking. This sign must be readable from a distance of at least 5 ft (1.5 m).
- Store liquid O_2 containers in a cool, well-ventilated area because of the venting of small amounts of O_2 from these low-pressure containers. The venting of O_2 prevents these containers from overpressurizing because liquid O_2 is continuously converting to gaseous O_2.

Cylinder Transport. The following guidelines apply to cylinder transport:

- Use cylinder carts with a securing mechanism for transportation of cylinders.
- Keep the protective cylinder caps in place during transportation of cylinders.
- Protect gas cylinders from striking other cylinders or objects to avoid damaging the safety devices, valve stems, or the cylinder itself.
- Avoid dropping, dragging, or rolling cylinders in transport.
- Do not transport cylinders for use that are not appropriately labeled.

Cylinder Use. The following guidelines apply to cylinder use:

- Secure gas cylinders at the patient's bedside in a way that prevents them from falling. Secure cylinders to the wall with a chain, bind or chain them to a suitable cart, or support the cylinder with a stand.
- Do not use flammable materials, especially oil or grease, on regulators, cylinders, fittings, or valves. This restriction includes oily hands, rags, and gloves.
- Never cover a cylinder with any material, including bed linens or hospital gowns.
- Open the cylinder valve slightly to remove dust and dirt before attaching the regulator. When slightly opening the valve, ensure no one is in front of the valve. "Crack" the cylinder before bringing it to the patient's bedside.
- Never use cylinder valves or regulators that need repair.
- Do not alter or deface cylinder markings or color.
- Never place cylinders near sources of heat.
- Never secure cylinders to movable objects unless the object has an apparatus that can contain the cylinder safely.
- Ensure that the connection between the regulator and the cylinder valve is an **American standard safety system (ASSS)** for H and G cylinders and a **pin-index safety system (PISS)** for E cylinders.
- When O_2 is in use, post a "No Smoking" sign unless signs in the entrances are posted that prohibit smoking in the facility.

Bulk Oxygen

Large acute care facilities use large volumes of O_2 every day. To meet these needs, a centralized bulk storage and delivery system is required. By definition, bulk O_2 storage systems hold at least 20,000 cubic ft of gas, including the unconnected reserves that are on site.[2] Bulk O_2 may be stored in either gaseous or liquid form, but liquid storage is most common. When needed, the O_2 flows from this central source throughout the facility through a piping system with outlets conveniently located.

A bulk O_2 system has several advantages over portable cylinders. Although initially expensive to construct, bulk O_2 systems are far less expensive over the long-term. Bulk O_2 systems are less prone to interruption. These systems eliminate the inconvenience and hazard of transporting and storing numerous cylinders. Bulk O_2 systems regulate delivery pressures centrally, eliminating the need for separate pressure-reducing valves at each outlet. These systems also operate at low pressures, making them much safer than high-pressure cylinders.

Safety standards for bulk O_2 systems are set by the NFPA and are subject to further control by local fire and building codes.[2] RTs should be familiar with both bulk units in general and the specific gas supply systems used in their facilities.

Gas Supply Systems

There are three types of centrally located gas supply systems: an alternating supply system or cylinder **manifold** system, a cylinder supply system with reserve supply, and a bulk gas system with a reserve.[2] The *alternating supply or cylinder manifold system* consists of large (normally H or K size) cylinders of compressed O_2 banked together in series (Figure 37-7). This alternating supply system has two sides: a primary bank and a reserve bank. When the pressure in the primary bank decreases to a set level, a control valve automatically switches over to the reserve bank. When this occurs, the primary bank is taken off-line, and the empty cylinders are replaced with full ones. The replenished primary bank becomes the reserve bank. Some large alternating supply systems are permanently fixed and are refilled on site by a supply truck. These cylinder manifold systems have pressure-reducing valves for regulation of delivered pressure and normally have low-pressure alarms. These alarms sound when reserve switchover occurs, and they warn of impending depletion or malfunction. Cylinder manifolds or alternating supply systems are used to supply O_2 from a central location in small facilities or to supply specialty gases, such as N_2O, to operating rooms (Figure 37-8).

A *cylinder supply system with a reserve* consists of a primary supply, a secondary supply, and a reserve supply. When the primary gas supply is depleted by the demand, this supply system automatically switches to the secondary supply. Master signal panels indicate that the changeover has occurred. This supply system operates in a manner similar to the alternating system except that this system has a reserve supply if primary and secondary supplies become depleted. Liquid containers may be used as the primary and secondary gas sources, but the reserve supply usually is high-pressure gas cylinders. Gas cylinders are used as the reserve supply because low-pressure liquid containers lose approximately 3% of the supply per day.[2]

For economy, safety, and convenience, most large health care facilities use a *liquid bulk O_2 system.* A small volume of liquid O_2 provides a very large amount of gaseous O_2 and minimizes space requirements. However, along with this advantage comes a major problem. O_2 has a critical temperature well below room temperature (−118.6° C [−181.4° F]).[1] Liquid O_2 must continually be stored below this temperature, or it reverts to its gaseous state.

To stay in liquid form, O_2 is stored in large stand tanks (Figure 37-9) at relatively low pressure (<250 psig). These stand tanks are similar to giant thermos bottles, consisting of inner and outer steel shells separated by an insulated vacuum chamber (Figure 37-10). Because it eliminates heat conduction, the vacuum keeps the liquid O_2 below its critical temperature without refrigeration. When it flows through vaporizer coils exposed to ambient temperature, the liquid O_2 quickly converts back to a gas. With the O_2 in its gaseous form, the pressure is decreased to the standard working pressure of 50 psi by a pressure-reducing valve. A safety vent allows vaporized liquid O_2 to escape if warming causes cylinder pressure to increase above a set limit.

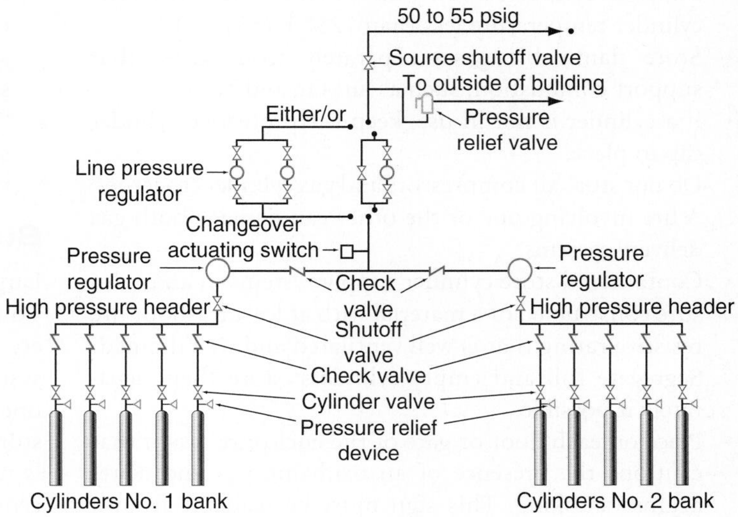

FIGURE 37-7 Gas cylinder manifold system. The alternating supply system is composed of primary and reserve banks, which alternate to charge the piping system. (Modified from Standard for nonflammable medical gas systems, NFPA No. 56F. Copyright 1973, National Fire Protection Association, Boston, MA.)

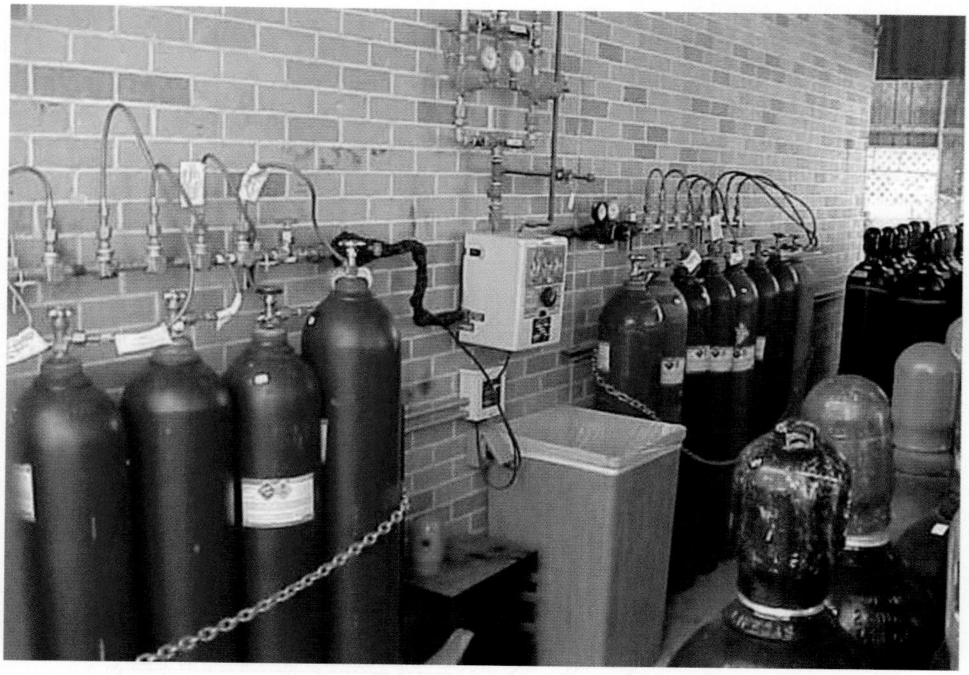

FIGURE 37-8 Alternating supply system of N_2O.

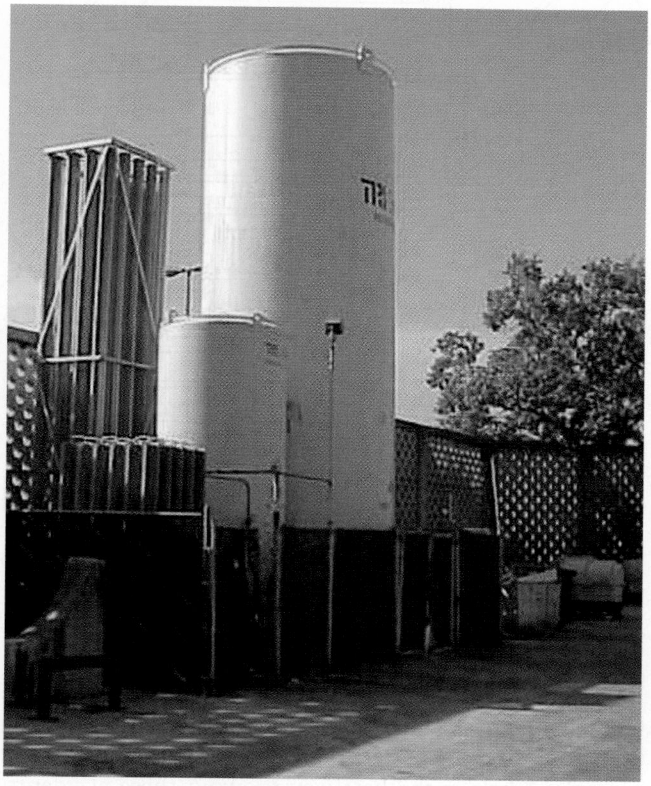

FIGURE 37-9 Large stand tank and reserve tank of liquid O_2 represents a typical bulk gas system with a reserve.

Smaller liquid cylinders are used for home O_2 supply. These cylinders come in several sizes and hold between ⅔ cubic ft and 1½ cubic ft of liquid O_2. Small liquid O_2 cylinders are refilled on site by means of transfer of liquid O_2 from a large cylinder. Chapter 51 describes the use of these small liquid O_2 cylinders in the home.

Bulk Oxygen Safety Precautions

The NFPA sets standards for the design, construction, placement, and use of bulk O_2 systems.[2] A key provision in these standards is the requirement for a reserve or backup gas supply to equal the average daily gas usage of the hospital. To meet this requirement, most large facilities have a second, smaller liquid stand tank. Smaller facilities may use a cylinder gas manifold as the backup.

Failure of bulk O_2 supply systems has been reported with resultant major problems.[13-15] Failure of a bulk O_2 supply can be life-threatening to any patient receiving O_2 or gas-powered ventilatory support. For this reason, the respiratory care staff must be prepared. Adherence to an established protocol is a quick way to identify and prioritize all affected patients. When affected patients are identified, staff members move appropriate backup equipment to the bedside (e.g., portable cylinders, bag-valve-mask resuscitators). Trained personnel bypass the failed system and provide needed patient support, while engineers determine the cause of the failure and correct it.

DISTRIBUTION AND REGULATION OF MEDICAL GASES

Before it can be administered to a patient, a medical gas must be delivered to the bedside and the pressure reduced to a workable level. This is the primary function of gas distribution and regulation systems. Modern hospital gas distribution systems deliver bulk O_2 and compressed air to patient rooms and special care areas through an elaborate piping network. This network may include a vacuum source and, for surgical areas, N_2O. Patient transport still requires the use of portable cylinders. Whether delivery

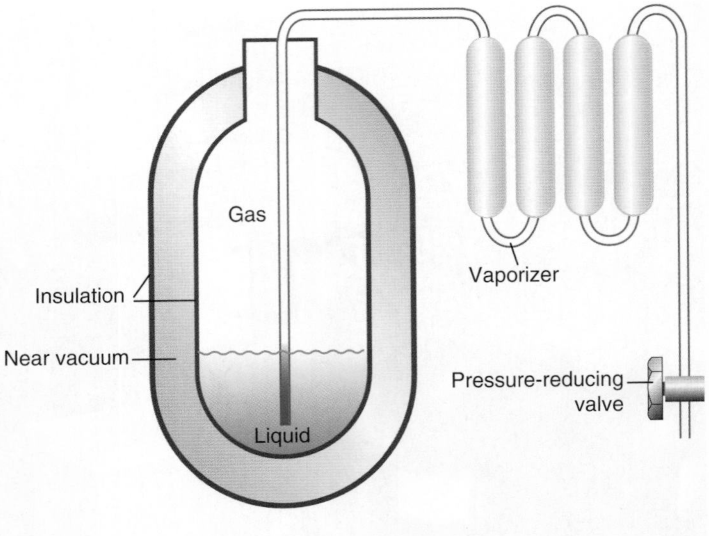

FIGURE 37-10 Liquid-O_2 stand tank (fixed station). (Modified from Cairo JM, Pilbeam SP: Mosby's respiratory care equipment, ed 8, St Louis, 2010, Mosby.)

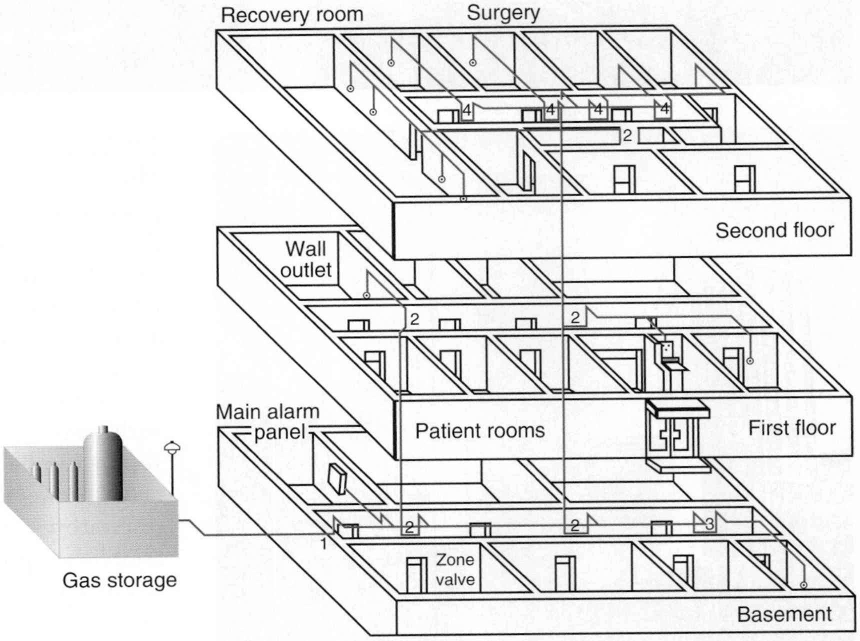

FIGURE 37-11 A hospital piping system. Numbers indicate zone valves.

occurs by central bulk supply or cylinder, patient safety is always the primary aim. For this reason, RTs must be proficient in the use of both delivery systems.

Central Piping Systems

Structural standards for piping systems are established by the NFPA and are described in more detail elsewhere.[2] Figure 37-11 shows a simple central piping gas system. The gas pressure in a central piping system normally is reduced to the standard working pressure of 50 psi at the bulk storage location. A main alarm warns of decreases in pressure or interruptions in flow from the source. **Zone valves** (Figure 37-12) throughout the system can be closed for system maintenance or in case of fire. Wall or station outlets at the delivery sites allow connection of various types of equipment to the gas distribution system. Because most delivery outlets include O_2, air, vacuum, and possibly N_2O, special safety connectors are used to help prevent accidental misconnections.

Safety Indexed Connector Systems

One of the greatest risks in medical gas therapy is giving the wrong gas to a patient. Carefully reading the cylinder or outlet labels is the best way to avoid these accidents. However, human error does occur. For this reason, the industry has developed indexed safety systems for gas delivery and regulation equipment. These safety systems make misconnection between pieces of equipment nearly impossible. For example, an indexed safety system normally prevents connecting a cylinder of N_2O to an O_2 delivery system. Three basic indexed safety systems are used in the delivery and regulation of medical gases: (1) the American National Standard/Compressed Gas Association Standard for Compressed Gas Cylinder Valve Outlet and Inlet Connections,

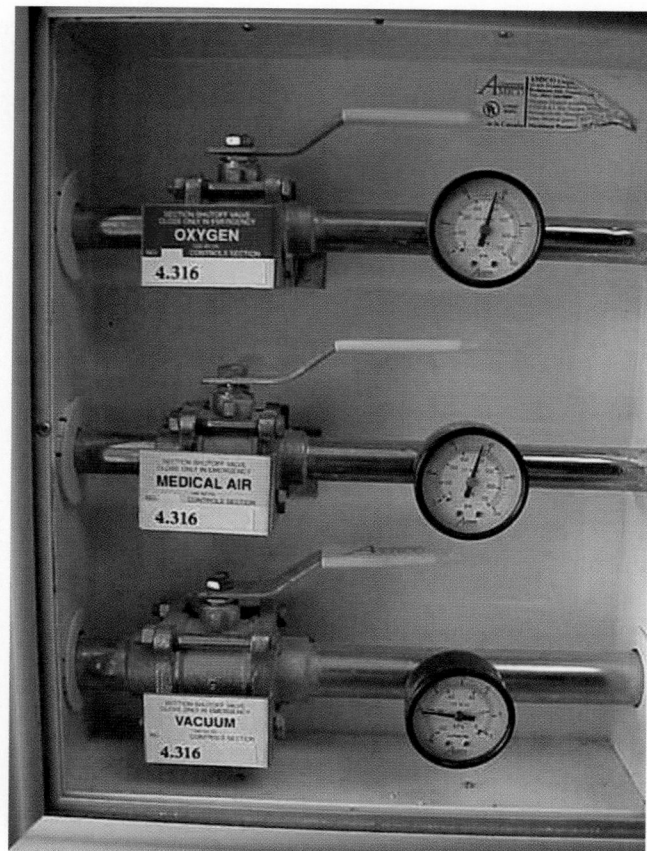

FIGURE 37-12 O_2, air, and vacuum zone valves.

or the ASSS; (2) the **diameter-index safety system (DISS);** and (3) the PISS.[16,17]

American Standard Safety System

Adopted in the United States and Canada, the ASSS provides standards for threaded high-pressure connections between large compressed gas cylinders (sizes F through H/K) and their attachments.[16] Specifications exist for more than 60 gases and gas mixtures. Figure 37-13 shows a typical ASSS connection between a threaded cylinder outlet and a pressure-reducing valve nipple. Use of the ASSS standards makes misconnections difficult because the size (bore) of the cylinder outlet and its threading differ based on the type of gas in the cylinder.

Because there are only 26 connections for the 62 listed gases and mixtures, each gas may not have a unique connection. Some gases have identical connections. Catalogs of cylinder equipment show the connection specifications for each type of cylinder and gas. A typical description for a large cylinder of O_2 is as follows: CGA-540 0.903-14NGO-RH-Ext. The connection for the threaded outlet of this cylinder is listed by the CGA as connection number 540. The outlet has a thread diameter (bore) of 0.903 inch; there are 14 threads per inch; and the threads are right-handed (RH) and external (Ext). It generally is necessary to use only one or two outlet connections because most of the gases that are used by RTs are grouped within a few connector

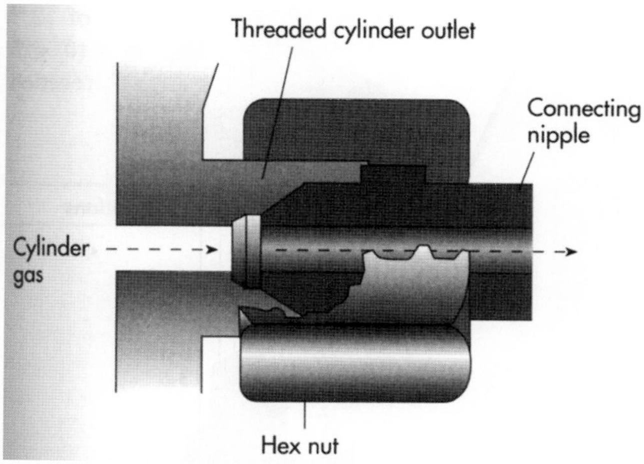

FIGURE 37-13 Typical ASSS connection used to attach a reducing valve to a large high-pressure cylinder. A hexagonal nut is held on the nipple of the reducing valve by a circular collar. The connection is made by (1) aligning the reducing valve nipple with the conical cylinder valve outlet and (2) tightening the reducing valve hex nut onto the threaded cylinder outlet. Different threading and cylinder outlet sizes make accidental misconnections difficult.

sizes. However, practitioners should be familiar with the classification scheme in general because expanding instrumentation and scope of services may bring RTs in contact with other gases and gas systems.

Pin-Index Safety System

Pin indexing is part of the ASSS but applies only to the valve outlets of small cylinders, up to and including size E. These cylinders have a yoke type of connection. Figure 37-14 illustrates the general structure of the pin-indexed yoke connection. The upper yoke fits over the lower valve stem. Two pins, projecting from the inner surface of the yoke connector, mate with two pinholes bored into the valve stem. Proper pin position aligns the small receiving nipple of the yoke with the recessed cylinder valve outlet. Tightening the hand screw on the yoke firmly seats the receiving nipple into the valve outlet. A nylon washer or bushing typically is used to ensure a leak-free connection.

Similar to the ASSS, the PISS helps prevent accidental misconnections between pieces of equipment. The exact positions of pins and pinholes vary for each gas. Unless the pins and holes align perfectly, the yoke nipple cannot seat in the recessed valve outlet. Six holes and pin positions constitute the total system. Because overlapping holes cannot be used, there are 10 possible pin combinations. Figure 37-15 is a diagram of the location of all six possible holes and their index numbers. Table 37-5 lists the gases included in the PISS system, including their index positions.

Diameter-Index Safety System

The ASSS and the PISS provide standards for high-pressure connections between cylinders and equipment; the DISS was established to prevent accidental interchange

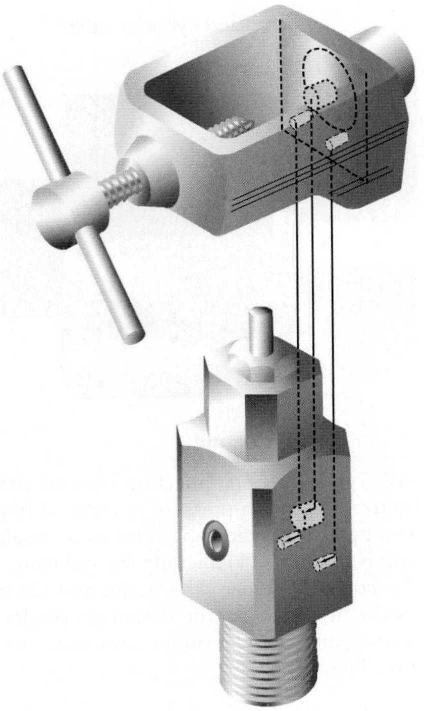

FIGURE 37-14 Yoke connector showing regulator inlet and pin-indexed safety system (for cylinders size AA to E).

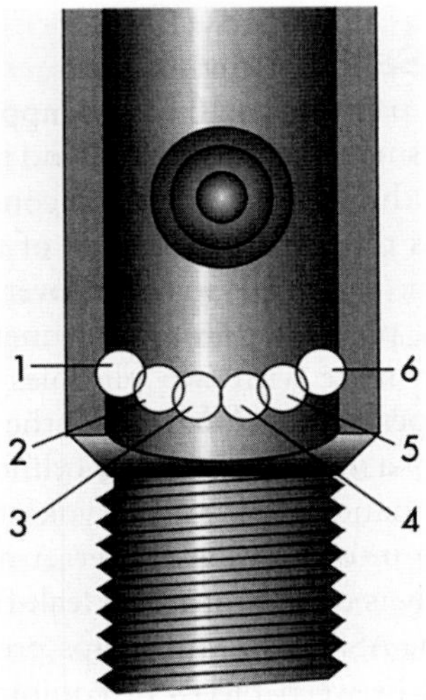

FIGURE 37-15 Location of the pin-index holes in the cylinder valve face for different gases. See Table 37-5 for pin-index hole locations for various gases.

of low-pressure (<200 psig) medical gas connectors.[17] RTs typically find DISS connections (1) at the outlets of pressure-reducing valves attached to cylinders; (2) at the station outlets of central piping systems; and (3) at the inlets of blenders, flowmeters, ventilators, and other pneumatic equipment.

As shown in Figure 37-16, the DISS connection consists of an externally threaded body and a mated nipple with a nut. As the two parts are joined, the shoulders of the nipple and the bores of the body mate, with the union held together by a hand-tightened hex nut. Indexing is achieved by varying the dimensions of the borings and shoulders. There are 11 indexed DISS connections and 1 connection for O_2, for a total of 12.[17] The standard threaded O_2 connector (0.5625 inch in diameter and 18 threads per inch) preceded adoption of this safety system. Nonetheless, it has been assigned a DISS number of 1240.

TABLE 37-5

Pin Index Hole Positions*

Gas	Pin Positions
O_2	2-5
O_2/CO_2 (CO_2 not >7%)	2-6
He/O_2 (He not >80%)	2-4
C_2H_4	1-3
N_2O	3-5
C_3H_6	3-6
He/O_2 (He >80%)	4-6
O_2/CO_2 (CO_2 >7%)	1-6
Air	1-5

C_2H_4, Ethylene; C_3H_6, cyclopropane.
*See Figure 37-15.

Although O_2 and air are generally used from a central outlet, it may be necessary to administer other gases that have different DISS connections. To avoid stocking a large variety of pressure regulators, flowmeters, and connectors for special gas use, adapters can be used to convert various DISS connections so that they can be used for different purposes. Using adapters to bypass a safety system carries the increased risk of misconnection. For this reason, RTs should exercise extreme caution when adapting equipment connections. Misconnections have occurred, with negative patient consequences.[13,18]

Quick-Connect Systems

Station outlets at the patient's bedside allow quick access to a bulk supply of O_2 and air or a vacuum source. Station outlets have DISS connections or quick-connect systems that are gas-specific or vacuum-specific. Various manufacturers have designed specially shaped connectors for each gas (Figure 37-17). Because each connector has a distinct shape, it does not fit into an outlet for another gas, and each manufacturer has its own unique design. For this reason, connectors from different manufacturers are not interchangeable. As long as a facility is standardized for a single quick-connect system, this incompatibility is seldom a problem.

A variety of safety systems help prevent inadvertent misconnections between medical delivery systems and equipment. Figure 37-18 summarizes the use of and relationships between the ASSS, PISS, and DISS systems as applied to cylinder gases. Proficiency in the proper use of these systems is a basic skill of RTs.

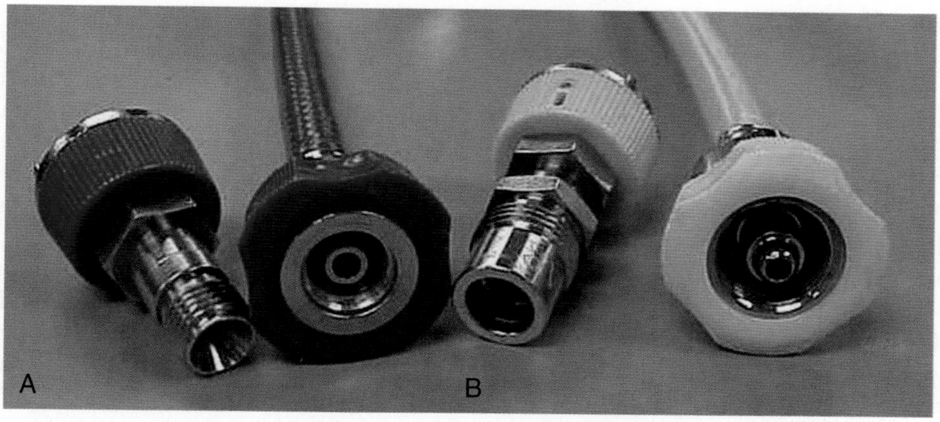

FIGURE 37-16 O_2 (A) and air (B) DISS connections. The two shoulders of the nipple allow the nipple to unite only with a body that has corresponding borings. If the match is incorrect, the nut does not engage the body threads. The difference in the shoulders and bore between the O_2 (A) and air (B) DISS connections is evident.

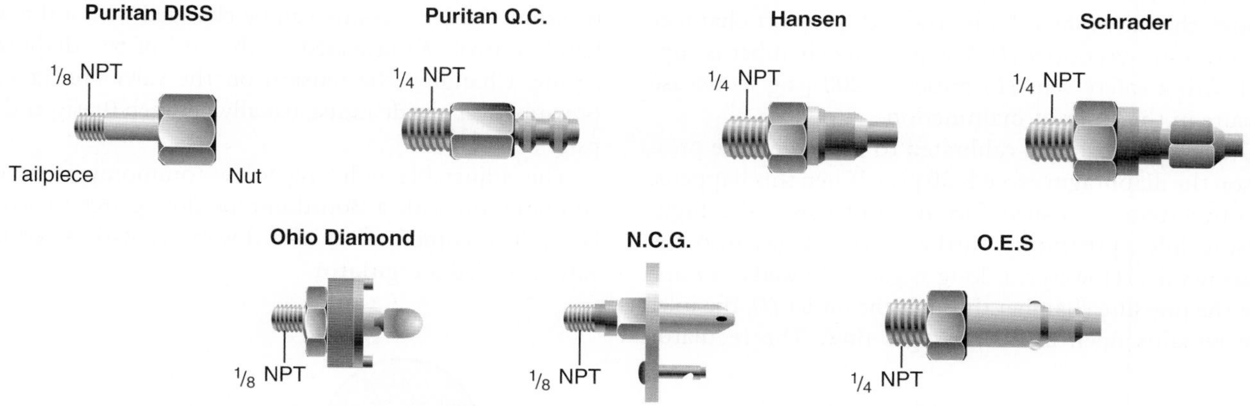

FIGURE 37-17 Common brands of quick connects. *NPT,* National pipe thread taper. (Courtesy Nellcor Puritan Bennett, Pleasanton, California.)

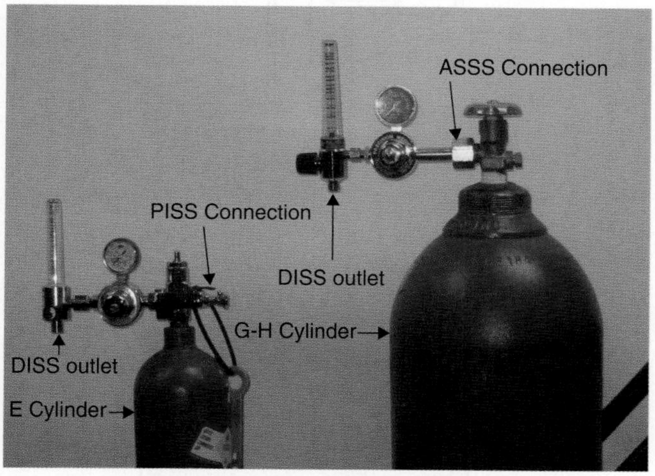

FIGURE 37-18 Comparison of safety systems used for compressed gases. The DISS connections are for low-pressure outlets (<200 psig). The ASSS provides for high-pressure connections with large cylinders. A variation of the ASSS entails a yoke and pin system (PISS) for connecting to small cylinders (AA through E).

Regulating Gas Pressure and Flow

Whatever the source of medical gas, for safe administration to a patient, the pressure and flow must be regulated. If the goal is solely a reduction in gas pressure, a **reducing valve** is used. For control of gas flow to a patient, a **flowmeter** is used. If control of both pressure and flow is needed, a regulator is used.

Cylinder gases such as O_2 and air exert a pressure that is much too high for use with respiratory care equipment. For use at the bedside, these high pressures must be reduced to a lower "working" level. In the United States, this working pressure is 50 psig. For bulk delivery systems with individual station outlets, built-in reducing valves decrease the delivered pressure to 50 psig. This standard pressure can be directly applied to power devices such as ventilators (see Chapter 42). However, if the goal is to control gas delivery to a patient for O_2 therapy or nebulized medication (see Chapters 36 and 38), a flowmeter must also be used.

High-Pressure Reducing Valves

There are two basic types of high-pressure reducing valves: single-stage and multiple-stage. Reducing valves are available as preset or adjustable. Although all of these valves function on the same principle, the design, features, and use are different. This section differentiates preset reducing valves and adjustable reducing valves and discusses multiple-stage reducing valves.

Preset Reducing Valve. Figure 37-19 shows the basic design of a high-pressure preset reducing valve. High-pressure gas (2200 psig for O_2) enters through the valve *(A)*, with the inlet pressure displayed on the pressure gauge *(B)*. The body of the valve is divided into a high-pressure chamber *(C)* and an ambient-pressure chamber *(D)* by a flexible diaphragm *(E)*. Attached to the diaphragm in the ambient-pressure chamber is a spring *(F)*, which is fixed to the other side of the chamber. Also attached to the diaphragm, but in the high-pressure chamber, is a valve stem *(G)* that sits on the high-pressure inlet *(H)*. Gas flows through the valve inlet *(H)* into the high-pressure chamber and on to the gas outlet *(I)*. The pressure chamber is supplied with a safety vent *(L)* preset to 200 psig to release pressure in the event of malfunction.

The spring tension is calibrated to give when the pressure on the diaphragm exceeds 50 psig. When this happens, the valve stem is pushed forward and closes the high-pressure inlet, preventing further entry of gas into the reducing valve. However, as long as gas is allowed to escape from the pressure chamber through the outlet *(I)*, the inlet valve remains open and allows gas flow. The regulator maintains a balance between outlet flow and inlet pressure. Automatic adjustment of the diaphragm-spring combination keeps the pressure in the high-pressure chamber at a near-constant 50 psig—hence the name *preset*. Preset reducing valves are normally used in conjunction with high-pressure gas cylinders to decrease the pressure to the standard 50 psig used with most respiratory care equipment.

Adjustable Reducing Valve. Although most respiratory care equipment works at the standard 50 psig, some devices need variable pressures. To provide variable outlet pressures from a high-pressure gas source, an adjustable reducing valve is needed. Figure 37-20 shows the basic design of a high-pressure adjustable reducing valve. As with the preset design, the inlet valve *(H)* remains open until the gas pressure exceeds the spring tension, displacing the diaphragm and blocking further gas entry. However, while the preset reducing valve provides a fixed pressure, the adjustable reducing valve allows a change in outlet pressure. Outlet pressure can be changed with a threaded hand control *(K)* attached to the end of the diaphragm spring. Changing the tension on the valve spring varies pressure over a wide range, usually between 0 psig and 100 psig.

The adjustable reducing valve commonly is used in combination with a Bourdon-type flow gauge (discussed later). The combination of a flowmeter with a reducing valve is called a **regulator.**

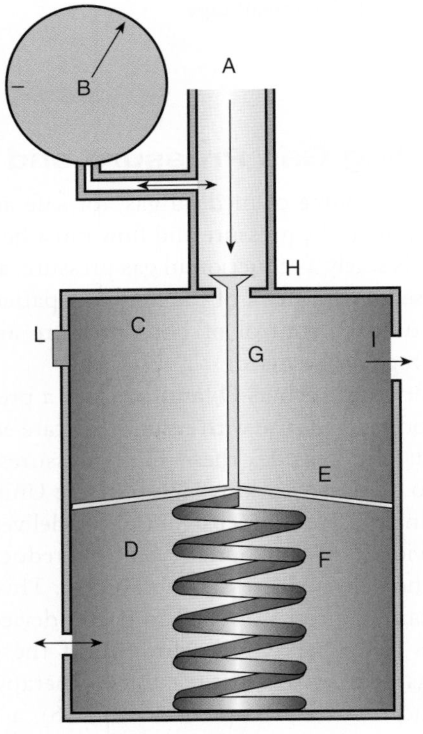

FIGURE 37-19 Preset high-pressure reducing valve.

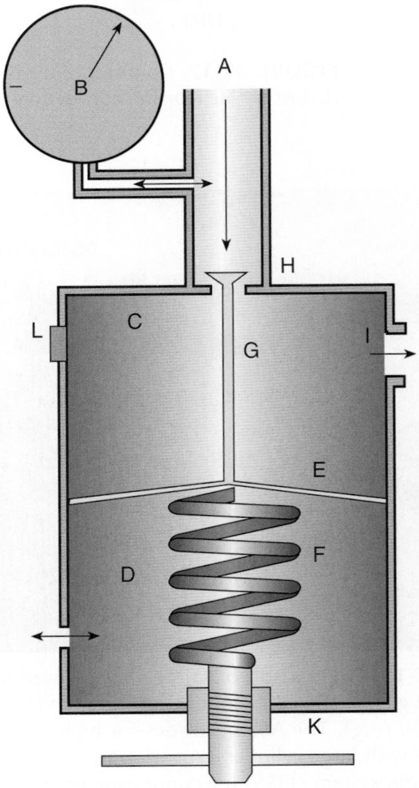

FIGURE 37-20 Adjustable high-pressure reducing valve.

Box 37-1 Safe Procedure for Setup of an Oxygen Cylinder and Reducing Valve or Regulator

1. Secure the cylinder according to the CGA guidelines. Verify the contents from the label that matches the color code and valve indexing.
2. Remove the protective cap or wrap, and inspect the cylinder valve to ensure that it is free of dirt, debris, and oil.
3. Warn any persons present that the cylinder valve is about to be "cracked" and that it will make some noise. Turn the cylinder valve away from persons present, stand to the side, and quickly open and close the valve. This removes any dust or small debris from the cylinder valve outlet.
4. Inspect the valve or regulator inlet for debris, dirt, and oil. Check the device label, and confirm that it is intended for high-pressure service and for use with the gas to be administered. O_2-reducing valves and regulators should have a label stating: *Oxygen: Use No Oil*.
5. After the valve or regulator inlet is confirmed to be free of contaminants, securely tighten (but do not force) the device onto the cylinder outlet. When making connections to the cylinder, use appropriate wrenches that are free of oil and grease. Never use pipe wrenches. Use only cylinder valve connections that conform to the ASSS and the PISS. Low-pressure connections must comply with the DISS or be noninterchangeable, low-pressure quick connects. Never connect fixed or adjustable orifices or metering devices directly to a cylinder without a pressure-reducing valve.
6. Confirm that the regulator or reducing valve is in the *off* or *closed* position, and slowly open the cylinder valve to pressurize the attached reducing valve or regulator. After pressurization has occurred, open the cylinder valve completely and turn it back one-fourth to one-half turn (this maneuver prevents a condition known as "valve freeze," in which the valve cannot be turned).

Multiple-Stage Reducing Valve. As the name suggests, a *multiple-stage reducing valve* reduces pressure in two or more steps. Multiple-stage reducing valves can be either preset or adjustable and can be combined with a flowmeter device as a true regulator. Two-stage reducing valves are used occasionally, and three-stage units are rarely needed. A two-stage reducing valve functions as two single-stage reducing valves working in series. Gas enters the first stage, where the pressure is reduced to an intermediate level (usually 200 to 700 psig). Gas then enters the second stage, where the pressure is decreased to working level (usually 50 psig). Because each pressure chamber has one safety relief vent, the user usually can determine the number of stages in a reducing valve by noting the number of relief vents present. Because they reduce pressure in multiple steps, these valves provide more precise and smooth flow control. However, they are larger and more expensive than single-stage reducing valves. For this reason, a multiple-stage reducing valve should be considered only if minimal fluctuations in pressure or flow are critical factors, as in research activities. For routine hospital work, single-stage reducing valves are satisfactory.

Proper Use of High-Pressure Reducing Valves. When a cylinder attached to a high-pressure reducing valve is open, gas undergoes rapid decompression followed by rapid recompression. Because the recompression is adiabatic (see Chapter 6), the gas temperature quickly increases. These rapid pressure and temperature changes are potentially hazardous. Rapid pressure swings can cause failure of reducing valve components.[19] Failed components can become high-velocity projectiles, endangering the practitioner and the patient. Rapid temperature changes can ignite combustible materials.[20] Ignition of combustible materials in the presence of 100% O_2 can cause an explosion. Box 37-1 provides guidelines for minimizing the risk associated with setting up O_2 cylinders with a high-pressure reducing valve or regulator.[1]

MINI CLINI

Leaky Connections

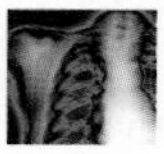

PROBLEM: Following standard procedure, the RT attaches a pressure-reducing valve to an O_2 cylinder. When the RT opens the cylinder valve, gas leaking at or near the connection can be heard.

SOLUTION: A leak usually indicates that the connection between the pressure-reducing valve and the cylinder outlet is not tight. If the cylinder outlet is a standard ASSS threaded connector, the connection is either cross-threaded or not properly seated and tightened. To solve this problem, the RT closes the cylinder valve and removes and reattaches the pressure-reducing valve, taking care to thread the connection properly and to tighten with a wrench. If the cylinder outlet is a pin-indexed connector, the RT closes the cylinder valve and removes the pressure-reducing valve. The RT checks to ensure that the nylon washer is present, in good condition, and properly fitted. The RT then reattaches the pressure-reducing valve, taking care to seat the connection properly and to hand tighten. If the leak continues after these corrective actions, it is likely that the pressure-reducing valve is malfunctioning and should be replaced.

Low-Pressure Gas Flowmeters

As with drugs, giving a medical gas to a patient requires knowledge of the dosage being delivered. Physicians often prescribe O_2 dosage as a flow, in liters per minute. In addition, certain gas-mixing equipment requires accurate knowledge of input flows, sometimes involving two or more gases. Flowmeters allow the rate of gas flow to a patient to be set and controlled. When the gas source is a high-pressure gas cylinder, a regulator (reducing valve plus flowmeter) is required. However, when the source is a bulk central supply system, the pressure has already been reduced to 50 psig by the time it reaches the outlet stations; this eliminates the need for pressure reduction and requires only a flowmeter.

Three categories of flowmeters are used in respiratory care: the flow restrictor, the **Bourdon gauge,** and the **Thorpe tube.** The Thorpe tube has two different designs: pressure compensated or not pressure compensated (uncompensated). Although uncompensated Thorpe tubes are rare, they may still be used at some institutions. For this reason, the principles underlying each of the four types of flow metering devices are compared and contrasted.

Flow Restrictor. The flow restrictor is the simplest and least expensive flowmeter device. As shown in Figure 37-21, a flow restrictor consists solely of a fixed orifice calibrated to deliver a specific flow at a constant pressure (50 psig). The operation of the flow restrictor is based on the principle of flow resistance, as described in Chapter 6. Specifically, the flow of gas through a tube can be quantified with the following equation:

$$R = \frac{P_1 - P_2}{V}$$

Rearranging the equation to solve for flow *(V)* yields the following:

$$V = \frac{P_1 - P_2}{R}$$

where *V* is the volumetric flow per unit time, P_1 is the pressure at the **upstream** point (point 1), P_2 is the pressure at the **downstream** point (point 2), and *R* is the total resistance to gas flow.

By design, a flow restrictor requires a source of constant pressure (usually 50 psig). As long as the source pressure remains fixed, $P_1 - P_2$ should stay constant. With a fixed-size orifice, the flow resistance *(R)* also remains constant. The rate of gas flow through a flow restrictor can be increased by increasing P_1 (upstream pressure) or by selecting a larger orifice size. Both fixed and adjustable orifice flow restrictors are used clinically. Commercially produced flow restrictors are calibrated at 50 psig. Table 37-6 summarizes the advantages and disadvantages of flow restrictors.

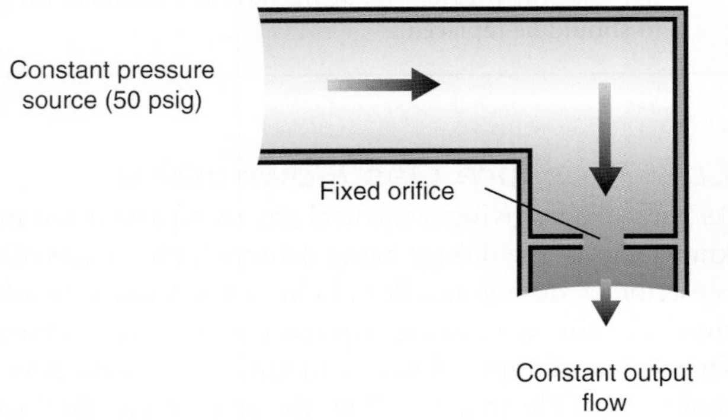

FIGURE 37-21 Flow restrictor.

Bourdon Gauge. A Bourdon gauge (Figure 37-22) is a flowmeter device that is always used in combination with an adjustable pressure-reducing valve. Similar to the flow restrictor, the Bourdon gauge uses a fixed orifice. In contrast to the flow restrictor, the Bourdon gauge operates under variable pressures, as adjusted with the pressure-reducing valve. The Bourdon gauge is a fixed-orifice, variable-pressure flowmeter, so increasing the upstream pressure increases gas flow out of the device unless downstream pressure also increases.

As shown in Figure 37-23, a Bourdon gauge has a calibrated fixed orifice *(A)*, which creates outflow resistance. The gauge itself is attached to the flow stream with a connector *(B)* located proximal to the orifice. Inside the gauge is a curved, hollow, closed tube *(C)* that responds to pressure changes by changing shape. The force of gas pressure tends to straighten the tube, causing its distal end to move. This motion is transmitted to a gear assembly and indicator needle *(D)*. A numbered scale is calibrated to read the needle movement in units of flow (liters per minute).

TABLE 37-6

Advantages and Disadvantages of Flow Restrictors

Advantages	Disadvantages
Low-cost, simple, reliable (no moving parts)	Different versions required for different flows
Cannot be set to incorrect flow	Accuracy varies with changes in source and downstream pressures
Can be used in any position (gravity-independent)	Cannot be used with high-resistance equipment

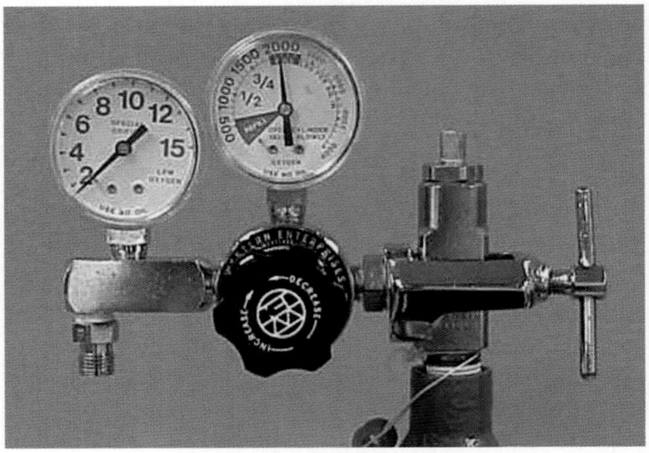

FIGURE 37-22 Bourdon gauge regulator.

As with the flow restrictor with fixed orifice, the output flow of the Bourdon gauge is proportional to the driving pressure. However, the Bourdon gauge provides a continuous range of flow, which the user adjusts by altering the driving pressure. Although the gauge actually measures pressure changes, it displays the corresponding flow.

As with a flow restrictor, gravity does not affect a Bourdon gauge. The Bourdon gauge is the best choice when a flowmeter cannot be maintained in an upright position. This situation is common when a patient is being transported with a portable O_2 source. In these instances, keeping the E cylinder upright is seldom easy, and movement of both the O_2 supply and the patient is common. Combined with its continuous range of flows, this feature makes the Bourdon gauge the metering device of choice for patient transport.

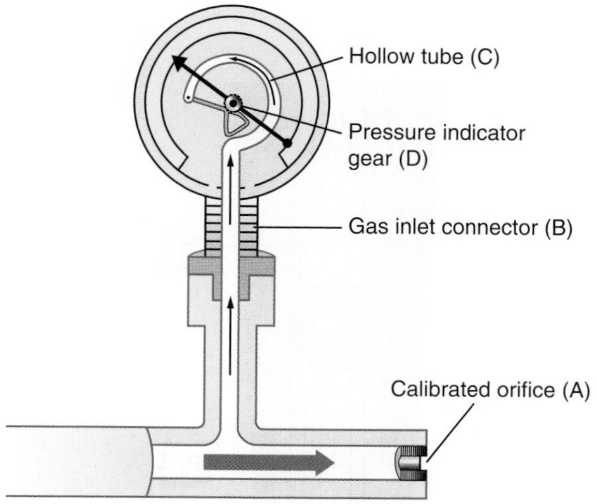

FIGURE 37-23 Components of a Bourdon pressure gauge. See text for more information.

The main disadvantage of the Bourdon gauge is its inaccuracy when pressure distal to the orifice (downstream pressures) changes. Specifically, if downstream pressure increases (as when high-resistance equipment is used), the pressure difference across the orifice and actual output flow decrease. However, the Bourdon gauge flow reading depends on upstream pressure, which stays constant. In this situation, the gauge reading is falsely higher than the actual delivered flow. Because it measures upstream pressure, the gauge registers flow even when the outlet is completely blocked (Figure 37-24). A user who needs accurate flow when using a device that creates high resistance should not select a Bourdon gauge. A compensated Thorpe tube should be used instead.

Integrated O_2 cylinders (Figure 37-25), including the Grab 'n Go System (Praxair, Inc, Danbury, Connecticut), have combined the O_2 cylinder with a pressure regulator and an adjustable flow restrictor to meter O_2 flow. These portable O_2 systems eliminate the need for separate O_2 tanks, Bourdon gauge regulators, and O_2 keys or wrenchs (needed to turn on standard E-cylinders). These integrated systems virtually eliminate problems and delays associated with incorrectly mounted regulators. The practitioner simply selects the flow on the flow-adjusting knob and connects the O_2 tubing to the system connection and the patient.

Thorpe Tube. The Thorpe tube flowmeter (Figure 37-26) is always attached to a 50-psig source, either a preset pressure-reducing valve or a bedside station outlet. Compared with the flow restrictor and the Bourdon gauge, the Thorpe tube functions as a variable-orifice, constant-pressure flowmeter, so increasing the size of the orifice

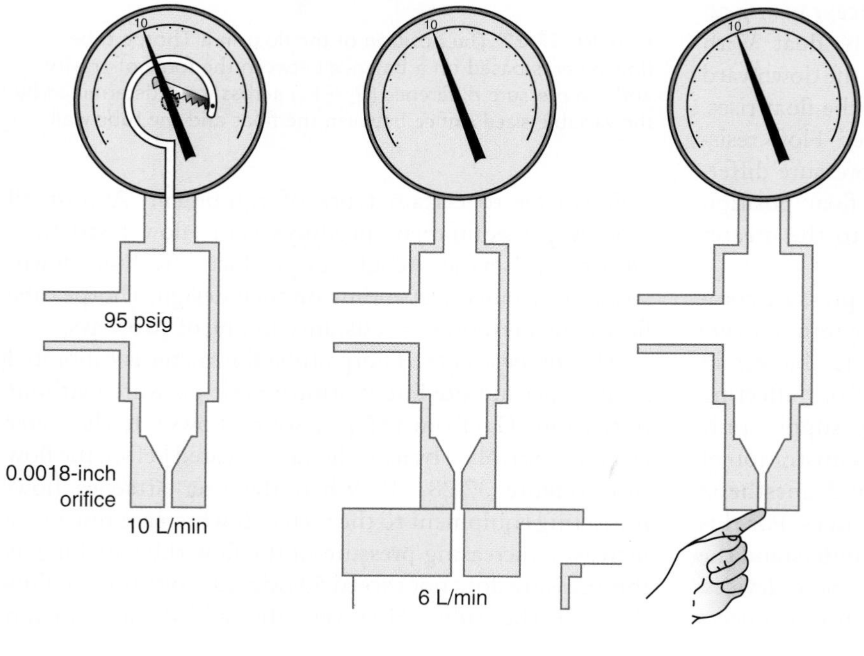

FIGURE 37-24 Bourdon performance when downstream pressures increase as a result of high-resistance equipment or blockage. *Left,* Normal state with fixed orifice and no downstream resistance results in an accurate flow reading. *Center,* High-resistance nebulizer increases downstream pressure, or back pressure. The result is a falsely high reading (10 L/min vs. actual flow of 6 L/min). *Right,* Complete blockage (zero flow) results in flow reading on gauge.

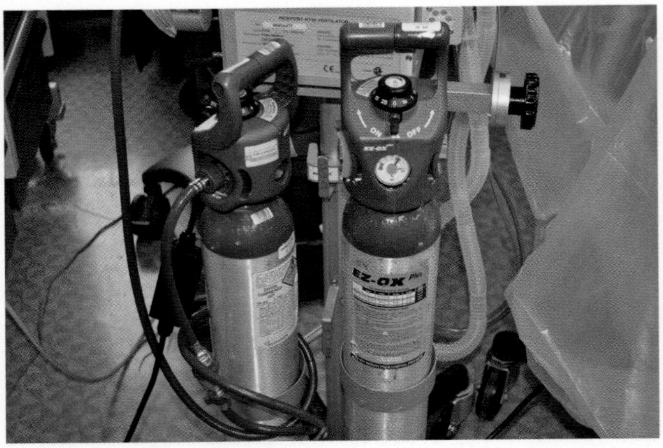

FIGURE 37-25 Grab 'n Go System (Praxair, Inc, Danbury, Connecticut).

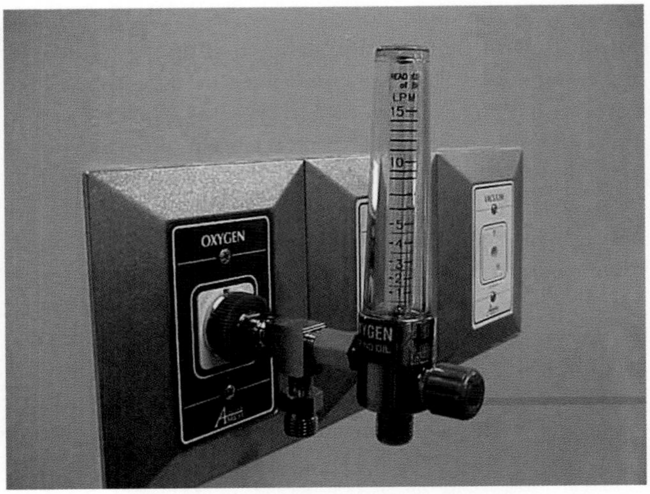

FIGURE 37-26 Thorpe tube flowmeter.

increases the gas flow. Figure 37-27 shows how a Thorpe tube works. The key component in this device is a tapered transparent tube that contains a float. The diameter of the tube increases from bottom to top. Gas flow suspends the float against the force of gravity. To read the flow, one simply compares the float position with an adjacent calibrated scale, normally calibrated in liters per minute.

Although the Bourdon gauge measures pressure, the Thorpe tube is used to measure true flow. Flow measurement involves the complex interaction of gravity and fluid dynamics. When gas begins to flow into a Thorpe tube, the initial pressure difference lifts the float. As the needle valve is opened, the float rises in the widening tube, the space available for flow around it increases, and resistance to flow decreases. The float ultimately stabilizes when the pressure difference across the float (an upward force) equals the opposing downward force of gravity.

As the needle valve of the flowmeter is opened, the increase in flow initially disrupts this balance, causing an increase in the pressure difference across the float. With the upward pressure difference greater than the downward force of gravity, the float rises. However, as the float rises, the available "orifice" increases in diameter. Flow resistance around the float decreases, and the pressure difference again equilibrates with gravity. The float position stabilizes at a higher level, proportionate to the greater flow around it.

Thorpe tubes come in two basic designs: pressure compensated and pressure uncompensated. The term *pressure compensation* refers to a design that prevents changes in downstream resistance, or back pressure, from affecting meter accuracy. All manufacturers now supply only pressure-compensated Thorpe tubes for administration of medical gas. However, some ventilators and anesthesia machines still use uncompensated Thorpe tubes. For this reason, clinicians using these devices must understand the effect of back pressure on the accuracy of these devices. Downstream resistance increases when the user connects

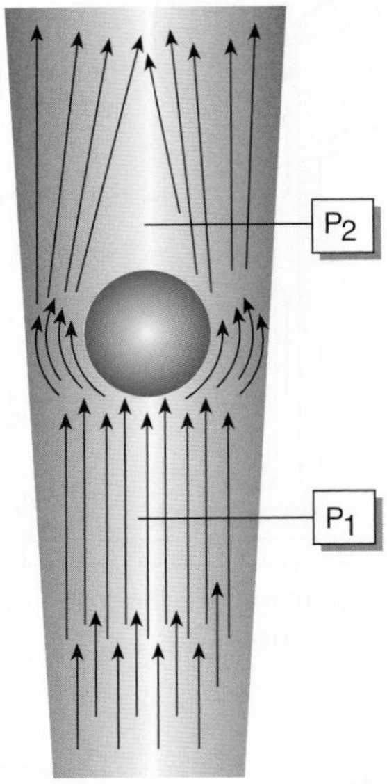

FIGURE 37-27 The position of the float in a Thorpe tube flowmeter is based on a balance between the force of gravity and the pressure difference ($P_2 - P_1$) across it, as determined by the variable-sized orifice between the float and the tube wall.

a flowmeter to certain types of equipment. Almost all therapy gas equipment produces some flow restriction. Devices such as jet nebulizers produce very high downstream resistance. Depending on their design, Thorpe tube flowmeters respond to resistance in one of two ways.

The *uncompensated* Thorpe tube flowmeter is calibrated in liters per minute but at atmospheric pressure (without restriction). Gas from a 50-psig source flows into the meter at a rate controlled by a needle valve located before the flow tube (Figure 37-28, *A*). When the user attaches flow-restricting equipment to the meter, downstream resistance increases, increasing pressure in the flow tube. As long as this pressure does not exceed 50 psig, gas continues to flow through the tube. However, the added downstream

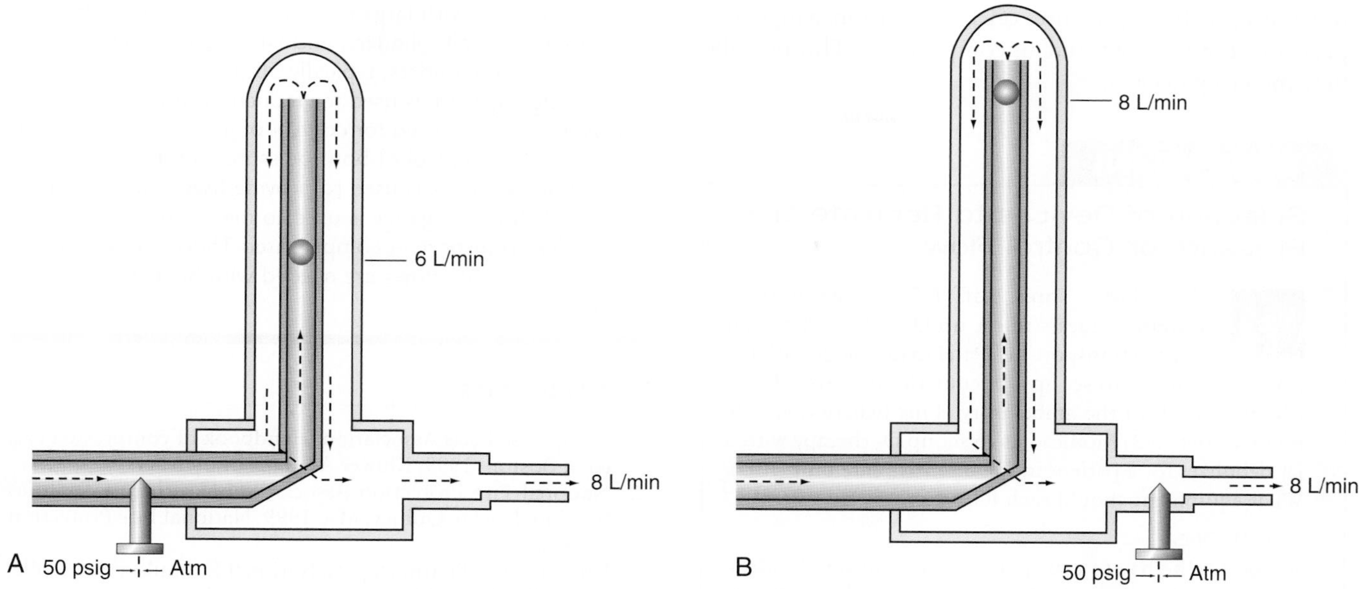

FIGURE 37-28 Comparison of pressure-uncompensated **(A)** and pressure-compensated **(B)** Thorpe tube flowmeters. In the pressure-uncompensated flowmeter, the flow-control valve is proximal to the meter, and the gauge records less than the actual output. In the pressure-compensated flowmeter, location of the valve distal to the meter correlates the gauge reading with the output.

resistance increases the pressure in the flow tube above atmospheric pressure. At higher pressures, a greater amount of gas flows through a given restriction than at atmospheric pressure. With the float at a given height, more gas flows through the tube than is indicated on the scale. Under these conditions, an uncompensated Thorpe tube falsely shows a flow lower than that actually delivered to the patient.[4]

In contrast, the scale of the compensated Thorpe tube flowmeter is calibrated at 50 psig instead of at atmospheric pressure. Its flow control needle valve is placed after (distal to) the flow tube (see Figure 37-28, *B*). The entire meter operates at constant 50-psig pressure. Knowing that the compensated Thorpe tube operates at 50 psig helps identify it. When a compensated Thorpe tube is connected to a 50-psig gas source with the needle valve closed, the float "jumps" and then returns to zero as the Thorpe tube is pressurized. Because the entire meter operates at constant pressure, an increase in downstream resistance increases pressure distal to the needle valve only. As long as the downstream pressure does not exceed 50 psig (in which case flow ceases), the position of the float accurately reflects actual outlet flow. For this reason, the pressure-compensated Thorpe tube is the preferred instrument in most clinical situations.

The only factor limiting the use of a pressure-compensated Thorpe tube is gravity. Because it is accurate only in an upright position, a Thorpe tube is not the ideal choice for patient transport. In these cases, the gravity-independent Bourdon gauge is a satisfactory alternative. Figure 37-29 summarizes the effects of downstream

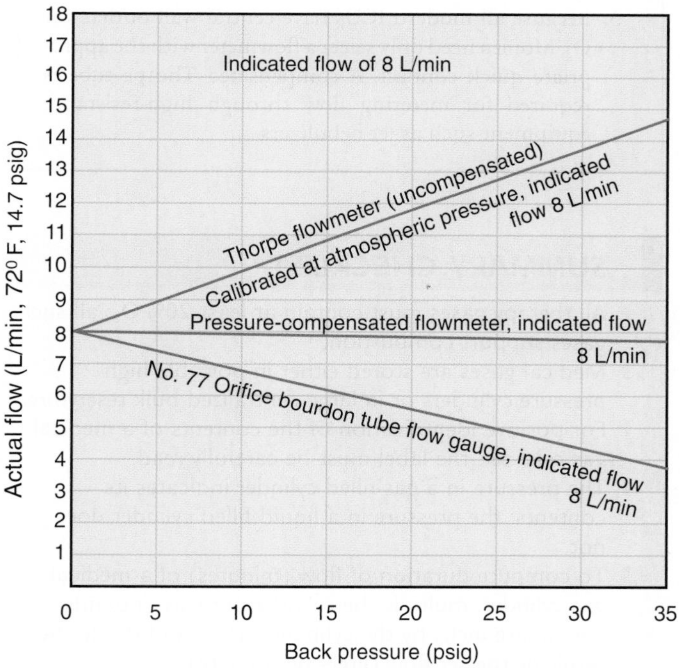

FIGURE 37-29 Comparative accuracy of flowmeter devices against increasing downstream pressure (back pressure). With the pressure-compensated Thorpe tube, indicated flow equals actual flow, regardless of downstream pressure. With the uncompensated Thorpe tube, indicated flow is progressively lower than actual flow as downstream pressure increases. With the Bourdon gauge, indicated flow is progressively higher than actual flow as downstream pressure increases. (Modified from McPherson SP, Spearman CB: Respiratory therapy equipment, ed 5, St Louis, 1995, Mosby. Modified from Puritan-Bennett Corp, Los Angeles, California.)

resistance, or back pressure, on the Bourdon gauge and pressure-compensated and uncompensated Thorpe tube flow metering devices.

MINI CLINI

Selection of Devices to Regulate Gas Pressure or Control Flow

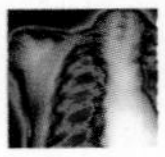

PROBLEM: Three staff RTs are given three separate requests to set up O_2. (1) Mark has an order to transport Ms. Patel to radiology with O_2. (2) Carmen needs to set up a pneumatically powered ventilator with O_2 in the ambulatory clinic (where there are no O_2 outlets). (3) Monica has to set up O_2 therapy with a jet nebulizer for a patient in the intensive care unit (ICU). What equipment should each RT select?

SOLUTIONS:

1. Because he has to transport a patient using O_2, Mark should select an E cylinder with an adjustable regulator that includes a Bourdon gauge (unaffected by gravity) or an integrated O_2 cylinder that includes an adjustable flow restrictor.
2. Because pneumatically powered ventilators require 50 psig and no central outlets are available, Carmen needs a preset (50 psig) reducing valve and a large G/H O_2 cylinder.
3. Because all modern ICUs have central wall outlets for O_2, Monica need only select a flowmeter with the appropriate quick connect. A compensated Thorpe tube is required for metering flow through high-resistance equipment such as jet nebulizers.

SUMMARY CHECKLIST

- All therapy gases must contain at least 20% O_2; all such gases support combustion.
- Medical gases are stored either in portable high-pressure cylinders or in large centralized bulk reservoirs.
- For positive identification of the contents of a medical gas cylinder, the label must be carefully read.
- The pressure in a gas-filled cylinder indicates its contents; the pressure in a liquid-filled cylinder does not.
- To compute duration of flow (minutes) of a medical gas cylinder, multiply the cylinder pressure (pounds per square inch) by the cylinder factor, and divide the result by the set flow (liters per minute).
- Gas supply systems provide gas at 50 psig to outlets throughout a facility through a network of pipes. Such a system must include both zone valves for repairs or fire and alarms to warn of failure.
- Failure of a bulk gas supply system can threaten the lives of patients receiving O_2 therapy or being supported with pneumatically powered devices. A protocol must exist to deal with this emergency.
- Indexed safety systems help prevent misconnections between equipment. The ASSS provides high-pressure connections with large cylinders; the PISS does the same for small cylinders; and DISS connections are for low-pressure outlets, typically 50 psig.
- A reducing valve is used for reduction of gas pressure. A flowmeter is used for control of gas flow. A regulator is used for control of both pressure and flow.
- A flow restrictor is used to provide fixed low flows of O_2. A Bourdon gauge is used to meter flow during patient transport. A compensated Thorpe tube is used when accurate flows are needed with high-resistance equipment.

References

1. Compressed Gas Association: Handbook of compressed gas, ed 4, Boston, 1999, Kluwer Academic Publishers.
2. National Fire Protection Association: Health care facilities handbook, ed 6, Quincy, MA, 1999, National Fire Protection Association.
3. United States Pharmacopeia/National Formulary, Rockville, MD: 2000, United States Pharmacopeial Convention.
4. Cairo JM, Pilbeam SP: Mosby's respiratory care equipment, ed 8, St Louis, 2010, Mosby.
5. Compressed Gas Association: Compressed air for human respiration (CGA G-7)/ANSI Z86.1), Arlington, VA, 1989, Compressed Gas Association.
6. American Academy of Pediatrics: Policy statement: use of inhaled nitric oxide. Pediatrics 106:344, 2000 (Reaffirmed December 2009, Pediatrics 125:e98, April 2010).
7. Finer NN, Barrington KJ: Nitric oxide for respiratory failure in infants born at or near term. Cochrane Database Syst Rev (4):CD000399, 2008.
8. Barrington KJ, Finer NN: Inhaled nitric oxide for respiratory failure in preterm infants. Cochrane Database of Syst Rev (12):CD000509, 2010.
9. United States Department of Transportation: Qualification, maintenance and use of cylinders, 180.213. Requalification markings (revised June 12, 2006), Washington, DC.
10. Compressed Gas Association: Standard color marking of compressed gas containers for medical use (CGA C-9), Arlington, VA, 1989, Compressed Gas Association.
11. Compressed Gas Association: Characteristics and safe handling of medical gases (P-2), Arlington, VA, 1989, Compressed Gas Association.
12. Cylinders with unmixed helium/oxygen. Health Devices 19:146, 1990.
13. Bernstein DB, Rosenberg AD: Intraoperative hypoxia from nitrogen tanks with oxygen fittings. Anesth Analg 1997; 84:225–227.
14. Stoller JK, Stefanak M, Orens D, et al: The hospital oxygen supply: an "O2K" problem. Respir Care 5:300–305, 2000.
15. Schumacher SD, Brockwell RC, Andrews J, et al: Bulk liquid oxygen supply failure. Anesthesiology 100:186, 2004.
16. Compressed Gas Association: Compressed gas cylinder valve outlet and inlet connections (ANSI/CGA V-1), Arlington, VA, 1989, Compressed Gas Association.
17. Compressed Gas Association: Diameter index safety systems (CGA V-5), Arlington, VA, 1989, Compressed Gas Association.
18. Mismating of precision brand medical gas fittings. Health Devices 19:333, 1990.
19. Allberry RA: Minireg failure (letter). Anaesth Intensive Care 17:234, 1989.
20. West GA, Primeau P: Nonmedical hazards of long-term oxygen therapy. Respir Care 28:906, 1983.

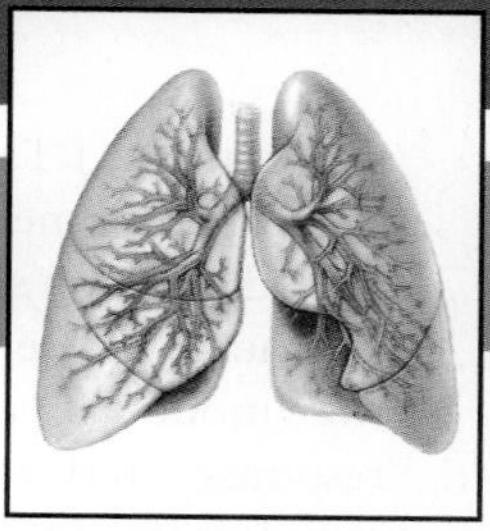

Chapter 38

Medical Gas Therapy

ALBERT J. HEUER

CHAPTER OBJECTIVES

After reading this chapter you will be able to:

- Describe when oxygen (O_2) therapy is needed.
- Assess the need for O_2 therapy.
- Describe what precautions and complications are associated with O_2 therapy.
- Select an O_2 delivery system appropriate for the respiratory care plan.
- Describe how to administer O_2 to adults, children, and infants.
- Describe how to check for proper function and to identify and correct malfunctions of O_2 delivery systems.
- Describe how to evaluate and monitor a patient's response to O_2 therapy.
- Describe how to modify or recommend modification of O_2 therapy on the basis of patient response.
- Describe how to implement protocol-based O_2 therapy.
- Identify what indications, complications, and hazards apply to hyperbaric O_2 therapy.
- Identify when and how to provide nitric oxide therapy.
- Identify when and how to administer helium-O_2 therapy.

CHAPTER OUTLINE

KEY TERMS

atmospheric pressure absolute (ATA)
bronchopneumonia
bronchopulmonary dysplasia
croup
cyclic guanosine 3′,5′-monophosphate (cGMP)
exudative
heliox therapy
high-flow system
hyperbaric oxygen (HBO) therapy
low-flow system
neovascularization
neutral thermal environment (NTE)
nitric oxide (NO)
reservoir system
retinopathy of prematurity (ROP)

Gas therapy is the most common mode of respiratory care. The origins of the field parallel the introduction of oxygen (O_2) as a medical treatment. Since that time, understanding of the various medical gases and methods to deliver them has changed. Of particular importance is the acknowledgment that most medical gases are drugs. As with any drug, respiratory therapists (RTs) recommend and administer a dosage, monitor the response, alter therapy accordingly, and record these steps in relation to the care plan in the patient record. In this context, RTs must have more than technical knowledge of equipment. In consultation with the physician, a skilled clinician should be able to assess the patient's need for therapy, determine the desired goals of therapy, select the mode of administration, monitor the patient's response, and recommend and implement timely and appropriate changes.

OXYGEN THERAPY

Consensus exists among clinicians about the proper use of O_2 therapy.[1-4] As the primary member of the health care team responsible for O_2 administration, the RT must be well versed in the goals and objectives of this therapy and its use in clinical practice.

General Goals and Clinical Objectives

The overall goal of O_2 therapy is to maintain adequate tissue oxygenation, while minimizing cardiopulmonary work. Specific clinical objectives for O_2 therapy are the following:

- Correct documented or suspected acute hypoxemia
- Decrease symptoms associated with chronic hypoxemia
- Decrease the workload hypoxemia imposes on the cardiopulmonary system

Correcting Hypoxemia

O_2 therapy corrects hypoxemia by increasing alveolar and blood levels of O_2. Correction of hypoxemia is the most tangible objective of O_2 therapy and the easiest to measure and document.

Decreasing Symptoms of Hypoxemia

In addition to relieving hypoxemia, O_2 therapy can help relieve the symptoms associated with certain lung disorders. Specifically, patients with chronic obstructive pulmonary disease (COPD) and some forms of interstitial lung disease report less dyspnea when receiving supplemental O_2.[5] O_2 therapy also may improve mental function among patients with chronic hypoxemia.[6]

Minimizing Cardiopulmonary Workload

The cardiopulmonary system compensates for hypoxemia by increasing ventilation and cardiac output. In cases of acute hypoxemia, supplemental O_2 can decrease demands on both the heart and the lungs. Patients with hypoxemia breathing air can achieve acceptable arterial oxygenation only by increasing ventilation. Increased ventilatory demand increases the work of breathing. In these cases, O_2 therapy can reduce both the high ventilatory demand and the work of breathing.

Patients with arterial hypoxemia can maintain acceptable tissue oxygenation only by increasing cardiac output. Because O_2 therapy increases blood O_2 content, the heart does not have to pump as much blood per minute to meet tissue demands. This reduced workload is particularly important when the heart is already stressed by disease or injury, as in myocardial infarction, sepsis, or trauma.

Hypoxemia causes pulmonary vasoconstriction and pulmonary hypertension. Pulmonary vasoconstriction and hypertension increase workload on the right side of the heart. For patients with chronic hypoxemia, this increased workload over the long-term can lead to right ventricular failure (cor pulmonale). O_2 therapy can reverse pulmonary vasoconstriction and decrease right ventricular workload.[7]

Clinical Practice Guideline

To guide practitioners in safe and effective patient care, the American Association for Respiratory Care (AARC) has developed and published clinical practice guidelines for O_2 therapy. Excerpts from the AARC guideline on O_2 therapy in acute care hospitals appear in Clinical Practice Guideline 38-1.[2] Additional AARC guidelines for O_2 therapy in the home or an extended care facility[3] and for selection of O_2 delivery devices for neonatal and pediatric patients[4] are provided in Chapters 48 and 51.

Assessing the Need for Oxygen Therapy

There are three basic ways to determine whether a patient needs O_2 therapy. The first is the use of laboratory measures to document hypoxemia. Second, a patient's need for O_2 therapy can be based on the specific clinical problem or condition. Third, hypoxemia has many manifestations, such as tachypnea, tachycardia, cyanosis, and distressed overall appearance. Astute bedside techniques of assessment for these and other symptoms can be used to determine the need for supplemental O_2.

Laboratory measures for documenting hypoxemia include hemoglobin saturation and partial pressure of oxygen (PO_2), as determined by either invasive or noninvasive means (see Chapter 18). Threshold criteria defining hypoxemia with these measures are described in the AARC clinical practice guideline (see Clinical Practice Guideline 38-1).[2]

O_2 therapy is needed for patients with disorders associated with hypoxemia. Examples are postoperative patients; patients with carbon monoxide or cyanide poisoning, shock, trauma, or acute myocardial infarction, and some premature infants.[1,2,8]

Careful bedside physical assessment can disclose a patient's need for O_2 therapy. Table 38-1 summarizes the common respiratory, cardiovascular, and neurologic signs used in the detection of hypoxia. The RT combines this information with more quantitative measures such as arterial blood gas results to confirm inadequate oxygenation. The patient care team often relies on the RT to recommend administration of supplemental O_2 based on quantitative and qualitative information.

38-1 Oxygen Therapy

AARC Clinical Practice Guideline (Excerpts)

INDICATIONS

- Documented hypoxemia as evidenced by
  - PaO_2 less than 60 mm Hg or SaO_2 less than 90% in subjects breathing room air
  - PaO_2 or SaO_2 below desirable range for a specific clinical situation
- Acute care situations in which hypoxemia is suspected
- Severe trauma
- Acute myocardial infarction
- Short-term therapy or surgical intervention (e.g., postanesthesia recovery)

CONTRAINDICATIONS

- With a few exceptions, no specific contraindications to O_2 therapy exist when indications are present.
- Certain delivery devices are contraindicated, such as nasal cannulas and nasopharyngeal catheters in pediatric and neonatal patients with nasal obstruction.

PRECAUTIONS AND/OR POSSIBLE COMPLICATIONS

- PaO_2 greater than or equal to 60 mm Hg; ventilator depression may occur rarely in spontaneously breathing patients with elevated $PaCO_2$
- With FiO_2 greater than 0.5, absorption atelectasis, O_2 toxicity, or depression of ciliary or leukocyte function may occur
- In premature infants, PaO_2 greater than 80 mm Hg may contribute to retinopathy of prematurity
- In infants with certain congenital heart lesions such as hypoplastic left heart syndrome, high PaO_2 can compromise the balance between pulmonary and systemic blood flow
- In infants, O_2 flow directed at the face may stimulate an alteration in respiratory pattern
- Increased FiO_2 can worsen lung injury in patients with paraquat poisoning or patients receiving bleomycin
- During laser bronchoscopy or tracheostomy, minimal FiO_2 should be used to avoid intratracheal ignition
- Fire hazard increased in the presence of high FiO_2
- Bacterial contamination can occur when nebulizers or humidifiers are used

ASSESSMENT OF NEED

Need is determined by measurement of inadequate PaO_2 or SaO_2, or both, by invasive or noninvasive methods and the presence of clinical indicators.

ASSESSMENT OF OUTCOME

Outcome is determined by clinical and physiologic assessment to establish adequacy of patient response to therapy.

MONITORING

Patient

- Clinical assessment including but not limited to cardiac, pulmonary, and neurologic status
- Assessment of physiologic parameters (PaO_2, SaO_2, SpO_2) in any patient treated with O_2 (consider need or indication to adjust FiO_2 for increased levels of activity and exercise) in conjunction with the initiation of therapy or
  - Within 12 hours of initiation with FiO_2 less than 0.40
  - Within 8 hours with FiO_2 of 0.40 or greater (including postanesthesia recovery)
  - Within 72 hours in acute myocardial infarction
  - Within 2 hours for any patient with principal diagnosis of COPD
  - Within 1 hour for the neonate
- Appropriate O_2 therapy use protocol is suggested as a method to decrease waste and to realize increased cost savings

Equipment

- All O_2 delivery systems should be checked at least once per day
- More frequent checks by calibrated analyzer are necessary in systems
  - Susceptible to variation in FiO_2 (e.g., hood, high-flow blending systems)
  - Applied to patients with artificial airways
  - Delivering a heated gas mixture
  - Applied to patients who are clinically unstable or who require FiO_2 greater than 0.50
  - Equipment supplying supplemental O_2 to newborn or premature infants

For complete guidelines, see American Association for Respiratory Care: Clinical practice guideline: selection of an oxygen delivery device for neonatal and pediatric patients, Respir Care 47:707, 2002; and American Association for Respiratory Care: Clinical practice guideline: oxygen therapy for adults in the acute care facility, Respir Care 47:717, 2002.

Precautions and Hazards of Supplemental Oxygen

Excerpts from the relevant AARC clinical practice guidelines (see Clinical Practice Guideline 38-1) outline the major precautions and hazards associated with administration of supplemental O_2.[2] Five of these hazards are common enough to warrant additional discussion.

TABLE 38-1

Clinical Signs of Hypoxia

Finding	Mild to Moderate	Severe
Respiratory	Tachypnea Dyspnea Paleness	Tachypnea Dyspnea Cyanosis
Cardiovascular	Tachycardia	Tachycardia, eventual bradycardia, arrhythmia
	Mild hypertension, peripheral vasoconstriction	Hypertension and eventual hypotension
Neurologic	Restlessness Disorientation Headaches Lassitude	Somnolence Confusion Distressed appearance Blurred vision Tunnel vision Loss of coordination Impaired judgment Slow reaction time Manic-depressive activity Coma

Oxygen Toxicity

O_2 toxicity primarily affects the lungs and the central nervous system (CNS).[9-11] Two primary factors determine the harmful effects of O_2: PO_2 and exposure time (Figure 38-1). The higher the PO_2 and the longer the exposure, the greater the likelihood of damage. Effects on the CNS, including tremors, twitching, and convulsions, tend to occur only when a patient is breathing O_2 at pressures greater than 1 atm (hyperbaric pressure). Pulmonary effects can also occur with enriched O_2 environments at normal atmospheric pressures.

Table 38-2 summarizes the physiologic response to breathing 100% O_2 at sea level. A patient exposed to a high PO_2 for a prolonged period has signs similar to **bronchopneumonia.** Patchy infiltrates appear on chest

TABLE 38-2

Physiologic Responses of Healthy Individuals to Exposure to 100% Inspired Oxygen

Exposure Time (hr)	Physiologic Response
0-12	Normal pulmonary function Tracheobronchitis Substernal chest pain
12-24	Decreasing vital capacity
25-30	Decreasing lung compliance Increasing $P(A-a)O_2$ Decreasing exercise PO_2
30-72	Decreasing diffusing capacity

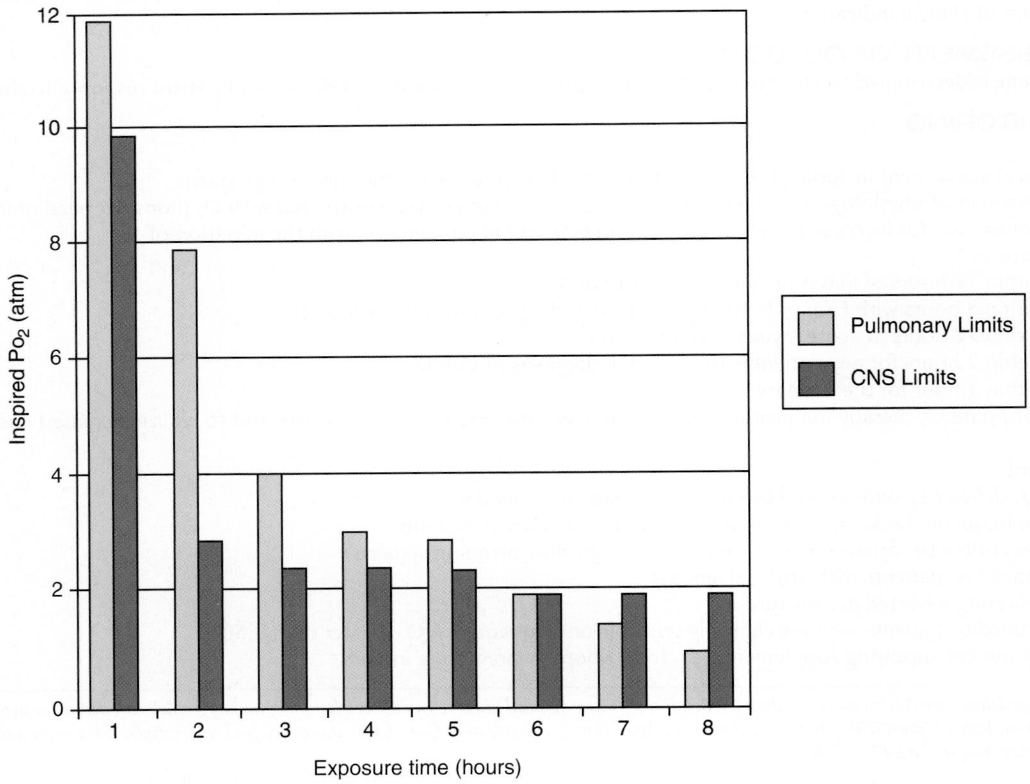

FIGURE 38-1 Relationship between PO_2 and exposure time causing O_2 toxicity.

radiographs and usually are most prominent in the lower lung fields.

Underlying the gross clinical signs is major alveolar injury. Exposure to high PO_2 first damages the capillary endothelium. Interstitial edema follows and thickens the alveolar-capillary membrane. If the process continues, type I alveolar cells are destroyed, and type II cells proliferate. An **exudative** phase follows, resulting from alveolar fluid buildup, which leads to a low ventilation/perfusion ratio, physiologic shunting, and hypoxemia. In the end stages, hyaline membranes form in the alveolar region, and pulmonary fibrosis and hypertension develop.

As the lung injury worsens, blood oxygenation deteriorates. If this progressive hypoxemia is managed with additional O_2, the toxic effects worsen (Figure 38-2). However, if the patient can be kept alive while fractional inspired oxygen concentration (FiO_2) is decreased, the pulmonary damage sometimes resolves.

The toxicity of O_2 is caused by overproduction of O_2 free radicals. O_2 free radicals are by-products of cellular metabolism. If unchecked, these radicals can severely damage or kill cells.[9] Normally, however, special enzymes such as superoxide dismutase inactivate the O_2 free radicals before they can do serious damage. Antioxidants such as vitamin E, vitamin C, and beta-carotene also can defend against O_2 free radicals.

These defenses normally are adequate to protect cells exposed to air. In the presence of high PO_2, however, free radicals can overwhelm the antioxidant system and cause cell damage. Cell damage provokes an immune response and causes tissue infiltration by neutrophils and macrophages. These scavenger cells release inflammatory mediators that worsen the initial injury. At the same time, local neutrophils and platelets may release more free radicals, which continue the process.

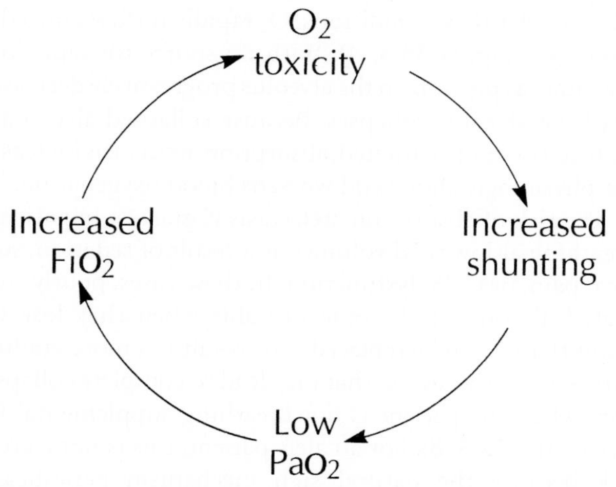

FIGURE 38-2 The vicious circle that can occur in managing hypoxemia with high FiO_2. High FiO_2 can be toxic to the lung parenchyma and cause further physiologic shunting. Increased shunting worsens the hypoxemia, necessitating higher FiO_2. (Modified from Flenley DC: Long-term oxygen therapy—state of the art. Respir Care 28:876, 1983.)

Exactly how much O_2 is safe is the subject of debate. Results of most studies indicate that adults can breathe up to 50% for extended periods without major lung damage.[12] Rather than applying strict cutoffs, one can weigh both FiO_2 and exposure time in assessing the risks of high PO_2 (see the accompanying Rule of Thumb).[13] The goal always should be to use the lowest possible FiO_2 compatible with adequate tissue oxygenation.

RULE OF THUMB

Avoiding Oxygen Toxicity

Limit patient exposure to 100% O_2 to less than 24 hours whenever possible. High FiO_2 is acceptable if the concentration can be decreased to 70% within 2 days and 50% or less in 5 days.

Because the growing lung may be more sensitive to O_2, more caution is needed with infants. High PO_2 also is associated with retinopathy of prematurity (ROP) and **bronchopulmonary dysplasia** in infants.

Regardless of approach, supplemental O_2 never should be withheld from hypoxic patients. Although the toxic effects of high O_2 concentrations can be serious, it is not FiO_2 but rather PO_2 that results in such harmful effects. If a patient needs a high FiO_2 to maintain adequate tissue O_2, the patient should receive it.

Depression of Ventilation

When breathing moderate to high O_2 concentrations, a very small percentage of patients with COPD and chronic hypercapnia tend to ventilate less.[14] Decreases in ventilation of nearly 20% have been observed in these patients with accompanying elevations in arterial partial pressure of carbon dioxide ($PaCO_2$) of 20 to 23 mm Hg.[15] However, this hypoventilation is not typical of patients with COPD, and although these patients should always be carefully monitored, appropriate management of hypoxemia should never be avoided because of concern for O_2-induced hypoventilation.

The primary reason some patients with COPD hypoventilate when given O_2 is most likely suppression of the hypoxic drive. In these patients, the normal response to high partial pressure of carbon dioxide (PCO_2) is blunted, the primary stimulus to breathe being lack of O_2 as sensed by the peripheral chemoreceptors. The increase in the blood O_2 level in these patients suppresses peripheral chemoreceptors, depresses ventilatory drive, and elevates the PCO_2.[16,17] High blood O_2 levels may disrupt the normal ventilation/perfusion balance and cause an increase in dead space-to-tidal volume ratio (V_D/V_T) and in $PaCO_2$.[18]

The fact that O_2 therapy can cause some patients to hypoventilate should never stop the RT from giving O_2 to a patient in need. Preventing hypoxia always is the first

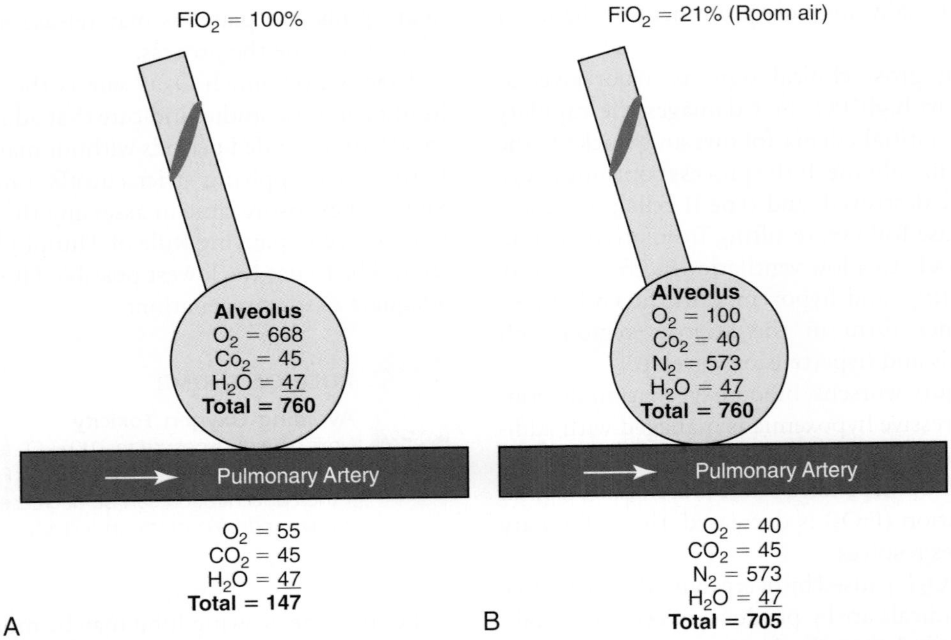

FIGURE 38-3 The development of atelectasis beyond blocked airways when breathing of 100% O_2 **(A)** and room air **(B).** In each case, the sum of the gas pressures in mixed venous blood (pulmonary artery) is less than in the alveoli. The pressure gradient is much greater when breathing 100% O_2 **(A),** causing more rapid diffusion from the alveoli. *Note:* The gas pressures in the room air alveolus will change slightly over time, but the total will remain close to 760 mm Hg.

priority. Avoiding depression of ventilation is discussed in more detail later in this chapter.

Retinopathy of Prematurity

Retinopathy of prematurity (ROP), also called *retrolental fibroplasia,* is an abnormal eye condition that occurs in some premature or low-birth-weight infants who receive supplemental O_2. An excessive blood O_2 level causes retinal vasoconstriction, which leads to necrosis of the blood vessels. In response, new vessels form and increase in number. Hemorrhage of these delicate new vessels causes scarring behind the retina. Scarring often leads to retinal detachment and blindness.[19] ROP most often affects neonates up to approximately 1 month of age, by which time the retinal arteries have sufficiently matured. Excessive O_2 is not the only factor associated with ROP; other factors associated with ROP include hypercapnia, hypocapnia, intraventricular hemorrhage, infection, lactic acidosis, anemia, hypocalcemia, and hypothermia.

Because premature infants often need supplemental O_2, the risk of ROP poses a serious management problem. The American Academy of Pediatrics recommends keeping arterial PO_2 in an infant less than 80 mm Hg as the best way to minimize the risk of ROP.[8]

Absorption Atelectasis

FiO_2 greater than 0.50 presents a significant risk of absorption atelectasis.[20] Nitrogen normally is the most plentiful gas in both the alveoli and the blood. Breathing high levels of O_2 quickly depletes body nitrogen levels. As blood nitrogen levels decrease, the total pressure of venous gases rapidly decreases. Under these conditions, gases that exist at atmospheric pressure within any body cavity rapidly diffuse into the venous blood. This principle is used for removing trapped air from body cavities. Giving patients high levels of O_2 can help clear trapped air from the abdomen or thorax.

This same phenomenon can cause lung collapse, especially if the alveolar region becomes obstructed (Figure 38-3). Under these conditions, O_2 rapidly diffuses into the blood (see Figure 38-3, *A*). With no source for repletion, the total gas pressure in the alveolus progressively decreases until the alveolus collapses. Because collapsed alveoli are perfused but not ventilated, absorption atelectasis increases the physiologic shunt and worsens blood oxygenation.[20]

The risk of absorption atelectasis is greatest in patients breathing at low tidal volumes as a result of sedation, surgical pain, or CNS dysfunction. In these cases, poorly ventilated alveoli may become unstable when they lose O_2 faster than it can be replaced. The result is a more gradual shrinking of the alveoli that may lead to complete collapse, even when the patient is not breathing supplemental O_2 (see Figure 38-3, *B*). For an alert patient, this is not a great risk because the natural sigh mechanism periodically hyperinflates the lung.

Fire Hazard

Despite numerous preventive measures, fires involving enriched O_2 environments continue to occur in health care facilities. Fires seem to pose the greatest risk in operating rooms and in association with selected respiratory procedures. During surgery and procedures such as tracheotomies, electronic scalpels and similar devices are often used while the patient is receiving supplemental O_2. To complicate matters, even higher O_2 concentrations may exist under surgical drapes.[21] Other situations associated with increased fire risk involve home care patients smoking while receiving low-flow O_2 and the use of aluminum O_2 regulators. Additionally, hyperbaric oxygen (HBO) therapy or therapy at increased atmospheric pressures (discussed later in this chapter) often involves the administration of supplemental O_2 and greatly increases fire risk.

Some simple strategies can be used to reduce the fire risk in health care facilities. Effectively managing the fire triangle of O_2, heat, and fuel is key. An essential component is always using the lowest effective FiO_2 for a given clinical situation. In addition, using scavenging systems to minimize O_2 buildup beneath sterile drapes during surgery or while performing tracheostomies can help reduce fire risk. Avoiding the use of inappropriate or outdated equipment such as aluminum gas regulators and educating clinicians, patients and caregivers on safe O_2 use are also important measures. Additionally, fire prevention protocols for HBO therapy should be strictly followed.[21]

Oxygen Delivery Systems: Design and Performance

RTs can select from an array of systems for administering O_2 and other therapeutic gases. Proper device selection requires in-depth knowledge of both the general performance characteristics of these systems and the individual capabilities.[22] O_2 delivery devices traditionally are categorized by design. Three basic designs exist: **low-flow systems, reservoir systems,** and **high-flow systems.** Enclosures, commonly identified as a fourth category, are reservoirs that surround the head or body. The design categories share functional characteristics, capabilities, and limitations.

Although design plays an important role in the selection of these devices, clinical performance ultimately determines how the device is used. The user judges the performance of an O_2 delivery system by answering two key questions: (1) How much O_2 can the system deliver (FiO_2 or FiO_2 range)? (2) Does the delivered FiO_2 remain fixed or vary under changing patient demands?[22]

Regarding the FiO_2 range, O_2 systems can be broadly divided into systems designed to deliver a low (<35%), moderate (35% to 60%), or high (>60%) O_2 concentration. Some designs can deliver O_2 across the full range of concentrations (21% to 100%).

Whether a device delivers a fixed or variable FiO_2 depends on how much of the patient's inspired gas it supplies. If the system provides all of the patient's inspired gas, FiO_2 remains stable, even under changing demands. If the device provides only some of the inspired gas, the patient must draw the remainder from the surrounding air. In this case, the more the patient breathes, the more air dilutes the delivered O_2, and FiO_2 is lower. If the patient breathes less with this type of device, less air dilutes the O_2, and FiO_2 increases. A system that supplies only a portion of the inspired gas always provides a variable FiO_2.[23] FiO_2 supplied with such systems can vary widely from minute to minute and even from breath to breath.

Figure 38-4 shows these concepts as applied to low-flow, reservoir, and high-flow systems. With the low-flow system (see Figure 38-4, *A*) the patient's inspiratory flow often

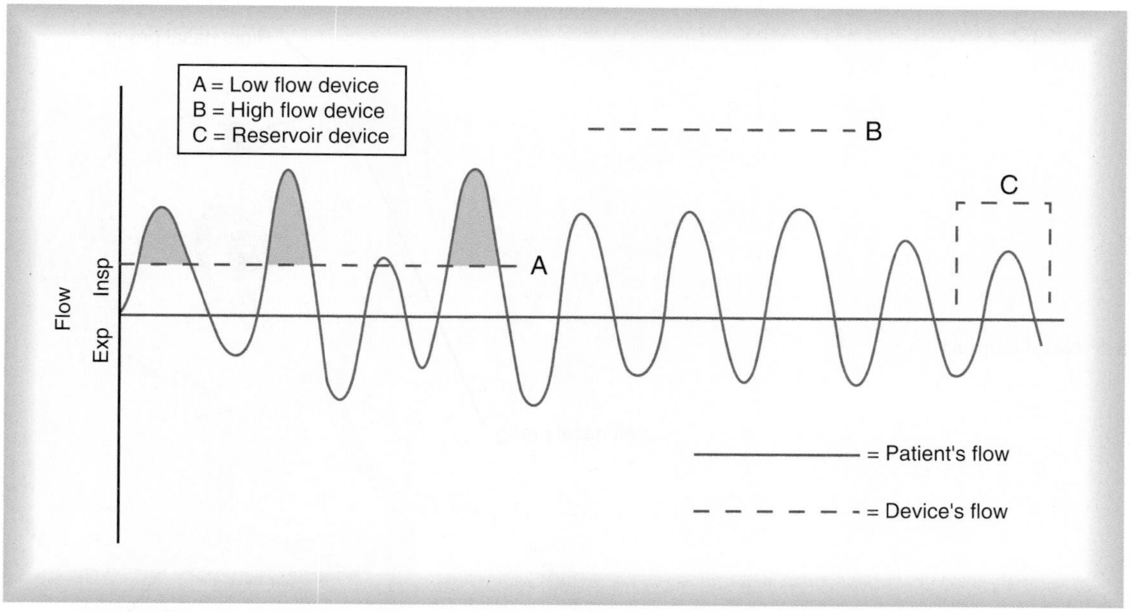

FIGURE 38-4 Differences between O_2 delivery systems. *A*, Low-flow device. *B*, High-flow device. *C*, Reservoir device.

exceeds the flow delivered by the device; the result is air dilution *(shaded areas)*. The greater the patient's inspiratory flow, the more air is breathed, and FiO_2 is lower. The high-flow system (see Figure 38-4, *B*) always exceeds the patient's flow and provides a fixed FiO_2. A fixed FiO_2 can be achieved with a reservoir system (see Figure 38-4, *C*), which stores a reserve volume (flow × time) that equals or exceeds the patient's tidal volume. For a reservoir system to provide a fixed FiO_2, the reservoir volume must always exceed the patient's tidal volume, and there cannot be any air leaks in the system. Table 38-3 outlines the general specifications for the common O_2 therapy systems in current use.

Low-Flow Systems

Typical low-flow systems provide supplemental O_2 directly to the airway at a flow of 8 L/min or less. Because the inspiratory flow of a healthy adult exceeds 8 L/min, the O_2 provided by a low-flow device is always diluted with air; the result is a low and variable FiO_2. Low-flow O_2 delivery systems include nasal cannula, nasal catheter, and transtracheal catheter.

Nasal Cannula. A nasal cannula is a disposable plastic device consisting of two tips or prongs approximately 1 cm long that are connected to several feet of small-bore O_2 supply tubing (Figure 38-5). The user inserts the prongs directly into the vestibule of the nose while attaching the supply tubing either directly to a flowmeter or to a bubble humidifier. In most cases, a humidifier is used only when the input flow is greater than 4 L/min.[2] Even with extra humidity, flow greater than 6 to 8 L/min can cause patient discomfort, including nasal dryness and bleeding.[22] Cannulas should not be used in newborns and infants if their nasal passages are obstructed, and flows generally should be limited to 2 L/min unless a specialized high-flow cannula system is being used.[2] A high-flow nasal cannula, which is a variation of a standard nasal cannula, is discussed in more detail later in this chapter. Table 38-3 lists the FiO_2 range, FiO_2 stability, advantages, disadvantages, and best use of a nasal cannula.

Nasal Catheter. Although use is generally limited to short-term O_2 administration during specialized procedures such as a bronchoscopy, a nasal catheter is another low-flow O_2 delivery device. A nasal catheter is a soft plastic tube with several small holes at the tip that is inserted by gently advancing it along the floor of either nasal passage and visualizing it just behind and above the uvula (Figure 38-6). Once in position, the catheter is taped to the bridge of the nose. If direct visualization is impossible, the catheter may be blindly inserted to a depth equal to the distance from the nose to the earlobe.

When placed too deep, the catheter can provoke gagging or swallowing of gas, which increases the likelihood of aspiration. Nasal catheters also affect the production of secretions; for this reason, a nasal catheter should be replaced with a new one (placed in the opposite naris) at least every 8 hours. Nasal catheters should be avoided in most patients with maxillofacial trauma, basal skull fracture, nasal obstruction, and coagulation problems. It has also been determined that nasal catheters are inappropriate for neonatal patients. As a result of these notable limitations, nasal catheters are rarely used today.[4]

Transtracheal Catheter. A transtracheal O_2 catheter was first described by Heimlich in 1982.[24] A physician surgically inserts this thin polytetrafluoroethylene (Teflon) catheter with a guidewire directly into the trachea between the second and third tracheal rings (Figure 38-7). A

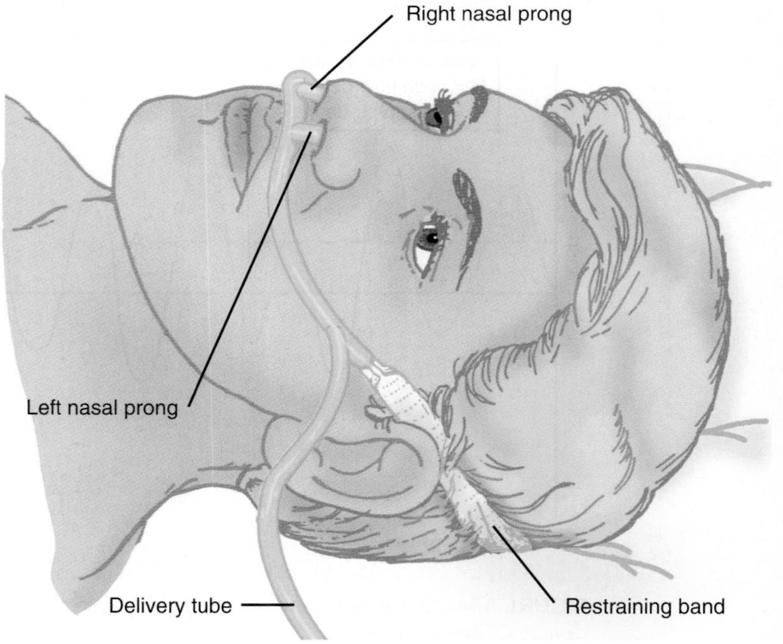

FIGURE 38-5 Nasal cannula.

TABLE 38-3

Overview of Oxygen Therapy Systems

Category	Device	Flow	FiO_2 Range	FiO_2 Stability	Advantages	Disadvantages	Best Use
Low flow	Nasal cannula	¼-8 L/min (adults) ≤2 L/min (infants)	22%-40%	Variable	Use on adults, children, infants; easy to use; disposable; low cost; well tolerated	Unstable, easily dislodged; high flow uncomfortable; can cause dryness, bleeding; polyps; deviated septum and mouth breathing may reduce FiO_2	Patient in stable condition who needs low FiO_2; home care patient who needs long-term therapy, low to moderate FiO_2 while eating
	Nasal catheter	¼-8 L/min	22%-45%	Variable	Use on adults, children, infants; good stability; disposable; low cost	Difficult to insert; high flow increases back pressure; needs regular changing; polyps, deviated septum may block insertion; may provoke gagging, air swallowing, aspiration	Procedures in which cannula is difficult to use (bronchoscopy); long-term care of infants
	Transtracheal catheter	¼-4 L/min	22%-35%	Variable	Lower O_2 use and cost; eliminates nasal and skin irritation; improved compliance; increased exercise tolerance; increased mobility; enhanced image	High cost; surgical complications; infection; mucous plugging; lost tract	Home care or ambulatory patients who need increased mobility or do not accept nasal O_2
	Reservoir cannula	¼-4 L/min	22%-35%	Variable	Lower O_2 use and cost; increased mobility; less discomfort because of lower flow	Unattractive, cumbersome; poor compliance; must be regularly replaced; breathing pattern affects performance	Home care or ambulatory patients who need increased mobility
	Simple mask	5-10 L/min	35%-50%	Variable	Use on adults, children, infants; quick, easy to apply; disposable; inexpensive	Uncomfortable; must be removed for eating; prevents radiant heat loss; blocks vomitus in unconscious patients	Emergencies; short-term therapy requiring moderate FiO_2; mouth breathing patients requiring moderate FiO_2
	Partial rebreathing mask	Minimum of 10 L/min (prevent bag collapse on inspiration)	40%-70%	Variable	Same as simple mask; moderate to high FiO_2	Same as simple mask; potential suffocation hazard	Emergencies; short-term therapy requiring moderate to high FiO_2
	Nonrebreathing mask	Minimum of 10 L/min (prevent bag collapse on inspiration)	60%-80%	Variable	Same as simple mask; high FiO_2	Same as simple mask; potential suffocation hazard	Emergencies; short-term therapy requiring high FiO_2
	Nonrebreathing circuit (closed)	$3 \times V_E$ (prevent bag collapse on inspiration)	21%-100%	Fixed	Full range of FiO_2	Potential suffocation hazard; requires 50 psi air/O_2; blender failure common	Patients who need precise FiO_2 at any level (21%-100%)

Continued

TABLE 38-3

Overview of Oxygen Therapy Systems—cont'd

Category	Device	Flow	FiO_2 Range	FiO_2 Stability	Advantages	Disadvantages	Best Use
High flow	AEM	Varies; should provide output flow >60 L/min	24%-50%	Fixed	Easy to apply; disposable, inexpensive; stable, precise FiO_2	Limited to adult use; uncomfortable, noisy; must be removed for eating; FiO_2 >0.40 not ensured; FiO_2 varies with back pressure	Patients in unstable condition who need precise low FiO_2
	Air-entrainment nebulizer	10-15 L/min input; should provide output flow of at least 60 L/min	28%-100%	Fixed	Provides temperature control and extra humidification	FiO_2 < 0.28 or >0.40 not ensured; FiO_2 varies with back pressure; high infection risk	Patients with artificial airways who need low to moderate FiO_2
	Blending system (open)	Should provide output flow of at least 60 L/min	21%-100%	Fixed	Full range of FiO_2	Requires 50 psi air/O_2; blender failure or inaccuracy common	Patients with high V_E who need high FiO_2
	High-flow nasal cannula system	Up to 40 L/min (depending on system)	35%-90%	Variable or fixed depending on system and input flow	Wide range of FiO_2 and relative/absolute humidity; use on adults, children, infants	FiO_2 not ensured depending on input flow and patient breathing pattern; infection risk	Patients of all ages with high or variable V_E who need supplemental O_2, positive pressure, or humidity
Enclosure	Oxyhood	≥7 L/min	21%-100%	Fixed	Full range of FiO_2	Difficult to clean, disinfect	Infants who need supplemental O_2
	Isolette	8-15 L/min	40%-50%	Variable	Provides temperature control	Expensive, cumbersome, unstable FiO_2 (leaks); difficult to clean, disinfect; limits patient mobility; fire hazard	Infants who need supplemental O_2 and precise thermal regulation
	Tent	12-15 L/min	40%-50%	Variable	Provides concurrent aerosol therapy	Expensive, cumbersome, unstable FiO_2 (leaks); requires cooling; difficult to clean, disinfect; limits patient mobility; fire hazard	Toddlers or small children who need low to moderate FiO_2 and aerosol

V_E, Minute volume.

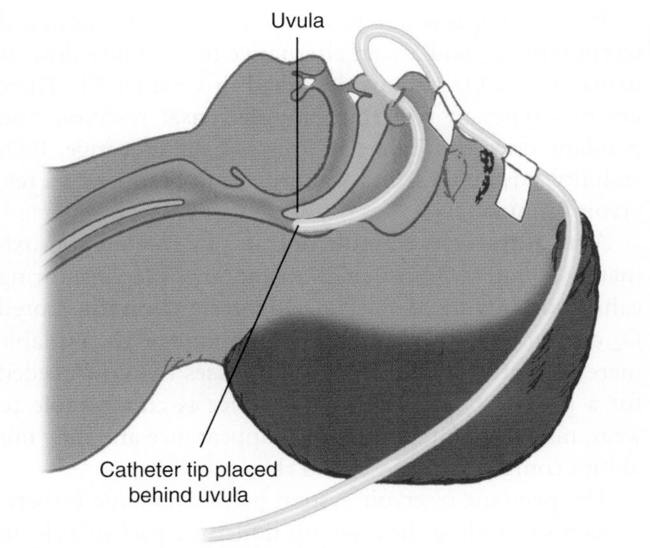

FIGURE 38-6 Placement of nasal catheter in the nasopharynx.

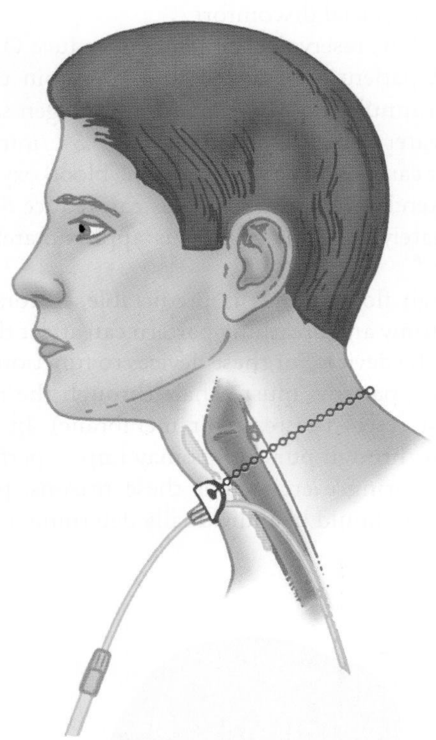

FIGURE 38-7 Transtracheal O_2 catheter.

custom-sized chain necklace secures the catheter in position. Standard tubing connected directly to a flowmeter provides the O_2 source flow.[25] Because flow is so low, no humidifier is needed.

Because the transtracheal catheter resides directly in the trachea, O_2 builds up both there and in the upper airway during expiration. This process effectively expands the anatomic reservoir and increases the FiO_2 at any given flow. Compared with a nasal cannula, a transtracheal catheter needs about half of the O_2 flow to achieve a given arterial partial pressure of oxygen (PaO_2).[25] Some patients need a flow of only 0.25 L/min to achieve adequate oxygenation. This reduced flow can be of great economic and practical benefit to patients needing continuous long-term O_2 therapy because it can greatly increase the duration of flow of portable O_2 systems. Transtracheal O_2 therapy can pose problems and risks, however, and these devices have not received widespread acceptance. Careful patient selection, rigorous patient education, and ongoing self-care with professional follow-up evaluation can help minimize these risks. Chapter 51 provides details on these aspects of transtracheal O_2 therapy. Table 38-3 lists the FiO_2 range, FiO_2 stability, advantages, disadvantages, and best use of a transtracheal catheter.

TABLE 38-4

Variables Affecting FiO_2 of Low-Flow Oxygen Systems

Increases FiO_2	Decreases FiO_2
Higher O_2 input	Lower O_2 input
Mouth-closed breathing*	Mouth-open breathing*
Low inspiratory flow	High inspiratory flow
Low tidal volume	High tidal volume
Slow rate of breathing	Fast rate of breathing
Small minute ventilation	Large minute ventilation
Long inspiratory time	Short inspiratory time
High I : E ratio	Low I : E ratio

I:E, Inspiratory/expiratory.
*Cannula only.

Performance Characteristics of Low-Flow Systems

Research studies on nasal low-flow systems show O_2 concentration ranging from 22% at 1 L/min to 60% at 15 L/min.[2,3,22] The range of 22% to 45% cited in Table 38-3 is based on 8 L/min as the upper limit of comfortable flow. These wide FiO_2 ranges occur because the O_2 concentration delivered by a low-flow system varies with the amount of air dilution. The amount of air dilution depends on several patient and equipment variables. Table 38-4 summarizes these key variables and how they affect FiO_2 provided by low-flow systems.

Simple formulas exist for estimating FiO_2 provided by low-flow systems (see the accompanying Rule of Thumb). Given the large number of variables affecting FiO_2, however, the RT can never know precisely how much O_2 a patient is receiving with these systems. Even if it were possible to measure the exact FiO_2, this value could change from

RULE OF THUMB

Estimating FiO_2 Provided by Low-Flow Systems

For patients with a normal rate and depth of breathing, each 1 L/min of nasal O_2 increases FiO_2 approximately 4%. For example, a patient using a nasal cannula at 4 L/min has an estimated FiO_2 of approximately 37% (21 + 16).

minute to minute and even from breath to breath with certain breathing patterns. Without knowing the patient's exact FiO_2, the RT must rely on assessing the actual response to O_2 therapy.

Troubleshooting Low-Flow Systems

Common problems with low-flow O_2 delivery systems include inaccurate flow, system leaks and obstructions, device displacement, and skin irritation. The problem of inaccurate flow is greatest when low-flow flowmeters (≤3 L/min) are used. Given the trend toward assessment of outcome of O_2 therapy (with either blood gases or pulse oximetry), ensuring the absolute accuracy of O_2 input flow generally is not essential. Nonetheless, similar to all respiratory care equipment, flowmeters should be subjected to regular preventive maintenance and testing for accuracy. Equipment that fails preventive maintenance standards should be removed from service and repaired or replaced. Table 38-5 provides guidance on troubleshooting the most common clinical problems with nasal cannulas. Details on troubleshooting transtracheal catheters are provided in Chapter 51.

Reservoir Systems

Reservoir systems incorporate a mechanism for gathering and storing O_2 between patient breaths. Patients draw on this reserve supply whenever inspiratory flow exceeds O_2 flow into the device. Because air dilution is reduced, reservoir devices generally provide higher FiO_2 than low-flow systems. Reservoir devices can decrease O_2 use by providing FiO_2 comparable with nonreservoir systems but at lower flow. Reservoir systems in use at the present time include reservoir cannulas, masks, and nonrebreathing circuits. In principle, enclosure systems, such as tents and hoods, operate as reservoirs surrounding the head or body.

TABLE 38-5

Troubleshooting Common Problems With a Nasal Oxygen Cannula

Problem or Clue	Cause	Solution
No gas flow can be felt coming from the cannula	Flowmeter not on	Adjust flowmeter
	System leak	Check connections
Humidifier pop-off is sounding	Obstruction distal to humidifier	Find and correct the obstruction
	Flow is set too high	Use alternative device
	Obstructed naris	Use alternative device
Patient reports soreness over lip or ears	Irritation or inflammation caused by appliance straps	Loosen straps
		Place cotton balls at pressure points
		Use a different device
Mouth breathing	Habitual mouth breathing, blocked nasal passages	Switch to simple mask or Venturi mask

Reservoir Cannula. Reservoir cannulas are designed to conserve O_2 and are an alternative to the pulse-dose or demand-flow O_2 systems described in Chapter 51. There are two types of reservoir cannula: nasal reservoir and pendant reservoir. Table 38-3 lists the FiO_2 range, FiO_2 stability, advantages, disadvantages, and best use of a reservoir cannula.

A nasal reservoir cannula operates by storing approximately 20 ml of O_2 in a small membrane reservoir during exhalation (Figure 38-8). The patient draws on this stored O_2 during early inspiration. The amount of O_2 available increases with each breath and decreases the flow needed for a given FiO_2. Although the device is comfortable to wear, many patients object to its appearance and may not always comply with prescribed therapy.

The pendant reservoir system helps overcome esthetic concerns by hiding the reservoir under the patient's clothing on the anterior chest wall (Figure 38-9). Although the device is less visible, the extra weight of the pendant can cause ear and facial discomfort.

At low flow, reservoir cannulas can reduce O_2 use 50% to 75%. A patient at rest who needs 2 L/min through a standard cannula to achieve an arterial oxygen saturation (SaO_2) greater than 90% may need only 0.5 L/min through a reservoir cannula to achieve the same blood oxygenation. During exercise, reservoir cannulas can reduce flow needs approximately 66%; the savings is approximately 50% at high flow.[26]

Although flow savings is predictable, factors such as nasal anatomy and breathing pattern can affect the performance of the device. For these devices to function properly at low flow, patients must exhale through the nose (this reopens or resets the reservoir membrane). In addition, exhalation through pursed lips may impair performance, especially during exercise. For these reasons, prescribed flow settings should be individually determined by means

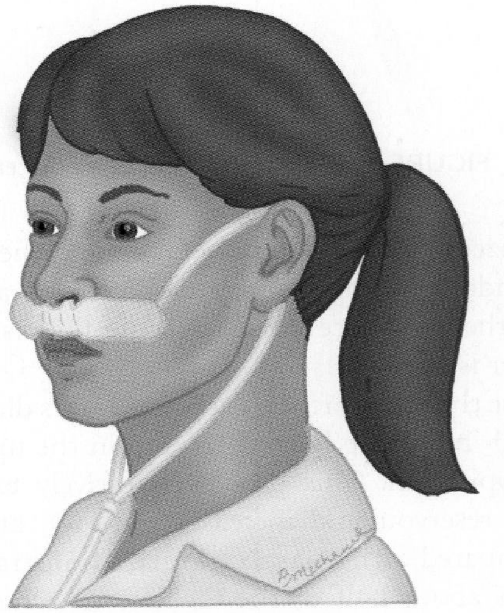

FIGURE 38-8 Reservoir cannula.

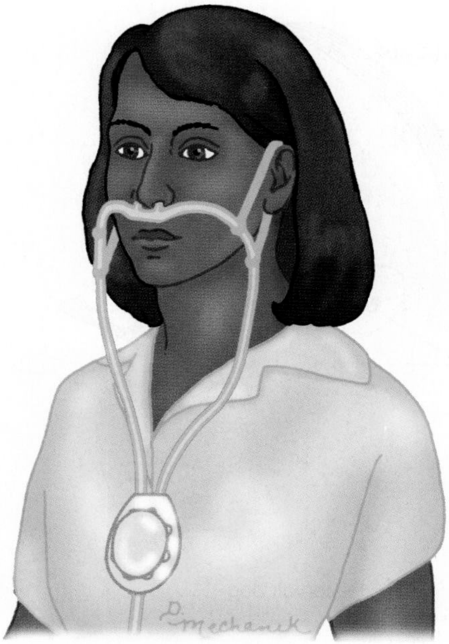

FIGURE 38-9 Pendant reservoir cannula.

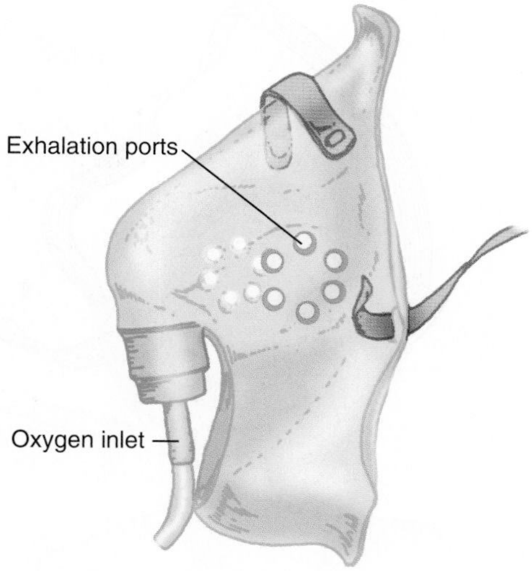

FIGURE 38-10 Simple O_2 mask.

of clinical assessment, including SaO_2 monitoring, during rest and exercise.[26]

The low flow at which the reservoir cannula operates makes humidification unnecessary. Excess moisture can hinder proper action of the reservoir membrane.[26] Even regular use can cause membrane wear. For this reason, patients should replace the reservoir cannula approximately every 3 weeks. Replacement needs partially offset the O_2 cost savings afforded by these devices.

Reservoir Masks. Masks are the most commonly used reservoir systems. There are three types of reservoir masks: (1) simple mask, (2) partial rebreathing mask, and (3) nonrebreathing mask. Table 38-3 lists the FiO_2 range, FiO_2 stability, advantages, disadvantages, and best use of each of these devices.

A simple mask is a disposable plastic unit designed to cover both the mouth and the nose (Figure 38-10). The body of the mask itself gathers and stores O_2 between patient breaths. The patient exhales directly through open holes or ports in the mask body. If O_2 input flow ceases, the patient can draw in air through these holes and around the mask edge.

The input flow range for an adult simple mask is 5 to 10 L/min. Generally, if flow greater than 10 L/min is needed for satisfactory oxygenation, use of a device capable of a higher FiO_2 should be considered. At a flow less than 5 L/min, the mask volume acts as dead space and causes carbon dioxide (CO_2) rebreathing.[27]

Because air dilution easily occurs during inspiration through its ports and around its body, a simple mask provides a variable FiO_2. How much FiO_2 varies depends on the O_2 input flow, the mask volume, the extent of air leakage, and the patient's breathing pattern.[28]

As shown in Figure 38-11, a partial rebreathing mask and a nonrebreathing mask have a similar design. Each has a 1-L flexible reservoir bag attached to the O_2 inlet. Because the bag increases the reservoir volume, both masks provide higher FiO_2 capabilities than a simple mask. The key difference between these designs is the use of valves. A partial rebreathing mask has no valves (see Figure 38-11, *A*). During inspiration, source O_2 flows into the mask and passes directly to the patient. During exhalation, source O_2 enters the bag. However, because no valves separate the mask and the bag, some of the patient's exhaled gas also enters the bag (approximately the first third). Because it comes from the anatomic dead space, the early portion of exhaled gas contains mostly O_2 and little CO_2. As the bag fills with both O_2 and dead space gas, the last two-thirds of exhalation (high in CO_2) escapes out the exhalation ports of the mask. As long as the O_2 input flow keeps the bag from collapsing more than about one-third during inhalation, CO_2 rebreathing is negligible.

Although it can provide a higher FiO_2 than a simple mask (see Table 38-3), a standard disposable partial rebreathing mask is subject to considerable air dilution. The result is delivery of a moderate but variable FiO_2 dependent on the same factors as with a simple mask.

A nonrebreathing mask prevents rebreathing with one-way valves (see Figure 38-11, *B*). An inspiratory valve sits on top of the bag, and expiratory valves cover the exhalation ports on the mask body. During inspiration, slight negative mask pressure closes the expiratory valves, preventing air dilution. At the same time, the inspiratory valve on top of the bag opens, providing O_2 to the patient. During exhalation, valve action reverses the direction of flow. Slight positive pressure closes the inspiratory valve, which prevents exhaled gas from entering the bag. Concurrently, the one-way expiratory valves open and divert exhaled gas out to the atmosphere.

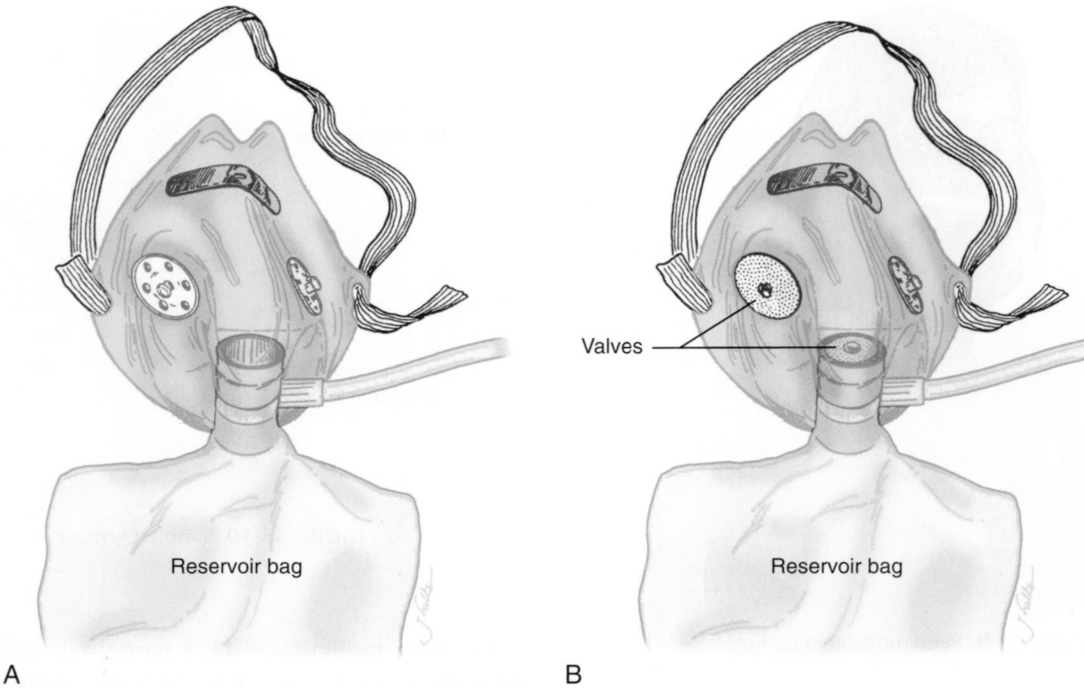

FIGURE 38-11 **A,** Partial rebreathing mask. **B,** Nonrebreathing mask.

Because it is a closed system, a leak-free nonrebreathing mask with competent valves and enough flow to prevent more than one-third bag collapse during inspiration can deliver 100% source gas. As indicated in Table 38-3, however, modern disposable nonrebreathing masks normally do not provide much more than approximately 70% O_2.[22]

Large air leaks are the primary problem. Air leakage occurs both around the mask body and through the open (nonvalved) exhalation port. This open exhalation port is a common safety feature designed to allow air breathing if the O_2 source fails. The port also allows air dilution whenever inspiratory flow or volume is high. Although a disposable nonrebreathing mask can deliver moderate to high O_2 concentration, FiO_2 still varies with the amount of air leakage and the patient's breathing pattern.

Nonrebreathing Reservoir Circuit. A nonrebreathing circuit operates with the same design principles as a nonrebreathing mask. Although the nonrebreathing circuit requires an elaborate combination of equipment and supplies, it can be more versatile than a nonrebreathing mask because it provides a full range of FiO_2 (21% to 100%) and can be used for both intubated and nonintubated patients.[22] As shown in Figure 38-12, a typical nonrebreathing circuit incorporates a blending system to premix air and O_2. The gas mixture is warmed and humidified, ideally with a servo-controlled heated humidifier. Gas flows through large-bore tubing into an inspiratory volume reservoir, which includes a fail-safe inlet valve. The patient breathes through a closed airway appliance, in this case, a mask with one-way valves. A valved T tube also can be used in the care of a patient with an endotracheal or a tracheostomy tube.

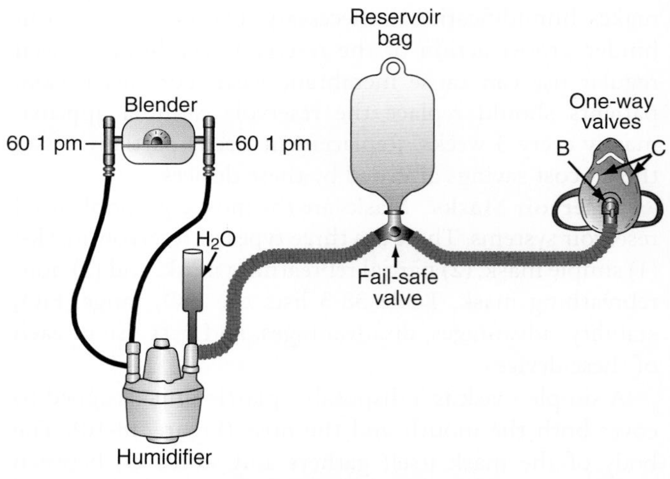

FIGURE 38-12 Nonrebreathing reservoir circuit with a valved face mask. Reservoir bag in combination with high-flow (0 to 100 L/min) flowmeters ensures delivery of set FiO_2. (Modified from Foust GN, Potter WA, Wilons MD, et al: Shortcomings of using two jet nebulizers in tandem with an aerosol face mask for optimal oxygen therapy, Chest 99:1346, 1991.)

Troubleshooting Reservoir Systems. Common problems with reservoir masks include device displacement, system leaks and obstructions, improper flow adjustment,

TABLE 38-6

Troubleshooting Common Problems With Reservoir Masks

Problem or Clue	Cause	Solution
Patient constantly removes mask	Claustrophobia	Use alternative device
	Confusion	Restrain patient
No gas flow can be detected	Flowmeter not on	Adjust flowmeter
	System leak	Check connections
Humidifier pop-off is sounding	Obstruction distal to humidifier	Find and correct obstruction
	High input flow	Omit humidifier if therapy is short-term
	Jammed inspiratory valve	Fix or replace valve
Reservoir bag collapses when the patient inhales	Flow is inadequate	Increase flow
Reservoir bag remains inflated throughout inhalation	Large mask leak	Correct leak
	Inspiratory valve jammed or reversed	Repair or replace mask
Erythema develops over face or ears	Irritation or inflammation owing to appliance or straps	Reposition mask or straps Place cotton balls over ear pressure points Provide skin care

and skin irritation. Table 38-6 provides guidance on troubleshooting the most common clinical problems with reservoir masks.

High-Flow Systems

High-flow systems supply a given O_2 concentration at a flow equaling or exceeding the patient's peak inspiratory flow. An air-entrainment or a blending system is used. As long as the delivered flow exceeds the patient's flow, both systems can ensure a fixed FiO_2. The accompanying Rule of Thumb can help determine which devices truly qualify as high-flow systems.

RULE OF THUMB

High-Flow Devices

To qualify as a high-flow device, a system should provide at least 60 L/min total flow. This flow criterion is based on the fact that the average adult peak inspiratory flow during tidal ventilation is approximately three times the minute volume. Because 20 L/min is close to the upper limit of sustainable minute volume for an ill person, a flow of 3 × 20, or 60 L/min, should suffice in most situations. In a few rare circumstances, flow must reach or exceed 100 L/min.

Box 38-1 Equations for Computing Oxygen Percentage, Ratio, and Flow*

1. To compute the O_2 percentage of a mixture of air and O_2:

$$\%O_2 = \frac{(\text{Air flow} \times 21) + (O_2\ \text{flow} \times 100)}{\text{Total flow}} \quad \text{(Eq. 38-1)}$$

2. To compute the air-to-O_2 ratio needed to obtain a given O_2 percentage:

$$\frac{\text{Liters air}}{\text{Liters } O_2} = \frac{(100 - \%O_2)}{(\%O_2 - 21)} \quad \text{(Eq. 38-2)}$$

3. To compute the total output flow from an air-entrainment device (given the O_2 input):
   a. Compute the air-to-O_2 ratio (see Equation 38-2).
   b. Add the air-to-O_2 ratio parts.
   c. Multiply the sum of the ratio parts by the O_2 input flow.
4. To compute the flow of O_2 and air needed to obtain a given O_2 percentage at a given total flow:
   a. Compute the O_2 flow:

$$O_2\ \text{flow} = \frac{\text{Total flow} \times (O_2\% - 21)}{79} \quad \text{(Eq. 38-3)}$$

   b. Compute the air flow:

$$\text{Air flow} = \text{Total flow} - O_2\ \text{flow}$$

*For simplicity, in all equations, percentage concentration (0 to 100) is used instead of decimal-based FiO_2. To convert a computed percentage to the corresponding FiO_2, divide by 100.

Principles of Gas Mixing. All high-flow systems mix air and O_2 to achieve a given FiO_2. These gases are mixed with air-entrainment devices or blending systems. Computations involving mixtures of air and O_2 are based on a modified form of the dilution equation for solutions:

$$V_F C_F = V_1 C_1 + V_2 C_2$$

In this equation, V_1 and V_2 are the volumes of the two gases being mixed; C_1 and C_2, the O_2 concentration in these two volumes; and V_F and C_F, the final volume and concentration of the resulting mixture.

Box 38-1 shows how to apply variations of this equation to compute (1) the final concentration of a mixture of air and O_2, (2) the air-to-O_2 ratio needed to obtain a given FiO_2, (3) the total output flow from an air-entrainment device, and (4) the amount of O_2 that must be added to a volume of air to obtain a given FiO_2. Clinical examples of these computations are provided in the accompanying Mini Clini boxes.

Air-Entrainment Systems. Air-entrainment systems direct a high-pressure O_2 source through a small nozzle or jet surrounded by air-entrainment ports (Figure 38-13). The amount of air entrained at these ports varies directly with

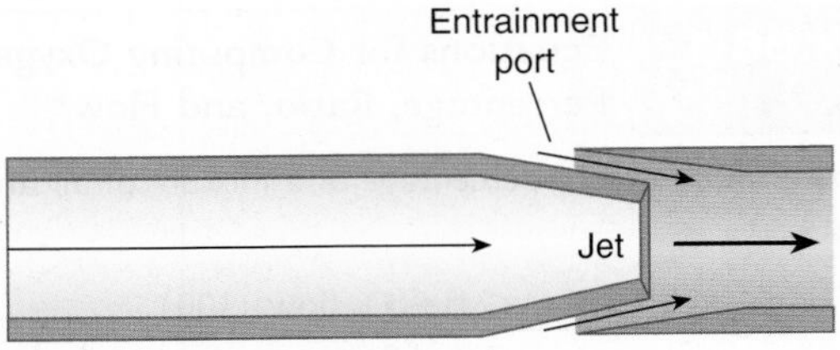

FIGURE 38-13 Basic components of an air-entrainment system. Pressurized gas passes through a nozzle or jet, beyond which are air-entrainment ports. Shear forces at the jet orifice entrain air into the primary gas stream, diluting the O_2 and increasing the total flow output of the device.

MINI CLINI

Conflicting Assessment Information

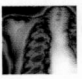

PROBLEM: A disoriented postoperative male patient breathing room air exhibits tachypnea, tachycardia, and mild cyanosis of the mucous membranes. Using a pulse oximeter, the RT measures the patient's oxyhemoglobin saturation as 93%. What should the RT recommend to the patient's surgeon?

DISCUSSION: This is a classic example of how monitoring data and results of bedside assessment can conflict. Both the patient's condition and the observed clinical signs indicate hypoxemia, but the pulse oximeter indicates adequate oxygenation. In situations such as this, it is always better to err on the side of the patient and recommend O_2 therapy—treat the patient, not the monitor. This concept is particularly important in the use of monitoring technologies known to have limited accuracy, such as pulse oximetry (see Chapter 18).

MINI CLINI

Determining FiO_2 of an Air-Oxygen Mixture

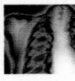

PROBLEM: An air-entrainment device mixes at a fixed ratio of three volumes of air to each volume of O_2 (3 : 1 ratio). What is the resulting FiO_2?

SOLUTION: Substituting air, O_2, and total (air + O_2) volumes into Equation 38-1:

$$\%O_2 = \frac{(\text{Air flow} \times 21) + (O_2\ \text{flow} \times 100)}{\text{Total flow}}$$

$$\%O_2 = \frac{(3 \times 21) + (1 \times 100)}{3+1}$$

$$\%O_2 = 41$$

An air-entrainment device that mixes three volumes of air with one volume of O_2 provides a gas mixture with FiO_2 of approximately 0.40.

MINI CLINI

Computing Total Flow Output of an Air-Entrainment Device

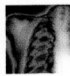

PROBLEM: A patient is receiving O_2 through an air-entrainment device set to deliver 50% O_2. The input O_2 flow is set to 15 L/min. What is the total output flow of this system?

SOLUTION: Step 1: Compute the air-to-O_2 ratio by substituting 50 for the $\%O_2$ in Equation 38-2:

$$\frac{\text{Liters air}}{\text{Liters } O_2} = \frac{(100 - \%O_2)}{(\%O_2 - 21)}$$

$$\frac{\text{Liters air}}{\text{Liters } O_2} = \frac{(100 - 50)}{(50 - 21)}$$

$$\frac{\text{Liters air}}{\text{Liters } O_2} = \frac{50}{29}$$

$$\frac{\text{Liters air}}{\text{Liters } O_2} \approx \frac{1.7}{1}$$

Step 2: Add the air-to-O_2 ratio parts:

$$1.7 + 1 = 2.7$$

Step 3: Multiply the sum of the ratio parts times the O_2 input flow:

$$2.7 \times 15\ \text{L/min} = 41\ \text{L/min}$$

An air-entrainment device set to deliver 50% O_2 that has an input flow of 15 L/min provides a total output flow of approximately 41 L/min.

the size of the port and the velocity of O_2 at the jet. The larger the intake ports and the higher the gas velocity at the jet, the more air is entrained.

Because they dilute source O_2 with air, entrainment devices always provide less than 100% O_2. The more air they entrain, the higher is the total output flow, but the delivered FiO_2 is lower. High flow is possible only when low O_2 concentration is delivered. For these reasons, air-entrainment devices function as true high-flow systems only at low FiO_2. If the flow output from an air-entrainment device decreases to less than a patient's inspiratory flow, air dilution occurs, and FiO_2 becomes variable.

FiO_2 provided by air-entrainment devices depends on two key variables: the air-to-O_2 ratio and the amount of flow resistance downstream from the mixing site. Changing the input flow of an air-entrainment device alters the total output flow but has little effect on delivered FiO_2. Generally, FiO_2 remains within 1% to 2% of that specified by the manufacturer, regardless of input flow.[29]

The size of the jet and entrainment ports of a device determines the air-to-O_2 ratio and the delivered FiO_2. The accompanying Mini Clini entiled Determing FiO_2 of an Air-Oxygen Mixture shows how to compute the FiO_2

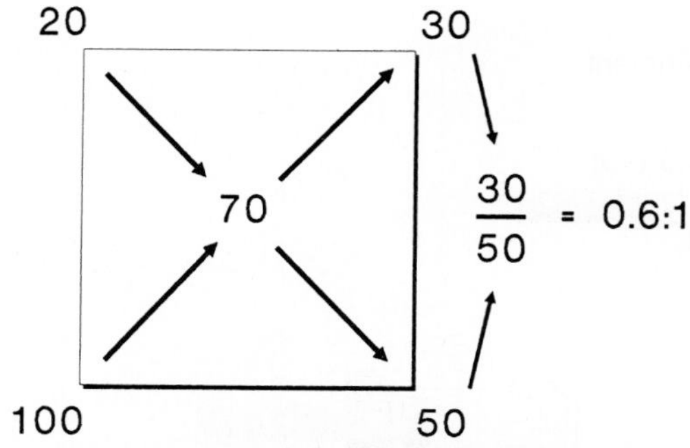

FIGURE 38-14 The magic box used to estimate air-to-O_2 ratio.

provided by an air-entrainment system if the air-to-O_2 ratio is known.

A more common clinical problem arises when the total output flow from an air-entrainment system must be determined. As described in the previous Rule of Thumb, the total flow output of a system determines whether it truly performs as a high-flow device. The accompanying Mini Clini entitled Computing Total Flow Output of an Air-Entrainment Device shows how to determine the total output flow of an air-entrainment system.

Rather than using Equation 38-2 in Box 38-1 to compute air-to-O_2 ratio, many RTs derive quick estimates by using a simple mathematical aid called the *magic box* (Figure 38-14). To use the magic box, one draws a square and places 20 in the top left corner and 100 in the bottom left corner. One places the desired O_2 percentage in the center of the box (in this case, 70%). One subtracts diagonally from lower left to the upper right (disregard the sign). One subtracts diagonally again from upper left to lower right (disregard the sign). The resulting numerator (30) is the value for air, and the denominator (50) is the value for O_2.

By convention, the air-to-O_2 ratio is expressed with the denominator (liters of O_2) set to 1. An air-entrainment device with a 7:1 ratio mixes 7 L of air with 1 L of O_2. To reduce any ratio to a ratio of x:1, one divides both the numerator and the denominator by the denominator. In the magic box example (also see Figure 38-14):

$$\frac{30}{50}=\frac{30/50}{50/50}=\frac{0.61}{1}$$

The magic box can be used only for estimation of air-to-O_2 ratio. For absolute accuracy, Equation 38-2 always should be used. Based on Equation 38-2, Table 38-7 lists the approximate air-to-O_2 ratios for several common O_2 percentages.

The other major factor determining the O_2 concentration provided by an air-entrainment device is downstream flow resistance. In the presence of flow resistance distal to the jet, the volume of air entrained always decreases. With less air being entrained, total flow output decreases, and the delivered O_2 concentration increases.

Although the delivered O_2 concentration increases, the actual FiO_2 received by the patient may decrease,

TABLE 38-7

Approximate Air-to-Oxygen Ratios for Common Oxygen Concentrations*

Percentage O_2	Approximate Air-to-O_2 Ratio	Total Ratio Parts
100	0:1	1
80	0.3:1	1.3
70	0.6:1	1.6
60	1:1	2
50	1.7:1	2.7
45	2:1	3
40	3:1	4
35	5:1	6
30	8:1	9
29	10:1	11
24	25:1	26

*Total output flow (air + O_2) in L/min can be calculated by multiplying the total ratio parts by the O_2 input flow (L/min).

especially on devices set to deliver 30% to 50% O_2.[29] This phenomenon is caused mainly by the decrease in total output flow. As the total output flow decreases below the flow needed to meet the patient's inspiratory needs, room air is inhaled. A similar event occurs if the air intake ports surrounding the jet are blocked. Under both conditions, these high-flow systems begin to behave as low-flow devices. The two most common O_2 delivery systems in which air entrainment is used are the air-entrainment mask (AEM) and the air-entrainment nebulizer.

Air-Entrainment (Venturi) Mask. The use of an O_2 mask for provision of controlled FiO_2 by means of air entrainment was first reported in 1941 by Barach and Eckman.[30] The system provided relatively high FiO_2 (>40%) through the use of adjustable air-entrainment ports that controlled the amount of air mixed with O_2. Almost 20 years later, Campbell[31] developed an entrainment mask that provided controlled, low FiO_2 and called the device a *Venturi mask* or *venti-mask*.

As the name *venti-mask* suggests, the operating principle behind these devices has often been attributed to the Venturi principle (see Chapter 6). This assumption is incorrect.[32] Rather than having an actual Venturi tube that entrains air, these devices have a simple restricted orifice or jet through which O_2 flows at high velocity. Air is entrained by shear forces at the boundary of jet flow, not by low lateral pressures. The smaller the orifice, the greater the velocity of O_2, and more air is entrained.

Figure 38-15 depicts a typical AEM, designed to deliver a range of low to moderate FiO_2 (0.24 to 0.40). The mask consists of a jet orifice or nozzle around which is an air-entrainment port *(top drawing)*. The body of the mask has several large ports, which allow escape of both excess flow from the device and exhaled gas from the patient. In this design, FiO_2 is regulated by selection and changing of the jet adapter. The smallest jet provides the highest O_2 velocity, the most air entrainment, and the lowest FiO_2 (0.24).

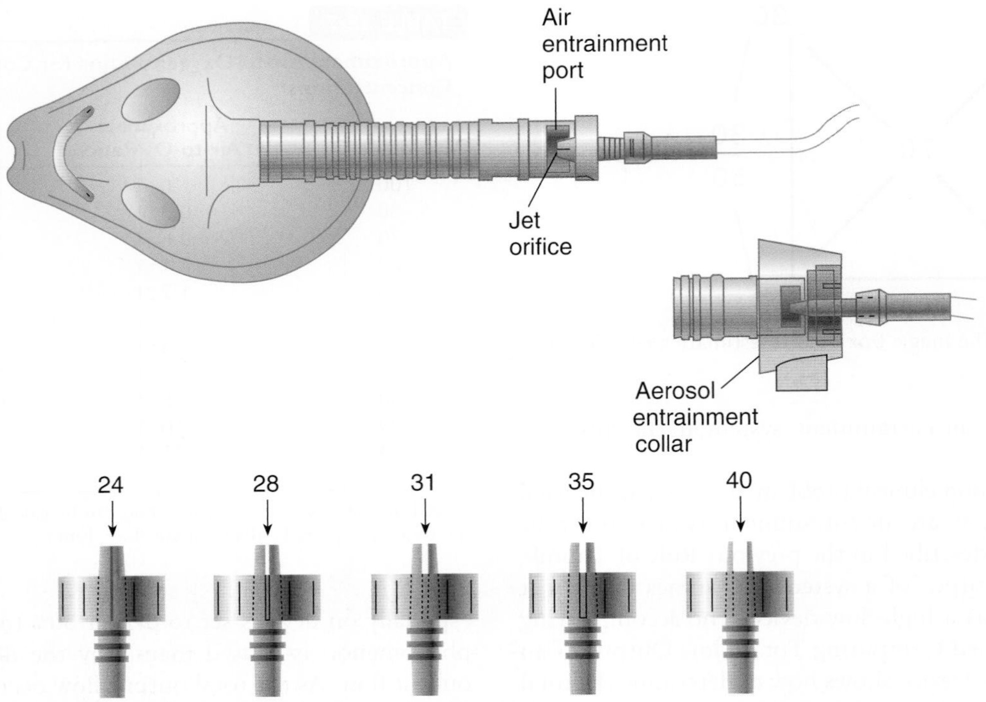

FIGURE 38-15 Typical AEM. FiO_2 is regulated by changing a jet adapter. The aerosol collar allows high humidity or aerosol entrainment from an air source. (Modified from Kacmarek RM: In-hospital O_2 therapy. In Kacmarek RM, Stoller J, editors: Current respiratory care, Toronto, 1988, BC Decker.)

The largest jet provides the lowest O_2 velocity, the least air entrainment, and the highest FiO_2 (0.40). Other AEM designs may vary both jet and entrainment port size to provide an even broader range up to 50% FiO_2. The aerosol entrainment collar fits over the air-entrainment ports (see later).

For controlled FiO_2 at flow high enough to prevent air dilution, the total output flow of an AEM must exceed the patient's peak inspiratory flow.[29] With an entrainment ratio exceeding 5:1, an AEM set to deliver less than 35% O_2 has little trouble meeting or exceeding the 60 L/min high-flow criterion (see previous Rule of Thumb). At settings greater than 35%, total AEM flow decreases significantly, and FiO_2 becomes variable. For example, when set to deliver 50% O_2, some AEMs provide 0.39 FiO_2.[32-34]

Air-Entrainment Nebulizer. Pneumatically powered air-entrainment nebulizers have most of the features of AEMs but have added capabilities, including additional humidification and temperature control. Humidification is achieved through production of aerosol at the nebulizer jet. Temperature control is provided by an optional heating element. In combination, these added features allow delivery of particulate water (in excess of needs for body temperature and pressure, saturated) to the airways. These devices are also widely known as *jet nebulizers* or *large volume nebulizers*.

Because of added humidification and heat control, air-entrainment nebulizers have been the traditional device of choice for delivering O_2 to patients with artificial tracheal airways. O_2 typically is delivered with a T tube or a tracheostomy mask. An alternative is to use an aerosol mask or a face tent to deliver an O_2 mixture via aerosol to patients with intact upper airways (Figure 38-16).[35]

AEMs can vary both jet and entrainment port size to obtain a given FiO_2; however, gas-powered nebulizers have a fixed orifice. Air-to-O_2 ratios can be altered only by varying entrainment port size. Disposable nebulizers usually have a continuous range of settings from 28% to 100%. Less commonly used nondisposable nebulizers have fixed entrainment settings, such as 100%, 70%, and 40%.[22]

Similar to AEMs, air-entrainment nebulizers perform as fixed-performance devices only when output flow meets or exceeds the patient's inspiratory demand. In contrast to AEMs, air-entrainment nebulizers do not allow easy increases in nebulizer output flow by means of an increase in O_2 input. With most nebulizer systems, the extremely small size of the jet needed for aerosol production limits the maximum O_2 input flow to 12 to 15 L/min at 50 psig. For example, the total output flow of an air-entrainment nebulizer set to deliver 40% O_2 ranges from 48 to 60 L/min. Although this amount may be adequate for most patients, it is insufficient for patients with very high inspiratory flow or minute volume.[35]

The actual FiO_2 received by patients may be affected by the choice of airway appliance. The FiO_2 delivered by face

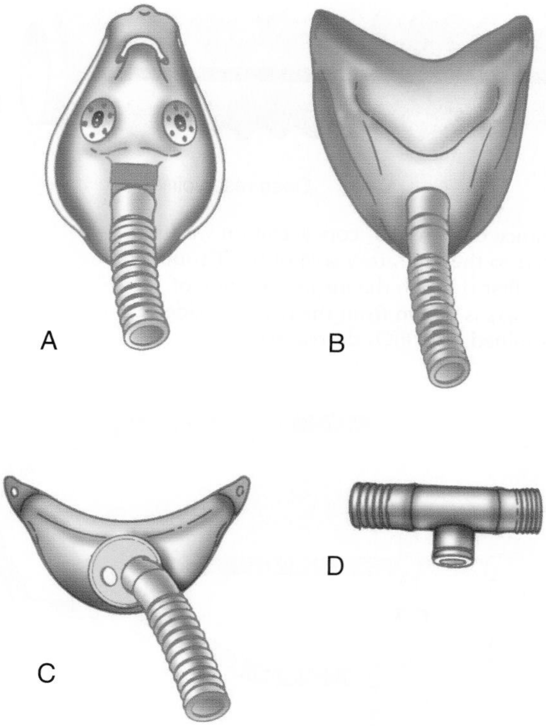

FIGURE 38-16 Devices for delivery of O_2 mixtures with aerosol. **A,** Aerosol mask. **B,** Face tent. **C,** Tracheostomy collar. **D,** T tube. (Modified from Kacmarek RM: In-hospital O_2 therapy. In Kacmarek RM, Stoller J, editors: Current respiratory care, Toronto, 1988, BC Decker.)

tent is consistently less than the set nebulizer concentration, especially at higher levels.[36]

Air-entrainment nebulizers should be treated as fixed-performance devices only when set to deliver low O_2 concentration (≤35%).[33] When a nebulizer is used to deliver a higher concentration of O_2, the RT must determine whether the flow is sufficient to meet patient needs. There are two ways to assess whether the flow of an air-entrainment nebulizer meets the patient's needs. The first method is simple visual inspection. With this approach (generally used only with a T tube), the RT sets up the device to deliver the highest possible flow at the prescribed FiO_2. After connecting the system to the patient, the RT observes the mist output at the expiratory side of the T tube. As long as mist can be seen escaping throughout inspiration, flow is adequate to meet the patient's needs, and the delivered FiO_2 is ensured.

The second way to assess the adequacy of nebulizer flow is to compare it with the patient's peak inspiratory flow. A patient's peak inspiratory flow during tidal breathing is approximately three times minute volume. As long as the nebulizer flow exceeds this value, the delivered FiO_2 is ensured. If the patient's peak flow exceeds that provided by the nebulizer, the device functions as a low-flow system with variable FiO_2 (see the accompanying Mini Clini for an example).[35]

MINI CLINI

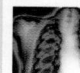

Computing Minimum Flow Needs

PROBLEM: A physician orders 40% O_2 through an air-entrainment nebulizer to a patient with a tidal volume of 0.6 L and a respiratory rate of 33 breaths/min. If maximum nebulizer input flow is 12 L/min, will the patient receive 40% O_2? If not, what total flow is needed to meet this patient's needs?

SOLUTION:

1. Estimate the patient's inspiratory flow:

$$\text{Peak inspiratory flow} = \dot{V}_E \times 3 = (0.6 \times 33) \times 3 = 59.4\ \text{L/min}$$

2. Compute the total flow of the nebulizer:

$$\text{Sum of ratio parts } (3:1) \times \text{Input flow } (12\ \text{L/min}) = 48\ \text{L/min}$$

3. Compare value 1 with value 2 (patient with nebulizer):

$$59.4\ \text{L/min (patient)} > 48\ \text{L/min (nebulizer)}$$

Under these conditions, the patient does not receive 40% O_2. To deliver a stable 40% O_2 concentration, the total flow would have to be at least 59.4 L/min.

Troubleshooting Air-Entrainment Systems. The major problem with air-entrainment systems is ensuring that the set FiO_2 actually is delivered to the patient. Problems usually do not occur when the devices are used to deliver low FiO_2 (<0.35). However, the design of these devices makes it difficult to provide even moderate FiO_2 at the high flow needed to ensure a set O_2 concentration. The performance of all air-entrainment devices is affected by downstream resistance. The result can be inaccurate FiO_2 that makes delivery of a low O_2 concentration difficult with air-entrainment nebulizers.

Providing Moderate to High FiO_2 at High Flow. AEMs and air-entrainment nebulizers differ in ratio settings and input and output flow capabilities. Most AEMs can be set to deliver no more than 50% O_2. When set according to the manufacturer's specifications to provide much more than 35% O_2, AEMs simply do not generate enough flow to ensure the set FiO_2. The solution is to boost the total output flow. With AEMs, total output flow can be boosted with a simple increase in input flow. For a 35% AEM (5:1 ratio) with an input flow of 8 L/min, the total output flow is 48 L/min. This flow is insufficient to ensure 35% O_2 delivery to all patients. Simply increasing the input flow to 12 L/min boosts the output flow of the AEM by 50%, to 72 L/min. The new high flow ensures delivery of the set O_2 concentration to essentially all patients.

This solution is impossible with most air-entrainment nebulizers. Because the small jets in many of these devices limit O_2 flow to 12 to 15 L/min, the input flow cannot be

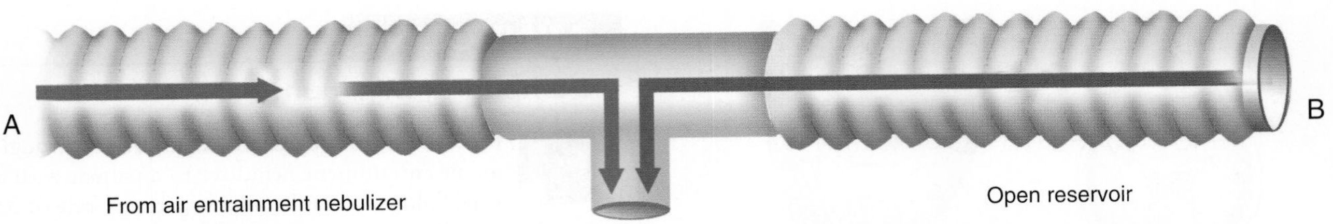

FIGURE 38-17 Use of an open volume reservoir to enhance delivered O_2 concentration with a T tube. From 50 to 150 ml of aerosol tubing is connected to the expiratory side of the T tube. **A,** When the patient inhales, gas at the set FiO_2 is drawn first through the inspiratory side of the circuit. **B,** If the patient's flow exceeds nebulizer flow, gas is drawn from the reservoir side. After the reservoir volume is fully tapped, room air is entrained, and FiO_2 decreases.

Box 38-2 Increasing FiO_2 Capabilities of Air-Entrainment Nebulizers

- Add open reservoir to expiratory side of T tube
- Provide inspiratory reservoir with one-way expiratory valve
- Connect two or more nebulizers together in parallel
- Set nebulizer to low concentration; bleed-in O_2; analyze and adjust
- Use a commercial dual-flow system

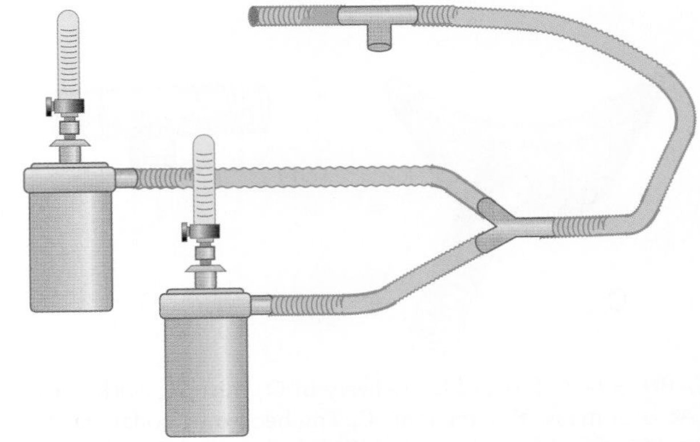

FIGURE 38-18 Use of two nebulizers in parallel to provide high FiO_2 at high flow.

increased beyond these levels. A few nebulizer models, such as the Thera-Mist Barrel Nebulizer (Smiths Medical, London, England), supposedly can provide moderately high output flows of 54 L/min at FiO_2 80%. However, most air-entrainment nebulizers cannot because of the total flow-to-FiO_2 tradeoff. The five alternatives for boosting the FiO_2 capabilities in these situations are presented in Box 38-2.

The simplest approach to achieving higher FiO_2 with these devices is to add a 50- to 150-ml aerosol tubing reservoir to the expiratory side of the T tube (Figure 38-17). Given its simplicity, adding an open volume reservoir to the expiratory side of T tubes is standard procedure in most clinical settings. This approach can be used only in the treatment of intubated patients. Even then, the small reservoir size limits the ability of this system to ensure stable FiO_2, especially greater than 40%, and larger reservoirs can cause rebreathing.

Rather than a simple open reservoir, a closed reservoir or nonrebreathing system similar to that shown in Figure 38-12 can be used. These systems combine an inspiratory volume reservoir (usually a compliant 3- to 5-L anesthesia bag) with a one-way expiratory valve. Whenever patient flow exceeds nebulizer flow, the expiratory valve closes, and the patient draws additional gas from the reservoir. Although they can ensure delivery of the set O_2 concentration, these systems pose considerable hazards. If source flow stops for any reason, the patient can suffocate. For this reason, these systems must be equipped with an emergency inlet valve that allows room air breathing in the event of source gas failure.

The third and most common approach to higher FiO_2 with air-entrainment nebulizers is to connect two or more devices together with a "wye" adapter (Figure 38-18).[22] Although a single air-entrainment nebulizer set at 60% (1:1 ratio) with a maximum input flow of 15 L/min has a total output flow of only 30 L/min, connecting two of these devices together doubles the total output flow to 60 L/min (the minimum needed for a high-flow device). This approach works well only for delivery of a concentration of 60% or less to patients with a minute volume less than 10 L/min.[35,37]

A fourth method for boosting FiO_2 provided by air-entrainment nebulizers is to set the device to a lower concentration than that prescribed (to generate high flow) while bleeding supplemental O_2 into the delivery tubing. This method increases both FiO_2 and total output flow. To achieve a specific FiO_2 in this type of system, the RT must analyze the delivered concentration and carefully adjust the supplemental O_2 input flow until the concentration is the desired value.

Commercial dual-flow systems entail a similar approach. One flow source powers the jet, while another flow source provides supplemental O_2. The Misty Ox (Vital Signs, Inc, Totowa, New Jersey) gas injection nebulizer is an example. This system is not an air-entrainment system because it does not depend on entrainment ports to increase total flow or O_2 concentration to the patient. Rather, it uses two

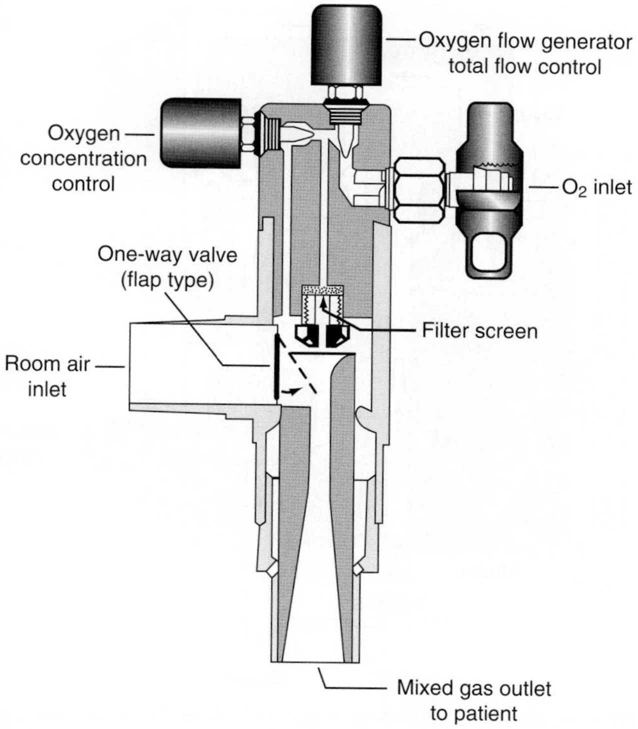

FIGURE 38-19 Downs adjustable flow generator (side view). O_2 source gas goes through two needle valves. One powers the jet and determines the amount of air entrained. The other provides supplemental O_2 to boost FiO_2.

flowmeters: one that operates the jet and one that feeds into the side of the jet manifold. The Misty Ox system can provide FiO_2 of 0.96 at a flow of 42 L/min and offers O_2 concentrations ranging from 0.21 to nearly 1.00.[35]

If aerosol is not needed, a simple dual-flow device such as the Downs flow generator (Figure 38-19) can be used. This device is attached to a 50-psig O_2 source and provides O_2 concentrations of 30% to 100% at a flow up to 100 L/min.[38]

Problems With Downstream Flow Resistance. Any increase in flow resistance downstream from (distal to) the point of air entrainment alters the performance of all air-entrainment systems. Increased downstream flow resistance causes back pressure. The back pressure decreases both the volume of entrained air and the total flow output of these devices. With less air entrained, the delivered O_2 concentration increases; however, because total flow output also decreases, the effect on FiO_2 varies. High downstream flow resistance usually turns air-entrainment systems from high-flow (fixed) O_2 delivery systems into low-flow (variable) O_2 delivery systems incapable of delivering a precise and constant FiO_2.[29]

This problem explains why it is extremely difficult to deliver less than 28% to 30% O_2 with an air-entrainment nebulizer. The 5 to 6 ft (1.5 to 1.8 m) of aerosol tubing normally used with these devices produces enough flow resistance to decrease air entrainment and prevent a lower FiO_2.

A similar situation can occur when the entrainment ports of an air-entrainment device become obstructed (most common with AEMs). Delivered O_2 concentration increases, but total output flow decreases. The net effect usually is a variable FiO_2. The accompanying Mini Clini is an example of the effect of increased downstream flow resistance on the performance of an air-entrainment device.

MINI CLINI

Effect of Downstream Flow Resistance on Performance of an Air-Entrainment Device

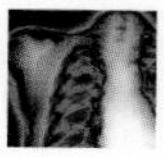

PROBLEM: A tracheostomy patient is receiving O_2 therapy through a T tube attached to an air-entrainment nebulizer set at 35% O_2 with an input flow of 10 L/min. Over the past 30 minutes, the patient's SpO_2 has decreased from 93% to 88%. When assessing the patient, the RT finds that the large-bore delivery tubing of the nebulizer is partially obstructed with condensate and that aerosol mist at the T tube is not visible throughout inspiration. What is the likely problem, and what is the best solution?

SOLUTION: The likely problem is a decrease in FiO_2 owing to the increased downstream resistance caused by the condensate. At 10 L/min input flow, the device was probably delivering approximately 60 L/min of 35% O_2 before the tubing became obstructed. Because aerosol mist is not visible at the T tube throughout inspiration, it is clear that the total output flow is no longer sufficient and that the patient is now diluting the delivered O_2 with room air. Draining the tubing restores the system flow and ensures delivery of the set FiO_2.

Blending Systems. When air-entrainment devices cannot provide a high enough O_2 concentration or flow, use of a gas blending system should be considered. With a blending system, separate pressurized air and O_2 sources are input, and the gases are mixed either manually or with a precision valve (blender). This system allows precise control over both FiO_2 and total flow output. Most blending systems can provide flow much greater than 60 L/min, qualifying them as true fixed-performance delivery devices. For adults, gas is delivered from the blender either through an open system, such as an aerosol mask or T tube, or with a closed nonrebreathing system. For many patients requiring high FiO_2 and breathing spontaneously, this is the ideal setup, provided that the gas is humidified. The use of high-flow blended systems with heated humidity as opposed to a heated aerosol are very well tolerated by most patients, including patients with tracheostomies.

Mixing Gases Manually. When gases are mixed manually, separate air and O_2 flowmeters must be adjusted for the desired FiO_2 and flow (see the accompanying Mini

Clini). For adults, this approach requires calibrated high-flow flowmeters (at least 60 L/min) and monitoring of delivered FiO_2.

MINI CLINI

Manually Mixing Air and Oxygen to Achieve Specified Concentration at a Given Flow

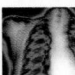

PROBLEM: To mix air and O_2 manually to provide a patient with 50% O_2 at a total flow of 60 L/min, what O_2 and air flow would the RT set?

SOLUTION:

1. Use Equation 38-3 to compute the O_2 flow:

$$O_2 \text{ flow} = \frac{\text{Total flow} \times (O_2\% - 21)}{79}$$

$$O_2 \text{ flow} = \frac{60 \times (50 - 12)}{79}$$

$$O_2 \text{ flow} = 22 \text{ L/min}$$

2. Compute the air flow:

$$\text{Air flow} = \text{Total flow} - O_2 \text{ flow}$$

$$\text{Air flow} = 60 - 22$$

$$\text{Air flow} = 38 \text{ L/min}$$

To provide a patient with 50% O_2 at a total flow of 60 L/min, blend 22 L of O_2 with 38 L of air.

Oxygen Blenders. Rather than manually mixing air and O_2, the RT can use an O_2 blender. Figure 38-20 shows the major components of a typical O_2 blender. Air and O_2 enter the blender and pass through dual pressure regulators that exactly match the two pressures. Gas flows to a precision proportioning valve. Because the two gas pressures at this point are equal, varying the size of the air and O_2 inlets provides precise control over the relative concentration.

An alarm system gives an audible warning when either source gas fails or the pressure decreases below a specified value. The alarm system usually has a crossover or bypass feature whereby failure of one gas source causes the blender system to switch to the other. If the air source fails when delivering 60% O_2, the alarm sounds, and the blender switches over to delivery of 100% O_2.

Although they allow ideal control over both FiO_2 and flow, blenders are especially prone to inaccuracy and failure.[39,40] To avoid these problems, the RT always should conduct an operational check of any blender before using it on a patient (Box 38-3). FiO_2 should be checked and confirmed with a calibrated O_2 analyzer at least once per shift.[2] As always, a device that does not perform according to expectations should be replaced immediately. When a blender is used in the care of a neonate, an O_2 analyzer should be kept in-line at all times. In the use of a nonrebreathing or closed delivery system, (1) all breathing valves should be inspected and tested before application to a patient, and (2) a fail-safe inspiratory valve should be included in the delivery system.

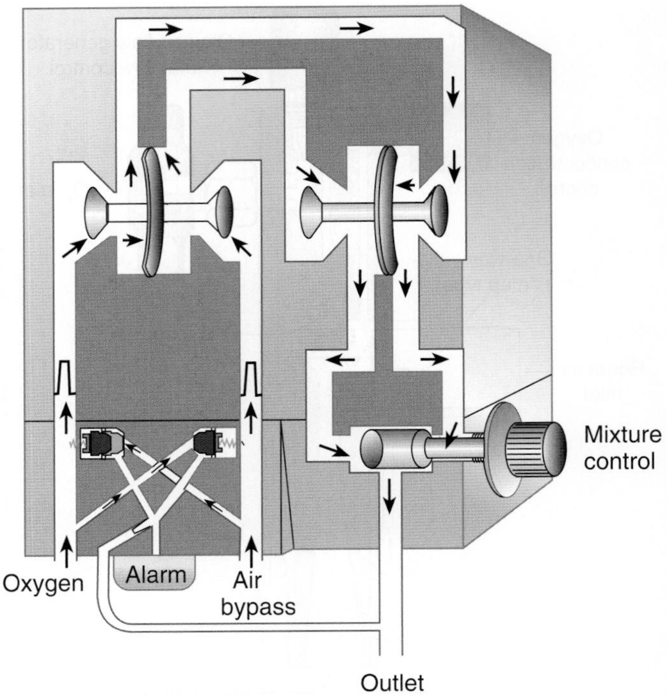

FIGURE 38-20 O_2 blending device. (Modified from McPherson SP: Respiratory therapy equipment, ed 3, St. Louis, 1985, Mosby.)

Box 38-3 Procedure for Confirming Operation of an Oxygen Blender

1. Confirm that inlet pressures of air and O_2 are within manufacturer's specifications.
2. Test low air and O_2 alarms by disconnecting each source; also confirm safety bypass or crossover system.
3. Analyze O_2 concentration at 100%, 21%, and specified FiO_2.

Enclosures. The concept of enclosing a patient in a controlled-O_2 atmosphere is among the oldest approaches to O_2 therapy. Entire rooms once were used for this purpose. With today's simpler airway devices, enclosures are generally used only in the care of infants and children. The primary types of O_2 enclosures used for infants and children are tents, incubators, and hoods.

Oxygen Tents. O_2 tents previously were the most common method of O_2 therapy in the treatment of both adults and children. Use of O_2 tents in both adults and children is rare at the present time. However, when they are used, it is common for tents to be air-conditioned or cooled with ice to provide a comfortable temperature within a plastic sheet canopy (Figure 38-21).

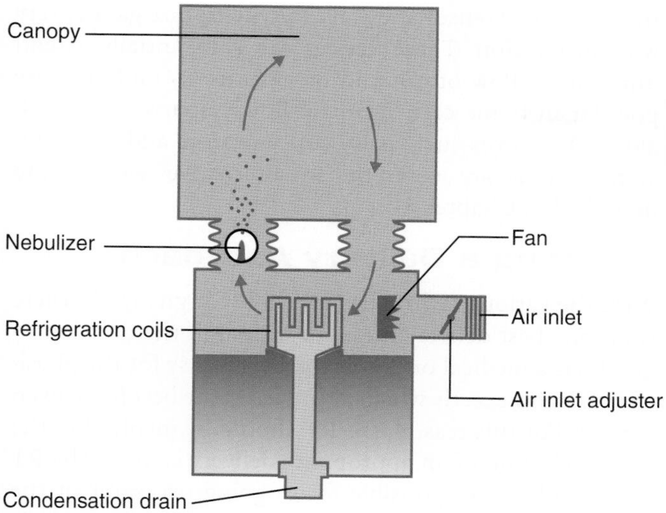

FIGURE 38-21 O_2 tent incorporating refrigeration coils for cooling. (Modified from Cairo JM, Pilbeam SP: Mosby's respiratory care equipment, ed 8, St. Louis, 2010, Mosby.)

The main problem with tents is that frequent opening and closing of the canopy cause wide swings in O_2 concentration. Constant leakage makes a high FiO_2 impossible. In large tents, O_2 input flow of 12 to 15 L/min can provide only 40% to 50% O_2 levels. Comparable FiO_2 can be achieved in smaller pediatric or croup tents with flow of 8 to 10 L/min. Because of these limitations, tents are used primarily for pediatric aerosol therapy in the care of children with **croup** or cystic fibrosis.

Hoods. An O_2 hood, also known as an *oxyhood,* is often the best method for administration of controlled O_2 therapy to infants. As shown in Figure 38-22, an O_2 hood covers only the head, leaving the infant's body free for nursing care. O_2 is delivered to the hood through either a heated air-entrainment nebulizer or a blending system with a heated humidifier. A minimum flow of 7 L/min should be set to prevent accumulation of CO_2.[41] Depending on the size of the hood, flow of 10 to 15 L/min may be needed to maintain stable high O_2 concentration. Higher flow generally is not needed and may produce a harmful noise level and additional stress on neonatal patients.[42]

In the care of premature infants, it is especially important to ensure that the gas mixture is properly warmed and humidified and not directed toward the patient's face or head. Low temperatures or convection cooling produced by high flow over the head can cause heat loss and cold stress. In premature infants, cold stress can increase O_2 consumption and cause apnea.[43]

The temperature of gases provided to an infant in an O_2 hood should be precisely set to maintain a **neutral thermal environment (NTE).** The NTE temperature varies according to an infant's age and weight. The NTE temperature for newborns weighing less than 1200 g is 95° F (35° C). For older infants weighing 2500 g or more, the NTE is lower, approximately 86° F (30° C).[43] The importance of temperature regulation in infants is discussed in more detail in Chapter 48.

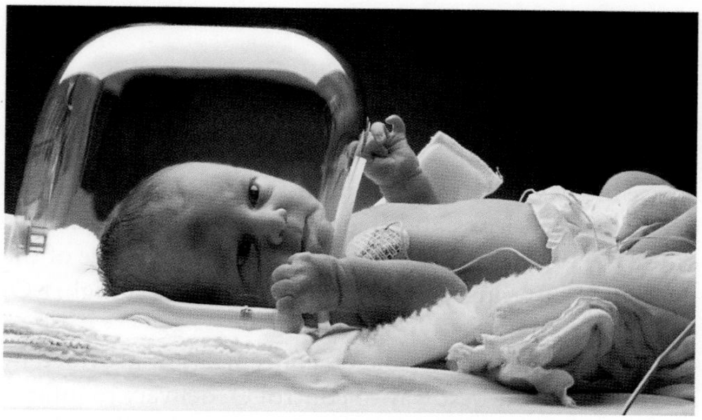

FIGURE 38-22 Infant O_2 hood. (Courtesy Utah Medical Products, Inc, Midvale, Utah.)

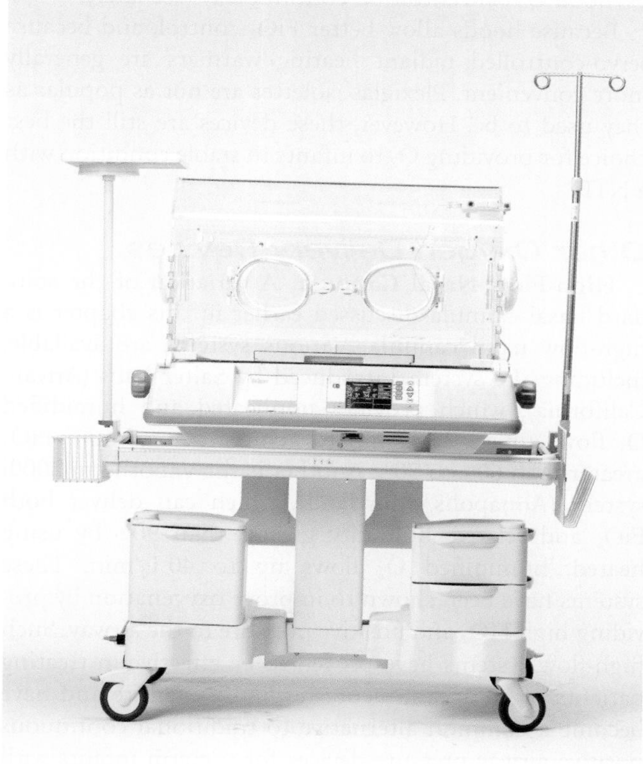

FIGURE 38-23 Infant isolette. (Courtesy Dräger Medical AG & Co, Lübeck, Germany.)

Incubators. Incubators, also known by the trade name Isolette (Dräger Medical AG & Co, Lübeck, Germany) are polymethyl methacrylate (Plexiglas) enclosures that combine servo-controlled convection heating with supplemental O_2 (Figure 38-23). In older models, humidification was provided with a blow-over water reservoir located under the patient platform. Because of the high infection risk associated with this design, these systems are no longer in common use. When it is needed, supplemental humidity usually is provided with an external heated humidifier or nebulizer.

Supplemental O_2 can be administered with a direct connection between the incubator and a flowmeter that has a heated humidifier. In some units, a filtered air-entrainment device limits the delivered concentration to approximately 0.40. However, leaks and frequent opening of the isolette dilute the O_2 levels to much less than 40%. Blockage of the inlet filter can cause less air entrainment and a higher O_2 concentration.[43]

Given the highly variable O_2 concentration provided by these devices, the best way to control O_2 delivery to infants in an isolette is with an oxyhood. The oxyhood is placed over the infant's head inside the isolette. The O_2 concentration and gas temperature within the oxyhood, not in the isolette, must be assessed. It is ideal to monitor isolette or oxyhood O_2 concentration continuously (see later).[2,4]

Because hoods allow better FiO_2 control, and because servo-controlled radiant heating warmers are generally more convenient, Plexiglas isolettes are not as popular as they used to be. However, these devices are still the best choice for providing O_2 to infants in stable condition with a NTE.[43]

Other Oxygen Delivery Devices

High-Flow Nasal Cannula. A variation of the standard nasal cannula discussed earlier in this chapter is a high-flow nasal cannula. Various systems are available, including the system introduced by Salter Labs (Arivan, California), which provides nonheated and humidified O_2 flows up to 15 L/min to achieve a maximum FiO_2 greater than 60% to 70%. Another is the Vapotherm 2000i system (Annapolis, Maryland), which can deliver both FiO_2 and relative humidity greater than 90% by using heated, humidified O_2 flows up to 40 L/min. These systems have been shown to improve oxygenation by providing high FiO_2 and positive pressure to the airway. Such high-flow systems have proven to be effective in treating patients of all ages in acute respiratory failure and have become a common alternative to traditional continuous positive airway pressure devices for preterm infants with disorders including apnea of prematurity and bronchopulmonary dysplasia. However, a major limitation of these devices is that it is generally impossible to determine precisely and monitor the level of positive pressure actually applied.[35]

Bag-Mask Devices. There are other ways to administer O_2 in selected settings in addition to the previously described systems. Bag-mask devices use a self-inflating bag and nonrebreathing valve features to provide up to 100% O_2. Bag-mask devices are often used in emergency life support and in critical care and are more completely discussed in Chapter 34.

Demand-Flow and Pulse-Dose Systems. Finally, specialized O_2 delivery systems are common in non–acute care settings. These include demand-flow or pulse-dose systems that use a flow sensor and valve to synchronize gas delivery with inspiration. These devices can substantially extend duration of flow of a liquid or gaseous O_2 tank and are popular in home care. Demand-flow systems and standalone O_2 sources such as O_2 concentrators and liquid O_2 systems that are common in alternative settings are described in Chapter 51.

Selecting a Delivery Approach

With the various techniques available for giving O_2, there is no one best delivery method. Although the decision to give O_2 is a medical one, it is not always easy for the physician to know exactly which approach is the best for a given patient. For this reason, the RT should be involved in the initial selection of an appropriate delivery system. The RT also should be responsible for ongoing oversight of the prescribed therapy. This responsibility should include making recommendations—on the basis of sound patient assessment—to change or discontinue the treatment regimen (see later section on Protocol-Based Oxygen Therapy).

The three Ps—*purpose, patient,* and *performance*—are used in the selection or recommendation of a change in O_2 delivery system. The goal is to match the performance characteristics of the equipment to both the objectives of therapy (purpose) and the patient's special needs.

Purpose

The general purpose or objective of all O_2 therapy is to increase FiO_2 sufficiently to correct arterial hypoxemia. Other objectives, including decreasing hypoxic symptoms and minimizing increased cardiopulmonary work, follow from this primary purpose.

Patient

Key patient considerations in selecting O_2 therapy equipment for use in acute care are summarized in Box 38-4. Knowledge of these factors helps guide the RT in selecting the appropriate equipment. For example, a simple mask at 5 to 6 L/min is probably more suitable than a nasal cannula at 4 L/min for a mouth breathing, mildly hypoxemic patient. An infant with moderate hypoxia and a normal airway usually needs an O_2 enclosure (hood or enclosed incubator).

Box 38-4 Patient Factors in Selecting Oxygen Therapy Equipment

- Severity and cause of hypoxemia
- Patient age group (infant, child, adult)
- Degree of consciousness and alertness
- Presence or absence of tracheal airway
- Stability of minute ventilation
- Mouth breathing vs. nose breathing patient

TABLE 38-8

Selection of an Oxygen Delivery System Based on Desired FiO_2 Level and Stability

	Desired FiO_2 Stability	
Desired FiO_2 Level	**Fixed**	**Variable**
Low (<35%)	AEM	Nasal cannula
	Air-entrainment nebulizer	Nasal catheter
	Blending system	Transtracheal catheter
	Isolette, incubator (infant)	
Moderate (35%-60%)	Air-entrainment nebulizer	Simple mask
	Blending system	Air-entrainment nebulizer
	Oxyhood (infant)	Tent (child)
High (>60%)	Blending system	Partial rebreather
	Oxyhood (infant)	Nonrebreather

Performance

O_2 systems vary according to actual FiO_2 delivered and stability of FiO_2 under changing patient demands. Generally, the more critically ill the patient, the greater the need for a stable, high FiO_2. Less acutely ill patients generally need a lower, less exact FiO_2. Table 38-8 lists guidelines for selecting an O_2 delivery system on the basis of the level and stability of the FiO_2 needed.

General Goals and Patient Categories

On the basis of overall consideration of the three *Ps*, general goals can be set for several patient categories. In emergencies in which tissue hypoxia is suspected, patients should be given the highest FiO_2 possible–ideally 100%. This level can be achieved with a true high-flow or a closed reservoir system. The goal is the highest possible blood O_2 content. Clinical examples include respiratory or cardiac arrest, severe trauma, shock, carbon monoxide poisoning, and cyanide poisoning. Carbon monoxide and cyanide poisoning may necessitate HBO therapy (see later).

A critically ill adult patient with moderate to severe hypoxemia needs either a reservoir or a high-flow system capable of at least 60% O_2. Thereafter, changes in FiO_2 (and device) should be based on results of assessment of physiologic values. The goal is a PaO_2 greater than 60 mm Hg or oxyhemoglobin saturation greater than 90%.

In the care of adult patients in more stable condition but who are acutely ill with mild to moderate hypoxemia, a system capable of low to moderate O_2 concentration can be used. In these cases, stability of FiO_2 is not critical. Applicable devices include a nasal cannula at moderate flow or a simple mask. Common examples include patients in the immediately postoperative phase and patients recovering from acute myocardial infarction.

Adult patients with chronic lung disease and accompanying acute-on-chronic hypoxemia present a special case. In the care of these patients, the goal is to ensure adequate arterial oxygenation without depressing ventilation. Adequate oxygenation of these patients generally means SaO_2 of 85% to 92% with PaO_2 of 50 to 70 mm Hg.[31,44] These values usually are achieved with either low-flow nasal O_2 or a low-concentration (24% to 28%) AEM. The less stable the patient's condition, the greater the need for a high-flow AEM.[22]

Because of size, discomfort, and appearance, AEMs are less well tolerated than nasal cannulas for long-term therapy. In contrast to a cannula, an AEM must be removed for eating and drinking. Because even a short break in O_2 therapy can cause a rapid decrease in PaO_2 in some patients, these patients should be taught to switch to a nasal cannula whenever they must remove the mask.[22]

Lastly, it is sometimes necessary to modify O_2 delivery systems to facilitate patient transport. An example is a spontaneously breathing patient with a tracheostomy tube receiving a moderate FiO_2 via a blended system or an air-entrainment nebulizer connected to a tracheostomy mask. Given the impracticalities of transporting a patient on an air-entrainment nebulizer, it may be more suitable to connect a Venturi adapter temporarily to provide the appropriate FiO_2 to the tracheostomy mask during the transport. It is important to remember to reconnect patients back to the original set-up immediately after the transport to avoid exposing them to dry gases for long time periods.

Protocol-Based Oxygen Therapy

O_2 therapy is ideally suited for a protocol. Bedside assessment of oxygenation by RTs and other clinicians has progressed to where it is more cost-effective and clinically appropriate to use a protocol rather than obtaining a new physician order for each change in FiO_2. An order for "O_2 therapy via protocol" permits O_2 therapy to be initiated, modified, or discontinued by the RT, provided that an assessment reveals that the patient meets previously approved clinical criteria. A well-designed O_2 protocol ensures the patient (1) undergoes initial assessment, (2) is evaluated for protocol criteria, (3) receives a treatment plan that is modified according to need, and (4) stops receiving therapy as soon as it is no longer needed.[45]

Figure 38-24 shows the decision algorithm underlying an O_2 therapy titration protocol developed at the Cleveland Clinic Foundation. In the algorithm, a pulse oximetry saturation (SpO_2) of 92% is the threshold value that indicates the need for therapy. As indicated in the algorithm, the titration is bypassed if a patient already has signs of hypoxemia, in which case the patient immediately receives supplemental O_2. Otherwise, the level of supplemental O_2 is adjusted, and the patient is reassessed on each shift for determination of continuing need. When the SpO_2 is 92% or greater on room air, therapy is discontinued.

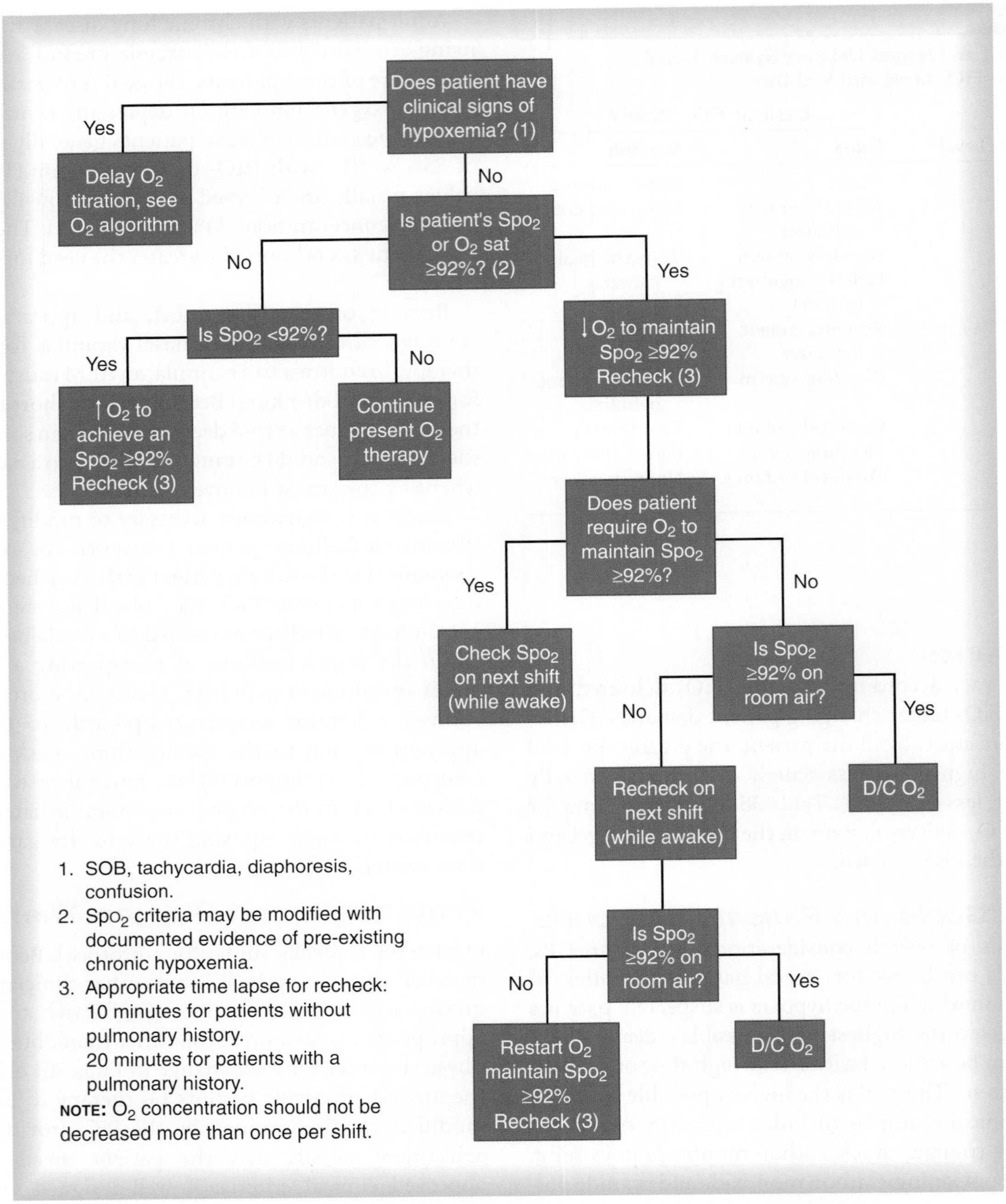

FIGURE 38-24 Protocol for titration of O_2 therapy. (Courtesy the Respiratory Therapy Section, Cleveland Clinic Foundation, Cleveland, Ohio.)

HYPERBARIC OXYGEN THERAPY

Hyperbaric oxygen (HBO) therapy is the therapeutic use of O_2 at pressures greater than 1 atm.[46-48] Pressures during HBO therapy usually are expressed in multiples of **atmospheric pressure absolute (ATA):** 1 ATA equals 760 mm Hg (101.32 kPa). Most HBO therapy is conducted at pressures between 2 ATA and 3 ATA, although other pressures may be used, often based on U.S. Navy diving treatment tables.[47-49]

Physiologic Effects

The known physiologic effects of HBO therapy are summarized in Box 38-5.[46] These effects are mainly due to either high pressure or high O_2 tension in body fluids and tissues. In conditions such as air embolism and decompression sickness, high pressure exerts a physical effect on air or nitrogen bubbles trapped in the blood or tissues. According to Boyle's law, high pressure decreases the size of these bubbles and minimizes potential harm. Because pressure is crucial in these cases, HBO treatments may be conducted at 6 ATA or more.[47,49]

Box 38-5 Physiologic Effects of Hyperbaric Oxygen Therapy

- Bubble reduction (Boyle's law)
- Hyperoxygenation of blood and tissue (Henry's law)
- Vasoconstriction
- Enhanced host immune function
- Neovascularization

The second beneficial effect of HBO is hyperoxia. When a patient is breathing room air, only a small amount of O_2 dissolves in the plasma (approximately 0.3 ml/dl). At 3 ATA, plasma contains nearly 7 ml/dl dissolved O_2, a level exceeding average resting tissue uptake.[47]

O_2 supply to the tissues affects the immune system, wound healing, and vascular tone. A tissue PO_2 of at least 30 mm Hg is necessary for normal cellular function. Damaged and infected tissues often have a lower PO_2. Increasing O_2 supply to these tissues can help restore both white blood cell function and antimicrobial activity.

Hyperoxia affects the cardiovascular system. HBO therapy causes generalized vasoconstriction and a small decrease in cardiac output. Although these changes may decrease blood flow to a region, this effect is more than offset by the increase in O_2 content. In conditions such as burns, cerebral edema, and crush injuries, vasoconstriction may be helpful because it reduces edema and tissue swelling while maintaining tissue oxygenation.

Hyperoxia also helps form new capillary beds, a process called **neovascularization.** Although the exact mechanism is unknown, neovascularization is an essential component of tissue repair, especially in radiation-induced injuries.[47,48]

Study results suggest that HBO may be useful in many other conditions, including the management of stroke, wound healing, and treating stubborn soft tissue infections. Because HBO has emerged as a highly effective therapy for various conditions, government and many private health insurance providers have expanded coverage for HBO. Likewise, many hospitals now offer HBO therapy, and opportunities in this area have increased for RTs.[50,51]

Methods of Administration

HBO is administered in either a multiplace or a monoplace chamber. A multiplace chamber is a large tank capable of holding a dozen or more people (Figure 38-25, *A*). Because patients are directly cared for by medical staff inside the tank, multiplace chambers have air locks that allow entry and exit without altering the pressure. The multiplace chamber is generally filled with air. If indicated, only the patient breathes supplemental O_2 (through a mask or another device). Because they can achieve pressures of 6 ATA or more, multiplace chambers are ideal for the management of decompression sickness and air embolism.[47-49]

Box 38-6 Indications for Hyperbaric Oxygen Therapy

ACUTE CONDITIONS

- Decompression sickness
- Air or gas embolism
- Carbon monoxide and cyanide poisoning
- Acute traumatic ischemia (compartment syndrome, crush injury)
- Acute peripheral arterial insufficiency
- Intracranial abscesses
- Crush injuries and suturing of severed limbs
- Clostridial gangrene
- Necrotizing soft tissue infection
- Ischemic skin graft or flap

CHRONIC CONDITIONS

- Diabetic wounds of the lower extremities and other nonhealing wounds
- Refractory osteomyelitis
- Actinomycosis (chronic systemic abscesses)
- Radiation necrosis (HBO as an adjunct to conventional treatment)

A typical monoplace chamber consists of a transparent Plexiglas cylinder large enough only for a single patient (see Figure 38-25, *B*). During therapy, the cylinder O_2 concentration is kept at 100%. The patient need not wear a mask. Because of the high O_2 concentration, most electronic equipment cannot be used in a monoplace chamber. In addition, many ventilators do not function properly under these conditions. However, monitoring systems and ventilators can be adapted to allow treatment of a critically ill patient with hyperbaric pressure. Additionally, artificial airways suited to function properly under hyperbaric conditions should be used.[46]

Indications

HBO has long been accepted as the primary treatment of divers with decompression sickness. Several other of the most common indications for HBO therapy are listed in Box 38-6.[46,48] The two most common acute conditions for which RTs administer HBO are air embolism and carbon monoxide poisoning.[46,49,52]

Air Embolism

Air embolism is a complication that can occur with certain cardiovascular procedures, lung biopsy, hemodialysis, and central line placement. Air bubbles that reach the cerebral or cardiac circulation can cause severe neurologic symptoms or sudden death. HBO decreases the volume of air bubbles and helps oxygenate local tissues. Typical therapy for air embolism involves immediate pressurization in air to 6 ATA for 15 to 30 minutes. This step is followed by decompression to 2.8 ATA with prolonged O_2 treatment.[47-49]

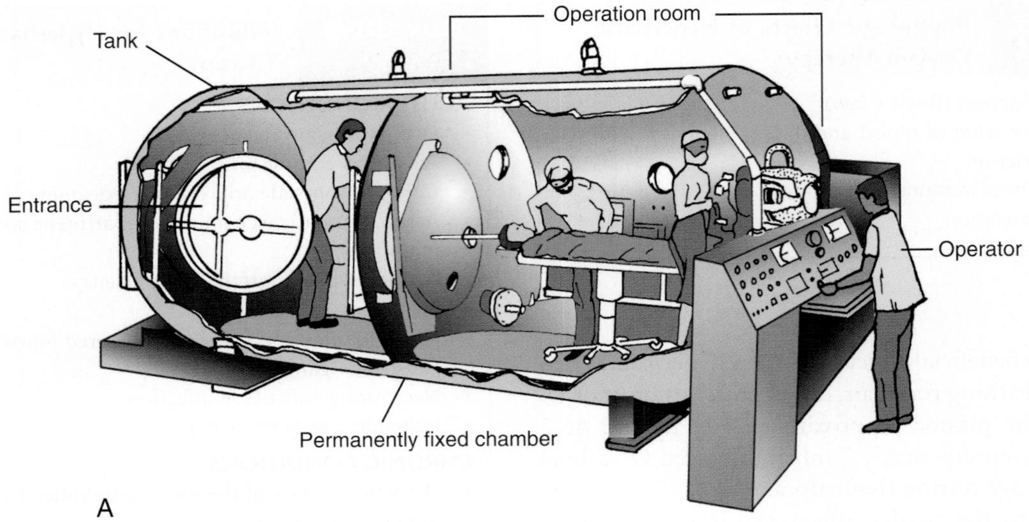

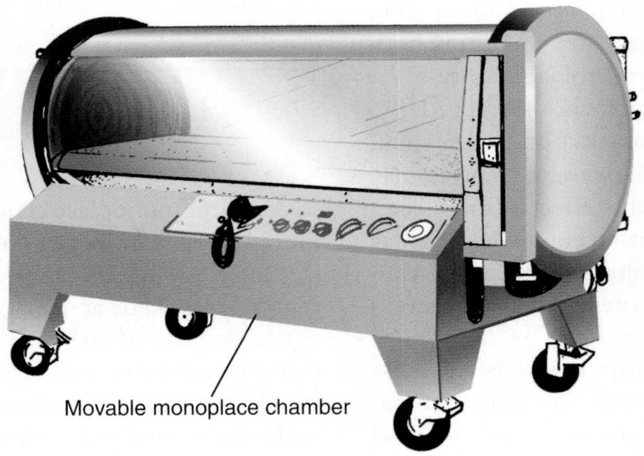

FIGURE 38-25 **A,** Fixed hyperbaric chamber. **B,** Monoplace chamber.

Carbon Monoxide Poisoning

Carbon monoxide poisoning accounts for about half of all poisoning deaths in the United States. The condition of a patient with carbon monoxide poisoning improves quickly with HBO treatment because this treatment is the fastest way to remove carbon monoxide from the blood.[52] If a patient breathes air, it takes more than 5 hours to remove only one half of the carboxyhemoglobin in the blood. Breathing 100% O_2 reduces this "half-life" to 80 minutes. The half-life of carboxyhemoglobin under HBO at 3 ATA is only 23 minutes. Box 38-7 lists the major criteria for selecting patients with acute carbon monoxide poisoning for treatment with HBO.[52]

Box 38-7 **Criteria for Hyperbaric Oxygen Therapy for Acute Carbon Monoxide Poisoning**

- History of unconsciousness
- Presence of neuropsychiatric abnormality
- Presence of cardiac instability or cardiac ischemia
- Carboxyhemoglobin level 25% (lower levels for children and pregnant women)

Complications and Hazards

Although the benefits of HBO are significant, this type of therapy also has significant risks. As a result, the benefits should be compared with the hazards before therapy is initiated. Common complications of HBO are listed in Box 38-8.[47] These complications are generally caused by high pressure, O_2 toxicity, fire, or worsening of certain existing conditions. The most frequent problems involve barotrauma to closed body cavities, such as the middle ear or sinuses. Pneumothorax and air embolism also are possible during HBO treatment but are rare in patients with normal lungs.

O_2 at high pressure can be neurotoxic. Early signs of impending CNS toxicity include twitching, sweating,

Box 38-8 Major Complications of Hyperbaric Oxygen Therapy

BAROTRAUMA
- Ear or sinus trauma
- Tympanic membrane rupture
- Alveolar overdistention and pneumothorax
- Gas embolism

OXYGEN TOXICITY
- CNS toxic reaction
- Pulmonary toxic reaction

OTHER
- Fire
- Sudden decompression
- Reversible visual changes
- Claustrophobia
- Decreased cardiac output

pallor, and restlessness. These signs usually are followed by seizures and convulsions. However, CNS toxicity rarely occurs with the pressures and treatment times commonly used for clinical HBO therapy.[48]

In terms of pulmonary O_2 toxicity, HBO treatments do not normally expose patients to high PO_2 long enough to cause damage. However, HBO may have an additive effect on critically ill patients who receive high FiO_2 between HBO treatments.[47,48]

Avoiding fire and sudden decompression are primary safety concerns. Only 100% cotton fabric should be used to avoid fire from a static electrical discharge. Other ignition sources such as matches or lighters should never be brought into HBO chambers, and alcohol or petroleum-based products, including makeup or deodorant, should never be used. Other potential hazards of HBO involve the aggravation of existing conditions, including diabetes, epilepsy, and hypertension. These concerns can be addressed by being aware of such preexisting conditions through an appropriate history and chart review, close patient monitoring, and appropriate adjustment of therapy.

There are numerous relative contraindications for HBO, many of which relate to the potential complications and hazards noted earlier. For patients with inner ear infections and seizure disorders, which represent relative contraindications, the risks of HBO should be carefully weighed against the benefits. Absolute contradictions include an untreated pneumothorax and congenital heart defects resulting in dependency on a patent ductus arteriosus for survival. Such patients generally should not receive HBO therapy.[48]

Troubleshooting

Although fire hazards restrict the use of certain electronic equipment, some state-of-the-art monitors and ventilators with solid-state circuitry can be used within the chamber. This equipment allows intensive care of critically ill patients.[46]

In regard to ventilator use, reductions in delivered tidal volume should be expected and corrected. Additionally, tracheostomy or endotracheal tubes with foam or fluid-filled cuffs should generally be used to preserve cuff integrity under pressure. If not accounted for, reduced tidal volumes and leaks can lead to respiratory hypercapnia and acidosis. Hypercapnia can result in respiratory acidosis and can worsen CNS toxicity owing to cerebral vasodilation.[48] Generally, pressure-regulating and flow-regulating equipment used in a hyperbaric chamber must be specifically designed for operation at chamber pressure or appropriately modified to the additional barometric pressure exerted.

OTHER MEDICAL GAS THERAPIES

O_2 is not the only medical gas administered by RTs. The potent pulmonary vasodilator, **nitric oxide (NO),** and helium-O_2 mixtures, used as an adjunct tool in certain forms of airway obstruction, are among other medical gases administered by RTs.

Nitric Oxide Therapy

Mode of Action

NO gas is a colorless, odorless, highly diffusible, and lipid-soluble free radical that oxidizes quickly to nitrogen dioxide (NO_2) in the presence of O_2. NO is normally produced in the human body from L-arginine in a reaction catalyzed by the enzyme NO synthase. NO activates guanylate cyclase, which catalyzes the production of **cyclic guanosine 3′,5′-monophosphate (cGMP).** The end result is that increased cGMP levels cause vascular smooth muscle relaxation.[53]

Because it relaxes capillary smooth muscle, the therapeutic benefit of inhaled NO stems from improved blood flow to ventilated alveoli. The result is a reduction in intrapulmonary shunting, improvement in arterial oxygenation, and a decrease in pulmonary vascular resistance and pulmonary arterial pressure.

The effects of inhaled NO are limited to the pulmonary circulation. After diffusing into the capillaries, free NO immediately binds to hemoglobin, forming nitrosylhemoglobin. Nitrosylhemoglobin is rapidly oxidized to methemoglobin, which eventually undergoes conversion to reduced hemoglobin.[53]

Indications

After several years of clinical testing, inhaled NO was approved in December 1999 by the U.S. Food and Drug Administration (FDA) for treating selected neonates. Specifically, NO, in conjunction with such therapies as ventilatory support, has been approved for the treatment of term and near-term (>34 weeks) neonates with hypoxic (type I) respiratory failure with associated pulmonary hypertension. As a result of the clinical benefits of reduced pulmonary vascular resistance, improved oxygenation, and less need for a highly invasive method for increasing tissue oxygenation known as *extracorporeal membrane oxygenation,* inhaled NO is emerging as the standard of care for near-term neonates with this type of respiratory failure.[54]

In adults, studies have shown that inhaled NO has been effective in treating pulmonary hypertension associated with acute respiratory distress syndrome (ARDS). However, these benefits seem to be short-lived, and no significant improvement in clinical outcomes, including mortality, has been shown to date. As a result of these findings and lower cost alternative drug therapies, including inhaled epoprostenol sodium (Flolan) and similar medications (discussed in Chapter 32), the use of inhaled NO in adults has neither been approved by the FDA nor gained widespread acceptance, However, potential indications and various delivery methods for inhaled NO continue to be examined. Potential indications for inhaled NO are listed in Box 38-9.[54,55]

Dosing

The amount of NO needed to improve oxygenation or decrease pulmonary vascular pressure in neonates is relatively low. The therapeutic range of NO is 2 to 20 ppm, and an initial dose of 20 ppm is commonly used. Treatment should be continued until underlying oxygenation desaturation has resolved. For many patients, dosages often can be reduced to less than 20 ppm at the end of 4 hours of initial treatment, as tolerated. At these levels, NO has minimal toxicity.[54] In clinical trials, higher doses were not shown to be more effective and placed the patient at a higher risk of complications.[53-55]

Toxicity and Adverse Effects

The toxicity of NO is caused by its own direct action and its chemical by-products. In high concentrations (5000 to 20,000 ppm), NO causes acute pulmonary edema that can be fatal. Inhalation of a lower concentration has been associated with direct cellular damage and impaired surfactant production.[55,56]

Most of the toxic effects of NO are caused by its chemical by-products, especially NO_2. NO_2 is produced spontaneously whenever NO is exposed to O_2. NO_2 is more toxic than NO. Levels greater than 10 ppm can cause cell damage, hemorrhage, pulmonary edema, and death. The U.S. Occupational Safety and Health Administration has set the safety limit for NO_2 exposure at 5 ppm. The clinical goal is to keep NO_2 exposure less than 2 ppm during administration of NO.[56]

Other harmful chemical by-products produced in reaction with NO include methemoglobin and peroxynitrite (produced when NO reacts with superoxide). Although it can occur with NO administration, methemoglobinemia probably is not a large problem considering the doses commonly used and the required monitoring systems discussed later in this section. Peroxynitrite is a potent oxidant that can cause severe cell damage; however, there is no hard evidence supporting its toxic effects during NO administration.

Potential adverse effects associated with NO therapy are listed in Box 38-10.[56] A poor or paradoxical response to NO has been observed in some patients. Of patients with ARDS, 40% do not have initial improvement in oxygenation with NO therapy, and some patients have experienced more severe hypoxemia (probably because of a worsening ventilation/perfusion imbalance when no shunt was present). NO inhibits platelet agglutination, and the result is an antithrombotic effect. However, no significant increase in bleeding time has been reported in NO trials with human subjects. Because it can quickly reduce right ventricular afterload, NO may increase left ventricular filling pressure in some patients. In the presence of congestive heart failure, this effect could cause or worsen pulmonary edema. Concerns involving increased left heart pressures also account for inhaled NO being contraindicated for neonates with certain cardiac and vascular anomalies such as coarctation of the aorta.[54] In certain patients, the withdrawal of NO has resulted in development of hypoxemia and pulmonary hypertension, perhaps worse than they were before therapy was started. This phenomenon is known as a *rebound effect.* This rebound effect occurs because the administration of nitric oxide depresses the body's normal production of NO. NO after use for more than a few hours should always be slowly weaned over hours. When NO is finally discontinued, FiO_2 frequently needs to be initially increased then slowly reduced to baseline over 1 or 2 hours.[53]

Box 38-9 Potential Uses for Inhaled Nitric Oxide

- ARDS
- Persistent pulmonary hypertension of the newborn
- Primary pulmonary hypertension
- Pulmonary hypertension after cardiac surgery
- Cardiac transplantation
- Acute pulmonary embolism
- COPD
- Congenital diaphragmatic hernia
- Sickle cell disease
- Testing pulmonary vascular responsiveness

Box 38-10 Adverse Effects Associated With Nitric Oxide Therapy

- Poor or paradoxical response
- Methemoglobinemia
- Increased left ventricular filling pressure
- Complications of certain cardiac anomalies (coarctation of the aorta)
- Rebound hypoxemia, pulmonary hypertension

Although NO has been used safely with other drugs and treatments such as dopamine, steroids, surfactant, and high-frequency ventilation, the interaction of NO with other medications is still being studied. One investigational area may involve the study of patients receiving both inhaled NO and other NO-related compounds such as nitroglycerin and the possible development of methemoglobinemia or systemic hypotension. Likewise, the carcinogenic, mutagenic, and other adverse effects of NO are still under investigation.[55]

Methods of Administration

Before inhaled NO administration, the patient ideally should be stabilized as much as possible. To stabilize the patient, thought must be given to clinical considerations such as FiO_2, blood pH, sedation, and possibly muscle relaxation. After the patient is prepared, NO is administered to mechanically ventilated patients through a system with the capability for operator-determined concentration of NO in the breathing gas, a constant concentration throughout the breathing cycle, and a concentration that does not cause generation of excessive inhaled NO_2. Features of an ideal NO delivery system are listed in Box 38-11.

The INOmax DS (Delivery System) (Ikaria, Clinton, New Jersey) shown in Figure 38-26 provides these features.[55,57] The INOmax DS delivers INOmax (NO for inhalation) into the inspiratory limb of the patient's breathing circuit in a manner that provides a constant concentration of NO, as preset by the clinician, throughout inspiration. Through a dual-channel design, the first channel uses a delivery mechanism, flow controller, and injector module to ensure precise delivery of NO. The highly specialized injector module allows tracking of the ventilator flow waveforms and the delivery of synchronized and proportional dose of NO. The second channel uses a separate monitoring mechanism, electrochemical gas sensors, and a graphically enhanced user interface to monitor O_2, NO_2, and NO continuously. The INOmax DS uses several alarm systems to alert clinicians when problems arise, including alarms for high and low NO, high NO_2, and high and low O_2. Other alarms can be set to notify clinicians of a significant decrease in source gas pressure, if the electrochemical cells fail, and when calibration is required.[58]

Box 38-11 Features of Ideal Nitric Oxide Delivery System

- Dependability and safety
- Delivery of a precise and stable dose of NO
- Limited production of nitrogen dioxide
- Accurate monitoring of NO and nitrogen dioxide levels
- Capability for scavenging of NO
- Maintenance of adequate patient ventilation

These systems entail use of cylinder mixtures of NO containing up to 800 ppm of NO in nitrogen. This high concentration of NO is diluted with nitrogen, air, or O_2 before delivery to the patient. Because adding NO to the circuit decreases the FiO_2, O_2 concentration must be continuously monitored downstream from the titration site.

The INOmax DS can also be interfaced with specialty ventilators including high-frequency oscillators and jet ventilators and anesthesia machines. Inhaled NO has also been used with noninvasive ventilation, but rebreathing inherent in this mode of ventilation can cause NO_2 levels to increase beyond acceptable levels. Other special considerations apply, and resources such as ventilator procedure manuals and department policy and procedures should be reviewed to help ensure proper setup and patient safety.[57]

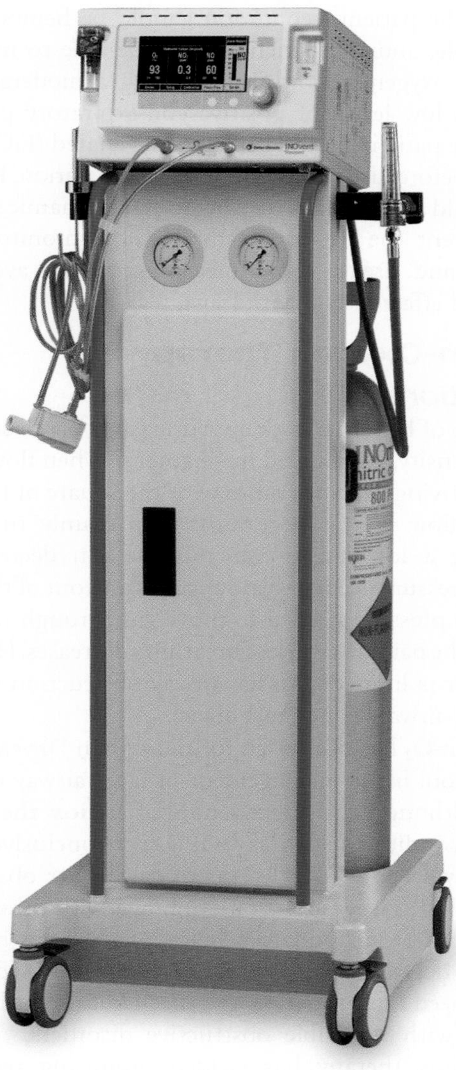

FIGURE 38-26 INOvent delivery system for administration of NO to mechanically ventilated patients. (Courtesy Ikaria, Clinton, New Jersey.)

The administration of inhaled NO to spontaneously breathing patients is also possible. This use and some other uses are described in the research literature but have not yet officially been approved by the FDA and are regarded as off-label use. INOmax DS can be used with a nasal cannula and a face mask. The maximum delivered NO via cannula is generally 20 ppm. When titrating NO via cannula, it is recommended that the concentration not be increased by more than 5 ppm in a 5-minute period, and the clinician should be aware that excessive flow can cause back pressure leading to monitoring failure alarms. Inhaled NO delivery via face mask is similar to a cannula setup except that it is important to use a tight-fitting mask and a flow sufficient to prevent entrainment of air into the mask.[57]

Withdrawing Therapy

Care must be taken when NO therapy is withdrawn to prevent the rebound effect. First, the NO level should be reduced to the lowest effective dose (ideally ≤5 ppm). Second, the patient's condition should be hemodynamically stable, and the patient should be able to maintain adequate oxygenation while breathing a moderate FiO_2 (≤0.4) on low levels of positive end-expiratory pressure. Third, the patient should be hyperoxygenated (FiO_2 0.6 to 0.7) just before discontinuation of NO inhalation. Preparation should also be made to provide hemodynamic support in the event the patient needs it. Close monitoring of patients and use of these measures usually avoid any untoward effect of NO withdrawal.[54]

Helium-Oxygen Therapy

Indications

The value of helium as a therapeutic gas is based solely on its low density. As detailed in Chapter 6, when flow is turbulent, driving pressure varies with the square of the flow. Because flow in the large airways is mainly turbulent, breathing a low-density gas mixture can decrease the driving pressure needed to move gas in and out of this area. With less pressure needed to move gas through the large airways, the patient's work of breathing decreases. However, this effect is limited to large airway obstruction (flow in the small airways is not turbulent).

Helium-O_2 has been used for more than 70 years as an adjunct tool in the management of large airway obstruction.[59] Although the effectiveness of **heliox therapy** in treating conditions such as COPD is inconclusive, it has been shown to be effective in treating other obstructive disorders.[60,61] Either alone or combined with other therapies such as bronchodilators, helium-O_2 therapy has been shown to decrease the respiratory rate, the level of dyspnea, and the need for intubation and mechanical ventilation in patients with reversible obstructive disorders.[62] Specifically, heliox therapy has yielded promising results in the management of acute upper airway obstruction of varying origin,[63] postextubation stridor in pediatric trauma patients,[64] acute severe asthma, and croup.[65]

Guidelines for Use

Because it is inert and unable to support life, helium always must be mixed with at least 20% O_2. The most common combination is 80% helium and 20% O_2. From the standpoint of its ability to oxygenate, this mixture is comparable to air, but helium is used in place of nitrogen. Although air has a density of 1.293 g/L, the density of an 80% helium mixture is 0.429 g/L. For a comparable flow through constricted large airways, this low-density mixture can dramatically decrease the work of breathing.

Heliox combinations can be prepared at the bedside, or commercially available cylinders of premixed gases can be used. The premixed cylinders are commonly available in an 80:20 or a 70:30 combination. The 70% helium and 30% O_2 mixture has a density of 0.554 g/L and can provide additional O_2 for the management of the hypoxemia that can occur with large airway obstruction. Other combinations such as 60:40 and 65:35 mixtures are being examined and show promising results.[62,66]

Several methods have been used to mix heliox at the bedside, although many are improvised setups. One method involves running a nebulizer connected to an O_2 flowmeter at 10 L/min or more, bleeding in 100% helium via a small-bore connection, and titrating the flow to achieve the desired FiO_2. An O_2 analyzer with active alarms should always be used to measure continuously the FiO_2 of the heliox mixture output flowing to the patient. Continued use of improvised setups or setups that are not approved by the FDA for heliox administration can place the patient, clinician, and hospital at risk. Devices cleared by the FDA for use with heliox should be integrated into clinical practice.[62,67]

The low-density benefit of heliox is the same attribute that presents challenges in selecting a delivery device. Because helium is highly diffusible, administration through low-flow systems such as a nasal cannula tends not to deliver sufficient concentrations to treat obstructive disorders in adults. However, heliox administered via cannulas with an adequate seal at the nares has shown to be effective in some infants.[68] Generally, however, heliox should be delivered to most spontaneously breathing patients via a tight-fitting nonrebreathing mask with a fully functional valved exhalation port. The delivery system should be high flow, sufficient to meet or exceed the patient's minute ventilation and peak inspiratory flow requirements. Closed systems with demand valves and reservoirs or the use of demand regulators has proved to be suitable for delivering heliox to patients with artificial airways.[67]

Helium mixtures can be given through a cuffed tracheal airway with a positive-pressure ventilator. However, the performance of ventilators in delivering heliox tends to vary significantly by model, and only some of them have received FDA clearance for such use. Consequently, RTs should ensure that an appropriate ventilator is being used to administer heliox, determine if a conversion factor is needed to adjust settings, and ensure that the patient is monitored closely while such an approach is being used.[69]

Other methods of heliox administration have been examined, including the use of large-volume enclosures, such as hoods. These devices have generally proven to be unsatisfactory because helium tends to concentrate at the top of the devices, and the much higher thermal conductivity of helium can cause excessive heat loss and hypothermia. Blenders have also been used to administer heliox, When a blender is used, the 80:20 heliox is generally attached to the air inlet, and an O_2 analyzer is placed downstream. However, because the accuracy of blenders tends to vary, the system's FiO_2 readings should first be tested, and the difference between the set and actual FiO_2 should be known.

Heliox has also been combined with bronchodilator therapy to treat acute obstructive disorders such as status asthmaticus. Heliox improves aerosol deposition mainly because of a reduction in turbulence and less impaction and medication loss. When administering such a therapeutic combination, the RT should be mindful that only certain nebulizers have been approved for such use and that output may vary because of the characteristics of heliox.

When a helium-O_2 mixture is given alone or as part of nebulization, the RT should realize that a typical hospital O_2 flowmeter is inaccurate because of the lower density of helium. Flowmeters calibrated for helium should be used to ensure accurate delivery. However, correction factors are available for O_2 flowmeters. The correction for an 80:20 helium-O_2 mixture is 1.8; this means that for every 10 L/min indicated flow, 10×1.8, or 18 L/min, of the 80:20 mixture actually leaves the flowmeter. For delivery of a specific flow from an 80:20 helium-O_2 source, the RT sets the flowmeter to the desired flow divided by 1.8. If a flow of 9 L/min of an 80:20 helium-O_2 mixture is needed, the RT sets the flowmeter to 9/1.8, or 5 L/min. Factors for any other mixture can be calculated if needed. The factor for a 70:30 helium-O_2 mixture is 1.6.

In addition to special flow considerations, the RT should use an O_2 analyzer to monitor heliox (actually O_2) concentrations continuously between the source of the mixture and the patient. The basis for this recommendation is that the gas is either helium or O_2, and if the FiO_2 is known, assuming there are no leaks, the remaining gas is helium. This monitoring helps ensure that the patient is receiving the therapeutic benefits of a less dense gas while maintaining the appropriate FiO_2.

Troubleshooting and Hazards

The low density of helium mixtures makes them poor vehicles for aerosol transport. High-density bland water aerosols are difficult to deliver with helium mixtures. The low density of helium mixtures also makes coughing less effective. An expulsive cough depends in part on the development of turbulent flow in the large airways. Because helium promotes laminar flow, clearance of secretions by coughing is impaired. If the patient can develop an effective cough, this problem can be rectified by means of washing out the helium before coughing.

The most common side effect of helium is a benign one. When a patient is breathing a helium mixture, the spoken word is badly distorted at a pitch so high as to make it almost unintelligible. This effect is caused by the passage of a low-density gas through the vocal cords on exhalation. The effect is important only to conscious, nonintubated patients, who should be warned of the effect and reassured that it disappears immediately after therapy is stopped.

A more serious problem is hypoxemia associated with breathing helium mixtures.[67,70] Although this problem may have been caused by using too low an O_2 concentration (20%), there is another possibility. Very rarely, some commercial helium-O_2 cylinders stored for long periods of time have been found to contain these gases in an unmixed, or separated, state. The only way to avoid this potential hazard is to analyze the O_2 concentration coming from the cylinder before administering the gas.

As clinical applications for heliox have expanded, other hazards have emerged. One potential problem is volume-induced lung injury when heliox is administered via a mechanical ventilator. This risk can be addressed by using only ventilators approved by the FDA for heliox administration. The use of heliox for bronchodilator nebulization may present another possible hazard. The lower density of helium-O_2 mixtures may result in greater variability in medication delivery to the airways. Careful patient monitoring during such therapy can help minimize this concern. Another rare but possible problem is hypothermia to infants receiving heliox via an oxyhood. This risk results from the high thermal conductivity of helium and can be avoided by warming and humidifying the heliox gas.[67]

Carbon Dioxide–Oxygen (Carbogen) Therapy

Although rarely used, CO_2-O_2 mixtures (carbogen) have been employed to treat hiccups and carbon monoxide poisoning and to prevent complete washout of CO_2 during cardiopulmonary bypass. More recently, it has been investigated as a treatment for hearing loss and seizures. However, the application of carbogen in clinical settings has been quite limited given the potential adverse effects of hypoxemia, premature ventricular contractions, hypertension, and muscle twitching.[71]

Carbogen is supplied in compressed gas cylinders as either 5%:95% or 7%:93% CO_2-O_2 mixtures. It can be administered to patients with a snug-fitting nonrebreathing mask, with a flow sufficient to prevent the reservoir from collapsing during inhalation. Because of the potential adverse effects, patients receiving carbogen should be monitored closely, especially at 7%:93% mixtures, with special attention paid to pulse, respiratory rate, pulse oximetry, blood pressure, and mental status. If any significant adverse effects are noted, the therapy should be stopped, and the patient should be monitored closely.[71]

SUMMARY CHECKLIST

- O_2 therapy is used to (1) correct acute hypoxemia, (2) decrease the symptoms of chronic hypoxemia, and (3) decrease cardiopulmonary workload.
- The need for supplemental O_2 can be assessed with laboratory measures, clinical history or status, and bedside patient evaluation.
- In the care of adults, children, and infants older than 28 days, O_2 therapy is indicated if PaO_2 is less than 60 mm Hg or SaO_2 is less than 90%.
- Exposure to 100% O_2 for more than 24 hours should be avoided whenever possible; high FiO_2 is acceptable if the concentration can be decreased to 0.70 within 2 days and to 0.50 or less in 5 days.
- Concern that O_2 therapy can cause hypoventilation should never preclude administration of O_2 to a patient in need. Prevention of hypoxia always is the first priority.
- If an O_2 delivery system provides all of a patient's inspired gas, FiO_2 remains stable. If the device provides only part of the inspired gas, air dilutes the O_2, and FiO_2 varies with breathing.
- O_2 provided with low-flow devices such as a nasal cannula always is diluted with air; the result is a low and variable FiO_2.
- Reservoir devices can provide higher FiO_2 than low-flow systems or can be used to conserve O_2.
- To avoid rebreathing, the RT must administer at least 5 L/min flow with a mask; for reservoir masks with bags, the flow must be sufficient to prevent bag collapse.
- A nonrebreathing reservoir circuit can provide a full range of FiO_2 (21% to 100%) at any needed flow to both intubated and nonintubated patients.
- High-flow systems supply a given O_2 concentration at a flow of at least 60 L/min.
- Because entrainment devices dilute source O_2 with air, they always provide less than 100% O_2. The more air entrained, the higher the total flow, but the delivered FiO_2 is lower.
- Air-entrainment nebulizers should be treated as fixed-performance devices only when set to deliver low O_2 concentration ($\leq$35%).
- One way to achieve high FiO_2 with air-entrainment nebulizers is to connect two or more devices together in parallel.
- Back pressure decreases both the volume of entrained air and the total flow output of air-entrainment devices.
- A blending system allows precise control over FiO_2 and total flow output; most blending systems qualify as true fixed-performance delivery devices.
- An operational check of an O_2 blender should always be conducted before the device is used to treat a patient.
- O_2 therapy enclosures are used mainly in the care of children and infants. Problems include limited and highly variable FiO_2 and temperature control.
- The three Ps—purpose, patient, and performance of the device—should be considered in the selection or recommendation of an O_2 delivery system.
- In HBO therapy, O_2 is administered at a pressure greater than 1 atm for management of conditions such as air embolism and carbon monoxide poisoning.
- Inhaled NO improves blood flow to ventilated alveoli, reduces intrapulmonary shunting, improves arterial oxygenation, and decreases pulmonary vascular resistance and pulmonary arterial pressure.
- An ideal NO delivery system provides precise and stable delivery of the NO dose; limits NO_2 production; and allows accurate monitoring, with alarms, of NO and NO_2 levels.
- When NO therapy is being withdrawn, care must be taken to prevent a rebound effect.

References

1. Fulmer JF, Snider GL: American College of Chest Physicians/National Heart, Lung and Blood Institute National Conference on Oxygen Therapy. Chest 86:224, 1984.
2. American Association for Respiratory Care: Clinical practice guideline: oxygen therapy for adults in the acute care facility. Respir Care 47:717, 2002.
3. American Association for Respiratory Care: Clinical practice guideline: oxygen therapy in the home or extended care facility—2007 revision and update. Respir Care 52:1063, 2007.
4. American Association for Respiratory Care: Clinical practice guideline: selection of an oxygen delivery device for neonatal and pediatric patients. Respir Care 47:707, 2002.
5. Stoller JK, Panos RJ, Krachman S, et al: Oxygen therapy for patients with COPD: current evidence and the long-term oxygen treatment trial. Chest 138:179, 2010.
6. Thakur N, Blanc PD, Julian LJ, et al: COPD and cognitive impairment: the role of hypoxemia and oxygen therapy. Int J Chron Obstruct Pulmon Dis 5:263, 2010.
7. Boutet K, Montani D, Jais X, et al: Therapeutic advances in pulmonary arterial hypertension. Ther Adv Respir Dis 2:249, 2008.
8. Tarnow-Mordi WO, Darlow B, Doyle L: Target ranges of oxygen saturation in extremely pre-term infants. N Engl J Med 363:1285, 2010.
9. Panayiotidis MI, Rancourt RC, Allen CB, et al: Hyperoxia-induced DNA damage causes decreased DNA methylation in human lung epithelial-like A549 cells. Antioxid Redox Signal 6:129, 2004.
10. Auten RL, Davis JM: Oxygen toxicity and reactive oxygen species: the devil is in the details. Pediatr Res 66:121, 2009.
11. Sola A: Oxygen in neonatal anesthesia: friend or foe? Curr Opin Anaesthesiol 21:332, 2008.
12. Eastwood GM, Peck L, Young H, et al: Oxygen administration and monitoring for ward adult patients in a teaching hospital. Intern Med J 16:332, 2010.
13. Moradkhan R, Sinoway LI: Revisiting the role of oxygen therapy in cardiac patients. J Am Coll Cardiol 56:1013, 2010.
14. New A: Oxygen: kill or cure? Prehospital hyperoxia in the COPD patient. Emerg Med J 23:144, 2006.
15. Wijesinghe M, Perrin K, Healy B, et al: Pre-hospital oxygen therapy in acute exacerbations of chronic obstructive pulmonary disease. Intern Med J 41:618, 2011.

16. Make B, Krachman S, Panos RJ, et al: Oxygen therapy in advanced COPD: in whom does it work? Semin Respir Crit Care Med 31:334, 2010.
17. Lima DF, Dela Coleta K, Tanni SE, et al: Potentially modifiable predictors of mortality in patients treated with long-term oxygen therapy. Respir Med 105:470, 2011.
18. Macnee W: Prescription of oxygen: still problems after all these years. Am J Respir Crit Care Med 172:517, 2005.
19. Chen ML, Guo L, Smith LE, et al: High or low oxygen saturation and severe retinopathy of prematurity: a meta-analysis. Pediatrics 125:e1483, 2010.
20. Nunn JF: Conscious volunteers developed hypoxemia and pulmonary collapse when breathing air and oxygen at reduced lung volumes. Anesthesiology 98:258, 2003.
21. Lypson ML, Stephens S, Colletti L: Preventing surgical fires: who needs to be educated? Jt Comm J Qual Patient Saf 31:522, 2005.
22. Holmes M: Evaluation of oxygen therapy devices. Anaesth Intensive Care 37:691, 2009.
23. Ayhan H, Iyigun E, Tastan S, et al: Comparison of two different oxygen delivery methods in early postoperative period: randomized trial. J Adv Nurs 65:1237, 2009.
24. Heimlich HJ: Respiratory rehabilitation with transtracheal oxygen system. Ann Otol Rhinol Laryngol 91:643, 1982.
25. Lenfant F, Pean D, Brisard L, et al: Oxygen delivery during transtracheal oxygenation: a comparison of two manual devices. Anesth Analg 111:922, 2010.
26. Dumont CP, Tiep BL: Using a reservoir nasal cannula in acute care. Crit Care Nurse 22:41, 2002.
27. Slessarev M, Somogyi R, Preiss D, et al: Efficiency of oxygen administration: sequential gas delivery versus "flow into cone" methods. Crit Care Med 34:829, 2006.
28. Sim MA, Dean P, Kinsella J, et al: Performance of oxygen delivery devices when the breathing pattern of respiratory failure is stimulated. Anaesthesia 63:938, 2008.
29. Hui DS, Chow BK, Chu LC, et al: Exhaled air and aerosolized droplet dispersion during application of a jet nebulizer. Chest 135:648, 2009.
30. Barach AL, Eckman M: A physiologically controlled oxygen mask apparatus. Anesthesiology 2:421, 1941.
31. Campbell EJM: A method of controlled oxygen administration which reduces the risk of carbon dioxide retention. Lancet 1:12, 1960.
32. Adcock CJ, Dawson JS: The venture mask: more than moulded plastic. Br J Hosp Med 68:28, 2007.
33. Redding JS, McAfee DD, Parham AM: Oxygen concentrations received from commonly used delivery systems. South Med J 71:169, 1978.
34. Woolner DF, Larkin J: An analysis of the performance of a variable Venturi-type oxygen mask. Anaesth Intensive Care 8:44, 1980.
35. Cairo JM, Pilbeam SP: Respiratory care equipment, ed 8, St. Louis, 2010, Mosby.
36. Caille V, Ehrmann S, Boissinot E, et al: Influence of jet nebulization and oxygen delivery on the fraction of inspired oxygen: an experimental model. J Aerosol Med Pulm Drug Del 22:255, 2009.
37. Foust GN, Potter WA, Wilons MD, et al: Shortcomings of using two jet nebulizers in tandem with an aerosol face mask for optimal oxygen therapy. Chest 99:1346, 1991.
38. Fried JL: A new Venturi device for administering continuous positive airway pressure (CPAP). Respir Care 26: 133, 1981.
39. Karmann U, Roth F: Prevention of accidents associated with air-oxygen mixers. Anaesthesia 37:680, 1982.
40. Inaccurate O_2 concentrations from oxygen-air proportioners. Health Devices 18:366, 1989.
41. Walsh BK, Brooks TM, Grenier BM: Oxygen therapy in the neonatal environment. Respir Care 54:1193, 2009.
42. Tin W, Gupta S: Optimum oxygen therapy in preterm babies. Arch Dis Child Fetal Neonatal Ed 92:143, 2007.
43. St Clair N, Touch SM, Greenspan JS: Supplemental oxygen delivery to the nonventilated neonate. Neonatal Netw 20:39, 2001.
44. Niewoehner DE: Clinical practice: outpatient management of severe COPD. N Engl J Med 362:1407, 2010.
45. Stoller JK: Implementing change in respiratory care. Respir Care 55:749, 2010.
46. Kuffler DP: Hyperbaric oxygen therapy: an overview. J Wound Care 19:77, 2010.
47. Bullock MR: Hyperbaric oxygen therapy. J Neurosurg 112:1078, 2010.
48. Savage S: New medical therapy: hyperbarics. Tenn Med 103:39, 2010.
49. Edsell ME, Kirk-Bayley J: Hyperbaric oxygen therapy for arterial gas embolism. Br J Anaesth 103:306, 2009.
50. Rollins MD, Gibson JJ, Hunt TK, et al: Wound oxygen levels during hyperbaric oxygen treatment in healing wounds. Undersea Hyperb Med 33:17, 2006.
51. Helms AK, Whelan HT, Torbey MT: Hyperbaric oxygen therapy of cerebral ischemia. Cerebrovasc Dis 20:417, 2005.
52. Chang DC, Lee JT, Lo CP, et al: Hyperbaric oxygen ameliorates delayed neuropsychiatric syndrome of carbon monoxide poisoning. Undersea Hyperb Med 37:23, 2010.
53. Griffiths MJ, Evans TW: Inhaled nitric oxide therapy in adults. N Engl J Med 353:2683, 2005.
54. Steinhorn RH: Neonatal pulmonary hypertension. Pediatr Crit Care Med 11(2 Suppl):S79, 2010.
55. Center for Drug Evaluation and Research: NO labeling, Washington, DC, 2004, U.S. Food and Drug Administration.
56. INOmax (nitric oxide) for inhalation package insert (revised), Clinton, NJ, 2007, INO Therapeutics.
57. Sosenko IR, Bancalari E: NO for preterm infants at risk for bronchopulmonary dysplasia. Lancet 376:308, 2010.
58. Lundberg JO, Weitzberg E: Extrapulmonary effects of nitric oxide inhalation therapy: time to consider new dosing regimes? Crit Care 12:406, 2008.
59. Hess DR, Fink JB, Venkataraman ST, et al: The history and physics of heliox. Respir Care 51:608, 2006.
60. Vorwerk C, Coats T: Heliox for croup in children. Cochrane Database Syst Rev (2):CD006822, 2010.
61. Hess DR: Heliox and noninvasive positive-pressure ventilation: a role for heliox in exacerbations of chronic obstructive pulmonary disease? Respir Care 51:640, 2006.
62. Bigham MT, Jacobs BR, Monaco MA, et al: Helium/oxygen-driven albuterol nebulization in the management of children with status asthmaticus: a randomized, placebo-controlled trial. Pediatr Crit Care Med 11:356, 2010.
63. Frazier MD, Cheifetz IM: The role of heliox in paediatric respiratory diseases. Paediatr Respir Rev 11:46, 2010.
64. Berkenbosch JW, Grueber RE, Graff GR, et al: Patterns of helium-oxygen (heliox) usage in the critical care environment. J Intensive Care Med 19:335, 2004.
65. Myers TR: Use of heliox in children. Respir Care 51:619, 2006.
66. Bathke P, Gallagher T: Respiratory problems in accident and emergency—the role of helium-oxygen mixtures. Anaesthesia 64:576, 2009.
67. Fink JB: Opportunities and risks of using heliox in your clinical practice. Respir Care 51:651, 2006.
68. Williams J, Stewart K, Tobias JD, et al: Therapeutic benefits of helium-oxygen delivery to infants via nasal cannula. Pediatr Emerg Care 20:574, 2004.

69. Hurford WE, Cheifetz IM: Respiratory controversies in the critical care setting: should heliox be used for mechanically ventilated patients? Respir Care 52:582, 2007.
70. Cylinders with unmixed helium/oxygen. Health Devices 19:146, 1990.
71. Malhotra N, Saini S, Kumar P, et al: Carbogen therapy: "old anaesthesia machine can still be gold". J Anaesth Clin Pharmacol 24:63, 2008.

Chapter 39

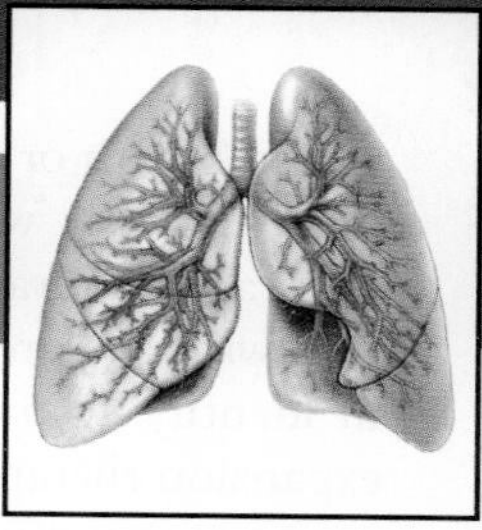

Lung Expansion Therapy

DANIEL F. FISHER

CHAPTER OBJECTIVES

After reading this chapter you will be able to:

- Describe the various causes of atelectasis.
- Identify which patients need lung expansion therapy.
- Define the clinical findings seen in atelectasis.
- Describe how lung expansion therapy works.
- List the indications, hazards, and complications associated with the various modes of lung expansion therapy.
- Describe the primary responsibilities of the respiratory therapist in planning, implementing, and evaluating lung expansion therapy.

CHAPTER OUTLINE

KEY TERMS

atelectasis
compression atelectasis
continuous positive airway pressure (CPAP)
deep breathing/directed cough
gas absorption atelectasis
incentive spirometry (IS)
intermittent positive airway pressure breathing (IPPB)
lobar atelectasis
noninvasive ventilation (NIV)
positive expiratory pressure (PEP)

Pulmonary complications are common serious problems seen in patients who have undergone thoracic or abdominal surgery.[1,2] Such complications include **atelectasis** (alveolar collapse), pneumonia, and acute respiratory failure. These respiratory problems can be minimized or avoided if proper respiratory care is implemented during the perioperative period. The most common form of therapy used in high-risk patients is lung expansion therapy.

Lung expansion therapy encompasses a variety of respiratory care modalities designed to prevent or correct atelectasis. The most common modalities include **deep breathing/directed cough, incentive spirometry (IS), continuous positive airway pressure (CPAP), positive expiratory pressure (PEP),** and **intermittent positive airway pressure breathing (IPPB).** The common purpose that all of these techniques share is to guide the patient into improving pulmonary function by maximizing alveolar recruitment and optimizing airway clearance.

Various lung expansion therapies can be effective in preventing or correcting atelectasis in selected patients.[1] However, the precise method to apply in a given situation is not always clear because no advantage of any one method has been established. The most efficient use of resources is a primary concern with any plan to apply lung expansion therapy.

If all of the following therapies were to be compared, the common factor they share is that they all are designed to increase functional residual capacity (FRC). In other words, these all are supplemental techniques to simulate a deep breath or sigh. In an uncompromised patient, this mechanism is working effectively. In this context, the respiratory therapist (RT) plays a vital role. In consultation with the prescribing physician, the RT should assist in identifying patients most likely to benefit from lung expansion therapy, recommend and initiate the appropriate and most efficient therapeutic approach, monitor the patient's response, and alter the treatment regimen as needed.

CAUSES AND TYPES OF ATELECTASIS

Although atelectasis can occur from a large variety of problems, this chapter focuses on the two primary types associated with postoperative or bedridden patients who are breathing spontaneously without mechanical assistance: (1) gas absorption atelectasis and (2) compression atelectasis. **Gas absorption atelectasis** can occur either when there is a complete interruption of ventilation to a section of the lung or when there is a significant shift in ventilation/perfusion ($\dot{V}/\dot{Q}$). Gas distal to the obstruction is absorbed by the passing blood in the pulmonary capillaries, which causes partial collapse of the nonventilated alveoli. When ventilation is compromised to a larger airway or bronchus, **lobar atelectasis** can develop.

Compression atelectasis results when the forces within the chest wall and lung–specifically, the pleural pressure–are exceeded by the transmural pressure, which is what distends and maintains the alveoli in an open state.[2-4] Compression atelectasis is primarily caused by persistent use of small tidal volumes by the patient. This situation is common when general anesthesia is given, with the use of sedatives and bed rest, and when deep breathing is painful, as when broken ribs are present or surgery has been performed on the upper abdominal region. Weakening or impairment of the diaphragm can also contribute to compression atelectasis. Compression atelectasis results when the patient does not periodically take a deep breath and expand the lungs fully. It is a common cause of atelectasis in hospitalized patients. It may occur in combination with gas absorption atelectasis in a patient with excessive airway secretions who breathes with small tidal volumes for a prolonged period.

Factors Associated With Causing Atelectasis

Atelectasis can occur in any patient who cannot or does not take deep breaths periodically and in patients who are restricted to bed rest for any reason.[5] Patients who have difficulty taking deep breaths without assistance include patients with significant obesity, patients with neuromuscular disorders or who are under heavy sedation, and patients who have undergone upper abdominal or thoracic surgery. Diaphragmatic position and function is the major contributor to the onset of atelectasis. In an anesthetized patient, there is a cephalad (toward the head) shift of the diaphragm. For patients who are supine, the lower, dependent portion of the diaphragm performs the most movement. The opposite occurs in patients who are paralyzed–the upper portion of the diaphragm is involved in movement.[3,4] Patients undergoing lower abdominal surgery are at less risk for atelectasis than patients undergoing upper abdominal or thoracic surgery, but they still may be at significant risk. Patients with spinal cord injury are prone to respiratory complications, the most common of which is atelectasis. Bedridden patients, such as patients recovering from major trauma, are particularly predisposed to developing atelectasis secondary to lack of mobility. Atelectasis is one of the most important determinants of hypoxemia after abdominal surgery and may account for 24% of deaths within 6 days of surgery.[6] It is clinically prudent to consider atelectasis in every assessment of postoperative patients.

Impairment of the function of pulmonary surfactant can also have an impact on the development of atelectasis. Surfactants decrease the surface tension of the walls of the alveoli. When there is deterioration of the function of this vital protein, the relative increase in surface tension can cause the walls of the alveoli to collapse.[4]

Most postoperative patients also have problems coughing effectively because of their reduced ability to take deep breaths. An ineffective cough impairs normal clearance mechanisms and increases the likelihood of retained secretions, which could lead to the development of gas absorption atelectasis in a patient with excessive mucus production. Patients with a history of lung disease that causes increased mucus production (e.g., chronic bronchitis) are most prone to develop complications in the postoperative period. Similarly, a significant history of cigarette smoking should alert the RT to the high risk for respiratory complications with surgery. Such patients must be identified in the preoperative period and considered strong candidates for airway clearance and lung expansion therapy. Elective surgery for these patients may need to be postponed in some cases until such therapies can be included in the treatment plan. Lung expansion therapy and chest physical therapy in the postoperative period may help improve clearance of secretions by improving the effectiveness of coughing and secretion removal.

RULE OF THUMB

The closer the incision is to the diaphragm, the greater the risk for postoperative atelectasis. Patients with a history of inadequate nutritional intake, as shown by an albumin level less than 3.2 mg/dl, have an increased risk for pulmonary complications in the postoperative period. This increased risk is most likely due to inadequate strength of the inspiratory muscles to maintain a normal FRC and VC.

MINI CLINI

Risk Factors for Atelectasis

PROBLEM: The RT is called to evaluate a 47-year-old obese man admitted to the hospital for upper abdominal surgery. He has a 60 pack-year smoking history and is scheduled for surgery tomorrow morning. Examination reveals bilateral inspiratory and expiratory coarse crackles and expiratory wheezes. He is alert and oriented with normal vital signs. His past medical history is positive for diabetes and kidney stones. What factors are present that predispose this patient for postoperative atelectasis, and what treatment plan should the RT recommend?

DISCUSSION: Several important risk factors are present in this patient. The three most important are positive smoking history, obesity, and the site of surgery (upper abdomen). The findings of adventitious lung sounds and positive smoking history are very suggestive of a current pulmonary problem that would probably require bronchial hygiene, humidity therapy, and bronchodilators before surgery. Delaying the surgery may be necessary if significant secretion retention is present. Postoperatively, this high-risk patient would need careful monitoring and IS to minimize the risk of atelectasis.

CLINICAL SIGNS OF ATELECTASIS

RTs must be able to recognize the clinical signs of atelectasis in patients so that appropriate therapy can be implemented in a timely fashion. The patient's medical history often provides the first clue in identifying atelectasis. Recent upper abdominal or thoracic surgery in any patient should suggest possible atelectasis. A history of chronic lung disease or cigarette smoking or both provides additional evidence that the patient is prone to respiratory complications after major surgery or prolonged bed rest.

The physical signs of atelectasis may be absent or very subtle if the patient has minimal atelectasis. When the atelectasis involves a more significant portion of the lungs, the patient's respiratory rate increases proportionally. Fine, late-inspiratory crackles may be heard over the affected lung region. These crackles are produced by the sudden opening of distal airways with deep breathing. Bronchial-type breath sounds may be present as the lung becomes more consolidated with atelectasis. Diminished breath sounds are common when excessive secretions block the airways and prevent transmission of breath sounds. Tachycardia may be present if atelectasis leads to significant hypoxemia. Patients with preexisting lung disease often present with significant abnormalities in respiratory and heart rates, even when atelectasis is not severe.

RULE OF THUMB

There is a direct relationship between the spontaneous respiratory rate and the degree of atelectasis present. Typically, as atelectasis progresses, respiratory rate increases proportionally.

The chest radiograph is often used to confirm the presence of atelectasis. The atelectatic region of the lung has increased opacity. Evidence of volume loss is present in patients with significant atelectasis. Direct signs of volume loss on the chest film include displacement of the interlobar fissures, crowding of the pulmonary vessels, and air bronchograms. Indirect signs include elevation of the diaphragm; shift of the trachea, heart, or mediastinum; pulmonary opacification; narrowing of the space between the ribs; and compensatory hyperexpansion of the surrounding lung.

LUNG EXPANSION THERAPY

All modes of lung expansion therapy increase lung volume by increasing the transpulmonary pressure (PL) gradient. As detailed elsewhere in this text, P_L gradient represents the difference between the alveolar pressure (Palv) and the pleural pressure (Ppl):

$$PL = Palv - Ppl$$

With all else being constant, the greater the PL gradient, the more that the alveoli expand.

As depicted in Figure 39-1, the PL gradient can be increased by either (1) decreasing the surrounding Ppl (see Figure 39-1, *A*) or (2) increasing the Palv (see Figure 39-1, *B*). A spontaneous deep inspiration increases the PL gradient by decreasing the Ppl. The application of positive pressure to the lungs increases the PL gradient by increasing the pressure inside the lung.

All lung expansion therapies use one of these two approaches. IS enhances lung expansion via a spontaneous and sustained decrease in Ppl. Positive airway pressure techniques increase Palv in an effort to expand the lung. Positive pressure lung expansion therapies may apply

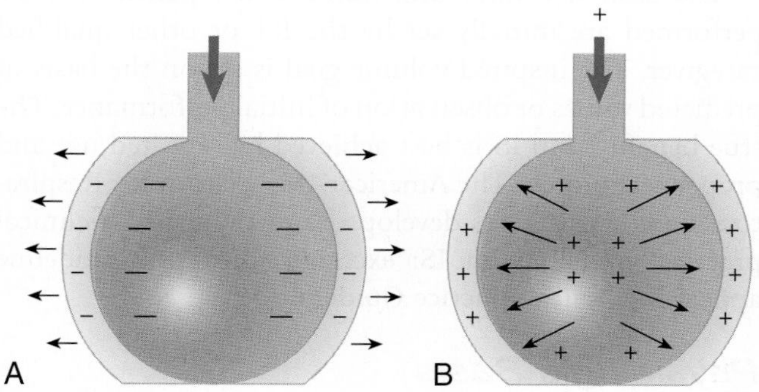

FIGURE 39-1 Transpulmonary pressure gradients with spontaneous inspiration **(A)** and positive pressure inspiration **(B)**.

pressure during inspiration only (as in IPPB), during expiration only (as in PEP and expiratory positive airway pressure [EPAP]), or during both inspiration and expiration (CPAP). Although all of these approaches are used in lung expansion therapy, the methods that decrease Ppl (e.g., IS) have more of a physiologic effect than the methods that increase Palv and often are most effective. However, they require an alert, cooperative patient who is capable of taking a deep breath.

The goal of any lung expansion therapy should be to implement a plan that provides an effective strategy in the most efficient manner. Staff time and equipment are the two major issues related to efficiency. For a patient with minimal risk of postoperative atelectasis, deep breathing exercises, frequent repositioning, and early ambulation are usually effective and can be done with minimal coaching and time from clinicians and without equipment.[4] For a patient at high risk for atelectasis (e.g., a patient undergoing upper abdominal surgery), IS is usually instituted. The additional staff time and equipment are justified in this high-risk group. Positive pressure therapy requires significantly more staff time and equipment and is reserved for high-risk patients who cannot perform IS techniques. The remainder of this chapter describes the use of IS and positive pressure therapy for the prevention or correction of atelectasis.

Incentive Spirometry

The purpose of IS is to guide the patient to take a sustained maximal inspiratory effort resulting in a decrease in Ppl and maintain the patency of airways at risk for closure. Because of its simplicity, IS has been the mainstay of lung expansion therapy for many years. IS devices are designed to mimic natural sighing by encouraging patients to take slow, deep breaths. IS can be performed using devices that provide visual cues to patients when the desired inspiratory flow or volume has been achieved. IS has been shown to be an efficient and effective prophylaxis against postoperative atelectasis in high-risk patients.[5] The first documented use of incentive spirometry as a therapy was in 1972, and this led to the development of a visual feedback device in 1973.[7]

The desired volume and number of repetitions to be performed are initially set by the RT or other qualified caregiver. The inspired volume goal is set on the basis of predicted values or observation of initial performance. The true benefit from IS is best achieved by repeated use and proper technique.[8] The American Association for Respiratory Care (AARC) has developed and published a clinical practice guideline on IS; excerpts from this guideline appear in Clinical Practice Guideline 39-1.

Physiologic Basis

The basic maneuver of IS is a sustained maximal inspiration (SMI). An SMI is a slow, deep inhalation from the functional residual capacity (FRC) up to (ideally) the total lung capacity, followed by a 5- to 10-second breath hold. An SMI is functionally equivalent to performing an inspiratory capacity (IC) maneuver, followed by a breath hold. Figure 39-2 compares the alveolar and Ppl changes occurring during a normal spontaneous breath and an SMI during IS.

During the inspiratory phase of spontaneous breathing, the decrease in Ppl caused by expansion of the thorax is transmitted to the alveoli. With Palv now negative, a pressure gradient is created between the airway opening and the alveoli. This transrespiratory pressure gradient causes gas to flow from the airway into the alveoli. Within certain limits, the greater the transrespiratory pressure gradient, the more that lung expansion occurs.

Indications

Indications for IS are listed in Box 39-1. The primary indication for IS is to treat existing atelectasis. IS may also be used as a preventive measure when conditions exist that make the development of atelectasis likely.[6]

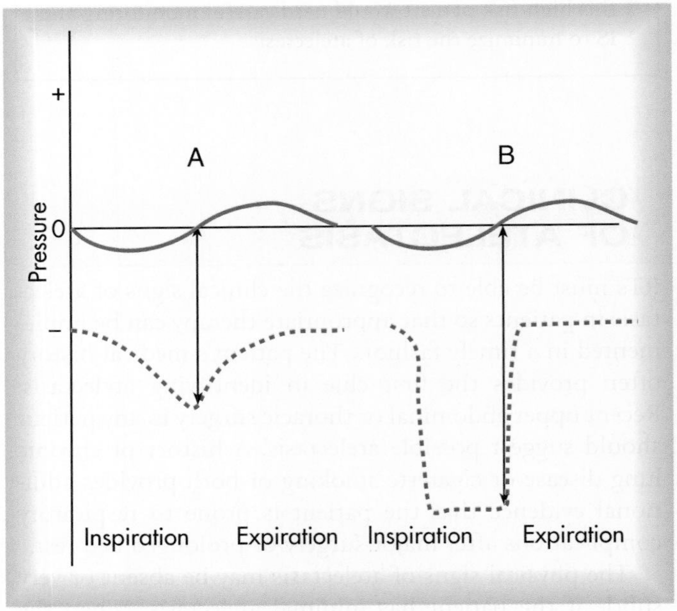

FIGURE 39-2 Alveolar *(solid lines)* and pleural *(dotted lines)* pressure changes during spontaneous breathing *(A)* and SMI *(B)*. Note the difference in PL gradients *(double arrows)*.

Box 39-1 Indications for Incentive Spirometry

- Presence of pulmonary atelectasis
- Presence of conditions predisposing to atelectasis
  - Upper abdominal surgery
  - Thoracic surgery
  - Surgery in patients with COPD
- Presence of a restrictive lung defect associated with quadriplegia or dysfunctional diaphragm

39-1 Incentive Spirometry

AARC Clinical Practice Guideline (Excerpts)*

INDICATIONS

- Presence of conditions predisposing to the development of pulmonary atelectasis (upper abdominal surgery, thoracic surgery, surgery in patients with COPD)
- Presence of pulmonary atelectasis
- Presence of restrictive lung defect associated with quadriplegia or dysfunctional diaphragm

CONTRAINDICATIONS

- Patient cannot be instructed or supervised to ensure appropriate use of device
- Patient cooperation is absent, or patient is unable to understand or demonstrate proper use of device
- Patient is unable to deep breathe effectively (e.g., with VC < 10 ml/kg or IC < ⅓ predicted)
- Presence of an open tracheal stoma is not a contraindication but requires adaptation of the spirometer

HAZARDS AND COMPLICATIONS

- Ineffective unless closely supervised or performed as ordered
- Inappropriate as sole treatment for major lung collapse or consolidation
- Hyperventilation
- Barotrauma (emphysematous lungs)
- Discomfort secondary to inadequate pain control
- Hypoxia owing to break in mask O_2 therapy
- Exacerbation of bronchospasm
- Fatigue

ASSESSMENT OF NEED

- Surgical procedure involving upper abdomen or thorax
- Conditions predisposing to atelectasis, including immobility, poor pain control, and abdominal binders
- Presence of neuromuscular disease involving respiratory musculature

ASSESSMENT OF OUTCOME

- Absence of or improvement in signs of atelectasis
- Decreased respiratory rate
- Resolution of fever
- Normal pulse rate
- Absence of crackles or presence of or improvement in previously absent or diminished breath sounds
- Normal chest radiograph
- Improved PaO_2 and decreased alveolar-arterial O_2 tension gradient
- Increased VC and peak expiratory flows
- Return of FRC or VC to preoperative values, in absence of lung resection
- Improved inspiratory muscle performance (e.g., attainment of preoperative flow and volume levels, increased FVC)

MONITORING

Direct supervision of every patient performance is unnecessary after the patient has demonstrated mastery of technique; however, preoperative instruction, volume goals, and feedback are essential to optimal performance.

- Observation of patient performance and use
- Frequency of sessions
- Number of breaths per session
- Inspiratory volume or flow goals achieved and 3- to 5-second breath hold maintained
- Effort and motivation
- Periodic observation of patient compliance with technique, with additional instruction as necessary
- Device within reach of patient and patient encouraged to perform independently
- New and increasing inspiratory volumes established each day
- Vital signs

**For complete guidelines, see American Association for Respiratory Care: Clinical practice guidelines: incentive spirometry. Respir Care 36:1402, 1991.*

Box 39-2 Contraindications for Incentive Spirometry

- Patient cannot be instructed or supervised to ensure appropriate use of device
- Patient cooperation is absent, or patient is unable to understand or demonstrate proper use of device
- Patients unable to deep breathe effectively (VC < 10 ml/kg *or* IC $< \frac{1}{3}$ predicted)

Box 39-3 Hazards and Complications of Incentive Spirometry

- Hyperventilation and respiratory alkalosis
- Discomfort secondary to inadequate pain control
- Pulmonary barotrauma
- Exacerbation of bronchospasm
- Fatigue

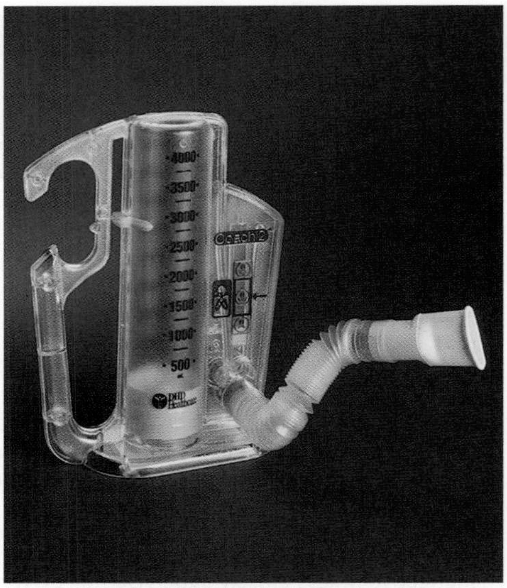

FIGURE 39-3 Volumetric incentive spirometer. (Courtesy DHE Healthcare, Canastota, NY.)

Contraindications

IS is a simple and safe modality. For this reason, contraindications are few (Box 39-2).

Hazards and Complications

Given its normal physiologic basis, IS presents few major hazards and complications; those that can occur are listed in Box 39-3. Acute respiratory alkalosis is the most common problem and occurs when the patient performs IS too rapidly. Dizziness and numbness around the mouth are the most frequently reported symptoms associated with respiratory alkalosis. This problem is easily corrected with careful instruction and monitoring of the patient. Discomfort with deep inspiratory efforts secondary to pain is usually the result of inadequate pain control in a postoperative patient. This problem can be rectified by ensuring appropriate analgesia. In addition, pain medication should be coordinated with IS activity.

Equipment

The equipment needed for IS is typically simple, portable, and inexpensive. Although advances in technology have produced more complex devices, there is no evidence that these devices produce any better outcomes than their lower cost, disposable counterparts.

IS devices can generally be categorized as volume-oriented or flow-oriented. True volume-oriented devices measure and visually indicate the volume achieved during an SMI. The most popular true volume-oriented IS devices employ a bellows that rises according to the inhaled volume. When the patient reaches a target inspiratory volume, a controlled leak in the device allows the patient to sustain the inspiratory effort for a short period (usually 5 to 10 seconds). Because the bellows types of IS devices are bulky and large, smaller devices that indirectly indicate volume based on flow through a fixed orifice have been developed. These devices sacrifice accurate measurement of the inhaled volume to achieve portability and smaller size (Figure 39-3).

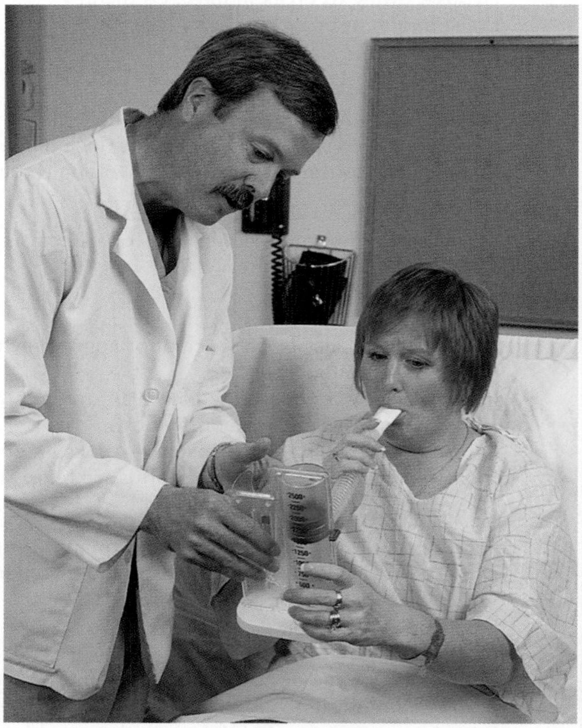

FIGURE 39-4 Flow-oriented incentive spirometer. (From DeWit, S: Fundamental concepts and skills for nursing, ed 2, St Louis, 2004, Saunders.)

Flow-oriented devices measure and visually indicate the degree of inspiratory flow (Figure 39-4). This flow can be equated with volume by assessing the duration of inspiration or time (flow × time = volume). Both flow-oriented and volume-oriented devices attempt to encourage the same goal for the patient: a sustained maximal inspiratory effort to prevent or correct atelectasis. No evidence to date indicates that one type is more beneficial than the other.

Administration

The successful application of IS involves three phases: planning, implementation, and follow-up. Because many of the components of this process are similar to those previously described, we highlight only the key points and differences in approach.

Preliminary Planning. During preliminary planning, the need for IS should be determined by careful patient assessment. Once the need is established, planning for IS should focus on selecting explicit therapeutic outcomes. Box 39-4 lists potential outcomes that can be considered for patients receiving IS.

The outcomes applicable to a specific patient depend on the diagnostic information that supports the need for IS. In this regard, the baseline patient assessment is critical. Patients scheduled for upper abdominal or thoracic surgery should be screened before undergoing the surgical procedure. Assessment conducted at this point helps identify patients at high risk for postoperative complications and allows determination of their baseline lung volumes and capacities. Also, this approach provides an opportunity to orient high-risk patients to the procedure before undergoing surgery, increasing the likelihood of success when IS is provided after surgery.

Implementation. Successful IS requires effective patient teaching. The RT should set an initial goal that is attainable to the patient yet requires a moderate effort. Setting an initial goal that is too low for the patient results in little incentive and an ineffective maneuver, at least initially. The patient should be instructed to inspire slowly and deeply to maximize the distribution of ventilation.

The RT should observe the patient perform the initial inspiratory maneuvers and ensure the patient uses correct technique. Correct technique calls for diaphragmatic breathing at slow to moderate inspiratory flows. Demonstration is probably the most effective way to assist patient understanding and cooperation. Both the operation of the device and the proper breathing technique can be explained easily when the RT uses himself or herself as an example, and much trial and error can be avoided.

The RT instructs the patient to sustain his or her maximal inspiratory effort for 5 to 10 seconds. Many patients have difficulty with this aspect of the maneuver. Nonetheless, patients should be encouraged to try not to breathe in too fast or slowly and to attempt a brief breath hold.

A normal exhalation should follow the breath hold, and the patient should be given the opportunity to rest as long as needed before the next SMI maneuver. Some patients in the early postoperative stage may need to rest for 30 seconds to 1 minute between maneuvers. This rest period helps avoid a common tendency by some patients to repeat the maneuver at rapid rates, causing respiratory alkalosis. The goal is not rapid, partial lung inflation but intermittent, maximal inspiration.

The exact number of sustained maximal inspirations needed to reverse or prevent atelectasis is not known and probably varies according to the patient's clinical status. However, because healthy individuals average about 6 sighs per hour, an IS regimen should probably aim to ensure a minimum of 5 to 10 SMI maneuvers each hour.[9]

Follow-up. Assessing the patient's performance is vital to ensuring achievement of goals. To do so, the RT should make return visits to monitor treatment sessions until the correct technique and appropriate effort are achieved. Suggested monitoring activities for IS are outlined in Box 39-5.

After the patient has demonstrated mastery of technique, IS may be performed with minimal supervision. Even when IS is self-administered, records of progress

Box 39-4 Potential Outcomes of Incentive Spirometry

- Absence of or improvement in signs of atelectasis
- Decreased respiratory rate
- Normal pulse rate
- Resolution of abnormal breath sounds
- Normal or improved chest radiograph
- Improved PaO_2 and decreased $PaCO_2$
- Increased SpO_2
- Increased VC and peak expiratory flows
- Restoration of preoperative FRC or VC
- Improved inspiratory muscle performance and cough
- Attainment of preoperative flow and volume levels
- Increased FVC

Box 39-5 Monitoring Patients Receiving Incentive Spirometry

Observe patient performance and use:

- Frequency of sessions
- Number of breaths per session
- Volume and flow goals achieved
- Breath hold maintained
- Effort and motivation
- Periodic observation of patient compliance, with additional instruction as needed
- Device within reach of patient and patient encouraged to perform independently
- New and increasing inspiratory volumes established each day
- Vital signs and breath sounds

pertaining to the patient's clinical status must be maintained throughout the course of treatment. The result of this assessment can guide the physician and RT in revising the respiratory care plan or terminating treatment after the goals are achieved. For patients with a neuromuscular disease or spinal injury, the use of a mechanical cough device (in-exsufflator) may provide a similar therapeutic objective. However, further study is needed to evaluate this approach.

Noninvasive Ventilation

Noninvasive ventilation (NIV) provides breathing support to patients with inadequate ability to ventilate. NIV has been documented to have beneficial effects for patients who may need periodic, short-term support or patients who are experiencing exacerbations of pulmonary disease. NIV offers some benefits over traditional, invasive ventilation owing to lower infection risk and reduced need for sedation because of the absence of an artificial airway. NIV is discussed in detail elsewhere in this text. In addition, variations of NIV, including IPPB and PEP therapy, can be potentially valuable lung expansion tools and are discussed in the following sections.

Intermittent Positive Airway Pressure Breathing

Physiologic Basis

IPPB is a specialized form of NIV used for relatively short treatment periods (approximately 15 minutes per treatment). The intent of IPPB is not to provide full ventilatory support as with some other forms of NIV but to provide some machine-assisted deep breaths assisting the patient to deep breathe and stimulate cough. This section emphasizes the intermittent use of IPPB as a modality for the treatment of atelectasis.

Positive pressure is transmitted from the alveoli to the pleural space during the inspiratory phase of an IPPB treatment, causing Ppl to increase during inspiration. Depending on the mechanical properties of the lung, Ppl may exceed atmospheric pressure during a portion of inspiration. As with spontaneous breathing, the recoil force of the lung, stored as potential energy during the positive pressure breath, causes a passive exhalation. As gas flows from the alveoli out to the airway opening, Palv decreases to atmospheric level, while Ppl is restored to its normal subatmospheric range (Figure 39-5). The AARC has developed and published a clinical practice guideline for IPPB; excerpts from this guideline appear in Clinical Practice Guideline 39-2.

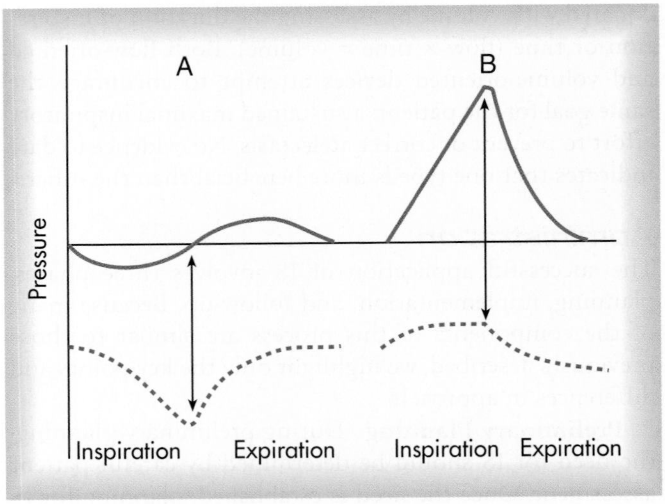

FIGURE 39-5 Alveolar *(solid lines)* and pleural *(dotted lines)* pressure changes during spontaneous breathing *(A)* and IPPB *(B)*. Note the difference in PL gradients *(double arrows)*.

Indications

There is little research supporting the use of IPPB as an aerosol delivery system. However, there is supporting evidence that periodic sessions of positive pressure ventilation provided noninvasively can be useful in the treatment of pulmonary complications or exacerbations of lung disease.[10-12] NIV, or, more specifically, IPPB, may be useful for patients with clinically diagnosed atelectasis unresponsive to other therapies, such as IS and chest physiotherapy. In addition, short-term use of NIV in the form of IPPB may be useful for patients who are at high risk for atelectasis and unable to participate in more patient-directed techniques such as IS or even deep breathing. IPPB should not be used as a single treatment modality for a patient with gas absorption atelectasis because of excessive airway secretions. In addition, the RT should be aware of potential complications, such as mucous plugging, which can be worsened owing to a humidity deficit that can occur with IPPB therapy. Because of the need for specialized machinery and training, IPPB itself should not be thought of as the first line of therapy. Applying positive pressure to the lung in such cases can cause overinflation of the lung regions not affected by secretions and minimal or no expansion of the affected lung segments. Airways clearance with humidity therapy should be considered in conjunction with IPPB for optimizing results in patients with retained secretions.

In concept, a correctly administered IPPB treatment should provide the patient with augmented tidal volumes, achieved with minimal effort. The optimal breathing pattern to reinflate collapsed lung units with IPPB consists of slow, deep breaths that are sustained or held at end-inspiration. This type of inspiratory maneuver increases the distribution of inspired gas to areas of the lung with low compliance—specifically, the atelectatic areas.

Contraindications

There are several clinical situations in which IPPB should not be used (Box 39-6). With the exception of untreated tension pneumothorax, most of these contraindications

39-2 Intermittent Positive Pressure Breathing

AARC Clinical Practice Guideline (Excerpts)*

INDICATIONS

- Need to improve lung expansion
- Presence of clinically significant pulmonary atelectasis when other forms of therapy (e.g., IS) have been unsuccessful or the patient cannot cooperate
- Inability to clear secretions adequately because of pathology that severely limits the ability to ventilate or cough effectively and failure to respond to other modes of treatment
- Need for short-term noninvasive ventilatory support for hypercapnic patients (as an alternative to intubation and continuous ventilatory support)
- Need to deliver aerosol medication
- Although some authors oppose the use of IPPB in the treatment of severe bronchospasm (e.g., acute asthma), we recommend a careful, closely supervised trial of IPPB when treatment using other techniques (metered dose inhaler [MDI] or nebulizer) has been unsuccessful
- IPPB may be used to deliver aerosol medications to patients with ventilatory muscle weakness or fatigue or chronic conditions in which intermittent noninvasive ventilatory support is indicated.

CONTRAINDICATIONS

Although no absolute contraindications to use of IPPB therapy (except tension pneumothorax) have been reported, a patient with any of the following should be carefully evaluated before a decision is made to initiate IPPB therapy:

- ICP >15 mm Hg
- Hemodynamic instability
- Recent facial, oral, or skull surgery
- Tracheoesophageal fistula
- Recent esophageal surgery
- Active hemoptysis
- Nausea
- Air swallowing
- Active, untreated tuberculosis
- Radiographic evidence of bleb
- Singultus (hiccups)

HAZARDS AND COMPLICATIONS

- Increased airway resistance
- Barotrauma, pneumothorax
- Nosocomial infection
- Hyperventilation or hypocapnia
- Hemoptysis
- Hyperoxia when O_2 is the gas source
- Gastric distention
- Secretion impaction (inadequate humidity)
- Psychological dependence
- Impedance of venous return
- Exacerbation of hypoxemia
- Hypoventilation
- Increased $\dot{V}/\dot{Q}$ mismatch
- Air trapping, auto-PEEP, overdistended alveoli

ASSESSMENT OF NEED

- Presence of clinically significant atelectasis
- Reduced timed volumes or VC (e.g., FEV_1 < 65% predicted, FVC < 70% predicted, maximum voluntary ventilation <50% predicted, or VC < 10 ml/kg) precluding an effective cough
- Neuromuscular or skeletal disorders associated with decrease in lung volumes and capacities
- Fatigue or muscle weakness with impending respiratory failure
- Presence of acute, severe bronchospasm or exacerbated COPD that fails to respond to other therapy (consider MDI with spacer or holding chamber first)
- With demonstrated effectiveness, the patient's preference for a positive pressure device should be honored

ASSESSMENT OF OUTCOME

- A minimum delivered tidal volume of at least one-third of predicted IC ($\frac{1}{3} \times 50$ ml/kg) has been suggested
- FEV_1 or peak flow increase
- Cough more effective with treatment

Continued

39-2 Intermittent Positive Pressure Breathing—cont'd

AARC Clinical Practice Guideline (Excerpts)*

- Secretion clearance enhanced as a consequence of deep breathing and coughing
- Chest radiograph improved
- Breath sounds improved
- Favorable patient subjective response

MONITORING

Items from the following list should be chosen as appropriate for the specific patient:

- Machine performance (trigger sensitivity, peak pressure, flow settings, FiO_2, inspiratory time, expiratory time, plateau pressure, PEEP)
- Respiratory rate and volume
- Peak flow or FEV_1/FVC
- Pulse rate and rhythm from electrocardiogram if available
- Patient subjective response to therapy (pain, discomfort, dyspnea)
- Sputum production (quantity, color, consistency, and odor)
- Mental function
- Skin color
- Breath sounds
- Blood pressure
- Arterial hemoglobin saturation by pulse oximetry (if hypoxemia is suspected)
- ICP in patients for whom ICP is of critical importance
- Chest radiograph

**For complete guidelines, see American Association for Respiratory Care: Intermittent positive pressure breathing—2003 revision and update. Respir Care 48:540, 2003.*

MINI CLINI

Importance of Air Bronchograms on the Chest Film

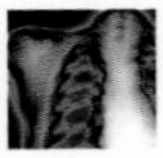

PROBLEM: The RT is called to evaluate a 59-year-old woman admitted to the hospital several days ago for cardiac surgery. The patient underwent surgery 2 days earlier and has developed complications. She is alert but disoriented and has decreased breath sounds bilaterally in the bases. The chest radiograph shows elevation of the right hemidiaphragm and air bronchograms in both lower lung fields. The attending physician wants to start IPPB and asks the RT's opinion about the treatment plan.

DISCUSSION: This patient needs lung expansion therapy, but IPPB alone could be harmful given the evidence of retained secretions. Air bronchograms are seen when air-filled airways are surrounded by portions of the distal lung regions impacted with mucus. The application of positive pressure to the lungs in this situation may be harmful because the pressure would shunt toward the unobstructed airways and may lead to overinflation of selected regions. This patient needs bronchial hygiene and humidity therapy in addition to lung expansion therapy.

are relative. As with all procedures, a sound knowledge of the patient's condition tempered with good clinical insight should guide the RT in the decision-making process. A patient with any of the conditions listed in Box 39-6 should be carefully evaluated before a decision is made to begin IPPB therapy.

Hazards and Complications

As with any clinical intervention, certain hazards and complications are associated with IPPB. These potential problems should be addressed in the initial stages of planning for IPPB. In addition, hazards and complications must be considered throughout the course of therapy as part of the process of assessing the patient for unwanted side effects. The most common complication associated with IPPB is the inducement of respiratory alkalosis. Respiratory alkalosis is induced when the patient hyperventilates during the treatment. Deep, fast breathing leads to a sharp decrease in PCO_2 and an equally marked increase in arterial pH. The patient usually feels light-headed and numb around the mouth. Arrhythmias are also possible if the alkalosis is severe or if the patient's heart is unstable. This problem is easily avoided through proper coaching of the patient before and during treatment.

Box 39-6 Clinical Situations Contraindicating Intermittent Positive Airway Pressure Breathing Therapy

- Tension pneumothorax
- ICP > 15 mm Hg
- Hemodynamic instability
- Active hemoptysis
- Tracheoesophageal fistula
- Recent esophageal surgery
- Active, untreated tuberculosis
- Radiographic evidence of blebs
- Recent facial, oral, or skull surgery
- Singultus (hiccups)
- Air swallowing
- Nausea

Box 39-7 Hazards and Complications of Intermittent Positive Airway Pressure Breathing

- Increased airway resistance and work of breathing
- Barotrauma, pneumothorax
- Nosocomial infection
- Hypocarbia
- Hemoptysis
- Gastric distention
- Impaction of secretions (associated with inadequately humidified gas mixture)
- Psychologic dependence
- Impedance of venous return
- Exacerbation of hypoxemia
- Hypoventilation or hyperventilation
- Increased mismatch of ventilation and perfusion
- Air trapping, auto-PEEP, overdistention

Another potential complication of IPPB is gastric distention; this occurs when gas from the IPPB device passes directly into the esophagus. Gastric distention is uncommon in an alert patient but is a significant risk for a neurologically obtunded patient. Normally, the esophagus does not open until a pressure of about 20 to 25 cm H_2O has been reached. Gastric distention represents the greatest risk in patients receiving IPPB at high pressures. The major hazards and complications of IPPB are listed in Box 39-7.

Administration

Effective IPPB requires careful preliminary planning, individualized patient assessment and implementation, and thoughtful follow-up. In all three phases of the process, the RT should work closely with the prescribing physician to determine patient need, select the appropriate therapeutic approach, and assess patient progress toward predefined clinical outcomes. Only by ensuring that these elements are combined as part of the overall respiratory care plan can the RT expect to achieve the desired results.

Box 39-8 Potential Outcomes of Intermittent Positive Airway Pressure Breathing Therapy

- Improved VC
- Increased FEV_1 or peak flow
- Enhanced cough and secretion clearance
- Improved chest radiograph
- Improved breath sounds
- Improved oxygenation
- Favorable patient subjective response

Preliminary Planning. During preliminary planning, the need for IPPB is determined, and desired therapeutic outcomes are established. The outcomes chosen for a patient are based on diagnostic information that supports the need for IPPB therapy. In addition, therapeutic outcomes should be as explicit and measurable as possible. Outcomes must also be consistent with the therapeutic indications previously described. Outcomes that are inconsistent with these indications are generally inappropriate. Box 39-8 lists potential accepted and desired outcomes of IPPB therapy. Not all the outcomes listed in Box 39-8 apply to every patient. For example, for a patient exhibiting clinical signs and symptoms of postoperative atelectasis, the following outcomes might be set: improved patient comfort, increased aeration on auscultation, decreased respiratory rate and work of breathing, and improvement in the chest radiograph.

Evaluating Alternatives. A key component in early planning must be consideration of alternative therapies. Specifically, before starting IPPB, the RT and prescribing physician must determine whether simpler and less costly methods might be as effective in achieving the desired outcomes. If this is the case, further consideration of IPPB should be postponed until the patient's response to the simpler therapy is assessed.

Baseline Assessment. Before beginning therapy, a baseline patient assessment should be conducted. This information helps individualize the treatment and allows objective evaluation of the patient's subsequent response to therapy. Together with the patient's medical history, this baseline assessment also alerts the RT to possible problems or hazards associated with administering IPPB to the patient. The baseline assessment includes a general evaluation of the patient's clinical status and a specific assessment related to the chosen therapeutic goals. The general assessment, common to all patients for whom IPPB is ordered, includes (1) measurement of vital signs, (2) observational assessment of the patient's appearance and sensorium, and (3) breathing pattern and chest auscultation.

MINI CLINI

Evaluating the Effectiveness of Lung Expansion Therapy

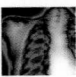

PROBLEM: The RT is the supervisor for the day shift in the surgical intensive care unit. The nursing supervisor asks for the RT's opinion on the best ways to evaluate the effectiveness of lung expansion therapy. She is developing a new documentation form for the nurses to use at the bedside and wants the RT's opinion on the parameters to list. How should the RT respond?

DISCUSSION: The RT should suggest numerous parameters that are useful. One of the best is observation of the patient's spontaneous respiratory rate at rest. There is a strong correlation between respiratory rate and degree of atelectasis. The more atelectasis present, the higher the spontaneous respiratory rate. If lung expansion therapy is preventing or correcting atelectasis, the respiratory rate would be at or near normal. Auscultation can also be useful and should document the presence of abnormal breath sounds and adventitious lung sounds. A reduction in late-inspiratory crackles and improvement in breath sounds suggest the treatment is effective. Findings on the most recent chest film can be very useful to document the presence or lack of atelectasis. The signs of volume loss disappear with effective lung expansion therapy. In addition, the patient may complain less of dyspnea when the lung is expanded to its healthy position.

Implementation. Implementation of IPPB involves equipment preparation, patient orientation, and careful adjustment of the treatment parameters according to the patient's response.

Equipment Preparation. Although all IPPB equipment should undergo a regular schedule of preventive maintenance and calibration, it is the responsibility of the RT to ensure that all components are in proper working order before any use in patients. Most respiratory care departments have standard protocols for this purpose. Because pressure-cycled IPPB devices do not end inspiration if leaks occur in the system, it is important to check the patency of the patient's breathing circuit before each use. This check can be done by aseptically occluding the patient connector and manually triggering a breath at a low-flow setting. If the system pressure increases and the machine cycles off, the circuit is free of any major leak.

Patient Orientation. Successful IPPB therapy depends mainly on the effectiveness of initial patient orientation. Before the first treatment, the RT must carefully explain to the patient the purpose of the therapy. This explanation should be tailored to the patient's level of understanding and address, at a minimum, the following points: (1) why the physician ordered the treatment, (2) what the treatment does, (3) how it will feel, and (4) what are the expected results.

The IPPB device should not be brought to the bedside until the RT believes that the patient adequately understands the procedure and the importance of cooperation. When the RT decides to bring the equipment to the bedside, a simple functional description may allay any fear or anxiety associated with the use of such an unfamiliar device. A simulated demonstration of the procedure can be particularly useful in this regard. This demonstration can be done effectively with a test lung or, if deemed necessary, by self-application using a separate breathing circuit kept for this purpose. For some patients, an effective demonstration can make the difference between success and failure in implementing the treatment regimen.

Patient Positioning. For best results, the patient should be in a semi-Fowler position. Slouching should be discouraged because it impairs diaphragm movement and decreases inspired volumes. The supine position may be acceptable in certain patients in whom an upright position is contraindicated.

Initial Application. To eliminate airway leaks in an alert patient, an initial trial of nose clips may be needed until the technique is understood and the treatment can be performed without them. The mouthpiece must be inserted well past the lips, and a tight seal must be encouraged to prevent gas leakage from the site. The use of a mask as an interface with IPPB is generally not recommended. To provide adequate therapy, the mask often needs to be held tightly to the patient's face and tends to be quite uncomfortable. If a mask is needed to provide lung expansion therapy, it is generally suggested to find another method such as CPAP or NIV.

The machine should be set so that a breath can be initiated with minimal patient effort. A sensitivity or trigger level of −1 to −2 cm H_2O is adequate for most patients. Initially, system pressure is set low enough for the patient to be able to trigger the IPPB machine for both inspiration and expiration. Resulting volumes should be measured, and the pressure or flow should be adjusted accordingly after the treatment has begun. If the device has a flow control, the RT should begin the treatment with a low-to-moderate flow and adjust it according to the patient's breathing pattern. Generally, the goal is to establish a breathing pattern consisting of about 6 breaths per minute, with an expiratory time of at least three to four times longer than inspiration (inspiratory-to-expiratory [I:E] ratio of ≤1:3 to 1:4). These settings may need to be adjusted according to individual needs and patient response. Careful monitoring of the breathing pattern and coaching to maintain it must be conducted throughout the treatment.

Adjusting Parameters. After the treatment begins and the patient's basic ventilatory pattern is established, the pressure and flow should be individually adjusted and monitored according to the goals of the therapy. IPPB therapy should be volume-oriented when used to treat atelectasis. In these situations, arbitrary pressure settings are unacceptable, and tidal volumes must be monitored. A tidal volume goal must be set for each individual patient, and the therapy must be delivered on the basis of these goals.

There are various ways of determining these volume goals. Most clinical centers strive to achieve an IPPB tidal volume of 10 to 15 ml/kg of body weight or at least 30% of the patient's predicted IC. If the initial volumes fall short of this goal and the patient can tolerate it, the pressure is gradually increased until the goal is achieved. Pressures of 30 to 35 cm H_2O may be needed to achieve this end when lung compliance is reduced. If high pressures are required, care needs to be taken to minimize the risk of gastric insufflation.

To achieve the largest inspiratory volumes during IPPB, the RT should encourage the patient to breathe actively during the positive pressure breath. However, no definitive studies exist that show the need to have the patient actively participate in inspiration. Regardless of the approach, IPPB is useful in the treatment of atelectasis only if the volumes delivered exceed the volumes achieved by the patient's spontaneous efforts.

Discontinuation and Follow-up

Depending on the goals of therapy and condition of the patient, IPPB treatments typically last 15 to 20 minutes. Follow-up activities include posttreatment assessment of the patient, recordkeeping, and equipment maintenance.

Posttreatment Assessment. At the end of a treatment session, the patient assessment is repeated. As with the baseline assessment, this follow-up evaluation has two components. The general follow-up evaluation of the patient's clinical status should focus on determining any pertinent changes in vital signs, sensorium, and breath sounds, with emphasis on identifying possible untoward effects. The more specific follow-up assessment provides information relevant to evaluating progress toward achieving the chosen goals of therapy.

Treatment frequency should be determined by assessing patient response to therapy. For acute care patients, orders should be reevaluated based on patient response to therapy at least every 72 hours or with any change of patient status.

Recordkeeping. A succinct but complete account of the treatment session, including the preassessment and postassessment results, must be entered in the patient's medical record according to the approved institutional protocol. Any untoward patient responses also must be reported immediately to responsible personnel, including at least the prescribing physician and attending nurse.

Monitoring and Troubleshooting

As indicated in Box 39-9, monitoring of IPPB therapy involves both patient response and machine performance. Information derived from monitoring allows for titration of therapy and can aid in the early identification of common problems.

Box 39-9 Monitoring Intermittent Positive Airway Pressure Breathing Therapy

MACHINE PERFORMANCE

- Sensitivity
- Peak pressure
- Flow setting
- FiO_2
- I:E ratio

PATIENT RESPONSE*

- Breathing rate and expired volume
- Peak flow or $FEV_1/FVC\%$
- Pulse rate and rhythm (from electrocardiogram if available)
- Sputum quantity, color, consistency, and odor
- Mental function
- Skin color
- Breath sounds
- Blood pressure
- SpO_2 (if hypoxemia is suspected)
- ICP (in patients for whom ICP is important)
- Chest radiograph (when appropriate)
- Subjective response to therapy

*Items should be chosen as appropriate for the specific patient.

Machine Performance. In terms of machine performance, large negative pressure swings early in inspiration indicate an incorrect sensitivity or trigger setting. In this case, the RT should increase the sensitivity or alter the trigger level until only 1 to 2 cm H_2O is needed to trigger the device into inspiration. If system pressure decreases after inspiration begins or fails to increase steadily until the very end of the machine breath, the problem is too low a flow. In this situation, the flow should be increased (as tolerated) until system pressure increases steadily and holds near the preset value.

Knowing proper IPPB machine operation is vital to being able to troubleshoot the most commonplace issues experienced. Some of these issues include premature transition into exhalation, inability to trigger the machine, or improper flow delivery. Checking the circuit and properly instructing the patient are the best ways to prevent or correct these problems.

Leaks pose a different problem. In the presence of leaks, a pressure-cycled IPPB device does not reach its preset cycling pressure and does not cycle off. This problem is evident when inspiration continues well beyond the expected time. To troubleshoot leaks, the RT needs to differentiate between the machine and patient interface. Machine leaks most commonly occur at connection points, such as the nebulizer or exhalation valve. In addition, a torn or improperly seated exhalation valve diaphragm causes a large system leak. Leaks at the patient interface usually occur at the mouth (loose seal around mouthpiece) or through the nose. If the problem is mouth leaks, additional instruction may help. If not, a flanged mouthpiece may be needed. Leaks through the nose are easily corrected with nose clips.

The last consideration regarding machine performance involves selecting an IPPB machine capable of providing the appropriate FiO_2. Some electrically powered IPPB machines are capable of providing only room air or slightly enriched oxygen (O_2) concentrations (<40%) and may cause or worsen hypoxemia in some patients needing supplemental O_2. To avoid this problem in such patients, an IPPB machine capable of providing a high FiO_2, such as the Bird Mark 7 (Care Fusion, Corp, San Diego), should be selected.

Patient Response. In monitoring the patient's response, the RT takes into account the intended purpose of the therapy and the patient's clinical conditions. These factors dictate exactly what must be monitored for a patient.

Positive Airway Pressure Therapy

Similar to IPPB, positive airway pressure (PAP) adjuncts use positive pressure to increase the PL gradient and enhance lung expansion. In contrast to IPPB, PAP therapy requires no complex machinery. Some methods do not even need a source of pressurized gas.

Physiologic Basis

There are three current approaches to PAP therapy: PEP, EPAP, and CPAP. All three techniques are effective in treating atelectasis in most postsurgical patients.[13,14] Because PEP and EPAP are used most often as part of airway clearance, they are described in Chapter 40. This chapter describes the intermittent use of CPAP for the treatment of atelectasis. Continuous use of CPAP is discussed elsewhere in this text.

PEP and EPAP create expiratory positive pressure only, whereas CPAP maintains a positive airway pressure throughout both inspiration and expiration. Figure 39-6 compares the alveolar and Ppl changes occurring during a normal spontaneous breath (Figure 39-6, *A*) and CPAP (see Figure 39-6, *B*). As can be seen, CPAP elevates and maintains high alveolar and airway pressures throughout the full breathing cycle; this increases PL gradient throughout both inspiration and expiration. Typically, a patient on CPAP breathes through a pressurized circuit against a threshold resistor, with pressures maintained between 5 cm H_2O and 20 cm H_2O. To maintain system pressure throughout the breathing cycle, CPAP requires a source of pressurized gas.

The following factors involving PAP, EPAP, and CPAP therapy contribute to the beneficial effects: (1) recruitment of collapsed alveoli via an increase in FRC, (2) decreased work of breathing secondary to increased compliance or elimination of intrinsic positive end expiratory pressure (PEEP), (3) improved distribution of ventilation through collateral channels (e.g., Kohn pores), and (4) increase in the efficiency of secretion removal.

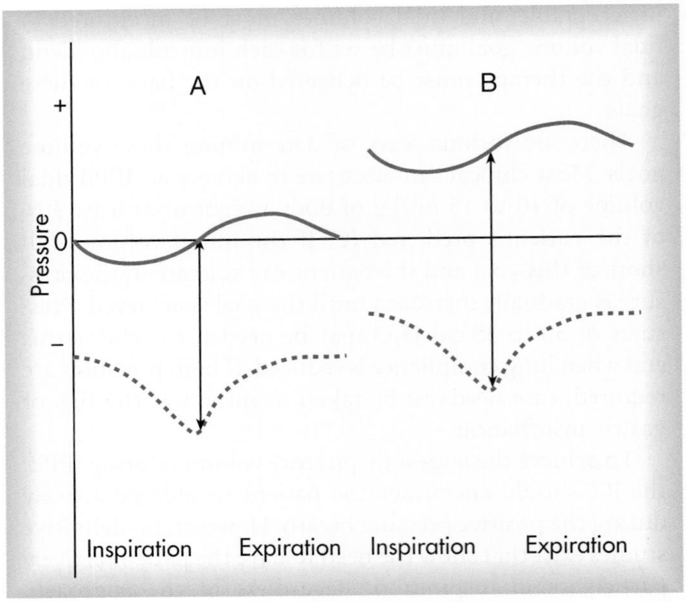

FIGURE 39-6 Alveolar *(solid lines)* and pleural *(dotted lines)* pressures during spontaneous breathing *(A)* and CPAP *(B)*. Note the difference in PL gradients *(double arrows)*.

Indications

Although evidence exists to support the use of CPAP therapy in the treatment of postoperative atelectasis, as with all mechanical techniques, the duration of beneficial effects appears limited. The corresponding increase in FRC may be lost within 10 minutes after the end of the treatment. For this reason, it has been suggested that CPAP should be used on a continuous basis until the patient recovers.

CPAP by mask also has been used to treat cardiogenic pulmonary edema. In such patients, CPAP reduces venous return and cardiac filling pressures, which is helpful in reducing pulmonary vascular congestion. Lung compliance is improved, and the work of breathing is decreased.

Contraindications

Intermittent use of CPAP for the correction of atelectasis is contraindicated when certain clinical situations exist. A patient who is hemodynamically unstable is unlikely to tolerate CPAP for even a short period. A patient who is suspected to have hypoventilation is not a good candidate for CPAP because it does not ensure ventilation, but the patient may be an ideal candidate for consideration of NIV. Other problems that may indicate CPAP is not an appropriate therapy include nausea, facial trauma, untreated pneumothorax, and elevated intracranial pressure (ICP).

Hazards and Complications

Most hazards and complications associated with CPAP are caused by either the increased pressure or the apparatus. The increased work of breathing caused by the apparatus

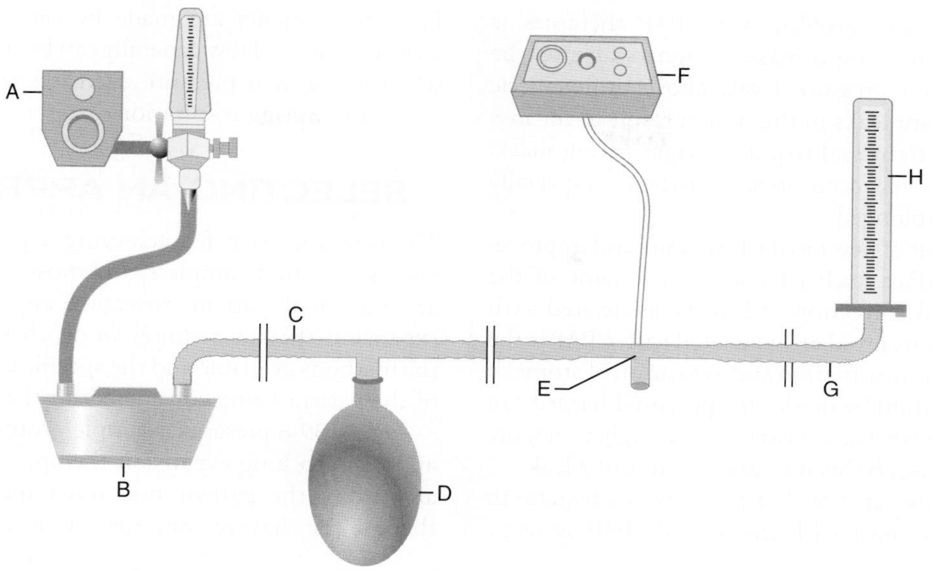

FIGURE 39-7 Continuous-flow CPAP system. See text for description. (Modified from Branson RD, Hurst JM, Dellayen CB: Mask CPAP: state of the art. Respir Care 30:846, 1985.)

can lead to hypoventilation and hypercapnia. In addition, because CPAP does not augment spontaneous ventilation, patients with an accompanying ventilatory insufficiency may hypoventilate during application. Barotrauma is a potential hazard of CPAP and is more likely to occur in a patient with emphysema and blebs. Gastric distention may occur especially if CPAP values greater than 15 cm H_2O are needed. This condition may lead to vomiting and aspiration in a patient with an inadequate gag reflex.

Equipment

Equipment used to deliver CPAP varies substantially in design and complexity. For purposes of illustration, the key elements of a simple continuous-flow CPAP circuit are shown in Figure 39-7. A breathing gas mixture from an O_2 blender *(A)* flows continuously through a humidifier *(B)* into the inspiratory limb of a breathing circuit *(C)*. A reservoir bag *(D)* provides reserve volume if the patient's inspiratory flow exceeds that of the system. The patient breathes in and out through a simple valveless T-piece connector *(E)*. A pressure alarm system with manometer *(F)* monitors the CPAP at the patient's airway. The alarm system can warn of either low (usually caused by a disconnection) or high system pressure. The expiratory limb of the circuit *(G)* is connected to a threshold resistor, in this case, a water column *(H)*.

As can be seen, the CPAP circuit is essentially the same as the EPAP circuit, with the exception of the closed reservoir and monitoring system. Because it is a closed system, the CPAP circuit should also have an emergency inlet valve (not shown). This emergency inlet valve ensures that atmospheric air is available to the patient should the primary gas source fail.

Administering Intermittent Continuous Positive Airway Pressure

As with all respiratory care, effective CPAP therapy requires careful planning, individualized patient assessment and implementation and thoughtful follow-up.

Planning. During planning, the need for PAP therapy should be determined, and desired therapeutic outcomes should be set. Specifically, an improvement in breath sounds, improvement in vital signs (e.g., lower respiratory rate), resolution of abnormal radiograph findings, and restoration of normal oxygenation all would indicate that the therapy has achieved its goal.

Procedures. Whether used on an intermittent or continuous basis, CPAP is a complex and potentially hazardous approach to patient management. As with all therapies, the appropriate CPAP level for a patient must be determined on an individual basis. Initial application and monitoring require a broader range of knowledge and skill than required for simpler modes of lung expansion therapy.

Monitoring and Troubleshooting

CPAP poses a danger of hypoventilation. Experience with long-term CPAP shows that patients must be able to maintain adequate excretion of carbon dioxide on their own if the therapy is to be successful. For these reasons, patients receiving CPAP must be closely and continuously monitored for untoward effects. In addition, it is vital that the CPAP device be equipped with a means to monitor the pressure delivered to the airways and alarms to indicate the loss of pressure owing to system disconnect or mechanical failure. There should also be a device allowing for excessive pressure to be released (pop-off). These are essential components of any CPAP device.

The most common problem with PAP therapies is system leaks. When using a mask, a tight seal must be maintained to keep pressure levels above atmospheric levels. Any significant leaks in the system result in the loss of PAP. Because a tight seal requires a tight-fitting mask, pain and irritation may occur in some patients, especially if the therapy is prolonged.

The development of new nasal CPAP units and improvement on the interface itself have addressed some of the comfort issues and correction of leakage associated with CPAP. A more serious problem associated with CPAP is the possibility of gastric insufflation and aspiration of stomach contents. As with IPPB by mask, this potential hazard can be eliminated by use of a nasogastric tube at higher pressure requirements, although this increases the risk of a leak.

The RT must also ensure that the flow is adequate to meet the patient's needs with the use of CPAP systems. Flow adjustments are made by carefully observing the airway pressure. Flow generally can be considered adequate when the system pressure decreases no more than 1 to 2 cm H_2O during inspiration.

SELECTING AN APPROACH

The best approach for achieving a given clinical goal is always the safest, simplest, and most effective method for an individual patient. Selecting an approach for lung expansion therapy requires in-depth knowledge of both the methods available and the specific condition and needs of the patient being considered for therapy.

Figure 39-8 presents a sample protocol for selecting an approach to lung expansion therapy. As indicated in the algorithm, the patient first must meet the criteria for therapy by having one or more of the indications

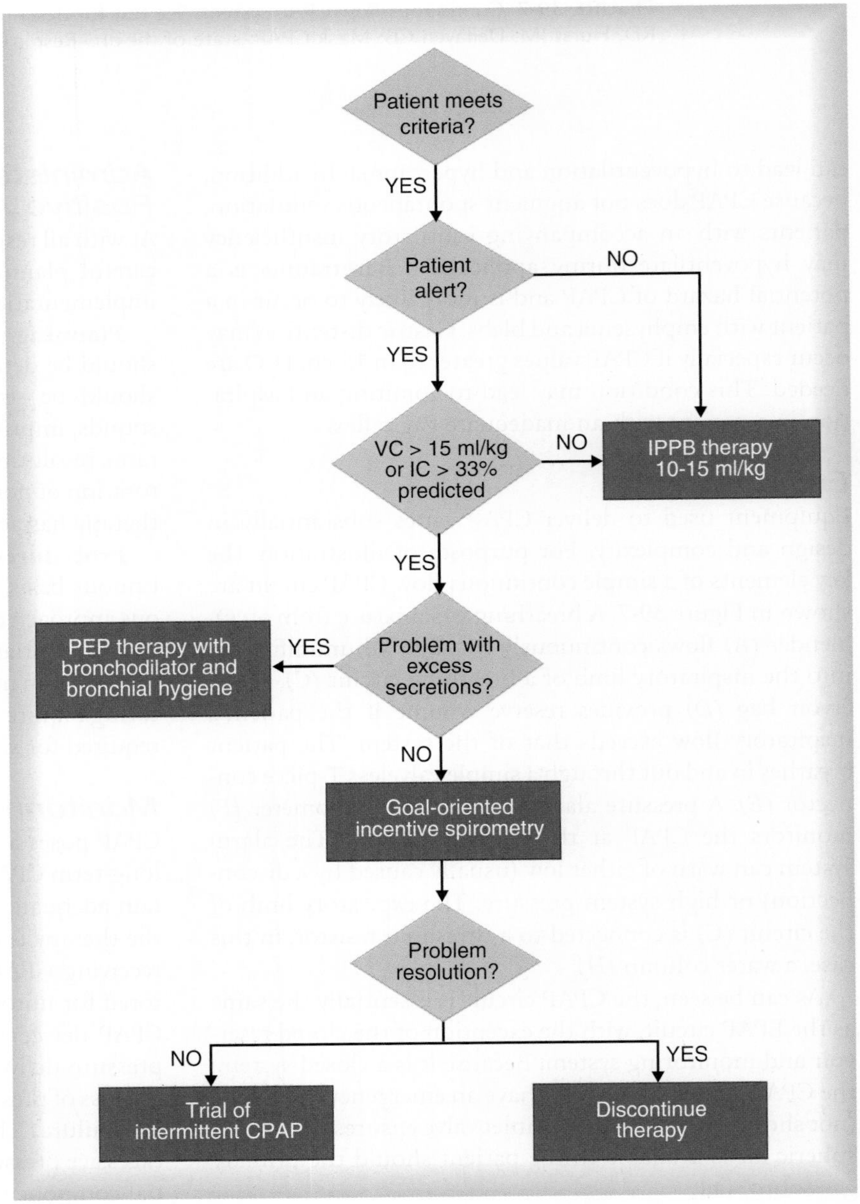

FIGURE 39-8 Example protocol for selecting an approach for lung expansion therapy. See text for details.

previously specified. For patients meeting the inclusion criteria, the RT first determines the degree of alertness. Because an obtunded patient cannot be expected to cooperate with IS or PEP or EPAP therapy, IPPB or NIV is initiated with appropriate monitoring. If the patient is alert, a bedside assessment is conducted. This assessment should include measurement of either the IC or vital capacity (VC) and evaluation of the volume and consistency of the patient's secretions.

For a patient having no difficulty with secretions, if the VC exceeds 15 ml/kg of lean body weight or the IC is greater than 33% of predicted, IS is given. If either the VC or the IC is less than these threshold levels, IPPB is initiated, with the pressure gradually manipulated from the initial setting to deliver at least 15 ml/kg.

If excessive sputum production is a compounding factor, a trial of PEP therapy is substituted for IS. Based on patient response, bronchodilator therapy and bronchial hygiene measures may be added to this regimen. If monitoring fails to reveal improvement and atelectasis persists, a trial of CPAP should be considered. Because evidence of the effectiveness of CPAP is still contradictory, its use should be limited to treating atelectasis after alternative approaches have been tried without success.

SUMMARY CHECKLIST

- Atelectasis is caused by persistent ventilation with small tidal volumes or by resorption of gas distal to obstructed airways.
- Patients who have undergone upper abdominal or thoracic surgery are at greatest risk for atelectasis. A history of lung disease or significant cigarette smoking increases the risk.
- Patients with atelectasis usually have rapid, shallow breathing; fine, late-inspiratory crackles; and abnormalities on chest radiograph.
- Lung expansion therapy corrects atelectasis by increasing the P_L gradient; this can be accomplished by deep spontaneous breaths or by the application of positive pressure.
- The most common problem associated with lung expansion therapy is the onset of respiratory alkalosis, which occurs when the patient breathes too fast.
- RTs are responsible for implementing, monitoring, and documenting results of lung expansion therapy.

References

1. Lawrence VA, Cornell JE, Smetana GW: Strategies to reduce postoperative pulmonary complications after noncardiothoracic surgery: systematic review for the American College of Physicians. Ann Intern Med 144:596, 2006.
2. Benditt JO: Esophageal and gastric pressure management. Respir Care 50:68, 2005.
3. Duggan M, Kavanagh BP: Atelectasis in the perioperative patient. Curr Opin Anesthesiol 20:37, 2007.
4. Duggan M, Kavanagh BP: Pulmonary atelectasis: a pathogenic perioperative entity. Anesthesiology 102:838, 2005.
5. Brower RG: Consequences of bed rest. Crit Care Med 37:S422, 2009.
6. Ferreyra GP, Baussano I, Squadrone V, et al: Continuous positive airway pressure for treatment of respiratory complications after abdominal surgery. Ann Surg 247:617, 2008.
7. Guimaraes MM, El Dib R, Smith AF, et al: Incentive spirometry for prevention of postoperative pulmonary complications in upper abdominal surgery. Cochrane Database Syst Rev (3):CD006058, 2009.
8. Westerdahl E: Deep-breathing exercises reduce atelectasis and improve pulmonary function after coronary artery bypass surgery. Chest 128:3482, 2005.
9. American Association for Respiratory Care: Clinical practice guidelines: incentive spirometry. Respir Care 36:1402, 1991.
10. American Association for Respiratory Care: Intermittent positive pressure breathing—2003 revision and update. Respir Care 48:540, 2003.
11. Narita M, Tanizawa K, Chin K, et al: Noninvasive ventilation improves the outcome of pulmonary complications after liver resection. Intern Med 49:1501, 2010.
12. Pessoa KC, Araujo GF, Pinheiro AN, et al: Noninvasive ventilation in the immediate postoperative of gastrojejunal derivation with Roux-en-Y gastric bypass. Rev Bras Fisioter 14:290, 2010.
13. Sehlin M, Ohberg F, Johansson G, et al: Physiological responses to positive expiratory pressure breathing: a comparison of the PEP bottle and PEP mask. Respir Care 52:1000, 2007.
14. Squadrone V, Coha M, Cerutti E, et al: Continuous positive airway pressure for treatment of postoperative hypoxemia: a randomized controlled trial. JAMA 293:589, 2005.

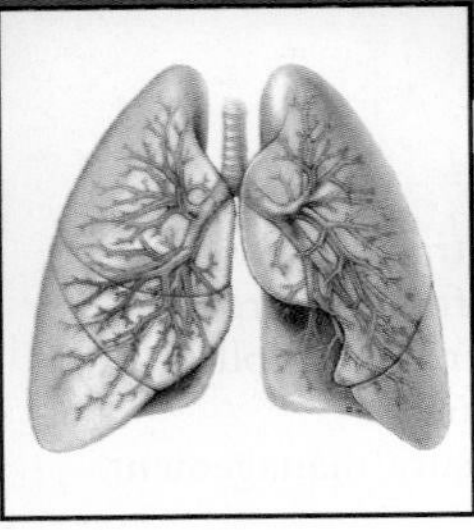

Chapter 40

Airway Clearance Therapy

CHRISTOPHER A. HIRSCH

CHAPTER OBJECTIVES

After reading this chapter you will be able to:

- Describe how normal airway clearance mechanisms work and the factors that can impair their function.
- Identify pulmonary diseases associated with abnormal clearance of secretions.
- State the goals and clinical indications for airway clearance therapy.
- Describe the proper technique and potential benefit of each of the following:
  - Postural drainage
  - Directed coughing and related expulsion techniques
  - Positive expiratory pressure therapy
  - High-frequency compression/oscillation methods
  - Mobilization and exercise
- Evaluate a patient's response to airway clearance therapy.
- Modify airway clearance therapies on the basis of patient response.

CHAPTER OUTLINE

KEY TERMS

active cycle of breathing technique (ACBT)
autogenic drainage (AD)
bronchiectasis
chest physical therapy (CPT)
ciliary dyskinetic syndromes
forced expiratory technique (FET)
Hertz (Hz)
high-frequency chest wall compression (HFCWC)
huff cough
inspissation
intrapulmonary percussive ventilation (IPV)
mechanical insufflation-exsufflation (MIE)
mucous plugging
oscillation
positive expiratory pressure (PEP)
splinting

Airway clearance therapy involves the use of noninvasive techniques designed to help mobilize and remove secretions and improve gas exchange.[1-6] Previously, airway clearance methods often were grouped under a broad category of techniques called **chest physical therapy (CPT).** CPT involves not only airway clearance techniques but also various exercise protocols and breathing retraining methods.[1,2] This chapter focuses on noninvasive airway clearance. The primary invasive method of airway clearance, suctioning, is discussed in Chapter 33.

Traditionally, airway clearance therapy has involved CPT *(postural drainage, percussion, and vibration [PDPV])* combined with cough instruction.[6] Over the years, several additional noninvasive airway clearance methods have been developed to augment or replace this traditional approach. These newer techniques include modified breathing and coughing routines, manual hyperinflation, and mechanical devices designed to augment secretion clearance.[2]

In the past, airway clearance methods were commonly used in medical practice without firm scientific knowledge regarding their effectiveness. One example was to order CPT for essentially all postoperative patients in the hope that its use would prevent the respiratory complications of surgery.[7-12] It is now known that this broad application of airway clearance therapy is both ineffective and costly. In an effort to address these types of issues, the American College of Chest Physicians (ACCP) conducted a formal systematic review of the evidence-based practice for nonpharmacologic airway clearance therapies.[3] The recommendations of the ACCP are included in this chapter.

As a result of evidence-based initiatives, it has been shown that combining certain airway clearance techniques with exercise can improve lung function in patients with cystic fibrosis (CF).[3,5,6] Another review of related research raised questions regarding the effectiveness of CPT in patients with acute and stable chronic obstructive pulmonary disease (COPD), chronic bronchitis, or **bronchiectasis.**[13,14] Successful outcomes in airway clearance techniques require knowledge of normal and abnormal physiology, careful patient evaluation and selection, a clear definition of therapeutic goals, rigorous application of the appropriate evidence-based methods, and ongoing assessment and follow-up.[15-18]

PHYSIOLOGY OF AIRWAY CLEARANCE

To apply airway clearance methods properly, one first must understand how normal airway clearance mechanisms work and what can impair their function.

Normal Clearance

Normal airway clearance requires a patent airway, a functional mucociliary escalator, and an effective cough.[5,19,20] Airways normally are kept open by structural support mechanisms (see Chapter 8) and kept clear by proper function of the ciliated mucosa. The mucociliary clearance mechanism operates from the larynx down to the respiratory bronchioles. The mucus itself originates from the goblet cells and submucosal glands, although Clara cells and tissue fluid transudation also contribute to airway secretions. Ciliated epithelial cells normally move this mucus via a coordinated wave of ciliary motion toward the trachea and larynx, where excess secretions can be swallowed or expectorated.

Although essentially a reserve clearance mechanism, cough is one of the most important protective reflexes.[21-23] By ridding the larger airways of excessive mucus and foreign matter, cough assists the normal mucociliary clearance and helps ensure airway patency.

As shown in Figure 40-1, there are four distinct phases to a normal cough: *irritation, inspiration, compression,* and *expulsion*. In the initial irritation phase, an abnormal stimulus provokes sensory fibers in the airways to send

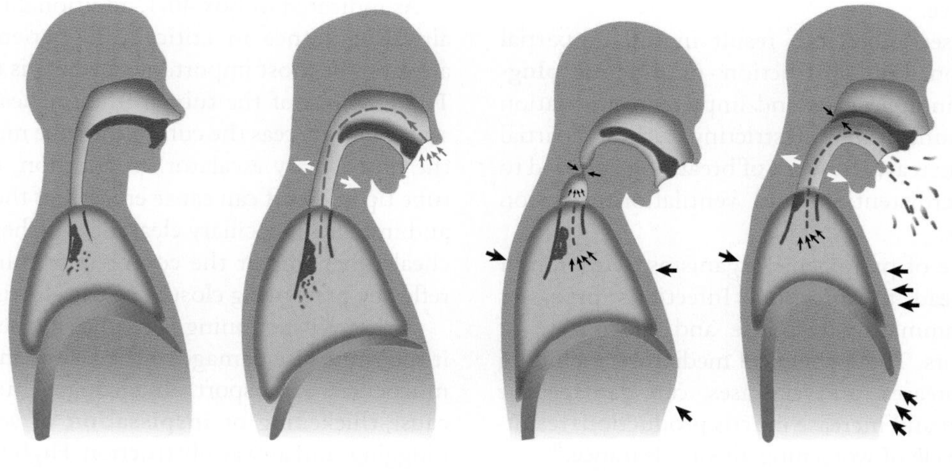

FIGURE 40-1 The cough reflex. (Modified from Cherniack RM, Cherniack L: Respiration in health and disease, ed 3, Philadelphia, 1983, WB Saunders.)

impulses to the medullary cough center in the brain. This stimulus normally is inflammatory, mechanical, chemical, or thermal. Infection is a good example of cough stimulation caused by an *inflammatory* process. Foreign bodies can provoke a cough through *mechanical* stimulation. *Chemical* stimulation can occur when irritating gases are inhaled (e.g., cigarette smoke). Finally, cold air may cause *thermal* stimulation of sensory nerves and produce a cough.

When these afferent impulses are received, the cough center generates a reflex stimulation of the respiratory muscles to initiate a deep inspiration (the second phase). In normal adults, this inspiration averages 1 to 2 L.

During the third, or compression, phase, reflex nerve impulses cause glottic closure and a forceful contraction of the expiratory muscles. This compression phase is normally about 0.2 second and results in a rapid increase in pleural and alveolar pressures, often greater than 100 mm Hg.

At this point, the glottis opens, initiating the expulsion phase. With the glottis open, a large pressure gradient between the intrathoracic airways and the atmospheric pressure is exposed. Together with the continued contraction of the expiratory muscles, this pressure gradient normally causes a violent, expulsive flow of air from the lungs, with velocities often 500 miles per hour. High-velocity gas flow, combined with dynamic airway compression, creates huge shear forces that displace mucus from the airway walls into the air stream. Mucus and foreign material are expelled from the lower airways to the upper airway, where they can be expectorated or swallowed.

Abnormal Clearance

Any abnormality that alters airway patency, mucociliary function, strength of the inspiratory or expiratory muscles, thickness of secretions, or effectiveness of the cough reflex can impair airway clearance and cause retention of secretions.[19,20,22,23] In addition, some therapeutic interventions, especially interventions used in critical care, can result in abnormal clearance.

Retention of secretions can result in full or partial airway obstruction. Full obstruction, or **mucous plugging,** can result in atelectasis and impaired oxygenation secondary to shunting. By restricting airflow, partial obstruction can increase the work of breathing and lead to air trapping, overdistention, and ventilation/perfusion ($\dot{V}/\dot{Q}$) imbalances.

In the presence of pathogenic organisms, retention of secretions can lead to infection. Infectious processes provoke an inflammatory response and the release of chemical mediators. These chemical mediators, including leukotrienes, proteases, and elastases, can damage the airway epithelium and increase mucus production, resulting in a vicious cycle of worsening airway clearance.[20]

Compounding these problems may be failure of the cough reflex. In patients with retained secretions, interference with any one of the four phases of cough can result in ineffective airway clearance. Table 40-1 provides examples of factors that can impair the normal cough reflex.

As indicated in Box 40-1, additional factors can impair airway clearance in critically ill patients with artificial airways, the most important of which is the airway itself.[16] The presence of the tube in the trachea increases mucus secretion, whereas the cuff of the tube mechanically blocks the mucociliary escalator. In addition, movement of the tube tip and cuff can cause erosion of the tracheal mucosa and impair mucociliary clearance further. Lastly, endotracheal tubes impair the compression phase of the cough reflex by preventing closure of the glottis (see Table 40-1).

Although suctioning is used to aid secretion clearance, it too can cause damage to the airway mucosa and impair mucociliary transport. Inadequate humidification can cause thickening or **inspissation** of secretions, mucous plugging, and airway obstruction. High fractional inspired oxygen (FiO_2) concentrations can impair mucociliary clearance, either directly or by causing acute tracheobronchitis. Several common drugs, including some general

TABLE 40-1

Mechanisms Impairing Cough Reflex

Phase	Examples of Impairments
Irritation	Anesthesia CNS depression Narcotic-analgesics
Inspiration	Pain Neuromuscular dysfunction Pulmonary restriction Abdominal restriction
Compression	Laryngeal nerve damage Artificial airway Abdominal muscle weakness Abdominal surgery
Expulsion	Airway compression Airway obstruction Abdominal muscle weakness Inadequate lung recoil (e.g., emphysema)

CNS, Central nervous system.

Box 40-1 Causes of Impaired Mucociliary Clearance in Intubated Patients

- Endotracheal or tracheostomy tube
- Tracheobronchial suction
- Inadequate humidification
- High FiO_2 values
- Drugs
- General anesthetics
- Opiates
- Narcotics
- Underlying pulmonary disease

anesthetics and narcotic-analgesics, can depress mucociliary transport. Lastly, several diseases commonly seen in critically ill patients are associated with poor secretion clearance; these are discussed in the following sections.[3,12]

Diseases Associated With Abnormal Clearance

Several diseases are associated with abnormal clearance, including diseases affecting airway patency, composition and production of mucus, ciliary structure and function, and normal cough reflex.[3,20,24] Internal obstruction or external compression of the airway lumen can impair airway clearance. Examples include foreign bodies, tumors, and congenital or acquired thoracic anomalies such as kyphoscoliosis. Internal obstruction also can occur with mucus hypersecretion, inflammatory changes, or bronchospasm, further narrowing the lumen. Examples include asthma, chronic bronchitis, and acute infections.

Diseases that alter normal mucociliary clearance can also cause retention of secretions. CF is a common disorder in this category. In CF, the solute concentration of the mucus is altered because of abnormal sodium and chloride transport.[25] This alteration increases the viscosity of mucus and impairs its movement up the respiratory tract. Although less common, there are several conditions in which the respiratory tract cilia do not function properly.[26] These **ciliary dyskinetic syndromes** also can contribute to ineffective airway clearance.

Chronic airway inflammation and infection can lead to bronchiectasis, a common finding in CF and ciliary dyskinetic syndromes. In bronchiectasis, the airway is permanently damaged, dilated, and prone to constant obstruction by retained secretions.[14] Other conditions that can lead to bronchiectasis include chronic obstructive lung diseases, foreign body aspiration, and obliterative bronchiolitis.[27]

As previously discussed, any condition that affects the four components of an effective cough also alters airway clearance. Mucociliary function may be normal, but without an effective cough, mucous plugs, obstruction, and atelectasis can occur. The most common conditions affecting the cough reflex are musculoskeletal and neurologic disorders, including muscular dystrophy, amyotrophic lateral sclerosis, spinal muscular atrophy, myasthenia gravis, poliomyelitis, and cerebral palsy (see Chapter 29).

GENERAL GOALS AND INDICATIONS

The primary goal of airway clearance therapy is to help mobilize and remove retained secretions, with the ultimate aim to improve gas exchange, promote alveolar expansion, and reduce the work of breathing. Box 40-2 lists general indications for airway clearance therapy.[3,5,12] More specific indications are described as each airway clearance technique is discussed.

Box 40-2 Indications for Airway Clearance Therapy

ACUTE CONDITIONS
- Copious secretions
- Acute respiratory failure with retained secretions
- Acute lobar atelectasis
- $\dot{V}/\dot{Q}$ abnormalities caused by unilateral lung disease

CHRONIC CONDITIONS
- CF
- Bronchiectasis
- Ciliary dyskinetic syndromes
- Chronic bronchitis

DISORDERS ASSOCIATED WITH RETENTION OF SECRETIONS
- Acute disease
- Immobile patients
- Postoperative patients—related to effect of general anesthetics, opiates, and narcotics
- Inadequate humidification
- Acute exacerbations: (1) COPD, (2) CF, (3) bronchiectasis
- Chronic disease: (1) CF, (2) neuromuscular disorders

Airway Clearance Therapy for Acute Conditions

Patients with acute conditions in whom airway clearance therapy may be indicated include (1) acutely ill patients with copious secretions; (2) patients in acute respiratory failure with clinical signs of retained secretions (audible abnormal breath sounds, deteriorating arterial blood gases, chest radiographic changes); (3) patients with acute lobar atelectasis; and (4) patients with $\dot{V}/\dot{Q}$ abnormalities owing to lung infiltrates or consolidation.[15-17] In treating acute respiratory conditions, inhaled bronchodilator therapy before airway clearance therapy may improve the overall effectiveness of the treatment both by opening the airways and by increasing the mucociliary activity. For acute pulmonary infections, inhaled antibiotics after airway clearance therapy can lead to improved deposition of the antibiotic.[2] Acute conditions for which airway clearance therapy is probably not indicated include (1) acute exacerbations of COPD, (2) pneumonia without clinically significant sputum production, and (3) uncomplicated asthma.[3,5]

Airway Clearance Therapy for Chronic Conditions

Airway clearance therapy has proved effective in aiding secretion clearance and improving pulmonary function in chronic conditions associated with copious sputum production, including CF, bronchiectasis, and chronic bronchitis in certain patients.[3,10,15-17] Generally, sputum production must exceed 25 to 30 ml/day for airway clearance therapy to improve secretion removal significantly.

MINI CLINI

Assessing a Patient's Cough Clearance

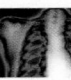

PROBLEM: The RT is called by a nurse to determine why her patient is having difficulty clearing secretions. The patient is an alert, obese, 45-year-old man who underwent general anesthesia and surgery for bowel obstruction 3 hours earlier. Physical signs indicate retention of secretions, but there is no history of lung disease. The patient is breathing through an endotracheal tube and receiving 40% O_2 with aerosol via T tube. Through visual clues, the patient has been indicating severe pain in the epigastric area. The patient was started on intravenous morphine 1 hour earlier.

DISCUSSION: Even without lung disease, it is no surprise that this patient is having difficulty clearing secretions via cough. Recent anesthesia and the narcotic-analgesic potentially are impairing his cough. In addition, obesity, abdominal restriction and weakness, and pain are impairing the inspiration, compression, and expulsion phases. Lastly, the presence of the endotracheal tube further impairs coughing and mucus clearance.

The patient should immediately be started on an aggressive airway clearance regimen. Judicious use of pain medication, coinciding with therapy, should continue. Cough instruction (with coaching in incisional splinting) should be part of the plan. Early mobilization should be considered. The head of the patient's bed should be elevated at least to 30 to 45 degrees, to minimize the risk of aspiration. The endotracheal tube should be removed as soon as possible. Until then, suctioning on an as-needed basis is required.

RULE OF THUMB

When obtaining information from patients regarding sputum production, use common measures they can understand. For example, copious production (25 to 30 ml/day) is about 1 fluid ounce or a "shot-glass full."

Airway Clearance Therapy to Prevent Retention of Secretions

Airway clearance therapy has been used as a preventive mode of respiratory care in various disorders. Current evidence is inclusive regarding the benefits of this approach. The best-documented preventive uses of airway clearance therapy include (1) body positioning and patient mobilization to prevent retained secretions in acutely ill patients and (2) CPT combined with physical activity to maintain lung function in patients with CF.[3,4,6,8,28] Other preventive applications of airway clearance therapy have not proved to be useful.[3,5]

Box 40-3 Initial Assessment of Need for Airway Clearance Therapy

MEDICAL RECORD

History of pulmonary problems causing increased secretions
Admission for upper abdominal or thoracic surgery; consider:
- Age (elderly)
- History of COPD
- Obesity
- Nature of procedure
- Type of anesthesia
- Duration of procedure

Presence of artificial tracheal airway
Chest radiograph indicating atelectasis or infiltrates
Results of pulmonary function testing
Arterial blood gas values or O_2 saturation

PATIENT

Posture, muscle tone
Effectiveness of cough
Sputum production
Breathing pattern
General physical fitness
Breath sounds
Vital signs, heart rate and rhythm

DETERMINING THE NEED FOR AIRWAY CLEARANCE THERAPY

Effective airway clearance therapy requires proper initial and ongoing patient assessment. All the key elements involved in determining the need for respiratory care apply, as detailed elsewhere in this book. Formulation of the respiratory care plan depends on review of the patient's medical history and interview for current symptoms, physical assessment, laboratory testing (including pulmonary function tests), and radiologic evaluation.

Box 40-3 lists the key factors that must be considered when assessing a patient's need for airway clearance therapy.[3,15-17] Physical findings such as a loose, ineffective cough, labored breathing pattern, decreased or bronchial breath sounds, coarse inspiratory and expiratory crackles, tachypnea, tachycardia, or fever may indicate a potential problem with retained secretions. A chest radiograph often shows atelectasis and areas of increased density in such cases.

AIRWAY CLEARANCE METHODS

Five general approaches to airway clearance therapy, which can be used alone or in combination, include (1) CPT; (2) coughing and related expulsion techniques (including manual insufflation-exsufflation [MIE]); (3) positive airway pressure (PAP) adjuncts (**positive expiratory pressure [PEP],** continuous PAP [CPAP], expiratory PAP [EPAP]); (4) high-frequency compression/oscillation methods; and (5) mobilization and physical activity. Appropriate use of these techniques requires an understanding of their underlying principles, relative efficacy, and methods of application.

Chest Physical Therapy

CPT (percussion, postural drainage, and vibration) has long been considered a standard of care in patients with CF and in some other patients with specific pulmonary conditions. Evidence suggests that these therapies benefit mucus transport and assist in the expectoration of secretions.[3,11,21]

Postural drainage involves the use of gravity and mechanical energy to help mobilize secretions. The various body positions assumed are intended to drain secretions from each of the patient's lung segments into the central airways, where they can be removed by cough or suctioning.[1,2,15,29-31] This drainage is accomplished by simply placing the segmental bronchus to be drained in a more vertical position, permitting gravity to assist in the process. Positions generally are held for 3 to 15 minutes (longer in special situations) and modified as the patient's condition and tolerance warrant.[15] Cough methods are used with postural drainage therapy and are discussed separately.

To guide practitioners in applying postural drainage techniques, the American Association for Respiratory Care (AARC) has developed and published a clinical practice guideline on postural drainage. Excerpts from the AARC guideline, including indications, contraindications, hazards and complications, assessment of need, assessment of outcome, and monitoring, appear in Clinical Practice Guideline 40-1.[15]

Postural drainage is most effective in conditions characterized by excessive sputum production (>25 to 30 ml/day). For maximum effect, head-down positions should exceed 25 degrees below horizontal.[1,2,30-33] Positions can be modified if a patient's condition presents a contraindication to treatment.[2] Postural drainage is not likely to succeed unless and until adequate systemic and airway hydration is ensured.[34,35] In patients in critical care, including patients on mechanical ventilation, postural drainage should be performed every 4 to 6 hours as indicated. In spontaneously breathing patients, frequency should be determined by assessing patient response to therapy.

Technique

On the basis of a preliminary assessment of the patient and review of the physician's order, the clinician should identify the appropriate lobes and segments for drainage. Also, on the basis of the preliminary assessment, it should be determined if the positions chosen need to be modified. The clinician may need to modify head-down positions in patients with unstable cardiovascular status, hypertension, cerebrovascular disorders, or dyspnea related to changes in position.

To avoid gastroesophageal reflux and the possibility of aspiration, treatment times should be scheduled before or at least 1½ to 2 hours after meals or tube feedings.[36,37] If the patient assessment indicates that pain may hinder treatment implementation, the clinician also should consider coordinating the treatment regimen with prescribed pain medication.

Before positioning, the procedure (including adjunctive techniques) should be explained to the patient. As necessary, clothing around the waist and neck should be loosened. Also, the clinician should inspect any monitoring leads, intravenous tubing, and oxygen (O_2) therapy equipment connected to the patient and, if necessary, make adjustments to ensure continued function during the procedure. Because postural drainage positioning predisposes patients to arterial desaturation, pulse oximetry should be considered if hypoxemia is suspected.[15] Before starting the procedure, the clinician should measure the patient's vital signs and auscultate the chest. These simple assessments serve as baseline measurements for monitoring the patient's response during the procedure and can assist in determining outcomes.

Figure 40-2 depicts the primary positions used to drain the various lung lobes and segments. Generally, to obtain the proper head-down position, the clinician must lower the head of the bed by at least 16 to 18 inches to achieve the desired 25-degree angle. In the ambulatory care setting, a tilt table can be used in lieu of a hospital bed. A tilt table allows precise positioning at head-down angles up to 45 degrees. When angles this large are used, shoulder supports must be provided to prevent the patient from sliding off the tilt table.

When the patient is in position, the clinician confirms the patient's comfort and ensures proper support of all joints and bony areas with pillows or towels. The indicated position is maintained for a minimum of 3 to 15 minutes if tolerated and longer if good sputum production results.[2] Between positions, pauses for relaxation and breathing control are useful and can help prevent hypoxemia. Because postural drainage therapy can increase O_2 consumption, critically ill patients at risk for hypoxemia should be given supplemental O_2 during the procedure.[32]

During the procedure, the patient is continually observed for any untoward effects or complications (see Clinical Practice Guideline 40-1). Moderate changes in vital signs are expected during treatment; however, as indicated in Table 40-2, significant problems may require immediate intervention.[15]

Also, the clinician should ensure that the patient uses appropriate coughing technique during and after positioning. When using the head-down position, the patient should avoid strenuous coughing because this markedly increases intracranial pressure. Rather, the patient should

40-1 Postural Drainage

AARC Clinical Practice Guideline (Excerpts)*

■ INDICATIONS

- Turning
- Inability or reluctance of patient to change body position
- Poor oxygenation associated with position (e.g., unilateral lung disease)
- Potential for or presence of atelectasis
- Presence of artificial airway
- Evidence or suggestion of difficulty with secretion clearance
- Difficulty clearing secretions, with expectorated sputum production greater than 25 to 30 ml/day (adult)
- Evidence or suggestion of retained secretions in the presence of an artificial airway
- Presence of atelectasis caused by or suspected to be caused by mucous plugging
- Diagnosis of diseases such as CF, bronchiectasis, or cavitating lung disease
- Presence of foreign body in airway
- External manipulation of the thorax: sputum volume or consistency suggesting a need for additional manipulation (e.g., percussion or vibration or both) to assist movement of secretions by gravity in a patient receiving postural drainage

■ CONTRAINDICATIONS

The decision to use postural drainage requires assessment of potential benefits vs potential risks. Therapy should be provided for no longer than necessary to obtain the desired therapeutic results. Listed contraindications are relative unless marked as absolute *(A)*.

Positioning: All positions are contraindicated for:

- Head and neck injury until stabilized *(A)*
- Active hemorrhage with hemodynamic instability *(A)*
- Intracranial pressure (ICP) greater than 20 mm Hg
- Recent spinal surgery or acute spinal injury
- Active hemoptysis
- Empyema
- Bronchopleural fistula
- Pulmonary edema associated with congestive heart failure
- Aged, confused, or anxious patients who do not tolerate position changes
- Pulmonary embolism
- Rib fracture, with or without flail chest
- Surgical wound or healing tissue
- Large pleural effusions

Trendelenburg position contraindicated for:

- Recent gross hemoptysis related to recent lung carcinoma treated surgically or with radiation therapy
- ICP greater than 20 mm Hg
- Uncontrolled hypertension
- Distended abdomen
- Patients in whom increased ICP is to be avoided (e.g., neurosurgery, aneurysms, eye surgery)
- Uncontrolled airway at risk for aspiration (tube feeding or recent meal)
- Esophageal surgery

External manipulation of the thorax (in addition to contraindications previously listed):

- Subcutaneous emphysema
- Recent epidural spinal infusion or spinal anesthesia
- Recently placed transvenous pacemaker or subcutaneous pacemaker
- Lung contusion
- Osteomyelitis of the ribs
- Coagulopathy
- Recent skin grafts, or flaps, on the thorax
- Burns, open wounds, and skin infections of the thorax
- Suspected pulmonary tuberculosis
- Bronchospasm
- Osteoporosis
- Complaint of chest wall pain

40-1 Postural Drainage—cont'd

AARC Clinical Practice Guideline (Excerpts)*

HAZARDS AND COMPLICATIONS

- Hypoxemia
- Increased ICP
- Acute hypotension during procedure
- Pulmonary hemorrhage
- Pain or injury to muscles, ribs, or spine
- Vomiting
- Aspiration
- Bronchospasm
- Arrhythmias

ASSESSMENT OF NEED

The following should be assessed together to establish a need for postural drainage:

- Excessive sputum production
- Effectiveness of cough
- History of problems treated successfully with postural drainage (e.g., bronchiectasis, CF)
- Decreased breath sounds or crackles or rhonchi suggesting secretions in the airway
- Change in vital signs
- Abnormal chest radiograph consistent with atelectasis, mucous plugging, or infiltrates
- Deterioration in arterial blood gas values or O_2 saturation

ASSESSMENT OF OUTCOME

The following items represent individual criteria that indicate a positive response to therapy (and support continuation of therapy). Not all criteria are required to justify continuation of therapy (e.g., a ventilated patient may not have sputum production >30 ml/day but have improvement in breath sounds, chest radiograph, or increased compliance or decreased resistance).

- Change in sputum production
- Change in breath sounds of lung fields being drained
- Patient subjective response to therapy
- Change in vital signs
- Change in chest radiograph
- Change in arterial blood gas values or O_2 saturation
- Change in ventilator variables

MONITORING

The following items should be chosen as appropriate for monitoring a patient's response to postural drainage before, during, and after therapy:

- Subjective response (pain, discomfort, dyspnea, response to therapy)
- Pulse rate, arrhythmia, and electrocardiogram if available
- Breathing pattern and rate, symmetric chest expansion, synchronous thoracoabdominal movement, flail chest
- Sputum production (quantity, color, consistency, odor) and cough effectiveness
- Mental function
- Skin color
- Breath sounds
- Blood pressure
- O_2 saturation by pulse oximetry (if hypoxemia is suspected)
- ICP

**For complete guidelines, see American Association for Respiratory Care: Clinical practice guideline: postural drainage therapy. Respir Care 36:1418, 1991.*

use the forced expiration technique (described later in this chapter). Generally, total treatment time should not exceed 30 to 40 minutes. Both the patient and the clinician should understand that postural drainage does not always result in the immediate production of secretions. More often, secretions are simply mobilized toward the trachea for easier removal by coughing. If the procedure causes vigorous coughing, have the patient sit up until the cough subsides.

After the procedure, the patient is restored to the pretreatment position, and the clinician ensures the patient's stability and comfort. Immediate posttreatment

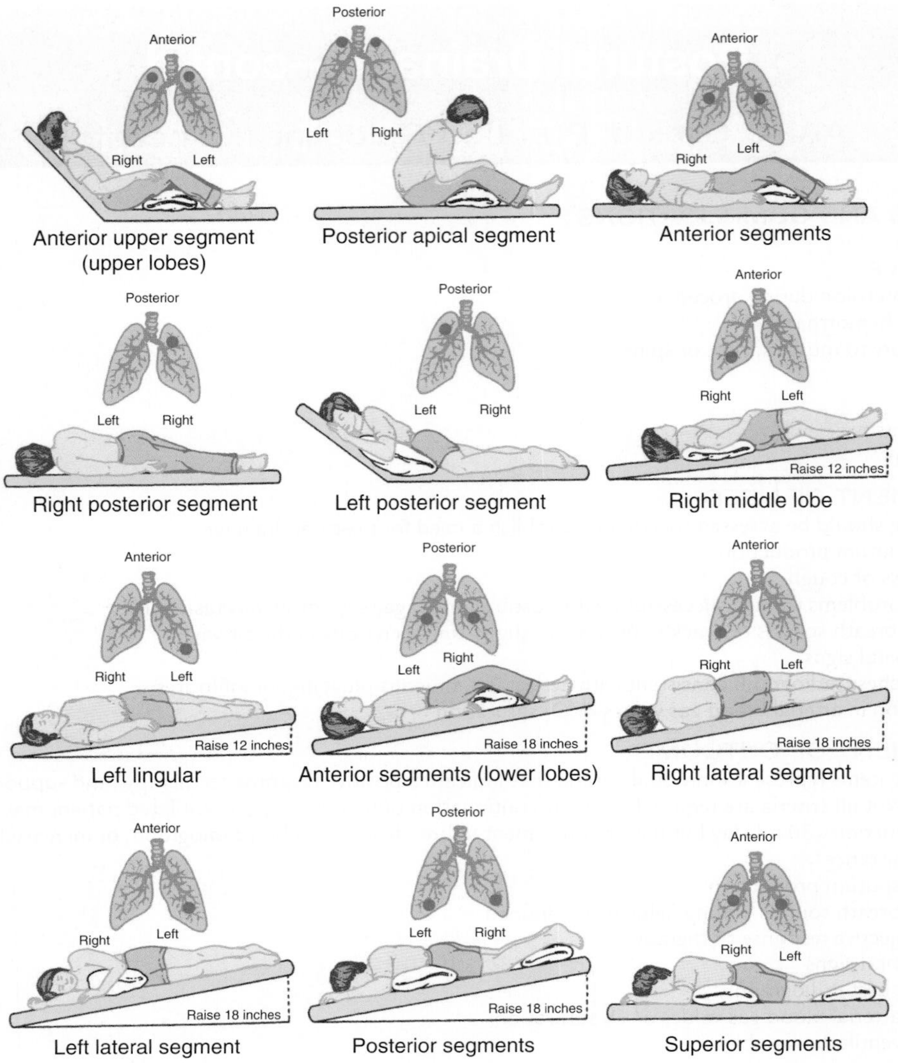

FIGURE 40-2 Patient positions for postural drainage. (Modified from Potter PA, Perry AG: Fundamentals of nursing: concepts, process and practice, ed 4, St Louis, 1997, Mosby.)

MINI CLINI

Postural Drainage, Percussion, and Vibration

PROBLEM: A physician's progress note indicates a potential bacterial pneumonia localized to a patient's right middle lobe. He orders PDPV four times daily "until radiograph clears." What positions should the RT select for postural drainage, and where should the RT provide percussion?

DISCUSSION: The correct position for draining the right middle lobe would be head down (foot of bed raised about 12 inches), with the patient rotated about 45 degrees left from supine (modified left side-lying position). Percussion should be performed on the right anterior chest wall, between the fourth and sixth ribs (see Chapter 15 for external anatomic landmarks).

assessment includes repeat vital signs, confirmation of satisfactory arterial saturation, chest auscultation, and questioning the patient regarding his or her subjective response to the procedure.

RULE OF THUMB

Generally, whenever you observe an untoward patient response during postural drainage, follow the "triple S rule": stop the therapy (return patient to original resting position) and stay with the patient until he or she is stabilized.

Outcome Assessment

Specific outcome criteria indicating a positive response to postural drainage are listed in the AARC clinical practice guideline excerpts that appear in Clinical Practice Guideline 40-1. Generally, achievement of one or more of these

TABLE 40-2

Complications of Postural Drainage Therapy and Recommended Interventions

Complication	Action to Be Taken/Possible Intervention
Hypoxemia	Administer higher FiO_2 during procedure if potential for or observed hypoxemia exists. If patient becomes hypoxemic during treatment, administer 100% O_2, stop therapy immediately, return patient to original position, and consult physician
Increased intracranial pressure	Stop therapy, return patient to original resting position, and consult physician
Acute hypotension during procedure	Stop therapy, return patient to original resting position, and consult physician
Pulmonary hemorrhage	Stop therapy, return patient to original resting position, and call physician immediately. Administer O_2 and maintain an airway until physician responds
Pain or injury to muscles, ribs, or spine	Stop therapy that appears directly associated with pain or problem, exercise care in moving patient, and consult physician
Vomiting and aspiration	Stop therapy, clear airway and suction as needed, administer O_2, maintain airway, return patient to previous resting position, and contact physician immediately
Bronchospasm	Stop therapy, return patient to previous resting position, and administer or increase O_2 delivery while contacting physician. Administer physician-ordered bronchodilators
Arrhythmias	Stop therapy, return patient to previous resting position, and administer or increase O_2 delivery while contacting physician

outcomes indicates that the therapy is meeting its objectives and should be continued. Not all criteria are required to justify continuing postural drainage.

Because secretion clearance is affected by patient hydration, the clinician may need to wait for at least 24 hours after optimal systemic hydration has been achieved to see any evidence of increased sputum production. In the interim, tracheobronchial clearance can be enhanced in some patients by the provision of bland aerosol therapy with an unheated jet nebulizer. Depending on the specific application, other aerosol generators may be deployed to deliver bland aerosol.[34,38]

Breath sounds may seem to "worsen" after therapy. Typically, the clinician may initially note diminished breath sounds and crackles before therapy that change to coarse crackles after treatment. This change is due to the loosening of secretions and their movement into the larger airways, an intended purpose of the therapy. These coarse crackles should clear after coughing or suctioning.

In terms of the patient's subjective response to therapy, the patient should be encouraged to report any pain, discomfort, shortness of breath, dizziness, or nausea during or after therapy. Any of these adverse effects may be grounds for either modifying or stopping treatment. Patient reports of easier clearance or increased volume of secretions after therapy support continuing therapy.

On the basis of assessment results, the postural drainage order should be reevaluated at least every 48 hours for patients in critical care and at least every 3 days for other hospitalized patients. Patients receiving home care should be reevaluated at least every 3 months or whenever their status changes.

Documentation and Follow-Up

The chart entry should include the positions used, time in position, patient tolerance, subjective and objective indicators of treatment effectiveness (including amount, color, and consistency of sputum produced), and any untoward effects observed. Because the effects of the procedure may not be immediately evident, the clinician should follow up with the patient, if possible, to determine any desired or adverse effects.

Percussion and Vibration

Percussion and vibration involve application of mechanical energy to the chest wall by the use of either hands or various electrical or pneumatic devices. Both methods are designed to augment secretion clearance.[3] In theory, percussion should help loosen secretions from the tracheobronchial tree, making them easier to remove by coughing or suctioning. Vibration should aid movement of secretions toward the central airways during exhalation.

The effectiveness of percussion and vibration as an adjunct to postural drainage is controversial. This controversy is partly due to the fact that there is no consensus regarding what represents the "right" force or frequency for either technique.[1,5] In addition, because percussion and vibration are often only a part of the treatment regimen in most clinical studies, it is hard to draw conclusions about the effect of these methods alone.[3] Both the types of patients studied and the outcome measures used often differ across studies. In studies that focus on patients who produce copious secretions, percussion generally is found to be effective in increasing sputum production.[39] When the outcome measure is not the volume of secretions produced, results are less positive.[3,5]

For these reasons, and in light of current knowledge, the routine use of these methods cannot be justified. However, because percussion and vibration may increase the volume of sputum production in some patients, the addition of these techniques to postural drainage may be appropriate in selected cases, especially if postural drainage alone fails to mobilize secretions.[15]

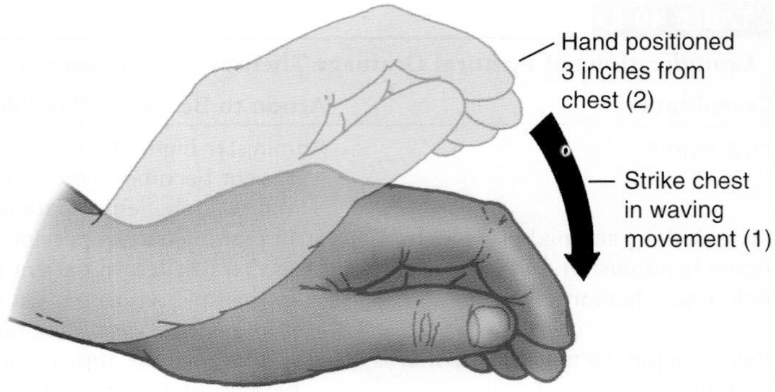

FIGURE 40-3 Movement of cupped hand at wrist, to percuss chest.

Manual Percussion and Vibration. The clinician performs manual percussion with his or her hands in a cupped position, with fingers and thumb closed (Figure 40-3). This position traps a cushion of air between the hand and chest wall.[2] The striking force may be against the bare skin, although a thin layer of cloth, such as a hospital gown or bed sheet, does not significantly impair transmission of the energy wave and is more comfortable for the patient.

The clinician rhythmically strikes the chest wall in a waving motion, using both hands alternately in sequence with the elbows partially flexed and wrists loose (see Figure 40-3). Slower, more relaxing rates are better tolerated by the patient and the clinician. It is not a difficult technique to master, but practice is needed to determine the appropriate force and to maintain a rhythmic pattern.

Ideally, the clinician should percuss back and forth in a circular pattern over the localized area for 3 to 5 minutes. Care should be taken to avoid tender areas or sites of trauma or surgery, and one should never percuss directly over bony prominences, such as the clavicles or vertebrae. Hands should be positioned parallel to the ribs.

Vibration sometimes is used together with percussion but is limited to application during exhalation. It may also be used as an alternative to percussion in acutely ill patients with chest wall discomfort or injury. To vibrate the chest wall, the clinician lays one hand on the patient's chest over the involved area and places the other hand on top of the first (Figure 40-4). Alternatively, the clinician places the hands on either side of the chest. After the patient takes a deep breath, the clinician exerts slight to moderate pressure on the chest wall and initiates a rapid vibratory motion of the hands throughout expiration.

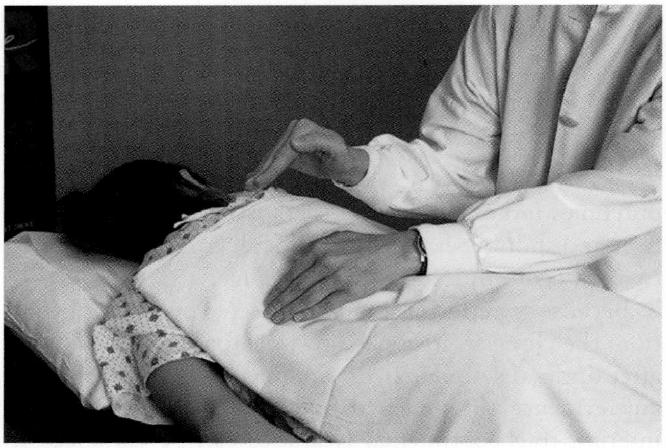

FIGURE 40-4 Hand placement for chest vibration. (From Harkreader H, Hogan M, Thobaben M: Fundamentals of nursing, caring and clinical judgment, ed 3, St Louis, 2007, Saunders.)

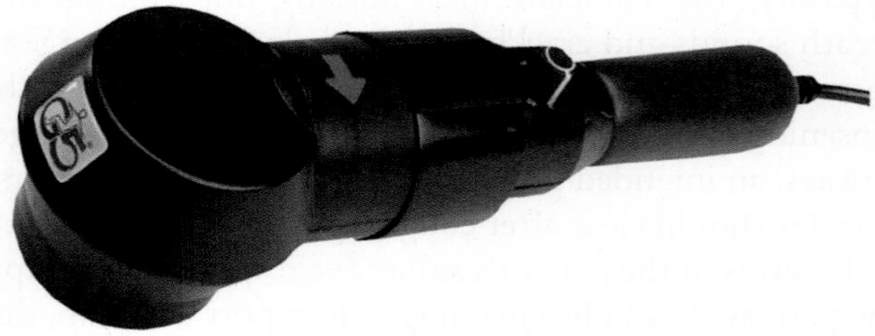

FIGURE 40-5 Example of an electrically powered mechanical percussor/vibrator. (Courtesy General Physiotherapy, Inc. St Louis, MO.)

Mechanical Percussion and Vibration. Various electrical and pneumatic devices have been developed to generate and apply the energy waves used during percussion and vibration. Typically, these devices have both a frequency and a percussion force control (Figure 40-5). Most units provide frequencies up to 20 to 30 cycles per second, or 20 to 30 Hz. Noise, excess force, and mechanical failure all are potential problems. Electrical devices also pose a potential shock hazard.

These devices have the advantage of reducing fatigue on the caregiver and can deliver consistent rates, rhythms, and impact forces.[1,2] However, there is no firm evidence that such devices are more effective than manual techniques. For this reason, the selection of manual or mechanical methods should be left to the patient in consultation with the care provider.[40]

Coughing and Related Expulsion Techniques

Most airway clearance therapies help only to move secretions into the central airways. Clearance of these secretions requires either coughing or suctioning. In this respect, an effective cough (or alternative expulsion measure) is an essential component of all airway clearance therapy. These expulsion methods are also useful in obtaining sputum specimens for diagnostic analysis.

RULE OF THUMB

Without an effective cough, most airway clearance techniques cannot succeed in fully clearing secretions. Clinicians must ensure an effective cough regimen in patients.[41]

Directed Cough

Directed cough is a deliberate maneuver that is taught, supervised, and monitored. It aims to mimic the features of an effective spontaneous cough in patients who are too weak to produce a forceful expiratory maneuver.

Although cough may stimulate mucociliary activity, it has little direct effect on secretion clearance in individuals who do not produce sputum.[40,41] In patients with copious secretions, directed coughing is as good at clearance as more complicated methods.[7,42-45] However, coughing is most effective in clearing secretions from the central, and not peripheral, airways.[46] To help practitioners apply this important technique, the AARC has developed and published a clinical practice guideline on directed cough. Excerpts from the AARC guideline, including indications, contraindications, hazards and complications, assessment of need, assessment of outcome, and monitoring, appear in Clinical Practice Guideline 40-2.[16]

Standard Technique. After the clinical need for directed coughing has been established, the respiratory therapist (RT) should assess the patient for any factors that could limit the success of directed cough. An effective directed cough regimen is generally impossible with obtunded, paralyzed, or uncooperative patients. In addition, some patients with advanced COPD or severe restrictive disorders (including neurologic, muscular, or skeletal abnormalities) may be unable to generate an effective spontaneous cough. Likewise, pain or fear of pain caused by coughing may limit the success of directed cough. Lastly, systemic dehydration; thick, tenacious secretions; artificial airways; or the use of central nervous system depressants can thwart efforts to implement an effective directed cough regimen. If any of these limitations exist, it is the responsibility of the RT to recommend alternative means to help expel secretions. Alternative secretion clearance strategies are discussed later.

Good patient teaching is crucial in developing an effective directed cough regimen. The three most important aspects involved in patient teaching are (1) instruction in proper positioning, (2) instruction in breathing control, and (3) exercises to strengthen the expiratory muscles.[7] These activities are modified according to the patient's underlying clinical problem.

40-2 Directed Cough

AARC Clinical Practice Guideline (Excerpts)*

INDICATIONS

- Need to aid in the removal of retained secretions from central airways
- Presence of atelectasis
- As prophylaxis against postoperative pulmonary complications
- As a routine part of bronchial hygiene in patients with CF, bronchiectasis, chronic bronchitis, necrotizing pulmonary infection, spinal cord injury
- As an integral part of other bronchial hygiene therapies, such as postural drainage therapy, PEP therapy, and incentive spirometry
- To obtain sputum specimens for diagnostic analysis

CONTRAINDICATIONS

Directed cough is rarely contraindicated. The contraindications listed must be weighed against potential benefit in deciding to eliminate cough from the care of the patient. Listed contraindications are relative:

- Inability to control possible transmission of infection from patients suspected or known to have pathogens transmittable by droplet nuclei (e.g., *Mycobacterium tuberculosis*)
- Presence of elevated ICP or known intracranial aneurysm
- Presence of reduced coronary artery perfusion, such as in acute myocardial infarction
- Acute unstable head, neck, or spine injury
- Manually assisted directed cough with pressure to the epigastrium may be contraindicated in the presence of increased potential for regurgitation or aspiration, acute abdominal pathology, abdominal aortic aneurysm, hiatal hernia, pregnancy, bleeding diathesis, or untreated pneumothorax
- Manually assisted directed cough with pressure to the thoracic cage may be contraindicated in the presence of osteoporosis or flail chest

Continued

40-2 Directed Cough—cont'd

AARC Clinical Practice Guideline (Excerpts)*

HAZARDS AND COMPLICATIONS
- Reduced coronary artery perfusion
- Reduced cerebral perfusion
- Incontinence
- Fatigue
- Rib or costochondral fracture
- Headache
- Visual disturbances, including retinal hemorrhage
- Bronchospasm
- Muscular damage or discomfort
- Incisional pain, evisceration
- Anorexia, vomiting
- Gastroesophageal reflux
- Spontaneous pneumothorax
- Pneumomediastinum
- Subcutaneous emphysema
- Cough paroxysms
- Chest pain
- Central line displacement
- Paresthesia

ASSESSMENT OF NEED
- Patients with spontaneous cough that fails to clear secretions from the airway
- Patients with ineffective spontaneous cough as judged by clinical observation, evidence of atelectasis, or results of pulmonary function testing
- Postoperative upper abdominal or thoracic surgery patients
- Long-term care of patients with tendency to retain airway secretions
- Patients with presence of endotracheal or tracheostomy tube

ASSESSMENT OF OUTCOME
- Presence of sputum specimen after a cough
- Clinical observation of improvement
- Patient's subjective response to therapy
- Stabilization of pulmonary hygiene in patients with COPD and history of secretion retention

MONITORING
The following items should be chosen as appropriate for monitoring a patient's response to cough technique:
- Patient response: pain, discomfort, dyspnea
- Sputum expectorated after cough: color, consistency, odor, volume
- Breath sounds
- Adverse neurologic signs or symptoms after cough
- Cardiac dysrhythmias
- Alterations in hemodynamics after coughing
- Measures of pulmonary mechanics, when indicated, may include vital capacity, peak inspiratory pressure, peak expiratory pressure, positive expiratory flow, and airway resistance

For complete guidelines, see American Association for Respiratory Care: Clinical practice guideline: directed cough. Respir Care 38:495, 1993.

First, patients are taught to assume a position that aids exhalation and allows easy thoracic compression. Because of abdominal muscle tension, it is difficult to generate an effective cough in the supine position. Rather, the patient should assume a sitting position with one shoulder rotated inward and the head and spine slightly flexed. The patient's feet should be supported to provide abdominal and thoracic support for the patient. If the patient is unable to sit up, the clinician should raise the head of the bed and ensure that the patient's knees are slightly flexed with the feet braced on the mattress.

Breathing control measures help ensure that the inspiration, compression, and expulsion phases of the cough are maximally effective and coordinated. For effective inspiration, the patient should be taught to inspire slowly and deeply through the nose, using the diaphragmatic method (discussed subsequently). In patients with copious amounts of sputum, such breaths alone may stimulate coughing by loosening secretions in the larger airways.

After confirming that the patient can take a good, deep inspiration, the clinician has the patient bear down against the glottis, in much the same manner as would occur with straining during a bowel movement. For patients with pain or patients subject to bronchiolar collapse, it is probably best that they be shown how to "stage" their expiratory effort into two or three short bursts. For these patients, this method is generally less fatiguing and more effective in producing sputum than a single violent expulsion. Effective breathing control is best taught via demonstration. The clinician demonstrates the various phases of the cough sequence while emphasizing the correct technique. The clinician explains how to avoid common errors, such as simple throat clearing.

Proper positioning and breathing control alone may not ensure an effective cough. This limitation often is due to weak breathing muscles. Muscle weakness is common in patients with neuromuscular disease, patients with COPD, and patients needing long-term ventilatory support. These muscles may atrophy from lack of use. In these cases, either suctioning or **mechanical insufflation-exsufflation (MIE)** may be required.

Modifications in Technique. Modifying the normal directed cough routine according to the needs of the individual patient may overcome any limitations. Good clinical examples of the need to modify directed cough are seen in surgical patients, patients with COPD, and patients with neuromuscular disorders.

In surgical patients, preoperative training in breathing control can help prepare the patient for the postoperative regimen. This preparation can minimize the anxiety related to pain that commonly impairs an effective cough in these patients. In addition, the postoperative regimen can be enhanced by coordinating the coughing sessions with prescribed pain medication and assisting the patient in **splinting** the operative site. The clinician can use his or her hands to support the area of incision during the expiratory phase of the cough. Eventually, the patient can learn to use a pillow or blanket roll to splint the incision site. The **forced expiratory technique (FET)** (discussed subsequently) may also be valuable in these patients.

In some patients with COPD, the high pleural pressures during a forced cough may compress the smaller airways and limit the cough's effectiveness. In this situation, the patient is placed in the sitting position previously described. The patient is instructed to take in a moderately deep breath slowly through the nose.

To help enhance expulsion, the patient should exhale with moderate force through pursed lips, while bending forward. This forward flexion of the thorax enhances expiratory flow by upward displacement of the abdominal contents. After three or four repetitions of this maneuver, the patient is encouraged to bend forward and initiate short staccato-like bursts of air. This technique relieves the strain of a prolonged hard cough, and the staccato rhythm at a relatively low velocity minimizes airway collapse. This technique has a modification called *huffing*, whereby the patient is instructed to make the sound of "huff, huff, huff" rapidly with the mouth open.[3] Alternatively, either FET or autogenic drainage (AD) may be used in these patients. Both of these clearance mechanisms are discussed later.

Patients with neuromuscular conditions present a special challenge in cough management. These patients typically are unable to generate the forceful expulsion needed to move secretions toward the trachea.[24] If this problem results in retained secretions, there are only three options: (1) placement of an artificial airway and removal of secretions by tracheobronchial suctioning (see Chapter 33), (2) manually assisted cough, and (3) MIE.

Manually assisted cough is external application of pressure to the thoracic cage or epigastric region, coordinated with forced exhalation.[16,22] In this technique, the patient takes as deep an inspiration as possible, assisted as needed by the application of positive pressure via a self-inflating bag or intermittent positive pressure breathing device. At the end of the patient's inspiration, the clinician begins exerting pressure on the lateral costal margins or epigastrium. This pressure increases the force of compression throughout expiration; this mimics the normal cough mechanism by generating an increase in the velocity of the expired air and may be helpful in moving secretions toward the trachea, where they can be removed by suctioning. Manually assisted cough with pressure to the lateral costal margins is contraindicated in patients with osteoporosis or flail chest.[16] Manually assisted cough using epigastric pressure is contraindicated in unconscious patients with unprotected airways, in pregnant women, and in patients with acute abdominal pathology, abdominal aortic aneurysm, or hiatal hernia.[16]

Forced Expiratory Technique

FET is a modification of the normal directed cough. FET, or **huff cough,** consists of one or two forced expirations of middle to low lung volume without closure of the glottis, followed by a period of diaphragmatic breathing and relaxation.[46,47] The goal of this method is to help clear secretions with less change in pleural pressure and less likelihood of bronchiolar collapse. To help keep the glottis open during FET, the patient is taught to phonate or "huff" during expiration. The period of diaphragmatic breathing and relaxation following the forced expiration is essential in restoring lung volume and minimizing fatigue.

Comparative clinical studies on the effectiveness of FET have shown favorable results. Generally, FET results in increased sputum production, especially when combined with postural drainage.[7,48] The technique is particularly useful in patients prone to airway collapse during normal coughing, such as patients with COPD, CF, or bronchiectasis. However, FET requires that patients generate high expiratory airflow, which may not be attainable in intubated patients with respiratory failure.

Active Cycle of Breathing Technique

To emphasize that FET always should include breathing exercises, the originators of this technique modified the procedure and renamed it the **active cycle of breathing technique (ACBT).**[2,20] ACBT consists of repeated cycles of breathing control, thoracic expansion, and FET (Box 40-4). *Breathing control* involves gentle diaphragmatic breathing at normal tidal volumes for 5 to 10 seconds with relaxation of the upper chest and shoulders. This phase is intended to help prevent bronchospasm. The thoracic expansion exercises involve deep inhalation, approaching vital capacity, with relaxed exhalation, which may be accompanied by percussion, vibration, or compression. The *thoracic expansion* phase is designed to help loosen secretions, improve the distribution of ventilation, and provide the volume needed for FET. The subsequent FET moves secretions into the central airways. Postoperative patients may require splinting at the thoracic or abdominal incision site. Patients with extreme airway sensitivity are susceptible to airway irritation during ACBT.

Although ACBT can be performed in the sitting position, it is most beneficial when combined with postural drainage. As an added benefit, ACBT seems to minimize or prevent the O_2 desaturation so common during postural drainage, at least in patients with CF.[49] When ACBT is compared with similar methods of secretion clearance, studies indicate that ACBT can provide comparable results in terms of both sputum production and distribution of ventilation.[5,6,20,50,51] ACBT is not useful with young children (<2 years old) or critically ill patients.

Box 40-4 Active Cycle of Breathing Technique Sequence

1. Relaxation and breathing control
2. Three or four thoracic expansion exercises
3. Relaxation and breathing control
4. Repeat three to four thoracic expansion exercises
5. Repeat relaxation and breathing control
6. Perform one or two FETs (huffs)
7. Repeat relaxation and breathing control

Autogenic Drainage

Autogenic drainage (AD) is another modification of directed coughing, designed as an airway clearance mechanism that can be performed independently by trained patients.[3,20] During AD, the patient uses diaphragmatic breathing to mobilize secretions by varying lung volumes and expiratory airflow in three distinct phases (Figure 40-6).[20] For maximum benefit, the patient should be in the sitting position. Patients are taught to control their expiratory flows to prevent airway collapse while trying to achieve a mucous "rattle" rather than a wheeze. Coughing should be suppressed until all three breathing phases are completed.

In patients with CF, AD provides sputum clearance comparable to PDPV but is less likely to produce O_2 desaturation. In addition, AD seems to be tolerated better by patients and has the advantage of being performed without assistance and in one position.[3,7,52-55]

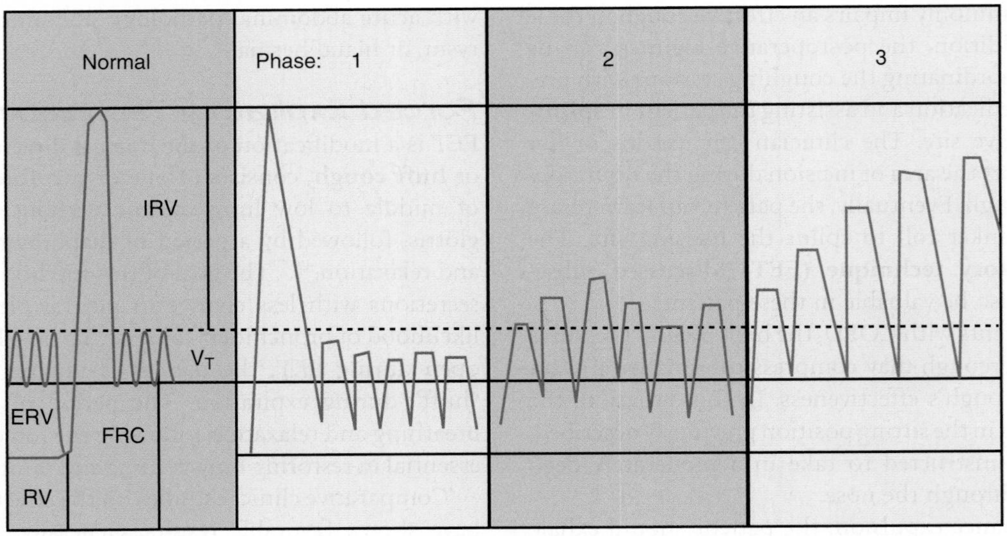

FIGURE 40-6 Spirogram of lung volumes during three phases of autogenic drainage. Phase 1 involves a full inspiratory capacity maneuver, followed by breathing at low lung volumes. This phase is designed to "unstick" peripheral mucus. Phase 2 involves breathing at low to middle lung volumes in order to collect mucus in the middle airways. Phase 3 is the evacuation phase, in which mucus is readied for expulsion from the large airways. (Modified from Hardy KA, Anderson BD: Respir Care Clin North Am 2:323, 1996.)

Mechanical Insufflation-Exsufflation

In the early 1950s, "artificial cough machines," or MIE devices, were used to help patients with polio clear secretions. Use of these machines continued until the mid-1960s, when artificial tracheal airways and suctioning became the method of choice for secretion clearance in patients unable to cough.

The use of MIE devices (also called *cough-assist device* or "coughlator") has experienced a resurgence more recently, especially in patients with certain neuromuscular disorders (Figure 40-7).[3,24] The reason is growing evidence that MIE helps prevent respiratory complications in patients with neuromuscular disorders by helping them generate sufficient expiratory flow rates needed for effective secretion clearance.[56-61]

The MIE device delivers a positive pressure breath of 30 to 50 cm H_2O over a 1- to 3-second period via a face mask or tracheal airway. The airway pressure is abruptly reversed to −30 to −50 cm H_2O and maintained for 2 to 3 seconds. Peak expiratory "cough" flows obtained with this device are in the normal range (mean 7.5 L/sec), far better than can be achieved with manually assisted coughing. Expiratory flows remain high in the immediate postexsufflation period, indicating that MIE does not promote airway collapse.

A typical treatment session consists of about five cycles of MIE followed by a period of normal spontaneous or assisted breathing (to avoid hyperventilation). This process is repeated five or more times until secretions are cleared and the vital capacity and SpO_2 return to baseline. Treatments may be required every 10 minutes during acute respiratory tract infections. Prior treatment with bland aerosol can aid clearance when secretions are inspissated. Patients tend to prefer MIE to suctioning because airway clearance occurs without the discomfort and trauma of tracheal aspiration.

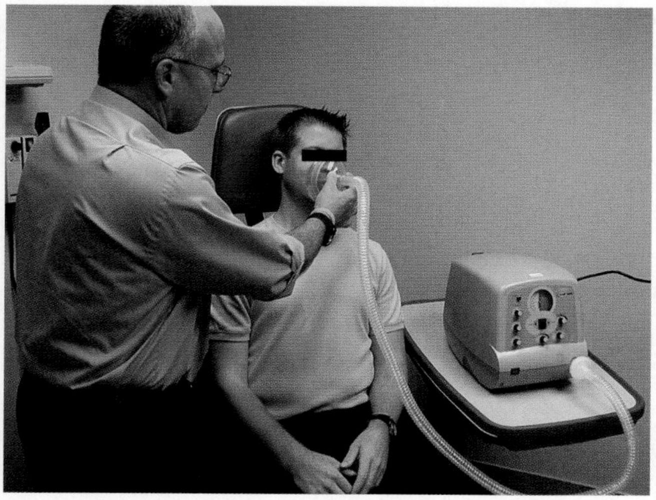

FIGURE 40-7 MIE devices. (From Mason R, Broaddus V, Martin T et al: Murray & Nadel's textbook of respiratory medicine, ed 10, Philadelphia, 2010, Saunders.)

MIE via an oronasal interface is effective, provided that there is no fixed airway obstruction or glottic collapse during exsufflation. For patients with severe restrictive disease who have not been taking deep breaths, insufflation pressures should be increased gradually to avoid chest wall muscle strains. Abdominal distention is infrequent and reduced by decreasing insufflation, not exsufflation, pressures. The effectiveness of MIE in persons with airway obstruction caused by disorders such as COPD is less clear, and MIE may be detrimental.[3,55]

Precautions should be observed using MIE with patients with known cardiac instability in whom it would be advisable to monitor heart rate and O_2 saturation very closely. MIE is contraindicated in patients with a history of bullous emphysema, known susceptibility to pneumothorax or pneumomediastinum, or recent barotraumas.

Positive Airway Pressure Adjuncts

PAP adjuncts are used to help mobilize secretions and treat atelectasis. As adjuncts for airway clearance, these methods are never used alone; they are always combined with directed cough or other airway clearance techniques.[17] One of three different approaches can be used: (1) CPAP, (2) EPAP, and (3) PEP.

The AARC has developed and published a clinical practice guideline on the use of PAP adjuncts with airway clearance therapy to guide practitioners in applying these techniques. Excerpts from the AARC guideline, including indications, contraindications, hazards and complications, assessment of need, assessment of outcome, and monitoring, appear in Clinical Practice Guideline 40-3.[17] Use of these methods to treat atelectasis is reviewed in Chapter 39. The following discussion focuses on the use of PEP therapy as an adjunct in secretion clearance.

PEP therapy involves active expiration against a variable flow resistance. In theory, PEP helps move secretions into the larger airways by (1) filling underaerated or nonaerated segments via collateral ventilation and (2) preventing airway collapse during expiration. A subsequent huff or FET maneuver allows the patient to generate the flows needed to expel mucus from blocked airways.

Most clinical studies of PEP therapy involved patients with CF, although its use in COPD and in preventing postoperative atelectasis has also been investigated.[3,62] Generally, compared with other airway clearance methods (PDPV, AD, ACBT) in patients with CF, PEP therapy provides comparable mucociliary clearance, with the added advantages of being potentially self-administered and cost-effective.[3,63-66] Patients generally prefer PEP over other methods. However, PEP therapy does not appear to be as useful in enhancing lung clearance in chronic bronchitis.[67] In regard to the prevention of postoperative atelectasis, studies provide conflicting results.[61-63] In addition, PEP therapy cannot be used in young children (<3 years old).

40-3 Use of Positive Airway Pressure Adjuncts to Bronchial Hygiene Therapy

AARC Clinical Practice Guideline (Excerpts)*

INDICATIONS
- To reduce air trapping in asthma and COPD
- To aid in mobilization of retained secretions (in CF and chronic bronchitis)
- To prevent or reverse atelectasis
- To optimize delivery of bronchodilators in patients receiving bronchial hygiene therapy

CONTRAINDICATIONS
Although no absolute contraindications to the use of PEP, CPAP, or EPAP mask therapy have been reported, the following should be carefully evaluated before initiating therapy:
- Patients unable to tolerate increased work of breathing (acute asthma, COPD)
- Intracranial pressure (ICP) greater than 20 mm Hg
- Hemodynamic instability
- Acute sinusitis
- Active hemoptysis
- Untreated pneumothorax
- Known or suspected tympanic membrane rupture or other middle ear pathology
- Recent facial, oral, or skull surgery or trauma
- Epistaxis
- Esophageal surgery
- Nausea

HAZARDS AND COMPLICATIONS
- Pulmonary barotraumas
- Increased ICP
- Cardiovascular compromise (myocardial ischemia, decreased venous return)
- Skin breakdown and discomfort from mask
- Air swallowing, vomiting, and aspiration
- Claustrophobia
- Increased work of breathing that may lead to hypoventilation and hypercapnia

ASSESSMENT OF NEED
The following items should be assessed together to establish a need for PAP therapy:
- Sputum retention not responsive to spontaneous or directed coughing
- History of pulmonary problems treated successfully with postural drainage therapy
- Decreased breath sounds or adventitious sounds suggesting secretions in the airway
- Change in vital signs (increase in breathing frequency, tachycardia)
- Abnormal chest radiograph consistent with atelectasis, mucous plugging, or infiltrates
- Deterioration in arterial blood gas (ABG) values or O_2 saturation

ASSESSMENT OF OUTCOME
- Change in sputum production
- Change in vital signs
- Change in breath sounds
- Change in chest radiograph
- Patient subjective response to therapy
- Change in ABG values or O_2 saturation

MONITORING
The following items should be chosen as appropriate for a specific patient's response:
- Patient subjective response: pain, discomfort, dyspnea
- Pulse rate and cardiac rhythm (if electrocardiogram is available)
- Mental function
- Breath sounds
- Pulse oximetry or ABG analysis (if indicated)
- Breathing pattern and rate, symmetric costal expansion, synchronous abdominal movement
- Sputum production
- Skin color
- Blood pressure
- ICP (if indicated)

**For complete guidelines, see American Association for Respiratory Care: Clinical practice guideline: use of PAP adjuncts to bronchial hygiene therapy, Respir Care 38:516, 1993.*

The clinical procedure for PAP therapy is presented in Box 40-5.[67] Equipment can be easily assembled from available parts in most respiratory care departments. Single-use commercial devices are available for purchase (Figure 40-8). Regardless of the equipment used, it is essential to monitor actual airway pressures (as opposed to set or intended pressures).[68]

Common strategies for PEP therapy vary from three to four times daily, with frequency determined by assessment of patient response. During acute exacerbations, therapy

Box 40-5 Clinical Procedure for Positive Airway Pressure Therapy

1. Assess need for PAP therapy and design a treatment program to accomplish treatment objectives.
   a. Bring equipment to bedside and provide initial therapy to patient, adjusting pressure settings to meet patient need.
   b. After initial patient treatment or training, communicate treatment plan to physician and nurse, and provide instruction to nursing staff if required.
2. Explain purpose of PAP therapy to patient; teach patient "huff" (directed cough procedure).
3. Instruct patient to:
   a. Sit comfortably.
   b. If using a mask, apply it tightly but comfortably over the nose and mouth. If mouthpiece is used, place lips firmly around it and breathe through mouth.
   c. Take in a breath that is larger than normal, but do not completely fill lungs.
   d. Exhale actively, but not forcefully, creating a PAP of 10 to 20 cm H_2O during exhalation (determined with manometer during initial therapy sessions). Length of inhalation should be approximately one-third of the total breathing cycle (inspiratory-to-expiratory ratio of 1:3 to 1:4).
   e. Perform 10 to 20 breaths.
   f. Remove the mask or mouthpiece, and perform two or three "huff" coughs; rest as needed.
   g. Repeat above cycle four to eight times, not to exceed 20 minutes.
4. Evaluate patient for the ability to self-administer.
5. When appropriate, teach patient to self-administer. Observations on several occasions of proper technique, uncoached, should precede allowing the patient to self-administer without supervision.
6. When patients are also receiving bronchodilator aerosol, administer in conjunction with PAP therapy by placing a nebulizer in line with the PAP device.
7. When PAP device is visibly soiled, rinse it with sterile water and shake or air dry; leave within reach at patient's bedside in a clear plastic bag.
8. Send the PAP device (if single-patient use) home with the patient, or discard it on discharge. If device is nondisposable, send in-house for high-level disinfection.
9. Document in the patient's medical record procedures performed (including device, settings used, pressure developed, number of breaths per treatment, and frequency); patient response to therapy; patient teaching provided; and patient ability to self-administer.

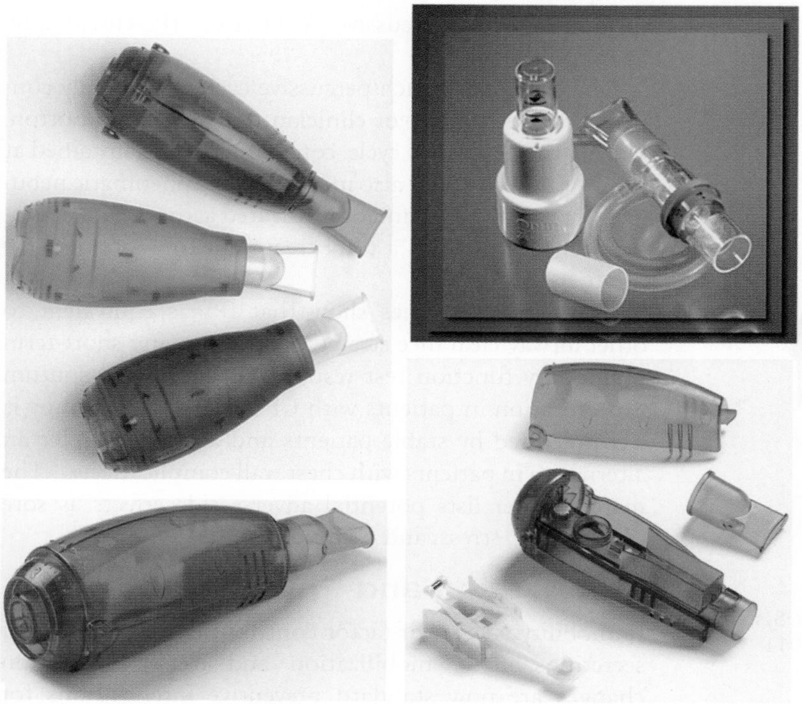

FIGURE 40-8 Positive expiratory devices: TheraPEP and Acapella. (From Frownfelter D, Dean E: Cardiovascular and pulmonary physical therapy, evidence and practice, ed 4, St Louis, 2007, Mosby.)

should be performed at decreasing intervals rather than extending the length of the therapy sessions. Aerosol drug therapy may be added to a PEP session using either an in-line hand-held nebulizer or a metered dose inhaler attached to the one-way valve inlet of the system (see Figure 40-8).[67] The combination of aerosol drug therapy with PEP seems to improve the efficacy of bronchodilator administration, probably because of better distribution to the peripheral airways.[62,67]

High-Frequency Compression/ Oscillation

As applied to airway clearance, **oscillation** refers to the rapid vibratory movement of small volumes of air back and forth in the respiratory tract. At high frequencies (12 to 25 Hz), these oscillations act as a physical "mucolytic," enhancing cough clearance of secretions.[69] There are two general approaches to oscillation: external (chest wall) application and airway application. External application is often called **high-frequency chest wall compression (HFCWC).** Airway application of oscillation methods includes (1) the flutter valve and (2) **intrapulmonary percussive ventilation (IPV).**

High-Frequency Chest Wall Oscillation

High-frequency chest wall oscillation is accomplished by using a two-part system: (1) a variable air-pulse generator and (2) a nonstretch inflatable vest that covers the patient's entire torso (Vest Airway Clearance System [Figure 40-9]).[2,70] Small gas volumes are alternately injected into and withdrawn from the vest by the air-pulse generator at a fast rate, creating an oscillatory motion against the patient's thorax. Typically, RTs perform 30-minute therapy sessions at oscillatory frequencies between 5 **Hertz (Hz)** and 25 Hz. Depending on need and response, one to six therapy sessions may occur per day.

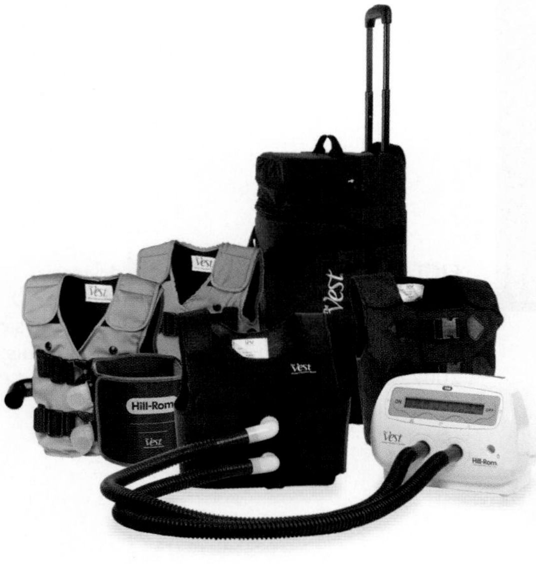

FIGURE 40-9 Patient using the Vest Airway Clearance System for high frequency chest wall oscillation. (Copyright 2011 Hill-Rom Services, Inc., Batesville, IN, Reprinted with permission. All rights reserved.)

Compression frequency and flow bias (inspiratory vs. expiratory) determine the effectiveness of therapy. Additionally, the oscillation frequency used affects both patient comfort and efficacy.[71-73] The current recommendation is to identify individually the frequency that produces optimal results and patient comfort.

Clinical studies of high-frequency chest wall oscillation and HFCWC have shown mixed results. Several studies concluded that when used in patients with CF, the two techniques are equivalent to other airway clearance techniques as measured by improved spirometry or sputum production.[3,70,71] Studies in other populations have shown some improvement, as measured by patient perception, increased compliance, or outcome.[70,73,74]

An alternative device to the vest, the Hayak oscillator (United Hayek Industries, Inc, San Diego, CA), uses a chest shield (turtle shell) strapped to the anterior chest wall. The shell is connected by a large hose to a negative/positive pressure generator that can provide oscillations at frequencies up to 15 Hz. This device is primarily considered a form of providing negative pressure ventilation, and research evaluating its effectiveness as an airway device is limited.[75]

Intrapulmonary Percussive Ventilation

IPV is an airway clearance technique that uses a pneumatic device to deliver a series of pressurized gas minibursts at rates of 100 to 225 cycles per minute (1.6 to 3.75 Hz) to the respiratory tract, usually via a mouthpiece (Figure 40-10). The device was approved by the U.S. Food and Drug Administration (FDA) in 1993 and is marketed as the Intrapulmonary Percussive Ventilator (Percussionaire, Sandpoint, Idaho).

The duration of each percussive cycle is manually controlled by the patient or clinician using a thumb button. During the percussive cycle, constant PAP is maintained at the airway. The device also incorporates a pneumatic nebulizer for delivery of bland or medicated aerosol. The manufacturer recommends a total treatment time of about 20 minutes.

Comparative studies show that IPV is equivalent to other airway clearance strategies in improving short-term pulmonary function test results and enhancing sputum expectoration in patients with CF.[3,33,70,71,76] The therapy is well tolerated by stable patients and appears to offer an alternative in patients with chest wall complications.[77] The manufacturer lists potential adverse side effects as sore ribs, fatigue, stress, and irritation.[71]

Mobilization and Physical Activity

Immobility is a major factor contributing to retention of secretions. Early mobilization and frequent position changes are now standard preventive interventions for

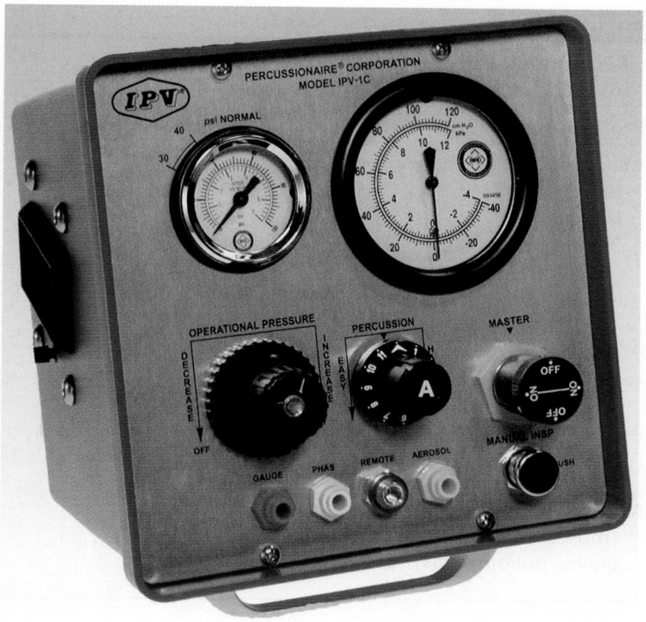

FIGURE 40-10 Intrapulmonary Percussive Ventilator (IPV). (Courtesy Percussionaire, SandPoint, Idaho.)

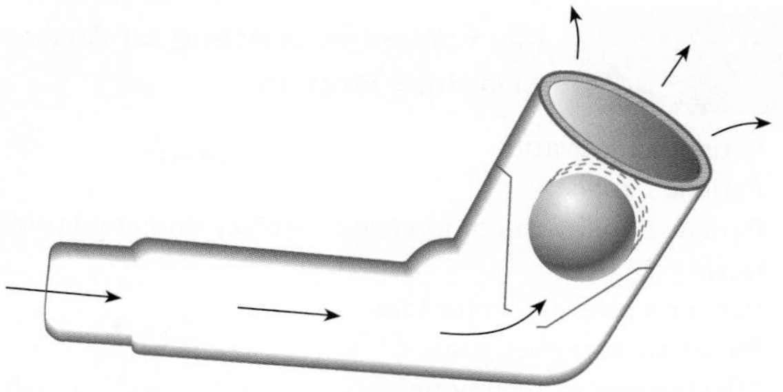

FIGURE 40-11 Cross section of a flutter valve. Exhalation through the device provides both positive expiratory pressure (PEP) and high-frequency oscillations.

atelectasis and pneumonia in postoperative patients.[28,78-80] Adding systematic physical activity to mobilization and coughing can enhance mucus clearance further.[4,44,53]

Frequent movement and physical activity also improve overall aeration and $\dot{V}/\dot{Q}$ matching.[12,79] In addition, frequent movement and daily physical activity can improve patients' general fitness, functional capacity, self-esteem, and quality of life within the limitations of their pulmonary disease or deficit.[28]

Frequent movement and physical activity can be fatiguing and result in O_2 desaturation among patients with significant pulmonary impairment.[12] For these reasons, it is probably wise to conduct an exercise evaluation on an ambulatory patient with severe lung disease being considered for exercise therapy (see Chapter 50). In addition, young children and patients with neuromuscular limitations may not be good candidates for airway clearance via exercise but should be evaluated for other forms of physical activity.

Airway Oscillating Devices

Airway oscillating devices produce PEP with oscillations in the airway during expiration. These devices are believed to work based on the principle of collateral ventilation, which suggests that airflow can occur between adjacent lung segments through the canals of Lambert and through the pores of Kohn. PEP studies have shown it to be as effective as other forms of airway clearance.[81,82] Patients appear to prefer techniques such as PEP that promote independence; this is important because it has been shown that compliance to airway clearance techniques and exercise is often poor.[83]

A popular approach to PEP therapy is the flutter valve. It combines the techniques of EPAP with high-frequency oscillations (HFOs) at the airway opening. The valve consists of a pipe-shaped device with a heavy steel ball sitting in an angled "bowl" (Figure 40-11). The pipe bowl is covered by a perforated cap. When the patient exhales actively into the pipe, the ball creates a positive expiratory pressure of between 10 cm H_2O and 25 cm H_2O. At the same time, the pipe angle causes the ball to flutter back and forth at about 15 Hz. When the valve is properly used, the oscillations created are transmitted down into the airways. Patients can control the pressure by changing their expiratory flows. Changing the angle of the device alters the oscillations.

Clinical trials of the flutter valve have produced mixed results in patients with CF compared with existing methods of airway clearance (PDPV or ACBT).[71,84,85] However, the flutter device can decrease viscoelasticity of mucus within the airways, modifying mucus and allowing it to be cleared more easily by cough.[86] Two studies have shown that the use of the flutter valve in patients with hyperproductive disorders showed equivalent or moderately improved pulmonary function values and secretion clearance.[87,88] Given that the flutter valve is readily accepted by patients, is inexpensive, is fully portable, and does not require caregiver assistance (after instruction is provided), additional clinical trials seem justified.[85]

Other devices include the RC-Cornet (Respan Products, Inc, Toronto, Canada), Pare Respiratory Equipment, and the Acapella (Smiths Medical ASD, Inc./Portex, Kent, UK). The RC-Cornet (currently available in Europe) appears to have an advantage over the flutter valve because it is position-independent and provides a more constant pressure and flow rate throughout expiration. The Acapella and the flutter valve have similar performance characteristics, but the Acapella appears to offer some advantages. It can customize, based on clinical needs, both the frequency and the flow resistance by adjusting the dial. Also, it can be used in any posture, including sitting, standing, or reclining.[89]

Box 40-6 Key Factors in Selecting an Airway Clearance Strategy

- Patient's motivation
- Patient's goals
- Patient's ability to comprehend—literacy and cognition levels
- Patient's physical limitations
- Physician/caregiver goals
- Effectiveness of technique
- Ease of learning and teaching
- Skill of therapists or teachers
- Fatigue associated or work required
- Need for assistants or equipment
- Limitations of technique based on disease type and severity
- Costs (direct and indirect)
- Desirability of combining methods

TABLE 40-3

Recommended Airway Clearance Techniques in Specific Conditions

Problem Area	Appropriate Techniques
CF, ciliary dyskinesia syndromes, bronchiectasis	
Infants	PDPV
3-12 yr	Exercise, PEP, PDPV, ACBT, HFO
>12 yr	Exercise, ACBT, AD, PEP, PDPV, HFO
Atelectasis	PEP, PDPV, ACBT
Asthma (with mucous plugging)	Exercise, PEP, PDPV, HFO (flutter valve)
Neurologic abnormalities (spasticity, bulbar palsy, aspiration-prone)	PDPV, suction, MIE
Musculoskeletal weakness (muscular dystrophy, myasthenia gravis, poliomyelitis)	PEP, MIE

SELECTING AIRWAY CLEARANCE TECHNIQUES

Selection Factors

Box 40-6 specifies the key factors clinicians should consider when selecting an airway clearance strategy. Motivation is crucial to routine performance of any procedure, especially for chronically ill patients in ambulatory or home care settings. No airway clearance strategy is successful if it is abandoned by the patient. Likewise, no routine strategy is likely to be followed without substantial results. In this regard, increased sputum production, although frequently shown not to be related to improved pulmonary function, is one of the few real outcomes clinicians can use to motivate the patient and gain his or her ongoing cooperation.

Age and patient preference often dictate available methods. Also, availability of specific airway clearance regimens is variable depending on the clinical site; as an independent variable, the regimen may not have a significant impact on outcome. If different methods are deemed equivalent, it makes sense to allow the patient to choose. Patient and caregiver goals for treatment should be discussed jointly, with the intent of choosing the method that best fits the patient's goals and lifestyle. The clinician's skill and patience in teaching all techniques is a major factor that determines success. The patient's learning needs and barriers to learning are significant factors to be considered.

Because patients reject methods that are fatiguing, this should be considered in method selection. In addition, the patient's disease either may suggest the best approach or may impose certain limitations that preclude using a particular method. Patients with some neuromuscular diseases may be unable to engage in therapeutic exercise. Lastly, cost is a critical factor in selecting all treatment strategies. Selecting the least expensive strategy is acceptable if the strategy is also effective. Increasingly, these strategies include therapies that are either self-administered or provided by unskilled caregivers outside the acute care setting. In this context, effective patient or caregiver education plays an increasingly important role (see Chapter 49).

MINI CLINI

Recommending Airway Clearance Strategies

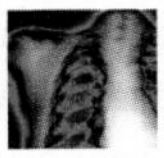

PROBLEM: The RT is asked to evaluate and recommend an appropriate ambulatory airway clearance therapy regimen for a 7-year-old active girl with CF who is being cared for in her home by elderly grandparents.

DISCUSSION: Generally, appropriate secretion clearance strategies for this patient include exercise, PEP, PDPV, ACBT, and HFO (Table 40-3). Because PDPV would be difficult to implement in this patient's home setting (elderly caregivers), emphasis should be placed on either PEP with ACBT or HFO (flutter valve) with ACBT. An exercise plan should also be incorporated into the overall strategy. Dietary and medication considerations are also important.

Clearance Strategies for Specific Conditions

Table 40-3 presents airway clearance techniques for the most common conditions associated with retained secretions. In some cases, a combination of methods may be needed to achieve desired results.

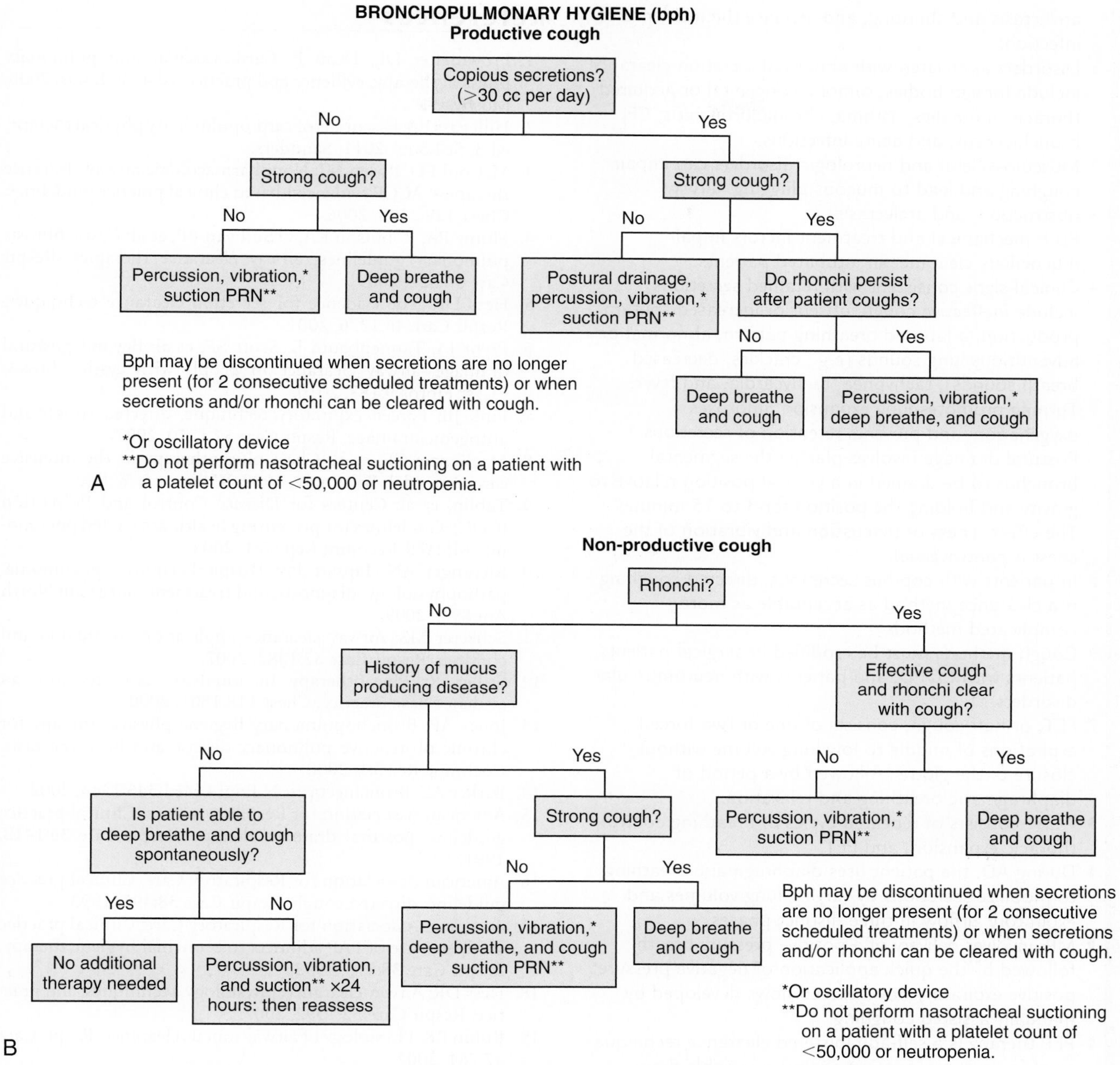

FIGURE 40-12 Example of algorithm underlying an airway clearance protocol. (Bronchial Hygiene Algorithm from the Cleveland Clinic Respiratory Therapy Consult Service Handbook. Courtesy of the Cleveland Clinic.)

Protocol-Based Airway Clearance

Numerous RT-driven protocols have been published for airway clearance therapy. All of these protocols involve rigorous assessment of the patient both to establish preliminary need and to determine continuation of or modification in therapy. Figure 40-12 is an algorithm used in one such protocol. Changes in therapy occur throughout and are based on the patient's response and the evaluation of the clinician.

SUMMARY CHECKLIST

- Normal airway clearance requires a patent airway, a functional mucociliary escalator, and an effective cough.
- The primary goal of airway clearance therapy is to help mobilize and remove retained secretions, improve gas exchange, and reduce the work of breathing.
- Retained secretions can increase the work of breathing, cause air trapping, worsen $\dot{V}/\dot{Q}$ imbalance, promote

Continued

atelectasis and shunting, and increase the incidence of infection.

- Disorders associated with abnormal secretion clearance include foreign bodies, tumors, congenital or acquired thoracic anomalies, asthma, chronic bronchitis, CF, bronchiectasis, and acute infections.
- Musculoskeletal and neurologic disorders can impair coughing and lead to mucous plugging, airway obstruction, and atelectasis.
- Both mechanical and treatment factors impair mucociliary clearance in intubated patients.
- Clinical signs consistent with retained secretions include ineffective cough, absent or increased sputum production, a labored breathing pattern, abnormal or adventitious lung sounds (e.g., crackles, decreased breath sounds), tachypnea, tachycardia, and fever.
- Turning promotes lung expansion, improves oxygenation, and prevents retention of secretions.
- Postural drainage involves placing the segmental bronchus to be drained in a vertical position relative to gravity and holding the position for 3 to 15 minutes.
- The effectiveness of percussion and vibration of the chest is controversial.
- In patients with copious secretions, directed coughing is a clearance method as acceptable as more complicated methods.
- Cough methods must be modified in surgical patients, patients with COPD, and patients with neuromuscular disorders.
- FET, or huff cough, consists of one or two forced expirations of middle to low lung volume without closure of the glottis, followed by a period of diaphragmatic breathing and relaxation.
- ACBT consists of repeated cycles of breathing control, thoracic expansion, and FET.
- During AD, the patient uses diaphragmatic breathing to mobilize secretions by varying lung volumes and expiratory airflow in three distinct phases.
- MIE involves delivery of a positive pressure breath followed by the quick application of negative pressure; positive expiratory flows exceed flows developed by manually assisted coughing.
- PEP therapy is a self-administered clearance technique involving active expiration against a variable-flow resistance, followed by FET; patients frequently prefer PEP over other methods.
- At high frequencies (12 to 25 Hz), airway oscillations enhance cough clearance of secretions.
- Airway oscillations can be created externally (HFCWC) or at the airway opening (flutter valve, IPV).
- Adding physical activity to mobilization and coughing enhances mucus clearance, improves overall aeration and $\dot{V}/\dot{Q}$ matching, and improves pulmonary function.
- Numerous factors must be considered in trying to select the best airway clearance strategy for a given patient.

References

1. Frownfelter DL, Dean E: Cardiovascular and pulmonary physical therapy, evidence and practice, ed 4, St. Louis, 2006, Mosby.
2. Hillegass EA: Essentials of cardiopulmonary physical therapy, ed 3, St Louis, 2011, Saunders.
3. McCool FD, Rosen MJ: Nonpharmacologic airway clearance therapies: ACCP evidenced-based clinical practice guidelines. Chest 129:250S, 2006.
4. Flume PA, Robinson KA, O'Sullivan BP, et al: Cystic fibrosis pulmonary guidelines: airway clearance therapies. Respir Care 54:522, 2009.
5. Hess DR: The evidence for secretion clearance techniques. Respir Care 46:1276, 2001.
6. Pryor JA, Tannenbaum E, Scott SF, et al: Beyond postural drainage: airway clearance in people with cystic fibrosis. J Cyst Fibros 9:187, 2010.
7. Fink JB: Forced expiratory technique, directed cough and autogenic drainage. Respir Care 52:1210, 2007.
8. MacKenzie CF, et al: Chest physiotherapy in the intensive care unit, ed 2, Baltimore, 1989, Williams & Wilkins.
9. Tablin, et al: Centers for Disease Control and Prevention (CDC): Guidelines for preventing health-associated pneumonia. MMWR Recomm Rep 53:1, 2004.
10. Kieninger AN, Lipsett PA: Hospital-acquired pneumonia: pathophysiology, diagnosis, and treatment. Surg Clin North Am 89:2, 2009.
11. Schecter MS: Airway clearance applications in infants and children. Respir Care 52:1382, 2007.
12. Stiller K: Physiotherapy in intensive care: towards an evidence-base practice. Chest 118:1801, 2000.
13. Jones AP: Bronchopulmonary hygiene physical therapy for chronic obstructive pulmonary disease and bronchiectasis. Cochrane Rev 3:1, 2000.
14. Barker AF: Bronchiectasis. N Engl J Med 346:1383, 2002.
15. American Association for Respiratory Care: Clinical practice guideline: postural drainage therapy. Respir Care 36:1418, 1991.
16. American Association for Respiratory Care: Clinical practice guideline: directed cough. Respir Care 38:495, 1993.
17. American Association for Respiratory Care: Clinical practice guideline: use of PAP adjuncts to bronchial hygiene therapy. Respir Care 38:516, 1993.
18. Hess DR: Airway clearance: physiology, techniques, and practice. Respir Care 52:1392, 2007.
19. Rubin BK: Physiology of airway mucus clearance. Respir Care 47:761, 2002.
20. Lapin CD: Airway physiology, autogenic drainage, and active cycle of breathing. Respir Care 47:778, 2002.
21. Haas CF, et al: Airway clearance applications in the elderly and in patients with neurologic or neuromuscular compromise. Respir Care 52:1362, 2007.
22. Langerson J: The cough: its effectiveness depends on you. Respir Care 24:142, 1979.
23. Irwin RS, et al: Cough: a comprehensive review. Arch Intern Med 137:1189, 1977.
24. Tzeng AC, Bach JR: Prevention of pulmonary morbidity for patients with neuromuscular disease. Chest 118:1390, 2000.
25. Hardy KA: Advances in our understanding and care of patients with cystic fibrosis. Respir Care 38:282, 1993.
26. Le Mauviel L: Primary ciliary dyskinesia. West J Med 155:280, 1991.
27. Setz AE, et al: Trends and burdens of bronchiectasis-associated hospitalizations in the United States, 1993-2006. Chest 138:944, 2010.

28. Perme C, Chandrashekar R: Early mobilization and walking program for patients in intensive care units: creating a standard of care. Am J Crit Care 18:212, 2009.
29. Oldenburg FA, et al: Effects of postural drainage, exercise, and cough on mucus clearance in chronic bronchitis. Am Rev Respir Dis 120:739, 1979.
30. Wong JW, et al: Effects of gravity on tracheal transport rates in normal subjects and in patients with cystic fibrosis. Pediatrics 60:146, 1977.
31. Fink JB: Positioning versus postural drainage. Respir Care 47:769, 2002.
32. Kigin C: Chest physical therapy. In Pierson DJ, Kacmarek RM, editors: Foundations of respiratory care, New York, 1992, Churchill Livingstone.
33. deBoeck K, Vermeulen F: Airway clearance techniques to treat acute respiratory disorders in previously healthy children: where is the evidence? Eur J Pediatr 167:607, 2008.
34. Conway JH, et al: Humidification as an adjunct to chest physiotherapy in aiding tracheobronchial clearance in patients with bronchiectasis. Respir Med 86:109, 1992.
35. Chopra SK, et al: Effects of hydration and physical therapy on tracheal transport velocity. Am Rev Respir Dis 115:1009, 1974.
36. Taylor CJ, Threlfall D: Postural drainage techniques and gastro-esophageal reflux in cystic fibrosis. Lancet 349:1567, 1997.
37. Farley, et al: Bronchiectasis: pathophysiology, presentation and management. Nurs Stand 23:50, 2008.
38. American Association for Respiratory Care: Clinical practice guideline: bland aerosol administration. Respir Care 48:529, 2003.
39. Gallon A: Evaluation of chest percussion in the treatment of patients with copious sputum production. Respir Med 85:45, 1991.
40. Bauer ML, McDougal J, Schoumacher RA: Comparison of manual and mechanical chest percussion in hospitalized patients with cystic fibrosis. J Pediatr 124:250, 1994.
41. Irwin RS, et al: Managing cough as a defense mechanism and as a symptom: a consensus panel of the American College of Chest Physicians. Chest 114:133S, 1998.
42 Cornacchia PG, et al: Chest physiotherapy with positive airway pressure: a pilot study of short-term effects on sputum clearance in patients with cystic fibrosis and severe airway obstruction. Respir Care 51:1145, 2006.
43. van der Schans C: Conventional chest physical therapy for obstructive lung disease. Respir Care 52:1198, 2007.
44. Garrod R, Lasseson T: Role of physiotherapy in the management of chronic lung diseases: an overview of systematic reviews. Respir Med 101:2429, 2007.
45. Gore DC: Perioperative maneuvers to avert postoperative respiratory failure in elderly patients. Gerontology 53:438, 2007.
46. Hasani A, et al: The effect of unproductive coughing/FET on regional mucus movement in the human lungs. Respir Med 85:23, 1991.
47. Hietpas BG, Roth RD, Jensen WM: Huff coughing and airway patency. Respir Care 24:710, 1979.
48. Olseni L, et al: Chest physiotherapy in chronic obstructive pulmonary disease: forced expiratory technique combined with either postural drainage or positive expiratory pressure breathing. Respir Med 88:435, 1994.
49. Pryor JA, Webber BA, Hodson ME: Effect of chest physiotherapy on oxygen saturation in patients with cystic fibrosis. Thorax 45:77, 1990.
50. Holland AE, Button BM: Is there a role for airway clearance techniques in chronic obstructive pulmonary disease? Chron Respir Dis 3:83, 2006.
51. Robinson KA, et al: Active cycle of breathing technique for cystic fibrosis. Cochrane Database Syst Rev 11:CD007862, 2007.
52. Miller S, et al: Chest physiotherapy in cystic fibrosis: a comparative study of autogenic drainage and the active cycle of breathing techniques with postural drainage. Thorax 50:165, 1995.
53. McIlwaine M: Chest physical therapy, breathing techniques and exercise in children with CF. Paediatr Respir Rev 8:8, 2007.
54. Savci S, et al: A comparison of autogenic drainage and the active cycle of breathing techniques in patients with chronic obstructive pulmonary diseases. J Cardiopulm Rehabil 20:37, 2000.
55. Giles DR, et al: Short-term effects of postural drainage with clapping vs. autogenic drainage on oxygen saturation and sputum recovery in patients with cystic fibrosis. Chest 108:952, 1995.
56. Homnick DN: Mechanical insufflation-exsufflation for airway mucus clearance. Respir Care 52:1296, 2007.
57. Finsterer J: Cardiopulmonary support in Duchenne muscular dystrophy. Lung 184:205, 2006.
58. Miske LJ, et al: Use of the mechanical in-exsufflator in pediatric patients with neuromuscular disease and impaired cough. Chest 125:1406, 2004.
59. Chatwin M, Simonds AK: The addition of mechanical insufflation/exsufflation shortens airway-clearance sessions in neuromuscular patients with chest infections. Respir Care 54:1473, 2009.
60. Gomez-Merino E, et al: Mechanical insufflation-exsufflation: pressure, volume, and flow relationships, Am J Phys Med Rehab 81:579, 2002.
61. Kang SW, Bach JR: Maximum insufflation capacity: vital capacity and cough flows in neuromuscular disease. Am J Phys Med Rehab 79:222, 2000.
62. Fink JB: Positive pressure techniques for airway clearance. Respir Care 47:786, 2002.
63. Myers TR: Positive expiratory pressure and oscillatory positive expiratory pressure therapies. Respir Care 52:1308, 2007.
64. Hristara-Papadopoulu A: Current devices of respiratory physiotherapy. Hippokratia 12:211, 2010.
65. Olseni L, et al: Chest physiotherapy in chronic obstructive pulmonary disease: forced expiratory technique combined with either postural drainage or positive expiratory pressure breathing. Respir Med 88:435, 1994.
66. Darbee JC, et al: Physiologic evidence for high frequency chest wall oscillation and positive expiratory pressure breathing in hospitalized subjects with cystic fibrosis. Phys Ther 85:1278, 2005.
67. Fink JB: Volume expansion therapy. In Burton GG, Hodgkin JE, Ward JJ, editors: Respiratory care: a guide to clinical practice, ed 4, Philadelphia, 1997, Lippincott.
68. Christensen EF, et al: Flow-dependent properties of positive expiratory pressure devices. Monaldi Arch Chest Dis 50:150, 1995.
69. Tomkiewicz RP, Biviji A, King M: Effects of oscillating air flow on the rheological properties and clearability of mucus gel simulants. Biorheology 31:511, 1994.
70. Chatburn RL: High-frequency assisted airway clearance. Respir Care 52:1224, 2007.
71. Fink JB, Mahlmeister MJ: High-frequency oscillation of the airway and chest wall. Respir Care 47:797, 2002.
72. Kempainen RR, et al: Comparison of settings used for high-frequency chest-wall compressions in cystic fibrosis. Respir Care 55:782, 2010.
73. Yuan, et al: Safety, tolerability, and efficacy of high-frequency chest wall oscillation in pediatric patients with cerebral palsy

and neuromuscular diseases: an exploratory randomized controlled trial. J Child Neurol 25:815, 2010.
74. Allan JS, et al: High-frequency chest-wall compression during the 48 hours following thoracic surgery. Respir Care 54:340, 2009.
75. Phillips GE, et al: Comparison of active cycle of breathing and high-frequency oscillation jacket in children with cystic fibrosis. Pediatr Pulmonol 37:71, 2004.
76. Newhouse PA, et al: The intrapulmonary percussive ventilator and flutter device compared to standard chest physiotherapy in patients with cystic fibrosis. Clin Pediatr 37:427, 1998.
77. McNally NG, et al: Use of intrapulmonary percussive ventilation (IPV) in the management of pulmonary complications of an infant with osteogenesis imperfecta. Pediatr Pulm 44:1151, 2009.
78. Baldwin DR, et al: Effect of addition of exercise to chest physiotherapy on sputum expectoration and lung function in adults with cystic fibrosis. Respir Med 88:49, 1994.
79. Tang CY, et al: Chest physiotherapy for patients admitted to hospital with an acute exacerbation of chronic obstructive pulmonary disease: a systematic review. Physiotherapy 96:243, 2009.
80. Hodgkin KE, et al: Physical therapy utilization in intensive care units: results from a national survey. Crit Care Med 37:561, 2009.
81 Elkins MR, Jones A, van der Schans C: Positive expiratory pressure physiotherapy for airway clearance in people with cystic fibrosis. The Cochrane Library, Issue 2, Chichester, 2004, Wiley.
82. Main E, Prasad A, van der Schans C: Conventional chest physiotherapy compared to other airway clearance techniques for cystic fibrosis. The Cochrane Library, Issue 1, Chichester, 2005, Wiley.
83. Kettler LJ, Sawyer SM, Winefield HR, et al: Determinants of adherence in adults with cystic fibrosis. Thorax 57:459, 2002.
84. Ambrosino N, et al: Clinical evaluation of oscillating positive expiratory pressure for enhancing expectoration in diseases other than cystic fibrosis. Monaldi Arch Chest Dis 50:269, 1995.
85. Konstan MW, Stern RC, Doershuk CF: Efficacy of the Flutter device for airway mucus clearance in patients with cystic fibrosis. J Pediatr 124:689, 1994.
86. App EM, et al: Sputum rheology changes in cystic fibrosis lung disease following two different types of physiotherapy: flutter vs. autogenic drainage. Chest 114:171, 1998.
87. Patterson JE: Acapella versus usual airway clearance during acute exacerbation in bronchiectasis: a randomized crossover trial. Chron Respir Dis 4:67, 2007.
88. Girard JP, Terki N: The Flutter VRP-1: a new personal pocket therapeutic device used as an adjunct to drug therapy in the management of bronchial asthma. J Invest Allergol Clin Immunol 4:23, 1994.
89. Volsko TA, et al: Performance characteristics of two oscillating positive expiratory pressure devices: Acapella versus flutter. Respir Care 48:124, 2003.

SECTION VI

ACUTE AND CRITICAL CARE

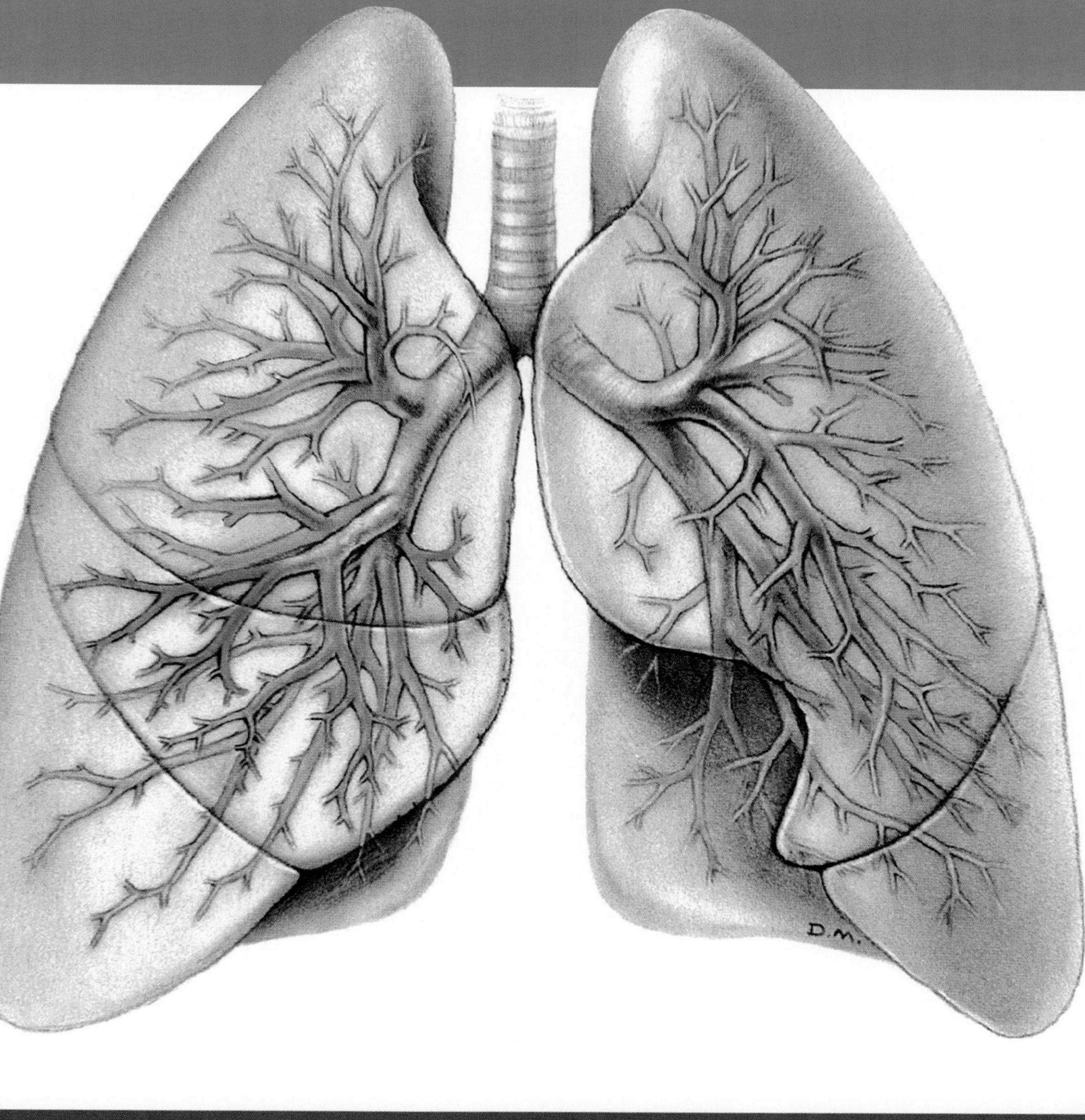

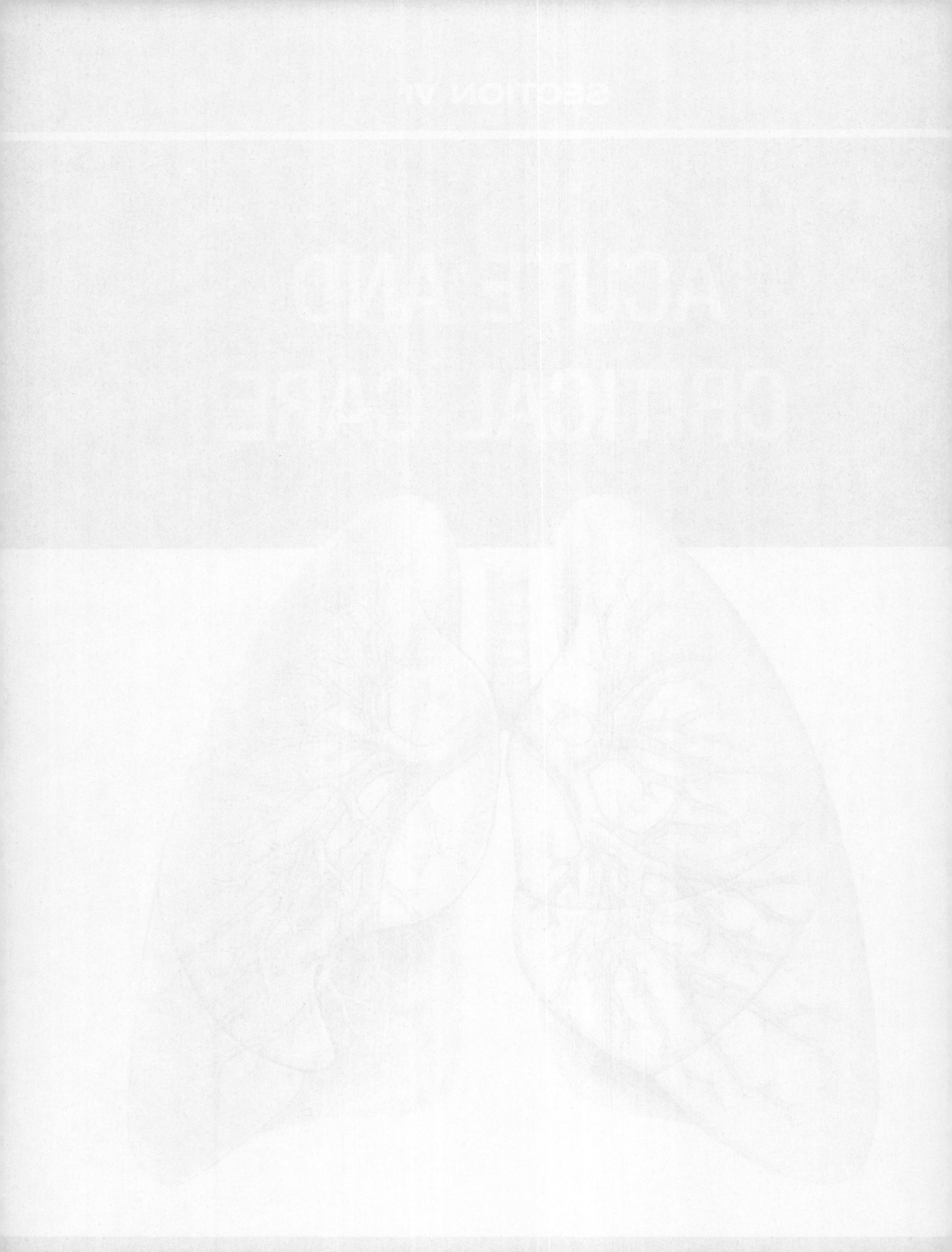

Chapter 41

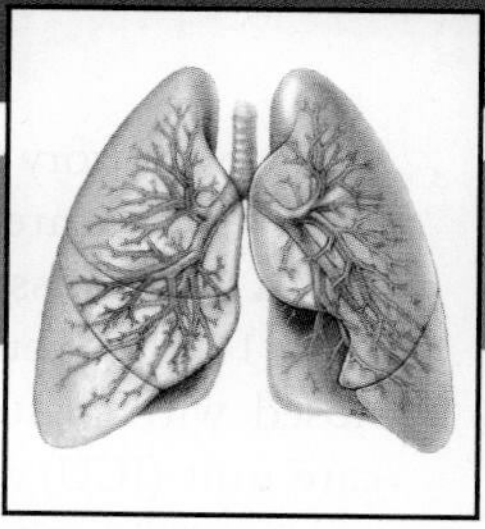

Respiratory Failure and the Need for Ventilatory Support

LOUTFI S. ABOUSSOUAN

CHAPTER OBJECTIVES

After reading this chapter you will be able to:

- Define acute respiratory failure.
- Differentiate between hypoxemic respiratory failure (type I) and hypercapnic respiratory failure (type II).
- Discuss the causes of acute respiratory failure.
- Discuss the differences between chronic respiratory failure and acute-on-chronic respiratory failure.
- Identify the complications of respiratory failure.
- Discuss the indication for ventilatory support.
- Discuss general management principles of hypoxemic and hypercapnic respiratory failure.
- Discuss indications for noninvasive ventilation.

CHAPTER OUTLINE

Hypoxemic Respiratory Failure (Type I)
- Ventilation/Perfusion Mismatch
- Shunt
- Alveolar Hypoventilation
- Diffusion Impairment
- Perfusion/Diffusion Impairment
- Decreased Inspired Oxygen
- Venous Admixture
- Differentiating the Causes of Acute Hypoxemic Respiratory Failure

Hypercapnic Respiratory Failure (Type II)
- Insidious Exposure
- Increased Carbon Dioxide Production
- Impairment in Respiratory Control
- Impairment in Respiratory Effectors

Chronic Respiratory Failure (Type I and Type II)
- Acute-on-Chronic Respiratory Failure
- Complications of Acute Respiratory Failure
- Clinical Presentation
- Indications for Ventilatory Support

Assessment of Respiratory Fatigue, Weakness, and Failure and Work of Breathing
- Respiratory Muscle Weakness
- Respiratory Muscle Fatigue
- Respiratory Failure
- Work of Breathing

Choosing a Ventilatory Support Strategy for Different Causes of Respiratory Failure
- Noninvasive Ventilation
- Noninvasive Ventilation in Acute Conditions
- Noninvasive Ventilation in Chronic Conditions
- Invasive Ventilatory Support

KEY TERMS

auto-PEEP
barotrauma
dynamic hyperinflation
high-frequency ventilation
hypercapnic respiratory failure (type II)
hypoxemic respiratory failure (type I)
maximum expiratory pressure (MEP)
maximum inspiratory pressure (MIP)
maximum voluntary ventilation (MVV)
muscle fatigue
noninvasive ventilation (NIV)
positive end-pertest expiratory pressure (PEEP)
pressure control ventilation
respiratory alternans
tension-time index
work of breathing

Respiratory failure is a clinical problem that all respiratory care practitioners must be skilled at identifying, assessing, and treating. A 1994 study of more than 1400 patients concluded that 44% of patients diagnosed with acute respiratory failure requiring intensive care unit (ICU) admission died in the hospital.[1] A review of hospital discharge records from 2005 in six states in the United States showed only marginal improvement, with hospital mortality of 34.5%.[2] The need for oxygen (O_2) delivery, mechanical ventilation, and other modalities makes the respiratory therapist (RT) indispensable in the treatment of this life-threatening condition.

Respiratory failure is the "inability to maintain either the normal delivery of O_2 to the tissues or the normal removal of carbon dioxide (CO_2) from the tissues"[3] and often results from an imbalance between respiratory workload and ventilatory strength or endurance. Criteria for respiratory failure based on arterial blood gases (ABGs) were established by Campbell[4] and generally define *failure* as arterial partial pressure of oxygen (PaO_2) less than 60 mm Hg or alveolar partial pressure of carbon dioxide ($PaCO_2$) greater than 50 mm Hg (or both) in otherwise healthy individuals breathing room air at sea level. Respiratory failure can be an acute or a chronic process. Additionally and classically, it has also been separated into two other categories to reflect the type of physiologic impairment. *Hypoxemic (type I) respiratory failure* occurs when the primary problem is inadequate O_2 delivery. *Hypercapnic (type II) respiratory failure* describes "bellows failure" of the lungs resulting in elevated CO_2 levels. Hypercapnic respiratory failure is also known as *ventilatory failure*. Patients with baseline acid-base derangement (e.g., chronic obstructive pulmonary disease [COPD], restrictive lung disease) may be chronically hypercapnic and in chronic ventilatory failure based on the guidelines. These individuals develop acute failure when their chronic state deteriorates significantly; this is sometimes referred to as *acute ventilatory failure superimposed on chronic ventilatory failure*.

Although ABG analysis is helpful in distinguishing hypoxemic (type I) and hypercapnic (type II) respiratory failure, many patients in acute respiratory failure develop both hypoxemia and hypercapnia. As noted earlier, patients with chronically elevated arterial $PaCO_2$ levels (chronic ventilatory failure) may develop a sudden, further increase in $PaCO_2$ associated with an acute exacerbation of their chronic condition (acute ventilatory failure superimposed on chronic ventilatory failure).

HYPOXEMIC RESPIRATORY FAILURE (TYPE I)

The primary causes of hypoxemia are the following:

- Ventilation/perfusion ($\dot{V}/\dot{Q}$) mismatch
- Shunt
- Alveolar hypoventilation
- Diffusion impairment
- Perfusion/diffusion impairment
- Decreased inspired O_2
- Venous admixture

These entities are briefly discussed here and are discussed in more detail in Chapters 10 and 11.

Ventilation/Perfusion Mismatch

There are regions in healthy lungs where ventilation and perfusion are not evenly matched, so it seems logical that this is the most common cause of hypoxemia. RTs are familiar with this concept through the work of West,[5] which described a high $\dot{V}/\dot{Q}$ ratio at the apex of the lungs and a low ratio at the bases. This concept can be oversimplified and stated as there being more air than blood at the apices and more blood than air at the bases.

Pathologic $\dot{V}/\dot{Q}$ mismatch occurs when disease disrupts this balance, and hypoxemia results (Figure 41-1, *A*). Most commonly, areas of low $\dot{V}/\dot{Q}$ ratio are seen in which ventilation is compromised despite adequate blood flow. Obstructive lung diseases are frequent causes. The bronchospasm, mucous plugging, inflammation, and premature airway closure that signal asthmatic or emphysematous exacerbations worsen ventilation and create $\dot{V}/\dot{Q}$ mismatch. Infection, heart failure, and inhalation injury may lead to partially collapsed or fluid-filled alveoli, also resulting in decreased ventilation and reduced blood O_2 levels.

Clinical Presentation

Because patients present with hypoxemia, the initial goal is always to treat the low PaO_2 or SpO_2 (arterial O_2 saturation by pulse oximeter). $\dot{V}/\dot{Q}$ mismatch responds to supplemental O_2 (see Figure 41-1, *B*). Hypoxemia commonly manifests with dyspnea, tachycardia, and tachypnea, but these are very nonspecific findings. However, patient observation is extremely valuable. The use of accessory muscles of respiration (scalene, pectoralis major, and sternomastoid) is an important sign that normal diaphragmatic inspiration is inadequate. In an elderly, cachectic, or barrel-chested individual who is leaning forward on his or her arms, COPD is the likely diagnosis. Nasal flaring may be present. Lower extremity edema is more indicative of cardiac failure as the cause of hypoxemia. Cyanosis may be peripheral and primarily due to decreased blood flow. Central cyanosis, seen most easily as a bluish tint around the lips, occurs when greater than 5 g/dl of unsaturated hemoglobin is present. This finding is more common in patients with polycythemia but may be subject to wide observer variability. More severe hypoxemia can lead to significant central nervous system (CNS) dysfunction, ranging from irritability to confusion to coma.

Auscultation is very useful when added to patient observation. Bilateral wheezing, especially in a young patient in respiratory distress, often identifies the bronchospasm of asthma. Upper airway disease or fluid-filled airways may also result in wheezing. Breath sounds that

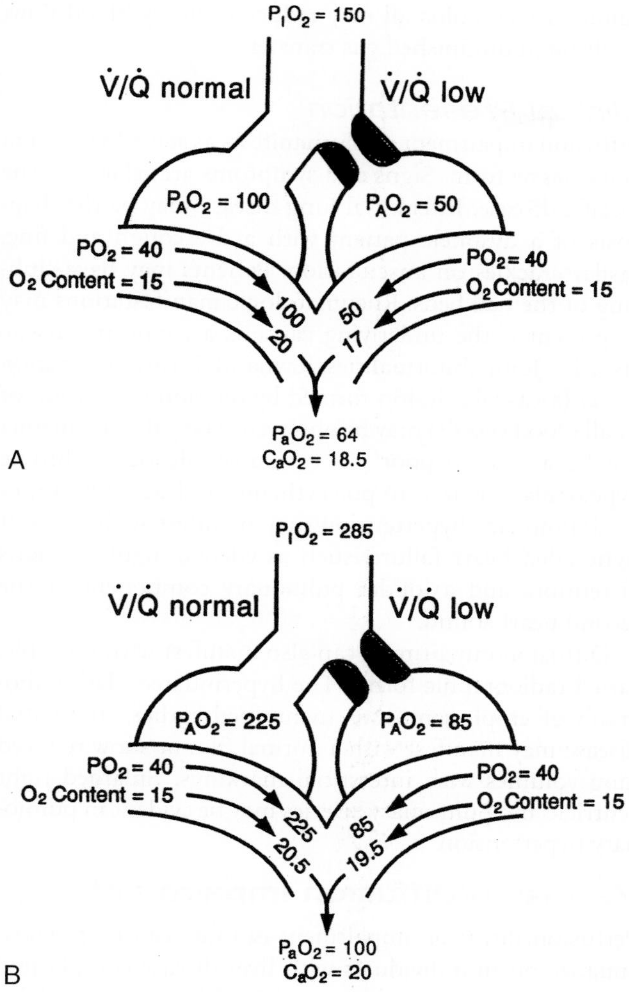

FIGURE 41-1 Hypoxemia caused by $\dot{V}/\dot{Q}$ mismatch showing the effect of supplemental O_2. $\dot{V}/\dot{Q}$ is normal on the left side of each idealized lung unit and low on the right. Only O_2 exchange is shown, and $P(A - a)O_2$ is assumed to be zero. **A,** With room air, not enough O_2 reaches the poorly ventilated alveolus to saturate its capillary blood fully. **B,** With 40% O_2, PaO_2 in this alveolus is increased enough to make capillary PO_2 nearly normal. PaO_2 in the mixed blood from the two capillaries is determined by the average of the O_2 contents of the two streams of blood, not by the PaO_2 values. (Modified from Pierson DJ, Kacmarek RM: Foundations of respiratory care, New York, 1992, Churchill Livingstone.)

are diminished bilaterally are common in emphysema. Unilateral abnormalities are significant. Wheezing in one lung may identify an endobronchial lesion, whereas the absence of breath sounds on one side of the chest may reveal collapse, infection, edema, or effusion as potential causes of $\dot{V}/\dot{Q}$ mismatch. Unilateral crackles generally indicate an alveolar filling process (mass, infection, fluid).

Radiographically, $\dot{V}/\dot{Q}$ mismatch can manifest as a "black" radiograph, with large or hyperinflated lungs as in the case of obstructive disease. A "white" chest radiograph is evident when alveoli are partially occluded. The "blackness" or "whiteness" of the lung fields on the plain chest radiograph has important diagnostic value in assessing a patient with acute respiratory failure.

Shunt

Shunt is an extreme version of $\dot{V}/\dot{Q}$ mismatch in which there is no ventilation to match perfusion ($\dot{V}/\dot{Q} = 0$). About 2% to 3% of the blood supply is shunted via the bronchial and thebesian veins that feed the lungs and heart; this is normal anatomic shunt. Pathologic anatomic shunt occurs as a result of right-to-left blood flow through cardiac openings (e.g., atrial or ventricular septal defects) or in pulmonary arteriovenous malformations. Physiologic shunt leads to hypoxemia when alveoli collapse or are filled with fluid or exudate. Common etiologies of physiologic shunting include atelectasis, pulmonary edema, and pneumonia. In contrast to $\dot{V}/\dot{Q}$ mismatch, shunt does not respond to supplemental O_2 because the gas exchange unit (the alveolus) is not open (Figure 41-2, *A*).

Clinical Presentation

The clinical presentation of shunt is very similar in many ways to the presentation of $\dot{V}/\dot{Q}$ mismatch. Patient observations are similar, although chest excursion occasionally may be asymmetric in shunt. Bilateral or unilateral crackles are common owing to the alveolar filling process. Unilateral absence of breath sounds may indicate significant collapse, mass, or effusion; these conditions require treatment before oxygenation can improve. Shunt usually manifests with a "white" chest radiograph. The most advanced example of this is the diffuse, bilateral haziness in acute respiratory distress syndrome (ARDS). Shunting can be diagnosed by using 100% O_2 breathing techniques, contrast-enhanced echocardiography, macroaggregated albumin scanning, or pulmonary angiography.[6] Shunt is differentiated from $\dot{V}/\dot{Q}$ mismatch by the lack of increase in PO_2 as fractional inspired oxygen (FiO_2) is increased (see Figure 41-2, *B*).

Alveolar Hypoventilation

Alveolar hypoventilation is discussed subsequently in the section on Hypercapnic Respiratory Failure (Type II).

Diffusion Impairment

Diffusion refers to movement of gas across the alveolar-capillary membrane secondary to a pressure gradient. Although diffusion is rarely a cause of significant hypoxemia at rest, its effects become more pronounced with exercise, which limits the time for gas exchange. This time limitation is normally not a problem, unless diffusion impairment is present, in which case hypoxemia results. Diffusion impairment in interstitial lung disease may contribute 20% to 30% of the widening in the alveolar-arterial O_2 gradient during exercise.[7] Diffusion impairment most commonly manifests in patients with interstitial lung disease (e.g., pulmonary fibrosis, asbestosis, sarcoidosis) in which the thickening and scarring of the interstitium

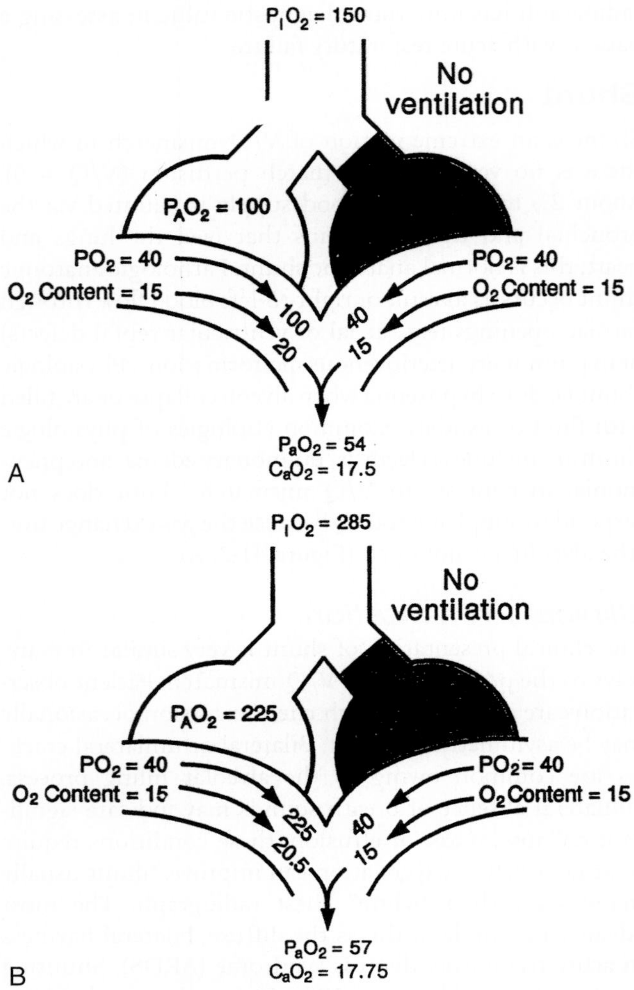

FIGURE 41-2 Alveolar-capillary diagram of intrapulmonary (capillary) shunting showing why supplemental O_2 fails to correct hypoxemia. Only O_2 exchange is shown, and $P(A - a)O_2$ is assumed to be zero. **A,** With room air, although blood leaving the normal alveolar-capillary unit is normally saturated, blood passing the capillary on the right "sees" no O_2 because its alveolus is unventilated, and it leaves the unit unsaturated. When the two streams of blood mix, the resulting PaO_2 is determined by the average of the O_2 contents, not by the PO_2 values. **B,** Addition of 40% O_2 fails to correct the hypoxemia because O_2 content is not significantly increased in the normal unit, and capillary blood in the unventilated unit still "sees" no O_2. Even 100% O_2 could not completely reverse the oxygenation defect in this example; this is very different from the effect with low $\dot{V}/\dot{Q}$ as illustrated in Figure 41-1. (Modified from Pierson DJ, Kacmarek RM: Foundations of respiratory care, New York, 1992, Churchill Livingstone.)

undermine normal gas exchange. Emphysema, with its inherent alveolar destruction, also has subnormal transfer of O_2 and CO_2 between the alveolus and the capillary. The reduced ventilation in both diseases implies that $\dot{V}/\dot{Q}$ mismatch also plays a role in the resulting hypoxemia.

Pulmonary vascular abnormalities can also lead to diffusion impairment. Anemia, pulmonary hypertension, and pulmonary embolus all may reduce capillary blood flow, resulting in diminished gas transfer.

Clinical Presentation

Diffusion impairment rarely manifests as acute hypoxemia in its classic form. Signs and symptoms are related to the specific disease. Interstitial lung disease may be the diagnosis of a dyspneic patient with a dry cough and fine, basilar crackles on auscultation. Patients may have clubbing of the nail beds. Rheumatologic manifestations may be present if the underlying cause is a connective tissue disorder. Joint abnormalities, Raynaud disease, and *telangiectasia* (a vascular lesion formed by dilation of a group of small blood vessels) may be observed. The pallor of anemia can be a clue to poor gas exchange, although chronic hypoxemia may lead to polycythemia and possibly cyanosis. Pulmonary hypertension may manifest with signs of right-sided heart failure, such as edema, jugular venous distention, and a louder pulmonary component of the second heart sound.

Diffusion impairment can also manifest with multiple, varied radiographic forms. The hyperinflated, dark radiograph of emphysema was mentioned earlier. Interstitial disease may manifest with a normal film or show reduced lung volumes with interstitial markings. Enlarged right ventricle and pulmonary arteries may be evident in pulmonary hypertension.

Perfusion/Diffusion Impairment

Perfusion/diffusion impairment is a rare cause of hypoxemia found in individuals with liver disease complicated by hepatopulmonary syndrome.[6] In this condition, right-to-left intracardiac shunt combines with dilated pulmonary capillaries resulting in impaired gas exchange. Specifically, the normal alveolar partial pressures of O_2 may be insufficient to drive the O_2 molecules to the center of the dilated pulmonary vasculature. Cirrhosis is the most common liver disease, and portal hypertension is usually present. Although shunt is a component of the syndrome, significant supplemental O_2 can overcome the gas transfer reduction owing to the dilated vessels, so this is commonly called a *perfusion/diffusion defect.*

Clinical Presentation

Obvious signs of liver disease (e.g., ascites, jaundice, and spider nevi) may or may not be present. Digital clubbing can occur in hepatopulmonary syndrome. *Platypnea,* which is the sensation of dyspnea when moving to the upright position from the supine position, may be a patient complaint. *Orthodeoxia,* an actual decrease in the measured O_2 level, may parallel this subjective sensation.

Decreased Inspired Oxygen

Also clinically uncommon, hypoxemia may develop when the inspired O_2 is less than body requirements. The most common situation is at high altitude, where barometric pressure decreases, which results in a decrease in the partial pressure of inspired O_2. Although airlines account for this decrease in barometric pressure by pressurizing their cabins, travelers with chronic hypoxemia may still need supplemental O_2.[8] Similarly, mountain climbers sometimes require O_2 masks. Cases of patient-O_2 disconnects and delivery of an incorrect gas source, which, it is hoped, occur rarely, are also included in this category.

Inspired O_2 less than 21% can be used diagnostically and therapeutically. The Hypoxia Altitude Simulation Test seeks to replicate inspired partial pressure of O_2 (PiO_2) during air travel by asking the potential traveler to inhale a hypoxic mixture. Inhaling at FiO_2 of 15% replicates the PiO_2 found at an altitude of 8000 feet (108 mm Hg). For a lower altitude of 5400 feet, an equivalent FiO_2 of 17% can be calculated.[8] Infants with certain cyanotic congenital heart defects (e.g., hypoplastic left ventricle) may benefit from FiO_2 below room air level. In the preoperative state, low FiO_2 helps to prevent pulmonary dilation and the excessive pulmonary blood flow, which could flood the lungs.

Clinical Presentation

The signs and symptoms of hypoxemia may be present, with the cause clearly related to the patient environment such as the altitude.

Venous Admixture

A decrease in mixed venous O_2 increases the gradient by which O_2 needs to be stepped up as it passes through the lungs and can contribute to the development of hypoxemia. Congestive heart failure with low cardiac output is the most common cause of low mixed venous O_2, owing to increased peripheral extraction of O_2. Other causes include low hemoglobin concentration and increased O_2 consumption. A low mixed venous O_2 may have a significant effect on the ultimate arterial O_2 tension in the presence of lung disease. There may be other, more important coexisting determinants of hypoxemia, such as $\dot{V}/\dot{Q}$ mismatch and shunting.[3]

Clinical Presentation

Signs and symptoms of congestive heart failure or underlying lung disease, or both, may be present and typically overshadow the clinical presentation.

Differentiating the Causes of Acute Hypoxemic Respiratory Failure

It is important to recognize the physiologic basis of each of the three main causes of hypoxemic respiratory failure (hypoventilation, $\dot{V}/\dot{Q}$ mismatch, and shunt). Hypoventilation differs from the other causes in manifesting with a normal alveolar-to-arterial PO_2 difference [$P(A - a)O_2$] indicating normal lung parenchyma (Table 41-1). A clinical determination of this difference is made by subtracting PaO_2 from PAO_2 (partial pressure of alveolar O_2) derived from the alveolar air equation:

TABLE 41-1

Differentiating the Cause of Hypoxemia

Cause	$P(A - a)O_2$	Response to Increased FiO_2
Hypoventilation	Normal	Marked
Shunt	Increased	Minimal
$\dot{V}/\dot{Q}$ mismatch	Increased	Marked

$$PAO_2 = FiO_2\,(P_B - P_{H_2O}) - PaCO_2/R$$

where P_B is barometric pressure, P_{H_2O} is water vapor tension, and R is the respiratory exchange ratio (0.8).

The $P(A - a)O_2$ ranges from 10 mm Hg in young patients to approximately 25 mm Hg in elderly patients while breathing room air (see the accompanying Rule of Thumb). In patients with hypoxemia caused by hypoventilation, treatment can be focused on improving ventilation because the hypoxemia is purely a result of alveolar displacement of O_2 by elevated CO_2.

RULE OF THUMB

The mean alveolar-to-arterial difference [$P(A - a)O_2$] in PO_2 increases slightly with age and can be estimated with the following equation:

$$\text{Mean age-specific } P(A - a)O_2 = (\text{age}/4) + 4$$

Example: A 76-year-old person living at sea level:

$$P(A - a)O_2 = (76/4) + 4 = 19 + 4 = 23 \text{ mm Hg}$$

A $\dot{V}/\dot{Q}$ mismatch and shunt both result in elevated $P(A - a)O_2$ levels, indicating that the resultant hypoxemia is due to an abnormality of lung tissue, requiring treatment to address that abnormality. When the RT encounters an increased $P(A - a)O_2$, a $\dot{V}/\dot{Q}$ mismatch and shunt can be differentiated by means of O_2 administration (see Figures 41-1 and 41-2). A significant response to applying even small amounts of O_2 identifies $\dot{V}/\dot{Q}$ mismatch as the cause of hypoxemia because altered $P(A - a)O_2$ has not been totally obliterated. True shunt shows little or no improvement in oxygenation even with 100% FiO_2 (see Table 41-1). As a result, treatment of intrapulmonary shunt must be directed toward opening collapsed alveoli or clearing fluid or exudative material before O_2 can be beneficial at below toxic levels. Testing to rule out anatomic shunt should be done in the right clinical setting (e.g., clear or black parenchyma on the chest radiograph).

HYPERCAPNIC RESPIRATORY FAILURE (TYPE II)

Hypercapnic respiratory failure (type II), also known as *pump failure* or *ventilatory failure,* is characterized by an elevated $PaCO_2$, creating an uncompensated respiratory acidosis (whether acute or acute-on-chronic). $PaCO_2$ and alveolar ventilation ($\dot{V}_A$) are inversely related, meaning that alveolar and arterial PCO_2 levels are doubled when alveolar ventilation is halved. This is illustrated by the relationship:

$$PaCO_2 = (0.863\ \dot{V}CO_2)/\dot{V}_A$$
$$\dot{V}_A = MV\ (1 - V_D/V_T)$$

where $\dot{V}_A$ is alveolar ventilation (L/min), MV is minute ventilation, V_D/V_T is dead space-to-tidal volume ratio, and $\dot{V}CO_2$ is CO_2 production (ml/min).

Similarly, this relationship shows that $PaCO_2$ may increase as dead space (V_D/V_T) rises or as CO_2 production ($\dot{V}CO_2$) increases. Additionally, a change in the $\dot{V}/\dot{Q}$ distribution of the lung toward lower ratios not only causes hypoxemia, as shown in Figures 41-1 and 41-2, but also to a lesser extent can cause an elevation of $PaCO_2$ by reducing the CO_2 discharge from the pulmonary circulation to the alveoli. However, increased dead space, increased $\dot{V}CO_2$, and shifts in the $\dot{V}/\dot{Q}$ distribution toward lower ratios all are usually matched by a corrective increase in ventilation because respiratory control mechanisms tend to maintain the $PaCO_2$ constant. The following sections describe mechanisms of hypercarbia caused by an imbalance between CO_2 exposure (external or internal) and CO_2 clearance (central and respiratory effector mechanisms). Hypoxemia may often accompany pump failure simply because of the displacement of alveolar PO_2 (PAO_2) by the increased $PaCO_2$. This situation is identified on a room air ABG assessment by a normal $P(A - a)O_2$ as discussed previously. This situation identifies alveolar hypoventilation as a cause of hypoxemic respiratory failure, as mentioned earlier. The presence of an increased $P(A - a)O_2$ indicates that concomitant hypoxemia is present, most likely as a result of $\dot{V}/\dot{Q}$ mismatch or shunt. The disorders responsible for hypercapnic respiratory failure (ventilatory failure) are discussed next.

Insidious Exposure

Although most cases of increased $PaCO_2$ are due to hypoventilation, an insidious exposure can occur in certain situations.

MINI CLINI

Differentiating Causes of Hypoxemia

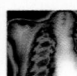

PROBLEM: Two patients present with the following ABG values at sea level:

Patient A		Patient B	
pH	7.45	pH	7.21
$PaCO_2$	33 mm Hg	$PaCO_2$	72 mm Hg
PaO_2	40 mm Hg	PaO_2	53 mm Hg
HCO_3^-	22 mEq/L	HCO_3^-	28 mEq/L
SaO_2	70%	SaO_2	81%
FiO_2	0.21	FiO_2	0.21

1. Define the respiratory condition indicated by each ABG analysis.
2. What is the $P(A - a)O_2$ for each blood gas?
3. Identify the type of respiratory failure in each case.
4. In which case would administration of 100% FiO_2 help determine therapy?

DISCUSSION

1. Patient A exhibits uncompensated respiratory alkalosis with hypoxemia. Patient B exhibits partially compensated respiratory acidosis with hypoxemia.
2. Patient A:
   $PaO_2 = 0.21\ (760 - 47) - 33/0.8 = 108$ mm Hg
   $PaO_2 = 40$ mm Hg
   $P(A - a)O_2 = 108 - 40 = 68$ mm Hg on room air
   Patient B:
   $PaO_2 = 0.21\ (760 - 47) - 72/0.8 = 60$ mm Hg
   $PaO_2 = 53$ mm Hg
   $P(A - a)O_2 = 60 - 53 = 7$ mm Hg on room air
   The normal values for $P(A - a)O_2$ range from 10 mm Hg in young people to approximately 25 mm Hg in elderly people while breathing room air.
3. Patient A has hypoxemic respiratory failure (type I) as characterized by below-normal PaO_2 (40 mm Hg). $PaCO_2$ is also below normal (33 mm Hg) indicating hyperventilation is occurring in an effort to improve the oxygenation. Patient B has hypercapnic respiratory failure (type II) as characterized by above-normal $PaCO_2$ (72 mm Hg) indicating hypoventilation (ventilatory failure) is occurring. This is also known as acute ventilatory failure superimposed on chronic ventilatory failure. This patient is also hypoxemic (53 mm Hg). There is a slight elevation of HCO_3^- (28 mEq/L) indicating an element of chronic respiratory failure may be present, which has now become acute.
4. Patient A has hypoxemic respiratory failure with $P(A - a)O_2$ of 68 mm Hg, which is well above normal, indicating an oxygenation defect. The administration of 100% O_2 in this case would help to determine the cause of the defect. Significant response to 100% FiO_2 would point to $\dot{V}/\dot{Q}$ mismatch as the cause, whereas shunt would be implicated if PaO_2 did not respond to the increase in delivered O_2. In the latter condition, some form of PEEP would be necessary to improve gas exchange by improving functional residual capacity. Patient B has hypercapnic respiratory failure (ventilatory failure) with hypoxemia, but with $P(A - a)O_2$ of 7 mm Hg, which is within the normal range. A pure ventilatory defect is the cause of hypoxemia, and administration of 100% FiO_2 would not help to determine therapy. Depending on the full patient scenario, this patient may require intubation and mechanical ventilation to restore normal acid-base status.

Clinical Presentation

These insidious exposures follow unusual clinical scenarios including defective CO_2 scrubbers in the settings of anesthesia machines or life-support systems in scuba units, airtight chambers, spacecrafts, or submersible crafts. Occupational exposures also occur in spelunkers in caves (from groundwater seepage), individuals who work with dry ice (dry-ice is a solid form of CO_2), miners, and firefighters.

Increased Carbon Dioxide Production

Fever, agitation, exertion, shivering, hypermetabolism, and excess caloric intake all can result in an increase in $\dot{V}CO_2$, with consequent hypercapnia in patients with additional impairment in respiratory control and effector mechanisms.

Clinical Presentation

The most common clinical scenario involving increases in CO_2 production probably involves mechanically ventilated patients with an already compromised lung function, in whom attempts to liberate from artificial ventilation are complicated by type II respiratory failure. Recognition and management of fever, agitation, and hypermetabolic states may contribute to a favorable outcome. One other important clinical consideration to recognize is excess caloric intake, in particular, carbohydrate-rich enteral solutions.

Impairment in Respiratory Control

Inspiratory muscles are innervated by the phrenic and intercostal nerves via spinal cord transmission from the CNS. Both central (medullary) and peripheral (aortic and carotid bodies) chemoreceptors responding to CO_2 tension and O_2 tension stimulate the drive to breathe.[9] This ventilatory drive can be diminished by various factors, such as drugs (overdose or sedation), bilateral carotid endarterectomy with incidental resection of the carotid bodies, brainstem lesions, diseases of the CNS such as multiple sclerosis or Parkinson disease, hypothyroidism, morbid obesity (e.g., obesity-hypoventilation), and sleep apnea. Other, less common potential causes include metabolic alkalosis, malnutrition, and sleep deprivation.[10] Patients with metabolic encephalopathy or elevated intracranial pressure (ICP) may develop a reduced drive to breathe. Patients at risk of having a decreased ventilatory drive usually can be identified by their clinical situation (e.g., CNS insult, overdose of sedative medications). Significantly, many causes of central depression are easily reversible with treatment, so the clinician should be attentive to reversible causes.

Clinical Presentation

The hallmark of the clinical scenario of decreased ventilatory drive is bradypnea and perhaps ultimately apnea. A respiratory rate less than 12 breaths/min is abnormal in adults. Drug overdose or a brain disorder can manifest with an altered level of consciousness ranging from merely lethargic to obtunded and comatose, with decreased respirations. Evidence of drug use by history or toxicity screen confirms the diagnosis of drug overdose. Evidence of head trauma and brain computed tomography (CT) scan abnormalities are important in the diagnosis of a brain disorder. Although hypothyroidism classically manifests with fatigue, weight gain, hyporeflexia, and constipation, it can progress to significant hypoventilation and myxedema coma. Patients with obesity-hypoventilation may have a rapid, shallow breathing pattern, which results from decreased compliance and microatelectasis. Although these patients may also have nighttime sleep apnea, daytime $PaCO_2$ is also elevated because of a decrease in the drive to breathe or an increase in the work of breathing.[11]

Impairment in Respiratory Effectors

Neurologic Diseases

The lung is basically a pump that inhales and exhales under the guidance of the CNS. In some patients, the CNS signal does not reach its goal, resulting in neuromuscular dysfunction. Examples include spinal trauma, motor neuron disease in which lesions of the anterior horn cells may gradually lead to progressive ventilatory failure (e.g., amyotrophic lateral sclerosis or poliomyelitis), motor nerve disorders (including Guillain-Barré syndrome and Charcot-Marie-Tooth disease), disorders of the neuromuscular junction (e.g., myasthenia gravis and botulism), and muscular diseases (including muscular dystrophy, myositis, critical care myopathy, and metabolic disorders).[12] These diseases range from irreversible and usually terminal (e.g., amyotrophic lateral sclerosis) to reversible and usually self-limiting (e.g., myasthenia and Guillain-Barré syndrome).[12]

Clinical Presentation. Although hypercapnia may be a common end point, these diseases have varied clinical presentations. Patient observation is a key skill. Drooling, dysarthria, and weak cough are common signs in amyotrophic lateral sclerosis. As muscle wasting and weakness become more severe, diaphragmatic insufficiency develops, and supine paradoxical breathing is common.[13] Guillain-Barré syndrome commonly manifests with lower extremity weakness progressing to the respiratory muscles in one-third of patients.[14] Weak cough and gag may be seen, which can threaten airway patency and lead to microatelectasis, hypoxemia, and uncompensated respiratory acidosis. Although myasthenia gravis commonly manifests with ocular muscle weakness, it also can exhibit bulbar weakness on its path to respiratory muscle fatigue. Myasthenia gravis does not always result in respiratory failure.[15] These diseases are quite different in clinical course, but there is much overlap in their presentations, and they commonly result in respiratory muscle fatigue and failure and elevated $PaCO_2$.

Increased Work of Breathing

Despite normal respiratory drive, nerve transmission, and neuromuscular response, hypercapnic respiratory failure can still occur if the imposed workload cannot be overcome.[3,16] Most commonly, this situation occurs when increased dead space accompanies COPD, or elevated airway resistance accompanies asthma. Both of these obstructive airway diseases may increase respiratory work requirements excessively secondary to the presence of intrinsic **positive end-expiratory pressure (PEEP).** Increased workload can also result from thoracic abnormalities such as pneumothorax, rib fractures with a flail chest, pleural effusions, and other conditions creating a restrictive burden on the lungs. Finally, requirements for increased minute ventilation can arise when increased CO_2 production accompanies hypermetabolic states, such as in extensive burns.

Clinical Presentation. The RT must be alert to the possibility of respiratory failure when a heavy load is imposed on the respiratory system. Patients with asthma or COPD should present with hyperventilation in an exacerbation, but if breathing becomes more rapid but shallow, it may indicate impending failure. This increased V_D/V_T ratio leads to hypercapnia because the significant airway obstruction does not resolve with treatment. Diminished breath sounds in a young patient with asthma likewise can be an ominous sign. Irritability, confusion, and ultimately coma are possible signs in worsening hypercapnia, as they are in hypoxemic respiratory failure. More subtle findings include muscle tremor owing to catecholamine release and papilledema resulting from cerebral vasodilation in states of elevated arterial PCO_2.[17]

In summary, hypercapnic (type II) respiratory failure, also known as ventilatory failure, develops when ventilation is impaired secondary to intrinsically or extrinsically increased CO_2 exposure; impairment in respiratory control; or impairment in respiratory effector mechanisms, including neurologic disease or pulmonary and chest wall disorders associated with increased work of breathing (Table 41-2).

CHRONIC RESPIRATORY FAILURE (TYPE I AND TYPE II)

For some patients with pulmonary disease and respiratory failure, the condition has developed over weeks to months to years and has become a chronic state, and this has allowed the body to develop compensatory mechanisms to

TABLE 41-2

Causes of Respiratory Failure

	Type II (Hypercapnic)			
Type I (Hypoxemic)	**Increased Exposure**	**Impaired Respiratory Control**	**Neurologic Disease**	**Increased Work of Breathing**
ARDS	Extrinsic	Drug overdose	Spinal cord trauma	Obstructive lung disease
Pulmonary embolism	Defective CO_2 scrubbers (anesthesia or life-support systems)	Bilateral endarterectomy with carotid body resection	Motor neuron	COPD
Pulmonary edema	Occupational exposure (miners, spelunkers, dry-ice workers, firemen)	Central sleep apnea	Poliomyelitis	Asthma
Septic shock	Intrinsic	Hypocapnia	Amyotrophic lateral sclerosis	Upper airway obstruction
Pulmonary infection	Fever	Cheyne-Stokes	Motor nerve	Obesity-hypoventilation
Viral	Shivering	Acromegaly	Phrenic nerve	Pneumothorax
Bacterial	Hypermetabolism	Hypothyroid	Guillain-Barré	Severe burns
Fungal	Agitation	Brainstem lesions	Charcot-Marie-Tooth	Chest wall disorders
Inhalation	Excess caloric intake	Cerebrovascular accident	Neuromuscular junction	Kyphoscoliosis
Smoke		Encephalitis	Myasthenia gravis	Ankylosing spondylitis
Chemical		Multiple sclerosis	Botulism	
Water		Parkinson disease	Muscular	
Pleural effusion		Metabolic alkalosis	Muscular dystrophy	
Interstitial lung disease		Primary alveolar hypoventilation	Myositis	
Obstructive lung disease		(Ondine's curse)	Myopathy	
Aspiration		Congenital central hypoventilation	Acid maltase	
Primary pulmonary hypertension		Carotid body resection	Metabolic	
		Obesity-hypoventilation		

adapt to the disease. Most commonly, chronic hypercapnic respiratory failure accompanying COPD or obesity-hypoventilation syndrome elicits a renal response, and the kidneys retain bicarbonate to elevate the blood pH. However, this compensatory metabolic alkalosis would not be expected to restore the pH to normal. Chronic hypercapnic respiratory failure is also known as *chronic ventilatory failure*.

RULE OF THUMB

Chronic and acute hypercapnic respiratory failure can be differentiated by the severity of change in pH.[16]

- *Acute hypercapnic failure (acute ventilatory failure)*: pH decreases 0.08 for every 10-mm Hg increase in $PaCO_2$
- *Chronic hypercapnic failure (chronic ventilatory failure)*: pH decreases 0.03 for every 10-mm Hg increase in $PaCO_2$

Similarly, polycythemia may result from prolonged hypoxemic respiratory failure (e.g., sleep apnea) when O_2 delivery to the tissues is compromised, and erythropoietin levels increase to elicit erythrocytosis. Hemoglobin also releases O_2 more easily as the O_2 dissociation curve shifts to the right in the face of acidosis. Finally, O_2 delivery to the brain is enhanced when hypercapnia results in increased cerebral blood flow.[17]

Acute-on-Chronic Respiratory Failure

Chronic respiratory failure can be complicated by acute setbacks that create acute-on-chronic respiratory failure. Patients with chronic hypercapnic respiratory failure (chronic ventilatory failure) are at significant risk for this condition, as indicated by the fact that COPD is now the fourth leading cause of death in the United States.[18] Acute-on-chronic respiratory failure can also be the presenting manifestation of neuromuscular disease in the setting of a concurrent pulmonary infection.[19] Most common precipitating factors include bacterial or viral infections, congestive heart failure, pulmonary embolus, chest wall dysfunction, and medical noncompliance.[19-21] In these patients, the presence of respiratory failure cannot be judged by the normal ABG criteria but by a significant change from the baseline $PaCO_2$ to a level having the potential for morbidity and mortality.

Treatment goals include normalizing pH (avoiding mechanical ventilation if possible), elevating SaO_2 to 90% (if hypoxemia is also present), improving airflow, treating infection, monitoring and maintaining fluid status, and preventing or treating complications as necessary.[16,20,21] Optimally treated patients with acute-on-chronic respiratory failure have shown improving hospital mortality rates despite the overall stagnant rates for respiratory failure in general.[22,23] Higher death rates are associated with factors such as significant baseline disease, a severe precipitating illness, severity of acidosis, and presence of complications.[23] The use of advance directives regarding a patient's desire for mechanical ventilation influences short-term mortality. Episodes of acute respiratory failure in these patients seem to have a significant long-term influence with mortality rates reaching 49% within 2 years of an acute exacerbation.[22]

Patients with chronic hypoxemic respiratory failure (type I) are at similar risk for acute deterioration of hypoxemia. Infection and heart failure can result in worsening of the tenuous oxygenation status of patients with interstitial pulmonary fibrosis or primary pulmonary hypertension.

Complications of Acute Respiratory Failure

Although respiratory failure is life-threatening by itself, complications frequently arise that can add significantly to morbidity and mortality. Especially in patients with ARDS, more deaths are due to complications (e.g., sepsis, multi-organ failure) than to the primary disease.[24] Modern ICUs with sophisticated mechanical ventilation can prolong but may not preserve life. Pulmonary complications such as emboli, **barotrauma,** and infection may be secondary to treatment strategies such as catheters, mechanical ventilation, and endotracheal tubes. A wide array of nonpulmonary complications exists, ranging from cardiac disorders (e.g., arrhythmias, hypotension) to gastrointestinal ailments (e.g., hemorrhage, dysmotility) to renal disturbances (e.g., acute renal failure, positive fluid balance). Bacteremia, malnutrition, and psychosis secondary to prolonged ICU stays can also seriously complicate an episode of acute respiratory failure.[24]

Clinical Presentation

Clinically, a patient with respiratory muscle fatigue shows an initially increased respiratory rate followed by *bradypnea* (slowed respiratory rate) and apnea as fatigue ensues. **Respiratory alternans,** which is a phasic alteration between rib cage and abdominal breathing, may also occur. Opinions vary on the sensitivity and specificity of abdominal motion paradox in patients with respiratory muscle weakness, but at least some investigators suggest that respiratory muscle paradox is an early sign (see Chapter 15). When ventilatory failure is full-blown, ABG results show hypercapnia with acidosis. As mentioned earlier, the presence of hypercapnia with acidosis can also indicate that the respiratory center is not responding properly.[25]

Tachypnea is the cardinal sign of increased work of breathing. Tachypnea occurs when the respiratory center increases breathing frequency in an attempt to lessen respiratory excursion and reduce the amount of work performed by the respiratory muscles.[26] Overall workload is reflected in the minute volume needed to maintain normocapnia.

MINI CLINI

Acute or Chronic Hypercapnic Respiratory Failure

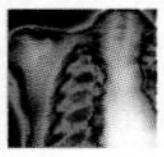

PROBLEM: A 55-year-old man presents to the emergency department complaining of increased shortness of breath and yellow-green sputum production for 1 week. He is alert and oriented. He has a 60 pack-year smoking history. Vital signs are blood pressure 165/90 mm Hg, pulse 120 beats/min, respirations 25 breaths/min, and temperature 100.5° F oral.

ABG values on room air are as follows:

pH	7.28
$PaCO_2$	70 mm Hg
PaO_2	35 mm Hg
HCO_3^-	36 mm Hg
SaO_2	66%

1. Define the respiratory condition indicated by the ABG results.
2. What is the $P(A - a)O_2$?
3. What type of respiratory failure is present?
4. What kind of therapy is indicated?

DISCUSSION

1. The ABG values indicate a partially compensated respiratory acidosis with hypoxemia.
2. $PAO_2 = 0.21\ (760 - 47) - 70/0.8 = 62$ mm Hg
   $PaO_2 = 35$ mm Hg
   $P(A - a)O_2 = 62 - 35 = 27$ mm Hg on room air
3. This is hypercapnic respiratory failure (type II), also known as ventilatory failure. However, in acute failure, the pH decreases 0.08 for every 10-mm Hg increase in $PaCO_2$. In this patient, $PaCO_2$ has increased 30 mm Hg (70 − 40), and the pH has decreased 0.12. The pH would be expected to decrease 0.24 (3 × 0.08) if this were acute ventilatory failure. This is a case of acute-on-chronic failure. HCO_3^- of 36 mEq/L (normal 22 to 26 mEq/L) also indicates renal compensation has occurred, which takes days to achieve. $P(A - a)O_2$ is 27 mm Hg, which is above normal, indicating that hypoxemia cannot be explained fully by hypoventilation.
4. Because the patient is alert, conservative therapy to improve lung function is indicated. O_2 administration to achieve SaO_2 of at least 90% is required. If PaO_2 does not respond to O_2 administration, shunt is present, and positive airway pressure may be necessary. Antibiotics are indicated for the probable infection (fever, discolored sputum), and bronchopulmonary hygiene (bronchodilators, steroids, cough assist) is indicated to improve ventilation.

Indications for Ventilatory Support

For each type of oxygenation and ventilatory failure, the goal of mechanical ventilation is either to support the patient until the underlying problem resolves or to maintain support of the patient with chronic ventilatory problems. These goals may be achieved by improving alveolar ventilation and arterial oxygenation, increasing lung volume, or reducing work of breathing.[27] This section discusses the indications for mechanical ventilation for hypoxemic (type I) and hypercapnic (type II) respiratory failure. Hypoxemic respiratory failure is divided into processes that require short-term and long-term ventilatory support. Hypercapnic respiratory failure is broken down into unstable ventilatory drive, muscle fatigue, excessive work of breathing, and alveolar hypoventilation. The relationship between work of breathing and the need for mechanical ventilation is discussed. Numerical indicators of the need for ventilatory support are reviewed. Management that is specific for each type of respiratory failure is described, including the indications for less commonly used modes of ventilation. Finally, the specific management of patients with obstructive lung disease and patients with head injury is discussed.

TABLE 41-3

Physiologic Indicators for Ventilatory Support, Classified by Mechanism Underlying Respiratory Failure

Mechanism	Normal Values	Support Indicated
Inadequate Alveolar Ventilation		
$PaCO_2$ (mm Hg)	35-45	>55
pH	7.35-7.45	<7.20
Inadequate Lung Expansion		
Tidal volume (V_T) ml/kg	5-8	<5
Vital capacity (VC) ml/kg	65-75	<10
Respiratory rate	12-20	>35
Inadequate Muscle Strength		
Maximum inspiratory pressure (cm H_2O)	−80-100	≥−20
Vital capacity (VC, ml/kg)	65-75	<10
Maximum voluntary ventilation (MVV, L/min)	120-180	<2× VE
Increased Work of Breathing		
Minute ventilation ($\dot{V}_E$)	5-6	>10
V_D/V_T (%)	0.25-0.40	>0.6
Hypoxemia		
$P(A - a)O_2$ on 100% O_2 (mm Hg)	25-65	>350
PaO_2/FiO_2	350-450	<200

VE, Minute ventilation.

Parameters Indicating Need for Ventilatory Support

Although various measurements have been proposed to help decide if a patient needs mechanical ventilation, the clinical status of the patient is the most important criterion. Table 41-3 and the discussion that follows review common physiologic indicators for initiating support by the underlying cause of respiratory failure.

Hypoxemic Respiratory Failure. Severe, refractory hypoxemia is a common indication for intubation and ventilator support. Table 41-3 lists different measures of hypoxemia that have been used to assess the need for ventilatory support. Most commonly, PaO_2 is compared with FiO_2 as with the PaO_2/FiO_2 ratio or the alveolar-arterial O_2 difference $[P(A - a)O_2]$. Indicators of profoundly impaired oxygenation suggesting the need for intubation, high inspired O_2 administration, and PEEP include $P(A - a)O_2$ value of 350 mm Hg on FiO_2 of 1.0 or a PaO_2/FiO_2 value of less than 200. These values are useful for all causes of **hypoxemic respiratory failure (type I)** but cannot help distinguish if the process is a readily reversible one, such as pulmonary edema or atelectasis, or a process, such as acute lung injury, that resolves more slowly. Frequently, patients have a combination of hypoxemic and hypercapnic respiratory failure.

Hypercapnic Respiratory Failure (Ventilatory Failure). As previously discussed, hypercapnic (type II) respiratory failure or ventilatory failure can be caused by increased ventilatory dead space, increased CO_2 production, or decreased alveolar ventilation. All of these processes cause an increase in $PaCO_2$.[25] Assessment of the pH allows a determination of whether the problem is acute or chronic. Chronic hypoventilation is compensated by the kidneys' retention of bicarbonate, although this response requires several days. The following example shows the importance of pH in interpreting the significance of elevated $PaCO_2$.

	Patient A	Patient B
$PaCO_2$	60 mm Hg	60 mm Hg
Serum HCO_3^-	25 mEq/L	36 mEq/L
pH	7.25	7.38

Although both patients in this example have the same level of hypercapnia, only patient A exhibits acute ventilatory failure with an elevated $PaCO_2$ but normal serum bicarbonate (25 mEq/L). Patient B has a compensated respiratory acidosis from chronic hypercapnic respiratory failure, as indicated by the normal pH and elevated serum bicarbonate (36 mEq/L). This condition is also known as *chronic ventilatory failure*. The distinction between acute and chronic ventilatory failure is very important in respiratory care and emphasizes the need to use both $PaCO_2$ and pH as indicators for ventilatory support. The trend in pH and $PaCO_2$ values is also useful in assessing the effects of therapies in correcting acute ventilatory failure.

Significance of Elevated Alveolar Partial Pressure of Carbon Dioxide. Because elevated $PaCO_2$ increases ventilatory drive in healthy subjects, the existence of hypoventilation suggests other problems with the respiratory apparatus. Specifically, the presence of acute respiratory acidosis indicates one of three major problems: (1) The respiratory center is not responding normally to elevated $PaCO_2$; (2) the respiratory center is responding normally, but the signal is not getting through to the respiratory muscles; or (3) despite normal neurologic response mechanisms, the lungs and chest bellows are incapable of providing adequate ventilation because of parenchymal lung disease or muscular weakness.[28]

ASSESSMENT OF RESPIRATORY FATIGUE, WEAKNESS, AND FAILURE AND WORK OF BREATHING

Respiratory Muscle Weakness

Respiratory muscle weakness refers to the decreased capacity of a rested muscle to generate force and decreased endurance.[29] Respiratory muscle weakness occurs most commonly in patients with neuromuscular disease. Other conditions that lead to muscle weakness by increasing demand include COPD, kyphoscoliosis, and obesity.

The most commonly used tests to assess respiratory muscle strength at the bedside are **maximum inspiratory pressure (MIP)** and **maximum expiratory pressure (MEP),**[30] forced vital capacity, and **maximum voluntary ventilation (MVV)** (see Table 41-3). MIP of −30 cm H_2O or less (more negative) usually indicates adequate respiratory muscle strength to continue spontaneous breathing, but the overall trend needs to be considered. This consideration is especially important in patients with myasthenic crisis or Guillain-Barré syndrome, where values of MIP that are becoming less negative may be the only clue to impending respiratory failure. The MVV maneuver can be performed at the bedside with a hand-held spirometer, but its use in the critical care setting is limited because substantial patient cooperation is required. The sniff nasal inspiratory pressure may also be used to assess inspiratory muscle strength. Advantages include ease of performance even in patients with advanced disease and its prognostic value.[31]

Respiratory Muscle Fatigue

Fatigue is usually defined as a condition in which there is loss of the capacity to develop force or velocity of a muscle resulting from muscle activity under load, which is reversible by rest.[32] Fatigue can be assessed by measuring the loss of force in response to repeated stimulations. It can be caused by both specific demands placed on the muscle and reduced supply of necessary nutrients. The demand on a muscle is increased by increased work of breathing, increased strength of muscle contraction, and decreased muscle efficiency. Hypoxemia, decreased inspiratory muscle blood flow, poor nutrition, and inability of a muscle to extract energy from supplied substrates can lead to fatigue as well.[29]

There are three types of respiratory **muscle fatigue.** (1) Central muscle fatigue is an exertion-induced, reversible decrease in central respiratory drive; (2) transmission muscle fatigue is an exertion-induced, reversible impairment in the transmission of neural impulses; and (3) contractile muscle fatigue is a reversible impairment in the contractile response to a neural impulse in an overloaded muscle.[28]

Respiratory Failure

Respiratory failure is an unfavorable imbalance between a respiratory workload, on the one hand, and ventilatory muscle strength and endurance, on the other hand. The **tension-time index** takes into account the fact that respiratory muscle endurance depends both on the size of the respiratory load in relation to respiratory strength (P_{di}/P_{dimax}) and on the duration of the inspiratory effort in relation to total breath time (the duty cycle, or T_i/T_{tot}). This index $(P_{di}/P_{dimax}) \times (T_i/T_{tot})$ determines whether a respiratory load can be tolerated without development of failure: Values less than 0.15 are generally tolerated for a long period, whereas indices greater than 0.18 usually result in fatigue and respiratory failure within 45 minutes.[33] Comparing the spontaneous minute ventilation with MVV is also a helpful index because fatigue and failure are both likely to occur if the minute ventilation exceeds 60% of MVV.[34]

These closely related concepts of weakness, fatigue, and failure usually overlap and can result in acute or chronic respiratory failure. Respiratory muscle weakness can predispose to ventilatory muscle fatigue. Whether fatigue consistently leads to failure has historically been the subject of much debate.[35] In one study, weaning failure was not accompanied by fatigue of the diaphragm despite the presence of diaphragm weakness.[36] Alternatively, fatigue of the diaphragm lasting for 24 hours is reliably present after hyperventilation at 60% of MVV or greater until task failure.[34,37]

Work of Breathing

Work of breathing is the amount of pressure needed to move a given volume into the lung with a relaxed chest wall. Excessive work of breathing is the most common cause of respiratory muscle fatigue. Work of breathing is due to physiologic work and imposed work. Physiologic work involves overcoming the elastic forces during inspiration and overcoming the resistance of the airways and lung tissue. Normal work of breathing is 0.3 to 0.6 J/L. Airway and pulmonary parenchymal abnormalities can increase the physiologic work of breathing. In intubated patients, sources of imposed work of breathing include the endotracheal tube, ventilator circuit, and **auto-PEEP** secondary to **dynamic hyperinflation** with airflow obstruction, as is commonly seen in a patient with COPD.[26] Increased work of breathing can also be an impediment to weaning.[38] Measurement of work of breathing with an esophageal balloon catheter and a flow transducer has been used to determine work of breathing and break it down into physiologic and imposed components.[38] Kirton and colleagues[39] showed that 96% of patients with a physiologic work of breathing less than 0.8 J/L were successfully weaned and extubated from ventilatory support.

CHOOSING A VENTILATORY SUPPORT STRATEGY FOR DIFFERENT CAUSES OF RESPIRATORY FAILURE

The remainder of this chapter briefly discusses current ventilatory strategies for hypoxemic and hypercapnic respiratory failure. The clinical application of specific modes of mechanical ventilation is described in Chapters 42 and 44, and noninvasive ventilation (NIV) is reviewed in more detail in Chapter 45. When it has been determined that the patient needs ventilatory support, the initial decision is whether to intubate or to ventilate noninvasively. In the acute setting, this decision is sometimes based on the underlying process, the type of respiratory failure, and how rapidly the underlying process can be reversed.

Noninvasive Ventilation

A consensus report supports the use of noninvasive support of ventilation to reduce the morbidity and possibly the mortality of both hypoxemic and hypercarbic respiratory failure.[40] In this context, **noninvasive ventilation (NIV)** can be defined as any mode of ventilatory support that is provided without endotracheal intubation, encompassing continuous positive airway pressure (CPAP) alone or in combination with any mode of pressure-limited or volume-limited ventilation.[40] NIV can improve hypoxemia and hypercarbia via several mechanisms including but not limited to (1) compensating for the inspiratory threshold load imposed by intrinsic PEEP,[41] (2) supplementing a reduced tidal volume,[42] (3) partial or complete unloading of the respiratory muscles,[42] (4) reducing venous return and left ventricular afterload,[43,44] (5) alveolar recruitment,[45] (6) preventing intermittent narrowing and collapse in patients with concomitant obstructive sleep apnea hypopnea syndrome by acting as a pneumatic splint during sleep,[46] and (7) improving lung function (particularly functional residual capacity) and daytime gas exchange in obstructive sleep apnea hypopnea syndrome.[47] NIV currently has indications in both acute[48] and chronic[49] respiratory failure.

Noninvasive Ventilation in Acute Conditions

Exacerbations of Chronic Obstructive Pulmonary Disease

NIV is considered to be a standard of care practice in patients with exacerbations of COPD.[50] A meta-analysis of eight randomized controlled trials showed that NIV combined with usual care in exacerbations of COPD resulted in a lower relative risk (RR) of treatment failure (defined as mortality, need for intubation, or intolerance) of 0.51 in favor of NIV (number needed to treat [NNT] to prevent 1 treatment failure was 5), reduced risk of intubation (RR 0.43, NNT = 5), reduction in mortality (RR 0.41,

NNT = 8), reduced risk of complications (RR 032, NNT = 3), and reduced hospital length of stay by about 3 days.[50]

Current recommendations are to initiate NIV before the development of severe acidosis in the course of a COPD exacerbation with $PaCO_2$ greater than 45 mm Hg.[50] Otherwise, in patients with mild COPD exacerbations (pH > 7.35), NIV was no more effective than standard medical therapy in preventing the occurrence of acute respiratory failure, improving mortality, or reducing length of hospitalization.[51] Nearly 50% of the patients did not tolerate NIV.[51]

Cardiogenic Pulmonary Edema

NIV is a recommended option in the management of acute respiratory failure in the setting of cardiogenic pulmonary edema. In the largest randomized trial comparing CPAP or NIV with standard O_2 therapy in acute pulmonary edema (N = 1156 patients), the combined noninvasive treatment arms (CPAP and NIV) significantly reduced dyspnea score, heart rate, acidosis, and hypercapnia within the first hour after the start of treatment.[52] However, there was no significant treatment effect compared with standard therapy in the 7-day or 30-day mortality in the rates of intubation, rate of admission to the critical care unit, or mean length of hospital stay.[52] The results of this large study are in contrast to smaller randomized trials and meta-analyses that showed decreased intubation and mortality rates with NIV.[53] Factors that may account for those differences include the much smaller intubation rates in the study by Gray and colleagues (2.9% overall vs. 20% with conventional therapy in other trials),[52] the higher mortality in the Gray study, and methodologic differences (patients failing standard therapy in the Gray study received rescue NIV). There was no difference in outcomes between CPAP and NIV devices in this setting.[52,53]

Acute Asthma

In a prospective study of episodes of asthma associated with acute respiratory failure, NIV progressively improved pH and $PaCO_2$ over 12 to 24 hours and reduced the respiratory rate.[54] In a subsequent controlled trial, NIV improved lung function, resolved the attack faster, and reduced the need for hospitalization.[55] Despite those promising results, the use of NIV in status asthmaticus remains controversial, and large, prospective, randomized controlled trials are needed to confirm the role of NIV in that setting.[56]

Acute Lung Injury and Acute Respiratory Distress Syndrome

NIV in the settings of acute lung injury and ARDS has been disappointing; a meta-analysis of the topic concluded that such an approach was associated with a 50% failure rate.[57] An earlier study that used CPAP in patients with acute respiratory failure predominantly caused by acute lung injury showed early physiologic improvements but no reduction in the need for intubation, no improvement in outcomes, and an increase in adverse events including cardiac arrest in patients randomly assigned to CPAP.[58] A prospective study showed that NIV was successful in improving gas exchange and avoiding intubation in 54% of patients, with consequent reduction in ventilator-associated pneumonia and lower ICU mortality rate.[59] Factors that may be associated with NIV failure in these settings include the presence of shock, metabolic acidosis, severe hypoxemia, a Simplified Acute Physiology Score (SAPS) II greater than 34, and a PaO_2/FiO_2 less than 175 after 1 hour of NIV.[59,60]

Noninvasive Ventilation in Chronic Conditions

Obesity-Hypoventilation Syndrome

Obesity-hypoventilation syndrome refers to the presence of daytime hypercapnia ($PaCO_2$ > 45 mm Hg) in obese individuals when no other cause of hypoventilation is present. In a meta-analysis, factors associated with daytime hypercapnia included body mass index, the presence of nocturnal apnea hypopnea, mean overnight O_2 saturation, and severity of restrictive pulmonary function.[61] In a study of patients with obesity-hypoventilation syndrome who failed initial CPAP treatment, average volume-assured pressure support, a form of NIV in which pressure support is automatically adjusted to reach a set tidal volume, was found to lower $PaCO_2$ compared with bilevel positive airway pressure alone but without improving oxygenation, sleep quality, or quality of life.[62]

Stable Chronic Obstructive Pulmonary Disease

A randomized controlled trial of NIV in patients with severe COPD and $PaCO_2$ greater than 46 mm Hg showed a survival benefit in favor of NIV and O_2 compared with O_2 alone (hazard ratio 0.6).[63] However, there was a low level of adherence to NIV, an apparent worsening in certain quality-of-life indices, and no reduction in hospitalization rates,[63] perhaps owing to selection of inspiratory pressures that were insufficient to reduce hypercapnia. In a randomized trial, compared with low-intensity NIV (mean inspiratory positive airway pressure 14 cm H_2O, backup rate 8/min), the use of settings that aimed to reduce $PaCO_2$ maximally (mean inspiratory positive airway pressure 29 cm H_2O with backup rate 17.5/min) increased the daily use of NIV by 3.6 hr/day and improved exercise-related dyspnea, daytime $PaCO_2$, forced expiratory volume in 1 second, vital capacity and health-related quality of life.[64]

Neuromuscular Diseases and Thoracic Cage Abnormalities

This condition most commonly applies to chronic neuromuscular disease, with several studies showing that even in progressive neuromuscular disorders, NIV can prolong survival, improve quality of life, enhance cognitive function, and reduce pneumonia and hospitalization rates.[12]

Other NIV techniques using rocking beds, pneumobelts, and negative pressure ventilation are much less frequently used and are becoming less easily available.

MINI CLINI

Indications for Continuous Positive Airway Pressure versus Continuous Mechanical Ventilation With Positive End Expiratory Pressure

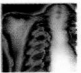

PROBLEM: A patient in the ICU is severely tachypneic and hypoxemic. The respiratory rate is 30 breaths/min. On approximately 50% O_2 by mask at sea level, PaO_2 is 50 mm Hg, $PaCO_2$ is 30 mm Hg, pH is 7.51, and HCO_3^- is 23 mEq/L. The patient is in distress but alert and able to cooperate and follow instructions.

1. What is this patient's $P(A - a)O_2$?
2. What type of respiratory failure is this?
3. What is the appropriate initial therapy?

DISCUSSION: This patient does not have hypercapnic respiratory failure, as is confirmed by $PaCO_2$ of 30 mm Hg. The patient does have a serious oxygenation defect, as confirmed by $P(A - a)O_2$.

$$PAO_2 = 0.50\ (713) - 30/0.8 = 318\ \text{mm Hg}$$
$$P(A-a)O_2 = 318 - 50 = 268\ \text{mm Hg}$$

The elevated $P(A - a)O_2$ indicates the presence of severe intrapulmonary shunt. Shunts this severe can occur only when significant airway closure and atelectasis are present. The mode of therapy should be aimed at reinflating collapsed alveoli and keeping the alveoli open throughout the breathing cycle. In this patient, alveolar ventilation is not impaired ($PaCO_2$ = 30 mm Hg). CPAP alone may be effective in reducing shunt. (CPAP does not ventilate the patient; all breaths are patient-initiated and spontaneous.) CPAP may be applied noninvasively via face mask, as would be indicated in this alert, cooperative patient. If hypercapnia and acidemia develop, mechanical ventilation with PEEP would be indicated.

Invasive Ventilatory Support

Patients with profound hypoxemia from a process that is expected to resolve slowly, such as acute lung injury, usually require intubation and mechanical ventilation. Other indications for intubation include conditions where NIV may be poorly tolerated or even deleterious, such as the presence of upper airway obstruction, inability to clear secretions and protect airway, inability to achieve a proper mask fit, and intolerance of the intervention. Both hypoxemic and hypercarbic types of respiratory failure can be managed effectively by invasive mechanical ventilation.

There are several ventilator variables, some independently set by the operators and others that are dependent on the set variables. Independent and dependent variables vary with the mode of ventilation. FiO_2 and PEEP are independently set variables regardless of mode of ventilation used to manage hypoxemia. In volume-controlled or flow-controlled ventilation, tidal volume, flow, and respiratory rate are independently set variables. In **pressure control ventilation,** driving pressure, inspiratory time, and respiratory rate are independently set variables. Other modes and strategies include inverse ratio ventilation, liquid ventilation, prone positioning, airway pressure release ventilation, and **high-frequency ventilation.** Considerations in selected cases of respiratory failure requiring invasive ventilatory support are briefly reviewed.

MINI CLINI

Acute Hypercapnic Respiratory Failure

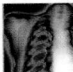

PROBLEM: A patient with COPD presents to the emergency department in moderate respiratory distress. He is alert and cooperative. Respiratory rate is 26 breaths/min. Lung examination shows poor air entry with expiratory wheezing. Room air ABGs show pH 7.24, $PaCO_2$ 60 mm Hg, and PaO_2 60 mm Hg.

1. What type of respiratory failure is this?
2. How should the patient be managed?

DISCUSSION: ABGs show an acute respiratory acidosis with normal $PaO_2 - PaO_2$ gradient.

$$PAO_2 = 0.21\ (713) - 60/0.8 = 74$$
$$P(A-a)O_2 = 74 - 60 = 14\ \text{mm Hg}$$

This patient has hypercapnic respiratory failure related to obstructive lung disease, also known as ventilatory failure. In addition to bronchodilators and corticosteroids, the RT should aim to improve ventilation to reverse the respiratory acidosis. In this patient, who is alert and cooperative, NIV via face mask may be tried. Initial mask ventilation can start in the pressure support ventilation mode with a level of support of 10 cm H_2O and 5 cm H_2O PEEP. Tidal volume should be maintained at approximately 6 to 8 ml/kg. If this patient deteriorates despite therapy, he would need to be intubated and mechanically ventilated.

Acute Respiratory Distress Syndrome

Profound hypoxemic respiratory failure is often due to severe pneumonia and ARDS. Patients with these conditions have very noncompliant lungs. Volume-cycled ventilation in patients with ARDS frequently leads to high peak airway and plateau pressures. It has been established that ventilating these patients with small tidal volumes (about 6 ml/kg) reduces complications associated with mechanical ventilation and improves survival.[65]

Increased Intracranial Pressure

Hyperventilation applied acutely and for short periods may be used to reduce ICP. The goal is to lower $PaCO_2$ to between 25 mm Hg and 30 mm Hg, which causes alkalosis, which in combination with hypocapnia helps reduce cerebral blood flow until ICP can be controlled by other measures. Ongoing ventilatory support should maintain PCO_2 in the range of 30 to 40 mm Hg. By maintaining PCO_2 in this range, sudden increases in ICP can be quickly controlled by short-term hyperventilation. Although reducing blood flow can reduce brain swelling and ICP, cerebral ischemia can also result. Another concern in ventilating patients with elevated ICP is using PEEP to manage hypoxemia. There is a concern that increased intrathoracic pressure secondary to PEEP would cause decreased cerebral venous return leading to increased ICP and that PEEP can decrease cerebral perfusion by limiting cardiac output. The use of PEEP in patients with elevated ICP may require invasive monitoring of ICP because the combination of decreased cerebral perfusion and elevated ICP can narrow cerebral perfusion pressure.[66] Elevation of the head of the bed can offset the increased ICP associated with the application of PEEP.

Obstructive Lung Disease

Patients with obstructive lung disease have markedly increased airway resistance that leads to a decrease in the rate of expiratory flow with resulting hyperinflation. These patients frequently have problems with elevated airway pressure or dynamic hyperinflation (auto-PEEP), which can cause barotrauma and increased dyssynchrony between the patient and ventilator.[67]

The management goal for patients with COPD with respiratory failure is to oxygenate and ventilate the patient successfully, while avoiding dyssynchrony and dynamic hyperinflation. In these patients, lower tidal volumes (6 to 8 ml/kg), moderate respiratory rates, and high sustained (square wave) inspiratory flow rates (70 to 100 L/min) are recommended to avoid dynamic hyperinflation.[68] These maneuvers reduce inspiratory time and prolong expiratory time, which allows a patient with obstructive lung disease to have a longer time to exhale.

Another consideration in patients with obstructive lung disease is the inspiratory threshold load imposed by auto-PEEP resulting in increased patient inspiratory work.[41] In this case, applied (or extrinsic) PEEP can compensate for this threshold load and reduce the work of breathing for patient-triggered breaths in any assisted ventilatory mode.[41]

Ventilatory Support in Chronic Hypercapnic Respiratory Failure

The goal of therapy in hypercapnic respiratory failure (acute ventilatory failure) is to guarantee a set minute ventilation. In treating patients with chronic ventilatory failure, the goal is to normalize the pH but not the $PaCO_2$. Correction of $PaCO_2$ in a patient with chronic hypoventilation from diverse causes can lead to a posthypercapnic metabolic alkalosis, which can produce hypokalemia, seizures, and arrhythmias.

SUMMARY CHECKLIST

- Acute respiratory failure is identified by PaO_2 less than 60 mm Hg or $PaCO_2$ greater than 50 mm Hg, or both, in otherwise healthy individuals at sea level.
- Hypoxemic respiratory failure is most commonly due to $\dot{V}/\dot{Q}$ mismatch, shunt, or hypoventilation.
- Hypercapnic respiratory failure, also known as ventilatory failure, results from decreased ventilatory drive, neurologic disease, or increased work of breathing.
- Chronic respiratory failure may manifest with hypercapnia and evidence of a compensatory metabolic alkalosis (chronic ventilatory failure) or with polycythemia reflecting chronic hypoxemia.
- The clinical status of the patient is the most important factor determining the need for ventilatory support.
- Excessive work of breathing is the most common cause of respiratory muscle fatigue.
- The beneficial role of NIV in the acute setting has been best established in acute exacerbations of COPD and in cardiogenic edema.
- Increased FiO_2 and PEEP are the main therapies for severe hypoxemia.
- The goal of therapy in hypercapnic respiratory failure (acute ventilatory failure) is to normalize the pH.

References

1. Vasilyev S, Schaap RN, Mortensen JD: Hospital survival rates of patients with acute respiratory failure in modern respiratory intensive care units: an international, multicenter, prospective survey. Chest 107:1083–1088, 1995.
2. Wunsch H, Linde-Zwirble WT, Angus DC, et al: The epidemiology of mechanical ventilation use in the United States. Crit Care Med. 38:1947–1953, 2010.
3. Greene KE, Peters JI: Pathophysiology of acute respiratory failure. Clin Chest Med 15:1–12, 1994.
4. Campbell EJ: Respiratory failure. BMJ 5448:1451–1460, 1965.
5. West JB: Respiratory physiology: the essentials, ed 7, Philadelphia, 2005, Lippincott Williams & Wilkins.
6. Aboussouan LS, Stoller JK: The hepatopulmonary syndrome. Baillieres Best Pract Res Clin Gastroenterol 14:1033–1048, 2000.
7. American Thoracic Society: Idiopathic pulmonary fibrosis: diagnosis and treatment. International consensus statement. American Thoracic Society (ATS), and the European Respiratory Society (ERS). Am J Respir Crit Care Med 161(2 Pt 1): 646–664, 2000.
8. Aboussouan LS, Stoller JK: Traveling with supplemental oxygen for patients with chronic lung disease. In Maurer JR, editor: Non-neoplastic advanced lung disease, New York, 2003, Marcel Dekker, pp 711–730.
9. Caruana-Montaldo B, Gleeson K, Zwillich CW: The control of breathing in clinical practice. Chest 117:205–225, 2000.
10. Dick CR, Sassoon CS: Patient-ventilator interactions. Clin Chest Med 17:423–438, 1996.
11. Rapoport DM, Garay SM, Epstein H, et al: Hypercapnia in the obstructive sleep apnea syndrome. A reevaluation of the "Pickwickian syndrome," Chest 89:627–635, 1986.

12. Aboussouan LS: Respiratory disorders in neurologic diseases. Cleve Clin J Med 72:511–520, 2005.
13. Kaplan LM, Hollander D: Respiratory dysfunction in amyotrophic lateral sclerosis. Clin Chest Med 15:675–681, 1994.
14. Teitelbaum JS, Borel CO: Respiratory dysfunction in Guillain-Barre syndrome. Clin Chest Med 15:705–714, 1994.
15. Zulueta JJ, Fanburg BL: Respiratory dysfunction in myasthenia gravis. Clin Chest Med 15:683–691, 1994.
16. Curtis JR, Hudson LD: Emergent assessment and management of acute respiratory failure in COPD. Clin Chest Med 15:481–500, 1994.
17. Jozefowicz RF: Neurologic manifestations of pulmonary disease. Neurol Clin 7:605–616, 1989.
18. Jemal A, Ward E, Hao Y, et al: Trends in the leading causes of death in the United States, 1970-2002. JAMA 294:1255–1259, 2005.
19. Chen R, Grand'Maison F, Strong MJ, et al: Motor neuron disease presenting as acute respiratory failure: a clinical and pathological study. J Neurol Neurosurg Psychiatry 60:455–458, 1996.
20. Derenne JP, Fleury B, Pariente R: Acute respiratory failure of chronic obstructive pulmonary disease. Am Rev Respir Dis 138:1006–1033, 1988.
21. Schmidt GA, Hall JB: Acute or chronic respiratory failure: assessment and management of patients with COPD in the emergency setting. JAMA 261:3444–3453, 1989.
22. Connors AF, Jr, Dawson NV, Thomas C, et al: Outcomes following acute exacerbation of severe chronic obstructive lung disease. The SUPPORT Investigators (Study to Understand Prognoses and Preferences for Outcomes and Risks of Treatments). Am J Respir Crit Care Med 154(4 Pt 1):959–967, 1996.
23. Hudson LD: Survival data in patients with acute and chronic lung disease requiring mechanical ventilation. Am Rev Respir Dis 140(2 Pt 2):S19–S24, 1989.
24. Pingleton SK: Complications of acute respiratory failure. Rev Respir Dis 137:1463–1493, 1988.
25. Roussos C: Respiratory muscle fatigue and ventilatory failure. Chest 97(3 Suppl):89S–96S, 1990.
26. Banner MJ: Respiratory muscle loading and the work of breathing. J Cardiothorac Vasc Anesth 9:192–204, 1995.
27. Slutsky AS: Consensus conference on mechanical ventilation—January 28-30, 1993 at Northbrook, Illinois, USA. Part I. European Society of Intensive Care Medicine, the ACCP and the SCCM. Intensive Care Med 20:64–79, 1994.
28. Mador MJ: Respiratory muscle fatigue and breathing pattern. Chest 100:1430–1435, 1991.
29. Stoller JK: Physiologic rationale for resting the ventilatory muscles. Respir Care 36:290–296, 1991.
30. Gibson GJ: Measurement of respiratory muscle strength. Respir Med 89:529–535, 1995.
31. Morgan RK, McNally S, Alexander M, et al: Use of Sniff nasal-inspiratory force to predict survival in amyotrophic lateral sclerosis. Am J Respir Crit Care Med 171:269–274, 2005.
32. NHLBI Workshop summary: Respiratory muscle fatigue. Report of the Respiratory Muscle Fatigue Workshop Group. Am Rev Respir Dis 142:474–480, 1990.
33. Bellemare F, Grassino A: Effect of pressure and timing of contraction on human diaphragm fatigue. J Appl Physiol 53:1190–1195, 1982.
34. Mador JM, Rodis A, Diaz J: Diaphragmatic fatigue following voluntary hyperpnea. Am J Respir Crit Care Med 154:63–67, 1996.
35. Macklem PT, Roussos CS: Respiratory muscle fatigue: a cause of respiratory failure? Clin Sci Mol Med 53:419–422, 1977.
36. Laghi F, Cattapan SE, Jubran A, et al: Is weaning failure caused by low-frequency fatigue of the diaphragm? Am J Respir Crit Care Med 167:120–127, 2003.
37. Laghi F, D'Alfonso N, Tobin MJ: Pattern of recovery from diaphragmatic fatigue over 24 hours. J Appl Physiol 79:539–546, 1995.
38. Petros AJ, Lamond CT, Bennett D: The Bicore pulmonary monitor: a device to assess the work of breathing while weaning from mechanical ventilation. Anaesthesia 48:985–988, 1993.
39. Kirton OC, DeHaven CB, Morgan JP, et al: Elevated imposed work of breathing masquerading as ventilator weaning intolerance. Chest 108:1021–1025, 1995.
40. International Consensus Conferences in Intensive Care Medicine: noninvasive positive pressure ventilation in acute respiratory failure. Am J Respir Crit Care Med 163:283–291, 2001.
41. MacIntyre NR, Cheng KC, McConnell R: Applied PEEP during pressure support reduces the inspiratory threshold load of intrinsic PEEP. Chest 111:188–193, 1997.
42. MacIntyre NR, Leatherman NE: Ventilatory muscle loads and the frequency-tidal volume pattern during inspiratory pressure-assisted (pressure-supported) ventilation. Am Rev Respir Dis 141:327–331, 1990.
43. Lenique F, Habis M, Lofaso F, et al: Ventilatory and hemodynamic effects of continuous positive airway pressure in left heart failure. Am J Respir Crit Care Med 155:500–505, 1997.
44. Naughton MT, Rahman MA, Hara K, et al: Effect of continuous positive airway pressure on intrathoracic and left ventricular transmural pressures in patients with congestive heart failure. Circulation 91:1725–1731, 1995.
45. De Michele M, Grasso S: Measurement of PEEP-induced alveolar recruitment: just a research tool? Crit Care 10:148, 2006.
46. Sullivan CE, Berthon-Jones M, Issa FG: Remission of severe obesity-hypoventilation syndrome after short-term treatment during sleep with nasal continuous positive airway pressure. Am Rev Respir Dis 128:177–181, 1983.
47. Verbraecken J, Willemen M, De Cock W, et al: Continuous positive airway pressure and lung inflation in sleep apnea patients. Respiration 68:357–364, 2001.
48. Aboussouan LS, Ricaurte B: Noninvasive positive pressure ventilation: increasing use in acute care. Cleve Clin J Med 77:307–316, 2010.
49. Theerakittikul T, Ricaurte B, Aboussouan LS: Noninvasive positive pressure ventilation for stable outpatients: CPAP and beyond. Cleve Clin J Med 77:705–710, 2010.
50. Lightowler JV, Wedzicha JA, Elliott MW, et al: Non-invasive positive pressure ventilation to treat respiratory failure resulting from exacerbations of chronic obstructive pulmonary disease: Cochrane systematic review and meta-analysis. BMJ 326:185, 2003.
51. Keenan SP, Sinuff T, Cook DJ, et al: Which patients with acute exacerbation of chronic obstructive pulmonary disease benefit from noninvasive positive-pressure ventilation? A systematic review of the literature. Ann Intern Med 138:861–870, 2003.
52. Gray A, Goodacre S, Newby DE, et al: Noninvasive ventilation in acute cardiogenic pulmonary edema. N Engl J Med 359:142–151, 2008.
53. Ho KM, Wong K: A comparison of continuous and bi-level positive airway pressure non-invasive ventilation in patients with acute cardiogenic pulmonary oedema: a meta-analysis. Crit Care 10:R49, 2006.
54. Meduri GU, Cook TR, Turner RE, et al: Noninvasive positive pressure ventilation in status asthmaticus. Chest 110:767–774, 1996.

55. Ram FS, Wellington S, Rowe B, et al: Non-invasive positive pressure ventilation for treatment of respiratory failure due to severe acute exacerbations of asthma. Cochrane Database Syst Rev CD004360, 2005.
56. Soroksky A, Stav D, Shpirer I: A pilot prospective, randomized, placebo-controlled trial of bilevel positive airway pressure in acute asthmatic attack. Chest 123:1018–1025, 2003.
57. Agarwal R, Aggarwal AN, Gupta D: Role of noninvasive ventilation in acute lung injury/acute respiratory distress syndrome: a proportion meta-analysis. Respir Care 55:1653–1660, 2010.
58. Delclaux C, L'Her E, Alberti C, et al: Treatment of acute hypoxemic nonhypercapnic respiratory insufficiency with continuous positive airway pressure delivered by a face mask: a randomized controlled trial. JAMA 284:2352–2360, 2000.
59. Rana S, Jenad H, Gay PC, et al: Failure of non-invasive ventilation in patients with acute lung injury: observational cohort study. Crit Care 10:R79, 2006.
60. Antonelli M, Conti G, Esquinas A, et al: A multiple-center survey on the use in clinical practice of noninvasive ventilation as a first-line intervention for acute respiratory distress syndrome. Crit Care Med 35:18–25, 2007.
61. Kaw R, Hernandez AV, Walker E, et al: Determinants of hypercapnia in obese patients with obstructive sleep apnea: a systematic review and metaanalysis of cohort studies. Chest 136:787–796, 2009.
62. Storre JH, Seuthe B, Fiechter R, et al: Average volume-assured pressure support in obesity hypoventilation: a randomized crossover trial. Chest 130:815–821, 2006.
63. McEvoy RD, Pierce RJ, Hillman D, et al: Nocturnal non-invasive nasal ventilation in stable hypercapnic COPD: a randomised controlled trial. Thorax 64:561–566, 2009.
64. Dreher M, Storre JH, Schmoor C, et al: High-intensity versus low-intensity non-invasive ventilation in patients with stable hypercapnic COPD: a randomised crossover trial. Thorax 65:303–308, 2010.
65. Acute Respiratory Distress Syndrome Network: Ventilation with lower tidal volumes as compared with traditional tidal volumes for acute lung injury and the acute respiratory distress syndrome. N Engl J Med 342:1301–1308, 2000.
66. Borel C, Hanley D, Diringer MN, et al: Intensive management of severe head injury. Chest 98:180–189, 1990.
67. Leatherman JW: Mechanical ventilation in obstructive lung disease. Clin Chest Med 17:577–590, 1996.
68. Shapiro JM: Management of respiratory failure in status asthmaticus. Am J Respir Med 1:409–416, 2002.

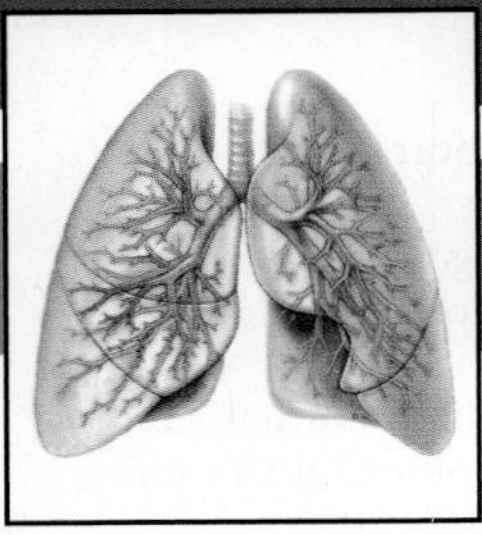

Chapter 42

Mechanical Ventilators

ROBERT L. CHATBURN AND TERESA A. VOLSKO

CHAPTER OBJECTIVES

After reading this chapter you will be able to:

- Discuss the basic design features of ventilators.
- Classify ventilators and describe how they work.
- Define what constitutes a mode of ventilation.
- Classify and discuss modes of ventilation.
- Classify and discuss types of mechanical ventilators.

CHAPTER OUTLINE

KEY TERMS

breath sequence
breathing pattern
closed loop control
compliance
continuous mandatory ventilation (CMV)
continuous spontaneous ventilation (CSV)
control variable
cycle variable
dual control
elastance
intermittent mandatory ventilation (IMV)
mandatory breath
open loop control
phase variable
pressure-controlled ventilation
resistance
spontaneous breath
target variable
targeting scheme
time constant
trigger variable
volume-controlled ventilation

To initiate and manage a mechanical ventilator safely and effectively, the respiratory therapist (RT) must thoroughly understand (1) ventilator design, classification, and operation; (2) appropriate clinical application of ventilatory modes (i.e., the proper matching of ventilator capability with physiologic need); and (3) the physiologic effects of mechanical ventilation, including gas exchange and pulmonary mechanics. This chapter focuses on the first and second of these. This chapter explains classification terminology and outlines a framework for understanding current and future ventilatory support devices.[1-3] For the application of ventilators, the specific indications and clinical use of the various modes of full and partial ventilatory support are outlined.

HOW VENTILATORS WORK

To understand how ventilators work, one must have some knowledge of basic mechanics. A ventilator is simply a *machine,* which is a system designed to alter, transmit, and direct applied energy in a predetermined manner to perform useful work.[4] Ventilators are provided with energy in the form of either electricity or compressed gas. The energy is transmitted or transformed (by the drive mechanism of the ventilator) in a predetermined manner (by the control circuit) to augment or replace the patient's muscles in performing the work of breathing (the desired output). To understand mechanical ventilators, the following four basic functions of ventilators must be understood:

- Input power
- Power transmission and conversion
- Control system
- Output (pressure, volume, and flow waveforms)

This simple outline format can be expanded to add as much detail about a given ventilator as desired.

Input Power

The power source for a ventilator is either electrical energy (energy = volts × amperes × time) or compressed gas (energy = pressure × volume).[5]

Electrical Energy

An electrically powered ventilator uses voltage from an electrical line outlet. In the United States, this line voltage is normally 110 to 115 V alternating current (AC) (60 Hz). In addition to powering the ventilator, this AC voltage may be reduced and converted to direct current (DC). This DC source can be used to power delicate electronic control circuits. Some ventilators, notably transport ventilators, have rechargeable batteries to be used as a source of power if AC is unavailable. In the home care setting, battery backup for electrically powered ventilators is an essential lifesaving feature in the event of a power outage.

Pneumatic Power

A pneumatically powered ventilator uses compressed gas as its power source. Most modern intensive care unit (ICU) ventilators are pneumatically powered. Ventilators powered by compressed gas usually have internal pressure-reducing valves so that the normal operating pressure is lower than the source pressure. Ventilators can operate without interruption from hospital-piped gas sources, which are usually regulated to 50 psi (pounds per square inch) but are subject to periodic fluctuations.

Most pneumatically powered ICU ventilators still require electrical power to support their control functions (see the following section on control mechanisms). However, a few pneumatically powered ventilators can function without electrical power. These devices are ideal in situations where electrical power is unavailable (e.g., during certain types of patient transport) or as a backup to electrically powered ventilators in case of power failures. They are also particularly useful where electrical power is undesirable, such as near magnetic resonance imaging (MRI) equipment.

> **RULE OF THUMB**
>
> For patient transport, you must use either a pneumatically powered ventilator or one that can run solely on batteries. Always take along a manually powered bag-valve mask, and for long transports be sure to have back-up power available (extra cylinders or batteries).

Power Transmission and Conversion

The power transmission and conversion system consists of the drive and output control mechanisms. The drive mechanism generates the actual force needed to deliver gas under pressure. The output control consists of one or more valves that regulate gas flow to the patient.

Drive Mechanism

The drive mechanism of the ventilator converts the input power to useful work. The characteristic flow and pressure patterns the ventilator produces are determined in part by the type of drive mechanism it contains. Drive mechanisms can be either (1) a direct application of compressed gas via a pressure-reducing valve or (2) an indirect application via an electrical motor or compressor. Descriptions of these devices are provided in textbooks devoted to respiratory care equipment.[6]

Output Control Valve

The output control valve regulates the flow of gas to the patient. It may be a simple on/off exhalation valve, as in the Newport E100i (Newport NMI Ventilators; Newport Medical Instruments, Newport Beach, CA). Alternatively, the output control valve can shape the output waveform, as in the Maquet SERVO-i (Maquet, Bridgewater, NJ). Commonly used output control valves include the pneumatic diaphragm, electromagnetic poppet/plunger valve, and proportional valve.[6]

Control System

Knowledge of the mechanics of breathing provides a good foundation for understanding how ventilators work. Specifically, the pressure needed to drive gas into the airway and inflate the lungs is important. The formula that relates these variables is known as the equation of motion for the respiratory system (Figure 42-1):[7]

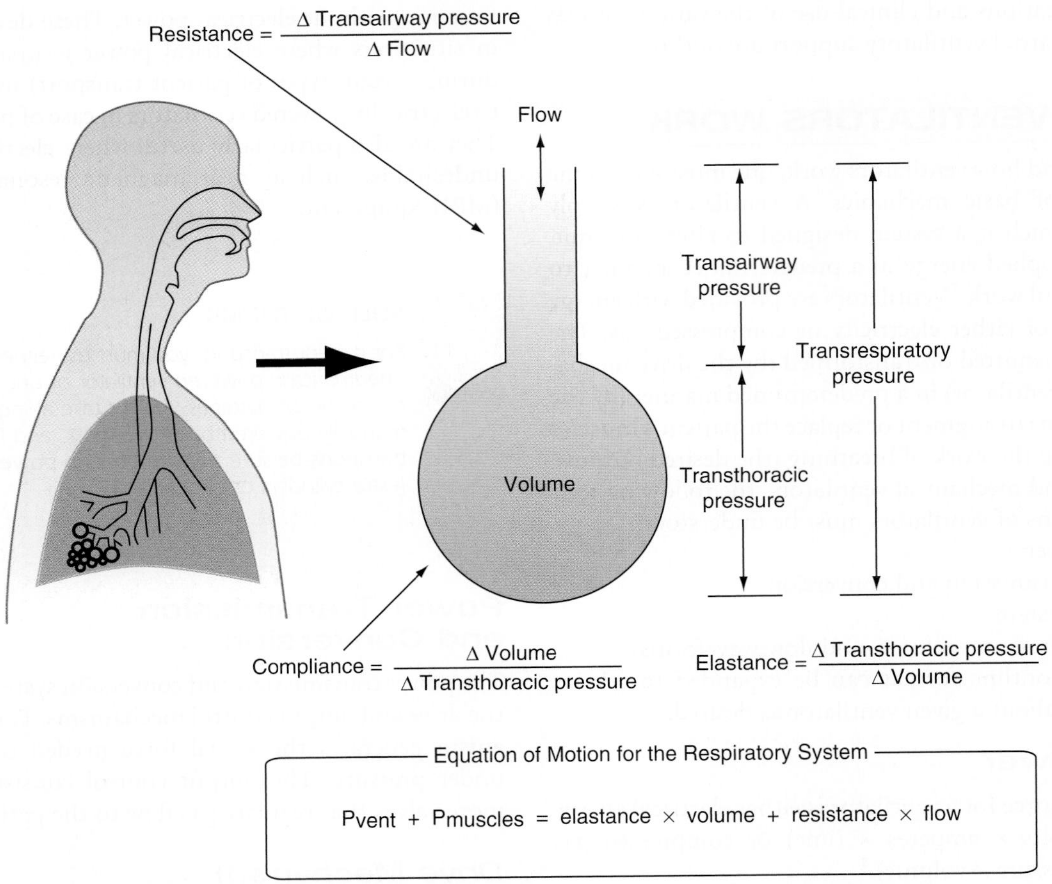

FIGURE 42-1 The respiratory system can be modeled as a single-flow conducting tube connected to a single elastic compartment. This physical model can be described by a mathematical model called the equation of motion for the respiratory system. In this model, pressure, volume, and flow are variables (i.e., functions of time), whereas resistance and elastance (or compliance) are constants.

$$P_{VENT} + P_{MUS} = (E \times V) + (R \times \dot{V}) + \text{auto-PEEP}$$

Equation 42-1, *A*

where P_{VENT} is the pressure generated by the ventilator above positive end expiratory pressure (PEEP), P_{MUS} is the pressure generated by the ventilatory muscles to expand the lungs and chest wall, E is respiratory system elastance, V is the change in lung volume above functional residual capacity (FRC), R is respiratory system resistance, and $\dot{V}$ is flow (usually zero unless auto-PEEP is present). Auto-PEEP is the difference between end expiratory airway pressure and end expiratory lung pressure. The combined muscle and ventilator pressures cause gas to flow into the lungs. **Elastance** (elastance = Δpressure/Δvolume) and **resistance** (resistance = Δpressure/Δflow) together constitute the impedance or load against which the muscles and ventilator do work. The equation of motion is sometimes expressed in terms of **compliance** (compliance = Δvolume/Δpressure) instead of elastance.

The auto-PEEP term in the equation of motion indicates that if auto-PEEP is present, more force is required by the ventilator or the muscles or both to generate a given tidal volume and flow. Under passive conditions (P_{MUS} = 0) for volume control ventilation, where the terms E × V and E × $\dot{V}$ are constant because of the preset values of tidal volume and inspiratory flow, as auto-PEEP increases, peak inspiratory pressure increases. For pressure control ventilation, the airway pressure waveform is constant because of the preset value of inspiratory pressure. As auto-PEEP increases, both inspired tidal volume and peak inspiratory flow decrease. If inspiration is unassisted (P_{VENT} = 0), the equation shows that P_{MUS} must exceed auto-PEEP before inspiratory flow can begin. If the patient is connected to a ventilator, P_{MUS} must be greater than auto-PEEP to trigger an assisted breath. In these cases, auto-PEEP increases the patient's work of breathing. However, auto-PEEP is not always undesirable, as in the application of airway pressure release ventilation where expiratory time is intentionally shortened to create gas trapping in the absence of a set PEEP. Auto-PEEP is also present as an unavoidable and perhaps desirable factor during high-frequency ventilation.

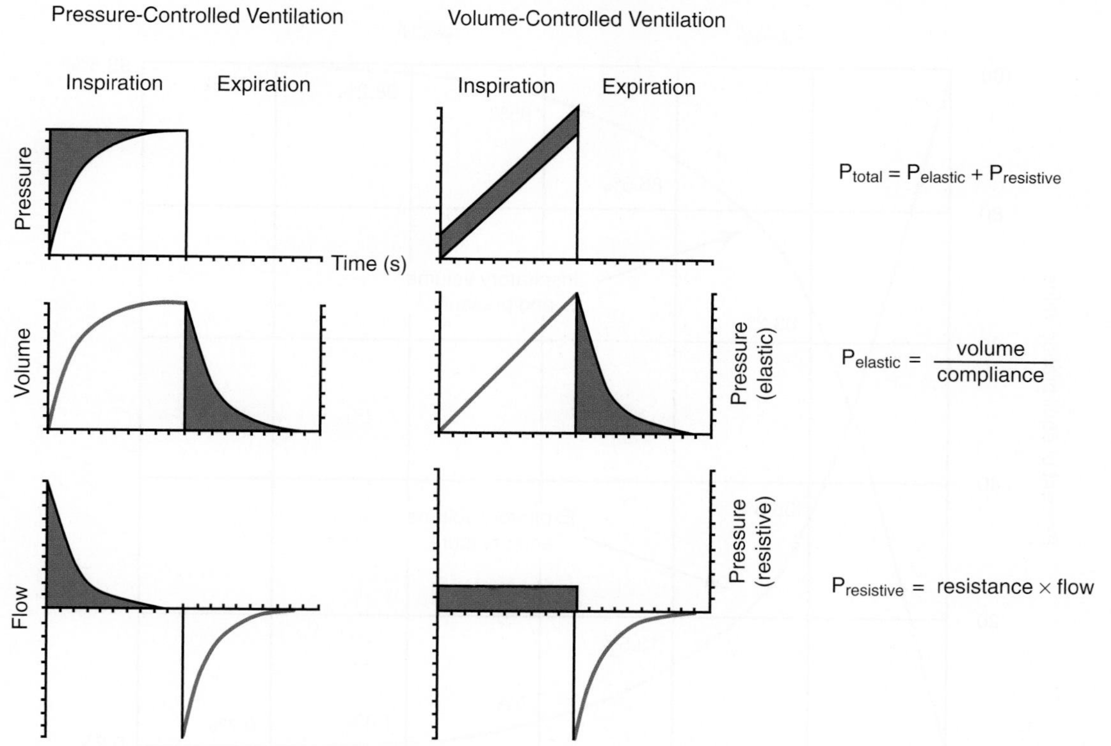

FIGURE 42-2 Characteristic waveforms for volume-controlled ventilation and pressure-controlled ventilation. The volume waveform has the same shape as the transthoracic or lung pressure waveform (i.e., pressure owing to elastic recoil). The flow waveform has the same shape as the transairway pressure waveform (i.e., pressure owing to airway resistance). *Shaded areas* represent pressure owing to resistance; *open areas* represent pressure owing to elastic recoil. The mean pressure at the airway is the same as that in the lung, and mean pressure for volume-controlled ventilation is less than that for pressure-controlled ventilation.

Pressure, volume, and flow all are changeable variables measured relative to their baseline or end expiratory values. When pressure, volume, and flow are plotted as functions of time, characteristic waveforms for **volume-controlled ventilation** and **pressure-controlled ventilation** are produced (Figure 42-2). The conventional order of presentation is pressure, volume, and flow from top to bottom. Convention also dictates that positive flow values (above the horizontal axis) correspond to inspiration and that negative flow values (below the horizontal axis) correspond to expiration. The vertical axes are in units of the measured variables (usually cm H_2O for pressure, L or ml for volume, and L/min or L/sec for flow). The horizontal axis of these graphs is time. Many ventilators have monitors that display pressure, volume, and flow waveforms, providing the clinician with information to evaluate ventilator-patient interaction.

Figure 42-2 shows that the expiratory lung pressure curves are the same shape for both volume and pressure control. This shape is called an *exponential decay waveform* (often called a *decelerating waveform*), and it is characteristic of passive emptying of the lungs (exhalation). Solving the equation of motion for lung pressure (assuming no auto-PEEP) provides the following expression:

$$P_L = \frac{V_T}{C} e^{-t/RC} \qquad \text{Equation 42-2}$$

where P_L is lung pressure during passive exhalation, V_T is tidal volume, *e* is the base of the natural logarithms (approximately 2.72), t is time (in this case, the time allowed for exhalation), R is respiratory system resistance, and C is respiratory system compliance. The product of R and C has units of time and is called the **time constant.** It is referred to as a "constant" because after a period of time

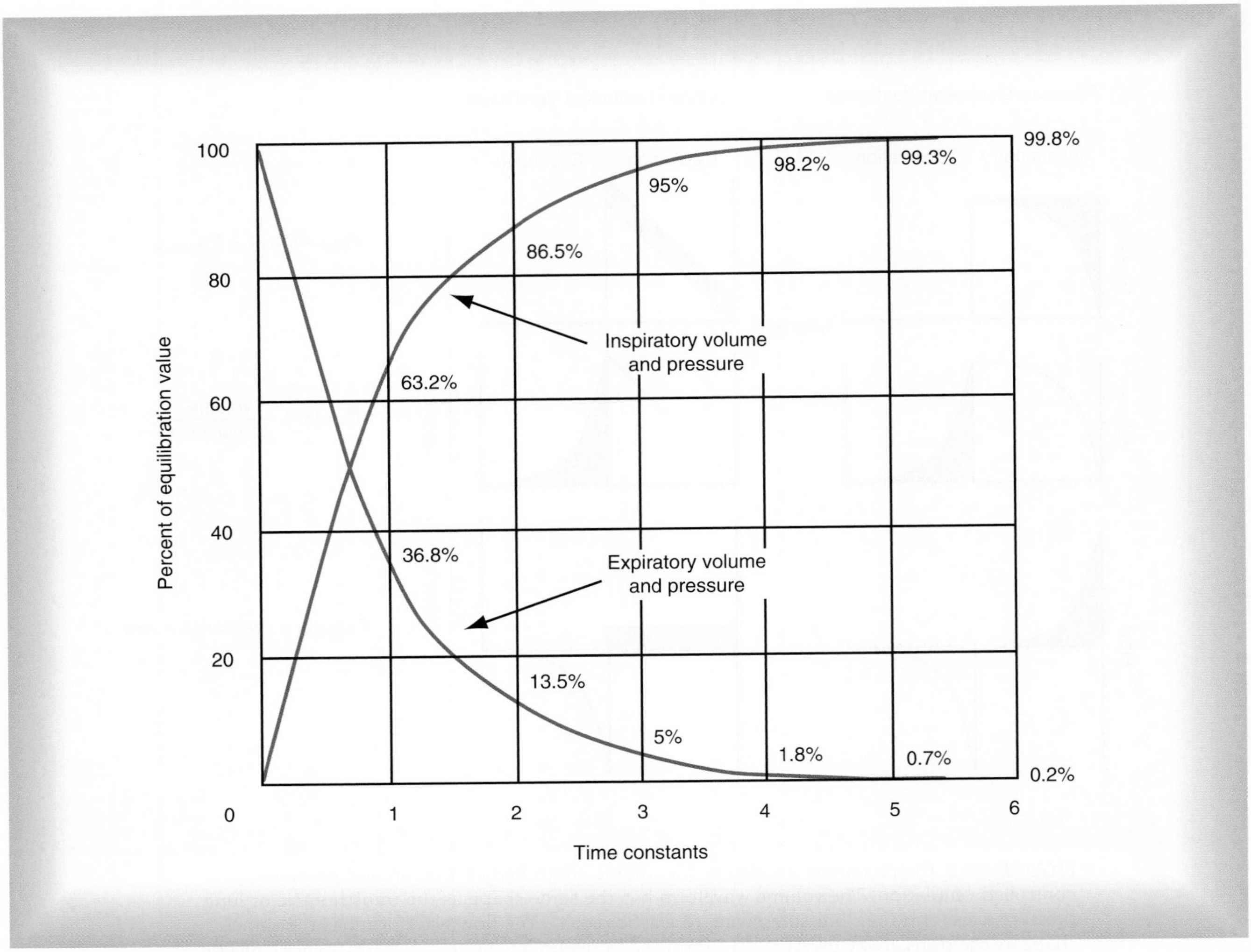

FIGURE 42-3 The time constant is a measure of how long the respiratory system takes to inflate or deflate passively in response to a sudden change in transrespiratory system pressure. The time constant is calculated as the product of resistance × compliance and is expressed in units of time, usually seconds.

equal to RC, the lung pressure changes by 63%. In the next period equal to RC, lung pressure changes another 63% and so on to infinity. When the expiratory time is equal to the time constant, the patient will have passively exhaled 63% of his or her tidal volume. This can be shown using Equation 42-2 by setting t equal to RC:

$$P_L = \frac{V_T}{C} e^{-RC/RC} = \frac{V_T}{C} 2.72^{-1} = \frac{V_T}{C} 0.37 \quad \text{Equation 42-3}$$

This expression shows that after an expiratory time equal to one time constant, only 37% of the lung pressure is left. Because volume is equal to pressure multiplied by compliance, multiplication of both sides of Equation 42-3 by compliance shows that only 37% of the tidal volume remains in the lungs. The implication is that 63% of the tidal volume has been exhaled. After two time constants (i.e., t = 2RC), exhalation is 86% completed, and after three time constants, exhalation is 95% complete. After five time constants, exhalation is considered to be 100% complete for practical purposes (Figure 42-3).

A similar expression can be derived for passive inhalation:

$$P_L = \frac{V_T}{C}(1 - e^{-t/RC}) \quad \text{Equation 42-4}$$

When this equation is graphed, it looks like the curved line showing lung pressure and volume during inhalation for pressure-controlled ventilation in Figure 42-2. These same equations govern the passive flow curves for volume-controlled and pressure-controlled ventilation. It is important to understand the concept of time constants to make appropriate ventilator setting adjustments. In any mode of ventilation, the expiratory time should be at least three time constants long to avoid clinically important gas trapping. Similarly, in pressure-controlled modes, inspiratory time (for passive inspiration) should be at least five time

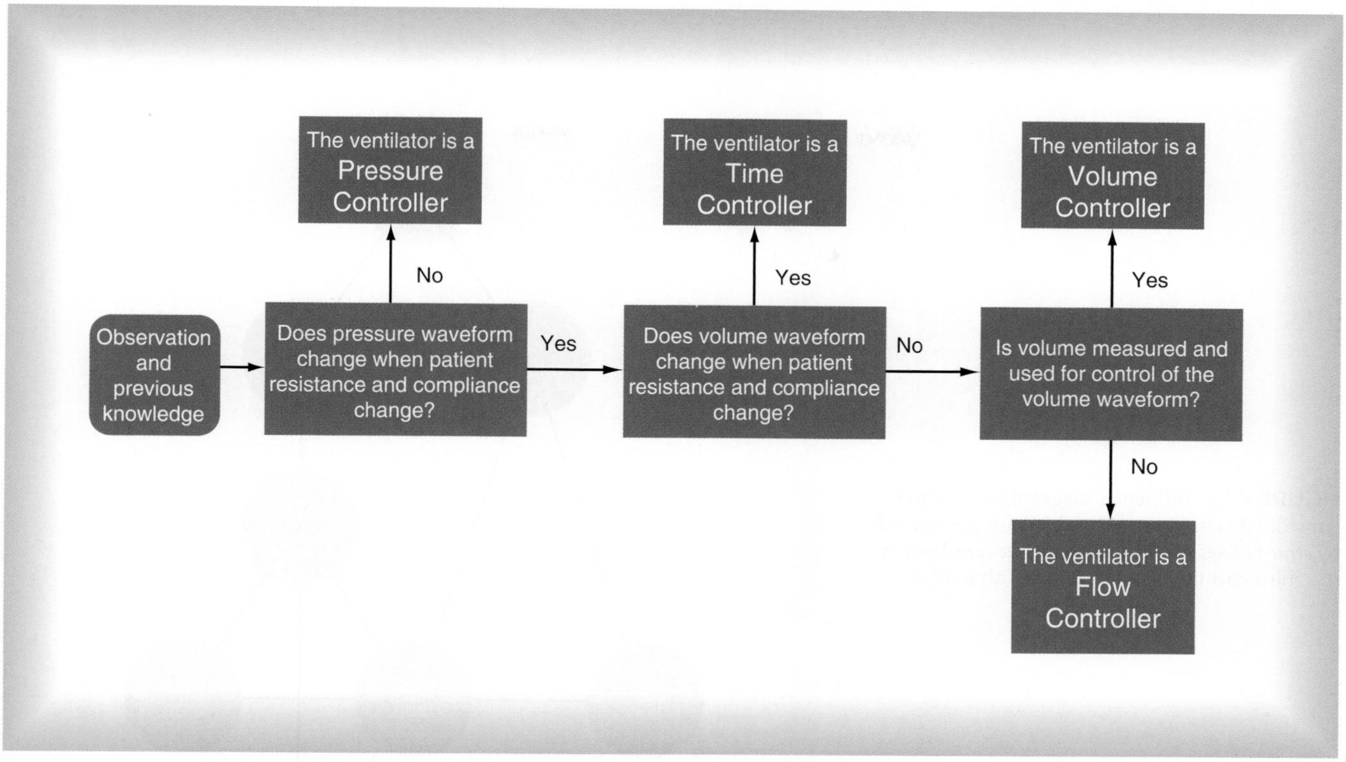

FIGURE 42-4 Criteria for determining the control variable during a ventilator-assisted inspiration.

constants long to get the maximum tidal volume from the set pressure gradient (i.e., peak inspiratory pressure [PIP] – end expiratory pressure).

Control Circuit

To manipulate pressure, volume, and flow, a ventilator must have a control circuit. A control circuit is a system of components that measures and directs the output of the ventilator to replace or assist the breathing efforts of the patient. A ventilator control circuit may include mechanical, pneumatic, electrical, electronic, or fluidic components. Most modern ventilators combine two or more of these subsystems to provide user control.

Mechanical control circuits use devices such as levers, pulleys, and cams. These types of circuits were used in the early manually operated ventilators illustrated in history books.[8] Pneumatic control is provided using gas-powered pressure regulators, needle valves, jet entrainment devices, and balloon-valves. Some transport ventilators use pneumatic control systems.

Electrical control circuits use only simple switches, rheostats (or potentiometers), and magnets to control ventilator operation. Electronic control circuits use devices such as resistors, capacitors, diodes, and transistors and combinations of these components in the form of integrated circuits. The most sophisticated electronic systems use preprogrammed microprocessors to control ventilator function.

Fluidic logic-controlled ventilators, such as the Bio-Med MVP-10 (Bio-Med Devices, Stanford, Connecticut) and Sechrist IV-100B (Sechrist, Anaheim, California), also use pressurized gas to regulate the parameters of ventilation. However, instead of simple pressurized valves and timers, these ventilators use fluidic logic circuits that function similar to electrical circuit boards.[9] Fluidic control mechanisms have no moving parts. In addition, fluidic circuits are immune to failure from surrounding electromagnetic interference, as can occur around MRI equipment.

Control Variables

A **control variable** is the primary variable that the ventilator manipulates to cause inspiration. There are only three explicit variables in the equation of motion that a ventilator can control: pressure, volume, and flow. Because only one of these variables can be the independent variable, the others are dependent variables. In other words, only one variable can be directly controlled at a time, and a ventilator must function as a pressure, volume, or flow controller. Time is implicit in the equation of motion and in some cases serves as a control variable. Figure 42-4 illustrates the criteria for determining what variable the ventilator controls at any given time.

Figure 42-5 illustrates the important variables for volume-controlled modes. It shows that the primary variable we wish to control is the patient's minute ventilation. A particular ventilator may allow the operator to set

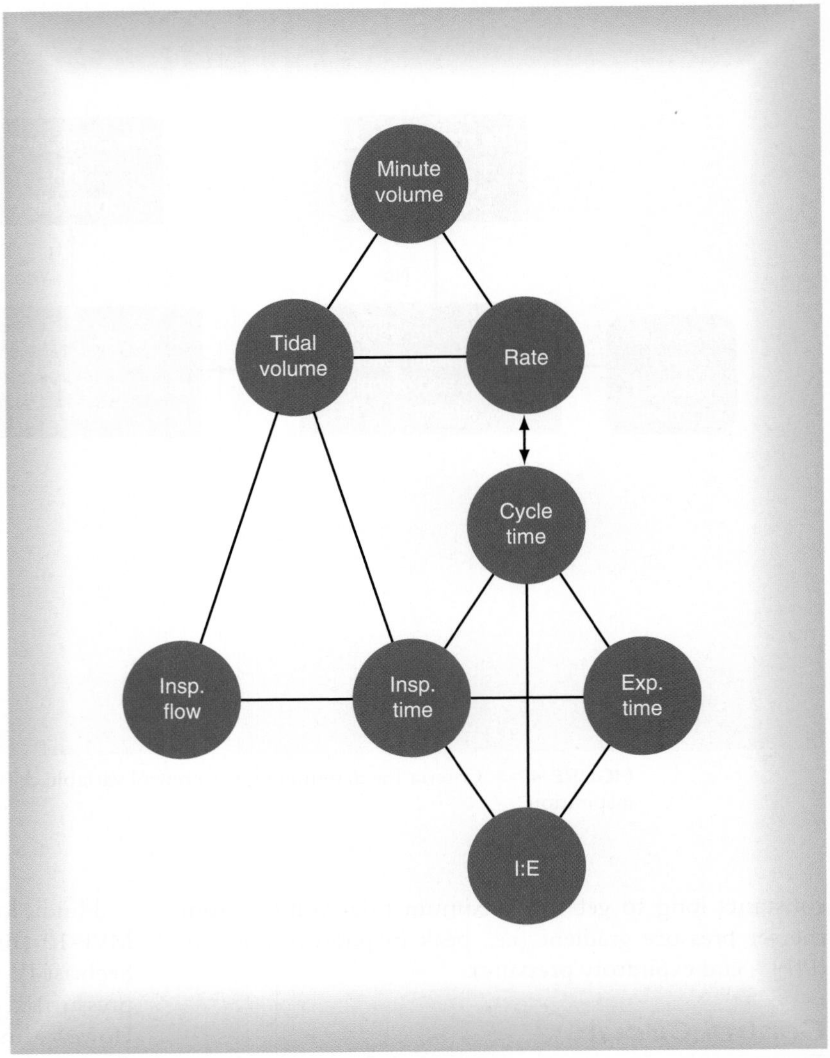

FIGURE 42-5 Influence diagram for volume-controlled ventilation. Variables are connected by *straight lines* such that if any two are known, the third can be calculated (see Table 42-2).

minute ventilation directly. More frequently, minute ventilation is adjusted by means of a set tidal volume and frequency. Tidal volume is a function of the set inspiratory flow and the set inspiratory time. Inspiratory time is affected by the set frequency and, if applicable, the set inspiratory-to-expiratory (I:E) ratio. The mathematical relationships among all these variables are shown in Table 42-1.

With pressure-controlled modes, the goal is also to maintain adequate minute ventilation. However (as the equation of motion shows), when pressure is controlled, tidal volume and minute ventilation are determined not only by the ventilator's pressure settings but also by the elastance and resistance of the patient's respiratory system. This additional variable makes minute ventilation (and gas exchange) less stable in pressure-controlled modes than in volume-controlled modes. Figure 42-6 shows the important variables for pressure-controlled modes. Tidal volume is not set on the ventilator. It is the result of the pressure settings and the patient's lung mechanics and the inspiratory time. On some ventilators, the speed with which the PIP is achieved (i.e., the pressure rise time) is adjustable. That adjustment affects the shape of the pressure waveform and the mean airway pressure. Mean airway pressure is important because, within reasonable limits, as the mean airway pressure increases, arterial O_2 tension increases. Mean airway pressure is higher for pressure-controlled modes than for volume-controlled modes (at the same tidal volume) owing to the differences in the shapes of the airway pressure waveforms.

Phase Variables

A complete ventilatory cycle or breath consists of four phases: (1) the initiation of inspiration, (2) inspiration itself, (3) the end of inspiration, and (4) expiration. To understand a breath cycle, the clinician must know how the ventilator starts, sustains, and stops inspiration and must know what occurs between breaths.

The **phase variable** is a variable that is measured and used by the ventilator to initiate some phase of the breath

TABLE 42-1

Equations Relating the Important Parameters for Volume-Controlled and Pressure-Controlled Ventilation

Mode	Parameter	Symbol	Equation
Volume-controlled	Tidal volume (L)	V_T	$V_T = \dot{V}_E \div f$ $V_T = \dot{V}_I \times T_I$
	Mean inspiratory flow (L/min)	$\bar{\dot{V}}_I$	$\bar{\dot{V}}_I = 60 \times V_T \div T_I$ $\bar{\dot{V}}_I = \frac{\dot{V}_E \times TCT}{T_I}$
Pressure-controlled	Tidal volume (L)	V_T	$V_T = \Delta P \times C \times (1 - e^{-t/\tau})$
	Instantaneous inspiratory flow (L/min)	$\dot{V}_I$	$\dot{V}_I = \left(\frac{\Delta P}{R}\right)e^{-t/\tau}$
	Pressure gradient (cm H_2O)	ΔP	$\Delta P = PIP - PEEP$
Both modes	Exhaled minute ventilation (L/min)	$\dot{V}_E$	$\dot{V}_E = V_T \times f$
	Total cycle time or ventilatory period (seconds)	TCT	$TCT = T_I + T_E = 60 \div f$
	I:E ratio	I:E	$I:E = T_I : T_E = \frac{T_I}{T_E}$
	Time constant (seconds)	τ	$\tau = R \times C$
	Resistance (cm H_2O/L/sec)	R	$R = \frac{\Delta P}{\Delta \dot{V}}$
	Compliance (L/cm H_2O)	C	$C = \frac{\Delta V}{\Delta P}$
	Elastance	E	$E = \frac{1}{C}$
	Mean airway pressure (cm H_2O)	$\bar{P}_{aw}$	$\bar{P}_{aw} = \left(\frac{1}{TCT}\right)\int_{t=0}^{t=TCT} P_{aw}dt$
Primary variables	Pressure (cm H_2O)	P	
	Volume (L)	V	
	Flow (cm H_2O/L/sec)	$\dot{V}$	
	Time (sec)	τ	
	Inspiratory time (sec)	T_I	
	Expiratory time (sec)	T_E	
	Frequency (breaths/min)	f	
	Base of natural logarithm (≈2.72)	e	

cycle. The variable causing a breath to begin is the **trigger variable.** The variable limiting the magnitude of any parameter during inspiration is the **target variable.** The variable causing a breath to end is the **cycle variable.** To describe what happens during expiration, the baseline variable that is in effect must be known. Figure 42-7 shows the criteria for determining phase variables.

Trigger Variable

On most modern ventilators, either the machine or the patient can initiate a breath. If the machine initiates the breath, the trigger variable is time. If the patient initiates the breath, pressure, flow, or volume may serve as the trigger variable. Manual or operator-initiated triggering is also available on most ventilators.

Time Triggering. When triggering by time, a ventilator initiates a breath according to a predetermined time interval, without regard to patient effort. In the past, time triggering was the only method available to initiate a ventilator cycle. At the present time, time triggering is most commonly seen when using the intermittent mandatory ventilation (IMV) mode.

Specific systems for setting a breathing rate vary from ventilator to ventilator. A rate control is the most common approach, which divides each minute into equal time segments, allotting one time segment for each full breath. When a rate control is used, inspiratory and expiratory times vary according to other control settings, such as flow and volume. An alternative approach is to provide separate timers for inspiration and expiration. Changing either or both of these timers alters the breathing rate.

Pressure Triggering. Pressure triggering occurs when a patient's inspiratory effort causes a decrease in pressure within the breathing circuit. When this pressure decrease reaches the pressure-sensing mechanism, the ventilator starts gas delivery. On most ventilators, the pressure

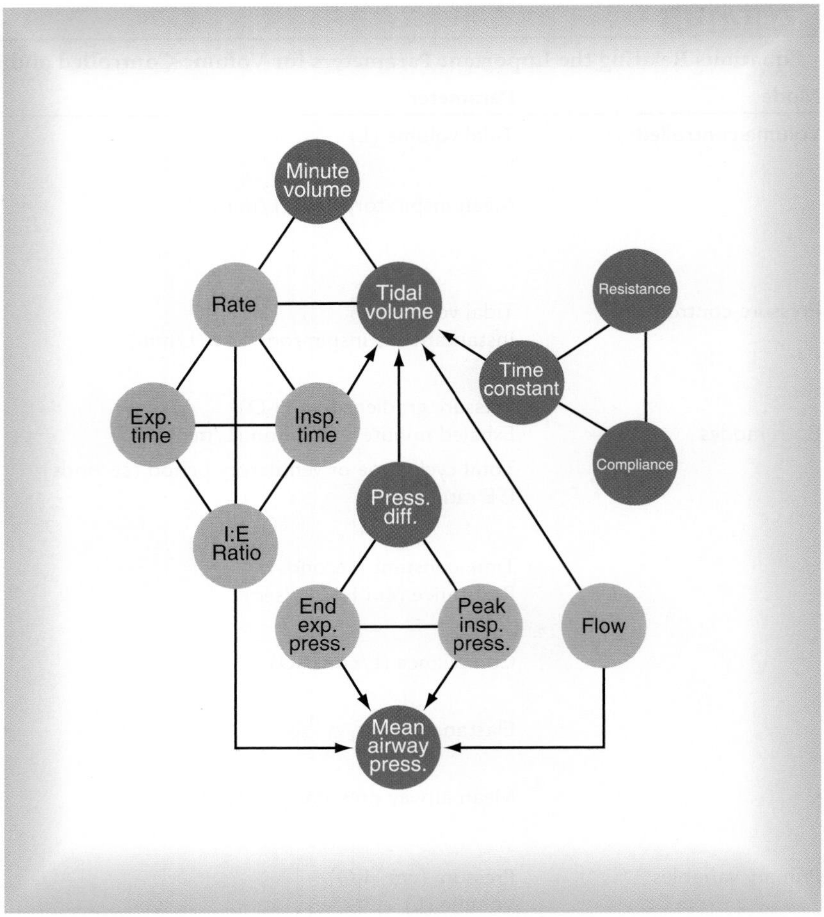

FIGURE 42-6 Influence diagram for pressure-controlled ventilation. Variables are connected by *straight lines* such that if any two are known, the third can be calculated (see Table 42-2). *Arrows* represent relationships that are more complex. *Purple circles* represent variables that are directly controlled by ventilator settings. *Gray circles* show indirectly controlled variables.

decrease needed to trigger a breath can be adjusted. The trigger level is often called the *sensitivity*. Typically, the trigger level is set 0.5 to 1.5 cm H_2O below the baseline expiratory pressure. Setting the trigger level to a higher number, such as 3 cm H_2O, makes the ventilator less sensitive and requires the patient to work harder to initiate inspiration. Conversely, setting the trigger level lower makes the ventilator more sensitive to patient effort. How fast the ventilator mechanism responds to patient effort is called the *response time*. It is important for the ventilator to have a short response time to maintain optimal synchrony with the patient's inspiratory efforts. Either a large pressure decrease (i.e., low sensitivity setting) or a delay in flow delivery can increase a patient's work of breathing.

Flow Triggering. Using flow as the trigger variable is more complex. A ventilator that uses flow triggering typically provides a continuous low flow of gas through its circuit. The ventilator measures the flow coming out of the main flow control valve and the flow through the exhalation valve. Between breaths, these two flows are equal (assuming no leaks in the patient circuit). When the patient makes an inspiratory effort, the flow through the exhalation valve falls below the flow from the output valve. The difference between these two flows is the *flow trigger variable*.

Flow Trigger Variable. To adjust the sensitivity of a flow-triggered system, the clinician usually sets both a base continuous flow and a trigger flow level. Typically, the trigger flow level is set to 1 to 3 L/min (below baseline). If the base continuous flow is set at 10 L/min and the trigger is set at 2 L/min, the ventilator triggers a breath when the output flow decreases to 8 L/min or less. An alternative approach used with some ventilators is simply to measure the flow at the "wye" connector and start breath delivery on that signal.

Compared with pressure, using flow as the trigger variable decreases a patient's work of breathing.[11,12] However, ventilators that use a flow-triggering mechanism tend to be highly susceptible to circuit leaks or movement caused by turbulence or gas flow through condensed water. Either of these conditions can cause spurious breaths, which can disrupt patient-ventilatory synchrony and increase the work of breathing. The perception exists, with regard to the most recent generation of ICU ventilators, that pressure and flow triggering are equally effective. Using volume

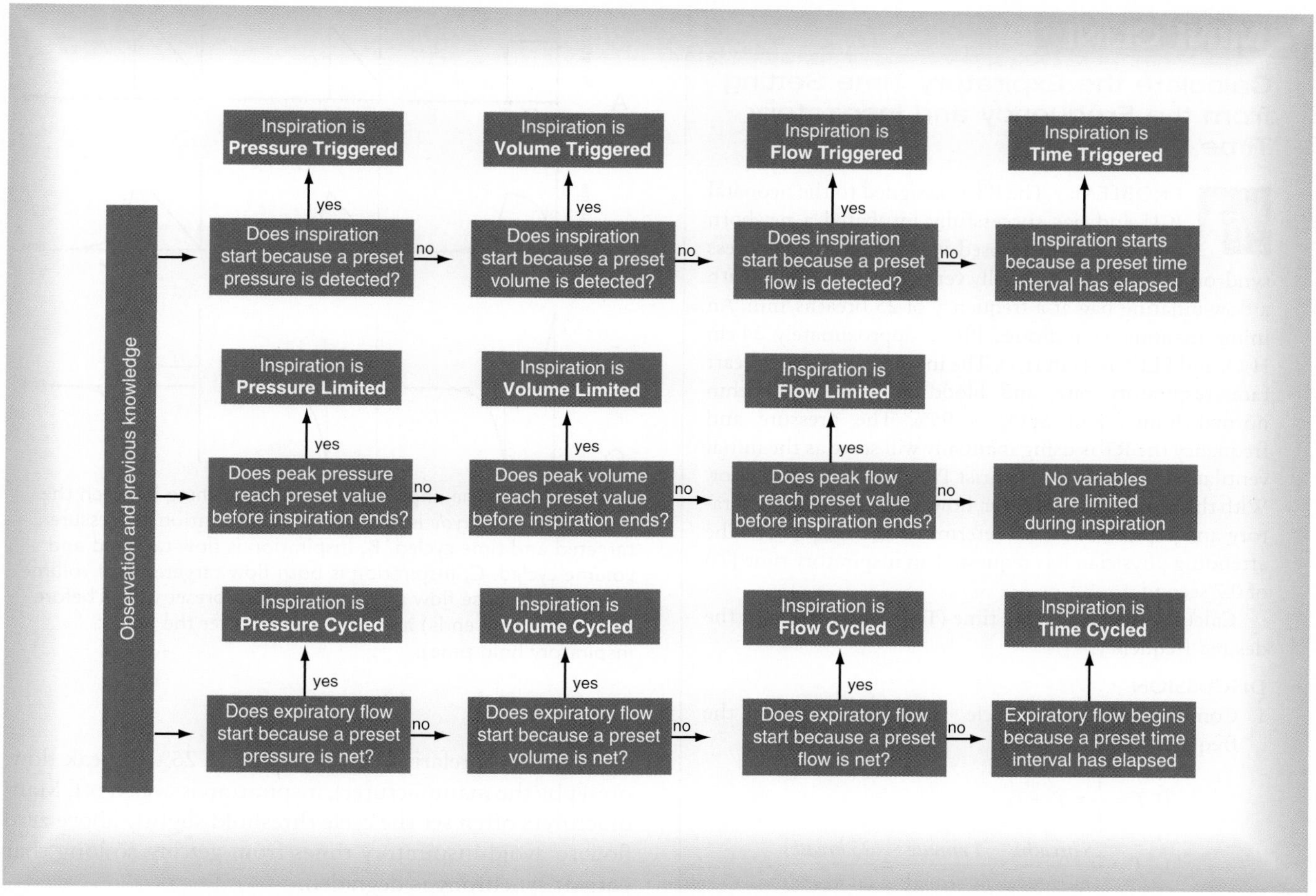

FIGURE 42-7 Criteria for determining the phase variables during a breath on a mechanical ventilator.

as the trigger can help overcome synchrony problems caused by circuit leaks, but at the present time only the Draeger Babylog (Draeger Medical, Telford, Pennsylvania) uses true volume triggering.

Other Trigger Variables. Other variables can be used to trigger inspiration, such as a decrease in total minute ventilation below a preset threshold (e.g., mandatory minute ventilation mode on the Draeger Evita XL ventilator) or the electrical signal generated by diaphragmatic contraction (e.g., neurally adjusted ventilatory assist mode on the Maquet SERVO-i ventilator).

Target Variable

A target variable is one that can reach and maintain a preset level before inspiration ends but does not terminate inspiration. Pressure, flow, or volume can serve as a target variable.

Clinicians often confuse target variables with cycle variables. A *cycle variable* always ends inspiration. A *target variable* does not terminate inspiration—it sets an upper bound only for pressure, volume, or flow. Figure 42-8 illustrates the importance of distinguishing between target and cycle variables.

Cycle Variable

The inspiratory phase always ends when some variable reaches a preset value. The variable that is measured and used to end inspiration is called the *cycle variable*. The cycle variable can be pressure, volume, flow, or time. Manual cycling is also available on some modern ventilators.

Pressure Cycling. When a ventilator is set to pressure cycle, it delivers flow until a preset pressure is reached. When the set pressure is achieved, inspiratory flow stops, and expiratory flow begins. The most common application of pressure cycling is for alarm settings. Intermittent positive pressure breathing therapy is usually performed with pressure cycled machines.

Volume Cycling. When a ventilator is set to volume cycle, it delivers flow until a preselected volume has been expelled from the device. As soon as the set volume is met, inspiratory flow stops, and expiratory flow begins. The volume that passes through the ventilator's output control valve is never exactly equal to the volume delivered to the patient because of the volume compressed in the patient circuit. Some ventilators use a sensor at the "wye" connector (e.g., the Hamilton Galileo, Hamilton Medical, Reno, NV) for accurate tidal volume measurement. Others

MINI CLINI

Calculate the Expiratory Time Setting from the Frequency and Inspiratory Time

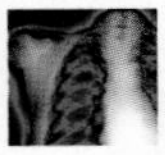

PROBLEM: The RT is assigned to the neonatal ICU and has successfully intubated a newborn term infant diagnosed with respiratory distress syndrome. The RT is manually ventilating the infant with a flow-inflating bag at a frequency of 25 breaths/min. An inline manometer indicates PIP is approximately 24 cm H_2O, and PEEP is 4 cm H_2O. The infant's vital signs (heart rate, respiratory rate, and blood pressure) are within normal limits, and SpO_2 is 95%. The pressure and frequency the RT is using manually will serve as the initial ventilator settings on a Sechrist IV100B infant ventilator. With this particular ventilator, however, setting the inspiratory and expiratory times determines the frequency. The attending physician has requested an inspiratory time (T_I) of 0.7 second.

Calculate the expiratory time (T_E) necessary to give the desired frequency.

DISCUSSION

1. Compute the total cycle time (TCT) using the frequency (f):

$$TCT = \frac{1}{f} = T_I + T_E$$

$$f = \frac{25\ breaths}{minute} \times \frac{1\ minute}{60\ seconds} = \frac{25\ breaths}{60\ seconds}$$

$$TCT = \frac{1}{25\ breaths/60\ seconds} = \frac{60\ seconds}{25\ breaths}$$

$$= \frac{2.4\ seconds}{breath}$$

2. Compute the expiratory time:

$$T_E = TCT - T_I = 2.4 - 0.7 = 1.7\ \text{seconds}$$

3. Check the digital display to verify the set frequency remains at 25 breaths/min.

measure volume at some point inside the ventilator and calculate the tubing compliance during operational checks, before connecting the patient to the ventilator circuit. It is imperative for the operator to know whether the ventilator compensates for compressed gas in its tidal volume readout.

Flow Cycling. When a ventilator is set to flow cycle, it delivers flow until a preset level is met, and then flow stops and expiration begins. The most frequent application of flow cycling is in the pressure support mode. In this mode, the control variable is pressure, and the ventilator provides the flow necessary to meet the inspiratory pressure limit. In doing so, flow starts out at a relatively high value and decays exponentially (see Figure 42-2). When flow has decreased to a relatively low value (e.g., 25% of peak flow, preset by the manufacturer), inspiration is cycled off. Manufacturers often set the cycle threshold slightly above zero flow to avoid inspiratory times from getting so long that patient synchrony is degraded.

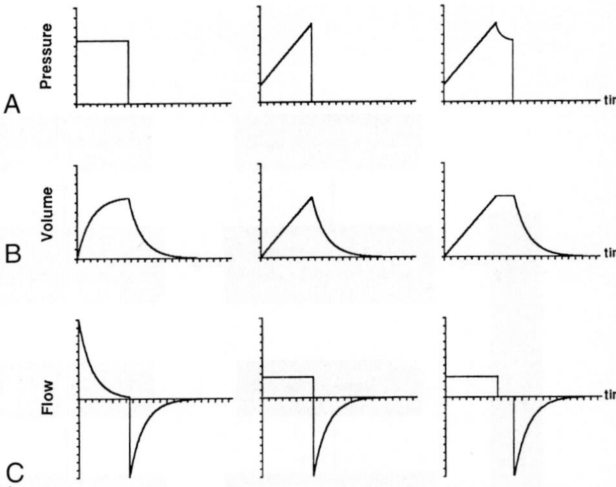

FIGURE 42-8 The importance of distinguishing between the terms *trigger* and *cycle* is illustrated. **A,** Inspiration is pressure targeted and time cycled. **B,** Inspiration is flow targeted and volume cycled. **C,** Inspiration is both flow targeted and volume targeted (because flow and volume reach preset values before inspiratory time ends) and time cycled (after the preset inspiratory hold time).

Time Cycling. Time cycling means that expiratory flow starts because a preset time interval has elapsed. There are several time intervals of interest during inspiration. One is the *inspiratory flow time.* As the name implies, this is the time during which inspiratory flow is delivered to the patient. Another interval is the *inspiratory hold time,* during which inspiratory flow has ceased but expiratory flow is not yet allowed. The sum of these two intervals is the *inspiratory time.* Time cycling occurs when the inspiratory time has elapsed. An inspiratory hold time may not be used. If it is used, it may be set directly, or it may occur indirectly if the set inspiratory time is longer than the inspiratory flow time (determined by the set tidal volume and flow; time = volume/flow).

Patient versus Machine Triggering and Cycling. Trigger and cycle signals can be grouped into two categories: patient-generated and machine-generated. The determination of whether the patient or the machine generated the signal is based on the equation of motion. However, this time the equation is expressed in another way:

$$P_{insp} = P_E + P_R \qquad \text{Equation 42-5}$$

where P_{insp} reflects the pressure required for inspiration, P_E is the pressure resisting inspiration by the elastance of the respiratory system, and P_R is the pressure resisting the inspiration by the resistance of the respiratory system. This equation can be expanded as follows:

MINI CLINI

Calculate Inspiratory Hold Time Given Set Inspiratory Time, Tidal Volume, and Flow When Using the Siemens Servo

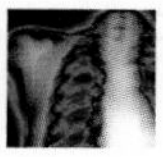

PROBLEM: The RT is performing a ventilator check on an ICU patient with a blunt chest trauma. The ventilator is set to volume-controlled IMV on a Draeger Evita 4. The physician wants the minimum mean airway pressure for the given level of ventilation to preserve the patient's already low cardiac output. The physician asks the RT to ensure the night shift therapist removed the inspiratory hold the patient had been on.

Determine from the ventilator settings alone whether there is an inspiratory hold, and if so, make the appropriate changes to eliminate it. Ventilator settings are:
Tidal volume: 500 ml = 0.5 L
Inspiratory flow: 60 L/min = 1 L/sec
Inspiratory time: 0.8 second
Frequency: 10 breaths/min

DISCUSSION

1. Calculate the inspiratory flow time (TIF) using appropriate unit conversions:

$$T_{IF} = \frac{\textit{tidal volume}}{\textit{inspiratory flow}} = \frac{500\ ml}{60\ L/minute} \times \frac{1\ L}{1000\ ml} \times \frac{60\ seconds}{1\ minute} = \frac{0.5\ L}{1\ L/second} = 0.5\ second$$

2. Compare the set inspiratory time (0.8 second) with the flow time resulting from the tidal volume and flow settings (0.5 second). Inspiratory time lasts longer than inspiratory flow. Because inspiration is time cycled, this means that there is an inspiratory hold of duration equal to 0.8 – 0.5 = 0.3 second.
3. You could eliminate the inspiratory hold either by decreasing the inspiratory flow or by decreasing the inspiratory time. The goal is to minimize the mean inspiratory pressure. You choose to decrease inspiratory time for two reasons: (1) It decreases the I:E ratio and may allow more time for spontaneous breaths to occur, lowering mean intrathoracic pressure; (2) decreasing inspiratory flow may make tidal volume delivery slower than the patient demands, decreasing patient-ventilator synchrony.

$$P_{vent} + P_{mus} = (P_{E,vent} + P_{R,vent}) + (P_{R,mus} + P_{R,mus}) \quad \text{Equation 42-6}$$

where P_{vent} is the pressure generated by the ventilator, independent of the patient, P_{mus} is the pressure generated by the patient's ventilatory muscles independent of the ventilator, $P_{E,vent}$ is the elastic load supported by the ventilator, $P_{E,mus}$ is the elastic load supported by the patient's muscles, $P_{R,vent}$ is the resistive load supported by the ventilator, and $P_{R,mus}$ is the resistive load supported by the patient's muscles. In this form of the equation, we can easily differentiate sources of patient versus machine trigger and cycle signals.

For the definition of *patient* trigger and cycle signals, the patient's ventilatory efforts are represented by P_{mus}, $P_{E,mus}$, and $P_{R,mus}$. Because $P_E = EV$ and $P_R = R\dot{V}$, it follows that patient trigger and cycle signals are based on three variables (P_{mus}, V_{mus}, and $\dot{V}_{mus}$) and two parameters (E and R). The ventilator can be triggered or cycled by a signal representing P_{mus} (e.g., the electrical signal of the diaphragm as with neurally adjusted ventilatory assist or a calculated estimate of P_{mus}) or the volume or flow generated by the patient's ventilatory muscles (V_{mus} and $\dot{V}_{mus}$ [e.g., volume triggering in the Draeger Babylog or flow triggering on many other ventilators]). The ventilator can be triggered or cycled by the patient's passive respiratory system mechanics (E and R). Examples are flow triggering with the AutoRelease feature on the Draeger Evita Infinity V500 ventilator and flow cycling during pressure support on any ventilator. Manufacturers may have specific marketing terms for flow cycling. For example, flow cycling on the Puritan Bennett 840 ventilator (Pleasanton, California) is termed *E-sensitivity*. Given the definition of *patient* trigger and cycle signals, we can define *machine* trigger and cycle signals as being anything else that starts or ends inspiration (excluding operator-generated manual signals).

Baseline Variable

The baseline variable is the parameter controlled during expiration. Although pressure, volume, or flow could serve as the baseline variable, pressure control is the most practical and is implemented by all modern ventilators.

Baseline or *expiratory pressure* is always measured and set relative to atmospheric pressure. For baseline pressure to equal atmospheric pressure, it is at zero. For baseline pressure to exceed atmospheric pressure, it is set at a positive value, called *positive end expiratory pressure (PEEP)*. Although seldom used, the baseline pressure could be set below atmospheric pressure, a technique called *negative end expiratory pressure (NEEP)*.

Zero end expiratory pressure (ZEEP) is the default baseline value during positive pressure ventilation, meaning that it is normally in effect unless purposely changed. Regardless of the mechanism by which gas is delivered to the lungs, it must leave before the next inspiration. Exhalation normally occurs by virtue of the stored pressure in the expanded lungs and thorax. With ZEEP in effect, when exhalation begins, the ventilator's expiratory valve simply opens to the atmosphere, exposing the patient's airway to a relative pressure of zero. At this point, alveolar pressure exceeds airway pressure, gas moves from alveoli out to the atmosphere, and the lungs and thorax passively recoil down to their resting volume, or functional residual capacity (FRC).

PEEP is the application of pressure above atmospheric pressure at the airway throughout expiration. PEEP elevates a patient's FRC and can help improve oxygenation

TABLE 42-2

Specifications for Some Modes Found on the Draeger Evita XL Ventilator

		Mandatory Breaths*				Spontaneous Breaths			
Draeger Mode Name	**Breathing Pattern**	**Targeting Scheme**	**Trigger†**	**Target‡**	**Cycle**	**Targeting Scheme**	**Trigger**	**Target**	**Cycle**
CMV	VC-CMV	Set-point	T	F, V	T	NA	NA	NA	NA
	Operational Logic: Every breath is volume controlled and mandatory. Every breath is machine triggered and cycled								
CMV + AutoFlow	PC-CMV	Adaptive	T, F	P	T	NA	NA	NA	NA
	Operational Logic: Mandatory breaths are pressure controlled, but patient may trigger breath. If target tidal volume is not met, pressure target is automatically adjusted								
CMV + Pressure Limited Ventilation	PC-CMV	Dual	T, F	F, V, P	T	NA	NA	NA	NA
	Operational Logic: Mandatory breath starts out in volume control but switches to pressure control if airway pressure reaches set Pmax								
SIMV	VC-IMV	Set-point	T, F	F, V	T	Set-point	P	P	P
	Operational Logic: Mandatory breaths are volume-controlled. Spontaneous breaths may occur within window determined by set rate and are not assisted (i.e., inspiratory pressure stays at baseline)								
PC+	PC-IMV	Set-point	T, F	P	T	Set-point	F	P	F
	Operational Logic: Mandatory breaths are pressure-controlled. Spontaneous breaths may occur within window determined by set rate and are not assisted (i.e., inspiratory pressure stays at baseline)								
SIMV + AutoFlow	PC-IMV	Adaptive	T, F	P	T	Set-point	P	P	P
	Operational Logic: Mandatory breaths are pressure-controlled and pressure target is automatically adjusted if target tidal volume is not met. Spontaneous breaths may occur with window determined by set rate and are not assisted (i.e., inspiratory pressure stays at baseline)								
CPAP	PC-CSV	NA	NA	NA	NA	Set-point	P	P	P
	Operational Logic: Spontaneous breaths are unassisted								
Pressure Support	PC-CSV	NA	NA	NA	NA	Set-point	F	P	F
	Operational Logic: Spontaneous breaths are assisted (i.e., inspiratory pressure increases above baseline)								
SmartCare	PC-CSV	NA	NA	NA	NA	Intelligent	F	P	F
	Operational Logic: Spontaneous breaths are assisted (i.e., inspiratory pressure increases above baseline). Pressure support level automatically adjusted by rule-based expert system								

CMV, Continuous mandatory ventilation (all breaths are mandatory); *CSV,* continuous spontaneous ventilation (all breaths are spontaneous); *F,* flow; *IMV,* intermittent mandatory ventilation (spontaneous breaths between mandatory breaths); *NA,* not available; *P,* pressure; *PC,* pressure-controlled; *T,* time; *V,* volume; *VC,* volume-controlled.

*Patient can take spontaneous breaths during mandatory breaths with PC and AutoFlow but not with Pressure Limited Ventilation.

†Flow trigger may be turned off. When off, mandatory breaths cannot be triggered, but spontaneous breaths are automatically pressure triggered with factory set sensitivity.

‡Volume target achieved if inspiratory time set longer than tidal volume/flow.

by preventing collapse of alveolar units that are made unstable by lack of surfactant or disease.

NEEP is the application of subatmospheric pressure to the airway during expiration. NEEP was originally developed to overcome the harmful cardiovascular effects of positive pressure ventilation. The assumption was that NEEP could offset the impedance to venous return created by the positive pressure during inspiration. NEEP has occasionally been promoted as a way to help patients overcome expiratory airway resistance. In this approach, negative pressure is applied only to help return airway pressure to baseline. Because NEEP can cause airway collapse and decrease the FRC if misapplied, great care must be taken in applying this technique.

Modes of Ventilation

The objective of mechanical ventilation is to ensure that the patient receives the minute volume of appropriate gases required to satisfy respiratory needs, while not damaging the lungs, impairing circulation, or increasing the patient's discomfort. *Mode of ventilation* is the manner in which a ventilator achieves this objective. A mode can be identified by specifying a combination of the following:

- *Control variable* (pressure or volume)
- *Breath sequence* (pattern of mandatory or spontaneous breaths, or both)
- **Targeting scheme** (for mandatory and spontaneous breaths)

An example of how this mode classification system can be applied is shown in Table 42-2. The key to understanding modes of ventilation is to link simple, defined terms in a way that allows descriptions of varying complexity to be built; this is much more practical than trying to memorize arbitrary names for every new feature a manufacturer wishes to promote. It is analogous to using an alphabet of several dozen letters to build words rather than memorizing tens of thousands of separate ideographs that each represents a word. One need only compare the English written language with the Chinese written language to appreciate the analogy.[3]

Control Variable

In the equation of motion, the control variable is the variable that is predetermined for a given inspiration (i.e., pressure or volume). *Predetermined* means that the operator presets the parameters of the variable's waveform independent of the patient's mechanics. In volume control, the operator may preset the inspiratory flow and tidal volume. In pressure control, the operator may preset the inspiratory pressure and inspiratory time. In a more exotic form of pressure control, such as proportional assist ventilation, the operator presets the parameters of elastance and resistance to be supported, and the ventilator delivers pressure according to the equation of motion.

There are clinical advantages and disadvantages to volume versus pressure control, which are discussed in Chapter 43. Briefly, volume control results in a more stable minute ventilation (and more stable blood gases) than pressure control if lung mechanics are unstable. Pressure control allows better patient-ventilatory synchrony with the patient because inspiratory flow is not constrained to a preset value. Although it is possible to control only one variable at a time, a ventilator can automatically switch between pressure control and volume control in an attempt to guarantee minute ventilation while maximizing patient synchrony. This feature is called **dual control**[13] and is discussed in the section on Targeting Schemes.

Pressure Control. If the ventilator controls pressure, the pressure waveform remains consistent, but volume and flow vary with changes in respiratory system mechanics. The ventilator can control either the airway pressure (causing it to increase above body surface pressure for inspiration) or the pressure on the body surface (causing it to decrease below airway opening pressure for inspiration). This pressure control is the basis for classifying ventilators as being either positive or negative pressure types. The Newport Wave would be classified as a positive pressure controller that generates a rectangular pressure waveform, whereas the Emerson Iron Lung is a negative pressure controller that produces a quasisinusoidal pressure waveform.

Volume Control. If the ventilator controls volume, the volume and flow waveforms remain consistent, but pressure varies with changes in respiratory mechanics. To qualify as a true volume controller, a ventilator must measure volume and use this signal to control the volume waveform. Volume can be controlled directly by the displacement of a device such as a piston or bellows. Volume can be controlled indirectly by controlling flow; this follows from the fact that volume and flow are inverse functions of time (i.e., volume is the integral of flow, and flow is the derivative of volume).

If the ventilator controls flow, the flow and volume waveforms remain consistent, but pressure varies with changes in respiratory mechanics. Flow can be controlled directly using something as simple as a flow meter or as complex as a proportional solenoid valve. Flow can be controlled indirectly by controlling volume.

Infant ventilators, such as the Sechrist, are the simplest examples of flow controllers. In this ventilator, flow is controlled directly by a flowmeter and an exhalation valve. As long as the airway pressure does not reach the set pressure limit, the resulting volume waveform remains constant.[10] Current-generation adult ICU ventilators typically function as flow controllers. However, these systems are much more complex than ventilators such as the Sechrist; flow is measured and adjusted hundreds of times per second through sophisticated computerized output control valves.

For simplicity in classifying modes of ventilation, we consider flow control to be volume control. It has been observed that direct control of flow is indirect control of volume because volume is the mathematical inverse of flow (i.e., volume is the integral of flow with respect to time).

RULE OF THUMB

Volume is the integral of flow. For constant flow, volume = flow × time. Any ventilator that controls flow controls volume. Think of using a water faucet to fill the sink: the greater the flow and the longer the time, the greater is the volume.

Breath Sequence

Specifying only the control variable for a mode, the clinician can distinguish only among pressure and volume control modes; this is often all that is needed to communicate. At the bedside, the clinician might simply have to indicate that the patient has become asynchronous with the ventilator, and the mode has been changed from "volume control" to "pressure control."

The second component of the mode classification scheme is the **breath sequence.** A *breath* is defined as a positive change in airway flow (inspiration) paired with a negative change in airway flow (expiration), both relative to baseline flow and associated with ventilation of the lungs. This definition excludes flow changes caused by hiccups or cardiogenic oscillations, but it allows the superimposition of a spontaneous breath on a mandatory breath or vice versa (these breath types are defined subsequently). Traditionally, the flow baseline is taken as flow = 0 L/min (i.e., end expiration). However, because "breaths" can be superimposed on existing flow in various circumstances (e.g., high-frequency ventilation), the inspiratory and expiratory movements of gas must be judged relative to the level of flow existing when these movements occur.

Typically, expiration immediately follows inspiration. However, with some modes, such as airway pressure release

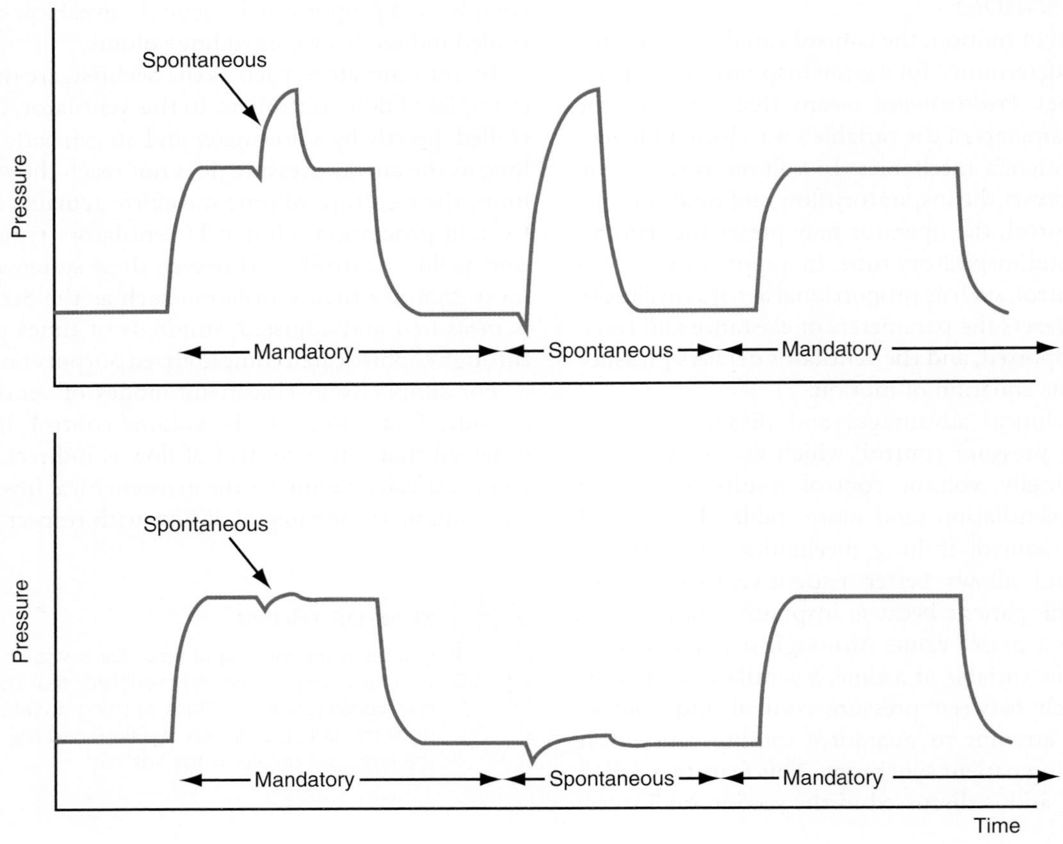

FIGURE 42-9 Pressure-time curves illustrate how a spontaneous breath (e.g., pressure triggered, flow cycled) can occur either between or during mandatory breaths (e.g., time triggered, time cycled). Spontaneous breaths may be assisted (pressure support in this figure but could be something else, such as proportional assist or tube compensation) as shown in the *top curve,* or unassisted, as shown in the *bottom curve*. As one example of this, the Puritan Bennett 840 ventilator allows all spontaneous breaths to be assisted during the bilevel mode.

ventilation, there can be a large inspiration, followed by several small inspirations and expirations, followed by a large expiration.

The classification of modes requires the definition of two basic categories of breaths: spontaneous and mandatory. A **spontaneous breath** is a breath for which the start and end of inspiration may be determined by the patient, independent of any machine settings for inspiratory time and expiratory time. In other words, the patient both triggers and cycles the breath. As a consequence, the patient retains substantial, if not complete, control over the timing (frequency and inspiratory time) and size (tidal volume) of the breath. A spontaneous breath may occur during a mandatory breath (Figure 42-9). A spontaneous breath may be assisted or unassisted. An *assisted breath* is a breath during which all or part of inspiratory or expiratory flow is generated by a change in transrespiratory pressure (i.e., airway pressure minus body surface pressure) owing to an external agent (e.g., manual or automatic resuscitator, mechanical ventilator).

A **mandatory breath** is a breath for which the start or end of inspiration (or both) is determined by the ventilator, independent of the patient; the machine triggers or cycles the breath. As a consequence, the patient substantially, if not completely, loses control over the timing (frequency and inspiratory time) and size (tidal volume) of the

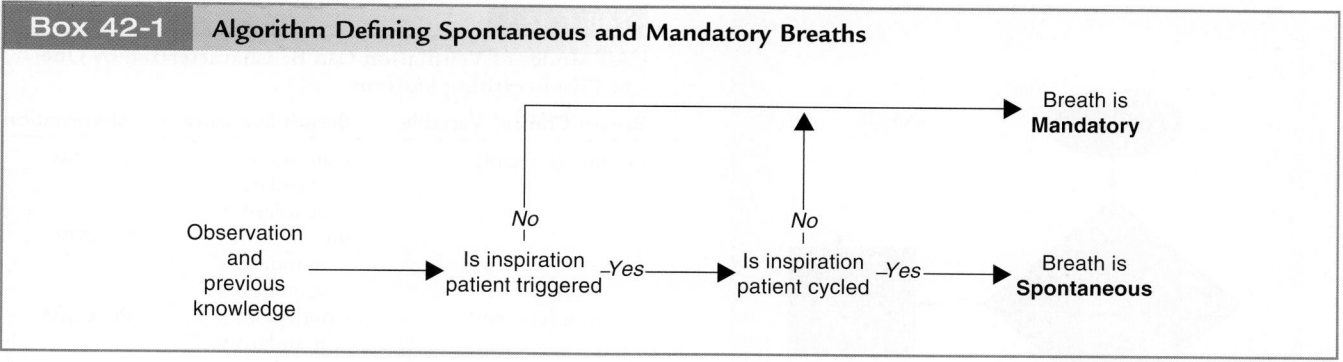

Box 42-1 Algorithm Defining Spontaneous and Mandatory Breaths

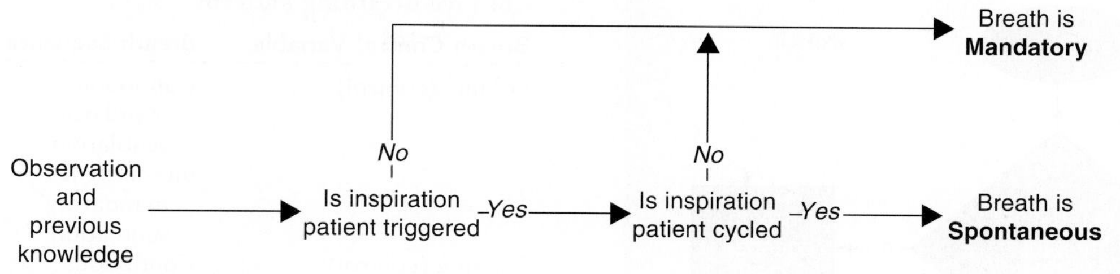

breath. Mandatory breaths are generally assisted. Box 42-1 shows an algorithm defining spontaneous and mandatory breaths.

Having defined spontaneous and mandatory breaths, there are three possible sequences of breaths, designated as follows:

- **Continuous mandatory ventilation (CMV)**
- **Intermittent mandatory ventilation (IMV)**
- **Continuous spontaneous ventilation (CSV)**

The abbreviation *CMV* has been used to mean a variety of things by ventilator manufacturers. The most logical use in this classification system is to represent *continuous mandatory ventilation* as part of a continuum from full ventilatory support to unassisted breathing. The abbreviation *IMV* has a long history of consistent use to mean *intermittent mandatory ventilation* (i.e., a combination of mandatory and spontaneous breaths). However, the development of the *active exhalation valve* and other innovations has made it possible for the patient to breathe spontaneously during a mandatory breath. This is primarily a feature used to help ensure synchrony between the ventilator and patient in the event that the mandatory breath parameters (e.g., preset inspiratory time, pressure, volume, or flow) do not match the patient's inspiratory demands. This feature blurs the historical distinction between CMV and IMV.

The key difference now between CMV and IMV is that with CMV, the clinical intent is to make every inspiration a mandatory breath, whereas with IMV, the clinical intent is to partition ventilatory support between mandatory and spontaneous breaths. This means that during CMV, if the operator decreases the ventilatory rate (often considered to be a safety "backup" rate in the event of apnea), the level of ventilatory support is unaffected, provided that the patient continues triggering mandatory breaths at the same rate (i.e., each breath is assisted to the same degree). With IMV, the rate setting directly affects the number of mandatory breaths and the level of ventilatory support (assuming that spontaneous breaths are not assisted to the same degree as mandatory breaths). CMV is normally considered a method of "full" ventilatory support, whereas IMV is usually viewed as a method of partial ventilatory support. For classification purposes, *if spontaneous breaths are not allowed between mandatory breaths, the breath sequence is CMV; otherwise, the sequence is IMV* (Figure 42-10). Given that almost every ventilator has a mechanism to synchronize breath delivery with patient effort, it is no longer necessary to add an *S* to designate *synchronized IMV (SIMV)*. The term *SIMV* was important in the early days of mechanical ventilation but is an anachronism now. Patient triggering can be specified in the description of mode phase variables.

There has been no consistent abbreviation to signify a **breathing pattern** composed of all spontaneous breaths. However, the logical progression would be from CMV to IMV to CSV.

When a breath sequence is added to the control variable in classifying a mode, the result is a breathing pattern. A breathing pattern provides a greater ability to discriminate between similar modes. For example, it is possible to distinguish between pressure-control IMV (PC-IMV) and pressure-control CSV (PC-CSV). By classifying modes based solely on the breathing pattern, there are only five possibilities in two groups (Table 42-3). The utility of this system is immediately obvious. A new mode, such as *airway pressure release ventilation (APRV),* can be explained as simply a form of PC-IMV. Assuming the clinician already understands the concept of PC-IMV, it takes little effort to understand the additional nuances of APRV (e.g., different labels for control settings, alarms). This level of description avoids the cumbersome verbal ad hoc definition for APRV, such as "a mode that allows spontaneously breathing patients to breathe at a positive-pressure level but drops briefly to a reduced pressure level for carbon dioxide (CO_2) elimination during each breathing cycle," or the misleading description of some authors who explain APRV as two levels of continuous positive airway pressure.

PC-IMV and PC-CSV can also be used to clarify what *bilevel positive airway pressure ventilation* means. For example, on the Respironics BiPAP S/T or BiPAP AVAPS (Phillips Healthcare, Andover, Massachusetts) noninvasive home ventilators, the "timed" mode is PC-IMV, whereas the "spontaneous" mode is PC-CSV. *BiPAP ventilation* and

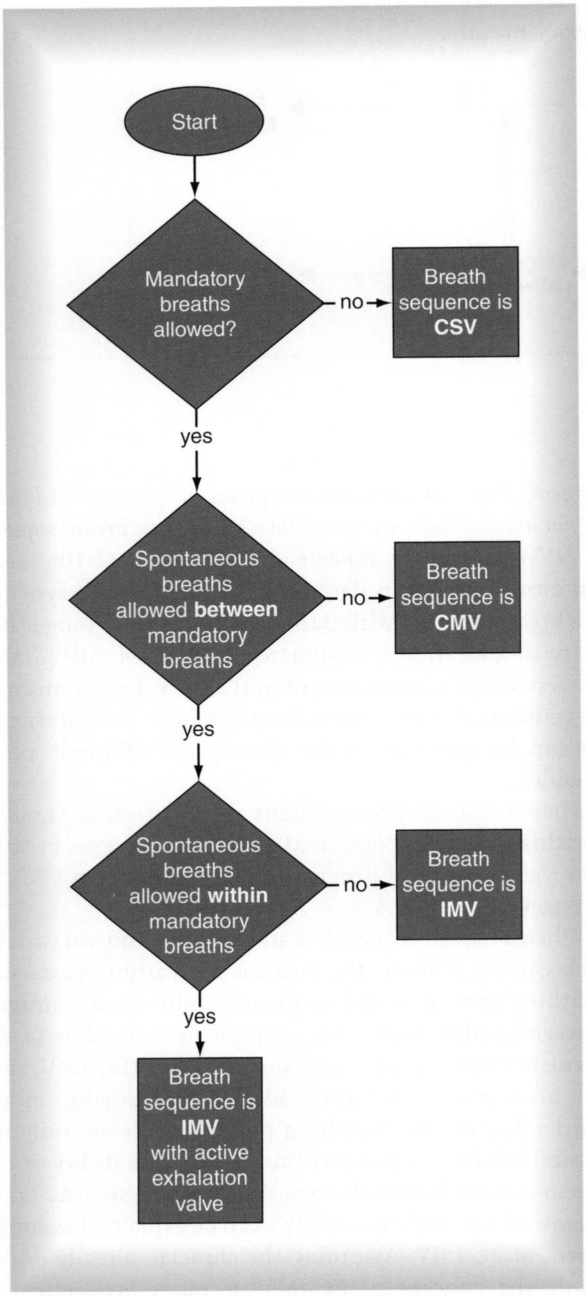

FIGURE 42-10 Algorithm distinguishing between CSV, CMV, and two forms of IMV.

bilevel ventilation are particularly ambiguous terms. To make matters even more confusing, the Puritan Bennett 840 ventilator has a "bilevel" mode that allows for additional pressure support during a pressure-limited, time-cycled, mandatory breath. With PEEP, the mandatory pressure limit, and the pressure support limit, the mode actually provides "trilevel" ventilation.

The specification of breathing pattern is also useful for grouping together modes that function the same way but are given different names. Both "CMV plus pressure limited ventilation" (Draeger Evita 4) and "volume-assured pressure support" (Bird 8400ST) are PC-IMV. It is also possible to group ventilators in terms of the number of breathing patterns they offer; some offer only one or two, whereas others offer all five. This grouping might be useful as an initial screening tool when planning ventilator purchases. Although the Bird 8400ST and 8400 STi may still be in use, this particular ventilator is not actively supported by the manufacturer (CareFusion, San Diego, California).

TABLE 42-3

All Modes of Ventilation Can Be Characterized by One of Five Breathing Patterns

Breath Control Variable	Breath Sequence	Abbreviation
Volume (control)	Continuous mandatory ventilation	VC-CMV
	Intermittent mandatory ventilation	VC-IMV
Pressure (control)	Continuous mandatory ventilation	PC-CMV
	Intermittent mandatory ventilation	PC-IMV
	Continuous spontaneous ventilation	PC-CSV

Targeting Schemes

Control variables and the differences between pressure and volume control have been discussed, but what is meant by *control* has not been explained. There are two general ways to control a variable: open loop control and closed loop control.[14]

Open Loop Control. Open loop control means that the control circuit makes no adjustments for external disturbances. The Percussionaire Intrapulmonary Percussive Ventilator (Percussionaire Corporation, Sandpoint, Idaho) generates pulses of gas flow without feedback control of pressure, volume, or flow. Flow into the patient is a function of the impedance of the respiratory system. Delivered pressures and volumes are affected by any disturbances in the system (e.g., changing lung mechanics, the patient's ventilatory efforts, and leaks).

Closed Loop Control. Closed loop control means that the delivered pressure, volume, and flow can be measured and used as feedback information to control the driving mechanism (similar to speed control in an automobile). Inspiratory volumes, flows, and pressures can be made to match specified input values despite disturbances such as changes in patient load and minor leaks in the system.

The basic concept of closed loop control has evolved into at least six different ventilator control systems or *targeting schemes*[14] (set-point, dual, servo, adaptive, optimal, and intelligent). These targeting schemes are the foundation that makes possible several dozen apparently different modes of ventilation. Once it is understood how these targeting schemes work, many of the apparent differences are seen to be similarities. A lot of the confusion surrounding ventilator marketing hype is avoided, and the true clinical capabilities of different ventilators are appreciated.

Set-point. Most ventilators use at least set-point targeting. The output is constrained to match a constant preset input (i.e., the set-point, such as a set maximum pressure or flow value). This matching makes possible the standard volume or pressure control modes. The operator sets either a fixed pressure or a flow target, and the ventilator maintains a consistent pressure or flow waveform output. This type of targeting scheme is similar to "cruise control" on an automobile.

Dual. Dual targeting is a more advanced version of set-point targeting. It gives the ventilator the decision of whether the breath will be volume controlled or pressure controlled according to the operator-set priorities. The breath may start out in pressure control and automatically switch to volume control, as in the Bird VAPS mode or, the reverse, as in the Draeger Pmax mode. The Maquet SERVO-i ventilator has a mode called volume control, and the operator presets both inspiratory time and tidal volume as would be expected with any conventional volume control mode. However, if the patient makes an inspiratory effort that decreases inspiratory pressure by 3 cm H_2O, the ventilator switches to pressure control and, if the effort lasts long enough, flow cycles the breath. If the tidal volume and inspiratory time are set relatively low and the inspiratory effort is relatively large, the resultant breath delivery is indistinguishable from pressure support. As a result, the tidal volume may be much larger than the expected, preset value. This occurrence highlights the need to understand dual targeting. Because both pressure and volume may be the control variables during dual targeting, by convention we designate the control variable as the one with which the breath initiates; the alternative control variable may never be implemented during the breath, depending on the other factors in the targeting scheme.

Servo. Set-point targeting attempts to maintain a constant output to match a constant input, whereas servo targeting is designed to track a moving input, similar to power steering on an automobile. Servo targeting was developed during World War II to aim ships' guns and radar equipment. It makes the proportional assist mode possible.[15] In this mode, the output of the ventilator follows and amplifies the patient's own flow pattern. The ventilator can support the abnormal load imposed by disease, while the patient's own muscles handle a normal load secondary to the respiratory system's natural resistance and compliance.

Adaptive. Adaptive targeting means automatic adjustment of one set-point to maintain a different operator-selected set-point. One of the first examples of a mode using adaptive control was pressure-regulated volume control on the Siemens Servo 300 ventilator (Siemens Corp, New York City, New York). Adaptive targeting is an evolutionary step because it gives the ventilator the capability to determine a set-point level independent of the operator. While set-point targeting operates within breaths, adaptive control introduces another feedback loop that operates between breaths (i.e., pressure targeting within breaths and volume targeting between breaths). Using feedback of volume allows the ventilator to adapt to changes in the patient's lung mechanics. Despite having various names for the specific modes it allows, adaptive targeting to date has been implemented most commonly as a way for the ventilator to adjust the inspiratory pressure of a breath automatically to meet an operator set volume target over several breaths. Another example would be adjustment of the mandatory breath frequency to achieve a minute ventilation target.

Optimal. Optimal targeting takes adaptive control a step further by allowing the ventilator to set both volume and pressure set-points. Optimal control takes its name from the fact that a mathematical model is used to find the best (e.g., highest or lowest) value of some performance function. Hamilton Medical makes the only commercially available ventilators with this feature. Optimal targeting allows the ventilator to make all subsequent adjustments after the operator sets the target minute ventilation. Hamilton Medical (and the authors who did the basic research published in the literature) refer to the optimal control mode as *adaptive support,* which confuses their more highly evolved targeting scheme, optimal control, with the simpler adaptive control described earlier.

Other forms of optimal control give the ventilator even more authority using exhaled CO_2 as a feedback signal.[16] In Europe, Hamilton Medical has introduced IntelliVent, a system for complete closed loop control of minute ventilation, fractional inspired oxygen (FiO_2), and PEEP using both CO_2 and SpO_2 as feedback signals.

Intelligent. The term *intelligent* refers to automatic targeting strategies that make use of artificial intelligence methods, such as "fuzzy logic," rule-based expert systems, and even neural networks.[14] This type of automatic targeting is yet another evolutionary step because it gives the ventilator more information than what may be contained in a simple, static, mathematical model. Knowledge-based targeting schemes attempt to capture the experience of human experts and expand the scope of control to potentially all parameters of the ventilatory mode. An experimental application of this type of control has been described for automatic adjustment of pressure support.[17] That system has now been commercialized as the Draeger SmartCare mode.

An even more sophisticated approach coupled a knowledge base with fuzzy logic.[18] In this case, the ventilator used both instantaneous measurements of physiologic values such as respiratory rate and saturation and their rates of change. Fuzzy logic[19] was used as a way to integrate the measurements with predefined ranges of values representing the patient status. When the patient's status was determined, appropriate expert rules were selected from a lookup table and used to adjust the ventilator. Although this was a limited application, it proved the concept.

The most convincing proof of concept was presented by East and colleagues.[20] These investigators used a rule-based expert system for ventilator management in a large, multicenter prospective randomized trial. Although survival and length of stay were not different between human and computer management, computer control resulted in a significant reduction in multiorgan dysfunction and lower incidence and severity of lung overdistention injury. However, the most important finding was that expert knowledge can be encoded and successfully shared with institutions that had no input into the model. The expert system did not directly control the ventilator but rather made suggestions for the human operator. Theoretically, the operator could be eliminated.

Perhaps the most exotic targeting scheme to date is the artificial neural network.[21] This experimental system (not yet commercially available) did not directly control the ventilator but acted as a decision support system. Snowden and coworkers[21] commented that the neural network was capable of learning, which offers significant advantages over static rule-based systems.

Neural networks are essentially data modeling tools used to capture and represent complex input-output relationships. A neural network learns by experience the same way a human brain does, by storing knowledge in the strengths of internode connections. As data modeling tools, neural networks have been used in many business and medical applications for both diagnosis and forecasting.[22] A neural network, similar to an animal brain, is composed of individual neurons. Signals *(action potentials)* appear at the unit's inputs *(synapses)*. The effect that each signal has may be approximated by multiplying the signal by some number or *weight* to indicate the strength of the synapse. The weighted signals are summed to produce overall unit activation. If this activation exceeds a certain threshold, the unit produces an output response. As the network learns, the weights change, affecting the final output.

Specifying the targeting scheme in a mode description can help to distinguish between modes that look nearly identical on a graphics monitor and present conceptual or verbal problems when trying to differentiate them. It might be difficult to appreciate the difference between pressure support and volume support on a Maquet SERVO-i ventilator, but consider these simple descriptions: Pressure support is PC-CSV with set-point targeting of inspiratory pressure. Volume support is PC-CSV with adaptive targeting of inspiratory pressure. If a clinician knows the definitions of these words and acronyms, he or she can immediately understand how different the modes are. Attention would also be directed to the clinical implications for the patient (e.g., what settings are required). Knowledge of targeting schemes also allows the clinician to see that something like Draeger's AutoFlow feature is not just a "supplement" or "extra setting" as the operator's manual indicates but creates a whole new mode. Operating the Draeger Evita 4 in CMV yields VC-CMV with set-point targeting of inspiratory volume and flow. However, activating AutoFlow when CMV is set yields PC-CMV with adaptive targeting of inspiratory pressure and vastly different clinical ramifications for the patient. These two modes are about as different as any two modes can be.

If the breath sequence is IMV, a complete description of the mode includes targeting schemes for both mandatory and spontaneous breaths. On the Puritan Bennett 840 ventilator, the mode called *synchronized intermittent mandatory ventilation* would be described as VC-IMV with set-point targeting of volume for mandatory breaths and set-point targeting of pressure for spontaneous breaths.

At the highest level of detail, a mode can be fully characterized by adding the phase variables, followed by detailing the operational logic programmed into the software control system. The specification of the breathing pattern that the mode can produce, the type of targeting, and the specific strategy (phase variable and operational logic) it uses for both mandatory and spontaneous breaths make up a complete classification for any mode of ventilation (see Table 42-2).

The AutoMode feature on the Draeger Evita XL ventilator illustrates one example of why it is important to separate mandatory from spontaneous breath descriptions. AutoMode is a form of IMV, and there are three different types, as follows:

1. Mandatory breaths are volume-controlled with set-point targeting, and spontaneous breaths are pressure-controlled with adaptive targeting (i.e., volume support).
2. Mandatory breaths are pressure-controlled with set-point targeting, and spontaneous breaths are pressure-controlled with set-point targeting (i.e., pressure support).
3. Mandatory breaths are pressure-controlled with adaptive targeting (e.g., pressure-regulated volume control), and spontaneous breaths are pressure-controlled with adaptive targeting (i.e., volume support).

Two important facts about current ventilators should be apparent. First, ventilators offer far more complex modes than in the past, so understanding how they work is no trivial task. Manufacturers are throwing together combinations of features that not only are difficult to comprehend but also strain rational justification, often with

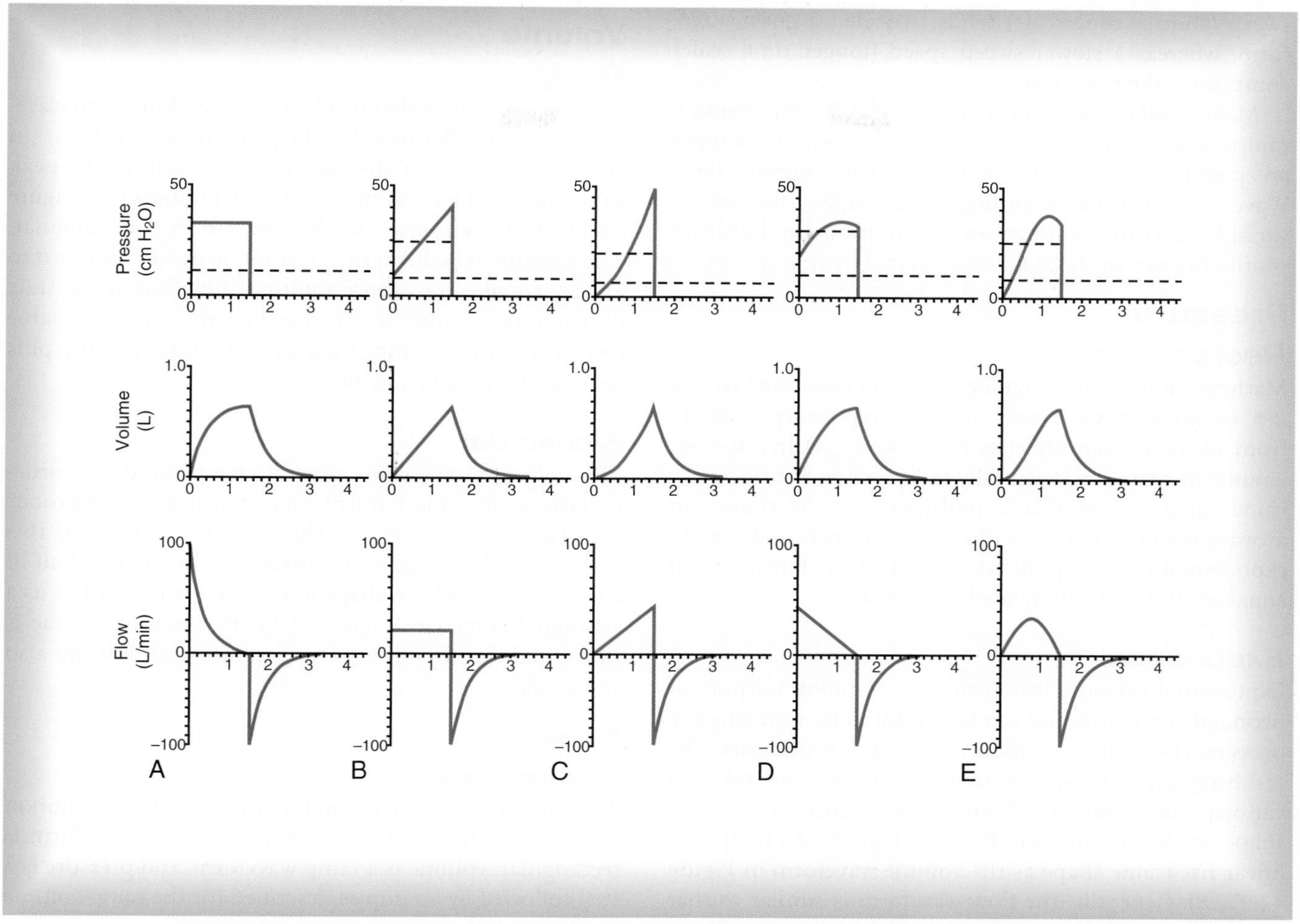

FIGURE 42-11 Model pressure, volume, and flow waveforms generated with a computer using the equation of motion. **A,** Pressure-controlled inspiration with a rectangular pressure waveform (identical to flow-controlled inspiration with an exponential decay flow waveform). **B,** Flow-controlled inspiration with a rectangular flow waveform (identical to volume-controlled inspiration with an ascending ramp volume waveform). **C,** Flow-controlled inspiration with an ascending ramp flow waveform. **D,** Flow-controlled inspiration with a descending ramp flow waveform. **E,** Flow-controlled inspiration with a sinusoidal flow waveform. *Short dotted lines* represent mean inspiratory pressure, and *long dotted lines* represent mean airway pressure (assuming zero PEEP). For the rectangular pressure waveform in **A,** the mean inspiratory pressure is the same as the PIP. For all waveforms, V_T = 644 ml, compliance = 20 ml/cm H_2O, and resistance = 20 cm H_2O/L/sec.

no clinical data to support their efficacy. Second, there is no agreement among ventilator manufacturers when it comes to nomenclature. Also, the names they create for modes are baffling.

OUTPUT WAVEFORMS

Electrocardiograms and blood pressure waveforms are studied to understand heart physiology. In the same way, to understand ventilator-patient interaction, output waveforms must be examined. The output waveforms of interest during ventilatory support are pressure, volume, and flow. For each control variable, current ventilators produce a limited number of waveforms. Basic waveforms are shown in Figure 42-11.

Because the waveforms in Figure 42-11 are models, they do not show the minor deviations, or "noise," often seen during actual ventilator use. Such noise can be caused by many factors, including vibration and turbulence. These waveforms also do not show the effect of expiratory circuit resistance because this varies depending on the ventilator and type of circuit. The waveforms do not show the various indicators of problems with ventilator-patient synchrony (e.g., improper sensitivity setting and gas trapping), which are beyond the scope of this chapter. Finally, waveform appearances change when the time scale is altered. A faster sweep (shorter time scale) tends to widen a given waveform, whereas a slower sweep speed (longer time scale) compresses the waveform.

Most ventilator waveforms are rectangular, exponential, ramp, or sinusoidal in shape. Although various subtypes are possible, we describe only the most common here. Waveforms are listed according to the shape of the control variable waveform. Any new waveforms produced by future ventilators can easily be accommodated by this system.

Pressure

Rectangular

Mathematically, a rectangular waveform is referred to as a *step* or *instantaneous change* in transrespiratory pressure from one value to another (see Figure 42-11, *A*). In response, volume increases exponentially from zero to a steady-state value equal to compliance multiplied by the change in airway pressure (i.e., PIP – PEEP). Inspiratory flow decreases exponentially from a peak value (at the start of inspiration) equal to (PIP – PEEP) divided by resistance.

Exponential

Exponential pressure waveforms are common outputs of neonatal ventilators and can be produced by adjusting the pressure rise control on some newer adult ventilators. The resulting pressure and volume waveforms can take on various shapes ranging from an exponential rise (same shape as the volume waveform in Figure 42-11, *A*) to a linear rise (same shape as the volume waveform in Figure 42-11, *B*). Generally, the flow waveform is similar to that seen in Figure 42-11, *A* except that peak inspiratory flow is reached gradually rather than instantaneously (resulting in a rounded rather than peaked waveform), and peak flow is lower than with a rectangular pressure waveform.

Sinusoidal

As previously described, a sinusoidal pressure waveform can be created by attaching a piston to a rotating crank. In addition, a linear drive motor driven by a microprocessor can produce a sine wave pressure pattern. In response, the volume and flow waveforms are also sinusoidal, but they attain their peak values at different times (see Figure 42-11, *E*).

Oscillating

Oscillating pressure waveforms can take on various shapes, from sinusoidal to ramp (SensorMedics 3100 Oscillator, Care Fusion Inc, Yorba Linda, CA) to roughly triangular (some jet ventilators). The distinguishing feature of a ventilator classified as an oscillator is that it can generate negative transrespiratory pressure. If the mean airway pressure is set equal to atmospheric pressure, the airway pressure waveform oscillates above and below zero. If the pressure waveform is sinusoidal, volume and flow are also sinusoidal but out of phase with each other (i.e., their peak values occur at different times).

Volume

Ramp

Volume controllers that produce an ascending ramp waveform (i.e., the Bennett MA-1) produce a linear rise in volume from zero at the start of inspiration to the peak value, or set tidal volume, at end-inspiration (see Figure 42-11, *B*). In response, the flow waveform is rectangular. The pressure waveform rises instantaneously from zero to a value equal to resistance multiplied by flow at the start of inspiration. From here, it rises linearly to its peak value (PIP) equal to elastance multiplied by tidal volume plus resistance multiplied by flow.

Sinusoidal

This volume waveform is most often produced by ventilators whose drive mechanism is a piston attached to a rotating crank (e.g., Emerson). The output waveform of this type of ventilator can be approximated by the first half of a cosine curve, whose shape in this case is referred to as a sigmoidal curve (see Figure 42-11, *E*). Because volume is sinusoidal during inspiration, pressure and flow are also sinusoidal.

Flow

Rectangular

A rectangular flow waveform is perhaps the most common output (see Figure 42-11, *B*). When the flow waveform is rectangular, volume is a ramp waveform, and pressure is a step followed by a ramp as described for the ramp volume waveform.

Ramp

Many respiratory care practitioners (and ventilator manufacturers) refer to ramp waveforms as either *accelerating* or *decelerating* flow patterns. The use of either of these terms is usually inappropriate. If a car slows, we do not say that its velocity decelerates; we say that the car decelerates. We do not say that a cyclotron is a velocity accelerator but that it is a particle accelerator. The rate of change of position of an object is the velocity of the object; analogously, the rate of change of volume is flow. The rate of change of velocity of an object is the acceleration of the object; likewise, the rate of change of flow is the acceleration of volume, not the acceleration of flow. So if we want to say that flow changes, we should simply talk about an increasing flow or a decreasing flow (or an accelerating volume or a decelerating volume), not an accelerating flow or a decelerating flow.

Ascending Ramp. A true ascending ramp waveform starts at zero and increases linearly to the peak value (see Figure 42-11, *C*). Actual ventilator flow waveforms may be truncated; inspiration starts with an initial instantaneous flow. The Bear-5 starts inspiration at 50% of the set peak flow. Flow increases linearly to the set peak flow rate. In response to an ascending ramp flow waveform, the pressure and volume waveforms are exponential with a concave upward shape. As previously described with the 8400 St and STi ventilators, this particular ventilator may still be in use, however, the current manufacturer does not actively produce or support this product.

Descending Ramp. A true descending ramp waveform starts at the peak value and decreases linearly to zero (see Figure 42-11, *D*). Ventilator flow waveforms are usually truncated; inspiratory flow rate decreases linearly from the set peak flow until it reaches some arbitrary threshold where flow drops immediately to zero (e.g., the Puritan Bennett 7200a ends inspiration when the flow rate decreases to 5 L/min). In response to a descending ramp flow waveform, the pressure and volume waveforms are exponential with a concave downward shape.

Sinusoidal

Some ventilators offer a mode in which the inspiratory flow waveform approximates the shape of the first half of a sine wave (see Figure 42-11, *E*). As with the ramp waveform, ventilators often truncate the sine waveform by starting and ending flow at some percentage of the set peak flow rather than start and end at zero flow. In response to a sinusoidal flow waveform, the pressure and volume waveforms are also sinusoidal but out of phase with each other.

Effects of Calibration Errors and the Patient Circuit

The pressure, volume, and flow the patient receives are never precisely the same as what the clinician sets on the ventilator. These differences sometimes are caused by instrument inaccuracies or calibration error. In addition, the patient delivery circuit contributes to discrepancies between the desired and actual patient values because the patient circuit has its own compliance and resistance. The pressure measured on the inspiratory side of a ventilator always is higher than the pressure at the airway opening owing to patient circuit resistance. In addition, the volume and flow coming out of the ventilator exceeds the volume and flow delivered to the patient because of the compliance of the patient circuit.

Using an analogy to electrical circuits, compliance of the delivery circuit can be shown to be connected in parallel with the compliance of the respiratory system (i.e., both elements sharing the same driving pressure). Consequently, the total compliance of the ventilator-patient system is simply the sum of the two compliances. The resistance of the delivery circuit is connected in series with the respiratory system resistance (i.e., both elements sharing the same flow) so that the total resistance is the sum of the two. Based on these assumptions, the relationship between the volume input to the patient (at the point of connection to the patient's airway opening) and the volume output from the ventilator (at the point of connection to the patient circuit) can be described by the following equation:

$$\text{Volume input to patient} = \frac{\text{Volume output from ventilator}}{1 + C_{pc}/C_{rs}}$$

Equation 42-7

where C_{pc} is the compliance of the patient circuit, and C_{rs} is the total compliance of the patient's respiratory system. The equation shows that the larger the patient circuit compliance compared with the patient's respiratory system, the larger the denominator on the right-hand side of the equation, and the smaller the delivered tidal volume is compared with the volume coming from the ventilator's drive mechanism.

Assuming that the volume exiting the ventilator is the set tidal volume, the patient circuit compliance (C_{pc}) is calculated as follows:

$$C_{pc} = \frac{\text{Set tidal volume}}{P_{plat} - \text{PEEP}}$$

Equation 42-8

where P_{plat} is the pressure measured during an inspiratory hold maneuver with the Y-piece of the patient circuit occluded (patient not connected), and PEEP is end expiratory pressure (i.e., baseline pressure). Most authors recommend the use of PIP for P_{plat} in this equation, which is acceptable but may lead to a slight underestimation of patient circuit compliance. P_{plat} is slightly lower than PIP because of the flow-resistive pressure decrease of the patient circuit if pressure is not measured at the Y-piece. This difference is greatest in small-bore, corrugated patient circuit tubing but is probably insignificant.

The effects of patient circuit compliance are most troublesome during volume-controlled ventilation. In neonatal ventilation, the patient circuit compliance can be three times that of the respiratory system, even with small-bore tubing and a small-volume humidifier. In an attempt to deliver a preset tidal volume, the volume delivered to the patient may be only 25% of that exiting the ventilator, whereas 75% is compressed in the patient circuit.

During pressure-controlled ventilation, the compliance of the patient circuit has the effect of rounding the leading edge of a rectangular pressure waveform (see Figure 39-9), which could reduce the volume delivered to the patient. This effect is prevented if the pressure limit is maintained for at least five time constants of the respiratory system.

For both pressure-controlled and volume-controlled ventilation, the patient circuit compliance and resistance, along with the resistance of the exhalation valve (in series with the patient circuit and respiratory system resistance) increase the expiratory time constant. A large circuit compliance coupled with a short expiratory time can lead to inadvertent PEEP or auto-PEEP. The set values for pressure, volume, and flow may be different from the output (from ventilator) values because of calibration errors and different from the input (to the patient) because of the effects of the patient circuit. These two general sources of error cause discrepancies between the desired and actual patient values.

OPERATOR INTERFACE

The ventilator's operator interface, or ventilator display, has undergone extensive evolution over the last 30 years. Originally, the displays on ventilators were "analog." Operator inputs, or settings, were accomplished with hard-wired knobs, buttons, and dials. The ventilator outputs, such as alarm conditions and ventilating pressure, were displayed with bulbs, light emitting diodes (LEDs), and meters. Some older home care ventilators still use analog displays (Figure 42-12). The development of inexpensive microprocessors has led manufacturers to use "digital" displays almost exclusively on all types of ventilators. Digital interfaces use LED or LCD screens for visual display of ventilator data along with some multipurpose hard-wired buttons. The simplest example would be the display of a bilevel positive airway pressure machine used for treating sleep apnea at home (Figure 42-13). A more advanced digital display uses dedicated special-purpose buttons and dials (Figure 42-14). The most advanced interfaces use the concept of the "virtual" instrument, meaning that knobs, buttons, dials, and meters are simulated on a computer screen (sometimes a touch screen) and often incorporating a single mechanical dial that is used to set multiple parameters (Figure 42-15). Computer screens allow graphic displays of alarm settings as bar graphs along with pressure, volume, and flow waveforms as scalars or loops.

Operator Inputs

The operator inputs include the parameters of the ventilatory pattern (i.e., mode and phase variables) and any desired alarm settings. We discuss some specific examples

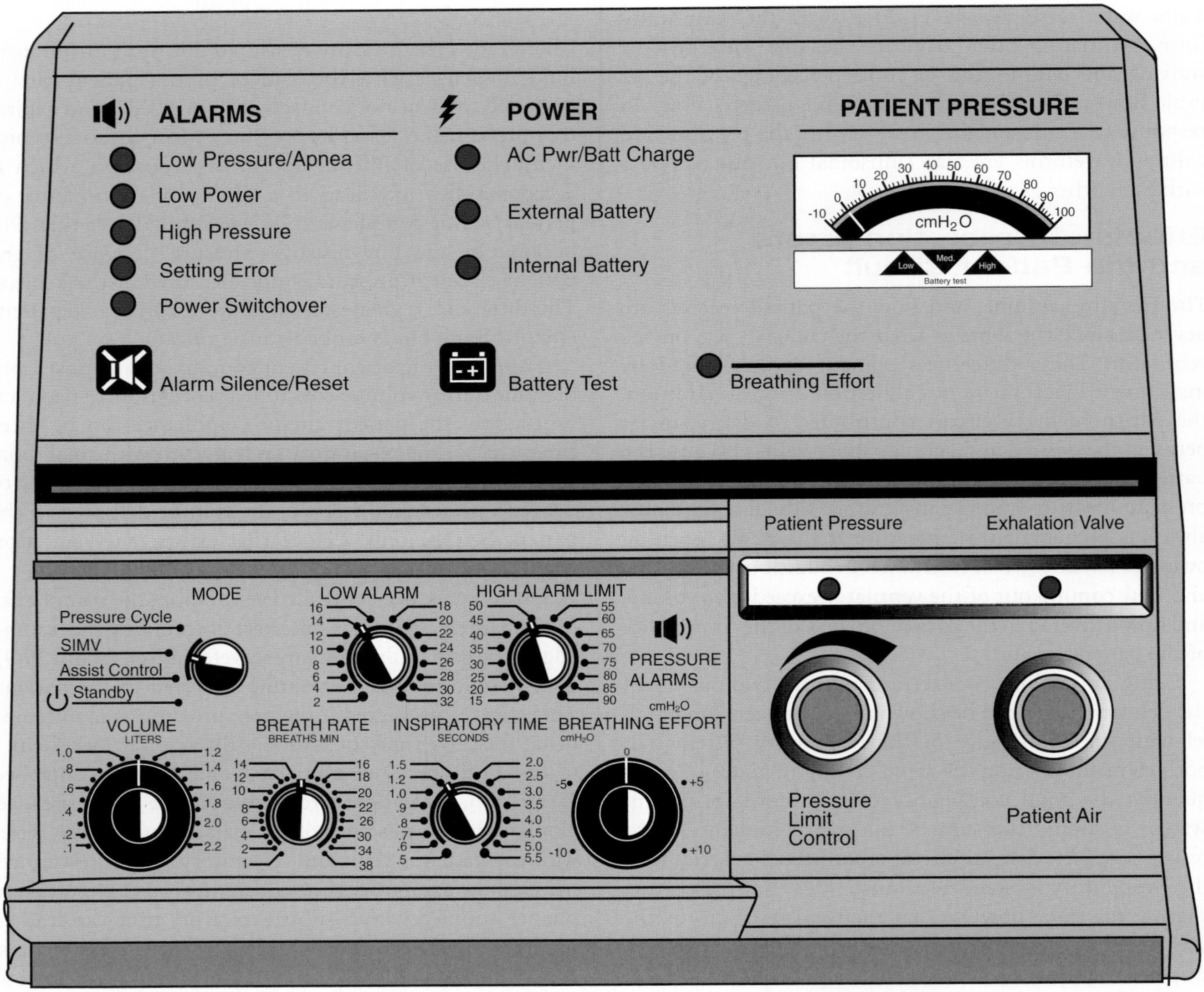

FIGURE 42-12 Control panel of the Puritan Bennett LP10 ventilator. (Courtesy Covidien Nellcor Puritan Bennett, Boulder, Colorado.)

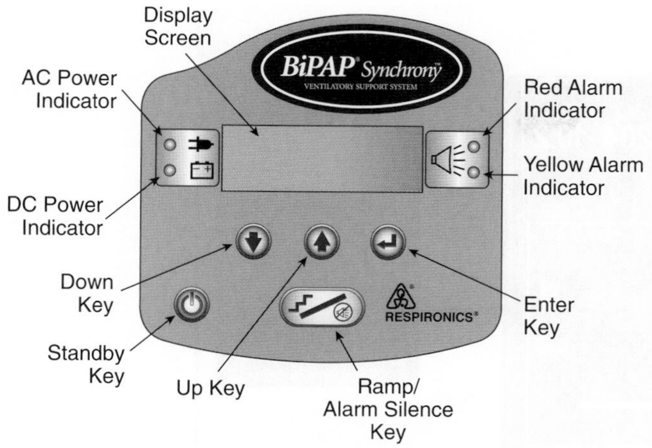

FIGURE 42-13 Control panel of the Respironics BiPAP Synchrony. (Courtesy Philips Respironics, Murrysville, Pennsylvania.)

of trigger, target, and cycle variables and an assortment of alarm parameters. Each ventilator has its own unique layout, so a complete description of all available devices is beyond the scope of this chapter.

Mode Settings

There is no standardization among ventilator manufacturers regarding the names of modes, their classification, or how the operator identifies and sets them on a given device. This requires the operator to learn the specific terminology and layout of each individual brand of ventilator for every function it provides. For clinical settings where many different ventilator brands are used, this can be a daunting and perhaps unachievable task. For an example of how different and confusing ventilator displays can be regarding mode selection, compare Figures 42-16 and 42-17.

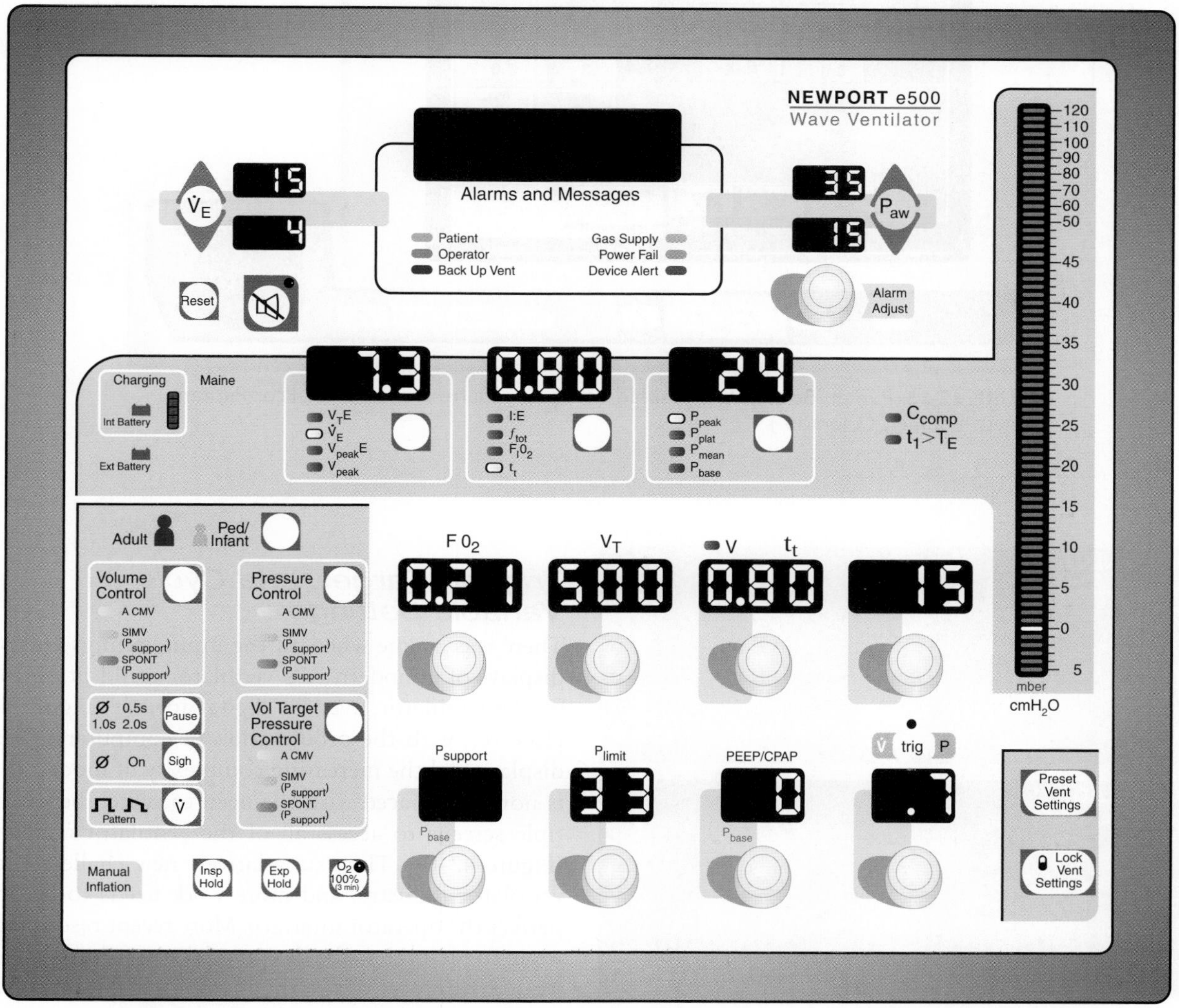

FIGURE 42-14 Control panel of the Newport e500 ventilator. (Courtesy Newport Medical, Newport, CA.)

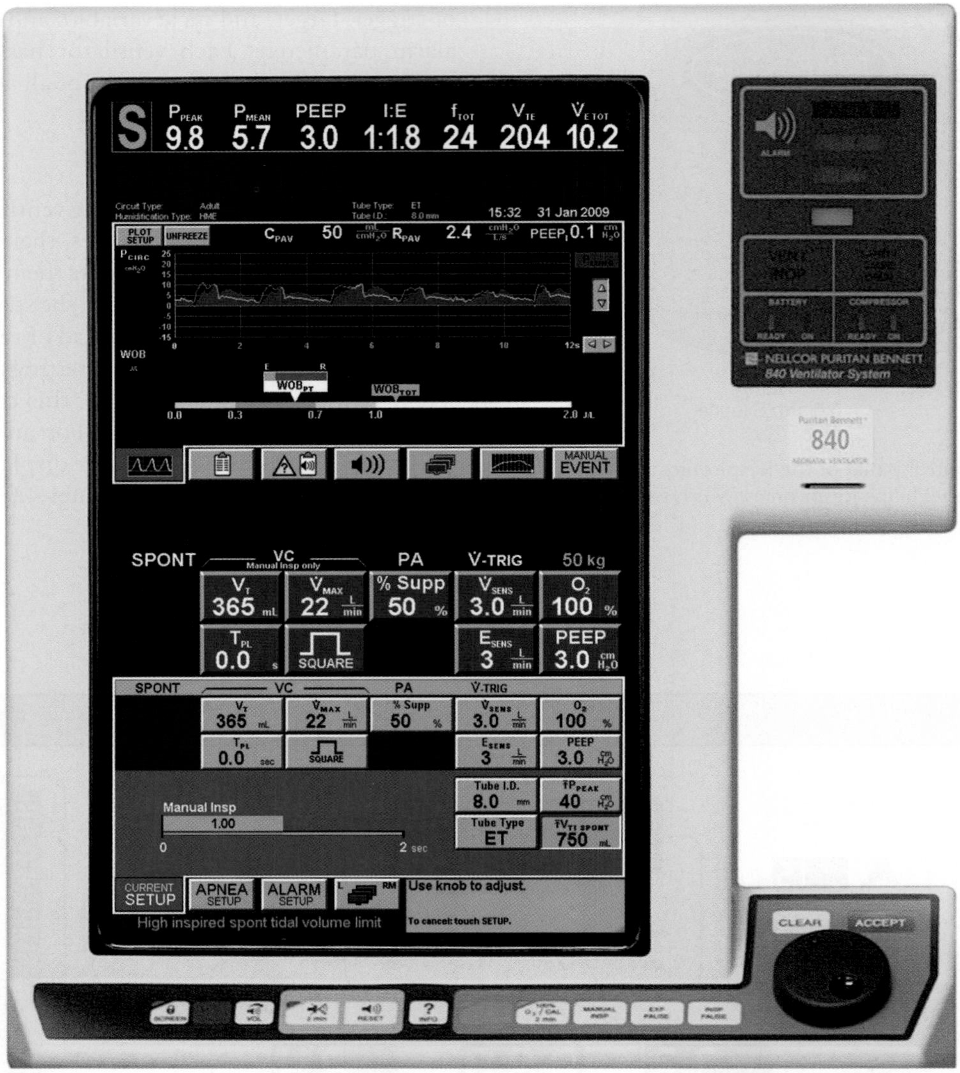

FIGURE 42-15 Puritan Bennett 840 graphic interface. (Courtesy Covidien Nellcor Puritan Bennett, Boulder, Colorado.)

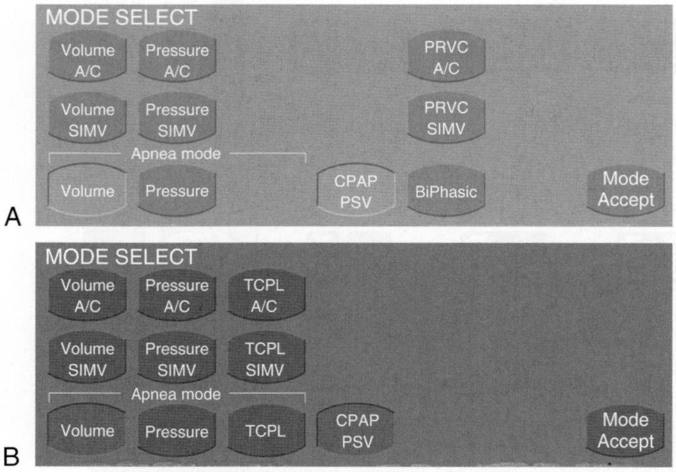

FIGURE 42-16 Mode selection screen for the CareFusion Avea ventilator. (Courtesy CareFusion Viasys, San Diego, California.)

Trigger, Target, and Cycle Variable Settings

There was a time when all the input settings and output displays of a modern ICU ventilator could fit on the face of the ventilator, even in digital format (Figure 42-18). However, with the proliferation of computer screens for displays and the increasing complexity of modes, the user is now often faced with the need to switch between multiple screens to access all of the ventilator's capabilities (Figure 42-19). This is a relatively new challenge for the ventilator industry, and more work needs to be done to perfect the operator interface. More recent research on the topic suggests that the design of the user interface is relevant to the occurrence of operational failures and that ventilator designers could optimize the user-interface design to reduce operational failures.[23]

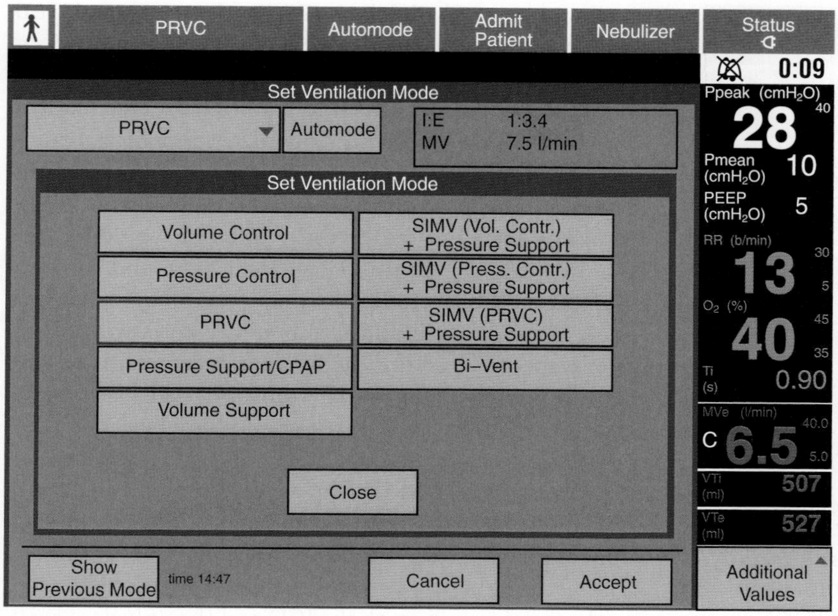

FIGURE 42-17 Mode selection screen for the Maquet SERVO-i ventilator. (Courtesy Maquet, Inc, Bridgewater, New Jersey.)

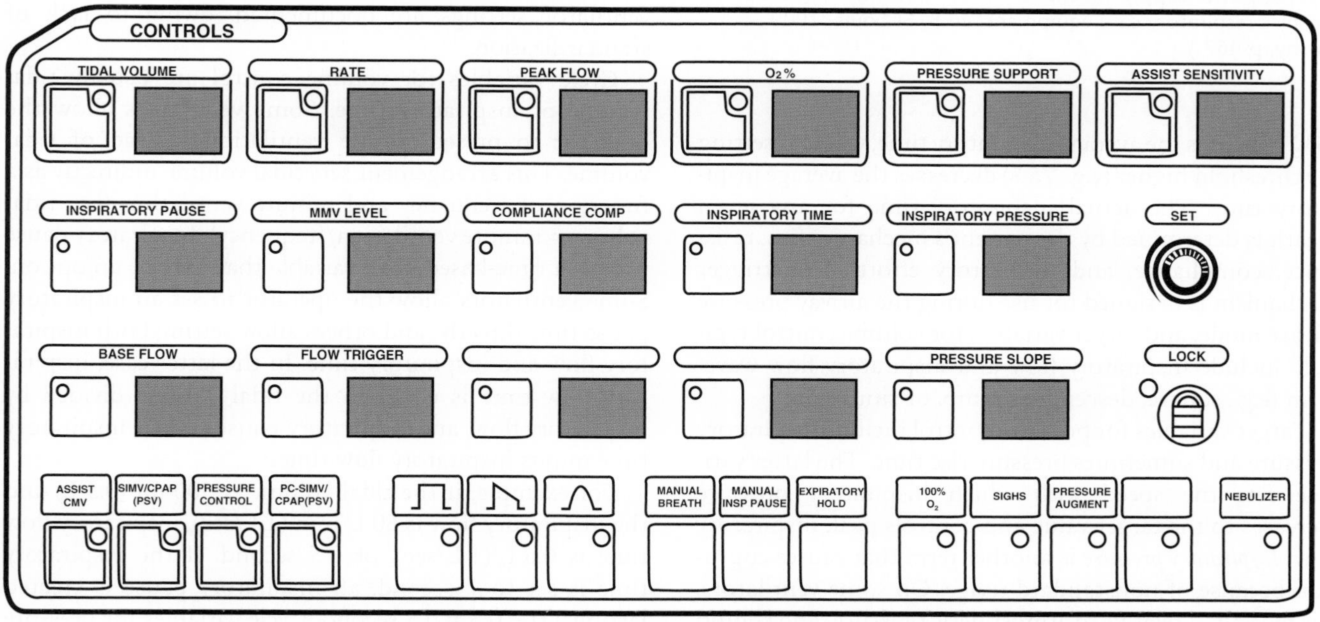

FIGURE 42-18 Control panel of the Bear 1000 ventilator. (Courtesy Cardinal Health, Palm Springs, California.)

Trigger variables include selection of either pressure or flow triggering and the trigger thresholds (in cm H_2O or L/min). Sometimes these variables are explicitly described, and sometimes they are just referred to as a *sensitivity* setting. Frequency is also a trigger variable, setting the time delay between time-triggered inspirations. A preset minute ventilation can also be a trigger variable in modes such as Draeger's mandatory minute ventilation mode and Hamilton's adaptive support mode; if the total minute ventilation from mandatory and spontaneous breaths falls below the preset value, the ventilator triggers mandatory breaths. Draeger has introduced a novel trigger mechanism (called AutoRelease on its Evita Infinity V500 ventilator) based on the percentage of peak expiratory flow. Mandatory pressure-controlled breaths are flow triggered when expiratory flow decays to the preset threshold, usually expressed as a percentage of the peak expiratory flow for the breath. Setting the cycle threshold at a lower value (e.g.,

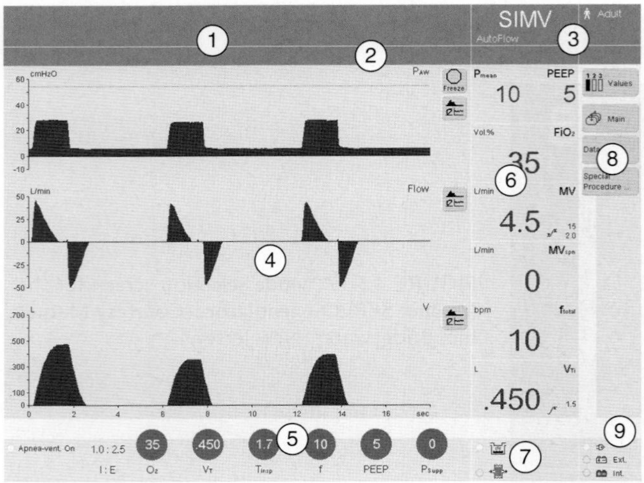

FIGURE 42-19 View of the typical screen display on the Draeger Evita XL ventilator: *1,* Space for display of alarm messages; *2,* space for display of operator prompts; *3,* mode of ventilation display; *4,* graphic display of waveforms, loops, and trends; *5,* digital display of set ventilation parameters; *6,* display of measured values; *7,* humidification type and status; *8,* touch-sensitive screen keys available for the currently selected page; *9,* power supply indicator. (From Cairo MJ, Pilbeam SP: Mosby's respiratory care equipment, ed 8, St Louis, 2009, Mosby, p 467.)

25%) increases the average inspiratory time, whereas setting the threshold higher (e.g., 75%) decreases the average inspiratory time. The actual inspiratory time for any given breath is determined by the patient's mechanics (i.e., resistance, compliance, and inspiratory effort). The trigger mechanism is designed for use during the airway pressure release mode, and target variables for volume control typically include inspiratory flow and inspiratory flow waveform (e.g., square, descending ramp, or sinusoidal).

Target variables for pressure control include inspiratory pressure and sometimes pressure rise time. The latter variable sets the speed with which inspiratory pressure increases to the target value and controls peak inspiratory flow. *Inspiratory pressure* is another term that causes confusion because of nonstandard usage. On some ventilators, it is measured relative to atmospheric pressure (and should be called *peak inspiratory pressure*), and on others it is measured relative to PEEP and should be called simply *inspiratory pressure.*[24] The problem is that when a patient is changed from one ventilator (or mode) using one convention to another ventilator (or mode) with the other convention, the risk of inadvertently setting the wrong inspiratory pressure increases and could lead to adverse events.

For example, imagine a ventilated patient with respiratory system resistance of 10 cm H_2O/L/sec and compliance of 0.035 L/cm H_2O. This patient is transported on a ventilator with set inspiratory pressure of 25 cm H_2O (relative to atmospheric pressure), PEEP of 10 cm H_2O, and inspiratory time of 1.0 second. Under the assumptions of passive ventilation and no intrinsic PEEP, the measured peak airway pressured with this particular ventilator is 25 cm H_2O, the ΔP is $25 - 10 = 15$ cm H_2O, and the tidal volume would be 495 ml. On arrival to the ICU, pressure-control ventilation is initiated with a ventilator in which inspiratory pressure is set relative to PEEP. If the same settings were used (inspiratory pressure 25 cm H_2O and PEEP 10 cm H_2O) the new peak airway pressure would be $25 + 10 = 35$ cm H_2O, ΔP would be 25 cm H_2O, and the tidal volume would 825 ml. In this example, the patient is put at risk of ventilator-induced lung injury and cardiac compromise because of the inadvertent increase in ΔP and mean airway pressure. If the transport had been in the opposite direction, the patient would have been at risk of hypoventilation because of a lower ΔP and loss of oxygenation owing to decreased mean airway pressure. One could argue that a knowledgeable clinician would not make such a mistake because of familiarity with the two ventilators. What if the patient was being manually ventilated during intrahospital transport to the ICU and the only data available were the inspiratory pressure and PEEP? The risk of confusion, if not actual harm, is inherent in the way ventilator settings are documented, owing to lack of standardization.

Cycle variables for volume control are usually tidal volume or inspiratory time. Some ventilators allow the operator to preset minute ventilation instead of tidal volume. This arrangement sets tidal volume indirectly as a function of frequency and minute ventilation (i.e., tidal volume = minute ventilation/frequency). Inspiratory pause time is a time-based cycle variable that may be an option. Some ventilators allow the operator to set an inspiratory pause time directly, and others allow setting both inspiratory flow and inspiratory time. In the latter case, inspiratory flow time is equal to the tidal volume divided by inspiratory flow, and inspiratory pause time is inspiratory time minus inspiratory flow time.

For example, if the tidal volume is 500 ml (0.5 L) and the inspiratory flow is 60 L/min (1 L/sec), inspiratory flow time is 0.5 L/(1 L/sec), or 0.5 second. If the inspiratory time is set to 1 second, an inspiratory pause is created lasting $1.0 - 0.5 = 0.5$ second. Cycle variables for pressure control generally include inspiratory time (or I : E ratio) for mandatory breaths and possibly flow cycle threshold for spontaneous (pressure support) breaths. Pressure support breaths are flow cycled when inspiratory flow decays to the preset threshold, usually expressed as a percentage of the peak inspiratory flow for the breath. Setting the cycle threshold at a lower value (e.g., 25%) increases the average inspiratory time, whereas setting the threshold higher (e.g., 75%) decreases the average inspiratory time. The actual inspiratory time for any given breath is determined by the patient's mechanics (i.e., resistance, compliance, and inspiratory effort). All ventilators except for some home care devices, allow adjustment of the baseline pressure, or PEEP.

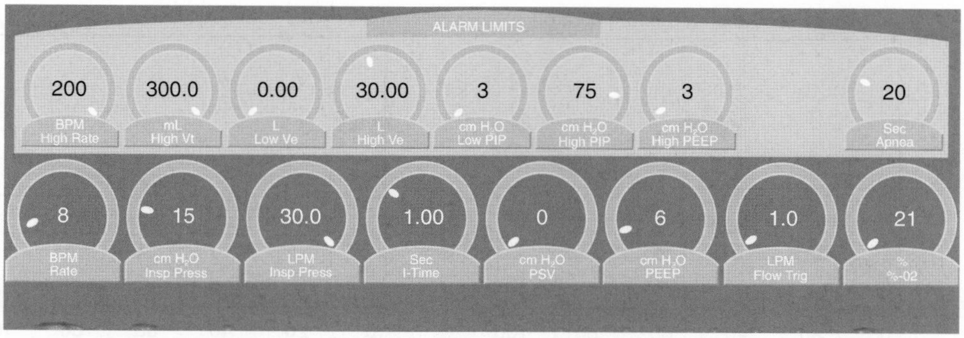

FIGURE 42-20 Alarm panel of CareFusion Viasys ventilator. (Courtesy CareFusion Viasys, San Diego, California.)

Alarm Settings

The purpose of ventilator alarms is to bring events to the attention of the clinician. Events are conditions or occurrences that require clinician awareness or intervention. Events can be classified according to four levels of priority.[25] Level 1 events are immediately life-threatening. These include insufficient or excessive gas delivery to the patient, exhalation valve failure, control circuit failure, or loss of power. Alarm indicators in this category should be mandatory (cannot be turned off by the operator), redundant, and noncanceling. Level 2 events range from mild irregularities in machine function to dangerous situations that could threaten patient safety if left unattended. These include failure of the air-O_2 blending system, inadequate or excessive PEEP, autotriggering, circuit leak, circuit occlusion, inappropriate I:E ratio, and failure of the humidification system. Alarms in this category are not redundant and may be self-canceling (i.e., automatically turned off if the event ceases). Level 3 events reflect changes in the level of ventilatory support. Examples include changes in the patient's ventilatory drive or respiratory system mechanics and the presence of auto-PEEP. Level 3 events often trigger the same alarms as levels 1 and 2. Level 4 events are focused entirely on the patient. These include changes in gas exchange, dead space, oxygenation, and cardiovascular functions. Many ventilators do not warn of these events, and external monitors are required for surveillance.

Ventilators do not display alarm settings in terms of levels of priority. Instead, they tend to lump them all together on the screen (Figures 42-20 and 42-21; see Figure 42-15). The setting of alarm thresholds is a complicated topic that has been studied but for which little information is available regarding mechanical ventilation. The basic problem is to maximize true alarms and minimize false alarms. A high false alarm rate leads to habituation and clinicians ignoring warnings. False alarms can also lead to inappropriate responses. In one 200-hour study of an ICU, 1214 alarms occurred, and 2344 tasks were performed. On average, alarms occurred six times per hour; 23% were effective, 36% were ineffective, and 41% were ignored.[26] In another ICU study, during 982 hours of observation, 5934 alarms occurred, corresponding to six per hour. About 40% of the alarms did not correctly describe the patient condition and were classified as technically false; 68% of those were caused by manipulation. Only 885 (15%) of all alarms were considered clinically relevant.[27]

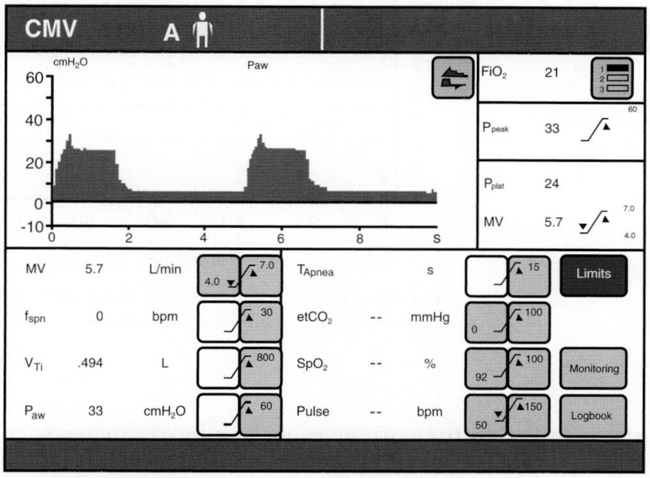

FIGURE 42-21 Alarm panel of Draeger Evita XL ventilator. (Courtesy Draeger Medical, Telford, Pennsylvania.)

Although these studies did not address mechanical ventilator alarms specifically, it is not hard to imagine similar results for such a study. Ventilator alarms are usually set by the operator (or as default values by the ventilator) as either a set value or a set percentage of the current value. Examples would be low and peak airway pressure alarms set at the current value ±5 cm H_2O or low and peak tidal volume and minute ventilation set at ±25% of the current value.[25] The problem is that the parameters we want to set alarms for, in particular, airway pressure, tidal volume, and minute ventilation, are highly variable, with significant portions at extreme values (Figure 42-22).[28] Limits set as absolute values or percentages may reduce safety for some extreme values, while increasing nuisance events for other values. An alternative approach might be to reference the

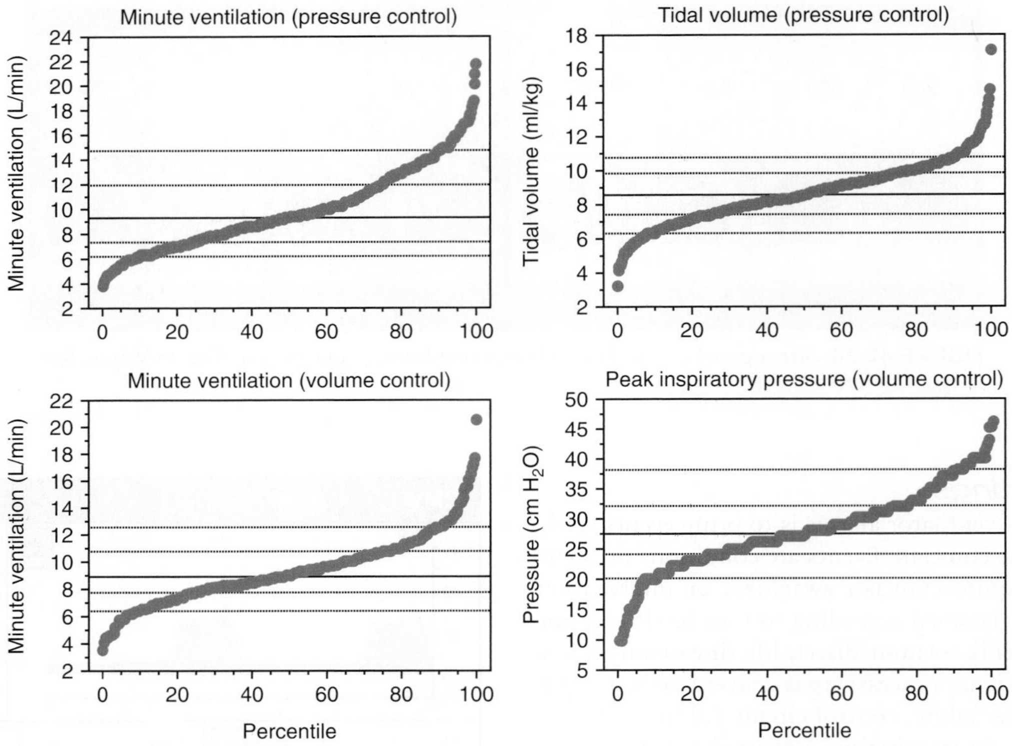

FIGURE 42-22 Distribution of alarmable ventilator parameters from intensive care ventilators in use in an academic medical center.

alarm limits to the current value of the parameter such that extreme values have tighter limits. Further research is needed to identify optimization algorithms (i.e., minimize both harmful and nuisance events) for intelligent targeting schemes to set alarms automatically during mechanical ventilation.

Ventilator Output Displays

Ventilator output displays are essentially the values of monitored parameters that result from the operator settings. There are four basic ways to present the monitored data: as numbers, as waveforms, as trend lines, and in the form of abstract graphic symbols.

Numeric Values

The most common data represented as numeric values are FiO_2; peak, plateau, mean, and baseline airway pressures; inhaled and exhaled tidal volume; minute ventilation; and frequency. Depending on the ventilator, a wide range of calculated parameters may also be displayed, including resistance, compliance, time constant, $P_{0.1}$, % leak, I:E ratio, and peak inspiratory/expiratory flow.

Waveforms and Loops

Most ICU ventilators display waveforms (sometimes called *scalars*) of airway pressure, volume, and flow as functions of time. Such displays are useful for identifying the effects of changes in settings or mechanics on the level of ventilation. They are also very useful for identifying sources of patient-ventilator asynchrony, such as missed triggers, flow asynchrony, and delayed or premature cycling.[29] They can also display one variable against another as an *x-y* or "loop" display. The most common loop displays show pressure on the horizontal axis and volume on the vertical axis or volume on the horizontal axis and flow on the vertical axis. Pressure-volume loop displays are useful for identifying optimal PEEP levels (quasistatic loops only) and overdistention. Flow-volume loops are useful for identifying the response to bronchodilators. An example of a composite display showing numeric values, waveforms, and loops is shown in Figure 42-23.

Trends

Many ventilators provide trend graphs of just about any parameter they measure or calculate. These graphs show how the monitored parameters change over long periods so that significant events or gradual changes in patient condition can be identified (Figure 42-24).

Picture Graphics

A new development in ventilator displays involves the use of picture graphics to represent useful information about the patient-ventilator system. A study[30] showed that subjects with graphic rather than conventional displays of obstructed endotracheal tubes and auto-PEEP problems were detected and treated faster. The investigators also

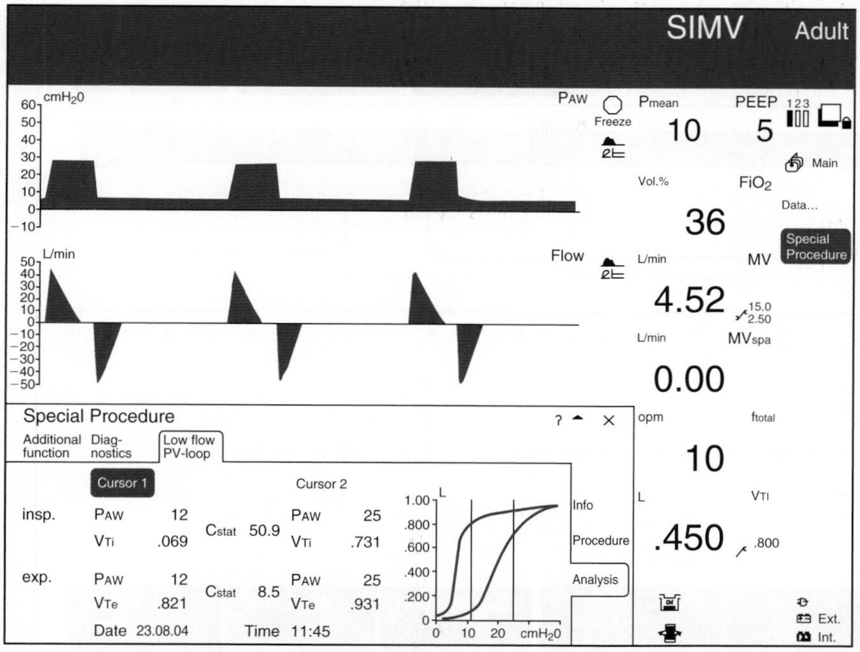

FIGURE 42-23 Portion of display screen on the Draeger Evita XL ventilator. (Courtesy Draeger Medical, Telford, Pennsylvania.)

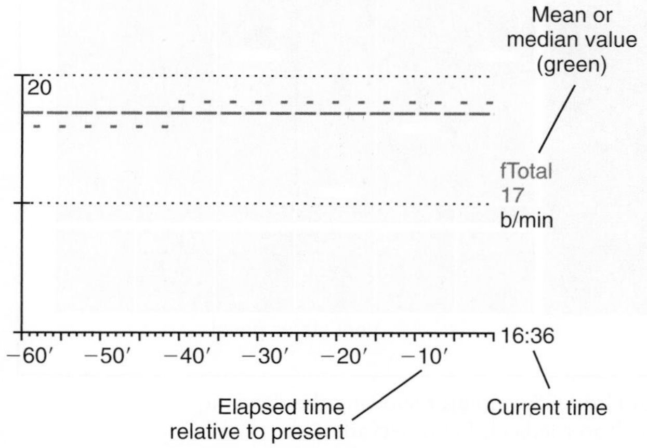

FIGURE 42-24 Trend screen display from the Hamilton G5 ventilator. (Courtesy Hamilton Medical, Reno, Nevada.)

reported significantly lower subjective workloads using the graphic display.

Hamilton Medical was the first manufacturer to use innovative picture graphics on their G5 ventilator. In particular, they created a graphic representation of the lungs, called a *dynamic lung panel,* which visually displayed information about resistance and compliance by the shape and color of the lungs and airways (Figure 42-25). In addition, Hamilton Medial created a unique graphic representation called the *vent status panel* that displays key parameters (e.g., oxygenation, ventilation, and spontaneous breathing activity) and shows when each item is in or out of an acceptable zone and for how long. This graphic display makes weaning status easy to identify. Draeger Medical followed with a similar graphic display called *Smart Pulmonary View,* which is a graphic display of respiratory system compliance and resistance and of the spontaneous and mandatory minute volume (Figure 42-26).

TYPES OF VENTILATORS

Ventilators may be divided into categories according to type and the setting in which the ventilator is to be used. The two types or classes ventilators may be divided into are conventional and nonconventional. *Conventional ventilators* produce breathing patterns that are at or near physiologic normal values for the intended population (e.g., adult, pediatric, and infant). There are also manufacturing limits on the maximum breath rate a conventional ventilator may deliver. The U.S. Food and Drug Administration (FDA) places a maximum breath rate limit of 150 breaths/min for conventional ventilators. Tidal volumes that are either operator-set or delivered to the patient as a result of a preset pressure through a conventional ventilator are sufficient or large enough to clear anatomic dead space. Conversely, high-frequency ventilators typically produce respiratory frequencies or breathing rates that are much higher than physiologically possible and tidal volumes that are less than anatomic dead space.

Ventilators may also be categorized by the setting in which they are used along the continuum of care—specifically critical care, subacute, home care and long-term care, and transport. The designs of the ventilators match the needs of the patient population and the unique characteristics of the setting in which they are used. Ventilator manufacturers have paid particular attention to economic constraints health care facilities are facing. Innovations in ventilator design have broadened their use

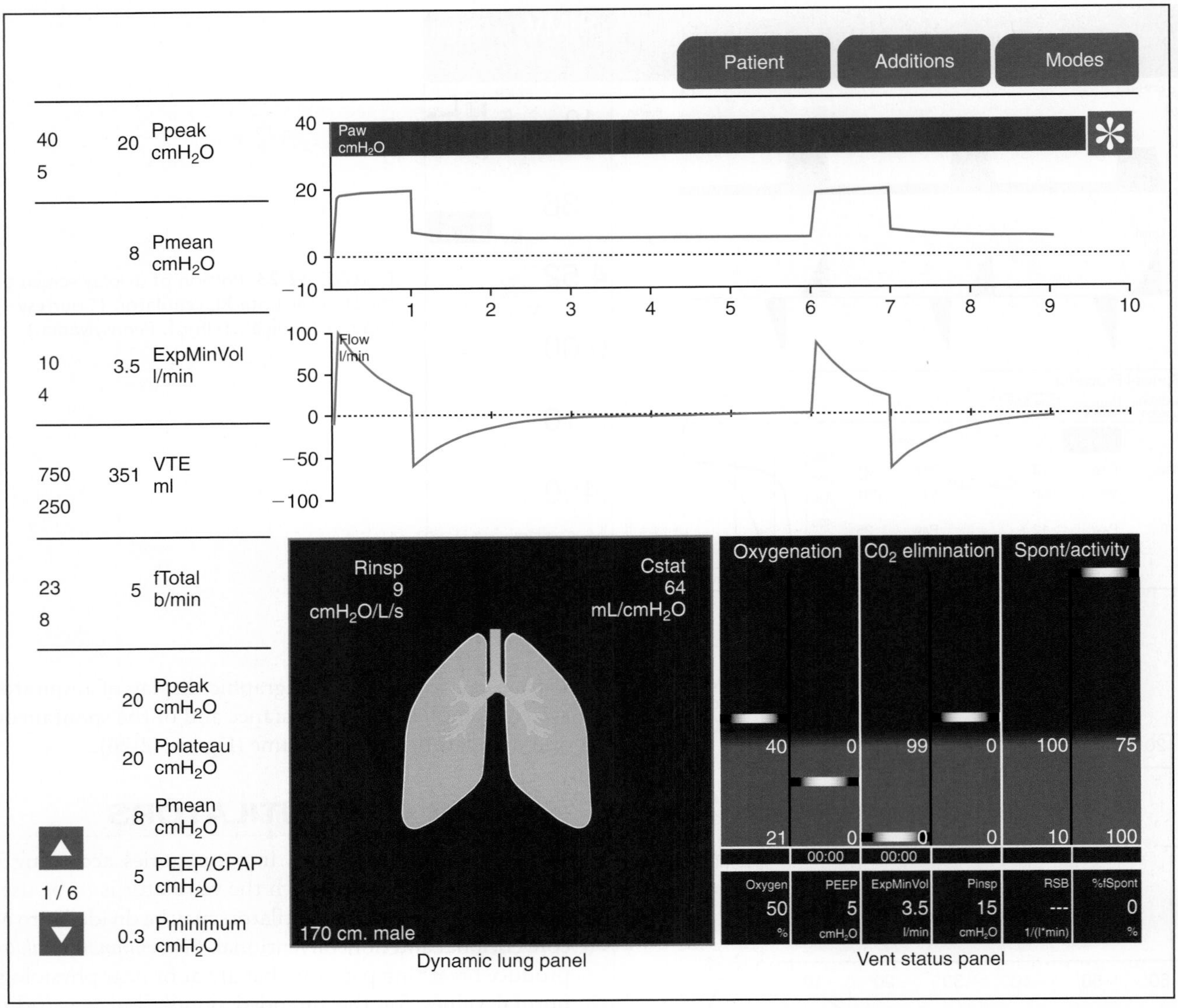

FIGURE 42-25 Picture graphic display from the Hamilton G5 ventilator showing the dynamic lung panel and the vent status panel. (Courtesy Hamilton Medical, Reno, Nevada.)

across settings. An example is the use of ventilators across a spectrum of ages. This innovation does not negate the need for specific ventilators for use with infants and children but provides a mechanism through which respiratory care departments can maximize the use of capital expenditures. Although ventilators are not subcategorized as adult or pediatric in this chapter, it is crucial for the practitioner to be aware of factors such as minimal tidal volume limits, trigger sensitivity, response time, and availability of leak compensation when selecting a ventilator for use with pediatric patients. A comprehensive listing of all ventilators available for use in the United States is not provided. Rather, a small sample representing some commercially available products and their specifications is provided. Comprehensive listings may be found in textbooks dedicated to respiratory care equipment.

Critical Care Ventilators

Critical care ventilators provide clinicians with sophisticated methods for breath delivery. This class of ventilators also provides advanced monitoring capabilities and tools that enable clinicians to assess the patient-ventilator interaction easily. Calculations of lung mechanics parameters, including auto-PEEP, static and dynamic compliance, inspiratory/expiratory resistance, rapid shallow breathing index, time constant, and work of breathing, are integrated into ventilators used in this environment. Integrated physiologic noninvasive and invasive assessment tools, such as esophageal pressure monitoring and end-tidal CO_2 monitoring, are also commercially available. The availability of these features equips bedside caregivers with the tools needed to assess patient-ventilator interaction and match

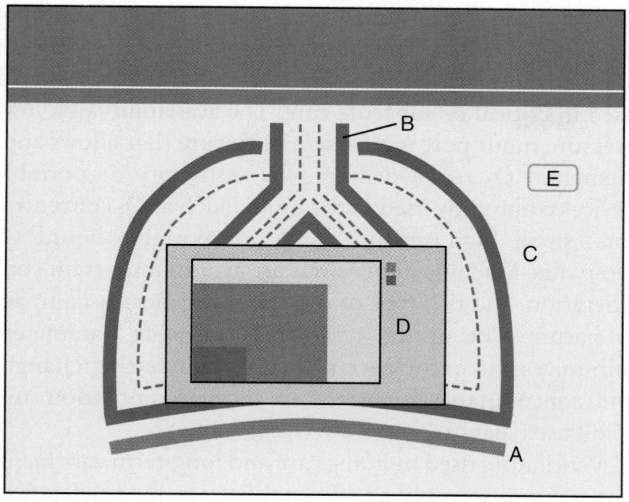

FIGURE 42-26 Picture graphic display from Draeger Evita Infinity V500 ventilator showing the Smart Pulmonary View. *A,* The movement of the diaphragm indicates synchronized mandatory breaths or supported (triggered) breaths. *B,* The blue line around the trachea indicates the resistance, R. The higher the resistance, the thicker the line. The numeric value is also displayed. *C,* The blue line around the lungs indicates the compliance, Cdyn. The higher the compliance, the thinner the line. The numeric value is also displayed. *D,* Diagram displaying the relationship between spontaneous breathing and mandatory ventilation. The following parameters are displayed in different colors: – $V_{T,spon}$ and RR_{spon} – $V_{T,mand}$ and RR_{mand}. (Courtesy Draeger Medical, Telford Pennsylvania.)

ventilator capability with physiologic need. Both high-frequency and conventional ventilators may be used in the critical care setting.

High-Frequency Ventilators

The availability of sophisticated devices, such as jet ventilators and high-frequency oscillators, facilitates ventilatory management of infants, children, and adults in the PC-IMV mode who fail to maintain adequate oxygenation and acid-base balance with conventional ventilatory support. High-frequency jet ventilators, such as the Bunnell Life Pulse (Bunnell Inc, Salt Lake City, Utah), deliver short bursts, or jet pulses, of mixed gas through a special adapter for endotracheal tubes or a specially designed endotracheal tube. The LifePort Endotracheal Tube Adapter (Bunnell Inc, Salt Lake City, Utah) is designed to replace the 15-mm outer diameter adapter on the proximal portion of a traditional endotracheal tube. This adapter has a high-frequency ventilator circuit connection port. The use of this adapter minimizes the need to reintubate the patient with a specially designed endotracheal tube. The connection port may be capped off or occluded when there is no longer a need for high-frequency ventilation. An endotracheal tube specially designed for use with high-frequency ventilation is similar in appearance to a conventional tube, with two additional small chambers molded into the wall. This triple-lumen design enables tracheal pressures to be monitored during the delivery of jet pulses.

High-frequency jet ventilators require a high pressure source (20 to 50 psig) to function. This type of ventilator consists of a system for regulating inlet pressure (psig) and a cycling mechanism and a device such as an air-O_2 blender for controlling FiO_2. The small volumes of gas are delivered at rapid rates (4 to 250 times the normal respiratory rate).[31] The benefits of rescue and elective use of high-frequency jet ventilation as a treatment for acute lung disease and acute respiratory distress syndrome (ARDS) are unclear.[31] However, the literature supports its effectiveness in maintaining alveolar ventilation and reducing morbidity during surgical repair of tracheal and airway anomalies.[32,33]

High-frequency oscillation also allows very small tidal volumes to be delivered at rapid frequencies (180 to 1200 cycles/minute). High-frequency oscillators use a piston-driven diaphragm to produce the airflow oscillations. Tidal volume depends on the force and distance the piston moves from baseline. A special endotracheal tube is not required to implement this form of PC-IMV. The SensorMedics 3100A and 3100B high-frequency oscillators (CareFusion) are approved and commercially available for use in neonatal/pediatric (<35 kg) and pediatric/adult (>35 kg) populations. There are independent reports of improved morbidity and mortality with the use of high-frequency oscillation in infants and children with diffuse alveolar and small airways disease.[34] Combined evidence from observational and clinical trials appears to be favorable with respect to improved mortality rates in patients with heterogeneous lung disease, such as ARDS.[35,36] In contrast to conventional ventilators, convention plays a minor role in gas transport with high-frequency jet ventilation and high-frequency oscillation. Rather, the mixing and diffusion of gases in the airways enhances fresh gas delivery to and elimination of CO_2 from the alveoli.

Conventional Ventilators

Conventional ventilators may be used with various interfaces in the critical care setting. Options are available on this type of ventilator for use with an artificial airway (endotracheal or tracheostomy tube) or noninvasively with assorted interfaces (e.g., nasal, oronasal, or full-face masks). The availability of the noninvasive option eliminates the need for a standalone noninvasive ventilator. However, standalone noninvasive ventilators do have application and are also used in the critical care setting. This type of ventilator is discussed in detail subsequently. Ventilators used in the critical care environment have the capability to assess and monitor complex ventilator-patient interactions. Work of breathing or the intricacies of breath delivery may be examined by evaluating numerically or graphically displayed data. Many ventilators also apportion automatic adjustments to breath delivery in response to changes in lung mechanics and parameters preset by the operator.

In addition to universal patient population applications, some critical care ventilators are manufactured with an internal battery. The SERVO-i has a plug-in battery module. This ventilator can provide at least 3 hours of uninterrupted power supply when six rechargeable 12-V batteries are used in the module. Uninterrupted ventilatory assistance may be provided not only in the critical care setting but also during interhospital transport. Minimizing circuit disconnections can enhance safety by reducing the risks for derecruitment,[37] hemodynamic instability,[38] and factors contributing to nosocomial infections.[39] The aforementioned features enable clinicians to optimize the patient-ventilator interaction.

Subacute Care Ventilators

Patients who have an acute illness, injury, or exacerbation of disease process receive subacute care. Generally, mechanically ventilated patients in this setting have a stable cardiopulmonary status. Their condition is such that the care provided in this setting does not depend heavily on high-technology monitoring or complex diagnostic procedures. Rather, the focus is on coordinated services aimed at managing complex medical conditions, liberation from ventilatory support, and rehabilitation services. Ventilators used in this care venue have less sophisticated monitoring systems and mode options. Subacute care may be rendered in freestanding facilities or within a specialized unit within a hospital. Consequently, the ventilators used in this environment bridge the gap between ventilators designed specifically for critical care and ventilators for home care or long-term care. The Savina (Draeger Medical) offers features germane to critical care ventilators, such as graphic display of pressure, volume, and flow waveforms and the availability of a noninvasive ventilation mode of operation. The availability of a low-pressure O_2 option enables O_2 delivery independent of a central gas supply. An O_2 concentrator can be used to supply O_2 to the patient breathing circuit; this is analogous to O_2 delivery methods used by ventilators in the home care or long-term care environment.

Home Care Ventilators

Patients with chronic respiratory failure from primary pulmonary disease, trauma, or neuromuscular disease may require ventilatory assistance to augment or replace spontaneous breathing and maintain life. Ventilators designed for use in the home or long-term care institutions facilitate the transition of patients from an acute or subacute care environment to one focused on enhancing the individual's quality of life and providing services to sustain or improve physical or physiologic function in a cost-efficient manner.[40] Ventilators must be able to support the ventilatory needs of the patient and provide supplemental O_2 in a venue where compressed gas resources are limited, power supply interruptions may occur, and patient mobility needs must be met. The interface on this type of ventilator is much simpler than the interface found on a ventilator used in critical or subacute care. The availability of a low-pressure input port is an essential feature that allows supplemental O_2 to be delivered by stationary or portable devices commonly used in the home, such as O_2 concentrators, small high-pressure tanks, or portable liquid O_2 reservoirs. Machine dimensions are also an important consideration, and this type of ventilator is generally compact in nature. The option to lock operator-set parameters minimizes the occurrence of inadvertent setting changes and concomitant alterations in alveolar ventilation and acid-base balance.

Ventilators used in home care and long-term care facilities require not only an internal battery for brief power interruptions but also connections for an external battery when the power supply is interrupted for extended periods as a result of natural disasters; man-made occurrences; or participation in academic, employment, or recreational activities. The Carina home ventilator (Draeger Medical) can provide invasive or noninvasive ventilation. Although the ventilator's primary power source is 100-V or 240-V AC, the internal battery provides patients with approximately 2 hours of power. There is also an external battery pack that offers an additional 10-hour power supply when fully charged.

Transport Ventilators

Transport ventilators share attributes common to ventilators used in the home and critical care environments. It is necessary for this ventilator type to be lightweight, compact, durable, and maintained on a reliable power supply and to have low compressed gas consumption. The ventilator interface should be easy to navigate, allowing the clinician to set or change parameters before or during movement to and from a prescribed destination. Operator-set and monitored data should be visible under optimal conditions or conditions of low ambient light. These characteristics enhance patient safety and minimize the potential for complications or adverse effects to occur during air or ground transport. Monitoring is also an important consideration. Clinical practice guidelines recommend the level of monitoring during patient transport be analogous with that provided to the patient during stationary care.[41,42] Modern transport ventilators provide the ability to display scalar waveforms and numerical data.

The BioMed Crossvent 4+ (BioMed Devices, Inc, Guilford, Connecticut) ventilator can be used to transport critically ill patients of any age, from infant to adult. This ventilator may be configured with a blender to allow for the delivery of a range of O_2 concentrations from 21% to 100% or with an air-entrainment unit that delivers either 50% or 100% O_2 without the need for an external air supply source. Pressure-controlled and volume-controlled ventilation may be provided in the CMV, IMV, or CSV mode. Tidal volumes may be adjusted from 5 to 2500 ml, and flow may be delivered at rates up to120 L/min. The internal battery offers 6 hours of uninterrupted power when fully charged. This unit is small (28 cm × 25.4 cm × 14 cm) and weighs less than 5 kg. The units main display screen is color and backlit for enhanced visibility.

Noninvasive Ventilators

Noninvasive ventilation is used across the continuum of care—from critical care to home care with individuals of any age. As previously mentioned, a noninvasive ventilation feature may be incorporated in critical care ventilators (e.g., SERVO-i and Puritan Bennett 840), subacute ventilators (Savina), and home care ventilators (Carina home). However, standalone noninvasive ventilators exist and are used extensively in various settings from the hospital to the home. In the acute and critical care setting, noninvasive ventilators have been used to reduce complications associated with diagnostic procedures, such as bronchoscopy,[43] and in the treatment of acute respiratory insufficiency and respiratory failure[44] and prevention of postextubation failure.[45] This technology has also been associated with positive outcomes in the outpatient setting. The literature reports the use of noninvasive ventilation to restore and maintain adequate alveolar ventilation with individuals compromised by neuromuscular disorders, congestive heart failure, chronic obstructive lung disease, and sleep-disordered breathing.[46]

Features common to home and hospital grade units enhance patient comfort and promote adherence to therapy. Ramp time allows the clinician to program a delay in the initiation of a delivered inspiratory pressure. Ramp time is usually adjustable (e.g., 0 to 45 minutes), during which the patient breathes at a preset or operator-set expiratory pressure (e.g., 4 cm H_2O). Likewise, rise time can be altered to reduce pressure overshoot and enhance breath delivery. An additional helpful tool is the ability to detect and quantify interface leak, estimated tidal volume, and minute ventilation delivery. Hospital-grade units have the capability to display patient data in graphic and numeric form. Clinicians are able to view pressure, flow, and scalar waveforms, such as on the BiPAP Vision (Respironics Inc, Murrysville, Pennsylvania). As with critical care ventilators, careful analysis of waveforms may assist clinicians in the identification and correction of patient-ventilator synchrony.

SUMMARY CHECKLIST

- Ventilators can be described in terms of their input power requirements (e.g., electrical or pneumatic) and how the input power is transformed into desired outputs of pressure, volume and flow.
- A key feature of a ventilator is the variety of modes of ventilation it offers.
- A mode of ventilation is a predetermined pattern of interaction with the patient. Modes are given many confusing names but they can be understood using a simple classification system.
- Mode classification is based on identifying 3 main components: the primary control variable, the breath sequence, and the targeting schemes used for mandatory and spontaneous breaths.
- Pressure control means that pressure delivery is predetermined by a targeting scheme such that inspiratory pressure is either proportional to patient effort or has a particular waveform regardless of respiratory system mechanics. Volume control means that inspiratory flow and volume delivery are predetermined by a targeting scheme to have particular waveforms independent of respiratory system mechanics.
- A spontaneous breath is one for which the timing and size of the breath is determined by the patient, i.e., inspiration is patient triggered and patient cycled. A mandatory breath is one for which the patient cannot determine the timing and/or size of the breath, i.e., inspiration is machine triggered and/or machine cycled.
- Spontaneous breaths may be assisted (meaning that the ventilator provides some portion of the work of breathing) or unassisted. Mandatory breaths are generally assisted.
- The breath sequence of a mode is the pattern of mandatory vs spontaneous breaths. Continuous spontaneous ventilation (CSV) means that all breath delivered by the ventilator are spontaneous. Intermittent mandatory ventilation (IMV) means that spontaneous breaths can occur between mandatory breaths. Continuous mandatory ventilation means that spontaneous breaths cannot occur between mandatory breaths.
- The targeting scheme is a description of the relation between operator settings and ventilator outputs for a mode. Currently, all modes can be classified as having one of 6 targeting schemes (set-point, dual, servo, adaptive, optimal, and intelligent).
- Ventilators can also be categorized by the settings in which they are used. Examples include: critical care, sub-acute care, home care, transport and noninvasive ventilators.

References

1. Chatburn RL, Primiano FP, Jr: A new system for understanding modes of mechanical ventilation. Respir Care 46:604, 2001.
2. Chatburn RL: Classification of ventilator modes: update and proposal for implementation. Respir Care 52:301–323, 2007.
3. Chatburn RL: Understanding mechanical ventilators. Expert Rev Respir Med 4:809–819, 2010.
4. Morris W: The American heritage dictionary of the English language, Boston, 1975, American Heritage and Houghton Mifflin.
5. Barnes TA: Core textbook of respiratory care practice, ed 2, St Louis, 1994, Mosby.

6. Cairo JM, Pilbean SP: Mosby's respiratory care equipment, ed 8, St Louis, 2009, Mosby.
7. Chatburn RL: Classification of mechanical ventilators. In Tobin MJ, editor: Principles and practice of mechanical ventilation, ed 2, New York, 2006, McGraw-Hill.
8. Morch ET: History of mechanical ventilation. In Kirby RR, Smith RA, Desautels DA, editors: Mechanical ventilation, New York, 1985, Churchill Livingstone.
9. Russell DF, Ross DG, Manson HJ: Fluidic cycling devices for inspiratory and expiratory timing in automatic ventilators. J Biomech Eng 5:227, 1983.
10. Hess D, Lind L: Nomograms for the application of the Bourns Model BP200 as a volume-constant ventilator. Respir Care 25:248, 1980.
11. Sassoon CS, Giron AE, Ely EA, et al: Inspiratory work of breathing on flow-by and demand-flow continuous positive airway pressure. Crit Care Med 17:1108, 1989.
12. Branson RD: Flow-triggering systems. Respir Care 42:138, 1994.
13. Branson RD, MacIntyre NR: Dual-control modes of mechanical ventilation. Respir Care 41:294, 1996.
14. Chatburn RL: Closed loop control of mechanical ventilation: description and classification of targeting schemes. Respir Care 56:85–98, 2011.
15. Younes M: Proportional assist ventilation, a new approach to ventilatory support. Am Rev Respir Dis 145:121–129, 1992.
16. Laubscher TP, Frutiger A, Fanconi S, et al: The automatic selection of ventilation parameters during the initial phase of mechanical ventilation. Intensive Care Med 22:199–207, 1996.
17. Dojat M, Harf A, Touchard D, et al: Clinical evaluation of a computer-controlled pressure support mode. Am J Respir Crit Care Med 161:1161–1166, 2000.
18. Nemoto T, Hatzakis G, Thorpe CW, et al: Automatic control of pressure support ventilation using fuzzy logic. Am J Respir Crit Care Med 160:550–556, 1999.
19. Bates JH, Hatzakis GE, Olivenstein R: Fuzzy logic and mechanical ventilation. Respir Care Clin North Am 7:363–377, 2001.
20. East TD, Heermann LK, Bradshaw RL, et al: Efficacy of computerized decision support for mechanical ventilation: results of a prospective multi-center randomized trial. Proc AMIA Symp 251–255, 1999.
21. Snowden S, Brownlee KG, Smye SW, et al: An advisory system for artificial ventilation of the newborn utilizing a neural network. Med Inform (Lond) 18:367–376, 1993.
22. Gottschalk A, Hyzer MC, Greet RT: A comparison of human and machine-based predictions of successful weaning from mechanical ventilation. Med Decis Making 20:243–244, 2000.
23. Uzawa Y, Yamada Y, Suzukawa M: Evaluation of the user interface simplicity in the modern generation of mechanical ventilators. Respir Care 53:329–337, 2008.
24. Chatburn RL, Volsko TA: Documentation issues for mechanical ventilation in pressure-control modes. Respir Care 55:1705–1716, 2011.
25. MacIntyre NR, Branson RD: Mechanical ventilation, ed 2, St Louis, 2009, Saunders.
26. Görges M, Markewitz BA, Westenskow DR: Improving alarm performance in the medical intensive care unit using delays and clinical context. Anesth Analg 108:1546–1552, 2009.
27. Siebig S, Kuhls S, Imhoff M, et al: Intensive care unit alarms—how many do we need? Crit Care Med 38:451–456, 2010.
28. Mullin R, Chatburn RL: Reference data for determining ventilator alarm limits. Respir Care 55:1520, 2010.
29. de Wit M: Monitoring of patient-ventilator interaction at the bedside. Respir Care 56:61–72, 2011.
30. Wachter SB, Johnson K, Albert R, et al: The evaluation of a pulmonary display to detect adverse respiratory events using high resolution human simulator. J Am Med Inform Assoc 13:635–642, 2006.
31. Wunsch H, Mapstone J: High frequency ventilation versus conventional ventilation for the treatment of acute lung injury and acute respiratory distress syndrome: a systematic review and Cochrane analysis. Anesth Analg 100:1765, 2005.
32. Rezaie-Majd A, Bigenzahn W, Denk DM, et al: Superimposed high frequency jet ventilation (SHFJV) for endoscopic laryngotracheal surgery in more than 1500 patients. Br J Anaesth 96:650–659, 2006.
33. Markus-Rodden MM, Bojko T, Hauck LC: Traumatic tracheal laceration in a pediatric patient medically managed with high-frequency oscillatory ventilation. Pediatr Emerg Care 24:236–237, 2008.
34. Slee-Wijffels FY, van der Vaart KR, Twisk JW, et al: High frequency oscillatory ventilation in children: a single-center of 53 cases. Crit Care 9:R274, 2005.
35. Bollen CW, Uiterwaal CSPM, van Vught AJ: Systematic review of determinants of mortality in high frequency oscillatory ventilation in acute respiratory distress syndrome. Crit Care 10:R34, 2006.
36. Sud S, Sud M, Friedrich JO, et al: High frequency oscillation in patients with acute lung injury and acute respiratory distress syndrome (ARDS): systematic review and meta-analysis. BMJ 340:c2327, 2010.
37. Chacko J, Rani U: Alveolar recruitment maneuvers in acute lung injury/acute respiratory distress syndrome. Indian J Crit Care Med 13:1–6, 2009.
38. Doring BL, Kerr ME, Lovasik DA, et al: Factors that contribute to complications during intrahospital transport of the critically ill. J Neurosci Nurs 31:80–86, 1999.
39. AARC Evidence Based Clinical Practice Guideline: Care of the ventilator circuit and its relation to ventilator-associated pneumonia. Respir Care 48:869–879, 2003.
40. AARC Clinical Practice Guideline: Long term invasive mechanical ventilation in the home—2007 revision and update. Respir Care 52:1056–1062, 2007.
41. Warren J, Fromm RE, Jr, Orr RA, et al: Guidelines for the inter- and intrahospital transport of critically ill patients. Crit Care Med 32:256–262, 2004.
42. AARC Clinical Practice Guideline: In-hospital transport of the mechanically ventilated patient—2002 revision and update. Respir Care 47:721–723, 2002.
43. Murgu SD, Pecson J, Colt HG: Bronchoscopy during noninvasive ventilation: indications and technique. Respir Care 55:595–600, 2010.
44. Calderini E, Chidini G, Pelosi P: What are the current indications for noninvasive ventilation in children? Curr Opin Anaesthesiol 23:368–374, 2010.
45. Eryüksel E, Karakurt S, Celikel T: Noninvasive positive pressure ventilation in unplanned extubation. Ann Thorac Med. 4:17–20, 2009.
46. Theerakittikul T, Ricaurte B, Aboussouan LS: Noninvasive positive pressure ventilation for stable outpatients: CPAP and beyond. Cleve Clin J Med 77:705–714, 2010.

Chapter 43

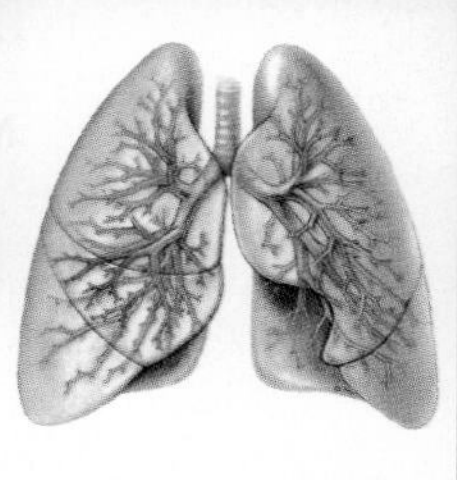

Physiology of Ventilatory Support

ROBERT M. KACMAREK AND TERESA A. VOLSKO

CHAPTER OBJECTIVES

After reading this chapter you will be able to:

- Discuss the pressures and pressure gradients that affect gas delivery during spontaneous breathing, negative pressure ventilation (NPV), and positive pressure ventilation (PPV).
- Identify the effects of mechanical ventilation on oxygenation, ventilation, and lung mechanics.
- Describe the currently available modes of mechanical ventilation.
- Discuss the indications and physiologic effect of positive end expiratory pressure (PEEP).
- Describe the cardiovascular effects of PPV and NPV.
- Describe the effects of PPV on other body systems.
- Identify and list the complications and hazards of providing mechanical ventilatory support.
- Discuss how to minimize adverse effects of mechanical ventilation.

CHAPTER OUTLINE

KEY TERMS

aerophagia
autoregulation
atelectrauma
barotrauma
biotrauma
mean airway pressure
passive
patient-ventilator asynchrony
time constant
transairway pressure
transalveolar pressure
trans-chest wall pressure
transdiaphragmatic pressure
transpulmonary pressure
transrespiratory pressure
transthoracic pressure
volutrauma

Mechanical ventilation can be beneficial or detrimental depending on how it is initially applied and modified as the patient's condition changes. Respiratory therapists (RTs) must be able to anticipate the physiologic effects of mechanical ventilation and respond appropriately when complications arise. This chapter familiarizes the reader with (1) the physiologic effects of mechanical ventilation on lung and cardiovascular function and other body systems, (2) the basic approaches to providing mechanical ventilation, and (3) the complications and hazards of mechanical ventilation. A solid understanding of the normal physiology of breathing is essential for all RTs, especially when working with patients receiving mechanical ventilation. RTs must understand intrathoracic pressure changes associated with spontaneous, negative pressure, and positive pressure breathing. Intrathoracic pressure changes are necessary for ventilation to occur; however, large changes in these pressures may also induce various physiologic changes in other systems.

PRESSURE AND PRESSURE GRADIENTS

For gas to flow through the airway, a pressure gradient must exist. The airways begin at the mouth and end at the alveoli, so mouth pressure (*pressure at the airway opening* [P_{awo}]) and *alveolar pressure* (P_{alv}) are important in describing gas flow, as are *intrapleural pressure* (P_{pl}) and *body surface pressure* or atmospheric pressure (P_{bs}). In addition, *intraabdominal pressure* (P_{ab}) affects the impact of P_{pl} change on diaphragm movement. P_{pl} is the pressure in the pleural space, the virtual space between the visceral and parietal pleurae, and is usually negative in relation to P_{alv}. Figure 43-1 shows a graphic model of the respiratory system with these pressures identified as points in space. Mathematical models relating pressure, volume, and flow corresponding to this graphic model are constructed using pressure differences. The various components of the graphic model are defined as everything that exists between these points in space. The respiratory system is everything that exists between the airway opening and the body surface. The associated pressure difference is **transrespiratory pressure** (P_{tr}), defined as $P_{awo} - P_{bs}$. The components of transrespiratory pressure correspond to the components of the graphic model. The airways are represented by **transairway pressure** (P_{ta}), defined as $P_{awo} - P_{alv}$. The lungs are represented by the **transalveolar pressure:** ($P_L = P_{alv} - P_{pl}$). The chest wall is represented by **trans-chest wall pressure:** ($P_{tcw} = P_{pl} - P_{bs}$). If the lungs and chest wall are lumped together, they can be represented by **transthoracic pressure:** ($P_{tt} = P_{alv} - P_{bs}$).

Another pressure gradient not defined in Figure 43-1 that also affects gas movement is the **transdiaphragmatic pressure** (P_{di}). This pressure gradient is the difference between intraabdominal pressure and pleural pressure and affects diaphragmatic movement: ($P_{pl} - P_{ab}$). Once these pressures and pressure gradients are understood, the differences between spontaneous ventilation, positive pressure ventilation (PPV), and negative pressure ventilation (NPV) become evident.

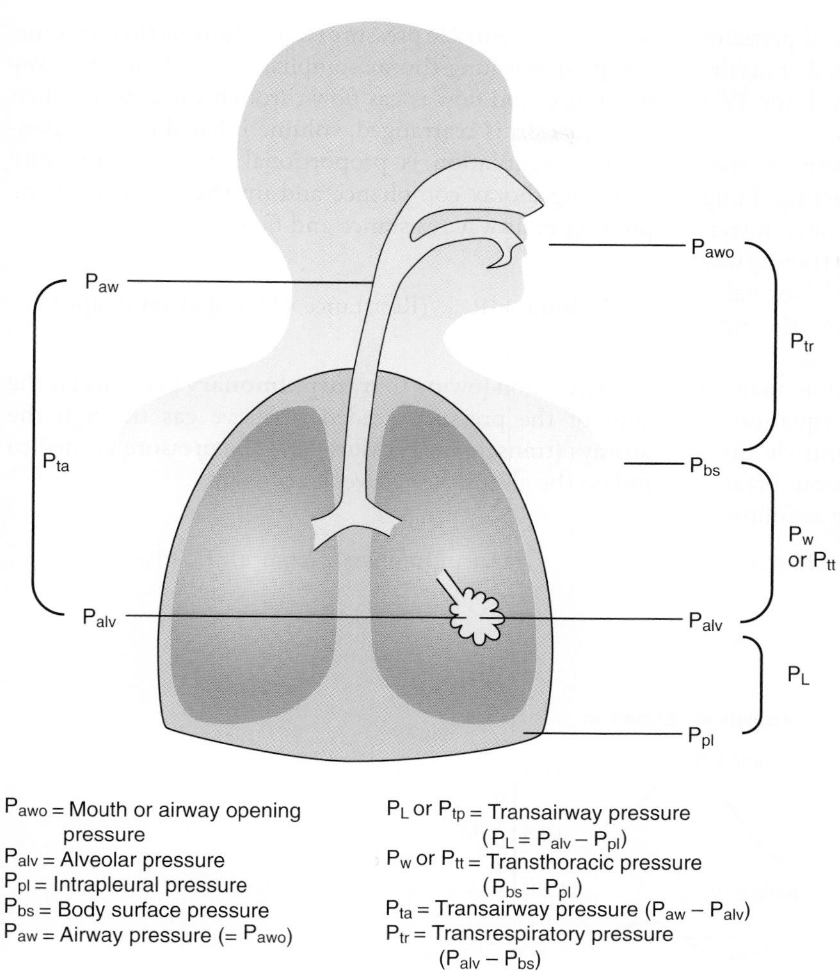

FIGURE 43-1 Pressures and pressure gradients in the lung. Airflow is a function of the transairway pressure (P_{ta}), which is the pressure gradient between the airway (P_{aw}) and the alveoli (P_{alv}). Transalveolar pressure (P_L) maintains alveolar inflation, and transpulmonary pressure (P_{tp}) is the pressure needed to expand the lungs and chest wall.

TABLE 43-1

Changes in Airway Pressure Gradients During Spontaneous, Negative, and Positive Pressure Ventilation

Pressure (cm H_2O) Ventilation Type	Transpulmonary Pressure	Transthoracic Pressure	Transairway Pressure	Transrespiratory Pressure
Spontaneous				
Inspiration	Small increase (+)	Increase (+)	Increase (+)	Constant (−)
Expiration	Small increase (−)	Increase (−)	Increase (−)	Constant (+)
Negative (NPV)				
Inspiration	Small increase (+)	Increase (+)	Increase (+)	Increase (−)
Expiration	Small increase (−)	Increase (−)	Increase (−)	Increase (+)
Positive (PPV)				
Inspiration	Small increase (+)	Increase (+)	Increase (+)	Increase (+)
Expiration	Small increase (−)	Decrease (−)	Decrease (−)	Decrease (−)

Airway, Alveolar, and Intrathoracic Pressure, Volume, and Flow During Spontaneous Ventilation

Spontaneous breathing is normally an autonomic phenomenon. In other words, we do not think about breathing; it is controlled by the autonomic nervous system. Not until our breathing is stressed do we consider the effort to breathe or the energy expended. At end-exhalation, intrapleural pressure is slightly negative. Alveolar, mouth, and body surface pressures are zero. The diaphragm contracts in response to stimulation of the phrenic nerve via the respiratory center in the medulla of the brain. When the diaphragm contracts, it descends into the abdominal cavity, decreasing intrapleural pressure. When intrapleural pressure becomes more negative, alveolar pressure becomes negative as well. The effects of spontaneous breathing on the pressure gradients are shown in Table 43-1. Under normal circumstances, a decrease in intrapleural pressure results in decreased alveolar pressure, increased transairway pressure, and inspiration of the tidal volume (V_T) (Figure 43-2).

At end-inspiration, alveolar pressure returns to zero when the muscles of inspiration stop contracting. Lung recoil causes a sudden increase in alveolar pressure in relation to pressure at the mouth, reversing the transairway pressure gradient, and air flows out of the lungs. Normally, there is a short end expiratory pause before the next inspiration.

V_T and flow during spontaneous ventilation may be described by the equation of motion.[1,2] The equation of motion describes the relationship between muscle pressure (analogous to pleural pressure in spontaneous breathing), compliance, resistance, flow, and volume as follows:

$$P_{musc} = \text{Volume/Compliance} + (\text{Resistance} \times \text{Flow})$$

where P_{musc} is muscle pressure (P_{tp}), volume is tidal volume, compliance is lung-thorax compliance, resistance is airway resistance, and flow is gas flow through the airway. When the equation is rearranged, volume inhaled during spontaneous ventilation is proportional to muscle pressure and lung-thorax compliance and inversely related to the product of airway resistance and flow:

$$\text{Volume} = [P_{musc}/(\text{Resistance} \times \text{Flow})] + \text{Compliance}$$

Ventilation (owing to **transpulmonary pressure**) is the sum of the pressure needed to move gas through the airways (transairway pressure) and the pressure needed to inflate the alveoli (transalveolar pressure):

$$\text{Transpulmonary pressure} = P_{ta} + P_{alv}$$

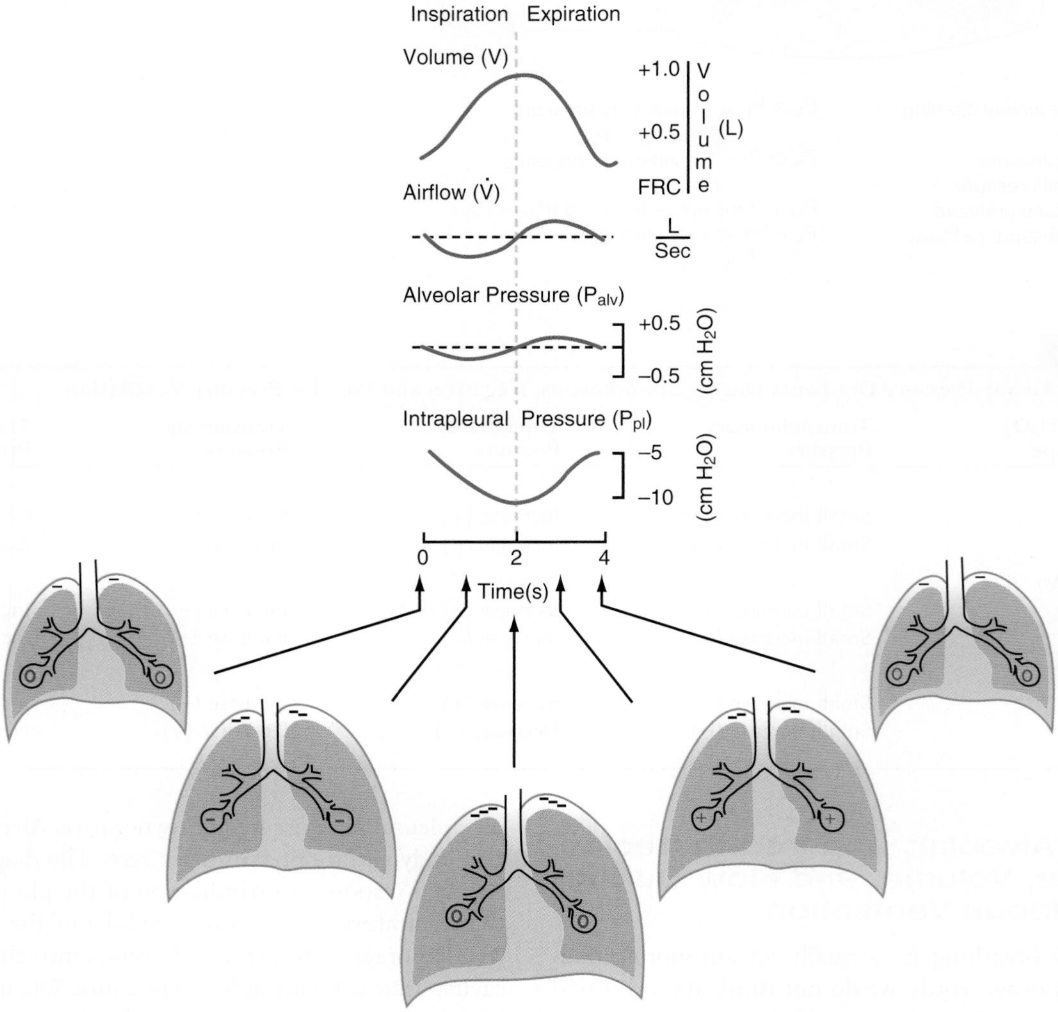

FIGURE 43-2 Changes in pressure, volume, and flow during a single spontaneous breath. (Modified from Martin L: Pulmonary physiology in clinical practice: the essentials for patient care and evaluation, St Louis, 1987, Mosby.)

Airway, Alveolar, and Intrathoracic Pressure, Volume, and Flow During Negative Pressure Mechanical Ventilation

Mechanical NPV is similar to spontaneous breathing. NPV decreases pleural pressure (P_{pl}) during inspiration by exposing the chest to subatmospheric pressure. Negative pressure at the body surface (P_{bs}) is transmitted first to the pleural space and then to the alveoli (P_{alv}). Because the airway opening remains exposed to atmospheric pressure during NPV, a transairway pressure gradient is created. Gas flows from the relatively high pressure at the airway opening (zero) to the relatively low pressure in the alveoli (negative). As with spontaneous breathing, alveolar expansion during NPV is determined by the magnitude of the transpulmonary pressure gradient. During expiration in both spontaneous breathing and NPV, the lungs and chest wall passively recoil to their resting end expiratory levels. As this recoil occurs, pleural pressure becomes less negative, and alveolar pressure increases above atmospheric pressure (Figure 43-3). This increase in alveolar pressure reverses the transairway pressure gradient. As P_{alv} becomes greater than P_{awo}, gas flows from the alveoli to the airway opening. The effects of NPV on the pressure gradients are shown in Table 43-1.

Volume and flow during NPV also are described by the equation of motion except transairway pressure developed by the ventilator fully or partially replaces the patient's respiratory muscle pressure as follows:

$$P_{musc} + P_{vent} = \text{Volume/Compliance} + (\text{Resistance} \times \text{Flow})$$

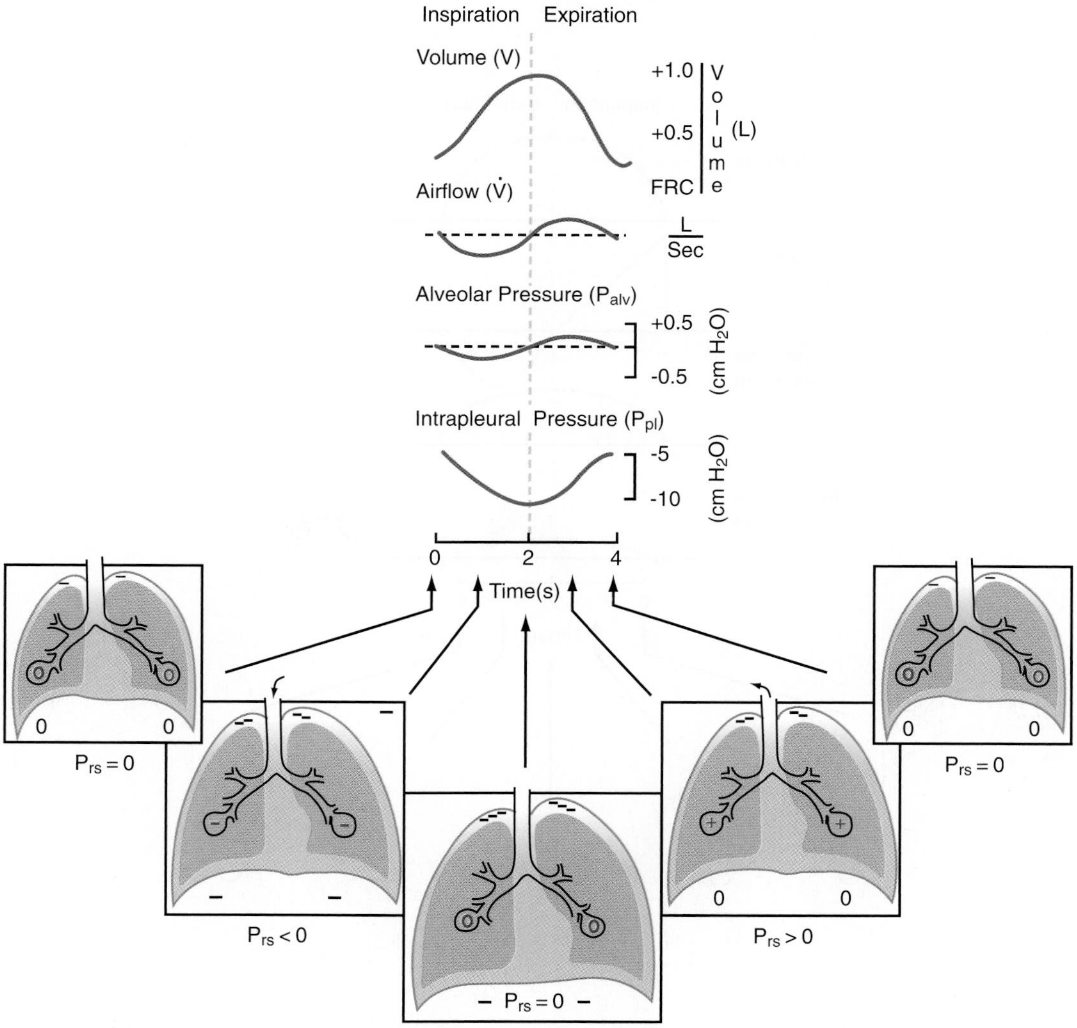

FIGURE 43-3 Changes in pressure, volume, and flow during a single mechanical negative pressure breath. The box surrounding the lungs represents the enclosure formed by the negative pressure ventilator. *Prs,* Pressure of the respiratory system. (Modified from Martin L: Pulmonary physiology in clinical practice: the essentials for patient care and evaluation, St Louis, 1987, Mosby.)

In this equation, P_{vent} is the pressure the ventilator develops to overcome the patient's lung-thorax elastance and airway resistance to deliver the V_T. In this case, P_{vent} is negative but is the driving force behind decreasing the intrapleural pressure and increasing the transairway and transpulmonary pressures.

Physiologic complications associated with NPV are uncommon because NPV simulates normal spontaneous breathing. The most common problems with NPV are related to interference with caring for the patient caused by the device surrounding the chest (the iron lung or chest cuirass). Supplemental oxygen (O_2) cannot be provided to the patient through the negative pressure ventilator. Depending on patient need, low-flow or high-flow O_2 delivery devices must be used to provide O_2 therapy. Immediate access to patients requiring routine or emergent medical care may be difficult in systems that enclose the entire thorax and lower body, such as the iron lung and Porta-Lung (Respironics Inc, Murrysville, PA). These systems may impede venous return by creating a negative pressure in the abdomen and lower half of the body, which may lead to hypotension, a phenomenon known as "tank shock." The risk of glottis closure and the development of obstructive sleep apnea have been reported in association with NPV of patients with chronic obstructive pulmonary disease (COPD) and neuromuscular dysfunction.

Airway, Alveolar, and Intrathoracic Pressure, Volume, and Flow During Positive Pressure Mechanical Ventilation

PPV causes air to flow into the lungs because of an increase in airway pressure, not a decrease in pleural pressure as occurs during spontaneous breathing and NPV (Figure 43-4). However, similar to spontaneous breathing and NPV, PPV causes an increase in P_{tp}, which allows gas to flow into the lungs. Gas flows into the lungs because pressure at the airway opening (P_{awo}) is positive, and alveolar

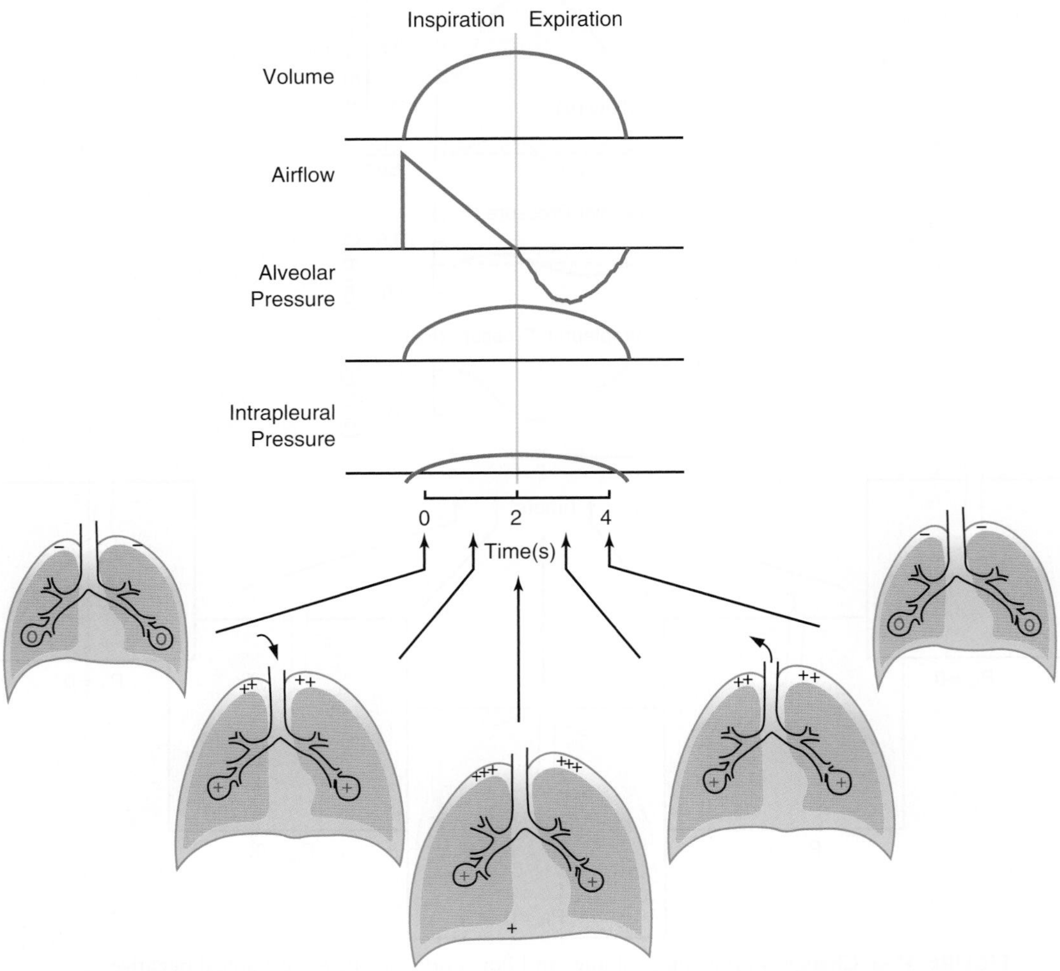

FIGURE 43-4 Changes in pressure, volume, and flow during a single decelerating flow, positive pressure breath. *Arrows* into and out of the trachea represent airflow. (Modified from Martin L: Pulmonary physiology in clinical practice: the essentials for patient care and evaluation, St Louis, 1987, Mosby.)

pressure (P_{alv}) is initially zero or less positive. Alveolar pressure rapidly increases during the inspiratory phase of PPV. The increased alveolar pressure expands the airways and alveoli. Because alveolar pressure is greater than pleural pressure (P_{pl}) during PPV, positive pressure is transmitted from the alveoli to the pleural space, causing pleural pressure to increase during inspiration. Depending on the compliance and resistance of the lungs, pleural pressure may markedly exceed atmospheric pressure during a portion of inspiration. These changes in pleural pressure during PPV can lead to significant physiologic changes (see later section). Pressure gradients during PPV are similar to pressure gradients during spontaneous breathing and NPV except that they are created by a positive pressure at the airway opening instead of a negative pressure in the pleural space (see Table 43-1). All pressure gradients change in the same direction as during NPV and spontaneous breathing except the transrespiratory pressure, which changes in the opposite direction.

Similar to spontaneous breathing, the recoil force of the lungs and chest wall, stored as potential energy during the positive pressure breath, causes passive exhalation. As gas flows from the alveoli to the airway opening, alveolar pressure decreases to atmospheric level, while pleural pressure is restored to its normal subatmospheric level (see Figure 43-4).

Volume and flow during PPV are also described by the equation of motion. The magnitude of P_{vent} not only depends on the patient's lung mechanics but also on the P_{musc} of the patient. If the patient makes no effort, P_{vent} is responsible for all volume and flow. During volume-controlled ventilation, as muscle effort increases, P_{vent} decreases, and V_T remains constant. During pressure-controlled ventilation, as P_{musc} increases, V_T increases, and P_{vent} remains unchanged.

RULE OF THUMB

Ideally, the transalveolar pressure should be as low as possible during mechanical ventilation. A transalveolar pressure less than about 28 to 30 cm H_2O minimized the development of ventilator-induced lung injury. If the plateau pressure is kept less than 28 to 30 cm H_2O, the transalveolar pressure can never exceed this level.

EFFECTS OF MECHANICAL VENTILATION ON VENTILATION

Increased Minute Ventilation

The primary indication for mechanical ventilation is *hypercapnic respiratory failure,* also known as *ventilatory failure.* For patients with acute ventilatory failure, the goal of mechanical ventilation is improving alveolar ventilation to compensate for the patient's inability to maintain normal $PaCO_2$. $PaCO_2$ is inversely related to alveolar ventilation, which is related to minute ventilation. Minute ventilation ($\dot{V}_E$) is the product of tidal volume (V_T) and ventilatory rate (f):

$$\dot{V} = V_T \times f$$

Use of a mechanical ventilator usually implies a change in V_T, ventilatory rate, or both from preintubation values. A normal spontaneous V_T is approximately 5 to 7 ml/kg. The currently accepted V_T for mechanical ventilation in acute respiratory failure is 4 to 8 ml/kg for patients with acute respiratory distress syndrome (ARDS) and 6 to 8 ml/kg for patients with normal lungs or with COPD; in some patients, a slightly larger V_T (up to 10 ml/kg) may be indicated. These volumes are based on ideal body weight. The mechanical ventilator rate depends on the patient's status. For postoperative ventilation, a rate of 12 to 20 breaths/min may be adequate. Conditions that necessitate a higher initial rate include ARDS, acutely increased intracranial pressure (ICP) (with caution; see later), and metabolic acidosis. Conditions that may necessitate a lower rate include acute asthma exacerbation, to allow an increased expiratory time to minimize air trapping. When an adequate V_T is established, the set rate is adjusted to achieve desired $PaCO_2$. Mechanical ventilation increases minute ventilation by increasing V_T, ventilator rate, or both.

Increased Alveolar Ventilation

Alveolar ventilation ($\dot{V}_A$) is inversely related to $PaCO_2$ as defined by the following relationship:

$$\dot{V}_A = (\dot{V}CO_2 \times 0.863)/PaCO_2$$

where $\dot{V}CO_2$ is carbon dioxide (CO_2) production.[2]

As alveolar ventilation decreases, $PaCO_2$ increases. As CO_2 production increases, alveolar ventilation must increase to maintain the same $PaCO_2$. Mechanical ventilation may be needed in either case. It is more useful to look at this equation solved for $PaCO_2$ because changes in $PaCO_2$ usually correlate with the need for mechanical ventilation:

$$PaCO_2 = (\dot{V}CO_2 \times 0.863)/\dot{V}_A$$

If $\dot{V}_A$ decreases or $\dot{V}CO_2$ increases, $PaCO_2$ increases, and hypercapnic respiratory failure follows; mechanical ventilation may be indicated in this setting. Because mechanical ventilation increases ventilation, $PaCO_2$ can be decreased to the desired level depending on the total ventilatory rate.

Decreased Ventilation/Perfusion Ratio

Spontaneous ventilation results in gas distribution mainly to the dependent and peripheral zones of the lungs. PPV tends to reverse this normal pattern of gas distribution, and most of the delivered volume is directed to nondependent lung zones (Figure 43-5). This phenomenon is

MINI CLINI

Alveolar, Transpulmonary, and Transalveolar Pressures

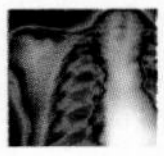

PROBLEM: Mr. Jones is 58 years old, 5 feet 8 inches tall, and weighs 410 lb and is being ventilated because of ARDS. His current ventilator settings are pressure control mode, peak pressure 35 cm H_2O, PEEP 20 cm H_2O, FiO_2 0.60, respiratory rate 30 breaths/min, and V_T 400 ml. At the end of expiration gas, flow returns to zero about 100 msec before the end of the breath. What are the alveolar, transpulmonary, and transalveolar pressures for Mr. Jones?

SOLUTION: Because there is a short end inspiratory pause, it is reasonable to assume that the peak airway pressure in pressure control is equal to the average peak alveolar pressure. The average is used because alveolar units have different time constants and as a result different peak pressure, but when there is end inspiratory equilibration of pressure, the resulting value is the average pressure across all lung units. To be more confident of this value, an additional end inspiratory pause can be added for a single breath to determine better the end inspiratory pause pressure or plateau pressure.

To determine the transpulmonary pressure ($P_{awo} - P_{pl}$) and transalveolar pressure ($P_{alv} - P_{pl}$), an estimate of pleural pressure must be made. The ideal method is to measure the esophageal pressure. Although not exactly equal to the pleural pressure, it accurately reflects changes in pleural pressure. Some authors have also recommended evaluation of bladder pressure, which changes in the same manner as esophageal pressure. The reading from the esophageal catheter at the time an end inspiratory pause was applied was 10 cm H_2O. The transpulmonary pressure and transalveolar pressure are the same—35 − 10 cm H_2O or 25 cm H_2O. This is because Mr. Jones was ventilated in pressure control, and there was a short end inspiratory pause, so both peak and plateau pressures were equal. However, if he was ventilated in volume ventilation and the peak airway pressure was 45 cm H_2O, while the plateau pressure remained 35 cm H_2O when an end inspiratory pause was added, the transalveolar pressure would be the same—35 − 10 cm H_2O or 25 cm H_2O—but the transpulmonary pressure during peak inspiration would be 45 − 10 cm H_2O or 35 cm H_2O.

Mr. Jones is receiving lung protective ventilation because his transalveolar pressure is only 25 cm H_2O. The high airway pressures are needed because of his stiff chest wall, which minimizes the transmission of pressure across the lung, reducing lung stretch.

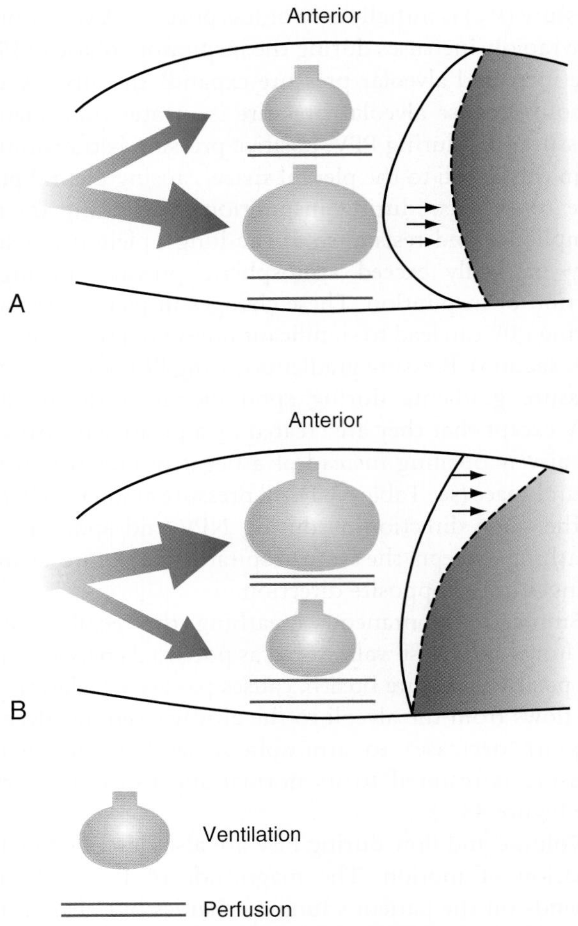

FIGURE 43-5 Effect of spontaneous ventilation and PPV on gas distribution in a supine subject. **A,** During spontaneous ventilation, diaphragmatic action distributes most ventilation to the dependent zones of the lungs, where perfusion is greatest. The result is a nearly normal $\dot{V}/\dot{Q}$ ratio. Partly because of diaphragmatic inactivity, PPV reverses this normal pattern of gas distribution, and most delivered volume is directed to the upper lung zones. **B,** An increase in ventilation to the upper lung zones, where there is less perfusion, increases the $\dot{V}/\dot{Q}$ ratio, effectively increasing physiologic dead space. At the same time, higher alveolar pressure in the better ventilated upper lung zones diverts blood flow away from these areas to the areas receiving the least ventilation. The result is areas of low $\dot{V}/\dot{Q}$ ratio and impaired oxygenation. (Modified from Kirby RR: Clinical application of ventilatory support, New York, 1990, Churchill Livingstone.)

caused partly by the inactivity of the diaphragm and chest wall during PPV. Although these structures actively facilitate gas movement during spontaneous breathing, inactivity of these structures during PPV impedes ventilation to dependent lung zones. An increase in ventilation to the nondependent zones of the lung, where there is less perfusion, increases the ventilation/perfusion ($\dot{V}/\dot{Q}$) ratio, effectively increasing physiologic dead space. The increase in $P(A - a)O_2$ often observed with PPV is caused by areas of low $\dot{V}/\dot{Q}$ ratio.

PPV decreases the $\dot{V}/\dot{Q}$ ratio in the bases and dependent lung zones mainly as a result of ventilation being primarily distributed to nondependent lung zones. The $\dot{V}/\dot{Q}$ ratio is also decreased in nondependent lung zones because of the effect of PPV on perfusion. PPV can compress the pulmonary capillaries. This compression increases pulmonary vascular resistance and decreases perfusion. Minimal blood flow perfuses the areas with the greatest V_T and contributes to a further increase in dead space. Conversely, blood intended for these areas is diverted to regions with lower vascular resistance—generally more dependent lung regions. Pulmonary blood flow during PPV tends to perfuse the least well-ventilated lung regions. This perfusion decreases the $\dot{V}/\dot{Q}$ ratio in those areas and increases the $P(A - a)O_2$.

Changes in Alveolar and Arterial Carbon Dioxide

Normal alveolar carbon dioxide tension (P_ACO_2) is 40 mm Hg, whereas mixed venous blood typically has a $P\bar{v}CO_2$ of 45 mm Hg. Under normal circumstances, CO_2 moves out of the blood at the pulmonary capillary interface; the result is a $PaCO_2$ of 40 mm Hg. In the event of a decrease in alveolar ventilation or an increase in CO_2 production, $PaCO_2$ increases. Mechanical ventilation can increase minute volume and alveolar ventilation and reduce P_ACO_2 and $PaCO_2$. With an increase in V_D/V_T, $PaCO_2$ increases if there is no change in minute volume; this may occur when alveolar blood flow is decreased by acute pulmonary embolism, an excessive level of positive end expiratory pressure (PEEP), or advanced dead space–producing disease such as emphysema or pulmonary embolism.

When excessive PEEP is used, blood flow is diverted from ventilated alveoli to hypoventilated alveoli; the result is an increased $\dot{V}/\dot{Q}$ ratio. In emphysema, formation of bullae is coincident with the destruction of pulmonary capillaries; the result is large areas of poorly perfused but ventilated alveoli. Pulmonary emboli may completely occlude pulmonary vessels; the result is lack of perfusion to alveoli distal to the blockage.

Changes in Acid-Base Balance

Respiratory acidemia, defined by a $PaCO_2$ greater than 45 to 50 mm Hg and a pH less than 7.35, occurs when minute ventilation and alveolar ventilation per minute ($\dot{V}_A$) are inadequate to meet the needs of the body. Respiratory acidemia can occur when the V_T is low, even though an accompanying mandatory rate is high.

Volume delivery also decreases if high airway pressures develop secondary to volume loss as a result of ventilator circuit tubing compliance (compressible volume loss). Ventilator circuits may have compliance of 3 ml/cm H_2O, which effectively reduces V_T:

$$\text{Volume lost} = \text{Tubing compliance} \times (\text{Peak pressure} - \text{PEEP})$$

Tubing compliance was a concern with older ventilators; however, most intensive care unit (ICU) ventilators in use at the present time allow the user to compensate for compressible volume loss as a result of tubing compliance. When activated, the volume set is the volume delivered to the patient. This issue is discussed in more detail later in the chapter.

An increase in V_D/V_T ratio can cause a reduction in alveolar ventilation, even though minute ventilation may be normal or increased. These problems emphasize the importance of proper selection of V_T and mandatory rate. When respiratory acidemia exists, the patient may become restless and anxious, resulting in **patient-ventilator asynchrony.** A communicative patient may complain of dyspnea. If these symptoms are observed, especially when $PaCO_2$ is increased, minute ventilation generally should be increased.

Respiratory alkalemia occurs if the minute ventilation is too high. It is recognized when $PaCO_2$ is less than 35 mm Hg and pH is greater than 7.45. A patient who is dyspneic, anxious, or in pain may develop this condition; the usual manifestations are an increased ventilatory rate or patient-ventilator asynchrony or both. The ventilator can cause respiratory alkalemia secondary to an inappropriately high V_T or rate. Regardless, the result is excessive minute and alveolar ventilation. This condition requires that the RT adjust the ventilator appropriately and address the patient's pain or anxiety to avoid the systemic effects of a prolonged alkalosis.

Metabolic acidemia in a patient receiving mechanical ventilation is recognized by a normal $PaCO_2$, with a decreased pH (<7.35), decreased bicarbonate level (<22 mEq/L), and increased base excess (<–2 mEq/L). With metabolic acidemia, the patient tries to compensate by increasing minute ventilation to blow off CO_2 in an effort to increase the pH. The resulting increase in work of breathing (WOB) may lead to ventilatory muscle fatigue and continued respiratory failure. The best therapy for metabolic acidosis is to manage the underlying cause while supporting the patient's ventilation as needed. Many patients cannot be liberated from mechanical ventilation until the underlying acidosis is controlled.

Bicarbonate has been used as therapy for metabolic acidosis. If it is administered, bicarbonate quickly combines with hydrogen ions and dissociates to form CO_2 and water, a reaction that may increase WOB. Generally, bicarbonate administration is not recommended until acidosis is severe (pH < 7.2). When necessary, bicarbonate is administered according to the following formula:[2]

$$NaHCO_3^- \text{ required} = \left[\tfrac{1}{4}\,\text{Body weight (kg)} \times \text{Base deficit}\right]/2$$

A temporary measure to compensate partially for metabolic acidosis is to increase minute ventilation during therapy to control the acidosis with the goal of a pH greater than 7.20.

Metabolic alkalemia is defined as a normal $PaCO_2$ with an elevated pH (>7.45) and an increased bicarbonate level (>26 mEq/L) and base excess (>+2 mEq/L). With metabolic alkalemia, in an effort to compensate for the increased pH, the patient tries to decrease minute ventilation. If weaning is attempted when the patient has a metabolic alkalemia, the patient may continue to hypoventilate, and weaning may fail. As with metabolic acidemia, the underlying cause should be determined and managed. Common causes of metabolic alkalosis include hypochloremia or hypokalemia secondary to gastrointestinal loss, diuretics, or steroid administration. See Chapter 13 for details on acid-base balance.

EFFECTS OF MECHANICAL VENTILATION ON OXYGENATION

Increased Inspired Oxygen

Mechanical ventilators usually deliver an increased fractional inspired oxygen (FiO_2) ranging from room air (0.21) to 100% O_2 (1.0). As a result, the alveolar partial pressure of oxygen (P_AO_2) and arterial partial pressure of oxygen (PaO_2) may be restored to normal with appropriate management. The effectiveness of increased FiO_2 in the management of hypoxemia depends on the cause of hypoxemia. Hypoxemia caused by a decrease in the $\dot{V}/\dot{Q}$ ratio or hypoventilation is more responsive to increased FiO_2 than hypoxemia caused by a diffusion defect or shunt. Hypoxemia caused by hypoventilation responds well to an increase in FiO_2, but alveolar ventilation can be restored only by improved ventilation. Hypoxemia caused by diffusion defect and shunt generally respond better to an increase in PEEP than to an increase in FiO_2. The fact that PaO_2 responds well to increased FiO_2 generally indicates that a low $\dot{V}/\dot{Q}$ ratio is the cause of hypoxemia. If the patient is receiving mechanical ventilation and has adequate alveolar ventilation, failure of the PaO_2 to respond to increased FiO_2 likely means that hypoxemia is due to a diffusion defect or shunt.

Mechanical ventilation increases alveolar ventilation, which increases PaO_2 if the underlying problem is hypoventilation. An increase in PaO_2 after an increase in FiO_2 likely means that the cause of hypoxemia is a low $\dot{V}/\dot{Q}$ ratio. In the event that PaO_2 is not restored by an increase in FiO_2, hypoxemia is probably due to a diffusion defect or shunt.

Alveolar Oxygen and Alveolar Air Equation

Increasing FiO_2 increases P_AO_2, according to the alveolar air equation:[2]

$$P_AO_2 = [FiO_2\,(P_B - 47)] - PaCO_2 \times [FiO_2 + (1 - FiO_2/R)]$$

where P_AO_2 is the partial pressure of oxygen in the alveoli; FiO_2 is the fractional inspired oxygen; P_B is the barometric pressure in mm Hg; 47 is the partial pressure of water vapor in the alveoli in mm Hg at 37° C; $PaCO_2$ is the partial pressure of carbon dioxide in arterial blood in mm Hg; and R is the respiratory exchange ratio ($\dot{V}CO_2/\dot{V}O_2$), normally 0.8.

When FiO_2 is increased, P_AO_2 increases as well, if there is no change in $PaCO_2$ or the respiratory exchange ratio. $PaCO_2$ may change with a change in alveolar ventilation or metabolic rate. O_2 consumption and CO_2 production increase with an increase in metabolic rate, such as with fever or overfeeding. If metabolic rate and alveolar ventilation are constant, an increase in FiO_2 results in a proportional increase in P_AO_2.

Arterial Oxygenation and Oxygen Content

Mechanical ventilation at FiO_2 of 0.21 may restore arterial oxygenation if the only cause of hypoxemia was hypoventilation. Hypoventilation may be the sole cause with central nervous system depression, apnea, and neuromuscular disease. With other causes of hypoxemia, an increase in FiO_2 is needed to increase arterial O_2 content.

O_2 content is directly related to arterial oxygenation and hemoglobin concentration, defined by the equation for arterial oxygen content (CaO_2):[2]

$$CaO_2\ (\text{vol\%}) = (1.34 \times Hb \times SaO_2) + (PaO_2 \times 0.003\ \text{ml}\ O_2/\text{mm Hg})$$

where 1.34 is a constant for the amount of O_2 carried by each fully saturated gram of hemoglobin (1.34 ml O_2/1 g hemoglobin), Hb is the hemoglobin concentration in g/dl, SaO_2 is the oxygen saturation of hemoglobin, and 0.003 is the amount of O_2 carried in the plasma in ml/mm Hg PaO_2. Under circumstances of normal diffusion, FiO_2, and hemoglobin concentration, the arterial content is normal at approximately 19.8 ml O_2/100 ml blood. As defined by this equation, CaO_2 decreases if hemoglobin concentration, arterial saturation, or PaO_2 decreases.

Decreased Shunt

Mechanical ventilation alone does not decrease shunt. Otherwise, it would be much easier to restore PaO_2 in patients with ARDS. Administration of PEEP with mechanical ventilation or to a spontaneously breathing patient in the form of continuous positive airway pressure (CPAP) helps to maintain open alveoli and stabilize small, collapsed, or fluid-filled alveoli. The results are an increase in alveolar surface area for diffusion and improvement in $\dot{V}/\dot{Q}$ matching and arterial oxygenation.

PEEP or CPAP should be used judiciously (see later in this chapter and Chapter 44). High pressure can overdistend alveoli and redistribute pulmonary blood flow to capillaries surrounding poorly ventilated alveoli resulting in increased shunt.

Increased Tissue Oxygen Delivery

When a mechanical ventilator is used to improve arterial oxygenation by increasing FiO_2 or PEEP, CaO_2 increases. However, the increase in CaO_2 represents only part of tissue O_2 delivery because O_2 delivery is defined by CaO_2 and cardiac output, as follows:[2]

$$DO_2 \text{ (tissue oxygen delivery in ml/min)} = CaO_2 \text{ (ml } O_2\text{/100 ml blood)} \times \text{Cardiac output (L/min)} \times 10$$

where 10 is a constant for converting deciliters to milliliters.

Normal tissue O_2 delivery is approximately 990 ml/min because the normal CaO_2 is approximately 20 vol%, and the normal cardiac output is approximately 5 L/min. When PaO_2, CaO_2, and cardiac output are adequate, so is tissue O_2 delivery. When PEEP is needed to improve PaO_2, it must be used cautiously because PEEP increases intrathoracic pressure. When intrathoracic pressure is increased, pleural pressure around the heart also increases, and the increase can affect the mechanical activity of the heart and impede venous return and decrease cardiac output. As discussed in Chapter 44, careful titration of PEEP must include monitoring the cardiovascular status of the patient. *Optimal PEEP* provides adequate arterial oxygenation and tissue O_2 delivery.

EFFECTS OF POSITIVE PRESSURE MECHANICAL VENTILATION ON LUNG MECHANICS

Time Constants

The time necessary for **passive** inflation and deflation of the lung or each alveolus is determined by the product of compliance and resistance. This product is the **time constant** of the lung or alveolar unit. The compliance of a "normal" lung is 0.1 L/cm H_2O, and resistance of a normal lung is 1 cm H_2O/L/sec. The time constant for a normal lung is 0.1 second (0.1 L/cm $H_2O \times 1$ cm H_2O/L/sec). For patients with normal lungs, 95% of the alveoli are inflated within three time constants (i.e., within 0.3 second). In four time constants (0.4 second), 98% of alveoli are inflated, and in five time constants (0.5 second), 99.3% of alveoli are inflated. The same numbers apply for exhalation.

The two major factors that affect alveolar time constants are changes in compliance and changes in resistance. If compliance or resistance decreases, the time constant for a given lung unit decreases, and the lung fills and empties faster. If compliance or resistance increases, the time constant increases, and it takes more time to fill and empty the lung.

There are clinical implications for patients with disorders consistent with abnormal time constants. A longer inspiratory time may be needed for patients with asthma because airway resistance is increased. Attempting to ventilate these patients with a normal inspiratory time may result in inadequate volume to affected lung units because the airways are obstructed, and volume is likely to travel to airways with the lowest resistance. Inspiratory time in severe asthma needs to be set between about 1.0 second to 1.5 seconds to ensure adequate gas delivery. The primary limiting factor is that the airways are also obstructed during exhalation. The expiratory time must also be longer to allow as complete an exhalation as possible.

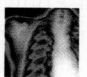

Asthma is very different from COPD, in which the inspiratory time constant is normal, but the expiratory time constant is long. In general, asthma requires very slow

MINI CLINI

Oxygen Delivery

PROBLEM: Oxygen delivery (DO_2) depends on PaO_2, hemoglobin concentration, and cardiac output. The formula for DO_2 is:

$$DO_2 = CaO_2 \times \text{Cardiac output (L/min)} \times 10$$

where CaO_2 is the arterial oxygen content, and 10 is the conversion factor between deciliters and milliliters. Normal DO_2 is 990 ml/min. DO_2 is normal when the hemoglobin concentration is 15 g/dl, cardiac output is 5.0 L/min, and PaO_2 is 100 mm Hg:

$$DO_2 = [15 \text{ g Hb} \times 1.34 \text{ ml } O_2/\text{g Hb} \times 0.97\ (SaO_2) + 0.003 \times 100 \text{ mm Hg}] \times (5.0 \text{ L/min}) \times 10 = 19.8\ (CaO_2) \times 5 \text{ (L/min)} \times 10 = 990 \text{ ml/min}$$

When the practitioner calculates DO_2 and determines it to be low, the component of the formula that is low denotes the problem and the therapeutic target. If CaO_2 is low because of a low hemoglobin concentration, increasing the hemoglobin concentration with blood transfusion is indicated. If CaO_2 is low because of low PaO_2 or SaO_2, increasing PaO_2 and SaO_2 with O_2 or PEEP is indicated. If cardiac output is low, the cause (decreased preload, increased afterload, decreased contractility, or bradycardia) is determined, and appropriate therapy is initiated. Frequently, a decrease in CaO_2 results in an increase in the cardiac output to compensate for decreased DO_2.

EXAMPLE: Given PaO_2 of 65 mm Hg, hemoglobin concentration of 10 g/dl, SaO_2 of 91%, and cardiac output of 4.8 L/min, what increase in cardiac output is necessary to maintain DO_2 of 900 ml/min?

$$DO_2 \text{ at given values is } [(1.34 \times 10 \times 0.97) + (0.003 \times 65)] \times 4.8 \times 10 = 633 \text{ ml/min}$$

An increase in cardiac output to 6.8 L/min results in DO_2 that is close to normal: $[(1.34 \times 10 \times 0.97) + (0.003 \times 65)] \times 6.8 \times 10 = 897$ ml/min. An increase in cardiac output to 6.8 L/min increases myocardial work. Because the cause of decreased DO_2 in this patient is hypoxemia and anemia, the goal of therapy should be to increase PaO_2. This strategy allows cardiac output and work to return to normal while adequate DO_2 is maintained. Increasing the hemoglobin concentration is normally not performed by transfusion unless the hemoglobin concentration is less than 8 to 10 g/dl because of the adverse effects associated with transfusions.

respiratory rates with longer than normal inspiratory and expiratory times to account for the altered time constants during both inspiration and expiration. Patients with COPD generally tolerate a more rapid rate because only the expiratory time constant is lengthened. In both of these situations, air trapping is very common because of the long time constants. In patients with COPD, inspiratory times are generally short (about 0.7 to 0.9 second). In patients with ARDS or acute lung injury (ALI), time constants are very short, and as a result inspiratory times can also be very short. Most patients with ARDS require an inspiratory time of only 0.5 to 0.6 second. Expiratory time constants are also short—hence the ability to ventilate these patients rapidly with small V_T. Respiratory rates greater than 30 breaths/min are frequently well tolerated by patients with ARDS. The major concern with patients with ARDS and their short time constants is that any disruption of the airway rapidly results in loss of lung volume. Atelectasis occurs with disconnections from the ventilator of only 1 or 2 seconds. As a result, *all* patients with ARDS should be suctioned *only* with inline suction catheters, and any circuit disconnection should be avoided. Ventilator management in the care of patients with COPD, asthma, and ARDS is described in detail in Chapter 44.

Increased Pressure

Peak inspiratory pressure (PIP) is the highest pressure produced during the inspiratory phase. It is the sum of the pressures necessary to overcome airway resistance and lung and chest wall compliance. PIP is also known as *peak pressure* or *peak airway pressure.*

Plateau pressure (P_{plat}) is the pressure observed during a period of inflation hold or end inspiratory pause. To obtain a plateau pressure, the RT initiates an inspiratory pause time of 0.5 to 2.0 seconds. During inspiration, the peak pressure is reached and then immediately followed by the inspiratory pause. During the pause, pressure decreases to a pressure plateau. When a valid plateau pressure value is obtained, the inspiratory pause time is returned to zero. Plateau pressure represents the average peak alveolar pressure (P_{alv}). In volume-controlled ventilation, plateau pressure is always lower than peak pressure because the peak pressure is the sum of the alveolar pressure and the pressure needed to overcome airway resistance. When flow is delivered by a square waveform, the difference between plateau pressure and peak pressure is the pressure necessary to overcome airway resistance. If the V_T is divided by the difference between the plateau pressure and PEEP, the quotient is the quasistatic lung-thorax compliance:[3]

$$C_{static} = V_T/(P_{plat} - PEEP)$$

This value is referred to as the lung-thorax compliance because the compliance of the lungs and the compliance of the rib cage are being calculated as a unit. The lung compliance cannot be determined without the use of an esophageal balloon.[3] Ideally, the volume lost owing to tubing compliance should be subtracted from the V_T if the ventilator has not compensated for it, making the equation:[3]

$$C_{static} = \text{Adjusted } V_T/(P_{plat} - PEEP)$$

It may be more useful to follow trends in lung compliance, rather than making judgments on only one calculation. A downward trend in compliance means that the lungs or chest wall is stiffer, as in ARDS.

Airway resistance (R_{aw}) during volume ventilation is estimated by the difference between PIP and P_{plat} divided by the inspiratory flow ($\dot{V}_I$) in L/sec, provided that the flow is constant (square waveform):[3]

$$R_{aw} = (PIP - P_{plat})/\dot{V}_I$$

During mechanical ventilation, the plateau pressure should be less than 30 cm H_2O.[4] At levels greater than 30 cm H_2O, alveolar damage from overdistention is likely. This form of *ventilator-induced lung injury (VILI)* is referred to as **volutrauma** (see later). This trauma can result in air leakage from alveoli, the release of inflammatory mediators, and multisystem organ failure (MSOF). When the plateau pressure approaches 30 cm H_2O during either volume or pressure ventilation, the pressure limit or the V_T should be decreased. This approach to ventilation is referred to as *lung protective ventilation.*[3]

> **RULE OF THUMB**
>
> When measuring lung mechanics, airway resistance and compliance always use the same ventilator settings to make comparisons from one point in time to another much easier. In adults, settings are volume ventilation, V_T 500 ml, square wave flow, and peak flow set at 60 L/min.

Mean Airway Pressure

Mean airway pressure is the average pressure across the total cycle time (TCT). The mean airway pressure ($P_{\overline{AW}}$) can be calculated manually if the flow is constant, as follows:[3]

$$P_{\overline{AW}} = \tfrac{1}{2}(PIP - PEEP) \times (\text{Inspiratory time}/TCT) + PEEP$$

Mean airway pressure is computed by the ventilator as the integral of the pressure signal over the total cycle time (as a rolling average), so the RT can record the ventilator computed value, rather than manually calculating it. Because expiratory (baseline) pressure is lower than inspiratory pressure, the mean pressure is between peak and end expiratory pressure. The variables affecting mean pleural and mean airway pressure are summarized in Box 43-1. For a given minute volume, partial ventilatory support modes such as synchronized intermittent mandatory ventilation (SIMV) result in lower mean airway and pleural pressures than continuous mandatory ventilation (CMV) modes. For a specific mandatory breath, as peak pressure increases, so does mean pressure. Likewise, long inspiratory times increase mean pressure. Prolonging expiratory time has the opposite effect on mean airway pressure. Generally, the harmful cardiovascular effects of PPV are more likely to occur when $P_{\overline{AW}}$ or inspiratory-to-expiratory (I:E) ratio increases (e.g., >1:1).

The pressure waveform of a mandatory breath affects mean pressure. In Figure 43-6, for a given inspiratory time, the constant pressure pattern (curve *A*) results in the greatest area under the airway pressure curve and the highest mean airway pressure. A constant pressure pattern is normally produced by a pressure targeted breath that provides decreasing (descending ramp) flow. The effect of PEEP on mean airway pressure is simple: Every 1 cm H_2O of applied PEEP increases the mean airway pressure 1 cm H_2O.

Effect of Peak Airway Pressure on Lung Recruitment

As peak airway pressure increases, previously collapsed, small, or fluid-filled alveoli are recruited, that is, reopened.[5] This reopening of alveoli increases alveolar surface area and restores functional residual capacity (FRC). At the alveolar level, the surface area available for diffusion is increased. As a result, PaO_2 increases, consistent with Fick's law. The use of extrinsic PEEP maintains the airways and recruited open alveoli. Extrinsic PEEP is controlled directly by the PEEP control on the ventilator, and the RT always knows how much extrinsic PEEP is present. Several factors, including inverse ratio ventilation (IRV), may add intrinsic PEEP or auto-PEEP by starting the next breath before the previous exhalation has ended. The amount of intrinsic PEEP added by IRV can be measured by implementing an end expiratory pause, which stops the next breath from being delivered. During this end expiratory pause, alveolar and mouth pressures equilibrate, and the total PEEP is now presented by the ventilator. The amount of auto-PEEP present is the difference between the total PEEP and the extrinsic PEEP:

Intrinsic PEEP (auto-PEEP) = Total PEEP − Extrinsic PEEP

Box 43-1 Factors That Increase Mean Airway Pressure

- Absence of spontaneous ventilation
- Increasing positive pressure
- Increasing duration of inspiration
- Decreasing duration of expiration
- Nature of inspiratory waveform
- Increasing level of PEEP
- Decreasing compliance, increasing airways resistance

Increased Lung Volume: Tidal Volume

The volume delivered during pressure-controlled modes varies with changes in set pressure, patient effort, and lung mechanics. For all pressure-targeted modes, the volume delivered at a given pressure decreases as compliance decreases. An increase in resistance, active exhalation, or muscle tensing by the patient during inspiration also decreases delivered volume in pressure ventilation.

If pressure serves as the limit variable instead of the cycle variable, changes in airway resistance during pressure-limited ventilation may or may not affect delivered volume. In this case, the key factor is the time available for pressure equilibration. Volume can remain constant even if airway resistance increases, as long as there is sufficient time for alveolar and airway pressures to equilibrate. However, if

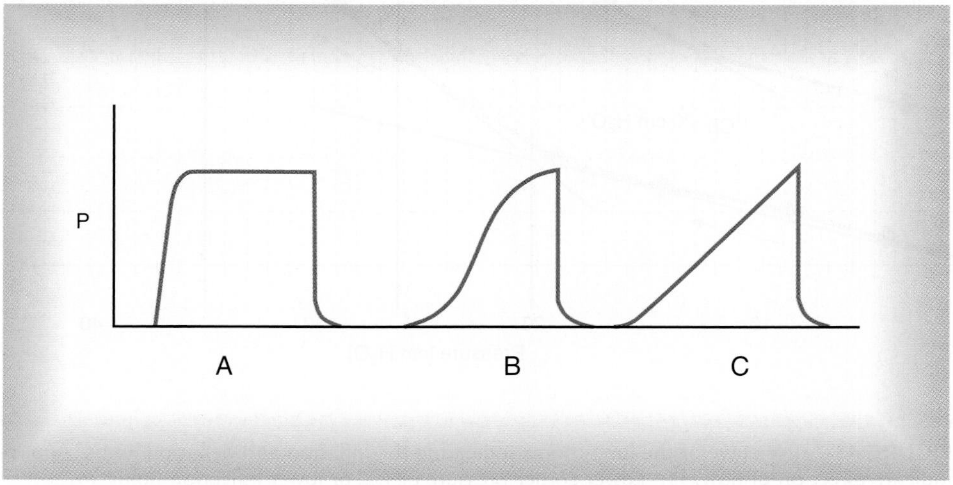

FIGURE 43-6 Pressure patterns resulting from a descending ramp flow waveform *(A)*, a sine wave flow waveform *(B)*, and a constant flow waveform *(C)*. Because waveform *A* has the highest pressure for the longest inspiratory time, it also has the greatest mean airway pressure.

insufficient time is available for pressure equilibration, delivered volume decreases as airway resistance increases. The length of time needed for pressure equilibration is usually at least three times greater than the time constant for the respiratory system. In pressure modes, ventilator-delivered flow varies with patient effort and lung mechanics; this tends to avoid patient-ventilator asynchrony.[6]

Increased Functional Residual Capacity

FRC is not known to change significantly with the application of PPV alone because passive exhalation allows the end expiratory pressure to return to atmospheric pressure with each breath. If an increase in FRC is to be achieved, end expiratory pressure must be increased. This increase is commonly achieved with PEEP or CPAP. PEEP or CPAP does not recruit collapsed lung units but prevents lung units that have been opened from collapsing at end expiration. Peak airway pressure recruits lung volume. The magnitude of the increase in FRC sustained by PEEP or CPAP is proportional to the lung-thorax compliance. With acute restriction, as PEEP is increased, lung compliance improves. Initially, FRC gain as PEEP is added is small. However, as FRC and compliance increase, additional increments of PEEP tend to result in larger increases in FRC up to the point at which overdistention occurs. At that point, as PEEP is increased, increases in FRC decline, as does compliance. There is no practical way of measuring FRC in all patients, so other methods of determining an increase in FRC are used, such as improving PaO_2 at a constant FiO_2, increasing PaO_2/FiO_2 ratio, decreasing shunt fraction, or decreasing FiO_2 while maintaining PaO_2. The management of PEEP is described in more detail in Chapter 44.

Pressure-Volume Curve and Lung Recruitment in Acute Respiratory Distress Syndrome

Figure 43-7 depicts the pressure-volume (P-V) relationship of the lung-thorax in an idealized patient with ARDS.[7] On the inflation P-V curve, there are two points of inflection: the lower inflection point referred to as P_{flex} or *lower corner pressure,* and an upper inflection point, also referred to as *upper corner pressure.* These two points represent defined changes in compliance. The lower inflection point represents an abrupt increase in lung-thorax compliance as collapsed or atelectatic lung begins to be recruited.[8] The upper deflection points represent the point where the rate of lung recruitment decreases and overinflation begins. It

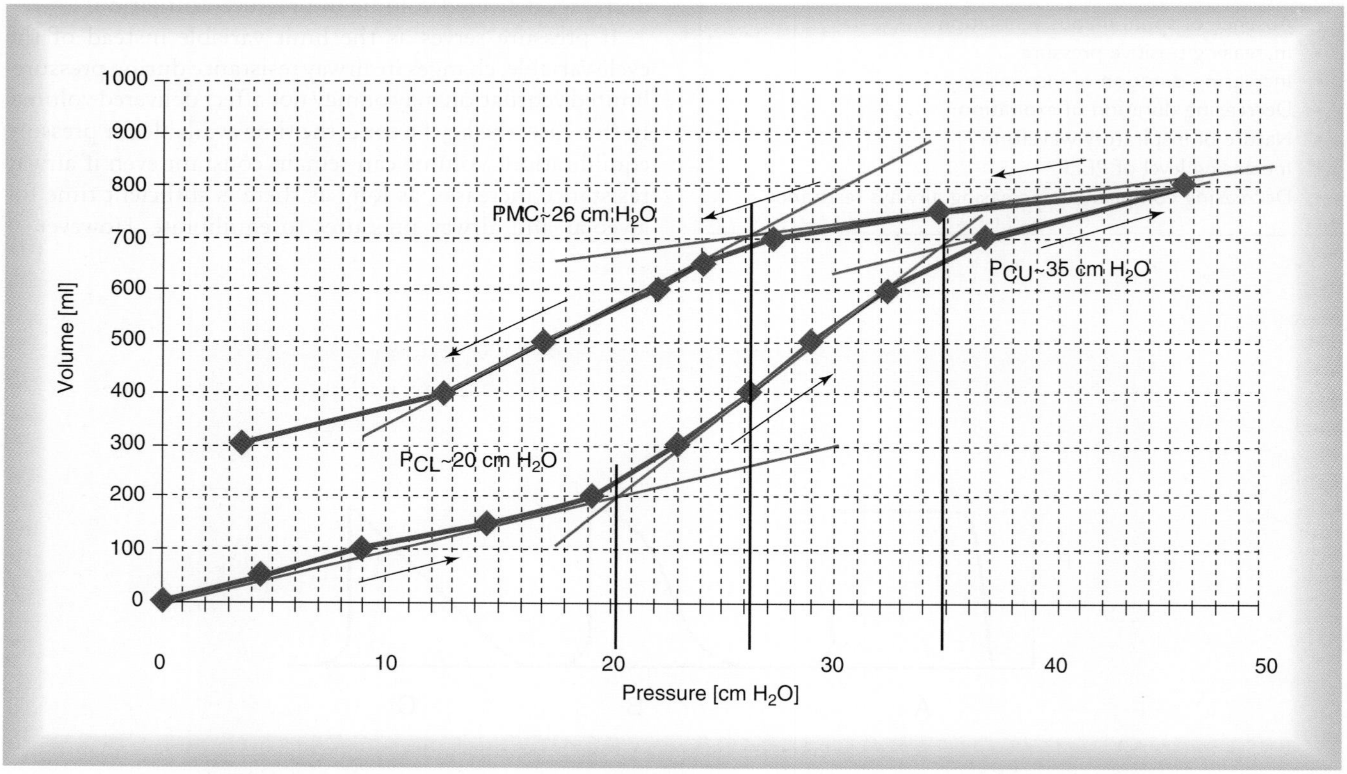

FIGURE 43-7 P-V curve of the lung-thorax indicating the inflation and deflation limbs. *Arrows* indicate direction of flow. P_{CL}, Lower corner pressure or P_{flex} or lower inflection point; P_{CU}, upper corner pressure or upper inflection point; P_{MG}, point of maximum compliance change. (Modified from Godon S, Fujino Y, Hromi JM, et al: Optimal mean airway pressure during high frequency oscillation. Anesthesiology 94:862–868, 2001.)

is most important to realize from this graph that the lung is recruited by pressure and that the higher the peak airway pressure, the greater the potential for lung to be recruited. The maximum pressure needed to recruit a given patient's lung is unknown; however, pressures up to 50 cm H_2O most likely are safe with most patients when applied for short (1 to 3 minutes) periods.[9-11] If these pressures were applied for longer periods, lung injury would most likely result.

The deflation limb of the P-V curve is similar in shape to the inflation limb but is separated from the inflation limb. This hysteresis (separation) is a result of surfactant and surface tension interactions. Basically, less pressure is required to keep the lung open on the deflation limb of the P-V curve than on the inflation limb; this is obvious on examination of the volume maintained in the lung at P_{flex}, or 20 cm H_2O. On the inflation limb, lung volume increases about 200 ml at 20 cm H_2O, but on the deflation limb, lung volume increases about 550 ml. The goal of an open lung approach to ventilation that has been proposed by many authors is to open the lung and then to ventilate the patient on the deflation limb of the P-V curve.[9-11]

Figure 43-7 is an idealized P-V curve; actual patient P-V curves in ARDS are not as well defined. In 10% to 20% of patients with ARDS, P_{flex} cannot be identified on the inflation P-V curve. As a result, despite two positive randomized controlled trials using P_{flex} to set PEEP,[12,13] the use of P-V curves clinically has not become common practice; a second reason for this is the difficulty measuring the P-V curve. However, many newer ICU ventilators are including algorithms that allow P-V curves to be performed by the ventilator with the ventilator identifying P_{flex}. This option may increase the use of the P-V curve for the management of patients with ARDS.

Box 43-2 Performance of Recruitment Maneuver and Decremental Positive End Expiratory Pressure Trial

Pressure control ventilation settings are:
- PEEP 20-30 cm H_2O
- Peak inspiratory pressure 40-50 cm H_2O
- Inspiratory time 1-2 sec
- Rate about 15-20 breaths/min
- Time 1-3 min

After completing RM, set PEEP at 20 cm H_2O, ventilate with VC, V_T 4 to 6 ml/kg ideal body weight, increase rate, avoid auto-PEEP.

Measure dynamic compliance after 3 to 5 minutes of stabilization.

Decrease PEEP 2 cm H_2O.

Measure dynamic compliance after 3 to 5 minutes of stabilization.

Repeat until maximum compliance is determined.

Optimal PEEP = maximum compliance PEEP + 2 cm H_2O.

Repeat RM and set PEEP at the identified settings; adjust ventilation.

After PEEP and ventilation are set and stabilized, decrease FiO_2 until PO_2 in target range.

If response is poor and the patient tolerates the procedure well, repeat RM with PEEP 25 cm H_2O and peak pressure 45 cm H_2O after a period of stabilization.

If response is still poor and the patient tolerates the procedure well, repeat RM with PEEP 30 cm H_2O and peak pressure 50 cm H_2O.

Do not exceed 50 cm H_2O peak airway pressure during RM.

An approach to setting PEEP that has been proposed more recently in association with an open lung approach to ARDS management is a decremental PEEP trial immediately after a lung recruitment maneuver (RM).[11,12,14] Many different approaches to performing lung RMs have been published, but the approach that is considered the safest and most efficacious is the use of pressure-controlled continuous mandatory ventilation (PV-CMV).[11,12,14] To perform a lung RM with PC-CMV, high enough PEEP must be set to avoid derecruitment after each inspiration. Essentially, a minimum of 20 cm H_2O PEEP is required during the RM. Peak pressure is usually started at 40 cm H_2O, and if the patient tolerates the pressure hemodynamically, it may be increased to 50 cm H_2O (Box 43-2). Inspiratory time is increased to about 1.5 to 2.0 seconds, and respiratory rate is decreased to about 15 to 20 breaths/min. The maneuver is applied for 1 to 3 minutes. During the RM, the patient must be sedated to apnea to avoid fighting the ventilator.

Before any RM, the patient must be hemodynamically stable. RMs should not be performed in patients with existing **barotrauma** or with a high likelihood of developing barotrauma (blebs or bullae) or in patients who are hemodynamically unstable. In addition, RMs are most effective and result in the least adverse reaction if performed early in the course of ARDS. During and after the RM, the patient must be carefully monitored for hemodynamic and oxygenation instability and the development of barotrauma.

After an RM, the best way to identify the minimum effective PEEP level that maintains the lung open is to perform a decremental PEEP trial.[11,12,14] This trial is performed by changing the mode from PC-CMV to volume-controlled continuous mandatory ventilation (VC-CMV), V_T 4 to 6 ml/kg, inspiratory time 1.0 second or less, PEEP 20 cm H_2O, and rate set at the maximum that does not cause auto-PEEP.[7] After stabilization (3 to 5 minutes), dynamic compliance is measured.[7] PEEP is then decreased 2 cm H_2O, the patient is stabilized (3 to 5 minutes), and measurement of dynamic compliance is repeated; this is continued until the PEEP level at which the compliance decreases is identified. Generally, compliance at 20 cm H_2O PEEP is low, and it increases as PEEP is decreased; compliance then decreases as PEEP is decreased further.

Open lung PEEP is the PEEP associated with the highest compliance. Set PEEP is open lung PEEP plus 2 cm H_2O.

After open lung PEEP is identified, the lung is again recruited because during the decremental PEEP trial derecruitment occurred. After recruitment, PEEP is set at the identified level, ventilation is adjusted using a lung protective V_T (4 to 8 ml/kg), and rate is adjusted to normalize PCO_2. After all is set, FiO_2 is decreased to the level that maintains PaO_2 in the range of 55 to 70 mm Hg. Repeat RMs may be needed if the patient did not respond to the initial RM or if the patient is disconnected from the ventilator and derecruitment occurs. A successful RM is one that allows the FiO_2 to be reduced to less than 0.5.

The use of RM has been documented in many case series. However, no data have been published indicating that outcome is improved as a result of RMs and decremental PEEP settings. Research is ongoing, but RM is mostly considered to be experimental at the present time.

RULE OF THUMB

A lung RM is most likely to be successful if it is performed early in the course of ARDS. Ideally, if indicated, a lung RM should be performed once the patient is fully stabilized after intubation and initiation of mechanical ventilation. The longer the patient is mechanically ventilated, the less likely the RM would be successful.

Increased Dead Space

The dead space fraction is increased with the institution of mechanical ventilation owing to inspiratory mechanical bronchodilation and the preferential ventilation of more apical, nondependent alveoli, the reduction of blood flow away from ventilated alveoli and the continued perfusion of basilar or dependent alveoli (see Figure 43-5). This increase is concurrent with a decrease in $\dot{V}/\dot{Q}$ ratio.

Decreased Work of Breathing

Although improper ventilator management can increase WOB, one of the primary objectives of mechanical ventilation is to decrease WOB. PPV can significantly reduce WOB in patients with actual or impending respiratory muscle fatigue. RTs frequently see patients relax as the ventilator assumes a major portion of their WOB. To lessen WOB, ventilation must be sufficient to meet the patient's needs. Otherwise, a spontaneously breathing patient tends to resist the ventilator, and an asynchronous breathing pattern develops. Inappropriately applied PPV can result in alveolar hypoventilation and consequently a considerable increase in the patient's WOB.

Mode, trigger setting, and inspiratory flow have an effect on WOB. WOB consists of two components: (1) ventilator work (WOB_{vent}) occurring as the ventilator forces gas into the lungs and (2) patient work (WOB_{pt}) as the inspiratory muscles draw gas into the lungs. The magnitude of WOB_{pt} depends on compliance, resistance, and ventilatory drive and on ventilator variables, such as trigger sensitivity, peak flow, cycling coordination, and V_T.[15,16]

Regardless whether flow or pressure triggering is selected, either should always be set as sensitive as possible without causing autotriggering. The less sensitive the setting, the greater the patient effort. In older generation ventilators, flow triggering was shown to require less effort than pressure triggering.[17] However, with the newest generation of ICU ventilators, both are equally effective.

As described in Chapter 42, a mode of ventilation is a ventilatory pattern that can be described by identifying the control variable, breath sequence, and targeting scheme. The breath sequence may be thought of as being on a continuum from assuming very little to assuming all WOB (Figure 43-8). As the breath sequence is changed from continuous spontaneous ventilation (CSV) to CMV, the ventilator assumes more WOB. An example of this transition would be from CPAP to pressure support to IMV to CMV. In CPAP, a continuous spontaneous mode

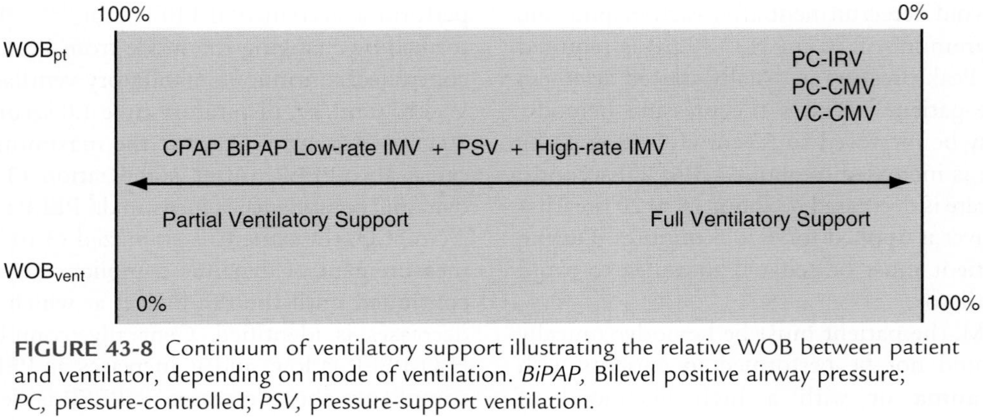

FIGURE 43-8 Continuum of ventilatory support illustrating the relative WOB between patient and ventilator, depending on mode of ventilation. *BiPAP,* Bilevel positive airway pressure; *PC,* pressure-controlled; *PSV,* pressure-support ventilation.

of ventilation, the patient assumes all WOB. The ventilator merely provides positive pressure throughout the patient's breathing cycle. The ventilator assumes more WOB during IMV and CMV. Pressure support is also an example of CSV. During pressure support ventilation (PSV), the patient determines breath timing (length of inspiration and expiration) and frequency. Depending on the set inspiratory pressure, the clinician may program the ventilator to provide a minimal to a maximal amount of WOB. In instances where the patient has no spontaneous efforts, all breaths during IMV or CMV are time triggered, and all work performed is WOB_{vent}. This situation commonly occurs when the diaphragmatic paralysis occurs as a result of pharmacologic intervention (sedation or paralysis), disease state (Guillain-Barré syndrome), or trauma (spinal cord injury). Although it may be advantageous for the ventilator to assume all WOB for a while, extended periods of passive ventilation may cause diaphragmatic atrophy, which may unnecessarily prolong the need for mechanical ventilation and delay weaning. At initiation of patient-triggered pressure or volume modes, WOB_{pt} resumes. With volume ventilation, this work is primarily associated with triggering the ventilator and inspiring the V_T at the set inspiratory flow. If the sensitivity, V_T, and inspiratory flow are set appropriately, WOB_{pt} is small. If flow or V_T are set too low, patient-ventilator asynchrony often occurs, and increased WOB_{pt} results.

During assisted ventilation, pressure-targeted modes are generally more capable of meeting patient ventilatory demands and minimizing WOB_{pt}.[18] As pressure level is increased, ventilatory muscles are unloaded, V_T increases for a given amount of patient effort, and WOB_{pt} decreases. Most clinicians increase pressure level until the breathing pattern approaches normal—that is, until the spontaneous ventilatory rate is 15 to 25 breaths/min and the spontaneous V_T is normal (5 to 8 ml/kg).

Measuring WOB is technically difficult. It is often accomplished by esophageal balloon monitoring, in which a balloon is placed in the distal third of the esophagus, and a pneumotachometer is attached to the airway. WOB is the integral of the esophageal pressure and V_T. Normal WOB is 0.6 to 0.8 J/L. One approach to pressure-controlled ventilation is titration of the inspiratory pressure level on the basis of measured WOB. If work is greater than 0.8 J/L, pressure is increased until work decreases to within normal limits (unloading the muscles of ventilation). If work is less than 0.6 J/L, pressure is decreased until work increases to within normal limits (loading the muscles of ventilation). Although it may be useful to titrate pressure level to WOB_{pt},[19] bedside measurement of WOB is rarely performed because it is technically difficult to perform. Respiratory rate, frequency, use of accessory muscles, airway pressure waveform, and patients' answers to questions about their breathing comfort help the RT determine whether WOB_{pt} is excessive.

MINIMIZING ADVERSE PULMONARY EFFECTS OF POSITIVE PRESSURE MECHANICAL VENTILATION

Decreasing Pressure

The main objective of mechanical ventilation is to provide a minute ventilation appropriate to achieve adequate alveolar ventilation and supplemental O_2 and PEEP to provide adequate arterial oxygenation.

MINI CLINI

Overcoming an Increase in the Work of Breathing

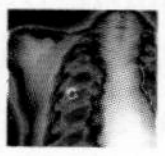

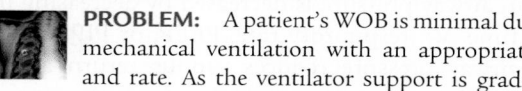

PROBLEM: A patient's WOB is minimal during mechanical ventilation with an appropriate V_T and rate. As the ventilator support is gradually discontinued and the patient is expected to take over more of WOB, airway resistance associated with breathing through an endotracheal tube may become clinically important. The RT must be able to recognize this problem readily and know how to correct it.

A patient has received mechanical ventilation in volume-controlled CMV mode for the past week. The patient's condition is now clinically stable, and ventilation is provided by PSV. As the PSV pressure level is reduced to 12 cm H_2O, the patient begins using accessory muscles to breathe, the spontaneous respiratory rate increases to 30 breaths/min, and the patient reports shortness of breath. Blood gas values are acceptable, and no abnormal lung sounds are present. What is the problem, and what should the RT do?

SOLUTION: The patient may be experiencing excessive WOB because of airway resistance associated with the endotracheal tube; a small sized tube or partial obstruction of the tube with secretions may be the problem. Other possibilities that should be considered include deterioration in the patient's cardiopulmonary disease, but the normal blood gas values and lung sounds suggest the problem is not the lungs. Passing a suction catheter through the tube may help to identify the problem. If the catheter does not pass easily, the tube may be partially obstructed. Two options exist: Change the tube or extubate the patient. Because the tube would need to be removed regardless of the choice, a trial extubation should be considered. Because this patient is at risk immediately after extubation, noninvasive ventilation should be started. If the patient cannot tolerate extubation, an appropriate-sized endotracheal tube can be reinserted.

Peak pressure is the result of the pressure required to overcome system resistance and compliance. Although there is no absolute maximum pressure, most practitioners try to avoid peak pressures greater than 40 cm H_2O. As the peak pressure approaches 40 cm H_2O, it is important to consider the causes. Factors that increase airway resistance include airway edema, bronchospasm, and secretions. The RT can manage or avoid these problems by ensuring adequate humidity, bronchial hygiene (suctioning, airway care), and administration of bronchodilators and antiinflammatory drugs. Factors that increase the pressure needed to inflate the lung and overcome compliance include alveolar and interstitial edema, atelectasis, fibrosis, and chest wall restriction.

Plateau pressure reflects mean maximum alveolar pressure. Plateau pressures of 30 cm H_2O or greater have an increased likelihood of causing lung injury. If plateau pressure approaches 30 cm H_2O during volume ventilation, the V_T should be decreased so that the plateau pressure is less than 30 cm H_2O, or with pressure ventilation, target pressure should be set less than 30 cm H_2O.[4,20]

Mean airway pressure is decreased by decreasing inspiratory time, V_T, respiratory rate, PEEP, or PIP. Increased mean airway pressure reduces venous return and may reduce cardiac output.

Positive End Expiratory Pressure or Continuous Positive Airway Pressure

PEEP is the application of positive pressure at end exhalation. PEEP is used primarily to improve oxygenation in patients with refractory hypoxemia. As a rule, refractory hypoxemia exists when PaO_2 cannot be maintained at greater than 50 to 60 mm Hg with FiO_2 0.60 or greater. PEEP improves oxygenation in these patients by maintaining alveoli open, restoring FRC, and decreasing physiologic shunting. The improved alveolar volume provided by PEEP allows a lower FiO_2. Other values such as lung compliance, shunt fraction, and PaO_2/FiO_2 ratio also may improve when PEEP is appropriately applied. PEEP may be indicated in the care of patients with COPD who have dynamic hyperinflation (auto-PEEP).[21,22] (See discussion later in this chapter.)

Beneficial and harmful effects are associated with the use of PEEP (Table 43-2). Detrimental effects of inappropriately high levels of PEEP include decreased cardiac output, increased pulmonary vascular resistance, and increased dead space. When one or more of these problems occur, PEEP is decreased to the previous level or to a value between the current level and the previous level. If cardiac output decreases and an increase in PEEP is necessary to maintain oxygenation, intravenous fluid, inotropic cardiac drugs, or both are administered to restore cardiac output.

PEEP is contraindicated in the presence of a tension pneumothorax. PEEP should be applied cautiously in patients with severe unilateral lung disease because PEEP would overinflate the lung with higher compliance. The result is lung overdistention and compression of adjacent pulmonary capillaries. Independent lung ventilation can be used to apply separate inspiratory and baseline pressures to the right and the left lung when severe unilateral lung disease is present.[23] PEEP is contraindicated in the care of patients with increased ICP only if the application of PEEP increases ICP further.

TABLE 43-2

Physiologic Effects of Positive End Expiratory Pressure

Beneficial Effects of Appropriate PEEP	Detrimental Effects of Inappropriate PEEP
Restored FRC, avoids derecruitment	Increased pulmonary vascular resistance
Decreased shunt fraction	Potential decrease in venous return and cardiac output
Increased lung compliance	Decreased renal and portal blood flow
Decreased WOB	Increased ICP
Increased PaO_2 for a given FiO_2	Increased dead space

RULE OF THUMB

Refractory hypoxemia exists when PaO_2 cannot be maintained at greater than 50 to 60 mm Hg with FiO_2 0.60 or greater. This situation is an indication for PPV with PEEP or CPAP because an increased end expiratory pressure with either of these modalities improves oxygenation by decreasing physiologic shunting.

Effects of Ventilatory Pattern

The most commonly used inspiratory flow patterns are constant or square and descending ramp during volume-controlled ventilation and exponential decay during pressure-controlled ventilation. In mechanical and computer models, a descending ramp (volume-controlled ventilation) flow pattern improves gas distribution to lung units with long-time constants. The literature often refers to the descending ramp as a decelerating flow pattern. Similar findings in humans have been reported. Compared with a square flow waveform, a descending ramp has been shown to reduce peak pressure, inspiratory work, V_D/V_T, and $P(A - a)O_2$ without affecting hemodynamic values.[24] Compared with volume-controlled ventilation with a square flow waveform, pressure-controlled ventilation with an exponential decay flow waveform may result in a higher PaO_2, lower $PaCO_2$, and lower PIPs. However, mean airway pressure is higher with pressure-controlled ventilation compared with volume-controlled ventilation because pressure increases to the set inspiratory pressure and remains constant throughout inspiration. During pressure-controlled ventilation, flow is responsive to patient demand. The ventilator delivers flow to the patient in proportion to patient need. Flow is also greater at the onset of inspiration, resulting in V_T delivery at a time when the lungs are most compliant, the beginning of the breath. As a breath ends, flow is least, and the volume delivered is small. The result is a lower peak airway pressure for any given V_T.

In most spontaneously breathing persons, lower inspiratory flows improve gas distribution. However, during PPV, low inspiratory flow may lead to lengthy inspiratory times and air trapping if expiratory time is too short. High ventilator inspiratory flow allows more time for exhalation and reduces the incidence of air trapping. Avoidance of air trapping improves gas exchange and reduces WOB in patients with high ventilatory demands.[16,25]

An inflation hold also affects gas exchange. By momentarily maintaining lung volume under conditions of no flow, an inflation hold allows additional time for gas redistribution between lung units with different time constants. In both animal and human studies, increasing the length of an inflation hold decreases the V_D/V_T, $PaCO_2$, and inert gas washout time. Adding an inflation hold effectively increases total inspiratory time, shortening the time available for exhalation. This step predisposes patients with airway obstruction to auto-PEEP. In practice, an inflation hold should be used only to obtain P_{plat} values. Because the technique prevents the onset of exhalation, asynchrony occurs if the patient is actively breathing.

Trigger Site and Work of Breathing

Studies have examined the effects of sensing a patient's inspiratory effort at the tip of the endotracheal tube rather than in the ventilator circuit, as is done with all ventilators. Triggering and managing gas delivery by measurement of pressure at the tip of the endotracheal tube decreases patient effort and improves synchrony; however, no practical system has been designed.[26] In addition, the efficiency of ventilator flow and pressure triggering seems to improve with each new generation of mechanical ventilator.

PHYSIOLOGIC EFFECTS OF VENTILATORY MODES

Volume-Controlled Ventilation versus Pressure-Controlled Ventilation

Figure 42-5 (see p. 1012) illustrates the important variables for volume ventilation modes. The figure shows that the primary variable to be controlled is the patient's minute ventilation. A particular ventilator may allow the operator to set minute ventilation directly. More frequently, minute ventilation is adjusted by means of a set V_T and frequency. V_T is a function of the set inspiratory flow and the set inspiratory time. Inspiratory time is affected by the set frequency and, if applicable, the set I:E ratio. The mathematical relationships among all these variables are shown in Table 43-3.

With pressure-controlled ventilation, the goal is also to maintain adequate minute ventilation. However (as the equation of motion shows), when pressure is controlled, V_T and minute ventilation are determined not only by the ventilator's pressure settings but also by the elastance and resistance of the patient's respiratory system. Minute ventilation and hence gas exchange are less stable in pressure-controlled modes than in volume-controlled modes. Figure 42-6 (see p. 1014) shows the important variables for pressure-controlled ventilation. V_T is not operator set on the ventilator. It is the result of the set inspiratory pressure, the patient's lung mechanics, and the inspiratory time. On most ventilators, the speed with which inspiratory pressure is achieved (i.e., the pressure rise time) is adjustable. That adjustment affects the shape of the pressure waveform and the mean airway pressure.

Continuous Mandatory Ventilation

CMV (also referred to as *assist/control*) is a mode of ventilation in which total ventilatory support is provided by the mechanical ventilator. All breaths are mandatory and delivered by the ventilator at a preset volume or pressure, breath rate, and inspiratory time. If the patient has spontaneous respiratory efforts, the ventilator delivers a patient-triggered breath. If patient efforts are absent, the ventilator delivers time-triggered breaths. The clinician needs to set an appropriate trigger level and flow rate for the patient in this mode of ventilation. There is a potential for the ventilator to autotrigger when the trigger level is set too sensitive. As a result, hyperventilation, air trapping, and patient anxiety often ensue. However, if the trigger level is not sensitive enough, the ventilator does not respond to the patient's inspiratory efforts, which results in increased WOB.

Occasionally, all attempts to optimize patient comfort, reduce WOB, and achieve the goals of this mode of ventilation are futile. In cases in which this mode is poorly tolerated and spontaneous triggering is counterproductive to the goals set for a particular patient, sedation or paralysis or both may be required. These agents may be used to minimize patient effort and normalize WOB.

Volume-Controlled Continuous Mandatory Ventilation

Volume-controlled continuous mandatory ventilation (VC-CMV) is indicated when a precise minute ventilation or blood gas parameter, such as $PaCO_2$, is therapeutically essential to the care of patients.[25] Theoretically, volume control (with a constant inspiratory flow) (Figure 43-9) results in a more even distribution of ventilation (compared with pressure control) among lung units with different time constants where the units have equal resistances but unequal compliances (e.g., ARDS).[26]

During VC-CMV, volume is guaranteed, but airway pressure varies depending on changes in the patient's lung mechanics. A reduction in lung compliance or an increase

TABLE 43-3

Equations Relating the Important Parameters for Volume-Controlled and Pressure-Controlled Ventilation

Mode	Parameter	Symbol	Equation
Volume-controlled	Tidal volume (L)	V_T	$V_T = \dot{V}_E \div f$ $V_T = \bar{\dot{V}}_I \times T_I$
	Mean inspiratory flow (L/min)	$\bar{\dot{V}}_I$	$\bar{\dot{V}}_I = 60 \times V_T \div T_I$ $\bar{\dot{V}}_I = \frac{\dot{V}_E \times TCT}{T_I}$
Pressure-controlled	Tidal volume (L)	V_T	$V_T = \Delta P \times C \times (1 - e^{-t/\tau})$
	Instantaneous inspiratory flow (L/min)	$\dot{V}_I$	$\dot{V}_I = \left(\frac{\Delta P}{R}\right) e^{-t/\tau}$
	Pressure gradient (cm H_2O)	ΔP	$\Delta P = PIP - PEEP$
Both modes	Exhaled minute ventilation (L/min)	$\dot{V}_E$	$\dot{V}_E = V_T \times f$
	Total cycle time or ventilatory period (sec)	TCT	$TCT = T_I + T_E = 60 \div f$
	I : E ratio	I : E	$I{:}E = T_I{:}T_E = \frac{T_I}{T_E}$
	Time constant (sec)	τ	$\tau = R \times C$
	Resistance (cm H_2O/L/sec)	R	$R = \frac{\Delta P}{\Delta \dot{V}}$
	Compliance (L/cm H_2O)	C	$C = \frac{\Delta V}{\Delta P}$
	Elastance	E	$E = \frac{1}{C}$
	Mean airway pressure (cm H_2O)	$\bar{P}_{aw}$	$\bar{P}_{aw} = \left(\frac{1}{TCT}\right) \int_{t=0}^{t=TCT} P_{aw} dt$
Primary variables	Pressure (cm H_2O)	P	
	Volume (L)	V	
	Flow (cm H_2O/L/sec)	$\dot{V}$	
	Time (sec)	τ	
	Inspiratory time (sec)	T_I	
	Expiratory time (sec)	T_E	
	Frequency (breaths/min)	f	
	Base of natural logarithm (≈2.72)	e	

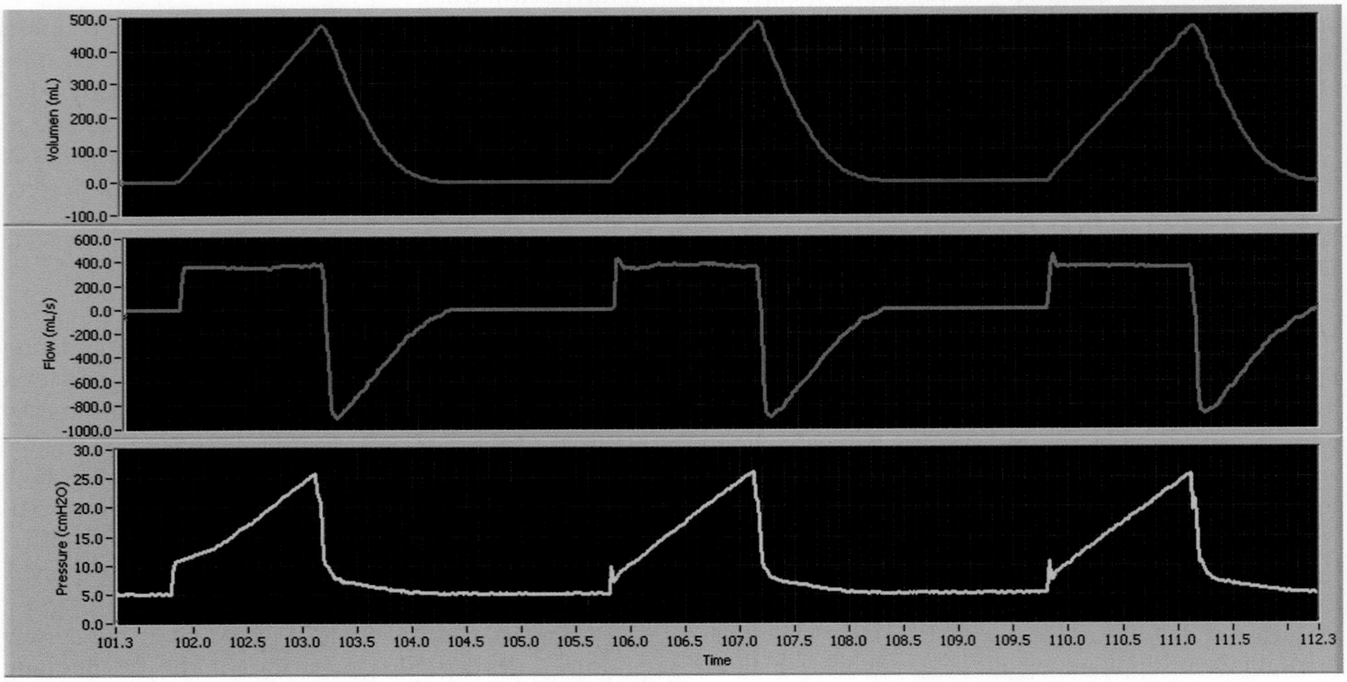

FIGURE 43-9 VC-CMV. *Top,* V_T; *middle,* flow; *bottom,* airway pressure waveform.

in resistance causes higher peak airway pressures. Care should also be taken when setting the inspiratory flow. Avoid setting a flow that fails to match patient needs or exceeds their demand. An insufficient flow rate would result in an imposed increase in the patient's WOB and a concomitant increase in O_2 consumption. The inspiratory phase may be prematurely shortened if the set inspiratory flow exceeds patient demands. Meticulous patient monitoring and use of VC-CMV allow the clinician to achieve precise and predictable physiologic results.

Example. Perhaps the most common application of VC-CMV is its use to ventilate patients in the immediate postoperative period. Patients are often sedated to minimize their response to noxious stimuli and ventilator asynchrony. VC-CMV can achieve fairly precise regulation of gas exchange.

Pressure-Controlled Continuous Mandatory Ventilation

Similar to VC-CMV, pressure-controlled continuous mandatory ventilation (CMV) can be used as a basic mode of ventilatory support. The primary difference between volume-controlled and pressure-controlled ventilation is the control variable with which the clinician is most concerned.[27,28] Theoretically, pressure control (with a constant inspiratory pressure) (Figure 43-10) results in a more even distribution of ventilation (compared with volume control) among lung units with different time constants when units have equal compliances but unequal resistances (e.g., status asthmaticus).[26] The instability of V_T caused by airway leaks can be minimized by using pressure-controlled rather than volume-controlled ventilation. Increased V_T stability may lead to better gas exchange and lower risk of pulmonary volutrauma.[29]

Use of a rectangular pressure waveform opens alveoli earlier in the inspiratory phase during PC-CMV and results in a higher mean airway pressure than VC-CMV with a rectangular flow waveform, allowing more time for oxygenation to occur.[30] In PC-CMV, however, inspiratory flow is not a parameter set by the clinician. It is variable and dependent on patient effort and lung mechanics, improving patient comfort and patient-ventilator synchrony. However, as lung mechanics or patient effort or both change, volume delivery (V_T and minute ventilation) changes, leading to poor control of blood gases.

Because V_T is not directly controlled, the pressure gradient (PIP – PEEP) is the primary parameter used to alter the breath size and CO_2 tensions. Typically, PIP is adjusted to provide the patient with a V_T within the desired range. PIPs may be adjusted to achieve target V_T.[31] As with VC-CMV, the mandatory breath rate set by the clinician depends on the presence of ventilatory muscle activity and the severity of lung disease. When higher mandatory breath rates are needed (>30 breaths/min), it is essential for the clinician to provide a sufficient expiratory time and prevent air trapping.

As long as lung mechanics and patient effort remain constant, the volume and peak flow delivered to the patient remain unchanged.[32] When a decrease in patient effort, decrease in compliance, or increase in resistance occurs, less volume is delivered for the preset pressure for each breath. Conversely, improvements in patient effort and

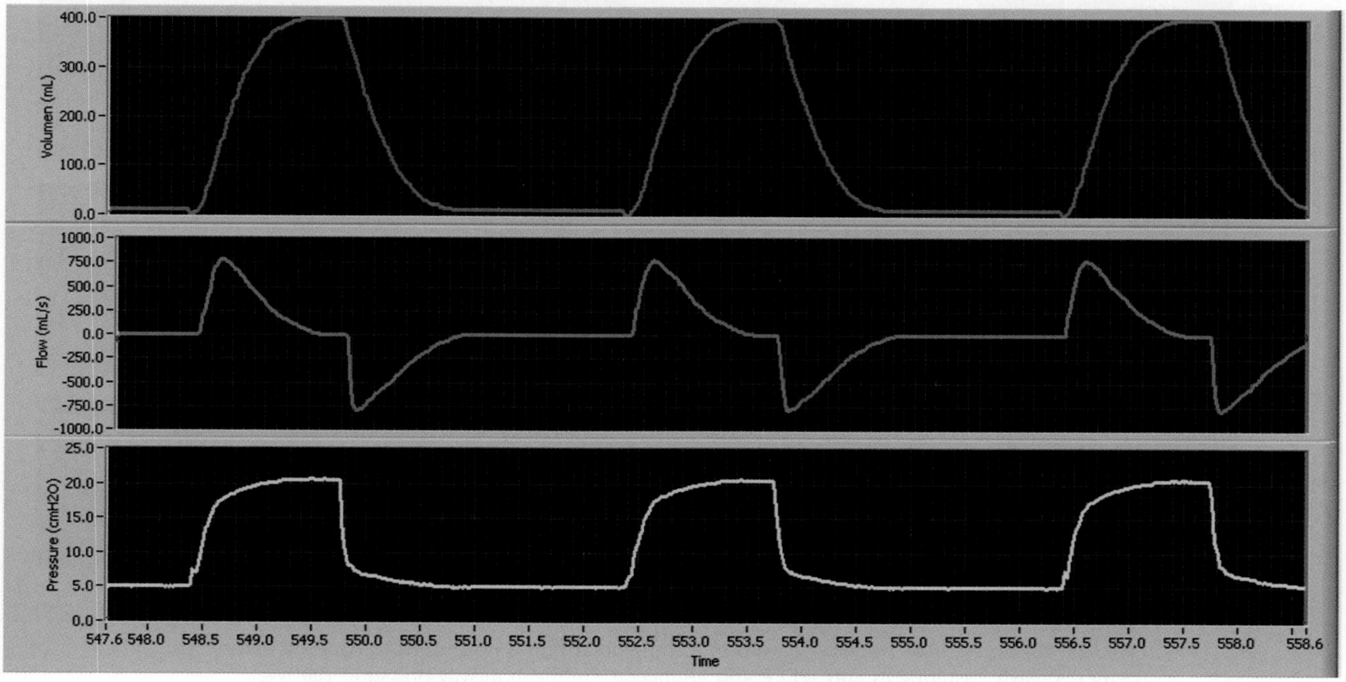

FIGURE 43-10 PC-CMV. *Top,* V_T; *middle,* flow; *bottom,* airway pressure waveform.

mechanics can dramatically increase the volume delivery to the patient in this mode. Close V_T monitoring is required to avoid ventilator-induced hyperventilation or hypoventilation.

Example. Perhaps the most common use of PC-CMV has been in patients with ARDS whose oxygenation status has failed to improve with the application of VC-CMV. Pressure-controlled ventilation is often touted as being superior to volume-controlled ventilation because it results in lower peak airway pressure, but this concept is often misunderstood. Peak airway pressure during volume control is higher because of the resistive pressure decrease across the endotracheal tube and upper airways (i.e., flow × resistance in the equation of motion). However, transalveolar pressure (alveolar pressure – pleural pressure), not airway pressure displayed by the ventilator (i.e., transrespiratory system pressure), leads to lung damage. If a patient has severely decreased chest wall compliance or a partially blocked endotracheal tube, the peak transrespiratory system pressures may be very high, but the transalveolar pressures might be normal. If V_T is the same for pressure-controlled and volume-controlled ventilation, both would produce the same peak alveolar pressure and, presumably, the same risk for overdistention. The only time there is a real clinical difference between the use of volume-controlled ventilation and pressure-controlled ventilation is in patients actively triggering ventilatory support. In this setting, pressure-controlled ventilation responds better to patient demand minimizing WOB and patient-ventilator asynchrony.

The patient's cardiac index and O_2 consumption should be closely monitored as well. Higher mean airway pressures may impair cardiac output. In addition, PC-CMV with IRV can lead to the development of auto-PEEP, which can impair venous return, compromise O_2 delivery to the tissues, and result in marked air trapping.[33]

Pressure-Controlled Inverse Ratio Ventilation

PC-CMV may be used to accomplish pressure-controlled inverse ratio ventilation (PC-IRV), by increasing the inspiratory time directly or by increasing the I:E ratio to the desired value. PC-IRV is defined as pressure-controlled ventilation with an I:E ratio greater than 1:1 (Figure 43-11). With PC-IRV, mean airway pressure increases as the I:E ratio increases. Pressure-controlled IRV has been suggested for severe hypoxemia when high FiO_2 and high PEEP have failed to improve oxygenation in ALI/ARDS. Because alveoli affected by ALI/ARDS have short time constants, more time is allotted for inspiration, and less time is allotted for expiration. The result is intrinsic PEEP and the maintenance of numerous alveoli open, improving arterial oxygenation.[26] Although some studies have shown improvement in oxygenation with PC-IRV versus CMV with PEEP, others have shown concurrent decreases in cardiac output.[27,34] Generally, if applied PEEP in normal ratio ventilation is equal to total PEEP (applied and intrinsic PEEP) in PC-IRV, the oxygenation benefits are equivalent without the marked depression in cardiac output.

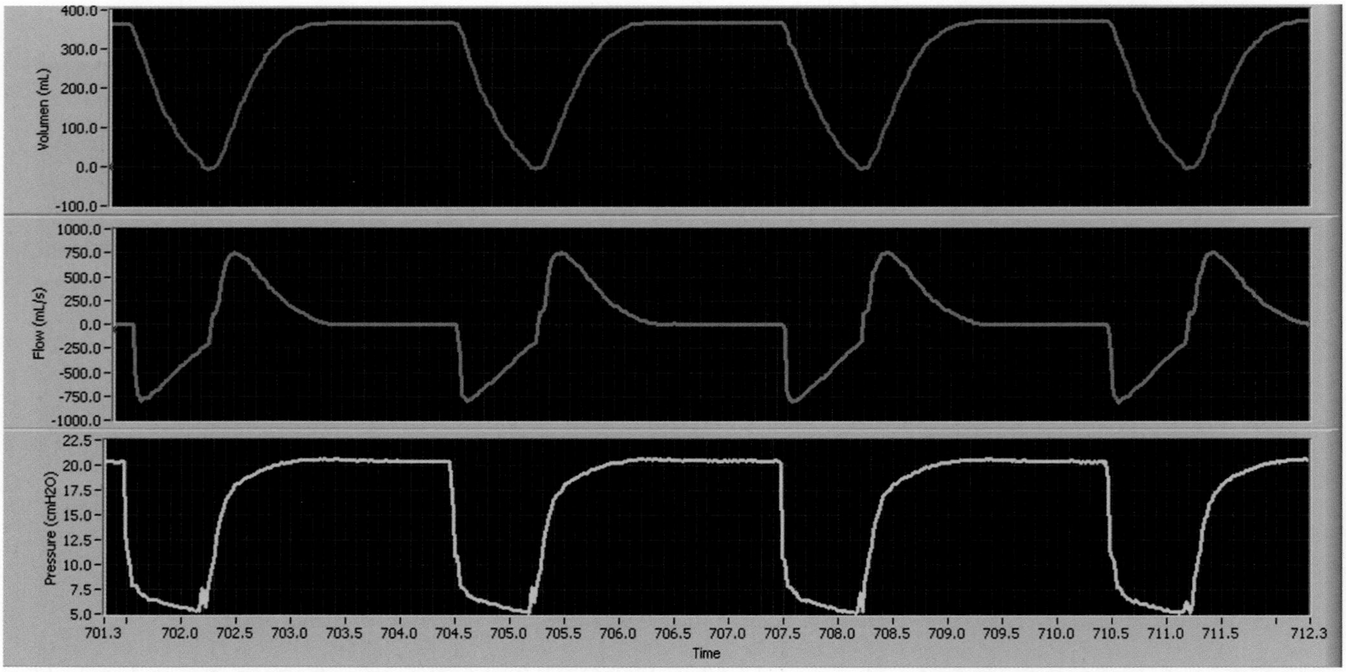

FIGURE 43-11 PC-IRV. The flow waveform for any breath does not return to baseline before the next breath, resulting in auto-PEEP and an increase in mean airway pressure. *Top,* V_T; *middle,* flow; *bottom,* airway pressure waveform.

MINI CLINI

Using Pressure-Controlled Ventilation

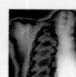

PROBLEM: The RT is caring for a 20-year-old patient with ARDS. The patient has no respiratory effort. Current ventilator settings are as follows:
Mode: VC-CMV
V_T: 400 ml
Frequency: 25 breaths/min
PEEP: 14 cm H_2O
FiO_2: 1
PIPs monitored on the ventilator: 40 to 50 cm H_2O
Mean airway pressure: 22 to 24 cm H_2O
Plateau pressure: 30 cm H_2O

An arterial blood gas is obtained, which reveals pH 7.28, PCO_2 41 mm Hg, and PO_2 50 mm Hg. The physician would like to employ pressure-controlled ventilation. What are the appropriate initial settings in PC-CMV mode to maintain the current minute ventilation?

SOLUTION: Initial ventilator setting would be as follows:
Ventilator frequency, PEEP, and FiO_2: the same
Frequency: 25 breaths/min
PEEP: 14 cm H_2O
FiO_2: 1

To keep the minute ventilation constant, the RT needs to set the PIP high enough to deliver the same V_T as in volume control (400 ml).

1. Calculate the patient's respiratory system compliance:

$$\begin{aligned} \text{Compliance} &= V_T/\text{Plateau pressure} - \text{PEEP} \\ &= 400\ \text{ml}/30\ \text{cm}\ H_2O - 14\ \text{cm}\ H_2O \\ &= 25\ \text{ml/cm}\ H_2O \end{aligned}$$

2. Calculate the pressure limit in PC-CMV mode to achieve the target V_T. Because the pressure limit is measured relative to PEEP on this ventilator, the equation is:

$$\begin{aligned} \text{Ventilating pressure} &= V_T/\text{Compliance} \\ &= 400\ \text{ml}/25\ \text{ml/cm}\ H_2O \\ &= 16\ \text{cm}\ H_2O \end{aligned}$$

$$\text{PIP} = \text{Ventilating pressure (PC setting 16 cm } H_2O) + \text{PEEP (14 cm } H_2O) \text{ or 30 cm } H_2O$$

A shortcut is to realize that the required pressure limit is the plateau pressure on VC-CMV. The PIP (relative to atmospheric pressure) is 30 cm H_2O.

MINI CLINI

Determining Appropriate Ventilator Rate

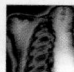

PROBLEM: A 36-year-old woman with TBI was intubated in the emergency department with a 7-mm endotracheal tube and transferred to the RT in the neurointensive care unit. She is paralyzed and sedated. Her current ventilator settings are as follows:
Mode: VC-CMV
V_T: 405 ml
Frequency: 15 breaths/min
FiO_2: 1.0

The pulse oximeter displays 97%, and end-tidal CO_2 monitor is reading 49. The patient's weight is estimated at 45 kg. End-tidal CO_2 is stable and 4 mm Hg higher than $PaCO_2$. The clinical goal is to minimize ICP. Because intracranial blood flow is inversely proportional to $PaCO_2$, ventilation should be increased to maintain $PaCO_2$ at about 35 mm Hg. The RT needs to make appropriate ventilator changes to achieve the target $PaCO_2$.

DISCUSSION: The current V_T is already large at 9 ml/kg. The increase in ventilation must be achieved by increasing frequency. Because the patient is paralyzed, the ventilation level is controlled by the set frequency, and $PaCO_2$ is predictable. The new frequency required is calculated using the following equation:

$$\text{Required frequency} = \text{Current frequency} \times \text{Current } PaCO_2/\text{Desired } PaCO_2$$

$$\begin{aligned} \text{Required frequency} &= 15\ \text{breaths/min} \times 49\ \text{mm Hg}/35\ \text{mm Hg} \\ &= 21\ \text{breaths/min} \end{aligned}$$

Intermittent Mandatory Ventilation

As a partial support mode, IMV allows or requires the patient to sustain some WOB. The level of mechanical support needed depends on the specific physiologic process causing the need for mechanical ventilation, presence or degree of ventilatory muscle weakness, and presence and severity of lung disease. In this mode, mandatory breaths are delivered at a set rate. Between the mandatory breaths, the patient can breathe spontaneously at his or her own V_T and rate (Figure 43-12). Breaths can occur separately (e.g., IMV); breaths can be superimposed on each other (e.g., spontaneous breaths superimposed on mandatory breaths, as in bilevel positive airway pressure [bilevel PAP] or airway pressure release ventilation [APRV]); or mandatory breaths can be superimposed on spontaneous breaths, as in high-frequency ventilation administered during spontaneous breathing. Spontaneous breaths may be assisted (e.g., PSV) (Figure 43-13) or unassisted (e.g., PEEP or CPAP).

When the mandatory breath is patient-triggered, modern-day ventilators deliver the mandatory breath in synchrony with the patient's inspiratory effort. If no spontaneous efforts occur, the ventilator delivers a time-triggered breath. This delivery is generally much more comfortable for the patient, and it is largely attributed to developments in ventilator design. Because spontaneous breaths decrease pleural pressure, ventilatory support with IMV usually results in a lower mean intrathoracic pressure than CMV, which can result in a higher cardiac output.[35]

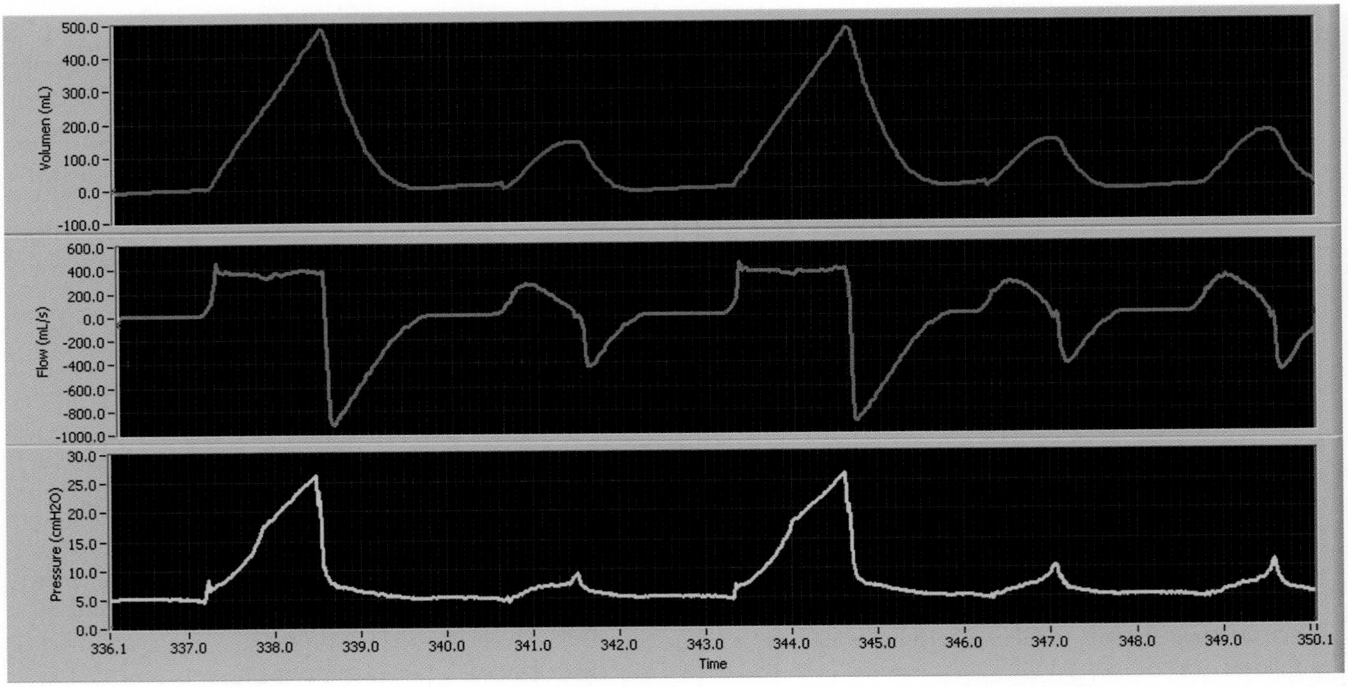

FIGURE 43-12 VC-SIMV + CPAP. *Top,* V_T; *middle,* flow; *bottom,* airway pressure waveform.

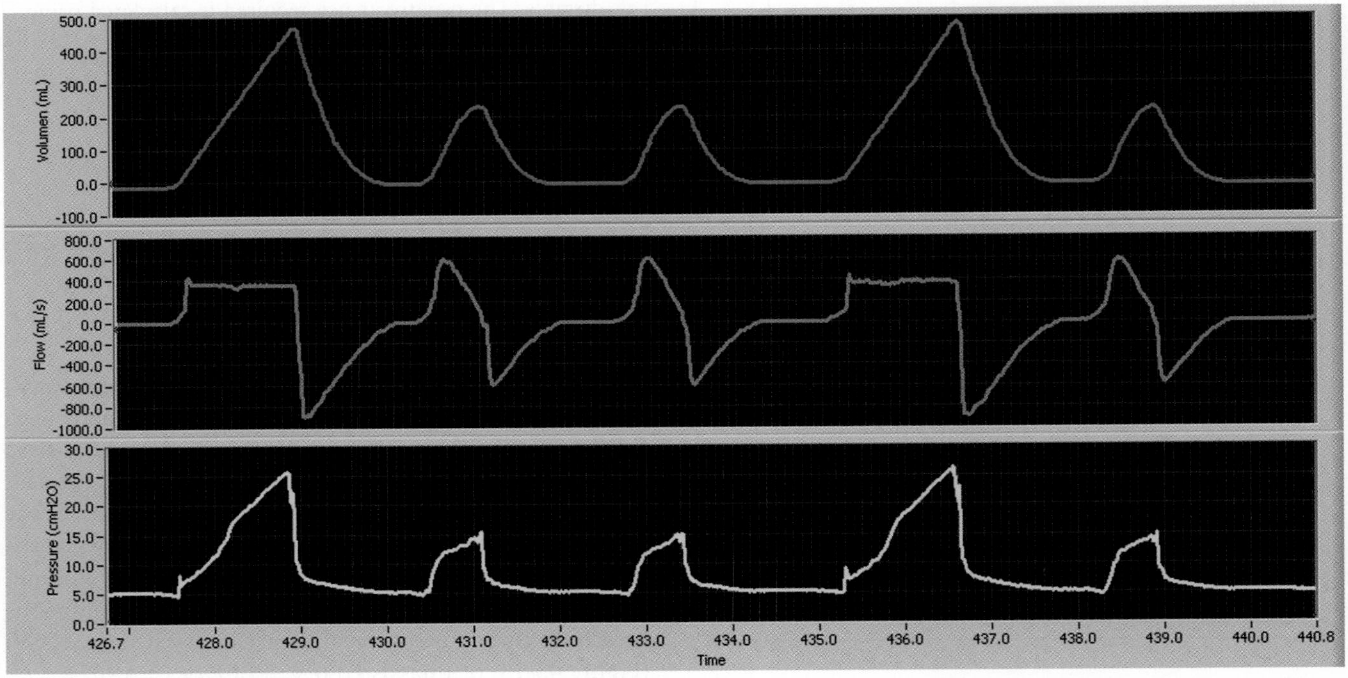

Figure 43-13 VC-SIMV + PSV. The addition of PSV to the spontaneous breaths increases spontaneous V_T. *Top,* V_T; *middle,* flow; *bottom,* airway pressure waveform.

When used to wean a patient from mechanical ventilation, the intent of IMV is to provide respiratory muscle rest during the mandatory breaths and exercise during spontaneous breaths. However, studies have shown that IMV weaning prolongs the duration of mechanical ventilation compared with PSV and spontaneous breathing trials.[36,37]

Volume-Controlled Intermittent Mandatory Ventilation

Volume-controlled intermittent mandatory ventilation (VC-IMV) has been advocated for patients with relatively normal lung function recovering from sedation or rapidly reversing respiratory failure.[38] However, the use of IMV has greatly decreased over the years in favor of VC-CMV, PC-CMV, and PSV.

As the patient is capable of providing more work, the level of ventilatory support can be decreased accordingly. Weaning from VC-IMV usually involves the gradual reduction of the mandatory breath rate, while maintaining a constant V_T. Frequency is decreased rather than V_T because the patient's spontaneous breaths tend to be shallow at first, and relatively large mandatory breaths tend to prevent atelectasis and preserve oxygenation. As the breath rate is reduced, the patient assumes more of the load. When the mandatory breath rate has been reduced enough (typically ≤4 breaths/min), the patient is assessed for either a spontaneous breathing trial or extubation. VC-IMV has been shown to delay weaning and increase the length of ventilatory support.

Example. VC-IMV is usually selected for patients with neuromuscular disorders, such as Guillain-Barré syndrome. Typically, normal lung function and an intact ventilatory drive characterize these patients. As the disease progresses, ascending muscle weakness eventually affects the patient's ventilatory muscles. Mechanical ventilation is considered when it is difficult for the patient to sustain V_T and minute ventilation. The degree of support depends on the patient's inherent muscle strength. Large V_T (8 to 10 ml/kg) and high peak flow (>80 L/min) may be needed to alleviate dyspnea and maximize patient comfort.[39] As respiratory muscle function improves, mandatory breath support can be reduced.

Pressure-Controlled Intermittent Mandatory Ventilation

Pressure-controlled intermittent mandatory ventilation (PC-IMV) is indicated when preservation of the patient's spontaneous efforts is important and patient-ventilatory synchrony is a concern.[40] PC-IMV has been traditionally associated with mechanical ventilation of infants not only because of their oxygenation problems but also because traditionally it had been difficult to control V_T at such small values.[41]

Liberation from this mode involves the gradual reduction of the PIP and the mandatory breath rate. As lung compliance improves, adjustments in PIP are necessary to prevent overdistention of the lung. Adjustments in PIP and set mandatory breath rate are critical to prevent hyperventilation.

Example. Perhaps the most familiar scenario is the application of PC-IMV in premature infants with respiratory distress syndrome. Initially, because of a noncompliant lung, compliant chest wall, and poor respiratory effort, the infant may require a relatively high PIP and high mandatory breath rate to achieve acceptable V_T and acid-base balance. Mandatory breath rates are set to provide adequate minute ventilation.

With PC-IMV, the infant can breathe spontaneously between or during the mandatory breaths, at his or her own rate and V_T. Liberation from this mode of partial support ventilation involves the gradual reduction of the PIP and mandatory breath rate. As the infant's lung compliance improves and spontaneous ventilatory efforts become more effective, lower PIPs and mandatory breath rates are needed to deliver adequate minute ventilation.

Airway Pressure Release Ventilation

A mode related to both PC-IRV and PC-IMV is APRV, in which the patient breathes spontaneously throughout periods of high and low applied CPAP (Figure 43-14).[42] APRV intermittently decreases or "releases" the airway pressure from an upper pressure (P_{high}) or CPAP level to a lower pressure (P_{low}) or CPAP level. The pressure release usually lasts about 0.2 to 1.5 seconds depending on whether or not air trapping is desired. In Figure 43-14, inspiratory time is longer than expiratory time, and spontaneous breaths are superimposed on this mandatory pattern of pressurization and release. Spontaneous breaths are supplemented by PSV. This is a feature of APRV available on some ventilators, where APRV is referred to as *bilevel ventilation.* In APRV, the I : E ratio is usually greater than 1 : 1, which is similar to PC-IRV, but APRV offers the advantage of allowing spontaneous breathing throughout the periods of inspiratory and expiratory positive pressure. Spontaneous breathing offers the benefits of lung recruitment, and improved ventilation of dependent lung zones, resulting in improved $\dot{V}/\dot{Q}$ matching with decreased shunt.[43]

APRV also provides ventilation and oxygenation without adversely affecting hemodynamic values because of the periodic reductions in intrathoracic pressure during the spontaneous breaths. Because patients receiving APRV are breathing spontaneously, less sedation is needed than during PC-IRV. In addition, peak airway pressure during APRV may be less than with VC-IRV for comparable oxygenation and ventilation.[44] In one study, VC-IRV was compared with APRV in patients with ALI. During APRV, peak airway pressure and venous admixture were lower than during VC-IRV, a finding that indicated progressive alveolar recruitment.[45] In a review of APRV in patients with ALI/ARDS by Fan and Stewart,[46] results of studies comparing APRV with conventional volume-controlled or pressure-controlled SIMV showed that with APRV there was a decrease in peak airway pressures, improved hemodynamics, and a decreased need for vasopressor and intropic support. However, the cost of these potential benefits is patient effort, and WOB is markedly increased during APRV. There are no data to indicate a better outcome with APRV than with other approaches to ventilatory support when a similar approach to managing oxygenation is used.

Specific indications for APRV are unclear. This modality was originally proposed as therapy for severe hypoxemia. APRV may be more effective in improving oxygenation than in improving alveolar ventilation.

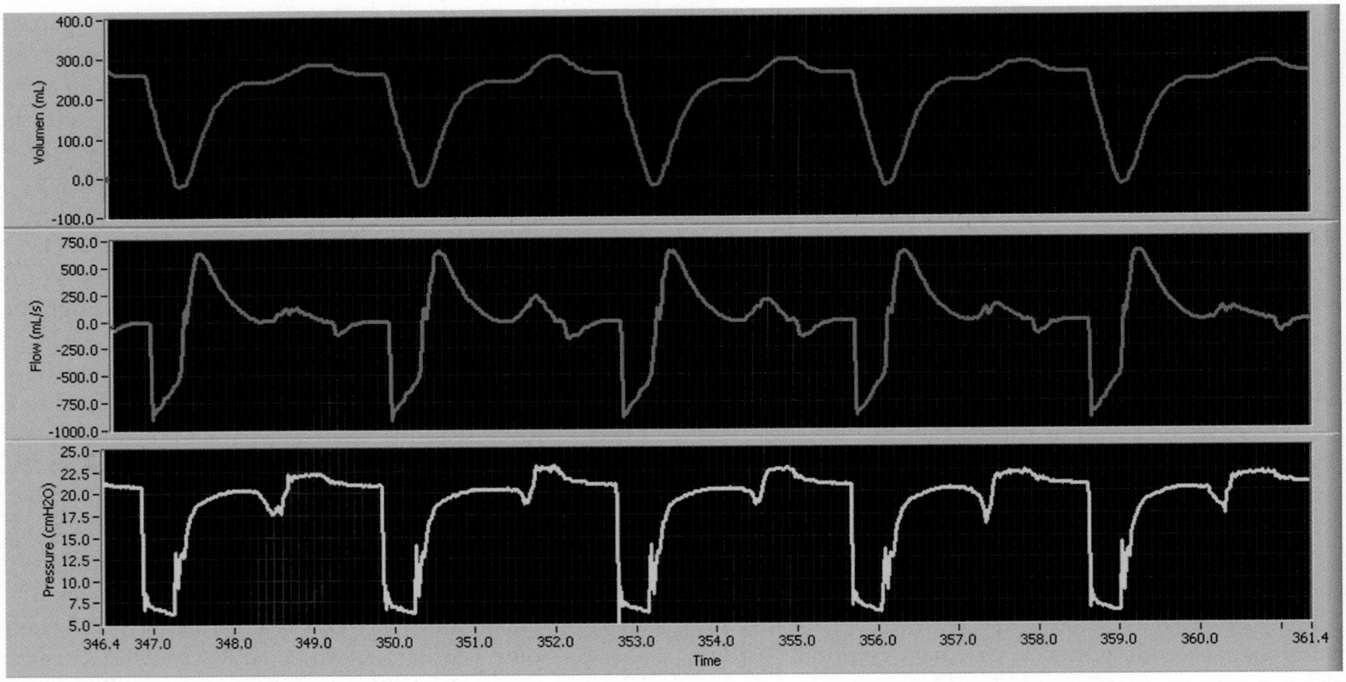

FIGURE 43-14 APRV. In APRV, the patient is able to breathe spontaneously throughout the total cycle time. *Top,* V_T; *middle,* flow; *bottom,* airway pressure waveform.

Continuous Spontaneous Ventilation

Spontaneous breath modes include modes in which all breaths are initiated and ended by the patient. The level of support these modes of ventilation provide determines the amount of WOB the patient ultimately assumes. CPAP, PSV, automatic tube compensation (ATC), proportional assist ventilation (PAV), and neurally assisted ventilatory assist (NAVA) are continuous spontaneous breath modes.

PSV (pressure-controlled continuous spontaneous ventilation [PC-CSV]) is indicated in any spontaneously breathing patient with an intact ventilatory drive, especially if patient-ventilator synchrony is a problem during CMV. As with all spontaneous breathing modes, PSV also improves or stabilizes oxygenation by reducing alveolar derecruitment in intubated patients who do not require full ventilatory support.[46,47]

CPAP provides no ventilatory assist or inspiratory muscle unloading (other than possibly improving lung compliance). Rather, it improves or stabilizes oxygenation by reducing alveolar derecruitment in patients who do not require ventilatory support. CPAP also reduces abnormalities in gas exchange that can be associated with the presence of an artificial airway in patients requiring no assisted mechanical ventilatory support. Low levels of CPAP (3 to 5 cm H_2O) maintain physiologic PEEP and prevent alveolar collapse at end expiration.[47]

PAV and NAVA are very similar modes of ventilation.[48] In both modes, pressure, flow, volume, and time are not set, and each mode augments patient effort by performing a defined proportion of total WOB (PAV) or providing a defined number of cm H_2O pressure assist for each microvolt of diaphragmatic electrical activity (NAVA). The primary differences between the two modes are that NAVA requires the placement of a specially designed nasogastric tube with built-in electromyographic (EMG) electrodes, and NAVA can unload the work associated with air trapping and auto-PEEP, whereas PAV cannot because its measurements are based on airway pressure, flow, and volume.

ATC is similar to PAV except it provides only flow assist based on the characteristics of the artificial airway. ATC is designed to eliminate WOB imposed by the artificial airway. Essentially, ATC attempts to maintain the tracheal pressure at baseline throughout inspiration and expiration or inspiration only.

If CPAP levels are set inappropriately high, alveolar overdistention and air trapping rather than alveolar recruitment result.[49] In addition to deleterious pulmonary effects, circulatory impairment may result from a decrease in left ventricular stroke volume. The reduction in cardiac output and arterial blood pressure also hinders adequate O_2 delivery.[50]

Continuous Positive Airway Pressure

CPAP is spontaneous breathing at an elevated baseline pressure (Figure 43-15). Breaths are patient-triggered and cycled. V_T depends on patient effort and lung mechanics. CPAP increases alveolar pressure and maintains alveoli open. In contrast to NPV and PPV, airway pressure with

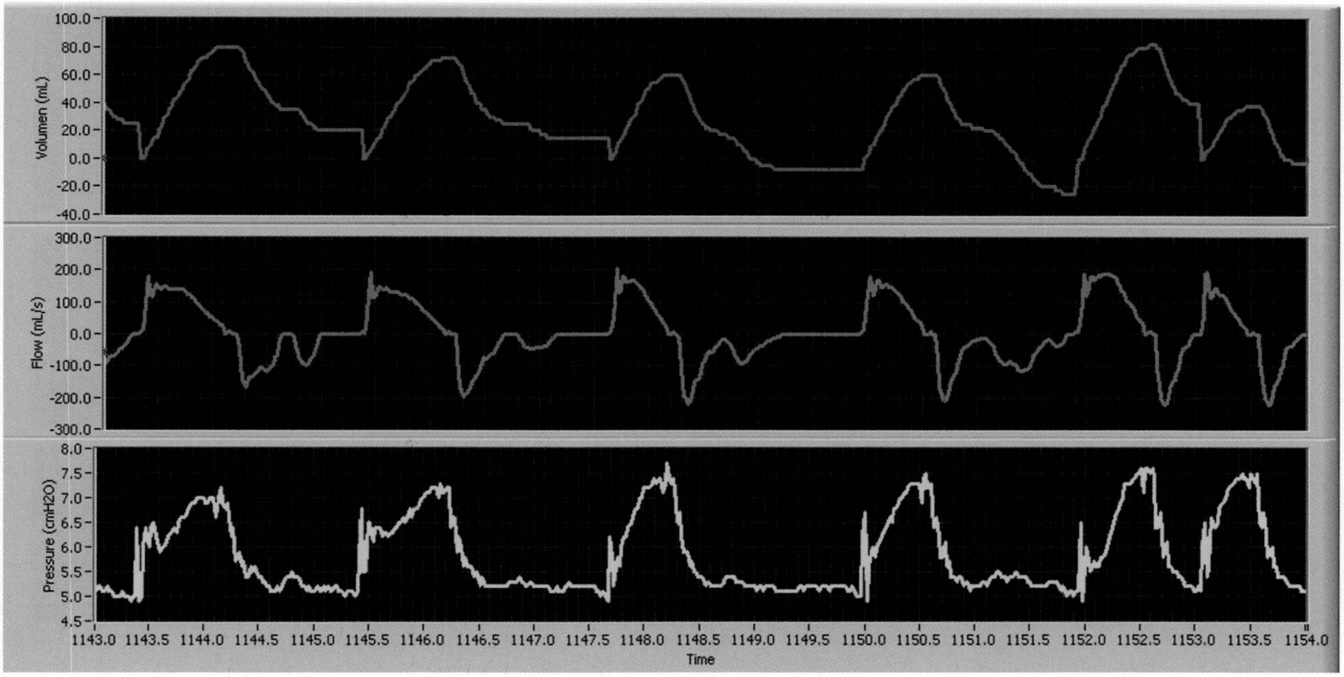

FIGURE 43-15 CPAP. *Top,* V_T scalar; *middle,* flow scalar; *bottom,* airway pressure scalar.

CPAP is theoretically constant (baseline pressure ±2 cm H_2O) throughout the respiratory cycle. Because airway pressure does not change, CPAP does not provide ventilation. For gas to move into the lungs during CPAP, the patient must create a spontaneous transairway pressure gradient. Although NPV and PPV produce the pressure gradients needed for gas flow into the lungs, CPAP maintains alveoli at greater inflation volume, restoring FRC. An important physiologic feature of CPAP is that as alveoli are maintained open, FiO_2 needed to maintain adequate PaO_2 may decrease. Oxygenation becomes more efficient at any given FiO_2, as measured by PaO_2/FiO_2 ratio and shunt fraction. The potential side effects associated with PPV also exist for CPAP but usually to a lesser degree.

Pressure Support Ventilation

PSV is a form of PC-CSV that assists the patient's inspiratory efforts (Figure 43-16). At very low levels of support, this mode unloads WOB the ventilator circuitry imposes on the respiratory muscles.[51] If the level of support is maximized, the ventilator may assume all WOB.[52] The result of high levels of support is a reduction in the respiratory rate, reduction in respiratory muscle activity and fatigue, reduction in O_2 consumption, and improvement or stabilization of spontaneous V_T.[53,54] However, the positive attributes of this mode of ventilation can be negated if ventilator parameters are not properly set. The ventilator must be able to detect spontaneous patient effort. It is critical for the clinician to adjust the trigger sensitivity correctly. Of equal importance is the clinician-set rise time, the time required for the ventilator to reach the inspiratory pressure limit, and termination criteria, the minimal flow resulting in cycling to exhalation. Ventilator graphics are often helpful when adjusting these parameters and optimizing patient-ventilator synchrony.

Regardless of the level of support provided, the patient has primary control over the breath rate and inspiratory time and flow rate delivered during this mode of assisted ventilation. PSV is designed to provide assisted ventilation with pressure as the only control variable. In addition, PSV overcomes airway resistance caused by an endotracheal tube, secretions, bronchospasm, or other imposed mechanical resistance. Regardless of the pressure support level provided, the patient has primary control over the breathing frequency, inspiratory time, and flow. The V_T resulting from a PSV breath depends on the preset pressure level, patient effort, and mechanical forces opposing ventilation (lung-chest wall compliance and airway resistance). Of all of the classic modes of ventilation, PSV exerts the least control over the patient's ventilatory pattern and as a result should improve patient-ventilator synchrony. Since the first description of PSV in 1982, it has been used either to overcome the imposed resistance associated with the artificial airway or to provide ventilatory support with minimal control.[55] PSV is useful in any patient with an intact ventilatory drive and a stable ventilatory demand.

Bilevel PAP (BiPAP; Respironics, Inc, Murrysville, PA) is simply PSV with PEEP applied noninvasively.[56] With bilevel PAP, inspiratory positive airway pressure (or PSV) and expiratory positive airway pressure (PEEP) are set. The duration of inspiratory positive airway pressure and expiratory positive airway pressure can be independently

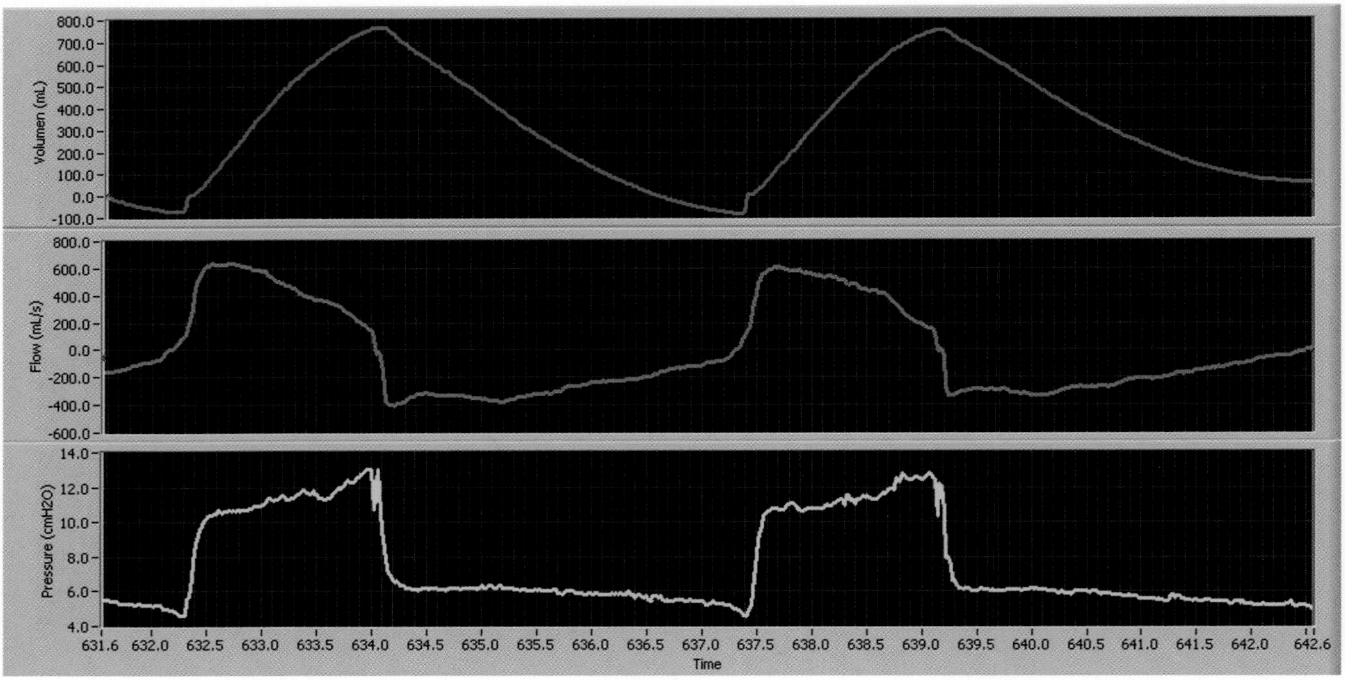

FIGURE 43-16 PSV. *Top,* V_T; *middle,* flow; *bottom,* airway pressure waveform.

adjusted to set the I:E ratio. Although it was originally developed to enhance the capabilities of home CPAP systems used for management of obstructive sleep apnea, bilevel PAP has been successfully used in the home and the hospital for noninvasive ventilatory support of patients with acute and chronic respiratory failure.[57]

Example. An example of the use of PC-CSV is noninvasive PSV and PEEP in the management of a patient with COPD in an acute exacerbation. As described in detail in Chapter 45, PSV has been shown in this setting to decrease the frequency of intubation, length of mechanical ventilation, development of ventilator-associated pneumonia, and patient mortality.

Proportional Assist Ventilation

PAV is based on both the mechanics of the total respiratory system and the resistive properties of the artificial airway; that is, the ventilator delivers a pressure assist in proportion to the patient's desired V_T (volume assist) and to the patient's instantaneous inspired flow (flow assist). The response of these two aspects of ventilatory assistance is automatically adjusted to meet changes in the patient's ongoing ventilatory demand. This algorithm is based on the law of motion as it applies to the respiratory system:

$$P_{musc} + P_{appl} = (\text{Volume} \times E) + (\text{Flow} \times R)$$

where P_{musc} is pressure generated by the respiratory muscles, P_{appl} is pressure applied by the ventilator, and E and R are elastic and resistance properties of the respiratory system. Assuming that E and R are linear during inspiration, the instantaneous flow and volume to be delivered are proportional to the resistive and elastic WOB. The ventilator continuously measures the instantaneous flow and volume and periodically measures the E and R. Using this information, the ventilator software adjusts gas delivery by estimating P_{musc} and assisting P_{musc} in a proportional manner. The patient is the determinant of the ventilatory pattern. Patients are given the freedom to select a ventilatory pattern that is rapid and shallow or slow and deep. If the patient desires a small V_T, a low level of pressure is applied, and if a large V_T is desired, a high pressure is applied. The ventilator does not force any control variable except the unloading of E and R in a proportional manner. See Chapter 42 for details on operation of PAV.

Numerous studies have evaluated the effect of PAV during noninvasive PPV.[58-62] Most of these comparisons were between PAV and PSV,[58,62] and in almost all of these comparisons the patients evaluated had chronic respiratory failure and were in an acute exacerbation. Patients managed with PAV had a lower refusal rate, had a more rapid reduction in respiratory rate, and developed fewer complications.[60,61] In these studies, gas exchange and respiratory pattern did not differ between PSV and PAV, but the patients ventilated with PAV were more comfortable. PAV has also been shown to be essentially equivalent to PSV in stable patients with chronic ventilatory failure[59] and in patients with acute cardiogenic pulmonary edema.[62]

PAV has been most widely studied during invasive mechanical ventilation.[63-65] As with the evaluation of PAV in other settings, most of the comparisons focused on the physiologic response observed when PSV is changed to PAV. Generally, during invasive ventilation, the change from PSV to PAV results in lower V_T, more rapid respiratory rate, lower peak airway pressure, and lower mean airway pressure without significant changes in gas exchange or hemodynamics.[66-68] Ranieri and colleagues[63] and Grasso and associates[64] were unable to identify a difference in patients' work and effort between PSV and PAV as ventilatory load was increased. The best long-term evaluation of PAV versus PSV randomly assigned the application of each for a 48-hour period in a series of critically ill patients.[65] The percentage of patients' failing the transition to PAV or PSV differed (P = .04): 11% failing PAV versus 22% failing PSV. In addition, the proportion of patients developing asynchrony was greater with PSV versus PAV (29% vs. 5.6%, P < .001). The primary reason for the asynchrony was missed triggers. This difference was a result of PSV forcing a larger V_T causing air trapping and preventing normal triggering. Trigger synchrony is generally better in PAV because a large V_T is not forced on the patient. The current data on PAV indicates it can sustain the same patients as PSV—patients who can breathe spontaneously and manage their ventilator drive normally.

Neurally Adjusted Ventilatory Assist

From a conceptual perspective, NAVA is essentially the same as PAV except that PAV responds to changes in airway pressure and flow, whereas NAVA responds to changes in diaphragmatic EMG activity. However, for NAVA to function properly, a specially designed nasogastric catheter with a 10-cm length of EMG electrodes must be in place. Both PAV and NAVA respond to patient effort providing ventilatory support in a proportional manner. The clinician does not set pressure, volume, flow, or time in either mode. The only parameter set is the proportion of effort unloaded by the ventilator; in NAVA, this is set as the number of cm H_2O applied per microvolt of diaphragmatic EMG activity.

Colombo and coworkers[69] matched the setting during NAVA and PSV by adjusting both to produce a V_T of 6 to 8 ml/kg. These investigators compared the two modes at these settings and setting 50% higher and 50% lower. At the initial and lowest setting, they found no differences in gas exchange, ventilatory pattern, ventilatory assistance, or respiratory drive between the modes. At the highest setting, V_T significantly increased, and ventilator response rate and peak diaphragmatic EMG activity significantly decreased during PSV resulting in air trapping and cycling asynchrony. The asynchrony index was greater than 10% in five of the six patients studied during PSV and 0.0% in all patients during NAVA even at the highest settings. Sgahija and coworkers[70] reported similar finding in a series of 12 patients with an acute exacerbation of COPD. The asynchrony index was 23% ± 12% of breaths during PSV but only 7% ± 2% during NAVA (P < .05). The authors cited air trapping as the cause of the cycling asynchrony during PSV.

The effect of PEEP titration during NAVA was reported by Passath and colleagues[71] in a series of 20 patients (only 1 with ARDS). These investigators titrated PEEP level up and down evaluating its effect on respiratory drive. They found that at adequate NAVA levels increasing PEEP reduced ventilatory drive and that monitoring V_T divided by diaphragmatic EMG activity during PEEP changes identified the PEEP level at which tidal breathing occurred at a minimal EMG activity cost.

NAVA application in neonates results in similar outcomes as observed in adults.[72,73] After the change to NAVA, V_T tends to decrease, respiratory rate to increase, and peak diaphragmatic EMG activity to decrease. In addition, despite the open ventilating system (uncuffed artificial airway), triggering and cycling were still primarily neurally activated. Beck and associates[72] reported no significant difference between triggering and cycling delays during invasive and noninvasive application of NAVA in 936-g, 26-week neonates. In a series of 21 mechanically ventilated children 2 days to 15 years old, Bengtsson and Edberg[73] noted that neural triggering occurred 68% of the time, and neural cycling occurred 88% of the time.

The most important advantage of PAV and NAVA over traditional modes of ventilation is improved synchrony. The specific indications for PAV and NAVA are not fully established; however, both can be reasonably used in any patient with an intact ventilatory drive. The primary indication would be a patient with a significant level of asynchrony.

Automatic Tube Compensation

ATC is similar to the flow assist aspect of PAV but considers only the resistance of the endotracheal tube.[74] ATC is an adjunct that automatically adjusts the airway pressure to compensate for endotracheal tube resistance to gas flow by maintaining tracheal pressure constant at the baseline level.[74] The goal is to eliminate WOB imposed by the endotracheal tube. In ATC, the RT inputs into the ventilator the type and size of artificial airway (endotracheal tube or tracheostomy tube) and the percent compensation desired (10% to 100%). The ventilator continuously measures flow and calculates the amount of pressure needed to overcome the resistance of the airway (pressure = resistance × flow). As a result, the greater the inspiratory demand, the greater the pressure applied. Pressure varies throughout the breath.

ATC may be applied during inspiration (positive airway pressure) or during both inspiration and expiration (negative airway pressure). However, expiratory ATC may result in early airway closure and increased air trapping. ATC has been referred to as *electronic extubation,* meaning that if the airway pressure is low during inspiration (5 to 7 cm H_2O), it is simply overcoming the resistance of the endotracheal tube with a normal inspiratory effort.[75] Consequently, many clinicians consider this an indication that spontaneous ventilation can be maintained without ventilatory support and the patient should be considered for extubation. Although in theory the use of ATC to wean patients appears ideal, no data to date have indicated that ATC weans patients faster than T-piece trials.

Adaptive Modes and Dual Control

The first adaptive control/dual control mode was described by Amato and colleagues.[76] Their major finding was that the ventilatory workload imposed on the inspiratory muscles during volume-assured PSV was significantly reduced by the use of dual control. In this mode, pressure support is combined with volume control. However, this benefit was due to the fact that inspiration started out in pressure support and stayed there unless the V_T target was not met. The improvement was mostly a result of the improved synchrony between the patient and the machine. These investigators did not show a specific benefit of the actual dual nature of the mode (i.e., switching from pressure support to volume control), and no evidence has been published in the literature since then supporting this mode. Anecdotal reports indicate that it is difficult to adjust pressure, volume, and flow settings to make the mode work properly, in particular, if the mechanical properties of the patient's respiratory system are changing rapidly.

Pressure-regulated volume control (PRVC), or PC-CMV, and *volume support (VS)*, or PC-CSV, are examples of adaptive control/dual control modes. PRVC is based on pressure-controlled ventilation, and VS is based on PSV. In both modes, the ventilator attempts to maintain a target V_T by adjusting the pressure level based on the previous breath. When a clinician places a patient in PRVC, a target V_T, breath rate, and maximum (i.e., alarm) pressure limit are clinician set, whereas for a patient placed in VS, a target V_T and maximum (i.e., alarm) pressure limit are clinician set. In both modes, once the patient is connected to the ventilator, the patient-ventilator interaction that occurs in the first few breaths is critical. Initially, the ventilator calculates total system compliance. On the succeeding three or four breaths, the ventilator monitors the peak airway pressures and expiratory V_T. The ventilator determines the pressure level necessary to deliver the clinician-set "target" V_T, for the given total system compliance. ("Target" is used because the ventilator aims to deliver it, over the course of several breaths, but may not hit the mark if the maximum pressure limit is set too low.)

The patient-ventilator interaction is monitored on a breath-by-breath basis. If the patient's lung compliance improves (or patient effort increases), the ventilator delivers subsequent mandatory breaths at a lower pressure level to maintain the target V_T. This adjustment by the ventilator reduces the risk of alveolar overdistention and volutrauma. Conversely, the ventilator responds to worsening pulmonary compliance (or decreasing patient effort) by increasing the pressure limit until the V_T is achieved. The ventilator makes pressure level changes in small increments, 1 to 3 cm H_2O per breath, and does not exceed the maximum pressure limit set by the clinician. These automatic ventilator responses to changes in a patient's lung mechanics minimize the risk of ventilator-induced hyperventilation or hypoventilation. The desired outcome is a stable or consistent minute ventilation and enhanced patient comfort. However, the major problem with these modes is that the ventilator cannot distinguish between the patient improving and heightened levels of ventilator demand. If patient demand results in a larger V_T, the ventilator ventilates less.[77]

In most ventilators, pressure can be decreased all the way to the PEEP level. This situation can lead to ventilatory failure.[75] Both RPVC and VS should be used very cautiously in all patients with a normal or increased ventilatory demand. Randomized comparison between these modes and other, more traditional, modes failed to show any outcome benefit.[78,79]

Example. PRVC or VS has been used in infants with respiratory distress syndrome.[80] Rapidly changing pulmonary mechanics from surfactant administration are associated with complications such as pulmonary air leaks, intraventricular hemorrhage, and bronchopulmonary dysplasia. These adaptive modes respond to changes in a patient's lung mechanics and may reduce the incidence of these common complications.

Adaptive support ventilation (ASV), or PC-IMV, is an example of optimal control in adaptive ventilation. Adaptive support ventilation is a pressure-targeted mode that optimizes the relationship between V_T and respiratory frequency based on lung mechanics as predicted by Otis.[81] ASV uses a pressure ventilation format establishing a ventilatory pattern that minimizes WOB and auto-PEEP, while limiting peak airway pressure. In this regard, ASV is similar to PC-CMV and PRVC in its gas delivery format. It differs from PC-CMV and PRVC by its additional algorithmic control of the ventilatory pattern.[82] ASV automatically determines the V_T and respiratory rate that best maintains the peak pressure below the target level.[83] The clinician inputs the patient's ideal body weight, high pressure limit, PEEP, FiO_2, inspiratory rise time, flow cycle percentage, and percentage of predicted minute volume desired. The ventilator periodically measures dynamic compliance and the respiratory time constant and determines the desired mandatory rate. Ideal body weight is used by the ventilator to calculate the minute volume, which is divided by the rate for determination of V_T.[84]

Tassaux and associates[85] compared VC-IMV with ASV in patients with respiratory failure of various causes. They concluded that ASV decreased inspiratory load and improved patient-ventilator synchrony. Sulzer and coworkers[86] showed that ASV resulted in a shorter duration of intubation than VC-IMV in postoperative cardiac patients with no complications. More recently, Belliato and colleagues[87] compared PC-IMV (optimal) in ventilated patients with acute respiratory failure, ventilated patients with chronic respiratory failure, and ventilated patients with normal lungs and in a physical lung model. Their results showed that the ventilator was able to differentiate between these types of patients and select appropriate settings. Using a lung model, Sulemanji and coworkers[89] determined that ASV could provide better lung protection than a fixed V_T of 6 ml/kg ideal body weight. ASV control has been adapted to respond to end-tidal CO_2 levels.[89] This new adaptation allows specific algorithms to be selected based on patient diagnosis: ARDS, COPD, brain injury, or healthy lung. This mode is the most sophisticated of the closed loop control modes available on ICU ventilators at the present time. However, additional study is needed to determine fully the type of patient in whom ASV is most useful. Current data would indicate ASV works very well in patients under controlled approaches to ventilatory support, but additional data in spontaneously ventilated patients are needed before it can be recommended in these patients.

RULE OF THUMB

Most patients requiring ventilatory support can be effectively ventilated with volume assist/control, pressure assist/control, and PSV modes.

Patient Positioning to Optimize Oxygenation and Ventilation

Patients receiving mechanical ventilation are turned frequently, usually at least every 2 hours, unless turning is contraindicated. Kinetic beds continually rotate patients and are designed to help prevent atelectasis, hypoxemia, secretion retention, and pressure sores. When patients are kept immobile, pooling of secretions in dependent lung zones can promote nosocomial pneumonia, and shrinking of dependent alveoli leads to decreases in ventilation and hypoxemia. However, the use of rotating kinetic beds is controversial in the prevention of nosocomial pneumonia.[90] No data are available to indicate that these very expensive beds improve patient outcome.

Patients with unilateral lung disease benefit from being placed in positions that promote matching of ventilation and perfusion. In unilateral lung disease, only one lung is affected by atelectasis, consolidation, or pneumonia. If the affected lung is placed in the dependent position, blood flow follows. The resultant poor $\dot{V}/\dot{Q}$ ratio in the affected lung contributes to venous admixture and hypoxemia. However, if the patient is rotated so that the good lung is in the dependent position, these relationships are reversed. With the good lung down, blood flows to well-ventilated alveoli, and $\dot{V}/\dot{Q}$ matching and arterial blood gas values improve. An added benefit of this maneuver is that the affected lung is placed in a postural drainage position, which promotes gravity drainage of retained secretions so that they can be removed.

A similar phenomenon has been described in ARDS. In a supine patient with ARDS, alveoli in the bases and posterior segments become atelectatic. Shunt increases, and the patient requires a high FiO_2 and PEEP for adequate oxygenation. If the patient is rotated into the prone position, several mechanisms have been proposed to improve oxygenation.[91] Blood flow is redistributed to areas that are better ventilated. This redistribution improves $\dot{V}/\dot{Q}$ relationships. Prone positioning removes the weight of the heart from its position over the lungs while the patient is supine. Pleural pressure in the now nondependent collapsed lung becomes more negative, improving alveolar recruitment. In addition, the stomach no longer lies over the dependent basilar posterior segments of the lower lobes.

In a review of 20 randomized clinical studies comprising 297 patients referred to as a "meta-analysis," Curley[92] found that oxygenation improved within 2 hours in 69% of cases, and improvements were cumulative and persistent. However, factors predictive of patients' responses were inconsistent, and patients' initial responses were not predictive of long-term response. An improvement in PaO_2 of 10 mm Hg within 30 minutes seemed to differentiate responders from nonresponders. However, patient positioning is not without complications. Several persons are needed to "flip" the patient while ensuring monitoring lines and catheters are not disrupted and the patient is not inadvertently extubated. Wound dehiscence, facial or upper chest wall necrosis despite extensive padding, cardiac arrest immediately after movement to the prone position, dependent edema of the face, and corneal abrasion have been reported.[93] A meta-analysis of existing randomized controlled trials indicated no outcome benefit from prone positioning in patients with ARDS.[94] However, this meta-analysis also found that patients with PaO_2/FiO_2 less than 100 mm Hg were the group most likely to benefit from prone positioning. Considering the complications associated with prone positioning, only patients with very severe hypoxemia (PaO_2/FiO_2 < 100 mm Hg) should be placed prone.

RULE OF THUMB

Patients who have unilateral or dependent consolidation or atelectasis and severe hypoxemia may benefit from positioning with the affected lung or segments in the nondependent position to promote improvement in $\dot{V}/\dot{Q}$ relationships. Prone positioning is indicated only if the PaO_2/FiO_2 is less than 100 mm Hg. When positioning the patient, great care should be taken to avoid the hazards associated with prone positioning.

CARDIOVASCULAR EFFECTS OF POSITIVE PRESSURE MECHANICAL VENTILATION

Thoracic Pump and Venous Return During Spontaneous and Mechanical Ventilation

The lungs and heart have a close functional relationship, and impaired performance of one affects the other. For this reason, the RT must fully understand what happens to cardiovascular function when a patient receives ventilatory support.

Early studies of the effect of PPV on the cardiovascular system showed an early, small, and transient increase in cardiac output that was followed almost immediately by a marked reduction in left ventricular outflow. Generally, the reduced cardiac output in these cases was directly related to the amount of pressure applied. More specifically, the decrease in left ventricular output corresponded to the increase in pleural pressure that occurred with PPV. Figure 43-17 compares the effects of spontaneous inspiration with the effect observed during PPV. Negative pleural pressure during spontaneous inspiration normally enhances venous return, increases right atrial filling, and improves pulmonary blood flow (see Figure 43-17, *A*). In combination, these factors increase left atrial and left ventricular filling and left ventricular stroke volume.

However, during PPV, pleural pressure can become positive (see Figure 43-17, *B*). Positive pleural pressure compresses the intrathoracic veins and increases central venous and right atrial filling pressures. As these pressures increase, venous return to the heart is impeded, and right ventricular preload and stroke volume decrease, as does pulmonary blood flow. Blood already in the pulmonary circulation is initially displaced into the left side of the heart and causes a transient increase in filling pressure and output. This initial effect lasts for only a few heartbeats. If positive pressure is continued, flow both to and from the left side of the heart decreases.

The high impedance encountered by blood returning to the right heart causes venous pooling, mainly in the capacitance vessels of abdominal viscera. This process effectively removes a large volume of blood from the circulation, which can further impair left ventricular output. These interactions are magnified when pleural pressure is increased further or circulating blood volume is low.[95] The venous impedance caused by PPV is not limited to blood flow coming from the abdomen. An increase in central venous pressure can restrict return flow from the brain. Impedance to venous return from the brain can increase ICP and reduce cerebral perfusion pressure (CPP). In combination with a decrease in left ventricular output, an increase in ICP during PPV can significantly impair cerebral perfusion and possibly result in cerebral ischemia and cerebral hypoxia.

In healthy individuals, the effects of PPV on cerebral blood flow (CBF) are minimized by autoregulatory mechanisms that maintain cranial perfusion pressures within a narrow range. However, patients with preexisting cerebrovascular problems and patients who already have an

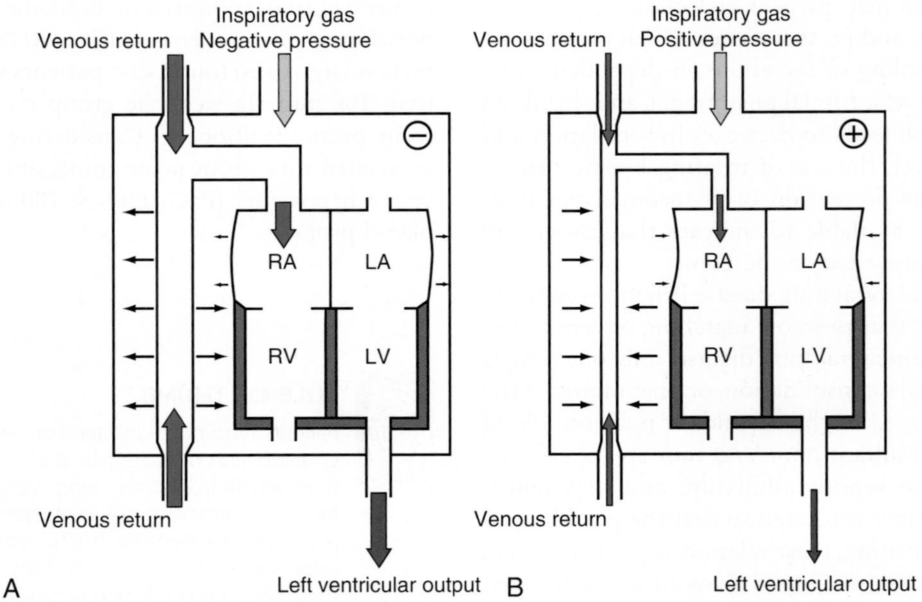

FIGURE 43-17 Relationship between pleural pressure and cardiac output in spontaneous **(A)** and positive pressure **(B)** breathing. *LA,* Left atrium; *LV,* left ventricle; *RA,* right atrium; *RV,* right ventricle.

elevation in ICP may be at risk of decreased cerebral perfusion with PPV. Examples include neurosurgical patients and patients with head injuries, intracranial tumors, or cerebral edema from any cause. ICP monitoring may be necessary in the care of these patients.

Compensation in Healthy Persons

A decrease in cardiac output or blood pressure is rare among individuals with a normal cardiopulmonary system who are receiving mechanical ventilation. Compensatory mechanisms used to counter the decrease in stroke volume include increased heart rate, increase in systemic vascular and peripheral venous resistance, and shunting of blood away from the kidneys and lower extremities, which results in a consistent blood pressure. Because these compensatory mechanisms function by reflexes, the reflexes must be intact. Factors that block or blunt these vascular reflexes include sympathetic blockade, spinal anesthesia, spinal cord transection, and polyneuritis.

Pulmonary Vascular Pressure, Blood Flow, and Pulmonary Vascular Resistance

In patients with a normal cardiopulmonary system who are receiving mechanical ventilation, there is no significant increase in pulmonary vascular pressure or pulmonary vascular resistance and no decrease in pulmonary blood flow. However, when alveoli are distended by increased V_T or high PEEP, pulmonary blood flow is impeded because the alveoli press against the pulmonary capillaries. The pressure increases right ventricular afterload and volume and decreases right ventricular output. The ventricular septum may be shifted to the left, but this effect is more consistent with a high PEEP. This condition decreases left ventricular filling and output. The magnitude of these changes is proportional to lung compliance. As lung compliance decreases, the stiffer lungs can retain the increased pressure imposed by PEEP. In other words, the increased pressure in the lung is not transmitted to the vasculature to impede right ventricular output. An increase in intrapleural pressure secondary to an increase in lung pressure impedes venous return and decreases cardiac output further.

Right and Left Ventricular Function

Under conditions of a normal cardiovascular system with normal ventilation values, there are no significant changes in right or left ventricular function. Otherwise, mechanical ventilation would be difficult to manage, and the mortality and morbidity among patients receiving ventilation would be much higher. Right or left ventricular dysfunction appears to occur if the patient is hypovolemic, is receiving an excessive V_T, or is receiving more than optimum PEEP. The common factor is excessive alveolar pressure, enough to overcome or impede pulmonary blood flow or venous return.

Effect With Left Ventricular Dysfunction

PPV can improve cardiac output in some patients. In patients with left ventricular failure, application of PPV can increase both the left ventricular ejection fraction and the cardiac output. These improvements occur because PPV decreases left ventricular afterload in these patients. Afterload is an important factor in determining cardiac output, as is the resistance of the systemic vasculature. When afterload increases, cardiac output decreases (heart failure). When afterload is decreased by PPV or pharmacologic therapy, cardiac output may increase. This phenomenon explains why the cardiovascular status of some patients deteriorates when PPV is discontinued or treatment is changed from full to partial ventilatory support.

Endocardial Blood Flow

Blood flow in the coronary arteries depends on the gradient between the systemic diastolic pressure and the left ventricular end-diastolic pressure (represented by the pulmonary capillary wedge pressure). Any factor that decreases systemic diastolic pressure or increases wedge pressure decreases endocardial perfusion pressure. The factors of PPV that may decrease the systemic diastolic pressure are high mean airway pressure owing to a high PEEP, high V_T, or long inspiratory time. Factors that may increase the wedge pressure include excessive PEEP and left ventricular failure.

Cardiac Output, Cardiac Index, and Systemic Blood Pressure

When the cardiovascular system is normal with normal ventilation values, there are no significant changes in cardiac output, cardiac index, or systemic blood pressure. Cardiac output can be affected by a decrease in stroke volume with PPV, but this decrease is compensated by an increase in heart rate. Because the cardiac index is the quotient of cardiac output and body surface area (cardiac index = cardiac output in liters per minute/body surface area in square meters), a change in cardiac output would be reflected in the cardiac index. Systemic arterial pressure remains stable because of reflex compensation, which increases systemic vascular resistance. Cardiac output, cardiac index, and arterial pressure decrease only when mean airway pressure is high and intrapleural pressure increases precipitously. Hypotension owing to PPV alone is rare because clinicians do all that is necessary to prevent it, including adequate fluid administration, proper management of mean airway pressure and PEEP, and use of vasoconstricting drugs. Most cases of hypotension during mechanical ventilation are caused by sepsis and the accompanying vascular collapse.

RULE OF THUMB

Patient most likely to experience hemodynamic effects of mechanical ventilation are patients with a normal or increased lung compliance associated with decreased chest wall compliance. In this setting, there is little lung stretch but maximum transmission of ventilating pressure to the intrathoracic space.

MINIMIZING CARDIOVASCULAR EFFECTS OF POSITIVE PRESSURE MECHANICAL VENTILATION

The effect of PPV on the circulatory system depends primarily on two major factors: mean pleural pressure and cardiovascular status.

Mean Pleural Pressure

Pleural pressure is the pressure in the virtual pleural space. At the bedside, pleural pressure usually is measured indirectly as the esophageal pressure through an esophageal balloon connected to a pressure transducer. Because the esophagus is close to the pleurae, separated by only the flexible esophageal wall, change in esophageal pressure reflects change in pleural pressure but does not equal actual pleural pressure. An alternative to measuring pleural pressure is measuring mean airway pressure. Mean airway pressure is linearly related to mean pleural pressure and can be used clinically for monitoring of pressure changes.[96]

The effect of PEEP on pleural pressure is complex and depends on the patient's lungs and thoracic mechanics. Some of the pressure generated by a ventilator reaches the alveoli, where it is transmitted across the alveolar walls to the pleural space. How much of this alveolar pressure is transmitted to the pleural space depends on lung and thoracic mechanics.

Generally, for a given alveolar pressure, the more compliant the lung, the greater is the increase in pleural pressure. A patient with a disease causing a loss of elastic tissue, such as emphysema, is more subject to the cardiovascular effects of positive pressure than a person with normal lungs. In contrast, a lung with low compliance transmits less pressure to the pleural space; this explains, in part, why high levels of PEEP often are used with minimal cardiovascular effects on patients with low lung compliance (e.g., ARDS).

When the compliance of the chest wall is reduced, expansion of the thorax is limited, and more alveolar pressure is transmitted to the pleural space. Patients who have normal lungs but have thoracic restriction, as caused by kyphoscoliosis and spondylitis, are more subject to the cardiovascular effects of positive pressure than individuals with normal chest wall compliance. A similar effect can occur in patients with normal thoracic compliance who actively oppose a mandatory breath by contracting the expiratory muscles (as might occur in patient-ventilator asynchrony). Contraction of the expiratory muscles effectively decreases thoracic compliance and causes more alveolar pressure to be transmitted to the pleural space.

If resistance to airflow is high, less of the pressure generated at the airway reaches the alveoli. The high peak airway pressure common in patients with obstructive disorders is not reflected in high pleural pressure.

The effects of moderate increases in pleural pressure on cardiac output in healthy persons are minimal. In healthy persons, as left ventricular stroke volume decreases, compensatory responses increase both the cardiac rate and the tone of the venous capacitance vessels. These normal responses ensure adequate blood flow and perfusion pressure. However, if the patient already is hypovolemic or has lost peripheral venomotor tone, cardiovascular compensation may be impossible. In these cases, even a small increase in pleural pressure may result in a marked decrease in cardiac output.

Decreasing Mean Airway Pressure

Mean airway pressure is affected by respiratory rate, V_T, inspiratory time, inspiratory pause, expiratory time, I:E ratio, peak pressure, baseline pressure (PEEP or CPAP), and inspiratory flow waveform. If a decrease in mean airway pressure is necessary, altering any factor that contributes to mean airway pressure has an effect. If the PaO_2 is high, one of the most effective changes is a decrease in PEEP because it has a 1:1 relationship with mean airway pressure. If a decrease in PEEP is indicated, the RT must ensure that desaturation does not occur when the decrease has been accomplished. If the patient is being hyperventilated, a decrease in mandatory rate or V_T also decreases mean airway pressure.

The best way to determine the magnitude of the change is to use the mean airway pressure monitor on the ventilator. The peak pressure usually decreases with a decrease in VT. In pressure-controlled modes, the peak pressure may be decreased directly. The plateau pressure is a reflection of mean peak alveolar pressure. In volume-controlled ventilation, a decrease in V_T decreases plateau pressure. In pressure-controlled ventilation, the pressure setting may be reduced to limit plateau pressure. Efforts that increase lung compliance, such as PEEP or administration of diuretics to decrease interstitial edema, also may affect plateau pressure. Inspiratory time, expiratory time, and I:E ratio affect mean airway pressure. As inspiratory time lengthens or expiratory time decreases, mean airway pressure increases.

Fluid Management and Cardiac Output

The relationship between cardiac output and preload (end-diastolic volume) is described by the Frank-Starling phenomenon, which states, "in the normal heart, the diastolic volume (preload) is the principal force that governs the strength of ventricular contraction."[97] As preload (stretch) increases, so does force and presumably stroke volume. Stroke volume continues to increase with preload until the heart is distended by excess preload, after which stroke volume decreases. Another cause of a decrease in stroke volume is the decrease in ventricular contractility that occurs when afterload increases as the result of hypertension. With hypertension comes dilation and distention of the ventricles, which make the heart structurally abnormal. In an abnormal heart, it takes much less preload to put the heart into failure. Failure in this case is defined as decreased stroke volume despite increased preload (Figure 43-18).

When a patient receives PPV, there is risk of a decrease in venous return (preload) because of the increase in intrapleural pressure. Stroke volume may decrease, but the decrease is compensated for by a reflex increase in heart rate and vasomotor tone. Because of these compensatory mechanisms, most patients with a normal cardiopulmonary status who receive mechanical ventilation do not need additional fluid to maintain cardiac output. However, certain conditions can increase the risk of relative or actual hypovolemia, and the increase can decrease stroke volume, even if normal reflex compensation is present. These conditions include hypovolemic shock (owing to trauma and blood loss), sepsis (in which the normal reflex compensation is not present), and high PEEP and high mean airway pressure. In these conditions, fluid or blood administration may be necessary to maintain cardiac output and end-organ perfusion. In some patients who receive PPV with PEEP, an increase in PEEP can decrease cardiac output as discussed earlier. In this case, the outcome of PEEP in terms of improved tissue oxygenation ($DO_2 = CaO_2 \times$ cardiac output) should be determined. If tissue O_2 delivery decreases because of a decrease in cardiac output, but CaO_2 increases, fluid administration may be indicated to restore cardiac output by increasing preload.

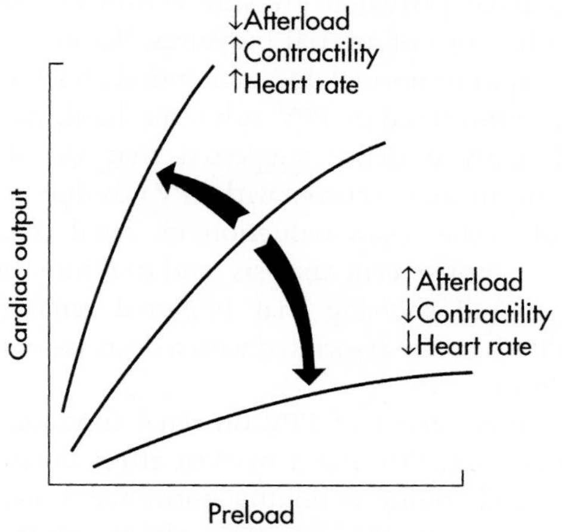

FIGURE 43-18 Effects of preload, afterload, contractility, and heart rate on cardiac output function curve. (Modified from Green JF: Fundamental cardiovascular and pulmonary physiology, ed 2, Philadelphia, 1987, Lea & Febiger.)

Pharmacologic Maintenance of Cardiac Output and Blood Pressure

First-line therapy for decreased cardiac output and blood pressure is fluid administration, unless the patient has congestive heart failure. In heart failure, inotropic therapy is indicated for decreased myocardial contractility, and vasodilators and diuretics are used to control hypertension, which decreases afterload. Diuretics are used to control fluid overload and to decrease preload to the distended heart. These factors in combination may return the heart to a more optimal portion of the Frank-Starling curve and improve stroke volume.

EFFECTS OF POSITIVE PRESSURE MECHANICAL VENTILATION ON OTHER BODY SYSTEMS

Increased Intracranial Pressure

Perfusion of the brain is quantified by the CPP. The CPP is the difference between mean arterial pressure (MAP) and ICP. CPP may decrease in any case in which MAP decreases or ICP increases. If CPP decreases, CBF decreases. The result is cerebral ischemia and a decrease in cerebral O_2 metabolism. The cerebral circulation has the ability to maintain CBF even when CPP changes, a process called *cerebral autoregulation*. Cerebral **autoregulation** is a function of cerebral vascular resistance. If CPP decreases, cerebral vascular resistance decreases to maintain CPP. Cerebral autoregulation functions as long as CPP is in the range of 60 to 150 mm Hg and is limited by the ability of the cerebral arterioles to constrict and dilate. Under normal conditions, cerebral O_2 delivery and CPP exceed the metabolic needs of the brain for O_2 and glucose.

Normal MAP is 93 mm Hg if arterial pressure is 120/80 mm Hg. Normal ICP is less than 10 mm Hg, so normal CPP is 83 to 93 mm Hg. CPP decreases when MAP decreases or ICP increases. Conditions leading to a decrease in MAP are shock, high PEEP, and high mean airway pressure. Increases in ICP are caused by traumatic brain injury (TBI), cerebral hemorrhage, cerebrovascular accident (stroke), and masses. Data have shown that a CPP greater than 60 mm Hg maintains CBF and cerebral O_2 metabolism.

CO_2 is a potent cerebral vasodilator and an important regulator of the cerebral arteriolar diameter. As $PaCO_2$

decreases from 40 mm Hg, systemic pH increases. CO_2 concurrently diffuses across the blood-brain barrier. The result is an increased cerebrospinal fluid (CSF) pH. Although $PaCO_2$ is monitored in patients with TBI, the CSF pH modulates cerebral vascular resistance in an effort to decrease the ICP. When mechanical hyperventilation is used, cerebral vascular resistance increases, and the result is decreased ICP; this is why hyperventilation has been used in the management of TBI and increased ICP. However, in the presence of an already decreased CPP, CBF may decrease to the point at which cerebral ischemia is likely; this is the problem with immediate hyperventilation of a patient with TBI. In addition, prolonged hyperventilation allows renal excretion of bicarbonate, which allows the CSF pH to return to normal and negates any positive effect of hyperventilation on ICP. The effect of hyperventilation on the reduction of ICP lasts 1 hour. If hyperventilation is withdrawn and arterial pH and $PaCO_2$ return to normal values, the CSF pH decreases. Subsequent CSF acidosis leads to cerebral vasodilation and a rebound increase in CBF and ICP that exceeds the values before hyperventilation. For these reasons, hyperventilation must be used cautiously in the treatment of patients with TBI.[98]

Treatment of a Patient With a Closed Head Injury

Guidelines for the management of severe TBI were developed by neurosurgeons in the Joint Section on Neurotrauma and Critical Care.[99] The recommendation is as follows: "The use of prophylactic hyperventilation ($PaCO_2$ < 35 mm Hg) during the first 24 hours after TBI should be avoided because it can compromise cerebral perfusion during a time when CBF is reduced. Hyperventilation therapy may be necessary for brief periods when there is acute neurologic deterioration or for longer periods if there is intracranial hypertension refractory to sedation, paralysis, CSF drainage, and osmotic diuretics." The Joint Section further noted that "in the absence of increased ICP, chronic, prolonged hyperventilation therapy ($PaCO_2$ < 35 mm Hg) should be avoided after TBI." These findings have resulted in several recommendations regarding the care of patients with TBI, as follows:

1. Patients with TBI may have transient, short periods of increased ICP, called *plateau waves*. Plateau waves may be caused by suctioning, repositioning, or other noxious stimuli. During a plateau wave, acute hyperventilation with a manual ventilator or by an increase in ventilator rate can control ICP until the pressure returns to baseline, at which time ventilation is resumed at the previous rate.
2. Hyperventilation should be used temporarily after TBI until other methods can be employed to decrease elevated ICP. These methods include ventriculostomy for drainage of CSF, craniotomy for removal of mass lesions, osmotic diuretics, sedation, placing the patient in the semi-Fowler position, and paralysis. CPP is maintained at greater than 70 mm Hg.
3. Hyperventilation is instituted with a moderate V_T (8 to 10 ml/kg) ensuring a plateau pressure less than 30 cm H_2O and an increased rate. A moderate V_T is used to avoid an increase in intrathoracic pressure, which can decrease MAP. Intubation should be attempted only after the patient has been sedated, to prevent the associated increase in ICP. Exhaled partial pressure of end-tidal carbon dioxide ($PETCO_2$) should be monitored to maintain a constant $PaCO_2$ after arterial blood gas values are determined to find the correlation between $PaCO_2$ and $PETCO_2$.
4. When ICP is less than 20 mm Hg, hyperventilation may be gradually discontinued through decreasing the mandatory rate. The rate of weaning must be individualized via monitoring the response to an increase in $PaCO_2$. If there is a subsequent increase in ICP, the new respiratory rate can be maintained until the CBF readjusts and ICP decreases.[99]

Effect on Renal Function

Some patients receiving long-term PPV retain salt and water. In critically ill patients, water retention usually is evident when rapid weight gain occurs. In addition, such patients may have a reduced hematocrit, which is also consistent with hypervolemia secondary to water retention. These early observations are attributed to the direct and indirect effects of PPV on renal function.

In terms of direct effect, PPV can reduce urinary output 30% to 50%. This reduced urinary output during PPV is associated with a simultaneous reduction in renal blood flow, glomerular filtration rate, and sodium and potassium excretion.

Decreases in MAP to less than 75 mm Hg reduce renal blood flow, glomerular filtration rate, and urinary output. However, MAP this low seldom is caused by PPV alone, and kidney autoregulatory mechanisms generally can keep renal perfusion pressure within normal limits over a wide range of arterial pressures. Because restoring cardiac output to normal does not entirely restore urinary output compromised by PPV, other mechanisms must be involved. Early evidence suggested that the decreased urinary output that occurred with PPV was due to redistribution of, rather than reduction in, renal blood flow. Results of a more recent analysis tend to refute this explanation, instead showing that impaired renal function during PPV is better associated with a decrease in intravascular volume.

The indirect effect of PPV on renal function may be most important. PPV has a marked effect on the water-retaining and sodium-retaining hormonal systems. Specifically, long-term PPV increases plasma renin activity, plasma aldosterone level, and level of vasopressin (urinary antidiuretic hormone). In addition, PPV decreases atrial natriuretic hormone levels (Figure 43-19).

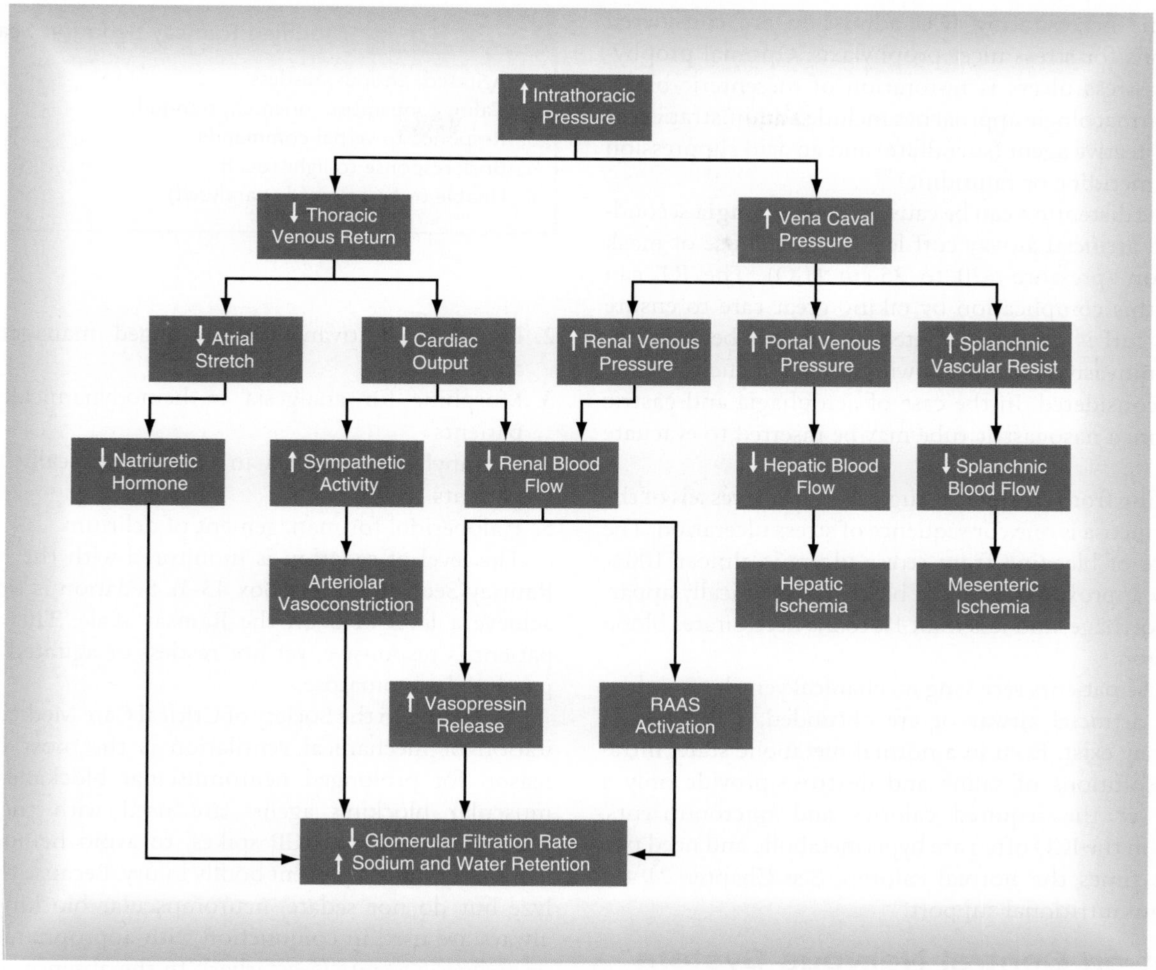

FIGURE 43-19 Cardiac, renal, hepatic, and splanchnic effects associated with increased intrathoracic pressure caused by PPV. *RAAS,* Renin-angiotensin-aldosterone system; ↑, increased; ↓, decreased. (Modified from Florete OG, Gammage GW: Complications of ventilatory support. In Kirby RR, Banner MI, Downs JB, editors: Clinical applications of ventilatory support, New York, 1990, Churchill Livingstone.)

Decreased right atrial transmural pressure is primarily responsible for the decrease in atrial natriuretic hormone, which leads to sodium retention. Similarly, vasopressin secretion may be enhanced by stimulation of the left atrial stretch receptors, which innervate the posterior pituitary gland. Increased secretion of vasopressin (antidiuretic hormone) and activation of the renin-angiotensin-aldosterone system lead to a decrease in urine output.

Decreased Liver and Splanchnic Perfusion

The effects of PPV on the liver and intestine are related to its effects on the cardiovascular system. Hepatic dysfunction with PPV can occur in patients with otherwise normal livers and manifests as an increase in serum bilirubin level. These effects appear to be directly related to the reduction in hepatic blood flow that occurs with PPV. Regardless of cause, these effects are aggravated by PEEP but can be reversed when cardiac output is returned to pre-PEEP levels with intravascular volume infusions.

Decreased Gastrointestinal Function

An increase in splanchnic resistance can contribute to gastric mucosal ischemia and helps explain the high incidence of gastrointestinal bleeding and stress ulceration in patients receiving long-term PPV. Stress ulcers (erosions of the gastric mucosa) are common among patients with life-threatening illness. Impaired blood flow inhibits the ability of the gastric mucosa to replace itself normally every 2 or 3 days. Stress ulcers are caused by impaired blood flow, not gastric acidity. Gastroduodenal motility also is severely impaired in mechanically ventilated patients.[100] These factors may result in translocation of bacteria from the intestine to the blood and nosocomial septicemia. Mechanical ventilation for more than 48 hours and most other conditions necessitating ICU admission are considered indications for stress ulcer prophylaxis. Optimal prophylaxis for stress ulcers is restoration of mesenteric blood flow. Pharmacologic approaches include administration of a cytoprotective agent (sucralfate) and an acid suppression agent (cimetidine or ranitidine).[97]

Gastric distention can be caused by **aerophagia** secondary to an artificial airway cuff leak or by the use of mask ventilation (pressure >20 to 25 cm H_2O). The RT can prevent this complication by taking great care to ensure that the cuff is properly inflated. If patients being ventilated noninvasively are swallowing air, an artificial airway may be considered. In the case of aerophagia and gastric distention, a nasogastric tube may be inserted to evacuate the air.

Bleeding from erosion through the surface vessels of the gastric mucosa is one consequence of stress ulceration. The incidence of bleeding from stress ulcers is almost 100%, but only approximately 5% of bleeding is clinically apparent hemorrhage, and less than 1% to 2% necessitates blood transfusion.

Because patients receiving mechanical ventilation often have an artificial airway or are obtunded, a nutritional deficit may exist. Even in a normal metabolic state, intravenous solutions of saline and dextrose provide only a fraction of the required calories and micronutrients. Patients in the ICU often are hypermetabolic and need two to three times the normal calories. See Chapter 21 for details on nutritional support.

Effect on Central Nervous System

Patients in the ICU are placed into an artificial environment over which they have little control. From the start, the patient loses autonomy. When mechanical ventilation is introduced, the patient is sedated and possibly paralyzed and may not return to a normal, awake level of consciousness until discharged from the ICU. Instead, the patient is kept somnolent (easily aroused and aware) or is stuporous (arousable with difficulty and impaired awareness) or comatose (arousable but unaware).[97] The presence of an artificial airway makes communication difficult. Caregivers should make a paper tablet and pen, communication board, or communication cards available to patients who are aware enough to write or use them.

Sedatives, Hypnotics, and Neuromuscular Blocking Agents

Sedation is necessary for the management of the nearly inevitable agitation, fear, and anxiety associated with the ICU environment, pain, invasive and noninvasive procedures, and loss of normal sleep pattern. The Society of Critical Care Medicine has published the following guidelines for sedation and analgesia in the care of critically ill patients:[101]

1. Midazolam (Versed) or propofol for short-term (<24 hours) management of anxiety
2. Lorazepam (Ativan) for prolonged management of anxiety
3. Morphine for analgesia in hemodynamically stable patients
4. Fentanyl for analgesia in hemodynamically unstable patients
5. Haloperidol for management of delirium

Box 43-3 Modified Ramsay Sedation Scale

1. Agitated, anxious, restless
2. Calm, cooperative, oriented, tranquil
3. Responds to verbal commands
4. Brisk response to light touch
5. Unable to be assessed (paralyzed)

The level of sedation is monitored with the Modified Ramsay Sedation Scale (Box 43-3). Sedation is titrated to achieve a level of 3 on the Ramsay scale. This way the patient is responsive, yet not restless or agitated and not paralyzed or comatose.

According to the Society of Critical Care Medicine, facilitation of mechanical ventilation is the most common reason for prolonged neuromuscular blockade. Neuromuscular blocking agents are used with mechanical ventilation to avoid ICP spikes, to avoid hemodynamic instability, and to prevent bodily injury. Because they paralyze but do not sedate, neuromuscular blocking agents always are used in conjunction with appropriate sedative or analgesic agents (see earlier). In the absence of a sedative, a patient under the influence of a neuromuscular blocking agent is paralyzed and fully aware of the surroundings. During neuromuscular blockade, patients should be assessed for the degree of blockade that is being sustained.[101] The patient is observed for ventilatory effort, and train-of-four stimulation is performed. Although it is commonly used in the operating room, use of train-of-four stimulation is uncommon in the ICU. Neuromuscular blockade should be allowed to dissipate daily so that clinical evaluation, assessment of concomitant sedation and analgesia, and evaluation of the need for continued paralysis can be conducted.

COMPLICATIONS OF MECHANICAL VENTILATION

Negative Pressure Ventilation

Pulmonary

Hypoventilation during NPV can be caused by a decrease in the transairway pressure owing to inadequate negative pressure or leaks in the ventilator or patient-ventilator interface. Iron lung negative pressure ventilators rely on a tight seal at the patient's neck and at all access ports in the tank. Chest cuirass ventilators rely on a tight seal between the cuirass and thorax. Poncho-type ventilators must remain free of leaks or tears. When there is a leak at any of these points, transairway pressure decreases, and the result is a decrease in minute ventilation.

Hyperventilation can occur if the pressure is more negative than is necessary. The results are increased transairway pressure, increased V_T, and increased minute ventilation.

Cardiovascular

Abdominal blood pooling can occur in patients receiving NPV in an iron lung. The negative pressure exerted on the thorax also is exerted on the more compliant abdominal wall. When the pressure in the iron lung becomes negative, the abdominal wall is pulled outward and with it the viscera and associated blood supply. Venous return to the heart, cardiac output, and systemic blood pressure decrease; the result is a condition called "tank shock."

Positive Pressure Ventilation: Artificial Airway Complications

Chapter 33 describes complications related to artificial airways.

Complications Related to Pressure

Ventilator-associated lung injury is the term used to define lung injury in humans owing to mechanical ventilation. These are complications resulting from high pressure, infection, and patient-ventilator asynchrony. High ventilation pressure has long been associated with barotrauma. Barotrauma is categorized as pneumothorax, pneumomediastinum, pneumopericardium, and subcutaneous emphysema (Figure 43-20). All of these complications are descriptions of extraalveolar air. High ventilatory pressure can cause gas to escape through ruptured alveoli. The eventual location of the escaping gas defines the type of barotrauma. If gas escapes through ruptured alveoli into the pleural space, pneumothorax occurs. Gas escaping along perivascular sheaths to the mediastinum produces pneumomediastinum. Further dissection from the mediastinum to tissue planes in the neck and chest wall results in subcutaneous emphysema and potentially pneumomediastinum and pneumoperitoneum.

Pneumothorax is identified by observation of a decrease in chest movement, hyperresonance on percussion, possible deviation of the trachea away from the affected side, and decreased or absent breath sounds over the affected side. In nonintubated patients, there may also be a decrease in vocal fremitus over the affected side. A line separating lung tissue from air is observed on the chest radiograph, although the line sometimes is difficult to see in a small (<20%) pneumothorax. Respiratory distress increases with increasing pneumothorax, as does hypoxemia. Normally, in spontaneously breathing patients, intrapulmonary and pleural pressures are equal in pneumothorax. PPV can cause intrapleural pressures to increase (tension pneumothorax).

Tension pneumothorax is life-threatening, because it tends to develop very rapidly in patients who are mechanically ventilated and shifts the mediastinum, heart, and great vessels; the results are a decrease in cardiac output and hypotension. Tension pneumothorax is a medical emergency; it is relieved by insertion of a large-bore needle into the pleural space through the anterior second or third interspace above the rib. This maneuver is followed by

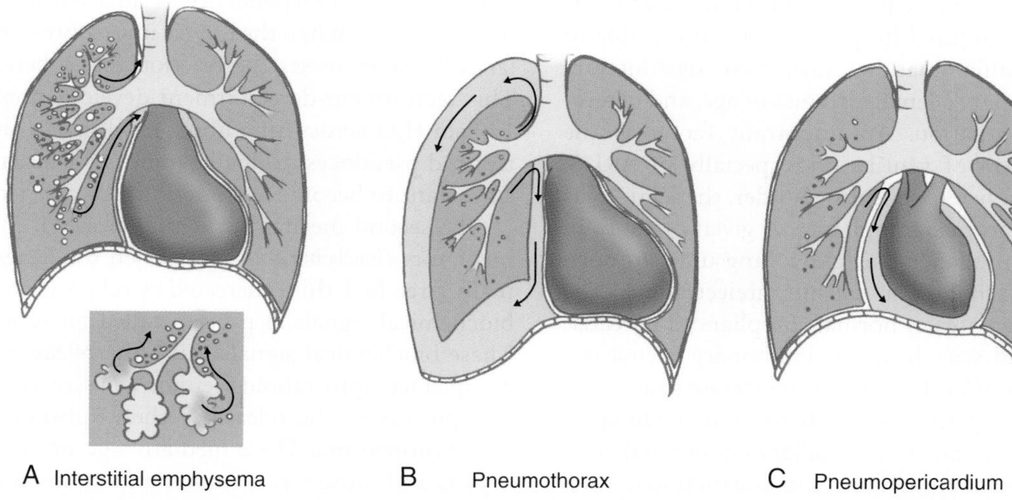

FIGURE 43-20 Pulmonary barotrauma. **A,** Ruptured alveoli are indicated in framed alveoli at bottom. Air dissects from alveoli along vascular sheaths to the hilum and then to the pleural space. **B,** Pneumothorax. Origin of air in lung tissue and its pathway to inflate the pleural space are indicated. The heart shifts to the left because of high pressure in the right side of the chest. **C,** Course of air from the lung to pericardial space. The distended pericardial space causes cardiac tamponade. (Modified from Korones SB: High-risk newborn infants, ed 4, St Louis, 1986, Mosby.)

chest tube insertion. While waiting for needle decompression, the patient may be ventilated with 100% O_2 at a low V_T and pressure. Pneumomediastinum and pneumoperitoneum are identified on a chest radiograph by the presence of air in these locations.

Complications Related to Volume

Ventilator-induced lung injury (VILI) has been defined as the application of pressure, positive or negative, to the lungs causing damage to the acinus. The damage has been described as an increase in permeability of the alveolar-capillary membrane, pulmonary edema, cell wounding and necrosis, and diffuse alveolar damage as the result of using an inappropriate ventilation strategy. Several more recent reviews summarize understanding of the mechanisms, effects, and means to prevent VILI.[102-104]

It has been shown that overdistention, as opposed to volume or pressure per se, is an important determinant of lung damage. Animals ventilated with large V_T (>30 ml/kg) develop severe injury—hence the term *volutrauma*. The degree of alveolar distention is determined by the transpulmonary pressure (plateau pressure minus the pleural pressure), which must be approximated by the esophageal pressure. As plateau pressure increases, so does transpulmonary pressure, increasing the likelihood of lung damage. Lung damage may also occur when ventilating at low V_T, if alveoli are allowed to deflate and reinflate repeatedly with each breath. This injury is called **atelectrauma.** These two factors have led to the recommendation that lungs should be opened ("recruited") and kept open by an appropriate PEEP level and ventilated to a plateau pressure of no more than 30 cm H_2O by decreasing V_T. This technique is called the *open lung technique* and is described in detail in Chapter 44.

Factors that predispose a patient to VILI include underlying lung disease (injured lungs are more susceptible to VILI), systemic inflammation, surfactant dysfunction, aspiration, pulmonary edema, extremes of age, and heterogeneous lung ventilation. An important factor is the uneven distribution of ventilation, especially in ARDS. Because ARDS is a heterogeneous disorder, there are areas of both low and normal compliance. A given pressure in an area of low compliance may allow lung units to open and close with each breath, causing atelectrauma. The same pressure in an area of normal compliance may cause overdistention and stretch injury. Pulmonary edema is a prominent feature of VILI, owing to an increase in alveolar-capillary membrane permeability. Microvascular damage is characterized by separation of capillary endothelial cells, disruption of alveolar epithelium, and destruction of alveolar type I cells.

VILI occurs via two mechanisms, as shown in Figure 43-21.[105] One mechanism is the physical disruption of tissues and cells *(biophysical injury)*. Physical disruption of the tissues occurs as air ruptures across the alveolar epithelial surface and tracks along the bronchovascular

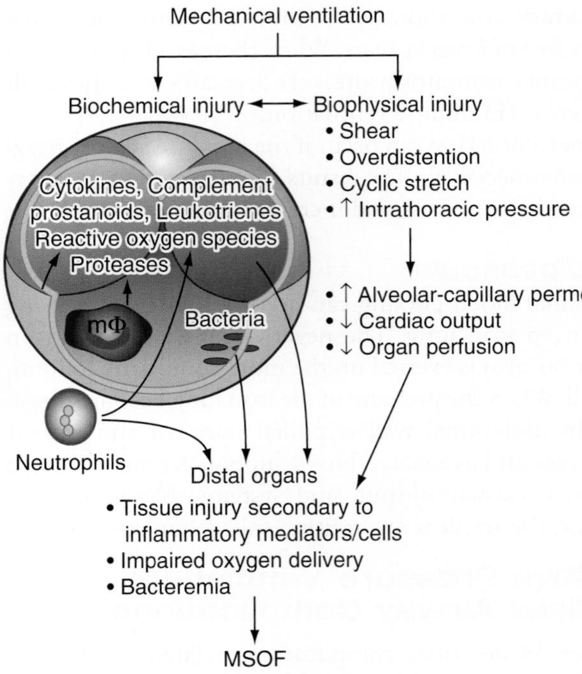

FIGURE 43-21 Mechanisms by which mechanical ventilation might contribute to MSOF. (From Mason RJ, Broaddus VC, Murray JF, et al: Murray and Nadel's textbook of respiratory medicine, ed 4, Philadelphia, 2005, Saunders.)

sheath. Air tracks into the interstitium causing pulmonary interstitial emphysema, into the pleural space causing pneumothorax, and into the pericardium causing pneumopericardium. The pulmonary capillary epithelium also fails in response to high-volume ventilation, resulting in hemorrhage and edema. Another factor in biophysical injury is the interdependence of adjacent alveoli and terminal bronchi. When the lung is unevenly expanded, alveolar collapse increases the traction forces between alveoli. This recruitment-derecruitment develops pressures up to 140 cm H_2O across lung units, resulting in air-filled cavities and pseudocysts. Finally, injurious ventilation, causes surfactant to become dysfunctional or deficient or both.

The second mechanism is the release of inflammatory mediators *(biochemical injury)*. When the lungs are abnormally stretched, this is detected by cells and converted into biochemical signals, a process called *mechanotransduction*. These biochemical signals cause the release of cytokines, complement, prostanoids, leukotrienes, reactive O_2 species, and proteases. The release of these substances has been called **biotrauma.** These mediators go on to the terminal organs and cause tissue inflammation, impairment of O_2 delivery, and bacteremia (see Figure 43-21), leading to MSOF. As mentioned earlier in the chapter, hyperinflation during mechanical ventilation causes bacteria to "spill over" from the gut into the bloodstream, a process called *translocation*. In this manner, translocation contributes to MSOF, as bacteria migrate into the blood and then to terminal organs. Other factors contributing to MSOF are an increase in circulating cell death (apoptotic) factors, suppression of the peripheral immune response, and individual genetic variability.

Alveolar distention occurs when the lungs are stiff and the chest wall is normal or when one or both lungs are ventilated with a high plateau pressure. Plateau pressure ideally should be maintained at less than 30 cm H_2O in all patients. However, in patients with a stiff chest wall (marked obesity, fluid overload, increased abdominal pressure), higher plateau pressure can be tolerated without injury because of the reduction in transpulmonary pressure caused by the stiff chest wall.

Human studies have compared high and low V_T ventilation, using ICU mortality, ventilator-free days, and overall mortality as outcome variables. The consensus is that a low V_T strategy, with PEEP adequate to keep lungs open to avoid atelectrauma, results in a significantly better outcome. In studies in which inflammatory mediators were also measured, high V_T groups had a higher level of inflammatory mediators.[106,107] VILI is related to both mechanical and chemical factors. On one hand, overstretch directly injures the alveolar epithelium and capillary endothelium. On the other hand, through mechanotransduction, cells release many inflammatory mediators into the blood, leading to MSOF.

Auto–Positive End Expiratory Pressure

Air trapping occurs with incomplete emptying of lung units. Lung units prone to air trapping are units with long-time constants (i.e., with high resistance or high compliance). Air trapping during PPV is often referred to as *dynamic hyperinflation, auto-PEEP, occult PEEP,* or *intrinsic PEEP*. The terms *occult* and *intrinsic* are more descriptive because this form of air trapping cannot be determined by simple observation of airway pressure. Auto-PEEP often goes unrecognized.

Figure 43-22, *A,* shows the generation of auto-PEEP. As long as airway resistance is normal and expiratory time is

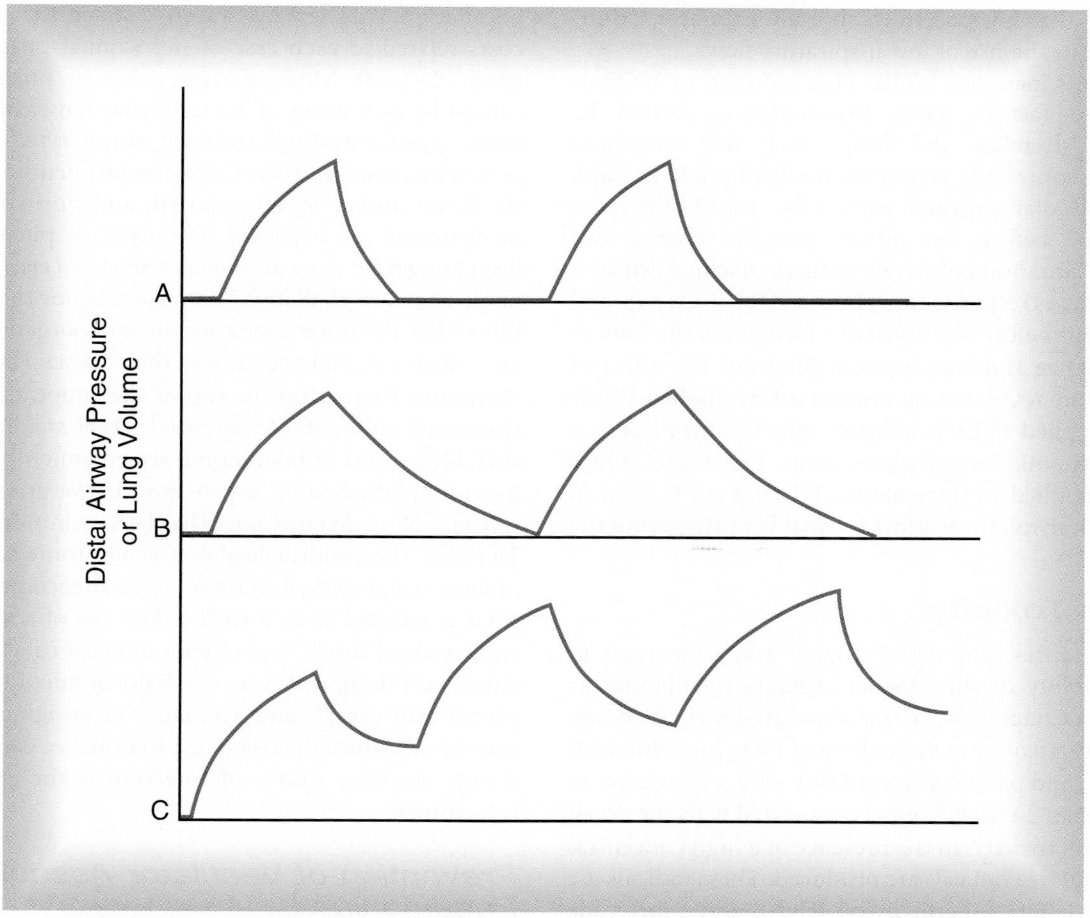

FIGURE 43-22 Causes of auto-PEEP. **A,** When airway resistance is normal and expiratory time is long enough, distal airway pressure and lung volume return to normal after a positive pressure breath. **B,** High expiratory resistance prolongs exhalation to the point at which air-trapping begins and causes auto-PEEP. **C,** Shortening the expiratory time aggravates the problem and worsens auto-PEEP. (Modified from Benson MS, Pierson DJ: Auto-PEEP during mechanical ventilation of adults, Respir Care 33:557, 1988.)

sufficiently long, distal airway pressure and lung volume return to baseline during PPV breaths. Alone or in combination, three factors account for the development of auto-PEEP. First, by effectively increasing the time constant of the lung, high expiratory resistance prolongs exhalation to the point at which air trapping begins (see Figure 43-22, *B*). Second, any increase in the minute ventilation increases the likelihood of auto-PEEP. Third, any shortening of the expiratory time (see Figure 43-22, *C*) aggravates the problem and increases both distal airway pressure and lung volume (auto-PEEP). By increasing FRC and alveolar pressure, auto-PEEP increases WOB and impedes venous return, the result being a decrease in cardiac output. Auto-PEEP also can increase pulmonary vascular resistance.

Patients at greatest risk for auto-PEEP are patients with high airway resistance who are being supported by modes that limit expiratory time. High-risk patient groups include patients with obstructive disease, any disease producing increased secretions, and any disease that increases lung compliance. High-risk ventilatory support techniques include any method that increases the I:E ratio, especially CMV at a high rate or in the assist-control mode, and approaches that purposefully shorten expiratory time, such as IRV or the use of low inspiratory flow.

Auto-PEEP increases WOB. This increase in WOB is due to two factors. First, hyperinflation caused by auto-PEEP stretches the lung, and the stretching impairs the contractile action of the diaphragm. Second, the high alveolar pressure caused by auto-PEEP must be overcome before any airway pressure change can occur. This situation effectively reduces machine sensitivity and increases response time. Increased effort is required by the patient before the ventilator recognizes the flow or pressure change and triggers to inspiration. The effect of auto-PEEP on WOB can be minimized by applied PEEP. However, applied PEEP is effective only if auto-PEEP is a result of dynamic airway obstruction. Essentially, PEEP should be applied in increments of 1 to 2 cm H_2O until every patient inspiratory effort is capable of triggering the ventilator.

Oxygen Toxicity

O_2 toxicity causes lung tissue damage and an increase in the permeability of the alveolar-capillary membrane. As suggested in Chapter 38, factors associated with the development of O_2 toxicity include elevated FiO_2, long duration of exposure, and patient susceptibility. FiO_2 of 0.6 or more for longer than 24 to 48 hours is associated with the development of O_2 toxicity. In the presence of a high concentration of O_2, O_2 free radicals are produced. These radicals are the hydroxyl (OH^-), perhydroxyl (HO_2), and superoxide (O_2^-) radicals. Free radicals normally are rapidly detoxified by the enzyme superoxide dismutase, which is produced by alveolar type II cells. With higher FiO_2, the presence of free radicals is greater, and type II cells are less likely to produce superoxide dismutase. The presence of free radicals increases the permeability of the alveolar-capillary membrane. The combination of direct injury by free radicals and decreased surfactant production leads to exudation of fluid into the alveoli and a subsequent decrease in compliance. Every effort should be made to decrease FiO_2 whenever it exceeds 0.6. The decrease usually is accomplished with application of PEEP or CPAP. However, the evidence supporting the development of O_2 toxicity in critically ill patients is poor, and oxygenation should never be sacrificed for the purpose of avoiding O_2 toxicity.

Ventilator-Associated (Nosocomial) Pneumonia

Pneumonia is the second most common nosocomial infection, primarily affecting infants and young children, adults older than 65 years, patients with severe underlying disease, immunosuppressed patients, patients who have depressed sensorium, patients with cardiopulmonary disease, and patients who have had thoracoabdominal surgery. RTs should be prepared to prevent this threat to respiratory patients, who are 6 to 21 times more susceptible to the development of nosocomial pneumonia than the general population. A review by Craven[108] stated that health care costs related to each case of nosocomial pneumonia are about $40,000. Most of these cases of pneumonia are caused by aspiration of bacteria that have colonized the upper gastrointestinal tract or oropharynx. Intubation greatly increases the risk of nosocomial pneumonia because the lower airway is left exposed, and normal protective mechanisms are bypassed. This type of pneumonia has been known for years as *ventilator-associated pneumonia*. This name has been challenged because it is not the ventilator, but rather the microaspiration of microorganisms in oral or gastrointestinal secretions, that causes the infection. Secretions that sit on the top of the endotracheal or tracheostomy tube cuff are aspirated via the small folds in the cuff. Most cases of pneumonia are polymicrobial, consisting of gram-negative organisms. However, methicillin-resistant *Staphylococcus aureus* has been common in the past 10 years. The endotracheal or tracheostomy tube is a site of bacterial growth, and these bacteria become encased in what is referred to as a *biofilm*. The use of a silver-coated endotracheal tube[109] use of endotracheal tubes with alternative cuff designs,[110] use of subglottic suction airways,[111] proper cuff care,[112] and avoidance of lavaging when suctioning all reduce the risk of aspiration. See Chapter 33 for details. Another source of infection is the endotracheal tube lumen.

Prevention of Ventilator-Associated Pneumonia

In addition to standard precautions, specific infection control procedures apply to the use of endotracheal tubes and ventilators. These ventilator bundles for prevention of ventilator-associated pneumonia include the following:[112]

- Perform appropriate hand hygiene. Hands should be disinfected with a sanitizer (e.g., Cal-Stat hand sanitizer) before entering any patient's room regardless of the reason and when leaving the patient's room regardless of the activities that occurred in the room.
- Perform gentle suctioning (presumably to help prevent coughing, aspiration, and sloughing of biofilm).
- Place the patient in a semirecumbent position (30- to 45-degree head elevation).
- Do not routinely change ventilator circuits.
- Drain and discard inspiratory tube condensate away from the patient, or prevent its formation by using heated wire circuits or heat and moisture exchangers.
- Use a metered dose inhaler rather than a nebulizer for medication administration. If a small volume nebulizer is used, it should be replaced after each treatment (i.e., one nebulizer = one treatment).
- Interrupt sedatives daily to evaluate patient readiness to wean from the ventilator—this is effective in decreasing the length of intubation and mechanical ventilation.
- Assess daily the ability of the patient to perform a spontaneous breathing trial.
- Use noninvasive ventilation whenever possible to avoid intubation.
- Perform regular oral hygiene at least every 4 hours.

Early tracheostomy has been evaluated as a possible preventive measure, but several studies and meta-analyses showed no advantage of tracheostomy in preventing ventilator-associated pneumonia.[108] Other measures that may decrease the likelihood of nosocomial infection include the use of closed suction systems (although the benefit remains unproved); use of disposable resuscitation bags; and high-level disinfection of ventilators, O_2 analyzers, and other equipment between patients.

Ventilator Malfunction

Ventilator malfunction can be categorized as a failure in the patient circuit or a failure in the ventilator. Failures in the patient circuit include failures related to the endotracheal tube: cuff rupture, main stem intubation, laryngeal intubation, esophageal intubation, soft tissue erosion because the cuff pressure is too high, and disconnection from the circuit (Figure 43-23). Failures in the tubing circuit include leaks anywhere there is a tubing connection; a leak at the site of a nebulizer or metered dose inhaler; humidifier malfunctions that include failure to fill the reservoir, overheating, or mechanical failure; and exhalation valve failure. These failures are recognized by the ventilator as changes in respiratory rate, airway pressure, or V_T outside the limits set on the alarms.

Airway and ventilator malfunctions can be avoided with proper care of the endotracheal tube (taping the tube snugly), ensuring equal breath sounds, checking to ensure the tubing is patent and free of leaks, and ensuring that all connections are firmly made. If patient activity is the cause of ventilator disconnection, patient teaching to refrain

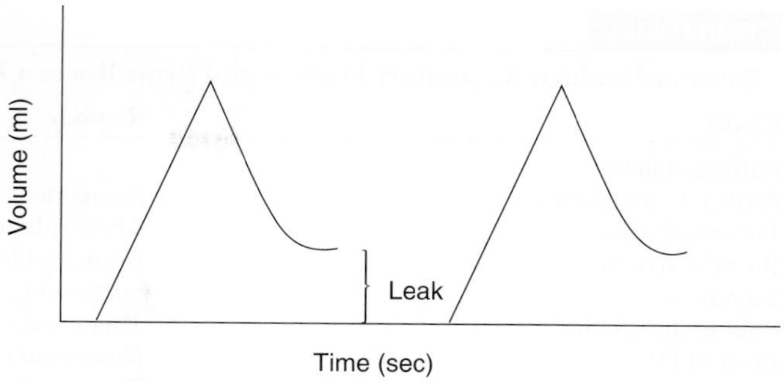

FIGURE 43-23 Volume-time waveform illustrating a leak in the ventilator circuit. Note the abrupt end of expiration before the tracing reaches the baseline.

from attempting to disconnect the ventilator or pulling on or biting the tube or sedation or restraint may be necessary. Failures related to the ventilator include electrical failure, microprocessor failure, exhalation valve failure, internal volume leakage, gas supply failure, and any failure that could result in an increase or decrease in minute ventilation or FiO_2. Ventilators have alarms that alert the RT to these dysfunctions.

Patient safety is always the primary concern when a malfunction is detected. For this reason, a manual resuscitator always should be placed near the bedside. If the reason for the patient's distress is clear, such as disconnection at the endotracheal tube, the connection is reestablished, and patient comfort and ventilation are ensured. If the reason is not obvious, the patient is ventilated with a manual ventilator while the cause of the malfunction is investigated. The steps for managing sudden distress in a patient receiving ventilatory support are listed in Table 43-4.

RULE OF THUMB

Always have a manual ventilator (bag-valve-mask device [Ambu bag]) at the bedside of a patient receiving mechanical ventilation. Ensure that the manual ventilator is connected to an O_2 source. If the patient is receiving PEEP, ensure that the manual ventilator is equipped with a PEEP valve that provides PEEP equivalent of that being administered to the patient with the ventilator. Keep the patient connection of the manual ventilator clean and covered and the valve free of secretions.

Operator Error

The provision of mechanical ventilation is highly complex, the equipment used is very sophisticated, and the potential options to be applied to a given patient increase each year. As a result, clinician error is an ongoing concern. To minimize the possibility of error, a clinician should never

TABLE 43-4

Causes of Sudden Respiratory Distress and Remedies in a Patient Receiving Ventilatory Support

Cause	Remedy
Patient Related	
Artificial airway problems	Assessment of cuff, airway position (see Chapter 33)
Pneumothorax	Chest tube insertion
Bronchospasm	Bronchodilator therapy
Secretions	Suctioning, tracheobronchial hygiene
Pulmonary edema	Therapy directed at cause of pulmonary edema
Auto-PEEP	Decreased minute volume, tracheobronchial hygiene, decrease in I : E
Abnormal respiratory drive	Therapy directed at cause, possible sedation or paralysis
Alteration in body posture	Repositioning of patient
Abdominal distention	Therapy directed at cause, insertion of nasogastric tube
Anxiety	Reassurance, anxiolytics, assessment of minute ventilation
Patient-ventilator asynchrony	Assessment of flow and sensitivity, auto-PEEP, change of mode to accommodate patient's pattern of ventilation
Ventilator Related	
System leak	Assessment of connections in the ventilator circuit
Circuit malfunction	Assessment of circuit with test lung, replace if necessary
Inadequate FiO_2	Assessment of SpO_2, assessment of FiO_2 with analyzer, increase in FiO_2, or replacement of blender or ventilator if malfunction is found
Inadequate ventilatory support	Review of therapeutic strategy for the patient (see Chapter 44)
Improper flow-trigger setting	Adjust trigger and flow to patient demand

make an adjustment to a mechanical ventilator unless he or she has been properly trained to operate the ventilator and the clinician's skills at using the machine have been assessed by an independent evaluator. It is essential for the operator to document ventilator settings in a consistent manner and to understand the terminology used when documenting the ventilator-patient interaction in a paper chart or electronic medical record. This attention to proper documentation is especially important when documenting ventilator settings during pressure control ventilation, where documentation errors can lead to hyperventilation or hypoventilation. Appropriate operation of the mechanical ventilator should be assessed on a regular basis based on the severity and criticality of the patient's clinical presentation. To minimize errors, any adjustment should be checked to ensure that the appropriate change was actually made and that the patient responded as expected. A clinician should never leave the bedside of a patient until the clinician is assured that the patient is being ventilated as ordered and that the ventilator is responding as expected. Patient safety should always be the primary concern of all RTs.

SUMMARY CHECKLIST

- Response to an increase in FiO_2 helps determine the cause of hypoxemia.
- Hypoxemia responsive to an increase in FiO_2 is likely caused by a low $\dot{V}/\dot{Q}$ ratio.
- Hypoxemia unresponsive to increased FiO_2 is likely caused by a diffusion defect or shunt.
- Alveolar ventilation and CO_2 production determine $PaCO_2$.
- Mechanical ventilation should increase alveolar ventilation and may decrease CO_2 production when WOB is relieved. These factors decrease $PaCO_2$.
- Mechanical ventilation with positive pressure increases dead space and decreases $\dot{V}/\dot{Q}$ ratio.
- Inspiratory or expiratory time can be manipulated to improve oxygenation and alveolar emptying in disorders that effect alveolar time constants.
- Physiologic benefits of PPV include improved oxygenation and ventilation, alveolar expansion, decreased WOB and cardiac work, and improved O_2 delivery.
- No outcome differences have been identified among the various modes of ventilation except that SIMV prolongs the weaning process. However, modes of ventilation that allow the patient control over the process of gas delivery have been shown to improve patient-ventilator synchrony.
- No single flow pattern has been shown to be the most physiologically beneficial. However, research results indicate better oxygenation, ventilation, and patient-ventilator synchrony with the decelerating flow compared with the square wave flow pattern.
- A decelerating flow waveform tends to have a lower peak and a higher mean airway pressure, whereas a square wave tends to have a higher peak and a lower mean airway pressure.
- Flow triggering appears to decrease WOB compared with pressure triggering on older generation ventilators.
- PEEP is used to restore FRC in acute restrictive disease and to splint the airways in obstructive disease.
- WOB is decreased by the appropriate application of mode, trigger variable, and flow.

- PPV is detrimental to the $\dot{V}/\dot{Q}$ ratio primarily by shifting ventilation to areas that are less perfused. PPV can cause hyperventilation, tissue damage, and barotraumas if not carefully managed.
- PPV can decrease venous return and cardiac output, especially when it increases intrapleural and mean airway pressures.
- PPV can cause renal, hepatic, and gastrointestinal malfunction primarily owing to decreased perfusion of the capillary tissue beds.
- Elevation of the head, osmotic diuretics, and CSF drainage are effective means of decreasing ICP in TBI. Acute hyperventilation should be used only temporarily until other, more effective means can be employed.
- Ventilator bundles should always be adhered to during mechanical ventilation to minimize the development of ventilator-associated pneumonia.
- Patient safety and error-free patient care are the first priority when caring for any patient.

References

1. Chatburn RL: Classification of mechanical ventilators. In Branson RD, et al, editors: Respiratory care equipment, ed 2, Philadelphia, 1999, Lippincott Williams & Wilkins.
2. Beachy W: Respiratory care anatomy and physiology: foundations for clinical practice, St Louis, 2007, Mosby.
3. Hess DR, Kacmarek RM: Essentials of mechanical ventilation, New York, 2002, McGraw-Hill.
4. The ARDSnet: Ventilation with low tidal volume compared with traditional tidal volumes for acute lung injury and the acute respiratory distress syndrome. N Engl J Med 342:1301-1308, 2000.
5. Lachman B: Open up the lung and keep it open. Intensive Care Med 18:319-321, 1992.
6. MacIntyre NR: Patient-ventilator interactions. In MacIntyre NR, Branson RD, editors: Mechanical ventilation, Philadelphia, 2001, Saunders.
7. Goddon S, Fujino Y, Hromi JM, et al: Optimal mean airway pressure during high frequency oscillation. Anesthesiology 94:862-868, 2001.
8. Hickling KG: Best compliance during a decremental, but not incremental, positive end-expiratory pressure trial is related to open-lung positive end expiratory pressure: a mathematical model of acute respiratory distress syndrome lungs. Am J Respir Crit Care Med 163:69-78, 2001.
9. Borges JB, Okamoto VN, Matos GFJ, et al: Reversibility of lung collapse and hypoxemia in early acute respiratory distress syndrome. Am J Respir Crit Care Med 174:268-278, 2006.
10. Kacmarek RM, Villar J: Lung recruitment maneuvers during acute respiratory distress syndrome: is it useful? Minerva Anestesiol 76:1-2, 2010.
11. Girgis K, Hamed H, Khater Y, et al: A decremental PEEP trial identifies the PEEP level that maintains oxygenation post lung recruitment. Respir Care 51:1132-1140, 2006.
12. Amato MBP, Barbas CSV, Medeiros DM, et al: Effect of a protective-ventilation strategy on mortality in the acute respiratory distress syndrome. N Engl J Med 338:347-354, 1998.
13. Villar J, Kacmarek RM, Perez-Mendez L, et al: ARIES Network: A high positive end-expiratory pressure, low tidal volume ventilatory strategy improves outcome in persistent acute respiratory distress syndrome: a randomized, controlled trial. Crit Care Med 34:1311-1318, 2006.
14. Suarez-Sipmann F, Bohm SH, Tusman G, et al: Use of dynamic compliance for open lung positive end-expiratory pressure titration in an experimental study. Crit Care Med 35:214-221, 2007.
15. Haas CF, et al: Patient-determined inspiratory flow during assisted mechanical ventilation. Respir Care 40:716, 1995.
16. Trille AW, Cabello B, Galia F, et al: Reduction of patient-ventilator asynchrony by reducing tidal volume during pressure support ventilation. Intensive Care Med 34:1477-1486, 2008.
17. Sassoon CS, et al: Influence of pressure and flow triggered synchronous intermittent mandatory ventilation on inspiratory muscle work. Crit Care Med 22:1933, 1994.
18. MacIntyre NR: Respiratory system mechanics. In MacIntyre NR, Branson RD, editors: Mechanical ventilation, Philadelphia, 2001, Saunders.
19. Banner MJ, et al: Partially and totally unloading respiratory muscles based on real-time measurements of work of breathing: a clinical approach. Chest 106:1835, 1994.
20. MacIntyre NR: Mechanical ventilation strategies for parenchymal lung injury. In MacIntyre NR, Branson RD, editors: Mechanical ventilation, Philadelphia, 2001, Saunders.
21. Ranieri VM, et al: Physiologic effects of positive end-expiratory pressure in patients with chronic obstructive pulmonary disease during acute ventilatory failure and controlled mechanical ventilation. Am Rev Respir Dis 147:5, 1993.
22. Chiumello D, Polli F, Tallarini F, et al: Effect of different cycling-off criteria and positive end-expiratory pressure during pressure support ventilation in patients with chronic obstructive pulmonary disease. Crit Care Med 35:2547-2552, 2007.
23. Ost D, Corbridge T: Independent lung ventilation. Clin Chest Med 17:591, 1996.
24. Al Saady N, Bennett ED: Decelerating inspiratory flow waveform improves lung mechanics and gas exchange in patients on intermittent positive-pressure ventilation. Intensive Care Med 11:68, 1985.
25. Rattenborg CC, Via-Reque E: Clinical use of mechanical ventilation, St Louis, 1981, Mosby.
26. Chatburn RL, El-Khatib MF, Smith PG: Respiratory system behavior during mechanical inflation with constant inspiratory pressure and flow. Respir Care 42:979, 1994.
27. Natalini G, et al: Pressure-controlled verses volume controlled ventilation with mask airway. J Clin Anesth 13:436, 2001.
28. Slutsky AS: Consensus conference on mechanical ventilation. Intensive Care Med 20:64, 1994.
29. Chatburn RL, Volsko TA, El-Khatib M: The effect of airway leak on tidal volume during pressure- or flow-controlled ventilation of the neonate: a model study. Respir Care 41:728, 1996.
30. Finney SJ, Evans TW: Mechanical ventilation in acute respiratory distress syndrome. Curr Opin Anesthesiol 14:165-171, 2001.
31. Gillette MA, Hess DR: Ventilator-induced lung injury and the evolution of lung protective strategies in acute respiratory distress syndrome. Respir Care 46:130, 2001.
32. Kacmarek RM, Dimas S, Mack C: Essentials of respiratory care, ed 4, St Louis, MO, 2005, Elsevier.
33. McCarthy MC, et al: Pressure control inverse ratio ventilation in the treatment of adult respiratory distress syndrome in patients with blunt chest trauma. Am Surg 6:1027, 1999.
34. Demling R, Riessen R: Pulmonary dysfunction after cerebral injury. Crit Care Med 18:768, 1990.

35. Weisman JM, et al: Intermittent mandatory ventilation. Am Rev Respir Dis 127:641, 1983.
36. Brochard L, et al: Comparison of three methods of gradual withdrawal from ventilatory support during weaning from mechanical ventilation. Am J Respir Crit Care Med 150:896, 1994.
37. Esteban A, Frutos F, Tobin MJ, et al: A comparison of four methods of weaning patients from mechanical ventilation. N Engl J Med 332:345–350, 1995.
38. Calzia E, et al: Stress response during weaning after cardiac surgery. Br J Anaesth 87:490, 2001.
39. Hahn AF: The challenge of respiratory dysfunction in Guillain-Barré syndrome. Arch Neurol 58:893, 2001.
40. Roze JC, et al: Oxygen cost of breathing and weaning process in newborn infants. Eur Respir J 10:2583, 1997.
41. Sinha SK, Donn SM: Volume-controlled ventilation: variations on a theme. Clin Perinatol 28:547, 2001.
42. Putensen C, Zech S, Wrigge H, et al: Long-term effects of spontaneous breathing during ventilatory support in patients with acute lung injury. Am J Respir Crit Care Med 164:43, 2001.
43. Newman P, Golisch J, Strohmeyer A, et al: Influence of different release times on spontaneous breathing pattern during pressure release ventilation. Intensive Care Med 28: 1742, 2002.
44. Davis K, et al: Airway pressure release ventilation. Arch Surg 128:1348, 1993.
45. Sydow M, et al: Long term effects of two different ventilatory modes on oxygenation in acute lung injury. Am J Respir Crit Care Med 149:1550, 1994.
46. Fan E, Stewart TE: New modalities of mechanical ventilation: high frequency oscillatory ventilation and airway pressure release ventilation. Clin Chest Med 27:615–625, 2006.
47. Tunsmann G, et al: Alveolar recruitment strategy improves arterial oxygenation during general anesthesia. Br J Anaesth 82:8, 1999.
48. Kacmarek RM: Proportional assist ventilation and neurally adjusted ventilatory support. Respir Care 56:140–148, 2011.
49. Klerk AM, Klerk RK: Nasal continuous positive airway pressure and outcomes or preterm infants. Neonatal Intensive Care 14:58, 2001.
50. Dinger J, et al: Effect of positive end expiratory pressure on functional residual capacity and compliance in surfactant-treated preterm infants. Neonat Intensive Care 14:26, 2001.
51. Brochard L, Pluskwa F, Lemaire F: Improved efficacy of spontaneous breathing with inspiratory pressure support. Am Rev Respir Dis 136:411, 1987.
52. MacIntyre NR: Pressure support ventilation: effects on ventilatory reflexes and ventilatory muscle workload. Respir Care 32:447, 1987.
53. Brochard L, et al: Pressure support decreases work of breathing and oxygen consumption during weaning from mechanical ventilation (abstract). Am Rev Respir Dis 135:A51, 1987.
54. Grande CM, Kahn RC: The effect of pressure support ventilation on ventilatory variables and work of breathing (abstract). Anesthesiology 65:A84, 1986.
55. MacIntyre NR: Respiratory function during pressure support ventilation. Chest 89:677–683, 1986.
56. Sassoon CSH, Mahutte CK, Light RW: Ventilator modes: old and new. Crit Care Clin 6:605, 1990.
57. Hill NS, Brennan J, Garpestad E, et al: Noninvasive ventilation in acute respiratory failure. Crit Care Med 35:2402–2407, 2007.
58. Gay PC, Hess DR, Hill NS: Noninvasive proportional assist ventilation for acute respiratory insufficiency: comparison with pressure support ventilation. Am J Respir Crit Care Med 164:1606–1611, 2001.
59. Porta R, Appendini L, Vitacca M, et al: Mask proportional assist vs. pressure support ventilation in patients in clinically stable condition with chronic ventilatory failure. Chest 122:479–488, 2002.
60. Wysocki M, Richard JC, Meshaka P: Noninvasive proportional assist ventilation compared with noninvasive pressure support ventilation in hypercapnic acute respiratory failure. Crit Care Med 30;323–329, 2002.
61. Serra A, Polese G, Braggion C, et al: Non-invasive proportional assist and pressure support ventilation in patients with cystic fibrosis and chronic respiratory failure. Thorax 57:50–54, 2002.
62. Rusterholtz T, Bollaert PE, Feissel M, et al: Continuous positive airway pressure vs. proportional assist ventilation for noninvasive ventilation in acute cardiogenic pulmonary edema. Intensive Care Med 34:840–846, 2008.
63. Ranieri VM, Grasso S, Mascia L, et al: Effects of proportional assist ventilation on inspiratory muscle effort in patients with chronic obstructive pulmonary disease and acute respiratory failure. Anesthesiology 86:79–91, 1997.
64. Grasso S, Puntillo F, Mascia L, et al: Compensation for increase in respiratory workload during mechanical ventilation. Am J Respir Crit Care Med 16:819–826, 2000.
65. Xirouchaki N, Kondili E, Vaporidi K, et al: Proportional assist ventilation with load-adjustable gain factors in critically ill patients: comparison with pressure support. Intensive Care Med 34:2026–2034, 2008.
66. Wrigge H, Golisch W, Zinserling J, et al: Proportional assist versus pressure support ventilation: effects on breathing pattern and respiratory work of patients with chronic obstructive pulmonary disease. Intensive Care Med 25:790–798, 1999.
67. Passam F, Hoing S, Prinianakis G, et al: Effect of different levels of pressure support and proportional assist ventilation on breathing pattern work of breathing and gas exchange in mechanically ventilated hypercapnic COPD patients with acute respiratory failure. Respiration 70:355–361, 2003.
68. Delaere S, Roeseler J, D'hoore W, et al: Respiratory muscle workload in intubated, spontaneously breathing patients without COPD: pressure support vs. proportional assist ventilation. Intensive Care Med 29:949–954, 2003.
69. Colombo D, Cammarota G, Bergamaschi V, et al: Physiologic response to varying levels of pressure support and neurally adjusted ventilatory assist in patients with acute respiratory failure. Intensive Care Med 34:1010–2018, 2008.
70. Sgahija J, de Marchie M, Albert M, et al: Patient-ventilator interaction during pressure support ventilation and neurally adjusted ventilatory assist. Crit Care Med 38:518–526, 2010.
71. Passath C, Takala J, Tuchscherer D, et al: Physiological response to changing positive end-expiratory pressure during neurally adjusted ventilatory assist in sedated, critically ill adults. Chest 138:578–587, 2010.
72. Beck J, Reilly M, Grasselli G, et al: Patient-ventilator interaction during neurally adjusted ventilatory assist in low birth weight infants. Pediatr Res 65:663–668, 2009.
73. Bengtsson JA, Edberg KE: Neurally adjusted ventilatory assist in children: an observational study. Pediatr Crit Care Med 11:253–257, 2010.
74. Gutman J, Eberhard L, Fabry B: Continuous calculation of intratracheal pressure in tracheally intubated patients. Anesthesiology 79:503–511, 1993.
75. Fabry B, Haberthur C, Zappe D: Breathing pattern and additional work of breathing in spontaneously breathing patients with different ventilatory demands during inspiratory pressure support and automatic tube compensation. Intensive Care Med 23:545–552, 1997.

76. Amato MB, et al: Volume assure pressure support ventilation: a new approach for reducing muscle workload during acute respiratory failure. Chest 102:1225, 1992.
77. Jaber S, Delay JM, Matecki S, et al: Volume-guaranteed pressure support ventilation facing acute changes in ventilatory demand. Intensive Care Med 31:1181–1188, 2005.
78. Piotrowski A, Sobala W, Kawczynski P: Patient-initiated, pressure-regulated, volume-controlled ventilation compared with intermittent mandatory ventilation in neonates: a prospective, randomised study. Intensive Care Med 23:975–981, 1987.
79. Randolph AG, Wypig D, Venkataraman S, et al: Effect of mechanical ventilator weaning protocols on respiratory outcomes in infants and children: a randomized controlled trial. JAMA 288:2561–2568, 2002.
80. McCallion N, Davis PG, Morley CJ: Volume-targeted versus pressure-limited ventilation in the neonate. Cochrane Database Syst Rev 3:CD003666, 2005.
81. Otis AB: The work of breathing. Physiol Rev 34:449–458, 1954.
82. Branson RD, Chatburn RL: Controversies in the critical care setting: should adaptive pressure control modes be utilized for virtually all patients receiving mechanical ventilation? Respir Care 52: 478–485, 2007.
83. Thompson BT, Hayden D, Matthay MA, et al: Clinicians' approaches to mechanical ventilation in acute lung injury and ARDS. Chest 120:1622–1627, 2001.
84. Hamilton Medical: Adaptive support ventilation. www.hamilton-medical.com, accessed August 2011.
85. Tassaux D, Dalmas E, Gratadour P, et al: Patient-ventilator interactions during partial ventilatory support: a preliminary study comparing the effects of adaptive support ventilation with synchronized intermittent mandatory ventilation plus inspiratory pressure support. Crit Care Med 30:801–807, 2002.
86. Sulzer CF, Chiolero R, Chassot PG, et al: Adaptive support ventilation for fast tracheal extubation after cardiac surgery: a randomized controlled study. Anesthesiology 95:1339–1345, 2001.
87. Belliato M, Palo A, Pasero D, et al: Evaluation of adaptive support ventilation in paralyzed patients and in a physical lung model. Int J Artif Organs 27:709–716, 2004.
88. Sulemanji D, Marchese A, Garbarini P, et al: Adaptive support ventilation: an appropriate mechanical ventilation strategy for acute respiratory distress syndrome? Anesthesiology 111:863–870, 2009.
89 Sulemanji DS, Marchese A, Wysocki M, et al. Adaptive support ventilation with end-tidal CO_2 closed loop control vs. conventional ventilation (in normal settings, ARDS, COPD and brain injury). Society of Critical Care Medicine 40th Critical Care Congress, January 2011, San Diego.
90. Guidelines for prevention of nosocomial pneumonia. MMWR Recomm Rep 46:1, 1997.
91. Taccone P, Pesenti A, Latini R, et al: Prone positioning in patients with moderate and severe acute respiratory distress syndrome: a randomized controlled trial. JAMA 302:1977–1984, 2009.
92. Curley MA: Prone positioning of patients with acute respiratory distress syndrome: a systematic review. Am J Crit Care 8:397, 1999.
93. Mancebo J, Fernandez R, Blanch L, et al: A multicenter trial of prolonged prone ventilation in severe acute respiratory distress syndrome. Am J Respir Crit Care Med 173:1233–1239, 2006.
94. Sud S, Friedrich JO, Taccone P, et al: Prone ventilation reduces mortality in patients with acute respiratory failure and severe hypoxemia: systematic review and meta-analysis. Intensive Care Med 36:585–599, 2010.
95. Pinsky MR: The effects of mechanical ventilation on the cardiovascular system. Crit Care Clin 6:663, 1990.
96. Marini JJ, Ravenscraft SA: Mean airway pressure: physiologic determinants and clinical importance, I: physiologic determinants and measurements. Crit Care Med 20:1461, 1992.
97. Marino PL: The ICU book, ed 3, Philadelphia, 2005, Lippincott Williams & Wilkins.
98. Yundt KD, Diringer MN: The use of hyperventilation and its impact on cerebral ischemia in the treatment of traumatic brain injury. Crit Care Clin 13:163, 1997.
99. Bullock R, et al: The use of hyperventilation in the acute management of severe traumatic brain injury. In Bullock R, et al, editors: Guidelines for the management of severe head injury, New York, 1995, Brain Trauma Foundation.
100. Dive A, et al: Gastroduodenal motility in mechanically ventilated critically ill patients: a manometric study. Crit Care Med 22:441, 1994.
101. Shapiro BA, et al: Practice parameters for intravenous analgesia and sedation for adult patients in the intensive care unit: an executive summary. Crit Care Med 23:1596, 1995.
102. Whitehead T, Slutsky AS: The pulmonary physician in critical care. 7: ventilator-induced lung injury. Thorax 57: 635–642, 2002.
103. Tremblay LN, Slutsky AS: Ventilator-induced lung injury: from the bench to the bedside. Intensive Care Med 32: 24–33, 2006.
104. Plötz FB, Slutzsky AS, van Vught AJ, et al: Ventilator-induced lung injury and multiple system organ failure: a critical review of facts and hypotheses. Intensive Care Med 30:1865–1872, 2004.
105. Slutzky AS, Tremblay LN: Multiple system organ failure: is mechanical ventilation a contributing factor? Am J Respir Crit Care Med 157:1721–1725, 1998.
106. Ranieri VM, Suter PM, Tortella C, et al: Effect of mechanical ventilation on inflammatory mediators in patients with acute respiratory distress syndrome: a randomized controlled trial. JAMA 282:54–61, 1999.
107. Parsons P, Eisner MD, Thompson T, et al: Lower tidal volume ventilation and plasma cytokine markers of inflammation in patients with acute lung injury. Crit Care Med 33:1–6, 2005.
108. Craven DE: Preventing ventilator associated pneumonia in adults. Chest 130:251–260, 2006.
109. Kollef MH, Bekele A, Anzueto A: Silver-coated endotracheal tubes and incidence of ventilator-associated pneumonia: the NASCENT randomized trial. JAMA 300:805–813, 2008.
110. Dezfulian C, Shojania K, Collard HR, et al: Subglottic secretion drainage preventing ventilator associated pneumonia: a meta-analysis. Am J Respir Crit Care Med 118:11–18, 2005.
111. Pitts R, Fisher D, Sulemanji D, et al: Variables affecting leakage past endotracheal tube cuffs: a bench study. Intensive Care Med 36:2066–2073, 2010.
112. Torres A, Ewig S, Lode H, et al: European HAP working group: Defining, treating and preventing hospital acquired pneumonia: European experience. Intensive Care Med 35:9–29, 2009.

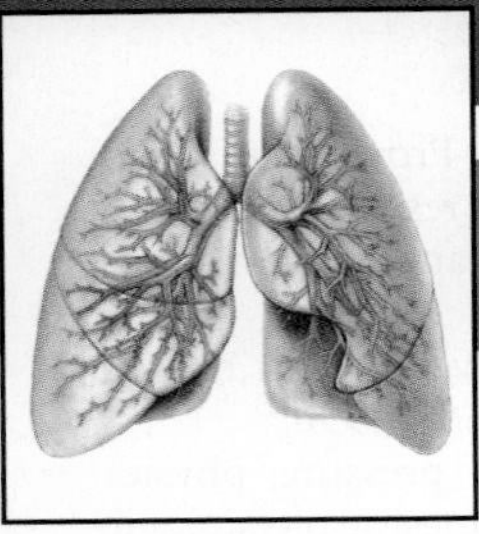

Chapter 44

Initiating and Adjusting Invasive Ventilatory Support

ROBERT M. KACMAREK

CHAPTER OBJECTIVES

After reading this chapter you will be able to:

- Discuss the goals of ventilatory support.
- Describe how to choose an appropriate ventilator to begin ventilatory support.
- Explain how to select an appropriate mode of ventilation given a patient's specific condition and ventilatory requirements.
- Choose appropriate initial ventilator settings, based on patient assessment.
- Describe how to assess a patient after initiation of ventilation.
- Discuss how to adjust ventilatory support based on oxygenation and ventilation status.
- Discuss how to ventilate using the concept of lung protective ventilation.
- Discuss asynchrony and how ventilator adjustments in pressure and volume ventilation improve asynchrony.
- Explain how to adjust the ventilator on the basis of the patient's response.

CHAPTER OUTLINE

KEY TERMS

- assist-control volume ventilation
- controlled ventilation
- full ventilatory support
- high-frequency oscillatory ventilation (HFOV)
- lung protective ventilatory strategy
- neurally adjusted ventilatory assistance (NAVA)
- partial ventilatory support
- plateau pressure (P_{plat})
- pressure-controlled ventilation (PCV)
- pressure-regulated volume control (PRVC)
- pressure support ventilation (PSV)
- proportional assist ventilation (PAV)
- synchronized intermittent mandatory ventilation (SIMV)
- transpulmonary pressure
- volume-controlled ventilation
- volume support

Mechanical ventilation entails the use of sophisticated life-support technology aimed at maintaining tissue oxygenation and removal of carbon dioxide (CO_2). At its most basic level, mechanical ventilation supports or replaces the normal ventilatory pump, moving air into and out of the lungs. The primary function of a mechanical ventilator is simply to ventilate. The main indication for mechanical ventilation is inadequate or absent spontaneous breathing.

Mechanical ventilation is not without risk, and the complications and hazards can be life-threatening. The decision to initiate mechanical ventilatory support is a serious one that requires sound clinical judgment and a clear understanding of the various approaches to ventilatory support. This chapter reviews and describes the initial setup of the ventilator. After ventilator initiation, adjustments in ventilatory support are made on the basis of the patient's response. Techniques for patient stabilization; methods for optimizing oxygenation, ventilation, synchrony, and acid-base balance; and methods for minimizing harmful side effects are described.

GOALS OF MECHANICAL VENTILATION

The goals of mechanical ventilatory support are to maintain adequate alveolar ventilation and oxygen (O_2) delivery, restore acid-base balance, and reduce the work of breathing (WOB) with minimum harmful side effects and complications.[1] Mechanical ventilation also may reduce increased myocardial work secondary to hypoxemia and an increased WOB.[1] Other physiologic objectives of mechanical ventilatory support include increasing or maintaining lung volume with positive end expiratory pressure (PEEP) and continuous positive airway pressure (CPAP) for promotion, improvement, or maintenance of lung recruitment.[1]

A **lung protective ventilatory strategy** is an approach to mechanical ventilation that includes the use of small tidal volume (V_T) and appropriate levels of PEEP.[2] This approach is usually employed in patients with acute lung injury (ALI) or the acute respiratory distress syndrome (ARDS). However, the concept of lung protection should be applied to all patients requiring ventilatory support for acute respiratory failure. Lung injury is primarily caused by an elevated transpulmonary pressure during positive pressure ventilation.[3] **Transpulmonary pressure** is the difference between alveolar pressure and pleural pressure. A safe transpulmonary pressure during mechanical ventilation is not firmly established, but most clinicians would agree that the lower the transpulmonary pressure, the less likely the development of ventilator-induced lung injury.[4] High transpulmonary pressures are associated with alveolar overdistention and lung injury.[3]

Plateau pressure (P_{plat}), the end inspiratory equilibration pressure, measures the mean peak alveolar pressure and is the best bedside clinical reflection of transpulmonary pressure.[2,4,5] Although P_{plat} is not an accurate measurement of transpulmonary pressure, the transpulmonary pressure never exceeds the P_{plat}.[4] P_{plat} provides an excellent bedside assessment of the level of potentially dangerous ventilating pressure. Limiting P_{plat} reduces the likelihood of ventilator-induced lung injury. Generally, the lower the P_{plat}, the better the patient outcome.[2,5] Ideally, P_{plat} should be less than 30 cm H_2O.[5] However, a P_{plat} greater than 30 cm H_2O may be applied in patients with a decreased thoracic compliance without resulting in overdistention[5] because a decrease in chest wall compliance (obesity, massive fluid resuscitation, abdominal distention, elevated bladder pressure) increases the pleural pressure, decreasing the transpulmonary pressure. Generally, the lowest possible P_{plat} is maintained by selecting a V_T of 4 to 8 ml/kg of ideal body weight (IBW). The higher the P_{plat}, the smaller the V_T should be. Generally, V_T greater than 10 ml/kg IBW is never indicated in critically ill patients.

Lung injury can also be caused by repetitive opening and closing of unstable lung units.[6] The application of an appropriate level of PEEP ensures that unstable lung units are maintained in the open position reducing the likelihood of additional lung injury.

Specific clinical objectives of mechanical ventilation include reversal of hypoxemia, hypercapnia, and associated respiratory acidosis and prevention or reversal of ventilatory muscle dysfunction. The general trajectory of pH,

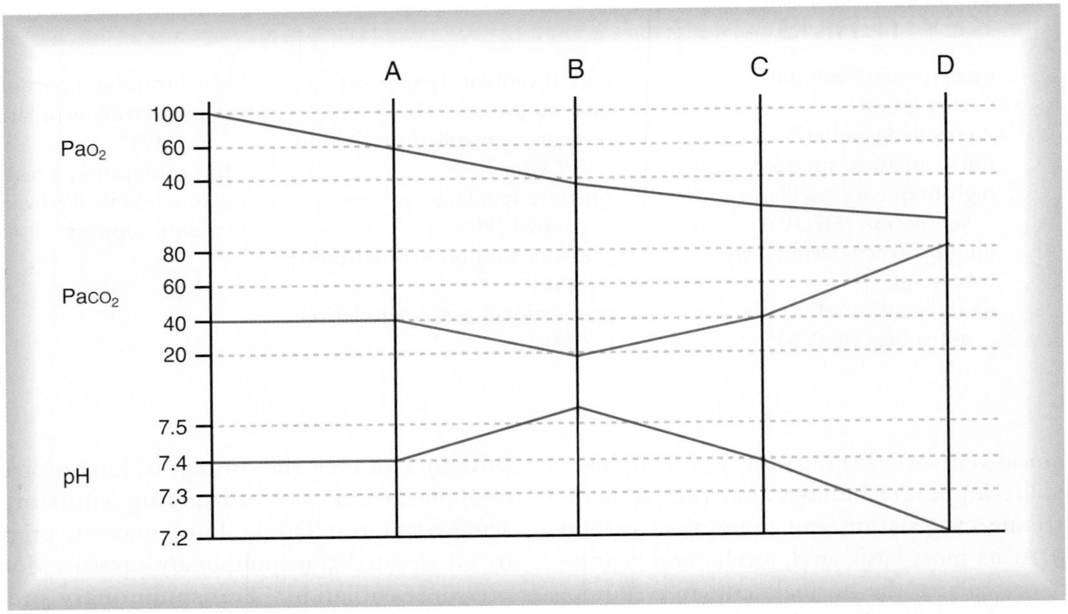

FIGURE 44-1 Typical progression of acute respiratory failure. Initially, there is a decline in arterial O_2 tension and saturation. When PaO_2 decreases to approximately 60 mm Hg *(A)*, the patient begins to breathe more, $PaCO_2$ decreases, and pH increases. Early in the progression, arterial blood gas results show acute alveolar hyperventilation (uncompensated respiratory alkalosis) secondary to hypoxemia. As the patient's condition worsens, increases in ventilatory workload typically lead to the adoption of a rapid, shallow breathing pattern; although minute ventilation may remain high, effective ventilation decreases, $PaCO_2$ begins to increase, and pH begins to decrease *(B)*. At point *C*, arterial blood gas results may show normal $PaCO_2$ and pH with moderate to severe hypoxemia. If mechanical ventilation is not initiated, the patient's condition may progress to acute ventilatory failure, severe hypoxemia, and corresponding severe respiratory acidosis *(D)*.

PCO_2, and PO_2 during the progression of acute respiratory failure is depicted in Figure 44-1. Mechanical ventilation may be used to allow sedation or paralysis for certain procedures, to decrease myocardial and ventilatory muscle O_2 consumption to maximize O_2 delivery to the tissues, to decrease intracranial pressure acutely in the presence of closed head injury or cerebral edema (by reducing $PaCO_2$ to 25 to 30 mm Hg for a short period and promoting cerebral vasoconstriction), to prevent or reverse atelectasis, and to stabilize the chest wall in the case of a massive flail or chest wall resection. Table 44-1 lists the most common causes of acute respiratory failure leading to ventilatory support in the United States and Canada. Hazards of mechanical ventilation include decreased venous return and cardiac output, patient-ventilatory asynchrony, and ventilatory muscle dysfunction owing to inappropriate ventilator settings, ventilator-associated pneumonia, and ventilator-induced lung injury.[1] Box 44-1 lists the goals of ventilatory support, and Box 44-2 lists specific objectives of mechanical ventilation.

TABLE 44-1

Most Common Causes of Acute Respiratory Failure Requiring Mechanical Ventilation in the United States and Canada

Condition	Rank	Percentage
Postoperative respiratory failure	1	17
Sepsis	1	17
Other	2	16
Heart failure	3	13
Pneumonia	3	13
Trauma	3	13
ARDS	4	9
Aspiration	5	3

Modified form Esteban A, Anzueto A, Alia I, et al: How is mechanical ventilation employed in the intensive care unit? An international utilization review. Am J Respir Crit Care Med 161:1450, 2000.

VENTILATOR INITIATION

When the decision to begin mechanical ventilatory support is made, one must choose the mode of ventilation, select an appropriate device, and establish the initial ventilator settings. In the selection of initial ventilator settings, the goal is to optimize the patient's oxygenation, ventilation, and acid-base balance, while avoiding harmful side effects. This goal is achieved by choosing an appropriate mode of ventilation, fractional inspired oxygen (FiO_2), V_T (volume ventilation) or pressure level (pressure ventilation), rate, peak flow and flow waveform, inspiratory time, and PEEP level. Appropriate trigger sensitivity, pressure limit, alarms,

Box 44-1 Physiologic Goals of Ventilatory Support

- Support or manipulate gas exchange
- Alveolar ventilation ($PaCO_2$ and pH)
- Arterial oxygenation (PaO_2, SaO_2, SpO_2, CaO_2, and DO_2)
- Increase lung volume
- End inspiratory and end expiratory lung inflation
- Functional residual capacity (FRC)
- Reduce or manipulate WOB
- Minimize cardiovascular impairment
- Ensure patient-ventilatory synchrony
- Avoid ventilator-induced lung injury

Box 44-2 Specific Clinical Objectives of Ventilatory Support

- To reverse hypoxemia
- To reverse acute respiratory acidosis
- To relieve respiratory distress
- To prevent or reverse atelectasis
- To reverse ventilatory muscle dysfunction
- To allow sedation and neuromuscular blockade
- To decrease systemic or myocardial O_2 consumption
- To maintain or improve cardiac output
- To reduce intracranial pressure
- To stabilize the chest

From Slutsky AS: Mechanical ventilation. American College of Chest Physicians' Consensus Conference. Chest 104:1833–1859, 1993.

Box 44-3 Initial Ventilator Setup

Initial ventilator setup includes the following key decisions:

- Noninvasive vs. invasive ventilation
- Type and method of establishment of an airway
- Partial vs. full ventilatory support
- Choice of ventilator
- Mode of ventilation
- Assist-control ventilation (volume vs. pressure) vs. SIMV (with or without pressure support)
- Pressure support
- Other newer modes and adjuncts to ventilation

Next, the clinician must consider key ventilatory values:

- Trigger method (pressure or flow trigger) and sensitivity
- V_T (volume ventilation) or pressure level (pressure support and PA/C)
- Rate
- Inspiratory flow, inspiratory time, expiratory time, or I : E ratio
- Inspiratory flow waveform
- FiO_2
- PEEP/CPAP

Last, the clinician must choose appropriate alarm and backup values:

- Low-pressure, low PEEP alarms
- High-pressure limit and alarm
- Volume alarms (low V_T/high V_T, high and low minute ventilation)
- High rate and low rate alarms
- Apnea alarm and apnea ventilation values
- High/low O_2 alarm
- High/low temperature alarm
- I : E ratio limit and alarm

backup ventilation, and humidification must be selected. After initial ventilator setup, adjustments must be made on the basis of the patient's response and the patient-specific clinical objectives of ventilatory support. Most patients who need mechanical ventilatory support receive invasive positive pressure ventilation; however, an increasing number of patients are being ventilated noninvasively (see Chapter 46). Next, the clinician must choose the mode of ventilation (e.g., volume assist/control [VA/C], pressure assist/control [PA/C], pressure support ventilation [PSV], **pressure regulated volume control [PRVC], volume support,** adaptive support ventilation, **proportional assist ventilation [PAV],** or **neurally adjusted ventilatory assist [NAVA]**) and initial ventilator settings (e.g., rate, V_T or pressure level, FiO_2, PEEP). Finally, the clinician must choose appropriate alarm and apnea settings. Box 44-3 summarizes key decisions that must be made as a part of initial ventilator setup.

Noninvasive Ventilation

Although more than 75% to 80% of all patients receiving ventilatory assistance receive it invasively, the use of noninvasive ventilation should be considered in select patients requiring ventilatory assistance. Noninvasive ventilation is preferred in some patients because the outcomes are better. Chapter 46 provides details on all aspects on noninvasive ventilation.

Establishment of the Airway

Conventional mechanical ventilatory support requires the establishment of an artificial airway. Initially, nearly 100% of patients receiving positive pressure ventilation are intubated, and of these, 99% have oral endotracheal tubes, and only about 1% are intubated nasally.[7] Approximately 5% to 10% of patients receiving mechanical ventilation have a tracheotomy performed at some point.[7] Airway management is described in detail in Chapter 33.

Pressure-Controlled versus Volume-Controlled Ventilation

The next decision to be made regarding initiation of mechanical ventilation is whether to use a primarily pressure-targeted or volume-targeted mode of ventilation. Volume-targeted ventilation essentially includes VA/C and synchronized intermittent mandatory ventilation (SIMV). Pressure ventilation includes PA/C, SIMV, PRVC, volume support, and airway pressure release ventilation. In addition, the clinician can select the patient controlled modes PAV or NAVA. However, most patients are initially ventilated with pressure or volume forms of ventilation. The operational capabilities of these modes are described in detail in Chapter 42, and the indications, benefits, and concerns regarding these modes are discussed in Chapter 43.

Full Ventilatory Support versus Partial Ventilatory Support

Full ventilatory support can be defined as the application of mechanical support such that all or most of the energy necessary for effective alveolar ventilation is provided by the ventilator.[8] When a ventilator is set to deliver full ventilatory support, the patient is either passive or simply triggers the breath to initiate inspiration allowing the ventilator to perform most of the work of breathing. However, it is very difficult to set the ventilator to assume all of the work of breathing without significantly sedating the patient. In most patient-triggered approaches to ventilatory support, patient-ventilatory synchrony is a major issue, and very careful titration of the ventilator settings is necessary to ensure synchrony and minimize patient WOB. Patient-ventilatory synchrony is discussed in detail later in the chapter.

Partial ventilatory support implies that only a percentage of the WOB is provided by the ventilator.[8] Normally, when partial ventilatory support is indicated, SIMV, PSV, volume support, PAV, and NAVA are the modes of choice. However, as with full ventilatory support, care in setting the ventilatory is critical to ensure that patient-ventilator synchrony is maximized. Partial ventilatory support strategies minimize the loss of ventilatory muscle function, require less sedation, assist in recruiting and stabilizing alveolar units, and generally move patients closer to ventilator discontinuance than full ventilatory support approaches.

Choice of a Ventilator

After the decision is made to initiate mechanical ventilator support, the clinician must select an appropriate ventilator. This decision should be guided by considering the features, modes available, pressure and flow capabilities, alarms and monitoring systems included, and reliability. However, the most important feature is the clinician's familiarity with the equipment. Only a ventilator with which the clinician is totally familiar with every feature should ever be used.

INITIAL VENTILATOR SETTINGS

Initial ventilator settings are chosen based on the patient's clinical presentation and the need to provide full or partial ventilator support.

Choice of Mode

Most modern critical care ventilators include VA/C, PA/C, SIMV, and PSV and many of the newer modes of ventilation. However, some modes of ventilation are found only on a specific type of ventilator, such as PAV PB 840 (Covidien-Nellcor, Boulder, Colorado), adaptive support ventilation Hamilton ventilators (Hamilton Medical, Bonaduz, Switzerland), NAVA Servo-i ventilator (Maquet, Inc, Wayne, New Jersey), and SmartCare Draeger XL (Draeger Medical, Inc, Telford, Pennsylvania).

Assist-Control Ventilation (Patient-Triggered or Time-Triggered Continuous Mandatory Ventilation)

Assist-control ventilation can be delivered in either pressure-targeted or volume-targeted ventilation. Suggested initial settings for **assist-control volume ventilation** in the care of adults are listed in Box 44-4. Advantages of assist-control volume ventilation include the assurance that a minimum safe level of ventilation is achieved, yet the patient can still set his or her own breathing rate. In the event of sedation or apnea, a minimum safe level of ventilation is guaranteed by the selection of an appropriate backup rate, usually approximately 4 to 6 breaths/min less than the patient's assist rate but not less than the rate necessary to provide a minimum safe level of ventilation (e.g., a backup rate of at least 12 to 14 breaths/min).[8]

Because assist-control ventilation usually provides full ventilatory support, it may result in less WOB than partial

Box 44-4 Typical Values for Ventilator Initiation for Adults Receiving Volume or Pressure Assist-Control Ventilation

- Trigger sensitivity: −0.5 to −1.5 cm H_2O or 2 to 3 L/min set to minimize trigger work without autocycling
- V_T: Volume ventilation 6 to 8 ml/kg IBW; pressure ventilation, pressure level to achieve 6 to 8 ml/kg IBW
- Rate: Backup rate of ≥12 to 14 breaths/min if providing controlled ventilation
- Inspiratory flow: Volume ventilation 60 to 80 L/min to achieve inspiratory time of approximately <1 second and I:E ratio of ≤1:2; inspiratory flow ≥80 L/min may be required in the care of some patients to meet or exceed the patient's spontaneous inspiratory flow demand
- Flow waveform volume ventilation: Decreasing ramp
- Inspiratory time pressure ventilation: <1.0 second
- PEEP: 5 cm H_2O
- Pressure limit: Start at 30 to 40 cm H_2O depending on approach (volume 40 cm H_2O, pressure 30 cm H_2O) and adjust after patient connection to 10 to 15 cm H_2O above PIP
- Humidification: Begin with heated humidifier to provide temperature 35° C at the airway connection or appropriate HME

MINI CLINI

Selecting Initial Ventilator Settings

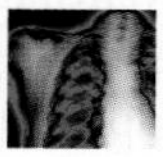

PROBLEM: A 52-year-old man, 5 ft 10 in (178 cm) tall and weighing 200 lb (91 kg), is being returned from the operating room after coronary artery bypass surgery. He is being manually (bag-tube) ventilated with supplemental O_2 by the anesthesiologist en route to the ICU. He is apneic at this time. The patient has no history of lung disease and has never smoked cigarettes. Heart rate and blood pressure are stable, and SpO_2 during manual ventilation is 99%. What initial mode, V_T, rate, and FiO_2 should the RT select when starting ventilatory support for this patient?

SOLUTION: The patient is apneic at this time but is likely to resume spontaneous breathing as the anesthetic wears off and sedation is reduced. Because the patient is expected to resume breathing spontaneously, volume ventilation or pressure ventilation in either assist-control or SIMV is appropriate.

Initial V_T and rate should be selected to provide full ventilatory support. Generally, initial V_T of approximately 6 to 8 ml/kg IBW or pressure control setting to establish this V_T with a rate of 12 to 20 breaths/min provides an adequate starting minute ventilation for most adult patients. The formulas for estimating IBW are:

$$\text{IBW in kilograms (men)} = [106 + 6(H - 60)]/2.2$$
$$\text{IBW in kilograms (women)} = [105 + 5(H - 60)]/2.2$$

where H is height in inches.

For this patient:

$$\text{IBW} = [106 + 6(70 - 60)]/2.2 = 75.5\ \text{kg}$$

On the basis of IBW of 75.5 kg, initial V_T can be set at about 600 ml. Initial inspiratory flow should be set at 60 L/min with a decreasing ramp flow waveform to achieve an inspiratory time of approximately 1 second. Initially, rate can be set at 12/min. Because the patient has a normal respiratory system and it is usual to return from the operating room with a below-normal body temperature, a low initial control rate is indicated. Trigger sensitivity (assist-control or SIMV) should be set so that minimal patient effort triggers the ventilator without autocycling.

Initial FiO_2 should be set at 1.0, but because of the patient's history and the presence of normal lung function, it is expected that it will be reduced rapidly as the patient recovers. Initial PEEP is set at 5 cm H_2O. If the SIMV mode is chosen, PSV should be started at 10 cm H_2O and adjusted as needed when the patient resumes spontaneous breathing.

In summary, appropriate initial ventilator settings for this patient are:

Mode: Assist-control (volume or pressure) or SIMV (volume or pressure) with PSV

V_T: 8 ml/kg, 600 ml

f_{mach}: 12 breaths/min

PSV: 10 cm H_2O (SIMV mode only)

FiO_2: 1.0 followed by immediate assessment and SpO_2 observation with titration downward as indicated

Inspiratory flow and time: 60 L/min, decreasing ramp, inspiratory time approximately 1 second

Pressure limit: 30 cm H_2O and adjust to 10 to 15 cm H_2O above PIP after patient connection

Humidification: Heated humidifier to achieve temperature >35° C at the airway or an appropriate HME

support modes. However, less WOB should not be assumed just because the patient is in assist-control ventilation. Trigger work may be significant if inappropriate sensitivity settings are selected. In addition, when a breath is triggered, inspiratory muscle activity persists.[9,10] If the inspiratory flow rate during volume ventilation does not meet or exceed the patient's inspiratory demand, or inspiratory time is too lengthy, the patient's WOB may be greater, equaling or exceeding the work of a spontaneous unassisted breath.[9,10] In pressure ventilation, lengthy inspiratory times, inadequate rise time, and improperly set pressure levels can also cause asynchrony. (See later sections focusing on patient-ventilator synchrony.)

If properly applied and tolerated by the patient, assist-control ventilation may provide ventilatory muscle rest that allows the ventilatory muscles to recover from ventilatory muscle dysfunction. Disadvantages of assist-control mode include an increase in WOB.[8,11] Assist control also may be poorly tolerated by awake, nonsedated patients. The patient may fight the ventilator, or asynchronous patient-to-ventilator breathing patterns may develop. Because flow is based on patient demand in pressure-targeted ventilation, synchrony is generally better achieved during PA/C than with VA/C ventilation. Advantages and disadvantages of **pressure-controlled ventilation (PCV)** are described in Box 44-5.

Assist-control volume ventilation is the most common ventilator mode used throughout the world as the primary initial mode of ventilatory support.[7,12] Regardless of the indication for ventilatory support or underlying disease, this mode is able when properly adjusted and the patient is properly managed to provide adequate ventilatory support for all indications for ventilatory support.[6,12]

Controlled Ventilation (Time-Triggered Continuous Mandatory Ventilation)

Controlled ventilation, pressure, or volume is achieved using the assist-control mode when the patient is apneic because of a medical condition, anesthesia, or use of sedative drugs and paralytic agents. Ventilators in use today do not prevent a patient with sufficient effort from triggering the ventilator, a situation always to be avoided. Controlled ventilation can be achieved only with pharmacologic agents. Advantages of controlled ventilation

Box 44-5 Advantages and Disadvantages of Pressure-Controlled Ventilation

ADVANTAGES

- Variable flow results in square pressure waveform and improves gas distribution
- Ensures that P_{plat} cannot exceed set pressure control level
- All alveoli are placed under the same sustained inspiratory pressure, which decreases hyperinflation of more compliant alveoli compared with volume ventilation square wave flow
- Sustained inspiratory pressure may result in more alveolar recruitment
- Improved gas distribution allows for lower V_T
- Lower PIP is achieved compared with that achieved with volume ventilation with a square flow waveform

DISADVANTAGES

- Higher mean airway pressure can decrease venous return and decrease cardiac output if preload is inadequate
- V_T varies depending on lung compliance, resistance, and patient effort
- If V_T or minute ventilation alarms are not set properly, alveolar hypoventilation and acidosis may not be detected

include eliminating WOB and complete control over the patient's ventilatory pattern. In cases in which WOB is high, controlled ventilation may allow for ventilatory muscle rest, reduce O_2 consumption of the ventilatory muscles, and "free up" O_2 for delivery to the tissues.[8]

Controlled ventilation is a common initial approach in situations of severe acute respiratory failure especially if the primary problem is hypoxemia. Figure 44-2 depicts the effects of inspiratory time on V_T during controlled ventilation. Disadvantages of controlled ventilation include the need for sedatives and perhaps paralytic drugs. All patients given paralytic drugs must be sedated adequately because paralysis does not alter the patients' perception of their surroundings. All patients' senses are active; none are affected by paralysis; only voluntary muscles are paralyzed. In addition, in the care of apneic patients, ventilator malfunction or disconnection can lead to death.

Synchronized Intermittent Mandatory Ventilation

Synchronized intermittent mandatory ventilation (SIMV) may be used as a means of providing partial or full ventilatory support.[8] With SIMV, the machine breath may be volume or pressure targeted; in adults, it is typically a volume-targeted breath. SIMV often is combined with pressure support to overcome the imposed work of

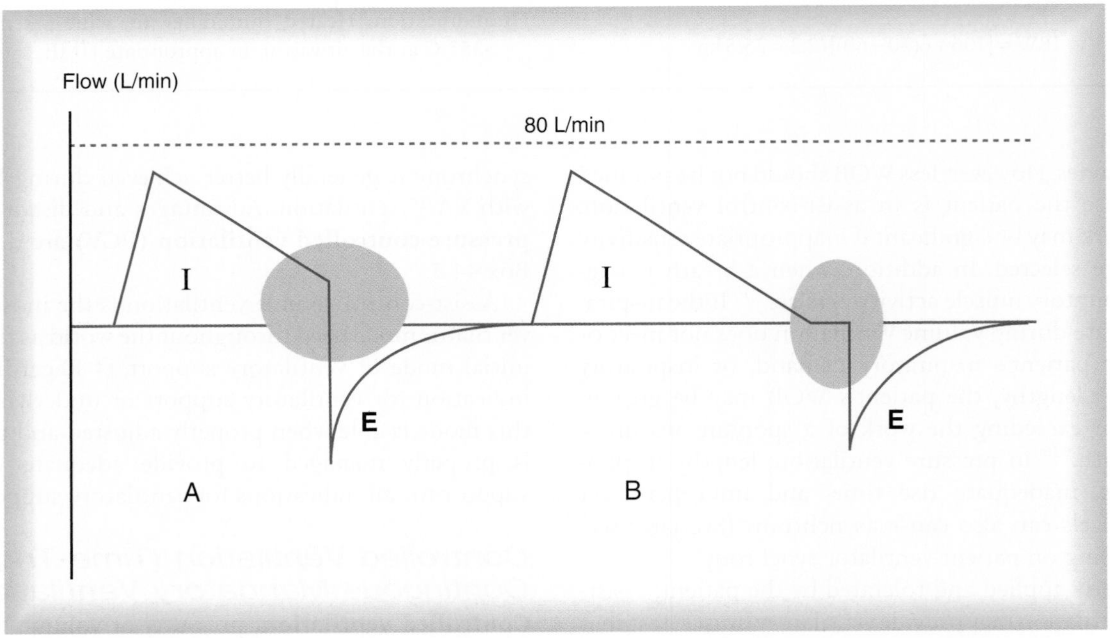

FIGURE 44-2 Flow versus time waveform during PCV. *Curve A* shows a flow pattern during controlled ventilation in which inspiratory time *(I)* is inadequate to ensure maximum V_T has been delivered. During inspiration, flow does not decrease to zero before exhalation occurs, so the preset pressure has not equilibrated to that in the lung. *Curve B* shows an increase in I from *curve A*. Inspiratory flow reaches zero maximizing V_T delivery and allows the preset pressure to equilibrate in the lungs. Exhaled V_T is greater for *curve B* than for *curve A* despite the pressure setting not changing.

breathing (WOB_I) during spontaneous breathing owing to the artificial airway. SIMV allows the clinician to vary the amount of support provided from minimal to full ventilatory support. Disadvantages of SIMV include possible development of respiratory muscle dysfunction, especially in patients with rapid, shallow spontaneous breathing patterns; acute hypoventilation with use of low rates if patients do not continue to do their share of breathing; and an increase in WOB secondary to lack of ventilatory support during spontaneous breaths unless pressure support is applied.[8] SIMV also delays weaning compared with spontaneous breathing trials or pressure support.[13,14] The advantages and disadvantages of assist-control and SIMV modes are summarized in Table 44-2. Outside of the United States, SIMV is an infrequently used mode of ventilation because of the above-mentioned problems.

Pressure Support Ventilation

Pressure support ventilation (PSV) assumes minimal control over the patient's ventilatory pattern. Specifically, only the level of pressure applied is controlled by the ventilator, and all other aspects of gas delivery are controlled by the patient. However, PSV is very similar to PA/C. The primary difference is that in PSV flow terminates the breath, whereas in PA/C time terminates the breath. Other than this, PA/C has a backup rate, and with pressure support an apnea mode of ventilation is set.[15] PSV can reduce work of breathing and may improve patient-ventilator synchrony by placing more control with the patient.[16] Many clinicians use PSV simply to overcome WOB imposed by the artificial airway.[16] The PSV level needed to overcome WOB_I may be estimated as follows:

$$PSV = \frac{(PIP - P_{plat}) \times \dot{V}_I \text{ spontaneous}}{\dot{V} \text{ ventilator}}$$

where PSV is the pressure support level needed to overcome WOB_I, PIP is the peak inspiratory pressure during a volume-control machine breath, P_{plat} is the plateau pressure after an inspiratory pause (usually >1 second), $\dot{V}_I$ is the patient's spontaneous peak inspiratory flow (L/sec), and $\dot{V}$ ventilator is the ventilator peak inspiratory flow rate (L/sec) with a square wave inspiratory flow waveform. An example of the calculations for PSV needed to overcome WOB_I is presented in Box 44-6.

PSV can and is increasingly being used as a primary mode of ventilation. PSV is essentially the only mode of ventilation used during noninvasive ventilation. It is also an acceptable mode of ventilation for any patients capable of triggering ventilatory support who have an intact ventilatory drive. Many clinicians use this mode in the initial phases of ventilatory support and following the most acute phase of ventilatory failure. The actual PSV level needed is based on the desired V_T. PSV is adjusted to ensure the

TABLE 44-2

Advantages and Disadvantages of Synchronized Intermittent Mandatory Ventilation

Advantages	Disadvantages
Lower mean airway pressure may result than is achieved with assist-control ventilation	SIMV with PSV may increase mean airway pressure
Ventilatory muscle activity, strength, and coordination are maintained	Ventilatory muscle fatigue may occur
Level of support to maintain adequate levels of alveolar ventilation is easy to titrate	Acute hypoventilation may occur, especially with lower machine rates (<8-10 breaths/min)
Weaning protocols are easy to apply	Weaning may be prolonged
Spontaneous breathing, which is physiologic, is incorporated	Addition of pressure support often is required to overcome WOB_I
Patients tend not to hyperventilate and may not fight the ventilator, as they may do with assist mode	Patients may have difficulty adjusting to the ventilator; breath stacking is possible with intermittent mandatory ventilation
Sedation or paralysis is not required, as it is in control mode	Patients may experience or continue a rapid, shallow breathing pattern or continue to make spontaneous breathing efforts during delivery of a "machine breath"
Full or partial ventilatory support and level of support can be titrated according to patient's need	Patient's workload increases considerably when SIMV rate decreases to approximately 50% of full ventilatory support value

Box 44-6 Calculation of Pressure Support Ventilation Level Needed to Overcome Imposed Work of Breathing and During Synchronized Intermittent Mandatory Ventilation

- Machine delivered V_T during VA/C: 450 ml
- Machine inspiratory flow rate: 50 L/min (1 L/sec)
- Flow pattern: Square wave
- PIP: 25 cm H_2O
- P_{plat}: 23 cm H_2O
- Patient's spontaneous inspiratory flow rate: 30 L/min (0.5 L/sec)

$$PSV = \frac{(PIP - P_{plat}) \times \dot{V}_I \text{ spontaneous}}{\text{Ventilator inspiratory flow}}$$
$$= \frac{(40 - 30 \text{ cm } H_2O) \times 0.5 \text{ L/s}}{1 \text{ L/s}}$$
$$= \frac{10 \text{ cm } H_2O \times 0.5 \text{ L/s}}{\text{L/s}} = 5 \text{ cm } H_2O$$

desired V_T is delivered, and rise time and termination criteria are set to avoid asynchrony. Few clinicians at the present time attempt to calculate PSV level based on the previously listed formula.

High-Frequency Oscillatory Ventilation

High-frequency oscillatory ventilation (HFOV) is the primary approach to high-frequency ventilation used in adults. Respiratory rates range from about 3 Hz (180/min) to about 8 Hz (480/min), and very small V_T, often approaching anatomic dead space, is delivered.[17] Gas transport during HFOV is due to conventional bulk flow, longitudinal (Taylor) dispersion, pendelluft, asymmetric velocity profiles, cardiogenic mixing, or enhanced molecular diffusion.[17] Although high-frequency ventilation has been shown to be safe and effective in maintaining oxygenation and ventilation in various patients,[17-19] HFOV has not been shown to be superior to conventional ventilation. The primary setting where HFOV has been used is in the treatment of ARDS, but randomized trials comparing the two indicate no difference in outcome. Most clinicians consider HFOV and conventional ventilation equivalent in their ability to manage ARDS. Many clinicians wait until the patient reaches a critical level of illness before instituting HFOV; however, if one considers HFOV the better approach to managing ARDS, it should be started early in the course of ARDS instead of waiting and using it only as a rescue technique. High-frequency ventilation may allow for reduction in airway pressure and may have value as part of a lung protective strategy for the management of ARDS.[19]

Initial Choice of Mode

Most patients who need mechanical ventilation in the acute care setting initially are managed with volume or pressure ventilation in the assist-control mode or with PSV.[7,12] SIMV may also be used, but it has no advantage over these modes, and it has considerable disadvantages. However, there is no evidence suggesting any of the modes are more beneficial in terms of patient outcomes except that weaning is delayed with SIMV.[13,14] Consequently, the choice of initial ventilator mode is primarily one of clinician preference and patient tolerance. Once the patient is stabilized on a ventilator mode, decisions can be made regarding the use of other, newer modes of ventilation, such as PRVC, volume support, adaptive support ventilation, PAV, or NAVA.

> **RULE OF THUMB**
>
> *For most patients, begin mechanical ventilatory support with VA/C, PA/C, or PSV. When the patient is stabilized, other modes of ventilation can be considered.*

Tidal Volume and Rate

V_T and machine rate should be chosen concurrently because these are the two major determinants of minute ventilation. Normal spontaneous V_T for unstressed adults is on average 6.3 ml/kg IBW (approximately 5 to 7 ml/kg IBW) with a respiratory rate of 12 to 18 breaths/min establishing a minute ventilation of approximately 100 ml/kg IBW per minute.[20] In the past, the Radford nomogram was used to estimate V_T and rate on the basis of estimated body weight (Figure 44-3). In modern practice, acceptable V_T for mechanical ventilation usually ranges from 4 to 10 ml/kg IBW,[1,5] although V_T larger than 8 ml/kg IBW is harmful in patients with ALI/ARDS[2,21,22] and is mostly harmful to any patient in acute respiratory failure regardless of the cause of the failure.

Generally, regardless of mode, an initial V_T of 6 to 8 ml/kg IBW with a rate of 12 to 16 breaths/min is suggested for patients without acute restrictive disease.[5,23] After initiation of ventilation, the P_{plat} can be assessed, and V_T can be adjusted downward, as needed, for maintenance of a P_{plat} less than 30 cm H_2O. A smaller initial V_T (4 to 6 ml/kg IBW) is appropriate for patients with ALI/ARDS[2,20,21] with high P_{plat} and is usually necessary in patients with severe acute asthma. Table 44-3 lists V_T values for men and women according to calculated IBW.

> **RULE OF THUMB**
>
> *When starting ventilatory support for most adult patients, use an initial V_T of 6 to 8 ml/kg (IBW) and a respiratory rate of 12 to 16 breaths/min.*

V_T times rate (f) determines minute ventilation ($\dot{V}_E$) As a rule, for adult patients, the resultant minute ventilation should be approximately 80 to 100 ml/kg IBW per minute.[8] A 70-kg adult (IBW) would have a minute ventilation of approximately 7000 ml/min. Patients with elevated CO_2 production ($\dot{V}CO_2$) or increased physiologic dead space (V_{Dphys}) need a larger minute ventilation to maintain acceptable $PaCO_2$. Minute volume should be increased by increasing the rate, not the V_T.

In SIMV, the total minute ventilation is composed of spontaneous tidal volume (V_{Tsp}), spontaneous rate (f_{sp}), machine tidal volume (V_{Tmach}), and machine rate (f_{mach}). For SIMV, total minute ventilation ($\dot{V}_{E\,TOT}$) is described as follows:

$$\dot{V}_{E\,TOT} = \dot{V}_E \text{ machine} + \dot{V}_E \text{ spontaneous}$$

and

$$\dot{V}_E = (V_{Tmach} \times f_{mach}) + (V_{Tsp\text{-}average} \times f_{sp})$$

For PA/C or PSV, the delivered V_T depends on the pressure limit, the inspiratory time, and the patient's lung

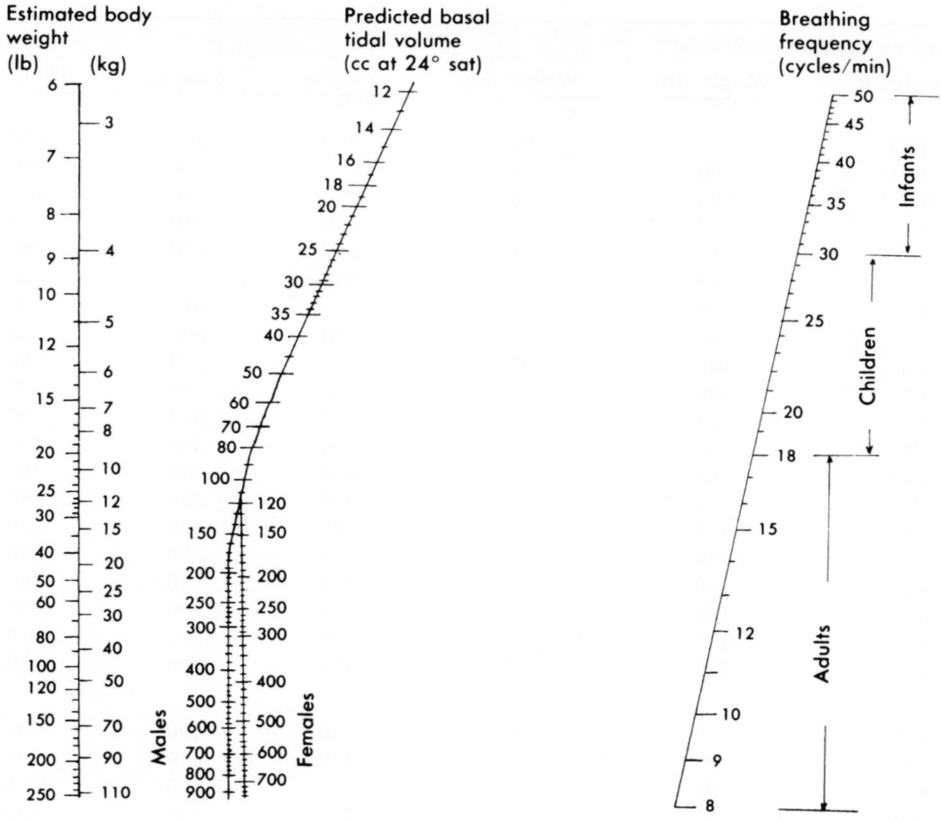

Corrections of predicted basal tidal volumes.

For patients not in coma: add 10%

Fever: add 5% for each °F above 99 (rectal)

add 9% for each °C above 37 (rectal)

Altitude: add 5% for each 2000 feet above sea level

add 8% for each 1000 meters above sea level

Intubation: subtract volume equal to one-half body weight in pounds

subtract 1 cc/kg of body weight

Dead space: add equipment dead space

FIGURE 44-3 Radford nomogram. Although first published in 1955, normal resting V_T can still be accurately predicted using this nomogram. (Modified from Radford EP Jr: Ventilation standards for use in artificial respiration. J Appl Physiol 7:451–460, 1955.)

mechanics. Generally, the pressure limit is increased or decreased to achieve a target V_T while a P_{plat} of less than 30 cm H_2O is maintained. A good initial pressure setting is to start at 15 cm H_2O (above baseline pressure) and observe the resulting V_T. Pressure is increased or decreased to achieve the desired volume. As with VA/C, minute ventilation with PA/C is simply rate multiplied by V_T ($\dot{V}_E = f \times V_T$). Recommended initial V_T and frequency for various patient types are described in Table 44-4.

Patients with ALI/ARDS may need lower V_T to avoid further lung injury and a higher rate to maintain effective alveolar ventilation while P_{plat} is maintained less than 30 cm H_2O. Results of multicenter studies suggest V_T of 4 to 8 ml/kg IBW for patients with ARDS.[2,20,21] In these studies, patients receiving a V_T of 4 to 8 ml/kg had lower mortality and morbidity than patients receiving a V_T of 10 to 12 ml/kg. For patients with ALI/ARDS, one may begin with V_T of 8 ml/kg and decrease the volume as needed to maintain P_{plat} less than 30 cm H_2O.[2] Machine rates of 25 to 35 breaths/min may be needed in patients with ALI/ARDS to maintain adequate minute ventilation. Box 44-7 summarizes the ARDS Clinical Network guidelines for initial ventilator setup.[2,24]

Trigger Sensitivity

Trigger sensitivity for patient-triggered ventilation should be set at the most sensitive level avoiding autotriggering to minimize trigger work and missed triggering. With flow

TABLE 44-3

Tidal Volume Based on Ideal Body Weight*

Height (in)	Height (ft)	Weight (lb)	Weight (kg)	6 ml/kg	8 ml/kg	10 ml/kg	12 ml/kg
Men							
58	4′10″	94	43	260	340	430	520
59	4′11″	100	45	270	360	450	540
60	5′0″	106	48	290	380	480	580
61	5′1″	112	51	310	410	510	610
62	5′2″	118	54	320	430	540	650
63	5′3″	124	56	340	450	560	670
64	5′4″	130	59	350	470	590	710
65	5′5″	136	62	370	500	620	740
66	5′6″	142	65	390	520	650	780
67	5′7″	148	67	400	540	670	800
68	5′8″	154	70	420	560	700	840
69	5′9″	160	73	440	580	730	880
70	5′10″	166	75	450	600	750	900
71	5′11″	172	78	470	620	780	940
72	6′0″	178	81	490	650	810	970
73	6′1″	184	84	500	670	840	1010
74	6′2″	190	86	520	690	860	1030
75	6′3″	196	89	530	700	890	1070
76	6′4″	202	92	550	740	920	1100
77	6′5″	208	95	570	760	950	1140
Women							
55	4′7″	80	36	220	290	360	430
56	4′8″	85	39	230	310	390	470
57	4′9″	90	41	250	330	410	500
58	4′10″	95	43	260	340	430	520
59	4′11″	100	45	270	360	450	540
60	5′0″	105	48	290	380	480	580
61	5′1″	110	50	300	400	500	600
62	5′2″	115	52	310	416	520	620
63	5′3″	120	55	330	440	550	660
64	5′4″	125	57	340	460	570	680
65	5′5″	130	59	350	470	590	710
66	5′6″	135	61	370	490	610	730
67	5′7″	140	64	380	510	640	770
68	5′8″	145	66	400	530	660	790
69	5′9″	150	68	410	540	680	820
70	5′10″	155	70	420	560	700	840
71	5′11″	160	73	440	580	730	876
72	6′0″	165	75	450	600	750	900

*Ideal body weight (lb): Men, 106 + [6(H – 60)]; women, 105 + [5(H – 60)], where H is height in inches.

triggering, the trigger should be set at 1 to 2 L/min, and with pressure triggering, the range is generally −0.5 to −1.5 cm H_2O. However, because of pin holes in disposable ventilator circuits, the sensitivity may need to be adjusted to 3 or 4 L/min or −2 cm H_2O to avoid autotriggering. The increased use of ventilator graphics packages has led to the recognition that patients' inspiratory efforts often are insufficient to trigger the ventilator.[8] Factors that can prolong ventilator response time include large V_T, low trigger sensitivity, auto-PEEP, high bias circuit flow, and abdominal paradox (Box 44-8). (See later discussion of asynchrony.)

Many ventilators offer the option of a pressure or a flow trigger. With older generation intensive care unit (ICU) ventilators, flow triggering offered slightly lower trigger work than pressure triggering,[25-27] although the gain in terms of the patient's total WOB was slight. Newer ventilators with fast pressure-triggering capabilities are as sensitive as flow-triggered devices.[28] However, no triggering mechanism can reduce the WOB that is a result of auto-PEEP. Auto-PEEP must be addressed by other means (see later section).[27] Flow-trigger settings vary by ventilator. Generally, for flow triggering, the trigger flow should be set 1 to 2 L/min below baseline or bias flow.

TABLE 44-4

Suggested Initial Tidal Volume and Frequency for Mechanical Ventilation Based on Disease State or Condition

Patient Type	Tidal Volume (ml/kg)	Frequency (breaths/min)
Adults		
Normal lungs	6-8	12-16
Neuromuscular disease, postoperative period, or with normal pulmonary mechanics in which maintaining lung volume is a concern	6-10	12-16
Acute restrictive disease, ALI/ARDS	4-8*	20-35
Obstructive lung disease (COPD)	6-8	10-12†
Acute severe asthma exacerbation	4-6	10-12
Children		
Age 8-16 yr	6-8	20-30
Age 0-8 yr	6-8	25-35

*For ALI/ARDS, maintain P_{plat} at ≤30 cm H_2O. V_T begins at 8 ml/kg and is gradually reduced to 6 ml/kg. V_T of 4 ml/kg may be required in the care of these patients to avoid ventilator-induced lung injury.

†For patients with obstructive disease, ensure a short inspiratory time and long expiratory time to avoid air trapping and minimize auto-PEEP. Lower V_T and rate may be necessary in acute asthma to avoid further lung overinflation.

Inspiratory Flow, Time, and Inspiratory-to-Expiratory Ratio for Volume Ventilation

Most modern critical care ventilators allow the clinician to select peak flow, V_T, and rate *or* inspiratory time (or percentage inspiratory time, V_T, and rate). For most adults, an initial inspiratory time of approximately 0.8 second (range 0.6 to 1.0 second) with a resultant inspiratory-to-expiratory (I:E) ratio of 1:2 or lower is a good starting point. This value corresponds to an initial peak flow setting of approximately 60 L/min (range 40 to 80 L/min) and a down ramp or square flow waveform.[29] Higher flow (≤100 L/min) may improve gas exchange in patients with chronic obstructive pulmonary disease (COPD), probably because of the resulting better synchrony and increase in expiratory time.[9,29]

Inspiratory flow rate should be adjusted to ensure that the flow provided meets or exceeds the patient's spontaneous inspiratory flow.[29] This rate can be achieved by observing the resultant pressure-time curve contour on a graphics monitor. Ideally, the pressure curve should show a linear increase during inspiration.[9,29] A large negative deflection indicates inadequate trigger sensitivity, and excessive scalloping of the waveform indicates inadequate ventilatory flow settings (Figure 44-4).[9,10] A less sensitive trigger level and lower ventilator inspiratory flow tend to increase the

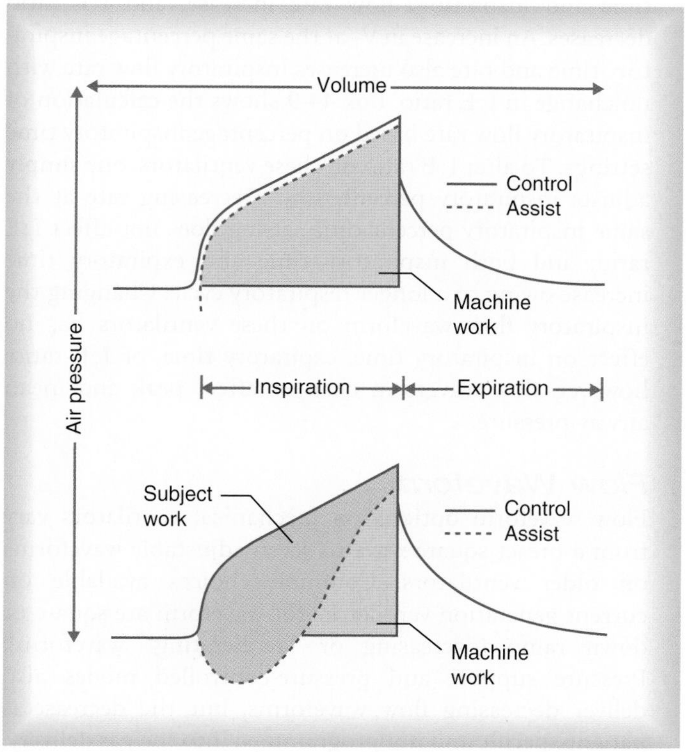

FIGURE 44-4 Plot of an ideal pressure-time waveform during volume-targeted ventilation *(top)*. Plot of actual pressure-time curve *(dotted line)* is superimposed on the ideal curve *(bottom)*. The scooped-out actual pressure waveform is evident. *Green area* reflects the work performed by the patient during assisted volume-targeted ventilation. This type of actual pressure waveform is indicative of inadequate peak inspiratory flow or too lengthy an inspiratory time. The peak flow should be increased, normally to between 60 L/min and 90 L/min to minimize patient effort during volume-limited ventilation. (Modified from Marini JJ, Rodriguez M, Lamb V: The inspiratory workload of patient-initiated mechanical ventilation. Am Rev Respir Dis 134:902, 1986.)

Box 44-7 Initial Ventilator Setup and Management of Oxygenation, Plateau Pressure, and pH

1. Calculate predicted (ideal) body weight as follows:
   - Men: Weight in kilograms = 50 + 2.3 (height in inches − 60)
   - Women: Weight in kilograms = 45.5 + 2.3 (height in inches − 60)
2. Select assist-control mode.
3. Set V_T to 8 ml/kg of predicted body weight.
4. Reduce V_T by 1 ml/kg at intervals of ≤2 hours until V_T is 6 ml/kg.
5. Set initial rate to achieve baseline minute ventilation ($\dot{V}_E$). Do not exceed 35 breaths/min.
6. Adjust V_T and rate to achieve pH of 7.30 to 7.45 while maintaining P_{plat} of ≤30 cm H_2O.
7. Set inspiratory flow rate above patient demand (may be >80 L/min).
8. For oxygenation to achieve PaO_2 of 55 to 80 mm Hg or SpO_2 88% to 95%, use the following incremental FiO_2/PEEP combinations. Higher PEEP options (lower row) decrease FiO_2 and may be preferred in patients with high FiO_2 who can tolerate higher PEEP (stable blood pressure, no barotrauma). Survival is similar with both PEEP approaches.

FiO_2	0.3	0.4	0.4	0.5	0.5	0.6	0.7	0.7
Low PEEP	5	5	8	8	10	10	10	12
High PEEP	12-14	14	16	16	18-20	20	20	20
FiO_2	0.7	0.8	0.9	0.9	0.9	1.0	1.0	1.0
Low PEEP	14	14	14	16	18	20	22	24
High PEEP	20	20-22	22	22	22	22	22	24

9. Check P_{plat}, SpO_2, respiratory rate, V_T, and pH (if available) at least every 4 hours and after each change in PEEP or V_T:
   - If P_{plat} is >28 cm H_2O, decrease V_T by 1-ml/kg steps (minimum 4 ml/kg)
   - If P_{plat} is <25 cm H_2O and V_T is <6 ml/kg, increase V_T by 1-ml/kg steps until P_{plat} is >25 cm H_2O or V_T is 6 ml/kg
   - If P_{plat} is <20 and breath stacking occurs, V_T may be increased in 1-ml/kg increments (maximum 8 ml/kg)
10. The pH goal is 7.30 to 7.45.
    For acidosis management (pH < 7.30):
    - If pH is 7.15 to 7.30, increase the rate until pH is >7.30 or $PaCO_2$ is <25 mm Hg (maximum 35); if rate is 35 and $PaCO_2$ is <25 mm Hg, $NaHCO_3$ may be given
    - If pH is <7.15, increase rate to 35; if pH remains <7.15 and $NaHCO_3$ is considered, V_T may be increased in 1-ml/kg steps until pH is >7.15 (P_{plat} target may be exceeded)

    For alkalosis management (pH > 7.45), decrease ventilator rate, if possible.

Adapted from National Institutes of Health (NIH) National Heart Lung and Blood Institute (NHLBI) ARDS Clinical Network Mechanical Ventilation Protocol Summary (Mechanical Ventilation Protocol Summary, revised 25 January 2005).

Box 44-8 Factors That Can Prolong Ventilator Response Time

- Low trigger sensitivity
- Large V_T (causing air trapping)
- Abdomen–rib cage paradox
- Auto-PEEP (dynamic hyperinflation)
- High tubing compliance
- High circuit dead space
- High bias flow in the circuit
- Mechanical malfunction

patient's WOB. Common ventilator configurations and related controls that determine inspiratory flow, time, and I:E ratio are described in Figure 44-5.

For ventilators with V_T, peak flow, and rate controls, inspiratory time is determined by V_T, peak flow, and flow pattern. To decrease inspiratory time, one may increase peak flow, decrease V_T, or change from a down ramp to a square wave flow pattern. Expiratory time and I:E ratio are determined by inspiratory time and rate. To increase expiratory time (and decrease I:E ratio), one may decrease the inspiratory time as described earlier or increase the expiratory time by decreasing the rate.[29]

For ventilators with V_T (or minute ventilation), percentage inspiratory time, and rate controls, the inspiratory time and V_T determine the inspiratory flow rate. On these ventilators, one can directly increase or decrease the percentage inspiratory time. At the same rate, as inspiratory time (or percentage inspiratory time) decreases, expiratory time and inspiratory flow rate increase, and I:E ratio decreases. An increase in V_T at the same percentage inspiratory time and rate also increases inspiratory flow rate with no change in I:E ratio. Box 44-9 shows the calculation of inspiratory flow rate based on percentage inspiratory time settings. To alter I:E ratio on these ventilators, one simply adjusts inspiratory percent time. Decreasing rate at the same inspiratory percent time setting does not affect I:E ratio, and both inspiratory time and expiratory time increase owing to a longer respiratory cycle. Changing the inspiratory flow waveform on these ventilators has no effect on inspiratory time, expiratory time, or I:E ratio; however, flow waveform changes affect peak and mean airway pressure.

Flow Waveform

Flow waveform options on mechanical ventilators vary from a preset square wave to seven adjustable waveforms on older ventilators. Common choices available on current generation ventilators for waveform are square or down ramp (decreasing or "decelerating" waveform). Pressure support and pressure-controlled modes also deliver decreasing flow waveforms, but the decrease is patient-specific and not programmed into the gas delivery.

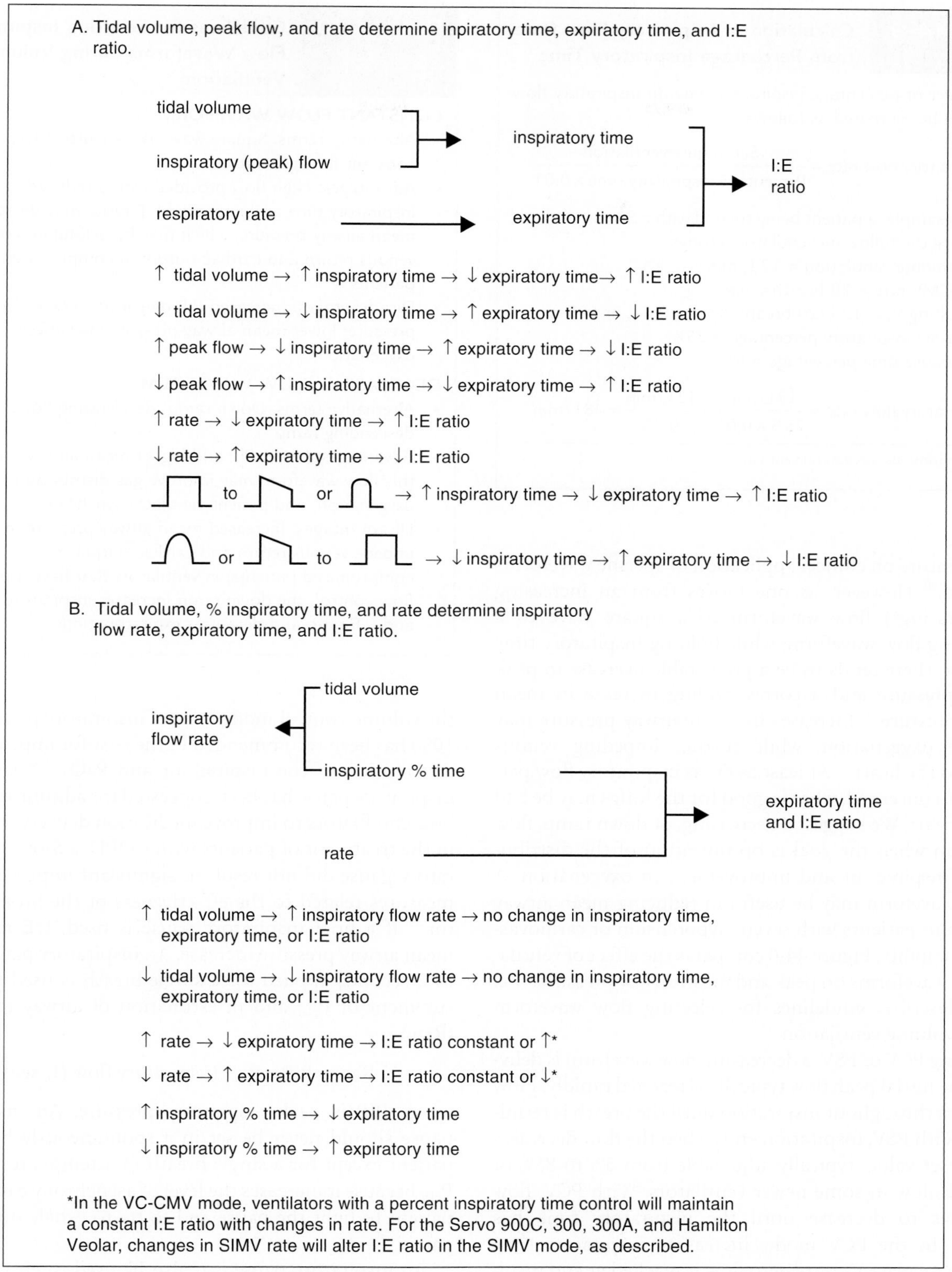

A. Tidal volume, peak flow, and rate determine inpiratory time, expiratory time, and I:E ratio.
tidal volume
inspiratory (peak) flow
respiratory rate
inspiratory time
expiratory time
I:E ratio
↑ tidal volume → ↑ inspiratory time → ↓ expiratory time→ ↑ I:E ratio
↓ tidal volume → ↓ inspiratory time → ↑ expiratory time → ↓ I:E ratio
↑ peak flow → ↓ inspiratory time → ↑ expiratory time → ↓ I:E ratio
↓ peak flow → ↑ inspiratory time → ↓ expiratory time → ↑ I:E ratio
↑ rate → ↓ expiratory time → ↑ I:E ratio
↓ rate → ↑ expiratory time → ↓ I:E ratio
to or → ↑ inspiratory time → ↓ expiratory time → ↑ I:E ratio
or to → ↓ inspiratory time → ↑ expiratory time → ↓ I:E ratio
B. Tidal volume, % inspiratory time, and rate determine inspiratory flow rate, expiratory time, and I:E ratio.
tidal volume
inspiratory flow rate
inspiratory % time
rate
expiratory time and I:E ratio
↑ tidal volume → ↑ inspiratory flow rate → no change in inspiratory time, expiratory time, or I:E ratio
↓ tidal volume → ↓ inspiratory flow rate → no change in inspiratory time, expiratory time, or I:E ratio
↑ rate → ↓ expiratory time → I:E ratio constant or ↑*
↓ rate → ↑ expiratory time → I:E ratio constant or ↓*
↑ inspiratory % time → ↓ expiratory time
↓ inspiratory % time → ↑ expiratory time
*In the VC-CMV mode, ventilators with a percent inspiratory time control will maintain a constant I:E ratio with changes in rate. For the Servo 900C, 300, 300A, and Hamilton Veolar, changes in SIMV rate will alter I:E ratio in the SIMV mode, as described.

FIGURE 44-5 Relationship between V_T, inspiratory flow, inspiratory time, expiratory time, and I:E ratio in various ventilator systems. *A,* Effects of V_T, flow, and respiratory rate on inspiratory time, expiratory time, and I:E ratio. Some ventilators provide V_T, inspiratory flow, and rate control in volume control (VC) and SIMV modes. *B,* Effects of volume, inspiratory time, and rate on inspiratory flow, expiratory time, and I:E ratio. Other ventilators provide controls for inspiratory time (or percentage inspiratory time), V_T (or minute ventilation), and rate in the VC and SIMV modes. In the VC mode (controlled ventilation), ventilators with a percentage inspiratory time control maintain a constant I:E ratio with changes in respiratory rate. In the SIMV mode, changes in SIMV rate alter I:E ratio on these machines.

Box 44-9 Calculation of Inspiratory Flow Rate from Percentage Inspiratory Time

The effect of percentage inspiratory time on inspiratory flow rate can be estimated as follows:

$$\text{Inspiratory flow rate} = \frac{\text{Set minute ventilation}}{\text{Percentage inspiratory time} \times 0.01}$$

For example, a patient being treated with a Servo ventilator may have the following ventilator settings:

- Set minute ventilation = 12 L/min
- Set CMV rate = 20 breaths/min
- Resulting V_T = 12 L/20 breaths/min = 0.6 L or 600 ml
- Set time inspiratory percentage = 25%
- Set pause time percentage = 0%

$$\text{Inspiratory flow rate} = \frac{12\,\text{L/min}}{25\% \times 0.01} = \frac{12\,\text{L/min}}{0.25} = 48\,\text{L/min}$$

CMN, Continuous mechanical ventilation.

Box 44-10 Guidelines for Selecting Inspiratory Flow Waveforms during Volume Ventilation

CONSTANT FLOW WAVEFORM

- Alternative terms: Square wave, rectangular wave, constant flow generator
- Advantages: High flow provided with a reduced inspiratory time and improved I : E ratio; may decrease mean airway pressure, which may be helpful in terms of venous return and cardiac output in compromised patients
- Disadvantages: Increased PIP may lead to excessive pressure; lower mean airway pressure may affect oxygenation

DECREASING FLOW WAVEFORM

- Alternative terms: Down ramp, decelerating flow, descending ramp
- Advantages: Lower PIP and higher mean airway pressure; this flow waveform may improve gas distribution, oxygenation, and patient-ventilator synchrony
- Disadvantages: Increased mean airway pressure may impede venous return and cardiac output in compromised patients; in ventilators that have a peak flow control, the down ramp increases inspiratory time and I : E ratio and decreases expiratory time

The literature on clinical application of specific waveforms is mixed.[30] However, as one moves from an increasing ("accelerating") flow waveform to a square wave to a decreasing flow waveform, while holding inspiratory time constant, there tends to be a predictable decrease in peak airway pressure and a corresponding increase in mean airway pressure.[30] Increases in mean airway pressure may improve oxygenation, while further impeding venous return to the heart.[30] At least as far as inspiratory flow patterns are concerned, what is good for the lungs may be bad for the heart. We suggest a decreasing, or down ramp, flow waveform when the goal is optimization of the distribution of inspired air and improvement in oxygenation. A square waveform may be useful in reducing mean airway pressure in patients with severe hypotension or cardiovascular instability. Figure 44-6 compares the effect of ventilator flow waveforms on peak and mean airway pressure. Box 44-10 describes guidelines for selecting flow waveform during volume ventilation.

During PCV or PSV, a decreasing flow waveform is delivered. The initial peak flow typically is reached rapidly. Flow decreases throughout inspiration until the breath is terminated. With PSV, inspiration ends when the flow decreases to a preset value, typically adjustable from 5% to 85% of the peak flow in some newer ventilators. With PCV, flow continues to decrease until the inspiratory time has elapsed. In the PCV mode, increasing inspiratory time tends to increase V_T until zero flow is reached at end inspiration. Further increases in inspiratory time do not increase V_T, although distribution of inspired air may improve, and mean airway pressure does increase.

Inspiratory Pause

In addition to inspiratory time or flow, most ventilators have an option for setting an inspiratory pause or hold in the volume-control mode. A brief inspiratory pause (up to 10%) has been recommended in the past for improving the distribution of the inspired air and PaO_2.[31,32] Use of an inspiratory pause has been suggested for administration of bronchodilators to improve medication delivery. However, in the treatment of patients with COPD, a 5-second inspiratory pause did not result in significant improvement in measures related to the effectiveness of the bronchodilator.[31] If a brief inspiratory pause is used, I:E ratio and mean airway pressure increase. An inspiratory pause of 0.5 to 2 seconds applied for a single breath is used for measurement of P_{plat} and in estimation of airway resistance (Raw):

$$\text{Raw} = \text{PIP} - P_{plat}/\text{Inspiratory flow (L/sec)}$$

where PIP is peak inspiratory pressure. An inspiratory pause should never be set in a spontaneously breathing patient except for a single breath in attempts to measure P_{plat} because it increases the level of asynchrony causing the patient to fight the pause and to try to exhale during the pause.

An inspiratory pause can also be used to ensure a full inspiration before a chest radiograph is obtained, and this step may improve the quality of the resulting radiograph.[33] Use of an extended inspiratory pause should be limited because of the resultant increase in mean airway pressure and risk of impeding venous return and cardiac output, especially in patients who are hypovolemic or hypotensive or whose condition is hemodynamically unstable.

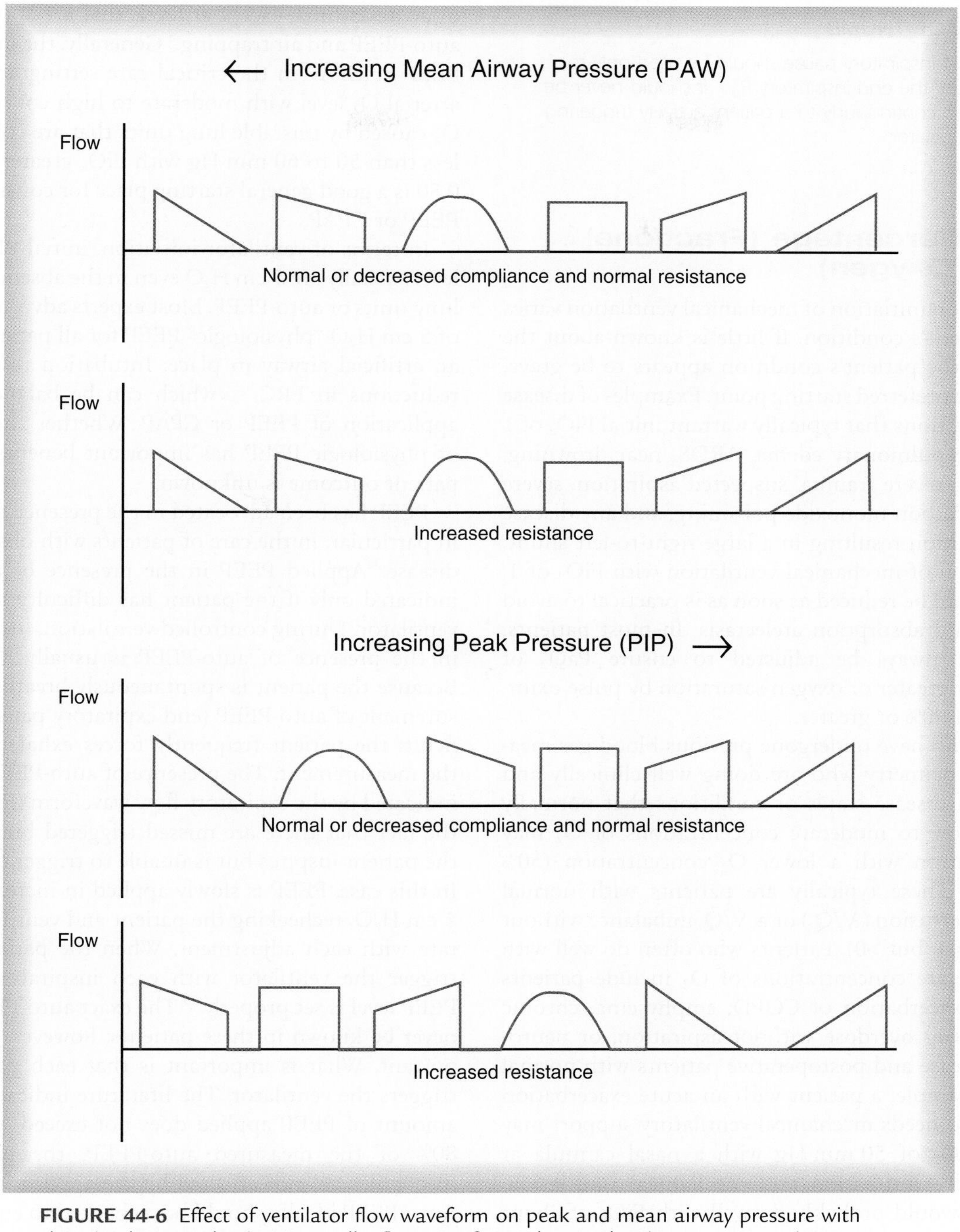

FIGURE 44-6 Effect of ventilator flow waveform on peak and mean airway pressure with changing lung mechanics. Generally, flow waveforms that tend to increase mean airway pressure also decrease peak pressure (PIP) and vice versa. Consequently, if increasing mean airway pressure is the goal, decelerating (down ramp) flow waveforms may be helpful. However, in the care of patients with cardiovascular compromise, in whom reducing mean airway pressure may be helpful, a square wave or accelerating flow (up ramp) may be valuable. Accelerating flow waveforms are no longer available on newer critical care ventilators. (Modified from Rau JL, Shelledy DC: The effect of varying inspiratory flow waveforms on peak and mean airway pressures with a time-cycled volume ventilator: a bench study. Respir Care 36:347, 1991.)

RULE OF THUMB

An end inspiratory pause should be used only to estimate the end inspiratory P_{plat}. It should never be applied continuously to a patient actively triggering the ventilator.

Oxygen Percentage (Fractional Inspired Oxygen)

FiO_2 selected on initiation of mechanical ventilation varies with the patient's condition. If little is known about the patient or if the patient's condition appears to be grave, 100% O_2 is the preferred starting point. Examples of disease states or conditions that typically warrant initial FiO_2 of 1 include acute pulmonary edema, ARDS, near drowning, cardiac arrest, severe trauma, suspected aspiration, severe pneumonia, carbon monoxide poisoning, and any disease state or condition resulting in a large right-to-left shunt. After initiation of mechanical ventilation with FiO_2 of 1, the FiO_2 should be reduced as soon as is practical to avoid O_2 toxicity and absorption atelectasis. In most patients, FiO_2 should always be adjusted to ensure PaO_2 of 60 mm Hg or greater or oxygen saturation by pulse oximeter (SpO_2) of 90% or greater.

Patients who have undergone previous blood gas measurement or oximetry who are doing well clinically and patients with disease states or conditions that normally respond to low to moderate concentrations of O_2 may begin ventilation with a lower O_2 concentration (50% to 70% O_2). These typically are patients with normal ventilation/perfusion ($\dot{V}/\dot{Q}$) or a $\dot{V}/\dot{Q}$ imbalance without shunt ($\dot{V}/\dot{Q} < 1$ but >0). Patients who often do well with low to moderate concentrations of O_2 include patients with acute exacerbation of COPD, emphysema, chronic bronchitis, drug overdose without aspiration, or neuromuscular disease and postoperative patients with normal lungs. For example, a patient with an acute exacerbation of COPD who needs mechanical ventilatory support may have had PaO_2 of 50 mm Hg with a nasal cannula at 4 L/min before intubation and mechanical ventilation. This patient would probably do well with FiO_2 of about 0.50 when adequate ventilation is restored. The patient can begin with 50% O_2 and be immediately assessed for assurance of adequate SpO_2. FiO_2 can be adjusted according to the patient's response.

Positive End Expiratory Pressure and Continuous Positive Airway Pressure

PEEP and CPAP are effective techniques for improving and maintaining lung volume and improving oxygenation for patients with acute restrictive disease such as ALI, pneumonia, pulmonary edema, and ARDS.[8,29] PEEP and CPAP should be cautiously applied in the treatment of patients with an already elevated FRC, such as patients with COPD or acute asthma, except at levels that are applied to offset auto-PEEP and air trapping.[8] Generally, the indications for PEEP or CPAP in the critical care setting are inadequate arterial O_2 level with moderate to high concentrations of O_2 caused by unstable lung units that are collapsed. PaO_2 less than 50 to 60 mm Hg with FiO_2 greater than 0.40 to 0.50 is a good general starting place for considering use of PEEP or CPAP.

In terms of ventilator initiation, initial PEEP or CPAP levels usually are 5 cm H_2O even in the absence of unstable lung units or auto-PEEP. Most experts advocate for the use of 5 cm H_2O "physiologic" PEEP for all patients who have an artificial airway in place. Intubation results in small reductions in FRC,[8,29] which can be balanced with the application of PEEP or CPAP. Whether the application of physiologic PEEP has important benefits in terms of patient outcome is unknown.

PEEP has been advocated in the presence of auto-PEEP, in particular, in the care of patients with obstructive lung disease.[34]Applied PEEP in the presence of auto-PEEP is indicated only if the patient has difficulty triggering the ventilator. During controlled ventilation, increasing PEEP in the presence of auto-PEEP is usually not indicated. Because the patient is spontaneously breathing, the measurement of auto-PEEP (end expiratory pause) is very difficult; the patient frequently forces exhalation negating the measurement. The presence of auto-PEEP is generally indicated by the expiratory flow waveform (Figure 44-7) or the fact that there are missed triggered breaths. That is, the patient inspires but is unable to trigger the ventilator. In this case, PEEP is slowly applied in increments of 1 to 2 cm H_2O, rechecking the patient and ventilator response rate with each adjustment. When the patient is able to trigger the ventilator with each inspiratory effort, the PEEP level is set properly.[29] The exact auto-PEEP level may never be known in these patients; however, this is unimportant. What is important is that each patient's effort triggers the ventilator. The literature indicates that if the amount of PEEP applied does not exceed approximately 80% of the measured auto-PEEP, the patients' lung mechanics are not affected by the application of PEEP.[35] Auto-PEEP ideally should be rechecked to ensure intrinsic PEEP does not increase as PEEP is applied. Box 44-11 summarizes methods for minimizing the effects of auto-PEEP. An absolute contraindication to PEEP is an uncontrolled tension pneumothorax. However, PEEP should be cautiously applied in any patient with severe intrinsic lung disease, hypotension, and elevated intracranial pressure.

Open Lung Strategy, Recruitment Maneuvers, and Positive End Expiratory Pressure

In the care of patients with ALI/ARDS, it is usually necessary to initiate PEEP at 10 to 15 cm H_2O.[21,22,35,36] However, many clinicians use the ARDS Clinical Network PEEP/FiO_2 tables to set PEEP initially during the establishment

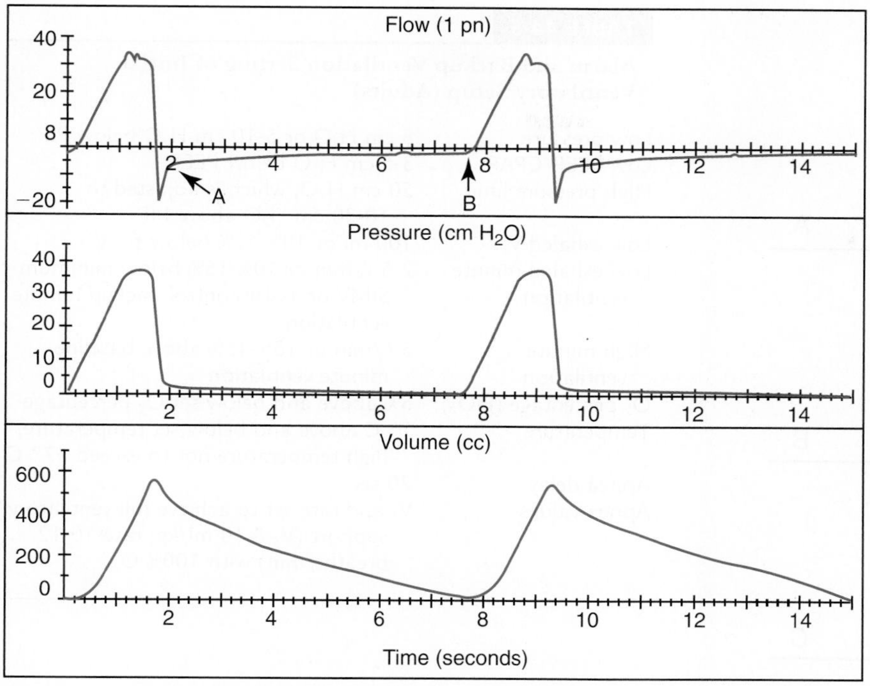

FIGURE 44-7 Airway flow, pressure, and volume in a patient with severe airflow obstruction and auto-PEEP. There is a rapid decrease in expiratory flow at the onset of exhalation because of the obstruction *(arrow A)*, and there is a lack of return of flow to baseline at the end of the breath *(arrow B)*. This type of expiratory flow pattern, regardless of the expiratory time, indicates auto-PEEP. The amount of auto-PEEP cannot be determined from this example, but anytime end expiratory flow is greater than zero, auto-PEEP is present.

Box 44-11 Techniques for Minimizing Effects of Auto-PEEP

- Decrease airflow obstruction
- Secretion management
- Aggressive bronchodilation
- Larger sized endotracheal tubes
- Modify ventilatory pattern
- Decrease inspiratory time
- Increase inspiratory flow (on ventilators with inspiratory peak flow control)
- Decrease percentage inspiratory time (on ventilators with $\%T_i$ control)
- Decrease VT
- Increase expiratory time
- Decrease rate
- Use low-compressible volume circuit
- Apply PEEP or CPAP to balance auto-PEEP

of ventilatory support (see Box 44-7). When patients are stabilized, the use of an open lung ventilation strategy in early-stage ARDS has been recommended.[5,29] Such a strategy incorporates V_T of 4 to 8 ml/kg IBW with either pressure-targeted or volume-targeted ventilation and a PEEP level set after a lung recruitment maneuver using a decremental PEEP trial.[5,29,37] The lung recruitment maneuver is intended to open collapsed lung units, and the setting of PEEP using a decremental PEEP trial is intended to apply PEEP based on the patient's lung mechanics to keep the lung units recruited open.

Although all patients with ARDS/ALI require PEEP, not all patients with ALI respond to PEEP, and patients with pulmonary (vs. nonpulmonary) causes of ALI/ARDS, such as pneumonia, may be less likely to respond to low to moderate levels of PEEP.[11] Nonpulmonary causes of ALI/ARDS (e.g., extrathoracic trauma, intraabdominal sepsis) seem to respond well to PEEP.[11] In practice, some authors have suggested that higher levels of PEEP (>15 cm H_2O) be reserved for patients with a high percentage of recruitable lung.[38] High levels of PEEP have been shown to improve outcomes in ARDS in patients with the most severe forms of ARDS ($PaO_2/FiO_2 < 150$ mm Hg).[39,40] (See later section on the performance of recruitment maneuvers and the setting of PEEP by decremental trial.)

Pressure Rise Time or Slope

Most newer critical care ventilators include an inspiratory pressure rise time or pressure slope. This control functions only with pressure-limited breaths (PSV, PCV, PRVC, volume support, airway pressure release ventilation, pressure SIMV). The purpose of this control is to adjust the rate at which flow increases from baseline to peak.[41-43] Generally, rise time should be set at a value that ensures adequate inspiratory gas flow (meeting or exceeding patient demand) without an excessive "overshoot" of the pressure at the beginning of inspiration. A slow or low rise time may increase the patient's WOB.[41-43] The effect of changing inspiratory rise time is described in Figure 44-8 and discussed more in the section on patient-ventilator synchrony.

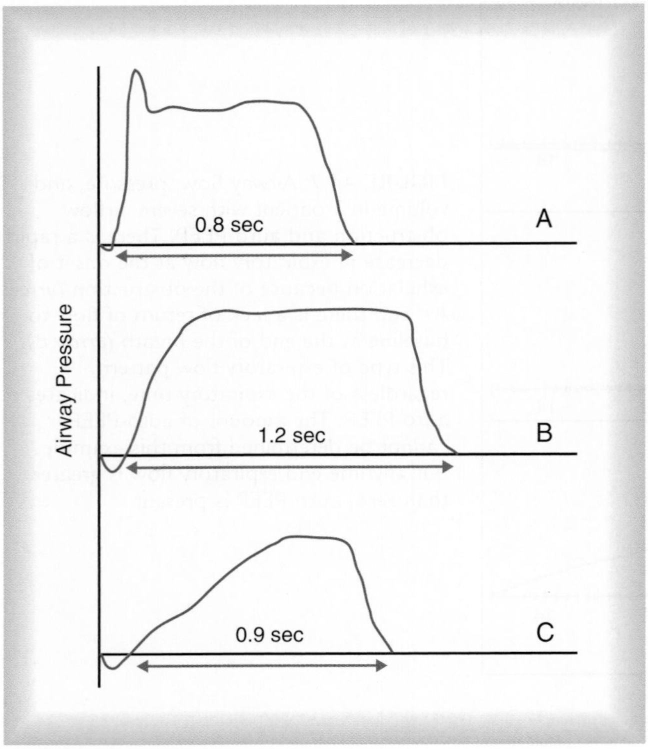

FIGURE 44-8 Effect of changing rise time during pressure-targeted breaths for a patient who prefers a moderate flow. *A,* Flow exceeds patient demand, and a pressure spike and short inspiratory time result. *B,* As flow is decreased, inspiratory time lengthens, and the pressure spike disappears. Machine output matches patient demand. *C,* When flow is reduced further, patient demand exceeds machine flow; the result is deformation of the pressure waveform and a decrease in inspiratory time. (Modified from Branson RD, Campbell RS, Davis K, et al: Altering flow rate during maximum pressure support ventilation (PSV_{max}): effect on cardiorespiratory function. Respir Care 35:1056-1069, 1990.)

Limits and Alarms

Ventilator alarms and limits warn of ventilator malfunction and changes in patient status. Ventilator malfunction alarms include power or gas supply loss and electronic or pneumatic malfunction. These alarms usually are preset by the manufacturer.

Patient status alarms usually are set by the respiratory therapist (RT). These include maximum inspiratory pressure, low-pressure and low-PEEP alarms, high-volume and low-volume and rate alarms, O_2 and humidification alarms, and apnea alarms. After initiation of ventilation, alarms and limits are readjusted as needed. Alarms usually are set so that they warn the clinician of important changes or problems. Without proper setting, these alarms can become a nuisance by falsely signaling problems that are not real.[8]

In volume ventilation, a pressure limit should be set. Generally, before the patient is connected to the ventilator, the limit should be set at 40 cm H_2O to avoid overpressuring the system when the patient is connected. After the patient is connected to the ventilator, the peak and plateau pressures should be assessed. If P_{plat} is greater than 30 cm H_2O, consideration should be given to decreasing the set V_T. If P_{plat} is less than 30 cm H_2O, the high pressure limit can be adjusted to 10 to 15 cm H_2O above PIP. One can decrease peak pressure by decreasing the peak flow rate, increasing the inspiratory time, changing the inspiratory flow waveform from a square to a down ramp, or decreasing the delivered V_T. For spontaneously breathing patients, inspiratory flow and time must meet or exceed the patient's inspiratory demand to ensure one does not increase the patient's WOB further (see the section on Patient-Ventilator Interaction). Preset or adjustable alarms common to most ventilators include pressure (high-low), volume (high-low V_T, minute ventilation), apnea, O_2 percentage, and temperature. Suggested initial settings for these alarms and backup ventilator settings are presented in Table 44-5.

TABLE 44-5

Alarm and Backup Ventilation Setting of Initial Ventilatory Setup (Adults)

Low pressure	8 cm H_2O or 5-10 cm H_2O below PIP
Low PEEP/CPAP	3-5 cm H_2O below PEEP
High pressure limit	50 cm H_2O, which is adjusted to 10-20 cm H_2O above PIP
Low exhaled V_T	100 ml or 10%-15% below set V_T
Low exhaled minute ventilation	2-5 L/min or 10%-15% below minimum SIMV or assist-control backup minute ventilation
High minute ventilation	5 L/min or 10%-15% above baseline minute ventilation
O_2 percentage (FiO_2)	5% above and below set O_2 percentage
Temperature	2° C above and below set temperature, high temperature not to exceed 37° C
Apnea delay	20 sec
Apnea values	V_T and rate set to achieve full ventilatory support (V_T 8-10 ml/kg; rate 10-12 breaths/min) with 100% O_2

Humidification

Humidification is required during both invasive and noninvasive mechanical ventilation. A heated humidifier or a heat and moisture exchanger (HME) should provide a minimum of 30 mg/L of water with a temperature of 30° C or greater.[44] Use of HMEs should be avoided in the care of patients with secretion problems and patients with low body temperature (<32° C), high spontaneous minute ventilation (>10 L/min), or air leaks in which exhaled V_T is less than 70% of delivered V_T.[44] Heated humidifiers may be used to deliver 100% body humidity at 37° C. Current clinical practice guidelines suggest an inspired gas temperature of 33° C ± 2° C, although inspiratory gas temperatures of 33° C to 37° C are acceptable in most patients.[44] We prefer an optimal humidity approach and use of a heated humidifier to deliver gas in the range of 33° C to 37° C at the airway in most intubated patients and at a temperature consistent with patient comfort during noninvasive ventilation. However, in patients without primary pulmonary dysfunction and short-term ventilation, HMEs are very useful; generally, these are postoperative patients after elective surgery, patients in the emergency department, and patients recovering from an overdose.

Periodic Sighs

Constant, monotonous tidal ventilation at a small volume (<7 ml/kg) may result in progressive atelectasis.[8,45] Periodic deep breaths or sighs taken every 6 to 10 minutes reverse this trend.[8,45] During the 1960s and 1970s, it was common to ventilate patients with a smaller V_T (5 to 7 ml/kg) and no PEEP. As a result, an intermittent sigh function was incorporated into most volume ventilators. Sighs were programmed at 1½ to 2 times the set V_T at an interval of every 6 to 10 minutes. Sometimes multiple sighs were included at a preset interval of up to 10 times per hour. Because of the use of PEEP, sighs are no longer routinely included. PEEP prevents the formation of atelectasis in a patient on ventilation with constant small V_T. This is the primary reason why 5 cm H_2O of PEEP is routinely used on patients, including patients with healthy lungs. General guidelines for the initial ventilator settings for most adult patients are described in Box 44-12.

Box 44-12 General Guidelines for Initial Ventilator Settings for Adult Patients

MODE
- Assist-control volume or pressure targeted
- Pressure support
- SIMV with or without pressure support volume or pressure targeted

TIDAL VOLUME
- 4 to 8 ml/kg IBW
- Avoid overdistention
- Maintain P_{plat} < 30 cm H_2O
- For COPD, V_T 6 to 8 ml/kg IBW in assist-control or pressure support mode with adequate expiratory time for reducing air trapping is suggested
- For ALI/ARDS, begin at 6 to 8 ml/kg IBW; adjust as indicated to maintain P_{plat} < 30 cm H_2O
- For acute asthma, V_T 4 to 6 ml/kg IBW is indicated to maintain P_{plat} < 30 cm H_2O

RATE
- 16 to 35 breaths/min
- Minimize auto-PEEP
- Set initial rate and V_T to maintain baseline minute ventilation (approximately 100 ml/kg IBW for most healthy adults)
- PEEP/CPAP
- 5 cm H_2O in most patients ventilated without acute lung injury
- 5 to 10 cm H_2O in patients with acute lung injury
- 10 to 15 cm H_2O in most patients with ARDS
- 5 cm H_2O in patients with COPD/asthma, adjust as indicated to offset effect of auto-PEEP on ventilator triggering
- Trigger sensitivity −0.5 to −1.5 cm H_2O or flow trigger 2 to 3 LPM; minimize trigger work without autocycle
- Inspiratory flow and time 60 to 100 L/min
- Inspiratory time 0.6 to 1.0 second; inspiratory flow must meet or exceed patient's spontaneous inspiratory flow demand
- Resultant I : E ratio should be ≤1 : 2

ADJUSTING VENTILATORY SUPPORT

After ventilator initiation, the patient should be carefully assessed and the ventilator adjusted so that patient-ventilator synchrony is ensured; WOB is minimized; and oxygenation, ventilation, and acid-base balance are optimized while harmful cardiovascular effects are minimized. Initial patient evaluation should include physical assessment, assessment of ventilator settings, cardiovascular assessment, oximetry, and measurement of arterial blood gases (Box 44-13).

Physical assessment should include general appearance, level of consciousness, signs of anxiety or dyspnea, color, extremities (temperature, edema, capillary refill), heart rate and blood pressure, respiratory rate and pattern, inspection of the neck for jugular venous distention, and chest examination. Cyanosis is associated with hypoxemia. Use of accessory muscles, tachypnea, retractions, or chest to abdomen asynchrony may indicate increased WOB. Unilateral or unequal lung expansion is associated with bronchial intubation, pneumothorax, and other unilateral disorders.

Breath sounds should be assessed for good aeration, and absent, diminished, or abnormal breath sounds should be documented. Palpation should be performed as appropriate for tracheal position, chest wall motion, and presence of subcutaneous air. Percussion of the chest should be performed for assessment of resonance, dullness, or

Box 44-13 Initial Assessment of Ventilatory Support

- Inspection, palpation, and auscultation
- Assessment of position of artificial airway and cuff inflation
- Assessment of pulse, blood pressure, oximetry, and electrocardiogram
- Inspection of patient-ventilator system breathing circuit, humidifier, ventilator settings, and findings
- Analysis of arterial blood gas values
- Inspection of chest radiograph

MINI CLINI

Humidification of the Airways during Mechanical Ventilation

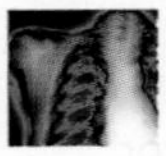

PROBLEM: A mechanically ventilated patient is in the medical ICU recovering from acute respiratory failure secondary to aspiration pneumonia. The patient currently needs airway suctioning every 30 to 60 minutes according to the RT and staff nurse caring for the patient. Both caregivers note that the secretions are thick and copious. Current ventilator settings are as follows:

Mode: Assist-control volume ventilation
V_T: 500 ml (6.8 ml/kg IBW)
Preset rate: 16 breaths/min
Total rate: 26 breaths/min
FiO_2: 0.50
PIP: 31 cm H_2O
V_E: 13 L/min

The RT is asked to place an HME on the ventilator circuit at the "wye." Is this an appropriate action?

SOLUTION: Humidification can be provided with either a heated humidifier or an HME unit. Although useful in some instances, placement of an HME would be contraindicated in this case for several reasons. Adequate humidification for a patient with an artificial airway is critical in preventing inspissation of airway secretions, injury to and destruction of the airway epithelium, and atelectasis.

The patient information in this clinical scenario points to several potential problems with use of an HME, the most obvious one being copious, thick airway secretions. The HME may not provide sufficient water vapor and heat output, and secretions could be retained. The airway secretions could be coughed into the HME, causing increased resistance to flow and possible obstruction. Because the patient has high ventilatory requirements, as evidenced by an elevated exhaled minute ventilation, it is important that the humidification system be able to maintain adequate heat and moisture output when demands dictate.

Other situations in which an HME should not be used are administration of aerosol treatments through the ventilator tubing circuit, high minute ventilation (>10 L/min), and body temperature less than 32° C.

hyperresonance. Key findings at initial assessment of a patient undergoing ventilation are described in Table 44-6.

Ventilator settings that should be assessed after initiation of mechanical ventilation include peak, plateau, and mean airway pressures; exhaled volumes (spontaneous and machine V_T, minute ventilation); respiratory rate (spontaneous and machine rate); baseline pressures (PEEP, CPAP, auto-PEEP); trigger effort; O_2 concentration; inspiratory time; flow; I:E ratio; humidification; and airway temperature. In addition, patient-ventilator interaction should be assessed to ensure that a spontaneously breathing patient

Box 44-14 Factors Affecting Patient-Ventilator Interaction

- Artificial airway
- Mode of ventilation
- Level of ventilatory support
- Inspiratory flow
- Trigger sensitivity
- Expiratory sensitivity (for PSV)
- Inspiratory time
- Flow-triggered system function
- Demand valve function
- Presence of auto-PEEP
- Humidification systems

is able to trigger a breath easily and that inspiratory flow and time are such that WOB is minimized. When using pressure ventilation, the patient should also be evaluated to ensure ease of cycling to expiration. Factors that may affect patient-ventilator interaction are listed in Box 44-14.

The artificial airway should be assessed for proper placement, patency, and cuff inflation. Size, position, and depth of the endotracheal tube and cuff pressure, including volume used to inflate the cuff, should be recorded. An extra endotracheal tube or tracheostomy tube of the correct size should be placed at the patient's bedside, and the equipment needed to replace the airway must be available and easily accessible. A clean, functioning manual resuscitator with O_2 supply and suction equipment including an appropriate supply of suction catheters, sterile water or saline solution, and sterile gloves also must be placed near the bedside. Patients requiring high levels of PEEP (>5 cm H_2O) should have PEEP valves attached to the manual ventilator.

Cardiovascular assessment should include observation of heart rate, blood pressure, and electrocardiogram for the presence of arrhythmias. Tachycardia, ST segment elevation, and frequent premature ventricular contractions may indicate myocardial ischemia. If the patient has a central venous line or pulmonary arterial catheter, hemodynamic variables may be assessed, including central venous pressure, pulmonary arterial pressure, wedge pressure, and cardiac output.

Continuous monitoring with pulse oximetry is recommended for patients receiving mechanical ventilatory support in the ICU, and arterial blood gases should be measured 30 to 60 minutes after initiation of mechanical ventilation. A chest radiograph should be obtained to verify proper endotracheal tube placement and to evaluate the chest. After the initial assessment, the method and level of ventilatory support are adjusted to optimize oxygenation, ventilation, WOB, acid-base balance, and cardiovascular status. The ventilatory adjustments for each of these areas are discussed next.

TABLE 44-6

Assessment of Ventilatory Support

Ancillary equipment in room	Crash cart (patient's condition unstable); cardiac monitor; chest tubes (pneumothorax, chest drainage, thoracic surgery); aortic balloon pump (heart failure); cooling blanket (fever); other
General appearance	Resting quietly, calm, relaxed (no distress); restless, anxious, distressed (pain, anxiety, inadequate oxygenation or ventilation)
Level of consciousness	Alert, awake, and oriented to person, place, and time (good mental status, neurologic function); confused (neurologic problems, hypoxia, low cardiac output, drugs); sleepy (tired, sedatives, narcotics); lethargic (exhaustion, impaired CNS status, sedation); somnolent (CNS impairment, sedation); coma (CNS malfunction, heavy sedation, severe hypoxia)
Extremities	Cyanosis (hypoxemia); pale, cold, and clammy (poor cardiac output, low blood pressure, shock); edema (fluid overload)
Respiratory rate and pattern	Normal (good cardiopulmonary status); tachypnea (pain, anxiety, hypoxemia, acidosis, CNS problems); bradypnea or apnea (severe hypoxia, CNS problems, heavy sedation, paralysis)
Head, eyes, ears, nose, and throat	Cyanotic lips and gums (hypoxemia); pupils dilated (drugs, severe hypoxia, low cardiac output, cardiac arrest); pupils dilated and fixed (brain death); pupils contracted (drugs, light); response to light (good if responsive)
Neck	Accessory muscle use (increased WOB, respiratory distress); jugular vein distention (right-sided heart failure, positive pressure impeding venous return)
Chest inspection	Right-left chest wall synchrony (normal); right-left chest wall asynchrony (right main stem intubation, pneumothorax, large unilateral pleural effusion, flail on one side); chest-diaphragm synchrony (normal); chest-diaphragm asynchrony—abdominal paradox (increased WOB, diaphragmatic fatigue)
Chest auscultation	Good bilateral breath sounds (normal); decreased breath sounds unilaterally (right main stem intubation, pneumothorax, unilateral lung disease); bilaterally decreased or absent breath sounds (inadequate or decreased ventilation, large leak, ventilator malfunction or disconnect, misplaced endotracheal tube); air leak around cuff (underinflation, cuff malfunction); wheezing (bronchospasm, tumor, narrowing of airway); bibasilar crackles in patients with congestive heart failure (pulmonary edema); rhonchi, coarse crackles (secretions in the larger airways); bronchial breath sounds (consolidation or microatelectasis)
Palpation	Subcutaneous air (pneumothorax, pneumomediastinum); tracheal shift (tension pneumothorax, large area of atelectasis); right-left chest motion symmetry (normal); right-left asymmetric breathing (unilateral disease, pneumothorax, bronchial intubation)
Percussion	Resonant over lung tissue (normal); dull (pleural effusion, lobar infiltrates, consolidation, atelectasis); hyperresonant (pneumothorax, overinflation—COPD, asthma exacerbation)
Vital signs	Normal heart rate and rhythm (normal); tachycardia (hypoxemia, pain, anxiety, distress); hypertension (anxiety, cardiovascular disease, head trauma); bradycardia (severe hypoxia, severe hypercapnia, cardiac disease); hypotension (blood loss, shock, gram-negative sepsis, heart failure)

CNS, Central nervous system.

Patient-Ventilator Interaction

Patient-ventilator interaction refers to patient comfort, WOB, and synchrony during ventilator-assisted breaths. Generally, ventilatory support should be initially adjusted to minimize the WOB and to allow the ventilatory muscles to rest.[46] Diaphragmatic dysfunction often accompanies ventilatory failure, and a sustained increase in workload can lead to structural injury to the muscle.[11] When the ventilatory muscles become fatigued, at least 24 hours is required for recovery.[58] Complete rest of the diaphragm, as in controlled ventilation, may lead to diaphragmatic deconditioning, weakness, and atrophy in 48 hours.[47] In the presence of spontaneous breathing, inappropriate ventilator settings may increase patient work and fatigue further.[11] However, careful selection of ventilator settings can reduce the workload to a normal range without resulting in deconditioning and atrophy of the respiratory muscles.[11]

Patient-ventilator synchrony is a critical issue for every patient triggering the ventilator for a mechanically supported inspiration. A lack of synchrony increases ventilatory effort, respiratory rate, and the patient's WOB because the ventilator is not providing flow to match the patient's inspiratory demand. Pressure-targeted modes of ventilation are generally better than volume-targeted modes at reducing the likelihood of asynchrony because pressure ventilation allows the ventilator to deliver a variable flow with each breath based on the patient's inspiratory demand.[48] In addition, most ventilators now allow adjustment of rise time to ensure gas delivery is matched to the patient's inspiratory flow demand.[48,49]

Patient-ventilator synchrony is also affected by the inspiratory time. The ventilator's inspiratory time and the patient's inspiratory time should be equal; that is, the ventilator should cycle to exhalation when the patient is ready to begin exhalation. Trigger sensitivity should always be set to be as sensitive as possible without causing spontaneous autotriggering. Generally, flow triggering is recommended over pressure triggering.[50] A final factor affecting patient-ventilator synchrony is auto-PEEP,[51] which normally is a problem only in patients with airways obstruction, although it is a potential concern in all patients. If the patient's inspiratory efforts fail to trigger the ventilator, the problem is usually auto-PEEP.[52,53]

Peak Flow and Flow Waveform and Volume Ventilation

If a patient is spontaneously triggering the ventilator, peak flow delivery during volume ventilation should match the patient's inspiratory flow demand.[9,10] Most adult patients with moderate to strong ventilatory demands require a peak flow of 80 L/min or greater. As shown by Marini and colleagues,[9,10] if the peak flow does not meet the patient's inspiratory demand, the WOB performed by the patient increases (see Figure 44-4). In this setting, the efficiency of the work may be greater than during spontaneous breathing, but the overall patient work may be similar.[9,10] In volume ventilation, there is always an indirect relationship between the work provided by the ventilator and the patient's WOB (Figure 44-9). In volume ventilation, the more work the patient does, the less work the ventilator performs for the patient.

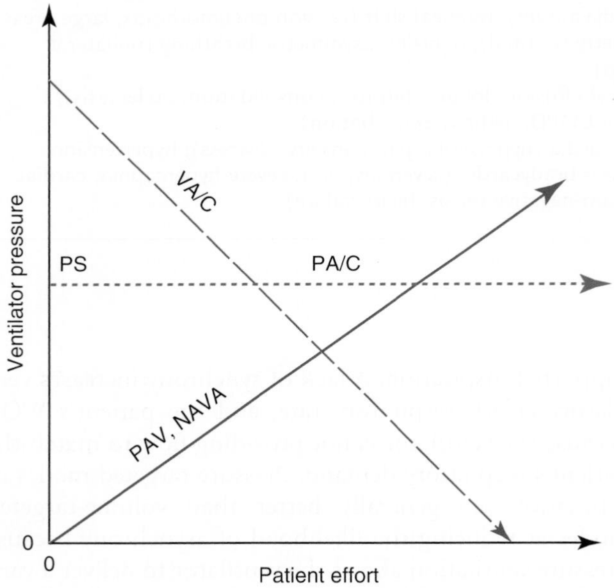

FIGURE 44-9 Relationship between ventilator pressure and patient effort during various forms of ventilatory support. During volume ventilation, there is always an indirect relationship between ventilator pressure and patient effort; the greater the patient effort, the less the ventilator pressure, and the greater the potential asynchrony. With pressure ventilation, airway pressure theoretically does not change as patient effort increases; there is equal ventilator work regardless of patient effort. During PAV and NAVA, ventilator pressure and patient effort are directly related. That is, as patient effort increases, ventilatory pressure increases. With PAV and NAVA, all the clinician sets is the slope of the relationship between ventilator and patient effort. (Modified from Younes M: Proportional assist ventilation, a new approach to ventilatory support. Theory. Am Rev Respir Dis 145:114–117, 1992.)

If the patient is triggering the positive pressure breaths, the WOB is shared between the patient and the ventilator. For this reason, patients initially receiving assisted ventilation show altered gas delivery patterns after they are sedated to apnea. With the transition to controlled ventilation, the peak airway and plateau pressures usually increase during volume ventilation, and V_T decreases in pressure ventilation.[29] Because the patient is no longer performing a portion of the WOB, the work performed by the ventilator must increase.

Most ventilators during volume ventilation mode can deliver gas flow in a decelerating or square wave flow pattern. If the patient is triggering inspiration, we recommend a decelerating flow pattern, especially when a small V_T is being delivered.[29,54] A decelerating flow pattern allows a high peak flow to be delivered but also ensures that the inspiratory time can be adequately set. In patients who are sedated and who are not triggering the ventilator, the choice of flow waveform is unimportant, and the setting of peak flow depends on the inspiratory time and V_T desired by the clinician.

Inspiratory Time and Volume Ventilation

In patients self-triggering every breath, the set inspiratory time should equal the patients' neuroinspiratory time.[55] As illustrated in Figure 44-10, when the inspiratory time is decreased to equal the patient's desired inspiratory time and peak flow is increased to match the patient's demand, the patient's WOB and effort correspondingly decrease. A patient with a moderate to high ventilatory demand rarely desires an inspiratory time greater than 1 second.[54] Many adults with moderate or high ventilatory demands desire an inspiratory time between 0.6 second and 0.9 second.[29] Carefully matching the ventilator's inspiratory time with the patient's inspiratory time generally markedly improves patient-ventilator synchrony.

In patients who are receiving controlled mechanical ventilation, inspiratory time is set based on the V_T and the clinician's perceived optimal time of inspiration. In most settings, an inspiratory time of about 1.0 second is ideal. In patients with severe asthma, the inspiratory time may need to be increased to 1.2 to 1.5 seconds to ensure ventilation passes beyond markedly obstructed airways.[29] In asthma, the airways resistance is increased not only during exhalation but also during inspiration. As a result, to ventilate patients with asthma, inspiratory time needs to be increased beyond the level normally required.

V_T can also affect synchrony during volume ventilation. Both too large and too small V_T adversely affects synchrony. Too large V_T frequently induces missed triggering (Figure 44-11).[56-58] This missed triggering occurs because V_T larger than a patient's respiratory center desires is delivered, and the allotted expiratory time of the respiratory center is not long enough for complete exhalation to occur. The result is air trapping and auto-PEEP. This problem can

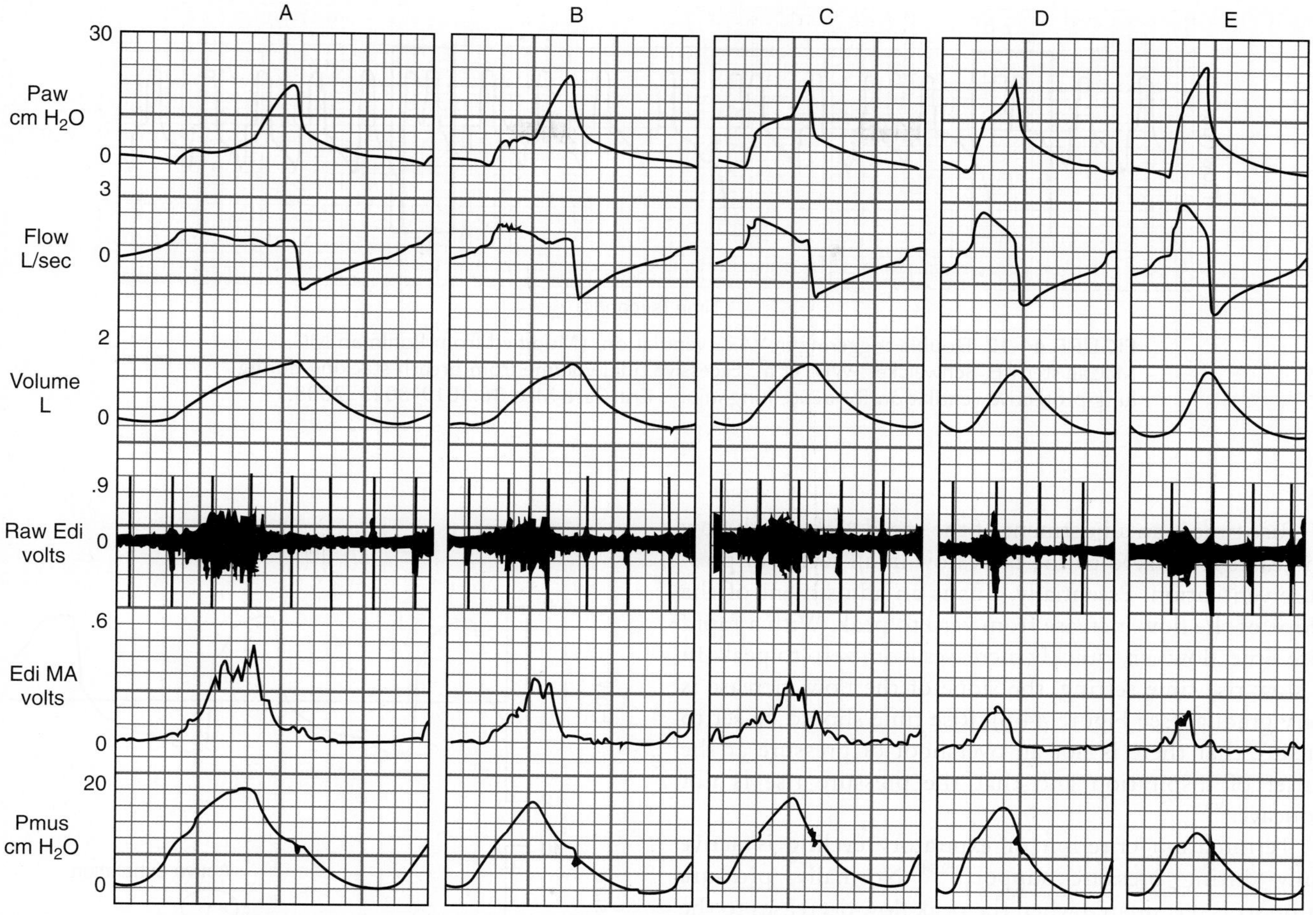

FIGURE 44-10 Airway pressure (P_{aw}), flow, volume, raw (R_{aw}) electromyographic activity of the diaphragm (E_{di}), integrated E_{di}, and muscular work of the diaphragm (P_{mus}) in volume ventilation during varying inspiratory flow and inspiratory time settings (columns *A, B, C, D, E*). As peak flow is increased and inspiratory time is decreased (left to right), indices of patient effort and work are decreased. Ideal settings of flow and inspiratory time generally can be identified by observing the airway pressure curve during volume ventilation. The closer the airway pressure curve is to the ideal curve (*D* and *E*), the less the patient's work. (From Fernandez R, Mendez M, Younes M: Effect of ventilator flow rate on respiratory timing in normal humans. Am J Respir Crit Care Med 159:710–719, 1999.)

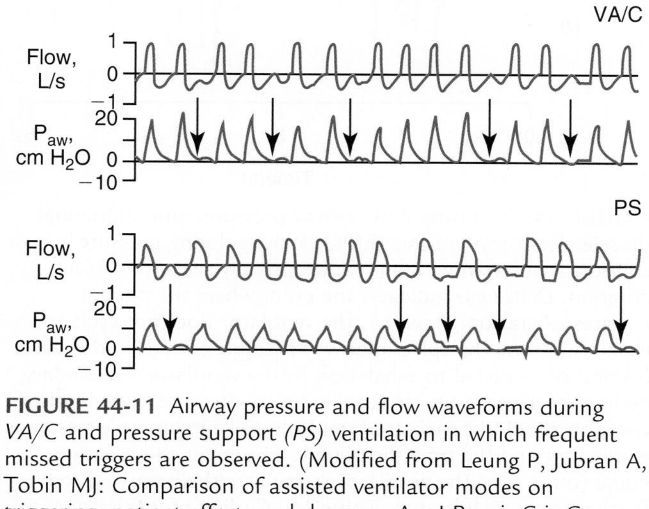

FIGURE 44-11 Airway pressure and flow waveforms during *VA/C* and pressure support *(PS)* ventilation in which frequent missed triggers are observed. (Modified from Leung P, Jubran A, Tobin MJ: Comparison of assisted ventilator modes on triggering, patient effort, and dyspnea. Am J Respir Crit Care Med 155:1387, 1997.)

be fixed easily by decreasing delivered V_T.[58] Too small V_T is frequently identified by double triggering (Figure 44-12).[59] This problem can be corrected by increasing V_T or appropriately sedating the patient.[59]

Rise Time, Termination Criteria (Inspiratory Time), and Pressure Ventilation

Generally, pressure-targeted modes of ventilation are more likely to improve patient ventilatory synchrony than volume-targeted modes because in pressure ventilation, increased patient demand results in greater flow and the ability to change V_T. This situation may be a concern for lung injury based on the size of V_T, but synchrony is generally better in pressure ventilation.[57,58] However, numerous factors can affect synchrony during pressure ventilation, rise time, termination criteria, inspiratory time, and pressure setting.

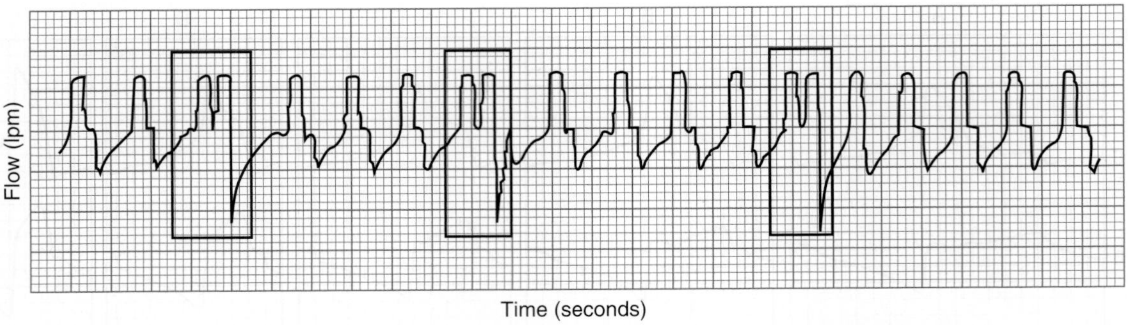

FIGURE 44-12 Double triggering in VA/C ventilation. (Modified from Pohlman MC, McCallister KE, Schweickert WD, et al: Excessive tidal volume from breath stacking during lung-protective ventilation for acute lung injury. Crit Care Med 36:3019–3023, 2008.)

Rise time is an adjustment of the speed with which flow increases from zero to the peak flow in all forms of pressure ventilation. Essentially, this is an adjustment of the slope of the flow increase from zero to peak. With a rapid rise time, flow very quickly increases from zero to peak. In a slow rise time setting, the slope of the flow increase is very gradual (see Figure 44-8). Rise time should be set to ensure that there is not an overshoot of pressure at the onset of inspiration and that the pressure rise is not concave.[29]

Termination criterion or expiratory cycling is active only during pressure support.[29,54] Normally, pressure support is terminated when the peak flow decreases to the predetermined level. Historically, this level is 25% of peak flow.[15] However, not all patients choose to terminate inspiration at this 25% setting. Patients with marked respiratory distress and patients with chronic pulmonary disease choose to end inspiration at high terminal flow.[58] In our experience, these patients require a termination criterion set at 50% or higher. Figure 44-13 depicts the problem encountered by patients if the termination criterion is set at a lower percentage than the patient chooses to end inspiration. Specifically, patients' neuroinspiratory time is shorter than the ventilator's inspiratory time[59]; when this happens, the patient activates accessory muscles of expiration to force the ventilator into exhalation.

In Figure 44-13, abdominal muscles activate midway through the ventilator inspiratory phase—the patient started to exhale in the middle of the ventilator's inspiratory phase. The clinician can identify that this is happening by an increase in the set pressure at the end of inspiration. This increase indicates that the breath is terminated by the second termination criterion, an increase in airway pressure above the set level. This level is ventilator-specific.[29,54] If the breath is ended by a spike in pressure, the termination criterion needs to be increased slowly until there is a smooth decrease in pressure. If the ventilator does not have the ability to adjust the termination criterion, the problem can be corrected by switching to PA/C. PA/C essentially operates during assisted breaths

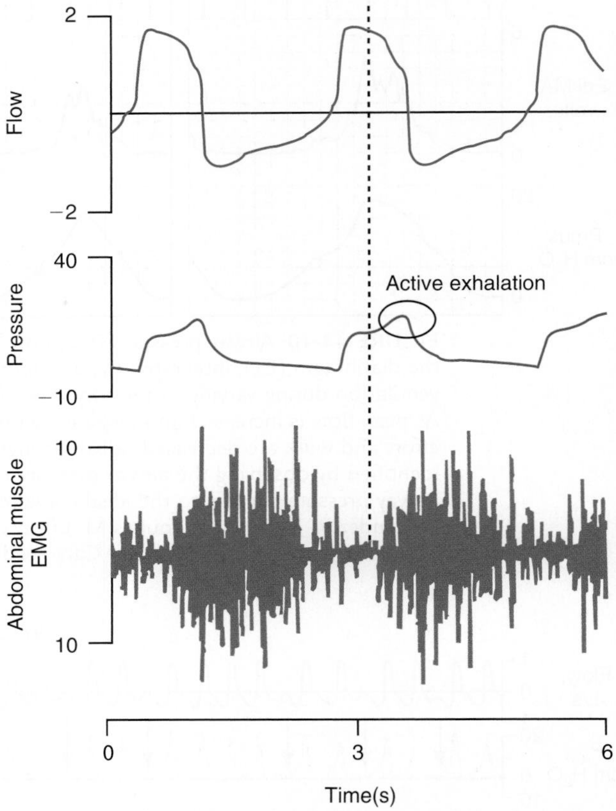

FIGURE 44-13 Airway flow, airway pressure, and abdominal muscle electromyographic (EMG) activity during pressure support ventilation with an inappropriately set termination criterion. *Dotted line* indicates the point where the patient initiates expiration. However, the ventilator does not cycle to exhalation until the spike in airway pressure *(circle)*. In this case, inspiration is cycled to exhalation by the ventilator's secondary cycling mechanism an increase in airway pressure. Termination criterion should be increased until the spike in airway pressure is eliminated and the time the patient terminates the breath is equal to the time the ventilator terminates the breath. (From Parthasarathy S, Jubran A, Tobin MJ: Cycling of inspiratory and expiratory muscle groups with the ventilator in airflow limitation. Am J Respir Crit Care Med 158:1471–1478, 1998.)

the same as PSV except that inspiration terminates at a set time.[15] If there is a spike in pressure at the end of a PA/C breath, the inspiratory time setting needs to be decreased until the spike disappears.

In addition, in all pressure-targeted modes of ventilation, the pressure level should be set to ensure that the resultant V_T is 4 to 8 ml/kg IBW. If too high a pressure is set, air trapping may occur resulting in missed triggering. Inappropriately set V_T is the primary cause of missed triggered breaths.[58]

OXYGENATION

Oxygen Concentration

Initiation of treatment for most patients in the acute care setting is with 100% O_2, unless detailed information identifying precise FiO_2 needed is available. FiO_2 is titrated to achieve PaO_2 of 60 to 80 mm Hg with SaO_2 or SpO_2 90% or greater. Pulse oximetry values always should be with simultaneous measurements of arterial blood gases to ensure correlation. Estimate of O_2 needs can be derived as follows:

$$FiO_2 = \left(\frac{PaO_2 \text{ desired}}{PaO_2/PAO_2 \text{ ratio}} + PaCO_2 \times 1.25 \right) \times \frac{1}{P_B - P_{H_2O}}$$

where FiO_2 required is the FiO_2 needed to achieve a desired PaO_2, PaO_2/PAO_2 is the initial PaO_2 divided by the initial alveolar partial pressure of oxygen (PAO_2), $PaCO_2$ is the initial $PaCO_2$, PB is barometric pressure, and P_{H_2O} is water vapor pressure. A simpler but less accurate calculation is the following:

$$\underset{\text{Initial}}{PaO_{2(1)}/FiO_2(1)} = \underset{\text{Desired}}{PaO_{2(2)}/FiO_2(2)}$$

Instead of a formula, a nomogram can be used to predict a patient's required FiO_2 (Figure 44-14). In either case, it is suggested that O_2 levels be titrated down from 100% to minimal FiO_2 required in decrements not to exceed 20%; titration is followed by oximetry or measurement of blood gases. When titrating FiO_2 downward, the clinician should wait at least 20 minutes between changes in FiO_2 to allow O_2 levels to stabilize. Patients with obstructive disease need a longer period for equilibration after a change in FiO_2.

When minimal FiO_2 is identified, further reduction in FiO_2 should be in steps of 5% to 10% followed by oximetry or measurement of blood gases. Box 44-15 lists a conservative method of titrating O_2 concentration down from an initial FiO_2 of 1 on the basis of PaO_2.

Once the desired PaO_2 and saturation are reached, monitoring should be continued. Generally, O_2 levels are titrated up and down as needed with adjustments in FiO_2 of 0.05 to 0.10 to maintain PaO_2 of 60 to 80 mm Hg with SpO_2 of 90% to 95%. Titration is followed by oximetry or measurement of blood gases. SpO_2 of 88% to 90% may be acceptable for patients who need FiO_2 of 0.80 or more.

Box 44-15 Titrating Fractional Inspired Oxygen Down from an Initial Starting Point of 1.0 According to Initial PaO_2 and Pulse Oximetry Findings

Initial PaO_2 on FiO_2 1.0 (mm Hg)	FiO_2 Step 1	Step 2	Step 3	Step 4	Step 5
>300	0.80	0.60	0.50	0.40	0.35*
200-300	0.80	0.60	0.50	0.40*	—
150-199	0.80	0.60*	—	—	—
100-149	0.80*	—	—	—	—

Decrease FiO_2 to the target value in steps, and perform pulse oximetry or arterial blood gas measurements. Patients should continue to receive a given FiO_2 long enough to ensure equilibration and acceptable SpO_2 before further reductions are made in FiO_2. This procedure takes 20 minutes per FiO_2 change for most patients and up to 30 minutes for patients with obstructive disease. It usually is safe to continue to decrease FiO_2 as long as SpO_2 is greater than 95% (which should correspond to a PaO_2 > 90 mm Hg) for most patients. When SpO_2 is less than 97%, increase or decrease FiO_2 in steps of 0.05 per change.

*Target FiO_2 based on initial PaO_2.

RULE OF THUMB

If a patient's oxygenation status is unknown, or if the patient's condition is unstable or critical, begin ventilatory support with FiO_2 of 1 until PaO_2, SaO_2, or SpO_2 can be assessed.

Positive End Expiratory Pressure and Continuous Positive Airway Pressure

Various approaches to adjusting PEEP or CPAP have been suggested over the years, including minimum PEEP, optimal or best PEEP, use of PEEP tables, PEEP titrated by compliance or pressure-volume curves, and decremental PEEP trials. With acute restrictive disease, as PEEP or CPAP levels are increased, PaO_2, SpO_2, and static compliance tend to improve until the point at which lung overinflation occurs.[60,61] As mean airway pressure increases, venous return decreases. The result may be a decrease in cardiac output. Figure 44-15 shows the physiologic factors that change during application of PEEP or CPAP. Several approaches to adjusting PEEP or CPAP are described later.

Minimum Positive End Expiratory Pressure

Minimum PEEP can be defined as the minimal PEEP needed to maintain recruited lung open and achieve adequate PaO_2 (and SpO_2) with FiO_2 less than 0.6. Generally, the PEEP level needed to achieve PaO_2 of at least 60 mm Hg (SpO_2 ≥ 90%) with FiO_2 of 0.40 to 0.50 or less is the

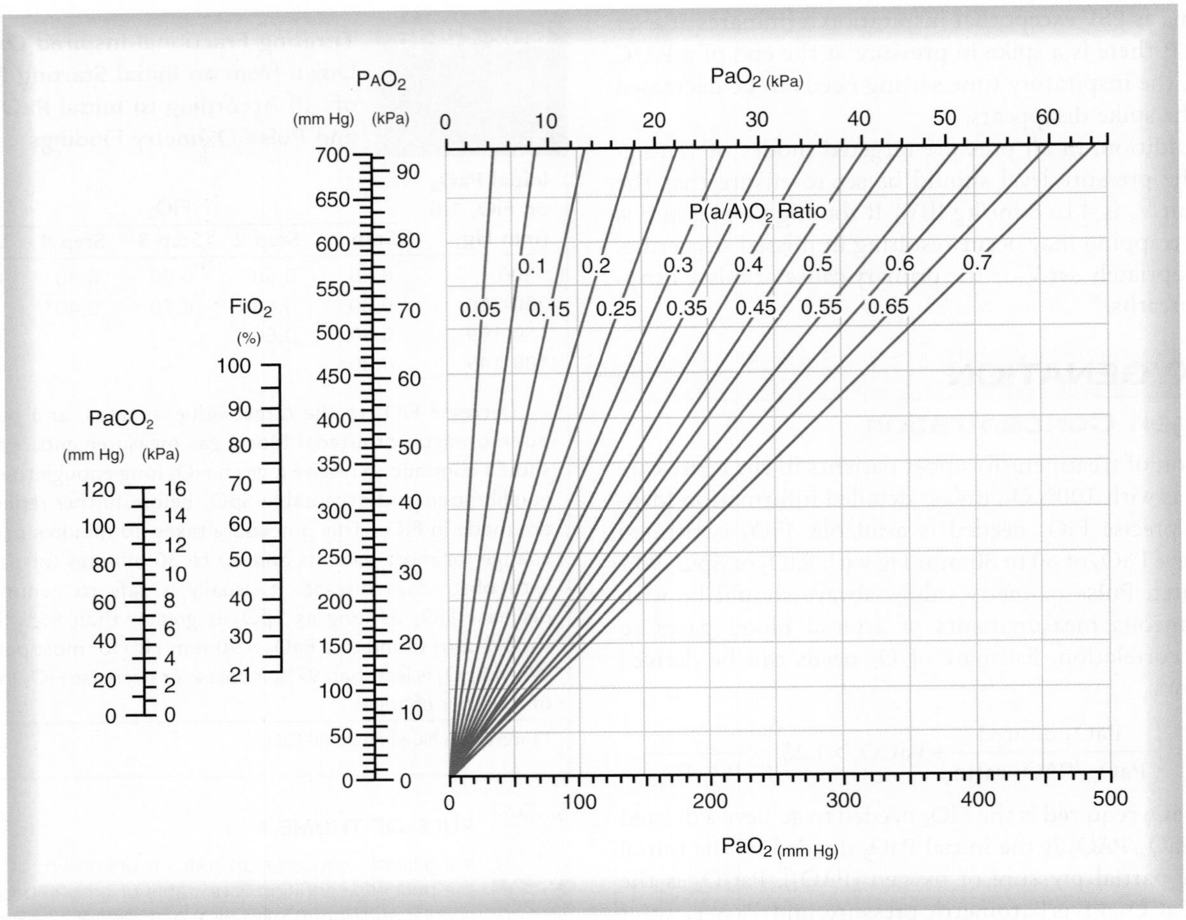

FIGURE 44-14 Nomogram for computing PaO_2/PAO_2 ratio and predicting FiO_2 required for desired PaO_2. To use the nomogram, first align the patient's current $PaCO_2$ and FiO_2 *(left two columns)* with a straight edge. This line intersects the vertical line corresponding to the patient's PAO_2 *(third column)*. Draw a horizontal line from this point to the vertical line corresponding to the patient's PaO_2. The diagonal line at this point (or one interpolated from the nearest diagonal lines bracketing it) is the PaO_2/PAO_2 ratio. $PaCO_2$ of 40 mm Hg and FiO_2 of 50% give PAO_2 of about 310 mm Hg. If PaO_2 is 50 mm Hg, PaO_2/PAO_2 is about 0.15. To predict FiO_2 required for PaO_2 of 70 mm Hg, follow the diagonal line representing 0.15 up to where it intersects the vertical line representing $PaO_2 = 70$ mm Hg. From this point, draw a horizontal line to the left intersecting the PAO_2 column at about 450 mm Hg. Connect this point to the present $PaCO_2$ (40 mm Hg) and note that the line passes through the required FiO_2 of about 70%. (From Chatburn RL, Lough MD: Handbook of respiratory care, Chicago, 1990, Year Book Medical Publishers.)

minimum PEEP. With this approach, the least PEEP or CPAP level needed to achieve this therapeutic end point is applied.[29]

Optimal or Best Positive End Expiratory Pressure Based on Oxygen Delivery

Optimal or best PEEP may be defined as the PEEP that maximizes oxygen delivery (DO_2). Oxygen delivery is calculated as cardiac output ($\dot{Q}_T$) multiplied by oxygen content (CaO_2):

$$DO_2 = \dot{Q}_T \times CaO_2$$

For the optimal PEEP level, PEEP is increased in increments of 2 cm H_2O. Blood pressure, mixed venous O_2 levels (partial pressure of oxygen in mixed venous blood [$P\bar{v}O_2$], mixed venous oxygen saturation [$S\bar{v}O_2$], arteriovenous oxygen content difference [$C(a-\bar{v})O_2$]) cardiac output, and cardiac index are assessed. PEEP is increased incrementally until there is a decline in O_2 delivery, at which point the best or optimal PEEP has been exceeded. PEEP is adjusted down to the previous level that represents the "best" PEEP. Table 44-7 shows an example of a PEEP study for determining optimal PEEP based on O_2 delivery. In Table 44-7, as PEEP is increased from 8 cm H_2O to 10 cm H_2O to 12 cm H_2O, $P\bar{v}O_2$, $S\bar{v}O_2$, and O_2

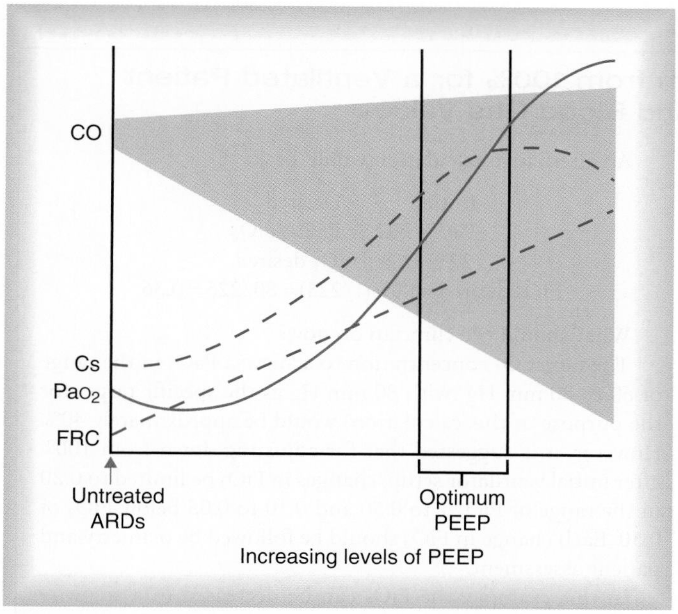

FIGURE 44-15 Curves represent the physiologic factors that change during the application of PEEP and CPAP. As PEEP level is increased, PaO_2, FRC, and static compliance (Cs) normally increase. Cardiac output (CO) *(shaded area)* can increase slightly, stay the same, or decrease. Optimum PEEP level can be expected to occur when PaO_2, FRC, and Cs are high. CO should be maintained near normal so that O_2 transport to the tissues remains high. (Modified from Pilbeam SP: Mechanical ventilation: physiological and clinical applications, ed 3, St Louis, 1998, Mosby.)

delivery increase with no decline in cardiac output ($\dot{Q}_T$) or blood pressure. However, when PEEP is increased to 14 cm H_2O, $S\bar{v}O_2$, O_2 delivery, $\dot{Q}_T$, and blood pressure decline, indicating that optimal PEEP for this patient has been exceeded. The best PEEP for this patient would be 12 cm H_2O. Before determining PEEP using this approach, it is critical that the patient's hemodynamic status is stabilized. Patients with a compromised hemodynamic status generally do not tolerate PEEP titration without further compromise.

Compliance-Titrated Positive End Expiratory Pressure

With the compliance-titrated technique, PEEP is increased in increments of 2 cm H_2O, and the patient's estimated static compliance (Cs) is measured:

$$Cs = \frac{\text{Volume delivered (ml)}}{P_{plat} - P_{baseline}\ (\text{PEEP/CPAP})}$$

where total PEEP equals the sum of applied PEEP plus auto-PEEP.

Best PEEP has been exceeded at the point where an increase in PEEP is followed by a decrease in compliance. PEEP is reduced to the previous level, and this is optimal PEEP based on compliance.[60] For the example shown in Table 44-7, the best PEEP based on compliance would be 12 cm H_2O. Regional lung overdistention and declines in cardiac output can occur at levels less than compliance-titrated best PEEP, and consequently hemodynamic status should be optimized before any PEEP trial.

Positive End Expiratory Pressure Titrated With Pressure-Volume Curves as Part of a Lung Protective Strategy

A lung protective strategy that has been shown to improve outcome in ALI/ARDS includes use of a low V_T (4 to 8 ml/kg) and PEEP set 2 cm H_2O above the lower inflection point (P_{flex}) on a pressure-volume curve.[21,22] This strategy requires the use of static pressure-volume curves or slow-flow pressure-volume curves to determine best PEEP. To obtain a static pressure-volume curve, the RT passively inflates the patient's lungs with varying volumes in increasing increments of 50 to 100 ml. At each end point, static pressure is obtained by means of application of an end inspiratory pause, and the resultant pressure-volume curve is plotted (Figure 44-16). Upper and lower inflection points typically can be determined. The lower inflection point is thought to be the point at which alveolar recruitment begins. The upper inflection point indicates lung overdistention. PEEP is set at approximately 2 cm H_2O above the lower inflection point (P_{flex}). Determining PEEP level using the P_{flex} value may be done after a lung recruitment maneuver (see later). V_T is adjusted to ensure that the upper inflection point is not exceeded during inspiration.

Calculating the static pressure-volume curve is technically difficult and time-consuming.[11] An alternative is to use the slow-flow pressure-volume curve. A slow-flow curve (≤6 L/min) may also identify the lower inflection point for the purposes of setting PEEP (Figure 44-17). However, in either case, some patients do not have a lower inflection point. In about 25% of patients, the P_{flex} cannot be identified from the pressure-volume curve.[22] In addition, observer variability in identifying the lower inflection point can be significant.[62]

Positive End Expiratory Pressure and Lung Recruitment Maneuvers

Various lung recruitment maneuvers have been suggested for improving $\dot{V}/\dot{Q}$ and reducing shunting in patients with ALI/ARDS. These maneuvers include several variations that incorporate CPAP[21,63,64] or the use of PCV with high PEEP levels.[61,65] Regardless of approach, before any lung recruitment maneuver is performed, the patient must be hemodynamically stable and sedated to apnea. Neuromuscular paralysis is unnecessary, but the patient must be accepting of passive ventilation at high pressures. Hemodynamic stability is crucial because of the high intrathoracic pressures established during all recruitment maneuvers, although the few data that are available indicate that pressure control recruitment maneuvers are

MINI CLINI

Adjustment of Oxygen Concentration Down from 100% for a Ventilated Patient According to Fractional Inspired Oxygen and Blood Gas Values

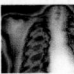

PROBLEM: At 9:00 AM, mechanical ventilation is initiated with the following settings for a 70-kg patient:

Mode: VA/C with the patient actively triggering the ventilator
V_T: 500 ml
Rate: 20 to 26 breaths/min
FiO_2: 1
PEEP: 5 cm H_2O

An arterial blood gas is obtained 20 minutes after ventilator initiation:

FiO_2: 1
PaO_2: 225 mm Hg
pH: 7.42
$PaCO_2$: 40 mm Hg
HCO_3: 24 mEq/L
Base excess: +1 mEq/L

Calculated alveolar PAO_2 and PaO_2/PAO_2 ratios are:

$$PAO_2 = FiO_2\,(PB - P_{H_2O}) - PaCO_2 \times 1.25 = 663$$
$$PaO_2/PAO_2 = 225/663 = 0.34$$

What FiO_2 is needed to achieve a target PaO_2 of 80 mm Hg?

SOLUTION: The following equation and normal barometric pressure ($P_B = 760$), lead to the calculation:

$$FiO_2 \text{ required} = \left(\frac{PaO_2 \text{ desired}}{PaO_2/PAO_2 \text{ ratio}} + PaCO_2 \times 1.25\right) \times \frac{1}{P_B - P_{H_2O}}$$
$$= \left(\frac{80}{0.34} + 40 \times 1.25\right) \times \frac{1}{760 - 47} = 0.40$$

An alternative calculation would be:

$$\text{Initial} \quad \text{Desired}$$
$$PaO_2/FiO_2 = PaO_2/FiO_2$$
$$225/1 = 80/FiO_2 \text{ desired}$$
$$FiO_2 \text{ desired} = 80 \times (1/225) = 80/225 = 0.36$$

What should the clinician do now?

The target O_2 concentration to achieve a PaO_2 in the range of 60 to 80 mm Hg (with 80 mm Hg as the specific target for the purpose of this calculation) would be approximately 40%. However, it is suggested that for adjusting down from 100% after initial ventilator setup, changes in FiO_2 be limited to 0.20 in the range of FiO_2 1 to 0.50 and 0.10 to 0.05 below FiO_2 of 0.50. Each change in FiO_2 should be followed by oximetry and patient assessment.

In this example, the FiO_2 can be decreased in a stepwise manner, as follows:

Time	FiO_2	SpO_2 (%)
9:30 AM	1	99
9:45 AM	0.80	99
10:00 AM	0.60	98
10:15 AM	0.50	97
10:30 AM	0.45	97
10:45 AM	0.40	95

Arterial blood gas on FiO_2 of 0.40 reveals a PaO_2 of 80 mm Hg.

better tolerated than CPAP recruitment maneuvers.[66,67] The original recruitment techniques applied 40 to 45 cm H_2O CPAP for 30 to 40 seconds.[21,63,64] For recruitment maneuvers to be successful, they should be performed as early as possible after the patient is stabilized on the ventilator.[63-65] The longer the length of mechanical ventilation before the recruitment maneuver, the greater the likelihood that the maneuver will fail. See Box 44-16 for details on the performance of lung recruitment maneuvers and decremental PEEP trials.

The most widely accepted approach to recruiting the lung is the use of PCV. With this approach, PEEP is set higher than levels needed to maintain the recruited lung open, usually between 20 cm H_2O and 25 cm H_2O; a pressure control level 15 to 20 cm H_2O above this is then set. Ventilation is provided with an I:E of 1:1 to 1:2 at a rate of 15 to 20 per minute. All recruitment maneuvers are preformed with 100% O_2. If this initial approach to lung recruitment does not open the lung, PEEP can be set higher in increments of 5 cm H_2O, and the recruitment is repeated after the patient has totally stabilized from the previous maneuver (>30 minutes). The maximum safe peak pressure during a recruitment maneuver is 50 cm H_2O. Peak pressures greater than 50 cm H_2O increase the likelihood of barotraumas during the maneuver.[64,65]

The best method of establishing optimal PEEP after recruitment is a decremental PEEP trial.[61,63,65,68] It is best to perform the trial in volume ventilation because the easiest bedside method of identifying the optimal PEEP is to determine the best compliance PEEP. The best oxygenation PEEP can also be determined. It takes only about 3 to 5 minutes for the compliance to stabilize when PEEP is changed, but at least 20 minutes is required for PaO_2 to stabilize after a PEEP adjustment.

MINI CLINI

Adjusting Fractional Inspired Oxygen

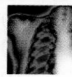

PROBLEM: A 70-kg patient in the ICU is receiving mechanical ventilation in the VA/C mode. The patient's arterial blood gas values and related ventilator settings are:

Mode: VA/C the patient is not breathing spontaneously
FiO_2: 0.40
PaO_2: 50 mm Hg
V_T: 450 ml
pH: 7.4
Rate: 22 breaths/min
$PaCO_2$: 40 mm Hg
PEEP: 10 cm H_2O
HCO_3: 24 mEq/L
Base excess: +1 mEq/L

What FiO_2 would be required to increase this patient's PaO_2 to 60 mm Hg?

SOLUTION: First, calculate the patient's current PAO_2 and PaO_2/PAO_2 ratio:

$$PAO_2 = FiO_2\,(PB - P_{H_2O}) - PaCO_2/0.8$$
$$= 0.40\,(760-47) - 40/0.8$$
$$= 285 - 50 = 235 \text{ mm Hg}$$
$$PaO_2/PAO_2 = 50/235 = 0.21$$

Next, calculate the FiO_2 needed to achieve the desired PaO_2 of 60 mm Hg:

$$FiO_2 \text{ required} = \left(\frac{PaO_2 \text{ desired} + PaCO_2 \times 1.25 \times 1}{PaO_2/PAO_2 \text{ ratio } P_B - P_{H_2O}}\right)$$
$$= \left(\frac{60 + (40 \times 1.25) \times 1}{0.21760 - 47}\right)$$
$$= \frac{335.7 \times 1}{713} = 0.47$$

For this patient, if the FiO_2 is increased from 0.40 to 0.50, the PaO_2 should increase from 50 to 60 mm Hg. An alternative calculation, based on PaO_2/FiO_2 ratio, would be:

$$\text{Actual} \quad \text{Desired}$$
$$PaO_2/FiO_2 = PaO_2/FiO_2$$

Solving for FiO_2, this becomes:

$$FiO_2 \text{ required} = PaO_2 \text{ desired} \times (FiO_2 \text{ actual}/PaO_2 \text{ actual})$$
$$= 60 \times (0.40/50) = 0.48$$

To increase this patient's PaO_2 to greater than 60 mm Hg would require increasing FiO_2 to approximately 0.50. Although FiO_2 of 0.50 or less is acceptable, as an alternative, the RT may consider increasing PEEP to 12 cm H_2O and then perform a clinical assessment, including evaluation of the effect of the increase on blood pressure, compliance, and arterial blood gases.

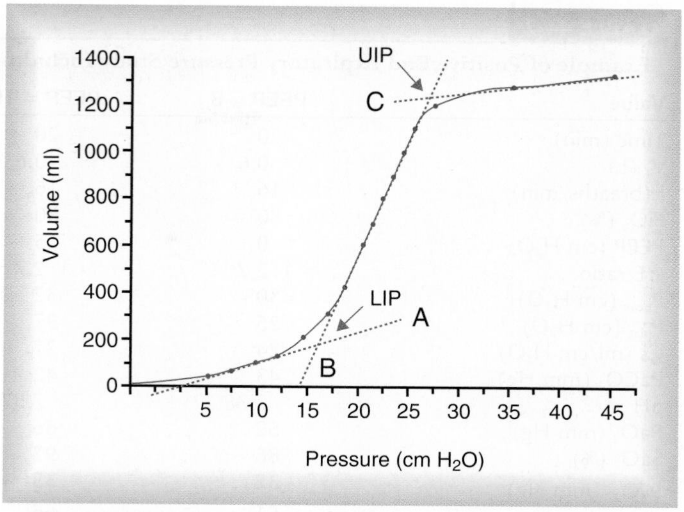

FIGURE 44-16 Static pressure-volume curve of a patient with ARDS. Volume is increased in increments of approximately 100 ml, inspiratory P_{plat} is measured, and a pressure-volume curve is plotted. Straight lines (*A, B,* and *C*) are drawn tangent to the curve, and the lower inflection point *(LIP)* and the upper inflection point *(UIP)* are identified. PEEP is adjusted to approximately 2 cm H_2O above the *LIP*.

Box 44-16 Performing a Lung Recruitment Maneuver and Decremental Positive End Expiratory Pressure Trial

- General approach: PCV
- PEEP: 20 to 25 cm H_2O
- Pressure control setting: 15 to 20 cm H_2O
- Inspiratory time: 1 to 2 seconds
- Rate: 15 to 20/min
- Duration 2 to 3 min

Immediately followed by a decremental PEEP trial

- Mode: Volume control
- PEEP: 20 to 25 cm H_2O
- V_T: 4 to 6 ml/kg IBW
- Rate: Highest rate avoiding auto-PEEP
- Ventilate until dynamic compliance stabilizes 3 to 5 minutes
- Record compliance
- Decrease PEEP by 2 cm H_2O
- Ventilate until dynamic compliance stabilizes 3 to 5 minutes
- Decrease PEEP by 2 cm H_2O
- Ventilate until dynamic compliance stabilizes 3 to 5 minutes
- Continue this until PEEP level that results in the best compliance is identified
- Repeat the recruitment maneuver
- Set PEEP at best compliance PEEP plus 2 to 3 cm H_2O

Before performing a recruitment maneuver, ensure that the patient is hemodynamically stable and sedated to apnea.

TABLE 44-7

Example of Positive End Expiratory Pressure Study Including Ventilation, Oxygenation, and Hemodynamic Data*

Value	PEEP = 8	PEEP = 10	PEEP = 12	PEEP = 14	PEEP = 16
Time (min)	0	20	40	60	80
V_T (L)	0.6	0.6	0.6	0.6	0.6
f (breaths/min)	16	16	16	16	16
FiO_2 (%)	80	80	80	80	80
PEEP (cm H_2O)	0	5	10	15	20
I:E ratio	1:2.7	1:2.7	1:2.7	1:2.7	1:2.7
P_{peak} (cm H_2O)	30	32	35	42	50
P_{plat} (cm H_2O)	25	27	29	36	43
Cs (ml/cm H_2O)	24	27	32	29	26
$PaCO_2$ (mm Hg)	43	42	43	42	44
pH	7.38	7.37	7.39	7.35	7.32
PaO_2 (mm Hg)	52	66	87	90	97
SaO_2 (%)	86	92	96	97	98
$P\bar{v}O_2$ (mm Hg)	32	35	37	37	36
$S\bar{v}O_2$ (mm Hg)	61	66	71	69	64
Blood pressure (mm Hg)	131/78	133/82	130/79	125/74	110/69
Cardiac output (L/min)	5.9	5.7	5.9	5.4	4.8
DO_2 (ml/min)	989	1022	1105	1021	917

*When first reviewing a PEEP study, observe changes in the following: (1) airway pressure, (2) blood pressure, (3) arterial oxygen (PaO_2, SaO_2) and mixed venous oxygenation ($P\bar{v}O_2$, $S\bar{v}O_2$), and (4) oxygen transport (DO_2). With increases in PEEP, PaO_2 and saturation improve; airway pressure increases; compliance improves and then decreases at higher levels of PEEP; and oxygen transport (DO_2) improves and then declines. Optimum PEEP for this patient is 10 cm H_2O because it provides the best arterial oxygenation (PaO_2, SaO_2) without a decline in DO_2 or cardiac output.

To perform the trial, PEEP should begin at 20 to 25 cm H_2O but always at PEEP higher than expected necessary to maintain the lung open. V_T during the decremental PEEP trial is usually set at 4 to 6 ml/kg IBW depending on P_{plat}. Inspiratory time is set at 0.6 to 0.8 second, and rate is at the highest level that does not result in auto-PEEP. First, the compliance is recorded at these settings after stabilization. Then the PEEP is decreased 2 cm H_2O, and the compliance again is allowed to stabilize. The process is continued until the best compliance PEEP can be identified. Generally, compliance is low at the starting PEEP (20 to 25 cm H_2O) because of overdistention. As PEEP is decreased, compliance improves until it peaks and then starts to decrease because of derecruitment and atelectasis.[61] The best compliance PEEP is increased by 2 to 3 cm H_2O because the best compliance PEEP underestimates the best oxygenation PEEP by 2 to 3 cm H_2O.[61] After identifying the optimal PEEP level, the lung must be recruited again because derecruitment occurred during the decremental PEEP trial. After this second recruitment, PEEP is set at the optimal level determined during the decremental trial.

A recruitment maneuver should be stopped if there is a decrease in SpO_2 to less than 85%, a significant change in heart rate (>140 beats/min or <60 beats/min), a significant change in mean arterial blood pressure (<60 mm Hg or a decrease >20 mm Hg from baseline), the development of cardiac arrhythmia, or any indication that barotraumas occurred.[63] More recent meta-analyses indicate that the use of high PEEP benefits patients with ARDS but does not benefit patients with ALI.[39,40]

Positive End Expiratory Pressure Tables

The ARDS Clinical Network study used an FiO_2-PEEP table to adjust PEEP levels.[2] Using this approach, PEEP and FiO_2 are alternately adjusted to obtain PaO_2 of 60 to 80 mm Hg or SpO_2 90% or greater (see Box 44-7). The table offers higher and lower PEEP options. For the lower PEEP option, PEEP is set at 5 to 10 cm H_2O with FiO_2 of 0.30 to 0.70; the higher PEEP option sets PEEP at 12 to 20 cm H_2O in the same FiO_2 range. The higher PEEP option should be reserved for patients who may benefit from higher PEEP in terms of lung recruitment and who have a stable blood pressure and no barotrauma. Of all the approaches to setting PEEP, this is the approach least based on the physiology of the patient. It is a reasonable approach to establish initial PEEP, but it is generally a poor choice for further adjustment of PEEP.

Other Techniques for Improving Oxygenation

The primary techniques for optimizing oxygenation in patients receiving mechanical ventilatory support are adjusting FiO_2 and PEEP. Other techniques that may be helpful in improving arterial O_2 levels include optimizing the patient's hemodynamic status, providing good bronchial hygiene, prone positioning, high-frequency

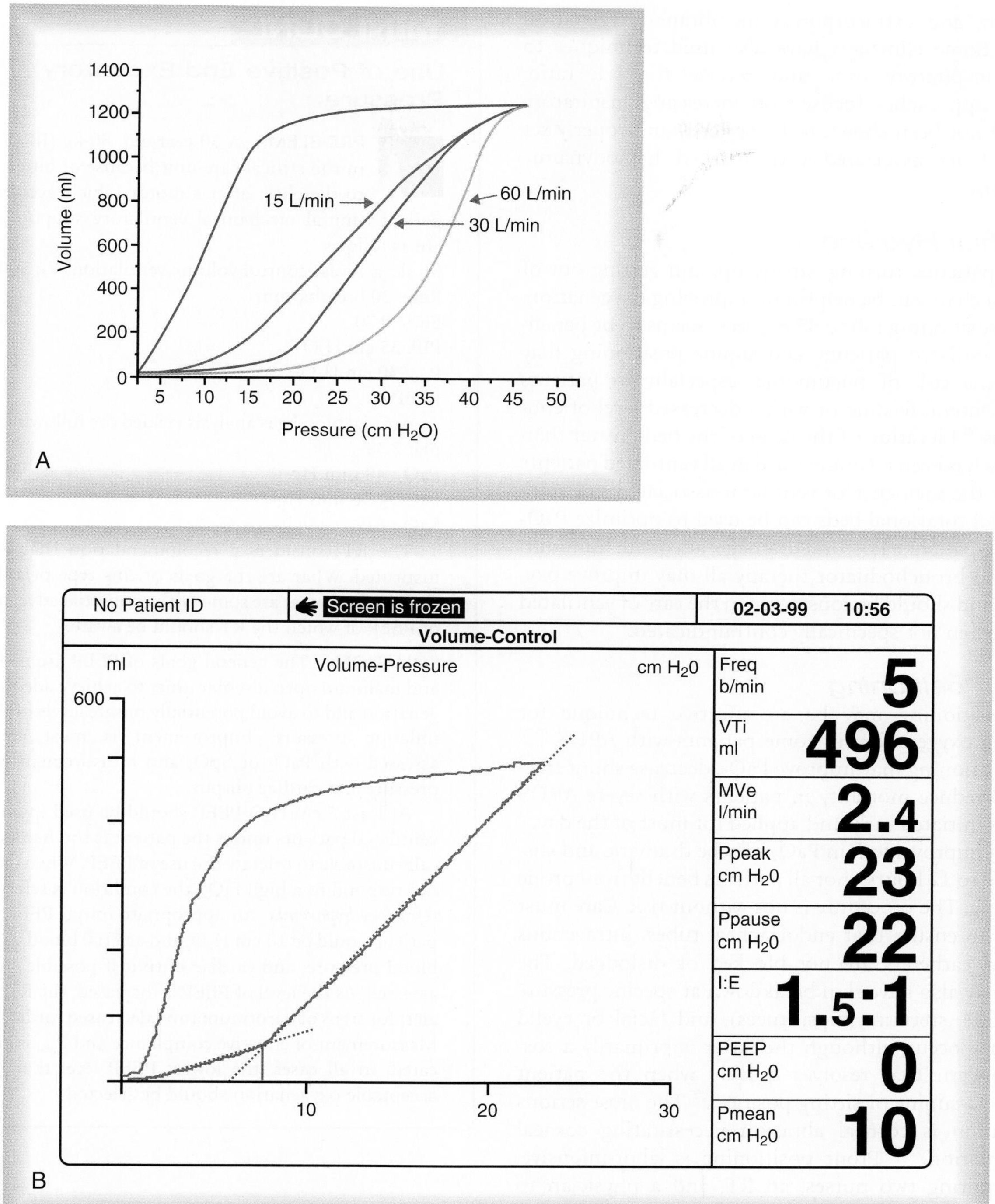

FIGURE 44-17 **A,** Pressure-volume curves generated by a ventilator graphics package with the flow set at 60 L/min, 30 L/min, and 15 L/min. As flow is decreased, the curve shifts to the left and more closely approximates a static pressure-volume curve. Flow of less than 6 L/min is recommended for substituting the lower inflection point *(LIP)* from a slow-flow pressure-volume curve for the static curve value. **B,** Slow-flow pressure-volume curve with use of a set rate of 5 breaths/min, I : E ratio of 1.5 : 1, and V_T of 500 ml. LIP is approximately 8 cm H_2O. The respiratory cycle time is 12 seconds (cycle time = 60/f = 60/5 = 12 seconds). An I : E ratio of 1.5 : 1 results in an inspiratory time of 4.8 seconds. Inspiratory flow is V_T/T_i = 0.5 L/4.8 sec = 0.104 L/sec, or approximately 6 L/min.

ventilation, and extracorporeal membrane oxygenation (ECMO). Some clinicians have also used techniques to prolong inspiratory time and reverse the I:E ratio. However, approaches focused on increasing inspiratory time have not been shown to be better than properly set PEEP and are associated with marked hemodynamic compromise.

Bronchial Hygiene

In many patients, turning, sitting up, and getting out of bed into a chair can be helpful in improving oxygenation. Upright positioning (30 to 45 degrees) seems to be beneficial for ventilated patients, and supine positioning may increase the risk of pneumonia, especially in patients receiving enteral feeding or with a decreased level of consciousness.[69] Elevation of the head of the bed greater than 30 degrees has been recommended in all ventilated patients to reduce the incidence of ventilator-associated pneumonia. Special rotational beds can be used to optimize PaO_2 in selected patients. Postural drainage, adequate humidification, and bronchodilator therapy all may improve oxygenation and should be considered in the care of ventilated patients when not specifically contraindicated.

Prone Positioning

Prone positioning may be an effective technique for improving oxygenation in some patients with ARDS.[70-73] Prone positioning may improve PaO_2, decrease shunt fraction, and reduce mortality in patients with severe ARDS when it is initiated early and applied for most of the day.[74] Although improvement in PaO_2 may be dramatic and sustained (up to 12 hours), not all patients benefit from prone positioning. The procedure is not without risk. Care must be taken to ensure that endotracheal tubes, intravenous lines, and catheters are not blocked or dislodged. The patient may also have skin breakdown at specific pressure points (face, sternum, hips, knees), and facial or eyelid edema may occur, although the latter is primarily a cosmetic concern that resolves quickly when the patient returns to a supine or sitting position.[75] The most serious complication is corneal abrasion necessitating corneal transplantation.[75,76] Prone positioning is labor-intensive, often requiring two nurses, an RT, and a physician to "flip" the patient. Numerous randomized controlled trials have evaluated the impact of prone positioning on survival in ARDS/ALI[70-73]; however, none of the trials have shown improved outcome. A more recent meta-analysis indicated improved survival in patients with the most severe lung injury—patients with PaO_2/FiO_2 ratio less than 100 mm Hg.[74] Similar to all lung protective approaches to ventilatory support, prone positioning should be used early in the course of ARDS if it is to be beneficial.

The mechanism of action of prone positioning is unclear. In ARDS, dorsal lung injury tends to increase shunt and decrease $\dot{V}/\dot{Q}$, resulting in hypoxemia. Supine positioning tends to increase regional pressure in the dependent, or dorsal, portions of the lungs. Prone positioning may improve $\dot{V}/\dot{Q}$ and reduce shunting by removing the pressure of the heart on the dorsal regions, causing regional dorsal traction, which may promote lung opening. The recommended technique for prone positioning is outlined in Box 44-17.

MINI CLINI

Use of Positive End Expiratory Pressure

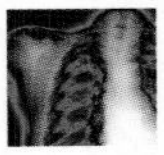

PROBLEM: A 30-year-old, 80-kg (IBW) man is in the critical care unit because of blunt trauma to the chest after a motor vehicle accident. The patient's initial mechanical ventilatory support settings are as follows:

Mode: = Assist-control volume ventilation, V_T: 500 ml
Rate: 20 breaths/min
FiO_2: 0.70
PIP: 35 cm H_2O
P_{plat}: 30 cm H_2O
PEEP: 0

Arterial blood gas analysis yielded the following results:

pH: 7.38
PaO_2: 48 mm Hg
$PaCO_2$: 36 mm Hg
SaO_2: 81%

The RT considers a recommendation that PEEP be instituted. What are the goals of this type of adjunctive therapy, and what are some of the potential adverse effects of PEEP of which the RT should be aware?

SOLUTION: The general goals of PEEP are to stabilize and maintain open alveolar units to achieve adequate oxygenation and to avoid potentially unsafe levels of FiO_2 and inflation pressure. Improvement is most commonly assessed with PaO_2 or SpO_2 and measurement of blood pressure and cardiac output.

At least 5 cm H_2O PEEP should be used in all acutely ventilated patients unless the patient is too hemodynamically unstable to tolerate the use of PEEP. When PaO_2 does not respond to a high FiO_2, the condition is referred to as *refractory hypoxemia*. An appropriate initial PEEP for this patient would be 10 cm H_2O, and arterial blood gases, P_{plat}, blood pressure, and cardiac output if possible should be assessed. As the level of PEEP is increased, the RT must be alert for signs of barotrauma and decreased cardiac output. Measurement of effective compliance and P_{plat} is also indicated. In all cases, the lowest PEEP level that provides acceptable oxygenation should be selected.

VENTILATION

Alveolar ventilation is determined by respiratory rate, V_T, and dead space and is described by the following equation:

Box 44-17 Prone Positioning

Preparation for prone positioning includes the following:

- Adequate sedation of patient
- Clear assignment of responsibilities between team members
- Moving the patient to one side of the bed
- Checking all lines for length
- Checking the security of the endotracheal tube
- Endotracheal suctioning
- Preoxygenation with 100% O_2
- Checking all vital signs

The turn includes:

- Tipping the patient to the side
- Securing electrocardiogram leads
- Turning the patient prone
- Turning the patient's head toward the ventilator

Care after the turn includes:

- Checking artificial airway
- Checking all lines
- Checking ventilator pressure and volume
- Monitoring vital signs
- Repositioning and recalibrating pressure transducers
- The patient needs supports (pillows) for each side of chest and forehead so that the endotracheal tube and head are not compromised.

$$\dot{V}_A = (V_T - V_{Dphys})f$$

where $\dot{V}_A$ is alveolar ventilation, V_T is tidal volume, V_{Dphys} is physiologic dead space, and f is respiratory frequency or rate. The relationship between arterial $PaCO_2$, alveolar ventilation ($\dot{V}_A$), and CO_2 production ($\dot{V}CO_2$) is described as follows:

$$PaCO_2 = (0.863)(\dot{V}CO_2)/\dot{V}_A$$

Arterial $PaCO_2$ is considered the best index of effective ventilation. Increases in $\dot{V}_A$ or decreases in $\dot{V}CO_2$ result in a decrease in $PaCO_2$, whereas increases in $\dot{V}CO_2$ or decreases in $\dot{V}_A$ result in an increase in $PaCO_2$. If there is no change in $\dot{V}CO_2$, the following relationships can be used to estimate the effect of changes in $\dot{V}_A$ on $PaCO_2$:

$$\begin{array}{cc} \text{Initial} & \text{Desired} \\ PaCO_{2(1)} \times \dot{V}_{A(1)} = & PaCO_{2(2)} \times \dot{V}_{A(2)} \end{array}$$

The foregoing predictive equation can be used during mechanical ventilation with the following modifications:

$$PaCO_{2(1)}(V_{T(1)} - V_{Dphys(1)})f_{(1)} = PaCO_{2(2)}(V_{T(2)} - V_{DSphys(2)})f_{(2)}$$

For changes in rate alone, if there is no change in $\dot{V}CO_2$ or V_{Dphys}, this becomes:

$$\begin{array}{cc} \text{Initial} & \text{Desired} \\ PaCO_{2(1)} \times f_{(1)} = & PaCO_{2(2)} \times f_{(2)} \end{array}$$

Box 44-18 Example of the Effect of Change in $\dot{V}_A$ on $PaCO_2$

If a patient has an initial $PaCO_2$ of 50 mm Hg with a corresponding alveolar ventilation ($\dot{V}_A$) of 4 L/min, what level of alveolar ventilation is required to decrease the $PaCO_2$ to 40 mm Hg (if there is no change in $\dot{V}_ACO_2$)?

If the patient's $\dot{V}_A$ is increased from 4 L/min to 5 L/min, the $PaCO_2$ should decrease from 50 mm Hg to 40 mm Hg.

For changes in VT alone, this becomes:

$$\begin{array}{cc} \text{Initial} & \text{Desired} \\ PaCO_{2(1)} \times V_{T(1)} = & PaCO_{2(2)} \times V_{T(2)} \end{array}$$

A major goal of mechanical ventilatory support is optimization of the patient's ventilation and $PaCO_2$; however, this does not mean normalization of $PaCO_2$. Acceptable arterial pH and alveolar pressure are maintained as assessed by P_{plat}. For many patients, the level of ventilatory support is adjusted to achieve a $PaCO_2$ of 35 to 45 mm Hg with a pH of 7.35 to 7.45. In the care of patients with acute exacerbation of COPD and accompanying chronic ventilatory failure, the clinician may target ventilatory support to achieve the patient's "normal" $PaCO_2$ and pH. For patients with COPD and chronic hypercapnia, the target $PaCO_2$ may be 50 to 60 mm Hg with a pH of 7.30 to 7.35. In patients with severe ARDS, a $PaCO_2$ of 70 mm Hg with an acidic pH may be have to be accepted to protect the lung from ventilator-induced lung injury. The sicker the patient, the more likely the clinician is to accept oxygenation and acid-base values that greatly deviate from normal. Regardless of the patient's condition, optimizing pH is more important than targeting a specific $PaCO_2$ value.[8,29,54] Box 44-18 presents an example of the effect of change in $\dot{V}_A$ on $PaCO_2$.

Adjusting Tidal Volume and Rate

V_T and rate may be adjusted for a desired level of ventilation as assessed by $PaCO_2$. V_T usually is based on specific patient considerations but ideally should never result in P_{plat} greater than 30 cm H_2O. Respiratory rate is adjusted to achieve the desired $PaCO_2$. Normal resting V_T of healthy individuals is 6.3 ml/kg IBW. In most critically ill patients, V_T should be in the range of 4 to 8 ml/kg IBW. In patients with improving respiratory function, V_T of 10 ml/kg IBW may be acceptable; however, V_T greater than 10 ml/kg IBW should never be selected for a critically ill patient.

Apnea (Controlled Ventilation)

In an apneic patient, precise control of $PaCO_2$ usually can be achieved with volume ventilation because the ventilator rate and V_T are determined by the clinician.

Rate. In the care of apneic patients, the clinician has complete control over the patient's rate, and changes in ventilator rate can be used precisely to alter $PaCO_2$. For rate changes alone (V_T held constant):

$$\begin{array}{c}\text{Initial} \qquad \text{Desired}\\ PaCO_{2(1)} \times f_{(1)} = PaCO_{2(2)} \times f_{(2)}\end{array}$$

For example, if a patient's initial rate was 18 breaths/min and resultant $PaCO_2$ was 50 mm Hg, the rate change needed to decrease the patient's $PaCO_2$ to 40 mm Hg could be calculated as follows:

$$\begin{array}{c}\text{Initial} \qquad \text{Desired}\\ PaCO_{2(1)} \times f_{(1)} = PaCO_{2(2)} \times f_{(2)}\\ 50 \times 8 = 40 \times f_{(2)}\\ f_{(2)} = (50 \times 8)/40 = 10 \text{ breaths/min}\end{array}$$

For this patient, an increase in machine rate from 18 to 23 breaths/min would decrease $PaCO_2$ from 50 mm Hg to 40 mm Hg. Two warnings must be kept in mind in the use of this predictive equation. First, it is assumed that $\dot{V}CO_2$ is constant. If there is an increase or decrease in $\dot{V}CO_2$, the resultant $PaCO_2$ would be different from the predicted value. Common causes of increased $\dot{V}CO_2$ in the ICU include pain, agitation, anxiety, fever, overfeeding, increased activity, and fighting the ventilator. Decreases in $\dot{V}CO_2$ may be caused by decreased activity, sedation, paralysis, anesthesia, or sleep. Second, the equation is based on the assumption that the patient is apneic. Patients who are triggering the ventilator in the assist-control mode determine their own $PaCO_2$ on the basis of the assist rate. Patients in the SIMV mode who are spontaneously breathing may simply increase or decrease their level of spontaneous breathing and make $PaCO_2$ prediction difficult.

Tidal Volume. Changes in V_T can be used to alter $PaCO_2$. For a patient 80 kg IBW receiving ventilation in the control mode with V_T of 600 ml (7.5 ml/kg) and resultant $PaCO_2$ of 30 mm Hg, the change in V_T to achieve a PaO_2 of 40 mm Hg would be calculated as follows:

$$\begin{array}{c}\text{Initial} \qquad \text{Desired}\\ PaCO_{2(1)} \times V_{T(1)} = PaCO_{2(2)} \times V_{T(2)}\\ 30 \times 600 = 40 \times V_{T(2)}\\ V_{T(2)} = (30 \times 600)/40 = 450 \text{ ml}\end{array}$$

For this patient, a decrease in V_T from 600 ml to 450 ml results in an increase in $PaCO_2$ from 30 mm Hg to 40 mm Hg. Several warnings should be kept in mind for changes in V_T. First, V_T should be within the preferred range for a given patient condition. In the example, new V_T (450 ml) represents 5.6 ml/kg IBW, which is an acceptable value. V_T should be small enough to avoid lung injury and maintain P_{plat} at less than 30 cm H_2O. Second, in this equation, $\dot{V}CO_2$ and V_{Dphys} are assumed to be constant because changes in $\dot{V}CO_2$ or V_{Dphys} affect $PaCO_2$. Activity, agitation, fever, and overfeeding may increase $\dot{V}CO_2$, whereas sedation, paralysis, or sleep may decrease $\dot{V}CO_2$. V_{Dphys} changes with changes in airway pressure, and increases in ventilator V_T may result in increased dead space. Development of pulmonary emboli or hemodynamic instability may abruptly increase V_{Dphys}.

Mechanical Dead Space. Mechanical dead space is defined as the volume of gas rebreathed as the result of a mechanical device. Large-bore tubing attached between the patient "wye" and the patient connection serves as mechanical dead space, and 6 inches (15 cm) of large-bore tubing represents a volume of approximately 50 to 70 ml.

For ventilation of tracheostomy patients, 6 inches (15 cm) of mechanical dead space often is used to keep the weight of the "wye" connection and tubing off of the tracheostomy tube and to give additional flexibility to the circuit for patient movement. Mechanical dead space usually is not used for endotracheally intubated patients, and the addition of mechanical dead space can serve as a cause for an increase in $PaCO_2$. Mechanical dead space is a primary concern in patients with severe ARDS in whom V_T is 4 to 6 ml/kg IBW, and as a result $PaCO_2$ is elevated. The simple removal of mechanical dead space in these patients in some cases can markedly improve CO_2 elimination. HME filters are another major cause of mechanical dead space. Depending on the brand, 80 ml of dead space can be added by these devices.

In healthy persons, V_{Dphys} and anatomic dead space are approximately the same and can be estimated at approximately 1 ml/lb or 2.2 ml/kg IBW. Although healthy persons have a dead space-to-tidal volume (V_D/V_T) ratio of approximately 0.20 to 0.40, a V_D/V_T ratio greater than 0.50 is common among ventilated patients.

Control of $PaCO_2$ in Synchronized Intermittent Mandatory Ventilation Mode

In the SIMV mode, machine breaths are interspersed with spontaneous breathing, and the spontaneous breaths may be PSV. $PaCO_2$ can be decreased by increasing V_T, increasing PSV for spontaneous breaths, or increasing the machine rate. Levels of $PaCO_2$ may be increased by reducing the machine rate, decreasing V_T, or decreasing the level of PSV for spontaneous breaths. As with apneic (control) ventilation, an appropriate V_T should be selected on the basis of the patient's condition and with the goal of keeping P_{plat} less than 30 cm H_2O with V_T ideally 4 to 8 ml/kg IBW depending on the patient's pulmonary status. PSV level in the SIMV mode should be adjusted to overcome WOB_I; the usual range is 5 to 15 cm H_2O, although higher levels may be needed by patients with high resistance or a high spontaneous inspiratory flow rate. PSV should be adjusted to ensure that during spontaneous breathing, WOB is not excessive. Accessory muscle use or suprasternal, intercostal, or substernal retractions during spontaneous breathing indicate the need to increase the PSV level. When appropriate V_T and PSV level are selected, the primary

MINI CLINI

Adjusting $PaCO_2$ During Volume Ventilation

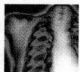

PROBLEM: A 22-year-old man, 5 ft 10 in (178 cm) tall, being treated for a drug overdose is being ventilated with the following settings:

Mode: VA/C
FiO_2: 0.40
V_T: 600 ml
Rate: 15 breaths/min
PIP: 20 cm H_2O
P_{plat}: 13 cm H_2O
PEEP: 5 cm H_2O

The patient's lungs are clear to auscultation, and there is no evidence of aspiration. Arterial blood gas values obtained 15 minutes ago were:

PaO_2: 80 mm Hg
$PaCO_2$: 30 mm Hg
SaO_2: 95%
HCO_3: 24 mEq/L
pH: 7.52
Base excess: +2 mEq/L

The physician asks the RT to normalize this patient's oxygenation and ventilatory status. What should the RT do?

SOLUTION: At this time, the patient is making no spontaneous breathing efforts. The patients' oxygenation status is fine, and no adjustments are needed. In the absence of spontaneous breathing in the VA/C mode, $PaCO_2$ can be adjusted by changing machine rate (f) or V_T. Because the V_T is large (600 ml), the correct adjustment would be to decrease the V_T.

For prediction of the needed change in V_T to increase $PaCO_2$ to 40 mm Hg, the following calculation could be performed:

$$\begin{array}{cc} \text{Actual} & \text{Desired} \\ V_{T(1)} \times PaCO_{2(1)} = & V_{T(2)} \times PaCO_{2(2)} \end{array}$$

$$V_{T(2)}\ \text{Desired} = (V_{T(1)} \times PaCO_{2(1)})/PaCO_{2(2)}$$

$$V_{T(2)}\ \text{Desired} = (600 \times 30)/40 = 458\ \text{ml}$$

If V_T is decreased to 450 ml, $PaCO_2$ and pH should normalize.

method for adjusting $PaCO_2$ is to increase or decrease SIMV rate.

After ventilator initiation, two different approaches may be taken. For full ventilatory support, an initial SIMV rate and V_T are selected to provide 100% of the patient's ventilatory requirements; for most adults, this means starting with V_T of 6 to 8 ml/kg IBW with SIMV rate of 15 to 20 breaths/min. Generally, a minute ventilation of approximately 100 ml/kg IBW is achieved with these initial settings. Arterial blood gas values are obtained 20 to 30 minutes after initiation of mechanical ventilation, and SIMV rate is titrated up or down in increments of 2 breaths/min until desired $PaCO_2$ is achieved. Monitoring is continued, and adjustments are made by increasing or decreasing SIMV rate to maintain full ventilatory support until the patient's condition improves and ventilator discontinuation is considered.

Partial ventilatory support in the SIMV mode requires a different initial approach. Ventilation begins with V_T and machine rate sufficient to provide full ventilatory support, and arterial blood gases are measured. If $PaCO_2$ is adequate, the patient is immediately challenged with a decrease in SIMV rate of 2 breaths/min. This procedure is followed by patient assessment and measurement of arterial blood gases, as indicated. If the resultant assessment values remain adequate, the patient continues to be challenged with decreases in SIMV rate until $PaCO_2$ increases. At that point, the patient's ventilatory capacity has been exceeded, and SIMV rate is returned to the previous value. Box 44-19 provides an example of titration of the SIMV rate for partial ventilatory support after ventilator initiation in a spontaneously breathing patient.

Assist-Control Mode Volume Ventilation and $PaCO_2$

Ventilator initiation in the VA/C mode begins with selection of initial V_T and backup control rate to ensure a safe minimum level of ventilation. In PA/C, a pressure control level sufficient to establish desired V_T is selected along with a backup as in VA/C. The patient is allowed to trigger the machine as often as desired above this backup rate, and the resultant assist rate is determined by the patient's ventilatory drive. If the respiratory drive is intact, patients tend to trigger the ventilator at an appropriate rate to achieve adequate $PaCO_2$ and pH. By allowing patients to set their own rates, the level of ventilation increases or decreases on the basis of the patient's physiologic needs. Should the patient become apneic owing to sedation or sleep, a minimum backup control rate is provided.

Because the patient determines the level of ventilation, $PaCO_2$ levels are regulated by the patient. However, problems arise when the patient triggers the ventilator at an inappropriately rapid rate. Pain, anxiety, hypoxemia, secretions in the airway, and metabolic acidosis may contribute to an excessive trigger rate. The result can be an inappropriate I:E ratio and an inadequate expiratory time. These abnormal values may increase mean airway pressure, reduce venous return, and result in auto-PEEP and overinflation and associated missed triggering of the ventilator, especially in patients with obstructive disease. Patients may fight the ventilator, resulting in high inspiratory pressure. In the event that a patient receiving ventilation in the assist-control mode is triggering the ventilator at an inappropriately high rate, the first step the RT should take is to identify the cause of the increased rate. Patient anxiety may be diminished with simple reassurance and

Box 44-19 Partial Ventilatory Support with Synchronized Intermittent Mandatory Ventilation

Mechanical ventilation is initiated in the SIMV mode for a 70-kg, spontaneously breathing 38-year-old man. Before initiation of ventilation, the patient's spontaneous rate was 30 breaths/min with a spontaneous V_T of 200 ml. Initial ventilator settings are:

V_T: 500 ml
SIMV rate: 14 breaths/min
FiO_2: 0.40
PSV: +8 cm H_2O
PIP: 24 cm H_2O
P_{plat}: 18 cm H_2O
PEEP: 8 cm H_2O

Arterial blood gases are obtained in 20 minutes, with the following results:

PaO_2: 88 mm Hg
SaO_2: 97%
pH: 7.38
$PaCO_2$: 40 mm Hg
HCO_3: 24 mEq/L
Base excess: +1 mEq/L

The decision is made to provide partial ventilatory support for this patient, and the SIMV rate is titrated as follows:

Time	V_T (ml)	SIMV Rate	Total Rate	$PaCO_2$ (mm Hg)
9:00 AM	600	14	20	40
9:30 AM	600	12	15	38
10:00 AM	600	10	18	38
10:30 AM	600	8	24	46
11:00 AM	600	10	18	42

The patient's condition should now be stabilized at a rate of 10 breaths/min with titration of SIMV to the patient's needs with observation and measurement of arterial blood gases. When the rate is decreased to 8 breaths/min, $PaCO_2$ begins to increase. The rate is increased to the previous setting of 10 breaths/min. Titrating the level of SIMV support to the patient's needs is not the same as weaning the patient. After improvement in the patient's condition, weaning may be tried (see Chapter 47) with a daily spontaneous breathing trial.

encouragement to relax and "let the machine breathe for you." Hypoxemia should be managed with appropriate O_2 therapy and PEEP, if indicated. Secretions should be removed by suctioning, and bronchial hygiene techniques should be applied. The cause of metabolic acidosis should be identified and managed, if possible.

In some patients, appropriate sedation improves the ventilatory rate. Patients who begin fighting the ventilator after a previous period of calm may have a new and potentially life-threatening complication. If a patient begins fighting the ventilator, a careful assessment should be made to identify the problem. Often, careful attention to the ventilator trigger sensitivity, flow rate, volume, and pressure is helpful, and administration of analgesic and sedative agents may be needed.[11] If sedation is required, the use of intermittent sedation with daily interruption using a sedation protocol may reduce the duration of mechanical ventilation.[77,78] A last resort is pharmacologic controlled ventilation.[11] In the presence of a metabolic acidosis, a sudden change from assisted ventilation at a rapid rate with the associated hyperventilation to controlled ventilation at a slower rate can result in severe acidosis, which can be life-threatening. Other problems with controlled ventilation include patient safety, ventilatory muscle atrophy, and prolonged muscle weakness if paralytic agents are used for a prolonged period.

Pressure Support Ventilation and $PaCO_2$

PSV is normally set at the level needed to establish a normal V_T of 4 to 8 ml/kg IBW. To increase or decrease V_T, the clinician simply increases or decreases the PSV level and observes the resultant V_T on the ventilator exhaled volume monitoring screen. Because PSV is an assist mode, the patient is allowed to trigger the ventilator as desired. The result should be an adequate $PaCO_2$ and pH. In patients with an unstable ventilatory drive or periods of apnea, PSV should be avoided.

Pressure-Controlled Ventilation and $PaCO_2$

Management of ventilation and $PaCO_2$ during PCV is similar to PSV; the only difference between these two modes in a spontaneously breathing patient is the method of breath termination. With PSV, the breath is terminated as a result of the patient's inspiratory flow decreasing to the termination cycling flow, whereas in PA/C, the breath is terminated when the inspiratory time is reached. No other real differences in these modes exist in a spontaneously breathing patient.

To increase or decrease $PaCO_2$ in the PCV mode, the RT can simply increase or decrease the pressure limit while observing the exhaled V_T on the ventilator display monitor until desired V_T is obtained. The most important problem with the use of V_T to adjust $PaCO_2$ in the PCV mode is that the pressure should not be increased greater than 30 cm H_2O to avoid ventilator-induced lung injury.

In a patient receiving PCV, a change in the rate affects $PaCO_2$ in the same manner as in **volume-controlled ventilation.** If VT remains constant, an increase in rate decreases $PaCO_2$ and vice versa. However, in the PCV mode, percent inspiratory time ($\%T_i$) and I:E ratio may be fixed. If $\%T_i$ is constant, and respiratory rate is increased, actual inspiratory time decreases, and V_T also may decrease. Decreases in rate ($\%T_i$ and pressure limit constant) may result in an increase in delivered V_T. The following example shows this principle.

A patient receiving ventilation in the PCV mode has an inspiratory pressure of 25 cm H_2O, PEEP of 5 cm H_2O, $\%T_i$

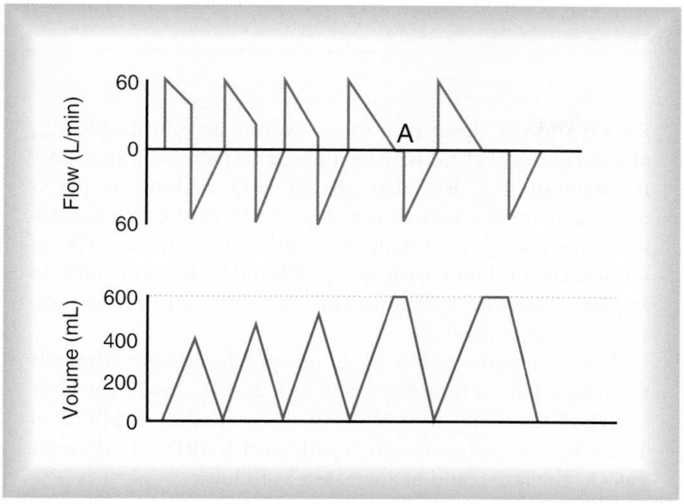

FIGURE 44-18 Effect of inspiratory time and inspiratory plateau on delivered V_T in the PCV mode. Initially, as inspiratory time is increased, V_T increases. When an inspiratory plateau *(A)* is achieved, a further increase in inspiratory time does not result in increased V_T. The same effect occurs as inspiratory time is decreased. Initially, with small decreases in inspiratory time, there would be no change in V_T as long as an end inspiratory plateau was maintained. When the inspiratory time is less than that needed for an inspiratory plateau, further decreases in inspiratory time result in a decrease in V_T at the same pressure.

of 50%, I:E ratio of 1:1, and rate of 20 breaths/min. In this example, respiratory cycle time can be calculated as follows:

$$\text{Respiratory cycle} = 60/f = 60/20 = 3 \text{ seconds}$$

Inspiratory time (T_i) would be:

$$T_i = \%T_i \times \text{Respiratory cycle} = 0.50 \times 3 = 1.5 \text{ seconds}$$

A pressure of 25 cm H_2O applied for 1.5 seconds might achieve V_T of 600 ml for this patient.

If the rate were increased to 30 breaths/min, what would happen to respiratory cycle time, inspiratory time, and delivered V_T? Respiratory cycle and inspiratory time are calculated for a rate of 30 breaths/min as follows:

$$\text{Respiratory cycle} = 60/f = 60/30 = 2 \text{ seconds}$$

$$T_i = \%T_i \times \text{Respiratory cycle} = 0.50 \times 2 = 1 \text{ second}$$

At a constant inspiratory pressure of 25 cm H_2O, a decrease in inspiratory time from 1.5 seconds to 1 second may reduce delivered V_T. An increase in respiratory rate may reduce delivered V_T and increase (rather than decrease) $PaCO_2$.

When using PCV, the RT should observe the effect of inspiratory time and pressure limit on the patient's flow and volume curves as displayed by a ventilator graphics monitoring package. Generally, as inspiratory time increases at a given pressure, volume also increases until an inspiratory plateau or hold is reached. This point can be identified by observing the inspiratory flow curve. If the inspiratory flow curve decreases to zero and holds that value for a time before exhalation begins, an inspiratory plateau is present (Figure 44-18). Further increases in inspiratory time do not result in additional V_T. Conversely, if an inspiratory plateau or hold is present, a decrease in inspiratory time does not decrease V_T (at the same pressure limit) until the inspiratory plateau is no longer present (see Figure 44-18). Table 44-8 summarizes methods of altering $PaCO_2$ during volume-controlled ventilation and PCV.

TABLE 44-8

Changing Ventilation and $PaCO_2$

Mode Increase	Ventilation (↓ $PaCO_2$)	Decrease Ventilation (↑ $PaCO_2$)
Volume-Controlled Ventilation		
VC-CMV control	↑ V_T; ↑ f; remove V_{Dmach}	↓ V_T; ↓ f; add V_{Dmach}
VC-CMV assist control	↑ V_T; ↑ f (to greater than assist rate); remove V_{Dmach}	↓ VT; ↓ f (may require sedation, control mode)
SIMV	↑ VT; ↑ f; add/increase PSV	↓ VT; ↓ f; reduce PSV
Pressure-Controlled Ventilation		
PCV*	↑ ΔP; ↑ f (maintaining same T_i)	↓ ΔP; ↓ f (maintaining same T_i)
PSV	↑ ΔP	↓ ΔP
Bilevel PAP	↑ IPAP (↑ ΔP)	↓ IPAP (↓ ΔP)
APRV	↑ ΔP ↑ release frequency	↓ ΔP ↓ release frequency

Note: In assist (patient-triggered) mode, the patient may simply alter the trigger rate after a ventilator change, and it becomes difficult to predict the results of a ventilator change on $PaCO_2$ in the assist mode.

APRV, Airway pressure release ventilation; *IPAP,* inspiratory positive airway pressure.

*In PCV, if $\%T_i$ is preset, an increase in respiratory rate results in a decrease in inspiratory time and may reduce V_T. If $\%T_i$ is set at 50% in PCV mode, an increase in rate from 15 to 20 breaths/min causes inspiratory time to decrease from 2 seconds (50% of 4 seconds) to 1.5 seconds (50% of 3 seconds). If the pressure limit is not changed, V_T is likely to decrease.

$PaCO_2$ When Using Lung Protective Strategies for Acute Lung Injury and Acute Respiratory Distress Syndrome

Ventilation strategies for lung protection include low V_T, rapid respiratory rates, and permissive hypercapnia if necessary to avoid overdistention (P_{plat} > 30 cm H_2O).

MINI CLINI

Adjusting Ventilation in PA/C Mode

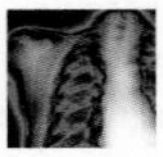

PROBLEM: A 70-kg (IBW) patient with ARDS is receiving PCV in the control mode with the following ventilator settings:

Pressure: 15 cm H_2O
Rate: 25 breaths/min
Inspiratory time: 0.8
FiO_2: 0.60
PEEP: 12 cm H_2O
V_T (exhaled): 425 ml

Arterial blood gas values with these ventilator settings are as follows:

PaO_2: 60 mm Hg
SaO_2: 90%
pH: 7.30
$PaCO_2$: 50 mm Hg
HCO_3: 23 mEq/L
Base excess: −2 mEq/L

The physician requests that the respiratory rate be increased to 18 breaths/min to decrease the patient's $PaCO_2$ to 40 mm Hg and normalize the pH. What should the RT do?

SOLUTION: This patient has a PaO_2/FiO_2 ratio of 100 (60/0.60), which is consistent with the diagnosis of ARDS. Special considerations for the ventilatory management of ARDS include maintaining P_{plat} less than 30 cm H_2O. V_T is started at 8 ml/kg IBW and gradually reduced to 6 ml/kg IBW to achieve this goal and minimize ventilator-induced lung injury. Respiratory rate may be increased to maintain $PaCO_2$ and pH closer to normal, as long as volume and P_{plat} are acceptable. $PaCO_2$ may be allowed to increase if necessary to maintain P_{plat} less than 30 cm H_2O as long as pH is acceptable for the patient (usually >7.25). Oxygenation problems are managed initially with PEEP to achieve PaO_2 of 60 mm Hg or more with acceptable FiO_2. If PEEP fails to improve PaO_2, lung recruitment maneuvers and prone positioning may be used.

For this patient, the V_T is acceptable at approximately 6 ml/kg (70 kg × 6 ml/kg = 420 ml), and P_{plat} is 27 cm H_2O. $PaCO_2$ (50 mm Hg) and pH (7.30) are acceptable, and PEEP of 12 cm H_2O is appropriate for a patient with ARDS. To decrease $PaCO_2$, the rate could be increased as follows:

Initial Desired

$$f_{(1)} \times PaCO_{2(1)} = f_{(2)} \times PaCO_2$$

$$25 \times 50 = f_{(2)} \times 40$$

$$f_{(2)}\ \text{Desired} = (25 \times 50/40) = 31.25$$

If V_T is maintained at 425 ml, a rate of 30 to 32 breaths/min should bring $PaCO_2$ and pH into normal range. However, if respiratory rate is increased, air trapping and auto-PEEP may develop. If auto-PEEP develops, V_T is likely to decrease. In pressure ventilation, an auto-PEEP increase is equal to an equivalent to a decrease in pressure control level, decreasing V_T. Rate should be increased cautiously, constantly evaluating the impact of the rate increase on V_T. More importantly, there is no reason to try to normalize $PaCO_2$ in this patient. $PaCO_2$ of 50 mm Hg with pH of 7.30 is acceptable.

Open Lung Approach

The use of a high PEEP, low V_T lung protective strategy using V_T of 4 to 8 ml/kg and PEEP set after a lung recruitment maneuver and decremental PEEP as discussed previously may improve mortality in patients with persistent ARDS.[21,22] Because V_T is reduced, respiratory rate should be increased incrementally up to 35 to 40 breaths/min. The limitation on rate is the development of auto-PEEP; if auto-PEEP does not develop, the rate can be increased. The primary concern in patients with severe ARDS is acidosis. However, most patients without severe sepsis, cardiovascular dysfunction, or renal failure can tolerate severe acidosis. The ARDS Clinical Network defined the limit for acidosis as pH less than 7.15.[2] $PaCO_2$, although important, should be allowed to increase before accepting V_T that results in P_{plat} greater than 30 mm Hg. The need to allow $PaCO_2$ to increase to avoid inducing lung injury is referred to as *permissive hypercapnia*. However, the goal is not to allow the $PaCO_2$ to increase but to avoid P_{plat} that may induce lung injury. With this approach in severe ARDS, V_T is frequently 4 to 5 ml/kg IBW, and $PaCO_2$ is greater than 60 mm Hg. Table 44-9 compares the effect of acute changes in $PaCO_2$ on pH.

TABLE 44-9

Effect of Acute Changes in $PaCO_2$ on pH

$PaCO_2$	pH
80	7.16
70	7.22
60	7.28
50	7.34
40	7.40
35	7.45
30	7.50
25	7.55
20	7.60

From Malley WJ: Clinical blood gases: assessment and intervention, ed 2, Philadelphia, 2005, Saunders.

When applying this approach, PEEP is set after it is determined by a lung recruitment maneuver and a decremental PEEP trial. V_T or pressure level is adjusted ensuring that P_{plat} or pressure control setting is less than 30 cm H_2O. Because V_T is small, inspiratory times can be short (frequently 0.5 to 0.8 second). The respiratory rate is set to achieve CO_2 elimination with its limit the development of auto-PEEP. Initially, FiO_2 is set to 1.0 but then titrated downward until PaO_2 is greater than 55 mm Hg. Generally, PEEP is sustained at the set level until FiO_2 is less than 0.5, and when PEEP is decreased, it should be decreased in increments of 2 cm H_2O no more frequently than about every 6 to 8 hours. If PaO_2 decreases when PEEP is decreased, the correct decision is to reestablish PEEP level, *not* increase FiO_2, because if this occurs, the lung derecruited, and lung volume needs to be reestablished.

When to repeat a recruitment maneuver is a difficult question to answer, and data are insufficient at this time to provide an answer. However, if the PaO_2 does not decrease after the lung recruitment maneuver, there is no reason to perform an additional recruitment maneuver. Suctioning may cause derecruitment and hypoxemia, and ventilator discontinuation always results in derecruitment. If either of these situations occurs, the lung needs to be recruited again, but PEEP is reestablished at the previous PEEP level because the hypoxemia was *not* a result of deterioration in lung function. A recruitment maneuver and decremental PEEP trial should be repeated only if the patient's lung function deteriorates.

In all patients with severe ARDS, mechanical dead space should be eliminated, in-line suction catheters should be in place, and airway suctioning should be performed only to the level of the main stem bronchus. In addition, ideally the ventilator circuit should not be disconnected.

Other Lung Protective Strategies

Alternative techniques for facilitating CO_2 removal during lung protective ventilation in patients with ARDS include extracorporeal CO_2 removal, ECMO, reduction of CO_2 production by control of fever, avoidance of overfeeding, and neuromuscular paralysis. A randomized controlled trial showed that in patients with severe ARDS (PaO_2 < 150 mm Hg), neuromuscular paralysis for the first 48 hours resulted in improved mortality all other factors being equal.[79] Other authors have advocated the use of HFOV; however, the data do not show any difference in outcome between HFOV and a lung protective approach to ventilatory support.[80-82] Overall, these approaches are equivalent; however, if a clinician has the expertise and equipment to perform HFOV and believes it to be better than conventional ventilation, it should be started ideally early in the course of ARDS and *not* used as a rescue therapy. The data on the use of HFOV as a rescue therapy showed poor overall outcome.

ECMO is effective in supporting newborns with acute respiratory failure; survival rates 80% or greater have been achieved.[83,84] The results of early studies of ECMO in the treatment of adult patients with ARDS were disappointing. The use of new, advanced ECMO technology may be beneficial in the care of adults with ARDS; however, only one randomized, controlled study that had very poor methodology for conventional ventilation showed the value of ECMO in adults.[85] Numerous case series of H1N1 influenza showed some promise for the use of ECMO in severe ARDS. Many newer systems are just entering the market that may dramatically change the pattern of ECMO use and the results of using ECMO.

SUMMARY CHECKLIST

- P_{plat} should ideally be maintained at less than 30 cm H_2O in all patients to prevent ventilator-induced lung injury.
- PEEP is used primarily to maintain lung volume resulting in improved oxygenation and lower FiO_2 in patients with severe oxygenation problems and refractory hypoxemia.
- Initially, all acutely ill patients should be ventilated with V_T of 4 to 8 ml/kg IBW with a respiratory rate to maintain adequate CO_2 removal.
- Patients with ALI/ARDS may begin mechanical ventilation with V_T of 8 ml/kg but may need volume adjusted to less than 6 ml/kg IBW to maintain P_{plat} less than 30 cm H_2O.
- Lung protective strategies in the management of ALI/ARDS include use of lower V_T (6 ml/kg), maintaining P_{plat} less than 30 cm H_2O, permissive hypercapnia, and PEEP set above the lower inflection point on the static pressure-volume curve.
- An open lung approach to mechanical ventilation includes the application of lung recruitment maneuvers, decremental PEEP trial, choosing V_T that maintains P_{plat} less than 30 cm H_2O, and accepting permissive hypercapnia.
- Inspiratory flow for most adult patients should be initially set at approximately 60 L/min or greater to achieve an inspiratory time of approximately 0.6 to 1 second.
- Patient ventilator synchrony is a major problem in patients during patient-triggered ventilation.
- Rise time should be adjusted to ensure that initial airway pressure does not exceed the target level.
- Termination criteria should be adjusted to ensure that the patient's neuroinspiratory time and the ventilator's inspiratory time are equal.
- In all modes of pressure ventilation, the pressure level should be set to ensure that V_T of 4 to 8 ml/kg IBW is delivered.
- When in doubt, initial FiO_2 should be set at 1.0.
- Auto-PEEP is a problem in patients with obstructive lung disease (COPD, asthma).
- In spontaneously triggering patients with COPD, PEEP should be added to ensure that all patient efforts result in triggering of the ventilator.
- An appropriate goal of PEEP would be to achieve PaO_2 60 to 80 mm Hg with FiO_2 less than 0.50.
- Alternative lung protective strategies in patients with ALI/ARDS include prone positioning, ECMO, and high-frequency ventilation.
- Careful attention to acid-base homeostasis and the effect of $PaCO_2$ on pH is an essential part of ventilator management.

References

1. American College of Chest Physicians: ACCP consensus conference: mechanical ventilation. Chest 104:1833, 1993.
2. The Acute Respiratory Distress Syndrome Network: Ventilation with lower tidal volumes as compared with traditional tidal volumes for acute lung injury and the acute respiratory distress syndrome. N Engl J Med 342:1301–1308, 2000.
3. Dreyfuss D, Saumon G: Ventilator-induced lung injury: lessons from experimental studies. Am J Respir Crit Care Med 157:294–323, 1998.
4. Chiumello D, Carlesso E, Cadringher P, et al: Lung stress and strain during mechanical ventilation for acute respiratory distress syndrome. Am J Respir Crit Care Med 178:346–355, 2008.
5. Kacmarek RM: The cost in some is an increase in the work of breathing: is it too high? (editorial). Respir Care 50:1624–1626, 2005.
6. Tremblay L, Valenza F, Riberiro S, et al: Injurious ventilatory strategies increases cytokines and c-fos mRNA expression in an isolated rat lung model. J Clin Invest 99:944–952, 1997.
7. Esteban A, Ferguson ND, Meade MO, et al; VENTILA Group: Evolution of mechanical ventilation in response to clinical research. Am J Respir Crit Care Med 177:170–177, 2008.
8. Tobin MJ: Principles and practice of mechanical ventilation, ed 2, New York, 2006, McGraw-Hill.
9. Marini JJ, Rodriguez RM, Lamb V: The inspiratory workload of patient-initiated mechanical ventilation. Am Rev Respir Dis 134:902, 1986.
10. Marini JJ, Capps JS, Culver BH: The inspiratory work of breathing during assisted mechanical ventilation. Chest 87:612, 1985.
11. Tobin MJ: Advances in mechanical ventilation. N Engl J Med 344:1986, 2001.
12. Esteban A, Anzueto A, Alia I, et al: How is mechanical ventilation employed in the intensive care unit? An international utilization review. Am J Respir Crit Care Med 161:1450, 2000.
13. Brochard L, Rauss A, Benito S, et al: Comparison of three methods of gradual withdrawal from ventilatory support during weaning from mechanical ventilation. Am J Respir Crit Care Med 150:896–903, 1994.
14. Estaban A, Frutos F, Tobin MJ, et al: A comparison of four methods of weaning patients from mechanical ventilation. N Engl J Med 332:345–350, 1995.
15. Williams P, Muelver M, Kratohvil J, et al: Pressure support and pressure assist/control: are there differences? An evaluation of the newest ICU ventilators. Respir Care 45:1169–1181, 2000.
16. Dekel B, Segal E, Perel A: Pressure support ventilation. Arch Intern Med 156:369, 1996.
17. Derdak S, Mehta S, Stewart TE, et al: High-frequency oscillatory ventilation for acute respiratory distress syndrome in adults: a randomized, controlled trial. Am J Respir Crit Care Med 166:801–808, 2002.
18. Bollen CW, Well G, Sherry T, et al: High frequency oscillatory ventilation compared with conventional mechanical ventilation in adult respiratory distress syndrome: a randomized controlled trial [ISRCTN2422669]. Crit Care 9:R430–R439, 2005.
19. Eastman A, Holland D, Higgins J, et al: High frequency percussive ventilation improves oxygenation in trauma patients with respiratory distress syndrome: a retrospective review. Am J Surg 192:191, 2006.
20. Jesus J, Kacmarek RM, Hedensternia G: From ventilator-induced lung injury to physician-induced lung injury: why the reluctance to use small tidal volumes? Acta Anesthesiol Scand 48:267–271, 2004.
21. Amato MBP, Barbas CSV, Medeiros DM, et al: Effect of a protective-ventilation strategy on mortality in the acute respiratory distress syndrome. N Engl J Med 338:347–354, 1998.
22. Villar J, Kacmarek RM, Perez-Mendez L, et al; ARIES Network: A high positive end-expiratory pressure, low tidal volume ventilatory strategy improves outcome in persistent acute respiratory distress syndrome: a randomized, controlled trial. Crit Care Med 34:1311–1318, 2006.
23. Gajic O, Dara SI, Mendez JL, et al: Ventilator associated lung injury in patients without acute lung injury at the onset of mechanical ventilation. Crit Care Med 32:1817–1824, 2004.
24. NIH/NHLBI ARDS Network: Ventilation with lower tidal volume as compared to traditional tidal volume for acute lung injury and the acute respiratory distress syndrome. N Engl J Med 342:1301–1308, 2000.
25. Hill LL, Pearl RG: Flow triggering, pressure triggering and auto triggering during mechanical ventilation. Crit Care Med 28:579, 2000.
26. Sassoon CSH: Mechanical ventilator design and function: the trigger variable. Respir Care 37:1056, 1992.
27. Branson RD: Flow-triggering systems. Respir Care 39:138, 1994.
28. Holbrook PJ, Guiles SP: Response time of four pressure support ventilators: effect of triggering method and bias flow. Respir Care 42:952, 1997.
29. Hess DR, Kacmarek RM: Essentials of mechanical ventilation, ed 2, New York, 2002, McGraw-Hill.
30. Rau JL, Shelledy DC: The effect of varying inspiratory flow waveforms on peak and mean airway pressures with a time-cycled volume ventilator: a bench study. Respir Care 36:347, 1991.
31. Pilbeam SP: Mechanical ventilation: physiological and clinical applications, St Louis, 1998, Mosby.
32. Lindahl S: Influence of an end inspiratory pause on pulmonary ventilation, gas distribution, and lung perfusion during artificial ventilation. Crit Care Med 7:540, 1979.
33. Langevin PB, Hellein V, Harms SM, et al: Synchronization of radiograph film exposure with the inspiratory pause: effect on the appearance of bedside chest radiographs in mechanically ventilated patients. Am J Respir Crit Care Med 160:2067, 1999.
34. Sethi J, Siegel MD: Mechanical ventilation in chronic obstructive lung disease. Clin Chest Med 21:799, 2000.
35. Mercat A, Richard JC, Vielle B, et al: Positive end-expiratory pressure setting in adults with acute lung injury and acute respiratory distress syndrome. JAMA 299:646–655, 2008.
36. Talmor D, Sarge T, Malhotra A, et al: Mechanical ventilation guided by esophageal pressure in acute lung injury. N Engl J Med 359:2095–2104, 2008.
37. Kacmarek RM, Villar J: Lung recruitment maneuvers during acute respiratory distress syndrome: is it useful? Minerva Anestesiol 77:85–89, 2011.
38. Gattinoni L, Caironi P, Cressoni M, et al: Lung recruitment in patients with acute respiratory distress syndrome. N Engl J Med 354:1175, 2006.
39. Phoenix SI, Paravastu S, Columb M, et al: Does a higher positive end expiratory pressure decrease mortality in acute respiratory distress syndrome? Anesthesiology 110:1098–1105, 2009.
40. Briel M, Meade M, Mercat A, et al: Higher vs lower positive end-expiratory pressure in patients with acute lung injury and acute respiratory distress syndrome: systematic review and meta-analysis. JAMA 303:865–873, 2010.
41. Bonmarchand G, Chevron V, Menard JF, et al: Effects of pressure ramp slope values on the work of breathing during

pressure support ventilation in restrictive patients. Crit Care Med 27:715, 1999.
42. Branson RD, Campbell RS, Davis K, et al: Altering flow rate during maximum pressure support ventilation (PSV_{max}): effect on cardiorespiratory function. Respir Care 35:1056-1069, 1990.
43. Branson RD, Campbell RS: Pressure support ventilation, patient-ventilatory synchrony and ventilator algorithms. Respir Care 43:1045-1053, 1998.
44. American Association for Respiratory Care: AARC clinical practice guideline: humidification during mechanical ventilation. Respir Care 37:887, 1992.
45. Bendixen HH, Egbert LD, Hedley-Whyte J, et al: Respiratory care, St Louis, 1965, Mosby.
46. MacIntyre N: Of Goldilocks and ventilatory muscle loading. Crit Care Med 28:588, 2000.
47. Laghi F, D'Alfonso N, Tobin MJ: Pattern of recovery from diaphragmatic fatigue over 24 hours. J Appl Physiol 79:539-546, 1995.
48. McIntyre NR, McConnell R, Cheng KC, et al: Patient-ventilator flow dyssynchrony: flow-limited versus pressure-limited breaths. Crit Care Med 25:1671-1677, 1997.
49. Hess DR, MacIntyre NR, Mishoe SC, et al: Respiratory care: principles and practice, Philadelphia, 2002, Saunders.
50. Chatburn RL: Mechanical ventilators. In Branson RD, Hess DR, Chatburn RL, editors: Respiratory Care Equipment, ed 2, St Louis, 1999, Mosby.
51. Goulet R, Hess D, Kacmarek RM: Pressure vs. flow triggering during pressure support ventilation. Chest 111:1649-1654, 1997.
52. Pepe PE, Marini JJ: Occult positive end-expiratory pressure in mechanically ventilated patients with airflow obstruction: the auto-PEEP effect. Am Rev Respir Dis 126:166-170, 1982.
53. Smith TC, Marini JJ: Impact of PEEP on lung mechanics and work of breathing in severe airflow obstruction. J Appl Phys 64:1488-1496, 1988.
54. Kacmarek RM, Dimas S, Mack C: Essentials of respiratory care, ed 4, St Louis, 2005, Mosby.
55. Fernandez R, Mendez M, Younes M: Effect of ventilator flow rate on respiratory timing in normal humans. Am J Respir Crit Care Med 159:710-719, 1999.
56. Leung P, Jubran A, Tobin MJ: Comparison of assisted ventilator modes on triggering, patient effort, and dyspnea. Am J Respir Crit Care Med 155:1387,1997.
57. Tassaux D, Gainnier M, Battisti A, et al: Impact of expiratory trigger setting on delayed cycling and inspiratory muscle workload. Am J Respir Crit Care Med 172:1283-1289, 2005.
58. Thille AW, Cabello B, Galia F: Reduction of patient-ventilator asynchrony by reducing tidal volume during pressure support ventilation. Intensive Care Med 34:1477-1486, 2008.
59. Parthasarathy S, Jubran A, Tobin MJ: Cycling of inspiratory and expiratory muscle groups with the ventilator in airflow limitation. Am J Respir Crit Care Med 158:1471-1478, 1998.
60. Hickling KD: Best compliance during a decremental, but not incremental, positive end-expiratory pressure trial is related to open-lung positive end-expiratory pressure: a mathematical model of acute respiratory distress syndrome lung. Am J Respir Crit Care Med 163:69-78, 2001.
61. Suarez-Sipmann F, Bohm SH, Tusman G, et al: Use of dynamic compliance for open lung positive end-expiratory pressure titration in an experimental study. Crit Care Med 35:214-221, 2007.
62. O'Keefe GE, Gentilello LM, Erford S, et al: Imprecision in lower "inflection point" estimation from static pressure-volume curves in patients at risk for acute respiratory distress syndrome. J Trauma 44:1064, 1998.
63. Girgis K, Hamed H, Khater Y, et al: A decremental PEEP trial identifies the PEEP level that maintains oxygenation after lung recruitment. Respir Care 51:1132, 2006.
64. Medoff BD, Harris SR, Kesselman H, et al: Use of recruitment maneuvers and high positive end expiratory pressure in a patient with acute respiratory distress syndrome. Crit Care Med 28:1210, 2000.
65. Borges JB, Okamoto V, Gustavo M, et al: Reversibility of lung collapse and hypoxemia in early acute respiratory distress syndrome. Am J Respir Crit Care Med 174:268-278, 2006.
66. Lin SC, Alander A, Simonson DA, et al: Transient hemodynamic effects of recruitment maneuvers in three experimental models of acute lung injury. Crit Care Med 32:2371-2384, 2004.
67. Toth I, Leiner T, Mikor A, et al: Hemodynamic and respiratory changes during lung recruitment and descending optimal positive end-expiratory pressure titration in patients with acute respiratory distress syndrome. Crit Care Med 35:787-793, 2007.
68. Tugrul A, Akinci O, Ozcan PE, et al: Effects of sustained inflation and postinflation positive end-expiratory pressure in acute respiratory distress syndrome: focusing on pulmonary and extrapulmonary forms. Crit Care Med 31:738-744, 2003.
69. Drakulovic MB, Mm Hges A, Bauer TT, et al: Supine body position was a risk factor for nosocomial pneumonia in mechanically ventilated patients: a randomized trial. Lancet 354:1851, 1999.
70. Chatte G, Sab JM, Dubois JM, et al: Prone position in mechanically ventilated patients with severe acute respiratory failure. Am J Respir Crit Care Med 155:473-478, 1997.
71. Gattinoni L, Tognoni G, Pesnti A, et al: Effect of prone positioning on the survival of patients with acute respiratory failure. N Engl J Med 345:568-573, 2001.
72. Mancebo J, Fernandez R, Blanch L, et al: A multicenter trial of prolonged prone ventilation in severe acute respiratory distress syndrome. Am J Respir Crit Care Med 173:1233-1239, 2006.
73. Taccone P, Pesenti A, Latini R, et al: Prone positioning in patients with moderate and severe acute respiratory distress syndrome: a randomized controlled trial. JAMA 302:1977-1984, 2009.
74. Sud S, Friedrich JO, Taccone P, et al: Prone ventilation reduces mortality in patients with acute respiratory failure and severe hypoxemia: systematic review and meta-analysis. Intensive Care Med 36:585-599, 2010.
75. Curley MA: Prone positioning in patients with acute respiratory distress syndrome: a systematic review. Am J Crit Care 8:397, 1999.
76. Hirvela E: Advances in the management of acute respiratory distress syndrome: protective ventilation. Arch Surg 135:126, 2000.
77. Izurieta R, Rabatin J: Sedation during mechanical ventilation: a systematic review. Crit Care Med 30: 2644-2648, 2002.
78. Girard TD, Kress JP, Fuchs BD, et al: Efficacy and safety of a paired sedation and ventilation weaning protocol for mechanically ventilated patients in intensive care (Awakening and Breathing Controlled trial): a randomized controlled trial. Lancet 371:126-134, 2008.
79. Papazian L, Forel JM, Gacouin A, et al: Neuromuscular blockers in early acute respiratory distress syndrome. N Engl J Med 363:1107-1116, 2010.
80. Derdak S, Mehta S, Stewart TE, et al: High-frequency oscillatory ventilation for acute respiratory distress syndrome in adults: a randomized, controlled trial. Am J Respir Crit Care Med 166:801-808, 2002.

81. Bollen CW, Well G, Sherry T, et al: High frequency oscillatory ventilation compared with conventional mechanical ventilation in adult respiratory distress syndrome: a randomized controlled trial [ISRCTN2422669]. Crit Care 9:R430–R439, 2005.
82. Mentzelopoulos SD, Malachias S, Tzoufi M, et al: High frequency oscillation and tracheal gas insufflation for severe acute respiratory distress syndrome. Intensive Care Med 33:S142, 2007.
83. Lewandowski K: Extracorporeal membrane oxygenation for severe acute respiratory failure. Crit Care 4:156, 2000.
84. Zwischenberger JB, Tao W, Bidani A: Intravascular membrane oxygenation and carbon dioxide removal devices: a review of performance improvements. ASAIO J 45:41, 1999.
85. Peek GJ, Elbourne D, Mugford M, et al: Efficacy of controlled ventilatory support vs. extracorporeal membrane oxygenation for severe acute respiratory distress syndrome (CESAR): a multicenter randomized controlled trial. Lancet 374:1330–1338, 2009.

Chapter 45

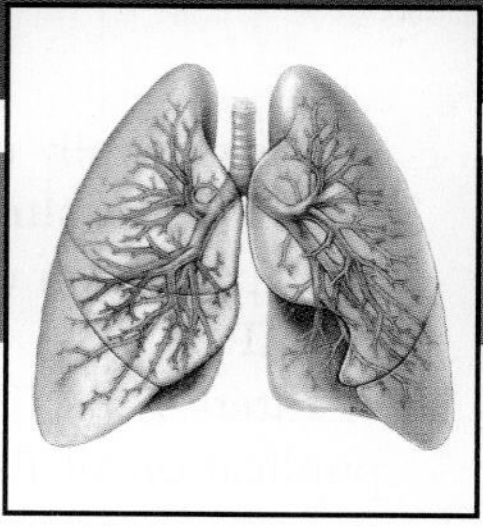

Noninvasive Ventilation

PURRIS F. WILLIAMS

CHAPTER OBJECTIVES

After reading this chapter you will be able to:
- Identify the goals and benefits of noninvasive ventilation (NIV).
- Discuss indications for NIV and the relative strength of the supporting evidence for each indication.
- List the selection and exclusion criteria for successful NIV.
- List the factors that predict successful NIV.
- Identify the types of patient interfaces available for NIV and how to choose an appropriate interface for a patient.
- Discuss the types of mechanical ventilators and ventilation modes used to provide NIV.
- Describe the role of the respiratory therapist during the initial application of NIV.
- Describe the ongoing ventilator management of NIV in the acute care setting.
- List potential complications associated with NIV, and suggest possible solutions.

CHAPTER OUTLINE

History and Development of Noninvasive Ventilation
Indications for Noninvasive Ventilation
- Goals and Benefits of Using Noninvasive Ventilation
- Acute Care Indications
- Long-Term Care Indications

Selecting Appropriate Patients for Noninvasive Ventilation
- Acute Care Setting
- Long-Term Care Setting

Equipment Used for Noninvasive Ventilation
- Patient Interfaces
- Types of Mechanical Ventilators and Modes of Ventilation
- Heated Humidifiers

Management of Noninvasive Ventilation
- Initial Application of Noninvasive Ventilation
- Clinical Assessment Criteria to Identify Success or Failure of Noninvasive Ventilation
- Adjusting Noninvasive Ventilator Settings
- Aerosolized Medication Delivery
- Safe Delivery of Noninvasive Ventilation
- Weaning from Noninvasive Ventilation

Complications of Noninvasive Ventilation
Time and Costs Associated With Noninvasive Ventilation

KEY TERMS

chest cuirass
continuous positive airway pressure (CPAP)
expiratory positive airway pressure (EPAP)
hypercapnic respiratory failure
hypoxemic respiratory failure
inspiratory positive airway pressure (IPAP)
iron lung
negative pressure ventilator
nocturnal hypoventilation
noninvasive positive pressure ventilation (NPPV)
noninvasive ventilation (NIV)
pneumobelt
rocking bed
Trendelenburg position

Noninvasive ventilation (NIV) is the delivery of ventilatory support without using an invasive artificial airway, such as an endotracheal or tracheostomy tube. NIV can be provided by applying either negative or positive pressure to the airways. Almost any type of mechanical ventilator can be used to deliver NIV in conjunction with many possible noninvasive patient interfaces. However, at the present time, NIV is almost always delivered via oronasal or nasal mask with a positive pressure ventilator designed specifically for noninvasive use.

NIV is generally understood to include both **noninvasive positive pressure ventilation (NPPV)** and the noninvasive application of **continuous positive airway pressure (CPAP).**

Interest in NIV has increased in recent years with the publication of findings from clinical trials using NIV in the management of respiratory failure. At the same time, technologically advanced noninvasive ventilators were introduced. Most intensive care unit (ICU) ventilators now include a specific noninvasive mode of ventilation. Improvements in the design of patient interfaces have made them more comfortable so that patients can tolerate NIV for longer periods. The net effect of these developments is that clinicians are using NIV more often than ever before in both acute and long-term care settings.[1] This chapter reviews the evidence supporting the use of NIV to manage various disease processes and makes recommendations on the types of patients and specific techniques for its successful application.

HISTORY AND DEVELOPMENT OF NONINVASIVE VENTILATORS

Some early devices used for NIV relied on the intermittent application of abdominal pressure and the force of gravity to accomplish inspiration and expiration. These devices are most effective when used for patients with neuromuscular or neurologic disease in the absence of primary pulmonary disease. They are capable of generating tidal volume (V_T) in the range of 4 to 6 ml/kg in appropriately selected patients.

First described in the 1930s, the **pneumobelt** consists of a rubber bladder that is strapped around the abdomen and connected to a positive pressure ventilator (Figure 45-1).[2] The pneumobelt is properly positioned above the pelvic arch and below the umbilicus. When inflated, the rubber bladder compresses the abdomen, pushes the diaphragm upward, and assists exhalation. On deflation of the rubber bladder, the abdominal contents and diaphragm move down, facilitating inspiration.[2] Because this device requires gravity to be effective, the patient must be sitting at an angle of at least 30 degrees.[3] Some abdominal mass is necessary for the pneumobelt to be effective. It does not work well in thin patients. Some patients with neuromuscular or neurologic disease and long-term dependence on a ventilator prefer to use a pneumobelt when they are out of bed and in a wheelchair.[4]

The **rocking bed** (Figure 45-2) periodically rocks from the **Trendelenburg position** to reverse Trendelenburg position, using gravity to produce exhalation and inspiration. Rocking beds were used in the 1950s to wean patients from negative pressure ventilators and to provide long-term ventilatory support to patients following recovery from polio.[2] A major problem with the rocking bed is

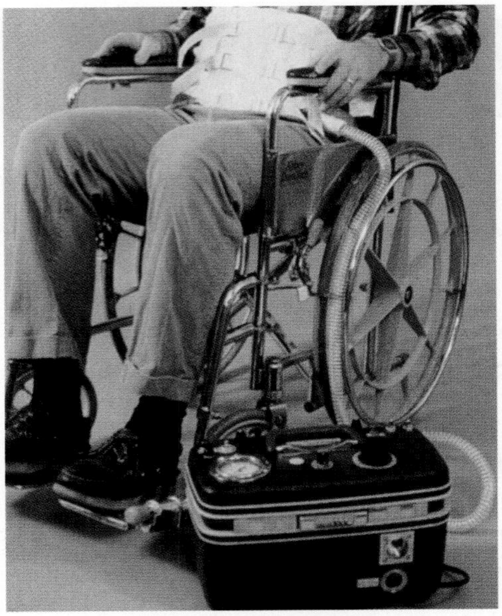

FIGURE 45-1 Pneumobelt, an intermittent abdominal pressure device. (From Albert RK, Spiro SG, Jett JR: Clinical respiratory medicine, ed 2, Philadelphia, 2004, Mosby.)

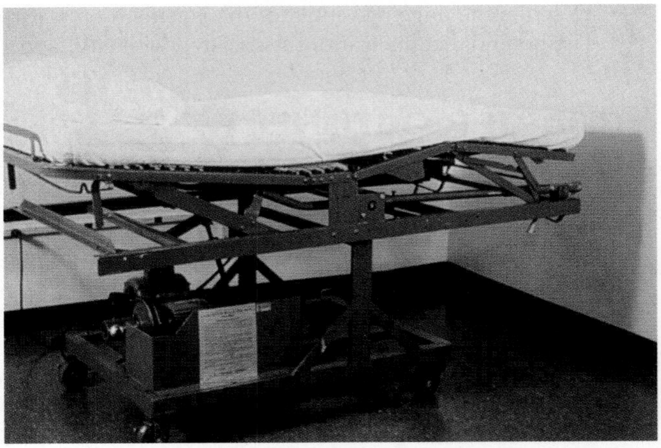

FIGURE 45-2 Rocking bed. (From Albert RK, Spiro SG, Jett JR: Clinical respiratory medicine, ed 2, Philadelphia, 2004, Mosby.)

motion sickness, which prevents some patients from tolerating the device despite adequate ventilation.

A **negative pressure ventilator** generates negative pressure within a chamber that surrounds the thorax. The chest wall expands owing to the decrease in pressure in the chamber, and intraalveolar pressure becomes negative, causing air to flow into the lung during inspiration. When the negative pressure is released, the lungs and chest wall return to their normal size owing to elastic recoil, resulting in passive exhalation. The first electrically powered negative pressure ventilator, known as the **iron lung** (Figure 45-3), surrounded the entire body from the neck down. Negative pressure ventilators were widely used from the late 1920s through the 1960s during the polio epidemic.[2] Other designs were developed during that time, including

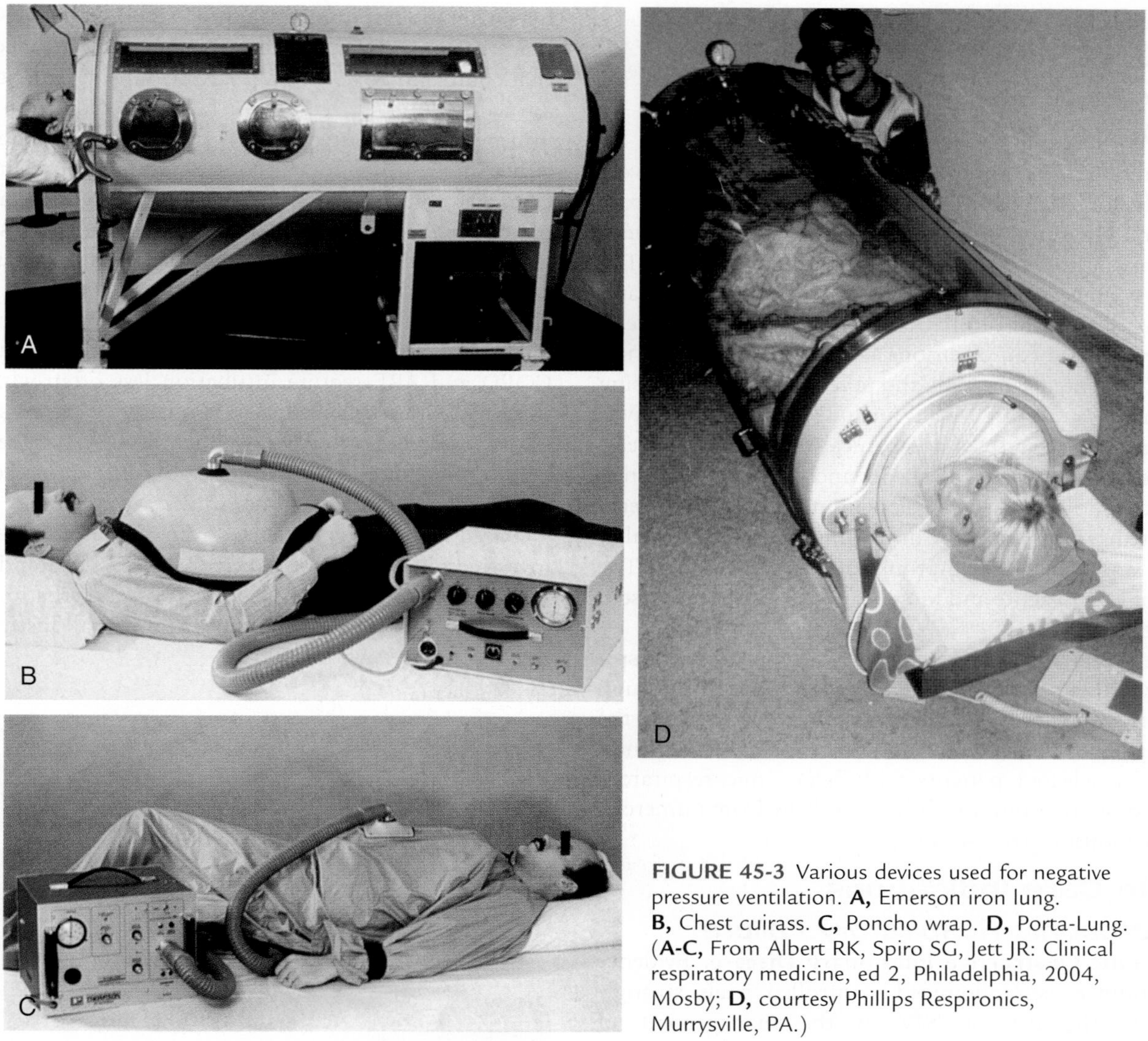

FIGURE 45-3 Various devices used for negative pressure ventilation. **A,** Emerson iron lung. **B,** Chest cuirass. **C,** Poncho wrap. **D,** Porta-Lung. (**A-C,** From Albert RK, Spiro SG, Jett JR: Clinical respiratory medicine, ed 2, Philadelphia, 2004, Mosby; **D,** courtesy Phillips Respironics, Murrysville, PA.)

the **chest cuirass,** which enclosed only the chest, the Porta-Lung, and the poncho wrap.[2] Effective negative pressure ventilation can be challenging to achieve if the device has air leaks or does not fit properly. Negative pressure ventilators that enclose the body limit caregiver access to the patient. In addition, collapse of the upper airway can occur during inspiration when excessive negative pressure is applied. With the development of positive pressure ventilators and the expanded use of NPPV, interest in negative pressure ventilation has greatly diminished.[2] Negative pressure ventilators are seldom seen in hospitals but continue to be used successfully in the home by patients with chronic respiratory failure from neuromuscular diseases, such as polio.

The first reported use of NPPV was in 1780, when Chaussier used a bag and face mask during resuscitation.[1] However, widespread clinical use of NPPV did not begin until much later, with the introduction of intermittent positive pressure breathing in 1947.[1,2] Intermittent positive pressure breathing was primarily used to deliver aerosolized medications. The use of intermittent positive pressure breathing declined significantly in the mid-1980s[2] after no benefit was found compared with aerosol medication delivery with a small volume nebulizer in a randomized, controlled trial involving the treatment of patients with chronic obstructive pulmonary disease (COPD).[5] Around this time, nasal mask CPAP was suggested as a therapy for obstructive sleep apnea.[6] Nasal masks also were used nocturnally in conjunction with positive pressure ventilators to provide rest for the respiratory muscles in patients with neuromuscular disorders.[7] In 1989, NPPV was used successfully to support 8 of 10 patients with acute respiratory failure (ARF).[8] Those positive findings renewed the interest in NIV that continues today. NIV has been used to treat a wide variety of clinical conditions in numerous trials during the past 20 years. The next section provides background and discussion focusing on the most relevant studies. Study findings are evaluated, and evidence-based recommendations for NIV are provided for each indication.

INDICATIONS FOR NONINVASIVE VENTILATION

Goals and Benefits of Using Noninvasive Ventilation

ARF causes impairment in gas exchange that is often severe enough for patients to require additional ventilatory support. The standard treatment for severe ARF is endotracheal intubation and mechanical ventilation. The primary goals of NIV are to improve gas exchange and avoid endotracheal intubation. If NIV is applied successfully, significant complications associated with intubation can be prevented. The goals and potential benefits of using NIV in the acute care setting include improving survival, decreasing the length of mechanical ventilation, decreasing the length of hospitalization, and decreasing the incidence of ventilator-associated pneumonia. In the long-term care setting, major goals are improving the patient's quality of life and relieving symptoms of hypoventilation. The goals of NIV in acute and long-term care settings are listed in Box 45-1.

The primary indication for NIV is **hypercapnic respiratory failure** secondary to COPD exacerbation. Although patients with acute hypercapnic respiratory failure are the most likely to benefit from the use of NIV, it is also indicated for selected patients with hypoxemic respiratory failure or with respiratory failure resulting from numerous other conditions (Box 45-2).[2,9]

Acute Care Indications

Hypercapnic Respiratory Failure

Chronic Obstructive Pulmonary Disease. Evidence from numerous randomized, controlled trials strongly supports the use of NIV in the management of hypercapnic respiratory failure secondary to COPD exacerbation.[10-15] Only one randomized, controlled trial that compared NIV with standard therapy in patients with an acute COPD exacerbation failed to show significant improvement in outcome.[16] In this study, no patients in either the treatment or the control group required intubation, and all of the patients survived. The average arterial pH was higher than in other studies,[11,12] and the resulting respiratory acidosis was less severe. This study has been criticized because the study patients, with only mild hypercapnic respiratory failure, were not sick enough to require NIV.[13] The results of four trials show that patients with COPD and ARF require intubation less often with NIV than with standard medical treatment.[10-13] Other studies have shown a reduction in hospital mortality,[11,13-15] reduced length of hospital stay,[11,12] and significantly fewer complications compared with standard therapy.[11]

Based on strong evidence from the aforementioned investigations, NIV should be considered the standard of care for treatment of an acute COPD exacerbation. NIV should be available as first-line therapy in all institutions treating patients with COPD.[17]

RULE OF THUMB

All patients with an acute COPD exacerbation should be evaluated for NIV as an alternative to intubation and conventional mechanical ventilation. NIV is the standard of care in these patients.

Box 45-1 Goals of Noninvasive Ventilation

ACUTE CARE SETTING
- Improve gas exchange
- Avoid intubation
- Decrease mortality
- Decrease length of time on ventilator
- Decrease length of hospitalization
- Decrease incidence of ventilator-associated pneumonia
- Relieve symptoms of respiratory distress
- Improve patient-ventilator synchrony
- Maximize patient comfort

LONG-TERM CARE SETTING
- Relieve or improve symptoms
- Enhance quality of life
- Avoid hospitalization
- Increase survival
- Improve mobility

Modified from Mehta S, Hill NS: Noninvasive ventilation. Am J Respir Crit Care Med 163:540, 2001.

Box 45-2 Acute and Chronic Disease Processes for Which Noninvasive Ventilation May Be Indicated

ACUTE CONDITIONS
- Hypercapnic respiratory failure
- COPD exacerbation
- Asthma
- Facilitation of extubation in COPD
- Hypoxemic respiratory failure
- Acute cardiogenic pulmonary edema
- Pneumonia
- ARDS/ALI
- Respiratory failure in immunocompromised patients
- End-of life care and DNI orders
- Postoperative respiratory failure
- Prevention of reintubation in high-risk patients
- Postextubation respiratory failure

CHRONIC CONDITIONS
- Nocturnal hypoventilation
- Restrictive thoracic disease
- ALS
- COPD
- OHS

Asthma

NIV has been used successfully in the management of ARF caused by severe asthma, but the supporting evidence is weak. Meduri and colleagues[18] reported positive results in an uncontrolled study using NIV in the care of 17 patients with status asthmaticus. The initial average arterial partial pressure of carbon dioxide ($PaCO_2$) was 65 mm Hg, and pH was 7.25. Within 2 hours after initiation of NIV, gas exchange (both ventilation and oxygenation) had markedly improved. Arterial blood gas measurements during this initial period showed significantly deceased $PaCO_2$, increased pH, and increased PaO_2. Respiratory rate also was significantly reduced from an average of 29 breaths/min to 22 breaths/min. These physiologic changes were achieved without using excessively high airway pressures. The average inspiratory pressure used in the study was 18 cm H_2O, and the maximum inspiratory pressure was 25 cm H_2O.[18] Only two of the patients in the study required intubation.

Several other studies have reported using NIV successfully to manage ARF in patients with asthma,[19-21] but this indication remains controversial. Without a randomized, controlled trial focusing on this patient population, routine management with NIV cannot be recommended in asthmatic patients. Frequently, patients with severe asthma are unable to tolerate the tight-fitting mask necessary to provide NIV. Effective NIV can be difficult to achieve in patients with severe asthma and high airways resistance. They may require ventilating pressures that exceed 20 to 25 cm H_2O, increasing the likelihood of failure. If patients with severe asthma receive a trial of NIV, they must be monitored closely. Significant improvement in the symptoms of respiratory failure should be evident within 1 to 2 hours, and if improvement is not evident, intubation should proceed without delay.

Facilitation of Weaning in Chronic Obstructive Pulmonary Disease

The use of NIV to facilitate weaning from mechanical ventilation has been primarily evaluated in patients with COPD. In two similar studies, patients who failed weaning trials were electively extubated to NIV. In one study, NIV reduced weaning time, length of ICU stay, nosocomial pneumonia rate, and 60-day mortality compared with conventional weaning with invasive pressure support ventilation (PSV).[15] A second study showed no benefit from NIV, but this study was criticized because patients with COPD did not receive NIV before intubation, which is inconsistent with the current standard of care. In a third study, Ferrer and colleagues[22] randomly assigned only patients who failed 3 consecutive days of spontaneous breathing trials and found that NIV was associated with faster weaning. A prospective case series of difficult-to-wean patients with COPD showed that both NIV and invasive PSV significantly reduced work of breathing and improved ventilation compared with a T-piece trial.[23] This study also showed that NIV was associated with greater respiratory pump efficiency and lower dyspnea scores than invasive PSV in this patient population.[23]

NIV can be used effectively to facilitate weaning from mechanical ventilation but only in a select group of difficult-to-wean patients. There is reasonable evidence that patients with COPD and hypercapnic respiratory failure who fail spontaneous breathing trials and are likely to receive a tracheostomy should be selectively extubated to NIV. The failure of NIV to prevent intubation does not preclude its successful use at a later time.

RULE OF THUMB

A trial extubation directly to NIV should be considered for patients with COPD and hypercapnic ARF who are likely to receive a tracheostomy for failure to wean.

Hypoxemic Respiratory Failure

Hypoxemic respiratory failure, defined by a PaO_2/fractional inspired oxygen (FiO_2) ratio less than 300, can result from several distinct causes. Clinical trials of NIV to manage acute hypoxemic respiratory failure have yielded conflicting results. The efficacy of NIV largely depends on the etiology of the hypoxemia. Further study is needed to determine clearly the types of patients who would benefit from NIV.

Acute Cardiogenic Pulmonary Edema

In 1991, mask CPAP was shown to improve hypoxemia and reduce the need for intubation in patients with severe cardiogenic pulmonary edema.[24] Similar findings in other randomized controlled trials provided strong evidence that both CPAP[25,26] and NPPV[27-29] improve outcomes in these patients compared with simple oxygen (O_2) therapy. NPPV seems to be superior to CPAP only if hypercapnia is present.[30-35] Mask CPAP of 8 to 12 cm H_2O and 100% O_2 is first-line therapy to treat hypoxemia associated with severe cardiogenic pulmonary edema. NPPV should be reserved only for patients who cannot adequately ventilate without assistance. Extra caution is recommended for patients who present with cardiac ischemia, hemodynamic instability, arrhythmias, or depressed mental status. Patients with these risk factors should be intubated and invasively ventilated.[31]

RULE OF THUMB

CPAP of 8 to 12 cm H_2O with 100% O_2 should be considered first-line therapy in acute pulmonary edema. NPPV should be used only when hypercapnia is present.

Pneumonia

Jolliet and associates[36] studied NIV in 24 patients with severe community-acquired pneumonia. None of the patients in the study had chronic lung disease. Although oxygenation initially improved with NIV, two-thirds of the patients went on to require intubation, and one-third died. A randomized, controlled trial of NIV in patients with severe community-acquired pneumonia showed significant decreases in intubation rate, number of days in the ICU, and 2-month mortality when patients received NIV. Subgroup analysis determined that these positive findings occurred only in patients with underlying COPD.[37] Further studies are needed to validate these findings. The current recommendation for the use of NIV in pneumonia is to limit its routine use to patients who also have COPD.[37]

Acute Lung Injury and Acute Respiratory Distress Syndrome

Several studies have reported failure rates greater than 50% when NIV is used to treat acute lung injury (ALI) and acute respiratory distress syndrome (ARDS).[38-40] Patients with risk factors such as hemodynamic instability, metabolic acidosis, or profound hypoxemia are more likely to fail NIV.[38] Survey data from centers in the United States and Europe with extensive experience using NIV indicate that more than 60% of patients with hypoxemic respiratory failure required intubation, with greater than 60% mortality.[40] More recently, positive findings were reported in a prospective multicenter survey that used NIV as the first-line intervention in selected patients with ALI/ARDS.[41] Results showed that 54% avoided intubation with improved outcome. Failure was predicted if PaO_2/FiO_2 ratio was less than 175 at 1 hour after initiation of NIV.[41] Three randomized controlled trials in patients with ALI/ARDS found that NIV decreased intubation rate and mortality, resulting in improved outcome.[40,42,43] However, a meta-analysis of these trials indicated that NIV did not decrease mortality despite a reduction in intubation rate,[44] and this analysis was consistent with other reports.[45]

Another randomized controlled trial[46] in patients with hypoxemic respiratory failure but no hypercapnia showed that mask CPAP significantly improved PaO_2/FiO_2 ratio within the first hour but failed to reduce the intubation rate, length of ICU stay, or hospital mortality. In this study, many patients who failed CPAP sustained cardiac arrest during intubation.[46] It is thought that clinicians did not readily accept the failure of NIV to correct hypoxemia in these patients, resulting in an unacceptable delay before intubation that contributed to the poor outcome in the failed CPAP group.

The evidence to date does not support routine NIV use in patients with ALI/ARDS, but randomized controlled trials focusing exclusively on ALI/ARDS are needed.[9] The data suggest that a closely monitored trial of NIV in carefully selected patients may be appropriate. If NIV does not markedly improve hypoxemia within 1 hour, patients should be intubated.

Respiratory Failure in Immunosuppressed Patients

The risk of developing nosocomial infections, including ventilator-associated pneumonia, is decreased when NIV is used compared with intubation and invasive mechanical ventilation. Randomized controlled trials involving immunosuppressed patients[47] and patients awaiting solid organ transplantation[48] who developed hypoxemic respiratory failure found decreased intubation rates and mortality with NIV compared with standard therapy. A nonrandomized trial of NIV in patients with AIDS and *Pneumocystis carinii* pneumonia showed similar results.[49] Despite the small numbers of patients in these single-center trials, NIV is accepted as first-line therapy in immunosuppressed patients because it avoids the risk of infection[50-52] associated with intubation in a setting where an infection can have devastating consequences.

Palliative Care and Do-Not-Intubate Orders

The use of NIV in patients with do-not-intubate (DNI) orders and end-stage disease remains controversial. Patients with DNI orders may receive NIV either for supportive treatment of a nonterminal, reversible event or for palliative care. There is evidence that NIV in patients with end-stage disease provides an effective method of support with some relief from associated symptoms.[53] Two more recent case series[54,55] support the use of NIV in the management of ARF in patients with DNI orders. Schettino and colleagues[54] and Levy and coworkers[55] showed that more than 65% of patients with COPD or cardiogenic pulmonary edema and DNI status were successfully managed with NIV. For palliative care application, the expectation is that NIV should make the process of dying more comfortable. If the patient is not more comfortable with NIV, it should be discontinued.

The primary controversy over the use of NIV in patients with DNI orders involves patient consent. Before consent is obtained, clinicians should take the time to discuss wishes for life-sustaining treatment with the patient and family and explain what NIV is and what it is intended to accomplish.[56] NIV is appropriate and can be beneficial in the care of patients with DNI orders if a patient understands that NIV is a form of life support and that its goal is either to reverse an acute disease process or to provide a comfort measure at the end of life.[56]

Postoperative Respiratory Failure

In one study, prophylactic use of NIV by obese patients who underwent gastroplasty markedly improved pulse oximetry oxygen saturation (SpO_2) and forced vital capacity (FVC), which allowed faster recovery of preoperative

MINI CLINI

Noninvasive Ventilation to Treat Hypoxemic Acute Respiratory Failure

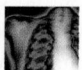

PROBLEM: A patient with acute hypoxemic respiratory failure is receiving NIV via nasal mask with a noninvasive ventilator. The ventilator is delivering PSV with peak inspiratory pressure set at 12 cm H_2O and end expiratory pressure set at 5 cm H_2O. O_2 at 6 L/min is flowing into the nasal mask. After 40 minutes on NIV, the patient continues to have signs of respiratory distress (dyspnea, tachypnea with respiratory rate 30, heart rate 120 beats/min, SpO_2 88% and cyanosis). The patient is having difficulty keeping his mouth closed, and there is a large air leak as a result. An arterial blood gas was drawn, and PaO_2 is 50 mm Hg.

SOLUTIONS

1. Change the interface to a full-face mask to prevent the air leak and provide more effective ventilator support. A chin strap could be tried but is not likely to be successful. Dyspneic patients tend to breathe through their mouths preferentially.
2. Change to a ventilator that can provide precise, high FiO_2; displays graphics; calculates exhaled volumes; and has alarms. Bleeding in O_2 to the mask or circuit provides only low, inconsistent FiO_2. Additional information from waveforms and calculated values can help provide better assessments and interventions. For a patient this sick, alarms are an important consideration.
3. Increase PEEP to 8 to 10 to maintain open alveoli in the lung and improve severe hypoxemia; 5 cm H_2O is probably inadequate in this situation.
4. If these interventions do not result in significant improvement in oxygenation within 30 to 45 minutes, the patient should be electively intubated and ventilated. Delaying intubation is associated with greater risk of death during intubation. Such delays can result if clinicians do not recognize an unsuccessful NIV trial in the setting of hypoxemia.

pulmonary function.[57] Two studies compared postoperative use of noninvasive CPAP with simple O_2 therapy. Squadrone and associates[58] found that patients receiving CPAP had lower intubation, pneumonia, overall infection, and sepsis rates after major abdominal surgery. Kindgen-Milles and coworkers[59] showed fewer pulmonary complications and a shorter hospital length of stay when patients received CPAP after thoracoabdominal aortic aneurysm repair. Although the results of these studies are encouraging, additional randomized trials are needed to identify specific postoperative populations that would benefit from NPPV or CPAP. At the present time, there is insufficient evidence to support routine postoperative use of NIV.

Prevention of Reintubation in High-Risk Patients

Reintubation has been associated with increased mortality, longer hospital stay, and a greater need for long-term care than in patients who are initially successfully extubated.[60] In more recent studies, Nava and colleagues[61] and Ferrer and coworkers[62] randomly assigned patients at risk for reintubation to NIV or standard care; both studies showed lower reintubation rates with NIV. Patients with hypercapnia gained the most benefit from NIV. Risk factors associated with extubation failure included a diagnosis of COPD or congestive heart failure, age older than 65 years, ineffective cough and excessive secretions, upper airway obstruction, history of one or more weaning failures, one or more comorbid conditions, and Acute Physiology and Chronic Health Evaluation (APACHE) II score greater than 12 on the day of extubation.

Patients who do not require reintubation have better outcomes than patients failing extubation. Sufficient evidence exists to support selective application of NIV to avoid reintubation and its associated risks, including higher mortality, longer hospital stay, and greater need for long-term care. NIV should be started after extubation of patients with multiple risk factors, especially patients with COPD, congestive heart failure, or hypercapnia. These patients should be monitored closely and reintubated promptly if NIV does not prevent respiratory distress.

Postextubation Respiratory Failure

The use of NIV to manage postextubation hypoxemic respiratory failure requires a cautious approach. Two randomized controlled trials[63,64] indicated no benefit or worse outcome when NIV was used to manage hypoxemic ARF. Keenan and associates[63] compared NIV and standard therapy in patients who developed respiratory failure during the first 2 days after extubation and observed a 70% reintubation rate in both groups. Esteban and colleagues[64] randomly assigned patients to standard therapy or NIV at the first sign of postextubation respiratory distress. Both groups had a 50% reintubation rate, but the group managed with NIV had higher mortality. This finding was attributed to the delay in reintubation that occurred in the NIV group. Relatively few patients with COPD were included in these two studies. The use of NIV to treat postextubation ARF generally should be reserved for patients with COPD and hypercapnic respiratory failure or patients with congestive heart failure. If hypoxemia does not significantly improve with NIV, these patients should be reintubated without delay.

RULE OF THUMB

Before using NIV in the management of ARF, be sure the process causing respiratory failure is reversible, selection criteria are met, and exclusion criteria are absent.

Long-Term Care Indications

Nocturnal Hypoventilation

Nocturnal hypoventilation is common with neuromuscular diseases, severe kyphoscoliosis, COPD, obesity, and central and obstructive sleep apnea.[65] Patients with these disorders are able to breathe spontaneously without assistance but typically have symptoms related to hypoventilation and sleep-disordered breathing. These symptoms may include excessive sleepiness during daytime hours; fatigue; morning headaches; and cognitive dysfunction, such as difficulty concentrating.[66]

Normally, the onset of sleep is characterized by a slight increase in $PaCO_2$ followed by a further increase in hypercapnia during rapid eye movement (REM) sleep. It is thought that the increased work of breathing associated with obesity and COPD or the muscle weakness caused by neuromuscular diseases results in greater levels of hypercapnia. Some of these patients are hyporesponsive to carbon dioxide (CO_2), which contributes to even more CO_2 retention. In response, the kidneys attempt to compensate by retaining bicarbonate, reducing respiratory drive further. This vicious cycle progressively worsens, leading to pulmonary hypertension, cor pulmonale, CO_2 narcosis, and eventually death.[65] There is strong evidence that the cycle can be stopped if breathing is assisted by NIV for 4 hours per night for 1 to 3 months.[65] One study suggested that NIV use during the daytime hours promotes similar improvement in gas exchange during periods of unassisted ventilation as seen when NIV is used at night.[67]

Three mechanisms have been proposed to explain the positive effects of NIV on nocturnal hypoventilation. First, it was thought that NIV rests fatigued respiratory muscles, improving their performance during the day.[68,69] Common sense supports this hypothesis, but few studies have been able to show significant or sustained improvement in muscle strength after using NIV.[70] Second, NIV reduces $PaCO_2$ and may reset the central ventilatory controller to a lower baseline $PaCO_2$. Current evidence suggests that NIV is effective because it prevents nocturnal hypoventilation and preserves ventilatory response to increases in CO_2 in patients with COPD or restrictive thoracic diseases.[67,71-73] Third, the improvements in lung compliance, lung volume, and dead space that result from NIV may be beneficial.[66]

Restrictive Thoracic Diseases

Restrictive thoracic diseases successfully managed with NIV include postpolio syndrome, neuromuscular diseases, chest wall deformities, spinal cord injuries, and severe kyphoscoliosis.[66] Patients with severe kyphoscoliosis showed improved nighttime and daytime gas exchange, fewer symptoms of hypoventilation, and increased spontaneous V_T and FVC after using NIV.[74] A study of eight patients with Pompe disease found that NIV corrected arterial blood gas abnormalities and resolved cor pulmonale 3 to 6 months after starting NIV.[75] Disease progression was not slowed by NIV. Diaphragmatic weakness is characteristic of this disease, in contrast to most other neuromuscular diseases. After starting NIV, pulmonary function tests improved slightly, but the improvement was not sustained for a long period.[75] Patients with Duchenne muscular dystrophy, a rapidly progressive neuromuscular disorder, were randomly assigned to either prophylactic nocturnal NIV or conventional treatment.[76] In this study, nocturnal NIV failed to slow progression of the disease and was associated with a higher mortality.[76]

The current recommendation for patients with restrictive thoracic disorders is to initiate NIV when patients develop symptoms of nocturnal hypoventilation. There is little evidence to support prophylactic NIV in patients with most restrictive thoracic diseases.

Amyotrophic Lateral Sclerosis

Amyotrophic lateral sclerosis (ALS), also known as *Lou Gehrig's disease,* is a neurodegenerative disease that affects motor neurons, resulting in progressive muscle weakness and paralysis. Mean survival time is 3 to 5 years after diagnosis. All patients with ALS eventually need full ventilatory support to survive. NIV is probably effective in prolonging the lives of patients with ALS.[77]

In a randomized controlled trial, Bourke and associates[78] found that patients with ALS who used NIV gained a median survival benefit of 205 days but only in the absence of bulbar dysfunction. Evidence suggests that using NIV slows the rate of lung function decline as indicated by FVC measurement.[78,79] Lung function decline occurs more slowly and survival benefit increases when NIV is used for more than 4 hours per day.[79] Several factors influencing compliance with NIV of patients with ALS have been identified. Early intervention[80] and orthopnea[81] correlated with better tolerance of NIV, whereas bulbar involvement[78,82] and the presence of cognitive or executive dysfunction[83] negatively affected compliance with NIV.

In contrast to other restrictive thoracic diseases, there may be a survival benefit when NIV is initiated earlier in the course of ALS. In one study, patients experiencing more than 15 episodes of nocturnal O_2 desaturation per hour were started on NIV.[80] This "early" intervention resulted in survival lasting 11 months longer and suggested that NIV may also provide some benefit in patients with bulbar involvement.[80] More studies are needed to assess the effects of early NIV initiation.

Clinicians in the acute care setting have conflicting feelings about initiating NIV in patients with ALS, often voicing concerns about the patient's quality of life and eventual dependence on NIV. Four studies found that NIV had a positive effect on patients' quality of life.[78,81,84,85] Positive changes associated with NIV included relief from dyspnea, increased energy and vitality, better concentration, less physical fatigue, and fewer symptoms of hypoventilation.[85] There was no difference in the perceived quality of life of patients using NIV compared with patients who received invasive mechanical ventilation through a tracheostomy.[86] However, invasive ventilation through a tracheostomy tube may have a negative effect on caregivers' quality of life. Most patients were comfortable with their decisions involving assisted ventilation with 94% of patients receiving NIV and 81% of patients with a tracheostomy indicating that they would choose ventilation again.[86]

There is good evidence that using NIV lengthens survival and slows the decline of lung function of patients with ALS. In its evidence-based Practice Parameters, the American Academy of Neurology recommended considering NIV for all patients with ALS and respiratory failure.[77] NIV is typically started when pulmonary function declines significantly (FVC < 50%). Although the evidence supporting early NIV initiation is weak, starting NIV at the first sign of nocturnal hypoventilation may be considered to improve compliance with NIV.

RULE OF THUMB

Patients with restrictive thoracic disorders should have symptoms of nocturnal hypoventilation before NIV is considered.

Chronic Obstructive Pulmonary Disease in Patients Needing Long-Term Care

There are two proposed hypotheses to explain how patients with severe COPD benefit from the use of NIV.[66] First, positive inspiratory pressure improves gas exchange and may unload the respiratory muscles, allowing them to recover, gain strength, and reduce fatigue resulting in improved quality of life. Second, NIV should decrease the symptoms of nocturnal hypoventilation and sleep-disordered breathing, improving sleep quality and daytime gas exchange.[66]

The use of NIV in the management of stable COPD is controversial. Four studies investigated the use of nocturnal NIV at varied levels of pressure support in stable, hypercapnic patients with COPD.[87-90] Only one of the studies showed improvement in gas exchange and quality of life.[89] The major criticism of this study was that its sample size was too small to draw any meaningful conclusions. A meta-analysis of the four trials found that NIV did not significantly improve gas exchange, lung function, or sleep quality when used nocturnally by patients with COPD.[70] In contrast, positive findings were reported in an Italian multicenter trial.[91] This study included 90 patients with COPD who were randomly assigned to nocturnal NIV with O_2 or O_2 therapy alone. After 2 years, the NIV group had lower $PaCO_2$, better quality of life, and fewer annual hospital days per patient.[91] A small retrospective study reported that when NIV was started on a group of patients who required frequent hospitalizations, the number of annual hospital days decreased significantly from 78 to 25 per patient.[92] Compliance with NIV therapy has been problematic in many studies involving patients with COPD.[93]

The role of NIV in the management of patients with stable, severe COPD has not been clearly established and remains controversial. A 1999 consensus conference report on indications for NIV recommended starting NIV in patients with stable COPD who have symptoms of hypoventilation plus $PaCO_2$ of at least 55 mm Hg or $PaCO_2$ of 50 to 54 mm Hg with nocturnal desaturation, or at least two hospitalizations for hypercapnic respiratory failure within the previous year.[66]

RULE OF THUMB

NIV should be considered for management of respiratory failure in patients with ALS because it probably slows the rate of decline of lung function and lengthens survival.

Obesity-Hypoventilation Syndrome

Obesity-hypoventilation syndrome (OHS) is defined as chronic daytime hypoventilation ($PaCO_2$ > 45 mm Hg) associated with obesity (body mass index >30 kg/m^2) when no other known cause for hypoventilation is present. Approximately 0.5% of women and 1% of men in the general population are estimated to have OHS.[94] Evidence suggests that OHS is a common yet underdiagnosed condition in extremely obese patients.[95] Obese patients consume many health care resources before a diagnosis of OHS is made,[96] which is a cause for concern as obesity becomes more prevalent in the United States. In a study of hospitalized obese patients, Nowbar and colleagues[97] found that hypercapnia with no other reason for hypoventilation was present in approximately one-third of patients with body mass index greater than 35 kg/m^2 and almost one-half of patients with body mass index greater than 50 kg/m^2.

Several studies showed improved daytime gas exchange and relief of symptoms associated with nocturnal hypoventilation within 1 to 4 months of initiation of NIV.[97-99] A randomized trial of CPAP versus NPPV in patients with OHS without severe nocturnal desaturations found that both modes were equally effective in decreasing daytime $PaCO_2$.[100] At the present time, nocturnal NPPV is recommended for OHS when nasal CPAP and other first-line therapies fail to alleviate the hypoventilation.[66,101]

SELECTING APPROPRIATE PATIENTS FOR NONINVASIVE VENTILATION

Acute Care Setting

The success or failure of NIV depends to a large degree on the clinician's clinical judgment in choosing appropriate patients. The primary selection criterion is the need for

MINI CLINI

Preventing a High-Risk Patient from Requiring Reintubation

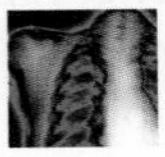

PROBLEM: A 74-year-old man was intubated for hypercapnic respiratory failure 3 days ago. Past medical history is significant for hypertension, coronary artery disease, COPD, and former cigarette smoker × 35 years (quit 10 years ago). He is currently on low-level PSV (PSV 8, PEEP 5 cm H_2O, FiO_2 0.3). Vital signs are heart rate 80 beats/min, blood pressure 130/70 mm Hg, respiratory rate 16 breaths/min, and SpO_2 95%. Endotracheal suctioning has been performed every 2 to 3 hours for moderate to large amounts of yellow secretions. Ipratropium MDI, 2 puffs every 6 hours, is ordered. He was placed on a spontaneous breathing trial this morning and passed; however, his ability to clear secretions is a concern. After much discussion among the patient care team, the decision was made not to extubate as planned, and antibiotics were started for presumed pneumonia.

SOLUTIONS

1. Extubate and immediately start NIV. Evidence supports using NIV to prevent reintubation in high-risk patients. Patients with hypercapnia are most likely to benefit. Other factors associated with high risk of extubation failure are age older than 65, COPD, and excessive secretions.
2. Continue aerosolized bronchodilators by delivering the MDI to a collapsible holding chamber added to the NIV circuit. Place the chamber between the exhalation port and the mask. Coordinate MDI actuation as closely as possible to the patient's own inspiration. Shake the MDI canister between each actuation to mix the propellant and the drug. These three points are important to deliver maximum medication to the patient.

ventilatory assistance resulting from ARF. Patients who are unable to ventilate adequately on their own typically show signs and symptoms of respiratory distress, including use of accessory muscles, paradoxical breathing, tachypnea, and dyspnea.[2,9] The feeling of dyspnea should be worse than usual for patients with COPD. In addition, these patients are unable to maintain normal gas exchange and usually develop respiratory acidosis or severe hypoxemia (Box 45-3).[2,9]

NIV exclusion criteria include apnea, hemodynamic or cardiac instability, lack of cooperation by the patient, conditions that preclude use of a noninvasive interface, copious amounts of secretions, and high risk of aspiration (Box 45-4).[2,9] Two studies of hypercapnic ARF in patients with COPD showed that NIV could be successful in patients with decreased level of consciousness or hypercapnic coma.[102,103] Decreased level of consciousness should not be considered an exclusion criterion for NIV in patients with COPD, but caution and monitoring are recommended when NIV is applied to these patients. The patient should be under constant observation until consciousness is regained. If the selection criteria are met and there are no contraindications, NIV should be considered.

It is important to consider the cause of ARF because the efficacy of NIV varies depending on the underlying condition being treated. In the acute care setting, most evidence supports the use of NIV in patients with COPD exacerbations or acute cardiogenic pulmonary edema. There is less evidence supporting NIV for the other indications discussed earlier; however, it is being used more frequently for patients with DNI orders, to facilitate extubation of high-risk patients, and as a means of preventing extubation failure and reintubation. Several studies identified potential predictors of success during NIV (Box 45-5). Patients with COPD and acute-on-chronic respiratory failure with comorbid conditions such as pneumonia are less likely to be managed successfully with NIV.[104] Early initiation of NIV is encouraged in patients with ARF because severe hypercapnia and acidosis are predictors of NIV failure.[104] Significant improvements in $PaCO_2$ and pH after 30 to 120 minutes of NIV is predictive of success.[105-107] In some cases, clinical judgment precludes an NIV trial based on the severity of the respiratory failure or other factors that increase the likelihood of failure to respond to NIV. However, in many situations, a reasonable plan would be

Box 45-3 Noninvasive Ventilation Selection Criteria for Patients With Acute Respiratory Failure

Two or more of the following should be present:

- Use of accessory muscles
- Paradoxical breathing
- Respiratory rate ≥25 breaths/min
- Moderate to severe dyspnea (increased dyspnea in COPD patients)
- $PaCO_2 > 45$ mm Hg with pH < 7.35
- PaO_2/FIO_2 ratio <200

Modified from Mehta S, Hill NS: Noninvasive ventilation. Am J Respir Crit Care Med 163:540, 2001.

Box 45-4 Exclusion Criteria for Noninvasive Ventilation in Patients With Acute Respiratory Failure

- Apnea
- Inability to protect airway/high aspiration risk
- Hemodynamic or cardiac instability
- Lack of patient cooperation
- Inability to use a noninvasive interface because of facial burns, trauma, or abnormal anatomy
- Excessive amounts of secretions

Modified from Mehta S, Hill NS: Noninvasive ventilation. Am J Respir Crit Care Med 163:540, 2001.

Box 45-5 Predictors of Noninvasive Ventilation Success in the Acute Care Setting

- Minimal air leak
- Low severity of illness
- Respiratory acidosis ($PaCO_2 > 45$ mm Hg but <92 mm Hg)
- pH < 7.35 but >7.22
- Improvement in gas exchange within 30 minutes to 2 hours of initiation
- Improvement in respiratory rate and heart rate

Modified from Mehta S, Hill NS: Noninvasive ventilation. Am J Respir Crit Care Med 163:540, 2001.

a trial of NIV for 1 to 2 hours, with periodic reassessment and plans to intubate if the patient's condition does not significantly improve. Successful application of NIV includes short-term goals of improving gas exchange and preventing endotracheal intubation and long-term goals of improved outcome, decreased length of stay, and decreased mortality.

Long-Term Care Setting

The current recommended selection guidelines for NIV in restrictive thoracic disease may be separated into two parts. First, patients should have symptoms of chronic hypoventilation and lack of sleep quality. Second, patients should meet one of the following measurable parameters: $PaCO_2$ 45 mm Hg or greater, nocturnal O_2 saturation less than 88% for 5 minutes, maximal inspiratory pressure less than 60 cm H_2O, or FVC less than 50% of predicted.[66] Although a decline in pulmonary function has been associated with CO_2 retention, more evidence is needed to support the use of a declining maximal inspiratory pressure or FVC as an indication for NIV.[2]

Recommendations for use of NIV in the management of nocturnal hypoventilation caused by disorders other than restrictive lung disease and COPD include documentation of a disorder that causes hypoventilation and failure of the disorder to respond to first-line therapy. First-line therapy includes weight loss, O_2 therapy, respiratory stimulants, and CPAP. NIV is recommended as the initial therapy for moderate to severe cases of nocturnal hypoventilation.[66]

Patients with COPD and signs and symptoms of chronic hypoventilation and poor quality of sleep should receive optimal medical treatment before NIV is recommended.[66] If symptoms remain despite optimal management, the presence of one of the following selection criteria indicates the need for NPPV: $PaCO_2$ 55 mm Hg or greater or $PaCO_2$ 50 to 54 mm Hg with recurrent hospitalizations or nocturnal desaturation.[66] Recurrent hospitalization is defined as two or more hospitalizations for hypercapnic respiratory failure in a 12-month period. Nocturnal desaturation is defined by a pulse oximeter reading of less than 89% for 5 minutes with administration of at least 2 L/min of O_2.[62]

In long-term care settings, a follow-up examination is suggested 1 month or so after starting NIV to help the patient acclimate to the device. A 2-month follow-up is recommended to determine compliance with NIV and to assess benefit.[66]

Exclusion Criteria for Noninvasive Ventilation in a Long-Term Care Setting

Relative contraindications for the use of NIV for restrictive thoracic disease, nocturnal hypoventilation, and chronic COPD include an unsupportive family, copious amounts of secretions, uncooperative behavior on the part of the patient, high risk of aspiration, and any anatomic abnormality that interferes with gas delivery.[2]

EQUIPMENT USED FOR NONINVASIVE VENTILATION

Many factors, including the choice of patient interface, ventilator, mode of ventilation, and initial ventilator settings, play a role in determining whether NIV will be successful in a given patient. This section discusses the equipment and modes of ventilation used in the application of NIV.

Patient Interfaces

Various devices are available to provide a noninvasive interface between the patient and the ventilator. When selecting an interface, clinicians should evaluate the fit and air leak associated with the interface. These factors have a major impact on the efficacy of NIV. Patient comfort is also an important consideration because it influences patient compliance with therapy, particularly in the long-term care setting. Other considerations include volume of dead space and position of the exhalation port in the interface and whether the interface functions properly with the type of ventilator to be used. The most common noninvasive patient interfaces used in the acute care setting are full-face or oronasal masks followed by nasal masks. An oronasal mask is usually the best choice when NIV is used to treat ARF.

Nasal and Oronasal Masks

Nasal and oronasal masks are typically manufactured in two parts. The body of these devices is made of clear, hard plastic. Surrounding the outer edge of the mask body is either a soft plastic or silicone lip or a cushion filled with hydrogel, silicone gel, or air. The best design has a soft inner lip that forms a seal with the patient's face. When a higher positive pressure is applied, the mask fits more closely to the face. The opposite effect occurs when resuscitation masks are used for positive pressure ventilation.

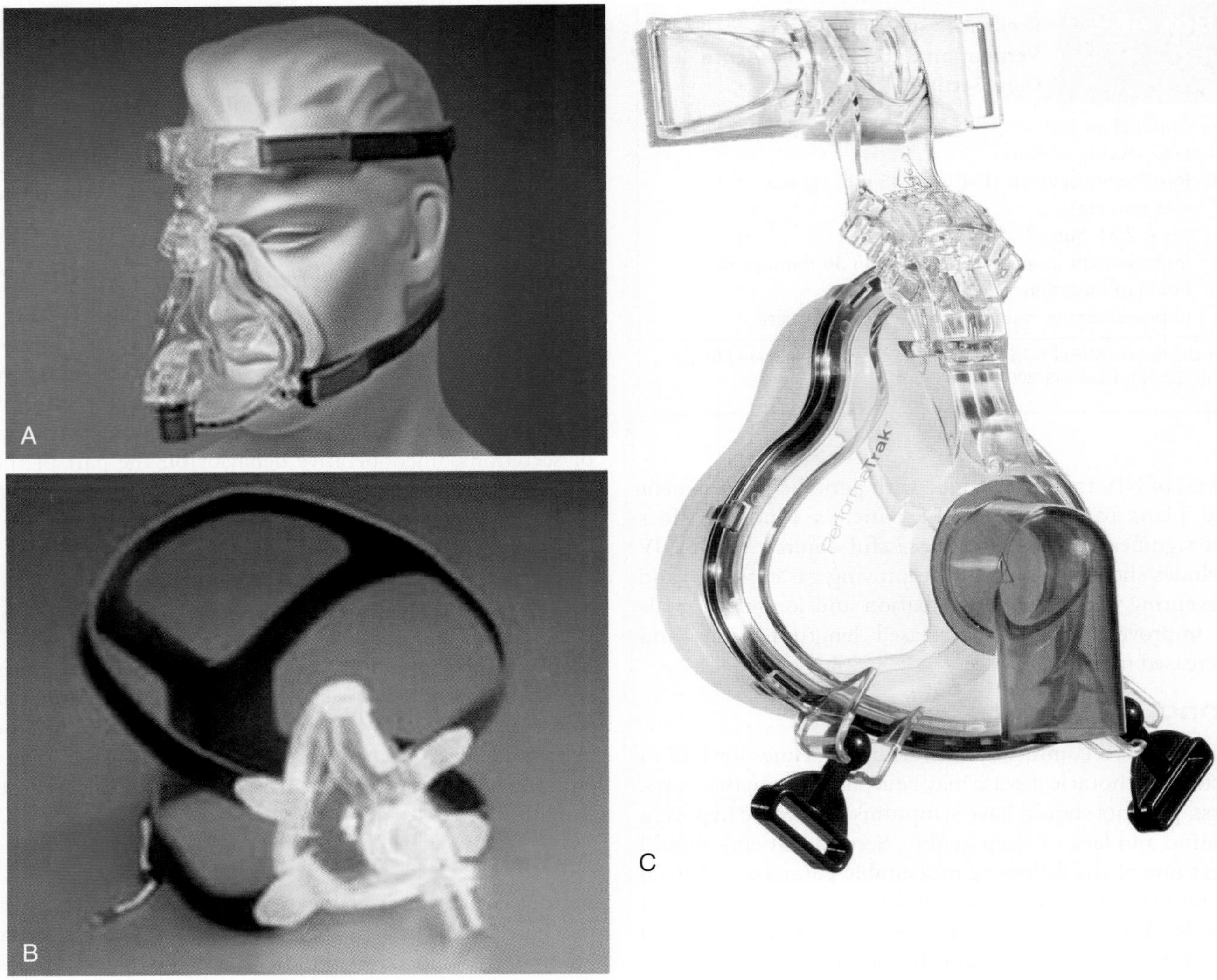

FIGURE 45-4 **A,** Nasal mask and head strap. Straps should be loosened if two fingers cannot be inserted between the cheek and the strap. **B,** Nasal mask and head strap. **C,** Nasal mask with adjustable forehead support to minimize pressure on the bridge of the nose. (**A,** Courtesy of Phillips Respironics, Murrysville, PA. **B,** From Albert R, Spiro S and Jett J: Clinical respiratory medicine, ed 2, Philadelphia, 2004, Mosby.)

Higher airway pressures tend to force this type of mask away from the face, increasing the air leak.

NIV masks incorporate straps and headgear to maintain and stabilize the mask's position on the face (Figure 45-4). It is important to avoid tightening the straps more than necessary. A perfect seal between the mask and the face is not required because ventilators used for NIV are designed to function properly in the presence of small air leaks. Pulling the straps excessively tight is likely to result in pressure-related damage to the skin on the bridge of the nose or sometimes on the cheeks. Clinicians must be vigilant for early signs of skin damage and take steps to minimize damage and prevent development of pressure ulcers. An area of reddened skin that persists after removal of the mask is usually the first sign of pressure-related skin damage. A liquid skin barrier and a hydrocolloid patch may be applied to protect the reddened area.

To address the problem of skin breakdown, most masks incorporate some means of minimizing pressure on the skin. These include foam wedges used as spacers and adjustable mechanical controls that prevent the apex of the mask from being pulled too close to the face. Some masks have foam pads that rest on the forehead to help maintain proper mask positioning. An easy way to check for excessive tightness is to insert two fingers between the straps and the patient's face. If the straps are too tight to do this easily, they should be loosened slightly. A strategy for minimizing the risk of pressure ulcer formation is to alternate the use of two or more masks with different points of facial contact.

A key factor in patient tolerance and NIV efficacy is the choice of an appropriately sized mask. Most masks include sizing templates that can be used before removing the mask from its packaging (Figure 45-5). Nasal masks should

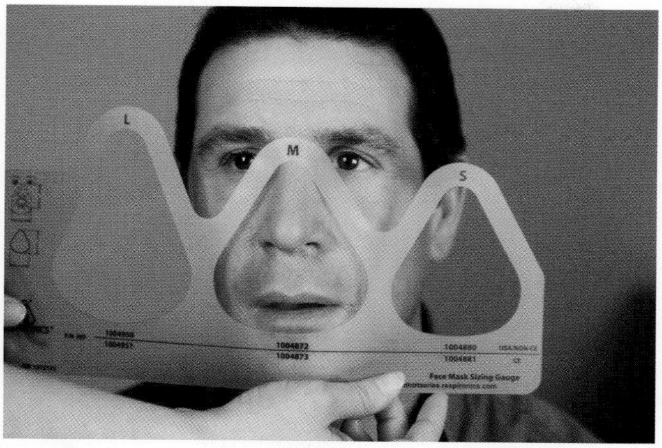

FIGURE 45-5 Templates help clinicians select an appropriately sized mask. Full face masks should rest on the bridge of the nose $\frac{1}{3}$ of the way from the top of the bridge of the nose and in the indentation between the chin and the lower lip. (Courtesy Phillips Respironics, Murrysville, PA.)

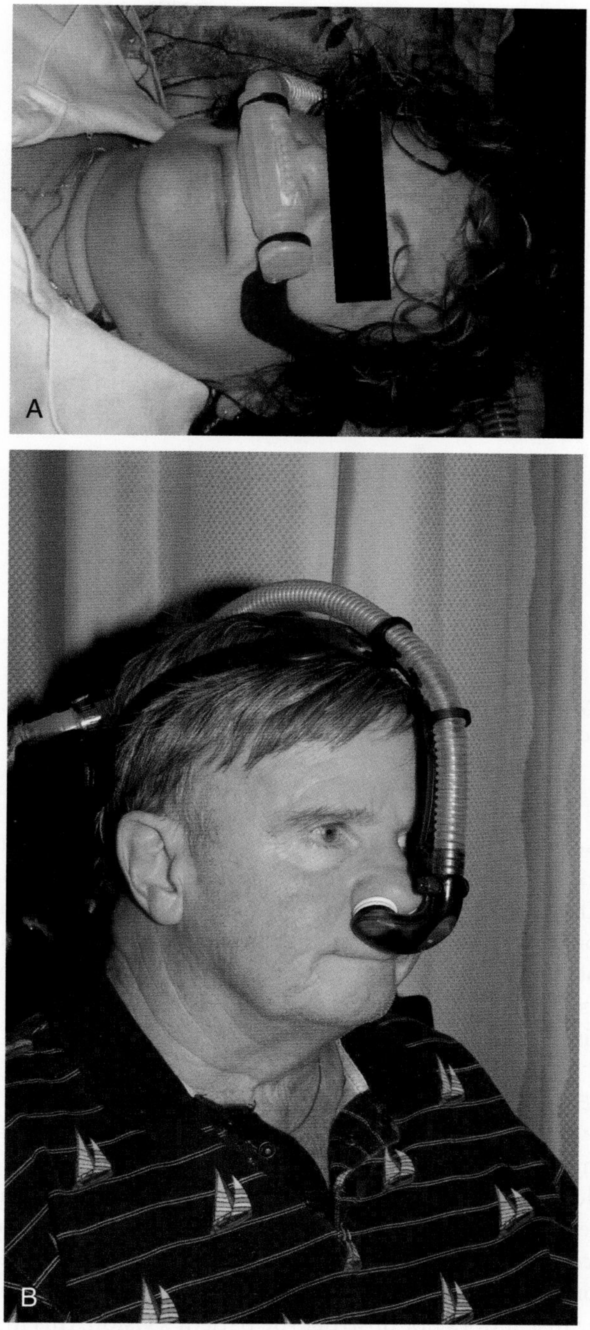

FIGURE 45-6 Nasal pillows are available in several designs and various sizes. (**A,** From Parillo J and Dellinger R: Critical care medicine: principles of diagnosis and management in the adult, ed 3, Philadelphia, 2007, Mosby. **B,** From Schapira A: Neurology and clinical neuroscience, Philadelphia, 2007, Mosby.)

be sized so that the cushion starts one-third of the way down from the top of the bridge of the nose and fits closely around the lateral aspects of the nose and rests above the upper lip, just under the nose. Full-face masks fit similarly except the bottom of the mask rests in the depression above the chin and just below the lower lip. Mask sizes range from extra small to large, but for many individuals, a small or medium-small mask is a good fit. Ill-fitting masks can allow air leaks into the eyes, leading to poor tolerance. Small leaks around the mouth are generally less problematic because most ventilators used for NIV are designed to function with a baseline leak.

Nasal masks are more prone to air leaks than full-face masks, especially for patients who are mouth breathers. Chin straps are available that provide tension to help keep the mouth closed, but in practice, they seldom work well. Full-face masks are less prone to mouth leaks because both the mouth and the nose are covered. Disadvantages associated with full-face masks include increases in dead space, risk of aspiration, and feelings of claustrophobia. Nasal masks may be better tolerated by patients with claustrophobia. Full-face masks interfere with patients' ability to communicate, eat, drink, and expectorate secretions without removing the mask.

In the past few years, new types of patient interfaces have been introduced in various designs, sizes, and shapes that are intended to promote more comfort and better tolerance. The respiratory therapist (RT) should be aware of all available designs to choose a relatively comfortable, well-tolerated, correctly fitted interface through which the needed level of ventilatory support can be delivered.

Nasal Pillows

Nasal pillows (Figure 45-6) are round, soft cushions that fit directly into the nares. Specially designed headgear holds the prongs in place. This interface is used most often during nasal CPAP by patients with chronic disease who do not tolerate a nasal mask. Nasal pillows are often a good option for patients with skin necrosis on the bridge of the nose or to deliver nocturnal CPAP to patients who prefer to sleep on their side. A newer design is the wedge-shaped mini-nasal mask that covers only the end of the nose.

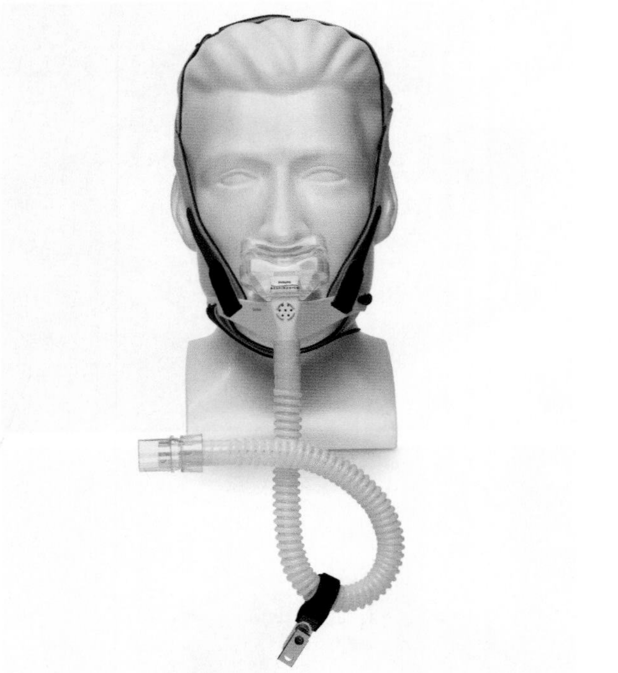

FIGURE 45-7 Hybrid mask does not apply pressure to the bridge of the nose. (Courtesy ResMed Corp, San Diego, CA.)

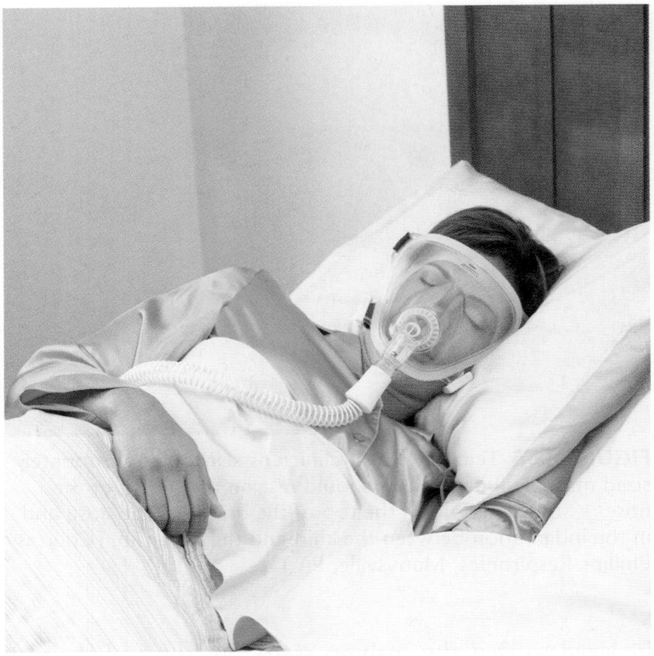

FIGURE 45-8 Total Face Mask. (Courtesy Phillips Respironics, Murrysville, PA.)

Another is the hybrid mask (Figure 45-7), which covers the mouth with a small mask and seals the nares with nasal pillows connected to the top. This interface allows ventilation with fewer leaks, similar to an oronasal mask that does not have contact with the skin on the bridge of the nose. Besides the advantage of decreased risk of tissue damage, this design allows patients to wear glasses during NIV.

Face Masks

A variation of the full-face mask is the total face mask, which surrounds the entire face (Figure 45-8). A soft, flexible layer around the edge of this mask forms a seal and prevents leaking when the mask is pressurized. The total face mask comes in one size, which allows quick application in the emergency department or critical care unit. Because it does not obstruct the patient's vision, this mask may help patients who feel claustrophobic when wearing other full-face or nasal masks. However, it has a large dead space and can interfere with triggering and cycling.

The helmet is an interface that is unavailable in the United States at the present time (Figure 45-9). This interface surrounds the entire head like a plastic bubble. The only point where the patient experiences stress is in the axillary area where the two straps holding the helmet in place cross. Numerous more recent studies discussed the effectiveness of the helmet during CPAP and NPPV.[108-112] Results indicated that the helmet is more effective for CPAP than NPPV.[111] However, CPAP must be applied with a high continuous flow to prevent CO_2 from accumulating inside the helmet.[112] If CPAP is provided by a ventilator, the patient is likely to rebreathe CO_2 because of the large capacitance of the helmet.[112] During NIV with the helmet, CO_2 is not eliminated as effectively compared with full-face masks, and triggering and cycling the ventilator can be adversely affected.[111]

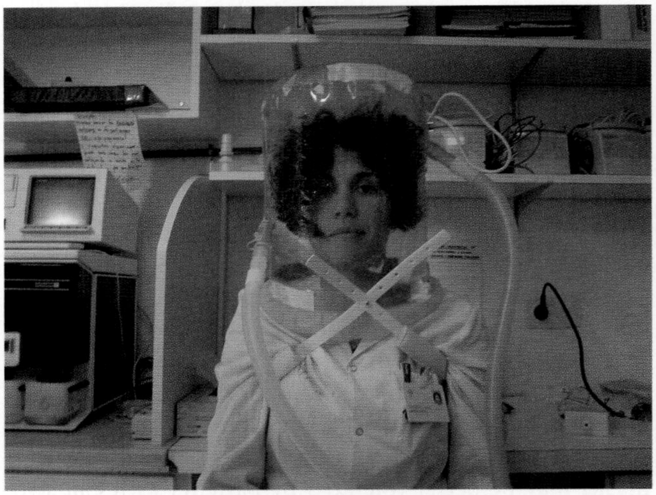

FIGURE 45-9 The best application for the helmet is providing continuous high-flow CPAP. (From Albert RK, Slutsky AS, Ranieri VM, et al: Clinical critical care medicine, Philadelphia, 2006, Mosby.)

Face masks are specifically designed for use with either ICU or noninvasive ventilators (Figure 45-10). Face masks for noninvasive ventilators have entrainment valves that prevent asphyxia if the ventilator fails or the tubing becomes disconnected. Full-face masks designed for ICU

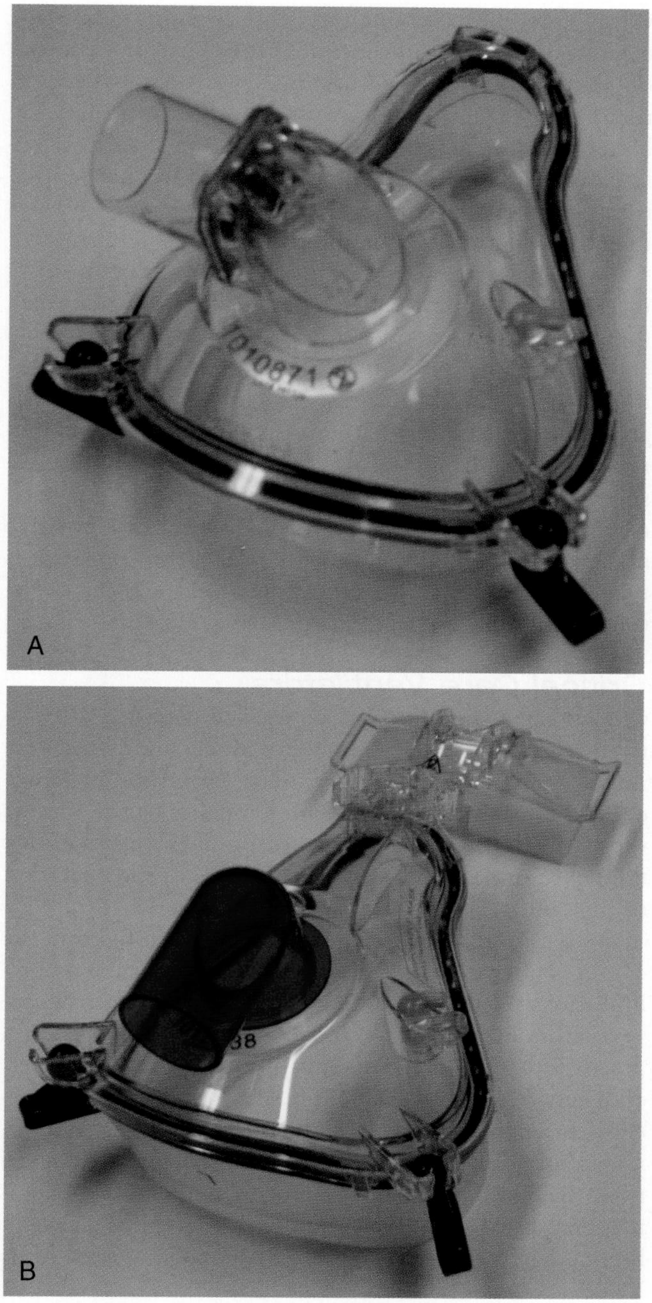

FIGURE 45-10 Full-face masks used for NIV. **A,** Noninvasive ventilator. **B,** Critical care ventilator.

ventilators do not have this feature. In addition, noninvasive ventilators using a single-limb circuit require a leak port either in the tubing or in the mask itself. Masks with leak ports should be used only with noninvasive ventilators because the leak interferes with the function of ICU ventilators.

Few data are available in the literature to help guide the choice of an interface for NIV. One study compared 30 minutes of full-face mask, nasal mask, and nasal pillows applied in random order to hypercapnic patients.[113] The investigators reported that the full-face mask and nasal pillows improved ventilation more than the nasal mask but that the nasal mask was better tolerated.[113] Use of a full-face mask also was associated with a significant increase in V_T compared with the nasal mask.[113] Similar findings were reported in a more recent study of 90 patients with hypercapnic ARF randomly assigned to full-face mask or nasal mask.[114] Both studies support the belief that full-face masks may be more effective for patients in the acute care setting.[113,114] There is no perfect NIV interface that meets the needs of every patient. Success is more likely if the interface can be tolerated for long periods and only a small air leak is present. A full-face mask is the interface of choice for patients requiring NIV for ARF. For patients who cannot tolerate a full-face mask, a nasal mask should be tried before accepting failure.

RULE OF THUMB

Use a full-face mask for patients in ARF. If the patient is unable to tolerate a full-face mask, try a nasal mask before accepting NIV failure.

Types of Mechanical Ventilators and Modes of Ventilation

Three types of ventilators are used for NIV: noninvasive ventilators, critical care ventilators, and portable home care ventilators. This section describes the characteristics and function of the three types of ventilators.

Noninvasive Ventilators

Most noninvasive ventilators are electrically powered, blower-driven, and microprocessor-controlled (Figure 45-11). These devices deliver a continuous but variable flow of gas to the patient through a single-limb circuit without an exhalation valve. To function properly, noninvasive ventilators must have a continuous air leak through one or more small ports either in the ventilator circuit or in the patient interface. The ports also provide the outlet through which the patient's exhaled gas is vented from the circuit. The main advantage of noninvasive ventilators over other types of ventilators is the ability to trigger and cycle appropriately when small to moderate air leaks are present.

The microprocessor controls gas delivery to the patient. Although flow and pressure are measured internally, noninvasive ventilators are sensitive to changes in flow and pressure and can rapidly respond to patient demands. The design of these ventilators maintains a low resistance between the patient and the ventilator at all times. Key factors are the absence of valves in the ventilator circuit, smooth internal lumen tubing for the circuit, and use of only low-resistance heated humidifiers.

Noninvasive ventilators used in the acute care setting for patients who would otherwise need intubation should meet a few minimum performance characteristics. They

MINI CLINI

Problems With Triggering During Noninvasive Ventilation

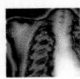

PROBLEM: A patient with COPD is receiving NIV with a noninvasive ventilator using a full-face mask. The ventilator settings are as follows: PSV mode, peak pressure 14 cm H_2O, PEEP 4 cm H_2O, backup rate 10 breaths/min. Arterial blood gas was obtained after 30 minutes on NIV. $PaCO_2$ was 75 mm Hg, essentially unchanged since NIV was initiated. The RT notices that the ventilator is not triggering with every patient effort, and his respiratory distress has not improved. What should the RT do?

SOLUTION

1. The problems of failure to trigger and ineffective ventilation could be caused by a large air leak. Determine if an air leak is present. If so, reposition, refit, or select a better fitting mask; adjust strap tension; and consider adding a forehead spacer to minimize the leak.
2. These two problems could be related to intrinsic PEEP. Carefully observe the patient and ventilator graphics, if available, for missed trigger attempts. The ventilator should trigger with every inspiratory effort by the patient. Try increasing PEEP slowly from 4 cm H_2O to 6 cm H_2O or 8 cm H_2O. If the applied PEEP from the ventilator is set to minimize the difference between end expiratory pressure and the patient's intrinsic PEEP, the ability to trigger should improve. In some ventilators, increasing or decreasing PEEP in pressure-targeted ventilation modes does not also affect the peak pressure. In this case, increasing PEEP could result in a decrease in the ventilating pressure and V_T. Check the peak pressure to determine if the ventilating pressure has changed, and increase the peak pressure by the same amount as PEEP increased. Effective ventilation is usually achieved if the exhaled V_T is about 4 to 6 ml/kg.

should be able to provide mandatory rates up to 30 breaths/min; inspiratory pressure up to 30 cm H_2O; positive end expiratory pressure (PEEP), or **expiratory positive airway pressure (EPAP),** up to 15 cm H_2O; and inspiratory flow rates up to 180 L/min at 20 cm H_2O. Safety requirements include minimal CO_2 rebreathing; potential antiasphyxia capabilities in the event of power loss or circuit disconnection; and alarms for circuit disconnection, loss of power, and battery failure if a battery is present.

Ideally, noninvasive ventilators should have an internal blending device, capable of providing FiO_2 ranging from 0.21 to about 1. Bleeding O_2 into the ventilator circuit or the interface results in maximum FiO_2 of about 0.5,[115] which is prone to wide fluctuations from variations in flow rates, patient effort, and leaks. Low baseline pressure settings have been associated with significant rebreathing of CO_2 in single-limb circuits.[116,117] These reports suggest the use of 3 to 5 cm H_2O PEEP or the use of a nonrebreathing valve to prevent rebreathing of CO_2.[117] For this reason, the expiratory pressure can be set no lower than 3 or 4 cm H_2O on many noninvasive ventilators. Newer noninvasive ventilators for use in acute care usually include an internal battery; include graphics monitoring; and display calculated volumes that estimate leak, V_T, and minute ventilation. Graphics are very useful when adjusting NIV settings to enhance patient-ventilator synchrony.

Modes available on noninvasive ventilators usually include CPAP, spontaneous (pressure support), and timed (pressure assist/control). With CPAP, the ventilator delivers no additional pressure to alleviate the work of breathing when the patient inspires. The patient simply breathes at an elevated baseline. With pressure support and spontaneous modes, inspiration is patient-triggered. With pressure assist/control, inspiration is either patient-triggered or time-triggered. Similar to PSV, **inspiratory positive airway pressure (IPAP),** equal to peak airway pressure, is typically pressure-limited and flow-cycled or time-cycled (Figure 45-12).

Critical Care Ventilators

Critical care ventilators can be used to deliver NIV effectively (Figure 45-13). The choices of modes and settings are important determinants of patient tolerance, but these choices often depend on the functionality of the specific ventilator to be used. For this reason, it is important for the RT to understand the actual change in the operation of the ventilator that occurs in the NIV mode.

With critical care ventilators, CO_2 rebreathing from the circuit is not a concern because the ventilators use a dual-limb circuit with a separate exhalation valve. Critical care ventilators have internal blenders capable of delivering a precise FiO_2 up to 1.0. This capability can make the difference between success and failure of NIV in severely hypoxemic patients. Critical care ventilators usually provide high inspiratory flows that meet any patient demand. In addition, they have extensive monitoring and alarm capabilities. Alarms are essential to patient safety, but they can become a nuisance when repeatedly actuated because of air leaks.

The main problem with using older critical care ventilators to provide NIV is their inability to compensate for leaks. Air leaks can cause problems with triggering and cycling. To minimize the risk of these problems, critical care ventilators should be used only with a full-face mask. State-of-the-art critical care ventilators now have ventilation modes designed for noninvasive application. With a few models, the NIV mode activates only new alarms (low pressure) and deactivates low V_T and minute volume alarms. However, most models incorporate some level of leak compensation during triggering, cycling, or both. A common feature of NIV modes is the ability to set a maximum inspiratory time during PSV. This setting does not deactivate flow cycling but provides an additional limit for inspiration in the presence of a large leak.

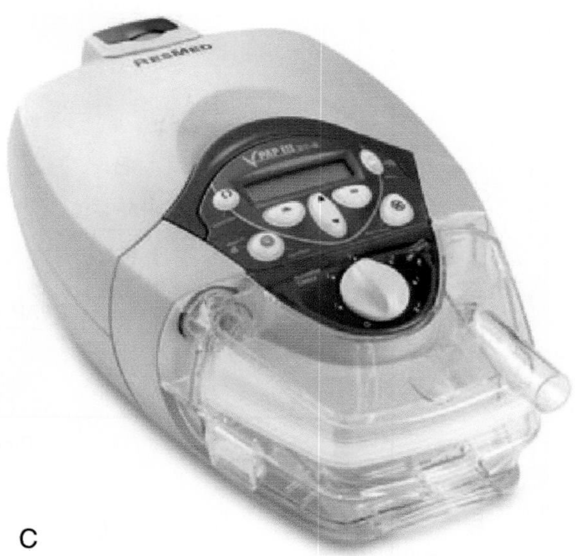

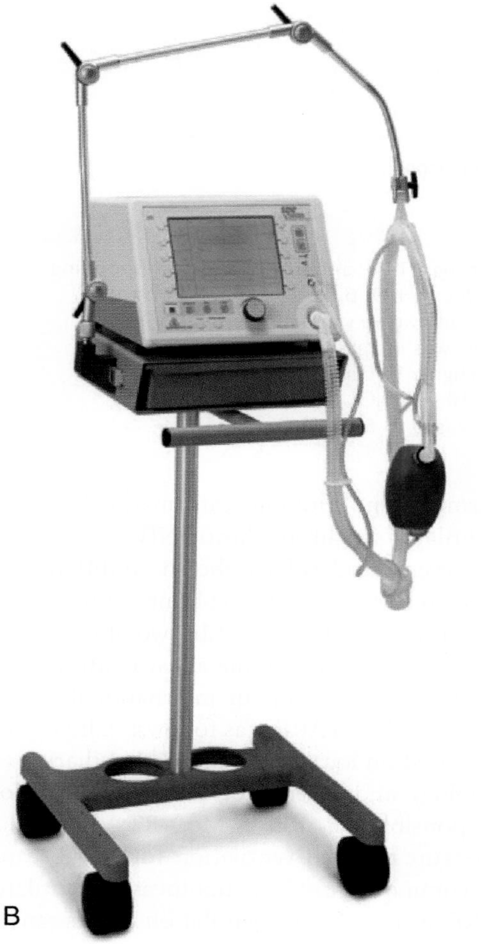

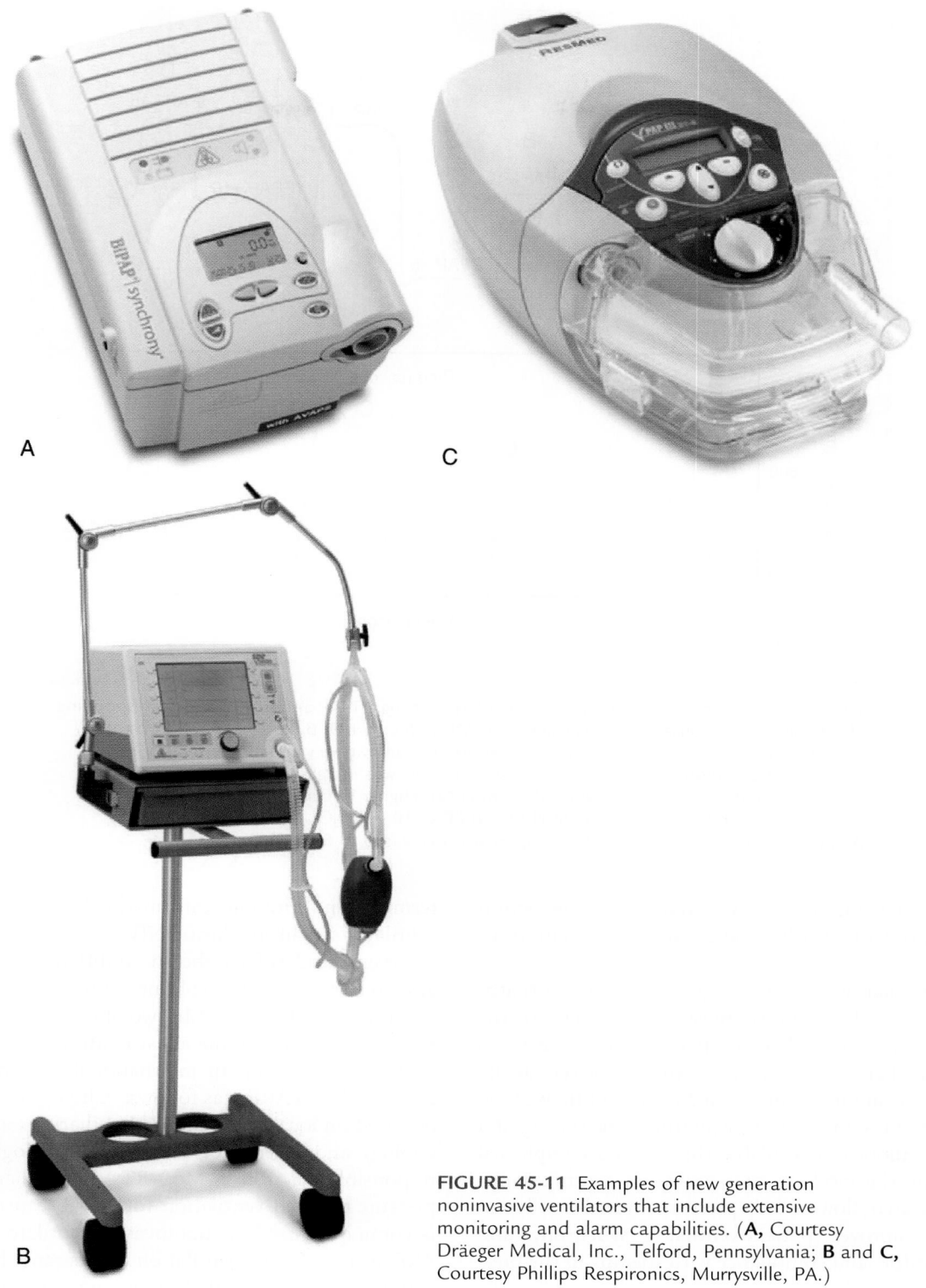

FIGURE 45-11 Examples of new generation noninvasive ventilators that include extensive monitoring and alarm capabilities. (**A,** Courtesy Dräeger Medical, Inc., Telford, Pennsylvania; **B** and **C,** Courtesy Phillips Respironics, Murrysville, PA.)

To deliver NIV, ICU ventilators can be set in PSV mode, which is a patient-triggered, pressure-limited, flow-cycled mode. During inspiration, a high gas flow is delivered until the preset pressure limit is achieved. At that point, the flow begins to decrease until a predetermined level of flow is reached, cycling the breath to exhalation. Depending on the specific ventilator used, this flow level can be a fixed flow rate (e.g., 5 L/min) or a percentage of the peak flow (e.g., 25%). The flow-cycling mechanism of PSV can cause problems during NIV if air leaks are present because the flow may not decrease to the level necessary to cycle the breath to expiration. In this case, the patient may have to exhale actively, using abdominal muscles to increase airway pressure to cycle the ventilator

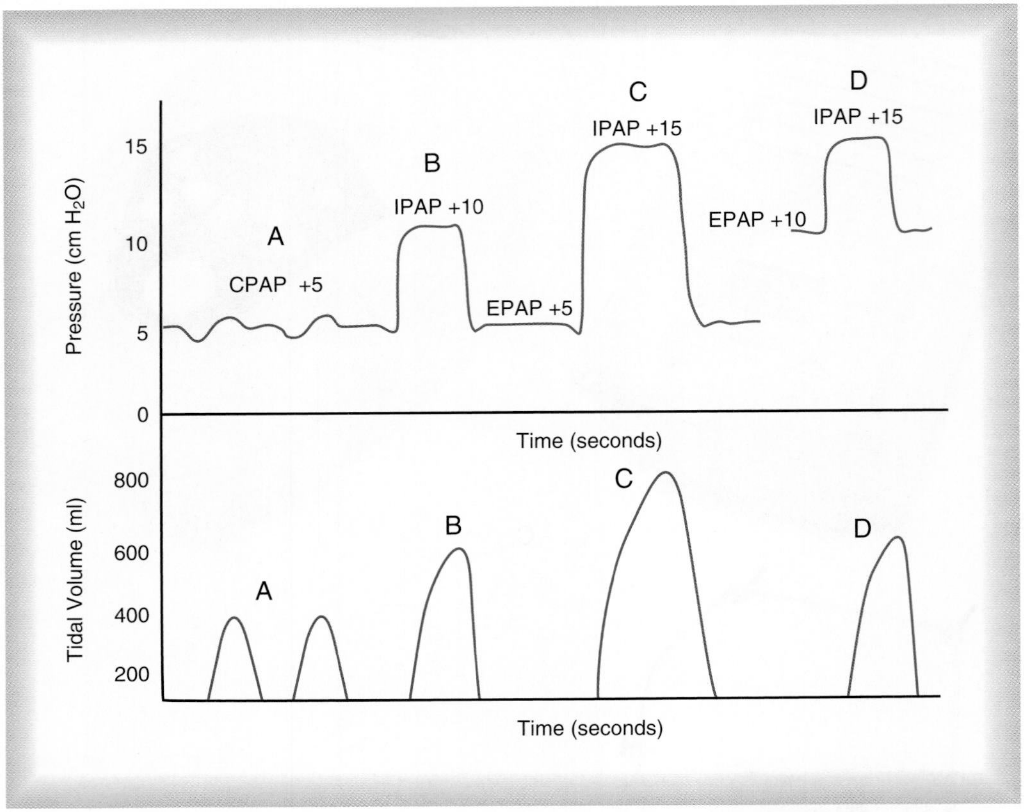

FIGURE 45-12 Changes in noninvasive ventilator settings (IPAP and EPAP) and corresponding effects on V_T. *A,* Spontaneous breathing on CPAP of 5 cm H_2O. *B,* Patient-triggered breath with the addition of 5 cm H_2O of pressure support (noninvasive ventilator settings are IPAP 10 cm H_2O and EPAP 5 cm H_2O). *C,* Pressure support was increased to 10 cm H_2O (NIV settings are IPAP 15 cm H_2O and EPAP 5 cm H_2O). Higher V_T occurs as pressure support is increased in *A* and *B*. *D,* IPAP 15 cm H_2O and EPAP 10 cm H_2O. Increasing EPAP setting results in lower V_T because pressure support was decreased to 5 cm H_2O.

to exhalation using secondary criteria.[118,119] This action increases work of breathing and can lead to failure of NIV.

Active exhalation can be recognized on the ventilator graphics by a spike in airway pressure at the end of the breath (Figure 45-14). There are two ways to correct this problem so that the patient can exhale passively again. First, inspiration can be time-cycled instead of flow-cycled by decreasing the maximum inspiratory time setting; if a noninvasive mode is unavailable, this can be accomplished by changing the mode to pressure assist/control. Time-cycled (instead of flow-cycled), pressure-limited ventilation markedly improves patient-ventilator synchrony and patient comfort and compliance with therapy in the presence of air leaks.[120]

The second option is to adjust the termination criterion[121] by changing the percentage of the peak inspiratory flow that terminates the breath. Most current generation ICU ventilators allow the termination criterion setting to range from 5% to 10% to 60% to 80% or more of the peak flow rate (Figure 45-15). To prevent active exhalation, the percentage is simply increased until the spike disappears from the pressure waveform. Proper adjustment of the termination criterion can markedly improve patient-ventilator synchrony during NIV.

Several studies have shown no difference in success or gas exchange between volume-controlled and pressure-controlled modes.[113,122,123] In two of these studies, patients preferred PSV to volume assist/control.[122,123] The current recommendation by an international consensus conference on NIV in ARF is as follows: "Choice of mode should be based on local expertise and familiarity, tailored to the etiology and severity of the pathophysiological process responsible for ARF."[124] Most RTs are familiar with using pressure-targeted ventilation for NIV because this mode is commonly used on noninvasive ventilators. In severe ARF, using pressure ventilation makes sense because leak compensation is provided, triggering and cycling can be adjusted to suit patient needs, and minute ventilation and end expiratory pressures are preserved. Volume-controlled modes are not recommended for NIV. Inability to compensate for the decrease in minute ventilation and loss of pressure caused by large leaks are major problems when volume targeted modes are used for NIV. Air leaks during volume-controlled ventilation can result in hypoventilation secondary to loss of the set V_T.

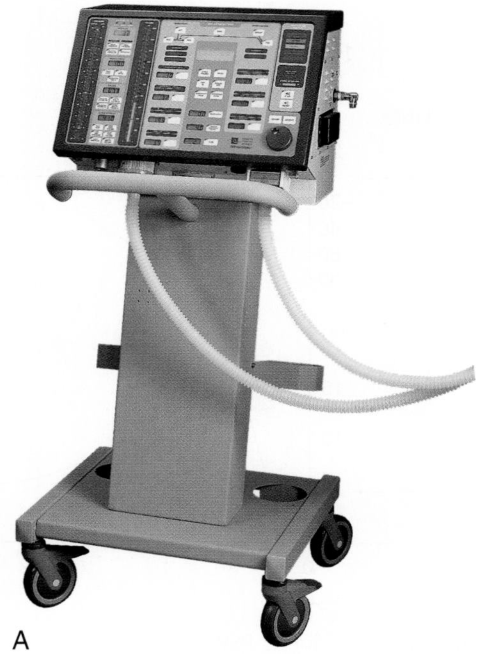
A

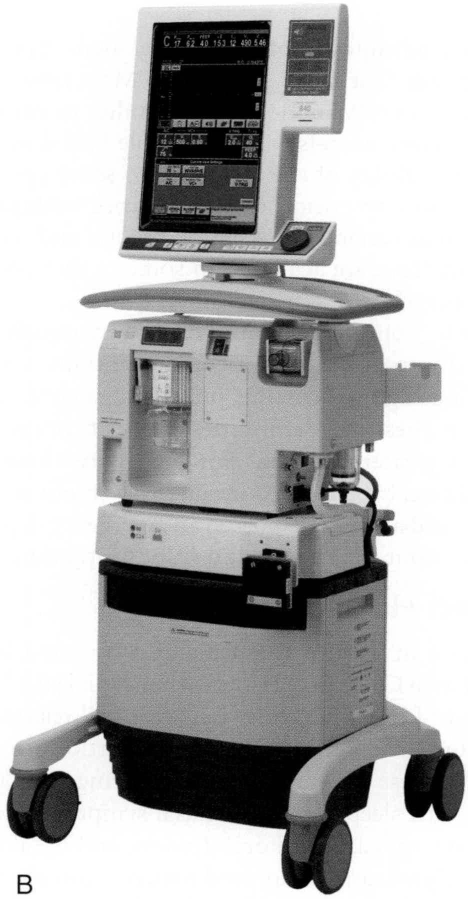
B

FIGURE 45-13 Examples of critical care ventilators that can be used to provide noninvasive ventilation. **A,** Puritan Bennett 760 Ventilation System. **B,** Puritan Bennett Ventilation System. (Images used by permission of Nellcor 840 Puritan Bennett LLC, Boulder, Colorado, doing business as Covidien.)

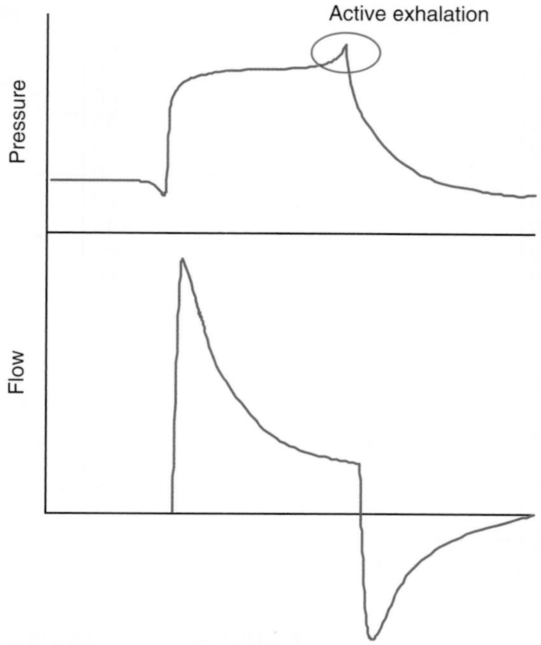

FIGURE 45-14 Active exhalation is recognized by the spike on the pressure waveform at the end of inspiration. The patient uses abdominal muscles to increase airway pressure and cycle the ventilator into exhalation.

In the long-term care setting, volume ventilation is sometimes used for patients with neuromuscular weakness.[3] Volume ventilation may allow a patient to stack breaths, increasing lung volume to near inspiratory capacity and resulting in improved cough peak flow. High cough peak flow should enhance secretion clearance. In patients with limited muscle strength, pressure-controlled ventilation does not allow breath stacking because inspiratory pressure is held constant, in contrast to volume ventilation, in which delivered V_T is constant. However, there is no proven advantage of one mode versus another in the long-term care setting.[2] Enhanced secretion clearance is easily provided using a mechanical cough assist device.

Portable Home Care or Transport Ventilators

Most portable home care ventilators (Figure 45-16) are electrically powered and microprocessor-controlled. These devices can operate from alternating current (AC) or, if equipped with internal or external batteries, direct current (DC) power sources. The batteries usually can provide power for several hours. Batteries add a measure of safety in areas where AC power outages occur regularly. They also allow the patient to be more mobile, which may improve their quality of life. These ventilators use a single-limb or double-limb ventilator circuit with an exhalation valve that prevents rebreathing of CO_2. Updated technology has improved the performance characteristics of these ventilators to a level comparable to critical care ventilators with

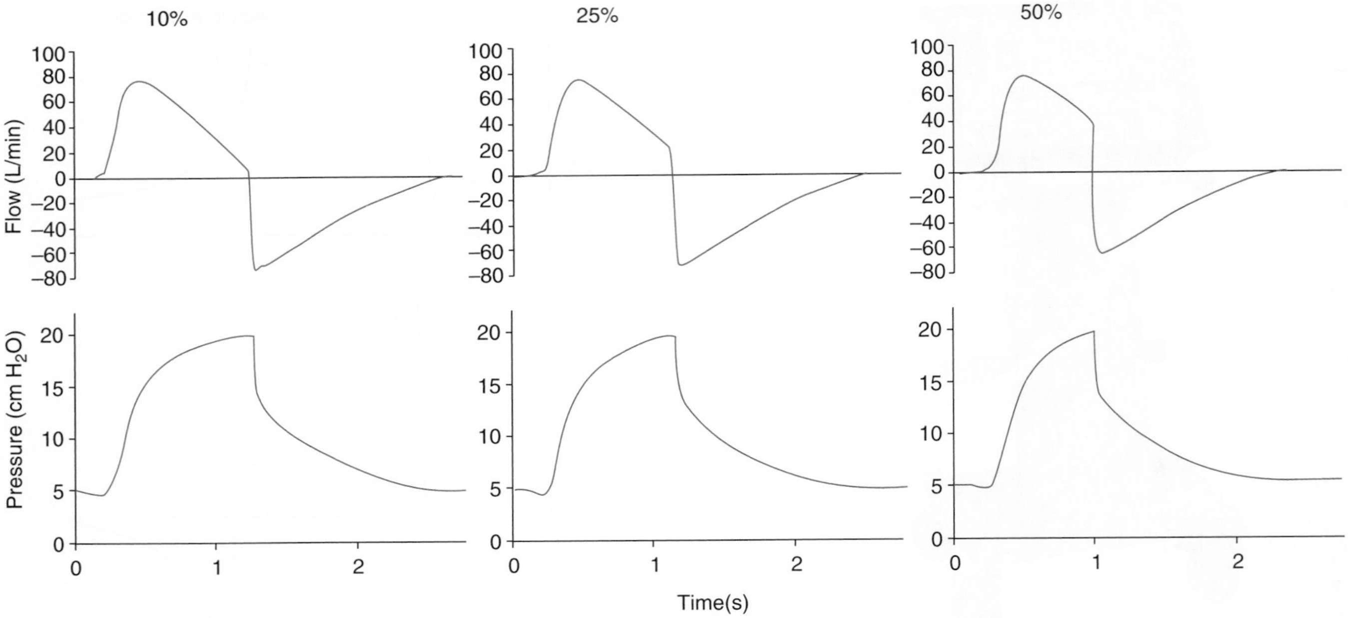

FIGURE 45-15 The effects of changing the termination criteria during PSV.

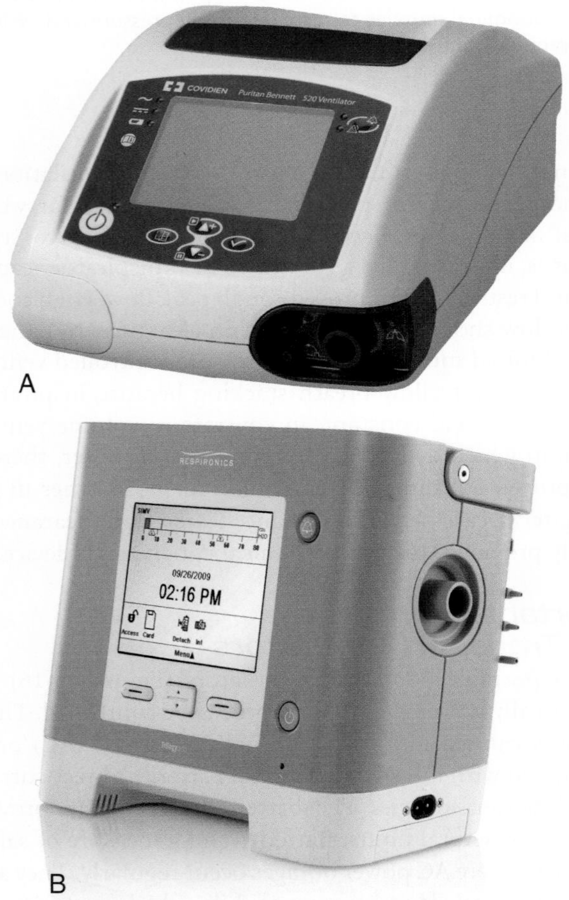

FIGURE 45-16 Two examples of new generation portable ventilators that can be used in acute care, home care, or transport settings. (**A,** Puritan Bennett 520 Portable Ventilator. Used by permission of Nellcor Puritan Bennett LLC, Boulder, Colorado, doing business as Covidien. **B,** Trilogy Portable Ventilator, courtesy Phillips Respironics, Murrysville, PA.)

the added advantages of small size, light weight, and battery power that allow portability. Most newer models incorporate an NIV mode with the ability to compensate for leaks. Some models with adjustable bias flow settings improve the ability of the ventilator to sense patient triggering. Similar to critical care ventilators, additional features, such as variable termination criteria and maximum inspiratory time, are available on some of these devices to enhance breath termination in PSV.

Portable home care ventilators are currently recommended for patients who need continuous ventilatory support or high ventilating pressures, such as patients with severe chest wall deformities or obesity or for patients who want greater mobility.[2] For acute care, these ventilators could easily be used to initiate NIV in nontraditional locations and allow transport to an emergency department or ICU without the need to interrupt ventilation.

Heated Humidifiers

An increase in nasal resistance and congestion has been reported with CPAP in patients with mouth leaks.[125,126] The addition of heated humidity relieves nasal resistance and congestion. Cold passover humidification does not provide relief.[125] The use of heated humidity during nasal CPAP in patients with sleep apnea and nasal symptoms (sneezing, nasal draining, nasal and oral dryness, and nasal obstruction) has significantly improved patients' compliance with this therapy.[127,128] It seems likely that the same effect would occur in NPPV. To avoid the negative effect on patient compliance caused by this common complaint and the accumulation of dried retained secretions in the back of the oral pharynx, humidified gas, heated to a temperature that is comfortable to the patient (usually about 30° C), should be the standard when using NIV.

RULE OF THUMB

Heated humidity (about 30° C) should always be provided with NIV to avoid nasal symptoms, to avoid the accumulation of secretions in the back of the oral pharynx, and to enhance patient tolerance.

MANAGEMENT OF NONINVASIVE VENTILATION

Initial Application of Noninvasive Ventilation

Starting NIV requires the selection of a ventilator and an interface and a significant time commitment from the RT. The time requirement includes gathering and assembling equipment. It also includes invaluable time spent at the bedside reassessing the patient on a frequent basis and providing instructions, encouragement, and coaching while making small adjustments to the ventilator settings, gradually increasing support to the level needed by the patient. The RT should always explain the procedure before placing the mask on the patient. Patients in ARF may feel anxious or frightened because of dyspnea and respiratory distress.

The patient should be seated in a chair or bed at an angle of 30 degrees or greater (Box 45-6).[2] When the mask is applied for the first time, the ventilating pressures should be set as low as possible. It is difficult for patients to acclimate to high airway pressures, and a strategy of starting with low pressures can help patients adjust more readily. As the patient becomes accustomed to the sensation of NIV, pressures can be adjusted in small increments until exhaled V_T is 4 to 6 ml/kg predicted body weight or respiratory distress improves. When applying the mask for the first time, the RT should hold the mask in place or allow the patient to hold it, if he or she is able to do so. Holding the mask allows rapid removal of the mask if the patient begins to panic or needs to communicate. The mask should not be strapped on until the patient is comfortable with the application of NIV and the RT has adjusted pressures to provide proper ventilation.

The actual final airway pressures required to support the patient during NIV are difficult or impossible to determine before NIV has been started. Some patients may need high pressures; others need low pressures—it is impossible to know until the process is begun. However, most patients require PEEP levels of 5 to 8 cm H_2O and ventilating pressure of 8 to 12 cm H_2O. Peak airway pressures greater than 20 cm H_2O are rarely needed. To avoid gastric distention, ventilating pressure should be less than the normal gastric opening pressures of 20 to 25 cm H_2O.[129] If the patient has a nasogastric tube in place, the probability of gastric distention increases dramatically, as does the probability of NIV failure.

Final adjustment of the ventilator should deliver a V_T of about 4 to 6 ml/kg ideal body weight with a respiratory rate less than 30 breaths/min. The goal of NIV is not to deliver a large V_T but rather to maintain normal ventilatory patterns with acceptable gas exchange and decrease the work of breathing. FiO_2 should be titrated to PaO_2 of at least 60 mm Hg or SpO_2 greater than 90%.

Box 45-6 Initiation of Noninvasive Ventilation

1. Choose a location with appropriate monitoring based on the severity of the patient's condition.
2. Position the patient with the head of the bed elevated ≥30 degrees.
3. Select a ventilator and an appropriately sized interface.
4. Turn on the ventilator and humidifier, and connect the interface.
5. Set initial settings at a low level of support: PEEP 0 to 4 cm H_2O, ventilatory pressure 2 to 4 cm H_2O.
6. Hold the mask on the patient's face or have the patient hold the mask until he or she is comfortable with the sensation of NIV.
7. Adjust FiO_2 or bleed-in O_2 flow to keep $SpO_2 > 90\%$.
8. After the patient becomes comfortable with the initial settings, increase inspiratory pressure until V_T is about 4 to 6 ml/kg predicted body weight or signs of respiratory distress improve. Increase PEEP to reduce asynchrony from air trapping or to improve oxygenation.
9. Check for air leaks, especially around the eyes; adjust mask as needed.
10. Reassess frequently for tolerance and efficacy of NIV (at least every 30 minutes) for the first 1 to 2 hours.

RULE OF THUMB

Most patients with ARF can be stabilized with an expiratory pressure setting of 5 to 8 cm H_2O and ventilating pressure of 8 to 12 cm H_2O. Avoid using peak pressures greater than 20 cm H_2O.

Clinical Assessment Criteria to Identify Success or Failure of Noninvasive Ventilation

Successful application of NIV is easy to define—gas exchange improves, $PaCO_2$ decreases, pH normalizes, and PaO_2 and SpO_2 increase. Along with improvement of these measured values, the patient's clinical presentation improves; respiratory rate decreases, V_T increases, accessory muscle use decreases or is eliminated, and pulse rate and blood pressure normalize. If the patient's clinical status improves within 1 to 2 hours, he or she may be on the way to successful application of NIV. NIV should be continued, but the patient needs to be monitored carefully. If clinical status and gas exchange have not improved after 1 to 2 hours of NIV, intubation should be considered; this is especially true if the indication for NIV was hypoxemic respiratory failure. Various reports indicate increased risk of cardiac arrest in patients with hypoxemic respiratory failure who do not improve after a trial of NIV for 1 to 2 hours.[46]

Adjusting Noninvasive Ventilator Settings

Ventilator settings may need to be adjusted after the patient stabilizes and acclimates or when arterial blood gas analysis reveals gas exchange problems. Hypercapnia is addressed by minimizing any significant air leaks and then by increasing the ventilating pressure. The result is an increase in the delivered V_T and minute ventilation and a decrease in $PaCO_2$. NIV is typically delivered in a spontaneous mode, where all breaths are patient-triggered and none are mandatory, so adjusting the ventilator frequency is not an option. For patients with chronic hypercapnia, ventilation should be adjusted to maintain an acceptable pH. No attempt should be made to normalize the $PaCO_2$ in such patients.

Increasing PEEP increases the patient's functional residual capacity, mean airway pressure, and PaO_2. Higher PEEP should also improve trigger synchrony in the setting of air trapping. Decreasing PEEP theoretically should cause the opposite effects. In clinical practice, decreasing PEEP may not affect PaO_2 as the disease process resolves and alveolar stability improves.

If the assist/control mode is used for NIV, the rate should be set at a level below the patient's spontaneous rate, allowing the patient to trigger the ventilator as needed. Setting the rate in this manner provides a backup rate for safety if apnea occurs and avoids overventilating the patient. If the patient's disease process limits the ability to trigger or breathe spontaneously, as in some neuromuscular disorders, the set rate has a direct relationship to minute ventilation and an inverse relationship to $PaCO_2$. These relationships may not always be the case in clinical practice and in a spontaneously breathing patient. Table 45-1 summarizes ventilator adjustments during NIV.

TABLE 45-1

Expected Results of Changing Noninvasive Ventilator Settings

Setting	Adjustment	Anticipated Result
IPAP	↑	↑ V_T, ↑ minute ventilation, ↓ $PaCO_2$
	↓	↓ V_T, ↓ minute ventilation, ↑ $PaCO_2$
EPAP	↑	↑ FRC, ↑ PaO_2, ↓ V_T If intrinsic PEEP is present, fewer missed trigger attempts and improved patient-ventilator synchrony
	↓	↓ FRC, ↓ PaO_2, ↑ V_T, ↓ $PaCO_2$ Possible rebreathing of CO_2 if EPAP < 4 cm H_2O
FiO_2	↑	↑ PaO_2; if bleeding O_2 into circuit, maximum expected FiO_2 is approximately 0.5; increasing O_2 flow >15 L/min may adversely affect triggering
	↓	↓ PaO_2
Rate control*	↑	↑ minute volume in timed modes, ↓ $PaCO_2$
	↓	↓ minute volume in timed modes, ↑ $PaCO_2$

FRC, Functional residual capacity.
*Rate control is generally set at 8 to 10 as a backup rate and not changed in spontaneous/timed mode.

Aerosolized Medication Delivery

For patients on intermittent NIV, aerosol medications are often administered while the patient is off the ventilator. Removal of assisted ventilation from patients in ARF makes little sense and is unnecessary. Aerosol therapy can be delivered in the usual manner through an ICU ventilator used for NIV. With a noninvasive ventilator, positioning the nebulizer between the exhalation port and mask maximizes drug delivery.[130] If the exhalation port is located in the mask or any other position distal to the nebulizer, much of the drug is lost via the exhalation port during both inspiration and expiration. A metered dose inhaler (MDI) can be administered by placing an adapter or collapsible holding chamber in the same position in the circuit. Drug delivery should improve because the MDI is actuated only during inspiration. However, dosing can safely be doubled and should be adjusted based on patient response to compensate for loss through leaks in the system and other inefficiencies.

Safe Delivery of Noninvasive Ventilation

Monitoring During Noninvasive Ventilation

In acute care or long-term care applications, clinicians must not lose sight of the goals of NIV.[2] The RT should confirm ventilator function and assess the patient on a regular basis for leaks, accessory muscle use, ventilator synchrony, comfort, and changes in vital signs and gas exchange. In the acute care setting, respiratory rate, heart rate, and gas exchange should improve within 1 to 2 hours after initiation of NIV. If there is no improvement after 30 to 60 minutes on optimal settings, intubation should be considered. At a minimum, SpO_2 must be continuously monitored. In the acute care setting, continuous monitoring of heart rate and blood pressure is the safest practice. A current consensus statement recommends a higher level of monitoring for patients with acute hypoxemia, worsening condition, involvement of nonrespiratory organ systems, or persistent acidosis.[124] If the patient cannot sustain ventilation independent of NIV for at least 1 hour,

MINI CLINI

Improving Patient-Ventilator Synchrony During Noninvasive Ventilation

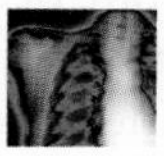

PROBLEM: An oncology patient with DNI orders is receiving NIV from a critical care ventilator with a full-face mask. The ventilator is set in the PSV mode. Peak inspiratory pressure is 15 cm H_2O, PEEP is 5 cm H_2O, and flow trigger is 2 L/min. The patient has a nasogastric tube in place that is causing a large leak. The ventilator is self-triggering and fails to cycle into expiration when the patient exhales. The patient is dyspneic and appears uncomfortable.

SOLUTION: Large leaks can cause patient-ventilator asynchrony with ventilators that do not have leak compensation. Triggering and cycling are affected because the ventilator is no longer sensitive to changes in flow or pressure changes generated by the patient.

1. Repositioning the mask and placing a flat piece of gauze or hydrocolloid dressing between the mask and the nasogastric tube and another between the nasogastric tube and the patient's face may help reduce the leak.
2. Change to a critical care ventilator with a noninvasive mode or a noninvasive ventilator designed for ICU use.
3. If switching ventilators is not feasible, and a large leak is still present, adjusting the termination criterion to a higher setting can shorten inspiratory time, allowing breath termination to occur at a higher percentage of the peak flow.
4. If termination criteria are not adjustable, change to pressure assist/control mode. Observe the ventilator graphics to determine the patient's desired inspiratory time, and set the inspiratory time on the ventilator accordingly. Typically, critically ill patients should have inspiratory times of about 0.7 to 1 second (in some cases, 0.5 second).

the same level of monitoring as any intubated patient should occur.

In the long-term care setting, improvement in gas exchange may require weeks to several months depending on daily use and compliance with the prescribed therapy.[2] Clinicians providing follow-up treatment in the long-term care setting should determine usage with the elapsed time indicator on the ventilator. The patient should be assessed for complications, symptoms of hypoventilation and poor sleep quality, patient-ventilator synchrony, and other factors that affect compliance.

Patient Location

NIV can be initiated in any acute care location, including the emergency department, ICU, or general care floor.[124] After NIV is initiated, patients should be transferred to an ICU or other inpatient location with continuous monitoring capabilities, skilled staff, and access to endotracheal intubation if needed.[2,124] Hypercapnic patients with COPD and a pH of 7.30 or greater[124] and patients who can sustain ventilation without NIV for at least 1 hour can be managed safely on a general care floor.[56] It is important that staff members be adequately trained before caring for patients on NIV. Another consensus conference recommendation calls for one-to-one monitoring of NIV patients for the first few hours by a trained, experienced RT, nurse, or physician.[124]

Weaning from Noninvasive Ventilation

At the present time, there is no proven or broadly accepted standard for weaning from NIV. A common weaning strategy is to decrease high levels of inspiratory and baseline pressure gradually to minimal settings as the acute disease process resolves. The length of time off the ventilator can be increased gradually as tolerated.

COMPLICATIONS OF NONINVASIVE VENTILATION

The reported failure rate of NIV ranges from 7% to 70%.[2] Serious complications such as aspiration or pneumothorax occur less than 5% of the time. The undesired side effects of NIV are less serious, although more common. These side effects can be grouped into categories related to the noninvasive interface and to gas flow and airway pressures. Table 45-2 lists the complications, frequency of occurrence, and suggested remedies.

Air leaks can cause several problems of various levels of concern, ranging from eye irritation and dry mouth to inability to trigger inspiration. Small air leaks should be expected during NIV. Large air leaks should be addressed immediately before they lead to patient-ventilator asynchrony or worsening gas exchange.[3] Air leaks often can be avoided by selecting an appropriately sized mask. If excessive airflow is leaking through the mouth, changing to a full-face mask should be helpful. If the problem persists, one can reposition the mask, add a forehead spacer, and readjust strap tension. Sometimes, ventilator settings must be adjusted if ventilation is adversely affected by the leak. Using a ventilator with leak compensation should resolve problems with leaks. If that option is unavailable, one can consider changing the termination criteria, using a time-cycled mode and adjusting the trigger sensitivity.

Mask-related side effects are the most common problems. Mask discomfort may be reported by 50%[2] of patients receiving NIV, and excessive discomfort decreases patient tolerance for NIV. Switching to a correctly sized mask or loosening the straps slightly is often all that it takes to resolve this issue. Skin damage is a problem that is only going to get worse if not addressed immediately for patients who need to continue using NIV. RTs should keep a watchful eye on reddened areas, usually on the bridge of the nose. A liquid skin barrier should be applied to protect

TABLE 45-2

Side Effects and Complications of Noninvasive Ventilation

	Incidence*	Possible Solutions
Interface-Related Side Effects		
Discomfort	Common	Loosen straps Refit, reposition, or change interface
Erythema	Common	Apply skin barrier or hydrocolloid dressing or both Loosen straps, adjust forehead support, or add spacer Alternate the use of 2 masks
Claustrophobia	Infrequent	Change interface Consider anxiolytic
Pressure ulcer	Infrequent	Apply hydrocolloid dressing Change interface
Skin rash	Infrequent	Apply topical steroid or antibiotic
Air Pressure–Related or Flow-Related Side Effects		
Nasal congestion	Common	Administer inhaled corticosteroid or decongestant
Nasal dryness	Common	Avoid by using heated humidification with NIV Administer saline nasal spray
Sinus or ear pain	Common	Decrease ventilating pressure
Eye irritation	Common	Refit, reposition, or change interface
Gastric distention	Infrequent	Administer simethicone Lower pressures
Serious Complications		
Aspiration	Rare	Avoid through careful patient selection Stop NIV, if status will allow
Pneumothorax	Rare	Decrease ventilating pressure Place chest tube, if indicated
Hypotension	Rare	Decrease inflation pressure

From Mehta S, Hill NS: Noninvasive ventilation. Am J Respir Crit Care Med 163:540, 2001.

**Common*—occurs in 30% to 50% of patients; *infrequent*—occurs in approximately 5% to 20% of patients; *rare*—occurs in <5% of patients.

the area. Applying "artificial skin" or a hydrocolloid dressing or patch is a good idea to provide further protection. These patches should also be used if a pressure ulcer forms. Taking steps to minimize pressure such as loosening the straps and adding a forehead spacer are important. Other strategies to reduce the risk of pressure ulcers include alternating use of two or more different masks and removing the mask every 4 to 6 hours for a few minutes if the patient can tolerate being off the ventilator without increased respiratory distress.

Complications related to air pressure and flow include nasal congestion, upper airway dryness, sinus and ear pain, eye irritation, and gastric insufflation.[2] Usually, nasal congestion and upper airway dryness can be prevented by using heated humidity whenever NIV is initiated. Decongestants and saline spray are sometimes needed to relieve symptoms of congestion. Sinus and ear pain may be related to high inspiratory pressure; use of the lowest effective inspiratory pressure may prevent or alleviate this problem.

Clinically significant gastric insufflation is a rare occurrence in patients using NIV.[2] Use of the lowest effective pressure may prevent gastric insufflation. Routine use of a nasogastric tube is not recommended. A nasogastric tube increases the risk of gastric insufflation, adversely affects mask fit, and usually causes a large air leak, increasing the likelihood of NIV failure.

Most major complications can be avoided with careful patient selection and use of the lowest inspiratory pressure that improves the patient's gas exchange and relieves symptoms. NIV should be avoided if the patient is a high aspiration risk or is hemodynamically unstable. The risk of aspiration increases if inspiratory pressures greater than 20 cm H_2O are used. In general, the head of the bed should be maintained at 30 degrees to reduce the risk of aspiration during NIV.

TIME AND COSTS ASSOCIATED WITH NONINVASIVE VENTILATION

The cost-effectiveness of NIV is linked to appropriate patient selection, familiarity of staff members with NIV, and the success or failure of NIV in preventing endotracheal intubation.[131,132] Staff time is one of the most valuable and expensive resources in hospitals. Time required by nurses and physicians during the first 48 hours of NIV is similar to the time required for invasive mechanical ventilation, but the time required by RTs for NIV is considerably greater than for invasive mechanical ventilation.[133] However, another study showed that the time required by RTs was significantly greater for the first 8 hours but significantly lower during the next 8 hours.[10] The increased time requirement associated with starting NIV is due to mask fitting, gradual upward adjustment of ventilator settings, and remaining at the bedside to provide coaching and encouragement to patients as they acclimate to NIV. After the patient begins to improve, the time required to maintain NIV should decrease to a level similar to invasive ventilation.

SUMMARY CHECKLIST

- NIV is the application of positive pressure ventilation or CPAP with a mask or other noninvasive interface to improve gas exchange or decrease the work of breathing.
- The use of NIV to manage ARF has improved patient outcomes.

- Evidence supports NIV as the standard of care for managing patients with COPD exacerbations and acute cardiogenic pulmonary edema. There is less evidence supporting other indications for NIV.
- NIV may be justified in the management of ARF if selection criteria (see Box 45-2) are present, exclusion criteria (see Box 45-3) are absent, and the disease process is reversible.
- Acute cardiogenic pulmonary edema should be managed initially with CPAP of 8 to 12 cm H_2O. NPPV should be considered only if hypercapnia is present.
- NIV is beneficial in the management of patients extubated but at risk of reintubation and patients with DNI orders.
- Patients with ALS should receive NIV because it probably prolongs their lives.
- Caution should be used in applying NIV to patients with acute hypoxemic respiratory failure.
- NIV is most successful in the acute care setting when air leaks are minimal, the patient's severity of illness is moderate, respiratory acidosis is present, and improvement in gas exchange and vital signs occurs within 30 minutes to 2 hours after NIV initiation.
- NIV is typically administered in the PSV mode with PEEP.
- Airway pressure during NIV should be kept as low as possible to achieve therapeutic goals (ideally <20 cm H_2O).
- Although any ventilator can be used for NIV, ventilators designed to compensate for leaks can be expected to perform best.
- Heated humidity (about 30° C) should always be provided with NIV.
- Aerosolized drugs can be administered without interrupting NIV.
- The initiation of NIV requires significant staff time, but after patients stabilize, the time required to maintain NIV is similar to invasive ventilation.

References

1. Pierson DJ: Noninvasive positive pressure ventilation: history and terminology. Respir Care 42:370, 1997.
2. Mehta S, Hill NS: Noninvasive ventilation. Am J Respir Crit Care Med 163:540, 2001.
3. Bach JR: The prevention of ventilatory failure due to inadequate pump function. Respir Care 42:403, 1997.
4. Bach JR, Alba AS: Intermittent abdominal pressure ventilation in a regimen of noninvasive ventilatory support. Chest 99:630, 1991.
5. Intermittent Positive Pressure Breathing Trial Group: Intermittent positive pressure breathing therapy of chronic obstructive pulmonary disease. Ann Intern Med 69:612, 1983.
6. Sullivan CE, Issa FG, Berthon-Jones M, et al: Reversal of obstructive sleep apnea by continuous positive airway pressure applied through the nares. Lancet 1:862–865, 1981.
7. Rideau Y, Gatin G, Bach J, et al: Prolongation of life in Duchenne's muscular dystrophy. Acta Neurol Belg 5:118–124, 1983.
8. Meduri GU, Conoscenti CC, Menashe P, et al: Noninvasive face mask ventilation in patients with acute respiratory failure. Chest 95:865–870, 1989.
9. Hill N, Brennan J, Garpestad E, et al: Noninvasive ventilation in acute respiratory failure. Crit Care Med 35:2402–2407, 2007.
10. Kramer N, Meyer TJ, Meharg J, et al: Randomized, prospective trial of noninvasive positive pressure ventilation in acute respiratory failure. Am J Respir Crit Care Med 151: 1799–1806, 1995.
11. Brochard L, Mancebo J, Wysocki M, et al: Noninvasive ventilation for acute exacerbations of chronic obstructive pulmonary disease. N Engl J Med 333:817–822, 1995.
12. Celikel T, Sungur M, Ceyhan B, et al: Comparison of noninvasive positive pressure ventilation with standard medical therapy in hypercapnic acute respiratory failure. Chest 114:1636–1642, 1998.
13. Plant PK, Owen JL, Elliott MW: Noninvasive ventilation for acute exacerbations of chronic obstructive pulmonary disease on general respiratory wards: a multicentre randomized, controlled trial. Lancet 355:1931, 2000.
14. Bott J, Carroll MP, Conway JH, et al: Randomized, controlled trial of nasal ventilation in acute ventilatory failure due to chronic obstructive airways disease. Lancet 341:1555–1557, 1993.
15. Nava S, Ambrosino N, Clini E, et al: Noninvasive mechanical ventilation in the weaning of patients with respiratory failure due to chronic obstructive pulmonary disease: a randomized, controlled trial. Ann Intern Med 128:721–728, 1998.
16. Barbe F, Togores B, Rubi M, et al: Noninvasive ventilatory support does not facilitate recovery from acute respiratory failure in chronic obstructive pulmonary disease. Eur Respir J 9:1240–1245, 1996.
17. Keenan SP, Sinuff T, Cook DJ, et al: Which patients with acute exacerbation of chronic obstructive pulmonary disease benefit from noninvasive positive-pressure ventilation? A systematic review of the literature. Ann Intern Med 138:I27, 2003.
18. Meduri GU, Cook TR, Turner RE, et al: Noninvasive positive pressure ventilation in status asthmaticus. Chest 110:767–774, 1996.
19. Carroll CL, Schramm CM: Noninvasive positive pressure ventilation for the treatment of status asthmaticus in children. Ann Allergy Asthma Immunol 96:454–459, 2006.
20. Ram FS, Wellington S, Row BH, et al: Noninvasive positive pressure ventilation for treatment of respiratory failure due to severe acute exacerbations of asthma. Cochrane Database Syst Rev (1):CD004360, 2005.
21. Rabatin JT, Gay PC: Noninvasive ventilation. Mayo Clin Proc 74:817–820, 1999.
22. Ferrer M, Esquinas A, Arancibia F, et al: Noninvasive ventilation during persistent weaning failure. Am J Respir Crit Care Med 168:70–76, 2003.
23. Vitacca M, Ambrosino N, Clini E, et al: Physiological response to pressure support ventilation delivered before and after extubation in patients not capable of totally spontaneous autonomous breathing. Am J Respir Crit Care Med 164:638–641, 2001.
24. Bersten AD, Holt AW, Vedig AE, et al: Treatment of severe cardiogenic pulmonary edema with continuous positive airway pressure delivered by face mask. N Engl J Med 325:1825–1830, 1991.
25. Lin M, Yang YF, Chiang HT, et al: Reappraisal of continuous positive airway pressure therapy in acute cardiogenic pulmonary edema. Chest 107:1379–1386, 1995.

26. Kelly CA, Newby DE, McDonagh TA, et al: Randomised controlled trial of continuous positive airway pressure and standard oxygen therapy in acute pulmonary oedema. Eur Heart J 23:1379–1386, 2002.
27. Masip J, Betbese AJ, Paez J, et al: Noninvasive pressure support ventilation versus conventional oxygen therapy in acute cardiogenic pulmonary oedema: a randomised trial. Lancet 356:2126–2132, 2000.
28. Levitt MA: A prospective, randomized trial of BiPAP in severe acute congestive heart failure. J Emerg Med 21:363–369, 2001.
29. Nava S, Carbone G, DiBattista N, et al: Noninvasive ventilation in cardiogenic pulmonary edema. Am J Respir Crit Care Med 168:1432–1437, 2003.
30. Mehta S, Jay GD, Woolard RH, et al: Randomized, prospective trial of bilevel versus continuous positive airway pressure in acute pulmonary edema. Crit Care Med 25:620–625, 1997.
31. Bellone A, Monari A, Cortellaro F, et al: Myocardial infarction rate in acute pulmonary edema: noninvasive pressure support ventilation versus continuous positive airway pressure. Crit Care Med 32:1860–1865, 2004.
32. Bellone A, Vettorello M, Monari A, et al: Noninvasive pressure support ventilation versus continuous positive airway pressure in acute hypercapnic pulmonary edema. Intensive Care Med 31:807–811, 2005.
33. Park M, Lorenzi-Filho G, Feltrim MI, et al: Oxygen therapy, continuous positive airway pressure, or noninvasive bilevel positive pressure ventilation in the treatment of acute cardiogenic pulmonary edema. Arq Bras Cardiol 76:221–230, 2001.
34. Crane SD, Elliott MW, Gilligan P, et al: Randomised controlled comparison of continuous positive airways pressure, bilevel noninvasive ventilation, and standard treatment in emergency department patients with acute cardiogenic pulmonary oedema. Emerg Med J 21:155–161, 2004.
35. Park M, Sangean MC, Volpe Mde S, et al: Randomized, prospective trial of oxygen, continuous positive airway pressure, and bilevel positive airway pressure by face mask in acute cardiogenic pulmonary edema. Crit Care Med 32:2407–2415, 2004.
36. Jolliet P, Abajo B, Pasquina P: Non-invasive pressure support ventilation in severe community-acquired pneumonia. Intensive Care Med 27:797–799, 2001.
37. Confalonieri M, Potena A, Carbone G, et al: Acute respiratory failure in patients with severe community acquired pneumonia. Am J Respir Crit Care Med 160:1585–1591, 1999.
38. Rana S, Jenad H, Gay P, et al: Failure of non-invasive ventilation in patients with acute lung injury: observational cohort study. Crit Care 10:R79, 2006.
39. Antonelli M, Conti G, Moro ML, et al: Predictors of failure of noninvasive positive pressure ventilation in patients with acute hypoxemic respiratory failure: a multi-center study. Intensive Care Med 27:1718–1728, 2001.
40. Ferrer M, Esquinas A, Leon M, et al: Noninvasive ventilation in severe hypoxemic respiratory failure. Am J Respir Crit Care Med 168:1438–1444, 2003.
41. Antonelli M, Conti G, Esquinas A, et al: A multiple-center survey on the use in clinical practice of noninvasive ventilation as a first-line intervention for acute respiratory distress syndrome. Crit Care Med 35:18–25, 2007.
42. Antonelli M, Conti G, Rocco M, et al: A comparison of noninvasive positive-pressure ventilation and conventional mechanical ventilation in patients with acute respiratory failure. N Engl J Med 339:429–435, 1998.
43. Martin TJ, Hovis JD, Costantino JP, et al: A randomized prospective evaluation of noninvasive ventilation for acute respiratory failure. Am J Respir Crit Care Med 161:807–813, 2000.
44. Keenan SP, Sinuff T, Cook DJ, et al: Does noninvasive positive pressure ventilation improve outcome in acute hypoxemic respiratory failure? A systematic review. Crit Care Med 32:2516–2523, 2004.
45. Schettino GPP, Hess D, Altobelli N, et al: Is noninvasive positive pressure ventilation (NPPV) effective outside of controlled trials? (abstract). Am J Respir Crit Care Med 165:A389, 2002.
46. Delclaux C, L'Her E, Alberti C, et al: Treatment of acute hypoxemic nonhypercapnic respiratory insufficiency with continuous positive airway pressure delivered by a face mask: a randomized, controlled trial. JAMA 284:2352–2360, 2000.
47. Hilbert G, Gruson D, Vargas F, et al: Noninvasive ventilation in immunosuppressed patients with pulmonary infiltrates, fever, and acute respiratory failure. N Engl J Med 344:481–487, 2001.
48. Antonelli M, Conti G, Bufi M, et al: Noninvasive ventilation for treatment of acute respiratory failure in patients undergoing solid organ transplantation. JAMA 283:235–241, 2000.
49. Confalonieri M, Calderini E, Terraciano S, et al: Noninvasive ventilation for treating acute respiratory failure in AIDS patients with Pneumocystis carinii pneumonia. Intensive Care Med 28:1233–1238, 2002.
50. Nourdine N, Combes P, Carton MJ, et al: Does noninvasive ventilation reduce the ICU nosocomial infection risk? A prospective clinical survey. Intensive Care Med 25:567–573, 1999.
51. Girou E, Schortgen F, Delclaux C, et al: Association of noninvasive ventilation with nosocomial infections and survival in critically ill patients. JAMA 284:2361–2367, 2000.
52. Hill N: Noninvasive ventilation for immunocompromised patients. N Engl J Med 344:522, 2001.
53. Meduri GU, Fox RC, Abou-Shala N, et al: Noninvasive mechanical ventilation via face mask in patients with acute respiratory failure who refused endotracheal intubation. Crit Care Med 22:1584–1590, 1994.
54. Schettino G, Altobelli N, Kacmarek RM: Noninvasive positive pressure ventilation reverses acute respiratory failure in select "do-not-intubate" patients. Crit Care Med 33:1976–1982, 2005.
55. Levy M, Tanios MA, Nelson D, et al: Outcomes of patients with do-not-intubate orders treated with noninvasive ventilation. Crit Care Med 32:2002–2007, 2004.
56. Curtis JR, Cook DJ, Sinuff T, et al: Noninvasive positive pressure ventilation in critical and palliative care settings: understanding the goals of therapy. Crit Care Med 35:932–939, 2007.
57. Joris JL, Sottiauz TM, Chiche JD, et al: Effect of bi-level positive airway pressure nasal ventilation on the postoperative pulmonary restrictive syndrome in obese patients undergoing gastroplasty. Chest 111:665–670, 1997.
58. Squadrone V, Coha M, Cerutti E, et al: Continuous positive airway pressure for treatment of postoperative hypoxemia. JAMA 293:589–595, 2005.
59. Kindgen-Milles D, Muller E, Buhl R, et al: Nasal-continuous positive airway pressure reduces pulmonary morbidity and length of hospital stay following thoracoabdominal aortic surgery. Chest 128:821–828, 2005.
60. Epstein SK, Ciubotaru RL, Wong JB: Effect of failed extubation on the outcome of mechanical ventilation. Chest 112:186, 1997.
61. Nava S, Gregoretti C, Fanfulla F, et al: Noninvasive ventilation or prevent respiratory failure after extubation in high-risk patients. Crit Care Med 33:2465–2470, 2005.

62. Ferrer M, Valencia M, Nicolas JM, et al: Early noninvasive ventilation averts extubation failure in patients at risk. Am J Respir Crit Care Med 173:164–170, 2006.
63. Keenan SP, Powers C, McCormack DG, et al: Noninvasive positive-pressure ventilation for postextubation respiratory distress. JAMA 287:3238–3244, 2002.
64. Esteban A, Frutos-Vivar F, Ferguson ND, et al: Noninvasive positive-pressure ventilation for respiratory failure after extubation. N Engl J Med 350:2452–2460, 2004.
65. Ozsancak A, D'Ambrosio C, Hill N: Nocturnal noninvasive ventilation. Chest 133:1275–1285, 2008.
66. Clinical indications for noninvasive positive pressure ventilation in chronic respiratory failure due to restrictive lung disease, COPD, and nocturnal hypoventilation: a consensus conference report. Chest 116:521, 1999.
67. Schonhofer B, Polkey MI, Suchi S, et al: Effect of home mechanical ventilation on inspiratory muscle strength in COPD. Chest 130:1834–1838, 2006.
68. When should respiratory muscles be exercised? Chest 84:76–84, 1983.
69. Hill N: Noninvasive ventilation: does it work, for whom, and how? Am Rev Respir Dis 147:1050–1055, 1993.
70. Wijkstra PJ, Lacasse Y, Guyatt GH, et al: A meta-analysis of nocturnal noninvasive positive pressure ventilation in patients with stable COPD. Chest 124:337–343, 2003.
71. Hill NS, Eveloff SE, Carlisle CC, et al: Efficacy of nocturnal nasal ventilation in patients with restrictive thoracic disease. Am Rev Respir Dis 145:365–371, 1992.
72. Annane D, Quera-Salva MA, Lofasa F, et al: Mechanisms underlying the effects of nocturnal ventilation on daytime blood gases in neuromuscular diseases. Eur Respir J 13:157–162, 1999.
73. Nickol AN, Hart N, Hopkinson NS, et al: Mechanisms of improvement of respiratory failure in patients with restrictive thoracic disease treated with non-invasive ventilation. Thorax 60:754–760, 2005.
74. Ferris G, Servera-Pieras E, Vergara P, et al: Kyphoscoliosis ventilatory insufficiency: noninvasive management outcomes. Am J Phys Med Rehabil 79:24–29, 2000.
75. Mellies U, Dohna-Schwake C, Ragette R, et al: Respiratory failure in Pompe disease: treatment with noninvasive ventilation. Neurology 64:1465–1467, 2005.
76. Raphael JC, Chevret S, Chastang C, et al: Randomized trial of preventive nasal ventilation in Duchenne muscular dystrophy. French Multicentre Cooperative Group on Home Mechanical Ventilation Assistance in Duchenne de Boulogne Muscular Dystrophy. Lancet 343:1600–1604, 1994.
77. Miller R, Jackson C, Kasarskis, E, et al: Practice parameter update: the care of the patient with amyotrophic lateral sclerosis (an evidence-based review). Report of the Quality Standards Subcommittee of the American Academy of Neurology. Neurology 73:1218–1226, 2009.
78. Bourke S, Tomlinson M, Williams T, et al: Effects of noninvasive ventilation on survival and quality of life in patients with amyotrophic lateral sclerosis: a randomized controlled trial. Lancet Neurol 5:140–146, 2006.
79. Kleopa KA, Sherman M, Neal B, et al: Bipap improves survival and rate of pulmonary function decline in patients with ALS. J Neurol Sci 164:82–88, 1999.
80. Pinto A, de Carvalho M, Evangelista T, et al: Nocturnal pulse oximetry: a new approach to establish the appropriate time for non-invasive ventilation in ALS patients. Amyotroph Lateral Scler Other Motor Neuron Disord 4:31–35, 2003.
81. Bourke SC, Bullock RE, Williams TL, et al: Noninvasive ventilation in ALS: indications and effect on quality of life. Neurology 61:171–177, 2003.
82. Gruis KL, Brown DL, Schoennemann A, et al: Predictors of noninvasive ventilation tolerance in patients with amyotrophic lateral sclerosis. Muscle Nerve 32:808–811, 2005.
83. Olney RK, Murphy J, Forshew D, et al: The effects of executive and behavioral dysfunction on the course of ALS. Neurology 65:1774–1777, 2005.
84. Lyall RA, Donaldson N, Fleming T, et al: A prospective study of quality of life in ALS patients treated with noninvasive ventilation. Neurology 57:153–156, 2001.
85. Butz M, Wollinsky KH, Wiedemuth-Catrinescu U, et al: Longitudinal effects of noninvasive positive-pressure ventilation in patients with amyotrophic lateral sclerosis. Am J Phys Med Rehabil 82:597–604, 2003.
86. Kaub-Wittemer D, Steinbuchel N, Wasner M, et al: Quality of life and psychosocial issues in ventilated patients with amyotrophic lateral sclerosis and their caregivers. J Pain Symptom Manage 26:890–896, 2003.
87. Strumpf DA, Millman RP, Carlisle CC, et al: Nocturnal positive-pressure ventilation via nasal mask in patients with severe chronic obstructive pulmonary disease. Am Rev Respir Dis 144:1234–1239, 1991.
88. Gay PC, Patel AM, Viggiano RW, et al: Nocturnal nasal ventilation for treatment of patients with hypercapnic respiratory failure. Mayo Clin Proc 66:695–703, 1991.
89. Meecham-Jones DJ, Paul EA, Jones PW: Nasal pressure support ventilation plus oxygen compared with oxygen therapy alone in hypercapnic COPD. Am J Respir Crit Care Med 152:538, 1995.
90. Casanova C, Celli BR, Tost L, et al: Long-term controlled trial of nocturnal nasal positive pressure ventilation in patients with severe COPD. Chest 118:1582–1590, 2000.
91. Clini E, Sturani C, Rossi A, et al: The Italian multicenter study on noninvasive ventilation in chronic obstructive pulmonary disease patients. Eur Respir J 20:529–538, 2002.
92. Tuggery JM, Plant PK, Elliott MW: Domiciliary non-invasive ventilation for recurrent acidotic exacerbations of COPD: an economic analysis. Thorax 58:867–871, 2003.
93. Criner GJ, Brennan K, Travaline JM, et al: Efficacy and compliance with noninvasive positive pressure ventilation in patients with chronic respiratory failure. Chest 116:667–675, 1999.
94. Casey KR, Ortiz KO, Brown LK: Sleep-related hypoventilation/hypoxemic syndromes. Chest 131:1936–1948, 2007.
95. Olson AL, Zwillich C: The obesity hypoventilation syndrome. Am J Med 118:948–956, 2005.
96. Berg G, Delaive K, Manfreda J, et al: The use of health-care resources in obesity-hypoventilation syndrome. Chest 120:377–383, 2001.
97. Nowbar S, Burkart KM, Gonzales R, et al: Obesity-associated hypoventilation in hospitalized patients: prevalence, effects and outcome. Am J Med 116:1–7, 2004.
98. Masa JF, Celli BR, Riesco JA, et al: The obesity hypoventilation syndrome can be treated with noninvasive mechanical ventilation. Chest 119:1102–1107, 2001.
99. Perez de Llano LA, Golpe R, Ortiz Piquer M, et al: Short-term and long-term effects of nasal intermittent positive pressure ventilation in patients with obesity-hypoventilation syndrome. Chest 128:587–594, 2005.
100. Piper AJ, Wang D, Yee BJ, et al: Randomized trial of CPAP vs bilevel support in the treatment of obesity hypoventilation syndrome without severe nocturnal desaturation. Thorax 63:395–401, 2008.
101. Mokhlesi B, Tulaimat A: Recent advances in obesity hypoventilation syndrome. Chest 132:1322–1336, 2007.
102. Diaz GG, Alcaraz AC, Talavera JC, et al: Noninvasive positive-pressure ventilation to treat hypercapnic coma secondary to respiratory failure. Chest 127:952–960, 2005.

103. Scala R, Naldi M, Archinucci I, et al: Noninvasive positive pressure ventilation in patients with acute exacerbations of COPD and varying levels of consciousness. Chest 128:1657–1666, 2005.
104. Soo Hoo GW, Santiago S, Williams AJ: Nasal mechanical ventilation for hypercapnic respiratory failure in chronic obstructive pulmonary disease: determinants of success and failure. Crit Care Med 22:1253–1261, 1994.
105. Ambrosino N, Foglio K, Rubini F, et al: Noninvasive mechanical ventilation in acute respiratory failure due to chronic obstructive pulmonary disease: correlates for success. Thorax 50:755–757, 1995.
106. Poponick JM, Renston JP, Bennett RP, et al: Use of a ventilatory support system (BiPAP) for acute respiratory failure in the emergency department. Chest 116:166–171, 1999.
107. Meduri GU, Turner RE, Abou-Shala N, et al: Noninvasive positive pressure ventilation via face mask: first line intervention in patients with acute hypercapnic and hypoxemic respiratory failure. Chest 109:179–193, 1996.
108. Codazzi D, Nacoti M, Passoni M, et al: Continuous positive airway pressure with modified helmet for treatment of hypoxemic acute respiratory failure in infants and a preschool population: a feasibility study. Pediatr Crit Care Med 7:455–460, 2006.
109. Chiumello D, Pelosi P, Carlesso E, et al: Noninvasive positive pressure ventilation delivered by helmet versus standard face mask. Intensive Care Med 29:1671–1679, 2003.
110. Patroniti N, Foti G, Manfio A, et al: Head helmet versus face mask for noninvasive continuous positive airway pressure: a physiological study. Intensive Care Med 29:1680–1687, 2003.
111. Antonelli M, Pennisi MA, Pelosi P, et al: Noninvasive positive pressure ventilation using a helmet in patients with acute exacerbation of chronic obstructive pulmonary disease: a feasibility study. Anesthesiology 100:16–24, 2004.
112. Taccone P, Hess D, Caironi P, et al: Continuous positive airway pressure delivered with a "helmet": effects on carbon dioxide rebreathing. Crit Care Med 32:2090–2096, 2004.
113. Navalesi P, Fanfulla F, Frigerio P, et al: Physiologic evaluation of noninvasive mechanical ventilation delivered with three types of mask in patients with chronic hypercapnic respiratory failure. Crit Care Med 28:1785–1790, 2000.
114. Girault C, Briel A, Benichou J, et al: Interface strategy during noninvasive positive pressure ventilation for hypercapnic acute respiratory failure. Crit Care Med 37:124–131, 2009.
115. Schwartz RA, Kacmarek RM, Hess DR: Factors affecting oxygen delivery with bi-level positive airway pressure. Respir Care 49:270–275, 2004.
116. Ferguson GT, Gilmartin M: CO_2 rebreathing during BiPAP ventilatory assistance. Am J Respir Crit Care Med 151:1126–1135, 1995.
117. Lofaso F, Brochard L, Touchard D, et al: Evaluation of carbon dioxide rebreathing during pressure support ventilation with airway management system (BiPAP) devices. Chest 108:772–778, 1995.
118. Jurban A, Van de Graaff WB, Tobin MJ: Variability of patient-ventilator interaction with pressure support ventilation in patients in patients with chronic obstructive pulmonary disease. Am J Respir Crit Care Med 152:129, 1995.
119. Parthasarathy S, Jubran A, Tobin MJ: Cycling of inspiratory and expiratory muscle groups with the ventilator in airflow limitation. Am J Respir Crit Care Med 158:1471–1478, 1998.
120. Calderini E, Confalonieri M, Puccio PG, et al: Patient-ventilator asynchrony during noninvasive ventilation: the role of expiratory trigger. Intensive Care Med 25:662–667, 1999.
121. Branson RD, Campell RS: Pressure support ventilation, patient-ventilator synchrony, and ventilator algorithms. Respir Care 43:1045–1047, 1998.
122. Vitacca M, Rubini F, Foglio K, et al: Noninvasive modalities of positive pressure ventilation improve the outcome of acute exacerbations in COLD patients. Intensive Care Med 19:450–455, 1993.
123. Girault C, Richard JC, Chevron V, et al: Comparative physiologic effects of noninvasive assist-control and pressure support ventilation in acute hypercapnic respiratory failure. Chest 111:1639–1648, 1997.
124. Evans TW: International Consensus Conference in Intensive Care Medicine: noninvasive positive pressure ventilation. Intensive Care Med 27:166–178, 2001.
125. Richards GN, Cistulli PA, Ungar RG, et al: Mouth leak with nasal continuous positive airway pressure increases nasal airway resistance. Am J Respir Crit Care Med 154:182–186, 1996.
126. Hayes MJ, McGregor FB, Roberts DN, et al: Continuous nasal positive airway pressure with a mouth leak: effect on nasal mucosal blood flux and nasal geometry. Thorax 50:1179–1182, 1995.
127. Massie CA, Hart RW, Peralez K, et al: Effects of humidification on nasal symptoms and compliance in sleep apnea patients using continuous positive airway pressure. Chest 116:403–408, 1999.
128. Rakotonanahary D, Pelletier-Fleury N, Gagnadoux F, et al: Predictive factors for the need for additional humidification during nasal continuous positive airway pressure therapy. Chest 119:460–465, 2001.
129. Ho-Tai LM, Devitt JH, Noel AG, et al: Gas leak and gastric insufflation during controlled ventilation: face mask versus laryngeal mask airway. Can J Anaesth 45:206–211, 1998.
130. Chatmongkolchart S, Schettino GP, Dillman C, et al: In vitro evaluation of aerosol bronchodilator delivery during noninvasive positive pressure ventilation: effect of ventilator settings and nebulizer position. Crit Care Med 30:2515–2519, 2002.
131. Keenan SP, Gregor J, Sibbald WJ, et al: Noninvasive positive pressure ventilation in the setting of severe, acute exacerbations of chronic obstructive pulmonary disease: more effective and less expensive. Crit Care Med 28:2094–2102, 2000.
132. Jasmer RM, Matthay MA: Cost-effectiveness of noninvasive ventilation for acute chronic obstructive pulmonary disease: cashing in too quickly. Crit Care Med 28:2170–2171, 2000.
133. Nava S, Evangelisti I, Rampulla C, et al: Human and financial costs of noninvasive mechanical ventilation in patients affected by COPD and acute respiratory failure. Chest 111:1631–1638, 1997.

Chapter 46

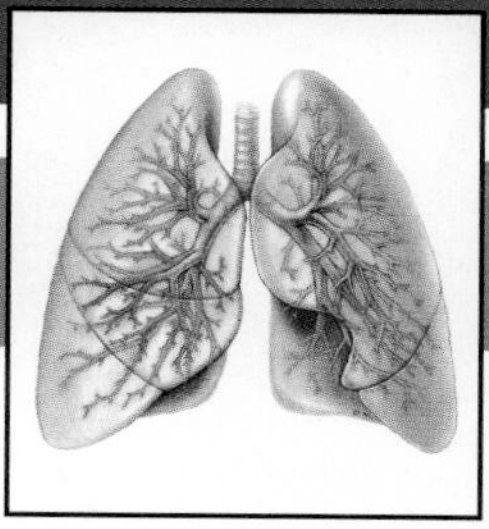

Monitoring the Patient in the Intensive Care Unit

ALEXANDER B. ADAMS

CHAPTER OBJECTIVES

After reading this chapter you will be able to:

- Discuss the principles of monitoring the respiratory system, cardiovascular system, neurologic status, renal function, liver function, and nutritional status of patients in intensive care.
- Identify the risks and benefits of intensive care unit (ICU) monitoring techniques.
- Explain why the caregiver is the most important monitor in the ICU.
- Describe how to evaluate measures of patient oxygenation in the ICU.
- Explain why $PaCO_2$ is the best index of ventilation for critically ill patients.
- Describe the approach used to evaluate changes in respiratory rate, tidal volume, minute ventilation, $PaCO_2$, and end-tidal PCO_2 values for monitoring purposes.
- Identify monitoring techniques used in the ICU to evaluate lung and chest wall mechanics and work of breathing.
- Discuss the importance of monitoring peak and plateau pressures in patients receiving mechanical ventilatory support.
- Identify monitoring techniques that have become available more recently, such as lung stress and strain, functional residual capacity, stress index, electrical impedance tomography, and acoustic respiratory monitoring.
- Describe the approach used to interpret the results of ventilator graphics monitoring.
- Describe the cardiovascular monitoring techniques used in the care of critically ill patients and how to interpret the results of hemodynamic monitoring.
- Discuss the importance of monitoring neurologic status in the ICU and the variables that should be monitored.
- Discuss evaluation of renal function, liver function, and nutritional status in the ICU.
- List and discuss the use of composite and global scores to measure patient status in the ICU, such as the Murray lung injury score and the APACHE severity of illness scoring system.
- Discuss monitoring and troubleshooting of the patient-ventilator system in the ICU.

CHAPTER OUTLINE

KEY TERMS

acoustic respiratory monitoring (ARM)
afterload
alveolar and arterial oxygen tension difference ($P(A - a)O_2$)
APACHE scoring system
artifacts
bladder pressure
capnography
capnometry
cardiac output
contractility
dead space/tidal volume (V_D/V_T) ratio
driving pressure
electrical impedance tomography (EIT)
esophageal balloon
factitious events
Fick equations
frequency/tidal volume (f/V_T) ratio
Glasgow Coma Scale (GCS)
Harris-Benedict equation
lung ultrasonography
lung stress and strain
maximal inspiratory pressure (MIP)
maximum voluntary ventilation (MVV)
mean airway pressure (MAP)
Murray lung injury score
oxygen consumption ($\dot{V}O_2$)
PaO_2/FiO_2 ratio
physiologic shunt ($\dot{Q}_S/\dot{Q}_T$)
preload
pressure-time product (PTP)
respiratory inductive plethysmography
stress index
Swan-Ganz catheter
systematic errors
tissue oxygen sensing
venous admixture
vital capacity (VC)

The concept and purposes of monitoring have evolved over the past 50 years. The importance of monitoring was established with the advent of the intensive care unit (ICU) during the polio epidemic in the 1950s.[1] Enhanced monitoring represents the main difference between a general hospital ward and the ICU. The purpose of monitoring is simple and clear: to measure in "real time" physiologic values that can change rapidly. The values can be analyzed and interpreted with the expectation that interventions such as fluid resuscitation, medication administration, or changes in ventilator settings can be made in time to prevent adverse consequences.

For the purposes of this chapter, monitoring emphasizes real-time measurements in the ICU and not intermittent diagnostic procedures such as radiographic imaging, electroencephalography, or angiography. The distinction between monitoring and diagnostic testing is not always well defined. Pulmonary function values are "monitored" over years in outpatient clinics with a concern for chronic disease management. In the ICU, data are monitored continuously or periodically over the course of the ICU admission. This chapter describes monitoring of the respiratory system, cardiovascular system, neurologic status, renal function, liver function, and nutritional status in the ICU.

PRINCIPLES OF MONITORING

Each monitoring test, procedure, or instrument carries certain risks and provides information that has value. There is an important balance between the risks and benefits of monitoring, especially when evaluating new monitoring techniques. Every test or monitoring technique should be continually judged for usefulness. Figure 46-1 depicts a continuum for judging the risk and benefit of tests, diagnostic procedures, and monitoring techniques. The most useful tests have little or no risk and high potential value. Less useful tests carry higher risk with little potential value. Use of a pulse oximeter probe carries little physical risk and provides valuable information about blood oxygenation (low risk-benefit ratio). However, there is a small but known risk of obtaining incorrect values with the instrument. Hemodynamic monitoring requires placement of a highly invasive **Swan-Ganz catheter** (pulmonary artery catheter) in the pulmonary artery to provide data that must be correctly interpreted. This type of monitoring should be undertaken only with an expectation of collecting important (high value) information. The risk-benefit ratio for pulmonary artery catheterization is high. For this reason and with fluid status data available from central venous pressure (CVP) monitoring, the widespread use of pulmonary arterial catheterization has markedly decreased.[2]

The measurements made during monitoring must be evaluated in the context of a patient's overall clinical presentation. All monitored variables have defined boundaries for acceptable values and indicators of abnormality that may require immediate attention. The fidelity of a measurement—the degree to which the instrument is actually correct in measuring the value—must be known. There often is nearly complete trust in a digital value

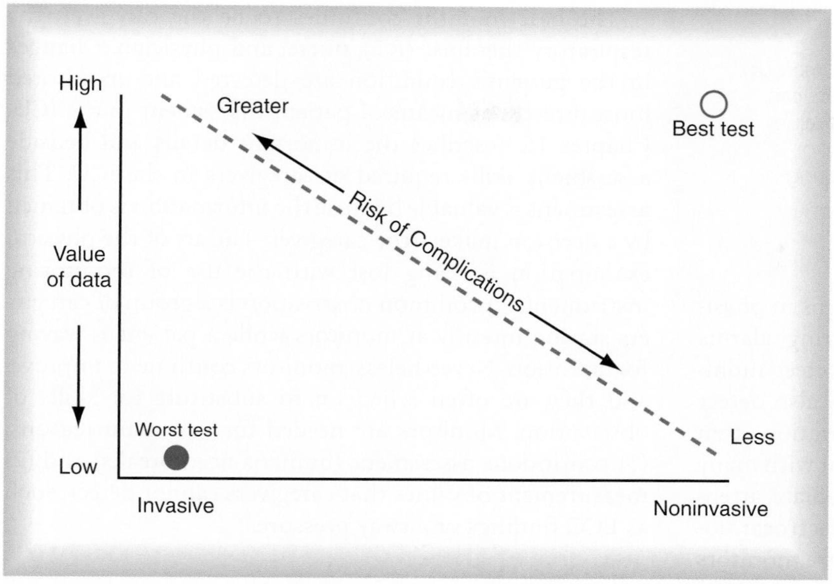

FIGURE 46-1 Balancing the value and risks of monitoring. A test or monitoring technique provides valuable data, but acquisition of the information may carry some risks. Generally, more invasive techniques have an increasing risk of complications; at the same time, the value of the data should be greater. The best monitoring test would be noninvasive, have little risk, and provide valuable data. In contrast, a poor test would be invasive with high risk and low value.

displayed, but the monitor may be displaying an incorrect value. When something looks wrong, the patient or the monitor may be the source of the abnormal value. Signals or values are susceptible to variability owing to **artifacts, factitious events,** physiologic variation, and instrument drift. Instrument software filtering may obscure the problem. Artifacts or nonphysiologic signals are frequently seen, such as when the patient or monitoring lines are moved. The artifacts usually are spikes or major shifts in values that are inconsistent with the patient's clinical status, or there are nonphysiologic changes. Factitious events are values that are real and "out of range" but often are temporary, such as the elevation in airway pressure during a cough. Factitious events, being real, may require attention, whereas artifacts are usually self-resolving. In addition, the signal itself can exhibit a random variability related to the inherent imprecision of the signal or because of normal physiologic variability in the patient. Blood pressure changes within a certain range for many reasons.

The measuring instrument can produce values that are shifted in a systematic way—consistently high or low or in error in relation to the magnitude of the signal. These shifts are referred to as either *parallel* or *slope shifts* (Figure 46-2). Generally, all values must be interpreted with a background of training and experience so that one can understand when a value is normal and when it should be considered abnormal.

Monitored values should be accurate or unbiased; that is, the measured values should correctly reflect the real values. Values should be precise; measurements should not vary widely when repeated (the standard deviation of repeated measurements should be low). **Systematic errors** can be parallel (constant) or slope (change with value) errors that should be correctable by calibrating the

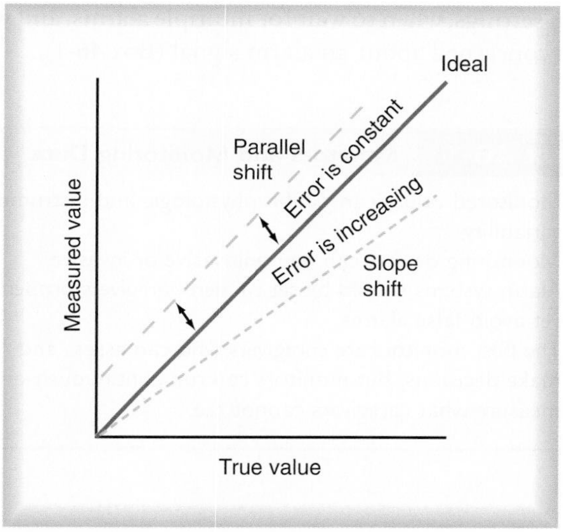

FIGURE 46-2 Errors in data obtained with a monitoring instrument. Under ideal circumstances, the measured values obtained with a monitoring instrument are correct, and the instrument displays the true values. In reality, there are two forms of shifting from the true values—a parallel shift and a slope shift. Parallel shifts have a constant difference from the true value; a 1-point calibration brings all values into line. A slope shift occurs when measured values have an increasing (or decreasing) difference from the true values. Slope shifts require 2-point calibration.

instrument (although many monitors now have regular autocalibration algorithms).

Several types of instruments and monitors are used for ICU monitoring. The equipment either is at the bedside (point of care) or is brought to the bedside, or the specimens are transported from the patient to instruments in the clinical laboratory. The monitors can be noninvasive—connected to the surface of the body—or invasive—connected to lines or catheters that penetrate the body.

RULE OF THUMB

The caregiver has the ability to interpret numerous monitored values and to intervene. Monitors can run continuously and be used to measure values that caregivers cannot "see." The best monitor is the caregiver who understands the monitoring equipment, alarms, and resulting data.

With the responsibility of detecting variations in physiologic data comes the responsibility of setting alarms appropriately. The alarms should be set to detect monitored values that require attention. Monitors also detect the artifacts, factitious events, and random variation often seen in the ICU. The ICU is a noisy environment with many alarms sounding that may not require immediate attention. Ventilators respond to coughs, and electrocardiographs (ECGs), oximeters, and vascular pressure monitors sound alarms with physical movements of the patient. Practitioners must develop mental filtering skills to evaluate true and false alarms and to know when to correct the alarm settings, when to wait for multiple alarms, and when to be concerned about an alarm signal (Box 46-1).

Box 46-1 Monitors and Monitoring Data

- Monitored values can exhibit physiologic and instrument variability.
- Monitoring devices can be noninvasive or invasive.
- Alarm systems should be set to alert caregivers properly yet avoid false alarms.
- The best monitors are caregivers who can assess and make decisions, but monitors can run continuously and measure what caregivers cannot see.

The best monitor continues to be the caregiver: the respiratory therapist (RT), nurse, and physician. Changes in the patient's condition are detected and monitored most directly by means of patient assessment in the ICU. Chapter 15 describes the important details and bedside assessment skills required of caregivers in the ICU. This assessment is valuable because the information is obtained by a decision maker—the caregiver. The art of the physical examination is being lost with the use of monitoring instruments. A common observation is a group of caregivers staring intently at monitors while a patient is waving for attention. Nevertheless, monitors continue to improve, and they are often relied on to substitute for skills of observation. Monitors are needed for two main reasons: (1) continuous assessment (humans need breaks) and (2) measurement of values that caregivers cannot detect, such as ECG findings or airway pressure.

PATHOPHYSIOLOGY AND MONITORING

Monitoring produces numbers from measurements. Fixing the numbers rather than managing the dysfunction often becomes the goal of treatment. A commonly occurring example is increasing the fractional inspired oxygen concentration (FiO_2) in response to reductions in pulse oximeter oxygen saturation (SpO_2). Whenever possible, the goals of monitoring and treatment should be based on managing and treating pathophysiology. For each organ or organ system, there is a conceptual framework for the disease process, and treatment should be based on correcting or adapting to the pathophysiologic condition.

The lungs contain 300 million alveoli, but a basic model of lung injury reduces a lung disorder to three types of injured lung units (Figure 46-3): (1) alveoli that are

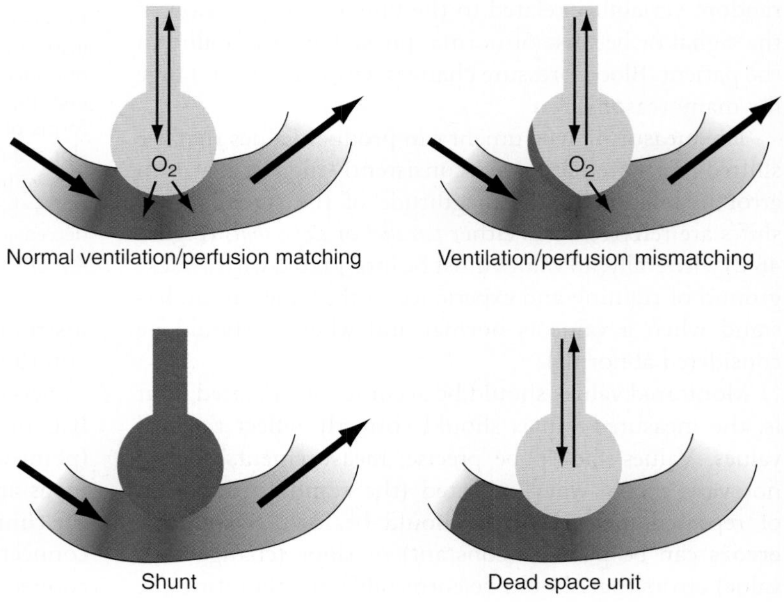

FIGURE 46-3 A model for the causes of uneven matching of gas and blood in the lung.

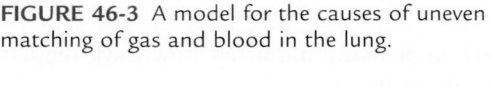

ventilated but not perfused (dead space units), (2) alveoli that are perfused but not ventilated (shunt units), and (3) alveoli that are receiving either partial ventilation or partial perfusion ($\dot{V}/\dot{Q}$ mismatch). In terms of treatment options, $\dot{V}/\dot{Q}$ mismatching is more responsive to oxygen (O_2) therapy than shunt or dead space units. However, all three forms of disordered lung units display reduced O_2 saturation. Within the context of this model, treatment should be aimed at the source of the disorder and not an attempt to "fix" the arterial partial pressure of oxygen (PaO_2) or SpO_2.

RESPIRATORY MONITORING

Gas Exchange

The most important function of the lungs is uptake of O_2 from air into the arterial blood and disposal of carbon dioxide (CO_2) from mixed venous or pulmonary artery blood into the environment. Arterial blood gas (ABG) values contain this gas exchange information. A typical ABG report includes PaO_2, $PaCO_2$, pH, a calculated HCO_3^-, and an estimated base excess or deficit. ABG samples can be obtained quickly and analyzed rapidly. The typical absolute values, predicted values, derangements including compensation, and basic interpretation of ABGs are described in Chapter 18. However, ABGs do not tell the complete story; other values assessing gas exchange that are actively obtained or calculated are discussed in this section.

Monitoring Oxygenation

Tissue oxygenation depends on FiO_2, inspired partial pressure of oxygen (PiO_2), alveolar oxygen tension (PAO_2), arterial oxygenation (PaO_2, SaO_2, oxygen content of arterial blood [CaO_2]), oxygen delivery, tissue perfusion, and O_2 uptake.

Arterial Pulse Oximetry. The goal of breathing and circulation is adequate tissue oxygenation. All organs require O_2 delivery that meets O_2 use demands; the brain and kidneys have particularly high requirements. An important innovation in monitoring is the use of oximetry—a color spectrum measurement of pulsing arterial blood is used for continuous assessment of arterial oxygenation (SpO_2). The human eye is not good at detecting or quantifying arterial hypoxemia. Frank cyanosis does not develop until there is at least 5 g/dl of deoxyhemoglobin in the blood.[3] The threshold at which cyanosis becomes apparent is affected by skin perfusion, skin pigmentation, and hemoglobin concentration. ABG analysis has been the accepted method of detecting hypoxemia in critically ill patients, but obtaining arterial blood can be painful and cause complications, and ABG analysis does not provide immediate or continuous data. For these reasons, SpO_2 has become the standard for a continuous, noninvasive assessment of SaO_2. SpO_2 does not measure $PaCO_2$, and patients breathing an elevated FiO_2 can build up CO_2 (increased $PaCO_2$), although SpO_2 values are acceptable. Ventilatory failure may go unnoticed unless ABGs are measured.

SpO_2 measurements are based on spectrophotometric principles, which are based on the law of Beer-Lambert. Lightweight probes direct filtered light of specific wavelengths (usually two) through a digit, the bridge of the nose, or an earlobe or reflected from a forehead sensor. The relative absorption of these spectrophotometric beams after passing through the tissue (which differs for O_2 saturated and desaturated blood) is converted into the appropriate saturation value with processor-stored algorithms.

Tissue O_2 sensors designed to measure SaO_2 of muscle or the brain were developed more recently.[4] Brain oxygenation is crucial, and deep muscle tissue in compartment syndromes can become deoxygenated. This **tissue oxygen sensing** technique involves positioning of an emitter and detector (of usually four wavelengths) on the skin surface over the tissue or organ of interest. Light from the emitter reflects from tissue at a depth of one-third the distance between the emitter and detector. The light received by the detector is read, and algorithms determine tissue oxygenation, not SpO_2.

RULE OF THUMB

SpO_2 values have been considered a fifth vital sign. There are two very important problems with relying on SpO_2 to monitor adequate respiratory function: (1) SpO_2 values reflect oxygenation, not ventilation; and (2) SpO_2 measurement is susceptible to numerous factors that can produce false values.

Although SpO_2 has been universally adopted, it does have limitations (Box 46-2).[5,6] Motion artifact is an important problem, resulting in inaccurate readings and false alarms. Motion artifacts are common because of shivering, seizure activity, pressure on the sensor, or transport of the patient. The choice of probe site may also affect accuracy. Finger probes appear to be more accurate than forehead, nose, or earlobe probes during low perfusion states. Intense daylight and fluorescent, incandescent, xenon, and infrared light sources have caused errors in SpO_2 readings. Anemia and deeply pigmented skin can affect the accuracy of SpO_2; however, the effect of anemia is not clinically

Box 46-2 Values Affecting Pulse Oximetry

- Motion artifact
- Environmental light (e.g., sunlight, fluorescence)
- Anemia
- Deeply pigmented skin
- Carboxyhemoglobin, methemoglobin
- Nail polish
- Blood-borne dyes

significant until the hemoglobin level is markedly reduced. Carboxyhemoglobin and methemoglobin can produce falsely high SpO_2 values, and some colors of nail polish, particularly blue, green, and black, interfere with light transmission and absorbency, as do some blood-borne dyes, such as indocyanine green and methylene blue, which tend to produce falsely low SpO_2 values. Although rare, exposure to numerous toxins and drugs, including topical benzocaine, can elevate methemoglobin and produce falsely elevated SpO_2 values.

MINI CLINI

Trusting the Pulse Oximeter

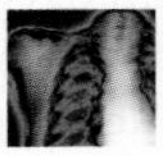

PROBLEM: A 32-week-gestation newborn is intubated and receiving CPAP therapy. The patient appears to be in mild to moderate respiratory distress, yet SpO_2 is 98%. Hurricane spray (20% benzocaine) had been used to reduce the irritation of the endotracheal tube. Analysis of ABG values reveals PaO_2 325 mm Hg, and the cooximeter shows a methemoglobin value of 38%.

SOLUTION: The most common problems with the fidelity of pulse oximeter readings are motion artifacts, interference by external light sources, or malposition of the sensor. Each of these problems can be easily and quickly assessed. In this case, the clinical symptoms did not correlate with an acceptable SpO_2 value. Because adequate O_2 delivery is the ultimate goal, CO and O_2-carrying ability must be considered as causes of the respiratory distress. The high methemoglobin value necessitates immediate therapy with methylene blue dye. Although the pulse oximeter has provided an excellent, safe means of monitoring blood oxygenation, there must be a wary vigilance about trusting the values.

Oxygen Consumption. Oxygen consumption ($\dot{V}O_2$) is the volume of O_2 consumed by the body in milliliters per minute. Normal resting $\dot{V}O_2$ is approximately 250 ml/min, and $\dot{V}O_2$ increases with activity, stress, and temperature. The acquisition of O_2 from the lungs into the circulatory system is described by the **Fick equations:**

$$\dot{V}O_2 = \dot{Q}_T\,(CaO_2 - C\bar{v}O_2)\ \textit{or}\ \dot{Q}_T = \dot{V}O_2/(CaO_2 - C\bar{v}O_2)$$

in which $\dot{Q}_T$ is cardiac output (CO), and CaO_2 and $C\bar{v}O_2$ are arterial and mixed venous oxygen contents. If the values for $\dot{Q}_T$, CaO_2, and $C\bar{v}O_2$ are normal, this becomes:

$$\begin{aligned}\dot{V}O_2 \text{ in ml/min}&\\ &= \dot{Q}_T\,(CaO_2 - C\bar{v}O_2)\\ &= (5000\text{ ml/min})\,(20\text{ ml/100 ml} - 15\text{ ml/100 ml})\\ &= (5000\text{ ml/min})\,(5\text{ ml/100 ml})\\ &= 250\text{ ml/min}\end{aligned}$$

To an engineer or systems analyst, the function of the lungs is summarized by the Fick equation—O_2 in the alveoli diffuses into mixed venous blood flowing by at the pace of CO. This process converts deoxygenated venous blood to oxygenated arterial blood.

An alternative calculation for $\dot{V}O_2$ that does not require an arterial or mixed venous blood sample or measurement of **cardiac output** (CO) is:

$$\dot{V}O_2 = [(FiO_2)\,(\dot{V}_I)] - [(F_{\bar{E}}O_2)\,(\dot{V}_E)]$$

where FiO_2 and $F_{\bar{E}}O_2$ are the mean inspired and expired fractional concentrations of oxygen, and $\dot{V}_I$ and $\dot{V}_E$ are the inspired and expired minute ventilations. If $\dot{V}_I$ equals $\dot{V}_E$ (normally $\dot{V}_I$ is slightly greater than $\dot{V}_E$, but the difference is small), this becomes:

$$\dot{V}O_2 = (FiO_2 - F_{\bar{E}}O_2)\,\dot{V}_E$$

If the values for minute ventilation and inspired and expired gas concentrations are normal, this becomes:

$$\dot{V}O_2 = (0.21 - 0.168)\,(6\text{ L/min}) = 0.252\text{ L/min},$$
$$\text{or approximately 250 ml/min}$$

A normal resting $\dot{V}O_2$ of 250 ml/min represents approximately 25% of normal O_2 delivery (1000 ml/min). The blood carries a large reservoir of O_2 that can diffuse into deoxygenated tissues under high O_2 demand conditions.

$\dot{V}O_2$ may be useful in determining nutritional requirements and adequacy of O_2 delivery and may occasionally help determine the cause of a high ventilation requirement. If there is a stable tissue demand for O_2, measurements of $\dot{V}O_2$ may be used to follow the hemodynamic response to therapeutic interventions.

Alveolar-Arterial Oxygen Tension Difference. The **alveolar and arterial oxygen tension difference ($P(A - a)O_2$)** is a useful measurement of the efficiency of gas exchange. A healthy person breathing room air has $P(A - a)O_2$ of approximately 5 to 15 mm Hg. This value increases with age to approximately 10 to 20 mm Hg in elderly adults. $P(A - a)O_2$ also increases normally with an increase in FiO_2. A healthy person has $P(A - a)O_2$ of 5 to 15 mm Hg while breathing room air; however, $P(A - a)O_2$ increases to 100 to 150 mm Hg when the person is breathing 100% O_2.

Most importantly, an abnormal increase in $P(A - a)O_2$ is associated with gas exchange problems. If PaO_2 is 80 mm Hg while the patient is breathing 100% O_2, a significant gas exchange problem is present even though oxygenation seems acceptable.

If PaO_2 is 80 mm Hg, $PaCO_2$ is 40 mm, FiO_2 is 1, and barometric pressure (PB) is 760 mm Hg, then:

$$\begin{gathered}PAO_2 = PiO_2 - (PaCO_2)\,(1.25)\\ PiO_2 = [(PB - P_{H_2O})\,(FiO_2)] = 713\\ PAO_2 = [(760 - 47)\,(1)] - (40)\,(1.25) = 663\text{ mm Hg}\\ P(A - a)O_2 = PAO_2 - PaO_2 = 663 - 80\\ P(A - a)O_2 = 583\text{ mm Hg}\end{gathered}$$

where P_{H2O} is water vapor pressure. $P(A - a)O_2$ is markedly elevated considering that normal $(A - a)O_2$ is 100 to

150 mm Hg while the patient is breathing 100% O_2. (A − a) O_2 also can be used to give a rough estimate of percentage shunt, where:

$$\text{Shunt} \cong \frac{(P(A-a)O_2 \text{ on } 100\%\ O_2)}{20}$$

In this example, percentage shunt would be approximately 29%: $P(A - a)O_2/20 = 583/20 = 29.2\%$.

$P(A - a)O_2$ takes into account $PaCO_2$ and eliminates hypoventilation and hypercapnia from consideration as the sole cause of hypoxemia. Although $P(A - a)O_2$ is infrequently calculated, astute experienced clinicians consciously or subconsciously estimate $P(A - a)O_2$ of every blood gas value.

PaO_2/FiO_2 Ratio. The **PaO_2/FiO_2 ratio** has become important for the determination of the extent of acute lung injury (ALI) and acute respiratory distress syndrome (ARDS) in multicenter collaborative studies.[7,8] A normal PaO_2/FiO_2 ratio while breathing room air is about 400 to 500 mm Hg. The PaO_2/FiO_2 ratio provides an index for the effect of O_2 on PaO_2 when a range of FiO_2 settings may be prescribed. The index allows comparisons of severity between patients or if FiO_2 is changed in the same patient. ARDS has been defined by a PaO_2/FiO_2 ratio less than 200 mm Hg. The PaO_2/FiO_2 ratio is easy to calculate and a reliable index of gas exchange when FiO_2 is greater than 0.5 and PaO_2 is less than 100 mm Hg—values often observed in critically ill patients. The level of applied **mean airway pressure (MAP),** which is strongly affected by PEEP, must also be considered as an independent factor that influences the PaO_2/FiO_2 ratio.

RULE OF THUMB

ALI/ARDS definitions include:
- Bilateral infiltrates on chest x-ray
- Absence of left ventricular failure with a pulmonary capillary wedge pressure less than 18 mm Hg
- PaO_2/FiO_2 less than 300 mm Hg for ALI
- PaO_2/FiO_2 less than 200 mm Hg for ARDS

Oxygenation Index. Calculation of oxygenation index (OI) by the following equation provides an index that accounts for FiO_2 and MAP:

$$OI = \frac{FiO_2 * MAP}{PaO_2}$$

Quantification of Shunt. The most accurate and reliable measure of oxygenation efficiency is direct computation of the **physiologic shunt ($\dot{Q}_S/\dot{Q}_T$)**. The physiologic shunt is computed as follows:

$$\dot{Q}_S/\dot{Q}_T = (CcO_2 - CaO_2)/(CcO_2 - C\bar{v}O_2)$$

where CcO_2 is the oxygen content of alveolar capillary blood, CaO_2 is the oxygen content of arterial blood, and $C\bar{v}O_2$ is the oxygen content of mixed venous blood, all expressed in milliliters of O_2 per 100 ml of blood. When the patient is breathing 100% O_2, $\dot{Q}_S/\dot{Q}_T$ can be estimated as follows:

$$\dot{Q}_S/\dot{Q}_T = [(P(A-a)O_2)][0.003]/[(P(A-a)O_2)][0.003] + [CaO_2 - C\bar{v}O_2]$$

For measurement of physiologic shunt, both an arterial and a mixed venous blood sample must be obtained. A true mixed venous blood sample can be obtained only from the distal sample port of an indwelling pulmonary arterial catheter. The total O_2 content of the arterial, mixed venous blood, and pulmonary capillary blood (CaO_2, $C\bar{v}O_2$, CcO_2) is calculated in the same manner as any O_2 content calculations:

$$O_2 \text{ content} = (1.34)\ (Hb)\ (SO_2) + (0.003)\ (PO_2)$$

where Hb is the hemoglobin concentration, SO_2 is the oxygen saturation, and PO_2 is the partial pressure of oxygen. If the patient is breathing 100% O_2, the capillary saturation is 100%, the PCO_2 (capillary PO_2) being the calculated PAO_2 value. Samples should be obtained and analyzed quickly to avoid error from continued metabolism. Similar to $P(A - a)O_2$, $\dot{Q}_S/\dot{Q}_T$ is influenced by $\dot{V}/\dot{Q}$ mismatching and by fluctuations in mixed venous oxygen saturation ($S\bar{v}O_2$) and FiO_2. A "shunt" calculation when FiO_2 is less than 1.0 is defined as **venous admixture.** If venous admixture is elevated but all alveoli are patent, venous admixture decreases toward the normal value (<5%) as FiO_2 is increased. Conversely, if increased venous admixture is caused by a true shunt such as an intracardiac defect, there would be no change in venous admixture as FiO_2 is increased.

Murray Lung Injury Score. ARDS is a syndrome of severe lung injury that was originally described by Ashbaugh and Petty in 1970.[9] Evaluating and treating a patient with ARDS is a primary challenge for the ICU clinician. To monitor the severity of this disease, Murray and colleagues[10] developed a lung injury score that is often calculated in studies of ALI/ARDS. The **Murray lung injury score** quantifies the injury level using the following four factors: chest radiographic findings, PaO_2/FiO_2 ratio, positive end expiratory pressure (PEEP) setting, and compliance. The Murray lung injury score is an example of a composite score that allows quantification of lung status according to different aspects of the injury—gas exchange, radiographic findings, and mechanics. This score is used as an index of the effectiveness of therapy or for interstudy comparisons. The method for calculating the Murray lung injury score is shown in Box 46-3. Other measures of lung injury are listed in Box 46-4.

Monitoring Ventilation

Similar to oxygenation, the adequacy and efficiency of ventilation is routinely evaluated in the ICU (Box 46-5). Monitoring of patients receiving mechanical ventilatory

Box 46-3 Murray Lung Scoring

Component	Value
1. Chest Radiograph	
No alveolar consolidation	0
Alveolar consolidation confined to 1 quadrant	1
Alveolar consolidation confined to 2 quadrants	2
Alveolar consolidation confined to 3 quadrants	3
Alveolar consolidation in all 4 quadrants	4
2. Hypoxemia Score	
$PaO_2/FiO_2 > 300$	0
PaO_2/FiO_2 225-299	1
PaO_2/FiO_2 175-224	2
PaO_2/FiO_2 100-174	3
$PaO_2/FiO_2 < 100$	4
3. PEEP Score (When Ventilated)	
PEEP ≤ 5 cm H_2O	0
PEEP 6-8 cm H_2O	1
PEEP 9-11 cm H_2O	2
PEEP 12-14 cm H_2O	3
PEEP > 15 cm H_2O	4
4. Respiratory System Compliance Score (When Available)	
Compliance ≥ 80 ml/cm H_2O	0
Compliance 60-79 ml/cm H_2O	1
Compliance 40-59 ml/cm H_2O	2
Compliance 20-39 ml/cm H_2O	3
Compliance ≤ 19 ml/cm H_2O	4

The final value is obtained by dividing the aggregate sum by the number of components used.

SCORE

No lung injury—0
Mild to moderate lung injury—0.1-2.5
Severe lung injury (ARDS)—>2.5

Box 46-4 Measures of Decreased Blood Oxygenation or Lung Injury

↓ SpO_2
↓ PaO_2
↑ $P(A-a)O_2$ – ($PAO_2 - PaO_2$)
↓ P/F ratio – (PaO_2/FiO_2)
↑ Shunt/venous admixture
↑ Murray lung injury score

Box 46-5 Monitoring the Adequacy of Ventilation

- Respiratory volume and rate (V_T, f, $\dot{V}_E$)
- $PaCO_2$
- V_D/V_T
- Capnometry (not for routine use but in special situations, such as ensuring tracheal intubation and cardiac blood flow in resuscitation efforts)

support in the ICU includes measurement of the patient's tidal volume (V_T), respiratory rate (f), and minute ventilation ($\dot{V}_E$) where:

$$\dot{V}_E = (f) * (V_T)$$

However, effective ventilation depends on alveolar ventilation ($\dot{V}_A$), as follows:

$$\dot{V}_A = (V_T - V_{Dphys})(f)$$

where V_{Dphys} is physiologic dead space, and:

$$\dot{V}_A = (0.863 * \dot{V}CO_2)/PaCO_2$$

where $\dot{V}CO_2$ is CO_2 production in milliliters per minute, and 0.863 is a conversion factor. With a normal $PaCO_2$ and $\dot{V}CO_2$, this becomes:

$$\dot{V}_A = (0.863 * 200 \text{ ml/min})/40 \text{ mm Hg} = 4.3 \text{ L/min}$$

Because of the relationship between alveolar ventilation and $PaCO_2$, the best index of effective ventilation is measurement of $PaCO_2$. $PaCO_2$ is the standard assessment for adequacy of ventilation in the ICU. Ventilation is adequate if $PaCO_2$ is associated with a normal arterial pH. For healthy persons, $PaCO_2$ is between 35 mm Hg and 45 mm Hg, resulting in an arterial pH of 7.35 to 7.45. An elevated $PaCO_2$ with normal pH is common in patients with chronic obstructive pulmonary disease (COPD).

Dead Space. The **dead space/tidal volume (V_D/V_T) ratio** is a measure of the efficiency of gas exchange. This ratio is an estimate of the proportion of ventilation participating in diffusion of CO_2. V_D/V_T can be calculated from the Enghoff modification of the Bohr equation as follows:

$$V_D/V_T = (PaCO_2 - P_{\bar{E}}CO_2)/PaCO_2$$

where $F_{\bar{E}}CO_2$ is the CO_2 concentration in mixed expired gas. A rapid response capnometry or exhaled flow analysis provides a volumetric CO_2 method for attaining $F_{\bar{E}}CO_2$ values.[11] When $F_{\bar{E}}CO_2$ is determined, a specimen of arterial blood should be drawn for ABG analysis. When the gas and blood samples are analyzed, the preceding formula can be used to calculate V_D/V_T.

In healthy persons who are sitting, the V_D/V_T ratio is 0.20 to 0.40. This value varies little with age, position, exercise, V_T, or breath holding. In the setting of critical illness, however, the V_D/V_T ratio commonly exceeds 0.6. Frequently, the V_D/V_T ratio is increased in patients with congestive heart failure, pulmonary embolism, ALI, or pulmonary hypertension and in patients undergoing mechanical ventilation. The V_D/V_T ratio has been used to evaluate patients being considered for weaning from mechanical ventilation. A V_D/V_T ratio greater than 0.60 requires continuation of ventilatory support. Increased V_D/V_T in the early phase of ARDS has been associated with an increased risk of death.[12]

Monitoring of Inspired and Exhaled Gas Volumes. Although the best index of effective ventilation is measurement of $PaCO_2$, measurement of inspired and expired gas volumes is an important aspect of monitoring patients receiving mechanical ventilatory support. For patients receiving controlled mechanical ventilation, minute ventilation ($\dot{V}_E$), respiratory rate (f), and V_T are assessed by:

$$\dot{V}_E = (V_T)(f) \textit{ and } V_T \text{ average} = \dot{V}_E/f$$

For patients receiving ventilation in the synchronized intermittent mandatory ventilation (SIMV) mode, total minute ventilation ($\dot{V}_{ETOT}$) is the sum of the patient's spontaneous minute ventilation ($\dot{V}_{Esp}$) and the machine minute ventilation ($\dot{V}_{Emach}$) provided:

$$\dot{V}_{ETOT} = \dot{V}_{Esp} + \dot{V}_{Emach} \textit{ and}$$
$$\dot{V}_{ETOT} = (V_{Tmach})(f_{mach}) + (V_{Tpatient})(f_{patient})$$

With an adequate V_T, increases in minute ventilation tend to increase alveolar ventilation and decrease $PaCO_2$, whereas decreases in minute ventilation tend to have the opposite effect. However, in the presence of rapid shallow breathing with normal or elevated minute ventilation, a decrease in effective ventilation can result in an increase in $PaCO_2$. This effect is caused by ineffective shallow tidal breaths that are at or below dead space volume. Spontaneous respiratory rate often is a sensitive indicator of the need for mechanical ventilation. Rates greater than 20 breaths/min may indicate distress, and a rate greater than 30 breaths/min with a spontaneous V_T of less than 300 ml often indicates the need for mechanical ventilatory support in adults because a large proportion of ventilatory effort is being expended to move dead space gases.

Inspired versus Expired Tidal Volume. Normal inspired V_T and expired V_T should be nearly the same. However, in the presence of an air leak, inspired V_T may be larger than expired V_T, and measurement of delivered V_T versus exhaled V_T may be useful in detecting and quantifying the size of a leak—a situation that may require immediate attention.

Capnography. Capnometry is the measurement of CO_2 at the airway opening during the ventilatory cycle. **Capnography** refers to plotting CO_2 concentration against time or against exhaled volume. The normal CO_2 waveform is displayed in Figure 46-4. The height of the capnogram (the peak value) indicates the end-tidal CO_2 value. $P_{ET}CO_2$ normally is 1 to 5 mm Hg less than $PaCO_2$, ranging between 35 mm Hg and 43 mm Hg. Because $P_{ET}CO_2$ in healthy persons closely approximates $PaCO_2$, this measure is a potentially useful noninvasive index of the adequacy of ventilation. Abnormal waveform contours can indicate changes in the distribution of ventilation and perfusion, or airway obstruction. These changes typically are an irregular increase in CO_2 level and a lower than normal end-tidal CO_2 level. Positive pressure ventilation (especially with PEEP), pulmonary embolism, cardiac arrest, and pulmonary hypoperfusion also may cause an increase in $PaCO_2$ to $P_{ET}CO_2$ difference [$P(a - ET)CO_2$]. Exercise and

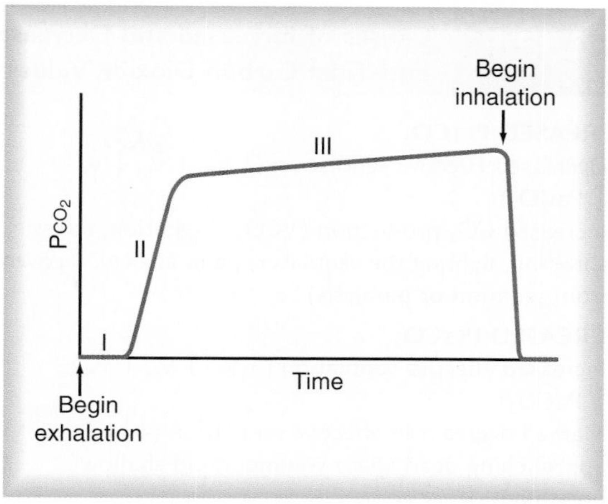

FIGURE 46-4 Time-based capnograph. *Phase I,* Anatomic dead space; *phase II,* transition from anatomic dead space to alveolar plateau; *phase III,* the alveolar plateau.

a large V_T can reverse the $P(a - ET)CO_2$ difference, and $P_{ET}CO_2$ can exceed $PaCO_2$ temporarily.

Patients for whom capnometry may be a useful monitoring tool include patients with normal lungs but an unstable ventilatory drive who are breathing spontaneously or receiving low-level ventilatory support. In these patients, capnometry readings should initially be validated by comparison with $PaCO_2$. Changes in $P_{ET}CO_2$ can be used to alert the clinician to potential changes in patient ventilation. Thereafter, periodic reevaluation should be performed as the patient's clinical state changes. Capnometry has been extremely useful in emergency situations, such as verification of endotracheal intubation and assessment of blood flow during or after cardiac arrest. Small in-line CO_2 monitors that employ colorimetry are now routinely used to verify endotracheal intubation.[13]

Although $P_{ET}CO_2$ and $PaCO_2$ values tend to correlate at a single point in time, correlation between changes in $P_{ET}CO_2$ and changes in $PaCO_2$ tend to be weaker.[14] Decreases in ventilation are reflected by increases in $P_{ET}CO_2$ and $PaCO_2$. However, with very small V_T, $PaCO_2$ increases, whereas $P_{ET}CO_2$ may decrease. Although the appropriate role of capnometry in critical care may be unclear, integration of capnometry into modern ventilators is reasonable because the primary role of the ventilator is CO_2 extraction. As a guide for clinicians, the American Association for Respiratory Care (AARC) has created clinical practice guidelines for the use of capnometry in ventilated patients. Box 46-6 lists common causes of changes in monitored $P_{ET}CO_2$ values.

With improvements in infrared capnometry response time and a simultaneous measure of exhaled volume, volumetric CO_2 monitoring holds promise in the continuous monitoring of ventilation efficiency. VCO_2, or the net volume of CO_2 eliminated from the lungs, can be continuously monitored in a patient being weaned from mechanical ventilation as an indicator of adequate or improving

Box 46-6 Causes of Increased and Decreased End-Tidal Carbon Dioxide Values

INCREASED $P_{ET}CO_2$

- Decreased effective ventilation ($\downarrow V_T$, $\downarrow \dot{V}_E$, $\downarrow \dot{V}_A$, $\uparrow PaCO_2$)
- Increased CO_2 production ($\dot{V}CO_2$) (agitation, stress, shivering, fighting the ventilator, pain, anxiety, recovery from sedation or paralysis)

DECREASED $P_{ET}CO_2$

- Increased effective ventilation ($\uparrow V_T$, $\uparrow \dot{V}_E$, $\uparrow \dot{V}_A$, $\downarrow PaCO_2$)
- Marked decrease in effective ventilation ($\downarrow\downarrow \dot{V}_T$ approaching dead space volume; rapid shallow breathing)
- Decreased CO_2 production ($\dot{V}CO_2$) (sedation, sleep, cooling)
- Decrease in lung perfusion (pulmonary embolus, decreased CO)

ABSENT $P_{ET}CO_2$

- Apnea
- Cardiac arrest
- Ventilator disconnect or malfunction
- Airway obstruction

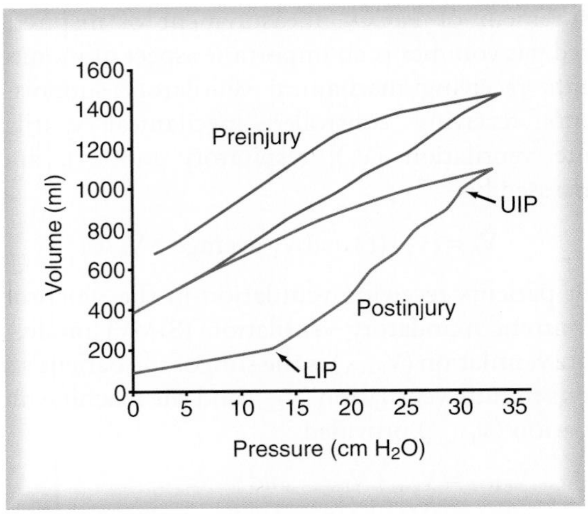

FIGURE 46-5 P-V curves generated by a normal lung (preinjury) and after oleic acid injury (postinjury). In the preinjury curve, the linear relationship between pressure and volume with minimal hysteresis is evident. The postinjury curve displays marked hysteresis and two changes in compliance on the inspiratory limb: a lower inflection point *(LIP)* and upper inflection point *(UIP)*.

ventilatory efficiency.[15] The volumetric capnogram has been examined as a potential tool for detecting a pulmonary embolism[16] and may be useful for tracking the efficiency of mechanical ventilation.[17]

Monitoring Lung and Chest Wall Mechanics

Ventilation of the lungs involves overcoming the flow-resistive, inertial, and elastic properties of the respiratory system. A reasonable model for the mechanics of the respiratory system is an analogy to an electrical circuit.[18] The circuit for gas flow is the pathway to the lungs with resistive elements interposed in series. The gas is collected or stored in a capacitor (the lungs) and discharged (exhaled) through the circuitry. Several assumptions are made with the acceptance of this model (a constant value for resistance and compliance and nonturbulent flow); however, this model serves to simplify and explain the dynamics of ventilation for at least a mechanical lung model.

Actual in vivo measurements of resistance and compliance of the lungs are not dependably constant during the respiratory cycle. Resistance can vary throughout the cycle, and compliance is a function of the pressure-volume (P-V) relationship of the respiratory system. In a ventilated patient, change in airway pressure during ventilation is used to determine the P-V relationship of the total respiratory system. Pressure changes measured by an esophageal balloon reflect P-V changes of the chest wall. The difference between the curves is the lung P-V relationship. P-V relationships can be determined for inflation and deflation. There is normally a difference in the P-V relationship of these curves because of the effects of surfactant on surface tension, producing a *hysteresis*—the separation of the inspiratory and expiratory curves.

A mechanical test lung displays a straight line during a P-V determination. An actual in vivo P-V relationship is curvilinear and displays hysteresis (Figure 46-5). To measure a static P-V curve of a ventilated patient from resting (at functional residual capacity [FRC]) to total lung capacity, a calibrated syringe, referred to as a *supersyringe* ranging from 1.5 to 3 L, was used until more recently to inject 50- to 100-ml increments into the lungs while airway pressure was recorded. Patients were usually sedated during the maneuver. A P-V curve can be measured more easily by the continuous delivery of a low flow of gas into the lung (<5 L/min) with the simultaneous recording of system pressure change. Current ICU ventilators allow the determination of an inflation P-V curve using this approach. The P-V curve is plotted as part of the ventilator graphics package with cursors available to identify specific points on the curve. However, the clinical utility of the P-V relationship of patients may not be directly related to the patient receiving mechanical ventilation owing to an effect on lung volume from tidal recruitment.[19]

The inflation P-V curve often, but not always, reveals two points at which the slope of the curve changes. The lower point at which the slope changes is called the *lower inflection point*. As depicted in Figure 46-5, a lower inflection point may occur over the lower range of volumes, indicating a pressure above which total respiratory system compliance is improved owing to the beginning of alveolar recruitment or the peripheralization of secretions.[20] A recommended strategy is to set PEEP slightly above the lower inflection point with the goal of maintaining recruitment and stabilization of dependent alveoli that may otherwise sustain injury from repetitive opening, closing, and reopening of lung units during tidal ventilation. The other pressure change in the slope, called an *upper deflection point,* may be seen at a higher volume, indicating where compliance decreases owing to alveolar overdistention or a slowing of lung recruitment. Although the risk of alveolar overdistention is generally reduced if the end inspiratory plateau pressure (P_{plat}) is less than 30 cm H_2O, deflection points in patients with ARDS may occur at pressures of 25 cm H_2O.[21]

Respiratory System Compliance

Respiratory system compliance during a tidal breath is an important measure of the stiffness of the lungs. Tidal compliance calculations should be routinely monitored in all ventilated patients. To attain an accurate assessment of compliance, two maneuvers must be performed because the alveolar pressures at end-inspiration and end-expiration are unavailable under dynamic conditions. An end inspiratory hold maneuver in a passive, ventilated patient allows equilibration of pressure across the lung and an estimation of peak alveolar pressure or the end inspiratory P_{plat}. Because compliance (C) is calculated as $C = \Delta V/\Delta P$, V_T (corrected for tubing compliance) is ΔV and ($P_{plat} - PEEP_T$) is ΔP. If auto-PEEP is present, it must be accounted for by adding the auto-PEEP level to the applied PEEP to attain a $PEEP_T$ value.

Normal compliance ranges from 60 to 100 ml/cm H_2O. Diseases of the lung parenchyma, such as pneumonia, pulmonary edema, and any chronic disease causing fibrosis, cause decreased effective compliance. Acute changes, such as atelectasis, pulmonary edema, ARDS, and lung compression, caused by tension pneumothorax cause a rapid decrease in compliance. Compliance is often less than 25 to 30 ml/cm H_2O in patients with ARDS. Common causes of changes in respiratory system compliance are listed in Box 46-7. Several ventilators report breath-to-breath compliance and resistance values dynamically without the use of pause maneuvers. Monitoring these estimates can indicate impedance problems, but they should be verified by static maneuver calculations.

Chest Wall Compliance

In a significant proportion of patients, chest wall or abdominal pathology can influence the P-V relationship during ventilation. The external effect on the lungs of a pleural effusion or abdominal fluid (ascites) can increase airway pressure in a ventilated patient. Although this elevated pressure might be considered detrimental, it may buffer the lung-damaging effect of elevated airway pressure by reducing transpulmonary pressure (Ptp). In a passively ventilated patient who may be vulnerable to lung damage from elevated airway pressure, measurement of the chest wall effect can be made by esophageal or **bladder pressure** determinations. If the bladder pressure is elevated, Ptp is reduced but usually at the expense of effective ventilation.

End inspiratory Ptp can be monitored to evaluate the potential for overdistention—usually allowing some liberty in accepting higher P_{plat} to deliver adequate ventilation. The monitoring of end expiratory Ptp has been used more recently as a rationale for setting PEEP. A negative Ptp probably indicates lung closure (dependent lobe) during expiration that can result in lung opening and closing during the ventilatory cycle. Adequate PEEP is the PEEP level that establishes a positive Ptp or dependent lobe recruitment. (See Chapter 44 for details.)

Box 46-7 Common Causes of Changes in Compliance and Resistance in Mechanically Ventilated Patients

DECREASED COMPLIANCE
↓ Lung compliance (atelectasis, pneumonia, pulmonary edema, ALI/ARDS, pneumothorax, fibrosis, bronchial intubation)
↓ Thoracic compliance (obesity, ascites, chest wall deformity)

INCREASED COMPLIANCE
↑ Lung compliance (improvement in any of the above-listed conditions, pulmonary emphysema)
↑ Thoracic compliance (improvement in any of the above-listed conditions; flail chest; position change—sitting patient up)

INCREASED RESISTANCE
Small endotracheal tube, secretions plugging endotracheal tube, biting on endotracheal tube
↑ Bronchospasm, mucosal edema
↑ Secretions
↑ Airway obstruction
High gas flow rate (or ↑ gas flow)

DECREASED RESISTANCE
↓ Improvement in any of the above-listed conditions
↓ Bronchodilator administration
↓ Suctioning and airway care
↓ Use of lower inspiratory gas flow rate

Resistance

Depending on the **driving pressure** measured, various resistances can be calculated, including airway, pulmonary, chest wall, and total respiratory system resistance. An airway resistance (Raw) can be determined dynamically from simultaneous measurements of airflow and the pressure difference between the airway opening (P_{ao}) and the alveoli (P_{alv}) by $Raw = (P_{ao} - P_{alv})/flow$. Because resistance changes throughout inspiration and expiration, and expiratory resistance generally is greater than inspiratory resistance, instantaneous measures of resistance are not performed clinically. Inspiratory resistance can be calculated simply during constant flow, volume ventilation. This allows monitoring of airway status over time or after the effects of bronchodilator therapy and is determined by dividing the pressure change by the flow rate (see previous equation).

$$Raw = \Delta P/\Delta F = (P_{peak} - P_{plat})/flow$$

where P_{peak} is peak airway pressure and P_{plat} is plateau pressure. Automated methods of measuring expiratory resistance have been integrated into some ventilators.

In ventilated patients, a significant component of the total flow resistance is from endotracheal tubes, which have highly curvilinear flow-resistive properties.[22] In healthy persons, flow is relatively laminar during tidal ventilation and becomes turbulent only with increasing ventilatory demands. The flow resistance offered by the endotracheal tube increases markedly with increasing flow and varies with the size of the tube. Normal airway resistance is approximately 1 to 2 cm H_2O/L per second; however, intubated patients receiving mechanical ventilatory support typically have an airway resistance of 5 to 10 cm H_2O/L per second or more. Automated tube compensation modes have been added to mechanical ventilators to deliver flow that accounts for the added resistance of the endotracheal tube. Common causes of changes in airway resistance in mechanically ventilated patients are listed in Box 46-7.

Peak and Plateau Pressures

The maximum value of airway pressure at the airway opening during a ventilatory cycle is routinely monitored in the ICU. Peak airway pressure greater than 50 to 60 cm H_2O is generally discouraged because high values of peak pressure carry increased risk of barotrauma and hypotension.[23] An increase in peak pressure results from increased resistive pressure or increased elastic pressure from decreased lung or chest wall compliance. Measurement of end inspiratory P_{plat} helps to differentiate between the resistive and elastic components. The P_{plat} level should be monitored for all ventilated patients. P_{plat} ideally should not exceed 30 cm H_2O because elevated P_{plat} increases the likelihood of developing ventilator-induced lung injury.

Auto–Positive End Expiratory Pressure (Intrinsic Positive End Expiratory Pressure)

PEEP is the pressure maintained in the airway by the ventilator at end-exhalation. An alveolar pressure that exists above the applied or extrinsic PEEP level at end-exhalation is termed *intrinsic PEEP* or *auto-PEEP*. At the bedside, *total PEEP* is the sum of extrinsic PEEP and intrinsic PEEP. Confusion exists when total PEEP is designated as intrinsic PEEP; however, when PEEP is increased to counterbalance intrinsic PEEP, they approach equivalency.

Numerous factors, both internal and external to the patient, contribute to the development of auto-PEEP. Expiratory muscle activity can increase auto-PEEP and may interfere with attempts at assessment of auto-PEEP based solely on dynamic hyperinflation. Patients receiving mechanical ventilation for obstructive airways disease have a large degree of inhomogeneity in the emptying of lung units, and auto-PEEP can develop even at relatively low minute ventilation. Auto-PEEP is common in mechanically ventilated patients receiving high minute ventilation and occurs in patients with ARDS.[24] The presence of auto-PEEP can underestimate the effect of mean alveolar pressure when MAP is being monitored to reflect mean alveolar pressure. An increase in mean alveolar pressure owing to auto-PEEP may exacerbate the hemodynamic effects of positive pressure ventilation and increase the likelihood of barotrauma in a manner similar to the application of PEEP. In addition, auto-PEEP alters the effective trigger sensitivity of the ventilator, making it more difficult for the patient to trigger a ventilator-assisted inspiration.

Finally, if unrecognized, auto-PEEP leads to erroneous calculation of static lung compliance by underestimation of total PEEP. Decreasing minute volume can reduce or eliminate auto-PEEP; however, minimal auto-PEEP can be benign. In addition, increasing expiratory time allows more time for airways to empty normally, decreasing auto-PEEP. The use of extrinsic PEEP can partially overcome the trigger sensitivity problem seen with auto-PEEP and may provide a "stent" to allow more complete lung emptying.[25]

Methods for Determining Auto–Positive End Expiratory Pressure. Dynamically, auto-PEEP varies throughout the lungs; however, all measurements of auto-PEEP reflect an average auto-PEEP level throughout the lungs. Assessment of auto-PEEP involves first its detection and then a measurement. Auto-PEEP is suspected if flow continues at end-expiration as seen on ventilator graphics monitoring. In this case, auto-PEEP must be present unless there is active contraction of the expiratory muscles producing end expiratory flow. The following methods are used to estimate auto-PEEP level.

End Expiratory Hold by the Ventilator. Either automated or manual, end expiratory hold by the ventilator closes the expiratory valve at end-exhalation. The hold period must extend until the end expiratory pressure is stabilized or the value is an underestimate of auto-PEEP.

Esophageal Balloon. An **esophageal balloon** is used to measure the esophageal pressure deflection required to trigger the ventilator. The change in esophageal pressure from baseline to the pressure initiating flow at the airway is equal to the total PEEP that must be overcome to trigger a breath.

Matching Auto–Positive End Expiratory Pressure with Positive End Expiratory Pressure. PEEP can be applied to a level (this is possible in some patients) that results in flow reaching zero at end exhalation. The concept involves stenting of the airways by PEEP to allow lung emptying.[25] This maneuver is essentially performed by slowly increasing applied PEEP until every patient effort triggers a ventilator breath.

Mean Airway Pressure

MAP represents the average airway pressure over the total ventilatory cycle. Correct measurement of this value requires continuous sampling of airway pressure at the airway opening—this is an automated feature of modern ventilators. MAP is related to mean lung volume, which correlates with oxygenation if perfusion is adequate. When MAP is increased, arterial O_2 levels often improve, but venous return and subsequently arterial pressure can be adversely affected.

In an effort to increase oxygenation while monitoring arterial pressure, the clinician can manage MAP by several means, including V_T, frequency, inspiratory-to-expiratory (I:E) ratio, and PEEP. The management of MAP relates to a concern for improving oxygenation balanced against its detrimental influence on venous return to the chest. Normally, expiratory resistance is greater than (twice) inspiratory resistance, and mean alveolar pressure normally is greater than MAP. For patients with COPD and elevated expiratory resistance, high mean alveolar volume can be significant during mechanical ventilation. For patients with ALI/ARDS, airway resistance is more typically low, so MAP and mean alveolar pressures may be similar. Mean alveolar volume is related to gas exchange, in particular, oxygenation, depending on regional lung perfusion. Mean alveolar pressure or mean alveolar volume cannot be easily measured, but with some reasonable assumptions about their relationships, MAP directly affects arterial oxygenation.

There is an understandable caution while increasing MAP, usually by increasing PEEP, yet two ventilator modes apply dramatic increases in MAP—high-frequency oscillation and airway pressure release ventilation. The marked improvements in oxygenation seen with these modes can be attributed to high MAP. In the case of high-frequency oscillation, the lungs are never allowed to derecruit between breaths. Airway pressure release ventilation is more complicated because the lung deflates to varying unknown alveolar volumes on exhalation. In the use of either mode, end expiratory alveolar lung volume status cannot be easily determined, but oxygenation is often improved.

Driving Pressure

Driving pressure is a measure of the pressure difference between P_{plat} and total PEEP (PEEP plus auto-PEEP). The swing in pressure from end-inspiration to end-expiration may be an independent stress factor on the lungs. Driving pressure monitors the roles of reducing P_{plat} and increasing PEEP.

Monitoring Breathing Effort and Patterns

Work of Breathing

Work of breathing (WOB) is often increased in critically ill patients. Commercially available systems are available for measuring WOB in ventilated patients. For computation of WOB, changes in Ptp must be measured. The procedure requires an assessment of pleural pressure, which is normally estimated by esophageal pressure after placement of an esophageal balloon catheter. The measurement is estimated from the esophageal pressure-versus-volume curve (Figure 46-6).

For healthy persons, average total WOB ranges from 0.030 to 0.050 kg/m/L (0.3 to 0.6 J/L).[26] Patients with severe obstructive or restrictive lung disease "work" at levels two to three times this normal value at rest, with marked increases in work at higher minute ventilation. How much work a patient can tolerate before the ventilatory muscles fatigue is unclear. Maintaining adequate spontaneous ventilation is impossible in many patients when the workload exceeds 0.15 kg/m/L (1.5 J/L).

Monitoring WOB may be valuable in certain situations, such as weaning. Clinicians are expected to assess a patient's WOB continually and to take appropriate action if WOB becomes excessive. Because a direct measurement of WOB requires esophageal manometry, simpler indicators are sought. Monitoring the patient's spontaneous

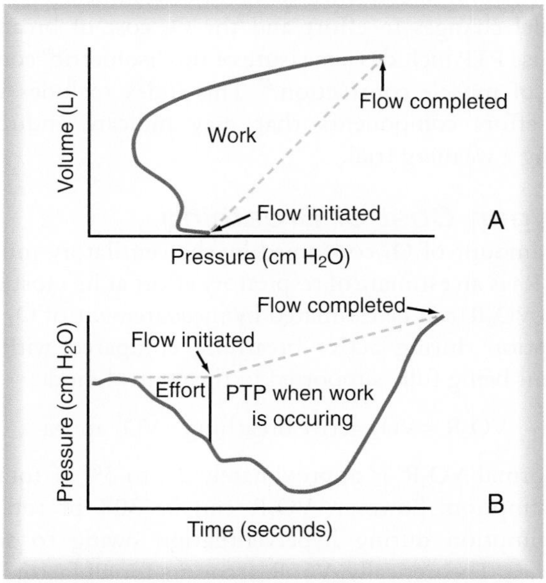

FIGURE 46-6 WOB **(A)** and PTP **(B)** from the same spontaneous breath of a patient receiving ventilatory support. *Dashed lines* represent a tracing of passive inflation by a ventilator-supported breath. Areas of work and PTP are not directly comparable because WOB units (P-V) and PTP units (pressure-time) differ. The area of effort in the total PTP area occurs before (and in addition to) the work measurement.

breathing rate, V_T, and **frequency/tidal volume (f/V_T) ratio** provides useful surrogates for WOB during ventilator weaning trials. Assessment of the patient's overall clinical presentation also is useful in assessing the WOB. Increased WOB is associated with a rapid shallow breathing pattern, rapid pulse rate, hypertension, and use of accessory muscles of ventilation.

Esophageal Pressure Monitoring

Esophageal pressure monitoring is used to reflect clinically intrapleural pressure change, or the distending pressure of the lungs and chest wall. Esophageal pressure monitoring allows calculation of WOB and measurement of Ptp. The thin esophageal catheter (approximately 2-mm diameter) used for monitoring esophageal pressure is not as uncomfortable as a nasogastric tube, is simple to insert, and poses little risk of esophageal perforation. Appropriate placement is achieved by first inflating the 10-cm long balloon with approximately 0.5 to 1.0 ml of air and passing it into the stomach. The catheter is carefully withdrawn until the final position of the balloon is within the lower third of the esophagus, as verified by the presence of cardiac oscillations within the pressure tracing. Proper placement can also be confirmed by occluding the airway and measuring the simultaneous deflections in pressure at the airway opening and esophageal pressure.

Pressure-Time Product. The **pressure-time product (PTP)** is the area encompassed by the esophageal pressure-time tracing during inspiration as shown in Figure 46-6. PTP is simpler to measure than WOB because it does not require simultaneous measurement of volume. PTP values parallel changes in effort and the O_2 cost of breathing because PTP includes a measure of the "isometric" component of muscle contraction.[27] This index includes work and effort components that may indicate endurance during a weaning trial.

Oxygen Cost of Breathing

The amount of O_2 consumed by the ventilatory muscles ($\dot{V}O_2R$) is an estimate of respiratory effort at its most basic level. $\dot{V}O_2R$ can be estimated by measurement of O_2 consumption during active breathing compared with the patient being fully supported in the control mode:

$$\dot{V}O_2R = \dot{V}O_2 \text{ active breathing} - \dot{V}O_2 \text{ apnea}$$

Normal $\dot{V}O_2R$ is approximately 2% to 5% of total O_2 consumption; however, $\dot{V}O_2R$ can be 30% of total O_2 consumption during hyperventilation owing to severe dyspnea. Theoretically, $\dot{V}O_2R$ accounts for all factors that tax the respiratory muscles—that is, the external workload and the efficiency of the conversion between cellular energy and useful work. $\dot{V}O_2R$ is difficult to measure if the patient's condition is unstable. Other measures of respiratory muscle function are sought to assess the cost of breathing.

Assessing Ventilatory Drive

Until more recently, little attention was paid to measurement of respiratory drive during critical illness. During machine-assisted breathing, ventilatory drive can play an important role in determining the energy expenditure of the patient. One study showed that patients not being weaned from mechanical ventilation often have an elevated drive to breathe and a limited ability to respond to increases in ventilatory load (e.g., increased $PaCO_2$).[28]

A measure that has been used to index drive is $P_{0.1}$. $P_{0.1}$ is the pressure recorded 100 msec after initiation of an inspiratory effort against an occluded airway. $P_{0.1}$ is influenced by muscle strength and lung volume but does not depend on respiratory mechanics. Elevated $P_{0.1}$ (>6 cm H_2O) indicates a continuing need for mechanical ventilation.

In a sophisticated, commercially available system, a direct measure of the neural drive to breathe from the phrenic nerve can be measured by a catheter positioned within the esophagus. This signal is integrated into a feedback circuit in a modern ventilator. As a mode within the ventilator, flow delivery is coordinated and augmented in response to the neural drive to breathe; this is known as *neurally adjusted ventilatory assist.* (See Chapters 42 and 44 for details.)

Rapid Shallow Breathing Index

When muscular strength is limited, patients tend to meet minute ventilation ($\dot{V}_E$) requirements by increasing frequency (f) while decreasing V_T. Although smaller breaths require less effort, rapid shallow breathing increases dead space ventilation causing a need for higher minute ventilation to eliminate CO_2. A very high and continuously increasing frequency (>30 breaths/min) is a sign of ventilatory muscle decompensation and, potentially, impending fatigue.

Considerable attention has been focused on the rapid shallow breathing index (f/V_T ratio), a simple bedside index that indicates whether mechanically ventilated patients can breathe without mechanical assistance.[29] The f/V_T ratio is easy to measure and is independent of the patient's effort and cooperation. Discontinuation of ventilator support is likely to prove successful if f/V_T ratio is less than 105 breaths/min per L within the first minute of a brief trial of fully spontaneous breathing.[29]

Respiratory Inductive Plethysmography

Respiratory inductive plethysmography is a noninvasive means of monitoring frequency, V_T, fractional duration of inspiration (T_i/T_{tot}), and respiratory muscle coordination. With this technique, loose elastic bands encircle the chest and abdomen. Band expansion and contraction during ventilation (spontaneous or supported) provides a volume-time plot that can also reflect short-term shifts in actual lung volume.

Monitoring Strength and Muscle Endurance

Two values commonly used for bedside assessment of respiratory muscle strength are **vital capacity (VC)** and **maximal inspiratory pressure (MIP).** A VC maneuver can be performed at the bedside with a simple respirometer connected to the patient's airway. Because VC is effort-dependent, accurate measurements can be obtained only when the patient is conscious and cooperative. Because of an expected variability in bedside VC, three measurements should be obtained, and the best result should be reported. Healthy persons are able to generate a VC of approximately 70 ml/kg. A VC less than 10 to 15 ml/kg indicates considerable muscle weakness, which indicates an inability to breathe spontaneously.

MIP is a more specific measure than VC. MIP provides information based solely on maximum output of the inspiratory muscles. A maximum stimulus is provided by total occlusion of the airway. In contrast to the VC maneuver, the MIP maneuver can be performed on unconscious or uncooperative patients. Measurement of MIP at the bedside requires an aneroid manometer with a maximum value indicator. In an effort to make the measurements more reliable, Marini and colleagues[30] described a modified technique in which a one-way valve is attached to the airway to ensure that inspiratory effort is made at a low lung volume. Maintaining an occlusion for 20 seconds, the values with the one-way valve in place were approximately one-third more negative than values without an occlusion (Figure 46-7).

Endurance: Maximum Voluntary Ventilation

Respiratory muscle fatigue (lack of endurance) may be a cause of respiratory failure. **Maximum voluntary ventilation (MVV)** is a measure used to assess respiratory muscle reserve, endurance, or fatigue. VC is measured to assess the patient's coordinated muscle function from a single breath; MVV is measured to determine the ability of a patient to sustain ventilation over time. Similar to the VC maneuver, the MVV procedure can be performed with a respirometer attached to the patient's airway as the patient is encouraged to breathe as deeply and as fast as possible over a predefined time interval (10 or 15 seconds). The value is extrapolated to a full minute.

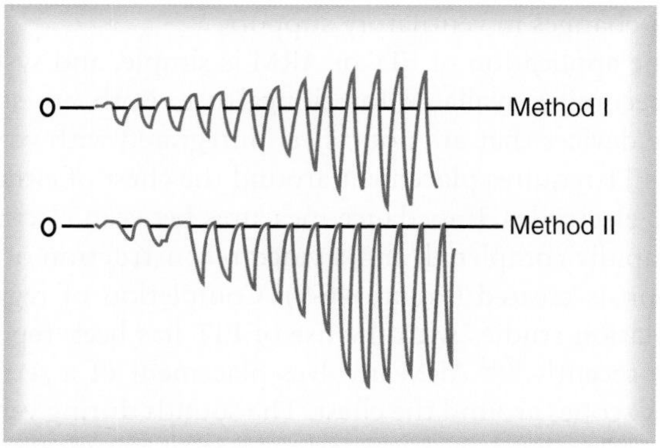

FIGURE 46-7 Measurement of MIP during 25 seconds of airway occlusion. *Method I* is occlusion by sealing the airway to allow no movement of air. *Method II* occludes inspiratory flow but allows expiratory flow through a unidirectional valve.

> **RULE OF THUMB**
>
> To wean from mechanical ventilation, the patient must have adequate gas exchange, respiratory muscle strength and endurance, and WOB that is not excessive. The original cause of respiratory failure must be partially, if not completely, resolved. Although numerous values have been studied to indicate the probability of successful weaning, a frequency-to-V_T ratio less than 105 has been the best index of ability to wean.

Normal MVV values for adults range from 120 to 180 L/min. Values less than twice the spontaneous minute ventilation are associated with difficulty in maintaining spontaneous ventilation without mechanical assistance.[31]

Lung Stress and Strain

During mechanical ventilation, the lungs are exposed to positive pressure that exerts more stress and strain on the lungs than experienced during spontaneous ventilation. This **lung stress and strain** may cause injury or extend existing lung injury along the injury/normal tissue border. When positive pressure becomes injurious, it is referred to as *ventilator-induced lung injury*. However, the concepts of stress and strain as applied to the lungs are not clearly defined. The physical definition of stress is a force per unit area. Strain is the deformation of a structure compared with its overall size. Hooke's law associates the two factors by the following relationship: stress = k * strain.

Working definitions for stress and strain applied to the lungs have been studied.[32] *Stress* is simply defined as Ptp ($P_{airway} - P_{esophageal}$). Driving pressure, as previously discussed, may be an alternative measure of stress. *Strain* has been defined as V_T (the deformation) divided by FRC (the resting size of the lungs). These definitions have been associated as stress = 13.5 * strain, predicting that a stress of 27 cm H_2O (Ptp of 27 cm H_2O) and a strain of 2 (V_T of twice the FRC) approach the limits of safe ventilation.[32] As previously discussed, Ptp requires placement of an esophageal catheter. To measure strain, automated FRC determinations have become available on some modern ventilators.[33] Stress can also occur at lower pressures if lung units are opening and closing during the ventilator cycle.

Stress Index

Another index involving the dynamic measurement of stress has been reported.[34] The **stress index** is a value derived from the airway pressure-time curve during

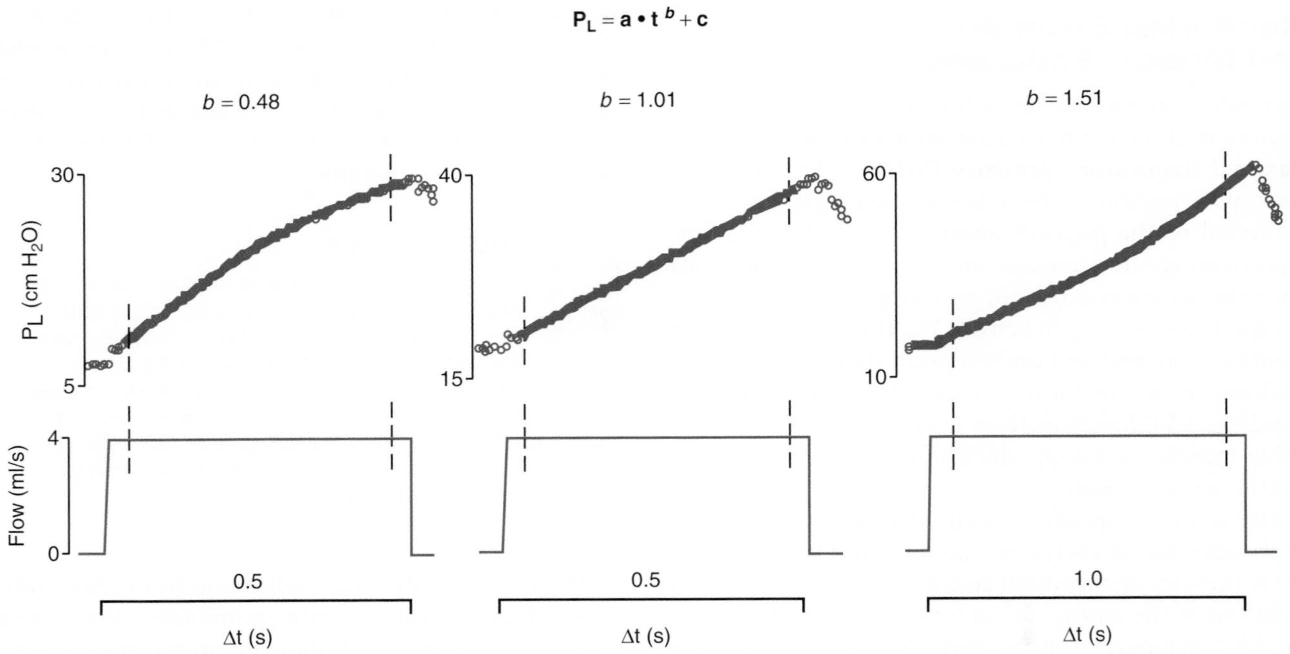

FIGURE 46-8 Conceptional illustration of the dynamic pressure-time (p-t) curve. *Left,* Convex curve indicating recruitment during the breath. *Center,* Linear relationship between pressure and time indicating no recruitment or overdistention. *Right,* Concave curve indicating overdistention. (From Formenti P, Graf J, Santos A, et al: Non-pulmonary factors strongly influence the stress index. Intensive Care Med 37:594–600, 2011.)

constant flow delivery of a tidal breath. During constant flow (when resistance is constant), the slope of the pressure-time tracing is analyzed to evaluate the elastic properties of the lungs. The index is calculated by performing a curve fit of the slope of the pressure-time tracing, where pressure = a * $time^b$ + c. Ideally, a slope (b) of 1 indicates normal filling during lung expansion, whereas a slope greater than 1 indicates overdistention, and a slope less than 1 indicates lung recruitment (Figure 46-8). This measure can be calculated for each delivered tidal breath, although an acceptance criterion should be used to exclude analysis of artifacts and factitious breaths. Although the index may not determine a threshold for excessive stress or strain, it may be a useful indicator of lung response to positive pressure. If the chest wall contributes variably to airway pressure, the calculated index can be altered and deceptive.[35]

Lung Mapping

The extent of gas exchange abnormalities is revealed by ABG values and SpO_2, but the location or source of the disorder remains unknown. The source, but not the extent or type of the pathologic process, can be assessed by auscultation. Localization of the disorder within the lungs is more precisely evaluated by static images obtained by radiographic techniques, such as chest x-ray or computed tomography (CT). These assessments are key to directing therapeutic approaches and for tracking changes in pathology. However, thorough imaging studies frequently require transportation of the patient to a radiology suite, and transport presents risks to the patient.[36] Also, the imaging is often static, not dynamically obtained throughout the ventilator cycle.

Mapping techniques that can actively locate regions of interest have been developed more recently. Two techniques are available that allow mapping of the lungs during ventilation: **electrical impedance tomography (EIT)** and **acoustic respiratory monitoring (ARM).** Each technique provides imaging of ventilation that allows localization of the injury and an assessment of the extent of injury. Each technique produces a two-dimensional video or graphic representation of ventilation; quiet regions without ventilation are not "seen." With EIT and ARM, there is an opportunity to perform at the bedside a real-time evaluation of the effects of PEEP, recruitment maneuvers, or other changes in ventilatory support.

The application of EIT or ARM is simple, and systems are becoming available for clinical use. Both are standalone devices that are not, as yet, integrated with ventilators. EIT requires placement around the chest of either 16 or 32 electrodes. Impedance measures between electrodes are rapidly completed, and a video reconstruction of ventilation is created (Figure 46-9). Completion of regional ventilation studies with the use of EIT has been reported more recently.[37,38] ARM involves placement of a series of stethoscopes around the chest. The sounds during ventilation are localized, and, similarly, a map of sounds (ventilation) is reconstructed. Specific characteristics of crackles from interstitial pulmonary fibrosis compared with congestive heart failure have been differentiated by ARM.[39]

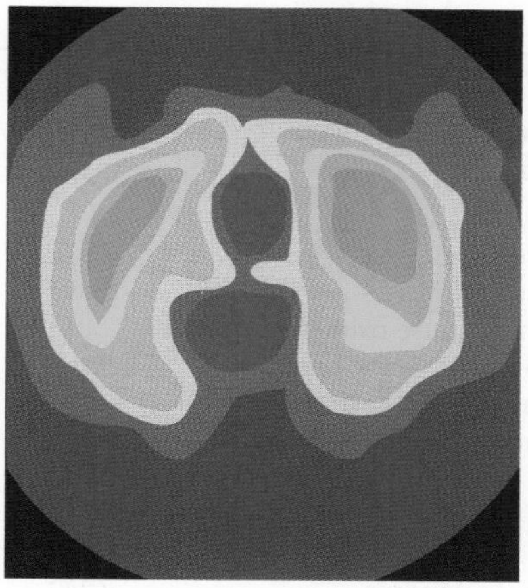

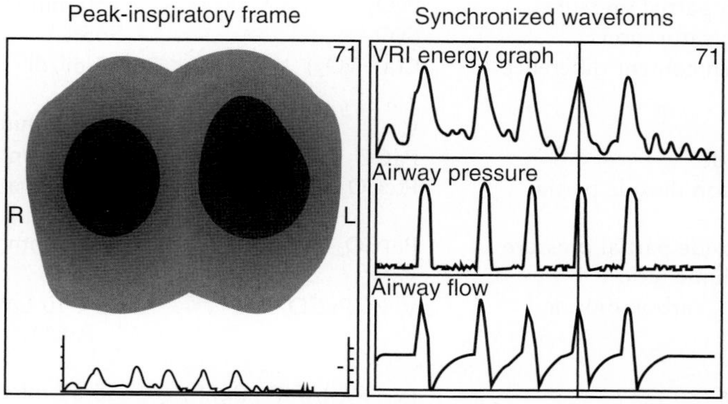

Sound energy distribution

	Right	Left
Upper	18%	25%
Middle	22%	25%
Lower	5%	5%
TOTAL	45%	55%

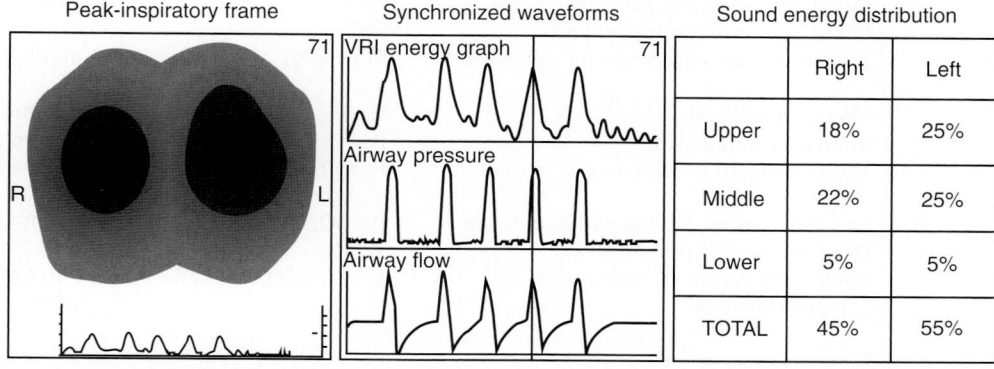

FIGURE 46-9 Mapping of ventilation by EIT. *Bottom,* Mapping of ventilation by acoustic respiratory monitoring.

Lung Ultrasonography

Bedside echocardiography has become routine within ICUs. An echocardiograph is obtained by skilled technicians interrogating the heart with an external ultrasound probe on the chest surface. The images obtained are two-dimensional dynamic videos that clearly display the chamber sizes, wall thicknesses, and cardiac performance. Ultrasound technology is not as helpful for imaging the lungs because air-filled lung tissue is not penetrated by ultrasound. However, pathologic processes outside the lungs can be seen by ultrasound, such as pleural fluids, air, or lesions. Pneumothorax, empyema, and pleural effusions are most frequently located by **lung ultrasonography;** their extent can be defined and treated with the use of ultrasound. As a diagnostic tool, lung ultrasonography is relatively inexpensive, can be performed in 15 minutes, and does not emit ionizing radiation. There is potential for ultrasonography to evaluate the lung expansion effects of recruitment maneuvers or high-frequency oscillation.

Monitoring Patient-Ventilator System

Monitoring of a patient during mechanical ventilatory support should include a physical examination (inspection, palpation, percussion, auscultation), assessment of oxygenation and ventilation, and assessment of ventilatory load and capacity. Table 46-1 lists key physiologic monitoring data and acceptable values for patients receiving mechanical ventilation. Monitoring of all aspects of the patient-ventilator system is an important responsibility that must be clearly delineated within the ICU. Monitoring a ventilated patient is the primary responsibility of the RT. Important areas of this responsibility include the following:

- Assessing the integrity of the airway and circuitry, including secretion clearance
- Maintaining the prescribed settings and assessing their appropriateness
- Ensuring acceptable gas exchange values
- Monitoring of respiratory system mechanics
- Evaluating the comfort and synchrony of breathing of the patient
- Setting of alarms
- Caring for any other safety issues, such as risk of extubation

A system of ensuring and documenting all aspects of safe and appropriate care must be in place. This system usually includes a manual or, more frequently, an electronic recording of all important settings, alarms, and ABG values at regular intervals. This monitoring process has been called *patient-ventilator assessments.* An example

TABLE 46-1

Physiologic Monitoring Data (Respiratory Values)

Function Assessed	Description of Value	Symbol/Formula	Acceptable Value
Oxygenation			
Lung exchange (external)			
Adequacy	Arterial oxygen pressure	PaO_2	60-100 mm Hg
	Arterial oxygen saturation	SaO_2	≥90%
	Oxygen saturation by pulse oximeter	SpO_2	≥90%
	Transcutaneous oxygen partial pressure	$PtcO_2$	60-100 mm Hg
Efficiency	Alveolar to arterial oxygen tension gradient	$P(A-a)O_2$	<350 mm Hg (100% O_2)
	Arterial to alveolar	PaO_2/PAO_2	>0.6
	Respiratory index	$P(A-a)O_2/PaO_2$	<5
	P/F ratio	PaO_2/FiO_2	>300
	Percentage shunt	$\dot{Q}_S/\dot{Q}_T$	<15%-20%
Time exchange (internal)	Mixed venous oxygen content	$C\bar{v}O_2$	>10.0 ml/dl
	Mixed venous oxygen partial pressure	$P\bar{v}O_2$	>30 mm Hg
	Mixed venous oxygen saturation	$S\bar{v}O_2$	>65%
	Arterial-venous oxygen content difference	$C(a-\bar{v}O_2)$	<7 ml/dl
Ventilation			
Adequacy	Minute ventilation	$\dot{V}_E$	5-10 L/min
	Arterial carbon dioxide	$PaCO_2$	35-45 mm Hg (normal pH)
	Transcutaneous carbon dioxide partial pressure	$PtcCO_2$	35-45 mm Hg (normal pH)
	End-tidal carbon dioxide partial pressure	$PETCO_2$	35-43 mm Hg (4.6%-5.6%)
Efficiency	Dead space/tidal volume ratio	V_D/V_T	<0.6
	Minute ventilation vs. carbon dioxide partial pressure	$\dot{V}_E$ vs. $PaCO_2$	$\dot{V}_E$ < 10 L/min with normal $PaCO_2$
Ventilatory Load			
Total impedance	Dynamic compliance	$(V_T-V_C)/(PIP-PEEP)$	35-50 ml/cm H_2O
Compliance	Effective compliance	$C_{eff}=\dfrac{(V_T-V_C)}{P_{plat}-PEEP}$	60-100 ml/cm H_2O
WOB	Work = kg × m/L or J/L	Work = P × V	<0.15 kg × m/L <1.5 J/L
Ventilatory Capacity			
Drive	Occlusion pressure	P0.1	<6 cm H_2O
	Mean inspiratory flow	V_T/T_i	Not established
Strength	Vital capacity	VC	>10-15 mL/kg
	Maximal inspiratory pressure	MIP; PI_{max}	<−20 to −30 cm H_2O
Endurance	Maximum voluntary ventilation	MVV	>20 L/min or 2 × $\dot{V}_E$
	Ratio of minute ventilation to MVV	$\dot{V}_E$/MVV	<1 : 2
	Pressure-time index	$(Pdi/Pmax)*TI/T_{tot}$	<0.15

of a recording form used for this purpose is shown in Figure 46-10. Increasingly, electronic transfer of ventilator settings and monitored data is being added to the electronic medical record. The responsibility of the RT is much greater than the task of recording values. This responsibility is care of a critically ill, vulnerable patient with respiratory failure who is being supported with a lifesaving machine. The procedure for performing a patient-ventilator system assessment is outlined in Table 46-2. Although the importance of monitoring the patient-ventilator system has increased, the necessity of entry and transcription of numbers into an assessment sheet is decreasing. The era of electronic transfer of monitored data directly to the patients' charts will soon become the standard. All modern ventilators have the capacity for data transfer, but until standardized transfer protocols, charting formats, and archiving methods are established, electronic monitoring of the patient-ventilator system will continue to be customized to the local setting.

Graphics Monitoring

Monitoring of graphic tracings generated during mechanical ventilation has become widely available and accepted in the ICU. A visual display of pressure, flow, and volume tracings is available on all modern ventilators. Graphic displays are possible through the development of improvements in sensing technology, integrated circuitry, and graphic-user interface. Ventilators measure inspiratory and expiratory flow and circuit pressure with pneumotachometers and transducers. The volume displays are generated through calculation of an integral of the flow tracings. All three values (flow, pressure, and volume) can

Adult Mechanical Ventilation Flow Sheet

Patient ______	Cuff pressure (volume) ______
Physician ______	☐ M.O.V. ☐ Minimal leak
Diagnosis ______	Ventilator ______ Vent. day ______
Age ______ Height ______	Circuit change (Date / Time) ______
Weight ______ Ideal body weight ______	Tape change (Date / Time) ______
ET tube / trach tube size ______	Other therapy ______
Tube Position (length) ______	______

Patient ID

Date							
Time							
Mode (A/C; SIMV, PSV, PCV, etc.)							
Set Tidal Volume / Delivered Tidal Volume							
Spontaneous Tidal Volume							
Machine Rate / Total Rate							
Minute Volume							
Peak Pressure / Static Pressure							
Mean Airway Pressure							
PEEP / CPAP [IPAP / EPAP]							
Auto PEEP							
Support / Pressure Control Level (cmH_2O)							
Sensitivity or Flowtrigger (Flowby)							
FIO2 Set / Analyzed							
Inspiratory Flow / Time							
Wave Form (⎍ |\ ⎍)							
I : E Ratio							
Sigh Volume / Sigh Frequency							
Airway Temperature							
Static Compliance / Dynamic Compliance							
Airway Resistance [(PIP - PLAT / Insp. Flow L/Sec)]							
Apnea Parameters Check (Y / N)							
ALARMS	Pressure High / Low						
	Low VT						
	High / Low VE						
	High rate						
BLOOD GASES	pH						
	PaO2						
	PaC02						
	Sa02 / Oximetry (Sp02)						
	Hb						
	HC03-						
	B.E.						
	Ca02						
	Pv02						
	Sv02						
	Ca02 - Cv02						
	Qs / Qt						
	Vd / Vt						
	P (ET) C02						
HEMO DYNAMICS	Pulse						
	Blood Pressure (Systolic / Diastolic)						
	CVP						
	PAP (Systolic / Diastolic)						
	PCWP						
	Cardiac Output / Cardiac Index						
	SVR						
	PVR						
SPONTANEOUS	MIP / MEP						
	Vital Capacity (VC)						
	Spontaneous Volumes (VT / VE)						
	Spontaneous Rate (f)						
	RSBI (f/VT)						
Other							
Initials							

A

FIGURE 46-10 Ventilator flow sheet.

Continued

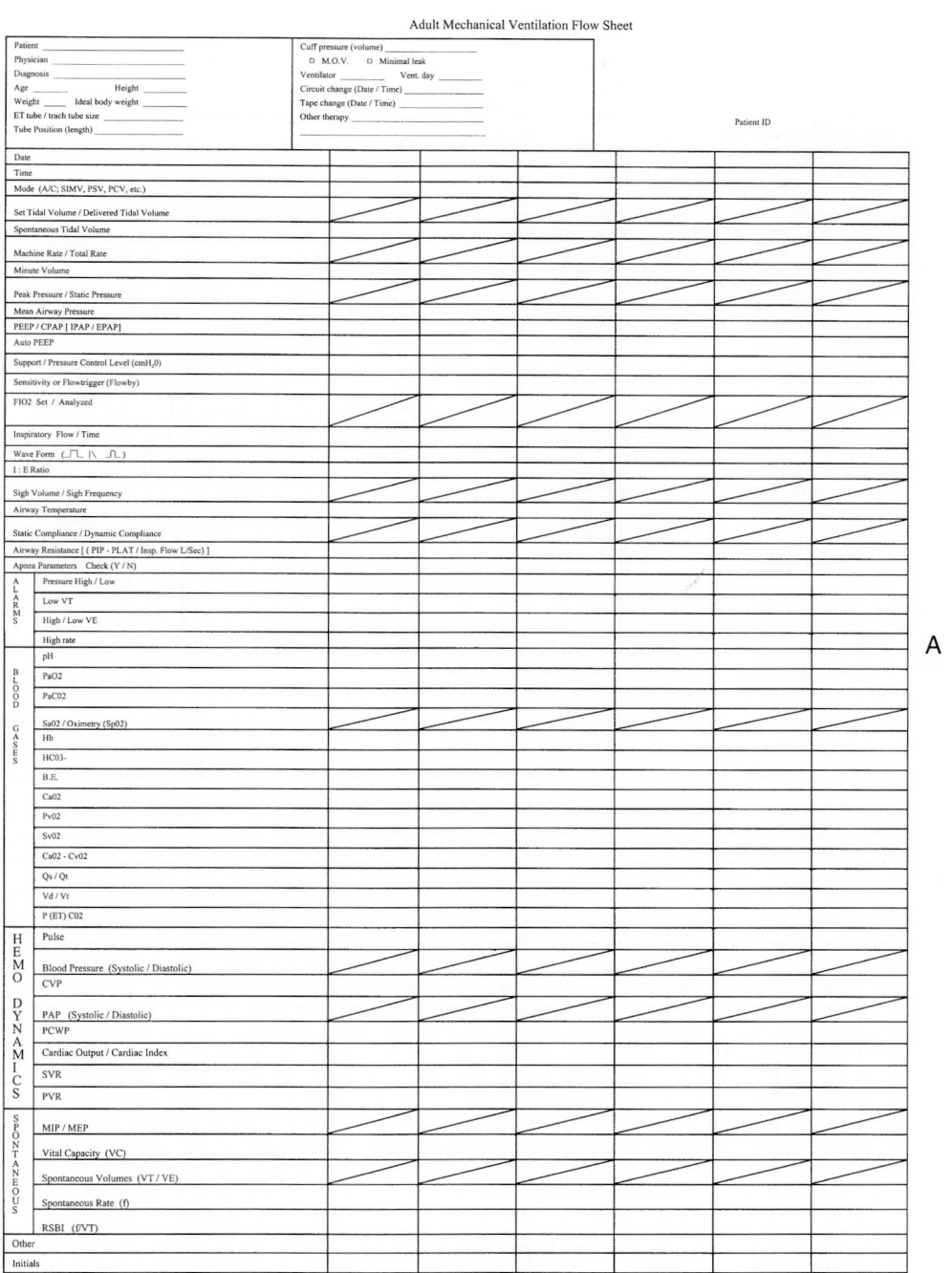

Adult Mechanical Ventilation Flow Sheet

Respiratory Care Progress Notes

S: (pt Awareness, response, sedations / paralytics) Responds ☐ Non-responsive ☐ Sedated ☐ Paralytics ☐ See comment ☐ ☐

O: (WOB, Color, Chest Expansion, BBS, Sputum Production, latest x-ray, pertinent pt assessment concerns, lab values, fluids)

General Skin Color
- ☐ Pink
- ☐ Ashy
- ☐ Cyanotic
- ☐ Jaundice

Skin Characteristics
- ☐ Warm
- ☐ Dry
- ☐ Diaphoretic
- ☐ Cool
- ☐ Moist

Mucous Membranes
- ☐ Pink
- ☐ Ashy
- ☐ Cyanotic

Work of Breathing
- ☐ Normal
- ☐ Mild
- ☐ Moderate
- ☐ High
- ☐ Absent

Chest Excursion
- ☐ Bilateral
- ☐ Unilateral
- ☐ Diminished
- ☐ Paradoxical/Flail

Chest Configuration
- ☐ Normal
- ☐ Other__________

- ☐ Subcutaneous Emphysema
- ☐ Tactile Fremitus
- ☐ Tracheal Deviation
- ☐ Abdominal Distention

Nailbeds
- ☐ Pink
- ☐ Ashy
- ☐ Cyanotic

Capillary Refill
- ☐ Rapid
- ☐ Sluggish

Anterior

Auscultation
1) Clear
2) Wheeze
3) Crackles
4) Rhonchi

Posterior
A. Good Aeration
B. Diminished
C. Absent

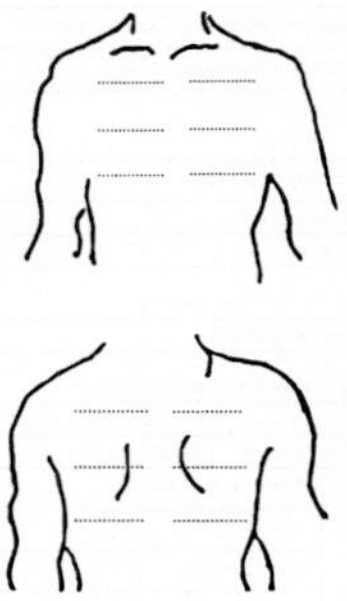

B

A: (Pt history, Admit dx. & date, events leading to intubation/trach/ventilation, significant problems, etc.)

P: (Care plan , standing orders, treatments)

WEANING MECHANICS		
TIME		
VC		
I/E FORCES		
VT		
RR		
VE		
f/VT		

Pt. EVENTS / CHANGES	Time	(Reasons for changes, significant pt. events, CT Scan, chest tube placement, BP problems, codes, etc.)

Signature ______________ Initials ______

FIGURE 46-10, cont'd.

TABLE 46-2

Performing a Patient-Ventilator System Assessment

Step	Key Points
Gather correct equipment and supplies	Respirometer, O_2 analyzer, stethoscope, and watch with second indicator are needed. *Note:* Most modern ventilators incorporate volume-measuring devices into the system Additional auxiliary equipment may include pulse oximeter, cuff pressure manometer, suction and airway equipment, and sterile distilled water
Review patient record	Note patient's admitting diagnosis or problem list, physician orders, medications, vital signs, history and physical examination findings, progress notes, results of laboratory studies, chest radiograph, blood gases, and respiratory care notes
Enter patient area; wash hands and put on gloves	Inattention to proper handwashing and poor aseptic technique are associated with nosocomial infection
Identify the patient	Wristbands sometimes may be attached to the patient's leg or to the foot of the bed If there is no attached name band, check with the patient's nurse
Explain what you are doing	Communication with the patient is important; even patients who appear unaware of their surroundings may be able to hear and understand Use broad terms, such as "I'm here to assess your breathing"
Observe overall situation and note general patient condition, including level of consciousness, condition of extremities, presence of pallor, skin color, capillary refill, airway patency, circuit connection and patency, and ECG findings	Note general appearance, sensorium, color, and level of activity Note equipment in use, including ventilator, circuit, airway type, humidification, manual resuscitation bag, and related equipment and supplies Ensure that the patient's condition appears stable and that ventilation is adequate
Drain tubing and service humidifier, if needed	This procedure should be done before the actual ventilator check, if possible
Attend to patient's airway, if necessary	Suctioning and other airway manipulation should be done before actual ventilator check, if possible; after suctioning, note volume and character of secretions Note endotracheal or tracheostomy tube stability and position; measure tube cuff pressure and volume to inflate If ventilator check is performed first and the patient circuit or airway is disrupted, errors may not be caught, and one of the purposes of ventilator monitoring, patient safety, is defeated
Inspect chest and note accessory muscle use, retractions, jugular vein engorgement, bilateral symmetric chest wall movement, symmetric diaphragm–chest wall movement, respiratory rate and rhythm, and chest wall stability (flail)	Be alert for signs of respiratory distress, increased WOB or patient-ventilatory asynchrony Observe patient effort to ensure adequate trigger sensitivity and inspiratory flow rate
Auscultate chest	Always move stethoscope from side to side to compare right and left sides of chest Note adventitious breath sounds (crackles, rhonchi, wheezing, bronchovesicular breath sounds) Note diminished or absent breath sounds; if breath sounds are absent, attempt to ascertain cause immediately Water in the tubing, use of chest tubes, or PEEP may result in adventitious sounds
Percuss chest for dullness, resonance, or hyperresonance	Dullness may be caused by pleural effusion, atelectasis, or consolidation Resonance is the percussion note found over normal lung tissue Hyperresonance is associated with excess air in the chest (pneumothorax, pulmonary hyperinflation)
Note location of trachea	Tracheal shift is associated with severe atelectasis and tension pneumothorax
Note peak pressure, static or plateau pressure (P_{plat}), baseline pressure (PEEP/CPAP), pressure support level, MAP, and presence of auto-PEEP	Sudden increase in peak airway pressure is associated with pneumothorax, secretions in the airway, bronchospasm, fighting the ventilator, biting the endotracheal tube, occlusion of the airway, and bronchial intubation

Continued

TABLE 46-2

Performing a Patient-Ventilator System Assessment—cont'd

Step	Key Points
	Sudden decrease in peak airway pressure is associated with reversal of any of the above-mentioned conditions, a leak in the system, or patient disconnection MAP may be useful in predicting a decrease in CO or barotraumas; the lowest possible MAP needed to achieve adequate ventilation and oxygenation should be used P_{plat} > 30-35 cm H_2O is associated with barotraumas; if P_{plat} is ≥30-35 cm H_2O, consider reducing delivered V_T
Record exhaled volume (ml/kg predicted body weight) and respiratory frequency	Ensure ventilator compensates for compressible volume If volume is measured at the exhalation valve, volume loss caused by tubing compliance may be calculated and subtracted from the measured volume
If intermittent mandatory ventilation (IMV)/SIMV system is in use, calculate delivered volume per machine breath, spontaneous volume between machine breaths, machine rate, total rate, patient spontaneous rate, and minute ventilation	For IMV/SIMV: $V_{ISP} = \frac{\dot{V}_{Etot} - \dot{V}_{Emech}}{f_{tot} - f_{mach}}$ For assist control: $\text{Average } V_T = \frac{\dot{V}_{Etot}}{f_{tot}}$
If a ventilator graphics package is in use, observe pressure-time, flow-time, volume-time, and P-V curves	Mode of ventilation, patient trigger, adequacy of machine inspiratory flow, and patient-ventilator synchrony can be evaluated with a ventilator graphics package Slow flow P-V curve can be used to assess lower and upper inflection points Overdistention can be elevated with use of dynamic P-V curve Flow-volume curve may be helpful in assessing effect of bronchodilator
Note delivered FiO_2	FiO_2 should be analyzed
Record other ventilatory values	Ventilatory values include inspiratory flow, inspiratory time, I:E ratio, inspiratory and expiratory positive airway pressures (IPAP and EPAP), sigh volume and rate, airway temperature, compliance and resistance, and alarm settings Many departments chart endotracheal tube size, tube length, cuff pressure or volume, use of minimal occluding volume or minimal leak, ventilator day, circuit change, and other therapy
Record blood gas values and related data, as appropriate	These data may include pH, PaO_2, $PaCO_2$, SaO_2, hemoglobin level, HCO_3^- level, IPAP, base excess, and CaO_2 Blood gas data should be recorded in such a way that the corresponding FiO_2, PEEP, V_T, frequency, mode, and other ventilator settings on which the sample was obtained are noted
Record results of other physiologic monitoring of cardiopulmonary system, as appropriate	These values may include SpO_2, $P_{ET}CO_2$, $PtcCO_2$, $PtcO_2$, $\dot{Q}_S/\dot{Q}_T$, and V_D/V_T
Record hemodynamic data, as appropriate	These values may include heart rate, blood pressure, CVP, PAP, PCWP, $\dot{Q}_T$, cardiac index, $S\bar{v}O_2$, $P\bar{v}O_2$, $CaO_2 - C\bar{v}O_2$, pulmonary vascular resistance, and systemic vascular resistance
Record weaning values as appropriate	These values may include spontaneous frequency, V_T, f/V_T ratio, $\dot{V}_E$, VC, and inspiratory force (MIP)
Return all alarm systems to optimal condition. Complete charting using appropriate departmental forms or computer entry systems	Alarms include low pressure, high pressure, disconnection, and volume Apnea values should be reviewed. Apnea values usually are set to deliver an adequate V_T, f_{mach}, and FiO_2 (100%) in the event of apnea development

be displayed and plotted against time or each other (Figure 46-11).

Ventilator manufacturers have developed the graphic displays that allow astute clinicians to base decisions on many more factors than gas exchange values (Box 46-8). However, the study and verification of features observed in ventilator graphics have not developed at the pace of the technology. Ventilator graphics show many important patient-ventilator interactions, such as presence of auto-PEEP, elevated airway pressure, presence of secretions, and general pattern and dependability of supported ventilation (Figure 46-12). The potential for expanded use of ventilator graphics awaits further investigation of the clinical importance of the graphic displays. For more details, see Chapter 44.

Monitoring During Lung Protective Ventilation

A lung protective ventilation strategy that reduces the risk of pressure injury to the lungs has evolved from numerous animal studies and several key clinical studies.[40] Meticulous monitoring of the status of patients with ALI/ARDS

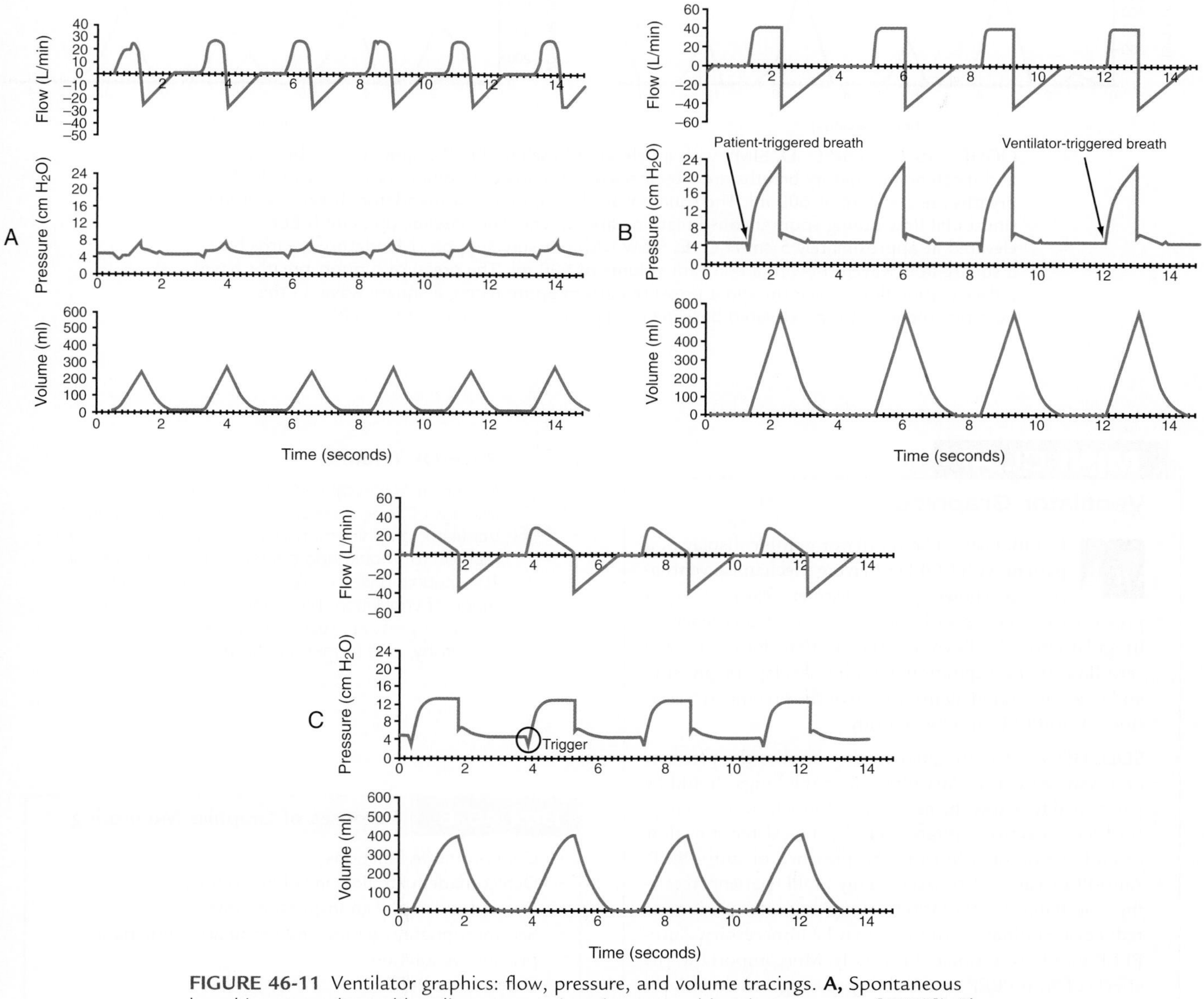

FIGURE 46-11 Ventilator graphics: flow, pressure, and volume tracings. **A,** Spontaneous breathing at an elevated baseline pressure (continuous positive airway pressure [CPAP]). Flow, pressure, and volume curves show spontaneous breathing with a CPAP level of approximately 5 cm H_2O. The flow curve is sinusoidal, the pressure curve fluctuates approximately 1 to 3 cm H_2O around the baseline pressure, and the volume delivered varies. These are typical observations during spontaneous breathing. **B,** Volume ventilation in the assist-control mode. Some breaths are time-triggered, and others are patient-triggered. There is a square wave flow pattern, and volume is constant, breath to breath. **C,** Pressure support breaths (pressure support ventilation). The patient trigger for each breath is evident. Flow is decelerating, and the pressure waveform approaches a square wave. *Continued*

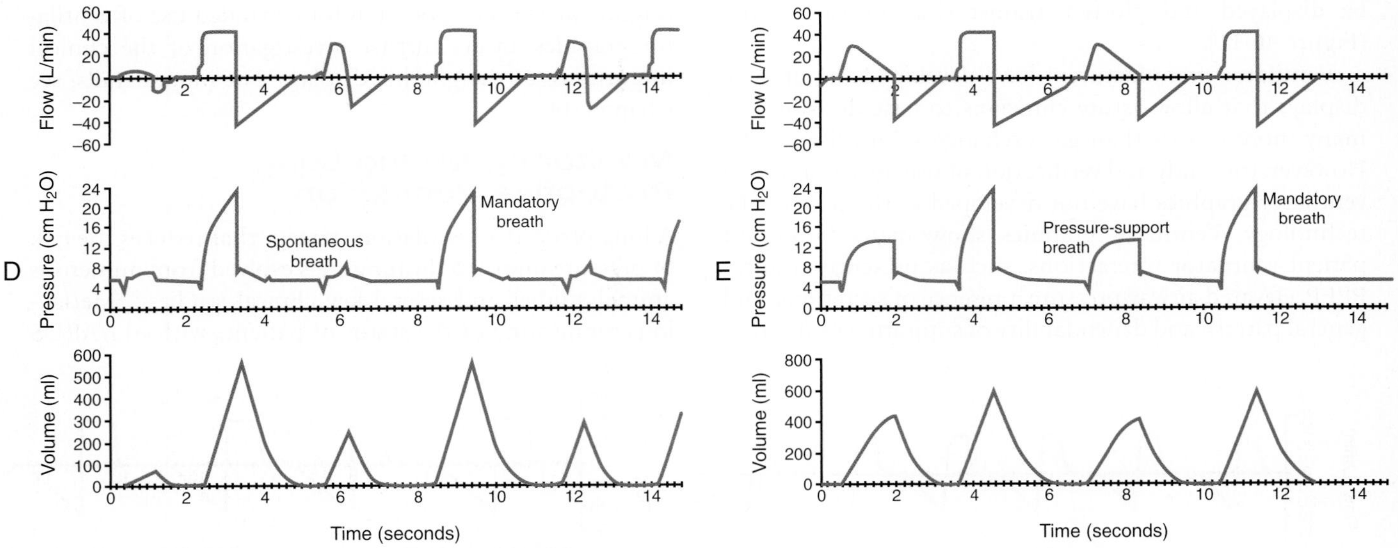

FIGURE 46-11, cont'd **D,** SIMV with an elevated baseline (PEEP). Spontaneous breathing and machine mandatory breaths are interspersed. Spontaneous volume varies, but the SIMV breaths are constant at 600 ml. The square wave flow pattern for mandatory breaths and the sinusoidal flow during spontaneous breathing are evident. The baseline pressure (PEEP) is elevated at approximately 5 cm H_2O. **E,** SIMV with pressure support. Mandatory breaths have a square flow waveform with a constant volume of 600 ml. The pressure support breaths have a decelerating flow waveform and a pressure pattern approaching a square wave. In this example, there is also an elevated baseline of approximately +5 cm H_2O (PEEP).

MINI CLINI

Ventilator Graphics

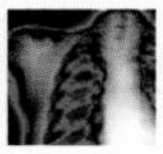

PROBLEM: The ventilator graphic display of a patient with COPD receiving mechanical ventilation is showing two distinct features: (1) a pressure-time tracing with spikes and dips that is generally irregular and (2) a flow-time tracing that does not reach zero flow at end expiration. Graphic displays of pressure and flow allow rapid identification of the presence of secretions, auto-PEEP, and asynchrony.

SOLUTION: The irregular tracing implies the presence of airway secretions. Auscultation of the lungs should be performed to assess the need for endotracheal suctioning. Without an active expiratory effort, the existence of flow at end expiration confirms the presence of auto-PEEP. Auto-PEEP can be detected in many COPD patients receiving mechanical ventilation. However, intervention to reduce or eliminate auto-PEEP may be unnecessary. Auto-PEEP should be estimated regularly. More important, the effects of auto-PEEP on the ability to trigger the ventilator or on cardiovascular dynamics (caused by reduced venous return) should be monitored. For reduction or elimination of auto-PEEP, adjusting the ventilator settings or bronchodilator therapy may be required. If the patient is unable to trigger every breath because of the auto-PEEP, apply PEEP in steps of 1 to 2 cm H_2O until the patient is able to trigger the ventilator with every inspiratory effort.

RULE OF THUMB

Modern mechanical ventilators routinely display tracings of flow, pressure, and volume versus time. Ventilator graphics monitoring is a convenient visual method for monitoring patient-ventilator interaction. The graphic patterns allow rapid determination of mode of ventilation, breathing pattern, auto-PEEP, excessive pressure, secretions in the airway, synchrony, and triggering efforts.

Box 46-8 Purposes of Graphics Monitoring

- Confirm mode functions
- Detect inadequate flow in volume ventilation
- Detect too lengthy an inspiratory time
- Set appropriate rise time and termination criteria in pressure ventilation
- Detect auto-PEEP
- Determine patient-ventilator synchrony
- Assess and adjust trigger levels
- Measure WOB
- Adjust V_T and minimize overdistention
- Assess effect of administration of bronchodilators
- Detect equipment malfunction
- Determine appropriate PEEP level

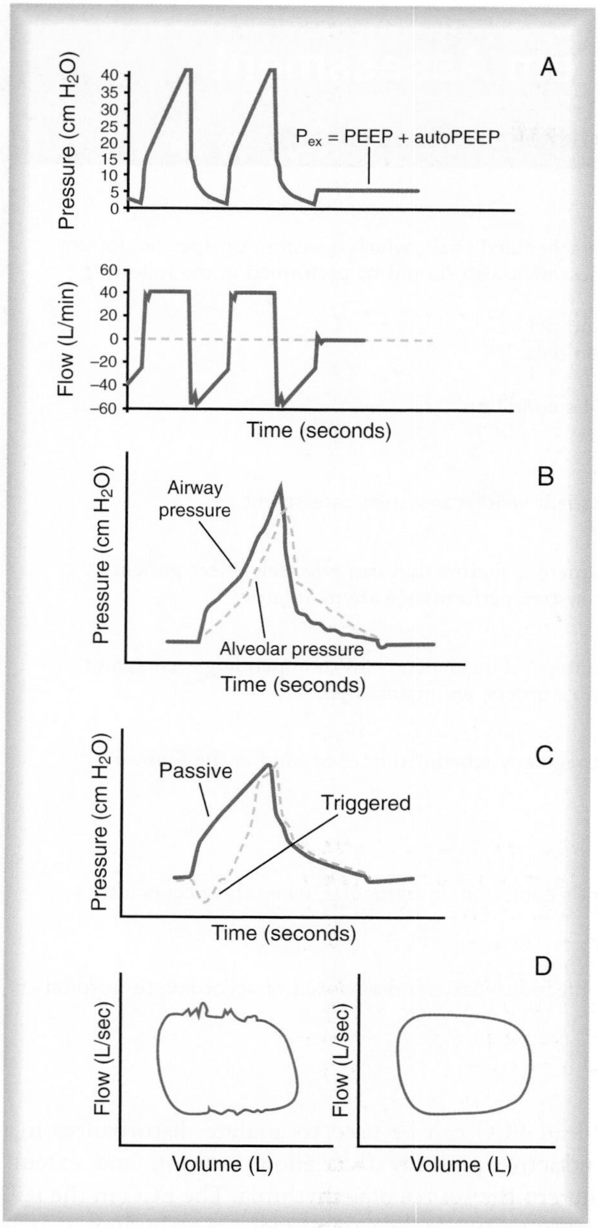

FIGURE 46-12 Patient-ventilator interactions easily identified from tracings of continuous monitoring of pressure, volume, and flow. **A,** Auto-PEEP. Flow and pressure tracings during ventilator-supported breaths and during end expiratory occlusion. The airway pressure during the end expiratory occlusion is an auto-PEEP estimate. **B,** Overdistention. The upper concavity of the airway pressure-time tracing is indicative of overdistention. This example also shows alveolar pressure and its corresponding overdistention. **C,** Patient effort. This is an example of mechanically ventilated passive inflation pressure and the airway pressure-time tracing deformation caused by effort by the patient. **D,** Presence of secretions. P-V tracing of a ventilator-supported breath displays the presence of secretions. The inspiratory and expiratory limbs are irregular (not smooth) when secretions are present. An irregular airflow-time tracing also can indicate the presence of secretions.

or patients at risk of ALI/ARDS is necessary to avoid ventilator-induced lung injury. Three principles have been confirmed: (1) reduce the risk of high-pressure exposure by limiting P_{plat} to less than 30 cm H_2O, (2) reduce V_T ventilation to 4 to 8 ml/kg, and (3) maintain adequate end expiratory lung volume with PEEP to avoid opening/closing injury. The AARC created a clinical practice guideline on patient-ventilator system assessment; excerpts from this guideline appear in Clinical Practice Guideline 46-1.

Other considerations have received attention in monitoring patients with ALI/ARDS. Although P-V curves have been automated in ventilator algorithms, the clinical significance of curves determined from PEEP of 0 cm H_2O is questionable. However, current recommendations are to maintain ventilation on the upper portion of the deflation limb of the P-V curve to avoid alveolar derecruitment even though this position with the P-V hysteresis curve of a patient may be difficult to determine. A primary concern is to achieve adequate oxygenation in patients with lung injury, but this target can be deceptive if the price of adequate oxygenation is pressure injury to the lungs. An acceptable practice in ventilating these patients is permissive hypercapnia or pressure-protective ventilation that allows $PaCO_2$ to drift upward. This strategy is a higher frequency–lower V_T approach with the predictable effect of decreasing pH that requires careful monitoring.

As previously discussed, elevated chest wall or abdominal compliance must also be considered during lung protective ventilation. This concern can be significant in obese patients. Essentially, the stiffer the chest wall or abdomen, the greater is the P_{plat} that can be established without inducing lung injury. In particularly challenging patients with ARDS, high-frequency ventilation has been considered.[41] The importance of setting an elevated PEEP level to maintain an open lung has been established in animal studies.[42] However, large multicenter studies designed to determine the effect of high PEEP on mortality in ALI/ARDS have reported conflicting results.[43,44] Nevertheless, setting PEEP levels greater than 15 cm H_2O is often necessary in patients with ARDS to maintain oxygenation. Elevated PEEP places greater importance on monitoring cardiovascular performance and development of barotrauma.

CARDIAC AND CARDIOVASCULAR MONITORING

The cardiovascular system is routinely monitored in the critical care setting because patient survival depends on reliable, competent cardiac and cardiovascular performance. There is little question about the importance of monitoring ECG, a noninvasive, continuous assessment of the performance of the conduction system of the heart. In the care of acutely ill patients, there may be clear justification for continuous monitoring of arterial blood pressure.

46-1 Patient-Ventilator System Assessment

AARC Clinical Practice Guideline (Excerpts)*

INDICATIONS

A patient-ventilator system assessment must be performed on a scheduled basis, which is institution-specific, for any patient requiring mechanical ventilation for life support. An assessment also should be performed in the following circumstances:

- Before obtaining blood samples for analysis of blood gases and pH
- Before obtaining hemodynamic or bedside pulmonary function data
- After any change in ventilator settings
- As soon as possible after an acute deterioration of the patient's condition
- Anytime ventilator performance is questionable

CONTRAINDICATIONS

There are no absolute contraindications to performance of a patient-ventilator system assessment.

ASSESSMENT OF NEED

Because of the complexity of mechanical ventilators and the numerous factors that can adversely affect patient-ventilator interaction, routine assessments of patient-ventilator system performance are mandatory.

ASSESSMENT OF OUTCOME

Routine patient-ventilator system assessments should prevent untoward incidents; warn of impending events; and ensure that proper ventilator settings, according to the physician's orders, are maintained.

FREQUENCY

A patient-ventilator system assessment should be performed at regularly scheduled intervals and in the following circumstances:

- After any change in ventilator settings
- Before obtaining any blood gas samples
- Before obtaining hemodynamic or pulmonary function data
- As soon as possible after an acute deterioration of the patient's condition, in particular, when this occurs after a violation of the ventilator alarm threshold

INFECTION CONTROL ISSUES

- Condensation from the patient circuit should be considered infectious waste and disposed of according to hospital policy.
- Universal precautions should be observed.

More controversial has been the assessment of left ventricular function by right heart catheterization with measurement of pulmonary capillary wedge pressure (PCWP) and continuous monitoring of pulmonary artery pressure (PAP). Although highly invasive, assessment of preload, contractility, and afterload (Figure 46-13) may be necessary to guide therapy. In addition to the invasive nature of pulmonary artery catheterization, improper interpretation of the pulmonary artery tracing can present problems.[2] Although direct monitoring of cardiac and cardiovascular function is performed at the bedside, assessment of troponins, cardiac enzymes, brain natriuretic peptide, or other serologic indicators of heart damage usually is conducted in the clinical laboratory. Table 46-3 summarizes cardiovascular monitoring criteria with normal ranges and abnormal values.

Electrocardiography

The conduction system of the heart is monitored in the ICU with a purpose different from that of the standard 12-lead ECG examination (see Chapter 17). The standard 12-lead ECG can be used to analyze disturbances in the conductive pathway that allow location and extent of injury or the source of arrhythmia. The ECG in the ICU is used primarily to detect and manage arrhythmias such as tachycardia, bradycardia, atrioventricular dissociation, ventricular tachycardia, atrial flutter, premature ventricular contractions, and ventricular fibrillation. For this purpose, there is a need for only three electrodes: right arm (or shoulder or right upper chest), left arm (or shoulder or left upper chest), and left lower chest. The deflections usually represent lead II of a standard 12-lead ECG. The direction or amplitude of the waves is of lesser concern than the rhythms being displayed.

When any arrhythmia is detected, therapy or intervention should be considered. The source of the arrhythmia often necessitates management of the underlying cause, such as O_2 therapy for hypoxia or changes or addition to infusion therapy for fluid and electrolyte disturbances. In the ICU, certain interventions may be necessary and must be immediately available. A defibrillator must be available when ventricular fibrillation is detected.

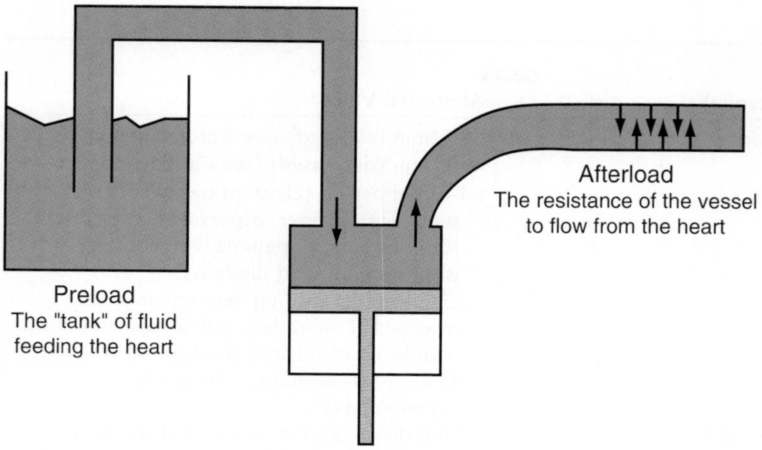
Afterload
The resistance of the vessel
to flow from the heart
Preload
The "tank" of fluid
feeding the heart
Contractility
The strength and rate
of cardiac contractions

FIGURE 46-13 Preload contractility and afterload.

TABLE 46-3
Cardiovascular Monitoring Criteria

Criterion	Normal Value (Range)	Abnormal Value
Heart rate (HR)	80 beats/min (60-100 beats/min)	>100 beats/min (tachycardia) <60 beats/min (bradycardia)
Arterial blood pressure (ABP)	120/80 mm Hg (90-140/60-90 mm Hg)	<140/90 mm Hg (hypertension) <90/60 mm Hg (hypotension)
Mean arterial blood pressure ($\overline{MAP}$)	90 mm Hg (80-100 mm Hg)	<80 mm Hg (hypotension) >100 mm Hg (hypertension)
ECG	Normal heart rate and rhythm	PR interval >0.2 sec (tachycardia, bradycardia, heart block [first, second, or third degree], premature ventricular contractions, premature atrial contractions, atrial fibrillation, atrial flutter, elevated ST segment, inverted T wave, ventricular tachycardia, ventricular fibrillation, asystole)
Central venous pressure (CVP)	2-6 mm Hg	>6 mm Hg (fluid overload, right ventricular failure, pulmonary hypertension, valvular stenosis, pulmonary embolus, cardiac tamponade, pneumothorax, positive pressure ventilation, PEEP, left ventricular failure) <2 mm Hg (hypovolemia, blood loss, shock, peripheral vasodilation, cardiovascular collapse)
Pulmonary artery pressure (PAP)	25/10 mm Hg (20-35/5-15 mm Hg)	>35/15 mm Hg (pulmonary hypertension, left ventricular failure, fluid overload) <20/5 mm Hg (pulmonary hypotension, hypovolemia, cardiovascular collapse)
Mean pulmonary artery pressure ($\overline{PAP}$)	15 mm Hg (10-20 mm Hg)	>20 mm Hg (same as ↑ PAP) <10 mm Hg (same as ↓ PAP)
Pulmonary capillary wedge pressure (PCWP)	5-10 mm Hg (<18 mm Hg)	>18 mm Hg (left ventricular failure, fluid overload) >20 mm Hg (interstitial edema) >25 mm Hg (alveolar filling) >30 mm Hg (frank pulmonary edema) <5 mm Hg (hypovolemia, shock, cardiovascular collapse)

Continued

TABLE 46-3

Cardiovascular Monitoring Criteria—cont'd

Criterion	Normal Value (Range)	Abnormal Value
Cardiac output ($\dot{Q}_T$ or CO)	5 L/min (4-8 L/min)	>8 L/min (elevated) (see Cardiac index) <4 L/min (decreased) (see Cardiac index)
Cardiac index (CI)	2.5-4 L/min per m^2	>4 L/min per m^2 (elevated owing to stress, septic shock, fever, hypervolemia, or drugs [dobutamine, dopamine, epinephrine, isoproterenol, and digitalis]) <2.5 L/min per m^2 (left ventricular failure, myocardial infarction, pulmonary embolus, high levels of positive pressure ventilation, PEEP, pneumothorax, blood loss, hypovolemia)
Systemic vascular resistance (SVR)	900-1400 dynes-sec/cm^5 (11.25-17.5 mm Hg/L per min)	>1400 dynes-sec/cm^5 (increased owing to vasoconstrictors [dopamine, norepinephrine, and epinephrine], hypovolemia, late septic shock) <900 dynes-sec/cm^5 (decreased owing to vasodilators [nitroglycerin, nitroprusside, and morphine] or early septic shock)
Pulmonary vascular resistance (PVR)	110-250 dynes-sec/cm^5 (1.38-3.13 mm Hg/L per min)	>250 dynes-sec/cm^5 (hypoxemia, ↓ pH, $PaCO_2$, vasopressors, emboli, emphysema, interstitial fibrosis, pneumothorax) <110 dynes-sec/cm^5 (pulmonary vasodilators, nitric oxide, O_2, calcium blockers)

CI = $\dot{Q}_T$/Body surface area.
SVR = $[(\overline{MAP} - CVP)/CO] \times 80$ = dynes-sec/cm^5.
PVR = $[(\overline{PAP} - PCWP)/CO] - 80$ = dynes-sec/cm^5.

Arterial Blood Pressure Monitoring

Arterial blood pressure is a crucial measurement for assessing the integrity of cardiovascular tone and the probability that O_2 delivery is dependable. Regulation of cardiovascular tone is under the influence of the autonomic nervous system, but there are other factors that affect blood pressure, such as fluid status or the effects of medications. Major concerns include the adequacy of O_2 delivery during hypotension and the risks of hypertension, such as increased hydrostatic pressure or stroke. Continuous monitoring of the actual blood pressure is performed by placement of a catheter usually in the femoral or radial artery. Because fluid is not compressible, the catheter and connecting tubing are filled with saline solution so that the arterial pressure is transmitted to a transducer that allows display of the arterial pressure tracing (Figure 46-14). The transducer must be properly zeroed and calibrated to reflect the true values of the deflections. The arterial line also provides access for obtaining arterial blood for ABG analysis.

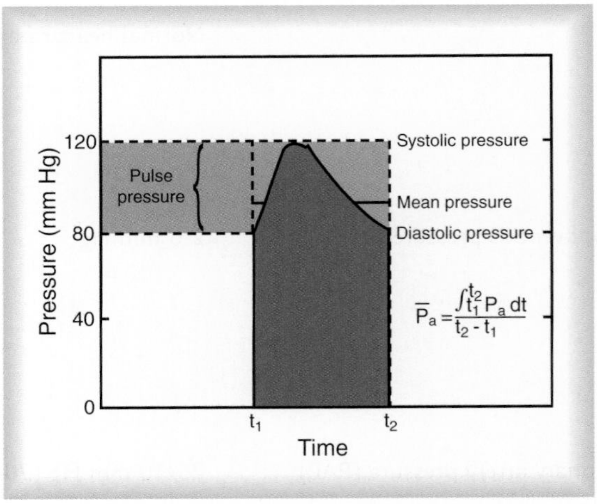

FIGURE 46-14 Arterial pressure wave form systolic pressure, diastolic pressure, MAP, and pulse pressure.

Central Venous Pressure–Right Atrial Pressure Monitoring

Right atrial pressure or CVP is monitored in the ICU by placement of a central venous catheter. Right atrial pressure normally is the lowest of all the heart chamber pressures, ranging from 2 to 6 mm Hg. Mean right atrial pressure is the same as CVP. CVP is a measure of right atrial preload. Atrial preload is determined by the balance between the capacity of the cardiovascular system, its circulating volume, and the amount of venous return to the heart (see Chapter 9). Right atrial pressure also is a reflection of right ventricular preload under normal circumstances. As a result, abnormally low right atrial pressure

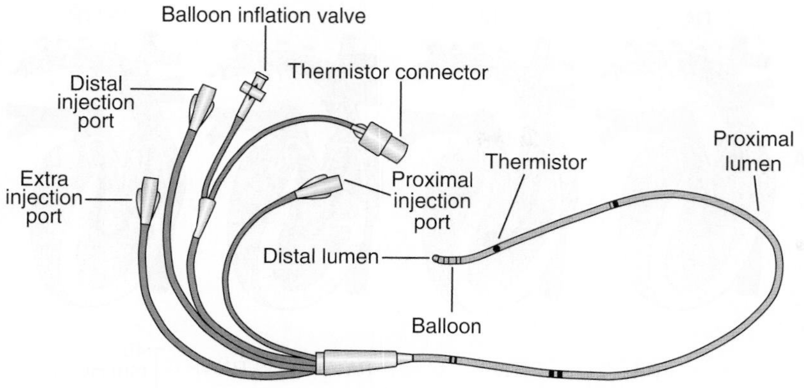

FIGURE 46-15 Quadruple-channel pulmonary artery catheter. The distalmost channel (distal injection port) is for measurement of PAP. Blood can be aspirated from this channel for mixed venous O_2 measurements. A second channel (balloon inflation valve) is used to inflate or deflate the distal balloon. A third channel (proximal injection port), which exits 30 cm from the catheter tip, is used for CVP (right atrial pressure) monitoring and fluid infusion. The fourth channel (extra injection port), which is not present on all catheters, can be used for continuous infusion of hyperalimentation fluid.

Box 46-9 Causes of Increased Right Atrial and Central Venous Pressure

- Right ventricular failure (myocardial infarction, cardiomyopathy)
- Pulmonary valvular stenosis
- Tricuspid stenosis and regurgitation
- Pulmonary hypertension
- Pulmonary embolism
- Volume overload
- Compression around the heart, constrictive pericarditis, cardiac tamponade
- Increased large vessel tone throughout the body, resulting in venoconstriction
- Arteriolar vasodilation, which increases blood supply to the venous system
- Increased intrathoracic pressure (positive pressure breath or pneumothorax)
- Placement of transducer below the patient's right atrial level
- Infusion of solution, especially with pressure infusion pumps, into CVP line
- Left-sided heart failure

suggests inadequate filling of the right ventricle and is common in hypovolemia. Causes of abnormal right atrial pressure or CVP are summarized in Box 46-9.

Pulmonary Artery Pressure Monitoring

Routine monitoring of PAP began in the 1970s, when the importance of understanding left heart failure became known.[45] Placement of a right heart/pulmonary artery catheter (Swan-Ganz catheter) is invasive and is associated with risk of pneumothorax, hemothorax, and arrhythmias. Placement of the balloon-tipped 7.5F catheter (Figure 46-15) must be performed aseptically by an experienced clinician. The catheter is guided into the pulmonary artery while the clinician visualizes waveforms with a fluid-filled system identical to the arterial pressure monitoring system (Figure 46-16).

Placement of a Swan-Ganz catheter allows determination of CVP, PAP, and PCWP. Data gathered with a Swan-Ganz catheter can be used to calculate thermodilution CO, pulmonary and arterial vascular resistance, and other associated indices (see Table 46-3). PAP monitoring may be helpful in the presence of shock (cardiogenic, hypovolemic, septic), left ventricular failure, myocardial infarction, pulmonary vascular disease, pulmonary edema, and ARDS. Measurement of PCWP is especially helpful in discriminating between cardiogenic and noncardiogenic pulmonary edema (e.g., ARDS). In ALI/ARDS, PCWP is generally less than 18 mm Hg, whereas PCWP is elevated in cardiogenic pulmonary edema. The reading and interpretation of Swan-Ganz catheter tracings can be inconsistent. There has been considerable controversy because of the risk-benefit ratio of the procedure.[2] The use of a pulmonary artery catheter in patients without primary cardiovascular disease has decreased markedly in more recent years.

Preload

Preload is defined as the pressure that stretches the ventricular walls at the onset of ventricular contraction. Preload can be approximated by measurement of PCWP. PCWP is an estimate of left atrial pressure, which reflects left ventricular end-diastolic pressure. During left-sided heart failure, preload increases; the increase is reflected in elevated PCWP. Symptoms of congestive heart failure usually can be controlled with diuretic therapy.

Contractility

Contractility is the forcefulness of the heart muscle contracting under a constant load. Numerous pharmacologic agents are used to cause a modest increase in ejection fraction (contractility) and are associated with improvement in symptoms in patients with congestive heart failure.

Afterload

Afterload usually is defined as the load against which the ventricles must contract. An increase in systemic vascular resistance increases left ventricular afterload. Although increased afterload usually is equated with increased blood

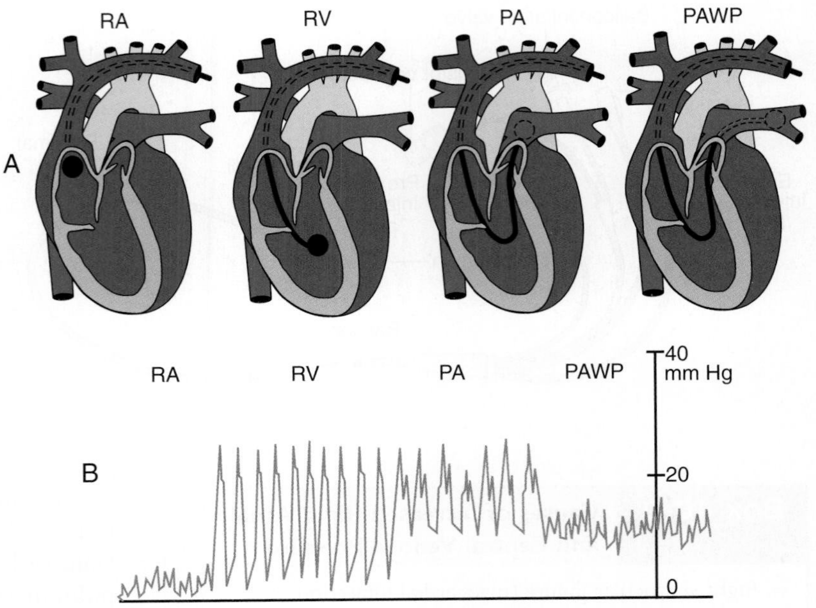

FIGURE 46-16 **A,** Position of pulmonary arterial catheter in the heart. **B,** As monitored by pressure tracings. *PA,* Pressure tracing from pulmonary artery; *PAWP,* pulmonary artery wedge pressure tracing; *RA,* pressure tracing from right atrium; *RV,* pressure tracing from right ventricle.

TABLE 46-4

Common Alterations in Hemodynamic Variables

	VARIABLE							
Condition	**Infiltrate on Chest Radiograph**	**BP**	**Cardiac Output**	**CVP**	**PAP**	**PCWP**	**$P\bar{v}O_2$ and $S\bar{v}O_2$**	**$C(a-\bar{v}O_2)$**
Shock								
Hypovolemic	—	↓	↓	↓	Variable	↓	↓	↑
Septic	None, one, or both sides	↓	↑	↓	N or ↓	N or ↓	N or ↑	N or ↑
Cardiogenic	One or both sides	↓	↓	↓↑	↑↑	↑↑	↓	↑
Left ventricular failure								
Mild	One or both sides	N or ↓	↓	N	↑	↑↑	↓	↑
Severe	One or both sides	↓	↓	N or ↑	↑↑	↑↑	↓	↑
Hypervolemic—fluid overload	One or both sides	N or ↑	N or ↑	N or ↑	↑	↑	N or ↑	N or ↓
Pulmonary embolus	None	N	Variable	↑	↑↑	N or ↓	Variable	Variable
ARDS	Both sides	Variable	Variable	Variable	Variable	N or ↓	Variable	Variable
Mechanical ventilation/PEEP	Variable	N or ↓	N or ↓	N or ↑	N or ↓	↑	N or ↓	N or ↑
Pulmonary hypertension	None	N or ↓	N or ↓	↑↑	↑↑	N	Variable	Variable

BP, Blood pressure; *N*, normal or little or no change.

pressure, the cause is better understood as the muscle tension required by the left ventricle to generate blood flow. Table 46-4 lists common conditions and associated alterations in hemodynamic variables. Table 46-5 summarizes steps to take in troubleshooting changes in monitored cardiovascular values and vital signs, including possible causes and appropriate corrective action.

Cardiac Output

Cardiac performance is affected by preload, contractility, and afterload and is evaluated by the measure of CO. The effect of cardiac pathology, medications, or mechanical ventilation on CO can be critical monitoring information. An accurate assessment of CO presents a challenge to the clinician. The physical examination (see Chapter 15) can reveal signs and symptoms of impaired cardiac performance, but a composite number provided by CO can provide more direct insight into problem and treatment options.

CO as determined by thermodilution via the use of a Swan-Ganz catheter was the primary method of CO assessment for 3 decades. The invasiveness of this method and inaccuracies in reading and interpretation led to a decrease in use of the Swan-Ganz catheter. Other methods of CO determination have become available based on algorithms that analyze the arterial pressure waveform and a Fick principle rebreathing method. The waveform analysis methods can be "calibrated" by lithium dilution or by thermodilution. Each technique has been studied and found to be accurate in relatively stable patients.[46-48]

TABLE 46-5

Troubleshooting Changes in Vital Signs

Clue	Possible Problem	Advice
Hypotension	Hypovolemia, pump failure	Evaluate fluid balance and possible need for intravenous fluids or inotropic agents
Hypertension	Anxiety; response to decreased PaO_2, decreased $PaCO_2$ or pain	Reassure, alleviate fear, check patient-ventilatory system; if not easily correctable, obtain and evaluate ABGs
Alteration of blood pressure with breathing	Decreased venous return (caused by changes in intrathoracic pressure)	If systolic/diastolic pressures are less than adequate perfusion levels, evaluate fluid balance; consider intravenous fluids
New arrhythmias, tachycardia, bradycardia	Anxiety	Reassure, alleviate fear
	Decreased PaO_2, decreased $PaCO_2$, increased $PaCO_2$	Check patient-ventilator system; if not quickly correctable, obtain and evaluate ABGs
Large swings in CVP or PCWP	Decreased venous return	Evaluate other hemodynamic values for adequacy of perfusion
Decreased urinary output	Decreased CO	Evaluate other hemodynamic values for adequacy of perfusion
	Hypovolemia	
Fever	Infection	Control infection; review preventive measures
	Atelectasis	Check patient-ventilator system for secretions, plugs, slippage of tube into right main stem bronchus
	Overheated humidifier	Check humidifier heater temperature
Weight gain	Fluid retention	Evaluate hemodynamic values for adequacy of perfusion; consider diuresis
Changes in respiratory rate	Altered settings	Check patient-ventilator settings
	Change in metabolic needs	Evaluate metabolic rate
	Anxiety	Reassure, alleviate fear
	Sleep	Normal; metabolic rate is decreased
Use of accessory muscles or paradoxical breathing	Increased WOB	Increase support level; check and change inspiratory flow
	Patient-ventilator asynchrony	Provide pressure support ventilation
		Increase sensitivity
	Auto-PEEP	Eliminate auto-PEEP

NEUROLOGIC MONITORING

Monitoring of the nervous system is most frequently overlooked in the ICU for several reasons. The first and most important reason is lack of knowledge of proper assessment of the nervous system of a ventilated, restrained, and often sedated patient in the ICU. Neurologic dysfunction is difficult to recognize in a sedated patient. Proper clinical assessment of the nervous system emphasizes neurologic history and examination (Box 46-10).

Box 46-10 Neurologic Monitoring

One of the most important, and frequently overlooked, areas of monitoring is the neurologic examination, which includes the following:

- History
- Assessment of mental status
- Pupillary response
- Eye movement assessment
- Corneal response
- Gag reflex
- Respiratory rate and pattern
- General motor and sensory evaluations

History

Obtaining a history from a critically ill patient, in particular, a patient with altered state of consciousness, can be difficult. However, attempting to obtain a history by speaking with the patient or family members can provide extremely useful information in the ICU.

Medical conditions with neurologic symptoms can be revealed through history and appropriate clinical tests. A history of an evolving focal deficit occurring over days to weeks before loss of consciousness suggests abscess, tumor, or subdural hematoma, whereas a progression to coma over minutes to hours favors a metabolic cause. Problems such as hypothyroidism, renal failure, cirrhosis, or psychiatric illness suggest greater likelihood of a metabolic cause. Uncontrolled hypertension can induce metabolic (e.g., hypertensive encephalopathy) or structural (e.g., intracerebral hemorrhage) coma.

Neurologic Examination

The neurologic examination of a patient in the ICU should address several key issues. In addition to determination of level of consciousness, the primary goal is to determine the presence of focal neurologic signs so that the clinician can

MINI CLINI

Hemodynamic Monitoring

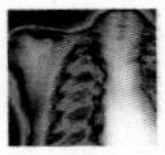

PROBLEM: A 55-year-old man with a history of congestive heart failure is admitted to the ICU in acute cardiorespiratory distress. A pulmonary artery catheter is placed for continuous monitoring of hemodynamic status. Initial CO is 3.2 L/min (decreased), cardiac index is 1.6 L/min per m^2 (decreased), heart rate is 135 beats/min (increased), stroke volume is 24 ml (decreased), systemic vascular resistance is 19.4 mm Hg/L per minute (unchanged), pulmonary vascular resistance is 2.3 mm Hg/L per minute (unchanged), arterial blood pressure is 90/60 mm Hg (decreased), PAP is 38/22 mm Hg (increased), PCWP is 20 mm Hg (increased), and CVP is 8 mm Hg or 11 cm H_2O (increased).

SOLUTION: The patient is being monitored for management of an exacerbation of congestive heart failure. The decreased CO, cardiac index, stroke volume, and arterial blood pressure accompanied by increases in PCWP and CVP indicate congestive heart failure caused by fluid overload to a weakened heart. Heart rate has increased to compensate for the reduction in stroke volume. The initial conservative treatment is preload reduction by fluid restriction, a diuretic, and CPAP therapy. The goals of this treatment are to reduce PCWP and CVP with an expected improvement in CO and index. A question currently under investigation is whether this management plan can be implemented and safely monitored with CVP, arterial blood pressure data, and clinical signs and symptoms alone without the use of a pulmonary artery catheter.

localize the lesion anatomically and generate a differential diagnosis and treatment plan.

Mental Status

The mental status examination should determine whether the patient has an altered state of consciousness. Terms such as *lethargy, confusion,* and *disorientation* lack precise definitions. A brief description of the applied stimulus and arousal pattern is preferred. The mental status examination in the ICU varies if the patient is intubated and cannot vocalize responses or speak. The earliest sign of abnormal mental status often is the patient's inability to follow a conversation or complex commands. Subtle changes in mental status often are the earliest signs of central nervous system dysfunction.

Pupillary Response

Pupil size, congruency, and response to light and accommodation should be described. Pupillary light reflexes provide information regarding the status of the brain and of the sympathetic and parasympathetic nervous systems. Pupillary function is controlled by the midbrain. If pupillary function is normal, the cause of coma is either metabolic or a structural lesion located above the midbrain. Small "pinpoint" pupils usually result from pontine hemorrhage or from ingestion of narcotics or organophosphates. Pupillary responses almost always remain intact in metabolic causes of coma. Dilated and fixed (unresponsive to light) pupils are seen in patients who have been given atropine. Midposition and fixed pupils often indicate severe cerebral damage.

Eye Movements

Abnormalities of extraocular movement have prognostic importance in the ICU. Normal movement of the eyes requires an intact pontomedullary-midbrain connection. The resting position of the gaze, the presence of nystagmus, and the response to head movements and cold tympanic membrane stimulation should be identified. Cervical spine stability must be ensured before oculocephalic maneuvers are performed. If rotation of the head (oculocephalic) and vestibular stimulation (calorics) produce no change in eye position, the pons is nonfunctional. If only the eye ipsilateral to the stimulus abducts, a lesion of the medial longitudinal fasciculus should be suspected.

Corneal Responses

The corneal reflex is used to test the afferent fifth and the efferent seventh cranial nerves. This test is performed by lightly touching the cornea with a cotton swab; the patient should blink both eyes in response. The presence of this response implies an intact ipsilateral fifth cranial nerve, intact central pons, and intact bilateral seventh cranial nerve. Testing must be performed bilaterally to evaluate both afferent components of the fifth cranial nerve.

Gag Reflex

The gag reflex is tested by using a tongue blade to stimulate one side of the posterior pharynx of an intubated patient. Each side should be tested separately. A normal response is bilateral movement of the posterior pharyngeal muscles and implies intact ninth and tenth cranial nerves. The ability to cough on suctioning can be tested in an intubated patient and implies an intact tenth cranial nerve. This test should not be attempted on nonintubated patients in the ICU because of the risk of aspiration.

Respiratory Rate and Pattern

The brainstem is the primary site of the central control of respiration. This control occurs at a subconscious level and results in rhythmic contraction and relaxation of the respiratory muscles. The most common abnormal respiratory pattern seen in patients with neurologic disorders is Cheyne-Stokes respiration, which consists of phases of hyperpnea that regularly alternate with episodes of apnea. Breathing waxes in a smooth crescendo and when a peak is reached wanes in an equally smooth decrescendo. Cheyne-Stokes respiration usually has an intracranial cause, although it can be caused by hypoxemia and cardiac failure. Ataxic breathing is a marker of severe brainstem dysfunction. Despite the nonspecificity of most breathing patterns, the respiratory pattern can provide valuable clues to the cause of coma.

Motor Evaluation

A thorough motor evaluation should be performed for all patients. The systematic approach described earlier is key to localization of the site of a pathologic process. The symmetry and pattern of the motor response to noxious stimuli and associated neurologic symptoms should be documented for all patients.

Sensory Evaluation

The assessment of light touch, pinprick, and temperature sensation can be achieved by applying a cotton swab, a clean pin, and a cold or warm object to various parts of the upper and lower extremities. Symmetry of responses between sides and between upper and lower extremities should be documented and is valuable in localizing the site of a pathologic process.

Intracranial Pressure Monitoring

There are three primary reasons to measure intracranial pressure (ICP): (1) to monitor patients at risk of life-threatening intracranial hypertension, (2) to monitor for evidence of infection, and (3) to assess the effects of therapy aimed at reducing ICP. Mean ICP of a supine patient is normally 10 to 15 mm Hg, and the ICP waveform normally undulates gently in time with the cardiac cycle. Fluctuations of the ICP waveform (>10 mm Hg) suggest a position near the critical inflection point of the cranial P-V curve. Elevations in ICP to 15 to 20 mm Hg compress the capillary bed and compromise microcirculation. At ICP levels of 30 to 35 mm Hg, venous drainage is impeded, and edema develops in uninjured tissue. Even when autoregulatory mechanisms are intact, cerebral perfusion cannot be maintained if ICP increases to within 40 to 50 mm Hg of the mean arterial pressure. When ICP approximates mean arterial pressure, perfusion stops, and the brain dies.

Two categories of ICP monitoring techniques are available at the present time. Fluid-filled systems have external transducers, such as an intraventricular catheter and subarachnoid bolts. Solid-state systems have miniature pressure transducers that can be inserted in the lateral ventricle, brain parenchyma, or subarachnoid or epidural space.

Glasgow Coma Scale Score

The most widely used scoring system for acute neurologic disorders is the **Glasgow Coma Scale (GCS)** (Table 46-6). The GCS score is used to test best motor response, best verbal response, and opening of the eyes. The scale goes from 3 to 15 and can be used for rapid triage. Patients with head injury and GCS scores of 13 to 15 often are admitted to a non-ICU observational unit unless neurologic examination or a CT scan reveals a lesion or abnormality that warrants ICU admission. Scores of 9 to 13 on the GCS signify a significant insult with depressed level of consciousness. Patients with head injury and GCS scores of 8 and less need monitoring of ICP.

TABLE 46-6
Glasgow Coma Scale

Eyes	Open	Spontaneous	4
		To verbal command	3
		To pain	2
		No response	1
Best motor response	To verbal command	Obeys	6
	To painful stimulus	Localized pain	5
		Flexion—withdrawal	4
		Flexion—decorticate	3
		Flexion—decerebrate	2
		No response	1
Best verbal response		Oriented, converses	5
		Disoriented, converses	4
		Inappropriate words	3
		Incomprehensible sounds	2
		No response	1
Total			*3-15*

MONITORING RENAL FUNCTION

The kidney is the main filter of waste products and the principal regulator of the volume and electrolyte composition of body fluid. Because the kidney is the primary excreter of nitrogenous waste, plasma concentrations of blood urea nitrogen (BUN) and creatinine are used to track renal function. As a general guideline, the BUN level increases 10 to 15 mg/dl per day, and the creatinine level increases 1 to 2.5 mg/dl per day after abrupt renal failure. The serum potassium level usually increases 0.5 mEq/L per day, and bicarbonate (HCO_3^-) level decreases approximately 1 mEq/L per day. Under the catabolic stress of burns, trauma, rhabdomyolysis (an acute and sometimes fatal disease in which products of skeletal muscle destruction produce acute renal failure), sepsis, or starvation, the rates of change in these values can double. In contrast to BUN, daily production of creatinine is relatively constant. An increasing creatinine level indicates that the rate of production exceeds clearance by means of glomerular filtration. A stable elevation in creatinine level implies a new steady state has been achieved at a decreased glomerular filtration rate. Until the creatinine level stabilizes, the severity of acute renal dysfunction cannot be assessed reliably. The most common method of estimating glomerular filtration rate (renal function) is measurement of plasma creatinine and creatinine clearance rate. Although calculation of creatinine clearance is more accurate, the procedure entails 24-hour urine collection. The most important factor is whether glomerular filtration rate is changing or stable, and plasma creatinine level is tracked for most patients.

Urine volume usually reflects kidney perfusion. *Polyuria* and *oliguria* refer to a daily urine output of more than 3 L and less than 0.4 L in average-sized adults. *Anuria* is present when urine output is less than 50 ml/day. Polyuria should not be confused with urinary frequency, in which multiple small voidings occur, but total output is less than 3 L/day.

MONITORING LIVER FUNCTION

Adequate liver function is essential for survival of critically ill patients. The liver must detoxify wastes from metabolism and digestion and process poisons. Elevated results of liver function tests reflect the occurrence of liver parenchymal damage. Hepatic dysfunction may precipitate or worsen ALI.[49] Routine indications for liver function testing in the treatment of critically ill patients include abdominal pain, jaundice, unexplained fever, nausea, malaise, failure to thrive, weight loss, and leukocytosis. Additional indications are facilitation of acuity scoring and definition of the contribution of the liver to multisystem organ failure.

Batteries of biochemical studies are routine in the evaluation of critically ill patients, but they reflect liver function minimally. Acute liver disease can develop in critically ill patients receiving total parenteral nutrition.[53] Liver disease may manifest as increased liver size and tenderness. When abnormal results of liver function tests have been obtained, it is essential to determine the cause. Elevations in levels of canalicular enzymes and bilirubin necessitate a search for mechanical obstruction and appropriate radiographic investigations. Elevations of transaminase levels are unusual in cholestatic processes, unless there is a superimposed ischemic event—a confounding factor in many critically ill patients. Elevated levels of aspartate aminotransferase and alanine aminotransferase suggest hepatic inflammation. Ischemia, viral hepatitis, and autoimmune hepatitis should be considered in the differential diagnosis.

NUTRITIONAL MONITORING

Assessment and monitoring of nutrition are required in the care of some critically ill patients because nutritional disorders are frequent and important determinants of outcome. Nutritional support is commonly needed by patients who have been critically ill for an extended period and patients with increased metabolic demands and limited nutritional reserve.

Assessment of Nutritional Status

Early detection of malnutrition in critically ill patients, whether preexisting or a result of acute illness, enables prompt and aggressive intervention with supplemental nutrition. No single measurement or assessment tool can adequately characterize nutritional status, and the diagnosis of malnutrition is subjective. However, both functional and biochemical factors should be examined to identify whether a patient is at increased risk of malnutrition and its complications.

Functional Assessment

The functional nutritional assessment consists of the medical history, physical examination, and appraisal of muscle and organ function. Identification of preexisting malnutrition should be attempted by careful attention to the history of present illness, the relevant medical and surgical history, medications, social habits, and a dietary history. Obtaining this information from a critically ill patient frequently is impossible, but the patient's family may be able to provide data on recent dietary habits and weight loss. Historical data should be used to estimate the nutritional consequences of the current hospitalization. Prehospitalization weight should be documented, and any weight changes since hospitalization should be documented and evaluated in the context of diuresis or fluid supplementation. Critically ill patients frequently have volume overload, which makes changes in dry weight difficult to assess.

The physical examination findings may suggest the presence of nutritional and metabolic deficiencies. Temporal muscle wasting, sunken supraclavicular fossae, and decreased adipose stores are easily recognized signs of starvation. Careful inspection of the hair, skin, eyes, mouth, and extremities can reveal protein-calorie malnutrition or vitamin and mineral deficiencies. An assessment of muscle mass and function can provide information about a patient's protein reserves and overall nutritional status. An estimation of muscle mass and fat stores can be obtained from anthropometric measurements such as arm circumference.

The function of the cardiovascular, respiratory, and gastrointestinal systems should be evaluated both for evidence of malnutrition-related dysfunction and because functional deficits may affect the ability of the patient to tolerate nutritional supplementation. The large fluid volumes associated with parenteral nutrition may not be tolerated in the setting of impaired cardiovascular function, and a distended abdomen makes tolerance of enteral supplementation less likely.

Metabolic Assessment

Serum albumin concentration is the most frequently used laboratory measure of nutritional status; a value less than 2.2 g/dl generally reflects severe malnutrition. Although albumin level is popular as an indicator of nutritional status, the reliability of albumin as a marker of visceral protein status is compromised by its long half-life of 14 to 20 days, making it less responsive to acute changes in nutritional status. Serum albumin concentration increases rapidly in response to exogenously administered albumin and is altered regardless of nutritional status in conditions such as dehydration, sepsis, trauma, and liver disease.

Serum chemistry values are important in determining the specifics of nutritional support but do not directly reflect nutritional status. Sodium, potassium, chloride, total CO_2, BUN, glucose, prothrombin time, partial thromboplastin time, iron, magnesium, calcium, and phosphate should be measured at admission and rechecked periodically.

Estimating Nutritional Requirements

The first step in calculating the nutritional prescription is to estimate the energy or caloric needs of the patient. Determining energy needs requires calculating basal energy expenditure (BEE). The BEE is the amount of energy required to perform metabolic functions at rest and is influenced by body size and illness. The BEE classically is estimated with the **Harris-Benedict equation,** as follows:[50]

$$\text{Men: BEE} = 66 + (13.7)(\text{Weight}) + (5)(\text{Height}) - (6.8)(\text{Age})$$

$$\text{Women: BEE} = 65 + (9.6)(\text{Weight}) + (1.8)(\text{Height}) - (4.7)(\text{Age})$$

where weight is expressed in kilograms; height, in centimeters; and age, in years.

The weight in these equations should be the usual or actual weight of a patient without significant weight loss, current weight for a patient with marked weight loss, and ideal body weight for an obese patient. The use of this measurement in the care of a critically ill patient has traditionally involved multiplication by a stress factor of 0.5 to 2.5. The use of the stress factor may result in overfeeding and may predispose the patient to fatty degeneration of the liver (steatosis), hyperglycemia, electrolyte imbalances, respiratory embarrassment owing to increased CO_2 production, and macrophage dysfunction. Use of the baseline Harris-Benedict equation without the stress factor in determining the BEE of critically ill patients yields an average estimate of 25 kcal/kg body weight.

GLOBAL MONITORING INDICES

Organizing the flood of information made available by monitoring instruments is a skill and responsibility of critical care practitioners. In the ICU, the immediate concern is the welfare of the patient. Decisions frequently are based on prognosis with respect to the appropriate tests, treatments, and medications prescribed. Guiding these decisions is the weighing of risks and benefits to the patient and the responsible use of resources. Although the physician makes such decisions with all current information, specific data on the probability of survival can be estimated. In the past 30 years, prognostic indices have been derived from large clinical data sets that provide an indication of the seriousness of the patient's condition. These indices (Acute Physiology and Chronic Health Evaluation [APACHE I, II, III, and IV], Acute Physiology Score, Therapeutic Intervention Scoring System, and Burns Weaning Assessment Program) are determinations of scores from numerous monitored values obtained from isolated observations of the patient's condition, usually during the first 24 hours after hospital admission. A score may be assigned for that patient at that time, and risk of mortality can be calculated (Box 46-11).

Box 46-11 Global Monitoring Indices

- Indices (scores) have been developed that take into account several monitored values.
- These scoring systems provide an estimate of illness acuity level and an estimate of the risk of mortality.
- For clinical studies, scoring systems are required to ensure that the control and experimental groups are similar.
- Scoring systems can be useful as a longitudinal monitor of acuity or a means of evaluating the effect of changes in services.
- At this time, scoring systems have little value in the care of individual patients. The most commonly used acuity of illness scoring system is APACHE II.

The value of severity of illness scoring for individual patients is limited, and the accuracy and usefulness of physiology scoring often are questioned. Imposing a scoring system to judge intent to treat places too much emphasis on the validity of the system. Scoring systems have not been clearly associated with important outcomes such as length of stay or time on mechanical ventilation. At the present time, as a bedside tool in the care of an individual patient, scoring systems have limited value. A specific condition may "score" a 17% risk of death, but a patient has two possible outcomes: life (0%) and death (100%). The decision to withdraw or limit care would rarely be based on a "score" because many other factors are involved in such a decision. Inaccuracies in predicting mortality are frequently reported. Discrepancies are probably due to patient mix differences, hospital factors, admission policies, data collection methods, and differences in quality of care. At the present time, the global indices have limited use in care of individual patients.

Global monitoring has a definite role in research. Global indices are valuable in the study of the effectiveness of new medications or therapy and the establishment of guidelines for care. When control and experimental (new treatment) groups are compared in a randomized, controlled trial, the severity scores of the groups must be similar, or differences in baseline condition may account for differences in results. As a tracking tool, scoring has significant value; the increasing severity of causes of ICU admissions can be followed over time with severity of illness scoring. The consequences of changes in services or policies or interhospital comparisons can be crudely tracked with the use of expected mortality calculations from APACHE

Box 46-12 Causes of Sudden Respiratory Distress in a Patient Receiving Ventilatory Support

PATIENT-RELATED CAUSES
- Artificial airway problems
- Movement of endotracheal tube
- Cuff herniation
- Cuff leak
- Kinking of endotracheal tube
- Foreign body
- Transesophageal fistula
- Innominate artery rupture
- Malpositioned nasogastric tube
- Secretions
- Bronchospasm
- Pneumothorax
- Pulmonary edema
- Pulmonary embolism
- Acute hypoxemia
- Blood in endotracheal tube
- Dynamic hyperinflation
- Abnormal respiratory drive
- Alteration in body posture
- Drug-induced problems
- Abdominal distention
- Agitation

VENTILATOR-RELATED CAUSES
- Ventilator malfunction
- Circuit malfunction
- Leaks or disconnects
- Condensate
- In-line nebulizers
- Inadequate ventilatory support
- Patient-ventilator asynchrony

From Tobin MJ, Alex CJ, Fahey PJ: Fighting the ventilator. In Tobin MJ, editor: Principles and practice of mechanical ventilation, New York, 2006, McGraw-Hill.

scores. Some institutions calculate severity of illness scores for all patients.

Acute Physiology and Chronic Health Evaluation (APACHE)

The **APACHE scoring system** was developed in 1981 to monitor severity of illness in clinical studies.[51] Studies have referenced a risk of mortality estimate as calculated from APACHE scoring, and the studies can be compared with similar studies in which the APACHE scoring system is used. The APACHE II scoring system assigns points to physiologic variables on the basis of whether the values are high abnormal, low abnormal, or normal. Variables rated include temperature, mean arterial pressure, heart rate, respiratory rate, PaO_2 [or $P(A - a)O_2$], pH, sodium level, potassium level, creatinine level, hematocrit, white blood cell count, and GCS score. Assigned points are added to derive a total APACHE score. There is an imprecision to estimating a risk of mortality. To emphasize the importance of the neurologic examination, the scoring system is weighted toward the importance of the GCS score. Refinements of APACHE are ongoing, although the APACHE II system continues to be used more often than other systems.[52]

TROUBLESHOOTING

Identification and correction of patient-related and ventilator-related problems during mechanical ventilatory support are primary responsibilities of the RT. Under ideal circumstances, potential problems are identified before they occur, or before they can cause harm to the patient. Potential problems with the patient include anxiety, agitation, altered mental status, fighting the ventilator, hypoxemia, hypoventilation, and development of metabolic acidosis. The patient may experience acute changes in respiratory rate, heart rate, blood pressure, and CO.

Box 46-13 Steps for Managing Sudden Distress in a Patient Receiving Ventilatory Support

1. Remove the patient from the ventilator.
2. Initiate manual ventilation with 100% O_2.
3. Patient improvement indicates that the ventilator is the cause of distress.
4. Lack of improvement indicates the problem is within the patient.
5. If death appears imminent, consider and manage the most likely causes, check for airway obstruction (by passing a suction catheter), a dislodged endotracheal tube, or a pneumothorax.
6. If death is not imminent, wait until the patient's condition is stable before attempting a more detailed assessment including a chest radiograph.

Modified from Tobin MJ, Alex CJ, Fahey PJ: Fighting the ventilator. In Tobin MJ, editor: Principles and practice of mechanical ventilation, New York, 2006, McGraw-Hill.

Other common patient-related problems include excessive secretions, bronchospasm, and other causes of decreased compliance or increased resistance. Recognition of signs of pneumothorax, pneumomediastinum or subcutaneous emphysema, airway malfunction or leaks, and chest tube leaks should lead to prompt attention to the problem.

Problems associated with the ventilator include leaks or malfunctions in the system, inappropriate ventilator settings (including trigger sensitivity and inspiratory flow rate), development of auto-PEEP, and improper humidification. Box 46-12 lists causes of sudden respiratory distress in patients receiving mechanical ventilatory support. Box 46-13 lists steps for managing sudden respiratory distress.

Table 46-7 summarizes troubleshooting of the patient-ventilator system.

If medical and mechanical problems have been excluded and the patient continues to fight the ventilator or exhibit high levels of agitation or distress, sedation should be considered. Agents commonly used for sedation in the ICU include benzodiazepines (lorazepam, midazolam), opiates (fentanyl, morphine), haloperidol, and propofol.

Pharmacologic paralysis should be considered only when no other alternatives are effective. The use of neuromuscular blocking agents can mask other patient problems, and ventilator malfunction or disconnection in the care of a paralyzed patient can be catastrophic. In addition, some patients receiving neuromuscular blocking agents in the ICU may experience prolonged neuropathy. Pharmacologic agents used to produce sedation or paralysis in the ICU are listed in Box 46-14.

TABLE 46-7

Troubleshooting the Patient-Ventilator System

Clue to Problem	Possible Cause	Corrective Action
Decreased minute ventilation or V_T	Leak around endotracheal or chest tube	Check all connections for leaks
	Decreased patient-triggered respiratory rate	Evaluate patient Check sensitivity Measure auto-PEEP Increase set rate Change mode
	Decreased lung compliance	Evaluate patient
	Airway secretions	Clear airway of secretions
	Altered settings	Check patient-ventilator system
	Malfunctioning volume monitor	Check with external respirometer
Increased minute ventilation or V_T	Increased patient-triggered respiratory rate	Check respiratory rate Check sensitivity Change mode
	Altered settings	Check patient-ventilator system
	Hypoxia	Evaluate patient Consider ABG and SpO_2 values
	Increased lung compliance	Decrease pressure Decrease inspiratory time
	Malfunctioning volume monitor	Check with external respirometer
Change in respiratory rate	Altered setting	Check patient-ventilator system
	Increased metabolic demand	Evaluate patient
	Hypoxia	Evaluate patient Consider ABG and SpO_2 values
Sudden increase in peak airway pressure	Coughing	Alleviate uncontrolled coughing
	Airway secretions or plugs	Clear airway secretions
	Ventilator tubing kinked or filled with water	Check for kinks and water
	Changes in patient position	Consider repositioning patient
	Endotracheal tube in right main stem bronchus	Verify position
	Patient-ventilator asynchrony	Correct asynchrony Check for adequate peak flow Verify with waveforms
	Bronchospasm	Identify cause and treat
	Pneumothorax	Insert chest tubes
Gradual increase in peak airway pressure	Diffuse, reactive, or obstructive process	Evaluate for problems, such as atelectasis, increasing lung water, bronchospasm
Sudden decrease in peak airway pressure	Volume loss from leaks in the system	Check patient-ventilator systems for leaks Verify with waveforms Check for active inspirations Evaluate patient
FiO_2 drift	O_2 analyzer error	Calibrate analyzer Change O_2 sensor
	Blender piping failure	Correct failure
	O_2 source failure	Correct failure
	O_2 reservoir leak	Check ventilator reservoir

Continued

TABLE 46-7

Troubleshooting the Patient-Ventilator System—cont'd

Clue to Problem	Possible Cause	Corrective Action
I : E ratio too high or too low	Altered inspiratory flow	Check flow setting and correct
	Alteration in other settings that control I : E ratio	Check settings and correct
	Alteration in sensitivity setting	Check setting and correct
	Airway secretions (pressure ventilator)	Clear airway of secretions
	Subtle leaks	Measure minute ventilation
Inspired gas temperature too high	Addition of cool water to humidifier	Wait
	Altered settings	Correct temperature control setting
	Adding cool gas by small-volume nebulizer treatment	Turn off heater during treatment
	Thermostat failure	Replace heater
Changes in PEEP	Change in V_T	Adjust PEEP level
	Change in compliance	Adjust PEEP level
	Altered settings	Check settings and correct
Changes in static pressure	Changes in lung compliance	Evaluate patient and correct if possible
Changes in ventilator setting	Changes in these settings resulting from deliberate or accidental adjustment of dials or knobs	Determine whether current settings are the intended ones

Modified from Martz K, Joiner JW, Shepherd RM: Management of the patient-ventilator system: a team approach, ed 2, St. Louis, 1994, Mosby.

Box 46-14 Pharmacologic Agents Used to Produce Sedation or Paralysis

I. Benzodiazepine tranquilizing agents
  A. Diazepam (Valium)
  B. Lorazepam (Ativan)
  C. Midazolam (Versed)
II. Sedative hypnotics and miscellaneous agents
  A. Sodium thiopental (Pentothal)
  B. Etomidate (Amidate)
  C. Haloperidol (Haldol)
  D. Propofol (Diprivan)
III. Narcotic analgesics
  A. Morphine
  B. Fentanyl (Sublimaze)
IV. Neuromuscular blocking agents
  A. Nondepolarizing (competitive)
    1. Steroidal agents
      Pancuronium (Pavulon)
      Pipecuronium (Arduan)
      Rocuronium (Zemuron)
      Vecuronium (Norcuron)
    2. Benzylisoquinolinium esters
      Atracurium (Tracrium)
      Cisatracurium (Nimbex)
      Doxacurium (Nuromax)
      Metocurine (Metubine)
      Mivacurium (Mivacron)
      Tubocurarine (Tubarine)
  B. Depolarizing
    1. Succinylcholine (Anectine, Quelicin)
    2. Decamethonium (Syncurine)

SUMMARY CHECKLIST

- Caregivers must be experienced at filtering the noise from the changes in monitored variables that require attention. Caregivers need to recognize false alarms. They also need to discriminate real pathophysiologic changes from normal physiologic variations and from variations inherent in the data.
- Because only caregivers can make choices about altering care, caregivers continue to be the most important monitors.
- Monitoring of the respiratory system includes assessment of ventilation, gas exchange, and respiratory system mechanics and function.
- Ventilation is monitored by measurement of V_T, respiratory rate, and minute ventilation and by assessment of dead space and alveolar ventilation.
- Gas exchange is routinely monitored with ABG analysis and pulse oximetry. Derived values such as V_D/V_T, $P(A - a)O_2$ difference, PaO_2/FiO_2 ratio, shunt, and lung injury score can clarify the nature and severity of gas exchange abnormality. Arterial $PaCO_2$ is the best index of alveolar ventilation.
- Respiratory system mechanics are routinely monitored by tracking peak pressure, P_{plat}, auto-PEEP, compliance, and resistance.
- Factors such as WOB, f/V_T, VC, MIP, and MVV can be extremely helpful in assessing the need to increase ventilatory support or in assessing the potential for weaning.
- Advanced monitoring techniques include EIT, ARM, lung stress and strain, stress index, and esophageal pressure monitoring.
- The most important responsibility of the RT in the ICU is monitoring of the patient-ventilator system.

- Monitoring of the patient-ventilator system includes overall assurance of the integrity and safety of the system. Monitoring requires complete knowledge of the ventilator settings; all aspects of ventilator function; the circuitry; airway status; gas exchange; ventilator graphics; lung mechanics; alarms; and the overall care, safety, and comfort of the patient.
- Acute changes in cardiac performance, cardiovascular status, or impulse conduction (ECG) can be life-threatening; some form of monitoring of the heart, vascular system, and ECG is necessary in the care of nearly all patients in the ICU.
- Hemodynamic monitoring requires the use of invasive pulmonary arterial, central venous, and arterial catheters. Values obtained with these monitoring lines must be carefully interpreted by experienced caregivers. All ICU patients should receive ECG monitoring.
- Monitoring of changes in neurologic status is extremely important and is more often overlooked than monitoring of other organ systems.
- The neurologic examination includes assessment of mental status, pupillary response, eye movements, corneal response, gag reflex, and respiratory rate and pattern and a general motor and sensory evaluation. ICP monitoring may be needed to detect or manage elevated ICP.
- Global index monitoring is calculation of an illness level score that is an estimate of the risk of mortality from numerous monitoring values. Illness scores are not used in the care plan for an individual patient, but scoring systems are widely used in clinical studies. The APACHE II system is among the most popular of these estimates.
- Troubleshooting the patient-ventilator system is aimed at identifying and correcting problems before they harm the patient.

References

1. Colice GL: A historical perspective on the development of mechanical ventilation. In Tobin MJ, editor: Principles and practice of mechanical ventilation, New York, 2006, McGraw-Hill, p 30.
2. Wiener RS, Welch HG: Trends in the use of the pulmonary artery catheter in the United States, 1993-2004. JAMA 298:423-429, 2007.
3. Feiner JR, Severinghaus JW, Bickler PE: Dark skin decreases the accuracy of pulse oximeters at low oxygen saturation: the effects of oximeter probe type and gender. Anesth Analg 105:S18-S23, 2007.
4. Cohn SM, Nathens AB, Moore FA, et al; StO2 in Trauma Patients Trial Investigators: Tissue oxygen saturation predicts the development of organ dysfunction during traumatic shock resuscitation. J Trauma 62:44-54, 2007.
5. Mendelson Y: Pulse oximetry: theory and applications for noninvasive monitoring. Clin Chem 38:1601-1607, 1992.
6. Cairo JN, Pilbeam SP: Mosby's respiratory care equipment, ed 7, St Louis, 2004, Mosby.
7. Girard TD, Bernard GR: Mechanical ventilation in ARDS: a state-of-the-art review. Chest 131:921-929, 2007.
8. Villar J, Blanco J, Kacmarek RM: Acute respiratory distress syndrome definition: do we need a change? Curr Opin Crit Care 17:13-17, 2011.
9. Petty TL, Ashbaugh DG: The adult respiratory distress syndrome: clinical features, factors influencing prognosis and principles of management. Chest 60:233-239, 1971.
10. Murray JF, Matthay MA, Luce JM, et al: An expanded definition of the adult respiratory distress syndrome. Am Rev Respir Dis 138:720-723, 1988.
11. Kallet RH: Capnography and respiratory care in the 21st century. Respir Care 53:860-861, 2008.
12. Nuckton TJ, Alonso JA, Kallet RH, et al: Pulmonary dead-space fraction as a risk factor for death in the acute respiratory distress syndrome. N Engl J Med 346:1281-1286, 2002.
13. Rabitsch W, Nikolic A, Schellongowski P, et al: Evaluation of an end-tidal portable ETCO2 colorimetric breath indicator (COLIBRI). Am J Emerg Med 22:4-9, 2004.
14. Hinkelbein J, Floss F, Denz C, et al: Accuracy and precision of three different methods to determine Pco2 (Paco2 vs. Petco2 vs. Ptcco2) during interhospital ground transport of critically ill and ventilated adults. J Trauma 65:10-18, 2008.
15. Anderson CT, Breen PH: Carbon dioxide kinetics and capnography during critical care. Crit Care 4:207-215, 2000.
16. Yem JS, Turner MJ, Baker AB: Sources of error in partial rebreathing pulmonary blood flow measurements in lungs with emphysema and pulmonary embolism. Br J Anaesth 97:732-741, 2006.
17. AARC Clinical practice guidelines: Capnography/capnometry during mechanical ventilation: revised 2003. Respir Care 48:534-539, 2003.
18. Bergman NA: Fourier analysis of effects of varying pressure waveforms in electrical lung analogs. Acta Anaesthesiol Scand 28:174-181, 1984.
19. Adams AB, Cakar N, Marini JJ: Static and dynamic pressure-volume curves reflect different aspects of respiratory mechanics in experimental acute respiratory distress syndrome. Respir Care 46:686-693, 2001.
20. Hubmayr RD: Perspective on lung injury and recruitment: a skeptical look at the opening and collapse story. Am J Respir Crit Care Med 165:1647-1653, 2002.
21. Villar J, Pérez-Méndez L, Basaldúa S, et al: A risk textiles model for predicting mortality in patients with acute respiratory distress syndrome: Age, plateau pressure and PaO2/FIO2 at ARDS onset predict outcome. Respir Care 56:420-428, 2011.
22. Schumann S, Haberthuer C, Guttmann J: Compensating for endotracheal tube resistance. Anesth Analg 110:639-640, 2010.
23. Stewart TE, Meade MO, Cook DJ, et al: Evaluation of a ventilation strategy to prevent barotrauma in patients at high risk for acute respiratory distress syndrome. Pressure- and Volume-Limited Ventilation Strategy Group. N Engl J Med 338:355-361, 1998.
24. Mughal MM, Culver DA, Minai OA, et al: Auto-positive end-expiratory pressure: mechanisms and treatment. Cleve Clin J Med 72:801-809, 2005.
25. Blanch L, Bernabé F, Lucangelo U: Measurement of air trapping, intrinsic positive end-expiratory pressure, and dynamic hyperinflation in mechanically ventilated patients. Respir Care 50:110-123, 2005.
26. Layon J, Banner MJ, Kirby RR, et al: Partially and totally unloading respiratory muscles based on real-time measurements. Chest 106:1835-1842A, 1994.
27. Kapasi M, Fujino Y, Kirmse M, et al: Effort and work of breathing in neonates during assisted patient-triggered ventilation. Pediatr Crit Care Med 2:9-16, 2001.
28. Purro A, Appendini L, De Gaetano A, et al: Physiologic determinants of ventilator dependence in long-term mechanically

ventilated patients. Am J Respir Crit Care Med 161:1115-1123, 2000.

29. Yang K, Tobin M: A prospective study of indexes predicting outcome of trials of weaning from mechanical ventilation. N Engl J Med 324:1445-1450, 1991.
30. Marini JJ, Smith TC, Lamb V: Estimation of inspiratory muscle strength in mechanically ventilated patients: the measurement of maximal inspiratory pressure. J Crit Care 191:323-326, 1986.
31. Adams A: Pulmonary function in the mechanically ventilated patient. Respir Care Clin North Am 3:322-331, 1997.
32. Chiumello D, Carlesso E, Cadringher P, et al: Lung stress and strain during mechanical ventilation for acute respiratory distress syndrome. Am J Respir Crit Care Med 178:346-355, 2008.
33. Graf J, Santos A, Dries D, et al: Functional residual capacity by nitrogen washin/washout and CT techniques agree in pleural effusion model. Respir Care 11:1464-1468, 2010.
34. Grasso S, Terragni P, Mascia L, et al: Airway pressure-time profile (stress index) detects tidal recruitment/hyperinflation in experimental acute lung injury. Crit Care Med 32:1018-1027, 2004.
35. Formenti P, Graf J, Santos A, et al: Non-pulmonary factors strongly influence the stress index. Intensive Care Med 37:594-600, 2011.
36. Kue R, Brown P, Ness C, et al: Adverse clinical events during intrahospital transport by a specialized team: a preliminary report. Am J Crit Care 20:153-161, 2011.
37. Lowhagen K, Lundin S, Stenqvist O: Regional intratidal gas distribution in acute lung injury and acute respiratory distress syndrome—assessed by electric impedance tomography. Minerva Anestesiol 76:1024-1035, 2010.
38. Bikker IG, Leonhardt S, Reis Miranda D, et al: Bedside measurement of changes in lung impedance to monitor alveolar ventilation in dependent and non-dependent parts by electrical impedance tomography during a positive end-expiratory pressure trial in mechanically ventilated intensive care unit patients. Crit Care 14:R100, 2010.
39. Vyshedskiy A, Ishikawa S, Murphy R: Crackle pitch and rate do not vary significantly during a single examining session in patients with pneumonia, congestive heart failure, and interstitial pulmonary fibrosis. Respir Care 56:806-817, 2011.
40. Yilmaz M, Gajic O: Optimal ventilator settings in acute lung injury and acute respiratory distress syndrome. Eur J Anaesthesiol 25:89-96, 2008.
41. Mehta S, Granton J, MacDonald RJ, et al: High-frequency oscillatory ventilation in adults: the Toronto experience. Chest 126:518-527, 2004.
42. Simonson DA, Adams AB, Wright LA, et al: Experimental ventilator induced lung injury: PEEP, inspiratory time and an early indicator of injury. Crit Care Med 32:781-786, 2004.
43. Brower RG, Lanken PN, MacIntyre NR, et al; ARDSNet NIH NHLBI: Higher versus lower positive end-expiratory pressures in patients with the acute respiratory distress syndrome. N Engl J Med 351:327-336, 2004.
44. Villar J, Kacmarek RM, Pérez-Méndez L, et al: A high positive end-expiratory pressure, low tidal volume ventilatory strategy improves outcome in persistent acute respiratory distress syndrome: a randomized, controlled trial. Crit Care Med 34:1311-1318, 2006.
45. Swan HJ, Ganz W, Forrester J, et al: Catheterization of the heart in man with use of a flow-directed balloon-tipped catheter. N Engl J Med 83:447-451, 1970.
46. Saraceni E, Rossi S, Persona P, et al: Comparison of two methods for cardiac output measurement in critically ill patients. Br J Anaesth 106:690-694, 2011.
47. Geerts B, de Wilde R, Aarts L, et al: Cardiothoracic pulse contour analysis to assess hemodynamic response to passive leg raising. Vasc Anesth 25:48-52, 2011.
48. Young BP, Low LL: Noninvasive monitoring cardiac output using partial CO(2) rebreathing. Crit Care Clin 26:383-392, 2010.
49. TenHoor T, Mannino DM, Moss M: Risk factors for ARDS in the United States: analysis of the 1993 National Mortality Followback Study. Chest 119:1179-1184, 2001.
50. MacArthur C: Nutritional assessment and support. In Respiratory care: principles and practice Boston, 2010, Jones & Bartlett, p 685.
51. Wong DT, Knaus WA: Predicting outcome in critical care: the current status of the APACHE prognostic scoring system. Can J Anesth 38:374-383, 1991.
52. Wheeler MM: APACHE: an evaluation. Crit Care Nurs Q 32:46-48, 2009.
53. Nussbaum MS, Fisher JE: Pathogenesis of hepatic steatosis during total parenteral nutrition. Surg Ann 223:1-11, 1991.

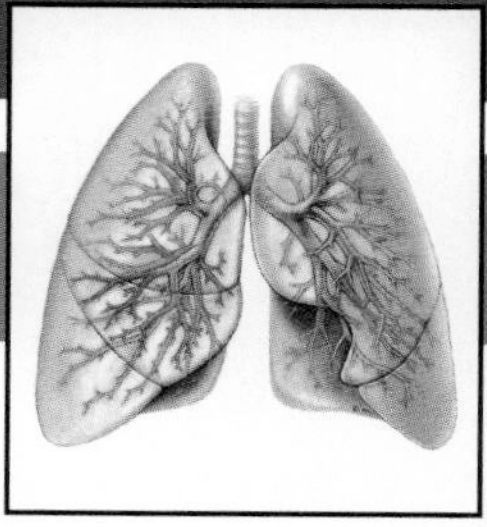

Chapter 47

Discontinuing Ventilatory Support

ROBERT M. KACMAREK

CHAPTER OBJECTIVES

After reading this chapter you will be able to:

- Discuss the relationship between ventilatory demand and ventilatory capacity as well as their relationship with ventilator discontinuance.
- List the factors associated with ventilator dependence.
- Explain how to evaluate a patient before attempting ventilator discontinuation or weaning.
- List acceptable values for specific weaning indices used to predict a patient's readiness for discontinuation of ventilatory support.
- Describe factors that should be optimized before an attempt is made at ventilator discontinuation or weaning.
- Describe techniques used in ventilator weaning, including daily spontaneous breathing trials, synchronized intermittent mandatory ventilation, pressure support ventilation, and other newer methods.
- Contrast the advantages and disadvantages associated with various weaning methods and techniques.
- Describe how to assess a patient for extubation.
- List the primary reasons why patients fail a ventilator discontinuance trial.
- Explain why some patients cannot be successfully weaned from ventilatory support.

CHAPTER OUTLINE

KEY TERMS

adaptive support ventilation (ASV)
airway occlusion pressure
automatic tube compensation (ATC)
continuous positive airway pressure (CPAP)
mandatory minute volume ventilation (MMV)
pressure support ventilation (PSV)
prolonged mechanical ventilation (PMV)
rapid, shallow breathing index (f/V_T)
spontaneous awaking trial (SAT)
spontaneous breathing trial (SBT)
synchronized intermittent mandatory ventilation (SIMV)

The purpose of mechanical ventilation is to support the patient until the disease state or condition that caused the need for support is alleviated or resolved.[1-3] Ventilatory support can sustain life, but it cannot cure disease. Further, many complications and hazards are associated with mechanical ventilation. Consequently, ventilatory support should be withdrawn as soon as the patient is able to adequately resume spontaneous breathing.[1-4] All patients who are mechanically ventilated should be evaluated on a daily basis for their ability to wean from ventilatory support.[5,6]

After the problem or condition that caused the need for mechanical ventilation is resolved, most patients can be quickly and easily removed from ventilatory support. For example, for most patients who need mechanical ventilation as a result of drug overdose or severe asthma, for those who are recovering from postoperative anesthesia, and for those who have received ventilation for 72 hours or less, one may simply discontinue ventilation when the precipitating condition has resolved.[1,5] However, some patients require mechanical ventilation for longer periods. The term *ventilator dependent* is usually reserved for patients who need ventilatory support for lengthy periods (i.e., 2 weeks or more) or who have not responded to attempts at ventilator discontinuation.[3] For these patients, a more formal ventilator discontinuation process is required.[3]

Ventilator discontinuation should be carefully timed.[4] Premature removal from the ventilator may severely stress the cardiopulmonary system and delay the patient's recovery.[4] Premature discontinuation also exposes the patient to the hazards of reintubation. However, delays in discontinuing ventilation expose the patient to an increased risk of complications, including nosocomial pneumonia, myocardial infarction, and death.[6]

There are three basic methods for discontinuing ventilatory support:

1. **Spontaneous breathing trials (SBTs)** alternating with mechanical ventilation
2. **Synchronized intermittent mandatory ventilation (SIMV)**
3. **Pressure support ventilation (PSV)**[4]

Other techniques that may facilitate ventilator discontinuation include the use of volume-support ventilation (VSV), **adaptive support ventilation (ASV)**; automatic tube compensation (ATC); proportional assist ventilation (PAV), which is also known as *proportional pressure support* (PPS); and **continuous positive airway pressure (CPAP).**[4,7-9] However, little data exist that support the use of any of these techniques except CPAP during the ventilator discontinuation process.

Techniques for predicting when patients are ready for ventilator discontinuation and weaning have been studied extensively.[6] Many weaning indices have been used, and a number of different weaning methods have been advocated. Despite this, there are no universally applicable rules for predicting success. Of all of the methods studied, SBTs and PSV have been shown to be the most effective methods for ventilator discontinuation and weaning. Evidence-based reviews recommend the use of at least daily SBTs.[3] Protocols for ventilator discontinuation administered by an interdisciplinary team of respiratory therapists, nurses, and physicians can be highly effective, and the use of ventilator discontinuation protocols has also been recommended.[3,6,10-13] Regardless of the method used, success is unlikely unless the precipitating problems that caused the ventilator dependency have been resolved.[1,3,7,14] After these problems are resolved, an organized plan or protocol should be followed, and variations should be based on each patient's response.[3,6,10]

Some patients cannot be successfully removed from mechanical ventilatory support. This group of ventilator-dependent patients poses clinical, economic, and ethical concerns.[15]

Many clinicians use the term *weaning* as a general term to refer to the process of discontinuing ventilatory support, regardless of the time frame or method involved.[7,8,16] The term has also been used to refer to reductions in fractional inspired oxygen concentration (FiO_2), PEEP, and CPAP.[8] Alternatively, the term *ventilator discontinuation* has been used to refer to the process of disconnecting a patient from mechanical ventilatory support. For the purposes of this chapter, the term *weaning* is defined as a gradual reduction in the level of ventilatory support,[1,7-9] whereas *discontinuing ventilatory support* refers to the overall process of removing the patient from the ventilator, regardless of the method used.[3] In general, patients who are being considered for removal from ventilatory support fall into one of four categories:

1. Those for whom removal is quick and routine, which is normally the vast majority of ventilated patients
2. Those who need a more systematic approach to discontinuing ventilatory support, which is normally about 15% to 20% of ventilated patients
3. Those who require days to weeks to wean from ventilatory support, which is usually less than 5% of ventilated patients
4. Those ventilator-dependent or "unweanable" patients, who compose less than 1% of patients who require ventilatory support[17]

Box 47-1 Factors That May Increase Ventilatory Workload

INCREASED VENTILATORY DEMAND: INCREASED LEVEL OF VENTILATION REQUIRED

- Increased CNS drive: hypoxia, acidosis, pain, fear, anxiety, and stimulation of J receptors (e.g., pulmonary edema)
- Increased metabolic rate: increased carbon dioxide production, fever, shivering, agitation, trauma, infection, and sepsis
- Increased dead space: COPD and pulmonary embolus

DECREASED COMPLIANCE

- Decreased lung compliance: atelectasis, pneumonia, fibrosis, pulmonary edema, and acute respiratory distress syndrome
- Decreased thoracic compliance: obesity, ascites, abdominal distention, and pregnancy

INCREASED RESISTANCE

- Increased airway resistance: bronchospasm, mucosal edema, and secretions
- Artificial airways: endotracheal tubes, tracheostomy tubes, and partial obstruction of the airway
- Other mechanical factors: ventilator circuits, demand flow systems, and inappropriate ventilator flow or sensitivity settings

REASONS FOR VENTILATOR DEPENDENCE

Patients may require mechanical ventilation because of apnea, acute or impending ventilatory failure, or severe oxygenation problems that necessitate high levels of PEEP or CPAP. Regardless of the reason for initiating mechanical ventilation, patients remain dependent on the ventilator because of respiratory, cardiovascular, neurologic, or psychologic factors.[3]

Ventilatory Workload or Demand

Patients who need mechanical ventilation often have a ventilatory workload or demand that exceeds their ventilatory capacity. This is the most common cause of ventilator dependence.[1,2] The term *ventilatory workload* refers to the amount of work that the respiratory muscles are asked to perform to provide an appropriate level of ventilation. A patient's total ventilatory workload is primarily determined by the following: (1) the level of ventilation needed; (2) the compliance of the lungs and thorax; (3) the resistance to gas flow through the airways, and (4) any imposed work of breathing (WOB_I) due to mechanical factors.[1,7]

The level of ventilation required is determined by the following: (1) the metabolic rate; (2) the central nervous system (CNS) drive; and (3) the ventilatory dead space. Common causes of an increased demand for ventilation include increased carbon dioxide production (i.e., fever, shivering, agitation, trauma, or sepsis) and increased dead space (i.e., pulmonary emboli or chronic obstructive pulmonary disease [COPD]). Other common causes of increased ventilatory demand include metabolic acidosis, severe hypoxemia, pain, and anxiety.

Compliance is determined by the elastic nature of the lung-thorax system. Resistance is largely related to the nature of the conducting airways. Common causes of decreased lung compliance include atelectasis, pneumonia, pulmonary edema, acute lung injury, and acute respiratory distress syndrome. Thoracic compliance may be reduced because of obesity, ascites, or abdominal distention. Airway resistance increases with bronchospasm, excessive secretions, and mucosal edema.

Mechanical factors that can increase the work of breathing include artificial airways (i.e., endotracheal and tracheotomy tubes), partial obstruction of the airway, ventilator circuits, demand flow systems, auto-PEEP, and inappropriate ventilator flow and sensitivity settings. Factors that may increase ventilatory workload are summarized in Box 47-1.

Ventilatory Capacity

Ventilatory capacity is determined by CNS drive, ventilatory muscle strength, and ventilatory muscle endurance.[18] Most patients who are being withdrawn from ventilatory support have a normal or an increased drive to breathe. Patients with neuromuscular disorders and those who are receiving sedatives, narcotics, or neuromuscular blocking

Box 47-2 Factors That May Reduce Ventilatory Drive

- Decreased $PaCO_2$ (respiratory alkalosis)
- Metabolic alkalosis
- Pain (visceral)
- Electrolyte imbalance
- Pharmacologic depressants (narcotics, sedatives)
- Fatigue
- Decreased metabolic rate
- Increased $PaCO_2$ associated with chronic carbon dioxide retention
- Neurologic or neuromuscular disease

agents may have a reduced drive to breathe or impaired neuromuscular transmission. Patients with metabolic alkalosis, hypothyroidism, and sleep deprivation also may have reduced ventilatory drive. Box 47-2 summarizes the factors that may reduce ventilatory drive.

Muscle strength is influenced by age, sex, muscle bulk, and overall health. Malnutrition, starvation, and electrolyte imbalances (especially involving calcium, magnesium, potassium, and phosphate) can lead to ventilatory muscle weakness.[18,19] Critical illness myopathy, critical illness polyneuropathy, and the prolonged use of neuromuscular blocking agents are major causes of the development of ventilatory muscle weakness in the intensive care unit (ICU).[20] Controlled ventilation for prolonged periods can result in ventilatory muscle discoordination and atrophy.[18] Ventilatory muscle endurance is a function of energy supply versus demand. Energy supply is related to nutrition, perfusion, and cell use, whereas demand is related to the amount of work performed and is a function of minute ventilation, compliance, and resistance. Figure 47-1 summarizes the relationship between ventilatory demands and capabilities.

Global Criteria for Discontinuing Ventilatory Support

Success with the discontinuation of ventilatory support is related to the patient's condition in four main areas[1,2,7]:

1. Ventilatory workload versus ventilatory capacity
2. Oxygenation status
3. Cardiovascular function
4. Psychologic factors

Simply put, when ventilatory workload or demand exceeds ventilatory capacity, successful ventilator discontinuation is unlikely.[1,2] Excessive ventilatory workload may lead to ventilatory muscle fatigue. When the ventilatory muscles fatigue, they must be rested for at least 24 hours to recover.[3,4,19] Ventilatory workload increases with decreased compliance, increased airway resistance, or an increased level of ventilation. Ventilatory capacity can be reduced by ventilatory muscle fatigue and by a loss of muscle strength and endurance.

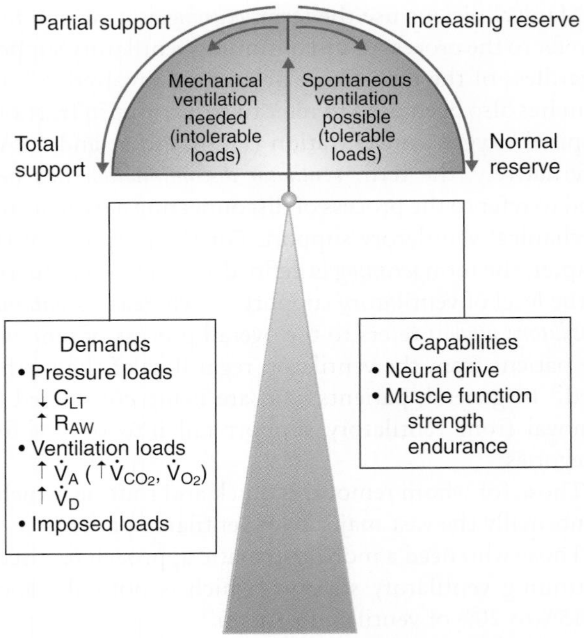

FIGURE 47-1 Ventilatory failure and the need for ventilatory support depend on the balance between ventilatory muscle demands (i.e., loads) and ventilatory muscle capabilities. C_{LT}, Lung-thorax compliance; *RAW,* airway resistance, $\dot{V}_A$, minute alveolar ventilation; $\dot{V}_D$, minute dead space ventilation. (Modified from MacIntyre NR: Respiratory factors in weaning from mechanical ventilatory support. Respir Care 40:244–259, 1995.)

Other factors that may contribute to ventilator dependence include inadequate arterial oxygenation, poor tissue oxygen delivery, myocardial ischemia, arrhythmias, low cardiac output, and cardiovascular instability.[7,16] Neurologic problems that may contribute to ventilator dependence include decreased central drive to breathe and impaired peripheral nerve transmission.[3] Psychologic issues that may contribute to ventilatory dependence include the fear of removal of the life support system, anxiety, stress, depression, and sleep deprivation.[3] Box 47-3 summarizes the major factors that contribute to ventilator dependence.

PATIENT EVALUATION

Careful patient assessment is required to determine which patients are ready to be removed from the ventilator quickly, which patients may need a prolonged ventilator discontinuation phase, and which patients are not yet ready for the discontinuation of ventilatory support.

An important factor to consider as part of this assessment is the length of time that the patient has been receiving mechanical ventilation. In general, those who receive support for 72 hours or less often can be removed quickly from the ventilator.[1,5,21] Those who need a longer period of support may need a more structured approach. Current guidelines recommend that patients who need mechanical ventilation for more than 48 to 72 hours be carefully

Box 47-3 Factors That Contribute to Ventilator Dependence

RESPIRATORY FACTORS
- Ventilatory workload exceeds ventilatory capacity
- Decreased compliance: lung or chest wall
- Increased resistance: artificial airways, bronchospasm, mucosal edema, secretions, and mechanical demand flow systems
- Increased dead space: pulmonary embolus and COPD
- Ventilatory muscle weakness or fatigue
- Oxygenation problems
  - $\downarrow \dot{V}/\dot{Q}$
  - $\downarrow \dot{Q}s/\dot{Q}t$
  - $\downarrow DO_2$
  - ↓ Oxygen extraction ratio

NONRESPIRATORY FACTORS
- Cardiovascular factors
- Myocardial ischemia
- Heart failure
- Hemodynamic instability, hypotension, and arrhythmias
- Neurologic factors
- Decreased or increased central drive to breathe
- Decreased peripheral nerve transmission
- Psychologic factors
- Fear and anxiety
- Stress
- Confusion or altered mental status
- Depression
- Poor nutrition
- Multiple-system organ failure
- Equipment shortcomings

Data from MacIntyre N: Respiratory factors in weaning from mechanical ventilatory support. Respir Care 40:244, 1995; Slutsky AS: Mechanical ventilation. American College of Chest Physicians' Consensus Conference. Chest 104:1833-1859, 1993; Pierson DJ: Nonrespiratory aspects of weaning from mechanical ventilation. Respir Care 40:263-270, 1995; MacIntyre NR, Cook DJ, Ely EW Jr, et al; American College of Chest Physicians; American Association for Respiratory Care; American College of Critical Care Medicine: Evidence-based guidelines for weaning and discontinuing ventilatory support: a collective task force facilitated by the American College of Chest Physicians; the American Association for Respiratory Care; and the American College of Critical Care Medicine. Chest 120(6 Suppl):375S-395S, 2001.

assessed to determine all of the possible causes of ventilator dependence.[3] These include the respiratory, cardiovascular, neurologic, and psychologic causes of ventilator dependence that are listed in Box 47-3. This recommendation is especially important for the care of patients who have had unsuccessful attempts at the discontinuation of ventilation.[3] Factors associated with readiness for the discontinuation of ventilatory support are summarized in Box 47-4.

The Most Important Criterion

The single most important criterion to consider when evaluating a patient for ventilator discontinuation or weaning is whether there has been significant alleviation or reversal

Box 47-4 Factors Associated With Readiness for the Discontinuation of Ventilatory Support

- Reversal or partial reversal of reason for instituting mechanical ventilation
- Good baseline functional status
- Ventilatory capacity that is capable of meeting ventilatory workload
- Good oxygenation status
- Good cardiovascular performance
- Good functional status of other organs and systems
- Short duration of the critical illness
- Short duration of mechanical ventilation
- No psychologic factors affecting the current status

Modified from Pierson DJ: Nonrespiratory aspects of weaning from mechanical ventilation. Respir Care 40:263-270, 1995.

of the disease state or condition that necessitated use of the ventilator in the first place.[3,7,14] The clinician should determine whether the patient's condition is improving, whether the initial reason for providing ventilatory support is improved or resolved, and whether the patient's clinical condition is stable. The following specific questions for patient evaluation have been suggested[3]:

1. Is there evidence of improvement or reversal of the disease state or condition that caused the need for mechanical ventilation?
2. Is the patient's oxygenation status adequate? Specific criteria may include the following: partial pressure of oxygen in the arteries PaO_2 of 60 mm Hg or more, FiO_2 of less than 0.40 to 0.50, PEEP of less than 5 to 8 cm H_2O; PaO_2/FiO_2 of 150 to 200 or more; and pH of 7.25 or more.
3. Is the patient medically and hemodynamically stable? Specific criteria may include the absence of acute myocardial ischemia or marked hypotension. Patients should have adequate blood pressure without vasopressor therapy or with only low-dose vasopressor therapy (i.e., less than 5 μg/kg/min of dopamine or dobutamine).
4. Can the patient breathe spontaneously? The patient must be able to breathe spontaneously and have a sufficient drive to breathe if ventilator discontinuation is being considered.

If the patient's condition is improving, if the alleviation or reversal of the precipitating disease state or condition has occurred, if the patient is capable of spontaneous breathing, and if the oxygenation status and hemodynamic values are stable, then a formal evaluation for ventilator discontinuation should be performed.[3]

Weaning Indices

Mechanical ventilation is hazardous, and unnecessary delays in ventilator discontinuation increase the associated complication rate.[3,4] Unfortunately, premature ventilator discontinuation may also cause serious problems, including difficulty with reestablishing the artificial airway and serious compromise of the patient's clinical status.[3,4] Clinical judgment has been found to be a poor guide to determining whether a patient is ready for ventilator discontinuation, and more specific indicators have been sought.[4] Ideally, specific indicators or weaning indices would clearly show whether a patient is ready to have the ventilator removed and would help to avoid inappropriate ventilator discontinuation. Unfortunately, none of the current weaning indices are capable of predicting readiness for ventilator discontinuance with a high level of accuracy.

Traditional discontinuation indices include the PaO_2/FiO_2 ratio, the alveolar-to-arterial partial pressure of oxygen difference [$P(A–a)O_2$], the maximum inspiratory pressure (MIP), the vital capacity (VC), the spontaneous minute ventilation (V_{Esp}), and the maximum voluntary ventilation (MVV).[5,21] Newer indices include the **rapid, shallow breathing index (f/V_T), airway occlusion pressure** ($P_{0.1}$), and measures of WOB.[6-8] Although all of these values can be useful, there are enormous discrepancies in the literature regarding their accuracy with regard to the prediction of "weanability."[3,6,7] With respect to the more traditional discontinuation indices, vital capacity and MIP can be highly variable, whereas minute ventilation, respiratory rate (f), and f/V_T tend to be more reliable.[22] However, these measures may not correlate well with discontinuation success among all patients and especially among those receiving long-term ventilatory support, the elderly, and those with major pulmonary abnormalities.[5,18,23]

A comprehensive evidence-based review identified a possible role for 66 specific measurements as predictors of weaning success.[6] Of these, eight values were found to be the most useful for the prediction of successful ventilator discontinuation.[3,6] Useful predictive measures included spontaneous respiratory rate, spontaneous tidal volume, f/V_T, minute ventilation, MIP, $P_{0.1}$, $P_{0.1}$/MIP, and a combined index called the *CROP score* that included compliance, rate, oxygenation, and MIP.[3,6] Unfortunately, these measures all have limitations and relatively high false-positive predictions in specific settings.

It is doubtful that a single index will be found that can be used for consistent discrimination between discontinuation success and failure.[7] Moreover, none of these traditional indicators alone has proved useful for the prediction of improvements in patient outcome or in the selection of a particular discontinuation method.[7,10] The likely explanation for this failure to identify any consistently powerful discontinuation predictor is that patients' conditions vary greatly and, for research purposes, clinicians already fully consider information from predictors when choosing patients for trials of the reduction or discontinuation of ventilatory support.[10,23]

Notwithstanding these limitations, the measurement of discontinuation indices in the difficult-to-wean patient may provide guidance with regard to the reasons that patients fail discontinuation trials. Many find it useful to trend these data on a daily basis for those patients who require lengthy weaning times.[15] Specific values for respiratory indices that are used to predict the successful discontinuation of ventilatory support are found in Table 47-1.

TABLE 47-1

Indices That Are Used to Predict the Success of Weaning and Ventilator Discontinuation

Measurement	Criterion
Oxygenation	
FiO_2	≤0.40 to 0.50
PEEP (cm H_2O)	≤5 to 8
PaO_2 (mm Hg)	≥60
SaO_2 (%)	≥90
SvO_2 (%)	≥60
PaO_2/PAO_2 ratio	≥0.35
PaO_2/FiO_2 ratio	>150 to 200
$P(A-a)O_2$ (mm Hg)	<350
$\dot{Q}s/\dot{Q}t$ (% shunt)	<15% to 20%
No lactic acidosis, adequate $\dot{Q}t$, blood pressure	
Ventilation	
$PaCO_2$ (mm Hg)	<50
pH	≥7.35
Ventilatory Mechanics	
Respiratory rate (f) (breaths/min)	12 to 30
Tidal volume (V_T) (ml/kg)	>5
Vital capacity (VC) (ml/kg)	>10 to 15
Static compliance (ml/cm H_2O)	>25
f/V_T	<105
Respiratory Muscle Strength	
Maximum inspiratory force (MIF) (cm H_2O)	<–20 to –30
Ventilatory Drive (Demand)	
Minute ventilation ($\dot{V}_E$) for	
Normal PCO_2 (L/min)	<10
V_{DS}/V_T	<0.55 to 0.60
$P_{0.1}$ (cm H_2O)	<6
$P_{0.1}$/MIP	<0.30
Work of Breathing	
Spontaneous work of breathing	<1.6 kg·m/min (<0.14 kg·m/L)
Pressure–time index	<0.15 to 0.18
Ventilatory Reserve	
Maximum voluntary ventilation (MVV) (L/min)	>20; more than twice the $\dot{V}_E$

Data from MacIntyre NR, Cook DJ, Ely EW, et al: Evidence-based guidelines for weaning and discontinuing ventilator support: a collective task force facilitated by the American College of Chest Physicians, the American Association for Respiratory Care, and the American College of Critical Care Medicine. Chest 120:375S–395S, 2001; AHRQ publication no. 01-E010, Rockville, MD, 2000, Agency for Healthcare Research and Quality; American College of Chest Physicians: Chest 104:1833, 1993; Burns SM et al: Am J Crit Care 4:4, 1995; Sharar S: Resp Care 40:239, 1995; Bassili HR, Deitel M: JPEN J Parenter Enteral Nutr 5:161, 1981.

Ventilation

Increased thoracic cage movement during spontaneous breathing and asynchronous chest-wall-to-diaphragm movement are related to an increased workload that may lead to ventilatory muscle fatigue and failure.[19] Tachypnea (i.e., more than 30 to 35 breaths/min) is a sensitive marker of respiratory distress, but it can prolong intubation if it is used as an exclusive criterion.[25] Irregular spontaneous breathing or periods of apnea indicate that the patient is at risk for weaning failure. Asynchronous and rapid, shallow breathing patterns—although not definitive—suggest respiratory decompensation.[19]

The evaluation of patients for the presence of palpable scalene muscle use during inspiration, an irregular ventilatory pattern, palpable abdominal muscle tensing during expiration, and the inability to alter the ventilatory pattern on command can be helpful for the assessment of the potential for prolonged spontaneous ventilation. Patients with none of these signs have a 90% chance of success.[26] Patients with one or two of these signs usually need continued support. The presence of three or more of these signs can mean that the patient's condition is unstable and that the patient has a poor prognosis for ventilator removal.

$P_{0.1}$ is the inspiratory pressure that is measured 100 milliseconds after airway occlusion.[21] The $P_{0.1}$ is effort independent, and it correlates well with central respiratory drive.[19] Ventilator-dependent patients with COPD who have a $P_{0.1}$ of more than 6 cm H_2O tend to be difficult to wean.[21]

The f/V_T is the ratio of spontaneous breathing frequency (breaths/min) to tidal volume (liters), and it has been found to be a good predictor of discontinuation success for the care of many patients who need mechanical ventilation.[4,6,23] The f/V_T has less predictive power for the care of patients who need ventilatory support for longer than 8 days, and it may be less useful for predicting discontinuation success among elderly patients.[8,23,27] Adjusting the threshold value for f/V_T to 130 or less measured at 3 hours was very effective for predicting discontinuation success among patients 70 years old and older. Despite these limitations, an f/V_T of less than 105 can be an accurate and early predictor of weaning outcome, and an f/V_T of 80 is associated with an almost 95% probability of successful discontinuation.[4,23] The ratio must be calculated during 1 minute of unsupported spontaneous breathing, and the addition of pressure support significantly reduces the predictive value of the ratio.[4]

RULE OF THUMB

Adult patients with respiratory rates in excess of 35 breaths/min and tidal volumes of less than 250 ml may be difficult to wean.

The $P_{0.1}$/MIP ratio has been found to be a good early predictor of discontinuation success,[3,19] and it may be more useful than the MIP by itself. The f/V_T also has been found to be a better predictor of discontinuation success than the MIP alone.[2,3] However, even with f/V_T of less than 105, as many as 20% of patients have false-positive results (i.e., they cannot be discontinued from ventilation despite a favorable index) as a result of unpredictable factors such as congestive heart failure, aspiration, or the development of a new pulmonary lesion.[28] However, some patients can be successfully discontinued from ventilatory support despite poor f/V_T values.[29]

MINI CLINI

Calculating and Interpreting the Rapid, Shallow Breathing Index

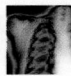

PROBLEM: You measure the following spontaneous breathing values for two patients who are being considered for weaning from mechanical ventilation:

Patient	Rate (f) (breaths/min)	V_T (L)
A	32	0.28
B	28	0.42

For which patient is successful weaning least likely?

SOLUTION: First, compute the rapid, shallow breathing index for each patient as follows:

Patient	Rate (f) (breaths/min)	V_T (L)	f/V_T
A	32	0.28	114
B	28	0.42	67

Patient A clearly exceeds the threshold criterion of 105 breaths/min per liter, whereas patient B falls well below this criterion. All else being equal, patient A is least likely to be successfully weaned.

WOB would seem to be an excellent way to gauge spontaneous ventilatory workload. Successful weaning has been found to be less likely among patients with spontaneous WOB levels of more than 1.6 kg/m/min (16 J/min) or 0.14 kg/m/L (1.4 J/L).[5] However, WOB may not be predictive of weaning success for specific patients.[7] This may be because WOB does not take into account ventilatory muscle capacity or fatigue. Consequently, WOB may be less accurate than other conventional discontinuation indices, and it is very difficult to measure at the bedside.[30]

Oxygen cost of breathing (OCB) is the difference between oxygen consumption during spontaneous breathing and oxygen consumption during apnea (i.e., during full ventilatory support), which is determined as follows:

$$OCB = VO_{2sp} - VO_2 \text{ (controlled ventilation)}$$

After the OCB has been estimated, the relative proportion of oxygen consumed by the respiratory muscles as compared with the body as a whole can be calculated as follows:

$$\%VO_2 \text{ (Resp)} = (OCB / VO_{2sp}) \times 100$$

Both OCB and $\%VO_2$ have been correlated with the number of days required to wean patients.[19] Patients with an OCB of 15% or less of the total VO_2 may be more likely to achieve discontinuation success. In one study,

OCB was a better predictor of discontinuation success than was f/V_T.[31]

Pressure-time product (i.e., the area under the inspiratory pressure-time curve) and pressure-time index (PTI) may be the best measures of ventilatory workload for the care of patients who are receiving mechanical support.[1] The PTI can be calculated as follows:

$$PTI = (\text{Mean inspiratory pressure}/MIP) \times T_i/T_{tot}$$

where MIP is maximum inspiratory pressure, T_i is the inspiratory time in seconds, and T_{tot} is the total respiratory cycle. The T_{tot} can be calculated by dividing 60 by the respiratory rate (f) (i.e., 60/f). A PTI of more than 0.15 to 0.18 has been associated with diaphragmatic fatigue,[32] and a PTI of more than 0.15 cannot be sustained indefinitely.[1] There is currently no well accepted and reliable way to measure ventilatory muscle fatigue for patients who are receiving mechanical ventilation.[5]

Oxygenation

Poor oxygenation status is associated with weaning failure.[3,7] Arterial blood gas (ABG) analysis, pulse oximetry, and continuous mixed venous oximetry have been used to monitor and assess the oxygenation status of patients before and during a discontinuation trial. In general, a PaO_2 of more than 60 mm Hg (or of more than 55 mm Hg for patients with COPD with carbon dioxide retention) with an FiO_2 of less than 0.40 to 0.50 and a PEEP of 5 to 8 cm H_2O or less should be adequate for ventilator discontinuation.[3,7] The PaO_2/FiO_2 ratio should be 150 to 200 mm Hg or more.[3] With these values, a normal hemoglobin level, a normal oxygen saturation (SaO_2), and adequate cardiac output and tissue perfusion are assumed. Specific indices used to assess oxygenation status are found in Table 47-1.

Acid-Base Balance

Ideally the patient should have a normal acid-base balance (i.e., a pH of 7.35 to 7.45), and abnormalities in acid-base status should be corrected, if possible, before weaning. Patients with metabolic acidosis often have an increased ventilatory drive that can make weaning difficult. Patients who have metabolic alkalosis or those who have been mechanically hyperventilated for several days may have a reduced ventilatory drive. In these cases, a gradual method of discontinuing ventilatory support should be considered.

Metabolic Factors

Metabolic factors primarily affect discontinuation in those patients who require long-term ventilatory support. Although nutritional factors are important for all patients, they are unlikely to affect discontinuation in those who only require short-term ventilatory support. Nutrition should be adequate to maintain respiratory muscle mass and contractile force.[16] Feeding should be adjusted according to individual patient needs; most patients need 1.5 to 2.0 times their resting energy expenditure.[33] In addition, protein intake should be between 1 and 1.5 g/kg per day. Excessive carbohydrate feeding can increase carbon dioxide production and may precipitate acute hypercapnic respiratory failure.[16] Parenteral nutrition solutions that contain amino acid formulations (e.g., arginine/lysine) can cause metabolic acidosis and thus increase ventilatory demand.[33] Metabolic rate can increase as a result of fever or sepsis. Increased WOB, shivering, seizures, and agitation can also increase oxygen demand and should be evaluated.

Renal Function and Electrolytes

Adequate renal function is required to maintain acid-base homeostasis, electrolyte concentrations, and fluid balance.[34] The patient ideally should have an adequate urine output (i.e., more than 1000 ml/day), and there should be no inappropriate weight gain or edema.

Renal insufficiency can lead to metabolic acidosis, which increases respiratory drive. Electrolyte disorders can impair ventilatory muscle function.[3,16] Key electrolytes should be normal (i.e., magnesium, 1.8 to 3 mEq/L; phosphate, 2.5 to 4.8 mEq/L; potassium, 3.5 to 5 mEq/L); see Chapter 16 for details. Fluid overload can lead to congestive heart failure and pulmonary edema, which may impair pulmonary gas exchange.

Cardiovascular Function

Adequate cardiovascular function is needed to provide sufficient oxygen delivery to the tissues. Cardiac rate and rhythm and blood pressure should be evaluated.[3,16] Tachycardia (i.e., a heart rate of more than 100 to 120 beats/min) and bradycardia (i.e., a heart rate of less than 60 to 70 beats/min) should be controlled. The presence of arrhythmias, hypotension (i.e., a blood pressure of less than 90/60 mm Hg), and severe hypertension (i.e., a blood pressure of more than 180/110 mm Hg) should be evaluated carefully before the discontinuation of ventilatory support is considered.[3,19]

Cardiac output and index measurements as well as central line and pulmonary arterial pressures (i.e., central venous pressure, pulmonary arterial pressure, and pulmonary capillary wedge pressure) may be helpful for the evaluation of cardiovascular function. Left ventricular dysfunction, myocardial ischemia, and cardiovascular instability are associated with decreased discontinuation success.[3,21] Table 47-2 provides criteria for confirming cardiovascular stability. However, very few patients without primary cardiovascular dysfunction have pulmonary artery catheters in place. The assessment of cardiac output is usually by noninvasive means, and only arterial and central venous pressures are generally available.

Psychologic Factors and Central Nervous System Assessment

Adequate CNS function is needed to ensure stable ventilatory drive, adequate secretion clearance (i.e., coughing and deep breathing), and the protection of the airway (i.e., gag

TABLE 47-2

Criteria for Confirming Cardiovascular Stability

Criterion	Normal Value	Values That May Be Inconsistent With Weaning
Heart rate (beats/min)	60 to 100	<60, >120
Blood pressure (mm Hg)	90/60 to 150/90	<90/60, >180/110
$\dot{Q}t$ (L/min)	4 to 8	
Cardiac index ($L/min^{-1} \cdot m^2$)	2.5 to 4	<2.1
Cardiac rhythm	No major arrhythmias present	Tachycardia, bradycardia, multiple premature ventricular contractions, heart block
Hemoglobin (g/dl)	12 to 15	Anemia, <10
Hematocrit	40% to 50%	
No angina present		
No lactic acidosis		

reflex and swallow). In addition, the level of consciousness, dyspnea, anxiety, depression, and motivation can affect discontinuation success.[3,5]

The patient ideally is awake and alert, free of seizures, and able to follow instructions.[3,34] Patients should have an intact central drive to breathe and peripheral nerve function. Brainstem strokes, electrolyte disturbances, sedation, neuromuscular blocking agents, and narcotic drugs can impair the central neurologic control of ventilation.[3] Mental status is a good predictor of discontinuation success, and patients who are not alert are at risk for upper airway obstruction, aspiration, and secretion retention. Obtunded patients should, at a minimum, have an adequate gag reflex and cough. Decreased levels of consciousness are associated with aspiration after extubation. The level of consciousness is affected by the use of narcotic, sedative, and analgesic drugs. Drugs with CNS depressant effects should be discontinued, if possible, before the withdrawal of ventilatory support and extubation.[16] Protocols to reduce sedation and the daily cessation of sedative drugs may reduce weaning time[12,35,36] (see the section on Spontaneous Awaking Trials). The use of neuromuscular blocking agents to allow for controlled ventilation should be avoided, because they may prolong mechanical ventilation.[37]

Psychologic factors may be among the most important nonrespiratory contributing factors that lead to ventilator dependence.[3] Fear, anxiety, and stress should be minimized, and frequent communication among the staff, the patient, and the patient's family can be helpful.[3] Box 47-5 summarizes nonrespiratory factors that affect discontinuation success.

Integrated Indices

Many factors are associated with discontinuation success. In an analysis of 217 patients, discontinuation success could be accurately predicted in about 75% of the patients when multiple predictors were combined.[24] For all patients, regardless of diagnosis, days of mechanical ventilation (DMV), f/V_T; MIP, $P_{0.1}$, maximum expiratory pressure, and VC—when used in combination—were the best predictors.[24] For patients with acute respiratory failure, the best predictors were DMV, $P_{0.1}$/MIP, MIP, f/V_T, and age (76.1% accurate); for patients with COPD, the best predictors were DMV, f/V_T, $P_{0.1}$, $P_{0.1}$/MIP, MIP, and age (93.9% accurate); and for patients with neuromuscular disease, MIP, maximum expiratory pressure, f/V_T, and $P_{0.1}$ were the best predictors (73.9% accurate).[24] Integrated indices improve prediction by combining several measures of ability to breathe without ventilatory support. Current examples of integrated indexes include the CROP score, the Adverse Factor/Ventilator Score, the weaning index, and the Burns Weaning Assessment Program.[7,19] The CROP score combines measures of ventilatory load, respiratory muscle strength, and gas exchange.[7,23]

The Adverse Factor/Ventilator Score combines ratings of 15 adverse factors, including hemodynamic values, infection, nutrition, and neurologic/psychiatric state, with ratings of six ventilator factors, including FiO_2, compliance, minute ventilation, and rate.[19] The weaning index combines measures of ventilatory strength, endurance, and efficiency of gas exchange.[19] A weaning index of

Box 47-5 Nonrespiratory Factors That Affect Weaning

- Acid-base status
- Metabolic alkalosis: decreased ventilatory drive
- Metabolic acidosis: increased ventilatory demand
- Mineral and electrolyte balance
- Hypophosphatemia: ventilatory muscle weakness
- Hypomagnesemia: ventilatory muscle weakness
- Hypokalemia: ventilatory muscle weakness
- Hypothyroidism: decreased ventilatory drive and impaired muscle function
- Medical stability of other organs and systems
- Cardiac: excessive preload (e.g., overall volume overload, increased preload on discontinuation of positive pressure ventilation) and impaired contractility
- Renal: renal insufficiency and metabolic acidosis
- Hepatic: encephalopathy and protein synthesis
- Gastrointestinal: stress-related hemorrhage and ability to take enteral nutrition
- Neurologic: level of consciousness, ability to protect the airway, and clear secretions
- Effects of drugs: narcotics, benzodiazepines, other sedatives and hypnotics, muscle relaxants, and aminoglycosides
- Nutritional status
- Ventilatory muscle function
- Ventilatory drive
- Immune defense system
- Psychologic and motivational factors

Modified from Pierson DJ: Nonrespiratory aspects of weaning from mechanical ventilation. Respir Care 40:289, 1995.

less than 4 suggests successful discontinuation from mechanical ventilation.[18,32] The Burns Weaning Assessment Program is a 26-item assessment that combines 12 general and 14 respiratory factors into a single score.[19] Although integrated indices appear promising, no single index has emerged as superior for use in diverse patient populations. Despite the success of these integrated indices in very specific settings, the best approach to determining if a patient can be successfully discontinued from ventilatory support is the patient's performance on spontaneous breathing trials. All patients should be assessed daily, and their ability to breathe spontaneously should be the primarily variable to determine if the ventilator can be discontinued.

MINI CLINI

Assessment of Readiness for a Spontaneous Breathing Trial

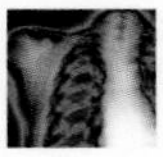

PROBLEM: A 64-year-old man who underwent a lung resection and who has a long history of COPD is now 24 hours postoperative, and he is being evaluated for readiness for an SBT. The data currently available for this patient include the following:

- Ventilator settings:
  - Mode volume assist/control)
  - VT 450 ml (6.5 ml/kg ideal body weight)
- Respiratory rate of 28 breaths/min
- FiO_2 of 0.40
- PEEP of 5 cm H_2O

The patient is alert, there is cooperative spontaneous breathing, and he is regularly triggering the ventilator.

The patient is not receiving any vasoactive drugs, and he is only receiving intermittent sedatives and narcotics.

Should this patient be placed on an SBT?

SOLUTION: By 24 hours, the patient should have initially recovered from the effects of the surgical procedure. The patient's ventilator settings are offering minimal support. Because the patient is alert and able to breathe spontaneously and because he requires only intermittent sedatives or narcotics, it is very appropriate to perform an SBT on this patient at this time.

Evaluation of the Airway

The ability to maintain a patent natural airway and the likelihood of aspiration should be evaluated as a part of the process of discontinuing ventilatory support.

It is important for the clinician to separate the decision to discontinue ventilatory support from the decision to extubate.[29] The clinician must also be aware that most weaning indices do not evaluate airway patency or protection (see the section on Extubation). The inability to protect or maintain the natural airway is a clear contraindication to extubation. Some patients who can be successfully removed from a ventilator should not be extubated.[29] Tracheotomy may be considered for the care of patients who need artificial airways for an extended period.

Tracheotomy may improve patient comfort, allow for more effective suctioning, decrease airway resistance, enhance mobility, and allow the patient to eat and speak.[3] Some patients also need high levels of sedation to tolerate the endotracheal tube.[3] Consequently, tracheotomy should be considered for the care of patients who are likely to benefit and for those who need prolonged mechanical ventilatory support.[3] See Chapter 33 for details about airway management and extubation.

Other patients with good airway patency and protection may be unable to maintain spontaneous breathing for prolonged periods without assistance.[29] These patients may be candidates for noninvasive ventilation (NIV) after extubation; see Chapter 46 for details.[18,38]

PREPARING THE PATIENT

Optimizing the Patient's Medical Condition

Before the removal of ventilatory support is attempted, the patient's oxygenation status, ventilation, cardiovascular status, and overall medical condition should be optimized. Disease-imposed ventilatory load is minimized with the management of infection, bronchospasm, and airway edema.[1] Bronchodilator therapy should be maximized and the appropriate use of anti-inflammatory agents considered.[1,29] Techniques to facilitate secretion clearance (e.g., suctioning, adequate humidification, bronchial hygiene techniques), good nutrition, and optimal positioning should be used.[29] The patient should be rested and not fatigued or sleep deprived, which can be common in the ICU. The patient should be allowed to sleep at night while maintained on a level of ventilatory support that ensures ventilatory muscle rest.[16,39]

The patient's ventilatory workload should be minimized with PSV.[29] Flow-trigger or flow-by ventilation or ATC may also be helpful for minimizing imposed ventilatory work. Intrinsic PEEP during mechanical ventilation may increase trigger work, and small amounts of PEEP or CPAP can help to overcome this problem.[1,2] Box 47-6 lists factors that should be optimized before ventilatory support is discontinued.

Patients' Psychologic and Communication Needs

As many as 47% of patients who spend more than 5 days in an ICU may experience psychologic disturbances.[38] The cause may be the stress of critical illness, the interruption of nighttime sleep, or the use of sedatives, tranquilizers, hypnotics, narcotics, and other drugs that affect the CNS.[39] The patient's environment should be optimized, anxiety and depression should be evaluated, and communication should be maximized.[3,19,21,39]

Box 47-6 Factors That Should Be Optimized Before the Discontinuation of Ventilatory Support Is Attempted

- Oxygenation
- PaO_2 and SaO_2
- Anemia, if present
- Atelectasis, pneumonia, and acute pulmonary disease
- Ventilation
- Humidification
- Secretion clearance (e.g., bronchial hygiene, suctioning)
- Bronchodilator therapy
- Respiratory alkalosis
- Imposed WOB
- Respiratory muscle fatigue or atrophy
- Acid-base balance and electrolytes
- Metabolic acidosis (e.g., lactic acidosis, ketoacidosis)
- Metabolic alkalosis (e.g., decreased serum potassium or chloride ions, nasogastric tube, vomiting)
- Low phosphate level
- Low magnesium level
- Cardiac and cardiovascular status
- Blood pressure and cardiac output
- Arrhythmias, if present
- Myocardial ischemia
- Left ventricular function
- Renal factors
- Kidney function
- Fluid balance
- Fever, infection, or sepsis
- Pain (i.e., minimize without oversedation)
- Sleep deprivation
- Exercise tolerance (up in a chair, if possible)
- Drugs (narcotics, sedatives, tranquilizers, hypnotics, aminoglycosides, and neuromuscular blocking agents can depress or block the ventilatory drive)
- Psychologic status
- Level of consciousness (e.g., delirium, coma)
- Agitation
- Motivation
- Fear and anxiety
- Psychologic dependence on the ventilator
- Depression
- ICU psychosis
- Hypothyroidism
- Nutritional factors
- Overfeeding (i.e., increased carbon dioxide production)
- Malnutrition or protein loss
- Consider a high-fat, low-carbohydrate diet to minimize the production of carbon dioxide
- Gastrointestinal bleeding or obstruction
- Abdominal distention or ascites
- Procedural factors that should be optimized
- Time of day (avoid evenings, nights, and shift changes)
- Adequate staffing
- Interruptions and disruptions
- Technical factors to consider
- Appropriate level of PSV to overcome endotracheal tube resistance
- Flow-trigger or flow-by ventilation
- PEEP/CPAP to balance intrinsic PEEP

Modified from Hess DR, Kacmarek RM: Essentials of mechanical ventilation, ed 2, New York, 2003, McGraw Hill; Kacmarek RM, Mack CW, Dimus S: Essentials of respiratory care, ed 4, St. Louis, 2005, Mosby; and Tobin MJ: Principles and practice of mechanical ventilation, ed 2, McGraw Hill, 2006, New York.

Environmental considerations that may improve the patient's sense of well-being and outlook include reducing extraneous noise and providing clocks, calendars, pictures, a radio, a television, and, if possible, a room with windows.[38] Daily mobility should be considered, including getting the patient up in a chair or placing the patient in the hall in a chair.[39] Patients whose condition has been stable can sometimes even be helped to walk with the use of an E cylinder for oxygen, a manual resuscitator bag, and two or more health care workers for support.

A method for the patient to communicate with staff and visitors should be devised, if possible. Writing tablets, picture boards, and alphabet boards have been used effectively by patients to communicate with staff and visitors.

Anxiety and agitation should be minimized, and communication and encouragement may be helpful.[39] The patient should be told what is planned and be given some control over the situation. Patients should be asked to participate and help in the weaning process. Depression or a lack of motivation may increase weaning time.[5,39] If depression is present, assessment and treatment by an appropriate health care provider should be considered.[39]

METHODS

There are three basic methods of discontinuing ventilatory support[4]:

1. Spontaneous breathing trials (via the mechanical ventilator or with a T-piece) alternating with mechanical ventilatory support
2. SIMV
3. PSV

Box 47-7 summarizes evidence-based criteria and related conclusions regarding methods for ventilator discontinuation.

Rapid Ventilator Discontinuation

When the precipitating disease state or condition that necessitates support has been significantly alleviated or reversed, most patients can be rapidly removed from

Box 47-7 Agency for Healthcare Research and Quality Summary of Evidence for Criteria for Weaning from Mechanical Ventilation

- Differences in clinicians' intuitive thresholds for the reduction or discontinuation of ventilatory support have a far greater impact on the failure of SBTs and on reintubation than do modes of discontinuation. When clinicians set a high threshold, many patients who could tolerate weaning remain on mechanical support longer than is necessary.
- There may be an interaction between the threshold and the mode of discontinuation; in other words, one mode may be superior when the threshold is high, whereas another may be superior when the threshold is low.
- Research to date suggests that the best answer to the question of when to start discontinuation trials is to develop a protocol that can be implemented by nurses and respiratory therapists that begins testing for the opportunity to reduce support immediately after intubation and reduces support at every opportunity.
- For stepwise reductions in mechanical support, pressure support mode or multiple daily spontaneous breathing trials may be superior to SIMV.
- For trials of unassisted breathing, low levels of pressure support may be beneficial.
- There may be substantial benefits to the use of noninvasive positive pressure ventilation during the discontinuation process.
- After cardiac surgery, early extubation is unequivocally achieved with a variety of anesthetic interventions and ICU protocols; however, the corresponding reduction in ICU stay is generally small, and the effect on complications, although rare, remains unclear.
- Although steroids can reduce postextubation stridor in children, the impact of steroids on reintubation in children and adults remains uncertain.
- Most theoretically plausible predictors of discontinuation and extubation success have no predictive power. Those with some predictive power include the rapid, shallow breathing index, which has been most intensively studied, the $P_{0.1}$/MIP ratio, and the CROP index. However, these are relatively weak predictors of discontinuation success.
- Tests are rarely useful for increasing the probability of discontinuation success; on occasion, the results can lead to moderate reductions in the probability of success.
- In general, discontinuation predictors are probably found to perform poorly because physicians have already considered the results when they select patients for studies.

Modified from the Agency for Healthcare Research and Quality: Evidence report/technology assessment Number 23 (AHRQ Publication No. 01-E010), Rockville, Md, 2000, Agency for Healthcare Research and Quality.

mechanical ventilation.[16,21] These patients typically have acceptable blood gas levels with mechanical ventilation, adequate myocardial function, and no underlying cardiovascular, pulmonary, neurologic, or neuromuscular disorders.[21]

After a careful evaluation, patients in stable condition who have been treated with a ventilator for less than 72 hours and who have a good spontaneous respiratory rate and minute ventilation may undergo an SBT on the ventilator or with a T-piece for 30 to 120 minutes.[3,7] If the patient does well, the endotracheal tube can then be removed if there is no reason to maintain an artificial airway.

Today, most SBTs are performed with the patient attached to a ventilator that is set on zero PSV and zero CPAP. This allows for a stable FiO_2 and ongoing monitoring. Others have recommended treating the patient with a low level of PSV (i.e., 5 to 7 cm H_2O) to overcome the resistance caused by the ventilator circuit, the demand flow system, and the artificial airway.[2] Others may prefer simply using CPAP (i.e., 5 to 7 cm H_2O).[2,3] These methods have the advantage of allowing the clinician to maintain ventilator alarm settings that can provide a margin of safety in the event of apnea or severe hypoventilation. Low levels of CPAP may be useful for maintaining lung volumes and overcoming intrinsic PEEP.[2] Some experts recommend PSV in combination with PEEP or CPAP.[2] However, the most widely accepted guidelines[3] recommend a simple spontaneous breathing trial for the first SBT using the ventilator at zero CPAP and zero PEEP or a T-piece.

Patients Who Need Progressive Weaning of Ventilatory Support

Patients who have been receiving mechanical ventilation for more than 72 hours and those with marginal oxygenation, ventilatory, cardiovascular, or medical statuses may need a more prolonged period for ventilator discontinuation.[19,21] The most common methods for accomplishing this are SBTs interspersed with continued ventilatory support, SIMV, and PSV.[4]

Spontaneous Breathing Trials

The oldest discontinuation method is an SBT via either the ventilator or T-piece, which allows for spontaneous breathing several times per day interspersed with periods of mechanical ventilatory support. For gradual weaning, initial SBTs may last only 5 to 10 minutes.[4,7] Full ventilatory support is resumed for a 1- to 4-hour rest period in the assist-control or pressure-support mode. The time off of the ventilator is gradually increased until the patient is able to stay off of the ventilator for an extended period. SBTs can progress rapidly to ventilator removal.

When weaning is very difficult, the process can last days or even weeks. When a T-piece is used instead of the ventilator, the patient must be more carefully monitored, because none of the ventilator alarms are active during the SBT. If distress occurs, mechanical ventilation is resumed.

In no case should the patient be overstressed during the SBT, because exhaustion can delay weaning.[2,8] An example of an SBT is presented in Box 47-8.

In one major multicenter study, one or more daily SBTs resulted in three times faster extubation than with SIMV and two times faster than with PSV[40] (Figure 47-2). Results of another study favored PSV over T-tube trials or SIMV[47] (Figure 47-3). In a third study, SBTs were more effective than SIMV for weaning quadriplegic patients.[41] Advantages of SBTs include the early and frequent testing of the patient's ability to breathe spontaneously without support.[2,3] The use of SBTs several times per day has become unpopular, because it requires a great deal of time on the part of ICU staff, and a single daily SBT seems to be just as effective for most patients.[3,4,10] PSV and CPAP are sometimes used during the SBT, and patients who tolerate spontaneous breathing with a low level of PSV (i.e., 7 cm H_2O or less) should be able to tolerate extubation.[42] Current recommendations suggest a single daily trial of spontaneous breathing may be preferable to other methods of weaning.[3] Results of randomized, controlled studies have shown SBTs to be faster than SIMV and at least as

Box 47-8 Steps for Spontaneous Breathing Trials

1. Prepare the patient psychologically.
2. Set the ventilator at zero PSV and zero CPAP.
3. Maintain the FiO_2 at the baseline FiO_2 that the patient is receiving.
4. Monitor the patient's appearance, pulse, oxygen saturation measured by pulse oximeter, and blood pressure; observe the cardiac monitor for arrhythmia. Use the ventilator to monitor respiratory rate, tidal volume, and minute ventilation.
5. If the patient tolerates the SBT for 30 to 120 minutes, consider extubation.
6. If the patient does not tolerate the SBT for at least 30 minutes, reestablish the ventilator settings, and allow the patient to rest for at least a few hours before reattempting another SBT.
7. If repeated SBTs over multiple days are needed, individualize the patient's schedule, depending on his or her condition. In general, the weaning schedule should be stopped during the night so that the patient can rest and sleep.

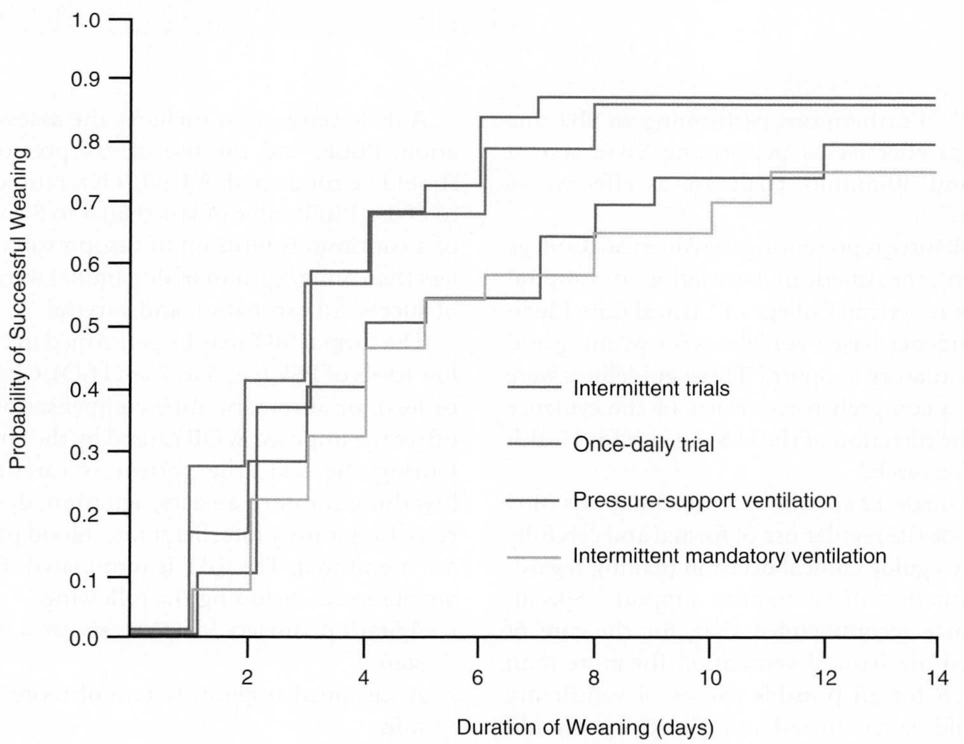

FIGURE 47-2 Kaplan-Meier curves of the probability of successful weaning with SIMV, PSV, intermittent trials of spontaneous breathing, and a once-daily trial of spontaneous breathing. After adjustment for baseline characteristics, the rate of successful weaning with a once-daily trial of spontaneous breathing was 2.83 times higher than that obtained with SIMV ($P < .006$) and 2.05 times higher than that of pressure support ($P < .04$). (Modified from Esteban A, Frutos F, Tobin M, et al: A comparison of four methods of weaning patients from mechanical ventilation. Spanish Lung Failure Collaborative Group. N Engl J Med 332:345-350, 1995.)

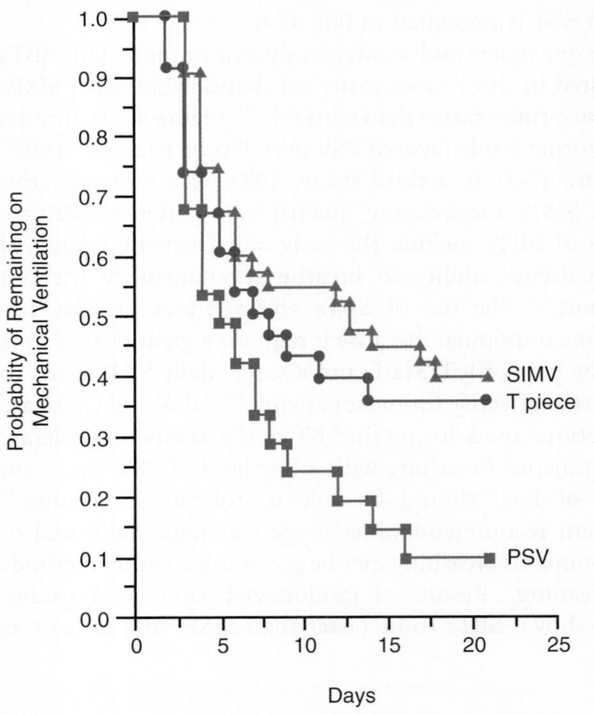

FIGURE 47-3 Probability of continuing mechanical ventilation for the care of patients with prolonged difficulties with tolerating spontaneous breathing. This probability was significantly lower for PSV than for SBT or SIMV (cumulative probability for 21 days, $P < .03$ with the log-rank test). (Modified from Brochard L, Rauss A, Bentio S, et al: Comparison of three methods of gradual withdrawal from ventilatory support during weaning from mechanical ventilation. Am J Respir Crit Care Med 150:896–903, 1994.)

effective as PSV.[3,4,10] Furthermore, performing an SBT one time per day is as effective as performing SBTs several times per day, and 30-minute trials are as effective as 120-minute trials.[4]

A collective task force representing the American College of Chest Physicians, the American Association for Respiratory Care, and the American College of Critical Care Medicine published evidence-based guidelines for weaning and discontinuing ventilatory support.[3] These guidelines were based in part on a comprehensive review of the evidence collected under the direction of the U.S. Agency for Health Care Policy and Research.[6]

The task force made 12 specific recommendations (Box 47-9). These include the regular use of formal and carefully monitored SBTs to guide clinical decision making regarding the discontinuation of ventilatory support.[3] Specifically, the task force recommended that, for the care of patients who need mechanical ventilation for more than 24 hours, a search for all possible causes of ventilatory dependence should be conducted and an attempt should be made to reverse or optimize each condition. Spontaneously breathing patients with evidence of reversal of the underlying condition that necessitated the ventilatory support, adequate oxygenation, and hemodynamic stability should be assessed with an SBT. Table 47-3 lists criteria to be used when determining whether patients who are receiving high levels of ventilatory support can be considered for SBTs.

A daily screen that includes the assessment of oxygenation, PEEP, and the use of vasopressors and sedatives should be conducted. A PaO_2/FiO_2 ratio of more than 150 to 200, a PEEP value of less than 5 to 8 cm H_2O, and a lack of a continuous infusion of vasopressors or sedatives (i.e., less than 5 mg/kg/min of dopamine) were good predictors of successful extubation and survival.[41]

The formal SBT may be performed in combination with low levels of PSV (i.e., 5 to 7 cm H_2O), CPAP (i.e., 5 cm H_2O or less), or automatic tube compensation applied to just offset the imposed WOB caused by the endotracheal tube.[3] During the SBT, the patient is carefully observed for breathing comfort, anxiety, agitation, dyspnea, or diaphoresis. Respiratory rate, heart rate, blood pressure, and SpO_2 are monitored. The SBT is terminated if signs of distress are observed, including the following:

- Agitation, anxiety, diaphoresis, or a change in mental status
- A sustained respiratory rate of more than 35 breaths/min
- A sustained SpO_2 of less than 90%
- A more than 20% increase or decrease in heart rate or a heart rate of more than 120 to 140 beats/min
- A systolic blood pressure of more than 180 mm Hg or of less than 90 mm Hg

Patients with unsuccessful results of an SBT are returned to full ventilatory support for 24 hours to allow the ventilatory muscles to recover. During this period, the causes of

Box 47-9 Evidence-Based Guidelines for Weaning and Discontinuing Ventilatory Support

Recommendation 1: For patients who need mechanical ventilation for more than 24 hours, a search for all of the causes that may be contributing to ventilatory dependence should be undertaken. This is particularly true for the patient who has failed attempts at withdrawing the mechanical ventilator. Reversing all possible ventilatory and nonventilatory issues should be an integral part of the ventilatory discontinuation process.

Recommendation 2: Patients who are receiving mechanical ventilation for respiratory failure should undergo a formal assessment of discontinuation potential if the following criteria are satisfied:

1. Evidence for some reversal of the underlying cause for respiratory failure;
2. Adequate oxygenation (e.g., PaO_2/FiO_2 ratio of more than 150 to 200; requiring PEEP of no more than 5 to 8 cm H_2O; FiO_2 of no more than 0.4 to 0.5) and pH of more than 7.25;
3. Hemodynamic stability as defined by the absence of active myocardial ischemia and the absence of clinically significant hypotension (i.e., a condition that necessitates no vasopressor therapy or therapy with only low-dose vasopressors such as dopamine or dobutamine [less than 5 μg/kg/min]); and
4. The capability to initiate an inspiratory effort.

The decision to use these criteria must be individualized. Some patients who are not satisfying all of these criteria (e.g., patients with chronic hypoxemia values of less than the thresholds cited) may be ready for attempts at the discontinuation of mechanical ventilation.

Recommendation 3: Formal discontinuation assessments for patients who are receiving mechanical ventilation for respiratory failure should be performed during spontaneous breathing rather than while the patient is still receiving substantial ventilatory support. An initial brief period of spontaneous breathing can be used to assess the capability of continuing onto a formal SBT. The criteria with which to assess patient tolerance during SBTs are the respiratory pattern, the adequacy of gas exchange, hemodynamic stability, and subjective comfort. The tolerance of SBTs that last 30 to 120 minutes should prompt consideration for permanent ventilatory discontinuation.

Recommendation 4: The removal of the artificial airway from a patient who has successfully been discontinued from ventilatory support should be based on assessments of airway patency and the ability of the patient to protect the airway.

Recommendation 5: Patients who are receiving mechanical ventilation for respiratory failure who fail an SBT should have the cause of the failed SBT determined. After any reversible causes of failure are corrected and if the patient still meets the criteria listed in Table 47-3, subsequent SBTs should be performed every 24 hours.

Recommendation 6: Patients who are receiving mechanical ventilation for respiratory failure who fail an SBT should receive a stable, nonfatiguing, and comfortable form of ventilatory support.

Recommendation 7: Anesthesia and sedation strategies and ventilatory management that are aimed at early extubation should be used for postsurgical patients.

Recommendation 8: Weaning and discontinuation protocols that are designed for nonphysician health care professionals should be developed and implemented by ICUs. Protocols that are aimed at optimizing sedation should also be developed and implemented.

Recommendation 9: Tracheotomy should be considered after an initial period of stabilization on the ventilator when it becomes apparent that the patient needs prolonged ventilatory assistance. Tracheotomy should then be performed when the patient appears to be likely to gain one or more of the benefits ascribed to the procedure. Patients who may derive particular benefit from early tracheotomy include the following:

- Those who need high levels of sedation to tolerate translaryngeal tubes;
- Those with marginal respiratory mechanics (often manifested as tachypnea) in whom a tracheostomy tube with lower resistance may reduce the risk of muscle overload;
- Those who may derive psychological benefit from the ability to eat orally, communicate by articulated speech, and experience enhanced mobility; and
- Those in whom enhanced mobility may assist with physical therapy efforts.

Recommendation 10: Unless there is evidence for clearly irreversible disease (e.g., high spinal cord injury, advanced amyotrophic lateral sclerosis), a patient who requires prolonged mechanical ventilatory support for respiratory failure should not be considered permanently ventilator dependent until 3 months of weaning attempts have failed.

Recommendation 11: Critical care practitioners should familiarize themselves with facilities in their communities or units in hospitals that they staff that specialize in managing patients who have prolonged dependence on mechanical ventilation. Such familiarization should include reviewing published peer-reviewed data from those units, if available. When they are medically stable for transfer, patients who have failed ventilatory discontinuation attempts in the ICU should be transferred to those facilities that have demonstrated success and safety with accomplishing ventilator discontinuation.

Recommendation 12: Weaning strategies in the patient who requires prolonged mechanical ventilation should be slow paced and should include gradually lengthening self-breathing trials.

Modified from MacIntyre NR, Cook DJ, Ely EW, Jr, et al; American College of Chest Physicians; American Association for Respiratory Care; American College of Critical Care Medicine: Evidence-based guidelines for weaning and discontinuing ventilatory support: a collective task force facilitated by the American College of Chest Physicians; the American Association for Respiratory Care; and the American College of Critical Care Medicine, Chest 120 (6 Suppl):375S–395S, 2001.

TABLE 47-3

Criteria Used to Determine Whether Patients Who Are Receiving Ventilatory Support Can Be Considered for Spontaneous Breathing Trials

Criteria	Description
Objective measurements	Adequate oxygenation (e.g., PO_2 of ≥60 mm Hg with an FiO_2 of ≤0.40 to 0.50; PEEP of ≤5 to 8 cm H_2O; PO_2/FiO_2 ratio of ≥150 to 200) Stable cardiovascular system (e.g., heart rate ≤140 beats/min; stable blood pressure; no [or minimal] pressors) Afebrile (i.e., temperature about 37° C) No significant respiratory acidosis Adequate hemoglobin (e.g., ≥8 to 10 g/dl) Adequate mentation (e.g., arousable, Glasgow coma score of ≥13, no continuous sedative infusions) Stable metabolic status (e.g., acceptable electrolyte levels)
Subjective clinical assessments	Resolution of acute phase of disease; physician believes discontinuation is possible; adequate cough

Modified from MacIntyre NR, Cook DJ, Ely EW, et al: Evidence-based guidelines for weaning and discontinuing ventilator support: a collective task force facilitated by the American College of Chest Physicians, the American Association for Respiratory Care, and the American College of Critical Care Medicine. Chest 120:375S–395S, 2001.

failure are identified and corrected, if possible, and the patient is then reevaluated. If the criteria listed in Table 47-3 continue to be met, SBTs are repeated every 24 hours.[3] Patients who tolerate the formal SBT for 30 to 120 minutes remain off of the ventilator, and extubation is considered. Box 47-10 is a sample protocol for an SBT for the discontinuation of ventilatory support.

Box 47-10 Weaning Protocol for a Spontaneous Breathing Trial

1. Verify that the patient is a candidate for ventilator discontinuation.
   a. Is there evidence of the reversal or alleviation of the disease state or condition that required mechanical ventilatory support?
   b. Is the patient able to breathe spontaneously?
   c. Has the patient's medical condition been optimized (i.e., afebrile, adequate hemoglobin, and acceptable electrolyte levels)?
   d. Are oxygenation, ventilation, and blood gas values adequate?
      - PaO_2 of at least 60 mm Hg with FiO_2 of no more than 0.40 to 0.50 with PEEP/CPAP of no more than 5 to 8 cm H_2O
      - PaO_2/FiO_2 ratio of 150 to 200 mm Hg or more
      - pH of 7.25 or more
   e. Is the patient awake and alert, free of seizures, and able to follow instructions?
   f. Is there evidence of hemodynamic stability? Are vasopressors only administered intermittently?
2. Prepare the patient for the SBT.
   a. Be sure that adequate personnel are present.
   b. Ensure that there are no other ongoing procedures or other major activities.
   c. Eliminate or minimize respiratory depressants (e.g., sedatives, narcotics).
   d. Suction the airway, as needed.
   e. Sit the patient up in bed, if possible.
3. Set the ventilator at zero CPAP and zero pressure support.
4. Continuously monitor the patient.
5. If any of the following occurs and are sustained, return the patient to mechanical ventilatory support:
   a. Respiratory rate of at least 35 breaths/min
   b. Oxygen saturation measured by pulse oximeter of less than 90%
   c. 20% increase or decrease in heart rate or heart rate of more than120 beats/min
   d. Systolic blood pressure of more than 180 mm Hg or of less than 90 mm Hg
   e. Agitation, diaphoresis, or anxiety
6. Continue the trial for at least 30 minutes but not more than 2 hours. If no signs of intolerance develop (see step 5), consider extubation.

Modified from MacIntyre NR, Cook DJ, Ely EW, Jr, et al; American College of Chest Physicians; American Association for Respiratory Care; American College of Critical Care Medicine: Evidence-based guidelines for weaning and discontinuing ventilatory support: a collective task force facilitated by the American College of Chest Physicians; the American Association for Respiratory Care; and the American College of Critical Care Medicine. Chest 120(6 Suppl):375S–395S, 2001.

Continuous Positive Airway Pressure

CPAP is used during an SBT in many facilities. CPAP has the advantages of maintaining the lung volume during the weaning phase and thus of improving the patient's oxygenation status. Minimal levels of CPAP may be useful for reducing WOB and compensating for auto-PEEP, particularly in patients with obstructive lung disease.[2] CPAP is usually provided through the use of the CPAP mode that is available on most mechanical ventilators. By using the ventilator in the CPAP mode, the clinician can take advantage of the alarm systems that are available. This may provide an improved margin of safety as compared with the use of a T-piece. However, in one study, CPAP was no more effective as compared with T-piece trials for the weaning of patients who were recovering from coronary artery bypass graft surgery.[43]

Synchronized Intermittent Mandatory Ventilation

SIMV has been advanced since the early 1970s as a method that can speed weaning and ventilator discontinuation.[8] SIMV can be used to provide full or partial ventilatory support. Weaning from SIMV involves the gradual reduction of the machine rate on the basis of the results of ABG analysis and patient assessment.[7] Early claims that SIMV allowed for faster weaning times[8] have not been substantiated by subsequent studies.[44] However, SIMV is a commonly used mode of ventilation throughout the United States.[45,46]

Patients who are receiving ventilation in the SIMV mode uncouple their breathing efforts from the support provided by the machine.[2] They continue to make spontaneous breathing efforts during the delivery of a "mandatory breath." Evidence also suggests that, once the machine cycling rate is reduced to approximately 50% of the full ventilatory support value, the patient breathes approximately as hard per cycle as when ventilatory support is completely withdrawn.[2] SIMV provides a higher-level of WOB than control[46] or assist-control[47] ventilation, although the increase in WOB is not always evident.[46] This additional work can be overcome with the use of pressure support (i.e., 5 to 10 cm H_2O). However, the addition of pressure support further complicates the weaning process. For initial ventilator setup, the SIMV rate and the tidal volume usually are set at values that are equivalent to those used during volume control-continuous manditory ventilation (VC-CMV) or pressure control-continuous mandatory ventilation (PC-CMV). When the patient's condition has been stabilized, one of two approaches can be used. Some clinicians prefer to continue at these settings until the patient's precipitating disease state or condition has improved considerably.[2] At that point, the rate is reduced in a stepwise manner until complete spontaneous breathing can be achieved.[2] Other clinicians prefer to immediately reduce the level of mechanical ventilation, thereby forcing the patient to perform additional WOB.[1,2] From the beginning, attempts are made to reduce the SIMV rate, and the patient is challenged to provide a portion of the required ventilation.[2] The clinician adjusts the ventilator to make up the difference between what the patient is able to do and the total ventilation needed.[2] The rationale for this partial ventilatory support approach is that only the minimal level of mechanical support should be provided. The level of partial ventilatory support is titrated up or down the entire time that the patient is ventilated on the basis of changes in the patient's condition.

Unfortunately, research indicates that SIMV prolongs ventilatory support and that it is the least effective method of weaning from ventilatory support as compared with either SBT or PSV.[6,10,40,49]

Pressure Support Ventilation

PSV is a mode of ventilatory support that allows the patient to have significant control over the process of ventilatory support. The only gas-delivery variable directly controlled by the ventilator is peak airway pressure; see Chapters 42 and 44 for details.

For initial ventilator setup in the PSV mode, the beginning pressure level can be adjusted to deliver an appropriate tidal volume, which is usually approximately 6 to 10 ml/kg of the ideal body weight based on the patient's condition and the desired tidal volume. PSV is then gradually reduced to a minimal value that only compensates for the WOB imposed by the artificial airway.[48-50] Generally this is about 5 to 8 cm H_2O. After this reduction is accomplished, extubation can be performed directly from the low level pressure support, or an SBT may be conducted for 30 to 120 minutes.[2,3]

PSV allows the clinician to manipulate the level of patient work, but the benefit of this to weaning is questionable.[1,2] In general, patients who can spontaneously breathe comfortably at 5 to 8 cm H_2O of PSV can be extubated without problems.[4] However, if upper airway edema is present, WOB after extubation may be about the same as that caused by the endotracheal tube.[4] In these cases, low levels of pressure support may give a false impression about the patient's ability to tolerate extubation[4] (Box 47-11).

Box 47-11 Protocol for Pressure Support Weaning

1. Verify that the patient is a candidate for ventilator discontinuation:
   - Evidence of alleviation or reversal of the disease state or condition that necessitated ventilatory support
   - Stable, spontaneous breathing pattern without irregular breathing or periods of apnea
   - Optimization of the patient's medical condition
   - Adequate oxygenation, ventilation, and acid-base balance
2. Begin with a PSV level that achieves a tidal volume of 6 to 10 ml/kg of the ideal body weight. A PSV of more than 20 cm H_2O rarely is needed. The need for a high level of PSV indicates that the patient may not be ready for ventilator discontinuation.
3. Reduce the PSV 2 to 4 cm H_2O as tolerated, ideally at least twice daily, and reassess the patient for signs of intolerance:
   - Rate of at least 25 to 30 breaths/min
   - 20% or greater increase in heart rate or a heart rate of more than 120 beats/min
   - 20% or greater increase in systolic blood pressure or systolic blood pressure of more than 180 mm Hg or of less than 90 mm Hg
   - Agitation, anxiety, and diaphoresis
4. If the patient does not tolerate a reduction in PSV, return to the previous value, and reassess.
5. Continue to reduce PSV as tolerated at least twice per day and more frequently if the patient does not have signs of distress.
6. Consider extubation when the patient is able to tolerate a PSV of 5 to 8 cm H_2O for 2 hours with no apparent distress.

Modified from Esteban A, Frutos F, Tobin M, et al: A comparison of four methods of weaning patients from mechanical ventilation. Spanish Lung Failure Collaborative Group, N Engl J Med 332:345-350, 1995; and Brochard L, Rauss A, Benito S, et al: Comparison of three methods of gradual withdrawal from ventilatory support during weaning from mechanical ventilation. Am J Respir Crit Care Med 150:896-903, 1994.

Synchronized Intermittent Mandatory Ventilation With Pressure Support Ventilation

With SIMV, the addition of pressure support can overcome the WOB imposed during "spontaneous" breaths because of the presence of endotracheal and tracheostomy tubes, demand flow systems, and ventilator circuits. In this setting, pressure support is set to achieve the desired tidal volume during the spontaneous breaths (i.e., 6 to 10 ml/kg of the ideal body weight).

MINI CLINI

Setting Pressure Support Levels

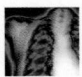

PROBLEM: An intubated patient is receiving mechanical ventilation in the SIMV mode with the following settings:

- V_T = 500 ml
- Rate = 12 breaths/min
- Peak inspiratory pressure = 40 cm H_2O
- Plateau pressure (P_{plat}) = 20 cm H_2O
- Ventilator inspiratory flow ($\dot{V}_{mach}$) = 60 L/min (1 L/s)

The patient is breathing spontaneously with a spontaneous rate of 12 breaths/min and a spontaneous peak inspiratory flow of 30 L/min (0.5 L/s). Find the level of PSV that is needed to overcome the imposed WOB.

SOLUTION:

$$PSV = ([PIP - P_{plat}]/\dot{V}_{mach}) \times \dot{V}_{Imax}$$
$$PSV = ([40 \text{ cm } H_2O - 20 \text{ cm } H_2O]/1 \text{ L/s}) \times 0.5 \text{ L/s} = 10 \text{ cm } H_2O$$

The calculated PSV level to overcome the imposed WOB for this patient is 10 cm.

Although it is clear that the addition of PSV during SIMV can reduce or eliminate imposed work caused by mechanical factors, it has not been shown how this affects weaning. In one study, SIMV with PSV increased tidal volume and reduced respiratory rate but did not significantly reduce weaning time or success as compared with SIMV alone.[51] On the basis of all of the weaning trials, it can be concluded that this approach to weaning can only increase the length of ventilatory support.[38,49] Current guidelines recommend the use of SBT to rapidly wean patients from ventilatory support.[3]

Spontaneous Awaking Trials

Concern regarding the use of sedation in critically ill patients has increased markedly during the last few years. This concern has focused on the issue of delirium.[52] The indiscriminate use of sedatives in the ICU is considered inappropriate patient management. In general, sedatives should always be considered last when trying to handle an agitated patient. Something has caused the patient's agitation, and it should be addressed and corrected, if possible, before sedation is administered. In addition, it is becoming clearer that the use of excessive sedation lengthens the time of mechanical ventilation. A recent clinical trial compared an SBT alone with SBT with a spontaneous awaking trial (SAT). The SAT required that all of the sedation that a patient was receiving be stopped at midnight and the patient reassessed. If the patient did continue to require sedation, it was restarted at half the dose that the patient previously received. The use of the SAT along with the daily SBT resulted in the faster weaning of patients from ventilatory support as well as a decrease in mortality.[53] The authors argued that the decrease in morality was a result of patients being exposed for a shorter time to the complications of mechanical ventilation. Throughout the course of mechanical ventilation, sedation should be kept to the bare minimum necessary; patient sedation should be periodically stopped and the patient carefully assessed before additional sedation is given.[53]

NEWER TECHNIQUES FOR FACILITATING VENTILATOR DISCONTINUANCE

Mandatory Minute Volume Ventilation

Mandatory minute volume ventilation (MMV) was described by Hewlett, Plott, and Terry and introduced in 1977 in Great Britain.[54] With this mode of ventilation, the total minute volume is set, and the patient may elect to inspire all of the minute volume, part of the minute volume, or none of the minute volume spontaneously. The ventilator would automatically provide a clinician set level of minute volume. It was originally assumed that, as the patient's status improved, he or she would assume a greater and greater percentage of the set minute volume, eventually inspiring it all spontaneously. However, this did not occur; patients generally settled into a ventilator pattern where the overall WOB was shared between the patient and the ventilator, and the patient never assumed a greater percentage of the work.[55] There is no data to support the use of MMV over SBT or PSV to wean patients from ventilatory support.

Adaptive Support Ventilation

ASV is a newer mode of ventilation that maintains a minimum minute ventilation with an optimal breathing pattern (tidal volume and rate) and that is based on the work of Otis;[56,57] see Chapters 42 and 44 for details. ASV automatically adjusts inspiratory pressure and ventilator breath rate to achieve the target minute volume set. As the patient's status improves, the target minute volume is reduced, and the level of pressure required each breath diminishes. When a minimal level is reached, the patient is considered weaned from ventilatory support and ready for extubation.

Preliminary studies of ASV for the care of patients who are recovering from cardiac surgery show a reduction in the duration of mechanical ventilation as compared with an SIMV weaning protocol.[57,58] The ASV weaning protocol used in the study incorporated two 50% reductions in minute ventilation. Each reduction was followed by an assessment of patient tolerance according to criteria that were similar to those suggested for SBTs. Additional data about ASV indicates that it works very well for patients who are under controlled ventilation,[59] but additional data from a large heterogeneous group of patients will be necessary to determine if AVS truly improves the speed of ventilator discontinuation.

Computer-Based Weaning

Current versions of MMV and ASV are examples of computer-controlled mechanical ventilation. Several more complex systems have been developed, including Ventilation Manager, VQ-attending, ESTER, Continuous Respiratory Evaluator (CORE), KUSIVAR, and WEAN-PRO.[19] The desire to develop computer-based weaning protocols is based on two factors. First, weaning is a time-consuming and labor-intensive process. If computer control can expedite or simplify this process, considerable time and money can be saved. Second, because most weaning decisions are based on objective data, computer-based weaning protocols are relatively easy to develop. In one study in which physician-directed weaning was compared with computer-based weaning, the computer-based system resulted in the less-frequent assessment of ABGs and shorter weaning times.[19] Another study showed that a handheld computer weaning protocol for use by respiratory therapists was more effective than a paper-based weaning protocol.[60]

The most successful computerized application for weaning is the Smart Care approach, which is based on data from Laurent Brochard's group.[61] The system adjusts pressure support on the basis of the patient's tidal volume, respiratory rate, and end-tidal carbon dioxide level. When the pressure support has been decreased to a predefined level, the ventilator automatically begins an SBT. If the patient fails the SBT, which is determined by changes in the patient's respiratory rate, tidal volume, and end-tidal carbon dioxide level, then the ventilator automatically reassumes ventilatory support. If the patient passes the SBT, the ventilator also returns to baseline ventilatory support but notifies the clinician that the patient is ready for ventilator discontinuation. In a randomized comparison with clinician-applied SBT, this system weaned patients faster and decreased the total number of days that patients were maintained in the ICU as well as the need for postextubation NIV. One criticism of this study was that the clinician-applied SBTs were not always performed properly; however, this is clinical reality, and if an automated system can wean patients faster, it will have a place in the care of critically ill patients.

Automatic Tube Compensation

ATC is an option on newer mechanical ventilators that compensates for the flow-dependent pressure decrease across the endotracheal tube during both inspiration and expiration; see Chapters 42 and 44 for details. ATC reduces WOB and may improve patient comfort.[62] Because it compensates for the imposed WOB caused by the artificial airway, ATC has been referred to as *electronic extubation.* Patients who are able to breathe adequately with the addition of ATC at low peak airway pressure (i.e., less than 8 cm H_2O) should tolerate extubation. ATC is similar to pressure support in that an inspiratory pressure is used to compensate for imposed WOB; however, ATC varies the pressure, depending on the size of the endotracheal tube and the patient's inspiratory flow rate. Alternatively, PSV delivers a preset inspiratory pressure that may overcompensate or undercompensate imposed WOB at any given point in time. However, no data is available to indicate that ATC weans patients faster than SBTs or PSV.

MINI CLINI

Response to a Spontaneous Breathing Trial

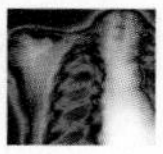

PROBLEM: A 70-year-old woman with a long history of congestive heart failure has been mechanically ventilated for 6 days. She has failed three previous SBTs, but today, at the end of a 45-minute SBT, her clinical presentation was as follows:

- Respiratory rate of 24 breaths/min
- Tidal volume of 300 ml (6 ml/kg ideal body weight)
- Pulse of 98 beats/min
- Blood pressure of 138/86 mm Hg

The patient did not appear to be short of breath, and she did not demonstrate excessive use of her accessory muscles of ventilation to breathe during the trial.

Should this patient's ventilatory support be discontinued?

SOLUTION: On the basis of the given data, this patient passed her SBT and should be discontinued from ventilatory support and extubated if there is no reason for her to remain intubated. However, because of her age, history of congestive heart failure, and multiple failures of SBT, she should ideally be placed on NIV immediately after she is extubated and slowly transitioned to independent spontaneous breathing over the next 12 to 48 hours.

Volume Support

VC is a newer mode of ventilation that combines pressure support and volume ventilation by allowing a level of pressure support that is automatically adjusted to maintain a preset tidal volume. In the VC mode, inspiration is initiated by the patient. During the inspiratory phase, the pressure level is regulated to a value that is based on the previous breath's pressure–volume relationship as compared with a preset tidal volume. The pressure-support level is automatically adjusted in a stepwise manner by ±3 cm H_2O from one breath to the next to maintain the preset tidal volume.

A major problem with VC is the excessive reduction of airway pressure in the presence of high ventilatory demand, thereby increasing patient effort.[63] With most ventilators offering this mode, no lower limit to ventilating airway pressure is set, and inspiratory airway pressure can decrease all the way to the PEEP level. Volume support may offer a sort of automatic weaning from pressure support. As the patient's spontaneous tidal volume improves, the level of pressure support is automatically reduced. Clinical trials indicate no benefit to the use of VC to wean patients.[64]

Noninvasive Ventilation

A number of groups have studied the use of NIV as an adjunct to ventilator discontinuance. Essentially, NIV has been used in this setting in three different manners:

1. Transitioning patients with COPD who failed SBTs from invasive ventilation to spontaneous breathing[65-67]
2. Supporting patients who passed SBTs but who were considered to be at high risk for failing the extubation[68-70]
3. Supporting patients who developed hypoxemic respiratory failure after extubation[71,72]

The literature strongly supports the first two indications but does not support the third application. Refer to Chapter 45 for details regarding the application of NIV during weaning and the use of NIV in general.

Respiratory-Therapist–Driven Protocols

A number of randomized, controlled clinical trials have demonstrated that patients are weaned faster with the use of protocols than with individual physician orders.[73-76] In all of these studies, the therapists, nurses, and physicians who normally manage patients in the unit developed the protocol. In addition, in the individual physician order group, the physicians who wrote the protocol also wrote the individual weaning orders. In all of these trials, patients who were randomized to the protocol group weaned faster and with less complications then the patients randomized to the individual physician group.[73-76]

What these results do not mean is that therapists wean patients better than physicians. However, what they do mean is that, when an evidence-based approach to patient management is developed and followed precisely, care is generally better than with individual physician orders. The reason for this is that protocols empower the clinician at the bedside to advance care when the patient meets specific criteria without waiting for the physician to come and write an order. In many community hospitals, the wait for the physician could be an hour or a whole shift or more. Thus, with protocols, care processes rapidly on the agreed-upon course. In addition, the individual bias of the caregiver does not affect the manner in which care is provided. Thus, the approach does not change from day to day depending on which physician is at the bedside. An example of a respiratory-therapist–directed ventilatory discontinuance protocol is presented in Box 47-12.

Box 47-12 Respiratory-Therapist–Directed Weaning Protocol

- The physician's written order identifies the patient as being eligible for the respiratory-therapist–directed weaning protocol.
- The timing of weaning initiation is defined as part of the protocol.
- All patients must undergo continuous oxyhemoglobin saturation monitoring by pulse oximetry.
- When the patient meets weaning criteria, the ventilator is set to zero CPAP and zero PEEP.
- The SBT continues for a minimum of 30 minutes to a maximum of 120 minutes if none of the following weaning failure conditions are present:
  - SaO_2 of less than 90% or diaphoresis
  - Spontaneous respiratory rate of at least 35 breaths/min that is sustained for at least 5 minutes
  - Agitation or a decreased level of consciousness
  - A heart rate increase of at least 20%
  - A blood pressure change of at least 20%
  - A cardiac output reduction of at least 30% or ventricular arrhythmia
- If the SBT is well tolerated and there is no reason not to extubate the patient, then the patient is extubated.

SELECTING AN APPROACH

Current evidence suggests that, for progressive weaning from mechanical support, it may be best to avoid SIMV.[3,6,10] It has also been suggested, regardless of the mode of weaning used, that protocols administered by respiratory therapists and other health care workers be developed.[3,6,10] These protocols should be designed to begin testing for the opportunity to reduce support very soon after intubation and to reduce the level of ventilatory support at every opportunity.[6,73] The approach to weaning that seems to wean patients most rapidly is the SBT. This should be the approach that is used to identify readiness for ventilator discontinuance in the vast majority of patients.[6] In addition, NIV should be considered as part of the total ventilator discontinuance process.[74]

One area that requires additional research is the role of ventilatory muscle conditioning in patients who require long-term ventilatory support. Endurance conditioning of the ventilatory muscles can be achieved by the continuous repetition of low levels of ventilatory work. Strength conditioning can be achieved by maximal ventilatory effort for short periods. In theory, PSV would allow for improving ventilatory muscle endurance, whereas intermittent SBTs would favor the development of muscle strength. Inspiratory resistive training to improve ventilatory muscle strength has been tried as an adjunct to weaning for the care of patients undergoing long-term ventilation.[19] Unfortunately, the role of ventilatory muscle rest and load in the care of difficult-to-wean patients has not been established.[19]

In summary, a single daily SBT that lasts from 30 minutes to 2 hours has been recommended as the primary approach to weaning.[3,4] If the trial is successful, extubation is considered. If the trial is unsuccessful, at least 24 hours of ventilatory support is provided before another trial is attempted.[3] There are advantages and disadvantages to each of the methods used to conduct ventilator weaning. Table 47-4 compares SBT, SIMV, and PSV as weaning techniques. The best approach may be the one with which a given clinician is most familiar.[8] It should be based on knowledge of the patient's condition, a sound rationale, and good clinical experience.[2,8] The method chosen should include careful patient assessment, and the patient's condition should be optimized before weaning. For the vast majority of patients, a protocolized approach to ventilator discontinuance is most efficient.

MONITORING THE PATIENT DURING WEANING

Ventilatory Status

Respiratory rate and pattern are easy to monitor and may be the most reliable indicators of patient progress during weaning.[1,5] Weaning may proceed as quickly as the patient's respiratory rate and subjective tolerance allow.[1] However, in no case should patients be pushed beyond their physiologic limits; to do so may result in diaphragmatic dysfunction and further delay the weaning process.[2,4,6] If the patient is allowed to fatigue during a weaning trial, it will require at least 24 hours for the muscles to recover.[77,78] Dyspnea should be monitored during weaning and may be quantified with a visual analog scale or a modified Borg scale[79] (Table 47-5). The onset or worsening of discomfort, respiratory distress, fatigue, sweating, signs of increased WOB (e.g., accessory muscle use, abdominal paradox), deterioration in vital signs, or changes in mental status (e.g., agitation, anxiety, somnolence, coma) may be signs of intolerance of a weaning trial.[3]

The single best index of ventilation remains the measurement of $PaCO_2$. However, the assessment of a patient's tolerance of an SBT should be based on clinical presentation rather than $PaCO_2$. A patient with a $PaCO_2$ of 40 mm Hg but a clinical presentation defined by a rapid, shallow breathing pattern with abdominal paradox,

TABLE 47-4

Comparison of Available Weaning Methods

Method	Advantages	Disadvantages
SBT	Tests patient's spontaneous breathing ability Allows periods of work and rest Weans faster than SIMV A single daily SBT may be as effective as multiple trials May be performed with 5 cm H_2O CPAP, 5 cm H_2O PSV, or both	More staff time Abrupt transition may be difficult for some patients May overstress the patient if not monitored carefully Requires careful supervision
SIMV	Less staff time Gradual transition Easy to use Minimum minute ventilation guaranteed Sophisticated alarm systems may be used May be used in combination with PSV or CPAP	Patient-ventilator asynchrony Prolongs weaning May worsen fatigue
PSV	Less staff time Gradual transition Prevents fatigue Maintains activity of diaphragm Increased patient comfort Weans faster than SIMV Overcomes resistive WOB caused by the following: • Endotracheal and tracheostomy tubes • Ventilator circuits • Demand flow systems Patient can control cycle length, rate, and inspiratory flow Every breath is supported	Large changes in minute ventilation can occur Increased mean airway pressure as compared with SBT Tidal volume not guaranteed; low tidal volumes possible May prolong weaning

TABLE 47-5

Modified Borg Scale for Dyspnea

Grade	Degree of Dyspnea
0	None
0.5	Very, very slight (just noticeable)
1	Very slight
2	Slight
3	Moderate
4	Somewhat severe
5	Severe
6	Very severe
7	
8	
9	Very, very severe (almost maximal)
10	Maximal

Modified from Mahler DA: Dyspnea, Mt. Kisco, NY, 1990, Futura.

TABLE 47-6

Changes During the Withdrawal of Ventilatory Support

Expected Change	Deleterious Change
Respiratory	
Respiratory rate minimally increased	Respiratory rate of ≥35 breaths/min
Stable $\dot{V}_E$	Large increase or decrease in $\dot{V}_E$
$SpO_2 \geq 90\%$	Decrease in SpO_2 to ≤90%
5 to 10 mm Hg swing in PaO_2	PaO_2 of <60 mm Hg
5 to 10 mm Hg swing in $PaCO_2$	An increase of >10 mm Hg in $PaCO_2$
pH of >7.30 and <7.50	pH of <7.30
Minimal use of accessory muscles	Increased use of accessory muscles
No paradoxical breathing	Paradoxical breathing
	Diaphoresis
	Dyspnea
Cardiovascular	
Heart rate increased by 15 to 20 beats/min	Persistent tachycardia of ≥120 to 140 beats/min
Blood pressure increased 10 to 15 mm Hg	Hypotension (blood pressure of <90/60 mm Hg)
	Hypertension (systolic blood pressure of >180 mm Hg)
Increased cardiac index	Decreased cardiac index
Increased stroke volume	Decreased stroke volume
	Angina
	New arrhythmias
	Increased pulmonary capillary wedge pressure
Other	
Mental status good (i.e., awake, alert, responsive)	Anxiety, agitation, somnolence, coma

tachycardia, and hypertension has not passed an SBT. The results of capnography should not be used to guide the weaning of patients with pulmonary parenchymal disease.[80] End-tidal PCO_2 values can be highly misleading as an estimate of effective ventilation in sick patients.[80] Gastric pH has been used as a predictor of patient status, and gastrointestinal acidosis may be an early sign of weaning failure.[81]

Oxygenation

Continuous pulse oximetric (SpO_2) monitoring can provide a sensitive indicator of oxygenation status during weaning.[5] Arterial blood gas analysis for PaO_2 and SaO_2 and the calculation of the oxygen content of the arterial blood (CaO_2) should be performed if doubt exists when assessing a patient's oxygenation status during weaning.

Cardiovascular Status

Pulse, blood pressure, and cardiac rhythm should be monitored, and arrhythmias should be assessed to determine whether weaning should be continued. Tachycardia, bradycardia, and abnormalities in blood pressure should be promptly evaluated and the patient returned to ventilatory support or a higher level of support, if indicated. Silent myocardial ischemia may occur frequently in some postoperative patients during weaning.[82] Table 47-6 summarizes changes that may occur during the withdrawal of ventilatory support.

EXTUBATION

Artificial Airways and Weaning

The effect on a patent of a properly sized artificial airway on WOB is controversial. In a study with 14 successfully extubated patients, at the end of a 2-hour SBT, there was no difference in WOB before and after extubation.[83] However, many endotracheal tubes are partially obstructed and as a result impose a significant increase in WOB. Removing the endotracheal tube may markedly improve the patients' clinical status.

There is little difference in the airway resistance of healthy adults with low minute ventilation (i.e., 8 L/min) breathing through endotracheal tubes with an internal diameter (ID) of 7, 8, or 9 mm.[84] Decreases in ID and increases in minute ventilation increase WOB. Adults have a critical increase in workload when the tube has an ID of less than 7 mm.[84] It is thought that the added work due to the presence of an artificial airway may contribute to ventilator dependency among patients with borderline pulmonary function or ventilatory muscle weakness.[84,85]

Endotracheal tubes themselves can cause reflex bronchoconstriction. Consequently, some experts believe that the routine use of bronchodilators is justified in the care of all intubated patients. Dried secretions in the endotracheal tube can cause dramatic increases in airway resistance, especially among infants and children.[84,85] Taking care to provide adequate humidification can help to avoid this problem.

Tracheotomy may substantially reduce the WOB of patients who need mechanical ventilatory support.[74] The short length of tracheotomy tubes results in an overall decrease in resistance as compared with the resistance of an endotracheal tube, even though the curvature of the tracheotomy tube is greater.[3] It appears that the performance of a tracheotomy improves airway resistance and reduces the load of the ventilatory muscles. The clinical benefit of this improvement in terms of weaning has not been established.[3]

Weaning and extubation should be separate decisions.[29] Weaning indices are not predictive of the adequacy of airway patency or the need for the protection of the airway.[29] The reintubation rate among patients with prolonged postoperative ventilation as a result of respiratory failure can range from 5% to 20%.[29]

Patients who have been successfully extubated generally have the following characteristics: (1) the resolution of the disease state or condition; (2) hemodynamic stability; (3) the absence of sepsis; (4) adequate oxygenation status with a decreased FiO_2 and decreased PEEP or CPAP; and (5) adequate ventilatory status and $PaCO_2$.[29] The decision to extubate should be based on the assessment of upper airway patency and protection.[29] No one indicator is 100% sensitive and specific with regard to the prediction of successful extubation.[29] Practical guidelines for extubation are presented in Box 47-13. Regardless of the weaning technique used, an SBT is recommended before extubation to ensure that the patient can sustain spontaneous unsupported ventilation.[2]

Some patients may be successfully extubated even if extubation criteria are not met.[29] If the patient is at risk, trained personnel who are able to perform reintubation must be immediately available before extubation is attempted. At a minimum, those who perform the extubation must be prepared to provide an airway and ventilatory support in the event that problems develop immediately after extubation. Extubation should be postponed when myocardial ischemia is present, when the patient has upper gastrointestinal hemorrhage, or when a procedure that necessitates reintubation is impending. If difficult reintubation is anticipated, trained personnel should be immediately available.[29]

Many patients report hoarseness and sore throat after extubation, and patients should be advised that these symptoms may occur. Other common problems after extubation include airway obstruction, increased risk of aspiration, and difficulty with secretion clearance.[29] Patients with neurologic or neuromuscular disorders and those with excessive secretions are at increased risk after extubation.[28] The compression of the airway as a result of a traumatic or postoperative hematoma of the neck, infectious masses or abscesses, and malignant tumors or compression after major head or neck surgery can lead to upper airway obstruction after extubation.[29] The cuff leak test may detect airway obstruction before extubation; however, results of studies addressing this are controversial.[86,87] An air leak of less than 11% to 12% or 110 to 130 ml has been shown to be predictive of stridor.[86,87] Box 47-14 describes the cuff leak test.

After extubation, glottic edema can result in partial airway obstruction, which can cause mild to severe stridor.[29] Postextubation stridor occurs in 2% to 16% of patients in the ICU and should be viewed with concern.[88] Severe edema after extubation can lead to complete airway obstruction.[29]

Box 47-13 Common Causes of Weaning Failure

- Poor respiratory mechanics or wheezing
- Untreated cardiac disease
- Electrolyte imbalances
- Anxiety
- Secretions
- Aspiration
- Alkalosis
- Neuromuscular weakness
- Sepsis
- Excessive sedation
- Inadequate nutrition
- Opiates
- Obesity
- Thyroid disease

Box 47-14 Practical Guidelines for Extubation

- There is no immediate need for mechanical ventilation or intubation.
- The medical course does not suggest impending respiratory failure or other indications for mechanical ventilation.
- Procedures that require intubation and general anesthesia are not immediately planned.
- There is an achievement of adequate oxygenation and ventilation with spontaneous ventilation.
- The patient's FiO_2 requirement can be achieved with a mask or a nasal cannula.
- The patient no longer needs mechanical ventilatory assistance.
- Weaning is successful.
- There is a minimal risk of upper airway obstruction.
- The patient has minimal edema or mass encroachment of the oropharynx and upper airway; oral and upper airway anatomy is otherwise normal.
- There is adequate airway protection and a minimal risk of aspiration.
- The level of consciousness and neuromuscular function allows for a gag reflex and an adequate cough.
- Gastric contents are minimized by the discontinuation of tube feedings for 4 to 6 hours before extubation.
- A positive gag reflex is present.
- There is adequate clearance of pulmonary secretions.
- The level of consciousness and muscular strength allow for an effective cough.
- Secretion volume and thickness are not worsening.

Children, patients with epiglottitis or angioedema (i.e., dermal, subcutaneous, or submucosal edema of the face or larynx), and patients who have sustained smoke inhalation are at greater risk.[29] Postextubation edema occurs in as many as 47% of children with trauma injuries or burns.[29] See Chapter 33 for detailed information about airway management and postextubation care.

MINI CLINI

Patient Who Requires Long-Term Weaning

PROBLEM: A 68-year-old man with a history of COPD was hospitalized after a motor vehicle accident. Over the course of the next 2 weeks, the patient became septic and developed acute respiratory distress syndrome. For the last week, the patient has met the criteria for an SBT, but he has failed every attempt. How should this patient's ventilator care progress from this point forward?

SOLUTION: This patient should be classified as a difficult-to-wean patient who would benefit from a program that has been designed specifically for patients who are failing to wean. This program should systematically evaluate all systems to determine the cause of weaning failure and include the assistance of other health care providers, specifically physical therapy, occupational therapy, and speech and language pathology; he may also benefit from the efforts of social services. Ideally, this should take place in a unit that has been specifically designed for the difficult-to-wean patient.

VENTILATOR DISCONTINUANCE FAILURE

As many as 25% of patients who have been removed from ventilatory support experience respiratory distress that is severe enough to necessitate the reinstitution of mechanical ventilation.[4] In patients who are unlikely to be successfully weaned, rapid, shallow breathing begins almost immediately after the ventilator is disconnected.[4] As spontaneous breathing continues, respiratory mechanics worsen in these patients for reasons that are not clearly understood.[4] Approximately half of patients who have poor results after the discontinuation of ventilation experience marked hypercapnia as a result of rapid, shallow breathing.[4] An unsuccessful SBT also causes considerable cardiovascular stress.[4] Myocardial ischemia may occur frequently among ventilator-dependent patients, and it has been associated with weaning failure.[89] Critical illness polyneuropathy has been cited as a frequent cause of neuromuscular weaning failure among critically ill patients.[19,90] Unsuspected neuromuscular disease may be an important factor in ventilator dependency.[19]

Inability to wean can sometimes be attributed to psychologic dependence, poor oxygenation status, or cardiovascular instability (i.e., congestive heart failure or ischemia).[2] However, the most common cause of the inability to wean is an imbalance between ventilatory capability and ventilatory demand.[2] Inability to wean is usually caused by a concurrent pathologic process that necessitates treatment.[2,3] Common causes of weaning failure are summarized in Box 47-13.

PROLONGED MECHANICAL VENTILATION

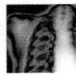

Prolonged mechanical ventilation (PMV) may be required for 3% to 7% of patients who are receiving mechanical ventilation.[3] Patients who require a lengthy course of ventilatory support after the acute phase of their disease has resolved may be suffering from some of the items listed in Box 47-14. Any patient who is repeatedly failing SBTs should undergo a complete review of all systems to determine if something had been overlooked that may add to the patient's workload, thereby preventing them from weaning. In many patients, their pulmonary mechanics have not been optimized and thus they are unable to assume the workload required of spontaneous breathing. In others, underlying cardiac disease may not have been properly treated. Always a concern is the patient's acid–base status. If a patient had baseline compensated respiratory acidosis, then he or she will not be able to wean if the compensation has been eliminated. Every time these patients are trialed on an SBT, their carbon dioxide levels will rise, and they will develop respiratory failure. If this is the problem, the baseline acid–base status must be slowly reestablished if these patients are to wean. In other patients, sedation, opiates, nutritional status, electrolytes, and other underlying issues many be the concern. The more carefully all systems are reviewed, the greater the likelihood that the problem will be identified and the patient weaned from ventilatory support.

CHRONICALLY VENTILATOR-DEPENDENT PATIENTS

Chronically ventilator-dependent patients (i.e., less than 1% of those requiring ventilatory support) present ethical, economic, and practical problems.[17,91] From an economic point of view, the long-term care of ventilator-dependent patients in an ICU is prohibitively expensive. Often these patients are transferred to subacute or long-term care facilities, where they can be cared for in an environment that is less intrusive and more like home.[91] For cases in which the family has adequate resources, the patient may be cared for in the home. Regional weaning centers have been developed and have reported success with weaning most patients who are undergoing long-term mechanical ventilation.[3,16,91] Current guidelines suggest that, unless there is clear evidence of an irreversible cause of ventilator dependency (e.g., a high spinal cord injury, amyotrophic lateral sclerosis), patients should not be considered permanently ventilator dependent until 3 months of weaning attempts have failed.[3] If the patient is unweanable, the goal should be to restore the patient to the highest level of independent function possible.[15] For example, portable wheelchair-mounted ventilators have been effective for providing a surprising level of mobility and independence to persons who are quadriplegic. Table 47-7 describes the management of common problems among difficult-to-wean patients. Box 47-15 lists the goals of weaning of patients who are receiving long-term ventilation.

TABLE 47-7

Management of Problems Among Difficult-to-Wean Patients

Problem	Management Strategy
Anemia	Transfuse when hemoglobin level is ≤10 g/dl and hematocrit level is ≤30% if these are thought to be factors in decreased tissue oxygenation.
Increased WOB	1. Tube related a. Apply pressure support or ATC. b. Change the size of the small endotracheal tube. c. Cut the length of endotracheal tube if it is 2 in (5 cm) past the mouth. d. Deflate the cuff if all breathing is spontaneous and the risk of aspiration is minimal. e. Consider tracheotomy. 2. Secretion related (see later) 3. Bronchospasm related a. Administer bronchodilators. • β_2-agonists with a nebulizer • Anticholinergics • Steroids • Methylxanthines b. Apply CPAP to reduce auto-PEEP. c. Manage the cause. 4. Ventilator related a. Assure synchrony for machine breaths. b. Eliminate auto-PEEP. c. Use flow-by or flow-trigger ventilation with or without pressure support.
Secretions, atelectasis, or plugging	1. Systemically hydrate. 2. Provide extra humidity (i.e., increase humidifier temperature to 35° C to 37° C at airway connection). 3. Maximally bronchodilate when necessary. 4. Perform coughing exercises. 5. Perform chest physiotherapy. 6. Suction.
Dyspnea	1. Use positioning (i.e., out of bed, dangling, and leaning forward). 2. Reassure and communicate with the patient. 3. Provide periodic bag insufflation while the patient is off of the ventilator. 4. Increase endurance. a. Alternate weaning with rest to promote endurance. b. Consider providing inspiratory resistive training. 5. Provide distraction.
Malposition	1. Position the patient to maximize diaphragmatic excursion and to improve lung volume and gas exchange (i.e., sitting or dangling). 2. Use a rocking chair. 3. Follow $\dot{V}_E$, V_T, rate, MIP, MVV, and ABG values for optimum positioning.
Respiratory muscle fatigue	1. Direct management at the cause. 2. Ensure adequate oxygen transport and cardiac output. 3. Nourish the patient. 4. Replace depleted electrolytes. 5. Decrease the WOB. a. Administer supplemental oxygen. b. Clear secretions. c. Decrease airway resistance. d. Use mechanical ventilation to rest fatigued muscles, and then rotate weaning and rest.
Hemodynamic and fluid problems	1. Administer volume replacement and drugs to increase contractility, increase or decrease preload, and decrease afterload. 2. Delay weaning until the patient's cardiovascular status is stable. 3. Use techniques and the mode of ventilation to decrease the mean airway pressure.

Continued

TABLE 47-7

Management of Problems Among Difficult-to-Wean Patients—cont'd

Problem	Management Strategy
Infection	1. Identify potential sites of infection. 2. Remove lines early, or replace them periodically. 3. Control infection. 4. Wash hands, and use gloves. 5. Nourish the patient.
Metabolic problems	1. Control the cause and postpone weaning if the patient has acidosis. 2. Keep the carbon dioxide level at baseline if the patient has COPD, or allow progressive renal compensation during long-term weaning. 3. Provide moderate carbohydrate loading with total parenteral nutrition.
Low magnesium level	4. Give supplements.
High magnesium level	5. Provide dialysis or calcium chloride.
Low calcium level	6. Control the cause before weaning.
Low phosphate level	7. Replace phosphate before weaning.
Nutrition	1. Assess weight, albumin, and total lymphocyte count at admission. 2. Label the degree of malnutrition, and calculate protein needs. 3. Nourish the patient.
Exercise	1. Provide exercise therapy to increase muscle function, prevent contracture, and maintain joint integrity (i.e., passive-to-active range of motion and sitting to walking). 2. Increase strength during activities of daily living. 3. Secure a physiotherapy consultation. 4. Consider the use of an exercise bicycle. 5. Encourage wheelchair rides or walks with a portable ventilator. 6. Provide breathing retraining.
Psychologic problems	1. Secure early psychiatric consultation. 2. Allow for patient control. 3. Demonstrate staff accountability and honesty. 4. Provide a communication method. 5. Decrease environmental stress. 6. Teach relaxation methods. 7. Provide mental stimulation. 8. Provide recreation. 9. Provide rewards for reaching short-term goals. 10. Encourage self-care. 11. Allow other patients to visit. 12. Provide flexible visiting hours 13. Take the patient out of the ICU environment.
Sleep disturbances	1. Provide a quiet environment (i.e., dim lights), reposition the patient, give a back rub, and administer sedation. 2. Provide for uninterrupted sleep. 3. Avoid weaning at night. 4. Provide relaxation method (e.g., hypnosis, biofeedback, progressive muscle relaxation). 5. Prescribe short-acting sedative hypnotics.
Pain	1. Administer minimal analgesia.

Modified from Norton LC, Neureuter A: Weaning the long-term ventilator-dependent patient: common problems and management. Crit Care Nurse 9:42–52, 1989.

Box 47-15 Goals for Weaning After Long-Term Mechanical Ventilation

- Reduce the amount of support.
- Decrease the invasiveness of any support.
- Increase independence from mechanical devices.
- Preserve function.
- Maintain medical stability.

From Pierson DJ: Nonrespiratory aspects of weaning from mechanical ventilation. Respir Care 40:289, 1995.

TERMINAL WEANING

The term *terminal weaning* has been used to refer to the discontinuation of mechanical ventilatory support in the face of a catastrophic and irreversible illness.[92] The decision to proceed with disconnecting the ventilator when such an act is likely to cause the death of a patient is fraught with ethical, emotional, and practical problems. The decision should be made by the family in consultation with the patient's physician and in accordance with established ethical and legal guidelines.[92]

Determinants of the decision to withdraw ventilation include the patient's desire to not continue with life support, the predictions of a low chance of survival in the ICU (i.e., less than 10%), the likelihood that future cognitive function would be severely impaired, and the continuous need for inotropes or vasopressors to maintain blood pressure.[93] After the decision has been made, the process is generally one of ventilator disconnection rather than weaning. The method of terminal weaning should be as humane and as comfortable as possible and should not be done in a way that further burdens the family.[92]

SUMMARY CHECKLIST

- The most common cause of ventilator dependence is a ventilatory workload that exceeds the patient's ventilatory capabilities.
- Other common causes of ventilator dependence include oxygenation problems, cardiovascular instability, and psychologic factors.
- The most important criterion for determining whether a patient is ready for ventilator discontinuation or weaning is a significant improvement or reversal of the disease state or condition that caused the patient to need ventilatory support.
- Factors that should be optimized before weaning include oxygenation, ventilation, acid-base balance and electrolyte levels, cardiovascular status, kidney function and fluid balance, sleep deprivation, psychologic status, nutrition, and overall medical condition.
- Weaning techniques include spontaneous breathing trials, SIMV, and PSV.
- Spontaneous breathing trials or PSV may result in the faster discontinuation of ventilatory support as compared with SIMV.
- The ideal approach to weaning the vast majority of patients is a therapist-driven protocol that makes use of an SBT.
- The monitoring of the patient during weaning should include physical, respiratory rate and pattern, dyspnea, pulse oximetry, cardiac rate and rhythm, and blood pressure assessments.
- The use of daily SATs not only improves the speed of weaning but has also been shown to improve mortality.
- Before extubation, patients should be assessed for the ability to maintain and protect their airway and for the presence of upper airway edema.
- Common causes of weaning failure include an excessive ventilatory workload in the presence of ventilatory muscle weakness or fatigue, oxygenation problems, cardiovascular instability, the inability to clear secretions, poor mental status, and the presence of an underlying concurrent pathologic condition that necessitates treatment.
- The goals of the weaning of long-term ventilator-dependent patients include reducing the amount of support, reducing the invasiveness of support, and increasing the patient's level of independent function.

References

1. MacIntyre N: Respiratory factors in weaning from mechanical ventilatory support. Respir Care 40:244–248, 1995.
2. Marini JJ: Weaning techniques and protocols. Respir Care 40:233–238, 1995.
3. MacIntyre NR, Cook DJ, Ely EW, et al: Evidence-based guidelines for weaning and discontinuing ventilator support: a collective task force facilitated by the American College of Chest Physicians, the American Association for Respiratory Care, and the American College of Critical Care Medicine. Chest 120:375S–395S, 2001.
4. Tobin M: Medical progress: advances in mechanical ventilation. N Engl J Med 344:1986–1996, 2001.
5. Clement JM, Buck EA: Weaning from mechanical ventilatory support. Dimens Crit Care Nurs 15:114–129, 1996.
6. Agency for Healthcare Research and Quality: Criteria for weaning from mechanical ventilation, evidence report/technology assessment No. 23 (AHRQ publication no. 01-E010), Rockville, MD, 2000, Agency for Healthcare Research and Quality.
7. Slutsky AS: Mechanical ventilation. American College of Chest Physicians' Consensus Conference. Chest 104:1833–1859, 1993.
8. Pierson DJ: Weaning from mechanical ventilation: why all the confusion? Respir Care 40:228–232, 1995.
9. Sassoon CSH, Machutte CK: What you need to know about the ventilator in weaning. Respir Care 40:249–256, 1995.
10. Meade MO, Guyalt H, Cook DJ: Weaning from mechanical ventilation: the evidence from clinical research. Respir Care 46:1408–1415, 2001.
11. Grap MJ, Strickland D, Tormey L, et al: Collaborative practice: development, implementation, and evaluation of a weaning protocol for patients receiving mechanical ventilation. Am J Crit Care 12:454–460, 2003.
12. Tonnelier JM: Impact of a nurses' protocol-directed weaning procedure on outcomes in patients undergoing mechanical ventilation for longer than 48 hours: a prospective cohort study with a matched historical control group. Crit Care 9:R83–R89, 2005.
13. Smyrnios NA, Connolly A, Wilson MM, et al: Effects of a multifaceted, multidisciplinary, hospital-wide quality improvement program on weaning from mechanical ventilation. Crit Care Med 30:1224–1230, 2002.
14. Ramachandran V, Grap MJ, Sessier CN: Protocol-directed weaning: a process of continuous performance improvement. Crit Care 9:138–140, 2005.
15. Pierson DJ: Long-term mechanical ventilation and weaning. Respir Care 40:289–295, 1995.
16. Pierson DJ: Nonrespiratory aspects of weaning from mechanical ventilation. Respir Care 40:263–270, 1995.
17. Bigatello LM, Stelfox HT, Berra L, et al: Outcome of patients undergoing prolonged mechanical ventilation after critical illness. Crit Care Med. 35:2491–2497, 2007
18. Marini JJ: The physiologic determinants of ventilator dependence. Respir Care 31:271–282, 1986.
19. Burns SM, Clochesy JM, Hannenman SK, et al: Weaning from long-term mechanical ventilation. Am J Crit Care 4:4–22, 1995.
20. Deem S: Intensive-care-unit-acquired muscle weakness. Respir Care 51:1042–1052, 2006.
21. Hanneman SK, Ingersoll GL, Knebel AR, et al: Weaning from short term mechanical ventilation: a review. Am J Crit Care 3:421–441, 1994.
22. Yang KL: Reproducibility of weaning parameters: a need for specialization. Chest 102:1829–1832, 1992.

23. Yang KL, Tobin MJ: A prospective study of indexes predicting the outcome of trials of weaning from mechanical ventilation. N Engl J Med 324:1445–1550, 1991.
24. Vallverdu I, Calaf N, Subirana M, et al: Clinical characteristics, respiratory functional parameters, and outcome of a two-hour T-piece trial in patients weaning from mechanical ventilation. Am J Respir Crit Care 158:1855–1862, 1998.
25. DeHaven CB, Kirton OC, Morgan JP, et al: Breathing measurement reduces false-negative classification of tachypneic preextubation trial failures. Crit Care Med 24:976–980, 1996.
26. Pardee NE, Winterbauer RH, Allen JD: Bedside evaluation of respiratory distress. Chest 85:203–206, 1984.
27. Krieger BP, Isber J, Breitenbucher A, et al: Serial measurements of the rapid-shallow breathing index as a predictor of weaning outcome in elderly medical patients. Chest 112:1029–1034, 1997.
28. Gandia F, Blanco J: Evaluation of indexes predicting outcome of ventilator weaning and value of adding supplemental inspiratory load. Intensive Care Med 18:327–333, 1992.
29. Sharar SS: Weaning and extubation are not the same. Respir Care 40:239–224, 19953.
30. Levy MM, Miyasaki A, Langston D: Work of breathing as a weaning parameter in mechanically ventilated patients. Chest 108:1018–1020, 1995.
31. Shikora PA, Benotti PN, Johannigman JA: The oxygen cost of breathing may predict weaning from mechanical ventilation better than respiratory rate to tidal volume ratio. Arch Surg 129:269–274, 1994.
32. Truwit J: Lung mechanics. In Dantzker DR, MacIntyre NR, Bakow ED, editors: Comprehensive respiratory care, Philadelphia, 1995, WB Saunders.
33. Bassili HR, Deitel M: Effect of nutritional support on weaning patients off mechanical ventilators. JPEN J Parenter Enteral Nutr 5:161–163, 1981.
34. Hess DR: Mechanical ventilation of the adult patient: initiation, management and weaning. In Burton GG, Hodgkin JE, Ward JJ, editors: Respiratory care: a guide to clinical practice, Philadelphia, 1997, Lippincott Williams & Wilkins.
35. Kress JP, Pohlman AS, O'Connor MF, et al: Daily interruption of sedative infusions in critically ill patients undergoing mechanical ventilation. N Engl J Med 342:1471–1477, 2000.
36. Sessler CN: Wake up and breathe. Crit Care Med 32:1413–1414, 2004.
37. Arroliga A, Frutos-Vivar F, Hall J, et al: Use of sedatives and neuromuscular blockers in a cohort of patients receiving mechanical ventilation. Chest 128:496–506, 2005.
38. Sassoon CSH: Noninvasive positive-pressure ventilation in acute respiratory failure: review of reported experience with special attention to use during weaning. Respir Care 40: 282–288, 1995.
39. MacIntyre NR: Psychological factors in weaning from mechanical ventilatory support. Respir Care 40:277–281, 1995.
40. Esteban A, Frutos F, Tobin MJ, et al: A comparison of four methods of weaning patients from mechanical ventilation. N Engl J Med 332:345–350, 1995.
41. Ely EW, Baker AM, Evans GW, et al: The prognostic significance of passing a daily screen of weaning parameters. Intensive Care Med 25:581–587, 1999.
42. Esteban A, Alia I, Gordo F, et al. Extubation outcome after spontaneous breathing trial with T-piece or pressure support ventilation. Am J Respir Crit Care Med 156:459–465, 1997.
43. Baily CR, Jones RM, Kelleher AA: The role of continuous positive airway pressure during weaning from mechanical ventilation in cardiac surgical patients. Anaesthesia 50: 677–681, 1995.
44. Schachter EN, Tucker D, Beck GJ: Does intermittent mandatory ventilation accelerate weaning? JAMA 246:1210–1214, 1981.
45. Esteban A, Anzueto A, Alia I, et al: How is mechanical ventilation employed in the intensive care unit? An international utilization review. Am J Respir Crit Care Med 161:1450–1458, 2000.
46. Groeger JS, Levinson MR, Carlon GC: Assist control versus synchronized intermittent mandatory ventilation during acute respiratory failure. Crit Care Med 17:607–612, 1989.
47. Prakash O, Meij SH: Oxygen consumption and blood gas exchange during controlled and intermittent mandatory ventilation after cardiac surgery. Crit Care Med 13:556–559, 1985.
48. Savino JA, Dawson JA, Agarwal N, et al: The metabolic cost of breathing in critical surgical patients. J Trauma 25:1126–1133, 1985.
49. Brochard L, Rauss A, Benito S, et al: Comparison of three methods of gradual withdrawal from ventilatory support during weaning from mechanical ventilation. Am J Respir Crit Care Med 150:896–903, 1994.
50. Shikora SA, MacDonald GF, Bistrian BR, et al: Could the oxygen cost of breathing be used to optimize the application pressure support? J Trauma 33:521–526, 1992.
51. Jounieaux V, Duran A, Levi-Valensi P: Synchronized intermittent mandatory ventilation with and without pressure support ventilation in weaning patients with COPD from mechanical ventilation. Chest 105:1204–1210, 1994.
52. Heymann A, Radtke F, Schiemann A, et al: Delayed treatment of delirium increases mortality rate in intensive care unit patients. J Int Med Res 38:1584–1595, 2010.
53. Girard TD, Kress JP, Fuchs BD, et al. Efficacy and safety of a paired sedation and ventilation weaning protocol for mechanically ventilated patients in intensive care (awaking and breathing control trial): a randomized controlled trial. Lancet 371–126–134, 2008.
54. Hewlett AW, Plott AS, Terry VG: Mandatory minute ventilation. Anesthesia 32:163–169, 1977.
55. Davis S, Potgieter PD, Linton DM: Mandatory minute volume weaning in patients with pulmonary pathology. Anaesth Intensive Care 17:170–174, 1989.
56. Campbell RS, Branson RD, Johannigman JA: Adaptive support ventilation. Respir Care Clin N Am 7:425–440, 2001.
57. Sulzer CF, Chiolero R, Chassot P, et al: Adaptive support ventilation for fast tracheal extubation after cardiac surgery: a randomized controlled study. Anesthesiology 95:1339–1345, 2001.
58. Cassina T, Chioléro R, Mauri R, Revelly JP: Clinical experience with adaptive support ventilation for fast tract anesthesia. J Cardiothorac Vasc Anesth 17:571–575, 2003.
59. Armal JC, Wysocki M, Nafati C, et al. Automatic selection of breathing pattern using adaptive support ventilation. Intensive Care Med 34:75–81, 2008
60. Iregui M, Ward S, Clinikscale D, et al: Use of a handheld computer by respiratory care practitioners to improve the efficiency of weaning patients from mechanical ventilation. Crit Care Med 30:2038–2043, 2002.
61. Lellouche F, Mancebo J, Jolliet P, et al: A multicenter randomized trial of computer-driven protocolized weaning from mechanical ventilation. Am J Respir Crit Care Med 174:849–851, 2006.
62. Guttmann J, Haberthur C, Mols G: Automatic tube compensation. Respir Care Clin N Am 7:475–501, 2001.
63. Jabar S, Delay JM, Matecki S, et al: Volume guaranteed pressure support ventilation facing acute changes in ventilatory demand. Intensive Care Med 31:1181–1188, 2005.

64. Randolph AJ, Wypij D, Venkataraman S, et al: Effects of mechanical ventilation on respiratory outcome in infants and children. JAMA 288:2561-2568, 2002
65. Nava S, Ambrosino N, Enrico C, et al: Noninvasive ventilation in the weaning of patients with respiratory failure due to chronic obstructive pulmonary disease: a randomized controlled trial. Ann Intern Med 128:721-728, 1998.
66. Girault C, Daudenthua I, Chevron V, et al: Noninvasive ventilation as a systematic extubation and weaning technique in acute-on-chronic respiratory failure: a prospective randomized controlled study. Am J Respir Crit Care Med 160:86-92, 1999.
67. Ferrer M, Esquinas A, Arancibia F et al: Noninvasive ventilation during persistent weaning failure. Am J Respir Crit Care Med 168:70-76, 2003
68. Nava S, Gregoretti C, Fanfulla F, et al: Noninvasive ventilation to prevent respiratory failure after extubation in high-risk patients. Crit Care Med 33:2465-2470, 2005.
69. Ferrer M, Valencia M, Nicolas JM et al: Early noninvasive ventilation averts extubation failure in patients at risk. Am J Respir Crit Care Med 173:164-170, 2006.
70. Ferrer M, Sellares J, Valencia M et al: Noninvasive ventilation after extubation in hypercarbic patients with chronic respiratory disorders: a randomized controlled trial. Lancet 374:1082-1088, 2009.
71. Keenan SP, Powers C, McCormack DG, Block G: Noninvasive positive pressure ventilation for post-extubation respiratory distress. JAMA 287:2338-2344, 2002.
72. Esteban A, Frutos-Vivar F, Ferguson ND et al: Noninvasive positive pressure ventilation for respiratory failure alter extubation. N Engl J Med 350:2452-2460, 2004.
73. Krishnan JA, Moore D, Robeson C: A prospective, controlled trial of a protocol-based strategy to discontinue mechanical ventilation. Am J Respir Crit Care Med 169:673-678, 2004.
74. Wood G, MacLeod B, Moffatt S: Weaning from mechanical ventilation: physician-directed vs a respiratory-therapist-directed protocol. Respir Care 40:219-224, 1995.
75. Ely W, Baker AM, Dunagan DP, et al: Effects on the duration of mechanical ventilation of identifying patients capable of breathing spontaneously. N Engl J Med 335:1864-1869, 1996.
76. Marlich G, Murin S, Battistella F et al: Protocol weaning of mechanical ventilation in medical and surgical patients by respiratory care practitioners and nurses. Chest 118:459-467, 2000.
77. Sassoon, C, Ehu Z, Caiozzo VJ: Assist-control mechanical ventilation attenuates ventilator-induced diaphragmatic dysfunction. Am J Respir Crit Care Med 170:626-632, 2004.
78. Jubran A: Critical illness and mechanical ventilation: effects on the diaphragm. Respir Care 51:1054-1061, 2006.
79. Marini JJ: Dyspnea during weaning. Respir Care 40:271-276, 1995.
80. Morley TF, Giaimo J, Maroszan E, et al: Use of capnography for assessment of the adequacy of alveolar ventilation during weaning. Am Rev Respir Dis 148:339-344, 1993.
81. Mohsenifar Z, Hay A, Hay J, et al: Gastric intramural pH as a predictor of success or failure in weaning patients from mechanical ventilation. Ann Intern Med 119:794-798, 1993.
82. Abalos A, Leibowitz AB, Distefano D, et al: Myocardial ischemia during the weaning period. Am J Crit Care 1:32-36, 1992.
83. Straus C, Louis B, Isabey D, et al: Contribution of the endotracheal tube and the upper airway to breathing workload. Am J Respir Crit Care Med 157:23-30, 1998.
84. Sharar S: The effects of artificial airways on airflow and ventilatory mechanics: basic concepts and clinical relevance. Respir Care 40:257-262, 1995.
85. Diehl JL, El Atrous S, Touchard D, et al: Changes in the work of breathing induced by tracheotomy in ventilatory-dependent patients. Am J Respir Crit Care Med 159:383-388, 1999.
86. Miller RL, Cole RP: Association between reduced cuff leak volume and postextubation stridor. Chest 110:1035-1040, 1996.
87. Sandhu RS, Pasquale MD, Miller K, et al: Measurement of endotracheal tube cuff leak to predict postextubation stridor and need for reintubation. J Am Coll Surg 190:682-687, 2000.
88. Jaber S, Chanques G, Matecki S, et al: Post-extubation stridor in intensive care unit patients. Risk factors evaluation and importance of the cuff-leak test. Intensive Care Med 29:69-74, 2003.
89. Hurford WE, Favorito F: Association of myocardial ischemia with failure to wean from mechanical ventilation. Crit Care Med 23:1475-1480, 1995.
90. Hund EF, Fogel W, Krieger D, et al: Critical illness polyneuropathy: clinical findings and outcomes of a frequent cause of neuromuscular weaning failure. Crit Care Med 24:1328-1333, 1996.
91. Management of patients requiring prolonged mechanical ventilation: report of a NAMDRC Consensus Conference. Chest 128:3937-3954, 2005.
92. Shekleton ME, Burns SM, Clochesy JM, et al: Terminal weaning from mechanical ventilation: a review. AACN Clin Issues Crit Care Nurs 5:523-533, 1994.
93. Cook D, Rocker G, Marshall J, et al: Withdrawal of mechanical ventilation in anticipation of death in the intensive care unit. N Engl J 349:1123-1132, 2003.

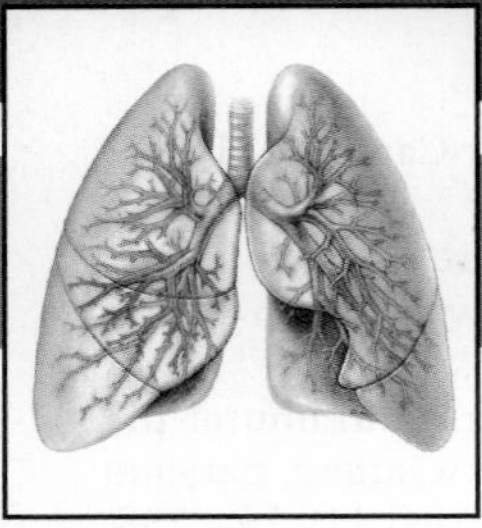

Chapter 48

Neonatal and Pediatric Respiratory Care

DANIEL W. CHIPMAN AND PATRICIA ENGLISH

CHAPTER OBJECTIVES

After reading this chapter you will be able to:

- Describe the correct approach to assessment of the fetus and newborn infant.
- Discuss the use of oxygen therapy, bronchial hygiene therapy, aerosol drug therapy, airway management, and resuscitation approaches in the care of infants and children.
- Describe the correct approach to assessment of the pediatric patient.
- Discuss the use of continuous positive airway pressure and the basics of mechanical ventilation including high-frequency ventilation in the care of infants and children.
- List clinical situations where nitric oxide and extracorporeal life support are used, and discuss the basic application of each.

CHAPTER OUTLINE

KEY TERMS

Apgar score
appropriate for gestational age (AGA)
continuous positive airway pressure (CPAP)
extracorporeal membrane oxygenation (ECMO)
extremely low birth weight (ELBW)
grunting, flaring, and retracting
high-frequency ventilation (HFV)
inhaled nitric oxide (INO)
large for gestational age (LGA)
meconium
patent ductus arteriosus (PDA)
primary pulmonary hypertension of the newborn (PPHN)
retinopathy of prematurity (ROP)
surfactant
very low birth weight (VLBW)

Caring for infants and children is one of the most challenging and rewarding aspects of respiratory care. Competent clinical practice in this area requires knowledge of the many pathophysiologic differences among infants, children, and adults. Understanding the unique pathophysiology involved in neonatal and pediatric respiratory disorders (see Chapter 31) can assist the respiratory therapist (RT) in providing quality care to infants and children. A thorough understanding of how the respiratory system develops in the fetus is the first step toward acquiring the specialized knowledge needed to practice neonatal respiratory care (see Chapter 8). This chapter begins with an overview of neonatal and pediatric patient assessment and then describes respiratory care modalities used to treat these patients.

ASSESSMENT OF THE NEWBORN

Assessment of the newborn begins before birth with assessment of the maternal history, the maternal condition, and the status of the fetus.

Maternal Factors

Maternal risk factors include many medical, physical, and social conditions. Maternal health and individual physiology, pregnancy complications, and maternal behaviors affect the health of the fetus. Any condition that causes an interference with placental blood flow or the transfer of oxygen (O_2) to the fetus can result in an adverse outcome. The clinician must be prepared for the possibility of resuscitation at delivery. This possibility is best anticipated by identifying risk factors that relate to neonatal compromise. Table 48-1 lists maternal risks and related outcomes of which the team preparing to receive the infant should be aware when the infant is delivered.

TABLE 48-1

Maternal Condition and Neonatal Outcomes

Maternal Condition	Fetal or Neonatal Outcome
Previous pregnancy complication	Same outcome as previous fetus
Diabetes mellitus	LGA, congenital malformations, RDS, hypoglycemia
Pregnancy-induced hypertension	Prematurity, SGA (preeclampsia)
Maternal age <17 years	Low birth weight, prematurity
Maternal age >35 years	Prematurity, chromosomal defects
Placenta previa	Prematurity, bleeding, SGA
Abruptio placentae	Fetal asphyxia, bleeding
Alcohol consumption	SGA, CNS dysfunction, mental retardation, facial dysmorphology
Smoking	SGA, prematurity, mental retardation, SIDS
Drug use	Placental abruption, IUGR, prematurity, CNS abnormalities, withdrawal disorders

IUGR, Intrauterine growth restriction; *RDS,* respiratory distress syndrome; *SIDS,* sudden infant death syndrome.

Fetal Assessment

Fetal assessment is performed with ultrasonography, amniocentesis, fetal heart rate monitoring, and fetal blood gas analysis. Ultrasonography uses high-frequency sound waves to obtain an image of the infant in utero. This image allows the physician to view the position of the fetus and placenta, measure fetal growth, identify possible anatomic anomalies, and assess the amniotic fluid qualitatively.

Amniocentesis involves direct sampling and quantitative assessment of amniotic fluid. Amniotic fluid may be inspected for **meconium** (fetal bowel contents) or blood. In addition, sloughed fetal cells can be analyzed for genetic normality. Lung maturation can be assessed with amniocentesis. The lecithin-to-sphingomyelin ratio (L:S ratio) involves measurement of two phospholipids, lethicin and sphingomyelin, synthesized by the fetus in utero. As shown in Figure 48-1, the L:S ratio increases with increasing gestational age. At approximately 34 to 35 weeks' gestation, this ratio abruptly increases to greater than 2:1. An L:S ratio greater than 2:1 indicates stable **surfactant** production and mature lungs. Phosphatidylglycerol is another lipid found in the amniotic fluid that is used to assess fetal lung maturity. Phosphatidylglycerol first appears at approximately 35 to 36 weeks' gestation. If phosphatidylglycerol is more than 1% of the total phospholipids, the risk of respiratory distress syndrome is less than 1%.

Fetal heart rate monitoring is the measurement of fetal heart rate and uterine contractions during labor. Examination of fetal heart rate changes related to uterine contractions identifies a fetus in distress. Fetal well-being is obtained by examining the variability and reactivity of the fetal heart rate. A normal fetal heart rate ranges from 120 to 160 beats/min. Fetal tachycardia can be a sign of fetal hypoxemia or could be related to other factors, such as prematurity or maternal fever. Temporary declines in fetal heart rate are called *decelerations* and can be mild (<15 beats/min), moderate (15 to 45 beats/min), or severe (>45 beats/min). Decelerations are classified by their occurrence in the uterine contraction cycle.

Figure 48-2 illustrates the three common patterns of early decelerations, late decelerations, and variable decelerations. Early decelerations occur when the fetal heart rate decreases in the beginning of a contraction. This type of deceleration is benign and in most cases is caused by a vagal response related to compression of the fetal head in the birth canal. A late deceleration occurs when the heart rate decreases 10 to 30 seconds after the onset of contractions. A late deceleration pattern indicates impaired maternal-placental blood flow, or uteroplacental insufficiency. With variable decelerations, there is no clear relationship between contractions and heart rate. This pattern is the most common of the three and probably related to umbilical cord compression. Short periods of

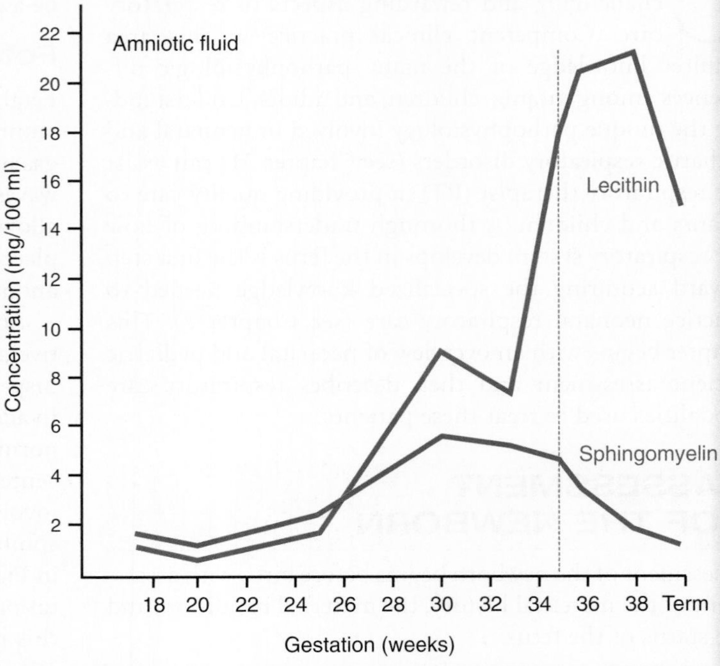

FIGURE 48-1 Lecithin *(red line)* and sphingomyelin *(blue line)* concentrations plotted against gestational age. L:S ratio rises to 1.2 at 28 weeks and to 2 or more at 35 weeks, indicating maturation of the fetal lung. (Modified from Gluck L, et al: Am J Obstet Gynecol 109:440, 1971.)

cord compression are generally benign, but prolonged periods of compression result in impaired umbilical blood flow and can lead to fetal distress. Fetal heart rate variability is the beat-to-beat variation in rate that occurs because of normal sympathetic or parasympathetic influences. A completely monotonous heart rate tracing may be indicative of fetal asphyxia. Fetal heart rate reactivity is the ability of the fetal heart rate to increase in response to movement or external stimuli. A healthy fetus has two accelerations within a 20-minute period.

In utero, the fetus receives its blood supply from the placenta. Only a small portion of the blood that enters the fetal right heart flows through the lungs. This is a result of fetal pulmonary blood vessels being constricted with a high resistance to blood flow. There are two openings in the fetal heart through which most fetal blood flows. These normal anatomic shunts in the fetus are called *patent foramen ovale* and *patent ductus arteriosus (PDA)*. Blood flows through these openings and into the umbilical vessels before returning to the mother. Pressure in the umbilical vessels is low. During the transition from fetal life to newborn life, the umbilical cord is clamped, and the infant's systemic blood pressure is increased. The infant begins to breathe, and O_2 enters the infant's blood. Oxygenated blood entering the pulmonary vessels causes the vessels to dilate and decreases pulmonary resistance. With higher systemic resistance and lower pulmonary resistance, less blood flows through the anatomic openings, and these openings begin to close. Evidence of normal transitional circulation is noted as the infant's skin turns from a bluish hue to pink over the first several minutes of life.

RULE OF THUMB

Infants presenting with a monotonous heart rate or a fetal scalp pH less than 7.2 may be experiencing asphyxia.

Fetal Blood Gas Analysis

When other factors indicate potential problems during labor and delivery, fetal blood pH can be used to determine severity. Normally, fetal blood is obtained from a capillary sample taken from the presenting body part, usually the scalp. Normal fetal capillary pH ranges from 7.35 to 7.25, with the lower values occurring late in labor. A pH less than 7.20 may indicate that the fetus is experiencing asphyxia. There is no direct correlation between fetal scalp and arterial blood pH; scalp pH should be used only to assist in interpreting clinical signs of fetal distress.

Evaluation of the Newborn

All newborns should be assessed immediately on delivery. Most newborns (>90%) do not need intervention when transitioning from intrauterine to extrauterine life. The two categories of newborns most likely to need intervention are infants born with evidence of meconium in their airway and premature infants. The need for intervention is determined by assessing for the presence of meconium, breathing or crying, muscle tone, color, and gestational age.

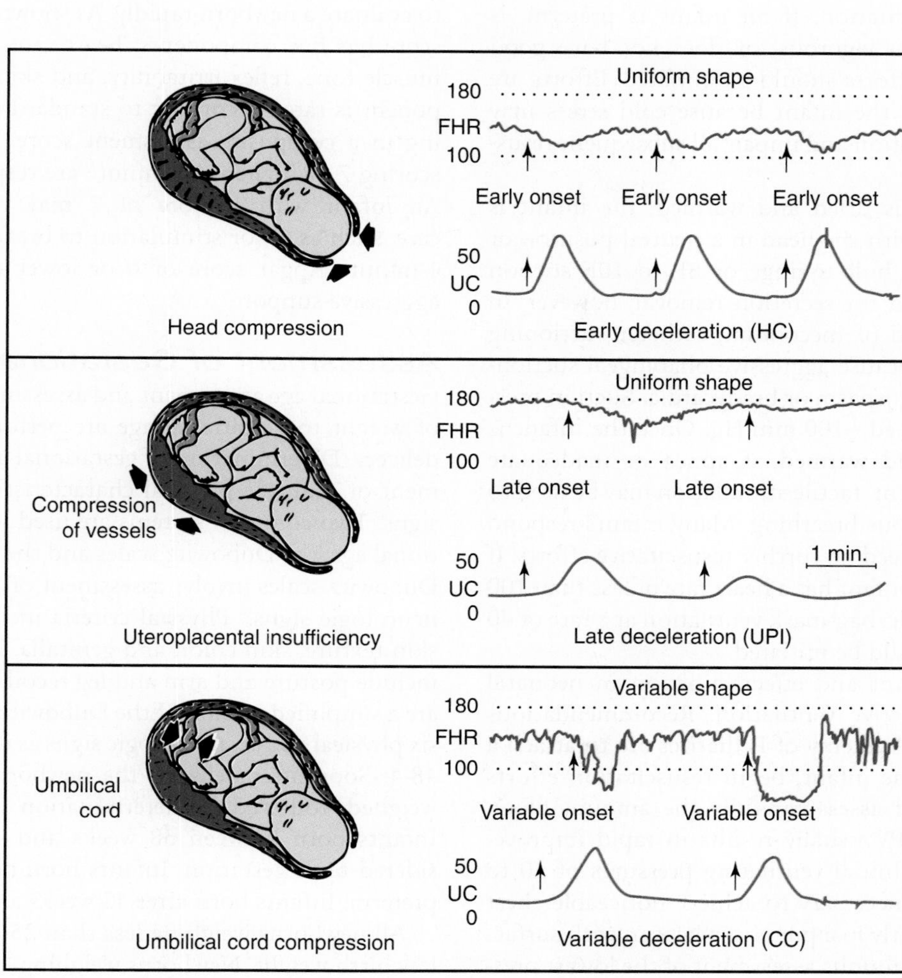

FIGURE 48-2 Fetal heart rate patterns. (Modified from Avery GB, editor: Neonatology: pathophysiology and management of the newborn, ed 2, Philadelphia, 1981, JB Lippincott.)

Meconium is the medical term for the infant's first stools. It is a sticky green-black substance that if inhaled by the infant can cause significant respiratory problems. It is most likely present in a term or postterm newborn. Term infants delivered without evidence of meconium who are crying or breathing and have good tone should not routinely be separated from the mother. They should be dried, covered, and given to the mother and observed for breathing, activity, and color. If meconium is present and the infant is vigorous, pharyngeal suctioning with a bulb suction is appropriate. Simultaneously the infant should be dried and placed under a warmer and assessed for signs of respiratory distress. See later section on Respiratory Assessment of the Infant. If meconium is present in a nonvigorous infant, stimulation should be avoided.

Immediate endotracheal intubation before positive pressure ventilation (PPV) is indicated as a means to clear meconium from the airway. The endotracheal tube should be attached to a meconium aspirator, and a suction device should be regulated for −70 to −100 mm Hg. As soon as the endotracheal tube is inserted, suction should be applied to the tube, and then the endotracheal tube is withdrawn. Reintubation and repeat suctioning may be necessary if meconium is still visible in the airway. Frequent assessment of the heart rate is indicated during this process, and if bradycardia is present, bag-mask ventilation should be considered. Intubation of the trachea is not recommended in a vigorous infant with meconium. Preterm infants frequently need intervention. The more preterm the infant, the more likely the infant will need some level of resuscitation. If an infant is preterm, is not breathing, is not vigorous, or does not have good tone, resuscitation efforts should be initiated. Efforts are directed at warming the infant because cold stress may increase O_2 consumption and impair all subsequent resuscitation efforts.

After the infant is dried and warmed, the infant is positioned supine, with the head in a neutral position or slightly extended. A bulb syringe or 8F to 10F suction catheter may be used for secretion removal; however, in the absence of blood or meconium, catheter suctioning should be limited because aggressive pharyngeal suctioning may cause laryngospasm or bradycardia. Suction pressure should not exceed −100 mm Hg. Once the infant is suctioned, dried, and warmed, if apnea or inadequate respirations are present, tactile stimulation may be used to encourage spontaneous breathing. Many infants respond to stimulation and need no further resuscitative efforts. If after 30 seconds the infant has a heart rate of less than 100 beats/min or is apneic, bag-mask ventilation at a rate of 40 to 60 beats/min should be initiated.

The *most* important and effective action in neonatal resuscitation is effective ventilation. Recommendations from the American Academy of Pediatrics are to attach a pulse oximeter to the infant, begin resuscitation efforts using room air, and assess carefully the amount of O_2 needed.[1] Effective PPV usually results in rapid improvement of heart rate. Initial ventilating pressures of 30 to 40 cm H_2O may be necessary to achieve noticeable chest movement, particularly in a preterm newborn with surfactant deficiency. Continuous assessment of the lowest pressure needed to observe the chest rise is essential throughout the resuscitation. After application of PPV for 30 seconds, the heart rate is reassessed. If the heart rate is less than 60 beats/min, chest compressions are begun, and PPV is maintained. If the heart rate remains less than 60 beats/min after adequate ventilation with 100% O_2 and chest compressions for 30 seconds, appropriate medications are given. As soon as the heart rate is noted to be greater than 100 beats/min, compressions are discontinued. If spontaneous breathing is present, PPV may be gradually reduced and then discontinued. If spontaneous breathing remains inadequate or if heart rate remains less than 100 beats/min, assisted ventilation is continued via bag-mask or endotracheal tube. Figure 48-3 outlines a newborn resuscitation algorithm and includes the targeted saturation levels for the first 10 minutes of life.

RULE OF THUMB

The most *important and effective action in neonatal resuscitation is to ventilate.*

Apgar Score

An Apgar score is assigned at 1 minute and 5 minutes of life. The **Apgar score** is an objective scoring system used to evaluate a newborn rapidly. As shown in Table 48-2, the score has five components: heart rate, respiratory effort, muscle tone, reflex irritability, and skin color. Each component is rated according to standard definitions, resulting in a composite assessment score. Generally, infants scoring 7 or higher at 1 minute are responding normally. An infant with a score of 7 may require supportive care, such as O_2 or stimulation to breathe. Infants with a 1-minute Apgar score of 6 or lower may require more aggressive support.

Assessment of Gestational Age

Gestational age assessment and assessment of relationship of weight to gestational age are performed shortly after delivery. Determination of gestational age involves assessment of multiple physical characteristics and neurologic signs. Two common systems are used to determine gestational age: the Dubowitz scales and the Ballard scales. The Dubowitz scales involve assessment of 11 physical and 10 neurologic signs.[2] Physical criteria include assessment of skin texture, skin color, and genitalia. Neurologic criteria include posture and arm and leg recoil. The Ballard scales are a simplified version of the Dubowitz scales and include six physical and six neurologic signs as illustrated in Figure 48-4. Soon after delivery, the newborn is stabilized and weighed, followed by determination of gestational age. Infants born between 38 weeks and 42 weeks are considered term gestation. Infants born before 38 weeks are preterm. Infants born after 42 weeks are postterm.

All newborns weighing less than 2500 g are considered low birth weight. Newborns weighing less than 1500 g are considered **very low birth weight (VLBW).** Newborns weighing less than 1000 g are considered **extremely low birth weight (ELBW).** A newborn with a weight that is either too large or too small or who has been born preterm or postterm has a higher risk of morbidity and mortality. As shown in Figure 48-5, by plotting the infant's gestational age against weight, the newborn's relative developmental status can be classified. Infants whose weight falls between the 10th and 90th percentiles are **appropriate for gestational age (AGA).** Infants whose weight is above the 90th percentile are **large for gestational age (LGA).** Infants whose weight is below the 10th percentile are small for gestational age (SGA).

RULE OF THUMB

Infants weighing less than 2500 g are normally considered low birth weight neonates. Infants weighing less than 1500 g are considered VLBW neonates, and neonates weighing less than 1000 g are considered ELBW neonates.

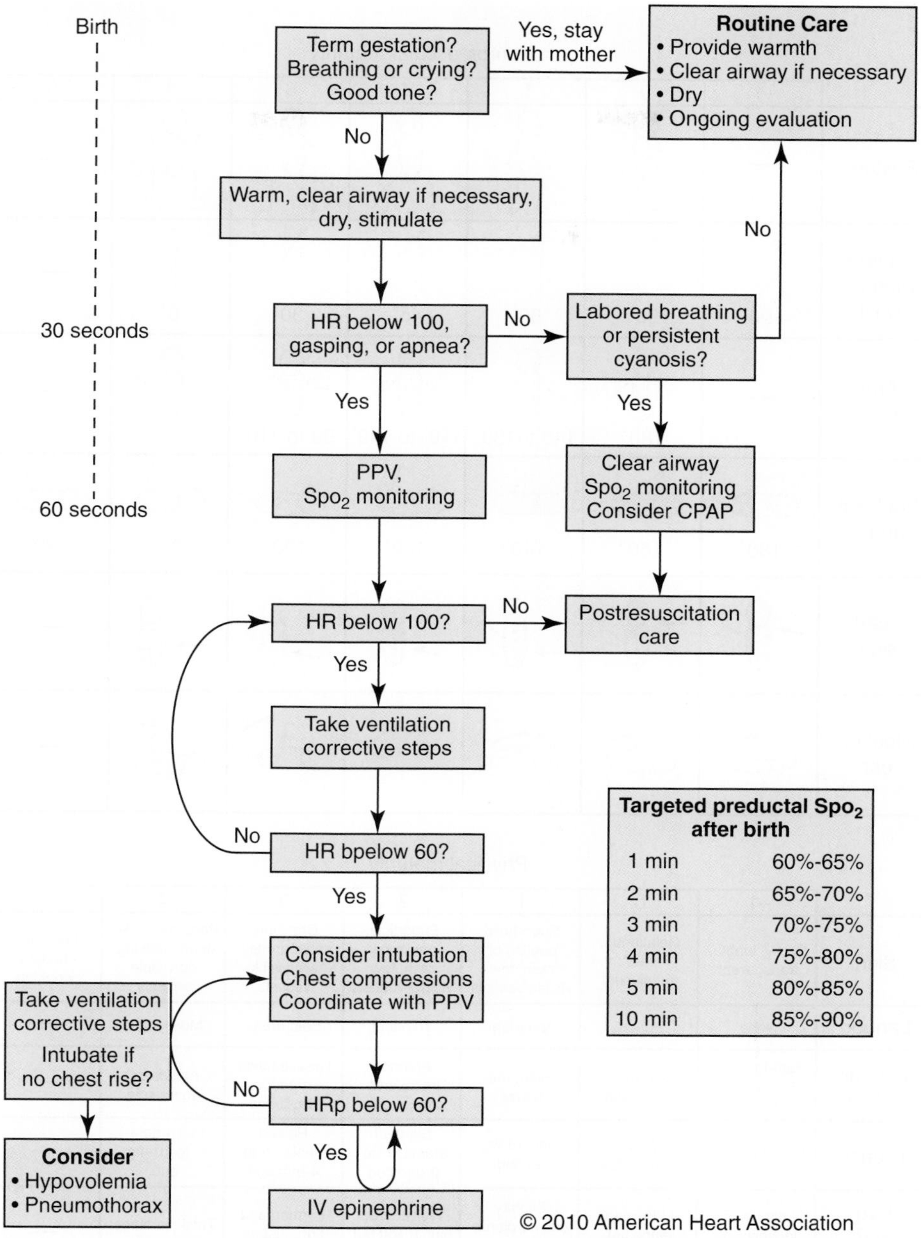

FIGURE 48-3 Neonatal resuscitation algorithm. Neonatal Resuscitation: 2010. American Heart Association Guidelines for Cardiopulmonary Resuscitation and Emergency Cardiovascular Care. © 2010 American Heart Association, Inc.

TABLE 48-2

Apgar Scoring System for Newborn Assessment

	Score		
Sign	**0**	**1**	**2**
Heart rate	Absent	<100/min	>100/min
Respirations	Absent	Slow, irregular	Good, crying
Muscle tone	Limp	Some flexion	Active motion
Reflex irritability (catheter in nares, tactile stimulation)	No response	Grimace	Cough, sneeze, cry
Color	Blue or pale	Pink body with completely blue extremities	Pink

From Koff PB, Eitzman DV, Neu J: Neonatal and pediatric respiratory care, ed 2, St Louis, 1993, Mosby.

Neuromuscular maturity

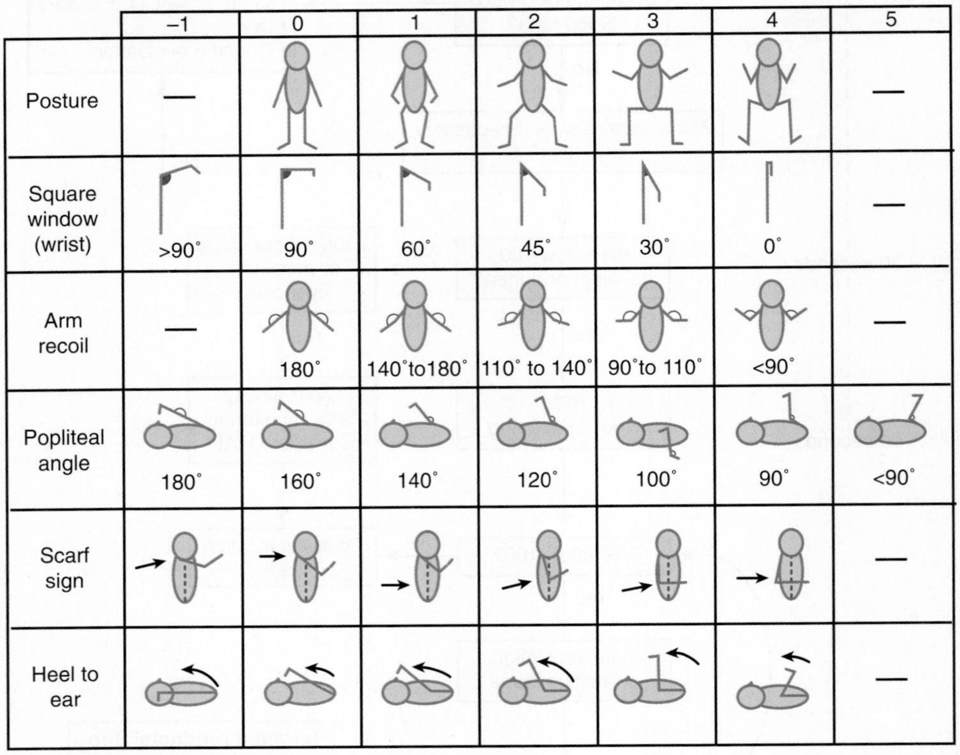
-1
0
1
2
3
4
5
Posture
Square window (wrist)
>90°
90°
60°
45°
30°
0°
Arm recoil
180°
140° to 180°
110° to 140°
90° to 110°
<90°
Popliteal angle
180°
160°
140°
120°
100°
90°
<90°
Scarf sign
Heel to ear

Physical maturity

	–1	0	1	2	3	4	5
Skin	Sticky, friable, transparent	Gelatinous, red, translucent	Superficial peeling or rash; few visible vessels	Superficial peeling or rash; few visible vessels	Cracking; pale areas; rare visible vessels	Parchment-like; deep cracking; no visible vessels	Leathery, cracked, wrinkled
Lanugo	None	Sparse	Abundant	Thinning	Bald areas	Mostly bald	—
Plantar surface	Heel-toe 40 to 50 mm: –1; <40mm: –2	>50 mm; no crease	Faint, red marks	Anterior transverse crease only	Creases over anterior two-thirds	Creases over entire sole	—
Breast	Imperceptible	Barely perceptible	Flat areola; no bud	Stippled areola; 1- to 2-mm bud	Raised areola; 3- to 4-mm bud	Full areola; 5- to 10-mm bud	—
Eye and ear	Lids fused, loosely: –1; tightly: –2	Lids open; pinna flat, stays folded	Slightly curved pinna; soft, slow recoil	Well curved pinna; soft but ready recoil	Formed and firm; instant recoil	Thick cartilage; ear stiff	—
Genitalia, male	Scrotum flat, smooth	Scrotum empty; faint rugae	Testes in upper canal; rare rugae	Testes descending; few rugae	Testes down; good rugae	Testes pendulous; deep rugae	—
Genitalia, female	Clitoris prominent; labia flat	Prominent clitoris; small labia minora	Prominent clitoris; enlarging minora	Major and minora equally prominent	Majora large; minora small	Majora cover clitoris and minora	—

Maturity rating

Score	–10	–5	0	5	10	15	20	25	30	35	40	45	50
Weeks	20	22	24	26	28	30	32	34	36	38	40	42	44

FIGURE 48-4 The Ballard gestational age assessment. (Modified from Ballard JL, et al: J Pediatr 95:769, 1979.)

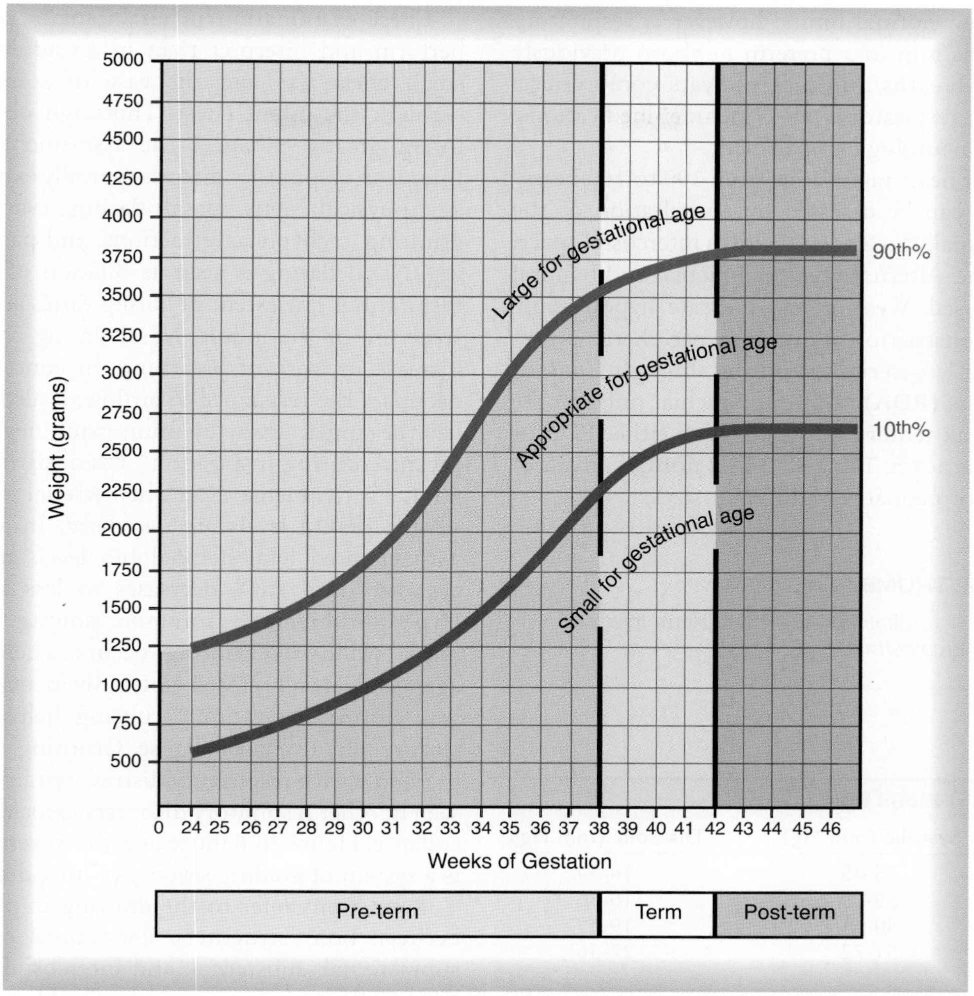

FIGURE 48-5 Colorado intrauterine growth chart. (Modified from Avery GB, editor: Neonatology: pathophysiology and management of the newborn, ed 4, Philadelphia, 1994, JB Lippincott.)

By classifying infants into one of the combined categories, such as "preterm, AGA," the clinician can help identify infants at highest risk and predict the nature of the risks involved and the likely mortality rate. Small, preterm infants are at highest risk. Compared with term infants, the lungs of these infants are not yet fully prepared for gas exchange. In addition, their digestive tracts cannot normally absorb fat, and their immune systems are not yet capable of warding off infection. Small, preterm infants also have a very large surface area-to-body weight ratio; this increases heat loss and impairs thermoregulation. Finally, the vasculature of these small infants is less well developed, increasing the likelihood of hemorrhage (especially in the ventricles of the brain).

RULE OF THUMB

Infants born before 38 weeks' gestation are considered preterm.

Respiratory Assessment of the Infant

Not all respiratory problems occur at birth; many respiratory disorders develop after birth and may develop slowly or suddenly. RTs are commonly called on to help assess and treat infants who develop respiratory distress after birth.

Physical Assessment

Physical assessment of the infant begins with measurement of vital signs. A normal newborn respiratory rate is 40 to 60 breaths/min. The lower the gestational age, the higher the normal respiratory rate will be. A 28-week gestational age infant may normally breathe 60 times a minute, whereas the rate more typical of a term newborn is 40 breaths/min. Tachypnea (>60 breaths/min) can occur because of hypoxemia, acidosis, anxiety, or pain. Respiratory rates less than 40 breaths/min should be interpreted with previous trends of the newborn's respiratory rate. A baseline respiratory rate of 36 breaths/min in a term newborn is within normal limits; however, a respiratory rate of 36 breaths/min in a preterm newborn previously breathing at 70 breaths/min may indicate compromise. Causes of slow respiratory rates include medications, hypothermia, or neurologic impairment.

Normal infant heart rates range from 100 to 160 beats/min. Heart rate can be assessed by auscultation of the apical pulse, normally located at the fifth intercostal space, midclavicular line. Alternatively, the brachial and femoral pulses may be used. Weak pulses indicate hypotension, shock, or vasoconstriction. Bounding peripheral pulses occur with major left-to-right shunting through a **patent ductus arteriosus (PDA).**[3] A strong brachial pulse in the presence of a weak femoral pulse suggests either PDA or coarctation of the aorta. Table 48-3 lists normal ranges of blood pressure for neonates of different sizes.

RULE OF THUMB

The normal respiratory rate for a full-term infant is 40 to 60 breaths/min.

TABLE 48-3

Normal Neonatal Blood Pressures

Weight (g)	Systolic (mm Hg)	Diastolic (mm Hg)
750	35-45	14-34
1000	39-59	16-36
1500	40-61	19-39
3000	51-72	27-46

From Whitaker K: Comprehensive perinatal and pediatric respiratory care, ed 3, Albany, NY, 2001, Delmar.

Chest examination in an infant is more difficult to perform and interpret than in an adult because of the small chest size and the ease of sound transmission through the infant chest. Thorough observation of the infant greatly enhances the assessment data obtained. Infants in respiratory distress typically exhibit one or more key physical signs: nasal flaring, cyanosis, expiratory grunting, tachypnea, retractions, and paradoxical breathing. Nasal flaring is seen as dilation of the ala nasi on inspiration. The extent of flaring varies according to facial structure of the infant. Nasal flaring coincides with an increase in work of breathing. In concept, nasal flaring decreases the resistance to airflow. It also may help stabilize the upper airway by minimizing negative pharyngeal pressure during inspiration.[4] Cyanosis may be absent in infants with anemia, even when arterial partial pressure of oxygen (PaO_2) levels are decreased. In addition, infants with elevated fetal hemoglobin levels may not become cyanotic until PaO_2 decreases to less than 30 mm Hg. Hyperbilirubinemia, common among newborns, may mask cyanosis. Grunting occurs when infants exhale against a partially closed glottis. By increasing airway pressure during expiration, grunting helps prevent airway closure and alveolar collapse. Grunting is most common in infants with respiratory distress syndrome, but it is also seen in other respiratory disorders associated with alveolar collapse. Figure 48-6 illustrates the Silverman score, which is a system of grading severity of lung disease.

Retractions refer to the drawing in of chest wall skin between bony structures. Retractions can occur in the suprasternal, substernal, and intercostal regions. Retractions indicate an increase in work of breathing, especially because of decreased pulmonary compliance. Paradoxical

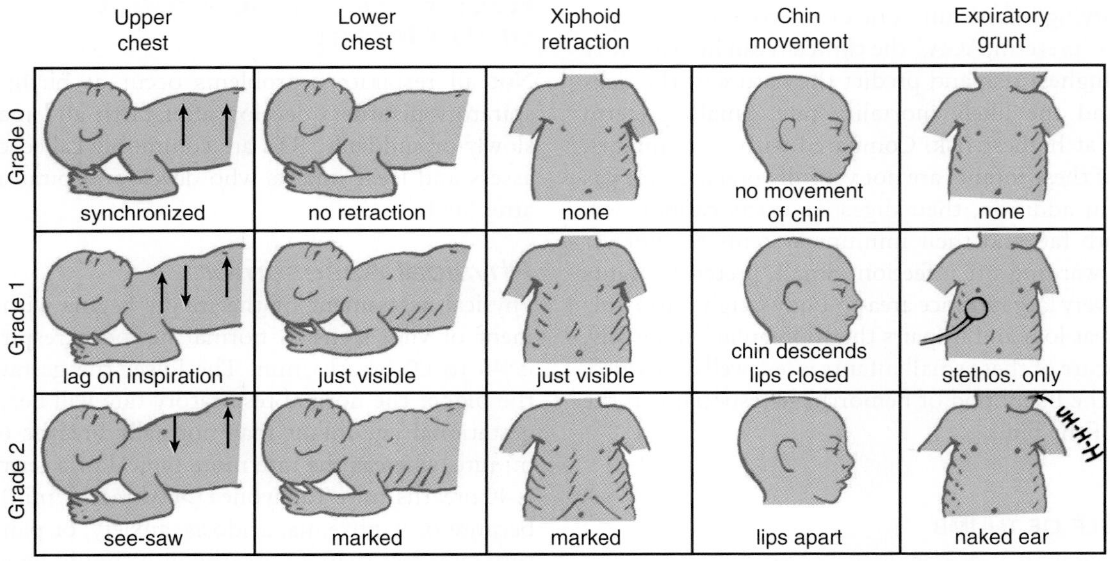

FIGURE 48-6 Silverman score—a system for grading severity of underlying lung disease. (Modified from Silverman WA, Anderson DH: Pediatrics 17:1, 1956.)

breathing in infants differs from paradoxical breathing normally seen in adults. Instead of drawing the abdomen in during inspiration, an infant with paradoxical breathing tends to draw in the chest wall. This inward movement of the chest wall may range in severity. As with retractions, paradoxical breathing indicates an increase in ventilatory work. Applying continuous positive airway pressure (CPAP) to a newborn exhibiting signs of respiratory distress including **grunting, flaring, and retracting** may help to increase lung volume and improve gas exchange. The benefits of CPAP in children are discussed in more detail later.

Surfactant

Surfactant production begins around the 24th week of gestation and continues through gestation. Surfactant contributes to the stability of the alveolar sacs by reducing the surface tension of the fluids that coat the alveoli. Surfactant deficiency places an infant at increased risk for respiratory distress. By about 34 weeks' gestation, most infants have produced enough surfactant to keep the alveoli from collapsing. There are two specific approaches to preventing and treating surfactant deficiency. Surfactant deficiency is due to lung immaturity. When a premature delivery is anticipated, steroids are given to the mother to help promote lung maturation. In addition, infants born before 35 weeks' gestation, especially infants born very prematurely (<30 weeks), should be assessed for the need to receive exogenous surfactant. The need for surfactant is determined by assessing the infant's lung volume on chest x-ray, evaluating the inspired O_2 concentration to maintain O_2 saturations greater than approximately 88%, and clinically assessing the infant's work of breathing. Once surfactant deficiency is determined, administering exogenous surfactant as soon as possible has been found to be most beneficial.[5]

Surfactant administration has also been shown to be useful in conditions in which surfactant function has been altered. These conditions include meconium aspiration, neonatal pneumonia, and pulmonary hemorrhage. Administration of surfactant requires intubation. It is essential to ensure the endotracheal tube is properly positioned, approximately 0.5 to 1 cm above the carina, before delivering surfactant. The dose depends on the specific brand of surfactant being administered. Close monitoring of the infant's vital signs, O_2 saturation, and compliance is necessary during and after surfactant administration. Soon after surfactant is delivered, the infant's compliance should begin to increase resulting in improved gas exchange. Ventilating pressures and fractional inspired oxygen (FiO_2) need to be decreased to avoid lung injury and excessive partial pressure of O_2. The ventilating pressure should be decreased to the level that maintains a tidal volume (V_T) of 5 to 7 ml/kg. FiO_2 should be decreased to maintain an oxygen saturation level (SpO_2) of approximately 88% to 92% in preterm infants and to the lowest FiO_2 possible to maintain SpO_2 greater than 95% in term or postterm infants.

Blood Gas and Pulse Oximetry Analysis

Blood gas analysis is helpful in assessing respiratory distress in an infant. Many noninvasive techniques, such as transcutaneous partial pressure of oxygen ($PtcO_2$), transcutaneous partial pressure of carbon dioxide ($PtcCO_2$), end tidal carbon dioxide (CO_2), and pulse oximetry (SpO_2), are used to obtain comparable data, although blood gas analysis is more precise when results are critical. An infant blood gas sample can be obtained from an artery or capillary. Chapter 18 summarizes the advantages, disadvantages, and complications of these sampling methods. Care must be taken in assessing the results of capillary sampling. Capillary blood gases provide only information regarding ventilation and acid-base status, and accuracy is highly dependent on technique.[6] Normal values for infant blood gases are listed in Table 48-4.

Monitoring O_2 saturation using a pulse oximeter is a standard of care for sick newborns. Saturation probes must be carefully placed on the newborn; the most common sites are the wrist, the medial surface of the palm, or the foot. Sufficient cardiac output and skin blood flow are essential to provide an accurate saturation value. The pulse rate indicated on the oximeter should correlate with the infant's actual pulse before any conclusions regarding

TABLE 48-4

Age-Related Values Commonly Reported for Normal Blood Gases

	Normal Preterm Infants (at 1-5 Hours)	Normal Term Infants (at 5 Hours)	Normal Preterm Infants (at 5 Days)	Children, Adolescents, and Adults
pH (range)	7.33 (7.29-7.37)	7.34 (7.31-7.37)	7.38 (7.34-7.42)	7.40 (7.35-7.45)
PCO_2 (range)	47 (39-56)	35 (32-39)	36 (32-41)	40 (35-45)
PO_2 (range)	60 (52-68)	74 (62-86)	76 (62-92)	95 (85-100)
HCO_3^- range	25 (22-23)	19 (18-21)	21 (19-23)	24 (22-26)
BE range	−4 (−5 to −2.2)	−5 9 (−6 to −2)	−3 (−5.8 to −1.2)	0 (−2 to +2)

Modified from Orzalesi MM, Mendicini M, Bucci G, et al: Arterial oxygen studies in premature newborns with and without mild respiratory disorders. Arch Dis Child 42:174, 1967. From Koff PB, Eitzman DV, Neu J: Neonatal and pediatric respiratory care, ed 2, St Louis, 1993, Mosby.
BE, Base excess; *HCO_3^-*, bicarbonate.

saturation can be drawn. Intracardiac shunting and intrapulmonary shunting are causes of decreased saturation in sick infants. When interpreting saturation levels in a newborn, it is important to consider where the saturation is being monitored. Saturation probes placed on the right hand assess preductal saturations. Probes placed on other extremities indicate postductal saturation levels. Infants at risk for pulmonary hypertension should have saturation probes placed to monitor preductal and postductal saturations. A large difference (>5%) between the two readings should prompt the clinician to consider pulmonary hypertension as a potential concern. Conditions that prevent the closing of the ductus arteriosus and foramen ovale result in decreased saturation. Many congenital heart defects result in significant intracardiac shunting. Interpreting adequate saturation for a newborn requires knowledge of any cardiac defect along with the infant's pulmonary condition.

Respiratory Assessment of the Pediatric Patient

Normal breathing in children is evidenced by quiet inspiration and passive expiration at an age-appropriate rate. Respiratory rates are rapid in neonates and decrease in toddlers and older children. Table 48-5 lists normal respiratory rates. The initial assessment of a pediatric patient starts with evaluating airway patency. Normal heart rates are higher in younger children and decrease with age. In assessing a pediatric patient, establishing if the airway is patent or has any obstructive component is essential. Signs that suggest upper airway obstruction include increased inspiratory effort with retractions or inspiratory efforts with no airway or breath sounds.

The clinician observes for movement of the chest or abdomen. The clinician listens for breath sounds focusing on both inspiratory sounds and expiratory sounds. Chest or abdominal movement without breath sounds may indicate total airway obstruction, and basic life support maneuvers are indicated. High-pitched sounds heard on inspiration (stridor) are often indicative of upper airway conditions, whereas expiratory noises are more often associated with lower airway obstruction.

Causes of stridor in children can be infections, such as croup; foreign body aspiration, particularly in a small child; congenital or acquired airway abnormalities; allergic reactions; or edema after a procedure. Inhaled epinephrine via nebulizer and intravenous steroids are commonly used to treat stridor. Common causes of lower airway obstruction are bronchiolitis and asthma. When wheezing is noted, inhaled bronchodilators are indicated. If the patient is able to use a metered dose inhaler (MDI),

TABLE 48-5

Normal Respiratory and Heart Rates by Age

Age	Breaths/Minute	Heart Rates
Infants (<1 yr)	30-60	90-120
Toddler (1-3 yr)	24-40	80-100
Preschooler (4-5 yr)	22-34	70-90
School age (6-12 yr)	18-30	70-90
Adolescent (13-18 yr)	16-22	60-80

MINI CLINI

Neonatal Ventilation

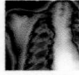

PROBLEM: A 1.8-kg, 28-week newborn is transported from the delivery room to the neonatal ICU. The patient was intubated immediately after delivery with a 3.0 uncuffed endotracheal tube and has been manually ventilated with PIP of 25 cm H_2O and PEEP approximately 3 to 5 cm H_2O during transport. When the neonate is admitted to the neonatal ICU, the RT is asked to recommend appropriate ventilator settings.

SOLUTION

- Mode—A/C pressure ventilation
- PIP—20 cm H_2O
- PEEP—5 cm H_2O
- Set respiratory rate—40 breaths/min
- Inspiratory time—0.3 sec
- FiO_2—0.4

Because the patient was manually ventilated during transport, it is unclear what V_T has been delivered. Initial PIP of 20 cm H_2O and PEEP of 5 cm H_2O are safe and common settings. Immediate observation of the chest would allow the RT to evaluate chest expansion and adjust PIP as required. Over the next several minutes if V_T monitoring is available, targeting V_T of 6 to 8 ml/kg would guide subsequent settings.

Set respiratory rate of 40 breaths/min is at the lower end of the normal range for this patient; however, use of the A/C mode with appropriately set trigger sensitivity would allow the patient to establish a more comfortable respiratory rate. Adjustment of the inspiratory time may also be necessary to increase patient comfort and improve patient ventilator synchrony. Further adjustments may be guided by $PaCO_2$. Because this patient was born prematurely, rapid assessment of SpO_2 is essential, and FiO_2 should be adjusted to maintain SpO_2 between 88% and 92%.

This patient should receive surfactant replacement therapy. The clinician may consider volume-targeted, pressure-limited ventilation (e.g., pressure-regulated volume control, volume guarantee) during and immediately after surfactant delivery. This modality may help prevent lung overdistention until compliance has stabilized.[44,45]

repeated inhalations can act quickly to improve aeration. When the patient is unable to use the MDI appropriately or when severe symptoms are present, delivering a bronchodilator with a nebulizer can bring relief. More than one nebulizer treatment often is necessary to relieve airway inflammation. A common approach is to deliver three consecutive treatments. If the patient continues to be symptomatic, continuous bronchodilator therapy may be delivered with a nebulizer attached to an infusion pump set to administer a bronchodilator continuously. Tachycardia secondary to the beta-1 effect of inhaled bronchodilators can be seen. Frequent reassessment of any patient receiving continuous bronchodilator therapy is essential. Heliox, an inhaled mixture of helium and O_2 (described in the section on specialty gases), has been shown to be beneficial in cases of some airways conditions in children.

As noted in the section describing newborn assessment, use of accessory muscles, grunting, flaring, and retracting all can be signs of respiratory distress. Head bobbing, noted by chin up and neck extended during inspiration with chin falling during expiration, and seesaw respirations, indicated by the chest retracting and the abdomen expanding during inspiration, are signs of impending respiratory failure. Assessing the child's level of alertness is essential. Levels of alertness range from fully awake, agitated, minimally responsive, to unresponsive. A child's ability to protect his or her airway should be questioned in a minimally responsive or unresponsive child.

RESPIRATORY CARE

Respiratory care of infants and children incorporates approaches taken from adult practice. Important physiologic and age-related differences between adults and children require variations in the provision of respiratory care. This section focuses on neonatal and pediatric O_2 therapy, bronchial hygiene, humidity and aerosol therapy, airway management, and resuscitation.

Oxygen Therapy

Goals and Indications

O_2 should be administered as any other drug, using the lowest dose necessary to achieve the intended goal. The goal of O_2 therapy is to provide adequate tissue oxygenation. However, O_2 therapy is most frequently adjusted according to O_2 saturation levels. A clear understanding of the limitation of O_2 saturation is needed to interpret the saturation reading and make appropriate decisions. Infants and children receiving O_2 therapy have variable O_2 saturation target ranges depending on age and underlying condition.

Lower saturation levels are targeted in infants less than 32 weeks' gestation. There is evidence that exposure to supplemental O_2 in a premature infant is a risk factor for the development of **retinopathy of prematurity (ROP).** ROP is caused by an abnormal vascularization of the retina, which in the most severe cases leads to retinal detachment. Preterm neonates weighing less than 1500 g are most susceptible. Hyperoxia is not the only factor associated with ROP, but close monitoring and adjusting of O_2 therapy to avoid hyperoxia is crucial to decrease the risk of ROP. Specific saturation goals for this age group should be established, and O_2 should be adjusted to maintain the intended target. Avoiding very high or very low saturation levels is critical. Adjusting the delivered O_2 concentration by small increments avoids large swings in saturation levels.[7-11]

In a term infant with **primary pulmonary hypertension of the newborn (PPHN),** a higher targeted saturation level is desired to avoid further pulmonary constriction associated with hypoxemia. The position of the saturation probe needs to be considered when interpreting saturation. Intracardiac shunting can occur in the presence of PPHN. One saturation probe positioned on the upper right extremity represents preductal saturations and is indicative of the saturation of blood being delivered to the brain. O_2 saturation measured on other extremities is considered postductal and represents saturation to other parts of the body.

Newborns with certain cardiac anomalies are dependent on their intracardiac shunt through the ductus arteriosus to survive. An increased saturation in newborns promotes constriction of the ductus arteriosus. Although this constriction is normally a positive response, it may cause premature closure of the ductus arteriosus in infants with ductal-dependent congenital heart defects. An infant born with hypoplastic left heart syndrome, a defect in which the left-sided heart structures are poorly developed, relies on the patency of the ductus arteriosus for systemic blood supply. In addition, hyperoxia can increase aortic pressures and systemic vascular resistance, decreasing the cardiac index and O_2 transport in children with acyanotic congenital heart disease. The emphasis for O_2 therapy for all newborns should be to provide only as much O_2 as indicated by the infant's condition. O_2 therapy should be administered using a written care plan with specified clinical outcomes (e.g., titrate flow/FiO_2 to maintain SpO_2 88% to 92%, notify physician if FiO_2 is >0.40).

Methods of Administration

The effectiveness of O_2 devices depends on the performance characteristics of the device (delivered FiO_2, flow rate, relative humidity), the interface of the device, and the tolerance of the patient for using the device. Children are often frightened and combative, making it impractical to use some O_2 administration devices. Selection of an O_2 device must be based on the degree of hypoxemia and the emotional and physical needs of the child and family. O_2 can be administered to infants and children by mask, cannula, high-flow nasal cannulas, or oxyhood. Table 48-6

TABLE 48-6

Oxygen Delivery Devices

Device	Age	FDO_2	Advantages	Disadvantages
Air entrainment mask	≥3 yr	High flow; 0.24-1	Precise FiO_2; good for transport; ease of application	Low relative humidity; pressure necrosis to face; difficult to fit and maintain on active child, not recommended for infants; risk of aspiration
Nasal cannula	Premature infants to adult	Low flow; 25 ml/min–6.0 L/min	Tolerated well by all ages	Inaccurate FiO_2; low relative humidity; excessive flows may cause inadvertent CPAP in infants; precise FiO_2 may be achieved with O_2 blender
Incubator	Newborns ≤28 days	<0.40 FiO_2, combine use with cannula or hood for precise FiO_2	Low FiO_2 for stable infants; neutral thermal environment for premature infants	Varying FiO_2; long stabilization time; limits access to child for patient care
Oxyhood	Premature infants to ≤6 mo	0.21-1 FiO_2 with O_2 blender maintained at 30° C to 34° C	Warmed and humidified gas at stable FiO_2 during routine patient care	Overheating may cause apnea and dehydration; underheating may cause O_2 consumption; inadequate flow causes CO_2 buildup; noise produced by humidification device may cause hearing loss
Mist tent	Infants to toddlers	High flow; 0.21-0.40 FiO_2	Allows child movement, high humidity, cool temperatures	Isolation of child from family; wet bedding and clothes; difficult to maintain stable FiO_2; risk of cross-contamination; limits patient care

FDO_2, Delivered oxygen concentration.

compares the advantages and disadvantages of standard O_2 delivery methods.

Secretion Clearance Techniques

Secretion clearance techniques that can be applied to infants and children include chest physiotherapy, positive expiratory pressure therapy, autogenic drainage, flutter therapy, and mechanical insufflation-exsufflation.[12,13] Secretion clearance techniques are considered when accumulated secretions impair pulmonary function and an infiltrate is visible on a chest radiograph. Secretion retention is common in children who have pneumonia, bronchopulmonary dysplasia, cystic fibrosis, bronchiectasis, and some neuromuscular diseases. Figure 48-7 shows postural drainage and percussion positions for infants and children.

Methods

Infants and young children cannot cough on command. For this reason, secretions often must be removed by suctioning. For older children with excessive secretions, directed deep breathing and coughing may help improve pulmonary clearance. The use of mechanical insufflation-exsufflation in children with neuromuscular disease can be helpful in clearing secretions. Adjunctive therapy devices such as positive expiratory pressure, flutter, or intermittent percussive ventilation therapy have been effective in secretion clearance in patients with cystic fibrosis.[14]

Monitoring

Given the instability of most critically ill infants and children, a thorough initial assessment and ongoing patient evaluation during and after treatment are mandatory. Traditional assessment of vital signs, blood pressure, color, and breath sounds before, during, and after treatment should be supplemented with pulse oximetry monitoring if hypoxemia is suspected.

Humidity and Aerosol Therapy

Key differences in humidity and aerosol therapy in infants and children include assessment of patient response to therapy, age-related physiologic changes, and equipment application.

Humidity Therapy

In children with an intact upper airway, O_2 therapy devices, such as low-flow nasal cannulas, do not routinely need to be humidified When the upper airway is bypassed by intubation, supplemental humidification must be provided using a heated humidifier. Humidification of inspired gases for infants and children receiving mechanical ventilation is commonly provided by a servo-controlled humidifier. Ideal features for these systems include the following: (1) low internal volume and constant water level to minimize compressed volume loss; (2) closed, continuous feed water supply to avoid contamination; (3) distal airway temperature sensor and high/low alarms. Common problems

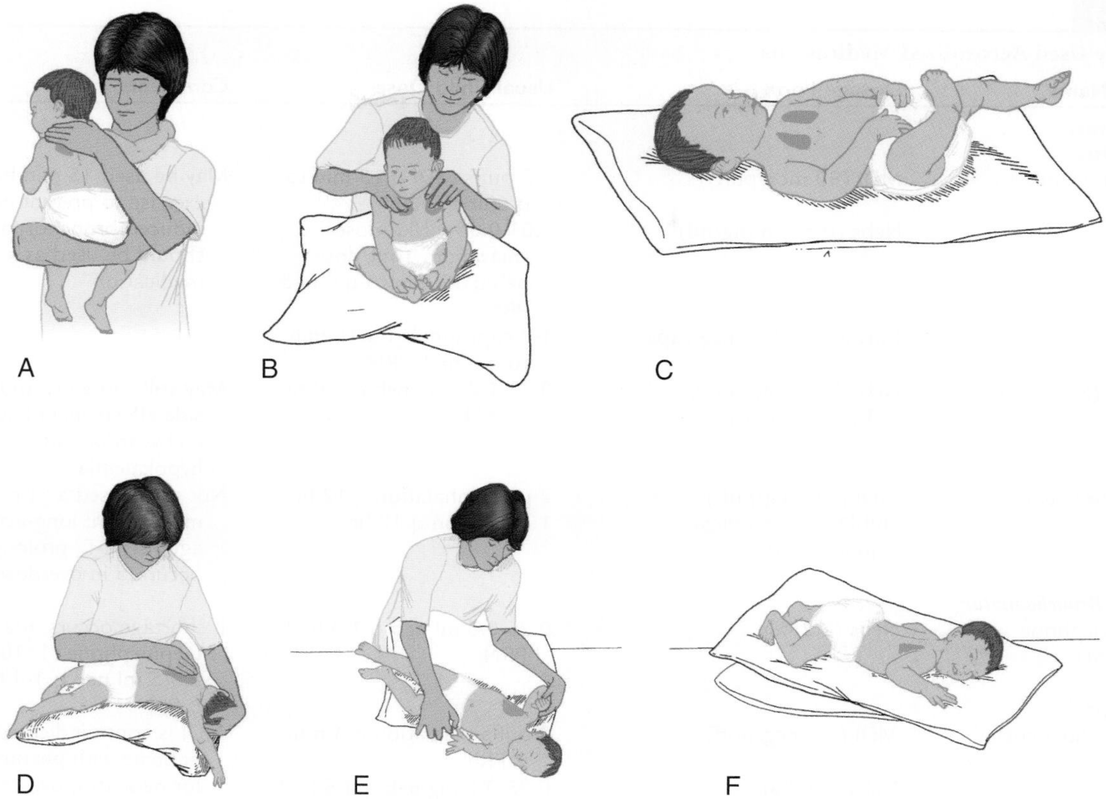

FIGURE 48-7 Postural drainage and percussion positions for infant and child. Angles of drainage for infant are not as obtuse as those for child. **A,** Posterior segments of right and left upper lobes are drained with patient in upright position at 30-degree angle forward. Percuss over upper posterior thorax. **B,** Apical segments of right and left upper lobes are drained with patient in upright position, leaning forward 30 degrees. Percuss over area between clavicle and tip of scapula on each side. **C,** Anterior segments of right and left upper lobes are drained with patient in flat, supine position. Percuss anterior side of chest directly under clavicles to around nipple area *(shaded)*. Avoid direct pressure on sternum. **D,** Right and left lateral basal segments of lower lobes are drained at 30 degrees Trendelenburg. Patient lies on appropriate side, rotated 30 degrees forward. Percuss over uppermost portions of lower ribs. **E,** Right and left anterior basal segments of lower lobes are drained at 30 degrees Trendelenburg. Patient lies on appropriate side with a 20-degree turn backward. Percuss above anterior lower margin of ribs. **F,** Right and left superior segments of lower lobes are drained at 15 degrees Trendelenburg, with patient in prone position. Percuss below scapula in midback area.

with humidifier systems include condensation in the tubing, inadequate humidification, and hazards associated with the heating coil.[15,16] Using heated wire circuits can also reduce condensation in the circuit. Frequent evaluation of the humidification system is necessary to increase the potential of adequate humidity delivered to the airway. Inadequate humidification occurs in nonheated circuits when the humidifier temperature probe is placed too far upstream from the airway connector. Variable humidification problems occur when ventilator circuits pass through an environment and then into a warmed enclosure, such as an incubator or radiant warmer.

Aerosol Drug Therapy

Drug action in infants and children differs significantly from drug action in adults because of differences in physiology, which may include immature enzyme systems, immature receptors, and variable gastrointestinal absorption. Dosing may be imprecise, and systemic effects may be hard to predict. Table 48-7 lists aerosolized medications commonly used in children.

Small volume nebulizers (SVNs), MDIs, and dry powder inhalers (DPIs) can be used to deliver aerosolized drugs via mouthpiece or face mask to infants and children.[17] Continuous aerosol drug therapy is also used for patients unresponsive to intermittent SVN treatments. Aerosol drug administration to intubated infants and children is challenging because of the decreased deposition from baffling of small endotracheal tubes in these patients, which prevents approximately 90% of the drug from entering the lungs, regardless of delivery system. In addition, careful adjustments must be made to the ventilator so that

TABLE 48-7

Commonly Used Aerosolized Medications

Medication Name	Dosage Form	Usual Child Dose	Comments
Bronchodilators			
Beta-2 Agonists			
Albuterol (Proventil, Ventolin)	MDI (90 mcg/puff)	1-2 puffs MDI q 15 min to q 6 hr ± PRN	May be used 15 min before exercise to prevent exercise-induced bronchospasm; should be used as a rescue medication
	Nebs (0.5%, 5 mg/ml)	0.01-0.05 ml/kg/dose (maximum 1 ml/dose) neb q 15 min to q 6 hr ± PRN	
	Rotohaler (200 mcg caps)	1-2 caps inhaled q 15 min to q 6 hr ± PRN	
Levalbuterol (Xopenex)	Nebs (0.63 mg/3 ml, 1.25 mg/3 ml)	0.32-1.25 mg neb q 6-8 hr ± PRN	May still cause extrapulmonary side effects including tachycardia and hypokalemia
Salmeterol (Serevent)	MDI (21 mcg/puff)	2 puffs inhalation q 12 hr	Not to be used as a rescue medication; long-acting beta-2 agonist; QT_C prolongation has occurred in overdose
	DPI-Diskus (50 mcg/inhalation)	1 inhalation q 12 hr	
Nonselective Bronchodilator			
Racemic epinephrine (Vaponefrin)	Nebs (2.25%)	0.25-0.5 ml neb q 1-4 hr ± PRN	If shortage occurs, may use L-epinephrine (1:1000) 2.5-5 ml neb q 1-4 hr ± PRN
Anticholinergic			
Ipratropium (Atrovent)	MDI (18 mcg/puff)	2 puffs inhalation q 4-6 hr ± PRN	MDI is contraindicated in patients with peanut allergy; for neonates, use 25 mcg/kg/dose neb tid; may cause mydriasis if aerosolized drug gets into the eye
	Nebs (0.02%)	0.25-0.5 mg neb q 4-6 hr ± PRN	
Antiinflammatory Agents			
Corticosteroids			
Beclomethasone (Beclovent, Vanceril)	MDI (42 mcg/puff)	1-2 puffs inhalation qid or 2-4 puffs inhalation bid	Start at lower end of dosing range if patient not previously on steroids; titrate to lowest dose that is effective; always rinse mouth after each treatment
	MDI double strength (84 mcg/puff)	2 puffs inhalation bid	
Budesonide (Pulmicort)	DPI-Turbuhaler (200 mcg/inhalation)	1-2 puffs inhalation bid	May take several weeks to see benefit; not to be used as a rescue medication
	Nebs-Respules (0.25 mg/2 ml, 0.5 mg/2 ml)	0.25-0.5 mg neb bid *or* 0.5-1 mg neb qd	
Flunisolide (Aerobid, Aerobid-M)	MDI (250 mcg/puff)	2-3 puffs inhalation bid	
Fluticasone (Flovent)	MDI (44 mcg/puff, 110 mcg/puff, 220 mcg/puff)	2 puffs inhalation bid (maximum 880 mcg/day)	
	Rotadisk (50 mcg/blister)	50-100 mcg inhalation bid	
Triamcinolone (Azmacort)	MDI (100 mcg/puff)	1-2 puffs inhal qid	
Mast Cell Stabilizers			
Cromolyn (Intal)	MDI (800 mcg/puff)	2 puffs inhalation qid	May take several weeks to see benefit; not to be used as a rescue medication
	Nebs (20 mg/2 ml)	20 mg neb qid	
Nedocromil (Tilade)	MDI (1.75 mg/puff)	2 puffs inhalation qid	
Mucolytics			
N-acetylcysteine (Mucomyst)	Nebs (20%, 200 mg/ml)	3-5 ml neb qid	Consider pretreatment with albuterol 15 min before *N*-acetylcysteine secondary to bronchospasm
Dornase alfa (Pulmozyme)	Nebs (2.5 mg/2.5 ml)	2.5 mg neb qid-bid	May cause hemoptysis

Neb, Nebulizer.

TABLE 48-7

Commonly Used Aerosolized Medications—cont'd

Medication Name	Dosage Form	Usual Child Dose	Comments
Antiinfectives			
Pentamidine (Pentam)	Nebs (300 mg)	8 mg/kg/dose (maximum 300 mg/dose) neb q month	Used for PCP prophylaxis
Ribavirin (Virazole)	Powder (6 g vial)	2 g over 2 hr neb q 8 hr × 3-7 days *or* 6 g over 12-18 hr neb q 24 hr × 3-7 days	Used for RSV treatment; mutagenic, teratogenic
Tobramycin (TOBI)	Nebs (300 mg/5 ml)	300 mg neb q 12 hr	Used for pseudomonal infection of the lungs

PCP, Pneumocystis jiroveci pneumonia; *RSV,* respiratory syncytial virus.

nebulizer flows do not alter delivered V_T and inspiratory pressure and interfere with triggering efforts.[18]

Airway Management

Airway management methods in infants and children are unique because of the anatomic differences between neonates and adults. Specifically, equipment and technique must be tailored to each child according to his or her size, weight, and postpartum age. Masks, oral airways, suction catheters, laryngoscope blades, and endotracheal tubes in a wide selection of infant and child sizes are needed to account for variations in patient age and weight. Table 48-8 provides recommendations regarding endotracheal tube and suction catheter sizes for infants and children.

Intubation

Endotracheal intubation is a generally safe method of airway management in infants and children, even when used for extended periods.[19,20] Complications and hazards associated with intubation in these age groups are listed in Box 48-1. The infant's age or weight can be used to estimate proper endotracheal tube size and depth of insertion. If the tube is too small in diameter, a leak may result, decreasing delivered minute ventilation. Small endotracheal tubes have high inspiratory resistance, increasing the spontaneous work of breathing for the child. An inappropriately large endotracheal tube can cause mucosal and laryngeal damage that is evident after extubation, resulting in upper airway obstruction.[21]

Most neonatal and pediatric endotracheal tubes are uncuffed. The narrowest point of the airway in an infant and small child is the cricoid cartilage. When an appropriately sized uncuffed tube is positioned in the airway, the fit of the tube in the airway "seals" the airway enough so that adequate ventilation can usually be maintained. Cuffed endotracheal tubes are an option if a large leak persists around the tube and stable ventilation cannot be maintained. Similar to with adults when a cuffed tube is used, careful attention to the pressure of the cuff on the tracheal wall is essential. Because the tongue is large and the epiglottis is anatomically high in infants and small children, practitioners generally find the Miller (straight) laryngoscope blade best for intubation. Infant endotracheal tubes are small and can be easily kinked or obstructed. In addition, slight changes in the position of the endotracheal tube in movement can result in bronchial intubation.[22]

Once a tube is inserted, immediate securing of the tube to the infant's face and ongoing evaluation of the security of the tube are essential. Proper head positioning and avoidance of cumbersome connecting apparatus help reduce the potential of accidental extubation. Estimates of the distance the tube should be inserted into the airway based on patient weight are provided in Table 48-9. Further confirmation of correct tube position should be evaluated with a chest x-ray. Noting the infant's head position when the chest x-ray is obtained is helpful in assessing appropriate tube position in the airway. Slight changes in head position can result in the tube position sitting too high or too low in the airway. In very small infants, light flexion of the head can move the tube into the right main stem bronchus.

Breath sounds may be of limited value in infants and small children for evaluation of tube position. Portable end tidal CO_2 monitoring devices may be used to help assess the tube in the airway, although these should be used as only additional assessment tools with recognition of their limitations. Factors associated with accidental extubation of infants include tension on the tube from the ventilator circuit, patient agitation, suctioning, head turning, chest physiotherapy, too short a tube distance between lip and adapter, moving the patient during procedures, and inadequately taped endotracheal tube.[23]

Laryngeal mask airways (LMAs) are available as an alternative to intubation. LMAs are typically used in children during periods when a short-term airway is indicated, such as during some surgical procedures or when endotracheal intubation cannot be accomplished and an

TABLE 48-8

Endotracheal Tube and Suction Catheter Sizes for Infants and Children

Age or Weight	Endotracheal Tube ID (mm)	Oral Tube Length (cm)	Nasal Tube Length (cm)	Suction Catheter (F)
Newborn				
<1000 g	2.5	9-11	11-12	6
1000-2000 g	3	9-11	11-12	6
2000-3000 g	3.5	10-12	12-14	6
>3000 g	4	11-12	13-14	8
Children				
6 mo	3-4	11-12	12-14	6-8
18 mo	3.5-4.5	11-13	13-15	8
2 yr	4-5	12-14	14-16	8-10
3-5 yr	4.5-5.5	12-15	14-17	8-10
6 yr	5.5-6	14-16	16-18	10
8 yr	6-6.5	15-17	17-19	10-12
12 yr	6-7	17-19	19-21	10-12
16 yr	6.5-7.5	19-21	21-23	10-12

Estimating formula for tube internal diameter (ID) in mm:
Tube ID = (Age + 16)/4
Tube ID = Height (cm)/20
Estimating formula for tube length in cm:
Oral: 12 + (Age/2)
Nasal: 15 + (Age/2)

Box 48-1 Complications and Hazards of Endotracheal Intubation in Infants and Children

- Palatal grooving (neonates)
- Incisal enamel hypoplasia (neonates)
- Accidental extubation
- Tube blockage
- Tracheal stenosis
- Esophageal perforation
- Tracheal perforation

TABLE 48-9

Approximate Distance from Infant's Lip to End of Inserted Oral Endotracheal Tube

Weight (kg)	Mark at Lip (cm)
<1	6.5
1	7
2	8
3	9
4	10

airway needs to be established. Table 48-10 outlines appropriate sizes and maximum cuff volumes of LMAs for varying weights.

TABLE 48-10

Appropriate Sizes and Maximum Cuff Volumes of Laryngeal Mask Airways for Varying Weights

LMA Size	Patient Weight (kg)	Maximum Cuff Volume
1	1-5	4
1.5	5-10	7
2	10-20	10
2.5	20-30	14
3	30-40	20

Suctioning Intubated Pediatric Patients

The goal of suctioning is to remove secretions from large airways and stimulate a cough. Although suctioning can be beneficial, significant risks are associated with the procedure, including lung derecruitment, hypoxia, hypertension, increased intracranial pressure, tracheal trauma, and infection. Absolute and relative indications for suctioning are listed in Box 48-2.

Additional considerations include the use of closed suction catheters for all mechanically ventilated patients. The closed suctioning technique helps to minimize derecruitment, which is more likely to occur during ventilator disconnections. An increase in O_2 concentration after suctioning may be necessary but should be evaluated for each patient. To reduce the risk of tracheal trauma, suction catheters should not be inserted further than 1 cm beyond the tip of the endotracheal tube or tracheostomy tube. Routine instillation of normal saline is not recommended. Increasing ventilator support to regain volume lost during the procedure may be necessary but should be assessed each time the patient is suctioned. Because of the risks associated with suctioning, the procedure should be performed only when a clinical indication exists, not on a fixed interval.

Box 48-2 Indications for Suctioning

ABSOLUTE INDICATIONS
- Secretions visible in endotracheal tube
- Aspiration of gastrointestinal or oropharyngeal contents
- Inadvertent water aspiration from ventilator circuit
- Physician order to suction patient

RELATIVE INDICATIONS
- Rhonchi noted during auscultation raising suspicion of retained secretions
- Change in compliance (↓ V_T at same peak pressure or ↑ pressure for same V_T)
- ↑ Work of breathing
- ↓ SpO_2 with same or ↑ FiO_2

Box 48-3 Complications and Hazards of Tracheal Suctioning in Infants and Small Children

- Infection
- Lung derecruitment
- Accidental extubation
- Atelectasis
- Blood pressure instability
- Increased intracranial pressure
- Cerebral vasodilation or increased blood volume
- Arterial hypoxemia
- Cerebral hypoxemia
- Hypercapnia
- Bradycardia
- Pneumothorax
- Mucosal damage

Suctioning. Nasopharyngeal and tracheal suctioning helps minimize aspiration, prevents endotracheal tube occlusion, and reduces airway resistance in infants and children.[24] Suctioning is a hazardous procedure, and complications can occur. Box 48-3 lists the common complications and hazards associated with tracheal suctioning of infants and children. Tracheal suctioning of preterm infants and neonates should be performed only when clinical signs indicate a need.[25,26]

Oral and pharyngeal suctioning of infants can be done with a bulb syringe. A DeLee trap or a mechanical vacuum source with catheter may be used for nasopharyngeal and nasotracheal suctioning of neonates. Equipment for suctioning larger infants and children is similar to the equipment used with adults with modifications in vacuum pressure and catheter size. Recommended suction pressures for neonates range from approximately −60 to −80 mm Hg. With large infants and children, pressures in the range of −80 to −100 mm Hg are generally safe and effective. Catheter sizes are chosen according to the age of the patient and the size of the tracheal airway (see Table 48-8). Other techniques for averting hypoxemia include use of endotracheal tube adapters that allow preoxygenation and suctioning without disconnection of the ventilator and use of closed tracheal suction systems.[27,28]

Box 48-4 Indications for Continuous Positive Airway Pressure in Children

RESPIRATORY DISTRESS
- Tachypnea
- Retractions or accessory muscle use
- Grunting
- Nasal flaring
- Head bobbing

ABNORMAL BREATHING PATTERNS
- Apnea of prematurity
- Obstructive sleep apnea

LUNG DISEASE
- Decreased lung volumes on chest radiograph
- Pneumonia
- Tracheomalacia
- Pulmonary edema
- $PaO_2 < 50$ mm Hg with $FiO_2 \geq 0.60$

OTHER
- Postextubation failure

CONTINUOUS POSITIVE AIRWAY PRESSURE

Spontaneous breathing can be supported with **continuous positive airway pressure (CPAP),** a breathing mode that maintains a constant pressure above baseline throughout inspiration and expiration. CPAP maintains inspiratory and expiratory pressures above ambient, which improves functional residual capacity (FRC) and static lung compliance.[29] It is essential that the patient is able to maintain adequate minute volume while breathing spontaneously because ventilatory support is not provided.

CPAP is indicated when arterial oxygenation is inadequate despite elevated FiO_2. This condition is usually accompanied by certain signs of respiratory distress. CPAP is commonly used when PaO_2 is less than 50 mm Hg while the infant is breathing FiO_2 of 0.60 or greater, provided that the $PaCO_2$ is less than or equal to 50 mm Hg and the pH is greater than 7.25. The indications for CPAP are described in Box 48-4.

Methods of Administration

The application of CPAP is most commonly accomplished noninvasively. In preterm and term neonates, nasal prongs or nasopharyngeal tubes were traditionally used. However, the more recent introduction of improved interface devices has led to more consistent CPAP delivery and better

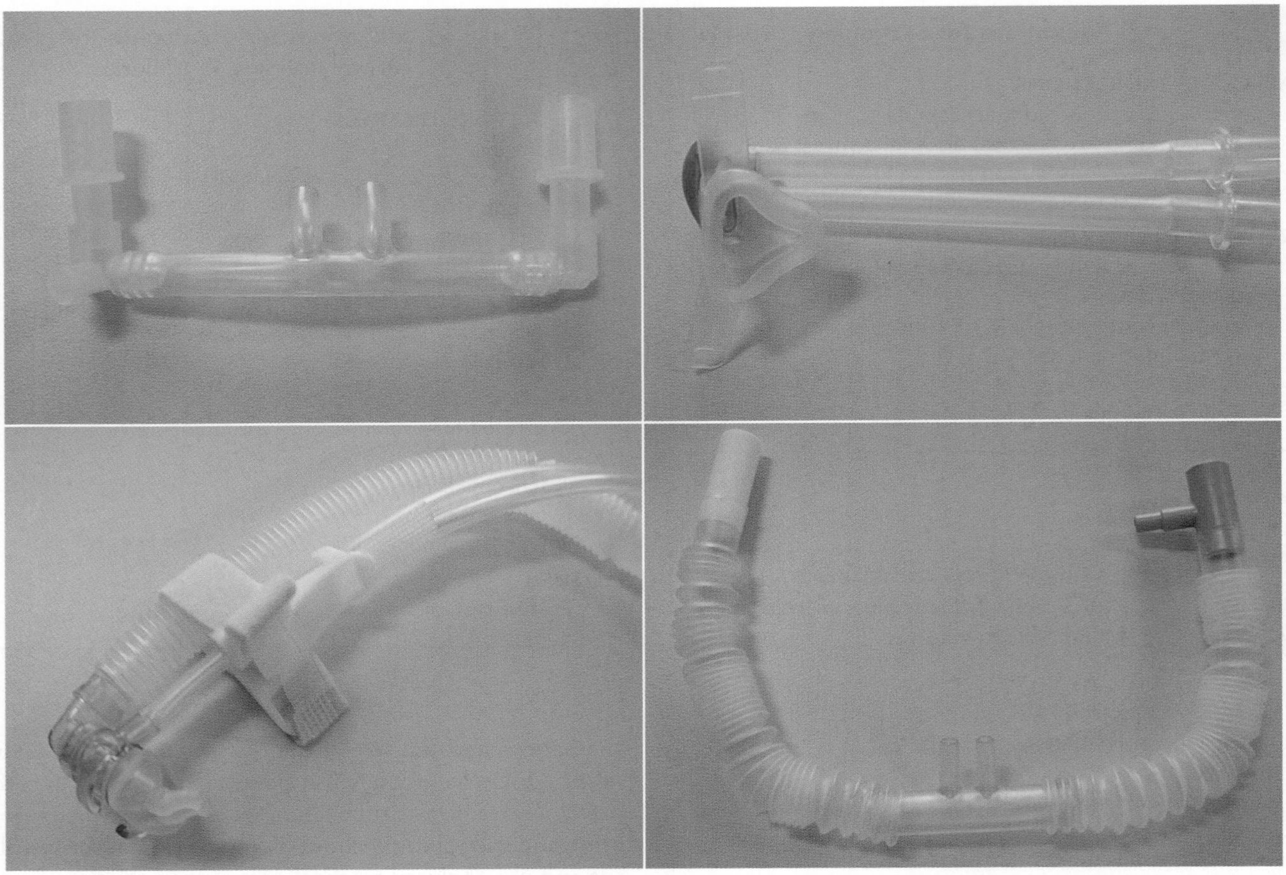

FIGURE 48-8 Patient interfaces for CPAP or NPPV.

patient comfort (Figure 48-8). These interfaces include nasal masks and soft, pliable nasal cannulas that provide a comfortable interface without applying excessive pressure to maintain a tight fitting seal. The American Association for Respiratory Care (AARC) has published Clinical Practice Guideline: Application of CPAP to Neonates via Nasal Prongs, Nasopharyngeal Tube, or Nasal Mask. Excerpts from this guideline appear in Clinical Practice Guideline 48-1.

For larger children, nasal masks, oronasal masks, nasal pillows, and other interfaces similar to interfaces used in adults may be used. In all patients, it is important to assess the patient-device interface at regular intervals to allow prevention or early detection and intervention in the event of pressure ulcers.

The appliance or interface is connected to either a mechanical ventilator set in the CPAP mode or a stand-alone CPAP device The complexity of stand-alone devices ranges from a simple continuous flow of gas against a fixed resistance or threshold to sophisticated CPAP generators that adjust flow and trigger sensitivity in the presence of a leak or increased patient demand. CPAP levels are selected based on clinical observation. Initial CPAP levels are usually 5 to 6 cm H_2O and are adjusted in increments of 1 to 2 cm H_2O. The patient's SpO_2, respiratory rate, work of breathing, breath sounds, and blood pressure are monitored. The appropriate CPAP level is achieved when the respiratory rate decreases to near-normal ranges, signs of respiratory distress are lessened, and SpO_2 increases while O_2 requirements are reduced. Arterial and capillary blood gas analysis may provide additional information in determining the effectiveness of CPAP, and chest radiographs are obtained to determine the degree of lung inflation.

Weaning and eventually discontinuing CPAP is considered when oxygenation is adequate at FiO_2 less than 0.30 to 0.40, there is a sustained reduction in work of breathing, and chest radiograph and clinical assessment indicate resolution of the underlying disorder. The use of CPAP for prolonged periods in preterm infants helps reduce the work of breathing and prevent intubation. Long-term and intermittent use of CPAP is indicated in children with obstructive airway problems, chronic lung disease, and neuromuscular disorders.

High-Flow Nasal Cannula

Supplemental O_2 administration by nasal cannula is the most comfortable and simplest means of providing O_2 for infants and children. Evidence in preterm and term neonates indicates that using a nasal cannula at flow rates of

48-1 Application of Continuous Positive Airway Pressure to Neonates via Nasal Prongs, Nasopharyngeal Tube, or Nasal Mask

AARC Clinical Practice Guideline (Excerpts)*

■ INDICATIONS

- Abnormalities on physical examination—tachypnea, substernal and suprasternal retractions, grunting, and nasal flaring; the presence of pale or cyanotic skin color; agitation
- Inadequate oxygenation (PaO_2 < 50 mm Hg with $FiO_2 \leq 0.60$, provided that VE is adequate as indicated by $PaCO_2$ 50 mm Hg and pH ≥ 7.25)
- Presence of poorly expanded or infiltrated lung fields on chest radiograph
- Presence of a condition thought to be responsive to CPAP, including
  - Respiratory distress syndrome
  - Recent extubation
  - Pulmonary edema
  - Transient tachypnea of the newborn
  - Atelectasis
  - Apnea of prematurity
  - Tracheomalacia or other similar abnormality of the lower airways

■ CONTRAINDICATIONS

- Although nasal CPAP has been used in bronchiolitis, this application may be contraindicated
- Need for intubation or mechanical ventilation or both as evidenced by the presence of
  - Upper airway abnormalities that contraindicate nasal CPAP (e.g., choanal atresia, tracheoesophageal fistula)
  - Severe cardiovascular instability and impending arrest
  - Unstable respiratory drive with frequent apneic episodes resulting in desaturation or bradycardia or both
  - Ventilatory failure as indicated by the inability to maintain $PaCO_2$ < 60 mm Hg and pH > 7.25
- Application of nasal CPAP to patients with untreated congenital diaphragmatic hernia may lead to gastric distention and further compromise of thoracic organs

■ HAZARDS AND COMPLICATIONS

Hazards and complications associated with equipment include the following:

- Obstruction of nasal prongs from mucous plugging or kinking may interfere with delivery of CPAP and result in a decrease in FiO_2 through entrainment of room air via opposite naris or mouth.
- Inactivation of airway pressure alarms
  - High resistance through nasal appliances can maintain pressure in the system even after decannulation; this can result in failure of low airway pressure or disconnect alarms to respond
  - Complete obstruction of nasal prongs and nasopharyngeal tubes results in continued pressurization of CPAP system without activation of low or high airway pressure alarms
- Activation of a manual breath (commonly available on infant ventilators) may cause gastric insufflation and patient discomfort, particularly if the peak pressure is set inappropriately high

Hazards and complications associated with the patient's clinical condition include the following:

- Lung overdistention causing barotrauma, $\dot{V}/\dot{Q}$ mismatch, hypercapnia, including work of breathing
- Impedance of pulmonary blood flow (increased pulmonary vascular resistance, decreased cardiac output)
- Gastric insufflation and abdominal distention potentially leading to aspiration
- Nasal irritation with septal distortion
- Skin irritation and pressure necrosis
- Nasal mucosal damage owing to inadequate humidification

■ ASSESSMENT OF OUTCOME

CPAP is initiated at levels of 4 to 5 cm H_2O and may be gradually increased up to 10 cm H_2O to provide the following:

- Stabilization of FiO_2 requirement ≤0.60 with PaO_2 levels >50 mm Hg or the presence of clinically acceptable noninvasive monitoring of O_2 ($PtcO_2$), while maintaining an adequate VE as indicated by $PaCO_2$ of ≤50 to 60 mm Hg and pH ≥ 7.25
- Reduced work of breathing as indicated by decreased respiratory rate, retractions, grunting, nasal flaring
- Improvement in lung volumes and appearance of lung as indicated by chest radiograph
- Improvement in patient comfort as assessed by bedside caregiver

Continued

48-1 Application of Continuous Positive Airway Pressure to Neonates via Nasal Prongs, Nasopharyngeal Tube, or Nasal Mask—cont'd

AARC Clinical Practice Guideline (Excerpts)*

MONITORING

Patient-ventilator system assessments should be performed at least every 2 to 4 hours and should include documentation of ventilator settings and patient assessments as recommended by the AARC clinical practice guideline on patient-ventilator system checks (see Chapter 46) and the clinical practice guideline on humidification during mechanical ventilation (see Chapter 35). Monitoring should include the following:

- O_2 and CO_2 monitoring, including periodic sampling of ABG values and continuous noninvasive monitoring (e.g., transcutaneous O_2 and CO_2 monitoring, pulse oximetry)
- Continuous monitoring of electrocardiogram and respiratory rate
- Continuous monitoring of proximal airway pressure, PEEP, and $\overline{P}aw$
- Continuous monitoring of FiO_2
- Periodic physical assessment of breath sounds and signs of increased work of breathing
- Periodic evaluation of chest radiographs

VE, *Minute ventilation.*

**For complete guideline, see American Association for Respiratory Care: Clinical practice guideline: application of continuous positive airway pressure to neonates via nasal prongs, nasopharyngeal tune, nasal mask: 2004 revision and update. Respir Care 49:1100, 2004.*

2 to 8 L/min may be as effective as and is easier to apply than a nasal CPAP system.[30,31]

Specially designed humidification systems have been developed and allow the use of nasal cannulas at flow rates of 2 to 30 L/min.[32] These devices maximize humidification and minimize condensation accumulating in the small diameter supply tubing. High-flow nasal cannula systems have been used successfully in neonates for the same indications that CPAP has been used. Instead of titrating levels of CPAP, the flow rate is incrementally adjusted. However, the amount of positive pressure that the high-flow nasal cannula potentially produces cannot be measured, and inadvertent high levels may occur, particularly if the nasal cannula fits snugly in the nares.[33-35]

High-flow nasal cannula systems have the potential for maximizing supplemental O_2 administration because the O_2 concentration delivered to the patient should approximate the set FiO_2. This approximation occurs because the anatomic reservoir of the upper airway is continuously flushed, greatly reducing the entrainment of room air. High-flow nasal cannula systems may be beneficial in stabilizing acute respiratory failure caused by hypoxemia, which may reduce the need for noninvasive or invasive assisted ventilation, such as in the case of a pulmonary exacerbation in a patient with cystic fibrosis or a patient experiencing congestive heart failure.

MECHANICAL VENTILATION

Early attempts to provide assisted ventilation to infants and children were largely derived from the experiences gained in adults, including the type of ventilators used and the associated techniques. Recognition of the physiologic differences of neonates and children led to further advances in ventilator design and modes and a wider range of capabilities. Although the classic "infant ventilator" is still widely used, modern microprocessor ventilators offer an ever-evolving array of options capable of supporting the full range of patient sizes and physiologic conditions.[36] RTs caring for infants and children need to be familiar with their physiologic differences to select and modify the appropriate ventilator strategy.[37-39]

Basic Principles

Conventional mechanical ventilation is the delivery of a bulk flow of humidified gas into and out of the lungs. The removal of CO_2, typically measured by PCO_2, is directly related to alveolar ventilation (frequency $\times$ V_T). Gas moves from the ventilator across an artificial airway in response to a change in pressure or pressure gradient. The magnitude of pressure required to move a particular amount of volume is derived from the compliance of the pulmonary system and the resistance of the airways.

Compliance is a measure of the distensibility of the lungs and is expressed as the volume change per unit of pressure change ($C = \Delta V/\Delta P$). *Resistance* is the tendency for airflow across the tracheobronchial tree to be impeded at a particular pressure per unit of gas flow ($R = \Delta P/\text{flow}$). The product of compliance and resistance is the respiratory time constant, or the measure of time necessary for the equilibration of a change in airway pressure ($TC = C \times R$). A patient with stiff or noncompliant lungs, such as a preterm infant with surfactant deficiency, has short time constants, meaning less time is required for equilibration,

Box 48-5 Indications for Mechanical Ventilation

APNEA

Respiratory Failure

- $PaO_2 < 50$ mm Hg
- $PaCO_2 > 65$ mm Hg

Pulmonary Disease

- Respiratory distress syndrome
- PPHN
- Meconium aspiration syndrome
- Pneumonia
- ARDS

NEUROLOGIC AND NEUROMUSCULAR

- Asphyxia
- Head trauma
- Spinal muscle atrophy
- Muscular dystrophy

CONGENITAL ABNORMALITIES

- Congenital diaphragmatic hernia
- Congenital heart disease

POSTSURGERY

- Thoracic surgery

and filling and emptying of lungs occur faster, which means shorter inspiratory and expiratory times. A patient with a disease characterized by impaired airflow or high resistance, such as a child with asthma, has longer time constants, in which more time is required for filling and emptying, meaning longer inspiratory and expiratory times are needed.

Goals of Mechanical Ventilation

The basic goals of mechanical ventilation are to improve O_2 delivery to meet metabolic demand and eliminate CO_2, while reducing the work of breathing.[38,39] The basic aim of assisted ventilation is to meet the goals while minimizing the associated deleterious effects. One approach to mechanical ventilation begins with the selection of an appropriate breath type, either pressure-controlled or volume-controlled, and a mode that best meets the physiologic needs of the patient's condition.[40] Box 48-5 lists the indications for mechanical ventilation in infants and children.

Modes of Ventilation and Breath Delivery Types

Historically, the most common mode of ventilation used in neonates and children was intermittent mandatory ventilation. Because early infant ventilators were unable to respond to the small triggering efforts of these patients, mandatory timed breaths were superimposed over a continuous flow of gas. These asynchronous, mandatory breaths provided most of the ventilation, while the patient was allowed to breathe spontaneously from the continuous gas source. Eventually, technologic improvements resulted in triggering devices that provided synchronization of the mandatory breaths with patient effort (synchronized intermittent mandatory ventilation [SIMV]) followed by the ability to provide assist control (A/C) and pressure support ventilation (PSV). Despite evidence that SIMV is more likely to result in patient-ventilator asynchrony,[41,42] most neonatal and pediatric patients are managed by using one of these three modes or a combination (i.e., SIMV + PSV). The most common triggering device for infant ventilators is a pneumotachygraph placed in the ventilator circuit, often proximal to the airway, which in many cases also serves as a monitoring device. The pneumotachygraph allows for the integration of a flow signal, which can be displayed as inhaled and exhaled V_T and minute ventilation. Figure 48-9 displays graphic representations of A/C, SIMV, and PSV.

In almost all cases of neonatal ventilation, the mechanical breaths delivered during SIMV and A/C are time-cycled, pressure-limited breaths.[43] Inspiration is initiated by patient effort or as a result of the set respiratory rate (whichever comes first). Based on the available flow—continuous, demand, or both—the set inspiratory pressure is reached early in the inspiratory phase and maintained throughout the remainder of the inspiratory time, after which the ventilator cycles to expiration. Most current-generation ventilators are capable of providing volume-targeted, pressure-limited ventilation, often referred to as *pressure-regulated volume control* or *volume guarantee*. In this dual mode of ventilation, the inspiratory V_T is compared with a preset target V_T, and the inspiratory pressure on the next breath is adjusted up or down in an attempt to meet the target volume. True volume-controlled breaths are rarely used for ventilating neonatal patients. (See Chapter 42 for details.)

RULE OF THUMB

When ventilating neonates, choose time-cycled, pressure-limited mechanical breaths.

Pediatric patients may be ventilated with either volume-controlled or pressure-controlled breaths. The choice may be based on health care team or institutional preference, prior experience, and equipment availability or may be evidence-based for specific diseases (e.g., asthma).

Ventilator Settings and Parameters

After the mode of ventilation is selected, the RT begins to adjust the various settings associated with the mode, while keeping in mind the goals of ventilation and the patient's weight, underlying problem, and reason for mechanical ventilation. The RT often can get a sense of the patient's compliance by manually ventilating the patient and observing the pressure needed to make the chest rise.

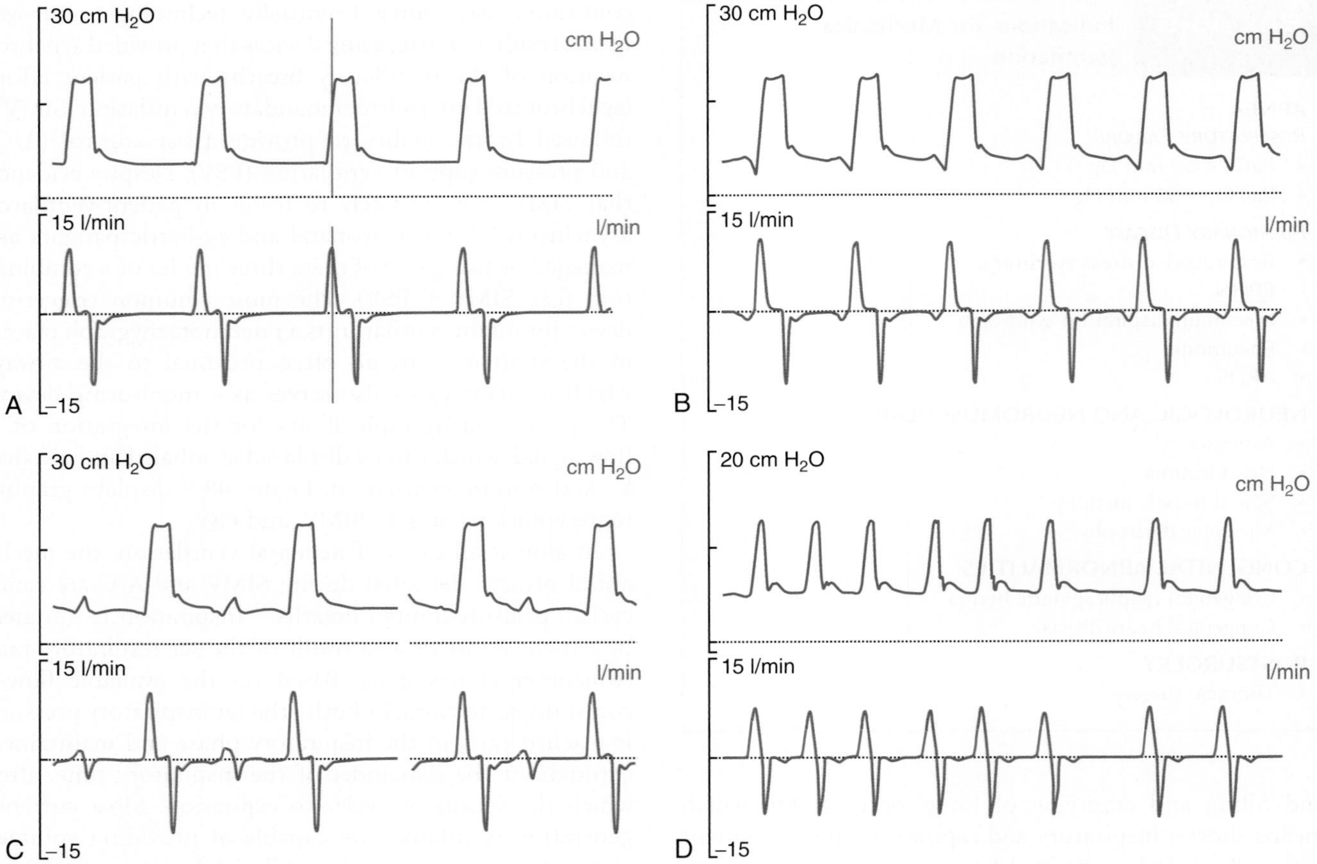

FIGURE 48-9 Airway graphics. **A,** Patient is apneac. Regardless of SIMV or A/C mode all breaths are mandatory at set rate. **B,** A/C mode. Total respiratory rate is determined by patient's spontaneous rate. **C,** SIMV mode. Mechanical breaths are delivered at a set rate. Patient is allowed to breathe spontaneously in between mandatory breaths. **D,** PSV mode. There are no set mandatory breaths. All breaths are pressure supported at patient's spontaneous rate.

Peak Inspiratory Pressure

For time-cycled, pressure-limited breaths, the peak inspiratory pressure (PIP) is set according to predetermined criteria (e.g., 20 to 25 cm H_2O) or by observing the pressure required to move the chest during manual ventilation with a flow inflating bag. The delivered V_T is monitored, and adjustments may be made. Increasing the PIP normally results in an increase in V_T, whereas a decrease in PIP results in decreased V_T. In the absence of V_T monitoring, PIP may be adjusted based on subjective assessment of chest movement and auscultation of breath sounds. Efforts should be made to maintain the lowest possible PIP that delivers the target V_T because PIP greater than 30 cm H_2O in pressure ventilators has been shown to increase the likelihood of ventilator-induced lung injury.

RULE OF THUMB

Always strive to maintain PIP less than 30 cm H_2O.

Positive End Expiratory Pressure

Positive end expiratory pressure (PEEP), often referred to as the *baseline pressure,* is used to prevent alveolar collapse at end-expiration. PEEP results in improved oxygenation for a given O_2 concentration. If the PEEP is set too low, alveolar collapse may occur, resulting in decreased FRC, altered ventilation/perfusion ($\dot{V}/\dot{Q}$ matching), and hypoxemia. If the PEEP is set too high, overdistention may occur, increasing the likelihood of lung injury. Typically, PEEP is set between 3 cm H_2O and 6 cm H_2O, although higher levels may be used if necessary. PEEP is set in conjunction with PIP, and the difference between the two is often referred to as the delta P or *ventilating pressure.* As the delta P is increased, either by increasing PIP or decreasing PEEP, the V_T is most likely to increase as well (unless overdistention occurs) Conversely, decreasing the delta P results in lower V_T.

Tidal Volume

When selecting V_T, the clinician must consider a volume that provides adequate lung inflation without overstretching the alveoli. Setting V_T that is too high most likely

MINI CLINI

Pediatric Ventilation

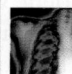

PROBLEM: A 12-year-old girl with asthma is admitted to the emergency department. She was intubated in the field by paramedics and is currently ventilated with a transport ventilator at the following settings:

- Mode–SIMV
- V_T–12 ml/kg
- PIP–90 cm H_2O
- PEEP–0 cm H_2O
- Set respiratory rate–16 breaths/min
- Total respiratory rate–20 breaths/min
- Inspiratory time–0.25 sec
- FiO_2–1.0

The paramedics inform the RT that since the patient has been placed on the mechanical ventilator, PIP has steadily increased, blood pressure has begun to decrease, and breaths sounds consisting of bilateral inspiratory and expiratory wheezes have become increasingly diminished. What should the RT recommend?

SOLUTION: The ventilator circuit should be immediately disconnected from the endotracheal tube allowing the patient to exhale fully. This patient should be fully sedated and possibly paralyzed to allow the RT to set and control ventilation. The ventilator settings should be set as follows:

- Mode–A/C
- Breath delivery type–volume controlled
- V_T–4 to 6 ml/kg
- Plateau pressure–maintain at ≤30 cm H_2O
- Respiratory rate–set at whatever rate allows ventilation without development of auto-peep or increased plateau pressure or both
- Inspiratory time–1.0 sec
- PEEP–5 cm H_2O
- FiO_2–1.0

Patients with severe status asthmaticus are among the most challenging patients to ventilate. The pulmonary time constants are increased such that it is equally difficult to inflate the lungs as it is for the patient to exhale. The inspiratory flow rate must be controlled by the clinician by means of volume-controlled ventilation, and sufficient time must be provided to allow the lungs to inflate. Expiratory time must be sufficient to allow exhalation, preventing the accumulation of trapped gas or auto-PEEP. The result is a decrease in minute ventilation, which leads to permissive hypercapnia as a lung protective strategy. $PaCO_2$ should be allowed to increase as long as the pH is greater than or equal to 7.10.

The inspiratory time must be increased (up to 1 second for this patient and longer in older teenagers) to allow inspiratory gas flow to the patient. Although this increase in inspiratory time may seem counterproductive in a patient with prolonged expiratory time constants, it is necessary to deliver gas on inspiration. Decreasing the inspiratory time by less than 1 second does little to prevent the development of auto-PEEP.

In the presence of an elevated $PaCO_2$ and decreased pH, a higher FiO_2 is required to maintain SpO_2 greater than 90% owing to shifting of the oxyhemoglobin dissociation curve. FiO_2 should be initially set at 1.0 and titrated to maintain SpO_2 within acceptable range.

Box 48-6 Interrelationship of Tidal Volume, Flow, and Time

V_T = Flow in L/sec × Inspiratory time
Inspiratory time = V_T/Flow rate

would result in lung injury. V_T of 6 to 8 ml/kg is generally considered safe in most patients. However, in some patients with extremely low lung compliance, such as patients with severe acute respiratory distress syndrome (ARDS), it may be necessary to reduce V_T to 4 to 5 ml/kg.

If the clinician chooses to deliver volume-controlled breaths, V_T is set as a control variable. Every mechanical breath delivers an identical V_T at either a preset inspiratory time or a preset flow rate. Set V_T, inspiratory time, and flow all are interrelated. If V_T is set at 300 ml, and flow rate is 30 L/min (0.5 L/sec), the inspiratory time is 0.6 second. See formulas in Box 48-6.

When ventilating patients with pressure-controlled breaths, V_T is not set, but it should be monitored. The clinician must compare the monitored V_T with a predetermined target and adjust the delta P to meet that target.

Regardless of whether the clinician chooses volume-controlled or pressure-controlled breaths, he or she must recognize that some of the V_T is compressed in the circuit and not delivered to the patient; this is referred to as *compressible volume loss*. Most current-generation ventilators automatically compensate for compressible volume loss and adjust the delivered and displayed (monitored) V_T accordingly. With older ventilators, during volume-controlled breaths, the clinician must calculate the compressible volume loss and increase the set V_T to deliver the desired volume to the patient. During volume-controlled and pressure-controlled breaths, the calculated compressible volume loss must be subtracted from the ventilator displayed exhaled V_T. See Box 48-7 for calculation of compressible volume loss.

RULE OF THUMB

Large V_T (>8 ml/kg) is likely to overstretch the lung, resulting in acute lung injury, and should be avoided. Patients with severe ARDS may require even lower V_T (4 to 5 ml/kg).

Box 48-7 Determining Effective or Corrected Tidal Volume

$$\text{Effective } V_T = \text{Delivered } V_T - \text{Compressible volume}$$
$$\text{Compressible volume} = \text{Compressible factor} \times (\text{PIP} - \text{PEEP})$$

Example: A 12-year-old child weighing 28 kg requires assisted ventilation. V_T is set at 240 ml, PIP is 25 cm H_2O, and PEEP is 5 cm H_2O. The compressible factor for the ventilator is 2 ml/cm H_2O.

$$\text{Compressible volume} = (2 \text{ ml/cm } H_2O) \times (25 - 5 \text{ cm } H_2O) = 40 \text{ ml}$$
$$\text{Effective } V_T = 240 \text{ ml} - 40 \text{ ml} = 200 \text{ ml}$$
$$\text{Effective } V_T/\text{kg} = 200 \text{ ml} \div 28 \text{ kg} = 7.1 \text{ ml/kg}$$

MINI CLINI

Pediatric Ventilation

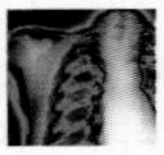

PROBLEM: A 10-year-old boy with a complex medical history including history of trisomy 21, intractable infantile spasms, seizure disorder, and developmental delay (nonverbal), is admitted with increased difficulty breathing and found to be positive for respiratory syncytial virus. His home regimen includes nocturnal NIV via nasal mask with an inspiratory pressure of 8 cm H_2O, 3 cm PEEP, and 2 L/min of O_2 added to the breathing circuit. On admission, the patient complains of shortness of breath. His respiratory rate is 40 breaths/min, and SpO_2 is 88% on a nonrebreathing mask. What should the RT suggest?

SOLUTION:

- NIV—consider beginning NIV via oronasal mask
- PIP—10 to 12 cm H_2O
- PEEP—3 to 5 cm H_2O
- Set respiratory rate—12 breaths/min
- FiO_2—1.0

Although this patient receives NIV for nocturnal support when stable, he currently has an acute infection superimposed on chronic restrictive lung disease. Beginning NIV now may provide sufficient support to prevent intubation during this acute condition. Initial PIP of 10 to 12 cm H_2O titrated to patient comfort may provide additional support, increasing V_T and allowing respiratory rate to return to baseline. Choosing an oronasal mask may prove to be a more efficient interface than the patient's usual nasal mask at this time. The set respiratory rate of 12 breaths/min is intended to be a backup rate because this patient is spontaneously breathing and should be allowed to establish his own breathing pattern. FiO_2 should be adjusted to maintain an acceptable SpO_2.

To guide practitioners in providing quality care, the AARC has published Clinical Practice Guideline: Neonatal Time-Triggered, Pressure-Limited, Time-Cycled Mechanical Ventilation. Excerpts from this guideline appear in Clinical Practice Guideline 48-2.

Ventilator Rate

The ventilator rate is the set number of breaths delivered in 1 minute. During A/C ventilation, the set respiratory rate is the minimum number of breaths the patient will receive and is increased if the patient triggers the ventilator at a respiratory rate faster than that which is set. The actual or total respiratory rate multiplied by V_T determines the minute ventilation, which is directly related to alveolar ventilation and PCO_2. Because V_T is usually set according to the patient's ideal or calculated body weight, adjusting minute ventilation is most often accomplished by changing the respiratory rate. The clinician must be aware of the total respiratory rate when making changes to adjust minute ventilation. If the set respiratory rate is 16, but the total respiratory rate is 22 because of patient triggering, decreasing the set rate to 12 would have no effect on minute ventilation.

Inspiratory Time

The inspiratory time is often defined as the time required to deliver V_T; however, this may be misleading. As described earlier, with volume-controlled breaths, the inspiratory time is determined by V_T and inspiratory flow rate and is the time required to deliver the preset V_T at the preset flow rate. However, with pressure-controlled breaths, the inspiratory time is set by the clinician and may be shorter, longer, or equal to the time required to deliver the breath. In the case of increased airway resistance, such as a patient with asthma, if the inspiratory time is not set long enough, flow delivery to the patient may not decelerate to zero by the end of the set inspiratory time. Under these circumstances, increasing inspiratory time would result in an increase in delivered V_T. Conversely, under the same conditions, shortening the inspiratory time would result in a decrease in delivered V_T. In the case of decreased compliance, as in pneumonia, increasing inspiratory time beyond the time necessary to allow full flow deceleration would result in an inspiratory pause or breath hold, which may not be tolerated by the patient.

RULE OF THUMB

Inspiratory time is usually set between 0.2 second and 0.4 second for neonates and up to 1.0 second in teenagers. With patients who are awake and have spontaneous breathing efforts, inspiratory time must be set at a level that matches patient demand to avoid patient-ventilator asynchrony.

Oxygen Concentration

The O_2 concentration or FiO_2 is kept as low as possible to avoid the risk of O_2 toxicity. Although the precise mechanisms are not understood, the best approach is to maintain the lowest FiO_2 possible. The immature lung is particularly susceptible to O_2 toxicity, which can result in the development of bronchopulmonary dysplasia. In a preterm infant, FiO_2 is titrated to a narrow SpO_2 range

48-2 Neonatal Time-Triggered, Pressure-Limited, Time-Cycled Mechanical Ventilation

AARC Clinical Practice Guideline (Excerpts)*

INDICATIONS

- Apnea
- Hypoxemic (PaO_2 < 50 mm Hg) or hypercapnic (pH < 7.20-7.25) respiratory acidosis despite use of CPAP and supplemental O_2 (i.e., $FiO_2 \geq 0.60$)
- Abnormalities on physical examination
  - Increased work of breathing shown by grunting, nasal flaring, tachypnea, and sternal and intercostal retractions
  - Presence of pale or cyanotic skin
  - Agitation
- Alterations in neurologic status that compromise the central drive to breathe
  - Apnea of prematurity
  - Intracranial hemorrhage
  - Congenital neuromuscular disorders
- Impaired respiratory function resulting in a compromised FRC owing to decreased lung compliance or increased airways resistance or both, including but not limited to
  - Respiratory distress syndrome
  - Bronchiolitis
  - Meconium aspiration syndrome
  - Congenital diaphragmatic hernia
  - Pneumonia
  - Sepsis
  - Bronchopulmonary dysplasia
  - Radiographic evidence of decreased lung volume
- Impaired cardiovascular function
  - PPHN
  - Postresuscitation
  - Congenital heart disease
  - Shock
- Postoperative state characterized by impaired ventilatory function

CONTRAINDICATIONS

There are no specific contraindications when indications are judged to be present.

HAZARDS AND COMPLICATIONS

- Air leak syndromes secondary to barotrauma or volume overinflation (i.e., volutrauma) including pneumothorax, pneumomediastinum, pneumopericardium, pneumoperitoneum, subcutaneous emphysema, and pulmonary interstitial emphysema
- Chronic lung disease associated with prolonged PPV and O_2 toxicity (e.g., bronchopulmonary dysplasia)
- Airway complications associated with endotracheal intubation
  - Laryngotracheobronchomalacia
  - Unplanned extubation
  - Damage to upper airway structures
  - Air leak around uncuffed endotracheal tube
  - Malpositioning of endotracheal tube
  - Subglottic stenosis
  - Obstruction of endotracheal tube with mucus
  - Main stem intubation
  - Kinking of endotracheal tube
  - Pressure necrosis
- Increased work of breathing (during spontaneous breaths) owing to the high resistance of small endotracheal tubes
- Nosocomial pulmonary infection (e.g., pneumonia)
- Decreased venous return, decreased cardiac output, increased intracranial pressure leading to intraventricular hemorrhage
- Supplemental O_2 may lead to increased risk of ROP
- Complications associated with endotracheal suctioning
- Failure of ventilator, alarms, circuit, humidifier; loss of or inadequate gas supply
- Patient-ventilator asynchrony
- Inappropriate ventilator settings leading to auto-PEEP, hypoventilation or hyperventilation, hypoxemia or hyperoxemia, and increased work of breathing

Continued

48-2 Neonatal Time-Triggered, Pressure-Limited, Time-Cycled Mechanical Ventilation—cont'd

AARC Clinical Practice Guideline (Excerpts)*

ASSESSMENT OF NEED

Determination that valid indications are present

ASSESSMENT OF OUTCOME

Establishment of neonatal assisted ventilation should result in improvement in the patient's condition or reversal of indications:

- Reduction in work of breathing as evidenced by decreases in respiratory rate, severity of retractions, nasal flaring, and grunting
- Radiographic evidence of improved lung volume
- Subjective improvement in lung volume as indicated by increased chest excursion and aeration by chest auscultation
- Improved gas exchange
  - Ability to maintain a $PaO_2 \geq 50$ mm Hg with $FiO_2 < 0.60$
  - Ability to reverse respiratory acidosis and maintain pH > 7.23
- Subjective improvement as indicated by decrease in grunting, nasal flaring, sternal and intercostal retraction, and respiratory rate

MONITORING

Patient-ventilator system assessments should be performed every 2 to 4 hours and should include documentation of ventilator settings and patient assessments as recommended by the AARC clinical practice guideline on patient-ventilator system assessments (see Chapter 46) and AARC clinical practice guideline on humidification during mechanical ventilation (see Chapter 35). Monitoring should include the following:

- O_2 and CO_2 monitoring
  - Periodic sampling of blood gas values; keep $PaO_2 < 80$ mm Hg in preterm infants to avoid ROP
  - An unstable infant should be monitored continuously by transcutaneous O_2 monitor or pulse oximeter
  - An unstable infant should be monitored continuously by transcutaneous or end-tidal CO_2 monitoring
  - Fractional concentration of O_2 delivered by the ventilator should be monitored continuously
- Continuous monitoring of cardiac activity (via electrocardiograph) and respiratory rate
- Monitoring of blood pressure by indwelling arterial line or by periodic cuff measurements
- Continuous monitoring of airway pressures including PIP, PEEP, and mean pressure ($\overline{P}aw$)
  - Higher Paw may improve oxygenation; however, Paw > 12 cm H_2O may lead to barotrauma
  - The difference between PIP and PEEP (ΔP) in conjunction with patient mechanics determines V_T; as ΔP changes, V_T varies
  - PIP should be adjusted initially to achieve adequate V_T as reflected by chest excursion and adequate breath sounds or by V_T measurement
  - PEEP increases FRC and may improve oxygenation (PEEP is typically adjusted at 4-7 cm H_2O—higher levels may cause hyperinflation, particularly in obstructive airways disease [e.g., meconium aspiration syndrome or bronchiolitis])
- Many neonatal ventilators provide continuous monitoring of ventilator rate, inspiratory time, and inspiratory-to-expiratory (I : E) ratio; if only two of these variables are directly monitored, the third should be calculated
  - Lengthening inspiratory time increases Paw and should improve oxygenation
  - I : E ratio >1 : 1 may lead to auto-PEEP and hyperinflation
  - Rates of 30 to 60/min with shorter inspiratory times (e.g., I : E ratio 1 : 2) are commonly used in patients with respiratory distress syndrome
- Depending on the internal diameter of the ventilator circuit, excessive flows can cause expiratory resistance that leads to increased work of breathing and increased PEEP. Some ventilators have demand-flow systems that permit the use of lower baseline flow rates but provide the patient with additional flow as needed
- Because of the possibility of complete obstruction or kinking of the endotracheal tube and the inadequacy of ventilator alarms in these situations, continuous V_T monitoring via an appropriately designed (minimum dead space) proximal airway flow sensor is recommended
- Periodic physical assessment of chest excursion and breath sounds and for signs of increased work of breathing and cyanosis
- Periodic evaluation of chest radiographs to follow the progress of the disease, identify possible complications, and verify endotracheal tube placement

**For complete guideline, see American Association for Respiratory Care: Clinical practice guideline: neonatal time-triggered, pressure-limited, time-cycled mechanical ventilation. Respir Care 39:808, 1994.*

(e.g., 88% to 94%) so that retinal damage (ROP), which is caused by elevated PO_2, does not develop.[11]

RULE OF THUMB

O_2 is considered a drug and should be used appropriately. High O_2 concentrations are potentially injurious and may cause O_2 toxicity in the immature lung and retinal damage in preterm infants.

Mean Airway Pressure

Mean airway pressure ($\bar{P}$aw) is the average airway pressure during a 1-minute period. It is affected by changes in PIP, PEEP, inspiratory time, and respiratory rate. An increase in $\bar{P}$aw is often associated with improved oxygenation but is not without hazards. Increasing PEEP would result in increased $\bar{P}$aw and potentially increased oxygenation. However, if the PEEP is set too high, the alveoli may become overinflated resulting in worsening $\dot{V}/\dot{Q}$ matching, and lung injury may occur.

Noninvasive Ventilation

Noninvasive ventilation (NIV), also known as *noninvasive positive pressure ventilation,* has become more popular recently in neonatal patients. In the past, use of NIV was limited by the lack of available interfaces; however, these are becoming more readily available. Figure 48-8 shows various interfaces that may be used for NIV (or CPAP) in neonates. More recent evidence supports the use of both synchronized and nonsynchronized NIV in the neonatal intensive care unit (ICU).[46] It is hoped that future research will clarify which patients are most likely to benefit from this form of support.

NIV has been used extensively in patients of all ages, including pediatric patients.[47-50] Indications may include short-term support of hypoxemic respiratory failure, such as that seen with pulmonary edema associated with left-sided heart failure; prevention of intubation; postextubation support; and long-term support of patients with neuromuscular disease. Some limitation of available interfaces persists, particularly in smaller patients; however, most patients can be fitted without too much difficulty. As with CPAP and other noninvasive interface devices, care must be taken to prevent or minimize patient injury owing to iatrogenic pressure ulcers from a tight or poorly fitted device.

NIV may be provided with simple, single-limb devices such as bilevel positive airway pressure generators, or sophisticated ICU ventilators. Care must be taken whenever a single-limb circuit is employed to provide sufficient PEEP in the system to prevent rebreathing of gases (see Chapter 46).

Monitoring Mechanical Ventilation

The RT should develop a systematic approach to monitoring the effects of mechanical ventilation. Components of a ventilator assessment should include an evaluation of the artificial airway, physical examination, assessment of patient-ventilator interaction,[51] analysis of laboratory and radiographic data, adjunct ventilator monitoring, and a systematic ventilator safety assessment including alarm function and assessment of humidification. Alarms should be connected to a central monitoring system to alert appropriately clinicians away from the bedside of a change the patient's condition.

A flow sheet is used to prompt the user and guide the clinician through the process of assessing the patient, while serving as documentation of the ventilator settings and outputs. In the past, these flow sheets were paper and were maintained as part of the patient's medical record. It is becoming more common to have the flow sheet integrated into an electronic medical record that is readily available to the entire patient care team. Although many elements of the patient-ventilator assessment are automatically entered via an electronic interface and require validation only by the clinician, some data must still be entered by hand. It is hoped that as these systems become more sophisticated and standardization improves, all of the data, including ventilator information, laboratory values, and radiographic and other imaging data, will automatically download, eliminating transcription errors, providing a more comprehensive assessment, and allowing the clinician to focus on the patient and patient-ventilator interaction.

Physical Examination

Examination of the patient can yield quick and useful information. The chest is examined for adequacy of chest rise, the presence of asymmetric movement and deformities, and signs of increased work of breathing such as retractions. Breath sounds are helpful in gauging the degree of air entry, verifying bilateral aeration, and identifying airflow problems and areas of diminished aeration. Skin appearance can also give the clinician a sense of the patient's perfusion—an indirect measure of cardiac output. A mottled appearance, poor capillary refill, and pale or gray color indicate poor perfusion.

Patient-Ventilator Interaction

The patient-ventilator interaction is the assessment used to determine the ease with which the patient can trigger the ventilator and is made by simultaneously observing the trigger indicator and the patient. Refinements in the trigger threshold may need to be made if there is a leak present or the work to trigger or initiate a breath is too great. The manner in which the breath is terminated is also assessed. Together, patient synchrony and comfort are determined. Patient-ventilator asynchrony occurs when the patient's efforts to breathe are unmatched with the preselected ventilator support. Airway graphics are also helpful in identifying nuances and refining ventilator settings.[52] Airway graphics routinely displayed are scalar

MINI CLINI

Pediatric Mechanical Ventilation

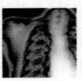

PROBLEM: A 14-month-old child, who weighs 13 kg and has a history of chronic lung disease (bronchopulmonary dysplasia), requires mechanical ventilation after surgery for correction of gastric reflux. The surgeon requests that the RT select ventilator parameters and develop a weaning plan for this child. The child has an uncuffed 4.5 oral endotracheal tube in place. SpO_2 is 100% with manual ventilation and 100% O_2. Sedation is prescribed to keep the child comfortable but allow spontaneous breathing.

This child needs a ventilatory strategy that takes into account his age, disease process, amount of sedation, and current ventilation needs. What would be the appropriate choices for his initial ventilator management in terms of mode, V_T, set rate, FiO_2, and PEEP level?

SOLUTION:

- Mode—A/C
- V_T—6 to 8 ml/kg or 100 to 130 ml in this case
- FiO_2—1.0 then titrated to an acceptable SpO_2
- PEEP—5 cm H_2O

If this child had previously been mechanically ventilated, reviewing the presurgery settings may be helpful in deciding a ventilator plan. If not, a rationale for the suggested parameters follows.

By using the mode A/C, patient-ventilator synchrony can be more easily achieved; this reduces the need for sedation later, after the pain of surgery has dissipated. The initial V_T is based on current recommendations. The ventilator rate is determined by the normal respiratory rate for the age of the child, the desired PCO_2 level, and the number of assisted or triggered breaths the child is having. Because this child has chronic lung disease, a higher PCO_2 may be optimal at this time. A younger child with a higher PCO_2 and with a decreased respiratory rate may have a higher set rate. Initial FiO_2 is usually reflective of the amount currently being delivered with hand ventilation but quickly titrated to maintain normal SpO_2. FiO_2 of 0.40 after surgery would not be unusual in the child.

waveforms of flow, airway pressure, and volume. Additionally, each of these parameters can be plotted against each other. Pressure-volume and flow-volume loops can be particularly helpful in assessing alterations in work of breathing, overdistention of the lung, and compliance.

Additional Monitoring

The use of noninvasive monitors, particularly measurements of end tidal CO_2 and SpO_2, has become routine. Periodic blood gas analysis is a useful tool to quantify acid-base status and to refine ventilator settings further. Other laboratory data, such as electrolytes and hematologic information, are also assessed. Periodic chest radiographs are obtained to identify suspected problems and to assess the progress of lung disease.

Patient-Ventilator Periodic Assessment

A systematic patient-ventilator assessment should be conducted periodically.[53] Prescribed ventilator settings are confirmed and documented along with verification of ventilator outputs. Measurements of mandatory and spontaneous V_T values are made and expressed per the patient's weight to determine if targets are being achieved. Alarms are set and tested and should minimally detect loss of pressure, high pressure, and patient disconnection.

The humidification system is evaluated including airway temperature and the presence of condensation in the ventilator circuit. Some visible condensation or "rainout" is important because a completely dry circuit may be a sign of inadequate humidification.

RULE OF THUMB

Routine monitoring of ventilated patients is essential and should include an assessment of the patient's physiologic status including vital signs and a systematic assessment of the patient-ventilator interaction.

Weaning from Mechanical Ventilation

Weaning or, more appropriately, liberation from mechanical ventilation is a topic that until more recently has received little attention in pediatric and neonatal patients. Clear guidelines for "assessment of readiness to extubate" and "spontaneous breathing trials" are standard practice in adults. However, this assessment has not yet become standard practice in pediatric and neonatal patients even though there are resources available to guide the pediatric/neonatal clinician in this area.[54] Nevertheless, these patients should be assessed daily to determine their readiness for liberation from mechanical ventilation. Some general considerations for extubation are presented in Box 48-8; however, distinct differences exist among

Box 48-8 Considerations for Extubation

- Spontaneous respiratory rate appropriate for age and weight
- Presence of apnea or periodic breathing
- FiO_2 requirement ≤ 0.4
- Ability to protect airway
- Normal work of breathing
- Acceptable amount and consistency of respiratory secretions
- Normal vital signs
- Minimal sedation needs
- $SpO_2 > 90\%$
- Spontaneous $V_T > 4$-5 ml/kg

Box 48-9 Pediatric Ventilator Discontinuance Protocol

STEP 1

Exclusion Criteria

- Brain death, ICP > 15 mm Hg, suspected high ICP, or difficult to control ICP
- Neuromuscular blockade
- Significant hemoptysis (significant amounts of blood from endotracheal tube or tracheostomy)
- Hemodynamic instability
- Unstable airway
- $FiO_2 > 0.6$
- PEEP ≥ 8 cm H_2O
- Pediatric ICU team consensus says no
- Extracorporeal life support
- Chronic disease requiring ventilation

Issues to Address Before Extubation

- Fluid overload
- Secretions
- Neurologic impairment
- Medication requirement precludes safe extubation
- NPO time insufficient
- Unstable, unsafe, swollen airway
- Imminent procedure
- Psychosocial factors (e.g., unclear code status, assent)

STEP 2

If none of the above conditions exist, the pediatric ICU team discusses the feasibility of extubation.

Consider the Following

- Stage of ventilation
  I—initial or acute stage (escalation)
  II—ventilator management stage (plateau)
  III—discontinuance stage (deescalation)
- Immediate extubation (may include reversal of sedation)
- Spontaneous breathing trial (may include some level of pressure support)
- Reduction of ventilator settings

If Spontaneous Breathing Trial Is Performed, Stop Trial at Any Point for the Following

- Tachypnea, bradypnea, apnea (age appropriate)
- Excessive use of accessory muscles, nasal flaring present, subjective dyspnea (consider baseline)
- Significant, unresolved change in agitation or anxiety
- Unacceptable decrease in SpO_2

STEP 3

Critical care team discusses extubation plan.

ICP, Intracranial pressure; *NPO,* nothing per mouth.

these various patients, and it is reasonable to develop an age-specific, multidisciplinary approach to this task. One alternative would be to begin with existing adult guidelines and modify them to meet the needs of pediatric and neonatal patients. Two sets of guidelines, one for pediatric patients and one for neonates, are presented in Boxes 48-9 and 48-10. (See Chapter 47 for details on weaning.)

Box 48-10 Neonatal Ventilator Discontinuance Protocol

STEP 1

Exclusion Criteria

- Suspected high or difficult to control ICP
- Neuromuscular blockade
- Recent pulmonary hemorrhage or significant blood from endotracheal tube or tracheostomy
- Hemodynamic instability
- Unstable airway
- Neonatal ICU team consensus not in favor of extubation at this time
- Extracorporeal life support

Issues to Address Before Extubation

- Fluid overload
- Secretions
- Neurologic impairment
- Medication requirement precludes safe extubation
- NPO time insufficient
- Unstable, unsafe, edematous airway
- Imminent procedure
- Psychosocial factors (e.g., unclear code status, assent)
- Imminent transport to home hospital

STEP 2

If none of the above conditions exist, the neonatal ICU team discusses the feasibility of extubation.

Consider the Following

- Stage of ventilation
  I—initial or acute stage (escalation)
  II—ventilator management stage (plateau)
  III—discontinuance stage (deescalation)
- Immediate extubation (may include reversal of sedation)
- Spontaneous breathing trial—must include some level of pressure support
- Reduction of ventilator settings

If Spontaneous Breathing Trial Is Performed, Stop Trial at Any Point for the Following

- Tachypnea, bradypnea, apnea above baseline (age appropriate)
- Excessive use of accessory muscles, nasal flaring present (consider baseline)
- Tachycardia or bradycardia above baseline
- Hemodynamic changes
- Significant, unresolved change in agitation
- Increased number of desaturations or sustained decrease in SpO_2 requiring increase in FiO_2

STEP 3

Neonatal ICU team discusses extubation plan.

ICP, Intracranial pressure; *NPO,* nothing per mouth.

High-Frequency Ventilation

High-frequency ventilation (HFV) is a form of invasive mechanical ventilation that uses small V_T values (less than dead space) at rapid frequencies, sometimes greater than 900 breaths/min (15 Hz). The primary goal of HFV is to provide adequate ventilation and oxygenation, while limiting the incidence of lung injury. HFV has been used as a primary mode of ventilation and a rescue therapy for patients determined to be failing conventional mechanical ventilation. Although early studies showed a beneficial effect compared with conventional ventilation, there has been no demonstrated improvement in outcome compared with current lung protective strategies.[55-61] HFV remains an acceptable mode of ventilation for patients of any age but should be used only by clinicians expert in its clinical application and knowledgeable about its physiologic effects.

There are three basic types of HFV: high-frequency oscillatory ventilation, high-frequency jet ventilation, and high-frequency percussive ventilation. High-frequency oscillatory ventilation is the most common form of HFV. Oxygenation is achieved by inflating the patient's lungs to a high resting level, or FRC, by establishing a high $\bar{P}aw$, similar to CPAP, at levels typically ranging from 16 to 30 cm H_2O. This "recruitment" improves the $\dot{V}/\dot{Q}$ ratio by opening previously collapsed alveoli. Ventilation is provided by the to-and-fro movement of a large piston in the ventilator circuit that results in high-frequency oscillations in the patient's airways. Gas exchange results from a combination of six mechanisms: bulk flow of gas, longitudinal dispersion, pendelluft, asymmetric velocity profiles, cardiogenic mixing, and molecular diffusion.

Cardiovascular Effects

The cardiovascular effects of HFV vary with the strategy employed. Using the high lung volume strategy, lung volume is recruited, and $\bar{P}aw$ can be slowly reduced while maintaining alveolar ventilation. This strategy limits the adverse side effects of PPV on cardiovascular performance and may result in increased systemic blood flow. However, if $\bar{P}aw$ greater than that used during conventional ventilation is required during HFV, cardiovascular compromise may occur. Increases in intravascular volume and use of vasoactive drugs help support mean arterial blood pressure, cardiac output, and O_2 delivery. Increases in central venous pressure or decreases in mean arterial pressure indicate decreases in systemic blood flow as a result of overdistention of the lung and inappropriately high $\bar{P}aw$ after adequate intravascular volume has been established.

Weaning from High-Frequency Ventilation

When FiO_2 is equal to or less than 0.6, $\bar{P}aw$ is weaned slowly. When $\bar{P}aw$ is less than 15 to 18 cm H_2O, the patient may be trialed off or transitioned to conventional ventilation.

Complications of Mechanical Ventilation

Box 48-11 summarizes the most common complications associated with mechanical ventilation in newborns and other pediatric patients.

Box 48-11 Complications of Mechanical Ventilation in Infants and Children

- Ventilator-induced injuries
- Air leak syndromes
- Pneumothorax
- Pneumomediastinum
- Pneumopericardium
- Pneumoperitoneum
- Pulmonary interstitial emphysema
- Subcutaneous emphysema
- Parenchymal lung damage
- Bronchopulmonary dysplasia
- Cardiovascular complications
- Decreased venous return
- Decreased cardiac output
- Increased pulmonary vascular resistance
- Increased intracranial pressure
- Increased incidence of intraventricular hemorrhage
- O_2-induced injuries
- O_2 toxicity
- ROP
- Airway complications
- Accidental extubation
- Atelectasis
- Inadequate humidification
- Endobronchial intubation
- Equipment contamination
- Postintubation stridor
- Endotracheal tube plugging or kinking
- Tracheal lesions
- Infection
- Ventilator-associated pneumonia

Box 48-12 Indications for Inhaled Nitric Oxide

Hypoxic respiratory failure
Term and near-term neonates (>34 weeks' gestation) with PPHN
  Gradient between preductal and postductal SpO_2
  Echocardiographic evidence
Congenital diaphragmatic hernia
Oxygenation index (OI) >25
  $OI = (\bar{P}aw \times FiO_2/PaO_2)$

SPECIALTY GASES

Inhaled Nitric Oxide

Inhaled nitric oxide (INO) is a selective pulmonary vasodilator used to treat newborns who require mechanical ventilation for hypoxic respiratory failure.[62,63] INO improves oxygenation and reduces the need for extracorporeal membrane oxygenation (ECMO), the more invasive and complication-prone alternative. The approved indications for INO are listed in Box 48-12. INO has also been studied in preterm infants with the aim to reduce

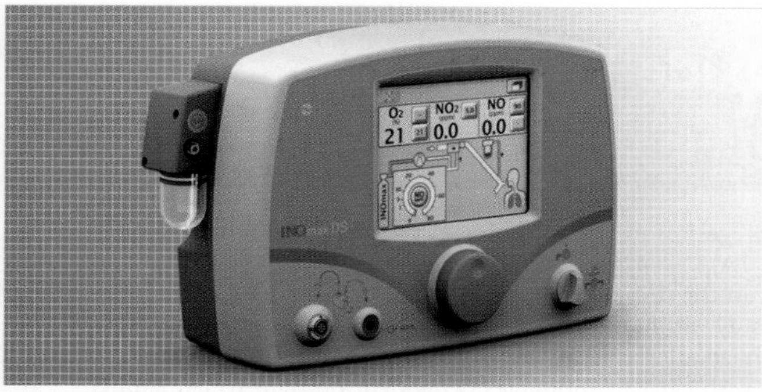

FIGURE 48-10 Nitric oxide delivery system (Ikaria INOmax DS_{ir} Operator's Manual, Ikaria, Inc. 2010).

the incidence of chronic lung disease. These clinical investigations showed a modest improvement in pulmonary outcomes, but other problems associated with prematurity, such as intracranial hemorrhage, were unchanged. At the present time, INO is not routinely used in the management of respiratory failure associated with prematurity.

INO is administered in conjunction with mechanical ventilation via a specially designed delivery and monitoring system that provides precision drug dosing and safety features (Figure 48-10). The recommended INO dose is 20 parts per million (ppm) with an optimal response achieved when lung inflation is maximized.[64,65] When a response has been achieved and sustained, the INO dose is gradually reduced, typically by 50% each step, to a final dose of 1 ppm, at which point the drug is discontinued. During withdrawal of INO, FiO_2 is increased to minimize any recurrence of pulmonary hypertension.[66]

During INO therapy, concentrations of nitric oxide and O_2 are continuously monitored. The combined exposure of nitric oxide and O_2 lead to the formation of nitrogen dioxide, which is potentially toxic and is continuously monitored. INO doses typically used are considered to be very low and have a good safety profile. A metabolite of INO is the formation of methemoglobin as the nitric oxide molecule is bound to the red blood cell. During INO administration, the patient's ability to metabolize methemoglobin is assessed by periodically monitoring methemoglobin levels.

INO should be available in any hospital that has a level III intensive care nursery. INO should be an integral part of any high-risk transport team, and it is important that non-ECMO centers have a plan for treatment failure that takes into account the distance to an ECMO center.[67] INO therapy has also been used for diagnosing and treating certain congenital heart diseases; although used in the management of ARDS, it seems to have less of a sustained effect in this setting.[68] The AARC has published a clinical practice guideline on INO therapy. Excerpts from this guideline appear in Clinical Practice Guideline 48-3.[69]

Heliox

Heliox is gas mixture of O_2 and helium. Typical concentration of a tank of heliox is 80%/20% or 70%/30%. Helium is less dense than air. Inhaling a less dense gas can reduce airway resistance and result in decreased work of breathing. In patients with a high O_2 requirement, helium is less effective. Heliox has been used in conjunction with other therapies in the treatment of partial airway obstruction and asthma where airway resistance is high. It can be used to help deliver bronchodilators and serve as a temporizing measure while steroids are administered to reduce airway swelling. When high O_2 concentrations are necessary, heliox is not likely to be effective as the amount of inspired helium is diminished. Signs of decreased work of breathing, decreased use of accessory muscles, improved aeration, and decreased respiratory rate after initiating heliox are indications of its effectiveness.

EXTRACORPOREAL MEMBRANE OXYGENATION

Extracorporeal membrane oxygenation (ECMO) is a modified form of cardiopulmonary bypass used to provide relatively long-term pulmonary or cardiopulmonary life support when maximum medical interventions have failed.[70] There are two types of ECMO support: venoarterial (VA), in which both heart and lung function is supported, and venovenous (VV), in which only the lungs are supported.

During VA ECMO, a cannula is inserted into the right internal jugular vein and advanced to the right atrium. Blood is drained from the right heart to a circuit where it is pumped through an artificial lung. The blood is oxygenated, and CO_2 is removed by the artificial lung and returned to the patient through a cannula inserted most often into the carotid artery. The blood is warmed to body temperature before reinfusion to the patient (Figure 48-11). VV ECMO differs technically in that blood is drained and reinfused to the right side of the heart through a specially designed double-lumen cannula, one larger lumen for draining blood and a smaller lumen for reinfusion, or through two cannulas each inserted into a vein. The veins commonly cannulated are the right internal jugular vein and the right femoral vein. The blood traverses the same circuitry as with VA ECMO, but the arterial circulation is not invaded. When heart function is adequate, VV support can accomplish the goal of providing adequate oxygenation, while reducing the risk of lung injury from the ventilator. Box 48-13 outlines the advantages and disadvantages of VA and VV support. Arterial and venous access may also be achieved transthoracically (e.g., postoperative cardiac patients) or through femoral vessels (e.g., pediatric applications).

ECMO has been shown to improve survival in newborns with hypoxic respiratory failure associated with PPHN,

48-3 Inhaled Nitric Oxide Therapy

AARC Clinical Practice Guideline (Excerpts)*

1. A trial of INO is recommended in newborns (>34 weeks' gestation, 14 days of age) with PaO_2 100 mm Hg on FiO_2 1.0 or an oxygenation index >25, or both. (Grade 1A)
2. It is recommended that INO therapy be instituted early in the disease course, which potentially reduces the length of mechanical ventilation, O_2 requirement, and stay within the ICU. (Grade 1A)
3. INO should not be used routinely in newborns with congenital diaphragmatic hernia. (Grade 1A)
4. INO therapy should not be used routinely in newborns with cardiac anomalies dependent on right-to-left shunts, congestive heart failure, and lethal congenital anomalies. (Grade 2C)
5. There are insufficient data to support the routine use of INO therapy in postoperative management of hypoxic term or near-term infants with congenital heart disease. (Grade 2C)
6. The recommended starting dose for INO is 20 ppm. (Grade 1A)
7. Response to a short trial (30-60 minutes) of INO should be judged by an improvement in PaO_2 or oxygenation index; if there is no response, INO should be discontinued. (Grade 1A)
8. For a newborn with parenchymal lung disease, optimal alveolar recruitment should be established before initiation of INO therapy. (Grade 1A)
9. For newborns with a response to INO therapy, the dose should be weaned to the lowest dose that maintains that response. (Grade 1A)
10. It is recommended that INO should not be discontinued until there is an appreciable clinical improvement, that the INO dose should be weaned to 1 ppm before an attempt is made to discontinue, and that FiO_2 should be increased before discontinuation of INO therapy. (Grade 1A)
11. INO delivery systems approved by the U.S. Food and Drug Administration should be used to ensure consistent and safe gas delivery during therapy. (Grade 1C)
12. During conventional mechanical ventilation, the INO gas injector module should be placed on the dry side of the humidifier. (Grade 2C)
13. During conventional ventilation, the sampling port should be placed in the inspiratory limb of the ventilator, downstream from the site of injection, no greater than 15 cm proximal to the patient connection/interface. (Grade 2C)
14. FiO_2 should be measured downstream from the injection of INO into the circuit. (Grade 2C)
15. The patient-ventilator system should be continuously monitored for changes in ventilation parameters, with adjustments to maintain desired settings during INO therapy. (Grade 2C)
16. The lowest effective doses of INO and O_2 should be used to avoid excessive exposure to nitric oxide, nitrogen dioxide (NO_2), and methemoglobinemia. (Grade 2C)
17. The INO delivery system should be properly purged before use to minimize inadvertent exposure to NO_2. (Grade 2C)
18. The high NO_2 alarm should be set at 2 ppm on the delivery system to prevent toxic gas exposure to the lungs. (Grade 2C)
19. Methemoglobin should be monitored approximately 8 hours and 24 hours after therapy initiation and daily thereafter. (Grade 2C)
20. The INO dose should be weaned or discontinued if methemoglobin increases to >5%. (Grade 2C)
21. It is suggested that continuous pulse oximetry and hemodynamic monitoring be used to assess patient response to INO therapy. (Grade 2C)
22. Scavenging of exhaled and unused gases during INO therapy is *not* necessary. (Grade 2C)

**For complete guideline, see DiBlasi RM, Myers TR, Hess DR: Evidence based clinical practice guideline: inhaled nitric oxide for neonates with acute hypoxic respiratory failure. Respir Care 55:1741, 2010.*

meconium aspiration syndrome, sepsis, and, to a lesser extent, congenital diaphragmatic hernia. However, advances in newborn medicine, such as surfactant replacement therapy, approaches to mechanical ventilation, and INO, have greatly reduced the need for ECMO in this population. ECMO has become an important adjunct in the management of patients with cardiac failure as a bridge to heart transplantation, during resuscitative efforts, and in perioperative management of patients with complex congenital heart disease. ECMO has also been used to support pediatric patients with severe respiratory failure. Although the criteria for neonatal ECMO are well established, the criteria for pediatric patients are not well defined. Box 48-14 outlines criteria for newborns. ECMO is highly invasive and associated with numerous complications. Bleeding and clot formation are two major concerns. As blood circulates through the ECMO circuit, it comes in contact with a foreign surface. The normal response to this contact is for blood to form clots. To minimize clot formation, the patient receives significant doses of anticoagulant and is at risk for bleeding. Frequent monitoring of the patient's coagulation status is essential. Mechanical failures of the

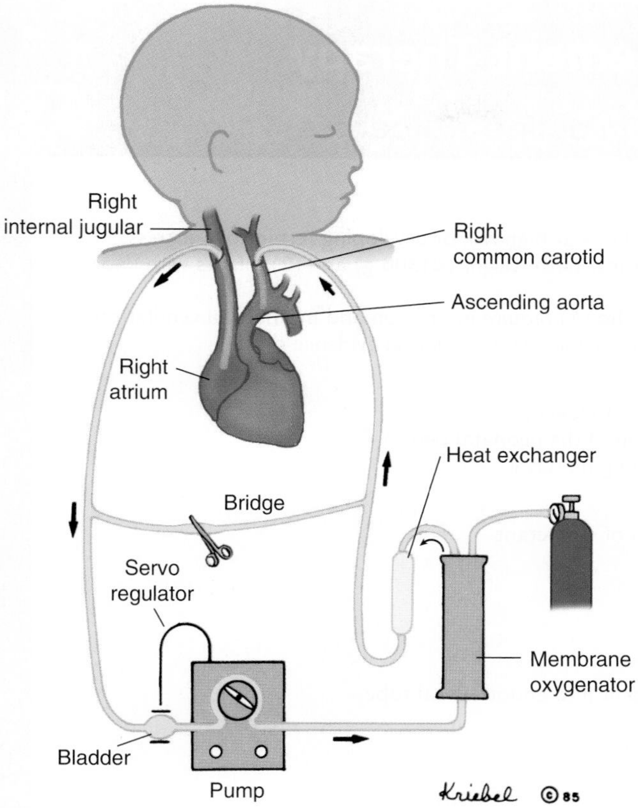

FIGURE 48-11 Venoarterial ECMO circuit. Venous blood is removed from the right atrium, oxygenated by passage thru a diffusing membrane, and then returned to the patient. (Modified from O'Rourke PP: Respir Care 36:7, 1991).

system are also risks associated with ECMO support. Successful outcome is related to the reversibility of the patient's underlying condition and minimizing the complications during the ECMO course.

The AARC has published a clinical practice guideline on surfactant replacement therapy. Excerpts from this guideline appear in Clinical Practice Guideline 48-4.

NEONATAL AND PEDIATRIC TRANSPORT

Treatment of a critically ill infant or child is usually provided at a tertiary care facility. Many of these facilities have established transport teams and go to the referring facility, initiate ICU-type support, and transport the patient back to the tertiary care center. The composition of transport teams varies from one institution to another; however, typical team members include some combination of registered nurse, RT, paramedic, nurse practitioner, and physician. Regardless of the composition of the team, there are some characteristics that all transport teams should have in common.[71] All members should have exquisite assessment and critical thinking skills. They should be technically adept and have good communication skills. Each team develops minimum criteria that a team member must possess. Many teams cross-train in multiple disciplines to perform certain technical tasks. Establishing proficiency and maintaining proficiency with all skills is a must for team members.

The team essentially functions as an extension of the ICU. To do this, much of the same equipment used in the

Box 48-13 Advantages and Disadvantages of Venovenous and Venoarterial Support

ADVANTAGES OF VENOVENOUS SUPPORT
- No carotid ligation
- Using double-lumen cannula, only single-vessel cannulation
- Better coronary O_2
- Decreased risk of air embolization
- Pulsatile flow maintained

DISADVANTAGES OF VENOVENOUS SUPPORT
- No cardiac support
- Recirculation
- Cannula position critical
- Achieve SaO_2 of 80%-90%
- Higher circuit pressures

ADVANTAGES OF VENOARTERIAL SUPPORT
- Provides circulatory support
- Achieves SpO_2 of 90%-100%
- No recirculation
- Less ventilator support required

DISADVANTAGES OF VENOARTERIAL SUPPORT
- Carotid ligation likely
- Increased risk of air embolization
- Decreased coronary O_2
- Loss of pulsatile flow

Box 48-14 Extracorporeal Life Support Organization Guidelines for Neonatal Extracorporeal Membrane Oxygenation

INDICATIONS
- OI = Mean airway pressure × FiO_2 × 100
- Postductal PaO_2
- OI = 20, consider ECLS; OI = 40, ECLS indicated

CONTRAINDICATIONS
- Lethal chromosomal disorder
- Irreversible brain damage
- Grade III or greater intraventricular hemorrhage

RELATIVE CONTRAINDICATIONS
- Irreversible organ damage (unless considered for organ transplant)
- Weight <2 kg and <34 weeks' postmenstrual age because of increased incidence of increased intracranial hemorrhage
- Disease states with a high probability of poor prognosis

48-4 Surfactant Replacement Therapy

AARC Clinical Practice Guideline (Excerpts)*

INDICATIONS

- Prophylactic surfactant administration is indicated in (1) infants at high risk of developing respiratory distress syndrome (RDS) because of short gestation (<32 weeks) or low birth weight (<1300 g) and (2) infants with known surfactant deficiency
- Rescue therapy is indicated in preterm or full-term infants who (1) require intubation and mechanical ventilation secondary to increased work of breathing and O_2 requirements and (2) have clinical evidence of RDS

CONTRAINDICATIONS

Relative contraindications to surfactant administration are the following:
- Presence of congenital anomalies incompatible with life beyond the neonatal period
- Respiratory distress in infants with laboratory evidence of lung maturity

HAZARDS AND COMPLICATIONS

- Procedural complications resulting from the administration of surfactant
  - Plugging of endotracheal tube by surfactant
  - Administration of surfactant to only one lung
  - Hemoglobin desaturation or need for extra O_2
  - Drug dosing errors
  - Bradycardia secondary to hypoxia
  - Tachycardia secondary to agitation, with reflux of surfactant into endotracheal tube
  - Pharyngeal deposition of surfactant
- Physiologic complications of surfactant replacement therapy
  - Apnea
  - Increased necessity for treatment for PDA
  - Pulmonary hemorrhage
  - Marginal increase in ROP
  - Mucous plugs
  - Barotrauma with increased lung compliance

ASSESSMENT OF NEED

Determine that valid indications are present:
- Assess lung immaturity before prophylactic administration of surfactant (see Contraindications)
- Establish the diagnosis of RDS in the presence of short gestation or low birth weight

ASSESSMENT OF OUTCOME

- Reduction of FiO_2 requirement or work of breathing or both
- Improvement in lung volumes and lung fields as indicated by chest radiograph
- Improvement in pulmonary mechanics (e.g., compliance, airway resistance, V_T, VE, FRC, transpulmonary pressure)
- Reduction in ventilator requirements (PIP, PEEP, Paw)
- Improvement in ratio of arterial to alveolar PO_2 (a/A PO_2), oxygenation index

MONITORING

The following should be monitored as part of surfactant replacement therapy:
- Variables to be monitored during surfactant administration
  - Proper placement of delivery device
  - Position of patient (i.e., head direction)
  - FiO_2 and ventilator settings
  - Chest wall movement
  - Reflux of surfactant into endotracheal tube
  - O_2 saturation by pulse oximetry
  - Heart and respiratory rate, chest expansion, skin color, and vigor
- Variables to be monitored after surfactant administration
  - Arterial blood gases
  - Pulmonary mechanics and volumes
  - Chest radiography
  - Breath sounds
  - Ventilator PIP, PEEP, Paw, FiO_2
  - Blood pressure
  - Heart and respiratory rate, chest expansion, skin color, and vigor

VE, *Minute ventilation.*

**For complete guideline, see American Association for Respiratory Care: Clinical practice guideline: surfactant replacement therapy. Respir Care 39:824, 1994.*

Box 48-15 Equipment and Supplies Needed to Provide Respiratory Care during Neonatal and Pediatric Transport

EQUIPMENT

- Adequate supply of O_2 and compressed air
- Air-O_2 blender
- Mechanical ventilator with circuit
- Manual resuscitator capable of giving 100% O_2 with PEEP
- Noninvasive O_2 monitor (SpO_2 or $PtcO_2$)
- O_2 analyzer
- Airway pressure monitor (electronic or mechanical)
- Electrocardiograph monitor
- Portable suction apparatus
- Laryngoscope handle
- Laryngoscope blades (sizes newborn to adult)
- Extra laryngoscope bulbs and batteries
- Stethoscope

SUPPLIES

- Resuscitation masks (sizes 0, 1, 2, 3, 4)
- Feeding tubes (sizes 6F, 8F, and 10F)
- Disposable O_2 hood
- O_2 connecting tubing
- Disposable hand-held nebulizer with tubing (for bronchodilators)
- Cloth adhesive tape for taping endotracheal tubes
- Tincture of benzoin for taping endotracheal tubes
- Pulse oximeter probes (at least two, in case one fails)
- Endotracheal tubes (sizes 2.5-7)
- Stylet
- Forceps
- Suction apparatus

ICU is taken to the referring hospital. Establishing responsibility for assessing function and maintaining appropriate inventory is essential. Many centers use elaborate checklists to be certain not to be without necessary equipment, disposables, or medications. Teams generally prepare for the worst. Many times when the team arrives at the referring facility, the patient's condition is not the same as when the initial call for help was made. Being prepared for the worst helps in stabilizing the patient for transport. The American Academy of Pediatrics has guidelines for all ages and common conditions requiring transport to a tertiary facility. Box 48-15 lists the basic equipment and supplies needed to provide respiratory care during neonatal and pediatric transport.

RULE OF THUMB

A high-risk transport team must be prepared to provide the same level of care and highly trained personnel as would be available in the ICUs they are transporting patients to and from.

SUMMARY CHECKLIST

- Neonatal and pediatric care is one of the most sophisticated specialty areas in the field of respiratory care. Competent practice in this area requires a firm understanding of the many anatomic and physiologic differences between infants, children, and adults.
- A critical component in the respiratory management of infants and children is thorough clinical assessment. Because of the significant anatomic and physiologic differences between adults and infants, many of the assessment techniques useful with adults do not apply to infants.
- General assessment of the infant begins before birth and involves the maternal history and the fetal and newborn status. As a child grows and develops, more of the assessment methods used with adults become applicable.
- Respiratory care plan development is based on accurate patient information, detailed knowledge of the disease process, and current treatment guidelines and recommendations.
- Respiratory care modalities can provide O_2, aerosol and humidity, airway care, and mechanical ventilation to neonates.
- CPAP is commonly used in neonates to overcome atelectasis and oxygenation problems.
- Using high-flow nasal cannulas in neonates may result in the delivery of higher than expected levels of CPAP.
- Noninvasive ventilation has become an acceptable choice of ventilation for neonates.
- Improved design of nasal masks and nasal prongs should help prevent the development of pressure ulcers during CPAP and noninvasive ventilation in neonates.
- For mechanically ventilated patients, plateau pressure should be not exceed 30 cm H_2O.
- V_T should be maintained between 6 ml/kg and 8 ml/kg.
- Compressible volume loss may account for a significant portion of the small V_T used for infants and small children.
- Most infants and children can be managed with conventional ventilation; however, HFV is an acceptable alternative for specific diseases.
- Mechanically ventilated infants and children should be assessed daily for readiness for liberation from mechanical ventilation.
- Nitric oxide is now considered standard therapy for the management of term infants who present with PPHN and should be available in all level III neonatal ICUs.
- ECMO is useful in the management of severely ill infants who do not respond to other forms of respiratory care.
- Surfactant replacement has become the standard of care for preterm (gestation <32 weeks) or low birth weight infants (<1300 g) and infants with known surfactant deficiency.
- Highly specialized transport teams are available to transport newborn and pediatric patients to tertiary care facilities.

References

1. American Association of Pediatrics: Guidelines for cardiopulmonary resuscitation and emergency cardiovascular care. Pediatrics 126:e1400, 2010.
2. Dubowitz LMS, Dubowitz D, Goldberg C: Clinical assessment of gestational age in the newborn infant. J Pediatr 77:110, 1970.
3. Shenoi A, Narang A, Bhakoo ON, et al: Clinical profile and management of symptomatic patent ductus arteriosus in premature newborns. Ind J Pediatr 28:125, 1991.
4. Carlo WA, Martin RJ, Bruce EN, et al: Alae nasi activation (nasal flaring) decreases nasal resistance in preterm infants. Pediatrics 72:338, 1983.
5. Engle WA; American Academy of Pediatrics Committee on Fetus and Newborn: Surfactant-replacement therapy for respiratory distress in the preterm and term neonate. Pediatrics 121:419, 2008.
6. Courtney SE, Weber KR, Breakie LA, et al: Capillary blood gases in the neonate: a reassessment and review of the literature. Am J Dis Child 144:168, 1990.
7. American Association for Respiratory Care: Clinical practice guideline: infant/toddler pulmonary function tests. Respir Care 40:761, 1995.
8. American Association for Respiratory Care: Clinical practice guideline. Oxygen therapy in the acute care hospital. Respir Care Clin North Am 36:1410, 1991.
9. Walsh M: Oxygen therapy through nasal cannula to preterm infants: can practice be improved. Pediatrics 116:857, 2005.
10. Chow LC, Wright KW, Sola A: Can changes in clinical practice decrease the incidence of severe retinopathy of prematurity in very low birth weight infants? Pediatrics 111:339, 2003.
11. Minghua L, Chen H, Guo L: High or low oxygen saturation and severe retinopathy of prematurity: a meta-analysis. Pediatrics 125:e1483, 2010.
12. Perrotta C, Ortiz Z, Roque M: Chest physiotherapy for acute bronchiolitis in pediatric patients between 0 and 24 months old. Cochrane Database Syst Rev (1):CD004873, 2007.
13. Hess DR: The evidence for secretion clearance techniques. Respir Care 46:1276, 2001.
14. Mahlmeister MJ, Fink JB, Hoffman GL, et al: Positive expiratory pressure mask therapy: theoretical and practical considerations and a review of the literature. Respir Care Clin N Am 36:1218, 1991.
15. Emergency Care Research Institute: Heated wires can melt disposable breathing circuits. Health Devices 18:174, 1989.
16. Levy H, Simpson Q, Duval D: Hazards of humidifiers with heated wires. Crit Care Med 21:477, 1993.
17. Mellon M, Leflein B, Walton-Bowen C, et al: Comparable efficacy of administration with face mask or mouthpiece of nebulized budesonide inhalation suspension for infants and young children with persistent asthma. Am J Respir Crit Care Med 162:593, 2000.
18. Cole CH: Special problems in aerosol delivery: neonatal and pediatric considerations. Respir Care 45:646, 2000.
19. Veldman A, Trautschold T, Weib K, et al: Characteristics and outcome of unplanned extubation in ventilated preterm and term newborns on a neonatal intensive care unit. Pediatr Anesth 16:968, 2006.
20. McMillan DD, Rademaker AW, Buchan KA, et al: Benefits of orotracheal and nasotracheal intubation in neonates requiring ventilatory assistance. Pediatrics 77:39, 1986.
21. Black AE, Hatch DJ, Nauth-Misir N: Complications of tracheal intubation in neonates, infants and children: a review of 4 years' experience in a children's hospital. Br J Anaesth 65:461, 1990.
22. Roopchand R, Roopnarinesingh S, Ramsewak S: Instability of the tracheal tube in neonates: a postmortem study. Anaesthesia 44:107, 1989.
23. Brown MS: Prevention of accidental extubation in newborns. Am J Dis Child 142:1240, 1988.
24. Prendiville A, Thomson A, Silverman M: Effect of tracheobronchial suction on respiratory resistance in intubated preterm babies. Arch Dis Child 61:1178, 1986.
25. Gardner D, Shirland L: Neonatal evidence-based guideline for suctioning the intubated neonate and infant. Neonatal Netw 28:281–302, 2009.
26. Shah AR, Kurth CD, Gwiazdowski B, et al: Fluctuations in cerebral oxygenation and blood volume during endotracheal suctioning in premature infants. J Pediatr 120:769, 1992.
27. Kalyn A, Blatz S, Feuerstake S, et al: Closed suctioning of intubated neonates maintains better physiologic stability: a randomized trial. J Perinatol 23:218–222, 2003.
28. El Masry A, Williams PF, Chipman DW, et al: The impact of closed endotracheal suctioning systems on mechanical ventilator performance. Respir Care 50:345–353, 2005.
29. American Association for Respiratory Care: Clinical practice guideline: application of continuous positive airway pressure to neonates via nasal prongs, nasopharyngeal tune, nasal mask: 2004 revision and update. Respir Care 49:1100, 2004.
30. Juretschke R, Spoula R: High flow nasal cannula in the neonatal population. Neonatal Intensive Care 17:20, 2004.
31. Sreenan C, Lemke RP, Hudson-Mason A, et al: High-flow nasal cannulae in the management of apnea of prematurity: a comparison with conventional nasal continuous positive airway pressure. Pediatrics 107:1081, 2001.
32. Locke RG, Wolfson MR, Shaffer TH, et al: Inadvertent administration of positive end-distending pressure during nasal cannula flow. Pediatrics 91:135, 1993.
33. Waugh JB, Granger WM: An evaluation of 2 new devices for high-flow gas therapy. Respir Care 49:902, 2004.
34. Sreenan C, Lemke RP, Hudson-Mason A, et al: High-flow nasal cannulae in the management of apnea of prematurity: a comparison with nasal continuous positive airway pressure. Pediatrics 107:1081–1083, 2001.
35. Holleman-Duray D, Kaupie D, Weiss M: Heated humidified high-flow nasal cannula: use and a neonatal early extubation protocol. J Perinatol 27:772–775, 2007.
36. Marchese AD, Chipman D, de le Oliva P, et al: Adult ICU ventilators to provide neonatal ventilation: a lung simulator study. Intensive Care Med 35:631, 2009.
37. Donn SM, Sinha SK: Invasive and noninvasive neonatal mechanical ventilation. Respir Care 48:426, 2003.
38. Cheifetz IM: Invasive and noninvasive pediatric mechanical ventilation. Respir Care 48:442, 2003.
39. Cannon ML, Cornell J, Tripp-Hamel DS, et al: Tidal volumes for ventilated infants should be determined with a pneumotachometer placed at the endotracheal tube. Am J Respir Crit Care Med 162:2109, 2000.
40. Mehta NM, Arnold JH: Mechanical ventilation in children with acute respiratory failure. Curr Opin Crit Care 10:7, 2004.
41. Greenough A, Milner AD, Dimitriou G: Synchronized mechanical ventilation for respiratory support in newborn infants. Cochrane Database Syst Rev (3):CD000456, 2005.
42. Kapasi M, Fujino Y, Kirmse M, et al: Effort and work of breathing in neonates during assisted patient-triggered ventilation. Pediatr Crit Care Med 2:9, 2001.
43. American Association for Respiratory Care: Clinical practice guideline: neonatal time-triggered, pressure-limited, time-cycled mechanical ventilation. Respir Care 39:808, 1994.
44. Mrozek JD, Bendel-Stenzel EM, Meyers PA, et al: Randomized controlled trial of volume-targeted synchronized

ventilation and conventional intermittent ventilation following initial exogenous surfactant therapy. Pediatr Pulmonol 29:11, 2000.
45. Cheema IU, Ahluwailia JS: Feasibility of tidal volume-guided ventilation in newborn infants: a randomized, crossover trial using the volume guaranteed modality. Pediatrics 107:1323, 2001.
46. Bhandari V, Finer NN, Ehrenkranz RA, et al: Synchronized nasal intermittent positive-pressure ventilation and neonatal outcomes. Pediatrics 124:517, 2009.
47. Hess DR: The evidence for non-invasive positive-pressure ventilation in the care of patients in acute respiratory failure: a systematic review of the literature. Respir Care 49:810, 2004.
48. Hess DR: Noninvasive ventilation in neuromuscular disease: equipment and application. Respir Care 51:896, 2006.
49. Panitch HB: Respiratory issues in the management of children with neuromuscular disease. Respir Care 51:885, 2006.
50. Padman R, Lawless ST, Kettrick RG: Noninvasive ventilation via bilevel positive airway support in pediatric practice. Crit Care Med 26:169, 1998.
51. Nilsestuen JO, Hargett KD: Using airway graphics to identify patient-ventilator asynchrony. Respir Care 50:202, 2005.
52. Wilson BG: Using airway graphics to optimize mechanical ventilation in neonates with respiratory distress syndrome. Neonatal Netw 16:71, 1997.
53. AARC Clinical Practice Guideline: Patient-ventilator system checks. Respir Care 37:882, 1992.
54. Randolph AG; Pediatric Acute Lung Injury and Sepsis Investigators Network: Effects of mechanical ventilator weaning protocols on respiratory outcomes in infants and children. JAMA 288:2561, 2002.
55. Henderson-Smart DJ, Bhuta T, Cools F: Elective high frequency oscillatory ventilation versus conventional ventilation for acute pulmonary dysfunction in preterm infants. Cochrane Database Syst Rev (3):CD000104, 2005.
56. Bhuta T, Henderson-Smart DJ: Elective high frequency jet ventilation versus conventional ventilation for respiratory distress syndrome in preterm infants. Cochrane Database Syst Rev (3):CD000328, 2005.
57. Arnold JH, Anas NG, Luckett P: High-frequency oscillatory ventilation in pediatric respiratory failure: a multicenter experience. Crit Care Med 28:3913, 2000.
58. Thome UH, Carlo WA, Pohlandt F: Ventilation strategies and outcome in randomized trials of high frequency ventilation. Arch Dis Fetal Neonatal Ed 90:F466, 2005.
59. Courtney SE, Durand DJ, Asselin JM: High-frequency oscillatory ventilation versus conventional ventilation for very-low-birthweight infants. N Engl J Med 347:643, 2002.
60. Grenier B, Thompson J: High-frequency oscillatory ventilation in pediatric patients. Respir Care Clin North Am 2:545, 1996.
61. Bollen CW, Uiterwaal CS, van Vught AJ: Cumulative meta-analysis of high-frequency versus conventional ventilation in premature neonates. Am J Respir Crit Care Med 168:1150, 2003.
62. Ichinose F, Roberts JD, Zapol WM: Inhaled nitric oxide: a selective pulmonary vasodilator: current uses and therapeutic potential. Circulation 109:3106, 2004.
63. Finer NN, Barrington KJ: Nitric oxide for respiratory failure in infants born at term or near term. Cochrane Database Syst Rev (3), 2009.
64. Christou H, VanMarter LJ, Wessel DL, et al: Inhaled nitric oxide reduces the need for extracorporeal membrane oxygenation in infants with persistent pulmonary hypertension of the newborn. Crit Care Med 28:3722, 2000.
65. Guthrie SO, Walsh WF, Clarke RH, et al: Initial dosing of inhaled nitric oxide in infants with hypoxic respiratory failure. J Perinatol 24:387, 2004.
66. Sokol GM, Fineberg NS, Wright LL, et al: Changes in arterial oxygen tension when weaning neonates from inhaled nitric oxide. Pediatr Pulmonol 32:14, 2001.
67. American Academy of Pediatrics Committee on Fetus and Newborn: Use of inhaled nitric oxide. Pediatrics 2:344, 2000.
68. Sebald M, Friedlich P, Burns C, et al: Risk of the need for extracorporeal membrane oxygenation in neonates with congenital diaphragmatic hernia treated with inhaled nitric oxide. J Perinatol 24:143, 2004.
69. DiBlasi RM, Myers TR, Hess DR: Evidence based clinical practice guideline: inhaled nitric oxide for neonates with acute hypoxic respiratory failure. Respir Care 55:1741, 2010.
70. Hansel DR: Extracorporeal membrane oxygenation for perinatal and pediatric patients. Respir Care 48:352, 2003.
71. Waren J, From R, Orr RA, et al: American College of Critical Care Medicine: guidelines for the inter- and intrahospital transport of critically ill patients. Crit Care Med 32:256, 2004.

SECTION VII

PATIENT EDUCATION AND LONG-TERM CARE

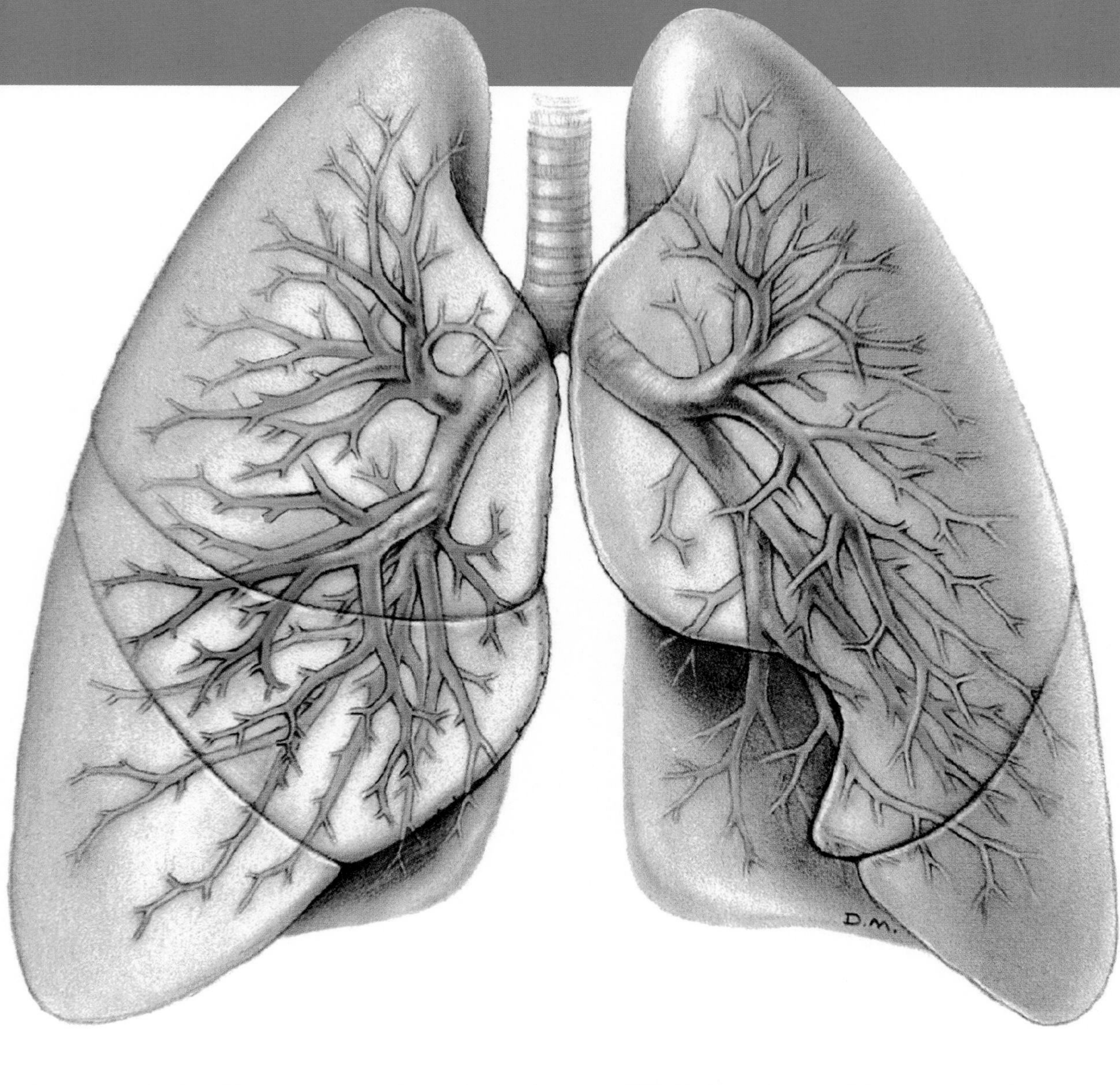

Chapter 49

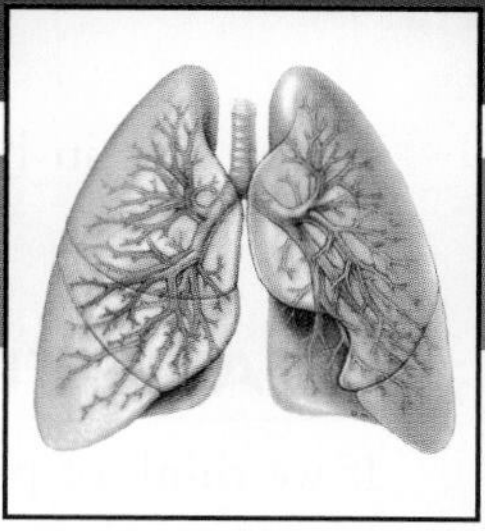

Patient Education and Health Promotion

DONNA D. GARDNER

CHAPTER OBJECTIVES

After reading this chapter you will be able to:
- Write learning objectives in the cognitive, affective, and psychomotor domains.
- Compare and contrast how adults and children learn.
- Describe the methods that are used to evaluate patient education.
- Explain the importance of health education.
- Identify the settings that are appropriate for the implementation of health promotion activities.
- Describe the respiratory therapist's role in a disease management program.

CHAPTER OUTLINE

KEY TERMS

affective domain
cognitive domain
disease management
health education
health promotion
psychomotor domain

Effective health education is invaluable to the health care of society. Respiratory therapists (RTs) educate patients by providing information about disease processes, medications, and treatment procedures. They teach patients how to perform diagnostic tests like basic spirometry, and they educate patients about health promotion issues such as tobacco cessation. RTs educate patients in all age groups, including geriatric, adult, adolescent, and pediatric patients. In certain situations, RTs educate the parents or the spouse of the patient in the home-care setting. RTs are also frequently called on to provide educational programs to patients with asthma and cystic fibrosis.

For these reasons, this chapter reviews important issues related to patient education, disease management, and health promotion.

The top five causes of death in the United States are heart disease, cancer, cerebrovascular disease, chronic obstructive lung disease (i.e., bronchitis and emphysema), and accidents.[1] It is believed by most experts in health care that the majority of these illnesses are preventable. Public education about risk factors is the key to the prevention of these diseases and probably has the greatest potential for making an impact on health care in this country. Therefore, the emphasis in health care should be on health promotion and disease prevention. RTs will play a greater role in health promotion and prevention in the future.

PATIENT EDUCATION

If we think of patient care as customer service—which it indeed is—then we cannot ignore education as a crucial component of that service. Whether we buy a car or a television set, we expect the salesperson to educate us about the essential aspects of our purchase. We also expect this information to be provided in writing. Likewise, education is an essential component of patient care. For patients to assume or resume control of their health, they must be educated. Because they rely on the health care practitioner to provide this education, every respiratory care education program should include instruction regarding patient education.

Performance Objectives

Initially it is helpful for the RT to develop learning objectives that are appropriate for the specific patient education topic to be addressed. These learning objectives will help to clarify the teaching strategies that are needed for patient education sessions. Objectives should be stated in measurable terms so that the RT and the patient can recognize when the objective has been accomplished. Clear objectives describe what is to be accomplished and how evaluation will occur.

The format for writing an objective is as follows:

1. Begin with the phrase, "At the end of the lesson, the patient will . . . ."
2. Write the action verb (e.g., "list," "describe," "demonstrate").
3. Write a condition, if needed (e.g., with or without the use of notes).
4. Write a standard, if needed (e.g., how fast, how accurate).

For example: At the end of the session, the patient will be given a metered-dose inhaler and spacer and be able to demonstrate the correct technique for using the metered-dose inhaler in 5 minutes or less.

Action verb: "demonstrate" (from the psychomotor domain; the relevant domains are discussed later in this chapter)

Condition: "given a metered-dose inhaler and spacer"

Standard: "in 5 minutes or less"

Learning Domains

Learning occurs in three domains: **cognitive, psychomotor,** and **affective.** Some learning sessions will involve only one domain, whereas others may involve all three. The cognitive domain is very important, because it will address the knowledge that a patient needs regarding his or her illness and how to manage it. The psychomotor domain addresses the skills that the patient will need to acquire to perform specific treatment modalities (e.g., the use of metered-dose inhalers). The affective domain involves teaching patients about the necessary attitudes and motivations for successfully living with their diseases.

MINI CLINI

Developing Learning Objectives for the Use of an Albuterol Metered-Dose Inhaler

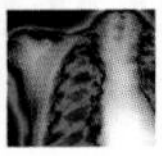

PROBLEM: Your 31-year-old patient is newly diagnosed with asthma, and she is being discharged tomorrow. She requires instruction regarding how to properly use her albuterol metered-dose inhaler. Develop learning objectives for her, and address each learning domain.

SOLUTION: Use a variety of learning objectives, including the following:

Cognitive domain: Describe the action of albuterol on the bronchial smooth muscle; recognize when it is necessary to seek medical attention.

Affective domain: Agree that it is important not to skip a dose; verbalize willingness to use the metered-dose inhaler; feel satisfaction by controlling the disease.

Psychomotor domain: Demonstrate the ability to assemble the metered-dose inhaler and spacer; inhale slowly and deeply with an inspiratory hold.

Cognitive Domain

The cognitive domain is probably the easiest to translate into learning objectives because it involves the facts and concepts that the RT wants the patient to know and apply by the end of the education session. Objectives for the cognitive domain might include the following:

1. List the indications for oxygen therapy.
2. Discuss the importance of using the prescribed liter flow.
3. Explain the relationship between oxygen and combustion.

Any factual information that you expect the patient to understand and apply falls under the cognitive domain. Action verbs for the cognitive domain are included in Table 49-1.[2]

Psychomotor Domain

Repetition and active involvement are important when teaching a psychomotor skill. RTs who teach new skills to patients need to provide plenty of opportunity for the patient to practice the activity. Simple demonstration of the skill to the patient is not enough. To confirm performance in the psychomotor domain, have your patients provide a return demonstration. Be sure to provide help and encouragement as needed. Be patient; not everyone develops skills at the same rate.

Examples of action verbs for the psychomotor domain are included in Table 49-2.[2]

TABLE 49-1
Verbs for the Cognitive Domain

Purpose	Example Verbs
1. Knowledge	Cite, define, read, identify, list, label, name, outline, recognize, select, state
2. Comprehension	Convert, describe, defend, explain, illustrate, interpret, give examples of, predict, paraphrase, summarize, translate
3. Application	Apply, compute, construct, demonstrate, change, calculate, use, estimate, modify, present, prepare, solve, proceed, relate, utilize
4. Analysis	Analyze, associate, compare, contrast, determine, diagram, differentiate, discriminate, distinguish, outline, illustrate, separate
5. Synthesis	Categorize, combine, compile, compose, create, design, develop, devise, integrate, modify, organize, plan, propose, rearrange, reorganize, revise, rewrite, translate, write
6. Evaluation	Appraise, assess, compare, conclude, contrast, critique, discriminate, make a decision, support, evaluate, judge, weigh

Modified from French D, Olrech N, Hale C, et al: Blended learning: an ongoing process for Internet integration, Victoria, Canada, 2003, Trafford Publishing.

TABLE 49-2
Verbs for the Psychomotor Domain

Purpose	Example Verbs
1. Perception: prepares and recognizes sensory cues to want to respond	Detect, distinguish, differentiate, identify, isolate, relate, recognize, observe, perceive, see, watch
2. Ready to act and respond	Begin, explain, move, react, show, state, establish a body position, place, posture, assume a stance, sit, stand, position
3. Guided response: imitate and practice; rough sequencing of events	Copy, duplicate, imitate, manipulate, operate, try, practice, dismantle
4. Efficiency: smooth sequencing of events	Assemble, calibrate, construct, display, fasten, fix, grind, manipulate, measure, mix, sketch, demonstrate, execute, increase speed, improve, make, show dexterity, pace, produce
5. Perform alone: modifies, responds as needed	Act habitually, advance confidently, control, excel, guide, manage, master, organize, perform quickly and more accurately
6. Creates a new or original model	Adapt, alter, rearrange, reorganize, revise

Modified from French D, Olrech N, Hale C, et al: Blended learning: an ongoing process for Internet integration, Victoria, Canada, 2003, Trafford Publishing.

RULE OF THUMB

People learn by doing. Get the learner involved.

Affective Domain

The patient's attitudes and motivations influence his or her ability to learn. It is important to remember that, with patient education, timing is everything. Patients who have recently been given a poor prognosis or who are in pain are not in an optimal position to learn. Maslow suggested a hierarchy of needs, and he identified physiologic needs as the most basic of human needs, followed by safety, love, esteem, and self-actualization.[3] Lower-level needs must first be satisfied before moving on to higher-level needs. For example, if a patient is dyspneic or in pain, he or she will probably not be receptive to learning the steps that are involved in cleaning a small-volume nebulizer. It is important for RTs to assess a patient's readiness to learn by talking with the patient and his or her family and by listening to the patient's concerns. It is important to develop a relationship of trust and to be empathetic with the patient.

The RT should begin with easy-to-master facts and skills. After the patient conquers these, motivation should increase, and the patient will have a feeling of accomplishment. Motivation is also enhanced by presenting material clearly with the use of a variety of teaching methods and by relating the facts and skills to practical applications. Getting patients to see how these skills will benefit them is the key to motivation. Communicating to the patient that there is something that he or she can do to maintain or improve his or her health and sense of well-being is important.

Objectives in the affective domain—using the oxygen therapy example mentioned earlier—might include the following:

1. Demonstrate genuine concern for yourself by using your oxygen therapy correctly.
2. Demonstrate a willingness to learn by being an active participant in the program.

Affective domain action verbs are included in Table 49-3.[2]

Teaching Tips

Following is a list of time-honored suggestions for improving patient education:

- Address the patient's immediate concerns first.
- Create an optimal learning environment. Teach in a quiet and relaxed setting.
- Have patients use as many of their senses as possible during their learning session. Whenever possible, include hearing, seeing, smelling, speaking, touching, and doing.
- Keep sessions short. If the material is complex, break it down into brief segments.
- Repeat, repeat, repeat!

TABLE 49-3

Verbs for the Affective Domain

Purpose	Example Verbs
1. Receive: becoming aware of	Accept, acknowledge, alert, choose, give, attend, notice, perceive, tolerate, select
2. Respond: interested in or doing something about something	Agree, assist with, aid, answer, assist, comply, conform, communicate, consent, label, obey, cooperate, follow, read, report, visit, volunteer, study
3. Value: concerned about, developing an attitude	Adopt, assume, behave, choose, demonstrate, commit, desire, initiate, join, exhibit, express, prefer, seek, share
4. Organize: arranging systematically, confirming	Adapt, adjust, arrange, classify, conceptualize, group, rank, validate, verify, strengthen, substantiate, corroborate, confirm
5. Characterize: internalizing a set of values, championing	Demonstrate a change in lifestyle, discriminate, defend, influence, invite, listen, preach, qualify, question, serve, act upon, advocate, devote, expose, justify, support

Modified from French D, Olrech N, Hale C, et al: Blended learning: an ongoing process for Internet integration, Victoria, Canada, 2003, Trafford Publishing.

Box 49-1 Learning Differences Between Children and Adults

CHILD
- Motivated by external factors like grades
- Directed by others
- Learning is a big part of his or her life
- Trusts teacher
- Has limited experience
- Learns for the future
- Learns quickly
- Tends to learn in accordance with his or her developmental stage
- Has no problem with a slow pace of learning
- Subject oriented

ADULT
- Motivated internally
- Is self-directed
- Learning is only one part of his or her life
- Questions the teacher
- Has rich life experiences
- Learns for the present
- May learn more slowly
- Varies with regard to learning ability
- Dislikes a slow pace of learning
- Problem oriented

- Provide many opportunities for the patient to practice psychomotor skills.
- Be prepared.
- Be organized. People learn more quickly when they are presented with information that is well organized.
- Demonstrate enthusiasm for what you are doing. The learner can always sense your level of motivation.
- Evaluate in a nonthreatening manner, and provide helpful feedback. Use evaluation as a learning tool.

Teaching Children As Compared With Teaching Adults

Teaching children is often very different than teaching adults. Children are more motivated by external factors (e.g., prizes) as compared with adults, who tend to have internal motivating factors. This suggests that adults will learn quicker if they can easily see the intrinsic value of knowing more about their illness. Alternatively, children may need a more obvious reward system in place before learning can take place. They have no problem taking instruction from adults, because they are often dependent on such instruction. Adults, however, are more independent, and they do not like being dependent on others. This suggests that adults should be more involved in setting program goals and that they will readily learn skills that make them more independent. Other important issues related to differences between children and adult learners are listed in Box 49-1, and allocated time for teaching is given by age in Box 49-2.[4]

Box 49-2 Attention Spans for Different Ages

- Toddlers: about 2 to 3 minutes
- School-aged children: about 10 to 15 minutes
- Adolescents and adults: about 20 to 30 minutes

Evaluation of Patient Education

The critical question that remains when all of the patient education sessions are complete is, "Has the patient learned?" Evaluation is the process that answers that question. The method used to evaluate learning is determined by the measurable learning objectives (i.e., cognitive, affective, or psychomotor). Cognitive objectives are often evaluated with the use of a written examination. Objectives in the affective and psychomotor domains are evaluated with the use of performance checklists.

Informal evaluation should occur during the educational process. The RT can ask simple questions along the way to identify whether the patient has comprehended the information. If the patient provides an answer that is not correct, the RT should view this as an opportunity to repeat previous discussions or to present the material with a new approach. The RT must never convey disappointment or frustration when patients are having trouble learning new material.

MINI CLINI

Metered-Dose Inhaler Instruction for a Pediatric Patient

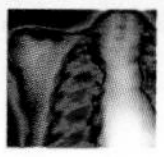

PROBLEM: How would you change the approach to the metered-dose inhaler situation described in the previous Mini Clini if your patient was a 7-year-old boy with asthma?

SOLUTION: Although the learning objectives may remain the same, the methods may be different. You may compare the slow, deep inspiration to getting ready to blow out the candles on a birthday cake. You may use swimming under water as an image to encourage breath holding. Use simple diagrams to show how the medication will act on the patient's lungs. If he likes sports, tell him about athletes who compete well despite having asthma (you may also use this illustration to stress the importance of controlling asthma). An abundance of resource materials are available for children with asthma; make use of them. Many local, state, and national lung associations (www.ala.org) offer such learning aids as age-appropriate books, coloring books, and puppets to make the learning process more fun for children.

RULE OF THUMB

Evaluation results reflect the quality of instruction as much as the degree of learning.

HEALTH EDUCATION

Health education may have been the earliest form of organized health promotion in the United States. Health programs in schools may be the result of Lemuel Shattuck's report in 1850 to the Sanitary Commission of Massachusetts, which described the value of schools helping to contain communicable diseases. However, it was not until 1875 that health education became widespread. During that year, the Women's Christian Temperance Union lobbied for alcohol education in the schools. As a result of these efforts, 38 states passed legislation to require this education, which later turned into tobacco, alcohol, and drug education. From that time, health education has been enhanced and expanded in schools. There are public health agencies at the local, state, national, and international levels that provide health education and care for those who would otherwise have none.

Health education is a process of planned learning that is designed to enable individuals to make informed decisions and to take responsible actions regarding their health. The primary goal of health education is behavior change, and it is designed to promote, maintain, and improve both individual and community health. Health education covers the continuum between health and disease and between prevention and treatment.

Box 49-3 American Association for Respiratory Care Health Promotion and Disease Prevention Statement

HEALTH PROMOTION AND DISEASE PREVENTION

- The AARC acknowledges that respiratory therapists in both the civilian and uniformed/military services are integral members of the health care team, in hospitals, home health care settings, pulmonary laboratories, rehabilitation programs and all other environments (including ICUs and critical care transport) where respiratory care is practiced.
- The AARC recognizes that education and training of the respiratory therapist is the best method by which to instill the ability to improve the patient's quality and longevity of life, and that such information should be included in their formal education and training in CoARC accredited programs.
- The AARC recognizes the respiratory therapist's responsibility to participate in pulmonary disease teaching, smoking cessation programs, pulmonary function studies for the public, air pollution alerts, allergy warnings, and sulfite warnings in restaurants, as well as research in those and other areas where efforts could promote improved health and disease prevention. Furthermore, the respiratory therapist is in a unique position to provide leadership in determining health promotion and disease prevention activities for students, faculty, practitioners, patients, and the general public in both civilian and uniformed service environments.
- The AARC recognizes the need to 1) provide and promote consumer education related to the prevention and control of pulmonary disease; 2) establish a strong working relationship with other health agencies, educational institutions, Federal and state government, businesses, military and other community organizations; and 3) monitor such activities. Furthermore, the AARC supports efforts to develop personal and professional wellness models and action plans that will inspire and encourage all respiratory therapists to cooperate on health promotion and cardiorespiratory disease prevention.

Effective 1985
Revised 2000
Revised 2005

From the American Association for Respiratory Care: *Position statement* (website): www.aarc.org/resources/position_statements/rms.html.

Health promotion helps people change their lifestyles in a variety of settings, from the home or school to the workplace or the health care agency or institution. To be effective, health education must be combined with strategies for health promotion; the two are strongly linked. The American Association for Respiratory Care has created a statement for health promotion and disease prevention (Box 49-3).[5]

Although individuals must ultimately assume responsibility for their own health, promoting healthy behaviors

49-1 Providing Patient and Caregiver Training

AARC Clinical Practice Guideline (Excerpts)*

American Association for Respiratory Care Clinical Practice Guideline (Excerpts)* updated June of 2010. www.rcjournal.com/cpgs/pdf/06.10.0765.pdf

■ INDICATIONS

Patients who need to increase knowledge and understanding of health status and therapy; improve skills needed for safe and effective health care; and develop a positive attitude, strong motivation, and increased compliance. Patients need to know the answers to "Ask Me 3": What is my main problem? What do I need to do? Why is it important for me to do this?

■ CONTRAINDICATIONS

None.

■ COMPLICATIONS

Omission of essential steps concerning care, presentation of inconsistent information, or failure to validate the learning process can lead to unfavorable results. Lack of cultural competence, and information appropriate in the language other than English will result in less than desirable outcomes. Lack of trust.

■ LIMITATIONS

- For the patient: Lack of motivation; impairment (physical, mental, or emotional); inability to understand instruction; illiteracy; language barriers; religious and/or cultural beliefs that are at odds with the material presented. Lack of health literacy, despite educational completed and conflicts of religious and/or cultural practices.
- For the RT: Lack of a positive attitude or flexibility; limited knowledge of skill being taught; inadequate assessment of patient's readiness to learn; cultural or religious practices that may affect learning; inability to personalize the material; insufficient time; inadequate communication skills, and inadequate knowledge of cultural or religious practice.
- For the system: Hospital stay too brief; lack of interdisciplinary communication and/or cooperation; inconsistent information presented; lack of an interpreter.
- Other factors: Lack of support system for the patient; reimbursement issues; interruptions, distractions, or noise; inadequate lighting, heat, or space; poorly chosen resources including inappropriate reading level and vocabulary.

■ ASSESSMENT OF NEED

Determine the knowledge gap between what the patient knows and what he or she needs to know. Apply this to cognitive, psychomotor, and affective domains.

■ ASSESSMENT OF OUTCOME

Evaluate knowledge gained, skills mastered, patient should return demonstration without assistance, reassess patient outlook, attitude and life style changes.

■ RESOURCES

Access trained interpreters, ensure the written materials are readable at a fifth or sixth grade level, materials should be available in variety of formats (audio and visual), use demonstration models, reevaluate the skills.

■ MONITORING

The monitoring of the training processes should include awareness of the patient's verbal and nonverbal responses, including eye contact, listening skills, and participation in discussion.

**For the complete guideline, see the American Association for Respiratory Care: AARC Clinical Practice Guidelines. Providing patient and caregiver training 2010. Respir Care 55(6):765-769, 2010.*

through education is an important part of being an RT. In this capacity, the RT should serve as a role model for the public. Unless health care professionals model healthy behaviors, successful health outcomes cannot be expected from the public. To this end, the American Association for Respiratory Care has created a role-model statement to encourage RTs to set a positive example for the public (Box 49-4).[6]

Providing a good example is not enough to ensure successful health education programming. For the desired outcomes to be achieved, certain conditions must first be met. The components are remarkably similar to patient education requirements. The essential components of effective health education are as follows:

1. Program participants must be actively engaged in the learning process.

49-2 Training of the Health Care Professional (HCP) for the Role of Patient and Caregiver Educator

AARC Clinical Practice Guideline (Excerpts)*

American Association for Respiratory Care Clinical Practice Guideline (Excerpts)*

INDICATIONS

- HCPs who must educate patients and caregivers about knowledge, skills, and motivation necessary to effectively participate in health care
- Evidence that HCPs lack the knowledge about educational principles and practices needed to:
  - Assess educational needs
  - Prepare educational objectives tailored to individuals or groups
  - Accomplish learning objectives
  - Prepare educational materials
  - Supervise practice of skills
  - Give feedback and assess outcomes
  - Modify educational efforts according to individual or group response

CONTRAINDICATIONS

None.

COMPLICATIONS

Inadequate training of the HCP may cause harm to the patient or inhibit the patient's ability to participate in the management of his or her own health.

LIMITATIONS

- Of the HCP: Lack of educational preparation; unreceptive or inept; lack of interdisciplinary cooperation; inability to modify learning objectives based on age, culture, or religion; inability to communicate effectively
- Of the system: Inadequate time, space, or financial resources; insufficient faculty for training program; inconsistent information provided to the HCP
- Of the patient or caregiver: Negative attitude; lack of basic education; presence of a language barrier or perception of cultural conflict

ASSESSMENT OF NEED

HCPs who provide education should be periodically assessed for adequate knowledge and skills by observation in a patient education setting and by a specialist.

ASSESSMENT OF OUTCOME

Evaluate verbally and in writing; observe HCP in teaching setting; evaluate whether goals set concerning knowledge, skills, compliance, and attitude have been met; evaluate long-term through institutional quality improvement indicators.

MONITORING

HCP training should include evidence of classes and in-service training; availability of written and audiovisual resources; and evaluation of training effectiveness.

**For complete guideline, see Training the health care professional for the role of patient and caregiver educator Respir Care 41(7):654-657, 1996; or www.rcjournal.com/cpgs/thcpcpg.html.*

2. Activities must incorporate the values and beliefs of the learner. Familial, cultural, societal, and economic factors must be considered.
3. The role of the health educator is to facilitate behavioral change. Thus, the learning process should be approached together by both the learner and the educator.
4. The process of predisposing an individual toward improved health as well as enabling and reinforcing health attitudes requires effort, which will only reap results over time.
5. The health care educator must be willing to listen nonjudgmentally to the concerns of the learners. Empathy and understanding are necessary to foster a trusting relationship.
6. The level of the learners' self-esteem and self-concept may either enhance or inhibit their ability to make decisions about their own health. The health care educator should be willing to provide emotional support as necessary.
7. The health care educator's personal characteristics have a direct impact on the outcome of the

Box 49-4 American Association for Respiratory Care Role Model Statement

- As health care professionals engaged in the performance of cardiopulmonary care, RTs must strive to maintain the highest personal and professional standards.
- In addition to upholding the code of ethics, the RT shall serve as a leader and advocate of public health.
- The RT shall participate in activities leading to awareness of the causes and prevention of pulmonary disease and the problems associated with the cardiopulmonary system. The RT shall support the development and promotion of pulmonary disease awareness programs, to include smoking cessation programs, pulmonary function screenings, air pollution monitoring, allergy warnings, and other public education programs.
- The RT shall support research to improve health and prevent disease.
- The RT shall provide leadership in determining health promotion and disease prevention activities for students, faculty, practitioners, patients, and the general public.
- The RT shall serve as a physical example of cardiopulmonary health by abstaining from tobacco use and shall make a special personal effort to eliminate smoking and the use of other tobacco products from the home and work environment.
- The RT shall strive to be a model for all members of the health care team by demonstrating responsibility and cooperating with other health care professionals to meet the health needs of the public.

Effective 3/90
Revised 3/00

From the American Association for Respiratory Care: *Position statement* (website): www.aarc.org/resources/position_statements/rms.html.

educational program. Generally, successful outcomes occur as a result of a confident and professional approach.

For RTs to assist patients, caregivers, or the public with regard to the development healthier lifestyles, greater emphasis must be placed on health promotion and disease prevention strategies.

HEALTH PROMOTION AND DISEASE PREVENTION

In 2008, the United States spent $2.3 trillion on health care.[7] Four of the five major causes of death in the United States are heart disease, cancer, cerebrovascular disease (stroke), and chronic obstructive pulmonary disease (COPD). These diseases have four central causes that, in large part, are preventable: tobacco use, poor diet, physical inactivity, and excessive alcohol use.[8]

Current medical practice is designed to respond to the acute problems of patients; its focus is on diagnosing and treating the presenting symptoms rather than focusing on the prevention of disease by identifying risk factors and providing methods for behavioral changes. Only focusing on the acute or episodic health problems creates a discrepancy when using this model of care to care for chronic conditions that may be prevented or managed. Preventative health care is very different from chronic care.

With this in mind, a quote from Rufus Howe is appropriate: "What a rare privilege it is to be in a position to improve the lives of others."[9]

A patient with asthma goes to the emergency department and is treated effectively and efficiently. The patient received good quality care, and, in many people's minds, the patient was "fixed." However, asthma is manageable to the point that the patient should not have to be in the emergency department. There are excellent national guidelines that outline how to manage asthma, and there are medications that control asthma and keep the patient out of this situation. Usually the reason for the emergency visit is that the patient's asthma is not in control; this may occur because the patient is not using inhaled steroids, because he or she has a poor understanding of the disease and how to treat it, because the national guidelines are not being used, or because of a combination of all of these issues. Either way, this chronic disease can be self-managed by a patient with the proper multidisciplinary education and follow up.

However, the public health model attempts to reduce disease in the nation as a whole through mass education campaigns. Examples include education about the hazards of drinking and driving, tobacco use (both smokeless and smoking) education, and food labeling to indicate fat and cholesterol content. This is known as *health promotion and disease prevention.* By participating in public education programs, RTs have the potential to affect the health of individuals and of the population as a whole.

Recent efforts such as Healthy People 2010 have attempted to place the focus on the health of the population rather than on that of the individual.[10] The two broad goals of this plan are as follows: (1) to increase the quality and years of healthy life; and (2) to eliminate health disparities. These goals encompass the essential elements of health promotion and disease prevention, which are the prevention of premature death, disease, and disability as well as the improvement of the quality of life.

The recognition that allied health professionals such as RTs play vital roles in these activities prompted professional organizations to develop policy statements about health promotion and disease prevention. The American Association for Respiratory Care policy statement appears in Box 49-5.[5]

RTs can take an active role in the development of educational materials to assist both the public and other health professionals with regard to health promotion activities. Many medical manufacturers have also developed asthma education kits of various types that include

Box 49-5 Health Promotion and Disease Prevention

- The AARC submits this paper to identify and illustrate the involvement of the RT in the promotion of health and prevention of disease and supports these activities. The AARC realizes that RTs are integral members of the health care team, in hospitals, home health care settings, pulmonary laboratories, rehabilitation programs, and all other environments where respiratory care is practiced.
- The AARC recognizes that education and training of the RT is the best method by which to instill the ability to improve the patient's quality and longevity of life, and that such information should be included in their formal education and training.
- The AARC recognizes the RT responsibility to participate in pulmonary disease teaching, smoking cessation programs, pulmonary function studies for the public, air pollution alerts, allergy warnings, and sulfite warnings in restaurants, as well as research in those and other areas where efforts could promote improved health and disease prevention. Furthermore, the RT is in a unique position to provide leadership in determining health promotion and disease prevention activities for students, faculty, practitioners, patients, and the general public.
- The AARC recognizes the need to provide and promote consumer education related to the prevention and control of pulmonary disease and to establish a strong working relationship with other health agencies, educational institutions, federal and state government, businesses and other community organizations and to monitor such. Furthermore, the AARC supports efforts to develop personal and professional wellness models and action plans that will inspire and encourage all RT to cooperate on health promotion and disease prevention.

Effective 7/85
Revised 3/00

From the American Association for Respiratory Care: *Position statement* (website): www.aarc.org/resources/position_statements/hpdp.html.

peak flow meters, spacers, and educational materials. These kits are generally developed with input from the medical community and in particular from RTs. An example of an asthma program is given in Table 49-4.[11] Respiratory care educational programs need to be diligent when incorporating health promotion and disease prevention activities into all learning domains as part of their curricula.

Another specific area of health promotion that receives much attention in both hospital and public health settings is nicotine intervention. Nicotine intervention is a progressive, comprehensive program that incorporates a series of steps from risk identification to maintenance support. Seventy percent of smokers report that they would like to quit but cannot.[12] Smoking cessation aids such as nicotine gum and nicotine patches are now available over the counter. Nicotine replacement therapy combined with behavioral therapy is often more effective for tobacco cessation. Varenicline tartrate (Chantix) received U.S. Food and Drug Administration approval for patients who are attempting smoking cessation.[13] It is not a nicotine replacement medication; rather, it acts at the sites in the brain that are affected by nicotine.

National, state, and local agencies such as the American Cancer Society, the American Lung Association, and the American Heart Association offer educational materials and behavioral counseling. The educational materials that these agencies offer are available via mail, telephone, and the Internet. In 2004, the U.S. Department of Health and Human Services established a nationwide toll-free number (800-QUIT-NOW [800-784-8669]) to serve as an access point for smokers who are seeking assistance with quitting. Components of the Office of Surgeon General's tobacco cessation program are included in Tables 49-5 and 49-6.[14]

DISEASE MANAGEMENT

The most recent data show that more than 145 million people—which is approximately half of all Americans—live with chronic disease.[15] Half of those with chronic illness have more than one chronic condition or comorbidity. These chronic diseases are extremely expensive and lead to unnecessary admissions. Chronic care models have been used since the 1990s. A chronic care model is patient centered; it encourages multidisciplinary focus on self-management and continuous quality control. Wagner presented the chronic care model that is illustrated in Figure 49-1.[16]

Wagner explains the model as follows: "[P]atients and families who struggle with chronic illness require planned, regular interactions with their caregivers, with a focus on function and prevention of exacerbations. This interaction includes systematic assessments, attention to treatment guidelines, and behaviorally sophisticated support for the patient's role as a self manager. These interactions must be linked through time by clinically relevant information and continuing follow-up."[16]

As with **disease management,** which is a method of applying the best health care practices to a population with a chronic illness one person at a time,[9] the goals of this type of program include improving the health of the person, improving patient satisfaction, reducing mortality, improving quality of life, and eliminating unnecessary medical treatment to reduce the cost of health care.[9] There is no one definition of disease management. However, the Care Continuum Alliance defines disease management as a coordinated system of interventions for people who have conditions that require significant self-care.[17] Disease management is measured by its impact on costs, clinical outcomes, and quality of life. The programs have similar components, including a coordinated comprehensive

TABLE 49-4

Components of an Asthma Disease Management Program

Component 1: Assessment and monitoring	Assessment: • Detailed patient history • Thorough physical examination • Spirometry to document the reversibility of airflow obstruction Monitoring: Periodic assessment and ongoing monitoring of asthma to determine if goals are being met • Minimal or no chronic and troublesome symptoms, day or night • Normal or near-normal pulmonary function • No limitations on activities • Minimal or no recurrent exacerbations of asthma • Optimal medications with minimal or no adverse side effects • Satisfaction with asthma care
Component 2: Control of the factors that contribute to asthma	Identify the allergens and irritants • House dust mites, cockroach feces, molds, and animal dander • Tobacco smoke, emissions from wood-burning stoves, strong odors and sprays such as perfume and hairspray • Nitrogen dioxide and sulfur dioxide • Rhinitis and sinusitis • Gastroesophageal reflux disease • Viral respiratory infections • Aspirin • Sulfites Reduce exposure to the allergens and irritants, and provide medications or immunotherapy
Component 3: Pharmacologic therapy: managing asthma for the long term	Classify the asthma severity into one of the four levels on the basis of the severity of recurrent symptoms and lung function Prescribe medications for the level of asthma • All patients with asthma need a quick-relief medication (i.e., short-acting β_2-agonists) • Those with persistent asthma need daily long-term control medications to achieve control (e.g., an inhaled corticosteroid) • Start treatment in a stepwise approach (i.e., begin at a higher level to achieve rapid control; when control is achieved and sustained, cautiously step down treatment)

Component 4: Patient education for a partnership in asthma care	Patient education begins at the time of diagnosis.
	• Provide basic facts about asthma
	• Identify the roles of the medications
	• Skills: correct use of the medication delivery devices, the peak flow meter, and the symptom diary
	• Discuss environmental control measures
	• Discuss when and how to take rescue actions
	Education techniques
	• Basic facts about asthma
	  • Describe the contrast between asthmatic and normal airways
	  • Describe what happens to the airways during an asthma attack
	• Describe the roles of the medications
	  • How the medications work
	  • Long-term control: medications that prevent symptoms, often by reducing inflammation
	  • Quick relief: short-acting bronchodilators relax muscles around the airways
	Stress the importance of long-term control medications, and emphasize that the patient should not expect quick relief
	• Skills
	  • Inhaler use (patient demonstration)
	  • Spacer and holding chamber use
	  • Symptom monitoring, peak flow monitoring, and recognizing early signs of deterioration
	• Environmental control measures
	  • Identifying and avoiding environmental precipitants or exposures
	  • When and how to take rescue actions
	• Responding to changes in asthma severity (i.e., daily self-management plan and action plan)

TABLE 49-5

The "5 As" Model for Treating Tobacco Use and Dependence as a Chronic Disease

Ask about tobacco use	Identify and document the tobacco use status of every patient at every visit • Expand the vital signs to include tobacco use
Advise to quit	Strongly urge all tobacco users to quit Advice should be clear, strong, and personalized
Assess every tobacco user's willingness to make a quit attempt	Ask every tobacco user if he or she is willing to make a quit attempt: "Are you willing to give quitting a try?" • If the patient is willing, provide assistance • If the patient is unwilling, provide a motivational intervention • If the patient is a member of a special population (e.g., pregnant, adolescent, minority), consider providing him or her with additional information
Assist by providing counseling and medication	• Set a quit date that is ideally within 2 weeks • Tell family and friends about quitting • Anticipate challenges, including nicotine withdrawal symptoms • Remove tobacco products from the environment Recommend the use of approved medications, except when they are contraindicated or if the patient is a member of a specific population (e.g., pregnant women, smokeless tobacco users, adolescents) • Explain how the medications work to increase success with quitting and to reduce withdrawal symptoms The medications approved for this purposed by the U.S. Food and Drug Administration include the following: • Bupropion SR • Nicotine gum • Nicotine inhaler • Nicotine lozenge • Nicotine nasal spray • Nicotine patch • Varenicline Provide practical counseling (i.e., problem solving, skills training): • Abstinence: striving for total abstinence is essential (i.e., "not one puff after the quit date") • Anticipate triggers and challenges: determine how the patient will successfully overcome these (i.e., avoid the triggers) • Alcohol should be avoided because it is associated with relapse (however, reducing alcohol intake could precipitate withdrawal in alcohol-dependent persons) • Other smokers in the home: quitting is more difficult when there is another smoker in the home; patients should encourage all to quit with them or to not smoke in their presence Provide intratreatment social support • Provide a supportive clinical environment while encouraging the patient in his or her quit attempt (i.e., "My office staff and I are here to assist you") Help the patient to obtain extra social support during treatment • Help the patient to develop social support in his or her environment outside of the treatment by asking the patient's spouse or partner, friends, and coworkers to support the quit attempt Provide supplementary materials, including information about quit lines • Sources: Federal agencies, nonprofit agencies, national quit line network (1-800-QUIT-NOW), and local/state/tribal health departments and quit lines • Type: culturally, racially, educationally, and age appropriate for the patient • Location: readily available Recommend counseling (there are three types): Practical counseling (i.e., problem solving, skills training) • Recognize danger situations • Develop coping skills • Provide basic information Supportive treatment counseling • Encourage the patient to quit • Communicate caring and concern • Encourage the patient to talk about quitting
Arrange for follow-up contacts, either in person or via the telephone	Timing: Follow-up contact should begin soon after the quit date, preferably during the first week; a second follow up is recommended within the first month, and follow up should be scheduled as indicated • Actions to take during the follow-up contacts: for all patients, identify problems that have been encountered, and anticipate challenges Assess the medication use and any associated problems: • Remind the patient of the support offered by quit lines • Address tobacco use at the next clinical visit • When patients have been abstinent, congratulate them on their success

TABLE 49-6

Components of a Tobacco Education Program for Those Who Are Unwilling to Quit Enhancing Motivation to Quit Tobacco: The "5 Rs"

Relevance	Encourage the patient to indicate why quitting is personally relevant and to be as specific as possible. Motivational information has the greatest impact if it is relevant to a patient's disease status or risk, to a family or social situation (e.g., having children in the home), or to health concerns, age, gender, and other important patient characteristics (e.g., prior quitting experience, personal barriers to cessation).
Risk	Ask the patient to identify potential negative consequences of tobacco use and suggest those that seem to be the most relevant to the patient. Emphasize that smoking low-tar or low-nicotine cigarettes or using other forms of tobacco (e.g., smokeless tobacco, cigars, pipes) will not eliminate these risks. Examples of risks include the following: • Acute risks: shortness of breath, exacerbation of asthma, harm to a pregnancy, impotence, infertility • Long-term risks: heart attack, stroke, lung and other cancers, chronic obstructive pulmonary disease, disability, need for extended care • Environmental risks: increased risk of lung cancer and heart disease in spouse, increased rates of smoking among children of tobacco users, sudden infant death syndrome, respiratory infections in the children of smokers
Rewards	Ask the patient to identify the potential benefits of stopping tobacco use: • Improved health • Food will taste better • Save money • Feel better • Home, car, clothing, and breath will smell better • Can stop worrying about quitting • Set an example for children • Have healthier babies and children • Reduce wrinkling and aging of skin
Roadblocks	Ask the patient to identify barriers to quitting: • Withdrawal symptoms • Fear of failure • Weight gain • Lack of support • Depression • Enjoyment of tobacco
Repetition	Repeat the motivational intervention information every time that an unmotivated patient is seen.

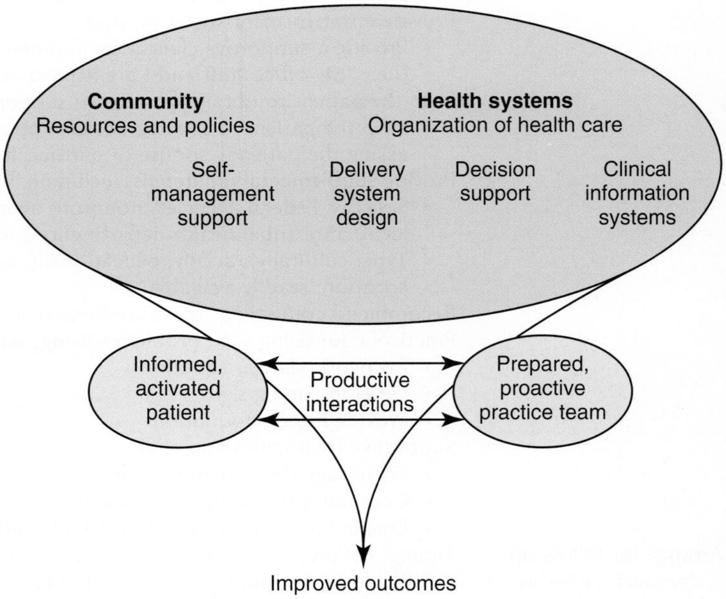

FIGURE 49-1 Illustration of a chronic care model that is focused on productive interactions and improved patient outcomes. (Modified from Wagner E: System changes and interventions: delivery system design. Improving chronic illness care, Orlando, Fl, 2001, Institute for Healthcare Improvement National Forum.)

interdisciplinary care team with a process for measuring improvement. Health insurance companies, pharmaceutical companies, and the federal government all pay for disease management programs.[9] Most programs have the following attributes:

- The provision of interdisciplinary comprehensive care (i.e., health promotion, prevention, and acute care)
- A population-identification process (for a specific disease or condition)

- The use of evidence-based guidelines, protocols, and pathways
- Collaborative and coordinated components of care
- Active patient self-management and education (e.g., empowerment, behavior modification)
- Quality improvement methods
- The use of information technology to create a feedback loop

If you were interested in creating a disease management program, you would want to make sure to include these components. There are many disease management programs offered to patients with chronic diseases such as COPD, asthma, amyotrophic lateral sclerosis, and cystic fibrosis. RTs are ideal members of a disease management program. The patients whom RTs care for have chronic diseases, and these individuals need to be taught about the health risks associated with the disease, the prophylactic measures used to maintain quality health, and disease-specific respiratory therapy. For example, in a disease management program for a patient with COPD, RTs would provide one-on-one counseling for tobacco cessation education (if the patient continued to use these products); discuss pulmonary rehabilitation that included exercise as well as strength and endurance training; and recognize and manage an acute situation and appropriate medication. The RT would work with the patient to establish personal goals, including changing the person's behaviors and reducing the risks associated with the chronic disease.

Implications for the Respiratory Therapist

Because the RT is able to function as both an individual counselor and a public health advocate, depending on the setting or circumstances, it is useful to examine the most likely settings in which the RT's health promotion and disease prevention knowledge can be put to good use.

Health Care Institutions

Health care institutions in which RTs provide both health education and promotion include inpatient facilities (e.g., hospitals, skilled nursing facilities) as well as ambulatory care centers (e.g., physicians' offices, clinics, health insurance organizations). RTs may participate in wellness programs for staff and patients that are aimed at improving cardiopulmonary wellness through exercise (e.g., pulmonary rehabilitation, asthma management education programs).

Work Site

Healthier workers are absent from work less often; they are also more satisfied with their jobs and more productive. This all translates into a more cost-effective workplace. RTs may find themselves involved in work-site wellness by participating in the following: (1) performing pulmonary function or blood pressure screenings; (2) developing and implementing stress management or nicotine intervention programs; and (3) consulting on policies related to smoking and occupational or environmental exposure to foreign dusts (e.g., silica, asbestos) or noxious fumes (e.g., smog).

Home

Home health care continues to be a rapidly growing segment of the health care industry. It has been proved repeatedly to be more cost-effective than hospital care. RTs can perform a wide variety of services in the patient's home, including oxygen therapy and mechanical ventilation on either a temporary or long-term basis. Generally the focus is on tertiary prevention (i.e., preventing further decline). Patient education is of primary importance in the home in so that the patient may become as self-reliant as possible (see Chapters 50 and 51).

Community

Most of the health promotion activities described earlier pertain to the individual. At the community level, the focus is on the group. Community health promotion activities provided by the RT may include the following: pulmonary function screening at health fairs, smoking cessation programs, family asthma management education programs, and COPD (i.e., better breathing) support groups. RTs, who are certified in basic cardiac life support instruction, may also volunteer to perform certification in this practice for various groups.

Educational Institutions

Because many unhealthy behaviors begin during early childhood or adolescence, elementary, middle, and secondary schools are excellent places to begin health education activities. Education about smoking is one example.

Cigarette smoking is a primary risk factor that is associated with many of today's leading causes of death. Because most smoking begins during late childhood or early adolescence, schools provide the best setting in which to educate children about the dangers of tobacco. RTs are trained to provide these educational experiences. It is never too early to begin sending the antismoking message.

SUMMARY CHECKLIST

- Patient education and general approaches to health promotion are key issues in health care today.
- Educators should use learning objectives to direct teaching strategies toward individuals or large groups of patients.
- Learning objectives call for the use of an action verb to define the performance that is expected of the patient at the end of instruction.
- Learning occurs in three domains: cognitive (knowledge), psychomotor (skills), and affective (attitudes).

Continued

- Patients tend to learn by doing. Passive participation usually does not cause a change in behavior.
- Evaluate the cognitive domain objectives with written tests. Evaluate psychomotor and affective domain objectives with a skills checklist.
- The clinician should evaluate his or her teaching in an effort to improve.
- The RT can have an impact on several areas of health education and health promotion, including tobacco cessation programs, asthma education programs, and community health screenings.
- RTs can be a key player involved in disease management programs because of their understanding of the manifestations of the chronic cardiopulmonary diseases and their abilities to teach patients self-management with the use of the patient education tools discussed in this chapter.

References

1. National Vital Statistics Report, Vol 54, No 19, June 28, 2006. In Minino AM, Heron MP, Smith BL, editors: Deaths: preliminary data for 2004. National vital statistics reports; vol 54 no 19, Hyattsville, MD, 2006, National Center for Health Statistics.
2. French D, Olrech N, Hale C, et al: Blended learning: an ongoing process for Internet integration, Victoria, Canada, 2003, Trafford Publishing.
3. Maslow AH: A theory of human motivation. Psychol Review 50:370–385, 1943.
4. The American Academy of Allergy, Asthma & Immunology: Pediatric asthma: promoting best practices; patient education. Retrieved March 14, 2007, from http://www.aaaai.org/members/resources/initiatives/pediatricasthmaguidelines/default.stm.
5. American Association for Respiratory Care: Position statement: Health promotion and disease prevention. Retrieved on March 14, 2007, from http://www.aarc.org/resources/position_statements/hpdp.html.
6. American Association for Respiratory Care: Position statement: AARC role model statement, Dallas, March 2000, American Association for Respiratory Care.
7. Centers for Medicare and Medicaid Services, Office of the Actuary, National Health Statistics Group, National Health Care Expenditures Data, January 2010. http://www.cms.gov/nationalhealthexpenddata/01_overview.asp?
8. Danaei G, Ding EL, Mozaffarian D, Taylor B, Rehm J, et al: The Preventable Causes of Death in the United States: Comparative Risk Assessment of Dietary, Lifestyle, and Metabolic Risk Factors. PLoS Med 6:e1000058, 2009. doi:10.1371/journal.pmed.1000058
9. Howe R: The Disease Manager's Handbook, Boston, 2005, Jones and Bartlett.
10. U.S. Department of Health and Human Services. Healthy People 2010: understanding and improving health, ed 2, Washington, DC, November 2000, U.S. Government Printing Office. Retrieved from http://www.healthypeople.gov/document/pdf/uih/2010uih.pdf.
11. U.S. Department of Health and Human Services: Making a difference in the management of asthma: a guide for respiratory therapists, Bethesda, May 2003, National Institutes of Health, NIH publication No. 02-1964, May 2003.
12. Centers for Disease Control and Prevention: Cigarette smoking among adults–United States, 1999, MMWR Morb Mortal Wkly Rep 50:869-878, 2001.
13. National Institute on Drug Abuse; Research Report: Tobacco addiction, Bethesda, July 2006, National Institutes of Health, NIH publication No. 06-4342.
14. Fiore MC, Jaén CR, Baker TB, et al: Treating Tobacco Use and Dependence: 2008 Update. Quick Reference Guide for Clinicians. Rockville, MD, April 2009, U.S. Department of Health and Human Services. Public Health Service. http://www.ahrq.gov/clinic/tobacco/tobaqrg.htm#table4.
15. Centers for Disease Control and Prevention: Public health and aging: trends in aging-United States and worldwide. MMWR 52(06):101-106, 2003.
16. Wagner E: System changes and interventions: delivery system design. Improving Chronic Illness Care, Orlando, FL, 2001, IHI National Forum.
17. Care Continuum Alliance (CCA) Definition of Disease Management. Available at http://www.carecontinuum.org/dm_definition.asp.

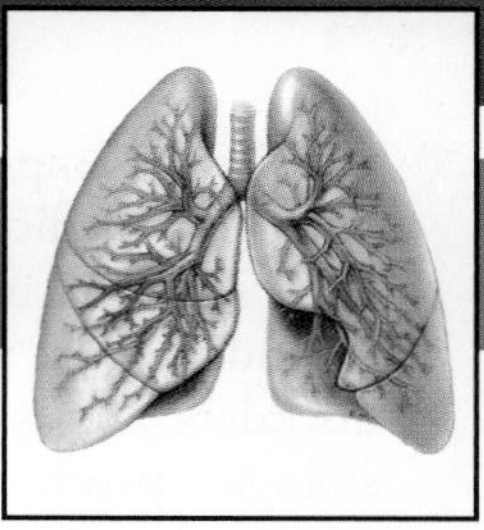

Chapter 50

Cardiopulmonary Rehabilitation

KENNETH A. WYKA

CHAPTER OBJECTIVES

After reading this chapter you will be able to:

- State the definition and general goals of pulmonary rehabilitation programs.
- Explain the rationale for exercise conditioning and psychosocial support of patients with chronic pulmonary disease.
- Describe how to evaluate and select patients for pulmonary rehabilitation.
- Describe pulmonary rehabilitation program design including format and content.
- List the educational content to be addressed in a pulmonary rehabilitation program.
- Describe the implementation of a pulmonary rehabilitation program, including staffing, facilities, scheduling, class size, equipment, costs, and reimbursement.
- Discuss the outcome measures that can be used to evaluate pulmonary rehabilitation programs.
- Identify the potential hazards associated with pulmonary rehabilitation.

CHAPTER OUTLINE

Definitions and Goals
Historical Perspective
Scientific Basis
  Physical Reconditioning
  Psychosocial Support
Structure of a Pulmonary Rehabilitation Program
  Program Goals and Objectives
  Patient Evaluation and Selection
  Program Design
  Program Implementation
  Cost, Fees, and Reimbursement
  Program Results
  Potential Hazards
Cardiac Rehabilitation
Conclusion

KEY TERMS

6- or 12-minute walk
aerobic exercises
cardiopulmonary exercise evaluation
comprehensive outpatient rehabilitative facilities (CORFs)
Karvonen's formula
onset of blood lactate accumulation (OBLA)
progressive resistance
psychosocial support needs
pulmonary rehabilitation
reconditioning
target heart rate
ventilatory threshold

Steady improvements in acute care are presenting new medical and social problems. As more patients survive acute illnesses, there are increasing numbers of individuals with chronic disorders. These chronic disorders are associated with a wide spectrum of physiologic, psychologic, and social disabilities. Foremost among these individuals with chronic disorders are individuals with chronic cardiopulmonary disease. Chronic obstructive pulmonary disease (COPD) is expected to be the third leading cause of death in the United States by 2020.[1]

Although differences in diagnoses can have an impact on treatment outcomes and survival, patients with chronic pulmonary disorders have much in common. All of these patients have difficulty coping with the physiologic limitations of their diseases, and these physiologic limitations result in many psychosocial problems. The end result often is an unsatisfactory quality of life. The high incidence of repeated hospitalizations and the progressive disability of these patients require well-organized programs of rehabilitative care. This chapter provides foundational knowledge regarding the goals, methods, and issues involved in providing planned programs of rehabilitation for individuals with chronic pulmonary disorders.

DEFINITIONS AND GOALS

The Council on Rehabilitation defines *rehabilitation* as "the restoration of the individual to the fullest medical, mental, emotional, social, and vocational potential of which he or she is capable."[2] The overall goal is to maximize functional ability and to minimize the impact the disability has on the individual, the family, and the community. **Pulmonary rehabilitation** is the "art of medical practice wherein an individually tailored, multidisciplinary program is formulated, which through accurate diagnosis, therapy, emotional support, and education stabilizes or reverses both the physio- and psychopathology of pulmonary diseases and attempts to return the patient to the highest possible functional capacity allowed by his or her pulmonary handicap and overall life situation."[3]

The general goals of pulmonary rehabilitation are to control and alleviate symptoms, restore functional capabilities as much as possible, and improve quality of life.[4] Pulmonary rehabilitation does not reverse or stop progression of the disease, but it can improve a patient's overall quality of life. Health care providers from various disciplines are needed to reach these goals.

HISTORICAL PERSPECTIVE

Pulmonary rehabilitation is not a new concept. In 1952, Barach and colleagues[5] recommended reconditioning programs for patients with chronic lung disease to help improve their ability to walk without dyspnea. Decades passed before clinicians paid any attention to this concept. Instead of having their patients participate in reconditioning programs, most physicians simply prescribed oxygen (O_2) therapy and bed rest. The result was a vicious cycle of skeletal muscle deterioration, progressive weakness and fatigue, and increasing levels of dyspnea including at rest. Patients became homebound, then roombound, and eventually bed-bound. Improved avenues of therapy and rehabilitation were needed.

In 1962, Pierce and associates[6] published results confirming Barach's insight into the value of **reconditioning.** They observed that patients with COPD who participated in physical reconditioning exhibited lower pulse rates, respiratory rates, minute volumes, and carbon dioxide (CO_2) production during exercise. However, they also found that these benefits occurred without significant changes in pulmonary function. Soon thereafter, Paez and associates[7] showed that reconditioning could improve both the efficiency of motion and O_2 use in patients with COPD. Subsequently, Christie[8] showed that the benefits of reconditioning could be achieved on an outpatient basis with minimal supervision. Since Christie's work in 1968, other investigators have continued to research the benefits of pulmonary rehabilitation.

The available evidence at the present time consistently indicates that pulmonary rehabilitation benefits patients with chronic obstructive and restrictive pulmonary disease.[9-12] When combined with smoking cessation, optimization of blood gases, and proper medication use, pulmonary rehabilitation offers the best treatment option for patients with symptomatic pulmonary disease. Programs for pulmonary rehabilitation must be founded on the sound application of current knowledge in the clinical and social sciences. In fall 2006, the American College of Chest Physicians (ACCP) and the American Association of Cardiovascular and Pulmonary Rehabilitation (AACVPR) released their evidence-based guidelines relating to pulmonary rehabilitation aimed at improving the way pulmonary rehabilitation programs are designed, implemented, and evaluated through patient outcomes.[13]

SCIENTIFIC BASIS

Rehabilitation must focus on the patient as a whole and not solely on the underlying disease. For this reason, effective pulmonary rehabilitation programs combine knowledge from both the clinical and the social sciences. Knowledge from the clinical sciences can help quantify the degree of physiologic impairment and establish outcome expectations for reconditioning. Application of the social sciences is helpful in determining the psychological, social, and vocational impact of the disability on the patient and family and in establishing ways to improve the patient's quality of life.

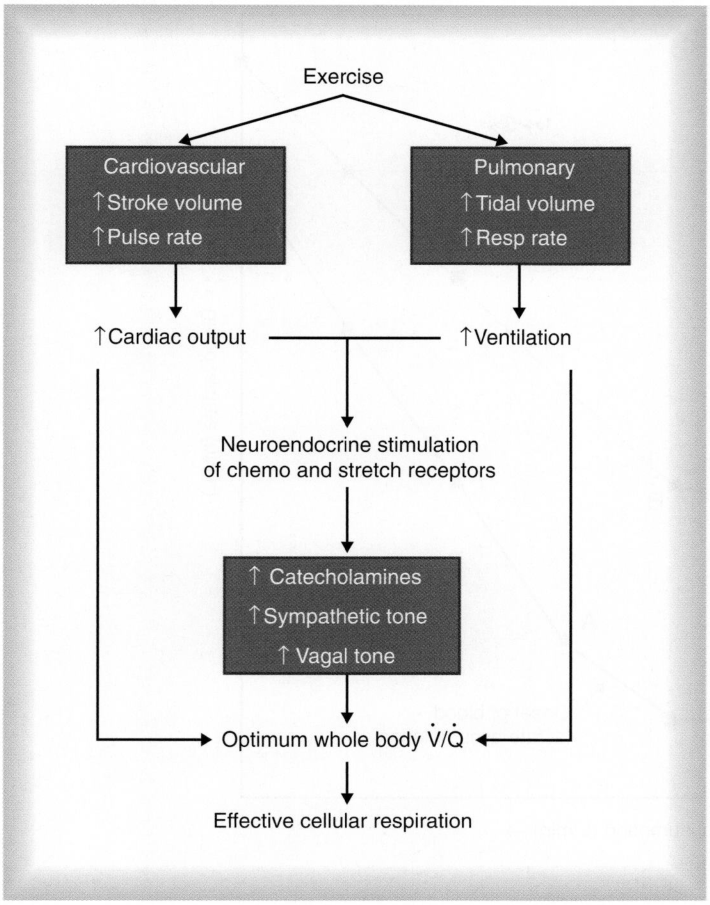

FIGURE 50-1 The body's response to increased levels of activity such as exercise.

Physical Reconditioning

At rest, an individual maintains homeostasis by balancing external, internal, and cellular respiration. Physical activity, such as exercise, increases energy demands. To maintain homeostasis during exercise, the cardiorespiratory system must keep pace. Figure 50-1 shows how the body responds to exercise. Ventilation and circulation increase to supply tissues and cells with additional O_2 and to eliminate the higher levels of CO_2 produced by metabolism.

As depicted in Figure 50-2, O_2 consumption and CO_2 production also increase in linear fashion as exercise intensity increases. If the body cannot deliver sufficient O_2 to meet the demands of energy metabolism, blood lactate levels increase above normal. In exercise physiology, this point is called the **onset of blood lactate accumulation (OBLA).** As this excess lactic acid is buffered, CO_2 levels increase, and the stimulus to breathe increases. The result is an abrupt upswing in both CO_2 and $\dot{V}_E$ (referred to as the **ventilatory threshold**). Beyond this point, metabolism becomes anaerobic, the efficiency of energy production decreases, lactic acid accumulates, and fatigue sets in.

Patients with COPD who lack adequate pulmonary function have severe limitations to their exercise capabilities. Their high rate of CO_2 production during exercise results in respiratory acidosis and a shortness of breath out of proportion to the level of activity. In addition, as ventilation increases, the rate of O_2 consumption in a patient with COPD increases significantly (Figure 50-3). Together, these factors limit patient tolerance for any significant increase in physical activity.

Pulmonary rehabilitation must include efforts to recondition patients physically and increase their exercise tolerance. Reconditioning involves strengthening essential muscle groups, improving overall O_2 use, and enhancing the body's cardiovascular response to physical activity (Box 50-1).

RULE OF THUMB

A good estimate of a patient's maximum voluntary ventilation (MVV) is derived by multiplying the FEV_1 (forced expiratory volume in 1 second) by a factor of 35. To estimate the MVV of a patient with FEV_1 of 1.5 L, multiply 1.5 L by 35:

$$MVV = FEV_1 \times 35$$

$$MVV = 1.5\ L \times 35 = 52.5\ L/min$$

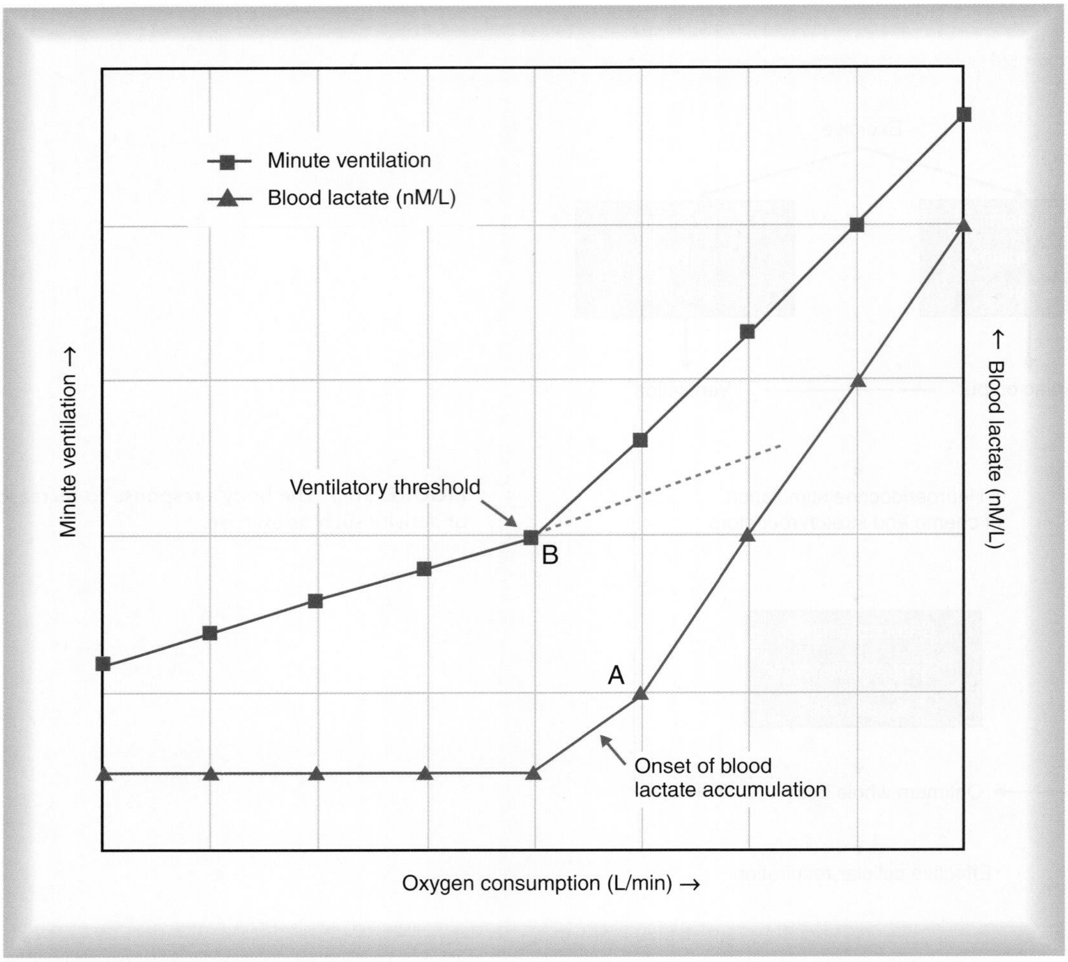

FIGURE 50-2 Minute ventilation, blood lactate, CO_2 production, and O_2 consumption during graded exercise to maximum. The *dashed line* represents the linear extrapolation between $\dot{V}E$ and $\dot{V}O_2$ during submaximal exercise. *Point A* represents OBLA. At the same time, $\dot{V}E$ and $\dot{V}CO_2$ "break" from their extrapolated rate of increase and abruptly rise *(point B)*. This is referred to as the ventilatory threshold. (Modified from McArdle WD, Katch FI, Katch VL: Exercise physiology: energy, nutrition and human performance, ed 6, Baltimore, 2007, Williams & Wilkins.)

FIGURE 50-3 Changes in O_2 consumption with increasing ventilation in a normal subject and in a patient with emphysema. *BTPS,* Body temperature, body pressure saturated; *STPD,* volume of dry gas at 0° C and 760 mm Hg atmospheric pressure. (Modified from Cherniack RM, Cherniack L, Naimark A: Respiration in health and disease, ed 3, Philadelphia, 1984, Saunders.)

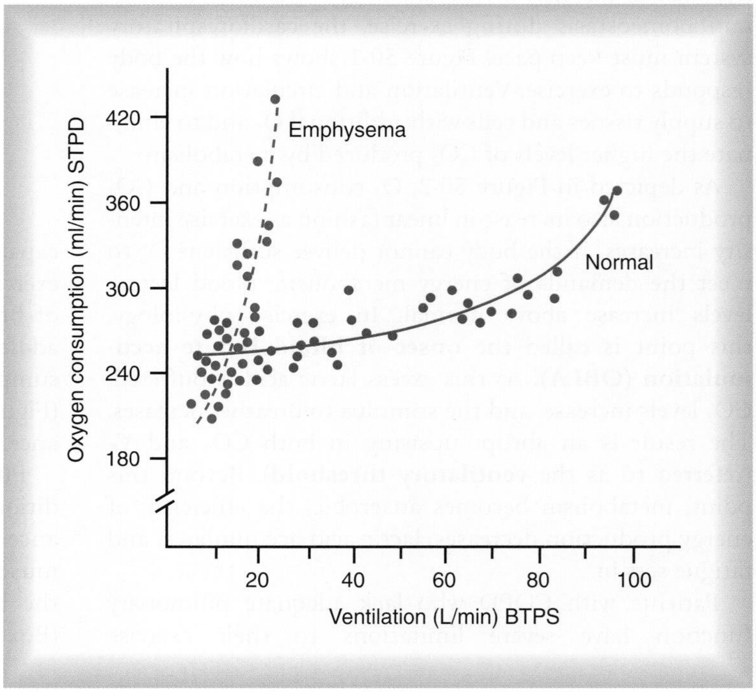

Box 50-1 Benefits from Exercise Reconditioning

ACCEPTED BENEFITS
- Increased physical endurance
- Increased maximum O_2 consumption
- Increased activity levels with:
  - Decreased ventilation
  - Decreased $\dot{V}O_2$
  - Decreased heart rate
  - Increased ventilatory threshold
  - Improved blood lipids

POTENTIAL BENEFITS
- Increased sense of well-being
- Improved secretion clearance
- Increased hypoxic drive
- Improved cardiac function

UNPROVEN BENEFITS
- Prolonged survival
- Improved pulmonary function test results
- Decreased pulmonary artery pressure
- Improved blood gases
- Change in muscle O_2 extraction
- Change in step desaturation

Data from references 15 and 16.

Psychosocial Support

If the overall goal of pulmonary rehabilitation is to improve the quality of patients' lives, physical reconditioning alone is insufficient. Psychosocial indicators generally are good predictors of morbidity in patients with COPD. Studies show that the relative success of reconditioning plays less of a role in determining whether patients complete a program than meeting their **psychosocial support needs.**[14]

There is a well-established relationship between physical, mental, and social well-being in humans. Everyday life is full of such relationships, such as the physical fatigue that follows a period of emotional tension. Many of these associations are part of normal human behavior. However, emotional states such as stress can cause or aggravate an existing physical problem. Likewise, physical manifestations of disease, such as recurrent dyspnea, can worsen stress.

The progressive nature of COPD can negatively affect the patient's overall outlook on his or her disease and reduce motivation to adapt to its consequences. The best medical care available can be negated, and a patient can experience a progressively downhill course because of an unfavorable mental state. Patients with COPD often have a tendency to develop severe anxiety, hostility, and stress as a direct consequence of their disability. Because patients are fearful of economic loss and death, they can develop hostility toward the disease and often toward the people around them.

In terms of social function, the physiologic impairment of chronic lung disease combined with other variables can severely restrict a patient's ability to perform routine tasks requiring physical exertion. Intolerance for physical exertion lessens patients' social activity. More important, however, is patients' potential loss of confidence in their ability to care for themselves that can accompany such impairments, followed by resultant loss of feelings of dignity and self-worth.

Figure 50-4 presents elements of how chronic lung disease and other variables can have an impact on a patient's quality of life. It is here that the link between the physical reconditioning and psychosocial support components of rehabilitation becomes most evident. By reducing exercise intolerance and enhancing the body's cardiovascular response to physical activity, patients can develop a more independent and active lifestyle. For some patients, simply being able to walk to the market or play with their grandchildren can contribute to a greater feeling of social importance and self-worth. For others, physical conditioning may allow a return to near-normal levels of activity, including vocational pursuits.

Many patients disabled with pulmonary disease are in their economically productive years and are anxious to return to economic self-sufficiency. For these patients, *occupational retraining* and *job placement* are key ingredients in a good rehabilitation program. An occupational therapist can play a vital role here and should be included, if possible, as a member of the interdisciplinary rehabilitation team and in the pulmonary rehabilitation program. The pulmonary rehabilitation program should be based on the individual needs and expectations of each patient. Each patient's physical ability and his or her education, past experience, aptitude, and personality should be considered. Evaluation and placement of the rehabilitation patient require the skills of vocational counselors and occupational therapists and the cooperation of business and industry.

STRUCTURE OF A PULMONARY REHABILITATION PROGRAM

Program Goals and Objectives

Pulmonary rehabilitation programs vary in their design and implementation but generally share common goals. Examples of these common goals are listed in Box 50-2. These general goals assist planners in formulating more specific program objectives. When determining objectives, both patients and members of the rehabilitation team should have input. These objectives should always be stated in measurable terms because this helps facilitate the determination of both patient outcomes and the therapeutic success and value of pulmonary rehabilitation. Depending on the specific needs of

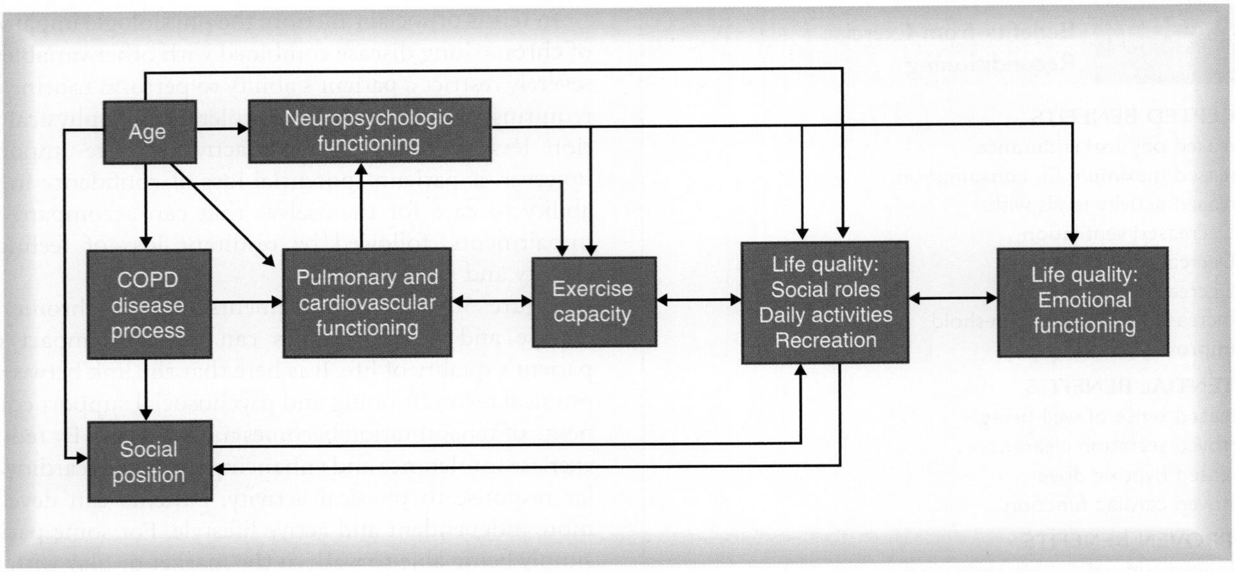

FIGURE 50-4 Model describing the relationship between physical and psychologic dysfunction in patients with chronic lung disease. (Modified from McSweeney AJ, Grant I, Heaton RK, et al: Life quality of patients with chronic obstructive pulmonary disease. Arch Intern Med 142:473, 1982.)

Box 50-2 Common Goals for Pulmonary Rehabilitation Programs

- Control of respiratory infections
- Basic airway management
- Improvement in ventilation and cardiac status
- Improvement in ambulation and other types of physical activity
- Reduction in overall medical costs
- Reduction in hospitalizations
- Psychosocial support
- Occupational retraining and placement (when and where possible)
- Family education, counseling, and support
- Patient education, counseling, and support
- Control of respiratory infections

the participants, program objectives can include the following:

- Development of diaphragmatic breathing skills
- Development of stress management and relaxation techniques
- Involvement in a daily physical exercise regimen to condition both skeletal and respiratory-related muscles
- Adherence to proper hygiene, diet, and nutrition
- Smoking cessation (if applicable)
- Proper use of medications, O_2, and breathing equipment (if applicable)
- Application of airway clearance techniques (when indicated)
- Focus on group support
- Provisions for individual and family counseling

When program objectives are specifically defined and structured in a measurable way, strategies can be tailored to ensure the maximum results and benefit. Demonstration of program effectiveness also becomes easier and more acceptable by the medical community. However, benefits realized by participating patients are not always easy to identify and may be controversial.

Patient Evaluation and Selection

Before beginning a pulmonary rehabilitation program, clinicians need to define and establish criteria for entry or selection. Patient selection requires comprehensive evaluation and testing.

Patient Evaluation

Pulmonary rehabilitation programs must have a qualified medical director, usually a pulmonologist, to provide overall medical direction of the program and to screen prospective patients.[17] Patient evaluation begins with a complete patient history—medical, psychologic, vocational, and social. A well-designed patient questionnaire and interview form assist with this step. The patient history should be followed by a complete physical examination (see Chapter 15). A recent chest film, resting electrocardiogram (ECG), complete blood count, serum electrolytes, and urinalysis provide additional information on the patient's current medical status (see Chapter 16).

To determine the patient's cardiopulmonary status and exercise capacity, both pulmonary function testing and a **cardiopulmonary exercise evaluation** may be performed. Pulmonary function testing includes assessment of pulmonary ventilation, lung volume determinations, diffusing capacity (DLCO), and spirometry before and after bronchodilator use (see Chapter 19).

The cardiopulmonary exercise evaluation serves two key purposes in pulmonary rehabilitation. First, it quantifies the patient's initial exercise capacity. This quantification provides the basis for the exercise prescription (including setting a **target heart rate**) and yields the baseline data for assessing a patient's progress over time. In addition, the evaluation helps determine the degree of hypoxemia or desaturation that can occur with exercise; this provides the objective basis for titrating O_2 therapy during the exercise program. To guide practitioners in implementing exercise evaluation, the American Association for Respiratory Care (AARC) has published clinical practice guidelines on exercise testing for evaluation of hypoxemia or desaturation or both[18] and pulmonary rehabilitation. Excerpts from these guidelines appear in Clinical Practice Guidelines 50-1 and 50-2.[19]

50-1 Exercise Testing for Evaluation of Hypoxemia, Desaturation, or Both

AARC Clinical Practice Guideline (Excerpts)*

INDICATIONS

- The need to assess and quantify arterial oxyhemoglobin (HbO_2) levels during exercise in patients with suspected desaturation
- The need to quantify the response to therapeutic intervention
- The need to titrate the optimum level of O_2 therapy during activity
- The need for preoperative assessment for lung resection or transplant
- The need to assess the degree of impairment for disability evaluation

CONTRAINDICATIONS

Absolute contraindications include the following:

- Acute ECG changes indicating myocardial ischemia or serious cardiac dysrhythmias
- Unstable angina
- Acute pericarditis
- Aneurysm of the heart or aorta
- Uncontrolled systemic hypertension
- Recent (within prior 4 weeks) myocardial infarction or myocarditis
- Second-degree or third-degree heart block
- Recent systemic or pulmonary embolus
- Acute thrombophlebitis or deep venous thrombosis

Relative contraindications to exercise testing include the following:

- Inability or unwillingness of patient to perform the test
- Severe pulmonary hypertension or cor pulmonale
- Known electrolyte disturbances (hypokalemia, hypomagnesemia)
- Resting diastolic blood pressure >110 mm Hg or resting systolic blood pressure >200 mm Hg
- Neuromuscular, musculoskeletal, or rheumatoid disorders exacerbated by exercise
- Uncontrolled metabolic disease (e.g., diabetes)
- SaO_2 or $SpO_2 < 85\%$ with the subject breathing room air
- Untreated or unstable asthma

PRECAUTIONS AND POSSIBLE COMPLICATIONS

Indications for ending testing include the following:

- ECG abnormalities (e.g., dangerous dysrhythmias, ventricular tachycardia, ST-T wave changes)
- Severe desaturation ($SaO_2 < 80\%$ or $SpO_2 < 83\%$ or 10% fall from baseline values)
- Angina
- Hypotensive responses
- Decrease of >20 mm Hg in systolic pressure, occurring after the normal exercise increase
- Decrease in systolic blood pressure below preexercise level
- Lightheadedness
- Request from patient to terminate test

Abnormal responses that may require discontinuation of exercise include (1) increase in systolic blood pressure to >250 mm Hg or diastolic pressure to >120 mm Hg, (2) increase in systolic pressure of >20 mm Hg from resting level, (3) mental confusion or headache, (4) cyanosis, (5) nausea or vomiting, (6) muscle cramping.

Continued

50-1 Exercise Testing for Evaluation of Hypoxemia, Desaturation, or Both—cont'd

AARC Clinical Practice Guideline (Excerpts)*

ASSESSMENT OF NEED

Indications for exercise testing to evaluate hypoxemia or desaturation or both include the following:
- History and physical examination indicators suggesting hypoxemia or desaturation or both
- The presence of abnormal diagnostic test results (e.g., DLCO, FEV_1, arterial blood gases)
- The need to titrate or adjust a therapy

MONITORING

The following should be monitored during testing:
- Physical assessment (chest pain, leg cramps, color, perceived exertion, dyspnea)
- Respiratory rate
- SpO_2
- Cooperation and effort level
- Borg or Modified Borg Dyspnea Scale
- Blood gas sampling site and technique
- Heart rate, rhythm, and ST-T wave changes
- Blood pressure

**For the complete guidelines, see American Association for Respiratory Care: AARC clinical practice guideline: exercise testing for evaluation of hypoxemia and/or desaturation. Respir Care 46:514, 2001.*
Refer to the Modified Borg Dyspnea Scale (immediately following).

Modified Borg Dyspnea Scale (With Dyspnea Descriptors)

10	Maximal (worst possible you can imagine)
9	Very, very severe
8	Very, very severe
7	Very severe
6	Very severe
5	Severe
4	Somewhat severe
3	Moderate
2	Slight
1	Very slight
0.5	Very, very slight (just noticeable)
0	None at all

Box 50-3 Common Physiologic Parameters Measured During Exercise Evaluation

- Blood pressure
- Heart rate
- ECG
- Respiratory rate
- Arterial blood gases/O_2 saturation
- Maximum ventilation ($\dot{V}Emax$)
- O_2 consumption (either absolute $\dot{V}O_2$ or METS)
- CO_2 production ($\dot{V}CO_2$)
- Respiratory quotient (RQ)
- O_2 pulse ($\dot{V}O_2$:heart rate)

METS, Metabolic equivalents of O_2 consumption.

The exercise evaluation procedure involves serial or continuous measurements of several physiologic parameters during various graded levels of exercise on either an ergometer or a treadmill (Box 50-3). To allow for steady-state equilibration, these graded levels are usually spaced at 3-minute intervals. Work levels are increased progressively until either (1) the patient cannot tolerate a higher level or (2) an abnormal or hazardous response occurs.

Blood gas and arterial saturation measures are obtained at rest and at peak exercise. Samples from single arterial punctures are as good as samples drawn from indwelling catheters. If the peak exercise puncture is unsuccessful, a sample drawn within 10 to 15 seconds of test termination usually suffices. Owing to inherent problems, pulse oximetry has a limited but nonetheless important role in exercise evaluation. The best use of pulse oximetry is as a monitor to warn clinicians of gross desaturation events during testing. In addition, the pulse oximeter can be used to assess the patient's response to supplemental O_2 during exercise.

Relative contraindications to exercise testing include the following:
- Inability or unwillingness of patient to perform the test
- Severe pulmonary hypertension or cor pulmonale
- Known electrolyte disturbances (hypokalemia, hypomagnesemia)
- Resting diastolic blood pressure greater than 110 mm Hg or resting systolic blood pressure greater than 200 mm Hg

50-2 Pulmonary Rehabilitation

AARC Clinical Practice Guideline (Excerpts)*

■ SETTINGS

Pulmonary rehabilitation (PR) may take place in any of the following sites:

- Inpatient setting, including medical center, skilled nursing facility, or rehabilitation hospital
- Outpatient setting, including outpatient hospital-based clinic, CORF, physician's office, alternative or extended care facility, or patient's home

■ INDICATIONS

Indications for PR include any of the following:

- Dyspnea during rest or exertion
- Hypoxemia or hypercapnia
- Reduced exercise tolerance
- Unexpected deterioration or worsening of symptoms against a background of chronic dyspnea and reduced but stable exercise tolerance
- Need for surgical intervention
- Chronic respiratory failure
- Ventilator dependence
- Increasing need for acute care intervention (i.e., emergency department visits, hospitalizations, or unscheduled physician office visits)

■ CONTRAINDICATIONS

Contraindications for PR include any of the following:

- Ischemic cardiac disease
- Acute cor pulmonale
- Severe pulmonary hypertension
- Significant hepatic dysfunction
- Metastatic cancer
- Renal failure
- Severe cognitive deficit
- Psychiatric disease affecting memory and compliance
- Substance abuse without the desire to cease use of substance
- Physical limitations, such as poor eyesight, impaired hearing, speech impediment, or orthopedic impairment, that may require modification of the PR setting but should not interfere with participation in the program

■ HAZARDS AND COMPLICATIONS

Hazards and complications are primarily related to the exercise portion of the program. During exercise, the cardiovascular and ventilatory systems must be able to respond to increased demands. Also, exercise can lead to muscle or ligament injuries.

■ ASSESSMENT OF NEED

Patients should be under the care of a physician for the pulmonary condition requiring PR. Appropriate members of the PR team participate in patient assessment. The initial evaluation should include medical history; diagnostic tests; assessment of current symptoms; physical assessment; determination of psychological, social, and vocational needs; assessment of nutritional status; assessment of exercise tolerance; determination of educational needs; and assessment of the patient's ability to carry out activities of daily living.

■ MONITORING

Patients should be monitored at baseline and at appropriate intervals to ensure validity of results and appropriateness of intervention. Monitoring should include the following:

- Patient's response to progressive and general reconditioning exercises in conjunction with breathing techniques
- Patient's O_2 requirements at rest and with exercise
- Knowledge and skills acquisition
- Patient's subjective comments
- Progress in achieving goals
- Patient appearance
- Vital signs
- Cardiac telemetry (if needed)
- Perceived exertion and dyspnea (use of Borg or Modified Borg Dyspnea Scale)

For the complete guidelines, see American Association for Respiratory Care: AARC clinical practice guideline: pulmonary rehabilitation. Respir Care 47:617, 2002.

TABLE 50-1

Exercise Parameters Distinguishing Cardiac and Ventilatory (Chronic Obstructive Pulmonary Disease) Limitations

Parameter*	Cardiac†	COPD†
Maximum $\dot{V}O_2$	↓	↓
Maximum HR	N or ↓	↓
O_2 pulse	↓	N
Maximum $\dot{Q}$	↓	↓
$\dot{Q}/\dot{V}O_2$	↓	N
PaO_2	N	↓
$PaCO_2$	↓	↑
$\dot{V}E/\dot{V}CO_2$	↑	↑
VT	↓	N

Modified from Lane EE, Walker JF: Clinical arterial blood gas analysis, St Louis, 1987, Mosby.
**HR,* Heart rate; $\dot{Q}$, cardiac output; $\dot{V}E/\dot{V}CO_2$, ratio of ventilation to CO_2 production; $\dot{V}O_2$, oxygen consumption; *VT,* ventilatory threshold.
†*N,* Normal; ↑, increased; ↓, decreased.

Box 50-4 Indications and Contraindications for Pulmonary Rehabilitation

INDICATIONS

Symptomatic patients with COPD—usually GOLD stage III (severe) and stage IV (very severe), but stage II (moderate) may also be considered

Patients with bronchial asthma and associated bronchitis (asthmatic bronchitis)

Patients with combined obstructive and restrictive ventilatory defects

Patients with chronic mucociliary clearance problems

Patients with exercise limitations because of severe dyspnea

CONTRAINDICATIONS

Cardiovascular instability requiring cardiac monitoring (consider cardiac rehabilitation)

Malignant neoplasms involving the respiratory system

Severe arthritis or neuromuscular abnormalities (a relative contraindication—refer to physical therapy for case-by-case review)

- Neuromuscular, musculoskeletal, or rheumatoid disorders exacerbated by exercise
- Uncontrolled metabolic disease (e.g., diabetes)
- SaO_2 or SpO_2 less than 85% with the subject breathing room air
- Untreated or unstable asthma
- Angina with exercise

Exercise evaluation also can help differentiate among patients with primary respiratory or cardiac limitations to increased work capacity. Table 50-1 summarizes these key similarities and differences. Besides helping to differentiate between the underlying cause of exercise intolerance, test results can assist in placing patients in the appropriate type of rehabilitation program.

To minimize patient risk during exercise evaluation, certain safety measures are implemented. First, the patient should undergo a physical examination just before the test, including a resting ECG. Second, a qualified physician should be present throughout the entire test. Third, emergency resuscitation equipment (cardiac crash cart with monitor, defibrillator, O_2, cardiac drugs, suction equipment, and airway equipment) must be readily available. Fourth, staff conducting and assisting with the procedure should be certified in basic and advanced life-support techniques. Last, the test should be terminated promptly whenever indicated.

With regard to test preparation, patients should fast 8 hours before the procedure. If the purpose of the test is to formulate an exercise prescription, the patient can take his or her regular medications. The patient should wear comfortable, loose-fitting clothing and footwear with adequate traction for treadmill or ergometer activity. The mouthpiece or face mask used during the test should be sized properly and fit comfortably with no leaks. Test conditions should be as standardized as possible to allow for comparison of results before and after rehabilitation periodically from year to year as the patient is treated and followed.

Patient Selection

Patients most likely to benefit from participation in pulmonary rehabilitation are patients with persistent symptoms caused by COPD who have low maximum O_2 uptakes at baseline. Pulmonary rehabilitation should be a part of the discharge planning process when a patient is released from the hospital after an exacerbation of the existing chronic respiratory condition. The feasibility of rehabilitation should be reviewed with the patient, physician, and respiratory therapist (RT). Other indications for pulmonary rehabilitation are listed in Box 50-4. Regardless of underlying conditions, patients also should be ex-smokers. Any patients who smoke should enroll in a smoking cessation program before starting pulmonary rehabilitation. Patients are excluded from pulmonary rehabilitation activities if (1) concurrent problems limit or preclude participation in exercise or (2) their condition is complicated by malignant neoplasms, such as lung cancer (see Box 50-4).

Objectively, candidates considered for inclusion in a pulmonary rehabilitation program generally fall into one of the following groups:[20]

- Patients in whom there is a respiratory limitation to exercise resulting in termination at a level less than 75% of the predicted maximum O_2 consumption ($\dot{V}O_2max$)
- Patients in whom there is significant irreversible airway obstruction with a forced expiratory volume in 1 second (FEV_1) of less than 2 L or an $FEV_{1\%}$ (ratio of FEV_1 to forced vital capacity [FVC]) of less than 60% (consider the Global Initiative on Obstructive Lung Disease [GOLD] standards for COPD severity here)
- Patients in whom there is significant restrictive lung disease with a total lung capacity (TLC) of less than 80%

of predicted and single breath carbon monoxide diffusing capacity (DLCO) of less than 80% of predicted
- Patients with pulmonary vascular disease in whom single breath DLCO is less than 80% of predicted or in whom exercise is limited to less than 75% of maximum predicted O_2 consumption (predicted $\dot{V}O_2max$)

Groups or classes for pulmonary rehabilitation should be kept homogeneous. Placing individuals in a program who are at different stages of cardiopulmonary disability can be very defeating. Individuals with mild to moderate impairment may become discouraged on how severe lung disease can become, and individuals with severe impairment may feel they cannot keep up with or maintain the level of activity exhibited by others with less severe impairment. It is best to group patients together on the basis of severity and overall ability. In this way, patients can participate, compete, and progress together in the program without frustration, fear, or loss of motivation.

Program Design

A good design helps achieve specific programming objectives with the selected group of participating patients. Key design considerations involve both format and content, with emphasis on patient reconditioning and education.

Format

Programs can use either an open-ended or a closed design, with or without planned follow-up sessions. With an *open-ended format,* patients enter the program and progress through it until they achieve certain predetermined objectives. There is no set time frame. Depending on his or her condition, needs, motivation, and performance, an individual patient can complete an open-ended program over weeks or months. This format is good for self-directed patients or patients with scheduling difficulties. It also may be the best format for patients requiring individual attention. The major drawback of the open-ended format is the lack of group support and involvement. In addition, insurance reimbursement may be a factor when the program is open-ended.

The more traditional *closed design* uses a set time period to cover program content. These programs usually run 6 to 16 weeks, with classes meeting one to three times a week. However, insurance coverage may dictate how many sessions make up the program. Medicare covers 36 initial sessions with possible coverage of another 36 sessions if the patient qualifies and would benefit from the additional rehabilitation sessions. Class sessions usually last up to 2 hours. Presentations are more formal, and group support and involvement is encouraged. A major drawback to this format is that the schedule determines program completion, rather than the objectives. However, most programs allow patients to reenroll if the anticipated improvements are not achieved.

Regardless of the format used, long-term improvements cannot be expected without planned follow-up.[21] Follow-up must be ongoing and available to all patients who complete the program. Frequently, this essential element of the process is difficult, especially when it is not covered by most insurance plans, but program coordinators must ensure that it is routinely scheduled. Follow-up or reinforcement could be open-ended (available during regular rehabilitation sessions and offering open attendance) or could be scheduled weekly, monthly, bimonthly, or quarterly. The important thing is to have some type of follow-up available.[22,23]

Content

The content of the rehabilitation program usually combines physical reconditioning with education activities. Table 50-2 outlines a sample session incorporating these two complementary components. Programs providing reconditioning or education alone are unlikely to be effective.

As shown in Table 50-2, the ideal rehabilitation session should last about 2 hours. Group size, available equipment, and group interaction dictate session length. Patients should arrive 10 to 15 minutes before a scheduled session to allow for informal group interaction and support. Classes should begin on time and conclude promptly as scheduled. Educational presentations should be brief and to the point. The use of audiovisuals or demonstrations should enhance understanding. To facilitate patient comprehension, the language should be simple, and unnecessary technical terms or concepts should be avoided. Handouts that enhance certain points made during a presentation are both useful and desirable. A folder or notebook in which program activities may be recorded and handout materials kept should be maintained by each patient.

Physical Reconditioning

The physical reconditioning component of the pulmonary rehabilitation program consists primarily of an exercise prescription with target heart rate based on the results of

TABLE 50-2

Sample Pulmonary Rehabilitation Session

Component	Focus	Time Frame
Educational	Welcome (group interaction)	5 min
	Review of program diaries (activities of past week)	20 min
	Presentation of educational topic	20 min
	Questions, answers, and group discussion	15 min
Physical reconditioning	Physical activity and reconditioning	45 min
	Individual goal setting and session summary	15 min
Total session		120 min (2 hr)

the patient's initial exercise evaluation. For most patients, an initial target heart rate is set using **Karvonen's formula,** or estimated as 20 beats/min greater than resting rate. Because of the severity of ventilatory impairment, some patients begin exercise reconditioning without a prescribed target heart rate.

RULE OF THUMB

To set a target heart rate for patient exercise, use Karvonen's formula:

$$\text{Target heart rate} = [(MHR - RHR) \times (50\% - 70\%)] + RHR$$

where MHR is maximum heart rate at limit of exercise tolerance and RHR is resting heart rate.

A good target exercise heart rate for a patient with COPD with MHR of 150 beats/min and RHR of 90 beats/min would be $[(150 - 90) \times 0.60] + 90 = 126$ beats/min.

MINI CLINI

Patient Selection for Pulmonary Rehabilitation

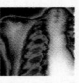

PROBLEM: A patient is being evaluated for possible inclusion in a pulmonary rehabilitation program. The patient undergoes a complete history and physical examination and pulmonary function testing, arterial blood gas analysis, and exercise evaluation. During the exercise test, the patient develops severe hypertension and premature ventricular contractions. The physician recommends that the patient be admitted to pulmonary rehabilitation and prescribes a modified exercise routine. The RT performing the test disagrees. How should the RT proceed?

SOLUTION: The RT should contact the department medical director for intervention. Although this patient could possibly be admitted to pulmonary rehabilitation, there is a high risk that some type of adverse response might occur during the exercise component of the program. The best direction would be to treat the cardiac manifestations first. After identifying the causes of the exercise-induced hypertension and arrhythmia, these problems can be properly treated. When the patient's cardiac manifestations are under control, the patient may be admitted to pulmonary rehabilitation and safely participate in and complete the program. Any underlying condition should be treated and managed first before pulmonary rehabilitation begins.

Typically, the exercise prescription includes the following four related components:[24,25]

1. Lower extremity (leg) **aerobic exercises**
2. Timed walking **(6- or 12-minute walk)**
3. Upper extremity (arm) aerobic exercises
4. Ventilatory muscle training

To ensure success with physical reconditioning, patients must actively participate both at the rehabilitation facility and at home. While exercising at the facility, patients should be monitored by pulse oximetry. Blood pressure measurements may also be made, but these are usually done at the start and end of each session unless a patient's condition dictates otherwise. In addition, exercise sessions should be upbeat. Lively music helps to maintain a positive atmosphere. Clinicians must remember that these patients are ill and require a nurturing attitude from team members, family, and the group itself.

To ensure compliance with the program, a daily log or diary sheet is completed. Figure 50-5 depicts a sample log sheet that makes up a section of the patient manual. These log or diary forms are reviewed each time the patient attends a session. Based on this information, further individualized reconditioning goals are set.

Patient Log   Week # _______

Day	Flow Resistive Device	6-min or 12-min Walk	Exercycle	Other Activity	Remarks
	Setting ______ Duration ______	Distance ______ No. of stops ______	Distance ______ Duration ______	Type ______ Duration ______	
	Setting ______ Duration ______	Distance ______ No. of stops ______	Distance ______ Duration ______	Type ______ Duration ______	
	Setting ______ Duration ______	Distance ______ No. of stops ______	Distance ______ Duration ______	Type ______ Duration ______	
	Setting ______ Duration ______	Distance ______ No. of stops ______	Distance ______ Duration ______	Type ______ Duration ______	
	Setting ______ Duration ______	Distance ______ No. of stops ______	Distance ______ Duration ______	Type ______ Duration ______	
	Setting ______ Duration ______	Distance ______ No. of stops ______	Distance ______ Duration ______	Type ______ Duration ______	
	Setting ______ Duration ______	Distance ______ No. of stops ______	Distance ______ Duration ______	Type ______ Duration ______	

FIGURE 50-5 Sample log or diary form on which a patient in a pulmonary rehabilitation program records daily physical reconditioning activities and exercises.

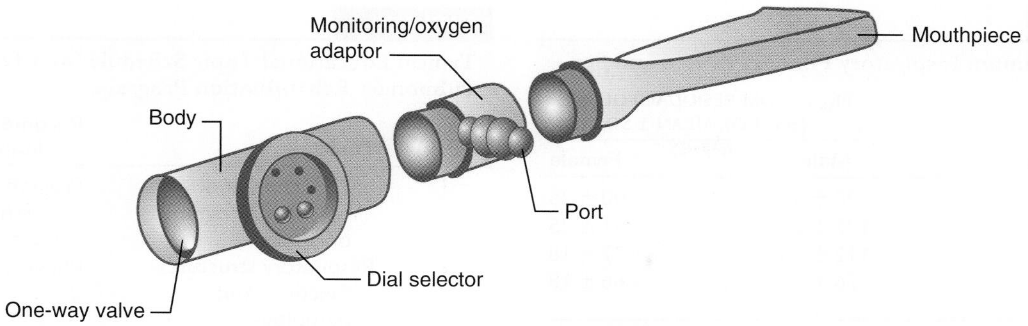

FIGURE 50-6 Flow-resistive breathing device.

Lower extremity exercises may include either walking or bicycling. Patients can walk on a stationary treadmill (with set goals for distance or time and grade) or on a flat, smooth surface. Patients can bicycle on an exercise cycle. With the treadmill or stationary bicycle, patients are required to cover a certain distance or duration every day that they are in the program. Commonly, the duration is set to 30 minutes daily, with patients encouraged to increase both their distance and equipment tension or resistance as tolerated. Patients with significant orthopedic disabilities can participate in aerobic aquatic exercises.

Walking also improves overall conditioning; this usually takes the form of a 6- or 12-minute walk performed once a day, depending on the patient's condition and tolerance. These walk exercises are a convenient way for patients to carry out a well-defined amount of activity with increasing vigor and results over a number of weeks. During the 6 or 12 minutes, patients should walk on flat ground for as far as possible. If severe dyspnea occurs, they should stop and rest, with the rest time included as part of the time interval. After resting briefly, they should try to continue walking at a comfortable pace. The objective is to walk as far as possible during the allotted time. Landmarks such as telephone poles, city blocks, or actual distance measures can be used to quantify progress. Under adverse weather conditions, walking can be done indoors in shopping malls, stores, or long hallways. Patients should record their progress in their manuals or diaries.

Aerobic upper extremity exercises improve rehabilitation outcomes for patients whose regular activities involve lifting or raising the arms.[24,26] Arm ergometers or rowing machines are available for this purpose; however, simple calisthenics using either a broomstick or free weights (by prescription and with training) are a satisfactory alternative. Upper body endurance generally is more limited, with many patients capable of only 2 to 3 minutes of daily activity to start. This limitation usually is related to the fact that patients may revert to using accessory muscles for breathing while doing the upper body exercise. Patients need to breathe diaphragmatically and perform the exercises at the same time. Arm exercises should get progressively longer, up to 20 minutes if possible. Upper body conditioning helps patients perform numerous useful activities at home and can increase overall physical endurance. As with other activity, patients should record daily results in their logs or manuals.

Although controversy exists, ventilatory muscle training probably can enhance the benefits of these more traditional exercises.[27] Ventilatory muscle training is based on the concept of **progressive resistance.** By imposing progressively greater loads on the inspiratory muscles (mainly the diaphragm) over time, the patient's strength and endurance should increase. These improvements should increase the patient's exercise tolerance.

Figure 50-6 shows a typical inspiratory resistance breathing device. The device is an adjustable flow resistor with a one-way breathing valve. The inspiratory load is created by forcing the patient to inhale through a restricted orifice. Varying the size of this orifice varies the inspiratory load, as do changes in the patient's inspiratory flow. During expiration, gas flows unimpeded out the one-way exhalation valve. Other types of devices are also available. One model replaces the variable size orifice with an adjustable spring-loaded valve. This valve ensures a constant load regardless of how quickly or slowly the patient breathes.

Because variations in breathing strategy during ventilatory muscle training can affect outcomes, proper patient evaluation, training, and follow-up are required. The RT initially measures the patient's maximum inspiratory pressure (PI_{max}) using a calibrated pressure manometer. The RT next compares the patient's maximum with established norms (Table 50-3). This preliminary measure of inspiratory pressure helps to establish initial loads and provides the basis for the subsequent monitoring of patient progress.

Before beginning ventilatory muscle training, the patient should assume a position that relaxes the abdominal muscles, such as the position used for cough training. If using a flow resistive device, the RT begins at the maximum orifice setting, while measuring the inspiratory pressure generated through the monitoring or O_2 adapter (a second adapter may be needed if the patient is receiving supplemental O_2). The RT encourages the patient to

TABLE 50-3

Normal Maximum Inspiratory Pressure by Age and Sex

Age Group (yr)	PI_{MAX} FROM RESIDUAL VOLUME ($cm\ H_2O$), MEAN ± SD Male	Female
9-18	96 ± 35	90 ± 25
19-50	127 ± 28	91 ± 25
51-70	112 ± 20	77 ± 18
>70	76 ± 27	66 ± 18

From Rochester DF, Hyatt RE: Respiratory muscle failure, Med Clin North Am 67:573, 1983.

breathe slowly through the device, at a rate no greater than 10 to 12 breaths/min. If the patient's inspiratory pressure is less than 30% of the measured PI_{max}, the next smaller orifice is selected, with this procedure repeated until the 30% effort is consistently achieved.

At this point, the RT instructs the patient to exercise with the device in one or two regular daily sessions lasting 10 to 15 minutes. As the level of resistance becomes more tolerable over time, the patient should progressively increase session duration up to 30 minutes. A self-maintained log of treatment times can help motivate the patient and assist the RT in subsequent progress monitoring.

Educational Component

The educational portion of the program covers topics that are both useful and necessary to the patient. Table 50-4 lists examples of topics covered during a 12-week rehabilitation program. Recommendations regarding the best facilitators for each session are included. Naturally, other topics can be included depending on the program schedule, but in terms of relative importance, the ones listed in Table 50-4 generally have the highest priority.

The actual content of these sessions follows. These topics should be presented in an orderly, coherent fashion using supplementary audiovisual tools and demonstrations, where appropriate. Team members should allocate sufficient time both for the class sessions themselves and for setup and breakdown of equipment.

The program facilitator or leader must ensure that sessions begin on time and encourage maximum participation by each patient. If available, health care professionals such as dietitians, occupational therapists, physical therapists, and psychologists should be invited to present their respective topics and discuss the subject matter with the group. In addition to technical knowledge, session leaders must possess group facilitation skills and be able to motivate patients to participate both in class and at home and to adhere to program guidelines. This task is not an easy one, but it can be accomplished with patience and persistence. The desired end result is to help patients lead more productive lives with decreased hospitalizations.

TABLE 50-4

Typical Educational Topic Schedule for a 12-Week Pulmonary Rehabilitation Program

Session (Week)	Topic(s)	Recommended Facilitator(s)
1	Introduction and welcome; program orientation	Program administrator or rehabilitation team
2	Respiratory structure, function, and pathology	Physician or RT
3	Breathing control methods	PT or RT
4	Relaxation and stress management	Clinical psychologist
5	Proper exercise techniques and personal routines	PT or RT
6	Methods to aid secretion clearance (bronchial hygiene)	PT or RT
7	Home oxygen and aerosol therapy	RT
8	Medications—their use and abuse	Pharmacist, physician, or nurse practitioner
9	Medications—use of MDIs and spacers	RT
10	Dietary guidelines and good nutrition	Dietitian or nutritionist
11	Recreation and vocational counseling Activities of daily living	Occupational therapist
12	Follow-up planning and program evaluation Graduation	Rehabilitation team

MDIs, Metered dose inhalers; *PT,* physical therapist; *RT,* respiratory therapist.

Respiratory Structure, Function, and Pathology, Including a Discussion of Dyspnea. This presentation lays the groundwork for the program and gives each patient some basic information about the cardiorespiratory system and related disorders. The causes of shortness of breath are presented.

Breathing Control Methods. This presentation serves as the cornerstone for the physical reconditioning effort. Patients must learn how to control their breathing efforts to ensure maximum result (ventilation) at a minimum of effort (energy expenditure). Diaphragmatic breathing with pursed lips helps to accomplish this, but this technique requires daily practice on the part of the patient and continued reinforcement throughout the entire program by the group facilitator.

Methods of Relaxation and Stress Management. Patients must learn to avoid aggravation and upsetting circumstances and to adopt a more relaxed attitude about their particular life circumstances. This attitude can help to reduce unnecessary O_2 use, conserve energy, and avoid undesirable cardiovascular and nervous responses to stress.

Exercise Techniques and Personal Routines. The rationale for and value of exercise should be discussed with suggestions for the adoption of personal exercise routines after the rehabilitation program is over.

Secretion Clearance and Bronchial Hygiene Techniques. This topic is especially helpful to patients who have secretion clearance problems associated with chronic bronchitis and bronchiectasis. Family members and friends may be invited to attend this session to acquire basic skills with these procedures.

Home Oxygen and Aerosol Therapy. An RT with home care experience should provide this session. The focus should be on the care and use of home care equipment and self-administration of therapy. Patients who have not yet been prescribed this type of therapeutic regimen may have questions or fears and be unreceptive to the concept. Presenting the modalities available and having patients discuss their positive experiences with respiratory home care personnel can help alleviate the fears and anxieties of others.

Medications. This is another topic about which patients have numerous questions and concerns. Content should emphasize proper use of medications, along with possible abuses and adverse effects. Participants' current prescriptions should dictate which specific drugs to cover. Common categories include beta-adrenergic agents, anticholinergic agents, steroids, diuretics, and methylxanthines. The session leader should demonstrate proper use of metered dose inhalers including spacers or holding chambers, dry powder inhalers, and hand-held nebulizers. Sufficient time should be provided for questions and answers. Two sessions should be allotted for this topic.

Dietary Guidelines. This subject focuses on weight management and good nutrition as it relates to cardiopulmonary health. Emphasis should be on the importance of a sound high-protein, low-carbohydrate diet. The facilitator also should cover proper eating habits, methods of gaining and losing weight, foods to avoid, ways to increase appetite, and daily menu planning. This session can stimulate patients to eat better and supply their bodies with the necessary fuel for increased energy production.

Recreational and Vocational Counseling. This session should motivate participants to participate in recreational activities and, according to ability, return to work. This topic is often presented at the end of the program when patients have increased their physical endurance and are preparing for a more active and productive lifestyle. The class may brainstorm ideas for recreational or physical activities, from which members can generate action plans.

Psychosocial and Behavioral Components

Psychologic and emotional stress is a common problem for patients with moderate to severe chronic lung disease. Pulmonary rehabilitation programs can bring in experts to implement psychosocial and behavioral therapies that provide patients with the opportunity to learn coping strategies. This component is most useful for patients with anxiety or depression or both.

Program Implementation

In 1987, the AARC and the AACVPR jointly conducted the first national survey of pulmonary rehabilitation programs. This National Pulmonary Rehabilitation Survey was published in 1988 and showed the variation existing in rehabilitation program structure, content, staffing, and cost throughout the United States.[28] In 2006, the ACCP, in conjunction with the AACVPR, released new evidence-based guidelines pertaining to the design and implementation of pulmonary rehabilitation programs.[13]

Staffing

Pulmonary rehabilitation is a multidisciplinary endeavor. Team care is enhanced by involving various health care professionals in the planning, implementation, and evaluation components of the program (Figure 50-7). It is recommended that any staff conducting pulmonary rehabilitation program sessions be certified in basic life support or advanced cardiac life support through the American Heart Association. In addition to professional involvement, family members are needed to provide feedback and ensure that instructions and the exercise prescription are carried out at home.

Facilities

Location and quality of facilities can directly affect patient attendance. Patients are less likely to attend programs that are inaccessible to public transportation, have poor parking arrangements, or are physically difficult to reach. The facility must be wheelchair accessible. For elderly patients who do not drive, arrangements can be made with community organizations to provide transportation to and from the program. Ideally, the facility should provide two separate rooms for the program—one room for educational activities and one room for physical reconditioning. Rooms should be spacious and comfortable with adequate lighting, ventilation, and temperature control. Chairs should be comfortable with good back support. Restroom facilities need to be readily accessible. A room for individual counseling is helpful, but any private office would suffice. It is also preferable to have pulmonary function testing and blood gas analysis capabilities on site. If this space is used by other departments for other functions, proper scheduling of rehabilitation sessions needs to be considered.

Scheduling

Another aspect of program implementation involves timely scheduling of the rehabilitation sessions. With the open-ended format, patients can attend rehabilitation at a time convenient to them as long as the facility is open and

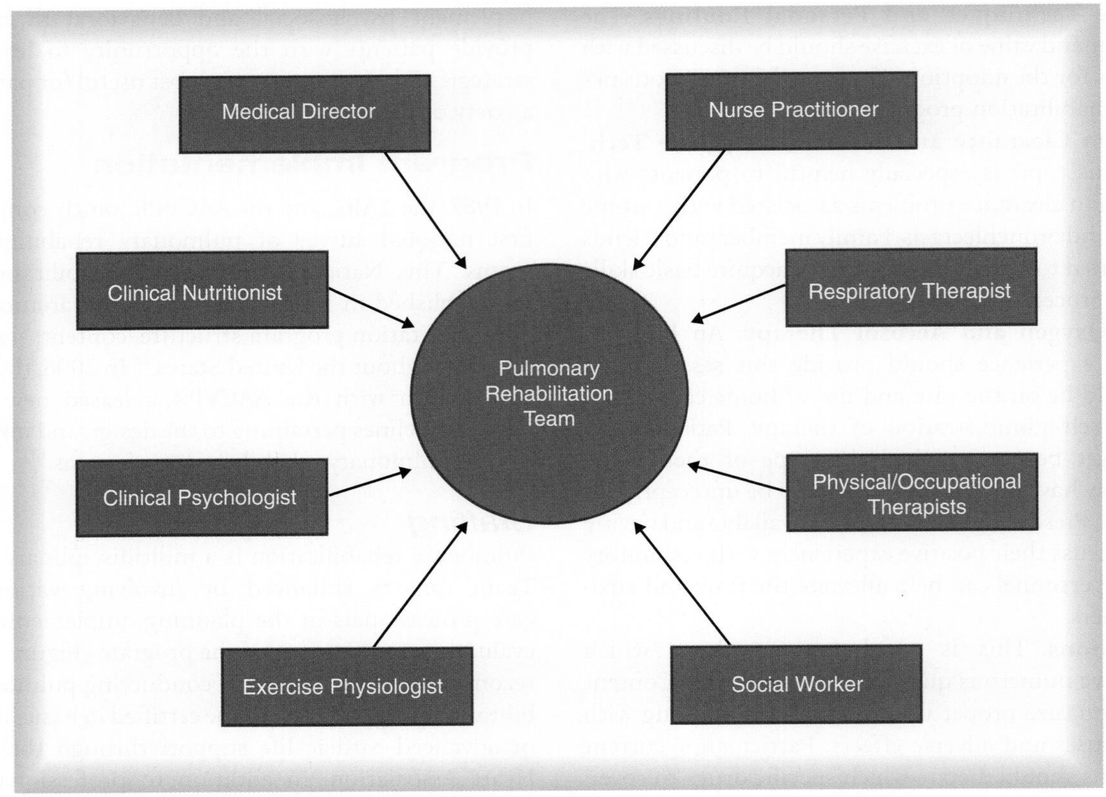

FIGURE 50-7 Multidisciplinary nature of pulmonary rehabilitation.

staffed accordingly. With the closed format, sessions are scheduled one to three times per week for 1 to 3 hours, with programs running 8 to 16 weeks. The length of the program often depends on insurance coverage and expected reimbursement for sessions attended. Class times need to be scheduled when the largest number of patients can attend. Traffic patterns, bus schedules, and availability of rides are concerns that need to be discussed. The ideal situation involves a separate area set aside for pulmonary rehabilitation with a dedicated staff of professionals conducting the program; this makes scheduling for either open-ended or closed programs easier and more manageable. Sessions can be conducted in the morning, afternoon, or evening and on weekends if necessary. Proper scheduling helps to encourage participation and removes potential stumbling blocks, which could undermine the rehabilitation process.

Class Size

Class size is another issue that must be addressed. Theoretically, a rehabilitation program could be conducted with 1 participant or 15 or more, depending on available space, equipment, and staff. However, to foster group identity, interaction, and support, small group discussions are encouraged. The ideal class size should range from 3 to 10 participants. Keeping the class size manageable facilitates vital group interaction processes and allows for more individualized attention. These factors help sustain motivation, reducing the likelihood of participant attrition.

Naturally, economic concerns surface when class size is considered. Although program quality must be the first priority, program viability realistically depends on the number of participants. Programs generally should be conducted with a class size that is comfortable with regard to space and staffing and that is economically feasible. Such an approach helps ensure that programs produce meaningful patient outcomes.

Equipment

Both the instruction and the reconditioning component of the program require equipment. To meet the educational needs of the program, a blackboard or flipchart along with a PowerPoint projector, screen, overhead projector, and cassette or CD tape player are needed. A videotape or DVD player with monitor may also be helpful, especially if individualized instruction or commercially available programs are used. Also, slides, tapes, videos, and formal learning packages dealing with the educational topics covered during the rehabilitation program should be available for group and individualized presentation. These can be purchased from outside sources or designed and developed in-house.

For physical reconditioning, stationary bicycles, treadmills, rowing machines, upper extremity ergometers, weights, pulse oximeters, and inspiratory resistance

MINI CLINI

Facilities Planning for Pulmonary Rehabilitation

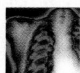

PROBLEM: The RT has been asked to assist in the planning process for starting a pulmonary rehabilitation program to support a 350-bed, full-service hospital. According to the strategic plan, the physical location of the rehabilitation center is about 3 blocks away from the hospital. The RT has not seen the proposed site but was asked to approve a recommendation that the facility be used. What factors should the RT take into account before making a decision on site selection?

SOLUTION: Because the hospital is currently in the planning process for starting a pulmonary rehabilitation program and has not made a final facility selection, the RT is in a key position to assess, among other areas, issues related to the proposed site. Patient attendance and participation would be adversely affected if the facility is unreachable, such as at the top of a hill. If the location is in a high crime or unsafe area with little or no security, this too would discourage patients from attending. As is true with any program, public transportation that does not permit accessibility to the proposed facility would be a limiting factor, as would little or no available parking. Numerous other facility considerations outside the actual physical location of the rehabilitation center would also need to be addressed. The current square footage of available space and room for future expansion would need to be evaluated relative to anticipated needs, as would whether the facility itself is wheelchair accessible with no barriers present.

breathing devices constitute the minimum equipment requirements. The quantity of equipment needed depends on class size, scheduling, and available space. Sufficient equipment should be on hand to keep all patients exercising and to monitor their activity. Emergency O_2 and bronchodilator medications should also be maintained in the rehabilitation area. Equipment guidelines for a class of 6 to 10 participants include the following: five stationary bicycles, two treadmills, two rowing machines, two upper extremity ergometers, five pulse oximeters for monitoring heart rate and O_2 saturation, one emergency O_2 cylinder (E), and bronchodilator medications. In addition, each patient should be supplied with an inspiratory resistance breathing device.

Because equipment can be expensive, care must be taken in its selection and purchase. Devices and appliances should be durable, easy and safe to use, simple to maintain, and not overly expensive. Initially, basic items are purchased. As a program develops and expands, equipment resources can be enhanced. Other program needs include the following:

- Maintaining individual patient manuals, including daily log forms or activity diaries

Box 50-5 Factors Affecting Pulmonary Rehabilitation Program Costs

- Marketing and program promotion
- Number of personnel involved in program facilitation and administration
- Space and utility expenses
- Audiovisual, exercise, and monitoring equipment (purchase and maintenance)
- Production and duplication of course materials
- Patient supplies
- Office supplies
- Refreshments
- Miscellaneous expenses

- Providing light refreshments for program participants
- Developing a communication network to announce schedule changes because of emergencies or cancellation of class sessions because of illness or weather
- Identifying available durable medical equipment providers for participants in need of specialized home care equipment
- Developing a system of charges and mechanism for patient payment

By considering all of the factors needed for effective implementation of pulmonary rehabilitation, programs have lower patient attrition and a greater chance for overall success. As programs are conducted, regular evaluations must be made by both patients and staff. Needed changes should be implemented on an ongoing basis. Only in this manner can one expect continued refinement of the process and improvement in patient outcomes.

Cost, Fees, and Reimbursement

Rehabilitation programs usually project their fees based on the average cost per participant. According to regional labor and material prices, costs vary throughout the United States. Several factors must be considered when projecting program costs (Box 50-5). The larger the class size and the more participants involved in the overall program, the lower the cost would be per patient. The aim should be to offer and conduct the highest quality program possible at a reasonable cost that meets any existing budgetary constraints.

When determining patient charges, consideration must also be given to the type and amount of funding that has been received to offset program expenses and available insurance reimbursement. Preprogram and postprogram testing and evaluations naturally generate revenues but should not be included in the formulation of program charges. However, payments for pulmonary function testing, exercise testing, arterial blood gas analysis, and other evaluations may help to keep a pulmonary rehabilitation program financially viable.

Charges for an entire program or for each session must be structured in a way that does not deter patient attendance. Many patients with a chronic pulmonary disease are on a fixed income and have other living and medical expenses. A happy medium between a patient's ability to pay and program expenses must be identified. Funding from local charitable organizations, foundations, or agencies such as the American Lung Association can help ease the financial burden. The most comprehensive and effective program available can have no impact if patients are unwilling or unable to attend and participate because of financial limitations.

Along with health care costs in general, the cost of providing pulmonary rehabilitation has increased over the years. Nationwide charges for pulmonary rehabilitation vary, depending on program length and, most importantly, insurance coverage. With most insurance plans reimbursing programs at 80% after a deductible, each patient would be responsible for the remaining 20% or copayment. Additional or supplemental medical coverage may cover this balance.

Charges for participation in these programs and inpatient rehabilitation reimbursement policies vary throughout the United States. In 1982, the Centers for Medicare and Medicaid Services (CMS, formerly the Health Care Financing Administration) published the final rules for Medicare reimbursement guidelines for **comprehensive outpatient rehabilitative facilities (CORFs).** Under Part B of Medicare, the scope of services of a CORF includes reimbursement for outpatient activities and one home visit. Reimbursement requires that the CORF meet the conditions of participation established in section 933 of Public Law 96-499; this also includes provisions for certification of the program. To establish reimbursement mechanisms, each CORF must present its program description and anticipated results to local third-party payers. The AACVPR also has developed guidelines for program design, implementation, and recognition.

By following recognized guidelines, Medicare has established an allowable charge for pulmonary rehabilitation and reimburses 80% of this rate after the patient meets the annual prescribed deductible. In the past, inpatient and outpatient pulmonary rehabilitation programs obtained reimbursement from third-party payers by charging for rehabilitation sessions as physical therapy exercises for COPD, reconditioning exercise sessions, office visits with therapeutic exercises, serial pulse oximetry determinations, or physician office visits. The goal was to obtain as much insurance reimbursement as possible, decreasing the financial burden on the patient. Box 50-6 lists all possible sources of reimbursement.[29,30]

There is now a national coverage policy for pulmonary rehabilitation under Medicare, which took effect on January 1, 2010, as a result of the passage of HR 6331. Programs have to obtain reimbursement for their Medicare beneficiaries following accepted protocol, policies, and provisions specified by Medicare. Coverage is for patients with stage II, III, and IV COPD (moderate to very severe according to the GOLD standards). Pulmonary rehabilitation programs must include five components, and these must be documented in the patient's medical record. The five components include the following:

1. Physician-prescribed exercise, including aerobic exercise, which is performed during each session
2. Education and training that relate to an individual patient's needs
3. Psychosocial assessment
4. Outcomes assessment
5. Treatment plan that details how these components are used for each individual patient

Box 50-6 Sources of Reimbursement for Pulmonary Rehabilitation Programs

- Nongovernment health insurance programs—private, single, or group health insurance plans
  - Health maintenance organizations (HMOs)
  - Preferred provider organizations (PPOs)
  - Medicare supplement
- Federal and state health insurance programs
  - Medicare
  - Medicaid
  - Uncompensated services (Hill-Burton)
  - CORF
  - Veterans Administration benefits
  - Civilian Health and Medical Programs of the Uniformed Services (CHAMPUS)
  - Federal workers insurance
- Ancillary liability and casualty insurance programs
  - Automobile insurance—related to automobile accidents
  - Workers' compensation—related to accidents on the job
  - Business insurance coverage—related to injuries sustained on business premises
  - Homeowner's insurance—related to injuries sustained on the owner's premises
  - Malpractice insurance on providers of health care
  - Product and service liability insurance—related to injuries caused by a product or service
- Other options of reimbursement
  - Senior care
  - Rehabilitation hospitals
  - Grants

RULE OF THUMB

To help ensure adequate reimbursement for pulmonary rehabilitation, identify patient goals and objectives; formulate and implement an effective exercise prescription for each patient; use diagnostic codes from the International Classification of Diseases, Ninth Revision, Clinical Modification (ICD-9-CM)*; use current and proper CPT* (Current Procedural Terminology) *coding; and document, document, document.*

According to CMS, claims for Medicare patients should be submitted to Medicare Part A for any component of pulmonary rehabilitation performed during a hospital stay, and claims for rehabilitation components provided on an outpatient basis must be submitted to Medicare Part B. As with other forms of therapy covered by CMS, other insurance providers have already or will follow Medicare policy for reimbursement of pulmonary rehabilitation. This payment mechanism has already undergone changes, and it is anticipated that Medicare will continue to change its reimbursement policy for pulmonary rehabilitation in the future. It is incumbent on clinicians who provide pulmonary rehabilitation to stay abreast of any changes in reimbursement policy and procedure and to make necessary adjustments to receive payment.

At the present time, there is provision to reimburse pulmonary rehabilitation programs for two 1-hour rehabilitation sessions per patient per day up to 36 sessions. An additional 36 sessions over an extended period can be approved by the individual Medicare contractor based on patient need for continued rehabilitation and physician referral. Documentation of programs is essential for payment of services rendered. In 2010, coding for pulmonary rehabilitation under Medicare Part B uses the HCPCS G0424 code. Provision has been made for face-to-face patient sessions and for group (two or more patients) sessions. Individual sessions must be at least 31 minutes in length. If two sessions are performed on the same day, services may be reported only if the duration of the combined treatments is at least 91 minutes. It is essential that the practitioner who conducts pulmonary rehabilitation is familiar with all current practices so that therapy provided and billed for complies with current Medicare policy, is properly documented for each patient, and is submitted in a timely fashion.[31,32]

Program Results

Patient and program outcomes must be evaluated at the conclusion of the program and periodically thereafter (Box 50-7). Evaluation results must compare patient status before the program with current patient status and may include physiologic, psychologic, and sociologic data. Common outcome measures include exercise tolerance, levels of dyspnea at rest and with exertion, and quality-of-life surveys.

Results of pulmonary rehabilitation must be communicated to the patient, family, referring physician, and home care company, if appropriate. Further goals and objectives for continued improvement may be established to provide the basis for follow-up and reinforcement activities. Quality of life for patients with chronic lung diseases is an outcome measure that many pulmonary rehabilitation programs are documenting.[33] A major predictor for improvement in health-related quality of life of a patient with COPD is frequent attendance in a maintenance program.[3,34]

MINI CLINI

Obtaining Insurance Payment for Pulmonary Rehabilitation

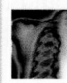

PROBLEM: The RT is asked to design and implement a pulmonary rehabilitation program on an outpatient basis at her hospital. After completing the first class that ran for 12 weeks, the hospital scheduled another one. However, although the institution had been submitting bills on a timely basis to numerous insurance providers, including Medicare, no payment has been received. What is the problem, and how can it be corrected?

SOLUTION: The insurance companies apparently either have denied claims or have not responded to the claims being submitted. This problem is often associated with improper or inaccurate claim filing. The RT should work closely with the billing department at the hospital to ensure that all information is complete for each patient (e.g., correct patient identification numbers), that the hospital has the correct addresses to submit claims, and that diagnosis and procedures have been properly coded. Some insurance companies have their own coding schemes, and these must be followed accordingly. Managed care companies also require preauthorization, and this must be obtained before entering any patient with a managed care plan into pulmonary rehabilitation. Finally, follow-up telephone calls are always helpful and should be conducted if payment is not received in a timely fashion.

Box 50-7 Evaluation of Rehabilitation Program Outcomes

- Changes in exercise tolerance
- Before and after 6- or 12-minute walking distance
- Before and after pulmonary exercise stress test
- Review of patient home exercise logs
- Strength measurement
- Flexibility and posture
- Performance on specific exercises (e.g., ventilatory muscle, upper extremity)
- Changes in symptoms
- Dyspnea measurement comparison
- Frequency of cough, sputum production, or wheezing
- Weight loss or gain
- Psychologic test instruments
- Other changes
- Activities of daily living changes
- Postprogram follow-up questionnaires
- Preprogram and postprogram knowledge tests
- Compliance improvement with pulmonary rehabilitation medical regimen
- Frequency and duration of respiratory exacerbations
- Frequency and duration of hospitalizations
- Frequency of emergency department visits
- Return to productive employment

If no improvements in physical or psychosocial measures occur within a class or group, program deficiencies are the most likely cause. Specifically, insufficient professional training in rehabilitation methods, a lack of uniformity in approach, inadequate program length, and lack of follow-up are the major reasons for unsatisfactory outcomes.

Finally, pulmonary rehabilitation has become recognized as a prerequisite for certain patients with emphysema who are able to undergo lung volume reduction surgery. Physical reconditioning and patient education before the procedure help to increase the chances for a successful outcome. Pulmonary rehabilitation appears to have favorable results with this specific patient population because of added patient and practitioner commitment and focus. Patients who do not complete the presurgical rehabilitation protocol are at higher risk for postsurgical complications.[35-38]

Potential Hazards

Although most patients with COPD can expect to realize benefits through physical reconditioning and pulmonary rehabilitation, certain potential hazards do exist, as follows:

I. Cardiovascular abnormalities
 A. Cardiac arrhythmias (can be reduced with supplemental O_2 during exercise)
 B. Systemic hypotension and hypertension

II. Blood gas abnormalities
 A. Arterial desaturation
 B. Hypercapnia
 C. Acidosis

III. Muscular abnormalities
 A. Functional or structural injuries
 B. Diaphragmatic fatigue and failure
 C. Exercise-induced muscle contracture

IV. Miscellaneous
 A. Exercise-induced asthma (more common in young patients with asthma than in patients with COPD)
 B. Hypoglycemia
 C. Dehydration

Proper patient selection, education, supervision, and monitoring are key factors in reducing possible hazards.

MINI CLINI

What to Expect from Pulmonary Rehabilitation

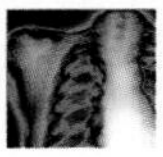

PROBLEM: The RT is asked to consult on a 63-year-old man hospitalized with severe COPD for possible participation in an outpatient pulmonary rehabilitation program. During the patient interview, the patient tells the RT that if the program will not cure him, he sees no reason to participate. How should the RT respond to the patient, keeping in mind his expectations of what pulmonary rehabilitation should accomplish?

SOLUTION: It is crucial for all RTs and other caregivers involved in pulmonary rehabilitation to recognize that the focus of any program should attempt to treat the patient as a whole and not solely the underlying disease. A well-constructed pulmonary rehabilitation program should be able both to quantify the extent of physiologic impairment and to assist in establishing outcome expectations for physical reconditioning. Regardless of setting or design, such programs must address the psychologic, social, and vocational impact of the disability on the patient and family and seek ways to improve the patient's quality of life. In this case, the RT should describe the benefits of pulmonary rehabilitation outside the traditional measures of pulmonary function. Although pulmonary rehabilitation cannot affect the progressive deterioration in lung function that occurs with COPD, both education and exercise may improve the patient's ability to perform activities of daily living and exercise tolerance. In addition, effective breathing techniques may lessen the frequency and severity of "panic breathing" episodes.

CARDIAC REHABILITATION

Patients with primary cardiac disease are often referred to cardiac rehabilitation programs where the focus is on improving cardiovascular fitness. *Cardiac rehabilitation* is defined as a comprehensive exercise and educational program designed for patients with cardiovascular diseases. Similar to pulmonary rehabilitation, good cardiac rehabilitation programs are multidisciplinary in approach and focus. Goals include patient education promoting heart-healthy living, physical reconditioning to improve work capacity, weight loss, and a return to work.

Enrollment in a cardiac rehabilitation program is based on a thorough cardiovascular evaluation and related parameters. The goal of a structured cardiac rehabilitation program is to assist patients in developing a regular pattern of safe exercise to achieve greater cardiovascular performance during activity. Most cardiac rehabilitation programs are conducted within a hospital facility, and the programs are generally divided into monitored and maintenance segments, with home options available. Exercise prescriptions are individualized for participating patients to maximize outcomes and reduce the likelihood of adverse effects.

Pulmonary and cardiac rehabilitation share many similarities and differences. Similarities include the need for patient evaluation before program enrollment, patient education, the focus on exercises to increase fitness and stamina, and the need to monitor patients during exercise and for compliance. Differences include disease focus, patient age (most cardiac patients range in age from late 30s to 60s and 70s, whereas pulmonary patients for the most part are ≥50 years), and exercises used within the program. Many cardiac patients can walk for up to 1 hour, whereas this may be virtually impossible for most pulmonary patients. Breathing exercises to improve ventilation are essential to the pulmonary patient but not that important to cardiac patients.

Reimbursement variables between the two types of programs also exist with cardiac rehabilitation being more recognized by insurance payers, including Medicare. Because cardiac rehabilitation has existed longer than pulmonary rehabilitation and because outcomes tend to have greater validity and acceptance, insurance reimbursement has been more readily available. There are four phases to cardiac rehabilitation from program introduction to the ongoing fitness aspect. Patient reimbursement depends on the phase of cardiac rehabilitation the patient is in. This division into phases does not currently exist for patients in pulmonary rehabilitation.

Finally, respiratory involvement in cardiac rehabilitation is significantly less. For the most part, the RT is involved with instruction on O_2 use and may assist with patient exercise sessions during cardiac rehabilitation. Most often, the cardiologist and cardiac nurse specialist are involved with program facilitation and administration. Other health care providers who may be involved include a dietitian; physical therapist, occupational therapist, or both; and psychologist.

MINI CLINI

Reacting to Adverse Outcomes

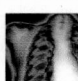

PROBLEM: A 73-year-old man with stage III COPD was accepted into a pulmonary rehabilitation program. Because of the severity of his disease, his preprogram cardiopulmonary exercise evaluation was stopped after 5 minutes because of excessive dyspnea and oxygen desaturation. He was placed on O_2 but was unable to complete the study. However, because of the desire of the patient's physician to get him into a program of pulmonary rehabilitation and the patient's desire to participate, the patient was put on home O_2 and admitted to the program. While exercising on a treadmill with supplemental O_2, the patient complained of headache and nausea. The RT stopped the exercise session and documented a significant increase in the patient's blood pressure (220/130 mm Hg). How should the RT proceed in this case?

SOLUTION: The RT should document the elevated blood pressure and notify the physician overseeing the pulmonary rehabilitation program and the patient's prescribing physician (if different) immediately. It is likely that the preprogram cardiopulmonary exercise test was stopped before the excessive increase in blood pressure was noted. While in pulmonary rehabilitation, the patient (on supplemental O_2) was able to exercise to a level greater than that during the exercise test. This elevated blood pressure will result in the patient going on some type of antihypertensive therapy and being reevaluated during another exercise test to determine the extent of his hypertensive condition. Depending on the instability of the patient's hypertension, it is also possible that this patient will be admitted to cardiac rehabilitation first before returning to the pulmonary rehabilitation program. This case shows the importance of a thorough and complete assessment of a patient's status before any admission to pulmonary rehabilitation.

CONCLUSION

A properly planned and implemented pulmonary rehabilitation program can produce positive and measurable patient outcomes. Goals and objectives of pulmonary rehabilitation should be written in these measurable terms and explained to the patient in a clear, concise fashion to achieve optimum therapeutic outcomes. The success of pulmonary rehabilitation depends on this along with careful application of current clinical knowledge and the use of a multidisciplinary approach throughout all phases of program organization, implementation, and evaluation. Within this context, pulmonary rehabilitation will continue to gain greater acceptance, and the role of the RT in pulmonary rehabilitation will be increasingly more important.

SUMMARY CHECKLIST

- Pulmonary rehabilitation has two major aims: (1) to control and alleviate disease symptoms and (2) to help patients achieve optimal levels of activity.
- Patients best able to benefit from pulmonary rehabilitation are patients with symptomatic COPD; patients with unstable cardiovascular disorders should be referred for cardiac rehabilitation.
- Effective rehabilitation programming requires a multidisciplinary approach and combines physical reconditioning with education and psychosocial support.
- Rehabilitation does not alter the progressive deterioration in pulmonary function that occurs with chronic lung disease.
- Increased exercise tolerance, decreased intensity of symptoms, and improved activity levels are the best-documented benefits of pulmonary rehabilitation.
- The exercise evaluation provides the basis for the exercise prescription, yields the baseline data needed to assess a patient's progress, and helps determine the degree of hypoxemia or need for supplemental O_2 during exercise.
- Reconditioning should combine lower extremity and upper extremity aerobic exercises with ventilatory muscle training.
- The educational portion of a rehabilitation program should provide patients with knowledge they can use to help cope with their disease and manage symptoms better.

Continued

- Decisions regarding facilities, scheduling, class size, and equipment all can affect rehabilitation program outcomes.
- Patient charges should be based on projected costs, as offset by external funding or available insurance reimbursement.
- Cardiac rehabilitation should be considered first if a patient with pulmonary disease also has an underlying cardiac condition that needs to be addressed and appropriately managed.

References

1. COPD International: COPD statistics. COPD International.com. Accessed March 16, 2004.
2. Council on Rehabilitation: Definition of rehabilitation, Chicago, 1942, Council on Rehabilitation.
3. Petty TL: Pulmonary rehabilitation. Basics RD 4:1, 1975.
4. Harris PL: A guide to prescribing pulmonary rehabilitation. Prim Care 12:253, 1985.
5. Barach AL, Bickerman HA, Beck G: Advances in the treatment of nontuberculous pulmonary disease. Bull N Y Acad Med 28:353, 1952.
6. Pierce AK, et al: Responses to exercise training in patients with emphysema. Arch Intern Med 113:28, 1964.
7. Paez PN, et al: The physiological basis of training patients with emphysema. Am Rev Respir Dis 95:944, 1967.
8. Christie D: Physical training in chronic obstructive lung disease. BMJ 2:150, 1968.
9. Jastrzebski D, Gumola A, Gawlik R, et al: Dyspnea and quality of life in patients with pulmonary fibrosis after six weeks of respiratory rehabilitation. J Physiol Pharmacol 4:139–148, 2006.
10. Guell R, Resqueti V, Sangenis M: Impact of pulmonary rehabilitation on psychosocial morbidity in patients with severe COPD. Chest 129:899–904, 2006.
11. Naji NA, Conner MC, Donnelly SC, et al: Effectiveness of pulmonary rehabilitation in restrictive lung disease. J Cardiopulm Rehabil 26:237–243, 2006.
12. Lacasse Y, Goldstein R, Lasserson TJ: Pulmonary rehabilitation for chronic pulmonary disease. Cochrane Database Syst Rev (4):CD003793, 2006.
13. Ries AL, Bauldoff GS, Carlin BW, et al: Pulmonary rehabilitation. Joint ACCP/AACVPR evidence-based clinical practice guidelines. Chest 131:1S–42S, 2007.
14. California Pulmonary Rehabilitation Collaborative Group: Effects of pulmonary rehabilitation on dyspnea, quality of life, and health care costs in California. J Cardiopulm Rehabil 24:52–62, 2004.
15. Hughes RL, Davison R: Limitations of exercise in COPD. Chest 83:241, 1983.
16. Stoedefalke K: Effects of exercise training on blood lipids and lipoproteins in children and adolescents. J Sports Sci Med 6:313–318, 2007.
17. Hill NS: Pulmonary rehabilitation. Proc Am Thorac Soc 3:66–74, 2006.
18. American Association for Respiratory Care: AARC clinical practice guideline: exercise testing for evaluation of hypoxemia and/or desaturation. Respir Care 46:514, 2001.
19. American Association for Respiratory Care: AARC clinical practice guideline: pulmonary rehabilitation. Respir Care 47:617, 2002.
20. Porszasz J, Emtner M, Whipp BJ, et al: Endurance training decreases exercise-induced dynamic hyperinflation in patients with COPD. Eur Respir J 22:205s, 2003.
21. Wijkstra PJ, Ten Vergert EM, van Altena R, et al: Long-term benefits of rehabilitation at home on quality of life and exercise tolerance in patients with chronic obstructive pulmonary disease. Thorax 50:824, 1995.
22. Heppner PS, Morgan C, Kaplan RM, et al: Regular walking and long-term maintenance of outcomes after pulmonary rehabilitation. J Cardiopulm Rehabil 26:44–53, 2006.
23. Cockram J, Cecins N, Jenkins S: Maintaining exercise capacity and quality of life following pulmonary rehabilitation. Respirology 11:98–104, 2006.
24. Nici L, Donner C, Wouters E, et al: American Thoracic Society/European Respiratory Society statement on pulmonary rehabilitation. Am J Respir Crit Care Med 173:1390–1413, 2006.
25. Global strategy for diagnosis, management, and prevention of chronic obstructive pulmonary disease. 2008. www.globalcopd.com/guidelineitem.asp?1=2&12=1&intld=2003, Accessed November 23, 2009.
26. Lake FR, Henderson K, Briffa T, et al: Upper-limb and lower-limb exercise training in patients with chronic airflow obstruction. Chest 97:1077, 1990.
27. Weiner P, Azgad Y, Ganam R: Inspiratory muscle training combined with general exercise reconditioning in patients with COPD. Chest 102:1351, 1992.
28. Bickford LS, Hodgkin JE: National pulmonary rehabilitation survey. Respir Care Clin N Am 33:1030, 1988.
29. Hilling LR: Reimbursement for pulmonary rehabilitation remains elusive, RT for Decision Makers in Respir Care, editorial, 2005. www.rtmagazine.com/issues/articles/2005-12_06.asp. Accessed on March 15, 2010.
30. Mackaman D: New Medicare Part B services for 2010: pulmonary rehabilitation, HCPro, Medicare Find, 2010. blogs.hcpro.com/medicarefind/2010/01/new-medicare-part-b-services. Accessed on March 15, 2010.
31. American Thoracic Society: Pulmonary rehabilitation: final rule sets Medicare coverage and reimbursement policy. www.thoracic.org/sections/about-ats/advocacy/washington-letter/letters/September-7-2009.html.
32. CMS: Correction notice to the OPSS final rule (for pulmonary rehabilitation). Federal Register, December 31, 2009.
33. Kaplan RM, Ries AL: Quality of life as an outcome measure in pulmonary diseases. J Cardiopulm Rehabil 25:321–331, 2005.
34. Nishiyama O, Taniguchi H, Kondoh Y, et al: Factors in maintaining long-term improvements in health-related quality of life after pulmonary rehabilitation for COPD. Qual Life Res 14:2315–2321, 2005.
35. Varnell M: Therapists may benefit from NETT's rehab project. Ad J Respir Care Pract 12:7, 1999.
36. Foss CM: Lung volume reduction surgery: what's up with "NETT"? AARC Times 25:42, 2001.
37. National Emphysema Treatment Trial Research Group: A randomized trial comparing lung volume reduction surgery with medical therapy for severe emphysema. N Engl J Med 348:2059–2073, 2003.
38. National Emphysema Treatment Trial Research Group: Cost-effectiveness of lung volume reduction surgery for patients with severe emphysema. N Engl J Med 348:2092–2102, 2003.

Chapter 51

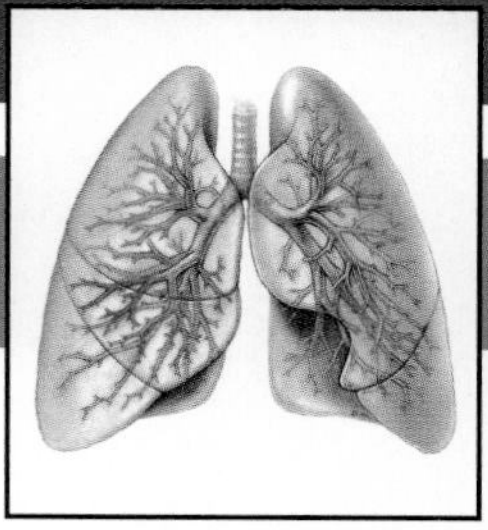

Respiratory Care in Alternative Settings

ALBERT J. HEUER

CHAPTER OBJECTIVES

After reading this chapter you will be able to:

- Describe alternative care settings in which respiratory care is often performed.
- Discuss more recent developments and trends in respiratory care at alternative sites.
- Identify who regulates alternative care settings.
- List the standards that apply to the delivery of respiratory care in alternative settings.
- Describe how to help formulate an effective discharge plan.
- List factors to evaluate when assessing alternative care sites and support services.
- Discuss how to justify, provide, evaluate, and modify oxygen (O_2) therapy in alternative care settings.
- Explain how to select, assemble, monitor, and maintain O_2 therapy equipment in alternative settings.
- Identify the special challenges that exist in providing ventilatory support outside an acute care hospital.
- Describe how to instruct patients or caregivers and confirm their ability to provide care in alternative settings.
- Identify which patients benefit the most from ventilatory support outside acute care hospitals.
- Explain how to select, assemble, monitor, and maintain portable ventilatory support and continuous positive airway pressure equipment, including applicable interfaces or appliances.
- Describe proper documentation regarding patient evaluation and progress in alternative settings.
- State how to ensure safety and infection control in alternative patient care settings.

CHAPTER OUTLINE

More Recent Developments and Trends
Relevant Terms and Goals
- Long-Term Subacute Care Hospitals
- Subacute Care
- Home Care

Standards
- Regulations
- Private Sector Accreditation

Traditional Acute Care versus Alternative Setting Care
Discharge Planning
- Multidisciplinary Team
- Site and Support Service Evaluation

Oxygen Therapy in Alternative Settings
- Oxygen Therapy Prescription
- Supply Methods
- Delivery Methods

Ventilatory Support in Alternative Settings
- Patient Selection
- Settings and Approaches
- Standards and Guidelines
- Special Challenges in Providing Home Ventilatory Support
- Invasive versus Noninvasive Ventilatory Support
- Equipment
- Evaluation and Follow-Up

Other Modes of Respiratory Care in Alternative Settings
- Bland Aerosol Therapy
- Aerosol Drug Administration
- Airway Care and Clearance Methods
- Nasal Continuous Positive Airway Pressure Therapy
- Apnea Monitoring

Patient Assessment and Documentation
- Institutional Long-Term Care
- Home Care

Equipment Disinfection and Maintenance
Palliative Care

KEY TERMS

alternative (nonacute) care
capped-rental
Centers for Medicare and Medicaid Services (CMS)
conditions of participation
durable medical equipment (DME) supplier
inexsufflator
molecular sieve
noninvasive ventilation (NIV)
O_2-conserving device
skilled nursing facility (SNF)
transtracheal oxygen therapy (TTOT)

With the introduction of Medicare in 1965, the cost savings and patient welfare benefits associated with home care and other nonacute care settings were recognized. This legislation established a reimbursement structure for health care services in alternative settings, including services provided at home. Since its adoption, Medicare is credited with substantial increases in the number of patients cared for at home. From 1967-1985, the number of home care agencies certified to participate in Medicare tripled to almost 6000. This figure peaked to slightly more 10,000 in 1997, the year in which the Balanced Budget Act (BBA) was introduced. The BBA of 1997, which is discussed in more detail in the following section, and other subsequent legislation had a monumental impact on health care reimbursement by reducing payments to durable medical equipment (DME) companies, home health agencies, and other alternative sites. Despite this reduction in reimbursement, however, approximately 10 million Americans continued to receive health care at home in 2007 at an estimated cost of approximately \$50 million.[1]

Although home care remains the most common alternative site for providing health care, numerous other **alternative (nonacute) care** settings, including subacute facilities, rehabilitation facilities, and **skilled nursing facilities (SNFs),** provide respiratory care to patients. Many patients in alternative settings require respiratory services, including supplemental oxygen (O_2), assisted ventilation, aerosol therapy, respiratory monitoring, pulmonary rehabilitation, and patient and caregiver education for asthma and other respiratory disorders.

Alternative health care settings offer the advantage of lower costs and enhanced patient comfort compared with acute care facilities. In 2007, the average daily acute care hospital charges were more than \$4000 versus less than \$1000 for SNFs.[1] However, improper or premature discharging of patients to alternative care settings and poor care plan implementation can erase these benefits and result in short-term readmission. This problem is particularly relevant to respiratory care because it has been found that the short-term readmission rate for patients with chronic obstructive pulmonary disease (COPD) is almost 20%.[2,3] Proper patient screening and evaluation and appropriate discharge planning, including a multidisciplinary care plan, proper care plan implementation, and patient follow-up, can minimize the risk of readmission.[4]

This chapter provides relevant definitions, discusses more recent policy developments, discusses aspects of optimal discharge and patient care planning, and reviews various therapeutic respiratory modalities in alternative care sites. A major alternative site is the sleep laboratory where respiratory therapists (RTs) conduct polysomnography, or sleep studies; this facet of respiratory care is covered in Chapter 30, which focuses exclusively on the pathophysiology, diagnosis, and treatment of disorders of sleep.

MORE RECENT DEVELOPMENTS AND TRENDS

Over the past decade, there have been several developments in the area of respiratory care in alternative sites. Some of these changes are simply enhancements to respiratory equipment used in such settings and are discussed later in this chapter. Additional developments involve complex government initiatives affecting reimbursement for such equipment and services. Other changes stem from the outcomes of research studies and demographic changes. These developments illustrate the dynamic nature of respiratory care in alternative settings.

One of the most notable changes is the introduction of Medicare's prospective payment system (PPS). Until the introduction of the PPS in the 1990s, Medicare mainly reimbursed providers such as home care agencies for "reasonable" charges up to a maximum monthly or one-time amount. However, under the PPS, reimbursement for many types of respiratory equipment in alternative sites is based on a predetermined monthly payment, adjusted for factors such as the health condition and geography. Additionally, certain types of respiratory equipment are categorized as **capped-rental** items. Capped-rental items are items eligible for reimbursement under the PPS for only a predetermined number of months, after which the equipment is deemed owned by the patient and rental payments cease. Other legislation that has substantially affected Medicare reimbursement includes the BBA of 1997 and the Deficit Reduction Act of 2005. Among other things, the BBA reduced reimbursement for home O_2 by 25% in 1998 and another 5% in 1999. The Deficit Reduction Act modified the PPS further by again reducing monthly payment for selected respiratory equipment and adding to the list of capped-rental items. Under this legislation, modalities such as home O_2 and bilevel positive airway pressure (bilevel PAP) with timed respiratory rate backup are capped at 36 months (O_2) and 13 months (bilevel PAP). The net effect of these and subsequent reimbursement reductions has been much lower reimbursement for respiratory care equipment in alternative sites. This unfavorable trend continues to present challenges to agencies and facilities attempting to provide quality care to patients in such settings.[5]

At the time of the writing of this chapter, other policy and legislative changes have been enacted but not yet fully implemented. Most notable of these is the Patient Protection and Affordable Care Act of 2010. There are many facets to this bill ranging from the expansion of health care coverage to many uninsured Americans, prohibiting the exclusion of preexisting conditions, and increasing the scope of coverage for certain types of preventive care. However, the provisions of this bill are still being closely examined, and modifications are likely. The exact impact of this bill and any related legislation on the U.S. health care system and the field of respiratory care remains to be seen.[6]

Another area that has been under review for some time is reimbursement for reasonable time spent by RTs in administering care and patient education in alternative care settings such as the home. Reimbursement under federal Medicare and state Medicaid programs applies only to respiratory equipment, such as home O_2 and mechanical ventilators, and RT time is not covered. Although a few states have piloted programs to reimburse for certain therapies and education done by RTs in alternative settings, widespread acceptance has not occurred. Although Medicare provides limited payment for nursing and physical therapy at home, it generally does not reimburse for RTs in such a setting. The American Association for Respiratory Care (AARC), through its Government Affairs initiatives, continues to promote legislation and sponsor efforts to expand the recognition of RTs. As a result of the delicate balance among factors such as increasing health care costs, limited resources, and patient care, it appears that the PPS and other related policies will continue to be reviewed and modified by government agencies such as the Centers for Medicare and Medicaid Services (CMS).[7]

A further development stemming mainly from the aging U.S. population is a significant increase in the popularity of another form of alternative care site known as *assisted living facilities*. These facilities permit residents, who are generally elderly or disabled, to live in their own unit either alone or with a companion. Generally, routine health care and other support services are available through an on-site nursing and health aide staff. These arrangements permit residents to live relatively independently with the convenience and safety of routine health services nearby. A growing number of home care and other alternative site RTs are providing care to patients at such locations.

Other changes affecting RTs in alternative sites have resulted from research study outcomes. In 1999, a report from Muse and Associates to the AARC found that Medicare beneficiaries treated by RTs had better outcomes and lower cost in such facilities.[8] More recently, other research projects have shown cost and quality benefits when RTs are involved in the management of patients receiving home O_2 therapy and in outpatient asthma education programs.[9] It is hoped that the Muse Report and the growing body of evidence stemming from other initiatives will help public agencies and private health care payers recognize the value of RTs in alternative care settings and shape policies accordingly.

RELEVANT TERMS AND GOALS

As the elderly population increases and managed care becomes the dominant delivery model, more health care services are being provided outside the acute care hospital. These alternative, or non–acute care, settings include long-term acute care hospitals (LTACHs), subacute care facilities, rehabilitation facilities, SNFs, and the home. However, rather than representing distinct entities, these approaches are part of an evolving continuum of care and share the common goal of providing appropriate medical services in a cost-effective manner and at settings suitable to a patient's condition.

Similar to the acute care setting, alternative care settings accomplish this goal by focusing on the whole person rather than simply a disease process through a coordinated team effort among many disciplines. The patient care team in alternative settings uses various specialized respiratory care services and equipment, including continuous O_2 therapy, long-term mechanical ventilation, aerosol drug administration, airway care, sleep apnea treatment, sleep apnea home monitoring, and pulmonary rehabilitation. Each of the major alternative settings, the respiratory equipment and services used within them, and other relevant considerations including patient and family education are discussed in subsequent sections of this chapter.

Long-Term Subacute Care Hospitals

Advances in technology, research, and clinical specialization have permitted more acutely ill patients to be treated outside of large-scale, acute care hospitals. Over the past decade, LTACHs have become more prevalent. These facilities provide highly focused care to patients with complex medical conditions, including patients who have been ventilator-dependent and difficult to wean. Generally, LTACHs employ a highly experienced clinical staff, including RTs, to provide integrated interdisciplinary care using the latest equipment and specialized treatment protocols. During the 20- to 30-day typical length of stay at an LTACH, patients commonly experience significant improvement, including successful weaning from mechanical ventilation and increased tolerance for activities of daily living.[10]

Subacute Care

According to the National Association of Subacute/Post Acute Care, *subacute care* is a comprehensive level of inpatient care for stable patients who (1) have experienced an acute event resulting from injury, illness, or exacerbation of a disease process; (2) have a determined course of treatment; and (3) require diagnostic or invasive procedures but not those requiring acute care.[10] Typically, the severity of the patient's condition requires active physician direction with frequent on-site visits, professional nursing care, significant ancillary services, and an outcomes-focused interdisciplinary approach employing a professional team.

The goal of acute care is to apply intensive resources to stabilize patients after severe episodic illness, whereas subacute care aims to restore the whole patient back to the highest practical level of function—ideally self-care. This holistic approach requires goal-oriented interdisciplinary team care, with frequent assessment of progress and a time-limited plan of care.[11]

Although most patients receiving subacute care are elderly, all age groups can be found at these sites. Pediatric, adolescent, and adult patients requiring ventilatory support or extensive care, depending on their diagnosis, are also cared for at these sites. Some patient conditions include neurologic disorders or injuries, musculoskeletal deformities, genetic defects, and any type of chronic pulmonary disease.

Home Care

Currently, most respiratory care in the alternative setting is provided in the home. Home care generally should be the first choice, but when patients have multiple ailments and are unable to care for themselves, when adequate patient support is unavailable, or when the home environment is unsuitable, an alternative care site must be selected.

The AARC defines *respiratory home care* as specific forms of respiratory care provided in the patient's place of residence by personnel trained in respiratory care working under medical supervision.[12] The primary goal of home care is to provide quality health care services to patients in their home setting, minimizing their dependence on institutional care. In regard to respiratory home care, several specific objectives are evident. Respiratory home care can contribute to the following:

- Supporting and maintaining life
- Improving patients' physical, emotional, and social well-being
- Promoting patient and family self-sufficiency
- Ensuring cost-effective delivery of care
- Maximizing patient comfort near the end of life

Most patients for whom respiratory home care is considered have chronic respiratory diseases. Applicable categories of disorders include the following:

- COPD
- Cystic fibrosis
- Chronic neuromuscular disorders
- Chronic restrictive conditions
- Carcinomas of the lung

Although not all aspects of respiratory home care have proven effective, various studies have shown that carefully selected treatment regimens can be of significant benefit to patients. These benefits include increased longevity, improved quality of life, increased functional performance, and a reduction in the individual and societal costs associated with hospitalization.[13,14]

STANDARDS

Standards for the delivery of respiratory care in the subacute and home settings are derived from several different sources. First, the Clinical Practice Guidelines published by the AARC offer RTs a clinical framework for performing numerous respiratory procedures, including many procedures used in alternative care settings. Several of these guidelines are described throughout this chapter. Other standards are established by federal and state laws and private-sector accreditation.

Regulations

Most reimbursement for care in alternative settings is through either the federal Medicare program or federal or state Medicaid programs. As the largest purchaser of health services, the federal government (in connection with state and local governments) plays a major role in setting standards and regulating this industry. The federal agency responsible for the overall administration of Medicare and Medicaid is the **Centers for Medicare and Medicaid Services (CMS).** Created in 1997, CMS oversees the framework for providing health coverage to elderly adults, disabled adults, and many disadvantaged young children in the United States.[5,6]

As part of this structure, CMS created the Medicare Provider Certification Program. This program ensures that institutional providers that serve Medicare beneficiaries, including hospitals, SNFs, LTACHs, home health agencies, and assisted living facilities, meet minimum health and safety requirements. These requirements are called **conditions of participation.** Current conditions of participation emphasize quality indicators, outcome measures, and cost efficiency designed to improve the quality and effectiveness of care provided to beneficiaries.[5,6] Institutions undergo certification surveys to determine their compliance with the applicable conditions of participation. These surveys are conducted by either state survey agencies or private accrediting organizations, such as The Joint

Commission (TJC), which is discussed in more detail in the following section.[15,16]

State survey agencies are partners with the federal government and principal agents in performing institutional certification. Typically, a state survey agency is either the state department of health or state licensing authority for health care facilities. The main function of the state survey agency is to ensure that facilities providing Medicare or Medicaid services comply with state and federal health, safety, and quality standards. Compliance is determined by periodic on-site inspections. Inspection reports are public information and can be obtained by contacting the applicable state survey agency.

In addition to federal Medicare and Medicaid conditions of participation, most states set additional regulations that govern licensing of providers of care in alternative settings. Because these regulations are different in each state, readers should contact their state health department for details.

Private Sector Accreditation

The primary organization responsible for standard setting and voluntary accreditation of care providers in alternative settings is TJC. To assist hospitals and health care organizations with the accreditation process and overall performance improvement, TJC develops and publishes standards and National Patient Safety Goals for long-term and subacute care, home care, and assisted living facilities. The standards cover general functional categories relating to quality patient care and the process and structure of the organization. These categories include patient rights, ethics, and assessment and organizational leadership and management of information. The patient safety goals target for improvement common problem areas for health care organizations, such as proper patient identification, medication safety, and infection control.[15,16]

Approximately 90% of all hospitals and other health care organizations voluntarily subscribe to TJC accreditation. Approximately 5000 of these alternative care organizations and facilities are surveyed at least every 3 years. There are several accreditation decision categories ranging from *accreditation* to *denial of accreditation*. A provider's accreditation status depends on the level of compliance with an array of *elements of performance,* which are rated by the surveyors as *insufficient compliance, partial compliance,* or *satisfactory compliance*. Insufficient or unsatisfactory compliance is flagged and requires formal follow-up to ensure correction. In certain circumstances, such unfavorable results may translate into a facility or an organization failing to maintain TJC accreditation.

In regard to home care, TJC applies different protocols to assess different types of home care agencies. The home equipment management protocol pertains only to companies that rent or sell home medical equipment. In most cases, this type of provider is involved only with basic O_2 and aerosol therapy setups and does not provide in-depth visits for patient assessment or evaluation. Agencies involved with clinical respiratory services perform periodic home visits with patient assessment. Agencies applying for accreditation at this level are involved with more sophisticated forms of home care that require routine follow-up visits, such as management of artificial airways and ventilator-dependent patients. The standards for this type of home care accreditation are more extensive and rigorous.[15,16]

TRADITIONAL ACUTE CARE VERSUS ALTERNATIVE SETTING CARE

For the RT, working in the alternative care setting is distinctly different from working in an acute care hospital. Key differences involve resource availability, supervision and work schedules, documentation and assessment, and provider-patient interaction (Table 51-1).[17] Although some practitioners do not like the alternative work settings, many find the greater independence, professional team orientation, creativity, and higher level of patient and family interaction quite rewarding. In addition, most RTs working in the alternative care environment argue that only in these settings is their full scope of training really used.

DISCHARGE PLANNING

Effective discharge planning provides the foundation for quality care in the alternative care setting. A properly designed and implemented discharge plan guides the multidisciplinary team in successfully transferring a respiratory care patient from the health care facility to an alternative site of care.[18] Effective implementation of the discharge plan also ensures the safety and efficacy of the patient's continuing care.

To guide practitioners in providing quality care, the AARC has published Clinical Practice Guideline: Discharge Planning for the Respiratory Care Patient.[19] Excerpts from this guideline appear in Clinical Practice Guideline 51-1.

Multidisciplinary Team

Although a physician normally initiates an order to discharge a patient to an alternative site, many other health care professionals are involved in the discharge process. Table 51-2 identifies these key professionals and their major responsibilities.[18] As with pulmonary rehabilitation (see Chapter 50), a team approach produces the best patient results. Communication and mutual respect for the talents and abilities of each team member are two key elements in making patient care in the alternative care setting work. Any breakdown in the system may delay or adversely affect patient discharge and the patient's physical health and mental well-being.

TABLE 51-1

Major Differences Between Traditional Acute Care Setting and Alternative Settings for Delivery of Respiratory Care Services

Area	Traditional Setting (Acute Care Hospital)	Alternative Settings (Long-Term Acute Care, Subacute, Home Care)
Diagnostic resources	In-house laboratory, x-ray, ABG analysis, PFT	Must rely on outside vendors to provide diagnostic tests
Equipment support	Extensive; supported by piped-in O_2 and suctioning	Limited availability; must use portable O_2 and suctioning systems
Travel requirements	None; remain in one facility	Must travel between facilities or residences
Level of supervision	Direct supervision	Respiratory care provider works independently with minimal supervision
Patient assessment	Moderate—primarily provided by attending physician or residents	Heavy—core responsibility related to care planning
Documentation requirements	Moderate—limited to medical recordkeeping	Heavy—includes initial justification, ongoing follow-up, and often detailed financial recordkeeping
Work schedule	Specific hours	Varied work schedule, often including "on-call" off hours coverage
Time constraints	More than one shift to deliver therapy	Must complete all therapy during shift or visit
Patient-family interaction	Limited treatment time available; little family interaction	One-on-one therapy; intensive family interaction
Provider interaction	Primarily attending physicians and patient's nurses	Continuous interaction with all members of professional team

ABG, Arterial blood gas; *PFT,* pulmonary function testing.

51-1 Discharge Planning for the Respiratory Care Patient

AARC Clinical Practice Guideline (Excerpts)*

INDICATIONS

Discharge planning is indicated for all respiratory care patients being considered for discharge or transfer to alternative sites. The plan should be developed and implemented as early as possible before transfer.

CONTRAINDICATIONS

There are no contraindications to the development of a discharge plan.

PRECAUTIONS AND POSSIBLE COMPLICATIONS

Undesirable or unexpected outcomes may occur if the patient is discharged before the full implementation of the plan. Undesirable or unexpected patient outcomes may also occur because of (1) the natural course of the disease or (2) other factors beyond the control of the discharge planning process.

METHOD

Discharge planning and implementation should begin as early as possible. The complexity of the plan is determined by the patient's medical condition, needs, and goals. The steps in the planning process are:

- Patient evaluation
  - Patient's medical condition
  - Psychosocial condition of patient and family
  - Respiratory and ventilatory support required
  - Desires for medical and ventilator care of patient and family
  - Patient's physical and functional ability and activities of daily living
  - Goals of care (patient and family, physician, health care professionals, bedside caregivers)
- Site evaluation for continuing care
  - Personnel
  - Physical environment (safety and suitability)
  - Equipment and supplies
  - Financial resources

51-1 Discharge Planning for the Respiratory Care Patient—cont'd

AARC Clinical Practice Guideline (Excerpts)*

- Development of multidisciplinary plan of care based on the patient's needs and goals
  - Plan for integration into the community
  - Medication administration
  - Plan for patient self-care as appropriate
  - Method for ongoing assessment of outcomes
  - Roles and responsibilities of team members for daily care management
  - Method to assess growth and development of pediatric patients
  - Documented mechanism for securing and training additional caregivers
  - Mechanism for communication among all members of health care team
  - Alternative emergency and contingency plan
  - Follow-up (e.g., medical, respiratory care) plans
  - Plan for use, maintenance, and troubleshooting of equipment
  - Plan for monitoring and appropriately responding to changes in patient's medical condition
  - Time frame for implementation
- Education and training with clear demonstration and documentation of competencies must occur before discharge and address key elements of the plan of care

ASSESSMENT OF NEED

All patients with a respiratory diagnosis should be assessed for a discharge plan.

ASSESSMENT OF OUTCOME

The desired outcome of the discharge plan is determined by the following:

- No readmission occurs because of discharge plan failure
- The equipment meets the patient's needs
- All treatments and modalities are performed satisfactorily by caregivers as instructed
- Caregivers are able to assess the patient, troubleshoot, and solve problems as they arise
- The treatment meets the patient's needs and goals
- The patient and family are satisfied
- The site provides the necessary services

MONITORING

The discharge plan coordinator and the physician should monitor the progress of the discharge plan. Each team member should participate in regularly scheduled team conferences to assess the progress of the discharge plan. Modifications may be made according to the goals and needs of the individual patient.

**For the complete guideline, see American Association for Respiratory Care: Clinical practice guideline: discharge planning for the respiratory care patient. Respir Care Clin N Am 40:1308, 1995.*

TABLE 51-2

Members of Patient Care Team in Alternative Settings

Discipline	Responsibilities
Utilization review	Advises or recommends consideration of patient discharge. Documents patient's in-hospital care
Discharge planning (social service or community or public health)	Brings all the needed elements together and ensures that a patient can be discharged to alternative care sites. Makes contacts with outside agencies that may assist with patient care
Physician	Writes order for patient discharge. Evaluates patient's condition and prescribes needed care. Establishes therapeutic objectives
Respiratory care	Evaluates patient and recommends appropriate respiratory care. Provides care and follow-up
Nursing	Writes and implements nursing care plan for patient. Assesses patient's status and provides necessary follow-up
Dietary and nutrition	Assesses patient's nutritional needs and writes dietary plan for patient. Makes arrangements for meals as necessary
Physical and occupational therapy	Provides necessary physical therapy and recommends any additional modalities or procedures
Psychiatry or psychology	Assesses patient's emotional status and provides any needed counseling or support
DME supplier or home care company	Provides needed equipment and supplies and handles any emergency situations involving delivery or equipment operation

Site and Support Service Evaluation

The primary factors determining the appropriate site for discharge are the goals and needs of the patient. These goals and needs should be met in an optimal and cost-effective manner using the resources available at the proposed site. In terms of institutional personnel, the staff of the selected facility must have all the competencies required to meet the patient's respiratory needs, be able to provide other needed health care services (e.g., physical therapy), and provide adequate 24-hour coverage.[17,19]

For discharge to the home, it is essential that the ability of caregivers to learn and perform the required care be evaluated before transfer. Caregivers must clearly demonstrate and have documented the competencies required to care for the specific patient and, in combination, provide 24-hour coverage.[17,19]

> **RULE OF THUMB**
>
> To confirm that a nonprofessional caregiver can perform a particular skill, the RT must go beyond demonstration and verbal confirmation of the caregiver's understanding. The RT must observe a return demonstration, whereby the caregiver properly performs the same procedural steps the RT demonstrated. In addition, providing the caregiver with written information relating to the procedural sets and equipment setup, maintenance, and basic troubleshooting can help reinforce key areas and ensure caregiver mastery of the competency.

Beyond the performance of a particular skill, it is imperative for the discharge team to ensure that an adequate number of professional and nonprofessional caregivers are part of the care plan to provide appropriate patient care coverage; this is particularly true when more complicated modes, such as mechanical ventilation, or multiple therapies are required by the patient. Common discharge planning mistakes are the reliance on too few individuals and overestimation of caregiver capabilities in alternative settings. Generally, substantial caregiver strain is associated with the care of patients in alternative settings. Proper assessment of the capabilities and number of potential caregivers in light of the therapy needed at home and appropriate training of such individuals can help address this concern.

Equipment support and selected clinical services for patients receiving respiratory home care are often provided by a **durable medical equipment (DME) supplier.** DME suppliers range in size from multimillion-dollar national corporations offering a broad range of services to small local companies. Both large and small companies usually provide the following services:

- Service 24 hours, 7 days a week
- Third-party insurance processing
- Home instruction and follow-up by an RT
- Most forms of respiratory care

When selecting a DME supplier from the available choices, the patient and family members and other members of the discharge planning team should consider the company's accreditation status, cost and scope of services, dependability, location, personnel, past track record, and availability. To help ensure a basic level of quality, one should select a DME supplier that is accredited. In addition, the service should be problem-free and provided by reliable, experienced, professional, and courteous staff. Charges should be reasonable and competitive, and clinical respiratory services should be provided by credentialed RTs.[17]

Finally, the selected site must meet basic safety standards and be suitable for managing the patient's specific condition. It should be free of fire, health, and safety hazards; provide adequate heating, cooling, and ventilation; provide adequate electrical service; and provide for patient access and mobility with adequate patient space (room to house medical and adaptive equipment) and storage facilities. The selected site must be capable of operating, maintaining, and supporting all equipment needed by the patient; including both respiratory and ancillary equipment and supplies as needed, such as the ventilator, suction, O_2, intravenous therapy, nutritional therapy, and adaptive equipment.[17,19] Box 51-1 lists key factors one should assess in planning the discharge of a respiratory care patient to the home environment.

A variety of equipment is available when a patient with a pulmonary disorder is discharged to an alternative setting. The most common types of respiratory therapy equipment used in alternative settings are discussed in the following sections.

Box 51-1 Assessing the Home Environment

ACCESSIBILITY
- In and out of house or apartment
- Accessibility between rooms
- Doorway width and threshold heights
- Stairways
- Wheelchair mobility
- Bathroom
- Kitchen
- Carpeting

EQUIPMENT
- Available space
- Electrical power supply
- Amperage
- Grounded outlets
- Presence of hazardous appliances

ENVIRONMENT
- Heating and ventilation
- Humidity
- Lighting
- Living space

OXYGEN THERAPY IN ALTERNATIVE SETTINGS

O_2 therapy is the most common mode of respiratory care in alternative care settings. This high use is based on the fact that O_2 therapy improves both survival and quality of life in selected patient groups, especially patients with advanced COPD.[20,21] In particular, studies have shown improved nocturnal O_2 saturation, reduced pulmonary artery pressure, and lower pulmonary vascular resistance with appropriate outpatient O_2 therapy.[22,23]

To guide practitioners in providing quality care, the AARC has published a Practice Guideline on Oxygen Therapy in the Home or Extended Care Facility.[24] Excerpts from the AARC guideline, including the indications, contraindications, precautions and possible complications, method, assessment of need, assessment of outcome, and monitoring, appear in Clinical Practice Guideline 51-2.

Oxygen Therapy Prescription

As indicated in Clinical Practice Guideline 51-2, O_2 prescriptions must be based on documented hypoxemia, as determined by either arterial blood gas analysis or oximetry. Prescriptions for O_2 therapy no longer can be based simply on patient diagnosis or signs and symptoms. In addition, as-needed O_2 therapy is no longer acceptable in the alternative care setting.

When the need for O_2 therapy is established, the physician writes a prescription. A prescription for O_2 therapy in the alternative care setting must include the following elements:[25]

- Flow rate in L/min or concentration or both
- Frequency of use in hours per day and minutes per hour (if applicable)
- Duration of need
- Diagnosis (severe primary lung disease, secondary conditions related to lung disease and hypoxia, related conditions or symptoms that may improve with O_2)
- Laboratory evidence (arterial blood gas analysis or oximetry under the appropriate testing conditions); home care companies cannot provide this testing
- Additional medical documentation (no acceptable alternatives to home O_2 therapy)

For home use, the ordering physician must authorize O_2 therapy using the CMS Certification of Medical Necessity form for O_2 (Figure 51-1). After the need for long-term therapy is documented, repeat arterial blood gas analysis or SpO_2 measurements are not needed. However, blood O_2 levels may still be measured when the need arises to assess changes in the patient's condition.[26]

MINI CLINI

Assessing the Home Environment

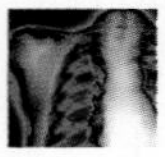

PROBLEM: A wheelchair-bound patient with a tracheostomy who requires mechanical ventilation is being discharged to the home care setting. Inspection of the two-story home reveals front and rear elevated porch entrances with all bedrooms upstairs. All room floors (except the kitchen and bathrooms) are covered with high pile carpeting. The largest bedroom is 12 ft × 14 ft. The electrical service is rated at 75 amps, and the only grounded outlets are in the kitchen and garage. Heating is provided by a forced hot-air system; there is a single window air conditioner in the patient's bedroom.

What problems do you see, and what changes would you recommend to provide the proper home environment for this patient?

SOLUTION: Although wheelchair-bound, this patient is still mobile. Both the elevated porch entrances and the high pile carpeting restrict mobility. A ramp entrance needs to be constructed, and the carpeting needs to be removed or covered with a flat, hard surface material. Given the size of the patient's upstairs room and the obstacle of the stairwell, it would be best to identify a large first-story room for conversion to a bedroom. Because the patient is likely to need at least an electrical bed, ventilator, and suction machine, the electrical service capacity is inadequate and needs upgrading to ensure at least 15 to 20 amps in the patient area, with 200 amps overall. Appliance, counter, sink, and toilet heights need to be assessed for easy patient access.

Supply Methods

Most alternative care sites do not have bulk O_2 storage or delivery systems. In these settings, O_2 normally is supplied from one of the following three sources:[27] (1) compressed O_2 cylinders, (2) liquid O_2 systems, or (3) O_2 concentrators. Table 51-3 summarizes the major advantages and disadvantages of each system.

Compressed Oxygen Cylinders

The primary use of compressed O_2 cylinders in alternative settings is either for ambulation (small cylinders) or as a backup to liquid or concentrator supply systems (H/K cylinders). Safety measures for cylinder O_2 are the same as those discussed in Chapters 37 and 38. For home use, the RT should thoroughly review these safety measures with both the patient and family members. After instruction, the RT should always confirm and document abilities of caregivers to use the delivery system safely.

In addition to the cylinder gas, a pressure-reducing valve with flowmeter is needed to deliver O_2 at the prescribed flow. Standard clinical flowmeters deliver flows up to 15 L/min; flows used in alternative settings are typically in the 0.25 to 5 L/min range. For this reason, the RT should select a calibrated low-flow flowmeter whenever possible. Alternatively, a preset flow restrictor can be used (see Chapter 37).

As in the hospital, there is usually no need to humidify nasal O_2 at flows of 4 L/min or less.[24] If humidification is

51-2 Oxygen Therapy in the Home or Alternative Site Health Care Facility

AARC Clinical Practice Guideline (Excerpts)*

■ INDICATIONS

- Documented hypoxemia
- Adults, children, and infants >28 days old: $PaO_2 \leq 55$ mm Hg or $SaO_2 \leq 88\%$ (room air)
- PaO_2 56 to 59 mm Hg or $SaO_2 \leq 89\%$ in association with specific clinical conditions (e.g., cor pulmonale, congestive heart failure, or erythrocythemia with hematocrit >56%)
- Patients who do not qualify for O_2 therapy at rest may qualify during ambulation, sleep, or exercise if SaO_2 decreases to <89% during these specific activities

■ CONTRAINDICATIONS

No absolute contraindications to O_2 therapy exist when indications are present.

■ PRECAUTIONS AND POSSIBLE COMPLICATIONS

- In spontaneously breathing hypoxemic patients with COPD, O_2 therapy may increase $PaCO_2$
- Problems may occur if the patient fails to comply with the physician's orders or receives inadequate instruction
- Complications may result from use of nasal cannulas or transtracheal catheters
- Fire hazard is increased in the presence of increased O_2 concentrations
- Bacterial contamination associated with certain nebulizers and humidifiers may occur
- Physical hazards include unsecured cylinders, ungrounded equipment, and liquid O_2 burns
- Power or equipment failure can lead to an inadequate O_2 supply

■ ASSESSMENT OF NEED

- Initial need is determined by documented hypoxemia at rest or during activity (see Indications)
- Additional measurements of blood gas tension or saturation by invasive or noninvasive methods may be indicated whenever there is a major change in clinical status that may be cardiopulmonary related
- Blood gases should be repeated after 1 to 3 months to determine the need for long-term O_2 therapy
- Once the need for long-term O_2 therapy has been documented, repeated measures are unnecessary other than to follow the course of the disease, to assess changes in clinical status, or to facilitate changes in the O_2 prescription

■ ASSESSMENT OF OUTCOME

Outcome is determined by clinical and physiologic assessment to establish adequacy of patient response to therapy.

■ MONITORING

- Patient
  - Initial and ongoing clinical assessment of patient's need for O_2 therapy should be performed by licensed or credentialed RTs (RRT or CRT) or other professional persons with equivalent training and documented ability to perform the tasks as part of a patient-specific plan of care/plan of service
  - Care plans should be developed at the initiation of O_2 therapy based on the needs of the individual patient and updated as necessary
  - Measurement of baseline O_2 tension or saturation is essential before O_2 therapy is begun. Measurements should be repeated when clinically indicated or to follow the course of the disease, as determined by the attending physician
  - Measurements of O_2 saturation also should be made to determine appropriate O_2 flow for ambulation, exercise, or sleep
- Equipment
  - All O_2 delivery equipment should be checked at least once daily by the patient or caregiver. Facets to be assessed include proper function of the equipment, prescribed flow rates, remaining liquid or compressed gas content, and backup supply
  - O_2 equipment should be serviced and maintained in accordance with the manufacturer's specification and consistent with all federal, state, and local laws and regulations
  - In the event there are no manufacturer specifications or guidance, O_2 equipment should be checked for proper function and performance by an appropriately trained or credentialed person no less than once per year

For the complete guideline, see American Association for Respiratory Care: Clinical practice guideline: oxygen therapy in the home or alternate site health care facility. Respir Care 52:1063, 2007.

DEPARTMENT OF HEALTH AND HUMAN SERVICES
CENTERS FOR MEDICARE & MEDICAID SERVICES

Form Approved
OMB No. 0938-0534

CERTIFICATE OF MEDICAL NECESSITY
CMS-484 — OXYGEN

DME 484.03

SECTION A **Certification Type/Date: INITIAL ___/___/___ REVISED ___/___/___ RECERTIFICATION___/___/___**

PATIENT NAME, ADDRESS, TELEPHONE and HIC NUMBER (_ _ _) _ _ _ - _ _ _ _ HICN ________		SUPPLIER NAME, ADDRESS, TELEPHONE and NSC or applicable NPI NUMBER/LEGACY NUMBER (_ _ _) _ _ _ - _ _ _ _ NSC or NPI #________
PLACE OF SERVICE________	HCPCS CODE	PT DOB ___/___/___ Sex ___ (M/F)
NAME and ADDRESS of FACILITY *if applicable (see reverse)*	______ ______ ______ ______	PHYSICIAN NAME, ADDRESS, TELEPHONE and applicable NPI NUMBER or UPIN (_ _ _) _ _ _ - _ _ _ _ UPIN or NPI #________

SECTION B **Information in This Section May Not Be Completed by the Supplier of the Items/Supplies.**

EST. LENGTH OF NEED (# OF MONTHS): ____ 1–99 *(99=LIFETIME)*	DIAGNOSIS CODES (ICD-9): ____ ____ ____ ____
ANSWERS	ANSWER QUESTIONS 1–9. (Circle Y for Yes, N for No, or D for Does Not Apply, unless otherwise noted.)
a)_____mm Hg b)_____% c)___/___/___	1. Enter the result of most recent test taken on or before the certification date listed in Section A. Enter (a) arterial blood gas PO2 and/or (b) oxygen saturation test; (c) date of test.
1 2 3	2. Was the test in Question 1 performed (1) with the patient in a chronic stable state as an outpatient, (2) within two days prior to discharge from an inpatient facility to home, or (3) under other circumstances?
1 2 3	3. Circle the one number for the condition of the test in Question 1: (1) At Rest; (2) During Exercise; (3) During Sleep
Y N D	4. If you are ordering portable oxygen, is the patient mobile within the home? If you are not ordering portable oxygen, circle D.
______LPM	5. Enter the highest oxygen flow rate ordered for this patient in liters per minute. If less than 1 LPM, enter a "X".
a)_____mm Hg b)_____% c)___/___/___	6. If greater than 4 LPM is prescribed, enter results of most recent test taken on 4 LPM. This may be an (a) arterial blood gas PO2 and/or (b) oxygen saturation test with patient in a chronic stable state. Enter date of test (c).
	ANSWER QUESTIONS 7-9 **ONLY** IF PO2 = 56–59 OR OXYGEN SATURATION = 89 IN QUESTION 1
Y N	7. Does the patient have dependent edema due to congestive heart failure?
Y N	8. Does the patient have cor pulmonale or pulmonary hypertension documented by P pulmonale on an EKG or by an echocardiogram, gated blood pool scan or direct pulmonary artery pressure measurement?
Y N	9. Does the patient have a hematocrit greater than 56%?

NAME OF PERSON ANSWERING SECTION B QUESTIONS, IF OTHER THAN PHYSICIAN (Please Print):
NAME: ____________ TITLE: __________ EMPLOYER: __________

SECTION C **Narrative Description of Equipment and Cost**

(1) Narrative description of all items, accessories and options ordered; (2) Supplier's charge and (3) Medicare Fee Schedule Allowance for each item, accessory and option. (See instructions on back.)

SECTION D **Physician Attestation and Signature/Date**

I certify that I am the treating physician identified in Section A of this form. I have received Sections A, B and C of the Certificate of Medical Necessity (including charges for items ordered). Any statement on my letterhead attached hereto, has been reviewed and signed by me. I certify that the medical necessity information in Section B is true, accurate and complete, to the best of my knowledge, and I understand that any falsification, omission, or concealment of material fact in that section may subject me to civil or criminal liability.

PHYSICIAN'S SIGNATURE ________________ DATE ___/___/___

Signature and Date Stamps Are Not Acceptable.

Form CMS-484 (09/05)

FIGURE 51-1 Certificate of Medical Necessity from the Centers for Medical and Medicaid Services (CMS) used to certify the medical necessity for home oxygen therapy.

Continued

INSTRUCTIONS FOR COMPLETING THE CERTIFICATE OF MEDICAL NECESSITY FOR OXYGEN (CMS-484)

SECTION A:	**(May be completed by the supplier)**
CERTIFICATION TYPE/DATE:	If this is an initial certification for this patient, indicate this by placing date (MM/DD/YY) needed initially in the space marked "INITIAL." If this is a revised certification (to be completed when the physician changes the order, based on the patient's changing clinical needs), indicate the initial date needed in the space marked "INITIAL," and indicate the recertification date in the space marked "REVISED." If this is a recertification, indicate the initial date needed in the space marked "INITIAL," and indicate the recertification date in the space marked "RECERTIFICATION." Whether submitting a REVISED or a RECERTIFIED CMN, be sure to always furnish the INITIAL date as well as the REVISED or RECERTIFICATION date.
PATIENT INFORMATION:	Indicate the patient's name, permanent legal address, telephone number and his/her health insurance claim number (HICN) as it appears on his/her Medicare card and on the claim form.
SUPPLIER INFORMATION:	Indicate the name of your company (supplier name), address and telephone number along with the Medicare Supplier Number assigned to you by the National Supplier Clearinghouse (NSC) or applicable National Provider Identifier (NPI). If using the NPI Number, indicate this by using the qualifier XX followed by the 10-digit number. If using a legacy number, e.g. NSC number, use the qualifier 1C followed by the 10-digit number. (For example. 1Cxxxxxxxxxx)
PLACE OF SERVICE:	Indicate the place in which the item is being used, i.e., patient's home is 12, skilled nursing facility (SNF) is 31, End Stage Renal Disease (ESRD) facility is 65, etc. Refer to the DMERC supplier manual for a complete list.
FACILITY NAME:	If the place of service is a facility, indicate the name and complete address of the facility.
HCPCS CODES:	List all HCPCS procedure codes for items ordered. Procedure codes that do not require certification should not be listed on the CMN.
PATIENT DOB, HEIGHT, WEIGHT AND SEX:	Indicate patient's date of birth (MM/DD/YY) and sex (male or female); height in inches and weight in pounds, if requested.
PHYSICIAN NAME, ADDRESS:	Indicate the PHYSICIAN'S name and complete mailing address.
PHYSICIAN INFORMATION:	Accurately indicate the treating physician's Unique Physician Identification Number (UPIN) or applicable National Provider Identifier (NPI). If using the NPI Number, indicate this by using the qualifier XX followed by the 10-digit number. If using UPIN number, use the qualifier 1G followed by the 6-digit number. (For example. 1Gxxxxxx)
PHYSICIAN'S TELEPHONE NO:	Indicate the telephone number where the physician can be contacted (preferably where records would be accessible pertaining to this patient) if more information is needed.
SECTION B:	**(May not be completed by the supplier. While this section may be completed by a non-physician clinician, or a Physician employee, it must be reviewed, and the CMN signed (in Section D) by the treating practitioner.)**
EST. LENGTH OF NEED:	Indicate the estimated length of need (the length of time the physician expects the patient to require use of the ordered item) by filling in the appropriate number of months. If the patient will require the item for the duration of his/her life, then enter "99".
DIAGNOSIS CODES:	In the first space, list the ICD9 code that represents the primary reason for ordering this item. List any additional ICD9 codes that would further describe the medical need for the item (up to 4 codes).
QUESTION SECTION:	This section is used to gather clinical information to help Medicare determine the medical necessity for the item(s) being ordered. Answer each question which applies to the items ordered, circling "Y" for yes, "N" for no, or "D" for does not apply.
NAME OF PERSON ANSWERING SECTION B QUESTIONS:	If a clinical professional other than the treating physician (e.g., home health nurse, physical therapist, dietician) or a physician employee answers the questions of Section B, he/she must print his/her name, give his/her professional title and the name of his/her employer where indicated. If the physician is answering the questions, this space may be left blank.
SECTION C:	**(To be completed by the supplier)**
NARRATIVE DESCRIPTION OF EQUIPMENT & COST:	Supplier gives (1) a narrative description of the item(s) ordered, as well as all options, accessories, supplies and drugs; (2) the supplier's charge for each item(s), options, accessories, supplies and drugs; and (3) the Medicare fee schedule allowance for each item(s), options, accessories, supplies and drugs, if applicable.
SECTION D:	**(To be completed by the physician)**
PHYSICIAN ATTESTATION:	The physician's signature certifies (1) the CMN which he/she is reviewing includes Sections A, B, C and D; (2) the answers in Section B are correct; and (3) the self-identifying information in Section A is correct.
PHYSICIAN SIGNATURE AND DATE:	After completion and/or review by the physician of Sections A, B and C, the physician's must sign and date the CMN in Section D, verifying the Attestation appearing in this Section. The physician's signature also certifies the items ordered are medically necessary for this patient.

According to the Paperwork Reduction Act of 1995, no persons are required to respond to a collection of information unless it displays a valid OMB control number. The valid OMB control number for this information collection is 0938-0534. The time required to complete this information collection is estimated to average 12 minutes per response, including the time to review instructions, search existing resources, gather the data needed, and complete and review the information collection. If you have any comments concerning the accuracy of the time estimate or suggestions for improving this form, please write to: CMS, Attn: PRA Reports Clearance Officer, 7500 Security Blvd. Baltimore, Maryland 21244.

DO NOT SUBMIT CLAIMS TO THIS ADDRESS. Please see http://www.medicare.gov/ for information on claim filing.

Form CMS-484 (09/05) INSTRUCTIONS

FIGURE 51-1, cont'd.

TABLE 51-3

Advantages and Disadvantages of Major Alternative Oxygen Supply Systems

System	Advantages	Disadvantages
Compressed O_2	Good for small volume user No waste or loss Stores O_2 indefinitely Widespread availability Portability (small cylinders)	Large cylinders are heavy and bulky High-pressure safety hazard Provides limited volume Requires frequent deliveries Tight valves can be a problem
Liquid O_2 system	Provides large volumes Low-pressure system (20-25 psi) Portable units can be refilled from reservoir (up to 8-hr supply at 2 L/min) Valuable for rehabilitation	Must be delivered as needed Loss of O_2 because of venting of system when not in use Low temperature safety hazard Cannot operate ventilators or other high-pressure devices Some difficulty in filling portable unit
O_2 concentrator	No waste or loss Low-pressure system (15 psi) Cost-effective when continual supply of O_2 is needed Eliminates need for deliveries	Disruption in electrical service renders system inoperable Backup O_2 is needed Cannot operate ventilators or other high-pressure devices FiO_2 decreases with increasing flow High electrical costs possible

needed, a simple unheated bubble humidifier can be used. Because the mineral content of tap water may be high (hard water), water used in these humidifiers should be distilled. Otherwise, the porous diffusing element may become occluded. Although complete blockage is unlikely, occlusion of the diffusing element can impair humidification and alter flow.

Liquid Oxygen Systems

Because 1 cubic ft of liquid O_2 equals 860 cubic ft of gas, liquid O_2 systems can store large quantities of O_2 in small spaces; this is ideal for the high-volume user. As shown in Figure 51-2, a typical personal liquid O_2 system is a miniature version of a hospital stand tank. Similar to its larger counterpart, this system consists of a reservoir unit similar in design to a thermos bottle. The inner container of liquid O_2 is suspended in an outer container, with a vacuum in between. The liquid O_2 is kept at approximately −300° F. Because of constant vaporization, gaseous O_2 always exists above the liquid. When the cylinder is not in use, this vaporization maintains pressures between 20 psi and 25 psi. When pressures increase above this level, gas vents out the pressure relief valve.

When flow is turned on, gaseous O_2 passes through a vaporizing coil, where it is warmed by exposure to room temperature. It leaves the system through an outlet, where it is metered by a flow control valve. These metering devices are usually calibrated in 0.5-L/min units and limited to a maximum flow of 5 to 8 L/min.

If the cylinder pressure decreases below a preset level during use (usually 20 psi), an economizer valve closes, causing the liquid O_2 to move up the center tube and into the vaporizing coil. When in the vaporizing coil, the liquid O_2 is converted to a gas.

Depending on manufacturer and model, small liquid O_2 cylinders hold 45 to 100 lb of liquid O_2. To calculate duration of flow of a liquid O_2 system, one first converts the weight of liquid O_2 in pounds to the equivalent volume of gaseous O_2 in liters. At normal liquid cylinder operating pressures, 1 lb of liquid O_2 equals approximately 344 L of gaseous O_2. The accompanying Mini Clini provides an example of how the clinician can compute the duration of flow in a liquid O_2 system.

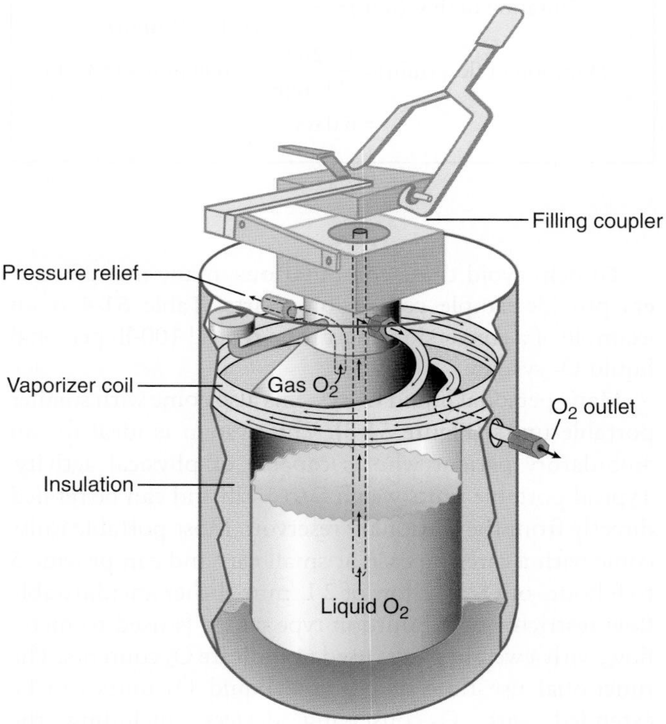

FIGURE 51-2 Diagram of a personal liquid oxygen supply system. (Modified from Lampton LM: Home and outpatient oxygen therapy. In Brashear RE, Rhodes ML, editors: Chronic obstructive lung disease, St Louis, 1978, Mosby.)

MINI CLINI

Computing Duration of Flow of a Liquid Oxygen System

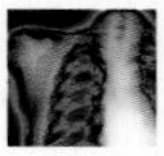

PROBLEM: A home care patient receives nasal O_2 at 2 L/min from a 100-lb liquid O_2 system. The system gauge indicates that the cylinder is half full. Approximately how long will this system last until empty?

SOLUTION

Step 1: Compute the available liquid O_2 (in lb)

$$100 \times 0.5 = 50 \text{ lb}$$

Step 2: Compute the available gaseous O_2

$$\text{Weight (lb) remaining} \times \text{factor}$$
$$50 \text{ lb} \times 344 \text{ L/lb} = 17{,}200 \text{ L}$$

Step 3: Divide the available volume of gaseous O_2 by the prescribed liter flow

$$\text{Duration of flow (min)} = \frac{\text{Volume of gaseous } O_2 \text{ (L)}}{\text{Liter flow (L/min)}}$$

$$\text{Duration of flow (min)} = \frac{17{,}200 \text{ L}}{2 \text{ L/min}} = 8600 \text{ min} = 143.3 \text{ hr}$$
$$= 6 \text{ days}$$

To help avoid these computations, many manufacturers provide simple conversion charts. Table 51-4 is an example of a conversion chart for a typical 100-lb personal liquid O_2 system.

Many personal liquid O_2 systems also come with smaller portable units (Figure 51-3). This system is ideal for an ambulatory patient who is capable of physical activity. Typical portable units weigh 5 to 14 lb and can be refilled directly from the stationary reservoir. Most portable units come with a carrying case or small cart and can provide 5 to 8 hours of O_2 at a flow of 2 L/min. Either an adjustable flow restrictor or a Bourdon-type gauge is used to meter flow, with a weight gauge used to indicate O_2 contents. The functional use time of portable liquid O_2 units can be extended with O_2-conserving devices, including the demand-flow systems discussed later in this chapter.

Because of the extremely low temperature of liquid O_2, patients and caregivers must be extremely careful when refilling these portable systems. Box 51-2 lists the steps needed to fill a portable liquid O_2 unit from a reservoir.[27] The procedure takes approximately 1 to 2 minutes, depending on the size of the portable tank. Wearing gloves can help prevent liquid O_2 skin burns.

Oxygen Concentrators

An O_2 concentrator is an electrically powered device that physically separates the O_2 in room air from nitrogen. The most common type of concentrator uses a **molecular sieve** to extract O_2.[27] Concentrators using membrane technology also exist, but they are not in common use.

The molecular sieve concentrator uses a pump to compress and deliver filtered room air to one of two sets of sieves (Figure 51-4). These sieves contain sodium-aluminum silicate pellets that absorb nitrogen, carbon dioxide (CO_2), and water vapor. To remove these unwanted gases from the pellets, an automatic pressure swing cycle switches back and forth between the sieve sets. One set is pressurized to produce O_2, and the other is depressurized to purge nitrogen, CO_2, and water vapor.

Gas leaving the sieves is stored in a small accumulator. At flows of 1 to 2 L/min, the typical molecular sieve concentrator provides between 92% and 95% O_2. At 5 L/min or greater, O_2 concentrations are between 85% and 93%.[27] The output of many concentrator models has been limited to

TABLE 51-4

Conversion Chart for Computing Duration of Flow for 100-lb (40-L) Liquid Oxygen Reservoir

Gauge reading	1	2	3	4	4
Weight (lb)	12.5	25	50	75	100
Liquid liters	5	10	20	30	40
Gaseous liters	4303	8606	17,212	25,818	34,424
Duration of Flow (Hours)					
Flow (L/min)					
1	72	143	287	430	574
2	36	72	143	215	287
3	24	48	96	143	191
4	18	36	72	108	143
5	14	29	57	86	115

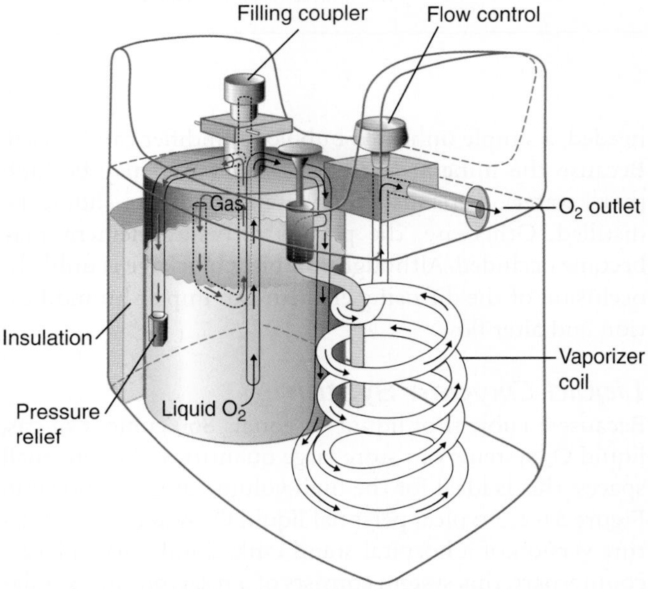

FIGURE 51-3 Diagram of a portable liquid oxygen unit. (Modified from Lampton LM: Home and outpatient oxygen therapy. In Brashear RE, Rhodes ML, editors: Chronic obstructive lung disease, St Louis, 1978, Mosby.)

5 L/min. However, more recently, models capable of delivering 10 L/min, such as the Respironics Millennium M10 (Phillips-Respironics, Murrysville, PA) have been introduced. In addition, technologic advances have accounted for other enhancements to O_2 production and delivery devices in alternative care settings. One such device is the Inogen One G2 System (Inogen Inc., Goleta, CA), which is a portable battery-powered concentrator with demand-flow conserving capabilities. The Inogen unit affords patients receiving low-flow O_2 increased mobility and has been approved for use in most commercial aircraft.

O_2 concentrators are the most cost-efficient supply method for patients in alternative care settings who need continuous low-flow O_2. For home use, a concentrator running 24 hours/day increases the average monthly electrical bill by only 5% to 10%. Depending on the season, heat given off by the concentrator's compressor can also affect energy usage by increasing room temperature. Nonetheless, when used with patients receiving low-flow O_2, concentrators are just as effective in increasing blood O_2 levels as more traditional supply systems (e.g., 100% cylinder gas with a cannula).

Box 51-2 Steps for Filling a Portable Liquid Oxygen Unit from the Reservoir

1. Check the gauge on the reservoir unit to ensure there is enough liquid O_2 in the reservoir to fill the portable unit.
2. Check the connectors on both units to ensure that they are clean and dry. Moisture on these connectors could cause the connectors to freeze together.
3. Connect the portable unit to the reservoir according to the manufacturer's instructions, generally by engaging the fittings on the portable unit and reservoir, then carefully twisting the portable unit until it "seats." The flow-rate controller should be turned off.
4. Open the portable unit vent. Allow the portable unit to fill. The portable unit is filled when excess O_2 begins being vented and the sound emitted from the unit changes. Close the vent valve.
5. Disengage the portable unit according to the manufacturer's instructions, generally by carefully twisting the portable tank until it is released from the liquid reservoir.

Problem Solving and Troubleshooting

Technical problems with O_2 supply systems in alternative settings are similar to problems encountered in the acute care hospital (see Chapter 37). In addition to these technical problems, situations can arise when patients or caregivers fail to follow instructions properly or respond as needed to simple incidents. To avoid communication problems, verbal instructions should always be reinforced by providing simple written instructions for subsequent reference. In addition, the clinician should always confirm and document the ability of caregivers to use the delivery system safely, including how to troubleshoot simple problems. The ability of caregivers and patients to give an adequate return demonstration on proper equipment usage should also be recorded.[24]

To avoid problems before they occur, the patient or caregiver should be instructed to check all O_2 delivery equipment at least once a day.[18] The proper function of all equipment, including liter flow and connections, should also be confirmed. In addition, the remaining liquid or compressed gas content of the supply system should be checked. Last, concentrator air inlet filters must be cleaned weekly. In the home setting, providing the patient or caregiver with a simple checklist form can help ensure that these important tasks are performed regularly.

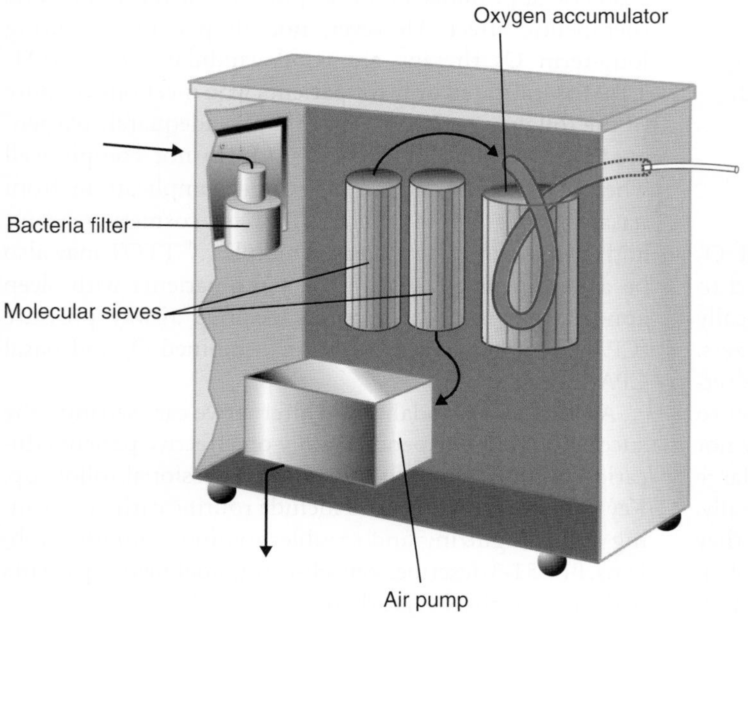

FIGURE 51-4 A molecular sieve oxygen concentrator.

In contrast to the hospital setting, O_2 supply problems in the alternative care setting cannot always be addressed immediately. For this reason, the clinician must ensure that all such systems have an emergency backup supply. This backup supply is normally provided by a large H/K cylinder, or at least an E cylinder for patients requiring lower flows. If the primary O_2 supply of a home care patient is by concentrator, the home care RT should notify the electric power company in writing that life-support equipment is in use at that location. In the event of a power outage, utility companies may try to restore service to that location first. For patients in more remote geographic areas, an emergency gasoline electrical generator can provide backup power for a concentrator.

Possible physical hazards to patients and caregivers include unsecured cylinders, ungrounded equipment, mishandling of liquid (resulting in burns), and fire.[24] Careful preliminary instruction, followed by ongoing assessment of the environment, can help minimize these problems. Bacterial contamination of nebulizer or humidification systems is another potential problem.[24] Infection control procedures designed to minimize this problem are discussed in detail on p. 1336.

Inaccurate O_2 flows or concentrations can also occur. Accurate flow output of O_2 systems should be confirmed by the supplier (using calibrated laboratory meters) before equipment is placed in alternative settings.[28] In the home, O_2 concentrator fractional inspired oxygen (FiO_2) levels should be checked and confirmed as part of a routine monthly maintenance visit.[29] Routine maintenance of these devices should include cleaning and replacing filters, checking the alarm system, and confirming FiO_2 levels using either the unit's O_2 sensor or a separate calibrated O_2 analyzer. If the concentration is less than the manufacturer's specification at the given flow, the pellet canisters are probably exhausted and should be replaced.

RULE OF THUMB

If an O_2 concentrator cannot supply at least 85% O_2 at 5 L/min, the pellet canisters are probably exhausted and should be replaced.

Because both concentrators and personal liquid O_2 systems operate at low pressures, they cannot be used to drive equipment needing 50 psi, such as pneumatically powered ventilators and large volume jet nebulizers. However, because many ventilators in alternative care settings are electrically powered and some use a flowmeter to provide supplementary O_2, this limitation is generally not a problem. Nonetheless, when 50 psi O_2 is needed, large gas cylinders are the storage system of choice. Additionally, many patients using liquid O_2 express concern when they hear gas venting from their system. The RT should explain to patients that venting is a normal feature of liquid O_2 systems. Venting does not occur during continual use because system pressures never build up to activate the relief valve.

Delivery Methods

The most common O_2 delivery system for long-term care is the nasal cannula. Simple O_2 masks and air entrainment masks may also be used but are much less common. Reservoir masks are also rare in alternative settings. To decrease O_2 use and costs, numerous O_2-conserving devices have been developed, including transtracheal O_2 catheter, reservoir cannula, and demand or pulsed-dose O_2 delivery systems.

RULE OF THUMB

O_2-conserving devices exhibit performance comparable to a nasal cannula at approximately one-third to one-half the flow. Based on this knowledge, when switching a patient from a nasal cannula at 2 L/min to an O_2-conserving device, the RT would start out at half the original flow, in this case, 1 L/min. The RT would then assess the response using a pulse oximeter and adjust the flow accordingly.

The performance characteristics, advantages, and disadvantages of transtracheal O_2 catheters and reservoir cannulas are described in detail in Chapter 38. We focus here on the application of the transtracheal O_2 catheter and the technical aspects of demand-flow systems.

Transtracheal Oxygen Therapy

Transtracheal oxygen therapy (TTOT) is O_2 delivered via a catheter with a small orifice that is inserted through the skin and neck tissue into the trachea. Although uncommon, this delivery method offers advantages of improved cosmetic appearance and lower flows to achieve the same therapeutic effect. However, not all patients requiring long-term O_2 therapy are good candidates for TTOT. TTOT is indicated only for patients who meet one or more of the following criteria: (1) cannot be adequately oxygenated with standard approaches, (2) do not comply well when using other devices, (3) exhibit complications from nasal cannula use, (4) prefer TTOT for cosmetic reasons, and (5) have need for increased mobility.[30] TTOT may also be a treatment alternative for some patients with sleep apnea when nasal continuous positive airway pressure (CPAP) is not tolerated or when combined O_2 and nasal CPAP are required.

As with most modalities in alternative care settings, the success of TTOT depends mainly on effective patient education and ongoing self-care with professional follow-up. Key patient responsibilities include routine catheter cleaning and recognizing and troubleshooting common problems. Box 51-3 describes key self-care guidelines for patients with transtracheal O_2 catheters.

Box 51-3 Self-Care Guidelines for Patients with Transtracheal Oxygen Catheters

- Never remove the catheter for more than a few minutes to avoid tract closure.
- Always keep the catheter clean.
- If you believe the catheter is not working properly even after cleaning it or if you cannot reinsert it, put on a nasal cannula and call your physician.
- If your humidifier pop-off is sounding, clear any hose blockage and clean the catheter.
- Never remove or insert the catheter while O_2 is flowing.
- Do not use antibiotics or other ointments at the site of catheter insertion.
- Try to keep the O_2 hose under your shirt, blouse, T-shirt, or pajama top and clipped to the top of your pants, skirt, or pajama bottom.
- Treat the O_2 hose as your lifeline by avoiding abuse or damage.
- If the equipment becomes split or broken or develops a permanent kink or foul odor, immediately discard and replace it. Catheters and hoses should be routinely replaced every 3 months.
- Always take catheter cleaning supplies, a nasal cannula, and a spare catheter when traveling.

Demand-Flow Oxygen Systems

A demand-flow O_2 delivery device, also known as a pulsed-dose **O_2-conserving device,** uses a flow sensor and valve to synchronize gas delivery with the beginning of inspiration.[31] As indicated in Figure 51-5, *A,* with continuous O_2 flow, most of the effective O_2 delivery occurs during the first half of inspiration. All the O_2 delivered during the latter half of inspiration and throughout most of expiration is wasted. Figure 51-5, *B,* shows the effect of a synchronized pulse of O_2 delivered at the beginning of inspiration. Ideally, this O_2 pulse should occur during the first quarter of inspiration. Under these conditions, a pulsed O_2 system can produce SaO_2 levels equal to levels seen with continuous flow, while using 60% less O_2.[32]

In theory, demand-flow O_2 systems provide the greatest savings in O_2 use for a given level of arterial saturation. In addition, there is generally no need for humidification. Demand-flow systems also have been successfully adapted for use with transtracheal catheters, resulting in even more efficient O_2 delivery. Current Medicare reimbursement guidelines provide no significant additional payments to cover the additional cost of demand delivery systems. Also, some patients receiving demand-flow O_2 desaturate during exercise.[31,33]

More recently, improvements to demand-flow systems have made them more reliable and user-friendly,

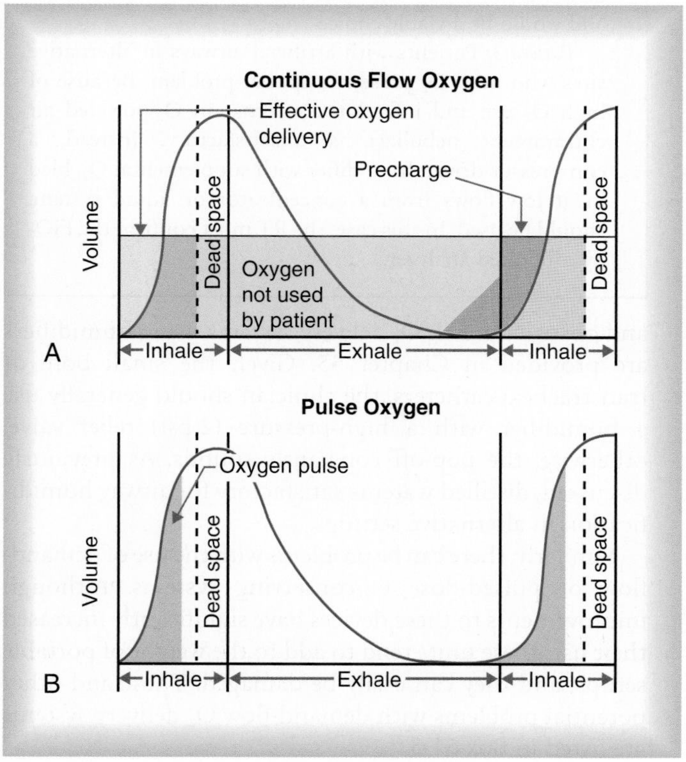

FIGURE 51-5 Demand-flow oxygen delivery. With continuous flow **(A),** most oxygen is delivered during the first half of inhalation, with the remainder wasted. With a coordinated pulse **(B),** most oxygen is delivered during the first 25% of inspiration, and no waste occurs. (Modified from O'Donohue WJ: The future of home oxygen therapy. Respir Care 33:1125, 1988.)

addressing the major disadvantages of earlier versions. As a result of these improvements and the ability of these devices to increase the duration of flow by two or three times, they have now gained wide acceptance. Demand-flow systems are considered a standard of practice for ambulatory patients using compressed or liquid O_2 in alternative sites.

Selecting a Long-Term Oxygen Delivery System

As when selecting hospital-based O_2 therapy systems, the "three P's" should always be considered when selecting a long-term O_2 system: purpose, patient, and performance. The goal is always to match the *performance* of the equipment to both the objectives of therapy *(purpose)* and the *patient's* special needs. Patients requiring low-flow home O_2 and enhanced mobility should be considered for a liquid O_2 setup with a pulsed-dose O_2-conserving device or the Inogen One System portable concentrator, maximizing portability and duration of flow.

Problem Solving and Troubleshooting

Most problems with long-term O_2 delivery systems are related to people. Patients and caregivers often fail to follow instructions or comply with the prescribed therapeutic or maintenance regimen.[24] Generally, caregivers should be allowed to operate and maintain O_2 delivery devices only after they have been instructed by credentialed RTs and have demonstrated the appropriate level of skill. In no case should the patient or caregiver be allowed or instructed to alter flow settings. Instead, when in doubt, they should be taught to switch to the backup supply at the same liter flow.

Technical problems are most common with TTOT and demand-flow systems. Most problems with TTOT are related to initial catheter insertion or ongoing maintenance. Most problems with demand-flow systems are based on the current limits of this technology.

The most common complications of TTOT are listed in Box 51-4. Although these problems occur infrequently, the clinician must be on constant guard for their occurrence. In particular, the RT should immediately report any evidence of tract tenderness, fever, excessive cough, increased dyspnea, or subcutaneous emphysema to the patient's physician.

To avoid complications or product failure, catheters and their tubing should be replaced every 3 months, at which time a checkup by the physician is also recommended. The patient or caregiver should clean the catheter every day, per the self-care guidelines listed on p. 1336. Patients should be instructed always to put on a nasal cannula and to call the physician if any major problem occurs.

Because transtracheal catheters are normally used with humidifiers, the clinician also must be prepared to troubleshoot this equipment. Guidelines for dealing with leaks and obstructions in O_2 delivery systems using humidifiers are provided in Chapter 35. Given the small bore of transtracheal catheters, the clinician should generally use a humidifier with a high-pressure (2 psi) relief valve; otherwise, the pop-off constantly sounds. As previously discussed, distilled water is satisfactory for airway humidification in alternative settings.

Similarly, there can be problems with the use of demand-flow or pulsed-dose O_2-conserving systems. Although improvements to these devices have significantly increased their use, these units tend to add to the weight of portable setups, and they can easily be damaged. These and other potential problems with demand-flow O_2 delivery systems are listed in Box 51-5.[33]

MINI CLINI

Selecting a Long-Term Oxygen Delivery System

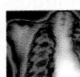

PROBLEM: The following three patients require long-term O_2: (1) a stable home care patient with restricted activity needing low FiO_2; (2) an active home care patient with low FiO_2 needs who desires increased mobility; and (3) a patient in a long-term care facility with a tracheostomy who needs moderate levels of O_2 and high humidity. Select the best O_2 delivery system for each patient.

SOLUTION

Patient 1: Because most home care patients who need O_2 are relatively stable, and because FiO_2 needs are minimal, traditional low-flow therapy by nasal cannula (using either a concentrator or a liquid reservoir) is the most common and accepted approach. When combined with a portable gas cylinder (for backup and limited walking), this combination is ideal for patients with restricted activity.

Patient 2: For an active patient with low FiO_2 needs who desires increased mobility, a conserving device used in conjunction with a portable liquid O_2 system (with the large reservoir used inside the home) is the ideal choice. Although a portable liquid O_2 unit can provide 5 to 8 hours of O_2 at 2 L/min by standard nasal cannula, use of a conserving device can double or even triple this time frame. Given that selected models of reservoir cannulas are poorly accepted by some patients, the choice of device usually narrows to a transtracheal catheter or a demand-flow/pulse-dosed system. Patients who meet the criteria for TTOT and can provide meticulous self-care should be considered for TTOT. Alternatively, demand-flow/pulsed-dose systems have been made less bulky and more reliable and would be a viable choice.

Patient 3: Patients with artificial airways in alternative sites who need O_2 present a special problem. Because of high O_2 use and infection concerns, an O_2-powered air entrainment nebulizer is unsatisfactory. Instead, a compressor-driven humidifier with supplemental O_2, bled in at low flows from a concentrator or liquid system, should be used. In this case, the RT must confirm the FiO_2 by calibrated analyzer.

Box 51-4 Complications of Transtracheal Oxygen Therapy

- Bleeding*
- Pneumothorax*
- Bronchospasm*
- Subcutaneous emphysema
- Catheter dislodgment or lost tract
- Increased sputum production
- Blockage by inspissated mucus
- Infection or abscess
- Extensive self-care and cleaning to avoid infection or blockage
- Tract tenderness

*Complications associated mainly with insertion.

Box 51-5 Potential Problems with Demand-Flow Oxygen Delivery Systems

- The devices can be cumbersome and cosmetically unattractive.
- The initial and maintenance costs of equipment can be high and not fully reimbursed.
- Earlier devices may possess poor response times and delays in valve opening or closing.
- The devices tend to be fragile and can be damaged easily if they fall.
- Most units require a battery, which needs to be charged or replaced.
- The catheters and sensors may malfunction because of sensor dislodgment or plugging or changes in breathing problems.

TABLE 51-5 Profiles of Patient Groups Requiring Ventilatory Support in Alternative Settings

Group Description	Diseases Involved
Profile 1	
Mainly composed of neuromuscular and thoracic wall disorders; particular stage of disease process allows patient certain periods of spontaneous breathing time during day; generally requires only nocturnal mechanical support	Amyotrophic lateral sclerosis Multiple sclerosis Kyphoscoliosis and related chest wall deformities Diaphragmatic paralysis Myasthenia gravis
Profile 2	
Requires continuous mechanical ventilatory support associated with long-term survival rates	High spinal cord injuries Apneic encephalopathies Severe COPD Late-stage muscular dystrophy
Profile 3	
Usually returns home at request of patient and family; patient's condition is terminal, life expectancy is short, and patient and family wish to spend remaining time at home; patients usually pose management problems in the home because of their rapidly deteriorating conditions	Lung cancer End-stage COPD Cystic fibrosis

VENTILATORY SUPPORT IN ALTERNATIVE SETTINGS

Providing successful ventilatory support outside the acute care hospital requires careful patient selection and good discharge planning.[34] Key factors include an interdisciplinary team approach, effective caregiver and family education, thorough assessment and preparation of the environment, and careful selection of needed equipment and supplies. Properly planned ventilatory support delivered in alternative settings can provide major benefits for both the patient and family, with substantial savings in health care costs.[35]

Patient Selection

Most patients needing ventilatory support outside the acute care hospital fall into one of the following three broad categories:[36]

1. Patients unable to maintain adequate ventilation over prolonged periods (in particular, noninvasive nocturnal or intermittent use)
2. Patients requiring continuous mechanical ventilation for long-term survival
3. Patients who are terminally ill with short life expectancies

Table 51-5 provides more detailed profiles of these patient groups. In addition to adults, a growing number of ventilator-assisted children are being managed in alternative settings. The same basic principles of discharge planning and patient care for adult patients should be followed for ventilator-assisted children.[37]

Regardless of diagnosis, patients being considered for ventilatory support in alternative settings must be medically and psychologically stable. In regard to assessing patient stability, Box 51-6 outlines the criteria developed by the American College of Chest Physicians (ACCP).[38]

Settings and Approaches

The most common setting for ventilatory support outside the acute care hospital is the home. Additional sites include LTACHs and long-term care facilities, including specialized long-term units designed specifically for ventilator patients.[38,39]

Based on individual evaluation of patient need, one of the following two major support approaches may be considered: (1) invasive or (2) noninvasive support. In alternative settings, invasive ventilatory support always involves

Box 51-6 Criteria to Determine Patient Stability for Ventilatory Support in Alternative Care Settings

- Ability to tolerate mechanical ventilation
- Acceptable arterial blood gas results and other blood chemistry (e.g., complete blood count)
- Relatively low FiO_2 needs (generally ≤40%)
- Psychologic stability
- Absence of life-limiting comorbidities, including cardiac dysfunction and arrhythmias
- PEEP should not exceed 10 cm H_2O
- Ability to clear airway secretions by cough, suction, or cough-assist device
- Tracheostomy tube, as opposed to endotracheal tube, for invasive ventilation
- No readmissions expected for >1 month

application of positive pressure ventilation by tracheotomy. Noninvasive approaches include positive pressure and negative pressure ventilation via an intact upper airway or abdominal displacement methods.[40,41]

Standards and Guidelines

Standards and guidelines for ventilatory support outside the acute care hospital continue to evolve. In the late 1980s, both the ACCP and the AARC developed and published recommendations for the care of ventilator-assisted individuals in the home and alternative care sites.[38,42] More recently, the AARC developed a clinical practice guideline on long-term invasive mechanical ventilation in the home.[43] Excerpts from these guidelines appear in Clinical Practice Guideline 51-3.

Special Challenges in Providing Home Ventilatory Support

Institutions that provide ventilatory support in alternative settings differ from acute care facilities mainly in their level of technology support. The home setting not only lacks this support but also must depend extensively on nontechnical, nonprofessional caregivers. For these reasons, providing ventilatory support in the home presents many special challenges.

Prerequisites

For home ventilatory support to be successful, several prerequisites must be met, including the following:[44]

- Willingness of family to accept responsibility
- Adequacy of family and professional support
- Overall viability of the home care plan
- Stability of patient
- Adequacy of home setting

In regard to the home setting, the same factors listed in Box 51-1 should be evaluated for patients being considered for home ventilatory support.

Planning

Successful home ventilatory support requires extensive planning, education, and follow-up by all members of the home care team. Basic steps in the discharge process for a ventilator-dependent patient include the following:

1. Family is consulted regarding feasibility.
2. Physician writes appropriate orders.
3. Discharge planner coordinates efforts of team members and discharge plan is formulated.
4. Physician and other team members discuss plan with family and caregivers.
5. Education and training are initiated and completed.
6. Patient and family are prepared for discharge.
7. Home layout is assessed with necessary changes made.
8. Equipment and supplies are readied.
9. Discharge planner meets with team and makes final preparations.
10. Patient is discharged (with trial period, if necessary).
11. Local power company is notified regarding the presence of life-support equipment; appropriate backup power (battery or compressed gas source) is made available.
12. Ongoing and follow-up care is provided by visiting nurse, RT, and other health care professionals (as necessary).

Caregiver Education

To prepare patients, family members, and other caregivers properly for home discharge, a comprehensive educational program must be undertaken and completed. Essential skills that must be taught include the following:[34]

- Simple patient assessment
- Airway management, including tracheostomy and stoma care, cuff care, suctioning, cough-assist, changing artificial airways or ties
- Chest physical therapy techniques, including percussion, vibration, and coughing
- Medication administration, including oral and aerosol
- Patient movement and ambulation
- Equipment operation and maintenance
- Equipment troubleshooting
- Cleaning and disinfection
- Emergency procedures

Emergency situations that caregivers must be trained to recognize and deal with properly include the following:

- Ventilator or power failure
- Ventilator circuit problems
- Airway emergencies
- Cardiac arrest

All caregivers should successfully complete this educational process. The specific time frame varies depending on caregiver ability and availability for training sessions. Training generally requires a minimum of 1 to 2 weeks, over which time several education sessions can take place and cover instruction, demonstration, caregiver practice, and evaluation. Caregivers should be strongly encouraged

51-3 Long-Term Invasive Mechanical Ventilation in the Home

AARC Clinical Practice Guideline (Excerpts)*

INDICATIONS

Patients requiring invasive long-term ventilatory support have shown:
- Inability to be completely weaned from invasive ventilatory support *or*
- Progression of disease etiology that requires increasing ventilatory support

Conditions that meet these criteria may include but are not limited to:
- Ventilatory muscle disorders
- Alveolar hypoventilatory syndrome
- Primary respiratory disorders
- Obstructive diseases
- Restrictive diseases
- Cardiac disorders including congenital anomalies

CONTRAINDICATIONS

Contraindications to long-term home mechanical ventilation include:
- Unstable condition that requires a level of care or resources unavailable in the home
  - FiO_2 requirement >0.40
  - PEEP > 10 cm H_2O
  - Need for continuous invasive monitoring (adults)
  - Lack of mature tracheostomy
- Patient's choice not to receive home mechanical ventilation
- Lack of an appropriate discharge plan
- Unsafe physical environment as determined by the patient's discharge planning team
  - Presence of fire, health, or safety hazards, including unsanitary conditions
  - Inadequate basic utilities (e.g., heat, air conditioning, electricity)
- Inadequate resources for care in the home
  - Financial
  - Personnel (e.g., inadequate medical follow-up, inability of patient to care for self, inadequate respite care for caregivers, inadequate numbers of competent caregivers)

PRECAUTIONS AND POSSIBLE COMPLICATIONS

Deterioration or acute change in clinical status of patient. The following may cause death or require rehospitalization for acute treatment:
- *Medical:* Hypocapnia, respiratory alkalosis, hypercapnia, respiratory acidosis, hypoxemia, barotrauma, seizures, hemodynamic instability, airway complications, respiratory infection, bronchospasm, exacerbation of underlying disease, or natural course of the disease
- *Equipment-related:* Failure of the ventilator, malfunction of equipment, inadequate warming and humidification of the inspired gases, inadvertent changes in ventilator settings, accidental disconnection from ventilator, accidental decannulation
- *Psychosocial:* Depression, anxiety, loss of resources (caregiver or financial), detrimental change in family structure or coping capacity

ASSESSMENT OF NEED

- Determination that indications are present and contraindications are absent
- Determination that one or more of the following goals can be met
  - To sustain and extend life and enhance quality of life
  - To reduce mortality
  - To improve or sustain physical and psychological function and enhance growth and development of pediatric patients
  - To provide cost-effective care
- Determination that no continued need exists for higher level of services
- Determination that frequent changes to the plan of care will not be needed

ASSESSMENT OF OUTCOME

At least the following aspects of patient management and condition should be evaluated periodically as long as the patient receives mechanical ventilation in the home:
- Implementation and adherence to plan of care
- Quality of life
- Patient satisfaction
- Resource satisfaction
- Growth and development in the pediatric patient

Continued

51-3 Long-Term Invasive Mechanical Ventilation in the Home—cont'd

AARC Clinical Practice Guideline (Excerpts)*

- Change in prognosis
- Unanticipated morbidity, including need for higher level site of care
- Unanticipated mortality

■ MONITORING

Frequency of monitoring should be determined by the ongoing individualized care plan and be based on the patient's current medical condition. The ventilator settings, proper function of equipment, and the patient's physical condition should be monitored and verified (1) with each initiation of invasive ventilation to the patient, including altering the source of ventilation, as from one ventilator or resuscitation bag to another ventilator; (2) with each ventilator setting change; (3) after moving the patient; (4) on a regular basis as specified by individualized plan of care.

All appropriately trained caregivers, both professional and appropriately trained lay caregivers, should follow the care plan and implement the monitoring that has been prescribed. After being trained and evaluated on their level of knowledge and ability to respond to each intervention, lay caregivers, with documented competency, may operate equipment, perform routine maintenance tasks, monitor equipment, and perform personal care required.

After completing training and demonstrating competency and if directed in the plan of care, lay caregivers should monitor the following:

- Patient's physical condition
  - Respiratory rate
  - Heart rate
  - Color changes
  - Chest excursion
  - Diaphoresis
  - Lethargy
  - Blood pressure
  - Body temperature
- Ventilator settings (frequency should be specified in the plan of care)
  - Peak pressures
  - PEEP level (if applicable)
  - Preset tidal volume
  - Appropriate humidification of inspired gases
  - Frequency of ventilator breaths
  - Temperature of inspired gases (if applicable)
  - Verification of FiO_2
  - Heat and moisture exchanger function
- Equipment function (frequency should be specified in the plan of care)
  - Appropriate configuration of circuit
  - Internal and external battery power levels
  - Alarm function
  - Overall condition of all equipment
  - Cleanliness of filters—according to manufacturer's recommendation
  - Self-inflating bag-valve-mask—cleanliness and function

Health care professionals should perform a thorough, comprehensive assessment of the patient and the patient-ventilator system on a regular basis as prescribed by the plan of care. In addition, the health care professional should implement, monitor, and assess results of other interventions as indicated by the clinical situation and anticipated in the care plan.

- Pulse oximetry—should be used to assess patients requiring a change in prescribed FiO_2 or in patients with a suspected change in condition; a physician's order for pulse oximetry must be obtained before testing is performed
- End-tidal CO_2—may be useful for establishing trends in CO_2 levels; a physician's order for end-tidal CO_2 monitoring must be obtained before it is performed
- Ventilator settings
- Exhaled tidal volume
- Analysis of fraction of inspired O_2

Health care professionals are also responsible for maintaining interdisciplinary communication concerning the plan of care. Health care professionals should integrate the respiratory plan of care into the patient's total care plan. The plan of care should include:

- All aspects of patient's respiratory care
- Ongoing assessment and education of the caregivers involved

**For the complete guideline, see American Association for Respiratory Care: Clinical practice guideline: long-term invasive mechanical ventilation in the home—2007 revision and update. Respir Care 52:1056, 2007.*

to complete a course in basic life support, such as offered by the American Heart Association, before the patient is discharged. Ideally, the patient should have a trial period on the actual home ventilator before discharge. In the early stages after discharge, patient follow-up by an RT likely should occur every day. As patient and caregivers become more familiar with the equipment and procedures, follow-up visits generally decrease to about once per month.[45,46]

Invasive versus Noninvasive Ventilatory Support

Until more recently, invasive positive pressure ventilation by tracheostomy was the default standard for long-term mechanical ventilation, especially for patients requiring 24-hour support. However, long-term tracheostomy is associated with many serious complications, including secretion retention, infection, aspiration, and ventilator-associated pneumonia. In addition, a permanent tracheostomy poses significant communication problems between caregivers and patients. Because many long-term care facilities treat a tracheostomy as an open wound, patient placement at certain sites is prohibited.[47] Last, invasive ventilation by tracheostomy poses significant limits on the patient's quality of life. For these reasons, noninvasive support is becoming increasingly popular. Noninvasive ventilatory support involves any method designed to augment alveolar ventilation without an endotracheal airway. **Noninvasive ventilation (NIV)** is usually the first choice. Any individual requiring mechanical ventilation can be supported with NIV if the following conditions are met:[47]

- The patient is mentally competent, cooperative, and not using heavy sedation or narcotics.
- Supplemental O_2 therapy is generally minimal ($FiO_2 \leq 40\%$).
- SaO_2 can be maintained at greater than 90% by aggressive airway clearance techniques.
- Bulbar muscle function is adequate for swallowing without potentially dangerous aspiration.
- No history exists of substance abuse or uncontrollable seizures.
- Unassisted or manually assisted peak expiratory flows during coughing exceed about 3 L/sec.
- No conditions are present that interfere with NIV interfaces (e.g., facial trauma, inadequate bite for mouthpiece, presence of orogastric or nasogastric tube, or facial hair that can hamper an airtight seal).

Patients who can benefit from NIV generally fall into one of two categories.[48] Patients in the first category have conditions in which cessation of ventilation could lead to imminent death. This category includes both acutely ill patients (patients with asthma, acute exacerbation of COPD, or pulmonary edema) and patients requiring long-term, 24-hour support (some patients with quadriplegia or patients with certain neuromuscular disorders). Patients in the second category have conditions in which NIV may offer clinical benefit, but cessation is not life-threatening. These patients generally require only intermittent or nocturnal support. Patients in this category include patients with chronic neuromuscular and chest wall diseases, such as muscular dystrophy and kyphoscoliosis. The application of long-term NIV for patients with obstructive disorders such as end-stage COPD or cystic fibrosis is less well documented, although some favorable results have been reported.[48] Relative contraindications to NIV include severe upper airway dysfunction, copious secretions that cannot be cleared by spontaneous or assisted cough, and O_2 concentration requirements exceeding 40%.[48]

Previously popular in alternative settings, negative pressure ventilation is now considered a second-line strategy for noninvasive ventilatory support. Compared with NIV, negative pressure ventilation is harder to apply, more cumbersome, and less well tolerated (because of poor breath synchronization). Negative pressure ventilation tends to limit patient mobility and can worsen upper airway obstruction in susceptible patients. Nonetheless, negative pressure ventilation may be appropriate in patients who are unable to use NIV or who have failed NIV trials.[41] Negative pressure ventilation may also be considered for patients who require frequent airway access for suctioning or patients with severe nasal congestion.[47]

Equipment

Box 51-7 lists the essential equipment and supplies needed for ventilator-dependent patients in alternative settings.[34,37]

Selecting Appropriate Ventilator

The choice of ventilator for a patient in an alternative care setting should be based on the patient's clinical need and the available support resources. In some cases, patient needs may dictate that more than one ventilator be provided.[43] A second backup ventilator should be provided for patients who cannot maintain spontaneous ventilation for more than 4 consecutive hours, for patients living in an area where a replacement ventilator cannot be secured within about 2 hours, and for patients whose care plan requires mechanical ventilation during mobility.[48]

Generally, ventilators chosen for care in alternative settings must be dependable and easy for caregivers to operate. If mobility is an essential element of the patient's care plan, the ventilator system selected should be portable. For these reasons, electrically powered devices (that run on both AC and DC battery power) are the best choice for ventilatory support in alternative settings. If the patient is receiving continuous ventilatory support in any alternative setting, external battery backup is required, and emergency AC power by way of a generator is recommended.

If invasive ventilation by tracheostomy is the selected approach, the best choice is a positive pressure ventilator. The invasive route also requires a humidification system,

Box 51-7 Essential Equipment and Supplies for Ventilator-Dependent Patients in Alternative Care Settings

EQUIPMENT
- Ventilator(s)
- Manual resuscitator (bag-valve-mask unit)
- Heated ventilator humidifier with thermostat or heat and moisture exchanger
- Monitoring or alarm devices (including remote where necessary)
- 12-V battery and battery charger
- Air compressor
- O_2 source
- Power strip or surge protector
- Suction machine with backup (manual or battery)
- Stethoscope or sphygmomanometer
- O_2 analyzer
- Pulse oximeter
- Hospital bed with table
- Patient lift
- Bedside commode, urinal, or bedpan
- Wheelchair

SUPPLIES
- O_2
- O_2 delivery devices, including manual resuscitator
- Airway interface (masks, mouthpieces, tracheostomy tubes)
- Tracheostomy tube inner cannulas
- Extra tracheostomy tubes including a tube one size smaller
- Tracheostomy care kits
- Ventilator circuits
- Bacterial filters
- Connecting tubing (aerosol, O_2, suction)
- Suction catheters
- Disposable gloves
- Distilled or sterile water
- Small volume nebulizer or metered dose inhaler with ventilator adapters, if appropriate
- Cleaning and disinfection supplies (10-ml syringe, 15- to 22-mm tubing adapters)

preferably a servo-controlled heated humidifier with alarms. Patients with a tracheostomy without retained secretions may use a heat and moisture exchanger during transport or to enhance their mobility.[43] For patients with an intact upper airway, a device capable of NIV is the first choice, unless contraindicated (Box 51-8 lists the absolute contraindications against using NIV).[49] In patients with an intact upper airway for whom NIV is contraindicated or unsuccessful, a negative pressure ventilator may be considered.

Positive Pressure Ventilators

Table 51-6 lists the essential, recommended, and optional features of positive pressure ventilators used in alternative care settings. An *essential* feature is basic to safe and effective operation in most patient care settings. A *recommended* feature helps provide optimal patient management. An *optional* feature is possibly useful in limited situations but not needed for most patients.[42,50]

Box 51-8 Absolute Contraindications Against Using Noninvasive Ventilation

- Need for immediate intubation
- Hemodynamic instability
- Uncooperative patient
- Facial burns or trauma
- Inadequate airway protection
- Patent tracheoesophageal fistula

TABLE 51-6
Essential, Recommended, and Optional Features of a Positive Pressure Ventilator for Use in an Alternative Care Setting

Feature	Necessity
Positive pressure tidal breaths	Essential
Mandatory rate	Essential
Flow or inspiratory-to-expiratory or inspiratory time	Recommended*
Expiratory pressure (PEEP)	Optional
FiO_2 to 1	Optional
Patient spontaneous breath (e.g., CPAP, intermittent mandatory ventilation)	Optional
Breath-triggering mechanism (flow or pressure sensors to initiate ventilator breath)	Recommended*
Flow-timing interaction (e.g., pressure support)	Optional
Feedback control (e.g., mandatory minute ventilation)	Optional

*Essential if the patient has intact ventilatory drive and respiratory muscles or if the possibility of partial or complete ventilator independence is anticipated.

As in the acute care setting, the use of volume-cycled versus pressure-limited ventilators is debated in alternative settings. Although volume-cycled ventilation has been the predominant mode of support in these settings, pressure-limited ventilation is gaining popularity for use in selected patients.

As shown in Figure 51-6, there are many new positive pressure ventilators designed for use in alternative settings. These ventilators can be used on adults or pediatric patients weighing at least 5 kg. Some are approximately the size and weight of a laptop computer and have many of the capabilities of much larger mechanical ventilators used in alternative sites and in acute care. These new ventilators offer ventilator-dependent patients the advantages of greater mobility and space conservation. Many of these models also offer pressure support to augment spontaneous breaths and can provide positive end expiratory

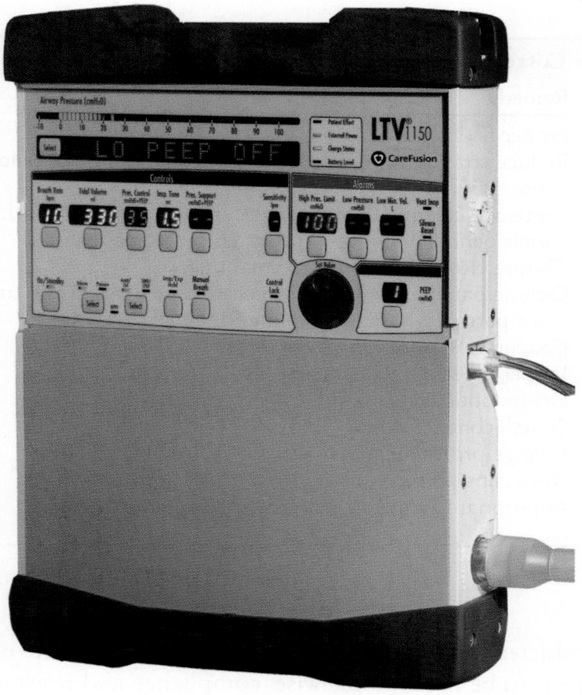

FIGURE 51-6 Pulmonetic Systems LTV 1150 ventilator. (Courtesy CareFusion, Viasys HealthCare, San Diego, CA.)

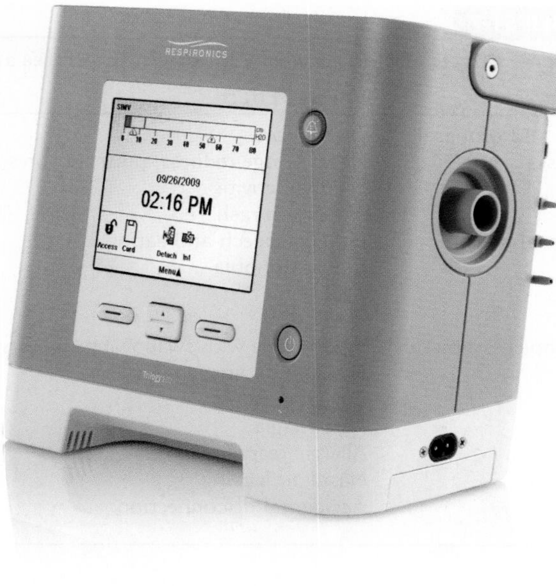

FIGURE 51-7 Philips-Respironics Trilogy 200 ventilator. (Used with permission of Philips Respironics, Murrysville, PA.)

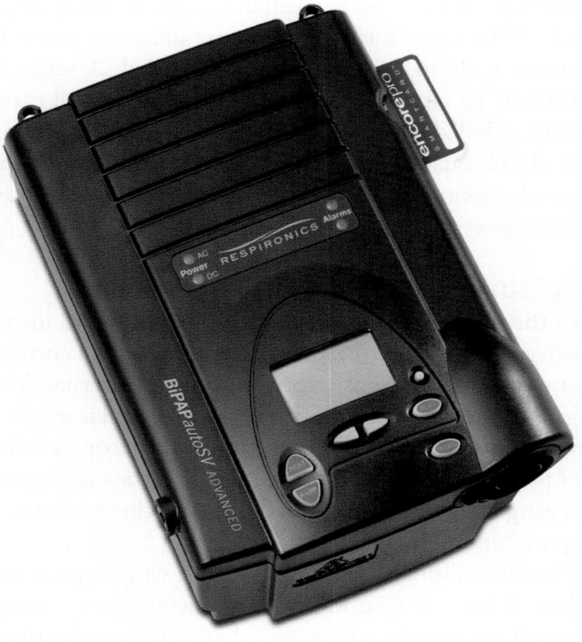

FIGURE 51-8 Respironics BiPAP autoSV. (Used with permission of Philips Respironics, Murrysville, PA.)

pressure (PEEP) without having to add an adapter to the ventilator circuit.[51-53]

Many new positive pressure ventilators designed for alternative care settings (Figure 51-7; see Figure 51-6) have an internal battery, which can provide 6 hours of use should AC line power fail. For longer periods of use away from AC line power, many of these devices can run for 10 to 12 hours using a 12-V deep-cell (marine) battery.

Additionally, time-triggered or patient-triggered, pressure-limited, flow-cycled devices (pressure support with timed backup) have been successfully applied in alternative settings.[41,54,55] Many units are currently available (Figure 51-8) that are specifically designed to provide this type of support, usually noninvasively by nasal or oronasal (full-face) masks.[41,56,57]

Any existing positive pressure ventilator essentially can be used to provide NIV.[48,58] Many patients, especially patients with COPD, prefer pressure-limited over volume-cycled ventilation. However, patients with neuromuscular or neurologic disorders often favor the consistent high inflations provided by volume ventilation, which enhance coughing and phonation. In addition, the alarm capabilities and internal battery backup provided with current portable volume ventilators make them the best choice for patients who cannot sustain any spontaneous breathing.[56]

The biggest challenge with NIV is not selecting the right ventilator but getting a good, comfortable, minimal leak interface. Interfaces commonly found in alternative care settings include oronasal (full-face) masks; nasal masks; nasal "pillows"; and simple, flanged, or custom mouthpieces. For long-term use, some patients prefer alternating between devices. A patient may prefer a simple mouthpiece for easy accessibility during the day, with a nasal mask providing support at night.[48] Table 51-7 summarizes common problems associated with NIV interfaces and how to correct them.[41,59]

All positive-pressure ventilators used in alternative settings must have an alarm to indicate loss of power (pneumatic or electrical). Portable volume-cycled ventilators should also incorporate a high-pressure alarm or cycle

TABLE 51-7

Adverse Effects of Noninvasive Ventilation Interfaces and Possible Corrective Actions

Interface	Adverse Effect	Remedy
Nasal and oronasal masks	Discomfort	Proper fit, adjust strap tension, change mask type
	Nasal bridge redness, pressure sores, conjunctivitis	Reduce strap tension, use forehead spacer, try nasal pillow, use artificial skin
	Acneiform rash	Cortisone cream, alternative (gel) mask
Oronasal masks	Impede speech and eating	Permit periodic removal if tolerated by the patient
	Claustrophobia	Choose clear masks with minimal bulk
	Aspiration	Exclude patients unable to protect airway; nasogastric tubes for patient with nausea and abdominal distention
Mouthpieces/lip seals	Interference with swallowing, salivary retention	Coaching, adaptation
	Pressure on lips, cheeks	Proper fit, strap adjustment
	Dental deformity	Orthodontic consultation
	Aerophagia	Simethicone, coaching
	Allergic reactions	Change prosthetic materials
	Nasal air leaking	Nose clips
	Accidental disconnection	Appropriate alarms in ventilator-dependent patients

override. For patients with conditions in which cessation of ventilation would cause death, a patient-disconnect alarm (low-pressure or low-exhaled volume) must be provided.[43,48] In some settings, a remote alarm or secondary disconnect alarm, or both, may be needed. A secondary alarm may be based on chest wall impedance and cardiac activity, exhaled volume, end-tidal CO_2, or pulse oximetry with alarm capabilities.[43] For patients in alternative settings who require only intermittent NIV, a loss of power alarm is generally sufficient.[48]

Negative Pressure Ventilators

With the increased popularity of noninvasive and invasive positive pressure ventilation, negative pressure ventilators are rarely used for ventilatory support in alternative settings.[41,60] The original negative pressure ventilator was the *iron lung,* used for patients needing ventilator assistance after poliomyelitis. For practical reasons, the cumbersome iron lung was essentially replaced by the chest cuirass and wrap or "pneumosuit."

The chest cuirass (a rigid shell) and wrap-type systems (nylon fabric surrounding a semicylindrical tentlike support) are simply enclosures that allow application of negative pressure to the thorax. These devices require a separate electrically powered negative pressure generator. An example of a negative pressure generator used to power cuirass or wrap-type systems is the Philips-Respironics NEV-100 (Phillips-Respironics, Murrysville, PA).[60]

Evaluation and Follow-Up

Patient parameters to be monitored during positive pressure ventilation are essentially the same parameters that are assessed in the acute care setting, with an emphasis on simplicity.[61] The caregiver should assess the patient's vital signs, lung sounds, and sputum production on a daily basis; arterial blood gas analysis (by the RT) may be conducted monthly or only when changes in the care plan appear to be needed. Likewise, compliance and resistance measures are performed only when other evidence indicates the need.

Routine follow-up visits by the RT help ensure the success of patient management within the home. Equipment must be checked and cleaned as necessary. The patient's status should be carefully assessed, and appropriate recommendations for change should be made to the primary or prescribing physician. Any prescribed respiratory therapy should be administered during the visit, and all necessary supply items should be left with the patient's caregivers. After each visit, a report documenting the status of the patient and equipment and progress toward care plan goals should be completed and maintained as part of the patient record. Subsequent follow-up visits should occur regularly (approximately monthly) and whenever needed.

OTHER MODES OF RESPIRATORY CARE IN ALTERNATIVE SITES

In addition to O_2 therapy and ventilatory support, other modes of respiratory care are now common in the alternative care setting. These may represent the primary therapy or may be used to supplement other modes of care. Included for discussion here are bland aerosol therapy, aerosol drug administration, airway care and clearance methods, nasal CPAP or bilevel PAP, and apnea monitoring.

Bland Aerosol Therapy

The delivery of bland aerosols has been common in alternative sites for many years. According to the AARC's Clinical Practice Guideline, bland aerosol therapy includes the delivery of sterile water or various concentrations of saline solution in aerosol form.[62] The aerosol can be produced by either an ultrasonic or jet (large volume) nebulizer. If using a jet nebulizer, a 50-psi air compressor is also required. Supplemental O_2 is provided by either a concentrator or liquid supply system.

Depending on the patient's condition and therapeutic objectives, bland aerosol therapy may be either continuous or intermittent. Historically, this approach was used for patients with tracheostomies because of their bypassed upper airway. Current knowledge suggests that bland aerosol therapy alone has little effect on the properties of mucus or its clearance.[62] However, it may be useful as an adjunct to airway clearance procedures in patients who regularly produce large amounts of sputum.[63]

The potential problem is infection from contaminated equipment. To reduce the incidence of infection, equipment and patient delivery systems must be cleaned and changed regularly. Disinfection procedures are discussed on p. 1336.

Aerosol Drug Administration

As in the acute care setting, the aerosol route is popular for drug administration to respiratory patients in alternative care settings. Drug categories commonly administered by the aerosol route include beta-adrenergic bronchodilators, anticholinergic agents, and antiinflammatory drugs.

Most pulmonary drugs are available in either metered dose inhaler or dry powder inhaler form. Alternatively, the caregiver can use a small volume nebulizer powered by a low output diaphragm compressor.[64] Guidelines on selecting the best delivery method for aerosolized drugs are discussed in Chapter 36. Regarding reimbursement for home use of small volume nebulizer or compressor systems, Medicare limits reimbursement by (1) requiring a certificate of medical necessity and (2) capping rental costs. Consequently, the reimbursable expenses related to aerosol drug administration in the home is quite limited.[5]

Airway Care and Clearance Methods

Patients in alternative care settings with tracheostomies require both daily stoma care and tracheobronchial secretion clearance. Tracheostomy care can be provided by any trained caregiver, but tube changes should be performed only by a nurse, physician, or RT.

In most alternative care settings, tracheobronchial clearance is often accomplished by suctioning using a portable electrically powered suction pump with collection bottle and connection tubing. In accordance with the AARC Clinical Practice Guideline for suctioning of the patient at home, some patients may be taught to suction themselves. Proper suctioning procedures should also be taught to caregivers. Education and training on proper suctioning methods may begin before patient discharge from the acute care setting, with reinforcement and follow-up as needed.[65] Because many of these systems measure pressure in inches of mercury (in Hg), care must be taken to teach proper adjustment according to patient age. Daily maintenance and cleaning are required. In an alternative care setting, a single suction catheter commonly may be used for 24 hours and then discarded. This measure helps control supply costs. To prevent bacterial growth, catheters are placed in a disinfecting solution such as hydrogen peroxide or 2.5% acetic acid between suctioning attempts.

RULE OF THUMB

For portable suction units calibrated in inches of mercury (in Hg), the following vacuum ranges are recommended (adjustment may be needed based on volume and viscosity of secretions):

Patient Category	Vacuum Setting (in Hg)
Infants	5-7
Children	7-12
Adults	12-15

Numerous methods are available for patients in an alternative care setting with an intact upper airway who need help with secretion clearance. These methods include both patient-independent and caregiver-dependent techniques.[66] Patients can be taught to apply independently coughing, forced exhalation, active cycle of breathing, and autogenic drainage methods. Caregiver assistance is required with traditional postural drainage, percussion and vibration, and directed or assisted cough. Additional assistance can be provided by mechanical devices such as positive expiratory pressure mask, flutter valve, intrapulmonary percussive ventilator, and high-frequency chest compression vest, which are routinely used for patients with cystic fibrosis.

Another airway clearance method involves the use of cough-assist devices such as the Emerson mechanical **inexsufflator,** or "coughlator." These devices have been on the market since the 1950s but have gained more widespread acceptance only more recently. The inexsufflator uses alternating positive and negative pressure as a form of lung expansion and airway clearance therapy. These devices can be especially effective with patients receiving NIV. The application of secretion clearance devices or techniques by nonprofessional caregivers should involve good preliminary instruction and ongoing follow-up by the RT working in any alternative site.[66] See Chapter 33 for more in-depth discussion of the inexsufflator.

Nasal Continuous Positive Airway Pressure Therapy

Nasal CPAP therapy has become an accepted form of home care used to treat sleep apnea-hypopnea syndrome. For Medicare reimbursement of home nasal CPAP equipment,

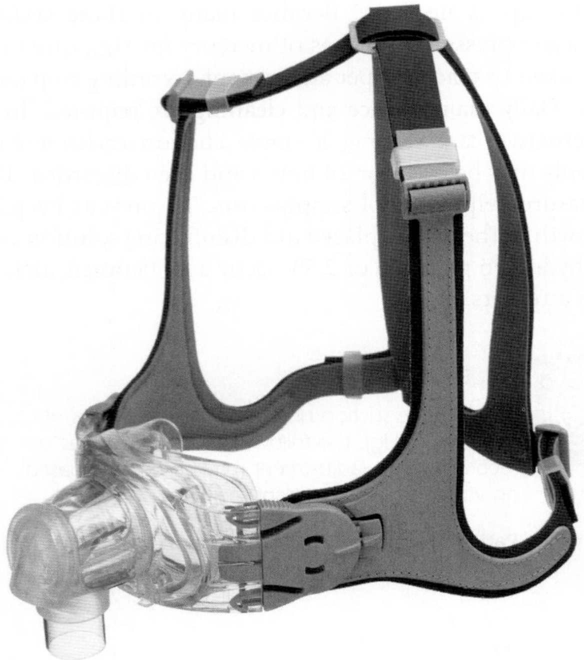

FIGURE 51-9 An Example of a nasal mask. (Mirage Kidsta Mask, Courtesy ResMed Inc, Phoenix, AZ, 2009.)

the diagnosis of sleep apnea must be confirmed by polysomnography, also known as a *sleep study*. With proper application and patient compliance, CPAP therapy can dramatically lessen or resolve the many problems associated with sleep apnea-hypopnea syndrome (morning headaches, daytime hypersomnolence, cognitive impairment). The patient's quality of life can be enhanced, and the incidence of more severe complications, such as systemic and pulmonary hypertension and cor pulmonale, may be reduced.[67]

Equipment

A typical nasal CPAP apparatus consists of a flow generator capable of establishing varying levels of PEEP or CPAP, a circuit, and a patient interface (e.g., nasal mask, nasal pillows). One of the most common interfaces in alternative settings is the nasal mask (Figure 51-9). Most systems provide manually adjustable pressures in the range of 2.5 to 20 cm H_2O. Many units now have a ramp feature that gradually increases the pressure to the prescribed level over a time interval. This feature helps some patients fall asleep and may increase therapy compliance.

A variation of nasal CPAP therapy is bilevel PAP. CPAP uses a single pressure level, whereas bilevel PAP uses two levels: (1) inspiratory positive airway pressure (IPAP) and (2) expiratory positive airway pressure (EPAP). In some patients, independent adjustment of IPAP and EPAP achieves the same results as conventional nasal CPAP therapy but at lower levels of expiratory pressure. In other patients, the difference in IPAP and EPAP aids the patient's inspiratory effort, improving ventilation. In this respect, bilevel PAP may be used as a form of NIV for patients with ventilatory insufficiency. Bilevel PAP may also reduce the adverse effects associated with nasal CPAP therapy and improve patient tolerance.[68]

Determining Proper Continuous Positive Airway Pressure Level

The proper CPAP level for a patient is determined by one of several methods. The most common method is to conduct the sleep study, titrating different levels of CPAP. Observed changes in the apnea-hypopnea index are correlated with the various CPAP levels. The prescribed level of CPAP is the lowest pressure at which apneic episodes are reduced to an acceptable frequency and duration.

CPAP units were developed more recently that automatically adjust the pressures to maintain airway patency, despite physiologic changes such as those affecting airway muscle tone or weight gain or loss. These self-titrating or auto-CPAP devices generally result in use of the lowest effective pressures and better patient compliance, while reducing the need for a sleep study and titration. As a result of such benefits, these devices are gaining widespread acceptance.[69]

Alternatively, CPAP may be titrated against pulse oximetry data (Figure 51-10). In this case, the goal is to use the lowest CPAP that prevents arterial desaturation (SpO_2 <90%).

Use and Maintenance

Once proper CPAP level is determined, the patient is fitted for a mask and trained in the proper use, cleaning, and maintenance of the equipment. Typical patient instructions for self-administration of nasal CPAP therapy are provided in Box 51-9.

Problem Solving and Troubleshooting

Patient problems associated with nasal CPAP therapy include skin irritation, conjunctivitis, epistaxis, and nasal discomfort (dryness, burning, and congestion). Skin irritation is usually because of tight mask straps or a dirty patient interface. Persistent redness on the face or around the nose is the primary sign. Adjusting the straps (while maintaining a good mask seal) can help prevent irritation. In addition, the patient interface should be cleaned daily to remove dirt and facial oils. Even with proper care, most interfaces such as masks harden over time, causing problems with irritation and leaks. For this reason, masks and nasal pillows should be replaced approximately every 3 to 6 months or sooner if leakage or discomfort occurs.

Conjunctivitis probably is the result of mask leakage around the bridge of the nose, which is easily corrected by ensuring a good seal in this area. Epistaxis and nasal discomfort are associated with drying of the nasal mucosa—a particular problem in cold, dry winter climates. Methods used to overcome excessive drying include in-line humidifiers, room vaporizers, chin straps (to decrease loss of upper

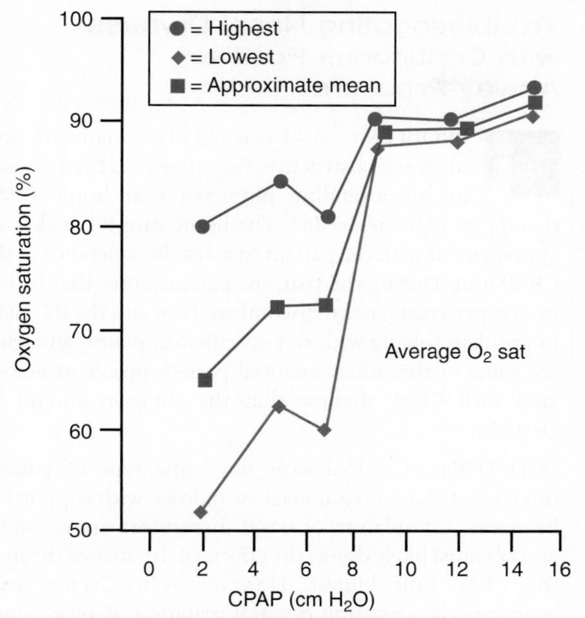

FIGURE 51-10 A realistic illustration of CPAP levels and corresponding oxygen saturations taken while the patient was asleep and using nasal CPAP. (Modified from Sleeper GP, Strohl KP, Armeni MA: Nasal CPAP for at-home treatment of obstructive sleep apnea: a case report, Respir Care Clin N Am 30:90, 1985.)

Box 51-9 Typical Patient Instructions for Self-Administration of Nasal Continuous Positive Airway Pressure Therapy

EQUIPMENT PREPARATION

1. Place blower unit on a level surface (table or nightstand) close to where you sleep.
2. Ensure that the air exhaust and inlet vents are not obstructed.
3. Plug machine into a standard grounded (three-prong) electrical outlet.
4. Check air inlet filter to ensure it is in place and free of dust.
5. Connect one end of the tubing to the interface (e.g., mask, nasal pillows).
6. Attach interface to the nose or face.
7. Adjust headgear strap tightness to seat interface firmly onto the nose or face.
8. Turn on the blower and verify a flow of air.
9. Ensure proper fit and adjustment of mask and headgear. Air should not be leaking out around the bridge of the nose into the eyes or from the mask to upper lip.
10. CPAP therapy is now fully functional, but minor adjustments may be needed as use continues.

IN THE MORNING

1. Remove mask by slipping strap off back of head (you may leave the head strap connected between cleaning).
2. Turn off blower.
3. Wash interface every morning with a mild detergent, then rinse it with water.
4. Once dry, store interface in a plastic bag to keep it clean.

WEEKLY

1. Wipe off the blower unit with a clean, damp cloth.
2. Wash the head strap and circuit tubing.
3. Service the filters according to the instructions in your patient manual.

airway moisture), and saline nasal sprays.[70] Because none of these methods have proved satisfactory for all patients, selection should be based on individual patient acceptance and observed improvement in comfort. However, almost all patients receiving nocturnal CPAP therapy benefit from the addition of an in-line humidifier.

The most common problem with the CPAP apparatus is an inability to reach or maintain the set pressure. This problem is usually due to either inadequate flow or, more commonly, system leaks. Common causes of leaks include inappropriate patient interface (mask vs. nasal pillows) or pressure loss through an open mouth. As part of their initial training, patients and caregivers should be taught how to recognize and correct these common problems. Box 51-10 outlines the procedures patients or caregivers can use to troubleshoot inadequate flows and system leaks.[71]

Follow-up with patients soon after they begin CPAP therapy is important to resolve complications promptly. If left unresolved, these issues often discourage the patient

Box 51-10 Patient and Caregiver Instructions for Troubleshooting Continuous Positive Airway Pressure Equipment

INADEQUATE FLOW

1. Ensure that unit is plugged into a working electrical outlet.
2. Confirm that unit is turned on.
3. Ensure all connections are tight.
4. Confirm that airflow is coming from blower.
5. Ensure that the intake/exhaust vents are not obstructed.
6. Check the blower inlet filter to confirm that air can easily enter unit. If the filter appears obstructed, wash or replace it.
7. If there is still no flow, contact your home care provider.

AIR LEAKS

1. Check interface fit, and readjust mask or headgear if necessary.
2. Request a chin strap to help keep mouth closed.
3. If problem is not resolved, contact the home care provider for adjustments or a different interface such as nasal pillows.

and result in decreased compliance and a return of original symptoms.[71]

Apnea Monitoring

Apnea monitors alert clinicians and caregivers of certain life-threatening events, most notably recurrent apnea, bradycardia, and hypoxemia. At-risk infants are frequently set up on apnea monitors while they are in the hospital. After extensive family instruction in both equipment use and resuscitation, some of these infants may be discharged to the home with this equipment.[72]

Most apnea monitors detect both respirations and heart rate and activate audio and visual alarms when preset high or low limits are reached. Follow-up visits by the RT or a nurse are usually frequent at first but occur less often as the family becomes skilled with the equipment and monitoring routine. Some models record each alarm event and can be useful in monitoring the patient's progress. The "memory" of such monitors generally requires periodic downloading during a follow-up visit or via a cable or telephone modem. Apnea monitors are usually discontinued after an infant has a negative pneumocardiogram (sleep study) or when recorded memory reveals no events during a prescribed time frame. Generally, apnea monitors are needed for 2 to 4 months for many of these patients.[72]

PATIENT ASSESSMENT AND DOCUMENTATION

Alternative care sites demand extensive patient assessment and documentation. These requirements are based on both stringent reimbursement criteria and the rehabilitation orientation characterizing these settings.

MINI CLINI

Troubleshooting Nasal Dryness with Continuous Positive Airway Pressure

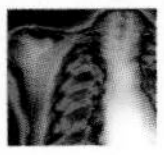

PROBLEM: A 43-year-old obese man with documented obstructive sleep apnea has been advised by his attending physician that home CPAP therapy at night is needed. The home care RT makes an appointment with the patient to assess his tolerance to the CPAP unit. During the visit, the patient notes that he has been experiencing nasal discomfort. How can the RT assist in problem solving with this specific complaint, and what are some of the other potential patient problems associated with CPAP therapy that the clinician should be alerted to?

SOLUTION: CPAP devices use some type of patient interface such as a nasal mask or pillows, with supporting headgear. Complaints of nasal discomfort are common and are most likely due to the effects of dry airflow through the CPAP unit blower. However, other factors may aggravate the sensation of nasal irritation. Poor systemic hydration could worsen nasal mucosal drying. In addition, environmental humidity may be a factor. Cold, dry, winter climates can aggravate symptoms, as can dry, forced-air heating systems. In these cases, the RT might recommend increasing oral intake of fluids (if no restrictions on fluid intake), the installation of a room or heating system humidifier or the as-needed use of a saline nasal spray. Also, almost all patients receiving nocturnal CPAP therapy benefit from the addition of an in-line humidifier.

In addition to the above-mentioned factors, large leaks in the system can significantly increase flows and worsen the drying effect of these devices. Often such leaks originate from a poorly fitting patient interface. Consequently, these problems can be remedied by ensuring a proper fit via repositioning the interface or switching to one of the many alternative masks or nasal pillows available today.

Institutional Long-Term Care

In institutions providing long-term care, the assessment and documentation process involves four key components: screening, treatment planning, ongoing assessment, and discharge (Figure 51-11).

Screening

On admission to a long-term care facility, all patients with a respiratory-related admitting diagnosis should be screened by an RT.[17] This screening is often accomplished solely by chart review, without direct contact with the newly admitted patient or resident. During screening, the RT reviews the pertinent respiratory diagnosis, onset and severity of symptoms (including the impressions of the resident's nurse), current radiograph results, pulmonary function tests, arterial blood gas values, and other nonrespiratory treatment orders (e.g., physical therapy).

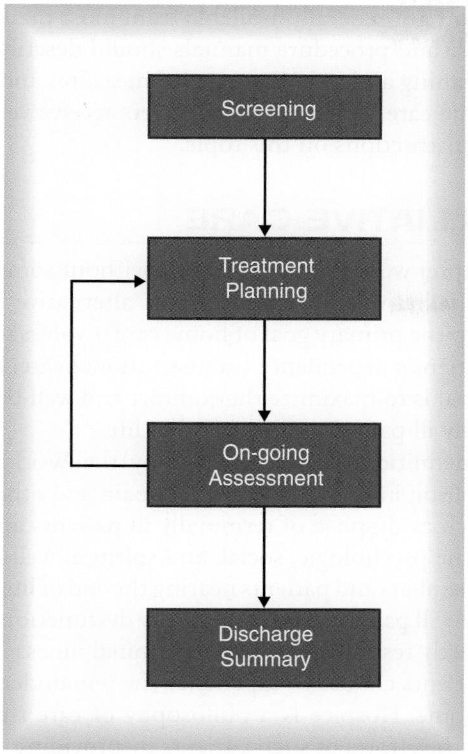

FIGURE 51-11 The assessment and documentation process in institutional subacute or long-term care.

If the review indicates the need for a more in-depth assessment, the RT can recommend a more complete evaluation. On receipt of the appropriate orders, the RT interviews the patient and conducts a physical assessment, including inspection, palpation, auscultation, and percussion. Key clinical findings include description of breath sounds; rate, depth, and pattern of respirations; heart rate; signs of dyspnea; cough; sputum production; level of consciousness; and ability of the resident to understand and follow commands. Also noteworthy are the resident's prior respiratory status, use of supplemental O_2, skin turgor, and medications. Where indicated, a pulse oximetry test is performed during the evaluation.[17,18]

Treatment Planning and Ongoing Assessment

Based on the information obtained during the initial screening process, the RT designs a specific treatment plan. A typical treatment plan includes patient demographics, assessment information, short-term and long-term goals reflective of overall rehabilitation potential, and measures to be used to achieve such goals. A treatment plan for a resident of a long-term care facility with moderate to severe COPD would likely reflect the treatment goal of correcting hypoxemia through the use of low-flow O_2 and patient monitoring.[17,18]

After therapy has been initiated, the RT uses several other tools to monitor a patient's progress. In addition to regular treatment documentation, the RT should document a regular summary on each patient. This summary provides a synopsis of residents' progress toward goal attainment, including changes in respiratory status, results of any additional tests, explanation of any patient education, and recommendations for additional therapy. These summaries become part of the resident's permanent record, with a copy going to the attending physician. Additionally, treatment plans and progress summaries are often required documentation for third-party reimbursement.[17,18]

Discharge Summary

When a patient reaches his or her maximum potential, has attained all set goals, or is discharged, the RT must complete a discharge summary. The discharge summary describes the complete course of respiratory therapy, including its success or failure.[17-19]

Home Care

A home care plan must specify not only the types of care provided but also a strategy for patient follow-up. The individual making the follow-up visits could be the attending physician but more commonly is the visiting nurse, a physical therapist, or an RT. For patients receiving respiratory care at home, follow-up by a home care team member should occur regularly, particularly for patients on "hi-tech" equipment such as ventilators and apnea monitors.[12] Some patients may require more frequent follow-up, especially patients recently discharged or patients requiring ventilatory support. Factors relevant to the frequency of home visits include the following:

- Patient's condition and therapeutic needs (objectives)
- Level of family or caregiver support available
- Type and complexity of home care equipment
- Overall home environment
- Ability of the patient to provide self-care
- Third-party reimbursement for such visits

When a visit is made by the RT, numerous functions must be performed, including the following:

- Patient assessment (objective and subjective data), including pretreatment and posttreatment clinical assessment
- Patient's compliance with prescribed respiratory home care
- Equipment assessment (operation, cleanliness, and need for related supplies)
- Identification of any problem areas or patient concerns
- Statement related to patient goals and therapeutic plan

A standard written report, consistent with the care plan, should be completed by the visiting RT. Copies are often sent to the patient's physician, the home care referral source, and any other member of the team requiring this information. The report should become part of the patient's medical record and should be referred to when following the patient's course and overall progress.[12,16]

EQUIPMENT DISINFECTION AND MAINTENANCE

With more and more patients receiving respiratory care outside the hospital, the danger of infection caused by direct contact with caregivers and visitors or indirect contact with contaminated articles and equipment has grown. To help minimize home-related infection, guidelines for disinfecting home respiratory care equipment have been established. Accepted infection control techniques are based on clinical evidence, such as the evidence outlined in several of the AARC Clinical Practice Guidelines that pertain to respiratory care provided in alternative settings.[24,43,62,65,73]

Collectively, these guidelines focus on sources of infection, basic principles of infection control, patients at high risk, disinfection methods, equipment processing, and care of solutions and medications. Procedures focus significantly on surveillance, prevention, and control of infection.[15,16]

In regard to infection control, all guidelines and procedures mandate proper hand hygiene techniques by all caregivers—either proper handwashing or use of antiseptic hand lotions. In addition, visits to the patient by friends or relatives with respiratory infections are discouraged. Relating to medical equipment suppliers, the guidelines suggest that all permanent equipment (e.g., ventilator circuits, O_2 delivery equipment, and aerosol systems) be sterilized or receive high-level disinfection before being supplied to another patient. Disposable or single-patient use equipment must be used by one patient only. It is recommended that all equipment be completely disassembled and washed first in water, followed by a soak in warm soapy water for several minutes, with equipment scrubbed as needed to remove any remaining organic material. Following this step, the equipment must be thoroughly rinsed to remove any residual soap and drained of excess water. Air drying on a clean surface or rack is recommended to minimize recontamination.

The use of quaternary ammonium compounds ("quats") or acetic acid to disinfect home care equipment is acceptable given that the infection risk is significantly lower in most homes than in a hospital setting. Additionally, individual differences in patient risk and the broader bactericidal activity exhibited by some new disinfectants should be taken into account. Issues such as infection risk, cost, and safety must be considered by the provider and the patient before selecting the best disinfectant technique.

In regard to using water for humidification or nebulization, it is recommended that distilled water be used as a first choice. However, boiled water, cooled in a refrigerator and discarded after 24 hours, is also generally acceptable. It is recommended that manufacturers' guidelines for the proper handling of specific medications be strictly followed. Detailed instructions for patients and caregivers on how to clean and disinfect selected respiratory care equipment are generally available from most manufacturers. Policy and procedure manuals should describe equipment cleaning and infection control measures and require that home care patients and caregivers receive verbal and written instructions on this topic.[73,74]

PALLIATIVE CARE

This chapter would not be complete without some discussion of palliative respiratory care in alternative settings. Although the primary goal of home care involves minimizing a patient's dependence on institutional care, an additional goal is to maximize the comfort and well-being of a terminally ill patient near the end of life.

The definition of *palliative care* by the World Health Organization involves the control of pain and other symptoms such as dyspnea of terminally ill patients and maximizing the psychologic, social, and spiritual well-being of family members and patients nearing the end of life.[75] Many terminally ill patients have respiratory dysfunction directly or indirectly resulting from their terminal illness. Some of these patients choose to experience the remainder of their life at home. Hospice is a philosophy of care that helps support the efforts of such patients by providing clinician coverage and equipment to these patients at home.[75]

Respiratory modalities, such as O_2 therapy and mechanical ventilation or aerosol drug administration, can be combined with other therapies, such as pain management, to increase patients' comfort and permit them to die at home with their family and friends nearby. The RT can help such patients and families by providing training on the proper use and maintenance of such equipment. The presence of the RT can also be a supportive influence for patients and their families. Although such cases can place a psychologic strain on the RT, maximizing the comfort of terminally ill patients can be rewarding, and such experiences are unforgotten by all involved.

SUMMARY CHECKLIST

- More health services are being provided in alternative care settings (i.e., subacute, rehabilitation, and skilled nursing facilities and the home).
- Subacute care aims to restore the whole patient back to the highest level of function—ideally self-care.
- Standards for subacute and home health care derive from federal and state laws and private-sector accreditation, mainly TJC.
- Acute and alternative care settings differ in regard to resource availability, supervision and work schedules, documentation and assessment, and professional-patient interaction.
- Effective discharge planning (1) guides the multidisciplinary team in transferring patients from acute care facilities to alternative sites of care and (2) ensures the safety and efficacy of the patient's continuing care.

- Whether in an institution or the home, caregivers must have all the competencies required to meet the patient's ventilatory and respiratory needs and provide adequate 24-hour coverage. The selected site also must meet basic safety standards and be suitable for managing the patient's specific condition.
- O_2 prescriptions for patients in alternative settings must be based on documented hypoxemia, as determined by either blood gas analysis or oximetry.
- In most alternative care sites, O_2 normally is supplied using either liquid O_2 systems or concentrators. Gaseous cylinders serve as backup supplies for portable use.
- Most patients in alternative care settings needing O_2 use a nasal cannula; conserving devices such as transtracheal catheter, reservoir cannula, and demand-flow O_2 system can decrease O_2 use and costs and provide greater patient mobility.
- Because most problems with long-term O_2 therapy are "people" problems, caregivers should be allowed to operate and maintain O_2 delivery devices only after they have been instructed by credentialed RTs and have demonstrated the appropriate skill level.
- Key factors needed for successful ventilatory support in alternative sites include (1) careful patient selection, (2) effective discharge planning, (3) interdisciplinary team approach, (4) effective caregiver and family education, (5) thorough assessment and preparation of the environment, and (6) careful selection of needed equipment and supplies.
- Patients being considered for ventilatory support in alternative settings must be medically and psychologically stable.
- Most patients requiring mechanical ventilation in alternative settings can be supported with noninvasive positive pressure ventilation if they are alert and cooperative, can maintain acceptable oxygenation without high FiO_2, have intact airway reflexes and adequate clearance mechanisms, and can be fitted with an appropriate NIV interface.
- Positive pressure ventilators used in alternative settings should be electrically powered, dependable, easy to operate, and portable (run on both AC and DC power). Loss-of-power alarms are essential, high-pressure alarms are needed on volume-cycled ventilators, and patient-disconnect alarms must be provided for any patients who cannot breathe on their own.
- Negative pressure ventilators, such as the chest cuirass and "pneumosuit," are now a second-line choice for ventilatory support in alternative care settings.
- Bland aerosols may aid airway clearance in patients who produce large amounts of sputum; delivery is usually by an ultrasonic nebulizer or a jet nebulizer driven by an air compressor; supplemental O_2 is provided by either a concentrator or liquid supply system; infection control with these systems is a must.
- Patients with tracheostomies in alternative care settings require both daily stoma care and tracheobronchial suctioning; tube changes should be performed only by a qualified health professional.
- A typical nasal CPAP system consists of a flow-generator or blower, PEEP or CPAP valve, and nasal mask; some units can increase pressure to the prescribed level over time (ramping); others can autoadjust the CPAP level in response to apnea, hypopnea, airflow limitation, or snoring.
- The proper CPAP level can be determined by polysomnography, continuous monitoring of hemoglobin saturation, or by an auto-CPAP system.
- A common problem with nasal CPAP systems is an inability to reach or maintain the set pressure, usually because of either inadequate flow or system leaks.
- In institutions providing subacute or long-term care, the assessment and documentation process involves four key components: screening, treatment planning, ongoing assessment, and discharge.
- Proper caregiver hand hygiene, limiting visits by persons with respiratory infections, providing sterile or disposable clean equipment, and proper equipment processing are the keys to infection control in the alternative care setting.
- Providing palliative care to keep terminally ill patients as comfortable as possible is an important aspect of respiratory care in alternative sites.

References

1. National Association for Home Care & Hospice: Basic statistics about home care, Washington, DC, 2008, National Association for Home Care & Hospice.
2. Jencks SF, Williams MV, Coleman EA: Rehospitalizations among patients in the Medicare fee-for-service program. N Engl J Med 360:1418, 2009.
3. Lawlor M, et al: Early discharge care with ongoing follow-up support may reduce hospital readmissions in COPD. Int J Chron Obstruct Pulmon Dis 4:55, 2009.
4. Sharma G, et al: Outpatient follow-up visit and 30-day emergency department visit and readmission in patients hospitalized for chronic obstructive pulmonary disease. Arch Intern Med 170:1664, 2010.
5. U.S. Department of Health and Human Services, Centers for Medicare & Medicaid Services: Skilled nursing facility prospective payment system. Fact Sheet. Washington, DC, 2010, USDHHS.
6. Dinan MA, Simmons LA, Snyderman R: Personalized health planning and the Patient Protection and Affordability Act: an opportunity for academic medicine to lead health care reform. Acad Med 85:1665, 2010.
7. Teenier P: 2008 refinements to the medical home health prospective system. Home Healthc Nurse 26:181, 2008.
8. Bunch D: 1999 Muse study shows respiratory therapists' positive impact on SNF patient outcomes and Medicare cost savings, AARC Times 23:20-27, 1999.
9. Shelledy DC, et al: The effect of a pediatric asthma management program provided by respiratory therapists on patient outcomes and cost. Heart Lung 34:423, 2005.
10. National Association of Subacute/Post Acute Care: NASPAC frequently asked questions, Washington, DC, 2010, National Association of Subacute/Post Acute Care.
11. Murer CG: Post-acute care bundling plan. Rehab Manag 22:32, 2009.
12. American Association for Respiratory Care: Home respiratory care services. An official position statement by the AARC,

American Association for Respiratory Care—Revised, Irving TX, 2010, AARC.
13. Coultas D, et al: A randomized trial of two types of nurse-assisted home care for patients with COPD. Chest 128:2017, 2005.
14. Utens CM, et al: Effectiveness and cost-effectiveness of early assisted discharge for chronic obstructive pulmonary disease exacerbations: the design of a randomized controlled trial. BMC Public Health 10:618, 2010.
15. Joint Commission on Accreditation of Healthcare Organizations: 2011 Comprehensive accreditation manual for long term care, Oakbrook Terrace, IL, 2010, The Joint Commission.
16. Joint Commission on Accreditation of Healthcare Organizations: 2011 Standards for home medical equipment and clinical respiratory, Oakbrook Terrace, IL, 2010, The Joint Commission.
17. Tearl DK, Cox TJ, Hertzog JH: Hospital discharge of respiratory-technology-dependent children: role of a dedicated respiratory care discharge coordinator. Respir Care 51:744, 2006.
18. Abad-Corpa E, et al: Effectiveness of planning hospital discharge and follow-up in primary care for patients with chronic obstructive pulmonary disease: research protocol. J Adv Nurs 66:1365, 2010.
19. American Association for Respiratory Care: Clinical practice guideline: discharge planning for the respiratory care patient. Respir Care Clin N Am 40:1308, 1995.
20. Dunne PJ: The clinical impact of new long-term oxygen therapy technology. Respir Care 54:1100, 2009.
21. Schultz MZ: Outpatient management of severe COPD. N Engl J Med 363:494, 2010.
22. Pierson DJ: Clinical practice guidelines for chronic obstructive pulmonary disease: a review and comparison of current resources. Respir Care 51:277, 2006.
23. Lynnes D, Kelly C: Domiciliary oxygen therapy: assessment and management. Nurs Stand 23:50, 2009.
24. American Association for Respiratory Care: Clinical practice guideline: oxygen therapy in the home or alternate site health care facility. Respir Care 52:1063, 2007.
25. Mason RH, Suntharalingam J: Long-term oxygen therapy (LTOT)—is it always appropriately prescribed? Clin Med 6:634, 2009.
26. U.S. Department of Health and Human Services, Centers for Medicare & Medicaid Services: Certificate of medical necessity CMS 484 oxygen, Fed Reg 71:44082, 2007.
27. Stoller JK, et al: Oxygen therapy for patients with COPD: current evidence and the long-term oxygen treatment trial. Chest 138:179, 2010.
28. Dougherty DE, Petty TL: Recommendations of the 6th Long-Term Oxygen Therapy Consensus Conference. Respir Care 51:519, 2006.
29. Oba Y: Cost-effectiveness of long-term oxygen therapy for chronic obstructive disease. Am J Manag Care 15:97, 2009.
30. Lenfant F, et al: Oxygen delivery during transtracheal oxygenation: a comparison of two manual devices. Anesth Analg 111:922, 2010.
31. Palwai A, et al: Critical comparisons of the clinical performance of oxygen-conserving devices. Am J Respir Crit Care Med 181:1061, 2010.
32. Tiep B, Carter R: Oxygen conserving devices and methodologies. Chron Respir Dis 5:109, 2008.
33. Chatburn RL, Lewarski JS, McCoy RW: Nocturnal oxygenation using pulsed-dose oxygen-conserving device compared to continuous flow. Respir Care 51:252, 2006.
34. Aloe K, et al: Creation of an intermediate respiratory care unit to decrease intensive care utilization. J Nurs Admin 39:494, 2009.
35. Goldberg AI: Home mechanical ventilation. Am J Nurs 110:13, 2010.
36. Murphy P, Hart N: Who benefits from home mechanical ventilation? Clin Med 9:160, 2009.
37. Kun SS, et al: How much do primary care givers know about tracheostomy and home mechanical ventilation emergency care? Pediatr Pulmonol 45:270, 2010.
38. American Association for Respiratory Care: Delivery of respiratory therapy services in skilled nursing facilities providing ventilator and/or high acuity respiratory care. An official position statement by the AARC, American Association for Respiratory Care—Revised, Irving TX, 2010, AARC.
39. Munoz-Price LS: Long-term acute care hospitals. Clin Infect Dis 49:438, 2009.
40. Hamel DS, Klonin H: The role of noninvasive ventilation for acute respiratory failure. Respir Care Clin N Am 12:421, 2006.
41. Hess DR: Noninvasive ventilation in neuromuscular disease: equipment and application. Respir Care 51:896, 2006.
42. MacIntyre NR, et al: Management of patients requiring prolonged mechanical ventilation: report from NAMDRC consensus conference. Chest 128:3937, 2005.
43. American Association for Respiratory Care: Clinical practice guideline: long-term invasive mechanical ventilation in the home—2007 revision and update. Respir Care 52:1056, 2007.
44. Guentner K, et al: Preferences for mechanical ventilation among survivors of prolonged mechanical ventilation and tracheostomy. Am J Crit Care 15:65, 2006.
45. Evers G, Loey CV: Monitoring patient/ventilator interaction: manufacturer's perspective. Open Respir Med J 12:17, 2009.
46. Ballangrud R, Bogsti WB, Johansson IS: Clients' experiences of living at home with a mechanical ventilator. J Adv Nurs 65:425, 2009.
47. Chang AY, et al: Long-term community non-invasive ventilation. Intern Med J 11:123, 2010.
48. Partab D: Principles of non-invasive ventilation: a critical review of practice issues. Br J Nurs 23:1004, 2009.
49. Honrubia T, et al: Noninvasive vs conventional mechanical ventilation in acute respiratory failure: a multicenter, randomized controlled trial. Chest 128:3916, 2005.
50. Senent C, et al: Home mechanical ventilators: the point of view of the patients. J Eval Clin Pract 16:832, 2010.
51. Cairo JM, Pilbeam SP: Mosby's respiratory equipment, ed 8, St Louis, 2010, Mosby.
52. Dybwik K, et al: Why does the provision of home mechanical ventilation vary so widely? Chron Respir Dis 7:67, 2009.
53. LTV 1200/1150 ventilator user manual, Minneapolis, MN, 2009, Pulmonetic Systems, Inc.
54. Storre JH, et al: Average volume-assured pressure support in obesity hypoventilation: a randomized crossover trial. Chest 130:815, 2006.
55. Theerakittikul T, Ricaurte B, Aboussouan LS: Noninvasive positive pressure ventilation for stable outpatients: CPAP and beyond. Cleve Clin J Med 77:705, 2010.
56. Farre R, et al: Performance of mechanical ventilators at the patient's home: a multicentre quality control study. Thorax 61:400, 2006.
57. Gonzalez-Bermejo J, et al: Evaluation of the user-friendliness of 11 home mechanical ventilators. Eur Respir J 27:1236, 2006.
58. Schonhofer B: Non-invasive positive pressure ventilation in patients with stable hypercapnic COPD: light at the end of the tunnel? Thorax 65:765, 2010.

59. Ryan S, et al: Nasal pillows as an alternative interface in patients with obstructive sleep apnoea syndrome initiating continuous positive airway pressure therapy. J Sleep Res 28:114, 2010.
60. Grasso F, et al: Negative-pressure ventilation: better oxygenation and less lung injury. Am J Respir Crit Care Med 177:412, 2008.
61. Simmons FM, Ferro J, Thomas-Nelson S: Discharging the ventilator-dependent patient to home—part 1. Prof Case Manag 15:296, 2010.
62. American Association for Respiratory Care: Clinical practice guideline: bland aerosol administration. Respir Care 48:529, 2003.
63. Rea H, et al: The clinical utility of long-term humidification therapy in chronic airway disease. Respir Med 104:525, 2010.
64. Dolovich MB, et al: Device selection and outcomes of aerosol therapy: evidence-based guidelines. Chest 127:335, 2005.
65. American Association for Respiratory Care: Clinical practice guideline: suctioning of the patient at home. Respir Care 44:99, 1999.
66. McCool FD, Rosen MJ: Nonpharmacologic airway clearance therapies: ACCP evidence-based clinical practice guidelines. Chest 129(suppl):250S, 2006.
67. Kakkar RK, Berry RB: Positive airway pressure treatment for obstructive sleep apnea. Chest 132:1057, 2007.
68. Antonescu-Turcu A, Parthasarathy S: CPAP and bi-level PAP therapy: new and established roles. Respir Care 55:1216, 2010.
69. Drummond F, et al: Empiric auto-titrating CPAP in people with suspected obstructive sleep apnea. J Clin Sleep Med 15:140, 2010.
70. Worsnop CJ, Miseski S, Rochford PD: Routine use of humidification with nasal continuous positive airway pressure. Intern Med J 40:650, 2010.
71. Ruhle KH, et al: Quality of life, compliance, sleep and nasopharyngeal side effects during CPAP therapy with and without controlled heated humidification. Sleep Breath 26:92, 2010.
72. Silvestri JM: Indications for home apnea monitoring (or not). Clin Perinatol 36:87, 2009.
73. Busa T, et al: Hygiene of nasal masks used at home for non-invasive ventilation in children. J Hosp Infect 76:187, 2010.
74. McGoldrick M: Preventing infections in patients using respiratory therapy equipment in the home. Home Healthc Nurse 28:212, 2010.
75. Brown-Saltzman K, et al: An intervention to improve respiratory therapists' comfort with end-of-life care. Respir Care 55:858, 2010.

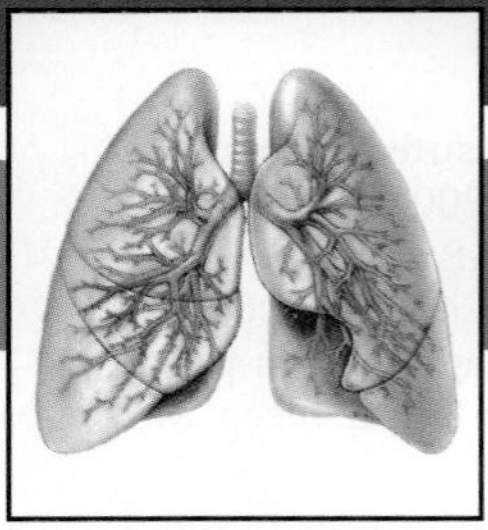

Glossary

A

AARC abbreviation for the *American Association for Respiratory Care,* the primary voluntary professional association for respiratory therapists. (Chapter 1)

abdominal compartment syndrome the abdomen has become a fixed compartment with increased pressure resulting in ischemia and organ dysfunction. (Chapter 15)

abdominal paradox abnormal breathing pattern seen as a sinking inward motion of the abdomen with each inspiratory effort; a sign of diaphragm fatigue. (Chapter 15)

abdominal thrust external pressure forcefully exerted on the abdomen, under the diaphragm, to expel obstructing objects from the upper airway. (Chapter 34)

absolute humidity actual mass or content of water in a measured volume of air, usually expressed in grams per cubic meter or pounds. (Chapter 6)

absorption atelectasis atelectasis resulting from the absorption of O_2 from obstructed or partially obstructed alveoli with high O_2 concentrations. (Chapter 39)

A/C alternative abbreviation for *assist/control ventilation;* see *assist/control.* (Chapter 42)

accessory muscles of breathing muscles of the neck, back, and abdomen that may assist the diaphragm and the internal and external intercostal muscles in respiration, especially in some breathing disorders or during exercise. (Chapter 8)

acid compound that yields hydrogen ions (H^+) when dissolved in an aqueous solution. (Chapter 12)

acidemia state in which arterial blood is more acidic than normal (pH < 7.35). (Chapter 13)

acid-fast of or pertaining to a bacterial stain that does not decolorize easily when washed with an acid solution; also refers to certain bacteria (especially mycobacteria) that retain red dyes after an acid wash.

acid-fast bacterium type of bacteria that resists decolorizing by acid after accepting a stain. (Chapter 16)

acinus any small, saclike structure, particularly one found in a gland. (Chapter 8)

acoustic respiratory monitoring (ARM) provides imaging of ventilation that allows localization of the injury and an assessment of the extent of injury. The technique produces a two-dimensional video or graphic representation of ventilation; quiet regions without ventilation are not "seen." With this technique there is an opportunity at the bedside to perform a real-time evaluation of the effects of positive end expiratory pressure, recruitment maneuvers, or other changes in ventilatory support. (Chapter 46)

active cycle of breathing (ACB) airway clearance strategy consisting of repeated cycles of breathing control and thoracic expansion, followed by the forced expiratory technique. (Chapter 40)

active transport movement of molecules across membranes in a direction opposite that expected because of diffusion or osmotic pressure. (Chapter 12)

acute chest syndrome a syndrome developed in patients with sickle cell disease. The chief complaints are acute chest pain, cough and shortness of breath caused by the sickling of red blood cells. (Chapter 11)

acute exacerbation of COPD state of worsening of chronic obstructive pulmonary disease (COPD), often defined by the need to increase medication or to escalate care. (Chapter 23)

acute lung injury (ALI) condition characterized by alveolar flooding caused by an acute insult (e.g., sepsis). Normally a rapidly developing bilateral pulmonary process of non-cardiac origin with a PaO_2 to FiO_2 ratio greater than 200 mm Hg but less than or equal to 300 mm Hg. (Chapter 27)

acute respiratory distress syndrome (ARDS) respiratory disorder characterized by respiratory insufficiency and hypoxemia; triggers include gram-negative sepsis, O_2 toxicity, trauma, pneumonia, and systemic inflammatory responses. (Chapter 27)

adaptive support ventilation (ASV) mode of ventilation guided by evaluation of the patient's lung mechanics; the ventilator tries to impose a ventilatory pattern that results in the least amount of patient work. (Chapter 47)

adenocarcinoma type of cancer characterized by glandular structures. (Chapter 28)

adhesion band of scar tissue that binds anatomic surfaces that normally are separate from each other. Adhesions most commonly form in the abdomen, after abdominal surgery, inflammation, or injury. (Chapter 6)

adrenergic of or pertaining to the sympathetic nerve fibers of the autonomic nervous system that use epinephrine or epinephrine-like substances as neurotransmitters; any chemical or drug that mimics the effect of these neurotransmitters. Also called a *sympathomimetic drug; catecholamine.* (Chapter 32)

advanced cardiac life support (ACLS) emergency medical procedures beyond basic life support; includes intravenous fluid line establishment, possible defibrillation, drug administration, control of cardiac arrhythmias, and use of ventilation equipment. ACLS usually requires direct or indirect supervision by a physician. (Chapter 34)

advanced directive document in which an individual specifies what medical care he or she desires to receive in the future, should he or she no longer be able to make decisions about medical treatment; may be in the form of a living will or durable power of attorney. (Chapters 5, 15)

adventitious lung sounds abnormal lung sounds superimposed on the basic underlying breath sounds. (Chapter 15)

aerobic exercise any physical activity that requires increased cardiac output and ventilation to meet the increased O_2 demands of the skeletal muscles. (Chapter 50)

aerophagia swallowing of air. (Chapter 43)

aerosol suspension of solid or liquid particles in a gas. (Chapter 36)

aerosol medications any medication that is delivered by aerosol via the respiratory tract. (Chapter 1)

aerosol output weight or mass of aerosol particles produced by a nebulizer per unit time or volume. (Chapter 36)

affective domain a learning domain addressing the area of emotion, mood, or feeling. (Chapter 49)

afterload load against which an activated muscle must try to shorten; greater afterloads result in lower velocities. (Chapters 9, 46)

agonist of or pertaining to a chemical substance or drug that has affinity for a receptor and exerts a desired or expected effect (as opposed to an antagonist). (Chapter 32)

air bronchograms lucent tubular shadows running through areas of consolidation. (Chapter 20)

airway hyperresponsiveness state of airways that causes them to constrict abnormally in response to stress or insults (e.g., exercise, inhaled materials such as dust or allergens). (Chapter 23)

airway inflammation localized protective response to pathogens occurring within the routes for passage of air into and out of the lungs and involving the release of mediators including mast cells, eosinophils, macrophages, epithelial cells, and T lymphocytes. (Chapter 23)

airway management the process of insuring that the upper airway is free of foreign substances and patent to gas flow. (Chapter 1)

airway obstruction state of abnormally slowed expiration, characterized most commonly by a decrease in FEV_1. (Chapter 23)

airway occlusion pressure (P0.1) inspiratory pressure generated 100 msec after airway occlusion; P0.1 is effort-independent and is thought to be a good measure of central respiratory drive. (Chapter 47)

airway pressure release ventilation (APRV) form of pressure ventilation that uses two levels of continuous positive airway pressure in an intermittent mandatory ventilation breathing pattern. (Chapter 27)

airway resistance measure of the impedance to ventilation caused by the movement of gas through the airways; abbreviated as Raw, airway resistance is computed as the change in pressure along a tube divided by the flow. (Chapter 10)

algorithm predetermined group of directions to solve a problem in a finite number of steps. (Chapter 2)

alkalemia a decreased hydrogen ion concentration in the blood; as applied to arterial blood, denotes pH greater than 7.45. (Chapter 13)

alveolar-arterial oxygen tension difference ($P(A - a)O_2$) difference between the alveolar and arterial PO_2, usually about 5 to 10 mm Hg when breathing room air. (Chapter 46)

alveolar-capillary membrane tissue that separates air from blood in the lung; consists of alveolar epithelium, basement membrane, and capillary endothelium, along with their associated structures. (Chapter 7)

alveolar dead space alveoli that are ventilated but are not perfused. The condition may exist when pulmonary circulation is obstructed, as by a thromboembolus. (Chapter 10)

alveolar shunt alveolar units that are closed to ventilation but are still perfused. (Chapter 11)

alveoli small outpouching of walls of alveolar space through which gas exchange between alveolar air and pulmonary capillary blood occurs. (Chapter 8)

ambulation process of helping a bedridden patient begin to sit up, stand, and walk around independently. (Chapter 3)

American Society for Testing and Materials (ASTM) nongovernment agency that establishes performance standards for various equipment and materials. (Chapters 33, 35)

American Standard Safety System (ASSS) specifications adopted in the United States and Canada for threaded high-pressure connections between compressed gas cylinders and their attachments. (Chapter 37)

amniocentesis process of direct sampling and quantitative assessment of the amniotic fluid. (Chapter 48)

ampere basic unit of electrical energy current; equivalent to the amount of electrons flowing when 1 V of electromotive force is applied to a circuit with 1 ohm of resistance. (Chapter 3)

amyotrophic lateral sclerosis (ALS) degenerative disease of the motor neurons often characterized by atrophy of the muscles of the hands, forearms, and legs and eventually involving most of the body, including the muscles of respiration. (Chapter 29)

anemia abnormal condition characterized by a reduction in the number of circulating red blood cells or the amount of normal hemoglobin available to carry O_2. (Chapter 16)

anergy lack of activity; an immunodeficient condition characterized by a lack of or diminished reaction to an antigen or group of antigens. This state may be seen in advanced tuberculosis and other serious infections, AIDS, and some malignancies. (Chapter 21)

angina spasmodic, cramplike choking feeling. (Chapter 15)

angle of Louis slightly oblique angle where the manubrium articulates with the body of the sternum. (Chapter 8)

anion a negative ion that migrates to the anode (positive electrode) in an electrolyte solution; a negative ion. (Chapter 12)

ankylosing spondylitis chronic inflammatory disease of unknown origin, first affecting the spine and adjacent structures and commonly leading to eventual fusion (ankylosis) of the involved joints. (Chapter 29)

antagonist in pharmacology, a drug that has affinity but produces no effect; an antagonist can be competitive (forms reversible bond with receptor) or noncompetitive (forms irreversible bond). (Chapter 32)

anterior nares opening to the nose. (Chapter 8)

anthropometry science of measuring the human body—height, weight, and size of component parts, including skin folds—to study and compare the relative proportions under normal and abnormal conditions. Also called *anthropometric measurement.* (Chapter 21)

antiadrenergic pertaining to blocking of the effects of impulses transmitted by the adrenergic postganglionic fibers of the sympathetic nervous system. (Chapter 32)

antibiotic therapy treatment of infections with an antimicrobial agents, such as the penicillins. (Chapter 22)

anticholinergic of or pertaining to blockade of acetylcholine receptors that results in the inhibition of transmission of parasympathetic nerve impulses. (Chapter 32)

antiseptic tending to inhibit growth and reproduction of microorganisms. (Chapter 4)

APACHE scoring system *Acute Physiology and Chronic Health Evaluation* scoring system; severity of illness scoring system used with critically ill patients. (Chapter 46)

Apgar score evaluation of an infant's physical condition, usually performed 1 minute and 5 minutes after birth, based on a rating of five factors that reflect the infant's ability to adjust to extrauterine life. (Chapter 48)

apices uppermost portions of the lungs. (Chapter 8)

apnea absence of spontaneous breathing. (Chapter 14)

apnea of prematurity disorder of preterm infants, probably of central nervous system origin, characterized by frequent apneic pauses lasting longer than 20 seconds and often associated with cyanosis, pallor, hypotonia, or bradycardia. (Chapter 31)

apneustic breathing pattern of respirations characterized by a prolonged inspiratory phase followed by expiratory apnea. (Chapters 14, 29)

apneustic center localized collection of neurons in the pons located at the level of the vestibular area that moderates the rhythmic activity of the medullary respiratory centers. (Chapter 14)

appropriate for gestational age (AGA) refers to a newborn whose size, growth, and maturation are normal for gestational age, whether delivered prematurely, at term, or later than term. (Chapter 48)

ARCF abbreviation for *American Respiratory Care Foundation,* a philanthropic agency that promotes the field of respiratory care through grants and awards. (Chapter 1)

arteriovenous anastomosis communication between an artery and a vein, either as a congenital anomaly or as a surgically produced link between vessels. (Chapter 9)

asbestosis restrictive lung disease caused by prolonged exposure to asbestos fibers; associated with a high incidence of malignant lung tumors and pleural abnormalities. (Chapter 24)

assault any conduct that creates a reasonable apprehension of being touched in an injurious manner; no actual touching is required to prove assault. (Chapter 5)

assist/control (A/C or ACV) continuous mandatory ventilation (CMV) in which the minimum breathing rate is predetermined, but the patient can initiate mechanical ventilation at an increased rate. (Chapter 44)

asthma respiratory disorder characterized by recurring episodes of paroxysmal dyspnea, wheezing on expiration or inspiration caused by constriction of the bronchi, coughing, and viscous mucoid bronchial secretions. The episodes may be precipitated by inhalation of allergens or pollutants, infection, cold air, vigorous exercise, or emotional stress. Also called *bronchial asthma.* (Chapter 23)

ataxic breathing type of breathing associated with a lesion in the medullary respiratory center and characterized by a series of increasing and decreasing inspirations and expirations. (Chapter 29)

atelectasis collapse of distal lung parenchyma. (Chapter 39)

atelectrauma lung injury as a result of alveolar collapse secondary to inappropriate mechanical ventilation settings. (Chapter 43)

atmospheric pressure absolute (ATA) measure of pressure used in hyperbaric medicine; 1 ATA equals 760 mm Hg or 101.32 kPa. (Chapter 38)

atomizer device that produces an aerosol suspension of liquid particles without using baffles to control particle size. (Chapter 36)

ATPS abbreviation for *ambient temperature, ambient pressure, saturated* (with water vapor). (Chapter 6)

atypical pathogens select organisms in *Legionella* species, *Chlamydophila pneumoniae,* and *Mycoplasma pneumoniae* that cause pneumonia. (Chapter 22)

auditory pertaining to the sense of hearing. (Chapter 3)

autogenic drainage (AD) modification of directed coughing, beginning with low lung volume breathing, inspiratory breath holds, and controlled exhalation and progressing to increased inspired volumes and expiratory flows. (Chapter 40)

automatic external defibrillator (AED) portable automatic device to perform defibrillation on patients outside a hospital. (Chapter 34)

automatic tube compensation (ATC) mode of ventilation that attempts to maintain tracheal pressure equal to end expiratory pressure during both inspiration during both inspiration and expiration. (Chapter 47)

automaticity refers to the heart's ability to generate its own intrinsic electrical rhythm. (Chapters 9, 16)

autonomy quality of having the ability or tendency to function independently. (Chapter 5)

auto-PEEP pressure above atmospheric remaining in the alveoli at end-exhalation due to air trapping. Also called *intrinsic PEEP.* (Chapter 41)

autoregulation automatic control of a mechanical or physiologic system; necessitates both a sensing mechanism (to measure what is regulated) and a feedback loop (to respond to changes). (Chapter 43)

Avogadro's law law in physics stating that equal volumes of all gases at a given temperature and pressure contain the identical number of molecules. (Chapter 5)

azotemia buildup of excess nitrogenous waste products in the blood, usually secondary to renal failure. (Chapter 21)

B

bactericidal substances with the ability to kill micro-organisms. (Chapter 4)

bacteriostatic ability to restrain the growth of micro-organisms. (Chapter 4)

baffle surface in a nebulizer designed specifically to cause impaction of large aerosol particles, causing either further fragmentation or removal from the suspension via condensation back into the reservoir. (Chapter 36)

baffling process of removing large water particles from suspension in a jet nebulizer so that the particles entering the patient's airways are of a uniform therapeutic size. (Chapter 35)

bands bundle of fibers, as seen in striated muscle, that encircles a structure or binds one part of the body to another. (Chapter 16)

baroreceptor one of the pressure-sensitive nerve endings in the walls of the atria of the heart, the vena cava, the aortic arch, and the carotid sinus. (Chapter 9)

barotrauma physical injury sustained as a result of exposure to ambient pressures above normal, most commonly secondary to positive pressure ventilation (e.g., pneumothorax, pneumomediastinum). (Chapters 27, 41, 43)

barrel chest abnormal increase in the anteroposterior diameter of the chest caused by hyperinflation of the lungs. (Chapter 15)

basal metabolic rate (BMR) amount of energy used in a unit of time by a fasting, resting subject. BMR, determined by the amount of O_2 used, is expressed in calories consumed per hour per square meter of body surface area or per kilogram of body weight. Also called *basal energy expenditure (BEE).* (Chapter 21)

base compound that yields hydroxyl ions [OH^-] when dissolved in an aqueous solution. (Chapter 12)

base excess (BE) difference between the normal buffer base (NBB) and the actual buffer base (BB) in a whole-blood sample, expressed in mEq/L; a normal BE is +2 mEq/L. (Chapter 13)

basic chemistry panel (BCP) or basic metabolic panel includes the predominant electrolytes sodium (Na^+), potassium (K^+), chloride (Cl^-), and total CO_2/bicarbonate (CO_2) and glucose. (Chapter 16)

basic life support (BLS) cardiopulmonary resuscitation designed to reinstitute either circulatory or respiratory function without equipment or drugs. (Chapter 34)

battery (legal) an unconsented touching of an individual that causes injury. (Chapter 5)

Becker muscular dystrophy chronic degenerative disease of the muscles, characterized by progressive weakness; occurs in children 8 to 20 years old. (Chapter 29)

benchmarking establishing the relationship between an organizations' ability to perform at a given level to that of other standard organizations. (Chapter 7)

beneficence principle that requires that health providers go beyond doing no harm and actively contribute to the health and well-being of their patients. (Chapter 5)

benevolent deception actions in which the truth is withheld from the patient for his or her own good. (Chapter 5)

bias the state of having your opinion markedly affected by past experience or knowledge; an oblique or a diagonal line. (Chapter 18)

bilevel positive airway pressure (bilevel PAP) spontaneous breath mode of ventilatory support, which allows separate regulation of the inspiratory and expiratory pressures. (Chapter 30)

biotrauma inflammation of the lungs in response to inappropriate mechanical ventilation that promotes alveolar overdistention in inspiration and derecruitment on exhalation. (Chapter 43)

Biot respiration breathing characterized by irregular periods of apnea alternating with periods in which four or five breaths of identical depth are taken. (Chapter 14)

bladder pressure pressure that is established in the bladder. (Chapter 46)

blood-brain barrier anatomic-physiologic feature of the brain thought to consist of walls of capillaries in the central nervous system and surrounding astrocytic glial membranes. The barrier separates the parenchyma of the central nervous system from blood. The blood-brain barrier prevents or slows the passage of some drugs and other chemical compounds, radioactive ions, and disease-causing organisms such as viruses from the blood into the central nervous system. (Chapter 14)

body humidity absolute humidity in a volume of gas saturated at a body temperature of 37° C; equivalent to 43.8 mg/L of water in the air. (Chapter 35)

body mass index (BMI) formula for determining obesity, calculated by dividing a person's weight in kilograms by the square of the person's height in meters. (Chapter 21)

Bohr effect effect of variations in blood pH on the affinity of hemoglobin for O_2. (Chapter 11)

BOMA abbreviation for the *Board of Medical Advisors,* the medical advisory group for the American Association for Respiratory Care. (Chapter 1)

Borg dyspnea scale validated scale used by patients to quantify the severity of dyspnea. (Chapter 50)

Bourdon gauge fixed orifice, variable pressure flowmeter (Chapter 37)

BPF abbreviation for *bronchopleural fistula*. (Chapter 25)

bradycardia abnormally decreased heart rate. (Chapter 15)

bradypnea abnormal decrease in breathing rate. (Chapter 15)

breach of contract failure, without legal excuse, to carry out the terms of a legal agreement. (Chapter 5)

breath-actuated nebulizer aerosol device that is responsive to the patient's inspiratory effort and reduces or eliminates aerosol generation during exhalation. (Chapter 36)

breath-enhanced nebulizer nebulizers that entrain room air in direct relationship to the inspiratory flow of the patient. (Chapter 36)

breathing pattern the ventilation pattern assumed by a patient during normal or mechanical ventilation. (Chapter 42)

breathlessness distressful sensation of uncomfortable breathing that may be caused by certain heart conditions, strenuous exercise, or anxiety. (Chapter 15)

bronchiectasis abnormal condition of the bronchial tree characterized by irreversible dilation and destruction of the bronchial walls. (Chapters 23, 40)

bronchiolitis acute infection of the lower respiratory tract causing expiratory wheezing, respiratory distress, inflammation, and obstruction of the bronchioles; bronchiolitis is usually caused by respiratory syncytial virus (RSV) and is most common in infants younger than 2 years old. (Chapter 31)

bronchodilator substance, especially a drug, that relaxes contractions of the smooth muscle of the bronchioles to improve ventilation to the lungs. Pharmacologic bronchodilators are prescribed to improve aeration in asthma, bronchiectasis, bronchitis, and emphysema. (Chapter 23)

bronchophony abnormal voice sounds heard over lung consolidation. (Chapter 15)

bronchopleural fistula any air communication from the lung to the pleural space. (Chapter 25)

bronchopneumonia acute inflammation of the lungs and bronchioles, characterized by chills, fever, high pulse and respirator rates, bronchial breathing, cough with purulent bloody sputum, and chest pain. (Chapter 38)

bronchopulmonary dysplasia (BPD) chronic respiratory disorder characterized by scarring of lung tissue, thickened pulmonary arterial walls, and mismatch between lung ventilation and perfusion. It often occurs in infants who have been dependent on long-term artificial pulmonary ventilation. (Chapters 31, 38)

bronchoscopy process of passing a bronchoscope into the airways for diagnostic testing or therapeutic purposes. (Chapter 33)

bronchospasm abnormal contraction of the smooth muscle of the bronchi, resulting in acute narrowing and obstruction. (Chapter 23)

BTPS abbreviation for *body temperature, ambient pressure, saturated* (with water vapor). (Chapter 6)

buffer base total blood buffer capable of binding hydrogen ions; normal buffer base (NBB) ranges from 48 to 52 mEq/L. (Chapter 13)

buffering the process of removing H^+ or OH^- in solution in order to minimize change in pH. (Chapter 12)

C

cachexia general ill health and malnutrition characterized by weakness and emaciation. (Chapter 15)

cachexic the state of being of general ill health and suffering from malnutrition. (Chapter 21)

calibration media types of equipment used to test and ensure that the output of an analyzer (blood gas) is both accurate and linear across the range of measured values. (Chapter 18)

capnography process of obtaining a tracing of the proportion of CO_2 in expired air using a capnograph. (Chapter 46)

capnometry measurement of CO_2 in a volume of gas, usually by methods of infrared absorption or mass spectrometry. (Chapter 46)

capped-rental items eligible for reimbursement under the Medicare prospective payment system for only a predetermined number of months, after which the equipment is deemed owned by the patient and rental payments cease. (Chapter 51)

carboxyhemoglobin compound produced by the chemical combination of hemoglobin with carbon monoxide. (Chapter 11)

cardiac output volume of blood pumped per minute by the heart. (Chapters 9, 46)

cardiac tamponade compression of the heart caused by the collection of blood, fluid, or gas under pressure in the pericardium. (Chapter 9)

cardiopulmonary exercise evaluation exercise-based assessment of a patient before pulmonary rehabilitation designed to determine the patient's exercise capacity and risk for desaturation. (Chapter 50)

cardiopulmonary resuscitation (CPR) basic emergency procedure for life support, consisting of artificial respiration and manual external cardiac massage. (Chapter 34)

cardiopulmonary system the combination of the respiratory and cardiac systems. (Chapter 1)

carina bifurcation of the trachea into the right and left main stem bronchi. (Chapter 8)

catecholamine any one of a group of sympathomimetic compounds composed of a catechol molecule and the aliphatic portion of an amine. (Chapter 32)

cation positively charged ion. (Chapter 12)

Centers for Medicare and Medicaid Services (CMS) previously known as the Health Care Financing Administration (HCFA), a federal agency within the U.S. Department of Health and Human Services that administers the Medicare program and works in partnership with state governments to administer Medicaid, the State Children's Health Insurance Program (SCHIP), and health insurance portability standards. (Chapter 51)

central neurogenic hyperinflation hyperinflation caused by a neurologic progress generally resulting in a markedly increased minute ventilation. (Chapter 29)

central sleep apnea absence of breathing as the result of medullary depression that inhibits respiratory movement, which becomes more pronounced during sleep. (Chapter 30)

cephalization refers to increased visualization of pulmonary blood vessels on a chest x-ray in the nondependent regions of the lung; often a sign of left heart failure. (Chapter 20)

channel passageway or groove that conveys fluid, such as the central channels that connect the arterioles with the venules. (Chapter 3)

chemoreceptor sensory nerve cell activated by changes in the chemical environment surrounding it; the chemoreceptors in the carotid artery are sensitive to PCO_2 in the blood, signaling the respiratory center in the brain to increase or decrease ventilation. (Chapters 9, 14)

chemotherapy treatment of infections and other diseases with chemical agents. (Chapter 28)

chest cuirass device to deliver negative pressure ventilation that fits over the thorax. (Chapter 45)

chest physical therapy (CPT) collection of therapeutic techniques designed to aid clearance of secretions, improve ventilation, and enhance the conditioning of the respiratory muscles; includes positioning techniques, chest percussion and vibration, directed coughing, and various breathing and conditioning exercises. (Chapter 40)

chest radiograph x-ray image of the chest; a posteroanterior view and a lateral, or side, view are routinely obtained. (Chapter 20)

Cheyne-Stokes respiration Abnormal breathing pattern with periods of progressively deeper breaths alternating with periods of shallow breathing and apnea. (Chapters 14, 29)

CHF abbreviation for *congestive heart failure;* an abnormal condition that reflects impaired cardiac output, caused by myocardial infarction, ischemic heart disease, or cardiomyopathy.

chlorofluorocarbons (CFCs) gaseous chemical compounds that were originally used to power metered dose inmhalers but currently phased out of use. (Chapter 36)

cholinergic of or pertaining to nerve fibers that elaborate acetylcholine at the myoneural junctions. (Chapter 32)

chronic bronchitis common debilitating pulmonary disease, characterized by greatly increased production of mucus by the glands of the trachea and bronchi that results in a cough with expectoration for at least 3 months of the year for more than 2 consecutive years. (Chapter 23)

chyle cloudy liquid products of digestion taken up by the small intestine. Consisting mainly of emulsified fats, chyle passes through finger-like projections in the small intestine, called *lacteals,* and into the lymphatic system for transport to the venous circulation at the thoracic duct in the neck. (Chapter 25)

chylothorax pleural fluid collection that is high in triglycerides, usually from disruption of the thoracic duct. (Chapter 25)

cilia tiny hair like projections that line mucus producing structures. Generally they operate in a wave-like motion moving mucous along the structure. (Chapter 8)

ciliary dyskinetic syndromes conditions in which respiratory tract cilia do not function properly. (Chapter 40)

clinical decision support system that matches the characteristics of individual patients and clinical interventions, drugs, and diagnostic tests to databases of scientific evidence and drug calculations to generate tailored recommendations, reminders, or standing orders. (Chapter 7)

clinical queries search filter in PubMed effective in retrieving valid research studies. (Chapter 7)

clinical simulation the simulation of an actual clinical scenario using actors, manikins and paper and pencil. (Chapter 7)

closed buffer system buffer system in which all components of acid-base reactions remain in the system. Products accumulate and reach equilibrium with reactants, and chemical activity ceases (no further buffering activity can take place). Closed buffer systems in the body include nonbicarbonate buffers, such as plasma proteins, hemoglobin, and phosphates. (Chapter 13)

closed-loop control control circuit that receives feedback from a measured variable that automatically adjusts a gas delivery variable based on the feedback. (Chapter 42)

clubbing bulbous swelling of the terminal phalanges of the fingers and toes, often associated with certain chronic lung diseases. (Chapter 15)

Coanda effect phenomenon in hydrodynamics whereby a fluid in motion may be attracted or held to a wall. (Chapter 6)

CoARC acronym for *Committee on Accreditation for Respiratory Care;* establishes standards and oversees approval of educational programs in respiratory care. (Chapters 1, 2)

cognitive domain area of the mental processes of comprehension, judgment, memory, and reasoning. (Chapter 49)

cohesion attractive force between like molecules. (Chapter 6)

cohorting grouping individuals who share a common characteristic, such as the same age or the same sex or a common infection. (Chapter 4)

colloid substance that contains large molecules that attract and hold water; also a dispersion or a gel. (Chapter 12)

community-acquired pneumonia acute inflammation of the lungs contracted from the environment (as distinguished from nosocomial, or hospital-acquired, pneumonia). (Chapter 22)

compensatory justice calls for the recovery of damages that were a result of the action of others. (Chapter 5)

complete blood count a determination of the number of red and white blood cells per cubic millimeter of blood. A complete blood count is one of the most routinely performed tests in a clinical laboratory and one of the most valuable screening and diagnostic techniques. (Chapter 16)

compliance volume change per unit in applied pressure. (Chapters 10, 19, 27, 42)

Comprehensive Outpatient Rehabilitation Facility (CORF) Medicare-approved facility that provides a broad scope of ambulatory rehabilitation services as defined in section 933 of Public Law 96-499. (Chapter 50)

compressed volume volume of gas compressed in the ventilator circuit and not delivered to the patient during a positive pressure breath. (Chapter 42)

compression atelectasis collapse of a part of the lung as a result of an external force compressing the lung. (Chapter 39)

computed tomography (CT) radiographic technique that produces a film that represents a detailed cross section of tissue structure. (Chapters 20, 28)

condensation change of state from gas to liquid, as with water vapor condensation. (Chapter 6)

conditions of participation a certificate awarded institutions that meet specific standards of quality and safety as determined by the Centers for Medicare and Medicaid Services. (Chapter 51)

conduction transfer of heat by the direct interaction of atoms or molecules in a hot area that contact atoms or molecules in a cooler area. (Chapter 6)

confidentiality nondisclosure of certain information except to another authorized person. (Chapter 5)

congestive heart failure (CHF) abnormal condition that reflects impaired cardiac pumping; caused by myocardial infarction, ischemic heart disease, or cardiomyopathy that results in either pulmonary or systemic edema. (Chapters 9, 27)

conjugate base the base associated with the weak acid in a buffer system. (Chapter 13)

conjunctivitis inflammation of the conjunctiva, caused by bacterial or viral infection, allergy, or environmental factors. (Chapter 45)

connective tissue disease group of acquired disorders that have in common diffuse immunologic and inflammatory changes in small blood vessels and connective tissue. The cause of most of these diseases is unknown. Also called *collagen vascular disease.* (Chapter 24)

consequentialism idea of judging an act to be right; an ethical viewpoint in which decisions are based on the assessment of consequences. (Chapter 5)

contact precautions safeguards designed to reduce the risk of transmission of epidemiologically important microorganisms by direct or indirect contact. (Chapter 4)

continuous mandatory ventilation (CMV) system of mechanical ventilation in which the patient is allowed to initiate breathing, but the ventilator delivers a set volume or pressure with each breath. The ventilator can also be programmed to initiate breathing if the patient's breathing slows beyond a certain point or stops altogether. (Chapter 42)

continuous positive airway pressure (CPAP) method of ventilatory support whereby the patient breathes spontaneously without mechanical assistance against threshold resistance, with pressure above atmospheric maintained at the airway throughout breathing. (Chapters 30, 39, 45, 47, 48)

continuous spontaneous ventilation (CSV) method of delivering ventilatory support where the patient determines when a breath is initiated and when it is terminated. (Chapter 42)

contractility property of muscle tissue to shorten in response to a stimulus, usually electrical. (Chapters 9, 46)

control variable primary variable that the ventilator controls to provide inspiration: pressure, volume time, or flow. (Chapter 42)

control ventilation use of an intermittent positive pressure breathing unit or other respirator that has an automatic cycling device that replaces spontaneous respiration. (Chapter 44)

convection heat transfer through the mixing of fluid molecules at different temperature states via thermal currents. (Chapter 6)

corticosteroid any one of the natural or synthetic hormones associated with the adrenal cortex, which influences or controls key processes of the body, such as carbohydrate and protein metabolism, electrolyte and water balance, and function of the cardiovascular system and kidneys. (Chapter 24)

costal cartilages fibrous tissues that connect the ribs to the sternum and to each other anteriorly. (Chapter 8)

costophrenic angle acute angle where the costal pleura meets the diaphragm. (Chapter 8)

cough forceful expiratory effort designed to expel mucus and other foreign material from the upper airway. (Chapter 15)

crackles discontinuous type of adventitious lung sound. (Chapter 15)

cricoid cartilage ring of cartilage that forms the lower border of the larynx. (Chapter 8)

critical illness myopathy a heterogeneous constellation of symptoms commonly occurring in the ICU in which patients develop flaccid weakness of proximal muscles. Risk factors include corticosteroids, use of paralytic agents, hyperglycemia, hyperthyroidism, and possibly a systemic inflammatory response without sepsis. (Chapter 29)

critical illness polyneuropathy the development of muscle weakness and atrophy, loss of deep tendon reflexes and loss of peripheral sensation to pinprick and touch in patients with severe sepsis. (Chapter 29)

critical pressure pressure exerted by a vapor in an evacuated container at its critical temperature. (Chapter 6)

critical temperature highest temperature at which a substance can exist as a liquid, regardless of pressure. (Chapter 6)

critical test value a test result that reqires immediate communication of the result with a physician. (Chapter 16)

cross-training process of providing health care professionals with multiple skills in areas that span disciplines; for example, training a respiratory care practitioner to take chest radiographs. (Chapter 2)

croup infectious disorder of the upper airway occurring chiefly in infants and children that normally results in subglottic swelling and obstruction. (Chapters 31, 38)

CRT abbreviation for *certified respiratory therapist;* a respiratory therapist who has successfully completed the technician (entry-level) certification examination of the NBRC. (Chapter 1)

cryogenic related to very low temperature. (Chapter 37)

current a flowing or streaming movement; a flow of electrons along a conductor in a closed circuit; an electric current. (Chapter 3)

cuvette small transparent tube or container with specific optical properties. The chemical composition of the container determines the vessel's use, such as Pyrex glass for examining materials in the visible spectrum or silica for examining materials in the ultraviolet range. (Chapter 18)

cyanosis abnormal bluish discoloration of the skin or mucous membranes. (Chapter 15)

cycle variable variable that terminates inspiration during mechanical ventilation. (Chapter 42)

cyclic guanosine 3,5-monophosphate (cGMP) substance that mediates the action of certain hormones in a manner similar to cyclic adenosine monophosphate. (Chapter 38)

cystic fibrosis autosomal recessive disease characterized by pancreatic insufficiency, abnormally thick secretions from the exocrine glands, and increased concentration of sodium and chloride in the sweat glands; known in Europe as *mucoviscidosis.* (Chapters 23, 31)

D

Dalton's law in physics, law stating that the total pressure exerted by a mixture of gases is equal to the sum of the pressures exerted by the individual gases if they were present alone in the container. (Chapter 6)

DataArc secure, password-protected, Web-based database management system for documenting and reporting clinical educational activities for nursing and allied health professions, including respiratory care. (Chapter 7)

dead space respired gas volume that does not participate in gas exchange; may be anatomic, alveolar, or mechanical. (Chapter 11)

dead space/tidal volume ratio (V_D/V_T) percentage of tidal volume that does not participate in gas exchange, usually about 30% to 35%. (Chapter 46)

decannulation removal of a cannula or tube that may have been inserted during a therapeutic or surgical procedure. (Chapter 33)

deep breathing/directed cough movements used to improve pulmonary gas exchange or to maintain respiratory function, especially after prolonged inactivity or general anesthesia. (Chapter 39)

deep venous thrombosis (DVT) blood clot forming in the deep veins, usually of the legs. (Chapter 26)

defendant person denying the party against whom relief or recovery is sought in an action or suit; also, the accused in a criminal case. (Chapter 5)

defibrillation termination of ventricular fibrillation by delivering a direct electrical countershock to the patient's precordium. (Chapter 34)

depolarization reduction of a membrane potential to a less negative value; in cardiac fibers, this results in the release of calcium ions into the myofibrils and activates the contractile process. (Chapter 17)

deposition testimony of a witness taken on interrogatories, either oral or in writing. (Chapter 36)

dew point temperature at which water vapor condenses back to its liquid form. (Chapter 6)

diameter-indexed safety system (DISS) specifications established to prevent accidental interchange of low-pressure (<200 psig) medical gas connectors. DISS is used in respiratory care to connect equipment to a low-pressure gas source. (Chapter 37)

diaphoresis secretion of sweat, especially profuse secretion associated with an elevated body temperature, physical exertion, exposure to heat, and mental or emotional stress. (Chapter 15)

diaphragm large dome-shaped muscle that separates the thorax from the abdomen; the primary muscle of ventilation. (Chapter 8)

diastolic blood pressure baseline blood pressure in the arteries during ventricular relaxation. (Chapter 15)

diffusing capacity of the lung (DL) number of milliliters of gas that transfer from the lungs to the pulmonary blood per minute for each 1 mm Hg partial pressure difference between the alveoli and pulmonary capillary blood. (Chapter 19)

diffusing capacity of the lung to alveolar volume ratio ($DLCO/V_A$) index of the diffusing capacity for each 1 L of lung volume and an index of the functional alveolar surface area available for diffusion. (Chapter 19)

diluent substance, generally a fluid, that makes a solution or mixture less concentrated, less viscous, or more liquid. (Chapter 12)

dilute solution a solution that contains a small amount of solute in relation to solvent. (Chapter 12)

dilution equation an equation used to determine the final concentration of a solution where the original volume multiplied by the original concentration are equal to the final volume multiplied by the final concentration. (Chapter 12)

disease management an integrated process for the care of patients with a particular chronic disease. Generally, a multidisciplinary group of practitioners providing care, most of which are non-physicians. (Chapter 49)

disinfection process of destroying at least the vegetative phase of pathogenic microorganisms by physical or chemical means. (Chapter 4)

distributive justice refers to proper allotment of the benefits and burdens in a society, such as taxes and subsidies. (Chapter 5)

dorsal respiratory groups (DRGs) groupings of cells in the medulla oblongata that are active in controlling inspiration. (Chapter 14)

double effect the understanding that many good actions have both a good and bad effect. (Chapter 5)

downstream relative reference to a point more distal from the source in a stream of flowing fluid. (Chapter 37)

driving pressure the pressure that is driving a fluid from one point to another. (Chapter 46)

droplet nuclei residue of evaporated water droplets; owing to their small size (0.5 to 12 mm), droplet nuclei can remain suspended in the air for long periods. (Chapter 4)

droplet precautions safeguards designed to reduce the risk of droplet transmission of infectious agents. (Chapter 4)

drug signaling mechanism by which a drug exerts its effect on receptors. (Chapter 32)

dual-control mode of ventilation in which the control variable (pressure, volume, flow) switches during a breath. (Chapter 42)

Duchenne muscular dystrophy (DMD) abnormal congenital condition characterized by progressive symmetric wasting of the leg and pelvic muscles; predominantly affects males and accounts for 50% of all muscular dystrophy diseases. (Chapter 29)

ductus arteriosus vascular channel in the fetus that joins the pulmonary artery directly to the descending aorta; it normally closes after birth. (Chapters 8, 31)

ductus venosus vascular channel in the fetus passing through the liver and joining the umbilical vein with the inferior vena cava; before birth, it carries highly oxygenated blood from the placenta to the fetal circulation. (Chapter 8)

durable medical equipment (DME) supplier a company that provides medical equipment to patients in the home. (Chapter 51)

dynamic compression collapse of airways caused by a pressure gradient that occurs with breathing or forced breathing and normally occurs in diseased airways. (Chapter 10)

dynamic hyperinflation increase in functional residual capacity (FRC) above the elastic equilibrium volume of the respiratory system; causes include increased flow resistance, short inspiratory time, and increased postinspiratory muscle activity; see also *auto-PEEP*. (Chapters 10, 41)

dysoxia abnormal metabolic state in which the tissues are unable to use properly the O_2 made available to them. (Chapter 11)

dyspnea difficult or labored breathing as perceived by the patient. (Chapter 15)

E

ectopic beat impulse that originates in the heart at a site other than the sinus node. (Chapter 17)

ectopic focus origination of a heartbeat from some place in the heart other than the sinoatrial node. (Chapter 17)

edema excess fluid in the interstitial spaces between cells; in the lungs, edema fluid may also be present in the airways and alveolar spaces.

effective total lung capacity (V_A) single-breath technique distributes a gas mixture through unobstructed airways to an alveolar volume. (Chapter 19)

eHealth emerging computer applications in clinical care, diagnostics, management, education, and research. (Chapter 7)

elastance tendency of matter to resist a stretching force and recoil or return to its original size or form after deformation or expansion; the reciprocal of compliance. Also called *elasticity*. (Chapters 10, 42)

elasticity ability of tissue to regain its original shape and size after being stretched, squeezed, or otherwise deformed. Muscle tissue is generally regarded as elastic because it is able to change size and shape and return to its original condition. (Chapter 10)

electrical impedance tomography (EIT) the process where mapping of the lung is obtained by a series of electrodes placed around the chest that sequentially emit low level current. The variability among the impedance to the current between electrodes is used to map lung volume. (Chapter 46)

electronic health records information systems that make patients' medical records available across the continuum of care in all geographic locations. (Chapter 7)

emitted dose describes the mass of drug leaving the mouthpiece of a nebulizer or inhaler as aerosol. (Chapter 36)

emphysema destructive process of the lung parenchyma leading to permanent enlargement of the distal air spaces; classified as either centrilobular (CLE), which mainly involves the respiratory bronchioles, or panlobular (PLE), which can involve the entire terminal respiratory unit. (Chapter 23)

empyema pus within the pleural space. A pleural fluid Gram stain that shows bacteria. (Chapters 20, 25)

end-diastolic volume (EDV) volume of blood remaining in the ventricles just prior to contraction. (Chapter 9)

end-systolic volume (ESV) volume of blood in the ventricles at the end of contraction, or systole. (Chapter 9)

endotracheal tubes artificial airways that pass through the oropharynx or nasopharynx into the trachea. (Chapter 33)

epiglottis flat cartilage that extends from the base of the tongue backward and upward. (Chapter 8)

epiglottitis acute, often life-threatening infection of the upper airway, which causes severe obstruction secondary to supraglottic swelling; caused primarily by *Haemophilus influenzae* type B and affecting mainly children younger than 5 years old. (Chapter 31)

equal pressure point (EPP) during forced exhalation, the point along an airway where the pressure inside its wall equals the intrapleural pressure; upstream beyond this point, the pleural pressure exceeds the pressure inside the airway, tending to promote bronchiolar collapse. (Chapter 10)

equilibrium constant a constant determined by the amount of a buffer that dissociates in solution. Identifies the pH where the buffer is most effective. (Chapter 13)

equivalent weight weight of an element in any given unit (e.g., grams) that displaces a unit weight of hydrogen from a compound or combines with or replaces a unit weight of hydrogen. (Chapter 12)

erythrocyte red blood cell. (Chapter 16)

esophageal balloon catheter a catheter with an elongated balloon placed in the esophagus used to measure pressure change. (Chapter 46)

eustachian tubes bilateral tubes that connect the nasopharynx to the middle ear and mastoid sinus. (Chapter 8)

evaporation change in state of a substance from liquid to gaseous form occurring below its boiling point. (Chapter 6)

expiratory positive airway pressure (EPAP) application of positive pressure to the airway during exhalation. Compare with *inspiratory positive airway pressure*. (Chapter 45)

expiratory reserve volume (ERV) total amount of gas that can be exhaled from the lung after a quiet exhalation. (Chapter 19)

external nares the external opening of the nasal passages. (Chapter 8)

external oblique abdominal muscle group that functions as an accessory muscle of ventilation. (Chapter 8)

external respiration part of the respiratory process that involves the exchange of gases in the alveoli of the lungs. (Chapter 8)

extracorporeal carbon dioxide removal ($ECCO_2R$) procedure whereby blood is passed from the patient through an external membrane, which filters CO_2 to support ventilation. (Chapter 27)

extracorporeal membrane oxygenation (ECMO) procedure whereby venous blood is pumped outside the body to a heart-lung machine for oxygenation and returned to the body. (Chapters 27, 46)

extremely low birth weight (ELBW) a neonate weighting less than 1.0 kilogram at birth. (Chapter 48)

extubation process of withdrawing a tube from an orifice or cavity of the body. (Chapter 32)

exudative relating to the oozing of fluid and other materials from cells and tissues, usually as a result of inflammation or injury. (Chapter 38)

exudative pleural effusion any pleural effusion high in protein or lactate dehydrogenase, which implies inflammation or vascular injury on the pleural surface. (Chapter 25)

ex vivo pertaining to outside of the body. (Chapter 18)

F

factitious events values that are real and "out-of-range" but often are temporary, such as the elevation in airway pressure during a cough. (Chapter 46)

false ribs of the 12 pairs of ribs forming a large part of the thoracic skeleton, the first 7 are called true ribs, and the next 5 are called false ribs; the first 3 attach to the ribs above, and the last 2 are free. (Chapter 8)

febrile to have a fever. (Chapter 15)

feedback in communication theory, information produced by a receiver and perceived by a sender that informs the sender of the receiver's reaction to the message. Feedback is a cyclic part of the process of communication that regulates and modifies the content of messages. (Chapter 3)

fenestrated an opening into a structure; from the Latin *fenestra*, meaning "window." (Chapter 33)

fetal hemoglobin (HbF) hemoglobin variant that has a greater affinity for O_2 than adult hemoglobin; HbF is gradually replaced over the first year of life by HbA. (Chapter 11)

fetid foul-smelling. (Chapter 15)

fever abnormal elevation of body temperature owing to disease. (Chapter 15)

Fick formula formula for computing cardiac output based on knowledge of O_2 consumption and the arterial-venous O_2 content difference. (Chapters 11, 46)

Fick's law of diffusion law for determining the rate of gaseous diffusion across biologic membranes. (Chapter 11)

filling density ratio between the weight of liquid gas put into a cylinder and the weight of water the cylinder could contain if full. (Chapter 37)

fine-particle fraction particles that are small enough to reach the lower respiratory tract. (Chapter 36)

fissures narrow clefts or slits; the lines that divide or separate the lobes of the lung glottis. (Chapter 8)

fixed acid titratable, nonvolatile acid representing the by-product of protein catabolism; examples include phosphoric acid and sulfuric acid. (Chapter 13)

flail chest traumatic chest injury in which a portion of the rib cage becomes unstable because of multiple rib fractures or costochondral separation; typically, the flail region exhibits paradoxical movement during inspiration, contributing to a maldistribution of ventilation. (Chapter 29)

flange rim used to strengthen an object, to help guide it, and to facilitate its attachment to another object. (Chapter 33)

flexible bronchoscopy a bronchoscopy that is flexible in structure allowing it to be placed deep into the respiratory tract. (Chapter 28)

floating ribs last two rib pairs that are free at their ventral extremities. (Chapter 8)

flow resistance difference in pressure between the two points along a tube, divided by the actual flow. (Chapter 6)

flowmeter device operated by a needle valve that controls and measures gas flow according to the principles of viscosity and density. (Chapter 37)

fluid entrainment use of the Bernoulli effect to draw a second fluid into a stream of flow. (Chapter 6)

fomite nonliving material, such as bed linens or equipment, which may transmit pathogenic organisms to a person who comes into contact with the object. (Chapters 4, 22)

foramen ovale opening in the septum between the right and the left atria in the fetal heart. This opening provides a bypass for blood that would otherwise flow to the fetal lungs. After birth, the foramen ovale functionally closes. (Chapter 8)

forced expiration technique (FET) modification of the normal cough sequence designed to facilitate clearance of bronchial secretions, while minimizing the likelihood of bronchiolar collapse. (Chapter 40)

forced expiratory flow between 200 ml and 1200 ml ($FEF_{200\text{-}1200}$) measure of average expiratory flow during the early phase of exhalation; specifically, it is a measure of the flow rate for the 1000 ml of expired gas immediately following the first 200 ml of expired gas. Formerly called *maximum expiratory flow rate (MEFR)*. (Chapter 19)

forced expiratory flow between 25% and 75% of forced vital capacity ($FEF_{25\%\text{-}75\%}$) measure of average expiratory flow during the middle half of forced vital capacity. (Chapter 19)

forced expiratory flow between 75% and 85% of forced vital capacity ($FEF_{75\%\text{-}85\%}$) measure of average expiratory flow during the end of forced vital capacity. (Chapter 19)

forced expiratory volume in half of a second ($FEV_{0.5}$) maximum volume of gas that the patient can exhale during the first one half second of a forced vital capacity maneuver. (Chapter 19)

forced expiratory volume in 1 second (FEV_1) maximum volume of gas that the patient can exhale during the first second of the forced vital capacity maneuver. (Chapter 19)

forced expiratory volume in 1 second-to-vital capacity ratio (%FEV_1/FVC) percent of the measured forced vital capacity that can be exhaled in 1 second. (Chapter 19)

forced vital capacity (FVC) maximum volume of gas that the subject can exhale as forcefully and as quickly as possible. (Chapter 19)

formalism ethical viewpoint that relies on rules and principles. (Chapter 5)

fractional distillation process of separating the components of a liquid mixture according to their boiling points via the application of heat; the primary commercial process used to produce O_2. (Chapter 37)

Frank-Starling principle the more a muscle fiber is stretched, the greater is the tension the muscle fiber generates when contracted. (Chapter 9)

frequency/tidal volume ratio (f/V_T) ratio of the tidal volume in ml divided by the respiratory rate. (Chapter 46)

full ventilatory support ventilatory support modes in which the ventilator provides all the minute ventilation requirements of the patient. (Chapter 44)

functional residual capacity (FRC) total amount of gas left in the lungs after a resting expiration. (Chapter 19)

G

gallop rhythm abnormal heart sound that resembles the gallop of a horse, most often indicates heart failure. (Chapter 15)

gantry examination table used for computed tomography (CT) scans. (Chapter 20)

gasping the process of breathing periodically with a labored forced inspiration. (Chapter 29)

gastric inflation introduction of air into the stomach and intestines. (Chapter 34)

gastroesophageal reflux disease (GERD) condition characterized by abnormal movement of stomach contents into the esophagus or mouth; acid from the stomach may be aspirated into the lung and cause asthma-like symptoms. (Chapter 31)

geometric standard deviation (GSD) describes the variability of particle describes the variability in particle size in an aerosol distribution set at one standard deviation above and below the median. (Chapter 36)

gladiolus the body of the sternum. (Chapter 8)

Glasgow Coma Scale scale used to provide a score to classify the level of conscious awareness in patients suspected to have an acute brain injury. (Chapter 46)

glottis variable opening between the vocal cords. (Chapter 8)

Graham's law law stating that the rate of diffusion of a gas through a liquid (or the alveolar-capillary membrane) is directly proportional to its solubility coefficient and inversely proportional to the square root of its density. (Chapter 6)

ground connection between the electrical circuit and the ground, which becomes a part of the circuit. (Chapter 3)

grunting, flaring, and retracting (GFR) the respiratory pattern observed in infants in marked respiratory distress. The neonate makes a grunting sound during breathing with flaring of the nostrils. (Chapter 48)

Guillain-Barré syndrome idiopathic, peripheral polyneuritis characterized by lower extremity weakness that progresses to the upper extremities and face; may lead to flaccid paraplegia and marked respiratory muscle weakness. (Chapter 29)

H

Haldane effect influence of hemoglobin saturation with O_2 on CO_2 dissociation. (Chapter 11)

Hamburger phenomenon the shifting of chloride ions out of the red blood cell as HCO ion is formed in the cell by hydrolysis (combination of CO_2 with H_2O). (Chapter 11)

Harris-Benedict equation equation used to estimate the caloric expenditure in normal individuals under conditions of minimal activity. (Chapter 46)

health care–associated pneumonia (HCAP) pneumonia occurring in any patient hospitalized for 2 or more days in the past 90 days in an acute care setting or who, in the past 30 days, has resided in a long-term care or nursing facility; attended a hospital or hemodialysis clinic; or received intravenous antibiotics, chemotherapy, or wound care. (Chapter 22)

Health Care Infection Control Practices Advisory Committee (HICPAC) federal advisory committee composed of 14 external infection control experts who provide advice and guidance to the U.S. Centers for Disease Control and Prevention (CDC) and the Secretary of the Department of Health and Human Services regarding the practice of health care infection control and strategies for surveillance and prevention and control of health care–associated infections in U.S. health care facilities. (Chapter 4)

health education process of planned learning opportunities designed to enable individuals to make informed decisions about and act to promote their own health. (Chapter 49)

health promotion combination of educational, organizational, economic, and environmental support necessary for behavior conducive to health; includes both disease prevention and wellness activities. (Chapter 49)

heart rate (HR) number of heartbeats per unit of time, usually expressed as beats per minute (beats/min). (Chapter 9)

heliox low-density therapeutic mixture of helium with at least 20% O_2; used in some centers to treat large airway obstruction. (Chapter 37)

heliox therapy used to reduce the work of breathing, especially in patients with severe acute asthma or upper airway obstructions, until the primary problem can be resolved. (Chapter 38)

hematemesis vomiting blood. (Chapter 15)

hematology branch of medicine involved in the study of blood morphology, physiology, and pathology. (Chapter 16)

hemolysis rupture of red blood cells. (Chapter 15)

Henry's law in physics, law stating that the solubility of a gas in a liquid is proportional to the pressure of the gas if the temperature is constant and if the gas does not chemically react with the liquid. (Chapter 6)

HEPA (high-efficiency particulate air/aerosol) filter filtration device, usually capable of 99.99% efficacy on particulate matter down to 0.3 mm in size. (Chapter 4)

hepatomegaly abnormal enlargement of the liver; usually a sign of disease. (Chapter 15)

Hering-Breuer inflation reflex parasympathetic inflation reflex mediated via the lung's stretch receptors that appears to influence the duration of the expiratory pause occurring between breaths. (Chapter 14)

heterodisperse referring to an aerosol consisting of particles of varying diameters and sizes. (Chapter 36)

high-flow system O_2 therapy equipment that supplies inspired gases at a consistent preset O_2 concentration. (Chapter 38)

high-frequency chest wall compression (HFCC) mechanical technique for augmenting secretion clearance; small gas volumes are alternately injected into and withdrawn from a vest by an air-pulse generator at a fast rate, creating an oscillatory motion against the patient's thorax. (Chapter 40)

high-frequency ventilation (HFV) ventilatory support provided at rates significantly higher than normal breathing frequencies. (Chapters 27, 41, 48)

hilum vertical opening on either side of the mediastinum through which all the airways and pulmonary vessels pass. (Chapter 8)

homeostasis relative constancy in the internal environment of the body, naturally maintained by adaptive responses that promote healthy survival. (Chapter 16)

Hoover sign inward movement of the lower lateral margins of the chest wall with each inspiratory effort owing to a low, flat diaphragm as seen in emphysema. (Chapter 15)

hospital-acquired or nosocomial infection infection acquired at least 72 hours after hospitalization, often caused by *Candida albicans, Escherichia coli,* hepatitis viruses, herpes zoster virus, *Pseudomonas,* or *Staphylococcus.* (Chapter 4)

hospital-acquired pneumonia (HAP) lower respiratory tract infection that develops in hospitalized patients more than 48 hours after admission and excludes community-acquired infections that are incubating at the time of admission. (Chapter 22)

huff cough type of forced expiration with an open glottis to replace coughing when pain limits normal coughing. (Chapter 40)

humidifier device that adds molecular water to gas. (Chapter 35)

hydrofluoroalkane (HFA) the current gaseous chemical compound used to power metered dose inhalers. (Chapter 36)

hydrophobic pertaining to the property of repelling water molecules, a quality possessed by nonpolar radicals or molecules that are more soluble in organic solvents than in water. (Chapter 35)

hydropneumothorax a pneumothorax that is partially fluid filled. (Chapter 20)

hydrostatic relating to the pressure of fluids or to their properties when in equilibrium. (Chapter 27)

hydrostatic pressure pressure caused by the weight of fluid; related to the volume of fluid in a container and the effects of gravity. (Chapter 12)

hydrostatic pulmonary edema pulmonary edema that is caused by an increase in hydrostatic (water) pressure. (Chapter 27)

hydrothorax noninflammatory accumulation of serous fluid in one or both pleural cavities. (Chapter 20)

hygrometer instrument that directly measures relative humidity of the atmosphere or the proportion of water in a specific gas or gas mixture, without extracting the moisture. (Chapter 35)

hygroscopic attracting or absorbing moisture from the air. (Chapters 35, 36)

hyperbaric oxygen therapy therapeutic application of O_2 at pressures greater than 1 atm (or 760 mm Hg). Also called *hyperbaric oxygenation.* (Chapter 38)

hypercalcemia greater than normal amounts of calcium in the blood, most often resulting from excessive bone resorption and release of calcium, as occurs in hyperparathyroidism, metastatic tumors of bone, Paget disease, and osteoporosis. (Chapter 15)

hypercapnia abnormal presence of excess amounts of CO_2 in the blood (in arterial blood, PCO_2 > 45 mm Hg). (Chapter 13)

hypercapnic respiratory failure inability to maintain normal removal of CO_2 from the tissues; may be indicated by $PaCO_2$ greater than 50 mm Hg in an otherwise healthy individual. see *ventilatory failure.* (Chapter 45)

hyperkalemia greater than normal amounts of potassium in the blood. (Chapters 12, 16)

hypernatremia greater than normal concentration of sodium in the blood, caused by excessive loss of water and electrolytes secondary to polyuria, diarrhea, excessive sweating, or inadequate water intake. (Chapter 16)

hypersensitivity pneumonitis inflammatory form of interstitial pneumonia that results from an immunologic reaction in a hypersensitive person. The reaction may be provoked by various inhaled organic dusts, often containing fungal spores. The disease can be prevented by avoiding contact with the causative agents. Also called *extrinsic allergic alveolitis.* (Chapter 24)

hypertension persistently high blood pressure. (Chapter 15)

hyperventilation ventilation greater than necessary to meet metabolic needs; signified by PCO_2 less than 35 mm Hg in the arterial blood. (Chapter 10)

hypocapnia presence of lower than normal amounts of CO_2 in the blood (in arterial blood, PCO_2 < 35 mm Hg). (Chapter 13)

hypoglycemia less than normal amount of glucose in the blood, usually caused by administration of too much insulin, excessive secretion of insulin by the islet cells of the pancreas, or dietary deficiency (normal blood glucose levels range from 70 to 105 mg/dl). (Chapter 16)

hypokalemia condition in which an inadequate amount of potassium, the major intracellular cation, is found in the circulating bloodstream. (Chapter 16)

hyponatremia less than normal concentration of sodium in the blood, caused by inadequate excretion of water or by excessive water in the circulating bloodstream. (Chapter 16)

hypopharynx lower portion of the upper airway between the oropharynx and the larynx. (Chapter 8)

hypotension abnormal condition in which the blood pressure is inadequate for normal perfusion and oxygenation of the tissues. (Chapter 15)

hypothermia abnormal and dangerous condition in which the temperature of the body is less than 32° C, usually caused by prolonged exposure to cold. (Chapters 15, 35)

hypotonic having a tonicity less than normal saline (0.9% NaCl). (Chapter 12)

hypoventilation ventilation less than necessary to meet metabolic needs; signified by PCO_2 greater than 45 mm Hg in the arterial blood. (Chapter 10)

hypovolemia abnormally low circulating blood volume. (Chapter 15)

hypoxemia abnormal deficiency of O_2 in the arterial blood. (Chapter 11)

hypoxemic respiratory failure inability to maintain normal oxygenation in the arterial blood. (Chapters 41, 45)

hypoxia abnormal condition in which the O_2 available to the body cells is inadequate to meet metabolic needs. (Chapter 11)

hysteresis failure of two associated phenomena to coincide, as in the observed difference between the inflation and deflation volume-pressure curves of the lung. (Chapter 10)

I

idiopathic pulmonary fibrosis formation of scar tissue in the connective tissue of the lungs without known cause resulting in severe chronic restrictive lung disease. (Chapter 24)

imprecision implying a level of inaccuary in a particular measurement. (Chapter 18)

impulse-conducting system Purkinje fibers within the heart muscle that conduct impulses controlling the contractions of the atria and ventricles. (Chapter 16)

incentive spirometry process of encouraging a bedridden patient to take deep breaths to avoid atelectasis; most often done with the use of an incentive spirometer that provides feedback to the patient when a predetermined lung volume is reached during an inspiratory breath. (Chapter 39)

inclusion body myosis inflammatory myopathy of unknown cause. (Chapter 29)

indirect calorimetry measurement of the amount of energy a body consumes (in kcal) by determining the consumption of O_2 and production of CO_2. (Chapter 21)

inertial impaction deposition of particles by collision with a surface; primary mechanism for pulmonary deposition of particles greater than 5 mm in diameter. (Chapter 36)

insufflator-exsufflator mechanical device that provides an artificial cough by alternately applying positive pressure and negative pressure to the airway. (Chapter 51)

infiltrate fluid that passes through body tissues into a space or virtual space as seen in the lung. (Chapter 20)

inhaled mass the mass of the particles inhaled from an aerosol. (Chapter 36)

inhaled nitric oxide (INO) gas that is administered to decrease pulmonary hypertension. (Chapter 48)

inspiratory capacity (IC) maximum amount of air that can be inhaled from the resting end expiratory level or FRC; sum of the tidal volume and inspiratory reserve volume. (Chapter 19)

inspiratory positive airway pressure (IPAP) application of positive pressure to the airway during inspiration. (Chapter 45)

inspiratory reserve volume (IRV) maximum volume of air that can be inhaled after a normal quiet inspiration. (Chapter 19)

inspissated (of a fluid) thickened or hardened through the absorption or evaporation of the liquid portion, as can occur with respiratory secretions when the upper airway is bypassed. (Chapters 35, 40)

intercostal of or pertaining to the space between two ribs. (Chapter 8)

intercostals referring to the muscle groups between the ribs. (Chapter 8)

intermittent mandatory ventilation (IMV) mode of mechanical ventilatory support in which the patient receives a preset number of machine breaths per minute set by time. The patient is allowed to breathe spontaneously as often as desired in between machine breaths. Depending on the base rate, IMV can provide partial or full ventilatory support. (Chapter 42)

intermittent positive pressure breathing (IPPB) application of positive pressure breaths to a patient for a relatively short period (10 to 20 minutes). (Chapter 39)

internal oblique abdominal muscle group that functions as an accessory muscle of ventilation. (Chapter 8)

internal respiration the exchange of O_2 and CO_2 at the tissue level. (Chapter 8)

International Council for Respiratory Care (ICRC) comprising governors from various countries, diverse group of worldwide health professionals addressing issues affecting educational, medical, and professional trends in the global respiratory care community. (Chapter 1)

International Standards Organization (ISO) nongovernment agency that sets standards for various technical equipment and procedures. (Chapter 35)

interstitial fluid fluid between cells but outside of the vascular spaces. (Chapter 12)

interstitial lung disease (ILD) respiratory disorder characterized by a dry, unproductive cough and dyspnea on exertion. X-rays usually show fibrotic infiltrates in the lung tissue, usually in the lower lobes. (Chapters 20, 24)

intrapulmonary percussive ventilation (IPV) airway clearance technique that uses a pneumatic device to deliver a series of pressurized small volume breaths at high rates (1.6 to 3.75 Hz) to the respiratory tract, usually via a mouthpiece; usually combined with aerosolized bronchodilator therapy. (Chapter 40)

intubation passage of a tube into a body aperture; commonly refers to the insertion of an endotracheal tube within the trachea. (Chapter 33)

intuitionism an ethical viewpoint that holds that there are certain self-evident truths, usually based on moral maxims such as "treat others fairly." (Chapter 5)

invasive characterized by a tendency to spread or infiltrate; also refers to the use of diagnostic or therapeutic methods requiring access to the inside of the body. (Chapter 18)

in vivo (of a biological reaction) occurring in a living organism. (Chapter 18)

ionic electrovalent; relating to or containing matter in the form of charged atoms or groups of atoms. (Chapter 12)

iron lung full-body negative pressure ventilator. (Chapter 45)

isohydric buffering a buffering process where the H ion produced by one buffer system is immediately buffered by another, such as the buffering of H ion by hemoglobin when H ion is formed by the combination of CO_2 and H_2O in the red blood cell. (Chapter 13)

isothermic saturation boundary (ISB) point at which inspired gas becomes fully saturated to 100% relative humidity at body temperature. (Chapter 35)

isotonic (of a solution) having the same concentration of solute as another solution and exerting the same amount of osmotic pressure as that solution, such as an isotonic saline solution that contains an amount of salt equal to that found in the extracellular fluid. (Chapter 12)

J

J-receptors vagal sensory sites that are located in the alveolar units; so named because they are found primarily in juxtaposition to the pulmonary capillaries. (Chapter 14)

The Joint Commission private nongovernment agency that establishes guidelines for the operation of hospitals and other health care facilities, conducts accreditation programs and surveys, and encourages the attainment of high standards of institutional medical care in the United States; formerly Joint Commission on Accreditation of Healthcare Organizations (JCAHO). (Chapter 2)

jugular venous distention abnormal distention of the jugular veins, most often caused by heart failure. (Chapter 15)

justice principle of fair and equal treatment for all, with due reward and honor. (Chapter 5)

K

Karvonen's formula simple formula used to set a target heart rate for patients during exercise. (Chapter 50)

Kerley B-lines thin lines seen near the pleural edge on a chest film as a result of increased pulmonary capillary pressures. (Chapter 20)

kinetic energy energy a body possesses by virtue of its motion. (Chapter 6)

Kussmaul respiration hyperpnea associated with diabetic ketoacidosis. (Chapter 15)

Kussmaul sign paradoxical increase in venous pressure with distention of the jugular veins during inspiration, as seen in constrictive pericarditis or mediastinal tumor. (Chapter 15)

kwashiorkor protein-energy malnutrition resulting from the stress of disease and the resulting increase in catabolic rate. (Chapter 21)

kyphoscoliosis abnormal condition characterized by anteroposterior and lateral curvature of the spine. (Chapter 29)

L

lactate anion of lactic acid. (Chapter 16)

Lambert-Eaton syndrome disorder of neuromuscular conduction commonly associated with an underlying malignancy that leads to muscle weakness frequently with sensory deficits that can often be improved by repetitive muscle contraction against pressure. (Chapter 29)

laminar flow pattern of flow consisting of concentric layers of fluid flowing parallel to the tube wall at linear velocities that increase toward the center. (Chapter 6)

Laplace's law principle of physics that the tension on the wall of a sphere is the product of the pressure times the radius of the chamber, and the tension is inversely related to the thickness of the wall. (Chapter 6)

large cell carcinoma type of lung cancer characterized by large cells on microscopy. (Chapter 28)

large for gestational age (LGA) refers to an infant whose fetal growth was accelerated and whose size and weight at birth are above the 90th percentile of appropriate-for-gestational-age infants, whether delivered prematurely, at term, or later than term. (Chapter 48)

laryngopharynx one of the three regions of the throat, extending from the hyoid bone to the esophagus. (Chapter 8)

larynx organ of the voice that is part of the upper air passage connecting the pharynx with the trachea. It accounts for a large bump in the neck called the *Adam's apple* and is larger in men than in women, although it remains the same size in boys and girls until puberty. (Chapter 8)

latent heat of fusion the amount of heat at a substances melting point required to change 1 gram of the substance from a solid to a liquid. (Chapter 6)

latent heat of vaporization the amount of heat at a substances boiling point required to change 1 gram of the substance from a liquid to a gas. (Chapter 6)

law of continuity velocity of a fluid moving through a tube and constant flow varies inversely with the available cross-sectional area. (Chapter 6)

law of mass action states that acids and bases in solution freely dissociate and re-associate in a solution at a constant rate relative to the structure of the acid and the temperature of the solution. (Chapter 12)

laws of thermodynamics laws that describe the relation between temperature and the kinetics of matter changing its state. (Chapter 6)

leukocyte white blood cell. (Chapter 16)

leukocytopenia abnormal decrease in white blood cells. (Chapter 16)

leukocytosis abnormal increase in the number of circulating white blood cells. (Chapter 16)

leukotriene class of biologically active compounds that occur naturally in leukocytes and produce allergic and inflammatory reactions similar to histamine. They are thought to play a role in the development of allergic and autoallergic diseases such as asthma, rheumatoid arthritis, inflammatory bowel disease, and psoriasis. (Chapter 32)

libel false accusation written, printed, or typewritten or presented in a picture or a sign that is made with malicious intent to defame the reputation of a person who is living or the memory of a person who is dead, resulting in public embarrassment, contempt, ridicule, or hatred. (Chapter 5)

living will advance declaration by a patient that, if determined to be hopelessly and terminally ill, the person does not want to be connected to life-support equipment; written agreement between a patient and physician to withhold heroic measures if the patient's condition is found to be irreversible. (Chapter 5)

lobes major divisions of the lungs; the right lung has three lobes, and the left lung has two lobes. (Chapter 8)

loud P-2 abnormally loud closure of the pulmonic valve as part of S_2; usually caused by pulmonary hypertension. (Chapter 15)

Lou Gehrig disease popular name for amyotrophic lateral sclerosis (ALS), a disease characterized by progressive muscle weakness secondary to nerve deterioration. (Chapter 29)

low-flow system variable performance O_2 therapy device that delivers O_2 at a flow that provides only a portion of the patient's inspired gas needs. Also called *variable performance system*. (Chapter 38)

lower respiratory tract infection any infectious disease of the left and right bronchi and the alveoli. (Chapter 22)

L/T ratio refers to aerosol, it is the lung availability of an aerosol divided by the total system availability of the aerosol. (Chapter 32)

lung protective ventilatory strategy approach to mechanical ventilation that attempts to avoid overdistention of the lung and recruitment and derecruitment of unstable lung units with each breath. (Chapter 44)

lung strain is the deformation of a structure compared to it overall size. As applied to the respiratory it is equal to the driving pressure during ventilation. (Chapter 46)

lung stress is the force applied per unit area. As applied to the respiratory system it is equal to transpulmonary pressure. (Chapter 46)

lung ultrasonography the use of ultrasound technology to view lung structures. (Chapter 46)

lymphadenopathy of or pertaining to a disease of the lymph nodes; refers also to the visualization of enlarged lymph nodes on radiographs. (Chapter 15)

lymphangioleiomyomatosis (LAM) lung abnormality most commonly observed in women and characterized by abnormal proliferation of smooth muscle cells in the interstitium, dyspnea, abnormal radiographic findings, and commonly pneumothorax. (Chapter 24)

lymphatic drainage system the main conduit for the removal of filtered fluid and protein from the lung. (Chapter 27)

M

macroshock shock from an electrical current of 1 mA or greater that is applied externally to the skin. (Chapter 3)

magnetic resonance imaging (MRI) imaging technique using magnetic disturbance of tissue to obtain images. (Chapter 28)

malpractice in law, professional negligence that is the proximate cause of injury or harm to a patient, resulting from a lack of professional knowledge, experience, or skill that can be expected in others in the profession or from a failure to exercise reasonable care or judgment in the application of professional knowledge, experience, or skill. (Chapter 5)

mandatory breath ventilatory support breath either initiated or ended by the machine. (Chapter 42)

mandatory minute volume ventilation (MMV) variation of the intermittent mandatory ventilation mode of ventilatory support in which the ventilator keeps the total minute volume constant. (Chapter 47)

manifold pipe with many connections; in medical gas storage, a collection of gas cylinders linked together for purposes of bulk storage and usually including at least one reserve bank and other safety systems, such as low-pressure alarms. (Chapter 37)

manubrium upper triangular portion of the sternum. (Chapter 8)

marasmus protein-energy malnutrition caused by starvation. (Chapter 21)

mass physical property of matter that gives it weight and inertia; aggregate of cells clumped together, such as a tumor. (Chapter 28)

mass median aerodynamic diameter (MMAD) measure of central tendency that describes the particle diameter in micrometers in medical aerosols and pertains to cascade impaction. (Chapter 36)

maximal inspiratory pressure (MIP) the median diameter of an aerosol particle expressed in grams. (Chapter 46)

maximum expiratory pressure (MEP) measure of the output of the expiratory muscles against a maximum stimulus, measured in cm H_2O positive pressure. (Chapter 41)

maximum inspiratory pressure (MIP) measure of the output of the inspiratory muscles against a maximum stimulus, measured in cm H_2O negative pressure. Also known as *negative inspiratory force (NIF)* or *maximum inspiratory force (MIF)*. (Chapter 41)

maximum voluntary ventilation (MVV) maximum volume of air in L/min that a subject can breathe during a 12- to 15-second period. It is a very patient-dependent test. Formerly called the maximum breathing capacity (MBC). (Chapters 19, 41, 46)

mean airway pressure average pressure applied to the airway. (Chapters 43, 46)

mechanical insufflation-exsufflation mechanical device that provides an artificial cough by alternately applying positive pressure and negative pressure to the airway, also referred to as an *in-exsufflator*. (Chapter 40)

mechanical ventilation an artificial device to assist a patient to breathe. (Chapter 1)

meconium material that collects in the intestines of a fetus and forms the first stools of a newborn. (Chapter 48)

meconium aspiration syndrome inhalation of meconium by a fetus or newborn; can block the air passages and cause failure of the lungs to expand. (Chapter 31)

mediastinum portion of the thoracic cavity lying in the middle of the thorax (between the two pleural cavities); extends from the vertebral column to the sternum and contains the trachea, esophagus, heart, and great vessels of the circulatory system. (Chapter 8)

melting point characteristic temperature at which the solid and liquid forms of a substance are in equilibrium. (Chapter 6)

metabolic acidosis nonrespiratory processes resulting in acidemia. (Chapter 13)

metabolic alkalosis nonrespiratory processes resulting in alkalemia. (Chapter 13)

methemoglobin abnormal form of hemoglobin in which the iron component has been oxidized from the ferrous to the ferric state. (Chapter 11)

methemoglobinemia abnormal condition characterized by high levels of methemoglobin in the blood and reduction in O_2-carrying capacity; may be caused by nitrite poisoning or ingestion of a certain oxidizing agent or a genetic defect in the enzyme NADH methemoglobin reductase (an autosomal dominant trait). (Chapter 11)

micrognathia underdevelopment of the jaw, especially the mandible. (Chapter 31)

microshock shock from a usually imperceptible electrical current (<1 mA) that is allowed to bypass the skin and follow a direct, low-resistance pathway into the body. (Chapter 3)

minute ventilation total lung ventilation per minute, the product of tidal volume and respiration rate. It is measured by expired gas collection for a period of 1 to 3 minutes; normal rate is 5 to 10 L/min. (Chapter 19)

misallocation process of prescribing diagnostic or treatment services when not indicated, consisting both of overordering and underordering services. (Chapter 2)

modified Allen test most common technique to determine the adequacy of ulnar circulation. (Chapter 18)

molecular sieve crystalline chemical separation device with molecular size pores that adsorbs small but not large molecules. (Chapter 51)

monitor to observe and evaluate a function of the body closely and constantly; mechanical device that provides a visual or audible signal or a graphic record of a particular function, such as a cardiac monitor or a fetal monitor. (Chapter 18)

monodisperse referring to an aerosol in which particles are of uniform size.(Chapter 36)

mucociliary escalator a term used to define the process where the cilia of the airways continually move mucus from the lower respiratory tract to the oral cavity. (Chapter 8)

mucoid resembling mucus. (Chapter 15)

mucous plugging the partial or complete occlusion of the airway by thick mucous. (Chapter 40)

multiple organ dysfunction syndrome (MODS) condition in which dysfunction of many different organs occurs, usually accompanying acute lung injury. (Chapter 27)

murmur abnormal heart sound created by turbulent blood flow through a narrowed or incompetent heart valve. (Chapter 15)

Murray lung injury score a score used to define the severity of injury in patients with ARDS. (Chapter 46)

muscarinic stimulating the postganglionic parasympathetic receptor; pertaining to the poisonous activity of muscarine (Chapter 32)

muscle fatigue condition involving loss of the capacity to develop force or velocity of a muscle resulting from muscle activity overload, which is reversible by rest. (Chapter 41)

myasthenia gravis disorder of neuromuscular conduction that leads to muscle weakness of the skeletal muscles, particularly the muscles of the face, throat, and respiratory system. Weakness and respiratory failure can occur rapidly as muscle strength decreases with repetitive contraction against a load. (Chapter 29)

mydriasis dilation of the pupil of the eye. (Chapter 32)

myopathy abnormal condition of skeletal muscle leading to muscle weakness, wasting, and histologic changes in the muscle tissue, as seen in muscular dystrophies. (Chapter 29)

myositis inflammation of the muscle. (Chapter 29)

myotonic dystrophy type of muscular dystrophy. (Chapter 29)

N

nanomole a quantity equal to 10^{-9} of a mole. (Chapter 12)

nasal flaring dilation of the alar nasi on inspiration; an early sign of an increase in ventilatory demands and the work of breathing, especially in infants. (Chapter 31)

nasopharynx upper portion of the airway behind the nasal and oral cavities. (Chapter 8)

National Board of Respiratory Care (NBRC) national credentialing agency for respiratory care practitioners and pulmonary function technologists. (Chapters 1, 2)

nebulizer device that produces an aerosol suspension of liquid particles in a gaseous medium using baffling to control particle size. (Chapters 35, 36)

needle-capping device safety device used to prevent or minimize needlestick injuries when capping a syringe needle (as required after blood gas sampling). (Chapter 18)

negative feedback loop when the output of a system acts to oppose changes to the input of the system, with the result that the changes are attenuated and output is balanced. (Chapter 9)

negative inotropism decrease in contractility of the heart. (Chapter 9)

negative-pressure ventilator approach to ventilation in which negative pressure is intermittently applied to the chest surface in an effort to cause inflation of the lungs. (Chapter 45)

negligence omission to do something that a reasonable person, guided by ordinary considerations, would do. (Chapter 5)

neovascularization formation of new capillary beds. (Chapter 38)

neurally adjusted ventilatory assistance (NAVA) an approach to ventilation based on the EMG activity of the diaphragm. Airway pressure is increased proportional to the change in EMG activity. No control variable is set. (Chapter 44)

neuropathy refers to abnormal conditions characterized by inflammation or degeneration of the nerves. (Chapter 29)

neutral thermal environment (NTE) ambient environment that prevents or minimizes the loss of body heat. (Chapter 38)

neutropenia abnormal decrease in the number of neutrophils in the blood. (Chapters 16, 32)

nitric oxide an inhaled gas used as inhaled therapy to reduce pulmonary artery pressure and improve arterial oxygenation. (Chapter 38)

nocturnal hypoventilation elevated $PaCO_2$ and accompanying decline in O_2 saturation that occurs in response to a progressive decrease in minute ventilation occurring during sleep, most often in the REM stage. (Chapter 45)

nodule small node; small nodelike structure. (Chapter 28)

nonflammable unable to support combustion. (Chapter 37)

nonhydrostatic pulmonary edema pulmonary edema that is caused by something other than an increase in blood pressure. (Chapter 27)

noninvasive pertaining to a diagnostic or therapeutic technique that does not require the skin to be broken or a cavity or organ of the body to be entered, such as obtaining a blood pressure reading by auscultation with a stethoscope and sphygmomanometer. (Chapter 18)

noninvasive positive pressure ventilation (NPPV) (also referred to as **noninvasive ventilation** or **NIV)** positive pressure ventilation without endotracheal intubation or tracheotomy, usually via a form-fitting nasal face mask. (Chapters 41, 45)

noninvasive ventilation mechanical ventilation performed without intubation or tracheostomy, usually with mask ventilation. (Chapters 23, 39, 45, 51)

nonmaleficence principle that obligates health care providers to avoid harming patients and actively to prevent harm where possible. (Chapter 5)

non–small cell carcinoma major category of histologic types of lung carcinomas, including adenocarcinoma of the lung, large cell carcinoma, and squamous cell carcinoma. Treatment depends on the stage of development of the cancer at the time of initial presentation. The treatment of choice for otherwise physically fit patients with early stages of disease is resection. (Chapter 28)

normal solution solution that contains the gram-equivalent weight of a reagent per liter; denoted by the symbols *N/I* or *N*. (Chapter 12)

normometabolic the normal level of metabolic function in a health individual. (Chapter 21)

nosocomial pneumonia infectious inflammatory process of the lung parenchyma that is contracted in the hospital. (Chapter 22)

O

O_2-conserving device an oxygen delivery system that minimizes the amount of oxygen actually delivered to a patient while also maintaining the FiO_2. (Chapter 51)

obesity-hypoventilation syndrome general syndrome involving chronic hypercapnia and hypoxemia, sleep apnea, and decreased respiratory center responsiveness to CO_2. Complications, primarily owing to chronic hypoxemia, include polycythemia, pulmonary hypertension, and cor pulmonale. (Chapter 30)

obstructive pulmonary disease any respiratory disease characterized by decreased airway size and increased airway secretions. (Chapter 19)

obstructive sleep apnea (OSA) condition in which five or more apneic periods (lasting at least 10 seconds each) occur per hour of sleep and characterized by occlusion of the oropharyngeal airway with continued efforts to breathe. (Chapter 30)

obturator device used to block a passage or a canal or to fill in a space, such as the obturator used to insert a tracheostomy tube. (Chapter 33)

occupational ILD interstitial lung disease resulting from an occupational exposure; asbestosis is a common example. (Chapter 24)

ohm unit of measurement to report the resistance to the flow of electricity. (Chapter 3)

Ondine curse apnea caused by loss of automatic control of respiration (derived from the name of a fabled water nymph). (Chapter 29)

onset of blood lactate accumulation (OBLA) point where blood lactate levels increase above normal when the body cannot deliver sufficient O_2 to meet the demands of energy metabolism; term used in exercise physiology. (Chapter 50)

open buffer system the bicarbonate buffer system is an open buffer system because H_2CO_3 can removed as CO_2, is broken down into H_2O and CO_2 as long as ventilation removes CO_2. The bicarbonate system is an example. (Chapter 13)

open loop control system in which there is no control over the delivered variable. (Chapter 42)

optical fluorescence the use of fluorescent dyes that are illuminated with light of a specific wavelength for the measurement of respiratory gases. (Chapter 18)

optode fluorescent chemosensor useful in measuring pH or gas tensions in arterial or mixed venous blood. (Chapter 18)

organizing pneumonia (OP) is the new term for bronchiolitis obliterans organizing pneumonia, that generally occurs in the setting of connective tissue disease. (Chapter 24)

orthodeoxia decrease in PaO_2 owing to changes in position. (Chapter 15)

orthopnea labored breathing in the reclining position. (Chapter 15)

oscillation back-and-forth motion; vibration or the effects of mechanical or electrical vibration. (Chapter 40)

OSHA abbreviation for the Occupational Safety and Health Administration, a branch of the U.S. Department of Labor responsible for regulation pertaining to on-the-job safety. (Chapter 4)

osmolarity osmotic pressure of a solution expressed in osmoles or mOsm/kg of the solution. (Chapter 12)

osmotic pressure force produced by solvent particles across semipermeable membranes. (Chapter 12)

oxidizing to combine or cause to combine with O_2, to remove hydrogen, or to increase the valence of an element through the loss of electrons. (Chapter 37)

oxygen therapy any procedure in which O_2 is administered to a patient to relieve hypoxemia. (Chapter 1)

oxyhemoglobin chemical combination resulting from the covalent bonding of O_2 to the ferrous iron pigment in hemoglobin. (Chapter 11)

P

pack-years a method of determining the quantity of cigarettes a patient smoked over time. The number of packs of cigarettes a person smoked divided by the number of years they smoked. (Chapter 15)

palate bony plate that separates the nasal cavity from the oral cavity. (Chapter 8)

Pancoast syndrome combination of signs associated with a tumor in the apex of the lung; signs include neuritic pain in the arm, atrophy of the muscles of the arm and the hand, and Horner syndrome and are caused by the damaging effects of the tumor on the brachial plexus and sympathetic ganglia. (Chapter 28)

PaO_2/FiO_2 ratio the PaO_2 divided by the FiO_2, indicative of the severity of lung injury. (Chapter 46)

paradoxical motion movement of the thoracic cavity where the cavity bows out with expiration and collapses inward during a spontaneous breath. The movement is associated with a decreased pressure gradient to drive inspiration and expiration and can result in respiratory failure. (Chapter 29)

paraneoplastic syndrome effect of tumors remote from the tumor site and often mediated by reactions to tumor products or immune response to the tumor. (Chapter 28)

paresthesia any subjective sensation, experienced as numbness, tingling, or a "pins and needles" feeling. (Chapter 13)

parietal pleura thin membrane covering the surface of the chest wall, mediastinum, and diaphragm that is continuous with the visceral pleura around the lung hilum. (Chapters 8, 25)

partial ventilatory support modes of ventilatory support in which the patient must contribute to the total minute volume with spontaneous breathing. (Chapter 44)

Pascal's principle law stating that a confined liquid transmits pressure equally in all directions. (Chapter 6)

patent ductus arteriosus (PDA) common cardiovascular anomaly of infants in which the ductus arteriosus either fails to close or reopens after birth. (Chapter 48)

patient-ventilator asynchrony lack of coordinated gas delivery between the patient and the ventilator. (Chapter 43)

peak expiratory flow rate (PEFR) maximum expiratory flow rate in L/sec. (Chapter 19)

pedal edema swelling of the ankles usually secondary to heart failure. (Chapter 15)

pericardium fibrous, serous sac that surrounds the heart and roots of the great vessels. (Chapter 9)

periodic breathing abnormal pattern of respiration, characterized by alternating periods of apnea and deep, rapid breathing. (Chapter 29)

persistent pulmonary hypertension of the newborn (PPHN) clinical syndrome seen in infants soon after birth and characterized by abnormally increased pulmonary vascular resistance. (Chapter 31)

pharmacodynamic phase mechanisms of drug action that cause effects on the body. (Chapter 32)

pharmacokinetic phase time, course, and disposition of a drug in the body. (Chapter 32)

pharyngeal airways devices that maintain the patency of the pharyngeal structure. (Chapter 33)

pharynx the throat—tubular structure about 13 cm long that extends from the base of the skull to the esophagus and is situated immediately in front of the cervical vertebrae. The pharynx serves as a passageway for the respiratory and digestive tracts and changes shape to allow the formation of various vowel sounds. (Chapter 8)

phase variable signal that is measured and used by the ventilator to begin some part (phase) of the breathing cycle. (Chapter 42)

phlegm mucus from the tracheobronchial tree. (Chapter 15)

phrenic nerves paired nerves that originate as branches of spinal nerves C3-5, pass down along the mediastinum, and innervate the diaphragm. (Chapter 8)

physician assistant (PA) individual academically and clinically prepared to practice medicine under the supervision of a licensed doctor of medicine or osteopathy. Within the physician-PA relationship, PAs exercise autonomy in medical decisions and provide a wide range of diagnostic and therapeutic services. Training programs average 25 to 27 months. National certification is available to graduates of approved training programs. (Chapter 1)

physiologic dead space area in the respiratory system that includes the anatomic dead space together with the space in the alveoli occupied by air that does not contribute to the O_2-CO_2 exchange. (Chapter 10)

physiologic shunt ($\dot{Q}_S / \dot{Q}_T$) percentage of the cardiac output that does not participate in gas exchange in the lung. (Chapter 46)

piezoelectric crystal transducer capable of converting electrical energy into the physical energy of high-frequency vibrations. (Chapter 35)

pin-indexed safety system (PISS) part of the American standard safety system, these specifications apply only to the valve outlets of small cylinders, up to and including size E, which use a yoke-type connection. (Chapter 37)

plaintiff person who brings an action; a person who seeks remedial relief for an injury to his or her rights. (Chapter 5)

plasma watery, colorless fluid portion of the blood and lymph in which cellular elements are suspended. (Chapter 12)

plasma colloid osmotic pressure (oncotic pressure) osmotic pressure exerted by the colloid suspended in the blood. (Chapter 12)

plateau pressure (P_{plat}) pressure in the patient's airway during mechanical ventilation resulting from the application of an end inspiratory hold. This is equal to the average peak alveolar pressure. (Chapter 44)

plate (or plate-like) atelectasis lung collapse that appears in distinct plate like structures. (Chapter 20)

platypnea opposite of orthopnea; an abnormal condition characterized by difficult breathing in the standing position, which is relieved in the lying or recumbent position. (Chapter 15)

plethysmograph device for measuring pressure; in pulmonary physiology, a chamber in which the subject sits to measure lung pressures and volumes. (Chapter 10)

pleural effusion abnormal collection of fluid in the pleural space. (Chapter 25)

pleurisy pain that comes from the pleural surface; usually a direct result of viral infections but has been generalized to any condition (e.g., pulmonary embolism) causing pleural pain. Synonymous with *pleurodynia*. (Chapter 25)

pleurodesis procedure of fusing the parietal and visceral pleura to prevent formation of pleural fluid or recurrence of pneumothorax. (Chapter 25)

pneumobelt ventilatory assist device that applies positive pressure to the abdominal contents during expiration. (Chapter 45)

pneumomediastinum presence of air or gas in the mediastinal tissues, which may lead to pneumothorax or pneumopericardium. (Chapter 20)

pneumonia inflammatory process of the lung parenchyma, usually infectious in origin. (Chapter 22)

pneumotachometer any device for measuring gas flow. (Chapter 10)

pneumotaxic center center in the upper part of the pons that rhythmically inhibits inspiration independently of the vagi. (Chapter 14)

pneumothorax presence of air or gas in the pleural space of the thorax; if this air or gas is trapped under pressure, tension pneumothorax exists. (Chapters 15, 20, 25)

point-of-care testing analysis of body fluids at the bedside, as opposed to conventional laboratory testing. (Chapter 18)

polycythemia abnormal increase in the number of erythrocytes in the blood; termed *secondary* if attributable to defined causes other than direct stimulation of the bone marrow, such as occurs in chronic hypoxemia. (Chapter 16)

polymyositis condition characterized by inflammation of many muscles. (Chapter 29)

pores of Kohn openings between adjacent alveoli. (Chapter 8)

positive end expiratory pressure (PEEP) application and maintenance of pressure above atmospheric at the airway throughout the expiratory phase of positive pressure mechanical ventilation. (Chapters 27, 41)

positive expiratory pressure (PEP) airway clearance technique in which the patient exhales against a fixed-orifice flow resistor to help move secretions into the larger airways for expectoration via coughing or swallowing. (Chapters 39, 40)

positive inotropism increase in the contractility of muscle tissue. (Chapter 9)

positron emission tomography (PET) computerized radiographic technique that uses radioactive substances to examine the metabolic activity of various body structures. The patient either inhales or is injected with a metabolically important substance such as glucose, carrying a radioactive element that emits positively charged particles, or positrons. When the positrons combine with electrons normally found in the cells of the body, gamma rays are emitted. The electronic circuitry and computers of the PET device detect the gamma rays and construct color-coded images that indicate the intensity of metabolic activity throughout the organ involved. (Chapter 28)

postural hypotension sudden decrease in arterial blood pressure caused by a change in position; most often occurs when a hypovolemic patient moves from the reclining position to the upright position. (Chapter 15)

potential energy energy contained in a body as a result of its position in space, internal structure, and stresses imposed on it. (Chapter 6)

preanalytic error error that occurs outside of that actual testing procedure. (Chapter 18)

precision the accuracy of an instrument during the measurement of a particular substance. (Chapter 18)

preload pressure stretching the ventricular walls at the onset of ventricular contraction. (Chapters 9, 46)

preoperative of or pertaining to the period of time preceding a surgical procedure. (Chapter 39)

pressure-controlled ventilation (PCV) mode of ventilatory support in which mandatory support breaths are delivered to the patient at a set inspiratory pressure. (Chapters 41, 42, 44)

pressure gradient the pressure difference between 2 points in a system. (Chapter 10)

pressure-regulated volume control (PRVC) pressure limited ventilation in which inspiratory time and a backup rate are set and a tidal volume is targeted. (Chapter 44)

pressure support ventilation (PSV) mode of ventilatory support designed to augment spontaneous breathing; patient-triggered, pressure-limited, flow-cycled ventilation. (Chapters 44, 47)

pressure-time product product of pressure over a time interval, usually pleural pressure times inspiratory time during breathing. (Chapter 46)

primary lobule the terminal bronchiole and the cluster of respiratory bronchioles that it supplies. (Chapter 8)

primary pulmonary hypertension form of pulmonary hypertension that occurs in the absence of other heart or lung diseases and is characterized by diffuse narrowing of the pulmonary arterioles without obvious reason. (Chapter 48)

primary spontaneous pneumothorax pneumothorax that occurs without underlying lung disease. (Chapter 25)

problem-oriented medical record (POMR) method of recording data about the health status of a patient in a problem system. (Chapter 3)

prodrug inactive or partially active drug that is metabolically changed in the body to an active drug. (Chapter 32)

proficiency testing (PT) process of comparing measurements of a known value from different sources to establish a level of accuracy. (Chapter 18)

progressive resistance method of increasing the strength of a weak or injured muscle by gradually increasing the resistance against which the muscle works, such as by using graduated weights over a period. Also called *graduated resistance*. (Chapter 50)

prolonged mechanical ventilation a lengthy process of mechanical ventilatory support. No precise length has been determined but most would consider >2 weeks prolonged ventilatory support. (Chapter 47)

propellant something that propels or provides thrust, as the propellant in a metered dose inhaler. (Chapter 36)

proportional assist ventilation (PAV) mode of ventilation without any control variable that delivers gas in proportion to the patient's actual inspiratory effort. (Chapter 44)

protein-energy malnutrition (PEM) wasting condition resulting from a diet deficient in either protein or energy (calories) or both. (Chapter 21)

pseudostratified of or pertaining to an epithelial cell type that appears to be organized in layers but in which each cell actually contacts the basement membrane. (Chapter 8)

psig abbreviation for pounds per square inch-gauge—the pressure above atmospheric registered on a meter or gauge. (Chapter 37)

psychomotor domain area of observable performance of skills that require some degree of neuromuscular coordination. (Chapter 49)

psychosocial of or pertaining to the mental, emotional, and social aspects of human existence or development. (Chapter 50)

pulmonary edema condition in which excessive amounts of plasma enter the pulmonary interstitium and alveoli; usually accompanied by severe respiratory distress, tachypnea, and hypoxemia. (Chapter 27)

pulmonary embolism blockage of a pulmonary artery by foreign matter. The obstruction may be fat, air, tumor tissue, or a thrombus that usually arises from a peripheral vein (most frequently arising from the deep veins of the legs). Pulmonary embolism is detected by chest x-ray, pulmonary angiography, and radioscanning of the lung fields. (Chapter 26)

pulmonary function testing (PFT) procedure for determining the capacity of the lungs to exchange O_2 and CO_2 efficiently. There are two general kinds of pulmonary function tests: one measures ventilation, or the ability of the bellows action of the chest and lungs to move gas in and out of alveoli; the other kind measures the diffusion of gas across the alveolar capillary membrane and the perfusion of the lungs by blood. (Chapters 1, 19)

pulmonary hypertension condition characterized by abnormally high pulmonary artery pressures (i.e., mean pulmonary artery pressures >22 mm Hg). (Chapter 26)

pulmonary Langerhans cell histiocytosis (PLCH) condition characterized by abnormal proliferation of Langerhans cells, accompanied by interstitial markings on the chest film and dyspnea. (Chapter 24)

pulmonary rehabilitation an organized multidisciplinary approach to improve the functional status of patients with COPD, usually including education, exercise, aerosolized medication and oxygen therapy. (Chapter 50)

pulse cooximetry a pulse oximetry that is capable of measuring carboxhemoglobin and methemoglobin. (Chapter 18)

pulse deficit discrepancy between the ventricular rate auscultated at the apex of the heart and the arterial rate of the radial pulse. (Chapter 15)

pulse pressure difference between systolic blood pressure and diastolic blood pressure. (Chapter 15)

pulsus alternans alternating between strong and weak heartbeats. (Chapter 15)

pulsus paradoxus abnormal decrease in pulse pressure with each inspiratory effort. (Chapter 15)

purulent consisting of or containing pus. (Chapter 15)

Q

quality assurance any evaluation of services provided and the results achieved compared with accepted standards. (Chapter 2)

quality control planned, systematic approach to designing, measuring, assessing, and improving performance. (Chapter 18)

R

radiation therapy treatment of neoplastic disease by using x-rays or gamma rays, usually from a cobalt source, to deter the proliferation of malignant cells by decreasing the rate of mitosis or impairing deoxyribonucleic acid synthesis. (Chapter 6)

radiograph x-ray image. (Chapter 20)

radiolucent of or pertaining to a substance or tissue that readily permits the passage of x-rays or other radiant energy. Compare with *radiopaque*. (Chapter 20)

radiopaque of or pertaining to a substance or tissue that does not readily permit the passage of x-rays or other radiant energy. Compare with *radiolucent*. (Chapters 20, 33)

radiotherapy treatment with radiation. (Chapter 28)

random error variability of a measurement outside of accepted limits that occurs in a nonreproducible fashion. (Chapter 18)

rapid shallow breathing index (f/V_T) patient's spontaneous respiratory rate (f) in breaths/min divided by the spontaneous tidal volume in liters. Values greater than 100 are associated with poor weaning outcomes. (Chapter 47)

reconditioning physical activity to strengthen essential muscle groups, improve overall O_2 use, and enhance the cardiovascular response of the body to physical activity. (Chapter 50)

rectus abdominis abdominal muscle group that functions as an accessory muscle of ventilation. (Chapter 8)

reducing valve valve that reduces gas pressure. (Chapter 37)

reexpansion pulmonary edema pulmonary edema that forms after rapid reexpansion of a lung that has been compressed with pleural fluid or pneumothorax. (Chapter 25)

reference range the acceptable range for a laboratory value measured during calibration or validation of operation. (Chapter 16)

regulator device that controls both pressure and flow. (Chapter 37)

regurgitation backward flow of blood through an incompetent valve of the heart. (Chapter 9)

relative humidity (RH) amount of moisture in the air compared with the maximum the air could contain at the same temperature. (Chapter 6)

repolarization process by which the cell is restored to its resting potential. (Chapter 16)
reservoir system O_2 delivery system that provides a reservoir O_2 volume that the patient taps into when the patient's inspiratory flow exceeds the device flow. (Chapter 38)
residual drug volume medication that remains in a small volume nebulizer after the device is no longer producing mist. (Chapter 36)
residual volume (RV) volume of gas remaining in the lungs after a complete exhalation. (Chapter 19)
res ipsa loquitur "the thing speaks for itself"; rule of evidence whereby negligence of an alleged wrongdoer may be inferred from the fact that the accident happened. (Chapter 5)
resistance impedance to flow in a tube or conduit; quantified as ratio of the difference in pressure between the two points. (Chapter 3)
respirable mass proportion of aerosolized drug of the proper particle size to reach the lower respiratory tract. (Chapters 36, 42)
respiratory acidosis hypoventilation resulting in acidemia. (Chapter 13)
respiratory alternans alternating between use of the diaphragm for short periods and use of the accessory muscles to breathe; indicative of end-stage respiratory muscle fatigue. (Chapters 15, 41)
respiratory care health care discipline that specializes in the promotion of optimal cardiopulmonary function and health. Also called *respiratory therapy*. (Chapter 1)
respiratory care management information systems an information system specifically designed for managing data regarding the respiratory care provided to patients. (Chapter 7)
respiratory care practitioner health professional with special training and experience in the treatment and rehabilitation of patients with respiratory disorders. The respiratory care practitioner typically does not diagnose but must be competent with patient assessment in various clinical settings. (Chapter 1)
respiratory care protocol specification of actions that allows respiratory care practitioners to initiate and adjust therapy independently, within guidelines previously established by medical staff. Also called *therapist-driven protocol*. (Chapter 2)
respiratory distress syndrome (RDS) condition of respiratory distress in newborns, usually caused by inadequate surfactant production (owing to immaturity). (Chapter 31)
respiratory inductive plethysmography device that, by measuring the change in the diameter of the chest and abdomen, can estimate inhaled and exhaled tidal volume. (Chapter 46)
respiratory therapist (RT) graduate of a CAAHEP/CoARC accredited school designed to qualify the graduate for the registry examination of the National Board for Respiratory Care (NBRC). (Chapter 1)
respiratory therapy any treatment that maintains or improves the ventilatory function of the respiratory tract. (Chapter 1)
respiratory therapy consult service program in which respiratory care services are determined by respiratory care practitioners based on prescribed guidelines or algorithms. Also called *evaluate-and-treat program*. (Chapter 2)
respondeat superior "let the master answer"; the master is liable in certain cases for the wrongful acts of his servant, meaning that a physician may be liable for the wrongful acts of someone working under the physician's supervision. The doctrine is inapplicable where injury occurs while the servant is acting outside the legitimate scope of authority. (Chapter 5)
resting energy expenditure (REE) caloric needs of the body estimated from O_2 consumption and CO_2 production, usually expressed in kcal/24 hr. (Chapter 21)
restrictive lung disease broad category of disorders with widely variable etiologies but all resulting in a reduction in lung volumes, particularly the inspiratory and vital capacities; categorized according to origin—skeletal/thoracic, neuromuscular, pleural, interstitial, and alveolar. (Chapter 19)
retinopathy of prematurity (ROP) abnormal ocular condition that occurs in some premature or low-birth-weight infants who receive O_2. Previously called retrolental fibroplasias. (Chapters 38, 48)
retractions sinking inward of the skin around the chest cage with each inspiratory effort. (Chapter 15)
Reynold's number a dimensionless number used to determine if flow is laminar or turbulent. If the reynold's number is above 2000 flow is turbulent. It is determined by multiplying the diameter of the system by the velocity of gas flow times the density of the gas divided by the viscosity of the gas. (Chapter 6)
right-to-left shunt anatomic bypass in which blood flows from the venous to the arterial side of the circulation, bypassing the lungs; this lowers both the O_2 content and PO_2 of the arterial blood. (Chapter 11)
rocking bed bed that rocks back and forth moving the abdominal contents up and down facilitating inspiration and expiration. (Chapter 45)
roentgenogram an x-ray image. (Chapter 20)
rule utilitarianism moral reasoning approach based not on which act has the greatest utility but on which rule would promote the greatest good if it were generally followed. (Chapter 5)

S

sarcoidosis chronic disorder of unknown origin characterized by the formation of tubercles of nonnecrotizing epithelioid tissue. (Chapter 24)
saturated solution solution in which the solvent contains the

maximum amount of solute it can take up. (Chapter 12)

scalenes referring to the three muscles arising from the cervical vertebrae, inserting into the first and second ribs; accessory muscles of ventilation. (Chapter 8)

scintigraphy photograph showing the distribution and intensity of radioactivity in various tissues and organs after administration of a radiopharmaceutical. (Chapter 36)

screening preliminary procedure, such as a test or examination, to detect the most characteristic sign or signs of a disorder that may require further investigation. (Chapter 28)

secondary spontaneous pneumothorax pneumothorax that occurs because of underlying lung disease. (Chapter 25)

sedimentation primary mechanism for deposition of particles 1 to 5 mm in diameter in the central airways, when particles slow and settle out of suspension. (Chapter 36)

segments minor divisions of the lung; each segment is associated with a major branch of the airway. (Chapter 8)

segs refers to segmented neutrophils the mature form of circulating neutrophils. (Chapter 16)

sensorium general term referring to the relative state of a patient's consciousness or alertness. (Chapter 15)

servo-controlled heating system in a humidifier, heating unit that monitors the temperature of gas delivered to the patient, adjusting the power to the heater based on the difference between the temperature setting and the temperature monitored by a thermistor probe placed downstream from the humidifier, at or near the patient airway connection. (Chapter 35)

shock condition in which perfusion to vital organs is inadequate to meet metabolic needs; includes hypovolemic, cardiogenic, septic, anaphylactic, and neurogenic forms. (Chapter 15)

sickle cell hemoglobin the presence of hemoglobin S causing the hemoglobin cell to form a sickle shape. (Chapter 11)

silicosis lung disorder caused by continued, long-term exposure to the dust of an inorganic compound, silicon dioxide, which is found in sands, quartzes, and many other stones; chronic silicosis is marked by widespread fibrotic nodular lesions in both lungs. (Chapter 24)

skilled nursing facility (SNF) institution or part of an institution that meets criteria for accreditation established by the sections of the Social Security Act that determine the basis for Medicaid and Medicare reimbursement for skilled nursing care. Skilled nursing care includes rehabilitation and various medical and nursing procedures. (Chapter 51)

slander any words spoken with malice that are untrue and prejudicial to the reputation, professional practice, commercial trade, office, or business of another person. (Chapter 5)

sleep-disordered breathing periods of an absence of attempts to breathe during sleep. (Chapter 30)

small cell cancer malignant, usually bronchogenic epithelial neoplasm consisting of small; tightly packed; round, oval, or spindle-shaped epithelial cells that stain darkly and contain neurosecretory granules and little or no cytoplasm. Many malignant tumors of the lung are of this type. Also called *oat cell carcinoma* or *small cell carcinoma*. (Chapter 28)

SOAP in a problem-oriented medical record, abbreviation for *subjective, objective, assessment,* and *plan,* the four parts of a written account of the health problem. (Chapter 3)

soft palate structure composed of mucous membrane, muscular fibers, and mucous glands, suspended from the posterior border of the hard palate forming the roof of the mouth. (Chapter 8)

solitary pulmonary nodule (SPN) a pulmonary parenchymal opacity smaller than 3 cm in diameter that is totally surrounded by aerated lung. (Chapter 20)

solubility coefficient (gas) volume of gas that can be dissolved in 1 ml of a given liquid at standard pressure and specified temperature. (Chapter 6)

solute substance dissolved in a solution. (Chapter 12)

solution mixture of one or more substances dissolved in another substance. The molecules of each of the substances disperse homogeneously and do not change chemically. A solution may be a gas, a liquid, or a solid. (Chapter 12)

solvent any liquid in which another substance can be dissolved. (Chapter 12)

specific gravity ratio of the density of a substance to the density of another substance accepted as a standard. The usual standard for liquids and solids is water. A liquid or solid with a specific gravity of 4 is as dense as water at the same temperature. Hydrogen is the usual standard for gases. (Chapter 6)

spectrophotometry measurement of color in a solution by determining the amount of light absorbed in the ultraviolet, infrared, or visible spectrum, widely used in clinical chemistry to calculate the concentration of substances in solution. (Chapter 18)

splinting process of immobilizing, restraining, or supporting a body part. (Chapter 40)

spontaneous awaking trial a trial of sedation removal or reduction preformed prior to a spontaneopus breathing trial. (Chapter 47)

spontaneous breath ventilatory support breaths initiated and ended by the patient. (Chapter 42)

spontaneous breathing trial (SBT) trial of spontaneous breathing independent of the ventilator. (Chapter 47)

sporicidal destructive to the spore form of bacteria. (Chapter 4)

sputum mucus from the respiratory tract that has passed through the mouth. (Chapter 15)

squamous cell carcinoma type of lung cancer characterized by cells that appear platelike. (Chapter 28)

staging system See *TNM staging.* (Chapter 28)

standard bicarbonate plasma concentration of HCO_3^- in mEq/L that would exist if PCO_2 were normal (40 mm Hg). (Chapter 13)

standard precautions guidelines recommended by the U.S. Centers for Disease Control and Prevention to reduce the risk of transmission of blood-borne and other pathogens in hospitals. Standard precautions apply to (1) blood; (2) all body fluids, secretions, and excretions, excluding sweat, regardless of whether they contain blood; (3) nonintact skin; and (4) mucous membranes. (Chapter 4)

Starling equilibrium the filtration of fluid across a membrane is a result of equilibration of osmotic and hydrostatic forces across the membrane. (Chapter 12)

stenosis narrowing of a valve or vessel. (Chapters 9, 33)

sterilization complete destruction of all microorganisms, usually by heat or chemical means. (Chapter 4)

sternal angle the fused connection between the manubrium and the body of the sternum is known as the sternal angle or angle of Louis. (Chapter 8)

sternocleidomastoid muscle muscle of the neck that is attached to the mastoid process of the temporal bone and superior nuchal line and by separate heads to the sternum and clavicle; sternocleidomastoid muscles function together to flex the head. (Chapter 8)

sternum elongated flattened bone forming the middle portion of the anterior thorax. (Chapter 8)

stomata small holes within the parietal pleura that are the main route for pleural fluid to exit. (Chapter 25)

STPD conditions of a volume of gas at 0° C and 760 mm Hg and containing no water vapor (dry). It should contain a calculable number of moles of a particular gas. (Chapter 6)

strain-gauge pressure transducers a pressure measuring device that records pressures by the expansion and contraction of a flexible metal diaphragm connected to electrical wires. (Chapter 6)

stress index an index used to determine if during mechanical controlled inhalation there is over distension or recruitment of collapse lung; determined by the slope change in the airway pressure curve during volume controlled square wave ventilation. (Chapter 46)

strict liability theory in tort law that can be used to impose liability without fault, even in situations where injury occurs under conditions of reasonable care; the most common cases of strict liability involve the use of dangerous products or techniques. (Chapter 5)

stridor high-pitched, continuous type of adventitious lung sound heard from the upper airway. (Chapter 15)

stroke condition characterized by the sudden onset of a neurologic deficit. (Chapter 29)

stroke volume volume of blood ejected by the left ventricle during each contraction. (Chapter 9)

subatmospheric below atmospheric; used to describe pressures below ambient. (Chapter 10)

subcutaneous emphysema accumulation of air in the subcutaneous tissues owing to leakage from the lung. (Chapter 15)

suctioning process of mechanically aspirating airway secretions. (Chapter 33)

sudden infant death syndrome (SIDS) leading cause of death in infants less than 1 year old in the United States. Commonly called *crib death.* (Chapter 31)

supplemental oxygen O_2 delivered at concentrations exceeding 21% to increase the amount of oxygen circulating in the blood. (Chapter 23)

suprasternal above the sternum. (Chapter 8)

surface tension tendency of a liquid to minimize the area of its surface by contracting. This property causes liquids to rise in a capillary tube, effects the exchange of gases in the pulmonary alveoli, and alters the ability of various liquids to wet another surface. (Chapter 10)

surfactant surface-acting agent that forms a monomolecular layer over pulmonary alveolar surfaces. These agents prevent alveolar collapse at lower lung volumes by reducing alveolar surface tension. (Chapter 48)

surgical resection the partial removal of an organ of tissues by surgical means. (Chapter 28)

surveillance (bacteriologic) ongoing process designed to ensure that infection control procedures are working; generally involves equipment, microbiologic identification, and epidemiologic investigation. (Chapter 4)

suspension dispersion of large particles suspended in a fluid medium; without physical agitation, the particles eventually settle out. (Chapter 12)

Swan-Ganz catheter catheter that is positioned in the pulmonary artery to measure pressures in the heart and pulmonary circulation and can be used to determine the patient's circulatory status. (Chapter 46)

synchronized cardioversion countershock synchronized with the heart's electrical activity. (Chapter 34)

synchronous intermittent mandatory ventilation (SIMV) mode of ventilatory support using periodic assisted ventilation with spontaneous breathing in between. Assisted breaths are responsive to patient demand. (Chapters 44, 46)

syncope temporary unconsciousness; fainting. (Chapter 15)

systematic error nonrandom statistical error that affects the mean of a population of data and defines the bias between the means of two populations. (Chapters 18, 47)

systolic blood pressure peak blood pressure occurring in the arteries during ventricular contraction. (Chapter 15)

T

tachycardia abnormally elevated heart rate. (Chapter 15)

tachyphylaxis phenomenon in which the repeated administration of some drugs results in a marked decrease in effectiveness. (Chapter 32)

tachypnea abnormal elevation of breathing rate. (Chapter 15)

target heart rate heart rate achieved at 65% of a patient's maximum O_2 consumption during an exercise evaluation, used for aerobic conditioning. (Chapter 50)

target variable a variable that can be reached and maintained at a preset level before inspiration ends but does not terminate inspiration. (Chapter 42)

targeting scheme the approach used by a particular mode to achieve the various targets active during ventilation. (Chapter 42)

telemedicine use of telecommunication equipment and information technology to provide clinical care to patients at distant sites and the transmission of medical and surgical information and images needed to provide that care. (Chapter 7)

tension pneumothorax air in the pleural space that exceeds atmospheric pressure causing outward expansion of the ribs, downward depression of the diaphragm, mediastinal shift, and hypotension. (Chapter 25)

tension-time index product of contractile force (ratio of diaphragmatic pressure to maximum diaphragmatic pressure) and contractile duration (ratio of inspiratory time to total breathing cycle time) used to indicate a level of contraction associated with fatigue. (Chapter 41)

tetralogy of Fallot congenital cardiac anomaly that consists of four defects: pulmonic stenosis, ventricular septal defect, malposition of the aorta so that it arises from the septal defect or the right ventricle, and right ventricular hypertrophy. (Chapter 31)

therapeutic index difference between the minimum therapeutic and minimum toxic concentrations of a drug. (Chapter 36)

therapist-driven protocol specification of actions that allow respiratory care practitioners to initiate and adjust therapy independently, within guidelines previously established by medical staff. Also called *respiratory care protocol.* (Chapter 2)

thermal conductivity measure of gas concentrations in a sample calculated by detecting the rate at which different gases conduct heat. (Chapter 6)

thermodynamics science of the interconversion of heat and work. (Chapter 6)

thoracentesis surgical perforation of the chest wall and pleural space with a needle for diagnostic or therapeutic purposes or for the removal of a specimen for biopsy. (Chapter 25)

thoracic gas volume (TGV) technique that measures lung volume. (Chapter 19)

Thorpe tube variable orifice, constant pressure flowmeter. (Chapter 37)

thrill fine palpable vibration felt accompanying a cardiac or vascular murmur. (Chapter 15)

thrombocytes smallest cells in the blood; they are formed in the red bone marrow, and some are stored in the spleen. Platelets are disc-shaped, contain no hemoglobin, and are essential for the coagulation of blood and in maintenance of hemostasis. (Chapter 16)

thrombocytopenia abnormal condition in which the number of blood platelets is reduced, usually associated with neoplastic diseases or an immune response to a drug. (Chapter 16)

tidal volume (V_T) volume of air that is inhaled or exhaled from the lungs during effortless breath. (Chapters 10, 19)

time constant mathematical expression describing the relative efficacy of lung unit filling and emptying and computed as the product of compliance times resistance (measured in seconds). (Chapters 10, 42, 43)

tissue oxygen sensing the monitoring of the oxygen saturation or PO_2 at the tissue level. (Chapter 46)

TNM staging staging system based on a size of the tumor *(T)*, the presence and position of abnormal lymph nodes *(N)*, and the presence or absence of metastasis (or spread beyond the primary tumor site) *(M)*. (Chapter 28)

tort legal wrong committed on a person or property independent of contract. (Chapter 5)

total lung capacity (TLC) total amount of gas in the lungs after a maximum inspiration. (Chapter 19)

trachea large main intrathoracic airway. (Chapter 8)

tracheal tugging effect of an aortic aneurysm in which the trachea is pulled downward with each heart contraction. (Chapter 15)

tracheoesophageal fistula a congenital malformation or an abnormality associated with disease in which there is an abnormal tubelike passage between the trachea and the esophagus. (Chapter 33)

tracheoinnominate fistula a fistula (connection between the trachea and the innominate artery). (Chapter 33)

tracheomalacia softening of the tracheal cartilages. (Chapter 33)

tracheostomy opening through the neck into the trachea, through which an indwelling tube may be inserted. (Chapter 33)

tracheostomy tubes artificial airways that are surgically placed directly into the trachea. (Chapter 33)

tracheotomy procedure by which an incision is made into the trachea through the neck below the larynx to gain access to the lower airways. (Chapter 33)

transairway pressure difference between airway pressure and alveolar pressure. (Chapters 10, 43)

transalveolar pressure difference between alveolar pressure and pleural pressure. (Chapters 10, 43)

transbronchial needle aspiration technique of sampling lung tissue through a bronchoscope that involves passing a thin needle through a bronchus. (Chapter 28)

trans–chest wall pressure difference between the pleural space and the body surface. Also called *transthoracic pressure.* (Chapters 10, 43)

transdiaphragmatic pressure (P_{di}) the pressure change across the diaphragm associated with breathing. (Chapter 43)

transient tachypnea of the newborn (TTN) the periodic increase in respiratory rate that is commonly observed in low birth weight infants. (Chapter 31)

transposition of the great arteries congenital cardiac condition characterized by an anatomic abnormality in which the aorta arises from the right ventricle, and the pulmonary artery arises from the left ventricle. (Chapter 31)

transpulmonary of or pertaining to the difference in a parameter (e.g., pressure) between the alveoli and pleural space. (Chapter 10)

transpulmonary pressure difference difference between intraalveolar and intrapleural pressure, or the pressure acting across the ling from the pleural space to the alveoli. (Chapters 10, 43, 44)

transrespiratory across the respiratory system; of or pertaining to the difference in a parameter (e.g., pressure) between the alveoli and the body surface. (Chapter 10)

transrespiratory pressure gradient pressure differential between the mouth and the alveoli that causes gas to flow in and out of the lungs. (Chapters 10, 43)

transthoracic across the thorax; of or pertaining to the difference in a parameter (e.g., pressure) between the pleural space and body surface. (Chapter 10)

transthoracic needle biopsy technique of obtaining a biopsy specimen of lung tissue by which a needle is passed into the chest, often guided by imaging. (Chapter 28)

transthoracic pressure of or pertaining to the difference in a parameter (such as pressure) between the pleural space and body surface. (Chapter 43)

transthoracic pressure difference (P_{TT}) difference between the pleural space and the body surface. Also called *trans–chest wall pressure.* (Chapter 10)

transtracheal oxygen therapy (T_{TOT}) administration of O_2 via a low-flow catheter inserted directly into the trachea. (Chapter 51)

transudative pleural effusion pleural effusion low in protein and lactate dehydrogenase, usually caused by congestive heart failure, nephrosis, or cirrhosis. (Chapter 25)

traumatic brain injury general term referring to any class of either focal or diffuse lesions that can result from head trauma; these lesions include injury to the nerve body (axon), hypoxic brain damage, swelling, hemorrhage, contusions, laceration, and infection. (Chapter 29)

Trendelenburg position position in which the head is low and the body and legs are on an inclined plane. (Chapter 45)

trigger variable variable that initiates inspiration during mechanical ventilation. (Chapter 42)

tripodding breathing technique most often used by patients with chronic obstructive pulmonary disease (COPD) in which they lean forward and place their elbows on a table or arms of a chair to support breathing with the accessory muscles. (Chapter 15)

troponin protein in the striated cell ultrastructure that modulates the interaction between actin and myosin molecules. It is believed to be part of the calcium-binding complex of the thin myofilaments. The level of blood troponin is used to identify the presence of a myocardial infarction. (Chapter 16)

troponin I protein similar to CPK-2; troponin I levels peak 12 to 16 hours after myocardial infarction. It is associated with cardiac muscle damage. (Chapter 16)

true ribs the first seven ribs on each side of the thorax are called true ribs. (Chapter 8)

tuberculosis chronic granulomatous infection caused by an acid-fast bacillus, *Mycobacterium tuberculosis.* It is generally transmitted by the inhalation or ingestion of infected droplets and usually affects the lungs, although infection of multiple organ systems occurs. (Chapter 22)

turbinates bony structures that extend from the lateral walls of the interior nasal passages. (Chapter 8)

turbulent flow flow of a fluid that does not occur in a straight line; flow in which molecules the tumble over each other. (Chapter 6)

12-minute walk usually a part of a pulmonary rehabilitation program, performed once a day for the duration of the program. The objective is for the patient to walk on a flat, smooth surface as far as possible during the 12 minutes, stopping as necessary and quantifying the total distance covered. (Chapter 50)

type I pneumocyte cuboidal, secretory epithelia that line the blind tubules of the acinus cells. (Chapter 8)

type II pneumocyte pneumocyte granular cells that are highly active forms part of the lining of the alveoli. These cells secrete surfactant and other substances. (Chapter 8)

U

ultrasonic nebulizer (USN) humidifier in which an electrical signal is used to produce high-frequency vibrations in a container of fluid.

The vibrations break up the fluid into aerosol particles. (Chapter 35)

upstream relative reference to a point closer to the source in a stream of flowing fluid. (Chapter 37)

uvula small cone-shaped process suspended in the mouth from the middle of the posterior border of the soft palate. (Chapter 8)

uvulopalatopharyngoplasty (UVPPP) surgical procedure used in treating severe obstructive sleep apnea, which involves shortening of the soft palate and removal of the uvula and tonsils. (Chapter 30)

V

vagovagal reflexes reflexes caused by stimulation of parasympathetic receptors in the airways that can result in laryngospasm, bronchoconstriction, hyperpnea, and bradycardia; often associated with mechanical stimulation, as during procedures such as tracheobronchial aspiration, intubation, or bronchoscopy. (Chapter 14)

vaporization process whereby matter in its liquid form is changed into its vapor or gaseous form. (Chapter 6)

vasoconstriction narrowing of the blood vessels. (Chapter 9)

vasodilation widening or distention of blood vessels, particularly arterioles, usually caused by nerve impulses or certain drugs that relax smooth muscle in the walls of the blood vessels. (Chapter 9)

VCV acronym for *volume-controlled ventilation,* a mode of ventilatory support in which volume (or flow × time) serves as the cycle variable. (Chapter 32)

venous admixture mixing of venous blood with arterial blood, resulting in a decrease in the O_2 content of the latter; occurs in anatomic and physiologic shunting. (Chapters 11, 46)

venous thromboembolism clot that spreads from one venous bed to another, such as from the leg veins to the lung. (Chapter 26)

ventilation molecular exchange of O_2 and CO_2 within the body's tissues. (Chapter 10)

ventilation/perfusion ($\dot{V}/\dot{Q}$) ratio ratio of pulmonary alveolar ventilation to pulmonary capillary perfusion, both measured quantities being expressed in the same units. (Chapter 11)

ventilator-associated pneumonia lower respiratory tract infection that develops more than 48 to 72 hours after endotracheal intubation. (Chapter 22)

ventilatory threshold during exercise, the point where increased levels of lactic acid result in increased CO_2 production and minute ventilation; the respiratory quotient equals or exceeds 1.0, indicating that CO_2 production equals or exceeds O_2 consumption; at this point, metabolism becomes anaerobic, decreasing energy production and increasing muscle fatigue. (Chapter 50)

ventral respiratory groups (VRGs) groupings of cells in the medulla oblongata that are active in controlling both inspiration and expiration. (Chapter 14)

veracity principle that binds the health provider and the patient to tell the truth, creating an environment of trust and mutual sharing of information. (Chapter 5)

very low birth weight (VLBW) a newborn who weights less than the 95% percentile of weight for newborns. (Chapter 48)

virtue ethics viewpoint that asks what a virtuous person would do in a similar circumstance; it is based on personal attributes of character or virtue, rather than on rules or consequences. (Chapter 5)

virucidal agent that destroys or inactivates viruses. (Chapter 4)

visceral pleura thin membrane covered by mesothelial cells that covers the entire surface of the lung, dipping into the lobar fissures. (Chapter 8)

viscosity internal force that opposes flow of a fluid, either liquids or gases. (Chapter 6)

vital capacity (VC) total amount of air that can be exhaled after a maximum inspiration; the sum of the inspiratory reserve volume, the tidal volume, and the expiratory reserve volume. (Chapters 19, 46)

volatile acid acid that can be excreted in its gaseous form; physiologically, carbonic acid is a volatile acid; approximately 24,000 mmol/L CO_2 is eliminated from the body daily via normal ventilation. (Chapter 13)

voltage expression of electromotive force in terms of volts. (Chapter 3)

volume-controlled ventilation (CMV) a mode of ventilatory support in which a specific tidal volume is set and delivered each breath under control ventilation conditions. (Chapters 3, 27, 42, 44)

volume-limited ventilation same as CMV, the primary control variable is tidal volume. (Chapter 27)

volume-median diameter (VMD) the median diameter of an aerosol particle measured in units of volume. (Chapter 36)

volume support pressure-limited ventilation where tidal volume is targeted. (Chapter 44)

volutrauma alveolar overdistention and damage caused by ventilation with high peak inflation pressures. (Chapter 43)

W

water vapor pressure the pressure exerted by water in its gaseous state. (Chapter 6)

wheezes high-pitched, continuous type of adventitious lung sound. (Chapter 15)

work of breathing (WOB) amount of force needed to move a given volume into the lung with a relaxed chest wall; mathematically, work is the integral of pressure times volume. (Chapter 41)

X

xiphoid process pointed lower portion of the sternum. (Chapter 8)

Z

zone valve on/off piping valve that controls medical gas distribution to a prespecified zone of a building. (Chapter 37)

Index

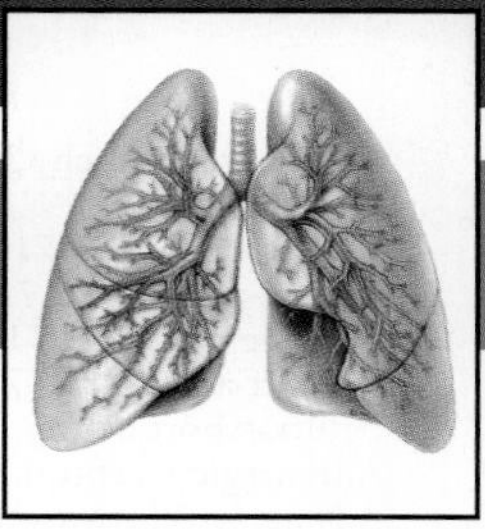

Note: Page numbers followed by "f" refer to illustrations; page numbers followed by "t" refer to tables; page numbers followed by "b" refer to boxes.

D

J

P

S

P_{100}	pressure on inspiration measured at 100 msec
Pa	arterial pressure
PA	pulmonary artery
$P(A\text{-}a)O_2$	alveolar-to-arterial partial pressure of oxygen
P(A-awo)	pressure gradient from alveolus to airway opening
$PACO_2$	partial pressure of carbon dioxide in the alveoli
$PaCO_2$	partial pressure of carbon dioxide in the arteries
P_{al}	alveolar pressure
PAO_2	partial pressure of oxygen in the alveoli
PaO_2	partial pressure of oxygen in the arteries
PaO_2/FiO_2	ratio of arterial PO_2 to FiO_2
PaO_2/PAO_2	ratio of arterial PO_2 to alveolar PO_2
PAOP	pulmonary artery occlusion pressure
PAP	pulmonary artery pressure
$\overline{PAP}$	mean pulmonary artery pressure
$P(a\text{-}et)CO_2$	arterial-to-end-tidal partial pressure of carbon dioxide
PAGE	perfluorocarbon associated gas exchange
P_{aug}	pressure augmentation
PAV	proportional assist ventilation
P_{aw}	airway pressure
$P_{\overline{aw}}$	mean airway pressure
P_{awo}	airway opening pressure
PAWP	pulmonary artery wedge pressure
PB	barometric pressure
P_{bs}	pressure at the body's surface
PC-CMV	pressure-controlled continuous mandatory ventilation
PCEF	peak cough expiratory flow
PCIRV	pressure control inverse ratio ventilation
PCO_2	partial pressure of carbon dioxide
PC-IMV	pressure-controlled intermittent mandatory ventilation
PC-SIMV	pressure-controlled synchronized intermittent mandatory ventilation
PCV	pressure-controlled ventilation
PCWP	pulmonary capillary wedge pressure
$PCWP_{tm}$	transmural pulmonary capillary wedge pressure
PDA	patent ductus arteriosus
PE	pulmonary embolism
PE_{max}	maximal expiratory pressure
PEA	pulseless electrical activity
$P_{\bar{E}}CO_2$	partial pressure of mixed expired carbon dioxide
PEEP	positive end expiratory pressure
$PEEP_E$	extrinsic PEEP(set-PEEP)
$PEEP_I$	intrinsic PEEP (auto-PEEP)
$PEEP_{total}$	total PEEP (sum of intrinsic and extrinsic PEEP)
PEFR	peak expiratory flow rate
P_{es}	esophageal pressure
$PetCO_2$	partial pressure of end-tidal carbon dioxide
P_{flex}	pressure at the inflection point of a pressure/volume curve
PFT	pulmonary function test(ing)
P_{ga}	gastric pressure
pH	relative acidity or alkalinity of a solution
P_{high}	high pressure during APRV
PHY	permissive hypercapnia
PIE	pulmonary interstitial edema
PIF	pulmonary interstitial fibrosis
PI_{max}	maximum inspiratory pressure (also MIP, MIF, NIF)
P_{inside}	inside pressure
$P_{intrapleural}$	intrapleural pressure (also Ppl)
PiO_2	partial pressure of inspired oxygen
PIP	peak inspiratory pressure (also P_{peak})
PISS	pin-indexed safety system
P_L	transpulmonary pressure
P_{low}	low pressure during APRV
PLV	partial liquid ventilation
P_M	mouth pressure
pMDI	pressurized metered dose inhaler
P_{mus}	muscle pressure
PO_2	partial pressure of oxygen
$P_{outside}$	pressure outside
P_{peak}	peak inspiratory pressure (also PIP)
PPHN	primary pulmonary hypertension of the neonate
P_{pl}	intrapleural pressure
$P_{plateau}$	plateau pressure
ppm	parts per million
PPST	premature pressure support termination
PPV	positive pressure ventilation
PRA	plasma renin activity
PRVC	pressure regulated volume control
PS	pressure support
PSB	protected specimen brush
P_{set}	set pressure
psi	pounds per square inch
psig	pounds per square inch gauge
PS_{max}	maximum pressure support
P_{st}	static transpulmonary pressure at a specified lung volume
PSV	pressure support ventilation
P_{TA}	transairway pressure
$PtcCO_2$	transcutaneous PCO_2
$PtcO_2$	transcutaneous PO_2
P_{tm}	transmural pressure
P_{TR}	transrespiratory pressure
PTSD	posttraumatic stress disorder
P_{TT}	transthoracic pressure (also Pw)
P-V	pressure-volume
PV	pressure ventilation
PVC(s)	premature ventricular contraction(s)
$P\bar{v}O_2$	partial pressure of oxygen in mixed venous blood
PVR	pulmonary vascular resistance
PVS	partial ventilatory support
P_w	transthoracic pressure (also P_{TT})
Q	blood volume
$\dot{Q}$	blood flow
$\dot{Q}_{c'}$	pulmonary capillary blood flow
q2h	every 2 hours
Q_T	cardiac output
$\frac{\dot{Q}_s}{\dot{Q}_t}$	shunt
$\dot{Q}sp$	physiologic shunt flow (total venous admixture)
R	resistance (i.e., pressure per unit flow)
$\bar{R}$	mean total resistance
RAM	random access memory
RAP	right atrial pressure
R_{aw}	airway resistance
rb	rebreathing
RCP	respiratory care practitioner
Rds	resistance of the airway on the oral side (downstream)
RDS	respiratory distress syndrome
Re	Reynolds number